DRUG INFORMATION HANDBOOK for DENTISTRY

Including Oral Medicine for Medically Compromised Patients & Specific Oral Conditions

19th Edition

Lexicomp®

DRUG INFORMATION HANDBOOK for DENTISTRY

Including Oral Medicine for Medically-Compromised Patients & Specific Oral Conditions

Richard L. Wynn, BSPharm, PhD
Professor of Pharmacology
Baltimore College of Dental Surgery
Dental School
University of Maryland Baltimore
Baltimore, Maryland

Timothy F. Meiller, DDS, PhD
Professor
Oncology and Diagnostic Sciences
Baltimore College of Dental Surgery
Professor of Oncology
Marlene and Stewart Greenebaum Cancer Center
University of Maryland Medical System
Baltimore, Maryland

Harold L. Crossley, DDS, PhD
Professor Emeritus
Baltimore College of Dental Surgery
Dental School
University of Maryland Baltimore
Baltimore, Maryland

Lexicomp®

NOTICE

This data is intended to serve the user as a handy reference and not as a complete drug information resource. It does not include information on every therapeutic agent available. The publication covers over 1700 commonly used drugs and is specifically designed to present important aspects of drug data in a more concise format than is typically found in medical literature or product material supplied by manufacturers.

The nature of drug information is that it is constantly evolving because of ongoing research and clinical experience and is often subject to interpretation. While great care has been taken to ensure the accuracy of the information and recommendations presented, the reader is advised that the authors, editors, reviewers, contributors, and publishers cannot be responsible for the continued currency of the information or for any errors, omissions, or the application of this information, or for any consequences arising therefrom. Therefore, the author(s) and/or the publisher shall have no liability to any person or entity with regard to claims, loss, or damage caused, or alleged to be caused, directly or indirectly, by the use of information contained herein. Because of the dynamic nature of drug information, readers are advised that decisions regarding drug therapy must be based on the independent judgment of the clinician, changing information about a drug (eg, as reflected in the literature and manufacturer's most current product information), and changing medical practices. Therefore, this data is designed to be used in conjunction with other necessary information and is not designed to be solely relied upon by any user. The user of this data hereby and forever releases the authors and publishers of this data from any and all liability of any kind that might arise out of the use of this data. The editors are not responsible for any inaccuracy of quotation or for any false or misleading implication that may arise due to the text or formulas as used or due to the quotation of revisions no longer official.

Certain of the authors, editors, and contributors have written this book in their private capacities. No official support or endorsement by any federal or state agency or pharmaceutical company is intended or inferred.

The publishers have made every effort to trace any third party copyright holders, if any, for borrowed material. If they have inadvertently overlooked any, they will be pleased to make the necessary arrangements at the first opportunity.

If you have any suggestions or questions regarding any information presented in this data, please contact our drug information pharmacists at (330) 650-6506. Book revisions are available at our website at http://www.lexi.com/home/revisions/.

This manual was produced using Lexi-Comp's Information Management System™ (LIMS) — a complete publishing service of Lexi-Comp, Inc.

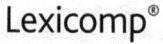

Lexicomp®

1100 Terex Road • Hudson, Ohio • 44236
(330) 650-6506

ISBN 978-1-59195-322-7

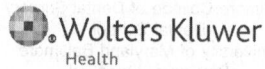

Wolters Kluwer
Health

TABLE OF CONTENTS

ABOUT THE EDITORS

Richard L. Wynn, BSPharm, PhD

Richard L. Wynn, PhD, is Professor of Pharmacology at the Baltimore College of Dental Surgery, Dental School, University of Maryland Baltimore. Dr Wynn has served as a dental educator, researcher, and teacher of dental pharmacology and dental hygiene pharmacology for his entire professional career. He holds a BS (pharmacy; registered pharmacist, Maryland), an MS (physiology) and a PhD (pharmacology) from the University of Maryland. Dr Wynn chaired the Department of Pharmacology at the University of Maryland Dental School from 1980 to 1995. Previously, he chaired the Department of Oral Biology at the University of Kentucky College of Dentistry.

Dr Wynn has to his credit over 380 publications, including original research articles, textbooks, textbook chapters, monographs, and articles in continuing education journals. He has given over 600 continuing education seminars to dental professionals in the U.S., Canada, and Europe. Dr Wynn has been a consultant to the drug industry for 29 years and his research laboratories have contributed to the development of new analgesics and anesthetics. He is a consultant to the Academy of General Dentistry, the American Dental Association, and a former consultant to the Council on Dental Education, Commission on Accreditation. He is a featured columnist and his drug review articles, entitled *Pharmacology Today*, appear in each issue of *General Dentistry*, a journal published by the Academy. One of his primary interests continues to be keeping dental professionals informed on all aspects of drug use in dental practice.

Timothy F. Meiller, DDS, PhD

Dr Meiller is Professor of Oncology and Diagnostic Sciences at the Baltimore College of Dental Surgery and Professor of Oncology at the Marlene and Stewart Greenebaum Cancer Center, University of Maryland Medical Systems in Baltimore. He is Director of the Oral Medicine Program in both the dental school and the cancer center. He has held his position at the Dental School for 36 years.

Dr Meiller is a Diplomate of the American Board of Oral Medicine and a graduate of Johns Hopkins University and the University of Maryland Dental and Graduate Schools, holding a DDS and a PhD in Immunology/Virology. He has over 200 publications to his credit, maintains an active general dental practice, and is a consultant to the National Institutes of Health and the Veterans Administration. He is currently engaged in ongoing investigations into cellular immune dysfunction in premalignant oral lesions, oral diseases associated with AIDS, in patients receiving therapies for cancer, and in other medically-compromised patients.

Harold L. Crossley, DDS, PhD

Dr Crossley is Professor Emeritus at the University of Maryland Dental School. A native of Rhode Island, Dr Crossley received a Bachelor of Science degree in Pharmacy from the University of Rhode Island in 1964. He later was awarded the Master of Science (1970) and Doctorate degrees (1972) in Pharmacology. The University of Maryland Dental School in Baltimore awarded Dr Crossley the DDS degree in 1980. The liaison between the classroom and his dental practice, which he mentored on a part-time basis in the Dental School Intramural Faculty Practice, produced a practical approach to understanding the pharmacology of drugs used in the dental office.

Dr Crossley has coauthored a number of articles and four books dealing with a variety of topics within the field of pharmacology. Other areas of expertise include the pharmacology of street drugs and chemical dependency. He serves on the Maryland State Dental Association's Well-Being Committee. He is an active member of Phi Kappa Phi, Omicron Kappa Upsilon Honorary Dental Society, the American College of Dentists, and International College of Dentists. He was the recipient of the 2008 Gordon Christensen Lecturer Recognition award presented by the Chicago Dental Society. He has been a consultant for the United States Drug Enforcement Administration and other law enforcement agencies since 1974. Drawing on this unique background, Dr Crossley has become nationally and internationally recognized as an expert on street drugs and chemical dependency as well as the clinical pharmacology of dental drugs.

EDITORIAL ADVISORY PANEL

Collin A. Hovinga, PharmD
Director of Research and *Associate Professor*
Dell Children's Medical Center
UT Austin School of Pharmacy

Darrell T. Hulisz, PharmD
Associate Professor
Department of Family Medicine
Case Western Reserve University

Douglas L. Jennings, PharmD, BCPS
Clinical Specialist
Cardiac Intensive Care Unit and
Advanced Heart Failure and Cardiothoracic
ICU/Ventricular-Assist Device Team
Henry Ford Hospital

Michael A. Kahn, DDS
Professor and Chairman
Department of Oral and Maxillofacial Pathology
Tufts University School of Dental Medicine

Jeannette Kaiser, MT, MBA
Medical Technologist
Akron General Medical Center

Julie J. Kelsey, PharmD
Clinical Specialist
Women's Health and Family Medicine
Department of Pharmacy Services
University of Virginia Health System

Patrick J. Kiel, PharmD, BCPS, BCOP
Clinical Pharmacy Specialist
Hematology and Stem Cell Transplant
Indiana University Simon Cancer Center

Polly E. Kintzel, PharmD, BCPS, BCOP
Clinical Pharmacy Specialist-Oncology
Spectrum Health

Michael Klepser, PharmD, FCCP
Professor of Pharmacy
Department of Pharmacy Practice
Ferris State University

Daren Knoell, PharmD
Associate Professor of Pharmacy Practice and
Internal Medicine
Davis Heart and Lung Research Institute
The Ohio State University

David Knoppert, MScPhm, FCCP,
MSc, FCSHP
Clinical Leader - Paediatrics
Pharmacy Services
London Health Sciences Centre
Children's Health Research Institute

Sandra Knowles, RPh, BScPhm
Drug Safety Pharmacist
Sunnybrook and Women's College HSC

Jill M. Kolesar, PharmD, FCCP, BCPS
Associate Professor
School of Pharmacy
University of Wisconsin
Paul P. Carbone Comprehensive Cancer Center

Susannah E. Koontz, PharmD, BCOP
Principal and Consultant
Pediatric Hematology/Oncology and
Stem Cell Transplantation/Cellular Therapy
Koontz Oncology Consulting, LLC

Donna M. Kraus, PharmD, FAPhA, FPPAG, FCCP
Associate Professor of Pharmacy Practice
and *Pediatric Clinical Pharmacist*
Departments of Pharmacy Practice and Pediatrics
University of Illinois

Daniel L. Krinsky, RPh, MS
Manager, MTM Services
Giant Eagle Pharmacy
Assistant Professor
Department of Pharmacy Practice
Northeast Ohio Medical University (NEOMED)

Tim T.Y. Lau, PharmD, ACPR, FCSHP
Pharmacotherapeutic Specialist in Infectious Diseases
Pharmaceutical Sciences
Vancouver General Hospital

Mandy C. Leonard, PharmD, BCPS
Assistant Professor
Cleveland Clinic Lerner College of
Medicine of Case Western University
Assistant Director, Drug Information Services
The Cleveland Clinic Foundation

John J. Lewin III, PharmD, BCPS
Clinical Specialist, Neurosciences Critical Care
The Johns Hopkins Hospital

Jeffrey D. Lewis, PharmD, MACM
Associate Dean and Associate Professor of
Pharmacy Practice
Cedarville University School of Pharmacy

John Lindsley, PharmD, BCPS
Cardiology Clinical Pharmacy Specialist
The Johns Hopkins Hospital

Nicholas A. Link, PharmD, BCOP
Clinical Specialist, Oncology
Hillcrest Hospital

Jennifer Fisher Lowe, PharmD, BCOP
Pharmacotherapy Contributor
Lexi-Comp, Inc

Sherry Luedtke, PharmD
Associate Professor
Department of Pharmacy Practice
Texas Tech University HSC School of Pharmacy

Melissa Makii, PharmD, BCPS
Clinical Pharmacy Specialist
Pediatric Oncology
Rainbow Babies & Children's Hospital

Vincent F. Mauro, BS, PharmD, FCCP
Professor of Clinical Pharmacy
and *Adjunct Professor of Medicine*
Colleges of Pharmacy and Medicine
The University of Toledo

Barrie McCombs, MD, FCFP
Medical Information Service Coordinator
The Alberta Rural Physician Action Plan

6

Chasity M. Shelton, PharmD, BCPS, BCNSP
Assistant Professor of Clinical Pharmacy
Department of Clinical Pharmacy
Neonatal Clinical Pharmacy Specialist
University of Tennessee Health Science Center

Grant Sklar, PharmD, BCPS
Assistant Professor, Department of Pharmacy
and *Principal Clinical Pharmacist, General Medicine*
National University Hospital of Singapore

Joseph Snoke, RPh, BCPS
Manager
Core Pharmacology Group
Lexi-Comp, Inc

Joni Lombardi Stahura, BS, PharmD, RPh
Pharmacotherapy Specialist
Lexi-Comp, Inc

Kim Stevens, RN
Home Care
Samaritan Regional Health System

Stephen Marc Stout, PharmD, MS, BCPS
Pharmacotherapy Specialist
Lexi-Comp, Inc

Dan Streetman, PharmD, RPh
Pharmacotherapy Specialist
Lexi-Comp, Inc

Darcie-Ann Streetman, PharmD, RPh
Clinical Pharmacist
University of Michigan Health System

Carol K. Taketomo, PharmD
Director of Pharmacy and Nutrition Services
Children's Hospital Los Angeles

Mary Temple-Cooper, PharmD
Pediatric Clinical Research Specialist
Hillcrest Hospital

Kelan Thomas, PharmD, MS, BCPS, BCPP
Pharmacotherapy Contributor
Lexi-Comp, Inc

Elizabeth A. Tomsik, PharmD, BCPS
Manager
Adverse Drug Reactions Group
Lexi-Comp, Inc

Dana Travis, RPh
Pharmacotherapy Specialist
Lexi-Comp, Inc

Jennifer Trofe-Clark, PharmD
Clinical Transplant Pharmacist
Hospital of The University of Pennsylvania

John N. van den Anker, MD, PhD, FCP, FAAP
Vice Chair of Pediatrics for Experimental Therapeutics
and *Chief and Professor of Evan and Cindy Jones Pediatric Clinical Pharmacology*
Children's National Medical Center
Professor of Pediatrics, Pharmacology & Physiology
George Washington University School of Medicine and Health Sciences

Heather L. VandenBussche, PharmD
Professor of Pharmacy, Pediatrics
Pharmacy Practice
Ferris State University College of Pharmacy

Amy Van Orman, PharmD, BCPS
Pharmacotherapy Specialist
Lexi-Comp, Inc

Kristin Watson, PharmD, BCPS
Assistant Professor, Cardiology
and *Clinical Pharmacist, Cardiology Service*
Heart Failure Clinic
University of Maryland Medical Center

David M. Weinstein, PhD, RPh
Manager
Metabolism, Interactions, and Genomics Group
Lexi-Comp, Inc

Anne Marie Whelan, PharmD
Associate Professor
College of Pharmacy
Dalhousie University

Greg Wiggers, PharmD, PhD
Pharmacotherapy Contributor
Lexi-Comp, Inc

Sherri J. Willard Argyres, MA, PharmD
Medical Science Pharmacist
Lexi-Comp, Inc

John C. Williamson, PharmD, BCPS
Pharmacy Clinical Coordinator, Infectious Diseases
Wake Forest Baptist Health

Nathan Wirick, PharmD
Infectious Disease and Antibiotic Management
Clinical Specialist
Hillcrest Hospital

Richard L. Wynn, BSPharm, PhD
Professor of Pharmacology
Baltimore College of Dental Surgery
University of Maryland

Sallie Young, PharmD, BCPS, AQ Cardiology
Clinical Pharmacy Specialist, Cardiology
Penn State Milton S. Hershey Medical Center

Jennifer Zimmer-Young, PharmD, CCRP
Educator, Clinical Pharmacist
ThedaCare

PREFACE TO THE NINETEENTH EDITION

The editors of the 19th edition of the *Drug Information Handbook for Dentistry* are extremely proud that the book remains as popular and as successful as its readers have affirmed. We thank each practitioner and student who has made the previous editions so widely accepted in the field of dentistry. In this new 19th edition, we have continued, as always, to respond to all of the comments and creative suggestions that come from our readership each year. We know that our text remains the premier companion to the daily practice of dentistry and that it complements Oral Medicine and medical reference libraries that every clinician has available in their office.

In addition to the extensive information presented, we are confident that the dental practitioners and dental hygienists who utilize the text will find the new size format to be easy to navigate. Their pharmacotherapeutics and oral medicine knowledge will be enhanced by its use. The complete cross-referencing of generic and brand names along with the foreign brands, makes the text the truly complete drug reference guide for dental practice.

The monographs now include over 1700 drugs and these have been updated in the 19th edition with the fields expanded in common monographs to make them easier to read and identify for all of the drugs. The fields most important to practicing dentists have been enhanced. The drugs most commonly used in dentistry have the added fields regarding specific use considerations in dentistry. Medical drugs also include dosing and dose formulation information. In addition, the adverse reaction section and the important uses and effects on dental treatment for all drugs have been updated throughout the text.

As in each previous edition, the Oral Medicine section has been updated offering a selection of prescription choices for management of common oral conditions often encountered during patient care. Stand-alone sections have been updated for the crucial topics of Antiplatelet and Anticoagulation Considerations in Dentistry, Clinical Risk Related to Drugs Prolonging QT Interval, and Osteonecrosis of the Jaw. Recommended readings have been edited for most chapter subsections. Sections have been expanded and added related to the latest Guidelines for Managing Patients with Joint Prostheses, Managing Alveolar Osteitis, prescribing medications with acetaminophen, and Sarcoidosis. Example prescriptions have been updated and remain in a stand-alone section for quicker reference. Prescribing information options are outlined and are available for easy cross reference for the dental practitioner. The subsection for Probiotics to Reduce Symptoms During Long-Term Antibiotic Therapy has been enhanced.

The alphabetical index at the back of the text continues to guide the reader through the text. The natural products section; drug synonyms; and U.S., Canadian, and Mexican brand names have all been updated. We hope that the active general dentist, the specialist, the dental hygienist, and the advanced student of dentistry remain better prepared for patient care while using this new 19th edition of the DIHD.

Richard L. Wynn

Timothy F. Meiller

Harold L. Crossley

DESCRIPTION OF SECTIONS AND FIELDS USED IN THIS HANDBOOK

The *Drug Information Handbook for Dentistry, 19th Edition* is organized into six sections: Introductory text; alphabetical listing of drug monographs; natural products; oral medicine topics; appendix; and indexes which include pharmacologic categories and alphabetical listings containing generic product names and index terms, as well as U.S., Canadian, and Mexican brand names.

INTRODUCTORY TEXT

Helpful guides to understanding the organization and format of the information in this handbook.

DRUG MONOGRAPHS

This alphabetical listing of drugs contains comprehensive monographs for medications commonly prescribed in dentistry and concise monographs for other popular drugs which dental patients may be taking. Monographs may contain the following fields:

Generic Name	U.S. adopted name
Pronunciation	Phonetic pronunciation guide
Related Information	Cross-reference(s) to pertinent information in other sections of this handbook
Related Sample Prescriptions	Cross-reference(s) to sample prescriptions.
Brand Names: U.S.	Trade name(s) (manufacturer-specific) found in the United States. The symbol [DSC] appears after trade names that have been recently discontinued.
Brand Names: Canada	Trade names found in Canada.
Generic Availability (U.S.)	Indicates availability of generic products in the United States
Pharmacologic Category	Indicates one or more systematic classifications of the drug
Dental Use	Information in the **Dental Use** field indicates when a drug has an established use specific to dentistry and/or oral medicine. In some cases, these uses are considered to be unlabeled, as they are not included in the FDA-approved product labeling (see Description of Dental Use).
Use	Statements under the **Use** field reflect the approved labeling by the FDA based on accepted clinical evaluation on safety and efficacy of the drug as submitted in the New Drug Application (NDA). The "gold standard" of clinical testing of a new drug requires a randomly-selected cohort of subjects, using a double-blind and placebo controlled protocol and an acceptable method of assessment to test differences between test compound and placebo. It is assumed that by their approval of the labeling, the FDA considers the new drug "safe and effective" for treating a particular condition in a given patient population.
Unlabeled Use	Statements under the **Unlabeled** use field refer to other conditions, dosages, or routes of administration which are decided by the prescriber, where such uses have not been officially approved by the FDA. Such "off label" use usually occurs in response to published studies supporting a drug's effectiveness in a new use and/or alternative dosing strategy. It is important to note that individual reports do not necessarily indicate in and of themselves that the safety and effectiveness of the drug in question has been established for the new use. If an individual report is one of many studies, the clinician is encouraged to read and critically review all of the studies in order to arrive at a decision on the safety and efficacy for the "off label" use.
Local Anesthetic/Vasoconstrictor Precautions	Specific information to prevent potential drug interactions related to anesthesia
Effects on Dental Treatment	Includes significant side effects of drug therapy which may directly or indirectly affect dental treatment or diagnosis; may also contain suggested management approaches and patient handling or care.
Effects on Bleeding	How the product affects bleeding during dental procedures
Adverse Effects	Side effects are grouped by percentage of incidence (if known) and/or body system
Dental Usual Dosage	The amount of the drug to be typically given or taken during dental treatment for children and adults

Dosage — The amount of the drug to be typically given or taken during therapy for children and adults; also includes any dosing adjustment/comments for renal impairment or hepatic failure; **Note:** For General Dosage Range: The range of dosing typically used during therapy in children and adults based upon route of administration. The information included is useful for confirming the dose is within the range but should not be used for prescribing purposes. Medications with a variety of indication-specific doses that cannot be encompassed by a range will not have a dose.

Mechanism of Action — How the drug works in the body to elicit a response

Contraindications — Information pertaining to inappropriate use of the drug as dictated by the approved labeling

Warnings/Precautions — Precautionary considerations, hazardous conditions related to use of the drug, and disease states or patient populations in which the drug should be cautiously used. Boxed warnings, when present, are clearly identified and are adapted from the FDA approved labeling. Consult the product labeling for the exact black box warning through the manufacturer's or the FDA website.

Drug Interactions

Metabolism/Transport Effects — If a drug has demonstrated involvement with cytochrome P450 enzymes, or other metabolism or transport proteins, this field will identify the drug as an inhibitor, inducer, or substrate of the specific enzyme(s) (eg, CYP1A2 or UGT1A1). CYP450 isoenzymes are identified as substrates (minor or major), inhibitors (weak, moderate, or strong), and inducers (weak or strong).

Avoid Concomitant Use — Designates drug combinations which should not be used concomitantly, due to an unacceptable risk:benefit assessment. Frequently, the concurrent use of the agents is explicitly prohibited or contraindicated by the product labeling.

Increased Effect/Toxicity — Drug combinations that result in an increased or toxic therapeutic effect between the drug listed in the monograph and other drugs or drug classes.

Decreased Effect — Drug combinations that result in a decreased therapeutic effect between the drug listed in the monograph and other drugs or drug classes.

Ethanol/Nutrition/Herb Interactions — Information regarding potential interactions with food, nutritionals, herbal products, vitamins, or ethanol

Dietary Considerations — Includes information on how the medication should be taken relative to meals or food

Pharmacodynamics/Kinetics

Onset of Action — The time after drug administration when therapeutic effect is observed; may also include time for peak therapeutic effect.

Duration of Action — Length of therapeutic effect.

Half-life Elimination — The reported half-life of elimination for the parent or metabolites of the drug

Time to Peak — Describes the relative time after ingestion when concentration achieves the highest serum concentration

Pregnancy Risk Factor — Five categories established by the FDA to indicate the potential of a systemically absorbed drug for causing risk to fetus.

Pregnancy Considerations — A summary of human and/or animal information pertinent to or associated with the use of the drug as it relates to clinical effects on the fetus, newborn, or pregnant women.

Lactation — Indicates if the drug listed in the monograph is present in breast milk and the manufacturers' recommendation for use while breast-feeding (where recommendation of American Academy of Pediatrics differs, notation is made).

Breast-Feeding Considerations — Information pertinent to or associated with the human use of the drug as it relates to clinical effects on the nursing infant or postpartum woman.

Product Availability — Provides availability information on products that have been approved by the FDA, but not yet available for use. Estimates for when a product may be available are included, when this information is known. May also provide any unique or critical drug availability issues.

Controlled Substance	Contains controlled substance schedule information as assigned by the United States Drug Enforcement Administration (DEA) or Canadian Controlled Substance Act (CDSA). CDSA information is only provided for drugs available in Canada and not available in the U.S.
Prescribing and Access Restrictions	Provides information on any special requirements regarding the prescribing, obtaining or dispensing of drugs, including access restrictions pertaining to drugs with REMS elements and those drugs whose access restrictions are not REMS-related.
Dosage Forms	Information with regard to form, strength, and availability of the drug in the United States. **Note:** Please consult individual product labeling for additional formulation information (eg, excipients, preservatives).
Dosage Forms: Canada	Information with regard to form, strength, and availability of products that are uniquely available in Canada, but currently not available in the United States.
Dental Comment	Pharmacology-related comments and considerations relevant to the dental professional
References	Sources and literature where the user may find additional information

NATURAL PRODUCTS: HERBAL AND DIETARY SUPPLEMENTS

The natural product content is adapted from *The Review of Natural Products* a Facts & Comparisons online database. This section consists of a clinical overview that summarizes the use, dosing, contraindications, pregnancy/lactation, interactions, adverse reactions, and toxicology information for each natural product. The dental-specific information is also included to further assist the dental professional in patient care.

ORAL MEDICINE TOPICS

This section is divided into three major parts and contains text on Oral Medicine topics. In each subsection, the systemic condition or the oral disease state is described briefly, followed by the pharmacologic considerations with which the dentist must be familiar.

I. **Dental Management and Therapeutic Considerations in Medically-Compromised Patients:** Focuses on common medical conditions and their associated drug therapies with which the dentist must be familiar. Patient profiles with commonly associated drug regimens are described.

II. **Dental Management and Therapeutic Considerations in Patients With Specific Oral Conditions:** Focuses on therapies the dentist may choose to prescribe for patients suffering from oral disease or who are in need of special care. Some overlap between these sections has resulted from systemic conditions that have oral manifestations and vice-versa. Cross-references to the descriptions and the monographs for individual drugs described elsewhere in this handbook allow for easy retrieval of information. Example prescriptions for each condition are presented so that the clinician can evaluate alternate approaches to treatment. Seldom is there a single drug of choice.
    Note: Prescriptions listed represent prototype drugs and popular prescriptions and are examples only. The pharmacologic category index is available for cross-referencing if alternatives or additional drugs are sought.

III. **Sample Prescriptions:** Examples provided for prototype drugs and popular prescriptions. Prescriptions included for the following uses: Bacterial endocarditis (prevention), prosthetic joint late infections (prevention), oral pain, bacterial infections and periodontal diseases, sinus infections treatment, antimicrobial rinses, fungal infections, viral infections, ulcerative and erosive disorders, sedation (prior to dental treatment).

APPENDIX

The appendix is broken down into various sections for easy use and offers a compilation of tables and guidelines which can often be helpful when considering patient care.

INDEXES

This section includes a pharmacologic category index with an easy-to-use classification system in alphabetical order and an alphabetical index which provides a quick reference for generic names, index terms, U.S., Canadian, and Mexican brand names. From this index, the reader can cross-reference to the monographs.

DESCRIPTION OF DENTAL USE

Unlabeled Use and Routes of Administration in Dentistry and Oral Medicine

The off-label use of a medication may involve differences in either the intended purpose or the route of administration of a particular medication. In dentistry, there are some situations which are common (clindamycin for endocarditis prophylaxis), and uncommon (application of Oralone® paste to the oral mucosa) which may be termed "unlabeled use". Depending on the degree of familiarity, the prescription of a drug for an off-label purpose may create concern on the part of healthcare professionals who are less familiar with the dental use of these medications. For example, a pharmacist may note the statement "for external use only" on the label of a tube of topical cream and question whether the drug should be applied to the oral mucosa. Usually, reinforcement of the use of a drug as well as an analysis of the likely systemic exposure/toxicity, can address these concerns.

The dentist who prescribes a drug bears the responsibility for deciding on the purpose of the prescription and the detail of the dosing regimen. These professional decisions are based on information from a variety of sources, including (but not limited to) the official labeling, sound scientific evidence, expert medical judgment, or published literature. In selected situations, these sources may justify the use of a drug in an off-label manner. Accepted professional standards indicate off-label use of a drug must be initiated in good faith, serve the best interest of the patient, and must be undertaken without fraudulent intent. Healthcare providers should recognize that the approved labeling is not intended to limit the practitioners in the exercise of his or her best professional judgment in serving the interest of patients. In addition, the purpose of labeling is not intended to impose liability for off-label use. However, it should be noted that a practitioner may be accountable for the negligent use in a civil action regardless of whether the FDA has approved the use of the drug in question. Based on these assertions, at least one medical organization (the American Academy of Pediatrics) has published in an official policy statement that the practice of medicine may actually require a practitioner to use drugs in an off-label manner in order to provide the most appropriate treatment for a given patient. Off-label use in dentistry and oral medicine is a frequently encountered issue. A discussion of the off-label use of drugs in dentistry appears in the *ADA Guide to Dental Therapeutics*, 3rd Edition, edited by Sebastian G. Ciancio, DDS in cooperation with the ADA Council on Scientific Affairs.

CONTROLLED SUBSTANCES

Schedule I = C-I

The drugs and other substances in this schedule have no legal medical uses except research. They have a **high** potential for abuse. They include selected opiates such as heroin, opium derivatives, and hallucinogens.

Schedule II = C-II

The drugs and other substances in this schedule have legal medical uses and a **high** abuse potential which may lead to severe dependence. They include former "Class A" narcotics, amphetamines, barbiturates, and other drugs.

Schedule III = C-III

The drugs and other substances in this schedule have legal medical uses and a **lesser** degree of abuse potential which may lead to **moderate** dependence. They include former "Class B" narcotics and other drugs.

Schedule IV = C-IV

The drugs and other substances in this schedule have legal medial uses and **low** abuse potential which may lead to **moderate** dependence. They include barbiturates, benzodiazepines, propoxyphenes, and other drugs.

Schedule V = C-V

The drugs and other substances in this schedule have legal medical uses and **low** abuse potential which may lead to **moderate** dependence. They include narcotic cough preparations, diarrhea preparations, and other drugs.

Note: These are federal classifications. Your individual state may place a substance into a more restricted category. When this occurs, the more restricted category applies. Consult your state law.

PREGNANCY CATEGORIES

Pregnancy Categories (sometimes referred to as pregnancy risk factors) are a letter system currently required under the *Teratogenic Effects* subsection of the product labeling. The system was initiated in 1979. The categories are required to be part of the package insert for prescription drugs that are systemically absorbed.

The categories are defined as follows:

A	Adequate and well-controlled studies in pregnant women have not shown that the drug increases the risk of fetal abnormalities.
B	Animal reproduction studies show no evidence of impaired fertility or harm to the fetus; however, no adequate and well-controlled studies have been conducted in pregnant women. **or** Animal reproduction studies have shown adverse events; however, studies in pregnant women have not shown that the drug increases the risk of abnormalities.
C	Animal reproduction studies have shown an adverse effect on the fetus. There are no adequate and well-controlled studies in humans and the benefits from the use of the drug in pregnant women may be acceptable, despite its potential risks. **or** Animal reproduction studies have not been conducted.
D	Based on human data, the drug can cause fetal harm when administered to pregnant women, but the potential benefits from the use of the drug may be acceptable, despite its potential risks.
X	Studies in animals or humans have demonstrated fetal abnormalities (or there is positive evidence of fetal risk based on reports and/or marketing experience) and the risk of using the drug in pregnant women clearly outweighs any possible benefit (for example, safer drugs or other forms of therapy are available).

The categories do not take into consideration nonteratogenic effects (that information is currently presented separately). In 2008, the Food and Drug Administration (FDA) proposed new labeling requirements which would eliminate the use of the pregnancy category system and replace it with scientific data and other information specific to the use of the drug in pregnant women. These proposed changes were suggested because the current category system may be misleading. For instance, some practitioners may believe that risk increases from category A to B to C to D to X, which is not the intent. In addition, practitioners may not be aware that some medications are categorized based on animal data, while others are based on human data. When the new labeling requirements are approved, product labeling will contain pregnancy and lactation subsections, each describing a risk summary, clinical considerations, and section for specific data.

For full descriptions of the current and proposed labeling requirements, refer to the following websites:

Labeling Requirements for Prescription Drugs and/or Insulin (Code of Federal Regulations, Title 21, Volume 4, Revised April 1, 2010). Available at http://www.accessdata.fda.gov/scripts/cdrh/cfdocs/cfCFR/CFRSearch.cfm?fr=201.57

Content and Format of Labeling for Human Prescription Drug and Biological Products; Requirements for Pregnancy and Lactation Labeling (Federal Register, May 29, 2008). Available at http://frwebgate.access.gpo.gov/cgi-bin/getdoc.cgi?dbname=2008_register&docid=fr29my08-33.pdfPregnancy Risk Factors

FDA NAME DIFFERENTIATION PROJECT: THE USE OF TALL-MAN LETTERS

Confusion between similar drug names is an important cause of medication errors. For years, The Institute For Safe Medication Practices (ISMP), has urged generic manufacturers to use a combination of large and small letters as well as bolding (ie, chlorpro**MAZINE** and chlorpro**PAMIDE**) to help distinguish drugs with look-alike names, especially when they share similar strengths. Recently the FDA's Division of Generic Drugs began to issue recommendation letters to manufacturers suggesting this novel way to label their products to help reduce this drug name confusion. Although this project has had marginal success, the method has successfully eliminated problems with products such as diphenhydr-**AMINE** and dimenhy**DRINATE**. Hospitals should also follow suit by making similar changes in their own labels, preprinted order forms, computer screens and printouts, and drug storage location labels.

Lexi-Comp, Inc. Medical Publishing will use "Tall-Man" letters for the drugs suggested by the FDA or recommended by ISMP.

The following is a list of generic and brand name product names and recommended revisions.

Drug Product	Recommended Revision
acetazolamide	aceta**ZOLAMIDE**
alprazolam	**ALPRAZ**olam
amiloride	a**MIL**oride
amlodipine	am**LODIP**ine
aripiprazole	**ARIP**iprazole
atomoxetine	ato**MOX**etine
atorvastatin	atorva**STAT**in
Avinza	**AVIN**za
azacitidine	aza**CITID**ine
azathioprine	aza**THIO**prine
bupropion	bu**PROP**ion
buspirone	bus**PIR**one
carbamazepine	car**BAM**azepine
carboplatin	**CARBO**platin
cefazolin	ce**FAZ**olin
cefotetan	cefo**TET**an
cefoxitin	cef**OX**itin
ceftazidime	cef**TAZ**idime
ceftriaxone	cef**TRIAX**one
Celebrex	Cele**BREX**
Celexa	Cele**XA**
chlordiazepoxide	chlordiaze**POXIDE**
chlorpromazine	chlorpro**MAZINE**
chlorpropamide	chlorpro**PAMIDE**
cisplatin	**CIS**platin
clobazam	clo**BAZ**am
clomiphene	clomi**PHENE**
clomipramine	clomi**PRAMINE**
clonazepam	clonaze**PAM**
clonidine	clo**NID**ine
clozapine	clo**ZAP**ine
cycloserine	cyclo**SERINE**
cyclosporine	cyclo**SPORINE**
dactinomycin	**DACTIN**omycin
daptomycin	**DAPTO**mycin
daunorubicin	**DAUNO**rubicin
dimenhydrinate	dimenhy**DRINATE**
diphenhydramine	diphenhydr**AMINE**
dobutamine	**DOBUT**amine
docetaxel	**DOCE**taxel
dopamine	**DOP**amine
doxorubicin	**DOXO**rubicin

Drug Product	Recommended Revision
duloxetine	DULoxetine
ephedrine	ePHEDrine
epinephrine	EPINEPHrine
epirubicin	EPIrubicin
eribulin	eriBULin
fentanyl	fentaNYL
flavoxate	flavoxATE
fluoxetine	FLUoxetine
fluphenazine	fluPHENAZine
fluvoxamine	fluvoxaMINE
glipizide	glipiZIDE
glyburide	glyBURIDE
guaifenesin	guaiFENesin
guanfacine	guanFACINE
Humalog	HumaLOG
Humulin	HumuLIN
hydralazine	hydrALAZINE
hydrocodone	HYDROcodone
hydromorphone	HYDROmorphone
hydroxyzine	hydrOXYzine
idarubicin	IDArubicin
infliximab	inFLIXimab
Invanz	INVanz
isotretinoin	ISOtretinoin
Klonopin	KlonoPIN
Lamictal	LaMICtal
Lamisil	LamISIL
lamivudine	lamiVUDine
lamotrigine	lamoTRIgine
levetiracetam	LevETIRAcetam
levocarnitine	levOCARNitine
lorazepam	LORazepam
medroxyprogesterone	medroxyPROGESTERone
metformin	metFORMIN
methylprednisolone	methylPREDNISolone
methyltestosterone	methylTESTOSTERone
metronidazole	metroNIDAZOLE
mitomycin	mitoMYcin
mitoxantrone	MitoXANtrone
Nexavar	NexAVAR
Nexium	NexIUM
nicardipine	niCARdipine
nifedipine	NIFEdipine
nimodipine	niMODipine
Novolin	NovoLIN
Novolog	NovoLOG
olanzapine	OLANZapine
oxcarbazepine	OXcarbazepine
oxycodone	oxyCODONE
Oxycontin	OxyCONTIN
paclitaxel	PACLitaxel
paroxetine	PARoxetine
pemetrexed	PEMEtrexed
penicillamine	penicillAMINE
pentobarbital	PENTobarbital
phenobarbital	PHENobarbital
pralatrexate	PRALAtrexate

Drug Product	Recommended Revision
prednisolone	predniso**LONE**
prednisone	predni**SONE**
Prilosec	Pri**LOSEC**
Prozac	**PRO**zac
quetiapine	**QUE**tiapine
quinidine	qui**NID**ine
quinine	qui**NINE**
rabeprazole	**RABE**prazole
Risperdal	Risper**DAL**
risperidone	risperi**DONE**
rituximab	ri**TUX**imab
romidepsin	romi**DEP**sin
romiplostim	romi**PLOS**tim
ropinirole	r**OPINIR**ole
Sandimmune	sand**IMMUNE**
Sandostatin	Sando**STATIN**
Seroquel	**SERO**quel
Sinequan	**SINE**quan
sitagliptin	sita**GLIP**tin
Solu-Cortef	Solu-**CORTEF**
Solu-Medrol	Solu-**MEDROL**
sorafenib	**SORA**fenib
sufentanil	**SUF**entanil
sulfadiazine	sulf**ADIAZINE**
sulfasalazine	sulfa**SALA**zine
sumatriptan	**SUMA**triptan
sunitinib	**SUN**Itinib
Tegretol	**TEG**retol
tiagabine	tia**GAB**ine
tizanidine	ti**ZAN**idine
tolazamide	**TOLAZ**amide
tolbutamide	**TOLBUT**amide
tramadol	tra**MAD**ol
trazodone	tra**ZOD**one
Trental	**TREN**tal
valacyclovir	val**ACY**clovir
valganciclovir	val**GAN**ciclovir
vinblastine	vin**BLAS**tine
vincristine	vin**CRIS**tine
zolmitriptan	**ZOLM**itriptan
Zyprexa	Zy**PREXA**
Zyrtec	Zyr**TEC**

"FDA and ISMP Lists of Look-Alike Drug Names with Recommended Tall Man Letter." Available at http://www.ismp.org/tools/tallmanletters.pdf. Last accessed January 6, 2011.
"Name Differentiation Project." Available at http://www.fda.gov/Drugs/DrugSafety/MedicationErrors/ucm164587.htm. Last accessed January 6, 2011.
U.S. Pharmacopeia, "USP Quality Review: Use Caution-Avoid Confusion," March 2001, No. 76. Available at http://www.usp.org

PRESCRIPTION WRITING

Doctor's Name
Address
Phone Number

Patient's Name/Date

Patient's Address/Age

Rx

Drug Name/Dosage Size
Disp: Number of tablets, capsules, ounces to be dispensed (roman numerals added as precaution for abused drugs)
Sig: Direction on how drug is to be taken

Doctor's signature
State license number
DEA number (if required)

PRESCRIPTION REQUIREMENTS

1. Date

2. Full name and address of patient

3. Name and address of prescriber

4. Signature of prescriber

If Class II drug, Drug Enforcement Agency (DEA) number necessary.

If Class II and Class III narcotic, a triplicate prescription form (in the state of California) is necessary and it must be handwritten by the prescriber.

Please turn to appropriate oral medicine chapters for examples of prescriptions.

PREVENTING PRESCRIBING ERRORS

Prescribing errors account for the majority of reported medication errors and have prompted healthcare professionals to focus on the development of steps to make the prescribing process safer. Prescription legibility has been attributed to a portion of these errors and legislation has been enacted in several states to address prescription legibility. However, eliminating handwritten prescriptions and ordering medications through the use of technology [eg, computerized prescriber order entry (CPOE)] has been the primary recommendation. Whether a prescription is electronic, typed, or hand-printed, additional safe practices should be considered for implementation to maximize the safety of the prescribing process. Listed below are suggestions for safer prescribing:

- Ensure correct patient by using at least 2 patient identifiers on the prescription (eg, full name, birth date, or address). Review prescription with the patient or patient's caregiver.

- If pediatric patient, document patient's birth date or age and most recent weight. If geriatric patient, document patient's birth date or age.

- Prevent drug name confusion: For more information, see http://www.ismp.org/tools/confuseddrugnames.pdf.

    - Use TALLman lettering (eg, buPROPion, busPIRone, predniSONE, prednisoLONE). For more information, see http://www.fda.gov/drugs/drugsafety/medicationerrors/default.htm.

    - Avoid abbreviated drug names (eg, MSO_4, $MgSO_4$, MS, HCT, 6MP, MTX), as they may be misinterpreted and cause error.

    - Avoid investigational names for drugs with FDA approval (eg, FK-506, CBDCA).

    - Avoid chemical names such as 6-mercaptopurine or 6-thioguanine, as sixfold overdoses have been given when these were not recognized as chemical names. The proper names of these drugs are mercaptopurine or thioguanine.

    - Use care when prescribing drugs that look or sound similar (eg, look- alike, sound-alike drugs). Common examples include: Celebrex® vs Celexa®, hydroxyzine vs hydralazine, Zyprexa® vs Zyrtec®.

- Avoid dangerous, error-prone abbreviations (eg, regardless of letter-case: U, IU, QD, QOD, µg, cc, @). Do not use apothecary system or symbols. Additionally, text messaging abbreviations (eg, "2Day") should never be used.

    - For more information, see http://www.ismp.org/tools/errorproneabbreviations.pdf.

- Always use a leading zero for numbers less than 1 (0.5 mg is correct and .5 mg is **incorrect**) and never use a trailing zero for whole numbers (2 mg is correct and 2.0 mg is **incorrect**).

- Always use a space between a number and its units as it is easier to read. There should be no periods after the abbreviations mg or mL (10 mg is correct and 10mg is **incorrect**).

- For doses that are greater than 1,000 dosing units, use properly placed commas to prevent 10-fold errors (100,000 units is correct and 100000 units is **incorrect**).

- Do not prescribe drug dosage by the type of container in which the drug is available (eg, do not prescribe "1 amp", "2 vials", etc).

- Do not write vague or ambiguous orders which have the potential for misinterpretation by other healthcare providers. Examples of vague orders to avoid: "Resume pre-op medications," "give drug per protocol," or "continue home medications."

- Review each prescription with patient (or patient's caregiver) including the medication name, indication, and directions for use.

- Take extra precautions when prescribing *high alert drugs* (drugs that can cause significant patient harm when prescribed in error). Common examples of these drugs include: Anticoagulants, chemotherapy, insulins, opioids, and sedatives.

    - For more information, see http://www.ismp.org/tools/institutionalhighalert.asp or http://www.ismp.org/communityRx/tools/ambulatoryhighalert.asp.

To Err Is Human: Building a Safer Health System, Kohn LT, Corrigan JM, and Donaldson MS, eds, Washington, D.C.: National Academy Press, 2000.

A Complete Outpatient Prescription[1]

A complete outpatient prescription can prevent the prescriber, the pharmacist, and/or the patient from making a mistake and can eliminate the need for further clarification. The complete outpatient prescription should contain:

- Patient's full name
- Medication indication
- Allergies
- Prescriber name and telephone or pager number
- For pediatric patients: Their birth date or age and current weight
- For geriatric patients: Their birth date or age
- Drug name, dosage form and strength
- For pediatric patients: Intended daily weight-based dose so that calculations can be checked by the pharmacist (ie, mg/kg/day or units/kg/day)
- Number or amount to be dispensed
- Complete instructions for the patient or caregiver, including the purpose of the medication, directions for use (including dose), dosing frequency, route of administration, duration of therapy, and number of refills.
- Dose should be expressed in convenient units of measure.
- When there are recognized contraindications for a prescribed drug, the prescriber should indicate knowledge of this fact to the pharmacist (ie, when prescribing a potassium salt for a patient receiving an ACE inhibitor, the prescriber should write "K serum leveling being monitored").

Upon dispensing of the final product, the pharmacist should ensure that the patient or caregiver can effectively demonstrate the appropriate administration technique. An appropriate measuring device should be provided or recommended. Household teaspoons and tablespoons should not be used to measure liquid medications due to their variability and inaccuracies in measurement; oral medication syringes are recommended.

For additional information, see http://www.ismp.org/Newsletters/acutecare/articles/20020601.asp

[1]Levine SR, Cohen MR, Blanchard NR, et al, "Guidelines for Preventing Medication Errors in Pediatrics," *J Pediatr Pharmacol Ther*, 2001, 6:426-42.

ALPHABETICAL LISTING OF DRUGS

Abacavir (a BAK a veer)

Related Information
HIV Infection and AIDS *on page 1520*
Brand Names: U.S. Ziagen®
Brand Names: Canada Ziagen®
Pharmacologic Category Antiretroviral Agent, Reverse Transcriptase Inhibitor (Nucleoside)
Use Treatment of HIV infections in combination with other antiretroviral agents
Local Anesthetic/Vasoconstrictor Precautions No information available to require special precautions
Effects on Dental Treatment No significant effects or complications reported
Effects on Bleeding No information available to require special precautions relative to altered hemostasis
Adverse Effects Hypersensitivity reactions (which may be fatal) occur in ~5% of patients. Symptoms may include anaphylaxis, fever, rash (including erythema multiforme), fatigue, diarrhea, abdominal pain; respiratory symptoms (eg, pharyngitis, dyspnea, cough, adult respiratory distress syndrome, or respiratory failure); headache, malaise, lethargy, myalgia, myolysis, arthralgia, edema, paresthesia, nausea and vomiting, mouth ulcerations, conjunctivitis, lymphadenopathy, hepatic failure, and renal failure.

Note: Rates of adverse reactions were defined during combination therapy with other antiretrovirals (lamivudine and efavirenz **or** lamivudine and zidovudine). Only reactions which occurred at a higher frequency in adults (except where noted) than in the comparator group are noted. Adverse reaction rates attributable to abacavir alone are not available.

>10%:
 Central nervous system: Headache (7% to 13%)
 Gastrointestinal: Nausea (7% to 19%, children 9%)
1% to 10%:
 Central nervous system: Depression (6%), fever/chills (6%, children 9%), anxiety (5%)
 Dermatologic: Rash (5% to 6%, children 7%)
 Endocrine & metabolic: Triglycerides increased (2% to 6%)
 Gastrointestinal: Diarrhea (7%), vomiting (children 9%), amylase increased (2%)
 Hematologic: Thrombocytopenia (1%)
 Hepatic: AST increased (6%)
 Neuromuscular & skeletal: Musculoskeletal pain (5% to 6%)
 Miscellaneous: Hypersensitivity reactions (2% to 9%; may include reactions to other components of antiretroviral regimen), infection (ENT 5%)
General Dosage Range Dosage adjustment recommended in patients with hepatic impairment
 Oral:
 Infants and Children ≥3 months to <16 years: 8 mg/kg twice daily (maximum: 300 mg twice daily)
 Adolescents ≥16 years and Adults: 600 mg/day in 1-2 divided doses (maximum: 600 mg/day)
Mechanism of Action Nucleoside reverse transcriptase inhibitor. Abacavir is a guanosine analogue which is phosphorylated to carbovir triphosphate which interferes with HIV viral RNA-dependent DNA polymerase resulting in inhibition of viral replication.
Pharmacodynamics/Kinetics
 Half-life Elimination 1.5 hours
 Time to Peak 0.7-1.7 hours
Pregnancy Risk Factor C

Pregnancy Considerations Adverse events have been observed in some animal reproduction studies. Abacavir crosses the human placenta. No increased risk of overall birth defects has been observed following first trimester exposure according to data collected by the antiretroviral pregnancy registry. Cases of lactic acidosis/hepatic steatosis syndrome related to mitochondrial toxicity have been reported in pregnant women with prolonged use of nucleoside analogues. It is not known if pregnancy itself potentiates this known side effect; however, women may be at increased risk of lactic acidosis and liver damage. In addition, these adverse events are similar to other rare but life-threatening syndromes which occur during pregnancy (eg, HELLP syndrome). Hepatic enzymes and electrolytes should be monitored in women receiving nucleoside analogues and clinicians should watch for early signs of the syndrome. In addition, mitochondrial dysfunction may develop in infants following *in utero* exposure. The pharmacokinetics of abacavir are not significantly changed by pregnancy and dose adjustment is not needed for pregnant women. The DHHS Perinatal HIV Guidelines consider abacavir to be an alternative NRTI in dual nucleoside combination regimens.

Regardless of CD4 count or HIV RNA copy number, all HIV-infected pregnant women should receive a combination antepartum antiretroviral (ARV) drug regimen; this includes women who require therapy for their own health, as well as women who do not yet require therapy for their own health. ARV therapy should be started as soon as possible if required for the woman's health. Although earlier initiation may be more effective in reducing the perinatal transmission of HIV, also consider maternal conditions (eg, nausea and vomiting) and the potential risks of first trimester fetal exposure for specific agents. Plasma HIV RNA levels should be assessed at ~34-36 weeks gestation in order to help determine mode of delivery. If ARV therapy must be interrupted for <24 hours during the peripartum period, stop then restart all medications simultaneously in order to decrease the chance of developing resistance. Long-term follow-up is recommended for all infants exposed to ARV medications.

Healthcare providers are encouraged to enroll pregnant women exposed to antiretroviral medications in the Antiretroviral Pregnancy Registry (1-800-258-4263 or www.APRegistry.com). Healthcare providers caring for HIV-infected women and their infants may contact the National Perinatal HIV Hotline (888-448-8765) for clinical consultation (DHHS [perinatal], 2012).

Abacavir and Lamivudine
(a BAK a veer & la MI vyoo deen)

Related Information
Abacavir *on page 22*
LamiVUDine *on page 791*
Brand Names: U.S. Epzicom®
Brand Names: Canada Kivexa™
Pharmacologic Category Antiretroviral Agent, Reverse Transcriptase Inhibitor (Nucleoside)
Use Treatment of HIV infections in combination with other antiretroviral agents
Local Anesthetic/Vasoconstrictor Precautions No information available to require special precautions
Effects on Dental Treatment No significant effects or complications reported

Effects on Bleeding No information available to require special precautions relative to altered hemostasis

Adverse Effects See individual agents.

General Dosage Range Oral: *Adults:* One tablet (abacavir 600 mg and lamivudine 300 mg) once daily

Mechanism of Action Nucleoside reverse transcriptase inhibitor combination.

Abacavir is a guanosine analogue which is phosphorylated to carbovir triphosphate which interferes with HIV viral RNA-dependent DNA polymerase resulting in inhibition of viral replication.

Lamivudine is a cytosine analog. After lamivudine is triphosphorylated, the principle mode of action is inhibition of HIV reverse transcription via viral DNA chain termination; inhibits RNA-dependent DNA polymerase activities of reverse transcriptase.

Pregnancy Risk Factor C

Pregnancy Considerations See individual agents.

Abacavir, Lamivudine, and Zidovudine
(a BAK a veer, la MI vyoo deen, & zye DOE vyoo deen)

Related Information
Abacavir *on page 22*
HIV Infection and AIDS *on page 1520*
LamiVUDine *on page 791*
Zidovudine *on page 1419*

Brand Names: U.S. Trizivir®

Brand Names: Canada Trizivir®

Pharmacologic Category Antiretroviral Agent, Reverse Transcriptase Inhibitor (Nucleoside)

Use Treatment of HIV infection (either alone or in combination with other antiretroviral agents) in patients whose regimen would otherwise contain the components of Trizivir®

Local Anesthetic/Vasoconstrictor Precautions No information available to require special precautions

Effects on Dental Treatment No significant effects or complications reported

Effects on Bleeding No information available to require special precautions relative to altered hemostasis

Adverse Effects Fatal hypersensitivity reactions have occurred in patients taking abacavir (in Trizivir®). If Trizivir® is to be restarted following an interruption in therapy, first evaluate the patient for previously unsuspected symptoms of hypersensitivity. Do not restart if hypersensitivity is suspected or if hypersensitivity cannot be ruled out.

The following information is based on CNA3005 study data concerning effects noted in patients receiving abacavir, lamivudine, and zidovudine. See individual agents for additional information.

>10%:
Central nervous system: Headache (13%), malaise (12%), fatigue (12%)
Gastrointestinal: Nausea (19%)
1% to 10%:
Central nervous system: Fever/chills (6%), depression (6%), anxiety (5%)
Dermatologic: Rash (5%)
Endocrine & metabolic: Triglycerides increased (2% grade 3-4)
Gastrointestinal: Nausea and vomiting (10%), diarrhea (7%), amylase increased (2%)
Hematologic: Neutropenia (5%)

Hepatic: ALT increased (6%)
Neuromuscular & skeletal: CPK increased (7%)
Otic: Ear infection (5%)
Respiratory: Nose/throat infection (5%)
Miscellaneous: Hypersensitivity (2% to 9% based on abacavir component), viral infection (5%)
Other (frequency unknown): Pancreatitis, GGT increased, fat redistribution, immune reconstitution syndrome

General Dosage Range Oral: *Adolescents ≥40 kg and Adults:* One tablet twice daily

Mechanism of Action The combination of abacavir, lamivudine, and zidovudine is believed to act synergistically to inhibit reverse transcriptase via DNA chain termination after incorporation of the nucleoside analogue as well as to delay the emergence of mutations conferring resistance.

Pregnancy Risk Factor C

Pregnancy Considerations See individual agents.

Abatacept (ab a TA sept)

Related Information
Rheumatoid Arthritis, Osteoarthritis, and Osteoporosis *on page 1526*

Brand Names: U.S. Orencia®

Brand Names: Canada Orencia®

Pharmacologic Category Antirheumatic, Disease Modifying; Selective T-Cell Costimulation Blocker

Use
Treatment of moderately- to severely-active adult rheumatoid arthritis (RA); may be used as monotherapy or in combination with other DMARDs
Treatment of moderately- to severely-active juvenile idiopathic arthritis (JIA); may be used as monotherapy or in combination with methotrexate
Note: Abatacept should **not** be used in combination with anakinra or TNF-blocking agents

Local Anesthetic/Vasoconstrictor Precautions No information available to require special precautions

Effects on Dental Treatment No significant effects or complications reported

Effects on Bleeding No information available to require special precautions

Adverse Effects Note: Percentages not always reported; COPD patients experienced a higher frequency of COPD-related adverse reactions (COPD exacerbation, cough, dyspnea, pneumonia, rhonchi)

>10%:
Central nervous system: Headache (≤18%)
Gastrointestinal: Nausea
Respiratory: Nasopharyngitis (12%), upper respiratory tract infection
Miscellaneous: Infection (adults 54%; children 36%), antibody formation (2% to 41%)
1% to 10%:
Cardiovascular: Hypertension (7%)
Central nervous system: Dizziness (9%), fever
Dermatologic: Rash (4%)
Gastrointestinal: Dyspepsia (6%), abdominal pain, diarrhea
Genitourinary: Urinary tract infection (6%)
Local: Injection site reaction (3%)
Neuromuscular & skeletal: Back pain (7%), limb pain (3%)
Respiratory: Cough (8%), bronchitis, pneumonia, rhinitis, sinusitis
Miscellaneous: Infusion-related reactions (≤9%), herpes simplex, immunogenicity (1% to 2%), influenza

General Dosage Range
I.V.: Repeat dose at 2 weeks and 4 weeks, then every 4 weeks thereafter
Children ≥6 years and <75 kg: 10 mg/kg/dose
Children ≥6 years and 75-100 kg: 750 mg/dose
Children ≥6 years and >100 kg: 1000 mg/dose
Adults <60 kg: 500 mg/dose
Adults 60-100 kg: 750 mg/dose
Adults >100 kg: 1000 mg/dose
SubQ: *Adults:* 125 mg/dose once weekly
Mechanism of Action Selective costimulation modulator; inhibits T-cell (T-lymphocyte) activation by binding to CD80 and CD86 on antigen presenting cells (APC), thus blocking the required CD28 interaction between APCs and T cells. Activated T lymphocytes are found in the synovium of rheumatoid arthritis patients.
Pharmacodynamics/Kinetics
Half-life Elimination 8-25 days
Pregnancy Risk Factor C
Pregnancy Considerations Teratogenic effects were not observed in animal studies. There are no adequate and well-controlled studies in pregnant women. Due to the potential risk for development of autoimmune disease in the fetus, use during pregnancy only if clearly needed. A pregnancy registry has been established to monitor outcomes of women exposed to abatacept during pregnancy (1-877-311-8972).

Abciximab (ab SIK si mab)

Related Information
Cardiovascular Diseases *on page 1492*
Brand Names: U.S. Reopro®
Brand Names: Canada ReoPro®
Pharmacologic Category Antiplatelet Agent, Glycoprotein IIb/IIIa Inhibitor
Use Prevention of cardiac ischemic complications in patients undergoing percutaneous coronary intervention (PCI); prevention of cardiac ischemic complications in patients with unstable angina (UA)/non-ST-elevation myocardial infarction (NSTEMI) unresponsive to conventional therapy when PCI is scheduled within 24 hours

Note: Intended for use with aspirin and heparin, at a minimum.
Unlabeled Use To support PCI during ST-elevation myocardial infarction (STEMI) (administered at the time of primary PCI)
Local Anesthetic/Vasoconstrictor Precautions No information available to require special precautions
Effects on Dental Treatment Key adverse event(s) related to dental treatment: Bleeding is a potential adverse effect of abciximab during dental surgery. See Effects on Bleeding.
Effects on Bleeding As with all antiplatelet drugs, bleeding is a potential adverse effect of abciximab during dental surgery; risk is dependent on multiple variables, including the intensity of anticoagulation and patient susceptibility. Medical consult is suggested. It is unlikely that ambulatory patients presenting for dental treatment will be taking intravenous antiplatelet therapy such as abciximab.
Adverse Effects As with all drugs which may affect hemostasis, bleeding is associated with abciximab. Hemorrhage may occur at virtually any site. Risk is dependent on multiple variables, including the concurrent use of multiple agents which alter hemostasis and patient susceptibility.

>10%:
Cardiovascular: Hypotension (14%), chest pain (11%)
Gastrointestinal: Nausea (14%)
Hematologic: Minor bleeding (4% to 17%)
Neuromuscular & skeletal: Back pain (18%)
1% to 10%:
Cardiovascular: Bradycardia (5%), peripheral edema (2%)
Central nervous system: Headache (7%)
Gastrointestinal: Vomiting (7%), abdominal pain (3%)
Hematologic: Major bleeding (1% to 14%), thrombocytopenia: <100,000 cells/mm^3 (3% to 6%); <50,000 cells/mm^3 (0.4% to 2%)
Local: Injection site pain (4%)
General Dosage Range I.V.: *Adults:* Bolus: 0.25 mg/kg; Infusion: 0.125 mcg/kg/minute (maximum: 10 mcg/minute)
Mechanism of Action Fab antibody fragment of the chimeric human-murine monoclonal antibody 7E3; this agent binds to platelet IIb/IIIa receptors, resulting in steric hindrance, thus inhibiting platelet aggregation
Pharmacodynamics/Kinetics
Onset of Action Rapid; platelet aggregation reduced to <20% of baseline at 10 minutes
Duration of Action Up to 72 hours for restoration of normal hemostasis (Schror, 2003)
Half-life Elimination Plasma: ~30 minutes; dissociation half-life from GP IIb/IIIa receptors: up to 4 hours (Schror, 2003). Note: 29% and 13% of abciximab estimated to remain on GP IIb/IIIa receptors at 8 and 15 days, respectively (Mascelli, 1998). Platelet function may remain abnormal for up to 7 days post infusion (Osende, 2001).
Time to Peak Platelet inhibition: ~30 minutes (Mascelli, 1998)
Pregnancy Risk Factor C
Pregnancy Considerations Animal reproduction studies have not been conducted. *In vitro* studies have shown only small amounts of abciximab to cross the placenta. It is not known whether abciximab can cause fetal harm when administered to a pregnant woman or can affect reproduction capacity.

Abiraterone Acetate (a bir A ter one AS e tate)

Brand Names: U.S. Zytiga®
Brand Names: Canada Zytiga®
Pharmacologic Category Antiandrogen; Antineoplastic Agent, Antiandrogen
Use Treatment of metastatic, castration-resistant prostate cancer (in combination with prednisone)
Local Anesthetic/Vasoconstrictor Precautions No information available to require special precautions
Effects on Dental Treatment No significant effects or complications reported
Effects on Bleeding No information available to require special precautions
Adverse Effects Note: Adverse reactions reported for use in combination with prednisone.
>10%:
Cardiovascular: Edema (25% to 27%), hypertension (9% to 22%; grades 3/4: 1% to 4%)
Central nervous system: Fatigue (39%), insomnia (14%)
Dermatologic: Bruising (13%)

Endocrine & metabolic: Triglycerides increased (63%), hyperglycemia (57%), hypernatremia (33%), hypokalemia (17% to 28%; grades 3/4: 3% to 5%), hypophosphatemia (24%; grades 3/4: 7%), hot flush (19% to 22%)

Gastrointestinal: Constipation (23%), diarrhea (18% to 22%), dyspepsia (6% to 11%)

Genitourinary: Urinary tract infection (12%)

Hematologic: Lymphopenia (38%; grades 3/4: 9%)

Hepatic: ALT increased (11% to 42%; grades 3/4: 1% to 6%), AST increased (31% to 37%; grades 3/4: 2% to 3%)

Neuromuscular & skeletal: Joint swelling/discomfort (30%), muscle discomfort (26%)

Respiratory: Cough (11% to 17%), upper respiratory infection (5% to 13%), dyspnea (12%), nasopharyngitis (11%)

1% to 10%:

Cardiovascular: Arrhythmia (7%), chest pain/discomfort (4%), heart failure (2%)

Central nervous system: Fever (9%)

Dermatologic: Rash (8%)

Genitourinary: Hematuria (10%), polyuria (7%), nocturia (6%)

Hepatic: Bilirubin increased (7%; grades 3/4: <1%)

Neuromuscular & skeletal: Groin pain (7%), falling (6%), fractures (6%)

General Dosage Range Dosage adjustment recommended in patients with hepatic impairment or who develop toxicity.

Oral: *Adults:* 1000 mg once daily

Mechanism of Action Selectively and irreversibly inhibits CYP17 (17 alpha-hydroxylase/C17,20-lyase), an enzyme required for androgen biosynthesis which is expressed in testicular, adrenal, and prostatic tumor tissues. Inhibits the formation of the testosterone precursors dehydroepiandrosterone (DHEA) and androstenedione.

Pharmacodynamics/Kinetics

Half-life Elimination 14.4-16.5 hours (Acharya, 2012)

Time to Peak 2 hours (Acharya, 2012)

Pregnancy Risk Factor X

Pregnancy Considerations Adverse effects were observed in animal reproduction studies at doses resulting in less systemic exposure than in humans. Adverse effects were also observed in the reproductive system of animals during toxicology and pharmacology studies. Based on the mechanism of action, abiraterone may cause fetal harm or fetal loss if administered during pregnancy. Abiraterone is not indicated for use in women and is specifically contraindicated in women who are or may become pregnant. It is not known if abiraterone is excreted in semen, therefore, men should use a condom and another method of birth control during treatment and for 1 week following therapy if having intercourse with a woman of reproductive age. Women who are or may become pregnant should wear gloves if contact with tablets may occur.

AbobotulinumtoxinA
(aye bo BOT yoo lin num TOKS in aye)

Brand Names: U.S. Dysport™

Pharmacologic Category Neuromuscular Blocker Agent, Toxin

Use Treatment of cervical dystonia in both toxin-naive and previously treated patients; temporary improvement in the appearance of moderate-severe glabellar lines associated with procerus and corrugator muscle activity

Local Anesthetic/Vasoconstrictor Precautions No information available to require special precautions

Effects on Dental Treatment Key adverse event(s) related to dental treatment: Xerostomia (normal salivary flow resumes upon discontinuation) and facial paresis.

Effects on Bleeding No information available to require special precautions

Adverse Effects

>10%:

Cervical dystonia:

Central nervous system: Dysphonia (≤28%), fatigue (12%), headache (11%)

Gastrointestinal: Dysphagia (15% to 39%), xerostomia (13% to 39%)

Local: Injection site discomfort/pain (5% to 22%)

Neuromuscular & skeletal: Weakness (11% to 56%), facial paresis (≤11%)

Ocular: Eye disorders (≤17%, includes accommodation disorder, blurred vision, diplopia, dryness, pain, pruritus, visual acuity decreased)

Miscellaneous: Infection (13%)

1% to 10%:

Cervical dystonia:

Cardiovascular: Heart rate decreased

Central nervous system: Dizziness (≤4%)

Endocrine & metabolic: Blood glucose increased

Neuromuscular & skeletal: Pain (7%), muscle atrophy (1%)

Respiratory: Breathing difficulties/dyspnea (~3%; onset: ~1 week; duration: ~3 weeks)

Miscellaneous: Antibody formation (3%)

Glabellar lines:

Central nervous system: Headache (9%)

Dermatologic: Contact dermatitis (2% to 3%)

Gastrointestinal: Nausea (2%)

Local: Injection site pain/reaction (2% to 3%)

Ocular: Eyelid edema (2%), eyelid ptosis (2%)

Renal: Hematuria (2%)

Respiratory: Nasopharyngitis (10%), upper respiratory tract infection (3%), cough (2% to 3%), pharyngolaryngeal pain (2% to 3%), bronchitis (2% to 3%), sinusitis (2%)

Miscellaneous: Flu-like syndrome (2% to 3%)

General Dosage Range I.M.:

Adults: Cervical dystonia: Initial: 500 units/treatment; subsequent doses: 250-1000 units

Adults <65 years: Reduction of glabellar lines: 10 units (0.05 mL or 0.08 mL) into each site (total dose: 50 units)

Mechanism of Action AbobotulinumtoxinA (previously known as botulinum toxin type A) is a neurotoxin produced by *Clostridium botulinum*, spore-forming anaerobic bacillus, which appears to affect only the presynaptic membrane of the neuromuscular junction in humans, where it prevents calcium-dependent release of acetylcholine and produces a state of denervation. Muscle inactivation persists until new fibrils grow from the nerve and form junction plates on new areas of the muscle-cell walls.

Pharmacodynamics/Kinetics

Onset of Action Peak effect: Cervical dystonia: 2-4 weeks

Duration of Action Cervical dystonia: Up to 4 months

Pregnancy Risk Factor C

Pregnancy Considerations Embryo-fetal toxicity has been observed in animal studies. There are no adequate and well-controlled studies in pregnant women. Use during pregnancy only if benefits justify the risk to the fetus.

Acamprosate (a kam PROE sate)

Brand Names: U.S. Campral®
Brand Names: Canada Campral®
Pharmacologic Category GABA Agonist/Glutamate Antagonist
Use Maintenance of alcohol abstinence
Local Anesthetic/Vasoconstrictor Precautions No information available to require special precautions
Effects on Dental Treatment Key adverse event(s) related to dental treatment: Xerostomia and changes in salivation (normal salivary flow resumes upon discontinuation) and taste perversion.
Effects on Bleeding No information available to require special precautions
Adverse Effects Note: Many adverse effects associated with treatment may be related to alcohol abstinence; reported frequency range may overlap with placebo.

>10%: Gastrointestinal: Diarrhea (10% to 17%)
1% to 10%:
Cardiovascular: Chest pain, edema (peripheral), hypertension, palpitation, syncope, vasodilatation
Central nervous system: Insomnia (6% to 9%), anxiety (5% to 8%), depression (4% to 8%), dizziness (3% to 4%), pain (2% to 4%), paresthesia (2% to 3%), abnormal thinking, amnesia, chills, headache, somnolence, tremor
Dermatologic: Pruritus (3% to 4%), rash
Endocrine & metabolic: Libido decreased
Gastrointestinal: Anorexia (2% to 5%), nausea (3% to 4%), flatulence (1% to 4%), xerostomia (1% to 3%), abdominal pain, appetite increased, constipation, dyspepsia, taste perversion, vomiting, weight gain
Genitourinary: Impotence
Neuromuscular & skeletal: Weakness (5% to 7%), arthralgia, back pain, myalgia
Ocular: Abnormal vision
Respiratory: Bronchitis, cough increased, dyspnea, pharyngitis, rhinitis
Miscellaneous: Diaphoresis (2% to 3%), flu-like syndrome, infection, suicide attempt
General Dosage Range Dosage adjustment recommended in patients with renal impairment.
Oral: *Adults:* 666 mg 3 times/day (maximum: 1998 mg/day)
Mechanism of Action Mechanism not fully defined. Structurally similar to gamma-amino butyric acid (GABA), acamprosate appears to increase the activity of the GABA-ergic system, and decreases activity of glutamate within the CNS, including a decrease in activity at N-methyl D-aspartate (NMDA) receptors; may also affect CNS calcium channels. Restores balance to GABA and glutamate activities which appear to be disrupted in alcohol dependence. During therapeutic use, reduces alcohol intake, but does not cause a disulfiram-like reaction following alcohol ingestion. Insignificant CNS activity, outside its effect on alcohol dependence, was observed including no anxiolytic, anticonvulsant, or antidepressant activity.
Pharmacodynamics/Kinetics
Half-life Elimination 20-33 hours
Pregnancy Risk Factor C
Pregnancy Considerations Teratogenic effects have been observed in animal studies. No adequate or well-controlled studies in pregnant women; use only if potential benefit outweighs possible risk to the fetus.

Acarbose (AY car bose)

Related Information
Endocrine Disorders and Pregnancy *on page 1517*
Brand Names: U.S. Precose®
Brand Names: Canada Glucobay™
Pharmacologic Category Antidiabetic Agent, Alpha-Glucosidase Inhibitor
Use Adjunct to diet and exercise to lower blood glucose in patients with type 2 diabetes mellitus (noninsulin dependent, NIDDM)
Local Anesthetic/Vasoconstrictor Precautions No information available to require special precautions
Effects on Dental Treatment No significant effects or complications reported
Effects on Bleeding No information available to require special precautions
Adverse Effects >10%:
Gastrointestinal: Diarrhea (31%) and abdominal pain (19%) tend to return to pretreatment levels over time; frequency and intensity of flatulence (74%) tend to abate with time
Hepatic: Transaminases increased (≤4%)
General Dosage Range Dosage adjustment recommended in patients on concomitant therapy
Oral: *Adults:* Initial: 25 mg 1-3 times/day; Maintenance: 75-300 mg/day in 3 divided doses (maximum: ≤60 kg: 150 mg/day; >60 kg: 300 mg/day)
Mechanism of Action Competitive inhibitor of pancreatic α-amylase and intestinal brush border α-glucosidases, resulting in delayed hydrolysis of ingested complex carbohydrates and disaccharides and absorption of glucose; dose-dependent reduction in postprandial serum insulin and glucose peaks; inhibits the metabolism of sucrose to glucose and fructose
Pharmacodynamics/Kinetics
Half-life Elimination ~2 hours
Time to Peak Active drug: ~1 hour
Pregnancy Risk Factor B
Pregnancy Considerations Adverse events have not been reported in animal reproduction studies; therefore, acarbose is classified as pregnancy category B. Low amounts of acarbose are absorbed systemically which should limit fetal exposure. Maternal hyperglycemia can be associated with adverse effects in the fetus, including macrosomia, neonatal hyperglycemia, and hyperbilirubinemia; the risk of congenital malformations is increased when the Hb A_{1c} is above the normal range. Diabetes can also be associated with adverse effects in the mother. Poorly-treated diabetes may cause end-organ damage that may in turn negatively affect obstetric outcomes. Physiologic glucose levels should be maintained prior to and during pregnancy to decrease the risk of adverse events in the mother and the fetus. Acarbose has been studied for its potential role in treating GDM; however, only limited information is available describing pregnancy outcomes. Until additional safety and efficacy data are obtained, the use of oral agents is generally not recommended as routine management of GDM or type 2 diabetes mellitus during pregnancy. Insulin is the drug of choice for the control of diabetes mellitus during pregnancy.

Acebutolol (a se BYOO toe lole)

Related Information
Cardiovascular Diseases *on page 1492*
Brand Names: U.S. Sectral®

Brand Names: Canada Apo-Acebutolol®; Ava-Acebutolol; Mylan-Acebutolol; Mylan-Acebutolol (Type S); Nu-Acebutolol; Rhotral; Sandoz-Acebutolol; Sectral®; Teva-Acebutolol

Pharmacologic Category Antiarrhythmic Agent, Class II; Beta-Blocker With Intrinsic Sympathomimetic Activity

Use Treatment of hypertension; management of ventricular arrhythmias

Unlabeled Use Treatment of chronic stable angina (**Note:** Not recommended for patients with prior MI)

Local Anesthetic/Vasoconstrictor Precautions No information available to require special precautions. Local anesthetic with vasoconstrictor can be safely used in patients medicated with acebutolol.

Effects on Dental Treatment Acebutolol is a cardioselective beta-blocker. Local anesthetic with vasoconstrictor can be safely used in patients medicated with acebutolol. Nonselective beta-blockers (ie, propranolol, nadolol) enhance the pressor response to epinephrine, resulting in hypertension and bradycardia; this has not been reported for acebutolol. Many nonsteroidal anti-inflammatory drugs, such as ibuprofen and indomethacin, can reduce the hypotensive effect of beta-blockers after 3 or more weeks of therapy with the NSAID. Short-term NSAID use (ie, 3 days) requires no special precautions in patients taking beta-blockers.

Effects on Bleeding No information available to require special precautions

Adverse Effects

>10%: Central nervous system: Fatigue (11%)

1% to 10%:
Cardiovascular: Chest pain (2%), edema (2%), bradycardia, hypotension, CHF
Central nervous system: Headache (6%), dizziness (6%), insomnia (3%), depression (2%), abnormal dreams (2%), anxiety, hyper-/hypoesthesia
Dermatologic: Rash (2%), pruritus
Gastrointestinal: Constipation (4%), diarrhea (4%), dyspepsia (4%), nausea (4%), flatulence (3%), abdominal pain, vomiting
Genitourinary: Micturition frequency (3%), dysuria, impotence, nocturia
Neuromuscular & skeletal: Myalgia (2%), back pain, joint pain
Ocular: Abnormal vision (2%), conjunctivitis, dry eyes, eye pain
Respiratory: Dyspnea (4%), rhinitis (2%), cough (1%), pharyngitis, wheezing

Potential adverse effects (based on experience with other beta-blocking agents) include agranulocytosis, allergic reactions, alopecia (reversible), catatonia, claudication, depression (reversible), disorientation, emotional lability, erythematous rash, ischemic colitis, laryngospasm, mesenteric artery thrombosis, Peyronie's disease, purpura, respiratory distress, short-term memory loss, slightly clouded sensorium, thrombocytopenia

General Dosage Range Dosage adjustment recommended in patients with renal impairment

Oral:
Adults: 200-1200 mg/day in 2 divided doses (maximum: 1200 mg/day)
Elderly: 200-800 mg/day in 2 divided doses (maximum: 800 mg/day)

Mechanism of Action Competitively blocks beta$_1$-adrenergic receptors with little or no effect on beta$_2$-receptors except at high doses; exhibits membrane stabilizing and intrinsic sympathomimetic activity

Pharmacodynamics/Kinetics
Onset of Action 1-2 hours
Duration of Action 12-24 hours
Half-life Elimination Parent drug: 3-4 hours; Metabolite: 8-13 hours
Time to Peak 2-4 hours
Pregnancy Risk Factor B
Pregnancy Considerations Adverse effects were not observed in animal reproduction studies; therefore, acebutolol is classified as pregnancy category C. Acebutolol and diacetolol (active metabolite) cross the placenta. In a cohort study, an increased risk of cardiovascular defects was observed following maternal use of beta-blockers during pregnancy. Intrauterine growth restriction (IUGR), small placentas, as well as fetal/neonatal bradycardia, hypoglycemia, and/or respiratory depression have been observed following *in utero* exposure to beta-blockers as a class. Adequate facilities for monitoring infants at birth should be available. Untreated chronic maternal hypertension and pre-eclampsia are also associated with adverse events in the fetus, infant, and mother. The plasma elimination half-life of acebutolol is longer in pregnant women at term. Acebutolol has been evaluated for the treatment of hypertension in pregnancy, but other agents may be more appropriate for use.

Acetaminophen (a seet a MIN oh fen)

Related Information
Antiplatelet and Anticoagulation Considerations in Dentistry *on page 1503*
Oral Pain *on page 1558*

Related Sample Prescriptions
Mild/Moderate Oral Pain *on page 1606*

Brand Names: U.S. Acephen™ [OTC]; APAP 500 [OTC]; Aspirin Free Anacin® Extra Strength [OTC]; Cetafen® Extra [OTC]; Cetafen® [OTC]; Excedrin® Tension Headache [OTC]; Feverall® [OTC]; Infantaire [OTC]; Little Fevers™ [OTC]; Mapap® Arthritis Pain [OTC]; Mapap® Children's [OTC]; Mapap® Extra Strength [OTC]; Mapap® Infant's [OTC]; Mapap® Junior Rapid Tabs [OTC]; Mapap® [OTC]; Non-Aspirin Pain Reliever [OTC]; Nortemp Children's [OTC]; Ofirmev™; Pain & Fever Children's [OTC]; Pain Eze [OTC]; Q-Pap Children's [OTC]; Q-Pap Extra Strength [OTC]; Q-Pap Infant's [OTC]; Q-Pap [OTC]; RapiMed® Children's [OTC]; RapiMed® Junior [OTC]; Silapap Children's [OTC]; Silapap Infant's [OTC]; Triaminic™ Children's Fever Reducer Pain Reliever [OTC]; Tylenol® 8 Hour [OTC]; Tylenol® Arthritis Pain Extended Relief [OTC]; Tylenol® Children's Meltaways [OTC]; Tylenol® Children's [OTC]; Tylenol® Extra Strength [OTC]; Tylenol® Infant's Concentrated [OTC] [DSC]; Tylenol® Jr. Meltaways [OTC]; Tylenol® [OTC]; Valorin Extra [OTC]; Valorin [OTC]

Brand Names: Canada Abenol®; Apo-Acetaminophen®; Atasol®; Novo-Gesic; Pediatrix; Tempra®; Tylenol®

Generic Availability (U.S.) Yes: Excludes extended release products; injectable formulation

Pharmacologic Category Analgesic, Miscellaneous

Dental Use Treatment of postoperative pain

Use Treatment of mild-to-moderate pain and fever (analgesic/antipyretic)
I.V.: Additional indication: Management of moderate-to-severe pain when combined with opioid analgesia

Local Anesthetic/Vasoconstrictor Precautions No information available to require special precautions

◄ Effects on Dental Treatment No significant effects or complications reported (see Dental Comment)

Effects on Bleeding As a single agent, acetaminophen does not appear to affect bleeding or platelet aggregation. Acetaminophen may prolong the INR and increase bleeding in patients taking warfarin (Coumadin®). For patients taking warfarin, single acetaminophen doses or acetaminophen therapy of short duration should be safe, but if large (>1.3 g/day) doses are administered for longer than 10-14 days, then the INR should be monitored (see Dental Comment).

Adverse Effects Oral, Rectal: Frequency not defined:

Dermatologic: Rash

Endocrine & metabolic: May increase chloride, uric acid, glucose; may decrease sodium, bicarbonate, calcium

Hematologic: Anemia; blood dyscrasias (neutropenia, pancytopenia, leukopenia)

Hepatic: Bilirubin increased, alkaline phosphatase increased

Renal: Ammonia increased, nephrotoxicity with chronic overdose, analgesic nephropathy

Miscellaneous: Hypersensitivity reactions (rare)

I.V.:
>10%: Gastrointestinal: Nausea (adults 34%; children ≥5%), vomiting (adults 15%; children ≥5%)

1% to 10%:

Cardiovascular: Edema (peripheral), hypervolemia, hypo/hypertension, tachycardia

Central nervous system: Headache (adults 10%; children ≥1%), insomnia (adults 7%; children ≥1%), agitation (children ≥5%), anxiety, fatigue

Dermatologic: Pruritus (children ≥5%), rash

Endocrine & metabolic: Hypoalbuminemia, hypokalemia, hypomagnesemia, hypophosphatemia

Gastrointestinal: Constipation (children ≥5%), abdominal pain, diarrhea

Hematologic: Anemia

Hepatic: Transaminases increased

Local: Infusion site pain

Neuromuscular & skeletal: Muscle spasms, pain in extremity, trismus

Ocular: Periorbital edema

Renal: Oliguria (children ≥1%)

Respiratory: Atelectasis (children ≥5%), breath sounds abnormal, dyspnea, hypoxia, pleural effusion, pulmonary edema, stridor, wheezing

Dental Usual Dosage Postoperative pain: Oral, rectal: Children <12 years: 10-15 mg/kg/dose every 4-6 hours as needed; do **not** exceed 5 doses (2.6 g) in 24 hours

Adults: 325-650 mg every 4-6 hours or 1000 mg 3-4 times/day; do **not** exceed 4 g/day

Dosage Note: No dose adjustment required if converting between different acetaminophen formulations. Limit acetaminophen dose from all sources (prescription and OTC) to <4 g daily.

Oral: Note: OTC dosing recommendations may vary by product and/or manufacturer.

Infants and Children <12 years: 10-15 mg/kg/dose every 4-6 hours as needed; do **not** exceed 5 doses (2.6 g) in 24 hours; alternatively, the following age-based doses may be used; see table.

Children ≥12 years, Adolescents, and Adults:
Regular release: 325-650 mg every 4-6 hours or 1000 mg 3-4 times daily (maximum: 4 g daily)
Extended release: 1300 mg every 8 hours (maximum: 3.9 g daily)

Acetaminophen Pediatric Dosing (Oral)[1]

Weight (kg)	Weight (lbs)	Age	Dosage (mg)
2.7-5.3	6-11	0-3 mo	40
5.4-8.1	12-17	4-11 mo	80
8.2-10.8	18-23	1-2 y	120
10.9-16.3	24-35	2-3 y	160
16.4-21.7	36-47	4-5 y	240
21.8-27.2	48-59	6-8 y	320
27.3-32.6	60-71	9-10 y	400
32.7-43.2	72-95	11 y	480

[1]Manufacturer's recommendations; use of weight to select dose is preferred; if weight is not available, then use age. Manufacturer's recommendations are based on weight in pounds (OTC labeling); weight in kg listed here is derived from pounds and rounded; kg weight listed also is adjusted to allow for continuous weight ranges in kg. OTC labeling instructs consumer to consult with physician for dosing instructions in children under 2 years of age.

Rectal:
Infants and Children <12 years: 10-20 mg/kg/dose every 4-6 hours as needed; do **not** exceed 5 doses (2.6 g) in 24 hours. **Note:** Although the perioperative use of high-dose rectal acetaminophen (eg, 25-45 mg/kg/dose) has been investigated in several studies, its routine use remains controversial; optimal doses and dosing frequency to ensure efficacy and safety have not yet been established (Buck, 2001).

Children ≥12 years, Adolescents, and Adults: 325-650 mg every 4-6 hours or 1000 mg 3-4 times daily (maximum: 4 g daily)

I.V.:
Children 2-12 years: 15 mg/kg every 6 hours **or** 12.5 mg/kg every 4 hours; maximum single dose: 15 mg/kg/dose; maximum daily dose: 75 mg/kg/day (≤3.75 g daily)

Adolescents and Adults:
<50 kg: 15 mg/kg every 6 hours or 12.5 mg/kg every 4 hours; maximum single dose: 750 mg/dose; maximum daily dose: 75 mg/kg/day (≤3.75 g daily)
≥50 kg: 650 mg every 4 hours or 1000 mg every 6 hours; maximum single dose: 1000 mg/dose; maximum daily dose: 4 g daily

Dosing interval in renal impairment:
Oral (Aronoff, 2007):
Children:
Cl$_{cr}$ <10 mL/minute: Administer every 8 hours
Intermittent hemodialysis or peritoneal dialysis: Administer every 8 hours
CRRT: No adjustments necessary
Adults:
Cl$_{cr}$ 10-50 mL/minute: Administer every 6 hours
Cl$_{cr}$ <10 mL/minute: Administer every 8 hours
Intermittent hemodialysis or peritoneal dialysis: No adjustment necessary
CRRT: Administer every 8 hours
I.V.: Cl$_{cr}$ ≤30 mL/minute: Use with caution; consider decreasing daily dose and extending dosing interval

Dosing adjustment/comments in hepatic impairment:
Oral: Use with caution. Limited, low-dose therapy is usually well tolerated in hepatic disease/cirrhosis. However, cases of hepatotoxicity at daily acetaminophen dosages <4 g daily have been reported. Avoid chronic use in hepatic impairment.

I.V.:

Mild-to-moderate impairment: Use with caution in hepatic impairment or active liver disease; manufacturer's labeling suggests a reduced total daily dosage may be warranted, although no specific dosage adjustments are provided.

Severe impairment: Use is contraindicated.

Mechanism of Action Although not fully elucidated, believed to inhibit the synthesis of prostaglandins in the central nervous system and work peripherally to block pain impulse generation; produces antipyresis from inhibition of hypothalamic heat-regulating center

Contraindications Hypersensitivity to acetaminophen or any component of the formulation; severe hepatic impairment or severe active liver disease (Ofirmev™)

Warnings/Precautions Limit acetaminophen dose from all sources (prescription and OTC) to <4 g/day. May cause severe hepatotoxicity on acute overdose; in addition, chronic daily dosing in adults has resulted in liver damage in some patients; hepatotoxicity is usually associated with excessive acetaminophen intake (>4 g/day). Use with caution in patients with alcoholic liver disease; consuming ≥3 alcoholic drinks/day may increase the risk of liver damage. Use caution in patients with hepatic impairment or active liver disease. Use of intravenous formulation is contraindicated in patients with severe hepatic impairment or severe active liver disease. Use caution in patients with known G6PD deficiency; rare reports of hemolysis have occurred. Use caution in patients with chronic malnutrition and hypovolemia (intravenous formulation). Use caution in patients with severe renal impairment; consider dosing adjustments. Hypersensitivity and anaphylactic reactions have been reported; discontinue immediately if symptoms of allergic or hypersensitivity reactions occur.

OTC labeling: When used for self-medication, patients should be instructed to contact healthcare provider if used for fever lasting >3 days or for pain lasting >10 days in adults or >5 days in children. OTC labeling limits the maximum daily dose to ≤3250 mg (dosage form specific).

Drug Interactions

Metabolism/Transport Effects Substrate of CYP1A2 (minor), CYP2A6 (minor), CYP2C9 (minor), CYP2D6 (minor), CYP2E1 (minor), CYP3A4 (minor); **Note:** Assignment of Major/Minor substrate status based on clinically relevant drug interaction potential; **Inhibits** CYP3A4 (weak)

Avoid Concomitant Use

Avoid concomitant use of Acetaminophen with any of the following: Pimozide

Increased Effect/Toxicity

Acetaminophen may increase the levels/effects of: ARIPiprazole; Busulfan; Dasatinib; Imatinib; Lomitapide; Mipomersen; Pimozide; Prilocaine; SORAfenib; Vitamin K Antagonists

The levels/effects of Acetaminophen may be increased by: Dasatinib; Imatinib; Isoniazid; Metyrapone; Probenecid; SORAfenib

Decreased Effect

The levels/effects of Acetaminophen may be decreased by: Anticonvulsants (Hydantoin); Barbiturates; CarBAMazepine; Cholestyramine Resin; Peginterferon Alfa-2b

Ethanol/Nutrition/Herb Interactions

Ethanol: Excessive intake of ethanol may increase the risk of acetaminophen-induced hepatotoxicity. Avoid ethanol or limit to <3 drinks/day.

Food: Rate of absorption may be decreased when given with food.

Herb/Nutraceutical: St John's wort may decrease acetaminophen levels.

Dietary Considerations Some products may contain phenylalanine and/or sodium.

Pharmacodynamics/Kinetics

Onset of Action

Oral: <1 hour

I.V.: Analgesia: 5-10 minutes; Antipyretic: Within 30 minutes

Peak effect: I.V.: Analgesic: 1 hour

Duration of Action

I.V., Oral: Analgesia: 4-6 hours

I.V.: Antipyretic: ≥6 hours

Half-life Elimination Prolonged following toxic doses

Neonates: 7 hours (range: 4-10 hours)

Infants: ~4 hours (range: 1-7 hours)

Children: 3 hours (range: 2-5 hours)

Adolescents: ~3 hours (range: 2-4 hours)

Adults: ~2 hours (range: 2-3 hours); may be slightly prolonged in severe renal insufficiency (Cl_{cr}<30 mL/minute): 2-5.3 hours

Time to Peak Serum: Oral: Immediate release: 10-60 minutes (may be delayed in acute overdoses); I.V.: 15 minutes

Pregnancy Risk Factor C (intravenous)

Pregnancy Considerations Animal reproduction studies have not been conducted with intravenous acetaminophen, therefore, acetaminophen I.V. is classified as pregnancy category C. Acetaminophen crosses the placenta and can be detected in cord blood, newborn serum, and urine immediately after delivery. An increased risk of teratogenic effects has not been observed following maternal use of acetaminophen during pregnancy. Prenatal constriction of the ductus arteriosus has been noted in case reports following maternal use during the third trimester. The use of acetaminophen in normal doses during pregnancy is not associated with an increased risk of miscarriage or still birth; however, an increase in fetal death or spontaneous abortion may be seen following maternal overdose if treatment is delayed. Frequent maternal use of acetaminophen during pregnancy may be associated with wheezing and asthma in early childhood. The absorption may be delayed and the bioavailability of acetaminophen may be decreased in some women during pregnancy due to delayed gastric emptying.

Lactation Enters breast milk/use caution (AAP rates "compatible"; AAP 2001 update pending)

Breast-Feeding Considerations Low concentrations of acetaminophen are excreted into breast milk and can be detected in the urine of nursing infants. Adverse reactions have generally not been observed; however, a rash caused by acetaminophen exposure was reported in one breast-feeding infant.

Dosage Forms

Caplet, oral: 500 mg

Cetafen® Extra [OTC]: 500 mg

Mapap® Extra Strength [OTC]: 500 mg

Pain Eze [OTC]: 650 mg

Tylenol® [OTC]: 325 mg

Tylenol® Extra Strength [OTC]: 500 mg

Caplet, extended release, oral:

Mapap® Arthritis Pain [OTC]: 650 mg

Tylenol® 8 Hour [OTC]: 650 mg

Tylenol® Arthritis Pain Extended Relief [OTC]: 650 mg

Capsule, oral:

Mapap® Extra Strength [OTC]: 500 mg

Captab, oral: 500 mg

Elixir, oral:
Mapap® Children's [OTC]: 160 mg/5 mL (118 mL, 480 mL)
Gelcap, oral: 500 mg
Mapap® [OTC]: 500 mg
Gelcap, rapid release, oral: 500 mg
Tylenol® Extra Strength [OTC]: 500 mg
Geltab, oral: 500 mg
Excedrin® Tension Headache [OTC]: 500 mg
Injection, solution [preservative free]:
Ofirmev™: 10 mg/mL (100 mL)
Liquid, oral: 160 mg/5 mL (120 mL, 473 mL); 500 mg/5 mL (240 mL)
APAP 500 [OTC]: 500 mg/5 mL (237 mL)
Mapap® Extra Strength [OTC]: 500 mg/5 mL (237 mL)
Q-Pap Children's [OTC]: 160 mg/5 mL (118 mL, 473 mL)
Silapap Children's [OTC]: 160 mg/5 mL (118 mL, 237 mL, 473 mL)
Tylenol® Extra Strength [OTC]: 500 mg/15 mL (240 mL)
Solution, oral: 160 mg/5 mL (5 mL, 10 mL, 20 mL, 118 mL, 473 mL)
Infantaire [OTC]: 80 mg/0.8 mL (15 mL, 30 mL)
Little Fevers™ [OTC]: 80 mg/mL (30 mL)
Mapap® [OTC]: 80 mg/0.8 mL (15 mL)
Pain & Fever Children's [OTC]: 160 mg/5 mL (118 mL, 473 mL)
Q-Pap Infant's [OTC]: 80 mg/0.8 mL (15 mL)
Silapap Infant's [OTC]: 80 mg/0.8 mL (15 mL, 30 mL)
Suppository, rectal: 120 mg (12s, 50s, 100s); 325 mg (12s); 650 mg (12s, 50s, 100s)
Acephen™ [OTC]: 120 mg (12s, 50s, 100s); 325 mg (6s, 12s, 50s, 100s); 650 mg (12s, 50s, 100s)
Feverall® [OTC]: 80 mg (6s, 50s); 120 mg (6s, 50s); 325 mg (6s, 50s); 650 mg (50s)
Suspension, oral: 160 mg/5 mL (5 mL, 10 mL, 10.15 mL, 20 mL, 20.3 mL)
Mapap® Children's [OTC]: 160 mg/5 mL (118 mL)
Mapap® Infant's [OTC]: 160 mg/5 mL (59 mL); 80 mg/0.8 mL (15 mL, 30 mL)
Nortemp Children's [OTC]: 160 mg/5 mL (118 mL)
Pain & Fever Children's [OTC]: 160 mg/5 mL (60 mL)
Q-Pap Children's [OTC]: 160 mg/5 mL (118 mL)
Tylenol® Children's [OTC]: 160 mg/5 mL (60 mL, 120 mL)
Syrup, oral:
Triaminic™ Children's Fever Reducer Pain Reliever [OTC]: 160 mg/5 mL (118 mL)
Tablet, oral: 325 mg, 500 mg
Aspirin Free Anacin® Extra Strength [OTC]: 500 mg
Cetafen® [OTC]: 325 mg
Mapap® [OTC]: 325 mg
Non-Aspirin Pain Reliever [OTC]: 325 mg
Q-Pap [OTC]: 325 mg
Q-Pap Extra Strength [OTC]: 500 mg
Tylenol® [OTC]: 325 mg
Tylenol® Extra Strength [OTC]: 500 mg
Valorin [OTC]: 325 mg
Valorin Extra [OTC]: 500 mg
Tablet, chewable, oral: 80 mg
Mapap® Children's [OTC]: 80 mg
Tablet, orally disintegrating, oral: 80 mg, 160 mg
Mapap® Children's [OTC]: 80 mg
Mapap® Junior Rapid Tabs [OTC]: 160 mg
RapiMed® Children's [OTC]: 80 mg
RapiMed® Junior [OTC]: 160 mg
Tylenol® Children's Meltaways [OTC]: 80 mg
Tylenol® Jr. Meltaways [OTC]: 160 mg

Dental Comment Hepatotoxicity caused by acetaminophen is potentiated by chronic alcohol consumption. People who are taking acetaminophen, even at therapeutic doses, and consume alcohol are at risk of developing hepatotoxicity.

Acetaminophen may increase the levels and enhance the anticoagulant effects of vitamin K antagonists acenocoumarol and warfarin (Coumadin®). Studies have reported that acetaminophen has increased the INR in warfarin treated patients with daily acetaminophen doses as low as 2 g, particularly when taking acetaminophen for >1 week (Antlitz, 1968; Boeijinga, 1982; Gebauer, 2003; Hylek, 1998; Rubin, 1984). In addition, case reports of bleeding as a result of increased INR have been published (Bagheri, 1999; Bartle, 1991). There is no known mechanism of the interaction; furthermore, some studies have failed to demonstrate this interaction (Gadisseur, 2003; Kwan, 1995; van den Bemt, 2002). In terms of risk, the data suggest that acetaminophen and warfarin could interact in some clinically significant manner but that the benefits of concomitant use of acetaminophen for pain control in dental patients taking warfarin usually outweigh the risks. An appropriate monitoring plan should be in place to identify potential negative effects and dosage adjustments may be necessary in a minority of patients. The interaction may be more likely to occur with daily acetaminophen doses of >1.3 g for >1 week.

There are no reports of acetaminophen interacting with antiplatelet drugs such as aspirin, clopidogrel (Plavix®), or prasugrel (Effient™). Also, there are no reports of acetaminophen in combination with hydrocodone, codeine, or oxycodone interacting with warfarin (Coumadin®).

References
Ahmad N, Grad HA, Haas DA, et al, "The Efficacy of Nonopioid Analgesics for Postoperative Dental Pain: A Meta-Analysis," *Anesth Prog*, 1997, 44(4):119-26.
Antlitz AM, Mead JA Jr, and Tolentino MA, "Potentiation of Oral Anticoagulant Therapy by Acetaminophen," *Curr Ther Res Clin Exp*, 1968, 10(10):501-7.
Bagheri H, Bernhard NB, and Montastruc JL, "Potentiation of the Acenocoumarol Anticoagulant Effect by Acetaminophen," *Ann Pharmacother*, 1999, 33(4):506.
Bartle WR and Blakely JA, "Potentiation of Warfarin Anticoagulation by Acetaminophen," *JAMA*, 1991, 265(10):1260.
Bell WR, "Acetaminophen and Warfarin: Undesirable Synergy," *JAMA*, 1998, 279(9):702-3.
Boeijinga JJ, Boerstra EE, Ris P, et al, "Interaction Between Paracetamol and Coumarin Anticoagulants," *Lancet*, 1982, 1(8270):506.
Dionne R, "Additive Analgesia Without Opioid Side Effects," *Compend Contin Educ Dent*, 2000, 21(7):572-4, 576-7.
Gadisseur AP, Van Der Meer FJ, and Rosendaal FR, "Sustained Intake of Paracetamol (Acetaminophen) During Oral Anticoagulant Therapy With Coumarins Does Not Cause Clinically Important INR Changes: A Randomized Double-Blind Clinical Trial," *J Thromb Haemost*, 2003, 1(4):714-7.
Gebauer MG, Nyfort-Hansen K, Henschke PJ, et al, "Warfarin and Acetaminophen Interaction," *Pharmacotherapy*, 2003, 23(1):109-12.
Hylek EM, Heiman H, Skates SJ, et al, "Acetaminophen and Other Risk Factors for Excessive Warfarin Anticoagulation," *JAMA*, 1998, 279(9):657-62.
Kwan D, Bartle WR, and Walker SE, "The Effects of Acetaminophen on Pharmacokinetics and Pharmacodynamics of Warfarin," *J Clin Pharmacol*, 1999, 39(1):68-75.
Kwan D, Bartle WR, and Walker SE, "The Effects of Acute and Chronic Acetaminophen Dosing on the Pharmacodynamics and Pharmacokinetics of (R)- and (S)-Warfarin," *Clin Pharmacol Ther*, 1995, 57:212.
Lee WM, "Drug-Induced Hepatotoxicity," *N Engl J Med*, 1995, 333(17):1118-27.
McClain CJ, Price S, Barve S, et al, "Acetaminophen Hepatotoxicity: An Update," *Curr Gastroenterol Rep*, 1999, 1(1):42-9.
Mehlisch DR, Aspley S, Daniels SE, et al, "Comparison of the Analgesic Efficacy of Concurrent Ibuprofen and Paracetamol With Ibuprofen or Paracetamol Alone in the Management of Moderate to Severe Acute Postoperative Dental Pain in Adolescents and Adults: A Randomized, Double-Blind, Placebo-Controlled, Parallel-Group, Single-Dose, Two-Center, Modified Factorial Study," *Clin Ther*, 2010, 32(5):882-95.
Rubin RN, Mentzer RL, and Budzynski AZ, "Potentiation of Anticoagulant Effect of Warfarin by Acetaminophen (Tylenol®)," *Clin Res*, 1984, 32:698a.

Shek KL, Chan LN, and Nutescu E, "Warfarin-Acetaminophen Drug Interaction Revisited," *Pharmacotherapy*, 1999, 19(10):1153-8.

Tanaka E, Yamazaki K, and Misawa S, "Update: The Clinical Importance of Acetaminophen Hepatotoxicity in Nonalcoholic and Alcoholic Subjects," *J Clin Pharm Ther*, 2000, 25(5):325-32.

van den Bemt PM, Geven LM, Kuitert NA, et al, "The Potential Interaction Between Oral Anticoagulants and Acetaminophen in Everyday Practice," *Pharm World Sci*, 2002, 24(5):201-4.

Acetaminophen and Codeine
(a seet a MIN oh fen & KOE deen)

Related Information
Acetaminophen *on page 27*
Codeine *on page 344*

Related Sample Prescriptions
Moderate/Moderately Severe Oral Pain *on page 1606*

Brand Names: U.S. Capital® and Codeine; Tylenol® with Codeine No. 3; Tylenol® with Codeine No. 4

Brand Names: Canada ratio-Emtec; ratio-Lenoltec; Triatec-30; Triatec-8; Triatec-8 Strong; Tylenol Elixir with Codeine; Tylenol No. 1; Tylenol No. 1 Forte; Tylenol No. 2 with Codeine; Tylenol No. 3 with Codeine; Tylenol No. 4 with Codeine

Generic Availability (U.S.) Yes

Pharmacologic Category Analgesic Combination (Opioid)

Dental Use Treatment of postoperative pain

Use Relief of mild-to-moderate pain

Local Anesthetic/Vasoconstrictor Precautions No information available to require special precautions

Effects on Dental Treatment No significant effects or complications reported (see Dental Comment)

Effects on Bleeding As a single agent, acetaminophen does not appear to affect bleeding or platelet aggregation. Acetaminophen may prolong the INR and increase bleeding in patients taking warfarin (Coumadin®). For patients taking warfarin, single acetaminophen doses or acetaminophen therapy of short duration should be safe, but if large (>1.3 g/day) doses are administered for longer than 10-14 days, then the INR should be monitored (see Dental Comment).

Adverse Effects
>10%:
Central nervous system: Dizziness, lightheadedness, sedation
Gastrointestinal: Nausea, vomiting
Respiratory: Dyspnea
1% to 10%:
Central nervous system: Dysphonia, euphoria
Dermatologic: Pruritus
Gastrointestinal: Abdominal pain, constipation
Miscellaneous: Histamine release

Dental Usual Dosage Postoperative pain: Adults: Analgesic: Based on codeine (30-60 mg/dose) every 4-6 hours (maximum: 4000 mg/24 hours based on acetaminophen component)

Dosage Doses should be adjusted according to severity of pain and response of the patient. Adult doses ≥60 mg codeine fail to give commensurate relief of pain but merely prolong analgesia and are associated with an appreciably increased incidence of side effects. Oral:

Children: Analgesic:
Codeine: 0.5-1 mg codeine/kg/dose every 4-6 hours
Acetaminophen: 10-15 mg/kg/dose every 4 hours up to a maximum of 2.6 g/24 hours for children <12 years; **alternatively, the following can be used:**
3-6 years: 5 mL 3-4 times/day as needed of elixir
7-12 years: 10 mL 3-4 times/day as needed of elixir
>12 years: 15 mL every 4 hours as needed of elixir

Adults:
Antitussive: Based on codeine (15-30 mg/dose) every 4-6 hours (maximum: 360 mg/24 hours based on codeine component)
Analgesic: Based on codeine (30-60 mg/dose) every 4-6 hours (maximum: 4000 mg/24 hours based on acetaminophen component)
1-2 tablets every 4 hours to a maximum of 12 tablets/24 hours

Dosing adjustment in renal impairment: See individual agents.

Dosing adjustment in hepatic impairment: Use with caution. Limited, low-dose therapy is usually well tolerated in hepatic disease/cirrhosis; however, cases of hepatotoxicity at daily acetaminophen dosages <4 g/day have been reported. Avoid chronic use in hepatic impairment.

Mechanism of Action Inhibits the synthesis of prostaglandins in the central nervous system and peripherally blocks pain impulse generation; produces antipyresis from inhibition of hypothalamic heat-regulating center; binds to opiate receptors in the CNS, causing inhibition of ascending pain pathways, altering the perception of and response to pain; causes cough supression by direct central action in the medulla; produces generalized CNS depression. Caffeine (contained in some non-U.S. formulations) is a CNS stimulant; use with acetaminophen and codeine increases the level of analgesia provided by each agent.

Contraindications Hypersensitivity to acetaminophen, codeine, or any component of the formulation; significant respiratory depression (in unmonitored settings); acute or severe bronchial asthma; hypercapnia; paralytic ileus

Warnings/Precautions Use with caution in patients with hypersensitivity reactions to other phenanthrene-derivative opioid agonists (morphine, hydrocodone, hydromorphone, levorphanol, oxycodone, oxymorphone); tablets contain metabisulfite which may cause allergic reactions. Tolerance or drug dependence may result from extended use. Use caution in patients with two or more copies of the variant CYP2D6*2 allele; may have extensive conversion to morphine and thus increased opioid-mediated effects.

[U.S. Boxed Warning]: Acetaminophen may cause severe hepatotoxicity, potentially requiring liver transplant or resulting in death; hepatotoxicity is usually associated with excessive acetaminophen intake (>4 g/day). Risk is increased with alcohol use, pre-existing liver disease, and intake of more than one source of acetaminophen-containing medications. Chronic daily dosing in adults has also resulted in liver damage in some patients. Hypersensitivity and anaphylactic reactions have been reported with acetaminophen use; discontinue immediately if symptoms of allergic or hypersensitivity reactions occur. Use caution in patients with known G6PD deficiency.

This combination should be used with caution in elderly or debilitated patients, hypotension, adrenocortical insufficiency, abdominal conditions, hepatic impairment, renal impairment, respiratory disease, thyroid disorders, prostatic hyperplasia, urethral stricture, seizure disorder, CNS depression, head injury or increased intracranial pressure. Causes sedation; caution must be used in performing tasks which require alertness (eg, operating machinery or driving). Safety and efficacy in pediatric patients have not been established. Effects may be potentiated when used with other sedative drugs or ethanol.

Note: Some non-U.S. formulations (including most Canadian formulations) may contain caffeine as an additional ingredient. Caffeine may cause CNS and cardiovascular stimulation, as well as GI irritation in high doses. Use with caution in patients with a history of peptic ulcer or GERD; avoid in patients with symptomatic cardiac arrhythmias.

Drug Interactions

Metabolism/Transport Effects Refer to individual components.

Avoid Concomitant Use

Avoid concomitant use of Acetaminophen and Codeine with any of the following: Azelastine (Nasal); Paraldehyde; Pimozide

Increased Effect/Toxicity

Acetaminophen and Codeine may increase the levels/ effects of: Alcohol (Ethyl); Alvimopan; ARIPiprazole; Azelastine (Nasal); Busulfan; CNS Depressants; Dasatinib; Desmopressin; Imatinib; Lomitapide; Metyrosine; Mipomersen; Mirtazapine; Paraldehyde; Pimozide; Pramipexole; Prilocaine; ROPINIRole; Rotigotine; Selective Serotonin Reuptake Inhibitors; SORAfenib; Thiazide Diuretics; Vitamin K Antagonists; Zolpidem

The levels/effects of Acetaminophen and Codeine may be increased by: Amphetamines; Antipsychotic Agents (Phenothiazines); Dasatinib; Droperidol; HydrOXYzine; Imatinib; Isoniazid; Magnesium Sulfate; Metyrapone; Perampanel; Probenecid; Sodium Oxybate; Somatostatin Analogs; SORAfenib; Succinylcholine

Decreased Effect

Acetaminophen and Codeine may decrease the levels/ effects of: Pegvisomant

The levels/effects of Acetaminophen and Codeine may be decreased by: Ammonium Chloride; Anticonvulsants (Hydantoin); Barbiturates; CarBAMazepine; Cholestyramine Resin; CYP2D6 Inhibitors (Moderate); CYP2D6 Inhibitors (Strong); Mixed Agonist / Antagonist Opioids; Peginterferon Alfa-2b

Ethanol/Nutrition/Herb Interactions Ethanol: Excessive intake of ethanol may increase the risk of acetaminophen-induced hepatotoxicity. Avoid ethanol or limit to <3 drinks/day.

Dietary Considerations May be taken with food.

Pregnancy Risk Factor C

Pregnancy Considerations Animal reproduction studies have not been conducted with this combination. Refer to individual monographs.

Lactation Enters breast milk/use caution

Breast-Feeding Considerations Refer to individual monographs.

Controlled Substance C-III; C-V

Dosage Forms

Solution, oral [C-V]: Acetaminophen 120 mg and codeine 12 mg per 5 mL

Suspension, oral [C-V]: Acetaminophen 120 mg and codeine 12 mg per 5 mL

Capital® and Codeine [C-V]: Acetaminophen 120 mg and codeine 12 mg per 5 mL

Tablet, oral [C-III]: Acetaminophen 300 mg and codeine 15 mg; acetaminophen 300 mg and codeine 30 mg; acetaminophen 300 mg and codeine 60 mg

Tylenol® with Codeine No. 3: Acetaminophen 300 mg and codeine 30 mg

Tylenol® with Codeine No. 4: Acetaminophen 300 mg and codeine 60 mg

Dosage Forms: Canada Note: In countries outside of the U.S., some formulations of Tylenol® with Codeine include caffeine.

Caplet:

ratio-Lenoltec No. 1, Tylenol No. 1: Acetaminophen 300 mg, codeine 8 mg, and caffeine 15 mg

Tylenol No. 1 Forte: Acetaminophen 500 mg, codeine 8 mg, and caffeine 15 mg

Solution, oral:

Tylenol Elixir with Codeine: Acetaminophen 160 mg and codeine 8 mg per 5 mL

Tablet:

ratio-Emtec, Triatec-30: Acetaminophen 300 mg and codeine 30 mg

ratio-Lenoltec No. 1: Acetaminophen 300 mg, codeine 8 mg, and caffeine 15 mg

ratio-Lenoltec No. 2, Tylenol No. 2 with Codeine: Acetaminophen 300 mg, codeine 15 mg, and caffeine 15 mg

ratio-Lenoltec No. 3, Tylenol No. 3 with Codeine: Acetaminophen 300 mg, codeine 30 mg, and caffeine 15 mg

ratio-Lenoltec No. 4, Tylenol No. 4 with Codeine: Acetaminophen 300 mg and codeine 60 mg

Triatec-8: Acetaminophen 325 mg, codeine 8 mg, and caffeine 30 mg

Triatec-8 Strong: Acetaminophen 500 mg, codeine 8 mg, and caffeine 30 mg

Dental Comment Hepatotoxicity caused by acetaminophen is potentiated by chronic alcohol consumption. People who are taking acetaminophen, even at therapeutic doses, and consume alcohol are at risk of developing hepatotoxicity.

Acetaminophen may increase the levels and enhance the anticoagulant effects of vitamin K antagonists acenocoumarol and warfarin (Coumadin®). Studies have reported that acetaminophen has increased the INR in warfarin treated patients with daily acetaminophen doses as low as 2 g, particularly when taking acetaminophen for >1 week (Antlitz, 1968; Boeijinga, 1982; Gebauer, 2003; Hylek, 1998; Rubin, 1984). In addition, case reports of bleeding as a result of increased INR have been published (Bagheri, 1999; Bartle, 1991). There is no known mechanism of the interaction; furthermore, some studies have failed to demonstrate this interaction (Gadisseur, 2003; Kwan, 1995; van den Bemt, 2002). In terms of risk, the data suggest that acetaminophen and warfarin could interact in some clinically significant manner but that the benefits of concomitant use of acetaminophen for pain control in dental patients taking warfarin usually outweigh the risks. An appropriate monitoring plan should be in place to identify potential negative effects and dosage adjustments may be necessary in a minority of patients. The interaction may be more likely to occur with daily acetaminophen doses of >1.3 g for >1 week.

There are no reports of acetaminophen interacting with antiplatelet drugs such as aspirin, clopidogrel (Plavix®), or prasugrel (Effient™). Also, there are no reports of acetaminophen in combination with hydrocodone, codeine, or oxycodone interacting with warfarin (Coumadin®).

References

Antlitz AM, Mead JA Jr, and Tolentino MA, "Potentiation of Oral Anticoagulant Therapy by Acetaminophen," *Curr Ther Res Clin Exp*, 1968, 10(10):501-7.

Bagheri H, Bernhard NB, and Montastruc JL, "Potentiation of the Acenocoumarol Anticoagulant Effect by Acetaminophen," *Ann Pharmacother*, 1999, 33(4):506.

Bartle WR and Blakely JA, "Potentiation of Warfarin Anticoagulation by Acetaminophen," *JAMA*, 1991, 265(10):1260.

Bell WR, "Acetaminophen and Warfarin: Undesirable Synergy," *JAMA*, 1998, 279(9):702-3.

Boeijinga JJ, Boerstra EE, Ris P, et al, "Interaction Between Paracetamol and Coumarin Anticoagulants," *Lancet*, 1982, 1(8270):506.

Chang DJ, Fricke JR, Bird SR, et al, "Rofecoxib Versus Codeine/Acetaminophen in Postoperative Dental Pain: A Double-Blind, Randomized, Placebo- and Active Comparator-Controlled Clinical Trial," *Clin Ther*, 2001, 23(9):1446-55.

Dionne RA, "New Approaches to Preventing and Treating Postoperative Pain," *J Am Dent Assoc*, 1992, 123(6):26-34.

Forbes JA, Butterworth GA, Burchfield WH, et al, "Evaluation of Ketorolac, Aspirin, and an Acetaminophen-Codeine Combination in Postoperative Oral Surgery Pain," *Pharmacotherapy*, 1990, 10(6 Pt 2):77S-93S.

Gadisseur AP, Van Der Meer FJ, and Rosendaal FR, "Sustained Intake of Paracetamol (Acetaminophen) During Oral Anticoagulant Therapy With Coumarins Does Not Cause Clinically Important INR Changes: A Randomized Double-Blind Clinical Trial," *J Thromb Haemost*, 2003, 1(4):714-7.

Gebauer MG, Nyfort-Hansen K, Henschke PJ, et al, "Warfarin and Acetaminophen Interaction," *Pharmacotherapy*, 2003, 23(1):109-12.

Hylek EM, Heiman H, Skates SJ, et al, "Acetaminophen and Other Risk Factors for Excessive Warfarin Anticoagulation," *JAMA*, 1998, 279(9):657-62.

Kwan D, Bartle WR, and Walker SE, "The Effects of Acute and Chronic Acetaminophen Dosing on the Pharmacodynamics and Pharmacokinetics of (R)- and (S)-Warfarin," *Clin Pharmacol Ther*, 1995, 57:212.

Mullican WS and Lacy JR, "Tramadol/Acetaminophen Combination Tablets and Codeine/Acetaminophen Combination Capsules for the Management of Chronic Pain: A Comparative Trial," *Clin Ther*, 2001, 23(9):1429-45.

Rubin RN, Mentzer RL, and Budzynski AZ, "Potentiation of Anticoagulant Effect of Warfarin by Acetaminophen (Tylenol®)," *Clin Res*, 1984, 32:698a.

van den Bemt PM, Geven LM, Kuitert NA, et al, "The Potential Interaction Between Oral Anticoagulants and Acetaminophen in Everyday Practice," *Pharm World Sci*, 2002, 24(5):201-4.

Wynn RL, "Narcotic Analgesics for Dental Pain: Available Products, Strengths, and Formulations," *Gen Dent*, 2001, 49(2):126-8, 130, 132 passim.

Acetaminophen and Diphenhydramine

(a seet a MIN oh fen & dye fen HYE dra meen)

Related Information

Acetaminophen *on page 27*

DiphenhydrAMINE (Systemic) *on page 433*

Brand Names: U.S. Aceta-Gesic®; Excedrin PM® [OTC]; Goody's PM® [OTC]; Legatrin PM® [OTC]; Mapap PM [OTC]; Percogesic® Extra Strength [OTC]; TopCare® Pain Relief PM [OTC]; Tylenol® PM [OTC]; Tylenol® Severe Allergy [OTC]

Pharmacologic Category Analgesic, Miscellaneous

Use Aid in the relief of insomnia accompanied by minor pain

Local Anesthetic/Vasoconstrictor Precautions No information available to require special precautions

Effects on Dental Treatment Key adverse event(s) related to dental treatment: Xerostomia (normal salivary flow resumes upon discontinuation). See Dental Comment.

Effects on Bleeding As a single agent, acetaminophen does not appear to affect bleeding or platelet aggregation. Acetaminophen may prolong the INR and increase bleeding in patients taking warfarin (Coumadin®). For patients taking warfarin, single acetaminophen doses or acetaminophen therapy of short duration should be safe, but if large (>1.3 g/day) doses are administered for longer than 10-14 days, then the INR should be monitored (see Dental Comment).

Adverse Effects See individual agents.

General Dosage Range Oral: *Children ≥12 years and Adults:* 50 mg of diphenhydramine HCl (76 mg diphenhydramine citrate) at bedtime

Dental Comment Hepatotoxicity caused by acetaminophen is potentiated by chronic alcohol consumption. People who are taking acetaminophen, even at therapeutic doses, and consume alcohol are at risk of developing hepatotoxicity.

Acetaminophen may increase the levels and enhance the anticoagulant effects of vitamin K antagonists acenocoumarol and warfarin (Coumadin®). Studies have reported that acetaminophen has increased the INR in warfarin treated patients with daily acetaminophen doses as low as 2 g, particularly when taking acetaminophen for >1 week (Antlitz, 1968; Boeijinga, 1982; Gebauer, 2003; Hylek, 1998; Rubin, 1984). In addition, case reports of bleeding as a result of increased INR have been published (Bagheri, 1999; Bartle, 1991). There is no known mechanism of the interaction; furthermore, some studies have failed to demonstrate this interaction (Gadisseur, 2003; Kwan, 1995; van den Bemt, 2002). In terms of risk, the data suggest that acetaminophen and warfarin could interact in some clinically significant manner but that the benefits of concomitant use of acetaminophen for pain control in dental patients taking warfarin usually outweigh the risks. An appropriate monitoring plan should be in place to identify potential negative effects and dosage adjustments may be necessary in a minority of patients. The interaction may be more likely to occur with daily acetaminophen doses of >1.3 g for >1 week.

There are no reports of acetaminophen interacting with antiplatelet drugs such as aspirin, clopidogrel (Plavix®), or prasugrel (Effient™). Also, there are no reports of acetaminophen in combination with hydrocodone, codeine, or oxycodone interacting with warfarin (Coumadin®).

Acetaminophen and Phenylephrine

(a seet a MIN oh fen & fen il EF rin)

Related Information

Acetaminophen *on page 27*

Phenylephrine (Systemic) *on page 1087*

Brand Names: U.S. Cetafen Cold® [OTC]; Contac® Cold + Flu Maximum Strength Non-Drowsy [OTC]; Excedrin® Sinus Headache [OTC]; Mapap® Sinus PE [OTC]; Robitussin® Peak Cold Nasal Relief [OTC]; Sinus Pain & Pressure [OTC]; Sudafed PE® Pressure + Pain [OTC]; Tylenol® Sinus Congestion & Pain Daytime [OTC]; Vicks® DayQuil® Sinex® Daytime Sinus [OTC]

Pharmacologic Category Analgesic, Miscellaneous; Decongestant

Use Temporary relief of sinus/nasal congestion and pressure, headache, and minor aches and pains

Local Anesthetic/Vasoconstrictor Precautions Use with caution since phenylephrine is a sympathomimetic amine which could interact with epinephrine to cause a pressor response.

Effects on Dental Treatment Key adverse event(s) related to dental treatment: Tachycardia, palpitations (use vasoconstrictor with caution), and xerostomia (normal salivary flow resumes upon discontinuation). See Dental Comment.

Effects on Bleeding As a single agent, acetaminophen does not appear to affect bleeding or platelet aggregation. Acetaminophen may prolong the INR and increase bleeding in patients taking warfarin (Coumadin®). For patients taking warfarin, single acetaminophen doses or acetaminophen therapy of short duration should be safe, but if large (>1.3 g/day) doses are administered for longer than 10-14 days, then the INR should be monitored (see Dental Comment).

Adverse Effects See individual agents.

General Dosage Range Oral: *Children ≥12 years and Adults:* Acetaminophen 325 mg and phenylephrine 5 mg/caplet: Take 2 caplets every 4 hours as needed (maximum: 12 caplets/24 hours; maximum acetaminophen: 4 g/day)

Mechanism of Action Acetaminophen inhibits the synthesis of prostaglandins in the central nervous system and peripherally blocks pain impulse generation. Phenylephrine causes vasoconstriction of the arterioles of the nasal mucosa.

Dental Comment Hepatotoxicity caused by acetaminophen is potentiated by chronic alcohol consumption. People who are taking acetaminophen, even at therapeutic doses, and consume alcohol are at risk of developing hepatotoxicity.

Acetaminophen may increase the levels and enhance the anticoagulant effects of vitamin K antagonists acenocoumarol and warfarin (Coumadin®). Studies have reported that acetaminophen has increased the INR in warfarin treated patients with daily acetaminophen doses as low as 2 g, particularly when taking acetaminophen for >1 week (Antlitz, 1968; Boeijinga, 1982; Gebauer, 2003; Hylek, 1998; Rubin, 1984). In addition, case reports of bleeding as a result of increased INR have been published (Bagheri, 1999; Bartle, 1991). There is no known mechanism of the interaction; furthermore, some studies have failed to demonstrate this interaction (Gadisseur, 2003; Kwan, 1995; van den Bemt, 2002). In terms of risk, the data suggest that acetaminophen and warfarin could interact in some clinically significant manner but that the benefits of concomitant use of acetaminophen for pain control in dental patients taking warfarin usually outweigh the risks. An appropriate monitoring plan should be in place to identify potential negative effects and dosage adjustments may be necessary in a minority of patients. The interaction may be more likely to occur with daily acetaminophen doses of >1.3 g for >1 week.

There are no reports of acetaminophen interacting with antiplatelet drugs such as aspirin, clopidogrel (Plavix®), or prasugrel (Effient™). Also, there are no reports of acetaminophen in combination with hydrocodone, codeine, or oxycodone interacting with warfarin (Coumadin®).

Acetaminophen and Phenyltoloxamine
(a seet a MIN oh fen & fen il to LOKS a meen)

Related Information
Acetaminophen *on page 27*
Brand Names: U.S. RhinoFlex™ [DSC]; RhinoFlex™-650 [DSC]; Zgesic
Pharmacologic Category Analgesic, Miscellaneous
Use Relief of mild-to-moderate pain
Local Anesthetic/Vasoconstrictor Precautions No information available to require special precautions
Effects on Dental Treatment No significant effects or complications reported (see Dental Comment)
Effects on Bleeding As a single agent, acetaminophen does not appear to affect bleeding or platelet aggregation. Acetaminophen may prolong the INR and increase bleeding in patients taking warfarin (Coumadin®). For patients taking warfarin, single acetaminophen doses or acetaminophen therapy of short duration should be safe, but if large (>1.3 g/day) doses are administered for longer than 10-14 days, then the INR should be monitored (see Dental Comment).
Adverse Effects Frequency not defined.

Central nervous system: Dizziness, drowsiness, lassitude
Dermatologic: Pruritus, rash
Gastrointestinal: Nausea
Ocular: Blurred vision
Miscellaneous: Diaphoresis

General Dosage Range Oral: Based on acetaminophen component:
Children <12 years: 10-15 mg/kg/dose every 4-6 hours as needed (maximum: 2.6 g/day)
Children ≥12 years and Adults: 325-650 mg every 4-6 hours as needed (maximum: 4 g/day)

Mechanism of Action Acetaminophen inhibits the synthesis of prostaglandins in the central nervous system and peripherally blocks pain impulse generation; produces antipyresis from inhibition of hypothalamic heat-regulating center. Phenyltoloxamine is an antihistamine (H_1-blocking agent) which acts primarily to inhibit secretions in the nose, mouth, and pharynx, as well as causing CNS depression.

Pregnancy Risk Factor C

Pregnancy Considerations Reproduction studies have not been conducted with this combination.

Dental Comment Hepatotoxicity caused by acetaminophen is potentiated by chronic alcohol consumption. People who are taking acetaminophen, even at therapeutic doses, and consume alcohol are at risk of developing hepatotoxicity.

Acetaminophen may increase the levels and enhance the anticoagulant effects of vitamin K antagonists acenocoumarol and warfarin (Coumadin®). Studies have reported that acetaminophen has increased the INR in warfarin treated patients with daily acetaminophen doses as low as 2 g, particularly when taking acetaminophen for >1 week (Antlitz, 1968; Boeijinga, 1982; Gebauer, 2003; Hylek, 1998; Rubin, 1984). In addition, case reports of bleeding as a result of increased INR have been published (Bagheri, 1999; Bartle, 1991). There is no known mechanism of the interaction; furthermore, some studies have failed to demonstrate this interaction (Gadisseur, 2003; Kwan, 1995; van den Bemt, 2002). In terms of risk, the data suggest that acetaminophen and warfarin could interact in some clinically significant manner but that the benefits of concomitant use of acetaminophen for pain control in dental patients taking warfarin usually outweigh the risks. An appropriate monitoring plan should be in place to identify potential negative effects and dosage adjustments may be necessary in a minority of patients. The interaction may be more likely to occur with daily acetaminophen doses of >1.3 g for >1 week.

There are no reports of acetaminophen interacting with antiplatelet drugs such as aspirin, clopidogrel (Plavix®), or prasugrel (Effient™). Also, there are no reports of acetaminophen in combination with hydrocodone, codeine, or oxycodone interacting with warfarin (Coumadin®).

Acetaminophen and Pseudoephedrine
(a seet a MIN oh fen & soo doe e FED rin)

Related Information
Acetaminophen *on page 27*
Pseudoephedrine *on page 1159*
Brand Names: U.S. Ornex® Maximum Strength [OTC]; Ornex® [OTC]

Brand Names: Canada Contac® Cold and Sore Throat, Non Drowsy, Extra Strength; Dristan® N.D.; Dristan® N.D., Extra Strength; Sinutab® Non Drowsy; Sudafed® Head Cold and Sinus Extra Strength; Tylenol® Decongestant; Tylenol® Sinus

Pharmacologic Category Alpha/Beta Agonist; Analgesic, Miscellaneous

Use Temporary relief of nasal congestion, and minor aches and pains associated with colds, flu, sinusitis, or allergies

Local Anesthetic/Vasoconstrictor Precautions Use with caution since pseudoephedrine is a sympathomimetic amine which could interact with epinephrine to cause a pressor response

Effects on Dental Treatment Key adverse event(s) related to dental treatment: Pseudoephedrine: Xerostomia (normal salivary flow resumes upon discontinuation). See Dental Comment.

Effects on Bleeding As a single agent, acetaminophen does not appear to affect bleeding or platelet aggregation. Acetaminophen may prolong the INR and increase bleeding in patients taking warfarin (Coumadin®). For patients taking warfarin, single acetaminophen doses or acetaminophen therapy of short duration should be safe, but if large (>1.3 g/day) doses are administered for longer than 10-14 days, then the INR should be monitored (see Dental Comment).

Adverse Effects See individual agents.

General Dosage Range Oral:
Children 6-11 years: Acetaminophen 325 mg/pseudoephedrine 30 mg every 4-6 hours (maximum: 120 mg/day pseudoephedrine)
Children ≥12 years and Adults: Acetaminophen 625-1000 mg/pseudoephedrine 60 mg every 4-6 hours (maximum: 240 mg/day pseudoephedrine)

Dental Comment Hepatotoxicity caused by acetaminophen is potentiated by chronic alcohol consumption. People who are taking acetaminophen, even at therapeutic doses, and consume alcohol are at risk of developing hepatotoxicity.

Acetaminophen may increase the levels and enhance the anticoagulant effects of vitamin K antagonists acenocoumarol and warfarin (Coumadin®). Studies have reported that acetaminophen has increased the INR in warfarin treated patients with daily acetaminophen doses as low as 2 g, particularly when taking acetaminophen for >1 week (Antlitz, 1968; Boeijinga, 1982; Gebauer, 2003; Hylek, 1998; Rubin, 1984). In addition, case reports of bleeding as a result of increased INR have been published (Bagheri, 1999; Bartle, 1991). There is no known mechanism of the interaction; furthermore, some studies have failed to demonstrate this interaction (Gadisseur, 2003; Kwan, 1995; van den Bemt, 2002). In terms of risk, the data suggest that acetaminophen and warfarin could interact in some clinically significant manner but that the benefits of concomitant use of acetaminophen for pain control in dental patients taking warfarin usually outweigh the risks. An appropriate monitoring plan should be in place to identify potential negative effects and dosage adjustments may be necessary in a minority of patients. The interaction may be more likely to occur with daily acetaminophen doses of >1.3 g for >1 week.

There are no reports of acetaminophen interacting with antiplatelet drugs such as aspirin, clopidogrel (Plavix®), or prasugrel (Effient™). Also, there are no reports of acetaminophen in combination with hydrocodone, codeine, or oxycodone interacting with warfarin (Coumadin®).

Acetaminophen and Tramadol
(a seet a MIN oh fen & TRA ma dole)

Related Information
Acetaminophen *on page 27*
Oral Pain *on page 1558*
TraMADol *on page 1346*

Related Sample Prescriptions
Moderate/Moderately Severe Oral Pain *on page 1606*

Brand Names: U.S. Ultracet®

Brand Names: Canada Apo-Tramadol/Acet®; CO Tramadol/Acet; JAMP-ACET-Tramadol; Mar-Tramadol/Acet; Pat-Tramadol/Acet; TEVA-Tramadol/Acetaminophen; Tramacet; Tramaphen-Odan

Generic Availability (U.S.) Yes

Pharmacologic Category Analgesic Combination (Opioid); Analgesic, Miscellaneous

Dental Use Treatment of postoperative pain (≤5 days)

Use Short-term (≤5 days) management of acute pain

Local Anesthetic/Vasoconstrictor Precautions No information available to require special precautions

Effects on Dental Treatment Key adverse event(s) related to dental treatment: Xerostomia and changes in salivation (normal salivary flow resumes upon discontinuation). See Dental Comment.

Effects on Bleeding As a single agent, acetaminophen does not appear to affect bleeding or platelet aggregation. Acetaminophen may prolong the INR and increase bleeding in patients taking warfarin (Coumadin®). For patients taking warfarin, single acetaminophen doses or acetaminophen therapy of short duration should be safe, but if large (>1.3 g/day) doses are administered for longer than 10-14 days, then the INR should be monitored (see Dental Comment).

Adverse Effects 1% to 10%:
Central nervous system: Somnolence (6%), dizziness (3%), insomnia (2%), anxiety, confusion, euphoria, fatigue, headache, nervousness, somnolence, tremor
Dermatologic: Pruritus (2%), rash
Endocrine & metabolic: Hot flashes
Gastrointestinal: Constipation (6%), anorexia (3%), diarrhea (3%), nausea (3%), dry mouth (2%), abdominal pain, dyspepsia, flatulence, vomiting
Genitourinary: Prostatic disorder (2%)
Neuromuscular & skeletal: Weakness
Miscellaneous: Diaphoresis increased (4%)

Dental Usual Dosage Acute postoperative pain (≤5 days): Adults: Oral: Two tablets every 4-6 hours as needed for pain relief (maximum: 8 tablets/day); treatment should not exceed 5 days

Dosage Oral: Adults: Acute pain: Two tablets every 4-6 hours as needed for pain relief (maximum: 8 tablets/day); treatment should not exceed 5 days

Dosage adjustment in renal impairment: Cl_{cr} <30 mL/minute: Maximum of 2 tablets every 12 hours; treatment should not exceed 5 days

Dosage adjustment in hepatic impairment: Use is not recommended.

Mechanism of Action
Based on **acetaminophen** component: Inhibits the synthesis of prostaglandins in the central nervous system and peripherally blocks pain impulse generation; produces antipyresis from inhibition of hypothalamic heat-regulating center

◀ Based on **tramadol** component: Binds to μ-opiate receptors in the CNS causing inhibition of ascending pain pathways, altering the perception of and response to pain; also inhibits the reuptake of norepinephrine and serotonin, which also modifies the ascending pain pathway

Contraindications Hypersensitivity to acetaminophen, tramadol, opioids, or any component of the formulation; opioid-dependent patients; acute intoxication with ethanol, hypnotics, narcotics, centrally-acting analgesics, opioids, or psychotropic drugs; hepatic dysfunction

Note: Based on Canadian product labeling: Tramadol is contraindicated during or within 14 days following MAO inhibitor therapy

Warnings/Precautions See individual agents.

Drug Interactions

Metabolism/Transport Effects Refer to individual components.

Avoid Concomitant Use

Avoid concomitant use of Acetaminophen and Tramadol with any of the following: Azelastine (Nasal); CarBAMazepine; Conivaptan; Paraldehyde

Increased Effect/Toxicity

Acetaminophen and Tramadol may increase the levels/effects of: Alcohol (Ethyl); Alvimopan; Azelastine (Nasal); Busulfan; CarBAMazepine; CNS Depressants; Dasatinib; Desmopressin; Imatinib; Lomitapide; MAO Inhibitors; Metoclopramide; Metyrosine; Mipomersen; Paraldehyde; Pramipexole; Prilocaine; ROPINIRole; Rotigotine; Selective Serotonin Reuptake Inhibitors; Serotonin Modulators; SORAfenib; Thiazide Diuretics; Vitamin K Antagonists; Zolpidem

The levels/effects of Acetaminophen and Tramadol may be increased by: Amphetamines; Antipsychotic Agents (Phenothiazines); Antipsychotics; Conivaptan; Cyclobenzaprine; CYP3A4 Inhibitors (Moderate); CYP3A4 Inhibitors (Strong); Dasatinib; HydrOXYzine; Imatinib; Isoniazid; Ivacaftor; Magnesium Sulfate; Metyrapone; Mifepristone; Perampanel; Probenecid; Selective Serotonin Reuptake Inhibitors; Sodium Oxybate; SORAfenib; Succinylcholine; Tricyclic Antidepressants

Decreased Effect

Acetaminophen and Tramadol may decrease the levels/effects of: CarBAMazepine; Pegvisomant

The levels/effects of Acetaminophen and Tramadol may be decreased by: Ammonium Chloride; Anticonvulsants (Hydantoin); Antiemetics (5HT3 Antagonists); Barbiturates; CarBAMazepine; Cholestyramine Resin; CYP2D6 Inhibitors (Moderate); CYP2D6 Inhibitors (Strong); CYP3A4 Inducers (Strong); Deferasirox; Mixed Agonist / Antagonist Opioids; Peginterferon Alfa-2b; Tocilizumab

Ethanol/Nutrition/Herb Interactions

Ethanol: Avoid ethanol (increased liver toxicity with concomitant use).

Food: May delay time to peak plasma levels, however, the extent of absorption is not affected.

Herb/Nutraceutical:

Acetaminophen: Avoid St John's wort (may decrease acetaminophen levels).

Tramadol: Avoid valerian, St John's wort, kava kava, gotu kola (may increase CNS depression).

Dietary Considerations May be taken with or without food.

Pregnancy Risk Factor C

Pregnancy Considerations Adverse events were observed in some animal reproduction studies using this combination. Acetaminophen and tramadol cross the placenta. Refer to individual monographs for additional information.

Lactation Enters breast milk/not recommended

Breast-Feeding Considerations Acetaminophen and tramadol can be detected in breast milk. The manufacturer does not recommend this combination for use as a preoperative medication or for postdelivery analgesia in nursing mothers. Refer to individual monographs for additional information.

Dosage Forms

Tablet: Acetaminophen 325 mg and tramadol 37.5 mg
Ultracet®: Acetaminophen 325 mg and tramadol 37.5 mg

Dental Comment Hepatotoxicity caused by acetaminophen is potentiated by chronic alcohol consumption. People who are taking acetaminophen, even at therapeutic doses, and consume alcohol are at risk of developing hepatotoxicity.

Acetaminophen may increase the levels and enhance the anticoagulant effects of vitamin K antagonists acenocoumarol and warfarin (Coumadin®). Studies have reported that acetaminophen has increased the INR in warfarin treated patients with daily acetaminophen doses as low as 2 g, particularly when taking acetaminophen for >1 week (Antlitz, 1968; Boeijinga, 1982; Gebauer, 2003; Hylek, 1998; Rubin, 1984). In addition, case reports of bleeding as a result of increased INR have been published (Bagheri, 1999; Bartle, 1991). There is no known mechanism of the interaction; furthermore, some studies have failed to demonstrate this interaction (Gadisseur, 2003; Kwan, 1995; van den Bemt, 2002). In terms of risk, the data suggest that acetaminophen and warfarin could interact in some clinically significant manner but that the benefits of concomitant use of acetaminophen for pain control in dental patients taking warfarin usually outweigh the risks. An appropriate monitoring plan should be in place to identify potential negative effects and dosage adjustments may be necessary in a minority of patients. The interaction may be more likely to occur with daily acetaminophen doses of >1.3 g for >1 week.

There are no reports of acetaminophen interacting with antiplatelet drugs such as aspirin, clopidogrel (Plavix®), or prasugrel (Effient™). Also, there are no reports of acetaminophen in combination with hydrocodone, codeine, or oxycodone interacting with warfarin (Coumadin®).

References

Antlitz AM, Mead JA Jr, and Tolentino MA, "Potentiation of Oral Anticoagulant Therapy by Acetaminophen," *Curr Ther Res Clin Exp*, 1968, 10(10):501-7.

Bagheri H, Bernhard NB, and Montastruc JL, "Potentiation of the Acenocoumarol Anticoagulant Effect by Acetaminophen," *Ann Pharmacother*, 1999, 33(4):506.

Bartle WR and Blakely JA, "Potentiation of Warfarin Anticoagulation by Acetaminophen," *JAMA*, 1991, 265(10):1260.

Boeijinga JJ, Boerstra EE, Ris P, et al, "Interaction Between Paracetamol and Coumarin Anticoagulants," *Lancet*, 1982, 1(8270):506.

Fricke JR Jr, Hewitt DJ, Jordan DM, et al, "A Double-Blind Placebo-Controlled Comparison of Tramadol/Acetaminophen and Tramadol in Patients With Postoperative Dental Pain," *Pain*, 2004, 109 (3):250-7.

Fricke JR Jr, Karim R, Jordan D, et al, "A Double-Blind, Single-Dose Comparison of the Analgesic Efficacy of Tramadol/Acetaminophen Combination Tablets, Hydrocodone/Acetaminophen Combination Tablets, and Placebo After Oral Surgery," *Clin Ther*, 2002, 24 (6):953-68.

Gadisseur AP, Van Der Meer FJ, and Rosendaal FR, "Sustained Intake of Paracetamol (Acetaminophen) During Oral Anticoagulant Therapy With Coumarins Does Not Cause Clinically Important INR Changes: A Randomized Double-Blind Clinical Trial," *J Thromb Haemost*, 2003, 1(4):714-7.

Gebauer MG, Nyfort-Hansen K, Henschke PJ, et al, "Warfarin and Acetaminophen Interaction," *Pharmacotherapy*, 2003, 23(1):109-12.

Hylek EM, Heiman H, Skates SJ, et al, "Acetaminophen and Other Risk Factors for Excessive Warfarin Anticoagulation," *JAMA*, 1998, 279(9):657-62.

Kwan D, Bartle WR, and Walker SE, "The Effects of Acute and Chronic Acetaminophen Dosing on the Pharmacodynamics and Pharmacokinetics of (R)- and (S)-Warfarin," *Clin Pharmacol Ther*, 1995, 57:212.

Medve RA, Wang J, and Karim R, "Tramadol and Acetaminophen Tablets for Dental Pain," *Anesth Prog*, 2001, 48(3):79-81.

Rubin RN, Mentzer RL, and Budzynski AZ, "Potentiation of Anticoagulant Effect of Warfarin by Acetaminophen (Tylenol®)," *Clin Res*, 1984, 32:698a.

Smith AB, Ravikumar TS, Kamin M, et al, "Combination Tramadol Plus Acetaminophen for Postsurgical Pain,' *Am J Surg*, 2004, 187 (4):521-7.

van den Bemt PM, Geven LM, Kuitert NA, et al, "The Potential Interaction Between Oral Anticoagulants and Acetaminophen in Everyday Practice," *Pharm World Sci*, 2002, 24(5):201-4.

Wynn RL, "NSAIDS and Cardiovascular Effects, Celecoxib for Dental Pain, and a New Analgesic - Tramadol with Acetaminophen," *Gen Dent*, 2002, 50(3):218-222.

Acetaminophen, Aspirin, and Caffeine
(a seet a MIN oh fen, AS pir in, & KAF een)

Related Information
Acetaminophen *on page 27*
Aspirin *on page 135*
Caffeine *on page 229*

Brand Names: U.S. Anacin® Advanced Headache Formula [OTC]; Excedrin® Extra Strength [OTC]; Excedrin® Migraine [OTC]; Fem-Prin® [OTC]; Goody's® Extra Strength Headache Powder [OTC]; Goody's® Extra Strength Pain Relief [OTC]; Pain-Off [OTC]; Vanquish® Extra Strength Pain Reliever [OTC]

Pharmacologic Category Analgesic, Miscellaneous

Use Relief of mild-to-moderate pain; mild-to-moderate pain associated with migraine headache

Local Anesthetic/Vasoconstrictor Precautions No information available to require special precautions

Effects on Dental Treatment Key adverse event(s) related to dental treatment: Aspirin component: As with all drugs which may affect hemostasis, bleeding is associated with aspirin. Hemorrhage may occur at virtually any site; risk is dependent on multiple variables including dosage, concurrent use of multiple agents which alter hemostasis, and patient susceptibility. Many adverse effects of aspirin are dose related, and are rare at low dosages. Other serious reactions are idiosyncratic, related to allergy or individual sensitivity (see Effects on Bleeding).

Effects on Bleeding As a single agent, acetaminophen does not appear to affect bleeding or platelet aggregation. Acetaminophen may prolong the INR and increase bleeding in patients taking warfarin (Coumadin®). For patients taking warfarin, single acetaminophen doses or acetaminophen therapy of short duration should be safe, but if large (>1.3 g/day) doses are administered for longer than 10-14 days, then the INR should be monitored (see Dental Comment).

Aspirin irreversibly inhibits platelet aggregation which can prolong bleeding. Upon discontinuation, normal platelet function returns only when new platelets are released (~7-10 days). However, in the case of dental surgery, there is no scientific evidence to support discontinuation of aspirin. The discontinuation of aspirin may place the patient at risk for a thrombotic event or other cardiovascular complication. In particular, aspirin should NOT be discontinued in patients with cardiac stents that have not completed their full course of dual antiplatelet therapy (eg, aspirin and clopidogrel [prasugrel or ticagrelor]); patient-specific situations need to be discussed with cardiologist. When feasible, postponement of dental surgery until the completion of dual antiplatelet therapy should be considered. Any modification of aspirin therapy should be discussed with the prescribing physician.

Adverse Effects See individual agents.

General Dosage Range Oral: *Children >12 years and Adults:* 1-2 doses every 4-6 hours as needed (maximum: 4 g/day [based on acetaminophen and aspirin component])

Pregnancy Considerations See individual agents.

Dental Comment There is no scientific evidence to warrant discontinuation of aspirin prior to dental surgery. Patients taking one aspirin tablet daily as an antithrombotic and who require dental surgery should be given special consideration in consultation with the physician before removal of the aspirin relative to prevention of postoperative bleeding.

Hepatotoxicity caused by acetaminophen is potentiated by chronic alcohol consumption. People who are taking acetaminophen, even at therapeutic doses, and consume alcohol are at risk of developing hepatotoxicity.

Acetaminophen may increase the levels and enhance the anticoagulant effects of vitamin K antagonists acenocoumarol and warfarin (Coumadin®). Studies have reported that acetaminophen has increased the INR in warfarin treated patients with daily acetaminophen doses as low as 2 g, particularly when taking acetaminophen for >1 week (Antlitz, 1968; Boeijinga, 1982; Gebauer, 2003; Hylek, 1998; Rubin, 1984). In addition, case reports of bleeding as a result of increased INR have been published (Bagheri, 1999; Bartle, 1991). There is no known mechanism of the interaction; furthermore, some studies have failed to demonstrate this interaction (Gadisseur, 2003; Kwan, 1995; van den Bemt, 2002). In terms of risk, the data suggest that acetaminophen and warfarin could interact in some clinically significant manner but that the benefits of concomitant use of acetaminophen for pain control in dental patients taking warfarin usually outweigh the risks. An appropriate monitoring plan should be in place to identify potential negative effects and dosage adjustments may be necessary in a minority of patients. The interaction may be more likely to occur with daily acetaminophen doses of >1.3 g for >1 week.

There are no reports of acetaminophen interacting with antiplatelet drugs such as aspirin, clopidogrel (Plavix®), or prasugrel (Effient™). Also, there are no reports of acetaminophen in combination with hydrocodone, codeine, or oxycodone interacting with warfarin (Coumadin®).

Acetaminophen, Caffeine, and Dihydrocodeine
(a seet a MIN oh fen, KAF een, & dye hye droe KOE deen)

Related Information
Acetaminophen *on page 27*
Caffeine *on page 229*

Brand Names: U.S. Trezix™

Generic Availability (U.S.) Yes: Tablet

Pharmacologic Category Analgesic Combination (Opioid)

Dental Use Relief of moderate to moderately-severe dental pain

Use Relief of moderate to moderately-severe pain

Local Anesthetic/Vasoconstrictor Precautions No information available to require special precautions

Effects on Dental Treatment No significant effects or complications reported (see Dental Comment)

Effects on Bleeding As a single agent, acetaminophen does not appear to affect bleeding or platelet aggregation. Acetaminophen may prolong the INR and increase bleeding in patients taking warfarin (Coumadin®). For patients taking warfarin, single acetaminophen doses or acetaminophen therapy of short duration should be safe, but if large (>1.3 g/day) doses are administered for longer than 10-14 days, then the INR should be monitored (see Dental Comment).

Adverse Effects Frequency not defined. Most common reactions with this combination include:

Central nervous system: Dizziness, drowsiness, light-headedness, sedation
Dermatologic: Pruritus, skin reactions
Gastrointestinal: Constipation, nausea, vomiting

Dental Usual Dosage Relief of moderate-to-moderately severe dental pain: Adults: Oral:
Capsule (acetaminophen 356.4 mg, caffeine 30 mg, and dihydrocodeine bitartrate 16 mg): Two capsules every 4 hours as needed; adjust dose based on severity of pain (maximum dose: 10 capsules/24 hours)
Tablet (acetaminophen 712.8 mg, caffeine 60 mg, and dihydrocodeine bitartrate 32 mg): One tablet every 4 hours as needed; adjust dose based on severity of pain (maximum dose: 5 tablets/24 hours)

Dosage Oral: Adults: Relief of pain:
Capsule (acetaminophen 356.4 mg, caffeine 30 mg, and dihydrocodeine bitartrate 16 mg): Two capsules every 4 hours as needed; adjust dose based on severity of pain (maximum dose: 10 capsules/24 hours)
Tablet (acetaminophen 712.8 mg, caffeine 60 mg, and dihydrocodeine bitartrate 32 mg): One tablet every 4 hours as needed; adjust dose based on severity of pain (maximum dose: 5 tablets/24 hours)

Mechanism of Action
Acetaminophen inhibits the synthesis of prostaglandins in the central nervous system and peripherally blocks pain impulse generation; produces antipyresis from inhibition of hypothalamic heat-regulating center.
Caffeine is a CNS stimulant; use with acetaminophen and dihydrocodeine increases the level of analgesia provided by each agent.
Dihydrocodeine binds to opiate receptors in the CNS, causing inhibition of ascending pain pathways, altering the perception of and response to pain; produces generalized CNS depression.

Contraindications Hypersensitivity to acetaminophen, caffeine, dihydrocodeine, codeine, or any component of the formulation; significant respiratory depression (in unmonitored settings); acute or severe bronchial asthma; hypercapnia; paralytic ileus

Warnings/Precautions [U.S. Boxed Warning]: Acetaminophen may cause severe hepatotoxicity, potentially requiring liver transplant or resulting in death; hepatotoxicity is usually associated with excessive acetaminophen intake (>4 g/day). Risk is increased with alcohol use, pre-existing liver disease, and intake of more than one source of acetaminophen-containing medications. Chronic daily dosing in adults has also resulted in liver damage in some patients. Hypersensitivity and anaphylactic reactions have been reported with acetaminophen use; discontinue immediately if symptoms of allergic or hypersensitivity reactions occur. Use caution in patients with known G6PD deficiency. Caffeine may cause CNS and cardiovascular stimulation as well as GI irritation in high doses. Dihydrocodeine should be used with caution in patients with

hypersensitivity reactions to other phenanthrene-derivative opioid agonists (morphine, hydrocodone, hydromorphone, levorphanol, oxycodone, oxymorphone), respiratory diseases including asthma, emphysema, COPD, history of drug abuse or severe hepatic or renal insufficiency. Use caution with MAO inhibitors.

This combination should be used with caution in elderly or debilitated patients, hypotension, adrenocortical insufficiency, thyroid disorders, prostatic hyperplasia, urethral stricture, seizure disorder, CNS depression, head injury or increased intracranial pressure. Causes sedation; caution must be used in performing tasks which require alertness (eg, operating machinery or driving). Safety and efficacy in pediatric patients have not been established.

Drug Interactions

Metabolism/Transport Effects Refer to individual components.

Avoid Concomitant Use
Avoid concomitant use of Acetaminophen, Caffeine, and Dihydrocodeine with any of the following: Azelastine (Nasal); Iobenguane I 123; Paraldehyde; Pimozide

Increased Effect/Toxicity
Acetaminophen, Caffeine, and Dihydrocodeine may increase the levels/effects of: Alcohol (Ethyl); Alvimopan; ARIPiprazole; Azelastine (Nasal); Busulfan; CNS Depressants; Dasatinib; Desmopressin; Formoterol; Imatinib; Indacaterol; Lomitapide; Metyrosine; Mipomersen; Mirtazapine; Paraldehyde; Pimozide; Pramipexole; Prilocaine; ROPINIRole; Rotigotine; Selective Serotonin Reuptake Inhibitors; SORAfenib; Sympathomimetics; Thiazide Diuretics; Vitamin K Antagonists; Zolpidem

The levels/effects of Acetaminophen, Caffeine, and Dihydrocodeine may be increased by: Abiraterone Acetate; Amphetamines; Antipsychotic Agents (Phenothiazines); AtoMOXetine; CYP1A2 Inhibitors (Moderate); CYP1A2 Inhibitors (Strong); Dasatinib; Deferasirox; Droperidol; HydrOXYzine; Imatinib; Isoniazid; Linezolid; Magnesium Sulfate; Metyrapone; Perampanel; Probenecid; Quinolone Antibiotics; Sodium Oxybate; SORAfenib; Succinylcholine

Decreased Effect
Acetaminophen, Caffeine, and Dihydrocodeine may decrease the levels/effects of: Adenosine; Iobenguane I 123; Pegvisomant; Regadenoson

The levels/effects of Acetaminophen, Caffeine, and Dihydrocodeine may be decreased by: Ammonium Chloride; Anticonvulsants (Hydantoin); Barbiturates; CarBAMazepine; Cholestyramine Resin; Mixed Agonist / Antagonist Opioids; Peginterferon Alfa-2b; QuiNIDine; Teriflunomide

Ethanol/Nutrition/Herb Interactions Ethanol: Excessive intake of ethanol may increase the risk of acetaminophen-induced toxicity. Ethanol may also increase CNS depression; monitor for increased effects with coadministration. Caution patients about effects.

Pregnancy Risk Factor C

Pregnancy Considerations Animal reproduction studies have not been conducted with this combination. Birth defects, including some heart defects, have been associated with maternal use of opioid analgesics during the first trimester of pregnancy (Broussard, 2011). Use of opioids during pregnancy may produce physical dependence in the neonate (Rathmell, 1997). Dihydrocodeine is a semisynthetic analogue of codeine; it has been shown to cause respiratory depression in the fetus when administered to women during labor (Leppert, 2010; Myers, 1958; Sliom, 1970). Also refer to the acetaminophen and caffeine monographs for additional information.

Lactation Enters breast milk/not recommended

Breast-Feeding Considerations Acetaminophen, caffeine, and dihydrocodeine are excreted in breast milk. Also refer to the acetaminophen and caffeine monographs for additional information.

Controlled Substance C-III

Dosage Forms

Capsule:

Trezix™: Acetaminophen 356.4 mg, caffeine 30 mg, and dihydrocodeine 16 mg

Tablet: Acetaminophen 712.8 mg, caffeine 60 mg, and dihydrocodeine bitartrate 32 mg

Dental Comment Hepatotoxicity caused by acetaminophen is potentiated by chronic alcohol consumption. People who are taking acetaminophen, even at therapeutic doses, and consume alcohol are at risk of developing hepatotoxicity.

Acetaminophen may increase the levels and enhance the anticoagulant effects of vitamin K antagonists acenocoumarol and warfarin (Coumadin®). Studies have reported that acetaminophen has increased the INR in warfarin treated patients with daily acetaminophen doses as low as 2 g, particularly when taking acetaminophen for >1 week (Antlitz, 1968; Boeijinga, 1982; Gebauer, 2003; Hylek, 1998; Rubin, 1984). In addition, case reports of bleeding as a result of increased INR have been published (Bagheri, 1999; Bartle, 1991). There is no known mechanism of the interaction; furthermore, some studies have failed to demonstrate this interaction (Gadisseur, 2003; Kwan, 1995; van den Bemt, 2002). In terms of risk, the data suggest that acetaminophen and warfarin could interact in some clinically significant manner but that the benefits of concomitant use of acetaminophen for pain control in dental patients taking warfarin usually outweigh the risks. An appropriate monitoring plan should be in place to identify potential negative effects and dosage adjustments may be necessary in a minority of patients. The interaction may be more likely to occur with daily acetaminophen doses of >1.3 g for >1 week.

There are no reports of acetaminophen interacting with antiplatelet drugs such as aspirin, clopidogrel (Plavix®), or prasugrel (Effient™). Also, there are no reports of acetaminophen in combination with hydrocodone, codeine, or oxycodone interacting with warfarin (Coumadin®).

References

Antlitz AM, Mead JA Jr, and Tolentino MA, "Potentiation of Oral Anticoagulant Therapy by Acetaminophen," *Curr Ther Res Clin Exp*, 1968, 10(10):501-7.

Bagheri H, Bernhard NB, and Montastruc JL, "Potentiation of the Acenocoumarol Anticoagulant Effect by Acetaminophen," *Ann Pharmacother*, 1999, 33(4):506.

Bartle WR and Blakely JA, "Potentiation of Warfarin Anticoagulation by Acetaminophen," *JAMA*, 1991, 265(10):1260.

Boeijinga JJ, Boerstra EE, Ris P, et al, "Interaction Between Paracetamol and Coumarin Anticoagulants," *Lancet*, 1982, 1(8270):506.

Gadisseur AP, Van Der Meer FJ, and Rosendaal FR, "Sustained Intake of Paracetamol (Acetaminophen) During Oral Anticoagulant Therapy With Coumarins Does Not Cause Clinically Important INR Changes: A Randomized Double-Blind Clinical Trial," *J Thromb Haemost*, 2003, 1(4):714-7.

Gebauer MG, Nyfort-Hansen K, Henschke PJ, et al, "Warfarin and Acetaminophen Interaction," *Pharmacotherapy*, 2003, 23(1):109-12.

Hylek EM, Heiman H, Skates SJ, et al, "Acetaminophen and Other Risk Factors for Excessive Warfarin Anticoagulation," *JAMA*, 1998, 279(9):657-62.

Kwan D, Bartle WR, and Walker SE, "The Effects of Acute and Chronic Acetaminophen Dosing on the Pharmacodynamics and Pharmacokinetics of (R)- and (S)-Warfarin," *Clin Pharmacol Ther*, 1995, 57:212.

Rubin RN, Mentzer RL, and Budzynski AZ, "Potentiation of Anticoagulant Effect of Warfarin by Acetaminophen (Tylenol®)," *Clin Res*, 1984, 32:698a.

van den Bemt PM, Geven LM, Kuitert NA, et al, "The Potential Interaction Between Oral Anticoagulants and Acetaminophen in Everyday Practice," *Pharm World Sci*, 2002, 24(5):201-4.

Acetaminophen, Chlorpheniramine, Phenylephrine, and Phenyltoloxamine

(a seet a MIN oh fen, klor fen IR a meen, fen il EF rin, & fen il tole LOKS a meen)

Related Information

Acetaminophen *on page 27*

Chlorpheniramine *on page 292*

Phenylephrine (Systemic) *on page 1087*

Brand Names: U.S. norel® SR

Pharmacologic Category Alkylamine Derivative; Alpha-Adrenergic Agonist; Analgesic, Miscellaneous; Decongestant; Ethanolamine Derivative; Histamine H_1 Antagonist; Histamine H_1 Antagonist, First Generation

Use Temporary relief of cold, allergy, or sinus symptoms caused from inhalation of airborne irritants

Local Anesthetic/Vasoconstrictor Precautions Use with caution since phenylephrine is a sympathomimetic amine which could interact with epinephrine to cause a pressor response.

Effects on Dental Treatment Key adverse event(s) related to dental treatment:

Chlorpheniramine: Prolonged use will cause significant xerostomia (normal salivary flow resumes upon discontinuation).

Phenylephrine: Up to 10% of patients could experience tachycardia, palpitations, and xerostomia (normal salivary flow resumes upon discontinuation); use vasoconstrictor with caution.

See Dental Comment

Effects on Bleeding As a single agent, acetaminophen does not appear to affect bleeding or platelet aggregation. Acetaminophen may prolong the INR and increase bleeding in patients taking warfarin (Coumadin®). For patients taking warfarin, single acetaminophen doses or acetaminophen therapy of short duration should be safe, but if large (>1.3 g/day) doses are administered for longer than 10-14 days, then the INR should be monitored (see Dental Comment).

Adverse Effects Frequency not defined.

Cardiovascular: Chest tightness

Central nervous system: Fever, fatigue, psychotic episodes

Dermatologic: Bruising

Hematologic: Anemia, bleeding

Neuromuscular & skeletal: Weakness

Miscellaneous: Allergic reactions

General Dosage Range Oral: *Children >12 years and Adults:* One tablet every 12 hours

Pregnancy Risk Factor C

Pregnancy Considerations Animal reproduction studies have not been conducted with this combination. Refer to individual agents.

Dental Comment Hepatotoxicity caused by acetaminophen is potentiated by chronic alcohol consumption. People who are taking acetaminophen, even at therapeutic doses, and consume alcohol are at risk of developing hepatotoxicity.

Acetaminophen may increase the levels and enhance the anticoagulant effects of vitamin K antagonists acenocoumarol and warfarin (Coumadin®). Studies have reported that acetaminophen has increased the INR in warfarin treated patients with daily acetaminophen

◀ doses as low as 2 g, particularly when taking acetaminophen for >1 week (Antlitz, 1968; Boeijinga, 1982; Gebauer, 2003; Hylek, 1998; Rubin, 1984). In addition, case reports of bleeding as a result of increased INR have been published (Bagheri, 1999; Bartle, 1991). There is no known mechanism of the interaction; furthermore, some studies have failed to demonstrate this interaction (Gadisseur, 2003; Kwan, 1995; van den Bemt, 2002). In terms of risk, the data suggest that acetaminophen and warfarin could interact in some clinically significant manner but that the benefits of concomitant use of acetaminophen for pain control in dental patients taking warfarin usually outweigh the risks. An appropriate monitoring plan should be in place to identify potential negative effects and dosage adjustments may be necessary in a minority of patients. The interaction may be more likely to occur with daily acetaminophen doses of >1.3 g for >1 week.

There are no reports of acetaminophen interacting with antiplatelet drugs such as aspirin, clopidogrel (Plavix®), or prasugrel (Effient™). Also, there are no reports of acetaminophen in combination with hydrocodone, codeine, or oxycodone interacting with warfarin (Coumadin®).

Acetaminophen, Dextromethorphan, and Phenylephrine
(a seet a MIN oh fen, deks troe meth OR fan, & fen il EF rin)

Related Information
Acetaminophen *on page 27*
Dextromethorphan *on page 406*
Phenylephrine (Systemic) *on page 1087*
Brand Names: U.S. Alka-Seltzer Plus® Day Cold [OTC]; Comtrex® Maximum Strength, Non-Drowsy Cold & Cough [OTC]; Daytime Cold & Flu Relief Multi-Symptom [OTC] [DSC]; Mapap® Multi-Symptom Cold [OTC]; Theraflu Warming Relief® Daytime Multi-Symptom Cold [OTC]; Theraflu Warming Relief® Daytime Severe Cold & Cough [OTC]; Theraflu® Daytime Severe Cold & Cough [OTC]; Tylenol® Cold Head Congestion Daytime [OTC]; Tylenol® Cold Multi-Symptom Daytime [OTC]; Vicks® DayQuil® Cold & Flu Multi-Symptom [OTC]; Vicks® Nature Fusion™ Cold & Flu Multi-Symptom Relief [OTC]
Pharmacologic Category Analgesic, Miscellaneous; Antitussive; Decongestant
Use Temporary relief of common cold and flu symptoms (eg, pain, fever, cough, congestion)
Local Anesthetic/Vasoconstrictor Precautions Use with caution since phenylephrine is a sympathomimetic amine which could interact with epinephrine to cause a pressor response.
Effects on Dental Treatment Key adverse event(s) related to dental treatment: Tachycardia, palpitations (use vasoconstrictor with caution), and xerostomia (normal salivary flow resumes upon discontinuation). See Dental Comment.
Effects on Bleeding As a single agent, acetaminophen does not appear to affect bleeding or platelet aggregation. Acetaminophen may prolong the INR and increase bleeding in patients taking warfarin (Coumadin®). For patients taking warfarin, single acetaminophen doses or acetaminophen therapy of short duration should be safe, but if large (>1.3 g/day) doses are administered for longer than 10-14 days, then the INR should be monitored (see Dental Comment).
Adverse Effects See individual agents.

General Dosage Range Oral: *Children ≥6 years and Adults:* Dosage varies greatly depending on product
Dental Comment Hepatotoxicity caused by acetaminophen is potentiated by chronic alcohol consumption. People who are taking acetaminophen, even at therapeutic doses, and consume alcohol are at risk of developing hepatotoxicity.

Acetaminophen may increase the levels and enhance the anticoagulant effects of vitamin K antagonists acenocoumarol and warfarin (Coumadin®). Studies have reported that acetaminophen has increased the INR in warfarin treated patients with daily acetaminophen doses as low as 2 g, particularly when taking acetaminophen for >1 week (Antlitz, 1968; Boeijinga, 1982; Gebauer, 2003; Hylek, 1998; Rubin, 1984). In addition, case reports of bleeding as a result of increased INR have been published (Bagheri, 1999; Bartle, 1991). There is no known mechanism of the interaction; furthermore, some studies have failed to demonstrate this interaction (Gadisseur, 2003; Kwan, 1995; van den Bemt, 2002). In terms of risk, the data suggest that acetaminophen and warfarin could interact in some clinically significant manner but that the benefits of concomitant use of acetaminophen for pain control in dental patients taking warfarin usually outweigh the risks. An appropriate monitoring plan should be in place to identify potential negative effects and dosage adjustments may be necessary in a minority of patients. The interaction may be more likely to occur with daily acetaminophen doses of >1.3 g for >1 week.

There are no reports of acetaminophen interacting with antiplatelet drugs such as aspirin, clopidogrel (Plavix®), or prasugrel (Effient™). Also, there are no reports of acetaminophen in combination with hydrocodone, codeine, or oxycodone interacting with warfarin (Coumadin®).

Acetaminophen, Diphenhydramine, and Phenylephrine
(a seet a MIN oh fen, dye fen HYE dra meen, & fen il EF rin)

Related Information
Acetaminophen *on page 27*
DiphenhydrAMINE (Systemic) *on page 433*
Phenylephrine (Systemic) *on page 1087*
Brand Names: U.S. Benadryl® Allergy and Cold [OTC]; Benadryl® Allergy and Sinus Headache [OTC]; Benadry® Maximum Strength Severe Allergy and Sinus Headache [OTC]; Cold Control PE [OTC]; One Tab™ Allergy & Sinus [OTC]; One Tab™ Cold & Flu [OTC]; Robitussin® Peak Cold Nighttime Multi-Symptom Cold [OTC]; Sudafed PE® Nighttime Cold [OTC]; Sudafed PE® Severe Cold [OTC]; Theraflu® Nighttime Severe Cold & Cough [OTC]; Theraflu® Sugar-Free Nighttime Severe Cold & Cough [OTC]; Theraflu™ Warming Relief™ Flu & Sore Throat [OTC]; Theraflu™ Warming Relief™ Nighttime Severe Cold & Cough [OTC]; Tylenol® Allergy Multi-Symptom Nighttime [OTC]; Tylenol® Children's Plus Cold and Allergy [OTC]
Pharmacologic Category Alpha-Adrenergic Agonist; Analgesic, Miscellaneous; Decongestant; Ethanolamine Derivative; Histamine H_1 Antagonist; Histamine H_1 Antagonist, First Generation
Use Temporary relief of symptoms of hay fever and the common cold, including sinus/nasal congestion and pain/pressure, headache, sneezing, runny nose, itchy/watery eyes, sore throat, fever, cough, and minor aches and pains

Local Anesthetic/Vasoconstrictor Precautions
Use with caution since phenylephrine is a sympathomimetic amine which could interact with epinephrine or mepivacaine and levonordefrin (Carbocaine® 2% with Neo-Cobefrin®) to cause a pressor response.

Effects on Dental Treatment Key adverse event(s) related to dental treatment:
Acetaminophen: See Dental Comment.
Diphenhydramine: Prolonged use will cause significant xerostomia (normal salivary flow resumes upon discontinuation).
Phenylephrine: Up to 10% of patients could experience tachycardia, palpitations, and xerostomia.

Effects on Bleeding As a single agent, acetaminophen does not appear to affect bleeding or platelet aggregation. Acetaminophen may prolong the INR and increase bleeding in patients taking warfarin (Coumadin®). For patients taking warfarin, single acetaminophen doses or acetaminophen therapy of short duration should be safe, but if large (>1.3 g/day) doses are administered for longer than 10-14 days, then the INR should be monitored (see Dental Comment).

Adverse Effects See individual agents.

General Dosage Range Oral:
Caplet:
Children 6-11 years: One caplet every 4 hours as needed (maximum: 5 doses/caplets)
Children ≥12 years and Adults: Two caplets every 4 hours as needed (maximum: 12 caplets/24 hours)
Liquid: *Children 6-11 years and 48-95 lbs:* 10 mL every 4 hours as needed (maximum: 5 doses/24 hours)
Powder for solution: *Children ≥12 years and Adults:* One packet every 4 hours as needed (maximum: 6 doses/24 hours)
Syrup: *Children ≥12 years and Adults:* 30 mL every 4 hours as needed (maximum: 6 doses/24 hours)

Mechanism of Action
Acetaminophen inhibits the synthesis of prostaglandins in the central nervous system and peripherally blocks pain impulse generation.
Diphenhydramine is an H_1-receptor antagonist.
Phenylephrine causes vasoconstriction of the arterioles of the nasal mucosa.

Dental Comment Hepatotoxicity caused by acetaminophen is potentiated by chronic alcohol consumption. People who are taking acetaminophen, even at therapeutic doses, and consume alcohol are at risk of developing hepatotoxicity.

Acetaminophen may increase the levels and enhance the anticoagulant effects of vitamin K antagonists acenocoumarol and warfarin (Coumadin®). Studies have reported that acetaminophen has increased the INR in warfarin treated patients with daily acetaminophen doses as low as 2 g, particularly when taking acetaminophen for >1 week (Antlitz, 1968; Boeijinga, 1982; Gebauer, 2003; Hylek, 1998; Rubin, 1984). In addition, case reports of bleeding as a result of increased INR have been published (Bagheri, 1999; Bartle, 1991). There is no known mechanism of the interaction; furthermore, some studies have failed to demonstrate this interaction (Gadisseur, 2003; Kwan, 1995; van den Bemt, 2002). In terms of risk, the data suggest that acetaminophen and warfarin could interact in some clinically significant manner but that the benefits of concomitant use of acetaminophen for pain control in dental patients taking warfarin usually outweigh the risks. An appropriate monitoring plan should be in place to identify potential negative effects and dosage adjustments may be necessary in a minority of patients. The interaction may be more likely to occur with daily acetaminophen doses of >1.3 g for >1 week.

There are no reports of acetaminophen interacting with antiplatelet drugs such as aspirin, clopidogrel (Plavix®), or prasugrel (Effient™). Also, there are no reports of acetaminophen in combination with hydrocodone, codeine, or oxycodone interacting with warfarin (Coumadin®).

Acetaminophen, Isometheptene, and Dichloralphenazone
(a seet a MIN oh fen, eye soe me THEP teen, & dye KLOR al FEN a zone)

Related Information
Acetaminophen *on page 27*
Pharmacologic Category Analgesic, Miscellaneous; Sedative; Sympathomimetic
Use Relief of migraine and tension headache
Local Anesthetic/Vasoconstrictor Precautions No information available to require special precautions
Effects on Dental Treatment No significant effects or complications reported (see Dental Comment)
Effects on Bleeding As a single agent, acetaminophen does not appear to affect bleeding or platelet aggregation. Acetaminophen may prolong the INR and increase bleeding in patients taking warfarin (Coumadin®). For patients taking warfarin, single acetaminophen doses or acetaminophen therapy of short duration should be safe, but if large (>1.3 g/day) doses are administered for longer than 10-14 days, then the INR should be monitored (see Dental Comment).

Adverse Effects Frequency not defined.
Central nervous system: Dizziness (transient)
Dermatological: Rash
General Dosage Range Oral: *Adults:* 2 capsules initially, then 1 capsule every hour until relief; alternatively, 1-2 capsules every 4 hours (maximum: 5 capsules/12 hours or 8 capsules/day)

Mechanism of Action
Acetaminophen: Although not fully elucidated, believed to inhibit the synthesis of prostaglandins in the central nervous system and work peripherally to block pain impulse generation; produces antipyresis from inhibition of hypothalamic health-regulating center
Dichloralphenazone: Prodrug, converted to chloral hydrate (sedative) and antipyrine (analgesic/antipyretic) that reduces patient's emotional response to painful stimuli
Isometheptene: A sympathomimetic that reduces stimuli leading to vascular headaches via constriction of dilated cranial and cerebral arterioles

Controlled Substance C-IV

Dental Comment Hepatotoxicity caused by acetaminophen is potentiated by chronic alcohol consumption. People who are taking acetaminophen, even at therapeutic doses, and consume alcohol are at risk of developing hepatotoxicity.

Acetaminophen may increase the levels and enhance the anticoagulant effects of vitamin K antagonists acenocoumarol and warfarin (Coumadin®). Studies have reported that acetaminophen has increased the INR in warfarin treated patients with daily acetaminophen doses as low as 2 g, particularly when taking acetaminophen for >1 week (Antlitz, 1968; Boeijinga, 1982; Gebauer, 2003; Hylek, 1998; Rubin, 1984). In addition, case reports of bleeding as a result of increased INR have been published (Bagheri, 1999; Bartle, 1991).

There is no known mechanism of the interaction; furthermore, some studies have failed to demonstrate this interaction (Gadisseur, 2003; Kwan, 1995; van den Bemt, 2002). In terms of risk, the data suggest that acetaminophen and warfarin could interact in some clinically significant manner but that the benefits of concomitant use of acetaminophen for pain control in dental patients taking warfarin usually outweigh the risks. An appropriate monitoring plan should be in place to identify potential negative effects and dosage adjustments may be necessary in a minority of patients. The interaction may be more likely to occur with daily acetaminophen doses of >1.3 g for >1 week.

There are no reports of acetaminophen interacting with antiplatelet drugs such as aspirin, clopidogrel (Plavix®), or prasugrel (Effient™). Also, there are no reports of acetaminophen in combination with hydrocodone, codeine, or oxycodone interacting with warfarin (Coumadin®).

AcetaZOLAMIDE (a set a ZOLE a mide)

Brand Names: U.S. Diamox® Sequels®
Brand Names: Canada Acetazolam; Diamox®
Pharmacologic Category Anticonvulsant, Miscellaneous; Carbonic Anhydrase Inhibitor; Diuretic, Carbonic Anhydrase Inhibitor; Ophthalmic Agent, Antiglaucoma
Use Treatment of glaucoma (chronic simple open-angle, secondary glaucoma, preoperatively in acute angle-closure); drug-induced edema or edema due to congestive heart failure (adjunctive therapy; I.V. and immediate release dosage forms); centrencephalic epilepsies (I.V. and immediate release dosage forms); prevention or amelioration of symptoms associated with acute mountain sickness (immediate and extended release dosage forms)
Unlabeled Use Metabolic alkalosis; respiratory stimulant in stable hypercapnic COPD
Local Anesthetic/Vasoconstrictor Precautions No information available to require special precautions
Effects on Dental Treatment Key adverse event(s) related to dental treatment: Metallic taste (resolves upon discontinuation)
Effects on Bleeding No information available to require special precautions
Adverse Effects Frequency not defined.
Cardiovascular: Flushing
Central nervous system: Ataxia, confusion, convulsions, depression, dizziness, drowsiness, excitement, fatigue, fever, headache, malaise
Dermatologic: Allergic skin reactions, photosensitivity, Stevens-Johnson syndrome, toxic epidermal necrolysis, urticaria
Endocrine & metabolic: Electrolyte imbalance, growth retardation (children), hyperglycemia, hypoglycemia, hypokalemia, hyponatremia, metabolic acidosis
Gastrointestinal: Appetite decreased, diarrhea, melena, nausea, taste alteration, vomiting
Genitourinary: Crystalluria, glycosuria, hematuria, polyuria, renal failure
Hematologic: Agranulocytosis, aplastic anemia, leukopenia, thrombocytopenia, thrombocytopenic purpura
Hepatic: Cholestatic jaundice, fulminant hepatic necrosis, hepatic insufficiency, liver function tests abnormal
Local: Pain at injection site
Neuromuscular & skeletal: Flaccid paralysis, paresthesia
Ocular: Myopia

Otic: Hearing disturbance, tinnitus
Miscellaneous: Anaphylaxis
General Dosage Range Dosage adjustment recommended in patients with renal impairment
I.V.: *Adults:* 250-1000 mg/day
Oral:
Immediate release:
Children: 8-30 mg/kg/day divided in 1-4 doses (maximum: 30 mg/kg/day or 1 g/day)
Adults: 250-1000 mg/day **or** 8-30 mg/kg/day in 1-4 divided doses (maximum: 30 mg/kg/day or 1 g/day) **or** 125-250 mg every 4 hours
Elderly: Initial: 250-500 mg/day
Extended release:
Adults: 500-1000 mg/day
Mechanism of Action Reversible inhibition of the enzyme carbonic anhydrase resulting in reduction of hydrogen ion secretion at renal tubule and an increased renal excretion of sodium, potassium, bicarbonate, and water. Decreases production of aqueous humor and inhibits carbonic anhydrase in central nervous system to retard abnormal and excessive discharge from CNS neurons.
Pharmacodynamics/Kinetics
Onset of Action Capsule (extended release), tablet (immediate release): 2 hours; I.V.: 5-10 minutes
Peak effect: Capsule (extended release): 8-18 hours; I.V.: 15 minutes; Tablet: 2-4 hours
Duration of Action Inhibition of aqueous humor secretion: Capsule (extended release): 18-24 hours; I.V.: 4-5 hours; Tablet: 8-12 hours
Time to Peak Plasma: Capsule (extended release): 3-6 hours; Tablet: 1-4 hours
Pregnancy Risk Factor C
Pregnancy Considerations Teratogenic effects have been observed in animal reproduction studies.

Acetic Acid, Propylene Glycol Diacetate, and Hydrocortisone
(a SEE tik AS id, PRO pa leen GLY kole dye AS e tate, & hye droe KOR ti sone)

Brand Names: U.S. Acetasol® HC; VoSol® HC
Pharmacologic Category Otic Agent, Anti-infective
Use Treatment of superficial infections of the external auditory canal caused by organisms susceptible to the action of the antimicrobial, complicated by swelling
Local Anesthetic/Vasoconstrictor Precautions No information available to require special precautions
Effects on Dental Treatment No significant effects or complications reported
Effects on Bleeding No information available to require special precautions
Adverse Effects Frequency not defined: Otic: Transient burning or stinging may be noticed occasionally when the solution is first instilled into the acutely inflamed ear
General Dosage Range Otic: *Children ≥3 years and Adults:* Instill 3-5 drops in ear(s) every 4-6 hours

Acetohydroxamic Acid
(a SEE toe hye droks am ik AS id)

Brand Names: U.S. Lithostat®
Brand Names: Canada Lithostat®
Pharmacologic Category Urinary Tract Product
Use Adjunctive therapy in chronic urea-splitting urinary infection
Local Anesthetic/Vasoconstrictor Precautions No information available to require special precautions

Effects on Dental Treatment No significant effects or complications reported

Effects on Bleeding Has been associated with bone marrow suppression and hemolytic anemia. No information to require specific precautions related to dental procedures.

Adverse Effects

>10%:

Central nervous system: Headache (30%), malaise (20% to 25%), anxiety (20%), depression (20%), nervousness (20%), tremulousness (20%)

Gastrointestinal: Anorexia (20 to 25%), nausea (20% to 25%), vomiting (20% to 25%)

Hematologic: Hemolytic anemia (3% to 15%)

≤1% to 10%:

Cardiovascular: Deep vein thrombosis (rare), flushing, palpitation

Dermatologic: Alopecia, macular skin rash

Hematologic: Reticulocytosis (5% to 6%)

Local: Phlebitis

Respiratory: Embolism

General Dosage Range Dosage adjustment recommended in patients with renal impairment.

Oral:

Children: Initial: 10 mg/kg/day in 2 or 3 divided doses

Adults: 250 mg 3-4 times daily maximum: 1500 mg daily)

Mechanism of Action Acetohydroxamic acid inhibits bacterial urease enzymes, decreasing the formation of ammonia in the urine by urea-splitting organisms. A reduction in urinary ammonia and decreased pH may increase the activity of some antimicrobial agents.

Pharmacodynamics/Kinetics

Half-life Elimination 5-10 hours (increased in patients with reduced renal function)

Time to Peak 0.25-1 hour

Pregnancy Risk Factor X

Pregnancy Considerations Teratogenic effects were observed in animal reproduction studies. Use is contraindicated in pregnant women.

Acetylcholine (a se teel KOE leen)

Brand Names: U.S. Miochol®-E

Brand Names: Canada Miochol®-E

Pharmacologic Category Cholinergic Agonist; Ophthalmic Agent, Miotic

Use Produces complete miosis in cataract surgery, keratoplasty, iridectomy, and other anterior segment surgery where rapid miosis is required

Local Anesthetic/Vasoconstrictor Precautions No information available to require special precautions

Effects on Dental Treatment No significant effects or complications reported

Effects on Bleeding No information available to require special precautions

Adverse Effects Frequency not defined.

Cardiovascular: Bradycardia, flushing, hypotension

Ocular: Clouding, corneal edema, decompensation

Respiratory: Dyspnea

Miscellaneous: Diaphoresis

General Dosage Range Intraocular: *Adults:* Instill 0.5-2 mL of 1% injection (5-20 mg)

Mechanism of Action Causes contraction of the sphincter muscles of the iris, resulting in miosis and contraction of the ciliary muscle, leading to accommodation spasm

Pharmacodynamics/Kinetics

Onset of Action Rapid

Duration of Action ~6 hours

Acetylcysteine (a se teel SIS teen)

Brand Names: U.S. Acetadote®

Brand Names: Canada Acetylcysteine Injection; Acetylcysteine Solution; Mucomyst®; Parvolex®

Pharmacologic Category Antidote; Mucolytic Agent

Use Antidote for acute acetaminophen poisoning; repeated supratherapeutic ingestion (RSTI) of acetaminophen; adjunctive mucolytic therapy in patients with abnormal or viscid mucous secretions in acute and chronic bronchopulmonary diseases; pulmonary complications of surgery and cystic fibrosis; diagnostic bronchial studies

Unlabeled Use Prevention of contrast-induced renal dysfunction (oral, I.V.); distal intestinal obstruction syndrome (DIOS, previously referred to as meconium ileus equivalent)

Local Anesthetic/Vasoconstrictor Precautions No information available to require special precautions

Effects on Dental Treatment Key adverse event(s) related to dental treatment: Stomatitis, bronchospasm, rhinorrhea

Effects on Bleeding No information available to require special precautions

Adverse Effects

Inhalation: Frequency not defined.

Central nervous system: Drowsiness, chills, fever

Gastrointestinal: Vomiting, nausea, stomatitis

Local: Irritation, stickiness on face following nebulization

Respiratory: Bronchospasm, rhinorrhea, hemoptysis

Miscellaneous: Acquired sensitization (rare), clamminess, unpleasant odor during administration

Intravenous:

>10%: Miscellaneous: Anaphylactoid reaction (8% to 18%; shorter infusion periods [eg, <60 minutes] associated with increased incidence)

1% to 10%:

Cardiovascular: Flushing (1% to 8%), tachycardia (1% to 4%), edema (1% to 2%)

Dermatologic: Urticaria (6% to 8%), rash (2% to 4%), pruritus (1% to 4%)

Gastrointestinal: Vomiting (2% to 10%), nausea (1% to 6%)

Respiratory: Pharyngitis (≤1%), rhinorrhea (≤1%), rhonchi (≤1%), throat tightness (≤1%)

General Dosage Range

Inhalation:

Nebulization:

Infants: 1-2 mL of 20% solution or 2-4 mL 10% solution 3-4 times/day

Children and Adults: 1-10 mL of 20% solution or 2-20 mL of 10% solution every 2-6 hours

Direct instillation: *Adults:* 1-4 mL of 10% or 1-2 mL of 20% solution every 1-4 hours

I.V.: Acetadote®:

Children and Adults: 21-hour regimen: Consists of 3 doses; total dose delivered: 300 mg/kg

Loading dose: 150 mg/kg (maximum: 15 g) infused over 60 minutes

Second dose: 50 mg/kg (maximum: 5 g) infused over 4 hours

Third dose: 100 mg/kg (maximum: 10 g) infused over 16 hours

Oral:
Children and Adults: Acetaminophen poisoning: 72-hour regimen: Consists of 18 doses; total dose delivered: 1330 mg/kg
Loading dose: 140 mg/kg
Maintenance dose: 70 mg/kg every 4 hours

Mechanism of Action Exerts mucolytic action through its free sulfhydryl group which opens up the disulfide bonds in the mucoproteins thus lowering mucous viscosity.

In patients with acetaminophen toxicity, acetylcysteine acts as a hepatoprotective agent by restoring hepatic glutathione, serving as a glutathione substitute, and enhancing the nontoxic sulfate conjugation of acetaminophen.

The presumed mechanism in preventing contrast-induced nephropathy is its ability to scavenge oxygen-derived free radicals and improve endothelium-dependent vasodilation.

Pharmacodynamics/Kinetics
Onset of Action Inhalation: 5-10 minutes
Duration of Action Inhalation: >1 hour
Half-life Elimination Reduced acetylcysteine: 2 hours; Total acetylcysteine: Adults: 5.6 hours, Newborns: 11 hours
Time to Peak Plasma: Oral: 1-2 hours
Pregnancy Risk Factor B
Pregnancy Considerations Based on limited reports using acetylcysteine to treat acetaminophen poisoning in pregnant women, acetylcysteine has been shown to cross the placenta and may provide protective levels in the fetus.

Aclidinium (a kli DIN ee um)

Related Information
Respiratory Diseases *on page 1514*
Brand Names: U.S. Tudorza™ Pressair™
Pharmacologic Category Anticholinergic Agent; Anticholinergic Agent, Long-Acting
Use Long-term maintenance treatment of bronchospasm associated with COPD (including bronchitis and emphysema)
Local Anesthetic/Vasoconstrictor Precautions No information available to require special precautions
Effects on Dental Treatment Key adverse event(s) related to dental treatment: Cough, nasopharyngitis, rhinitis, sinusitis, and toothache have been reported.
Effects on Bleeding No information available to require special precautions
Adverse Effects 1% to 10%:
Central nervous system: Headache (7%)
Gastrointestinal: Diarrhea (3%), vomiting (1%)
Neuromuscular & skeletal: Fall (1%)
Respiratory: Nasopharyngitis (6%), cough (3%), rhinitis (2%), sinusitis (2%)
Miscellaneous: Toothache (1%)
General Dosage Range Inhalation, oral: *Adults:* 400 mcg twice daily
Mechanism of Action Competitively and reversibly inhibits the action of acetylcholine at type 3 muscarinic (M_3) receptors in bronchial smooth muscle causing bronchodilation
Pharmacodynamics/Kinetics
Half-life Elimination 5-8 hours (following inhalation)
Time to Peak Plasma: Within 10 minutes (steady state, following inhalation)
Pregnancy Risk Factor C

Pregnancy Considerations Adverse events were observed in animal reproduction studies.

Acrivastine and Pseudoephedrine
(AK ri vas teen & soo doe e FED rin)

Related Information
Pseudoephedrine *on page 1159*
Brand Names: U.S. Semprex®-D
Pharmacologic Category Alkylamine Derivative; Alpha/Beta Agonist; Decongestant; Histamine H_1 Antagonist; Histamine H_1 Antagonist, Second Generation
Use Relief of symptoms associated with seasonal allergic rhinitis
Local Anesthetic/Vasoconstrictor Precautions Use with caution since pseudoephedrine is a sympathomimetic amine which could interact with epinephrine to cause a pressor response
Effects on Dental Treatment Key adverse event(s) related to dental treatment: Pseudoephedrine: Xerostomia (normal salivary flow resumes upon discontinuation).
Effects on Bleeding No information available to require special precautions
Adverse Effects Also refer to Pseudoephedrine monograph.
>10%: Central nervous system: Headache (19%), somnolence (12%)
1% to 10%:
Central nervous system: Insomnia (4%), dizziness (3%), nervousness (3%)
Endocrine & metabolic: Dysmenorrhea (2%)
Gastrointestinal: Xerostomia (7%), dyspepsia (2%), nausea (2%)
Respiratory: Pharyngitis (3%), cough (2%)
General Dosage Range Oral: *Children ≥12 years and Adults:* One capsule every 4-6 hours (maximum: 4 doses/24 hours)
Mechanism of Action Refer to Pseudoephedrine; acrivastine is an analogue of triprolidine and it is considered to be relatively less sedating than traditional antihistamines; believed to involve competitive blockade of H_1-receptor sites resulting in the inability of histamine to combine with its receptor sites and exert its usual effects on target cells
Pharmacodynamics/Kinetics
Half-life Elimination
Acrivastine: ~2-4 hours
Acrivastine propionic acid metabolite (active): ~4 hours
Time to Peak Acrivastine: ~1.1 hours
Pregnancy Risk Factor B
Pregnancy Considerations Teratogenic effects were not observed in animal reproduction studies with this combination; therefore, the manufacturer classifies acrivastine/pseudoephedrine as pregnancy category B. The use of antihistamines for the treatment of rhinitis during pregnancy is generally considered to be safe at recommended doses. Information related to the use of acrivastine during pregnancy is limited; therefore, other agents are preferred. Also refer to the Pseudoephedrine monograph for additional information.

Acyclovir (Systemic) (ay SYE kloe veer)

Related Information
Systemic Viral Diseases *on page 1537*
ValACYclovir *on page 1375*
Viral Infections *on page 1575*

Related Sample Prescriptions
Herpes Simplex (Primary) *on page 1616*
Shingles (Varicella-Zoster Virus) *on page 1616*

Brand Names: U.S. Zovirax®

Brand Names: Canada Apo-Acyclovir®; Mylan-Acyclovir; Nu-Acyclovir; ratio-Acyclovir; Teva-Acyclovir; Zovirax®

Generic Availability (U.S.) Yes

Pharmacologic Category Antiviral Agent

Dental Use Treatment of initial and prophylaxis of recurrent mucosal and cutaneous herpes simplex (HSV-1 and HSV-2) infections in immunocompromised patients

Use Treatment of genital herpes simplex virus (HSV) and HSV encephalitis

Unlabeled Use Prevention of HSV reactivation in HIV-positive patients; prevention of HSV reactivation in hematopoietic stem cell transplant (HSCT); prevention of HSV reactivation during periods of neutropenia in patients with cancer; prevention of varicella zoster virus (VZV) reactivation in allogenic HSCT; prevention of CMV reactivation in low-risk allogeneic HSCT; treatment of disseminated HSV or VZV in immunocompromised patients with cancer; empiric treatment of suspected encephalitis in immunocompromised patients with cancer; treatment of initial and prophylaxis of recurrent mucosal and cutaneous herpes simplex (HSV-1 and HSV-2) infections in immunocompromised patients

Local Anesthetic/Vasoconstrictor Precautions No information available to require special precautions

Effects on Dental Treatment No significant effects or complications reported

Effects on Bleeding No information available to require special precautions

Adverse Effects
Oral:
>10%: Central nervous system: Malaise (≤12%)
1% to 10%:
Central nervous system: Headache (≤2%)
Gastrointestinal: Nausea (2% to 5%), vomiting (≤3%), diarrhea (2% to 3%)

Parenteral:
1% to 10%:
Dermatologic: Hives (2%), itching (2%), rash (2%)
Gastrointestinal: Nausea/vomiting (7%)
Hepatic: Liver function tests increased (1% to 2%)
Local: Inflammation at injection site or phlebitis (9%)
Renal: BUN increased (5% to 10%), creatinine increased (5% to 10%), acute renal failure

Dental Usual Dosage
Mucocutaneous HSV: Adults:
Immunocompromised (unlabeled use): Oral: 400 mg 5 times a day for 7-14 days

Dosage Note: Obese patients should be dosed using ideal body weight

Genital herpes simplex virus (HSV) infection:
I.V.: Children ≥12 years and Adults (immunocompetent): Initial episode, severe: 5 mg/kg/dose every 8 hours for 5-7 days **or** 5-10 mg/kg/dose every 8 hours for 2-7 days, follow with oral therapy to complete at least 10 days of therapy (CDC, 2010)

Oral:
Children, immunocompetent:
Initial episode (unlabeled use): 40-80 mg/kg/day divided into 3-4 doses for 5-10 days (maximum: 1000 mg daily)
Chronic suppression (unlabeled use; limited data): 80 mg/kg/day in 3 divided doses (maximum: 1000 mg daily), re-evaluate after 12 months of treatment
Children, immunocompromised (unlabeled use; CDC, 2009): Initial episode:
Children <45 kg: 60 mg/kg/day divided into 3 doses for 5-14 days (maximum: 1200 mg daily)
Adolescents: 400 mg twice daily for 5-14 days
Adults:
Initial episode: 200 mg 5 times daily while awake for 10 days **or** 400 mg 3 times daily for 7-10 days (CDC, 2010)
Recurrence: 200 mg 5 times daily while awake for 5 days (per manufacturer's labeling; begin at earliest signs of disease)
Alternatively, the following regimens are also recommended by the CDC: 400 mg 3 times daily for 5 days; 800 mg twice daily for 5 days; 800 mg 3 times daily for 2 days (CDC, 2010)
Chronic suppression: 400 mg twice daily or 200 mg 3-5 times daily, for up to 12 months followed by re-evaluation (per manufacturer's labeling)

Herpes zoster (shingles):
Oral: Adults (immunocompetent): 800 mg 5 times daily for 7-10 days
I.V.:
Children <12 years (immunocompromised): 20 mg/kg/dose every 8 hours for 7 days
Children ≥12 years and Adults (immunocompromised): 10 mg/kg/dose or 500 mg/m²/dose every 8 hours for 7 days

HSV encephalitis: I.V.:
Children 3 months to 12 years: 20 mg/kg/dose every 8 hours for 10 days (per manufacturer's labeling); dosing for 14-21 days also reported
Children ≥12 years and Adults: 10 mg/kg/dose every 8 hours for 10 days (per manufacturer's labeling); 10-15 mg/kg/dose every 8 hours for 14-21 days also reported

Mucocutaneous HSV:
I.V.:
Children <12 years (immunocompromised): Treatment: 10 mg/kg/dose every 8 hours for 7 days
Children ≥12 years and Adults (immunocompromised): Treatment: 5-10 mg/kg/dose every 8 hours for 7 days (Leflore, 2000); dosing for up to 14 days also reported
Oral (unlabeled use): Adults (immunocompromised): 400 mg 5 times daily for 7 days (Leflore, 2000)

Neonatal HSV: I.V.: Infants: Birth to 3 months:
10 mg/kg/dose every 8 hours for 10 days (manufacturer's labeling); 20 mg/kg/dose every 8 hours for 14 (skin and mucous membrane disease) to 21 days (CNS disease) (CDC, 2010)

Orolabial HSV (unlabeled use): Oral:
Children 1-6 years (immunocompetent, gingivostomatitis): Treatment of primary infection: 15 mg/kg/dose (maximum: 200 mg per dose) 5 times daily for 7 days, initiated within 72 hours of symptom onset (Amir, 1997)

Adults (immunocompetent):
Treatment: 200-400 mg 5 times daily for 5 days (Cernik, 2008; Leflore, 2000; Spruance, 1990) for episodic/recurrent treatment; for initial treatment, limited data are available, 200 mg 5 times daily or 400 mg 3 times daily for 7-10 days has been recommended by some clinicians.
Chronic suppression: 400 mg 2 times daily (has been clinically evaluated for up to 1 year) (Cernik, 2008; Rooney, 1993)

Varicella-zoster (chickenpox): Begin treatment within the first 24 hours of rash onset:
Oral: **Note:** The CDC HIV guidelines recommended duration of therapy is 7-10 days or until no new lesions for 48 hours (for patients with mild varicella and no or moderate immune suppression).
Children ≥2 years and ≤40 kg (immunocompetent): 20 mg/kg/dose (maximum: 800 mg per dose) 4 times daily for 5 days
Children >40 kg and Adults (immunocompetent): 800 mg 4 times daily for 5 days
I.V.:
Manufacturer's labeling (immunocompromised):
Children <12 years: 20 mg/kg/dose every 8 hours for 7 days
Children ≥12 years and Adults: 10 mg/kg/dose every 8 hours for 7 days
CDC HIV guidelines (immunocompromised):
Children <1 year: 10 mg/kg/dose every 8 hours for 7-10 days or until no new lesions for 48 hours
Children ≥1 year: 10 mg/kg/dose or 500 mg/m^2/dose every 8 hours for 7-10 days or until no new lesions for 48 hours
Adolescents and Adults: 10-15 mg/kg/dose every 8 hours for 7-10 days

Varicella-zoster acute retinal necrosis infection in HIV-exposed/-positive (unlabeled use; CDC, 2009):
I.V.: Infants and Children: 10-15 mg/kg/dose every 8 hours for 10-14 days, followed by valacyclovir for 4-6 weeks

Prevention of HSV reactivation in HIV-positive patient (unlabeled use): Oral:
Children: 20 mg/kg/dose twice daily (maximum: 400 mg per dose) (CDC, 2009)
Adults: 400-800 mg 2-3 times daily (CDC, 2010)

Prevention of HSV reactivation in HSCT (unlabeled use): *CDC recommendations:* **Note:** Start at the beginning of conditioning therapy and continue until engraftment or until mucositis resolves (~30 days)
Oral: Adults: 200 mg 3 times daily
I.V.:
Children: 250 mg/m^2/dose every 8 hours or 125 mg/m^2/dose every 6 hours
Adults: 250 mg/m^2/dose every 12 hours

Prevention of VZV reactivation in allogeneic HSCT (unlabeled use): *NCCN guidelines:* Oral: Adults: 800 mg twice daily

Prevention of CMV reactivation in low-risk allogeneic HSCT (unlabeled use): *NCCN guidelines:* **Note:** Requires close monitoring (due to weak activity); not for use in patients at high risk for CMV disease: Oral: Adults: 800 mg 4 times daily

Treatment of disseminated HSV or VZV or empiric treatment of suspected encephalitis in immunocompromised patients with cancer: (unlabeled use): *NCCN guidelines:* I.V.: Adults: 10-12 mg/kg/dose every 8 hours

Treatment of episodic HSV infection in HIV-positive patient (unlabeled use): Oral: Adults: 400 mg 3 times daily for 5-10 days (CDC, 2010)

Dosage adjustment in renal impairment:
Oral:
Cl_{cr} 10-25 mL/minute/1.73 m^2: Normal dosing regimen 800 mg 5 times daily: Administer 800 mg every 8 hours
Cl_{cr} <10 mL/minute/1.73 m^2:
Normal dosing regimen 200 mg 5 times daily or 400 mg every 12 hours: Administer 200 mg every 12 hours
Normal dosing regimen 800 mg 5 times daily: Administer 800 mg every 12 hours
I.V.:
Cl_{cr} 25-50 mL/minute/1.73 m^2: Administer recommended dose every 12 hours
Cl_{cr} 10-25 mL/minute/1.73 m^2: Administer recommended dose every 24 hours
Cl_{cr} <10 mL/minute/1.73 m^2: Administer 50% of recommended dose every 24 hours
Intermittent hemodialysis (IHD) (administer after hemodialysis on dialysis days): Dialyzable (60% reduction following a 6-hour session): I.V.: 2.5-5 mg/kg every 24 hours (Heintz, 2009). **Note:** Dosing dependent on the assumption of 3 times weekly, complete IHD sessions.
Peritoneal dialysis (PD): Administer 50% of normal dose once daily; no supplemental dose needed
Continuous renal replacement therapy (CRRT) (Heintz, 2009; Trotman, 2005): Drug clearance is highly dependent on the method of renal replacement, filter type, and flow rate. Appropriate dosing requires close monitoring of pharmacologic response, signs of adverse reactions due to drug accumulation, as well as drug concentrations in relation to target trough (if appropriate). The following are general recommendations only (based on dialysate flow/ultrafiltration rates of 1-2 L/hour and minimal residual renal function) and should not supersede clinical judgment:
CVVH: I.V.: 5-10 mg/kg every 24 hours
CVVHD/CVVHDF: I.V.: 5-10 mg/kg every 12-24 hours
Note: The higher end of dosage range (eg, 10 mg/kg every 12 hours for CVVHDF) is recommended for viral meningoencephalitis and varicella-zoster virus infections.
Dosage adjustment in hepatic impairment: Oral, I.V.: No dosage adjustment provided in manufacturer's labeling; use caution in patients with severe impairment.

Mechanism of Action Acyclovir is converted to acyclovir monophosphate by virus-specific thymidine kinase then further converted to acyclovir triphosphate by other cellular enzymes. Acyclovir triphosphate inhibits DNA synthesis and viral replication by competing with deoxyguanosine triphosphate for viral DNA polymerase and being incorporated into viral DNA.

Contraindications Hypersensitivity to acyclovir, valacyclovir, or any component of the formulation

Warnings/Precautions Use with caution in immunocompromised patients; thrombocytopenic purpura/hemolytic uremic syndrome (TTP/HUS) has been reported. Use caution in the elderly, pre-existing renal disease (may require dosage modification), or in those receiving other nephrotoxic drugs. Renal failure (sometimes fatal) has been reported. Maintain adequate hydration during oral or intravenous therapy. Use I.V. preparation with caution in patients with underlying neurologic abnormalities, serious hepatic or electrolyte abnormalities, or substantial hypoxia.

Varicella-zoster: Treatment should begin within 24 hours of appearance of rash; oral route not recommended for routine use in otherwise healthy children with varicella, but may be effective in patients at increased risk of moderate-to-severe infection (>12 years of age, chronic cutaneous or pulmonary disorders, long-term salicylate therapy, corticosteroid therapy).

Drug Interactions

Metabolism/Transport Effects None known.

Avoid Concomitant Use

Avoid concomitant use of Acyclovir (Systemic) with any of the following: Zoster Vaccine

Increased Effect/Toxicity

Acyclovir (Systemic) may increase the levels/effects of: Mycophenolate; Tenofovir; Zidovudine

The levels/effects of Acyclovir (Systemic) may be increased by: Mycophenolate

Decreased Effect

Acyclovir (Systemic) may decrease the levels/effects of: Zoster Vaccine

Ethanol/Nutrition/Herb Interactions Food: Does not affect absorption of oral acyclovir.

Dietary Considerations May be taken with or without food. Some products may contain sodium.

Pharmacodynamics/Kinetics

Half-life Elimination Terminal: Neonates: 4 hours; Children 1-12 years: 2-3 hours; Adults: 3 hours

Time to Peak Serum: Oral: Within 1.5-2 hours

Pregnancy Risk Factor B

Pregnancy Considerations Teratogenic effects were not observed in animal reproduction studies. Acyclovir has been shown to cross the human placenta (Henderson, 1992). Results from a pregnancy registry, established in 1984 and closed in 1999, did not find an increase in the number of birth defects with exposure to acyclovir when compared to those expected in the general population. However, due to the small size of the registry and lack of long-term data, the manufacturer recommends using during pregnancy with caution and only when clearly needed. Acyclovir may be appropriate for the treatment of genital herpes in pregnant women (CDC, 2010).

Lactation Enters breast milk/use with caution (AAP rates "compatible"; AAP 2001 update pending)

Breast-Feeding Considerations Acyclovir is excreted in breast milk. The manufacturer recommends that caution be exercised when administering acyclovir to nursing women. Limited data suggest exposure to the nursing infant of ~0.3 mg/kg/day following oral administration of acyclovir to the mother. Nursing mothers with herpetic lesions near or on the breast should avoid breast-feeding (Gartner, 2005).

Dosage Forms

Capsule, oral: 200 mg
Zovirax®: 200 mg

Injection, powder for reconstitution: 500 mg, 1000 mg

Injection, solution [preservative free]: 50 mg/mL (10 mL, 20 mL)

Suspension, oral: 200 mg/5 mL (473 mL)
Zovirax®: 200 mg/5 mL (473 mL)

Tablet, oral: 400 mg, 800 mg
Zovirax®: 400 mg, 800 mg

Acyclovir (Topical) (ay SYE kloe veer)

Related Information

Systemic Viral Diseases *on page 1537*
Viral Infections *on page 1575*

Related Sample Prescriptions

Herpes Simplex (Primary) *on page 1616*
Herpes Simplex (Recurrent) *on page 1616*

Brand Names: U.S. Zovirax®

Brand Names: Canada Zovirax®

Generic Availability (U.S.) Yes: Excludes cream

Pharmacologic Category Antiviral Agent, Topical

Dental Use Treatment of initial and prophylaxis of recurrent mucosal and cutaneous herpes simplex (HSV-1 and HSV-2) infections in immunocompromised patients

Use Treatment of herpes labialis (cold sores), mucocutaneous HSV in immunocompromised patients

Local Anesthetic/Vasoconstrictor Precautions No information available to require special precautions

Effects on Dental Treatment Key adverse event(s) related to dental treatment: Topical (Zovirax® cream): Dry/cracked lips and dry/flaky skin were reported in fewer than 1 in 100 patients in clinical studies.

Effects on Bleeding No information available to require special precautions

Adverse Effects

>10%: Dermatologic: Mild pain, burning, or stinging (ointment 30%)

1% to 10%: Dermatologic: Pruritus (ointment 4%), itching

Dental Usual Dosage

Herpes labialis (cold sores): Children ≥12 years and Adults: Topical: Cream: Apply 5 times/day for 4 days
Mucocutaneous HSV: Adults: Nonlife-threatening, immunocompromised: Topical: Ointment: 1/2" ribbon of ointment for a 4" square surface area every 3 hours (6 times/day) for 7 days

Dosage Topical:
Genital HSV: Adults (immunocompromised): Ointment: Initial episode: 1/2" ribbon of ointment for a 4" square surface area every 3 hours (6 times/day) for 7 days
Herpes labialis (cold sores): Children ≥12 years and Adults: Cream: Apply 5 times/day for 4 days
Mucocutaneous HSV: Ointment: Adults (non-life-threatening, immunocompromised): 1/2" ribbon of ointment for a 4" square surface area every 3 hours (6 times/day) for 7 days

Mechanism of Action Acyclovir is converted to acyclovir monophosphate by virus-specific thymidine kinase then further converted to acyclovir triphosphate by other cellular enzymes. Acyclovir triphosphate inhibits DNA synthesis and viral replication by competing with deoxyguanosine triphosphate for viral DNA polymerase and being incorporated into viral DNA.

Contraindications Hypersensitivity to acyclovir, valacyclovir, or any component of the formulation

Warnings/Precautions

Genital herpes: Physical contact should be avoided when lesions are present; transmission may also occur in the absence of symptoms. Treatment should begin with the first signs or symptoms.

Herpes labialis: For external use only to the lips and face; do not apply to eye or inside the mouth or nose. Treatment should begin with the first signs or symptoms.

Drug Interactions

Metabolism/Transport Effects None known.

Avoid Concomitant Use There are no known interactions where it is recommended to avoid concomitant use.

Increased Effect/Toxicity There are no known significant interactions involving an increase in effect.

Decreased Effect There are no known significant interactions involving a decrease in effect.

Pregnancy Risk Factor B

Pregnancy Considerations Teratogenic effects were not observed in animal studies. When administered orally, acyclovir crosses the placenta. Refer to the Acyclovir (Systemic) monograph for details. The amount of acyclovir available systemically following topical application of the cream or ointment is significantly less in comparison to oral doses.

Breast-Feeding Considerations When administered orally, acyclovir enters breast milk. Refer to the Acyclovir (Systemic) monograph for details. The amount of acyclovir available systemically following topical application of the cream or ointment is significantly less in comparison to oral doses. Nursing mothers with herpetic lesions near or on the breast should avoid breast-feeding.

Dosage Forms
Cream, topical:
Zovirax®: 5% (2 g, 5 g)
Ointment, topical: 5% (15 g)
Zovirax®: 5% (15 g, 30 g)

Acyclovir and Hydrocortisone
(ay SYE kloe veer & hye droe KOR ti sone)

Related Information
Acyclovir (Topical) on page 47
Hydrocortisone (Topical) on page 699

Brand Names: U.S. Xerese™

Generic Availability (U.S.) No

Pharmacologic Category Antiviral Agent, Topical; Corticosteroid, Topical

Use Treatment of recurrent herpes labialis (cold sores)

Local Anesthetic/Vasoconstrictor Precautions No information available to require special precautions

Effects on Dental Treatment No significant effects or complications reported

Effects on Bleeding No information available to require special precautions

Adverse Effects <1%: Dermatologic: Burning, contact dermatitis, dryness, erythema, flaking, pigmentation changes, sensitization, signs/symptoms of inflammation, tingling

Dosage Topical: Herpes labialis (cold sores): Children ≥12 years and Adults: Apply 5 times/day for 5 days

Mechanism of Action See individual agents.

Contraindications There are no contraindications listed within the manufacturer's labeling.

Warnings/Precautions Treatment should begin with the first signs or symptoms. For external use only to the lips and around the mouth; do not apply to eye, inside the mouth or nose, or on the genitals. Contact healthcare provider if cold sore fails to heal in 2 weeks. Use with caution in immunocompromised patients. Use has been associated with local sensitization (irritation).

Drug Interactions

Metabolism/Transport Effects Refer to individual components.

Avoid Concomitant Use
Avoid concomitant use of Acyclovir and Hydrocortisone with any of the following: Aldesleukin

Increased Effect/Toxicity
Acyclovir and Hydrocortisone may increase the levels/ effects of: Deferasirox

The levels/effects of Acyclovir and Hydrocortisone may be increased by: Telaprevir

Decreased Effect
Acyclovir and Hydrocortisone may decrease the levels/ effects of: Aldesleukin; Corticorelin; Hyaluronidase; Telaprevir

Pregnancy Risk Factor B

Pregnancy Considerations Animal reproduction studies and studies in pregnant women have not been conducted with Xerese™. Systemic exposure of acyclovir and hydrocortisone after topical administration is minimal. See individual agents.

Lactation Excretion in breast milk unknown/use caution

Breast-Feeding Considerations Systemic exposure of acyclovir and hydrocortisone after topical administration is minimal. See individual agents.

Dosage Forms
Cream, topical:
Xerese®: Acyclovir 5% and hydrocortisone 1% (5 g)

Adalimumab (a da LIM yoo mab)

Related Information
Rheumatoid Arthritis, Osteoarthritis, and Osteoporosis on page 1526

Brand Names: U.S. Humira®; Humira® Pen

Brand Names: Canada Humira®

Pharmacologic Category Antirheumatic, Disease Modifying; Gastrointestinal Agent, Miscellaneous; Monoclonal Antibody; Tumor Necrosis Factor (TNF) Blocking Agent

Use
Treatment of active rheumatoid arthritis (moderate-to-severe) and active psoriatic arthritis; may be used alone or in combination with other nonbiologic disease-modifying antirheumatic drugs (DMARDs)
Treatment of ankylosing spondylitis
Treatment of moderately- to severely-active Crohn's disease in patients with inadequate response to conventional treatment, or patients who have lost response to or are intolerant of infliximab
Treatment of moderately- to severely-active ulcerative colitis in patients unresponsive to immunosuppressants (**Note:** Efficacy in patients that are intolerant or no longer responsive to other TNF blockers has not been established.)
Treatment of moderate-to-severe plaque psoriasis
Treatment of moderately- to severely-active juvenile idiopathic arthritis

Local Anesthetic/Vasoconstrictor Precautions No information available to require special precautions

Effects on Dental Treatment No significant effects or complications reported

Effects on Bleeding Rare reports of pancytopenia (including aplastic anemia), as well as medically significant thrombocytopenia, have been reported with tumor necrosis factor-alpha therapy; in patients undergoing active treatment, a medical consult is recommended

Adverse Effects
>10%:
Central nervous system: Headache (12%)
Dermatologic: Rash (6% to 12%)
Local: Injection site reaction (12% to 20%; includes erythema, itching, hemorrhage, pain, swelling)
Neuromuscular & skeletal: CPK increased (15%)

Respiratory: Upper respiratory tract infection (17%), sinusitis (11%)

Miscellaneous: Serious infection (adults 1.4-6.7 events/100 person years, children 2 events/100 person years [Burmester, 2012]), antibodies to adalimumab (3% to 26%; significance unknown), positive ANA (12%)

5% to 10%:

Cardiovascular: Hypertension (5%)

Endocrine & metabolic: Hyperlipidemia (7%), hypercholesterolemia (6%)

Gastrointestinal: Nausea (9%), abdominal pain (7%)

Genitourinary: Urinary tract infection (8%)

Hepatic: Alkaline phosphatase increased (5%)

Local: Injection site reaction (8%; other than erythema, itching, hemorrhage, pain, swelling)

Neuromuscular & skeletal: Back pain (6%)

Renal: Hematuria (5%)

Miscellaneous: Accidental injury (10%), flu-like syndrome (7%), hypersensitivity reactions (children 6%; adults <1%)

1% to 5%:

Cardiovascular: Arrhythmia, atrial fibrillation, chest pain, CHF, coronary artery disorder, deep vein thrombosis, heart arrest, MI, palpitation, pericardial effusion, pericarditis, peripheral edema, syncope, tachycardia, vascular disorder

Central nervous system: Confusion, fever, hypertensive encephalopathy, multiple sclerosis, subdural hematoma

Dermatologic: Alopecia, cellulitis, erysipelas

Endocrine & metabolic: Dehydration, menstrual disorder, parathyroid disorder

Gastrointestinal: Diverticulitis, esophagitis, gastroenteritis, gastrointestinal hemorrhage, vomiting

Genitourinary: Cystitis, pelvic pain

Hematologic: Agranulocytosis, granulocytopenia, leukopenia, pancytopenia, paraproteinemia, polycythemia

Hepatic: Cholecystitis, cholelithiasis, hepatic necrosis

Neuromuscular & skeletal: Arthralgia, arthritis, bone fracture, bone necrosis, joint disorder, muscle cramps, myasthenia, pain in extremity, paresthesia, pyogenic arthritis, synovitis, tendon disorder, tremor

Ocular: Cataract

Renal: Kidney calculus, pyelonephritis

Respiratory: Asthma, bronchospasm, dyspnea, lung function decreased, pleural effusion, pneumonia

Miscellaneous: Adenoma, allergic reactions (1%), carcinoma (including breast, gastrointestinal, skin, urogenital), healing abnormality, herpes zoster, ketosis, lupus erythematosus syndrome, lymphoma, melanoma, postsurgical infection, sepsis, tuberculosis (reactivation of latent infection; miliary, lymphatic, peritoneal and pulmonary)

General Dosage Range SubQ:

Children ≥4 years: 15 kg to <30 kg: 20 mg every other week; ≥30 kg: 40 mg every other week

Adults: Initial: 40-160 mg; Maintenance: 40 mg every other week (maximum: 40 mg every week)

Mechanism of Action Adalimumab is a recombinant monoclonal antibody that binds to human tumor necrosis factor alpha (TNF-alpha), thereby interfering with binding to TNFα receptor sites and subsequent cytokine-driven inflammatory processes. Elevated TNF levels in the synovial fluid are involved in the pathologic pain and joint destruction in immune-mediated arthritis. Adalimumab decreases signs and symptoms of psoriatic arthritis, rheumatoid arthritis, and ankylosing spondylitis. It inhibits progression of structural damage of rheumatoid and psoriatic arthritis. Reduces signs and symptoms and maintains clinical remission in Crohn's disease and ulcerative colitis; reduces epidermal thickness and inflammatory cell infiltration in plaque psoriasis.

Pharmacodynamics/Kinetics

Half-life Elimination Terminal: ~2 weeks (range: 10-20 days)

Time to Peak Serum: SubQ: 131 ± 56 hours

Pregnancy Risk Factor B

Pregnancy Considerations Teratogenic effects were not observed in animal studies, however, there are no adequate and well-controlled studies in pregnant women. Use during pregnancy only if clearly needed. A pregnancy registry has been established to monitor outcomes of women exposed to adalimumab during pregnancy (877-311-8972).

Adapalene (a DAP a leen)

Brand Names: U.S. Differin®

Brand Names: Canada Differin®; Differin® XP

Pharmacologic Category Acne Products; Topical Skin Product, Acne

Use Treatment of acne vulgaris

Local Anesthetic/Vasoconstrictor Precautions No information available to require special precautions

Effects on Dental Treatment No significant effects or complications reported

Effects on Bleeding No information available to require special precautions

Adverse Effects

>10%: Dermatologic: Dryness (≤45%), scaling (≤44%), erythema (≤38%), burning/stinging (≤29%)

1% to 10%: Dermatologic: Skin discomfort (1% to 6%), desquamation (2%), pruritus (≤2%), skin irritation (1% to 2%), sunburn (1% to 2%)

General Dosage Range Topical: *Children >12 years and Adults:* Apply once daily at bedtime

Mechanism of Action Retinoid-like compound which is a modulator of cellular differentiation, keratinization, and inflammatory processes, all of which represent important features in the pathology of acne vulgaris

Pharmacodynamics/Kinetics

Onset of Action 8-12 weeks

Pregnancy Risk Factor C

Pregnancy Considerations Adverse effects were observed in animal reproduction studies. Retinoids may cause harm when administered during pregnancy. A case report described maternal use of adapalene 1 month prior to pregnancy and through 13 weeks gestation; cerebral and ocular malformations were reported in the exposed fetus which resulted in termination of pregnancy (Autret, 1997). In clinical trials, women of childbearing potential were required to have a negative pregnancy test prior to therapy.

Adapalene and Benzoyl Peroxide
(a DAP a leen & BEN zoe il peer OKS ide)

Related Information

Adapalene *on page 49*

Benzoyl Peroxide *on page 180*

Brand Names: U.S. Epiduo®

Brand Names: Canada Tactuo™

Pharmacologic Category Acne Products; Topical Skin Product; Topical Skin Product, Acne

Use Topical treatment of acne vulgaris

◀ Local Anesthetic/Vasoconstrictor Precautions No information available to require special precautions

Effects on Dental Treatment No significant effects or complications reported

Effects on Bleeding No information available to require special precautions

Adverse Effects 1% to 10%: Dermatologic: Dry skin (<1% to 10%), scaling (<1% to 9%), erythema (1% to 8%), burning (1% to 7%), stinging (1% to 7%), contact dermatitis (3%), skin irritation (1%)

General Dosage Range Topical: *Children ≥9 years, Adolescents, and Adults:* Apply once daily

Mechanism of Action

Benzoyl peroxide releases free-radical oxygen which oxidizes bacterial proteins in the sebaceous follicles decreasing the number of anaerobic bacteria and decreasing irritating-type free fatty acids.

Adapalene is a retinoid-like compound which is a modulator of cellular differentiation, keratinization, and inflammatory processes, all of which represent important features in the pathology of acne vulgaris.

Pregnancy Risk Factor C

Pregnancy Considerations There are no well-controlled studies in pregnant women. Use only if benefit outweighs the potential risk to fetus.

Adefovir (a DEF o veer)

Related Information

HIV Infection and AIDS *on page 1520*

Systemic Viral Diseases *on page 1537*

Brand Names: U.S. Hepsera®

Brand Names: Canada Hepsera™

Pharmacologic Category Antiretroviral Agent, Reverse Transcriptase Inhibitor (Nucleotide)

Use Treatment of chronic hepatitis B with evidence of active viral replication (based on persistent elevation of ALT/AST or histologic evidence), including patients with lamivudine-resistant hepatitis B

Local Anesthetic/Vasoconstrictor Precautions No information available to require special precautions

Effects on Dental Treatment No significant effects or complications reported

Effects on Bleeding No information available to require special precautions

Adverse Effects

>10%:

Central nervous system: Headache (24% to 25%)

Gastrointestinal: Abdominal pain (15%), diarrhea (up to 13%)

Hepatic: Hepatitis exacerbation (up to 25% within 12 weeks of adefovir discontinuation)

Neuromuscular & skeletal: Weakness (up to 25%)

Renal: Hematuria (grade ≥3: 11%)

1% to 10%:

Dermatologic: Rash, pruritus

Endocrine & metabolic: Hypophosphatemia (<2 mg/dL: 1% and 3% in pre-/post-liver transplant patients, respectively)

Gastrointestinal: Flatulence (up to 8%), dyspepsia (5% to 9%), nausea, vomiting

Neuromuscular & skeletal: Back pain (up to 10%)

Renal: Serum creatinine increased (≥0.5 mg/dL: 2% to 3% in compensated liver disease; incidence may be higher in patients with decompensated cirrhosis or in liver transplant recipients), renal failure

Note: In liver transplant patients with baseline renal dysfunction, frequency of increased serum creatinine has been observed to be as high as 32% to 51% at 48 and 96 weeks post-transplantation, respectively; considering the concomitant use of other potentially nephrotoxic medications, baseline renal insufficiency, and predisposing comorbidities, the role of adefovir in these changes could not be established.

Respiratory: Cough (6% to 8%), rhinitis (up to 5%)

General Dosage Range Dosage adjustment recommended in patients with renal impairment

Oral: *Children ≥12 years and Adults:* 10 mg once daily

Mechanism of Action Acyclic nucleotide reverse transcriptase inhibitor (adenosine analog) which interferes with HBV viral RNA-dependent DNA polymerase resulting in inhibition of viral replication.

Pharmacodynamics/Kinetics

Half-life Elimination 7.5 hours; prolonged in renal impairment

Time to Peak 1.75 hours

Pregnancy Risk Factor C

Pregnancy Considerations Teratogenic effects were not observed in animal studies. There are no adequate and well-controlled studies in pregnant women. Use in pregnancy only when clearly needed. Pregnant women exposed to adefovir should be registered with the pregnancy registry (800-258-4263).

Adenosine (a DEN oh seen)

Brand Names: U.S. Adenocard® IV; Adenoscan®

Brand Names: Canada Adenocard®; Adenosine Injection, USP; PMS-Adenosine

Pharmacologic Category Antiarrhythmic Agent, Miscellaneous; Diagnostic Agent

Use

Adenocard®: Treatment of paroxysmal supraventricular tachycardia (PSVT) including that associated with accessory bypass tracts (Wolff-Parkinson-White syndrome); when clinically advisable, appropriate vagal maneuvers should be attempted prior to adenosine administration; **not effective for conversion of atrial fibrillation, atrial flutter, or ventricular tachycardia**

Adenoscan®: Pharmacologic stress agent used in myocardial perfusion thallium-201 scintigraphy

Unlabeled Use

ACLS/PALS Guidelines (2010): Stable, narrow-complex regular tachycardias; unstable narrow-complex regular tachycardias while preparations are made for synchronized direct-current cardioversion; stable regular monomorphic, wide-complex tachycardia as a therapeutic (if SVT) and diagnostic maneuver

Adenoscan®: Acute vasodilator testing in pulmonary artery hypertension

Local Anesthetic/Vasoconstrictor Precautions No information available to require special precautions

Effects on Dental Treatment No significant effects or complications reported

Effects on Bleeding No information available to require special precautions

Adverse Effects Note: Frequency varies based on use; higher frequency of infusion-related effects, such as flushing and lightheadedness, were reported with continuous infusion (Adenoscan®).

>10%:

Cardiovascular: Transient new arrhythmia (eg, atrial premature contractions, atrial fibrillation, PVCs) after cardioversion (55%), facial flushing (18% to 44%)

Central nervous system: Headache (2% to 18%), dizziness/lightheadedness (2% to 12%)

Gastrointestinal: GI discomfort (13%)

Neuromuscular & skeletal: Discomfort of neck, throat, jaw (<1% to 15%)

Respiratory: Chest pressure/discomfort (7% to 40%), dyspnea (12% to 28%)

1% to 10%:

Cardiovascular: AV block (infusion 6%; third-degree <1%), ST segment depression (3%), hypotension (<1% to 2%), chest pain, palpitation

Central nervous system: Nervousness (2%), apprehension

Gastrointestinal: Nausea (3%)

Neuromuscular & skeletal: Upper extremity discomfort (≤4%), numbness (≤2%), paresthesia (≤2%)

Respiratory: Hyperventilation

Miscellaneous: Diaphoresis

General Dosage Range I.V.:

Children <50 kg: Initial: 0.05-0.1 mg/kg/dose (maximum initial dose: 6 mg); repeat: 0.05-0.3 mg/kg/dose (maximum: 0.3 mg/kg/dose or 12 mg/dose)

Children ≥50 kg and Adults: Initial: 6 mg; if not effective, 12 mg may be given; may repeat 12 mg if needed (maximum: 12 mg/dose)

Mechanism of Action

Antiarrhythmic actions: Slows conduction time through the AV node, interrupting the re-entry pathways through the AV node, restoring normal sinus rhythm

Myocardial perfusion scintigraphy: Adenosine also causes coronary vasodilation and increases blood flow in normal coronary arteries with little to no increase in stenotic coronary arteries; thallium-201 uptake into the stenotic coronary arteries will be less than that of normal coronary arteries revealing areas of insufficient blood flow.

Pharmacodynamics/Kinetics

Onset of Action Rapid

Duration of Action Very brief

Half-life Elimination <10 seconds

Pregnancy Risk Factor C

Pregnancy Considerations Animal reproduction studies have not been conducted. Adenosine is an endogenous substance and adverse fetal effects would not be anticipated. Case reports of administration during pregnancy have indicated no adverse effects on fetus or newborn attributable to adenosine. ACLS guidelines suggest use is safe and effective in pregnancy.

Adenovirus (Types 4, 7) Vaccine
(ad e noh VYE rus typs for SEV en vak SEEN)

Pharmacologic Category Vaccine, Live (Viral)

Use Prevention of acute febrile respiratory disease caused by adenovirus types 4 and 7 (approved for use in military populations)

Local Anesthetic/Vasoconstrictor Precautions No information available to require special precautions

Effects on Dental Treatment No significant effects or complications reported

Effects on Bleeding No information available to require special precautions

Adverse Effects All serious adverse reactions must be reported to the U.S. Department of Health and Human Services (DHHS) Vaccine Adverse Event Reporting System (VAERS) at 1-800-822-7967 or online at https://vaers.hhs.gov/esub/index.

>10%:

Central nervous system: Headache (7% to 30%)

Gastrointestinal: Nausea (5% to 14%)

Respiratory: Nasal congestion (8% to 15%), pharyngolaryngeal pain (12% to 13%), cough (10% to 12%)

1% to 10%:

Central nervous system: Fever (≤1%)

Gastrointestinal: Diarrhea (3% to 10%)

Neuromuscular & skeletal: Limb pain (4%)

Respiratory: Rhinorrhea (4%)

General Dosage Range Oral: *Adolescents ≥17 years and Adults ≤50 years:* One tablet each of type 4 and type 7 as a single vaccine dose

Mechanism of Action Nonattenuated preparation of live adenovirus types 4 and 7 designed to release the live viruses in the intestine and replicate (in the intestinal tract) to induce immunity in individuals without (or with low) existing neutralizing antibodies to adenovirus types 4 and 7.

Pharmacodynamics/Kinetics

Onset of Action Viral shedding in the stool begins at 7 days; seroconversion occurs ~26 days following vaccination

Duration of Action Viral shedding no longer detected at 28 days

Pregnancy Considerations Use in pregnancy is contraindicated. Naturally-occurring adenovirus infections are associated with fetal harm. Information following inadvertent use during pregnancy is limited. Women of childbearing potential should avoid becoming pregnant for 6 weeks following vaccination. Healthcare providers are encouraged to enroll women exposed to adenovirus vaccine during pregnancy (or pregnancies occurring within 6 weeks of vaccination) in the Adenovirus Pregnancy Registry at 1-866-790-4549. Pregnant women should use caution if in close contact with vaccinated individuals for 28 days following vaccine administration.

Prescribing and Access Restrictions Product is approved for use in military populations

Ado-Trastuzumab Emtansine
(a do tras TU zoo mab em TAN seen)

Brand Names: U.S. Kadcyla™

Pharmacologic Category Antineoplastic Agent, Anti-HER2; Antineoplastic Agent, Antimicrotubular; Antineoplastic Agent, Monoclonal Antibody

Use Treatment of HER2-positive, metastatic breast cancer in patients who previously received trastuzumab and a taxane, separately or in combination, and have either received prior therapy for metastatic disease or developed disease recurrence during or within 6 months of completing adjuvant therapy.

Local Anesthetic/Vasoconstrictor Precautions No information available to require special precautions

Effects on Dental Treatment Key adverse event(s) related to dental treatment: Abnormal taste, oral discomfort, xerostomia and changes in salivation (normal salivary flow resumes upon discontinuation)

Effects on Bleeding Chemotherapy may result in significant myelosuppression, thrombocytopenia (31%; grades 3/4: 15%; Asians grades 3/4: 45%), anemia (14%; grades 3/4: 4%), neutropenia (7%; grades 3/4: 2%). In patients who are under active treatment with these agents, medical consult is suggested.

Adverse Effects

>10%:

Central nervous system: Fatigue (36%), headache (28%), fever (19%), insomnia (12%)

Dermatologic: Skin rash (12%)

Gastrointestinal: Nausea (40%), constipation (27%), diarrhea (24%), abdominal pain (19%), vomiting (19%), xerostomia (17%), stomatitis (14%)

Hematologic: Thrombocytopenia (31%; grades 3/4: 15%; Asians grades 3/4: 45%), anemia (14%; grades 3/4: 4%)

Hepatic: Increased serum aspartate aminotransferase (98%; grades 3/4: <8%), increased serum alanine aminotransferase (82%; grades 3/4: <6%), increased serum transaminases (29%), increased serum bilirubin (17%)

Neuromuscular & skeletal: Musculoskeletal pain (36%), peripheral neuropathy (21%; grades 3/4: 2%), arthralgia (19%), weakness (18%), myalgia (14%)

Respiratory: Epistaxis (23%), cough (18%), dyspnea (12%)

1% to 10%:

Cardiovascular: Peripheral edema (7%), hypertension (5%; grades 3/4: 1%), left ventricular systolic dysfunction (2%)

Central nervous system: Dizziness (10%), chills (8%)

Dermatologic: Pruritus (6%)

Endocrine & metabolic: Hypokalemia (10%; grades 3/4: 3%)

Gastrointestinal: Dyspepsia (9%), dysgeusia (8%)

Genitourinary: Urinary tract infection (9%)

Hematologic: Neutropenia (7%; grades 3/4: 2%)

Hepatic: Increased serum alkaline phosphatase (5%)

Local: Infusion related reaction (1%)

Ocular: Blurred vision (5%), conjunctivitis (4%), dry eye syndrome (4%), lacrimation (3%)

Respiratory: Pneumonitis (≤1%)

Miscellaneous: Antibody development (5%), hypersensitivity (2%)

General Dosage Range Dosage reduction recommended in patients who develop toxicities.

I.V.: *Adults:* 3.6 mg/kg every 3 weeks; maximum dose: 3.6 mg/kg

Mechanism of Action Ado-trastuzumab emtansine is a HER2-antibody drug conjugate which incorporates the HER2 targeted actions of trastuzumab with the microtubule inhibitor DM1 (a maytansine derivative). The conjugate, which is linked via a stable thioether linker, allows for selective delivery into HER2 overexpressing cells, resulting in cell cycle arrest and apoptosis.

Pharmacodynamics/Kinetics

Half-life Elimination ~4 days

Time to Peak Near the end of the infusion

Pregnancy Risk Factor D

Pregnancy Considerations Animal reproduction studies have not been conducted. **[U.S. Boxed Warning]: Exposure to ado-trastuzumab emtansine may cause embryo-fetal death. Effective contraception must be used in women of reproductive potential.** Oligohydramnios, pulmonary hypoplasia, skeletal malformations and neonatal death were observed following trastuzumab exposure during pregnancy (trastuzumab is the antibody component of ado-trastuzumab emtansine). The DM1 component of the ado-trastuzumab emtansine formulation is toxic to rapidly dividing cells and is also expected to cause fetal harm. Pregnancy status should be verified prior to therapy. Effective contraception is recommended during therapy and for 6 months after treatment for women of childbearing potential.

If ado-trastuzumab emtansine exposure occurs during pregnancy, healthcare providers should report the exposure to the Genentech Adverse Event Line (888-835-2555). Women exposed to ado-trastuzumab emtansine during pregnancy are encouraged to enroll in MotHER Pregnancy Registry (1-800-690-6720).

Aflibercept (Ophthalmic) (a FLIB er sept)

Brand Names: U.S. Eylea™

Pharmacologic Category Ophthalmic Agent; Vascular Endothelial Growth Factor (VEGF) Inhibitor

Use Treatment of neovascular (wet) age-related macular degeneration (AMD); treatment of macular edema following central retinal vein occlusion (CRVO)

Local Anesthetic/Vasoconstrictor Precautions No information available to require special precautions

Effects on Dental Treatment No significant effects or complications reported

Effects on Bleeding No information available to require special precautions

Adverse Effects

>10%: Ocular: Conjunctival hemorrhage (12% to 25%), eye pain (9% to 13%)

1% to 10%:

Local: Injection site pain (3%), injection site hemorrhage (1%)

Ocular: Intraocular pressure increased (5% to 8%), cataract (7%), vitreous detachment (6%), vitreous floaters (5% to 6%), conjunctival hyperemia (4% to 5%), corneal erosion (4% to 5%), foreign body sensation (3%), lacrimation increased (3%), retinal pigment epithelium detachment (3%), blurred vision (1% to 2%), retinal pigment epithelium tear (2%), eyelid edema (1%), corneal edema (1%)

Miscellaneous: Aflibercept antibodies (1% to 3%)

General Dosage Range Intravitreal: *Adults:* 2 mg (0.05 mL) every 4-8 weeks

Mechanism of Action Aflibercept is a recombinant fusion protein that acts as a decoy receptor for vascular endothelial growth factor-A (VEGF-A) and placental growth factor (PIGF). Decoy receptor binding prevents VEGF-A and PIGF from binding and activating endothelial cell receptors, thereby suppressing neovascularization and slowing vision loss.

Pharmacodynamics/Kinetics

Half-life Elimination Plasma: 5-6 days

Pregnancy Risk Factor C

Pregnancy Considerations Adverse events were observed in animal reproduction studies.

Agalsidase Alfa (aye GAL si days AL fa)

Brand Names: Canada Replagal®

Pharmacologic Category Enzyme

Use Replacement therapy for Fabry disease

Local Anesthetic/Vasoconstrictor Precautions No information available to require special precautions

Effects on Dental Treatment No significant effects or complications reported

Effects on Bleeding No information available to require special precautions

Adverse Effects Note: The most common and serious adverse reactions are infusion reactions (symptoms may include chills, dyspnea, facial flushing, fever, hypertension, nausea, rigors, tachycardia, urticaria, and vomiting).

>10%:
Cardiovascular: Flushing (24%)
Central nervous system: Fever (20%), headache (11%)
Neuromuscular & skeletal: Rigors (20%)
Miscellaneous: IgG antibody formation (55%), infusion-related reactions (13%)
1% to 10%:
Cardiovascular: Chest tightness (7%), hypertension (4%), tachycardia (4%), chest pain (2%), edema (2%), peripheral coldness (2%), peripheral edema (2%)
Central nervous system: Dizziness (9%), fatigue (9%), fatigue aggravated (7%), pain/discomfort (7%), hypersomnia (2%), hypoesthesia (2%), panic attack (2%), somnolence (2%), vertigo (2%)
Dermatologic: Acne (9%), erythema (7%), mottled skin (4%), pruritus (4%), dry skin (2%), eczema (2%), rash (2%)
Gastrointestinal: Nausea (9%), dysgeusia (6%), diarrhea (4%), vomiting (4%), abdominal pain (2%), dyspepsia (2%), gastrointestinal upset (2%), stomach cramps (2%), stomach discomfort (2%)
Neuromuscular & skeletal: Myalgia (6%), neuropathic pain (6%), tremor (4%), musculoskeletal discomfort (2%), back pain (2%), limb pain (2%), paraesthesia (2%), weakness (2%)
Ocular: Lacrimation increased (2%), periorbital edema (2%)
Respiratory: Hoarseness (6%), throat tightness (6%), cough (4%), dyspnea (4%), nasopharyngitis (4%), pharyngitis (4%), nasal congestion (2%), snoring (2%), throat irritation (2%)
Miscellaneous: Feeling hot (4%), influenza-like syndrome (2%), parosmia (2%)
General Dosage Range I.V.: *Children and Adults:* 0.2 mg/kg every 2 weeks
Mechanism of Action Agalsidase alfa is a recombinant form of the enzyme alpha-galactosidase-A, which catalyzes the hydrolysis of globotriaosylceramide (Gb-3) and other glycosphingolipids. These compounds may accumulate (over many years) within the tissues of patients with Fabry disease, leading to renal and cardiovascular complications. Agalsidase has been noted to reduce cellular levels of Gb-3 within the liver, heart, kidney, blood vessels, and in plasma.
Pharmacodynamics/Kinetics
Half-life Elimination ~1.5-2 hours
Pregnancy Considerations Adverse events were not observed in animal studies. There are no adequate and well-controlled studies in pregnant women. The benefits versus risks should be considered carefully before initiating agalsidase alfa therapy in pregnant women.
Product Availability Not available in U.S.

Agalsidase Beta (aye GAL si days BAY ta)

Brand Names: U.S. Fabrazyme®
Brand Names: Canada Fabrazyme®
Pharmacologic Category Enzyme
Use Replacement therapy for Fabry disease
Local Anesthetic/Vasoconstrictor Precautions No information available to require special precautions
Effects on Dental Treatment No significant effects or complications reported
Effects on Bleeding No information available to require special precautions

Adverse Effects Note: The most common and serious adverse reactions are infusion reactions (symptoms may include fever, tachycardia, hyper-/hypotension, throat tightness, dyspnea, chills, abdominal pain, paresthesia, pruritus, urticaria, vomiting).
>10%:
Cardiovascular: Peripheral edema (21%)
Central nervous system: Chills (43%), fever (39%), headache (39%), fatigue (24%), dizziness (21%), pain (16%)
Local: Infusion site reactions (50% to 55%; severe: ≥5%), procedural pain (25%)
Neuromuscular & skeletal: Paresthesia (31%), pain in extremity (19%), back pain (16%)
Respiratory: Upper respiratory tract infection (44%), cough (33%), nasal congestion (19%), lower respiratory infection (18%)
Miscellaneous: IgG antibody formation (69% to 79%), feeling cold (11%)
1% to 10%:
Cardiovascular: Hypertension (14%), tachycardia (9%), bradycardia (≥5%), chest pain/discomfort (≥5%), facial edema (≥5%), flushing (≥5%), hypotension (≥5%), pallor (≥5%), ventricular wall thickening (5%)
Central nervous system: Hypoesthesia (9%), anxiety (6%), depression (6%)
Dermatologic: Rash (20%), pruritus (10%), excoriation (9%), urticaria (≥5%), bruising (4%)
Gastrointestinal: Toothache (6%), abdominal pain (≥5%), diarrhea (≥5%), nausea (≥5%), vomiting (≥5%), xerostomia (4%)
Local: Postprocedural complication (10%), thermal burn (4%)
Neuromuscular & skeletal: Myalgia (14%), burning sensation (6%), fall (6%), muscle spasms (5%)
Otic: Tinnitus (8%), hearing impairment (5%)
Renal: Creatinine increased (9%)
Respiratory: Sinusitis (9%), congestion (8%), dyspnea (8%), pharyngitis (6%), wheezing (6%), throat tightness (≥5%)
Miscellaneous: Viral infection (5%), fungal infection (5%)
Other reported severe reactions (frequency not established): Anaphylaxis, allergic reactions, arrhythmia, ataxia, cardiac arrest, cardiac output decreased, nephrotic syndrome, stroke, vertigo
General Dosage Range I.V.: *Children ≥8 years and Adults:* 1 mg/kg every 2 weeks
Mechanism of Action Agalsidase beta is a recombinant form of the enzyme alpha-galactosidase-A, which is required for the hydrolysis of GL-3 and other glycosphingolipids. The compounds may accumulate (over many years) within the tissues of patients with Fabry disease, leading to renal and cardiovascular complications. In clinical trials of limited duration, agalsidase been noted to reduce tissue inclusions of a key sphingolipid (GL-3). It is believed that long-term enzyme replacement may reduce clinical manifestations of renal failure, cardiomyopathy, and stroke. However, the relationship to a reduction in clinical manifestations has not been established.
Pharmacodynamics/Kinetics
Half-life Elimination Children: 86-151 minutes; Adults: 45-119 minutes
Pregnancy Risk Factor B

53

◄ **Pregnancy Considerations** Animal reproduction studies have not demonstrated adverse effects. There are no adequate and well-controlled studies in pregnant women. Women of childbearing potential are encouraged to enroll in Fabry registry (www.fabryregistry.com or 1-800-745-4447).

Albendazole (al BEN da zole)

Brand Names: U.S. Albenza®
Pharmacologic Category Anthelmintic
Use Treatment of parenchymal neurocysticercosis caused by *Taenia solium* and cystic hydatid disease of the liver, lung, and peritoneum caused by *Echinococcus granulosus*
Unlabeled Use Albendazole has activity against *Ascaris lumbricoides* (roundworm); *Ancylostoma caninum*; *Ancylostoma duodenale* and *Necator americanus* (hookworms); cutaneous larva migrans; *Enterobius vermicularis* (pinworm); *Giardia duodenalis* (giardiasis); *Gnathostoma spinigerum*; *Gongylonema* sp; *Mansonella perstans* (filariasis); *Oesophagostomum bifurcum*; *Opisthorchis sinensis* (liver fluke); *Trichinella spiralis* (Trichinellosis); visceral larva migrans (toxocariasis); activity has also been shown against the liver fluke *Clonorchis sinensis*, *Giardia lamblia*, *Cysticercus cellulosae*, and *Echinococcus multilocularis*. Albendazole has also been used for the treatment of intestinal microsporidiosis (*Encephalitozoon intestinalis*), disseminated microsporidiosis (*E. hellem, E. cuniculi, E. intestinalis*, *Pleistophora* sp, *Trachipleistophora* sp, *Brachiola vesicularum*), and ocular microsporidiosis (*E. hellem, E. cuniculi, Vittaforma corneae*).
Local Anesthetic/Vasoconstrictor Precautions No information available to require special precautions
Effects on Dental Treatment No significant effects or complications reported
Effects on Bleeding No information available to require special precautions
Adverse Effects
>10%:
  Central nervous system: Headache (11% neurocysticercosis; 1% hydatid)
  Hepatic: LFTs increased (16% hydatid; <1% neurocysticercosis)
1% to 10%:
  Central nervous system: Intracranial pressure increased (≤2%), dizziness (≤1%), fever (≤1%), vertigo (≤1%), meningeal signs (1%)
  Dermatologic: Alopecia (<1% to 2%)
  Gastrointestinal: Abdominal pain (≤6%), nausea/vomiting (4% to 6%)
General Dosage Range Oral:
Children and Adults <60 kg: 15 mg/kg/day in 2 divided doses (maximum: 800 mg/day)
Children and Adults ≥60 kg: 800 mg/day in 2 divided doses (maximum: 800 mg/day)
Mechanism of Action Active metabolite, albendazole sulfoxide, causes selective degeneration of cytoplasmic microtubules in intestinal and tegmental cells of intestinal helminths and larvae; glycogen is depleted, glucose uptake and cholinesterase secretion are impaired, and desecratory substances accumulate intracellulary. ATP production decreases causing energy depletion, immobilization, and worm death.
Pharmacodynamics/Kinetics
Half-life Elimination 8-12 hours
Time to Peak Serum: 2-5 hours
Pregnancy Risk Factor C

Pregnancy Considerations Albendazole has been shown to be teratogenic in laboratory animals and should not be used during pregnancy, if at all possible. Women should be advised to avoid pregnancy for at least 1 month following therapy. Discontinue if pregnancy occurs during treatment.

Albuterol (al BYOO ter ole)

Related Information
Respiratory Diseases *on page 1514*
Brand Names: U.S. AccuNeb®; ProAir® HFA; Proventil® HFA; Ventolin® HFA; VoSpire ER®
Brand Names: Canada Airomir™; Apo-Salvent®; Apo-Salvent® AEM; Apo-Salvent® CFC Free; Apo-Salvent® Sterules; Dom-Salbutamol; Mylan-Salbutamol Respirator Solution; Mylan-Salbutamol Sterinebs P.F.; Novo-Salbutamol HFA; Nu-Salbutamol; PHL-Salbutamol; PMS-Salbutamol; ratio-Ipra-Sal; ratio-Salbutamol; Sandoz-Salbutamol; Teva-Salbutamol; Teva-Salbutamol Sterinebs P.F.; Ventolin®; Ventolin® Diskus; Ventolin® HFA; Ventolin® I.V. Infusion; Ventolin® Nebules P.F.
Generic Availability (U.S.) Yes: Excludes aerosol
Pharmacologic Category Beta$_2$ Agonist
Use Treatment or prevention of bronchospasm in patients with reversible obstructive airway disease; prevention of exercise-induced bronchospasm
Local Anesthetic/Vasoconstrictor Precautions No information available to require special precautions
Effects on Dental Treatment Key adverse event(s) related to dental treatment: Xerostomia (normal salivary flow resumes upon discontinuation)
Effects on Bleeding No information available to require special precautions
Adverse Effects Incidence of adverse effects is dependent upon age of patient, dose, and route of administration.

Cardiovascular: Angina, atrial fibrillation, arrhythmias, chest discomfort, chest pain, extrasystoles, flushing, hyper-/hypotension, palpitation, supraventricular tachycardia, tachycardia
Central nervous system: CNS stimulation, dizziness, drowsiness, headache, insomnia, irritability, lightheadedness, migraine, nervousness, nightmares, restlessness, seizure
Dermatologic: Angioedema, rash, urticaria
Endocrine & metabolic: Hyperglycemia, hypokalemia, lactic acidosis
Gastrointestinal: Diarrhea, dry mouth, dyspepsia, gastroenteritis, nausea, unusual taste, vomiting
Genitourinary: Micturition difficulty
Local: Injection: Pain, stinging
Neuromuscular & skeletal: Muscle cramps, musculoskeletal pain, tremor, weakness
Otic: Otitis media, vertigo
Respiratory: Asthma exacerbation, bronchospasm, cough, epistaxis, laryngitis, oropharyngeal drying/irritation, oropharyngeal edema, pharyngitis, rhinitis, upper respiratory inflammation, viral respiratory infection
Miscellaneous: Allergic reaction, anaphylaxis, diaphoresis, lymphadenopathy

Dosage

Oral:

Children: Bronchospasm:

2-6 years: 0.1-0.2 mg/kg/dose 3 times/day; maximum dose not to exceed 12 mg/day (divided doses)

6-12 years: 2 mg/dose 3-4 times/day; maximum dose not to exceed 24 mg/day (divided doses)

Extended release: 4 mg every 12 hours; maximum dose not to exceed 24 mg/day (divided doses)

Children >12 years and Adults: Bronchospasm (treatment): 2-4 mg/dose 3-4 times/day; maximum dose not to exceed 32 mg/day (divided doses)

Extended release: 8 mg every 12 hours; maximum dose not to exceed 32 mg/day (divided doses). A 4 mg dose every 12 hours may be sufficient in some patients, such as adults of low body weight.

Elderly: Bronchospasm (treatment): 2 mg 3-4 times/day; maximum: 8 mg 4 times/day

Metered-dose inhaler (90 mcg/puff):

Children ≤4 years *(NIH Guidelines, 2007)*:

Quick relief: 2 puffs every 4-6 hours as needed

Exacerbation of asthma (acute, severe): 4-8 puffs every 20 minutes for 3 doses, then every 1-4 hours as needed

Exercise-induced bronchospasm (prevention): 1-2 puffs 5 minutes prior to exercise

Children 5-11 years *(NIH Guidelines, 2007)*:

Bronchospasm, quick relief: 2 puffs every 4-6 hours as needed

Exacerbation of asthma (acute, severe): 4-8 puffs every 20 minutes for 3 doses, then every 1-4 hours as needed

Exercise-induced bronchospasm (prevention): 2 puffs 5-30 minutes prior to exercise

Children ≥12 years and Adults:

Bronchospasm, quick relief *(NIH Guidelines, 2007)*: 2 puffs every 4-6 hours as needed

Exacerbation of asthma (acute, severe) *(NIH Guidelines, 2007)*: 4-8 puffs every 20 minutes for up to 4 hours, then every 1-4 hours as needed

Exercise-induced bronchospasm (prevention) *(NIH Guidelines, 2007)*: 2 puffs 5-30 minutes prior to exercise

Metered-dose inhaler (100 mcg/puff): Airomir™ (Canadian availability):

Children 6-11 years:

Bronchospasm:

Acute treatment: 1 puff; additional puffs may be necessary if inadequate relief however patients should be advised to promptly consult healthcare provider or seek medical attention if no relief from acute treatment

Maintenance: 1 puff; may increase to maximum of 1 puff 4 times daily

Exercise-induced bronchospasm (prevention): 1 puff 30 minutes prior to exercise

Children ≥12 years and Adults:

Bronchospasm:

Acute treatment: 1-2 puffs; additional puffs may be necessary if inadequate relief however patients should be advised to promptly consult healthcare provider or seek medical attention if no relief from acute treatment

Maintenance: 1-2 puffs 3-4 times daily (maximum: 8 puffs daily)

Exercise-induced bronchospasm (prevention): 2 puffs 30 minutes prior to exercise

Solution for nebulization:

Children 2-12 years (AccuNeb®): Bronchospasm: 0.63-1.25 mg 3-4 times daily as needed

Children ≤4 years *(NIH Guidelines, 2007)*:

Quick relief: 0.63-2.5 mg every 4-6 hours as needed

Exacerbation of asthma (acute, severe): 0.15 mg/kg (minimum: 2.5 mg) every 20 minutes for 3 doses, then 0.15-0.3 mg/kg (maximum: 10 mg) every 1-4 hours as needed **or** 0.5 mg/kg/hour by continuous nebulization

Children 5-11 years *(NIH Guidelines, 2007)*:

Quick relief: 1.25-5 mg every 4-8 hours as needed

Exacerbation of asthma (acute, severe): 0.15 mg/kg (minimum: 2.5 mg) every 20 minutes for 3 doses, then 0.15-0.3 mg/kg (maximum: 10 mg) every 1-4 hours as needed **or** 0.5 mg/kg/hour by continuous nebulization

Children ≥12 years and Adults:

Bronchospasm: 2.5 mg 3-4 times daily as needed

Quick relief *(NIH Guidelines, 2007)*: 1.25-5 mg every 4-8 hours as needed

Exacerbation of asthma (acute, severe) *(NIH Guidelines, 2007)*: 2.5-5 mg every 20 minutes for 3 doses then 2.5-10 mg every 1-4 hours as needed, **or** 10-15 mg/hour by continuous nebulization

I.V. continuous infusion: Adults (Canadian labeling; product not available in U.S.): Severe bronchospasm and status asthmaticus: Initial: 5 mcg/minute; may increase up to 10-20 mcg/minute at 15- to 30-minute intervals if needed

Dosage adjustment in renal impairment: Use with caution in patients with renal impairment. No dosage adjustment required (including patients on hemodialysis, peritoneal dialysis, or CRRT; Aronoff, 2007).

Dosage adjustment in hepatic impairment: No dosage adjustment provided in manufacturer's labeling.

Mechanism of Action Relaxes bronchial smooth muscle by action on beta$_2$-receptors with little effect on heart rate

Contraindications Hypersensitivity to albuterol or any component of the formulation

Injection formulation (Canadian labeling; product not available in U.S.): Hypersensitivity to albuterol or any component of the formulation; tachyarrhythmias; risk of abortion during first or second trimester

Warnings/Precautions Optimize anti-inflammatory treatment before initiating maintenance treatment with albuterol. Do not use as a component of chronic therapy without an anti-inflammatory agent. Only the mildest forms of asthma (Step 1 and/or exercise-induced) would not require concurrent use based upon asthma guidelines. Patient must be instructed to seek medical attention in cases where acute symptoms are not relieved or a previous level of response is diminished. The need to increase frequency of use may indicate deterioration of asthma, and treatment must not be delayed.

Use caution in patients with cardiovascular disease (arrhythmia or hypertension or HF), convulsive disorders, diabetes, glaucoma, hyperthyroidism, or hypokalemia. Beta-agonists may cause elevation in blood pressure, heart rate, and result in CNS stimulation/excitation. Beta$_2$-agonists may increase risk of arrhythmia, increase serum glucose, or decrease serum potassium.

◀ Immediate hypersensitivity reactions (urticaria, angioedema, rash, bronchospasm) have been reported. Do not exceed recommended dose; serious adverse events, including fatalities, have been associated with excessive use of inhaled sympathomimetics. Rarely, paradoxical bronchospasm may occur with use of inhaled bronchodilating agents; this should be distinguished from inadequate response. All patients should utilize a spacer device or valved holding chamber when using a metered-dose inhaler; in addition, face masks should be used in children <4 years of age.

Drug Interactions

Metabolism/Transport Effects None known.

Avoid Concomitant Use

Avoid concomitant use of Albuterol with any of the following: Beta-Blockers (Nonselective); Iobenguane I 123

Increased Effect/Toxicity

Albuterol may increase the levels/effects of: Atosiban; Loop Diuretics; Sympathomimetics; Thiazide Diuretics

The levels/effects of Albuterol may be increased by: AtoMOXetine; Cannabinoids; MAO Inhibitors; Tricyclic Antidepressants

Decreased Effect

Albuterol may decrease the levels/effects of: Iobenguane I 123

The levels/effects of Albuterol may be decreased by: Alpha-/Beta-Blockers; Beta-Blockers (Beta1 Selective); Beta-Blockers (Nonselective); Betahistine

Ethanol/Nutrition/Herb Interactions

Food: Avoid or limit caffeine (may cause CNS stimulation).

Herb/Nutraceutical: Avoid ephedra, yohimbe (may cause CNS stimulation). Avoid St John's wort (may decrease the levels/effects of albuterol).

Dietary Considerations Oral forms should be taken with water 1 hour before or 2 hours after meals.

Pharmacodynamics/Kinetics

Onset of Action Peak effect:

Nebulization/oral inhalation: 0.5-2 hours
CFC-propelled albuterol: 10 minutes
Ventolin® HFA: 25 minutes

Oral: 2-3 hours

Duration of Action Nebulization/oral inhalation: 3-4 hours; Oral: 4-6 hours

Half-life Elimination Inhalation: 3.8 hours; Oral: 3.7-5 hours

Pregnancy Risk Factor C

Pregnancy Considerations Adverse events were observed in some animal reproduction studies. Albuterol crosses the placenta (Boulton, 1997). Congenital anomalies (cleft palate, limb defects) have rarely been reported following maternal use during pregnancy. Multiple medications were used in most cases, no specific pattern of defects has been reported, and no relationship to albuterol has been established. The amount of albuterol available systemically following inhalation is significantly less in comparison to oral doses.

Uncontrolled asthma is associated with adverse events on pregnancy (increased risk of perinatal mortality, preeclampsia, preterm birth, low birth weight infants). Albuterol is the preferred short acting beta agonist when treatment for asthma is needed during pregnancy (NAEPP, 2005; NAEPP, 2007).

Albuterol may affect uterine contractility. Maternal pulmonary edema and other adverse events have been reported when albuterol was used for tocolysis.

Albuterol is not approved for use as a tocolytic; use caution when needed to treat bronchospasm in pregnant women. Use of the injection (Canadian product; not available in the U.S.) is specifically contraindicated in women during the first or second trimester who may be at risk of threatened abortion.

Lactation Excretion in breast milk unknown/not recommended

Breast-Feeding Considerations It is not known if albuterol is excreted into breast milk. The amount of albuterol available systemically following inhalation is significantly less in comparison to oral doses. According to the manufacturer, the decision to continue or discontinue breast-feeding during therapy should take into account the risk of exposure to the infant and the benefits of treatment to the mother. The use of beta-2-receptor agonists are not considered a contraindication to breast feeding (NAEPP, 2005).

Dosage Forms

Aerosol, for oral inhalation:

ProAir® HFA: 90 mcg/inhalation (8.5 g)
Proventil® HFA: 90 mcg/inhalation (6.7 g)
Ventolin® HFA: 90 mcg/inhalation (8 g, 18 g)

Solution, for nebulization: 0.083% [2.5 mg/3 mL] (30s, 60s); 0.5% [100 mg/20 mL] (1s)

Solution, for nebulization [preservative free]: 0.021% [0.63 mg/3 mL] (25s); 0.042% [1.25 mg/3 mL] (25s, 30s); 0.083% [2.5 mg/3 mL] (25s, 30s, 60s); 0.5% [2.5 mg/0.5 mL] (30s)

AccuNeb®: 0.021% [0.63 mg/3 mL] (25s); 0.042% [1.25 mg/3 mL] (25s)

Syrup, oral: 2 mg/5 mL (473 mL, 480 mL)

Tablet, oral: 2 mg, 4 mg

Tablet, extended release, oral: 4 mg, 8 mg

VoSpire ER®: 4 mg, 8 mg

Dosage Forms: Canada

Aerosol, for oral inhalation:

Airomir™: 100 mcg/inhalation (3.7 g, 6.7 g)

Injection, solution:

Ventolin® I.V.: 1 mg/1mL (5 mL)

Alcaftadine (al KAF ta deen)

Brand Names: U.S. Lastacaft™

Pharmacologic Category Histamine H_1 Antagonist; Histamine H_1 Antagonist, Second Generation; Mast Cell Stabilizer

Use Prevention of itching associated with allergic conjunctivitis

Local Anesthetic/Vasoconstrictor Precautions No information available to require special precautions

Effects on Dental Treatment No significant effects or complications reported

Effects on Bleeding No information available to require special precautions

Adverse Effects 1% to 10%:

Central nervous system: Headache (<3%)

Ocular: Ocular reactions (<4%; includes burning, pruritus, irritation, redness, stinging)

Respiratory: Nasopharyngitis (<3%)

Miscellaneous: Influenza (<3%)

General Dosage Range Ophthalmic: *Children ≥2 years and Adults:* Instill 1 drop into each eye once daily

Mechanism of Action Direct H_1-receptor antagonist and inhibitor of histamine release from mast cells

Pharmacodynamics/Kinetics

Half-life Elimination Carboxylic acid: ~2 hours

Pregnancy Risk Factor B

Pregnancy Considerations There are no well-controlled studies in pregnant women. Animal studies showed no evidence of teratogenicity or harm to the fetus.

Alclometasone (al kloe MET a sone)

Brand Names: U.S. Aclovate®
Generic Availability (U.S.) Yes
Pharmacologic Category Corticosteroid, Topical
Dental Use Treatment of inflammation of corticosteroid-responsive dermatosis (low to medium potency topical corticosteroid)
Use Treatment of inflammation of corticosteroid-responsive dermatosis (low to medium potency topical corticosteroid)
Local Anesthetic/Vasoconstrictor Precautions No information available to require special precautions
Effects on Dental Treatment No significant effects or complications reported
Effects on Bleeding No information available to require special precautions
Adverse Effects
Dermatologic: Acne, allergic dermatitis, hypopigmentation, perioral dermatitis, skin atrophy, striae, miliaria
Endocrine & metabolic: HPA axis suppression, Cushing's syndrome, growth retardation
Local: Dryness (2%), irritation (2%), papular rash (2%), burning (1% to 2%), erythema (1% to 2%), itching (1% to 2%), folliculitis
Miscellaneous: Secondary infection
Dosage Note: Therapy should be discontinued when control is achieved; if no improvement is seen within 2 weeks, reassessment of diagnosis may be necessary.
Topical:
Children ≥1 year: Apply thin film to affected area 2-3 times/day; do not use for >3 weeks
Adults: Apply a thin film to the affected area 2-3 times/day
Mechanism of Action Stimulates the synthesis of enzymes needed to decrease inflammation, suppress mitotic activity, and cause vasoconstriction
Contraindications Hypersensitivity to alclometasone or any component of the formulation
Warnings/Precautions Topical corticosteroids may be absorbed percutaneously. Absorption may cause manifestations of Cushing's syndrome, hyperglycemia, or glycosuria. Absorption is increased by the use of occlusive dressings, application to denuded skin, or application to large surface areas. May cause hypercorticism or suppression of hypothalamic-pituitary-adrenal (HPA) axis, particularly in younger children or in patients receiving high doses for prolonged periods. HPA axis suppression may lead to adrenal crisis.

Prolonged treatment with corticosteroids has been associated with the development of Kaposi's sarcoma (case reports); if noted, discontinuation of therapy should be considered. Prolonged use may result in fungal or bacterial superinfection; discontinue if dermatological infection persists despite appropriate antimicrobial therapy. Local sensitization (redness, irritation) may occur; discontinue if sensitization is noted. Allergic contact dermatitis can occur, it is usually diagnosed by failure to heal rather than clinical exacerbation.

Safety and efficacy have not been established in children <1 year of age. Safety and efficacy for use >3 weeks has not been established. Children may absorb proportionally larger amounts after topical application and may be more prone to systemic effects. HPA axis suppression, intracranial hypertension, and Cushing's syndrome have been reported in children receiving topical corticosteroids. Prolonged use may affect growth velocity; growth should be routinely monitored in pediatric patients. Not for the treatment of diaper dermatitis.

Avoid use of topical preparations with occlusive dressings or on weeping or exudative lesions. If no improvement is seen within 2 weeks, reassessment of diagnosis may be necessary. Avoid contact with eyes. Generally not for routine use on the face, underarms, or groin area (including diapered area).
Drug Interactions
Metabolism/Transport Effects None known.
Avoid Concomitant Use
Avoid concomitant use of Alclometasone with any of the following: Aldesleukin
Increased Effect/Toxicity
Alclometasone may increase the levels/effects of: Deferasirox

The levels/effects of Alclometasone may be increased by: Telaprevir
Decreased Effect
Alclometasone may decrease the levels/effects of: Aldesleukin; Corticorelin; Hyaluronidase; Telaprevir
Pregnancy Risk Factor C
Pregnancy Considerations Some corticosteroids were found to be teratogenic following topical application in animal reproduction studies. Topical products are not recommended for extensive use, in large quantities, or for long periods of time in pregnant women.
Lactation Excretion in breast milk unknown/use caution
Breast-Feeding Considerations Systemic corticosteroids are excreted in human milk. It is not known if sufficient quantities of alclometasone are absorbed following topical administration to produce detectable amounts in breast milk.
Dosage Forms
Cream, topical: 0.05% (15 g, 45 g, 60 g)
Aclovate®: 0.05% (15 g, 60 g)
Ointment, topical: 0.05% (15 g, 45 g, 60 g)

Aldesleukin (al des LOO kin)

Brand Names: U.S. Proleukin®
Brand Names: Canada Proleukin®
Pharmacologic Category Antineoplastic Agent, Miscellaneous; Biological Response Modulator
Use Treatment of metastatic renal cell cancer, metastatic melanoma
Unlabeled Use Treatment of acute myeloid leukemia (AML)
Local Anesthetic/Vasoconstrictor Precautions No information available to require special precautions
Effects on Dental Treatment Key adverse event(s) related to dental treatment: Stomatitis
Effects on Bleeding Chemotherapy may result in significant myelosuppression, including thrombocytopenia. In patients who are under active treatment, a medical consult is suggested.
Adverse Effects
>10%:
Cardiovascular: Hypotension (71%; grade 4: 3%), peripheral edema (28%), tachycardia (23%), edema (15%), vasodilation (13%), supraventricular tachycardia (12%; grade 4: 1%), cardiovascular disorder (11%; includes blood pressure changes, HF and ECG changes)

Central nervous system: Chills (52%), confusion (34%; grade 4: 1%), fever (29%; grade 4: 1%), malaise (27%), somnolence (22%), anxiety (12%), pain (12%), dizziness (11%)

Dermatologic: Rash (42%), pruritus (24%), exfoliative dermatitis (18%)

Endocrine & metabolic: Acidosis (12%; grade 4: 1%), hypomagnesemia (12%), hypocalcemia (11%)

Gastrointestinal: Diarrhea (67%; grade 4: 2%), vomiting (19% to 50%; grade 4: 1%), nausea (19% to 35%), stomatitis (22%), anorexia (20%), weight gain (16%), abdominal pain (11%)

Hematologic: Thrombocytopenia (37%; grade 4: 1%), anemia (29%), leukopenia (16%)

Hepatic: Hyperbilirubinemia (40%; grade 4: 2%), AST increased (23%; grade 4: 1%)

Neuromuscular & skeletal: Weakness (23%)

Renal: Oliguria (63%; grade 4: 6%), creatinine increased (33%; grade 4: 1%)

Respiratory: Dyspnea (43%; grade 4: 1%), lung disorder (24%; includes pulmonary congestion, rales, and rhonchi), cough (11%), respiratory disorder (11%; includes acute respiratory distress syndrome, infiltrates and pulmonary changes)

Miscellaneous: Antibody formation (66% to 74%), infection (13%; grade 4: 1%)

1% to 10%:

Cardiovascular: Arrhythmia (10%), cardiac arrest (grade 4: 1%), MI (grade 4: 1%), ventricular tachycardia (grade 4: 1%)

Central nervous system: Coma (grade 4: 2%), stupor (grade 4: 1%), psychosis (grade 4: 1%)

Gastrointestinal: Abdomen enlarged (10%)

Hematologic: Coagulation disorder (grade 4: 1%; includes intravascular coagulopathy)

Hepatic: Alkaline phosphatase increased (10%)

Renal: Anuria (grade 4: 5%), acute renal failure (grade 4: 1%)

Respiratory: Rhinitis (10%), apnea (grade 4: 1%)

Miscellaneous: Sepsis (grade 4: 1%)

General Dosage Range Dosage adjustment recommended in patients who develop toxicities

I.V.: *Adults:* 600,000 units/kg every 8 hours (maximum: 14 doses); may repeat after 9 days for a total of 28 doses/course

Mechanism of Action Aldesleukin is a human recombinant interleukin-2 product which promotes proliferation, differentiation, and recruitment of T and B cells, natural killer (NK) cells, and thymocytes; causes cytolytic activity in a subset of lymphocytes and subsequent interactions between the immune system and malignant cells; can stimulate lymphokine-activated killer (LAK) cells and tumor-infiltrating lymphocytes (TIL) cells.

Pharmacodynamics/Kinetics

Half-life Elimination I.V.: Initial: 6-13 minutes; Terminal: 80-120 minutes

Pregnancy Risk Factor C

Pregnancy Considerations Maternal toxicity and embryocidal effects were noted in animal studies. There are no adequate and well-controlled studies in pregnant women; use during pregnancy only if benefits to the mother outweigh potential risk to the fetus. Contraception is recommended for fertile males or females using this medication.

Alemtuzumab (ay lem TU zoo mab)

Brand Names: U.S. Campath® [DSC]
Brand Names: Canada MabCampath®

Pharmacologic Category Antineoplastic Agent, Monoclonal Antibody; Monoclonal Antibody

Use Campath®: Treatment (as a single agent) of B-cell chronic lymphocytic leukemia (B-CLL)

Unlabeled Use Conditioning regimen in stem cell transplant; prophylaxis of graft-versus-host disease (GVHD); treatment of steroid-refractory GVHD; treatment of T-cell prolymphocytic leukemia; treatment of autoimmune hemolytic anemia (CLL-induced); immunosuppressant in solid organ transplant (induction and steroid-refractory rejection); treatment of relapsed-remitting multiple sclerosis

Local Anesthetic/Vasoconstrictor Precautions No information available to require special precautions

Effects on Dental Treatment Key adverse event(s) related to dental treatment: Stomatitis and mucositis.

Effects on Bleeding Chemotherapy may result in significant myelosuppression, including thrombocytopenia. In patients who are under active treatment, a medical consult is suggested.

Adverse Effects Adverse reactions reported with Campath®:

>10%:

Cardiovascular: Hypotension (16%), hypertension (14%), dysrhythmia (14%)

Central nervous system: Fever (69%), chills (53%), headache (14%), dysthesias, fatigue

Dermatologic: Urticaria (16%), rash (13%)

Gastrointestinal: Abdominal pain, anorexia, mucositis, nausea, vomiting

Hematologic: Lymphopenia (grades 3/4: 97%), neutropenia (77%; grade 3/4: 42% to 64% [median onset: 31 days, median duration: 28-37 days]), anemia (76%; grade 3/4: 12% to 38% [median onset: 31 days, median duration 8 days]), thrombocytopenia (71%; grade 3/4: 13% to 52% [median onset: 9 days; median duration: 14-21 days])

Local: Injection site reaction (SubQ administration: 90%)

Neuromuscular & skeletal: Musculoskeletal pain

Respiratory: Dyspnea (14%)

Miscellaneous: Infection (50% to 74%; grades 3/4: 5% to 21%; includes bacterial, fungal, protozoan, viral), CMV viremia (55%), infusion reactions (grades 3/4: 10% to 35%), CMV infection (16%), sepsis (grades 3/4/5: 3% to 10%)

1% to 10%:

Cardiovascular: Tachycardia (10%)

Central nervous system: Insomnia (10%), anxiety (8%)

Dermatologic: Erythema (4%)

Gastrointestinal: Diarrhea (10%)

Hematologic: Neutropenic fever (grades 3/4: 5% to 10%)

Neuromuscular & skeletal: Tremor (3%)

Respiratory: Bronchospasm

General Dosage Range Dosage adjustment recommended in patients who develop toxicities

I.V. (infusion): *Adults:* Initial: 3 mg/day, then 10 mg/day; Maintenance: 30 mg/day 3 times/week on alternate days; Maximum dose: 30 mg/day; 90 mg/week (cumulative)

Mechanism of Action Binds to CD52, a nonmodulating antigen present on the surface of B and T lymphocytes, a majority of monocytes, macrophages, NK cells, and a subpopulation of granulocytes. After binding to CD52+ cells, an antibody-dependent lysis of malignant cells occurs.

Pharmacodynamics/Kinetics
Half-life Elimination I.V.: 11 hours (following first 30 mg dose; range: 2-32 hours); 6 days (following the last 30 mg dose; range: 1-14 days)

Pregnancy Risk Factor C

Pregnancy Considerations Human IgG is known to cross the placental barrier; therefore, alemtuzumab may also cross the barrier and cause fetal B- and T-lymphocyte depletion. Use during pregnancy only if the benefit to the mother outweighs the potential risk to the fetus. Effective contraception is recommended during and for at least 6 months after treatment for women of child-bearing potential and men of reproductive potential.

Prescribing and Access Restrictions As of September 4, 2012, alemtuzumab (Campath®) is no longer commercially available in the United States (or Europe); a restricted distribution program will allow access (free of charge) for appropriate patients. Information on necessary documentation and requirements is available at Campath Distribution Program (1-877-422-6728) or Genzyme Medical Information (1-800-745-4447, option 2).

Alendronate (a LEN droe nate)

Related Information
Osteonecrosis of the Jaw *on page 1529*
Rheumatoid Arthritis, Osteoarthritis, and Osteoporosis *on page 1526*

Brand Names: U.S. Binosto™; Fosamax®

Brand Names: Canada Alendronate-FC; Apo-Alendronate®; CO Alendronate; Dom-Alendronate; Fosamax®; JAMP-Alendronate; Mylan-Alendronate; PHL-Alendronate; PMS-Alendronate; PMS-Alendronate-FC; Q-Alendronate; ratio-Alendronate; Riva-Alendronate; Sandoz-Alendronate; Teva-Alendronate

Generic Availability (U.S.) Yes: Excludes tablet for solution

Pharmacologic Category Bisphosphonate Derivative

Use Treatment of osteoporosis in postmenopausal females (Fosamax®, Binosto™); prevention of osteoporosis in postmenopausal females (Fosamax®); treatment of osteoporosis in males (Fosamax®, Binosto™); Paget's disease of the bone in patients who are symptomatic, at risk for future complications, or with alkaline phosphatase ≥2 times the upper limit of normal (Fosamax®); treatment of glucocorticoid-induced osteoporosis in males and females with low bone mineral density who are receiving a daily dosage ≥7.5 mg of prednisone (or equivalent) (Fosamax®)

Local Anesthetic/Vasoconstrictor Precautions No information available to require special precautions

Effects on Dental Treatment Osteonecrosis of the jaw (ONJ), generally associated with local infection and/or tooth extraction and often with delayed healing, has been reported in patients taking bisphosphonates. Symptoms included nonhealing extraction socket or an exposed jawbone. Most reported cases of bisphosphonate-associated osteonecrosis have been in cancer patients treated with intravenous bisphosphonates. However, some have occurred in patients with postmenopausal osteoporosis taking oral bisphosphonates. The risk of developing ONJ in patients taking oral bisphosphonates remains low with an estimated prevalence of 0.1% (one out of every 1000 cases of patients exposed to oral bisphosphonates). The benefits of using the oral bisphosphonates to prevent osteoporosis significantly outweighs the small risk of developing bisphosphonate-associated ONJ. Also, at the present

time, there are no validated diagnostic techniques to determine which patients are at increased risk of developing ONJ. ONJ in patients taking these drugs can occur spontaneously. In addition, the risk of ONJ increases with specific procedures that increase bone trauma, particularly tooth extractions. Other factors that increase risk of ONJ in patients taking these drugs are age (>65 years of age), periodontitis, use of bisphosphonates for >2 years, smoking, wearing dentures, and diabetes. Patients who develop ONJ while on bisphosphonate therapy should receive care by an oral surgeon. See Dental Comment.

Effects on Bleeding No information available to require special precautions

Adverse Effects Note: Incidence of adverse effects (mostly GI) increases significantly in patients treated for Paget's disease at 40 mg/day.

>10%: Endocrine & metabolic: Hypocalcemia (transient, mild, 18%); hypophosphatemia (transient, mild, 10%)

1% to 10%:
Central nervous system: Headache (up to 3%)
Gastrointestinal: Abdominal pain (1% to 7%), acid reflux (1% to 4%), dyspepsia (1% to 4%), nausea (1% to 4%), flatulence (up to 4%), diarrhea (1% to 3%), gastroesophageal reflux disease (1% to 3%), constipation (up to 3%), esophageal ulcer (up to 2%), abdominal distension (up to 1%), gastritis (up to 1%), vomiting (up to 1%), dysphagia (up to 1%), gastric ulcer (1%), melena (1%)
Neuromuscular & skeletal: Musculoskeletal pain (up to 6%), muscle cramps (up to 1%)

Dosage Oral: Adults: **Note:** Patients should receive supplemental calcium and vitamin D if dietary intake is inadequate.

Osteoporosis in postmenopausal females:
Prophylaxis: 5 mg once daily **or** 35 mg once weekly
Treatment: 10 mg once daily **or** 70 mg once weekly

Osteoporosis in males: 10 mg once daily **or** 70 mg once weekly

Osteoporosis secondary to glucocorticoids in males and females: Treatment: 5 mg once daily; a dose of 10 mg once daily should be used in postmenopausal females who are not receiving estrogen.

Paget's disease of bone in males and females: 40 mg once daily for 6 months

Retreatment: Relapses during the 12 months following therapy occurred in 9% of patients who responded to treatment. Specific retreatment data are not available. Following a 6-month post-treatment evaluation period, retreatment with alendronate may be considered in patients who have relapsed based on increases in serum alkaline phosphatase, which should be measured periodically. Retreatment may also be considered in those who failed to normalize their serum alkaline phosphatase.

Elderly: Refer to adult dosing.

Dosage adjustment in renal impairment:
Cl_{cr} ≥35 mL/minute: No dosage adjustment necessary.
Cl_{cr} <35 mL/minute: Use not recommended.

Dosage adjustment in hepatic impairment: No dosage adjustment necessary.

Mechanism of Action A bisphosphonate which inhibits bone resorption via actions on osteoclasts or on osteoclast precursors; decreases the rate of bone resorption, leading to an indirect increase in bone mineral density. In Paget's disease, characterized by disordered resorption and formation of bone, inhibition of resorption leads to an indirect decrease in bone formation; but the newly-formed bone has a more normal architecture.

◀ **Contraindications** Hypersensitivity to alendronate, other bisphosphonates, or any component of the formulation; hypocalcemia; abnormalities of the esophagus which delay esophageal emptying such as stricture or achalasia; inability to stand or sit upright for at least 30 minutes; increased risk of aspiration (effervescent tablets; oral solution)

Warnings/Precautions Use caution in patients with renal impairment (not recommended for use in patients with Cl$_{cr}$ <35 mL/minute); hypocalcemia must be corrected before therapy initiation; ensure adequate calcium and vitamin D intake. May cause irritation to upper gastrointestinal mucosa. Esophagitis, dysphagia, esophageal ulcers, esophageal erosions, and esophageal stricture (rare) have been reported; risk increases in patients unable to comply with dosing instructions. Use with caution in patients with dysphagia, esophageal disease, gastritis, duodenitis, or ulcers (may worsen underlying condition). Discontinue use if new or worsening symptoms develop.

Osteonecrosis of the jaw (ONJ) has been reported in patients receiving bisphosphonates. Risk factors include invasive dental procedures (eg, tooth extraction, dental implants, boney surgery); a diagnosis of cancer, with concomitant chemotherapy or corticosteroids; poor oral hygiene, ill-fitting dentures; and comorbid disorders (anemia, coagulopathy, infection, pre-existing dental disease). Most reported cases occurred after I.V. bisphosphonate therapy; however, cases have been reported following oral therapy. A dental exam and preventative dentistry should be performed prior to placing patients with risk factors on chronic bisphosphonate therapy. The manufacturer's labeling states that discontinuing bisphosphonates in patients requiring invasive dental procedures may reduce the risk of ONJ. However, other experts suggest that there is no evidence that discontinuing therapy reduces the risk of developing ONJ (Assael, 2009). The benefit/risk must be assessed by the treating physician and/or dentist/surgeon prior to any invasive dental procedure. Patients developing ONJ while on bisphosphonates should receive care by an oral surgeon.

Atypical femur fractures have been reported in patients receiving bisphosphonates for treatment/prevention of osteoporosis. The fractures include subtrochanteric femur (bone just below the hip joint) and diaphyseal femur (long segment of the thigh bone). Some patients experience prodromal pain weeks or months before the fracture occurs. It is unclear if bisphosphonate therapy is the cause for these fractures, although the majority have been reported in patients taking bisphosphonates. Patients receiving long-term (>3-5 years) therapy may be at an increased risk. Discontinue bisphosphonate therapy in patients who develop a femoral shaft fracture.

Severe (and occasionally debilitating) bone, joint, and/or muscle pain have been reported during bisphosphonate treatment. The onset of pain ranged from a single day to several months. Consider discontinuing therapy in patients who experience severe symptoms; symptoms usually resolve upon discontinuation. Some patients experienced recurrence when rechallenged with same drug or another bisphosphonate; avoid use in patients with a history of these symptoms in association with bisphosphonate therapy.

Each effervescent tablet contains 650 mg of sodium (NaCl 1650 mg); use with caution in patients following a sodium-restricted diet.

Drug Interactions
Metabolism/Transport Effects None known.
Avoid Concomitant Use There are no known interactions where it is recommended to avoid concomitant use.
Increased Effect/Toxicity
Alendronate may increase the levels/effects of: Deferasirox; Phosphate Supplements; SUNItinib

The levels/effects of Alendronate may be increased by: Aminoglycosides; Aspirin; Nonsteroidal Anti-Inflammatory Agents
Decreased Effect
The levels/effects of Alendronate may be decreased by: Antacids; Calcium Salts; Iron Salts; Magnesium Salts; Multivitamins/Minerals (with ADEK, Folate, Iron); Proton Pump Inhibitors
Ethanol/Nutrition/Herb Interactions
Ethanol: May increase risk of osteoporosis and gastric irritation. Management: Avoid ethanol.
Food: All food and beverages interfere with absorption. Coadministration with caffeine may reduce alendronate efficacy. Coadministration with dairy products may decrease alendronate absorption. Beverages (especially orange juice and coffee) and food may reduce the absorption of alendronate as much as 60%. Management: Alendronate must be taken first thing in the morning and ≥30 minutes before the first food, beverage (except plain water), or other medication of the day.

Dietary Considerations Ensure adequate calcium and vitamin D intake; women and men ≥50 years of age should consume 1200-1500 mg/day of elemental calcium and 800-1000 units/day of vitamin D. Alendronate must be taken first thing in the morning and at least 30 minutes before the first food, beverage (except plain water), or medication/supplement of the day. Effervescent tablets contain sodium.
Pharmacodynamics/Kinetics
Half-life Elimination Exceeds 10 years
Pregnancy Risk Factor C
Pregnancy Considerations Safety and efficacy have not been established in pregnant women. Animal studies have shown delays in delivery and fetal/neonatal death (secondary to hypocalcemia). Bisphosphonates are incorporated into the bone matrix and gradually released over time. Theoretically, there may be a risk of fetal harm when pregnancy follows the completion of therapy. Based on limited case reports with pamidronate, serum calcium levels in the newborn may be altered if administered during pregnancy.
Lactation Excretion in breast milk unknown/use caution
Dosage Forms
Tablet, oral: 5 mg, 10 mg, 35 mg, 40 mg, 70 mg
  Fosamax®: 70 mg
Tablet for solution, oral:
  Binosto™: 70 mg
Dental Comment A review of 2408 published cases of bisphosphonate-associated osteonecrosis of the jaw bone (BP-associated ONJ) was done by Filleul, 2010. BP therapy was associated with 89% of the cases to treat malignancies and 11% of the cases to treat nonmalignant conditions. Information on the specific bisphosphonate used was available for 1694 of the patients. Intravenous therapy (primarily zoledronic acid) was received by 88% of the patients and 12% received oral treatment (primarily alendronate). Of all the cases of BP-associated ONJ, 67% were preceded by tooth extraction and for 26% of patients, there was no predisposing factor identified.

A 2010 retrospective case review reported the prevalence of BP-associated ONJ in patients using alendronate-type drugs was one out of 952 patients or ~0.1% (Lo, 2010). Of the 8572 respondents, nine cases of ONJ were identified; five had developed ONJ spontaneously and four developed ONJ after tooth extraction. When extrapolated to patient-years of bisphosphonate exposure, this prevalence rate of 0.1% equates to a frequency of 28 cases per 100,000 person-years of oral bisphosphonate treatment. An Australian group (Mavrokokki, 2007), identified the frequency of BP-associated ONJ in osteoporotic patients, mainly taking weekly oral alendronate, was 1 in 8470 to 1 in 2260 (0.01% to 0.04%) patients. If extractions were carried out, the calculated frequency was 1 in 1130 to 1 in 296 (0.09% to 0.34%) patients. The median time to onset of ONJ in alendronate patients was 24 months.

According to the 2011 report by the American Dental Association (ADA), the incidence of BP-associated ONJ remains low and the benefits of using oral bisphosphonates significantly outweighs the risk of developing BP-associated ONJ for treatment and prevention of osteoporosis and cancer treatment (Hellstein, 2011). The full 47 page report can be accessed at http://www.ada.org/sections/professionalResources/pdfs/topics_ARONJ_report.pdf.

The ADA review of 2011 stated the incidence of oral BP-associated ONJ was one case for every 1000 individuals exposed to oral bisphosphonates (0.1%) (Hellstein, 2011).

References

Durie BG, Katz M, and Crowley J, "Osteonecrosis of the Jaw and Bisphosphonates," *N Engl J Med*, 2005, 353(1):99-102.

Filleul O, Crompot E, and Saussez S, "Bisphosphonate-Induced Osteonecrosis of the Jaw: A Review of 2,400 Patient Cases," *J Cancer Res Clin Oncol*, 2010, 136(8):1117-24.

Hellstein JW, Adler RA, Edwards B, et al, "Managing the Care of Patients Receiving Antiresorptive Therapy for Prevention and Treatment of Osteoporosis: Executive Summary of Recommendations From the American Dental Association Council on Scientific Affairs," *J Am Dent Assoc*, 2011, 142(11):1243-51.

Hellstein JW, Adler RA, Edwards B, et al, "Managing the Care of Patients Receiving Antiresorptive Therapy for Prevention and Treatment of Osteoporosis: Recommendations From the American Dental Association Council on Scientific Affairs," 2011, Available at http://www.ada.org/sections/professionalResources/pdfs/topics_ARONJ_report.pdf. Accessed February 2013.

Lo JC, O'Ryan FS, Gordon NP, et al, "Prevalence of Osteonecrosis of the Jaw in Patients With Oral Bisphosphonate Exposure," *J Oral Maxillofac Surg*, 2010, 68(2):243-53.

Marx RE, Sawatari Y, Fortin M, et al, "Bisphosphonate-Induced Exposed Bone (Osteonecrosis/Osteopetrosis) of the Jaws: Risk Factors, Recognition, Prevention, and Treatment," *J Oral Maxillofac Surg*, 2005, 63(11):1567-75.

Mavrokokki T, Cheng A, Stein B, et al, "Nature and Frequency of Bisphosphonate-Associated Osteonecrosis of the Jaws in Australia," *J Oral Maxillofac Surg*, 2007, 65(3):415-23.

Ruggiero SL, Dodson TB, Assael LA, et al, "American Association of Oral and Maxillofacial Surgeons Position Paper on Bisphosphonate-Related Osteonecrosis of the Jaws-2009 Update," *J Oral Maxillofac Surg*, 2009, 67(5 Suppl):2-12.

Ruggiero S, Gralow J, Marx RE, et al, "Practical Guidelines for the Prevention, Diagnosis, and Treatment of Osteonecrosis of the Jaw in Patients With Cancer," *J Clin Oncol*, 2006, 2(1):7-14.

Alendronate and Cholecalciferol
(a LEN droe nate & kole e kal SI fer ole)

Related Information

Alendronate *on page 59*

Cholecalciferol *on page 298*

Brand Names: U.S. Fosamax Plus D®

Brand Names: Canada Fosavance

Pharmacologic Category Bisphosphonate Derivative; Vitamin D Analog

Use Treatment of osteoporosis in postmenopausal females; increase bone mass in males with osteoporosis

Local Anesthetic/Vasoconstrictor Precautions No information available to require special precautions

Effects on Dental Treatment Osteonecrosis of the jaw (ONJ), generally associated with local infection and/or tooth extraction and often with delayed healing, has been reported in patients taking bisphosphonates. Symptoms included nonhealing extraction socket or an exposed jawbone. Most reported cases of bisphosphonate-associated osteonecrosis have been in cancer patients treated with intravenous bisphosphonates. However, some have occurred in patients with postmenopausal osteoporosis taking oral bisphosphonates. The risk of developing ONJ in patients taking oral bisphosphonates remains low with an estimated prevalence of 0.1% (one out of every 1000 cases of patients exposed to oral bisphosphonates). The benefits of using the oral bisphosphonates to prevent osteoporosis significantly outweighs the small risk of developing bisphosphonate-associated ONJ. Also, at the present time, there are no validated diagnostic techniques to determine which patients are at increased risk of developing ONJ. ONJ in patients taking these drugs can occur spontaneously. In addition, the risk of ONJ increases with specific procedures that increase bone trauma, particularly tooth extractions. Other factors that increase risk of ONJ in patients taking these drugs are age (>65 years of age), periodontitis, use of bisphosphonates for >2 years, smoking, wearing dentures, and diabetes. Patients who develop ONJ while on bisphosphonate therapy should receive care by an oral surgeon. See Dental Comment.

Effects on Bleeding No information available to require special precautions

Adverse Effects See individual agents.

General Dosage Range Oral: *Adults:* One tablet (alendronate 70 mg/cholecalciferol 2800-5600 units) once weekly

Mechanism of Action See individual agents.

Pregnancy Risk Factor C

Pregnancy Considerations Animal studies have shown delays in delivery and fetal/neonatal death (secondary to hypocalcemia). Bisphosphonates are incorporated into the bone matrix and gradually released over time. Theoretically, there may be a risk of fetal harm when pregnancy follows the completion of therapy. Adverse events were observed in animals when high maternal doses of vitamin D were administered during pregnancy. Vitamin D crosses the placenta but the transfer to the fetus from the mother is low. Maternal supplementation has not been shown to affect pregnancy outcomes. Vitamin D requirements are the same in pregnant and nonpregnant females (IOM, 2011).

Dental Comment See Alendronate monograph.

Alfacalcidol (Al fa CAL ce dol)

Brand Names: Canada One-Alpha®

Pharmacologic Category Vitamin D Analog

Use Management of hypocalcemia, secondary hyperparathyroidism, and osteodystrophy in patients with chronic renal failure

Local Anesthetic/Vasoconstrictor Precautions No information available to require special precautions

Effects on Dental Treatment Key adverse event(s) related to dental treatment: Xerostomia (normal salivary flow resumes upon discontinuation) or abnormal taste.

Effects on Bleeding No information available to require special precautions

Adverse Effects Frequency not defined; as associated with Hypervitaminosis D:

Cardiovascular: Cardiac arrhythmia, hypertension

Central nervous system: Headache, hyperthermia, psychosis (rare), somnolence

Dermatologic: Pruritus

Genitourinary: Nocturia

Endocrine & metabolic: Hypercalcemia, hypercholesterolemia, hyperphosphatemia, libido decreased, polydipsia

Gastrointestinal: Anorexia, constipation, nausea, pancreatitis, taste abnormal, vomiting, weight loss, xerostomia

Hepatic: ALT increased, AST increased

Neuromuscular & skeletal: Bone pain, muscle pain, weakness

Ocular: Conjunctivitis, corneal calcification, photophobia

Renal: BUN increased, polyuria

Respiratory: Rhinorrhea

General Dosage Range Individualize dosage:

Oral: *Adults:* 0.25-3 mcg/day

I.V.: *Adults:* 1-12 mcg/week (with dialysis)

Mechanism of Action Alfacalcidol is rapidly converted to the active metabolite of vitamin D (1,25-dihydroxyvitamin D_3) in the liver, effectively bypassing renal metabolic conversion; promotes intestinal absorption of calcium and phosphorous, resorption of calcium from the bone, and possibly renal reabsorption of calcium

Pharmacodynamics/Kinetics

Onset of Action 6 hours

Duration of Action Effect on intestinal calcium absorption levels: 1,25-$(OH)_2$ D_3: 48 hours

Half-life Elimination Renal insufficiency: 3 hours

Time to Peak Active vitamin D levels: Oral: 12 hours; I.V.: 4 hours

Pregnancy Considerations A decrease in litter size and birth weights has been observed in animal studies. Safety has not been established in pregnant women.

Product Availability Not available in the U.S.

Alfentanil (al FEN ta nil)

Brand Names: U.S. Alfenta®

Brand Names: Canada Alfentanil Injection, USP; Alfenta®

Pharmacologic Category Analgesic, Opioid; Anilidopiperidine Opioid

Use Analgesic adjunct for the induction and maintenance of general anesthesia; analgesic component for monitored anesthesia care (MAC)

Local Anesthetic/Vasoconstrictor Precautions No information available to require special precautions

Effects on Dental Treatment Key adverse event(s) related to dental treatment: Orthostatic hypotension. Erythromycin inhibits the liver metabolism of alfentanil resulting in increased sedation and prolonged respiratory depression. Clarithromycin may act similarly.

Effects on Bleeding No information available to require special precautions

Adverse Effects

>10%:

Cardiovascular: Bradycardia, peripheral vasodilation

Central nervous system: Drowsiness, sedation, intracranial pressure increased

Gastrointestinal: Nausea, vomiting, constipation

Endocrine & metabolic: Antidiuretic hormone release

Ocular: Miosis

1% to 10%:

Cardiovascular: Cardiac arrhythmia, orthostatic hypotension

Central nervous system: Confusion, CNS depression

Ocular: Blurred vision

General Dosage Range I.V.:

Anesthetic induction: *Children ≥12 years and Adults:* Initial: 130-245 mcg/kg; Maintenance: 0.5-1.5 mcg/kg/minute

Continuous infusion: *Children ≥12 years and Adults:* Initial: 50-75 mcg/kg; Maintenance: 0.5-3 mcg/kg/minute

Incremental injection: *Children ≥12 years and Adults:*

≤30 minutes anesthesia: Initial: 8-20 mcg/kg; Maintenance: 3-5 mcg/kg **or** 0.5-1 mcg/kg/minute (maximum: 40 mcg/kg total dose)

≥30 minutes anesthesia: Initial: 20-50 mcg/kg; Maintenance: 5-15 mcg/kg (maximum: 75 mcg/kg total dose)

Mechanism of Action Binds with stereospecific receptors at many sites within the CNS, increases pain threshold, alters pain perception, inhibits ascending pain pathways; is an ultra short-acting narcotic

Pharmacodynamics/Kinetics

Onset of Action Rapid

Duration of Action Dose dependent: 30-60 minutes

Half-life Elimination Newborns, premature: 5.33-8.75 hours; Children: 40-60 minutes; Adults: 83-97 minutes

Pregnancy Risk Factor C

Pregnancy Considerations Alfentanil is known to cross the placenta, which may result in respiratory or CNS depression in the newborn. Use during labor and delivery is not recommended.

Controlled Substance C-II

Alfuzosin (al FYOO zoe sin)

Related Information

Clinical Risk Related to Drugs Prolonging QT Interval *on page 1510*

Brand Names: U.S. Uroxatral®

Brand Names: Canada Apo-Alfuzosin®; Sandoz-Alfuzosin; Teva-Alfuzosin PR; Xatral

Pharmacologic Category Alpha$_1$ Blocker

Use Treatment of the functional symptoms of benign prostatic hyperplasia (BPH)

Unlabeled Use Facilitation of expulsion of ureteral stones

Local Anesthetic/Vasoconstrictor Precautions Alfuzosin is one of the drugs confirmed to prolong the QT interval and is accepted as having a risk of causing torsade de pointes. The risk of drug-induced torsade de pointes is extremely low when a single QT interval prolonging drug is prescribed. In terms of epinephrine, it is not known what effect vasoconstrictors in the local anesthetic regimen will have in patients with a known history of congenital prolonged QT interval or in patients taking any medication that prolongs the QT interval. Until more information is obtained, it is suggested that the clinician consult with the physician prior to the use of a vasoconstrictor in suspected patients, and that the vasoconstrictor (epinephrine, mepivacaine and levonordefrin [Carbocaine® 2% with Neo-Cobefrin®]) be used with caution.

Effects on Dental Treatment No significant effects or complications reported

Effects on Bleeding No information available to require special precautions

Adverse Effects 1% to 10%:
Central nervous system: Dizziness (6%), fatigue (3%), headache (3%), pain (1% to 2%)
Gastrointestinal: Abdominal pain (1% to 2%), constipation (1% to 2%), dyspepsia (1% to 2%), nausea (1% to 2%)
Genitourinary: Impotence (1% to 2%)
Respiratory: Upper respiratory tract infection (3%), bronchitis (1% to 2%), pharyngitis (1% to 2%), sinusitis (1% to 2%)
General Dosage Range Oral: *Adults:* 10 mg once daily
Mechanism of Action An antagonist of alpha$_1$-adrenoreceptors in the lower urinary tract. Smooth muscle tone is mediated by the sympathetic nervous stimulation of alpha$_1$-adrenoreceptors, which are abundant in the prostate, prostatic capsule, prostatic urethra, and bladder neck. Blockade of these adrenoreceptors can cause smooth muscles in the bladder neck and prostate to relax, resulting in an improvement in urine flow rate and a reduction in BPH symptoms.
Pharmacodynamics/Kinetics
Half-life Elimination 10 hours
Time to Peak Plasma: 8 hours following a meal
Pregnancy Risk Factor B
Pregnancy Considerations Teratogenic effects were not observed in animal studies.
Dental Comment Alfuzosin is known to prolong the QT interval. The QT interval is measured as the time and distance between the Q point of the QRS complex and the end of the T wave in the ECG tracing. After adjustment for heart rate, the QT interval is defined as prolonged if it is more than 450 msec in men and 460 msec in women. A long QT syndrome was first described in the 1950s and 60s as a congenital syndrome involving QT interval prolongation and syncope and sudden death. Some of the congenital long QT syndromes were characterized by a peculiar electrocardiographic appearance of the QRS complex involving a premature atria beat followed by a pause, then a subsequent sinus beat showing marked QT prolongation and deformity. This type of cardiac arrhythmia was originally termed "torsade de pointes" (translated from the French as "twisting of the points"). Alfuzosin is considered as having a risk of causing torsade de pointes. Since it is not known what effect vasoconstrictors in the local anesthetic regimen will have in patients with a known history of congenital prolonged QT interval or in patients taking any medication that prolongs the QT interval, a medical consult is suggested.

Aliskiren (a lis KYE ren)

Related Information
Cardiovascular Diseases *on page 1492*
Brand Names: U.S. Tekturna®
Brand Names: Canada Rasilez®
Pharmacologic Category Renin Inhibitor
Use Treatment of hypertension, alone or in combination with other antihypertensive agents
Unlabeled Use Treatment of persistent proteinuria in patients with type 2 diabetes mellitus, hypertension, and nephropathy despite administration of optimized recommended renoprotective therapy (eg, angiotensin II receptor blocker)
Local Anesthetic/Vasoconstrictor Precautions No information available to require special precautions
Effects on Dental Treatment No significant effects or complications required

Effects on Bleeding No information available to require special precautions
Adverse Effects 1% to 10%:
Dermatologic: Rash (1%)
Endocrine & metabolic: Hyperkalemia (monotherapy ≤1%; may be increased with concurrent ACE inhibitor or ARB)
Gastrointestinal: Diarrhea (2%)
Hematologic: Creatine kinase increased (>300%: 1%)
Renal: BUN increased (≤7%), serum creatinine increased (≤7%)
Respiratory: Cough (1%)
General Dosage Range Oral: *Adults:* 150-300 mg once daily (maximum: 300 mg daily)
Mechanism of Action Aliskiren is a direct renin inhibitor, resulting in blockade of the conversion of angiotensinogen to angiotensin I. Angiotensin I suppression decreases the formation of angiotensin II (Ang II), a potent blood pressure-elevating peptide (via direct vasoconstriction, aldosterone release, and sodium retention). Ang II also functions within the Renin-Angiotensin-Aldosterone System (RAAS) as a negative inhibitory feedback mediator within the renal parenchyma to suppress the further release of renin. Thus, reductions in Ang II levels suppress this feedback loop, leading to further increased plasma renin concentrations (PRC) and subsequent activity (PRA). This disinhibition effect can be potentially problematic for ACE inhibitor and ARB therapy, as increased PRA could partially overcome the pharmacologic inhibition of the RAAS. As aliskiren is a direct inhibitor of renin activity, blunting of PRA despite the increased PRC (from loss of the negative feedback) may be clinically advantageous. The effect of aliskiren on bradykinin levels is unknown.
Pharmacodynamics/Kinetics
Onset of Action Maximum antihypertensive effect: Within 2 weeks
Half-life Elimination ~24 hours (range: 16-32 hours)
Time to Peak 1-3 hours
Pregnancy Risk Factor D
Pregnancy Considerations [U.S. Boxed Warning]: Drugs that act on the renin-angiotensin system can cause injury and death to the developing fetus. Discontinue as soon as possible once pregnancy is detected. The use of drugs which act on the renin-angiotensin system are associated with oligohydramnios. Oligohydramnios, due to decreased fetal renal function, may lead to fetal lung hypoplasia and skeletal malformations. Use is also associated with anuria, hypotension, renal failure, skull hypoplasia, and death in the fetus/neonate. The exposed fetus should be monitored for fetal growth, amniotic fluid volume, and organ formation. Infants exposed *in utero* should be monitored for hyperkalemia, hypotension, and oliguria.

Aliskiren, Amlodipine, and Hydrochlorothiazide
(a lis KYE ren, am LOE di peen, & hye droe klor oh THYE a zide)

Related Information
Aliskiren *on page 63*
AmLODIPine *on page 88*
Hydrochlorothiazide *on page 687*
Brand Names: U.S. Amturnide™
Pharmacologic Category Antianginal Agent; Calcium Channel Blocker; Calcium Channel Blocker, Dihydropyridine; Diuretic, Thiazide; Renin Inhibitor
Use Treatment of hypertension (not for initial therapy)

63

Local Anesthetic/Vasoconstrictor Precautions No information available to require special precautions

Effects on Dental Treatment Key adverse event(s) related to dental treatment: Hydrochlorothiazide: Orthostatic hypotension.

Fewer reports of gingival hyperplasia with amlodipine than with other CCBs (usually resolves upon discontinuation); consultation with physician is suggested.

Effects on Bleeding No information available to require special precautions

Adverse Effects Frequencies reported with combination product. See individual monographs for additional adverse effects reported with each agent.

1% to 10%:

Cardiovascular: Peripheral edema (7%)

Central nervous system: Dizziness (4%), headache (4%)

Respiratory: Nasopharyngitis (3%)

General Dosage Range Oral: *Adults:* Aliskiren 150-300 mg and Amlodipine 5-10 mg and Hydrochlorothiazide 12.5-25 mg once daily (maximum recommended daily dose: Aliskiren 300 mg; amlodipine 10 mg; hydrochlorothiazide 25 mg)

Mechanism of Action

Aliskiren: Direct renin inhibitor, resulting in blockade of the conversion of angiotensinogen to angiotensin I. Angiotensin I suppression decreases the formation of angiotensin II (Ang II), a potent blood pressure-elevating peptide (via direct vasoconstriction, aldosterone release, and sodium retention). Ang II also functions within the Renin-Angiotensin-Aldosterone System (RAAS) as a negative inhibitory feedback mediator within the renal parenchyma to suppress the further release of renin. Thus, reductions in Ang II levels suppress this feedback loop, leading to further increased plasma renin concentrations (PRC) and subsequent activity (PRA). This disinhibition effect can be potentially problematic for ACE inhibitor and ARB therapy, as increased PRA could partially overcome the pharmacologic inhibition of the RAAS. As aliskiren is a direct inhibitor of renin activity, blunting of PRA despite the increased PRC (from loss of the negative feedback) may be clinically advantageous. The effect of aliskiren on bradykinin levels is unknown.

Amlodipine: Inhibits calcium ion from entering the "slow channels" or select voltage-sensitive areas of vascular smooth muscle and myocardium during depolarization, producing a relaxation of coronary vascular smooth muscle and coronary vasodilation; increases myocardial oxygen delivery in patients with vasospastic angina. Amlodipine directly acts on vascular smooth muscle to produce peripheral arterial vasodilation reducing peripheral vascular resistance and blood pressure.

Hydrochlorothiazide: Inhibits sodium reabsorption in the distal tubules causing increased excretion of sodium and water as well as potassium and hydrogen ions.

Pregnancy Risk Factor D

Pregnancy Considerations [U.S. Boxed Warning]: Drugs that act on the renin-angiotensin system can cause injury and death to the developing fetus. Discontinue as soon as possible once pregnancy is detected. Also see individual agents.

Aliskiren and Amlodipine

(a lis KYE ren & am LOE di peen)

Related Information

Aliskiren *on page 63*

AmLODIPine *on page 88*

Brand Names: U.S. Tekamlo™

Pharmacologic Category Antianginal Agent; Calcium Channel Blocker; Calcium Channel Blocker, Dihydropyridine; Renin Inhibitor

Use Treatment of hypertension, alone or in combination with other antihypertensive agents

Local Anesthetic/Vasoconstrictor Precautions No information available to require special precautions

Effects on Dental Treatment Fewer reports of gingival hyperplasia with amlodipine than with other calcium channel blockers (usually resolves upon discontinuation); consultation with physician is suggested.

Effects on Bleeding No information available to require special precautions

Adverse Effects Frequencies reported with combination product. See individual monographs for additional adverse effects reported with each agent.

1% to 10%: Cardiovascular: Peripheral edema (6% to 9%)

General Dosage Range Oral: *Adults:* Aliskiren 150-300 mg and amlodipine 5-10 mg once daily (maximum: 300 mg daily [aliskiren]; 10 mg daily [amlodipine])

Mechanism of Action

Aliskiren: Direct renin inhibitor, resulting in blockade of the conversion of angiotensinogen to angiotensin I. Angiotensin I suppression decreases the formation of angiotensin II (Ang II), a potent blood pressure-elevating peptide (via direct vasoconstriction, aldosterone release, and sodium retention). Ang II also functions within the Renin-Angiotensin-Aldosterone System (RAAS) as a negative inhibitory feedback mediator within the renal parenchyma to suppress the further release of renin. Thus, reductions in Ang II levels suppress this feedback loop, leading to further increased plasma renin concentrations (PRC) and subsequent activity (PRA). This disinhibition effect can be potentially problematic for ACE inhibitor and ARB therapy, as increased PRA could partially overcome the pharmacologic inhibition of the RAAS. As aliskiren is a direct inhibitor of renin activity, blunting of PRA despite the increased PRC (from loss of the negative feedback) may be clinically advantageous. The effect of aliskiren on bradykinin levels is unknown.

Amlodipine: Inhibits calcium ion from entering the "slow channels" or select voltage-sensitive areas of vascular smooth muscle and myocardium during depolarization, producing a relaxation of coronary vascular smooth muscle and coronary vasodilation; increases myocardial oxygen delivery in patients with vasospastic angina. Amlodipine directly acts on vascular smooth muscle to produce peripheral arterial vasodilation reducing peripheral vascular resistance and blood pressure.

Pregnancy Risk Factor D

Pregnancy Considerations [U.S. Boxed Warning]: Drugs that act on the renin-angiotensin system can cause injury and death to the developing fetus. Discontinue as soon as possible once pregnancy is detected. Also see individual agents.

Aliskiren and Hydrochlorothiazide
(a lis KYE ren & hye droe klor oh THYE a zide)

Related Information
Aliskiren on page 63
Hydrochlorothiazide on page 687
Brand Names: U.S. Tekturna HCT®
Brand Names: Canada Rasilez HCT®
Pharmacologic Category Diuretic, Thiazide; Renin Inhibitor
Use Treatment of hypertension, including use as initial therapy in patients likely to need multiple antihypertensives for adequate control
Local Anesthetic/Vasoconstrictor Precautions No information available to require special precautions
Effects on Dental Treatment Key adverse event(s) related to dental treatment: Orthostatic hypotension
Effects on Bleeding No information available to require special precautions
Adverse Effects Frequencies reported with combination product. See individual monographs for additional adverse effects reported with each agent.
>10%: Renal: BUN increased (12%)
1% to 10%:
Central nervous system: Dizziness (2%), vertigo (1%)
Endocrine & metabolic: Hypokalemia (2%), uric acid level increased (2%), hyperkalemia (1%)
Gastrointestinal: Diarrhea (2%)
Hepatic: ALT increased (1%)
Neuromuscular & skeletal: Arthralgia (1%), weakness (1%)
Respiratory: Cough (1%)
Miscellaneous: Flu-like syndrome (2%)
Note: Angioedema, periorbital edema, and peripheral edema have been reported with aliskiren. Severe dermatologic reactions and pancreatitis have been reported with hydrochlorothiazide.
General Dosage Range Oral: *Adults:* Aliskiren 150-300 mg and hydrochlorothiazide 12.5-25 mg once daily (maximum: 300 mg daily [aliskiren]; 25 mg daily [hydrochlorothiazide])
Mechanism of Action Aliskiren is a direct renin inhibitor, resulting in blockade of the conversion of angiotensinogen to angiotensin I. Angiotensin I suppression decreases the formation of angiotensin II (Ang II), a potent blood pressure-elevating peptide (via direct vasoconstriction, aldosterone release, and sodium retention). Hydrochlorothiazide inhibits sodium reabsorption in the distal tubules causing increased excretion of sodium and water as well as potassium and hydrogen ions.
Pregnancy Risk Factor D
Pregnancy Considerations [U.S. Boxed Warning]: Drugs that act on the renin-angiotensin system can cause injury and death to the developing fetus. Discontinue as soon as possible once pregnancy is detected. Also see individual agents.

Aliskiren and Valsartan
(a lis KYE ren & val SAR tan)

Related Information
Aliskiren on page 63
Valsartan on page 1381
Brand Names: U.S. Valturna® [DSC]
Pharmacologic Category Angiotensin II Receptor Blocker; Renin Inhibitor
Use Treatment of hypertension, including use as initial therapy in patients likely to need multiple antihypertensives for adequate control
Local Anesthetic/Vasoconstrictor Precautions No information available to require special precautions
Effects on Dental Treatment Key adverse event(s) related to dental treatment: Angioedema has been reported for both aliskiren and valsartan
Effects on Bleeding No information available to require special precautions
Adverse Effects Frequencies reported with combination product. See individual monographs for additional adverse effects reported with each agent.
1% to 10%:
Central nervous system: Fatigue (3%), vertigo (1%)
Endocrine & metabolic: Hyperkalemia (4%)
Respiratory: Nasopharyngitis (3%)
Miscellaneous: Influenza (1%)
Note: Angioedema, periorbital edema, and peripheral edema have been reported with aliskiren.
General Dosage Range Oral: *Adults:* Aliskiren 150-300 mg and valsartan 160-320 mg once daily (maximum: 300 mg/day [aliskiren]; 320 mg/day [valsartan])
Mechanism of Action Aliskiren is a direct renin inhibitor, resulting in blockade of the conversion of angiotensinogen to angiotensin I. Angiotensin I suppression decreases the formation of angiotensin II (Ang II), a potent blood pressure-elevating peptide (via direct vasoconstriction, aldosterone release, and sodium retention).

Valsartan produces direct antagonism of the angiotensin II (AT2) receptors, unlike the ACE inhibitors. It displaces angiotensin II from the AT1 receptor and produces its blood pressure-lowering effects by antagonizing AT1-induced vasoconstriction, aldosterone release, catecholamine release, arginine vasopressin release, water intake, and hypertrophic responses. This action results in more efficient blockade of the cardiovascular effects of angiotensin II and fewer side effects than the ACE inhibitors.
Pregnancy Risk Factor D
Pregnancy Considerations [U.S. Boxed Warning]: Drugs that act on the renin-angiotensin system can cause injury and death to the developing fetus. Discontinue as soon as possible once pregnancy is detected. Also see individual agents.

Alitretinoin (a li TRET i noyn)

Brand Names: U.S. Panretin®
Brand Names: Canada Toctino
Pharmacologic Category Antineoplastic Agent, Miscellaneous; Retinoic Acid Derivative
Use Orphan drug: Topical treatment of cutaneous lesions in AIDS-related Kaposi's sarcoma
Unlabeled Use Cutaneous T-cell lymphomas
Local Anesthetic/Vasoconstrictor Precautions No information available to require special precautions
Effects on Dental Treatment No significant effects or complications reported
Effects on Bleeding No information available to require special precautions
Adverse Effects
>10%:
Central nervous system: Pain (0% to 34%)
Dermatologic: Rash (25% to 77%), pruritus (8% to 11%)
Neuromuscular & skeletal: Paresthesia (3% to 22%)

5% to 10%:
Cardiovascular: Edema (3% to 8%)
Dermatologic: Exfoliative dermatitis (3% to 9%), skin disorder (0% to 8%)

General Dosage Range Topical: *Adults:* Apply twice daily

Mechanism of Action Binds to retinoid receptors to inhibit growth of Kaposi's sarcoma

Pregnancy Risk Factor D

Pregnancy Considerations Potentially teratogenic and/or embryotoxic; limb, craniofacial, or skeletal defects have been observed in animal models. If used during pregnancy or if the patient becomes pregnant while using alitretinoin, the woman should be advised of potential harm to the fetus. Women of childbearing potential should avoid becoming pregnant.

Allopurinol (al oh PURE i nole)

Brand Names: U.S. Aloprim®; Zyloprim®

Brand Names: Canada Alloprin®; Novo-Purol; Zyloprim®

Pharmacologic Category Antigout Agent; Xanthine Oxidase Inhibitor

Use

Oral: Management of primary or secondary gout (acute attack, tophi, joint destruction, uric acid lithiasis, and/or nephropathy); management of hyperuricemia associated with cancer treatment for leukemia, lymphoma, or solid tumor malignancies; management of recurrent calcium oxalate calculi (with uric acid excretion >800 mg/day in men and >750 mg/day in women)

I.V.: Management of hyperuricemia associated with cancer treatment for leukemia, lymphoma, or solid tumor malignancies

Local Anesthetic/Vasoconstrictor Precautions No information available to require special precautions

Effects on Dental Treatment No significant effects or complications reported

Effects on Bleeding No information available to require special precautions

Adverse Effects

Dermatologic: Rash
Endocrine & metabolic: Gout (acute)
Gastrointestinal: Diarrhea, nausea
Hepatic: Alkaline phosphatase increased, liver enzymes increased

General Dosage Range Dosage adjustment recommended in patients with renal impairment

I.V.:

Children: Initial: 200 mg/m^2/day as a single infusion or in equally divided doses at 6-, 8-, or 12-hour intervals
Adults: 200-400 mg/m^2/day as a single infusion or in equally divided doses at 6-, 8-, or 12-hour intervals (maximum: 600 mg/day)

Oral:

Children <6 years: 150 mg/day
Children 6-10 years: 10 mg/kg/day
Children >10 years and Adults: 100-800 mg/day in 1-3 divided doses (maximum: 800 mg/day)

Mechanism of Action Allopurinol inhibits xanthine oxidase, the enzyme responsible for the conversion of hypoxanthine to xanthine to uric acid. Allopurinol is metabolized to oxypurinol which is also an inhibitor of xanthine oxidase; allopurinol acts on purine catabolism, reducing the production of uric acid without disrupting the biosynthesis of vital purines.

Pharmacodynamics/Kinetics

Onset of Action Peak effect: 1-2 weeks

Half-life Elimination

Normal renal function: Parent drug: 1-3 hours; Oxypurinol: 18-30 hours
End-stage renal disease: Prolonged

Time to Peak Plasma: Oral: 30-120 minutes

Pregnancy Risk Factor C

Pregnancy Considerations There are few reports describing the use of allopurinol during pregnancy; no adverse fetal outcomes attributable to allopurinol have been reported in humans; use only if potential benefit outweighs the potential risk to the fetus.

Almotriptan (al moh TRIP tan)

Related Information

Temporomandibular Dysfunction (TMD), Chronic Pain, and Fibromyalgia *on page 1590*

Brand Names: U.S. Axert®

Brand Names: Canada Axert®

Generic Availability (U.S.) No

Pharmacologic Category Antimigraine Agent; Serotonin 5-HT$_{1B, 1D}$ Receptor Agonist

Use Acute treatment of migraine with or without aura in adults (with a history of migraine) and adolescents (with a history of migraine lasting ≥4 hours when left untreated)

Local Anesthetic/Vasoconstrictor Precautions No information available to require special precautions

Effects on Dental Treatment Key adverse effect(s) related to dental treatment: Xerostomia (normal salivary flow resumes upon discontinuation)

Effects on Bleeding No information available to require special precautions

Adverse Effects 1% to 10%:

Central nervous system: Somnolence (≤5%), dizziness (≤4%), headache (≤2%)
Gastrointestinal: Nausea (1% to 3%), vomiting (≤2%), xerostomia (1%)
Neuromuscular & skeletal: Paresthesia (≤1%)

Dosage Oral: Children ≥12 years and Adults: Migraine: Initial: 6.25-12.5 mg in a single dose; if the headache returns, repeat the dose after 2 hours (maximum daily dose: 25 mg)

Note: The safety of treating more than 4 migraines/month has not been established.

Dosage adjustment with concomitant use of an enzyme inhibitor:

Patients receiving a potent CYP3A4 inhibitor: Initial: 6.25 mg in a single dose; maximum daily dose: 12.5 mg
Patients with renal impairment and concomitant use of a potent CYP3A4 inhibitor: Avoid use
Patients with hepatic impairment and concomitant use of a potent CYP3A4 inhibitor: Avoid use

Dosage adjustment in renal impairment: Severe renal impairment (Cl$_{cr}$ ≤30 mL/minute): Initial: 6.25 mg in a single dose; maximum daily dose: 12.5 mg

Dosage adjustment in hepatic impairment: Initial: 6.25 mg in a single dose; maximum daily dose: 12.5 mg

Mechanism of Action Selective agonist for serotonin (5-HT$_{1B}$ and 5-HT$_{1D}$ receptors) in cranial arteries; causes vasoconstriction and reduces sterile inflammation associated with antidromic neuronal transmission correlating with relief of migraine

Contraindications Hypersensitivity to almotriptan or any component of the formulation; hemiplegic or basilar migraine; known or suspected ischemic heart disease (eg, angina pectoris, MI, documented silent ischemia, coronary artery vasospasm, Prinzmetal's variant angina); cerebrovascular syndromes (eg, stroke, transient ischemic attacks); peripheral vascular disease (eg, ischemic bowel disease); uncontrolled hypertension; use within 24 hours of another 5-HT$_1$ agonist; use within 24 hours of ergotamine derivatives and/or ergotamine-containing medications (eg, dihydroergotamine, ergotamine)

Warnings/Precautions Almotriptan is only indicated for the treatment of acute migraine headache; not indicated for migraine prophylaxis, or the treatment of cluster headaches, hemiplegic migraine, or basilar migraine. If a patient does not respond to the first dose, the diagnosis of acute migraine should be reconsidered.

Almotriptan should not be given to patients with documented ischemic or vasospastic CAD. Patients with risk factors for CAD (eg, hypertension, hypercholesterolemia, smoker, obesity, diabetes, strong family history of CAD, menopause, male >40 years of age) should undergo adequate cardiac evaluation prior to administration; if the cardiac evaluation is "satisfactory," the first dose of almotriptan should be given in the healthcare provider's office (consider ECG monitoring). All patients should undergo periodic evaluation of cardiovascular status during treatment. Cardiac events (coronary artery vasospasm, transient ischemia, myocardial infarction, ventricular tachycardia/fibrillation, cardiac arrest, and death), cerebral/subarachnoid hemorrhage, stroke, peripheral vascular ischemia, and colonic ischemia have been reported with 5-HT$_1$ agonist administration. Patients who experience sensations of chest pain/pressure/tightness or symptoms suggestive of angina following dosing should be evaluated for coronary artery disease or Prinzmetal's angina before receiving additional doses; if dosing is resumed and similar symptoms recur, monitor with ECG. Significant elevation in blood pressure, including hypertensive crisis, has also been reported on rare occasions following 5-HT$_1$ agonist administration in patients with and without a history of hypertension.

Transient and permanent blindness and partial vision loss have been reported (rare) with 5-HT$_1$ agonist administration. Almotriptan contains a sulfonyl group which is structurally different from a sulfonamide. Cross-reactivity in patients with sulfonamide allergy has not been evaluated; however, the manufacturer recommends that caution be exercised in this patient population. Use with caution in liver or renal dysfunction. Symptoms of agitation, confusion, hallucinations, hyperreflexia, myoclonus, shivering, and tachycardia (serotonin syndrome) may occur with concomitant proserotonergic drugs (ie, SSRIs/SNRIs or triptans) or agents which reduce almotriptan's metabolism. Concurrent use of serotonin precursors (eg, tryptophan) is not recommended. If concomitant administration with SSRIs is warranted, monitor closely, especially at initiation and with dose increases. Efficacy has not been demonstrated in improvement of migraine-associated symptoms (eg, phonophobia, nausea, photophobia) in patients aged 12-17 years (Linder, 2008).

Drug Interactions

Metabolism/Transport Effects Substrate of CYP2D6 (minor), CYP3A4 (minor); **Note:** Assignment of Major/Minor substrate status based on clinically relevant drug interaction potential

Avoid Concomitant Use
Avoid concomitant use of Almotriptan with any of the following: Ergot Derivatives; MAO Inhibitors

Increased Effect/Toxicity
Almotriptan may increase the levels/effects of: Ergot Derivatives; Metoclopramide; Serotonin Modulators

The levels/effects of Almotriptan may be increased by: Antipsychotics; CYP3A4 Inhibitors (Strong); Ergot Derivatives; MAO Inhibitors

Decreased Effect
The levels/effects of Almotriptan may be decreased by: Peginterferon Alfa-2b

Dietary Considerations May be taken without regard to meals.

Pharmacodynamics/Kinetics
Half-life Elimination 3-4 hours
Time to Peak Plasma: 1-3 hours

Pregnancy Risk Factor C

Pregnancy Considerations There are no adequate and well-controlled studies in pregnant women. Use in pregnancy should be limited to situations where benefit outweighs risk to fetus. In some (but not all) animal studies, administration was associated with embryolethality, fetal malformations, and decreased pup weight.

Lactation Excretion in breast milk unknown/use caution

Dosage Forms
Tablet, oral:
Axert®: 6.25 mg, 12.5 mg

Alosetron (a LOE se tron)

Brand Names: U.S. Lotronex®
Pharmacologic Category Selective 5-HT$_3$ Receptor Antagonist

Use Treatment of women with severe diarrhea-predominant irritable bowel syndrome (IBS) who have failed to respond to conventional therapy

Local Anesthetic/Vasoconstrictor Precautions No information available to require special precautions

Effects on Dental Treatment No significant effects or complications reported

Effects on Bleeding No information available to require special precautions

Adverse Effects
>10%: Gastrointestinal: Constipation (dose related; 9% to 29%)

1% to 10%:
Central nervous system: Fatigue (≥3%), headache (≥3%)
Gastrointestinal: Abdominal discomfort and pain (1% to 7%), nausea (6%), gastrointestinal discomfort and pain (5%), gastroenteritis (≥3%), vomiting (≥3%), diarrhea (2% to 3%), flatulence (1% to 3%), hemorrhoids (1% to 3%), abdominal distention (2%), regurgitation and reflux (2%)
Genitourinary: Urinary tract infection (≥3%)
Neuromuscular & skeletal: Muscle spasm (≥3%)
Respiratory: Cough (≥3%), nasopharyngitis (≥3%), upper respiratory tract infection (≥3%)

General Dosage Range Oral: *Adults:* Initial: 0.5 mg twice daily; may increase to 1 mg twice daily if needed (maximum: 2 mg/day)

Mechanism of Action Alosetron is a potent and selective antagonist of a subtype of the serotonin 5-HT$_3$ receptor. 5-HT$_3$ receptors are ligand-gated ion channels extensively distributed on enteric neurons in the human gastrointestinal tract, as well as other peripheral and central locations. Activation of these channels affect the regulation of visceral pain, colonic transit, and gastrointestinal secretions. In patients with irritable bowel syndrome, blockade of these channels may reduce pain, abdominal discomfort, urgency, and diarrhea.

Pharmacodynamics/Kinetics

Half-life Elimination 1.5 hours

Time to Peak 1 hour

Pregnancy Risk Factor B

Pregnancy Considerations There are no adequate and well-controlled studies in pregnant women. Alosetron should be used in pregnant women only if clearly needed.

Prescribing and Access Restrictions As a requirement of the REMS program, access to the medication is restricted. Physicians must enroll in the Prometheus Prescribing Program for Lotronex® (www.lotronexppl.com or 1-888-423-5227) in order to prescribe this medication. Program stickers must be affixed to all prescriptions; no phone, fax, or computerized prescriptions are permitted with this program.

Alpha₁-Proteinase Inhibitor
(al fa won PRO tee in ase in HI bi tor)

Brand Names: U.S. Aralast NP; Glassia™; Prolastin®-C; Zemaira®

Brand Names: Canada Prolastin®-C

Pharmacologic Category Antitrypsin Deficiency Agent; Blood Product Derivative

Use Replacement therapy in congenital alpha₁-proteinase inhibitor (alpha₁-antitrypsin, A₁-PI) deficiency with clinical emphysema

Local Anesthetic/Vasoconstrictor Precautions No information available to require special precautions

Effects on Dental Treatment Key adverse event(s) related to dental treatment: Pharyngitis

Effects on Bleeding No information available to require special precautions

Adverse Effects Frequency not defined. Actual incidence may vary by product.

Cardiovascular: Chest pain, peripheral edema, vasodilation

Central nervous system: Chills, dizziness, fever, headache, lightheadedness, malaise, migraine, pain, somnolence

Dermatologic: Bruising, pruritus, rash

Endocrine & metabolic: Hot flushes

Gastrointestinal: Abdominal pain, bloating, cholangitis, diarrhea, dyspepsia, nausea, sore throat

Genitourinary: Urinary tract infection

Hematologic: Hemorrhage

Hepatic: Transaminases increased

Local: Injection site reactions (including hemorrhage and pain)

Neuromuscular & skeletal: Arthralgia, back pain, musculoskeletal discomfort, paresthesia, weakness

Ocular: Vision changes

Respiratory: Asthma exacerbation, bronchitis, bronchospasm, COPD exacerbation, cough, dyspnea, pharyngitis, respiratory tract infection (lower/upper), rhinitis, sinusitis

Miscellaneous: Flu-like syndrome, infection

General Dosage Range I.V.: *Adults:* 60 mg/kg once weekly

Mechanism of Action Alpha₁-antitrypsin (AAT) is the principle protease inhibitor in serum. Its major physiologic role is to render proteolytic enzymes (secreted during inflammation) inactive. A decrease in AAT, as seen in congenital AAT deficiency, leads to increased elastic damage in the lung, causing emphysema.

Pharmacodynamics/Kinetics

Half-life Elimination Metabolic: ~5-6 days

Time to Peak Serum: ~1 hour; threshold levels achieved after 3 weeks

Pregnancy Risk Factor C

Pregnancy Considerations Reproduction studies have not been conducted.

ALPRAZolam (al PRAY zoe lam)

Related Information

Management of the Patient With Anxiety or Depression *on page 1594*

Temporomandibular Dysfunction (TMD), Chronic Pain, and Fibromyalgia *on page 1590*

Related Sample Prescriptions

Sedation (Prior to Dental Treatment) *on page 1621*

Brand Names: U.S. Alprazolam Intensol™; Niravam™; Xanax XR®; Xanax®

Brand Names: Canada Apo-Alpraz®; Apo-Alpraz® TS; Mylan-Alprazolam; NTP-Alprazolam; Nu-Alpraz; Teva-Alprazolam; Xanax TS™; Xanax®

Generic Availability (U.S.) Yes: Excludes oral solution

Pharmacologic Category Benzodiazepine

Dental Use Preoperative anxiety

Use Treatment of anxiety disorder (GAD); short-term relief of symptoms of anxiety; panic disorder, with or without agoraphobia; anxiety associated with depression

Unlabeled Use Anxiety in children

Local Anesthetic/Vasoconstrictor Precautions No information available to require special precautions

Effects on Dental Treatment Key adverse event(s) related to dental treatment: Significant xerostomia and changes in salivation (normal salivary flow resumes upon discontinuation)

Effects on Bleeding No information available to require special precautions

Adverse Effects

>10%:

Central nervous system: Abnormal coordination, cognitive disorder, depression, drowsiness, fatigue, irritability, lightheadedness, memory impairment, sedation, somnolence

Endocrine & metabolic: Libido decreased

Gastrointestinal: Appetite increased/decreased, constipation, weight gain/loss, xerostomia

Genitourinary: Micturition difficulty

Neuromuscular & skeletal: Dysarthria

Respiratory: Nasal congestion

1% to 10%:

Cardiovascular: Chest pain, hypotension, palpitation, sinus tachycardia

Central nervous system: Agitation, akathisia, ataxia, attention disturbance, confusion, depersonalization, derealization, disorientation, disinhibition, dizziness, dream abnormalities, fear, hallucination, headache, hypersomnia, hypoesthesia, insomnia, lethargy, malaise, mental impairment, nervousness, nightmares, restlessness, seizure, syncope, talkativeness, vertigo

Dermatologic: Dermatitis, rash

Endocrine & metabolic: Dysmenorrhea, libido increased, menstrual disorders, sexual dysfunction

Gastrointestinal: Abdominal pain, anorexia, diarrhea, dyspepsia, nausea, salivation increased, vomiting

Genitourinary: Incontinence

Hepatic: Bilirubin increased, jaundice, liver enzymes increased

Neuromuscular & skeletal: Arthralgia, back pain, dyskinesia, dystonia, muscle cramps, muscle twitching, myalgia, paresthesia, tremor, weakness

Ocular: Blurred vision

Respiratory: Allergic rhinitis, dyspnea, hyperventilation, upper respiratory infection

Miscellaneous: Diaphoresis

Dental Usual Dosage Preoperative anxiety (unlabeled use) Adults: Oral: 0.5 mg 60-90 minutes before procedure (De Witte, 2002)

Dosage Oral: **Note:** Treatment >4 months should be re-evaluated to determine the patient's continued need for the drug

Children: Anxiety (unlabeled use): Immediate release: Initial: 0.005 mg/kg/dose or 0.125 mg/dose 3 times/day; increase in increments of 0.125-0.25 mg, up to a maximum of 0.02 mg/kg/dose or 0.06 mg/kg/day (range of doses reported in one study: 0.375-3 mg/day) (Pfefferbaum, 1987). See "Dose Reduction" comment below.

Adults:

Anxiety: Immediate release: Initial: 0.25-0.5 mg 3 times/day; titrate dose upward every 3-4 days; usual maximum: 4 mg/day. Patients requiring doses >4 mg/day should be increased cautiously. Periodic reassessment and consideration of dosage reduction is recommended.

Panic disorder:

Immediate release: Initial: 0.5 mg 3 times/day; dose may be increased every 3-4 days in increments ≤1 mg/day. Mean effective dosage: 5-6 mg/day; some patients may require much as 10 mg/day

Extended release: 0.5-1 mg once daily; may increase dose every 3-4 days in increments ≤1 mg/day (range: 3-6 mg/day)

Switching from immediate release to extended release: Patients may be switched to extended release tablets by taking the total daily dose of the immediate release tablets and giving it once daily using the extended release preparation.

Preoperative anxiety (unlabeled use): 0.5 mg 60-90 minutes before procedure (De Witte, 2002)

Dose reduction: Abrupt discontinuation should be avoided. Daily dose may be decreased by 0.5 mg every 3 days; however, some patients may require a slower reduction. If withdrawal symptoms occur, resume previous dose and discontinue on a less rapid schedule.

Elderly: **Note:** Elderly patients may be more sensitive to the effects of alprazolam including ataxia and oversedation. The elderly may also have impaired renal function leading to decreased clearance. Titrate gradually, if needed and tolerated.

Immediate release: Initial: 0.25 mg 2-3 times/day

Extended release: Initial: 0.5 mg once daily

Dosing adjustment in renal impairment: No dosage adjustment provided in manufacturer's labeling; however, use caution

Dosing adjustment in hepatic impairment: Advanced liver disease:

Immediate release: 0.25 mg 2-3 times/day; titrate gradually if needed and tolerated

Extended release: 0.5 mg once daily; titrate gradually if needed and tolerated

Mechanism of Action Binds to stereospecific benzodiazepine receptors on the postsynaptic GABA neuron at several sites within the central nervous system, including the limbic system, reticular formation. Enhancement of the inhibitory effect of GABA on neuronal excitability results by increased neuronal membrane permeability to chloride ions. This shift in chloride ions results in hyperpolarization (a less excitable state) and stabilization.

Contraindications Hypersensitivity to alprazolam or any component of the formulation (cross-sensitivity with other benzodiazepines may exist); narrow-angle glaucoma; concurrent use with ketoconazole or itraconazole

Warnings/Precautions Rebound or withdrawal symptoms, including seizures, may occur following abrupt discontinuation or large decreases in dose (more common in patients receiving >4 mg/day or prolonged treatment); the risk of seizures appears to be greatest 24-72 hours following discontinuation of therapy. Breakthrough anxiety may occur at the end of dosing interval. Use with caution in patients receiving concurrent CYP3A4 inhibitors, moderate or strong CYP3A4 inducers, and major CYP3A4 substrates; consider alternative agents that avoid or lessen the potential for CYP-mediated interactions. Use with caution in renal impairment or predisposition to urate nephropathy; has weak uricosuric properties. In older adults, benzodiazepines increase the risk of impaired cognition, delirium, falls, fractures, and motor vehicle accidents. Due to increased sensitivity in this age group, avoid use for treatment of insomnia, agitation, or delirium (Beers Criteria). Use with caution in or debilitated patients, patients with hepatic disease (including alcoholics) or respiratory disease, or obese patients.

Causes CNS depression (dose related) which may impair physical and mental capabilities. Patients must be cautioned about performing tasks that require mental alertness (eg, operating machinery or driving). Effects with other sedative drugs or ethanol may be potentiated. Benzodiazepines have been associated with falls and traumatic injury and should be used with extreme caution in patients who are at risk of these events.

Use caution in patients with depression, particularly if suicidal risk may be present. Episodes of mania or hypomania have occurred in depressed patients treated with alprazolam. May cause physical or psychological dependence. Acute withdrawal may be precipitated in patients after administration of flumazenil.

Benzodiazepines have been associated with anterograde amnesia. Paradoxical reactions have been reported with benzodiazepines, particularly in adolescent/pediatric or psychiatric patients. Does not have analgesic, antidepressant, or antipsychotic properties.

Drug Interactions

Metabolism/Transport Effects Substrate of CYP3A4 (major); **Note:** Assignment of Major/Minor substrate status based on clinically relevant drug interaction potential

Avoid Concomitant Use

Avoid concomitant use of ALPRAZolam with any of the following: Azelastine (Nasal); Conivaptan; Indinavir; OLANZapine; Paraldehyde; Sodium Oxybate

Increased Effect/Toxicity

ALPRAZolam may increase the levels/effects of: Alcohol (Ethyl); Azelastine (Nasal); Buprenorphine; CloZAPine; CNS Depressants; Methotrimeprazine; Metyrosine; Mirtazapine; Paraldehyde; Pramipexole; ROPINIRole; Rotigotine; Selective Serotonin Reuptake Inhibitors; Sodium Oxybate; Zolpidem

The levels/effects of ALPRAZolam may be increased by: Antifungal Agents (Azole Derivatives, Systemic); Aprepitant; Boceprevir; Calcium Channel Blockers (Nondihydropyridine); Cimetidine; Conivaptan; Contraceptives (Estrogens); Contraceptives (Progestins); CYP3A4 Inhibitors (Moderate); CYP3A4 Inhibitors (Strong); Dasatinib; Droperidol; Fosaprepitant; Grapefruit Juice; HydrOXYzine; Indinavir; Isoniazid; Ivacaftor; Macrolide Antibiotics; Magnesium Sulfate; Methotrimeprazine; Mifepristone; OLANZapine; Perampanel; Protease Inhibitors; Proton Pump Inhibitors; Selective Serotonin Reuptake Inhibitors; Telaprevir

Decreased Effect

The levels/effects of ALPRAZolam may be decreased by: CarBAMazepine; CYP3A4 Inducers (Strong); Deferasirox; Rifamycin Derivatives; St Johns Wort; Theophylline Derivatives; Tocilizumab; Yohimbine

Ethanol/Nutrition/Herb Interactions

Cigarette: Smoking may decrease alprazolam concentrations up to 50%.

Ethanol: Ethanol may increase CNS depression. Management: Avoid ethanol.

Food: Alprazolam serum concentration is unlikely to be increased by grapefruit juice because of alprazolam's high oral bioavailability. The C_{max} of the extended release formulation is increased by 25% when a high-fat meal is given 2 hours before dosing. T_{max} is decreased 33% when food is given immediately prior to dose and increased by 33% when food is given ≥1 hour after dose.

Herb/Nutraceutical: St John's wort may decrease alprazolam levels. Valerian, kava kava, and gotu kola may increase CNS depression. Management: Avoid St John's wort. Avoid valerian, kava kava, and gotu kola.

Dietary Considerations

Extended release tablet should be taken once daily in the morning.

Pharmacodynamics/Kinetics

Onset of Action Immediate release and extended release formulations: 1 hour

Duration of Action Immediate release: 5.1 ± 1.7 hours; Extended release: 11.3 ± 4.2 hours

Half-life Elimination

Adults: 11.2 hours (Immediate release range: 6.3-26.9 hours; Extended release range: 10.7-15.8 hours); Orally-disintegrating tablet range: 7.9-19.2 hours)

Elderly: 16.3 hours (range: 9-26.9 hours)

Alcoholic liver disease: 19.7 hours (range: 5.8-65.3 hours)

Obesity: 21.8 hours (range: 9.9-40.4 hours)

Race: Asians: Increased by ~25% (as compared to Caucasians)

Time to Peak

Immediate release: 1-2 hours

Extended release: ~9 hours (Glue, 2006); decreased by 1 hour when administered at bedtime (as compared to morning administration); decreased by 33% when administered with a high-fat meal; increased by 33% when administered ≥1 hour after a high-fat meal

Orally-disintegrating tablet: 1.5-2 hours; occurs ~15 minutes earlier when administered with water; decreased by 2 hours when administered with a high-fat meal

Pregnancy Risk Factor D

Pregnancy Considerations Benzodiazepines have the potential to cause harm to the fetus. Alprazolam and its metabolites cross the human placenta. Teratogenic effects have been observed with some benzodiazepines; however, additional studies are needed. The incidence of premature birth and low birth weights may be increased following maternal use of benzodiazepines; hypoglycemia and respiratory problems in the neonate may occur following exposure late in pregnancy. Neonatal withdrawal symptoms may occur within days to weeks after birth and "floppy infant syndrome" (which also includes withdrawal symptoms) has been reported with some benzodiazepines.

Lactation Enters breast milk/not recommended (AAP rates "of concern"; AAP 2001 update pending)

Breast-Feeding Considerations In a study of eight postpartum women, peak concentrations of alprazolam were found in breast milk ~1 hour after the maternal dose and the half-life was ~14 hours. Samples were obtained over 36 hours following a single oral dose of alprazolam 0.5 mg. Metabolites were not detected in breast milk. In this study, the estimated exposure to the breast-feeding infant was ~3% of the weight-adjusted maternal dose. Drowsiness, lethargy, or weight loss in nursing infants have been observed in case reports following maternal use of some benzodiazepines.

Controlled Substance C-IV

Dosage Forms

Solution, oral:

Alprazolam Intensol™: 1 mg/mL (30 mL)

Tablet, oral: 0.25 mg, 0.5 mg, 1 mg, 2 mg

Xanax®: 0.25 mg, 0.5 mg, 1 mg, 2 mg

Tablet, extended release, oral: 0.5 mg, 1 mg, 2 mg, 3 mg

Xanax XR®: 0.5 mg, 1 mg, 2 mg, 3 mg

Tablet, orally disintegrating, oral: 0.25 mg, 0.5 mg, 1 mg, 2 mg

Niravam™: 0.25 mg, 0.5 mg, 1 mg, 2 mg

Alprostadil (al PROS ta dill)

Brand Names: U.S. Caverject Impulse®; Caverject®; Edex®; Muse®; Prostin VR Pediatric®

Brand Names: Canada Alprostadil Injection USP; Caverject®; Muse® Pellet; Prostin® VR

Pharmacologic Category Prostaglandin; Vasodilator

Use

Prostin VR Pediatric®: Temporary maintenance of patency of ductus arteriosus in neonates with ductal-dependent congenital heart disease until surgery can be performed. These defects include cyanotic (eg, pulmonary atresia, pulmonary stenosis, tricuspid atresia, Fallot's tetralogy, transposition of the great vessels) and acyanotic (eg, interruption of aortic arch, coarctation of aorta, hypoplastic left ventricle) heart disease.

Caverject®: Treatment of erectile dysfunction of vasculogenic, psychogenic, or neurogenic etiology; adjunct in the diagnosis of erectile dysfunction

Edex®, Muse®: Treatment of erectile dysfunction of vasculogenic, psychogenic, or neurogenic etiology

Unlabeled Use Treatment of pulmonary hypertension in infants and children with congenital heart defects with left-to-right shunts

Local Anesthetic/Vasoconstrictor Precautions No information available to require special precautions

Effects on Dental Treatment No significant effects or complications reported

Effects on Bleeding No information available to require special precautions

Adverse Effects

Intraurethral:

>10%: Genitourinary: Penile pain, urethral burning

2% to 10%:

Central nervous system: Headache, dizziness, pain

Genitourinary: Vaginal itching (female partner), testicular pain, urethral bleeding (minor)

Intracavernosal injection:

>10%: Genitourinary: Penile pain

1% to 10%:

Cardiovascular: Hypertension

Central nervous system: Headache, dizziness

Genitourinary: Prolonged erection (>4 hours, 4%), penile fibrosis, penis disorder, penile rash, penile edema

Local: Injection site hematoma and/or bruising

Intravenous:

>10%:

Cardiovascular: Flushing

Central nervous system: Fever

Respiratory: Apnea

1% to 10%:

Cardiovascular: Bradycardia, hyper-/hypotension, tachycardia, cardiac arrest, edema

Central nervous system: Seizure, headache, dizziness

Endocrine & metabolic: Hypokalemia

Gastrointestinal: Diarrhea

Hematologic: Disseminated intravascular coagulation

Neuromuscular & skeletal: Back pain

Respiratory: Upper respiratory infection, flu syndrome, sinusitis, nasal congestion, cough

Miscellaneous: Sepsis, localized pain in structures other than the injection site

General Dosage Range

I.V.: *Neonates:* Initial: 0.05-0.1 mcg/kg/minute; Maintenance: 0.01-0.4 mcg/kg/minute

Intracavernous: *Adults:* Initial: 1.25-2.5 mcg; Maintenance: Increase to effective dose no more than 3 times/week with at least 24 hours between doses (maximum: 40 mcg/dose [Edex®]; 60 mcg/dose [Caverject®])

Intraurethral: *Adults:* Initial: 125-250 mcg; Maintenance: As needed (maximum: 2 doses/day)

Mechanism of Action Causes vasodilation by means of direct effect on vascular and ductus arteriosus smooth muscle; relaxes trabecular smooth muscle by dilation of cavernosal arteries when injected along the penile shaft, allowing blood flow to and entrapment in the lacunar spaces of the penis (ie, corporeal veno-occlusive mechanism)

Pharmacodynamics/Kinetics

Onset of Action Rapid

Duration of Action <1 hour

Half-life Elimination 5-10 minutes

Pregnancy Risk Factor X/C (Muse®)

Pregnancy Considerations Alprostadil is embryotoxic in animal studies. It is not indicated for use in women. The manufacturer of Muse® recommends a condom barrier when being used during sexual intercourse with a pregnant women.

Alteplase (AL te plase)

Related Information

Cardiovascular Diseases *on page 1492*

Brand Names: U.S. Activase®; Cathflo® Activase®

Brand Names: Canada Activase® rt-PA; Cathflo® Activase®

Pharmacologic Category Thrombolytic Agent

Use Management of ST-elevation myocardial infarction (STEMI) for the lysis of thrombi in coronary arteries; management of acute ischemic stroke (AIS); management of acute pulmonary embolism (PE)

Recommended criteria for treatment:

STEMI (ACCF/AHA; O'Gara, 2013): Ischemic symptoms within 12 hours of treatment or evidence of ongoing ischemia 12-24 hours after symptom onset with a large area of myocardium at risk or hemodynamic instability.

STEMI ECG definition: New ST-segment elevation at the J point in at least 2 contiguous leads of ≥2 mm (0.2 mV) in men or ≥1.5 mm (0.15 mV) in women in leads V_2-V_3 and/or of ≥1 mm (0.1 mV) in other contiguous precordial leads or limb leads. New or presumably new left bundle branch block (LBBB) may interfere with ST-elevation analysis and should not be considered diagnostic in isolation.

At non-PCI-capable hospitals, the ACCF/AHA recommends thrombolytic therapy administration when the anticipated first medical contact (FMC)-to-device time at a PCI-capable hospital is >120 minutes due to unavoidable delays.

AIS: Onset of stroke symptoms within 3 hours of treatment

Acute pulmonary embolism: Age ≤75 years: Documented massive PE (defined as acute PE with sustained hypotension [SBP <90 mm Hg for ≤15 minutes or requiring inotropic support], persistent profound bradycardia [HR <40 bpm with signs or symptoms of shock], or pulselessness); alteplase may be considered for submassive PE with clinical evidence of adverse prognosis (eg, new hemodynamic instability, worsening respiratory insufficiency, severe RV dysfunction, or major myocardial necrosis) and low risk of bleeding complications. **Note:** Not recommended for patients with low-risk PE (eg, normotensive, no RV dysfunction, normal biomarkers) or submassive acute PE with minor RV dysfunction, minor myocardial necrosis, and no clinical worsening (Jaff, 2011).

Cathflo® Activase®: Restoration of central venous catheter function

Unlabeled Use Acute ischemic stroke presenting 3-4.5 hours after symptom onset; acute peripheral arterial occlusion; infected parapneumonic effusion (with [adult] or without [pediatric] dornase alfa); prosthetic valve thrombosis; intra-arterial administration for patients who have contraindications to I.V. use (**Note:** Intra-arterial administration requires patient to be at an experienced stroke center with rapid access to cerebral angiography and qualified interventionalists)

Local Anesthetic/Vasoconstrictor Precautions No information available to require special precautions

Effects on Dental Treatment Key adverse event(s) related to dental treatment: As with all drugs which may affect hemostasis, bleeding is the major adverse effect associated with alteplase. Hemorrhage may occur at virtually any site; risk is dependent on multiple variables, including the dosage administered, concurrent use of multiple agents which alter hemostasis, and patient predisposition. Rapid lysis of coronary artery thrombi by thrombolytic agents may be associated with reperfusion-related atrial and/or ventricular arrhythmias. See Effects on Bleeding.

Effects on Bleeding Bleeding is the major adverse effect associated with thrombolytic agents, such as alteplase. It is unlikely that ambulatory patients presenting for dental treatment will be taking parenteral thrombolytic therapy.

Adverse Effects As with all drugs which may affect hemostasis, bleeding is the major adverse effect associated with alteplase. Hemorrhage may occur at virtually any site. Risk is dependent on multiple variables, including the dosage administered, concurrent use of multiple agents which alter hemostasis, and patient predisposition. Rapid lysis of coronary artery thrombi by thrombolytic agents may be associated with reperfusion-related atrial and/or ventricular arrhythmia. **Note:** Lowest rate of bleeding complications expected with dose used to restore catheter function.

1% to 10%:
Cardiovascular: Hypotension
Central nervous system: Fever
Dermatologic: Bruising (1%)
Gastrointestinal: GI hemorrhage (5%), nausea, vomiting
Genitourinary: GU hemorrhage (4%)
Hematologic: Bleeding (0.5% major, 7% minor; GUSTO trial)
Local: Bleeding at catheter puncture site (15.3%, accelerated administration)

Additional cardiovascular events associated **with use in STEMI:** AV block, cardiogenic shock, heart failure, cardiac arrest, recurrent ischemia/infarction, myocardial rupture, electromechanical dissociation, pericardial effusion, pericarditis, mitral regurgitation, cardiac tamponade, thromboembolism, pulmonary edema, asystole, ventricular tachycardia, bradycardia, ruptured intracranial AV malformation, seizure, hemorrhagic bursitis, cholesterol crystal embolization

Additional events associated **with use in pulmonary embolism:** Pulmonary re-embolization, pulmonary edema, pleural effusion, thromboembolism

Additional events associated **with use in stroke:** Cerebral edema, cerebral herniation, seizure, new ischemic stroke

General Dosage Range
Intracatheter:
Children <30 kg: 110% of the internal lumen volume of the catheter; retain in catheter for 0.5-2 hours; may repeat once (maximum: 2 mg/2 mL/dose)
Children ≥30 kg and Adults: 2 mg (2 mL) retain in catheter for 0.5-2 hours; may repeat once
I.V. infusion: *Adults:* Dosage varies greatly depending on indication

Mechanism of Action Initiates local fibrinolysis by binding to fibrin in a thrombus (clot) and converts entrapped plasminogen to plasmin

Pharmacodynamics/Kinetics
Duration of Action >50% present in plasma cleared ~5 minutes after infusion terminated; ~80% cleared within 10 minutes

Pregnancy Risk Factor C

Pregnancy Considerations Teratogenic effects were not observed in animal studies. There are no adequate and well-controlled studies in pregnant women. The risk of bleeding may be increased in pregnant women. Use during pregnancy is limited; administer to pregnant women only if the potential benefits justify the risk to the fetus.

Altretamine (al TRET a meen)

Brand Names: U.S. Hexalen®
Brand Names: Canada Hexalen®
Pharmacologic Category Antineoplastic Agent, Miscellaneous
Use Palliative treatment of persistent or recurrent ovarian cancer
Local Anesthetic/Vasoconstrictor Precautions No information available to require special precautions
Effects on Dental Treatment No significant effects or complications reported
Effects on Bleeding Chemotherapy may result in significant myelosuppression, including thrombocytopenia. In patients who are under active treatment, a medical consult is suggested.
Adverse Effects
>10%:
Gastrointestinal: Nausea/vomiting (33%; severe 1%)
Hematologic: Anemia (33%), leukopenia (5% to 15%; grade 4: <1%)
Neuromuscular & skeletal: Peripheral sensory neuropathy (31%; mild: 9%; moderate-to-severe: 9%)
1% to 10%:
Central nervous system: Fatigue, seizure
Gastrointestinal: Anorexia
Hematologic: Thrombocytopenia
Hepatic: Alkaline phosphatase increased
Renal: BUN increased, serum creatinine increased
General Dosage Range Dosage adjustment recommended in patients who develop toxicities
Oral: *Adults:* 260 mg/m^2/day in 4 divided doses for 14 or 21 days of a 28-day cycle
Mechanism of Action Altretamine structurally resembles alkylating agents, although has demonstrated activity in tumors resistant to classic alkylating agents. Cytotoxic effect not fully characterized, however it is theorized that metabolically activated oxidative N-demethylation intermediates bind to and damage DNA.
Pharmacodynamics/Kinetics
Half-life Elimination ~7 hours (range: 2-10 hours)
Time to Peak Plasma: 0.5-3 hours
Pregnancy Risk Factor D
Pregnancy Considerations Teratogenic effects were noted in animal studies. There are no adequate and well-controlled studies in pregnant women. May cause fetal harm if administered during pregnancy. Women of childbearing potential should avoid becoming pregnant while on therapy.

Aluminum Chloride (a LOO mi num KLOR ide)

Related Information
Antiplatelet and Anticoagulation Considerations in Dentistry *on page 1503*
Brand Names: U.S. Hemodent™
Generic Availability (U.S.) No
Pharmacologic Category Astringent; Hemostatic Agent
Dental Use Hemostatic; gingival retraction; to control bleeding created during a dental procedure
Use Hemostatic
Local Anesthetic/Vasoconstrictor Precautions No information available to require special precautions
Effects on Dental Treatment No significant effects or complications reported
Effects on Bleeding No information available to require special precautions

Adverse Effects No data reported.

Dental Usual Dosage Control of dental bleeding: Apply retraction cord as directed

Dosage Control of bleeding: Apply retraction cord as directed

Dosage adjustment in renal impairment: No dosage adjustment provided in manufacturer's labeling.

Dosage adjustment in hepatic impairment: No dosage adjustment provided in manufacturer's labeling.

Mechanism of Action Precipitates tissue and blood proteins causing a mechanical obstruction to hemorrhage from injured blood vessels

Contraindications No data reported

Warnings/Precautions Since large amounts of astringents may cause tissue irritation and possible damage, only small amounts should be applied.

Drug Interactions

Metabolism/Transport Effects None known.

Avoid Concomitant Use There are no known interactions where it is recommended to avoid concomitant use.

Increased Effect/Toxicity There are no known significant interactions involving an increase in effect.

Decreased Effect There are no known significant interactions involving a decrease in effect.

Dosage Forms

Liquid, oral topical:
Hemodent™: 21% (10 mL, 20 mL, 40 mL)

Aluminum Hydroxide
(a LOO mi num hye DROKS ide)

Brand Names: U.S. ALternaGel® [OTC]; Dermagran® [OTC]

Brand Names: Canada Amphojel®; Basaljel®

Pharmacologic Category Antacid; Antidote; Protectant, Topical

Use Treatment of hyperacidity; hyperphosphatemia; temporary protection of minor cuts, scrapes, and burns

Local Anesthetic/Vasoconstrictor Precautions No information available to require special precautions

Effects on Dental Treatment Key adverse event(s) related to dental treatment: Chalky taste. Aluminum and magnesium ions prevent GI absorption of tetracycline by forming a large ionized chelated molecule with the aluminum ion and tetracyclines in the stomach. Aluminum hydroxide prevents GI absorption of ketoconazole and itraconazole by increasing the pH in the GI tract. Any of these drugs should be administered at least 1 hour before $Al(OH)_3$.

Effects on Bleeding No information available to require special precautions

Adverse Effects Frequency not defined.

Gastrointestinal: Constipation, discoloration of feces (white speckles), fecal impaction, nausea, stomach cramps, vomiting

Endocrine & metabolic: Hypomagnesemia, hypophosphatemia

General Dosage Range

Oral:

Children: 50-150 mg/kg/day in divided doses every 4-6 hours

Adults: 300-1200 mg 3-4 times/day

Topical: *Children and Adults:* Apply to affected area as needed; reapply at least every 12 hours

Mechanism of Action Neutralizes hydrochloride in stomach to form Al $(Cl)_3$ salt + H_2O

Pregnancy Considerations Most aluminum-containing antacids are considered low risk during pregnancy (Mahadevan, 2006).

Aluminum Hydroxide and Magnesium Carbonate
(a LOO mi num hye DROKS ide & mag NEE zhum KAR bun nate)

Related Information

Aluminum Hydroxide *on page 73*

Brand Names: U.S. Acid Gone Extra Strength [OTC]; Acid Gone [OTC]; Gaviscon® Extra Strength [OTC]; Gaviscon® Liquid [OTC]

Pharmacologic Category Antacid

Use Temporary relief of symptoms associated with gastric acidity

Local Anesthetic/Vasoconstrictor Precautions No information available to require special precautions

Effects on Dental Treatment Key adverse event(s) related to dental treatment: Chalky taste. Aluminum and magnesium ions prevent GI absorption of tetracycline by forming a large ionized chelated molecule with the tetracyclines in the stomach. Aluminum hydroxide prevents GI absorption of ketoconazole and itraconazole by increasing the pH in the GI tract. Any of these drugs should be administered at least 1 hour before aluminum hydroxide.

Effects on Bleeding No information available to require special precautions

Adverse Effects 1% to 10%:

Endocrine & metabolic: Hypermagnesemia, aluminum intoxication (prolonged use and concomitant renal failure), hypophosphatemia

Gastrointestinal: Constipation, diarrhea

Neuromuscular & skeletal: Osteomalacia

General Dosage Range Oral: *Adults:* 15-30 mL **or** 2-4 tablets 4 times/day

Pregnancy Considerations Most aluminum- and magnesium-containing antacids are considered low risk during pregnancy (Mahadevan, 2006).

Aluminum Hydroxide and Magnesium Hydroxide
(a LOO mi num hye DROKS ide & mag NEE zhum hye DROK side)

Related Information

Aluminum Hydroxide *on page 73*

Magnesium Hydroxide *on page 852*

Brand Names: U.S. Alamag [OTC]; Mag-Al Ultimate [OTC]; Mag-Al [OTC]

Brand Names: Canada Diovol®; Diovol® Ex; Gelusil® Extra Strength; Mylanta™

Pharmacologic Category Antacid

Use Antacid for symptoms related to hyperacidity associated with heartburn, hiatal hernia, upset stomach, peptic ulcer, peptic esophagitis, or gastritis

Local Anesthetic/Vasoconstrictor Precautions No information available to require special precautions

Effects on Dental Treatment Key adverse event(s) related to dental treatment: Chalky taste. Aluminum and magnesium ions prevent GI absorption of tetracycline by forming a large ionized chelated molecule with the tetracyclines in the stomach. Aluminum hydroxide prevents GI absorption of ketoconazole and itraconazole by increasing the pH in the GI tract. Any of these drugs should be administered at least 1 hour before aluminum hydroxide.

Effects on Bleeding No information available to require special precautions

Adverse Effects Frequency not defined.

Gastrointestinal: Constipation, chalky taste, cramping, fecal discoloration (white speckles), fecal impaction, nausea, vomiting

Endocrine & metabolic: Hypophosphatemia (rare), hypermagnesemia (rare)

General Dosage Range Oral: *Children ≥12 years and Adults:* 10-20 mL 4 times/day (maximum: magnesium hydroxide 4500 mg/day; aluminum hydroxide 4500 mg/day) **or** 1-2 tablets as needed (maximum: 16 tablets)

Pregnancy Considerations See individual agents.

Aluminum Hydroxide and Magnesium Trisilicate
(a LOO mi num hye DROKS ide & mag NEE zhum trye SIL i kate)

Related Information
Aluminum Hydroxide *on page 73*

Brand Names: U.S. Gaviscon® Tablet [OTC]

Pharmacologic Category Antacid

Use Temporary relief of hyperacidity

Local Anesthetic/Vasoconstrictor Precautions No information available to require special precautions

Effects on Dental Treatment Key adverse event(s) related to dental treatment: Chalky taste. Aluminum and magnesium ions prevent GI absorption of tetracycline by forming a large ionized chelated molecule with the tetracyclines in the stomach. Aluminum hydroxide prevents GI absorption of ketoconazole and itraconazole by increasing the pH in the GI tract. Any of these drugs should be administered at least 1 hour before aluminum hydroxide.

Effects on Bleeding No information available to require special precautions

General Dosage Range Oral: *Adults:* 2-4 tablets 4 times/day

Pregnancy Considerations Most aluminum-containing antacids are considered low risk during pregnancy; however, use of antacids containing magnesium trisilicate should be avoided (Mahadevan, 2006).

Aluminum Hydroxide, Magnesium Hydroxide, and Simethicone
(a LOO mi num hye DROKS ide, mag NEE zhum hye DROKS ide, & sye METH i kone)

Related Information
Aluminum Hydroxide *on page 73*
Magnesium Hydroxide *on page 852*
Simethicone *on page 1236*

Brand Names: U.S. Alamag Plus [OTC]; Aldroxicon I [OTC]; Aldroxicon II [OTC]; Almacone® Double Strength [OTC]; Almacone® [OTC]; Gelusil® [OTC]; Maalox® Advanced Maximum Strength [OTC]; Maalox® Advanced Regular Strength [OTC]; Mi-Acid Maximum Strength [OTC] [DSC]; Mi-Acid [OTC]; Mintox Plus [OTC]; Mylanta® Classic Maximum Strength Liquid [OTC]; Mylanta® Classic Regular Strength Liquid [OTC]; Rulox [OTC]

Brand Names: Canada Diovol Plus®; Gelusil®; Mylanta® Double Strength; Mylanta® Extra Strength; Mylanta® Regular Strength

Pharmacologic Category Antacid; Antiflatulent

Use Temporary relief of hyperacidity associated with gas; may also be used for indications associated with other antacids

Local Anesthetic/Vasoconstrictor Precautions No information available to require special precautions

Effects on Dental Treatment Key adverse event(s) related to dental treatment: Chalky taste. Aluminum and magnesium ions prevent GI absorption of tetracycline by forming a large ionized chelated molecule with the tetracyclines in the stomach. Aluminum hydroxide prevents GI absorption of ketoconazole and itraconazole by increasing the pH in the GI tract. Any of these drugs should be administered at least 1 hour before aluminum hydroxide.

Effects on Bleeding No information available to require special precautions

Adverse Effects

>10%: Gastrointestinal: Chalky taste, stomach cramps, constipation, bowel motility decreased, fecal impaction, hemorrhoids

1% to 10%: Gastrointestinal: Nausea, vomiting, discoloration of feces (white speckles)

General Dosage Range Oral: *Adults:* 10-20 mL or 2-4 tablets 4-6 times/day

Pregnancy Considerations See individual agents.

Aluminum Sulfate and Calcium Acetate
(a LOO mi num SUL fate & KAL see um AS e tate)

Related Information
Calcium Acetate *on page 231*

Brand Names: U.S. Domeboro® [OTC]; Gordon Boro-Packs [OTC]; Pedi-Boro® [OTC]

Pharmacologic Category Topical Skin Product

Use Astringent wet dressing for relief of inflammatory conditions of the skin; reduce weeping that may occur in dermatitis

Local Anesthetic/Vasoconstrictor Precautions No information available to require special precautions

Effects on Dental Treatment No significant effects or complications reported

Effects on Bleeding No information available to require special precautions

General Dosage Range Topical: *Adults:* Soak affected area or wet dressing in the solution 2-4 times/day

Alvimopan (al VI moe pan)

Brand Names: U.S. Entereg®

Pharmacologic Category Gastrointestinal Agent, Miscellaneous; Opioid Antagonist, Peripherally-Acting

Use Accelerate the time to upper and lower GI recovery following partial large or small bowel resection surgery with primary anastomosis

Local Anesthetic/Vasoconstrictor Precautions No information available to require special precautions

Effects on Dental Treatment No significant effects or complications reported

Effects on Bleeding No information available to require special precautions

Adverse Effects 1% to 10%: **Note:** Incidence reported limited to bowel resection patients only.

Endocrine & metabolic: Hypokalemia (10%)

Gastrointestinal: Dyspepsia (7%)

Genitourinary: Urinary retention (3%)

Hematologic: Anemia (5%)

Neuromuscular & skeletal: Back pain (3%)

General Dosage Range Oral: *Adults:* Initial: 12 mg prior to surgery; Maintenance: 12 mg twice daily (maximum: 15 doses)

Mechanism of Action An opioid receptor antagonist which blocks opioid binding at the mu receptor; alvimopan has restricted ability to cross the blood-brain barrier at therapeutic doses. It selectively and competitively binds to the GI tract mu opioid receptors and antagonizes the peripheral effects of opioids on gastrointestinal motility and secretion. Does not affect opioid analgesic effects or induce opioid withdrawal symptoms.

Pharmacodynamics/Kinetics
Half-life Elimination 10-17 hours
Time to Peak Plasma: Parent drug: ~2 hours; Metabolite: 36 hours

Pregnancy Risk Factor B

Pregnancy Considerations Animal studies have not shown teratogenic effects to the fetus. However, there are no adequate and well-controlled studies in pregnant women; use during pregnancy only if clearly needed.

Prescribing and Access Restrictions As a requirement of the REMS program, access to this medication is restricted. Only hospitals enrolled in the ENTEREG Access Support and Education (E.A.S.E.™) Program may administer this medication. Hospital staff must be educated on the need to limit to short-term (no more than 15 doses) and inpatient use. Hospitals may contact the E.A.S.E.™ program at 1-866-423-6567 (1-866-4ADOLOR).

Amantadine (a MAN ta deen)

Related Information
Systemic Viral Diseases *on page 1537*

Brand Names: Canada Dom-Amantadine; Mylan-Amantadine; PHL-Amantadine; PMS-Amantadine

Pharmacologic Category Anti-Parkinson's Agent, Dopamine Agonist; Antiviral Agent; Antiviral Agent, Adamantane

Use Prophylaxis and treatment of influenza A viral infection (per manufacturer labeling; also refer to current ACIP guidelines for recommendations during current flu season); treatment of parkinsonism; treatment of drug-induced extrapyramidal symptoms

Local Anesthetic/Vasoconstrictor Precautions No information available to require special precautions

Effects on Dental Treatment Key adverse event(s) related to dental treatment: Xerostomia (prolonged use may cause significant xerostomia; normal salivary flow resumes upon discontinuation) and orthostatic hypotension.

Effects on Bleeding No information available to require special precautions

Adverse Effects 1% to 10%:
Cardiovascular: Orthostatic hypotension, peripheral edema
Central nervous system: Agitation, anxiety, ataxia, confusion, delirium, depression, dizziness, dream abnormality, fatigue, hallucinations, headache, insomnia, irritability, lightheadedness, nervousness, somnolence
Dermatologic: Livedo reticularis
Gastrointestinal: Anorexia, constipation, diarrhea, nausea, xerostomia
Respiratory: Dry nose

General Dosage Range Dosage adjustment recommended in patients with renal impairment
Oral:
Children 1-9 years: 4.4-8.8 mg/kg/day in 2 divided doses (maximum: 150 mg/day)

Children ≥10 years and <40 kg: 5 mg/kg/day in 2 divided doses
Children ≥10 years and ≥40 kg: 100 mg twice daily (maximum: 200 mg/day)
Adults: 200-400 mg/day in 2 divided doses (maximum: 400 mg/day)
Elderly: 100-400 mg/day in 2 divided doses (maximum: 400 mg/day)

Mechanism of Action As an antiviral, blocks the uncoating of influenza A virus preventing penetration of virus into host; antiparkinsonian activity may be due to its blocking the reuptake of dopamine into presynaptic neurons or by increasing dopamine release from presynaptic fibers

Pharmacodynamics/Kinetics
Onset of Action Antidyskinetic: Within 48 hours
Half-life Elimination Normal renal function: 16 ± 6 hours (9-31 hours); Healthy, older (≥60 years) males: 29 hours (range: 20-41 hours); End-stage renal disease: 7-10 days
Time to Peak Plasma: 2-4 hours

Pregnancy Risk Factor C

Pregnancy Considerations Teratogenic effects were observed in animal studies and in case reports in humans.

Influenza infection may be more severe in pregnant women. Untreated influenza infection is associated with an increased risk of adverse events to the fetus and an increased risk of complications or death to the mother. Oseltamivir and zanamivir are currently recommended for the treatment or prophylaxis influenza in pregnant women and women up to 2 weeks postpartum. Antiviral agents are currently recommended as an adjunct to vaccination and should not be used as a substitute for vaccination in pregnant women (consult current CDC guidelines).

Healthcare providers are encouraged to refer women exposed to influenza vaccine, or who have taken an antiviral medication during pregnancy to the Vaccines and Medications in Pregnancy Surveillance System (VAMPSS) by contacting The Organization of Teratology Information Specialists (OTIS) at (877) 311-8972

Ambenonium (am be NOE nee um)

Brand Names: U.S. Mytelase® [DSC]
Pharmacologic Category Cholinergic Agonist
Use Treatment of myasthenia gravis

Local Anesthetic/Vasoconstrictor Precautions No information available to require special precautions

Effects on Dental Treatment No significant effects or complications reported

Effects on Bleeding No information available to require special precautions

Adverse Effects Frequency not defined.
Central nervous system: Anxiety, malaise, vertigo
Gastrointestinal: Abdominal cramps, diarrhea, nausea, salivation, vomiting
Genitourinary: Urinary urgency
Neuromuscular & skeletal: Fasciculations, muscle cramps
Ocular: Lacrimation, miosis
Respiratory: Bronchial secretions increased
Miscellaneous: Diaphoresis increased

General Dosage Range Oral: *Adults:* Usual dose: 5-25 mg 3-4 times/day; some patients may require as much as 50-75 mg/dose

Mechanism of Action Increases acetylcholine concentration at transmission sites in parasympathetic neurons and skeletal muscles by inhibiting acetylcholinesterase

Pregnancy Considerations Safety in pregnancy has not been established.

Ambrisentan (am bri SEN tan)

Brand Names: U.S. Letairis®
Brand Names: Canada Volibris®
Pharmacologic Category Endothelin Antagonist; Vasodilator
Use Treatment of pulmonary artery hypertension (PAH) World Health Organization (WHO) Group I to improve exercise ability and decrease the rate of clinical deterioration
Local Anesthetic/Vasoconstrictor Precautions No information available to require special precautions
Effects on Dental Treatment Key adverse event(s) related to dental treatment: Endothelin antagonists have caused bleeding gums; there have been no specific reports for ambrisentan
Effects on Bleeding No information available to require special precautions
Adverse Effects
>10%:
 Cardiovascular: Peripheral edema (17%)
 Central nervous system: Headache (15%)
1% to 10%:
 Cardiovascular: Palpitation (5%), flushing (4%)
 Gastrointestinal: Constipation (4%), abdominal pain (3%)
 Hematologic: Hemoglobin decreased (7% to 10%)
 Respiratory: Nasal congestion (6%), dyspnea (4%), nasopharyngitis (3%), sinusitis (3%)
General Dosage Range Dosage adjustment recommended in patients on concomitant therapy.
Oral: *Adults:* Initial: 5 mg once daily (maximum: 10 mg/day)
Mechanism of Action Blocks endothelin receptor subtypes ET_A and ET_B on vascular endothelium and smooth muscle. Stimulation of ET_A receptors, located primarily in pulmonary vascular smooth muscle cells is associated with vasoconstriction and cellular proliferation. Stimulation of ET_B receptors, located in both pulmonary vascular endothelial cells and smooth muscle cells is associated with vasodilation, antiproliferative effects, and endothelin clearance. Although ambrisentan blocks both ET_A and ET_B receptors, the affinity is greater for the ET_A receptor (>4000 fold higher affinity).
Pharmacodynamics/Kinetics
Half-life Elimination ~9 hours
Time to Peak ~2 hours
Pregnancy Risk Factor X
Pregnancy Considerations [U.S. Boxed Warning]: Use in pregnancy is contraindicated. Based on animal studies, ambrisentan is likely to produce major birth defects if used by pregnant women. Pregnancy must be excluded prior to initiation of therapy and follow-up pregnancy tests should be obtained monthly. Two reliable methods of contraception must be used throughout treatment and for one month after stopping treatment unless the patient has undergone a tubal ligation or the insertion of an intrauterine device (Copper T 380A or LNg 20). No other contraceptive measures are required for these patients.
Prescribing and Access Restrictions As a requirement of the REMS program, access to this medication is restricted. Ambrisentan (Letairis®) is only available

through Letairis Education and Access Program (LEAP). Only prescribers and pharmacies registered with LEAP may prescribe and dispense ambrisentan. Further information may be obtained from the manufacturer, Gilead Sciences, Inc (1-866-664-5327).

Amcinonide (am SIN oh nide)

Brand Names: Canada Amcort®; Cyclocort®; ratio-Amcinonide; Taro-Amcinonide
Pharmacologic Category Corticosteroid, Topical
Use Relief of the inflammatory and pruritic manifestations of corticosteroid-responsive dermatoses (high potency corticosteroid)
Local Anesthetic/Vasoconstrictor Precautions No information available to require special precautions
Effects on Dental Treatment No significant effects or complications reported
Effects on Bleeding No information available to require special precautions
Adverse Effects Frequency not defined.
 Dermatologic: Acne, hypopigmentation, allergic dermatitis, maceration of the skin, miliaria, skin atrophy, striae, telangiectasia
 Endocrine & metabolic: Cushing's syndrome, growth retardation (long-term use), HPA axis suppression, hyperglycemia; these reactions occur more frequently with occlusive dressings
 Local: Burning, dryness, folliculitis, hypertrichosis, itching, irritation
 Miscellaneous: Secondary infection
General Dosage Range Topical: *Adults:* Apply in a thin film 2-3 times/day
Mechanism of Action Stimulates the synthesis of enzymes needed to decrease inflammation, suppress mitotic activity, and cause vasoconstriction
Pregnancy Risk Factor C
Pregnancy Considerations Teratogenic effects have been observed in animals administered potent topical corticosteroids. Topical products are not recommended for extensive use, in large quantities, or for long periods of time in pregnant women.

Amifostine (am i FOS teen)

Brand Names: U.S. Ethyol®
Brand Names: Canada Ethyol®
Pharmacologic Category Adjuvant, Chemoprotective Agent (Cytoprotective); Antidote
Use Reduce the incidence of moderate-to-severe xerostomia in patients undergoing postoperative radiation treatment for head and neck cancer, where the radiation port includes a substantial portion of the parotid glands; reduce the cumulative renal toxicity associated with repeated administration of cisplatin
Unlabeled Use Prevention of radiation proctitis in patients with rectal cancer
Local Anesthetic/Vasoconstrictor Precautions No information available to require special precautions
Effects on Dental Treatment No significant effects or complications reported
Effects on Bleeding No information available to require special precautions
Adverse Effects
>10%:
 Cardiovascular: Hypotension (15% to 61%; grades 3/4: 3% to 8%; dose dependent)
 Gastrointestinal: Nausea/vomiting (53% to 96%; grades 3/4: 8% to 30%; dose dependent)

1% to 10%: Endocrine & metabolic: Hypocalcemia (clinically significant: 1%)

General Dosage Range I.V.: *Adults:* 910 mg/m^2 once daily 30 minutes prior to cytotoxic therapy **or** 200 mg/m^2/day 15-30 minutes prior to radiation therapy

Mechanism of Action Prodrug that is dephosphorylated by alkaline phosphatase in tissues to a pharmacologically-active free thiol metabolite. The free thiol is available to bind to, and detoxify, reactive metabolites of cisplatin; and can also act as a scavenger of free radicals that may be generated (by cisplatin or radiation therapy) in tissues.

Pharmacodynamics/Kinetics

Half-life Elimination ~8-9 minutes

Pregnancy Risk Factor C

Pregnancy Considerations Animal studies have demonstrated embryotoxicity. There are no adequate and well-controlled studies in pregnant women.

Amikacin (am i KAY sin)

Brand Names: Canada Amikacin Sulfate Injection, USP; Amikin®

Pharmacologic Category Antibiotic, Aminoglycoside

Use Treatment of serious infections (bone infections, respiratory tract infections, endocarditis, and septicemia) due to organisms resistant to gentamicin and tobramycin, including *Pseudomonas*, *Proteus*, *Serratia*, and other gram-negative bacilli; documented infection of mycobacterial organisms susceptible to amikacin

Unlabeled Use Bacterial endophthalmitis; *Mycobacterium avium* complex (MAC; fibrocavitary or severe nodular/bronchiectatic disease)

Local Anesthetic/Vasoconstrictor Precautions No information available to require special precautions

Effects on Dental Treatment No significant effects or complications reported

Effects on Bleeding No information available to require special precautions

Adverse Effects 1% to 10%:
Central nervous system: Neurotoxicity
Otic: Ototoxicity (auditory), ototoxicity (vestibular)
Renal: Nephrotoxicity

General Dosage Range Dosage adjustment recommended in patients with renal impairment

I.M.: *Infants, Children, and Adults:* 5-7.5 mg/kg/dose every 8 hours (maximum: 20 mg/kg/day)

I.V.:
Infants and Children: 5-7.5 mg/kg/dose every 8 hours (maximum: 20 mg/kg/day)
Adults: 5-7.5 mg/kg/dose every 8 hours **or** 15-20 mg/kg as a single daily dose (maximum: 20 mg/kg/day)

Mechanism of Action Inhibits protein synthesis in susceptible bacteria by binding to 30S ribosomal subunits

Pharmacodynamics/Kinetics

Half-life Elimination Renal function and age dependent:
Infants: Low birth weight (1-3 days): 7-9 hours; Full-term >7 days: 4-5 hours
Children: 1.6-2.5 hours
Adults: Normal renal function: 1.4-2.3 hours; Anuria/end-stage renal disease: 28-86 hours

Time to Peak Serum: I.M.: 45-120 minutes

Pregnancy Risk Factor D

Pregnancy Considerations Adverse events were not observed in the initial animal reproduction studies; however, renal toxicity has been reported in additional

studies. Amikacin crosses the placenta, produces detectable serum levels in the fetus, and concentrates in the fetal kidneys. Because of several reports of total irreversible bilateral congenital deafness in children whose mothers received another aminoglycoside (streptomycin) during pregnancy, the manufacturer classifies amikacin as pregnancy risk factor D. Although serious side effects to the fetus have not been reported following maternal use of amikacin, a potential for harm exists.

Due to pregnancy-induced physiologic changes, some pharmacokinetic parameters of amikacin may be altered. Pregnant women have an average-to-larger volume of distribution which may result in lower peak serum levels than for the same dose in nonpregnant women. Serum half-life may also be shorter.

AMILoride (a MIL oh ride)

Related Information
Cardiovascular Diseases *on page 1492*

Brand Names: Canada Apo-Amiloride®; Midamor

Pharmacologic Category Diuretic, Potassium-Sparing

Use Counteracts potassium loss induced by other diuretics in the treatment of hypertension or edematous conditions including CHF, hepatic cirrhosis, and hypoaldosteronism; usually used in conjunction with more potent diuretics such as thiazides or loop diuretics

Unlabeled Use Cystic fibrosis; reduction of lithium-induced polyuria; pediatric hypertension

Local Anesthetic/Vasoconstrictor Precautions No information available to require special precautions

Effects on Dental Treatment No significant effects or complications reported

Effects on Bleeding No information available to require special precautions

Adverse Effects 1% to 10%:
Central nervous system: Headache, fatigue, dizziness
Endocrine & metabolic: Hyperkalemia (up to 10%; risk reduced in patients receiving kaliuretic diuretics), hyperchloremic metabolic acidosis, dehydration, hyponatremia, gynecomastia
Gastrointestinal: Nausea, diarrhea, vomiting, abdominal pain, gas pain, appetite changes, constipation
Genitourinary: Impotence
Neuromuscular & skeletal: Muscle cramps, weakness
Respiratory: Cough, dyspnea

General Dosage Range Dosage adjustment recommended in patients with renal impairment

Oral:
Adults: 5-10 mg/day in 1-2 divided doses (maximum: 20 mg/day)
Elderly: Initial: 5 mg once daily or every other day

Mechanism of Action Blocks epithelial sodium channels in the late distal convoluted tubule (DCT), and collecting duct which inhibits sodium reabsorption from the lumen. This effectively reduces intracellular sodium, decreasing the function of Na+/K+ATPase, leading to potassium retention and decreased calcium, magnesium, and hydrogen excretion. As sodium uptake capacity in the DCT/collecting duct is limited, the natriuretic, diuretic, and antihypertensive effects are generally considered weak.

Pharmacodynamics/Kinetics

Onset of Action 2 hours

Duration of Action 24 hours

Half-life Elimination Normal renal function: 6-9 hours; End-stage renal disease: 8-144 hours

Time to Peak Serum: 6-10 hours

Pregnancy Risk Factor B
Pregnancy Considerations Teratogenic effects were not observed in animal studies.

Amiloride and Hydrochlorothiazide
(a MIL oh ride & hye droe klor oh THYE a zide)

Related Information
AMILoride *on page 77*
Hydrochlorothiazide *on page 687*
Brand Names: Canada Ami-Hydro; Apo-Amilzide®; Gen-Amilazide; Moduret; Novamilor; Nu-Amilzide
Pharmacologic Category Diuretic, Combination
Use Potassium-sparing diuretic; antihypertensive
Local Anesthetic/Vasoconstrictor Precautions No information available to require special precautions
Effects on Dental Treatment No significant effects or complications reported
Effects on Bleeding No information available to require special precautions
Adverse Effects See individual agents.
General Dosage Range Dosage adjustment recommended in patients with renal impairment
Oral:
Adults: 1-2 tablets (amiloride 5 mg/HCTZ 50 mg per tablet) once daily (maximum: 2 tablets/day)
Elderly: Initial: 1/2 to 1 tablet/day (maximum: 2 tablets/day)
Pregnancy Risk Factor B
Pregnancy Considerations Refer to Hydrochlorothiazide.

Aminocaproic Acid (a mee noe ka PROE ik AS id)

Related Information
Antiplatelet and Anticoagulation Considerations in Dentistry *on page 1503*
Brand Names: U.S. Amicar®
Pharmacologic Category Antifibrinolytic Agent; Antihemophilic Agent; Hemostatic Agent; Lysine Analog
Use To enhance hemostasis when fibrinolysis contributes to bleeding (causes may include cardiac surgery, hematologic disorders, neoplastic disorders, abruptio placentae, hepatic cirrhosis, and urinary fibrinolysis)
Unlabeled Use Treatment of traumatic hyphema; control bleeding in thrombocytopenia; control oral bleeding in congenital and acquired coagulation disorders; topical treatment (mouth rinse) of bleeding associated with dental procedures in patients on oral anticoagulant therapy; prevention of perioperative bleeding associated with cardiac surgery; prevention of bleeding associated with extracorporeal membrane oxygenation (ECMO); prevention of perioperative bleeding associated with spinal surgery (eg, idiopathic scoliosis)
Local Anesthetic/Vasoconstrictor Precautions No information available to require special precautions
Effects on Dental Treatment No significant effects or complications reported (see Effects on Bleeding)
Effects on Bleeding Used as an off-label indication to prevent or treat dental bleeding in patients with Hemophilia A; may cause thrombocytopenia
Adverse Effects Frequency not defined.
Cardiovascular: Arrhythmia, bradycardia, edema, hypotension, intracranial hypertension, peripheral ischemia, syncope, thrombosis
Central nervous system: Confusion, delirium, dizziness, fatigue, hallucinations, headache, malaise, seizure, stroke

Dermatologic: Rash, pruritus
Gastrointestinal: Abdominal pain, anorexia, cramps, diarrhea, GI irritation, nausea, vomiting
Genitourinary: Dry ejaculation
Hematologic: Agranulocytosis, bleeding time increased, leukopenia, thrombocytopenia
Local: Injection site necrosis, injection site pain, injection site reactions
Neuromuscular & skeletal: CPK increased, myalgia, myositis, myopathy, rhabdomyolysis (rare), weakness
Ophthalmic: Vision decreased, watery eyes
Otic: Tinnitus
Renal: BUN increased, intrarenal obstruction (glomerular capillary thrombosis), myoglobinuria (rare), renal failure (rare)
Respiratory: Dyspnea, nasal congestion, pulmonary embolism
Miscellaneous: Allergic reaction, anaphylactoid reaction, anaphylaxis
General Dosage Range
I.V.: *Adults:* Dosage varies greatly depending on indication
Oral: *Adults:* Initial: Loading dose: 4-5 g for first hour; Maintenance: 1 g/hour (or 1.25 g/hour using oral solution) for 8 hours or until bleeding controlled (maximum: 30 g/day)
Mechanism of Action Binds competitively to plasminogen; blocking the binding of plasminogen to fibrin and the subsequent conversion to plasmin, resulting in inhibition of fibrin degradation (fibrinolysis).
Pharmacodynamics/Kinetics
Onset of Action ~1-72 hours
Half-life Elimination ~2 hours
Time to Peak Oral: Within 2 hours
Pregnancy Risk Factor C
Pregnancy Considerations Animal reproduction studies have not been conducted.

Aminolevulinic Acid (a MEE noh lev yoo lin ik AS id)

Brand Names: U.S. Levulan® Kerastick®
Brand Names: Canada Levulan® Kerastick®
Pharmacologic Category Photosensitizing Agent, Topical; Topical Skin Product
Use Treatment of minimally to moderately thick actinic keratoses (grade 1 or 2) of the face or scalp; to be used in conjunction with blue light illumination
Unlabeled Use Photodynamic treatment of low-risk superficial basal cell skin cancer and low-risk squamous cell skin cancer *in situ* (Bowen's disease)
Local Anesthetic/Vasoconstrictor Precautions No information available to require special precautions
Effects on Dental Treatment Key adverse event(s) related to dental treatment: Bleeding/hemorrhage (limited to application/treatment site).
Effects on Bleeding Bleeding/hemorrhage at application or treatment site.
Adverse Effects Transient stinging, burning, itching, erythema, and edema result from the photosensitizing properties of this agent. Symptoms subside between 1 minute and 24 hours after turning off the blue light illuminator. Severe stinging or burning was reported in at least 50% of patients from at least 1 lesional site during treatment.

>10%: Dermatologic: Stinging or burning (most patients; severe: ≥50%), erythema (99%), scaling/crusted skin (64% to 71%), hyper-/hypopigmentation (22% to 36%), edematous lesions (35%), itching (14% to 25%), erosion (2% to 14%), skin disorder (5% to 12%)

1% to 10%:
Central nervous system: Dysesthesia (≤2%)
Dermatologic: Vesiculation (4% to 5%), skin ulceration (2% to 4%), pustular drug eruption (≤4%)
Hematologic: Bleeding/hemorrhage (2% to 4%)
Local: Wheal/flare (2% to 7%), scabbing (≤2%), tenderness (1% to 2%), edema (≤1%), excoriation (≤1%), local pain (≤1%), oozing (≤1%)

General Dosage Range Topical: *Adults:* Apply to actinic keratoses once; may repeat after 8 weeks

Mechanism of Action Aminolevulinic acid is a metabolic precursor of the photosensitizer protoporphyrin IX (PpIX). Photosensitization following local application of aminolevulinic acid occurs through the metabolic conversion to PpIX. When exposed to light of appropriate wavelength and energy, accumulated PpIX produces a photodynamic reaction resulting in local cytotoxicity. Precancerous and cancerous cells exhibit a higher rate of porphyrin induction compared to normal cells.

Pharmacodynamics/Kinetics
Onset of Action Peak fluorescence intensity of protoporphyrin IX (PpIX): Actinic keratosis: 11 hours ± 1 hour; Perilesional skin: 12 hours ± 1 hour
Half-life Elimination Mean fluorescence clearance half-life of PpIX for lesions: 30 ± 10 hours

Pregnancy Risk Factor C

Pregnancy Considerations Animal reproduction studies have not been conducted, and there are no adequate and well-controlled studies in pregnant women. Use during pregnancy only if clearly needed.

Aminophylline (am in OFF i lin)

Related Information
Respiratory Diseases *on page 1514*
Theophylline *on page 1315*
Brand Names: Canada Aminophylline Injection; JAA-Aminophylline
Pharmacologic Category Phosphodiesterase Enzyme Inhibitor, Nonselective
Use Treatment of symptoms and reversible airway obstruction due to asthma or other chronic lung diseases (eg, emphysema, chronic bronchitis)

Note: The National Heart, Lung, and Blood Institute Guidelines (2007) do not recommend aminophylline I.V. for the treatment of asthma exacerbations.

Unlabeled Use Reversal of adenosine-, dipyridamole-, or regadenoson-induced adverse reactions (eg, angina, hypotension) during nuclear cardiac stress testing

Local Anesthetic/Vasoconstrictor Precautions No information available to require special precautions

Effects on Dental Treatment Prescribe erythromycin products with caution to patients taking theophylline products. Erythromycin will delay the normal metabolic inactivation of theophyllines leading to increased blood levels; this has resulted in nausea, vomiting, and CNS restlessness.

Effects on Bleeding No information available to require special precautions

Adverse Effects Frequency not defined. Adverse events observed at therapeutic serum levels:
Cardiovascular: Flutter, tachycardia
Central nervous system: Behavior alterations (children), headache, insomnia, irritability, restlessness, seizures
Dermatologic: Allergic skin reactions, exfoliative dermatitis
Gastrointestinal: Diarrhea, nausea, vomiting
Neuromuscular & skeletal: Tremor
Renal: Diuresis (transient)

General Dosage Range
I.V.:
Infants to Adults: Loading dose: 5.7 mg/kg
Children 6 weeks to 1 year: Maintenance: Dose (mg/kg/hour) = [(0.008 x age in weeks) + 0.21] divided by 0.79
Children 1-9 years: Maintenance: 1.01 mg/kg/hour
Children 9-12 years: Maintenance: 0.89 mg/kg/hour
Adolescents 12-16 years (smokers): Maintenance: 0.89 mg/kg/hour
Adolescents 12-16 years (nonsmokers): Maintenance: 0.63 mg/kg/hour
Adolescents >16 years and Adults ≤60 years (nonsmokers): Maintenance: 0.51 mg/kg/hour (maximum: 900 mg/day)
Adults >60 years (nonsmokers): Maintenance: 0.38 mg/kg/hour (maximum: 400 mg/day)
Oral:
Children 1-15 years and <45 kg (without risk factors for impaired clearance): Initial: 15.2-17.7 mg/kg/day divided every 4-6 hours for 3 days (maximum: 380 mg), then increase to 20.3 mg/kg/day divided every 4-6 hours for 3 days (maximum: 400 mg/day); Maintenance: 25.3 mg/kg/day divided every 4-6 hours (maximum: 760 mg/day)
Children ≥45 kg and Adults: Initial: 380 mg/day divided every 6-8 hours for 3 days, then 507 mg/day divided every 6-8 hours for 3 days; Maintenance: 760 mg/day divided every 6-8 hours

Mechanism of Action Causes bronchodilatation, diuresis, CNS and cardiac stimulation, and gastric acid secretion by blocking phosphodiesterase which increases tissue concentrations of cyclic adenine monophosphate (cAMP) which in turn promote catecholamine stimulation of lipolysis, glycogenolysis, and gluconeogenesis and induce release of epinephrine from adrenal medulla cells

Pharmacodynamics/Kinetics
Half-life Elimination Theophylline: Highly variable and dependent upon age, liver function, cardiac function, lung disease, and smoking history
Premature infants, postnatal age 3-15 days: 30 hours (range: 17-43 hours)
Premature infants, postnatal age 25-57 days: 20 hours (range: 9.4-30.6 hours)
Children 1-4 yrs: 3.4 hours (range: 1.2-5.6 hours); 6-17 years: 3.7 hours (range: 1.5-5.9 hours)
Adults 16-60 years with asthma, nonsmoking, otherwise healthy: 8.7 hours (range: 6.1-12.8 hours)
Time to Peak Oral: 1-2 hours; I.V.: Within 30 minutes
Pregnancy Risk Factor C
Pregnancy Considerations Refer to Theophylline monograph.

Aminosalicylic Acid (a mee noe sal i SIL ik AS id)

Brand Names: U.S. Paser®
Pharmacologic Category Antitubercular Agent
Use Adjunctive treatment of tuberculosis used in combination with other antitubercular agents
Local Anesthetic/Vasoconstrictor Precautions No information available to require special precautions
Effects on Dental Treatment NSAID formulations are known to reversibly decrease platelet aggregation via mechanisms different than observed with aspirin. The dentist should be aware of the potential of abnormal coagulation. Caution should also be exercised in the use of NSAIDs in patients already on anticoagulant therapy with drugs such as warfarin (Coumadin®).

Effects on Bleeding No information available to require special precautions

Adverse Effects Frequency not defined.

Cardiovascular: Pericarditis, vasculitis

Central nervous system: Encephalopathy, fever

Dermatologic: Skin eruptions (including exfoliative dermatitis)

Endocrine & metabolic: Goiter (with or without myxedema), hypoglycemia, hypothyroidism

Gastrointestinal: Abdominal pain, diarrhea, nausea, vomiting

Hematologic: Agranulocytosis, anemia (hemolytic), leukopenia, thrombocytopenia

Hepatic: Hepatitis, jaundice

Ocular: Optic neuritis

Respiratory: Eosinophilic pneumonia

General Dosage Range Dosage adjustment recommended in patients with renal impairment

Oral:

Children: 200-300 mg/kg/day in 2-4 divided doses

Adults: 8-12 g/day in 2-3 divided doses

Mechanism of Action Aminosalicylic acid (PAS) is a highly-specific bacteriostatic agent active against *M. tuberculosis*. Structurally related to para-aminobenzoic acid (PABA) and its mechanism of action is thought to be similar to the sulfonamides, a competitive antagonism with PABA; disrupts plate biosynthesis in sensitive organisms.

Pharmacodynamics/Kinetics

Half-life Elimination Reduced with renal impairment

Time to Peak Serum: 6 hours

Pregnancy Risk Factor C

Pregnancy Considerations Teratogenic effects have been reported in animal reproduction studies. Salicylates have been noted to cross the placenta and enter fetal circulation. Aminosalicylic acid has been used safely during pregnancy; however, it should only be used if there are no alternatives for the treatment of multidrug-resistant tuberculosis (*MMWR*, 2003).

Amiodarone (a MEE oh da rone)

Related Information

Clinical Risk Related to Drugs Prolonging QT Interval *on page 1510*

Brand Names: U.S. Cordarone®; Nexterone®; Pacerone®

Brand Names: Canada Amiodarone Hydrochloride Injection; Apo-Amiodarone®; Ava-Amiodarone; Cordarone®; Dom-Amiodarone; Mylan-Amiodarone; PHL-Amiodarone; PMS-Amiodarone; PRO-Amiodarone; ratio-Amiodarone; Riva-Amiodarone; Sandoz-Amiodarone; Teva-Amiodarone

Generic Availability (U.S.) Yes

Pharmacologic Category Antiarrhythmic Agent, Class III

Use Management of life-threatening recurrent ventricular fibrillation (VF) or hemodynamically-unstable ventricular tachycardia (VT) refractory to other antiarrhythmic agents or in patients intolerant of other agents used for these conditions

Unlabeled Use

Atrial fibrillation (AF): Pharmacologic conversion of AF to and maintenance of normal sinus rhythm; treatment of AF in patients with heart failure [no accessory pathway] who require heart rate control (ACC/AHA/ESC Practice Guidelines) or in patients with hypertrophic cardiomyopathy (ACCF/AHA Practice Guidelines); prevention of postoperative AF associated with cardiothoracic surgery

Paroxysmal supraventricular tachycardia (SVT) (not initial drug of choice)

Ventricular tachyarrhythmias (ACLS/PALS guidelines): Cardiac arrest with persistent VT or VF if defibrillation, CPR, and vasopressor administration have failed; control of hemodynamically-stable monomorphic VT, polymorphic VT with a normal baseline QT interval, or wide-complex tachycardia of uncertain origin; control of rapid ventricular rate due to accessory pathway conduction in pre-excited atrial arrhythmias (ACLS guidelines) or stable narrow-complex tachycardia (ACLS guidelines)

Adjunct to ICD therapy to suppress recurrent ventricular tachyarrhythmias in otherwise optimally-treated patients with heart failure (ACC/AHA/ESC Practice Guidelines)

Local Anesthetic/Vasoconstrictor Precautions Amiodarone is one of the drugs confirmed to prolong the QT interval and is accepted as having a risk of causing torsade de pointes. The risk of drug-induced torsade de pointes is extremely low when a single QT interval prolonging drug is prescribed. In terms of epinephrine, it is not known what effect vasoconstrictors in the local anesthetic regimen will have in patients with a known history of congenital prolonged QT interval or in patients taking any medication that prolongs the QT interval. Until more information is obtained, it is suggested that the clinician consult with the physician prior to the use of a vasoconstrictor in suspected patients, and that the vasoconstrictor (epinephrine, mepivacaine and levonordefrin [Carbocaine® 2% with Neo-Cobefrin®]) be used with caution.

Effects on Dental Treatment Key adverse event(s) related to dental treatment: Oral: Abnormal salivation and taste

Effects on Bleeding No information available to require special precautions

Adverse Effects In a recent meta-analysis, adult patients taking lower doses of amiodarone (152-330 mg daily for at least 12 months) were more likely to develop thyroid, neurologic, skin, ocular, and bradycardic abnormalities than those taking placebo (Vorperian, 1997). Pulmonary toxicity was similar in both the low-dose amiodarone group and in the placebo group, but there was a trend towards increased toxicity in the amiodarone group. Gastrointestinal and hepatic events were seen to a similar extent in both the low-dose amiodarone group and placebo group. As the frequency of adverse events varies considerably across studies as a function of route and dose, a consolidation of adverse event rates is provided by Goldschlager, 2000.

>10%:

Cardiovascular: Hypotension (I.V. 16%, refractory in rare cases)

Central nervous system (3% to 40%): Abnormal gait/ataxia, dizziness, fatigue, headache, malaise, impaired memory, involuntary movement, insomnia, poor coordination, peripheral neuropathy, sleep disturbances, tremor

Dermatologic: Photosensitivity (10% to 75%)

Endocrine & Metabolic: Hypothyroidism (1% to 22%)

Gastrointestinal: Nausea, vomiting, anorexia, and constipation (10% to 33%)

Hepatic: AST or ALT level >2x normal (15% to 50%)

Ocular: Corneal microdeposits (>90%; causes visual disturbance in <10%)

1% to 10%:

Cardiovascular: CHF (3%), bradycardia (3% to 5%), AV block (5%), conduction abnormalities, SA node dysfunction (1% to 3%), cardiac arrhythmia, flushing, edema. Additional effects associated with I.V. administration include asystole, atrial fibrillation, cardiac arrest, electromechanical dissociation, pulseless electrical activity (PEA), ventricular tachycardia, and cardiogenic shock.

Dermatologic: Slate blue skin discoloration (<10%)

Endocrine & metabolic: Hyperthyroidism (3% to 10%; more common in iodine-deficient regions of the world), libido decreased

Gastrointestinal: Abdominal pain, abnormal salivation, abnormal taste (oral), diarrhea, nausea (I.V.)

Hematologic: Coagulation abnormalities

Hepatic: Hepatitis and cirrhosis (<3%)

Local: Phlebitis (I.V., with concentrations >3 mg/mL)

Ocular: Visual disturbances (2% to 9%), halo vision (<5% occurring especially at night), optic neuritis (1%)

Respiratory: Pulmonary toxicity has been estimated to occur at a frequency between 2% and 7% of patients (some reports indicate a frequency as high as 17%). Toxicity may present as hypersensitivity pneumonitis; pulmonary fibrosis (cough, fever, malaise); pulmonary inflammation; interstitial pneumonitis; or alveolar pneumonitis. ARDS has been reported in up to 2% of patients receiving amiodarone, and postoperatively in patients receiving oral amiodarone.

Miscellaneous: Abnormal smell (oral)

Dosage Note: Lower loading and maintenance doses are preferable in women and all patients with low body weight.

Oral:

Children: Arrhythmias (unlabeled use):

Loading dose: 10-20 mg/kg/day in 1-2 doses for 4-14 days or until adequate control of arrhythmia or prominent adverse effects occur; alternative loading dose in children <1 year: 600-800 mg/1.73 m^2/day in 1-2 divided doses/day

Maintenance dose: Dose may be reduced to 5 mg/kg/day for several weeks (or 200-400 mg/1.73 m^2/day given once daily); if no recurrence of arrhythmia, dose may be further reduced to 2.5 mg/kg/day; maintenance doses may be given 5-7 days/week

Adults:

Ventricular arrhythmias: 800-1600 mg/day in 1-2 doses for 1-3 weeks, then when adequate arrhythmia control is achieved, decrease to 600-800 mg/day in 1-2 doses for 1 month; maintenance: 400 mg/day. Lower doses are recommended for supraventricular arrhythmias.

Atrial fibrillation:

Pharmacologic cardioversion (unlabeled use): ACC/AHA/ESC Practice Guidelines: *Inpatient:* 1.2-1.8 g/day in divided doses until 10 g total, then 200-400 mg/day maintenance. *Outpatient:* 600-800 mg/day in divided doses until 10 g total, then 200-400 mg/day maintenance; although not supported by clinical evidence, a maintenance dose of 100 mg/day is commonly used especially for the elderly or patients with low body mass (Fuster, 2006; Zimetbaum, 2007). **Note:** Other regimens have been described and may be used clinically:

400 mg 3 times/day for 5-7 days, then 400 mg/day for 1 month, then 200 mg/day

or

10 mg/kg/day for 14 days, followed by 300 mg/day for 4 weeks, followed by maintenance dosage of 200 mg/day (Roy, 2000)

Prophylaxis following open heart surgery (unlabeled use): Starting in postop recovery: 400 mg twice daily for up to 7 days. Alternative regimen of amiodarone: 600 mg/day for 7 days prior to surgery, followed by 200 mg/day until hospital discharge, has also been shown to decrease the risk of postoperative atrial fibrillation. **Note:** A variety of regimens have been used in clinical trials.

I.V.:

Children:

Arrhythmias (unlabeled use, dosing based on limited data): Loading dose: 5 mg/kg over 30 minutes; may repeat up to 3 times if no response. Maintenance dose: Continuous infusion: 10-20 mg/kg/day followed by conversion to oral therapy as appropriate. **Note:** Maximum recommended total daily dose in adolescents is 2.2 g.

Note: I.V. administration at low flow rates (potentially associated with use in pediatrics) may result in leaching of plasticizers (DEHP) from intravenous tubing. DEHP may adversely affect male reproductive tract development. Alternative means of dosing and administration (1 mg/kg aliquots) may need to be considered.

Pulseless VT or VF (PALS dosing): I.V., I.O.: 5 mg/kg (maximum: 300 mg/dose) rapid bolus; may repeat up to a maximum total dose of 15 mg/kg during acute treatment.

Perfusing tachycardias (PALS dosing): I.V., I.O.: Loading dose: 5 mg/kg (maximum: 300 mg/dose) over 20-60 minutes; may repeat up to maximum total dose of 15 mg/kg during acute treatment.

Adults:

Atrial fibrillation:

Pharmacologic cardioversion (ACC/AHA/ESC Practice Guidelines) (unlabeled use): 5-7 mg/kg over 30-60 minutes, then 1.2-1.8 g/day continuous infusion until 10 g total. Maintenance: See oral dosing.

Prophylaxis following open heart surgery (unlabeled use): Starting at postop recovery: 1000 mg infused over 24 hours for 2 days has been shown to reduce the risk of postoperative atrial fibrillation. **Note:** A variety of regimens have been used in clinical trials.

Pulseless VT or VF (ACLS, 2010): I.V. push, I.O.: Initial: 300 mg rapid bolus; if pulseless VT or VF continues after subsequent defibrillation attempt or recurs, administer supplemental dose of 150 mg. **Note:** In this setting, administering **undiluted** is preferred (Dager, 2006; Skrifvars, 2004). *The*

Handbook of Emergency Cardiovascular Care (Hazinski, 2010) and the 2010 ACLS guidelines, do not make any specific recommendations regarding dilution of amiodarone in this setting. Experience limited with I.O. administration of amiodarone (ACLS, 2010).

Upon return of spontaneous circulation, follow with an infusion of 1 mg/minute for 6 hours, then 0.5 mg/minute for 18 hours (mean daily doses >2.1 g/day have been associated with hypotension).

Stable VT or SVT (unlabeled use): First 24 hours: 1050 mg according to following regimen

Step 1: 150 mg (100 mL) over first 10 minutes (mix 3 mL in 100 mL D_5W)

Step 2: 360 mg (200 mL) over next 6 hours (mix 18 mL in 500 mL D_5W): 1 mg/minute

Step 3: 540 mg (300 mL) over next 18 hours: 0.5 mg/minute

Note: After the first 24 hours: 0.5 mg/minute utilizing concentration of 1-6 mg/mL

Breakthrough stable VT or SVT: 150 mg supplemental doses in 100 mL D_5W or NS over 10 minutes (mean daily doses >2.1 g/day have been associated with hypotension)

I.V. to oral therapy conversion: Use the following as a guide:

<1-week I.V. infusion: 800-1600 mg/day
1- to 3-week I.V. infusion: 600-800 mg/day
>3-week I.V. infusion: 400 mg/day

Note: Conversion from I.V. to oral therapy has not been formally evaluated. Some experts recommend a 1-2 day overlap when converting from I.V. to oral therapy especially when treating ventricular arrhythmias.

Recommendations for conversion to intravenous amiodarone after oral administration: During long-term amiodarone therapy (ie, ≥4 months), the mean plasma-elimination half-life of the active metabolite of amiodarone is 61 days. Replacement therapy may not be necessary in such patients if oral therapy is discontinued for a period <2 weeks, since any changes in serum amiodarone concentrations during this period may **not** be clinically significant.

Elderly: No specific guidelines available. Dose selection should be cautious, at low end of dosage range, and titration should be slower to evaluate response. Although not supported by clinical evidence, a maintenance dose of 100 mg/day is commonly used especially for the elderly or patients with low body mass (Fuster, 2006; Zimetbaum, 2007).

Dosing adjustment in renal impairment: No dosage adjustment necessary

Hemodialysis: Not dialyzable (0% to 5%); supplemental dose is not necessary.

Peritoneal dialysis: Not dialyzable (0% to 5%); supplemental dose is not necessary.

Dosing adjustment in hepatic impairment: Dosage adjustment is probably necessary in substantial hepatic impairment. No specific guidelines available. If hepatic enzymes exceed 3 times normal or double in a patient with an elevated baseline, consider decreasing the dose or discontinuing amiodarone.

Mechanism of Action Class III antiarrhythmic agent which inhibits adrenergic stimulation (alpha- and beta-blocking properties), affects sodium, potassium, and calcium channels, prolongs the action potential and refractory period in myocardial tissue; decreases AV conduction and sinus node function

Contraindications Hypersensitivity to amiodarone, iodine, or any component of the formulation; severe sinus-node dysfunction; second- and third-degree heart block (except in patients with a functioning artificial pacemaker); bradycardia causing syncope (except in patients with a functioning artificial pacemaker); cardiogenic shock

Warnings/Precautions [U.S. Boxed Warning]: Only indicated for patients with life-threatening arrhythmias because of risk of toxicity. Alternative therapies should be tried first before using amiodarone. Patients should be hospitalized when amiodarone is initiated. Currently, the 2005 ACLS guidelines recommend I.V. amiodarone as the preferred antiarrhythmic for the treatment of pulseless VT/VF, both life-threatening arrhythmias. In patients with non-life-threatening arrhythmias (eg, atrial fibrillation), amiodarone should be used only if the use of other antiarrhythmics has proven ineffective or are contraindicated.

[U.S. Boxed Warning]: Lung damage (abnormal diffusion capacity) may occur without symptoms. Monitor for pulmonary toxicity. Evaluate new respiratory symptoms; pre-existing pulmonary disease does not increase risk of developing pulmonary toxicity, but if pulmonary toxicity develops then the prognosis is worse. The lowest effective dose should be used as appropriate for the acuity/severity of the arrhythmia being treated. **[U.S. Boxed Warning]: Liver toxicity is common, but usually mild with evidence of increased liver enzymes. Severe liver toxicity can occur and has been fatal in a few cases.**

[U.S. Boxed Warning]: Amiodarone can exacerbate arrhythmias, by making them more difficult to tolerate or reverse; other types of arrhythmias have occurred, including significant heart block, sinus bradycardia new ventricular fibrillation, incessant ventricular tachycardia, increased resistance to cardioversion, and polymorphic ventricular tachycardia associated with QT_c prolongation (torsade de pointes [TdP]). Risk may be increased with concomitant use of other antiarrhythmic agents or drugs that prolong the QT_c interval. Proarrhythmic effects may be prolonged.

Monitor pacing or defibrillation thresholds in patients with implantable cardiac devices (eg, pacemakers, defibrillators). Use very cautiously and with close monitoring in patients with thyroid or liver disease. May cause hyper- or hypothyroidism. Hyperthyroidism may result in thyrotoxicosis and may aggravate or cause breakthrough arrhythmias. If any new signs of arrhythmia appear, hyperthyroidism should be considered. Thyroid function should be monitored prior to treatment and periodically thereafter.

May cause optic neuropathy and/or optic neuritis, usually resulting in visual impairment. Corneal microdeposits occur in a majority of patients, and may cause visual disturbances in some patients (blurred vision, halos); these are not generally considered a reason to discontinue treatment. Corneal refractive laser surgery is generally contraindicated in amiodarone users. Avoid excessive exposure to sunlight; may cause photosensitivity.

Amiodarone is a potent inhibitor of CYP enzymes and transport proteins (including p-glycoprotein), which may lead to increased serum concentrations/toxicity of a number of medications. Particular caution must be used when a drug with QT_c-prolonging potential relies on metabolism via these enzymes, since the effect of elevated concentrations may be additive with the effect of amiodarone. Carefully assess risk:benefit of coadministration of other drugs which may prolong QT_c interval. Patients may still be at risk for amiodarone–related drug interactions after the drug has been discontinued. The pharmacokinetics are complex (due to prolonged duration of action and half-life) and difficult to predict. Correct electrolyte disturbances, especially hypokalemia or hypomagnesemia, prior to use and throughout therapy. Use caution when initiating amiodarone in patients on warfarin. Cases of increased INR with or without bleeding have occurred in patients treated with warfarin; monitor INR closely after initiating amiodarone in these patients.

In the treatment of atrial fibrillation in older adults, avoid antiarrhythmics as first-line treatment. In older adults, data suggests rate control may provide more benefits than risks compared to rhythm control for most patients (Beers Criteria).

May cause hypotension and bradycardia (infusion-rate related). Hypotension with rapid administration has been attributed to the emulsifier polysorbate 80. Commercially-prepared premixed solutions do not contain polysorbate 80 and may have a lower incidence of hypotension. Caution in surgical patients; may enhance hemodynamic effect of anesthetics; associated with increased risk of adult respiratory distress syndrome (ARDS) postoperatively. Vials for injection contain benzyl alcohol, which has been associated with "gasping syndrome" in neonates. Commercially-prepared premixed solutions do not contain benzyl alcohol. Commercially-prepared premixed infusion contains the excipient cyclodextrin (sulfobutyl ether beta-cyclodextrin), which may accumulate in patients with renal insufficiency.

Drug Interactions

Metabolism/Transport Effects **Substrate** of CYP1A2 (minor), CYP2C19 (minor), CYP2C8 (major), CYP2D6 (minor), CYP3A4 (major), P-glycoprotein; **Note:** Assignment of Major/Minor substrate status based on clinically relevant drug interaction potential; **Inhibits** CYP1A2 (weak), CYP2A6 (moderate), CYP2B6 (weak), CYP2C9 (moderate), CYP2D6 (moderate), CYP3A4 (moderate), P-glycoprotein

Avoid Concomitant Use

Avoid concomitant use of Amiodarone with any of the following: Agalsidase Alfa; Agalsidase Beta; Azithromycin (Systemic); Bosutinib; Conivaptan; Fingolimod; Grapefruit Juice; Highest Risk QTc-Prolonging Agents; Ivabradine; Lomitapide; Mifepristone; Moderate Risk QTc-Prolonging Agents; Pomalidomide; Propafenone; Protease Inhibitors; Silodosin; Thioridazine; Tolvaptan; Topotecan; VinCRIStine (Liposomal)

Increased Effect/Toxicity

Amiodarone may increase the levels/effects of: Antiarrhythmic Agents (Class Ia); ARIPiprazole; Avanafil; Beta-Blockers; Bosutinib; Budesonide (Systemic, Oral Inhalation); Cardiac Glycosides; Colchicine; CycloSPORINE (Systemic); CYP2A6 Substrates; CYP2C9 Substrates; CYP2D6 Substrates; CYP3A4 Substrates; Dabigatran Etexilate; Eplerenone; Everolimus; FentaNYL; Fesoterodine; Flecainide; Fosphenytoin; Highest Risk QTc-Prolonging Agents; HMG-CoA Reductase Inhibitors; Ivacaftor; Lidocaine (Systemic); Lidocaine (Topical); Lomitapide; Loratadine; Lurasidone; Metoprolol; Mipomersen; P-glycoprotein/ABCB1 Substrates; Phenytoin; Pimecrolimus; Pomalidomide; Porfimer; Propafenone; Prucalopride; Rivaroxaban; Salmeterol; Saxagliptin; Silodosin; Thioridazine; Tolvaptan; Topotecan; Vilazodone; VinCRIStine (Liposomal); Vitamin K Antagonists

The levels/effects of Amiodarone may be increased by: Azithromycin (Systemic); Boceprevir; Calcium Channel Blockers (Nondihydropyridine); Cimetidine; Conivaptan; CYP2C8 Inhibitors (Moderate); CYP2C8 Inhibitors (Strong); CYP3A4 Inhibitors (Moderate); CYP3A4 Inhibitors (Strong); Dasatinib; Deferasirox; EriBULin; Fingolimod; Grapefruit Juice; Ivabradine; Ivacaftor; Lidocaine (Topical); Mifepristone; Moderate Risk QTc-Prolonging Agents; P-glycoprotein/ABCB1 Inhibitors; Protease Inhibitors; QTc-Prolonging Agents (Indeterminate Risk and Risk Modifying); Telaprevir

Decreased Effect

Amiodarone may decrease the levels/effects of: Agalsidase Alfa; Agalsidase Beta; Clopidogrel; Codeine; Ifosfamide; Sodium Iodide I131; Tamoxifen; TraMADol

The levels/effects of Amiodarone may be decreased by: Bile Acid Sequestrants; CYP2C8 Inducers (Strong); CYP3A4 Inducers (Strong); Deferasirox; Etravirine; Fosphenytoin; Grapefruit Juice; Herbs (CYP3A4 Inducers); Orlistat; Peginterferon Alfa-2b; P-glycoprotein/ABCB1 Inducers; Phenytoin; Rifamycin Derivatives; Tocilizumab

Ethanol/Nutrition/Herb Interactions

Food: Increases the rate and extent of absorption of amiodarone. Grapefruit juice increases bioavailability of oral amiodarone by 50% and decreases the conversion of amiodarone to N-DEA (active metabolite); altered effects are possible. Management: Take consistently with regard to meals; grapefruit juice should be avoided during therapy.

Herb/Nutraceutical: St John's wort may decrease amiodarone levels or enhance photosensitization. Ephedra may worsen arrythmia. Management: Avoid St John's wort, ephedra and dong quai.

Dietary Considerations Take consistently with regard to meals. Amiodarone is a potential source of large amounts of inorganic iodine; ~3 mg of inorganic iodine per 100 mg of amiodarone is released into the systemic circulation. Recommended daily allowance for iodine in adults is 150 mcg.

Grapefruit juice is not recommended.

Pharmacodynamics/Kinetics

Onset of Action Oral: 2 days to 3 weeks; I.V.: May be more rapid; Peak effect: 1 week to 5 months

Duration of Action After discontinuing therapy: 7-50 days

Note: Mean onset of effect and duration after discontinuation may be shorter in children than adults

Half-life Elimination Terminal: 40-55 days (range: 26-107 days); shorter in children

Time to Peak Serum: 3-7 hours

Pregnancy Risk Factor D

Pregnancy Considerations May cause fetal harm when administered to a pregnant woman, leading to congenital goiter and hypo- or hyperthyroidism.

Lactation Enters breast milk/not recommended (AAP rates "of concern"; AAP 2001 update pending)

Breast-Feeding Considerations Hypothyroidism may occur in nursing infants. Both amiodarone and its active metabolite are excreted in human milk. Breast-feeding may lead to significant infant exposure and potential toxicity.

Dosage Forms
Infusion, premixed iso-osmotic dextrose solution: Nexterone®: 150 mg (100 mL); 360 mg (200 mL)
Injection, solution: 50 mg/mL (3 mL, 9 mL, 18 mL)
Tablet, oral: 200 mg, 400 mg
  Cordarone®: 200 mg
  Pacerone®: 100 mg, 200 mg, 400 mg

Dental Comment Amiodarone is known to prolong the QT interval. The QT interval is measured as the time and distance between the Q point of the QRS complex and the end of the T wave in the ECG tracing. After adjustment for heart rate, the QT interval is defined as prolonged if it is more than 450 msec in men and 460 msec in women. A long QT syndrome was first described in the 1950s and 60s as a congenital syndrome involving QT interval prolongation and syncope and sudden death. Some of the congenital long QT syndromes were characterized by a peculiar electrocardiographic appearance of the QRS complex involving a premature atria beat followed by a pause, then a subsequent sinus beat showing marked QT prolongation and deformity. This type of cardiac arrhythmia was originally termed "torsade de pointes" (translated from the French as "twisting of the points"). Amiodarone is considered as having a risk of causing torsade de pointes. Since it is not known what effect vasoconstrictors in the local anesthetic regimen will have in patients with a known history of congenital prolonged QT interval or in patients taking any medication that prolongs the QT interval, a medical consult is suggested.

Amitriptyline (a mee TRIP ti leen)

Related Information
Temporomandibular Dysfunction (TMD), Chronic Pain, and Fibromyalgia *on page 1590*
Vasoconstrictor Interactions With Antidepressants *on page 1650*

Brand Names: Canada Bio-Amitriptyline; Dom-Amitriptyline; Elavil; Levate®; Novo-Triptyn; PMS-Amitriptyline

Generic Availability (U.S.) Yes

Pharmacologic Category Antidepressant, Tricyclic (Tertiary Amine)

Dental Use Management of chronic neuropathic pain in temporomandibular dysfunction (TMD)

Use Relief of symptoms of depression

Unlabeled Use Analgesic for certain chronic and neuropathic pain (including diabetic neuropathy); prophylaxis against migraine headaches; treatment of depressive disorders in children; post-traumatic stress disorder (PTSD)

Local Anesthetic/Vasoconstrictor Precautions Amitriptyline is one of the drugs confirmed to prolong the QT interval and is accepted as having a risk of causing torsade de pointes. In terms of epinephrine, it is not known what effect vasoconstrictors in the local anesthetic regimen will have in patients with a known history of congenital prolonged QT interval or in patients taking any medication that prolongs the QT interval. Until more information is obtained, it is suggested that the clinician consult with the physician prior to the use of a vasoconstrictor in suspected patients, and that the vasoconstrictor (epinephrine, mepivacaine and levonordefrin [Carbocaine® 2% with Neo-Cobefrin®]) be used with caution. See Dental Comment.

Effects on Dental Treatment Key adverse event(s) related to dental treatment: Xerostomia and changes in salivation (normal salivary flow resumes upon discontinuation), orthostatic hypotension, stomatitis, peculiar taste, and black tongue. Amitriptyline is the most anticholinergic and sedating of the antidepressants; has pronounced effects on the cardiovascular system. Long-term treatment with TCAs such as amitriptyline increases the risk of caries by reducing salivation and salivary buffer capacity. In a study by Rundergren, et al, pathological alterations were observed in the oral mucosa of 72% of 58 patients; 55% had new carious lesions after taking TCAs for a median of 5¹/₂ years. Current research is investigating the use of the salivary stimulant pilocarpine (Salagen®) to overcome the xerostomia from amitriptyline.

Effects on Bleeding May cause thrombocytopenia

Adverse Effects Anticholinergic effects may be pronounced; moderate to marked sedation can occur (tolerance to these effects usually occurs).

Frequency not defined.
Cardiovascular: Orthostatic hypotension, tachycardia, ECG changes (nonspecific), AV conduction changes, cardiomyopathy (rare), MI, stroke, heart block, arrhythmia, syncope, hypertension, palpitation
Central nervous system: Restlessness, dizziness, insomnia, sedation, fatigue, anxiety, cognitive function (impaired), seizure, extrapyramidal symptoms, coma, hallucinations, confusion, disorientation, coordination impaired, ataxia, headache, nightmares, hyperpyrexia
Dermatologic: Allergic rash, urticaria, photosensitivity, alopecia
Endocrine & metabolic: Syndrome of inappropriate ADH secretion
Gastrointestinal: Weight gain, xerostomia, constipation, paralytic ileus, nausea, vomiting, anorexia, stomatitis, peculiar taste, diarrhea, black tongue
Genitourinary: Urinary retention
Hematologic: Bone marrow depression, purpura, eosinophilia
Neuromuscular & skeletal: Numbness, paresthesia, peripheral neuropathy, tremor, weakness
Ocular: Blurred vision, mydriasis, ocular pressure increased
Otic: Tinnitus
Miscellaneous: Diaphoresis, withdrawal reactions (nausea, headache, malaise)

Dental Usual Dosage Chronic neuropathic pain in temporomandibular dysfunction (TMD) (unlabeled use): Adults: Oral: Initial: 25 mg at bedtime; may increase as tolerated to 100 mg/day

Dosage
Children:
  Chronic pain management (unlabeled use): Oral: Initial: 0.1 mg/kg at bedtime, may advance as tolerated over 2-3 weeks to 0.5-2 mg/kg at bedtime
  Depressive disorders (unlabeled use): Oral: Initial doses of 1 mg/kg/day given in 3 divided doses with increases to 1.5 mg/kg/day have been reported in a small number of children (n=9) 9-12 years of age; clinically, doses up to 3 mg/kg/day (5 mg/kg/day if monitored closely) have been proposed
  Migraine prophylaxis (unlabeled use): Oral: Initial: 0.25 mg/kg/day, given at bedtime; increase dose by 0.25 mg/kg/day to maximum 1 mg/kg/day. Reported dosing ranges: 0.1-2 mg/kg/day; maximum suggested dose: 10 mg.
Adolescents: Depressive disorders: Oral: Initial: 25-50 mg/day; may administer in divided doses; increase gradually to 100 mg/day in divided doses

Adults:

Depression: Oral: 50-150 mg/day single dose at bedtime or in divided doses; dose may be gradually increased up to 300 mg/day

Chronic pain management (unlabeled use): Oral: Initial: 25 mg at bedtime; may increase as tolerated to 100 mg/day

Diabetic neuropathy (unlabeled use): Oral: 25-100 mg/day (Bril, 2011)

Migraine prophylaxis (unlabeled use): Oral: Initial: 10-25 mg at bedtime; usual dose: 150 mg; reported dosing ranges: 10-400 mg/day

Post-traumatic stress disorder (PTSD) (unlabeled use): Oral: 75-200 mg/day

Elderly: Depression: Oral: Initial: 10-25 mg at bedtime; dose should be increased in 10-25 mg increments every week if tolerated; dose range: 25-150 mg/day

Dosing interval in hepatic impairment: Use with caution and monitor plasma levels and patient response

Hemodialysis: Nondialyzable

Mechanism of Action Increases the synaptic concentration of serotonin and/or norepinephrine in the central nervous system by inhibition of their reuptake by the presynaptic neuronal membrane

Contraindications Hypersensitivity to amitriptyline or any component of the formulation (cross-sensitivity with other tricyclics may occur); use of MAO inhibitors within past 14 days; acute recovery phase following myocardial infarction; concurrent use of cisapride

Warnings/Precautions [U.S. Boxed Warning]: Antidepressants increase the risk of suicidal thinking and behavior in children, adolescents, and young adults (18-24 years of age) with major depressive disorder (MDD) and other psychiatric disorders; consider risk prior to prescribing. Short-term studies did not show an increased risk in patients >24 years of age and showed a decreased risk in patients ≥65 years. Closely monitor for clinical worsening, suicidality, or unusual changes in behavior; the patient's family or caregiver should be instructed to closely observe the patient and communicate condition with healthcare provider. Such observation would generally include at least weekly face-to-face contact with patients or their family members or caregivers during the first 4 weeks of treatment, then every other week visits for the next 4 weeks, then at 12 weeks, and as clinically indicated beyond 12 weeks. Additional contact by telephone may be appropriate between face-to-face visits. Adults treated with antidepressants should be observed similarly for clinical worsening and suicidality, especially during the initial few months of a course of drug therapy, or at times of dose changes, either increases or decreases. A medication guide should be dispensed with each prescription. **Amitriptyline is not FDA-approved for use in children <12 years of age.**

The possibility of a suicide attempt is inherent in major depression and may persist until remission occurs. Monitor for worsening of depression or suicidality, especially during initiation of therapy (generally first 1-2 months) or with dose increases or decreases. Worsening depression and severe abrupt suicidality that are not part of the presenting symptoms may require discontinuation or modification of drug therapy. The patient's family or caregiver should be alerted to monitor patients for the emergence of suicidality and associated behaviors (such as agitation, irritability, hostility, impulsivity, and hypomania) and notify healthcare provider.

May worsen psychosis in some patients or precipitate a shift to mania or hypomania in patients with bipolar disorder. Patients presenting with depressive symptoms should be screened for bipolar disorder. Monotherapy in patients with bipolar disorder should be avoided. **Amitriptyline is not FDA approved for bipolar depression.**

The degree of sedation, anticholinergic effects, orthostasis, and conduction abnormalities are high relative to other antidepressants. Amitriptyline often causes drowsiness/sedation, resulting in impaired performance of tasks requiring alertness (eg, operating machinery or driving). Sedative effects may be additive with other CNS depressants and/or ethanol. Use with caution in patients with a history of cardiovascular disease (including previous MI, stroke, tachycardia, or conduction abnormalities). Use with caution in patients with urinary retention, benign prostatic hyperplasia, narrow-angle glaucoma, xerostomia, visual problems, constipation, or a history of bowel obstruction.

TCAs may rarely cause bone marrow suppression; monitor for any signs of infection and obtain CBC if symptoms (eg, fever, sore throat) evident. May alter glucose control - use with caution in patients with diabetes. Consider discontinuing, when possible, prior to elective surgery. Therapy should not be abruptly discontinued in patients receiving high doses for prolonged periods. May lower seizure threshold - use caution in patients with a previous seizure disorder or condition predisposing to seizures such as brain damage, alcoholism, or concurrent therapy with other drugs which lower the seizure threshold. Hyperpyrexia has been observed with TCAs in combination with anticholinergics and/or neuroleptics, particularly during hot weather. May increase the risks associated with electroconvulsive therapy. Use with caution in hyperthyroid patients or those receiving thyroid supplementation. Use with caution in patients with hepatic or renal dysfunction. Avoid use in the elderly due to its potent anticholinergic and sedative properties, and potential to cause orthostatic hypotension. In addition, may cause or exacerbate syndrome of inappropriate antidiuretic hormone secretion or hyponatremia; monitor sodium closely with initiation or dosage adjustments in older adults (Beers Criteria).

Drug Interactions

Metabolism/Transport Effects Substrate of CYP1A2 (minor), CYP2B6 (minor), CYP2C19 (minor), CYP2C9 (minor), CYP2D6 (major), CYP3A4 (minor); **Note:** Assignment of Major/Minor substrate status based on clinically relevant drug interaction potential; **Inhibits** CYP1A2 (weak), CYP2C19 (weak), CYP2C9 (weak), CYP2D6 (weak), CYP2E1 (weak)

Avoid Concomitant Use

Avoid concomitant use of Amitriptyline with any of the following: Aclidinium; Cisapride; Iobenguane I 123; Ipratropium (Oral Inhalation); Linezolid; MAO Inhibitors; Methylene Blue; Tiotropium

Increased Effect/Toxicity

Amitriptyline may increase the levels/effects of: Alpha-/Beta-Agonists (Direct-Acting); Alpha1-Agonists; Amphetamines; Anticholinergics; Aspirin; Beta2-Agonists; Cisapride; Desmopressin; Highest Risk QTc-Prolonging Agents; Methylene Blue; Metoclopramide; Moderate Risk QTc-Prolonging Agents; NSAID (COX-2 Inhibitor); NSAID (Nonselective); QuiNIDine; Serotonin Modulators; Sodium Phosphates; Sulfonylureas; Tiotropium; TraMADol; Vitamin K Antagonists; Yohimbine

▶

The levels/effects of Amitriptyline may be increased by: Abiraterone Acetate; Aclidinium; Altretamine; Antipsychotics; BuPROPion; Cimetidine; Cinacalcet; Cobicistat; CYP2D6 Inhibitors (Moderate); CYP2D6 Inhibitors (Strong); Dexmethylphenidate; Divalproex; DULoxetine; Ipratropium (Oral Inhalation); Linezolid; Lithium; MAO Inhibitors; Methylphenidate; Metoclopramide; Metyrosine; Mifepristone; Pramlintide; Protease Inhibitors; QuiNIDine; Selective Serotonin Reuptake Inhibitors; Terbinafine (Systemic); Valproic Acid

Decreased Effect

Amitriptyline may decrease the levels/effects of: Acetylcholinesterase Inhibitors (Central); Alpha2-Agonists; Iobenguane I 123

The levels/effects of Amitriptyline may be decreased by: Acetylcholinesterase Inhibitors (Central); Barbiturates; CarBAMazepine; Peginterferon Alfa-2b; St Johns Wort

Ethanol/Nutrition/Herb Interactions

Ethanol: May increase CNS depression; monitor for increased effects with coadministration. Caution patients about effects.

Food: Grapefruit juice may inhibit the metabolism of some TCAs and clinical toxicity may result.

Herb/Nutraceutical: St John's wort may decrease amitriptyline levels. Avoid valerian, St John's wort, kava kava, gotu kola (may increase CNS depression).

Pharmacodynamics/Kinetics

Onset of Action Migraine prophylaxis: 6 weeks, higher dosage may be required in heavy smokers because of increased metabolism; Depression: 4-6 weeks, reduce dosage to lowest effective level

Half-life Elimination Adults: 9-27 hours (average: 15 hours)

Time to Peak Serum: ~4 hours

Pregnancy Risk Factor C

Pregnancy Considerations Teratogenic effects have been observed in animal studies. Amitriptyline crosses the human placenta; CNS effects, limb deformities and developmental delay have been noted in case reports.

Lactation Enters breast milk/not recommended (AAP rates "of concern"; AAP 2001 update pending)

Breast-Feeding Considerations Based on information from six mother/infant pairs, following maternal use of amitriptyline 75-175 mg/day, the estimated exposure to the breast-feeding infant would be 0.2% to 1.9% of the weight-adjusted maternal dose. Adverse events have not been reported in nursing infants (four cases). Infants should be monitored for signs of adverse events; routine monitoring of infant serum concentrations is not recommended.

Dosage Forms

Tablet, oral: 10 mg, 25 mg, 50 mg, 75 mg, 100 mg, 150 mg

Dental Comment Amitriptyline is known to prolong the QT interval. The QT interval is measured as the time and distance between the Q point of the QRS complex and the end of the T wave in the ECG tracing. After adjustment for heart rate, the QT interval is defined as prolonged if it is more than 450 msec in men and 460 msec in women. A long QT syndrome was first described in the 1950s and 60s as a congenital syndrome involving QT interval prolongation and syncope and sudden death. Some of the congenital long QT syndromes were characterized by a peculiar electrocardiographic appearance of the QRS complex involving a premature atria beat followed by a pause, then a subsequent sinus beat showing marked QT prolongation and deformity. This type of cardiac arrhythmia was

originally termed "torsade de pointes" (translated from the French as "twisting of the points"). Amitriptyline is considered as having a risk of causing torsade de pointes. Since it is not known what effect vasoconstrictors in the local anesthetic regimen will have in patients with a known history of congenital prolonged QT interval or in patients taking any medication that prolongs the QT interval, a medical consult is suggested.

References

Boakes AJ, Laurence DR, Teoh PC, et al, "Interactions Between Sympathomimetic Amines and Antidepressant Agents in Man," *Br Med J*, 1973, 1(849):311-5.

Friedlander AH and Mahler ME, "Major Depressive Disorder. Psychopathology, Medical Management, and Dental Implications," *J Am Dent Assoc*, 2001, 132(5):629-38.

Ganzberg S, "Psychoactive Drugs," *ADA Guide to Dental Therapeutics*, 2nd ed, Chicago, IL: ADA Publishing, a Division of ADA Business Enterprises, Inc, 2000, 376-405.

Jastak JT and Yagiela JA, "Vasoconstrictors and Local Anesthesia: A Review and Rationale for Use," *J Am Dent Assoc*, 1983, 107 (4):623-30.

Rundegren J, van Dijken J, Mörnstad H, et al, "Oral Conditions in Patients Receiving Long-Term Treatment With Cyclic Antidepressant Drugs," *Swed Dent J*, 1985, 9(2):55-64.

Yagiela JA, "Adverse Drug Interactions in Dental Practice: Interactions Associated With Vasoconstrictors. Part V of a Series," *J Am Dent Assoc*, 1999, 130(5):701-9.

Amitriptyline and Chlordiazepoxide
(a mee TRIP ti leen & klor dye az e POKS ide)

Related Information

Amitriptyline *on page 84*

ChlordiazePOXIDE *on page 288*

Vasoconstrictor Interactions With Antidepressants *on page 1650*

Pharmacologic Category Antidepressant, Tricyclic (Tertiary Amine); Benzodiazepine

Use Treatment of moderate-to-severe anxiety and/or agitation and depression

Local Anesthetic/Vasoconstrictor Precautions
Use with caution; epinephrine or mepivacaine and levonordefrin (Carbocaine® 2% with Neo-Cobefrin®) have been shown to have an increased pressor response in combination with TCAs

Effects on Dental Treatment Key adverse event(s) related to dental treatment:

Amitriptyline: Xerostomia and changes in salivation (normal salivary flow resumes upon discontinuation), orthostatic hypotension, stomatitis, peculiar taste, and black tongue. Amitriptyline is the most anticholinergic and sedating of the antidepressants; has pronounced effects on the cardiovascular system. Long-term treatment with TCAs such as amitriptyline increases the risk of caries by reducing salivation and salivary buffer capacity. In a study by Rundergren, et al, pathological alterations were observed in the oral mucosa of 72% of 58 patients; 55% had new carious lesions after taking TCAs for a median of 5½ years. Current research is investigating the use of the salivary stimulant pilocarpine (Salagen®) to overcome the xerostomia from amitriptyline.

Chlordiazepoxide: Over 10% of patients will experience xerostomia which disappears with cessation of drug therapy.

Effects on Bleeding May cause thrombocytopenia

Adverse Effects See individual agents.

General Dosage Range Oral: *Adults:* 2-6 tablets (amitriptyline 12.5-25 mg/chlordiazepoxide 5-10 mg per tablet)/day (maximum: 6 tablets/day)

Mechanism of Action See individual agents.

Pregnancy Considerations See individual agents.

Controlled Substance C-IV

Amitriptyline and Perphenazine
(a mee TRIP ti leen & per FEN a zeen)

Related Information
Amitriptyline *on page 84*
Perphenazine *on page 1078*
Vasoconstrictor Interactions With Antidepressants *on page 1650*

Brand Names: Canada PMS-Levazine

Pharmacologic Category Antidepressant, Tricyclic (Tertiary Amine); Antipsychotic Agent, Typical, Phenothiazine

Use Treatment of patients with moderate-to-severe anxiety and/or agitation and depression; schizophrenia with depressive symptoms

Local Anesthetic/Vasoconstrictor Precautions
Amitriptyline: Use with caution; epinephrine or mepivacaine and levonordefrin (Carbocaine® 2% with Neo-Cobefrin®) have been shown to have an increased pressor response in combination with TCAs

Perphenazine: No information available to require special precautions

Effects on Dental Treatment
Key adverse event(s) related to dental treatment:

Amitriptyline: Xerostomia and changes in salivation (normal salivary flow resumes upon discontinuation), orthostatic hypotension, stomatitis, peculiar taste, and black tongue. Amitriptyline is the most anticholinergic and sedating of the antidepressants; has pronounced effects on the cardiovascular system. Long-term treatment with TCAs such as amitriptyline increases the risk of caries by reducing salivation and salivary buffer capacity. In a study by Rundergren, et al, pathological alterations were observed in the oral mucosa of 72% of 58 patients; 55% had new carious lesions after taking TCAs for a median of 5$1/2$ years. Current research is investigating the use of the salivary stimulant pilocarpine (Salagen®) to overcome the xerostomia from amitriptyline.

Perphenazine: Extrapyramidal symptoms (pseudoparkinsonism, akathisia, dystonias, tardive dyskinesia), dizziness, seizures, headache, drowsiness, paradoxical excitement, restlessness, and hyperactivity.

Tardive dyskinesia: Prevalence rate may be 40% in elderly; development of the syndrome and the irreversible nature are proportional to duration and total cumulative dose over time. Extrapyramidal reactions are more common in elderly with up to 50% developing these reactions after 60 years of age. Drug-induced Parkinson's syndrome occurs often; akathisia is the most common extrapyramidal reaction in elderly.

Increased confusion, memory loss, psychotic behavior, and agitation frequently occur as a consequence of anticholinergic effects. Antipsychotic associated sedation in nonpsychotic patients is extremely unpleasant due to feelings of depersonalization, derealization, and dysphoria.

Effects on Bleeding
May cause thrombocytopenia

Adverse Effects See individual agents.

General Dosage Range Oral: *Adults:* Initial: Amitriptyline 25 mg/perphenazine 2-4 mg 3-4 times/day **or** amitriptyline 50 mg/perphenazine 4-8 mg 2-3 times/day; Maintenance: Amitriptyline 25 mg/perphenazine 2-4 mg 2-4 times/day **or** amitriptyline 50 mg/perphenazine 4 mg 2 times/day; maximum daily dose: amitriptyline 200 mg/perphenazine 16 mg

Mechanism of Action
Amitriptyline increases the synaptic concentration of serotonin and/or norepinephrine in the central nervous system by inhibition of their reuptake by the presynaptic neuronal membrane.

Perphenazine is a piperazine phenothiazine antipsychotic which blocks postsynaptic mesolimbic dopaminergic receptors in the brain; exhibits alpha-adrenergic blocking effect and depresses the release of hypothalamic and hypophyseal hormones.

Pregnancy Considerations See individual agents.

Amlexanox (am LEKS an oks)

Related Information
Ulcerative, Erosive, and Painful Oral Mucosal Disorders *on page 1578*

Related Sample Prescriptions
Recurrent Aphthous Stomatitis *on page 1618*

Brand Names: U.S. Aphthasol®

Generic Availability (U.S.) No

Pharmacologic Category Anti-inflammatory, Locally Applied

Dental Use Treatment of aphthous ulcers (ie, canker sores)

Use Treatment of aphthous ulcers (ie, canker sores)

Unlabeled Use Allergic disorders

Local Anesthetic/Vasoconstrictor Precautions
No information available to require special precautions

Effects on Dental Treatment
Key adverse event(s) related to dental treatment: Allergic contact dermatitis and oral irritation. Discontinue therapy if rash or contact mucositis develops (see Dental Comment).

Effects on Bleeding
No information available to require special precautions

Adverse Effects 1% to 2%:
Dermatologic: Allergic contact dermatitis
Gastrointestinal: Oral irritation

Dosage Topical: Administer ~$1/4$ inch (0.5 cm) directly on ulcers 4 times/day following oral hygiene, after meals, and at bedtime

Dosage adjustment in renal impairment: No dosage adjustment provided in manufacturer's labeling.

Dosage adjustment in hepatic impairment: No dosage adjustment provided in manufacturer's labeling.

Mechanism of Action As a benzopyrano-bipyridine carboxylic acid derivative, amlexanox has anti-inflammatory and antiallergic properties; it inhibits chemical mediatory release of the slow-reacting substance of anaphylaxis (SRS-A) and may have antagonistic effects on interleukin-3

Contraindications Hypersensitivity to amlexanox or any component of the formulation

Warnings/Precautions Discontinue therapy if rash or contact mucositis develops. Safety and efficacy have not been established in children.

Drug Interactions
Metabolism/Transport Effects None known.

Avoid Concomitant Use There are no known interactions where it is recommended to avoid concomitant use.

Increased Effect/Toxicity There are no known significant interactions involving an increase in effect.

Decreased Effect There are no known significant interactions involving a decrease in effect.

Pharmacodynamics/Kinetics
Half-life Elimination 3.5 hours
Time to Peak Serum: 2 hours

◀ **Pregnancy Risk Factor** B

Pregnancy Considerations Due to lack of data, avoid use in pregnancy, if possible.

Lactation Excretion in breast milk unknown/use caution

Dosage Forms

Paste, oral:
Aphthasol®: 5% (3 g)

Dental Comment Treatment of canker sores with amlexanox showed a 76% median reduction in ulcer size compared to a 40% reduction with placebo. Greer, et al, reported an overall mean reduction in ulcer size of 1.82 mm^2 for patients treated with 5% amlexanox versus an average reduction of 0.52 mm^2 for the control group. Recent studies in over thousands of patients have confirmed that amlexanox accelerates the resolution of pain and healing of aphthous ulcers more significantly than vehicle and no treatment.

References

Barrons RW, "Treatment Strategies for Recurrent Oral Aphthous Ulcers," *Am J Health Syst Pharm*, 2001, 58(1):41-50.

Binnie WH, Curro FA, Khandwala A, et al, "Amlexanox Oral Paste: A Novel Treatment That Accelerates the Healing of Aphthous Ulcers," *Compend Contin Educ Dent*, 1997, 18(11):1116-8, 1120-2, 1124 passim.

Greer RO Jr, Lindenmuth JE, Juarez T, et al, "A Double-Blind Study of Topically Applied 5% Amlexanox in the Treatment of Aphthous Ulcers," *J Oral Maxillofac Surg*, 1993, 51(3):243-8.

Khandwala A, Van Inwegen RG, and Alfano MC, "5% Amlexanox Oral Paste, A New Treatment for Recurrent Minor Aphthous Ulcers: I. Clinical Demonstration of Acceleration of Healing and Resolution of Pain," *Oral Surg Oral Med Oral Pathol Oral Radiol Endod*, 1997, 83 (2):222-30.

Khandwala A, Van Inwegen RG, Charney MR, et al, "5% Amlexanox Oral Paste, A New Treatment for Recurrent Minor Aphthous Ulcers: II. Pharmacokinetics and Demonstration of Clinical Safety," *Oral Surg Oral Med Oral Pathol Oral Radiol Endod*, 1997, 83(2):231-8.

AmLODIPine (am LOE di peen)

Related Information

Calcium Channel Blockers and Gingival Hyperplasia *on page 1640*

Cardiovascular Diseases *on page 1492*

Brand Names: U.S. Norvasc®

Brand Names: Canada Accel-Amlodipine; Amlodipine-Odan; Apo-Amlodipine®; CO Amlodipine; Dom-Amlodipine; GD-Amlodipine; JAMP-Amlodipine; Manda-Amlodipine; Mint-Amlodipine; Mylan-Amlodipine; Norvasc®; PHL-Amlodipine; PMS-Amlodipine; Q-Amlodipine; RAN™-Amlodipine; ratio-Amlodipine; Riva-Amlodipine; Sandoz Amlodipine; Septa-Amlodipine; Teva-Amlodipine; ZYM-Amlodipine

Generic Availability (U.S.) Yes

Pharmacologic Category Antianginal Agent; Calcium Channel Blocker; Calcium Channel Blocker, Dihydropyridine

Use Treatment of hypertension; treatment of symptomatic chronic stable angina, vasospastic (Prinzmetal's) angina (confirmed or suspected); prevention of hospitalization due to angina with documented CAD (limited to patients without heart failure or ejection fraction <40%)

Local Anesthetic/Vasoconstrictor Precautions No information available to require special precautions

Effects on Dental Treatment Fewer reports of gingival hyperplasia with amlodipine than with other CCBs (usually resolves upon discontinuation); consultation with physician is suggested.

Effects on Bleeding No information available to require special precautions

Adverse Effects

>10%:
Cardiovascular: Peripheral edema (2% to 11% dose related; female 15%; male 6%; HF patients 27% [Packer, 1996])

Respiratory: Pulmonary edema (HF patients 27% [Packer, 1996])

1% to 10%:
Cardiovascular: Palpitations (1% to 5% dose related), flushing (1% to 3% dose related, more frequent in females)

Central nervous system: Fatigue (5%), dizziness (1% to 3% dose related), somnolence (1%)

Dermatologic: Pruritus (1% to 2%), rash (1% to 2%)

Endocrine & metabolic: Male sexual dysfunction (1% to 2%)

Gastrointestinal: Nausea (3%), abdominal pain (2%)

Neuromuscular & skeletal: Muscle cramps (1% to 2%), weakness (1% to 2%)

Respiratory: Dyspnea (1% to 2%)

Dosage Oral:

Children 6-17 years: Hypertension: 2.5-5 mg once daily

Adults:

Hypertension: Initial dose: 5 mg once daily; maximum dose: 10 mg once daily. In general, titrate in 2.5 mg increments over 7-14 days. Usual dosage range (JNC 7): 2.5-10 mg once daily.

Angina: Usual dose: 5-10 mg; most patients require 10 mg for adequate effect

Elderly: Dosing should start at the lower end of dosing range and titrated to response due to possible increased incidence of hepatic, renal, or cardiac impairment. Elderly patients also show decreased clearance of amlodipine.

Hypertension: 2.5 mg once daily

Angina: 5 mg once daily

Dosage adjustment in renal impairment: Dialysis: Hemodialysis and peritoneal dialysis do not enhance elimination. Supplemental dose is not necessary.

Dosage adjustment in hepatic impairment:

Angina: Administer 5 mg once daily.

Hypertension: Administer 2.5 mg once daily.

Mechanism of Action Inhibits calcium ion from entering the "slow channels" or select voltage-sensitive areas of vascular smooth muscle and myocardium during depolarization, producing a relaxation of coronary vascular smooth muscle and coronary vasodilation; increases myocardial oxygen delivery in patients with vasospastic angina. Amlodipine directly acts on vascular smooth muscle to produce peripheral arterial vasodilation reducing peripheral vascular resistance and blood pressure.

Contraindications Hypersensitivity to amlodipine or any component of the formulation

Warnings/Precautions Increased angina and/or MI has occurred with initiation or dosage titration of calcium channel blockers. Symptomatic hypotension with or without syncope can rarely occur; blood pressure must be lowered at a rate appropriate for the patient's clinical condition. Use caution in severe aortic stenosis and/or hypertrophic cardiomyopathy with outflow tract obstruction. Use caution in patients with hepatic impairment; may require lower starting dose; titrate slowly with severe hepatic impairment. The most common side effect is peripheral edema; occurs within 2-3 weeks of starting therapy. Reflex tachycardia may occur with use. Peak antihypertensive effect is delayed; dosage titration should occur after 7-14 days on a given dose. Initiate at a lower dose in the elderly.

Drug Interactions

Metabolism/Transport Effects Substrate of CYP3A4 (major); **Note:** Assignment of Major/Minor substrate status based on clinically relevant drug interaction potential; **Inhibits** CYP1A2 (moderate),

CYP2A6 (weak), CYP2B6 (weak), CYP2C8 (weak), CYP2C9 (weak), CYP2D6 (weak), CYP3A4 (weak)

Avoid Concomitant Use

Avoid concomitant use of AmLODIPine with any of the following: Conivaptan; Pimozide; Pirfenidone

Increased Effect/Toxicity

AmLODIPine may increase the levels/effects of: Amifostine; Antihypertensives; ARIPiprazole; Atosiban; Beta-Blockers; Calcium Channel Blockers (Nondihydropyridine); CYP1A2 Substrates; Fosphenytoin; Hypotensive Agents; Lomitapide; Magnesium Salts; Neuromuscular-Blocking Agents (Nondepolarizing); Nitroprusside; Phenytoin; Pimozide; Pirfenidone; QuiNIDine; RiTUXimab; Simvastatin; Tacrolimus (Systemic)

The levels/effects of AmLODIPine may be increased by: Alpha1-Blockers; Antifungal Agents (Azole Derivatives, Systemic); Calcium Channel Blockers (Nondihydropyridine); Conivaptan; CycloSPORINE (Systemic); CYP3A4 Inhibitors (Moderate); CYP3A4 Inhibitors (Strong); Dasatinib; Diazoxide; Fluconazole; Grapefruit Juice; Herbs (Hypotensive Properties); Ivacaftor; Macrolide Antibiotics; Magnesium Salts; MAO Inhibitors; Mifepristone; Pentoxifylline; Phosphodiesterase 5 Inhibitors; Prostacyclin Analogues; Protease Inhibitors; QuiNIDine

Decreased Effect

AmLODIPine may decrease the levels/effects of: Clopidogrel; QuiNIDine

The levels/effects of AmLODIPine may be decreased by: Barbiturates; Calcium Salts; CarBAMazepine; CYP3A4 Inducers (Strong); Deferasirox; Herbs (CYP3A4 Inducers); Herbs (Hypertensive Properties); Melatonin; Methylphenidate; Nafcillin; Rifamycin Derivatives; Tocilizumab; Yohimbine

Ethanol/Nutrition/Herb Interactions

Food: Grapefruit juice may modestly increase amlodipine levels.

Herb/Nutraceutical: St John's wort may decrease amlodipine levels. Avoid herbs with *hypertensive* properties (bayberry, blue cohosh, cayenne, ephedra, ginger, ginseng [American], kola, licorice). Avoid herbs with *hypotensive* properties (black cohosh, California poppy, coleus, garlic, goldenseal, hawthorn, mistletoe, periwinkle, quinine, shepherd's purse).

Dietary Considerations May be taken without regard to meals.

Pharmacodynamics/Kinetics

Duration of Action Antihypertensive effect: 24 hours

Half-life Elimination Terminal: 30-50 hours; increased with hepatic dysfunction

Time to Peak Plasma: 6-12 hours

Pregnancy Risk Factor C

Pregnancy Considerations Embryotoxic effects have been demonstrated in animal studies. No well-controlled studies have been conducted in pregnant women. Use in pregnancy only when clearly needed and when the benefits outweigh the potential hazard to the fetus.

Lactation Excretion in breast milk unknown/not recommended

Dosage Forms

Tablet, oral: 2.5 mg, 5 mg, 10 mg
Norvasc®: 2.5 mg, 5 mg, 10 mg

References

Jorgensen MG, "Prevalence of Amlodipine-Related Gingival Hyperplasia," *J Periodontol*, 1997, 68(7):676-8.
Wynn RL, "Calcium Channel Blockers and Gingival Hyperplasia-An Update," *Gen Dent*, 2009, 57(2):105-7.

Amlodipine and Atorvastatin

(am LOW di peen & a TORE va sta tin)

Related Information

AmLODIPine *on page 88*
AtorvaSTATin *on page 145*

Brand Names: U.S. Caduet®

Brand Names: Canada Caduet®

Generic Availability (U.S.) Yes

Pharmacologic Category Antianginal Agent; Antilipemic Agent, HMG-CoA Reductase Inhibitor; Calcium Channel Blocker; Calcium Channel Blocker, Dihydropyridine

Use For use when treatment with both amlodipine and atorvastatin is appropriate:

Amlodipine: Treatment of hypertension; treatment of chronic stable angina, vasospastic (Prinzmetal's) angina (confirmed or suspected); prevention of hospitalization or to decrease coronary revascularization procedure due to angina with documented CAD (limited to patients without heart failure or ejection fraction <40%)

Atorvastatin: Treatment of dyslipidemias or primary prevention of cardiovascular disease (atherosclerotic) as detailed here:

Primary prevention of cardiovascular disease (high-risk for CVD): To reduce the risk of MI or stroke in patients without evidence of coronary heart disease who have multiple CVD risk factors or type 2 diabetes; also reduces the risk for angina or revascularization procedures in patients with multiple CVD risk factors without evidence of coronary heart disease

Secondary prevention of cardiovascular disease: To reduce the risk of MI, stroke, revascularization procedures, angina, and hospitalization for heart failure

Treatment of dyslipidemias: To reduce elevations in total cholesterol, LDL-C, apolipoprotein B, and triglycerides in patients with elevations of one or more components, and/or to increase low HDL-C as present in heterozygous familial/nonfamilial hypercholesterolemia and mixed dyslipidemia (Fredrickson type IIa and IIb hyperlipidemias); treatment of primary dysbetalipoproteinemia (Fredrickson type III), elevated serum TG levels (Fredrickson type IV), and homozygous familial hypercholesterolemia

Treatment of heterozygous familial hypercholesterolemia (HeFH) in adolescent patients (10-17 years of age, females >1 year postmenarche) having LDL-C ≥190 mg/dL or LDL-C ≥160 mg/dL with positive family history of premature cardiovascular disease (CVD) or with two or more CVD risk factors.

Local Anesthetic/Vasoconstrictor Precautions No information available to require special precautions

Effects on Dental Treatment Key adverse event(s) related to dental treatment: Fewer reports of gingival hyperplasia with amlodipine than with other calcium channel blockers (usually resolves upon discontinuation); consultation with physician is suggested.

Effects on Bleeding No information available to require special precautions

Adverse Effects See individual agents.

Dosage Oral: **Note:** Dose is individualized; combination product may be used as initial therapy or substituted for individual components in patients currently maintained on both agents separately or in patients not adequately controlled with monotherapy (using one of the agents or an agent within same pharmacologic class).

Children 10-17 years (females >1 year postmenarche): Hypertension and hyperlipidemia:

Initial therapy: Amlodipine 2.5 mg and atorvastatin 10 mg once daily; dose may be titrated after 1-2 weeks (amlodipine component) and after 2-4 weeks (atorvastatin component) to a maximum daily dose: Amlodipine 5 mg; atorvastatin 20 mg

Add-on therapy/replacement therapy: Amlodipine 2.5-5 mg and atorvastatin 10-20 mg once daily; dose may be titrated after 1-2 weeks (amlodipine component) and after 2-4 weeks (atorvastatin component) to a maximum daily dose: Amlodipine 5 mg; atorvastatin 20 mg

Adults: Hypertension, angina, and hyperlipidemia:

Initial therapy: Amlodipine 5 mg and atorvastatin 10-20 mg once daily; dose may be titrated after 1-2 weeks (amlodipine component) and after 2-4 weeks (atorvastatin component) to a maximum daily dose: Amlodipine 10 mg; atorvastatin 80 mg

Add-on therapy/replacement therapy: Amlodipine 5-10 mg and atorvastatin 10-80 mg once daily; dose may be titrated after 1-2 weeks (amlodipine component) and after 2-4 weeks (atorvastatin component) to a maximum daily dose: Amlodipine 10 mg; atorvastatin 80 mg

Elderly: Consider starting amlodipine at the lower end of dosing range due to increased incidence of hepatic, renal, or cardiac impairment. Elderly patients also show decreased clearance of amlodipine.

Dosage adjustment for atorvastatin with concomitant medications:

Boceprevir, nelfinavir: Use lowest effective atorvastatin dose (not to exceed 40 mg daily)

Clarithromycin, itraconazole, fosamprenavir, ritonavir (plus darunavir, fosamprenavir, or saquinavir): Use lowest effective atorvastatin dose (not to exceed 20 mg daily)

Dosage adjustment in renal impairment: No dosage adjustment is necessary

Dosage adjustment in hepatic impairment: Contraindicated in patients with active liver disease

Mechanism of Action

Amlodipine: Inhibits calcium ion from entering the "slow channels" or select voltage-sensitive areas of vascular smooth muscle and myocardium during depolarization, producing a relaxation of coronary vascular smooth muscle and coronary vasodilation; increases myocardial oxygen delivery in patients with vasospastic angina. Amlodipine directly acts on vascular smooth muscle to produce peripheral arterial vasodilation reducing peripheral vascular resistance and blood pressure.

Atorvastatin: Inhibitor of 3-hydroxy-3-methylglutaryl coenzyme A (HMG-CoA) reductase, the rate limiting enzyme in cholesterol synthesis (reduces the production of mevalonic acid from HMG-CoA); this then results in a compensatory increase in the expression of LDL receptors on hepatocyte membranes and a stimulation of LDL catabolism

Contraindications Hypersensitivity to amlodipine, atorvastatin, or any component of the formulation; active liver disease; unexplained persistent elevations of serum transaminases; pregnancy; breast-feeding

Note: Telaprevir Canadian product monograph contraindicates use with atorvastatin.

Warnings/Precautions See individual agents.

Drug Interactions

Metabolism/Transport Effects Refer to individual components.

Avoid Concomitant Use

Avoid concomitant use of Amlodipine and Atorvastatin with any of the following: Bosutinib; Conivaptan; CycloSPORINE (Systemic); Fusidic Acid; Gemfibrozil; Pimozide; Pirfenidone; Pomalidomide; Posaconazole; Red Yeast Rice; Telaprevir; Tipranavir; Topotecan; VinCRIStine (Liposomal)

Increased Effect/Toxicity

Amlodipine and Atorvastatin may increase the levels/effects of: Aliskiren; Amifostine; Antihypertensives; ARIPiprazole; Atosiban; Beta-Blockers; Bosutinib; Calcium Channel Blockers (Nondihydropyridine); CYP1A2 Substrates; DAPTOmycin; Digoxin; Diltiazem; Everolimus; Fosphenytoin; Hypotensive Agents; Ketoconazole (Systemic); Lomitapide; Magnesium Salts; Midazolam; Neuromuscular-Blocking Agents (Nondepolarizing); Nitroprusside; Pazopanib; P-glycoprotein/ABCB1 Substrates; Phenytoin; Pimozide; Pirfenidone; Pomalidomide; Prucalopride; QuiNIDine; RiTUXimab; Rivaroxaban; Simvastatin; Tacrolimus (Systemic); Topotecan; Trabectedin; Verapamil; VinCRIStine (Liposomal)

The levels/effects of Amlodipine and Atorvastatin may be increased by: Alpha1-Blockers; Amiodarone; Antifungal Agents (Azole Derivatives, Systemic); Bezafibrate; Boceprevir; Calcium Channel Blockers (Nondihydropyridine); Cobicistat; Colchicine; Conivaptan; CycloSPORINE (Systemic); CYP3A4 Inhibitors (Moderate); CYP3A4 Inhibitors (Strong); Cyproterone; Danazol; Dasatinib; Diazoxide; Diltiazem; Dronedarone; Eltrombopag; Fenofibrate; Fenofibric Acid; Fluconazole; Fusidic Acid; Gemfibrozil; Grapefruit Juice; Herbs (Hypotensive Properties); Itraconazole; Ivacaftor; Ketoconazole (Systemic); Macrolide Antibiotics; Magnesium Salts; MAO Inhibitors; Mifepristone; Niacin; Niacinamide; Pentoxifylline; P-glycoprotein/ABCB1 Inhibitors; Phosphodiesterase 5 Inhibitors; Posaconazole; Prostacyclin Analogues; Protease Inhibitors; QuiNIDine; QuiNINE; Red Yeast Rice; Sildenafil; Telaprevir; Tipranavir; Verapamil; Voriconazole

Decreased Effect

Amlodipine and Atorvastatin may decrease the levels/effects of: Clopidogrel; Dabigatran Etexilate; Lanthanum; QuiNIDine

The levels/effects of Amlodipine and Atorvastatin may be decreased by: Antacids; Barbiturates; Bexarotene (Systemic); Bile Acid Sequestrants; Bosentan; Calcium Salts; CarBAMazepine; CYP3A4 Inducers (Strong); Deferasirox; Efavirenz; Etravirine; Fosphenytoin; Herbs (Hypertensive Properties); Melatonin; Methylphenidate; Nafcillin; P-glycoprotein/ABCB1 Inducers; Phenytoin; Rifamycin Derivatives; St Johns Wort; Tocilizumab; Yohimbine

Ethanol/Nutrition/Herb Interactions See individual agents.

Dietary Considerations May take with food if desired; may take without regard to time of day. Before initiation of therapy with atorvastatin, patients should be placed on a standard cholesterol-lowering diet for 3-6 months and the diet should be continued during drug therapy. Red yeast rice contains an estimated 2.4 mg lovastatin per 600 mg rice.

Pregnancy Risk Factor X

Pregnancy Considerations Use is contraindicated in pregnant women. See individual agents.

Lactation Excretion in breast milk unknown/contraindicated

Breast-Feeding Considerations Use is contraindicated in nursing women. See individual agents.

Dosage Forms

Tablet, oral: Amlodipine 2.5 mg and atorvastatin 10 mg; Amlodipine 2.5 mg and atorvastatin 20 mg; Amlodipine 2.5 mg and atorvastatin 40 mg; Amlodipine 5 mg and atorvastatin 10 mg; Amlodipine 5 mg and atorvastatin 20 mg; Amlodipine 5 mg and atorvastatin 40 mg; Amlodipine 5 mg and atorvastatin 80 mg; Amlodipine 10 mg and atorvastatin 10 mg; Amlodipine 10 mg and atorvastatin 20 mg; Amlodipine 10 mg and atorvastatin 40 mg; Amlodipine 10 mg and atorvastatin 80 mg

Caduet®:
  2.5/10: Amlodipine 2.5 mg and atorvastatin 10 mg;
  2.5/20: Amlodipine 2.5 mg and atorvastatin 20 mg;
  2.5/40: Amlodipine 2.5 mg and atorvastatin 40 mg
  5/10: Amlodipine 5 mg and atorvastatin 10 mg; 5/20: Amlodipine 5 mg and atorvastatin 20 mg; 5/40: Amlodipine 5 mg and atorvastatin 40 mg; 5/80: Amlodipine 5 mg and atorvastatin 80 mg
  10/10: Amlodipine 10 mg and atorvastatin 10 mg; 10/20: Amlodipine 10 mg and atorvastatin 20 mg; 10/40: Amlodipine 10 mg and atorvastatin 40 mg; 10/80: Amlodipine 10 mg and atorvastatin 80 mg

---

Amlodipine and Benazepril
(am LOE di peen & ben AY ze pril)

Related Information
AmLODIPine *on page 88*
Benazepril *on page 173*

Brand Names: U.S. Lotrel®

Generic Availability (U.S.) Yes

Pharmacologic Category Angiotensin-Converting Enzyme (ACE) Inhibitor; Antianginal Agent; Calcium Channel Blocker; Calcium Channel Blocker, Dihydropyridine

Use Treatment of hypertension

Local Anesthetic/Vasoconstrictor Precautions No information available to require special precautions

Effects on Dental Treatment Fewer reports of gingival hyperplasia with amlodipine than with other CCBs (usually resolves upon discontinuation); consultation with physician is suggested.

Effects on Bleeding No information available to require special precautions

Adverse Effects See individual agents.

Dosage Oral: **Note:** Dose is individualized; combination product may be substituted for individual components in patients currently maintained on both agents separately or in patients not adequately controlled with monotherapy (using one of the agents or an agent within same antihypertensive class).

Adults: 2.5-10 mg (amlodipine) and 10-40 mg (benazepril) once daily; maximum: Amlodipine: 10 mg/day; benazepril: 80 mg/day

Elderly: Initial dose: 2.5 mg based on amlodipine component

Dosage adjustment in renal impairment: Cl_{cr} ≤30 mL/minute: Use of combination product is not recommended.

Dosage adjustment in hepatic impairment: Initial dose: 2.5 mg based on amlodipine component

Mechanism of Action
Amlodipine is a dihydropyridine calcium channel antagonist that inhibits transmembrane influx of calcium ions into vascular smooth muscle and cardiac muscle producing relaxation of coronary vascular smooth muscle and coronary vasodilation; amlodipine directly acts on vascular smooth muscle to produce peripheral arterial vasodilation reducing peripheral vascular resistance and blood pressure.

Benazepril lowers blood pressure by suppressing the renin-angiotensin-aldosterone system; benazepril has an antihypertensive effect even in patients with low-renin hypertension.

Contraindications Hypersensitivity to amlodipine, benazepril, other ACE inhibitors, or any component of the formulation; history of angioedema, with or without previous ACE inhibitor treatment; concomitant use with aliskiren in patients with diabetes mellitus

Warnings/Precautions Used as a replacement for separate dosing of components or combination therapy when response to single agent is suboptimal. The fixed combination is not indicated for initial treatment of hypertension. See individual agents for additional Warnings/Precautions.

Drug Interactions

Metabolism/Transport Effects Refer to individual components.

Avoid Concomitant Use

Avoid concomitant use of Amlodipine and Benazepril with any of the following: Conivaptan; Pimozide; Pirfenidone

Increased Effect/Toxicity

Amlodipine and Benazepril may increase the levels/effects of: Allopurinol; Amifostine; Antihypertensives; ARIPiprazole; Atosiban; AzaTHIOprine; Beta-Blockers; Calcium Channel Blockers (Nondihydropyridine); CycloSPORINE (Systemic); CYP1A2 Substrates; Ferric Gluconate; Fosphenytoin; Gold Sodium Thiomalate; Hypotensive Agents; Iron Dextran Complex; Lithium; Lomitapide; Magnesium Salts; Neuromuscular-Blocking Agents (Nondepolarizing); Nitroprusside; Nonsteroidal Anti-Inflammatory Agents; Phenytoin; Pimozide; Pirfenidone; QuiNIDine; RiTUXimab; Simvastatin; Sodium Phosphates; Tacrolimus (Systemic)

The levels/effects of Amlodipine and Benazepril may be increased by: Aliskiren; Alpha1-Blockers; Angiotensin II Receptor Blockers; Antifungal Agents (Azole Derivatives, Systemic); Calcium Channel Blockers (Nondihydropyridine); Canagliflozin; Conivaptan; CycloSPORINE (Systemic); CYP3A4 Inhibitors (Moderate); CYP3A4 Inhibitors (Strong); Dasatinib; Diazoxide; DPP-IV Inhibitors; Eplerenone; Everolimus; Fluconazole; Grapefruit Juice; Herbs (Hypotensive Properties); Hydrochlorothiazide; Ivacaftor; Loop Diuretics; Macrolide Antibiotics; Magnesium Salts; MAO Inhibitors; Mifepristone; Pentoxifylline; Phosphodiesterase 5 Inhibitors; Potassium Salts; Potassium-Sparing Diuretics; Prostacyclin Analogues; Protease Inhibitors; QuiNIDine; Sirolimus; Temsirolimus; Thiazide Diuretics; TiZANidine; Tolvaptan; Trimethoprim

Decreased Effect

Amlodipine and Benazepril may decrease the levels/effects of: Clopidogrel; Hydrochlorothiazide; QuiNIDine

The levels/effects of Amlodipine and Benazepril may be decreased by: Antacids; Aprotinin; Barbiturates; Calcium Salts; CarBAMazepine; CYP3A4 Inducers (Strong); Deferasirox; Herbs (CYP3A4 Inducers); Herbs (Hypertensive Properties); Icatibant; Lanthanum; Melatonin; Methylphenidate; Nafcillin; Nonsteroidal Anti-Inflammatory Agents; Rifamycin Derivatives; Salicylates; Tocilizumab; Yohimbine

Ethanol/Nutrition/Herb Interactions

Food: Grapefruit juice may modestly increase amlodipine levels.

Herb/Nutraceutical: St John's wort may decrease amlodipine levels. Avoid herbs with *hypertensive* properties (bayberry, blue cohosh, cayenne, ephedra, ginger, ginseng [American], kola, licorice). Avoid herbs with *hypotensive* properties (black cohosh, California poppy, coleus, garlic, goldenseal, hawthorn, mistletoe, periwinkle, quinine, shepherd's purse).

Pregnancy Risk Factor D

Pregnancy Considerations [U.S. Boxed Warning]: Drugs that act on the renin-angiotensin system can cause injury and death to the developing fetus. Discontinue as soon as possible once pregnancy is detected. Also see individual agents.

Lactation
Amlodipine: Excretion in breast milk unknown/not recommended
Benazepril: Enters breast milk

Dosage Forms
Capsule, oral: 2.5/10: Amlodipine 2.5 mg and benazepril 10 mg; 5/10: Amlodipine 5 mg and benazepril 10 mg; 5/20: Amlodipine 5 mg and benazepril 20 mg; 5/40: Amlodipine 5 mg and benazepril hydrochloride 40 mg; 10/20: Amlodipine 10 mg and benazepril 20 mg; 10/40: Amlodipine 10 mg and benazepril hydrochloride 40 mg
Lotrel®: 2.5/10: Amlodipine 2.5 and benazepril 10 mg; 5/10: Amlodipine 5 mg and benazepril 10 mg; 5/20: Amlodipine 5 mg and benazepril 20 mg; 5/40: Amlodipine 5 mg and benazepril 40 mg; 10/20: Amlodipine 10 mg and benazepril 20 mg; 10/40: Amlodipine 10 mg and benazepril 40 mg

References
Jorgensen MG, "Prevalence of Amlodipine-Related Gingival Hyperplasia," *J Periodontol*, 1997, 68(7):676-8.
Wynn RL, "Calcium Channel Blockers and Gingival Hyperplasia-An Update," *Gen Dent*, 2009, 57(2):105-7.

Amlodipine and Olmesartan
(am LOE di peen & olme SAR tan)

Related Information
AmLODIPine *on page 88*
Olmesartan *on page 1004*

Brand Names: U.S. Azor™

Pharmacologic Category Angiotensin II Receptor Blocker; Antianginal Agent; Calcium Channel Blocker; Calcium Channel Blocker, Dihydropyridine

Use Treatment of hypertension, including initial treatment in patients who will require multiple antihypertensives for adequate control

Local Anesthetic/Vasoconstrictor Precautions No information available to require special precautions

Effects on Dental Treatment Fewer reports of gingival hyperplasia with amlodipine than with other CCBs (usually resolves upon discontinuation); consultation with physician is suggested.

Effects on Bleeding No information available to require special precautions

Adverse Effects Reactions/percentages reported with combination product; also see individual agents
>10%: Cardiovascular: Peripheral edema (dose related: 18% to 26%)
Frequency not defined (limited to important or life-threatening): Anaphylaxis, hypotension, nocturia, orthostatic hypotension, palpitation, pruritus, rash, urinary frequency

General Dosage Range Oral: *Adults:* Amlodipine 5-10 mg and olmesartan 20-40 mg once daily (maximum: 10 mg/day [amlodipine]; 40 mg/day [olmesartan])

Mechanism of Action
Amlodipine inhibits calcium ion from entering the "slow channels" or select voltage-sensitive areas of vascular smooth muscle and myocardium during depolarization, producing a relaxation of coronary vascular smooth muscle and coronary vasodilation; increases myocardial oxygen delivery in patients with vasospastic angina. Amlodipine directly acts on vascular smooth muscle to produce peripheral arterial vasodilation reducing peripheral vascular resistance and blood pressure.

As a selective and competitive, nonpeptide angiotensin II receptor antagonist, olmesartan blocks the vasoconstrictor and aldosterone-secreting effects of angiotensin II; olmesartan interacts reversibly at the AT1 and AT2 receptors of many tissues and has slow dissociation kinetics; its affinity for the AT1 receptor is 12,500 times greater than the AT2 receptor. Angiotensin II receptor antagonists may induce a more complete inhibition of the renin-angiotensin system than ACE inhibitors, they do not affect the response to bradykinin, and are less likely to be associated with nonrenin-angiotensin effects (eg, cough and angioedema). Olmesartan increases urinary flow rate and, in addition to being natriuretic and kaliuretic, increases excretion of chloride, magnesium, uric acid, calcium, and phosphate.

Pregnancy Risk Factor D

Pregnancy Considerations [U.S. Boxed Warning]: Drugs that act on the renin-angiotensin system can cause injury and death to the developing fetus. Discontinue as soon as possible once pregnancy is detected. Also see individual agents.

Amlodipine and Valsartan
(am LOE di peen & val SAR tan)

Related Information
AmLODIPine *on page 88*
Valsartan *on page 1381*

Brand Names: U.S. Exforge®

Generic Availability (U.S.) No

Pharmacologic Category Angiotensin II Receptor Blocker; Antianginal Agent; Calcium Channel Blocker; Calcium Channel Blocker, Dihydropyridine

Use Treatment of hypertension

Local Anesthetic/Vasoconstrictor Precautions No information available to require special precautions

Effects on Dental Treatment Key adverse event(s) related to dental treatment: Fewer reports of gingival hyperplasia with amlodipine than with other calcium channel blockers (usually resolves upon discontinuation); consultation with physician is suggested.

Effects on Bleeding No information available to require special precautions

Adverse Effects Reactions/percentages reported with combination product; also see individual agents
>10%: Central nervous system: Headache (11%)
1% to 10%:
Cardiovascular: Peripheral edema (5% to 8%)
Central nervous system: Anxiety (3%), somnolence (3%), dizziness (≤2%)
Endocrine & metabolic: Hyperkalemia (3% to 10%)
Gastrointestinal: Abdominal pain (upper; 3%), diarrhea (3%), nausea (3%)
Renal: BUN increased (6% to 17%)
Respiratory: Nasopharyngitis (4%), upper respiratory tract infection (3%), cough (2%)
Miscellaneous: Influenza (2%)

Frequency not defined, but occurred at ≥0.2% incidence (limited to important or life-threatening): Abdominal discomfort/distension, arthralgia, chest pain, colitis, constipation, depression, diabetes, dyspepsia, dyspnea, edema (including pitting), epistaxis, erectile dysfunction, erythema, fever, flushing, gastritis, gout, hematuria, hypercholesterolemia, hypoesthesia, LFTs increased, lymphadenopathy, muscle spasm, myalgia, nephrolithiasis, palpitation, paresthesia, pharyngitis, pollakiuria, pruritus, rash, sinus congestion, somnolence, tachycardia, vomiting, weakness, xerostomia

Dosage Oral: Dose is individualized; combination product may be used as initial therapy or substituted for individual components in patients currently maintained on both agents separately or in patients not adequately controlled with monotherapy (using one of the agents or an agent within same antihypertensive class).

Adults: Hypertension:
Initial therapy: Amlodipine 5 mg and valsartan 160 mg once daily, dose may be titrated after 1-2 weeks of therapy. Maximum recommended doses: Amlodipine 10 mg daily; valsartan 320 mg daily

Add-on/replacement therapy: Amlodipine 5-10 mg and valsartan 160-320 mg once daily; dose may be titrated after 3-4 weeks of therapy. Maximum recommended doses: Amlodipine 10 mg daily; valsartan 320 mg daily

Elderly: Use of lower initial doses should be considered.

Dosing adjustment in renal impairment:
Cl_{cr} ≥30 mL/minute: No dosage adjustment necessary.
Cl_{cr} <30 mL/minute: No dosage adjustment provided in manufacturer's labeling; safety and efficacy has not been established.

Dosing adjustment in hepatic impairment:
Mild-to-moderate impairment: Use with caution; amlodipine elimination prolonged and valsartan exposure doubled in patients with mild-to-moderate chronic disease compared to healthy volunteers. No dosage adjustment for valsartan is necessary; however, a lower initial amlodipine dose may be required (possibly requiring use of the individual agents).

Severe impairment: No dosage adjustment provided in manufacturer's labeling; however, similar to patients with mild to moderate impairment, a lower initial amlodipine dose may be required (possibly requiring use of the individual agents); titrate slowly.

Mechanism of Action Amlodipine inhibits calcium ion from entering the "slow channels" or select voltage-sensitive areas of vascular smooth muscle and myocardium during depolarization, producing a relaxation of coronary vascular smooth muscle and coronary vasodilation; increases myocardial oxygen delivery in patients with vasospastic angina. Amlodipine directly acts on vascular smooth muscle to produce peripheral arterial vasodilation reducing peripheral vascular resistance and blood pressure.

Valsartan produces direct antagonism of the angiotensin II (AT2) receptors, unlike the ACE inhibitors. It displaces angiotensin II from the AT1 receptor and produces its blood pressure-lowering effects by antagonizing AT1-induced vasoconstriction, aldosterone release, catecholamine release, arginine vasopressin release, water intake, and hypertrophic responses. This action results in more efficient blockade of the cardiovascular effects of angiotensin II and fewer side effects than the ACE inhibitors.

Contraindications Hypersensitivity to amlodipine, valsartan, or any component of the formulation; concomitant use with aliskiren in patients with diabetes mellitus

Warnings/Precautions See individual agents.

Drug Interactions
Metabolism/Transport Effects Refer to individual components.

Avoid Concomitant Use
Avoid concomitant use of Amlodipine and Valsartan with any of the following: Conivaptan; Pimozide; Pirfenidone

Increased Effect/Toxicity
Amlodipine and Valsartan may increase the levels/effects of: ACE Inhibitors; Amifostine; Antihypertensives; ARIPiprazole; Atosiban; Beta-Blockers; Calcium Channel Blockers (Nondihydropyridine); CycloSPORINE (Systemic); CYP1A2 Substrates; Fosphenytoin; Hydrochlorothiazide; Hypotensive Agents; Lithium; Lomitapide; Magnesium Salts; Neuromuscular-Blocking Agents (Nondepolarizing); Nitroprusside; Nonsteroidal Anti-Inflammatory Agents; Phenytoin; Pimozide; Pirfenidone; Potassium-Sparing Diuretics; QuiNIDine; RiTUXimab; Simvastatin; Sodium Phosphates; Tacrolimus (Systemic)

The levels/effects of Amlodipine and Valsartan may be increased by: Aliskiren; Alpha1-Blockers; Antifungal Agents (Azole Derivatives, Systemic); Calcium Channel Blockers (Nondihydropyridine); Canagliflozin; Conivaptan; CycloSPORINE (Systemic); CYP3A4 Inhibitors (Moderate); CYP3A4 Inhibitors (Strong); Dasatinib; Diazoxide; Eltrombopag; Eplerenone; Fluconazole; Grapefruit Juice; Herbs (Hypotensive Properties); Hydrochlorothiazide; Ivacaftor; Macrolide Antibiotics; Magnesium Salts; MAO Inhibitors; Mifepristone; Pentoxifylline; Phosphodiesterase 5 Inhibitors; Potassium Salts; Prostacyclin Analogues; Protease Inhibitors; QuiNIDine; Tolvaptan; Trimethoprim

Decreased Effect
Amlodipine and Valsartan may decrease the levels/effects of: Clopidogrel; QuiNIDine

The levels/effects of Amlodipine and Valsartan may be decreased by: Barbiturates; Calcium Salts; CarBAMazepine; CYP3A4 Inducers (Strong); Deferasirox; Herbs (CYP3A4 Inducers); Herbs (Hypertensive Properties); Melatonin; Methylphenidate; Nafcillin; Nonsteroidal Anti-Inflammatory Agents; Rifamycin Derivatives; Tocilizumab; Yohimbine

Ethanol/Nutrition/Herb Interactions
Food: Decreases rate and extent of valsartan absorption by 50% and 40%, respectively.
Herb/Nutraceutical: Avoid dong quai if using for hypertension (has estrogenic activity). Avoid ephedra, yohimbe, ginseng (may worsen hypertension). Avoid garlic (may have increased antihypertensive effects).

Dietary Considerations Avoid salt substitutes which contain potassium. May be taken with or without food.

Pregnancy Risk Factor D

Pregnancy Considerations [U.S. Boxed Warning]: Drugs that act on the renin-angiotensin system can cause injury and death to the developing fetus. Discontinue as soon as possible once pregnancy is detected. Also see individual agents.

Lactation Excretion in breast milk unknown/not recommended

Breast-Feeding Considerations See individual agents.

Dosage Forms
Tablet:
  Exforge®: 5/160: Amlodipine 5 mg and valsartan 160 mg; 5/320 mg: Amlodipine 5 mg and valsartan 320 mg; 10/160: Amlodipine 10 mg and valsartan 160 mg; 10/320: Amlodipine 10 mg and valsartan 320 mg

References
Jorgensen MG, "Prevalence of Amlodipine-Related Gingival Hyperplasia," *J Periodontol*, 1997, 68(7):676-8.
Wynn RL, "Calcium Channel Blockers and Gingival Hyperplasia-An Update," *Gen Dent*, 2009, 57(2):105-7.

Amlodipine, Valsartan, and Hydrochlorothiazide
(am LOE di peen, val SAR tan, & hye droe klor oh THYE a zide)

Related Information
AmLODIPine *on page 88*
Hydrochlorothiazide *on page 687*
Valsartan *on page 1381*
Brand Names: U.S. Exforge HCT®
Pharmacologic Category Angiotensin II Receptor Blocker; Antianginal Agent; Calcium Channel Blocker; Calcium Channel Blocker, Dihydropyridine; Diuretic, Thiazide
Use Treatment of hypertension (not for initial therapy)
Local Anesthetic/Vasoconstrictor Precautions No information available to require special precautions
Effects on Dental Treatment Key adverse event(s) related to dental treatment: Fewer reports of gingival hyperplasia with amlodipine than with other calcium channel blockers (usually resolves upon discontinuation); consultation with physician is suggested.
Effects on Bleeding No information available to require special precautions
Adverse Effects Reactions/percentages reported with combination product; also see individual agents.
>10%: Renal: BUN increased (30%)
2% to 10%:
  Cardiovascular: Edema (7%)
  Central nervous system: Dizziness (8%), headache (5%), fatigue (2%)
  Endocrine & metabolic: Hypokalemia (7%), hyperkalemia (4%)
  Gastrointestinal: Dyspepsia (2%), nausea (2%)
  Neuromuscular & skeletal: Back pain (2%), muscle spasms (2%)
  Renal: Serum creatinine increased (2%)
  Respiratory: Nasopharyngitis (2%)
General Dosage Range Oral: *Adults:* Amlodipine 5-10 mg and valsartan 160-320 mg and hydrochlorothiazide 12.5-25 mg once daily (maximum: 10 mg daily [amlodipine]; 25 mg daily [hydrochlorothiazide]; 320 mg daily [valsartan])
Mechanism of Action
Amlodipine inhibits calcium ion from entering the "slow channels" or select voltage-sensitive areas of vascular smooth muscle and myocardium during depolarization, producing a relaxation of coronary vascular smooth muscle and coronary vasodilation; increases myocardial oxygen delivery in patients with vasospastic angina. Amlodipine directly acts on vascular smooth muscle to produce peripheral arterial vasodilation reducing peripheral vascular resistance and blood pressure.

Valsartan produces direct antagonism of the angiotensin II (AT2) receptors, unlike the ACE inhibitors. It displaces angiotensin II from the AT1 receptor and produces its blood pressure-lowering effects by antagonizing AT1-induced vasoconstriction, aldosterone release, catecholamine release, arginine vasopressin release, water intake, and hypertrophic responses. This action results in more efficient blockade of the cardiovascular effects of angiotensin II and fewer side effects than the ACE inhibitors.

Hydrochlorothiazide inhibits sodium reabsorption in the distal tubules causing increased excretion of sodium and water as well as potassium and hydrogen ions.
Pregnancy Risk Factor D
Pregnancy Considerations [U.S. Boxed Warning]: Drugs that act on the renin-angiotensin system can cause injury and death to the developing fetus. Discontinue as soon as possible once pregnancy is detected. Also see individual agents.

Ammonia Spirit (Aromatic)
(a MOE nee ah SPEAR it, air oh MAT ik)

Generic Availability (U.S.) Yes
Pharmacologic Category Respiratory Stimulant
Dental Use Emergency use in syncope
Use Prevention or treatment of fainting
Local Anesthetic/Vasoconstrictor Precautions No information available to require special precautions
Effects on Dental Treatment No significant effects or complications reported
Effects on Bleeding No information available to require special precautions
Adverse Effects Frequency not defined.
  Central nervous system: Headache
  Gastrointestinal: Diarrhea, vomiting
  Respiratory: Dyspnea, cough, irritation to nasal mucosa
Dosage Inhalation: Children >12 and Adults: Fainting: Slowly inhale the vapors of one crushed ampul or opened bottle of solution until fainting resolves
Contraindications Hypersensitivity to ammonia or any component of the formulation
Warnings/Precautions Use with caution in patients with asthma, bronchitis, emphysema, or other chronic lung conditions. Use with caution in patients with diseases of the eye; conditions may worsen. Patients should be evaluated for the cause of fainting, especially when accompanied by flushed face.
Drug Interactions
  Metabolism/Transport Effects None known.
  Avoid Concomitant Use There are no known interactions where it is recommended to avoid concomitant use.
  Increased Effect/Toxicity There are no known significant interactions involving an increase in effect.
  Decreased Effect There are no known significant interactions involving a decrease in effect.
Dosage Forms
Solution, for inhalation: 1.7% to 2.1% (0.33 mL, 60 mL)

Ammonium Chloride (a MOE nee um KLOR ide)

Pharmacologic Category Electrolyte Supplement, Parenteral
Use Treatment of hypochloremic states or metabolic alkalosis
Local Anesthetic/Vasoconstrictor Precautions No information available to require special precautions
Effects on Dental Treatment No significant effects or complications reported
Effects on Bleeding No information available to require special precautions

Adverse Effects Frequency not defined.

Central nervous system: Coma, drowsiness, EEG abnormalities, headache, mental confusion, seizure

Dermatologic: Rash

Endocrine & metabolic: Calcium-deficient tetany, hyperchloremia, hypokalemia, metabolic acidosis, potassium may be decreased, sodium may be decreased

Gastrointestinal: Abdominal pain, gastric irritation, nausea, vomiting

Hepatic: Ammonia may be increased

Local: Pain at site of injection

Neuromuscular & skeletal: Twitching

Respiratory: Hyperventilation

Mechanism of Action Increases acidity by increasing free hydrogen ion concentration

Pregnancy Risk Factor C

Pregnancy Considerations Reproduction studies have not been conducted.

Amobarbital (am oh BAR bi tal)

Brand Names: U.S. Amytal®

Brand Names: Canada Amytal®

Pharmacologic Category Barbiturate

Use Hypnotic in short-term treatment of insomnia; reduce anxiety and provide sedation preoperatively

Unlabeled Use Therapeutic or diagnostic "Amytal® Interviewing"; Wada test

Local Anesthetic/Vasoconstrictor Precautions No information available to require special precautions

Effects on Dental Treatment No significant effects or complications reported

Effects on Bleeding No information available to require special precautions

Adverse Effects Frequency not defined and is reported as barbiturate use (not specifically amobarbital).

Cardiovascular: Bradycardia, hypotension, syncope

Central nervous system: Agitation, anxiety, ataxia, confusion, CNS depression, dizziness, fever, hallucinations, headache, insomnia, nightmares, nervousness, psychiatric disturbances, somnolence, thinking abnormal

Gastrointestinal: Constipation, nausea, vomiting

Hematologic: Megaloblastic anemia (following chronic phenobarbital use)

Hepatic: Liver damage

Local: Injection site reaction

Neuromuscular & skeletal: Hyperkinesia

Respiratory: Apnea, atelectasis (postoperative), hypoventilation

Miscellaneous: Hypersensitivity reaction (including angioedema, rash, and exfoliative dermatitis)

General Dosage Range Dosage adjustment recommended in patients with hepatic or renal impairment

I.M., I.V.:

Children 6-12 years: Sedative: 65-500 mg/dose

Adults:

Hypnotic: 65-200 mg at bedtime (maximum single dose: 1000 mg)

Sedative: 30-50 mg 2-3 times/day (maximum single dose: 1000 mg)

Mechanism of Action Interferes with transmission of impulses from the thalamus to the cortex of the brain resulting in an imbalance in central inhibitory and facilitatory mechanisms

Pharmacodynamics/Kinetics

Onset of Action I.V.: Within 5 minutes

Half-life Elimination 15-40 hours (mean: 25 hours)

Pregnancy Risk Factor D

Pregnancy Considerations Barbiturates cross the placenta and distribute in fetal tissue. Teratogenic effects have been reported with 1st trimester exposure. Exposure during the 3rd trimester may lead to symptoms of acute withdrawal following delivery; symptoms may be delayed up to 14 days.

Controlled Substance C-II

Amoxapine (a MOKS a peen)

Related Information

Vasoconstrictor Interactions With Antidepressants *on page 1650*

Pharmacologic Category Antidepressant, Tricyclic (Secondary Amine)

Use Treatment of depression (including endogenous, neurotic, psychotic, and reactive depression); treatment of depression accompanied by anxiety or agitation

Local Anesthetic/Vasoconstrictor Precautions Use with caution; epinephrine and levonordefrin have been shown to have an increased pressor response in combination with TCAs. Amoxapine is one of the drugs confirmed to prolong the QT interval and is accepted as having a risk of causing torsade de pointes. The risk of drug-induced torsade de pointes is extremely low when a single QT interval prolonging drug is prescribed. In terms of epinephrine, it is not known what effect vasoconstrictors in the local anesthetic regimen will have in patients with a known history of congenital prolonged QT interval or in patients taking any medication that prolongs the QT interval. Until more information is obtained, it is suggested that the clinician consult with the physician prior to the use of a vasoconstrictor in suspected patients, and that the vasoconstrictor (epinephrine, mepivacaine and levonordefrin [Carbocaine® 2% with Neo-Cobefrin®]) be used with caution.

Effects on Dental Treatment Key adverse event(s) related to dental treatment: Xerostomia and changes in salivation (normal salivary flow resumes upon discontinuation). Long-term treatment with TCAs, such as amoxapine, increases the risk of caries by reducing salivation and salivary buffer capacity.

Effects on Bleeding May cause thrombocytopenia

Adverse Effects

>10%:

Central nervous system: Drowsiness (14%)

Gastrointestinal: Xerostomia (14%), constipation (12%)

1% to 10%:

Cardiovascular: Palpitations

Central nervous system: Anxiety, ataxia, confusion, dizziness, EEG abnormalities, excitement, fatigue, headache, insomnia, nervousness, nightmares, restlessness

Dermatologic: Edema, skin rash

Endocrine: Prolactin levels increased

Gastrointestinal: Appetite increased, nausea

Neuromuscular & skeletal: Tremor, weakness

Ocular: Blurred vision (7%)

Miscellaneous: Diaphoresis

General Dosage Range Oral:

Adults: 50 mg 2-3 times/day; usual effective dose: 200-300 mg/day; maximum: 600 mg/day (inpatient); 400 mg/day (outpatient)

Elderly: 25 mg 2-3 times/day; usual effective dose: 100-150 mg/day; maximum: 300 mg/day

Mechanism of Action Reduces the reuptake of serotonin and norepinephrine. The metabolite, 7-OH-amoxapine has significant dopamine receptor blocking activity similar to haloperidol.

Pharmacodynamics/Kinetics

Onset of Action Antidepressant effect: Usually occurs after 1-2 weeks, but may require 4-6 weeks

Half-life Elimination 8 hours; 7-hydroxyamoxapine metabolite: 4-6 hours; 8-hydroxyamoxapine metabolite: 30 hours

Time to Peak Serum: ~90 minutes

Pregnancy Risk Factor C

Pregnancy Considerations Teratogenic effects were not observed in animal reproduction studies; however, fetotoxic and embryotoxic effects were seen in some studies.

Dental Comment Amoxapine is known to prolong the QT interval. The QT interval is measured as the time and distance between the Q point of the QRS complex and the end of the T wave in the ECG tracing. After adjustment for heart rate, the QT interval is defined as prolonged if it is more than 450 msec in men and 460 msec in women. A long QT syndrome was first described in the 1950s and 60s as a congenital syndrome involving QT interval prolongation and syncope and sudden death. Some of the congenital long QT syndromes were characterized by a peculiar electrocardiographic appearance of the QRS complex involving a premature atria beat followed by a pause, then a subsequent sinus beat showing marked QT prolongation and deformity. This type of cardiac arrhythmia was originally termed "torsade de pointes" (translated from the French as "twisting of the points"). Amoxapine is considered as having a risk of causing torsade de pointes. Since it is not known what effect vasoconstrictors in the local anesthetic regimen will have in patients with a known history of congenital prolonged QT interval or in patients taking any medication that prolongs the QT interval, a medical consult is suggested.

Amoxicillin (a moks i SIL in)

Related Information

Antibiotic Prophylaxis *on page 1542*
Bacterial Infections *on page 1562*
Gastrointestinal Disorders *on page 1512*
Osteonecrosis of the Jaw *on page 1529*
Periodontal Diseases *on page 1570*

Related Sample Prescriptions

Bacterial Infections and Periodontal Diseases *on page 1609*
Infective Endocarditis (Prevention) *on page 1604*
Prosthetic Joint Late Infections (Prevention) *on page 1605*
Sinus Infection Treatment *on page 1611*

Brand Names: U.S. Moxatag™

Brand Names: Canada Apo-Amoxi®; Mylan-Amoxicillin; Novamoxin®; NTP-Amoxicillin; Nu-Amoxi; PHL-Amoxicillin; PMS-Amoxicillin; Pro-Amox-250; Pro-Amox-500

Generic Availability (U.S.) Yes: Excludes extended-release formulation

Pharmacologic Category Antibiotic, Penicillin

Dental Use Antibiotic for standard prophylactic regimen for dental patients who are at risk for infective endocarditis; prophylaxis in total joint replacement patients undergoing dental procedures; antibiotic used to treat orofacial infections. Useful (as amoxicillin or amoxicillin/clavulanic acid) in combination with metronidazole in addition to scaling and root planing in the treatment of periodontitis associated with the presence of *Actinobacillus actinomycetemcomitans* (AA). In aggressive periodontitis, greatest benefit is seen after 3 months of therapy. No benefit was seen after 6 months of therapy (Varela, 2011).

Use Treatment of otitis media, sinusitis, and infections caused by susceptible organisms involving the upper and lower respiratory tract, skin, and urinary tract; prophylaxis of infective endocarditis in patients undergoing surgical or dental procedures; as part of a multidrug regimen for *H. pylori* eradication; periodontitis

Unlabeled Use Postexposure prophylaxis for anthrax exposure with documented susceptible organisms; chronic oral antimicrobial suppression of prosthetic joint infection

Local Anesthetic/Vasoconstrictor Precautions No information available to require special precautions

Effects on Dental Treatment Prolonged use of penicillins may lead to development of oral candidiasis

Effects on Bleeding No information available to require special precautions

Adverse Effects Frequency not defined.

Central nervous system: Agitation, anxiety, behavioral changes, confusion, dizziness, headache, hyperactivity (reversible), insomnia, seizure

Dermatologic: Acute exanthematous pustulosis, erythematous maculopapular rash, erythema multiforme, exfoliative dermatitis, hypersensitivity vasculitis, mucocutaneous candidiasis, Stevens-Johnson syndrome, toxic epidermal necrolysis, urticaria

Gastrointestinal: Black hairy tongue, diarrhea, hemorrhagic colitis, nausea, pseudomembranous colitis, tooth discoloration (brown, yellow, or gray; rare), vomiting

Hematologic: Agranulocytosis, anemia, eosinophilia, hemolytic anemia, leukopenia, thrombocytopenia, thrombocytopenia purpura

Hepatic: Acute cytolytic hepatitis, ALT increased, AST increased, cholestatic jaundice, hepatic cholestasis

Renal: Crystalluria

Miscellaneous: Anaphylaxis, serum sickness-like reaction

Dental Usual Dosage Oral:

Children >3 months and <40 kg: Prophylaxis against infective endocarditis: 50 mg/kg 30-60 minutes before procedure. **Note:** American Heart Association (AHA) guidelines now recommend prophylaxis only in patients undergoing invasive procedures and in whom underlying cardiac conditions may predispose to a higher risk of adverse outcomes should infection occur. As of April 2007, routine prophylaxis for GI/GU procedures is no longer recommended by the AHA.

Adults:

Periodontitis (aggressive) (in combination with metronidazole) associated with presense of *Actinobacillus actinomycetemcomitans* (AA): 500 mg every 8 hours for 10 days used in addition to scaling and root planing (Varela, 2011)

Prophylaxis against infective endocarditis: 2 g 30-60 minutes before procedure. **Note:** American Heart Association (AHA) guidelines now recommend prophylaxis only in patients undergoing invasive procedures and in whom underlying cardiac conditions may predispose to a higher risk of adverse outcomes should infection occur. As of April 2007, routine prophylaxis for GI/GU procedures is no longer recommended by the AHA.

Orofacial infection: 250-500 mg every 8 hours or 500-875 mg twice daily

Prophylaxis in total joint replacement patients undergoing dental procedures which produce bacteremia: 2 g 1 hour prior to procedure

Dosage

Usual dosage range:

Children ≤3 months: Oral: 20-30 mg/kg/day divided every 12 hours

Children >3 months and <40 kg: Oral: 20-100 mg/kg/day in divided doses every 8-12 hours

Children >3 months and ≥40 kg: Refer to adult dosing

Children ≥12 years: Oral: Extended-release tablet: 775 mg once daily

Adults: Oral: 250-500 mg every 8 hours or 500-875 mg twice daily

Extended-release tablet: 775 mg once daily

Indication-specific dosing:

Children >3 months and <40 kg: Oral: **Note:** In general, children >3 months and ≥40 kg should be dosed according to the adult recommendations except where indicated.

Acute otitis media: 80-90 mg/kg/day divided every 12 hours

Community-acquired pneumonia (CAP) (IDSA/PIDS, 2011): Note: In children ≥5 years, a macrolide antibiotic should be added if atypical pneumonia cannot be ruled out.

Empiric treatment or *S. pneumoniae* (MICs to penicillin ≤2.0 mcg/mL) (preferred): 90 mg/kg/day in 2-3 divided doses (maximum: 4 g/day). **Note:** Dividing in 3 doses is recommended for MIC = 2 mcg/mL.

Group A *Streptococcus* (moderate-to-severe) (preferred): 50-75 mg/kg/day in 2 divided doses (maximum: 4 g/day)

H. influenzae (beta-lactamase negative) mild infection (preferred): 75-100 mg/kg/day in 3 divided doses (maximum: 4 g/day)

Ear, nose, throat, genitourinary tract, or skin/skin structure infections: Note: Amoxicillin-clavulanate is preferred for first-line treatment of acute bacterial rhinosinusitis (Chow, 2012):

Mild-to-moderate: 25 mg/kg/day in divided doses every 12 hours **or** 20 mg/kg/day in divided doses every 8 hours

Severe: 45 mg/kg/day in divided doses every 12 hours **or** 40 mg/kg/day in divided doses every 8 hours

Tonsillitis and/or pharyngitis: Children ≥12 years: Extended-release tablet: 775 mg once daily

Lower respiratory tract infections: 45 mg/kg/day in divided doses every 12 hours **or** 40 mg/kg/day in divided doses every 8 hours

Lyme disease: 25-50 mg/kg/day divided every 8 hours (maximum: 500 mg)

Pharyngitis, group A streptococci (IDSA guidelines): 50 mg/kg once daily or alternatively, 25 mg/kg twice daily (maximum total daily dose: 1000 mg) for 10 days (Shulman, 2012)

Postexposure inhalational anthrax prophylaxis (ACIP recommendations): Children <40 kg: 45 mg/kg/day divided into 3 daily doses (maximum: 500 mg/dose) (ACIP, 2010). **Note:** The AAP recommends a higher dose (80 mg/kg/day divided into 3 daily doses [maximum: 500 mg/dose]) due to the lack of data on amoxicillin dosages for treating anthrax and the high mortality rate.

Note: Use **only** if isolates of the specific *B. anthracis* are sensitive to amoxicillin (MIC ≤0.125 mcg/mL). Duration of antibiotic postexposure prophylaxis (PEP) is ≥60 days in a previously-unvaccinated exposed person. Antimicrobial therapy should continue for 14 days after the third dose of PEP vaccine. Those who are partially or fully vaccinated should receive at least a 30-day course of antimicrobial PEP and continue with licensed vaccination regimen. Unvaccinated workers, even those wearing personal protective equipment with adequate respiratory protection, should receive antimicrobial PEP. Antimicrobial PEP is not required for fully-vaccinated people (five-dose I.M. vaccination series with a yearly booster) who enter an anthrax area clothed in personal protective equipment. If respiratory protection is disrupted, a 30-day course of antimicrobial therapy is recommended (ACIP, 2010).

Prophylaxis against infective endocarditis: 50 mg/kg 1 hour before procedure. **Note:** American Heart Association (AHA) guidelines now recommend prophylaxis only in patients undergoing invasive procedures and in whom underlying cardiac conditions may predispose to a higher risk of adverse outcomes should infection occur. As of April 2007, routine prophylaxis for GI/GU procedures is no longer recommended by the AHA.

Adults: Oral:

Chlamydial infection during pregnancy (unlabeled use): 500 mg 3 times/day for 7 days (CDC, 2010)

Ear, nose, throat, genitourinary tract, or skin/skin structure infections: Note: Amoxicillin-clavulanate is preferred for first-line treatment of acute bacterial rhinosinusitis (Chow, 2012):

Mild-to-moderate: 500 mg every 12 hours **or** 250 mg every 8 hours

Severe: 875 mg every 12 hours **or** 500 mg every 8 hours

Tonsillitis and/or pharyngitis: Extended-release tablet: 775 mg once daily

Helicobacter pylori eradication: 1000 mg twice daily; requires combination therapy with at least one other antibiotic and an acid-suppressing agent (proton pump inhibitor or H_2 blocker)

Lower respiratory tract infections: 875 mg every 12 hours **or** 500 mg every 8 hours

Lyme disease: 500 mg every 6-8 hours (depending on size of patient) for 21-30 days

Periodontitis (aggressive) (in combination with metronidazole) associated with presense of *Actinobacillus actinomycetemcomitans* (AA): Oral: 500 mg every 8 hours for 10 days used in addition to scaling and root planing (Varela, 2011)

Pharyngitis, group A streptococci (IDSA guidelines): 1000 mg once daily or 500 mg twice daily (maximum daily dose: 1000 mg) for 10 days (Shulman, 2012)

Postexposure inhalational anthrax prophylaxis (ACIP recommendations): 500 mg every 8 hours. **Note:** Use **only** if isolates of the specific *B. anthracis* are sensitive to amoxicillin (MIC ≤0.125 mcg/mL); may be administered to pregnant and breast-feeding women. Duration of antibiotic postexposure prophylaxis (PEP) is ≥60 days in a previously unvaccinated exposed person. Antimicrobial therapy should continue for 14 days after the third dose of PEP vaccine. Those who are partially or fully vaccinated should receive at least a 30-day course of antimicrobial PEP and continue with licensed vaccination regimen. Unvaccinated workers, even those wearing personal protective equipment with adequate respiratory protection, should receive antimicrobial PEP. Antimicrobial PEP is not required for fully vaccinated people (five-dose I.M. vaccination series with a yearly booster) who enter an anthrax area clothed in personal protective equipment. If respiratory protection is disrupted, a 30-day course of antimicrobial therapy is recommended (ACIP, 2010).

Prophylaxis against infective endocarditis: Oral: 2 g 30-60 minutes before procedure. **Note:** American Heart Association (AHA) guidelines now recommend prophylaxis only in patients undergoing invasive procedures and in whom underlying cardiac conditions may predispose to a higher risk of adverse outcomes should infection occur. As of April 2007, routine prophylaxis for GI/GU procedures is no longer recommended by the AHA.

Prophylaxis in total joint replacement patients undergoing dental procedures which produce bacteremia: 2 g 1 hour prior to procedure

Prosthetic joint infection, chronic antimicrobial suppression of prosthetic joint infection associated with beta-hemolytic streptococci, penicillin-susceptible Enterococcus spp, or Propionibacterium spp (unlabeled use): Oral: 500 mg 3 times daily (Osmon, 2013)

Dosage adjustment in renal impairment: Use of certain dosage forms (eg, extended-release 775 mg tablet and immediate-release 875 mg tablet) should be avoided in patients with Cl_{cr} <30 mL/minute or patients requiring hemodialysis.
Cl_{cr} 10-30 mL/minute: 250-500 mg every 12 hours
Cl_{cr} <10 mL/minute: 250-500 mg every 24 hours
Dialysis: Moderately dialyzable (20% to 50%) by hemo- or peritoneal dialysis; approximately 50 mg of amoxicillin per liter of filtrate is removed by continuous arteriovenous or venovenous hemofiltration; dose as per Cl_{cr} <10 mL/minute guidelines
Dosage adjustment in hepatic impairment: No dosage adjustment provided in manufacturer's labeling.

Mechanism of Action Inhibits bacterial cell wall synthesis by binding to one or more of the penicillin-binding proteins (PBPs) which in turn inhibits the final transpeptidation step of peptidoglycan synthesis in bacterial cell walls, thus inhibiting cell wall biosynthesis. Bacteria eventually lyse due to ongoing activity of cell wall autolytic enzymes (autolysins and murein hydrolases) while cell wall assembly is arrested.

Contraindications Hypersensitivity to amoxicillin, penicillin, other beta-lactams, or any component of the formulation

Warnings/Precautions In patients with renal impairment, doses and/or frequency of administration should be modified in response to the degree of renal impairment; in addition, use of certain dosage forms (eg, extended release 775 mg tablet and immediate release 875 mg tablet) should be avoided in patients with Cl_{cr} <30 mL/minute or patients requiring hemodialysis. A high percentage of patients with infectious mononucleosis have developed rash during therapy with amoxicillin; ampicillin-class antibiotics not recommended in these patients. Serious and occasionally severe or fatal hypersensitivity (anaphylactoid) reactions have been reported in patients on penicillin therapy, especially with a history

of beta-lactam hypersensitivity, history of sensitivity to multiple allergens, or previous IgE-mediated reactions (eg, anaphylaxis, angioedema, urticaria). Use with caution in asthmatic patients. Prolonged use may result in fungal or bacterial superinfection, including C. difficile-associated diarrhea (CDAD) and pseudomembranous colitis; CDAD has been observed >2 months postantibiotic treatment. Chewable tablets contain phenylalanine.

Drug Interactions

Metabolism/Transport Effects None known.

Avoid Concomitant Use
Avoid concomitant use of Amoxicillin with any of the following: BCG

Increased Effect/Toxicity
Amoxicillin may increase the levels/effects of: Methotrexate; Vitamin K Antagonists

The levels/effects of Amoxicillin may be increased by: Allopurinol; Probenecid

Decreased Effect
Amoxicillin may decrease the levels/effects of: BCG; Mycophenolate; Sodium Picosulfate; Typhoid Vaccine

The levels/effects of Amoxicillin may be decreased by: Fusidic Acid; Tetracycline Derivatives

Dietary Considerations May be taken with food. Some products may contain phenylalanine.
Moxatag™: Take within 1 hour of finishing a meal.

Pharmacodynamics/Kinetics

Half-life Elimination
Neonates, full-term: 3.7 hours
Infants and Children: 1-2 hours
Adults: Normal renal function: 0.7-1.4 hours
Cl_{cr} <10 mL/minute: 7-21 hours

Time to Peak Capsule: 2 hours; Extended-release tablet: 3.1 hours; Suspension: 1 hour

Pregnancy Risk Factor B

Pregnancy Considerations Adverse events have not been observed in animal reproduction studies. Maternal use of amoxicillin has generally not resulted in an increased risk of adverse fetal effects; however, an increased risk of cleft lip with cleft palate has been observed in some studies. It is the drug of choice for the treatment of chlamydial infections in pregnancy and for anthrax prophylaxis when penicillin susceptibility is documented. Amoxicillin may be used in certain situations prior to vaginal delivery in women at high risk for endocarditis.

Due to pregnancy-induced physiologic changes, oral amoxicillin clearance is increased during pregnancy resulting in lower concentrations and smaller AUCs. Oral ampicillin-class antibiotics are poorly absorbed during labor.

Lactation Enters breast milk/use caution (AAP rates "compatible"; AAP 2001 update pending)

Breast-Feeding Considerations Very small amounts of amoxicillin are excreted in breast milk. The manufacturer recommends that caution be exercised when administering amoxicillin to nursing women. Nondose-related effects could include modification of bowel flora and allergic sensitization of the infant.

Dosage Forms
Capsule, oral: 250 mg, 500 mg
Powder for suspension, oral: 125 mg/5 mL (80 mL, 100 mL, 150 mL); 200 mg/5 mL (50 mL, 75 mL, 100 mL); 250 mg/5 mL (80 mL, 100 mL, 150 mL); 400 mg/5 mL (50 mL, 75 mL, 100 mL)

Tablet, oral: 500 mg, 875 mg
Tablet, chewable, oral: 125 mg, 200 mg, 250 mg, 400 mg
Tablet, extended release, oral:
Moxatag™: 775 mg

References

American Dental Association Council on Scientific Affairs, "Combating Antibiotic Resistance," *J Am Dent Assoc*, 2004, 135(4):484-7.

Jevsevar DS and Abt E, "The New AAOS-ADA Clinical Practice Guideline on Prevention of Orthopaedic Implant Infection in Patients Undergoing Dental Procedures," *J Am Acad Orthop Surg*, 2013, 21 (3):195-7.

Wilson W, Taubert KA, Gewitz M, et al, "Prevention of Infective Endocarditis. Guidelines From the American Heart Association. A Guideline From the American Heart Association Rheumatic Fever, Endocarditis, and Kawasaki Disease Committee, Council on Cardiovascular Disease in the Young, and the Council on Clinical Cardiology, Council on Cardiovascular Surgery and Anesthesia, and the Quality of Care and Outcomes Research Interdisciplinary Working Group," *Circulation*, 2007, 115. Available at http://circ.-ahajournals.org/cgi/reprint/CIRCULATIONAHA.106.183095v1; last accessed July 26, 2007.

Wynn RL, Bergman SA, Meiller TF, et al, "Antibiotics in Treating Oral-Facial Infections of Odontogenic Origin: An Update", *Gen Dent*, 2001, 49(3):238-40, 242, 244 passim.

Amoxicillin and Clavulanate
(a moks i SIL in & klav yoo LAN ate)

Related Information
Amoxicillin *on page 96*
Bacterial Infections *on page 1562*

Related Sample Prescriptions
Bacterial Infections and Periodontal Diseases *on page 1609*
Sinus Infection Treatment *on page 1611*

Brand Names: U.S. Amoclan; Augmentin ES-600®; Augmentin XR®; Augmentin®

Brand Names: Canada Amoxi-Clav; Apo-Amoxi-Clav®; Clavulin®; Novo-Clavamoxin; ratio-Aclavulanate

Generic Availability (U.S.) Yes

Pharmacologic Category Antibiotic, Penicillin

Dental Use Treatment of orofacial infections when beta-lactamase-producing staphylococci and beta-lactamase-producing *Bacteroides* are present

Use Treatment of otitis media, sinusitis, and infections caused by susceptible organisms involving the lower respiratory tract, skin and skin structure, and urinary tract; spectrum same as amoxicillin with additional coverage of beta-lactamase producing *B. catarrhalis*, *H. influenzae*, *N. gonorrhoeae*, and *S. aureus* (not MRSA). The expanded coverage of this combination makes it a useful alternative when amoxicillin resistance is present and patients cannot tolerate alternative treatments.

Unlabeled Use Chronic antimicrobial suppression of prosthetic joint infection

Local Anesthetic/Vasoconstrictor Precautions No information available to require special precautions

Effects on Dental Treatment Prolonged use of penicillins may lead to development of oral candidiasis (see Dental Comment)

Effects on Bleeding No information available to require special precautions

Adverse Effects
>10%: Gastrointestinal: Diarrhea (3% to 34%; incidence varies upon dose and regimen used)
1% to 10%:
Dermatologic: Diaper rash, skin rash, urticaria
Gastrointestinal: Abdominal discomfort, loose stools, nausea, vomiting
Genitourinary: Vaginitis, vaginal mycosis
Miscellaneous: Moniliasis

Additional adverse reactions seen with **ampicillin-class antibiotics**: Agitation, agranulocytosis, alkaline phosphatase increased, anaphylaxis, anemia, angioedema, anxiety, behavioral changes, bilirubin increased, black "hairy" tongue, confusion, convulsions, crystalluria, dizziness, enterocolitis, eosinophilia, erythema multiforme, exanthematous pustulosis, exfoliative dermatitis, gastritis, glossitis, hematuria, hemolytic anemia, hemorrhagic colitis, indigestion, insomnia, hyperactivity, interstitial nephritis, leukopenia, mucocutaneous candidiasis, pruritus, pseudomembranous colitis, serum sickness-like reaction, Stevens-Johnson syndrome, stomatitis, transaminases increased, thrombocytopenia, thrombocytopenic purpura, tooth discoloration, toxic epidermal necrolysis

Dental Usual Dosage Orofacial infections: Children >40 kg and Adults: Oral: 250-500 mg every 8 hours or 875 mg every 12 hours

Dosage Note: Dose is based on the amoxicillin component; see "Augmentin® Product-Specific Considerations" table on next page.

Usual dosage range:
Infants <3 months: Oral: 30 mg/kg/day divided every 12 hours using the 125 mg/5 mL suspension
Children ≥3 months and <40 kg: Oral: 20-90 mg/kg/day divided every 8-12 hours
Children >40 kg and Adults: Oral: 250-500 mg every 8 hours or 875 mg every 12 hours

Indication-specific dosing:
Children ≥3 months and <40 kg: Oral:
Community-acquired pneumonia (CAP) (IDSA/PIDS, 2011): Infants >3 months and Children: **Note:** In children ≥5 years, a macrolide antibiotic should be added if atypical pneumonia cannot be ruled out.
Presumed bacterial (mild-to-moderate infection) (alternative to amoxicillin): 45 mg/kg/dose in 2 doses (maximum: 4000 mg daily)
H. influenzae (typeable or nontypeable; beta-lactamase producing), step-down therapy or mild infection (preferred): 15 mg/kg/dose in 3 doses **or** 45 mg/kg/dose in 2 doses
Group A streptococci, chronic carrier treatment (IDSA guidelines): Refer to adult dosing.
Lower respiratory tract infections, severe infections, sinusitis: 45 mg/kg/day divided every 12 hours **or** 40 mg/kg/day divided every 8 hours
Mild-to-moderate infections: 25 mg/kg/day divided every 12 hours or 20 mg/kg/day divided every 8 hours
Otitis media (amoxicillin 600 mg and clavulanate potassium 42.9 mg per 5 mL): 90 mg/kg/day divided every 12 hours for 10 days in children with severe illness and when coverage for β-lactamase-positive *H. influenzae* and *M. catarrhalis* is needed.
Children <16 years: Oral:
Acute bacterial rhinosinusitis: 45 mg/kg/day divided every 12 hours (preferred) for 10-14 days. **Note:** May use high-dose therapy (90 mg/kg/day divided every 12 hours) if initial therapy fails, in areas with high endemic rates of penicillin-nonsusceptible *S. pneumoniae*, those with severe infections, daycare attendance, age <2 years, recent hospitalization, antibiotic use within the past month, or who are immunocompromised (Chow, 2012).

Children ≥16 years and Adults: Oral:

Acute bacterial rhinosinusitis: Extended release tablet: 2000 mg every 12 hours for 10 days or 500 mg every 8 hours or 875 mg every 12 hours for 5-7 days **Note:** May use high-dose therapy (extended release: 2000 mg every 12 hours) if initial therapy fails, in areas with high endemic rates of penicillin-nonsusceptible *S. pneumoniae*, those with severe infections, age >65 years, recent hospitalization, antibiotic use within the past month, or who are immunocompromised (Chow, 2012).

Bite wounds (animal/human): 875 mg every 12 hours **or** 500 mg every 8 hours

Chronic obstructive pulmonary disease: 875 mg every 12 hours **or** 500 mg every 8 hours

Diabetic foot: Extended release tablet: Two 1000 mg tablets every 12 hours for 7-14 days

Diverticulitis, perirectal abscess: Extended release tablet: Two 1000 mg tablets every 12 hours for 7-10 days

Erysipelas: 875 mg every 12 hours **or** 500 mg every 8 hours

Febrile neutropenia: 875 mg every 12 hours

Group A streptococci, chronic carrier treatment (IDSA guidelines): 40 mg/kg/day divided every 8 hours (maximum: 2000 mg daily) for 10 days (Shulman, 2012)

Pneumonia:

Aspiration: 875 mg every 12 hours

Community-acquired: Extended release tablet: Two 1000 mg tablets every 12 hours for 7-10 days

Prosthetic joint infection, chronic antimicrobial suppression, oxacillin-susceptible *Staphylococci* (alternative to cephalexin or cefadroxil) (unlabeled use): 500 mg 3 times daily (Osmon, 2013)

Pyelonephritis (acute, uncomplicated): 875 mg every 12 hours **or** 500 mg every 8 hours

Skin abscess: 875 mg every 12 hours

Dosage adjustment in renal impairment:

Cl_{cr} <30 mL/minute: Do not use 875 mg tablet or extended release tablets

Cl_{cr} 10-30 mL/minute: 250-500 mg every 12 hours

Cl_{cr} <10 mL/minute: 250-500 every 24 hours

Hemodialysis: Moderately dialyzable (20% to 50%) 250-500 mg every 24 hours; administer dose during and after dialysis. Do not use extended release tablets.

Peritoneal dialysis: Moderately dialyzable (20% to 50%)

Amoxicillin: Administer 250 mg every 12 hours

Clavulanic acid: Dose for Cl_{cr} <10 mL/minute

Continuous arteriovenous or venovenous hemofiltration effects:

Amoxicillin: ~50 mg of amoxicillin/L of filtrate is removed

Clavulanic acid: Dose for Cl_{cr} <10 mL/minute

Augmentin® Product-Specific Considerations

Strength	Form	Consideration
125 mg	S	q8h dosing
	S	For adults having difficulty swallowing tablets, 125 mg/5 mL suspension may be substituted for 500 mg tablet.
200 mg	CT, S	q12h dosing
	CT	Contains phenylalanine
	S	For adults having difficulty swallowing tablets, 200 mg/5 mL suspension may be substituted for 875 mg tablet.
250 mg	S, T	q8h dosing
	T	Not for use in patients <40 kg
	S	For adults having difficulty swallowing tablets, 250 mg/5 mL suspension may be substituted for 500 mg tablet.
400 mg	CT, S	q12h dosing
	CT	Contains phenylalanine
	S	For adults having difficulty swallowing tablets, 400 mg/5 mL suspension may be substituted for 875 mg tablet.
500 mg	T	q8h or q12h dosing
600 mg	S	q12h dosing
		Not for use in adults or children ≥40 kg
		600 mg/5 mL suspension is not equivalent to or interchangeable with 200 mg/5 mL or 400 mg/5 mL due to differences in clavulanic acid.
875 mg	T	q12h dosing; not for use in Cl_{cr} <30 mL/minute
1000 mg	XR	q12h dosing
		Not for use in children <16 years of age
		Not interchangeable with two 500 mg tablets
		Not for use if Cl_{cr} <30 mL/minute or hemodialysis

Legend: CT = chewable tablet, S = suspension, T = tablet, XR = extended release.

Dosage adjustment in hepatic impairment: No dosage adjustment provided in manufacturer's labeling; use with caution. Use contraindicated in patients with a history of amoxicillin and clavulanate-associated hepatic dysfunction.

Mechanism of Action Clavulanic acid binds and inhibits beta-lactamases that inactivate amoxicillin resulting in amoxicillin having an expanded spectrum of activity. Amoxicillin inhibits bacterial cell wall synthesis by binding to one or more of the penicillin-binding proteins (PBPs) which in turn inhibits the final transpeptidation step of peptidoglycan synthesis in bacterial cell walls, thus inhibiting cell wall biosynthesis. Bacteria eventually lyse due to ongoing activity of cell wall autolytic enzymes (autolysins and murein hydrolases) while cell wall assembly is arrested.

Contraindications Hypersensitivity to amoxicillin, clavulanic acid, penicillin, or any component of the formulation; history of cholestatic jaundice or hepatic dysfunction with amoxicillin/clavulanate potassium therapy; Augmentin XR™: severe renal impairment (Cl_{cr} <30 mL/minute) and hemodialysis patients

Warnings/Precautions Hypersensitivity reactions, including anaphylaxis (some fatal), have been reported. Prolonged use may result in fungal or bacterial superinfection, including *C. difficile*-associated diarrhea (CDAD) and pseudomembranous colitis; CDAD has been observed >2 months postantibiotic treatment. In patients with renal impairment, doses and/or frequency of administration should be modified in response to the degree of renal impairment. High percentage of patients with infectious mononucleosis have developed rash during therapy; ampicillin-class antibiotics not recommended in these patients. Incidence of diarrhea is higher than with amoxicillin alone. Due to differing content of clavulanic acid, not all formulations are interchangeable. Low incidence of cross-allergy with cephalosporins exists. Some products contain phenylalanine.

Drug Interactions
Metabolism/Transport Effects None known.

Avoid Concomitant Use
Avoid concomitant use of Amoxicillin and Clavulanate with any of the following: BCG

Increased Effect/Toxicity
Amoxicillin and Clavulanate may increase the levels/ effects of: Methotrexate; Vitamin K Antagonists

The levels/effects of Amoxicillin and Clavulanate may be increased by: Allopurinol; Probenecid

Decreased Effect
Amoxicillin and Clavulanate may decrease the levels/ effects of: BCG; Mycophenolate; Sodium Picosulfate; Typhoid Vaccine

The levels/effects of Amoxicillin and Clavulanate may be decreased by: Fusidic Acid; Tetracycline Derivatives

Dietary Considerations May be taken with meals or on an empty stomach; take with meals to increase absorption and decrease GI upset; may mix with milk, formula, or juice. Extended release tablets should be taken with food. Some products may contain sodium. Some products contain phenylalanine; if you have phenylketonuria or PKU, avoid use. All dosage forms contain potassium.

Pharmacodynamics/Kinetics
Half-life Elimination Clavulanic acid: 1 hour
Time to Peak Clavulanic acid: Serum: 1 hour

Pregnancy Risk Factor B

Pregnancy Considerations Adverse events have not been observed in animal reproduction studies. Both amoxicillin and clavulanic acid cross the placenta. Maternal use of amoxicillin/clavulanate has generally not resulted in an increased risk of birth defects. A possible increased risk of necrotizing enterocolitis in neonates or bowel disorders in children exposed to amoxicillin/clavulanate *in utero* have been observed. In women with acute infections during pregnancy, amoxicillin/clavulanate may be given if an antibiotic is required and appropriate based on bacterial sensitivity; however, use is not recommended in the management of preterm premature rupture of membranes. Oral ampicillin-class antibiotics are poorly absorbed during labor. When used during pregnancy, pharmacokinetic changes have been observed with amoxicillin alone (refer to the Amoxicillin monograph for details).

Lactation Enters breast milk/use caution

Breast-Feeding Considerations Amoxicillin is found in breast milk. The manufacturer recommends that caution be used if administered to breast-feeding women. The use of amoxicillin/clavulanate may be safe while breast-feeding. However, the risk of adverse events in the infant may be increased when compared to the use of amoxicillin alone and the risk may be related to maternal dose. Nondose-related effects could include modification of bowel flora and allergic sensitization of the infant.

Dosage Forms
Powder for suspension, oral: 200: Amoxicillin 200 mg and clavulanate potassium 28.5 mg per 5 mL; 250: Amoxicillin 250 mg and clavulanate potassium 62.5 mg per 5 mL; 400: Amoxicillin 400 mg and clavulanate potassium 57 mg per 5 mL; 600: Amoxicillin 600 mg and clavulanate potassium 42.9 mg per 5 mL

Amoclan:
200: Amoxicillin 200 mg and clavulanate potassium 28.5 mg per 5 mL
400: Amoxicillin 400 mg and clavulanate potassium 57 mg per 5 mL
600: Amoxicillin 600 mg and clavulanate potassium 42.9 mg per 5 mL

Augmentin®:
125: Amoxicillin 125 mg and clavulanate potassium 31.25 mg per 5 mL
250: Amoxicillin 250 mg and clavulanate potassium 62.5 mg per 5 mL

Augmentin ES-600®:
600: Amoxicillin 600 mg and clavulanate potassium 42.9 mg per 5 mL (75 mL, 125 mL, 200 mL) [contains phenylalanine 7 mg/5 mL, potassium 0.23 mEq/5 mL; strawberry cream flavor]

Tablet, oral: 250: Amoxicillin 250 mg and clavulanate potassium 125 mg; 500: Amoxicillin 500 mg and clavulanate potassium 125 mg; 875: Amoxicillin 875 mg and clavulanate potassium 125 mg

Augmentin®:
500: Amoxicillin 500 mg and clavulanate potassium 125 mg
875: Amoxicillin 875 mg and clavulanate potassium 125 mg

Tablet, chewable, oral: 200: Amoxicillin 200 mg and clavulanate potassium 28.5 mg; 400: Amoxicillin 400 mg and clavulanate potassium 57 mg

Tablet, extended release, oral: Amoxicillin 1000 mg and clavulanate acid 62.5 mg

Augmentin XR®: 1000: Amoxicillin 1000 mg and clavulanate acid 62.5 mg

Dental Comment In maxillary sinus, anterior nasal cavity, and deep neck infections, beta-lactamase-producing staphylococci and beta-lactamase-producing *Bacteroides* usually are present. In these situations, antibiotics that resist the beta-lactamase enzyme are indicated. Amoxicillin and clavulanic acid is administered orally for moderate infections. Ampicillin sodium and sulbactam sodium (Unasyn®) is administered parenterally for more severe infections.

References
American Dental Association Council on Scientific Affairs, "Combating Antibiotic Resistance," *J Am Dent Assoc*, 2004, 135(4):484-7.
Wynn RL, Bergman SA, Meiller TF, et al, "Antibiotics in Treating Oral-Facial Infections of Odontogenic Origin: An Update," *Gen Dent*, 2001, 49(3):238-40, 242, 244 passim.

Amphotericin B Cholesteryl Sulfate Complex
(am foe TER i sin bee kole LES te ril SUL fate KOM plecks)

Brand Names: U.S. Amphotec®
Brand Names: Canada Amphotec®
Pharmacologic Category Antifungal Agent, Parenteral

Use Treatment of invasive aspergillosis in patients who have failed amphotericin B deoxycholate treatment, or who have renal impairment or experience unacceptable toxicity which precludes treatment with amphotericin B deoxycholate in effective doses.

Unlabeled Use Effective in patients with serious *Candida* species infections

Local Anesthetic/Vasoconstrictor Precautions No information available to require special precautions

Effects on Dental Treatment No significant effects or complications reported

Effects on Bleeding No information available to require special precautions

Adverse Effects

>10%:

Cardiovascular: Hypotension, tachycardia

Central nervous system: Chills, fever

Endocrine & metabolic: Hypokalemia

Gastrointestinal: Vomiting

Hepatic: Hyperbilirubinemia

Renal: Creatinine increased

5% to 10%:

Cardiovascular: Chest pain, facial edema, hypertension

Central nervous system: Abnormal thinking, headache, insomnia, somnolence, tremor

Dermatologic: Pruritus, rash, sweating

Endocrine & metabolic: Hyperglycemia, hypocalcemia, hypomagnesemia, hypophosphatemia

Gastrointestinal: Abdominal enlargement, abdominal pain, diarrhea, dry mouth, hematemesis, jaundice, nausea, stomatitis

Hematologic: Anemia, hemorrhage, thrombocytopenia

Hepatic: Alkaline phosphatase increased, liver function test abnormal

Neuromuscular & skeletal: Back pain, rigor

Respiratory: Cough increased, dyspnea, epistaxis, hypoxia, rhinitis

Note: Amphotericin B colloidal dispersion has an improved therapeutic index compared to conventional amphotericin B, and has been used safely in patients with amphotericin B-related nephrotoxicity; however, continued decline of renal function has occurred in some patients.

General Dosage Range I.V.: *Children and Adults:* 3-4 mg/kg/day

Mechanism of Action Binds to ergosterol altering cell membrane permeability in susceptible fungi and causing leakage of cell components with subsequent cell death. Proposed mechanism suggests that amphotericin causes an oxidation-dependent stimulation of macrophages (Lyman, 1992).

Pharmacodynamics/Kinetics

Half-life Elimination ~28 hours; prolonged with higher doses

Pregnancy Risk Factor B

Pregnancy Considerations Adverse events were not observed in animal reproduction studies. Amphotericin crosses the placenta and enters the fetal circulation. Amphotericin B is recommended for the treatment of serious systemic fungal diseases in pregnant women; refer to current guidelines (King, 1998).

Amphotericin B (Conventional)
(am foe TER i sin bee con VEN sha nal)

Related Information

Fungal Infections *on page 1573*

Brand Names: Canada Fungizone®

Generic Availability (U.S.) Yes

Pharmacologic Category Antifungal Agent, Parenteral

Use Treatment of severe systemic and central nervous system infections caused by susceptible fungi such as *Candida* species, *Histoplasma capsulatum*, *Cryptococcus neoformans*, *Aspergillus* species, *Blastomyces dermatitidis*, *Torulopsis glabrata*, and *Coccidioides immitis*; fungal peritonitis; irrigant for bladder fungal infections; used in fungal infection in patients with bone marrow transplantation, amebic meningoencephalitis, ocular aspergillosis (intraocular injection), candidal cystitis (bladder irrigation), chemoprophylaxis (low-dose I.V.), immunocompromised patients at risk of aspergillosis (intranasal/nebulized), refractory meningitis (intrathecal), coccidioidal arthritis (intra-articular/I.M.).

Low-dose amphotericin B has been administered after bone marrow transplantation to reduce the risk of invasive fungal disease.

Local Anesthetic/Vasoconstrictor Precautions No information available to require special precautions

Effects on Dental Treatment No significant effects or complications reported

Effects on Bleeding No information available to require special precautions

Adverse Effects

>10%:

Central nervous system: Fever, chills, headache, malaise, generalized pain

Endocrine & metabolic: Hypokalemia, hypomagnesemia

Gastrointestinal: Anorexia

Hematologic: Anemia

Renal: Nephrotoxicity

1% to 10%:

Cardiovascular: Hypotension, hypertension, flushing

Central nervous system: Delirium, arachnoiditis, pain along lumbar nerves

Gastrointestinal: Nausea, vomiting

Genitourinary: Urinary retention

Hematologic: Leukocytosis

Local: Thrombophlebitis

Neuromuscular & skeletal: Paresthesia (especially with I.T. therapy)

Renal: Renal tubular acidosis, renal failure

Dosage Premedication: For patients who experience infusion-related immediate reactions, premedicate with the following drugs 30-60 minutes prior to drug administration: NSAID ± diphenhydramine **or** acetaminophen with diphenhydramine **or** hydrocortisone. If the patient experiences rigors during the infusion, meperidine may be administered.

Usual dosage ranges:

Infants and Children:

Test dose: I.V.: 0.1 mg/kg/dose to a maximum of 1 mg; infuse over 30-60 minutes. Many clinicians believe a test dose is unnecessary.

Maintenance dose: 0.25-1 mg/kg/day given once daily; infuse over 2-6 hours. Once therapy has been established, amphotericin B can be administered on an every-other-day basis at 1-1.5 mg/kg/dose; cumulative dose: 1.5-2 g over 6-10 weeks.

Duration of therapy: Varies with nature of infection, usual duration is 4-12 weeks or cumulative dose of 1-4 g

Adults:

Test dose: 1 mg infused over 20-30 minutes. Many clinicians believe a test dose is unnecessary.

Maintenance dose: Usual: 0.3-1.5 mg/kg/day; 1-1.5 mg/kg over 4-6 hours every other day may be given once therapy is established; aspergillosis, rhinocerebral mucormycosis, often require 1-1.5 mg/kg/day; do not exceed 1.5 mg/kg/day

Indication-specific dosing:
Infants and Children:
Aspergillosis (HIV-exposed/-positive): I.V.: 1-1.5 mg/kg/day once daily (CDC, 2009)
Candidiasis (HIV-exposed/-positive):
Invasive: I.V.: 0.5-1.5 mg/kg/day once daily (CDC, 2009)
Esophageal: I.V.: 0.3-0.5 mg/kg/day once daily (CDC, 2009)
Oropharyngeal, refractory: I.V.: 0.3-0.5 mg/kg/day (CDC, 2009)
Coccidioidomycosis (HIV-exposed/-positive): I.V.: 0.5-1 mg/kg/day (CDC, 2009)
Cryptococcus, **CNS disease (HIV-exposed/-positive):** I.V.: 0.7-1 mg/kg/day plus flucytosine; **Note:** Minimum 2 week induction followed by consolidation and chronic suppressive therapy; may increase amphotericin dose to 1.5 mg/kg/day if flucytosine is not tolerated.
Cryptococcus, **disseminated (non-CNS disease) or severe pulmonary disease (HIV-exposed/-positive):** I.V.: 0.7-1 mg/kg/day once daily with or without flucytosine
Histoplasma, CNS or severe disseminated: I.V.: 1 mg/kg/day once daily (CDC, 2009)
Adults:
Aspergillosis, disseminated: I.V.: 0.6-0.7 mg/kg/day for 3-6 months
Bone marrow transplantation (prophylaxis): I.V.: Low-dose amphotericin B 0.1-0.25 mg/kg/day has been administered after bone marrow transplantation to reduce the risk of invasive fungal disease.
Candidemia (neutropenic or non-neutropenic): I.V.: 0.5-1 mg/kg/day until 14 days after first negative blood culture and resolution of signs and symptoms (Pappas, 2009)
Candidiasis, chronic, disseminated: I.V.: 0.5-0.7 mg/kg/day for 3-6 months and resolution of radiologic lesions (Pappas, 2009)
Dematiaceous fungi: I.V.: 0.7 mg/kg/day in combination with an azole
Endocarditis: I.V.: 0.6-1 mg/kg/day (with or without flucytosine) for 6 weeks after valve replacement; **Note:** If isolates susceptible and/or clearance demonstrated, guidelines recommend step-down to fluconazole; also for long-term suppression therapy if valve replacement is not possible (Pappas, 2009)
Endophthalmitis, fungal:
Intravitreal (unlabeled use): 10 mcg in 0.1 mL (in conjunction with systemic therapy)
I.V.: 0.7-1 mg/kg/day (with or without flucytosine) for at least 4-6 weeks (Pappas, 2009)
Esophageal candidiasis: I.V.: 0.3-0.7 mg/kg/day for 14-21 days after clinical improvement (Pappas, 2009)
Histoplasmosis: Chronic, severe pulmonary or disseminated: I.V.: 0.5-1 mg/kg/day for 7 days, then 0.8 mg/kg every other day (or 3 times/week) until total dose of 10-15 mg/kg; may continue itraconazole as suppressive therapy (lifelong for immunocompromised patients)
Meningitis:
Candidal: I.V.: 0.7-1 mg/kg/day (with or without flucytosine) for at least 4 weeks; **Note:** Liposomal amphotericin favored by IDSA guidelines based on decreased risk of nephrotoxicity and potentially better CNS penetration (Pappas, 2009)

Cryptococcal or Coccidioides: I.T.: Initial: 0.01-0.05 mg as single daily dose; may increase daily in increments of 0.025-0.1 mg as tolerated (maximum: 1.5 mg/day; most patients will tolerate a maximum dose of ~0.5 mg/treatment). Once titration to a maximum tolerated dose is achieved, that dose is administered daily. Once CSF improvement noted, may decrease frequency on a weekly basis (eg, 5 times/week, then 3 times/week, then 2 times/week, then once weekly, then once every other week, then once every 2 weeks, etc) until administration occurs once every 6 weeks. Typically, concurrent oral azole therapy is maintained (Stevens, 2001). **Note:** IDSA notes that the use of I.T. amphotericin for cryptococcal meningitis is generally discouraged and rarely necessary (Perfect, 2010).
Histoplasma: I.V.: 0.5-1 mg/kg/day for 7 days, then 0.8 mg/kg every other day (or 3 times/week) for 3 months total duration; follow with fluconazole suppressive therapy for up to 12 months
Meningoencephalitis, cryptococcal (Perfect, 2010): I.V.:
HIV positive: Induction: 0.7-1 mg/kg/day (plus flucytosine 100 mg/kg/day) for 2 weeks, then change to oral fluconazole for at least 8 weeks; alternatively, amphotericin (0.7-1 mg/kg/day) may be continued uninterrupted for 4-6 weeks; maintenance: amphotericin 1 mg/kg/week for ≥1 year may be considered, but inferior to use of azoles
HIV negative: Induction: 0.7-1 mg/kg/day (plus flucytosine 100 mg/kg/day) for 2 weeks (low-risk patients), ≥4 weeks (non-low-risk, but without neurologic complication, immunosuppression, underlying disease, and negative CSF culture at 2 weeks), >6 weeks (neurologic complication or patients intolerant of flucytosine) Follow with azole consolidation/maintenance treatment.
Oropharyngeal candidiasis: I.V.: 0.3 mg/kg/day for 7-14 days (Pappas, 2009)
Osteoarticular candidiasis: I.V.: 0.5-1 mg/kg/day for several weeks, followed by fluconazole for 6-12 months (osteomyelitis) or 6 weeks (septic arthritis) (Pappas, 2009)
Penicillium marneffei: I.V.: 0.6 mg/kg/day for 2 weeks
Pneumonia: Cryptococcal (mild-to-moderate): I.V.:
HIV positive: 0.5-1 mg/kg/day
HIV negative: 0.5-0.7 mg/kg/day (plus flucytosine) for 2 weeks
Sporotrichosis: Pulmonary, meningeal, osteoarticular, or disseminated: I.V.: Total dose of 1-2 g, then change to oral itraconazole or fluconazole for suppressive therapy
Urinary tract candidiasis (Pappas, 2009):
Fungus balls: I.V.: 0.5-0.7 mg/kg/day with or without flucytosine 25 mg/kg 4 times daily
Pyelonephritis: I.V.: 0.5-0.7 mg/kg/day with or without flucytosine 25 mg/kg 4 times daily for 2 weeks
Symptomatic cystitis: I.V.: 0.3-0.6 mg/kg/day for 1-7 days
Bladder irrigation: Irrigate with 50 mcg/mL solution instilled periodically or continuously for 5-10 days or until cultures are clear for fluconazole-resistant *Candida*

Dosing adjustment in renal impairment: If renal dysfunction is due to the drug, the daily total can be decreased by 50% or the dose can be given every other day; I.V. therapy may take several months

◀

Renal replacement therapy: Poorly dialyzed; no supplemental dose or dosage adjustment necessary, including patients on intermittent hemodialysis or CRRT.

Peritoneal dialysis (PD): Administration in dialysate: 1-2 mg/L of peritoneal dialysis fluid either with or without low-dose I.V. amphotericin B (a total dose of 2-10 mg/kg given over 7-14 days). Precipitate may form in ionic dialysate solutions.

Mechanism of Action Binds to ergosterol altering cell membrane permeability in susceptible fungi and causing leakage of cell components with subsequent cell death. Proposed mechanism suggests that amphotericin causes an oxidation-dependent stimulation of macrophages (Lyman, 1992).

Contraindications Hypersensitivity to amphotericin or any component of the formulation

Warnings/Precautions Anaphylaxis has been reported with amphotericin B-containing drugs. During the initial dosing, the drug should be administered under close clinical observation. May cause nephrotoxicity; usual risk factors include underlying renal disease, concomitant nephrotoxic medications and daily and/or cumulative dose of amphotericin. Avoid use with other nephrotoxic drugs; drug-induced renal toxicity usually improves with interrupting therapy, decreasing dosage, or increasing dosing interval. However permanent impairment may occur, especially in patients receiving large cumulative dose (eg, >5 g) and in those also receiving other nephrotoxic drugs. Hydration and sodium repletion prior to administration may reduce the risk of developing nephrotoxicity. Frequent monitoring of renal function is recommended. Acute reactions (eg, fever, shaking chills, hypotension, anorexia, nausea, vomiting, headache, tachypnea) are most common 1-3 hours after starting the infusion and diminish with continued therapy. Avoid rapid infusion to prevent hypotension, hypokalemia, arrhythmias, and shock. If therapy is stopped for >7 days, restart at the lowest dose recommended and increase gradually. Leukoencephalopathy has been reported following administration of amphotericin. Total body irradiation has been reported to be a possible predisposition.

[U.S. Boxed Warning]: Should be used primarily for treatment of progressive, potentially life-threatening fungal infections, not noninvasive forms of infection. [U.S. Boxed warning]: Verify the product name and dosage if dose exceeds 1.5 mg/kg.

Drug Interactions

Metabolism/Transport Effects None known.

Avoid Concomitant Use

Avoid concomitant use of Amphotericin B (Conventional) with any of the following: Gallium Nitrate

Increased Effect/Toxicity

Amphotericin B (Conventional) may increase the levels/effects of: Aminoglycosides; Colistimethate; CycloSPORINE (Systemic); Flucytosine; Gallium Nitrate

The levels/effects of Amphotericin B (Conventional) may be increased by: Corticosteroids (Orally Inhaled); Corticosteroids (Systemic)

Decreased Effect

Amphotericin B (Conventional) may decrease the levels/effects of: Saccharomyces boulardii

The levels/effects of Amphotericin B (Conventional) may be decreased by: Antifungal Agents (Azole Derivatives, Systemic)

Pharmacodynamics/Kinetics

Half-life Elimination Biphasic: Initial: 15-48 hours; Terminal: 15 days

Time to Peak Within 1 hour following a 4- to 6-hour dose

Pregnancy Risk Factor B

Pregnancy Considerations Adverse events were not observed in animal reproduction studies. Amphotericin crosses the placenta and enters the fetal circulation. No teratogenic or undue systemic toxicity (electrolyte imbalance or renal dysfunction) has been reported in the mother or fetus. Toxic maternal effects are to be expected and must be monitored (Perfect, 2010). Amphotericin B is recommended for the treatment of serious systemic fungal diseases in pregnant women. Refer to current guidelines (King, 1998).

Lactation Excretion in breast milk unknown/not recommended

Breast-Feeding Considerations It is not known if amphotericin is excreted into breast milk. Due to its poor oral absorption, systemic exposure to the nursing infant is expected to be decreased; however, because of the potential for toxicity, breast-feeding is not recommended (Mactal-Haaf, 2001).

Dosage Forms

Injection, powder for reconstitution: 50 mg

Amphotericin B (Lipid Complex)
(am foe TER i sin bee LIP id KOM pleks)

Brand Names: U.S. Abelcet®

Brand Names: Canada Abelcet®

Pharmacologic Category Antifungal Agent, Parenteral

Use Treatment of invasive fungal infection in patients who are refractory to or intolerant of conventional amphotericin B (amphotericin B deoxycholate) therapy

Local Anesthetic/Vasoconstrictor Precautions No information available to require special precautions

Effects on Dental Treatment No significant effects or complications reported

Effects on Bleeding No information available to require special precautions

Adverse Effects Nephrotoxicity and infusion-related hyperpyrexia, rigor, and chilling are reduced relative to amphotericin deoxycholate.

>10%:

Central nervous system: Chills (18%), fever (14%)

Renal: Serum creatinine increased (11%)

Miscellaneous: Multiple organ failure (11%)

1% to 10%:

Cardiovascular: Hypotension (8%), cardiac arrest (6%), hypertension (5%), chest pain (3%)

Central nervous system: Headache (6%), pain (5%)

Dermatologic: Rash (4%)

Endocrine & metabolic: Hypokalemia (5%), bilirubinemia (4%)

Gastrointestinal: Nausea (9%), vomiting (8%), diarrhea (6%), gastrointestinal hemorrhage (4%), abdominal pain (4%)

Hematologic: Thrombocytopenia (5%), anemia (4%), leukopenia (4%)

Renal: Renal failure (5%)

Respiratory: Respiratory failure (8%), dyspnea (6%), respiratory disorder (4%)

Miscellaneous: Sepsis (7%), infection (5%)

General Dosage Range I.V.: *Children and Adults:* 5 mg/kg once daily

Mechanism of Action Binds to ergosterol altering cell membrane permeability in susceptible fungi and causing leakage of cell components with subsequent cell death. Proposed mechanism suggests that amphotericin causes an oxidation-dependent stimulation of macrophages.

Pharmacodynamics/Kinetics

Half-life Elimination 173 hours following multiple doses

Pregnancy Risk Factor B

Pregnancy Considerations Adverse events were not observed in animal reproduction studies. Amphotericin crosses the placenta and enters the fetal circulation. Amphotericin B is recommended for the treatment of serious, systemic fungal diseases in pregnant women, refer to current guidelines (King, 1998).

Amphotericin B (Liposomal)
(am foe TER i sin bee lye po SO mal)

Brand Names: U.S. AmBisome®
Brand Names: Canada AmBisome®
Pharmacologic Category Antifungal Agent, Parenteral

Use Empirical therapy for presumed fungal infection in febrile, neutropenic patients; treatment of patients with *Aspergillus* species, *Candida* species, and/or *Cryptococcus* species infections refractory to amphotericin B desoxycholate (conventional amphotericin), or in patients where renal impairment or unacceptable toxicity precludes the use of amphotericin B desoxycholate; treatment of cryptococcal meningitis in HIV-infected patients; treatment of visceral leishmaniasis

Unlabeled Use Treatment of systemic *Histoplasmosis* infection; empiric treatment of fungal meningitis or osteoarticular infections

Local Anesthetic/Vasoconstrictor Precautions No information available to require special precautions

Effects on Dental Treatment Key adverse event(s) related to dental treatment: Facial swelling, postural hypotension, mucositis, stomatitis, and ulcerative stomatitis (see Dental Comment)

Effects on Bleeding No information available to require special precautions

Adverse Effects Percentage of adverse reactions is dependent upon population studied and may vary with respect to premedications and underlying illness. Incidence of decreased renal function and infusion-related events are lower than rates observed with amphotericin B deoxycholate.

>10%:
Cardiovascular: Peripheral edema (15%), edema (12% to 14%), tachycardia (9% to 19%), hypotension (7% to 14%), hypertension (8% to 20%), chest pain (8% to 12%), hypervolemia (8% to 12%)
Central nervous system: Chills (29% to 48%), insomnia (17% to 22%), headache (9% to 20%), anxiety (7% to 14%), pain (14%), confusion (9% to 13%)
Dermatologic: Rash (5% to 25%), pruritus (11%)
Endocrine & metabolic: Hypokalemia (31% to 51%), hypomagnesemia (15% to 50%), hyperglycemia (8% to 23%), hypocalcemia (5% to 18%), hyponatremia (9% to 12%)
Gastrointestinal: Nausea (16% to 40%), vomiting (11% to 32%), diarrhea (11% to 30%), abdominal pain (7% to 20%), constipation (15%), anorexia (10% to 14%)
Hematologic: Anemia (27% to 48%), blood transfusion reaction (9% to 18%), leukopenia (15% to 17%), thrombocytopenia (6% to 13%)

Hepatic: Alkaline phosphatase increased (7% to 22%), bilirubinemia (≤18%), ALT increased (15%), AST increased (13%), liver function tests abnormal (not specified) (4% to 13%)
Local: Phlebitis (9% to 11%)
Neuromuscular & skeletal: Weakness (6% to 13%), back pain (12%)
Renal: Nephrotoxicity (14% to 47%), creatinine increased (18% to 40%), BUN increased (7% to 21%), hematuria (14%)
Respiratory: Dyspnea (18% to 23%), lung disorder (14% to 18%), cough (2% to 18%), epistaxis (9% to 15%), pleural effusion (13%), rhinitis (11%)
Miscellaneous: Infusion reactions (4% to 21%), sepsis (7% to 14%), infection (11% to 13%)
2% to 10%:
Cardiovascular: Arrhythmia, atrial fibrillation, bradycardia, cardiac arrest, cardiomegaly, facial swelling, flushing, orthostatic hypotension, valvular heart disease, vascular disorder, vasodilation
Central nervous system: Agitation, abnormal thinking, coma, depression, dysesthesia, dizziness (7% to 9%), hallucinations, malaise, nervousness, seizure, somnolence
Dermatologic: Alopecia, bruising, cellulitis, dry skin, maculopapular rash, petechia, purpura, skin discoloration, skin disorder, skin ulcer, urticaria, vesiculobullous rash
Endocrine & metabolic: Acidosis, fluid overload, hypernatremia (4%), hyperchloremia, hyperkalemia, hypermagnesemia, hyperphosphatemia, hypophosphatemia, hypoproteinemia, lactate dehydrogenase increased, nonprotein nitrogen increased
Gastrointestinal: Abdomen enlarged, amylase increased, dyspepsia, dysphagia, eructation, fecal incontinence, flatulence, gastrointestinal hemorrhage (10%), hematemesis, hemorrhoids, gum/oral hemorrhage, ileus, mucositis, rectal disorder, stomatitis, ulcerative stomatitis, xerostomia
Genitourinary: Vaginal hemorrhage
Hematologic: Coagulation disorder, hemorrhage, prothrombin decreased
Hepatic: Hepatocellular damage, hepatomegaly, veno-occlusive liver disease
Local: Injection site inflammation
Neuromuscular & skeletal: Arthralgia, bone pain, dystonia, myalgia, neck pain, paresthesia, rigors, tremor
Ocular: Conjunctivitis, dry eyes, eye hemorrhage
Renal: Abnormal renal function, acute renal failure, dysuria, renal failure, toxic nephropathy, urinary incontinence
Respiratory: Asthma, atelectasis, dry nose, hemoptysis, hyperventilation, pharyngitis, pneumonia, pulmonary edema, respiratory alkalosis, respiratory insufficiency, respiratory failure, sinusitis, hypoxia (6% to 8%)
Miscellaneous: Allergic reaction, cell-mediated immunological reaction, flu-like syndrome, graft-versus-host disease, herpes simplex, hiccup, procedural complication (8% to 10%), diaphoresis (7%)

General Dosage Range I.V.: *Children and Adults:* 3-6 mg/kg/day as a single daily dose (maximum: 6 mg/kg/day)

Mechanism of Action Binds to ergosterol altering cell membrane permeability in susceptible fungi and causing leakage of cell components with subsequent cell death. Proposed mechanism suggests that amphotericin causes an oxidation-dependent stimulation of macrophages (Lyman, 1992).

◄

Pharmacodynamics/Kinetics
Half-life Elimination Terminal: 174 hours
Pregnancy Risk Factor B
Pregnancy Considerations Adverse events were not observed in animal reproduction studies. Amphotericin crosses the placenta and enters the fetal circulation. Amphotericin B is recommended for the treatment of serious systemic fungal diseases in pregnant women; refer to current guidelines (King, 1998).

Dental Comment Amphotericin B, liposomal is a true single bilayer liposomal drug delivery system. Liposomes are closed, spherical vesicles created by mixing specific proportions of amphophilic substances such as phospholipids and cholesterol so that they arrange themselves into multiple concentric bilayer membranes when hydrated in aqueous solutions. Single bilayer liposomes are then formed by microemulsification of multi-lamellar vesicles using a homogenizer. Amphotericin B, liposomal consists of these unilamellar bilayer liposomes with amphotericin B intercalated within the membrane. Due to the nature and quantity of amphophilic substances used, and the lipophilic moiety in the amphotericin B molecule, the drug is an integral part of the overall structure of the amphotericin B liposomes. Amphotericin B, liposomal contains true liposomes that are <100 nm in diameter.

Ampicillin (am pi SIL in)

Related Information
Antibiotic Prophylaxis *on page 1542*
Brand Names: Canada Ampicillin for Injection; Apo-Ampi®; Novo-Ampicillin; Nu-Ampi
Generic Availability (U.S.) Yes
Pharmacologic Category Antibiotic, Penicillin
Dental Use I.V. or I.M. administration for the prevention of infective endocarditis in patients not allergic to penicillin and unable to take oral amoxicillin; I.V. or I.M. administration for prophylaxis in total joint replacement patients not allergic to penicillin and unable to take oral medications undergoing dental procedures
Use Treatment of susceptible bacterial infections (non-beta-lactamase-producing organisms); treatment or prophylaxis of infective endocarditis; susceptible bacterial infections caused by streptococci, pneumococci, non-penicillinase-producing staphylococci, *Listeria*, meningococci; some strains of *H. influenzae*, *Salmonella*, *Shigella*, *E. coli*, *Enterobacter*, and *Klebsiella*

Local Anesthetic/Vasoconstrictor Precautions No information available to require special precautions

Effects on Dental Treatment Key adverse event(s) related to dental treatment: Oral candidiasis, black hairy tongue, glossitis, sore mouth or tongue, and stomatitis.

Effects on Bleeding No information available to require special precautions

Adverse Effects Frequency not defined.
Central nervous system: Fever, penicillin encephalopathy, seizure
Dermatologic: Erythema multiforme, exfoliative dermatitis, rash, urticaria
Note: Appearance of a rash should be carefully evaluated to differentiate (if possible) nonallergic ampicillin rash from hypersensitivity reaction. Incidence is higher in patients with viral infection, *Salmonella* infection, lymphocytic leukemia, or patients that have hyperuricemia.

Gastrointestinal: Black hairy tongue, diarrhea, enterocolitis, glossitis, nausea, oral candidiasis, pseudomembranous colitis, sore mouth or tongue, stomatitis, vomiting
Hematologic: Agranulocytosis, anemia, hemolytic anemia, eosinophilia, leukopenia, thrombocytopenia purpura
Hepatic: AST increased
Renal: Interstitial nephritis (rare)
Respiratory: Laryngeal stridor
Miscellaneous: Anaphylaxis, serum sickness-like reaction

Dental Usual Dosage
Infective endocarditis prophylaxis: I.M., I.V.: Dental, oral, or respiratory tract procedures:
Infants and Children: 50 mg/kg within 30-60 minutes prior to procedure in patients not allergic to penicillin and unable to take oral amoxicillin.
Adults: 2 g within 30-60 minutes prior to procedure in patients not allergic to penicillin and unable to take oral amoxicillin.
Note: Intramuscular injections should be avoided in patients who are receiving anticoagulant therapy. In these circumstances, orally administered regimens should be given whenever possible. Intravenously administered antibiotics should be used for patients who are unable to tolerate or absorb oral medications.
Note: American Heart Association (AHA) guidelines now recommend prophylaxis only in patients undergoing invasive procedures and in whom underlying cardiac conditions may predispose to a higher risk of adverse outcomes should infection occur.
Prophylaxis in total joint replacement patient: Adults: I.M., I.V.: 2 g 1 hour prior to the procedure
Dosage
Usual dosage range:
Infants and Children:
Oral: 50-100 mg/kg/day in doses divided every 6 hours (maximum: 2-4 g/day)
I.M., I.V.: 100-400 mg/kg/day in divided doses every 6 hours (maximum: 12 g/day)
Adults:
Oral: 250-500 mg every 6 hours
I.M., I.V.: 1-2 g every 4-6 hours or 50-250 mg/kg/day in divided doses (maximum: 12 g/day)
Indication-specific dosing:
Infants and Children:
Community-acquired pneumonia (CAP) (IDSA/PIDS, 2011): Infants >3 months and Children: I.V.:
Note: May consider addition of vancomycin or clindamycin to empiric therapy if community-acquired MRSA suspected. In children ≥ 5 years, a macrolide antibiotic should be added if atypical pneumonia cannot be ruled out.
Empiric treatment or *S. pneumoniae* (moderate-to-severe; MICs to penicillin ≤2.0 mcg/mL) or *H. influenzae* (beta-lactamase negative) (preferred): 150-200 mg/kg/day divided every 6 hours
Group A *Streptococcus* (moderate-to-severe) (preferred): 200 mg/kg/day divided every 6 hours
S. pneumoniae (moderate-to-severe; MICs to penicillin ≥4.0 mcg/mL) (alternative to ceftriaxone): 300-400 mg/kg/day divided every 6 hours
Prophylaxis against infective endocarditis:
Dental, oral, or respiratory tract procedures: I.M., I.V.: 50 mg/kg within 30-60 minutes prior to procedure in patients not allergic to penicillin and unable to take oral amoxicillin. Intramuscular injections should be avoided in patients who are receiving

anticoagulant therapy. In these circumstances, orally administered regimens should be given whenever possible. Intravenously administered antibiotics should be used for patients who are unable to tolerate or absorb oral medications.

Note: American Heart Association (AHA) guidelines now recommend prophylaxis only in patients undergoing invasive procedures and in whom underlying cardiac conditions may predispose to a higher risk of adverse outcomes should infection occur.

Genitourinary and gastrointestinal tract procedures: I.M., I.V.:

High-risk patients: 50 mg/kg (maximum: 2 g) within 30 minutes prior to procedure, followed by ampicillin 25 mg/kg (or amoxicillin 25 mg/kg orally) 6 hours later; must be used in combination with gentamicin. **Note:** As of April 2007, routine prophylaxis for GI/GU procedures is no longer recommended by the AHA.

Moderate-risk patients: 50 mg/kg within 30 minutes prior to procedure

Mild-to-moderate infections:

Oral: 50-100 mg/kg/day in doses divided every 6 hours (maximum: 2-4 g/day)

I.M., I.V.: 100-150 mg/kg/day in divided doses every 6 hours (maximum: 2-4 g/day)

Severe infections, meningitis: I.M., I.V.: 200-400 mg/kg/day in divided doses every 6 hours (maximum: 6-12 g/day)

Adults:

Cholangitis (acute): I.V.: 2 g every 4 hours with gentamicin

Diverticulitis: I.M., I.V.: 2 g every 6 hours with metronidazole

Endocarditis:

Infective: I.V.: 12 g/day via continuous infusion or divided every 4 hours

Prophylaxis: Dental, oral, or respiratory tract: I.M., I.V.: 2 g within 30-60 minutes prior to procedure in patients not allergic to penicillin and unable to take oral amoxicillin. Intramuscular injections should be avoided in patients who are receiving anticoagulant therapy. In these circumstances, orally administered regimens should be given whenever possible. Intravenously administered antibiotics should be used for patients who are unable to tolerate or absorb oral medications.

Note: American Heart Association (AHA) guidelines now recommend prophylaxis only in patients undergoing invasive procedures and in whom underlying cardiac conditions may predispose to a higher risk of adverse outcomes should infection occur.

Prophylaxis in total joint replacement patient: I.M., I.V.: 2 g 1 hour prior to the procedure

Genitourinary and gastrointestinal tract procedures: High-risk patients: I.M., I.V.: 2 g within 30 minutes prior to procedure, followed by ampicillin 1 g (or amoxicillin 1 g orally) 6 hours later; must be used in combination with gentamicin. **Note:** As of April 2007, routine prophylaxis for GI/GU procedures is no longer recommended by the AHA.

Moderate-risk patients: I.M., I.V.: 2 g within 30 minutes prior to procedure

Group B streptococcus (neonatal prophylaxis): I.V.: 2 g initial dose, then 1 g every 4 hours until delivery (CDC, 2010)

Listeria **infections:** I.V.: 2 g every 4 hours (consider addition of aminoglycoside)

Mild-to-moderate infections: Oral: 250-500 mg every 6 hours

Prosthetic joint infection, *Enterococcus* spp (penicillin-susceptible): I.V.: 12 g continuous infusion every 24 hours **or** 2 g every 4 hours for 4-6 weeks; consider addition of aminoglycoside (Osmon, 2013)

Sepsis/meningitis: I.M., I.V.: 150-250 mg/kg/day divided every 3-4 hours (range: 6-12 g/day)

Urinary tract infections (*Enterococcus* suspected): I.V.: 1-2 g every 6 hours with gentamicin

Dosage adjustment in renal impairment:

Cl_{cr} >50 mL/minute: Administer every 6 hours

Cl_{cr} 10-50 mL/minute: Administer every 6-12 hours

Cl_{cr} <10 mL/minute: Administer every 12-24 hours

Intermittent hemodialysis (IHD) (administer after hemodialysis on dialysis days): Dialyzable (20% to 50%): I.V.: 1-2 g every 12-24 hours (Heintz, 2009). **Note:** Dosing dependent on the assumption of 3 times/week, complete IHD sessions.

Peritoneal dialysis (PD): 250 mg every 12 hours

Continuous renal replacement therapy (CRRT) (Heintz, 2009): Drug clearance is highly dependent on the method of renal replacement, filter type, and flow rate. Appropriate dosing requires close monitoring of pharmacologic response, signs of adverse reactions due to drug accumulation, as well as drug concentrations in relation to target trough (if appropriate). The following are general recommendations only (based on dialysate flow/ultrafiltration rates of 1-2 L/hour and minimal residual renal function) and should not supersede clinical judgment:

CVVH: Loading dose of 2 g followed by 1-2 g every 8-12 hours

CVVHD: Loading dose of 2 g followed by 1-2 g every 8 hours

CVVHDF: Loading dose of 2 g followed by 1-2 g every 6-8 hours

Dosage adjustment in hepatic impairment: No dosage adjustment provided in manufacturer's labeling.

Mechanism of Action Inhibits bacterial cell wall synthesis by binding to one or more of the penicillin-binding proteins (PBPs) which in turn inhibits the final transpeptidation step of peptidoglycan synthesis in bacterial cell walls, thus inhibiting cell wall biosynthesis. Bacteria eventually lyse due to ongoing activity of cell wall autolytic enzymes (autolysins and murein hydrolases) while cell wall assembly is arrested.

Contraindications Hypersensitivity to ampicillin, any component of the formulation, or other penicillins

Warnings/Precautions Dosage adjustment may be necessary in patients with renal impairment. Serious and occasionally severe or fatal hypersensitivity (anaphylactoid) reactions have been reported in patients on penicillin therapy, especially with a history of beta-lactam hypersensitivity, history of sensitivity to multiple allergens, or previous IgE-mediated reactions (eg, anaphylaxis, angioedema, urticaria). Use with caution in asthmatic patients. High percentage of patients with infectious mononucleosis have developed rash during therapy with ampicillin; ampicillin-class antibiotics not recommended in these patients. Appearance of a rash should be carefully evaluated to differentiate a nonallergic ampicillin rash from a hypersensitivity reaction. Ampicillin rash occurs in 5% to 10% of children receiving ampicillin and is a generalized dull red, maculopapular rash, generally appearing 3-14 days after the start of therapy. It normally begins on the trunk and spreads over most of the body. It may be most intense at pressure areas, elbows, and knees. Prolonged use may result in fungal or bacterial superinfection, including

◀ *C. difficile*-associated diarrhea (CDAD) and pseudo-membranous colitis; CDAD has been observed >2 months postantibiotic treatment.

Drug Interactions

Metabolism/Transport Effects None known.

Avoid Concomitant Use

Avoid concomitant use of Ampicillin with any of the following: BCG

Increased Effect/Toxicity

Ampicillin may increase the levels/effects of: Methotrexate; Vitamin K Antagonists

The levels/effects of Ampicillin may be increased by: Allopurinol; Probenecid

Decreased Effect

Ampicillin may decrease the levels/effects of: Atenolol; BCG; Mycophenolate; Sodium Picosulfate; Typhoid Vaccine

The levels/effects of Ampicillin may be decreased by: Chloroquine; Fusidic Acid; Lanthanum; Tetracycline Derivatives

Ethanol/Nutrition/Herb Interactions Food: Food decreases ampicillin absorption rate; may decrease ampicillin serum concentration. Management: Take at equal intervals around-the-clock, preferably on an empty stomach (1 hour before or 2 hours after meals). Maintain adequate hydration, unless instructed to restrict fluid intake.

Dietary Considerations Take on an empty stomach 1 hour before or 2 hours after meals. Some products may contain sodium.

Pharmacodynamics/Kinetics

Half-life Elimination

Children and Adults: 1-1.8 hours

Anuria/end-stage renal disease: 7-20 hours

Time to Peak Oral: Within 1-2 hours

Pregnancy Risk Factor B

Pregnancy Considerations Adverse events have not been observed in animal reproduction studies. Ampicillin crosses the placenta, providing detectable concentrations in the cord serum and amniotic fluid. Maternal use of ampicillin has generally not resulted in an increased risk of birth defects. Ampicillin is recommended for use in pregnant women for the management of preterm premature rupture of membranes (PPROM) and for the prevention of early-onset group B streptococcal (GBS) disease in newborns. Ampicillin may also be used in certain situations prior to vaginal delivery in women at high risk for endocarditis.

The volume of distribution of ampicillin is increased during pregnancy and the half-life is decreased. As a result, serum concentrations in pregnant patients are approximately 50% of those in nonpregnant patients receiving the same dose. Higher doses may be needed during pregnancy. Although oral absorption is not altered during pregnancy, oral ampicillin is poorly absorbed during labor.

Lactation Enters breast milk/use caution

Breast-Feeding Considerations Ampicillin is excreted in breast milk. The manufacturer recommends that caution be exercised when administering ampicillin to nursing women. Due to the low concentrations in human milk, minimal toxicity would be expected in the nursing infant. Nondose-related effects could include modification of bowel flora and allergic sensitization.

Dosage Forms

Capsule, oral: 250 mg, 500 mg

Injection, powder for reconstitution: 125 mg, 250 mg, 500 mg, 1 g, 2 g, 10 g

Powder for suspension, oral: 125 mg/5 mL (100 mL, 200 mL); 250 mg/5 mL (100 mL, 200 mL)

References

American Dental Association Council on Scientific Affairs, "Combating Antibiotic Resistance," *J Am Dent Assoc*, 2004, 135(4):484-7.

Jevsevar DS and Abt E, "The New AAOS-ADA Clinical Practice Guideline on Prevention of Orthopaedic Implant Infection in Patients Undergoing Dental Procedures," *J Am Acad Orthop Surg*, 2013, 21 (3):195-7.

Wilson W, Taubert KA, Gewitz M, et al, "Prevention of Infective Endocarditis. Guidelines From the American Heart Association. A Guideline From the American Heart Association Rheumatic Fever, Endocarditis, and Kawasaki Disease Committee, Council on Cardiovascular Disease in the Young, and the Council on Clinical Cardiology, Council on Cardiovascular Surgery and Anesthesia, and the Quality of Care and Outcomes Research Interdisciplinary Working Group," *Circulation*, 2007, 115. Available at http://circ.-ahajournals.org/cgi/reprint/CIRCULATIONAHA.106.183095v1; last accessed July 26, 2007.

Wynn RL, Bergman SA, Meiller TF, et al, "Antibiotics in Treating Oral-Facial Infections of Odontogenic Origin: An Update", *Gen Dent*, 2001, 49(3):238-40, 242, 244 passim.

Ampicillin and Sulbactam

(am pi SIL in & SUL bak tam)

Related Information

Ampicillin *on page 106*

Brand Names: U.S. Unasyn®

Brand Names: Canada Unasyn®

Generic Availability (U.S.) Yes

Pharmacologic Category Antibiotic, Penicillin

Dental Use Parenteral beta-lactamase-resistant antibiotic combination to treat more severe orofacial infections where beta-lactamase-producing staphylococci and beta-lactamase-producing *Bacteroides* are present

Use Treatment of susceptible bacterial infections involved with skin and skin structure, intra-abdominal infections, gynecological infections; spectrum is that of ampicillin plus organisms producing beta-lactamases such as *S. aureus*, *H. influenzae*, *E. coli*, *Klebsiella*, *Acinetobacter*, *Enterobacter*, and anaerobes

Unlabeled Use Treatment of acute bacterial rhinosinusitis (ABRS); endocarditis; intravascular catheter-associated bloodstream infection caused by susceptible bacteria; community-acquired pneumonia; early-onset hospital-acquired pneumonia

Local Anesthetic/Vasoconstrictor Precautions No information available to require special precautions

Effects on Dental Treatment Prolonged use of penicillins may lead to development of oral candidiasis (see Dental Comment)

Effects on Bleeding No information available to require special precautions

Adverse Effects Also see Ampicillin.

>10%: Local: Pain at injection site (I.M.)

1% to 10%:

Dermatologic: Rash

Gastrointestinal: Diarrhea

Local: Pain at injection site (I.V.), thrombophlebitis

Miscellaneous: Allergic reaction (may include serum sickness, urticaria, bronchospasm, hypotension, etc)

Dental Usual Dosage Severe orofacial infections: Adults: I.M., I.V.: 1000-2000 mg ampicillin (1500-3000 mg Unasyn®) every 6 hours (maximum: 8 g ampicillin/day, 12 g Unasyn®)

Dosage Note: Unasyn® (ampicillin/sulbactam) is a combination product.

Usual dosage range:

Children and Adolescents: I.V.: 100-400 mg ampicillin/kg/day divided every 6 hours (maximum: 8 g ampicillin daily, 12 g Unasyn®). **Note:** The American Academy of Pediatrics recommends a dose of up to 300 mg ampicillin/kg/day for severe infection in infants >1 month of age.

Adults: I.M., I.V.: 1000-2000 mg ampicillin (1500-3000 mg Unasyn®) every 6 hours (maximum: 8 g ampicillin daily, 12 g Unasyn®)

Indication-specific dosing:

Infants, Children, and Adolescents:

Endocarditis (unlabeled use) (Baddour, 2005): *Enterococcus organism (resistant to penicillin/susceptible to aminoglycoside and vancomycin):* I.V.: 300 mg ampicillin/kg/day in 4 divided doses with concomitant gentamicin for 6 weeks

Intravascular catheter-associated bloodstream infection (unlabeled use) (IDSA, 2009):
Infants: I.V.: 100-150 mg ampicillin/kg/day in 4 divided doses

Children and Adolescents: I.V.: 100-200 mg ampicillin/kg/day in 4 divided doses

Children and Adolescents:

Epiglottitis: I.V.: 100-200 mg ampicillin/kg/day divided in 4 doses

Mild-to-moderate infections: I.V.: 100-200 mg ampicillin/kg/day (150-300 mg Unasyn®) divided every 6 hours (maximum: 8 g ampicillin daily, 12 g Unasyn®)

Peritonsillar and retropharyngeal abscess: I.V.: 200 mg ampicillin/kg/day in 4 divided doses

Severe infections: I.V.: 200-400 mg ampicillin/kg/day divided every 6 hours (maximum: 8 g ampicillin daily, 12 g Unasyn®)

Adults: Doses expressed as ampicillin/sulbactam combination:

Acute bacterial rhinosinusitis, severe infection requiring hospitalization (unlabeled use): I.V.: 1500-3000 mg every 6 hours for 5-7 days (Chow, 2012)

Amnionitis, cholangitis, diverticulitis, endomyometritis (with doxycycline), endophthalmitis, epididymitis/orchitis, liver abscess (with metronidazole), or peritonitis: I.V.: 3000 mg every 6 hours

Bite (human, canine/feline): *Pasteurella multocida:* I.V.: 1500-3000 mg every 6 hours

Endocarditis (unlabeled use) (Baddour, 2005): *Enterococcus organism (resistant to penicillin/susceptible to aminoglycoside and vancomycin):* I.V.: 3000 mg every 6 hours with concomitant gentamicin for 6 weeks. **Note:** If enterococcus is gentamicin resistant, then >6 weeks of ampicillin-sulbactam therapy needed.

HACEK organism: I.V.: 3000 mg every 6 hours for 4 weeks

Intravascular catheter-associated bloodstream infection, *Acinetobacter* **spp (unlabeled use) (IDSA, 2009):** I.V.: 3000 mg every 6 hours

Orbital cellulitis: I.V.: 3000 mg every 6 hours

Osteomyelitis (diabetic foot) (Lipsky, 2004): I.V.: 3000 mg every 6 hours

Pelvic inflammatory disease: I.V.: 3000 mg every 6 hours with doxycycline

Peritonitis associated with CAPD: Intraperitoneal:
Intermittent: 3000 mg added to one exchange every 12 hours; allow to dwell for at least 6 hours (Blackwell, 1990; Li, 2010)
Continuous: Loading dose: 1500 mg per liter of dialysate; maintenance dose: 150 mg per liter of dialysate (Li, 2010)

Pneumonia:
Aspiration or community-acquired: I.V.: 1500-3000 mg every 6 hours
Hospital-acquired: I.V.: 3000 mg every 6 hours

Urinary tract infections, pyelonephritis: I.V.: 3000 mg every 6 hours for 14 days

Dosage adjustment in renal impairment: Note: Estimation of renal function for the purpose of drug dosing should be done using the Cockcroft-Gault formula.

Cl_{cr} 15-29 mL/minute/1.73 m^2: 1500-3000 mg every 12 hours

Cl_{cr} 5-14 mL/minute/1.73 m^2: 1500-3000 mg every 24 hours

Intermittent hemodialysis (IHD) (administer after hemodialysis on dialysis days): 1500-3000 mg every 12-24 hours (Heintz, 2009). **Note:** Dosing dependent on the assumption of 3 times weekly, complete IHD sessions.

Peritoneal dialysis (PD): 3000 mg every 24 hours

Continuous renal replacement therapy (CRRT): Drug clearance is highly dependent on the method of renal replacement, filter type, and flow rate. Appropriate dosing requires close monitoring of pharmacologic response, signs of adverse reactions due to drug accumulation, as well as drug levels in relation to target trough (if appropriate). The following are general recommendations only (based on dialysate flow/ultrafiltration rates of 1-2 L/hour and minimal residual renal function) and should not supersede clinical judgment (Heintz, 2009; Trotman, 2005):

CVVH: Initial: 3000 mg; maintenance: 1500-3000 mg every 8-12 hours

CVVHD: Initial: 3000 mg; maintenance: 1500-3000 mg every 8 hours

CVVHDF: Initial: 3000 mg; maintenance: 1500-3000 mg every 6-8 hours

Dosage adjustment in hepatic impairment: No dosage adjustment provided in manufacturer's labeling.

Mechanism of Action Inhibits bacterial cell wall synthesis by binding to one or more of the penicillin-binding proteins (PBPs) which in turn inhibits the final transpeptidation step of peptidoglycan synthesis in bacterial cell walls, thus inhibiting cell wall biosynthesis. Bacteria eventually lyse due to ongoing activity of cell wall autolytic enzymes (autolysins and murein hydrolases) while cell wall assembly is arrested. The addition of sulbactam, a beta-lactamase inhibitor, to ampicillin extends the spectrum of ampicillin to include some beta-lactamase-producing organisms.

Contraindications Hypersensitivity to ampicillin, sulbactam, penicillins, or any component of the formulations

Warnings/Precautions Dosage adjustment may be necessary in patients with renal impairment. Serious and occasionally severe or fatal hypersensitivity (anaphylactoid) reactions have been reported in patients on penicillin therapy, especially with a history of beta-lactam hypersensitivity, history of sensitivity to multiple allergens, or previous IgE-mediated reactions (eg, anaphylaxis, angioedema, urticaria). High percentage of patients with infectious mononucleosis have developed rash during therapy with ampicillin; ampicillin-class antibiotics not recommended in these patients. Appearance of a rash should be carefully evaluated to differentiate a nonallergic ampicillin rash from a hypersensitivity reaction. Prolonged use may result in fungal or bacterial superinfection, including *C. difficile*-associated diarrhea (CDAD) and pseudomembranous colitis; CDAD has been observed >2 months postantibiotic treatment.

Drug Interactions

Metabolism/Transport Effects None known.

Avoid Concomitant Use

Avoid concomitant use of Ampicillin and Sulbactam with any of the following: BCG

Increased Effect/Toxicity
Ampicillin and Sulbactam may increase the levels/ effects of: Methotrexate; Vitamin K Antagonists

The levels/effects of Ampicillin and Sulbactam may be increased by: Allopurinol; Probenecid

Decreased Effect
Ampicillin and Sulbactam may decrease the levels/ effects of: Atenolol; BCG; Mycophenolate; Sodium Picosulfate; Typhoid Vaccine

The levels/effects of Ampicillin and Sulbactam may be decreased by: Chloroquine; Fusidic Acid; Lanthanum; Tetracycline Derivatives

Dietary Considerations Some products may contain sodium.

Pharmacodynamics/Kinetics
Half-life Elimination Sulbactam: Normal renal function: 1-1.3 hours; **Note:** Elimination kinetics of both ampicillin and sulbactam are similarly affected in patients with renal impairment, therefore, the blood concentration ratio is expected to remain constant regardless of renal function.

Pregnancy Risk Factor B

Pregnancy Considerations Adverse events have not been observed in animal reproduction studies. Both ampicillin and sulbactam cross the placenta. Maternal use of penicillins has generally not resulted in an increased risk of birth defects. When used during pregnancy, pharmacokinetic changes have been observed with ampicillin alone (refer to the Ampicillin monograph for details). Ampicillin/sulbactam may be considered for prophylactic use prior to cesarean delivery (consult current guidelines).

Lactation Enters breast milk/use caution

Breast-Feeding Considerations Ampicillin and sulbactam are both excreted into breast milk in low concentrations. The manufacturer recommends that caution be used if administering to lactating women. Nondose-related effects could include modification of bowel flora and allergic sensitization of the infant. The maternal dose of sulbactam does not need altered in the postpartum period. Also refer to the Ampicillin monograph.

Dosage Forms
Injection, powder for reconstitution: 1.5 g [ampicillin 1 g and sulbactam 0.5 g]; 3 g [ampicillin 2 g and sulbactam 1 g]; 15 g [ampicillin 10 g and sulbactam 5 g]

Unasyn®: 1.5 g [ampicillin 1 g and sulbactam 0.5 g]; 3 g [ampicillin 2 g and sulbactam 1 g]; 15 g [ampicillin 10 g and sulbactam 5 g]; 15 g [ampicillin 10 g and sulbactam 5 g

Dental Comment In maxillary sinus, anterior nasal cavity, and deep neck infections, beta-lactamase-producing staphylococci and beta-lactamase-producing *Bacteroides* usually are present. In these situations, antibiotics that resist the beta-lactamase enzyme should be administered. Amoxicillin and clavulanic acid is administered orally for moderate infections. Ampicillin sodium and sulbactam sodium (Unasyn®) is administered parenterally for more severe infections.

Amsacrine (AM sah kreen)

Brand Names: Canada AMSA PD
Pharmacologic Category Antineoplastic Agent
Use Refractory acute leukemia
Unlabeled Use Acute myeloid leukemia (AML)
Local Anesthetic/Vasoconstrictor Precautions No information available to require special precautions

Effects on Dental Treatment Key adverse event(s) related to dental treatment: Oral ulcerations and stomatitis

Effects on Bleeding Chemotherapy may result in significant myelosuppression, potentially including significant reduction in platelet counts and altered hemostasis. In patients who are under active treatment with these agents, medical consult is suggested.

Adverse Effects
>10%:
Gastrointestinal: Nausea (>10%), vomiting (>10%), stomatitis (>10%), diarrhea (>10%), perirectal abscess (>10%), abdominal pain (>10%)
Hematologic: Myelosuppression, leukopenia (nadir: 11-13 days; recovery: days 17-25)

Frequency not defined:
Cardiovascular: Atrial tachyarrhythmia, atrial tachycardia, atrial fibrillation, bradycardia, cardiomyopathy (rare), cardiopulmonary arrest, CHF (rare); ECG changes (QT prolongation, nonspecific ST segment or T wave changes); ejection fraction decreased, hypotension, sinus tachycardia, tachycardia, ventricular arrhythmia, ventricular extrasystoles, ventricular fibrillation, ventricular tachyarrhythmia
Central nervous system: Confusion, dizziness, emotional lability, fever, headache, hypoesthesia, lethargy, seizure
Dermatologic: Alopecia, cutaneous inflammatory reaction, dermatologic reaction, purpura, rash (purpuric or maculopapular), urticaria
Gastrointestinal: Anorexia, dysphagia, gingivitis, gum hemorrhage, hematemesis, weight changes
Genitourinary: Orange-red discoloration of the urine
Hematologic: Anemia, granulocytopenia, hemorrhage, pancytopenia, thrombocytopenia
Hepatic: Alkaline phosphatase increased, AST increased, bilirubin increased, hepatic insufficiency, hepatitis, hepatotoxicity, jaundice, progressive liver failure
Local: Injection site inflammation, phlebitis
Neuromuscular & skeletal: Musculoskeletal pain, paresthesia, weakness
Renal: BUN increased, creatinine increased, hematuria, proteinuria, renal failure
Respiratory: Dyspnea
Miscellaneous: Allergic reaction, infection

General Dosage Range Dosage adjustment recommended in patients with hepatic or renal impairment or patients who develop toxicities
I.V.: *Adults:* Induction: 75-125 mg/m^2/day for 5 days every 3-4 weeks; Maintenance: ~50% of induction dose every 4-8 weeks

Mechanism of Action Amsacrine has been shown to inhibit DNA synthesis by binding to, and intercalating with, DNA; inhibits topoisomerase II activity.

Pharmacodynamics/Kinetics
Half-life Elimination 1.4-5 hours; Terminal: 8-9 hours
Pregnancy Considerations Animal reproduction studies have not been conducted. Women of childbearing potential should avoid becoming pregnant while receiving treatment.

Product Availability Not available in U.S.

Amyl Nitrite (AM il NYE trite)

Pharmacologic Category Antianginal Agent; Antidote; Vasodilator
Use Coronary vasodilator in angina pectoris

Note: Given the widespread use of newer nitrate compounds, the use of amyl nitrite for patients experiencing angina pectoris has fallen out of favor.

Unlabeled Use Adjunct treatment of cyanide toxicity; produce changes in the intensity of heart murmurs; provocation of latent left ventricular outflow tract (LVOT) gradient during echocardiography in patients with hypertrophic cardiomyopathy (HCM)

Local Anesthetic/Vasoconstrictor Precautions No information available to require special precautions

Effects on Dental Treatment Key adverse event(s) related to dental treatment: Postural hypotension

Effects on Bleeding No information available to require special precautions

Adverse Effects Frequency not defined.

Cardiovascular: Cerebral ischemia, facial flushing, hypotension, orthostatic hypotension, pallor, shock, syncope, tachycardia, vasodilation

Central nervous system: Dizziness, headache, intracranial pressure increased, restlessness

Dermatologic: Dermatitis, irritation

Gastrointestinal: Fecal incontinence, nausea, vomiting

Genitourinary: Urinary incontinence

Hematologic: Hemolytic anemia, methemoglobinemia

Neuromuscular & skeletal: Weakness

Ocular: Intraocular pressure increased, irritation

Miscellaneous: Diaphoresis

General Dosage Range Inhalation: *Adults:* 2-6 nasal inhalations from 1 crushed ampul; may repeat in 3-5 minutes

Mechanism of Action Relaxes vascular smooth muscle; decreases venous ratios and arterial blood pressure; reduces left ventricular work; decreases myocardial O_2 consumption. When used for cyanide poisoning, amyl nitrite promotes the formation of methemoglobin which competes with cytochrome oxidase for the cyanide ion. Cyanide combines with methemoglobin to form cyanomethemoglobin, thereby freeing the cytochrome oxidase and allowing aerobic metabolism to continue.

Pharmacodynamics/Kinetics

Onset of Action Angina: Within 30 seconds

Duration of Action Angina: 3-15 minutes; Pharmacologic provocation of latent left ventricular outflow tract (LVOT) gradient in hypertrophic cardiomyopathy (HCM): ~30 seconds (Reagan, 2005)

Pregnancy Risk Factor C

Pregnancy Considerations Animal reproduction studies have not been conducted. Because amyl nitrate significantly decreases systemic blood pressure and therefore blood flow to the fetus, use is contraindicated in pregnancy (per manufacturer). In addition, fetal hemoglobin may be more susceptible methemoglobin conversion (Valenzuela, 1986).

Anagrelide (an AG gre lide)

Brand Names: U.S. Agrylin®

Brand Names: Canada Agrylin®; Dom-Anagrelide; Mylan-Anagrelide; PMS-Anagrelide; Sandoz-Anagrelide

Pharmacologic Category Phosphodiesterase-3 Enzyme Inhibitor; Phospholipase A_2 Inhibitor

Use Treatment of thrombocythemia associated with myeloproliferative disorders (eg, chronic myelogenous leukemia, essential thrombocythemia, polycythemia vera, myeloid metaplasia with myelofibrosis, or other myeloproliferative disorder) to reduce the risk of thrombosis and reduce associated symptoms (including thrombohemorrhagic events)

Local Anesthetic/Vasoconstrictor Precautions No information available to require special precautions

Effects on Dental Treatment Key adverse event(s) related to dental treatment: Orthostatic hypotension

Effects on Bleeding Anagrelide causes dose-related reduction in platelet production and could affect normal clotting; hemorrhage has been reported. Medical consult is suggested for patients under active treatment with anagrelide.

Adverse Effects

>10%:

Cardiovascular: Palpitation (26%), edema (21%)

Central nervous system: Headache (44%), dizziness (15%), pain (15%)

Gastrointestinal: Diarrhea (26%), nausea (17%), abdominal pain (16%)

Neuromuscular & skeletal: Weakness (23%)

Respiratory: Dyspnea (12%)

1% to 10%:

Cardiovascular: Peripheral edema (9%), chest pain (8%), tachycardia (8%), angina, arrhythmia, HF, hypertension, orthostatic hypotension, syncope, thrombosis, vasodilatation

Central nervous system: Fever (9%), malaise (6%), amnesia, chills, confusion, depression, insomnia, migraine, nervousness, somnolence

Dermatologic: Rash (8%), pruritus (6%), alopecia, bruising, photosensitivity, urticaria

Endocrine & skeletal: Dehydration

Gastrointestinal: Flatulence (10%), vomiting (10%), anorexia (8%), dyspepsia (5%), aphthous stomatitis, constipation, eructation, gastritis, GI distress, GI hemorrhage, melena

Genitourinary: Dysuria

Hematologic: Thrombocytopenia (9%; grades 3/4: 5%), anemia, hemorrhage

Neuromuscular & skeletal: Back pain (6%), paresthesia (6%), arthralgia, leg cramps, myalgia

Ocular: Amblyopia, diplopia, visual field abnormality

Otic: Tinnitus

Renal: Renal abnormality (2%), renal failure (1%), hematuria

Respiratory: Pharyngitis (7%), cough (6%), asthma, bronchitis, epistaxis, pneumonia, rhinitis, sinusitis

Miscellaneous: Flu-like syndrome, lymphadenopathy

General Dosage Range Dosage adjustment recommended in patients with hepatic impairment

Oral:

Children: Initial: 0.5 mg/day; Maintenance: 0.5 mg 1-4 times/day (maximum: 10 mg/day; 2.5 mg/dose)

Adults: Initial: 0.5 mg 4 times/day **or** 1 mg twice daily (maximum: 10 mg/day; 2.5 mg/dose)

Mechanism of Action Anagrelide appears to inhibit cyclic nucleotide phosphodiesterase and the release of arachidonic acid from phospholipase, possibly by inhibiting phospholipase A_2. It also causes a dose-related reduction in platelet production, which results from decreased megakaryocyte hypermaturation (disrupts the postmitotic phase of maturation).

Pharmacodynamics/Kinetics

Onset of Action Initial: Within 7-14 days; complete response (platelets ≤600,000/mm³): 4-12 weeks

Duration of Action 6-24 hours; upon discontinuation, platelet count begins to rise within 4 days

Half-life Elimination Plasma: 1.3 hours

Time to Peak Serum: 1 hour

Pregnancy Risk Factor C

◄ **Pregnancy Considerations** Teratogenic effects were not observed in animal studies; however, decreased pup survival was noted. Use of anagrelide during pregnancy is limited. The manufacturer recommends effective contraception in women of childbearing potential. Use during pregnancy only if potential benefit to mother outweighs possible risk to the fetus.

Anakinra (an a KIN ra)

Related Information
Rheumatoid Arthritis, Osteoarthritis, and Osteoporosis on page 1526

Brand Names: U.S. Kineret®

Brand Names: Canada Kineret®

Pharmacologic Category Antirheumatic, Disease Modifying; Interleukin-1 Receptor Antagonist

Use Treatment of moderately- to severely-active rheumatoid arthritis (RA) in adult patients who have failed one or more disease-modifying antirheumatic drugs (DMARDs; may be used alone or in combination with DMARDs [other than tumor necrosis factor-blocking agents]); treatment of neonatal-onset multisystem inflammatory disease (NOMID), which is a cryopyrin-associated periodic syndrome (CAPS)

Local Anesthetic/Vasoconstrictor Precautions No information available to require special precautions

Effects on Dental Treatment No significant effects or complications reported

Effects on Bleeding No information available to require special precautions

Adverse Effects
>10%:
Central nervous system: Headache (12% to 14%), fever (12%)
Gastrointestinal: Nausea (8%)
Local: Injection site reaction (RA: ≤71%; mild: 73%; moderate: 24%; severe: 3%; NOMID: 16%)
Neuromuscular & skeletal: Arthralgia (6% to 12%)
Respiratory: Nasopharyngitis (12%)
Miscellaneous: Infection (39% versus 37% in placebo; serious infection 2% to 3%)
1% to 10%:
Gastrointestinal: Diarrhea (7%)
Hematologic: Neutropenia (5% to 8%)

General Dosage Range Dosage adjustment recommended in patients with renal impairment
SubQ:
Infants, Children, and Adolescents: Initial: 1-2 mg/kg daily in 1-2 divided doses (maximum: 8 mg/kg daily)
Adults: 100 mg once daily **or** initial: 1-2 mg/kg daily in 1-2 divided doses (maximum: 8 mg/kg daily)

Mechanism of Action Antagonist of the interleukin-1 (IL-1) receptor. Endogenous IL-1 is induced by inflammatory stimuli and mediates a variety of immunological responses, including degradation of cartilage (loss of proteoglycans) and stimulation of bone resorption.

Pharmacodynamics/Kinetics
Half-life Elimination Terminal: 4-6 hours; Severe renal impairment (Cl_{cr} <30 mL/minute): ~7 hours; ESRD: 9.7 hours (Yang, 2003)
Time to Peak SubQ: 3-7 hours

Pregnancy Risk Factor B

Pregnancy Considerations Animal reproduction studies have not revealed any evidence of impaired fertility or harm to fetus. Women exposed to anakinra during pregnancy may contact the Organization of Teratology Information Services (OTIS), Rheumatoid Arthritis and Pregnancy Study at 1-877-311-8972.

Anastrozole (an AS troe zole)

Brand Names: U.S. Arimidex®

Brand Names: Canada Apo-Anastrozole®; Arimidex®; JAMP-Anastrozole; Mar-Anastrozole; PMS-Anastrozole; Riva-Anastrozole; Sandoz-Anastrozole; Taro-Anastrozole; Teva-Anastrozole

Pharmacologic Category Antineoplastic Agent, Aromatase Inhibitor

Use First-line treatment of locally-advanced or metastatic breast cancer (hormone receptor-positive or unknown) in postmenopausal women; treatment of advanced breast cancer in postmenopausal women with disease progression following tamoxifen therapy; adjuvant treatment of early hormone receptor-positive breast cancer in postmenopausal women

Unlabeled Use Treatment of recurrent or metastatic endometrial or uterine cancers, treatment of recurrent ovarian cancer

Local Anesthetic/Vasoconstrictor Precautions No information available to require special precautions

Effects on Dental Treatment Key adverse event(s) related to dental treatment: Xerostomia (normal salivary flow resumes upon discontinuation).

Effects on Bleeding No information available to require special precautions

Adverse Effects
>10%:
Cardiovascular: Vasodilatation (25% to 36%), ischemic cardiovascular disease (4%; 17% in patients with pre-existing ischemic heart disease), hypertension (2% to 13%), angina (2%; 12% in patients with pre-existing ischemic heart disease)
Central nervous system: Mood disturbance (19%), fatigue (19%), pain (11% to 17%), headache (9% to 13%), depression (5% to 13%)
Dermatologic: Rash (6% to 11%)
Endocrine & metabolic: Hot flashes (12% to 36%)
Gastrointestinal: Nausea (11% to 19%), vomiting (8% to 13%)
Neuromuscular & skeletal: Weakness (16% to 19%), arthritis (17%), arthralgia (2% to 15%), back pain (10% to 12%), bone pain (6% to 11%), osteoporosis (11%)
Respiratory: Pharyngitis (6% to 14%), cough increased (8% to 11%)
1% to 10%:
Cardiovascular: Peripheral edema (5% to 10%), chest pain (5% to 7%), edema (7%), venous thromboembolic events (2% to 4%), ischemic cerebrovascular events (2%), MI (1%)
Central nervous system: Insomnia (2% to 10%), dizziness (6% to 8%), anxiety (2% to 6%), fever (2% to 5%), malaise (2% to 5%), confusion (2% to 5%), nervousness (2% to 5%), somnolence (2% to 5%), lethargy (1%)
Dermatologic: Alopecia (2% to 5%), pruritus (2% to 5%)
Endocrine & metabolic: Hypercholesterolemia (9%), breast pain (2% to 8%)
Gastrointestinal: Diarrhea (8% to 9%), constipation (7% to 9%), abdominal pain (7% to 9%), weight gain (2% to 9%), anorexia (5% to 7%), xerostomia (6%), dyspepsia (7%), weight loss (2% to 5%)
Genitourinary: Urinary tract infection (2% to 8%), vulvovaginitis (6%), pelvic pain (5%), vaginal bleeding (1% to 5%), vaginitis (4%), vaginal discharge (4%), vaginal hemorrhage (2% to 4%), leukorrhea (2% to 3%), vaginal dryness (2% to 5%)

Hematologic: Anemia (2% to 5%), leukopenia (2% to 5%)

Hepatic: Liver function tests increased (1% to 10%), alkaline phosphatase increased (1% to 10%), gamma GT increased (≤5%)

Local: Thrombophlebitis (2% to 5%)

Neuromuscular & skeletal: Fracture (1% to 10%), arthrosis (7%), paresthesia (5% to 7%), joint disorder (6%), myalgia (2% to 6%), neck pain (2% to 5%), carpal tunnel syndrome (3%), hypertonia (3%)

Ocular: Cataracts (6%)

Respiratory: Dyspnea (8% to 10%), sinusitis (2% to 6%), bronchitis (2% to 5%), rhinitis (2% to 5%)

Miscellaneous: Lymphedema (10%), infection (2% to 9%), flu-like syndrome (2% to 7%), diaphoresis (2% to 5%), cyst (5%), neoplasm (5%), tumor flare (3%)

General Dosage Range Oral: *Adults:* 1 mg once daily

Mechanism of Action Potent and selective nonsteroidal aromatase inhibitor. By inhibiting aromatase, the conversion of androstenedione to estrone, and testosterone to estradiol, is prevented, thereby decreasing tumor mass or delaying progression in patients with tumors responsive to hormones. Anastrozole causes an 85% decrease in estrone sulfate levels.

Pharmacodynamics/Kinetics

Onset of Action Onset of estradiol reduction: 70% reduction after 24 hours; 80% after 2 weeks therapy

Duration of Action Duration of estradiol reduction: 6 days

Half-life Elimination ~50 hours

Time to Peak Plasma: ~2 hours without food; 5 hours with food

Pregnancy Risk Factor X

Pregnancy Considerations Fetotoxicity was observed in animal studies. Anastrozole is contraindicated in women who are or may become pregnant (may cause fetal harm if administered during pregnancy). Use in premenopausal women with breast cancer does not provide any clinical benefit.

Anidulafungin (ay nid yoo la FUN jin)

Related Information
Fungal Infections *on page 1573*

Brand Names: U.S. Eraxis™

Brand Names: Canada Eraxis™

Pharmacologic Category Antifungal Agent, Parenteral; Echinocandin

Use Treatment of candidemia and other forms of *Candida* infections (including those of intra-abdominal, peritoneal, and esophageal locus)

Unlabeled Use Treatment of infections due to *Aspergillus* spp.

Local Anesthetic/Vasoconstrictor Precautions No information available to require special precautions

Effects on Dental Treatment No significant effects or complications reported

Effects on Bleeding No information available to require special precautions

Adverse Effects

>10%:

Cardiovascular: Hypotension (15%), hypertension (12%), peripheral edema (11%)

Central nervous system: Fever (9% to 18%), insomnia (15%)

Endocrine & metabolic: Hypokalemia (≤25%), hypomagnesemia (12%)

Gastrointestinal: Nausea (7% to 24%), diarrhea (9% to 18%), vomiting (7% to 18%)

Genitourinary: Urinary tract infection (15%)

Hepatic: Alkaline phosphatase increased (12%)

Respiratory: Dyspnea (12%)

Miscellaneous: Bacteremia (18%)

2% to 10%:

Cardiovascular: Deep vein thrombosis (10%), chest pain (5%)

Central nervous system: Confusion (8%), headache (8%), depression (6%)

Dermatologic: Decubitus ulcer (5%)

Endocrine & metabolic: Hypoglycemia (7%), dehydration (6%), hyperglycemia (6%), hyperkalemia (6%)

Gastrointestinal: Constipation (8%), dyspepsia (7%), abdominal pain (6%), oral candidiasis (5%)

Hematologic: Anemia (8% to 9%), thrombocythemia (6%), leukocytosis (5% to 8%)

Hepatic: Transaminases increased (≤5%)

Neuromuscular & skeletal: Back pain (5%)

Renal: Creatinine increased (5%)

Respiratory: Pleural effusion (10%), cough (7%), pneumonia (6%), respiratory distress (6%)

Miscellaneous: Sepsis (7%)

General Dosage Range I.V.: *Adults:* Initial dose: 100-200 mg as a single dose; Subsequent dosing: 50-100 mg daily

Mechanism of Action Noncompetitive inhibitor of 1,3-beta-D-glucan synthase resulting in reduced formation of 1,3-beta-D-glucan, an essential polysaccharide comprising 30% to 60% of *Candida* cell walls (absent in mammalian cells); decreased glucan content leads to osmotic instability and cellular lysis

Pharmacodynamics/Kinetics

Half-life Elimination Terminal: 40-50 hours

Pregnancy Risk Factor B

Pregnancy Considerations Adverse effects were observed in animal reproduction studies.

Anthralin (AN thra lin)

Brand Names: U.S. Dritho-Creme®; Zithranol®-RR

Brand Names: Canada Anthraforte®; Anthranol®; Anthrascalp®; Micanol®

Pharmacologic Category Antipsoriatic Agent; Keratolytic Agent

Use Treatment of psoriasis (quiescent or chronic psoriasis)

Local Anesthetic/Vasoconstrictor Precautions No information available to require special precautions

Effects on Dental Treatment No significant effects or complications reported

Effects on Bleeding No information available to require special precautions

Adverse Effects Frequency not defined: Dermatologic: Transient primary irritation of uninvolved skin; temporary discoloration of skin, hair, and fingernails; contact allergic reactions; erythema

General Dosage Range Topical: *Adults:* Generally, apply once a day or as directed

Mechanism of Action Reduction of the mitotic rate and proliferation of epidermal cells in psoriasis by inhibiting synthesis of nucleic protein from inhibition of DNA synthesis to affected areas

Pregnancy Risk Factor C

Pregnancy Considerations Animal reproduction studies have not been conducted.

Anthrax Vaccine (Adsorbed)
(AN thraks vak SEEN ad SORBED)

Brand Names: U.S. BioThrax®

Pharmacologic Category Vaccine, Inactivated (Bacterial)

Use Immunization against *Bacillus anthracis* in persons at high risk for exposure.

The Advisory Committee on Immunization Practices (ACIP) recommends routine vaccination (pre-exposure vaccination) for the following (CDC, 2010):
• Persons who work directly with the organism in the laboratory
• Persons who handle animals or animal products only when
  - potentially infected in research settings;
  - in areas of high incidence of enzootic anthrax; or
  - where standards and restrictions are not sufficient to prevent exposure
• Military personnel deployed to areas with high risk of exposure as recommended by the Department of Defense (DoD)
• Persons engaged in environmental investigations or remediation efforts

Routine immunization for the general population is not recommended. Routine vaccination may be offered to emergency and other responders (police and fire departments, the National Guard, etc) on a voluntary basis under the direction of a comprehensive occupational health and safety program.

The ACIP recommends postexposure prophylaxis after inhalation exposure to aerosolized *Bacillus anthracis* spores for the following (in the absence of completing a pre-exposure, routine vaccination schedule):
• The general public, including pregnant and breast-feeding women
• Medical professionals
• Children ages 0-18 years as determined on an event-by-event basis
• Persons engaged in handling certain animals or animal products
• Persons who work directly with the organism in the laboratory (postexposure vaccination dependant upon pre-event vaccination status)
• Military personnel as recommended by the DoD
• Persons engaged in environmental investigations or remediation efforts (postexposure vaccination dependent upon pre-event vaccination status)
• Emergency and other responders (police and fire departments, the National Guard, etc)
• Persons working in postal facilities

Local Anesthetic/Vasoconstrictor Precautions No information available to require special precautions

Effects on Dental Treatment No significant effects or complications reported

Effects on Bleeding No information available to require special precautions

Adverse Effects All serious adverse reactions must be reported to the U.S. Department of Health and Human Services (DHHS) Vaccine Adverse Event Reporting System (VAERS) 1-800-822-7967 or online at https://vaers.hhs.gov/esub/index.

Note: Percentages reported with I.M. administration; the incidence of local reactions may be increased with SubQ administration.

>10%:
Central nervous system: Fatigue (4% to 12%)

Local: Injection site reactions: Tenderness (41% to 51%), erythema (15% to 48%), edema (5% to 30%), induration (7% to 23%), pain (13% to 20%), warmth (4% to 19%); arm motion limitation (9% to 15%)
Neuromuscular & skeletal: Muscle ache (3% to 13%)
Miscellaneous: Burning sensation (45% to 97%)
1% to 10%:
Central nervous system: Headache (4% to 9%)
Local: Injection site reactions: Itching (1% to 10%), nodule (3% to 9%), bruise (2% to 5%)
Miscellaneous: Tender/painful axillary adenopathy (≤1%)

General Dosage Range
I.M.: *Adults ≤65 years:* 0.5 mL
SubQ: *Adults:* 0.5 mL

Mechanism of Action Active immunization against *Bacillus anthracis*. The vaccine is prepared from a cell-free filtrate of *B. anthracis*, but no dead or live bacteria. Completion of the entire vaccination series is required for full protection; annual boosters are required to maintain immunity.

Pregnancy Risk Factor D

Pregnancy Considerations Adverse events were not observed in animal developmental toxicity studies. Data from the Department of Defense suggest the vaccine may be linked with a slightly increased number of atrial septal defects when given during the first trimester of pregnancy; however, when premature infants are excluded from analysis, the association is not statistically significant. Current ACIP guidelines recommend deferring pre-exposure vaccination when possible; however, postexposure prophylaxis is recommended in pregnant women. Male fertility is not affected by vaccine administration (CDC, 2010).

Prescribing and Access Restrictions Not commercially available in U.S.; presently, all anthrax vaccine lots are owned by the U.S. Department of Defense. The Center for Disease Control (CDC) does not currently recommend routine vaccination of the general public.

Antihemophilic Factor (Human)
(an tee hee moe FIL ik FAK tor HYU man)

Brand Names: U.S. Hemofil M; Koāte®-DVI; Monoclate-P®

Brand Names: Canada Hemofil M

Pharmacologic Category Antihemophilic Agent; Blood Product Derivative

Use Prevention and treatment of hemorrhagic episodes in patients with hemophilia A (classic hemophilia); perioperative management of hemophilia A; can be of significant therapeutic value in patients with acquired factor VIII inhibitors not exceeding 10 Bethesda units/mL

Local Anesthetic/Vasoconstrictor Precautions No information available to require special precautions

Effects on Dental Treatment No significant effects or complications reported

Effects on Bleeding Following large doses, an increased bleeding tendency has rarely been reported. Mild thrombocytopenia has been reported. Due to underlying hemophilia and complications of thrombotic events, a medical consultation is warranted.

General Dosage Range I.V.: *Children and Adults:* Dosage varies greatly depending on indication

Mechanism of Action Protein (factor VIII) in normal plasma which is necessary for clot formation and maintenance of hemostasis; activates factor X in conjunction with activated factor IX; activated factor X converts prothrombin to thrombin, which converts fibrinogen to fibrin, and with factor XIII forms a stable clot

Pharmacodynamics/Kinetics

Half-life Elimination Mean: 8-27 hours

Pregnancy Risk Factor C

Pregnancy Considerations Reproduction studies have not been conducted. Safety and efficacy in pregnant women have not been established. Use during pregnancy only if clearly needed. Parvovirus B19 or hepatitis A, which may be present in plasma-derived products, may affect a pregnant woman more seriously than nonpregnant women.

Antihemophilic Factor (Recombinant)
(an tee hee moe FIL ik FAK tor ree KOM be nant)

Brand Names: U.S. Advate; Helixate® FS; Kogenate® FS; Recombinate; Xyntha®; Xyntha® Solofuse™

Brand Names: Canada Advate; Helixate® FS; Kogenate® FS; Xyntha®

Pharmacologic Category Antihemophilic Agent

Use Prevention and treatment of hemorrhagic episodes in patients with hemophilia A (classic hemophilia or congenital factor VIII deficiency); perioperative management of hemophilia A; routine prophylaxis in patients with hemophilia A to prevent bleeding episodes (Advate, Helixate® FS, Kogenate® FS)

Note: Helixate® FS and Kogenate® FS are also approved in children with hemophilia A with no pre-existing joint damage to reduce risk of joint damage. In addition, Recombinate can be of therapeutic value in patients with acquired factor VIII inhibitors ≤10 Bethesda units/mL.

Local Anesthetic/Vasoconstrictor Precautions No information available to require special precautions

Effects on Dental Treatment Key adverse event(s) related to dental treatment: Taste perversion.

Effects on Bleeding Following large doses, an increased bleeding tendency has rarely been reported. Mild thrombocytopenia has been reported. Due to underlying hemophilia and complications of thrombotic events, a medical consultation is warranted.

Adverse Effects >1% (actual frequency may vary by product):
Central nervous system: Chills, dizziness, fever, headache, pain
Dermatologic: Pruritus, rash, urticaria
Gastrointestinal: Constipation, diarrhea, nausea, taste perversion, vomiting
Local: Injection/infusion site reactions
Neuromuscular & skeletal: Arthralgia, joint swelling, pain in extremity, weakness
Otic: Ear infection, ear pain
Respiratory: Cough, nasal congestion, nasopharyngitis, pharyngolaryngeal pain, rhinorrhea, sinusitis
Miscellaneous: Catheter thrombosis, catheter infection, factor VIII inhibitor formation, flu-like syndrome, influenza

General Dosage Range I.V.: *Children and Adults:* Dosage varies greatly depending on indication

Mechanism of Action Factor VIII replacement, necessary for clot formation and maintenance of hemostasis. It activates factor X in conjunction with activated factor IX; activated factor X converts prothrombin to thrombin, which converts fibrinogen to fibrin, and with factor XIII forms a stable clot.

Pharmacodynamics/Kinetics

Half-life Elimination Mean: ~11-15 hours

Pregnancy Risk Factor C

Pregnancy Considerations Animal reproduction studies have not been conducted. Safety and efficacy in pregnant women has not been established. Use during pregnancy only if clearly needed.

Antihemophilic Factor/von Willebrand Factor Complex (Human)
(an tee hee moe FIL ik FAK tor von WILL le brand FAK tor KOM plex HYU man)

Brand Names: U.S. Alphanate®; Humate-P®; Wilate®

Brand Names: Canada Humate-P®

Pharmacologic Category Antihemophilic Agent; Blood Product Derivative

Use
Factor VIII deficiency: Alphanate®, Humate-P®: Prevention and treatment of hemorrhagic episodes in patients with hemophilia A (classical hemophilia) or acquired factor VIII deficiency (Alphanate® only); **Note:** Wilate® is not approved for use in patients with hemophilia A or acquired factor VIII deficiency

von Willebrand disease (VWD):
Alphanate®: Prophylaxis with surgical and/or invasive procedures in patients with VWD when desmopressin is either ineffective or contraindicated; **Note:** Not indicated for patients with severe VWD undergoing major surgery
Humate-P®: Treatment of spontaneous or trauma-induced bleeding, as well as prevention of excessive bleeding during and after surgery in patients with severe VWD, including mild or moderate disease where use of desmopressin is known or suspected to be inadequate; **Note:** Not indicated for the prophylaxis of spontaneous bleeding episodes
Wilate®: Treatment of spontaneous and trauma-induced bleeding in patients with severe VWD, including mild or moderate disease where use of desmopressin is known or suspected to be inadequate or contraindicated; **Note:** Not indicated for prophylaxis of spontaneous bleeding or prevention of excessive bleeding during and after surgery)

Local Anesthetic/Vasoconstrictor Precautions No information available to require special precautions

Effects on Dental Treatment No significant effects or complications reported

Effects on Bleeding Following large doses, an increased bleeding tendency has rarely been reported. Mild thrombocytopenia has been reported. Due to underlying hemophilia and complications of thrombotic events, a medical consultation is warranted.

Adverse Effects Frequency not defined.
Cardiovascular: Cardiorespiratory arrest, chest tightness, edema, femoral venous thrombosis, flushing, hypervolemia, orthostatic hypotension, shock, thromboembolic events, vasodilation
Central nervous system: Chills, dizziness, fever, headache, lethargy, pain, seizure, somnolence
Dermatologic: Itching, pruritus, rash, urticaria
Endocrine & metabolic: Parotid gland swelling
Gastrointestinal: Nausea, vomiting

Hematologic: Hematocrit decreased (moderate), hemorrhage, hemolysis, pseudothrombocytopenia (severe)

Hepatic: ALT increased

Local: Injection site stinging, phlebitis

Neuromuscular & skeletal: Extremity pain, joint pain, paresthesia, rigors

Respiratory: Cough, dyspnea, pharyngitis, pulmonary embolus (large doses)

Miscellaneous: Allergic reactions, anaphylactic reactions, factor VIII inhibitor formation, hypersensitivity reactions, von Willebrand factor inhibitor formation

General Dosage Range I.V.: *Children and Adults:* Dosage varies greatly depending on indication

Mechanism of Action Factor VIII and von Willebrand factor (VWF), obtained from pooled human plasma, are used to replace endogenous factor VIII and VWF in patients with hemophilia or VWD. Factor VIII in conjunction with activated factor IX, activates factor X which converts prothrombin to thrombin and fibrinogen to fibrin. VWF promotes platelet aggregation and adhesion to damaged vascular endothelium and acts as a stabilizing carrier protein for factor VIII. (Circulating levels of functional VWF are measured as ristocetin cofactor activity [VWF:RCo].)

Pharmacodynamics/Kinetics

Onset of Action Shortening of bleeding time: Immediate

Duration of Action VWD: Shortening of bleeding time: <6 hours postinfusion; presence of VWF multimers detected in the plasma: ≥24 hours

Half-life Elimination

Factor VIII coagulant activity (FVIII:C): Range: 8-28 hours in patients with hemophilia A

VWF:RCo: Range: 3-34 hours in patients with VWD

Pregnancy Risk Factor C

Pregnancy Considerations Reproduction studies have not been conducted. Safety and efficacy in pregnant women have not been established. Use during pregnancy only if clearly needed. Parvovirus B19 or hepatitis A, which may be present in plasma-derived products, may affect a pregnant woman more seriously than nonpregnant women.

Anti-inhibitor Coagulant Complex
(an TEE in HI bi tor coe AG yoo lant KOM pleks)

Brand Names: U.S. Feiba NF

Brand Names: Canada Feiba NF

Pharmacologic Category Activated Prothrombin Complex Concentrate (aPCC); Antihemophilic Agent; Blood Product Derivative

Use Hemophilia A & B patients with inhibitors who are to undergo surgery or those who are bleeding

Unlabeled Use Acquired hemophilia with factor VIII or factor IX inhibitor titers >5 Bethesda units (BU)

Local Anesthetic/Vasoconstrictor Precautions No information available to require special precautions

Effects on Dental Treatment No significant effects or complications reported

Effects on Bleeding Due to underlying hemophilia and complications of thrombotic events, a medical consultation is warranted.

Adverse Effects Frequency not defined.

Cardiovascular: Blood pressure decreased, MI, thromboembolism

Central nervous system: Hypoesthesia (including facial)

Dermatologic: Rash, urticaria

Hematologic: DIC

Local: Injection site pain

Miscellaneous: Allergic reaction (including anaphylaxis), anamnestic response, hypersensitivity

General Dosage Range I.V.: *Children and Adults:* 50-100 units/kg every 6-12 hours (maximum: 200 units/kg/day)

Pregnancy Risk Factor C

Pregnancy Considerations Reproduction studies have not been conducted. Administer to pregnant women only if clearly indicated.

Antipyrine and Benzocaine
(an tee PYE reen & BEN zoe kane)

Related Information

Benzocaine *on page 176*

Brand Names: U.S. Aurodex®

Brand Names: Canada Auralgan®

Pharmacologic Category Otic Agent, Analgesic; Otic Agent, Cerumenolytic

Use Temporary relief of pain and reduction of swelling associated with acute congestive and serous otitis media; facilitates ear wax removal

Local Anesthetic/Vasoconstrictor Precautions No information available to require special precautions

Effects on Dental Treatment No significant effects or complications reported

Effects on Bleeding No information available to require special precautions

General Dosage Range Otic: *Children and Adults:* Instill drops 3 times/day (ear wax removal) or fill ear canal every 1-2 hours (otitis media)

Mechanism of Action Antipyrine has analgesic properties; benzocaine is a local anesthetic; the glycerin base provides decreased middle ear pressure by osmosis.

Pharmacodynamics/Kinetics

Onset of Action Pain relief: ~30 minutes

Pregnancy Risk Factor C

Pregnancy Considerations Animal reproduction studies have not been conducted with this combination.

Antithrombin (an tee THROM bin)

Brand Names: U.S. Atryn®; Thrombate III®

Brand Names: Canada Antithrombin III NF; Thrombate III®

Pharmacologic Category Anticoagulant; Blood Product Derivative

Use Prophylaxis (ATryn®, Thrombate III®) of thromboembolic events in patients with hereditary antithrombin (AT or AT-III) deficiency undergoing surgical or obstetrical procedures (eg, childbirth); treatment (Thrombate III®) of thromboembolism in patients with hereditary AT deficiency

Local Anesthetic/Vasoconstrictor Precautions No information available to require special precautions

Effects on Dental Treatment No significant effects or complications reported

Effects on Bleeding As with all anticoagulant drugs, bleeding is a potential adverse effect of antithrombin during dental surgery; risk is dependent on multiple variables, including the intensity of anticoagulation and patient susceptibility. Medical consult is suggested. It is unlikely that ambulatory patients presenting for dental treatment will be taking intravenous anticoagulant therapy such as antithrombin.

Adverse Effects 1% to 10%:

Cardiovascular: Chest pain (≤2%)

Central nervous system: Dizziness (2%)

Hematologic: Hemorrhage (≥5%), hematoma (≤2%)

Hepatic: Liver enzyme abnormalities (≤2%)
Neuromuscular & skeletal: Hemarthrosis (≤2%)
Renal: Hematuria (≤2%)
Local: Infusion site reaction (≥5%)

General Dosage Range I.V.: *Adults:* Dosage varies greatly depending on indication

Mechanism of Action Antithrombin is the primary physiologic inhibitor of *in vivo* coagulation. It is an alpha$_2$-globulin. Its principal actions are the inactivation of thrombin, plasmin, and other active serine proteases of coagulation, including factors IXa, Xa, XIa, and XIIa. The inactivation of proteases is a major step in the normal clotting process. The strong activation of clotting enzymes at the site of every bleeding injury facilitates fibrin formation and maintains normal hemostasis. Thrombosis in the circulation would be caused by active serine proteases if they were not inhibited by antithrombin after the localized clotting process.

Pharmacodynamics/Kinetics

Half-life Elimination

Plasma derived (Thrombate III®): Biologic: 2.5 days (immunologic assay); 3.8 days (functional AT assay). Half-life may be decreased following surgery, with hemorrhage, acute thrombosis, and/or during heparin administration.

Recombinant derived (Atryn®): 12-18 hours; surgery, childbirth hemorrhage, and/or concomitant heparin may shorten half-life

Pregnancy Risk Factor B (Thrombate III®); C (ATryn®)

Pregnancy Considerations
ATryn®: Adverse events were observed in some clinical studies, but not considered to be related to treatment. There are no adequate and well-controlled studies in pregnant women. An increased risk of fetal effects has not been observed in studies involving a limited number of pregnant women in their 3rd trimester. Pharmacokinetic studies in pregnant women using the recombinant product showed an increase in clearance and volume of distribution compared to nonpregnant patients. Therefore, distinct initial dosing recommendations are provided for pregnant women compared to nonpregnant patients.

Thrombate III®: Teratogenic effects were not observed in animal studies. Dosing recommendations do not differ for obstetric patients compared to nonpregnant patients.

Antithymocyte Globulin (Equine)
(an te THY moe site GLOB yu lin, E kwine)

Brand Names: U.S. Atgam®
Brand Names: Canada Atgam®
Pharmacologic Category Immune Globulin; Immunosuppressant Agent; Polyclonal Antibody
Use Prevention and treatment of acute renal allograft rejection; treatment of moderate-to-severe aplastic anemia in patients not considered suitable candidates for bone marrow transplantation
Unlabeled Use Prevention and treatment of other solid organ allograft rejection; prevention or treatment of graft-versus-host disease (GVHD) following allogeneic stem cell transplantation; treatment of myelodysplastic syndrome (MDS)
Local Anesthetic/Vasoconstrictor Precautions No information available to require special precautions
Effects on Dental Treatment Key adverse event(s) related to dental treatment: Stomatitis
Effects on Bleeding No information available to require special precautions

Adverse Effects

>10%:
Central nervous system: Chills, fever, headache
Dermatologic: Pruritus, rash, urticaria, wheal/flare
Hematologic: Leukopenia, thrombocytopenia
Neuromuscular & skeletal: Arthralgia

1% to 10%:
Cardiovascular: Bradycardia, cardiac irregularity, chest pain, edema, heart failure, hyper-/hypotension, myocarditis
Central nervous system: Agitation, encephalitis, lethargy, lightheadedness, listlessness, seizure, viral encephalopathy
Gastrointestinal: Diarrhea, nausea, stomatitis, vomiting
Hepatic: Hepatosplenomegaly, liver function tests abnormal
Local: Injection site reactions (pain, redness, swelling), phlebitis, thrombophlebitis, burning soles/palms
Neuromuscular & skeletal: Aches, back pain, joint stiffness, myalgia
Ocular: Periorbital edema
Renal: Proteinuria, renal function tests abnormal
Respiratory: Dyspnea, pleural effusion, respiratory distress
Miscellaneous: Anaphylactic reaction, diaphoresis, lymphadenopathy, night sweats, serum sickness, viral infection

General Dosage Range I.V.:
Children: Initial: 5-25 mg/kg/day administered daily for 8-14 days; may be followed by administration every other day (maximum: 21 doses in 28 days)
Adults: Initial: 10-20 mg/kg/day administered daily; may be followed by administration every other day (maximum: 21 doses in 28 days)

Mechanism of Action Immunosuppressant involved in the elimination of antigen-reactive T lymphocytes (killer cells) in peripheral blood or alteration in the function of T-lymphocytes, which are involved in humoral immunity and partly in cell-mediated immunity; induces complete or partial hematologic response in aplastic anemia

Pharmacodynamics/Kinetics

Half-life Elimination Plasma: 1.5-12 days

Pregnancy Risk Factor C

Pregnancy Considerations Reproduction studies have not been conducted; use during pregnancy is not recommended. Use in pregnant women is not recommended and should be considered only in exceptional circumstances. Women exposed to Atgam® during pregnancy may be enrolled in the National Transplantation Pregnancy Registry (877-955-6877).

Apixaban (a PIX a ban)

Related Information
Antiplatelet and Anticoagulation Considerations in Dentistry *on page 1503*

Brand Names: U.S. Eliquis®
Brand Names: Canada Eliquis®
Pharmacologic Category Factor Xa Inhibitor
Use
U.S. labeling: To reduce the risk of stroke and systemic embolism in patients with nonvalvular atrial fibrillation
Canadian labeling: Postoperative prophylaxis of venous thromboembolism (VTE) following elective knee or hip replacement surgery; to reduce the risk of stroke and systemic embolism in patients with nonvalvular atrial fibrillation

Unlabeled Use To reduce the risk of recurrent DVT and/or PE (in patients completing 6-12 months of standard anticoagulation for venous thromboembolism)

Local Anesthetic/Vasoconstrictor Precautions No information available to require special precautions

Effects on Dental Treatment Key adverse event(s) related to dental treatment: Surgical site bleeding may occur. See Effects on Bleeding.

Effects on Bleeding Apixaban inhibits platelet activation and fibrin clot formation via direct, selective, and reversible inhibition of factor Xa. As with all anticoagulants, bleeding is the major adverse effect of apixaban. Hemorrhage may occur at virtually any site; risk is dependent on multiple variables including the intensity of anticoagulation and patient susceptibility. Medical consult is suggested.

Adverse Effects Note: Includes adverse reactions from nonvalvular atrial fibrillation and hip/knee replacement surgery clinical trials.

>10%: Hematologic: Bleeding (5% to 12%; major: ≤2%; clinically-relevant non-major bleeding: 2% to 4%)

1% to 10%:
Dermatologic: Bruising (1%)
Gastrointestinal: Nausea (3%)
Hematologic: Anemia (3%), postprocedural hemorrhage (1%)
Hepatic: GGT increased (1%), transaminases increased (1%)

General Dosage Range Dosage adjustment recommended in patients with multiple risk factors for bleeding including renal impairment or patients on concomitant therapy.

Oral: *Adults:* 2.5-5 mg twice daily

Mechanism of Action Inhibits platelet activation and fibrin clot formation via direct, selective and reversible inhibition of free and clot-bound factor Xa (FXa). FXa, as part of the prothrombinase complex consisting also of factor Va, calcium ions, and phospholipid, catalyzes the conversion of prothrombin to thrombin. Thrombin both activates platelets and catalyzes the conversion of fibrinogen to fibrin.

Pharmacodynamics/Kinetics
Onset of Action 3-4 hours
Half-life Elimination 2.5 mg dose (repeated oral administration): ~8 hours; 5 mg single dose: ~15 hours (Frost, 2012)
Time to Peak 3-4 hours
Pregnancy Risk Factor B
Pregnancy Considerations Adverse events were not observed in animal reproduction studies. Data are insufficient to evaluate the safety of oral factor Xa inhibitors during pregnancy; use during pregnancy should be avoided (Bates, 2012).

Dental Comment At this time there are no coagulation parameters for apixaban to predict the extent of bleeding. Increased bleeding may occur during invasive dental procedures in patients taking a 10 mg daily dose of apixaban. Currently, postsurgical treatment with apixaban is ~12 days for knee replacement patients and ~35 days for hip replacement patients. Medical consult is suggested prior to dental invasive procedures. There are no reports of interactions between the anticoagulant and amoxicillin, cephalexin, cefazolin, ampicillin, or clindamycin; therefore, any of these preprocedural antibiotics can safely be used in patients taking apixaban.

Apomorphine (a poe MOR feen)

Brand Names: U.S. Apokyn®

Pharmacologic Category Anti-Parkinson's Agent, Dopamine Agonist

Use Treatment of hypomobility, "off" episodes with Parkinson's disease

Unlabeled Use Treatment of erectile dysfunction

Local Anesthetic/Vasoconstrictor Precautions Apomorphine is one of the drugs confirmed to prolong the QT interval and is accepted as having a risk of causing torsade de pointes. The risk of drug-induced torsade de pointes is extremely low when a single QT interval prolonging drug is prescribed. In terms of epinephrine, it is not known what effect vasoconstrictors in the local anesthetic regimen will have in patients with a known history of congenital prolonged QT interval or in patients taking any medication that prolongs the QT interval. Until more information is obtained, it is suggested that the clinician consult with the physician prior to the use of a vasoconstrictor in suspected patients, and that the vasoconstrictor (epinephrine, mepivacaine and levonordefrin [Carbocaine® 2% with Neo-Cobefrin®]) be used with caution.

Effects on Dental Treatment Key adverse event(s) related to dental treatment: Orthostatic hypotension has been reported in significant numbers of patients.

Effects on Bleeding No information available to require special precautions

Adverse Effects
>10%:
Cardiovascular: Chest pain/pressure or angina (15%)
Central nervous system: Drowsiness or somnolence (35%), dizziness or orthostatic hypotension (20%)
Gastrointestinal: Nausea and/or vomiting (30%)
Neuromuscular & skeletal: Falls (30%), dyskinesias (24% to 35%)
Respiratory: Yawning (40%), rhinorrhea (20%)
1% to 10%:
Cardiovascular: Edema (10%), vasodilation (3%), hypotension (2%), syncope (2%), CHF
Central nervous system: Hallucinations or confusion (10%), anxiety, depression, fatigue, headache, insomnia, pain
Dermatologic: Bruising
Endocrine & metabolic: Dehydration
Gastrointestinal: Constipation, diarrhea
Local: Injection site reactions
Neuromuscular & skeletal: Arthralgias, weakness
Miscellaneous: Diaphoresis increased

General Dosage Range Dosage adjustment recommended in patients with renal impairment
SubQ: *Adults:* Initial test dose: 2 mg; Starting dose: 2-3 mg/dose at time of "off" episode; Maintenance dose: 2-6 mg/dose at time of "off" episode (maximum: 20 mg/day; 6 mg/dose; 5 doses/day)

Mechanism of Action Stimulates postsynaptic D2-type receptors within the caudate putamen in the brain.

Pharmacodynamics/Kinetics
Onset of Action SubQ: Rapid
Half-life Elimination Terminal: 40 minutes
Time to Peak Plasma: Improved motor scores: 20 minutes
Pregnancy Risk Factor C
Pregnancy Considerations Reproduction studies have not been conducted; use only if clearly needed.
Prescribing and Access Restrictions Apokyn® is only available through a select group of specialty pharmacies and cannot be obtained through a retail pharmacy. Apokyn® may be obtained from the following specialty pharmacies: Accredo Nova Factor or

PharmaCare. To obtain the medication, contact the APOKYN Call Center at 1-877-7APOKYN (1-877-727-6596).

Dental Comment Apomorphine is known to prolong the QT interval. The QT interval is measured as the time and distance between the Q point of the QRS complex and the end of the T wave in the ECG tracing. After adjustment for heart rate, the QT interval is defined as prolonged if it is more than 450 msec in men and 460 msec in women. A long QT syndrome was first described in the 1950s and 60s as a congenital syndrome involving QT interval prolongation and syncope and sudden death. Some of the congenital long QT syndromes were characterized by a peculiar electrocardiographic appearance of the QRS complex involving a premature atria beat followed by a pause, then a subsequent sinus beat showing marked QT prolongation and deformity. This type of cardiac arrhythmia was originally termed "torsade de pointes" (translated from the French as "twisting of the points"). Apomorphine is considered as having a risk of causing torsade de pointes. Since it is not known what effect vasoconstrictors in the local anesthetic regimen will have in patients with a known history of congenital prolonged QT interval or in patients taking any medication that prolongs the QT interval, a medical consult is suggested.

Apraclonidine (a pra KLOE ni deen)

Brand Names: U.S. Iopidine®
Brand Names: Canada Iopidine®
Pharmacologic Category Alpha$_2$ Agonist, Ophthalmic
Use Prevention and treatment of postsurgical intraocular pressure (IOP) elevation; short-term, adjunctive therapy in patients who require additional reduction of IOP
Local Anesthetic/Vasoconstrictor Precautions No information available to require special precautions
Effects on Dental Treatment Key adverse event(s) related to dental treatment: Xerostomia (normal salivary flow resumes upon discontinuation)
Effects on Bleeding No information available to require special precautions
Adverse Effects
Ocular:
5% to 15%: Discomfort, hyperemia, pruritus
1% to 5%: Blanching, blurred vision, conjunctivitis, discharge, dry eye, foreign body sensation, lid edema, tearing
Other body systems:
1% to 10%: Gastrointestinal: Dry mouth (10%)
<3%:
Cardiovascular: Arrhythmia, chest pain, facial edema, peripheral edema
Central nervous system: Depression, dizziness, headache, insomnia, malaise, nervousness, somnolence
Dermatologic: Contact dermatitis, dermatitis
Gastrointestinal: Constipation, nausea, taste perversion
Neuromuscular & skeletal: Abnormal coordination, myalgia, paresthesia, weakness
Respiratory: Asthma, dry nose, dyspnea, parosmia, pharyngitis, rhinitis
General Dosage Range Ophthalmic: *Adults:* 0.5%: Instill 1-2 drops in the affected eye(s) 3 times/day; 1%: Instill 1 drop in operative eye 1 hour prior to and upon completion of surgery
Mechanism of Action Apraclonidine is a potent alpha-adrenergic agent similar to clonidine; relatively selective for alpha$_2$-receptors but does retain some binding to alpha$_1$-receptors; appears to result in reduction of aqueous humor formation; its penetration through the blood-brain barrier is more polar than clonidine which reduces its penetration through the blood-brain barrier and suggests that its pharmacological profile is characterized by peripheral rather than central effects.
Pharmacodynamics/Kinetics
Onset of Action 1 hour; Peak effect: Decreased intraocular pressure: 3-5 hours
Half-life Elimination Systemic: 8 hours
Pregnancy Risk Factor C
Pregnancy Considerations Embryocidal effects were observed in some animal studies. There are no adequate and well-controlled studies in pregnant women.

Aprepitant (ap RE pi tant)

Brand Names: U.S. Emend®
Brand Names: Canada Emend®
Generic Availability (U.S.) No
Pharmacologic Category Antiemetic; Substance P/Neurokinin 1 Receptor Antagonist
Use Prevention of acute and delayed nausea and vomiting associated with moderately- and highly-emetogenic chemotherapy (in combination with other antiemetics); prevention of postoperative nausea and vomiting (PONV)
Local Anesthetic/Vasoconstrictor Precautions No information available to require special precautions
Effects on Dental Treatment Key adverse event(s) related to dental treatment: Hiccups, stomatitis, and mucous membrane disorder.
Effects on Bleeding No information available to require special precautions
Adverse Effects Note: Adverse reactions reported as part of a combination chemotherapy regimen or with general anesthesia.

>10%:
Central nervous system: Fatigue (≤18%)
Gastrointestinal: Nausea (6% to 13%), constipation (9% to 10%)
Neuromuscular & skeletal: Weakness (≤18%)
Miscellaneous: Hiccups (11%)
1% to 10%:
Cardiovascular: Hypotension (≤6%), bradycardia (≤4%)
Central nervous system: Dizziness (≤7%)
Endocrine & metabolic: Dehydration (≤6%)
Gastrointestinal: Diarrhea (≤10%), dyspepsia (≤6%), abdominal pain (≤5%), epigastric discomfort (4%), gastritis (4%), stomatitis (3%)
Hepatic: ALT increased (≤6%), AST increased (3%)
Renal: Proteinuria (7%), BUN increased (5%)
Dosage
Prevention of chemotherapy-induced nausea/vomiting: Adults: Oral:
Highly-emetogenic chemotherapy: 125 mg 1 hour prior to chemotherapy on day 1, followed by 80 mg once daily on days 2 and 3 (in combination with a 5-HT$_3$ antagonist antiemetic on day 1 and dexamethasone on days 1-4)
Moderately-emetogenic chemotherapy: 125 mg 1 hour prior to chemotherapy on day 1, followed by 80 mg once daily on days 2 and 3 (in combination with a 5-HT$_3$ antagonist antiemetic and dexamethasone on day 1)
Prevention of PONV: Adults: Oral: 40 mg within 3 hours prior to induction

▶

Dosage adjustment in renal impairment: No dosage adjustment necessary.
ESRD undergoing dialysis: No dosage adjustment necessary.

Dosage adjustment in hepatic impairment:
Mild-to-moderate impairment (Child-Pugh class A or B): No dosage adjustment necessary
Severe impairment (Child-Pugh class C): Use with caution; no data available.

Mechanism of Action Prevents acute and delayed vomiting by inhibiting the substance P/neurokinin 1 (NK_1) receptor; augments the antiemetic activity of $5-HT_3$ receptor antagonists and corticosteroids to inhibit acute and delayed phases of chemotherapy-induced emesis.

Contraindications Hypersensitivity to aprepitant or any component of the formulation; concurrent use with cisapride or pimozide

Warnings/Precautions Potentially significant drug-drug interactions may exist, requiring dose or frequency adjustment, additional monitoring, and/or selection of alternative therapy. Use caution with severe hepatic impairment (Child-Pugh class C); has not been studied. Not studied for treatment of existing nausea and vomiting. Chronic continuous administration is not recommended.

Drug Interactions
Metabolism/Transport Effects Substrate of CYP1A2 (minor), CYP2C19 (minor), CYP3A4 (major); **Note:** Assignment of Major/Minor substrate status based on clinically relevant drug interaction potential; **Inhibits** CYP2C19 (weak), CYP2C9 (weak), CYP3A4 (moderate); **Induces** CYP2C9 (strong), CYP3A4 (weak/moderate)

Avoid Concomitant Use
Avoid concomitant use of Aprepitant with any of the following: Axitinib; Bosutinib; Cisapride; Conivaptan; Ivabradine; Lomitapide; Pimozide; Tolvaptan

Increased Effect/Toxicity
Aprepitant may increase the levels/effects of: ARIPiprazole; Avanafil; Benzodiazepines (metabolized by oxidation); Bosutinib; Budesonide (Systemic, Oral Inhalation); Cisapride; Colchicine; Corticosteroids (Systemic); CYP3A4 Substrates; Diltiazem; Eplerenone; Everolimus; FentaNYL; Halofantrine; Ivabradine; Ivacaftor; Lomitapide; Lurasidone; Pimecrolimus; Pimozide; Propafenone; Ranolazine; Salmeterol; Saxagliptin; Tolvaptan; Vilazodone; Zuclopenthixol

The levels/effects of Aprepitant may be increased by: Antifungal Agents (Azole Derivatives, Systemic); Conivaptan; CYP3A4 Inhibitors (Moderate); CYP3A4 Inhibitors (Strong); Dasatinib; Diltiazem; Ivacaftor; Mifepristone

Decreased Effect
Aprepitant may decrease the levels/effects of: ARIPiprazole; Axitinib; Contraceptives (Estrogens); Contraceptives (Progestins); CYP2C9 Substrates; Diclofenac (Systemic); Ifosfamide; PARoxetine; Saxagliptin; TOLBUTamide; Warfarin

The levels/effects of Aprepitant may be decreased by: CYP3A4 Inducers (Strong); Deferasirox; Herbs (CYP3A4 Inducers); PARoxetine; Rifamycin Derivatives; Tocilizumab

Ethanol/Nutrition/Herb Interactions
Food: Aprepitant serum concentration may be increased when taken with grapefruit juice; avoid concurrent use.
Herb/Nutraceutical: Avoid St John's wort (may decrease aprepitant levels).

Dietary Considerations May be taken with or without food.
Pharmacodynamics/Kinetics
Half-life Elimination Terminal: ~9-13 hours
Time to Peak Plasma: ~3-4 hours
Pregnancy Risk Factor B
Pregnancy Considerations Teratogenic effects were not observed in animal reproduction studies. Use during pregnancy only if clearly needed. Efficacy of hormonal contraceptive may be reduced; alternative or additional methods of contraception should be used both during treatment with fosaprepitant or aprepitant and for at least 1 month following the last fosaprepitant/aprepitant dose.

Lactation Excretion in breast milk unknown/not recommended

Breast-Feeding Considerations Due to the potential for adverse reactions in the nursing infant, the decision to discontinue aprepitant or to discontinue breast-feeding should take into account the benefits of treatment to the mother.

Dosage Forms
Capsule, oral:
Emend®: 40 mg, 80 mg, 125 mg
Combination package, oral:
Emend®: Capsule: 80 mg (2s) and Capsule: 125 mg (1s)

Aprotinin (a proe TYE nin)

Brand Names: Canada Trasylol®
Pharmacologic Category Blood Product Derivative; Hemostatic Agent
Use Prevention of perioperative blood loss in patients who are at increased risk for blood loss and blood transfusions in association with cardiopulmonary bypass in coronary artery bypass graft (CABG) surgery

Note: Aprotinin has been withdrawn from the worldwide market due to evidence demonstrating an increased risk of renal dysfunction, myocardial infarction, and mortality in patients undergoing cardiac surgery (Canada has lifted this suspension); use limited to investigational use in the U.S. only according to a special treatment protocol allowing for treatment in select patients at increased risk of blood loss and transfusion during CABG surgery when alternative therapies are unacceptable.

Local Anesthetic/Vasoconstrictor Precautions No information available to require special precautions
Effects on Dental Treatment No significant effects or complications reported
Effects on Bleeding This agent is not likely to be used in a setting where dental procedures are contemplated.
Adverse Effects
>10%:
Central nervous system: Fever (15%)
Gastrointestinal: Nausea (11%)
1% to 10%:
Cardiovascular: Atrial flutter (6%), ventricular extrasystoles (6%), ventricular tachycardia (1% to 5%), heart failure (1% to 5%), arrhythmia (4%), supraventricular tachycardia (4%), bradycardia (1% to 2%), thrombosis (1% to 2%), bundle branch block (1% to 2%), cardiac arrest (1% to 2%), heart block (1% to 2%), hemorrhage (1% to 2%), myocardial ischemia (1% to 2%), pericardial effusion (1% to 2%), ventricular fibrillation (1% to 2%), shock (<1% to 2%)
Central nervous system: Agitation (1% to 2%), anxiety (1% to 2%), dizziness (1% to 2%), seizure (1% to 2%)

Endocrine & metabolic: Creatine phosphokinase increase (2%), acidosis (1% to 2%), hyperglycemia (1% to 2%), hypervolemia (1% to 2%), hypokalemia

Gastrointestinal: Diarrhea (3%), dyspepsia (1% to 2%), gastrointestinal hemorrhage (1% to 2%)

Hematologic: Disseminated intravascular coagulation (DIC), leukocytosis (1% to 2%), prothrombin decreased (1% to 2%), thrombocytopenia (1% to 2%)

Hepatic: Jaundice (1% to 2%), hepatic failure (1% to 2%)

Neuromuscular & skeletal: Arthralgia (1% to 2%)

Renal: Serum creatinine increase of >0.5 mg/dL above baseline (high dose: 9%), oliguria (1% to 2%), tubular necrosis (1% to 2%), kidney failure (1%)

Respiratory: Hypoxia (2%), pulmonary hypertension (1% to 2%), pneumonia (1% to 2%), apnea (1% to 2%), cough increased (1% to 2%)

Miscellaneous: Sepsis (1% to 2%), multisystem organ failure (1% to 2%)

General Dosage Range I.V.: *Adults:* Test dose: 1 mL (1.4 mg) 10 minutes prior to loading dose; Loading dose: 1-2 million KIU (140-280 mg; 100-200 mL); Pump prime volume: 1-2 million KIU (140-280 mg, 100-200 mL); Infusion: 250,000-500,000 KIU/hour (35-70 mg/hour; 25-50 mL/hour)

Mechanism of Action Bleeding from CABG surgery is thought to result from a systemic inflammatory response induced by the procedure. Contact of blood cells with the cardiopulmonary bypass (CPB) equipment leads to deregulated activation of the coagulation and fibrinolysis systems, with concurrent upregulation of proinflammatory cytokines. Aprotinin is a broad spectrum serine protease inhibitor that attenuates the coagulation, fibrinolytic and inflammatory pathways by interfering with the chemical mediators (thrombin, plasmin, kallikrein). Additionally, it protects platelet-expressed glycoproteins from mechanical shear forces. This preserves normal hemostatic activity through protease receptor-independent mechanisms (eg, via ADP, IIb/IIIa), while blocking CPB-induced thrombin-mediated aggregation.

Pharmacodynamics/Kinetics

Half-life Elimination 2.5 hours (plasma); terminal: 10 hours

Pregnancy Risk Factor B

Pregnancy Considerations Teratogenic effects were not observed in animal studies. There are no adequate and well-controlled studies in pregnant women.

Prescribing and Access Restrictions Available in U.S. under an investigational new drug (IND) process. The program will provide aprotinin for the treatment of adult patients undergoing coronary artery bypass graft (CABG) surgery requiring cardiopulmonary bypass (CPB) who are at increased risk of bleeding and transfusion during CABG surgery with no acceptable therapeutic alternative. Healthcare providers using aprotinin for this situation must also ensure that the benefits outweigh the risks for their patient. Healthcare providers with patients who may qualify can access information and forms for enrollment at http://www.trasylol.com/main.htm or contact Bayer Medical Communications at (888) 842-2937.

Arformoterol (ar for MOE ter ol)

Related Information

Respiratory Diseases *on page 1514*

Brand Names: U.S. Brovana®

Pharmacologic Category Beta₂-Adrenergic Agonist; Beta₂-Adrenergic Agonist, Long-Acting

Use Long-term maintenance treatment of bronchoconstriction in chronic obstructive pulmonary disease (COPD), including chronic bronchitis and emphysema

Local Anesthetic/Vasoconstrictor Precautions No information available to require special precautions

Effects on Dental Treatment No significant effects or complications reported

Effects on Bleeding No information available to require special precautions

Adverse Effects 2% to 10%:

Cardiovascular: Chest pain (7%), peripheral edema (3%)

Central nervous system: Pain (8%)

Dermatologic: Rash (4%)

Gastrointestinal: Diarrhea (6%)

Neuromuscular & skeletal: Back pain (6%), leg cramps (4%)

Respiratory: Dyspnea (4%), sinusitis (5%), congestive conditions (2%)

Miscellaneous: Flu-like syndrome (3%)

General Dosage Range Nebulization: *Adults:* 5 mcg twice daily (maximum: 30 mcg/day)

Mechanism of Action Arformoterol, the (R,R)-enantiomer of the racemic formoterol, is a long-acting beta₂-agonist that relaxes bronchial smooth muscle by selective action on beta₂-receptors with little effect on cardiovascular system.

Pharmacodynamics/Kinetics

Onset of Action 7-20 minutes; Peak effect: 1-3 hours

Half-life Elimination 26 hours

Time to Peak 0.5-3 hours

Pregnancy Risk Factor C

Pregnancy Considerations Teratogenic effects, decreased fetal weight and increased fetal loss were observed in animal studies. There are no adequate and well-controlled studies in pregnant women. Beta-agonists may interfere with uterine contractility if administered during labor. Use in pregnancy and/or during labor should be limited to situations where benefit outweighs risk to fetus.

Argatroban (ar GA troh ban)

Related Information

Cardiovascular Diseases *on page 1492*

Pharmacologic Category Anticoagulant, Thrombin Inhibitor

Use Prophylaxis or treatment of thrombosis in patients with heparin-induced thrombocytopenia (HIT); adjunct to percutaneous coronary intervention (PCI) in patients who have or are at risk of thrombosis associated with HIT

Unlabeled Use To maintain extracorporeal circuit patency (prefilter administration) of continuous renal replacement therapy (CRRT) in critically-ill patients with HIT

Local Anesthetic/Vasoconstrictor Precautions No information available to require special precautions

Effects on Dental Treatment Key adverse event(s) related to dental treatment: Bleeding is a potential adverse effect of argatroban during dental surgery; it is unlikely that ambulatory patients presenting for dental treatment will be taking intravenous anticoagulant therapy. See Effects on Bleeding.

Effects on Bleeding As with all anticoagulants, bleeding is a potential adverse effect of argatroban during dental surgery; risk is dependent on multiple variables, including the intensity of anticoagulation and patient susceptibility. Medical consult is suggested. It is unlikely that ambulatory patients presenting for dental treatment will be taking intravenous anticoagulant therapy such as argatroban.

Adverse Effects As with all anticoagulants, bleeding is the major adverse effect of argatroban. Hemorrhage may occur at virtually any site. Risk is dependent on multiple variables, including the intensity of anticoagulation and patient susceptibility.

>10%:
Cardiovascular: Chest pain (PCI related: <1% to 15%), hypotension (7% to 11%)
Gastrointestinal: Gastrointestinal bleed (major: <1% to 3%; minor: 3% to 14%)
Genitourinary: Genitourinary bleed and hematuria (major: <1%; minor: 2% to 12%)

1% to 10%:
Cardiovascular: Vasodilation (1% to 10%), cardiac arrest (6%), ventricular tachycardia (5%), bradycardia (5%), myocardial infarction (PCI: 4%), atrial fibrillation (3%), angina (2%), CABG-related bleeding (minor, 2%), myocardial ischemia (2%), cerebrovascular disorder (<1% to 2%), thrombosis (<1% to 2%)
Central nervous system: Fever (<1% to 7%), headache (5%), pain (5%), intracranial bleeding (1% to 4%)
Dermatologic: Skin reactions (bullous eruption, rash; 1% to <10%)
Gastrointestinal: Nausea (5% to 7%), diarrhea (6%), vomiting (4% to 6%), abdominal pain (3% to 4%)
Genitourinary: Urinary tract infection (5%)
Hematologic: Hemoglobin decreased (<2 g/dL), hematocrit decreased (minor: 2% to 10%; major: <1%)
Local: Bleeding at injection or access site (minor: 2% to 5%)
Neuromuscular & skeletal: Back pain (PCI related: 8%)
Renal: Abnormal renal function (3%)
Respiratory: Dyspnea (8% to 10%), cough (3% to 10%), hemoptysis (minor: <1% to 3%), pneumonia (3%)
Miscellaneous: Sepsis (6%), infection (4%)

General Dosage Range Dosage adjustment recommended in patients with hepatic impairment
I.V.:
Children: Initial dose: 0.75 mcg/kg/minute; dosage may be adjusted in increments of 0.1-0.25 mcg/kg/minute
Adults: Bolus dose: 150-350 mcg/kg during procedure; Infusion: Initial: 2 mcg/kg/minute **or** 25 mcg/kg/minute during procedure; Maintenance: 0.5-10 mcg/kg/minute (maximum: 10 mcg/kg/minute) **or** 25-40 mcg/kg/minute during procedure
Adults (critically-ill): Initial: 0.2 mcg/kg/minute; Maintenance: 0.5-1.3 mcg/kg/minute
Mechanism of Action A direct, highly-selective thrombin inhibitor. Reversibly binds to the active thrombin site of free and clot-associated thrombin. Inhibits fibrin formation; activation of coagulation factors V, VIII, and XIII; and activation of protein C; and platelet aggregation.
Pharmacodynamics/Kinetics
Onset of Action Immediate
Half-life Elimination 39-51 minutes; Hepatic impairment: ≤181 minutes
Time to Peak Steady-state: 1-3 hours
Pregnancy Risk Factor B

Pregnancy Considerations Adverse events were not observed in animal studies. Information related to argatroban in pregnancy is limited. Use of parenteral direct thrombin inhibitors in pregnancy should be limited to those women who have severe allergic reactions to heparin, including heparin-induced thrombocytopenia, and who cannot receive danaparoid (Guyatt, 2012).

ARIPiprazole (ay ri PIP ray zole)

Brand Names: U.S. Abilify Discmelt®; Abilify Maintena™; Abilify®
Brand Names: Canada Abilify®
Generic Availability (U.S.) No
Pharmacologic Category Antipsychotic Agent, Atypical
Use
Oral: Acute and maintenance treatment of schizophrenia; acute (manic and mixed episodes) and maintenance treatment of bipolar I disorder as monotherapy or as an adjunct to lithium or valproic acid; adjunctive treatment of major depressive disorder; treatment of irritability associated with autistic disorder
Injection: Agitation associated with schizophrenia or bipolar I disorder (Abilify®); treatment of schizophrenia (Abilify Maintena™)
Unlabeled Use Depression with psychotic features; aggression (children); conduct disorder (children); Tourette syndrome (children); pervasive developmental disorder not otherwise specified (PDD-NOS) (children); Asperger's Disorder (children); psychosis/agitation related to Alzheimer's dementia
Local Anesthetic/Vasoconstrictor Precautions No information available to require special precautions
Effects on Dental Treatment Key adverse event(s) related to dental treatment: Extrapyramidal symptoms (similar to placebo) (see Dental Comment); xerostomia and changes in salivation (normal salivary flow resumes upon discontinuation).
Effects on Bleeding No information available to require special precautions
Adverse Effects Unless otherwise noted, frequency of adverse reactions is shown as reported for adult patients receiving oral administration. Spectrum and incidence of adverse effects similar in children; exceptions noted when incidence much higher in children.
>10%:
Central nervous system: Headache (27%; injection 12%), agitation (19%), insomnia (18%), anxiety (17%), EPS (dose related; 5% to 16%; children 6% to 26%), akathisia (dose related; 8% to 13%; injection 2%), sedation (dose related; 5% to 11%; children 8% to 24%; injection 3% to 9%)
Gastrointestinal: Weight gain (2% to 30%; highest frequency in patients with baseline BMI <23 and prolonged use), nausea (15%; injection 9%), constipation (11%), vomiting (11%; children 9% to 14%; injection 3%), dyspepsia (9%)
1% to 10%:
Cardiovascular: Orthostatic hypotension (1% to 4%; injection 1% to 3%), tachycardia (injection 2%), chest pain, hypertension, peripheral edema
Central nervous system: Dizziness (10%; injection 8%), pyrexia (children 5% to 9%), restlessness (5% to 6%), fatigue (dose related; 6%; children 8% to 17%; injection 2%), lethargy (children 2% to 5%), lightheadedness (4%), pain (3%), dystonia (children 1%), hypersomnia (1%), irritability (children 1%), coordination impaired, suicidal ideation

Dermatologic: Rash (children 2%), hyperhidrosis

Endocrine & metabolic: Dysmenorrhea (children 2%)

Gastrointestinal: Salivation increased (dose related; children 4% to 9%), appetite decreased (children 4% to 7%), appetite increased (children 7%), xerostomia (5%), toothache (4%), abdominal discomfort (3%), diarrhea (children 5%), weight loss

Local: Injection site reaction (injection)

Neuromuscular & skeletal: Tremor (dose related; 5% to 6%; children 6% to 10%), extremity pain (4%), stiffness (4%), myalgia (2%), spasm (2%), arthralgia (children 1%), dyskinesia (children 1%), CPK increased, weakness

Ocular: Blurred vision (3%; children 3% to 8%)

Respiratory: Nasopharyngitis (children 6%), pharyngolaryngeal pain (3%), cough (3%), rhinorrhea (children 2%), aspiration pneumonia, dyspnea, nasal congestion

Miscellaneous: Thirst (children 1%)

Dosage Note: Oral solution may be substituted for the oral tablet on a mg-per-mg basis, up to 25 mg. Patients receiving 30 mg tablets should be given 25 mg oral solution. Orally disintegrating tablets (Abilify Discmelt®) are bioequivalent to the immediate release tablets (Abilify®).

Children ≥6 years: Irritability associated with autistic disorder: Oral: Initial: 2 mg once daily for 7 days, followed by an increase to 5 mg once daily; subsequent dose increases may be made in 5 mg increments at intervals of ≥1 week as needed, up to a maximum of 15 mg/day. Efficacy of continued treatment >8 weeks has not been established; the need for ongoing treatment should be assessed periodically.

Children ≥10 years (U.S. labeling): Bipolar I disorder (acute manic or mixed episodes) Oral:

Stabilization: Initial: 2 mg once daily for 2 days, followed by 5 mg once daily for 2 days with a further increase to target dose of 10 mg once daily as monotherapy or as adjunct to lithium or valproic acid; subsequent dose increases may be made in 5 mg increments, up to a maximum of 30 mg/day

Maintenance: Continue stabilization dose for up to 6 weeks; efficacy of continued treatment >6 weeks has not been established.

Adolescents ≥13 years (Canadian labeling): Bipolar I disorder (acute manic or mixed episodes): Oral: Initial: 2 mg once daily for 2 days, followed by 5 mg once daily for 2 days with a further increase to target dose of 10 mg once daily as monotherapy; subsequent dose increases may be made in 5 mg increments, up to a maximum of 30 mg/day. **Note:** Not approved for maintenance or as adjunctive therapy.

Adolescents ≥13 years (U.S. labeling) or ≥15 years (Canadian labeling): Schizophrenia: Oral: Initial: 2 mg once daily for 2 days, followed by 5 mg once daily for 2 days with a further increase to target dose of 10 mg once daily; subsequent dose increases may be made in 5 mg increments up to a maximum of 30 mg/day (30 mg/day not shown to be more efficacious than 10 mg/day)

Adults:

Acute agitation (schizophrenia/bipolar mania): I.M.: 9.75 mg as a single dose (range: 5.25-15 mg); repeated doses may be given at ≥2-hour intervals to a maximum of 30 mg/day. **Note:** If ongoing therapy with aripiprazole is necessary, transition to oral therapy as soon as possible.

Bipolar I disorder (acute manic or mixed episodes): Oral:

Stabilization:

Monotherapy: Initial: 15 mg once daily. May increase to 30 mg once daily if clinically indicated; safety of doses >30 mg/day has not been evaluated

Adjunct to lithium or valproic acid: Initial: 10-15 mg once daily. May increase to 30 mg once daily if clinically indicated; safety of doses >30 mg/day has not been evaluated.

Maintenance: Continue stabilization dose for up to 6 weeks; efficacy of continued treatment >6 weeks has not been established

Depression (adjunctive with antidepressants): Oral: Initial: 2-5 mg/day (range: 2-15 mg/day); dose adjustments of up to 5 mg/day may be made in intervals of ≥1 week. **Note:** Dosing based on patients already receiving antidepressant therapy.

Schizophrenia:

Oral: 10-15 mg once daily; may be increased to a maximum of 30 mg once daily (efficacy at dosages above 10-15 mg has not been shown to be increased). Dosage titration should not be more frequent than every 2 weeks.

I.M, extended release (Abilify Maintena™): 400 mg once monthly (doses should be separated by ≥26 days); **Note:** Tolerability should be established using oral aripiprazole prior to initiation of parenteral therapy. Continue oral aripiprazole (or other oral antipsychotic) for 14 days during initiation of parenteral therapy.

Missed doses:

Second or third doses missed:

>4 weeks but <5 weeks since last dose: Administer next dose as soon as possible

>5 weeks since last dose: Administer oral aripiprazole for 14 days with next injection

Fourth or subsequent doses missed:

>4 weeks but <6 weeks since last dose: Administer next dose as soon as possible

>6 weeks since last dose: Administer oral aripiprazole for 14 days with next injection

Dosage adjustment for adverse effects: Consider reducing dose to 300 mg once monthly

Elderly: Refer to adult dosing

Dosage adjustment with concurrent CYP450 inducer or inhibitor therapy:

Oral:

CYP3A4 inducers (eg, carbamazepine): Aripiprazole dose should be doubled; dose should be subsequently reduced if concurrent inducer agent discontinued.

Strong CYP3A4 inhibitors (eg, ketoconazole): Aripiprazole dose should be reduced to 50% of the usual dose, and proportionally increased upon discontinuation of the inhibitor agent.

Strong CYP2D6 inhibitors (eg, fluoxetine, paroxetine): Aripiprazole dose should be reduced to 50% of the usual dose, and proportionally increased upon discontinuation of the inhibitor agent. **Note:** Dose reduction does not apply to patients with major depressive disorder; follow usual dosing recommendations.

CYP3A4 and CYP2D6 inhibitors: Aripiprazole dose should be reduced to 25% of the usual dose. In patients receiving inhibitors of differing (eg, moderate 3A4/strong 2D6) or same (eg, moderate 3A4/moderate 2D6) potencies (excluding concurrent strong inhibitors), further dosage adjustments can be made to achieve the desired clinical response. In patients receiving strong CYP3A4 and 2D6 inhibitors, aripiprazole dose is proportionally increased upon discontinuation of one or both inhibitor agents.

I.M., extended release (Abilify Maintena™): **Note:** Dosage adjustments are not recommended for concomitant use of CYP3A4 inhibitors, CYP2D6 inhibitors or CYP3A4 inducers for <14 days. In patients who had their aripiprazole dose adjusted for concomitant therapy, the aripiprazole dose may need to be increased if the CYP3A4 and/or CYP2D6 inhibitor is withdrawn.

CYP3A4 inducers: Avoid use; aripiprazole serum concentrations may fall below effective levels.

Strong CYP3A4 or CYP2D6 inhibitors:
Current aripiprazole dose of 300 mg once monthly: Reduce aripiprazole dose to 200 mg once monthly
Current aripiprazole dose of 400 mg once monthly: Reduce aripiprazole dose to 300 mg once monthly

Strong CYP3A4 inhibitors **and** CYPD2D6 inhibitors:
Current aripiprazole dose of 300 mg once monthly: Reduce aripiprazole dose to 160 mg once monthly
Current aripiprazole dose of 400 mg once monthly: Reduce aripiprazole dose to 200 mg once monthly

Dosage adjustment based on CYP2D6 metabolizer status:
Oral: Aripiprazole dose should be reduced to 50% of the usual dose in CYP2D6 poor metabolizers and to 25% of the usual dose in poor metabolizers receiving a concurrent strong CYP3A4 inhibitor; subsequently adjust dose for favorable clinical response.

I.M., extended release (Abilify Maintena™): Reduce aripiprazole dose to 300 mg once monthly in CYP2D6 poor metabolizers; reduce dose to 200 mg once monthly in CYP2D6 poor metabolizers receiving a concurrent CYP3A4 inhibitor for >14 days.

Dosage adjustment in renal impairment: No dosage adjustment necessary.

Dosage adjustment in hepatic impairment: No dosage adjustment necessary.

Mechanism of Action Aripiprazole is a quinolinone antipsychotic which exhibits high affinity for D_2, D_3, 5-HT$_{1A}$, and 5-HT$_{2A}$ receptors; moderate affinity for D_4, 5-HT$_{2C}$, 5-HT$_7$, alpha$_1$ adrenergic, and H_1 receptors. It also possesses moderate affinity for the serotonin reuptake transporter; has no affinity for muscarinic (cholinergic) receptors. Aripiprazole functions as a partial agonist at the D_2 and 5-HT$_{1A}$ receptors, and as an antagonist at the 5-HT$_{2A}$ receptor.

Contraindications Hypersensitivity to aripiprazole or any component of the formulation

Warnings/Precautions [U.S. Boxed Warning]: Elderly patients with dementia-related psychosis treated with antipsychotics are at an increased risk of death compared to placebo. Most deaths appeared to be either cardiovascular (eg, heart failure, sudden death) or infectious (eg, pneumonia) in nature. In addition, an increased incidence of cerebrovascular effects (eg, transient ischemic attack, cerebrovascular accidents) has been reported in studies of placebo-controlled trials of aripiprazole in elderly patients with dementia-related psychosis. Aripiprazole is not approved for the treatment of dementia-related psychosis.

[U.S. Boxed Warning]: Antidepressants increase the risk of suicidal thinking and behavior in children, adolescents, and young adults (18-24 years of age) with major depressive disorder (MDD) and other psychiatric disorders; consider risk prior to prescribing. The possibility of a suicide attempt is inherent in major depression and may persist until remission occurs. Patients treated with antidepressants should be observed for clinical worsening and suicidality, especially during the initial few months of a course of drug therapy, or at times of dose changes, either increases or decreases. Prescriptions should be written for the smallest quantity consistent with good patient care. The patient's family or caregiver should be alerted to monitor patients for the emergence of suicidality and associated behaviors; patients should be instructed to notify their healthcare provider if any of these symptoms or worsening depression or psychosis occur.

Leukopenia, neutropenia, and agranulocytosis (sometimes fatal) have been reported in clinical trials and postmarketing reports with antipsychotic use; presence of risk factors (eg, pre-existing low WBC or history of drug-induced leuko-/neutropenia) should prompt periodic blood count assessment. Discontinue therapy at first signs of blood dyscrasias or if absolute neutrophil count <1000/mm^3.

A medication guide concerning the use of antidepressants should be dispensed with each prescription. **Aripiprazole is not FDA approved for adjunctive treatment of depression in children.**

May cause extrapyramidal symptoms (EPS), including pseudoparkinsonism, acute dystonic reactions, akathisia, and tardive dyskinesia (risk of these reactions is very low relative to typical/conventional antipsychotics, frequencies reported are similar to placebo). Risk of dystonia (and probably other EPS) may be greater with increased doses, use of conventional antipsychotics, males, and younger patients. May be associated with neuroleptic malignant syndrome (NMS).

May be sedating, use with caution in disorders where CNS depression is a feature. May cause orthostatic hypotension (although reported rates are similar to placebo); use caution in patients at risk of this effect or those who would not tolerate transient hypotensive episodes (cerebrovascular disease, cardiovascular disease, or other medications which may predispose).

Use caution in patients with Parkinson's disease; predisposition to seizures; and severe cardiac disease. May alter cardiac conduction; life-threatening arrhythmias have occurred with therapeutic doses of antipsychotics. Esophageal dysmotility and aspiration have been associated with antipsychotic use; use caution in patients at risk of pneumonia (eg, Alzheimer's disease). May alter temperature regulation.

Atypical antipsychotics have been associated with metabolic changes including loss of glucose control, lipid changes, and weight gain (risk profile varies with product). Development of hyperglycemia in some cases, may be extreme and associated with ketoacidosis, hyperosmolar coma, or death. Reports of hyperglycemia with aripiprazole therapy have been few and specific risk associated with this agent is not known. Use caution in patients with diabetes or other disorders of glucose regulation; monitor for worsening of glucose control.

Use in elderly patients with dementia is associated with an increased risk of mortality and cerebrovascular accidents; avoid antipsychotic use for behavioral problems associated with dementia unless alternative nonpharmacologic therapies have failed and patient may harm self or others. In addition, use may cause or exacerbate syndrome of inappropriate antidiuretic hormone secretion or hyponatremia; monitor sodium closely with initiation or dosage adjustments in older adults (Beers Criteria).

Tablets contain lactose; avoid use in patients with galactose intolerance or glucose-galactose malabsorption.

Abilify Discmelt®: Use caution in phenylketonuria; contains phenylalanine.

There are two formulations available for intramuscular administration: Abilify® is an immediate release short-acting formulation and Abilify Maintena™ is an extended-release formulation. These products are **not** interchangeable.

Drug Interactions

Metabolism/Transport Effects Substrate of CYP2D6 (major), CYP3A4 (major); **Note:** Assignment of Major/Minor substrate status based on clinically relevant drug interaction potential

Avoid Concomitant Use

Avoid concomitant use of ARIPiprazole with any of the following: Azelastine (Nasal); Metoclopramide; Paraldehyde

Increased Effect/Toxicity

ARIPiprazole may increase the levels/effects of: Alcohol (Ethyl); Azelastine (Nasal); Buprenorphine; CNS Depressants; DULoxetine; FLUoxetine; Highest Risk QTc-Prolonging Agents; Methotrimeprazine; Methylphenidate; Moderate Risk QTc-Prolonging Agents; Paraldehyde; PARoxetine; Serotonin Modulators; Zolpidem

The levels/effects of ARIPiprazole may be increased by: Abiraterone Acetate; Acetylcholinesterase Inhibitors (Central); CYP2D6 Inhibitors (Moderate); CYP2D6 Inhibitors (Strong); CYP2D6 Inhibitors (Weak); CYP3A4 Inhibitors (Moderate); CYP3A4 Inhibitors (Strong); CYP3A4 Inhibitors (Weak); Dasatinib; Droperidol; DULoxetine; FLUoxetine; HydrOXYzine; Ivacaftor; Lithium formulations; Magnesium Sulfate; Methotrimeprazine; Methylphenidate; Metoclopramide; Metyrosine; Mifepristone; PARoxetine; Perampanel; Sodium Oxybate; Tetrabenazine

Decreased Effect

ARIPiprazole may decrease the levels/effects of: Amphetamines; Anti-Parkinson's Agents (Dopamine Agonist); Quinagolide

The levels/effects of ARIPiprazole may be decreased by: CYP3A4 Inducers; Deferasirox; Lithium formulations; Peginterferon Alfa-2b; Tocilizumab

Ethanol/Nutrition/Herb Interactions

Ethanol: May increase CNS depression; monitor for increased effects with coadministration. Caution patients about effects.

Food: Ingestion with a high-fat meal delays time to peak plasma level.

Herb/Nutraceutical: St John's wort may decrease aripiprazole levels. Avoid kava kava, gotu kola, valerian, St John's wort (may increase CNS depression).

Dietary Considerations May be taken with or without food. Some products may contain phenylalanine.

Pharmacodynamics/Kinetics

Onset of Action Initial: 1-3 weeks

Half-life Elimination

Aripiprazole: 75 hours; dehydro-aripiprazole: 94 hours; I.M., extended release (terminal): ~30-47 days (dose-dependent)

CYP2D6 poor metabolizers: Aripiprazole: 146 hours

Time to Peak Plasma:

I.M.:

Immediate release: 1-3 hours

Extended release: 5-7 days

Tablet: 3-5 hours

With high-fat meal: Aripiprazole: Delayed by 3 hours; dehydro-aripiprazole: Delayed by 12 hours

Pregnancy Risk Factor C

Pregnancy Considerations Aripiprazole demonstrated developmental toxicity and teratogenic effects in animal models. Antipsychotic use during the third trimester of pregnancy has a risk for abnormal muscle movements (extrapyramidal symptoms [EPS]) and withdrawal symptoms in newborns following delivery. Symptoms in the newborn may include agitation, feeding disorder, hypertonia, hypotonia, respiratory distress, somnolence, and tremor; these effects may be self-limiting or require hospitalization. Information specific to the use of aripiprazole in pregnancy is limited. Treatment algorithms have been developed by the ACOG and the APA for the management of depression in women prior to conception and during pregnancy (Yonkers, 2009). Healthcare providers are encouraged to enroll women 18-45 years of age exposed to aripiprazole during pregnancy in the Atypical Antipsychotics Pregnancy Registry (866-961-2388 or http://www.womensmentalhealth.org/pregnancyregistry).

Lactation Enters breast milk

Breast-Feeding Considerations Aripiprazole is excreted in breast milk. According to the manufacturer, the decision to continue or discontinue breast-feeding during therapy should take into account the risk of exposure to the infant and the benefits of treatment to the mother.

Dosage Forms

Injection, powder for suspension, extended release: Abilify Maintena™: 300 mg, 400 mg

Injection, solution: Abilify®: 7.5 mg/mL (1.3 mL)

Solution, oral: Abilify®: 1 mg/mL (150 mL)

Tablet, oral: Abilify®: 2 mg, 5 mg, 10 mg, 15 mg, 20 mg, 30 mg

Tablet, orally disintegrating, oral: Abilify Discmelt®: 10 mg, 15 mg

Dental Comment Aripiprazole works differently from the classic antipsychotics, such as chlorpromazine, in that it does not appear to block central dopaminergic receptors, but rather seems to be a stabilizer of dopamine-serotonin central systems. The risk of extrapyramidal reactions such as pseudoparkinsonism, acute dystonic reactions, akathisia, and tardive dyskinesia are low and the frequencies reported are similar to placebo. Aripiprazole may be associated with neuroleptic malignant syndrome (NMS).

Armodafinil (ar moe DAF i nil)

Brand Names: U.S. Nuvigil®

Pharmacologic Category Central Nervous System Stimulant

Use Improve wakefulness in patients with excessive daytime sleepiness associated with narcolepsy and shift work sleep disorder (SWSD); adjunctive therapy for obstructive sleep apnea/hypopnea syndrome (OSAHS)

Local Anesthetic/Vasoconstrictor Precautions Use vasoconstrictor with caution. Patients may experience heart palpitations and increased heart rate when taking armodafinil.

Effects on Dental Treatment Key adverse event(s) related to dental treatment: Xerostomia (normal salivary flow resumes upon discontinuation).

Effects on Bleeding No information available to require special precautions

Adverse Effects
>10%: Central nervous system: Headache (14% to 23%; dose-related)
1% to 10%:
Cardiovascular: Palpitation (2%), heart rate increased (1%)
Central nervous system: Dizziness (5%), insomnia (4% to 6%; dose related), anxiety (4%), depression (1% to 3%; dose related), fatigue (2%), agitation (1%), attention disturbance (1%), depressed mood (1%), migraine (1%), nervousness (1%), pain (1%), pyrexia (1%), tremor (1%)
Dermatologic: Rash (1% to 4%; dose related), contact dermatitis (1%), hyperhidrosis (1%)
Gastrointestinal: Nausea (6% to 9%; dose related), xerostomia (2% to 7%; dose related), diarrhea (4%), abdominal pain (2%), dyspepsia (2%), anorexia (1%), appetite decreased (1%), constipation (1%), loose stools (1%), vomiting (1%)
Genitourinary: Polyuria (1%)
Hepatic: GGT increased (1%)
Neuromuscular & skeletal: Paresthesia (1%)
Respiratory: Dyspnea (1%)
Miscellaneous: Flu-like syndrome (1%), seasonal allergy (1%), thirst (1%)
General Dosage Range
Oral: *Adults:* 150-250 mg once daily
Mechanism of Action The exact mechanism of action of armodafinil is unknown. It is the R-enantiomer of modafinil. Armodafinil binds to the dopamine transporter and inhibits dopamine reuptake, which may result in increased extracellular dopamine levels in the brain. However, it does not appear to be a dopamine receptor agonist and also does not appear to bind to or inhibit the most common receptors or enzymes that are relevant for sleep/wake regulation.
Pharmacodynamics/Kinetics
Half-life Elimination 15 hours; Steady state: ~7 days
Time to Peak 2 hours (fasted)
Pregnancy Risk Factor C
Pregnancy Considerations Adverse events have been observed in animal reproduction studies, including visceral and skeletal abnormalities and decreased fetal weight. Efficacy of steroidal contraceptives may be decreased; alternate means of contraception should be considered during therapy and for 1 month after armodafinil is discontinued. A pregnancy registry has been established for patients exposed to armodafinil; healthcare providers are encouraged to register pregnant patients or pregnant women may register themselves by calling 1-866-404-4106.
Controlled Substance C-IV

Artemether and Lumefantrine
(ar TEM e ther & loo me FAN treen)

Related Information
Clinical Risk Related to Drugs Prolonging QT Interval *on page 1510*
Brand Names: U.S. Coartem®
Pharmacologic Category Antimalarial Agent
Use Treatment of acute, uncomplicated malaria infections due to *Plasmodium falciparum*, including geographical regions where chloroquine resistance has been reported

Local Anesthetic/Vasoconstrictor Precautions
Artemether and lumefantrine is one of the drugs confirmed to prolong the QT interval and is accepted as having a risk of causing torsade de pointes. The risk of drug-induced torsade de pointes is extremely low when a single QT interval prolonging drug is prescribed. In terms of epinephrine, it is not known what effect vasoconstrictors in the local anesthetic regimen will have in patients with a known history of congenital prolonged QT interval or in patients taking any medication that prolongs the QT interval. Until more information is obtained, it is suggested that the clinician consult with the physician prior to the use of a vasoconstrictor in suspected patients, and that the vasoconstrictor (epinephrine, mepivacaine and levonordefrin [Carbocaine® 2% with Neo-Cobefrin®]) be used with caution.
Effects on Dental Treatment No significant effects or complications reported
Effects on Bleeding No information available to require special precautions
Adverse Effects
>10%:
Cardiovascular: Palpitation (18%)
Central nervous system: Headache (adults 56%; children 13%), dizziness (adults 39%; children 4%), fever (25% to 29%), chills (adults 23%; children 5%), sleep disturbances (22%), fatigue (adults 17%; children 3%)
Gastrointestinal: Anorexia (adults 40%; children 13%), nausea (adults 26%; children 5%), vomiting (17% to 18%), abdominal pain (adults 17%; children 8%)
Neuromuscular & skeletal: Weakness (adults 38%; children 5%), arthralgia (adults 34%; children 3%), myalgia (adults 32%; children 3%)
Respiratory: Cough (adults 6%; children 23%)
3% to 10%:
Central nervous system: Insomnia (5%), malaise (3%), vertigo (3%)
Dermatologic: Pruritus (4%), rash (3%)
Gastrointestinal: Splenomegaly (9%), diarrhea (7% to 8%)
Hematologic: Anemia (4% to 9%)
Hepatic: Hepatomegaly (6% to 9%), AST increased (4%)
Respiratory: Rhinitis (4%), nasopharyngitis (3%)
General Dosage Range Oral:
Children 2 months to ≤16 years:
5 to <15 kg: Artemether 20 mg/lumefantrine 120 mg twice daily (maximum: 6 tablets per treatment course)
15 to <25 kg: Artemether 40 mg/lumefantrine 240 mg twice daily (maximum: 12 tablets per treatment course)
25 to <35 kg: Artemether 60 mg/lumefantrine 360 mg twice daily (maximum: 18 tablets per treatment course)
≥35 kg: Artemether 80 mg/lumefantrine 480 mg twice daily (maximum: 24 tablets per treatment course)
Children >16 years and Adults:
25 to <35 kg: Artemether 60 mg/lumefantrine 360 mg twice daily (maximum: 18 tablets per treatment course)
≥35 kg: Artemether 80 mg/lumefantrine 480 mg twice daily (maximum: 24 tablets per treatment course)
Mechanism of Action A coformulation of artemether and lumefantrine with activity against *Plasmodium falciparum*. Artemether and major metabolite dihydroartemisinin (DHA) are rapid schizontocides with activity attributed to the endoperoxide moiety common to each substance. Artemether inhibits an essential calcium adenosine triphosphatase. The exact mechanism of

lumefantrine is unknown, but it may inhibit the formation of β-hematin by complexing with hemin. Both artemether and lumefantrine inhibit nucleic acid and protein synthesis. Artemether rapidly reduces parasite biomass and lumefantrine eliminates residual parasites.

Pharmacodynamics/Kinetics

Half-life Elimination Artemether: 1-2 hours; DHA: 2 hours; Lumefantrine: 72-144 hours

Time to Peak Plasma: Artemether: ~2 hours; Lumefantrine: ~6-8 hours

Pregnancy Risk Factor C

Pregnancy Considerations Animal studies have demonstrated increased fetal resorption and postimplantation loss during the period of organogenesis. Safety data from an observational pregnancy study included 500 pregnant women exposed to artemether/lumefantrine and did not show an increased in adverse outcomes or teratogenic effects over background rate. Approximately one-third of these patients were in the third trimester. Efficacy has not been established in pregnant patients. Treatment failures with standard doses have been reported in pregnant women in areas where drug resistant parasites are prevalent. This may be attributed to lower serum concentration of both artemether and lumefantrine in this population (McGready, 2008). Use during pregnancy only if potential benefit justifies potential risk to the fetus.

Dental Comment Artemether and lumefantrine is known to prolong the QT interval. The QT interval is measured as the time and distance between the Q point of the QRS complex and the end of the T wave in the ECG tracing. After adjustment for heart rate, the QT interval is defined as prolonged if it is more than 450 msec in men and 460 msec in women. A long QT syndrome was first described in the 1950s and 60s as a congenital syndrome involving QT interval prolongation and syncope and sudden death. Some of the congenital long QT syndromes were characterized by a peculiar electrocardiographic appearance of the QRS complex involving a premature atria beat followed by a pause, then a subsequent sinus beat showing marked QT prolongation and deformity. This type of cardiac arrhythmia was originally termed "torsade de pointes" (translated from the French as "twisting of the points"). Artemether and lumefantrine is considered as having a risk of causing torsade de pointes. Since it is not known what effect vasoconstrictors in the local anesthetic regimen will have in patients with a known history of congenital prolonged QT interval or in patients taking any medication that prolongs the QT interval, a medical consult is suggested.

Artesunate (ar TES oo nate)

Pharmacologic Category Antimalarial Agent; Artemisinin Derivative

Unlabeled Use Treatment of severe malaria

Local Anesthetic/Vasoconstrictor Precautions No information available to require special precautions

Effects on Dental Treatment Key adverse event(s) related to dental treatment: Metallic taste has been reported

Effects on Bleeding No information available to require special precautions

Adverse Effects Frequency not defined.

Cardiovascular: Hypotension

Central nervous system: Anxiety, dizziness, headache, restlessness, slurred speech

Dermatologic: Angioedema, erythema, pruritus, rash, urticaria

Endocrine & metabolic: Hypoglycemia

Gastrointestinal: Anorexia, diarrhea, metallic taste, nausea, vomiting

Hematologic: Anemia, hemolysis, neutropenia, reticulocytopenia

Hepatic: ALT increased

Neuromuscular & skeletal: Ataxia, hyperreflexia, tremor

Renal: BUN increased

Respiratory: Dyspnea

Miscellaneous: Hypersensitivity reaction

General Dosage Range I.V.: *Children and Adults:* 2.4 mg/kg/dose initially, followed by 2.4 mg/kg/dose at 12 hours, 24 hours, and 48 hours after the initial dose for a total of 4 doses

Mechanism of Action Artesunate, a semisynthetic derivative of artemisinin, is a prodrug which is converted to dihydroartemisinin (DHA). DHA is an antimalarial agent active against all of the erythrocytic stages of the parasite including gametocytes; inhibits parasite metabolism and enhances the clearance of infected erythrocytes.

Antiparasitic activity is hypothesized to involve cleavage of the Fe^{2+} of endoperoxide bridge, thereby producing free radicals and damaging parasite proteins. DHA may also inhibit calcium adenosine triphosphatase (cATP) of the sarcoplasmic endoplasmic reticulum and impair parasite protein folding.

Pharmacodynamics/Kinetics

Half-life Elimination Artesunate: Adults infected with severe malaria: 0.22 hours (range: 0.08-0.61 hours); Dihydroartesiminin (DHA): 0.34 hours (range: 0.14-0.87 hours) (Newton, 2006)

Time to Peak Dihyrdoartemisinin (DHA): Adults infected with severe malaria: Within 15 minutes (Newton, 2006)

Pregnancy Considerations Teratogenic effects have been observed in animal reproduction studies. Limited studies in pregnant women have not revealed an increased risk of congenital abnormalities in newborns (McGready, 1998; McGready, 2008). Malaria infection in pregnant women may be more severe than in nonpregnant women. Because *P. falciparum* malaria can cause maternal death, congenital malaria, and fetal loss, pregnant women traveling to malaria-endemic areas must use personal protection against mosquito bites.

Prescribing and Access Restrictions Investigational agent – not approved for use in the U.S.

Artesunate is available in the U.S. for I.V. use in patients with malaria through an Investigational New Drug (IND) protocol. To obtain artesunate via the IND protocol, clinicians must contact the Centers for Disease Control (CDC) Malaria Hotline at 770-488-7788 (business hours) or 770-488-7100 (nonbusiness hours) and request to speak with a CDC Malaria Branch clinician.

Eligibility criteria under the IND protocol include (Hess, 2010):
- **Patients must have malaria:** Diagnosis by microscopy or strong clinical suspicion of *Plasmodium falciparum* or other *Plasmodium* spp. infection
- **Patients must require parenteral therapy:** Unable to take oral medications, high-density parasitemia (eg, >5%), or diagnosis of severe malaria
- **I.V. artesunate must be the preferred treatment:** I.V. artesunate is at least as readily available as I.V. quinidine or the patient has experienced quinidine failure (eg, parasitemia >10% baseline after 48 hours of quinidine therapy), quinidine intolerance, or contraindications to quinidine

For medical access to I.V. artesunate in Canada, please refer to special access information on the Public Health Agency of Canada website, http://www.phac-aspc.gc.ca/tmp-pmv/quinine/.

Articaine and Epinephrine
(AR ti kane & ep i NEF rin)

Related Information
EPINEPHrine (Systemic, Oral Inhalation) *on page 482*
Oral Pain *on page 1558*
Brand Names: U.S. Articadent™; Orabloc™; Septocaine® with epinephrine 1:100,000; Septocaine® with epinephrine 1:200,000; Zorcaine™
Brand Names: Canada Astracaine® with epinephrine 1:200,000; Astracaine® with epinephrine forte 1:100,000; Posicaine N; Posicaine SP; Septanest® N; Septanest® SP; Ultracaine® DS; Ultracaine® DS Forte; Zorcaine™
Generic Availability (U.S.) No
Pharmacologic Category Local Anesthetic
Dental Use Local, infiltrative, or conductive anesthesia in both simple and complex dental and periodontal procedures
Use Local, infiltrative, or conductive anesthesia during simple and complex dental procedures
Local Anesthetic/Vasoconstrictor Precautions No information available to require special precautions (see Dental Comment)
Effects on Dental Treatment No significant effects or complications reported
Effects on Bleeding Epinephrine decreases bleeding
Adverse Effects Adverse reactions to Septocaine™ are characteristic of those associated with other amide-type local anesthetics; adverse reactions to this group of drugs may also result from excessive plasma levels which may be due to overdosage, unintentional intravascular injection, or slow metabolic degradation.

≥1% (in controlled trial of 882 patients):
Central nervous system: Headache (4%), paresthesia (1%)
Gastrointestinal: Gingivitis (1%)
Miscellaneous: Pain (body as a whole 13%), facial edema (1%)
Additional adverse reactions reported with articaine and epinephrine: Arrhythmia, myocardial depression, asthma, convulsions, allergic reactions, injection site reactions, tissue necrosis
Dental Usual Dosage Adults:
Infiltration: Injection volume of 4% solution: 0.5-2.5 mL; total dose: 20-100 mg
Nerve block: Injection volume of 4% solution: 0.5-3.4 mL; total dose: 20-136 mg

Oral surgery: Injection volume of 4% solution: 1-5.1 mL; total dose: 40-204 mg
Note: These dosages are guides only; other dosages may be used; however, do not exceed maximum recommended dose

Special populations: The clinician is reminded that these doses serve only as a guide to the amount of anesthetic required for most routine procedures. The actual volumes to be used depend upon a number of factors, such as type and extent of surgical procedure, depth of anesthesia, degree of muscular relaxation, and condition of the patient. In all cases, the smallest dose that will produce the desired result should be given. Dosages should be reduced for pediatric patients, elderly patients, and patients with cardiac and/or liver disease.
Dosage Summary of recommended volumes and concentrations for various types of anesthetic procedures; dosages (administered by submucosal injection and/or nerve block) apply to normal healthy adults:

Infiltration: Injection volume of 4% solution: 0.5-2.5 mL; total dose: 20-100 mg
Nerve block: Injection volume of 4% solution: 0.5-3.4 mL; total dose: 20-136 mg
Oral surgery: Injection volume of 4% solution: 1-5.1 mL; total dose: 40-204 mg
Note: These dosages are guides only; other dosages may be used; however, do not exceed maximum recommended dose

Special populations: The clinician is reminded that these doses serve only as a guide to the amount of anesthetic required for most routine procedures. The actual volumes to be used depend upon a number of factors, such as type and extent of surgical procedure, depth of anesthesia, degree of muscular relaxation, and condition of the patient. In all cases, the smallest dose that will produce the desired result should be given. Dosages should be reduced for pediatric patients, elderly patients, and patients with cardiac and/or liver disease.

Children <4 years: Safety and efficacy have not been established
Children 4-16 years (dosages in a clinical trial of 61 patients):
Simple procedures: 0.76-5.65 mg/kg (0.9-5.1 mL) was administered safely to 51 patients
Complex procedures: 0.37-7.48 mg/kg (0.7-3.9 mL) was administered safely to 10 patients
Note: Approximately 13% of the pediatric patients required additional injections for complete anesthesia
Geriatric patients (dosages in a clinical trial):
65-75 years:
Simple procedures: 0.43-4.76 mg/kg (0.9-11.9 mL) was administered safely to 35 patients
Complex procedures: 1.05-4.27 mg/kg (1.3-6.8 mL) was administered safely to 19 patients
≥75 years:
Simple procedures: 0.78-4.76 mg/kg (1.3-11.9 mL) was administered safely to 7 patients
Complex procedures: 1.12-2.17 mg/kg (1.3-5.1 mL) was administered safely to 4 patients
Note: Approximately 6% of the patients 65-75 years of age (none of the patients ≥75 years of age) required additional injections for complete anesthesia, compared to 11% of the patients 17-65 years of age who required additional injections.

Maximum recommended dosages:
Children (use in pediatric patients <4 years is not recommended): Not to exceed 7 mg/kg (0.175 mL/kg) **or** 3.2 mg/lb (0.0795 mL/lb) of body weight

Adults (normal, healthy): Submucosal infiltration and/or nerve block: Not to exceed 7 mg/kg (0.175 mL/kg) **or** 3.2 mg/lb (0.0795 mL/lb) of body weight

The following numbers of dental cartridges (1.7 mL) provide the indicated amounts of articaine hydrochloride 4% and epinephrine 1:100,000:
1 cartridge provides 68 mg articaine HCl (4%) and 0.017 mg vasoconstrictor (epinephrine 1:100,000)
2 cartridges provides 136 mg articaine HCl (4%) and 0.034 mg vasoconstrictor (epinephrine 1:100,000)
3 cartridges provides 204 mg articaine HCl (4%) and 0.051 mg vasoconstrictor (epinephrine 1:100,000)
4 cartridges provides 272 mg articaine HCl (4%) and 0.068 mg vasoconstrictor (epinephrine 1:100,000)
5 cartridges provides 340 mg articaine HCl (4%) and 0.085 mg vasoconstrictor (epinephrine 1:100,000)
6 cartridges provides 408 mg articaine HCl (4%) and 0.102 mg vasoconstrictor (epinephrine 1:100,000)
7 cartridges provides 476 mg articaine HCl (4%) and 0.119 mg vasoconstrictor (epinephrine 1:100,000)
8 cartridges provides 544 mg articaine HCl (4%) and 0.136 mg vasoconstrictor (epinephrine 1:100,000)

The following numbers of dental cartridges (1.7 mL) provide the indicated amounts of articaine hydrochloride 4% and epinephrine 1:200,000:
1 cartridge provides 68 mg articaine HCl (4%) and 0.0085 mg vasoconstrictor (epinephrine 1:200,000)
2 cartridges provides 136 mg articaine HCl (4%) and 0.017 mg vasoconstrictor (epinephrine 1:200,000)
3 cartridges provides 204 mg articaine HCl (4%) and 0.026 mg vasoconstrictor (epinephrine 1:200,000)
4 cartridges provides 272 mg articaine HCl (4%) and 0.034 mg vasoconstrictor (epinephrine 1:200,000)
5 cartridges provides 340 mg articaine HCl (4%) and 0.043 mg vasoconstrictor (epinephrine 1:200,000)
6 cartridges provides 408 mg articaine HCl (4%) and 0.051 mg vasoconstrictor (epinephrine 1:200,000)
7 cartridges provides 476 mg articaine HCl (4%) and 0.060 mg vasoconstrictor (epinephrine 1:200,000)
8 cartridges provides 544 mg articaine HCl (4%) and 0.068 mg vasoconstrictor (epinephrine 1:200,000)

Dosage adjustment in renal impairment: No dosage adjustment provided in manufacturer's labeling (has not been studied).
Dosage adjustment in hepatic impairment: No dosage adjustment provided in manufacturer's labeling (has not been studied). Use with caution in patients with severe liver disease.
Mechanism of Action Local anesthetics block the generation and conduction of nerve impulses, presumably by increasing the threshold for electrical excitation in the nerve, by slowing the propagation of the nerve impulse, and by reducing the rate of rise of the action potential. In general, the progression of anesthesia is related to the diameter, myelination, and conduction velocity of the affected nerve fibers. Clinically, the order of loss of nerve function is as follows: 1) pain, 2) temperature, 3) touch, 4) proprioception, and 5) skeletal muscle tone.
Contraindications Hypersensitivity to local anesthetics of the amide type or any component of the formulation
Warnings/Precautions Intravascular injections should be avoided; aspiration should be performed prior to administration; the needle must be repositioned until no return of blood can be elicited by aspiration; however, absence of blood in the syringe does not guarantee that intravascular injection has been avoided. **Accidental intravascular injection may be associated with convulsions, followed by CNS or cardiorespiratory depression and coma, ultimately progressing to respiratory arrest.** Dental practitioners and/or clinicians using local anesthetic agents should be well trained in diagnosis and management of emergencies that may arise from the use of these agents. Resuscitative equipment, oxygen, and other resuscitative drugs should be available for immediate use.

Contains epinephrine, which can cause local tissue necrosis or systemic toxicity, usual precautions for epinephrine administration should be observed. Administration of articaine HCl with epinephrine results in a three- to fivefold increase in plasma epinephrine concentrations compared to baseline; however, in healthy adults, it does not appear to be associated with marked increases in blood pressure or heart rate, except in the case of accidental intravascular injection.

Products may contain sodium metabisulfite, which may cause allergic-type reactions (including anaphylactic symptoms, and life-threatening or less severe asthmatic episodes) in certain susceptible patients. The overall prevalence of the sulfite sensitivity in the general population is unknown, and is seen more frequently in asthmatic than in nonasthmatic persons.

To avoid serious adverse effects and high plasma levels, the lowest dosage resulting in effective anesthesia should be administered. Repeated doses may cause significant increases in blood levels with each repeated dose due to the possibility of accumulation of the drug or its metabolites. Tolerance to elevated blood levels varies with patient status. Reduced dosages, commensurate with age and physical condition, should be given to debilitated patients, elderly patients, acutely-ill patients, and pediatric patients. Use caution in patients with heart block.

Local anesthetic solutions containing a vasoconstrictor should be used cautiously. Patients with peripheral vascular disease or hypertensive vascular disease may exhibit exaggerated vasoconstrictor response, possibly resulting in ischemic injury or necrosis. It should also be used cautiously in patients during or following the administration of a potent general anesthetic agent, since cardiac arrhythmias may occur under these conditions.

Systemic absorption of local anesthetics may produce CNS and cardiovascular effects. Changes in cardiac conduction, excitability, refractoriness, contractility, and peripheral vascular resistance are minimal at blood concentrations produced by therapeutic doses. However, toxic blood concentrations depress cardiac conduction and excitability, which may lead to AV block, ventricular arrhythmias, and cardiac arrest (sometimes resulting in death). In addition, myocardial contractility is depressed and peripheral vasodilation occurs, leading to decreased cardiac output and arterial blood pressure.

Careful and constant monitoring of cardiovascular and respiratory (adequacy of ventilation) vital signs and the patient's state of consciousness should be done following each local anesthetic injection; at such times, restlessness, anxiety, tinnitus, dizziness, blurred vision, tremors, depression, or drowsiness may be early warning signs of CNS toxicity. Methemoglobinemia has been reported with articaine. Treatment is primarily symptomatic and supportive. Methemoglobinemia may be treated with methylene blue, 1-2 mg/kg I.V. infused over several minutes.

▶

In vitro studies show that ~5% to 10% of articaine is metabolized by the human liver microsomal P450 isoenzyme system; however, no studies have been performed in patient with liver dysfunction, and caution should be used in patients with severe hepatic disease. Use with caution in patients with impaired cardiovascular function, since they may be less able to compensate for function changes associated with prolonged AV conduction produced by these drugs.

Small doses of local anesthetics injected into dental blocks may produce adverse reactions similar to systemic toxicity seen in unintentional intravascular injections at larger doses. Confusion, convulsions, respiratory depression and/or respiratory arrest, and cardiovascular stimulation or depression have been reported. These reactions may be due to intra-arterial injection of the local anesthetic with retrograde flow to the cerebral circulation. Patients receiving such blocks should be observed constantly with resuscitative equipment and personnel trained in treatment of adverse reactions immediately available. Dosage recommendations should not be exceeded. Safety and efficacy have not been established in children <4 years of age.

Drug Interactions
Metabolism/Transport Effects Refer to individual components.

Avoid Concomitant Use
Avoid concomitant use of Articaine and Epinephrine with any of the following: Ergot Derivatives; Iobenguane I 123; Lurasidone

Increased Effect/Toxicity
Articaine and Epinephrine may increase the levels/ effects of: Bromocriptine; Lurasidone; Sympathomimetics

The levels/effects of Articaine and Epinephrine may be increased by: Antacids; AtoMOXetine; Beta-Blockers; Cannabinoids; Carbonic Anhydrase Inhibitors; COMT Inhibitors; Ergot Derivatives; Hyaluronidase; Inhalational Anesthetics; MAO Inhibitors; Serotonin/Norepinephrine Reuptake Inhibitors; Tricyclic Antidepressants

Decreased Effect
Articaine and Epinephrine may decrease the levels/ effects of: Benzylpenicilloyl Polylysine; Iobenguane I 123

The levels/effects of Articaine and Epinephrine may be decreased by: Alpha1-Blockers; Promethazine; Spironolactone

Pharmacodynamics/Kinetics
Onset of Action 1-6 minutes
Duration of Action Complete anesthesia: ~1 hour
Half-life Elimination Articaine: 1.8 hours; Articainic acid: 1.5 hours
Pregnancy Risk Factor C
Pregnancy Considerations Teratogenic effects were not observed in animal studies. There are no adequate and well-controlled studies in pregnant women.
Lactation Excretion in breast milk unknown/use caution
Breast-Feeding Considerations It is not known whether articaine is excreted in human milk.

Dosage Forms
Injection, solution [for dental use]:
Articadent™: Articaine hydrochloride 4% [40 mg/mL] and epinephrine 1:100,000 (1.7 mL)
Articadent™: Articaine hydrochloride 4% [40 mg/mL] and epinephrine 1:200,000 (1.7 mL)
Orabloc™: Articaine hydrochloride 4% [40 mg/mL] and epinephrine 1:100,000 (1.8 mL)

Orabloc™: Articaine hydrochloride 4% [40 mg/mL] and epinephrine 1:200,000 (1.8 mL)
Septocaine® with epinephrine 1:100,000: Articaine 4% [40 mg/mL] and epinephrine 1:100,000 (1.7 mL)
Septocaine® with epinephrine 1:200,000: Articaine 4% [40 mg/mL] and epinephrine 1:200,000 (1.7 mL)
Zorcaine™: Articaine 4% [40 mg/mL] and epinephrine 1:100,000 (1.7 mL)

Dosage Forms: Canada
Injection, solution [for dental use]:
Astracaine® with epinephrine 1:200,000: Articaine 4% and epinephrine 1:200,000 (1.8 mL)
Astracaine® Forte with epinephrine forte 1:100,000: Articaine 4% and epinephrine 1:100,000 (1.8 mL)
Septanest® N: Articaine 4% and epinephrine 1:200,000 (1.7 mL)
Septanest® SP: Articaine 4% and epinephrine 1:100,000 (1.7 mL)
Ultracaine® DS: Articaine 4% and epinephrine 1:200,000 (1.7 mL)
Ultracaine® DS Forte: Articaine 4% and epinephrine 1:100,000 (1.7 mL)

Dental Comment Septocaine™ (articaine hydrochloride 4% and epinephrine 1:100,000) is the first FDA approval in 30 years of a new local dental anesthetic providing complete pulpal anesthesia for approximately 1 hour. Chemically, articaine contains both an amide linkage and an ester linkage, making it chemically unique in the class of local anesthetics. Since it contains the ester linkage, articaine HCl is rapidly metabolized by plasma carboxyesterase to its primary metabolite, articainic acid, which is an inactive product of this metabolism. According to the manufacturer, *in vitro* studies show that the human liver microsomal P450 isoenzyme system metabolizes approximately 5% to 10% of available articaine with nearly quantitative conversion to articainic acid. The elimination half-life of articaine is about 1.8 hours, and that of articainic acid is about 1.5 hours. Articaine is excreted primarily through urine with 53% to 57% of the administered dose eliminated in the first 24 hours following submucosal administration. Articainic acid is the primary metabolite in urine. A minor metabolite, articainic acid glucuronide, is also excreted in the urine. Articaine constitutes only 2% of the total dose excreted in urine.

The anesthetic efficacy of the articaine 4% with 1:200,000 epinephrine (A/200) was compared to that of articaine 4% with 1:100,000 (A/100) using electric pulp tester to assess anesthesia using 63 subjects after either maxillary infiltration (Moore, 2006) or inferior alveolar block (Hersh, 2006).

After maxillary infiltration of 1 mL of each formula, the onset times to anesthesia were 3.1 ± 2.3 minutes for articaine 4% and 1:200,000 epinephrine (A/200), 3 ± 2.1 minutes for articaine 4% and 1:100,000 epinephrine (A/100), 3 ± 2 minutes for articaine 4% with no epinephrine (A/no). These three mean times of onset were not statistically different. Durations of anesthesia were 41.6 ± 21.1 minutes A/200, 45 ± 23.6 minutes A/100, 13.3 ± 6.8 minutes for A/no. There was no statistically significant difference between the durations elicited by the A/200 and A/100 formulations (Moore, 2006). In the second trial of the study, also using 63 subjects, the investigators administered an inferior alveolar nerve block injection of one cartridge (1.7 mL) using a standard intra-oral injection technique for inferior alveolar block anesthesia. Pulpal anesthesia was measured again using the pulp tester.

The onset times to anesthesia were 4.7 ± 2.6 minutes A/ 200, 4.2 ± 2.8 minutes A/100, and 4.3 ± 2.5 minutes for A/no. There were no statistically significant differences in these times to onset. Durations of anesthesia were 51.2 ± 55.9 minutes A/200, 61.8 ± 59 minutes A/100, and 49.7 ± 44.6 minutes for A/no. There were no statistically significant differences in the duration between A/ 200, A/100, and A/no formulations (Hersh, 2006).

Oral paresthesia: The occurrence of oral paresthesia associated with 4% solutions of prilocaine or articaine, although rare, continue to be slightly more frequent than other local anesthetics. From 1999-2008, there were 182 cases of nonsurgical paresthesia (Gaffen, 2009). Of the cases, 172 involved mandibular block injection only. Another eight cases involved mandibular block combined with at least one other type of anesthetic injection. A single case involved infiltration around tooth number 35 and the final case involved infiltration and intraligamentary injection in the maxillary anterior region.

A 2010 report, reviewed adverse events submitted voluntarily over a 10-year period involving the dental local anesthetics articaine, bupivacaine, lidocaine, mepivacaine, and prilocaine in the United States. Articaine reported incidence: One case per 4,159,848 cartridges sold. The reported incidence of paresthesia was one case for 13,800,970 cartridges of all local anesthetics sold in the U.S. (Garisto, 2010).

References

Gaffen AS and Haas DA, "Retrospective Review of Voluntary Reports of Nonsurgical Paresthesia in Dentistry," *J Can Dent Assoc*, 2009, 75(8):579.

Garisto GA, Gaffen AS, Lawrence HP, et al, "Occurrence of Paresthesia After Dental Local Anesthetic Administration in the United States," *J Am Dent Assoc*, 2010, 141(7):836-44.

Hersh EV, Giannakopoulos H, Levin LM, et al, "The Pharmacokinetics and Cardiovascular Effects of High-Dose Articaine With 1:100,000 and 1:200,000 Epinephrine," *J Am Dent Assoc*, 2006, 137 (11):1562-71.

Malamed SF, Gagnon S, Leblanc D, "A Comparison Between Articaine HCl and Lidocaine HCl in Pediatric Dental Patients," *Pediatr Dent*, 2000, 22(4):307-11.

Malamed SF, Gagnon S, Leblanc D, "Articaine Hydrochloride: A Study of the Safety of a New Amide Local Anesthetic," *J Am Dent Assoc*, 2001, 132(2):177-85.

Moore PA, Boynes SG, Hersh EV, et al, "The Anesthetic Efficacy of 4 Percent Articaine 1:200,000 Epinephrine: Two Controlled Clinical Trials," *J Am Dent Assoc*, 2006, 137(11):1572-81.

Wynn RL, Bergman SA, and Meiller TF, "Paresthesia Associated With Local Anesthetics: A Perspective on Articaine," *Gen Dent*, 2003, 51 (6):498-501.

Artificial Tears (ar ti FISH il tears)

Brand Names: U.S. Advanced Eye Relief™ Dry Eye Environmental [OTC]; Advanced Eye Relief™ Dry Eye Rejuvenation [OTC]; Bion® Tears [OTC]; HypoTears [OTC]; Murine Tears® [OTC]; Soothe® Hydration [OTC]; Soothe® [OTC]; Systane® Ultra [OTC]; Systane® [OTC]; Tears Again® [OTC]; Tears Naturale® Forte [OTC]; Tears Naturale® Free [OTC]; Tears Naturale® II [OTC]; Viva-Drops® [OTC]

Brand Names: Canada Teardrops®

Pharmacologic Category Ophthalmic Agent, Miscellaneous

Use Ophthalmic lubricant; for temporary relief of burning and eye irritation due to dry eyes

Local Anesthetic/Vasoconstrictor Precautions No information available to require special precautions

Effects on Dental Treatment No significant effects or complications reported

Effects on Bleeding No information available to require special precautions

Adverse Effects Frequency not defined: Ocular: blurred vision, crusting of eyelids, mild stinging

General Dosage Range Ophthalmic: *Children and Adults:* 1-2 drops into eye(s) as needed

Mechanism of Action Products contain demulcents (ie, cellulose derivatives, dextran 70, gelatin, polyols, polyvinal alcohol, or povidone); usually a water-soluble polymer, applied topically to the eye to protect and lubricate mucous membrane surfaces and relieve dryness and irritation

Ascorbic Acid (a SKOR bik AS id)

Related Information

Viral Infections *on page 1575*

Brand Names: U.S. Acerola [OTC]; Asco-Caps-1000 [OTC]; Asco-Caps-500 [OTC]; Asco-Tabs-1000 [OTC]; Ascocid® [OTC]; Ascocid®-500 [OTC]; C-Gel [OTC]; C-Gram [OTC]; C-Time [OTC]; Cemill 1000 [OTC]; Cemill 500 [OTC]; Chew-C [OTC]; Dull-C® [OTC]; Mild-C® [OTC]; One Gram C [OTC]; Time-C® [OTC]; Vicks® Vitamin C [OTC]; Vita-C® [OTC]

Brand Names: Canada Proflavanol C™; Revitalose C-1000®

Pharmacologic Category Vitamin, Water Soluble

Use Prevention and treatment of scurvy; acidify the urine

Unlabeled Use In large doses, to decrease the severity of "colds"; dietary supplementation; a 20-year study was recently completed involving 730 individuals which indicates a possible decreased risk of death by stroke when ascorbic acid at doses ≥45 mg/day was administered

Local Anesthetic/Vasoconstrictor Precautions No information available to require special precautions

Effects on Dental Treatment No significant effects or complications reported

Effects on Bleeding No information available to require special precautions

Adverse Effects 1% to 10%: Renal: Hyperoxaluria with large doses

General Dosage Range

I.M., SubQ:
Children: 100-300 mg/day in divided doses
Adults: 100-250 mg 1-2 times/day

I.V., Oral:
Children: 100-300 mg/day in divided doses (maximum: 500 mg every 6-8 hours)
Adults: 100-250 mg 1-2 times/day (maximum: 4-12 g/ day in 3-4 divided doses)

Mechanism of Action Not fully understood; necessary for collagen formation and tissue repair; involved in some oxidation-reduction reactions as well as other metabolic pathways, such as synthesis of carnitine, steroids, and catecholamines and conversion of folic acid to folinic acid

Pregnancy Risk Factor A/C (dose exceeding RDA recommendation)

Pregnancy Considerations Animal reproduction studies have not been conducted.

Asenapine (a SEN a peen)

Related Information

Clinical Risk Related to Drugs Prolonging QT Interval *on page 1510*

Brand Names: U.S. Saphris®

Brand Names: Canada Saphris®

Pharmacologic Category Antimanic Agent; Antipsychotic Agent, Atypical

Use Acute and maintenance treatment of schizophrenia; treatment of acute mania or mixed episodes associated with bipolar I disorder (as monotherapy or in combination with lithium or valproate)

Local Anesthetic/Vasoconstrictor Precautions Asenapine is one of the drugs confirmed to prolong the QT interval and is accepted as having a risk of causing torsade de pointes. The risk of drug-induced torsade de pointes is extremely low when a single QT interval prolonging drug is prescribed. In terms of epinephrine, it is not known what effect vasoconstrictors in the local anesthetic regimen will have in patients with a known history of congenital prolonged QT interval or in patients taking any medication that prolongs the QT interval. Until more information is obtained, it is suggested that the clinician consult with the physician prior to the use of a vasoconstrictor in suspected patients, and that the vasoconstrictor (epinephrine, mepivacaine and levonordefrin [Carbocaine® 2% with Neo-Cobefrin®]) be used with caution.

Effects on Dental Treatment Key adverse event(s) related to dental treatment: Xerostomia and increase in salivation (normal salivary flow resumes upon discontinuation). Abnormal taste, toothache, and edema of the tongue have been reported. Many patients may experience orthostatic hypotension with asenapine; precautions should be taken. Asenapine may cause extrapyramidal symptoms including tardive dyskinesia; risk may be greater with increased doses.

Effects on Bleeding No information available to require special precautions

Adverse Effects Actual frequency may be dependent upon dose and/or indication.

>10%:

Central nervous system: Somnolence (13% to 24%), insomnia (6% to 16%), extrapyramidal symptoms (6% to 12%), headache (12%), akathisia (4% to 11%; dose related), dizziness (3% to 11%)

Endocrine & metabolic: Hypertriglyceridemia (13% to 15%)

Gastrointestinal: Weight gain (2% to 15%)

Neuromuscular and skeletal: Creatine kinase increased (6% to 11%)

1% to 10%:

Cardiovascular: Peripheral edema (3%), hypertension (2% to 3%)

Central nervous system: Hypoesthesia (4% to 7%), fatigue (3% to 4%), anxiety (4%), depression (2%), irritability (1% to 2%)

Endocrine & metabolic: Cholesterol increased (8% to 9%), glucose increased (5% to 7%), hyperprolactinemia (2% to 3%)

Gastrointestinal: Constipation (4% to 7%), vomiting (4% to 7%), dyspepsia (3% to 4%), appetite increased (≤4%), salivation increased (≤4%), abnormal taste (3%), toothache (3%), abdominal discomfort (≤3%), xerostomia (1% to 3%)

Hepatic: Transaminases increased (<1% to 3%)

Neuromuscular & skeletal: Arthralgia (3%), extremity pain (2%)

Dosage Sublingual: Adults: **Note:** Safety of doses >20 mg/day has not been evaluated:

Schizophrenia:

Acute treatment: Initial: 5 mg twice daily. Daily doses >20 mg/day in clinical trials did not appear to offer any additional benefits and increased risk of adverse effects.

Maintenance treatment: Initial: 5 mg twice daily; may increase to 10 mg twice daily after 1 week based on tolerability

Bipolar disorder:

Monotherapy: Initial: 10 mg twice daily; decrease to 5 mg twice daily if dose not tolerated

Combination therapy (with lithium or valproate): 5 mg twice daily; may increase to 10 mg twice daily based on tolerability

Dosing adjustment in renal impairment: No dosage adjustment is necessary

Dosing adjustment in hepatic impairment:

Mild-to-moderate hepatic impairment (Child-Pugh class A or B): No dosage adjustment is necessary

Severe hepatic impairment (Child-Pugh class C): Use is not recommended

Mechanism of Action Asenapine is a dibenzo-oxepino pyrrole atypical antipsychotic with mixed serotonin-dopamine antagonist activity. It exhibits high affinity for 5-HT$_{1A}$, 5-HT$_{1B}$, 5-HT$_{2A}$, 5-HT$_{2B}$, 5-HT$_{2C}$, 5-HT$_{5-7}$, D$_{1-4}$, H$_1$ and, alpha$_1$- and alpha$_2$-adrenergic receptors; moderate affinity for H$_2$ receptors. Asenapine has no significant affinity for muscarinic receptors. The binding affinity to the D$_2$ receptor is 19 times lower than the 5-HT$_{2A}$ affinity (Weber, 2009). The addition of serotonin antagonism to dopamine antagonism (classic neuroleptic mechanism) is thought to improve negative symptoms of psychoses and reduce the incidence of extrapyramidal side effects as compared to typical antipsychotics.

Contraindications Hypersensitivity to asenapine or any component of the formulation

Warnings/Precautions [U.S. Boxed Warning]: Elderly patients with dementia-related psychosis treated with atypical antipsychotics are at an increased risk of death compared to placebo. Most deaths appeared to be either cardiovascular (eg, heart failure, sudden death) or infectious (eg, pneumonia) in nature. In addition, an increased incidence of cerebrovascular effects (eg, transient ischemic attack, cerebrovascular accidents) has been reported in studies of placebo-controlled trials of antipsychotics in elderly patients with dementia-related psychosis. Asenapine is not approved for the treatment of dementia-related psychosis.

Use in elderly patients with dementia is associated with an increased risk of mortality and cerebrovascular accidents; avoid antipsychotic use for behavioral problems associated with dementia unless alternative nonpharmacologic therapies have failed and patient may harm self or others. In addition, use may cause or exacerbate syndrome of inappropriate antidiuretic hormone secretion or hyponatremia; monitor sodium closely with initiation or dosage adjustments in older adults (Beers Criteria). Pharmacokinetic studies showed a decrease in clearance in older adults (65-85 years of age) with psychosis compared to younger adults; increased risk of adverse effects and orthostasis may occur.

Leukopenia, neutropenia, and agranulocytosis (sometimes fatal) have been reported in clinical trials and postmarketing reports with antipsychotic use; presence of risk factors (eg, pre-existing low WBC or history of drug-induced leuko/neutropenia) should prompt periodic blood count assessment. Discontinue therapy at first signs of blood dyscrasias or if absolute neutrophil count <1000/mm^3.

May be sedating; use with caution in disorders where CNS depression is a feature. Use with caution in Parkinson's disease. Use with caution in patients at risk of seizures, including those with a history of seizures, head trauma, brain damage, alcoholism, or concurrent therapy with medications which may lower seizure threshold. Use is not recommended in severe hepatic impairment; increased drug concentrations may occur. Esophageal dysmotility and aspiration have been associated with antipsychotic use; use with caution in patients at risk of aspiration pneumonia (ie, Alzheimer's disease). Elevates prolactin levels; use with caution in breast cancer or other prolactin-dependent tumors. May alter temperature regulation.

Use with caution in patients with cardiovascular diseases (eg, heart failure, history of myocardial infarction or ischemia, cerebrovascular disease, conduction abnormalities). May cause orthostatic hypotension; use with caution in patients at risk of this effect (eg, concurrent medication use which may predispose to hypotension/bradycardia or presence of hypovolemia) or in those who would not tolerate transient hypotensive episodes. May result in QT$_c$ prolongation. Risk may be increased by conditions or concomitant medications which cause bradycardia, hypokalemia, and/or hypomagnesemia. Avoid use in combination with QT$_c$-prolonging drugs and in patients with congenital long QT syndrome or patients with history of cardiac arrhythmia.

May cause extrapyramidal symptoms (EPS), including pseudoparkinsonism, acute dystonic reactions, akathisia, and tardive dyskinesia. Risk of dystonia (and probably other EPS) may be greater with increased doses, use of conventional antipsychotics, males, and younger patients. Risk of neuroleptic malignant syndrome (NMS) may be increased in patients with Parkinson's disease or Lewy body dementia. May cause hyperglycemia; in some cases may be extreme and associated with ketoacidosis, hyperosmolar coma, or death. Use with caution in patients with diabetes or other disorders of glucose regulation; monitor for worsening of glucose control. Dyslipidemia has been reported with atypical antipsychotics; risk profile may differ between agents. In clinical trials, the incidence of hypertriglyceridemia observed with asenapine was greater than that observed with placebo, while total cholesterol elevations were similar. Significant weight gain has been observed with antipsychotic therapy; incidence varies with product. Monitor waist circumference and BMI. May cause anaphylaxis or hypersensitivity reactions.

The possibility of a suicide attempt is inherent in psychotic illness or bipolar disorder; use caution in high-risk patients during initiation of therapy. Prescriptions should be written for the smallest quantity consistent with good patient care.

Drug Interactions
Metabolism/Transport Effects Substrate of CYP1A2 (major), CYP2D6 (minor), CYP3A4 (minor); **Note:** Assignment of Major/Minor substrate status based on clinically relevant drug interaction potential; **Inhibits** CYP2D6 (weak)

Avoid Concomitant Use
Avoid concomitant use of Asenapine with any of the following: Azelastine (Nasal); Highest Risk QTc-Prolonging Agents; Ivabradine; Metoclopramide; Mifepristone; Moderate Risk QTc-Prolonging Agents; Paraldehyde

Increased Effect/Toxicity
Asenapine may increase the levels/effects of: Alcohol (Ethyl); ARIPiprazole; Azelastine (Nasal); Buprenorphine; CNS Depressants; Highest Risk QTc-Prolonging Agents; Methotrimeprazine; Methylphenidate; Paraldehyde; PARoxetine; Serotonin Modulators; Zolpidem

The levels/effects of Asenapine may be increased by: Abiraterone Acetate; Acetylcholinesterase Inhibitors (Central); CYP1A2 Inhibitors (Moderate); CYP1A2 Inhibitors (Strong); Deferasirox; FluvoxaMINE; HydrOXYzine; Ivabradine; Lithium formulations; Magnesium Sulfate; MAO Inhibitors; Methotrimeprazine; Methylphenidate; Metoclopramide; Metyrosine; Mifepristone; Moderate Risk QTc-Prolonging Agents; Perampanel; QTc-Prolonging Agents (Indeterminate Risk and Risk Modifying); Sodium Oxybate; Tetrabenazine

Decreased Effect
Asenapine may decrease the levels/effects of: Amphetamines; Anti-Parkinson's Agents (Dopamine Agonist); Quinagolide

The levels/effects of Asenapine may be decreased by: CYP1A2 Inducers (Strong); Cyproterone; Lithium formulations; Peginterferon Alfa-2b

Ethanol/Nutrition/Herb Interactions Ethanol: May increase CNS depression; monitor for increased effects with coadministration. Caution patients about effects.

Dietary Considerations Avoid eating or drinking for at least 10 minutes after administration.

Pharmacodynamics/Kinetics
Half-life Elimination Terminal: ~24 hours
Time to Peak 0.5-1.5 hours

Pregnancy Risk Factor C
Pregnancy Considerations Animal studies indicate an increased risk of fetal mortality. Antipsychotic use during the third trimester of pregnancy has a risk for abnormal muscle movements (extrapyramidal symptoms [EPS]) and withdrawal symptoms in newborns following delivery. Symptoms in the newborn may include agitation, feeding disorder, hypertonia, hypotonia, respiratory distress, somnolence, and tremor; these effects may be self-limiting or require hospitalization. There are no adequate and well-controlled studies in pregnant women. Use during pregnancy only if the benefits justify the risk to the fetus. Healthcare providers are encouraged to enroll women 18-45 years of age exposed to asenapine during pregnancy in the Atypical Antipsychotics Pregnancy Registry (866-961-2388 or http://www.womensmentalhealth.org/pregnancyregistry).

Lactation Excretion in breast milk unknown/not recommended

Dosage Forms
Tablet, sublingual:
Saphris®: 5 mg, 10 mg

Dental Comment Asenapine is known to prolong the QT interval. The QT interval is measured as the time and distance between the Q point of the QRS complex and the end of the T wave in the ECG tracing. After adjustment for heart rate, the QT interval is defined as prolonged if it is more than 450 msec in men and 460 msec in women. A long QT syndrome was first described in the 1950s and 60s as a congenital syndrome involving QT interval prolongation and syncope and sudden death. Some of the congenital long QT syndromes were characterized by a peculiar electrocardiographic appearance of the QRS complex involving a premature atria beat followed by a pause, then a

◀ subsequent sinus beat showing marked QT prolongation and deformity. This type of cardiac arrhythmia was originally termed "torsade de pointes" (translated from the French as "twisting of the points"). Asenapine is considered as having a risk of causing torsade de pointes. Since it is not known what effect vasoconstrictors in the local anesthetic regimen will have in patients with a known history of congenital prolonged QT interval or in patients taking any medication that prolongs the QT interval, a medical consult is suggested.

Asparaginase (*E. coli*) (a SPEAR a ji nase e ko lye)

Brand Names: U.S. Elspar®
Brand Names: Canada Kidrolase®
Pharmacologic Category Antineoplastic Agent, Miscellaneous; Enzyme
Use Treatment (in combination with other chemotherapy) of acute lymphoblastic leukemia (ALL)
Unlabeled Use Treatment of lymphoblastic lymphoma
Local Anesthetic/Vasoconstrictor Precautions No information available to require special precautions
Effects on Dental Treatment Key adverse event(s) related to dental treatment: Stomatitis
Effects on Bleeding Thrombotic and hemorrhagic events have been reported with asparaginase (*E. coli*). A medical consult is recommended.
Adverse Effects Note: Immediate effects: Fever, chills, nausea, and vomiting occur in 50% to 60% of patients.

>10%:
  Central nervous system: Fatigue, fever, chills, depression, agitation, seizure (10% to 60%), somnolence, stupor, confusion, coma (25%)
  Endocrine & metabolic: Hyperglycemia/glucose intolerance (10%)
  Gastrointestinal: Nausea, vomiting (50% to 60%), anorexia, abdominal cramps (70%), acute pancreatitis (15%, may be severe in some patients)
  Hematologic: Hypofibrinogenemia and depression of clotting factors V and VIII, variable decrease in factors VII and IX, severe protein C deficiency and decrease in antithrombin III (may be dose limiting or fatal)
  Hepatic: Transaminases, bilirubin, and alkaline phosphatase increased (transient)
  Hypersensitivity: Acute allergic reactions (fever, rash, urticaria, arthralgia, hypotension, angioedema, bronchospasm, anaphylaxis (15% to 35%); may be dose limiting in some patients, may be fatal)
  Renal: Azotemia (66%)
1% to 10%:
  Endocrine & metabolic: Hyperuricemia
  Gastrointestinal: Stomatitis
  Miscellaneous: Allergic reaction (including anaphylaxis), antibody formation/immunogenicity (~25%)
General Dosage Range
  I.M.: *Children and Adults:* 6000 units/m^2/dose 3 times/week **or** 6000 units/m^2 every ~3 days
  I.V.: *Children and Adults:* Dosage varies greatly depending on indication
  Intradermal: *Children and Adults:* Test dose: 0.1-0.2 mL of a 20-250 units/mL concentration
Mechanism of Action Asparaginase inhibits protein synthesis by hydrolyzing asparagine to aspartic acid and ammonia. Leukemia cells, especially lymphoblasts, require exogenous asparagine; normal cells can synthesize asparagine. Asparaginase is cycle-specific for the G$_1$ phase.

Pharmacodynamics/Kinetics
  Half-life Elimination I.M.: 39-49 hours; I.V.: 8-30 hours
  Time to Peak I.M.: 14-24 hours
Pregnancy Risk Factor C
Pregnancy Considerations Decreased weight gain, resorptions, gross abnormalities, and skeletal abnormalities were observed in animal studies. There are no adequate and well-controlled studies in pregnant women. Use during pregnancy only if clearly needed.

Asparaginase (*Erwinia*)
(a SPEAR a ji nase er WIN i ah)

Brand Names: U.S. Erwinaze™
Brand Names: Canada Erwinase®
Pharmacologic Category Antineoplastic Agent, Miscellaneous; Enzyme
Use Treatment (in combination with other chemotherapy) of acute lymphoblastic leukemia (ALL) in patients with hypersensitivity to *E. coli*-derived asparaginase
Local Anesthetic/Vasoconstrictor Precautions No information available to require special precautions
Effects on Dental Treatment No significant effects or complications reported
Effects on Bleeding Thrombotic and hemorrhagic events have been reported with asparaginase (*Erwinia*). A medical consult is recommended.
Adverse Effects
>10%: Miscellaneous: Allergic reaction/hypersensitivity (17%; grades 3/4: 5% to 9%; includes anaphylaxis, urticaria)
1% to 10%:
  Cardiovascular: Thrombosis (2%; grades 3/4: ≤1%)
  Central nervous system: Fever (3%), headache (1%), seizure (1%)
  Endocrine & metabolic: Glucose intolerance (2%), hyperglycemia (2%; grades 3/4: 2%), hyperammonemia (1%)
  Gastrointestinal: Pancreatitis (4%; grades 3/4: ≤1%), nausea (2%), vomiting (2%), abdominal pain (1%), diarrhea (1%)
  Hematologic: Coagulation abnormalities (3%; grades 3/4: ≤1%), hemorrhage (1%; grades 3/4: <1%)
  Hepatic: Transaminases increased (3%; grades 3/4: ≤2%), hyperbilirubinemia (1%)
General Dosage Range I.M.: *Children and Adults:* 25,000 units/m^2 3 times/week (Mon, Wed, Fri) for 6 doses for each planned pegaspargase dose **or** 25,000 units/m^2 for each planned asparaginase (*E. coli*) dose
Mechanism of Action Asparaginase catalyzes the deamidation of asparagine to aspartic acid and ammonia, reducing circulating levels of asparagine. Leukemia cells lack asparagine synthetase and are unable to synthesize asparagine. Asparaginase reduces the exogenous asparagine source for the leukemic cells, resulting in cytotoxicity specific to leukemic cells.
Pharmacodynamics/Kinetics
  Half-life Elimination I.M.: ~16 hours (Asselin, 1993; Avramis, 2005)
Pregnancy Risk Factor C
Pregnancy Considerations Animal reproduction studies have not been conducted. The effects on human pregnancy are unknown.
Prescribing and Access Restrictions Erwinaze™ is distributed through Accredo Health Group, Inc. (1-877-900-9223).

Aspirin (AS pir in)

Related Information

Antiplatelet and Anticoagulation Considerations in Dentistry *on page 1503*
Cardiovascular Diseases *on page 1492*
Oral Pain *on page 1558*
Rheumatoid Arthritis, Osteoarthritis, and Osteoporosis *on page 1526*

Brand Names: U.S. Ascriptin® Maximum Strength [OTC]; Ascriptin® Regular Strength [OTC]; Aspercin [OTC]; Aspergum® [OTC]; Aspir-low [OTC]; Aspirtab [OTC]; Bayer® Aspirin Extra Strength [OTC]; Bayer® Aspirin Regimen Adult Low Strength [OTC]; Bayer® Aspirin Regimen Children's [OTC]; Bayer® Aspirin Regimen Regular Strength [OTC]; Bayer® Genuine Aspirin [OTC]; Bayer® Plus Extra Strength [OTC]; Bayer® Women's Low Dose Aspirin [OTC]; Buffasal [OTC]; Bufferin® Extra Strength [OTC]; Bufferin® [OTC]; Buffinol [OTC]; Ecotrin® Arthritis Strength [OTC]; Ecotrin® Low Strength [OTC]; Ecotrin® [OTC]; Halfprin® [OTC]; St Joseph® Adult Aspirin [OTC]; Tri-Buffered Aspirin [OTC]

Brand Names: Canada Asaphen; Asaphen E.C.; Entrophen®; Novasen; Praxis ASA EC 81 Mg Daily Dose

Generic Availability (U.S.) Yes: Excludes gum

Pharmacologic Category Antiplatelet Agent; Salicylate

Dental Use Treatment of postoperative pain

Use Treatment of mild-to-moderate pain, inflammation, and fever; prevention and treatment of acute coronary syndromes (ST-elevation MI, non-ST-elevation MI, unstable angina), acute ischemic stroke, and transient ischemic episodes; management of rheumatoid arthritis, rheumatic fever, osteoarthritis; adjunctive therapy in revascularization procedures (coronary artery bypass graft [CABG], percutaneous transluminal coronary angioplasty [PTCA], carotid endarterectomy), stent implantation

Unlabeled Use Low doses have been used in the prevention of pre-eclampsia, complications associated with autoimmune disorders such as lupus or antiphospholipid syndrome; colorectal cancer; Kawasaki disease; alternative therapy for prevention of thromboembolism associated with atrial fibrillation in patients not candidates for warfarin; pericarditis including pericarditis associated with MI; thromboprophylaxis for aortic valve repair, Blalock-Taussig shunt placement, carotid artery stenosis, coronary artery disease, Fontan surgery, peripheral arterial occlusive disease, peripheral artery percutaneous transluminal angioplasty, peripheral artery bypass graft surgery, prosthetic valves, ventricular assist device (VAD) placement

Local Anesthetic/Vasoconstrictor Precautions No information available to require special precautions

Effects on Dental Treatment Key adverse event(s) related to dental treatment: As with all drugs which may affect hemostasis, bleeding is associated with aspirin. Hemorrhage may occur at virtually any site; risk is dependent on multiple variables including dosage, concurrent use of multiple agents which alter hemostasis, and patient susceptibility. Many adverse effects of aspirin are dose related, and are rare at low dosages. Other serious reactions are idiosyncratic, related to allergy or individual sensitivity (see Dental Comment).

Aspirin in combination with clopidogrel (Plavix®), prasugrel (Effient®), or ticagrelor (Brilinta™) is the primary prevention strategy against stent thrombosis after placement of drug-eluting metal stents in coronary patients. Premature discontinuation of combination antiplatelet therapy (ie, dual antiplatelet therapy) strongly increases the risk of a catastrophic event of stent thrombosis leading to myocardial infarction and/or death, so says a science advisory issued in January 2007 from the American Heart Association in collaboration with the American Dental Association and other professional healthcare organizations. The advisory stresses a 12-month therapy of dual antiplatelet therapy after placement of a drug-eluting stent in order to prevent thrombosis at the stent site. Any elective surgery should be postponed for 1 year after stent implantation, and if surgery must be performed, consideration should be given to continuing the antiplatelet therapy during the perioperative period in high-risk patients with drug-eluting stents.

This advisory was issued from a science panel made up of representatives from the American Heart Association (AHA), the American College of Cardiology, the Society for Cardiovascular Angiography and Interventions, the American College of Surgeons, the American Dental Association (ADA), and the American College of Physicians (Grines, 2007).

Effects on Bleeding Aspirin irreversibly inhibits platelet aggregation which can prolong bleeding. Upon discontinuation, normal platelet function returns only when new platelets are released (~7-10 days). However, in the case of dental surgery, there is no scientific evidence to support discontinuation of aspirin. A recent study compared blood loss after a single tooth extraction in coronary artery disease patients who were either on aspirin (100 mg daily) or off aspirin for the extraction. The mean volume of bleeding was not statistically different between the groups. Local hemostatic measures were sufficient to control bleeding and there were no reported episodes of hemorrhaging intra- or postoperatively (Medeiros, 2011).

The discontinuation of aspirin may place the patient at risk for a thrombotic event or other cardiovascular complication. In particular, aspirin should **not** be discontinued in patients with cardiac stents that have not completed their full course of dual antiplatelet therapy (eg, aspirin and clopidogrel [prasugrel or ticagrelor]); patient-specific situations need to be discussed with cardiologist. When feasible, postponement of dental surgery until the completion of dual antiplatelet therapy should be considered. Any modification of aspirin therapy should be discussed with the prescribing physician.

Adverse Effects As with all drugs which may affect hemostasis, bleeding is associated with aspirin. Hemorrhage may occur at virtually any site. Risk is dependent on multiple variables including dosage, concurrent use of multiple agents which alter hemostasis, and patient susceptibility. Many adverse effects of aspirin are dose related, and are rare at low dosages. Other serious reactions are idiosyncratic, related to allergy or individual sensitivity. Accurate estimation of frequencies is not possible. The reactions listed below have been reported for aspirin (frequency not defined).

Cardiovascular: Hypotension, tachycardia, dysrhythmias, edema
Central nervous system: Fatigue, insomnia, nervousness, agitation, confusion, dizziness, headache, lethargy, cerebral edema, hyperthermia, coma
Dermatologic: Rash, angioedema, urticaria
Endocrine & metabolic: Acidosis, hyperkalemia, dehydration, hypoglycemia (children), hyperglycemia, hypernatremia (buffered forms)

◀

Gastrointestinal: Nausea, vomiting, dyspepsia, epigastric discomfort, heartburn, stomach pain, gastrointestinal ulceration (6% to 31%), gastric erosions, gastric erythema, duodenal ulcers

Hematologic: Anemia, disseminated intravascular coagulation (DIC), prothrombin times prolonged, coagulopathy, thrombocytopenia, hemolytic anemia, bleeding, iron deficiency anemia

Hepatic: Hepatotoxicity, transaminases increased, hepatitis (reversible)

Neuromuscular & skeletal: Rhabdomyolysis, weakness, acetabular bone destruction (OA)

Otic: Hearing loss, tinnitus

Renal: Interstitial nephritis, papillary necrosis, proteinuria, renal impairment, renal failure (including cases caused by rhabdomyolysis), BUN increased, serum creatinine increased

Respiratory: Asthma, bronchospasm, dyspnea, laryngeal edema, hyperpnea, tachypnea, respiratory alkalosis, noncardiogenic pulmonary edema

Miscellaneous: Anaphylaxis, prolonged pregnancy and labor, stillbirths, low birth weight, peripartum bleeding, Reye's syndrome

Dental Usual Dosage Postoperative pain:

Analgesic and antipyretic: Oral, rectal:

Children: 10-15 mg/kg/dose every 4-6 hours, up to a total of 4 g/day

Adults: 325-650 mg every 4-6 hours up to 4 g/day

Anti-inflammatory: Oral: Initial:

Children: 60-90 mg/kg/day in divided doses; usual maintenance: 80-100 mg/kg/day divided every 6-8 hours; monitor serum concentrations

Adults: 2.4-3.6 g/day in divided doses; usual maintenance: 3.6-5.4 g/day; monitor serum concentrations

Dosage

Children:

Analgesic and antipyretic: Oral, rectal: 10-15 mg/kg/dose every 4-6 hours, up to a total of 4 g/day

Anti-inflammatory: Oral: Initial: 60-90 mg/kg/day in divided doses; usual maintenance: 80-100 mg/kg/day divided every 6-8 hours; monitor serum concentrations

Antiplatelet effects: Adequate pediatric studies have not been performed; pediatric dosage is derived from adult studies and clinical experience and is not well established. Doses are typically rounded to a convenient amount (eg, 1/2 of 81 mg tablet).

Acute ischemic stroke (AIS): Oral:

Noncardioembolic: 1-5 mg/kg/dose once daily for ≥2 years; patients with recurrent AIS or TIAs should be transitioned to clopidogrel, LMWH, or warfarin (Monagle, 2012)

Secondary to Moyamoya and non-Moyamoya vasculopathy: 1-5 mg/kg/dose once daily. **Note:** In non-Moyamoya vasculopathy, continue aspirin for 3 months, with subsequent use guided by repeat cerebrovascular imaging (Monagle, 2012).

Blalock-Taussig shunts, primary prophylaxis (unlabeled use): Oral: 1-5 mg/kg/dose once daily (Monagle, 2012)

Fontan surgery, primary prophylaxis: Oral: 5 mg/kg/dose once daily (Monagle, 2011)

Prosthetic heart valve: Oral:

Bioprosthetic aortic valve (in normal sinus rhythm): 1-5 mg/kg/dose once daily (Monagle, 2012; Guyatt, 2012)

Mechanical aortic and/or mitral valve: Low-dose aspirin (eg, 1-5 mg/kg/day) combined with vitamin K antagonist (eg, warfarin) is recommended as first-line antithrombotic therapy (Guyatt, 2012).

Alternative regimens: 6-20 mg/kg/dose once daily in combination with dipyridamole (Bradley, 1985; El Makhlouf, 1987; LeBlanc, 1993; Serra, 1987; Solymar, 1991)

Ventricular assist device (VAD) placement: Oral: 1-5 mg/kg/dose once daily initiated within 72 hours of VAD placement; should be used with heparin (initiated between 8-48 hours following implantation) (Monagle, 2012)

Kawasaki disease (unlabeled use): Oral: 80-100 mg/kg/day divided every 6 hours for up to 14 days (until fever resolves for at least 48 hours); then decrease dose to 3-5 mg/kg/day once daily; in patients without coronary artery abnormalities, give lower dose (ie, 3-5 mg/kg/day) for at least 6-8 weeks. In patients with coronary artery abnormalities, low-dose aspirin should be continued indefinitely (in combination with warfarin). **Note:** Combine with I.V. immune globulin treatment within 10 days of symptom onset (Newbuger, 2004).

Adults: **Note:** For most cardiovascular uses, typical maintenance dosing of aspirin is 81 mg once daily.

Acute coronary syndrome (ST-segment elevation myocardial infarction [STEMI], unstable angina (UA)/non-ST-segment elevation myocardial infarction [NSTEMI]): Oral: Initial: 162-325 mg given on presentation (patient should chew nonenteric-coated aspirin especially if not taking before presentation); for patients unable to take oral, may use rectal suppository (300-600 mg [Antman, 2004; Maalouf, 2009]). Maintenance (secondary prevention): 75-162 mg once daily indefinitely (Anderson, 2007) or 81-325 mg once daily; 81 mg once daily preferred (O'Gara, 2013). **Note:** When aspirin is used with ticagrelor, the recommended maintenance dose of aspirin is 81 mg/day (Jneid, 2012; O'Gara, 2013).

UA/NSTEMI: Concomitant antiplatelet therapy (Jneid, 2012):

If invasive strategy chosen: Aspirin is recommended in combination with either clopidogrel, ticagrelor, (or prasugrel if at the time of PCI) or an I.V. GP IIb/IIIa inhibitor (if given before PCI, eptifibatide and tirofiban are preferred agents).

If noninvasive strategy chosen: Aspirin is recommended in combination with clopidogrel or ticagrelor.

Analgesic and antipyretic:

Oral: 325-650 mg every 4-6 hours up to 4 g/day

Rectal: 300-600 mg every 4-6 hours up to 4 g/day

Anti-inflammatory: Oral: Initial: 2.4-3.6 g/day in divided doses; usual maintenance: 3.6-5.4 g/day; monitor serum concentrations

Aortic valve repair (unlabeled use): Oral: 50-100 mg once daily (Guyatt, 2012)

Atrial fibrillation (in patients not candidates for oral anticoagulation or at low risk of ischemic stroke) (unlabeled use): Oral: 75-325 mg once daily (Furie, 2011; Fuster, 2006). **Note:** Combination therapy with clopidogrel has been suggested over aspirin alone for those patients who are unsuitable for or choose not to take oral anticoagulant for reasons other than concerns for bleeding (Guyatt, 2012).

As an alternative to adjusted-dose warfarin in patients with atrial fibrillation and mitral stenosis: 75-325 mg once daily with (preferred) or without clopidogrel (Guyatt, 2012)

CABG: Oral: 100-325 mg once daily initiated either preoperatively or within 6 hours postoperatively; continue indefinitely (Hillis, 2011)

Carotid artery stenosis (unlabeled use): Oral: 75-100 mg once daily. **Note:** When symptomatic (including recent carotid endarterectomy), the use of clopidogrel or aspirin/extended-release dipyridamole has been suggested over aspirin alone (Guyatt, 2012).

Coronary artery disease (CAD), established (unlabeled use): Oral: 75-100 mg once daily (Guyatt, 2012)

PCI: Oral:

Non-emergent PCI: Preprocedure: 81-325 mg (325 mg [nonenteric coated] in aspirin-naive patients) starting at least 2 hours (preferably 24 hours) before procedure. Postprocedure: 81 mg once daily continued indefinitely (in combination with a $P2Y_{12}$ inhibitor [eg, clopidogrel, prasugrel, ticagrelor] up to 12 months) (Levine, 2011)

Primary PCI: Preprocedure: 162-325 mg as early as possible prior to procedure; 325 mg preferred followed by a maintenance dose of 81 mg once daily even when a stent is deployed (O'Gara, 2013).

Alternatively, in patients who have undergone elective PCI with either bare metal or drug-eluting stent placement: The American College of Chest Physicians recommends the use of 75-325 mg once daily (in combination with clopidogrel) for 1 month (BMS) or 3-6 months (dependent upon DES type) followed by 75-100 mg once daily (in combination with clopidogrel) for up to 12 months. For patients who underwent PCI but did not have stent placement, 75-325 mg once daily (in combination with clopidogrel) for 1 month is recommended. In either case, single antiplatelet therapy (either aspirin or clopidogrel) is recommended indefinitely (Guyatt, 2012).

Pericarditis (unlabeled use): Oral: Initial: 2.4-3.6 g daily in 3-4 divided doses; usual maintenance: 3.6-5.4 g daily in divided doses; gradually taper over 2- to 3-week period as appropriate (Imazio, 2004; Imazio, 2009). In the treatment of postmyocardial infarction pericarditis, an initial dose of 650 mg 4 times daily increased to 975 mg 4 times daily if necessary (after 24 hours) has been used (Berman, 1981; O'Gara, 2013).

Peripheral arterial disease (unlabeled use): Oral: 75-100 mg once daily (Guyatt, 2012) **or** 75-325 mg once daily; may use in conjunction with clopidogrel in those who are not at an increased risk of bleeding but are of high cardiovascular risk. **Note:** These recommendations also pertain to those with intermittent claudication or critical limb ischemia, prior lower extremity revascularization, or prior amputation for lower extremity ischemia (Rooke, 2011).

Peripheral artery percutaneous transluminal angioplasty (with or without stenting) or peripheral artery bypass graft surgery, postprocedure (unlabeled use): Oral: 75-100 mg once daily (Guyatt, 2012). **Note:** For below-knee bypass graft surgery with prosthetic grafts, combine with clopidogrel (Guyatt, 2012).

Pre-eclampsia prevention (women at risk) (unlabeled use): Oral: 75-100 mg once daily starting in the second trimester (Guyatt, 2012)

Primary prevention: Oral:

American College of Cardiology/American Heart Association: Prevention of myocardial infarction: 75-162 mg once daily. **Note:** Patients are most likely to benefit if their 10-year coronary heart disease risk is ≥6% (Antman, 2004).

American College of Chest Physicians: Prevention of myocardial infarction and stroke: Select individuals ≥50 years of age (without symptomatic cardiovascular disease): 75-100 mg once daily (Guyatt, 2012; Grade 2B, weak recommendation)

Prosthetic heart valve: Oral:

Bioprosthetic aortic valve (patient in normal sinus rhythm) (unlabeled use): 50-100 mg once daily; usual dose: 81 mg once daily. **Note:** If mitral bioprosthetic valve, oral anticoagulation with warfarin (instead of aspirin) is recommended for the first 3 months postoperatively, followed by aspirin alone (Guyatt, 2012).

Mechanical aortic or mitral valve (unlabeled use):

Low risk of bleeding: 50-100 mg once daily (in combination with warfarin) (Guyatt, 2012)

History of thromboembolism while receiving oral anticoagulants: 75-100 mg once daily (in combination with warfarin) (Furie, 2011)

Transcatheter aortic bioprosthetic valve (unlabeled use): 50-100 mg once daily (in combination with clopidogrel) (Guyatt, 2012)

Stroke/TIA: Oral:

Acute ischemic stroke/TIA: Initial: 160-325 mg within 48 hours of stroke/TIA onset, followed by 75-100 mg once daily (Guyatt, 2012). The AHA/ASA recommends an initial dose of 325 mg within 24-48 hours after stroke; do not administer aspirin within 24 hours after administration of alteplase (Jauch, 2013).

Cardioembolic, secondary prevention (oral anticoagulation unsuitable): 75-100 mg once daily (in combination with clopidogrel) (Guyatt, 2012).

Cryptogenic with patent foramen ovale (PFO) or atrial septal aneurysm: 50-100 mg once daily (Guyatt, 2012)

Noncardioembolic, secondary prevention: 75-325 mg once daily (Smith, 2011) **or** 75-100 mg once daily (Guyatt, 2012). **Note:** Combination aspirin/extended release dipyridamole or clopidogrel is preferred over aspirin alone (Guyatt, 2012).

Women at high risk, primary prevention: 81 mg once daily **or** 100 mg every other day (Goldstein, 2010)

Dosing adjustment in renal impairment: Cl_{cr} <10 mL/minute: Avoid use.

Hemodialysis: Dialyzable (50% to 100%)

Dosing adjustment in hepatic disease: Avoid use in severe liver disease.

Mechanism of Action Irreversibly inhibits cyclooxygenase-1 and 2 (COX-1 and 2) enzymes, via acetylation, which results in decreased formation of prostaglandin precursors; irreversibly inhibits formation of prostaglandin derivative, thromboxane A_2, via acetylation of platelet cyclooxygenase, thus inhibiting platelet aggregation; has antipyretic, analgesic, and anti-inflammatory properties

Contraindications Hypersensitivity to salicylates, other NSAIDs, or any component of the formulation; asthma; rhinitis; nasal polyps; inherited or acquired bleeding disorders (including factor VII and factor IX deficiency); do not use in children (<16 years of age) for viral infections (chickenpox or flu symptoms), with or without fever, due to a potential association with Reye's syndrome

Warnings/Precautions Use with caution in patients with platelet and bleeding disorders, renal dysfunction, dehydration, erosive gastritis, or peptic ulcer disease. Heavy ethanol use (>3 drinks/day) can increase bleeding risks. Avoid use in severe renal failure or in severe hepatic failure. Low-dose aspirin for cardioprotective

◄ effects is associated with a two- to fourfold increase in UGI events (eg, symptomatic or complicated ulcers); risks of these events increase with increasing aspirin dose; during the chronic phase of aspirin dosing, doses >81 mg are not recommended unless indicated (Bhatt, 2008). Use of safer agents for routine management of pain or headache throughout pregnancy should be considered. If possible, avoid use during the third trimester of pregnancy.

Discontinue use if tinnitus or impaired hearing occurs. Caution in mild-to-moderate renal failure (only at high dosages). Patients with sensitivity to tartrazine dyes, nasal polyps, and asthma may have an increased risk of salicylate sensitivity. In the treatment of acute ischemic stroke, avoid aspirin for 24 hours following administration of alteplase; administration within 24 hours increases the risk of hemorrhagic transformation (Jauch, 2013). Concurrent use of aspirin and clopidogrel is not recommended for secondary prevention of ischemic stroke or TIA in patients unable to take oral anticoagulants due to hemorrhagic risk (Furie, 2011). Surgical patients should avoid ASA if possible, for 1-2 weeks prior to surgery, to reduce the risk of excessive bleeding (except in patients with cardiac stents that have not completed their full course of dual antiplatelet therapy [aspirin, clopidogrel]; patient-specific situations need to be discussed with cardiologist; AHA/ACC/SCAI/ACS/ADA Science Advisory provides recommendations). When used concomitantly with ≤325 mg of aspirin, NSAIDs (including selective COX-2 inhibitors) substantially increase the risk of gastrointestinal complications (eg, ulcer); concomitant gastroprotective therapy (eg, proton pump inhibitors) is recommended (Bhatt, 2008).

Elderly: Avoid chronic use of doses >325 mg/day (unless alternative agents ineffective and patient can receive concomitant gastroprotective agent); nonselective oral NSAID use is associated with an increased risk of GI bleeding and peptic ulcer disease in older adults in high risk category (eg, >75 years or age or receiving concomitant oral/parenteral corticosteroids, anticoagulants, or antiplatelet agents) (Beers Criteria).

When used for self-medication (OTC labeling): Children and teenagers who have or are recovering from chickenpox or flu-like symptoms should not use this product. Changes in behavior (along with nausea and vomiting) may be an early sign of Reye's syndrome; patients should be instructed to contact their healthcare provider if these occur.

Drug Interactions

Metabolism/Transport Effects Substrate of CYP2C9 (minor); **Note:** Assignment of Major/Minor substrate status based on clinically relevant drug interaction potential

Avoid Concomitant Use

Avoid concomitant use of Aspirin with any of the following: Floctafenine; Influenza Virus Vaccine (Live/Attenuated); Ketorolac (Nasal); Ketorolac (Systemic); Omacetaxine

Increased Effect/Toxicity

Aspirin may increase the levels/effects of: Alendronate; Anticoagulants; Carbonic Anhydrase Inhibitors; Collagenase (Systemic); Corticosteroids (Systemic); Dabigatran Etexilate; Divalproex; Drotrecogin Alfa (Activated); Heparin; Hypoglycemic Agents; Ibritumomab; Methotrexate; NSAID (COX-2 Inhibitor); Omacetaxine; PRALAtrexate; Rivaroxaban; Salicylates; Thrombolytic Agents; Ticagrelor; Tositumomab and Iodine I 131 Tositumomab; Valproic Acid; Varicella Virus-Containing Vaccines; Vitamin K Antagonists

The levels/effects of Aspirin may be increased by: Agents with Antiplatelet Properties; Ammonium Chloride; Antidepressants (Tricyclic, Tertiary Amine); Calcium Channel Blockers (Nondihydropyridine); Dasatinib; Floctafenine; Ginkgo Biloba; Glucosamine; Herbs (Anticoagulant/Antiplatelet Properties); Influenza Virus Vaccine (Live/Attenuated); Ketorolac (Nasal); Ketorolac (Systemic); Loop Diuretics; Multivitamins/Minerals (with ADEK, Folate, Iron); NSAID (Nonselective); Omega-3 Fatty Acids; Pentosan Polysulfate Sodium; Pentoxifylline; Potassium Acid Phosphate; Prostacyclin Analogues; Selective Serotonin Reuptake Inhibitors; Serotonin/Norepinephrine Reuptake Inhibitors; Tipranavir; Treprostinil; Vitamin E

Decreased Effect

Aspirin may decrease the levels/effects of: ACE Inhibitors; Hyaluronidase; Loop Diuretics; Multivitamins/Minerals (with ADEK, Folate, Iron); NSAID (Nonselective); Probenecid; Ticagrelor; Tiludronate

The levels/effects of Aspirin may be decreased by: Corticosteroids (Systemic); Floctafenine; Ketorolac (Nasal); Ketorolac (Systemic); NSAID (Nonselective)

Ethanol/Nutrition/Herb Interactions

Ethanol: Avoid ethanol (may enhance gastric mucosal damage).

Food: Food may decrease the rate but not the extent of oral absorption.

Folic acid: Hyperexcretion of folate; folic acid deficiency may result, leading to macrocytic anemia.

Iron: With chronic aspirin use and at doses of 3-4 g/day, iron-deficiency anemia may result.

Sodium: Hypernatremia resulting from buffered aspirin solutions or sodium salicylate containing high sodium content. Avoid or use with caution in CHF or any condition where hypernatremia would be detrimental.

Benedictine liqueur, prunes, raisins, tea, and gherkins: Potential salicylate accumulation.

Fresh fruits containing vitamin C: Displace drug from binding sites, resulting in increased urinary excretion of aspirin.

Herb/Nutraceutical: Avoid cat's claw, dong quai, evening primrose, feverfew, garlic, ginger, ginkgo, red clover, horse chestnut, green tea, ginseng (all have additional antiplatelet activity). Limit curry powder, paprika, licorice; may cause salicylate accumulation. These foods contain 6 mg salicylate/100 g. An ordinary American diet contains 10-200 mg/day of salicylate.

Dietary Considerations Take with food or large volume of water or milk to minimize GI upset.

Pharmacodynamics/Kinetics

Duration of Action 4-6 hours

Half-life Elimination Parent drug: 15-20 minutes; Salicylates (dose dependent): 3 hours at lower doses (300-600 mg), 5-6 hours (after 1 g), 10 hours with higher doses

Time to Peak Serum: ~1-2 hours

Pregnancy Considerations Salicylates have been noted to cross the placenta and enter fetal circulation. Adverse effects reported in the fetus include mortality, intrauterine growth retardation, salicylate intoxication, bleeding abnormalities, and neonatal acidosis. Use of aspirin close to delivery may cause premature closure of the ductus arteriosus. Adverse effects reported in the mother include anemia, hemorrhage, prolonged gestation, and prolonged labor (Østensen, 1998). Aspirin has been used for the prevention of pre-eclampsia; however, the ACOG currently recommends that it not be used in low-risk women (ACOG, 2002). Low-dose aspirin is used to treat complications resulting from antiphospholipid syndrome in pregnancy (either primary or secondary to SLE) (Carp, 2004; Guyatt, 2012; Tincani, 2003). In general, low doses during pregnancy needed for the treatment of certain medical conditions have not been shown to cause fetal harm, however, discontinuing therapy prior to delivery is recommended (Østensen, 2006). Use of safer agents for routine management of pain or headache should be considered.

Lactation Enters breast milk (AAP recommends use "with caution"; AAP 2001 update pending)

Breast-Feeding Considerations Low amounts of aspirin can be found in breast milk. Milk/plasma ratios ranging from 0.03-0.3 have been reported. Peak levels in breast milk are reported to be at ~9 hours after a dose. Metabolic acidosis was reported in one infant following an aspirin dose of 3.9 g/day in the mother. The WHO considers occasional doses of aspirin to be compatible with breast-feeding, but to avoid long-term therapy and consider monitoring the infant for adverse effects (WHO, 2002). Other sources suggest avoiding aspirin while breast-feeding due to the theoretical risk of Reye's syndrome (Bar-Oz, 2003; Spigset, 2000). When used for vascular indications, breast-feeding may be continued during low-dose aspirin therapy (Guyatt, 2012).

Dosage Forms

Caplet, oral: 500 mg
Ascriptin® Maximum Strength [OTC]: 500 mg
Bayer® Aspirin Extra Strength [OTC]: 500 mg
Bayer® Genuine Aspirin [OTC]: 325 mg
Bayer® Plus Extra Strength [OTC]: 500 mg
Bayer® Women's Low Dose Aspirin [OTC]: 81 mg

Caplet, enteric coated, oral:
Bayer® Aspirin Regimen Regular Strength [OTC]: 325 mg

Gum, chewing, oral:
Aspergum® [OTC]: 227 mg (12s)

Suppository, rectal: 300 mg (12s); 600 mg (12s)

Tablet, oral: 325 mg
Ascriptin® Regular Strength [OTC]: 325 mg
Aspercin [OTC]: 325 mg
Aspirtab [OTC]: 325 mg
Bayer® Genuine Aspirin [OTC]: 325 mg
Buffasal [OTC]: 325 mg
Bufferin® [OTC]: 325 mg
Bufferin® Extra Strength [OTC]: 500 mg
Buffinol [OTC]: 324 mg
Tri-Buffered Aspirin [OTC]: 325 mg

Tablet, chewable, oral: 81 mg
Bayer® Aspirin Regimen Children's [OTC]: 81 mg
St Joseph® Adult Aspirin [OTC]: 81 mg

Tablet, enteric coated, oral: 81 mg, 325 mg, 650 mg
Aspir-low [OTC]: 81 mg
Bayer® Aspirin Regimen Adult Low Strength [OTC]: 81 mg
Ecotrin® [OTC]: 325 mg
Ecotrin® Arthritis Strength [OTC]: 500 mg
Ecotrin® Low Strength [OTC]: 81 mg
Halfprin® [OTC]: 81 mg, 162 mg
St Joseph® Adult Aspirin [OTC]: 81 mg

Dental Comment The Food and Drug Administration (FDA), has issued a letter updating information and considerations regarding the use of ibuprofen (400 mg doses) in patients who are taking low dose aspirin (81 mg, immediate release; not enteric coated) for cardioprotection and stroke prevention. Ibuprofen, at these doses, may interfere with aspirin's antiplatelet effect depending upon when it is administered. Patients initiated on aspirin first (for ~1 week) then ibuprofen (400 mg 3 times/day for 10 days) seem to maintain

aspirin's platelet effect (Cryer, 2005). Ibuprofen has the greatest impact on aspirin if administered less than 8 hours before aspirin (Catella-Lawson, 2001).

Patients may require counseling about the appropriate timing of ibuprofen dosing in relationship to aspirin therapy. With occasional use of ibuprofen, a clinically-significant interaction with aspirin in unlikely. To avoid interference during chronic dosing, a single dose of ibuprofen should be taken 30-120 minutes after aspirin ingestion or at least 8 hours should elapse after ibuprofen dosing before giving aspirin (FDA, 2006; Catella-Lawson, 2001).

The clinical implications of the interaction are unclear. There have not been any clinical endpoint studies conducted at this time. Avoidance of this interaction is potentially important because aspirin's vascular protection could be decreased or negated.

Other nonselective NSAIDs may have potential for a similar interaction with aspirin. Such has been described with naproxen (Capone, 2005). Acetaminophen does not appear to interfere with the antiplatelet effect of aspirin. Other clinical scenarios (use of smaller ibuprofen doses, other aspirin products, other doses of aspirin) have not been evaluated.

Additional information is available at: http://www.fda. gov/Drugs/DrugSafety/PostmarketDrugSafetyInformationforPatientsandProviders/ucm125222.htm

References

Capone ML, Sciulli MG, Tacconelli S, et al, "Pharmacodynamic Interaction of Naproxen With Low-Dose Aspirin in Healthy Subjects," J Am Coll Cardiol, 2005, 45(8):1295-1301.
Catella-Lawson F, Reilly MP, Kapoor SC, et al, "Cyclooxygenase Inhibitors and the Antiplatelet Effects of Aspirin," N Engl J Med, 2001, 345(25):1809-17.
Cryer B, Verlin RG, Cooper SA, et al, "Double-Blind, Randomized, Parallel, Placebo-Controlled Study of Ibuprofen Effects on Thromboxane B2 Concentrations in Aspirin-Treated Healthy Adult Volunteers," Clin Ther, 2005, 27(2):185-191.
Grines CL, Bonow RO, Casey DE, et al, "AHA/ACC/SCAI/ACS/ADA Science Advisory, Prevention of Premature Discontinuation of Dual Antiplatelet Therapy in Patients With Coronary Artery Stents. A Science Advisory From the American Heart Association, American College of Cardiology, Society of Cardiovascular Angiography and Interventions, American College of Surgeons, and American Dental Association With Representation From The Amercian College Of Physicians," Circulation, 2007, 115(6):813-8. Available at http:// www.acc.org/qualityandscience/clinical/pdfs/Final_Dual_Antiplatelet_Statement_010507.pdf.
Jeske AH, Suchko GD, ADA Council on Scientific Affairs and Division of Science, et al, "Lack of a Scientific Basis for Routine Discontinuation of Oral Anticoagulation Therapy Before Dental Treatment," J Am Dent Assoc, 2003, 134(11):1492-7.

Aspirin and Dipyridamole
(AS pir in & dye peer ID a mole)

Related Information
Aspirin on page 135
Dipyridamole on page 440

Brand Names: U.S. Aggrenox®

Brand Names: Canada Aggrenox®

Pharmacologic Category Antiplatelet Agent

Use Reduction in the risk of stroke in patients who have had transient ischemia of the brain or ischemic stroke due to thrombosis

Unlabeled Use Hemodialysis graft patency; symptomatic carotid artery stenosis (including recent carotid endarterectomy)

Local Anesthetic/Vasoconstrictor Precautions No information available to require special precautions

Effects on Dental Treatment Key adverse event(s) related to dental treatment: As with all drugs which may affect hemostasis, bleeding is associated with aspirin. Hemorrhage may occur at virtually any site; risk is dependent on multiple variables including dosage, concurrent use of multiple agents which alter hemostasis, and patient susceptibility. Many adverse effects of aspirin are dose related, and are rare at low dosages. Other serious reactions are idiosyncratic, related to allergy or individual sensitivity (see Dental Comment).

Effects on Bleeding Aspirin irreversibly inhibits platelet aggregation which can prolong bleeding. Upon discontinuation, normal platelet function returns only when new platelets are released (~7-10 days). However, in the case of dental surgery, there is no scientific evidence to support discontinuation of aspirin. The discontinuation of aspirin may place the patient at risk for a thrombotic event or other cardiovascular complication. In particular, aspirin should **not** be discontinued in patients with cardiac stents that have not completed their full course of dual antiplatelet therapy (eg, aspirin and clopidogrel [prasugrel or ticagrelor]); patient-specific situations need to be discussed with cardiologist. When feasible, postponement of dental surgery until the completion of dual antiplatelet therapy should be considered. Any modification of aspirin therapy should be discussed with the prescribing physician.

Adverse Effects

>10%:
Central nervous system: Headache (39%; tolerance usually develops)
Gastrointestinal: Abdominal pain (18%), dyspepsia (18%), nausea (16%), diarrhea (13%)

1% to 10%:
Cardiovascular: Cardiac failure (2%), syncope (1%)
Central nervous system: Fatigue (6%), pain (6%), amnesia (2%), malaise (2%), seizure (2%), confusion (1%), somnolence (1%)
Dermatologic: Purpura (1%)
Gastrointestinal: Vomiting (8%), GI bleeding (4%), melena (2%), rectal bleeding (2%), hemorrhoids (1%), GI hemorrhage (1%), anorexia (1%)
Hematologic: Hemorrhage (3%), anemia (2%)
Neuromuscular & skeletal: Arthralgia (6%), back pain (5%), weakness (2%), arthritis (2%), arthrosis (1%), myalgia (1%)
Respiratory: Cough (2%), epistaxis (2%), upper respiratory tract infection (1%)

General Dosage Range Oral: *Adults:* 1 capsule (200 mg dipyridamole, 25 mg aspirin) twice daily

Mechanism of Action The antithrombotic action results from additive antiplatelet effects. Dipyridamole inhibits the uptake of adenosine into platelets, endothelial cells, and erythrocytes. Aspirin inhibits platelet aggregation by irreversible inhibition of platelet cyclooxygenase and thus inhibits the generation of thromboxane A_2.

Pregnancy Risk Factor D

Pregnancy Considerations Animal reproduction studies have shown an increase in aspirin-related fetal toxicity with this combination. Refer to individual monographs.

Dental Comment The Food and Drug Administration (FDA), has issued a letter updating information and considerations regarding the use of ibuprofen (400 mg doses) in patients who are taking low dose aspirin (81 mg, immediate release; not enteric coated) for cardioprotection and stroke prevention. Ibuprofen, at these doses, may interfere with aspirin's antiplatelet effect depending upon when it is administered. Patients initiated on aspirin first (for ~1 week) then ibuprofen (400 mg 3 times/day for 10 days) seem to maintain aspirin's platelet effect (Cryer, 2005). Ibuprofen has the greatest impact on aspirin if administered less than 8 hours before aspirin (Catella-Lawson, 2001).

Patients may require counseling about the appropriate timing of ibuprofen dosing in relationship to aspirin therapy. With occasional use of ibuprofen, a clinically-significant interaction with aspirin in unlikely. To avoid interference during chronic dosing, a single dose of ibuprofen should be taken 30-120 minutes after aspirin ingestion or at least 8 hours should elapse after ibuprofen dosing before giving aspirin (Catella-Lawson, 2001; FDA, 2006).

The clinical implications of the interaction are unclear. There have not been any clinical endpoint studies conducted at this time. Avoidance of this interaction is potentially important because aspirin's vascular protection could be decreased or negated.

Other nonselective NSAIDs may have potential for a similar interaction with aspirin. Such has been described with naproxen (Capone, 2005). Acetaminophen does not appear to interfere with the antiplatelet effect of aspirin. Other clinical scenarios (use of smaller ibuprofen doses, other aspirin products, other doses of aspirin) have not been evaluated.

Additional information is available at: http://www.fda.gov/Drugs/DrugSafety/PostmarketDrugSafetyInformationforPatientsandProviders/ucm125222.htm

---

Atazanavir (at a za NA veer)

Related Information
HIV Infection and AIDS *on page 1520*
Brand Names: U.S. Reyataz®
Brand Names: Canada Reyataz®
Pharmacologic Category Antiretroviral Agent, Protease Inhibitor
Use Treatment of HIV-1 infections in combination with at least two other antiretroviral agents

Local Anesthetic/Vasoconstrictor Precautions No information available to require special precautions

Effects on Dental Treatment No significant effects or complications reported

Effects on Bleeding Increased bleeding has been noted with protease inhibitors, such as atazanavir, in patients with hemophilia A or B. Thrombocytopenia has been reported. No other information is available to require special precautions in other patients.

Adverse Effects Includes data from both treatment-naive and treatment-experienced patients. Percentages listed for adults unless otherwise specified.

>10%:
Dermatologic: Rash (3% to 21%; median onset 7 weeks)
Endocrine & metabolic: Cholesterol increased (≥240 mg/dL: 6% or 25%)
Gastrointestinal: Nausea (3% to 14%), amylase increased (≤14%)
Hepatic: Bilirubin increased (≥2.6 times ULN: 35% to 49%)
Neuromuscular & skeletal: CPK increased (6% to 11%)
Respiratory: Cough (children 21%)

2% to 10%:
Cardiovascular: AV block (first degree: 6%; second degree [children] 2%)
Central nervous system: Headache (1% to 6%; children 7%), peripheral neuropathy (<1% to 4%), insomnia (<1% to 3%), depression (2%), fever (2%; children 19%), dizziness (<1% to 2%)
Endocrine & metabolic: Triglycerides increased (<1% to 8%), hyperglycemia (≥251 mg/dL: 5%)

Gastrointestinal: Lipase increased (<1% to 5%), abdominal pain (4%), vomiting (3% to 4%; children 8%), diarrhea (1% to 3%; children 8%)

Hematologic: Neutropenia (3% to 7%), hemoglobin decreased (<1% to 5%), thrombocytopenia (2%)

Hepatic: Jaundice (5% to 9%; children 13%), ALT increased (>5 times ULN: 3% to 9%; 10% to 25% in patients seropositive for hepatitis B and/or C), AST increased (>5 times ULN: 2% to 7%; 9% to 10% in patients seropositive for hepatitis B and/or C)

Neuromuscular & skeletal: Myalgia (4%)

Respiratory: Rhinorrhea (children 6%)

General Dosage Range Dosage adjustment recommended in patients with hepatic or renal impairment or on concomitant therapy

Oral:

Children 6 to <18 years:
15 to <20 kg: Atazanavir 150 mg once daily
20 to <40 kg: Atazanavir 200 mg once daily
≥40 kg: Atazanavir 300 mg once daily

Children ≥13 years (≥40 kg) and Adults: 400 mg once daily (antiretroviral-naive) **or** atazanavir 300 mg once daily

Mechanism of Action Binds to the site of HIV-1 protease activity and inhibits cleavage of viral Gag-Pol polyprotein precursors into individual functional proteins required for infectious HIV. This results in the formation of immature, noninfectious viral particles.

Pharmacodynamics/Kinetics

Half-life Elimination Unboosted therapy: 7-8 hours; Boosted therapy (with ritonavir): 9-18 hours

Time to Peak Plasma: 2-3 hours

Pregnancy Risk Factor B

Pregnancy Considerations Teratogenic effects have not been observed in animal reproduction studies. Atazanavir crosses the placenta with cord blood concentrations reported as 13% to 21% of maternal serum concentrations at delivery. An increased risk of teratogenic effects has not been observed based on information collected by the antiretroviral pregnancy registry. A small increased risk of preterm birth has been associated with maternal use of protease inhibitor-based combination antiretroviral (ARV) therapy during pregnancy; however, the benefits of its use generally outweigh this risk and protease inhibitors (PIs) should not be withheld if otherwise recommended. Hyperglycemia, new onset of diabetes mellitus, or diabetic ketoacidosis have been reported with PIs; it is not clear if pregnancy increases this risk. Hyperbilirubinemia or hypoglycemia may occur in neonates following *in utero* exposure to atazanavir, although data are conflicting.

The DHHS Perinatal HIV Guidelines recommend atazanavir as a preferred PI when combined with low-dose ritonavir boosting. Pharmacokinetic studies suggest that standard dosing during pregnancy may provide decreased plasma concentrations and some experts recommend increased doses during the second and third trimesters. However, the manufacturer notes that dose adjustment is not required unless using concomitant H$_2$-receptor blockers or tenofovir or for ARV-naive pregnant women taking efavirenz. May give as once-daily dosing.

Regardless of CD4 count or HIV RNA copy number, all HIV-infected pregnant women should receive a combination antepartum ARV drug regimen; this includes women who require therapy for their own health, as well as women who do not yet require therapy for their own health. ARV therapy should be started as soon as possible if required for the woman's health Although earlier initiation may be more effective in reducing the perinatal transmission of HIV), also consider maternal conditions (eg, nausea and vomiting) and the potential risks of first trimester fetal exposure for specific agents. Plasma HIV RNA levels should be assessed at ~34-36 weeks gestation in order to help determine mode of delivery. If ARV therapy must be interrupted for <24 hours during the peripartum period, stop then restart all medications simultaneously in order to decrease the chance of developing resistance. Long-term follow-up is recommended for all infants exposed to ARV medications.

Healthcare providers are encouraged to enroll pregnant women exposed to antiretroviral medications in the Antiretroviral Pregnancy Registry (1-800-258-4263 or www.APRegistry.com). Healthcare providers caring for HIV-infected women and their infants may contact the National Perinatal HIV Hotline (888-448-8765) for clinical consultation (DHHS [perinatal], 2012).

Atenolol (a TEN oh lole)

Related Information
Cardiovascular Diseases *on page 1492*

Brand Names: U.S. Tenormin®

Brand Names: Canada Apo-Atenolol®; Ava-Atenolol; CO Atenolol; Dom-Atenolol; JAMP-Atenolol; Mint-Atenolol; Mylan-Atenolol; Nu-Atenol; PMS-Atenolol; RAN™-Atenolol; ratio-Atenolol; Riva-Atenolol; Sandoz-Atenolol; Septa-Atenolol; Tenormin®; Teva-Atenolol

Generic Availability (U.S.) Yes

Pharmacologic Category Antianginal Agent; Beta-Blocker, Beta-1 Selective

Use Treatment of hypertension, alone or in combination with other agents; management of angina pectoris; secondary prevention postmyocardial infarction

Unlabeled Use Acute ethanol withdrawal (in combination with a benzodiazepine), supraventricular and ventricular arrhythmias, and migraine headache prophylaxis

Local Anesthetic/Vasoconstrictor Precautions No information available to require special precautions

Effects on Dental Treatment Atenolol is a cardioselective beta-blocker. Local anesthetic with vasoconstrictor can be safely used in patients medicated with atenolol. Nonselective beta-blockers (ie, propranolol, nadolol) enhance the pressor response to epinephrine, resulting in hypertension and bradycardia; this has not been reported for atenolol. Many nonsteroidal anti-inflammatory drugs, such as ibuprofen and indomethacin, can reduce the hypotensive effect of beta-blockers after 3 or more weeks of therapy with the NSAID. Short-term NSAID use (ie, 3 days) requires no special precautions in patients taking beta-blockers.

Effects on Bleeding No information available to require special precautions

Adverse Effects 1% to 10%:

Cardiovascular: Persistent bradycardia, hypotension, chest pain, edema, heart failure, second- or third-degree AV block, Raynaud's phenomenon

Central nervous system: Dizziness, fatigue, insomnia, lethargy, confusion, mental impairment, depression, headache, nightmares

Gastrointestinal: Constipation, diarrhea, nausea

Genitourinary: Impotence

Miscellaneous: Cold extremities

Dosage Oral:

Children: Hypertension: 0.5-1 mg/kg/dose given daily; range of 0.5-1.5 mg/kg/day; maximum dose: 2 mg/kg/day up to 100 mg/day

Adults:
Hypertension: 25-50 mg once daily, may increase to 100 mg/day. Doses >100 mg are unlikely to produce any further benefit.

Angina pectoris: 50 mg once daily, may increase to 100 mg/day. Some patients may require 200 mg/day.

Postmyocardial infarction: 100 mg/day or 50 mg twice daily for 6-9 days postmyocardial infarction.

Thyrotoxicosis (unlabeled use): 25-100 mg once or twice daily (Bahn, 2011)

Elderly: Hypertension: Consider lower initial doses and titrate to response (Aronow, 2011).

Dosage adjustment in renal impairment:
Cl_{cr} >35 mL/minute/1.73 m²: No dosage adjustment necessary.

Cl_{cr} 15-35 mL/minute/1.73 m²: Maximum dose: 50 mg daily

Cl_{cr} <15 mL/minute/1.73 m²: Maximum dose: 25 mg daily

Hemodialysis: Moderately dialyzable (20% to 50%) via hemodialysis; administer dose postdialysis or administer 25-50 mg supplemental dose.

Peritoneal dialysis: Elimination is not enhanced; supplemental dose is not necessary.

Dosage adjustment in hepatic impairment: No dosage adjustment provided in the manufacturer's labeling; however, atenolol undergoes minimal hepatic metabolism.

Mechanism of Action Competitively blocks response to beta-adrenergic stimulation, selectively blocks beta₁-receptors with little or no effect on beta₂-receptors except at high doses

Contraindications Hypersensitivity to atenolol or any component of the formulation; sinus bradycardia; sinus node dysfunction; heart block greater than first-degree (except in patients with a functioning artificial pacemaker); cardiogenic shock; uncompensated cardiac failure; pulmonary edema; pregnancy

Warnings/Precautions Consider pre-existing conditions such as sick sinus syndrome before initiating. Administer cautiously in compensated heart failure and monitor for a worsening of the condition (efficacy of atenolol in heart failure has not been established). **[U.S. Boxed Warning]: Beta-blocker therapy should not be withdrawn abruptly (particularly in patients with CAD), but gradually tapered to avoid acute tachycardia, hypertension, and/or ischemia.** Chronic beta-blocker therapy should not be routinely withdrawn prior to major surgery. Beta-blockers should be avoided in patients with bronchospastic disease (asthma). Atenolol, with B₁ selectivity, has been used cautiously in bronchospastic disease with close monitoring. May precipitate or aggravate symptoms of arterial insufficiency in patients with PVD and Raynaud's disease; use with caution and monitor for progression of arterial obstruction. Use cautiously in patients with diabetes - may mask hypoglycemic symptoms. May mask signs of hyperthyroidism (eg, tachycardia); use caution if hyperthyroidism is suspected, abrupt withdrawal may precipitate thyroid storm. Alterations in thyroid function tests may be observed. Use cautiously in the renally impaired (dosage adjustment required). Caution in myasthenia gravis or psychiatric disease (may cause CNS depression). Bradycardia may be observed more frequently in elderly patients (>65 years of age); dosage reductions may be necessary. Adequate alpha-blockade is required prior to use of any beta-blocker for patients with untreated pheochromocytoma. May induce or exacerbate psoriasis. Use caution with history of severe anaphylaxis to allergens; patients taking beta-blockers may

become more sensitive to repeated challenges. Treatment of anaphylaxis (eg, epinephrine) in patients taking beta-blockers may be ineffective or promote undesirable effects. Use with caution in patients on concurrent digoxin, verapamil, or diltiazem; bradycardia or heart block can occur. Use with caution in patients receiving inhaled anesthetic agents known to depress myocardial contractility.

Drug Interactions

Metabolism/Transport Effects None known.

Avoid Concomitant Use
Avoid concomitant use of Atenolol with any of the following: Floctafenine; Methacholine

Increased Effect/Toxicity
Atenolol may increase the levels/effects of: Alpha-/Beta-Agonists (Direct-Acting); Alpha1-Blockers; Alpha2-Agonists; Amifostine; Antihypertensives; Bupivacaine; Cardiac Glycosides; Cholinergic Agonists; Ergot Derivatives; Fingolimod; Hypotensive Agents; Insulin; Lidocaine (Systemic); Lidocaine (Topical); Mepivacaine; Methacholine; Midodrine; RiTUXimab; Sulfonylureas

The levels/effects of Atenolol may be increased by: Acetylcholinesterase Inhibitors; Alpha2-Agonists; Amiodarone; Anilidopiperidine Opioids; Calcium Channel Blockers (Dihydropyridine); Calcium Channel Blockers (Nondihydropyridine); Diazoxide; Dipyridamole; Disopyramide; Dronedarone; Floctafenine; Glycopyrrolate; Herbs (Hypotensive Properties); MAO Inhibitors; Pentoxifylline; Phosphodiesterase 5 Inhibitors; Prostacyclin Analogues; Reserpine

Decreased Effect
Atenolol may decrease the levels/effects of: Beta2-Agonists; Theophylline Derivatives

The levels/effects of Atenolol may be decreased by: Ampicillin; Herbs (Hypertensive Properties); Methylphenidate; Nonsteroidal Anti-Inflammatory Agents; Yohimbine

Ethanol/Nutrition/Herb Interactions
Food: Atenolol serum concentrations may be decreased if taken with food.

Herb/Nutraceutical: Dong quai has estrogenic activity. Ephedra, yohimbe, and ginseng may worsen hypertension. Garlic may have increased antihypertensive effect. Management: Avoid dong quai, ephedra, yohimbe, ginseng, and garlic.

Dietary Considerations May be taken without regard to meals.

Pharmacodynamics/Kinetics

Onset of Action Peak effect: Oral: 2-4 hours

Duration of Action Normal renal function: 12-24 hours

Half-life Elimination Beta:
Neonates: ≤35 hours; Mean: 16 hours

Children: 4.6 hours; children >10 years may have prolonged half-life (>5 hours) compared to children 5-10 years (<5 hours)

Adults: Normal renal function: 6-7 hours, prolonged with renal impairment; End-stage renal disease: 15-35 hours

Time to Peak Plasma: Oral: 2-4 hours

Pregnancy Risk Factor D

Pregnancy Considerations Studies in pregnant women have demonstrated a risk to the fetus; therefore, the manufacturer classifies atenolol as pregnancy category D. Atenolol crosses the placenta and is found in cord blood. In a cohort study, an increased risk of cardiovascular defects was observed following maternal use of beta-blockers during pregnancy. Intrauterine growth restriction (IUGR), small placentas, as well as fetal/neonatal bradycardia, hypoglycemia, and/or respiratory depression have been observed following *in utero* exposure to beta-blockers as a class. Adequate facilities for monitoring infants at birth should be available. Untreated chronic maternal hypertension and preeclampsia are also associated with adverse events in the fetus, infant, and mother. The maternal pharmacokinetic parameters of atenolol during the second and third trimesters are within the ranges reported in nonpregnant patients. Although atenolol has shown efficacy in the treatment of hypertension in pregnancy, it is not the drug of choice due to potential IUGR in the infant.

Lactation Enters breast milk/use caution (AAP recommends "use with caution"; AAP 2001 update pending)

Breast-Feeding Considerations Atenolol is excreted in breast milk and has been detected in the serum and urine of nursing infants. Peak concentrations in breast milk have been reported to occur between 2-8 hours after the maternal dose and in some cases are higher than the peak maternal serum concentration. Although most studies have not reported adverse events in nursing infants, avoiding maternal use while nursing infants with renal dysfunction or infants <44 weeks postconceptual age has been suggested. Beta-blockers with less distribution into breast milk may be preferred. The manufacturer recommends that caution be exercised when administering atenolol to nursing women.

Dosage Forms
Tablet, oral: 25 mg, 50 mg, 100 mg
Tenormin®: 25 mg, 50 mg, 100 mg

References
Foster CA and Aston SJ, "Propranolol-Epinephrine Interaction: A Potential Disaster," *Plast Reconstr Surg*, 1983, 72(1):74-8.
Wong DG, Spence JD, Lamki L, et al, "Effect of Nonsteroidal Anti-inflammatory Drugs on Control of Hypertension of Beta-Blockers and Diuretics," *Lancet*, 1986, 1(8488):997-1001.
Wynn RL, "Epinephrine Interactions With Beta-Blockers," *Gen Dent*, 1994, 42(1):16, 18.

Atenolol and Chlorthalidone
(a TEN oh lole & klor THAL i done)

Related Information
Atenolol *on page 141*
Chlorthalidone *on page 297*
Brand Names: U.S. Tenoretic®
Brand Names: Canada Apo-Atenidone®; Novo-Atenolthalidone; Tenoretic®; Teva-Atenolol Chlorthalidone
Pharmacologic Category Beta-Blocker, Beta-1 Selective; Diuretic, Thiazide
Use Treatment of hypertension with a cardioselective beta-blocker and a diuretic
Local Anesthetic/Vasoconstrictor Precautions No information available to require special precautions
Effects on Dental Treatment Atenolol is a cardioselective beta-blocker. Local anesthetic with vasoconstrictor can be safely used in patients medicated with atenolol. Nonselective beta-blockers (ie, propranolol, nadolol) enhance the pressor response to epinephrine, resulting in hypertension and bradycardia; this has not been reported for atenolol. Many nonsteroidal anti-inflammatory drugs, such as ibuprofen and indomethacin, can reduce the hypotensive effect of beta-blockers after 3 or more weeks of therapy with the NSAID. Short-term NSAID use (ie, 3 days) requires no special precautions in patients taking beta-blockers.

Effects on Bleeding No information available to require special precautions
Adverse Effects See individual agents.
General Dosage Range Dosage adjustment recommended in patients with renal impairment.
Oral: *Adults:* Initial: Atenolol 50 mg and chlorthalidone 25 mg once daily; Maintenance: Atenolol 50-100 mg and chlorthalidone 25 mg once daily (maximum dose: Atenolol 100 mg/day; chlorthalidone 25 mg/day)
Pregnancy Risk Factor D
Pregnancy Considerations See individual agents.

AtoMOXetine (AT oh mox e teen)

Brand Names: U.S. Strattera®
Brand Names: Canada Apo-Atomoxetine®; Mylan-Atomoxetine; PMS-Atomoxetine; Sandoz-Atomoxetine; Strattera®; Teva-Atomoxetine
Generic Availability (U.S.) No
Pharmacologic Category Norepinephrine Reuptake Inhibitor, Selective
Use Treatment of attention deficit/hyperactivity disorder (ADHD)
Local Anesthetic/Vasoconstrictor Precautions Use vasoconstrictor with caution. Atomoxetine may increase heart rate or blood pressure in the presence of pressor agents. Pressor agents include the vasoconstrictors epinephrine or mepivacaine and levonordefrin (Carbocaine® 2% with Neo-Cobefrin®)
Effects on Dental Treatment Key adverse event(s) related to dental treatment: Xerostomia (normal salivary flow resumes upon discontinuation)
Effects on Bleeding No information available to require special precautions
Adverse Effects Percentages as reported in children and adults; some adverse reactions may be increased in "poor metabolizers" (CYP2D6).

>10%:
Central nervous system: Headache (2% to 19%), insomnia (2% to 15%), somnolence (4% to 11%)
Gastrointestinal: Xerostomia (21%), nausea (7% to 21%), abdominal pain (7% to 18%), appetite decreased (11% to 16%), vomiting (3% to 11%)
1% to 10%:
Cardiovascular: Systolic blood pressure increased (4% to 5%), diastolic pressure increased (≤4%), palpitation (3%), flushing (≥2%), tachycardia (≤2%), orthostatic hypotension (<2%)
Central nervous system: Fatigue/lethargy (6% to 9%), dizziness (5% to 6%), irritability (≤6%), chills (3%), sleep disturbance (3%), mood swings (1% to 2%)
Dermatologic: Hyperhidrosis (4%), rash (2%)
Endocrine & metabolic: Hot flashes (8%), dysmenorrhea (6%), libido decreased (4%), menstruation disturbance (2%), orgasm abnormal (2%)
Gastrointestinal: Constipation (1% to 9%), dyspepsia (4%), anorexia (<3%), weight loss (2% to 3%)
Genitourinary: Erectile disturbance (9%), urinary hesitation/retention (7%), dysuria (3%), ejaculatory disturbance (3%), prostatitis (2%)
Neuromuscular & skeletal: Paresthesia (3% adults; postmarketing observation in children), tremor (2%)
Ocular: Mydriasis (≥2%)
Respiratory: Sinus headache (3%)
Miscellaneous: Jittery feeling (2%)

◀ **Dosage** Oral: **Note:** Atomoxetine may be discontinued without the need for tapering dose.

ADHD:

U.S. labeling:

Children ≥6 years and ≤70 kg:

Initial: 0.5 mg/kg/day, increase after minimum of 3 days to ~1.2 mg/kg/day; may administer as either a single daily dose or 2 evenly divided doses in morning and late afternoon/early evening. Maximum daily dose: 1.4 mg/kg or 100 mg, whichever is less.

Dosage adjustment in patients receiving strong CYP2D6 inhibitors (eg, paroxetine, fluoxetine, quinidine) or patients known to be CYP2D6 poor metabolizers: Initial: 0.5 mg/kg/day; if tolerating therapy but inadequate response, may increase after minimum of 4 weeks to 1.2 mg/kg/day. Maximum daily dose: 1.2 mg/kg/day.

Children ≥6 years and >70 kg and Adults:

Initial: 40 mg/day, increased after minimum of 3 days to ~80 mg/day; may administer as either a single daily dose or two evenly divided doses in morning and late afternoon/early evening. May increase to 100 mg/day in 2-4 additional weeks to achieve optimal response. Maximum daily dose: 100 mg/day.

Dosage adjustment in patients receiving strong CYP2D6 inhibitors (eg, paroxetine, fluoxetine, quinidine) or patients known to be CYP2D6 poor metabolizers: Initial: 40 mg/day; if tolerating therapy but inadequate response, may increase after minimum of 4 weeks to 80 mg/day. Maximum daily dose: 80 mg/day.

Canadian labeling:

Children ≥6 years and ≤70 kg:

Initial: ~0.5 mg/kg/day for 7-14 days (Step 1); if tolerated, may increase to ~0.8 mg/kg/day for 7-14 days (Step 2), then to ~1.2 mg/kg/day (Step 3); re-evaluate after ≥30 days and adjust for response if necessary. Maximum daily dose: 1.4 mg/kg or 100 mg, whichever is less. **Note:** Children should weigh at least 20 kg at the time of initiation as 10 mg is the lowest available capsule strength and capsules are to be swallowed whole.

Dosing recommendations according to weight:

Initial (Step 1):
20-29 kg: 10 mg/day
30-44 kg: 18 mg/day
45-64 kg: 25 mg/day
65-70 kg: 40 mg/day

First titration (Step 2):
20-29 kg: 18 mg/day
30-44 kg: 25 mg/day
45-64 kg: 40 mg/day
65-70 kg: 60 mg/day

Second titration (Step 3):
20-29 kg: 25 mg/day
30-44 kg: 40 mg/day
45-64 kg: 60 mg/day
65-70 kg: 80 mg/day

Dosage adjustment in patients receiving strong CYP2D6 inhibitors: Initial: 0.5 mg/kg/day; may increase to next dosage level after 14 days if previous dose is well tolerated but response is inadequate. **Note:** Canadian labeling does not include specific dosing recommendations in regards to patients who are poor CYP2D6 metabolizers although similar dose reductions would appear necessary.

Children ≥6 years and >70 kg and Adults:

Initial: 40 mg/day for 7-14 days (Step 1); if tolerated, may increase dose at 7-14 day intervals to 60 mg/day (Step 2) then to 80 mg/day (Step 3). If optimal response is not obtained after 2-4 additional weeks, may increase to a maximum dose of 100 mg/day.

Dosage adjustment in patients receiving strong CYP2D6 inhibitors: Initial: 40 mg/day; may increase to next dosage level after 14 days if previous dose is well tolerated but response is inadequate. **Note:** Canadian labeling does not include specific dosing recommendations in regards to patients who are poor CYP2D6 metabolizers although similar dose reductions would appear necessary.

Elderly: Use has not been evaluated in the elderly

Dosage adjustment in renal impairment: No dosage adjustment necessary

Dosage adjustment in hepatic impairment:

Mild impairment (Child-Pugh class A): No dosage adjustment provided in manufacturer's labeling.

Moderate impairment (Child-Pugh class B): All doses should be reduced to 50% of normal.

Severe impairment (Child-Pugh class C): All doses should be reduced to 25% of normal.

Mechanism of Action Selectively inhibits the reuptake of norepinephrine (Ki 4.5nM) with little to no activity at the other neuronal reuptake pumps or receptor sites.

Contraindications Hypersensitivity to atomoxetine or any component of the formulation; use with or within 14 days of MAO inhibitors; narrow-angle glaucoma; current or past history of pheochromocytoma; severe cardiovascular disorders in which the condition would be expected to deteriorate with clinically relevant blood pressure or heart rate increases

Canadian labeling: Additional contraindications (not in U.S. labeling): Symptomatic cardiovascular diseases, moderate-to-severe hypertension; advanced arteriosclerosis; uncontrolled hyperthyroidism

Warnings/Precautions [U.S. Boxed Warning]: Use caution in pediatric patients; may be an increased risk of suicidal ideation. Closely monitor for clinical worsening, suicidality, or unusual changes in behavior; especially during the initial few months of a course of drug therapy, or at times of dose changes, either increases or decreases. The child's family or caregiver should be instructed to closely observe the patient and communicate condition with healthcare provider. New or worsening symptoms of hostility or aggressive behaviors have been associated with atomoxetine, particularly with the initiation of therapy. Use caution in patients with a history of psychotic illness or bipolar disorder; therapy may induce mixed/manic disorder or psychotic symptoms. Atomoxetine is not approved for major depressive disorder. Patients presenting with depressive symptoms should be screened for bipolar disorder. Recommended to be used as part of a comprehensive treatment program for attention deficit disorders. Atomoxetine does not worsen anxiety in patients with existing anxiety disorders or tics related to Tourette's disorder.

Use caution with hepatic disease (dosage adjustments necessary in hepatic impairment). Use may be associated with rare but severe hepatotoxicity; discontinue and do not restart if signs or symptoms of hepatotoxic reaction (eg, jaundice, pruritus, flu-like symptoms) or laboratory evidence of liver disease are noted. Use caution in patients who are poor metabolizers of CYP2D6 metabolized drugs ("poor metabolizers"), bioavailability increases; dosage adjustments are recommended in patients known to be CYP2D6 poor metabolizers.

Orthostasis can occur; use caution in patients predisposed to hypotension or those with abrupt changes in heart rate or blood pressure. CNS stimulant use has been associated with serious cardiovascular events including sudden death in patients with pre-existing structural cardiac abnormalities or other serious heart problems (sudden death in children and adolescents; sudden death, stroke, and MI in adults). These products should be avoided in patients with known serious structural cardiac abnormalities, cardiomyopathy, serious heart rhythm abnormalities, or other serious cardiac problems that could increase the risk of sudden death that these conditions alone carry. Patients should be carefully evaluated for cardiac disease prior to initiation of therapy. May cause increased heart rate or blood pressure; use caution with hypertension or other cardiovascular disease; CYP2D6 poor metabolizers may experience greater increases in blood pressure and heart rate effects. Use caution with renal impairment. May cause urinary retention/hesitancy; use caution in patients with history of urinary retention or bladder outlet obstruction. Priapism has been associated with use (rarely). Allergic reactions (including angioneurotic edema, urticaria, and rash) may occur (rare).

Growth should be monitored during treatment. Height and weight gain may be reduced during the first 9-12 months of treatment, but should recover by 3 years of therapy. Safety and efficacy have not been evaluated in pediatric patients <6 years of age.

Drug Interactions

Metabolism/Transport Effects Substrate of CYP2C19 (minor), CYP2D6 (major); **Note:** Assignment of Major/Minor substrate status based on clinically relevant drug interaction potential; **Inhibits** CYP2D6 (weak), CYP3A4 (weak)

Avoid Concomitant Use

Avoid concomitant use of AtoMOXetine with any of the following: Iobenguane I 123; MAO Inhibitors; Pimozide

Increased Effect/Toxicity

AtoMOXetine may increase the levels/effects of: ARIPiprazole; Beta2-Agonists; Lomitapide; Pimozide; Sympathomimetics

The levels/effects of AtoMOXetine may be increased by: Abiraterone Acetate; CYP2D6 Inhibitors (Moderate); CYP2D6 Inhibitors (Strong); Darunavir; MAO Inhibitors

Decreased Effect

AtoMOXetine may decrease the levels/effects of: Iobenguane I 123

The levels/effects of AtoMOXetine may be decreased by: Peginterferon Alfa-2b

Ethanol/Nutrition/Herb Interactions Ethanol: May increase CNS depression; monitor for increased effects with coadministration. Caution patients about effects.

Dietary Considerations May be taken with or without food.

Pharmacodynamics/Kinetics

Half-life Elimination Atomoxetine: 5 hours (up to 24 hours in poor metabolizers); Active metabolites: 4-hydroxyatomoxetine: 6-8 hours; N-desmethylatomoxetine: 6-8 hours (34-40 hours in poor metabolizers)

Time to Peak Plasma: 1-2 hours

Pregnancy Risk Factor C

Pregnancy Considerations Decreased pup weight and survival were observed in animal studies. There are no adequate and well-controlled studies in pregnant women. Use only if potential benefit to the mother outweighs possible risk to fetus.

Lactation Excretion in breast milk unknown/use caution

Dosage Forms

Capsule, oral:
Strattera®: 10 mg, 18 mg, 25 mg, 40 mg, 60 mg, 80 mg, 100 mg

AtorvaSTATin (a TORE va sta tin)

Related Information
Cardiovascular Diseases *on page 1492*

Brand Names: U.S. Lipitor®

Brand Names: Canada Apo-Atorvastatin®; Ava-Atorvastatin; CO Atorvastatin; Dom-Atorvastatin; GD-Atorvastatin; Lipitor®; Mylan-Atorvastatin; Novo-Atorvastatin; PMS-Atorvastatin; RAN™-Atorvastatin; ratio-Atorvastatin; Sandoz-Atorvastatin

Generic Availability (U.S.) Yes

Pharmacologic Category Antilipemic Agent, HMG-CoA Reductase Inhibitor

Use Treatment of dyslipidemias or primary prevention of cardiovascular disease (atherosclerotic) as detailed below:

Primary prevention of cardiovascular disease (high-risk for CVD): To reduce the risk of MI or stroke in patients without evidence of heart disease who have multiple CVD risk factors or type 2 diabetes. Treatment reduces the risk for angina or revascularization procedures in patients with multiple risk factors.

Secondary prevention of cardiovascular disease: To reduce the risk of nonfatal MI, nonfatal stroke, revascularization procedures, hospitalization for heart failure, and angina in patients with evidence of coronary heart disease.

Treatment of dyslipidemias: To reduce elevations in total cholesterol (C), LDL-C, apolipoprotein B, and triglycerides in patients with elevations of one or more components, and/or to increase low HDL-C as present in Fredrickson type IIa, IIb, III, and IV hyperlipidemias, heterozygous familial and nonfamilial hypercholesterolemia, and homozygous familial hypercholesterolemia

Treatment of heterozygous familial hypercholesterolemia (HeFH) in adolescent patients (10-17 years of age, females >1 year postmenarche) having LDL-C ≥190 mg/dL or LDL-C ≥160 mg/dL with positive family history of premature cardiovascular disease (CVD) or with two or more CVD risk factors.

Unlabeled Use Secondary prevention in patients who have experienced a noncardioembolic stroke/TIA or following an ACS event regardless of baseline LDL-C using intensive lipid-lowering therapy

Local Anesthetic/Vasoconstrictor Precautions No information available to require special precautions

Effects on Dental Treatment No significant effects or complications reported

Effects on Bleeding No information available to require special precautions

Adverse Effects

>10%:
Gastrointestinal: Diarrhea (5% to 14%)
Neuromuscular & skeletal: Arthralgia (4% to 12%)
Respiratory: Nasopharyngitis (4% to 13%)

2% to 10%:
Central nervous system: Insomnia (1% to 5%)
Gastrointestinal: Nausea (4% to 7%), dyspepsia (3% to 6%)
Genitourinary: Urinary tract infection (4% to 8%)
Hepatic: Transaminases increased (2% to 3% with 80 mg/day dosing)
Neuromuscular & skeletal: Limb pain (3% to 9%), myalgia (3% to 8%), muscle spasms (2% to 5%), musculoskeletal pain (2% to 5%)
Respiratory: Pharyngolaryngeal pain (1% to 4%)
Additional class-related events or case reports (not necessarily reported with atorvastatin therapy): Cataracts, cirrhosis, dermatomyositis, eosinophilia, erectile dysfunction, extraocular muscle movement impaired, fulminant hepatic necrosis, gynecomastia, hemolytic anemia, immune-mediated necrotizing myopathy (IMNM), interstitial lung disease, ophthalmoplegia, peripheral nerve palsy, polymyalgia rheumatica, positive ANA, renal failure (secondary to rhabdomyolysis), systemic lupus erythematosus-like syndrome, thyroid dysfunction, tremor, vasculitis, vertigo

Dosage Oral:
Primary prevention: Note: Doses should be individualized according to the baseline LDL-cholesterol concentrations, the recommended goal of therapy, and patient response; adjustments should be made at intervals of 2-4 weeks (4 weeks for children)
Children 10-17 years (females >1 year postmenarche): HeFH: 10 mg once daily (maximum: 20 mg/day)
Adults:
Hypercholesterolemia (heterozygous familial and nonfamilial) and mixed hyperlipidemia (Fredrickson types IIa and IIb): Initial: 10-20 mg once daily; patients requiring >45% reduction in LDL-C may be started at 40 mg once daily; range: 10-80 mg once daily
Homozygous familial hypercholesterolemia: 10-80 mg once daily
Secondary prevention:
Clinically-evident coronary heart disease: Initial: 80 mg once daily; adjust based on patient tolerability and recommended goal LDL-C (LaRosa, 2005)
Intensive lipid-lowering after an ACS event regardless of baseline LDL (unlabeled use): Initial: 80 mg once daily; adjust based on patient tolerability and recommended goal LDL-C (Cannon, 2004; Pederson, 2005; Schwartz, 2001). **Note:** Currently, the ACC/AHA guidelines for UA/NSTEMI do not specify which statin to use (Anderson, 2007).
Noncardioembolic stroke/TIA (unlabeled use): Initial: 80 mg once daily; adjust based on patient tolerability and recommended goal LDL-C (Adams, 2008; Amarenco, 2006)

Dosage adjustment for atorvastatin with concomitant medications:
Boceprevir, nelfinavir: Use lowest effective atorvastatin dose (not to exceed 40 mg daily)
Clarithromycin, itraconazole, fosamprenavir, ritonavir (plus darunavir, fosamprenavir, or saquinavir): Use lowest effective atorvastatin dose (not to exceed 20 mg daily)
Lomitapide: Consider atorvastatin dose reduction (per lomitapide manufacturer).

Dosing adjustment in renal impairment: No dosage adjustment is necessary.

Dosing adjustment in hepatic impairment: Contraindicated in active liver disease or in patients with unexplained persistent elevations of serum transaminases.

Mechanism of Action Inhibitor of 3-hydroxy-3-methylglutaryl coenzyme A (HMG-CoA) reductase, the rate-limiting enzyme in cholesterol synthesis (reduces the production of mevalonic acid from HMG-CoA); this then results in a compensatory increase in the expression of LDL receptors on hepatocyte membranes and a stimulation of LDL catabolism

Contraindications Hypersensitivity to atorvastatin or any component of the formulation; active liver disease; unexplained persistent elevations of serum transaminases; pregnancy; breast-feeding

Note: Telaprevir Canadian product monograph contraindicates use with atorvastatin.

Warnings/Precautions Secondary causes of hyperlipidemia should be ruled out prior to therapy. Atorvastatin has not been studied when the primary lipid abnormality is chylomicron elevation (Fredrickson types I and V). Liver function tests must be obtained prior to initiating therapy, repeat if clinically indicated thereafter. May cause hepatic dysfunction. Use with caution in patients who consume large amounts of ethanol or have a history of liver disease; use is contraindicated in patients with active liver disease or unexplained persistent elevations of serum transaminases. Monitoring is recommended. Patients with a history of hemorrhagic stroke may be at increased risk for another hemorrhagic stroke with use.

Rhabdomyolysis with acute renal failure has occurred. Risk is dose related and is increased with concurrent use of lipid-lowering agents which may cause rhabdomyolysis (fibric acid derivatives or niacin at doses ≥1 g/day) or during concurrent use with potent CYP3A4 inhibitors (including amiodarone, clarithromycin, erythromycin, itraconazole, ketoconazole, nefazodone, grapefruit juice in large quantities, verapamil, or protease inhibitors such as indinavir, nelfinavir, or ritonavir). Ensure patient is on the lowest effective atorvastatin dose. If concurrent use of clarithromycin or combination protease inhibitors (eg, lopinavir/ritonavir or ritonavir/saquinavir) is warranted consider dose adjustment of atorvastatin. Do not use with cyclosporine, gemfibrozil, tipranavir plus ritonavir, or telaprevir. Monitor closely if used with other drugs associated with myopathy. Weigh the risk versus benefit when combining any of these drugs with atorvastatin. Discontinue in any patient in which CPK levels are markedly elevated (>10 times ULN) or if myopathy is suspected/diagnosed. The manufacturer recommends temporary discontinuation for elective major surgery, acute medical or surgical conditions, or in any patient experiencing an acute or serious condition predisposing to renal failure (eg, sepsis, hypotension, trauma, uncontrolled seizures). However, based upon current evidence, HMG-CoA reductase inhibitor therapy should be continued in the perioperative period unless risk outweighs cardioprotective benefit. Use with caution in patients with advanced age, these patients are predisposed to myopathy. Immune-mediated necrotizing myopathy (IMNM), an autoimmune-mediated myopathy, has been reported (rarely) with HMG-CoA reductase inhibitor therapy.

IMNM presents as proximal muscle weakness with elevated CPK levels, which persists despite discontinuation of HMG-CoA reductase inhibitor therapy; additionally, muscle biopsy may show necrotizing myopathy with limited inflammation; immunosuppressive therapy (eg, corticosteroids, azathioprine) may be used for treatment.

Drug Interactions

Metabolism/Transport Effects Substrate of CYP3A4 (major), P-glycoprotein, SLCO1B1; **Note:** Assignment of Major/Minor substrate status based on clinically relevant drug interaction potential; **Inhibits** CYP3A4 (weak), P-glycoprotein

Avoid Concomitant Use

Avoid concomitant use of AtorvaSTATin with any of the following: Bosutinib; Conivaptan; CycloSPORINE (Systemic); Fusidic Acid; Gemfibrozil; Pimozide; Pomalidomide; Posaconazole; Red Yeast Rice; Silodosin; Telaprevir; Tipranavir; Topotecan; VinCRIStine (Liposomal)

Increased Effect/Toxicity

AtorvaSTATin may increase the levels/effects of: Aliskiren; ARIPiprazole; Bosutinib; DAPTOmycin; Digoxin; Diltiazem; Everolimus; Ketoconazole (Systemic); Lomitapide; Midazolam; Pazopanib; P-glycoprotein/ABCB1 Substrates; Pimozide; Pomalidomide; Prucalopride; Rivaroxaban; Silodosin; Topotecan; Trabectedin; Verapamil; VinCRIStine (Liposomal)

The levels/effects of AtorvaSTATin may be increased by: Amiodarone; Bezafibrate; Boceprevir; Cobicistat; Colchicine; Conivaptan; CycloSPORINE (Systemic); CYP3A4 Inhibitors (Moderate); CYP3A4 Inhibitors (Strong); Cyproterone; Danazol; Dasatinib; Diltiazem; Dronedarone; Eltrombopag; Fenofibrate; Fenofibric Acid; Fluconazole; Fusidic Acid; Gemfibrozil; Grapefruit Juice; Itraconazole; Ivacaftor; Ketoconazole (Systemic); Macrolide Antibiotics; Mifepristone; Niacin; Niacinamide; P-glycoprotein/ABCB1 Inhibitors; Posaconazole; Protease Inhibitors; QuiNINE; Red Yeast Rice; Sildenafil; Telaprevir; Tipranavir; Verapamil; Voriconazole

Decreased Effect

AtorvaSTATin may decrease the levels/effects of: Dabigatran Etexilate; Lanthanum

The levels/effects of AtorvaSTATin may be decreased by: Antacids; Bexarotene (Systemic); Bile Acid Sequestrants; Bosentan; CYP3A4 Inducers (Strong); Deferasirox; Efavirenz; Etravirine; Fosphenytoin; P-glycoprotein/ABCB1 Inducers; Phenytoin; Rifamycin Derivatives; St Johns Wort; Tocilizumab

Ethanol/Nutrition/Herb Interactions

Ethanol: Ethanol may enhance the potential of adverse hepatic effects. Management: Avoid excessive ethanol consumption.

Food: Atorvastatin serum concentrations may be increased by grapefruit juice. Management: Avoid concurrent intake of large quantities of grapefruit juice (>1 quart/day). Red yeast rice contains an estimated 2.4 mg lovastatin per 600 mg rice.

Herb/Nutraceutical: St John's wort may decrease atorvastatin levels.

Dietary Considerations May take with food if desired; may take without regard to time of day. Before initiation of therapy, patients should be placed on a standard cholesterol-lowering diet for 3-6 months and the diet should be continued during drug therapy. Red yeast rice contains an estimated 2.4 mg lovastatin per 600 mg rice. Atorvastatin serum concentration may be increased when taken with grapefruit juice; avoid concurrent intake of large quantities (>1 quart/day).

Pharmacodynamics/Kinetics

Onset of Action Initial changes: 3-5 days; Maximal reduction in plasma cholesterol and triglycerides: 2 weeks

Half-life Elimination Parent drug: 14 hours; Equipotent metabolites: 20-30 hours

Time to Peak Serum: 1-2 hours

Pregnancy Risk Factor X

Pregnancy Considerations Adverse events were observed in animal reproductions studies. There are reports of congenital anomalies following maternal use of HMG-CoA reductase inhibitors in pregnancy; however, maternal disease, differences in specific agents used, and the low rates of exposure limit the interpretation of the available data (Godfrey, 2012; Lecarpentier, 2012). Cholesterol biosynthesis may be important in fetal development; serum cholesterol and triglycerides increase normally during pregnancy. The discontinuation of lipid lowering medications temporarily during pregnancy is not expected to have significant impact on the long term outcomes of primary hypercholesterolemia treatment.

Use of atorvastatin is contraindicated in pregnancy. HMG-CoA reductase inhibitors should be discontinued prior to pregnancy (ADA, 2013). If treatment of dyslipidemias is needed in pregnant women or in women of reproductive age, other agents are preferred (Berglund, 2012; NCEP, 2002). The manufacturer recommends administration to women of childbearing potential only when conception is highly unlikely and patients have been informed of potential hazards.

Lactation Excretion in breast milk unknown/contraindicated

Breast-Feeding Considerations It is not known if atorvastatin is excreted into breast milk. Due to the potential for serious adverse reactions in a nursing infant, use while breast-feeding is contraindicated by the manufacturer.

Dosage Forms

Tablet, oral: 10 mg, 20 mg, 40 mg, 80 mg
Lipitor®: 10 mg, 20 mg, 40 mg, 80 mg

References

Siedlik PH, Olson, SC, Yang BB, et al, "Erythromycin Coadministration Increases Plasma Atorvastatin Concentrations," *J Clin Pharmacol*, 1999, 39(5):501-4.

Atovaquone (a TOE va kwone)

Related Information
Systemic Viral Diseases *on page 1537*

Brand Names: U.S. Mepron®

Brand Names: Canada Mepron®

Pharmacologic Category Antiprotozoal

Use Acute oral treatment of mild-to-moderate *Pneumocystis jirovecii* pneumonia (PCP) in patients who are intolerant to co-trimoxazole; prophylaxis of PCP in patients who are intolerant to co-trimoxazole

Unlabeled Use Treatment of babesiosis; treatment/suppression of *Toxoplasma gondii* encephalitis; primary prophylaxis of HIV-infected persons at high risk for developing *Toxoplasma gondii* encephalitis

Local Anesthetic/Vasoconstrictor Precautions No information available to require special precautions

Effects on Dental Treatment Key adverse event(s) related to dental treatment: Oral moniliasis

Effects on Bleeding No information available to require special precautions

◄ **Adverse Effects Note:** Adverse reaction statistics have been compiled from studies including patients with advanced HIV disease; consequently, it is difficult to distinguish reactions attributed to atovaquone from those caused by the underlying disease or a combination thereof.

>10%:
Central nervous system: Fever (14% to 40%), headache (16% to 31%), insomnia (10% to 19%), depression, pain
Dermatologic: Rash (22% to 46%), pruritus (5% to ≥10%)
Gastrointestinal: Diarrhea (19% to 42%), nausea (21% to 32%), vomiting (14% to 22%), abdominal pain (4% to 21%)
Neuromuscular & skeletal: Weakness (8% to 31%), myalgia
Respiratory: Cough (14% to 25%), rhinitis (5% to 24%), dyspnea (15% to 21%), sinusitis (7% to ≥10%)
Miscellaneous: Infection (18% to 22%), diaphoresis, flu-like syndrome

1% to 10%:
Cardiovascular: Hypotension (≤1%)
Central nervous system: Dizziness (3% to 8%), anxiety (≤7%)
Endocrine & metabolic: Hyponatremia (7% to 10%), hyperglycemia (≤9%), hypoglycemia (≤1%)
Gastrointestinal: Amylase increased (7% to 8%), anorexia (≤7%), dyspepsia (≤5%), constipation (≤3%), taste perversion (≤3%)
Hematologic: Anemia (4% to 6%), neutropenia (3% to 5%)
Hepatic: Liver enzymes increased (4% to 8%)
Renal: BUN increased (≤1%), creatinine increased (≤1%)
Respiratory: Bronchospasm (2% to 4%)
Miscellaneous: Oral moniliasis (5% to 10%)

General Dosage Range Oral: *Children 13-16 years and Adults:* 1500 mg/day in 1-2 divided doses
Mechanism of Action Inhibits electron transport in mitochondria resulting in the inhibition of key metabolic enzymes responsible for the synthesis of nucleic acids and ATP
Pharmacodynamics/Kinetics
Half-life Elimination 1.5-4 days
Pregnancy Risk Factor C
Pregnancy Considerations There are no adequate and well-controlled studies of atovaquone in pregnant women. Use in pregnant women only if the potential benefit outweighs the possible risk to the fetus.

Atovaquone and Proguanil
(a TOE va kwone & pro GWA nil)

Related Information
Atovaquone *on page 147*
Brand Names: U.S. Malarone®
Brand Names: Canada Malarone®; Malarone® Pediatric
Pharmacologic Category Antimalarial Agent
Use Prevention or treatment of acute, uncomplicated *P. falciparum* malaria
Local Anesthetic/Vasoconstrictor Precautions No information available to require special precautions
Effects on Dental Treatment No significant effects or complications reported
Effects on Bleeding No information available to require special precautions

Adverse Effects The following adverse reactions were reported in patients being treated for malaria. When used for prophylaxis, reactions are similar to those seen with placebo.

>10%:
Gastrointestinal: Abdominal pain (17%), nausea (12%), vomiting (children 10% to 13%, adults 12%)
Hepatic: Transaminase increases (ALT 27%, AST 17%; increased LFT values typically normalized after ~4 weeks)

1% to 10%:
Central nervous system: Headache (10%), dizziness (5%)
Dermatologic: Pruritus (children 6%)
Gastrointestinal: Diarrhea (children 6%, adults 8%), anorexia (5%)
Neuromuscular & skeletal: Weakness (8%)

General Dosage Range Oral:
Children 5-8 kg: Treatment: 125 mg/50 mg as a single daily dose
Children 9-10 kg: Treatment: 187.5 mg/75 mg as a single daily dose
Children 11-20 kg: Prophylaxis: 62.5 mg/25 mg; Treatment: 250 mg/100 mg as a single daily dose
Children 21-30 kg: Prophylaxis: 125 mg/50 mg; Treatment: 500 mg/200 mg as a single daily dose
Children 31-40 kg: Prophylaxis: 187.5 mg/75 mg; Treatment: 750 mg/300 mg as a single daily dose
Children >40 kg and Adults: Prophylaxis: 250 mg/100 mg; Treatment: 1 g/400 mg as a single daily dose

Mechanism of Action
Atovaquone: Selectively inhibits parasite mitochondrial electron transport.
Proguanil: The metabolite cycloguanil inhibits dihydrofolate reductase, disrupting deoxythymidylate synthesis. Together, atovaquone/cycloguanil affect the erythrocytic and exoerythrocytic stages of development.

Pharmacodynamics/Kinetics
Half-life Elimination Proguanil: 12-21 hours
Time to Peak Proguanil: Plasma: 2-4 hours
Pregnancy Risk Factor C
Pregnancy Considerations Teratogenic effects were not observed with the combination of atovaquone/proguanil in animal reproduction studies using concentrations similar to the estimated human exposure. The pharmacokinetics of atovaquone and proguanil are changed during pregnancy. Malaria infection in pregnant women may be more severe than in nonpregnant women. Because *P. falciparum* malaria can cause maternal death and fetal loss, pregnant women traveling to malaria-endemic areas must use personal protection against mosquito bites. Atovaquone/proguanil may be used as an alternative treatment of malaria in pregnant women; consult current CDC guidelines.

Atropine (A troe peen)

Related Information
Dentin Hypersensitivity, Acid Erosion, High Caries Index, Management of Alveolar Osteitis, and Xerostomia *on page 1582*
Brand Names: U.S. AtroPen®; Atropine Care™; Isopto® Atropine
Brand Names: Canada Dioptic's Atropine Solution; Isopto® Atropine
Generic Availability (U.S.) Yes

Pharmacologic Category Anticholinergic Agent; Anticholinergic Agent, Ophthalmic; Antidote; Antispasmodic Agent, Gastrointestinal; Ophthalmic Agent, Mydriatic

Dental Use Reduction of salivation and bronchial secretions

Use

Injection: Preoperative medication to inhibit salivation and secretions; treatment of symptomatic sinus bradycardia, AV block (nodal level); antidote for anticholinesterase poisoning (carbamate insecticides, nerve agents, organophosphate insecticides); adjuvant use with anticholinesterases (eg, edrophonium, neostigmine) to decrease their side effects during reversal of neuromuscular blockade

Note: Use is no longer recommended in the management of asystole or pulseless electrical activity (PEA) (ACLS, 2010).

Ophthalmic: Produce mydriasis and cycloplegia for examination of the retina and optic disc and accurate measurement of refractive errors; produce papillary dilation in inflammatory conditions (eg, uveitis)

Local Anesthetic/Vasoconstrictor Precautions No information available to require special precautions

Effects on Dental Treatment Key adverse event(s) related to dental treatment: Xerostomia and changes in salivation (normal salivary flow resumes upon discontinuation), dry throat, and nasal dryness

Effects on Bleeding No information available to require special precautions

Adverse Effects Severity and frequency of adverse reactions are dose related and vary greatly; listed reactions are limited to significant and/or life-threatening.

Cardiovascular: Arrhythmia, flushing, hypotension, palpitation, tachycardia

Central nervous system: Ataxia, coma, delirium, disorientation, dizziness, drowsiness, excitement, fever, hallucinations, headache, insomnia, nervousness

Dermatologic: Anhidrosis, urticaria, rash, scarlatiniform rash

Gastrointestinal: Bloating, constipation, delayed gastric emptying, loss of taste, nausea, paralytic ileus, vomiting, xerostomia, dry throat, nasal dryness

Genitourinary: Urinary hesitancy, urinary retention

Neuromuscular & skeletal: Weakness

Ocular: Angle-closure glaucoma, blurred vision, cycloplegia, dry eyes, mydriasis, ocular tension increased

Respiratory: Dyspnea, laryngospasm, pulmonary edema

Miscellaneous: Anaphylaxis

Dental Usual Dosage Inhibit salivation and secretions (preanesthesia): Adults (doses <0.5 mg have been associated with paradoxical bradycardia):

I.M., I.V., SubQ: 0.4-0.6 mg 30-60 minutes preop and repeat every 4-6 hours as needed

Dosage

Infants and Children: Doses <0.1 mg have been associated with paradoxical bradycardia.

Inhibit salivation and secretions (preanesthesia): I.M., I.V., SubQ:

<5 kg: 0.02 mg/kg/dose 30-60 minutes preop then every 4-6 hours as needed. Use of a minimum dosage of 0.1 mg in neonates <5 kg will result in dosages >0.02 mg/kg. There is no documented minimum dosage in this age group.

>5 kg: 0.01-0.02 mg/kg/dose to a maximum 0.4 mg/dose 30-60 minutes preop; minimum dose: 0.1 mg

Alternate dosing:
3-7 kg (7-16 lb): 0.1 mg
8-11 kg (17-24 lb): 0.15 mg

11-18 kg (24-40 lb): 0.2 mg
18-29 kg (40-65 lb): 0.3 mg
>30 kg (>65 lb): 0.4 mg

Bradycardia:

I.V., I.O.: 0.02 mg/kg, minimum dose recommended by PALS: 0.1 mg; however, use of a minimum dosage of 0.1 mg in patients <5 kg will result in dosages >0.02 mg/kg and is not recommended (Barrington, 2011); there is no documented minimum dosage in this age group; maximum single dose: 0.5 mg; may repeat once in 3-5 minutes; maximum total dose: 1 mg (PALS, 2010).

Endotracheal: 0.04-0.06 mg/kg; may repeat once if needed (PALS, 2010)

Children: Organophosphate or carbamate insecticide or nerve agent poisoning: **Note:** The dose of atropine required varies considerably with the severity of poisoning. The total amount of atropine used for carbamate poisoning is usually less than with organophosphate insecticide or nerve agent poisoning. Severely poisoned patients may exhibit significant tolerance to atropine; ≥2 times the suggested doses may be needed. Titrate to pulmonary status (decreased bronchial secretions); consider administration of atropine via continuous I.V. infusion in patients requiring large doses of atropine. Once patient is stable for a period of time, the dose/dosing frequency may be decreased. Pralidoxime is a component of the management of organophosphate insecticide and nerve agent toxicity.

I.V., I.M. (unlabeled dose): Initial: 0.05-0.1 mg/kg; repeat every 5-10 minutes as needed, doubling the dose if previous dose does not induce atropinization (Hegenbarth, 2008; Rotenberg, 2003). Maintain atropinization by administering repeat doses as needed for ≥2-12 hours based on recurrence of symptoms (Reigart, 1999).

I.V. infusion (unlabeled dose): Following atropinization, administer 10% to 20% of the total loading dose required to induce atropinization as a continuous I.V. infusion per hour; adjust as needed to maintain adequate atropinization without atropine toxicity (Eddleston, 2004b; Roberts, 2007).

I.M. (AtroPen®):

Mild symptoms (≥2 mild symptoms): Administer the weight-based dose listed below as soon as an exposure is known or strongly suspected. If severe symptoms develop after the first dose, 2 additional doses should be repeated in rapid succession 10 minutes after the first dose; do not administer more than 3 doses. If profound anticholinergic effects occur in the absence of excessive bronchial secretions, further doses of atropine should be withheld.

Severe symptoms (≥1 severe symptoms): Immediately administer **three** weight-based doses in rapid succession.

Weight-based dosing:
<6.8 kg (15 lb): 0.25 mg/dose
6.8-18 kg (15-40 lb): 0.5 mg/dose
18-41 kg (40-90 lb): 1 mg/dose
>41 kg (>90 lb): 2 mg/dose

Symptoms of insecticide or nerve agent poisoning, as provided by manufacturer in the AtroPen® product labeling, to guide therapy:

Mild symptoms: Blurred vision, bradycardia, breathing difficulties, chest tightness, coughing, drooling, miosis, muscular twitching, nausea, runny nose, salivation increased, stomach cramps, tachycardia, teary eyes, tremor, vomiting, or wheezing

◀ Severe symptoms: Breathing difficulties (severe), confused/strange behavior, defecation (involuntary), muscular twitching/generalized weakness (severe), respiratory secretions (severe), seizure, unconsciousness, urination (involuntary); **Note:** Infants may become drowsy or unconscious with muscle floppiness as opposed to muscle twitching.

Endotracheal (unlabeled route): Increase the dose by 2-3 times the usual I.V. dose. Mix with 3-5 mL of normal saline and administer. Flush with 3-5 mL of NS and follow with 5 assisted manual ventilations (Rotenberg, 2003).

Adults (doses <0.5 mg have been associated with paradoxical bradycardia):

Inhibit salivation and secretions (preanesthesia): I.M., I.V., SubQ: 0.4-0.6 mg 30-60 minutes preop and repeat every 4-6 hours as needed

Bradycardia: **Note:** Atropine may be ineffective in heart transplant recipients: I.V.: 0.5 mg every 3-5 minutes, not to exceed a total of 3 mg or 0.04 mg/kg (ACLS, 2010)

Neuromuscular blockade reversal: I.V.: 25-30 mcg/kg 30-60 seconds before neostigmine or 7-10 mcg/kg 30-60 seconds before edrophonium

Organophosphate or carbamate insecticide or nerve agent poisoning: **Note:** The dose of atropine required varies considerably with the severity of poisoning. The total amount of atropine used for carbamate poisoning is usually less than with organophosphate insecticide or nerve agent poisoning. Severely poisoned patients may exhibit significant tolerance to atropine; ≥2 times the suggested doses may be needed. Titrate to pulmonary status (decreased bronchial secretions); consider administration of atropine via continuous I.V. infusion in patients requiring large doses of atropine. Once patient is stable for a period of time, the dose/dosing frequency may be decreased. Pralidoxime is a component of the management of organophosphate insecticide and nerve agent toxicity.

I.V., I.M. (unlabeled dose): Initial: 1-6 mg (ATSDR, 2011; Roberts, 2007); repeat every 3-5 minutes as needed, doubling the dose if previous dose did not induce atropinization (Eddleston, 2004b; Roberts, 2007). Maintain atropinization by administering repeat doses as needed for ≥2-12 hours based on recurrence of symptoms (Reigart, 1999).

I.V. Infusion (unlabeled dose): Following atropinization, administer 10% to 20% of the total loading dose required to induce atropinization as a continuous I.V. infusion per hour; adjust as needed to maintain adequate atropinization without atropine toxicity (Eddleston, 2004b; Roberts, 2007)

I.M. (AtroPen®):

Mild symptoms (≥2 mild symptoms): Administer 2 mg as soon as an exposure is known or strongly suspected. If severe symptoms develop after the first dose, 2 additional doses should be repeated in rapid succession 10 minutes after the first dose; do not administer more than 3 doses. If profound anticholinergic effects occur in the absence of excessive bronchial secretions, further doses of atropine should be withheld.

Severe symptoms (≥1 severe symptoms): Immediately administer **three** 2 mg doses in rapid succession.

Symptoms of insecticide or nerve agent poisoning, as provided by manufacturer in the AtroPen® product labeling, to guide therapy:

Mild symptoms: Blurred vision, bradycardia, breathing difficulties, chest tightness, coughing, drooling, miosis, muscular twitching, nausea, runny nose, salivation increased, stomach cramps, tachycardia, teary eyes, tremor, vomiting, or wheezing

Severe symptoms: Breathing difficulties (severe), confused/strange behavior, defecation (involuntary), muscular twitching/generalized weakness (severe), respiratory secretions (severe), seizure, unconsciousness, urination (involuntary)

Mydriasis, cycloplegia (preprocedure): Ophthalmic (1% solution): Instill 1-2 drops 1 hour before procedure.

Uveitis: Ophthalmic:

1% solution: Instill 1-2 drops up to 4 times/day

Ointment: Apply a small amount in the conjunctival sac up to 3 times/day; compress the lacrimal sac by digital pressure for 1-3 minutes after instillation

Dosage adjustment in renal impairment: No dosage adjustment provided in manufacturer's labeling.

Dosage adjustment in hepatic impairment: No dosage adjustment provided in manufacturer's labeling.

Mechanism of Action Blocks the action of acetylcholine at parasympathetic sites in smooth muscle, secretory glands, and the CNS; increases cardiac output, dries secretions. Atropine reverses the muscarinic effects of cholinergic poisoning due to agents with acetylcholinesterase inhibitor activity by acting as a competitive antagonist of acetylcholine at muscarinic receptors. The primary goal in cholinergic poisonings is reversal of bronchorrhea and bronchoconstriction. Atropine has no effect on the nicotinic receptors responsible for muscle weakness, fasciculations, and paralysis.

Contraindications Hypersensitivity to atropine or any component of the formulation; narrow-angle glaucoma; adhesions between the iris and lens (ophthalmic product); pyloric stenosis; prostatic hypertrophy.

Note: No contraindications exist in the treatment of life-threatening organophosphate or carbamate insecticide or nerve agent poisoning.

Warnings/Precautions Heat prostration may occur in the presence of high environmental temperatures. Psychosis may occur in sensitive individuals or following use of excessive doses. Avoid use if possible in patients with obstructive uropathy or in other conditions resulting in urinary retention; use is contraindicated in patients with prostatic hypertrophy. Avoid use in patients with paralytic ileus, intestinal atony of the elderly or debilitated patient, severe ulcerative colitis, and toxic megacolon complicating ulcerative colitis. Use with caution in patients with autonomic neuropathy, hyperthyroidism, renal or hepatic impairment, myocardial ischemia, HF, tachyarrhythmias (including sinus tachycardia), hypertension, and hiatal hernia associated with reflux esophagitis. Treatment-related blood pressure increases and tachycardia may lead to ischemia, precipitate an MI, or increase arrhythmogenic potential. In heart transplant recipients, atropine will likely be ineffective in treatment of bradycardia due to lack of vagal innervation of the transplanted heart; cholinergic reinnervation may occur over time (years), so atropine may be used cautiously; however, some may experience paradoxical slowing of the heart rate and high-degree AV block upon administration (ACLS, 2010; Bernheim, 2004).

Avoid relying on atropine for effective treatment of type II second-degree or third-degree AV block (with or without a new wide QRS complex). Asystole or bradycardic pulseless electrical activity (PEA): Although no evidence exists for significant detrimental effects, routine use is unlikely to have a therapeutic benefit and is no longer recommended (ACLS, 2010).

AtroPen®: There are no absolute contraindications for the use of atropine in severe organophosphate or carbamate insecticide or nerve agent poisonings; however in mild poisonings, use caution in those patients where the use of atropine would be otherwise contraindicated. Formulation for use by trained personnel only. Clinical symptoms consistent with highly-suspected organophosphate or carbamate insecticides or nerve agent poisoning should be treated with antidote immediately; administration should not be delayed for confirmatory laboratory tests. Signs of atropinization include flushing, mydriasis, tachycardia, and dryness of the mouth or nose. Monitor effects closely when administering subsequent injections as necessary. The presence of these effects is not indicative of the success of therapy; inappropriate use of mydriasis as an indicator of successful treatment has resulted in atropine toxicity. Reversal of bronchial secretions is the preferred indicator of success. Adjunct treatment with a cholinesterase reactivator (eg, pralidoxime) may be required in patients with toxicity secondary to organophosphorus insecticides or nerve agents. Treatment should always include proper evacuation and decontamination procedures; medical personnel should protect themselves from inadvertent contamination. Antidotal administration is intended only for initial management; definitive and more extensive medical care is required following administration. Individuals should not rely solely on antidote for treatment, as other supportive measures (eg, artificial respiration) may still be required. Atropine reverses the muscarinic but not the nicotinic effects associated with anticholinesterase toxicity.

Children may be more sensitive to the anticholinergic effects of atropine; use with caution in children with spastic paralysis. May be inappropriate in older adults depending on comorbidities (eg, dementia, delirium) due to its potent anticholinergic effects (Beers Criteria).

Drug Interactions
Metabolism/Transport Effects None known.
Avoid Concomitant Use
Avoid concomitant use of Atropine with any of the following: Aclidinium; Ipratropium (Oral Inhalation); Potassium Chloride; Tiotropium
Increased Effect/Toxicity
Atropine may increase the levels/effects of: AbobotulinumtoxinA; Anticholinergics; Cannabinoids; Mirabegron; OnabotulinumtoxinA; Potassium Chloride; RimabotulinumtoxinB; Tiotropium; Topiramate

The levels/effects of Atropine may be increased by: Aclidinium; Ipratropium (Oral Inhalation); Pramlintide
Decreased Effect
Atropine may decrease the levels/effects of: Acetylcholinesterase Inhibitors (Central); Secretin

The levels/effects of Atropine may be decreased by: Acetylcholinesterase Inhibitors (Central)
Pharmacodynamics/Kinetics
Onset of Action I.M., I.V.: Rapid
Half-life Elimination 2-3 hours; Children <2 years of age: 7 hours; Elderly 65-75 years of age: 10 hours
Time to Peak I.M.: 3 minutes
Pregnancy Risk Factor B/C (manufacturer specific)

Pregnancy Considerations Animal reproduction studies have not been conducted. Atropine has been found to cross the human placenta.
Lactation Enters breast milk/use caution (AAP rates "compatible"; AAP 2001 update pending)
Breast-Feeding Considerations Trace amounts of atropine are excreted into breast milk. Anticholinergic agents may suppress lactation.
Prescribing and Access Restrictions The AtroPen® formulation is available for use primarily by the Department of Defense.
Dosage Forms
Injection, solution: 0.05 mg/mL (5 mL); 0.1 mg/mL (5 mL, 10 mL); 0.4 mg/mL (1 mL, 20 mL)
AtroPen®: 0.25 mg/0.3 mL (0.3 mL); 0.5 mg/0.7 mL (0.7 mL); 1 mg/0.7 mL (0.7 mL); 2 mg/0.7 mL (0.7 mL)
Injection, solution [preservative free]: 0.4 mg/mL (1 mL); 1 mg/mL (1 mL)
Ointment, ophthalmic: 1% (3.5 g)
Solution, ophthalmic: 1% (2 mL, 5 mL, 15 mL)
Atropine Care™: 1% (2 mL, 5 mL, 15 mL)
Isopto® Atropine: 1% (5 mL, 15 mL)
Dental Comment The possibility of the need for an initial dose in excess of 0.4 mg has been confirmed by the American Dental Association in its recommendation on the use of this medication to reduce salivation during dental procedures.

Attapulgite (at a PULL gite)

Related Information
Ulcerative, Erosive, and Painful Oral Mucosal Disorders *on page 1578*
Brand Names: Canada Kaopectate® Children's [OTC]; Kaopectate® Extra Strength [OTC]; Kaopectate® [OTC]
Pharmacologic Category Antidiarrheal
Use Symptomatic treatment of diarrhea and cramps
Local Anesthetic/Vasoconstrictor Precautions No information available to require special precautions
Effects on Dental Treatment No significant effects or complications reported
Effects on Bleeding No information available to require special precautions
General Dosage Range Oral:
Children 3-6 years: 300 mg/dose (maximum dose: 2100 mg/day)
Children 6-12 years: 600-750 mg/dose (maximum dose: 4500 mg/day)
Children >12 years and Adults: 1200-1500 mg/dose (maximum dose: 8400 mg/day)
Mechanism of Action Nonselectively absorbs excess intestinal fluid, thereby reducing stool liquidity. May interfere with absorption of nutrients and other drugs as well.
Product Availability Not available in U.S.

Auranofin (au RANE oh fin)

Related Information
Rheumatoid Arthritis, Osteoarthritis, and Osteoporosis *on page 1526*
Brand Names: U.S. Ridaura®
Brand Names: Canada Ridaura®
Pharmacologic Category Gold Compound

Use Management of active stage classic or definite rheumatoid arthritis in patients who do not respond to or tolerate other agents

Local Anesthetic/Vasoconstrictor Precautions No information available to require special precautions

Effects on Dental Treatment Key adverse event(s) related to dental treatment: Glossitis and stomatitis.

Effects on Bleeding Thrombocytopenia has been reported in 1% to 3% of patients.

Adverse Effects
>10%:
  Dermatologic: Rash (24%), pruritus (17%)
  Gastrointestinal: Diarrhea/loose stools (47%), abdominal pain (14%), stomatitis (13%)
1% to 10%:
  Dermatologic: Alopecia (1% to 3%), urticaria (1% to 3%)
  Gastrointestinal: Nausea (10%), vomiting (10%), anorexia (3% to 9%), dyspepsia (3% to 9%), flatulence (3% to 9%), constipation (1% to 3%), dysgeusia (1% to 3%), glossitis (1% to 3%)
  Hematologic: Anemia (1% to 3%), eosinophilia (1% to 3%), leukopenia (1% to 3%), thrombocytopenia (1% to 3%)
  Hepatic: Transaminases increased (1% to 3%)
  Ocular: Conjunctivitis (3% to 9%)
  Renal: Proteinuria (3% to 9%), hematuria (1% to 3%)

General Dosage Range Dosage adjustment recommended in patients with renal impairment

Oral: *Adults:* Initial: 6 mg/day; Maintenance: 6-9 mg/day (maximum: 9 mg/day)

Mechanism of Action The exact mechanism of action of gold is unknown; gold is taken up by macrophages which results in inhibition of phagocytosis and lysosomal membrane stabilization; other actions observed are decreased serum rheumatoid factor and alterations in immunoglobulins. Additionally, complement activation is decreased, prostaglandin synthesis is inhibited, and lysosomal enzyme activity is decreased.

Pharmacodynamics/Kinetics
Onset of Action Delayed; therapeutic response may require as long as 3-4 months
Duration of Action Prolonged
Half-life Elimination Single or multiple dosing dependent: 21-31 days
Time to Peak Serum: ~2 hours
Pregnancy Risk Factor C
Pregnancy Considerations Adverse events were observed in animal reproduction studies.

Avanafil (a VAN a fil)

Pharmacologic Category Phosphodiesterase-5 Enzyme Inhibitor

Use Treatment of erectile dysfunction (ED)

Local Anesthetic/Vasoconstrictor Precautions No information available to require special precautions

Effects on Dental Treatment No significant effects or complications reported

Effects on Bleeding No information available to require special precautions

Adverse Effects
>10%: Central nervous system: Headache (5% to 12%)
2% to 10%:
  Cardiovascular: Flushing (3% to 10%), ECG abnormal (1% to 3%)
  Central nervous system: Dizziness (1% to 2%)
  Neuromuscular & skeletal: Back pain (1% to 3%)

Respiratory: Nasopharyngitis (1% to 5%), nasal congestion (1% to 3%), upper respiratory infection (1% to 3%)

General Dosage Range Dosage adjustment recommended in patients on concomitant therapy.

Oral: *Adults:* Initial: 100 mg 30 minutes prior to sexual activity; to be given as one single dose and not given more than once daily; dosing range: 50-200 mg once daily

Mechanism of Action Does not directly cause penile erections, but affects the response to sexual stimulation. The physiologic mechanism of erection of the penis involves release of nitric oxide (NO) in the corpus cavernosum during sexual stimulation. NO then activates the enzyme guanylate cyclase, which results in increased levels of cyclic guanosine monophosphate (cGMP), producing smooth muscle relaxation and inflow of blood to the corpus cavernosum. Avanafil enhances the effect of NO by inhibiting phosphodiesterase type 5 (PDE-5), which is responsible for degradation of cGMP in the corpus cavernosum; when sexual stimulation causes local release of NO, inhibition of PDE-5 by avanafil causes increased levels of cGMP in the corpus cavernosum, resulting in smooth muscle relaxation and inflow of blood to the corpus cavernosum; at recommended doses, it has no effect in the absence of sexual stimulation.

Pharmacodynamics/Kinetics
Half-life Elimination Terminal: ~5 hours
Time to Peak Plasma: 30-45 minutes (fasting); 1.12-1.25 hours (high-fat meal)
Pregnancy Risk Factor C
Pregnancy Considerations Based on data from animal reproduction studies, avanafil is predicted to have a low risk for major developmental abnormalities in humans. This product is not indicated for use in women.
Product Availability Stendra™: FDA approved April 2012; availability currently undetermined.

Axitinib (ax I ti nib)

Brand Names: U.S. Inlyta®
Brand Names: Canada Inlyta®
Pharmacologic Category Antineoplastic Agent, Tyrosine Kinase Inhibitor; Vascular Endothelial Growth Factor (VEGF) Inhibitor

Use Treatment of advanced renal cell cancer (RCC) after failure of one prior systemic treatment

Local Anesthetic/Vasoconstrictor Precautions Significant hypertension can occur with the use of this drug; monitor for hypertension prior to using local anesthetic with vasoconstrictor; medical consult if necessary

Effects on Dental Treatment Key adverse event(s) related to dental treatment: Oral mucosal inflammation, stomatitis, and taste alteration have been reported

Effects on Bleeding Chemotherapy may result in significant myelosuppression, potentially including significant reduction in platelet counts and altered hemostasis. Hemorrhagic events have been reported. In patients who are under active treatment with axitinib, medical consult is suggested.

Adverse Effects
>10%:
  Cardiovascular: Hypertension (40%; grades 3/4: 16%)
  Central nervous system: Fatigue (39%), dysphonia (31%), headache (14%)
  Dermatologic: Palmar-plantar erythrodysesthesia syndrome (27%; grades 3/4: 5%), rash (13%; grades 3/4: <1%)

Endocrine & metabolic: Bicarbonate decreased (44%), hypocalcemia (39%), hyperglycemia (28%), hypothyroidism (19%; grades 3/4: <1%), hypernatremia (17%), hyperkalemia (15%), hypoalbuminemia (15%), hyponatremia (13%), hypophosphatemia (13%), hypoglycemia (11%)

Gastrointestinal: Diarrhea (55%; grades 3/4: 11%), appetite decreased (34%), nausea (32%; grades 3/4: 3%), lipase increased (3% to 27%), amylase increased (25%), weight loss (25%), vomiting (24%; grades 3/4: 3%), constipation (20%), mucosal inflammation (15%), stomatitis (15%), abdominal pain (8% to 14%), taste alteration (11%)

Hematologic: Anemia (4% to 35%; grades 3/4: <1%), lymphopenia (33%; grades 3/4: 3%), hemorrhage (16%; grades 3/4 1%), thrombocytopenia (15%; grades 3/4: <1%), leukopenia (11%)

Hepatic: Alkaline phosphatase increased (30%), ALT increased (22%; grades 3/4: <1%), AST increased (20%; grades 3/4: <1%)

Neuromuscular & skeletal: Weakness (21%), arthralgia (15%), limb pain (13%)

Renal: Creatinine increased (55%), proteinuria (11%; grade 3: 3%)

Respiratory: Cough (15%), dyspnea (15%)

1% to 10%:

Cardiovascular: Venous thrombotic events (grades 3/4: 3%), arterial thrombotic events (2%; grade 3/4: 1%), deep vein thrombosis (1%), transient ischemic attack (1%)

Central nervous system: Dizziness (9%)

Dermatologic: Dry skin (10%), pruritus (7%), alopecia (4%), erythema (2%)

Endocrine & metabolic: Dehydration (6%), hyperthyroidism (1%)

Gastrointestinal: Dyspepsia (10%), hemorrhoids (4%), rectal hemorrhage (2%), fistula (1%), gastrointestinal perforation (≤1%)

Hematologic: Hemoglobin increased (9%), polycythemia (1%)

Neuromuscular & skeletal: Myalgia (7%)

Ocular: Retinal vein occlusion/thrombosis (1%)

Otic: Tinnitus (3%)

Renal: Hematuria (3%)

Respiratory: Epistaxis (6%), hemoptysis (2%), pulmonary embolism (2%)

General Dosage Range Dosage adjustment recommended in patients with hepatic impairment, on concomitant therapy, or who develop toxicities.

Oral: *Adults:* 5 mg every 12 hours; maximum: 10 mg every 12 hours

Mechanism of Action Axitinib is a selective second generation tyrosine kinase inhibitor which blocks angiogenesis and tumor growth by inhibiting vascular endothelial growth factor receptors (VEGFR-1, VEGFR-2, and VEGFR-3).

Pharmacodynamics/Kinetics

Half-life Elimination 2.5-6 hours

Time to Peak 2.5-4 hours

Pregnancy Risk Factor D

Pregnancy Considerations Teratogenic, embryotoxic, and fetotoxic events were observed in animal reproduction studies when administered in doses less than the normal human dose. Based on its mechanism of action and because axitinib inhibits angiogenesis (a critical component of fetal development), adverse effects on pregnancy would be expected. Women of childbearing potential should be advised to avoid pregnancy during therapy.

Prescribing and Access Restrictions Available from select specialty pharmacies. Further information may be obtained at 877-744-5675 or www.inlytahcp.com.

AzaCITIDine (ay za SYE ti deen)

Brand Names: U.S. Vidaza®

Brand Names: Canada Vidaza®

Pharmacologic Category Antineoplastic Agent, DNA Methylation Inhibitor

Use Treatment of myelodysplastic syndrome (MDS)

Unlabeled Use Treatment of acute myelogenous leukemia (AML)

Local Anesthetic/Vasoconstrictor Precautions No information available to require special precautions

Effects on Dental Treatment Key adverse event(s) related to dental treatment: Mucositis, gingival bleeding, oral mucosal petechiae, stomatitis, oral hemorrhage, and tongue ulceration.

Effects on Bleeding Gingival bleeding is reported in 10% of patients. Thrombocytopenia is reported in 66% to 70% of patients receiving azacitidine subcutaneously.

Adverse Effects

>10%:

Cardiovascular: Peripheral edema (7% to 19%), chest pain (16%), pallor (16%), pitting edema (15%)

Central nervous system: Fever (30% to 52%), fatigue (13% to 36%), headache (22%), dizziness (19%), anxiety (5% to 13%), depression (12%), insomnia (9% to 11%), malaise (11%), pain (11%)

Dermatologic: Bruising (19% to 31%), petechiae (11% to 24%), erythema (7% to 17%), skin lesion (15%), rash (10% to 14%), pruritus (12%)

Endocrine & metabolic: Hypokalemia (6% to 13%)

Gastrointestinal: Nausea (48% to 71%), vomiting (27% to 54%), diarrhea (36%), constipation (34% to 50%), anorexia (13% to 21%), weight loss (16%), abdominal pain (11% to 16%), abdominal tenderness (12%)

Hematologic: Thrombocytopenia (66% to 70%; grades 3/4: 58%), anemia (51% to 70%; grades 3/4: 14%), neutropenia (32% to 66%; grades 3/4: 61%), leukopenia (18% to 48%; grades 3/4: 15%), febrile neutropenia (14% to 16%; grades 3/4: 13%), myelosuppression (nadir: days 10-17; recovery: days 28-31)

Local: Injection site reactions (14% to 29%): Erythema (35% to 43%; more common with I.V. administration), pain (19% to 23%; more common with I.V. administration), bruising (5% to 14%)

Neuromuscular & skeletal: Weakness (29%), rigors (26%), arthralgia (22%), limb pain (20%), back pain (19%), myalgia (16%)

Respiratory: Cough (11% to 30%), dyspnea (5% to 29%), pharyngitis (20%), epistaxis (16%), nasopharyngitis (15%), upper respiratory tract infection (9% to 13%), pneumonia (11%), crackles (11%)

Miscellaneous: Diaphoresis (11%)

5% to 10%:

Cardiovascular: Cardiac murmur (10%), hypertension (≤9%), tachycardia (9%), hypotension (7%), syncope (6%), chest wall pain (5%)

Central nervous system: Lethargy (7% to 8%), hypoesthesia (5%), postprocedural pain (5%)

Dermatologic: Cellulitis (8%), urticaria (6%), dry skin (5%), skin nodule (5%)

◄ Gastrointestinal: Gingival bleeding (10%), oral mucosal petechiae (8%), stomatitis (8%), weight loss (≤8%), dyspepsia (6% to 7%), hemorrhoids (7%), abdominal distension (6%), loose stools (6%), dysphagia (5%), oral hemorrhage (5%), tongue ulceration (5%)

Genitourinary: Dysuria (8%), urinary tract infection (8% to 9%)

Hematologic: Hematoma (9%), postprocedural hemorrhage (6%)

Local: Injection site reactions: Pruritus (7%), hematoma (6%), rash (6%), granuloma (5%), induration (5%), pigmentation change (5%), swelling (5%)

Neuromuscular & skeletal: Muscle cramps (6%)

Renal: Hematuria (≤6%)

Respiratory: Rhinorrhea (10%), rales (9%), wheezing (9%), breath sounds decreased (8%), pharyngolaryngeal pain (6%), pleural effusion (6%), postnasal drip (6%), rhinitis (6%), rhonchi (6%), nasal congestion (6%), atelectasis (5%), sinusitis (5%)

Miscellaneous: Lymphadenopathy (10%), herpes simplex (9%), night sweats (9%), transfusion reaction (7%), mouth hemorrhage (5%)

General Dosage Range Dosage adjustment recommended in patients who develop toxicities

I.V., SubQ: *Adults:* 75-100 mg/m^2/day for 7 days/28-day treatment cycle

Mechanism of Action Antineoplastic effects may be a result of azacitidine's ability to promote hypomethylation of DNA leading to direct toxicity of abnormal hematopoietic cells in the bone marrow.

Pharmacodynamics/Kinetics

Half-life Elimination I.V., SubQ: ~4 hours

Time to Peak SubQ: 30 minutes

Pregnancy Risk Factor D

Pregnancy Considerations Embryotoxicity, fetal death, and fetal abnormalities were observed in animal studies. There are no adequate and well-controlled studies in pregnant women. Women of childbearing potential should be advised to avoid pregnancy during treatment. In addition, males should be advised to avoid fathering a child while on azacitidine therapy.

AzaTHIOprine (ay za THYE oh preen)

Brand Names: U.S. Azasan®; Imuran®

Brand Names: Canada Apo-Azathioprine®; Imuran®; Mylan-Azathioprine; Teva-Azathioprine

Generic Availability (U.S.) Yes

Pharmacologic Category Immunosuppressant Agent

Dental Use Adjunct with prednisone for managing severe erosive lichen planus, major aphthous stomatitis, erythema multiforme, and benign mucous membrane pemphigoid

Use Adjunctive therapy in prevention of rejection of kidney transplants; management of active rheumatoid arthritis (RA)

Unlabeled Use Adjunct in prevention of rejection of solid organ (nonrenal) transplants; remission maintenance or reduction of steroid use in Crohn's disease (CD) and in ulcerative colitis (UC); dermatomyositis/polymyositis; erythema multiforme; pemphigus vulgaris, lupus nephritis (maintenance), chronic refractory immune (idiopathic) thrombocytopenic purpura, relapsed/remitting multiple sclerosis

Local Anesthetic/Vasoconstrictor Precautions No information available to require special precautions

Effects on Dental Treatment No significant effects or complications reported

Effects on Bleeding Thrombocytopenia and bleeding may occur.

Adverse Effects Frequency not always defined; dependent upon dose, duration, indication, and concomitant therapy.

Central nervous system: Fever, malaise

Gastrointestinal: Nausea/vomiting (RA 12%), diarrhea

Hematologic: Leukopenia (renal transplant >50%; RA 28%), thrombocytopenia

Hepatic: Alkaline phosphatase increased, bilirubin increased, hepatotoxicity, transaminases increased

Neuromuscular & skeletal: Myalgia

Miscellaneous: Infection (renal transplant 20%; RA <1%; includes bacterial, fungal, protozoal, viral), neoplasia (renal transplant 3% [other than lymphoma], 0.5% [lymphoma])

Dental Usual Dosage Adjunctive management of severe recurrent aphthous stomatitis (unlabeled use): Adults: Oral: 50 mg once daily in conjunction with prednisone

Dosage Note: Patients with intermediate TPMT activity may be at risk for increased myelosuppression; those with low or absent TPMT activity receiving conventional azathioprine doses are at risk for developing severe, life-threatening myelotoxicity. Dosage reductions are recommended for patients with reduced TPMT activity.

I.V. dose is equivalent to oral dose (dosing should be transitioned from I.V. to oral as soon as tolerated): Adults:

Renal transplantation (treatment usually started the day of transplant, however, has been initiated [rarely] 1-3 days prior to transplant): Oral, I.V.: Initial: 3-5 mg/kg/day usually given as a single daily dose, then 1-3 mg/kg/day maintenance

Rheumatoid arthritis: Oral:

Initial: 1 mg/kg/day (50-100 mg) given once daily or divided twice daily for 6-8 weeks; may increase by 0.5 mg/kg every 4 weeks until response or up to 2.5 mg/kg/day; an adequate trial should be a minimum of 12 weeks

Maintenance dose: Reduce dose by 0.5 mg/kg (~25 mg daily) every 4 weeks until lowest effective dose is reached; optimum duration of therapy not specified; may be discontinued abruptly

Crohn's disease, remission maintenance or reduction of steroid use (unlabeled use): Oral: 2-3 mg/kg/day (Lichtenstein, 2009)

Dermatomyositis/polymyositis, adjunctive management (unlabeled use): Oral: 50 mg/day in conjunction with prednisone; increase by 50 mg/week to total dose of 2-3 mg/kg/day (Briemberg, 2003); **Note:** Onset of beneficial effects may take 3-6 months; however, may be preferred over methotrexate in patients with pulmonary or hepatic toxicity.

Immune (idiopathic) thrombocytopenic purpura, chronic refractory (unlabeled use): Oral: Maintenance: 100-200 mg/day (Boruchov, 2007)

Lupus nephritis, maintenance (unlabeled use): Oral: Initial: 2 mg/kg/day; may reduce to 1.5 mg/kg/day after 1 month (if proteinuria <1 g/day and serum creatinine stable) (Moroni, 2006) **or** target dose: 2 mg/kg/day (Hahn, 2012; Houssiau, 2010)

Ulcerative colitis, remission maintenance or reduction of steroid use (unlabeled use): Oral: 1.5-2.5 mg/kg/day (Kornbluth, 2010)

Dosage adjustment for concomitant use with allopurinol: Reduce azathioprine dose to one-third or one-fourth the usual dose when used concurrently with allopurinol. Patients with low or absent TPMT activity may require further dose reductions or discontinuation.

Dosage adjustment for toxicity:

Rapid WBC count decrease, persistently low WBC count, or serious infection: Reduce dose or temporarily withhold treatment

Severe toxicity in renal transplantation: May require discontinuation

Hepatic sinusoidal obstruction syndrome (SOS; veno-occlusive disease): Permanently discontinue

Dosage adjustment in renal impairment: No dosage adjustment provided in manufacturer's labeling; however, the following adjustments have been recommended (Aronoff, 2007):

Cl_{cr} >50 mL/minute: No adjustment recommended

Cl_{cr} 10-50 mL/minute: Administer 75% of normal dose

Cl_{cr} <10 mL/minute: Administer 50% of normal dose

Hemodialysis (dialyzable; ~45% removed in 8 hours): Administer 50% of normal dose; supplement: 0.25 mg/kg

CRRT: Administer 75% of normal dose

Dosage adjustment in hepatic impairment: No dosage adjustment provided in manufacturer's labeling.

Mechanism of Action Azathioprine is an imidazolyl derivative of mercaptopurine; antagonizes purine metabolism and may inhibit synthesis of DNA, RNA, and proteins; may also interfere with cellular metabolism and inhibit mitosis. The 6-thioguanine nucleotides appear to mediate the majority of azathioprine's immunosuppressive and toxic effects.

Contraindications Hypersensitivity to azathioprine or any component of the formulation; pregnancy (in patients with rheumatoid arthritis); patients with rheumatoid arthritis and a history of treatment with alkylating agents (eg, cyclophosphamide, chlorambucil, melphalan) may have a prohibitive risk of neoplasia with azathioprine treatment

Warnings/Precautions Hazardous agent - use appropriate precautions for handling and disposal (NIOSH, 2012).

[U.S. Boxed Warning]: Immunosuppressive agents, including azathioprine, are associated with the development of lymphoma and other malignancies, especially of the skin. Hepatosplenic T-Cell Lymphoma (HSTCL), a rare white blood cell cancer that is usually fatal, has predominantly occurred in adolescents and young adults treated for Crohn's disease or ulcerative colitis and receiving TNF blockers (eg, adalimumab, certolizumab pegol, etanercept, golimumab), azathioprine, and/or mercaptopurine. Most cases have occurred in patients treated with a combination of immunosuppressant agents, although there have been reports of HSTCL in patients receiving azathioprine or mercaptopurine monotherapy. Renal transplant patients are also at increased risk for malignancy (eg, skin cancer, lymphoma); limit sun and ultraviolet light exposure and use appropriate sun protection. Dose-related hematologic toxicities (leukopenia, thrombocytopenia, and anemias, including macrocytic anemia, or pancytopenia) may occur; delayed toxicities may also occur. May be more severe with renal transplants undergoing rejection; dosage modification for hematologic toxicity may be necessary. Chronic immunosuppression increases the risk of serious infections; may require dosage reduction. Use with caution in patients with liver disease or renal impairment; monitor hematologic

function closely. Azathioprine is metabolized to mercaptopurine; concomitant use may result in profound myelosuppression and should be avoided. Patients with genetic deficiency of thiopurine methyltransferase (TPMT) or concurrent therapy with drugs which may inhibit TPMT may be sensitive to myelosuppressive effects. Patients with intermediate TPMT activity may be at risk for increased myelosuppression; those with low or absent TPMT activity are at risk for developing severe myelotoxicity. TPMT genotyping or phenotyping may assist in identifying patients at risk for developing toxicity. Consider TPMT testing in patients with abnormally low CBC unresponsive to dose reduction. TPMT testing does not substitute for CBC monitoring. Xanthine oxidase inhibitors may increase risk for hematologic toxicity; reduce azathioprine dose when used concurrently with allopurinol; patients with low or absent TPMT activity may require further dose reductions or discontinuation.

Hepatotoxicity (transaminase, bilirubin, and alkaline phosphatase elevations) may occur, usually in renal transplant patients and generally within 6 months of transplant; normally reversible with discontinuation; monitor liver function periodically. Rarely, hepatic sinusoidal obstruction syndrome (SOS; formerly called veno-occlusive disease) has been reported; discontinue if hepatic SOS is suspected. Severe nausea, vomiting, diarrhea, rash, fever, malaise, myalgia, hypotension, and liver enzyme abnormalities may occur within the first several weeks of treatment and are generally reversible upon discontinuation. [U.S. Boxed Warning]: Should be prescribed by physicians familiar with the risks, including hematologic toxicities and mutagenic potential. Immune response to vaccines may be diminished.

Drug Interactions

Metabolism/Transport Effects None known.

Avoid Concomitant Use

Avoid concomitant use of AzaTHIOprine with any of the following: BCG; Febuxostat; Mercaptopurine; Natalizumab; Pimecrolimus; Tacrolimus (Topical); Tofacitinib

Increased Effect/Toxicity

AzaTHIOprine may increase the levels/effects of: Leflunomide; Mercaptopurine; Natalizumab; Tofacitinib; Vaccines (Live)

The levels/effects of AzaTHIOprine may be increased by: 5-ASA Derivatives; ACE Inhibitors; Allopurinol; Denosumab; Febuxostat; Pimecrolimus; Ribavirin; Roflumilast; Sulfamethoxazole; Tacrolimus (Topical); Trastuzumab; Trimethoprim

Decreased Effect

AzaTHIOprine may decrease the levels/effects of: BCG; Coccidioidin Skin Test; Sipuleucel-T; Vaccines (Inactivated); Vitamin K Antagonists

The levels/effects of AzaTHIOprine may be decreased by: Echinacea

Ethanol/Nutrition/Herb Interactions Herb/Nutraceutical: Avoid cat's claw, echinacea (have immunostimulant properties).

Dietary Considerations May be taken with food.

Pharmacodynamics/Kinetics

Half-life Elimination Parent drug: 12 minutes; mercaptopurine: 0.7-3 hours; End-stage renal disease: Slightly prolonged

Time to Peak Plasma: Oral: 1-2 hours (including metabolites)

Pregnancy Risk Factor D

▶

◀ **Pregnancy Considerations** Azathioprine was found to be teratogenic in animal studies; temporary depression in spermatogenesis and reduction in sperm viability and sperm count were also reported in mice. Azathioprine crosses the placenta in humans; congenital anomalies, immunosuppression, hematologic toxicities (lymphopenia, pancytopenia), and intrauterine growth retardation have been reported. There are no adequate and well-controlled studies in pregnant women. Azathioprine should not be used to treat rheumatoid arthritis during pregnancy. The potential benefit to the mother versus possible risk to the fetus should be considered when treating other disease states. Women of child-bearing potential should avoid becoming pregnant during treatment.

The National Transplantation Pregnancy Registry (NTPR, Temple University) is a registry for pregnant women taking immunosuppressants following any solid organ transplant. The NTPR encourages reporting of all immunosuppressant exposures during pregnancy in transplant recipients at 877-955-6877.

Lactation Enters breast milk/not recommended

Breast-Feeding Considerations Due to risk of immunosuppression and serious adverse effects in the nursing infant, breast-feeding is not recommended.

Dosage Forms
Injection, powder for reconstitution: 100 mg
Tablet, oral: 50 mg
   Azasan®: 75 mg, 100 mg
   Imuran®: 50 mg

Azelaic Acid (a zeh LAY ik AS id)

Brand Names: U.S. Azelex®; Finacea®; Finacea® Plus™ [DSC]
Brand Names: Canada Finacea®
Pharmacologic Category Topical Skin Product, Acne
Use
Azelex®: Treatment of mild-to-moderate inflammatory acne vulgaris
Finacea®: Treatment of inflammatory papules and pustules of mild-to-moderate rosacea
Local Anesthetic/Vasoconstrictor Precautions No information available to require special precautions
Effects on Dental Treatment No significant effects or complications reported
Effects on Bleeding No information available to require special precautions
Adverse Effects
>10%: Dermatologic: Burning/stinging/tingling (1% to 16%)
1% to 10%: Dermatologic: Pruritus (gel: 1% to 6%), dry skin/peeling/scaling/xerosis (≤5), erythema (≤2%), irritation (≤2%), acne (gel: ≤1%), contact dermatitis (≤1%), edema (gel: ≤1%)
General Dosage Range
Topical: *Children ≥12 years and Adults:* Apply to the affected area(s) twice daily.
Mechanism of Action Azelaic acid is a dietary constituent normally found in whole grain cereals; can be formed endogenously. Exact mechanism is not known. *In vitro*, azelaic acid possesses antimicrobial activity against *Propionibacterium acnes* and *Staphylococcus epidermidis*. May decrease microcomedo formation.
Pharmacodynamics/Kinetics
Half-life Elimination Topical: Healthy subjects: 12 hours
Pregnancy Risk Factor B

Pregnancy Considerations Adverse events were observed in animal reproduction studies following oral administration. Minimal systemic absorption (<4%) occurs following topical administration.

Azelastine (Nasal) (a ZEL as teen)

Brand Names: U.S. Astelin®; Astepro®
Brand Names: Canada Astelin®
Pharmacologic Category Histamine H₁ Antagonist; Histamine H₁ Antagonist, Second Generation
Use Treatment of the symptoms of seasonal allergic rhinitis such as rhinorrhea, sneezing, and nasal pruritus; treatment of the symptoms of vasomotor rhinitis
Local Anesthetic/Vasoconstrictor Precautions No information available to require special precautions
Effects on Dental Treatment Key adverse event(s) related to dental treatment: Bitter taste, xerostomia (normal salivary flow resumes upon discontinuation), aphthous stomatitis, glossitis, and burning sensation in throat. Chronic use of antihistamines will inhibit salivary flow, particularly in elderly patients. May contribute to periodontal disease and oral discomfort.
Effects on Bleeding No information available to require special precautions
Adverse Effects Note: Adverse reactions may be dose-, indication-, or product-dependent:
>10%:
Central nervous system: Headache (Astelin® 8% to 15%; Astepro® 1% to 3%), somnolence (<1% to 12%)
Gastrointestinal: Bitter taste (Astelin® 8% to 20%; Astepro® 6% to 7%)
Respiratory: Cold symptoms/rhinitis (2% to 17%), cough (11%)
2% to 10%:
Central nervous system: Dysesthesia (8%), dizziness (2%), fatigue (2%)
Gastrointestinal: Nausea (3%), weight gain (2%), xerostomia (3%)
Neuromuscular & skeletal: Myalgia (≤2%)
Ocular: Conjunctivitis (<2% to 5%)
Respiratory: Asthma (5%), nasal burning (4%), pharyngitis (4%), paroxysmal sneezing (3%), sinusitis (3%), epistaxis (2% to 3%)
<2%:
Cardiovascular: Flushing, hypertension, tachycardia
Central nervous system: Abnormal thinking, anxiety, depersonalization, depression, drowsiness, fever, hypoesthesia, malaise, nervousness, sleep disorder, vertigo
Dermatologic: Contact dermatitis, eczema, furunculosis, hair and follicle infection, skin laceration
Endocrine & metabolic: Amenorrhea, breast pain
Gastrointestinal: Abdominal pain, aphthous stomatitis, appetite increased, constipation, diarrhea, gastroenteritis, glossitis, loss of taste, ulcerative stomatitis, toothache, vomiting
Genitourinary: Albuminuria, hematuria, polyuria
Hepatic: ALT increased
Neuromuscular & skeletal: Back pain, extremity pain, hyperkinesia, rheumatoid arthritis, temporomandibular dislocation
Ocular: Eye pain, watery eyes
Respiratory: Bronchitis, bronchospasm, laryngitis, nasal congestion, nocturnal dyspnea, pharyngolaryngeal pain, postnasal drip, sinus hypersecretion, throat burning

Miscellaneous: Allergic reactions, herpes simplex infection, viral infection

General Dosage Range Intranasal:
Children 5-11 years: 1 spray in each nostril twice daily
Children ≥12 years and Adults: 1-2 sprays in each nostril twice daily

Mechanism of Action Competes with histamine for H₁-receptor sites on effector cells and inhibits the release of histamine and other mediators involved in the allergic response; when used intranasally, reduces hyper-reactivity of the airways; increases the motility of bronchial epithelial cilia, improving mucociliary transport

Pharmacodynamics/Kinetics
Onset of Action Peak effect: 3 hours
Duration of Action 12 hours
Half-life Elimination Azelastine: 22-25 hours; Desmethylazelastine: 52-57 hours
Time to Peak Serum: 2-4 hours
Pregnancy Risk Factor C
Pregnancy Considerations Animal reproduction studies have shown toxic effects to the fetus at maternally toxic doses.

Azelastine and Fluticasone
(a ZEL as teen & floo TIK a sone)

Brand Names: U.S. Dymista™
Pharmacologic Category Corticosteroid, Nasal; Histamine H₁ Antagonist, Second Generation
Use Symptomatic relief of seasonal allergic rhinitis
Local Anesthetic/Vasoconstrictor Precautions No information available to require special precautions
Effects on Dental Treatment Key adverse event(s) related to dental treatment: Azelastine: Bitter taste, xerostomia (normal salivary flow resumes upon discontinuation), aphthous stomatitis, glossitis, and burning sensation in throat. Chronic use of antihistamines will inhibit salivary flow, particularly in elderly patients. May contribute to periodontal disease and oral discomfort.
Effects on Bleeding No information available to require special precautions
Adverse Effects Reactions/percentages reported with combination product; also see individual agents.
1% to 10%:
Central nervous system: Fever (≥2%), headache (≥2%), pain (≥2%)
Gastrointestinal: Abnormal taste (≥2% to 4%), diarrhea (≥2%)
Respiratory: Cough (≥2%), epistaxis (≥2%), nasal congestion (≥2%), pharyngitis (≥2%), rhinitis (≥2%), upper respiratory tract infection (≥2%)
Miscellaneous: Viral infection (≥2%)
General Dosage Range Intranasal: *Children ≥12 years and Adults:* 1 spray (137 mcg azelastine/50 mcg fluticasone) per nostril twice daily
Mechanism of Action Azelastine competes with histamine for H₁receptor sites on effector cells and inhibits the release of histamine and other mediators involved in the allergic response; when used intranasally, reduces hyper-reactivity of the airways; increases the motility of bronchial epithelial cilia, improving mucociliary transport.

Fluticasone belongs to a group of corticosteroids which utilizes a fluorocarbothioate ester linkage at the 17 carbon position; extremely potent vasoconstrictive and anti-inflammatory activity.
Pregnancy Risk Factor C

Pregnancy Considerations Adverse events were observed in animal reproduction studies. Refer to individual monographs.

Azilsartan (ay zil SAR tan)

Related Information
Cardiovascular Diseases *on page 1492*
Brand Names: U.S. Edarbi™
Brand Names: Canada Edarbi™
Pharmacologic Category Angiotensin II Receptor Blocker
Use Treatment of hypertension; may be used alone or in combination with other antihypertensives
Local Anesthetic/Vasoconstrictor Precautions No information available to require special precautions
Effects on Dental Treatment Key adverse event(s) related to dental treatment: Orthostatic hypotension
Effects on Bleeding No information available to require special precautions
Adverse Effects
Cardiovascular: Hypotension, orthostatic hypotension
Central nervous system: Dizziness, fatigue
Gastrointestinal: Diarrhea (2%), nausea
Hematologic: Hemoglobin decreased, hematocrit decreased, leukopenia (rare), RBC decreased, thrombocytopenia (rare)
Neuromuscular & skeletal: Muscle spasm, weakness
Renal: Serum creatinine increased
Respiratory: Cough
General Dosage Range Oral: *Adults:* 40-80 mg once daily
Mechanism of Action Angiotensin II (which is formed by enzymatic conversion from angiotensin I) is the primary pressor agent of the renin-angiotensin system. Effects of angiotensin II include vasoconstriction, stimulation of aldosterone synthesis/release, cardiac stimulation, and renal sodium reabsorption. Azilsartan inhibits angiotensin II's vasoconstrictor and aldosterone-secreting effects by selectively blocking the binding of angiotensin II to the AT₁ receptor in vascular smooth muscle and adrenal gland tissues (azilsartan has a stronger affinity for the AT₁ receptor than the AT₂ receptor). The action is independent of the angiotensin II synthesis pathways. Azilsartan does not inhibit ACE (kininase II), therefore it does not affect the response to bradykinin (the clinical relevance of this is unknown) and does not bind to or inhibit other receptors or ion channels of importance in cardiovascular regulation.
Pharmacodynamics/Kinetics
Half-life Elimination ~11 hours
Time to Peak Serum: 1.5-3 hours
Pregnancy Risk Factor D
Pregnancy Considerations [U.S. Boxed Warning]: Drugs that act on the renin-angiotensin system can cause injury and death to the developing fetus. Discontinue as soon as possible once pregnancy is detected. The use of drugs which act on the renin-angiotensin system are associated with oligohydramnios. Oligohydramnios, due to decreased fetal renal function, may lead to fetal lung hypoplasia and skeletal malformations. Use is also associated with anuria, hypotension, renal failure, skull hypoplasia, and death in the fetus/neonate. The exposed fetus should be monitored for fetal growth, amniotic fluid volume, and organ formation. Infants exposed *in utero* should be monitored for hyperkalemia, hypotension, and oliguria.

Azilsartan and Chlorthalidone
(ay zil SAR tan & klor THAL i done)

Brand Names: U.S. edarbyclor™

Pharmacologic Category Angiotensin II Receptor Blocker; Diuretic, Thiazide

Use Treatment of hypertension

Local Anesthetic/Vasoconstrictor Precautions No information available to require special precautions

Effects on Dental Treatment Key adverse event(s) related to dental treatment: Orthostatic hypotension

Effects on Bleeding No information available to require special precautions

Adverse Effects Reactions/percentages reported with combination product; also see individual agents.

1% to 10%:
Cardiovascular: Hypotension (2%)
Central nervous system: Dizziness (9%), fatigue (2%)
Renal: Serum creatinine increased (2%), BUN increased

General Dosage Range Oral: *Adults:* 40 mg (azilsartan) and 12.5-25 mg (chlorthalidone) once daily; (maximum: Azilsartan 40 mg/day; chlorthalidone 25 mg/day)

Mechanism of Action
Azilsartan: Angiotensin II (which is formed by enzymatic conversion from angiotensin I) is the primary pressor agent of the renin-angiotensin system. Effects of angiotensin II include vasoconstriction, stimulation of aldosterone synthesis/release, cardiac stimulation, and renal sodium reabsorption. Azilsartan inhibits angiotensin II's vasoconstrictor and aldosterone-secreting effects by selectively blocking the binding of angiotensin II to the AT1 receptor in vascular smooth muscle and adrenal gland tissues (azilsartan has a stronger affinity for the AT1 receptor than the AT2 receptor). The action is independent of the angiotensin II synthesis pathways. Azilsartan does not inhibit ACE (kininase II), therefore it does not affect the response to bradykinin (the clinical relevance of this is unknown) and does not bind to or inhibit other receptors or ion channels of importance in cardiovascular regulation.
Chlorthalidone: A sulfonamide-derived diuretic that inhibits sodium and chloride reabsorption in the cortical-diluting segment of the ascending loop of Henle.

Pregnancy Risk Factor D

Pregnancy Considerations [U.S. Boxed Warning]: Drugs that act on the renin-angiotensin system can cause injury and death to the developing fetus. Discontinue as soon as possible once pregnancy is detected. Also see individual agents.

Azithromycin (Systemic) (az ith roe MYE sin)

Related Information
Antibiotic Prophylaxis *on page 1542*
Bacterial Infections *on page 1562*
Clinical Risk Related to Drugs Prolonging QT Interval *on page 1510*
Periodontal Diseases *on page 1570*
Sexually-Transmitted Diseases *on page 1536*

Related Sample Prescriptions
Bacterial Infections and Periodontal Diseases *on page 1609*
Infective Endocarditis (Prevention) *on page 1604*
Sinus Infection Treatment *on page 1611*

Brand Names: U.S. Zithromax®; Zithromax® TRI-PAK™; Zithromax® Z-PAK®; Zmax®

Brand Names: Canada Apo-Azithromycin®; Ava-Azithromycin; Azithromycin for Injection; CO Azithromycin; Dom-Azithromycin; GD-Azithromycin; Mylan-Azithromycin; Novo-Azithromycin; PHL-Azithromycin; PMS-Azithromycin; PRO-Azithromycin; ratio-Azithromycin; Riva-Azithromycin; Sandoz-Azithromycin; Zithromax®; Zithromax® For Intravenous Injection; Zmax SR™

Generic Availability (U.S.) Yes: Excludes extended release microspheres

Pharmacologic Category Antibiotic, Macrolide

Dental Use Alternate oral antibiotic for prevention of infective endocarditis in individuals allergic to penicillins or ampicillin, when amoxicillin cannot be used; alternate antibiotic in the treatment of common orofacial infections caused by aerobic gram-positive cocci and susceptible anaerobes

Use Oral, I.V.: Treatment of acute otitis media due to *H. influenzae, M. catarrhalis,* or *S. pneumoniae*; pharyngitis/tonsillitis due to *S. pyogenes*, community-acquired pneumonia due to *Chlamydia pneumonia, H. influenzae, M. pneumoniae,* or *S. pneumoniae*; pelvic inflammatory disease (PID) due to *C. trachomatis, N. gonorrhoeae,* or *M. hominis*; genital ulcer disease (in men) due to *H. ducreyi* (chancroid); acute bacterial exacerbations of chronic obstructive pulmonary disease (COPD) due to *H. influenzae, M. catarrhalis,* or *S. pneumoniae*; acute bacterial sinusitis due to *H. influenzae, M. catarrhalis,* or *S. pneumoniae*; prevention of *Mycobacterium avium* complex (MAC) (alone or in combination with rifabutin) in patients with advanced HIV infection; treatment of disseminated MAC (in combination with ethambutol) in patients with advanced HIV infection; skin and skin structure infections (uncomplicated) due to *S. aureus, S. pyogenes,* or *S. agalactiae*; urethritis and cervicitis due to *C. trachomatis* or *N. gonorrhoeae*

Unlabeled Use Treatment of babesiosis; cat scratch disease; gonococcal infections of the pharynx or rectum (combination therapy) and expedited partner therapy; granuloma inguinale (donovanosis); *Mycoplasma genitalium* infections; pertussis; prophylaxis of infective endocarditis in select patients who are allergic to penicillin and undergoing dental procedures; prevention of pulmonary exacerbations in patients with noncystic fibrosis bronchiectasis; treatment of *Shigella dysenteriae* type 1

Local Anesthetic/Vasoconstrictor Precautions Azithromycin is one of the drugs confirmed to prolong the QT interval and is accepted as having a risk of causing torsade de pointes. The risk of drug-induced torsade de pointes is extremely low when a single QT interval prolonging drug is prescribed. In terms of epinephrine, it is not known what effect vasoconstrictors in the local anesthetic regimen will have in patients with a known history of congenital prolonged QT interval or in patients taking any medication that prolongs the QT interval. Until more information is obtained, it is suggested that the clinician consult with the physician prior to the use of a vasoconstrictor in suspected patients, and that the vasoconstrictor (epinephrine, mepivacaine and levonordefrin [Carbocaine® 2% with Neo-Cobefrin®]) be used with caution. See Dental Comment.

Effects on Dental Treatment No significant effects or complications reported

Effects on Bleeding No information available to require special precautions

Adverse Effects
>10%: Gastrointestinal: Diarrhea (4% to 9%; high single-dose regimens 12% to 14%), nausea (≤7%; high single-dose regimens 18%)

2% to 10%:

Dermatologic: Pruritus, rash

Gastrointestinal: Abdominal pain, anorexia, cramping, vomiting (especially with high single-dose regimens)

Genitourinary: Vaginitis

Local: (with I.V. administration): Injection site pain, inflammation

Dental Usual Dosage

Prophylaxis against infective endocarditis (unlabeled use): Oral:

Children: 15 mg/kg 30-60 minutes before procedure (maximum: 500 mg). **Note:** American Heart Association (AHA) guidelines now recommend prophylaxis only in patients undergoing invasive procedures and in whom underlying cardiac conditions may predispose to a higher risk of adverse outcomes should infection occur. As of April 2007, routine prophylaxis for GI/GU procedures is no longer recommended by the AHA.

Adolescents ≥16 years and Adults: 500 mg 30-60 minutes prior to the procedure. **Note:** American Heart Association (AHA) guidelines now recommend prophylaxis only in patients undergoing invasive procedures and in whom underlying cardiac conditions may predispose to a higher risk of adverse outcomes should infection occur. As of April 2007, routine prophylaxis for GI/GU procedures is no longer recommended by the AHA.

Bacterial sinusitis: Oral:

Children ≥6 months: 10 mg/kg once daily for 3 days (maximum: 500 mg/day)

Adolescents ≥16 years and Adults: 500 mg/day for a total of 3 days

Extended release suspension (Zmax®): 2 g as a single dose

Orofacial infections: Adolescents ≥16 years and Adults: Oral: 500 mg/day, then 250 mg days 2-5

Treatment of periodontal disease: 500 mg once daily for 4-7 days

Dosage Note: Extended release suspension (Zmax®) is not interchangeable with immediate release formulations. Use should be limited to approved indications. All doses are expressed as immediate release azithromycin unless otherwise specified.

Usual dosage range:

Children ≥6 months: Oral: 5-12 mg/kg given once daily (maximum: 500 mg daily) **or** 30 mg/kg as a single dose (maximum: 1500 mg)

Extended release suspension (Zmax®): 60 mg/kg as a single dose; **Note:** Extended release suspension (Zmax®): Dose in mL is equal to the weight in lbs for patients <75 lbs (34 kg). Pediatric patients ≥75 lbs should receive the adult dose.

Adolescents ≥16 years and Adults:

Oral: 250-600 mg once daily **or** 1-2 g as a single dose

Extended release suspension (Zmax®): 2 g as a single dose

I.V.: 250-500 mg once daily

Indication-specific dosing:

Children:

Bacterial sinusitis: Oral: 10 mg/kg once daily for 3 days (maximum: 500 mg daily)

Cat scratch disease (unlabeled use; Bass, 1998; Stevens, 2005): Oral:

<45.5 kg: 10 mg/kg as a single dose, then 5 mg/kg once daily for 4 additional days

>45.5 kg: 500 mg as a single dose, then 250 mg once daily for 4 additional days

Community-acquired pneumonia (CAP) (IDSA/ PIDS, 2011): Infants >3 months and Children: **Note:** A beta-lactam antibiotic should be added if typical bacterial pneumonia cannot be ruled out

Presumed mild infection or step-down therapy, atypical *(M. pneumoniae, C. pneumoniae, C. trachomatis)* (preferred): Oral: 10 mg/kg (maximum dose: 500 mg) as a single dose on the first day, followed by 5 mg/kg/day (maximum dose: 250 mg) on days 2 through 5.

Presumed moderate-to-severe infection, atypical *(M. pneumoniae, C. pneumoniae, C. trachomatis)*: I.V.: 10 mg/kg/day on days 1 and 2, then switch to oral azithromycin therapy if possible to finish the 5-day course

Alternative regimens for community-acquired pneumonia: Oral: 10 mg/kg (maximum dose: 500 mg) once daily for 3 days (Kogan, 2003)

Extended release suspension (Zmax®):

<75 lbs (34 kg): 60 mg/kg as a single dose

≥75 lbs (34 kg): Refer to adult dosing

Disseminated *M. avium* complex disease in patients with advanced HIV infection (unlabeled use; CDC, 2009):

Treatment: 10-12 mg/kg/day (maximum: 500 mg) in combination with ethambutol; patients with severe disease should also receive rifabutin

Primary prophylaxis: 20 mg/kg (maximum: 1200 mg) once weekly (preferred) or alternatively, 5 mg/kg/day once daily (maximum: 250 mg daily)

Secondary prophylaxis: 5 mg/kg/day once daily (maximum: 250 mg daily) in combination with ethambutol, with or without rifabutin

Otitis media: Oral:

1-day regimen: 30 mg/kg as a single dose (maximum: 1500 mg)

3-day regimen: 10 mg/kg once daily for 3 days (maximum: 500 mg daily)

5-day regimen: 10 mg/kg on day 1 (maximum: 500 mg daily) followed by 5 mg/kg/day once daily on days 2-5 (maximum: 250 mg daily)

Pertussis (unlabeled use; CDC, 2005):

Children <6 months: 10 mg/kg/day for 5 days

Children ≥6 months: 10 mg/kg on day 1 (maximum: 500 mg daily) followed by 5 mg/kg/day once daily on days 2-5 (maximum: 250 mg daily)

Pharyngitis (including susceptible group A streptococci), tonsillitis (IDSA guidelines): Children ≥2 years: Oral: 12 mg/kg/day once daily for 5 days (maximum: 500 mg daily). **Note:** Recommended by the Infectious Disease Society of America (IDSA) as an alternative agent for group A streptococcal pharyngitis in penicillin-allergic patients (Shulman, 2012)

Prophylaxis against infective endocarditis (unlabeled use): 15 mg/kg 30-60 minutes before procedure (maximum: 500 mg). **Note:** American Heart Association (AHA) guidelines now recommend prophylaxis only in patients undergoing invasive procedures and in whom underlying cardiac conditions may predispose to a higher risk of adverse outcomes should infection occur. As of April 2007, routine prophylaxis for GI/GU procedures is no longer recommended by the AHA.

Shigella dysentery type 1 (unlabeled use): Oral: 6-20 mg/kg/day for 1-5 days (WHO, 2005)

Uncomplicated chlamydial urethritis or cervicitis (unlabeled use): Children ≥45 kg: 1 g as a single dose (CDC, 2010)

Adolescents ≥16 years and Adults:

Babesiosis (unlabeled use): Oral: 500-1000 mg on day 1, followed by 250 mg once daily for 7-10 days with atovaquone; higher doses may be required in immunocompromised patients (600-1000 mg daily). **Note:** Relapsing infection may require at least 6 weeks of therapy (Vannier, 2012; Wormser, 2006).

Bacterial sinusitis: Oral: 500 mg daily for a total of 3 days

Extended release suspension (Zmax®): 2 g as a single dose

Cat scratch disease (unlabeled use): Oral: >45.5 kg: 500 mg as a single dose, then 250 mg once daily for 4 additional days (Bass, 1998; Stevens, 2005)

Chancroid due to *H. ducreyi*: Oral: 1 g as a single dose (CDC, 2010)

C. trachomatis **urethritis/cervicitis:** Oral: 1 g as a single dose

Community-acquired pneumonia:

Oral: 500 mg on day 1 followed by 250 mg once daily on days 2-5

Extended release suspension (Zmax®): 2 g as a single dose

I.V.: 500 mg as a single dose for at least 2 days, follow I.V. therapy by the oral route with a single daily dose of 500 mg to complete a 7- to 10-day course of therapy.

Disseminated *M. avium* complex disease in patients with advanced HIV infection: Oral:

Treatment: 600 mg daily in combination with ethambutol

Primary prophylaxis: 1200 mg once weekly (preferred), with or without rifabutin **or** alternatively, 600 mg twice weekly (CDC, 2009)

Secondary prophylaxis: 500-600 mg daily in combination with ethambutol (CDC, 2009)

Gonococcal infection, uncomplicated (cervix, rectum, urethra) (unlabeled regimen): Oral: 1 g as a single dose in combination with ceftriaxone (preferred) or cefixime (only if ceftriaxone unavailable); if cefixime is used, test-of-cure in 7 days is recommended (CDC, 2012). **Note:** Monotherapy with azithromycin single dose of 2 g has been associated with resistance and/or treatment failure; however, may be appropriate for treatment of a gonococcal infection in pregnant women who cannot tolerate a cephalosporin (CDC, 2010).

Patients with severe cephalosporin allergy: 2 g as a single dose and test-of-cure in 7 days (CDC, 2012)

Gonococcal infection, uncomplicated (pharynx) (unlabeled use): 1 g as a single dose in combination with ceftriaxone (CDC, 2012)

Gonococcal infection, expedited partner therapy (unlabeled use): Oral: 1 g as a single dose in combination with cefixime (CDC, 2012). **Note:** Only used if a heterosexual partner cannot be linked to evaluation and treatment in a timely manner; dose delivered to partner by patient, collaborating pharmacy, or disease investigation specialist.

Granuloma inguinale (donovanosis) (unlabeled use): Oral: 1 g once a week for at least 3 weeks (and until lesions have healed) (CDC, 2010)

Mild-to-moderate respiratory tract, skin, and soft tissue infections: Oral: 500 mg in a single loading dose on day 1 followed by 250 mg daily as a single dose on days 2-5

Alternative regimen: Bacterial exacerbation of COPD: 500 mg daily for a total of 3 days

M. genitalium **infections (unlabeled use)** (confirmed cases in males or females or clinically significant persistent urethritis in males): Oral: 1 g as a single dose or 500 mg on day 1, followed by 250 mg daily on days 2-5 (Manhart, 2011):

Note: Follow up patients on either regimen in 3-4 weeks for test of cure; consider moxifloxacin for treatment failures (Manhart, 2011)

Pelvic inflammatory disease (PID): I.V.: 500 mg as a single dose for 1-2 days, follow I.V. therapy by the oral route with a single daily dose of 250 mg to complete a 7-day course of therapy

Pertussis (unlabeled use; CDC, 2005): Oral: 500 mg on day 1 followed by 250 mg daily on days 2-5 (maximum: 500 mg daily)

Pharyngitis, group A streptococci in penicillin-allergic patients (IDSA guidelines): Oral: 12 mg/kg once daily (maximum: 500 mg daily) for 5 days. **Note:** Recommended by the Infectious Disease Society of America (IDSA) as an alternative agent for group A streptococcal pharyngitis in penicillin-allergic patients (Shulman, 2012).

Prophylaxis against infective endocarditis (unlabeled use): Oral: 500 mg 30-60 minutes prior to the procedure. **Note:** American Heart Association (AHA) guidelines now recommend prophylaxis only in patients undergoing invasive procedures and in whom underlying cardiac conditions may predispose to a higher risk of adverse outcomes should infection occur. As of April 2007, routine prophylaxis for GI/GU procedures is no longer recommended by the AHA.

Prophylaxis against sexually-transmitted diseases following sexual assault (unlabeled use): Oral: 1 g as a single dose (in combination with a cephalosporin and metronidazole) (CDC, 2010)

Shigella dysentery type 1 (unlabeled use): Oral: 1000-1500 mg once daily for 1-5 days (WHO, 2005)

Adults:

Prevention of pulmonary exacerbations in patients with noncystic fibrosis bronchiectasis (unlabeled use): Oral: 500 mg 3 days per week. **Note:** Duration of treatment in clinical trial was 6 months; durations >6 months have not been evaluated. Trial patients had ≥1 exacerbation in the past year, no macrolide treatment for >3 months in the past 6 months, and were screened for nontuberculous mycobacterial infection prior to treatment (Wong, 2012). A more selective approach for patients with functionally mild disease has been suggested (Wilson, 2012).

Dosage adjustment in renal impairment: Use with caution in patients with GFR <10 mL/minute (AUC increased by 35% compared to patients with normal renal function); however, no dosage adjustment is provided in the manufacturer's labeling.

No supplemental dose or dosage adjustment necessary, including patients on intermittent hemodialysis, peritoneal dialysis, or continuous renal replacement therapy (eg, CVVHD) (Aronoff, 2007; Heintz, 2009).

Dosage adjustment in hepatic impairment: Azithromycin is predominantly hepatically eliminated; however, there is no dosage adjustment provided in the manufacturer's labeling, Use with caution due to potential for hepatotoxicity (rare); discontinue immediately for signs or symptoms of hepatitis.

Mechanism of Action Inhibits RNA-dependent protein synthesis at the chain elongation step; binds to the 50S ribosomal subunit resulting in blockage of transpeptidation

Contraindications Hypersensitivity to azithromycin, other macrolide (eg, azalide or ketolide) antibiotics, or any component of the formulation; history of cholestatic jaundice/hepatic dysfunction associated with prior azithromycin use

Note: The manufacturer does not list concurrent use of pimozide as a contraindication; however, azithromycin is listed as a contraindication in the manufacturer's labeling for pimozide.

Warnings/Precautions Use with caution in patients with pre-existing liver disease; hepatocellular and/or cholestatic hepatitis, with or without jaundice, hepatic necrosis, failure and death have occurred. Discontinue immediately if symptoms of hepatitis occur (malaise, nausea, vomiting, abdominal colic, fever). Allergic reactions have been reported (rare); reappearance of allergic reaction may occur shortly after discontinuation without further azithromycin exposure. May mask or delay symptoms of incubating gonorrhea or syphilis, so appropriate culture and susceptibility tests should be performed prior to initiating a treatment regimen. Prolonged use may result in fungal or bacterial superinfection, including *C. difficile*-associated diarrhea (CDAD); CDAD has been observed >2 months postantibiotic treatment. Use caution with renal dysfunction. Macrolides (especially erythromycin) have been associated with rare QT_c prolongation and ventricular arrhythmias, including torsade de pointes; consider avoiding use in patients with prolonged QT interval, congenital long QT syndrome, history of torsade de pointes, bradyarrhythmias, uncorrected hypokalemia or hypomagnesemia, clinically significant bradycardia, uncompensated heart failure, or concurrent use of Class IA (eg, quinidine, procainamide) or Class III (eg, amiodarone, dofetilide, sotalol) antiarrhythmic agents or other drugs known to prolong the QT interval. A recent retrospective cohort study (under FDA review) demonstrated an increased cardiac risk with azithromycin relative to amoxicillin or ciprofloxacin, and similar risk compared to levofloxacin; notably, increased cardiac mortality (an estimated 47 additional deaths per 1 million 5-day courses of treatment compared to amoxicillin) was associated with higher baseline cardiovascular risk (Ray, 2012). Use with caution in patients with myasthenia gravis.

Oral suspensions (immediate release and extended release) are not interchangeable.

Drug Interactions

Metabolism/Transport Effects Substrate of CYP3A4 (minor); **Note:** Assignment of Major/Minor substrate status based on clinically relevant drug interaction potential; **Inhibits** CYP1A2 (weak), P-glycoprotein

Avoid Concomitant Use

Avoid concomitant use of Azithromycin (Systemic) with any of the following: Amiodarone; BCG; Highest Risk QTc-Prolonging Agents; Ivabradine; Mifepristone; Pimozide; QuiNINE; Terfenadine

Increased Effect/Toxicity

Azithromycin (Systemic) may increase the levels/effects of: Amiodarone; Cardiac Glycosides; CycloSPORINE (Systemic); Highest Risk QTc-Prolonging Agents; Ivermectin (Systemic); Moderate Risk QTc-Prolonging Agents; Pimozide; QuiNINE; Rivaroxaban; Tacrolimus (Systemic); Tacrolimus (Topical); Terfenadine; Vitamin K Antagonists

The levels/effects of Azithromycin (Systemic) may be increased by: Ivabradine; Mifepristone; Nelfinavir; QTc-Prolonging Agents (Indeterminate Risk and Risk Modifying)

Decreased Effect

Azithromycin (Systemic) may decrease the levels/effects of: BCG; Sodium Picosulfate; Typhoid Vaccine

Ethanol/Nutrition/Herb Interactions Food: Rate and extent of GI absorption may be altered depending upon the formulation. Azithromycin suspension, not tablet form, has significantly increased absorption (46%) with food.

Dietary Considerations

Some products may contain sodium and/or sucrose.

Oral suspension, immediate release, may be administered with or without food.

Oral suspension, extended release, should be taken on an empty stomach (at least 1 hour before or 2 hours following a meal).

Tablet may be administered with food to decrease GI effects.

Pharmacodynamics/Kinetics

Half-life Elimination Terminal: Oral, I.V.: Immediate release: 68-72 hours; Extended release: 59 hours

Time to Peak Oral: Serum: Immediate release: 2-3 hours; Extended release: 5 hours

Pregnancy Risk Factor B

Pregnancy Considerations Adverse events were not observed in animal reproduction studies. Azithromycin crosses the placenta. Fetal malformations have not been observed following maternal use of azithromycin. The maternal serum half-life of azithromycin is unchanged in early pregnancy and decreased at term; however, high concentrations of azithromycin are sustained in the myometrium and adipose tissue. Azithromycin is recommended for the treatment of several infections, including chlamydia, gonococcal infections, and *Mycobacterium avium* complex (MAC) in pregnant patients (consult current guidelines).

Lactation Enters breast milk/use caution

Breast-Feeding Considerations Azithromycin is excreted in low amounts into breast milk. The manufacturer recommends that caution be exercised when administering azithromycin to breast-feeding women. Nondose-related effects could include modification of bowel flora.

Dosage Forms

Injection, powder for reconstitution: 500 mg

Microspheres for suspension, extended release, oral:

Zmax®: 2 g/bottle (60 mL)

Powder for suspension, oral: 100 mg/5 mL (15 mL); 200 mg/5 mL (15 mL, 22.5 mL, 30 mL); 1 g/packet (3s, 10s)

Zithromax®: 100 mg/5 mL (15 mL); 200 mg/5 mL (15 mL, 22.5 mL, 30 mL); 1 g/packet (3s, 10s)

Tablet, oral: 250 mg, 500 mg, 600 mg

Zithromax®: 250 mg, 500 mg, 600 mg

Zithromax® TRI-PAK™: 500 mg

Zithromax® Z-PAK®: 250 mg

Dental Comment There is evidence that azithromycin is proarrhythmic and there are published reports of azithromycin-associated prolongation of the QT interval. The QT interval is measured as the time and distance between the Q point of the QRS complex and the end of the T wave in the ECG tracing. After adjustment for heart rate, the QT interval is defined as prolonged if it is more than 450 msec in men and 460 msec in women. A long QT syndrome was first described in the 1950s and 60s as a congenital syndrome involving QT interval prolongation and syncope and sudden death. Some of the congenital long QT syndromes were characterized by a peculiar electrocardiographic appearance of the QRS complex involving a premature atria beat followed by a pause, then a subsequent sinus beat showing marked QT prolongation and deformity. This type of cardiac arrhythmia was originally termed "torsade de pointes" (translated from the French as "twisting of the points"). Azithromycin is considered as having a risk of causing torsade de pointes. Since it is not known what effect vasoconstrictors in the local anesthetic regimen will have in patients with a known history of congenital prolonged QT interval or in patients taking any medication that prolongs the QT interval, a medical consult is suggested.

A recent large retrospective review of the cardiovascular risks of azithromycin was published. Researchers reviewed a Tennessee Medicaid cohort of patients to evaluate cardiovascular mortality in patients taking azithromycin, amoxicillin, ciprofloxacin, levofloxacin, or no antibiotic. The cohort included patients who took azithromycin (347,795 prescriptions); propensity-score-matched persons who took no antibiotics (1,391,180 control periods); and patients who took amoxicillin (1,348,672 prescriptions), ciprofloxacin (264,626 prescriptions), or levofloxacin (193,906 prescriptions). The risk of cardiovascular death was greater with azithromycin than with ciprofloxacin, but similar to levofloxacin. Amoxicillin showed no increase in risk of cardiovascular death. The estimated risk for azithromycin was 47 additional cardiovascular deaths per million courses of treatment (Ray, 2012).

References

American Dental Association Council on Scientific Affairs, "Combating Antibiotic Resistance," *J Am Dent Assoc*, 2004, 135(4):484-7.

Cotter CJ and Bierne JC, "Azithromycin for Odontogenic Infection," *J Oral Maxillofac Surg*, 2003, 61(10):1238.

Kim MH, Berkowitz C, and Trohman RG, "Polymorphic Ventricular Tachycardia With a Normal QT Interval Following Azithromycin," *Pacing Clin Electrophysiol*, 2005, 28(11):1221-2.

Ray WA, Murray KT, Hall K, et al, "Azithromycin and the Risk of Cardiovascular Death," *N Engl J Med*, 2012, 366(20):1881-90.

Wilson W, Taubert KA, Gewitz M, et al, "Prevention of Infective Endocarditis. Guidelines From the American Heart Association. A Guideline From the American Heart Association Rheumatic Fever, Endocarditis, and Kawasaki Disease Committee, Council on Cardiovascular Disease in the Young, and the Council on Clinical Cardiology, Council on Cardiovascular Surgery and Anesthesia, and the Quality of Care and Outcomes Research Interdisciplinary Working Group," *Circulation*, 2007, 115. Available at http://circ.ahajournals.org/cgi/reprint/CIRCULATIONAHA.106.183095v1; accessed August 6, 2007.

Aztreonam (AZ tree oh nam)

Brand Names: U.S. Azactam®; Cayston®
Brand Names: Canada Cayston®
Pharmacologic Category Antibiotic, Miscellaneous
Use
Injection: Treatment of patients with urinary tract infections, lower respiratory tract infections, septicemia, skin/skin structure infections, intra-abdominal infections, and gynecological infections caused by susceptible gram-negative bacilli
Inhalation: Improve respiratory symptoms in cystic fibrosis (CF) patients with *Pseudomonas aeruginosa*
Local Anesthetic/Vasoconstrictor Precautions No information available to require special precautions
Effects on Dental Treatment No significant effects or complications reported
Effects on Bleeding No information available to require special precautions

Adverse Effects
Inhalation:
>10%:
  Central nervous system: Fever (13%; more common in children)
  Respiratory: Cough (54%), nasal congestion (16%), pharyngeal pain (12%), wheezing (16%)
1% to 10%:
  Cardiovascular: Chest discomfort (8%)
  Dermatologic: Rash (2%)
  Gastrointestinal: Abdominal pain (7%), vomiting (6%)
  Respiratory: Bronchospasm (3%)

Injection:
>10%:
  Hematologic: Neutropenia (children 3% to 11%)
  Hepatic: ALT/AST increased (children 4% to 6%; >3 times ULN: 15% to 20%, high dose)
  Local: Pain at injection site (children 12%, adults 2%)
1% to 10%:
  Central nervous system: Fever (≤1%)
  Dermatologic: Rash (children 4%, adults 1%)
  Gastrointestinal: Diarrhea (1%), nausea (1%), vomiting (1%)
  Hematologic: Eosinophilia (children 6%, adults <1%), thrombocytosis (children 4%, adults <1%), neutropenia (adults <1%)
  Local: Injection site reactions (1% to 3%) (erythema, induration; more common in children), phlebitis/thrombophlebitis (2%)
  Renal: Serum creatinine increased (children 6%)

General Dosage Range Dosage adjustment recommended in patients with renal impairment
I.M.:
  Children >1 month: 30-50 mg/kg/dose every 6-8 hours (maximum: 8 g/day)
  Adults: 500 mg to 1 g every 8-12 hours
I.V.:
  Children >1 month: 30-50 mg/kg/dose every 6-8 hours (maximum: 8 g/day)
  Adults: 1-2 g every 6-12 hours (maximum: 8 g/day)
Oral inhalation: *Children ≥7 years and Adults:* 75 mg 3 times/day

Mechanism of Action Inhibits bacterial cell wall synthesis by binding to one or more of the penicillin-binding proteins (PBPs) which in turn inhibits the final transpeptidation step of peptidoglycan synthesis in bacterial cell walls, thus inhibiting cell wall biosynthesis. Bacteria eventually lyse due to ongoing activity of cell wall autolytic enzymes (autolysins and murein hydrolases) while cell wall assembly is arrested. Monobactam structure makes cross-allergenicity with beta-lactams unlikely.

Pharmacodynamics/Kinetics
Half-life Elimination Injection:
  Children 2 months to 12 years: 1.7 hours
  Adults: Normal renal function: 1.7-2.9 hours
  End-stage renal disease: 6-8 hours
Time to Peak I.M., I.V. push: Within 60 minutes; I.V. infusion: 1.5 hours
Pregnancy Risk Factor B
Pregnancy Considerations Adverse events have not been observed in animal reproduction studies; therefore, the manufacturer classifies aztreonam as pregnancy category B. Aztreonam crosses the placenta and enters cord blood during middle and late pregnancy. Distribution to the fetus is minimal in early pregnancy. The amount of aztreonam available systemically following inhalation is significantly less in comparison to doses given by injection.

Prescribing and Access Restrictions Cayston® (aztreonam inhalation solution) is only available through a select group of specialty pharmacies and cannot be obtained through a retail pharmacy. Because Cayston® may only be used with the Altera® Nebulizer System, it can only be obtained from the following specialty pharmacies: Cystic Fibrosis Services, Inc; IV Solutions; Foundation Care; and Pharmaceutical Specialties, Inc. This network of specialty pharmacies ensures proper access to both the drug and device. To obtain the medication and proper nebulizer, contact the Cayston Access Program at 1-877-7CAYSTON (1-877-722-9786) or at www.cayston.com.

Bacitracin (bas i TRAY sin)

Brand Names: U.S. Baciguent® [OTC]; BACiiM™
Brand Names: Canada Baciguent®; Baciject®
Pharmacologic Category Antibiotic, Miscellaneous; Antibiotic, Ophthalmic; Antibiotic, Topical
Use Treatment of susceptible bacterial infections mainly (has activity against gram-positive bacilli); due to toxicity risks, systemic and irrigant uses of bacitracin should be limited to situations where less toxic alternatives would not be effective
Unlabeled Use Oral administration: Treatment of *Clostridium difficile*-associated diarrhea; has been used for enteric eradication of vancomycin-resistant enterococci (VRE)
Local Anesthetic/Vasoconstrictor Precautions No information available to require special precautions
Effects on Dental Treatment No significant effects or complications reported
Effects on Bleeding No information available to require special precautions
Adverse Effects
1% to 10%:
  Cardiovascular: Hypotension, edema of the face/lips, chest tightness
  Central nervous system: Pain
  Dermatologic: Rash, itching
  Gastrointestinal: Anorexia, nausea, vomiting, diarrhea, rectal itching
  Hematologic: Blood dyscrasias
  Renal: Nephrotoxicity (with systemic administration)
  Miscellaneous: Diaphoresis
<1%: Rare cases of anaphylaxis have been reported in association with topical and intraoperative exposures.
General Dosage Range
I.M.:
  Infants ≤2.5 kg: 900 units/kg/day in 2-3 divided doses
  Infants >2.5 kg: 1000 units/kg/day in 2-3 divided doses
Ophthalmic: *Children and Adults:* Instill 1/4" to 1/2" ribbon every 3-4 hours (acute infections) or 2-3 times daily (mild-to-moderate infections)
Oral: *Adults:* 25,000 units 4 times daily
Topical: *Children and Adults:* Apply 1-3 times daily
Mechanism of Action Inhibits bacterial cell wall synthesis by preventing transfer of mucopeptides into the growing cell wall
Pharmacodynamics/Kinetics
Duration of Action 6-8 hours
Time to Peak Serum: I.M.: 1-2 hours

Pregnancy Considerations It is unknown if bacitracin crosses the placenta. The minimal absorption after topical use should limit the amount of medication available for transfer to the fetus. If ophthalmic agents are needed during pregnancy, the minimum effective dose should be used in combination with punctual occlusion to decrease potential exposure to the fetus.

Bacitracin and Polymyxin B
(bas i TRAY sin & pol i MIKS in bee)

Related Information
  Bacitracin *on page 163*
  Polymyxin B *on page 1112*
Brand Names: U.S. AK-Poly-Bac™; Polycin™; Polysporin® [OTC]
Brand Names: Canada LID-Pack®; Optimyxin®
Pharmacologic Category Antibiotic, Ophthalmic; Antibiotic, Topical
Use Treatment of superficial infections caused by susceptible organisms
Local Anesthetic/Vasoconstrictor Precautions No information available to require special precautions
Effects on Dental Treatment No significant effects or complications reported
Effects on Bleeding No information available to require special precautions
Adverse Effects 1% to 10%: Local: Rash, itching, burning, anaphylactoid reactions, swelling, conjunctival erythema
General Dosage Range
Ophthalmic: *Children and Adults:* Instill 1/2" ribbon in the affected eye(s) every 3-4 hours (acute infections) or 2-3 times/day (mild-to-moderate infections)
Topical: *Children and Adults:* Apply to affected area 1-4 times/day
Mechanism of Action See individual agents.
Pregnancy Risk Factor C
Pregnancy Considerations Animal reproduction studies have not been conducted with this combination. See individual agents.

Bacitracin, Neomycin, and Polymyxin B
(bas i TRAY sin, nee oh MYE sin, & pol i MIKS in bee)

Related Information
  Bacitracin *on page 163*
  Neomycin *on page 968*
  Polymyxin B *on page 1112*
Brand Names: U.S. Neo-Polycin™; Neosporin® Neo To Go® [OTC]; Neosporin® Topical [OTC]
Pharmacologic Category Antibiotic, Ophthalmic; Antibiotic, Topical
Use Helps prevent infection in minor cuts, scrapes, and burns; short-term treatment of superficial external ocular infections caused by susceptible organisms
Local Anesthetic/Vasoconstrictor Precautions No information available to require special precautions
Effects on Dental Treatment No significant effects or complications reported
Effects on Bleeding No information available to require special precautions
Adverse Effects Frequency not defined.
  Dermatologic: Reddening, allergic contact dermatitis
  Local: Itching, failure to heal, swelling, irritation
  Ophthalmic: Conjunctival edema
  Miscellaneous: Anaphylaxis

General Dosage Range
Ophthalmic: *Children and Adults:* Instill ¹/₂" every 3-4 hours
Topical: *Children and Adults:* Apply 1-3 times/day
Mechanism of Action See individual agents.
Pregnancy Risk Factor C
Pregnancy Considerations Animal reproduction studies have not been conducted with this combination. See individual agents.

Bacitracin, Neomycin, Polymyxin B, and Hydrocortisone
(bas i TRAY sin, nee oh MYE sin, pol i MIKS in bee, & hye droe KOR ti sone)

Related Information
Bacitracin *on page 163*
Hydrocortisone (Topical) *on page 699*
Neomycin *on page 968*
Polymyxin B *on page 1112*
Brand Names: U.S. Cortisporin® Ointment; Neo-Polycin™ HC
Brand Names: Canada Cortisporin® Topical Ointment
Pharmacologic Category Antibiotic, Ophthalmic; Antibiotic, Topical; Corticosteroid, Ophthalmic; Corticosteroid, Topical
Use Prevention and treatment of susceptible inflammatory conditions where bacterial infection (or risk of infection) is present
Local Anesthetic/Vasoconstrictor Precautions No information available to require special precautions
Effects on Dental Treatment No significant effects or complications reported
Effects on Bleeding No information available to require special precautions
Adverse Effects Frequency not defined. For additional information, see individual agents.
Ophthalmic ointment:
Dermatologic: Delayed wound healing, rash
Ocular: Cataracts, corneal thinning, glaucoma, irritation, keratitis (bacterial), intraocular pressure increase, optic nerve damage, scleral thinning
Miscellaneous: Hypersensitivity (including anaphylaxis), secondary infection, sensitization to kanamycin, paromomycin, streptomycin, and gentamicin
Topical ointment:
Dermatologic: Acneiform eruptions, allergic contact dermatitis, burning skin, dryness, folliculitis, hypertrichosis, hypopigmentation, irritation, maceration of skin, miliaria, ocular hypertension, perioral dermatitis, pruritus, skin atrophy, striae
Otic: Ototoxicity
Renal: Nephrotoxicity
Miscellaneous: Hypersensitivity (including anaphylaxis), secondary infection, sensitization to karamycin, paromomycin, streptomycin, and gentamicin
General Dosage Range
Ophthalmic: *Children and Adults:* Instill ¹/₂ inch every 3-4 hours
Topical: *Children and Adults:* Apply sparingly 2-4 times/day
Mechanism of Action See individual agents.
Pregnancy Risk Factor C
Pregnancy Considerations Adverse events have been observed with topical corticosteroids in animal reproduction studies. See individual agents.

Bacitracin, Neomycin, Polymyxin B, and Pramoxine
(bas i TRAY sin, nee oh MYE sin, pol i MIKS in bee, & pra MOKS een)

Related Information
Bacitracin *on page 163*
Neomycin *on page 968*
Polymyxin B *on page 1112*
Pramoxine *on page 1125*
Brand Names: U.S. Neosporin® + Pain Relief Ointment [OTC]; Tri Biozene [OTC]
Pharmacologic Category Antibiotic, Topical
Use Prevention and treatment of susceptible superficial topical infections and provide temporary relief of pain or discomfort
Local Anesthetic/Vasoconstrictor Precautions No information available to require special precautions
Effects on Dental Treatment No significant effects or complications reported
Effects on Bleeding No information available to require special precautions
General Dosage Range Topical: *Children ≥2 years and Adults:* Apply 1-3 times/day to infected areas

Baclofen (BAK loe fen)

Brand Names: U.S. Gablofen®; Lioresal®
Brand Names: Canada Apo-Baclofen®; Ava-Baclofen; Dom-Baclofen; Lioresal®; Lioresal® D.S.; Lioresal® Intrathecal; Med-Baclofen; Mylan-Baclofen; Novo-Baclofen; Nu-Baclo; PHL-Baclofen; PMS-Baclofen; ratio-Baclofen; Riva-Baclofen
Pharmacologic Category Skeletal Muscle Relaxant
Use Treatment of reversible spasticity associated with multiple sclerosis or spinal cord lesions
Orphan drug: Intrathecal: Treatment of intractable spasticity caused by spinal cord injury, multiple sclerosis, and other spinal disease (spinal ischemia or tumor, transverse myelitis, cervical spondylosis, degenerative myelopathy)
Unlabeled Use Intractable hiccups, intractable pain relief, bladder spasticity, trigeminal neuralgia, cerebral palsy, short-term treatment of spasticity in children with cerebral palsy, Huntington's chorea
Local Anesthetic/Vasoconstrictor Precautions No information available to require special precautions
Effects on Dental Treatment No significant effects or complications reported
Effects on Bleeding No information available to require special precautions
Adverse Effects
>10%:
Central nervous system: Drowsiness, vertigo, psychiatric disturbances, insomnia, slurred speech, ataxia, hypotonia
Neuromuscular & skeletal: Weakness
1% to 10%:
Cardiovascular: Hypotension
Central nervous system: Fatigue, confusion, headache
Dermatologic: Rash
Gastrointestinal: Nausea, constipation
Genitourinary: Polyuria

General Dosage Range

Intrathecal:

Children: Test dose: 25-100 mcg; Initial infusion: Infuse at a 24-hourly rate dosed at twice the test dose

Adults: Test dose: 50-100 mcg; Initial infusion: Infuse at a 24-hourly rate dosed at twice the test dose

Oral:

Adults: Initial: 5 mg 3 times/day; Maintenance: Up to 80 mg/day in 2-3 divided doses

Elderly: Initial: 5 mg 2-3 times/day, increasing gradually as needed

Mechanism of Action Inhibits the transmission of both monosynaptic and polysynaptic reflexes at the spinal cord level, possibly by hyperpolarization of primary afferent fiber terminals, with resultant relief of muscle spasticity

Pharmacodynamics/Kinetics

Onset of Action 3-4 days; Peak effect: 5-10 days

Half-life Elimination 3.5 hours

Time to Peak Serum: Oral: Within 2-3 hours

Pregnancy Risk Factor C

Pregnancy Considerations Adverse events were observed in animal reproduction studies. Withdrawal symptoms in the neonate were noted in a case report following the maternal use of oral baclofen 20 mg 4 times/day throughout pregnancy (Ratnayaka, 2001). Plasma concentrations following administration of intrathecal baclofen are significantly less than those with oral doses; exposure to the fetus is expected to be limited (Morton, 2009).

Balanced Salt Solution

(BAL anced salt soe LOO shun)

Brand Names: U.S. AquaLase®; BSS Plus®; BSS®

Brand Names: Canada BSS Plus®; BSS®; Eye-Stream®

Pharmacologic Category Irrigating Solution; Ophthalmic Agent, Miscellaneous

Use

Irrigation solution for ophthalmic surgery:

AquaLase®, BSS®: Intraocular or extraocular irrigating solution

BSS Plus®: Intraocular irrigating solution

Irrigation solution for eyes, ears, nose, or throat

Local Anesthetic/Vasoconstrictor Precautions No information available to require special precautions

Effects on Dental Treatment No significant effects or complications reported

Effects on Bleeding No information available to require special precautions

Adverse Effects

>10%: Ocular: Intraocular pressure increased (11% to 12%), cataract (7% to 11%)

1% to 10%:

Central nervous system: Headache (3%)

Ocular: Discomfort (3% to 5%), dry eyes (3% to 5%), macular edema (4%), conjunctival hyperemia (3% to 4%), posterior capsule opacification (2% to 3%), iritis (1% to 3%), retinal hemorrhage (1% to 3%), blurred vision (1% to 2%)

General Dosage Range Irrigation: *Children and Adults:* Based on standard for each surgical procedure

---

Balsalazide (bal SAL a zide)

Brand Names: U.S. Colazal®; Giazo™

Pharmacologic Category 5-Aminosalicylic Acid Derivative; Anti-inflammatory Agent

Use Treatment of mildly- to moderately-active ulcerative colitis

Giazo™: Only approved in males ≥18 years; effectiveness in females was not demonstrated

Local Anesthetic/Vasoconstrictor Precautions No information available to require special precautions

Effects on Dental Treatment No significant effects or complications reported

Effects on Bleeding No information available to require special precautions

Adverse Effects

>10%:

Central nervous system: Headache (children 15%; adults 8%)

Gastrointestinal: Abdominal pain (children 12% to 13%; adults ≤6%)

1% to 10%:

Central nervous system: Insomnia (adults 2%), fatigue (children 4%; adults ≤2%), fever (children 6%; adults 2%)

Endocrine & metabolic: Dysmenorrhea (children 3%)

Gastrointestinal: Vomiting (children 10%; adults ≤4%), diarrhea (children 9%; adults ≤5%), ulcerative colitis exacerbation (children 6%; adults 1%), nausea (children 4%; adults 5%), hematochezia (children 4%), stomatitis (children 3%), anorexia (adults 2%), dyspepsia (adults 2%), flatulence (adults ≤2%), cramps (adults 1%), constipation (adults ≤1%), xerostomia (adults ≤1%)

Genitourinary: Urinary tract infection (adults 1% to 4%)

Hematologic: Anemia (4%)

Neuromuscular & skeletal: Arthralgia (adults ≤4%), musculoskeletal pain (adults 2%), myalgia (adults ≤1%)

Respiratory: Respiratory infection (adults ≤4%), cough (children 3%; adults 2%), pharyngitis (children 6%; adults 2%), pharyngolaryngeal pain (children 3%; adults 4%), rhinitis (adults 2%)

Miscellaneous: Flu-like syndrome (children 4%; adults 1%)

General Dosage Range Oral:

Capsule:

Children ≥5 years: 750 mg **or** 2.25 g 3 times daily

Adults: 2.25 g 3 times daily

Tablet: *Adults: Males:* 3.3 g twice daily

Mechanism of Action Balsalazide is a prodrug, converted by bacterial azoreduction to 5-aminosalicylic acid (mesalamine, active), 4-aminobenzoyl-β-alanine (inert), and their metabolites. 5-aminosalicylic acid may decrease inflammation by blocking the production of arachidonic acid metabolites topically in the colon mucosa.

Pharmacodynamics/Kinetics

Onset of Action Delayed; may require several days to weeks

Half-life Elimination Primary effect is topical (colonic mucosa); therapeutic effect appears not to be influenced by the systemic half-life of balsalazide (1.9 hours) or its metabolites (5-ASA [9.5 hours], N-Ac-5-ASA [10.4 hours])

Time to Peak Balsalazide: Capsule: 1-2 hours; Tablet: 0.5 hours

Pregnancy Risk Factor B

Pregnancy Considerations Teratogenic effects were not observed in animal reproduction studies. Mesalamine (5-aminosalicylic acid) is the active metabolite of balsalazide; mesalamine is known to cross the placenta.

Barium (BA ree um)

Brand Names: U.S. Digibar™ 190; E-Z Cat® Dry; E-Z-Cat®; E-Z-Disk™; E-Z-Dose™ with Liquid Polibar Plus®; E-Z-HD™; E-Z-Paque®; E-Z-Paste®; Entero Vu™; Entero VU™ 24%; Entero-H™; Esopho-Cat®; Liquid Entero Vu™; Liquid Polibar Plus®; Liquid Polibar®; Maxibar™; Polibar® ACB; Readi-Cat®; Readi-Cat® 2; Sensatrast™; Tagitol™ V; Ultra-R®; Varibar® Honey; Varibar® Nectar; Varibar® Pudding; Varibar® Thin Honey; Varibar® Thin Liquid; VoLumen®

Pharmacologic Category Radiopaque Agents

Use Diagnostic aid for computed tomography or x-ray examinations of the GI tract

Local Anesthetic/Vasoconstrictor Precautions No information available to require special precautions

Effects on Dental Treatment No significant effects or complications reported

Effects on Bleeding No information available to require special precautions

Pregnancy Considerations Safety and efficacy for use during pregnancy have not been established. In general, elective radiography of the abdomen is avoided during pregnancy unless essential for diagnosis.

Basiliximab (ba si LIK si mab)

Brand Names: U.S. Simulect®
Brand Names: Canada Simulect®
Pharmacologic Category Immunosuppressant Agent; Monoclonal Antibody

Use Prophylaxis of acute organ rejection in renal transplantation (in combination with cyclosporine and corticosteroids)

Unlabeled Use Treatment of refractory acute graft-versus-host disease (GVHD); prevention of liver or cardiac transplant rejection

Local Anesthetic/Vasoconstrictor Precautions No information available to require special precautions

Effects on Dental Treatment Key adverse event(s) related to dental treatment: Facial edema and ulcerative stomatitis. Causes gingival hypertrophy (GH) similar to that caused by cyclosporine; early reports indicate that frequency/incidence of basiliximab-induced GH not as high as cyclosporine-induced GH.

Effects on Bleeding No information available to require special precautions

Adverse Effects Administration of basiliximab did not appear to increase the incidence or severity of adverse effects in clinical trials. Adverse events were reported in 96% of both the placebo and basiliximab groups.

>10%:
Cardiovascular: Hypertension, peripheral edema
Central nervous system: Fever, headache, insomnia, pain
Dermatologic: Acne, wound complications
Endocrine & metabolic: Hypercholesterolemia, hyperglycemia, hyper-/hypokalemia, hyperuricemia, hypophosphatemia
Gastrointestinal: Abdominal pain, constipation, diarrhea, dyspepsia, nausea, vomiting
Genitourinary: Urinary tract infection
Hematologic: Anemia
Neuromuscular & skeletal: Tremor
Respiratory: Dyspnea, infection (upper respiratory)
Miscellaneous: Viral infection

3% to 10%:
Cardiovascular: Abnormal heart sounds, angina, arrhythmia, atrial fibrillation, chest pain, generalized edema, heart failure, hypotension, tachycardia
Central nervous system: Agitation, anxiety, depression, dizziness, fatigue, hypoesthesia, malaise
Dermatologic: Cyst, hypertrichosis, pruritus, rash, skin disorder, skin ulceration
Endocrine & metabolic: Acidosis, dehydration, diabetes mellitus, fluid overload, glucocorticoids increased, hyper-/hypocalcemia, hyperlipemia, hypertriglyceridemia, hypoglycemia, hypomagnesemia, hyponatremia, hypoproteinemia
Gastrointestinal: Abdomen enlarged, esophagitis, flatulence, gastroenteritis, GI hemorrhage, gingival hyperplasia, melena, moniliasis, stomatitis (including ulcerative), weight gain
Genitourinary: Bladder disorder, dysuria, genital edema (male), impotence, ureteral disorder, urinary frequency, urinary retention
Hematologic: Hematoma, hemorrhage, leukopenia, polycythemia, purpura, thrombocytopenia, thrombosis
Neuromuscular & skeletal: Arthralgia, arthropathy, back pain, cramps, fracture, hernia, leg pain, myalgia, neuropathy, paresthesia, rigors, weakness
Ocular: Abnormal vision, cataract, conjunctivitis
Renal: Albuminuria, hematuria, nonprotein nitrogen increased, oliguria, renal function abnormal, renal tubular necrosis
Respiratory: Bronchitis, bronchospasm, cough, pharyngitis, pneumonia, pulmonary edema, sinusitis, rhinitis
Miscellaneous: Accidental trauma, cytomegalovirus (CMV) infection, herpes infection (simplex and zoster), infection, sepsis

General Dosage Range I.V.:
Children <35 kg: 10 mg within 2 hours prior to transplant surgery, followed by a second 10 mg dose 4 days after transplantation
Children ≥35 kg and Adults: 20 mg within 2 hours prior to transplant surgery, followed by a second 20 mg dose 4 days after transplantation

Mechanism of Action Chimeric (murine/human) immunosuppressant monoclonal antibody which blocks the alpha-chain of the interleukin-2 (IL-2) receptor complex; this receptor is expressed on activated T lymphocytes and is a critical pathway for activating cell-mediated allograft rejection

Pharmacodynamics/Kinetics
Duration of Action Mean: 36 days (determined by IL-2R alpha saturation)
Half-life Elimination Children 1-11 years: 9.5 days; Adolescents 12-16 years: 9.1 days; Adults: Mean: 7.2 days

Pregnancy Risk Factor B
Pregnancy Considerations Teratogenic effects were not observed in animal studies. IL-2 receptors play an important role in the development of the immune system. Use in pregnant women only when benefit exceeds potential risk to the fetus. Women of childbearing potential should use effective contraceptive measures before beginning treatment and for 4 months after completion of therapy with this agent. The National Transplantation Pregnancy Registry (NTPR, Temple University) is a registry for pregnant women taking immunosuppressants following any solid organ transplant. The NTPR encourages reporting all immunosuppressant exposures during pregnancy in transplant recipients at 877-955-6877.

BCG (bee see jee)

Brand Names: U.S. BCG Vaccine; TheraCys®; TICE® BCG

Brand Names: Canada BCG Vaccine; ImmuCyst®; Oncotice™

Pharmacologic Category Biological Response Modulator; Vaccine, Live (Bacterial)

Use

BCG intravesical: Treatment and prophylaxis of carcinoma *in situ* of the bladder; prophylaxis of primary or recurrent superficial or minimally invasive papillary tumors following transurethral resection

BCG vaccine: Immunization against *Mycobacterium tuberculosis* in persons not previously infected and who are at high risk for exposure

BCG vaccine is not routinely administered for the prevention of *M. tuberculosis* in the United States. The Advisory Committee on Immunization Practices (ACIP) recommends vaccination be considered for the following:
- Children with a negative tuberculin skin test who are continually exposed to (and cannot be separated from) adults who are untreated or ineffectively treated for TB disease when the child cannot be given long-term treatment for infection **or** if the adult has TB caused by strains resistant to isoniazid and rifampin.
- Healthcare workers with a high percentage of patients with *M. tuberculosis* strains resistant to both isoniazid and rifampin, if there is ongoing transmission of the resistant strains and subsequent infection is likely, or if comprehensive infection-control precautions have not been successful. In addition, healthcare workers should be counseled on the risks and benefits of vaccination and treatment of latent TB infection

Local Anesthetic/Vasoconstrictor Precautions No information available to require special precautions

Effects on Dental Treatment No significant effects or complications reported

Effects on Bleeding No information available to require special precautions

Adverse Effects Following vaccination, all serious adverse reactions must be reported to the U.S. Department of Health and Human Services (DHHS) Vaccine Adverse Event Reporting System (VAERS) 1-800-822-7967 or online at https://vaers.hhs.gov/esub/index. Adverse events following intravesicular administration should be reported to MEDWATCH (800-FDA-1088 or www.fda.gov/medwatch) or the manufacturer.

Adverse reactions associated with **intravesicular administration**:

>10%:
Central nervous system: Malaise (7% to 40%), fever (17% to 38%), chills (9% to 34%), pain (17%)
Gastrointestinal: Nausea/vomiting (3% to 16%), anorexia/weight loss (2% to 11%)
Genitourinary: Dysuria (52% to 60%), bladder irritation (50%), urinary frequency (40% to 50%), hematuria (26% to 39%), cystitis (6% to 30%), urinary urgency (6% to 18%), urinary tract infection (2% to 18%)
Hematological: Anemia (<21%)
Miscellaneous: Flu-like syndrome (24% to 33%)
1% to 10%:
Central nervous system: Headache (2%)
Dermatologic: Rash (2% to 3%)

Gastrointestinal: Diarrhea (6%), abdominal pain (2% to 3%)
Genitourinary: Genital pain (10%), hemorrhagic cystitis (9%), bladder cramps/pain (6% to 8%), urinary incontinence (2% to 6%), contracted bladder (5%), nocturia (5%), urinary debris (2%), genital inflammation/abscess (2%)
Hematological: Leukopenia (<6%)
Neuromuscular & skeletal: Arthralgia/myalgia (3% to 7%), cramps/pain (4%), rigors (3%)
Renal: Renal toxicity (10%)
Respiratory: Pulmonary infection (<3%)
Miscellaneous: Infection (<1% to 5%), diaphoresis (3%), allergy (2%)

General Dosage Range

Percutaneous:
Children <1 month: 0.2-0.3 mL (half-strength dilution)
Children >1 month and Adults: 0.2-0.3 mL (full-strength dilution)

Intravesicular: *Adults:*
TheraCys®: 1 dose instilled into bladder (retain for 2 hours) once weekly for 6 weeks followed by 1 treatment at 3, 6, 12, 18, and 24 months after initial treatment
TICE® BCG: 1 dose instilled into bladder (retain for 2 hours) once weekly for 6 weeks (may repeat cycle 1 time), followed by approximately once monthly for at least 6-12 months

Mechanism of Action BCG live is an attenuated strain of bacillus Calmette-Guérin (*Mycobacterium bovis*) used as a biological response modifier. BCG live, when used intravesicularly for treatment of bladder carcinoma *in situ*, is thought to cause a local, chronic inflammatory response involving macrophage and leukocyte infiltration of the bladder. By a mechanism not fully understood, this local inflammatory response leads to destruction of superficial tumor cells of the urothelium. BCG is active immunotherapy which stimulates the host's immune mechanism to reject the tumor. Evidence of systemic immune response is also commonly seen, manifested by a positive PPD tuberculin skin test reaction, however, its relationship to clinical efficacy is not well-established.

Pregnancy Risk Factor C

Pregnancy Considerations Animal reproduction studies have not been conducted. Both BCG intravesical and BCG vaccine are not recommended for use in pregnant women. Women of childbearing potential should be advised to avoid pregnancy while on intravesical therapy.

Becaplermin (be KAP ler min)

Brand Names: U.S. Regranex®

Pharmacologic Category Growth Factor, Platelet-Derived; Topical Skin Product

Use Adjunctive treatment of diabetic neuropathic ulcers occurring on the lower limbs and feet that extend into subcutaneous tissue (or beyond) and have adequate blood supply

Local Anesthetic/Vasoconstrictor Precautions No information available to require special precautions

Effects on Dental Treatment No significant effects or complications reported

Effects on Bleeding No information available to require special precautions

Adverse Effects 1% to 10%: Dermatologic: Erythematous rash (2%)

◄ **General Dosage Range Topical:** *Adults:* Apply once daily; to determine the length of gel to apply to the ulcer, measure the greatest length of the ulcer by the greatest width of the ulcer. Tube size and unit of measure will determine the formula used in the calculation. Recalculate amount of gel needed every 1-2 weeks, depending on the rate of change in ulcer area.

Centimeters: 15 g tube: [ulcer length (cm) x width (cm)] divided by 4 = length of gel (cm); 2 g tube: [ulcer length (cm) x width (cm)] divided by 2 = length of gel (cm)

Inches: 15 g tube: [length (in) x width (in)] x 0.6 = length of gel (in); 2 g tube: [length (in) x width (in)] x 1.3 = length of gel (in)

Mechanism of Action Recombinant B-isoform homodimer of human platelet-derived growth factor (rPDGF-BB) which enhances formation of new granulation tissue, induces fibroblast proliferation and differentiation to promote wound healing; also promotes angiogenesis.

Pharmacodynamics/Kinetics

Onset of Action Complete healing: 15% of patients within 8 weeks, 25% at 10 weeks

Pregnancy Risk Factor C

Pregnancy Considerations Animal reproduction studies have not been conducted. Use in pregnancy only if clearly needed.

Beclomethasone (Oral Inhalation)
(be kloe METH a sone)

Related Information
Respiratory Diseases *on page 1514*

Brand Names: U.S. QVAR®

Brand Names: Canada QVAR®

Generic Availability (U.S.) No

Pharmacologic Category Corticosteroid, Inhalant (Oral)

Use Oral inhalation: Maintenance and prophylactic treatment of asthma; includes those who require corticosteroids and those who may benefit from a dose reduction/elimination of systemically-administered corticosteroids. Not for relief of acute bronchospasm.

Local Anesthetic/Vasoconstrictor Precautions No information available to require special precautions

Effects on Dental Treatment Key adverse event(s) related to dental treatment: Oral candidiasis, xerostomia (normal salivary flow resumes upon discontinuation), nasal dryness, and dry throat. Localized infections with *Candida albicans* or *Aspergillus niger* occur frequently in the mouth and pharynx with repetitive use of an oral inhaler; may require treatment with appropriate antifungal therapy or discontinuance of inhaler use.

Effects on Bleeding No information available to require special precautions

Adverse Effects
>10%: Central nervous system: Headache (12%)
1% to 10%:
Central nervous system: Dysphonia (1% to 3%), pain (2%)
Endocrine & metabolic: Dysmenorrhea (1% to 3%)
Gastrointestinal: Nausea (1%)
Neuromuscular & skeletal: Back pain (1%)
Respiratory: Upper respiratory tract infection (9%), pharyngitis (8%), rhinitis (6%), sinusitis (3%), cough (1% to 3%)

Dosage Inhalation, oral: Asthma (doses should be titrated to the lowest effective dose once asthma is controlled):
U.S. labeling:
Children 5-11 years: Initial: 40 mcg twice daily; maximum dose: 80 mcg twice daily
Children ≥12 years and Adults:
Patients previously on bronchodilators only: Initial dose 40-80 mcg twice daily; maximum dose: 320 mcg twice day
Patients previously on inhaled corticosteroids: Initial dose 40-160 mcg twice daily; maximum dose: 320 mcg twice daily
NIH Asthma Guidelines (NIH, 2007):
Children 5-11 years:
"Low" dose: 80-160 mcg/day
"Medium" dose: >160-320 mcg/day
"High" dose: >320 mcg/day
Children ≥12 years and Adults:
"Low" dose: 80-240 mcg/day
"Medium" dose: >240-480 mcg/day
"High" dose: >480 mcg/day

Canadian labeling:
Children 5-11 years: Initial: 50 mcg twice daily; maximum dose: 100 mcg twice daily
Children ≥12 years and Adults:
Mild asthma: 50-100 mcg twice daily; maximum dose: 100 mcg twice daily
Moderate asthma: 100-250 mcg twice daily; maximum dose: 250 mcg twice daily
Severe asthma: 300-400 mcg twice daily; maximum dose: 400 mcg twice daily

Conversion from oral systemic corticosteroid to orally inhaled corticosteroid: Initiation of oral inhalation therapy should begin in patients whose asthma is reasonably stabilized on oral corticosteroids (OCS). A gradual dose reduction of OCS should begin ~7 days after starting inhaled therapy. U.S. labeling recommends reducing prednisone dose no more rapidly than ≤2.5 mg/day (or equivalent of other OCS) every 1-2 weeks. The Canadian labeling recommends decreasing the daily dose of prednisone by 1 mg (or equivalent of other OCS) every 7 days or more in closely monitored patients. If adrenal insufficiency occurs, temporarily increase the OCS dose and follow with a more gradual withdrawal. **Note:** When transitioning from systemic to inhaled corticosteroids, supplemental systemic corticosteroid therapy may be necessary during periods of stress or during severe asthma attacks.

Mechanism of Action Controls the rate of protein synthesis; depresses the migration of polymorphonuclear leukocytes, fibroblasts; reverses capillary permeability and lysosomal stabilization at the cellular level to prevent or control inflammation

Contraindications Hypersensitivity to beclomethasone or any component of the formulation; status asthmaticus, or other acute asthma episodes requiring intensive measures

Canadian labeling: Additional contraindications (not in U.S. labeling): Moderate-to-severe bronchiectasis requiring intensive measures; untreated fungal, bacterial, or tubercular infections of the respiratory tract

Warnings/Precautions May cause hypercorticism or suppression of hypothalamic-pituitary-adrenal (HPA) axis, particularly in younger children or in patients receiving high doses for prolonged periods. HPA axis suppression may lead to adrenal crisis. Withdrawal and discontinuation of a corticosteroid should be done slowly and carefully. Particular care is required when patients are transferred from systemic corticosteroids to inhaled products due to possible adrenal insufficiency or withdrawal from steroids, including an increase in allergic symptoms. Patients receiving >20 mg per day of prednisone (or equivalent) may be most susceptible. Fatalities have occurred due to adrenal insufficiency in asthmatic patients during and after transfer from systemic corticosteroids to aerosol steroids; aerosol steroids do **not** provide the systemic steroid needed to treat patients having trauma, surgery, or infections.

Bronchospasm may occur with wheezing after inhalation; if this occurs, stop steroid and treat with a fast-acting bronchodilator. Supplemental steroids (oral or parenteral) may be needed during stress or severe asthma attacks. Not to be used in status asthmaticus or for the relief of acute bronchospasm. Corticosteroid use may cause psychiatric disturbances, including depression, euphoria, insomnia, mood swings, and personality changes. Pre-existing psychiatric conditions may be exacerbated by corticosteroid use. Prolonged use of corticosteroids may also increase the incidence of secondary infection, mask acute infection (including fungal infections), prolong or exacerbate viral infections, or limit response to vaccines. Avoid use in patients with ocular herpes or untreated viral, fungal, parasitic or bacterial systemic infections (Canadian labeling contraindicates use with untreated respiratory infections). Exposure to chickenpox should be avoided. Close observation is required in patients with latent tuberculosis and/or TB reactivity; restrict use in active TB (only in conjunction with antituberculosis treatment). Prolonged treatment with corticosteroids has been associated with the development of Kaposi's sarcoma (case reports); if noted, discontinuation of therapy should be considered.

Use with caution in patients with thyroid disease, hepatic impairment, renal impairment, cardiovascular disease, diabetes, glaucoma, cataracts, myasthenia gravis, patients at risk for osteoporosis, patients at risk for seizures, or GI diseases (diverticulitis, peptic ulcer, ulcerative colitis) due to perforation risk. Use caution following acute MI (corticosteroids have been associated with myocardial rupture). Because of the risk of adverse effects, systemic corticosteroids should be used cautiously in the elderly in the smallest possible effective dose for the shortest duration.

Orally-inhaled corticosteroids may cause a reduction in growth velocity in pediatric patients (~1 centimeter per year [range: 0.3-1.8 cm per year]) and related to dose and duration of exposure). To minimize the systemic effects of orally-inhaled corticosteroids, each patient should be titrated to the lowest effective dose. Growth should be routinely monitored in pediatric patients. Safety and efficacy have not been established in children <5 years of age. There have been reports of systemic corticosteroid withdrawal symptoms (eg, joint/ muscle pain, lassitude, depression) when withdrawing oral inhalation therapy.

Drug Interactions

Metabolism/Transport Effects None known.

Avoid Concomitant Use

Avoid concomitant use of Beclomethasone (Oral Inhalation) with any of the following: Aldesleukin; BCG; Natalizumab; Pimecrolimus; Tacrolimus (Topical); Tofacitinib

Increased Effect/Toxicity

Beclomethasone (Oral Inhalation) may increase the levels/effects of: Amphotericin B; Deferasirox; Leflunomide; Loop Diuretics; Natalizumab; Thiazide Diuretics; Tofacitinib

The levels/effects of Beclomethasone (Oral Inhalation) may be increased by: Denosumab; Pimecrolimus; Tacrolimus (Topical); Telaprevir; Trastuzumab

Decreased Effect

Beclomethasone (Oral Inhalation) may decrease the levels/effects of: Aldesleukin; Antidiabetic Agents; BCG; Coccidioidin Skin Test; Corticorelin; Hyaluronidase; Sipuleucel-T; Telaprevir; Vaccines (Inactivated)

The levels/effects of Beclomethasone (Oral Inhalation) may be decreased by: Echinacea

Pharmacodynamics/Kinetics

Onset of Action Therapeutic effect: 1-4 weeks

Half-life Elimination 17-BMP: 3 hours

Time to Peak Plasma: Oral inhalation: BDP: 0.5 hours; 17-BMP: 0.7 hours

Pregnancy Risk Factor C

Pregnancy Considerations Teratogenic effects were observed in animal reproduction studies following SubQ administration but not with oral inhalation. A decrease in fetal growth has not been observed with inhaled corticosteroid use during pregnancy. Inhaled corticosteroids are recommended for the treatment of asthma (most information available using budesonide) during pregnancy (NAEPP, 2005).

Lactation Excretion in breast milk unknown/use caution

Breast-Feeding Considerations Other corticosteroids have been found in breast milk; however, information for beclomethasone is not available. Use of inhaled corticosteroids is not a contraindication to breast-feeding (NAEPP, 2005).

Dosage Forms

Aerosol, for oral inhalation:

QVAR®: 40 mcg/inhalation (8.7 g); 80 mcg/inhalation (8.7 g)

Dosage Forms: Canada

Aerosol, for oral inhalation:

QVAR™: 50 mcg/inhalation (6.5 g, 12.4 g); 100 mcg/ inhalation (6.5 g, 12.4 g)

Beclomethasone (Nasal) (be kloe METH a sone)

Brand Names: U.S. Beconase AQ®; Qnasl™

Brand Names: Canada Apo-Beclomethasone®; Mylan-Beclo AQ; Nu-Beclomethasone; Rivanase AQ

Generic Availability (U.S.) No

Pharmacologic Category Corticosteroid, Nasal

Use

Beconase AQ®: Symptomatic treatment of seasonal or perennial allergic rhinitis; nonallergic (vasomotor) rhinitis; prevent recurrence of nasal polyps following surgery

Qnasl™: Symptomatic treatment of seasonal or perennial allergic rhinitis

Unlabeled Use Adjunct to antibiotics in empiric treatment of acute bacterial rhinosinusitis (ABRS) (Chow, 2012)

Local Anesthetic/Vasoconstrictor Precautions No information available to require special precautions

Effects on Dental Treatment No significant effects or complications reported

Effects on Bleeding No information available to require special precautions

◀ **Adverse Effects** Frequency not defined.
Central nervous system: Headache, lightheadedness
Dermatologic: Angioedema, rash, urticaria
Endocrine & metabolic: Growth velocity reduction in children and adolescents, HPA function suppression (dose related), weight gain
Gastrointestinal: Dry/irritated nose, throat and mouth, hoarseness, localized *Candida* or *Aspergillus* infection, loss of smell, loss of taste, nausea, unpleasant smell, unpleasant taste, vomiting
Local: Burning, epistaxis, localized *Candida* infection, nasal septum perforation (rare), nasal stuffiness, nosebleeds, rhinorrhea, sneezing, transient irritation, ulceration of nasal mucosa (rare)
Ocular: Cataracts (rare), glaucoma (rare), intraocular pressure increased (rare), tearing
Respiratory: Cough, paradoxical bronchospasm (rare), pharyngitis, sinusitis, wheezing
Miscellaneous: Anaphylactic/anaphylactoid reactions, immediate and delayed hypersensitivity reactions

Dosage Inhalation, nasal:
Children 6-11 years (Beconase® AQ): Rhinitis, nasal polyps (postsurgical prophylaxis): Initial: One inhalation each nostril twice daily (total dose: 168 mcg/day); if response inadequate, may increase to 2 inhalations each nostril twice daily (total dose: 336 mcg/day)
Children ≥12 years and Adults:
Beconase® AQ: Rhinitis, nasal polyps (postsurgical prophylaxis): 1-2 inhalations each nostril twice daily; total dose: 168-336 mcg/day
Qnasl™: Allergic rhinitis: Two inhalations each nostril once daily; total dose: 320 mcg/day

Dosage adjustment in renal impairment: No dosage adjustment provided in manufacturer's labeling.
Dosage adjustment in hepatic impairment: No dosage adjustment provided in manufacturer's labeling.
Mechanism of Action Controls the rate of protein synthesis; depresses the migration of polymorphonuclear leukocytes, fibroblasts; reverses capillary permeability and lysosomal stabilization at the cellular level to prevent or control inflammation
Contraindications Hypersensitivity to beclomethasone or any component of the formulation
Warnings/Precautions Hypersensitivity reactions (including anaphylaxis, angioedema, rash, and urticaria) have been reported; discontinue for severe reactions. May cause hypercorticism or suppression of hypothalamic-pituitary-adrenal (HPA) axis, particularly in younger children or in patients receiving high doses for prolonged periods. HPA axis suppression may lead to adrenal crisis. Withdrawal and discontinuation of a corticosteroid should be done slowly and carefully. Particular care is required when patients are transferred from systemic corticosteroids to inhaled products due to possible adrenal insufficiency or withdrawal from steroids, including an increase in allergic symptoms. Patients receiving >20 mg per day of prednisone (or equivalent) may be most susceptible. Fatalities have occurred due to adrenal insufficiency in asthmatic patients during and after transfer from systemic corticosteroids to aerosol steroids; aerosol steroids do not provide the systemic steroid needed to treat patients having trauma, surgery, or infections.

Hypersensitivity reactions, including anaphylaxis, angioedema, rash and urticaria have been reported; discontinue for severe reactions. Avoid nasal corticosteroid use in patients with recent nasal septal ulcers, nasal surgery or nasal trauma until healing has occurred. Nasal septal perforation and localized Candida albicans infections of the nose and/or pharynx may occur (rarely).

Increased intraocular pressure, open-angle glaucoma, and cataracts have occurred with intranasal corticosteroid use; use with caution in patients with a history of increased intraocular pressure, cataracts and/or glaucoma. Consider routine eye exams in chronic users or in patients who report visual changes.

Prolonged use of corticosteroids may increase the incidence of secondary infections, mask an acute infection (including fungal infections), prolong or exacerbate viral infections, or limit response to vaccines; avoid exposure to chickenpox and/or measles, especially if not immunized. Avoid use or use with caution in patients with latent/active tuberculosis, untreated bacterial or fungal infections (local or systemic), viral or parasitic infections, or ocular herpes simplex.

Intranasal corticosteroids may cause a reduction in growth velocity in pediatric patients (~1 centimeter per year [range: 0.3-1.8 cm per year] and related to dose and duration of exposure). To minimize the systemic effects of intranasal corticosteroids, each patient should be titrated to the lowest effective dose. Growth should be routinely monitored in pediatric patients. There have been reports of systemic corticosteroid withdrawal symptoms (eg, joint/muscle pain, lassitude, depression) when withdrawing oral inhalation therapy.

Drug Interactions
Metabolism/Transport Effects None known.
Avoid Concomitant Use There are no known interactions where it is recommended to avoid concomitant use.
Increased Effect/Toxicity There are no known significant interactions involving an increase in effect.
Decreased Effect There are no known significant interactions involving a decrease in effect.
Pharmacodynamics/Kinetics
Half-life Elimination BDP: ~0.3 hours; 17-BMP: ~4.5 hours
Pregnancy Risk Factor C
Pregnancy Considerations Teratogenic effects were observed in animal reproduction studies following SubQ administration but not with oral inhalation. A decrease in fetal growth has not been observed with inhaled corticosteroid use during pregnancy. Inhaled corticosteroids are recommended for the treatment of allergic rhinitis during pregnancy (NAEPP, 2005).
Lactation Excretion in breast milk unknown/use caution
Breast-Feeding Considerations Other corticosteroids have been found in breast milk; however, information for beclomethasone is not available. Use of inhaled corticosteroids is not a contraindication to breast-feeding (NAEPP, 2005).
Dosage Forms
Aerosol, spray, intranasal:
Qnasl™: 80 mcg/inhalation (8.7 g)
Suspension, intranasal:
Beconase AQ®: 42 mcg/inhalation (25 g)

Bedaquiline (bed AK wi leen)

Related Information
Clinical Risk Related to Drugs Prolonging QT Interval *on page 1510*
Pharmacologic Category Antitubercular Agent

Use Treatment of pulmonary multidrug-resistant tuberculosis in combination therapy when other alternatives are not available; should not be used for latent, extrapulmonary or drug-sensitive tuberculosis

Local Anesthetic/Vasoconstrictor Precautions Bedaquiline is one of the drugs confirmed to prolong the QT interval and is accepted as having a risk of causing torsade de pointes. In terms of epinephrine, it is not known what effect vasoconstrictors in the local anesthetic regimen will have in patients with a known history of congenital prolonged QT interval or in patients taking any medication that prolongs the QT interval. Until more information is obtained, it is suggested that the clinician consult with the physician prior to the use of a vasoconstrictor in suspected patients, and that the vasoconstrictor (epinephrine, mepivacaine and levonordefrin [Carbocaine® 2% with Neo-Cobefrin®]) be used with caution. See Dental Comment.

Effects on Dental Treatment No significant effects or complications reported

Effects on Bleeding No information available to require special precautions

Adverse Effects
>10%:
  Cardiovascular: Chest pain (11%)
  Central nervous system: Headache (28%)
  Gastrointestinal: Nausea (38%)
  Hepatic: Transaminases increased (9%; ALT increased >3 x ULN: 11%; AST increased >3 x ULN: 11%)
  Neuromuscular & skeletal: Arthralgia (33%)
  Respiratory: Hemoptysis (18%)
1% to 10%:
  Dermatologic: Rash (8%)
  Gastrointestinal: Anorexia (9%), amylase increased (3%)
Frequency not defined: QT prolongation

General Dosage Range Oral: *Adults:*
Weeks 1-2: 400 mg once daily
Weeks 3-24: 200 mg 3 times weekly (total weekly dose: 600 mg)

Mechanism of Action As a diarylquinoline antimycobacterial, inhibits the proton transfer chain of mycobacterial ATP synthase required for energy generation in *M. tuberculosis*. It is not active against human ATP synthase.

Pharmacodynamics/Kinetics
Half-life Elimination Terminal: 5.5 months
Time to Peak Serum: Oral: 5 hours

Pregnancy Risk Factor B
Pregnancy Considerations Adverse events were not observed in animal reproduction studies.

Product Availability Sirturo™: FDA approved December 2012; anticipated availability second quarter 2013.

Dental Comment Bedaquiline is known to prolong the QT interval. The QT interval is measured as the time and distance between the Q point of the QRS complex and the end of the T wave in the ECG tracing. After adjustment for heart rate, the QT interval is defined as prolonged if it is more than 450 msec in men and 460 msec in women. A long QT syndrome was first described in the 1950s and 60s as a congenital syndrome involving QT interval prolongation and syncope and sudden death. Some of the congenital long QT syndromes were characterized by a peculiar electrocardiographic appearance of the QRS complex involving a premature atria beat followed by a pause, then a subsequent sinus beat showing marked QT prolongation and deformity. This type of cardiac arrhythmia was originally termed "torsade de pointes" (translated from the French as "twisting of the points"). Bedaquiline is considered as having a risk of causing torsade de pointes. Since it is not known what effect vasoconstrictors in the local anesthetic regimen will have in patients with a known history of congenital prolonged QT interval or in patients taking any medication that prolongs the QT interval, a medical consult is suggested.

Belatacept (bel AT a sept)

Brand Names: U.S. Nulojix®
Pharmacologic Category Selective T-Cell Costimulation Blocker
Use Prophylaxis of organ rejection concomitantly with basiliximab, mycophenolate, and corticosteroids in Epstein-Barr virus (EBV) seropositive kidney transplant recipients

Local Anesthetic/Vasoconstrictor Precautions No information available to require special precautions

Effects on Dental Treatment Key adverse event(s) related to dental treatment: Stomatitis has been reported

Effects on Bleeding No information available to require special precautions

Adverse Effects Incidences reported occurred during clinical trials using belatacept compared to a cyclosporine control regimen. All patients also received basiliximab induction, mycophenolate mofetil, and corticosteroids, and were followed up to 3 years.
>10%:
  Cardiovascular: Peripheral edema (34%), hypertension (32%), hypotension (18%)
  Central nervous system: Fever (28%), headache (21%), insomnia (15%)
  Endocrine & metabolic: Hypokalemia (21%), hyperkalemia (20%), hypophosphatemia (19%), dyslipidemia (19%), hyperglycemia (16%), hypocalcemia (13%), hypercholesterolemia (11%)
  Gastrointestinal: Diarrhea (39%), constipation (33%), nausea (24%), vomiting (22%), abdominal pain (19%)
  Genitourinary: Urinary tract infection (37%), dysuria (11%)
  Hematologic: Anemia (45%), leukopenia (20%)
  Neuromuscular & skeletal: Arthralgia (17%), back pain (13%)
  Renal: Proteinuria (16%; up to 33% 2+ proteinuria at 1 month post-transplant), renal graft dysfunction (25%), hematuria (16%), serum creatinine increased (15%)
  Respiratory: Cough (24%), upper respiratory infection (15%), nasopharyngitis (13%), dyspnea (12%)
  Miscellaneous: Infection (72% to 82%; serious infection: 24% to 36%), herpes (7% to 14%), CMV (11% to 13%), influenza (11%)
1% to 10%:
  Cardiovascular: Arteriovenous fistula thrombosis (<10%), atrial fibrillation (<10%)
  Central nervous system: Anxiety (10%), dizziness (9%)
  Dermatologic: Alopecia (<10%), hyperhidrosis (<10%), acne (8%)
  Endocrine & metabolic: New-onset diabetes (5% to 8%), hypomagnesemia (7%), hyperuricemia (5%)
  Gastrointestinal: Stomatitis (<10%), upper abdominal pain (9%)
  Genitourinary: Urinary incontinence (<10%)
  Hematologic: Hematoma (<10%), neutropenia (<10%)
  Neuromuscular & skeletal: Musculoskeletal pain (<10%), tremor (8%)

Renal: Chronic allograft nephropathy (<10%), hydronephrosis (<10%), renal impairment (<10%), renal artery stenosis (<10%), renal tubular necrosis (9%)
Respiratory: Bronchitis (10%)
Miscellaneous: Guillain-Barré syndrome (<10%), lymphocele (<10%), infusion reactions (5%), malignancy (4%), polyoma virus (3% to 4%), antibelatacept antibody development (2%), nonmelanoma skin cancer (2%), tuberculosis (1% to 2%), BK virus-associated nephropathy (1%)

General Dosage Range I.V.: *Adults:* Initial phase: 10 mg/kg/dose; maintenance phase: 5 mg/kg/dose

Mechanism of Action Fusion protein which acts as a selective T-cell (lymphocyte) costimulation blocker by binding to CD80 and CD86 receptors on antigen presenting cells (APC), blocking the required CD28 mediated interaction between APCs and T cells needed to activate T lymphocytes. T-cell stimulation results in cytokine production and proliferation, mediators in immunologic rejection associated with kidney transplantation.

Pharmacodynamics/Kinetics

Half-life Elimination ~10 days (healthy patients and kidney transplant patients)

Pregnancy Risk Factor C

Pregnancy Considerations Teratogenic effects were not observed in animal studies. There are no adequate and well-controlled studies in pregnant women. Due to the potential risk for development of autoimmune disease in the fetus, use during pregnancy only if clearly needed. A pregnancy registry has been established to monitor outcomes of women exposed to belatacept during pregnancy (1-877-955-6877).

Prescribing and Access Restrictions The ENLiST registry has been created to further determine the safety of belatacept, particularly the incidence of post-transplant lymphoproliferative disorder (PTLD) and progressive multifocal leukoencephalopathy (PML), in EBV-seropositive kidney transplant patients. Transplant centers are encouraged to participate (1-800-321-1335).

Belimumab (be LIM yoo mab)

Brand Names: U.S. Benlysta®
Brand Names: Canada Benlysta®
Pharmacologic Category Monoclonal Antibody
Use Treatment of autoantibody-positive (antinuclear antibody [ANA] and/or antidouble-stranded DNA [anti-ds-DNA]) active systemic lupus erythematosus (SLE) in addition to standard therapy
Local Anesthetic/Vasoconstrictor Precautions No information available to require special precautions
Effects on Dental Treatment No significant effects or complications reported
Effects on Bleeding No information available to require special precautions
Adverse Effects
>10%:
Gastrointestinal: Nausea (15%), diarrhea (12%)
Miscellaneous: Infusion-related reaction (17%), hypersensitivity (13%)
≥3% to 10%:
Central nervous system: Fever (10%), insomnia (6% to 7%), migraine (5%), depression (5% to 6%), anxiety (4%), headache (≥3%)

Dermatologic: Skin reactions (≥3%)
Gastrointestinal: Viral gastroenteritis (3%)
Genitourinary: Urinary tract infection (site not specified >5%), cystitis (4%)
Hematologic: Leukopenia (4%)
Neuromuscular & skeletal: Pain in extremity (6%)
Respiratory: Bronchitis (9%), nasopharyngitis (9%), pharyngitis (5%), sinusitis (>5%), upper respiratory infection (>5%)
Miscellaneous: Influenza (>5%)

General Dosage Range I.V.: *Adults:* 10 mg/kg every 2 weeks for 3 doses; Maintenance: 10 mg/kg every 4 weeks

Mechanism of Action Belimumab is an IgG1-lambda monoclonal antibody that prevents the survival of B lymphocytes by blocking the binding of soluble human B lymphocyte stimulator protein (BLyS) to receptors on B lymphocytes. This reduces the activity of B-cell mediated immunity and the autoimmune response.

Pharmacodynamics/Kinetics

Onset of Action B cells: 8 weeks; Clinical improvement (SLE Responder Index and flare reduction): 16 weeks (Navarra, 2011)

Half-life Elimination 19.4 days

Pregnancy Risk Factor C

Pregnancy Considerations Adverse events were observed in some animal reproduction studies. IgG molecules are known to cross the placenta (belimumab is an engineered IgG molecule). Effective contraception should be used during and for at least 4 months following treatment in women of childbearing potential. Healthcare providers are encouraged to enroll women exposed to belimumab during pregnancy in a pregnancy registry (877-681-6296); patients may also enroll themselves.

Belladonna and Opium
(bel a DON a & OH pee um)

Related Information
Opium Tincture *on page 1017*
Pharmacologic Category Analgesic Combination (Opioid); Antispasmodic Agent, Urinary
Use Relief of moderate-to-severe pain associated with ureteral spasms not responsive to nonopioid analgesics and to space intervals between injections of opiates
Local Anesthetic/Vasoconstrictor Precautions No information available to require special precautions
Effects on Dental Treatment Key adverse event(s) related to dental treatment: Xerostomia and changes in salivation (normal salivary flow resumes upon discontinuation), and dry throat and nose.
Effects on Bleeding No information available to require special precautions
Adverse Effects Frequency not defined.
Cardiovascular: Palpitation
Central nervous system: Dizziness, drowsiness
Dermatologic: Pruritus, urticaria
Gastrointestinal: Constipation, nausea, vomiting, xerostomia
Genitourinary: Urinary retention
Ocular: Blurred vision, photophobia
General Dosage Range Rectal: *Children >12 years and Adults:* 1 suppository 1-2 times/day (maximum: 4 doses/day)

Mechanism of Action The pharmacologically active agents present in the belladonna component are atropine and scopolamine. Atropine blocks the action of acetylcholine at parasympathetic sites in smooth muscle, secretory glands, and the CNS causing a relaxation of smooth muscle and drying of secretions. The principle agent in opium is morphine. Morphine binds to opiate receptors in the CNS, causing inhibition of ascending pain pathways, altering the perception of and response to pain.

Pregnancy Risk Factor C

Pregnancy Considerations Reproduction studies have not been conducted with this product. Refer to Atropine and Morphine Sulfate monographs for additional information.

Controlled Substance C-II

Benazepril (ben AY ze pril)

Related Information
Cardiovascular Diseases on page 1492
Brand Names: U.S. Lotensin®
Brand Names: Canada Lotensin®
Generic Availability (U.S.) Yes
Pharmacologic Category Angiotensin-Converting Enzyme (ACE) Inhibitor
Use Treatment of hypertension, either alone or in combination with other antihypertensive agents
Local Anesthetic/Vasoconstrictor Precautions No information available to require special precautions
Effects on Dental Treatment No significant effects or complications reported
Effects on Bleeding No information available to require special precautions
Adverse Effects
1% to 10%:
Cardiovascular: Postural dizziness (2%)
Central nervous system: Headache (6%), dizziness (4%), somnolence (2%)
Renal: Serum creatinine increased (2%), worsening of renal function may occur in patients with bilateral renal artery stenosis or hypovolemia
Respiratory: Cough (1% to 10%)
Eosinophilic pneumonitis, anaphylaxis, neutropenia, agranulocytosis, renal insufficiency, and renal failure have been reported with other ACE inhibitors. In addition, a syndrome including fever, myalgia, arthralgia, interstitial nephritis, vasculitis, rash, eosinophilia, and elevated ESR has been reported to be associated with ACE inhibitors.

Dosage Oral: Hypertension:
Children ≥6 years: Initial: 0.2 mg/kg/day (up to 10 mg/day) as monotherapy; dosing range: 0.1-0.6 mg/kg/day (maximum dose: 40 mg/day)
Adults: Initial: 10 mg/day in patients not receiving a diuretic; 20-80 mg/day as a single dose or 2 divided doses; the need for twice-daily dosing should be assessed by monitoring peak (2-6 hours after dosing) and trough responses.
Note: Patients taking diuretics should have them discontinued 2-3 days prior to starting benazepril. If they cannot be discontinued, then initial dose should be 5 mg; restart after blood pressure is stabilized if needed.
Elderly: Oral: Initial: 5-10 mg/day in single or divided doses; usual range: 20-40 mg/day; adjust for renal function; also see **"Note"** in adult dosing.

Dosage adjustment in renal impairment: Cl_{cr} <30 mL/minute:
Children: Use is not recommended.
Adults: Administer 5 mg/day initially; maximum daily dose: 40 mg.
Hemodialysis: Moderately dialyzable (20% to 50%); administer dose postdialysis or administer 25% to 35% supplemental dose.
Peritoneal dialysis: Supplemental dose is not necessary.
Dosage adjustment in hepatic impairment: No dosage adjustment provided in manufacturer's labeling (has not been studied); use with caution.

Mechanism of Action Competitive inhibition of angiotensin I being converted to angiotensin II, a potent vasoconstrictor, through the angiotensin I-converting enzyme (ACE) activity, with resultant lower levels of angiotensin II which causes an increase in plasma renin activity and a reduction in aldosterone secretion

Contraindications Hypersensitivity to benazepril or any component of the formulation; patients with a history of angioedema (with or without prior ACE inhibitor therapy); concomitant use with aliskiren in patients with diabetes mellitus

Warnings/Precautions Anaphylactic reactions may occur rarely with ACE inhibitors. At any time during treatment (especially following first dose) angioedema may occur rarely with ACE inhibitors. It may involve the head and neck (potentially compromising airway) or the intestine (presenting with abdominal pain). African-Americans and patients with idiopathic or hereditary angioedema may be at an increased risk. Prolonged frequent monitoring may be required especially if tongue, glottis, or larynx are involved as they are associated with airway obstruction. Patients with a history of airway surgery may have a higher risk of airway obstruction. Aggressive and appropriate management is critical. Contraindicated in patients with history of angioedema with or without prior ACE inhibitor therapy. Hypersensitivity reactions may be seen during hemodialysis (eg, CVVHD) with high-flux dialysis membranes (eg, AN69), and rarely, during low density lipoprotein apheresis with dextran sulfate cellulose. Rare cases of anaphylactoid reactions have been reported in patients undergoing sensitization treatment with hymenoptera (bee, wasp) venom while receiving ACE inhibitors.

Symptomatic hypotension with or without syncope can occur with ACE inhibitors (usually with the first several doses); effects are most often observed in volume depleted patients; close monitoring of patient is required especially with initial dosing and dosing increases; blood pressure must be lowered at a rate appropriate for the patient's clinical condition. Initiation of therapy in patients with ischemic heart disease or cerebrovascular disease warrants close observation due to the potential consequences posed by falling blood pressure (eg, MI, stroke). **[U.S. Boxed Warning]: Drugs that act on the renin-angiotensin system can cause injury and death to the developing fetus. Discontinue as soon as possible once pregnancy is detected.** Use with caution in hypertrophic cardiomyopathy with outflow tract obstruction, severe aortic stenosis, or before, during, or immediately after major surgery.

Hyperkalemia may occur with ACE inhibitors; risk factors include renal dysfunction, diabetes mellitus, concomitant use of potassium-sparing diuretics, potassium supplements and/or potassium-containing salts. Use cautiously, if at all, with these agents and monitor potassium periodically. Cough may occur with ACE inhibitors. Other causes of cough should be considered (eg, pulmonary congestion in patients with heart failure) and excluded prior to discontinuation. Use with caution in patients with diabetes receiving insulin or oral antidiabetic agents; may be at increased risk for episodes of hypoglycemia.

May be associated with deterioration of renal function and/or increases in serum creatinine, particularly in patients with low renal blood flow (eg, renal artery stenosis, heart failure) whose glomerular filtration rate (GFR) is dependent on efferent arteriolar vasoconstriction by angiotensin II; deterioration may result in oliguria, acute renal failure, and progressive azotemia. Small increases in serum creatinine may occur following initiation; consider discontinuation only in patients with progressive and/or significant deterioration in renal function. Use with caution in patients with unstented unilateral/bilateral renal artery stenosis. When unstented bilateral renal artery stenosis is present, use is generally avoided due to the elevated risk of deterioration in renal function unless possible benefits outweigh risks. Concomitant use of an angiotensin receptor blocker (ARB) or renin inhibitor (eg, aliskiren) is associated with an increased risk of hypotension, hyperkalemia, and renal dysfunction; concomitant use with aliskiren should be avoided in patients with GFR <60 mL/minute and is contraindicated in patients with diabetes mellitus (regardless of GFR).

Rare toxicities associated with ACE inhibitors include cholestatic jaundice (which may progress to fulminant hepatic necrosis), agranulocytosis, neutropenia, or leukopenia with myeloid hypoplasia. Patients with collagen vascular diseases (especially with concomitant renal impairment) or renal impairment alone may be at increased risk for hematologic toxicity; periodically monitor CBC with differential in these patients.

Drug Interactions
Metabolism/Transport Effects None known.

Avoid Concomitant Use There are no known interactions where it is recommended to avoid concomitant use.

Increased Effect/Toxicity
Benazepril may increase the levels/effects of: Allopurinol; Amifostine; Antihypertensives; AzaTHIOprine; CycloSPORINE (Systemic); Ferric Gluconate; Gold Sodium Thiomalate; Hypotensive Agents; Iron Dextran Complex; Lithium; Nonsteroidal Anti-Inflammatory Agents; RiTUXimab; Sodium Phosphates

The levels/effects of Benazepril may be increased by: Alfuzosin; Aliskiren; Angiotensin II Receptor Blockers; Canagliflozin; Diazoxide; DPP-IV Inhibitors; Eplerenone; Everolimus; Herbs (Hypotensive Properties); Hydrochlorothiazide; Loop Diuretics; MAO Inhibitors; Pentoxifylline; Phosphodiesterase 5 Inhibitors; Potassium Salts; Potassium-Sparing Diuretics; Prostacyclin Analogues; Sirolimus; Temsirolimus; Thiazide Diuretics; TiZANidine; Tolvaptan; Trimethoprim

Decreased Effect
Benazepril may decrease the levels/effects of: Hydrochlorothiazide

The levels/effects of Benazepril may be decreased by: Antacids; Aprotinin; Herbs (Hypertensive Properties); Icatibant; Lanthanum; Methylphenidate; Nonsteroidal Anti-Inflammatory Agents; Salicylates; Yohimbine

Ethanol/Nutrition/Herb Interactions
Food: Potassium supplements and/or potassium-containing salts may cause or worsen hyperkalemia. Management: Consult prescriber before consuming a potassium-rich diet, potassium supplements, or salt substitutes.

Herb/Nutraceutical: Some herbal medications may worsen hypertension (eg, licorice); others may increase the antihypertensive effect of benazepril (eg, shepherd's purse). Management: Avoid bayberry, blue cohosh, cayenne, ephedra, ginger, ginseng (American), kola, licorice, and yohimbe. Avoid black cohosh, California poppy, coleus, golden seal, hawthorn, mistletoe, periwinkle, quinine, and shepherd's purse.

Pharmacodynamics/Kinetics
Onset of Action
Reduction in plasma angiotensin-converting enzyme (ACE) activity: Peak effect: 1-2 hours after 2-20 mg dose
Reduction in blood pressure: Peak effect: Single dose: 2-4 hours; Continuous therapy: 2 weeks

Duration of Action Reduction in plasma angiotensin-converting enzyme (ACE) activity: >90% inhibition for 24 hours after 5-20 mg dose

Half-life Elimination Benazeprilat: Effective: 10-11 hours; Terminal: Children: 5 hours, Adults: 22 hours

Time to Peak Parent drug: 0.5-1 hour

Pregnancy Risk Factor D

Pregnancy Considerations [U.S. Boxed Warning]: Drugs that act on the renin-angiotensin system can cause injury and death to the developing fetus. Discontinue as soon as possible once pregnancy is detected. Benazepril crosses the placenta; teratogenic effects may occur following maternal use during pregnancy. Drugs that act on the renin-angiotensin system are associated with oligohydramnios. Oligohydramnios, due to decreased fetal renal function, may lead to fetal lung hypoplasia and skeletal malformations. Their use in pregnancy is also associated with anuria, hypotension, renal failure, skull hypoplasia, and death in the fetus/neonate. Chronic maternal hypertension itself is also associated with adverse events in the fetus/infant. ACE inhibitors are not recommended during pregnancy to treat maternal hypertension or heart failure. Use of an ACE inhibitor should also be avoided in any woman of reproductive age. Women who are planning a pregnancy should be considered for other medication options if an ACE inhibitor is currently prescribed or the ACE inhibitor should be discontinued as soon as possible once pregnancy is detected. The exposed fetus should be monitored for fetal growth, amniotic fluid volume, and organ formation. Infants exposed to an ACE inhibitor *in utero* should be monitored for hyperkalemia, hypotension, and oliguria.

Lactation Enters breast milk

Breast-Feeding Considerations Small amounts of benazepril and benazeprilat are found in breast milk.

Dosage Forms
Tablet, oral: 5 mg, 10 mg, 20 mg, 40 mg
Lotensin®: 10 mg, 20 mg, 40 mg

Benazepril and Hydrochlorothiazide
(ben AY ze pril & hye droe klor oh THYE a zide)

Related Information
Benazepril on page 173
Hydrochlorothiazide on page 687
Brand Names: U.S. Lotensin HCT®

Pharmacologic Category Angiotensin-Converting Enzyme (ACE) Inhibitor; Diuretic, Thiazide

Use Treatment of hypertension

Local Anesthetic/Vasoconstrictor Precautions No information available to require special precautions

Effects on Dental Treatment No significant effects or complications reported

Effects on Bleeding No information available to require special precautions

Adverse Effects See individual agents.

General Dosage Range Oral: *Adults:* Benazepril 5-20 mg and hydrochlorothiazide 6.25-25 mg daily

Mechanism of Action Benazepril is a competitive inhibitor of angiotensin-converting enzyme (ACE); prevents conversion of angiotensin I to angiotensin II, a potent vasoconstrictor. This results in lower levels of angiotensin II which causes an increase in plasma renin activity and a reduction in aldosterone secretion. Hydrochlorothiazide inhibits sodium reabsorption in the distal tubules causing increased excretion of sodium and water as well as potassium and hydrogen ions.

Pregnancy Risk Factor D

Pregnancy Considerations [U.S. Boxed Warning]: Drugs that act on the renin-angiotensin system can cause injury and death to the developing fetus. Discontinue as soon as possible once pregnancy is detected. Also see individual agents.

Bendamustine (ben da MUS teen)

Brand Names: U.S. Treanda®

Brand Names: Canada Treanda®

Pharmacologic Category Antineoplastic Agent; Antineoplastic Agent, Alkylating Agent; Antineoplastic Agent, Alkylating Agent (Nitrogen Mustard)

Use Treatment of chronic lymphocytic leukemia (CLL); treatment of progressed indolent B-cell non-Hodgkin's lymphoma (NHL)

Unlabeled Use Treatment of relapsed or refractory Hodgkin lymphoma; treatment of mantle cell lymphoma; salvage therapy for relapsed multiple myeloma; first-line therapy for follicular lymphoma; treatment of Waldenström's macroglobulinemia

Local Anesthetic/Vasoconstrictor Precautions No information available to require special precautions

Effects on Dental Treatment Key adverse event(s) related to dental treatment: Stomatitis, xerostomia (normal salivary flow resumes upon discontinuation).

Effects on Bleeding Thrombocytopenia has been reported in 77% to 86% (grade 3/4: 11% to 25%) of patients.

Adverse Effects

>10%:

Cardiovascular: Peripheral edema (≤13%)

Central nervous system: Fatigue (9% to 57%), fever (24% to 34%), headache (≤21%), chills (6% to 14%), dizziness (≤14%), insomnia (≤13%)

Dermatologic: Rash (8% to 16%; grades 3/4: ≤3%)

Endocrine & metabolic: Dehydration (≤14%)

Gastrointestinal: Nausea (20% to 75%), vomiting (16% to 40%), diarrhea (9% to 37%), constipation (≤29%), anorexia (≤23%), weight loss (7% to 18%), stomatitis (≤15%), abdominal pain (5% to 13%), appetite loss (≤13%), dyspepsia (≤11%)

Hematologic: Myelosuppression (nadir: in week 3), lymphopenia (68% to 99%; grades 3/4: 47% to 94%), leukopenia (61% to 94%; grades 3/4: 28% to 56%), anemia (88% to 89%; grades 3/4: 11% to 13%), thrombocytopenia (77% to 86%; grades 3/4: 11% to 25%), neutropenia (75% to 86%; grades 3/4: 43% to 60%)

Hepatic: Bilirubin increased (≤34%; grades 3/4: 3%)

Neuromuscular & skeletal: Back pain (≤14%), weakness (8% to 11%)

Respiratory: Cough (4% to 22%), dyspnea (≤16%)

1% to 10%:

Cardiovascular: Tachycardia (≤7%), hypotension (≤6%), chest pain (≤6%), hypertension aggravated (≤3%)

Central nervous system: Anxiety (≤8%), depression (≤6%), pain (≤6%)

Dermatologic: Pruritus (5% to 6%), dry skin (≤5%)

Endocrine & metabolic: Hypokalemia (≤9%), hyperuricemia (≤7%; grades 3/4: 2%), hyperglycemia (grades 3/4: ≤3%), hypocalcemia (grades 3/4: ≤2%), hyponatremia (grades 3/4: ≤2%)

Gastrointestinal: Gastroesophageal reflux disease (≤10%), xerostomia (9%), taste alteration (≤7%), oral candidiasis (≤6%), abdominal distention (≤5%)

Genitourinary: Urinary tract infection (≤10%)

Hematologic: Febrile neutropenia (3% to 6%)

Hepatic: ALT increased (grades 3/4: ≤3%), AST increased (grades 3/4: ≤1%)

Local: Infusion site pain (≤6%), catheter site pain (≤5%)

Neuromuscular & skeletal: Arthralgia (≤6%), bone pain (≤5%), limb pain (≤5%)

Renal: Creatinine increased (grades 3/4: ≤2%)

Respiratory: Upper respiratory infection (10%), sinusitis (≤9%), pharyngolaryngeal pain (≤8%), pneumonia (≤8%), nasopharyngitis (6% to 7%), wheezing (≤5%), nasal congestion (≤5%)

Miscellaneous: Herpes infection (3% to 10%), infection (≤6%; grades 3/4: 2%), hypersensitivity (≤5%; grades 3/4: 1%), diaphoresis (≤5%), night sweats (≤5%)

General Dosage Range Dosage adjustment recommended in patients who develop toxicities

I.V.: *Adults:* 100 mg/m^2 on days 1 and 2 of a 28-day treatment cycle **or** 120 mg/m^2 on days 1 and 2 of a 21-day treatment cycle

Mechanism of Action Bendamustine is an alkylating agent (nitrogen mustard derivative) with a benzimidazole ring (purine analog) which demonstrates only partial cross-resistance (*in vitro*) with other alkylating agents. It leads to cell death via single and double strand DNA cross-linking. Bendamustine is active against quiescent and dividing cells. The primary cytotoxic activity is due to bendamustine (as compared to metabolites).

Pharmacodynamics/Kinetics

Half-life Elimination Bendamustine: ~40 minutes; M3: ~3 hours; M4: ~30 minutes

Time to Peak At end of infusion

Pregnancy Risk Factor D

Pregnancy Considerations Teratogenic and nonteratogenic events were observed in animal reproduction studies following intraperitoneal dosing. May cause fetal harm if administered during pregnancy. For women and men of reproductive potential, the U.S. labeling recommends effective contraception during and for 3 months after treatment. The Canadian labeling recommends effective contraception beginning 2 weeks prior to treatment and for ≥1 month after treatment.

Bentoquatam (BEN toe kwa tam)

Brand Names: U.S. Ivy Block® [OTC]

Pharmacologic Category Topical Skin Product

Use Skin protectant for the prevention of allergic contact dermatitis to poison oak, ivy, and sumac

Local Anesthetic/Vasoconstrictor Precautions No information available to require special precautions

Effects on Dental Treatment No significant effects or complications reported

Effects on Bleeding No information available to require special precautions

General Dosage Range Topical: *Children >6 years and Adults:* Apply to skin 15 minutes prior to potential exposure to poison ivy, poison oak, or poison sumac, and reapply every 4 hours

Mechanism of Action An organoclay substance which is capable of absorbing or binding to urushiol, the active principle in poison oak, ivy, and sumac. Bentoquatam serves as a barrier, blocking urushiol skin contact/absorption.

Benzalkonium Chloride and Benzocaine
(benz al KOE nee um KLOR ide & BEN zoe kane)

Brand Names: U.S. Viroxyn®
Generic Availability (U.S.) No
Pharmacologic Category Topical Skin Product
Dental Use Topical treatment of cold sores
Use Topical treatment of cold sores

Local Anesthetic/Vasoconstrictor Precautions No information available to require special precautions

Effects on Dental Treatment No significant effects or complications reported

Effects on Bleeding No information available to require special precautions

Adverse Effects Frequency not defined: Local: Irritation, stinging (short-term)

Dental Usual Dosage Children >2 years, Adolescents, and Adults: Topical: Cold sore: Apply single dose to cold sore with applicator

Dosage Children >2 years, Adolescents, and Adults: Topical: Cold sore: Apply single dose to cold sore with applicator

Dosage adjustment in renal impairment: No dosage adjustment provided in manufacturer's labeling(has not been studied)

Dosage adjustment in hepatic impairment: No dosage adjustment provided in manufacturer's labeling (has not been studied)

Mechanism of Action Benzalkonium chloride is an antiseptic and disinfectant; benzocaine is an ester local anesthetic that blocks both the initiation and conduction of nerve impulses by decreasing the neuronal membrane's permeability to sodium ions, which results in inhibition of depolarization with resultant blockade of conduction

Contraindications Hypersensitivity to benzalkonium chloride, benzocaine, other ester-type local anesthetics, or any component of the formulation; ophthalmic use; use over a large area of body or >3 times daily; longer than 1 week unless directed by healthcare provider

Warnings/Precautions For topical use only.
Drug Interactions
Metabolism/Transport Effects None known.

Avoid Concomitant Use There are no known interactions where it is recommended to avoid concomitant use.

Increased Effect/Toxicity
Benzalkonium Chloride and Benzocaine may increase the levels/effects of: Prilocaine

Decreased Effect There are no known significant interactions involving a decrease in effect.

Ethanol/Nutrition/Herb Interactions Food: Fruit juices and soft drinks may deactivate the active ingredient. Avoid drinking fruit juices and soft drinks for at least 1 hour after application.

Prescribing and Access Restrictions Product only available to dental professionals.

Dosage Forms
Solution, topical:
Viroxyn®: Benzalkonium chloride 0.13% and benzocaine 7.5% (0.6 mL)

Benzocaine (BEN zoe kane)

Related Information
Oral Pain *on page 1558*
Related Sample Prescriptions
Recurrent Aphthous Stomatitis *on page 1618*
Brand Names: U.S. Americaine® Hemorrhoidal [OTC]; Anbesol® Baby [OTC]; Anbesol® Cold Sore Therapy [OTC]; Anbesol® Jr. [OTC]; Anbesol® Maximum Strength [OTC]; Anbesol® [OTC]; Benzodent® [OTC]; Bi-Zets [OTC]; Boil-Ease® Pain Relieving [OTC]; Cepacol® Fizzlers™ [OTC]; Cepacol® Sore Throat & Coating [OTC]; Cepacol® Sore Throat Plus Coating Relief [OTC]; Cepacol® Sore Throat [OTC]; Cepacol® Ultra Sore Throat [OTC]; Chiggerex® Plus [OTC]; Chigger-Tox® [OTC]; Dent's Extra Strength Toothache Gum [OTC]; Dentapaine [OTC]; Dermoplast® Antibacterial [OTC]; Dermoplast® Pain Relieving [OTC]; Detane® [OTC]; Foille® [OTC]; HDA® Toothache [OTC]; Hurri-Caine ONE™; Hurricaine® [OTC]; Ivy-Rid® [OTC]; Kank-A® Soft Brush [OTC]; Lanacane® Maximum Strength [OTC]; Lanacane® [OTC]; Little Teethers® [OTC]; Medicone® Hemorrhoidal [OTC]; Mycinettes® [OTC]; Orabase® with Benzocaine [OTC]; Orajel® Baby Daytime and Nighttime [OTC]; Orajel® Baby Teething Nighttime [OTC]; Orajel® Baby Teething [OTC]; Orajel® Cold Sore [OTC]; Orajel® Denture Plus [OTC]; Orajel® Maximum Strength [OTC]; Orajel® Medicated Mouth Sore [OTC]; Orajel® Medicated Toothache [OTC]; Orajel® Mouth Sore [OTC]; Orajel® Multi-Action Cold Sore [OTC]; Orajel® PM Maximum Strength [OTC]; Orajel® Ultra Mouth Sore [OTC]; Orajel® [OTC]; Outgro® [OTC]; Red Cross™ Canker Sore [OTC]; Rid-A-Pain Dental [OTC]; Sepasoothe® [OTC]; Skeeter Stik® [OTC]; Sore Throat Relief [OTC]; Sting-Kill® [OTC]; Tanac® [OTC]; Thorets [OTC]; Trocaine® [OTC]; Zilactin® Tooth & Gum Pain [OTC]; Zilactin®-B [OTC]

Brand Names: Canada Anbesol® Baby; Zilactin Baby®; Zilactin-B®

Generic Availability (U.S.) Yes: Lozenge, liquid

Pharmacologic Category Local Anesthetic

Dental Use Ester-type topical local anesthetic for temporary relief of pain associated with toothache, minor sore throat pain, and canker sore

Use Temporary relief of pain associated with pruritic dermatosis, pruritus, minor burns, acute congestive, bee stings, and insect bites; mouth and gum irritations (toothache, minor sore throat pain, canker sores, dentures, orthodontia, teething, mucositis, stomatitis); sunburn; hemorrhoids; anesthetic lubricant for passage of catheters and endoscopic tubes

Local Anesthetic/Vasoconstrictor Precautions No information available to require special precautions

Effects on Dental Treatment No significant effects or complications reported (see Dental Comment).

Effects on Bleeding No information available to require special precautions

Adverse Effects Frequency not defined.
Hematologic: Methemoglobinemia
Local: Burning, contact dermatitis, edema, erythema, pruritus, rash, stinging, tenderness, urticaria
Miscellaneous: Hypersensitivity

Dental Usual Dosage Relief of pain (toothache, minor sore throat pain, and canker sore): Children ≥2 years and Adults: Topical (oral): 10% to 20%: Apply thin layer to affected area up to 4 times daily

Dosage Note: These are general dosing guidelines; refer to specific product labeling for dosing instructions.

Children ≥4 months: Topical (oral): Teething pain: 7.5% to 10%: Apply to affected gum area up to 4 times daily
Children ≥2 years and Adults:
Topical:
Bee stings, insect bites, minor burns, sunburn: 5% to 20%: Apply to affected area 3-4 times daily as needed. In cases of bee stings, remove stinger before treatment.
Boils: 20%: Apply to affected area up to 2 times daily (maximum: 2 times/day)
Lubricant for passage of catheters and instruments: 20%: Apply evenly to exterior of instrument prior to use.
Topical (oral): Mouth and gum irritation: 10% to 20%: Apply thin layer to affected area up to 4 times daily
Children ≥5 years and Adults: Oral: Sore throat: Allow 1 lozenge (10-15 mg) to dissolve slowly in mouth; may repeat every 2 hours as needed
Children ≥6 years and Adults: Topical (oral) spray: 5%: Sore throat or mouth: One spray to affected area, then wait ≥1 minute and spit; may repeat up to 4 times daily.
Note: Children 6-11 years should only use under adult supervision.
Children ≥12 years and Adults: Rectal: Hemorrhoids: 5% to 20%: Apply externally to affected area up to 6 times daily

Mechanism of Action Ester local anesthetic blocks both the initiation and conduction of nerve impulses by decreasing the neuronal membrane's permeability to sodium ions, which results in inhibition of depolarization with resultant blockade of conduction

Contraindications Hypersensitivity to benzocaine, other ester-type local anesthetics, or any component of the formulation; secondary bacterial infection of area; ophthalmic use

Warnings/Precautions Methemoglobinemia has been reported following topical use, particularly with higher concentration (14% to 20%) spray formulations applied to the mouth or mucous membranes. When applied as a spray to the mouth or throat, multiple sprays (or sprays of longer than indicated duration) are not recommended. Use caution with breathing problems (asthma, bronchitis, emphysema, in smokers), inflamed/damaged mucosa, heart disease, and hemoglobin or enzyme abnormalities (glucose-6-phosphate dehydrogenase deficiency, hemoglobin-M disease, NADH-methemoglobin reductase deficiency, pyruvate-kinase deficiency). Alternatives to benzocaine sprays, such as topical lidocaine preparations, should be considered for patients at higher risk of this reaction. Due to the heightened risk of methemoglobinemia, not recommended for use in patients <2 years of age unless under the advice and supervision by a healthcare professional.

The classical clinical finding of methemoglobinemia is chocolate brown-colored arterial blood. However, suspected cases should be confirmed by co-oximetry, which yields a direct and accurate measure of methemoglobin levels. Standard pulse oximetry readings or arterial blood gas values are not reliable. Clinically significant methemoglobinemia requires immediate treatment.

When topical anesthetics are used prior to cosmetic or medical procedures, the lowest amount of anesthetic necessary for pain relief should be applied. High systemic levels and toxic effects (eg, methemoglobinemia, irregular heart beats, respiratory depression, seizures, death) have been reported in patients who (without supervision of a trained professional) have applied topical anesthetics in large amounts (or to large areas of the skin), left these products on for prolonged periods of time, or have used wraps/dressings to cover the skin following application.

When used for self-medication (OTC), notify healthcare provider if condition worsens or does not improve within the timeframe noted on the product labeling or if accompanied by additional symptoms (eg, swelling, rash, headache, nausea, vomiting, or fever). Do not use topical products on open wounds; avoid contact with the eyes.

Drug Interactions

Metabolism/Transport Effects None known.

Avoid Concomitant Use There are no known interactions where it is recommended to avoid concomitant use.

Increased Effect/Toxicity
Benzocaine may increase the levels/effects of: Prilocaine

Decreased Effect There are no known significant interactions involving a decrease in effect.

Dietary Considerations Some products may contain sodium.

Pregnancy Risk Factor C

Pregnancy Considerations Reproduction studies have not been conducted.

Lactation Excretion in breast milk unknown/use caution

Breast-Feeding Considerations It is not known if benzocaine is excreted in breast milk. The manufacturer recommends that caution be exercised when administering benzocaine to nursing women.

Dosage Forms
Aerosol, spray, oral:
Hurricaine® [OTC]: 20% (60 mL)
Aerosol, spray, topical:
Dermoplast® Antibacterial [OTC]: 20% (82.5 mL)
Dermoplast® Pain Relieving [OTC]: 20% (60 mL, 82.5 mL)
Ivy-Rid® [OTC]: 2% (85 g)
Lanacane® Maximum Strength [OTC]: 20% (120 mL)
Combination package, oral:
Orajel® Baby Daytime and Nighttime [OTC]: gel, oral (Daytime Regular formula): benzocaine 7.5% (5.3 g) [1 tube] and gel, oral (Nighttime formula): benzocaine 10% (5.3 g) [1 tube]
Cream, oral:
Benzodent® [OTC]: 20% (7.5 g, 30 g)
Orajel® PM Maximum Strength [OTC]: 20% (5.3 g, 7 g)
Cream, topical:
Lanacane® [OTC]: 6% (28 g, 60 g)
Lanacane® Maximum Strength [OTC]: 20% (28 g)
Gel, oral: 20% (15 g)
Anbesol® [OTC]: 10% (7.1 g)
Anbesol® Baby [OTC]: 7.5% (7.1 g)
Anbesol® Jr. [OTC]: 10% (7.1 g)
Anbesol® Maximum Strength [OTC]: 20% (7.1 g, 10 g)
Dentapaine [OTC]: 20% (11 g)
HDA® Toothache [OTC]: 6.5% (15 mL)

Hurricaine® [OTC]: 20% (30 g); 20% (5.25 g, 30 g)
Kank-A® Soft Brush [OTC]: 20% (2 g)
Little Teethers® [OTC]: 7.5% (9.4 g)
Orabase® with Benzocaine [OTC]: 20% (7 g)
Orajel® [OTC]: 10% (5.3 g, 7 g, 9.4 g)
Orajel® Baby Teething [OTC]: 7.5% (11.9 g);
7.5% (9.4 g)
Orajel® Baby Teething Nighttime [OTC]: 10% (5.3 g)
Orajel® Denture Plus [OTC]: 15% (9 g)
Orajel® Maximum Strength [OTC]: 20% (5.4 g, 7 g,
9.4 g, 11.9 g)
Orajel® Mouth Sore [OTC]: 20% (5.3 g, 9.4 g, 11.9 g)
Orajel® Multi-Action Cold Sore [OTC]: 20% (9.4 g)
Orajel® Ultra Mouth Sore [OTC]: 15% (9.4 g)
Zilactin®-B [OTC]: 10% (7.5 g)
Gel, topical:
Detane® [OTC]: 7.5% (15 g)
Liquid, oral: 20% (15 mL)
Anbesol® [OTC]: 10% (9.3 mL)
Anbesol® Maximum Strength [OTC]: 20% (9.3 mL)
Cepacol® Ultra Sore Throat [OTC]: 5% (22.2 mL)
HurriCaine ONE™: 20% (0.5 mL)
Hurricaine® [OTC]: 20% (30 mL)
Orajel® Baby Teething [OTC]: 7.5% (13.3 mL)
Orajel® Maximum Strength [OTC]: 20% (13.5 mL)
Rid-A-Pain Dental [OTC]: 6.3% (30 mL)
Tanac® [OTC]: 10% (13 mL)
Liquid, topical:
ChiggerTox® [OTC]: 2% (30 mL)
Outgro® [OTC]: 20% (9.3 mL)
Skeeter Stik® [OTC]: 5% (14 mL)
Lozenge, oral:
Bi-Zets [OTC]: 15 mg (10s)
Cepacol® Sore Throat [OTC]: 15 mg (16s)
Cepacol® Sore Throat & Coating [OTC]: 15 mg (16s)
Cepacol® Sore Throat Plus Coating Relief [OTC]:
15 mg (18s)
Mycinettes® [OTC]: 15 mg (12s)
Sepasoothe® [OTC]: 10 mg (6s, 24s, 100s,
250s, 500s)
Sore Throat Relief [OTC]: 10 mg (100s, 250s, 500s)
Thorets [OTC]: 18 mg (300s)
Trocaine® [OTC]: 10 mg (50s, 300s)
Ointment, oral:
Anbesol® Cold Sore Therapy [OTC]: 20% (7.1 g)
Red Cross™ Canker Sore [OTC]: 20% (7.5 g)
Ointment, rectal:
Americaine® Hemorrhoidal [OTC]: 20% (30 g)
Medicone® Hemorrhoidal [OTC]: 20% (28.4 g)
Ointment, topical:
Boil-Ease® Pain Relieving [OTC]: 20% (30 g)
Chiggerex® Plus [OTC]: 6% (50 g)
Foille® [OTC]: 5% (3.5 g, 14 g, 28 g)
Pad, topical:
Sting-Kill® [OTC]: 20% (8s)
Paste, oral:
Orabase® with Benzocaine [OTC]: 20% (6 g)
Swab, oral:
Hurricaine® [OTC]: 20% (8s, 72s)
Orajel® Baby Teething [OTC]: 7.5% (12s)
Orajel® Cold Sore [OTC]: 20% (12s)
Orajel® Medicated Mouth Sore [OTC]: 20% (8s, 12s)
Orajel® Medicated Toothache [OTC]: 20% (8s, 12s)
Zilactin® Tooth & Gum Pain [OTC]: 20% (8s)
Swab, topical:
Boil-Ease® Pain Relieving [OTC]: 20% (12s)
Sting-Kill® [OTC]: 20% (5s)

Tablet, orally dissolving, oral:
Cepacol® Fizzlers™ [OTC]: 6 mg (12s)
Wax, oral:
Dent's Extra Strength Toothache Gum [OTC]:
20% (1 g)
Dental Comment Health Canada has issued a
reminder to healthcare professionals that benzocaine
sprays must be used judiciously to minimize the risk of
methemoglobinemia. Almost all reported cases have
been associated with higher concentration (14% to
20% benzocaine) spray products used in the mouth
and on other mucous membranes. Alternatives to benzocaine sprays, such as topical lidocaine preparations,
should be considered for patients at higher risk of this
reaction.

Benzocaine, Butamben, and Tetracaine
(BEN zoe kane, byoo TAM ben, & TET ra kane)

Related Information
Benzocaine *on page 176*
Tetracaine (Topical) *on page 1307*
Brand Names: U.S. Cetacaine®; Exactacain®
Generic Availability (U.S.) No
Pharmacologic Category Local Anesthetic
Dental Use Topical anesthetic for accessible mucous
membranes
Use Topical anesthetic to control pain in surgical or
endoscopic procedures; anesthetic for accessible
mucous membranes except for the eyes
Local Anesthetic/Vasoconstrictor Precautions No
information available to require special precautions
Effects on Dental Treatment Key adverse event(s)
related to dental treatment: A patient history of allergy to
ester-type local anesthetics contraindicates the use of
this product (see Dental Comment).
Effects on Bleeding No information available to
require special precautions
Adverse Effects Frequency not defined. Also see individual monographs for Benzocaine and Tetracaine.
Dermatologic: Contact dermatitis (eg, erythema, pruritus, vesiculation, oozing); dehydration of the epithelium; escharotic effect
Miscellaneous: Hypersensitivity/anaphylaxis reaction (rare)
Dental Usual Dosage Topical anesthetic (Exacta-
cain™): Adults: 3 metered sprays (maximum dose: 6
metered sprays); each metered spray delivers 9.3 mg
benzocaine, 1.3 mg butamben, 1.3 mg tetracaine
Dosage Topical anesthetic: **Note:** Decrease dose in the
acutely-ill patient.
Children: Dose has not been established; dose reduction is suggested
Adults:
Cetacaine®:
Aerosol: Apply for ≤1 second; use of sprays >2
seconds is contraindicated
Gel: Apply ~1/2 inch (13 mm) x 3/16 inch (5 mm);
application of >1 inch (26 cm) x 3/16 inch (5 mm) is
contraindicated
Liquid: Apply 6-7 drops (0.2 mL); application of
>12-14 drops (0.4 mL) is contraindicated
Exactacain™: 3 metered sprays (use of >6 metered
sprays is contraindicated)
Elderly: Dose reduction is suggested
Mechanism of Action Reversible blockage of initiation
and conduction of nerve impulses by decreasing the
neuronal membrane's permeability to sodium ions

Contraindications Hypersensitivity to benzocaine, butamben, tetracaine, or any component of the formulation; ophthalmic use; cholinesterase deficiencies; large areas of denuded or inflamed tissue; administration in excess of product labeling

Warnings/Precautions For topical use only. Methemoglobinemia has been reported following topical benzocaine use (rare), particularly with higher concentration (14% to 20%) spray formulations applied to the mouth or mucous membranes. The classical clinical finding of methemoglobinemia is chocolate brown-colored arterial blood. However, suspected cases should be confirmed by co-oximetry, which yields a direct and accurate measure of methemoglobin levels. Standard pulse oximetry readings or arterial blood gas values are not reliable. Clinically-significant methemoglobinemia requires immediate treatment.

Use caution with breathing problems (asthma, bronchitis, emphysema, in smokers), inflamed/damaged mucosa, heart disease, children <6 months of age, and hemoglobin or enzyme abnormalities (glucose-6-phosphate dehydrogenase deficiency, hemoglobin-M disease, NADH-methemoglobin reductase deficiency, pyruvate-kinase deficiency). Alternatives to benzocaine sprays, such as topical lidocaine preparations, should be considered for patients at higher risk of this reaction.

When topical anesthetics are used prior to cosmetic or medical procedures, the lowest amount of anesthetic necessary for pain relief should be applied. High systemic levels and toxic effects (eg, methhemoglobinemia, irregular heart beats, respiratory depression, seizures, death) have been reported in patients who (without supervision of a trained professional) have applied topical anesthetics in large amounts (or to large areas of the skin), left these products on for prolonged periods of time, or have used wraps/dressings to cover the skin following application.

Use caution in debilitated, elderly, acutely ill, and very young patients; dose adjustment is suggested. Do not use under dentures or cotton rolls; retention of active ingredients may cause escharotic effect.

Drug Interactions

Metabolism/Transport Effects None known.

Avoid Concomitant Use There are no known interactions where it is recommended to avoid concomitant use.

Increased Effect/Toxicity There are no known significant interactions involving an increase in effect.

Decreased Effect There are no known significant interactions involving a decrease in effect.

Pharmacodynamics/Kinetics

Onset of Action ~30 seconds

Duration of Action 30-60 minutes

Pregnancy Considerations Safety has not been established; use is not recommended during early pregnancy unless the potential benefits outweigh the risks.

Dosage Forms

Aerosol, spray, topical [kit]:
Cetacaine®: Benzocaine 14%, butamben 2%, and tetracaine 2% (56 g)

Aerosol, spray, topical:
Cetacaine®: Benzocaine 14%, butamben 2%, and tetracaine 2% (56 g)
Exactacain®: Benzocaine 14%, butamben 2%, and tetracaine 2% (60 g)

Gel, topical:
Cetacaine®: Benzocaine 14%, butamben 2%, and tetracaine 2% (32 g)

Liquid, topical, kit:
Cetacaine®: Benzocaine 14%, butamben 2%, and tetracaine 2% (14 g)

Liquid, topical:
Cetacaine®: Benzocaine 14%, butamben 2%, and tetracaine 2% (14 g, 30 g)

Dental Comment Manufacturer indication for use is suppression of gag reflex for gastroenterological procedures.

Health Canada has issued a reminder to healthcare professionals that benzocaine sprays must be used judiciously to minimize the risk of methemoglobinemia. Almost all reported cases have been associated with higher concentration (14% to 20% benzocaine) spray products used in the mouth and on other mucous membranes. Alternatives to benzocaine sprays, such as topical lidocaine preparations, should be considered for patients at higher risk of this reaction.

Benzoin (BEN zoin)

Brand Names: U.S. Benz-Protect Swabs™ [OTC]; Sprayzoin™ [OTC]

Pharmacologic Category Antibiotic, Topical; Topical Skin Product

Use Protective application for irritations of the skin; sometimes used in boiling water as steam inhalants for its expectorant and soothing action

Local Anesthetic/Vasoconstrictor Precautions No information available to require special precautions

Effects on Dental Treatment No significant effects or complications reported

Effects on Bleeding No information available to require special precautions

General Dosage Range Topical: *Children and Adults:* Apply 1-2 times/day

Benzonatate (ben ZOE na tate)

Related Information
Management of Patients Undergoing Cancer Therapy *on page 1596*

Brand Names: U.S. Tessalon®; Zonatuss™

Generic Availability (U.S.) Yes: Capsule (softgel)

Pharmacologic Category Antitussive

Use Symptomatic relief of nonproductive cough

Local Anesthetic/Vasoconstrictor Precautions No information available to require special precautions

Effects on Dental Treatment No significant effects or complications reported

Effects on Bleeding No information available to require special precautions

Adverse Effects Frequency not defined.
Central nervous system: Confusion, dizziness, hallucinations, headache, sedation
Dermatologic: Pruritus, skin eruptions
Gastrointestinal: Constipation, GI upset, nausea
Neuromuscular & skeletal: Chest numbness
Ocular: Burning sensation in eyes
Respiratory: Nasal congestion
Miscellaneous: Chill sensation, hypersensitivity reactions (bronchospasm, laryngospasm, cardiovascular collapse)

Dosage Children >10 years and Adults: Oral: 100-200 mg 3 times/day as needed for cough; maximum dose: 600 mg/day

Dosage adjustment in renal impairment: No dosage adjustment provided in manufacturer's labeling.

Dosage adjustment in hepatic impairment: No dosage adjustment provided in manufacturer's labeling.

Mechanism of Action Tetracaine congener with antitussive properties; suppresses cough by topical anesthetic action on the respiratory stretch receptors

Contraindications Hypersensitivity to benzonatate, related compounds (such as tetracaine), or any component of the formulation

Warnings/Precautions Severe reactions, including bronchospasm, cardiovascular collapse and laryngospasm have been reported. May be related to localized anesthetic effects due to sucking or chewing the capsule. Isolated cases of abnormal behavior including mental confusion and visual hallucinations have been reported; may be related to prior sensitivity to related agents (eg, tetracaine, procaine) or interaction with concurrent medications. Accidental ingestion and potentially fatal overdose of benzonatate has been reported in children <10 years of age. Signs and symptoms of overdose (restlessness, tremors, convulsion, coma, cardiac arrest) may occur within 15-20 minutes after ingestion. Death has been reported within 1 hour. Not approved for use in children <10 years of age.

Drug Interactions

Metabolism/Transport Effects None known.

Avoid Concomitant Use There are no known interactions where it is recommended to avoid concomitant use.

Increased Effect/Toxicity There are no known significant interactions involving an increase in effect.

Decreased Effect There are no known significant interactions involving a decrease in effect.

Pharmacodynamics/Kinetics

Onset of Action Therapeutic: 15-20 minutes

Duration of Action 3-8 hours

Pregnancy Risk Factor C

Pregnancy Considerations Animal reproduction studies have not been conducted.

Lactation Excretion in breast milk unknown/use caution

Breast-Feeding Considerations It is not known if benzonatate is excreted in breast milk. The manufacturer recommends that caution be exercised when administering benzonatate to nursing women.

Dosage Forms

Capsule, oral:
Zonatuss™: 150 mg

Capsule, softgel, oral: 100 mg, 200 mg
Tessalon®: 100 mg, 200 mg

Benzoyl Peroxide (BEN zoe il peer OKS ide)

Brand Names: U.S. Acne Clear Maximum Strength [OTC]; BenzEFoam Ultra™; BenzEFoam™; Benziq™; BP Cleanser [OTC]; BP Cleansing Lotion [OTC]; BP Wash [OTC]; BPO; Clean & Clear® advantage® 3-in-1 [OTC]; Clean & Clear® continuous control® [OTC]; Clean & Clear® persa-gel® 10 [OTC]; Clearskin [OTC]; Desquam-X® 10 [OTC]; Desquam-X® 5 [OTC]; Inova®; Neutrogena® On The Spot® Acne Treatment [OTC]; OXY® Clinical Clearing Treatment [OTC]; OXY® Maximum Face Wash [OTC]; OXY® Maximum Spot Treatment [OTC]; Pacnex®; Pacnex® HP; Pacnex® LP; PanOxyl® Bar [OTC]; PanOxyl® [OTC]; Pan-Oxyl®-4 [OTC]; PanOxyl®-8 [OTC]; PR™ Wash; SE BPO; TL BPO MX; Zapzyt® [OTC]

Brand Names: Canada Acetoxyl®; Benoxyl®; Benzac AC®; Benzac W® Gel; Benzac W® Wash; Desquam-X®; Oxyderm™; PanOxyl®; Solugel®

Pharmacologic Category Acne Products; Topical Skin Product; Topical Skin Product, Acne

Use Treatment of mild-to-moderate acne vulgaris and acne rosacea

Local Anesthetic/Vasoconstrictor Precautions No information available to require special precautions

Effects on Dental Treatment No significant effects or complications reported

Effects on Bleeding No information available to require special precautions

Adverse Effects 1% to 10%: Dermatologic: Irritation, contact dermatitis, dryness, erythema, peeling, stinging

General Dosage Range Topical: *Children ≥12 years, Adolescents, and Adults:*
Cleanser: Wash once or twice daily
Topical formulations: Apply sparingly once daily; gradually increase to 2-3 times/day if needed

Mechanism of Action Releases free-radical oxygen which oxidizes bacterial proteins in the sebaceous follicles decreasing the number of anaerobic bacteria and decreasing irritating-type free fatty acids

Pregnancy Risk Factor C

Pregnancy Considerations Animal reproduction studies have not been conducted; ~2% of the applied dose is expected to be absorbed systemically (Akhavan, 2003).

Benzoyl Peroxide and Hydrocortisone
(BEN zoe il peer OKS ide & hye droe KOR ti sone)

Related Information
Benzoyl Peroxide *on page 180*
Hydrocortisone (Topical) *on page 699*

Brand Names: U.S. Vanoxide-HC®

Brand Names: Canada Vanoxide-HC®

Pharmacologic Category Acne Products; Topical Skin Product; Topical Skin Product, Acne

Use Treatment of acne vulgaris and oily skin

Local Anesthetic/Vasoconstrictor Precautions No information available to require special precautions

Effects on Dental Treatment No significant effects or complications reported

Effects on Bleeding No information available to require special precautions

Adverse Effects See individual agents.

General Dosage Range Topical: *Adolescents ≥12 years and Adults:* Apply thin film 1-3 times/day

Pregnancy Risk Factor C

Pregnancy Considerations Animal reproduction studies have not been conducted with this combination. See individual agents.

Benzphetamine (benz FET a meen)

Brand Names: U.S. Didrex®; Regimex™

Pharmacologic Category Anorexiant; Central Nervous System Stimulant; Sympathomimetic

Use Short-term (few weeks) adjunct to caloric restriction in exogenous obesity

Pharmacotherapy for weight loss is recommended only for obese patients with a body mass index ≥30 kg/m^2, or ≥27 kg/m^2 in the presence of other risk factors such as hypertension, diabetes, and/or dyslipidemia or a high waist circumference; therapy should be used in conjunction with a comprehensive weight management program.

Local Anesthetic/Vasoconstrictor Precautions Use with caution since amphetamines have actions similar to epinephrine and norepinephrine

Effects on Dental Treatment Key adverse event(s) related to dental treatment: Xerostomia (normal salivary flow resumes upon discontinuation) and metallic taste.

Effects on Bleeding No information available to require special precautions

Adverse Effects Frequency not defined.

Cardiovascular: Cardiomyopathy/ischemic events (with chronic amphetamine use), hypertension, palpitation, tachycardia

Central nervous system: Depression (with withdrawal), dizziness, headache, insomnia, psychosis (rare), restlessness

Dermatologic: Skin reactions, urticaria

Endocrine & metabolic: Libido changes

Gastrointestinal: Diarrhea, nausea, unpleasant taste, xerostomia

Neuromuscular & skeletal: Tremor

Miscellaneous: Diaphoresis, overstimulation

General Dosage Range Oral: *Children ≥12 years and Adults:* Initial: 25-50 mg once daily; Maintenance: 25-50 mg 1-3 times/day (maximum: 150 mg/day)

Mechanism of Action Benzphetamine is a sympathomimetic amine with pharmacologic properties similar to the amphetamines. The mechanism of action in reducing appetite appears to be secondary to CNS effects, including stimulation of the hypothalamus to release norepinephrine.

Pregnancy Risk Factor X

Pregnancy Considerations Benzphetamine may cause fetal harm when used during pregnancy. Amphetamines were found to be teratogenic and embryotoxic in animal studies. Use is contraindicated in patients who are or may become pregnant.

Controlled Substance C-III

Benztropine (BENZ troe peen)

Brand Names: U.S. Cogentin®

Brand Names: Canada Apo-Benztropine®; Benztropine Omega; PMS-Benztropine

Pharmacologic Category Anti-Parkinson's Agent, Anticholinergic; Anticholinergic Agent

Use Adjunctive treatment of Parkinson's disease; aid in the treatment of drug-induced extrapyramidal symptoms (except tardive dyskinesia)

Local Anesthetic/Vasoconstrictor Precautions No information available to require special precautions

Effects on Dental Treatment Key adverse event(s) related to dental treatment: Xerostomia and changes in salivation (normal salivary flow resumes upon discontinuation), dry throat, and nasal dryness (very prevalent).

Effects on Bleeding No information available to require special precautions

Adverse Effects Frequency not defined.

Cardiovascular: Tachycardia

Central nervous system: Confusion, depression, disorientation, exacerbation of preexisting psychotic symptoms, fever, listlessness, memory impairment, nervousness, toxic psychosis, visual hallucinations

Dermatologic: Rash

Endocrine & metabolic: Heat stroke, hyperthermia

Gastrointestinal: Constipation, nausea, paralytic ileus, vomiting, xerostomia

Genitourinary: Urinary retention, dysuria

Neuromuscular & skeletal: Numbness of fingers

Ocular: Blurred vision, mydriasis

General Dosage Range I.M., I.V., Oral: *Adults:* Range: 0.5-8 mg/day

Mechanism of Action Possesses both anticholinergic and antihistaminic effects. *In vitro* anticholinergic activity approximates that of atropine; *in vivo* it is only about half as active as atropine. Animal data suggest its antihistaminic activity and duration of action approach that of pyrilamine maleate. May also inhibit the reuptake and storage of dopamine, thereby prolonging the action of dopamine.

Pharmacodynamics/Kinetics

Onset of Action I.M., I.V.: Within a few minutes

Time to Peak Plasma: 7 hours

Pregnancy Considerations Animal reproduction studies have not been conducted. Paralytic ileus (which resolved rapidly) was reported in two newborns exposed to a combination of benztropine and chlorpromazine during the second and third trimesters and the last 6 weeks of pregnancy, respectively (Falterman, 1980).

Benzydamine (ben ZID a meen)

Brand Names: Canada Apo-Benzydamine®; Dom-Benzydamine; Novo-Benzydamine; PMS-Benzydamine; Tantum®

Pharmacologic Category Local Anesthetic, Oral

Dental Use Symptomatic treatment of pain associated with acute pharyngitis; treatment of pain associated with radiation-induced oropharyngeal mucositis

Use Symptomatic treatment of pain associated with acute pharyngitis; treatment of pain associated with radiation-induced oropharyngeal mucositis

Local Anesthetic/Vasoconstrictor Precautions No information available to require special precautions

Effects on Dental Treatment Key adverse event(s) related to dental treatment: Numbness, burning/stinging sensation, and xerostomia (normal salivary flow resumes upon discontinuation).

Effects on Bleeding No information available to require special precautions

Adverse Effects

Central nervous system: Drowsiness, headache

Gastrointestinal: Nausea and/or vomiting (2%), xerostomia

Local: Numbness (10%), burning/stinging sensation (8%)

Respiratory: Cough, pharyngeal irritation

Dental Usual Dosage

Acute pharyngitis: Adults: Oral rinse: Gargle with 15 mL every 1½-3 hours until symptoms resolve. Patient should expel solution from mouth following use; solution should not be swallowed.

Radiation-associated mucositis: Adults: Oral rinse: 15 mL as a gargle or rinse 3-4 times/day; contact between the liquid and the oral mucosa should be maintained for at least 30 seconds, followed by expulsion from the mouth.

Dosage Oral rinse: Adults:

Acute pharyngitis: Gargle with 15 mL of undiluted solution every 1½-3 hours until symptoms resolve. Patient should expel solution from mouth following use; solution should not be swallowed.

Mucositis: 15 mL of undiluted solution as a gargle or rinse 3-4 times/day; contact should be maintained for at least 30 seconds, followed by expulsion from the mouth

Dosage adjustment in renal impairment: No adjustment required.

Mechanism of Action Local anesthetic and anti-inflammatory, reduces local pain and inflammation. Does not interfere with arachidonic acid metabolism.

Contraindications Hypersensitivity to benzydamine or any component of the formulation

Warnings/Precautions May cause local irritation and/or burning sensation in patients with altered mucosal integrity. Dilution (1:1 in warm water) may attenuate this effect. Use caution in renal impairment.

Drug Interactions

Metabolism/Transport Effects None known.

Avoid Concomitant Use There are no known interactions where it is recommended to avoid concomitant use.

Increased Effect/Toxicity There are no known significant interactions involving an increase in effect.

Decreased Effect There are no known significant interactions involving a decrease in effect.

Pregnancy Considerations Safety has not been established in pregnant women. Use only when potential benefit outweighs possible risk to the fetus.

Lactation Excretion in breast milk unknown/use caution

Breast-Feeding Considerations It is not known if benzydamine is excreted in breast milk. The manufacturer recommends that caution be exercised when administering benzydamine peroxide to nursing women.

Product Availability Not available in U.S.

Dosage Forms: Canada
Oral rinse: 0.15% (100 mL, 250 mL)

Benzylpenicilloyl Polylysine
(BEN zil pen i SIL oyl pol i LIE seen)

Brand Names: U.S. Pre-Pen®

Pharmacologic Category Diagnostic Agent

Use Adjunct in assessing the risk of administering penicillin (penicillin G or benzylpenicillin) in patients suspected of clinical penicillin hypersensitivity

Unlabeled Use Adjunct in assessment of hypersensitivity to other beta-lactam antibiotics (penicillins and cephalosporins) to determine the safety of penicillin administration in patients with a history of reaction to cephalosporins

Local Anesthetic/Vasoconstrictor Precautions No information available to require special precautions

Effects on Dental Treatment No significant effects or complications reported

Effects on Bleeding No information available to require special precautions

Adverse Effects Frequency not defined.

Cardiovascular: Hypotension

Dermatologic: Angioneurotic edema, pruritus, erythema, urticaria

Local: Inflammation (intense; at skin test site), wheal (locally)

Respiratory: Dyspnea

Miscellaneous: Systemic allergic reactions (including anaphylaxis; rare)

General Dosage Range

Intradermal: *Children and Adults:* Inject a volume of skin test solution sufficient to raise a small intradermal bleb ~3 mm in diameter, in duplicate

Puncture test (first step): *Children and Adults:* Apply a small drop of solution to make a single shallow puncture of the epidermis

Mechanism of Action Benzylpenicilloyl polylysine, a conjugate of the benzylpenicilloyl structural group (hapten) and the poly-l-lysine carrier (protein), is an antigen which reacts with benzylpenicilloyl IgE antibodies to elicit the release of chemical mediators, thereby producing type I (immediate or accelerated) urticarial reactions in patients hypersensitive to penicillins.

Pregnancy Risk Factor C

Pregnancy Considerations Animal reproduction studies have not been conducted with benzylpenicilloyl polylysine. The Centers for Disease Control and Prevention (CDC) states that penicillin skin testing may be useful in assessing suspected penicillin hypersensitivity in pregnant women diagnosed with syphilis (of any stage) due to a lack of proven alternatives to the use of penicillin in this population (CDC, 2006).

Bepotastine (be poe TAS teen)

Brand Names: U.S. Bepreve®

Pharmacologic Category Histamine H$_1$ Antagonist; Histamine H$_1$ Antagonist, Second Generation; Mast Cell Stabilizer

Use Treatment of itching associated with allergic conjunctivitis

Local Anesthetic/Vasoconstrictor Precautions No information available to require special precautions

Effects on Dental Treatment Key adverse event(s) related to dental treatment: Taste abnormalities reported in ≤25% of patients

Effects on Bleeding No information available to require special precautions

Adverse Effects

Central nervous system: Headache

Gastrointestinal: Taste abnormality

Ocular: Irritation

Respiratory: Nasopharyngitis

General Dosage Range Ophthalmic: *Children ≥2 years and Adults:* Instill 1 drop into the affected eye(s) twice daily

Mechanism of Action Direct H$_1$-receptor antagonist and inhibits release of histamine from mast cells

Pharmacodynamics/Kinetics

Onset of Action Within 3 minutes (Macejko, 2010)

Duration of Action Up to 16 hours (Williams, 2011)

Time to Peak Serum: 1-2 hours

Pregnancy Risk Factor C

Pregnancy Considerations Teratogenic effects were not observed in most animal reproduction studies following oral administration; however, a decrease in fetal weight and a decrease in live births were observed in some studies. In humans, plasma concentrations are below the limit of quantification (<2 ng/mL) 24 hours after ophthalmic administration.

Beractant (ber AKT ant)

Brand Names: U.S. Survanta®

Brand Names: Canada Survanta®

Pharmacologic Category Lung Surfactant

Use Prevention and treatment of respiratory distress syndrome (RDS) in premature infants

Prophylactic therapy: Body weight <1250 g in infants at risk for developing, or with evidence of, surfactant deficiency (administer within 15 minutes of birth)

Rescue therapy: Treatment of infants with RDS confirmed by x-ray and requiring mechanical ventilation (administer as soon as possible - within 8 hours of age)

Local Anesthetic/Vasoconstrictor Precautions No information available to require special precautions

Effects on Dental Treatment No significant effects or complications reported

Effects on Bleeding No information available to require special precautions

Adverse Effects During the dosing procedure:
>10%: Cardiovascular: Transient bradycardia
1% to 10%: Respiratory: Oxygen desaturation

General Dosage Range Endotracheal: *Premature infants:* Administer 4 mL/kg (100 mg phospholipids/kg); may repeat if needed, no more frequently than every 6 hours to a maximum of 4 doses/48 hours

Mechanism of Action Replaces deficient or ineffective endogenous lung surfactant in neonates with respiratory distress syndrome (RDS) or in neonates at risk of developing RDS. Surfactant prevents the alveoli from collapsing during expiration by lowering surface tension between air and alveolar surfaces.

Pregnancy Considerations Beractant is only indicated for use in premature infants.

Besifloxacin (be si FLOX a sin)

Brand Names: U.S. Besivance™
Brand Names: Canada Besivance™
Pharmacologic Category Antibiotic, Ophthalmic; Antibiotic, Quinolone
Use Treatment of bacterial conjunctivitis
Local Anesthetic/Vasoconstrictor Precautions No information available to require special precautions
Effects on Dental Treatment No significant effects or complications reported
Effects on Bleeding No information available to require special precautions
Adverse Effects 1% to 2%:
Central nervous system: Headache
Ocular: Conjunctival redness (2%), blurred vision, irritation, pain, pruritus

General Dosage Range Ophthalmic: *Children ≥1 year and Adults:* 1 drop into affected eye(s) 3 times/day (4-12 hours apart)

Mechanism of Action Inhibits both DNA gyrase and topoisomerase IV. DNA gyrase is an essential bacterial enzyme required for DNA replication, transcription, and repair. Topoisomerase IV is an essential bacterial enzyme required for decatenation during cell division. Inhibition effect is bactericidal.

Pharmacodynamics/Kinetics
Half-life Elimination ~7 hours

Pregnancy Risk Factor C

Pregnancy Considerations Oral besifloxacin has been shown to be fetotoxic in animal studies at doses that were also maternally toxic. Quinolone exposure during human pregnancy has been reported with other agents (refer to Ciprofloxacin [Systemic], Ofloxacin [Systemic], and Norfloxacin monographs). The low plasma concentrations of besifloxacin following ophthalmic use (<1.3 ng/mL in nonpregnant patients) should limit fetal exposure.

Beta-Carotene (BAY ta KARE oh teen)

Brand Names: U.S. A-Caro-25 [OTC]; B-Caro-T™ [OTC]; Lumitene™ [OTC]
Pharmacologic Category Vitamin, Fat Soluble
Use Prophylaxis against photosensitivity reactions in erythropoietic protoporphyria (EPP)
Local Anesthetic/Vasoconstrictor Precautions No information available to require special precautions

Effects on Dental Treatment No significant effects or complications reported

Effects on Bleeding No information available to require special precautions

Adverse Effects Frequency not defined.
Central nervous system: Dizziness
Dermatologic: Carotenodermia (yellowing of palms, hands, or soles of feet, and to a lesser extent the face)

General Dosage Range Oral:
Children <14 years: 30-150 mg/day
Adults: 30-300 mg/day

Mechanism of Action The exact mechanism of action in erythropoietic protoporphyria has not as yet been elucidated; although patient must become carotenemic before effects are observed, there appears to be more than a simple internal light screen responsible for the drug's action. A protective effect was achieved when beta-carotene was added to blood samples. The concentrations of solutions used were similar to those achieved in treated patients. Topically applied beta-carotene is considerably less effective than systemic therapy.

Pregnancy Considerations Maternal intake of beta carotene influences cord blood concentrations (Scaife, 2006).

Betaine (BAY ta een)

Brand Names: U.S. Cystadane®
Brand Names: Canada Cystadane®
Pharmacologic Category Homocystinuria, Treatment Agent
Use Treatment of homocystinuria (eg, deficiencies or defects in cystathionine beta-synthase [CBS], 5,10-methylene tetrahydrofolate reductase [MTHFR], and cobalamin cofactor metabolism [CBL])
Local Anesthetic/Vasoconstrictor Precautions No information available to require special precautions
Effects on Dental Treatment No significant effects or complications reported
Effects on Bleeding No information available to require special precautions
Adverse Effects
Frequency not defined: Gastrointestinal: Diarrhea, dysgeusia, GI distress, nausea
Postmarketing and/or case reports: Alopecia, anorexia, agitation, cerebral edema (associated with hypermethioninemia), dental disorders, depression, hives, glossitis, irritability, personality disorder, sleep disturbances, skin odor abnormalities, urinary incontinence, vomiting

General Dosage Range Oral:
Children <3 years: Initial: 100 mg/kg/day, then increase weekly by 50 mg/kg increments, as needed
Children ≥3 years and Adults: 3 g twice daily (maximum: 20 g/day)

Mechanism of Action Betaine acts as a methyl group donor in the remethylation of homocysteine to methionine. Homocystinuria is an inborn error of metabolism in which elevated plasma homocysteine levels can lead to mental retardation, ocular abnormalities, osteoporosis, premature atherosclerosis and thromboembolic disease. Remethylation is one of the two divergent pathways in the metabolism of homocysteine. The second pathway involves transulfuration of homocysteine to produce cysteine. A number of enzymes and cofactors are also involved in these pathways.

Pregnancy Risk Factor C

Pregnancy Considerations Animal reproduction studies have not been conducted with betaine. It is not known whether betaine can cause fetal harm when administered to a pregnant woman or can affect reproductive capacity. Betaine should be given to a pregnant woman only if needed.

Prescribing and Access Restrictions Cystadane® may be obtained by contacting Accredo Health Group Inc at 1-888-454-8860.

Betamethasone (bay ta METH a sone)

Related Information
Respiratory Diseases *on page 1514*

Related Sample Prescriptions
Mild Lichen Planus *on page 1618*
Recurrent Aphthous Stomatitis *on page 1618*

Brand Names: U.S. Celestone®; Celestone® Soluspan®; Diprolene®; Diprolene® AF; Luxiq®

Brand Names: Canada Betaderm; Betaject™; Betnesol®; Betnovate®; Celestone® Soluspan®; Diprolene®; Diprolene® Glycol; Diprosone®; Ectosone; Prevex® B; ratio-Ectosone; Ratio-Topilene; ratio-Topilene; Ratio-Topisone; ratio-Topisone; Rivasone; Rolene; Rosone; Taro-Sone; Valisone® Scalp Lotion

Generic Availability (U.S.) Yes: Excludes solution

Pharmacologic Category Corticosteroid, Systemic; Corticosteroid, Topical

Dental Use Treatment of a variety of oral diseases of allergic, inflammatory, or autoimmune origin

Use Inflammatory dermatoses such as seborrheic or atopic dermatitis, neurodermatitis, anogenital pruritus, psoriasis, inflammatory phase of xerosis

Unlabeled Use Accelerate fetal lung maturation in patients with preterm labor

Local Anesthetic/Vasoconstrictor Precautions No information available to require special precautions

Effects on Dental Treatment No significant effects or complications reported

Effects on Bleeding Variable effects on anticoagulant therapy are observed with glucocorticoids such as betamethasone.

Adverse Effects
Systemic:
Cardiovascular: Congestive heart failure, edema, hyper-/hypotension
Central nervous system: Dizziness, headache, insomnia, intracranial pressure increased, lightheadedness, nervousness, pseudotumor cerebri, seizure, vertigo
Dermatologic: Ecchymoses, facial erythema, fragile skin, hirsutism, hyper-/hypopigmentation, perioral dermatitis (oral), petechiae, striae, wound healing impaired
Endocrine & metabolic: Amenorrhea, Cushing's syndrome, diabetes mellitus, growth suppression, hyperglycemia, hypokalemia, menstrual irregularities, pituitary-adrenal axis suppression, protein catabolism, sodium retention, water retention
Local: Injection site reactions (intra-articular use), sterile abscess
Neuromuscular & skeletal: Arthralgia, muscle atrophy, fractures, muscle weakness, myopathy, osteoporosis, necrosis (femoral and humeral heads)
Ocular: Cataracts, glaucoma, intraocular pressure increased
Miscellaneous: Anaphylactoid reaction, diaphoresis, hypersensitivity, secondary infection

Topical:
Dermatologic: Acneiform eruptions, allergic dermatitis, burning, dry skin, erythema, folliculitis, hypertrichosis, irritation, miliaria, pruritus, skin atrophy, striae, vesiculation
Endocrine and metabolic effects have occasionally been reported with topical use.

Dental Usual Dosage Allergic or inflammatory diseases: Topical: Gel: Apply small quantity with Q-tip to affected area 3-4 times/day

Dosage Base dosage on severity of disease and patient response

Children: Use lowest dose listed as initial dose for adrenocortical insufficiency (physiologic replacement)
I.M.: ≤12 years: 0.0175-0.125 mg base/kg/day divided every 6-12 hours **or** 0.5-7.5 mg base/m²/day divided every 6-12 hours
Oral: ≤12 years: 0.0175-0.25 mg/kg/day divided every 6-8 hours **or** 0.5-7.5 mg/m²/day divided every 6-8 hours
Topical:
≤12 years: Use is not recommended.
≥13 years: Use minimal amount for shortest period of time to avoid HPA axis suppression
Gel, augmented formulation: Apply once or twice daily; rub in gently. **Note:** Do not exceed 2 weeks of treatment or 50 g/week.
Lotion: Apply a few drops twice daily
Augmented formulation: Apply a few drops once or twice daily; rub in gently. **Note:** Do not exceed 2 weeks of treatment or 50 mL/week.
Cream/ointment: Apply once or twice daily.
Augmented formulation: Apply once or twice daily. **Note:** Do not exceed 2 weeks of treatment or 45 g/week.

Adolescents and Adults:
Oral: 2.4-4.8 mg/day in 2-4 doses; range: 0.6-7.2 mg/day
I.M.: Betamethasone sodium phosphate and betamethasone acetate: 0.6-9 mg/day (generally, $\frac{1}{3}$ to $\frac{1}{2}$ of oral dose) divided every 12-24 hours
Adults:
Intrabursal, intra-articular, intradermal: 0.25-2 mL
Intralesional: Rheumatoid arthritis/osteoarthritis:
Very large joints: 1-2 mL
Large joints: 1 mL
Medium joints: 0.5-1 mL
Small joints: 0.25-0.5 mL
I.M.: Antenatal fetal maturation (unlabeled use): 12 mg every 24 hours for a total of 2 doses apart (ACOG, 2011). **Note:** Recommended for pregnant women with premature labor (24-34 weeks gestation) who are expected to deliver within 7 days.
Topical:
Foam: Apply to the scalp twice daily, once in the morning and once at night
Gel, augmented formulation: Apply once or twice daily; rub in gently. **Note:** Do not exceed 2 weeks of treatment or 50 g/week.
Lotion: Apply a few drops twice daily
Augmented formulation: Apply a few drops once or twice daily; rub in gently. **Note:** Do not exceed 2 weeks of treatment or 50 mL/week.
Cream/ointment: Apply once or twice daily
Augmented formulation: Apply once or twice daily. **Note:** Do not exceed 2 weeks of treatment or 45 g/week.

Dosing adjustment in hepatic impairment: Adjustments may be necessary in patients with liver failure because betamethasone is extensively metabolized in the liver

Mechanism of Action Controls the rate of protein synthesis; depresses the migration of polymorphonuclear leukocytes, fibroblasts; reverses capillary permeability and lysosomal stabilization at the cellular level to prevent or control inflammation

Contraindications Hypersensitivity to betamethasone, other corticosteroids, or any component of the formulation; systemic fungal infections; I.M. administration contraindicated in idiopathic thrombocytopenia purpura

Warnings/Precautions Very high potency topical products are not for treatment of rosacea, perioral dermatitis; not for use on face, groin, or axillae; not for use in a diapered area. Avoid concurrent use of other corticosteroids.

May cause hypercorticism or suppression of hypothalamic-pituitary-adrenal (HPA) axis, particularly in younger children or in patients receiving high doses for prolonged periods. HPA axis suppression may lead to adrenal crisis. Withdrawal and discontinuation of a corticosteroid should be done slowly and carefully. Particular care is required when patients are transferred from systemic corticosteroids to inhaled products due to possible adrenal insufficiency or withdrawal from steroids, including an increase in allergic symptoms. Patients receiving >20 mg per day of prednisone (or equivalent) may be most susceptible. Fatalities have occurred due to adrenal insufficiency in asthmatic patients during and after transfer from systemic corticosteroids to aerosol steroids; aerosol steroids do not provide the systemic steroid needed to treat patients having trauma, surgery, or infections. In stressful situations, HPA axis-suppressed patients should receive adequate supplementation with natural glucocorticoids (hydrocortisone or cortisone) rather than betamethasone (due to lack of mineralocorticoid activity).

Topical corticosteroids may be absorbed percutaneously. Absorption of topical corticosteroids may cause manifestations of Cushing's syndrome, hyperglycemia, or glycosuria. Absorption is increased by the use of occlusive dressings, application to denuded skin, or application to large surface areas.

Acute myopathy has been reported with high dose corticosteroids, usually in patients with neuromuscular transmission disorders; may involve ocular and/or respiratory muscles; monitor creatine kinase; recovery may be delayed. Corticosteroid use may cause psychiatric disturbances, including depression, euphoria, insomnia, mood swings, and personality changes. Pre-existing psychiatric conditions may be exacerbated by corticosteroid use. Prolonged use of corticosteroids may also increase the incidence of secondary infection, mask acute infection (including fungal infections), prolong or exacerbate viral infections, or limit response to vaccines. Exposure to chickenpox should be avoided; corticosteroids should not be used to treat ocular herpes simplex. Corticosteroids should not be used for cerebral malaria or viral hepatitis. Close observation is required in patients with latent tuberculosis and/or TB reactivity; restrict use in active TB (only in conjunction with antituberculosis treatment). Prolonged treatment with corticosteroids has been associated with the development of Kaposi's sarcoma (case reports); if noted, discontinuation of therapy should be considered. High-dose corticosteroids should not be used to manage acute head injury.

Use with caution in patients with thyroid disease, hepatic impairment, renal impairment, cardiovascular disease, diabetes, glaucoma, cataracts, myasthenia gravis, patients at risk for osteoporosis, patients at risk for seizures, or GI diseases (diverticulitis, peptic ulcer, ulcerative colitis) due to perforation risk. Use caution following acute MI (corticosteroids have been associated with myocardial rupture). Because of the risk of adverse effects, systemic corticosteroids should be used cautiously in the elderly in the smallest possible effective dose for the shortest duration. Discontinue if skin irritation or contact dermatitis should occur; do not use in patients with decreased skin circulation. Withdraw therapy with gradual tapering of dose.

Topical use in patients ≤12 years of age is not recommended. Children may absorb proportionally larger amounts after topical application and may be more prone to systemic effects. HPA axis suppression, intracranial hypertension, and Cushing's syndrome have been reported in children receiving topical corticosteroids. Prolonged use may affect growth velocity; growth should be routinely monitored in pediatric patients.

Drug Interactions

Metabolism/Transport Effects None known.

Avoid Concomitant Use

Avoid concomitant use of Betamethasone with any of the following: Aldesleukin; BCG; Mifepristone; Natalizumab; Pimecrolimus; Tacrolimus (Topical); Tofacitinib

Increased Effect/Toxicity

Betamethasone may increase the levels/effects of: Acetylcholinesterase Inhibitors; Amphotericin B; Deferasirox; Leflunomide; Loop Diuretics; Natalizumab; NSAID (COX-2 Inhibitor); NSAID (Nonselective); Thiazide Diuretics; Tofacitinib; Vaccines (Live); Warfarin

The levels/effects of Betamethasone may be increased by: Antifungal Agents (Azole Derivatives, Systemic); Aprepitant; Calcium Channel Blockers (Nondihydropyridine); Denosumab; Estrogen Derivatives; Fluconazole; Fosaprepitant; Indacaterol; Macrolide Antibiotics; Mifepristone; Neuromuscular-Blocking Agents (Nondepolarizing); Pimecrolimus; Quinolone Antibiotics; Roflumilast; Salicylates; Tacrolimus (Topical); Telaprevir; Trastuzumab

Decreased Effect

Betamethasone may decrease the levels/effects of: Aldesleukin; Antidiabetic Agents; BCG; Calcitriol; Coccidioidin Skin Test; Corticorelin; Hyaluronidase; Isoniazid; Salicylates; Sipuleucel-T; Telaprevir; Vaccines (Inactivated)

The levels/effects of Betamethasone may be decreased by: Aminoglutethimide; Antacids; Barbiturates; Bile Acid Sequestrants; Echinacea; Mifepristone; Mitotane; Primidone; Rifamycin Derivatives

Ethanol/Nutrition/Herb Interactions

Ethanol: Avoid ethanol (may enhance gastric mucosal irritation).

Food: Betamethasone interferes with calcium absorption.

Herb/Nutraceutical: Avoid cat's claw, echinacea (have immunostimulant properties).

Dietary Considerations May be taken with food to decrease GI distress.

Pharmacodynamics/Kinetics

Half-life Elimination 6.5 hours

Time to Peak Serum: I.V.: 10-36 minutes

Pregnancy Risk Factor C

◀ **Pregnancy Considerations** Adverse events have been observed with corticosteroids in animal reproduction studies. Betamethasone crosses the placenta; approximately 25% is metabolized by placental enzymes to an inactive metabolite. Due to its positive effect on stimulating fetal lung maturation, a single course of the injection is often used in patients with premature labor (24-34 weeks gestation) who are expected to deliver within 7 days. Topical products are not recommended for extensive use, in large quantities, or for long periods of time in pregnant women. Some studies have shown an association between first trimester systemic corticosteroid use and oral clefts; adverse events in the fetus/neonate have been noted in case reports following large doses of systemic corticosteroids during pregnancy. Women exposed to betamethasone during pregnancy for the treatment of an autoimmune disease may contact the OTIS Autoimmune Diseases Study at 877-311-8972.

Lactation Excretion in breast milk unknown/use caution

Breast-Feeding Considerations Corticosteroids are excreted in human milk. The onset of milk secretion after birth may be delayed and the volume of milk produced may be decreased by antenatal betamethasone therapy; this affect was seen when delivery occurred 3-9 days after the betamethasone dose in women between 28 and 34 weeks gestation. Antenatal betamethasone therapy did not affect milk production when birth occurred <3 days or >10 days of treatment. It is not known if systemic absorption following topical administration results in detectable quantities in human milk. Use with caution while breast-feeding; do not apply to nipples.

Dosage Forms
Aerosol, foam, topical: 0.12% (50 g, 100 g)
Luxiq®: 0.12% (50 g, 100 g)
Cream, topical: 0.05% (15 g, 45 g, 50 g); 0.1% (15 g, 45 g)
Diprolene® AF: 0.05% (15 g, 50 g)
Gel, topical: 0.05% (15 g, 50 g)
Injection, suspension: Betamethasone sodium phosphate 3 mg and betamethasone acetate 3 mg per 1 mL (5 mL)
Celestone® Soluspan®: Betamethasone sodium phosphate 3 mg and betamethasone acetate 3 mg per 1 mL (5 mL)
Lotion, topical: 0.05% (30 mL, 60 mL); 0.1% (60 mL)
Diprolene®: 0.05% (30 mL, 60 mL)
Ointment, topical: 0.05% (15 g, 45 g, 50 g); 0.1% (15 g, 45 g)
Diprolene®: 0.05% (15 g, 50 g)
Solution, oral:
Celestone®: 0.6 mg/5 mL (118 mL)

Betamethasone and Clotrimazole
(bay ta METH a sone & kloe TRIM a zole)

Related Information
Betamethasone *on page 184*
Clotrimazole (Topical) *on page 340*
Brand Names: U.S. Lotrisone®
Brand Names: Canada Lotriderm®
Generic Availability (U.S.) Yes
Pharmacologic Category Antifungal Agent, Topical; Corticosteroid, Topical
Dental Use Treatment of a variety of oral diseases of allergic, inflammatory, or autoimmune origin

Use Topical treatment of various dermal fungal infections (including tinea pedis, cruris, and corpora in patients ≥17 years of age)

Local Anesthetic/Vasoconstrictor Precautions No information available to require special precautions

Effects on Dental Treatment No significant effects or complications reported

Effects on Bleeding Variable effects on anticoagulant therapy are observed with glucocorticoids such as betamethasone.

Adverse Effects Also see individual agents. 1% to 10%:
Dermatologic: Dry skin (2%)
Local: Burning (2%)
Neuromuscular & skeletal: Paresthesia (2%)
Other reactions reported with topical corticosteroid use: Acneiform eruption dermatitis, bruising, folliculitis, hypertrichosis, hypopigmentation, striae, telangiectasia

Dental Usual Dosage Allergic or inflammatory diseases: Children ≥17 years and Adults: Topical: Apply to affected area twice daily, morning and evening

Dosage
Children <17 years: Do not use
Children ≥17 years and Adults:
Allergic or inflammatory diseases: Topical: Apply to affected area twice daily, morning and evening
Tinea corporis, tinea cruris: Topical: Massage into affected area twice daily, morning and evening; do not use for longer than 2 weeks; re-evaluate after 1 week if no clinical improvement; do not exceed 45 g cream/week or 45 mL lotion/week
Tinea pedis: Topical: Massage into affected area twice daily, morning and evening; do not use for longer than 4 weeks; re-evaluate after 2 weeks if no clinical improvement; do not exceed 45 g cream/week or 45 mL lotion/week
Elderly: Use with caution; skin atrophy and skin ulceration (rare) have been reported in patients with thinning skin; do not use for diaper dermatitis or under occlusive dressings

Mechanism of Action Betamethasone dipropionate is a corticosteroid which controls the rate of protein synthesis; depresses the migration of polymorphonuclear leukocytes, fibroblasts; reverses capillary permeability and lysosomal stabilization at the cellular level to prevent or control inflammation. Clotrimazole is an antifungal agent that binds to phospholipids in the fungal cell membrane altering cell wall permeability resulting in loss of essential intracellular elements.

Contraindications Hypersensitivity to betamethasone, clotrimazole, other corticosteroids or imidazoles, or any component of the formulation

Warnings/Precautions For topical use only; discontinue use if irritation occurs. Systemic absorption of topical corticosteroids may cause hypothalamic-pituitary-adrenal (HPA) axis suppression (reversible) particularly in younger children. HPA axis suppression may lead to adrenal crisis. Risk is increased when used over large surface areas, for prolonged periods, or with occlusive dressings. Adverse systemic effects including hyperglycemia, glycosuria, fluid and electrolyte changes, and HPA suppression may occur when used on large surface areas, for prolonged periods, or with an occlusive dressing. Prolonged treatment with corticosteroids has been associated with the development of Kaposi's sarcoma (case reports); if noted, discontinuation of therapy should be considered. Use with caution in the elderly. Not for use in pediatric patients <17 years of age. Do not use for diaper dermatitis.

Drug Interactions
Metabolism/Transport Effects None known.
Avoid Concomitant Use
Avoid concomitant use of Betamethasone and Clotrimazole with any of the following: Aldesleukin; BCG; Mifepristone; Natalizumab; Pimecrolimus; Tacrolimus (Topical); Tofacitinib
Increased Effect/Toxicity
Betamethasone and Clotrimazole may increase the levels/effects of: Acetylcholinesterase Inhibitors; Amphotericin B; Deferasirox; Leflunomide; Loop Diuretics; Natalizumab; NSAID (COX-2 Inhibitor); NSAID (Nonselective); Thiazide Diuretics; Tofacitinib; Vaccines (Live); Warfarin

The levels/effects of Betamethasone and Clotrimazole may be increased by: Antifungal Agents (Azole Derivatives, Systemic); Aprepitant; Calcium Channel Blockers (Nondihydropyridine); Denosumab; Estrogen Derivatives; Fluconazole; Fosaprepitant; Indacaterol; Macrolide Antibiotics; Mifepristone; Neuromuscular-Blocking Agents (Nondepolarizing); Pimecrolimus; Quinolone Antibiotics; Roflumilast; Salicylates; Tacrolimus (Topical); Telaprevir; Trastuzumab
Decreased Effect
Betamethasone and Clotrimazole may decrease the levels/effects of: Aldesleukin; Antidiabetic Agents; BCG; Calcitriol; Coccidioidin Skin Test; Corticorelin; Hyaluronidase; Isoniazid; Salicylates; Sipuleucel-T; Telaprevir; Vaccines (Inactivated)

The levels/effects of Betamethasone and Clotrimazole may be decreased by: Aminoglutethimide; Antacids; Barbiturates; Bile Acid Sequestrants; Echinacea; Mifepristone; Mitotane; Primidone; Rifamycin Derivatives
Pregnancy Risk Factor C
Pregnancy Considerations There are no adequate and well-controlled studies using topical betamethasone during pregnancy. However, intrauterine growth retardation has been reported with another topical steroid. Avoid use in large amounts for long periods of time during pregnancy. Clotrimazole is poorly absorbed when used topically.
Lactation Excretion in breast milk unknown/use caution
Breast-Feeding Considerations Betamethasone: Systemic corticosteroids are excreted in human milk. The extent of topical absorption is variable. Use with caution while breast-feeding; do not apply to nipples.
Dosage Forms
Cream: Betamethasone 0.05% and clotrimazole 1% (15 g, 45 g)
Lotrisone®: Betamethasone 0.05% and clotrimazole 1% (15 g, 45 g)
Lotion: Betamethasone 0.05% and clotrimazole 1% (30 mL)
Lotrisone®: Betamethasone 0.05% and clotrimazole 1% (30 mL)

Betaxolol (Systemic) (be TAKS oh lol)

Related Information
Cardiovascular Diseases *on page 1492*
Brand Names: U.S. Kerlone®
Pharmacologic Category Beta-Blocker, Beta-1 Selective
Use Management of hypertension
Unlabeled Use Treatment of coronary artery disease
Local Anesthetic/Vasoconstrictor Precautions No information available to require special precautions

Effects on Dental Treatment Betaxolol is a cardioselective beta-blocker. Local anesthetic with vasoconstrictor can be safely used in patients medicated with betaxolol. Nonselective beta-blockers (ie, propranolol, nadolol) enhance the pressor response to epinephrine, resulting in hypertension and bradycardia; this has not been reported for betaxolol. Many nonsteroidal anti-inflammatory drugs, such as ibuprofen and indomethacin, can reduce the hypotensive effect of beta-blockers after 3 or more weeks of therapy with the NSAID. Short-term NSAID use (ie, 3 days) requires no special precautions in patients taking beta-blockers.
Effects on Bleeding No information available to require special precautions
Adverse Effects 2% to 10%:
Cardiovascular: Bradycardia (6% to 8%; symptomatic bradycardia: <1% to 2%; dose-dependent), chest pain (2% to 7%), palpitation (2%), edema ($\leq$2%; similar to placebo)
Central nervous system: Fatigue (3% to 10%), insomnia (1% to 5%), lethargy (3%)
Gastrointestinal: Nausea (2% to 6%), dyspepsia (4% to 5%), diarrhea (2%)
Neuromuscular & skeletal: Arthralgia (3% to 5%), paresthesia (2%)
Respiratory: Dyspnea (2%), pharyngitis (2%)
Miscellaneous: Antinuclear antibody positive (5%), cold extremities (2%)
General Dosage Range Dosage adjustment recommended in patients with renal impairment
Oral:
Adults: 5-20 mg/day
Elderly: Initial dose: 5 mg/day
Mechanism of Action Competitively blocks beta$_1$-receptors, with little or no effect on beta$_2$-receptors
Pharmacodynamics/Kinetics
Onset of Action 1-1.5 hours
Half-life Elimination 14-22 hours; prolonged in hepatic disease and/or chronic renal failure
Time to Peak 1.5-6 hours
Pregnancy Risk Factor C
Pregnancy Considerations Teratogenic were effects were not observed in animal reproduction studies; therefore, the manufacturer classifies betaxolol as pregnancy category C. Betaxolol crosses the placenta and can be detected in the amniotic fluid as well as umbilical cord blood. Measurable concentrations of betaxolol can also be found in the newborn blood and urine. In a cohort study, an increased risk of cardiovascular defects was observed following maternal use of beta-blockers during pregnancy. Intrauterine growth restriction (IUGR), small placentas, as well as fetal/neonatal bradycardia, hypoglycemia, and/or respiratory depression have been observed following *in utero* exposure to beta-blockers as a class. Following maternal use of betaxolol, the beta-blocker effects may persist in the neonate for several days after birth. Adequate facilities for monitoring infants at birth should be available. Untreated chronic maternal hypertension and pre-eclampsia are also associated with adverse events in the fetus, infant, and mother. The half-life and serum concentration of betaxolol immediately postpartum are not significantly different than what is observed in nonpregnant women. Betaxolol is currently not recommended for the initial treatment of hypertension in pregnancy.

Bethanechol (be THAN e kole)

Brand Names: U.S. Urecholine®

◄ **Brand Names: Canada** Duvoid®; PHL-Bethanechol; PMS-Bethanechol

Pharmacologic Category Cholinergic Agonist

Use Treatment of acute postoperative and postpartum nonobstructive (functional) urinary retention; treatment of neurogenic atony of the urinary bladder with retention

Unlabeled Use Gastroesophageal reflux

Local Anesthetic/Vasoconstrictor Precautions No information available to require special precautions

Effects on Dental Treatment This is a cholinergic agent similar to pilocarpine; expect to see salivation and sweating in patients.

Effects on Bleeding No information available to require special precautions

Adverse Effects Frequency not defined.
Cardiovascular: Hypotension, tachycardia, flushed skin
Central nervous system: Headache, malaise, seizure
Gastrointestinal: Abdominal cramps, belching, borborygmi, colicky pain, diarrhea, nausea, vomiting, salivation
Genitourinary: Urinary urgency
Ocular: Lacrimation, miosis
Respiratory: Asthmatic attacks, bronchial constriction
Miscellaneous: Diaphoresis

General Dosage Range Oral: *Adults:* 10-100 mg 2-4 times/day

Mechanism of Action Due to stimulation of the parasympathetic nervous system, bethanechol increases bladder muscle tone causing contractions which initiate urination. Bethanechol also stimulates gastric motility, increases gastric tone and may restore peristalsis.

Pharmacodynamics/Kinetics
Onset of Action 30-90 minutes
Duration of Action Up to 6 hours

Pregnancy Risk Factor C

Pregnancy Considerations Reproduction studies have not been conducted.

Bevacizumab (be vuh SIZ uh mab)

Brand Names: U.S. Avastin®
Brand Names: Canada Avastin®

Pharmacologic Category Antineoplastic Agent, Monoclonal Antibody; Vascular Endothelial Growth Factor (VEGF) Inhibitor

Use Treatment of metastatic colorectal cancer (first-or second-line treatment and second-line after progression on a first-line treatment containing bevacizumab); treatment of unresectable, locally advanced, recurrent or metastatic nonsquamous, nonsmall cell lung cancer; treatment of progressive glioblastoma; treatment of metastatic renal cell cancer (not an approved use in Canada)

Note: Not indicated for the adjuvant treatment of colorectal cancer. For the treatment of glioblastoma, effectiveness is based on improvement in objective response rate.

Unlabeled Use Treatment of metastatic breast cancer, recurrent cervical cancer, recurrent advanced ovarian cancer (platinum-sensitive), soft tissue sarcomas (angiosarcoma or hemangiopericytoma/solitary fibrous tumor), age-related macular degeneration (AMD)

Local Anesthetic/Vasoconstrictor Precautions No information available to require special precautions

Effects on Dental Treatment Key adverse event(s) related to dental treatment: Xerostomia (normal salivary flow resumes upon discontinuation), stomatitis, taste disorder, and gingival bleeding.

Cases of osteonecrosis of the jaw (ONJ) have been associated with bevacizumab exposure. ONJ presents clinically as exposed necrotic bone of at least 8 weeks duration with or without the presence of pain, infection, or previous trauma in a patient who has not received radiation to the jaw. Since ONJ is also associated with bisphosphonate exposure and bisphosphonates are known to have antiangiogenic properties, inhibition of angiogenesis may play a role in ONJ associated with these two classes of drugs. Patients developing ONJ while on bevacizumab therapy should receive care by an oral surgeon. See Dental Comment.

Effects on Bleeding Minor gum bleeding has been reported in 2% to 4% of patients. Thrombocytopenia has been reported. A medical consult is suggested.

Adverse Effects Percentages reported as monotherapy and as part of combination chemotherapy regimens. Some studies only reported hematologic toxicities grades ≥4 and nonhematologic toxicities grades ≥3.
>10%:
Cardiovascular: Hypertension (12% to 34%; grades 3/4: 5% to 18%), thromboembolic event (≤21%; grades 3/4: 15%; venous thrombus/embolus: 8%; grades 3/4: 5% to 7%; arterial thrombosis 6%; grades 3/4: 3%), hypotension (7% to 15%)
Central nervous system: Pain (8% to 62%), headache (24% to 37%; grades 3/4: 2% to 4%), dizziness (19% to 26%), fatigue (≤45%; grades 3/4: 4% to 19%), sensory neuropathy (grades 3/4: 1% to 17%; in combination with paclitaxel: 24%)
Dermatologic: Alopecia (6% to 32%), dry skin (7% to 20%), exfoliative dermatitis (3% to 19%), skin discoloration (2% to 16%)
Gastrointestinal: Abdominal pain (8% to 61%; grades 3/4: 8%), vomiting (47% to 52%; grades 3/4: ≤11%), anorexia (35% to 43%), constipation (4% to 40%), diarrhea (grades 3/4: 1% to 34%), stomatitis (30% to 32%), gastrointestinal hemorrhage (19% to 24%), dyspepsia (17% to 24%), taste disorder (14% to 21%), weight loss (15% to 20%), flatulence (11% to 19%), nausea (grades 3/4: ≤12%)
Hematologic: Hemorrhage (≤40%; grades 3/4: 1% to 5%), leukopenia (grades 3/4: 37%), neutropenia (grade 4: 21% to 27%)
Neuromuscular & skeletal: Myalgia (8% to 19%), back pain (≤12%)
Renal: Proteinuria (4% to 36%; grades 3/4: ≤7%; median onset: 5.6 months; median time to resolution: 6.1 months)
Respiratory: Upper respiratory infection (40% to 47%), epistaxis (19% to 35%), dyspnea (25% to 26%), rhinitis
Miscellaneous: Infection (≤55%; serious: 7% to 14%; pneumonia, catheter, or wound infections)
1% to 10%:
Cardiovascular: DVT (6% to 9%; grades 3/4: 9%), HF (grades 3/4: 1% to 4%), syncope (grades 3/4: 3%), intra-abdominal venous thrombosis (grades 3/4: 3%), cardio-/cerebrovascular arterial thrombotic event (2% to 4%), left ventricular dysfunction (grades 3/4: 1%)
Central nervous system: CNS hemorrhage (1% to 5%; grades 3/4: 1%), dysphonia (≤5%)
Dermatologic: Skin ulcer (≤6%), wound dehiscence (1% to 6%), acne (≤1%)
Endocrine & metabolic: Dehydration (grades 3/4: ≤10%), hyponatremia (grades 3/4: 4%)

Gastrointestinal: Xerostomia (4% to 7%), colitis (1% to 6%), ileus (grades 3/4: 4% to 5%), gingival bleeding (2% to 4%), fistula (1%), gastrointestinal perforation (≤4%), gastroesophageal reflux (≤2%), gingivitis (≤2%), mouth ulceration (≤2%), tooth abscess (≤2%), intra-abdominal abscess (1%), gastritis (≤1%), gingival pain (≤1%)

Genitourinary: Vaginal hemorrhage (4%)

Hematologic: Neutropenic fever/infection (5%; grades 3 and/or 4: 4% to 5%), thrombocytopenia (5%)

Neuromuscular & skeletal: Weakness (10%), neuropathy (other than sensory: grades 3/4: 1% to 5%)

Ocular: Blurred vision (≤2%)

Otic: Tinnitus (≤2%), deafness (≤1%)

Respiratory: Voice alteration (5% to 9%), pneumonitis/pulmonary infiltrates (grades 3/4: 5%), hemoptysis (nonsquamous histology 2%), pulmonary embolism (≤1%)

Miscellaneous: Infusion reactions (<3%)

General Dosage Range I.V.: *Adults:* 5 or 10 mg/kg every 2 weeks **or** 15 mg/kg every 3 weeks

Mechanism of Action Bevacizumab is a recombinant, humanized monoclonal antibody which binds to, and neutralizes, vascular endothelial growth factor (VEGF), preventing its association with endothelial receptors, Flt-1 and KDR. VEGF binding initiates angiogenesis (endothelial proliferation and the formation of new blood vessels). The inhibition of microvascular growth is believed to retard the growth of all tissues (including metastatic tissue).

Pharmacodynamics/Kinetics

Half-life Elimination ~20 days (range: 11-50 days)

Pregnancy Risk Factor C

Pregnancy Considerations Teratogenic effects have been observed in animal reproduction studies. Angiogenesis is of critical importance to human fetal development, and bevacizumab inhibits angiogenesis. Adequate contraception during therapy is recommended (and for ≥6 months following last dose of bevacizumab). Patients should also be counseled regarding prolonged exposure following discontinuation of therapy due to the long half-life of bevacizumab.

Based on animal studies, bevacizumab may disrupt normal menstrual cycles and impair fertility by several effects, including reduced endometrial proliferation and follicular developmental arrest. Some parameters do not recover completely, or recover very slowly following discontinuation.

Dental Comment Three case reports describe the development of ONJ in association with bevacizumab therapy. All three cases were cancer patients treated with bevacizumab 10 mg/kg every 2 weeks and 15 mg/kg every 3 weeks (Estilo, 2009; Greuter, 2008). Another report showed that a combination of bisphosphonates and antiangiogenic factors (primarily bevacizumab) induces ONJ more frequently than bisphosphonates alone. Of the 25 patients receiving concurrent treatment with bisphosphonates and the antiangiogenic drug bevacizumab, four developed ONJ (16%). Of the 91 patients receiving bisphosphonates without antiangiogenic factors, one developed ONJ (1.1%), a significant statistical difference (Christodoulou, 2009).

Bexarotene (Systemic) (beks AIR oh teen)

Brand Names: U.S. Targretin®

Pharmacologic Category Antineoplastic Agent, Miscellaneous; Retinoic Acid Derivative

Use Treatment of cutaneous manifestations of cutaneous T-cell lymphoma in patients who are refractory to at least one prior systemic therapy

Local Anesthetic/Vasoconstrictor Precautions No information available to require special precautions

Effects on Dental Treatment Key adverse event(s) related to dental treatment: Xerostomia (normal salivary flow resumes upon discontinuation) and gingivitis.

Effects on Bleeding No information available to require special precautions

Adverse Effects

>10%:

Cardiovascular: Peripheral edema (11% to 13%)

Central nervous system: Headache (30% to 42%), fever (5% to 17%), chills (10% to 13%), insomnia (5% to 11%)

Dermatologic: Rash (17% to 23%), exfoliative dermatitis (10% to 28%), dry skin (9% to 11%), alopecia (4% to 11%)

Endocrine & metabolic: Hyperlipidemia (79%), hypercholesteremia (32% to 62%), hypothyroidism (29% to 53%)

Gastrointestinal: Diarrhea (7% to 42%), anorexia (2% to 23%), nausea (8% to 16%), vomiting (4% to 13%), abdominal pain (4% to 11%)

Hematologic: Leukopenia (17% to 47%), anemia (6% to 25%), hypochromic anemia (4% to 13%)

Hepatic: LDH increased (7% to 13%)

Neuromuscular & skeletal: Weakness (20% to 45%), back pain (2% to 11%)

Miscellaneous: Infection (13% to 23%; bacterial: 1% to 13%), flu-like syndrome (4% to 13%)

<10%:

Cardiovascular: Angina pectoris, cerebrovascular accident, chest pain, heart failure (right), hypertension, syncope, tachycardia

Central nervous system: Agitation, ataxia, confusion, depression, dizziness, hyperesthesia, subdural hematoma

Dermatologic: Acne, cellulitis, cheilitis, maculopapular rash, photosensitivity, pustular rash, serous drainage, skin nodule, skin rash, skin sensitivity, sunburn, vesicular bullous rash

Endocrine & metabolic: Breast pain, hypoproteinemia, hyperglycemia

Gastrointestinal: Amylase increased, colitis, constipation, dyspepsia, flatulence, gastroenteritis, gingivitis, melena, pancreatitis, weight loss/gain, xerostomia

Genitourinary: Dysuria, hematuria, urinary incontinence, urinary tract infection, urinary urgency

Hematologic: Coagulopathy, eosinophilia, hemorrhage, lymphocytosis, thrombocythemia, thrombocytopenia

Hepatic: ALT increased, AST increased, bilirubin increased, hepatic failure

Neuromuscular & skeletal: Arthralgia, arthrosis, bone pain, myalgia, myasthenia, neuropathy

Ocular: Blepharitis, cataracts (new and worsening), conjunctivitis, corneal lesion, dry eyes, keratitis, visual field defects

Otic: Ear pain, otitis externa

Renal: Albuminuria, creatinine increased, renal function abnormal

Respiratory: Bronchitis, cough, dyspnea, hemoptysis, hypoxia, pharyngitis, pleural effusion, pneumonia, pulmonary edema, rhinitis

Miscellaneous: Monilia, sepsis

General Dosage Range Dosage adjustment recommended in patients who develop toxicities.

Oral: *Adults:* 300-400 mg/m^2 once daily

Mechanism of Action Selectively binds to and activates retinoid X receptors (RXRs). Once activated, RXRs function as transcription factors to regulate the expression of genes which control cellular differentiation and proliferation. Bexarotene inhibits the growth *in vitro* of some tumor cell lines of hematopoietic and squamous cell origin and induces tumor regression *in vivo* in some animal models.

Pharmacodynamics/Kinetics

Half-life Elimination ~7 hours

Time to Peak ~2 hours

Pregnancy Risk Factor X

Pregnancy Considerations [U.S. Boxed Warning]: Bexarotene is a retinoid, a drug class associated with birth defects in humans; do not administer during pregnancy. Bexarotene caused birth defects when administered orally to pregnant rats. It must not be given to a pregnant woman or a woman who intends to become pregnant. If a woman becomes pregnant while taking the drug, it must be stopped immediately and appropriate counseling be given. In women of childbearing potential, therapy should be started on the second or third day of a normal menstrual period. Either abstinence or two forms of reliable contraception (one should be nonhormonal) must be used for at least 1 month before initiating therapy, during therapy, and for 1 month following discontinuation of bexarotene. A negative pregnancy test (sensitivity of at least 50 mIU/mL) within 1 week prior to beginning therapy, and monthly thereafter is required for women of childbearing potential. A maximum 1 month supply is recommended so that pregnancy tests may be evaluated. Male patients must use a condom during any sexual contact with women of childbearing age during therapy, and for at least 1 month following discontinuation of bexarotene.

Bexarotene (Topical) (beks AIR oh teen)

Brand Names: U.S. Targretin®

Pharmacologic Category Antineoplastic Agent, Miscellaneous

Use Treatment of cutaneous lesions in patients with refractory cutaneous T-cell lymphoma (stage 1A and 1B) or who have not tolerated other therapies

Local Anesthetic/Vasoconstrictor Precautions No information available to require special precautions

Effects on Dental Treatment No significant effects or complications reported

Effects on Bleeding No information available to require special precautions

Adverse Effects

Cardiovascular: Edema (10%)

Central nervous system: Headache (14%), weakness (6%), pain (30%)

Dermatologic: Rash (14% to 72%), pruritus (6% to 40%), contact dermatitis (14%), exfoliative dermatitis (6%)

Endocrine & metabolic: Hyperlipidemia (10%)

Hematologic: Leukopenia (6%), lymphadenopathy (6%)

Neuromuscular & skeletal: Paresthesia (6%)

Respiratory: Cough (6%), pharyngitis (6%)

Miscellaneous: Diaphoresis (6%), infection (18%)

General Dosage Range Topical: *Adults:* Initial: Apply once every other day for first week; Maintenance: Apply 1-4 times/day

Mechanism of Action The exact mechanism is unknown. Binds and activates retinoid X receptor subtypes. Once activated, these receptors function as transcription factors that regulate the expression of genes which control cellular differentiation and proliferation.

Pregnancy Risk Factor X

Pregnancy Considerations Bexarotene is a retinoid, a drug class associated with birth defects in humans; do not administer during pregnancy. Bexarotene caused birth defects when administered orally to pregnant rats. It must not be given to a pregnant woman or a woman who intends to become pregnant. If a woman becomes pregnant while using the gel, it must be stopped immediately and appropriate counseling be given. In women of childbearing potential, therapy should be started on the second or third day of a normal menstrual period. Either abstinence or two forms of reliable contraception (one should be nonhormonal) must be used for at least 1 month before initiating therapy, during therapy, and for 1 month following discontinuation of bexarotene. A negative pregnancy test (sensitivity of at least 50 mIU/mL) within 1 week prior to beginning therapy, and monthly thereafter is required for women of childbearing potential. Males patients must use a condom during any sexual contact with women of childbearing age during therapy, and for 1 month following discontinuation of bexarotene

Bicalutamide (bye ka LOO ta mide)

Brand Names: U.S. Casodex®

Brand Names: Canada Apo-Bicalutamide®; Ava-Bicalutamide; Casodex®; CO Bicalutamide; Dom-Bicalutamide; JAMP-Bicalutamide; Mylan-Bicalutamide; Novo-Bicalutamide; PHL-Bicalutamide; PMS-Bicalutamide; PRO-Bicalutamide; ratio-Bicalutamide; Sandoz-Bicalutamide

Pharmacologic Category Antineoplastic Agent, Antiandrogen

Use Treatment of metastatic prostate cancer (in combination with an LHRH agonist)

Unlabeled Use Monotherapy for locally-advanced prostate cancer

Local Anesthetic/Vasoconstrictor Precautions No information available to require special precautions

Effects on Dental Treatment Key adverse event(s) related to dental treatment: Xerostomia (normal salivary flow resumes upon discontinuation).

Effects on Bleeding No information available to require special precautions

Adverse Effects Adverse reaction percentages reported as part of combination regimen with an LHRH analogue unless otherwise noted.

>10%:

Cardiovascular: Peripheral edema (13%)

Central nervous system: Pain (35%)

Endocrine & metabolic: Hot flashes (53%), breast pain (6%; monotherapy [150 mg]: 39% to 85%), gynecomastia (9%; monotherapy [150 mg]: 38% to 73%)

Gastrointestinal: Constipation (22%), nausea (15%), diarrhea (12%), abdominal pain (11%)

Genitourinary: Pelvic pain (21%), hematuria (12%), nocturia (12%)

Hematologic: Anemia (11%)

Neuromuscular & skeletal: Back pain (25%), weakness (22%)

Respiratory: Dyspnea (13%)

Miscellaneous: Infection (18%)

≥2% to 10%:

Cardiovascular: Chest pain (8%), hypertension (8%), angina pectoris (2% to <5%), cardiac arrest (2% to <5%), CHF (2% to <5%), edema (2% to <5%), MI (2% to <5%), coronary artery disorder (2% to <5%), syncope (2% to <5%)

Central nervous system: Dizziness (10%), headache (7%), insomnia (7%), anxiety (5%), depression (4%), chills (2% to <5%), confusion (2% to <5%), fever (2% to <5%), nervousness (2% to <5%), somnolence (2% to <5%)

Dermatologic: Rash (9%), alopecia (2% to <5%), dry skin (2% to <5%), pruritus (2% to <5%), skin carcinoma (2% to <5%)

Endocrine & metabolic: Hyperglycemia (6%), dehydration (2% to <5%), gout (2% to <5%), hypercholesterolemia (2% to <5%), libido decreased (2% to <5%)

Gastrointestinal: Dyspepsia (7%), weight loss (7%), anorexia (6%), flatulence (6%), vomiting (6%), weight gain (5%), dysphagia (2% to <5%), gastrointestinal carcinoma (2% to <5%), melena (2% to <5%), periodontal abscess (2% to <5%), rectal hemorrhage (2% to <5%), xerostomia (2% to <5%)

Genitourinary: Urinary tract infection (9%), impotence (7%), polyuria (6%), urinary retention (5%), urinary impairment (5%), urinary incontinence (4%), dysuria (2% to <5%), urinary urgency (2% to <5%)

Hepatic: LFTs increased (7%), alkaline phosphatase increased (5%)

Neuromuscular & skeletal: Bone pain (9%), paresthesia (8%), myasthenia (7%), arthritis (5%), pathological fracture (4%), hypertonia (2% to <5%), leg cramps (2% to <5%), myalgia (2% to <5%), neck pain (2% to <5%), neuropathy (2% to <5%)

Ocular: Cataract (2% to <5%)

Renal: BUN increased (2% to <5%), creatinine increased (2% to <5%), hydronephrosis (2% to <5%)

Respiratory: Cough (8%), pharyngitis (8%), bronchitis (6%), pneumonia (4%), rhinitis (4%), asthma (2% to <5%), epistaxis (2% to <5%), sinusitis (2% to <5%)

Miscellaneous: Flu-like syndrome (7%), diaphoresis (6%), cyst (2% to <5%), hernia (2% to <5%), herpes zoster (2% to <5%), sepsis (2% to <5%)

General Dosage Range Oral: *Adults:* 50 mg once daily

Mechanism of Action Androgen receptor inhibitor; pure nonsteroidal antiandrogen that binds to androgen receptors; specifically a competitive inhibitor for the binding of dihydrotestosterone and testosterone; prevents testosterone stimulation of cell growth in prostate cancer

Pharmacodynamics/Kinetics

Half-life Elimination Active enantiomer: ~6 days, ~10 days in severe liver disease

Time to Peak Active enantiomer: ~31 hours

Pregnancy Risk Factor X

Pregnancy Considerations Animal studies have demonstrated teratogenicity. Bicalutamide use is contraindicated in women. Androgen receptor inhibition during pregnancy may affect fetal development.

Bimatoprost (bi MAT oh prost)

Brand Names: U.S. Latisse®; Lumigan®

Brand Names: Canada Latisse®; Lumigan®; Lumigan® RC

Pharmacologic Category Ophthalmic Agent, Antiglaucoma; Prostaglandin, Ophthalmic

Use Reduction of intraocular pressure (IOP) in patients with open-angle glaucoma or ocular hypertension; hypotrichosis treatment of the eyelashes

Local Anesthetic/Vasoconstrictor Precautions No information available to require special precautions

Effects on Dental Treatment No significant effects or complications reported

Effects on Bleeding No information available to require special precautions

Adverse Effects Adverse reactions and percentages are for Lumigan® unless noted:

>10%: Ocular: Conjunctival hyperemia (25% to 45%; Latisse®: <4%), growth of eyelashes, ocular pruritus (>10%; Latisse®: <4%)

1% to 10%:

Central nervous system: Headache (1% to 5%)

Dermatologic: Skin hyperpigmentation (Latisse®: <4%), abnormal hair growth

Hepatic: Liver function tests abnormal (1% to 5%)

Neuromuscular & skeletal: Weakness (1% to 5%)

Ocular: Dry eyes (1% to 10%; Latisse®: <4%), erythema (eyelid/periorbital region; 1% to 10%; Latisse®: <4%), irritation (1% to 10%; Latisse®: <4%), allergic conjunctivitis, asthenopia, blepharitis, burning, cataract, conjunctival edema, conjunctival hemorrhage, discharge, eyelash darkening, foreign body sensation, iris pigmentation increased (may be delayed), pain, photophobia, pigmentation of periocular skin, superficial punctate keratitis, tearing, visual disturbance

Miscellaneous: Infections (10% [primarily colds and upper respiratory tract infections])

General Dosage Range

Ophthalmic: *Adults:* Instill 1 drop into affected eye(s) once daily

Ophthalmic, topical: *Adults:* Place 1 drop on applicator and apply evenly along the skin of the upper eyelid at base of eyelashes once daily

Mechanism of Action As a synthetic analog of prostaglandin with ocular hypotensive activity, bimatoprost decreases intraocular pressure by increasing the outflow of aqueous humor. Bimatoprost may increase the percent and duration of hairs in the growth phase, resulting in eyelash growth.

Pharmacodynamics/Kinetics

Onset of Action Reduction of IOP: ~4 hours; Peak effect: Maximum reduction of IOP: ~8-12 hours

Half-life Elimination I.V.: ≤45 minutes

Time to Peak ≤10 minutes

Pregnancy Risk Factor C

Pregnancy Considerations Decreased gestation, decreased body weight, increased late resorptions, and increased mortality were observed in animal reproduction studies with oral doses achieving serum levels >33 times human exposure.

Bisacodyl (bis a KOE dil)

Brand Names: U.S. Alophen® [OTC]; Bisac-Evac™ [OTC]; Biscolax™ [OTC]; Correctol® Tablets [OTC]; Dacodyl™ [OTC]; Doxidan® [OTC]; Dulcolax® [OTC]; ex-lax® Ultra [OTC]; Femilax™ [OTC]; Fleet® Bisacodyl [OTC]; Fleet® Stimulant Laxative [OTC]; Veracolate® [OTC]

Brand Names: Canada Apo-Bisacodyl® [OTC]; Bisacodyl-Odan [OTC]; Bisacolax [OTC]; Carter's Little Pills® [OTC]; Codulax [OTC]; Dulcolax® [OTC]; PMS-Bisacodyl [OTC]; ratio-Bisacodyl [OTC]; Silver Bullet

Suppository [OTC]; Soflax [OTC]; The Magic Bullet [OTC]; Woman's Laxative [OTC]

Pharmacologic Category Laxative, Stimulant

Use Treatment of constipation; colonic evacuation prior to procedures or examination

Local Anesthetic/Vasoconstrictor Precautions No information available to require special precautions

Effects on Dental Treatment No significant effects or complications reported

Effects on Bleeding No information available to require special precautions

General Dosage Range
Oral:
Children >6 years: 5-10 mg (0.3 mg/kg) once daily
Adults: 5-15 mg as a single dose (maximum: 30 mg)
Rectal:
Children <2 years: 5 mg as a single dose
Children ≥2 years and Adults: 10 mg as a single dose

Mechanism of Action Stimulates peristalsis by directly irritating the smooth muscle of the intestine, possibly the colonic intramural plexus; alters water and electrolyte secretion producing net intestinal fluid accumulation and laxation

Pharmacodynamics/Kinetics
Onset of Action Oral: 6-10 hours; Rectal: 0.25-1 hour; V_d: BHPM: 289 L (after multiple doses) (Friedrich, 2011)
Half-life Elimination BHPM: ~8 hours (Friedrich, 2011)

Pregnancy Considerations Plasma concentrations of BHPM (the active metabolite of bisacodyl) are low (median: 61 ng/mL; range: 21-194 ng/mL) following doses of 10 mg/day for 7 days (Friedrich, 2011). Although not first choice for the treatment of constipation in pregnant women, short-term use of stimulant laxatives is generally considered safe in pregnancy; long-term use should be avoided (Cullen, 2007; Prather, 2004; Wald, 2003).

Bismuth (BIZ muth)

Related Information
Gastrointestinal Disorders *on page 1512*
Brand Names: U.S. Bismatrol Maximum Strength [OTC]; Bismatrol [OTC]; Diotame [OTC]; Kao-Tin [OTC]; Kaopectate® Extra Strength [OTC]; Kaopectate® [OTC]; Peptic Relief [OTC]; Pepto Relief [OTC]; Pepto-Bismol® Maximum Strength [OTC]; Pepto-Bismol® [OTC]

Pharmacologic Category Antidiarrheal

Use Subsalicylate formulation: Symptomatic treatment of mild, nonspecific diarrhea; control of traveler's diarrhea (enterotoxigenic *Escherichia coli*); as part of a multidrug regimen for *H. pylori* eradication to reduce the risk of duodenal ulcer recurrence

Local Anesthetic/Vasoconstrictor Precautions No information available to require special precautions

Effects on Dental Treatment Key adverse event(s) related to dental treatment: Darkening of tongue.

Effects on Bleeding No information available to require special precautions

Adverse Effects Frequency not defined; subsalicylate formulation:
Central nervous system: Anxiety, confusion, headache, mental depression, slurred speech

Gastrointestinal: Discoloration of the tongue (darkening), grayish black stools, impaction may occur in infants and debilitated patients
Neuromuscular & skeletal: Muscle spasms, weakness
Otic: Hearing loss, tinnitus

General Dosage Range Oral:
Subsalicylate based on 262 mg/5 mL liquid or 262 mg tablet (diarrhea):
Children 3-6 years: 1/3 tablet **or** 5 mL every 30 minutes to 1 hour as needed (maximum: 8 doses/day)
Children 6-9 years: 2/3 tablet **or** 10 mL every 30 minutes to 1 hour as needed (maximum: 8 doses/day)
Children 9-12 years: 1 tablet **or** 15 mL every 30 minutes to 1 hour as needed (maximum: 8 doses/day)
Subsalicylate based on 262 mg/15 mL liquid or 262 mg tablet:
Children >12 years: Diarrhea: 2 tablets **or** 30 mL every 30 minutes to 1 hour as needed (maximum: 8 doses/day)
Adults:
Diarrhea: 2 tablets **or** 30 mL every 30 minutes to 1 hour as needed (maximum: 8 doses/day)
H. pylori eradication: 524 mg 4 times/day

Mechanism of Action Bismuth subsalicylate exhibits both antisecretory and antimicrobial action. This agent may provide some anti-inflammatory action as well. The salicylate moiety provides antisecretory effect and the bismuth exhibits antimicrobial directly against bacterial and viral gastrointestinal pathogens.

Pharmacodynamics/Kinetics
Half-life Elimination Terminal: Bismuth: Highly variable

Pregnancy Considerations Following oral administration, bismuth and salicylates cross the placenta. The use of salicylates in pregnancy may adversely affect the newborn (Lione, 1988). Use during pregnancy is not recommended (Mahadevan, 2007).

Bismuth, Metronidazole, and Tetracycline
(BIZ muth, me troe NI da zole, & tet ra SYE kleen)

Related Information
Bismuth *on page 192*
MetroNIDAZOLE (Systemic) *on page 911*
Tetracycline *on page 1308*
Brand Names: U.S. Helidac®; Pylera™

Pharmacologic Category Antibiotic, Miscellaneous; Antibiotic, Tetracycline Derivative; Antidiarrheal

Use As part of a multidrug regimen for *H. pylori* eradication to reduce the risk of duodenal ulcer recurrence in combination with an H_2 agonist (Helidac®) or omeprazole (Pylera™)

Local Anesthetic/Vasoconstrictor Precautions No information available to require special precautions

Effects on Dental Treatment Tetracyclines are not recommended for use during pregnancy since they can cause enamel hypoplasia and permanent teeth discoloration; long-term use associated with oral candidiasis.

Effects on Bleeding No information available to require special precautions

Adverse Effects Also see individual agents.
Helidac® (includes studies with/without concomitant acid-suppression therapy):
>10%: Gastrointestinal: Nausea (12%)

1% to 10%:
  Central nervous system: Dizziness (2%), headache (2%), insomnia (1%), pain (1%)
  Gastrointestinal: Abdominal pain (7%), diarrhea (7%), melena (3%), anorexia (2%), constipation (2%), dyspepsia (2%), tongue discoloration (2%), vomiting (2%), abnormal stools (1%), anal discomfort (1%), duodenal ulcer (1%), flatulence (1%), GI hemorrhage (1%), taste perversion (1%)
  Neuromuscular & skeletal: Weakness (2%), paresthesia (1%)
  Respiratory: Upper respiratory infection (2%), sinusitis (1%)

Pylera™ (with concomitant omeprazole):
>10%: Gastrointestinal: Abnormal stools (16%)
1% to 10%:
  Cardiovascular: Chest pain (1%), palpitation (1%)
  Central nervous system: Headache (8%), dizziness (3%), pain (2%), anxiety (1%)
  Dermatologic: Maculopapular rash (1%)
  Gastrointestinal: Abdominal pain (9%), diarrhea (9%), dyspepsia (9%), nausea (8%), taste perversion (5%), gastritis (1%), gastroenteritis (1%), vomiting (1%), xerostomia (1%)
  Genitourinary: Vaginitis (4%), urine abnormality (2%)
  Hepatic: ALT increased (2%), AST increased (1%)
  Neuromuscular & skeletal: Weakness (4%), back pain (2%)
  Respiratory: Pharyngitis (2%), rhinitis (1%)
  Miscellaneous: Flu-like syndrome (5%), infection (1% to 2%)

General Dosage Range Oral: *Adults:*
  Helidac®: 2 bismuth subsalicylate 262.4 mg tablets, 1 metronidazole 250 mg tablet, and 1 tetracycline 500 mg capsule 4 times/day at meals and bedtime
  Pylera™: 3 capsules 4 times/day after meals and at bedtime

Mechanism of Action Bismuth, metronidazole, and tetracycline individually have demonstrated *in vitro* activity against most susceptible strains of *H. pylori* isolated from patients with duodenal ulcers. Resistance to metronidazole is increasing in the U.S.; an alternative regimen, not containing metronidazole, if *H. pylori* is not eradicated follow therapy.

Pregnancy Risk Factor D

Pregnancy Considerations See individual agents.

Bisoprolol (bis OH proe lol)

Related Information
  Cardiovascular Diseases *on page 1492*
Brand Names: U.S. Zebeta®
Brand Names: Canada Apo-Bisoprolol®; Ava-Bisoprolol; Mylan-Bisoprolol; Novo-Bisoprolol; PHL-Bisoprolol; PMS-Bisoprolol; PRO-Bisoprolol; Sandoz-Bisoprolol
Pharmacologic Category Beta-Blocker, Beta-1 Selective
Use Treatment of hypertension, alone or in combination with other agents
Unlabeled Use Chronic stable angina, supraventricular arrhythmias, PVCs, heart failure (HF)
Local Anesthetic/Vasoconstrictor Precautions No information available to require special precautions
Effects on Dental Treatment Bisoprolol is a cardioselective beta-blocker. Local anesthetic with vasoconstrictor can be safely used in patients medicated with bisoprolol. Nonselective beta-blockers (ie, propranolol, nadolol) enhance the pressor response to epinephrine, resulting in hypertension and bradycardia; this has not

been reported for bisoprolol. Many nonsteroidal anti-inflammatory drugs, such as ibuprofen and indomethacin, can reduce the hypotensive effect of beta-blockers after 3 or more weeks of therapy with the NSAID. Short-term NSAID use (ie, 3 days) requires no special precautions in patients taking beta-blockers.

Effects on Bleeding No information available to require special precautions

Adverse Effects 1% to 10%:
  Cardiovascular: Chest pain (1% to 2%)
  Central nervous system: Fatigue (dose related; 6% to 8%), insomnia (2% to 3%), hypoesthesia (1% to 2%)
  Gastrointestinal: Diarrhea (dose related; 3% to 4%), nausea (2%), vomiting (1% to 2%)
  Neuromuscular & skeletal: Arthralgia, weakness (dose related; ≤2%)
  Respiratory: Upper respiratory infection (5%), rhinitis (3% to 4%), sinusitis (dose related; 2%), dyspnea (1% to 2%)

General Dosage Range Dosage adjustment recommended in patients with renal impairment
Oral: *Adults and Elderly:* Initial: 2.5-5 mg once daily; Maintenance: 2.5-20 mg once daily

Mechanism of Action Selective inhibitor of beta$_1$-adrenergic receptors; competitively blocks beta$_1$-receptors, with little or no effect on beta$_2$-receptors at doses ≤20 mg

Pharmacodynamics/Kinetics
Onset of Action 1-2 hours
Half-life Elimination Normal renal function: 9-12 hours; Cl$_{cr}$ <40 mL/minute: 27-36 hours; Hepatic cirrhosis: 8-22 hours
Time to Peak 2-4 hours

Pregnancy Risk Factor C

Pregnancy Considerations Adverse events were observed in animal reproduction studies; therefore, the manufacturer classifies bisoprolol as pregnancy category C. In a cohort study, an increased risk of cardiovascular defects was observed following maternal use of beta-blockers during pregnancy. Intrauterine growth restriction (IUGR), small placentas, as well as fetal/neonatal bradycardia, hypoglycemia, and/or respiratory depression have been observed following *in utero* exposure to beta-blockers as a class. Adequate facilities for monitoring infants at birth should be available. Untreated chronic maternal hypertension and pre-eclampsia are also associated with adverse events in the fetus, infant, and mother. Limited information is available related to the use of bisoprolol for the treatment of hypertension in pregnancy; other agents may be more appropriate for use.

Bisoprolol and Hydrochlorothiazide
(bis OH proe lol & hye droe klor oh THYE a zide)

Related Information
  Bisoprolol *on page 193*
  Hydrochlorothiazide *on page 687*
Brand Names: U.S. Ziac®
Brand Names: Canada Ziac®
Pharmacologic Category Beta-Blocker, Beta-1 Selective; Diuretic, Thiazide
Use Treatment of hypertension
Unlabeled Use Treatment of hypertension in the pediatric patient
Local Anesthetic/Vasoconstrictor Precautions No information available to require special precautions

Effects on Dental Treatment Bisoprolol is a cardioselective beta-blocker. Local anesthetic with vasoconstrictor can be safely used in patients medicated with bisoprolol. Nonselective beta-blockers (ie, propranolol, nadolol) enhance the pressor response to epinephrine, resulting in hypertension and bradycardia; this has not been reported for bisoprolol. Many nonsteroidal antiinflammatory drugs, such as ibuprofen and indomethacin, can reduce the hypotensive effect of beta-blockers after 3 or more weeks of therapy with the NSAID. Short-term NSAID use (ie, 3 days) requires no special precautions in patients taking beta-blockers.

Effects on Bleeding No information available to require special precautions

Adverse Effects See individual agents.

General Dosage Range Oral: *Adults:* Initial: Bisoprolol 2.5 mg and hydrochlorothiazide 6.25 mg once daily; Maintenance: Bisoprolol 2.5-20 mg and hydrochlorothiazide 6.25-12.5 mg once daily; Maximum dose (manufacturer recommended): Bisoprolol 20 mg and hydrochlorothiazide 12.5 mg once daily

Mechanism of Action See individual agents.

Pregnancy Risk Factor C

Pregnancy Considerations See individual agents.

Bivalirudin (bye VAL i roo din)

Related Information
Cardiovascular Diseases *on page 1492*

Brand Names: U.S. Angiomax®

Brand Names: Canada Angiomax®

Pharmacologic Category Anticoagulant, Thrombin Inhibitor

Use Anticoagulant used in conjunction with aspirin for patients with unstable angina undergoing percutaneous transluminal coronary angioplasty (PTCA) or percutaneous coronary intervention (PCI) with provisional glycoprotein IIb/IIIa inhibitor; anticoagulant used in conjunction with aspirin for patients undergoing PCI with (or at risk of) heparin-induced thrombocytopenia (HIT) / thrombosis syndrome (HITTS)

Canadian labeling: Additional uses (not in U.S. labeling): In conjunction with aspirin for treatment of patients with ST-elevation myocardial infarction (STEMI) undergoing primary PCI; anticoagulant with or without aspirin in patients undergoing cardiac surgery with (or at risk of) heparin-induced thrombocytopenia (HIT) / thrombosis syndrome (HITTS)

Unlabeled Use Heparin-induced thrombocytopenia (HIT); ST-elevation myocardial infarction (STEMI) undergoing primary PCI

Local Anesthetic/Vasoconstrictor Precautions No information available to require special precautions

Effects on Dental Treatment Key adverse event(s) related to dental treatment: Bleeding is the major adverse effect of bivalirudin. Additional adverse effects are often related to idiosyncratic reactions, the frequency is difficult to estimate. Adverse reactions reported were generally less than those seen with heparin. See Effects on Bleeding.

Effects on Bleeding As with all anticoagulants, bleeding is a potential adverse effect of bivalirudin during dental surgery; risk is dependent on multiple variables, including the intensity of anticoagulation and patient susceptibility. Medical consult is suggested. It is unlikely that ambulatory patients presenting for dental treatment will be taking intravenous anticoagulant therapy such as bivalirudin.

Adverse Effects As with all anticoagulants, bleeding is the major adverse effect of bivalirudin. Hemorrhage may occur at virtually any site. Risk is dependent on multiple variables, including the intensity of anticoagulation, concurrent use of a glycoprotein IIb/IIIa inhibitor, and patient susceptibility. Additional adverse effects are often related to idiosyncratic reactions, and the frequency is difficult to estimate. Adverse reactions reported were generally less than those seen with heparin.

>10%:
Cardiovascular: Hypotension (≤12%)
Central nervous system: Pain (≤15%), headache (≤12%)
Gastrointestinal: Nausea (≤15%)
Hematologic: Minor hemorrhage (REPLACE-2 study: Protocol defined: 14%, compared to 26% with heparin; TIMI defined: 1%, compared to 3% with heparin)
Neuromuscular & skeletal: Back pain (9% to 42%)
1% to 10%:
Cardiovascular: Hypertension (6%), bradycardia (5%), angina (≤5%)
Central nervous system: Insomnia (7%), anxiety (6%), fever (5%), nervousness (5%)
Gastrointestinal: Vomiting (≤6%), dyspepsia (5%), abdominal pain (5%)
Genitourinary: Urinary retention (4%)
Hematologic: Major hemorrhage (Protocol defined: 2% to 4%, compared to 4% to 9% with heparin; REPLACE-2 Study: TIMI defined: 0.6%, compared to 0.9% with heparin), transfusion required (1% to 2%, compared to 2% to 6% with heparin)
Local: Injection site pain (≤8%)
Neuromuscular & skeletal: Pelvic pain (6%)

General Dosage Range
I.V.: *Adults:* Bolus: 0.75 mg/kg; may repeat at 0.3 mg/kg if necessary; Infusion: 1.75 mg/kg/hour for duration of procedure and up to 4 hours postprocedure if needed; after 4 hours may continue 0.2 mg/kg/hour for up to 20 hours if needed
Dosage adjustment recommended in patients with renal impairment

Mechanism of Action Bivalirudin acts as a specific and reversible direct thrombin inhibitor; it binds to the catalytic and anionic exosite of both circulating and clot-bound thrombin. Catalytic binding site occupation functionally inhibits coagulant effects by preventing thrombin-mediated cleavage of fibrinogen to fibrin monomers, and activation of factors V, VIII, and XIII. Shows linear dose- and concentration-dependent prolongation of ACT, aPTT, PT, and TT.

Pharmacodynamics/Kinetics

Onset of Action Immediate

Duration of Action Coagulation times return to baseline ~1 hour following discontinuation of infusion

Half-life Elimination Normal renal function (Cl_{cr} ≥90 mL/minute): 25 minutes; Severe renal impairment (Cl_{cr} 10-29 mL/minute): 57 minutes; Dialysis-dependent patients (off dialysis): 3.5 hours

Pregnancy Risk Factor B

Pregnancy Considerations Adverse events have not been observed in animal reproduction studies. Bivalirudin is used in conjunction with aspirin, which may lead to maternal or fetal adverse effects, especially during the third trimester. Use of parenteral direct thrombin inhibitors in pregnancy should be limited to those women who have severe allergic reactions to heparin, including heparin-induced thrombocytopenia, and who cannot receive danaparoid (Guyatt, 2012).

Bleomycin (blee oh MYE sin)

Brand Names: Canada Blenoxane®; Bleomycin Injection, USP

Pharmacologic Category Antineoplastic Agent, Antibiotic

Use Treatment of squamous cell carcinomas of the head and neck, penis, cervix, or vulva, testicular carcinoma, Hodgkin's lymphoma, and non-Hodgkin's lymphoma; sclerosing agent for malignant pleural effusion

Unlabeled Use Treatment of ovarian germ cell tumors

Local Anesthetic/Vasoconstrictor Precautions No information available to require special precautions

Effects on Dental Treatment Key adverse event(s) related to dental treatment: Stomatitis and mucositis.

Effects on Bleeding No information available to require special precautions

Adverse Effects

>10%:
  Dermatologic: Pain at the tumor site, phlebitis. About 50% of patients develop erythema, rash, striae, induration, hyperkeratosis, vesiculation, and peeling of the skin, particularly on the palmar and plantar surfaces of the hands and feet. Hyperpigmentation (50%), alopecia, nailbed changes may also occur. These effects appear dose related and reversible with discontinuation.

  Gastrointestinal: Stomatitis and mucositis (30%), anorexia, weight loss

  Respiratory: Tachypnea, rales, acute or chronic interstitial pneumonitis, and pulmonary fibrosis (5% to 10%); hypoxia and death (1%). Symptoms include cough, dyspnea, and bilateral pulmonary infiltrates. The pathogenesis is not certain, but may be due to damage of pulmonary, vascular, or connective tissue. Response to steroid therapy is variable and somewhat controversial.

  Miscellaneous: Acute febrile reactions (25% to 50%)

1% to 10%:
  Dermatologic: Skin thickening, diffuse scleroderma, onycholysis, pruritus

  Miscellaneous: Anaphylactoid-like reactions (characterized by hypotension, confusion, fever, chills, and wheezing; onset may be immediate or delayed for several hours); idiosyncratic reactions (1% in lymphoma patients)

General Dosage Range Dosage adjustment recommended in patients with renal impairment or who develop toxicities.

  I.V.: *Adults:* Dosage varies greatly depending on indication

  Intrapleural: *Adults:* 60 units as a single instillation

Mechanism of Action Inhibits synthesis of DNA; binds to DNA leading to single- and double-strand breaks; also inhibits (to a lesser degree) RNA and protein synthesis

Pharmacodynamics/Kinetics

  Half-life Elimination Biphasic: Renal function dependent:
    Normal renal function: Initial: 1.3 hours; Terminal: 9 hours
    End-stage renal disease: Initial: 2 hours; Terminal: 30 hours

  Time to Peak Serum: I.M.: Within 30 minutes

  Pregnancy Risk Factor D

Pregnancy Considerations Animal studies have demonstrated teratogenic and abortifacient effects. There are no adequate and well-controlled studies in pregnant women. Women of childbearing potential should avoid becoming pregnant during treatment.

Boceprevir (boe SE pre vir)

Related Information
Systemic Viral Diseases *on page 1537*

Brand Names: U.S. Victrelis®

Brand Names: Canada Victrelis®

Generic Availability (U.S.) No

Pharmacologic Category Antiviral Agent; Protease Inhibitor

Use Treatment of chronic hepatitis C (CHC) genotype 1 (in combination with peginterferon alfa and ribavirin) in patients with compensated liver disease (including cirrhosis) who were previously untreated or have failed prior therapy with peginterferon alfa and ribavirin therapy including prior null responders, partial responders, and relapsers

Local Anesthetic/Vasoconstrictor Precautions No information available to require special precautions

Effects on Dental Treatment Key adverse event(s) related to dental treatment: Xerostomia (normal salivary flow resumes upon discontinuation) and abnormal taste.

Effects on Bleeding No information available to require special precautions

Adverse Effects

>10%:
  Central nervous system: Fatigue (55% to 58%), chills (33% to 34%), insomnia (30% to 34%), irritability (21% to 22%), dizziness (16% to 19%), headache

  Dermatologic: Alopecia (22% to 27%), dry skin (18% to 22%), rash (16% to 17%)

  Gastrointestinal: Nausea (43% to 46%), abnormal taste (35% to 44%), appetite decreased (25% to 26%), diarrhea (24% to 25%), vomiting (15% to 20%), xerostomia (11% to 15%)

  Hematologic: Anemia (45% to 50%), neutropenia (14% to 31%)

  Neuromuscular & skeletal: Arthralgia (19% to 23%), weakness (15% to 21%)

  Respiratory: Dyspnea (8% to 11%)

1% to 10%: Hematologic: Thrombocytopenia

Dosage Oral: Adults: 800 mg 3 times daily (in combination with peginterferon alfa and ribavirin). *Missed doses:* If a dose is missed, skip dose if it is <2 hours before the next dose; if ≥2 hours before next dose is due, take dose with food and resume normal dosing schedule.

Treatment-naive patients without cirrhosis (interferon-responsive [≥1-log$_{10}$ HCV-RNA decline in viral load] at week 4):

  Weeks 1-4: Peginterferon alfa with concomitant ribavirin only

  Weeks 5-8: Boceprevir 800 mg 3 times daily with continued peginterferon alfa and ribavirin

  Weeks 9-24 (based on HCV-RNA results at week 8):
    HCV-RNA **undetectable** or **detectable** at a level of <100 units/mL: Boceprevir 800 mg 3 times daily with continued peginterferon alfa and ribavirin
    HCV-RNA ≥100 units/mL: Boceprevir 800 mg 3 times daily with continued peginterferon alfa and ribavirin. Recheck HCV-RNA at week 12. If HCV-RNA ≥100 units/mL at week 12 (treatment futility), discontinue treatment (boceprevir, peginterferon alfa, and ribavirin).

Weeks ≥24:
HCV-RNA **undetectable** at week 8 and week 24: Boceprevir 800 mg 3 times daily with continued peginterferon alfa and ribavirin for 4 additional weeks (through week 28)
HCV-RNA **detectable** at Week 8 and **undetectable** at week 24:
U.S. labeling: Boceprevir 800 mg 3 times daily with continued peginterferon alfa and ribavirin for 12 additional weeks (through week 36), followed by peginterferon alfa and ribavirin for additional 12 weeks (through week 48)
Canadian labeling: Boceprevir 800 mg 3 times daily with continued peginterferon alfa and ribavirin for 4 additional weeks (through week 28), followed by peginterferon alfa and ribavirin for additional 20 weeks (through week 48)
HCV-RNA **detectable** at week 24: Discontinue treatment (boceprevir, peginterferon alfa, and ribavirin)
Treatment-naive patients (interferon nonresponsive [<0.5-log$_{10}$ HCV-RNA decline in viral load] at week 4): **Note:** Manufacturer also recommends consideration of treatment of poor responders [<1-log$_{10}$ HCV-RNA decline in viral load at week 4] in order to maximize rate of sustained virologic response (SVR):
Weeks 1-4: Peginterferon alfa with concomitant ribavirin only
Weeks 5-48: Boceprevir 800 mg 3 times daily with continued peginterferon alfa and ribavirin
Previously-treated patients without cirrhosis (partial response or relapser): **Note:** Previously treated does not include prior treatment with boceprevir. "Partial response" includes patients with a ≥2-log$_{10}$ HCV-RNA decrease by week 12, but a nonsustained virologic response thereafter. "Relapser" includes patients with an undetectable HCV-RNA upon completion of previous treatment, but with detectable HCV-RNA during the follow-up period.
Weeks 1-4: Peginterferon alfa with concomitant ribavirin only
Weeks 5-8: Boceprevir 800 mg 3 times daily with continued peginterferon alfa and ribavirin
Weeks 9-24 (based on HCV-RNA results at week 8):
HCV-RNA **undetectable** or <100 units/mL: Boceprevir 800 mg 3 times daily with continued peginterferon alfa and ribavirin
HCV-RNA ≥100 units/mL: Boceprevir 800 mg 3 times daily with continued peginterferon alfa and ribavirin. Recheck HCV-RNA at week 12. If HCV-RNA ≥100 units/mL at week 12, discontinue treatment (boceprevir, peginterferon alfa, and ribavirin)
Weeks ≥24:
HCV-RNA **undetectable** at week 8 and week 24: Boceprevir 800 mg 3 times daily with continued peginterferon alfa and ribavirin for 12 additional weeks (through week 36)
HCV-RNA **detectable** at Week 8 and **undetectable** at week 24: Boceprevir 800 mg 3 times daily with continued peginterferon alfa and ribavirin for 12 additional weeks (through week 36), followed by peginterferon alfa and ribavirin for additional 12 weeks (through week 48)
HCV-RNA **detectable** at week 24: Discontinue treatment (boceprevir, peginterferon alfa, and ribavirin)
Previously treated patients with <2-log$_{10}$ HCV-RNA decline by week 12 (prior null responders):
Weeks 1-4: Peginterferon alfa with concomitant ribavirin only
Weeks 5-8: Boceprevir 800 mg 3 times daily with continued peginterferon alfa and ribavirin

Weeks 9-24 (based on HCV-RNA results at week 8):
HCV-RNA **undetectable** or <100 units/mL: Boceprevir 800 mg 3 times daily with continued peginterferon alfa and ribavirin
HCV-RNA **detectable**: Boceprevir 800 mg 3 times daily with continued peginterferon alfa and ribavirin. Recheck HCV-RNA at week 12. If HCV-RNA ≥100 units/mL at week 12, discontinue treatment (boceprevir, peginterferon alfa, and ribavirin).
Weeks ≥24:
HCV-RNA **undetectable** at week 24: Boceprevir 800 mg 3 times daily with continued peginterferon alfa and ribavirin for 24 additional weeks (through week 48)
HCV-RNA **detectable** at week 24: Discontinue treatment (boceprevir, peginterferon alfa, and ribavirin)
Cirrhosis, compensated:
Weeks 1-4: Peginterferon alfa with concomitant ribavirin only
Weeks 5-48: Boceprevir 800 mg 3 times daily with continued peginterferon alfa and ribavirin

Dosage adjustment in renal impairment:
Mild-to-severe impairment: No dosage adjustment necessary.
ESRD requiring hemodialysis: No dosage adjustment necessary. Not removed by hemodialysis.

Dosage adjustment in hepatic impairment:
Mild, moderate, or severe impairment: No dosage adjustment necessary.
Decompensated cirrhosis: No dosage adjustment provided in manufacturer's labeling (has not been studied); not approved for use in decompensated cirrhosis (safety/efficacy not established). Also refer to Peginterferon Alfa and Ribavirin individual monographs.

Mechanism of Action Binds reversibly to nonstructural protein 3 (NS 3) serine protease and inhibits replication of the hepatitis C virus. Considered a direct-acting antiviral treatment for HCV, also called a specifically targeted antiviral therapy for HCV (STAT-C).

Contraindications Hypersensitivity to boceprevir or any component of the formulation; pregnancy; male partners of pregnant women

Coadministration with CYP3A4/5 highly-dependent substrates (alfuzosin, cisapride, drospirenone, ergot derivatives, lovastatin, midazolam [oral], pimozide, sildenafil/tadalafil [when used for treatment of pulmonary arterial hypertension], simvastatin, triazolam) or strong CYP3A4/5 inducers (carbamazepine, phenobarbital, phenytoin, rifampin, St John's wort)

Refer to Peginterferon Alfa and Ribavirin monographs for individual product contraindications.

Canadian labeling: Additional contraindications (not in U.S. labeling): Autoimmune hepatitis, hepatic decompensation (Child-Pugh class B or C); coadministration with amiodarone, astemizole, propafenone, quinidine, terfenadine

Warnings/Precautions Avoid pregnancy in female patients and female partners of male patients, during therapy, and for at least 6 months after treatment; two forms of contraception should be used. Hypersensitivity reactions, angioedema and urticaria have been reported with boceprevir, peginterferon alfa, and ribavirin combination therapy. Discontinuation of combination therapy and institution of supportive measures may be necessary. Safety and efficacy have not been established in patients who have uncompensated cirrhosis, received organ transplants, or been coinfected with hepatitis B or HIV. Monotherapy is not effective for chronic hepatitis C infection. Safety and efficacy have not been established in patients documented to have less than a 2-log$_{10}$ HCV-RNA decline by treatment week 12 with prior peginterferon alfa and ribavirin therapy. Patients who have less than 0.5-log$_{10}$ HCV-RNA decline at treatment week 4 with peginterferon alfa and ribavirin when **initiating** boceprevir therapy are predicted to have less than a 2-log$_{10}$ HCV-RNA decline by treatment week 12. Those poor responders treated with boceprevir will likely not have a sustained virologic response (SVR) and have a predisposition to viral resistance at treatment failure.

Anemia has been reported with peginterferon alfa and ribavirin; addition of boceprevir is associated with further hemoglobin decreases. With anemia management, average hemoglobin decrease in clinical trials was ~1 g/dL. Dose reduction of ribavirin therapy is recommended for the initial management of anemia if hemoglobin <10 g/dL; permanent discontinuation of ribavirin treatment is recommended if hemoglobin <8.5 g/dL. The addition of boceprevir to peginterferon alfa and ribavirin therapy is also associated with a higher incidence of neutropenia. Dose modifications of peginterferon alfa and ribavirin were needed more often in patients also taking boceprevir. Complete blood counts should be obtained pretreatment and at weeks 2, 4, 8, and 12, as well as other times during treatment. May be severe or life-threatening (rare); discontinuation of therapy may be necessary. If ribavirin is permanently discontinued, boceprevir and peginterferon alfa must also be discontinued.

Drug Interactions
Metabolism/Transport Effects Substrate of BCRP, CYP3A4 (major), P-glycoprotein; **Note:** Assignment of Major/Minor substrate status based on clinically relevant drug interaction potential; **Inhibits** CYP3A4 (strong), P-glycoprotein

Avoid Concomitant Use
Avoid concomitant use of Boceprevir with any of the following: Ado-Trastuzumab Emtansine; Alfuzosin; Apixaban; Astemizole; Avanafil; Axitinib; Bosutinib; Cabozantinib; CarBAMazepine; Cisapride; Conivaptan; Crizotinib; Dihydroergotamine; Dronedarone; Drospirenone; Efavirenz; Eplerenone; Ergoloid Mesylates; Ergonovine; Ergotamine; Everolimus; Fluticasone (Oral Inhalation); Fosphenytoin; Halofantrine; Ivabradine; Lapatinib; Lomitapide; Lovastatin; Lurasidone; Methylergonovine; Midazolam; Nilotinib; Nisoldipine; PHENobarbital; Phenytoin; Pimozide; Pomalidomide; Primidone; Ranolazine; Red Yeast Rice; Regorafenib; Rifabutin; Rifampin; Rivaroxaban; RomiDEPsin; Salmeterol; Sildenafil; Silodosin; Simvastatin; St Johns Wort; Tamsulosin; Terfenadine; Ticagrelor; Tolvaptan; Toremifene; Triazolam; VinCRIStine (Liposomal)

Increased Effect/Toxicity
Boceprevir may increase the levels/effects of: Ado-Trastuzumab Emtansine; Alfuzosin; Almotriptan; Alosetron; ALPRAZolam; Amiodarone; Apixaban; ARIPiprazole; Astemizole; AtorvaSTATin; Avanafil; Axitinib; Bedaquiline; Bepridil [Off Market]; Bortezomib; Bosentan; Bosutinib; Brentuximab Vedotin; Brinzolamide; Budesonide (Nasal); Budesonide (Systemic, Oral Inhalation); Buprenorphine; Cabozantinib; Cisapride; Clarithromycin; Colchicine; Conivaptan; Contraceptives (Progestins); Corticosteroids (Orally Inhaled); Crizotinib; CycloSPORINE (Systemic); CYP3A4 Substrates; Desipramine; Dienogest; Digoxin; Dihydroergotamine; Dronedarone; Drospirenone; Dutasteride; Efavirenz; Enzalutamide; Eplerenone; Ergoloid

Mesylates; Ergonovine; Ergotamine; Everolimus; FentaNYL; Fesoterodine; Flecainide; Fluticasone (Nasal); Fluticasone (Oral Inhalation); Fluvastatin; GuanFACINE; Halofantrine; Iloperidone; Itraconazole; Ivabradine; Ivacaftor; Ixabepilone; Ketoconazole (Systemic); Lapatinib; Lomitapide; Lovastatin; Lumefantrine; Lurasidone; Maraviroc; Methadone; Methylergonovine; MethylPREDNISolone; Midazolam; Mifepristone; Nilotinib; Nisoldipine; Ospemifene; Paricalcitol; Pazopanib; Pimecrolimus; Pimozide; Pitavastatin; Pomalidomide; Ponatinib; Posaconazole; Pravastatin; Propafenone; QuiNIDine; Ranolazine; Red Yeast Rice; Regorafenib; Rifabutin; Rivaroxaban; RomiDEPsin; Rosuvastatin; Ruxolitinib; Salmeterol; Saxagliptin; Sildenafil; Silodosin; Simvastatin; Sirolimus; SORAfenib; Tacrolimus (Systemic); Tadalafil; Tamsulosin; Terfenadine; Ticagrelor; Tofacitinib; Tolterodine; Tolvaptan; Toremifene; TraZODone; Triazolam; Vardenafil; Vemurafenib; Vilazodone; VinCRIStine (Liposomal); Voriconazole; Warfarin; Zuclopenthixol

The levels/effects of Boceprevir may be increased by: Clarithromycin; CycloSPORINE (Systemic); Itraconazole; Ketoconazole (Systemic); Posaconazole; Voriconazole

Decreased Effect
Boceprevir may decrease the levels/effects of: Buprenorphine; Contraceptives (Estrogens); Escitalopram; Ifosfamide; Methadone; Prasugrel; Protease Inhibitors; Ritonavir; Ticagrelor; Warfarin

The levels/effects of Boceprevir may be decreased by: Bosentan; CarBAMazepine; CYP3A4 Inducers (Strong); Deferasirox; Efavirenz; Fosphenytoin; PHENobarbital; Phenytoin; Primidone; Protease Inhibitors; Rifabutin; Rifampin; Ritonavir; St Johns Wort; Tocilizumab

Dietary Considerations Take with food. The type or timing of a meal is not important as long as dose is taken with food.

Pharmacodynamics/Kinetics
Half-life Elimination Plasma: Adults: ~3 hours
Time to Peak Serum: 2 hours
Pregnancy Risk Factor B / X (in combination with ribavirin)
Pregnancy Considerations Adverse events were not observed with boceprevir in animal reproduction studies; however, boceprevir must not be used as monotherapy (must be used in combination with peginterferon alfa and ribavirin). Adverse events have been observed with ribavirin in animal reproduction studies. Use of ribavirin is contraindicated in pregnant women and males whose female partners are pregnant. A negative pregnancy test is required before initiation of therapy and pregnancy testing should be conducted monthly during treatment and for 6 months after therapy has ended. Women of childbearing potential and males must use at least 2 effective forms of contraception during treatment and continue contraceptive measures for at least 6 months after completion of therapy. One of the two forms of effective contraception may be a combined oral contraceptive product with at least 1 mg of norethindrone; oral contraceptives with <1 mg of norethindrone and other forms of hormonal contraception are contraindicated because they have not been studied. If patient or female partner becomes pregnant during treatment, she should be counseled about potential risks of exposure. If pregnancy occurs during use or within 6 months after treatment, report to the ribavirin pregnancy registry (800-593-2214).

Lactation Excretion in breast milk unknown/not recommended

Breast-Feeding Considerations It is not known if boceprevir is excreted into breast milk. According to the manufacturer, due to the potential for serious adverse reactions in the nursing infant, a decision should be made whether to discontinue nursing or to discontinue the drug, taking into account the importance of treatment to the mother.

Breast-feeding is not linked to the spread of hepatitis C virus; however, if nipples are cracked or bleeding, breast-feeding is not recommended (CDC, 2010).

Dosage Forms
Capsule, oral:
Victrelis®: 200 mg

Bortezomib (bore TEZ oh mib)

Brand Names: U.S. Velcade®
Brand Names: Canada Velcade®
Pharmacologic Category Antineoplastic Agent; Proteasome Inhibitor

Use Treatment of multiple myeloma; treatment of relapsed or refractory mantle cell lymphoma

Unlabeled Use Treatment of relapsed/refractory cutaneous T-Cell lymphomas (mycosis fungoides), relapsed/refractory follicular lymphoma, relapsed/refractory peripheral T-cell lymphoma, systemic light-chain amyloidosis, relapsed/refractory Waldenström's macroglobulinemia

Local Anesthetic/Vasoconstrictor Precautions No information available to require special precautions

Effects on Dental Treatment Key adverse event(s) related to dental treatment: Abnormal taste and stomatitis.

Effects on Bleeding Dose-related thrombocytopenia (~35%; nadir: day 11; recovery: by day 21) is most common hematological event with platelet counts usually returning to baseline following active therapy each cycle. A medical consult is suggested.

Adverse Effects Adverse reactions and incidences reported are associated with monotherapy.
>10%:
Central nervous system: Fatigue (7% to 52%), fever (8% to 35%), headache (10% to 19%), dizziness (10% to 18%; excludes vertigo)
Dermatologic: Rash (12% to 23%)
Gastrointestinal: Diarrhea (19% to 52%), nausea (16% to 52%), constipation (25% to 30%), vomiting (9% to 29%), anorexia (14% to 21%), abdominal pain (11%), appetite decreased (11%)
Hematologic: Thrombocytopenia (30% to 34%; grade 3: 5% to 24%; grade 4: 3% to 7%; nadir: Day 11; recovery: By day 21), neutropenia (10% to 27%; grade 3: 8% to 14%; grade 4: 2% to 4%; nadir: Day 11; recovery: By day 21), anemia (19% to 23%; grade 3: 4% to 6%; grade 4: <1%), leukopenia (18% to 20%; grade 3: 5%; grade 4: 1%)
Neuromuscular & skeletal: Peripheral neuropathy (SubQ 37%; I.V. 35% to 54%; grade ≥2: 24% to 39%; grade 3: SubQ 5%; I.V. 7% to 14%; grade 4: 1%), neuralgia (23%), paresthesia (7% to 19%), weakness (7% to 16%)
Respiratory: Dyspnea (11%)
1% to 10%:
Cardiovascular: Cardiac disorder (treatment emergent; 8%), hypotension (8%; grades 3/4: 2%), heart failure (≤1%; includes acute pulmonary edema, cardiac failure, congestive cardiac failure, cardiogenic shock)

Endocrine & metabolic: Dehydration (2%)
Hematologic: Bleeding (≥grade 3: 2%)
Local: Injection site irritation (SubQ 6%; I.V. 5%)
Respiratory: Pneumonia (1%)
Miscellaneous: Herpes zoster (1% to 2%)

General Dosage Range Dosage adjustment recommended in patients with hepatic impairment or who develop toxicities.
I.V., SubQ: *Adults:* Dosage varies greatly depending on indication

Mechanism of Action Bortezomib inhibits proteasomes, enzyme complexes which regulate protein homeostasis within the cell. Specifically, it reversibly inhibits chymotrypsin-like activity at the 26S proteasome, leading to activation of signaling cascades, cell-cycle arrest, and apoptosis.

Pharmacodynamics/Kinetics
Half-life Elimination Single dose: I.V.: 9-15 hours; multiple dosing: 1 mg/m^2: 40-193 hours; 1.3 mg/m^2: 76-108 hour

Pregnancy Risk Factor D

Pregnancy Considerations Adverse effects (fetal loss and decreased fetal weight) were observed in animal reproduction studies at doses less than the equivalent human dose (based on BSA). Women of reproductive potential should avoid becoming pregnant and should use effective contraception during treatment.

Bosentan (boe SEN tan)

Brand Names: U.S. Tracleer®
Brand Names: Canada CO Bosentan; Mylan-Bosentan; PMS-Bosentan; Sandoz-Bosentan; Tracleer®
Pharmacologic Category Endothelin Antagonist; Vasodilator

Use Treatment of pulmonary artery hypertension (PAH) (WHO Group I) in patients with NYHA Class II, III, or IV symptoms to improve exercise capacity and decrease the rate of clinical deterioration

Local Anesthetic/Vasoconstrictor Precautions No information available to require special precautions

Effects on Dental Treatment Key adverse event(s) related to dental treatment: Endothelin antagonists have caused bleeding gums; there have been no specific reports for bosentan

Effects on Bleeding No information available to require special precautions

Adverse Effects
>10%:
Cardiovascular: Edema (11%)
Central nervous system: Headache (15%)
Endocrine & metabolic: Spermatogenesis inhibition (25%)
Hematologic: Hemoglobin decreased (≥1 g/dL in up to 57%; <11 g/dL: 3% to 6%; typically in first 6 weeks of therapy)
Hepatic: Transaminases increased (≥3 times ULN; up to 12%; dose-related)
Respiratory: Respiratory tract infection (22%)
1% to 10%:
Cardiovascular: Chest pain (5%), syncope (5%), flushing (4%), hypotension (4%), palpitation (4%)
Dermatologic: Pruritus (2%)
Hematologic: Anemia (3%)
Hepatic: Abnormal hepatic function (4%)
Neuromuscular & skeletal: Arthralgia (4%)
Respiratory: Sinusitis (4%)

General Dosage Range Dosage adjustment recommended in patients with hepatic impairment or on concomitant therapy

Oral:
  Children >12 years and Adults <40 kg: Initial: 62.5 mg twice daily; Maintenance: 62.5 mg twice daily
  Children >12 years and Adults ≥40 kg: Initial: 62.5 mg twice daily; Maintenance: 125 mg twice daily

Mechanism of Action Blocks endothelin receptors on vascular endothelium and smooth muscle. Stimulation of these receptors is associated with vasoconstriction. Although bosentan blocks both ET_A and ET_B receptors, the affinity is higher for the A subtype.

Pharmacodynamics/Kinetics
  Half-life Elimination 5 hours; prolonged with heart failure, possibly with PAH
  Time to Peak Plasma: 3-5 hours

Pregnancy Risk Factor X

Pregnancy Considerations [U.S. Boxed Warning]: May cause birth defects; use in pregnancy is contraindicated. Exclude pregnancy prior to initiation of therapy and obtain pregnancy tests monthly during treatment. Reliable contraception must be used during therapy and for 1 month after stopping treatment. Hormonal contraceptives (oral, injectable, transdermal, or implantable) may not be effective and a second method of contraception (nonhormonal) is required. Patients with tubal ligation or an implanted IUD (Copper T 380A or LNg 20) do not need additional contraceptive measures. When a hormonal or barrier contraceptive is used, one additional method of contraception is still needed if a male partner has had a vasectomy. When initiating treatment for women of reproductive potential, a negative pregnancy test should be documented within the first 5 days of a normal menstrual period and ≥11 days after the last unprotected intercourse. A missed menses or suspected pregnancy should be reported to a healthcare provider and prompt immediate pregnancy testing. Sperm counts may be reduced in men during treatment. Women of childbearing potential should avoid splitting, crushing, or handling broken tablets and exposure to the generated dust (tablet splitting is currently outside of product labeling).

Prescribing and Access Restrictions As a requirement of the REMS program, access to this medication is restricted. Bosentan (Tracleer®) is only available through Tracleer® Access Program (T.A.P.). Only prescribers and pharmacies registered with T.A.P. may prescribe and dispense bosentan. Further information may be obtained from the manufacturer, Actelion Pharmaceuticals (1-866-228-3546 or http://www.tracleer.com/hcp/prescribing-tracleer.asp).

Brentuximab Vedotin (bren TUX i mab ve DOE tin)

Brand Names: U.S. Adcetris™
Brand Names: Canada Adcetris™
Pharmacologic Category Antineoplastic Agent, Monoclonal Antibody
Use Treatment of Hodgkin lymphoma after failure of at least 2 prior chemotherapy regimens (in patients ineligible for transplant) or after stem cell transplant failure; treatment of systemic anaplastic large cell lymphoma (sALCL) after failure of at least 1 prior chemotherapy regimen

Local Anesthetic/Vasoconstrictor Precautions No information available to require special precautions

Effects on Dental Treatment No significant effects or complications reported

Effects on Bleeding Thrombocytopenia occurred in 16% to 28% of patients. A medical consult is suggested.

Adverse Effects
  >10%:
    Cardiovascular: Peripheral edema (4% to 16%)
    Central nervous system: Fatigue (41% to 49%), fever (29% to 38%), pain (7% to 28%), headache (16% to 19%), insomnia (14% to 16%), dizziness (11% to 16%), chills (12% to 13%), anxiety (7% to 11%)
    Dermatologic: Rash (27% to 31%), pruritus (17% to 19%), alopecia (13% to 14%)
    Gastrointestinal: Nausea (38% to 42%), diarrhea (29% to 36%), abdominal pain (9% to 25%), vomiting (17% to 22%), constipation (16% to 19%), appetite decreased (11% to 16%), weight loss (6% to 12%)
    Hematologic: Neutropenia (54% to 55%; grade 4: 6% to 9%); anemia (33% to 52%; grade 4: ≤2%), thrombocytopenia (16% to 28%; grade 4: 2% to 5%)
    Neuromuscular & skeletal: Peripheral sensory neuropathy (52% to 53%; grade 3: 8% to 10%), arthralgia (9% to 19%), myalgia (16% to 17%), peripheral motor neuropathy (7% to 16%; grade 3: 3% to 4%), back pain (10% to 14%)
    Respiratory: Upper respiratory tract infection (12% to 47%), cough (17% to 25%), dyspnea (13% to 19%), oropharyngeal pain (9% to 11%)
    Miscellaneous: Infusion reactions (grades 1/2: 12%), night sweats (9% to 12%), lymphadenopathy (10% to 11%)
  1% to 10%:
    Cardiovascular: Supraventricular arrhythmia
    Dermatologic: Dry skin
    Genitourinary: Urinary tract infection
    Neuromuscular & skeletal: Limb pain, muscle spasms
    Renal: Pyelonephritis
    Respiratory: Pneumonitis, pneumothorax, pulmonary embolism
    Miscellaneous: Antibrentuximab antibody formation, septic shock

General Dosage Range Dosage adjustment recommended in patients who develop toxicities.
  I.V.: *Adults:* 1.8 mg/kg every 3 weeks (maximum dose: 180 mg)

Mechanism of Action Brentuximab vedotin is an antibody drug conjugate (ADC) directed at CD30 consisting of 3 components: 1) a CD30-specific chimeric IgG1 antibody cAC10; 2) a microtubule-disrupting agent, monomethylauristatin E (MMAE); and 3) a protease cleavable dipeptide linker (which covalently conjugates MMAE to cAC10). The conjugate binds to cells which express CD30, and forms a complex which is internalized within the cell and releases MMAE. MMAE binds to the tubules and disrupts the cellular microtubule network, inducing cell cycle arrest (G2/M phase) and apoptosis.

Pharmacodynamics/Kinetics
  Half-life Elimination Terminal: ADC: ~4-6 days
  Time to Peak ADC: At end of infusion; MMAE: ~1-3 days

Pregnancy Risk Factor D

Pregnancy Considerations Embryo-fetal toxicities and fetal malformations were noted in animal reproduction studies. Based on the mechanism of action, may cause fetal harm if administered to a pregnant woman.

Brimonidine (bri MOE ni deen)

Brand Names: U.S. Alphagan® P
Brand Names: Canada Alphagan®; Apo-Brimonidine P®; Apo-Brimonidine®; PMS-Brimonidine Tartrate; ratio-Brimonidine; Sandoz-Brimonidine
Pharmacologic Category Alpha$_2$ Agonist, Ophthalmic; Ophthalmic Agent, Antiglaucoma
Use Lowering of intraocular pressure (IOP) in patients with open-angle glaucoma or ocular hypertension
Local Anesthetic/Vasoconstrictor Precautions No information available to require special precautions
Effects on Dental Treatment Key adverse event(s) related to dental treatment: Xerostomia (normal salivary flow resumes upon discontinuation).
Effects on Bleeding No information available to require special precautions
Adverse Effects Actual frequency of adverse reactions may be formulation dependent; percentages reported with Alphagan® P:

>10%:
  Central nervous system: Somnolence (adults 1% to 4%; children 25% to 83%)
  Ocular: Allergic conjunctivitis, conjunctival hyperemia, eye pruritus
1% to 10% (unless otherwise noted 1% to 4%):
  Cardiovascular: Hypertension (5% to 9%), hypotension
  Central nervous system: Alertness decreased (children), dizziness, fatigue, headache, insomnia
  Dermatologic: Rash
  Endocrine & metabolic: Hypercholesterolemia
  Gastrointestinal: Xerostomia (5% to 9%), dyspepsia
  Neuromuscular & skeletal: Weakness
  Ocular: Burning sensation (5% to 9%), conjunctival folliculosis (5% to 9%), ocular allergic reaction (5% to 9%), visual disturbance (5% to 9%), blepharitis, blepharoconjunctivitis, blurred vision, cataract, conjunctival edema, conjunctival hemorrhage, conjunctivitis, dry eye, epiphora, eye discharge, eyelid disorder, eyelid edema, eyelid erythema, follicular conjunctivitis, foreign body sensation, irritation, keratitis, pain, photophobia, stinging, superficial punctate keratopathy, visual acuity worsened, visual field defect, vitreous detachment, vitreous floaters, watery eyes
  Respiratory: Bronchitis, cough, dyspnea, pharyngitis, rhinitis, sinus infection, sinusitis
  Miscellaneous: Allergic reaction, flu-like syndrome, infection
General Dosage Range Ophthalmic: *Children ≥2 years and Adults:* Instill 1 drop in affected eye(s) 3 times/day
Mechanism of Action Selective agonism for alpha$_2$-receptors; causes reduction of aqueous humor formation and increased uveoscleral outflow
Pharmacodynamics/Kinetics
  Onset of Action Peak effect: 2 hours
  Half-life Elimination ~2 hours
  Time to Peak Plasma: 0.5-2.5 hours
Pregnancy Risk Factor B
Pregnancy Considerations Teratogenic effects were not observed in animal studies. There are no adequate and well-controlled studies in pregnant women.

Brinzolamide (brin ZOH la mide)

Brand Names: U.S. Azopt®

Brand Names: Canada Azopt®
Pharmacologic Category Carbonic Anhydrase Inhibitor; Ophthalmic Agent, Antiglaucoma
Use Treatment of elevated intraocular pressure in patients with ocular hypertension or open-angle glaucoma
Local Anesthetic/Vasoconstrictor Precautions No information available to require special precautions
Effects on Dental Treatment Key adverse event(s) related to dental treatment: Taste disturbances.
Effects on Bleeding No information available to require special precautions
Adverse Effects 1% to 10%:
  Cardiovascular: Hyperemia (1% to 5%)
  Central nervous system: Headache (1% to 5%)
  Dermatologic: Dermatitis (1% to 5%)
  Gastrointestinal: Taste disturbances (5% to 10%)
  Ocular: Ocular: Blurred vision (5% to 10%), blepharitis (1% to 5%), dry eye (1% to 5%), eye discharge (1% to 5%), eye discomfort (1% to 5%), eye pain (1% to 5%), foreign body sensation (1% to 5%), itching of eye (1% to 5%), keratitis (1% to 5%)
  Respiratory: Rhinitis (1% to 5%)
General Dosage Range Ophthalmic: *Adults:* Instill 1 drop in affected eye(s) 3 times/day
Mechanism of Action Brinzolamide inhibits carbonic anhydrase, leading to decreased aqueous humor secretion. This results in a reduction of intraocular pressure.
Pregnancy Risk Factor C
Pregnancy Considerations Adverse effects have been observed in animal reproduction studies.

Brinzolamide and Timolol
(brin ZOH la mide & TIM oh lol)

Related Information
  Brinzolamide *on page 200*
  Timolol (Ophthalmic) *on page 1326*
Brand Names: Canada Azarga™
Pharmacologic Category Beta-Blocker, Nonselective; Carbonic Anhydrase Inhibitor; Ophthalmic Agent, Antiglaucoma
Use Treatment of elevated intraocular pressure in patients with ocular hypertension or open-angle glaucoma
Local Anesthetic/Vasoconstrictor Precautions No information available to require special precautions
Effects on Dental Treatment Key adverse event(s) related to dental treatment: Taste perversion has been reported.
Effects on Bleeding No information available to require special precautions
Adverse Effects Percentages as reported with combination product. Also see individual agents.
1% to 10%:
  Gastrointestinal: Taste perversion (2%)
  Ocular: Blurred vision (6%), eye irritation (4%), eye pain (3%), foreign body sensation in eyes (1%)
General Dosage Range Ophthalmic: *Adults:* Instill 1 drop twice daily
Mechanism of Action
  Brinzolamide inhibits carbonic anhydrase, leading to decreased aqueous humor secretion. This results in a reduction of intraocular pressure.
  Timolol: Blocks both beta$_1$- and beta$_2$-adrenergic receptors, reduces intraocular pressure by reducing aqueous humor production or possibly outflow.

Pregnancy Considerations There are no adequate and well-controlled studies in pregnant women with the combination product. Use only if benefit outweighs risk. Bradycardia and arrhythmia have been reported in an infant following ophthalmic administration of timolol during pregnancy. See individual agents.

Product Availability Not available in U.S.

Bromazepam (broe MA ze pam)

Brand Names: Canada Apo-Bromazepam®; Lectopam®; Mylan-Bromazepam; Novo-Bromazepam; Nu-Bromazepam; PRO-Doc Limitee Bromazepam

Pharmacologic Category Benzodiazepine

Use Short-term, symptomatic treatment of anxiety

Local Anesthetic/Vasoconstrictor Precautions No information available to require special precautions

Effects on Dental Treatment Key adverse event(s) related to dental treatment: Xerostomia (normal salivary flow resumes upon discontinuation).

Effects on Bleeding No information available to require special precautions

Adverse Effects Frequency not defined.

Cardiovascular: Cardiac arrest, hypotension, palpitation, tachycardia

Central nervous system: Anterograde amnesia, ataxia, confusion, depression, dizziness, drowsiness, euphoria, headache, lethargy, physical and psychological dependence, seizure. In addition, paradoxical reactions (including aggression, agitation, excitation, hallucinations, nightmares, release of hostility, restlessness, and psychosis) are known to occur with benzodiazepines.

Dermatologic: Pruritus, rash

Endocrine & metabolic: Hyperglycemia, hypoglycemia, libido changes

Gastrointestinal: Gastritis (rare), nausea, vomiting, xerostomia

Genitourinary: Incontinence

Hematologic: Hemoglobin decreased, hematocrit decreased, WBCs increased/decreased

Hepatic: Transaminases increased, alkaline phosphatase increased, bilirubin increased

Neuromuscular & skeletal: Weakness, muscle spasm

Ocular: Blurred vision, diplopia

Respiratory: Respiratory depression

Miscellaneous: Allergic reactions including anaphylaxis have been reported with benzodiazepines

General Dosage Range Oral:

Adults: Initial: 6-18 mg/day in divided doses; Maintenance: 6-30 mg/day in divided doses

Elderly: Initial: 3 mg/day in divided doses

Mechanism of Action Binds to stereospecific benzodiazepine receptors on the postsynaptic GABA neuron at several sites within the central nervous system, including the limbic system, reticular formation. Enhancement of the inhibitory effect of GABA on neuronal excitability results by increased neuronal membrane permeability to chloride ions. This shift in chloride ions results in hyperpolarization (a less excitable state) and stabilization.

Pharmacodynamics/Kinetics

Half-life Elimination 20 hours

Time to Peak Serum: ≤2 hours (may be delayed by food)

Pregnancy Considerations An increased risk of fetal malformations may be associated with first trimester exposure (malformations of the heart, cleft lip/palate). Maternal use later in pregnancy may be associated with adverse events in the fetus (irregular heart beat) and neonate (hypothermia, hypotonia, respiratory depression, poor feeding, withdrawal).

Product Availability Not available in U.S.

Bromfenac (BROME fen ak)

Brand Names: U.S. Bromday®

Pharmacologic Category Nonsteroidal Anti-inflammatory Drug (NSAID), Ophthalmic

Use Treatment of postoperative inflammation and reduction in ocular pain following cataract removal

Local Anesthetic/Vasoconstrictor Precautions No information available to require special precautions

Effects on Dental Treatment The dentist should be aware of the potential of abnormal coagulation. Caution should also be exercised in the use of NSAIDs in patients already on anticoagulant therapy with drugs such as warfarin (Coumadin®). See Effects on Bleeding.

Effects on Bleeding Bromfenac is marketed in the U.S. only as an ophthalmic drop. It is a nonselective NSAID which is known to reversibly inhibit platelet aggregation. However, there is no scientific evidence to warrant discontinuation of topical NSAIDs prior to dental surgery.

Adverse Effects 2% to 7%:

Central nervous system: Headache

Ocular: Abnormal sensation, conjunctival hyperemia, iritis, irritation (burning/stinging), pain, pruritus, redness

General Dosage Range Ophthalmic: *Adults:* Instill 1 drop into affected eye(s) once daily

Mechanism of Action Inhibits prostaglandin synthesis by decreasing the activity of the enzyme, cyclooxygenase, which results in decreased formation of prostaglandin precursors.

Pharmacodynamics/Kinetics

Half-life Elimination 0.5-4 hours (following oral administration)

Pregnancy Risk Factor C

Pregnancy Considerations In animal reproduction studies, at exposures much higher than those which would result from ophthalmic use, embryo-fetal lethality and increased postimplantation loss occurred. Exposure to nonsteroidal anti-inflammatory drugs late in pregnancy may lead to premature closure of the ductus arteriosus and may inhibit uterine contractions.

Product Availability Prolensa™ 0.07% ophthalmic solution: FDA approved April 2013; anticipated availability currently unknown. Consult prescribing information for additional information.

Bromocriptine (broe moe KRIP teen)

Brand Names: U.S. Cycloset®; Parlodel®; Parlodel® SnapTabs®

Brand Names: Canada Dom-Bromocriptine; PMS-Bromocriptine

Pharmacologic Category Anti-Parkinson's Agent, Dopamine Agonist; Antidiabetic Agent, Dopamine Agonist; Ergot Derivative

Use Treatment of hyperprolactinemia associated with amenorrhea with or without galactorrhea, infertility, or hypogonadism; treatment of prolactin-secreting adenomas; treatment of acromegaly; treatment of Parkinson's disease

Cycloset®: Management of type 2 diabetes mellitus (noninsulin dependent, NIDDM) as an adjunct to diet and exercise

◀ **Unlabeled Use** Neuroleptic malignant syndrome

Local Anesthetic/Vasoconstrictor Precautions
Bromocriptine is a semisynthetic ergot alkaloid derivative; there is a possibility that it has vasoconstricting effects; use vasoconstrictor with caution

Effects on Dental Treatment Key adverse event(s) related to dental treatment: Orthostatic hypotension.

Effects on Bleeding No information available to require special precautions

Adverse Effects Note: Frequency of adverse effects may vary by dose and/or indication.

>10%:

Central nervous system: Dizziness, fatigue, headache
Gastrointestinal: Constipation, nausea
Neuromuscular & skeletal: Weakness
Respiratory: Rhinitis

1% to 10%:

Cardiovascular: Hypotension (including postural/orthostatic), Raynaud's syndrome exacerbation, syncope
Central nervous system: Drowsiness, lightheadedness, somnolence
Endocrine & metabolic: Hypoglycemia (4%; in combination with sulfonylureas or other antidiabetic agents: 7% to 9%)
Gastrointestinal: Abdominal cramps, anorexia, diarrhea, dyspepsia, GI bleeding, vomiting, xerostomia
Neuromuscular & skeletal: Digital vasospasm
Ocular: Amblyopia
Respiratory: Nasal congestion, sinusitis
Miscellaneous: Infection, flu-like syndrome

General Dosage Range Oral:

Children 11-15 years: Initial: 1.25-2.5 mg daily; Maintenance: 2.5-10 mg/day

Children ≥16 years: Initial: 1.25-2.5 mg daily; Maintenance: 2.5-15 mg/day

Adults: Dosage varies greatly depending on indication

Mechanism of Action Semisynthetic ergot alkaloid derivative and a dopamine receptor agonist which activates postsynaptic dopamine receptors in the tuberoinfundibular (inhibiting pituitary prolactin secretion) and nigrostriatal pathways (enhancing coordinated motor control).

In the treatment of type 2 diabetes mellitus, the mechanism of action is unknown; however, bromocriptine is believed to affect circadian rhythms which are mediated, in part, by dopaminergic activity, and are believed to play a role in obesity and insulin resistance. It is postulated that bromocriptine (when administered during the morning and released into the systemic circulation in a rapid, 'pulse-like' dose) may reset hypothalamic circadian activities which have been altered by obesity, thereby resulting in the reversal of insulin resistance and decreases in glucose production, without increasing serum insulin concentrations.

Pharmacodynamics/Kinetics

Onset of Action Parlodel®: Prolactin decreasing effect: 1-2 hours

Half-life Elimination Cycloset®: ~6 hours; Parlodel®: ~5 hours

Time to Peak Serum: Cycloset®: 53 minutes; Parlodel®: 0.5-4.5 hours

Pregnancy Risk Factor B

Pregnancy Considerations No evidence of teratogenicity or fetal toxicity in animal studies. Bromocriptine is used for ovulation induction in women with hyperprolactinemia. In general, therapy should be discontinued if pregnancy is confirmed unless needed for treatment of macroprolactinoma. Data collected from women taking bromocriptine during pregnancy suggest the incidence of birth defects is not increased with use. However, the majority of women discontinued use within 8 weeks of pregnancy. Women not seeking pregnancy should be advised to use appropriate contraception.

Brompheniramine (brome fen IR a meen)

Brand Names: U.S. Bromax [DSC]; J-Tan PD [OTC]; LoHist-12 [DSC]

Pharmacologic Category Alkylamine Derivative; Histamine H_1 Antagonist; Histamine H_1 Antagonist, First Generation

Use Symptomatic relief of perennial and seasonal allergic rhinitis, vasomotor rhinitis, and other respiratory allergies

Local Anesthetic/Vasoconstrictor Precautions No information available to require special precautions

Effects on Dental Treatment Key adverse event(s) related to dental treatment: Xerostomia (normal salivary flow resumes upon discontinuation). Chronic use of antihistamines will inhibit salivary flow, particularly in elderly patients; this may contribute to periodontal disease and oral discomfort.

Effects on Bleeding No information available to require special precautions

Adverse Effects Frequency not defined.

Cardiovascular: Angina, blood pressure increased, chest tightness, circulatory collapse, extrasystoles, hypotension, palpitation, tachycardia
Central nervous system: Anxiety, chills, confusion, coordination impaired, dizziness, drowsiness, euphoria, excitation, fatigue, headache, hysteria, insomnia, irritability, nervousness, neuritis, restlessness, sedation, seizure, stimulation, tension, vertigo
Dermatologic: Photosensitivity, rash, urticaria
Endocrine & metabolic: Early menses
Gastrointestinal: Abdominal cramps, anorexia, constipation, diarrhea, dry throat, epigastric distress, heartburn, nausea, vomiting, xerostomia
Genitourinary: Dysuria, polyuria, urinary retention
Hematologic: Agranulocytosis, hemolytic anemia, hypoplastic anemia, thrombocytopenia
Neuromuscular & skeletal: Paresthesia, tremor, weakness
Ocular: Blurred vision, diplopia, mydriasis
Otic: Labyrinthitis (acute), tinnitus
Respiratory: Dry nose, nasal congestion, thickening of bronchial secretions, wheezing
Miscellaneous: Anaphylactic shock, diaphoresis

General Dosage Range Oral:

Children 2 to <6 years: J-Tan PD: 1 mg (1 mL) every 4-6 hours (maximum: 6 mg [6 mL]/24 hours)

Children 6-12 years:

J-Tan PD: 2 mg (2 mL) every 4-6 hours (maximum: 12 mg [12 mL]/24 hours)

LoHist-12: One tablet every 12 hours (maximum: 2 tablets/day)

Children >12 years and Adults:

Bromax: One tablet twice daily

LoHist-12: 1-2 tablets every 12 hours (maximum: 4 tablets/day)

Mechanism of Action Competes with histamine for H_1-receptor sites on effector cells

Pharmacodynamics/Kinetics

Half-life Elimination Children: ~12 hours (Simons, 1999); Adults: ~25 hours (Simons, 1982)

Time to Peak Serum: Children: 3-3.5 hours (Simons, 1999); Adults: 2-4 hours (Simons, 1982)

Pregnancy Risk Factor C

Pregnancy Considerations Maternal antihistamine use has generally not resulted in increased risk of birth defects; however, information specific to brompheniramine is limited. Brompheniramine may cause severe reactions (convulsions) in newborns and premature infants; the manufacturer recommends avoiding use in the third trimester. Antihistamines are recommended for the treatment of rhinitis, urticaria, and pruritus with rash in pregnant women (although second generation antihistamines may be preferred). Antihistamines are not recommended for treatment of pruritus associated with intrahepatic cholestasis in pregnancy.

Brompheniramine and Pseudoephedrine
(brome fen IR a meen & soo doe e FED rin)

Related Information
Brompheniramine on page 202
Pseudoephedrine on page 1159
Brand Names: U.S. Brotapp [OTC]; J-Tan D PD [OTC]; Lodrane® D [OTC]; LoHist PSB [OTC]; Q-Tapp Cold & Allergy [OTC]
Pharmacologic Category Alkylamine Derivative; Alpha/Beta Agonist; Decongestant; Histamine H_1 Antagonist; Histamine H_1 Antagonist, First Generation
Use Temporary relief of symptoms associated with seasonal and perennial allergic rhinitis, the common cold, or sinusitis
Local Anesthetic/Vasoconstrictor Precautions Use with caution since pseudoephedrine is a sympathomimetic amine which could interact with epinephrine to cause a pressor response
Effects on Dental Treatment Key adverse event(s) related to dental treatment:
Brompheniramine: Prolonged use may decrease salivary flow.
Pseudoephedrine: Xerostomia (normal salivary flow resumes upon discontinuation).
Effects on Bleeding No information available to require special precautions
Adverse Effects Frequency not defined.
Cardiovascular: Arrhythmias, flushing, hypertension, pallor, palpitation, tachycardia
Central nervous system: Convulsions, CNS stimulation, dizziness, excitability (children; rare), giddiness, hallucinations, headache, insomnia, irritability, lassitude, nervousness, sedation
Gastrointestinal: Anorexia, diarrhea, dyspepsia, nausea, vomiting, xerostomia
Genitourinary: Dysuria, urinary retention (with BPH)
Neuromuscular skeletal: Tremors, weakness
Ocular: Diplopia
Renal: Polyuria
Respiratory: Respiratory difficulty
General Dosage Range Oral: Children ≥2 years and Adults: Dosage varies greatly depending on product
Mechanism of Action Brompheniramine maleate is an antihistamine with H_1-receptor activity; pseudoephedrine, a sympathomimetic amine and isomer of ephedrine, acts as a decongestant in respiratory tract mucous membranes with less vasoconstrictor action than ephedrine in normotensive individuals.

Budesonide (Systemic, Oral Inhalation)
(byoo DES oh nide)

Related Information
Respiratory Diseases on page 1514
Brand Names: U.S. Entocort® EC; Pulmicort Flexhaler®; Pulmicort Respules®; Uceris™
Brand Names: Canada Entocort®; Pulmicort Turbuhaler®
Generic Availability (U.S.) Yes: Capsule; suspension for nebulization
Pharmacologic Category Corticosteroid, Inhalant (Oral); Corticosteroid, Systemic
Use
Nebulization: Maintenance and prophylactic treatment of asthma
Oral capsule: Treatment of active Crohn's disease (mild-to-moderate) involving the ileum and/or ascending colon; maintenance of remission (for up to 3 months) of Crohn's disease (mild-to-moderate) involving the ileum and/or ascending colon
Oral inhalation: Maintenance and prophylactic treatment of asthma; includes patients who require oral corticosteroids and those who may benefit from systemic dose reduction/elimination
Oral tablet: Induction of remission in patients with active ulcerative colitis (mild-to-moderate)
Local Anesthetic/Vasoconstrictor Precautions No information available to require special precautions
Effects on Dental Treatment Key adverse event(s) related to dental treatment: Xerostomia (normal salivary flow resumes upon discontinuation), dry throat, abnormal taste, and herpes simplex. Localized infections with Candida albicans or Aspergillus niger have occurred frequently in the mouth and pharynx with repetitive use of oral inhaler of corticosteroids. These infections may require treatment with appropriate antifungal therapy or discontinuance of treatment with corticosteroid inhaler.
Effects on Bleeding Variable effects on anticoagulant therapy are observed with glucocorticoids such as budesonide (systemic, oral inhalation).
Adverse Effects
Oral capsules:
>10%:
Central nervous system: Headache (21%)
Dermatologic: Bruising (5% to 15%), acne (<5% to 15%)
Gastrointestinal: Nausea (11%)
Respiratory: Respiratory infection (11%)
Miscellaneous: Fat redistribution (moon face, buffalo hump; 3% to 11%)
1% to 10%:
Cardiovascular: Edema (<5% to 7%), chest pain (<5%), facial edema (<5%), flushing (<5%), hypertension (<5%), palpitation (<5%), tachycardia (<5%)
Central nervous system: Dizziness (<5% to 7%), agitation (<5%), amnesia (<5%), confusion (<5%), fever (<5%), insomnia (<5%), malaise (<5%), nervousness (<5%), sleep disorder (<5%), somnolence (<5%), vertigo (<5%)
Dermatologic: Hirsutism (5%), alopecia (<5%), dermatitis (<5%), eczema (<5%), purpura (<5%), skin disorder (<5%), striae (2%)
Endocrine & metabolic: Hypokalemia (<5%), intermenstrual bleeding (<5%), menstrual disorder (<5%), adrenal insufficiency (≥1%)

Gastrointestinal: Diarrhea (10%), dyspepsia (6%), anus disorder (<5%), appetite increased (<5%), Crohn's disease exacerbation (<5%), enteritis (<5%), epigastric pain (<5%), gastrointestinal fistula (<5%), glossitis (<5%), hemorrhoids (<5%), intestinal obstruction (<5%), oral candidiasis (<5%), tongue edema (<5%), tooth disorder (<5%), weight gain (<5%)

Genitourinary: Dysuria (<5%), micturition frequency (<5%), nocturia (<5%), hematuria (≥1%), pyuria (≥1%), urinary tract infection (<5%)

Hematologic: Leukocytosis (<5%), anemia (≥1%), neutrophils abnormal (≥1%)

Hepatic: Alkaline phosphatase increased (≥1%)

Neuromuscular & skeletal: Arthralgia (5%), arthritis (<5%), hyperkinesia (<5%), muscle cramping (<5%), myalgia (<5%), paresthesia (<5%), tremor (<5%), weakness (<5%)

Ocular: Eye abnormality (<5%), vision abnormal (<5%)

Otic: Ear infection (<5%)

Respiratory: Sinusitis (8%), bronchitis (<5%), dyspnea (<5%), pharynx disorder (<5%), rhinitis (<5%)

Miscellaneous: Viral infection (6%), abscess (<5%), C-reactive protein increased (<5%), diaphoresis (<5%), flu-like syndrome (<5%), erythrocyte sedimentation rate increased (≥1%)

Postmarketing and/or case reports: Anaphylaxis, intracranial hypertension (benign), mood swings

Oral inhaler (Pulmicort Flexhaler®):

1% to 10%:

Cardiovascular: Syncope (1% to 3%)

Central nervous system: Fever (≥3%), headache (≥3%), pain (≥3%), insomnia (1% to 3%)

Dermatologic: Bruising (1% to 3%)

Gastrointestinal: Dyspepsia (≥5%), nausea (2% to ≥5%), abdominal pain (1% to 3%), taste perversion (1% to 3%), vomiting (1% to 3%), weight gain (1% to 3%), xerostomia (1% to 3%), gastroenteritis (viral; 2%), oral candidiasis (1%)

Neuromuscular & skeletal: Arthralgia (≥5%), weakness (≥5%), back pain (≥3%), fracture (1% to 3%), hypertonia (1% to 3%), myalgia (1% to 3%), neck pain (1% to 3%)

Otic: Otitis media (1%)

Respiratory: Nasopharyngitis (9%), cough (≥5%), rhinitis (≥5%), respiratory infection (≥3%), sinusitis (≥3%), nasal congestion (3%), pharyngitis (3%), allergic rhinitis (2%), upper respiratory tract infection (viral; 2%)

Miscellaneous: Infection (1% to 3%), voice alteration (1% to 3%)

Postmarketing and/or case reports: Aggressiveness, anxiety, cataracts, depression, glaucoma, hypercorticism, hypersensitivity reactions (immediate and delayed [includes rash, contact dermatitis, angioedema, bronchospasm, urticaria]), hypocorticism, intraocular pressure increased, irritability, nervousness, psychosis, restlessness, throat irritation, wheezing (patients with severe milk allergy)

Oral tablets:

>10%: Central nervous system: Headache (11%)

1% to 10%:

Central nervous system: Mood swings (7%), fatigue (3%)

Dermatologic: Acne (2% to 5%), hirsutism (<1% to 5%)

Endocrine & metabolic: Cortisol decreased (4%)

Gastrointestinal: Nausea (5%), upper abdominal pain (4%), flatulence (3%), abdominal distension (2%), constipation (2%)

Genitourinary: Urinary tract infection (2%)

Neuromuscular & skeletal: Arthralgia (2%)

Postmarketing and/or case reports: Anaphylaxis, intracranial hypertension (benign), mood swings

Suspension for nebulization:

>10%:

Otic: Otitis media (12%)

Respiratory: Respiratory infection (38%), rhinitis (11% to 12%)

1% to 10%:

Cardiovascular: Chest pain (1% to <3%)

Central nervous system: Dysphonia (1% to <3%), fatigue (1% to <3%), mood swings (1% to <3%)

Dermatologic: Rash (4%), contact dermatitis (1% to <3%), eczema (1% to <3%), pruritus (1% to <3%), purpura (1% to <3%), pustular rash (1% to <3%)

Gastrointestinal: Gastroenteritis (5%), diarrhea (4%), vomiting (4%), abdominal pain (3%), anorexia (1% to <3%)

Hematologic: Cervical lymphadenopathy (1% to <3%)

Neuromuscular & skeletal: Fracture (1% to <3%), hyperkinesia (1% to <3%), myalgia (1% to <3%)

Ocular: Conjunctivitis (4%), eye infection (1% to <3%)

Otic: Ear infection (5%), earache (1% to <3%), otitis externa (1% to <3%)

Respiratory: Cough (8% to 9%), epistaxis (2% to 4%), stridor (1% to <3%)

Miscellaneous: Viral infection (4% to 5%), moniliasis (4% to 5%), allergic reaction (1% to <3%), flu-like syndrome (1% to <3%), herpes simplex (1% to <3%), infection (1% to <3%)

Postmarketing and/or case reports: Aggressiveness, anxiety, avascular necrosis of the femoral head, bronchitis, bruising, cataracts, depression, facial skin irritation, fever, glaucoma, growth suppression, headache, hypercorticism, hypersensitivity reactions (immediate and delayed [includes angioedema, bronchospasm, urticaria]), hypocorticism, intraocular pressure increased, irritability, nervousness, osteoporosis, pain, pharyngitis, psychosis, restlessness, sinusitis, throat irritation

Dosage

Nebulization: Asthma: Pulmicort Respules®: Children 12 months to 8 years: Titrate to lowest effective dose once patient is stable; start at 0.25 mg/day or use as follows:

Previous therapy of bronchodilators alone: 0.5 mg/day administered as a single dose or divided twice daily (maximum daily dose: 0.5 mg)

Previous therapy of inhaled corticosteroids: 0.5 mg/day administered as a single dose or divided twice daily (maximum daily dose: 1 mg)

Previous therapy of oral corticosteroids: 1 mg/day administered as a single dose or divided twice daily (maximum daily dose: 1 mg)

NIH Asthma Guidelines (NIH, 2007):

Children 0-4 years:

"Low" dose: 0.25-0.5 mg/day

"Medium" dose: >0.5-1 mg/day

"High" dose: >1 mg/day

Children 5-11 years:

"Low" dose: 0.5 mg/day

"Medium" dose: 1 mg/day

"High" dose: 2 mg/day

Oral inhalation: Asthma: Titrate to lowest effective dose once patient is stable.

U.S. labeling: Pulmicort Flexhaler®: **Note:** May increase dose after 1-2 weeks of therapy in patients who are not adequately controlled.

Children ≥6 years: Initial: 180 mcg twice daily (some patients may be initiated at 360 mcg twice daily); maximum: 360 mcg twice daily

NIH Asthma Guidelines (NIH, 2007) (administer in divided doses twice daily):

Children 5-11 years:

"Low" dose: 180-400 mcg/day

"Medium" dose: >400-800 mcg/day

"High" dose: >800 mcg/day

Children ≥12 years: Refer to adult dosing.

Adults: Initial: 360 mcg twice daily (selected patients may be initiated at 180 mcg twice daily); maximum: 720 mcg twice daily

NIH Asthma Guidelines (NIH, 2007) (administer in divided doses twice daily):

"Low" dose: 180-600 mcg/day

"Medium" dose: >600-1200 mcg/day

"High" dose: >1200 mcg/day

Canadian labeling: Pulmicort® Turbuhaler®:

Children 6-11 years:

Initial (or during periods of severe asthma or when switching from oral corticosteroid therapy): 200-400 mcg daily in 2 divided doses

Maintenance: Individualized, lowest effective dose in 2 divided doses

Children ≥12 years and Adults:

Initial (or during periods of severe asthma or when switching from oral corticosteroid therapy): 400-2400 mcg daily in 2-4 divided doses

Maintenance: 200-400 mcg twice daily (higher doses may be needed for some patients). Patients taking 400 mcg/day may take as a single daily dose.

Conversion from oral systemic corticosteroid to orally inhaled corticosteroid: Initiation of oral inhalation therapy should begin in patients whose asthma is reasonably stabilized on oral corticosteroids (OCS). A gradual dose reduction of OCS should begin ~7-10 days after starting inhaled therapy. U.S. labeling recommends reducing prednisone dose by 2.5 mg/day (or equivalent of other OCS) on a weekly basis (patients using inhaler) or by ≤25% every 1-2 weeks (patients using respules). The Canadian labeling recommends decreasing the daily dose of prednisone by 2.5 mg (or equivalent of other OCS) every 4 days in closely monitored patients or every 10 days if not closely monitored. If adrenal insufficiency occurs, temporarily increase the OCS dose and follow with a more gradual withdrawal. **Note:** When transitioning from systemic to inhaled corticosteroids, supplemental systemic corticosteroid therapy may be necessary during periods of stress or during severe asthma attacks.

Oral:

Capsule: Crohn's disease (active): Adults: 9 mg once daily in the morning for up to 8 weeks; recurring episodes may be treated with a repeat 8-week course of treatment

Maintenance of remission: Following treatment of active disease (control of symptoms with CDAI <150), treatment may be continued at a dosage of 6 mg once daily for up to 3 months. If symptom control is maintained for 3 months, tapering of the dosage to complete cessation is recommended. Continued dosing beyond 3 months has not been demonstrated to result in substantial benefit.

Tablet: Ulcerative colitis (active): Adults: 9 mg once daily in the morning for up to 8 weeks

Dosage adjustment in renal impairment: Inhalation, Nebulization, Oral: No dosage adjustment provided in manufacturer's labeling (has not been studied).

Dosage adjustment in hepatic impairment: Inhalation, Nebulization, Oral: No specific dosage adjustment provided in the manufacturer's labeling (has not been studied). Manufacturer labeling for oral budesonide suggests a dosage reduction may be necessary with moderate to severe impairment. Budesonide undergoes hepatic metabolism; bioavailability increased in cirrhosis; monitor closely for signs and symptoms of hypercorticism.

Mechanism of Action Controls the rate of protein synthesis; depresses the migration of polymorphonuclear leukocytes, fibroblasts; reverses capillary permeability and lysosomal stabilization at the cellular level to prevent or control inflammation. Has potent glucocorticoid activity and weak mineralocorticoid activity.

Contraindications Hypersensitivity to budesonide or any component of the formulation; primary treatment of status asthmaticus, acute episodes of asthma; not for relief of acute bronchospasm

Canadian labeling: Additional contraindications (not in U.S. labeling): Moderate-to-severe bronchiectasis, pulmonary tuberculosis (active or quiescent), untreated respiratory infection (bacterial, fungal, or viral)

Warnings/Precautions May cause hypercorticism or suppression of hypothalamic-pituitary-adrenal (HPA) axis, particularly in younger children, in patients receiving high doses for prolonged periods, or with concomitant CYP3A4 inhibitor use. HPA axis suppression may lead to adrenal crisis. Withdrawal and discontinuation of a corticosteroid should be done slowly and carefully. Particular care is required when patients are transferred from systemic corticosteroids to inhaled products or corticosteroids with lower systemic effect due to possible adrenal insufficiency or withdrawal from steroids, including an increase in allergic symptoms. Patients receiving >20 mg per day of prednisone (or equivalent) may be most susceptible. Fatalities have occurred due to adrenal insufficiency in asthmatic patients during and after transfer from systemic corticosteroids to aerosol steroids; aerosol steroids do not provide the systemic steroid needed to treat patients having trauma, surgery, or infections. Do not use this product to transfer patients directly from oral corticosteroid therapy.

Bronchospasm may occur with wheezing after inhalation; if this occurs stop steroid and treat with a fast-acting bronchodilator (eg, albuterol). Supplemental steroids (oral or parenteral) may be needed during stress or severe asthma attacks. Not to be used in status asthmaticus or for the relief of acute bronchospasm. Acute myopathy has been reported with high-dose corticosteroids, usually in patients with neuromuscular transmission disorders; may involve ocular and/or respiratory muscles; monitor creatine kinase; recovery may be delayed. Corticosteroid use may cause psychiatric disturbances, including depression, euphoria, insomnia, mood swings, and personality changes. Pre-existing psychiatric conditions may be exacerbated by corticosteroid use. Prolonged use of corticosteroids may also increase the incidence of secondary infection, mask acute infection (including fungal infections), prolong or exacerbate viral infections, or limit response to vaccines. Exposure to chickenpox should be avoided; corticosteroids should not be used to treat ocular herpes simplex. Corticosteroids should not be used for viral hepatitis. Close observation is required in patients with latent tuberculosis and/or TB reactivity; restrict use in active TB (only in conjunction with antituberculosis ▶

treatment). *Candida albicans* infections may occur in the mouth and pharynx; rinsing (and spitting) with water after inhaler use may decrease risk. Prolonged treatment with corticosteroids has been associated with the development of Kaposi's sarcoma (case reports); if noted, discontinuation of therapy should be considered.

Use with caution in patients with thyroid disease, hepatic impairment, renal impairment, cardiovascular disease, diabetes, glaucoma, cataracts, myasthenia gravis, patients at risk for osteoporosis, patients at risk for seizures, or GI diseases (diverticulitis, peptic ulcer, ulcerative colitis) due to perforation risk. Use caution following acute MI (corticosteroids have been associated with myocardial rupture). Because of the risk of adverse effects, systemic corticosteroids should be used cautiously in the elderly in the smallest possible effective dose for the shortest duration.

Potentially significant interactions may exist, requiring dose or frequency adjustment, additional monitoring, and/or selection of alternative therapy. Consult drug interactions database for more detailed information.

Orally-inhaled corticosteroids may cause a reduction in growth velocity in pediatric patients (~1 centimeter per year [range: 0.3-1.8 cm per year] and related to dose and duration of exposure). To minimize the systemic effects of orally-inhaled corticosteroids, each patient should be titrated to the lowest effective dose. Growth should be routinely monitored in pediatric patients. Withdraw systemic therapy with gradual tapering of dose. There have been reports of systemic corticosteroid withdrawal symptoms (eg, joint/muscle pain, lassitude, depression) when withdrawing oral inhalation therapy. Pulmicort Flexhaler® contains lactose; very rare anaphylactic reactions have been reported in patients with severe milk protein allergy.

Drug Interactions

Metabolism/Transport Effects Substrate of CYP3A4 (major); **Note:** Assignment of Major/Minor substrate status based on clinically relevant drug interaction potential

Avoid Concomitant Use

Avoid concomitant use of Budesonide (Systemic, Oral Inhalation) with any of the following: Aldesleukin; BCG; Grapefruit Juice; Natalizumab; Pimecrolimus; Tacrolimus (Topical); Tofacitinib

Increased Effect/Toxicity

Budesonide (Systemic, Oral Inhalation) may increase the levels/effects of: Amphotericin B; Deferasirox; Leflunomide; Loop Diuretics; Natalizumab; Thiazide Diuretics; Tofacitinib

The levels/effects of Budesonide (Systemic, Oral Inhalation) may be increased by: CYP3A4 Inhibitors (Moderate); CYP3A4 Inhibitors (Strong); Dasatinib; Denosumab; Grapefruit Juice; Ivacaftor; Mifepristone; Pimecrolimus; Tacrolimus (Topical); Telaprevir; Trastuzumab

Decreased Effect

Budesonide (Systemic, Oral Inhalation) may decrease the levels/effects of: Aldesleukin; Antidiabetic Agents; BCG; Coccidioidin Skin Test; Corticorelin; Hyaluronidase; Sipuleucel-T; Vaccines (Inactivated)

The levels/effects of Budesonide (Systemic, Oral Inhalation) may be decreased by: Antacids; Bile Acid Sequestrants; Echinacea

Ethanol/Nutrition/Herb Interactions

Food: Grapefruit juice may double systemic exposure of orally administered budesonide. Administration of

capsules with a high-fat meal delays peak concentration, but does not alter the extent of absorption; administration of tablets with a high-fat meal decreases peak concentration (~27%). Management: Avoid grapefruit juice when using oral capsules or tablets.

Herb/Nutraceutical: Echinacea may diminish the therapeutic effect of budesonide. Management: Avoid echinacea.

Dietary Considerations Oral capsules, tablets: Avoid grapefruit juice.

Pharmacodynamics/Kinetics

Onset of Action Nebulization: 2-8 days; Inhalation: 24 hours

Peak effect: Nebulization: 4-6 weeks; Inhalation: 1-2 weeks

Half-life Elimination 2-3.6 hours

Time to Peak Capsule: 0.5-10 hours (variable in Crohn's disease); Nebulization: 10-30 minutes; Inhalation: 1-2 hours; Tablet: 7.4-19.2 hours

Pregnancy Risk Factor C (capsule, tablet)/B (inhalation)

Pregnancy Considerations Adverse events have been observed with corticosteroids in animal reproduction studies. Some studies of pregnant women have shown an association between first trimester systemic corticosteroid use and oral clefts; adverse events in the fetus/neonate have been noted in case reports following large doses of systemic corticosteroids during pregnancy. Studies of pregnant women using inhaled budesonide have not demonstrated an increased risk of abnormalities. Inhaled corticosteroids are recommended for the treatment of asthma during pregnancy; budesonide is preferred (ACOG, 2008; NAEPP, 2005)

Lactation Enters breast milk/use caution

Breast-Feeding Considerations Following use of the powder for oral inhalation, ~0.3% to 1% of the maternal dose was found in breast milk. The maximum concentration appeared within 45 minutes of dosing. Plasma budesonide levels obtained from infants ~90 minutes after breast-feeding (~140 minutes after maternal dose) were below the limit of quantification. Concentrations of budesonide in breast milk are expected to be higher following administration of oral capsules/tablets than after an inhaled dose. The use of inhaled corticosteroids is not considered a contraindication to breast-feeding (NAEPP, 2005).

Dosage Forms

Capsule, enteric coated, oral: 3 mg

Entocort® EC: 3 mg

Powder, for oral inhalation:

Pulmicort Flexhaler®: 90 mcg/inhalation (165 mg); 180 mcg/inhalation (225 mg)

Suspension, for nebulization: 0.25 mg/2 mL (30s); 0.5 mg/2 mL (30s)

Pulmicort Respules®: 0.25 mg/2 mL (30s); 0.5 mg/2 mL (30s); 1 mg/2 mL (30s)

Tablet, extended release, oral:

Uceris™: 9 mg

Dosage Forms: Canada

Powder for oral inhalation:

Pulmicort® Turbuhaler®: 100 mcg/inhalation, 200 mcg/inhalation, 400 mcg/inhalation

---

Budesonide (Nasal) (byoo DES oh nide)

Brand Names: U.S. Rhinocort Aqua®

Brand Names: Canada Mylan-Budesonide AQ; Rhinocort® Aqua®; Rhinocort® Turbuhaler®

Generic Availability (U.S.) No

Pharmacologic Category Corticosteroid, Nasal

Use Management of symptoms of seasonal or perennial rhinitis

Canadian labeling: Additional use (not in U.S. labeling): Prevention and treatment of nasal polyps

Unlabeled Use Adjunct to antibiotics in empiric treatment of acute bacterial rhinosinusitis (ABRS) (Chow, 2012)

Local Anesthetic/Vasoconstrictor Precautions No information available to require special precautions

Effects on Dental Treatment No significant effects or complications reported

Effects on Bleeding No information available to require special precautions

Adverse Effects 1% to 10%:

Respiratory: Epistaxis (8%), pharyngitis (4%), bronchospasm (2%), coughing (2%), nasal irritation (2%)

Miscellaneous: Although reported at higher rates with systemic administration, symptoms of HPA axis suppression and/or hypercorticism may occur rarely (<1%) following administration via methods which result in lower exposures (nasal).

Dosage Nasal inhalation:

U.S. labeling (Rhinocort® Aqua®): Rhinitis: Children ≥6 years and Adults: 64 mcg/day as a single 32 mcg spray in each nostril. Some patients who do not achieve adequate control may benefit from increased dosage. A reduced dosage may be effective after initial control is achieved.

Maximum dose: Children <12 years: 128 mcg/day; Adults: 256 mcg/day

Canadian labeling:

Rhinocort® Aqua®: Children ≥6 years and Adults:

Nasal polyps: 256 mcg/day administered as a single 64 mcg spray in each nostril twice daily

Rhinitis: Initial: 256 mcg/day administered as two 64 mcg sprays in each nostril once daily or a single 64 mcg spray in each nostril twice daily; Maintenance: Individualize, lowest effective dose

Maximum dose: 256 mcg/day

Rhinocort® Turbuhaler®: Children ≥6 years and Adults:

Nasal polyps: 100 mcg into each nostril twice daily (maximum: 400 mcg/day)

Rhinitis: Initial: 200 mcg into each nostril once daily; Maintenance: Individualize, lowest effective dose (maximum: 400 mcg/day)

Dosage adjustment in renal impairment: No dosage adjustment provided in manufacturer's labeling (has not been studied).

Dosage adjustment in hepatic impairment: No dosage adjustment provided in manufacturer's labeling. Systemic availability of budesonide may be increased in patients with cirrhosis; monitor closely for signs and symptoms of hypercorticism; dosage reduction may be required.

Mechanism of Action Controls the rate of protein synthesis; depresses the migration of polymorphonuclear leukocytes, fibroblasts; reverses capillary permeability and lysosomal stabilization at the cellular level to prevent or control inflammation. Has potent glucocorticoid activity and weak mineralocorticoid activity.

Contraindications Hypersensitivity to budesonide or any component of the formulation

Canadian labeling: Additional contraindications (not in U.S. labeling): Pulmonary tuberculosis (active or quiescent), untreated respiratory infection (bacterial, fungal, or viral); use in patients <6 years of age

Warnings/Precautions May delay wound healing; avoid nasal corticosteroid use in patients with recent nasal septal ulcers, nasal surgery or nasal trauma until healing has occurred. Localized *Candida albicans* infections of the nose and/or pharynx may occur (rarely). Prolonged use of corticosteroids may also increase the incidence of secondary infection, mask acute infection (including fungal infections), prolong or exacerbate viral infections, or limit response to vaccines. Exposure to chickenpox should be avoided. Close observation is required in patients with latent tuberculosis and/or TB reactivity restrict use in active TB (only in conjunction with antituberculosis treatment).

Intranasal corticosteroids may cause a reduction in growth velocity in pediatric patients (~1 centimeter per year [range 0.3-1.8 cm per year] and related to dose and duration of exposure). To minimize the systemic effects of orally-inhaled and intranasal corticosteroids, each patient should be titrated to the lowest effective dose. Growth should be routinely monitored in pediatric patients.

Drug Interactions

Metabolism/Transport Effects Substrate of CYP3A4 (minor); **Note:** Assignment of Major/Minor substrate status based on clinically relevant drug interaction potential

Avoid Concomitant Use There are no known interactions where it is recommended to avoid concomitant use.

Increased Effect/Toxicity

The levels/effects of Budesonide (Nasal) may be increased by: CYP3A4 Inhibitors (Strong); Telaprevir

Decreased Effect There are no known significant interactions involving a decrease in effect.

Pharmacodynamics/Kinetics

Onset of Action Rhinocort® Aqua®: ~10 hours

Peak effect: Rhinocort® Aqua®: ~2 weeks

Half-life Elimination 2-3.6 hours

Time to Peak Nasal: 1 hour

Pregnancy Risk Factor B

Pregnancy Considerations Adverse events have been observed with corticosteroids in animal reproduction studies. Studies of pregnant women using intranasal budesonide have not demonstrated an increased risk of abnormalities. Intranasal corticosteroids may be used in the treatment of rhinitis during pregnancy; budesonide is preferred (Wallace, 2008)

Lactation Enters breast milk/use caution

Breast-Feeding Considerations Following use of the powder for oral inhalation, ~0.3% to 1% of the maternal dose was found in breast milk. The maximum concentration appeared within 45 minutes of dosing. Plasma budesonide levels obtained from infants ~90 minutes after breast-feeding (~140 minutes after maternal dose) were below the limit of quantification. Milk concentrations following the use of the nasal inhaler are expected to be similar. The use of inhaled corticosteroids is not considered a contraindication to breast feeding (NAEPP, 2005).

Dosage Forms

Suspension, intranasal:

Rhinocort Aqua®: 32 mcg/inhalation (8.6 g)

Dosage Forms: Canada

Powder for nasal inhalation:

Rhinocort® Turbuhaler®: 100 mcg/inhalation

Suspension, intranasal [spray]:

Rhinocort® Aqua®: 64 mcg/inhalation

Budesonide and Formoterol
(byoo DES oh nide & for MOH te rol)

Related Information
Budesonide (Systemic, Oral Inhalation) *on page 203*
Formoterol *on page 629*

Brand Names: U.S. Symbicort®

Brand Names: Canada Symbicort®

Pharmacologic Category Beta$_2$ Agonist; Beta$_2$-Adrenergic Agonist, Long-Acting; Corticosteroid, Inhalant (Oral)

Use Treatment of asthma in patients ≥12 years of age where combination therapy is indicated; maintenance treatment of airflow obstruction associated with chronic obstructive pulmonary disease (COPD; including chronic bronchitis and emphysema)

Unlabeled Use Treatment of asthma in children 5-11 years of age where combination therapy is indicated

Local Anesthetic/Vasoconstrictor Precautions No information available to require special precautions

Effects on Dental Treatment Key adverse event(s) related to dental treatment: Formoterol: Xerostomia (normal salivary flow resumes upon discontinuation). Localized infections with *Candida albicans* or *Aspergillus niger* have occurred frequently in the mouth and pharynx with repetitive use of oral inhaler of corticosteroids. These infections may require treatment with appropriate antifungal therapy or discontinuance of treatment with corticosteroid inhaler.

Effects on Bleeding No information available to require special precautions

Adverse Effects Note: Percentage of adverse events may be dose related; causation not established. Also see individual agents.

>10%:
Central nervous system: Headache (7% to 11%)
Respiratory: Nasopharyngitis (7% to 11%), upper respiratory tract infections (4% to 11%)

1% to 10%:
Central nervous system: Dizziness (<3%)
Gastrointestinal: Stomach discomfort (1% to 7%), oral candidiasis (1% to 6%), vomiting (1% to 3%)
Neuromuscular & skeletal: Back pain (2% to 3%)
Respiratory: Pharyngolaryngeal pain (6% to 9%), lower respiratory tract infection (3% to 8%), sinusitis (4% to 6%), bronchitis (5%), nasal congestion (3%)
Miscellaneous: Influenza (2% to 3%)

General Dosage Range Inhalation:
Children 5-11 years: Symbicort® 80/4.5: Two inhalations twice daily (maximum: 4 inhalations/day)
Children ≥12 years: 2 inhalations once or twice daily (maximum: 4 inhalations/day)
Adults: 2 inhalations twice daily (maximum: 4 inhalations/day)

Mechanism of Action Formoterol relaxes bronchial smooth muscle by selective action on beta$_2$ receptors with little effect on heart rate. Formoterol has a long-acting effect. Budesonide is a corticosteroid which controls the rate of protein synthesis, depresses the migration of polymorphonuclear leukocytes/fibroblasts, and reverses capillary permeability and lysosomal stabilization at the cellular level to prevent or control inflammation.

Pharmacodynamics/Kinetics
Onset of Action Asthma: 15 minutes; maximum benefit: May take ≥2 weeks

Pregnancy Risk Factor C

Pregnancy Considerations Teratogenic and embryocidal effects were observed in animal studies when administered by inhalation at doses less than the maximum equivalent human dose. Also see individual agents.

Bumetanide (byoo MET a nide)

Related Information
Cardiovascular Diseases *on page 1492*

Brand Names: Canada Burinex®

Pharmacologic Category Diuretic, Loop

Use Management of edema secondary to heart failure or hepatic or renal disease (including nephrotic syndrome)

Unlabeled Use Treatment of hypertension

Local Anesthetic/Vasoconstrictor Precautions No information available to require special precautions

Effects on Dental Treatment No significant effects or complications reported

Effects on Bleeding No information available to require special precautions

Adverse Effects
>10%:
Endocrine & metabolic: Hyperuricemia (18%), hypochloremia (15%), hypokalemia (15%)
Renal: Azotemia (11%)

1% to 10%:
Central nervous system: Dizziness (1%)
Endocrine & metabolic: Hyponatremia (9%), hyperglycemia (7%), phosphorus altered (5%), CO_2 content altered (4%), bicarbonate altered (3%), calcium altered (2%)
Neuromuscular & skeletal: Muscle cramps (1%)
Renal: Serum creatinine increased (7%)
Miscellaneous: LDH altered (1%)

General Dosage Range
I.M., I.V.:
Infants and Children: 0.015-0.1 mg/kg/dose every 6-24 hours (maximum: 10 mg/day)
Adults: 0.5-1 mg/dose; may repeat in 2-3 hours for up to 2 doses (maximum: 10 mg/day)

Oral:
Infants and Children: 0.015-0.1 mg/kg/dose every 6-24 hours (maximum: 10 mg/day)
Adults: 0.5-2 mg 1-2 times/day; may repeat in 4-5 hours for up to 2 doses (maximum: 10 mg/day)

Mechanism of Action Inhibits reabsorption of sodium and chloride in the ascending loop of Henle and proximal renal tubule, interfering with the chloride-binding cotransport system, thus causing increased excretion of water, sodium, chloride, magnesium, phosphate, and calcium; it does not appear to act on the distal tubule

Pharmacodynamics/Kinetics
Onset of Action Oral, I.M.: 0.5-1 hour; I.V.: 2-3 minutes
Peak effect: Oral: 1-2 hours; I.V.: 15-30 minutes

Duration of Action 4-6 hours

Half-life Elimination Neonates: ~6 hours; Infants (1 month): ~2.4 hours; Adults: 1-1.5 hours

Pregnancy Risk Factor C

Pregnancy Considerations Adverse events have been observed in some animal reproduction studies.

Bupivacaine (byoo PIV a kane)

Related Information
Oral Pain *on page 1558*
Brand Names: U.S. Bupivacaine Spinal; Marcaine®; Marcaine® Spinal; Sensorcaine®; Sensorcaine®-MPF; Sensorcaine®-MPF Spinal
Brand Names: Canada Marcaine®; Sensorcaine®
Pharmacologic Category Local Anesthetic
Use Local or regional anesthesia; spinal anesthesia; diagnostic and therapeutic procedures; obstetrical procedures (only 0.25% and 0.5% concentrations):
  0.25%: Local infiltration, peripheral nerve block, sympathetic block, caudal or epidural block
  0.5%: Peripheral nerve block, caudal and epidural block
  0.75% **(not for obstetrical anesthesia)**: Retrobulbar block, epidural block. **Note:** Reserve for surgical procedures where a high degree of muscle relaxation and prolonged effect are necessary
Local Anesthetic/Vasoconstrictor Precautions No information available to require special precautions
Effects on Dental Treatment No significant effects or complications reported
Effects on Bleeding No information available to require special precautions
Adverse Effects Note: Incidence of adverse reactions is difficult to define. Most effects are dose related, and are often due to accelerated absorption from the injection site, unintentional intravascular injection, or slow metabolic degradation. The development of any central nervous system symptoms may be an early indication of more significant toxicity (seizure).

Cardiovascular: Hypotension, bradycardia, palpitation, heart block, ventricular arrhythmia, cardiac arrest
Central nervous system: Restlessness, anxiety, dizziness, seizure (0.1%); rare symptoms (usually associated with unintentional subarachnoid injection during high spinal anesthesia) include persistent anesthesia, paresthesia, paralysis, headache, septic meningitis, and cranial nerve palsies
Gastrointestinal: Nausea, vomiting; rare symptoms (usually associated with unintentional subarachnoid injection during high spinal anesthesia) include fecal incontinence and loss of sphincter control
Genitourinary: Rare symptoms (usually associated with unintentional subarachnoid injection during high spinal anesthesia) include urinary incontinence, loss of perineal sensation, and loss of sexual function
Neuromuscular & skeletal: Chondrolysis (continuous intra-articular administration), weakness
Ocular: Blurred vision, pupillary constriction
Otic: Tinnitus
Respiratory: Apnea, hypoventilation (usually associated with unintentional subarachnoid injection during high spinal anesthesia)
Miscellaneous: Allergic reactions (urticaria, pruritus, angioedema), anaphylactoid reactions

General Dosage Range
Caudal block: *Children >12 years and Adults:* 15-30 mL of 0.25% or 0.5%
Epidural block: *Children >12 years and Adults:* 10-20 mL of 0.25% or 0.5% in 3-5 mL increments **or** 10-20 mL of 0.75% if high degree of muscle relaxation and prolonged effects needed
Infiltration (local): *Children >12 years and Adults:* 0.25% (maximum: 175 mg)

Nerve block: *Children >12 years and Adults:*
  Peripheral: 5 mL of 0.25% or 0.5% (maximum: 400 mg/day)
  Sympathetic: 20-50 mL of 0.25%
Retrobulbar anesthesia: *Children >12 years and Adults:* 2-4 mL of 0.75%
Spinal: *Adults:* Preservative free solution of 0.75% bupivacaine in 8.25% dextrose:
  Cesarean section: 1-1.4 mL
  Lower abdominal procedures: 1.6 mL
  Lower extremity and perineal procedures: 1 mL
  Normal vaginal delivery: 0.8 mL (higher doses may be required in some patients)
Mechanism of Action Blocks both the initiation and conduction of nerve impulses by decreasing the neuronal membrane's permeability to sodium ions, which results in inhibition of depolarization with resultant blockade of conduction
Pharmacodynamics/Kinetics
Onset of Action Anesthesia (route and dose dependent): 1-17 minutes
Duration of Action Route and dose dependent: 2-9 hours
Half-life Elimination Age dependent: Neonates: 8.1 hours; Adults: 2.7 hours
Time to Peak Plasma: Caudal, epidural, or peripheral nerve block: 30-45 minutes
Pregnancy Risk Factor C
Pregnancy Considerations Decreased pup survival and embryocidal effects were observed in animal studies. Bupivacaine is approved for use at term in obstetrical anesthesia or analgesia. **[U.S. Boxed Warning]: The 0.75% is not recommended for obstetrical anesthesia.** Bupivacaine 0.75% solutions have been associated with cardiac arrest following epidural anesthesia in obstetrical patients and use of this concentration is not recommended for this purpose. Use in obstetrical paracervical block anesthesia is contraindicated.

Bupivacaine and Epinephrine
(byoo PIV a kane & ep i NEF rin)

Related Information
Bupivacaine *on page 209*
EPINEPHrine (Systemic, Oral Inhalation) *on page 482*
Oral Pain *on page 1558*
Brand Names: U.S. Marcaine® with Epinephrine; Sensorcaine® with Epinephrine; Sensorcaine®-MPF with Epinephrine; Vivacaine™
Brand Names: Canada Sensorcaine® with Epinephrine
Generic Availability (U.S.) Yes
Pharmacologic Category Local Anesthetic
Dental Use Local anesthesia
Use Local anesthetic (injectable) for peripheral nerve block, infiltration, sympathetic block, caudal or epidural block, retrobulbar block
Local Anesthetic/Vasoconstrictor Precautions No information available to require special precautions
Effects on Dental Treatment It is common to misinterpret psychogenic responses to local anesthetic injection as an allergic reaction. Intraoral injections are perceived by many patients as a stressful procedure in dentistry. Common symptoms to this stress are diaphoresis, palpitations, and hyperventilation. Patients may exhibit hypersensitivity to bisulfites contained in local anesthetic solution to prevent oxidation of epinephrine. In general, patients reacting to bisulfites have a history of

asthma and their airways are hyper-reactive to asthmatic syndrome.

Degree of adverse effects in the CNS and cardiovascular system is directly related to the blood levels of bupivacaine: Bradycardia, hypersensitivity reactions (rare; may be manifest as dermatologic reactions and edema at injection site), asthmatic syndromes.

High blood levels: Anxiety, restlessness, disorientation, confusion, dizziness, tremors, seizures, CNS depression (resulting in somnolence, unconsciousness and possible respiratory arrest), nausea, and vomiting.

Effects on Bleeding Epinephrine reduces bleeding

Adverse Effects See individual agents.

Dental Usual Dosage

Infiltration and nerve block in maxillary and mandibular area: Children >12 years and Adults: 9 mg (1.8 mL) of bupivacaine as a 0.5% solution with epinephrine 1:200,000 per injection site. A second dose may be administered if necessary to produce adequate anesthesia after allowing up to 10 minutes for onset. Up to a maximum of 90 mg of bupivacaine hydrochloride per dental appointment. The effective anesthetic dose varies with procedure, intensity of anesthesia needed, duration of anesthesia required, and physical condition of the patient; always use the lowest effective dose along with careful aspiration.

The following numbers of dental carpules (1.8 mL) provide the indicated amounts of bupivacaine hydrochloride 0.5% and vasoconstrictor (epinephrine 1:200,000). See table.

# of Cartridges (1.8 mL)	mg Bupivacaine (0.5%)	mg Vasoconstrictor (Epinephrine 1:200,000)
1	9	0.009
2	18	0.018
3	27	0.027
4	36	0.036
5	45	0.045
6	54	0.054
7	63	0.063
8	72	0.072
9	81	0.081
10	90	0.090

Note: Adult and children doses of bupivacaine hydrochloride with epinephrine cited from USP Dispensing Information (USP DI), 17th ed, The United States Pharmacopeial Convention, Inc, Rockville, MD, 1997, 134.

Dosage Dose varies with procedure, depth of anesthesia, vascularity of tissues, duration of anesthesia, and condition of patient. Do not use solutions containing preservatives for caudal or epidural block.

Children >12 years and Adults:

Caudal block (preservative free): 15-30 mL of 0.25% or 0.5%

Epidural block (other than caudal block, preservative free): 10-20 mL of 0.25% or 0.5%. Administer in 3-5 mL increments, allowing sufficient time to detect toxic manifestations of inadvertent I.V. or I.T. administration.

Surgical procedures requiring a high degree of muscle relaxation and prolonged effects only: 10-20 mL of 0.75% (**Note:** Not to be used in obstetrical cases)

Local anesthesia: Infiltration: 0.25% infiltrated locally (maximum: 175 mg of bupivacaine)

Peripheral nerve block: 5 mL of 0.25% or 0.5% (maximum: 400 mg/day of bupivacaine)

Retrobulbar anesthesia: 2-4 mL of 0.75%

Sympathetic nerve block: 20-50 mL of 0.25%

Infiltration and nerve block in maxillary and mandibular area: 9 mg (1.8 mL) of bupivacaine as a 0.5% solution with epinephrine 1:200,000 per injection site. A second dose may be administered if necessary to produce adequate anesthesia after allowing up to 10 minutes for onset. Up to a maximum of 90 mg of bupivacaine hydrochloride per dental appointment. The effective anesthetic dose varies with procedure, intensity of anesthesia needed, duration of anesthesia required, and physical condition of the patient; always use the lowest effective dose along with careful aspiration.

Note: Adult and children doses of bupivacaine hydrochloride with epinephrine cited from USP Dispensing Information (USP DI), 17th ed, The United States Pharmacopeial Convention, Inc, Rockville, MD, 1997, 134.

Dosage adjustment in renal impairment: No dosage adjustments provided in manufacturer's labeling; use with caution.

Dosage adjustment in hepatic impairment: No dosage adjustments provided in manufacturer's labeling; use with caution.

Mechanism of Action Local anesthetics bind selectively to the intracellular surface of sodium channels to block influx of sodium into the axon. As a result, depolarization necessary for action potential propagation and subsequent nerve function is prevented. The block at the sodium channel is reversible. When drug diffuses away from the axon, sodium channel function is restored and nerve propagation returns.

Epinephrine prolongs the duration of the anesthetic actions of bupivacaine by causing vasoconstriction (alpha-adrenergic receptor agonist) of the vasculature surrounding the nerve axons. This prevents the diffusion of bupivacaine away from the nerves resulting in a longer retention in the axon

Contraindications Hypersensitivity to bupivacaine, epinephrine, amide-type local anesthetics, or any component of the formulation

Warnings/Precautions Some commercially available formulations contain sodium metabisulfite, which may cause allergic-type reactions. Do not use solutions containing preservatives for caudal or epidural block. Intravascular injections should be avoided. Local anesthetics have been associated with rare occurrences of sudden respiratory arrest. Convulsions due to systemic toxicity leading to cardiac arrest have also been reported, presumably following unintentional intravascular injection. **[U.S. Boxed Warning]: The 0.75% is not recommended for obstetrical anesthesia.** A test dose is recommended prior to epidural administration and all reinforcing doses with continuous catheter technique. Use caution with cardiovascular dysfunction, hepatic impairment, or patients with compromised blood supply. Bupivacaine-containing products have been associated with rare occurrences of arrhythmias, cardiac arrest, and death. Use caution in debilitated, elderly, or acutely ill patients; dose reduction may be required. Dental practitioners and/or clinicians using local anesthetic agents should be well trained in diagnosis and management of emergencies that may arise from the use of these agents. Resuscitative equipment, oxygen, and other resuscitative drugs should be available for immediate use. Not recommended for use in children <12 years of age.

Continuous intra-articular infusion of local anesthetics after arthroscopic or other surgical procedures is **not** an approved use; chondrolysis (primarily shoulder joint) has occurred following infusion, with some requiring arthroplasty or shoulder replacement.

Drug Interactions

Metabolism/Transport Effects Refer to individual components.

Avoid Concomitant Use

Avoid concomitant use of Bupivacaine and Epinephrine with any of the following: Ergot Derivatives; Iobenguane I 123; Lurasidone

Increased Effect/Toxicity

Bupivacaine and Epinephrine may increase the levels/ effects of: Bromocriptine; Lurasidone; Sympathomimetics

The levels/effects of Bupivacaine and Epinephrine may be increased by: Antacids; AtoMOXetine; Beta-Blockers; Cannabinoids; Carbonic Anhydrase Inhibitors; COMT Inhibitors; Ergot Derivatives; Hyaluronidase; Inhalational Anesthetics; MAO Inhibitors; Serotonin/Norepinephrine Reuptake Inhibitors; Tricyclic Antidepressants

Decreased Effect

Bupivacaine and Epinephrine may decrease the levels/effects of: Benzylpenicilloyl Polylysine; Iobenguane I 123

The levels/effects of Bupivacaine and Epinephrine may be decreased by: Alpha1-Blockers; Promethazine; Spironolactone

Pregnancy Risk Factor C

Pregnancy Considerations See individual agents.

Lactation Enters breast milk/not recommended

Dosage Forms

Injection, solution [preservative free]: Bupivacaine 0.25% and epinephrine 1:200,000 (10 mL, 30 mL); bupivacaine 0.5% and epinephrine 1:200,000 (10 mL, 30 mL)

Marcaine® with Epinephrine: Bupivacaine 0.25% and epinephrine 1:200,000 (10 mL, 30 mL); bupivacaine 0.5% and epinephrine 1:200,000 (10 mL, 30 mL)

Sensorcaine® MPF with Epinephrine: Bupivacaine 0.25% and epinephrine 1:200,000 (10 mL, 30 mL); bupivacaine 0.5% and epinephrine 1:200,000 (10 mL, 30 mL); bupivacaine 0.75% and epinephrine 1:200,000 (30 mL)

Injection, solution: Bupivacaine 0.25% and epinephrine 1:200,000 (50 mL); bupivacaine 0.5% and epinephrine 1:200,000 (50 mL)

Marcaine® with Epinephrine, Sensorcaine® with Epinephrine: Bupivacaine 0.25% and epinephrine 1:200,000 (50 mL); bupivacaine 0.5% and epinephrine 1:200,000 (50 mL)

Injection, solution [for dental use]:

Marcaine® with Epinephrine, Vivacaine™: Bupivacaine 0.5% and epinephrine 1:200,000 (1.8 mL)

Dental Comment Oral paresthesia: The occurrence of oral paresthesia associated with 4% solutions of prilocaine or articaine, although rare, continue to be slightly more frequent than other local anesthetics. From 1999-2008, there were 182 cases of nonsurgical

paresthesia (Gaffen, 2009). Of the cases, 172 involved mandibular block injection only. Another eight cases involved mandibular block combined with at least one other type of anesthetic injection. A single case involved infiltration around tooth number 35 and the final case involved infiltration and intraligamentary injection in the maxillary anterior region.

A 2010 report, reviewed adverse events submitted voluntarily over a 10-year period involving the dental local anesthetics articaine, bupivacaine, lidocaine, mepivacaine, and prilocaine in the United States. Bupivacaine reported incidence: One case per 124,286,050 cartridges sold. The reported incidence of paresthesia was one case for 13,800,970 cartridges of all local anesthetics sold in the U.S. (Garisto, 2010).

References

Finder RL and Moore PA, "Adverse Drug Reactions to Local Anesthesia," *Dent Clin North Am*, 2002, 46(4):747-57, x.
Jastak JT and Yagiela JA, "Vasoconstrictors and Local Anesthesia: A Review and Rationale for Use," *J Am Dent Assoc*, 1983, 107 (4):623-30.
MacKenzie TA and Young ER, "Local Anesthetic Update," *Anesth Prog*, 1993, 40(2):29-34.
Malamed SF, "Allergy and Toxic Reactions to Local Anesthetics," *Dent Today*, 2003, 22(4):114-6, 118-21.
Yagiela JA, "Local Anesthetics," *Anesth Prog*, 1991, 38(4-5):128-41.

Bupivacaine (Liposomal)

(byoo PIV a kane lye po SO mal)

Brand Names: U.S. Exparel™

Pharmacologic Category Analgesic, Nonopioid

Use Injected into the surgical site (eg, bunionectomy, hemorrhoidectomy) to provide postoperative analgesia

Local Anesthetic/Vasoconstrictor Precautions No information available to require special precautions

Effects on Dental Treatment No significant effects or complications reported

Effects on Bleeding No information available to require special precautions

Adverse Effects

>10%: Gastrointestinal: Nausea (2% to 40%), vomiting (28%), constipation (2% to ≥10%)

1% to 10%:

Cardiovascular: Hypotension (2% to 10%), peripheral edema (2% to 10%), tachycardia (4%), bradycardia (2%), syncope (<2%), edema (<2%), hypertension (<2%), pallor (<2%), palpitation (<2%), sinus bradycardia (<2%), supraventricular extrasystoles (<2%), ventricular extrasystoles (<2%), ventricular tachycardia (<2%)

Central nervous system: Insomnia (2% to 10%), dizziness (6%), somnolence (2% to 5%), headache (4%), fever (2%), hypoesthesia (2%), agitation (<2%), anxiety (<2%), chills (<2%), confusion (<2%), depression (<2%), pain (<2%), restlessness (<2%), tremor (<2%), lethargy (1%)

Dermatologic: Pruritus (3%), erythema (<2%), hyperhidrosis (<2%), pruritic rash (<2%), urticaria (<2%)

Genitourinary: Urinary incontinence (<2%), urinary retention (<2%)

Hematologic: Anemia (hemorrhagic, postoperative; 2% to 10%)

Hepatic: AST increased (3%), ALT increased (1%)

Local: Incision site edema (2%)

Neuromuscular & skeletal: Back pain (2% to 10%), muscle spasm (2% to 10%), neck pain (<2%), paresthesia (<2%), weakness (<2%), chondrolysis (continuous intra-articular administration; develops months after surgery)

Ocular: Blurred vision (<2%)

Otic: Tinnitus (<2%)

Renal: Creatinine increased (2%)
Respiratory: Apnea (<2%), hypoxia (<2%), laryngospasm (<2%), respiratory depression/failure (<2%)
Miscellaneous: Feeling of warmth (2%), fungal infection (2%), anaphylactoid reactions (<2%), diaphoresis (<2%), hypersensitivity reactions (<2%)
Frequency not defined:
Cardiovascular: Cardiac arrest, heart block
Central nervous system: Persistent anesthesia, paralysis, seizures
Ocular: Pupillary constriction
General Dosage Range Infiltration (local): *Adults:* 8 mL (106 mg) to 20 mL (266 mg) as a single dose (maximum total dose: 266 mg)
Mechanism of Action Blocks both the initiation and conduction of nerve impulses by decreasing the neuronal membrane's permeability to sodium ions, which results in inhibition of depolarization with resultant blockade of conduction.
Pharmacodynamics/Kinetics
Duration of Action Local: ~24 hours; Systemic: 96 hours
Half-life Elimination Apparent: 24-34 hours
Time to Peak Bunionectomy: 2 hours: Hemorrhoidectomy: 30 minutes
Pregnancy Risk Factor C
Pregnancy Considerations Animal studies have demonstrated teratogenic effects. Use during pregnancy only if the benefits justify the risk to the fetus. Use in obstetrical paracervical block anesthesia is contraindicated.

Buprenorphine (byoo pre NOR feen)

Brand Names: U.S. Buprenex®; Butrans®
Brand Names: Canada Butrans®
Generic Availability (U.S.) Yes: Excludes patch
Pharmacologic Category Analgesic, Opioid; Analgesic, Opioid Partial Agonist
Use
Injection: Management of moderate-to-severe pain
Sublingual tablet: Treatment of opioid dependence
Transdermal patch: Management of moderate-to-severe chronic pain in patients requiring an around-the-clock opioid analgesic for an extended period of time
Unlabeled Use Injection: Management of opioid withdrawal in heroin-dependent hospitalized patients
Local Anesthetic/Vasoconstrictor Precautions No information available to require special precautions
Effects on Dental Treatment No significant effects or complications reported
Effects on Bleeding No information available to require special precautions
Adverse Effects
Injection:
>10%: Central nervous system: Sedation (≤66%)
1% to 10%:
Cardiovascular: Hypotension (1% to 5%)
Central nervous system: Dizziness/vertigo (5% to 10%), headache (1% to 5%)
Gastrointestinal: Nausea (5% to 10%), vomiting (1% to 5%)
Ocular: Miosis (1% to 5%)
Respiratory: Respiratory depression (1% to 5%)
Miscellaneous: Diaphoresis (1% to 5%)

Tablet:
>10%:
Central nervous system: Headache (30%), pain (24%), insomnia (21% to 25%), anxiety (12%), depression (11%)
Gastrointestinal: Nausea (10% to 14%), abdominal pain (12%), constipation (8% to 11%)
Neuromuscular & skeletal: Back pain (14%), weakness (14%)
Respiratory: Rhinitis (11%)
Miscellaneous: Withdrawal syndrome (18% to 22%; placebo 37%), infection (12% to 20%), diaphoresis (12% to 13%)
1% to 10%:
Central nervous system: Chills (6%), nervousness (6%), somnolence (5%), dizziness (4%), fever (3%)
Gastrointestinal: Vomiting (5% to 8%), diarrhea (5%), dyspepsia (3%)
Local: Abscess formation (2%)
Ocular: Lacrimation (5%)
Respiratory: Cough (4%), pharyngitis (4%)
Miscellaneous: Flu-like syndrome (6%)

Transdermal patch:
>10%:
Central nervous system: Headache (3% to 14%), dizziness (2% to 15%), somnolence (2% to 13%)
Gastrointestinal: Nausea (6% to 23%), constipation (3% to 13%)
Local: Application site pruritus (4% to 15%)
1% to 10%:
Cardiovascular: Chest pain (1% to <5%), hypertension (1% to <5%), peripheral edema (1% to <5%)
Central nervous system: Anxiety (1% to <5%), depression (1% to <5%), fatigue (1% to 5%), fever (1% to <5%), hypoesthesia (1% to <5%), insomnia (1% to <5%), migraine (1% to <5%), pain (1% to <5%)
Dermatologic: Hyperhydrosis (1% to <5%), pruritus (1% to <5%), rash (1% to <5%)
Gastrointestinal: Vomiting (4% to 9%), xerostomia (6%), anorexia (1% to <5%), diarrhea (1% to <5%), dyspepsia (1% to <5%), upper abdominal pain (1% to <5%), abdominal discomfort (2%)
Genitourinary: Urinary tract infection (1% to <5%)
Local: Application site erythema (3% to 10%), application site irritation (1% to 6%), application site rash (3% to 8%)
Neuromuscular & skeletal: Arthralgia (1% to <5%), back pain (1% to <5%), joint swelling (1% to <5%), muscle spasms (1% to <5%), musculoskeletal pain (1% to <5%), myalgia (1% to <5%), neck pain (1% to <5%), pain in extremity (1% to <5%), paresthesia (1% to <5%), tremor (1% to <5%), weakness (1% to <5%)
Respiratory: Bronchitis (1% to <5%), cough (1% to <5%), dyspnea (1% to <5%), nasopharyngitis (1% to <5%), pharyngolaryngeal pain (1% to <5%), sinusitis (1% to <5%), upper respiratory tract infection (1% to <5%)
Miscellaneous: Flu-like syndrome (1% to <5%)
Dosage
I.M., I.V.: Acute pain (moderate-to-severe): **Note: Long-term use is not recommended.** The following recommendations are guidelines and do not represent the maximum doses that may be required in all patients. Doses should be titrated to pain relief/prevention. In high-risk patients (eg, elderly, debilitated, presence of respiratory disease) and/or concurrent CNS depressant use, reduce dose by one-half. Buprenorphine has an analgesic ceiling.

Children 2-12 years: I.M., slow I.V.: 2-6 **mcg**/kg every 4-6 hours

Children ≥13 years and Adults:

I.M.: Initial: Opiate-naive: 0.3 mg every 6-8 hours as needed; initial dose (up to 0.3 mg) may be repeated once in 30-60 minutes after the initial dose if needed; usual dosage range: 0.15-0.6 mg every 4-8 hours as needed

Slow I.V.: Initial: Opiate-naive: 0.3 mg every 6-8 hours as needed; initial dose (up to 0.3 mg) may be repeated once in 30-60 minutes after the initial dose if needed

Adults: I.V. infusion: Opiate withdrawal in heroin-dependent hospitalized patients (unlabeled): 0.3-0.9 mg (diluted in 50-100 mL of NS) over 20-30 minutes every 6-12 hours (Welsh, 2002)

Sublingual tablet: Children ≥16 years and Adults: Opioid dependence: **Note:** The combination product, buprenorphine and naloxone, is preferred therapy over buprenorphine monotherapy for induction treatment (and stabilization/maintenance treatment) for short-acting opioid dependence (U.S. Department of Health and Human Services, 2005).

Manufacturer's labeling:

Induction: Day 1: 8 mg; Day 2 and subsequent induction days: 16 mg; usual induction dosage range: 12-16 mg/day (induction usually accomplished over 3-4 days). Treatment should begin at least 4 hours after last use of heroin or other short-acting opioids, preferably when first signs of withdrawal appear. Titrating dose to clinical effectiveness should be done as rapidly as possible to prevent undue withdrawal symptoms and patient drop-out during the induction period. There is little controlled experience with induction in patients on methadone or other long-acting opioids; consult expert physician experienced with this procedure.

Maintenance: Target dose: 16 mg daily; in some patients 12 mg daily may be effective; patients should be switched to the buprenorphine/naloxone combination product for maintenance and unsupervised therapy

Transdermal patch: Adults: Chronic pain (moderate-to-severe):

Opioid-naive patients: Initial: 5 **mcg**/hour applied once every 7 days

Opioid-experienced patients (conversion from other opioids to buprenorphine): Taper the current around-the-clock opioid for up to 7 days to ≤30 mg/day of oral morphine or equivalent before initiating therapy. Short-acting analgesics as needed may be continued until analgesia with transdermal buprenorphine is attained. There is a potential for buprenorphine to precipitate withdrawal in patients already receiving opioids.

Patients who were receiving daily dose of <30 mg of oral morphine equivalents: Initial: 5 **mcg**/hour applied once every 7 days

Patients who were receiving daily dose of 30-80 mg of oral morphine equivalents: Initial: 10 **mcg**/hour applied once every 7 days

Patient who were receiving daily dose of >80 mg of oral morphine equivalents: Buprenorphine transdermal patch, even at the maximum dose of 20 **mcg**/hour applied once every 7 days, may not provide adequate analgesia; **consider the use of an alternate analgesic.**

Dose titration (opioid-naive or opioid-experienced patients): May increase dose, based on patient's supplemental short-acting analgesic requirements,

with a minimum titration interval of 72 hours (maximum dose: 20 **mcg**/hour applied once every 7 days; risk for QT$_c$ prolongation increases with doses ≥20 **mcg**/hour patch).

Discontinuation of therapy: Taper dose gradually every 7 days to prevent withdrawal in the physically dependent patient; consider initiating immediate-release opioids, if needed.

Elderly:

I.M., slow I.V.: 0.15 mg every 6 hours; elderly patients are more likely to suffer from confusion and drowsiness compared to younger patients

Transdermal patch: Chronic pain (moderate-to-severe): No specific dosage adjustments required; use caution due to potential for increased risk of adverse events. Refer to adult dosing.

Dosage adjustment in renal impairment: Injection, sublingual, transdermal: No dosage adjustment provided in manufacturer's labeling (has not been adequately studied); use with caution.

Dosage adjustment in hepatic impairment:

Injection: No dosage adjustment provided in manufacturer's labeling; undergoes extensive hepatic metabolism; use with caution, especially in severe impairment.

Sublingual: Moderate-to-severe impairment: Dosage adjustments recommended; however, no specific recommendations are provided in the manufacturer's labeling.

Transdermal patch:

Mild-to-moderate impairment: Initial: 5 **mcg**/hour applied once every 7 days

Severe impairment: Not studied; consider alternative therapy with more flexibility for dosing adjustments.

Mechanism of Action Buprenorphine exerts its analgesic effect via high affinity binding to μ opiate receptors in the CNS; displays partial mu agonist and weak kappa antagonist activity

Contraindications Hypersensitivity to buprenorphine or any component of the formulation

Transdermal patch: Additional contraindications: Significant respiratory depression; acute or severe asthma; known or suspected paralytic ileus

Warnings/Precautions An opioid-containing analgesic regimen should be tailored to each patient's needs and based upon the type of pain being treated (acute versus chronic), the route of administration, degree of tolerance for opioids (naive versus chronic user), age, weight, and medical condition. The optimal analgesic dose varies widely among patients. Doses should be titrated to pain relief/prevention.

May cause CNS depression, which may impair physical or mental abilities; patients must be cautioned about performing tasks which require mental alertness (eg, operating machinery or driving). Effects with other sedative drugs or ethanol may be potentiated. Elderly may be more sensitive to CNS depressant and constipating effects. May cause respiratory depression - use caution in patients with respiratory disease or pre-existing respiratory depression. Hypersensitivity reactions, including bronchospasm, angioneurotic edema, and anaphylactic shock, have also been reported. Potential for drug dependency exists, abrupt cessation may precipitate withdrawal. Use caution in elderly, debilitated, cachectic, pediatric patients, depression or suicidal tendencies. Tolerance, psychological and physical dependence may occur with prolonged use. Partial antagonist activity may precipitate acute narcotic withdrawal in opioid-dependent individuals.

Hepatitis has been reported with buprenorphine use; hepatic events ranged from transient, asymptomatic transaminase elevations to hepatic failure; in many cases, patients had preexisting hepatic dysfunction. Monitor liver function tests in patients at increased risk for hepatotoxicity (eg, history of alcohol abuse, pre-existing hepatic dysfunction, I.V. drug abusers) prior to and during therapy. Use with caution in patients with hepatic impairment; dosage adjustments are recommended in hepatic impairment.

Use with caution in patients with pulmonary or renal function impairment. Also use caution in patients with head injury or increased ICP, biliary tract dysfunction, patients with history of hyperthyroidism, morbid obesity, adrenal insufficiency, prostatic hyperplasia, urinary stricture, CNS depression, toxic psychosis, pancreatitis, alcoholism, delirium tremens, or kyphoscoliosis. May cause hypotension; use with caution in patients with hypovolemia, cardiovascular disease (including acute MI), or drugs which may exaggerate hypotensive effects (including phenothiazines or general anesthetics). May obscure diagnosis or clinical course of patients with acute abdominal conditions. Use with caution in patients with a history of ileus or bowel obstruction; use of transdermal patch is contraindicated in patients with known or suspected paralytic ileus. Opioid therapy may lower seizure threshold; use caution in patients with a history of seizure disorders.

Transdermal patch: Indicated for the management of chronic moderate-to-severe pain when around the clock pain control is needed for an extended time period; should not be used for as-needed pain relief or for the treatment of mild pain, acute pain, or postoperative pain requiring short-term opioid analgesia. **[U.S. Boxed Warning]: May cause potentially life-threatening respiratory depression even with therapeutic use. Ensure proper dosing and titration; monitor for respiratory depression, especially within the first 24-72 hours of initiation or dose escalation. Buprenorphine transdermal patches should only be prescribed by healthcare professionals familiar with the use of potent opioids for chronic pain.** Do not exceed one 20 **mcg**/hour transdermal patch due to the risk of QTc-interval prolongation. Avoid using in patients with history of long QT syndrome or in patients with predisposing factors increasing the risk of QT abnormalities (eg, concurrent medications such as antiarrhythmics, hypokalemia, unstable heart failure, unstable atrial fibrillation). **[U.S. Boxed Warning]: Healthcare provider should be alert to problems of abuse, misuse, and diversion.** Risk of opioid abuse is increased in patients with a history or family history of alcohol or drug abuse or mental illness. **[U.S. Boxed Warning]: Proper storage, handling, and disposal of used patches are essential to prevent accidental exposures, especially in children; accidental exposure may result in a fatal overdose.** To properly dispose of Butrans® patch, fold it over on itself and flush down the toilet; alternatively, seal the used patch in the provided Patch-Disposal Unit and dispose of in the trash. Avoid exposure of application site and surrounding area to direct external heat sources. Buprenorphine release from the patch is temperature-dependent and may result in overdose. Patients who experience fever or increase in core temperature should be monitored closely. Application site reactions, including rare cases of severe reactions (eg, vesicles, discharge,"burns"), have been observed with use; onset varies from days to months after initiation; patients should be instructed to report severe reactions promptly. Therapy with the transdermal patch is not appropriate for use in the management of addictions.

Concurrent use of agonist/antagonist analgesics may precipitate withdrawal symptoms and/or reduced analgesic efficacy in patients following prolonged therapy with mu opioid agonists. Abrupt discontinuation following prolonged use may also lead to withdrawal symptoms and is not recommended; taper dose gradually when discontinuing.

Sublingual tablets, which are used for induction treatment of opioid dependence, should not be started until effects of withdrawal are evident.

Drug Interactions
Metabolism/Transport Effects Substrate of CYP3A4 (major); **Note:** Assignment of Major/Minor substrate status based on clinically relevant drug interaction potential; **Inhibits** CYP1A2 (weak), CYP2A6 (weak), CYP2C19 (weak), CYP2D6 (weak)

Avoid Concomitant Use
Avoid concomitant use of Buprenorphine with any of the following: Atazanavir; Azelastine (Nasal); Conivaptan; MAO Inhibitors; Paraldehyde

Increased Effect/Toxicity
Buprenorphine may increase the levels/effects of: Alvimopan; ARIPiprazole; Azelastine (Nasal); Desmopressin; MAO Inhibitors; Metyrosine; Mirtazapine; Paraldehyde; Pramipexole; ROPINIRole; Rotigotine; Selective Serotonin Reuptake Inhibitors; Thiazide Diuretics; Zolpidem

The levels/effects of Buprenorphine may be increased by: Alcohol (Ethyl); Amphetamines; Antipsychotic Agents (Phenothiazines); Atazanavir; Boceprevir; CNS Depressants; Conivaptan; CYP3A4 Inhibitors (Moderate); CYP3A4 Inhibitors (Strong); Dasatinib; Droperidol; HydrOXYzine; Ivacaftor; Magnesium Sulfate; Mifepristone; Perampanel; Sodium Oxybate; Succinylcholine

Decreased Effect
Buprenorphine may decrease the levels/effects of: Analgesics (Opioid); Atazanavir; Pegvisomant

The levels/effects of Buprenorphine may be decreased by: Ammonium Chloride; Boceprevir; CYP3A4 Inducers (Strong); Deferasirox; Efavirenz; Etravirine; Herbs (CYP3A4 Inducers); Mixed Agonist / Antagonist Opioids; Tocilizumab

Ethanol/Nutrition/Herb Interactions
Ethanol: May increase CNS depression; monitor for increased effects with coadministration. Caution patients about effect.

Herb/Nutraceutical: Avoid valerian, St John's wort, kava kava, gotu kola (may increase CNS depression).

Pharmacodynamics/Kinetics
Onset of Action Analgesic: I.M: Within 15 minutes; Peak effect: I.M.: ~1 hour; Transdermal patch: Steady state achieved by day 3

Duration of Action I.M.: ≥6 hours

Half-life Elimination I.V.: 2.2-3 hours; Apparent terminal half-life: Sublingual tablet: ~37 hours; Transdermal patch: ~26 hours. **Note:** Extended elimination half-life for sublingual administration may be due to depot effect (Kuhlman, 1996).

Time to Peak Plasma: Sublingual: 30 minutes to 1 hour (Kuhlman, 1996)

Pregnancy Risk Factor C

Pregnancy Considerations Adverse effects have been observed in animal reproduction studies following buprenorphine subcutaneous and transdermal administration. In humans, withdrawal has been reported in infants of women receiving buprenorphine during pregnancy. Onset of symptoms ranged from day 1 to day 8 of life, most occurring on day 1.

Lactation Enters breast milk/not recommended

Controlled Substance C-III

Prescribing and Access Restrictions Prescribing of tablets for opioid dependence is limited to physicians who have met the qualification criteria and have received a DEA number specific to prescribing this product. Tablets will be available through pharmacies and wholesalers which normally provide controlled substances.

Dosage Forms

Injection, solution: 0.3 mg/mL (1 mL)
  Buprenex®: 0.3 mg/mL (1 mL)

Injection, solution [preservative free]: 0.3 mg/mL (1 mL)

Patch, transdermal:
  Butrans®: 5 mcg/hr (4s); 10 mcg/hr (4s); 20 mcg/hr (4s)

Tablet, sublingual: 2 mg, 8 mg

Buprenorphine and Naloxone
(byoo pre NOR feen & nal OKS one)

Related Information
  Buprenorphine *on page 212*
  Naloxone *on page 955*

Brand Names: U.S. Suboxone®

Brand Names: Canada Suboxone®

Pharmacologic Category Analgesic, Opioid; Analgesic, Opioid Partial Agonist

Use Maintenance treatment for opioid dependence

Local Anesthetic/Vasoconstrictor Precautions No information available to require special precautions

Effects on Dental Treatment No significant effects or complications reported

Effects on Bleeding No information available to require special precautions

Adverse Effects Also see individual agents.
>10%:
  Central nervous system: Headache (36%), pain (22%)
  Gastrointestinal: Vomiting (8%), erythema (oral mucosa; film), glossodynia (film), oral hypoesthesia (film)
  Miscellaneous: Withdrawal syndrome (25%; placebo 37%), diaphoresis (14%)
1% to 10%:
  Cardiovascular: Vasodilation (9%)
  Gastrointestinal: Vomiting (7%)

General Dosage Range Sublingual: *Children ≥16 years and Adults:* 4-24 mg daily (target dose: 16 mg daily)

Mechanism of Action See individual agents.

Pharmacodynamics/Kinetics

Half-life Elimination Film: Buprenorphine: 24-42 hours; Naloxone: 2-12 hours

Pregnancy Risk Factor C

Pregnancy Considerations Withdrawal has been reported in infants of women receiving buprenorphine during pregnancy. Onset of symptoms ranged from day 1 to day 8 of life, most occurring on day 1.

Controlled Substance C-III

Prescribing and Access Restrictions Prescribing of tablets for opioid dependence is limited to physicians who have met the qualification criteria and have received a DEA number specific to prescribing this product. Tablets will be available through pharmacies and wholesalers which normally provide controlled substances.

BuPROPion (byoo PROE pee on)

Related Information
  Vasoconstrictor Interactions With Antidepressants *on page 1650*

Brand Names: U.S. Aplenzin™; Budeprion SR®; Budeprion XL® [DSC]; Buproban®; Forfivo™ XL; Wellbutrin SR®; Wellbutrin XL®; Wellbutrin®; Zyban®

Brand Names: Canada Ava-Bupropion SR; Bupropion SR®; Novo-Bupropion SR; PMS-Bupropion SR; ratio-Bupropion SR; Sandoz-Bupropion SR; Wellbutrin® SR; Wellbutrin® XL; Zyban®

Generic Availability (U.S.) Yes: Excludes bupropion hydrobromide tablet, extended release bupropion hydrochloride 450 mg tablet, sustained release hydrochloride tablet

Pharmacologic Category Antidepressant, Dopamine-Reuptake Inhibitor; Smoking Cessation Aid

Use Treatment of major depressive disorder, including seasonal affective disorder (SAD); adjunct in smoking cessation (Buproban®, Zyban®)

Unlabeled Use Attention-deficit/hyperactivity disorder (ADHD); depression associated with bipolar disorder

Local Anesthetic/Vasoconstrictor Precautions Part of the mechanism of bupropion is to block reuptake of norepinephrine along with dopamine. Because of the potential for norepinephrine elevation within CNS synapses, it is suggested that vasoconstrictor be administered with caution and to monitor vital signs in dental patients taking antidepressants that affect norepinephrine in this way.

Effects on Dental Treatment Key adverse event(s) related to dental treatment: Abnormal taste, significant xerostomia (normal salivary flow resumes with discontinuation).

Effects on Bleeding Thrombocytopenia (<1%) as been reported.

Adverse Effects Frequencies, when reported, reflect highest incidence reported with sustained release product.

>10%:
  Cardiovascular: Tachycardia (11%)
  Central nervous system: Headache (25% to 34%), insomnia (11% to 20%), dizziness (6% to 11%)
  Gastrointestinal: Xerostomia (17% to 26%), weight loss (14% to 23%), nausea (1% to 18%)
  Respiratory: Pharyngitis (3% to 13%)
1% to 10%:
  Cardiovascular: Palpitation (2% to 6%), arrhythmias (5%), chest pain (3% to 4%), hypertension (2% to 4%; may be severe), flushing (1% to 4%), hypotension (3%)
  Central nervous system: Agitation (2% to 9%), confusion (8%), anxiety (5% to 7%), hostility (6%), nervousness (3% to 5%), sleep disturbance (4%), sensory disturbance (4%), migraine (1% to 4%), abnormal dreams (3%), irritability (2% to 3%), somnolence (2% to 3%), pain (2% to 3%), memory decreased (≤3%), fever (1% to 2%), CNS stimulation (1% to 2%), depression

Dermatologic: Rash (1% to 5%), pruritus (2% to 4%), urticaria (1% to 2%)

Endocrine & metabolic: Menstrual complaints (2% to 5%), hot flashes (1% to 3%), libido decreased (3%)

Gastrointestinal: Constipation (5% to 10%), abdominal pain (2% to 9%), diarrhea (5% to 7%), flatulence (6%), anorexia (3% to 5%), appetite increased (4%), taste perversion (2% to 4%), vomiting (2% to 4%), dyspepsia (3%), dysphagia (≤2%)

Genitourinary: Polyuria (2% to 5%), urinary urgency (≤2%), vaginal hemorrhage (≤2%), UTI (≤1%)

Neuromuscular & skeletal: Tremor (3% to 6%), myalgia (2% to 6%), weakness (2% to 4%), arthralgia (1% to 4%), arthritis (2%), akathisia (≤2%), paresthesia (1% to 2%), twitching (1% to 2%), neck pain

Ocular: Blurred vision (2% to 3%), amblyopia (2%)

Otic: Tinnitus (3% to 6%), auditory disturbance (5%)

Respiratory: Upper respiratory infection (9%), cough increased (1% to 4%), sinusitis (1% to 5%)

Miscellaneous: Infection (8% to 9%), diaphoresis (5% to 6%), allergic reaction (including anaphylaxis, pruritus, urticaria)

Dosage Oral:

Children and Adolescents: ADHD (unlabeled use): Hydrochloride salt: 1.4-6 mg/kg/day (Barrickman, 1995; Conners, 1996)

Adults:

Depression: **Note:**Treatment should be periodically evaluated at appropriate intervals to ensure lowest effective dose is used.

Immediate release hydrochloride salt: Initial: 100 mg twice daily; after 3 days may increase to the usual dose of 100 mg 3 times a day; if no clinical improvement after several weeks, may increase to a maximum dose of 150 mg 3 times daily

Sustained release hydrochloride salt: Initial: 150 mg daily in the morning; if tolerated, as early as day 4, may increase to a target dose of 150 mg twice daily; if no clinical improvement after several weeks, may increase to a maximum dose of 200 mg twice daily

Extended release:

Hydrochloride salt: Initial: 150 mg once daily in the morning; if tolerated, as early as day 4, may increase to 300 mg once daily; if no clinical improvement after several weeks, may increase to a maximum dose 450 mg once daily. **Note:** Forfivo™ XL may only be used after initial dose titration with other bupropion products.

Hydrochloride salt (Forfivo™ XL): *Switching from Wellbutrin® immediate release, SR®, or XL® to Forfivo™ XL:* Patients receiving 300 mg daily of bupropion hydrochloride for at least 2 weeks and requiring a dose increase or patients already taking 450 mg daily of bupropion hydrochloride may switch to Forfivo™ XL 450 mg once daily.

Hydrobromide salt (Aplenzin™): Initial: 174 mg once daily in the morning; may increase as early as day 4 of dosing to 348 mg once daily (target dose); maximum dose: 522 mg daily. **Note:** In patients receiving 348 mg once daily, taper dose down to 174 mg once daily prior to discontinuing.

Switching from hydrochloride salt formulation (eg, Wellbutrin® immediate release, SR®, XL®, or Forfivo™ XL) to hydrobromide salt formulation (Aplenzin™):

Bupropion hydrochloride 150 mg daily is equivalent to bupropion hydrobromide 174 mg once daily

Bupropion hydrochloride 300 mg daily is equivalent to bupropion hydrobromide 348 mg once daily

Bupropion hydrochloride 450 mg daily is equivalent to bupropion hydrobromide 522 mg once daily

SAD: Initial: 150 mg once daily (Wellbutrin XL®) or 174 mg once daily (Aplenzin™) in the morning; if tolerated, may increase after 1 week to 300 mg once daily (Wellbutrin XL®) or 348 mg once daily (Aplenzin™) in the morning.

Note: Prophylactic treatment should be reserved for those patients with frequent depressive episodes and/or significant impairment. Initiate treatment in the Autumn prior to symptom onset, and discontinue in early Spring with dose tapering to 150 mg once daily for 2 weeks (Wellbutrin XL®) or 174 mg once daily (Aplenzin™), then discontinue. Doses >300 mg daily (Wellbutrin XL®) or >348 mg daily (Aplenzin™) have not been studied in SAD.

Smoking cessation (Zyban®, Buproban®): Initial: 150 mg once daily for 3 days; increase to 150 mg twice daily; treatment should continue for 7-12 weeks

Note: Therapy should begin at least 1 week before target quit date. Target quit dates are generally in the second week of treatment. If patient successfully quits smoking after 7-12 weeks, may consider ongoing maintenance therapy based on individual patient risk:benefit. Efficacy of maintenance therapy (300 mg daily) has been demonstrated for up to 6 months. Conversely, if significant progress has not been made by the seventh week of therapy, success is unlikely and treatment discontinuation should be considered.

Elderly:

Depression: Oral (hydrochloride salt): Initial: 37.5 mg of immediate release tablets twice daily or 100 mg daily of sustained release tablets; increase by 37.5-100 mg every 3-4 days as tolerated to a maximum dose of 300 mg/day (in divided doses). There is evidence that the elderly respond at 150 mg daily in divided doses, but some may require a higher dose. **Note:** Patients with Alzheimer's dementia-related depression may require a lower starting dosage of 37.5 mg once or twice daily (100 mg daily sustained release), increased as needed up to 300 mg daily in divided doses (300 mg daily for sustained release) (Rabins, 2007).

Smoking cessation: Refer to adult dosing.

Dosing conversion between hydrochloride salt immediate (Wellbutrin®), sustained (Wellbutrin SR®), and extended release (Wellbutrin XL®, Forfivo™ XL) products: Convert using same total daily dose (up to the maximum recommended dose for a given dosage form), but adjust frequency as indicated for sustained (twice daily) or extended (once daily) release products.

MAO inhibitor recommendations:

Switching to or from an MAO inhibitor antidepressant:

Allow 14 days to elapse between discontinuing an MAO inhibitor intended to treat depression and initiation of bupropion.

Allow 14 days to elapse between discontinuing bupropion and initiation of an MAO inhibitor intended to treat depression.

Use with reversible MAO inhibitors (such as linezolid or I.V. methylene blue):

Do not initiate bupropion in patients receiving linezolid or I.V. methylene blue; consider other interventions for psychiatric condition.

If urgent treatment with linezolid or I.V. methylene blue is required in a patient already receiving bupropion and potential benefits outweigh potential risks, discontinue bupropion promptly and administer linezolid or I.V. methylene blue. Monitor for increased risk of hypertensive reactions for 2 weeks or until 24 hours after the last dose of linezolid or I.V. methylene blue, whichever comes first. May resume bupropion 24 hours after the last dose of linezolid or I.V. methylene blue.

Dosing adjustment/comments in renal impairment: Use with caution and consider a reduction in dosing frequency; limited pharmacokinetic information suggests elimination of bupropion and/or the active metabolites may be reduced.

Moderate-to-severe renal impairment: Bupropion exposure was approximately twofold higher compared to normal subjects following a 150 mg single dose administration.

End-stage renal failure: Per the manufacturer, the elimination of hydroxybupropion and threohydrobupropion are reduced in patients with end-stage renal failure.

Forfivo™ XL: Use is not recommended.

Dosing adjustment in hepatic impairment:
Note: The mean AUC increased by ~1.5-fold for hydroxybupropion and ~2.5-fold for erythro/threohydrobupropion; median T_{max} was observed 19 hours later for hydroxybupropion, 31 hours later for erythro/threohydrobupropion; mean half-life for hydroxybupropion increased fivefold, and increased twofold for erythro/threohydrobupropion in patients with severe hepatic cirrhosis compared to healthy volunteers.

Mild-to-moderate hepatic impairment: Use with caution; consider a reduced dose and/or frequency.

Forfivo™ XL: Use is not recommended.

Severe hepatic cirrhosis: Use with extreme caution; maximum dose:

Aplenzin™: 174 mg every other day

Buproban®, Zyban®: 150 mg every other day

Forfivo™ XL: Use is not recommended.

Wellbutrin®: 75 mg once daily

Wellbutrin SR®: 100 mg once daily or 150 mg every other day

Wellbutrin XL®: 150 mg every other day

Mechanism of Action Aminoketone antidepressant structurally different from all other marketed antidepressants; like other antidepressants the mechanism of bupropion's activity is not fully understood. Bupropion is a relatively weak inhibitor of the neuronal uptake of norepinephrine and dopamine, and does not inhibit monoamine oxidase or the reuptake of serotonin. Metabolite inhibits the reuptake of norepinephrine. The primary mechanism of action is thought to be dopaminergic and/or noradrenergic.

Contraindications Hypersensitivity to bupropion or any component of the formulation; seizure disorder; history of anorexia/bulimia; patients undergoing abrupt discontinuation of ethanol or sedatives, including benzodiazepines; use of MAO inhibitors or MAO inhibitors intended to treat psychiatric disorders (concurrently or within 14 days of discontinuing either bupropion or the MAO inhibitor); initiation of bupropion in a patient receiving linezolid or intravenous methylene blue; patients receiving other dosage forms of bupropion

Aplenzin™: Additional contraindications: Other conditions that increase seizure risk, including arteriovenous malformation, severe head injury, severe stroke, CNS

tumor, CNS infection, or abrupt discontinuation of barbiturates or antiepileptics

Warnings/Precautions [U.S. Boxed Warning]: Use in treating psychiatric disorders: Antidepressants increase the risk of suicidal thinking and behavior in children, adolescents, and young adults (18-24 years of age) with major depressive disorder (MDD) and other psychiatric disorders; consider risk prior to prescribing. Short-term studies did not show an increased risk in patients >24 years of age and showed a decreased risk in patients ≥65 years. All patients must be closely monitored for clinical worsening, suicidality, or unusual changes in behavior, especially during the initiation of therapy (generally first 1-2 months) or following an increase or decrease in dosage. The patient's family or caregiver should be instructed to closely observe the patient and communicate condition with healthcare provider. A medication guide should be dispensed with each prescription. **Bupropion is not FDA approved for use in children.**

[U.S. Boxed Warning]: Use in smoking cessation: Serious neuropsychiatric events, including depression, suicidal thoughts, and suicide, have been reported with use; some cases may have been complicated by symptoms of nicotine withdrawal following smoking cessation. Smoking cessation (with or without treatment) is associated with nicotine withdrawal symptoms and the exacerbation of underlying psychiatric illness; however, some of the behavioral disturbances were reported in treated patients who continued to smoke. These neuropsychiatric symptoms (eg, mood disturbances, psychosis, hostility) have occurred in patients with and without pre-existing psychiatric disease; many cases resolved following therapy discontinuation although in some cases, symptoms persisted. Monitor all patients for behavioral changes and psychiatric symptoms (eg, agitation, depression, suicidal behavior, suicidal ideation); inform patients to discontinue treatment and contact their healthcare provider immediately if they experience any behavioral and/or mood changes.

The possibility of a suicide attempt is inherent in major depression and may persist until remission occurs. Use caution in high-risk patients. Worsening depression and severe abrupt suicidality that are not part of the presenting symptoms may require discontinuation or modification of drug therapy. The patient's family or caregiver should be alerted to monitor patients for the emergence of suicidality and associated behaviors (such as agitation, irritability, hostility, impulsivity, and hypomania) and notify the healthcare provider.

May worsen psychosis in some patients or precipitate a shift to mania or hypomania in patients with bipolar disorder. Patients presenting with depressive symptoms should be screened for bipolar disorder. Monotherapy in patients with bipolar disorder should be avoided. **Bupropion is not FDA approved for bipolar depression.**

May cause a dose-related risk of seizures. Use is contraindicated in patients with a history of seizures or certain conditions with high seizure risk (eg, arteriovenous malformation, severe head injury, severe stroke, CNS tumor, or CNS infection, history of anorexia/bulimia, or patients undergoing abrupt discontinuation of ethanol, benzodiazepines, barbiturates, or antiepileptic drugs). Use caution with concurrent use of antipsychotics, antidepressants, theophylline, systemic corticosteroids, stimulants (including cocaine), anorectants, or hypoglycemic agents, or with excessive use of ethanol, ▶

◀ benzodiazepines, sedative/hypnotics, or opioids. Use with caution in seizure-potentiating metabolic disorders (hypoglycemia, hyponatremia, severe hepatic impairment, and hypoxia). The dose-dependent risk of seizures may be reduced by gradual dose increases and limiting the daily dose to bupropion hydrochloride ≤450 mg or bupropion hydrobromide ≤522 mg. Use of multiple bupropion formulations is contraindicated. Permanently discontinue if seizure occurs during therapy. Chewing, crushing, or dividing long-acting products may increase seizure risk.

May cause CNS stimulation (restlessness, anxiety, insomnia) or anorexia. May increase the risks associated with electroconvulsive therapy (ECT). Consider discontinuing, when possible, prior to ECT. May cause weight loss; use caution in patients where weight loss is not desirable. The incidence of sexual dysfunction with bupropion is generally lower than with SSRIs.

Use caution in patients with cardiovascular disease, history of hypertension, or coronary artery disease; treatment-emergent hypertension (including some severe cases) has been reported, both with bupropion alone and in combination with nicotine transdermal systems. All children diagnosed with ADHD who may be candidates for stimulant medications should have a thorough cardiovascular assessment to identify risk factors for sudden cardiac death prior to initiation of drug therapy. Use with caution in patients with hepatic or renal dysfunction and in elderly patients; reduced dose and/or frequency may be recommended. Elderly patients may be at greater risk of accumulation during chronic dosing. May cause motor or cognitive impairment in some patients; use with caution if tasks requiring alertness such as operating machinery or driving are undertaken. Anaphylactoid/anaphylactic reactions have occurred, with symptoms of pruritus, urticaria, angioedema, and dyspnea. Serious reactions have been (rarely) reported, including Stevens-Johnson syndrome and anaphylactic shock. Arthralgia, myalgia, and fever with rash and other symptoms suggestive of delayed hypersensitivity resembling serum sickness have been reported. Potentially significant interactions may exist, requiring dose or frequency adjustment, additional monitoring, and/or selection of alternative therapy.

Extended release tablet: Insoluble tablet shell may remain intact and be visible in the stool.

Drug Interactions

Metabolism/Transport Effects Substrate of CYP1A2 (minor), CYP2A6 (minor), CYP2B6 (major), CYP2C9 (minor), CYP2D6 (minor), CYP2E1 (minor), CYP3A4 (minor); **Note:** Assignment of Major/Minor substrate status based on clinically relevant drug interaction potential; **Inhibits** CYP2D6 (strong)

Avoid Concomitant Use
Avoid concomitant use of BuPROPion with any of the following: MAO Inhibitors; Methylene Blue; Pimozide; Tamoxifen; Thioridazine

Increased Effect/Toxicity
BuPROPion may increase the levels/effects of: Alcohol (Ethyl); ARIPiprazole; AtoMOXetine; CYP2D6 Substrates; Fesoterodine; Iloperidone; Lorcaserin; Methylene Blue; Metoprolol; Nebivolol; Pimozide; Propafenone; Tetrabenazine; Thioridazine; Tricyclic Antidepressants

The levels/effects of BuPROPion may be increased by: Alcohol (Ethyl); CYP2B6 Inhibitors (Moderate); CYP2B6 Inhibitors (Strong); MAO Inhibitors; Mifepristone; Quazepam

Decreased Effect
BuPROPion may decrease the levels/effects of: Codeine; Iloperidone; Ioflupane I 123; Tamoxifen; TraMADol

The levels/effects of BuPROPion may be decreased by: CYP2B6 Inducers (Strong); Efavirenz; Lopinavir; Peginterferon Alfa-2b; Ritonavir

Ethanol/Nutrition/Herb Interactions
Ethanol: May increase CNS depression; monitor for increased effects with coadministration. Caution patients about effects.
Herb/Nutraceutical: Avoid valerian, St John's wort, SAMe, gotu kola, kava kava (may increase CNS depression).

Pharmacodynamics/Kinetics

Half-life Elimination
Distribution: 3-4 hours
Elimination: ~14 hours (range: 8-24 hours); Metabolites: Hydroxybupropion: 20 ± 5 hours; Erythrohydrobupropion: 33 ± 10 hours; Threohydrobupropion: 37 ± 13 hours
Extended release (Aplenzin™): 21 ± 7 hours; Metabolites: Hydroxybupropion: 24 ± 5 hours; Erythrohydrobupropion: 31 ± 8 hours; Threohydrobupropion: 51 ± 9 hours

Time to Peak
Bupropion: Immediate release: Within 2 hours; Sustained release: Within 3 hours; Extended release: ~5 hours (Forfivo™ XL: 5 hours [fasting]; 12 hours [fed])
Metabolite: Hydroxybupropion: Immediate release: ~3 hours; Extended release, sustained release: ~6-7 hours

Pregnancy Risk Factor C
Pregnancy Considerations Due to adverse events observed in some animal studies, bupropion is classified as pregnancy category C. A significant increase in major teratogenic effects has not been observed following exposure to bupropion during pregnancy; however, the risk of spontaneous abortions may be increased (additional studies are needed to confirm). The long-term effects on development and behavior have not been studied.

Pregnancy itself does not provide protection against depression. The ACOG recommends that therapy with antidepressants during pregnancy be individualized and should incorporate the clinical expertise of the mental health clinician, obstetrician, primary care provider, and pediatrician. If treatment is needed, consider gradually stopping antidepressants 10-14 days before the expected date of delivery to prevent potential withdrawal symptoms in the infant. If this is done and the woman is considered to be at risk of relapse from her major depressive disorder, the medication can be restarted following delivery, although the dose should be readjusted to that required before pregnancy. Bupropion has also been evaluated for smoking cessation during pregnancy; current recommendations suggest that pharmacologic treatments be considered only after other therapies have failed. Treatment algorithms have been developed by the ACOG and the APA for the management of depression in women prior to conception and during pregnancy (Yonkers, 2009).

Lactation Enters breast milk/use caution (AAP rates "of concern"; AAP 2001 update pending)
Breast-Feeding Considerations Bupropion and its metabolites are excreted into breast milk, although neither bupropion nor its metabolites have been detected in the plasma of breast-fed infants. Adverse events have not been reported in older breast-fed

infants; however, a seizure was noted in one 6-month old infant (a causal effect could not be confirmed). In a study of 10 women, estimated infant exposure was 2% of the weight-adjusted maternal dose. Use caution and consider risks of discontinuing therapy in nursing mothers.

Dosage Forms

Tablet, oral: 75 mg, 100 mg
  Wellbutrin®: 75 mg, 100 mg
Tablet, extended release, oral: 100 mg, 150 mg, 200 mg, 300 mg
  Aplenzin™: 174 mg, 348 mg, 522 mg
  Budeprion SR®: 100 mg, 150 mg
  Buproban®: 150 mg
  Forfivo™ XL: 450 mg
  Wellbutrin XL®: 150 mg, 300 mg
Tablet, sustained release, oral:
  Wellbutrin SR®: 100 mg, 150 mg, 200 mg
  Zyban®: 150 mg

Buserelin (BYOO se rel in)

Brand Names: Canada Suprefact®; Suprefact® Depot
Pharmacologic Category Gonadotropin Releasing Hormone Agonist
Use Palliative treatment in patients with hormone-dependent advanced prostate cancer (stage D); treatment of endometriosis in women who do not require surgical intervention as first-line therapy (length of therapy is usually 6 months, but no longer than 9 months)
Unlabeled Use Diagnostic test for hypogonadotropic hypogonadism in males with delayed puberty
Local Anesthetic/Vasoconstrictor Precautions Buserelin may cause hypertension and palpitations. Monitor blood pressure prior to dental procedures if using local anesthesia with vasoconstrictor. There have been no reports of any direct interaction with buserelin and vasoconstrictor.
Effects on Dental Treatment No significant effects or complications reported
Effects on Bleeding No information available to require special precautions
Adverse Effects Note: Adverse reaction profile differs based on population/medication and route of administration.
Depot:
>10%:
  Endocrine & metabolic: Hot flushes (14% to 23%)
  Genitourinary: Impotence (2% to 23%)
  Neuromuscular & skeletal: Weakness (<1% to 14%)
1% to 10%:
  Cardiovascular: Hypertension (2% to 9%), palpitation (5%), edema (1%)
  Central nervous system: Dizziness (5%), insomnia (<1% to 5%), depression (2%), pain (2%)
  Endocrine & metabolic: Libido decreased (2% to 5%)
  Gastrointestinal: Appetite increased (5%), nausea (5%)
  Local: Injection site reaction (1% to 5%)
  Neuromuscular & skeletal: Arthralgia (5%), myalgia (5%)

SubQ or intranasal:
>10%:
  Central nervous system: Headache (20% to 29%)
  Endocrine & metabolic: Libido decreased (12% to 85%), hot flushes (66% to 72%), vaginal dryness (29%), menorrhagia (24%)
  Genitourinary: Impotence (75% to 80%)
  Local: Injection site reaction: (8% to 12%)

1% to 10%:
  Cardiovascular: Edema (1% to 5%), palpitation (1% to 5%)
  Central nervous system: Dizziness (9%), depression (8%), emotional lability (7%), anxiety (1% to 5%), hostility (1% to 5%), insomnia (1% to 5%), migraine (1% to 5%), nervousness (1% to 5%), pain (1% to 5%), malaise, sleep disorder
  Dermatologic: Acne (5%), dry skin (1% to 5%), purpura (1% to 5%), skin disorder (1% to 5%), flare reaction (1% to 2%), pruritus
  Endocrine & metabolic: Breast pain (1% to 5%), hirsutism (1% to 5%), menstrual disorder (1% to 5%), gynecomastia (1% to 2%), premenstrual syndrome
  Gastrointestinal: Nausea (5% to 7%), constipation (1% to 5%), diarrhea (1% to 5%), gastrointestinal fullness (1% to 5%), taste perversion (1% to 5%), weight loss/gain (1% to 5%), xerostomia (1% to 2%), flatulence, sore throat, vomiting
  Genitourinary: Dyspareunia (1% to 5%), vaginitis (1% to 5%), leukorrhea, pelvic pain, vaginal discharge, vaginal discomfort
  Neuromuscular & skeletal: Weakness (7%), arthralgia (1% to 5%), myalgia (1% to 5%), neck rigidity (1% to 5%), paresthesia (1% to 5%), back pain
  Respiratory: Upper respiratory infection (1% to 5%), rhinitis (1% to 5%), dry nose (1% to 2%)
  Miscellaneous: Diaphoresis (1% to 2%), infection

General Dosage Range
Intranasal: *Adults*: 400 mcg (200 mcg into each nostril) 3 times/day
SubQ: *Adults*:
  Implants: 6.3 mg every 8 weeks **or** 9.45 mg every 12 weeks
  Injection: Initial: 500 mcg every 8 hours for 7 days; maintenance: 200 mcg once daily
Mechanism of Action Synthetic peptide analog of Gonadotropin hormone releasing hormone (GnRH) with substitutions at positions 6 and 10; altered peptide structure results in a significantly magnified GnRH agonist effect with an extended duration of activity. Following an initial rise in the pituitary gonadotropins luteinizing hormone (LH) and follicle-stimulating hormone (FSH), chronic administration of buserelin results in a sustained suppression of LH and FSH and an interference with the production of ovarian and testicular steroids. Eventually, a decline in gonadal steroids to castration levels is observed.
Pharmacodynamics/Kinetics
Half-life Elimination 70-80 minutes; Depot implants: 20-30 Days
Time to Peak Depot: <1 day
Pregnancy Considerations Buserelin is contraindicated in pregnant women. Patients should employ a nonhormonal method of contraception during therapy. Ovulation may occur with a missed dose; in the event a patient conceives, therapy should be discontinued.
Product Availability Not available in U.S.

BusPIRone (byoo SPYE rone)

Related Information
  Management of the Patient With Anxiety or Depression *on page 1594*
Brand Names: Canada Apo-Buspirone®; BuSpar®; Bustab®; Dom-Buspirone; Novo-Buspirone; Nu-Buspirone; PMS-Buspirone; Riva-Buspirone
Generic Availability (U.S.) Yes

Pharmacologic Category Antianxiety Agent, Miscellaneous

Use Management of generalized anxiety disorder (GAD)

Unlabeled Use Management of aggression in mental retardation and secondary mental disorders; major depression; potential augmenting agent for antidepressants; premenstrual syndrome

Local Anesthetic/Vasoconstrictor Precautions No information available to require special precautions

Effects on Dental Treatment Key adverse event(s) related to dental treatment: Xerostomia (normal salivary flow resumes upon discontinuation).

Effects on Bleeding No information available to require special precautions

Adverse Effects

>10%: Central nervous system: Dizziness (12%)

1% to 10%:
Cardiovascular: Chest pain (≥1%)
Central nervous system: Drowsiness (10%), headache (6%), nervousness (5%), lightheadedness (3%), anger/hostility (2%), confusion (2%), excitement (2%), dream disturbance (≥1%)
Dermatologic: Rash (1%)
Gastrointestinal: Nausea (8%), diarrhea (2%)
Neuromuscular & skeletal: Numbness (2%), weakness (2%), incoordination (1%), musculoskeletal pain (1%), paresthesia (1%), tremor (1%)
Ocular: Blurred vision (2%)
Otic: Tinnitus (≥1%)
Respiratory: Nasal congestion (≥1%), sore throat (≥1%)
Miscellaneous: Diaphoresis (1%)

Dosage Oral:

Generalized anxiety disorder (GAD): Adults: Oral: Initial: 7.5 mg twice daily; may increase every 2-3 days in increments of 2.5 mg twice daily to a maximum of 30 mg twice daily; a dose of 10-15 mg twice daily was most often used in clinical trials that allowed for dose titration

Augmentation agent for antidepressants (unlabeled use): Adults: Oral: Initial: 7.5 mg twice daily; may increase weekly in increments of 7.5 mg twice daily to a maximum of 30 mg twice daily (Trivedi, 2006).

Dosing adjustment in renal impairment: Patients with impaired renal function demonstrated increased plasma levels and a prolonged half-life of buspirone. Use in patients with severe renal impairment not recommended.

Dosing adjustment in hepatic impairment: Patients with impaired hepatic function demonstrated increased plasma levels and a prolonged half-life of buspirone. Use in patients with severe hepatic impairment not recommended.

Mechanism of Action The mechanism of action of buspirone is unknown. Buspirone has a high affinity for serotonin $5\text{-}HT_{1A}$ and $5\text{-}HT_2$ receptors, without affecting benzodiazepine-GABA receptors. Buspirone has moderate affinity for dopamine D_2 receptors.

Contraindications Hypersensitivity to buspirone or any component of the formulation

Warnings/Precautions Use in severe hepatic or renal impairment is not recommended; does not prevent or treat withdrawal from benzodiazepines. Low potential for cognitive or motor impairment. Use with MAO inhibitors may result in hypertensive reactions. Restlessness syndrome has been reported in small number of patients; monitor for signs of any dopamine-related movement disorders. Buspirone does not exhibit cross-tolerance with benzodiazepines or other sedative/hypnotic agents. If substituting buspirone for any of these agents, gradually withdraw the drug(s) prior to initiating buspirone. Safety and efficacy of buspirone have not been established in children <6 years of age; no long-term safety/efficacy data available in children.

Drug Interactions

Metabolism/Transport Effects Substrate of CYP2D6 (minor), CYP3A4 (major); **Note:** Assignment of Major/Minor substrate status based on clinically relevant drug interaction potential

Avoid Concomitant Use

Avoid concomitant use of BusPIRone with any of the following: Azelastine (Nasal); Conivaptan; MAO Inhibitors; Methylene Blue; Paraldehyde

Increased Effect/Toxicity

BusPIRone may increase the levels/effects of: Alcohol (Ethyl); Antidepressants (Serotonin Reuptake Inhibitor/Antagonist); Azelastine (Nasal); Buprenorphine; CNS Depressants; MAO Inhibitors; Methylene Blue; Metoclopramide; Metyrosine; Paraldehyde; Pramipexole; ROPINIRole; Rotigotine; Selective Serotonin Reuptake Inhibitors; Serotonin Modulators; Zolpidem

The levels/effects of BusPIRone may be increased by: Antifungal Agents (Azole Derivatives, Systemic); Antipsychotics; Calcium Channel Blockers (Nondihydropyridine); Conivaptan; CYP3A4 Inhibitors (Moderate); CYP3A4 Inhibitors (Strong); Dasatinib; Grapefruit Juice; HydrOXYzine; Ivacaftor; Macrolide Antibiotics; Magnesium Sulfate; Mifepristone; Perampanel; Selective Serotonin Reuptake Inhibitors; Sodium Oxybate

Decreased Effect

BusPIRone may decrease the levels/effects of: Ioflupane I 123

The levels/effects of BusPIRone may be decreased by: CYP3A4 Inducers (Strong); Deferasirox; Peginterferon Alfa-2b; Rifamycin Derivatives; Tocilizumab; Yohimbine

Ethanol/Nutrition/Herb Interactions

Ethanol: Ethanol may increase CNS depression. Management: Monitor for increased effects with coadministration. Caution patients about effects.

Food: Food may decrease the absorption of buspirone, but it may also decrease the first-pass metabolism, thereby increasing the bioavailability of buspirone. Grapefruit juice may cause increased buspirone concentrations. Management: Avoid intake of large quantities of grapefruit juice.

Herb/Nutraceutical: St John's wort may decrease buspirone levels or increase CNS depression. Kava kava, valerian, and gotu kola may increase CNS depression; yohimbe may diminish the therapeutic effect of buspirone. Management: Avoid St John's wort, kava kava, valerian, gotu kola, and yohimbe.

Dietary Considerations Avoid large quantities of grapefruit juice.

Pharmacodynamics/Kinetics

Half-life Elimination 2-3 hours

Time to Peak Serum: 40-90 minutes

Pregnancy Risk Factor B

Pregnancy Considerations Adverse events have not been observed in animal reproduction studies.

Lactation Excretion in breast milk unknown/not recommended

Breast-Feeding Considerations It is not known if buspirone is excreted in breast milk. Breast-feeding is not recommended by the manufacturer.

Dosage Forms

Tablet, oral: 5 mg, 7.5 mg, 10 mg, 15 mg, 30 mg

Busulfan (byoo SUL fan)

Brand Names: U.S. Busulfex®; Myleran®
Brand Names: Canada Busulfex®; Myleran®
Pharmacologic Category Antineoplastic Agent, Alkylating Agent
Use Palliative treatment of chronic myelogenous leukemia (CML) (oral); conditioning regimen prior to allogeneic hematopoietic progenitor cell transplantation (I.V.) for CML
Unlabeled Use Conditioning regimen prior to hematopoietic stem cell transplant (HSCT) (oral); treatment of polycythemia vera and essential thrombocytosis
Local Anesthetic/Vasoconstrictor Precautions No information available to require special precautions
Effects on Dental Treatment Key adverse event(s) related to dental treatment: Xerostomia (normal salivary flow resumes upon discontinuation), mucositis/stomatitis.
Effects on Bleeding Thrombocytopenia is a dose-limiting toxicity of busulfan. A medical consult is suggested.
Adverse Effects

I.V.:

>10%:
Cardiovascular: Tachycardia (44%), hypertension (36%; grades 3/4: 7%), edema (28% to 79%), thrombosis (33%), chest pain (26%), vasodilation (25%), hypotension (11%; grades 3/4: 3%)
Central nervous system: Insomnia (84%), fever (80%), anxiety (72% to 75%), headache (69%), chills (46%), pain (44%), dizziness (30%), depression (23%), confusion (11%)
Dermatologic: Rash (57%), pruritus (28%), alopecia (17%)
Endocrine & metabolic: Hypomagnesemia (77%), hyperglycemia (66% to 67%; grades 3/4: 15%), hypokalemia (64%), hypocalcemia (49%), hypophosphatemia (17%)
Gastrointestinal: Vomiting (43% to 100%), nausea (83% to 98%), mucositis/stomatitis (79% to 97%; grades 3/4: 26%), anorexia (85%), diarrhea (84%; grades 3/4: 5%), abdominal pain (72%), dyspepsia (44%), constipation (38%), xerostomia (26%), rectal disorder (25%), abdominal fullness (23%)
Hematologic: Myelosuppression (≤100%), neutropenia (100%; onset: 4 days; median recovery: 13 days [with G-CSF support]), thrombocytopenia (98%; median onset: 5-6 days), lymphopenia (children: 79%), anemia (69%)
Hepatic: Hyperbilirubinemia (49%; grades 3/4: 30%), ALT increased (31%; grades 3/4: 7%), hepatic sinusoidal obstruction syndrome (SOS; veno-occlusive disease) (adults: 8% to 12%; children: 21%), alkaline phosphatase increased (15%), jaundice (12%)
Local: Injection site inflammation (25%), injection site pain (15%)
Neuromuscular & skeletal: Weakness (51%), back pain (23%), myalgia (16%), arthralgia (13%)
Renal: Creatinine increased (21%), oliguria (15%)
Respiratory: Rhinitis (44%), lung disorder (34%), cough (28%), epistaxis (25%), dyspnea (25%), pneumonia (children: 21%), hiccup (18%), pharyngitis (18%)

Miscellaneous: Infection (51%; includes severe bacterial, viral [CMV], and fungal infections), allergic reaction (26%)
1% to 10%:
Cardiovascular: Arrhythmia (5%), cardiomegaly (5%), atrial fibrillation (2%), ECG abnormal (2%), heart block (2%), heart failure (grade 3/4: 2%), pericardial effusion (2%), tamponade (children with thalassemia: 2%), ventricular extrasystoles (2%), hypervolemia (2%)
Central nervous system: Lethargy (7%), hallucination (5%), agitation (2%), delirium (2%), encephalopathy (2%), seizure (2%), somnolence (2%), cerebral hemorrhage (1%)
Dermatologic: Vesicular rash (10%), vesiculobullous rash (10%), skin discoloration (8%), maculopapular rash (8%), acne (7%), exfoliative dermatitis (5%), erythema nodosum (2%)
Endocrine & metabolic: Hyponatremia (2%)
Gastrointestinal: Ileus (8%), weight gain (8%), esophagitis (grade 3: 2%), hematemesis (2%), pancreatitis (2%)
Hematologic: Prothrombin time increased (2%)
Hepatic: Hepatomegaly (6%)
Renal: Hematuria (8%), dysuria (7%), hemorrhagic cystitis (grade 3/4: 7%), BUN increased (3%; grades 3/4: 2%)
Respiratory: Asthma (8%), alveolar hemorrhage (5%), hyperventilation (5%), hemoptysis (3%), pleural effusion (3%), sinusitis (3%), atelectasis (2%), hypoxia (2%)

Oral: Frequency not defined:
Dermatologic: Hyperpigmentation of skin (5% to 10%), rash
Endocrine & metabolic: Amenorrhea, ovarian suppression
Gastrointestinal: Xerostomia
Hematologic: Myelosuppression (anemia, leukopenia, thrombocytopenia)
General Dosage Range
I.V.:
Children ≤12 kg: HSCT: 1.1 mg/kg (actual body weight) every 6 hours for 16 doses
Children >12 kg: HSCT: 0.8 mg/kg (actual body weight) every 6 hours for 16 doses
Adults: HSCT: 0.8 mg/kg every 6 hours for 16 doses (use ideal body weight or actual body weight, whichever is lower; use adjusted body weight if obese)
Oral: Dosage adjustment is recommended in patients who experience toxicity:
Children: Induction: 60 mcg/kg/day or 1.8 mg/m²/day; Maintenance: Resume induction dose or 1-3 mg/day
Adults: Induction: 60 mcg/kg/day or 1.8 mg/m²/day; usual range: 4-8 mg/day; Maintenance: Resume induction dose or 1-3 mg/day
Mechanism of Action Busulfan is an alkylating agent which reacts with the N-7 position of guanosine and interferes with DNA replication and transcription of RNA. Busulfan has a more marked effect on myeloid cells than on lymphoid cells and is also very toxic to hematopoietic stem cells. Busulfan exhibits little immunosuppressive activity. Interferes with the normal function of DNA by alkylation and cross-linking the strands of DNA.
Pharmacodynamics/Kinetics
Half-life Elimination 2-3 hours
Time to Peak Serum: Oral: ~1 hour; I.V.: Within 5 minutes
Pregnancy Risk Factor D

◀ **Pregnancy Considerations** Animal studies have demonstrated teratogenic effects. There are no adequate and well-controlled studies in pregnant women. May cause fetal harm if administered during pregnancy. The solvent in I.V. busulfan, DMA, is also associated with teratogenic effects and may impair fertility. Women of childbearing potential should avoid pregnancy while receiving busulfan treatment.

Butabarbital (byoo ta BAR bi tal)

Brand Names: U.S. Butisol Sodium®
Pharmacologic Category Barbiturate
Use Sedative; hypnotic
Local Anesthetic/Vasoconstrictor Precautions No information available to require special precautions
Effects on Dental Treatment No significant effects or complications reported
Effects on Bleeding No information available to require special precautions
Adverse Effects
1% to 3%: Central nervous system: Somnolence
Frequency not defined, postmarketing, and/or case reports: Agranulocytosis, anaphylaxis, angioedema, complex sleep-related activities, dependence, exfoliative dermatitis, fever, headache, hypersensitivity reactions, liver damage, megaloblastic anemia, rash, respiratory depression, Stevens-Johnson syndrome, thrombocytopenia, thrombophlebitis
General Dosage Range Oral:
Children: 2-6 mg/kg preoperatively (maximum: 100 mg)
Adults: 15-30 mg 3-4 times/day **or** 50-100 mg as a single dose
Mechanism of Action Interferes with transmission of impulses from the thalamus to the cortex of the brain resulting in an imbalance in central inhibitory and facilitatory mechanisms
Pharmacodynamics/Kinetics
Onset of Action 45-60 minutes
Duration of Action 6-8 hours
Half-life Elimination ~100 hours
Pregnancy Risk Factor D
Pregnancy Considerations Barbiturates cross the placenta and can be found in fetal tissues. Acute withdrawal symptoms may occur in the neonate following *in utero* exposure near term. Withdrawal symptoms may include seizures and hyperirritability and may be delayed for up to 14 days after birth.
Controlled Substance C-III

Butalbital, Acetaminophen, and Caffeine (byoo TAL bi tal, a seet a MIN oh fen, & KAF een)

Related Information
Acetaminophen *on page 27*
Caffeine *on page 229*
Brand Names: U.S. Alagesic LQ; Anolor 300; Dolgic® Plus; Esgic-Plus™; Esgic®; Fioricet®; Margesic; Orbivan™; Repan®; Zebutal®
Pharmacologic Category Barbiturate
Use Relief of the symptomatic complex of tension or muscle contraction headache
Local Anesthetic/Vasoconstrictor Precautions No information available to require special precautions
Effects on Dental Treatment No significant effects or complications reported (see Dental Comment)

Effects on Bleeding As a single agent, acetaminophen does not appear to affect bleeding or platelet aggregation. Acetaminophen may prolong the INR and increase bleeding in patients taking warfarin (Coumadin®). For patients taking warfarin, single acetaminophen doses or acetaminophen therapy of short duration should be safe, but if large (>1.3 g/day) doses are administered for longer than 10-14 days, then the INR should be monitored (see Dental Comment).
Adverse Effects Note: Specific percentages not reported.
Frequently observed:
Central nervous system: Dizziness, drowsiness, light-headedness, sedation
Gastrointestinal: Abdominal pain, nausea, vomiting
Respiratory: Dyspnea
Miscellaneous: Intoxicated feeling
General Dosage Range Oral: *Adults:* 1-2 tablets/capsules or 15-30 mL every 4 hours (maximum: 6 tablets/capsules daily; 180 mL/day)
Mechanism of Action
Butalbital is a short- to intermediate-acting barbiturate. Barbiturates depress the sensory cortex, decrease motor activity, alter cerebellar function, and produce drowsiness, sedation, hypnosis, and dose-dependent respiratory depression.
Acetaminophen inhibits the synthesis of prostaglandins in the central nervous system and peripherally blocks pain impulse generation; produces antipyresis from inhibition of hypothalamic heat-regulating center
Caffeine increases levels of 3'5' cyclic AMP by inhibiting phosphodiesterase; CNS stimulant which increases medullary respiratory center sensitivity to carbon dioxide, stimulates central inspiratory drive, and improves skeletal muscle contraction (diaphragmatic contractility)
Pharmacodynamics/Kinetics
Half-life Elimination Butalbital: 35 hours
Pregnancy Risk Factor C
Pregnancy Considerations Animal reproduction studies have not been conducted with this combination. Withdrawal seizures were reported in an infant 2 days after birth following maternal use of a butalbital product during the last 2 months of pregnancy; butalbital was detected in the newborns serum. Also refer to individual monographs for information specific to acetaminophen or caffeine.
Dental Comment Hepatotoxicity caused by acetaminophen is potentiated by chronic alcohol consumption. People who are taking acetaminophen, even at therapeutic doses, and consume alcohol are at risk of developing hepatotoxicity.

Acetaminophen may increase the levels and enhance the anticoagulant effects of vitamin K antagonists acenocoumarol and warfarin (Coumadin®). Studies have reported that acetaminophen has increased the INR in warfarin treated patients with daily acetaminophen doses as low as 2 g, particularly when taking acetaminophen for >1 week (Antlitz, 1968; Boeijinga, 1982; Gebauer, 2003; Hylek, 1998; Rubin, 1984). In addition, case reports of bleeding as a result of increased INR have been published (Bagheri, 1999; Bartle, 1991). There is no known mechanism of the interaction; furthermore, some studies have failed to demonstrate this interaction (Gadisseur, 2003; Kwan, 1995; van den Bemt, 2002). In terms of risk, the data suggest that acetaminophen and warfarin could interact in some clinically significant manner but that the benefits of concomitant use of acetaminophen for pain control in dental patients taking warfarin usually outweigh the risks. An appropriate monitoring plan should be in place to identify potential negative effects and dosage adjustments may be necessary in a minority of patients. The interaction may be more likely to occur with daily acetaminophen doses of >1.3 g for >1 week.

There are no reports of acetaminophen interacting with antiplatelet drugs such as aspirin, clopidogrel (Plavix®), or prasugrel (Effient™). Also, there are no reports of acetaminophen in combination with hydrocodone, codeine, or oxycodone interacting with warfarin (Coumadin®).

Butalbital, Acetaminophen, Caffeine, and Codeine

(byoo TAL bi tal, a seet a MIN oh fen, KAF een, & KOE deen)

Related Information

Acetaminophen *on page 27*
Caffeine *on page 229*
Codeine *on page 344*
Brand Names: U.S. Fioricet® with Codeine
Generic Availability (U.S.) Yes
Pharmacologic Category Analgesic Combination (Opioid); Barbiturate
Use Relief of symptoms of complex tension (muscle contraction) headache
Local Anesthetic/Vasoconstrictor Precautions No information available to require special precautions
Effects on Dental Treatment Key adverse event(s) related to dental treatment: Xerostomia (normal salivary flow resumes upon discontinuation). See Dental Comment.
Effects on Bleeding As a single agent, acetaminophen does not appear to affect bleeding or platelet aggregation. Acetaminophen may prolong the INR and increase bleeding in patients taking warfarin (Coumadin®). For patients taking warfarin, single acetaminophen doses or acetaminophen therapy of short duration should be safe, but if large (>1.3 g/day) doses are administered for longer than 10-14 days, then the INR should be monitored (see Dental Comment).
Adverse Effects Frequency not defined.
Cardiovascular: Syncope, tachycardia
Central nervous system: Agitation, depression, dizziness, drowsiness, euphoria, excitement, fatigue, fever, headache, high energy, intoxicated feeling, lightheadedness, mental confusion, sedation, seizure, sluggishness
Dermatologic: Hyperhidrosis, pruritus
Endocrine & metabolic: Hot flashes
Gastrointestinal: Abdominal pain, constipation, dysphagia, flatulence, heartburn, nausea, vomiting, xerostomia
Neuromuscular & skeletal: Leg pain, muscle fatigue, numbness, paresthesia, shaky feeling
Ocular: Heavy eyelids
Otic: Earache, tinnitus
Renal: Diuresis
Respiratory: Dyspnea, nasal congestion
Miscellaneous: Allergic reaction
Note: Potential reactions associated with components of Fioricet® with Codeine include agranulocytosis, cardiac stimulation, dependence, erythema multiforme, hyperglycemia, irritability, nephrotoxicity, rash, thrombocytopenia, toxic epidermal necrolysis, tremor
Dosage Oral: Adults: 1-2 capsules every 4 hours. Total daily dosage should not exceed 6 capsules.

Dosage adjustment in renal impairment: No dosage adjustments recommended. Use with caution due to increased risk of adverse effects.
Dosing adjustment in hepatic impairment: No dosage adjustments recommended; use with caution. Limited, low-dose therapy usually well tolerated in hepatic disease/cirrhosis. However, cases of hepatotoxicity at daily acetaminophen dosages <4 g/day have been reported.
Mechanism of Action Combination product for the treatment of tension headache. Contains codeine (narcotic analgesic), butalbital (barbiturate), caffeine (CNS stimulant), and acetaminophen (nonopiate, nonsalicylate analgesic).
Contraindications Hypersensitivity to butalbital, codeine, caffeine, acetaminophen, or any component of the formulation; porphyria
Warnings/Precautions May cause CNS depression, which may impair physical or mental abilities; patients must be cautioned about performing tasks which require mental alertness (eg, operating machinery or driving). Effects may be potentiated when used with other sedative drugs or ethanol. **[U.S. Boxed Warning]: Acetaminophen may cause severe hepatotoxicity, potentially requiring liver transplant or resulting in death; hepatotoxicity is usually associated with excessive acetaminophen intake (>4 g/day).** Risk is increased with alcohol use, pre-existing liver disease, and intake of more than one source of acetaminophen-containing medications. Chronic daily dosing in adults has also resulted in liver damage in some patients. Hypersensitivity and anaphylactic reactions have been reported with acetaminophen use; discontinue immediately if symptoms of allergic or hypersensitivity reactions occur.

Use with caution in patients with hypersensitivity reactions to other phenanthrene-derivative opioid agonists (eg, morphine, hydrocodone, oxycodone). Use caution with Addison's disease, known G6PD deficiency, severe renal or hepatic impairment. Use caution in patients with head injury or other intracranial lesions, acute abdominal conditions, urethral stricture of BPH, thyroid dysfunction, or in patients with respiratory diseases. Use caution in patients with two or more copies of the variant CYP2D6*2 allele; may have extensive conversion from codeine to morphine and thus increased opioid-mediated effects. Elderly (not recommended for use) and/or debilitated patients may be more susceptible to CNS depressants, as well as constipating effects of narcotics. Tolerance or drug dependence may result from extended use. Caffeine may cause CNS and cardiovascular stimulation, as well as GI irritation in high doses. Use with caution in patients with a history of peptic ulcer or GERD; avoid in patients with symptomatic cardiac arrhythmias. Safety and efficacy in pediatric patients have not been established.
Drug Interactions
Metabolism/Transport Effects Refer to individual components.
Avoid Concomitant Use
Avoid concomitant use of Butalbital, Acetaminophen, Caffeine, and Codeine with any of the following: Azelastine (Nasal); Iobenguane I 123; Paraldehyde; Pimozide; Voriconazole
Increased Effect/Toxicity
Butalbital, Acetaminophen, Caffeine, and Codeine may increase the levels/effects of: Alcohol (Ethyl); Alvimopan; ARIPiprazole; Azelastine (Nasal); Busulfan; CNS Depressants; Dasatinib; Desmopressin;

Formoterol; Fosphenytoin; Imatinib; Indacaterol; Lomitapide; Meperidine; Methadone; Metyrosine; Mipomersen; Mirtazapine; Paraldehyde; Pimozide; Pramipexole; Prilocaine; QuiNIDine; ROPINIRole; Rotigotine; Selective Serotonin Reuptake Inhibitors; SORAfenib; Sympathomimetics; Thiazide Diuretics; Vitamin K Antagonists; Zolpidem

The levels/effects of Butalbital, Acetaminophen, Caffeine, and Codeine may be increased by: Abiraterone Acetate; Amphetamines; Antipsychotic Agents (Phenothiazines); AtoMOXetine; Chloramphenicol; CYP1A2 Inhibitors (Moderate); CYP1A2 Inhibitors (Strong); Dasatinib; Deferasirox; Divalproex; Droperidol; Felbamate; Fosphenytoin; HydrOXYzine; Imatinib; Isoniazid; Magnesium Sulfate; Metyrapone; Perampanel; Phenytoin; Primidone; Probenecid; Quinolone Antibiotics; Sodium Oxybate; Somatostatin Analogs; SORAfenib; Succinylcholine; Valproic Acid

Decreased Effect

Butalbital, Acetaminophen, Caffeine, and Codeine may decrease the levels/effects of: Acetaminophen; Adenosine; Beta-Blockers; Calcium Channel Blockers; Chloramphenicol; Contraceptives (Estrogens); Contraceptives (Progestins); Corticosteroids (Systemic); CycloSPORINE (Systemic); Disopyramide; Divalproex; Doxycycline; Etoposide; Etoposide Phosphate; Felbamate; Fosphenytoin; Griseofulvin; Iobenguane I 123; LamoTRIgine; Methadone; Pegvisomant; Phenytoin; Propafenone; QuiNIDine; Regadenoson; Teniposide; Theophylline Derivatives; Tricyclic Antidepressants; Valproic Acid; Vitamin K Antagonists; Voriconazole

The levels/effects of Butalbital, Acetaminophen, Caffeine, and Codeine may be decreased by: Ammonium Chloride; Anticonvulsants (Hydantoin); Barbiturates; CarBAMazepine; Cholestyramine Resin; CYP2D6 Inhibitors (Moderate); CYP2D6 Inhibitors (Strong); Mixed Agonist / Antagonist Opioids; Multivitamins/Minerals (with ADEK, Folate, Iron); Peginterferon Alfa-2b; Pyridoxine; Rifamycin Derivatives; Teriflunomide

Ethanol/Nutrition/Herb Interactions Ethanol: Avoid ethanol (may increase CNS depression).

Pregnancy Risk Factor C

Pregnancy Considerations Animal reproduction studies have not been conducted with this combination. Withdrawal seizures were reported in an infant 2 days after birth following maternal use of a butalbital product during the last 2 months of pregnancy; butalbital was detected in the newborns serum. Also refer to individual monographs for information specific to acetaminophen, caffeine, or codeine.

Lactation Enters breast milk/not recommended

Breast-Feeding Considerations Barbiturates, acetaminophen, caffeine, and codeine are excreted in breast milk. Also refer to individual agents for information specific to acetaminophen, caffeine, or codeine.

Controlled Substance C-III

Dosage Forms

Capsule: Butalbital 50 mg, acetaminophen 325 mg, caffeine 40 mg, and codeine 30 mg

Fioricet® with Codeine: Butalbital 50 mg, acetaminophen 325 mg, caffeine 40 mg, and codeine 30 mg

Dental Comment Hepatotoxicity caused by acetaminophen is potentiated by chronic alcohol consumption. People who are taking acetaminophen, even at therapeutic doses, and consume alcohol are at risk of developing hepatotoxicity.

Acetaminophen may increase the levels and enhance the anticoagulant effects of vitamin K antagonists acenocoumarol and warfarin (Coumadin®). Studies have reported that acetaminophen has increased the INR in warfarin treated patients with daily acetaminophen doses as low as >2 g, particularly when taking acetaminophen for >1 week (Antlitz, 1968; Boeijinga, 1982; Gebauer, 2003; Hylek, 1998; Rubin, 1984). In addition, case reports of bleeding as a result of increased INR have been published (Bagheri, 1999; Bartle, 1991). There is no known mechanism of the interaction; furthermore, some studies have failed to demonstrate this interaction (Gadisseur, 2003; Kwan, 1995; van den Bemt, 2002). In terms of risk, the data suggest that acetaminophen and warfarin could interact in some clinically significant manner but that the benefits of concomitant use of acetaminophen for pain control in dental patients taking warfarin usually outweigh the risks. An appropriate monitoring plan should be in place to identify potential negative effects and dosage adjustments may be necessary in a minority of patients. The interaction may be more likely to occur with daily acetaminophen doses of >1.3 g for >1 week.

There are no reports of acetaminophen interacting with antiplatelet drugs such as aspirin, clopidogrel (Plavix®), or prasugrel (Effient™). Also, there are no reports of acetaminophen in combination with hydrocodone, codeine, or oxycodone interacting with warfarin (Coumadin®).

References

Antlitz AM, Mead JA Jr, and Tolentino MA, "Potentiation of Oral Anticoagulant Therapy by Acetaminophen," *Curr Ther Res Clin Exp*, 1968, 10(10):501-7.

Bagheri H, Bernhard NB, and Montastruc JL, "Potentiation of the Acenocoumarol Anticoagulant Effect by Acetaminophen," *Ann Pharmacother*, 1999, 33(4):506.

Bartle WR and Blakely JA, "Potentiation of Warfarin Anticoagulation by Acetaminophen," *JAMA*, 1991, 265(10):1260.

Boeijinga JJ, Boerstra EE, Ris P, et al, "Interaction Between Paracetamol and Coumarin Anticoagulants," *Lancet*, 1982, 1(8270):506.

Gadisseur AP, Van Der Meer FJ, and Rosendaal FR, "Sustained Intake of Paracetamol (Acetaminophen) During Oral Anticoagulant Therapy With Coumarins Does Not Cause Clinically Important INR Changes: A Randomized Double-Blind Clinical Trial," *J Thromb Haemost*, 2003, 1(4):714-7.

Gebauer MG, Nyfort-Hansen K, Henschke PJ, et al, "Warfarin and Acetaminophen Interaction," *Pharmacotherapy*, 2003, 23(1):109-12.

Hylek EM, Heiman H, Skates SJ, et al, "Acetaminophen and Other Risk Factors for Excessive Warfarin Anticoagulation," *JAMA*, 1998, 279(9):657-62.

Kwan D, Bartle WR, and Walker SE, "The Effects of Acute and Chronic Acetaminophen Dosing on the Pharmacodynamics and Pharmacokinetics of (R)- and (S)-Warfarin," *Clin Pharmacol Ther*, 1995, 57:212.

Rubin RN, Mentzer RL, and Budzynski AZ, "Potentiation of Anticoagulant Effect of Warfarin by Acetaminophen (Tylenol®)," *Clin Res*, 1984, 32:698a.

van den Bemt PM, Geven LM, Kuitert NA, et al, "The Potential Interaction Between Oral Anticoagulants and Acetaminophen in Everyday Practice," *Pharm World Sci*, 2002, 24(5):201-4.

Butalbital and Acetaminophen

(byoo TAL bi tal & a seet a MIN oh fen)

Related Information

Acetaminophen *on page 27*

PHENobarbital *on page 1080*

Brand Names: U.S. Bupap; Cephadyn [DSC]; Orviban® CF; Phrenilin® Forte; Promacet; Sedapap®

Pharmacologic Category Analgesic, Miscellaneous; Barbiturate

Use Relief of the symptomatic complex of tension or muscle contraction headache

Local Anesthetic/Vasoconstrictor Precautions No information available to require special precautions

Effects on Dental Treatment No significant effects or complications reported (see Dental Comment)

Effects on Bleeding As a single agent, acetaminophen does not appear to affect bleeding or platelet aggregation. Acetaminophen may prolong the INR and increase bleeding in patients taking warfarin (Coumadin®). For patients taking warfarin, single acetaminophen doses or acetaminophen therapy of short duration should be safe, but if large (>1.3 g/day) doses are administered for longer than 10-14 days, then the INR should be monitored (see Dental Comment).

Adverse Effects

Frequently observed:

Central nervous system: Dizziness, drowsiness, lightheadedness, sedation

Gastrointestinal: Abdominal pain, nausea, vomiting

Respiratory: Dyspnea

Miscellaneous: Intoxicated feeling

Infrequently observed:

Cardiovascular: Tachycardia

Central nervous system: Agitation, confusion, depression, euphoria, excitement, faintness, fever, headache, seizure

Dermatologic: Hyperhidrosis, pruritus

Endocrine & metabolic: Hot spells

Gastrointestinal: Constipation, dysphagia, heartburn, flatulence, xerostomia

Neuromuscular & skeletal: Leg pain, muscle fatigue, numbness, paresthesia

Ocular: Heavy eyelids

Otic: Earache, tinnitus

Renal: Diuresis

Respiratory: Nasal congestion

Miscellaneous: Allergic reaction, high energy, shaky feeling, sluggishness

General Dosage Range Oral: *Children ≥12 years and Adults:*

Butalbital 50 mg and acetaminophen 300-325 mg: 1-2 tablets every 4 hours as needed (maximum: 6 tablets/ 24 hours)

Butalbital 50 mg and acetaminophen 650 mg: One tablet/capsule every 4 hours as needed (maximum: 6 doses/24 hours)

Mechanism of Action

Butalbital is a short- to intermediate-acting barbiturate. Barbiturates depress the sensory cortex, decrease motor activity, alter cerebellar function, and produce drowsiness, sedation, hypnosis, and dose-dependent respiratory depression.

Acetaminophen inhibits the synthesis of prostaglandins in the central nervous system and peripherally blocks pain impulse generation; produces antipyresis from inhibition of hypothalamic heat-regulating center.

Pharmacodynamics/Kinetics

Half-life Elimination Butalbital: 35 hours

Pregnancy Risk Factor C

Pregnancy Considerations Animal reproduction studies have not been conducted with this combination. Withdrawal seizures were reported in an infant 2 days after birth following maternal use of a butalbital product during the last 2 months of pregnancy; butalbital was detected in the newborns serum. Also refer to acetaminophen monograph for information specific to acetaminophen.

Dental Comment Hepatotoxicity caused by acetaminophen is potentiated by chronic alcohol consumption. People who are taking acetaminophen, even at therapeutic doses, and consume alcohol are at risk of developing hepatotoxicity.

Acetaminophen may increase the levels and enhance the anticoagulant effects of vitamin K antagonists acenocoumarol and warfarin (Coumadin®). Studies have reported that acetaminophen has increased the INR in warfarin treated patients with daily acetaminophen doses as low as 2 g, particularly when taking acetaminophen for >1 week (Antlitz, 1968; Boeijinga, 1982; Gebauer, 2003; Hylek, 1998; Rubin, 1984). In addition, case reports of bleeding as a result of increased INR have been published (Bagheri, 1999; Bartle, 1991). There is no known mechanism of the interaction; furthermore, some studies have failed to demonstrate this interaction (Gadisseur, 2003; Kwan, 1995; van den Bemt, 2002). In terms of risk, the data suggest that acetaminophen and warfarin could interact in some clinically significant manner but that the benefits of concomitant use of acetaminophen for pain control in dental patients taking warfarin usually outweigh the risks. An appropriate monitoring plan should be in place to identify potential negative effects and dosage adjustments may be necessary in a minority of patients. The interaction may be more likely to occur with daily acetaminophen doses of >1.3 g for >1 week.

There are no reports of acetaminophen interacting with antiplatelet drugs such as aspirin, clopidogrel (Plavix®), or prasugrel (Effient™). Also, there are no reports of acetaminophen in combination with hydrocodone, codeine, or oxycodone interacting with warfarin (Coumadin®).

Butalbital, Aspirin, and Caffeine
(byoo TAL bi tal, AS pir in, & KAF een)

Related Information

Aspirin *on page 135*

Caffeine *on page 229*

Brand Names: U.S. Fiorinal®

Brand Names: Canada Fiorinal®

Pharmacologic Category Barbiturate

Use Relief of the symptomatic complex of tension or muscle contraction headache

Local Anesthetic/Vasoconstrictor Precautions No information available to require special precautions

Effects on Dental Treatment Key adverse event(s) related to dental treatment: Aspirin: As with all drugs which may affect hemostasis, bleeding is associated with aspirin. Hemorrhage may occur at virtually any site; risk is dependent on multiple variables including dosage, concurrent use of multiple agents which alter hemostasis, and patient susceptibility. Many adverse effects of aspirin are dose related, and are rare at low dosages. Other serious reactions are idiosyncratic, related to allergy or individual sensitivity (see Effects on Bleeding).

Effects on Bleeding Aspirin irreversibly inhibits platelet aggregation which can prolong bleeding. Upon discontinuation, normal platelet function returns only when new platelets are released (~7-10 days). However, in the case of dental surgery, there is no scientific evidence to support discontinuation of aspirin.

Adverse Effects

>10%:

Central nervous system: Dizziness, lightheadedness, drowsiness, "hangover" effect

Gastrointestinal: Heartburn, stomach pain, dyspepsia, epigastric discomfort, nausea

1% to 10%:
Central nervous system: Confusion, mental depression, unusual excitement, nervousness, faint feeling, headache, insomnia, nightmares, fatigue
Dermatologic: Skin rash
Gastrointestinal: Constipation, vomiting, gastrointestinal ulceration
Hematologic: Hemolytic anemia
Neuromuscular & skeletal: Weakness
Respiratory: Troubled breathing
Miscellaneous: Anaphylactic shock

General Dosage Range Oral: *Adults:* 1-2 tablets/capsules every 4 hours (maximum: 6 tablets/capsules daily)

Pregnancy Risk Factor C

Pregnancy Considerations Animal reproduction studies have not been conducted with this combination. Withdrawal seizures were reported in an infant 2 days after birth following maternal use of a butalbital product during the last 2 months of pregnancy; butalbital was detected in the newborns serum. Also refer to individual monographs for information specific to aspirin or caffeine.

Controlled Substance C-III

Dental Comment There is no scientific evidence to warrant discontinuance of aspirin prior to dental surgery. Patients taking one aspirin tablet daily as an antithrombotic and who require dental surgery should be given special consideration in consultation with the physician before removal of the aspirin relative to prevention of postoperative bleeding.

Butalbital, Aspirin, Caffeine, and Codeine (byoo TAL bi tal, AS pir in, KAF een, & KOE deen)

Related Information
Aspirin *on page 135*
Caffeine *on page 229*
Codeine *on page 344*

Brand Names: U.S. Ascomp® with Codeine; Fiorinal® with Codeine

Brand Names: Canada Fiorinal®-C 1/2; Fiorinal®-C 1/4; Tecnal C 1/2; Tecnal C 1/4

Pharmacologic Category Analgesic Combination (Opioid); Barbiturate

Use Relief of symptoms of complex tension (muscle contraction) headache

Local Anesthetic/Vasoconstrictor Precautions No information available to require special precautions

Effects on Dental Treatment Key adverse event(s) related to dental treatment: Aspirin: As with all drugs which may affect hemostasis, bleeding is associated with aspirin. Hemorrhage may occur at virtually any site; risk is dependent on multiple variables including dosage, concurrent use of multiple agents which alter hemostasis, and patient susceptibility. Many adverse effects of aspirin are dose related, and are rare at low dosages. Other serious reactions are idiosyncratic, related to allergy or individual sensitivity (see Effects on Bleeding).

Effects on Bleeding Aspirin irreversibly inhibits platelet aggregation which can prolong bleeding. Upon discontinuation, normal platelet function returns only when new platelets are released (~7-10 days). However, in the case of dental surgery, there is no scientific evidence to support discontinuation of aspirin.

Adverse Effects 1% to 10%:
Central nervous system: Dizziness/lightheadedness (3%), drowsiness (2%), intoxicated feeling (1%)
Gastrointestinal: Abdominal pain/nausea (4%)

Note: Potential reactions associated with components of Fiorinal® with Codeine include acute airway obstruction, anemia, bleeding time prolonged, cardiac stimulation, dependence, hemolytic anemia, hepatitis, hyperglycemia, irritability, nephrotoxicity, occult blood loss, peptic ulcer, pruritus, renal toxicity (high doses, prolonged therapy) thrombocytopenia, tremor, urate excretion impaired

General Dosage Range Oral: *Adults:* 1-2 capsules every 4 hours as needed (maximum: 6 capsules/day)

Mechanism of Action Butalbital is a short-to-intermediate acting barbiturate; aspirin inhibits prostaglandin synthesis and has analgesic, antipyretic and anti-inflammatory actions; caffeine is a CNS stimulant; codeine is a narcotic analgesic and antitussive which produced generalized CNS depression. The combination product is for the treatment of tension headache; however, the role of each component in the relief of symptoms is not completely understood.

Pregnancy Risk Factor C

Pregnancy Considerations Animal reproduction studies have not been conducted with this combination. Lissencephaly, pachygyria, and heterotopic gray matter were noted in a premature infant whose mother took this combination throughout pregnancy; mild developmental delay and seizures were also observed at 1 year of age. Withdrawal seizures were reported in an infant 2 days after birth following maternal use of a butalbital product during the last 2 months of pregnancy; butalbital was detected in the newborn's serum. Also refer to the individual monographs for aspirin, caffeine, and codeine for additional information.

Controlled Substance C-III

Dental Comment There is no scientific evidence to warrant discontinuance of aspirin prior to dental surgery. Patients taking one aspirin tablet daily as an antithrombotic and who require dental surgery should be given special consideration in consultation with the physician before removal of the aspirin relative to prevention of postoperative bleeding.

Butenafine (byoo TEN a feen)

Brand Names: U.S. Lotrimin® ultra™ [OTC]; Mentax®

Pharmacologic Category Antifungal Agent, Topical

Use Topical treatment of tinea pedis (athlete's foot), tinea cruris (jock itch), tinea corporis (ringworm), and tinea versicolor

Local Anesthetic/Vasoconstrictor Precautions No information available to require special precautions

Effects on Dental Treatment No significant effects or complications reported

Effects on Bleeding No information available to require special precautions

Adverse Effects ≥1%: Dermatologic: Burning, contact dermatitis, erythema, irritation, pruritus, stinging

General Dosage Range Topical: *Children >12 years and Adults:* Apply to affected area once or twice daily

Mechanism of Action Butenafine exerts fungicidal activity against dermatophytes (eg trichophyton, epidermophyton) by blocking squalene epoxidation, resulting in inhibition of ergosterol synthesis and subsequent weakening of fungal cell membranes.

Pharmacodynamics/Kinetics
Half-life Elimination Biphasic: Alpha: 35 hours; Beta: >150 hours
Time to Peak Serum: 6-15 hours

Pregnancy Risk Factor C
Pregnancy Considerations Teratogenic effects were not observed in animal studies.

Butoconazole (byoo toe KOE na zole)

Brand Names: U.S. Gynazole-1®
Brand Names: Canada Femstat® One; Gynazole-1®
Pharmacologic Category Antifungal Agent, Vaginal
Use Local treatment of vulvovaginal candidiasis
Local Anesthetic/Vasoconstrictor Precautions No information available to require special precautions
Effects on Dental Treatment No significant effects or complications reported
Effects on Bleeding No information available to require special precautions
Adverse Effects Frequency not defined.
Gastrointestinal: Abdominal pain or cramping
Genitourinary: Pelvic pain; vulvar/vaginal burning, itching, soreness, and swelling
General Dosage Range Intravaginal: *Adults:* Insert 1 applicatorful at bedtime
Mechanism of Action Inhibits biosynthesis of ergosterol, damaging the fungal cell wall membrane, which increases permeability in susceptible fungi (*Candida*), causing leaking of nutrients
Pharmacodynamics/Kinetics
Time to Peak 12-24 hours
Pregnancy Risk Factor C
Pregnancy Considerations Adverse events have been observed in some animal reproduction studies. Butoconazole may be considered for the treatment of vulvovaginal candidiasis in pregnant women (CDC, 2010). Use may weaken rubber or latex condoms or diaphragms; separate use by 3 days.

Butorphanol (byoo TOR fa nole)

Brand Names: Canada Apo-Butorphanol®; PMS-Butorphanol
Pharmacologic Category Analgesic, Opioid; Analgesic, Opioid Partial Agonist
Use
Parenteral: Management of moderate-to-severe pain; preoperative medication; supplement to balanced anesthesia; management of pain during labor
Nasal spray: Management of moderate-to-severe pain, including migraine headache pain
Local Anesthetic/Vasoconstrictor Precautions No information available to require special precautions
Effects on Dental Treatment Key adverse event(s) related to dental treatment: Xerostomia (normal salivary flow resumes upon discontinuation) and unpleasant aftertaste.
Effects on Bleeding No information available to require special precautions
Adverse Effects
>10%:
Central nervous system: Somnolence (43%), dizziness (19%), insomnia (nasal spray 11%)
Gastrointestinal: Nausea/vomiting (13%)
Respiratory: Nasal congestion (nasal spray 13%)
1% to 10%:
Cardiovascular: Palpitation, vasodilation
Central nervous system: Anxiety, confusion, headache, lethargy, lightheadedness
Dermatologic: Pruritus

Gastrointestinal: Anorexia, constipation, stomach pain, unpleasant aftertaste, xerostomia
Neuromuscular & skeletal: Tremor, paresthesia, weakness
Ocular: Blurred vision
Otic: Ear pain, tinnitus
Respiratory: Bronchitis, cough, dyspnea, epistaxis, nasal irritation, pharyngitis, rhinitis, sinus congestion, sinusitis, upper respiratory infection
Miscellaneous: Diaphoresis increased
General Dosage Range Dosage adjustment recommended in patients with hepatic or renal impairment
I.M.:
Adults: Initial: 2 mg, may repeat every 3-4 hours as needed; Usual range: 1-4 mg every 3-4 hours as needed **or** 2 mg prior to surgery
Elderly: Initial: 1/2 of the recommended dose, repeated dosing generally should be at least 6 hours apart
I.V.:
Adults: Initial: 1 mg, may repeat every 3-4 hours as needed; Usual range: 0.5-2 mg every 3-4 hours as needed **or** 2 mg and/or an incremental dose of 0.5-1 mg (up to 0.06 mg/kg) as supplement to surgery
Elderly: Initial: 1/2 of the recommended dose, repeated dosing generally should be at least 6 hours apart
Intranasal:
Adults: Initial: 1 spray (~1 mg) in 1 nostril, may repeat in 60-90 minutes, then repeat initial dose sequence in 3-4 hours after last dose as needed; may use initial dose of 1 spray in each nostril (2 mg) in patients who will remain recumbent
Elderly: Initial: Should not exceed 1 mg, may repeat after 90-120 minutes
Mechanism of Action Agonist of kappa opiate receptors and partial agonist of mu opiate receptors in the CNS, causing inhibition of ascending pain pathways, altering the perception of and response to pain; produces analgesia, respiratory depression, and sedation similar to opioids
Pharmacodynamics/Kinetics
Onset of Action I.M.: 5-10 minutes; I.V.: <10 minutes; Nasal: Within 15 minutes
Peak effect: I.M.: 0.5-1 hour; I.V.: 4-5 minutes
Duration of Action I.M., I.V.: 3-4 hours; Nasal: 4-5 hours
Half-life Elimination 2.5-4 hours
Pregnancy Risk Factor C
Pregnancy Considerations Adverse events were observed in some animal reproduction studies. Butorphanol crosses the placenta. Apnea or respiratory distress in the newborn may occur following use during labor. Use caution if abnormal fetal heart rate patterns are present.
Controlled Substance C-IV

C1 Inhibitor (Human) (cee won in HIB i ter HYU man)

Brand Names: U.S. Berinert®; Cinryze®
Brand Names: Canada Berinert®
Pharmacologic Category Blood Product Derivative
Use
Berinert®: Treatment of acute abdominal, facial, or laryngeal attacks of hereditary angioedema (HAE)
Cinryze®: Routine prophylaxis against angioedema attacks in patients with HAE
Local Anesthetic/Vasoconstrictor Precautions No information available to require special precautions

◀ **Effects on Dental Treatment** No significant effects or complications reported

Effects on Bleeding Thrombotic events have been reported.

Adverse Effects

>10%:

Central nervous system: Headache

Gastrointestinal: Nausea

1% to 10%:

Central nervous system: Dizziness, fever

Dermatologic: Erythema, pruritus, rash

Gastrointestinal: Abdominal pain/discomfort, abnormal taste, vomiting, xerostomia

Genitourinary: Vulvovaginal fungal infection

Local: Infusion-related reactions

Respiratory: Nasopharyngitis,upper respiratory tract infection

Miscellaneous: Flu-like syndrome, hereditary angioedema attack symptoms exacerbated, viral infection

General Dosage Range Oral: *Adolescents and Adults:* Prophylaxis: 1000 units every 3-4 days **or** treatment: 20 units/kg

Mechanism of Action C1 inhibitor, one of the serine proteinase inhibitors found in human blood, plays a role in regulating the complement and intrinsic coagulation (contact system) pathway, and is also involved in the fibrinolytic and kinin pathways. C1 inhibitor therapy in patients with C1 inhibitor deficiency, such as HAE, is believed to suppress contact system activation via inactivation of plasma kallikrein and factor XIIa, thus preventing bradykinin production. Unregulated bradykinin production is thought to contribute to the increased vascular permeability and angioedema observed in HAE.

Pharmacodynamics/Kinetics

Onset of Action

Berinert®: Onset of symptom relief: Median: 15 minutes; Time to complete resolution of HAE symptoms: Median: 8.4 hours

Cinryze®: Increased plasma C1 inhibitor levels observed ~1 hour or less;

Half-life Elimination Adults (following a single dose):

Berinert®: 22 hours (range: 17-24 hours)

Cinryze®: 56 hours (range: 11-108 hours)

Time to Peak Cinryze®: ~4 hours

Pregnancy Risk Factor C

Pregnancy Considerations Animal reproduction studies have not been conducted. There are no adequate and well-controlled studies in pregnant women. Information related to use during pregnancy is limited. Pregnancy may increase the incidence of attacks in patients with HAE.

Prescribing and Access Restrictions Assistance with procurement and reimbursement of Cinryze® is available for healthcare providers and patients through the CINRYZE*Solutions*® program (telephone: 1-877-945-1000) or at http://www.cinryze.com/Cinryze_-Solutions/Default.aspx

---

Cabazitaxel (ca baz i TAKS el)

Brand Names: U.S. Jevtana®

Brand Names: Canada Jevtana®

Pharmacologic Category Antineoplastic Agent, Antimicrotubular; Antineoplastic Agent, Taxane Derivative

Use Treatment of hormone-refractory metastatic prostate cancer (in patients previously treated with a docetaxel-containing regimen)

Local Anesthetic/Vasoconstrictor Precautions No information available to require special precautions

Effects on Dental Treatment Key adverse event(s) related to dental treatment: Taste alteration

Effects on Bleeding Thrombocytopenia has been reported in ≤48% of patients. A medical consult is suggested.

Adverse Effects Note: Adverse reactions reported for combination therapy with prednisone.

>10%:

Central nervous system: Fatigue (37%), fever (12%)

Gastrointestinal: Diarrhea (47%; grades 3/4: 6%), nausea (34%), vomiting (22%), constipation (20%), abdominal pain (17%), anorexia (16%), taste alteration (11%)

Hematologic: Anemia (98%; grades 3/4: 11%), leukopenia (96%; grades 3/4: 69%), neutropenia (94%; grades 3/4: 82%; nadir: 12 days [range: 4-17 days]), thrombocytopenia (48%; grades 3/4: 4%)

Neuromuscular & skeletal: Weakness (20%), back pain (16%), peripheral neuropathy (13%; grades 3/4: <1%), arthralgia (11%)

Renal: Hematuria (17%)

Respiratory: Dyspnea (12%), cough (11%)

1% to 10%:

Cardiovascular: Peripheral edema (9%), arrhythmia (5%), hypotension (5%)

Central nervous system: Dizziness (8%), headache (8%), pain (5%)

Dermatologic: Alopecia (10%)

Endocrine & metabolic: Dehydration (5%)

Gastrointestinal: Dyspepsia (10%), weight loss (9%), mucosal inflammation (6%)

Genitourinary: Urinary tract infection (8%), dysuria (7%)

Hematologic: Neutropenic fever (grades 3/4: 7%)

Hepatic: ALT increased (grades 3/4: ≤1%), AST increased (grades 3/4: ≤1%), bilirubin increased (grades 3/4: ≤1%)

Neuromuscular & skeletal: Muscle spasm (7%)

General Dosage Range Dosage adjustment recommended in patients with hepatic impairment or who develop toxicities

I.V.: *Adults:* 25 mg/m^2 once every 3 weeks

Mechanism of Action Cabazitaxel is a taxane derivative which is a microtubule inhibitor; it binds to tubulin promoting assembly into microtubules and inhibiting disassembly which stabilizes microtubules. This inhibits microtubule depolymerization and cell division, arresting the cell cycle and inhibiting tumor proliferation. Unlike other taxanes, cabazitaxel has a poor affinity for multidrug resistance (MDR) proteins, therefore conferring activity in resistant tumors.

Pharmacodynamics/Kinetics

Half-life Elimination Terminal: 95 hours

Pregnancy Risk Factor D

Pregnancy Considerations Animal studies have demonstrated adverse effects (embryotoxicity, fetotoxicity and fetal loss) at doses significantly lower than human doses. There are no adequate and well-controlled studies in pregnant women. May cause fetal harm if administered during pregnancy. Pregnant women should avoid exposure to cabazitaxel.

Cabergoline (ca BER goe leen)

Brand Names: Canada CO Cabergoline; Dostinex®

Pharmacologic Category Ergot Derivative

Use Treatment of hyperprolactinemic disorders, either idiopathic or due to pituitary adenomas

Canadian labeling: Additional use (not in U.S. labeling): Prevention of the onset of physiological lactation in the puerperium when clinically indicated (eg, still born baby or neonatal death, conditions that interfere with suckling, severe acute or chronic mental illness). **Note:** Not indicated for suppression of established postpartum lactation.

Local Anesthetic/Vasoconstrictor Precautions Cabergoline is a semisynthetic ergot alkaloid derivative; there is a possibility that it has vasoconstricting effects; use vasoconstrictor with caution

Effects on Dental Treatment Key adverse event(s) related to dental treatment: Xerostomia (normal salivary flow resumes upon discontinuation), throat irritation, and toothache.

Effects on Bleeding No information available to require special precautions

Adverse Effects

>10%:
Central nervous system: Headache (26%), dizziness (15% to 17%)
Gastrointestinal: Nausea (27% to 29%)

1% to 10%:
Cardiovascular: Orthostatic hypotension (4%), hypotension (1%), dependent edema (1%), edema (peripheral 1%), palpitation (1%), syncope (1%)
Central nervous system: Fatigue (5% to 7%), vertigo (1% to 4%), depression (3%), somnolence (2% to 5%), nervousness (1% to 2%), anxiety (1%), insomnia (1%), concentration impaired (1%), malaise (1%)
Dermatologic: Acne (1%), pruritus (1%)
Endocrine: Hot flashes (1% to 3%), breast pain (1% to 2%), dysmenorrhea (1%)
Gastrointestinal: Constipation (7% to 10%), abdominal pain (5%), dyspepsia (2% to 5%), vomiting (2% to 4%), xerostomia (2%), diarrhea (2%), flatulence (2%), anorexia (1%), throat irritation (1%), toothache (1%)
Neuromuscular & skeletal: Weakness (6% to 9%), pain (2%), paresthesia (1% to 2%), arthralgia (1%)
Ocular: Abnormal vision (1%), periorbital edema (1%)
Respiratory: Rhinitis (1%)
Miscellaneous: Flu-like syndrome (1%)

General Dosage Range Oral: *Adults:* Initial: 0.25 mg twice weekly; Maintenance: Up to 1 mg twice weekly

Mechanism of Action Cabergoline is a long acting dopamine receptor agonist with a high affinity for D_2 receptors; prolactin secretion by the anterior pituitary is predominantly under hypothalamic inhibitory control exerted through the release of dopamine. It is a potent $5\text{-}HT_{2B}$-receptor agonist, which may contribute to observed fibrotic/valvulopathic events.

Pharmacodynamics/Kinetics

Half-life Elimination 63-69 hours

Time to Peak 2-3 hours

Pregnancy Risk Factor B

Pregnancy Considerations Teratogenic effects were not observed in most animal studies when administered in maternally nontoxic doses. Treatment of hyperprolactinemia may restore fertility in a previously infertile woman. Because information concerning the use of cabergoline in pregnancy is limited, bromocriptine is generally recommended to treat hyperprolactinemia in women who wish to conceive. Based on preliminary data, cabergoline has not been shown to increase the risk of congenital malformations or miscarriages when used early in pregnancy (treatment was generally stopped once pregnancy was diagnosed). Not recommended for use in patients with pregnancy-induced hypertension unless benefit outweighs potential risk.

Canadian labeling (not in U.S. labeling): Exclude pregnancy prior to use; prevent pregnancy for ≥1 month following discontinuation of treatment.

Caffeine (KAF een)

Brand Names: U.S. Cafcit®; Enerjets [OTC]; No Doz® Maximum Strength [OTC]; Vivarin® [OTC]

Pharmacologic Category Central Nervous System Stimulant; Phosphodiesterase Enzyme Inhibitor, Nonselective

Use
Caffeine citrate: Treatment of idiopathic apnea of prematurity
Caffeine and sodium benzoate: Treatment of acute respiratory depression (not a preferred agent)
Caffeine [OTC labeling]: Restore mental alertness or wakefulness when experiencing fatigue

Unlabeled Use Caffeine and sodium benzoate: Treatment of spinal puncture headache; CNS stimulant; diuretic; augmentation of seizure induction during electroconvulsive therapy (ECT)

Local Anesthetic/Vasoconstrictor Precautions No information available to require special precautions

Effects on Dental Treatment No significant effects or complications reported

Effects on Bleeding No information available to require special precautions

Adverse Effects Frequency not specified; primarily serum-concentration related.
Cardiovascular: Angina, arrhythmia (ventricular), chest pain, flushing, palpitation, sinus tachycardia, tachycardia (supraventricular), vasodilation
Central nervous system: Agitation, delirium, dizziness, hallucinations, headache, insomnia, irritability, psychosis, restlessness
Dermatologic: Urticaria
Gastrointestinal: Esophageal sphincter tone decreased, gastritis
Neuromuscular & skeletal: Fasciculations
Ocular: Intraocular pressure increased (>180 mg caffeine), miosis
Renal: Diuresis

General Dosage Range

I.M. (caffeine and sodium benzoate):
Children: 8 mg/kg every 4 hours as needed
Adults: 250 mg as a single dose; may repeat as needed (maximum: 500 mg/dose; 2500 mg/day)

I.V.:
Neonates (caffeine citrate): Loading dose: 10-20 mg/kg; Maintenance: 5 mg/kg once daily
Children (caffeine and sodium benzoate): 8 mg/kg every 4 hours as needed
Adults (caffeine and sodium benzoate): 250 mg as a single dose; may repeat as needed (maximum: 500 mg/dose; 2500 mg/day) **or** 300-2000 mg (electroconvulsive therapy)

Oral:
Neonates (caffeine citrate): Loading dose: 10-20 mg/kg; Maintenance: 5 mg/kg once daily
Children ≥12 years and Adults: 100-200 mg every 3-4 hours as needed (OTC labeling)

SubQ (caffeine and sodium benzoate): *Children:* 8 mg/kg every 4 hours as needed

◀ **Mechanism of Action** Increases levels of 3'5' cyclic AMP by inhibiting phosphodiesterase; CNS stimulant which increases medullary respiratory center sensitivity to carbon dioxide, stimulates central inspiratory drive, and improves skeletal muscle contraction (diaphragmatic contractility); prevention of apnea may occur by competitive inhibition of adenosine

Pharmacodynamics/Kinetics

Half-life Elimination

Neonates: 72-96 hours (range: 40-230 hours)
Children >9 months and Adults: 5 hours

Time to Peak Serum: Oral: Within 30 minutes to 2 hours

Pregnancy Risk Factor C

Pregnancy Considerations Caffeine crosses the placenta; serum levels in the fetus are similar to those in the mother. When large bolus doses are administered to animals, teratogenic effects have been reported. Similar doses are not probable following normal caffeine consumption and moderate consumption is not associated with congenital malformations, spontaneous abortions, preterm birth or low birth weight. According to one source, pregnant women who do not smoke or drink alcohol could consume ≤5 mg/kg of caffeine over the course of a day without reproductive risk. Other sources recommend limiting caffeine intake to <150-200 mg/day. The half-life of caffeine is prolonged during the second and third trimesters of pregnancy.

Calcipotriene (kal si POE try een)

Brand Names: U.S. Calcitrene™; Dovonex®; Sorilux™
Brand Names: Canada Dovonex®
Pharmacologic Category Topical Skin Product; Vitamin D Analog
Use Treatment of plaque psoriasis of the body (cream, foam, ointment) or of the scalp (foam, solution)
Local Anesthetic/Vasoconstrictor Precautions No information available to require special precautions
Effects on Dental Treatment No significant effects or complications reported
Effects on Bleeding No information available to require special precautions
Adverse Effects Frequency may vary with site of application.
>10%: Dermatologic: Burning, itching, rash, skin irritation, stinging, tingling
1% to 10%: Dermatologic: Application site pain, dermatitis, dry skin, erythema, peeling, pruritus, worsening of psoriasis
General Dosage Range Topical: *Adults:* Cream: Apply a thin film to affected area twice daily; Foam: Apply a thin film to the affected skin or scalp twice daily; Ointment: Apply a thin film to affected area 1-2 times daily; Solution: Apply to affected scalp twice daily
Mechanism of Action Synthetic vitamin D_3 analog which regulates skin cell production and proliferation
Pharmacodynamics/Kinetics
Onset of Action Improvement begins after 2 weeks; marked improvement seen after 8 weeks
Pregnancy Risk Factor C
Pregnancy Considerations Teratogenic effects have been observed in animal studies. There are no adequate or well-controlled studies in pregnant women.

Calcitonin (kal si TOE nin)

Brand Names: U.S. Fortical®; Miacalcin®

Brand Names: Canada Apo-Calcitonin®; Calcimar®; Caltine®; Miacalcin® NS; PRO-Calcitonin; Sandoz-Calcitonin
Pharmacologic Category Antidote; Hormone
Use Treatment of symptomatic Paget's disease of bone (osteitis deformans); adjunctive therapy for hypercalcemia; treatment of osteoporosis in women >5 years postmenopause
Local Anesthetic/Vasoconstrictor Precautions No information available to require special precautions
Effects on Dental Treatment No significant effects or complications reported
Effects on Bleeding No information available to require special precautions
Adverse Effects Unless otherwise noted, frequencies reported are with nasal spray.

>10%: Respiratory: Rhinitis (≤12%, including ulcerative)
1% to 10%:
Cardiovascular: Flushing (nasal spray: <1%; injection: 2% to 5%), angina (1% to 3%), hypertension (1% to 3%)
Central nervous system: Depression (1% to 3%), dizziness (1% to 3%), fatigue (1% to 3%)
Dermatologic: Erythematous rash (1% to 3%)
Gastrointestinal: Nausea (injection: 10%; nasal spray: 2%), abdominal pain (1% to 3%), constipation (1% to 3%), diarrhea (1% to 3%), dyspepsia (1% to 3%)
Genitourinary: Cystitis (1% to 3%)
Local: Injection site reactions (injection: 10%)
Neuromuscular & skeletal: Back pain (5%), arthrosis (1% to 3%), myalgia (1% to 3%), paresthesia (1% to 3%)
Ocular: Conjunctivitis (1% to 3%), lacrimation abnormality (1% to 3%)
Respiratory: Nasal ulcerations (3%), bronchospasm (1% to 3%), sinusitis (1% to 3%), upper respiratory tract infection (1% to 3%)
Miscellaneous: Flu-like syndrome (1% to 3%), infection (1% to 3%), lymphadenopathy (1% to 3%)
General Dosage Range
I.M., SubQ: *Adults:* Paget's disease/osteoporosis: 50-100 units every 1-2 days; Hypercalcemia: 4-8 units/kg every 12 hours (maximum: 8 units/kg every 6 hours)
Intranasal: *Adults:* 200 units (1 spray) in one nostril daily
Mechanism of Action Peptide sequence similar to human calcitonin; functionally antagonizes the effects of parathyroid hormone. Directly inhibits osteoclastic bone resorption; promotes the renal excretion of calcium, phosphate, sodium, magnesium, and potassium by decreasing tubular reabsorption; increases the jejunal secretion of water, sodium, potassium, and chloride
Pharmacodynamics/Kinetics
Onset of Action
Hypercalcemia: I.M., SubQ: ~2 hours
Paget's disease: Within a few months; may take up to 1 year for neurologic symptom improvement
Duration of Action Hypercalcemia: I.M., SubQ: 6-8 hours
Half-life Elimination Terminal: I.M. 58 minutes; SubQ 59-64 minutes; Nasal: ~18 minutes
Time to Peak Plasma: SubQ ~23 minutes; Nasal: ~13 minutes
Pregnancy Risk Factor C
Pregnancy Considerations Decreased birth weight was observed in animal reproduction studies. Calcitonin does not cross the placenta. The nasal spray formulations are not indicated for use in pregnancy.

Calcitriol (kal si TRYE ole)

Brand Names: U.S. Calcijex® [DSC]; Rocaltrol®; Vectical®

Brand Names: Canada Calcijex®; Rocaltrol®; Silkis™

Pharmacologic Category Vitamin D Analog

Use

Management of hypocalcemia in patients on chronic renal dialysis (oral, injection); management of secondary hyperparathyroidism in patients with chronic kidney disease (CKD) (oral); management of hypocalcemia in patients with hypoparathyroidism and pseudohypoparathyroidism (oral); management of mild-to-moderate plaque psoriasis (topical)

Canadian labeling: Additional uses (not in U.S. labeling): Vitamin D-resistant rickets (oral)

Unlabeled Use Vitamin D-dependent rickets type I/ pseudovitamin D deficiency rickets (PDDR)

Local Anesthetic/Vasoconstrictor Precautions No information available to require special precautions

Effects on Dental Treatment Key adverse event(s) related to dental treatment: Metallic taste and xerostomia (normal salivary flow resumes upon discontinuation).

Effects on Bleeding No information available to require special precautions

Adverse Effects

Oral, I.V.: Frequency not defined.

Cardiovascular: Cardiac arrhythmia, hypertension

Central nervous system: Apathy, headache, hyperthermia, psychosis, sensory disturbances, somnolence

Dermatologic: Erythema multiforme, erythematous skin disorders, pruritus, rash, urticaria

Endocrine & metabolic: Dehydration, growth suppression, hypercalcemia, hypercholesterolemia, libido decreased, polydipsia

Gastrointestinal: Abdominal pain, anorexia, constipation, metallic taste, nausea, pancreatitis, stomach ache, vomiting, weight loss, xerostomia

Genitourinary: Nocturia, urinary tract infection

Hepatic: ALT increased, AST increased

Local: Injection site pain (mild)

Neuromuscular & skeletal: Bone pain, myalgia, dystrophy, soft tissue calcification, weakness

Ocular: Conjunctivitis, photophobia

Renal: Albuminuria, BUN increased, creatinine increased, hypercalciuria, nephrocalcinosis, polyuria

Respiratory: Rhinorrhea

Miscellaneous: Allergic reaction, hypersensitivity reactions

Topical:

>10%: Endocrine: Hypercalcemia (24%)

1% to 10%:

Dermatologic: Psoriasis (4%), skin discomfort (3%), pruritus (1% to 3%)

Genitourinary: Urine abnormality (4%)

Renal: Hypercalciuria (3%)

General Dosage Range Dosage adjustment recommended in patients who develop toxicities

I.V.: Adults: 0.5-4 mcg 3 times weekly

Oral:

Children 1 to <3 years: 0.25-0.75 mcg daily **or** 0.01-0.015 mcg/kg/day (maximum: 0.5 mcg daily)

Children ≥3-5 years: 0.25-0.75 mcg daily

Children ≥6 years: 0.25-2 mcg daily

Adults: 0.25 mcg every other day to 2 mcg once daily

Topical: Adults: Apply to affected areas twice daily (maximum: 200 g weekly)

Mechanism of Action Calcitriol is a potent active metabolite of vitamin D. Vitamin D promotes absorption of calcium in the intestines and retention at the kidneys thereby increasing calcium levels in the serum; decreases excessive serum phosphatase levels, parathyroid hormone levels, and decreases bone resorption; increases renal tubule phosphate resorption

The mechanism by which calcitriol is beneficial in the treatment of psoriasis has not been established.

Pharmacodynamics/Kinetics

Duration of Action Oral, I.V.: 3-5 days

Half-life Elimination Children ~27 hours; Healthy adults: 5-8 hours; Hemodialysis: 16-22 hours

Time to Peak Oral: 3-6 hours; Hemodialysis: 8-12 hours

Pregnancy Risk Factor C

Pregnancy Considerations Teratogenic effects have been observed in some animal reproduction studies. Mild hypercalcemia has been reported in a newborn following maternal use of calcitriol during pregnancy. Adverse effects on fetal development were not observed with use of calcitriol during pregnancy in women (N=9) with pseudovitamin D-dependent rickets. Doses were adjusted every 4 weeks to keep calcium concentrations within normal limits (Edouard, 2011). If calcitriol is used for the management of hypoparathyroidism in pregnancy, dose adjustments may be needed as pregnancy progresses and again following delivery. Vitamin D and calcium levels should be monitored closely and kept in the lower normal range.

Calcium Acetate (KAL see um AS e tate)

Related Information

Rheumatoid Arthritis, Osteoarthritis, and Osteoporosis on page 1526

Brand Names: U.S. Eliphos™; PhosLo®; Phoslyra™

Brand Names: Canada PhosLo®

Pharmacologic Category Antidote; Calcium Salt; Phosphate Binder

Use Control of hyperphosphatemia in end-stage renal failure; does not promote aluminum absorption

Local Anesthetic/Vasoconstrictor Precautions No information available to require special precautions

Effects on Dental Treatment No significant effects or complications reported

Effects on Bleeding No information available to require special precautions

Adverse Effects

>10%:

Endocrine & metabolic: Hypercalcemia

Gastrointestinal: Diarrhea (oral solution)

1% to 10%: Gastrointestinal: Nausea, vomiting

General Dosage Range Oral: Adults: Initial: 1334 mg with each meal; Maintenance: 2001-2668 mg with each meal

Mechanism of Action Combines with dietary phosphate to form insoluble calcium phosphate which is excreted in feces

Pregnancy Risk Factor C

Pregnancy Considerations Animal reproduction studies have not been conducted. Calcium crosses the placenta. The amount of calcium reaching the fetus is determined by maternal physiological changes.

Intestinal absorption of calcium increases during pregnancy. If use is required in pregnant patients with end stage renal disease, fetal harm is not expected if maternal calcium concentrations are monitored and maintained within normal limits as recommended (IOM, 2011).

Calcium and Vitamin D
(KAL see um & VYE ta min dee)

Brand Names: U.S. Cal-CYUM [OTC]; Caltrate® 600+D [OTC]; Caltrate® 600+Soy™ [OTC]; Caltrate® ColonHealth™ [OTC]; Chew-Cal [OTC]; Citracal® Maximum [OTC]; Citracal® Petites [OTC]; Citracal® Regular [OTC]; Liqua-Cal [OTC]; Os-Cal® 500+D [OTC]; Oysco 500+D [OTC]; Oysco D [OTC]; Oyst-Cal-D 500 [OTC]

Generic Availability (U.S.) Yes

Pharmacologic Category Calcium Salt; Electrolyte Supplement, Oral; Vitamin, Fat Soluble

Use Dietary supplement, antacid

Local Anesthetic/Vasoconstrictor Precautions No information available to require special precautions

Effects on Dental Treatment No significant effects or complications reported

Effects on Bleeding No information available to require special precautions

Adverse Effects Frequency not defined; also see individual agents

Central nervous system: Headache

Endocrine & metabolic: Hypercalcemia, hypercalciuria

Gastrointestinal: Gastrointestinal discomfort

Dosage Oral: Adults: Refer to individual monographs for dietary reference intake.

Dosage adjustment in renal impairment: Use caution in severe renal impairment

Contraindications Hypersensitivity to any component of the formulation; hypophosphatemia, hypercalcemia, evidence of vitamin D toxicity; history of kidney stones

Warnings/Precautions Constipation, bloating, and gas are common with calcium supplements. Use with caution in patients with respiratory failure, renal impairment or respiratory acidosis. Use with caution in patients with renal failure to avoid hypercalcemia; frequent monitoring of serum calcium and phosphorus is necessary. Use caution when administering calcium supplements to patients with a history of kidney stones. Hypercalcemia and hypercalciuria are most likely to occur in hypoparathyroid patients receiving high doses of vitamin D. Calcium absorption is impaired in achlorhydria; common in elderly, use an alternate salt (eg, citrate) and administer with food. Calcium administration interferes with absorption of some minerals and drugs; use with caution. Taking calcium (≤500 mg) with food improves absorption.

Some products may contain soy, tartrazine, or phenylalanine, or may be derived from shellfish.

Drug Interactions

Metabolism/Transport Effects None known.

Avoid Concomitant Use

Avoid concomitant use of Calcium Carbonate and Vitamin D with any of the following: Calcium Acetate; Ponatinib

Increased Effect/Toxicity

Calcium Carbonate and Vitamin D may increase the levels/effects of: Alpha-/Beta-Agonists; Amphetamines; Calcium Acetate; Calcium Polystyrene Sulfonate; Dexmethylphenidate; Methylphenidate; QuiNIDine; Sodium Polystyrene Sulfonate; Vitamin D Analogs

The levels/effects of Calcium Carbonate and Vitamin D may be increased by: Multivitamins/Minerals (with ADEK, Folate, Iron); Thiazide Diuretics

Decreased Effect

Calcium Carbonate and Vitamin D may decrease the levels/effects of: ACE Inhibitors; Allopurinol; Anticonvulsants (Hydantoin); Antipsychotic Agents (Phenothiazines); Atazanavir; Bisacodyl; Bisphosphonate Derivatives; Bosutinib; Calcium Channel Blockers; Cefditoren; Cefpodoxime; Cefuroxime; Chloroquine; Corticosteroids (Oral); Dabigatran Etexilate; Dasatinib; Deferiprone; Delavirdine; DOBUTamine; Eltrombopag; Elvitegravir; Erlotinib; Estramustine; Gabapentin; HMG-CoA Reductase Inhibitors; Iron Salts; Isoniazid; Itraconazole; Ketoconazole (Systemic); Mesalamine; Methenamine; Multivitamins/Minerals (with ADEK, Folate, Iron); Mycophenolate; Nilotinib; PenicillAMINE; Phosphate Supplements; Ponatinib; Protease Inhibitors; Quinolone Antibiotics; Rilpivirine; Strontium Ranelate; Tetracycline Derivatives; Thyroid Products; Trientine; Vismodegib

The levels/effects of Calcium Carbonate and Vitamin D may be decreased by: Trientine

Ethanol/Nutrition/Herb Interactions

Ethanol: Avoid ethanol (may increase risk of osteoporosis).

Food: Food may increase calcium absorption. Calcium may decrease iron absorption. Bran, foods high in oxalates, or whole grain cereals may decrease calcium absorption.

Dietary Considerations Take (preferably with food) 2 hours before or after other medications to minimize GI upset. Some products may contain phenylalanine (avoid use in phenylketonurics).

Pregnancy Considerations Available evidence suggests safe use during pregnancy.

Breast-Feeding Considerations Available evidence suggests safe use during lactation.

Dosage Forms

Caplet, oral:

Citracal® Maximum [OTC]: Calcium 315 mg and vitamin D 250 units

Capsule, softgel, oral: Calcium 500 mg and vitamin D 500 units; calcium 600 mg and vitamin D 100 units; calcium 600 mg and vitamin D 200 units

Liqua-Cal [OTC]: Calcium 600 mg and vitamin D 200 units

Tablet, oral: Calcium 250 mg and vitamin D 125 units; calcium 500 mg and vitamin D 125 units; calcium 500 mg and vitamin D 200 units; calcium 600 mg and vitamin D 125 units; calcium 600 mg and vitamin D 200 units; calcium 600 mg and vitamin D 400 units

Caltrate® 600+D [OTC]: Calcium 600 mg and vitamin D 200 units

Caltrate® 600+Soy™ [OTC]: Calcium 600 mg and vitamin D 200 units

Caltrate® ColonHealth™ [OTC]: Calcium 600 mg and vitamin D 200 units

Citracal® Petites [OTC]: Calcium 200 mg and vitamin D 250 units

Citracal® Regular [OTC]: Calcium 250 mg and vitamin D 200 units

Oysco D [OTC]: Calcium 250 mg and vitamin D 125 units

Oysco 500+D [OTC]: Calcium 500 mg and vitamin D 200 units

Oyst-Cal-D 500 [OTC]: Calcium 500 mg and vitamin D 200 units

Tablet, chewable: Calcium 500 mg and vitamin D 100 units; calcium 500 mg and vitamin D 200 units; calcium 600 mg and vitamin D 400 units

Os-Cal® 500+D [OTC]: Calcium 500 mg and vitamin D 400 units

Wafer, chewable:

Cal-CYUM [OTC]: Calcium 519 mg and vitamin D 150 units (50s)

Chew-Cal [OTC]: Calcium 333 mg and vitamin D 40 units (100s, 250s)

Calcium Carbonate (KAL see um KAR bun ate)

Related Information

Rheumatoid Arthritis, Osteoarthritis, and Osteoporosis on page 1526

Brand Names: U.S. Alcalak [OTC]; Alka-Mints® [OTC]; Cal-Gest® [OTC]; Cal-Mint [OTC]; Calci-Chew® [OTC]; Calci-Mix® [OTC]; Caltrate® 600 [OTC]; Children's Pepto [OTC]; Chooz® [OTC]; Florical® [OTC]; Maalox® Children's [OTC]; Maalox® Regular Strength [OTC]; Nephro-Calci® [OTC]; Nutralox® [OTC]; Oysco 500 [OTC]; Oystercal™ 500 [OTC]; Rolaids® Extra Strength [OTC]; Super Calcium 600 [OTC]; Titralac™ [OTC]; Tums® E-X [OTC]; Tums® Extra Strength Sugar Free [OTC]; Tums® Quickpak [OTC]; Tums® Smoothies™ [OTC]; Tums® Ultra [OTC]; Tums® [OTC]

Brand Names: Canada Apo-Cal®; Calcite-500; Caltrate®; Caltrate® Select; Os-Cal®; Tums Extra Strength; Tums Smoothies; Tums® Chews Extra Strength; Tums® Regular Strength; Tums® Ultra Strength

Pharmacologic Category Antacid; Antidote; Calcium Salt; Electrolyte Supplement, Oral

Use As an antacid; treatment and prevention of calcium deficiency or hyperphosphatemia (eg, osteoporosis, osteomalacia, mild/moderate renal insufficiency, hypoparathyroidism, postmenopausal osteoporosis, rickets); has been used to bind phosphate

Local Anesthetic/Vasoconstrictor Precautions No information available to require special precautions

Effects on Dental Treatment Key adverse event(s) related to dental treatment: Xerostomia (normal salivary flow resumes upon discontinuation).

Effects on Bleeding No information available to require special precautions

Adverse Effects Well tolerated

1% to 10%:

Central nervous system: Headache

Endocrine & metabolic: Hypophosphatemia, hypercalcemia

Gastrointestinal: Constipation, laxative effect, acid rebound, nausea, vomiting, anorexia, abdominal pain, xerostomia, flatulence

Miscellaneous: Milk-alkali syndrome with very high, chronic dosing and/or renal failure (headache, nausea, irritability, weakness, alkalosis, hypercalcemia, renal impairment)

General Dosage Range Oral:

Children <2 years: 45-65 mg/kg/day in 4 divided doses

Children 1-6 months: Adequate intake: 200 mg/day

Children 7-12 months: Adequate intake: 260 mg/day

Children 1-3 years: RDA: 700 mg/day

Children 2-5 years (24-47 lbs): Antacid: 161 mg (elemental calcium) as needed (maximum: 483 mg/day); Hypocalcemia: 45-65 mg/kg/day in 4 divided doses

Children 4-8 years: RDA: 1000 mg/day

Children 6-11 years (48-95 lbs): Antacid: 322 mg (elemental calcium) as needed (maximum: 966 mg/day); Hypocalcemia: 45-65 mg/kg/day in 4 divided doses

Children 9-18 years: RDA: 1300 mg/day

Children >11 years: 45-65 mg/kg/day in 4 divided doses

Adults 19-50 years: RDA: 1000 mg/day

Adults ≤51 years: Antacid: 1-2 tablets or 5-10 mL every 2 hours (maximum: 7000 mg/day); Hypocalcemia/dietary: 500-2000 mg/day in 2-4 divided doses

Adults ≥51 years, females: RDA: 1200 mg/day

Adults >51 years: Antacid: 1-2 tablets or 5-10 mL every 2 hours (maximum: 7000 mg/day); Hypocalcemia/dietary: 500-2000 mg/day in 2-4 divided doses; Osteoporosis: 1200 mg/day

Adults 51-70 years, males: RDA: 1000 mg/day

Adults >70 years, males: RDA: 1200 mg/day

Mechanism of Action As dietary supplement, used to prevent or treat negative calcium balance; in osteoporosis, it helps to prevent or decrease the rate of bone loss. The calcium in calcium salts moderates nerve and muscle performance and allows normal cardiac function. Also used to treat hyperphosphatemia in patients with advanced renal insufficiency by combining with dietary phosphate to form insoluble calcium phosphate, which is excreted in feces. Calcium salts as antacids neutralize gastric acidity resulting in increased gastric and duodenal bulb pH; they additionally inhibit proteolytic activity of peptic if the pH is increased >4 and increase lower esophageal sphincter tone.

Pregnancy Considerations Calcium crosses the placenta. Intestinal absorption of calcium increases during pregnancy. The amount of calcium reaching the fetus is determined by maternal physiological changes. Calcium requirements are the same in pregnant and nonpregnant females (IOM, 2011). Calcium-based antacids are considered low risk during pregnancy; excessive use should be avoided (Mahadevan, 2006).

Calcium Carbonate and Magnesium Hydroxide
(KAL see um KAR bun ate & mag NEE zhum hye DROKS ide)

Related Information

Calcium Carbonate on page 233

Magnesium Hydroxide on page 852

Brand Names: U.S. Mi-Acid™ Double Strength [OTC]; Mylanta® Gelcaps® [OTC]; Mylanta® Supreme [OTC]; Mylanta® Ultra [OTC]; Rolaids® Extra Strength [OTC]; Rolaids® [OTC]

Pharmacologic Category Antacid

Use Hyperacidity

Local Anesthetic/Vasoconstrictor Precautions No information available to require special precautions

Effects on Dental Treatment No significant effects or complications reported

Effects on Bleeding No information available to require special precautions

General Dosage Range Oral: Adults: 2-4 tablets between meals and at bedtime

Pregnancy Considerations See individual agents.

Calcium Carbonate and Simethicone
(KAL see um KAR bun ate & sye METH i kone)

Related Information

Calcium Carbonate on page 233

Simethicone on page 1236

Brand Names: U.S. Gas Ban™ [OTC]; Maalox® Advanced Maximum Strength [OTC]; Maalox® Junior Plus Antigas [OTC]; Titralac® Plus [OTC]

Pharmacologic Category Antacid; Antiflatulent

Use Relief of acid indigestion, heartburn, bloating, pressure, and discomfort of gas

Local Anesthetic/Vasoconstrictor Precautions No information available to require special precautions

Effects on Dental Treatment Do not give tetracyclines concomitantly.

Effects on Bleeding No information available to require special precautions

Adverse Effects Frequency not defined: Gastrointestinal: Constipation

General Dosage Range Oral:

Children 6-11 years: Maalox® Junior Plus Antigas: Two tablets as symptoms occur or as directed by healthcare provider (maximum: 6 tablets/24 hours)

Children ≥12 years; Maalox® Advanced Maximum Strength: 1-2 tablets as symptoms occur or as directed by healthcare provider (maximum: 8 tablets/24 hours)

Adults: Maalox® Advanced Maximum Strength: 1-2 tablets as symptoms occur or as directed by healthcare provider (maximum: 8 tablets/24 hours); Titralac® Plus: Two tablets every 2-3 hours as needed (maximum: 19 tablets/24 hours)

Pregnancy Risk Factor C

Pregnancy Considerations See individual agents.

Calcium Chloride (KAL see um KLOR ide)

Pharmacologic Category Calcium Salt; Electrolyte Supplement, Parenteral

Use Treatment of hypocalcemia and conditions secondary to hypocalcemia (eg, tetany, seizures, arrhythmias); emergent treatment of severe hypermagnesemia

Unlabeled Use Calcium channel blocker overdose; beta-blocker overdose (refractory to glucagon and high-dose vasopressors); severe hyperkalemia (K+ >6.5 mEq/L with toxic ECG changes) [ACLS guidelines]; malignant arrhythmias (including cardiac arrest) associated with hypermagnesemia [ACLS guidelines]

Local Anesthetic/Vasoconstrictor Precautions No information available to require special precautions

Effects on Dental Treatment No significant effects or complications reported

Effects on Bleeding No information available to require special precautions

Adverse Effects Frequency not defined. I.V.:

Cardiovascular (following rapid I.V. injection): Arrhythmia, bradycardia, cardiac arrest, hypotension, syncope, vasodilation

Central nervous system: Sense of oppression (with rapid I.V. injection)

Endocrine & metabolic: Hypercalcemia

Gastrointestinal: Irritation, chalky taste

Hepatic: Serum amylase increased

Local (following extravasation): Tissue necrosis

Neuromuscular & skeletal: Tingling sensation (with rapid I.V. injection)

Renal: Renal calculi

Miscellaneous: Hot flashes (with rapid I.V. injection)

Postmarketing and/or case reports: Calcinosis cutis

General Dosage Range I.V.: *Infants, Children, and Adults:* Dosage varies greatly depending on indication

Mechanism of Action Moderates nerve and muscle performance via action potential excitation threshold regulation

Pregnancy Risk Factor C

Pregnancy Considerations Animal reproduction studies have not been conducted. Calcium crosses the placenta. The amount of calcium reaching the fetus is determined by maternal physiological changes. Calcium

requirements are the same in pregnant and nonpregnant females (IOM, 2011). Information related to use as an antidote in pregnancy is limited. In general, medications used as antidotes should take into consideration the health and prognosis of the mother (Bailey, 2003).

Calcium Citrate (KAL see um SIT rate)

Related Information

Rheumatoid Arthritis, Osteoarthritis, and Osteoporosis *on page 1526*

Brand Names: U.S. Cal-C-Caps [OTC]; Cal-Cee [OTC]; Cal-Citrate™ 225 [OTC]; Calcitrate [OTC]

Brand Names: Canada Osteocit®

Pharmacologic Category Calcium Salt

Use Dietary supplement

Local Anesthetic/Vasoconstrictor Precautions No information available to require special precautions

Effects on Dental Treatment No significant effects or complications reported

Effects on Bleeding No information available to require special precautions

Adverse Effects Frequency not defined:

Mild hypercalcemia (calcium: >10.5 mg/dL) may be asymptomatic or manifest itself as constipation, anorexia, nausea, and vomiting

More severe hypercalcemia (calcium: >12 mg/dL) is associated with confusion, delirium, stupor, and coma

Central nervous system: Headache

Endocrine & metabolic: Hypophosphatemia, hypercalcemia

Gastrointestinal: Nausea, anorexia, vomiting, abdominal pain, constipation

Miscellaneous: Thirst

General Dosage Range Oral:

Children 1-6 months: Adequate intake: 200 mg/day

Children 7-12 months: Adequate intake: 260 mg/day

Children 1-3 years: RDA: 700 mg/day

Children 4-8 years: RDA: 1000 mg/day

Children 9-18 years: RDA: 1300 mg/day

Adults: 500-2000 mg divided 2-4 times/day

Adults 19-50 years: RDA: 1000 mg/day

Adults ≥51 years, females: RDA: 1200 mg/day

Adults 51-70 years, males: RDA: 1000 mg/day

Adults >70 years, males: RDA: 1200 mg/day

Mechanism of Action Moderates nerve and muscle performance via action potential excitation threshold regulation

Pregnancy Considerations Calcium crosses the placenta. Intestinal absorption of calcium increases during pregnancy. The amount of calcium reaching the fetus is determined by maternal physiological changes. Calcium requirements are the same in pregnant and nonpregnant females (IOM, 2011).

Calcium Glubionate (KAL see um gloo BYE oh nate)

Related Information

Rheumatoid Arthritis, Osteoarthritis, and Osteoporosis *on page 1526*

Brand Names: U.S. Calcionate [OTC]

Pharmacologic Category Calcium Salt

Use Dietary supplement

Local Anesthetic/Vasoconstrictor Precautions No information available to require special precautions

Effects on Dental Treatment No significant effects or complications reported

Effects on Bleeding No information available to require special precautions

Adverse Effects Frequency not defined; symptoms reported with hypercalcemia:

Gastrointestinal: Abdominal pain, anorexia, constipation, nausea, thirst, vomiting, xerostomia

Genitourinary: Polyuria

General Dosage Range Oral:

Children 1-6 months: Adequate intake: 200 mg/day

Children 7-12 months: Adequate intake: 260 mg/day

Children 1-3 years: RDA: 700 mg/day

Children 4-8 years: RDA: 1000 mg/day

Children 9-18 years: RDA: 1300 mg/day

Adults 19-50 years: RDA: 1000 mg/day

Adults ≥51 years, females: RDA: 1200 mg/day

Adults 51-70 years, males: RDA: 1000 mg/day

Adults >70 years, males: RDA: 1200 mg/day

Mechanism of Action As dietary supplement, used to prevent or treat negative calcium balance. The calcium in calcium salts moderates nerve and muscle performance and allows normal cardiac function.

Pregnancy Considerations Calcium crosses the placenta. Intestinal absorption of calcium increases during pregnancy. The amount of calcium reaching the fetus is determined by maternal physiological changes. Calcium requirements are the same in pregnant and nonpregnant females (IOM, 2011).

Calcium Gluconate (KAL see um GLOO koe nate)

Related Information

Rheumatoid Arthritis, Osteoarthritis, and Osteoporosis *on page 1526*

Brand Names: U.S. Cal-G [OTC] [DSC]; Cal-GLU™ [OTC]

Pharmacologic Category Calcium Salt; Electrolyte Supplement, Oral; Electrolyte Supplement, Parenteral

Use

I.V.: Treatment of hypocalcemia and conditions secondary to hypocalcemia (eg, tetany, seizures, arrhythmias); treatment of cardiac disturbances secondary to hyperkalemia; adjunctive treatment of rickets, osteomalacia, and magnesium sulfate overdose; decrease capillary permeability in allergic conditions, nonthrombocytopenic purpura, and exudative dermatoses (eg, dermatitis herpetiformis, pruritus secondary to certain drugs)

Oral: Dietary calcium supplementation

Unlabeled Use Calcium channel blocker overdose; treatment of hydrofluoric acid exposure

Local Anesthetic/Vasoconstrictor Precautions No information available to require special precautions

Effects on Dental Treatment No significant effects or complications reported

Effects on Bleeding No information available to require special precautions

Adverse Effects Frequency not defined.

I.V.:

Cardiovascular (with rapid I.V. injection): Arrhythmia, bradycardia, cardiac arrest, hypotension, syncope, vasodilation

Central nervous system: Sense of oppression (with rapid I.V. injection)

Endocrine & metabolic: Hypercalcemia

Gastrointestinal: Chalky taste

Neuromuscular & skeletal: Tingling sensation (with rapid I.V. injection)

Miscellaneous: Heat waves (with rapid I.V. injection)

Postmarketing and/or case reports: Calcinosis cutis

Oral: Gastrointestinal: Constipation

General Dosage Range

I.V.: *Children and Adults:* Dosage varies greatly depending on indication

Oral:

Children 1-6 months: Adequate intake: 200 mg **elemental calcium** daily

Children 7-12 months: Adequate intake: 260 mg **elemental calcium** daily

Children 1-3 years: RDA: 700 mg **elemental calcium** daily

Children 4-8 years: RDA: 1000 mg **elemental calcium** daily

Children 9-18 years: RDA: 1300 mg **elemental calcium** daily

Adults 19-50 years: RDA: 1000 mg **elemental calcium** daily

Adults ≥51 years, females: RDA: 1200 mg **elemental calcium** daily

Adults 51-70 years, males: RDA: 1000 mg **elemental calcium** daily

Adults >70 years, males: RDA: 1200 mg **elemental calcium** daily

Mechanism of Action Moderates nerve and muscle performance via action potential threshold regulation. In hydrogen fluoride exposures, calcium gluconate provides a source of calcium ions to complex free fluoride ions and prevent or reduce toxicity; administration also helps to correct fluoride-induced hypocalcemia.

Pregnancy Risk Factor C

Pregnancy Considerations Animal reproduction studies have not been conducted. Calcium crosses the placenta. The amount of calcium reaching the fetus is determined by maternal physiological changes. Calcium requirements are the same in pregnant and nonpregnant females (IOM, 2011). Information related to use as an antidote in pregnancy is limited. In general, medications used as antidotes should take into consideration the health and prognosis of the mother (Bailey, 2003).

Calcium Lactate (KAL see um LAK tate)

Related Information

Rheumatoid Arthritis, Osteoarthritis, and Osteoporosis *on page 1526*

Pharmacologic Category Calcium Salt

Use Treatment and prevention of calcium depletion

Local Anesthetic/Vasoconstrictor Precautions No information available to require special precautions

Effects on Dental Treatment No significant effects or complications reported

Effects on Bleeding No information available to require special precautions

General Dosage Range Oral:

Children 1-6 months: Adequate intake: 200 mg/day

Children 7-12 months: Adequate intake: 260 mg/day

Children 1-3 years: RDA: 700 mg/day

Children 4-8 years: RDA: 1000 mg/day

Children 9-18 years: RDA: 1300 mg/day

Adults 19-50 years: RDA: 1000 mg/day

Adults ≥51 years, females: RDA: 1200 mg/day

Adults 51-70 years, males: RDA: 1000 mg/day

Adults >70 years, males: RDA: 1200 mg/day

Mechanism of Action As dietary supplement, used to prevent or treat negative calcium balance; in osteoporosis, it helps to prevent or decrease the rate of bone loss. The calcium in calcium salts moderates nerve and muscle performance and allows normal cardiac function.

Pregnancy Considerations Calcium crosses the placenta. Intestinal absorption of calcium increases during pregnancy. The amount of calcium reaching the fetus is determined by maternal physiological changes. Calcium requirements are the same in pregnant and nonpregnant females (IOM, 2011).

Calcium Phosphate (Tribasic)
(KAL see um FOS fate tri BAY sik)

Related Information
Rheumatoid Arthritis, Osteoarthritis, and Osteoporosis *on page 1526*
Brand Names: U.S. Posture® [OTC]
Pharmacologic Category Calcium Salt
Use Dietary supplement
Local Anesthetic/Vasoconstrictor Precautions No information available to require special precautions
Effects on Dental Treatment No significant effects or complications reported
Effects on Bleeding No information available to require special precautions
General Dosage Range Oral:
Children 1-6 months: Adequate intake: 200 mg/day
Children 7-12 months: Adequate intake: 260 mg/day
Children 1-3 years: RDA: 700 mg/day
Children 4-8 years: RDA: 1000 mg/day
Children 9-18 years: RDA: 1300 mg/day
Adults: 2 tablets daily
Adults 19-50 years: RDA: 1000 mg/day
Adults ≥51 years, females: RDA: 1200 mg/day
Adults 51-70 years, males: RDA: 1000 mg/day
Adults >70 years, males: RDA: 1200 mg/day
Mechanism of Action As dietary supplement, used to prevent or treat negative calcium balance; in osteoporosis, it helps to prevent or decrease the rate of bone loss. The calcium in calcium salts moderates nerve and muscle performance and allows normal cardiac function.
Pregnancy Considerations Calcium crosses the placenta. Intestinal absorption of calcium increases during pregnancy. The amount of calcium reaching the fetus is determined by maternal physiological changes. Calcium requirements are the same in pregnant and nonpregnant females (IOM, 2011).

Calfactant (kaf AKT ant)

Brand Names: U.S. Infasurf®
Pharmacologic Category Lung Surfactant
Use Prevention of respiratory distress syndrome (RDS) in premature infants at high risk for RDS and for the treatment ("rescue") of premature infants who develop RDS

Prophylaxis: Therapy at birth with calfactant is indicated for premature infants <29 weeks of gestational age at significant risk for RDS. Should be administered as soon as possible, preferably within 30 minutes after birth.
Treatment: For infants ≤72 hours of age with RDS (confirmed by clinical and radiologic findings) and requiring endotracheal intubation.
Local Anesthetic/Vasoconstrictor Precautions No information available to require special precautions
Effects on Dental Treatment No significant effects or complications reported
Effects on Bleeding No information available to require special precautions

Adverse Effects
Cardiovascular: Cyanosis (65%), bradycardia (34%)
Respiratory: Airway obstruction (39%), reflux (21%), requirement for manual ventilation (16%), reintubation (3%)
General Dosage Range Intratracheal: *Premature infants:* 3 mL/kg (body weight at birth) every 12 hours for a total of 3 doses
Mechanism of Action Endogenous lung surfactant is essential for effective ventilation because it modifies alveolar surface tension, thereby stabilizing the alveoli. Lung surfactant deficiency is the cause of respiratory distress syndrome (RDS) in premature infants and lung surfactant restores surface activity to the lungs of these infants.

Camphor and Phenol (KAM for & FEE nole)

Related Information
Phenol *on page 1082*
Brand Names: U.S. Campho-Phenique® [OTC]
Pharmacologic Category Topical Skin Product
Use Relief of pain and itching associated with minor burns, sunburn, minor cuts, insect bites, minor skin irritation; temporary relief of pain from cold sores
Local Anesthetic/Vasoconstrictor Precautions No information available to require special precautions
Effects on Dental Treatment No significant effects or complications reported
Effects on Bleeding No information available to require special precautions
General Dosage Range Topical: *Adults:* Apply 1-3 times/day
Pregnancy Risk Factor C
Pregnancy Considerations Following exposure to large concentrations (eg, oral ingestion observed with poisonings), camphor crosses the placenta and is toxic to the fetus (Rabl, 1997).

Canakinumab (can a KIN ue mab)

Brand Names: U.S. Ilaris®
Brand Names: Canada Ilaris™
Pharmacologic Category Interleukin-1 Beta Inhibitor; Interleukin-1 Inhibitor; Monoclonal Antibody
Use Treatment of Cryopyrin-Associated Periodic Syndromes (CAPS), including familial cold autoinflammatory syndrome (FCAS) and Muckle-Wells syndrome (MWS)
Local Anesthetic/Vasoconstrictor Precautions No information available to require special precautions
Effects on Dental Treatment No significant effects or complications reported
Effects on Bleeding No information available to require special precautions
Adverse Effects
>10%:
Central nervous system: Headache (14%), vertigo (9% to 14%)
Gastrointestinal: Diarrhea (20%), nausea (14%), gastroenteritis (11%), weight gain (11%)
Neuromuscular and skeletal: Musculoskeletal pain (11%)
Respiratory: Nasopharyngitis (34%), rhinitis (17%), bronchitis (11%), pharyngitis (11%)
Miscellaneous: Influenza (17%)
1% to 10%:
Endocrine & metabolic: Calcium decreased (4% to 8%)

Hematologic: Eosinophils increased (3% to 7%)

Hepatic: AST increased (3% to 6%), ALT increased (3%), ALP increased (3%), bilirubin increased (3% to 7%)

Local: Injection site reactions (7% to 9%)

Renal: Creatinine clearance decreased (3% to 8%), proteinuria (4% to 8%)

General Dosage Range SubQ:

Children ≥4 years and 15-40 kg: 2-3 mg/kg every 8 weeks

Children ≥4 years and Adults >40 kg: 150 mg every 8 weeks

Mechanism of Action Canakinumab reduces inflammation by binding to interleukin-1 beta (IL-1β) (no binding to IL-1 alpha or IL-1 receptor antagonist) and preventing interaction with cell surface receptors. Cryopyrin-associated periodic syndromes (CAPS) refers to rare genetic syndromes caused by mutations in the nucleotide-binding domain, leucine rich family (NLR), pyrin domain containing 3 (NLRP-3) gene or the cold-induced autoinflammatory syndrome-1 (CIAS1) gene. Cryopyrin, a protein encoded by this gene, regulates IL-1β activation. Deficiency of cryopyrin results in excessive inflammation.

Pharmacodynamics/Kinetics

Half-life Elimination 26 days

Time to Peak Serum: Children: 2-7 days; Adults: ~7 days

Pregnancy Risk Factor C

Pregnancy Considerations Animal reproduction studies have demonstrated fetal skeletal development delays. There are no adequate and well-controlled studies in pregnant women. Use during pregnancy only if potential benefit to the mother outweighs potential risk to the fetus.

Candesartan (kan de SAR tan)

Related Information

Cardiovascular Diseases *on page 1492*

Brand Names: U.S. Atacand®

Brand Names: Canada Apo-Candesartan®; Atacand®; CO Candesartan; JAMP-Candesartan; Mylan-Candesartan; PMS-Candesartan; Sandoz-Candesartan; Teva-Candesartan

Generic Availability (U.S.) No

Pharmacologic Category Angiotensin II Receptor Blocker; Antihypertensive

Use Alone or in combination with other antihypertensive agents in treating hypertension; treatment of heart failure (NYHA class II-IV)

Local Anesthetic/Vasoconstrictor Precautions No information available to require special precautions

Effects on Dental Treatment No significant effects or complications reported

Effects on Bleeding No information available to require special precautions

Adverse Effects

Cardiovascular: Angina, hypotension (heart failure 19%), MI, palpitation, tachycardia

Central nervous system: Anxiety, depression, dizziness, drowsiness, fever, headache, lightheadedness, somnolence, vertigo

Dermatologic: Angioedema, rash

Endocrine & metabolic: Hyperglycemia, hyperkalemia (heart failure <1% to 6%), hypertriglyceridemia, hyperuricemia

Gastrointestinal: Dyspepsia, gastroenteritis

Neuromuscular & skeletal: Back pain, CPK increased, myalgia, paresthesia, weakness

Renal: Serum creatinine increased (up to 13% in patients with heart failure with drug discontinuation required in 6%), hematuria

Respiratory: Dyspnea, epistaxis, pharyngitis, rhinitis, upper respiratory tract infection

Miscellaneous: Diaphoresis increased

Dosage Oral:

Hypertension:

Children 1 to <6 years: Initial: 0.2 mg/kg/day in 1-2 divided doses; titrate to response (within 2 weeks, antihypertensive effect usually observed); usual range: 0.05 to 0.4 mg/kg/day; maximum daily dose: 0.4 mg/kg/day

Children 6 to <17 years:

<50 kg: Initial: 4-8 mg/day in 1-2 divided doses; titrate to response (within 2 weeks, antihypertensive effect usually observed); usual range: 2-16 mg/day; maximum daily dose: 32 mg/day

>50 kg: Initial: 8-16 mg/day in 1-2 divided doses; titrate to response (within 2 weeks, antihypertensive effect usually observed); usual range: 4-32 mg/day; maximum daily dose: 32 mg/day

Adults: Dosage must be individualized. Initial: 16 mg once daily; titrate to response (within 2 weeks, antihypertensive effect usually observed); usual range: 8-32 mg/day in 1-2 divided doses; maximum daily dose: 32 mg/day

Heart failure: Adults: Initial: 4 mg once daily; double the dose at 2-week intervals, as tolerated; target dose: 32 mg once daily

Note: In selected cases, concurrent therapy with an ACE inhibitor may provide additional benefit.

Elderly: No initial dosage adjustment is necessary for elderly patients (although higher concentrations (C_{max}) and AUC were observed in these populations), for patients with mildly impaired renal function, or for patients with mildly impaired hepatic function.

Dosage adjustment in renal impairment:

Children 1 to <17 years: No dosage adjustment provided in manufacturer's labeling (has not been studied). Children with GFR <30 mL/minute/1.73 m² should not receive candesartan.

Adults: No initial dosage adjustment necessary; however, in patients with severe renal impairment (Cl_{cr} <30 mL/minute/1.73 m²) AUC and C_{max} were approximately doubled after repeated dosing.

Dosage adjustment in hepatic impairment:

Mild impairment: No initial dosage adjustment necessary.

Moderate impairment: Consider initiation at lower dosages (AUC increased by 145%).

Severe impairment: No dosage adjustment provided in manufacturer's labeling (has not been studied).

Mechanism of Action Candesartan is an angiotensin receptor antagonist. Angiotensin II acts as a vasoconstrictor. In addition to causing direct vasoconstriction, angiotensin II also stimulates the release of aldosterone. Once aldosterone is released, sodium as well as water are reabsorbed. The end result is an elevation in blood pressure. Candesartan binds to the AT1 angiotensin II receptor. This binding prevents angiotensin II from binding to the receptor thereby blocking the vasoconstriction and the aldosterone secreting effects of angiotensin II.

Contraindications Hypersensitivity to candesartan or any component of the formulation; concomitant use with aliskiren in patients with diabetes mellitus

◀ **Warnings/Precautions [U.S. Boxed Warning]: Drugs that act on the renin-angiotensin system can cause injury and death to the developing fetus. Discontinue as soon as possible once pregnancy is detected.** May cause hyperkalemia; avoid potassium supplementation unless specifically required by healthcare provider. Avoid use or use a smaller dose in patients who are volume depleted; correct depletion first. May be associated with deterioration of renal function and/or increases in serum creatinine, particularly in patients with low renal blood flow (eg, renal artery stenosis, heart failure) whose glomerular filtration rate (GFR) is dependent on efferent arteriolar vasoconstriction by angiotensin II. Use with caution in unstented unilateral/bilateral renal artery stenosis, pre-existing renal insufficiency, or significant aortic/mitral stenosis. Use with caution in patients with moderate hepatic impairment. Contraindicated with severe hepatic impairment and/or cholestasis. Use caution when initiating in heart failure; may need to adjust dose, and/or concurrent diuretic therapy, because of candesartan-induced hypotension. Hypotension may occur during major surgery and anesthesia; use cautiously before, during, and immediately after such interventions. Concomitant use of an angiotensin-converting enzyme (ACE) inhibitor or renin inhibitor (eg, aliskiren) is associated with an increased risk of hypotension, hyperkalemia, and renal dysfunction; concomitant use with aliskiren should be avoided in patients with GFR <60 mL/minute and is contraindicated in patients with diabetes mellitus (regardless of GFR). Pediatric patients with a GFR <30 mL/minute/1.73 m^2 or children <1 year of age should not receive candesartan; has not been evaluated.

Drug Interactions

Metabolism/Transport Effects Substrate of CYP2C9 (minor); **Note:** Assignment of Major/Minor substrate status based on clinically relevant drug interaction potential; **Inhibits** CYP2C8 (weak), CYP2C9 (weak)

Avoid Concomitant Use There are no known interactions where it is recommended to avoid concomitant use.

Increased Effect/Toxicity

Candesartan may increase the levels/effects of: ACE Inhibitors; Amifostine; Antihypertensives; CycloSPORINE (Systemic); Hypotensive Agents; Lithium; Nonsteroidal Anti-Inflammatory Agents; Potassium-Sparing Diuretics; RiTUXimab; Sodium Phosphates

The levels/effects of Candesartan may be increased by: Alfuzosin; Aliskiren; Canagliflozin; Diazoxide; Eplerenone; Herbs (Hypotensive Properties); MAO Inhibitors; Pentoxifylline; Phosphodiesterase 5 Inhibitors; Potassium Salts; Prostacyclin Analogues; Tolvaptan; Trimethoprim

Decreased Effect

The levels/effects of Candesartan may be decreased by: Herbs (Hypertensive Properties); Methylphenidate; Nonsteroidal Anti-Inflammatory Agents; Yohimbine

Ethanol/Nutrition/Herb Interactions

Food: Potassium supplements and/or potassium-containing salts may cause or worsen hyperkalemia. Management: Consult prescriber before consuming a potassium-rich diet, potassium supplements, or salt substitutes.

Herb/Nutraceutical: Dong quai has estrogenic activity. Ephedra, yohimbe, and ginseng may worsen hypertension. Garlic may increase antihypertensive effect of candesartan. Management: Avoid dong quai if using for hypertension. Avoid ephedra, yohimbe, ginseng, and garlic.

Pharmacodynamics/Kinetics

Onset of Action 2-3 hours; Peak effect: 6-8 hours

Duration of Action >24 hours

Half-life Elimination Dose dependent: 5-9 hours

Time to Peak 3-4 hours

Pregnancy Risk Factor D

Pregnancy Considerations [U.S. Boxed Warning]: Drugs that act on the renin-angiotensin system can cause injury and death to the developing fetus. Discontinue as soon as possible once pregnancy is detected. The use of drugs which act on the renin-angiotensin system are associated with oligohydramnios. Oligohydramnios, due to decreased fetal renal function, may lead to fetal lung hypoplasia and skeletal malformations. Use is also associated with anuria, hypotension, renal failure, skull hypoplasia, and death in the fetus/neonate. The exposed fetus should be monitored for fetal growth, amniotic fluid volume, and organ formation. Infants exposed *in utero* should be monitored for hyperkalemia, hypotension, and oliguria.

Lactation Excretion in breast milk unknown/not recommended

Dosage Forms

Tablet, oral:

Atacand®: 4 mg, 8 mg, 16 mg, 32 mg

Candesartan and Hydrochlorothiazide
(kan de SAR tan & hye droe klor oh THYE a zide)

Related Information

Candesartan *on page 237*

Hydrochlorothiazide *on page 687*

Brand Names: U.S. Atacand HCT®

Brand Names: Canada Apo-Candesartan HCTZ®; Atacand® Plus; Co-Candesartan/HCT; Mylan-Candesartan HCTZ; PMS-Candesartan HCTZ; Sandoz-Candesartan Plus

Pharmacologic Category Angiotensin II Receptor Blocker; Diuretic, Thiazide

Use Treatment of hypertension; combination product should not be used for initial therapy

Local Anesthetic/Vasoconstrictor Precautions No information available to require special precautions

Effects on Dental Treatment No significant effects or complications reported

Effects on Bleeding No information available to require special precautions

Adverse Effects Reactions which follow have been reported with the combination product; see individual drug agents for additional adverse reactions that may be expected from each agent.

1% to 10%:

Central nervous system: Dizziness (3%), headache (3%, placebo 5%)

Neuromuscular & skeletal: Back pain (3%)

Respiratory: Upper respiratory tract infection (4%)

Miscellaneous: Flu-like syndrome (2%)

General Dosage Range Oral: *Adults:* Candesartan 16-32 mg/day in 1-2 divided doses and hydrochlorothiazide 12.5-25 mg once daily

Mechanism of Action

Candesartan: Candesartan is an angiotensin receptor antagonist. Angiotensin II acts as a vasoconstrictor. In addition to causing direct vasoconstriction, angiotensin II also stimulates the release of aldosterone. Once aldosterone is released, sodium as well as water are reabsorbed. The end result is an elevation in blood pressure. Candesartan binds to the AT1 angiotensin II receptor. This binding prevents angiotensin II from binding to the receptor, thereby blocking the vaso-constriction and the aldosterone-secreting effects of angiotensin II.

Hydrochlorothiazide: Inhibits sodium reabsorption in the distal tubules causing increased excretion of sodium and water as well as potassium and hydrogen ions

Pregnancy Risk Factor D

Pregnancy Considerations [U.S. Boxed Warning]: Drugs that act on the renin-angiotensin system can cause injury and death to the developing fetus. Discontinue as soon as possible once pregnancy is detected. Also see individual agents.

Cantharidin (kan THAR e din)

Brand Names: Canada Canthacur®; Cantharone®
Pharmacologic Category Keratolytic Agent
Use Removal of common warts, molluscum contagiosum, and periungual warts

Local Anesthetic/Vasoconstrictor Precautions No information available to require special precautions

Effects on Dental Treatment No significant effects or complications reported

Effects on Bleeding No information available to require special precautions

Adverse Effects Frequency not defined.
Dermatologic: Annular warts, depigmentation (temporary)
Local: Blisters, burning, pain, tenderness, tingling
Miscellaneous: Chemical lymphangitis

General Dosage Range Topical:
Children, Adolescents, and Adults (Canthacur®): Apply directly to lesion; once dry, may cover with nonporous tape for up to 1 week; repeat if necessary.
Children ≥3 years, Adolescents, and Adults (Canthar-one®): Apply directly to lesion; once dry, may cover with nonporous tape for up to 1 week; repeat if necessary.

Mechanism of Action Cantharidin is a vesicant thought to cause wart exfoliation via its acantholytic actions.

Pregnancy Considerations Use is not recommended during pregnancy.

Product Availability Not available in U.S.

Cantharidin, Podophyllin Resin, and Salicylic Acid
(kan THAR e din, po DOF fil um REZ in & sal i SIL ik AS id)

Brand Names: Canada Canthacur-PS®; Cantharone® Plus
Pharmacologic Category Keratolytic Agent
Use For removal of warts especially plantar, mosaic, and periungual; recommended for resistant and heavily keratinized warts; useful where painless application is desired. Canthacur-PS® is also indicated for removal of molluscum contagiosum.

Local Anesthetic/Vasoconstrictor Precautions No information available to require special precautions

Effects on Dental Treatment No significant effects or complications reported

Effects on Bleeding No information available to require special precautions

Adverse Effects Frequency not defined.
Dermatologic: Annular warts
Local: Burning, extreme tenderness, pain, tingling
Miscellaneous: Chemical lymphangitis

General Dosage Range Topical: Children ≥12 years and Adults: Applied by physician only.

Mechanism of Action Salicylic acid is a keratolytic that produces desquamation of hyperkeratotic epithelium via dissolution of the intercellular cement which causes the cornified tissue to swell, soften, macerate, and desquamate. Podophyllin directly affects epithelial cell metabolism by arresting mitosis through binding to a protein subunit of spindle microtubules (tubulin). Cantharidin is a vesicant thought to cause wart exfoliation via its acantholytic actions.

Pregnancy Considerations Reports of podophyllin use in pregnant women have shown evidence of fetal abnormalities, fetal death, and stillbirth; use is not recommended.

Product Availability Not available in the U.S.

Capecitabine (ka pe SITE a been)

Related Information
Fluorouracil (Systemic) on page 608
Brand Names: U.S. Xeloda®
Brand Names: Canada Xeloda®
Pharmacologic Category Antineoplastic Agent, Antimetabolite; Antineoplastic Agent, Antimetabolite (Pyrimidine Analog)
Use Treatment of metastatic colorectal cancer; adjuvant therapy of Dukes' C colon cancer; treatment of metastatic breast cancer

Unlabeled Use Treatment of gastric cancer, pancreatic cancer, esophageal cancer, ovarian cancer, metastatic renal cell cancer, neuroendocrine tumors, metastatic CNS lesions

Local Anesthetic/Vasoconstrictor Precautions No information available to require special precautions

Effects on Dental Treatment Key adverse event(s) related to dental treatment: Stomatitis, abnormal taste, and taste disturbance.

Effects on Bleeding Bleeding has been reported in <6% of patients. Thrombocytopenia has been reported in 24% of patients and is severe (grade 4) in 1%. A medical consult is suggested.

Adverse Effects Frequency listed derived from monotherapy trials.
>10%:
Cardiovascular: Edema (9% to 15%)
Central nervous system: Fatigue (16% to 42%), fever (7% to 18%), pain (12%)
Dermatologic: Palmar-plantar erythrodysesthesia (hand-and-foot syndrome) (54% to 60%; grade 3: 11% to 17%; may be dose limiting), dermatitis (27% to 37%)
Gastrointestinal: Diarrhea (47% to 57%; may be dose limiting; grade 3: 12% to 13%; grade 4: 2% to 3%), nausea (34% to 53%), vomiting (15% to 37%), abdominal pain (7% to 35%), stomatitis (22% to 25%), appetite decreased (26%), anorexia (9% to 23%), constipation (9% to 15%)

Hematologic: Lymphopenia (94%; grade 4: 14%), anemia (72% to 80%; grade 4: <1% to 1%), neutropenia (2% to 26%; grade 4: 2%), thrombocytopenia (24%; grade 4: 1%)

Hepatic: Bilirubin increased (22% to 48%; grades 3/4: 11% to 23%)

Neuromuscular & skeletal: Paresthesia (21%)

Ocular: Eye irritation (13% to 15%)

Respiratory: Dyspnea (14%)

5% to 10%:

Cardiovascular: Venous thrombosis (8%), chest pain (6%)

Central nervous system: Headache (5% to 10%), lethargy (10%), dizziness (6% to 8%), insomnia (7% to 8%), mood alteration (5%), depression (5%)

Dermatologic: Nail disorder (7%), rash (7%), skin discoloration (7%), alopecia (6%), erythema (6%)

Endocrine & metabolic: Dehydration (7%)

Gastrointestinal: Motility disorder (10%), oral discomfort (10%), dyspepsia (6% to 8%), upper GI inflammatory disorders (colorectal cancer: 8%), hemorrhage (6%), ileus (6%), taste perversion (colorectal cancer: 6%)

Neuromuscular & skeletal: Back pain (10%), weakness (10%), neuropathy (10%), myalgia (9%), arthralgia (8%), limb pain (6%)

Ocular: Abnormal vision (colorectal cancer: 5%), conjunctivitis (5%)

Respiratory: Cough (7%)

Miscellaneous: Viral infection (colorectal cancer: 5%)

General Dosage Range Dosage adjustment recommended in patients with renal impairment or who develop toxicities

Oral: *Adults:* 1250 mg/m^2 twice daily for 2 weeks, every 21 days

Mechanism of Action Capecitabine is a prodrug of fluorouracil. It undergoes hydrolysis in the liver and tissues to form fluorouracil which is the active moiety. Fluorouracil is a fluorinated pyrimidine antimetabolite that inhibits thymidylate synthetase, blocking the methylation of deoxyuridylic acid to thymidylic acid, interfering with DNA, and to a lesser degree, RNA synthesis. Fluorouracil appears to be phase specific for the G_1 and S phases of the cell cycle.

Pharmacodynamics/Kinetics

Half-life Elimination 0.5-1 hour

Time to Peak 1.5 hours; Fluorouracil: 2 hours

Pregnancy Risk Factor D

Pregnancy Considerations Animal studies have demonstrated teratogenicity and fetal loss. There are no adequate and well-controlled studies in pregnant women; however, fetal harm may occur. Women of childbearing potential should avoid pregnancy.

Capreomycin (kap ree oh MYE sin)

Brand Names: U.S. Capastat® Sulfate

Pharmacologic Category Antibiotic, Miscellaneous; Antitubercular Agent

Use Treatment of tuberculosis in conjunction with at least one other antituberculosis agent

Local Anesthetic/Vasoconstrictor Precautions No information available to require special precautions

Effects on Dental Treatment No significant effects or complications reported

Effects on Bleeding No information available to require special precautions

Adverse Effects

>10%:

Otic: Ototoxicity (subclinical hearing loss: 11%; clinical loss: 3%)

Renal: Nephrotoxicity (36%, increased BUN)

1% to 10%: Hematologic: Eosinophilia (dose related, mild)

General Dosage Range Dosage adjustment recommended in patients with renal impairment

I.M., I.V.: *Adults:* 1 g/day (maximum: 20 mg/kg/day) for 60-120 days, followed by 1 g 2-3 times/week

Mechanism of Action Capreomycin is a cyclic polypeptide antimicrobial. It is administered as a mixture of capreomycin IA and capreomycin IB. The mechanism of action of capreomycin is not well understood. Mycobacterial species that have become resistant to other agents are usually still sensitive to the action of capreomycin. However, significant cross-resistance with viomycin, kanamycin, and neomycin occurs.

Pharmacodynamics/Kinetics

Half-life Elimination Normal renal function: 4-6 hours; Cl_{cr} 100-110 mL/minute: 5-6 hours; Cl_{cr} 50-80 mL/minute: 7-10 hours; Cl_{cr} 20-40 mL/minute: 12-20 hours; Cl_{cr} 10 mL/minute: 29 hours; Cl_{cr} 0 mL/minute: 55 hours

Time to Peak Serum: I.M.: 1-2 hours

Pregnancy Risk Factor C

Pregnancy Considerations Capreomycin has been shown to be teratogenic in animal studies. **[U.S. Boxed Warning]: Safety has not been established in pregnant women**; use during pregnancy only if the potential benefit to the mother outweighs the possible risk to the fetus.

Capsaicin (kap SAY sin)

Related Information

Capsicum Peppers *on page 1444*

Ulcerative, Erosive, and Painful Oral Mucosal Disorders *on page 1578*

Brand Names: U.S. Capzasin-HP® [OTC]; Capzasin-P® [OTC]; DiabetAid® Pain and Tingling Relief [OTC]; Qutenza™; Salonpas® Gel-Patch Hot [OTC]; Salonpas® Hot [OTC] [DSC]; Trixaicin HP [OTC]; Trixaicin [OTC]; Zostrix® Diabetic Foot Pain [OTC]; Zostrix® [OTC]; Zostrix®-HP [OTC]

Brand Names: Canada Zostrix®; Zostrix® H.P.

Generic Availability (U.S.) Yes: Cream

Pharmacologic Category Analgesic, Topical; Topical Skin Product; Transient Receptor Potential Vanilloid 1 (TRPV1) Agonist

Dental Use Potential use as topical agent in burning mouth syndrome and oral mucositis

Use

Topical patch (Qutenza™): Management of postherpetic neuralgia (PHN)

OTC labeling: Temporary treatment of minor pain associated with muscles and joints due to backache, strains, sprains, bruises, cramps, or arthritis; temporary relief of pain associated with diabetic neuropathy

Unlabeled Use Diabetic neuropathy; treatment of pain associated with psoriasis and intractable pruritus. Potential use as topical agent in burning mouth syndrome and oral mucositis.

Local Anesthetic/Vasoconstrictor Precautions No information available to require special precautions

Effects on Dental Treatment No significant effects or complications reported

Effects on Bleeding May have antiplatelet effects

Adverse Effects Topical patch (Qutenza™, capsaicin 8%):
>10%: Local: Erythema (63%), pain (42%)
1% to 10%:
Cardiovascular: Hypertension (2%; transient)
Dermatologic: Pruritus (2%)
Gastrointestinal: Nausea (5%), vomiting (3%)
Local: Pruritus (6%), papules (6%), edema (4%), dryness (2%), swelling (2%)
Respiratory: Nasopharyngitis (4%), sinusitis (3%), bronchitis (2%)

Dental Usual Dosage Topical: Apply cream or gel to affected area 3-4 times/day

Dosage Topical:
Children ≥12 years and Adults: Pain relief: OTC labeling: Patch (Salonpas®-Hot): Apply patch to affected area up to 3-4 times/day for 7 days. Patch may remain in place for up to 8 hours.
Adults:
Pain relief: OTC labeling: Topical products (cream, gel, liquid, lotion): Apply to affected area 3-4 times/day; efficacy may be decreased if used less than 3 times/day; best results seen after 2-4 weeks of continuous use
Postherpetic neuralgia: Patch (Qutenza™ [capsaicin 8%]): Apply patch to most painful area for 60 minutes. Up to 4 patches may be applied in a single application. Treatment may be repeated ≥3 months as needed for return of pain (do not apply more frequently than every 3 months). Area should be pretreated with a topical anesthetic prior to patch application.
Diabetic neuropathy (unlabeled use): Cream (0.075%): Apply 4 times/day (Bril, 2011)

Mechanism of Action Capsaicin, a transient receptor potential vanilloid 1 receptor (TRPV1) agonist, activates TRPV1 ligand-gated cation channels on nociceptive nerve fibers, resulting in depolarization, initiation of action potential, and pain signal transmission to the spinal cord; capsaicin exposure results in subsequent desensitization of the sensory axons and inhibition of pain transmission initiation. In arthritis, capsaicin induces release of substance P, the principal chemomediator of pain impulses from the periphery to the CNS, from peripheral sensory neurons; after repeated application, capsaicin depletes the neuron of substance P and prevents reaccumulation. The functional link between substance P and the capsaicin receptor, TRPV1, is not well understood.

Contraindications There are no contraindications listed in the manufacturer's labeling.

Warnings/Precautions
Topical high-concentration capsaicin patch (Qutenza™): Do not apply to face, scalp, or allow contact with eyes or mucous membranes. If an unintended area of skin is inadvertently exposed, the cleansing gel should be used. Post-application pain should be treated with local cooling methods and/or analgesics (opioids may be necessary). Avoid rapid removal of patches to decrease risk of aerosolization of capsaicin; inhalation of airborne capsaicin may result in coughing or sneezing; if shortness of breath occurs, medical care is required; remove patches gently and slowly to decrease risk of aerosolization. Use with caution in patients with uncontrolled hypertension, or a history of cardiovascular or cerebrovascular events; transient increases in blood pressure due to treatment-related pain have occurred during and after application of patch.

Topical OTC products: Apply externally; avoid contact with eyes or mucous membranes. Should not be applied to broken or irritated skin. Treated area should not be exposed to heat or direct sunlight. Affected area should not be bandaged. Transient burning may occur and generally disappears after several days; discontinue use if severe burning develops. Stop use and consult a healthcare provider if redness or irritation develops, symptoms get worse, or symptoms resolve and then recur.

Drug Interactions
Metabolism/Transport Effects Substrate of CYP2E1 (minor); **Note:** Assignment of Major/Minor substrate status based on clinically relevant drug interaction potential

Avoid Concomitant Use There are no known interactions where it is recommended to avoid concomitant use.

Increased Effect/Toxicity There are no known significant interactions involving an increase in effect.

Decreased Effect There are no known significant interactions involving a decrease in effect.

Pharmacodynamics/Kinetics
Half-life Elimination Half-life elimination: Topical patch (capsaicin 8%): 1.64 hours (Babbar, 2009)

Pregnancy Risk Factor B
Pregnancy Considerations Adverse events have not been observed in animal reproduction studies with capsaicin patch or liquid. Systemic absorption is limited following topical administration of the patch; plasma concentrations are below the limit of detection 3-6 hours after the patch is removed.

Lactation Excretion in breast milk unknown
Breast-Feeding Considerations Systemic absorption is limited following topical administration of the patch. When using the topical high concentration (capsaicin 8%) patch, Qutenza™, the manufacturer recommends not breast-feeding on the day of treatment after the patch has been applied to reduce any potential infant exposure.

Dosage Forms
Cream, topical: 0.025% (60 g)
Capzasin-HP® [OTC]: 0.1% (42.5 g)
Capzasin-P® [OTC]: 0.035% (42.5 g)
Trixaicin [OTC]: 0.025% (60 g)
Trixaicin HP [OTC]: 0.075% (60 g)
Zostrix® [OTC]: 0.025% (60 g)
Zostrix® Diabetic Foot Pain [OTC]: 0.075% (60 g)
Zostrix®-HP [OTC]: 0.075% (60 g)
Gel, topical:
Capzasin-P® [OTC]: 0.025% (42.5 g)
Liquid, topical:
Capzasin-P® [OTC]: 0.15% (29.5 mL)
Lotion, topical:
DiabetAid® Pain and Tingling Relief [OTC]: 0.025% (120 mL)
Patch, topical:
Qutenza™: 8% (1s, 2s)
Salonpas® Gel-Patch Hot [OTC]: 0.025% (3s, 6s)

References
Buchanan J and Zakrzewska J, "Burning Mouth Syndrome," *Clin Evid (online)*, March 14, 2008. Available at http://www.ncbi.nlm.nih.gov/pmc/articles/PMC2907957/pdf/2008-1301.pdf.
Mínguez Serra MP, Salort Llorca C, Silvestre Donat FJ, "Pharmacological Treatment of Burning Mouth Syndrome: A Review and Update," *Med Oral Patol Oral Cir Bucal*, 2007, 12(4):E299-304.

Captopril (KAP toe pril)

Related Information
Cardiovascular Diseases *on page 1492*

Brand Names: Canada Apo-Capto®; Capoten®; Dom-Captopril; Mylan-Captopril; Nu-Capto; PMS-Captopril; Teva-Captopril

Generic Availability (U.S.) Yes

Pharmacologic Category Angiotensin-Converting Enzyme (ACE) Inhibitor

Use Management of hypertension; treatment of heart failure, left ventricular dysfunction after myocardial infarction, diabetic nephropathy

Unlabeled Use To delay the progression of nephropathy and reduce risks of cardiovascular events in hypertensive patients with type 1 or 2 diabetes mellitus; treatment of hypertensive crisis, rheumatoid arthritis; diagnosis of anatomic renal artery stenosis, hypertension secondary to scleroderma renal crisis; diagnosis of aldosteronism, idiopathic edema, Bartter's syndrome, postmyocardial infarction for prevention of ventricular failure; increase circulation in Raynaud's phenomenon, hypertension secondary to Takayasu's disease

Local Anesthetic/Vasoconstrictor Precautions No information available to require special precautions

Effects on Dental Treatment Key adverse event(s) related to dental treatment: Loss or diminished perception of taste and orthostatic hypotension.

Effects on Bleeding No information available to require special precautions

Adverse Effects
Frequency not defined:
Cardiovascular: Angioedema, cardiac arrest, cerebrovascular insufficiency, rhythm disturbances, orthostatic hypotension, syncope, flushing, pallor, angina, MI, Raynaud's syndrome, CHF
Central nervous system: Ataxia, confusion, depression, nervousness, somnolence
Dermatologic: Bullous pemphigus, erythema multiforme, Stevens-Johnson syndrome, exfoliative dermatitis
Endocrine & metabolic: Alkaline phosphatase increased, bilirubin increased, gynecomastia
Gastrointestinal: Pancreatitis, glossitis, dyspepsia
Genitourinary: Urinary frequency, impotence
Hematologic: Anemia, thrombocytopenia, pancytopenia, agranulocytosis, anemia
Hepatic: Jaundice, hepatitis, hepatic necrosis (rare), cholestasis, hyponatremia (symptomatic), transaminases increased
Neuromuscular & skeletal: Asthenia, myalgia, myasthenia
Ocular: Blurred vision
Renal: Renal insufficiency, renal failure, nephrotic syndrome, polyuria, oliguria
Respiratory: Bronchospasm, eosinophilic pneumonitis, rhinitis
Miscellaneous: Anaphylactoid reactions
1% to 10%:
Cardiovascular: Hypotension (1% to 3%), tachycardia (1%), chest pain (1%), palpitation (1%)
Dermatologic: Rash (maculopapular or urticarial) (4% to 7%), pruritus (2%); in patients with rash, a positive ANA and/or eosinophilia has been noted in 7% to 10%
Endocrine & metabolic: Hyperkalemia (1% to 11%)
Hematologic: Neutropenia may occur in up to 4% of patients with renal insufficiency or collagen-vascular disease

Renal: Proteinuria (1%), serum creatinine increased, worsening of renal function (may occur in patients with bilateral renal artery stenosis or hypovolemia)
Respiratory: Cough (<1% to 2%)
Miscellaneous: Hypersensitivity reactions (rash, pruritus, fever, arthralgia, and eosinophilia) have occurred in 4% to 7% of patients (depending on dose and renal function); dysgeusia - loss of taste or diminished perception (2% to 4%)

Dosage Note: Titrate dose according to patient's response; use lowest effective dose. Oral:
Infants: Initial: 0.15-0.3 mg/kg/dose; titrate dose upward to maximum of 6 mg/kg/day in 1-4 divided doses
Children: Initial: 0.3-0.5 mg/kg/dose; titrate upward to maximum of 6 mg/kg/day in 2-4 divided doses (NHBPEP, 2004)
Older Children: Initial: 6.25-12.5 mg/dose every 12-24 hours; titrate upward to maximum of 6 mg/kg/day
Adolescents: Initial: 12.5-25 mg/dose; titrate to a maximum of 450 mg/day
Adults:
Acute hypertension (urgency/emergency): 12.5-25 mg, may repeat as needed (may be given sublingually, but no therapeutic advantage demonstrated)
Heart failure:
Initial dose: 6.25-12.5 mg 3 times/day in conjunction with cardiac glycoside and diuretic therapy; initial dose depends upon patient's fluid/electrolyte status
Target dose: 50 mg 3 times/day
Hypertension:
Initial dose: 25 mg 2-3 times/day (a lower initial dose of 12.5 mg 3 times/day may also be considered [VA Cooperative Study Group, 1984]); may increase by 12.5-25 mg/dose at 1- to 2-week intervals up to 50 mg 3 times/day; add thiazide diuretic, unless severe renal impairment coexists then consider loop diuretic, before further dosage increases or consider other treatment options; maximum dose: 150 mg 3 times/day
Usual dose range (JNC 7): 25-100 mg/day in 2 divided doses
LV dysfunction after MI: Initial: 6.25 mg; if tolerated, follow with 12.5 mg 3 times/day; then increase to 25 mg 3 times/day during next several days and then gradually increase over next several weeks to target dose of 50 mg 3 times/day (some dose schedules are more aggressive to achieve an increased goal dose within the first few days of initiation)
Diabetic nephropathy: Initial: 25 mg 3 times/day. May be taken with other antihypertensive therapy if required to further lower blood pressure.
Elderly: Hypertension: Consider lower initial doses and titrate to response (Aronow, 2011)

Dosage adjustment in renal impairment:
Manufacturers recommendations: Reduce initial daily dose and titrate slowly (1- to 2-week intervals) with smaller increments. Slowly back titrate to determine the minimum effective dose once the desired therapeutic effect has been reached.
Alternative recommendations (Aronoff, 2007): Adults:
Cl_{cr} 10-50 mL/minute: Administer at 75% of normal dose every 12-18 hours.
Cl_{cr} <10 mL/minute: Administer at 50% of normal dose every 24 hours.
Intermittent hemodialysis (IHD): Administer after hemodialysis on dialysis days
Peritoneal dialysis: Dose for Cl_{cr} 10-50 mL/minute; supplemental dose is not necessary

Dosage adjustment in hepatic impairment: No dosage adjustment provided in manufacturer's labeling.

Mechanism of Action Competitive inhibitor of angiotensin-converting enzyme (ACE); prevents conversion of angiotensin I to angiotensin II, a potent vasoconstrictor; results in lower levels of angiotensin II which causes an increase in plasma renin activity and a reduction in aldosterone secretion

Contraindications Hypersensitivity to captopril, any other ACE inhibitor, or any component of the formulation; angioedema related to previous treatment with an ACE inhibitor; concomitant use with aliskiren in patients with diabetes mellitus

Warnings/Precautions Anaphylactic reactions may occur rarely with ACE inhibitors. At any time during treatment (especially following first dose) angioedema may occur rarely with ACE inhibitors; may involve the head and neck (potentially compromising airway) or the intestine (presenting with abdominal pain). African-Americans and patients with idiopathic or hereditary angioedema may be at an increased risk. Prolonged frequent monitoring may be required especially if tongue, glottis, or larynx are involved as they are associated with airway obstruction. Patients with a history of airway surgery may have a higher risk of airway obstruction. Aggressive early and appropriate management is critical. Use in patients with previous angioedema associated with ACE inhibitor therapy is contraindicated. Severe anaphylactoid reactions may be seen during hemodialysis (eg, CVVHD) with high-flux dialysis membranes (eg, AN69), and rarely, during low density lipoprotein apheresis with dextran sulfate cellulose. Rare cases of anaphylactoid reactions have been reported in patients undergoing sensitization treatment with hymenoptera (bee, wasp) venom while receiving ACE inhibitors.

Symptomatic hypotension with or without syncope can occur with ACE inhibitors (usually with the first several doses); effects are most often observed in volume depleted patients; close monitoring of patient is required especially with initial dosing and dosing increases; blood pressure must be lowered at a rate appropriate for the patient's clinical condition. Initiation of therapy in patients with ischemic heart disease or cerebrovascular disease warrants close observation due to the potential consequences posed by falling blood pressure (eg, MI, stroke). Use with caution in hypertrophic cardiomyopathy with outflow tract obstruction, severe aortic stenosis, or before, during, or immediately after major surgery. **[U.S. Boxed Warning]: Drugs that act on the renin-angiotensin system can cause injury and death to the developing fetus. Discontinue as soon as possible once pregnancy is detected.**

Hyperkalemia may occur with ACE inhibitors; risk factors include renal dysfunction, diabetes mellitus, concomitant use of potassium-sparing diuretics, potassium supplements and/or potassium containing salts. Use cautiously, if at all, with these agents and monitor potassium closely. Cough may occur with ACE inhibitors. Other causes of cough should be considered (eg, pulmonary congestion in patients with heart failure) and excluded prior to discontinuation.

May be associated with deterioration of renal function and/or increases in serum creatinine, particularly in patients with low renal blood flow (eg, renal artery stenosis, heart failure) whose glomerular filtration rate (GFR) is dependent on efferent arteriolar vasoconstriction by angiotensin II; deterioration may result in oliguria, acute renal failure, and progressive azotemia. Small increases in serum creatinine may occur following initiation; consider discontinuation only in patients with progressive and/or significant deterioration in renal function. Use with caution in patients with unstented unilateral/bilateral renal artery stenosis. When unstented bilateral renal artery stenosis is present, use is generally avoided due to the elevated risk of deterioration in renal function unless possible benefits outweigh risks. Concomitant use of an angiotensin receptor blocker (ARB) or renin inhibitor (eg, aliskiren) is associated with an increased risk of hypotension, hyperkalemia, and renal dysfunction; concomitant use with aliskiren should be avoided in patients with GFR <60 mL/minute and is contraindicated in patients with diabetes mellitus (regardless of GFR).

Rare toxicities associated with ACE inhibitors include cholestatic jaundice (which may progress to fulminant hepatic necrosis), agranulocytosis, neutropenia, or leukopenia with myeloid hypoplasia. Patients with collagen vascular diseases (especially with concomitant renal impairment) or renal impairment alone may be at increased risk for hematologic toxicity; closely monitor CBC with differential for the first 3 months of therapy and periodically thereafter in these patients.

Drug Interactions

Metabolism/Transport Effects Substrate of CYP2D6 (major); **Note:** Assignment of Major/Minor substrate status based on clinically relevant drug interaction potential

Avoid Concomitant Use There are no known interactions where it is recommended to avoid concomitant use.

Increased Effect/Toxicity

Captopril may increase the levels/effects of: Allopurinol; Amifostine; Antihypertensives; AzaTHIOprine; CycloSPORINE (Systemic); Ferric Gluconate; Gold Sodium Thiomalate; Hypotensive Agents; Iron Dextran Complex; Lithium; Nonsteroidal Anti-Inflammatory Agents; RiTUXimab; Sodium Phosphates

The levels/effects of Captopril may be increased by: Abiraterone Acetate; Alfuzosin; Aliskiren; Angiotensin II Receptor Blockers; Canagliflozin; CYP2D6 Inhibitors (Moderate); CYP2D6 Inhibitors (Strong); Darunavir; Diazoxide; DPP-IV Inhibitors; Eplerenone; Everolimus; Herbs (Hypotensive Properties); Loop Diuretics; MAO Inhibitors; Pentoxifylline; Phosphodiesterase 5 Inhibitors; Potassium Salts; Potassium-Sparing Diuretics; Prostacyclin Analogues; Sirolimus; Temsirolimus; Thiazide Diuretics; TiZANidine; Tolvaptan; Trimethoprim

Decreased Effect

The levels/effects of Captopril may be decreased by: Antacids; Aprotinin; Herbs (Hypertensive Properties); Icatibant; Lanthanum; Methylphenidate; Nonsteroidal Anti-Inflammatory Agents; Peginterferon Alfa-2b; Salicylates; Yohimbine

Ethanol/Nutrition/Herb Interactions

Food: Captopril serum concentrations may be decreased if taken with food. Long-term use of captopril may lead to a zinc deficiency which can result in altered taste perception. Potassium supplements and/or potassium-containing salts may cause or worsen hyperkalemia. Management: Take on an empty stomach 1 hour before or 2 hours after meals. Consult prescriber before consuming a potassium-rich diet, potassium supplements, or salt substitutes.

Herb/Nutraceutical: Some herbal medications may worsen hypertension (eg, licorice); others may increase the antihypertensive effect of captopril (eg, shepherd's purse). Management: Avoid bayberry, blue cohosh, cayenne, ephedra, ginger, ginseng (American), kola, yohimbe, and licorice. Avoid black cohosh, california poppy, coleus, golden seal, hawthorn, mistletoe, periwinkle, quinine, and shepherd's purse.

Dietary Considerations Should be taken at least 1 hour before or 2 hours after eating.

Pharmacodynamics/Kinetics

Onset of Action Peak effect: Blood pressure reduction: 1-1.5 hours after dose

Duration of Action Dose related, may require several weeks of therapy before full hypotensive effect

Half-life Elimination Renal and cardiac function dependent: Adults: Healthy volunteers: 1.9 hours; Heart failure: 2.06 hours; Anuria: 20-40 hours

Time to Peak 1 hour

Pregnancy Risk Factor D

Pregnancy Considerations [U.S. Boxed Warning]: Drugs that act on the renin-angiotensin system can cause injury and death to the developing fetus. Discontinue as soon as possible once pregnancy is detected. Captopril crosses the placenta; teratogenic effects may occur following maternal use during pregnancy. Drugs that act on the renin-angiotensin system are associated with oligohydramnios. Oligohydramnios, due to decreased fetal renal function, may lead to fetal lung hypoplasia and skeletal malformations. Their use in pregnancy is also associated with anuria, hypotension, renal failure, skull hypoplasia, and death in the fetus/neonate. Chronic maternal hypertension itself is also associated with adverse events in the fetus/infant. ACE inhibitors are not recommended during pregnancy to treat maternal hypertension or heart failure. Use of an ACE inhibitor should also be avoided in any woman of reproductive age. Women who are planning a pregnancy should be considered for other medication options if an ACE inhibitor is currently prescribed or the ACE inhibitor should be discontinued as soon as possible once pregnancy is detected. The exposed fetus should be monitored for fetal growth, amniotic fluid volume, and organ formation. Infants exposed to an ACE inhibitor *in utero* should be monitored for hyperkalemia, hypotension, and oliguria.

Lactation Enters breast milk/not recommended (AAP rates "compatible"; AAP 2001 update pending)

Breast-Feeding Considerations Captopril is excreted in breast milk. Breast-feeding is not recommended by the manufacturer.

Dosage Forms

Tablet, oral: 12.5 mg, 25 mg, 50 mg, 100 mg

Captopril and Hydrochlorothiazide
(KAP toe pril & hye droe klor oh THYE a zide)

Related Information

Captopril *on page 242*

Hydrochlorothiazide *on page 687*

Pharmacologic Category Angiotensin-Converting Enzyme (ACE) Inhibitor; Diuretic, Thiazide

Use Management of hypertension

Local Anesthetic/Vasoconstrictor Precautions No information available to require special precautions

Effects on Dental Treatment No significant effects or complications reported

Effects on Bleeding No information available to require special precautions

Adverse Effects See individual agents.

General Dosage Range Oral: *Adults:* Captopril 25-150 mg and hydrochlorothiazide 15-50 mg once daily

Mechanism of Action Captopril is a competitive inhibitor of angiotensin-converting enzyme (ACE); prevents conversion of angiotensin I to angiotensin II, a potent vasoconstrictor. This results in lower levels of angiotensin II which causes an increase in plasma renin activity and a reduction in aldosterone secretion. Hydrochlorothiazide inhibits sodium reabsorption in the distal tubules causing increased excretion of sodium and water as well as potassium and hydrogen ions.

Pregnancy Risk Factor C/D (2nd and 3rd trimesters)

Pregnancy Considerations See individual agents.

Carbachol (KAR ba kole)

Brand Names: U.S. Isopto® Carbachol; Miostat®

Brand Names: Canada Isopto® Carbachol; Miostat®

Pharmacologic Category Cholinergic Agonist; Ophthalmic Agent, Antiglaucoma; Ophthalmic Agent, Miotic

Use Lowers intraocular pressure in the treatment of glaucoma; cause miosis during surgery

Local Anesthetic/Vasoconstrictor Precautions No information available to require special precautions

Effects on Dental Treatment Key adverse event(s) related to dental treatment: Increased salivation.

Effects on Bleeding No information available to require special precautions

Adverse Effects Frequency not defined.

Cardiovascular: Arrhythmia, flushing, hypotension, syncope

Central nervous system: Headache

Gastrointestinal: Abdominal cramps, diarrhea, epigastric distress, salivation, vomiting

Genitourinary: Urinary bladder tightness

Ocular: Bullous keratopathy, burning (transient), ciliary spasm, conjunctival injection, corneal clouding, irritation, postoperative iritis (following cataract extraction), retinal detachment, stinging (transient)

Respiratory: Asthma

Miscellaneous: Diaphoresis

General Dosage Range Ophthalmic: *Adults:* Instill 1-2 drops up to 3 times/day **or** 0.5 mL as a single dose

Mechanism of Action Synthetic direct-acting cholinergic agent that causes miosis by stimulating muscarinic receptors in the eye

Pharmacodynamics/Kinetics

Onset of Action

Ophthalmic instillation: Miosis: 10-20 minutes

Intraocular administration: Miosis: 2-5 minutes

Duration of Action

Ophthalmic instillation: Reduction in intraocular pressure: 4-8 hours

Intraocular administration: 24 hours

Pregnancy Risk Factor C

Pregnancy Considerations Reproduction studies have not been conducted.

CarBAMazepine (kar ba MAZ e peen)

Related Information

Temporomandibular Dysfunction (TMD), Chronic Pain, and Fibromyalgia *on page 1590*

Brand Names: U.S. Carbatrol®; Epitol®; Equetro®; TEGretol®; TEGretol®-XR

Brand Names: Canada Apo-Carbamazepine®; Dom-Carbamazepine; Mapezine®; Mylan-Carbamazepine CR; Nu-Carbamazepine; PMS-Carbamazepine; San-doz-Carbamazepine; Taro-Carbamazepine Chewable; Tegretol®; Teva-Carbamazepine

Generic Availability (U.S.) Yes

Pharmacologic Category Anticonvulsant, Miscellane-ous

Dental Use Pain relief of trigeminal or glossopharyngeal neuralgia

Use

Carbatrol®, Tegretol®, Tegretol®-XR: Partial seizures with complex symptomatology (psychomotor, temporal lobe), generalized tonic-clonic seizures (grand mal), mixed seizure patterns, trigeminal neuralgia, glosso-pharyngeal neuralgia

Equetro®: Acute manic or mixed episodes associated with bipolar 1 disorder

Unlabeled Use Treatment of restless leg syndrome and post-traumatic stress disorders

Local Anesthetic/Vasoconstrictor Precautions No information available to require special precautions

Effects on Dental Treatment Key adverse event(s) related to dental treatment: Xerostomia (normal salivary flow resumes upon discontinuation).

Effects on Bleeding No information available to require special precautions

Adverse Effects Frequency not defined, unless other-wise specified.

Cardiovascular: Hypertension (3%), arrhythmias, AV block, chills, coronary artery disease exacerbation, edema, heart failure, hypotension, syncope, throm-boembolism, thrombophlebitis

Central nervous system: Dizziness (44%), somnolence (32%), headache (22%), ataxia (15%), speech disor-der (6%), abnormal thinking (2%), vertigo (2%), agi-tation, amnesia, confusion, coordination impaired, depression, drowsiness, fatigue, fever, hallucinations, neuroleptic malignant syndrome (NMS), slurred speech, talkativeness

Dermatologic: Pruritus (8%), rash (7%), alopecia, alter-ations in skin pigmentation, erythema (multiforme and nodosum), exfoliative dermatitis, disseminated lupus erythematosus exacerbation, nail shedding, onycho-madesis, photosensitivity reaction, purpura, Stevens-Johnson syndrome, toxic epidermal necrolysis, urti-caria

Endocrine & metabolic: Hypocalcemia, hyponatremia, syndrome of inappropriate ADH secretion (SIADH), thyroid function tests abnormal

Gastrointestinal: Nausea (29%), vomiting (18%), con-stipation (10%), xerostomia (8%), abdominal pain, anorexia, diarrhea, dry throat, gastric distress, glossi-tis, pancreatitis, stomatitis

Genitourinary: Impotence, urinary frequency, urinary retention

Hematologic: Agranulocytosis, anemia, aplastic anemia, bone marrow suppression, eosinophilia, leukocytosis, leukopenia, pancytopenia, porphyria, thrombocyto-penia

Hepatic: Abnormal liver function tests, hepatic failure, hepatitis, jaundice

Neuromuscular & skeletal: Weakness (8%), tremor (3%), paresthesia (2%), twitching (2%), arthralgia, leg cramps, myalgia, osteoporosis, peripheral neuritis

Ocular: Blurred vision (6%), conjunctivitis, diplopia, intraocular pressure increased, lens opacities, nystag-mus, oculomotor disturbances

Otic: Hyperacusis, tinnitus

Renal: Albuminuria, azotemia, blood urea nitrogen increased, glycosuria, oliguria, renal failure

Miscellaneous: Diaphoresis, drug rash with eosinophilia and systemic symptoms (DRESS), hypersensitivity, lymphadenopathy

Dental Usual Dosage Trigeminal or glossopharyngeal neuralgia: Oral:

Adults: Initial: 200 mg/day in 2 divided doses (tablets, extended release tablets, or extended release capsu-les) or 4 divided doses (oral suspension) with food, gradually increasing in increments of 200 mg/day as needed

Maintenance: Usual: 400-800 mg daily in 2 divided doses (tablets, extended release tablets, or extended release capsules) or 4 divided doses (oral suspension); maximum dose: 1200 mg/day

Dosage Dosage must be adjusted according to patient's response and serum concentrations. Administer tablets (chewable or conventional) in 2-3 divided doses daily and suspension in 4 divided doses daily. Oral:

Epilepsy:

Children:

<6 years: Initial: 10-20 mg/kg/day divided twice or 3 times daily as tablets or 4 times/day as suspension; increase dose every week until optimal response and therapeutic levels are achieved

Maintenance dose: Divide into 3-4 doses daily (tab-lets or suspension); maximum recommended dose: 35 mg/kg/day

6-12 years: Initial: 200 mg/day in 2 divided doses (tablets or extended release tablets) or 4 divided doses (oral suspension); increase by up to 100 mg/day at weekly intervals using a twice daily regimen of extended release tablets or 3-4 times daily regimen of other formulations until optimal response and therapeutic levels are achieved

Maintenance: Usual: 400-800 mg/day; maximum rec-ommended dose: 1000 mg/day

Note: Children <12 years who receive ≥400 mg/day of carbamazepine may be converted to extended release capsules (Carbatrol®) using the same total daily dosage divided twice daily

Children >12 years and Adults: Initial: 400 mg/day in 2 divided doses (tablets or extended release tablets) or 4 divided doses (oral suspension); increase by up to 200 mg/day at weekly intervals using a twice daily regimen of extended release tablets or capsules, or a 3-4 times/day regimen of other formulations until opti-mal response and therapeutic levels are achieved; usual dose: 800-1200 mg/day

Maximum recommended doses:

Children 12-15 years: 1000 mg/day

Children >15 years: 1200 mg/day

Adults: 1600 mg/day; however, some patients have required up to 1.6-2.4 g/day

Trigeminal or glossopharyngeal neuralgia: Adults: Initial: 200 mg/day in 2 divided doses (tablets, extended release tablets, or extended release capsu-les) or 4 divided doses (oral suspension) with food, gradually increasing in increments of 200 mg/day as needed

Maintenance: Usual: 400-800 mg daily in 2 divided doses (tablets, extended release tablets, or extended release capsules) or 4 divided doses (oral suspen-sion); maximum dose: 1200 mg/day

Bipolar disorder: Adults: Initial: 400 mg/day in 2 div-ided doses (tablets, extended release tablets, or extended release capsules) or 4 divided doses (oral suspension), may adjust by 200 mg/day increments; maximum dose: 1600 mg/day.

◀ **Note:** Equetro® is the only formulation specifically approved by the FDA for the management of bipolar disorder.

Neuropathic pain, critically-ill patients (unlabeled use): Initial: 50-100 mg twice daily in combination with I.V. opioids; Maintenance: 100-200 mg every 4-6 hours; maximum dose: 1200 mg daily (Barr, 2013)

Dosing adjustment in renal impairment: Dosage adjustments are not required or recommended in the manufacturer's labeling; however, the following guidelines have been used by some clinicians (Aronoff, 2007):

Children and Adults:

GFR <10 mL/minute: Administer 75% of dose

Hemodialysis, peritoneal dialysis: Administer 75% of dose (postdialysis)

Continuous renal replacement therapy (CRRT):

Children: Administer 75% of dose

Adults: No dosage adjustment recommended

Dosing adjustment in hepatic impairment: Use with caution in hepatic impairment; metabolized primarily in the liver

Mechanism of Action In addition to anticonvulsant effects, carbamazepine has anticholinergic, antineuralgic, antidiuretic, muscle relaxant, antimanic, antidepressive, and antiarrhythmic properties; may depress activity in the nucleus ventralis of the thalamus or decrease synaptic transmission or decrease summation of temporal stimulation leading to neural discharge by limiting influx of sodium ions across cell membrane or other unknown mechanisms; stimulates the release of ADH and potentiates its action in promoting reabsorption of water; chemically related to tricyclic antidepressants

Contraindications Hypersensitivity to carbamazepine, tricyclic antidepressants, or any component of the formulation; bone marrow depression; with or within 14 days of MAO inhibitor use; concurrent use of nefazodone; concomitant use of delavirdine or other non-nucleoside reverse transcriptase inhibitors

Warnings/Precautions Hazardous agent - use appropriate precautions for handling and disposal (NIOSH, 2012). **[U.S. Boxed Warning]: The risk of developing aplastic anemia or agranulocytosis is increased during treatment. Monitor CBC, platelets, and differential prior to and during therapy; discontinue if significant bone marrow suppression occurs.** A spectrum of hematologic effects has been reported with use (eg, agranulocytosis, aplastic anemia, neutropenia, leukopenia, thrombocytopenia, pancytopenia, and anemias); patients with a previous history of adverse hematologic reaction to any drug may be at increased risk. Early detection of hematologic change is important; advise patients of early signs and symptoms including fever, sore throat, mouth ulcers, infections, easy bruising, and petechial or purpuric hemorrhage.

[U.S. Boxed Warning]: Severe and sometimes fatal dermatologic reactions, including toxic epidermal necrolysis (TENS) and Stevens-Johnson syndrome (SJS), may occur during therapy. The risk is increased in patients with the variant HLA-B*1502 allele, found almost exclusively in patients of Asian ancestry. Patients of Asian descent should be screened prior to initiating therapy. Avoid use in patients testing positive for the allele; discontinue therapy in patients who have a serious dermatologic reaction. The risk of SJS or TENS may also be increased if carbamazepine is used in combination with other antiepileptic drugs associated with these reactions. Presence of the HLA-B*1502 allele has not been found to predict the risk of less serious dermatologic reactions such as anticonvulsant hypersensitivity syndrome or nonserious rash. The risk of developing a hypersensitivity reaction may be increased in patients with the variant HLA-A*3101 allele. The HLA-A*3101 allele may occur more frequently patients of African-American, Asian, European, Indian, Latin American, and Native American ancestry. Hypersensitivity has also been reported in patients experiencing reactions to other anticonvulsants; the history of hypersensitivity reactions in the patient or their immediate family members should be reviewed. Approximately 25% to 30% of patients allergic to carbamazepine will also have reactions with oxcarbazepine. Potentially serious, sometimes fatal multiorgan hypersensitivity reactions (also known as drug reaction with eosinophilia and systemic symptoms [DRESS]) have been reported with some antiepileptic drugs including carbamazepine; monitor for signs and symptoms of possible disparate manifestations associated with lymphatic, hepatic, renal, and/or hematologic organ systems; gradual discontinuation and conversion to alternate therapy may be required.

Antiepileptics are associated with an increased risk of suicidal behavior/thoughts with use (regardless of indication); patients should be monitored for signs/symptoms of depression, suicidal tendencies, and other unusual behavior changes during therapy and instructed to inform their healthcare provider immediately if symptoms occur.

Administer carbamazepine with caution to patients with history of cardiac damage, ECG abnormalities (or at risk for ECG abnormalities), hepatic or renal disease. When used to treat bipolar disorder, the smallest effective dose is suggested to reduce the risk for overdose/suicide; high-risk patients should be monitored for suicidal ideations. Prescription should be written for the smallest quantity consistent with good patient care. May activate latent psychosis and/or cause confusion or agitation; elderly patients may be at an increased risk for psychiatric effects.

Carbamazepine is not effective in absence, myoclonic, or akinetic seizures; exacerbation of certain seizure types have been seen after initiation of carbamazepine therapy in children with mixed seizure disorders. Abrupt discontinuation is not recommended in patients being treated for seizures. Dizziness or drowsiness may occur; caution should be used when performing tasks which require alertness until the effects are known. Effects with other sedative drugs or ethanol may be potentiated. Carbamazepine has a high potential for drug interactions; use caution in patients taking strong CYP3A4 inducers or inhibitors or medications significantly metabolized via CYP1A2, 2B6, 2C9, 2C19, and 3A4. Coadministration of carbamazepine and nefazodone may lead to insufficient plasma levels of nefazodone; combination is contraindicated. Coadministration yields insufficient plasma levels of delavirdine and other non-nucleoside reverse transcriptase inhibitors to achieve a therapeutic effect; concurrent use is contraindicated. Carbamazepine has mild anticholinergic activity; use with caution in patients with increased intraocular pressure, or sensitivity to anticholinergic effects. Hyponatremia caused by the syndrome of inappropriate antidiuretic hormone secretion (SIADH) may occur during therapy. Risk may be increased in the elderly or in patients also taking diuretics and may be dose-dependent. Use caution in elderly patients; may cause or exacerbate syndrome of inappropriate antidiuretic hormone secretion or hyponatremia; monitor sodium closely with initiation or dosage adjustments in older adults (Beers Criteria).

Administration of the suspension will yield higher peak and lower trough serum levels than an equal dose of the tablet form; consider a lower starting dose given more frequently (same total daily dose) when using the suspension. The suspension may contain sorbitol; avoid use in patents with hereditary fructose intolerance.

Drug Interactions

Metabolism/Transport Effects Substrate of CYP2C8 (minor), CYP3A4 (major); **Note:** Assignment of Major/Minor substrate status based on clinically relevant drug interaction potential; **Induces** CYP1A2 (strong), CYP2B6 (strong), CYP2C19 (strong), CYP2C8 (strong), CYP2C9 (strong), CYP3A4 (strong), P-glycoprotein

Avoid Concomitant Use

Avoid concomitant use of CarBAMazepine with any of the following: Apixaban; Axitinib; Azelastine (Nasal); Bedaquiline; Boceprevir; Bortezomib; Bosutinib; Cabozantinib; CloZAPine; Conivaptan; Crizotinib; Dabigatran Etexilate; Dronedarone; Enzalutamide; Everolimus; Ivacaftor; Lapatinib; Lurasidone; MAO Inhibitors; Mifepristone; Nefazodone; Nilotinib; Paraldehyde; Pazopanib; Pirfenidone; Pomalidomide; Ponatinib; Praziquantel; Ranolazine; Regorafenib; Reverse Transcriptase Inhibitors (Non-Nucleoside); Rivaroxaban; Roflumilast; RomiDEPsin; SORAfenib; Telaprevir; Ticagrelor; Tofacitinib; Tolvaptan; Toremifene; TraMADol; Vandetanib; VinCRIStine (Liposomal); Voriconazole

Increased Effect/Toxicity

CarBAMazepine may increase the levels/effects of: Adenosine; Alcohol (Ethyl); Azelastine (Nasal); Buprenorphine; ClomiPRAMINE; CloZAPine; CNS Depressants; Desmopressin; Fosphenytoin; Ifosfamide; Lithium; MAO Inhibitors; Methotrimeprazine; Metyrosine; Mirtazapine; Paraldehyde; Phenytoin; Pramipexole; ROPINIRole; Rotigotine

The levels/effects of CarBAMazepine may be increased by: Allopurinol; Antifungal Agents (Azole Derivatives, Systemic); Calcium Channel Blockers (Nondihydropyridine); Carbonic Anhydrase Inhibitors; Cimetidine; Conivaptan; CYP3A4 Inhibitors (Moderate); CYP3A4 Inhibitors (Strong); Danazol; Darunavir; Dasatinib; Droperidol; Fluconazole; Grapefruit Juice; HydrOXYzine; Isoniazid; Ivacaftor; LamoTRIgine; Macrolide Antibiotics; Magnesium Sulfate; Methotrimeprazine; Mifepristone; Nefazodone; Protease Inhibitors; QuiNINE; Selective Serotonin Reuptake Inhibitors; Sodium Oxybate; Telaprevir; Thiazide Diuretics; TraMADol; Zolpidem

Decreased Effect

CarBAMazepine may decrease the levels/effects of: Acetaminophen; Apixaban; ARIPiprazole; Axitinib; Bedaquiline; Bendamustine; Benzodiazepines (metabolized by oxidation); Boceprevir; Bortezomib; Bosutinib; Brentuximab Vedotin; Cabozantinib; Calcium Channel Blockers (Dihydropyridine); Calcium Channel Blockers (Nondihydropyridine); Caspofungin; CloZAPine; Cobicistat; Contraceptives (Estrogens); Contraceptives (Progestins); Crizotinib; CycloSPORINE (Systemic); CYP1A2 Substrates; CYP2B6 Substrates; CYP2C19 Substrates; CYP2C8 Substrates; CYP2C9 Substrates; CYP3A4 Substrates; Dabigatran Etexilate; Dasatinib; Diclofenac (Systemic); Divalproex; Doxycycline; Dronedarone; Elvitegravir; Enzalutamide; Everolimus; Exemestane; Felbamate; Flunarizine; Fosphenytoin; Gefitinib; GuanFACINE; Haloperidol;

Imatinib; Irinotecan; Ivacaftor; Ixabepilone; Lacosamide; LamoTRIgine; Lapatinib; Linagliptin; Lopinavir; Lurasidone; Maraviroc; Mebendazole; Methadone; MethylPREDNISolone; Mifepristone; Nefazodone; Nilotinib; OXcarbazepine; Paliperidone; Pazopanib; Perampanel; P-glycoprotein/ABCB1 Substrates; Phenytoin; Pirfenidone; Pomalidomide; Ponatinib; Praziquantel; Protease Inhibitors; QuiNINE; Ranolazine; Regorafenib; Reverse Transcriptase Inhibitors (Non-Nucleoside); RisperiDONE; Rivaroxaban; Roflumilast; RomiDEPsin; Rufinamide; Saxagliptin; Selective Serotonin Reuptake Inhibitors; SORAfenib; SUNItinib; Tadalafil; Telaprevir; Temsirolimus; Theophylline Derivatives; Thyroid Products; Ticagrelor; Tofacitinib; Tolvaptan; Topiramate; Toremifene; TraMADol; Treprostinil; Tricyclic Antidepressants; Ulipristal; Valproic Acid; Vandetanib; Vecuronium; Vemurafenib; VinCRIStine (Liposomal); Vitamin K Antagonists; Voriconazole; Ziprasidone; Zolpidem; Zuclopenthixol

The levels/effects of CarBAMazepine may be decreased by: CYP3A4 Inducers (Strong); Deferasirox; Divalproex; Felbamate; Fosphenytoin; Herbs (CYP3A4 Inducers); Ketorolac (Nasal); Ketorolac (Systemic); Mefloquine; Methylfolate; Phenytoin; Reverse Transcriptase Inhibitors (Non-Nucleoside); Rufinamide; Theophylline Derivatives; Tocilizumab; TraMADol; Valproic Acid

Ethanol/Nutrition/Herb Interactions

Ethanol: Ethanol may increase CNS depression. Management: Avoid concurrent use of ethanol.

Food: Carbamazepine serum levels may be increased if taken with food and/or grapefruit juice. Management Avoid concurrent ingestion of grapefruit juice. Maintain adequate hydration, unless instructed to restrict fluid intake.

Herb/Nutraceutical: Evening primrose may decrease seizure threshold. Valerian, St John's wort, kava kava, and gotu kola may increase CNS depression. Management: Avoid evening primrose. Avoid valerian, St John's wort, kava kava, and gotu kola.

Dietary Considerations Drug may cause GI upset, take with large amount of water or food to decrease GI upset. May need to split doses to avoid GI upset.

Pharmacodynamics/Kinetics

Half-life Elimination Half-life is variable because of autoinduction which is usually complete 3-5 weeks after initiation of a fixed carbamazepine regimen.

Carbamazepine: Initial: 25-65 hours; Extended release: 35-40 hours; Multiple doses: Children: 8-14 hours; Adults: 12-17 hours

Epoxide metabolite: Initial: 25-43 hours

Time to Peak Unpredictable:

Immediate release: Suspension: 1.5 hour; tablet: 4-5 hours

Extended release: Carbatrol®, Equetro®: 12-26 hours (single dose), 4-8 hours (multiple doses); Tegretol®-XR: 3-12 hours

Pregnancy Risk Factor D

Pregnancy Considerations Studies in pregnant women have demonstrated a risk to the fetus. Carbamazepine and its metabolites can be found in the fetus and may be associated with teratogenic effects, including spina bifida, craniofacial defects, cardiovascular malformations, and hypospadias. The risk of teratogenic effects is higher with anticonvulsant polytherapy than monotherapy.

Developmental delays have also been observed following *in utero* exposure to carbamazepine (per manufacturer); however, socioeconomic factors, maternal and paternal IQ, and polytherapy may contribute to these findings. Pregnancy may cause small decreases of carbamazepine plasma concentrations in the second and third trimesters; monitoring should be considered. When used for the treatment of bipolar disorder, use of carbamazepine should be avoided during the first trimester of pregnancy if possible. The use of a single medication for the treatment of bipolar disorder or epilepsy in pregnancy is preferred. Carbamazepine may decrease plasma concentrations of hormonal contraceptives; breakthrough bleeding or unintended pregnancy may occur and alternate or back-up methods of contraception should be considered.

Patients exposed to carbamazepine during pregnancy are encouraged to enroll themselves into the AED Pregnancy Registry by calling 1-888-233-2334. Additional information is available at www.aedpregnancy-registry.org.

Lactation Enters breast milk/not recommended (AAP rates "compatible"; AAP 2001 update pending)

Breast-Feeding Considerations Carbamazepine and its active epoxide metabolite are found in breast milk. Carbamazepine can also be detected in the serum of nursing infants. Transient hepatic dysfunction has been observed in some case reports. Nursing should be discontinued if adverse events are observed. According to the manufacturer, the decision to continue or discontinue breast-feeding during therapy should take into account the risk of exposure to the infant and the benefits of treatment to the mother. Respiratory depression, seizures, nausea, vomiting, diarrhea, and/or decreased feeding have been observed in neonates exposed to carbamazepine *in utero* and may represent a neonatal withdrawal syndrome.

Dosage Forms
Capsule, extended release, oral: 100 mg, 200 mg, 300 mg
Carbatrol®: 100 mg, 200 mg, 300 mg
Equetro®: 100 mg, 200 mg, 300 mg
Suspension, oral: 100 mg/5 mL (5 mL, 10 mL, 450 mL)
TEGretol®: 100 mg/5 mL (450 mL)
Tablet, oral: 200 mg
Epitol®: 200 mg
TEGretol®: 200 mg
Tablet, chewable, oral: 100 mg
TEGretol®: 100 mg
Tablet, extended release, oral: 200 mg, 400 mg
TEGretol®-XR: 100 mg, 200 mg, 400 mg

Carbamide Peroxide (KAR ba mide per OKS ide)

Brand Names: U.S. Auraphene B® [OTC]; Auro® [OTC]; Cankaid® [OTC]; Debrox® [OTC]; E-R-O® [OTC]; Gly-Oxide® [OTC]; Murine® Ear Wax Removal Kit [OTC]; Murine® Ear [OTC]; Otix® [OTC]; Wax Away [OTC]

Generic Availability (U.S.) Yes

Pharmacologic Category Anti-inflammatory, Locally Applied; Otic Agent, Cerumenolytic

Dental Use Relief of minor inflammation of gums, oral mucosal surfaces, and lips (including canker sores and dental irritation)

Use Relief of minor inflammation of gums, oral mucosal surfaces, and lips including canker sores and dental irritation; emulsify and disperse ear wax

Local Anesthetic/Vasoconstrictor Precautions No information available to require special precautions

Effects on Dental Treatment No significant effects or complications reported

Effects on Bleeding No information available to require special precautions

Adverse Effects Frequency not defined.
Dermatologic: Rash
Local: Irritation, redness
Miscellaneous: Superinfection

Dental Usual Dosage Minor inflammation of gums, oral mucosal surfaces and lips: Children and Adults: Topical: Oral solution (should not be used for >7 days): Apply several drops undiluted on affected area 4 times/day after meals and at bedtime; expectorate after 2-3 minutes or place 10 drops onto tongue, mix with saliva, swish for several minutes, expectorate

Dosage Children and Adults:
Oral: Inflammation/dental irritation: Solution (should not be used for >7 days): Oral preparation should not be used in children <2 years of age; apply several drops undiluted on affected area 4 times/day and at bedtime; expectorate after 2-3 minutes or place 10 drops onto tongue, mix with saliva, swish for several minutes, expectorate

Otic:
Children <12 years: Tilt head sideways and individualize the dose according to patient size; 3 drops (range: 1-5 drops) twice daily for up to 4 days, tip of applicator should not enter ear canal; keep drops in ear for several minutes by keeping head tilted and placing cotton in ear
Children ≥12 years and Adults: Tilt head sideways and instill 5-10 drops twice daily up to 4 days, tip of applicator should not enter ear canal; keep drops in ear for several minutes by keeping head tilted and placing cotton in ear

Mechanism of Action Carbamide peroxide releases hydrogen peroxide which serves as a source of nascent oxygen upon contact with catalase; deodorant action is probably due to inhibition of odor-causing bacteria; softens impacted cerumen due to its foaming action

Contraindications Hypersensitivity to carbamide peroxide or any component of the formulation; otic preparation should not be used in patients with a perforated tympanic membrane; ear drainage, ear pain, or rash in the ear

Warnings/Precautions
Oral: With prolonged use of oral carbamide peroxide, there is a potential for overgrowth of opportunistic organisms, damage to periodontal tissues, and delayed wound healing; should not be used for longer than 7 days. Not for OTC use in children <2 years of age.
Otic: Do not use if ear drainage or discharge, ear pain, irritation, or rash in ear. Should not be used for longer than 4 days. Not for OTC use in children <12 years of age.

Drug Interactions
Metabolism/Transport Effects None known.
Avoid Concomitant Use There are no known interactions where it is recommended to avoid concomitant use.
Increased Effect/Toxicity There are no known significant interactions involving an increase in effect.
Decreased Effect There are no known significant interactions involving a decrease in effect.

Pharmacodynamics/Kinetics
Onset of Action ~24 hours

Dosage Forms
Liquid, oral: 10% (60 mL)
Cankaid® [OTC]: 10% (15 mL)
Gly-Oxide® [OTC]: 10% (15 mL, 60 mL)

Solution, otic: 6.5% (15 mL)
Auraphene B® [OTC]: 6.5% (15 mL)
Auro® [OTC]: 6.5% (22.2 mL)
Debrox® [OTC]: 6.5% (15 mL, 30 mL)
E-R-O® [OTC]: 6.5% (15 mL)
Murine® Ear [OTC]: 6.5% (15 mL)
Murine® Ear Wax Removal Kit [OTC]: 6.5% (15 mL)
Otix® [OTC]: 6.5% (15 mL)
Wax Away [OTC]: 6.5% (15 mL)

Carbidopa (kar bi DOE pa)

Brand Names: U.S. Lodosyn®
Pharmacologic Category Anti-Parkinson's Agent, Decarboxylase Inhibitor
Use Given with carbidopa-levodopa in the treatment of parkinsonism to enable a lower dosage of levodopa to be used and a more rapid response to be obtained and to decrease side effects; use with carbidopa-levodopa in patients requiring additional carbidopa; has no effect without levodopa
Local Anesthetic/Vasoconstrictor Precautions No information available to require special precautions
Effects on Dental Treatment Key adverse event(s) related to dental treatment: Orthostatic hypotension. Dopaminergic therapy in Parkinson's disease includes the use of carbidopa in combination with levodopa. Carbidopa/levodopa combination is associated with orthostatic hypotension. Patients medicated with this drug combination should be carefully assisted from the chair and observed for signs of orthostatic hypotension.
Effects on Bleeding No information available to require special precautions
Adverse Effects Adverse reactions are associated with concomitant administration with levodopa.
Cardiovascular: Arrhythmia, chest pain, edema, flushing, hypotension, hypertension, MI, orthostatic hypotension, palpitation, phlebitis, syncope
Central nervous system: Agitation, anxiety, ataxia, confusion, delusions, dementia, depression (with or without suicidal tendencies), disorientation, dizziness, dreams abnormal, EPS, euphoria, faintness, falling, fatigue, gait abnormalities, headache, hallucinations, impulse control symptoms, insomnia, malaise, memory impairment, mental acuity decreased, nervousness, neuroleptic malignant syndrome, nightmares, on-off phenomena, paranoid ideation, pathological gambling, psychosis, seizure (causal relationship not established), somnolence
Dermatologic: Alopecia, malignant melanoma, rash
Endocrine & metabolic: Hot flashes, hyperglycemia, hypokalemia, libido increased (including hypersexuality), uric acid increased
Gastrointestinal: Abdominal pain, abdominal distress, anorexia, bruxism, constipation, diarrhea, discoloration of saliva, duodenal ulcer, dyspepsia, dysphagia, flatulence, GI bleeding, heartburn, nausea, sialorrhea, taste alterations, tongue burning sensation, weight gain/loss, vomiting, xerostomia
Genitourinary: Discoloration of urine, glycosuria, urinary frequency, priapism, proteinuria, urinary incontinence, urinary retention, urinary tract infection
Hematologic: Agranulocytosis, anemia, Coombs' test abnormal, hematocrit decreased, hemoglobin decreased, hemolytic anemia, leukopenia, thrombocytopenia
Hepatic: Alkaline phosphatase abnormal, ALT abnormal, AST abnormal, bilirubin abnormal, LDH abnormal

Neuromuscular & skeletal: Back pain, dyskinesias (including choreiform, dystonic and other involuntary movements), leg pain, muscle cramps, muscle twitching, numbness, paresthesia, peripheral neuropathy, shoulder pain, tremor increased, trismus, weakness
Ocular: Blepharospasm, blurred vision, diplopia, Horner's syndrome reactivation, mydriasis, oculogyric crises (may be associated with acute dystonic reactions)
Renal: BUN increased, serum creatinine increased
Respiratory: Cough, dyspnea, hoarseness, pharyngeal pain, upper respiratory infection
Miscellaneous: Discoloration of sweat, diaphoresis increased, hiccups, hypersensitivity reactions (including angioedema, pruritus, urticaria, bullous lesions [including pemphigus-like reactions], Henoch-Schönlein purpura [IgA vasculitis])
General Dosage Range Oral: *Adults:* 25 mg 3-4 times/day (maximum: 200 mg carbidopa/day)
Mechanism of Action Carbidopa is a peripheral decarboxylase inhibitor with little or no pharmacological activity when given alone in usual doses. It inhibits the peripheral decarboxylation of levodopa to dopamine; and as it does not cross the blood-brain barrier, unlike levodopa, effective brain concentrations of dopamine are produced with lower doses of levodopa. At the same time, reduced peripheral formation of dopamine reduces peripheral side-effects, notably nausea and vomiting, and cardiac arrhythmias, although the dyskinesias and adverse mental effects associated with levodopa therapy tend to develop earlier.
Pregnancy Risk Factor C
Pregnancy Considerations Adverse events have not been observed in animal reproduction studies. Carbidopa has been found to cross the human placenta; absorption in fetal tissue was minimal.

Carbidopa and Levodopa
(kar bi DOE pa & lee voe DOE pa)

Related Information
Carbidopa *on page 249*
Brand Names: U.S. Parcopa®; Sinemet®; Sinemet® CR
Brand Names: Canada Apo-Levocarb®; Apo-Levocarb® CR; Dom-Levo-Carbidopa; Duodopa™; Levocarb CR; Nu-Levocarb; PRO-Levocarb; Sinemet®; Sinemet® CR; Teva-Levocarbidopa
Pharmacologic Category Anti-Parkinson's Agent, Decarboxylase Inhibitor; Anti-Parkinson's Agent, Dopamine Precursor
Use Idiopathic Parkinson's disease; postencephalitic parkinsonism; symptomatic parkinsonism

Duodopa™ intestinal gel: Canadian labeling (not available in U.S.): Treatment of advanced levodopa-responsive Parkinson's disease in which severe motor symptoms are not controlled by other Parkinson's agents
Unlabeled Use Restless leg syndrome
Local Anesthetic/Vasoconstrictor Precautions No information available to require special precautions
Effects on Dental Treatment Key adverse event(s) related to dental treatment: Xerostomia (normal salivary flow resumes upon discontinuation) and taste alterations. Dopaminergic therapy in Parkinson's disease (ie, treatment with levodopa and carbidopa combination) is associated with orthostatic hypotension. Patients medicated with this drug combination should be carefully assisted from the chair and observed for signs of orthostatic hypotension.

◄ **Effects on Bleeding** No information available to require special precautions

Adverse Effects Frequency not defined.

Cardiovascular: Arrhythmia, chest pain, edema, flushing, hypotension, hypertension, MI, orthostatic hypotension, palpitation, phlebitis, syncope

Central nervous system: Agitation, anxiety, ataxia, confusion, delusions, dementia, depression (with or without suicidal tendencies), disorientation, dizziness, dreams abnormal, EPS, euphoria, faintness, falling, fatigue, gait abnormalities, headache, hallucinations, impulse control symptoms, insomnia, malaise, memory impairment, mental acuity decreased, nervousness, neuroleptic malignant syndrome, nightmares, on-off phenomena, paranoid ideation, pathological gambling, psychosis, seizure (causal relationship not established), somnolence

Dermatologic: Alopecia, malignant melanoma, rash

Endocrine & metabolic: Hot flashes, hyperglycemia, hypokalemia, libido increased (including hypersexuality), uric acid increased

Gastrointestinal: Abdominal pain, abdominal distress, anorexia, bruxism, constipation, diarrhea, discoloration of saliva, duodenal ulcer, dyspepsia, dysphagia, flatulence, GI bleeding, heartburn, nausea, sialorrhea, taste alterations, tongue burning sensation, weight gain/loss, vomiting, xerostomia

Genitourinary: Discoloration of urine, glycosuria, urinary frequency, priapism, proteinuria, urinary incontinence, urinary retention, urinary tract infection

Hematologic: Agranulocytosis, anemia, Coombs' test abnormal, hematocrit decreased, hemoglobin decreased, hemolytic anemia, leukopenia

Hepatic: Alkaline phosphatase abnormal, ALT abnormal, AST abnormal, bilirubin abnormal, LDH abnormal

Neuromuscular & skeletal: Back pain, dyskinesias (including choreiform, dystonic and other involuntary movements), leg pain, muscle cramps, muscle twitching, numbness, paresthesia, peripheral neuropathy, shoulder pain, tremor increased, trismus, weakness

Ocular: Blepharospasm, blurred vision, diplopia, Horner's syndrome reactivation, mydriasis, oculogyric crises (may be associated with acute dystonic reactions)

Renal: Difficult urination

Respiratory: Cough, dyspnea, hoarseness, pharyngeal pain, upper respiratory infection

Miscellaneous: Discoloration of sweat, diaphoresis increased, hiccups, hypersensitivity reactions (angioedema, pruritus, urticaria, bullous lesions [including pemphigus-like reactions], Henoch-Schönlein purpura [IgA vasculitis])

General Dosage Range Oral: *Adults:* Immediate release: Initial: Carbidopa 25 mg/levodopa 100 mg 3 times/day (maximum: 8 tablets of any strength/day **or** 200 mg of carbidopa and 2000 mg of levodopa); Controlled release: *Adults:* Initial: Carbidopa 50 mg/levodopa 200 mg 2 times/day, at intervals not <6 hours (maximum: 8 tablets/day)

Mechanism of Action Parkinson's symptoms are due to a lack of striatal dopamine; levodopa circulates in the plasma to the blood-brain-barrier (BBB), where it crosses, to be converted by striatal enzymes to dopamine; carbidopa inhibits the peripheral plasma breakdown of levodopa by inhibiting its decarboxylation, and thereby increases available levodopa at the BBB

Pharmacodynamics/Kinetics

Half-life Elimination Immediate release: Levodopa (in presence of carbidopa): 1.5 hours; Half-life may be prolonged with controlled release formulations due to continuous absorption.

Time to Peak Immediate release: 0.5 hours; Controlled release: 2 hours; Intestinal gel: therapeutic plasma levels reached 10-30 minutes following morning bolus dose

Pregnancy Risk Factor C

Pregnancy Considerations Teratogenic effects were observed with levodopa and carbidopa in animal studies. There are case reports of levodopa crossing the placenta in humans.

Prescribing and Access Restrictions Duodopa™ intestinal gel (Canadian labeling; product not available in U.S.): In Canada, the Duodopa™ Education Program is a risk mitigation program established to provide safe and effective use of Duodopa™ in advanced Parkinson's patients. The program involves:

- Education of prescribing neurologists and other healthcare providers on suitable candidates for treatment, surgical procedures (PEG tube placement), and follow-up care including infusion device education.

- Distribution of educational materials to patients and caregivers describing Duodopa™ intestinal gel and its proper use, PEG tube placement, and complications associated with the mode of administration and/or PEG tube placement.

Carbinoxamine (kar bi NOKS a meen)

Brand Names: U.S. Arbinoxa™; Palgic®

Pharmacologic Category Ethanolamine Derivative; Histamine H$_1$ Antagonist; Histamine H$_1$ Antagonist, First Generation

Use Seasonal and perennial allergic rhinitis; vasomotor rhinitis; allergic conjunctivitis; mild manifestations of urticaria and angioedema; dermatographism; adjunct therapy for anaphylactic reactions (after acute manifestations controlled)

Local Anesthetic/Vasoconstrictor Precautions No information available to require special precautions

Effects on Dental Treatment Key adverse event(s) related to dental treatment: Xerostomia (normal salivary flow resumes upon discontinuation).

Effects on Bleeding No information available to require special precautions

Adverse Effects Frequency not defined.

Cardiovascular: Extrasystoles, hypotension, palpitation, tachycardia

Central nervous system: Chills, confusion, coordination impaired (most frequent), dizziness (most frequent), euphoria, excitability, fatigue, headache, hysteria, insomnia, irritability, nervousness, neuritis, restlessness, sedation (most frequent), seizure, sleepiness (most frequent), vertigo

Dermatologic: Photosensitivity, rash, urticaria

Endocrine & metabolic: Early menses

Gastrointestinal: Anorexia, constipation, diarrhea, epigastric distress (most frequent), nausea, vomiting, xerostomia

Genitourinary: Difficult urination, urinary frequency, urinary retention

Hematologic: Agranulocytosis, hemolytic anemia, thrombocytopenia

Neuromuscular & skeletal: Paresthesia, tremor

Ocular: Blurred vision, diplopia

Otic: Labyrinthitis, tinnitus

Respiratory: Bronchial secretions thickening (most frequent), chest tightness, nasal congestion, nasopharyngeal dryness, wheezing

Miscellaneous: Diaphoresis, hypersensitivity reactions (including anaphylactic shock)

General Dosage Range Oral:

Children 2-5 years: 0.2-0.4 mg/kg/day divided into 3-4 doses **or** 1-2 mg 3-4 times/day

Children 6-11 years: 2-4 mg 3-4 times/day

Adults: 4-8 mg 3-4 times/day

Mechanism of Action Carbinoxamine competes with histamine for H_1-receptor sites on effector cells in the gastrointestinal tract, blood vessels, and respiratory tract.

Pharmacodynamics/Kinetics

Duration of Action ~4 hours

Pregnancy Risk Factor C

Pregnancy Considerations Animal reproduction studies have not been conducted. Maternal antihistamine use has generally not resulted in an increased risk of birth defects; however, information specific for the use of carbinoxamine during pregnancy has not been located. Although antihistamines are recommended for some indications in pregnant women, the use of other agents with specific pregnancy data may be preferred.

Product Availability Karbinal™ ER (extended release) oral suspension: FDA approved March 2013; availability anticipated in the fall of 2013. Consult the prescribing information for additional information.

CARBOplatin (KAR boe pla tin)

Brand Names: Canada Carboplatin Injection; Carboplatin Injection - LIQ IV

Pharmacologic Category Antineoplastic Agent, Alkylating Agent; Antineoplastic Agent, Platinum Analog

Use Initial treatment of advanced ovarian cancer in combination with other established chemotherapy agents; palliative treatment of recurrent ovarian cancer after prior chemotherapy, including cisplatin-based treatment

Unlabeled Use Treatment of bladder cancer, breast cancer (metastatic), central nervous system tumors, cervical cancer (recurrent or metastatic), endometrial cancer, esophageal cancer, head and neck cancer, Hodgkin's lymphoma (relapsed or refractory), malignant pleural mesothelioma, melanoma (advanced or metastatic), merkel cell carcinoma, neuroendocrine tumors (adrenal gland and carcinoid tumors), non-Hodgkin's lymphomas (relapsed or refractory), nonsmall cell lung cancer, retinoblastoma, sarcomas (Ewing's sarcoma and osteosarcoma), small-cell lung cancer, testicular cancer, thymic malignancies, unknown primary adenocarcinoma, and as a conditioning regimen prior to hematopoietic stem cell transplantation

Local Anesthetic/Vasoconstrictor Precautions No information available to require special precautions

Effects on Dental Treatment Key adverse event(s) related to dental treatment: Stomatitis, mucositis, and taste dysgeusia.

Effects on Bleeding Hemorrhagic complication (ie, bleeding) has been reported in 5% of patients. Thrombocytopenia is one of the dose-limiting complications of carboplatin's myelosuppression. A medical consult is suggested.

Adverse Effects Percentages reported with single-agent therapy.

>10%:

Central nervous system: Pain (23%)

Endocrine & metabolic: Hyponatremia (29% to 47%), hypomagnesemia (29% to 43%), hypocalcemia(22% to 31%), hypokalemia (20% to 28%)

Gastrointestinal: Vomiting (65% to 81%), abdominal pain (17%), nausea (without vomiting: 10% to 15%)

Hematologic: Myelosuppression (dose related and dose limiting; nadir at ~21 days with single-agent therapy), anemia (71% to 90%; grades 3/4: 21%), leukopenia (85%; grades 3/4: 15% to 26%), neutropenia (67%; grades 3/4: 16% to 21%), thrombocytopenia (62%; grades 3/4: 25% to 35%)

Hepatic: Alkaline phosphatase increased (24% to 37%), AST increased (15% to 19%)

Neuromuscular & skeletal: Weakness (11%)

Renal: Creatinine clearance decreased (27%), BUN increased (14% to 22%)

Miscellaneous: Hypersensitivity/allergic reaction (2% to 16%)

1% to 10%:

Central nervous system: Neurotoxicity (5%)

Dermatologic: Alopecia (2% to 3%)

Gastrointestinal: Constipation (6%), diarrhea (6%), stomatitis/mucositis (1%), taste dysgeusia (1%)

Hematologic: Bleeding (5%), hemorrhagic complications (5%)

Hepatic: Bilirubin increased (5%)

Neuromuscular & skeletal: Peripheral neuropathy (4% to 6%)

Ocular: Visual disturbance (1%)

Otic: Ototoxicity (1%)

Renal: Creatinine increased (6% to 10%)

Miscellaneous: Infection (5%)

General Dosage Range Dosage adjustment recommended in renal impairment or who develop toxicities

I.V.: *Adults:* 300-360 mg/m^2 every 4 weeks **or** AUC of 4-6 (using Calvert formula)

Mechanism of Action Carboplatin is a platinum compound alkylating agent which covalently binds to DNA; interferes with the function of DNA by producing interstrand DNA cross-links

Pharmacodynamics/Kinetics

Half-life Elimination Cl_{cr} >60 mL/minute: Carboplatin: 2.6-5.9 hours (based on a dose of 300-500 mg/m^2); Platinum (from carboplatin): ≥5 days

Pregnancy Risk Factor D

Pregnancy Considerations Embryotoxicity and teratogenicity have been observed in animal reproduction studies. May cause fetal harm if administered during pregnancy. Women of childbearing potential should avoid becoming pregnant during treatment.

Carboprost Tromethamine
(KAR boe prost tro METH a meen)

Brand Names: U.S. Hemabate®

Brand Names: Canada Hemabate®

Pharmacologic Category Abortifacient; Prostaglandin

Use Termination of pregnancy during the second trimester between weeks 13 and 20 of gestation; treatment of refractory postpartum hemorrhage due to uterine atony

Local Anesthetic/Vasoconstrictor Precautions No information available to require special precautions

Effects on Dental Treatment No significant effects or complications reported

Effects on Bleeding No information available to require special precautions

Adverse Effects Frequency not defined. Effects due to increased smooth muscle contractility are most common and are generally transient and reversible upon discontinuation of therapy.

Cardiovascular: Chest pain, flushing, hypertension, syncope, palpitation, tachycardia, tightness of chest

Central nervous system: Anxiety, chills/shivering, dizziness, drowsiness, dystonia, faintness, headache, lethargy, lightheadedness, nervousness, sleep disturbance, temperature elevation (may be drug induced or due to postabortion endometritis), vasovagal syndrome, vertigo

Dermatologic: Rash

Endocrine & metabolic: Breast tenderness, dysmenorrhea-like pain, endometritis, hot flashes, thyroid storm

Gastrointestinal: Choking sensation, diarrhea (~2/3 patients), dry throat, epigastric pain, gagging/retching, hematemesis, nausea (~1/3 patients), taste alteration, thirst, throat fullness, vomiting (~2/3 patients), xerostomia

Genitourinary: Perforated uterus, posterior cervical perforation, urinary tract infection, uterine bleeding (excessive), uterine rupture, uterine sacculation

Local: Injection site pain

Neuromuscular & skeletal: Backache, leg cramps, muscular pain, paresthesia, torticollis, weakness

Ocular: Blurred vision, eye pain, eyelid twitching

Otic: Tinnitus

Respiratory: Asthma, cough, bronchospasm, dyspnea, epistaxis, hyperventilation, pulmonary edema, respiratory distress, upper respiratory tract infection, wheezing

Miscellaneous: Diaphoresis, hiccups, retained placental fragment, septic shock

General Dosage Range I.M.: *Adults (females):* Termination of pregnancy: 250 mcg at 1.5- to 3.5-hour intervals, a 500 mcg dose may be given if uterine response is not adequate after several 250 mcg doses (maximum total dose: 12 mg); Postpartum bleeding: 250 mcg; may repeat if needed (maximum total dose: 2 mg [8 doses])

Mechanism of Action Carboprost tromethamine is a tromethamine salt analog of naturally occurring prostaglandin F$_2$ alpha (dinoprost) except for the addition of a methyl group at the C-15 position. This substitution produces longer duration of activity than dinoprost; carboprost stimulates uterine contractility which usually results in expulsion of the products of conception and is used to induce abortion between 13-20 weeks of pregnancy. When used postpartum, hemostasis at the placentation site is achieved through the myometrial contractions produced by carboprost.

Pharmacodynamics/Kinetics

Time to Peak Serum: I.M.: 30 minutes

Pregnancy Risk Factor C

Pregnancy Considerations Teratogenic effects were not observed in animal reproduction studies. When used for termination of pregnancy, carboprost tromethamine is not considered feticidal, but is used to terminate pregnancy due to its ability to stimulate uterine contractions; use is not indicated if the fetus has reached a stage of viability *in utero*. Complete termination of pregnancy may not be induced in ~20% of cases and should therefore be completed in another way.

Carboxymethylcellulose
(kar boks ee meth il SEL yoo lose)

Brand Names: U.S. Optive™ [OTC]; Refresh Liquigel™ [OTC]; Refresh Plus® [OTC]; Refresh Tears® [OTC]; Tears Again® Night & Day™ [OTC]; Theratears® [OTC]

Brand Names: Canada Celluvisc™; Refresh Plus®; Refresh Tears®

Pharmacologic Category Ophthalmic Agent, Miscellaneous

Use Artificial tear substitute

Local Anesthetic/Vasoconstrictor Precautions No information available to require special precautions

Effects on Dental Treatment No significant effects or complications reported

Effects on Bleeding No information available to require special precautions

General Dosage Range Ophthalmic: *Adults:* Instill 1-2 drops into eye(s) 3-4 times/day

Carisoprodol (kar eye soe PROE dole)

Brand Names: U.S. Soma®

Generic Availability (U.S.) Yes

Pharmacologic Category Skeletal Muscle Relaxant

Dental Use Treatment of muscle spasms and pain associated with acute temporomandibular joint (TMJ) pain

Use Short-term (2-3 weeks) treatment of acute musculoskeletal pain

Local Anesthetic/Vasoconstrictor Precautions No information available to require special precautions

Effects on Dental Treatment No significant effects or complications reported

Effects on Bleeding No information available to require special precautions

Adverse Effects

>10%: Central nervous system: Drowsiness (13% to 17%)

1% to 10%: Central nervous system: Dizziness (7% to 8%), headache (3% to 5%)

Dental Usual Dosage Treatment of muscle spasms and pain associated with acute TMJ pain: Adults: Oral: 250-350 mg 3 times/day and at bedtime

Dosage Note: Carisoprodol should only be used for short periods (2-3 weeks) due to lack of evidence of effectiveness with prolonged use.

Oral: Children ≥16 years and Adults: 250-350 mg 3 times/day and at bedtime

Dosing adjustment in renal impairment: Use in renal impairment has not been studied; use with caution

Dialysis: Removed by hemo- and peritoneal dialysis

Dosing adjustment in hepatic impairment: Use in hepatic impairment has not been studied; use with caution

Mechanism of Action Precise mechanism is not yet clear, but many effects have been ascribed to its central depressant actions. In animals, carisoprodol blocks interneuronal activity and depresses polysynaptic neuron transmission in the spinal cord and reticular formation of the brain. It is also metabolized to meprobamate, which has anxiolytic and sedative effects.

Contraindications Hypersensitivity to carisoprodol, meprobamate, or any component of the formulation; acute intermittent porphyria

Warnings/Precautions Can cause CNS depression, which may impair physical or mental abilities. Patients must be cautioned about performing tasks which require mental alertness (eg, operating machinery or driving); postmarketing reports of motor vehicle accidents have been associated with use. Effects with other CNS-depressant drugs or ethanol may be potentiated. Use with caution in patients with hepatic/renal dysfunction. Tolerance or drug dependence may result from extended use. Limit use to 2-3 weeks; use caution in patients who may be prone to addiction. May precipitate withdrawal after abrupt cessation of prolonged use.

Idiosyncratic reactions and/or severe allergic reactions may occur. Idiosyncratic reactions occur following the initial dose and may include severe weakness, transient quadriplegia, euphoria, or vision loss (temporary). Has been associated (rarely) with seizures in patients with and without seizure history. Carisoprodol should be used with caution in patients who are poor CYP2C19 metabolizers; poor metabolizers have been shown to have a fourfold increase in exposure to carisoprodol and a 50% reduced exposure to the metabolite meprobamate compared to normal metabolizers. Muscle relaxants are poorly tolerated by the elderly due to potent anticholinergic effects, sedation, and risk of fracture. Efficacy is questionable at dosages tolerated by elderly patients; avoid use (Beers Criteria).

Drug Interactions

Metabolism/Transport Effects Substrate of CYP2C19 (major); **Note:** Assignment of Major/Minor substrate status based on clinically relevant drug interaction potential

Avoid Concomitant Use

Avoid concomitant use of Carisoprodol with any of the following: Azelastine (Nasal); Paraldehyde

Increased Effect/Toxicity

Carisoprodol may increase the levels/effects of: Alcohol (Ethyl); Azelastine (Nasal); Buprenorphine; CNS Depressants; Methotrimeprazine; Metyrosine; Mirtazapine; Paraldehyde; Pramipexole; ROPINIRole; Rotigotine; Selective Serotonin Reuptake Inhibitors; Zolpidem

The levels/effects of Carisoprodol may be increased by: CYP2C19 Inhibitors (Moderate); CYP2C19 Inhibitors (Strong); Droperidol; HydrOXYzine; Magnesium Sulfate; Methotrimeprazine; Perampanel; Sodium Oxybate

Decreased Effect

The levels/effects of Carisoprodol may be decreased by: CYP2C19 Inducers (Strong)

Ethanol/Nutrition/Herb Interactions Ethanol: May increase CNS depression; monitor for increased effects with coadministration. Caution patients about effects.

Dietary Considerations May be taken with or without food.

Pharmacodynamics/Kinetics

Onset of Action ~30 minutes

Duration of Action 4-6 hours

Half-life Elimination ~2 hours; Meprobamate: 10 hours

Time to Peak 1.5-2 hours

Pregnancy Risk Factor C

Pregnancy Considerations Animal data suggests that carisoprodol crosses placenta and adverse events have been observed in animal studies. Limited postmarketing data with meprobamate (the active metabolite) demonstrate a possible risk for congenital malformations. Use only if benefit outweighs the risk.

Lactation Enters breast milk/use caution

Breast-Feeding Considerations Carisoprodol levels in breast milk may be 2-4 times that of maternal plasma levels. The estimated dose to the infant was reported as 6.9% of the weight adjusted maternal dose in one case report and ~4% of the weight-adjusted maternal dose in another. In both cases, breast milk production was decreased requiring supplemental formula or cessation of breast-feeding. Other than slight sedation reported in one infant, no symptoms of withdrawal or other adverse events were noted in these 2 cases. Effects on long-term development are not known.

Controlled Substance C-IV

Dosage Forms

Tablet, oral: 350 mg

Soma®: 250 mg, 350 mg

Carisoprodol and Aspirin
(kar eye soe PROE dole & AS pir in)

Related Information

Aspirin *on page 135*

Carisoprodol *on page 252*

Generic Availability (U.S.) Yes

Pharmacologic Category Skeletal Muscle Relaxant

Dental Use Treatment of muscle spasms and pain associated with acute temporomandibular joint pain (TMJ)

Use Relief of discomfort associated with acute, painful skeletal muscle conditions

Local Anesthetic/Vasoconstrictor Precautions No information available to require special precautions

Effects on Dental Treatment Key adverse event(s) related to dental treatment: Aspirin: As with all drugs which may affect hemostasis, bleeding is associated with aspirin. Hemorrhage may occur at virtually any site; risk is dependent on multiple variables including dosage, concurrent use of multiple agents which alter hemostasis, and patient susceptibility. Many adverse effects of aspirin are dose related, and are rare at low dosages. Other serious reactions are idiosyncratic, related to allergy or individual sensitivity (see Effects on Bleeding).

Effects on Bleeding Aspirin irreversibly inhibits platelet aggregation which can prolong bleeding. Upon discontinuation, normal platelet function returns only when new platelets are released (~7-10 days). However, in the case of dental surgery, there is no scientific evidence to support discontinuation of aspirin.

Adverse Effects See individual agents.

Dental Usual Dosage Treatment of muscle spasms and pain associated with acute TMJ pain: Adults: Oral: 1-2 tablets 4 times/day

Dosage Oral:

Children ≥16 years and Adults: Acute skeletal muscle pain: 1-2 tablets 4 times/day for 2-3 weeks (maximum: 8 tablets/24 hours)

Elderly: Avoid use in the elderly due to risk of orthostatic hypotension and CNS depression

Dosing adjustment in renal impairment: Use in renal impairment has not been studied; use with caution

Dosing adjustment in hepatic impairment: Use in hepatic impairment has not been studied; use with caution

Mechanism of Action See individual agents.

Contraindications Hypersensitivity to a carbamate (eg, meprobamate); serious gastrointestinal complications (eg, bleeding, perforations, obstruction) due to aspirin use; aspirin-induced asthma; acute intermittent porphyria

Warnings/Precautions Can cause CNS depression, which may impair physical or mental abilities. Patients must be cautioned about performing tasks which require mental alertness (eg, operating machinery or driving); postmarketing reports of motor vehicle accidents have been associated with use. Sedative effects may be potentiated when used with other CNS-depressant drugs or ethanol. Serious GI effects (eg, bleeding, perforation, and intestinal obstruction) may occur (possibly fatal) with aspirin use. Idiosyncratic reactions may occur (rarely) following initial dosing and may include ▶

severe weakness, transient quadriplegia, euphoria, or temporary vision loss. Use with caution in patients with a history of GI bleeding from ulcers; history of poor baseline health; geriatric patients; patients taking high doses of aspirin; patients taking concurrent anticoagulants, NSAIDs, or large amounts of ethanol.

Patients with sensitivity to tartrazine dyes, nasal polyps, and asthma may have an increased risk of salicylate sensitivity. Carisoprodol has been associated (rarely) with seizures in patients with and without seizure history. Idiosyncratic reactions may occur (rarely) following initial dosing and may include severe weakness, transient quadriplegia, euphoria, or temporary vision loss. Use with caution in patients with a history of drug abuse or acute alcoholism; potential for drug dependency exists. Tolerance, psychological and physical dependence may occur with prolonged use. Abrupt discontinuation following prolonged use may lead to withdrawal symptoms; use >3 weeks not recommended.

Use with caution in patients with hepatic or renal impairment; not studied. Abrupt discontinuation following prolonged use may lead to withdrawal symptoms; use >3 weeks not recommended. Aspirin should be avoided (if possible) in surgical patients for 1-2 weeks prior to surgery, to reduce the risk of excessive bleeding. Carisoprodol should be used with caution in patients with reduced function alleles of CYP2C19; poor metabolizers have been shown to have a fourfold increase in exposure to carisoprodol and a 50% reduced exposure to the metabolite meprobamate compared to normal metabolizers. Muscle relaxants are poorly tolerated by the elderly due to potent anticholinergic effects, sedation, and risk of fracture. Efficacy is questionable at dosages tolerated by elderly patients; avoid use (Beers Criteria).

Drug Interactions

Metabolism/Transport Effects Refer to individual components.

Avoid Concomitant Use

Avoid concomitant use of Carisoprodol and Aspirin with any of the following: Azelastine (Nasal); Floctafenine; Influenza Virus Vaccine (Live/Attenuated); Ketorolac (Nasal); Ketorolac (Systemic); Omacetaxine; Paraldehyde

Increased Effect/Toxicity

Carisoprodol and Aspirin may increase the levels/ effects of: Alcohol (Ethyl); Alendronate; Anticoagulants; Azelastine (Nasal); Buprenorphine; Carbonic Anhydrase Inhibitors; CNS Depressants; Collagenase (Systemic); Corticosteroids (Systemic); Dabigatran Etexilate; Divalproex; Drotrecogin Alfa (Activated); Heparin; Hypoglycemic Agents; Ibritumomab; Methotrexate; Methotrimeprazine; Metyrosine; Mirtazapine; NSAID (COX-2 Inhibitor); Omacetaxine; Paraldehyde; PRALAtrexate; Pramipexole; Rivaroxaban; ROPINIRole; Rotigotine; Salicylates; Thrombolytic Agents; Ticagrelor; Tositumomab and Iodine I 131 Tositumomab; Valproic Acid; Varicella Virus-Containing Vaccines; Vitamin K Antagonists; Zolpidem

The levels/effects of Carisoprodol and Aspirin may be increased by: Agents with Antiplatelet Properties; Ammonium Chloride; Antidepressants (Tricyclic, Tertiary Amine); Calcium Channel Blockers (Nondihydropyridine); CYP2C19 Inhibitors (Moderate); CYP2C19 Inhibitors (Strong); Dasatinib; Droperidol; Floctafenine; Ginkgo Biloba; Glucosamine; Herbs (Anticoagulant/ Antiplatelet Properties); HydrOXYzine; Influenza Virus Vaccine (Live/Attenuated); Ketorolac (Nasal); Ketorolac (Systemic); Loop Diuretics; Magnesium Sulfate; Methotrimeprazine; Multivitamins/Minerals (with

ADEK, Folate, Iron); NSAID (Nonselective); Omega-3 Fatty Acids; Pentosan Polysulfate Sodium; Pentoxifylline; Perampanel; Potassium Acid Phosphate; Prostacyclin Analogues; Selective Serotonin Reuptake Inhibitors; Serotonin/Norepinephrine Reuptake Inhibitors; Sodium Oxybate; Tipranavir; Treprostinil; Vitamin E

Decreased Effect

Carisoprodol and Aspirin may decrease the levels/ effects of: ACE Inhibitors; Hyaluronidase; Loop Diuretics; Multivitamins/Minerals (with ADEK, Folate, Iron); NSAID (Nonselective); Probenecid; Ticagrelor; Tiludronate

The levels/effects of Carisoprodol and Aspirin may be decreased by: Corticosteroids (Systemic); CYP2C19 Inducers (Strong); Floctafenine; Ketorolac (Nasal); Ketorolac (Systemic); NSAID (Nonselective)

Ethanol/Nutrition/Herb Interactions Ethanol: May increase CNS depression; monitor for increased effects with coadministration. Caution patients about effects.

Pregnancy Risk Factor C

Pregnancy Considerations Animal reproduction studies have not been conducted with this combination. See individual agents.

Lactation Enters breast milk/not recommended

Breast-Feeding Considerations Carisoprodol and aspirin are excreted into breast milk. Refer to individual monographs for additional information.

Controlled Substance C-IV

Dosage Forms

Tablet: Carisoprodol 200 mg and aspirin 325 mg

Dental Comment There is no scientific evidence to warrant discontinuance of aspirin prior to dental surgery. Patients taking one aspirin tablet daily as an antithrombotic and who require dental surgery should be given special consideration in consultation with the physician before removal of the aspirin relative to prevention of postoperative bleeding.

Carisoprodol, Aspirin, and Codeine
(kar eye soe PROE dole, AS pir in, and KOE deen)

Related Information

Aspirin *on page 135*

Carisoprodol *on page 252*

Codeine *on page 344*

Generic Availability (U.S.) Yes

Pharmacologic Category Skeletal Muscle Relaxant

Dental Use Treatment of muscle spasms and pain associated with acute temporomandibular joint pain (TMJ)

Use Skeletal muscle relaxant

Local Anesthetic/Vasoconstrictor Precautions No information available to require special precautions

Effects on Dental Treatment Key adverse event(s) related to dental treatment: Aspirin: As with all drugs which may affect hemostasis, bleeding is associated with aspirin. Hemorrhage may occur at virtually any site; risk is dependent on multiple variables including dosage, concurrent use of multiple agents which alter hemostasis, and patient susceptibility. Many adverse effects of aspirin are dose related, and are rare at low dosages. Other serious reactions are idiosyncratic, related to allergy or individual sensitivity (see Effects on Bleeding).

Effects on Bleeding Aspirin irreversibly inhibits platelet aggregation which can prolong bleeding. Upon discontinuation, normal platelet function returns only when new platelets are released (~7-10 days). However, in the case of dental surgery, there is no scientific evidence to support discontinuation of aspirin.

Adverse Effects See individual agents.

Dental Usual Dosage Treatment of muscle spasms and pain associated with acute TMJ pain: Adults: Oral: 1 or 2 tablets 4 times/day

Dosage Oral:
Adults: 1 or 2 tablets 4 times/day (maximum: 8 tablets/day); treatment should be temporary (2-3 weeks)
Elderly: Avoid or use with caution in the elderly (>65 years of age); adverse effects (eg, orthostatic hypotension and CNS depression) may be potentiated.

Dosage adjustment in renal impairment: No dosage adjustment provided in manufacturer's labeling.

Dosage adjustment in hepatic impairment: No dosage adjustment provided in manufacturer's labeling.

Mechanism of Action See individual agents.

Contraindications Hypersensitivity to a carbamate (eg, meprobamate); serious gastrointestinal complications (eg, bleeding, perforations, obstruction) due to aspirin use; aspirin-induced asthma; acute intermittent porphyria

Warnings/Precautions Use with caution in patients with hypersensitivity reactions to other phenanthrene-derivative opioid agonists (hydrocodone, hydromorphone, levorphanol, oxycodone, oxymorphone); hepatic or renal dysfunction; cardiovascular disease; biliary tract impairment; gastrointestinal disease; respiratory disease. May obscure diagnosis or clinical course of patients with acute abdominal conditions. May cause CNS depression, which may impair physical or mental abilities; patients must be cautioned about performing tasks which require mental alertness (eg, operating machinery or driving). May cause hypotension; use with caution in patients with hypovolemia, cardiovascular disease (including acute MI), or drugs which may exaggerate hypotensive effects (including phenothiazines or general anesthetics). Carisoprodol has been associated (rarely) with seizures in patients with and without seizure history.

Patients with sensitivity to tartrazine dyes, nasal polyps, and asthma may have an increased risk of salicylate sensitivity. Effects with other sedatives or ethanol may be potentiated. Use caution with concomitant use of aspirin, NSAIDs, warfarin, or other drugs that affect coagulation; the risk of bleeding may be potentiated. Use caution in patients with two or more copies of the variant CYP2D6*2 allele. Muscle relaxants are poorly tolerated by the elderly due to potent anticholinergic effects, sedation, and risk of fracture. Efficacy is questionable at dosages tolerated by elderly patients; avoid use (Beers Criteria). Use with caution in elderly patients; adverse effects may be potentiated. Safety and efficacy have not been established in children <16 years of age. Tolerance or drug dependence may result from extended use; abrupt discontinuation may lead to withdrawal symptoms. Limit use to 2-3 weeks; use caution in patients who may be prone to addiction. Aspirin products should be avoided (if possible) for 1-2 weeks prior to surgery.

Drug Interactions
Metabolism/Transport Effects Refer to individual components.

Avoid Concomitant Use
Avoid concomitant use of Carisoprodol, Aspirin, and Codeine with any of the following: Azelastine (Nasal); Floctafenine; Influenza Virus Vaccine (Live/Attenuated); Ketorolac (Nasal); Ketorolac (Systemic); Omacetaxine; Paraldehyde

Increased Effect/Toxicity
Carisoprodol, Aspirin, and Codeine may increase the levels/effects of: Alcohol (Ethyl); Alendronate; Alvimopan; Anticoagulants; Azelastine (Nasal); Carbonic Anhydrase Inhibitors; CNS Depressants; Collagenase (Systemic); Corticosteroids (Systemic); Dabigatran Etexilate; Desmopressin; Divalproex; Drotrecogin Alfa (Activated); Heparin; Hypoglycemic Agents; Ibritumomab; Methotrexate; Metyrosine; Mirtazapine; NSAID (COX-2 Inhibitor); Omacetaxine; Paraldehyde; PRALatrexate; Pramipexole; Rivaroxaban; ROPINIRole; Rotigotine; Salicylates; Selective Serotonin Reuptake Inhibitors; Thiazide Diuretics; Thrombolytic Agents; Ticagrelor; Tositumomab and Iodine I 131 Tositumomab; Valproic Acid; Varicella Virus-Containing Vaccines; Vitamin K Antagonists; Zolpidem

The levels/effects of Carisoprodol, Aspirin, and Codeine may be increased by: Agents with Antiplatelet Properties; Ammonium Chloride; Amphetamines; Antidepressants (Tricyclic, Tertiary Amine); Antipsychotic Agents (Phenothiazines); Calcium Channel Blockers (Nondihydropyridine); CYP2C19 Inhibitors (Moderate); CYP2C19 Inhibitors (Strong); Dasatinib; Droperidol; Floctafenine; Ginkgo Biloba; Glucosamine; Herbs (Anticoagulant/Antiplatelet Properties); HydrOXYzine; Influenza Virus Vaccine (Live/Attenuated); Ketorolac (Nasal); Ketorolac (Systemic); Loop Diuretics; Magnesium Sulfate; Multivitamins/Minerals (with ADEK, Folate, Iron); NSAID (Nonselective); Omega-3 Fatty Acids; Pentosan Polysulfate Sodium; Pentoxifylline; Perampanel; Potassium Acid Phosphate; Prostacyclin Analogues; Selective Serotonin Reuptake Inhibitors; Serotonin/Norepinephrine Reuptake Inhibitors; Sodium Oxybate; Somatostatin Analogs; Succinylcholine; Tipranavir; Treprostinil; Vitamin E

Decreased Effect
Carisoprodol, Aspirin, and Codeine may decrease the levels/effects of: ACE Inhibitors; Hyaluronidase; Loop Diuretics; Multivitamins/Minerals (with ADEK, Folate, Iron); NSAID (Nonselective); Pegvisomant; Probenecid; Ticagrelor; Tiludronate

The levels/effects of Carisoprodol, Aspirin, and Codeine may be decreased by: Ammonium Chloride; Corticosteroids (Systemic); CYP2C19 Inducers (Strong); CYP2D6 Inhibitors (Moderate); CYP2D6 Inhibitors (Strong); Floctafenine; Ketorolac (Nasal); Ketorolac (Systemic); Mixed Agonist / Antagonist Opioids; NSAID (Nonselective)

Ethanol/Nutrition/Herb Interactions
Ethanol: May increase CNS depression; monitor for increased effects with coadministration. Caution patients about effects.
Herb/Nutraceutical: St John's wort may decrease codeine levels. Avoid valerian, St John's wort, kava kava, gotu kola (may increase CNS depression). Avoid cat's claw, dong quai, evening primrose, feverfew, garlic, ginger, ginkgo, red clover, horse chestnut, green tea, ginseng (all have additional antiplatelet activity). Limit curry powder, paprika, licorice; may cause salicylate accumulation (these foods contain 6 mg salicylate/100 g; an ordinary American diet contains 10-200 mg/day of salicylate).

Pregnancy Risk Factor C

Pregnancy Considerations Animal reproduction studies have not been conducted with this combination. Refer to individual monographs.

Lactation Enters breast milk/not recommended

Breast-Feeding Considerations Carisoprodol, aspirin, and codeine are excreted into breast milk. Refer to individual monographs for additional information.

Controlled Substance C-III

Dosage Forms

Tablet: Carisoprodol 200 mg, aspirin 325 mg, and codeine 16 mg

Dental Comment There is no scientific evidence to warrant discontinuance of aspirin prior to dental surgery. Patients taking one aspirin tablet daily as an antithrombotic and who require dental surgery should be given special consideration in consultation with the physician before removal of the aspirin relative to prevention of postoperative bleeding.

Carmustine (kar MUS teen)

Brand Names: U.S. BiCNU®; Gliadel®

Brand Names: Canada BiCNU®; Gliadel Wafer®

Pharmacologic Category Antineoplastic Agent; Antineoplastic Agent, Alkylating Agent; Antineoplastic Agent, Alkylating Agent (Nitrosourea)

Use

Injection: Treatment of brain tumors (glioblastoma, brainstem glioma, medulloblastoma, astrocytoma, ependymoma, and metastatic brain tumors), multiple myeloma, Hodgkin's lymphoma (relapsed or refractory), non-Hodgkin's lymphomas (relapsed or refractory)

Wafer (implant): Adjunct to surgery in patients with recurrent glioblastoma multiforme; adjunct to surgery and radiation in patients with newly-diagnosed high-grade malignant glioma

Unlabeled Use Treatment of mycosis fungoides (topical)

Local Anesthetic/Vasoconstrictor Precautions No information available to require special precautions

Effects on Dental Treatment Key adverse event(s) related to dental treatment: Stomatitis.

Effects on Bleeding Bone marrow suppression, notably thrombocytopenia, may contribute to bleeding. A medical consult is suggested.

Adverse Effects

I.V.: Frequency not defined:

Cardiovascular: Arrhythmia (with high doses), chest pain, flushing (with rapid infusion), hypotension, tachycardia

Central nervous system: Ataxia, dizziness

Central nervous system: Ethanol intoxication (with high doses), headache

Dermatologic: Hyperpigmentation/skin burning (after skin contact)

Gastrointestinal: Nausea (common; dose related), vomiting (common; dose related), mucositis (with high doses), toxic enterocolitis (with high doses)

Hematologic: Leukopenia (common; onset: 5-6 weeks; recovery: after 1-2 weeks), thrombocytopenia (common: onset: ~4 weeks; recovery: after 1-2 weeks), anemia, neutropenic fever, secondary malignancies (acute leukemia, bone marrow dysplasias)

Hepatic: Alkaline phosphatase increased, bilirubin increased, hepatic sinusoidal obstruction syndrome (SOS; veno-occlusive disease; with high doses), transaminases increased

Local: Injection site reactions (burning, erythema, necrosis, pain, swelling)

Ocular: Conjunctival suffusion (with rapid infusion), neuroretinitis

Renal: Kidney size decreased, progressive azotemia, renal failure

Respiratory: Interstitial pneumonitis (with high doses), pulmonary fibrosis, pulmonary hypoplasia, pulmonary infiltrates

Miscellaneous: Allergic reaction, infection (with high doses)

Wafer: ≥4% (percentages reported only where incidence was greater compared to placebo):

Cardiovascular: Deep thrombophlebitis (10%), facial edema (6%), chest pain (5%)

Central nervous system: Brain edema (4% to 23%), confusion (10% to 23%), depression (16%), headache (15%), somnolence (14%), fever (12%), speech disorder (11%), intracranial hypertension (9%), anxiety (7%), facial paralysis (7%), pain (7%), ataxia (6%), hypesthesia (6%), hallucination (5%), seizure (grand mal 5%), meningitis (4%)

Dermatologic: Abnormal wound healing (14% to 16%), rash (5% to 12%)

Endocrine: Diabetes (5%)

Gastrointestinal: Nausea (8% to 22%), vomiting (8% to 21%), constipation (19%), abdominal pain (8%), diarrhea (5%)

Genitourinary: Urinary tract infection (21%)

Hematologic: Hemorrhage (7%)

Local: Abscess (4% to 8%)

Neuromuscular & skeletal: Weakness (22%), back pain (7%)

General Dosage Range Dosage adjustment recommended in patients with renal impairment or who develop toxicity.

I.V.: *Adults:* 150-200 mg/m^2 every 6-8 weeks **or** 75-100 mg/m^2/day for 2 days every 6-8 weeks

Implantation: *Adults:* 8 wafers placed in the resection cavity (total dose: 61.6 mg)

Mechanism of Action Interferes with the normal function of DNA and RNA by alkylation and cross-linking the strands of DNA and RNA, and by possible protein modification; may also inhibit enzyme processes by carbamylation of amino acids in protein

Pharmacodynamics/Kinetics

Half-life Elimination Biphasic: Initial: 1.4 minutes; Secondary: 20 minutes (active metabolites: plasma half-life of 67 hours)

Pregnancy Risk Factor D

Pregnancy Considerations Teratogenicity and embryotoxicity have been demonstrated in animal studies. Carmustine can cause fetal harm if administered to a pregnant woman. There are no adequate and well-controlled studies in pregnant women. Women of childbearing potential should avoid becoming pregnant while on treatment.

Carteolol (Ophthalmic) (KAR tee oh lole)

Pharmacologic Category Ophthalmic Agent, Anti-glaucoma

Use Treatment of chronic open-angle glaucoma and intraocular hypertension

Local Anesthetic/Vasoconstrictor Precautions No information available to require special precautions

Effects on Dental Treatment No significant effects or complications reported

Effects on Bleeding No information available to require special precautions

Adverse Effects

>10%: Ocular: Conjunctival hyperemia

1% to 10%: Ocular: Anisocoria, corneal punctate keratitis, corneal sensitivity decreased, corneal staining, eye pain, vision disturbances

General Dosage Range Ophthalmic: *Adults:* Instill 1 drop in affected eye(s) twice daily

Mechanism of Action Blocks both beta$_1$- and beta$_2$-receptors and has mild intrinsic sympathomimetic activity; reduces intraocular pressure by decreasing aqueous humor production

Pregnancy Risk Factor C

Pregnancy Considerations Adverse events were observed in some animal studies at maternally toxic doses.

Carvedilol (KAR ve dil ole)

Related Information

Cardiovascular Diseases *on page 1492*

Brand Names: U.S. Coreg CR®; Coreg®

Brand Names: Canada Apo-Carvedilol®; Ava-Carvedilol; Dom-Carvedilol; JAMP-Carvedilol; Mylan-Carvedilol; Novo-Carvedilol; PMS-Carvedilol; RAN™-Carvedilol; ratio-Carvedilol; ZYM-Carvedilol

Generic Availability (U.S.) Yes: Tablet

Pharmacologic Category Beta-Blocker With Alpha-Blocking Activity

Use Mild-to-severe heart failure of ischemic or cardiomyopathic origin (usually in addition to standard therapy); left ventricular dysfunction following myocardial infarction (MI) (clinically stable with LVEF ≤40%); management of hypertension

Unlabeled Use Angina pectoris

Local Anesthetic/Vasoconstrictor Precautions No information available to require special precautions

Effects on Dental Treatment Key adverse event(s) related to dental treatment: Postural hypotension. Periodontitis has been reported in product labeling for carvedilol; no other reports have confirmed this effect; any possible mechanism for this effect is unknown. Many nonsteroidal anti-inflammatory drugs, such as ibuprofen and indomethacin, can reduce the hypotensive effect of beta-blockers after 3 or more weeks of therapy with the NSAID. Short-term NSAID use (ie, 3 days) requires no special precautions in patients taking beta-blockers.

Effects on Bleeding No information available to require special precautions

Adverse Effects Note: Frequency ranges include data from hypertension and heart failure trials. Higher rates of adverse reactions have generally been noted in patients with heart failure. However, the frequency of adverse effects associated with placebo is also increased in this population.

>10%:

Cardiovascular: Hypotension (9% to 20%)

Central nervous system: Dizziness (2% to 32%), fatigue (4% to 24%)

Endocrine & metabolic: Hyperglycemia (5% to 12%)

Gastrointestinal: Diarrhea (1% to 12%), weight gain (10% to 12%)

Neuromuscular & skeletal: Weakness (7% to 11%)

1% to 10%:

Cardiovascular: Bradycardia (2% to 10%), syncope (3% to 8%), peripheral edema (1% to 7%), generalized edema (5% to 6%), angina (1% to 6%), dependent edema (≤4%), AV block, cerebrovascular accident, hypertension, hyper-/hypovolemia, orthostatic hypotension, palpitation

Central nervous system: Headache (5% to 8%), depression, fever, hypoesthesia, hypotonia, insomnia, malaise, somnolence, vertigo

Endocrine & metabolic: Hypercholesterolemia (1% to 4%), hypertriglyceridemia (1%), diabetes mellitus, gout, hyperkalemia, hyperuricemia, hypoglycemia, hyponatremia

Gastrointestinal: Nausea (2% to 9%), vomiting (1% to 6%), abdominal pain, melena, periodontitis, weight loss

Genitourinary: Impotence

Hematologic: Anemia, prothrombin decreased, purpura, thrombocytopenia

Hepatic: Alkaline phosphatase increased (1% to 3%), GGT increased, transaminases increased

Neuromuscular & skeletal: Back pain (2% to 7%), arthralgia (1% to 6%), arthritis, muscle cramps, paresthesia

Ocular: Blurred vision (1% to 5%)

Renal: BUN increased (≤6%), nonprotein nitrogen increased (6%), albuminuria, creatinine increased, glycosuria, hematuria, renal insufficiency

Respiratory: Cough (5% to 8%), nasopharyngitis (4%), rales (4%), dyspnea (>3%), pulmonary edema (>3%), rhinitis (2%), nasal congestion (1%), sinus congestion (1%)

Miscellaneous: Injury (3% to 6%), allergy, flu-like syndrome, sudden death

Dosage Oral: Adults: Reduce dosage if heart rate drops to <55 beats/minute.

Hypertension:

Immediate release: 6.25 mg twice daily; if tolerated, dose should be maintained for 1-2 weeks, then increased to 12.5 mg twice daily. If necessary, dosage may be increased to a maximum of 25 mg twice daily after 1-2 weeks.

Extended release: Initial: 20 mg once daily, if tolerated, dose should be maintained for 1-2 weeks if necessary; increased to 40 mg once daily if necessary; maximum dose: 80 mg once daily

Heart failure:

Immediate release: 3.125 mg twice daily for 2 weeks; if this dose is tolerated, may increase to 6.25 mg twice daily. Double the dose every 2 weeks to the highest dose tolerated by patient. (Prior to initiating therapy, other heart failure medications should be stabilized and fluid retention minimized.)

Maximum recommended dose:

Mild-to-moderate heart failure:

<85 kg: 25 mg twice daily

>85 kg: 50 mg twice daily

Severe heart failure: 25 mg twice daily

Extended release: Initial: 10 mg once daily for 2 weeks; if the dose is tolerated, increase dose to 20 mg, 40 mg, and 80 mg over successive intervals of at least 2 weeks. Maintain on lower dose if higher dose is not tolerated.

Left ventricular dysfunction following MI: **Note:** Should be initiated only after patient is hemodynamically stable and fluid retention has been minimized.

Immediate release: Initial 3.125-6.25 mg twice daily; increase dosage incrementally (ie, from 6.25-12.5 mg twice daily) at intervals of 3-10 days, based on tolerance, to a target dose of 25 mg twice daily.

Extended release: Initial: 10-20 mg once daily; increase dosage incrementally at intervals of 3-10 days, based on tolerance, to a target dose of 80 mg once daily.

Angina pectoris (unlabeled use): Immediate release: 25-50 mg twice daily

Elderly: Hypertension: Consider lower initial dose and titrate to response (Aronow, 2011)

Conversion from immediate release to extended release (Coreg CR®):
Current dose immediate release tablets 3.125 mg twice daily: Convert to extended release capsules 10 mg once daily
Current dose immediate release tablets 6.25 mg twice daily: Convert to extended release capsules 20 mg once daily
Current dose immediate release tablets 12.5 mg twice daily: Convert to extended release capsules 40 mg once daily
Current dose immediate release tablets 25 mg twice daily: Convert to extended release capsules 80 mg once daily

Dosing adjustment in renal impairment: None necessary

Dosing adjustment in hepatic impairment: Use is contraindicated in severe liver dysfunction.

Mechanism of Action As a racemic mixture, carvedilol has nonselective beta-adrenoreceptor and alpha-adrenergic blocking activity. No intrinsic sympathomimetic activity has been documented. Associated effects in hypertensive patients include reduction of cardiac output, exercise- or beta-agonist-induced tachycardia, reduction of reflex orthostatic tachycardia, vasodilation, decreased peripheral vascular resistance (especially in standing position), decreased renal vascular resistance, reduced plasma renin activity, and increased levels of atrial natriuretic peptide. In CHF, associated effects include decreased pulmonary capillary wedge pressure, decreased pulmonary artery pressure, decreased heart rate, decreased systemic vascular resistance, increased stroke volume index, and decreased right arterial pressure (RAP).

Contraindications Serious hypersensitivity to carvedilol or any component of the formulation; decompensated cardiac failure requiring intravenous inotropic therapy; bronchial asthma or related bronchospastic conditions; second- or third-degree AV block, sick sinus syndrome, and severe bradycardia (except in patients with a functioning artificial pacemaker); cardiogenic shock; severe hepatic impairment

Warnings/Precautions Consider pre-existing conditions such as sick sinus syndrome before initiating. Heart failure patients may experience a worsening of renal function (rare); risk factors include ischemic heart disease, diffuse vascular disease, underlying renal dysfunction, and systolic BP <100 mm Hg. Initiate cautiously and monitor for possible deterioration in patient status (eg, symptoms of HF). Worsening heart failure or fluid retention may occur during upward titration; dose reduction or temporary discontinuation may be necessary. Adjustment of other medications (ACE inhibitors and/or diuretics) may also be required. Bradycardia may be observed more frequently in elderly patients (>65 years of age); dosage reductions may be necessary.

Symptomatic hypotension with or without syncope may occur with carvedilol (usually within the first 30 days of therapy); close monitoring of patient is required especially with initial dosing and dosing increases; blood pressure must be lowered at a rate appropriate for the patient's clinical condition. Initiation with a low dose, gradual up-titration, and administration with food may help to decrease the occurrence of hypotension or syncope. Patients should be advised to avoid driving or other hazardous tasks during initiation of therapy due to the risk of syncope. Beta-blocker therapy should not be withdrawn abruptly (particularly in patients with CAD), but gradually tapered to avoid acute tachycardia, hypertension, and/or ischemia. Chronic beta-blocker therapy should not be routinely withdrawn prior to major surgery.

In general, patients with bronchospastic disease should not receive beta-blockers; if used at all, should be used cautiously with close monitoring. May precipitate or aggravate symptoms of arterial insufficiency in patients with PVD and Raynaud's disease; use with caution and monitor for progression of arterial obstruction. Use caution with concurrent use of digoxin, verapamil or diltiazem; bradycardia or heart block can occur. Use with caution in patients receiving inhaled anesthetic agents known to depress myocardial contractility. Use cautiously in patients with diabetes because it can mask prominent hypoglycemic symptoms. In patients with heart failure and diabetes, use of carvedilol may worsen hyperglycemia; may require adjustment of antidiabetic agents. May mask signs of hyperthyroidism (eg, tachycardia); if hyperthyroidism is suspected, carefully manage and monitor; abrupt withdrawal may exacerbate symptoms of hyperthyroidism or precipitate thyroid storm. May induce or exacerbate psoriasis. Use with caution in patients with myasthenia gravis or psychiatric disease (may cause CNS depression). Use with caution in patients with mild-to-moderate hepatic impairment; use is contraindicated in patients with severe impairment. Manufacturer recommends discontinuation of therapy if liver injury occurs (confirmed by laboratory testing). Adequate alpha-blockade is required prior to use of any beta-blocker for patients with untreated pheochromocytoma. Use caution with history of severe anaphylaxis to allergens; patients taking beta-blockers may become more sensitive to repeated challenges. Treatment of anaphylaxis (eg, epinephrine) in patients taking beta-blockers may be ineffective or promote undesirable effects.

Intraoperative floppy iris syndrome has been observed in cataract surgery patients who were on or were previously treated with alpha$_1$-blockers; causality has not been established and there appears to be no benefit in discontinuing alpha-blocker therapy prior to surgery. Instruct patients to inform ophthalmologist of carvedilol use when considering eye surgery.

Drug Interactions

Metabolism/Transport Effects Substrate of CYP1A2 (minor), CYP2C9 (minor), CYP2D6 (major), CYP2E1 (minor), CYP3A4 (minor), P-glycoprotein; **Note:** Assignment of Major/Minor substrate status based on clinically relevant drug interaction potential; **Inhibits** P-glycoprotein

Avoid Concomitant Use

Avoid concomitant use of Carvedilol with any of the following: Beta2-Agonists; Bosutinib; Floctafenine; Methacholine; Pomalidomide; Topotecan; VinCRIStine (Liposomal)

Increased Effect/Toxicity

Carvedilol may increase the levels/effects of: Alpha-/Beta-Agonists (Direct-Acting); Alpha1-Blockers; Alpha2-Agonists; Amifostine; Antihypertensives; Antipsychotic Agents (Phenothiazines); Bosutinib; Bupivacaine; Cardiac Glycosides; Cholinergic Agonists; Colchicine; CycloSPORINE (Systemic); Dabigatran Etexilate; Digoxin; Ergot Derivatives; Everolimus; Fingolimod; Hypotensive Agents; Insulin; Lidocaine (Systemic); Lidocaine (Topical); Mepivacaine; Methacholine; Midodrine; P-glycoprotein/ABCB1 Substrates; Pomalidomide; Prucalopride; RiTUXimab; Rivaroxaban; Sulfonylureas; Topotecan; VinCRIStine (Liposomal)

The levels/effects of Carvedilol may be increased by: Abiraterone Acetate; Acetylcholinesterase Inhibitors; Alpha2-Agonists; Aminoquinolines (Antimalarial); Amiodarone; Anilidopiperidine Opioids; Antipsychotic Agents (Phenothiazines); Calcium Channel Blockers (Dihydropyridine); Calcium Channel Blockers (Nondihydropyridine); Cimetidine; CYP2C9 Inhibitors (Moderate); CYP2C9 Inhibitors (Strong); CYP2D6 Inhibitors (Moderate); CYP2D6 Inhibitors (Strong); Darunavir; Diazoxide; Digoxin; Dipyridamole; Disopyramide; Dronedarone; Floctafenine; Herbs (Hypotensive Properties); MAO Inhibitors; Pentoxifylline; P-glycoprotein/ABCB1 Inhibitors; Phosphodiesterase 5 Inhibitors; Propafenone; Prostacyclin Analogues; QuiNIDine; Reserpine; Selective Serotonin Reuptake Inhibitors

Decreased Effect

Carvedilol may decrease the levels/effects of: Beta2-Agonists; Theophylline Derivatives

The levels/effects of Carvedilol may be decreased by: Barbiturates; Herbs (Hypertensive Properties); Methylphenidate; Nonsteroidal Anti-Inflammatory Agents; Peginterferon Alfa-2b; P-glycoprotein/ABCB1 Inducers; Rifamycin Derivatives; Yohimbine

Ethanol/Nutrition/Herb Interactions

Food: Food decreases rate but not extent of absorption. Administration with food minimizes risks of orthostatic hypotension.

Herb/Nutraceutical: Avoid herbs with hypertensive properties (bayberry, blue cohosh, cayenne, ephedra, ginger, ginseng [American], kola, licorice); may diminish the antihypertensive effect of carvedilol. Avoid herbs with hypotensive properties (black cohosh, California poppy, coleus, golden seal, hawthorn, mistletoe, periwinkle, quinine, shepherd's purse); may enhance the hypotensive effect of carvedilol.

Dietary Considerations

Should be taken with food to minimize the risk of orthostatic hypotension.

Pharmacodynamics/Kinetics

Onset of Action 1-2 hours; Peak antihypertensive effect: ~1-2 hours

Half-life Elimination 7-10 hours

Time to Peak Extended release: 5 hours

Pregnancy Risk Factor C

Pregnancy Considerations

Because adverse events were not observed in animal reproduction studies, carvedilol is classified as pregnancy category C. In a cohort study, an increased risk of cardiovascular defects was observed following maternal use of beta-blockers during pregnancy. Intrauterine growth restriction (IUGR), small placentas, as well as fetal/neonatal bradycardia, hypoglycemia, and/or respiratory depression have been observed following *in utero* exposure to beta-blockers as a class. Adequate facilities for monitoring infants at birth should be available. Untreated chronic maternal hypertension and pre-eclampsia are also associated with adverse events in the fetus, infant, and mother. Carvedilol is not currently recommended for the initial treatment of maternal hypertension during pregnancy.

Lactation Excretion in breast milk unknown/not recommended

Breast-Feeding Considerations It is not known if carvedilol is excreted into human milk. The manufacturer suggests that a decision should be made to either discontinue nursing or discontinue the medication.

Dosage Forms

Capsule, extended release, oral:
Coreg CR®: 10 mg, 20 mg, 40 mg, 80 mg

Tablet, oral: 3.125 mg, 6.25 mg, 12.5 mg, 25 mg
Coreg®: 3.125 mg, 6.25 mg, 12.5 mg, 25 mg

References

Foster CA and Aston SJ, "Propranolol-Epinephrine Interaction: A Potential Disaster," *Plast Reconstr Surg*, 1983, 72(1):74-8.

Wong DG, Spence JD, Lamki L, et al, "Effect of Nonsteroidal Anti-inflammatory Drugs on Control of Hypertension of Beta-Blockers and Diuretics," *Lancet*, 1986, 1(8488):997-1001.

Wynn RL, "Epinephrine Interactions With Beta-Blockers," *Gen Dent*, 1994, 42(1):16, 18.

Caspofungin (kas poe FUN jin)

Related Information

Fungal Infections *on page 1573*

Brand Names: U.S. Cancidas®

Brand Names: Canada Cancidas®

Pharmacologic Category Antifungal Agent, Parenteral; Echinocandin

Use Treatment of invasive *Aspergillus* infections in patients who are refractory or intolerant of other therapies; treatment of candidemia and other *Candida* infections (intra-abdominal abscesses, peritonitis, pleural space); treatment of esophageal candidiasis; empirical treatment for presumed fungal infections in febrile neutropenic patients

Unlabeled Use Alternate agent in the prophylaxis against *Candida* infection in neutropenic cancer patients with substantial risk (eg, allogeneic transplant or undergoing induction therapy for acute leukemia)

Local Anesthetic/Vasoconstrictor Precautions No information available to require special precautions

Effects on Dental Treatment No significant effects or complications reported

Effects on Bleeding No information available to require special precautions

Adverse Effects

>10%:

Cardiovascular: Hypotension (3% to 20%), peripheral edema (6% to 11%), tachycardia (4% to 11%)

Central nervous system: Fever (6% to 30%), chills (9% to 23%), headache (5% to 15%)

Dermatologic: Rash (4% to 23%)

Endocrine & metabolic: Hypokalemia (5% to 23%)

Gastrointestinal: Diarrhea (6% to 27%), vomiting (6% to 17%), nausea (4% to 15%)

Hematologic: Hemoglobin decreased (18% to 21%), hematocrit decreased (13% to 18%), WBC decreased (12%), anemia (2% to 11%)

Hepatic: Serum alkaline phosphatase increased (9% to 22%), transaminases increased (2% to 18%), bilirubin increased (5% to 13%)

Local: Phlebitis/thrombophlebitis (18%)

Renal: Serum creatinine increased (3% to 11%)

Respiratory: Respiratory failure (2% to 20%), cough (6% to 11%), pneumonia (4% to 11%)

Miscellaneous: Infusion reactions (20% to 35%), septic shock (11% to 14%)

5% to 10%:
  Cardiovascular: Hypertension (5% to 6%; children 9% to 10%)
  Dermatologic: Erythema (4% to 9%), pruritus (6% to 7%)
  Endocrine & metabolic: Hypomagnesemia (7%), hyperglycemia (6%)
  Gastrointestinal: Mucosal inflammation (4% to 10%), abdominal pain (4% to 9%)
  Hepatic: Albumin decreased (7%)
  Local: Infection (1% to 9%, central line)
  Renal: Hematuria (10%), blood urea nitrogen increased (4% to 9%)
  Respiratory: Dyspnea (9%), pleural effusion (9%), respiratory distress (≤8%), rales (7%)
  Miscellaneous: Sepsis (5% to 7%)

General Dosage Range Dosage adjustment recommended in patients with hepatic impairment or on concomitant therapy
I.V.:
  Infants ≥3 months, Children, and Adolescents ≤17 years: 70 mg/m² on day 1, subsequent dosing: 50-70 mg/m² once daily (maximum dose loading or maintenance: 70 mg daily)
  Adults: Initial: 50-70 mg on day 1; subsequent dose: 50-70 mg once daily
Mechanism of Action Inhibits synthesis of β(1,3)-D-glucan, an essential component of the cell wall of susceptible fungi. Highest activity is in regions of active cell growth. Mammalian cells do not require β(1,3)-D-glucan, limiting potential toxicity.
Pharmacodynamics/Kinetics
  Half-life Elimination Beta (distribution): 9-11 hours; Terminal: 40-50 hours
Pregnancy Risk Factor C
Pregnancy Considerations Adverse events have been observed in animal reproduction studies. Caspofungin should be used during pregnancy only if potential benefit justifies the potential risk to the fetus.

Castor Oil (KAS tor oyl)

Pharmacologic Category Laxative, Miscellaneous
Use Preparation for rectal or bowel examination or surgery; rarely used to relieve constipation; also applied to skin as emollient and protectant
Local Anesthetic/Vasoconstrictor Precautions No information available to require special precautions
Effects on Dental Treatment No significant effects or complications reported
Effects on Bleeding No information available to require special precautions
Adverse Effects Frequency not defined.
  Cardiovascular: Hypotension
  Central nervous system: Dizziness
  Endocrine & metabolic: Electrolyte disturbance
  Gastrointestinal: Abdominal cramps, diarrhea, nausea
  Genitourinary: Pelvic congestion
General Dosage Range Oral:
  Children 2-11 years: 5-15 mL as a single dose
  Children ≥12 years and Adults: 15-60 mL as a single dose
Mechanism of Action Acts primarily in the small intestine; hydrolyzed to ricinoleic acid which reduces net absorption of fluid and electrolytes and stimulates peristalsis
Pharmacodynamics/Kinetics
  Onset of Action 2-6 hours

Pregnancy Considerations Ingestion of castor oil may be associated with induction of labor. Use of castor oil as a laxative during pregnancy should be avoided (Cullen, 2007; Hall, 2011; Wald, 2003).

Cefaclor (SEF a klor)

Related Information
  Bacterial Infections *on page 1562*
Brand Names: Canada Apo-Cefaclor®; Ceclor®; Novo-Cefaclor; Nu-Cefaclor; PMS-Cefaclor
Generic Availability (U.S.) Yes
Pharmacologic Category Antibiotic, Cephalosporin (Second Generation)
Dental Use Alternative antibiotic for treatment of orofacial infections in patients allergic to penicillins; susceptible bacteria including aerobic gram-positive bacteria and anaerobes
Use Treatment of susceptible bacterial infections including otitis media, lower respiratory tract infections, acute exacerbations of chronic bronchitis, pharyngitis and tonsillitis, urinary tract infections, skin and skin structure infections
Local Anesthetic/Vasoconstrictor Precautions No information available to require special precautions
Effects on Dental Treatment No significant effects or complications reported (see Dental Comment)
Effects on Bleeding No information available to require special precautions
Adverse Effects
1% to 10%:
  Dermatologic: Rash (maculopapular, erythematous, or morbilliform) (1% to 2%)
  Gastrointestinal: Diarrhea (3%)
  Genitourinary: Vaginitis (2%)
  Hematologic: Eosinophilia (2%)
  Hepatic: Transaminases increased (3%)
  Miscellaneous: Moniliasis (2%)
  Reactions reported with other cephalosporins: Fever, abdominal pain, superinfection, renal dysfunction, toxic nephropathy, hemorrhage, cholestasis
Dental Usual Dosage Orofacial infections: Adults: Oral: Dosing range: 250-500 mg every 8 hours
Dosage
  Usual dosage range:
    Children >1 month: Oral: 20-40 mg/kg/day divided every 8-12 hours (maximum dose: 1 g/day)
    Adults: Oral: 250-500 mg every 8 hours
  Indication-specific dosing:
    Children: Oral:
      Otitis media: 40 mg/kg/day divided every 12 hours
      Pharyngitis: 20 mg/kg/day divided every 12 hours
  Dosage adjustment in renal impairment:
    Cl$_{cr}$ 10-50 mL/minute: Administer 50% to 100% of dose
    Cl$_{cr}$ <10 mL/minute: Administer 50% of dose
    Hemodialysis: Moderately dialyzable (20% to 50%)
  Dosage adjustment in hepatic impairment: No dosage adjustment provided in manufacturer's labeling.
Mechanism of Action Inhibits bacterial cell wall synthesis by binding to one or more of the penicillin-binding proteins (PBPs) which in turn inhibits the final transpeptidation step of peptidoglycan synthesis in bacterial cell walls, thus inhibiting cell wall biosynthesis. Bacteria eventually lyse due to ongoing activity of cell wall autolytic enzymes (autolysins and murein hydrolases) while cell wall assembly is arrested.
Contraindications Hypersensitivity to cefaclor, any component of the formulation, or other cephalosporins

Warnings/Precautions Modify dosage in patients with severe renal impairment. Prolonged use may result in fungal or bacterial superinfection, including *C. difficile*-associated diarrhea (CDAD) and pseudomembranous colitis; CDAD has been observed >2 months postantibiotic treatment. Use with caution in patients with a history of penicillin allergy, especially IgE-mediated reactions (eg, anaphylaxis, urticaria). Beta-lactamase-negative, ampicillin-resistant (BLNAR) strains of *H. influenzae* should be considered resistant to cefaclor. Extended release tablets are not approved for use in children <16 years of age.

Drug Interactions

Metabolism/Transport Effects None known.

Avoid Concomitant Use

Avoid concomitant use of Cefaclor with any of the following: BCG

Increased Effect/Toxicity

Cefaclor may increase the levels/effects of: Aminoglycosides; Vitamin K Antagonists

The levels/effects of Cefaclor may be increased by: Probenecid

Decreased Effect

Cefaclor may decrease the levels/effects of: BCG; Sodium Picosulfate; Typhoid Vaccine

Ethanol/Nutrition/Herb Interactions Food: Cefaclor serum levels may be decreased slightly if taken with food. The bioavailability of cefaclor extended release tablets is decreased 23% and the maximum concentration is decreased 67% when taken on an empty stomach.

Dietary Considerations Capsule and suspension may be taken with or without food.

Pharmacodynamics/Kinetics

Half-life Elimination 0.5-1 hour; prolonged with renal impairment

Time to Peak Capsule: 60 minutes; Suspension: 45 minutes

Pregnancy Risk Factor B

Pregnancy Considerations Adverse events were not observed in animal reproduction studies. An increased risk of teratogenic effects has not been observed following maternal use of cefaclor.

Lactation Enters breast milk/use caution

Breast-Feeding Considerations Small amounts of cefaclor are excreted in breast milk. The manufacturer recommends that caution be exercised when administering cefaclor to nursing women. Nondose-related effects could include modification of bowel flora.

Dosage Forms

Capsule, oral: 250 mg, 500 mg

Powder for suspension, oral: 125 mg/5 mL (150 mL); 250 mg/5 mL (150 mL); 375 mg/5 mL (100 mL)

Tablet, extended release, oral: 500 mg

Dental Comment Patients allergic to penicillins can use a cephalosporin; the incidence of cross-reactivity between penicillins and cephalosporins is 1% when the allergic reaction to penicillin is delayed. Cefaclor is effective against anaerobic bacteria, but the sensitivity of alpha-hemolytic *Streptococcus* varies; approximately 10% of strains are resistant. Nearly 70% are intermediately sensitive. If the patient has a history of immediate reaction to penicillin, the incidence of cross-reactivity is 20%; cephalosporins are contraindicated in these patients.

Cefadroxil (sef a DROKS il)

Related Information

Bacterial Infections *on page 1562*

Brand Names: Canada Apo-Cefadroxil®; PRO-Cefadroxil; Teva-Cefadroxil

Generic Availability (U.S.) Yes

Pharmacologic Category Antibiotic, Cephalosporin (First Generation)

Dental Use Alternative antibiotic for treatment of orofacial infections in patients allergic to penicillins; susceptible bacteria including aerobic gram-positive bacteria and anaerobes

Use Treatment of susceptible bacterial infections, including those caused by group A beta-hemolytic *Streptococcus*

Unlabeled Use Chronic oral antimicrobial suppression of prosthetic joint infection with *Staphylococci* (oxacillin-susceptible)

Local Anesthetic/Vasoconstrictor Precautions No information available to require special precautions

Effects on Dental Treatment No significant effects or complications reported

Effects on Bleeding No information available to require special precautions

Adverse Effects

1% to 10%: Gastrointestinal: Diarrhea

Reactions reported with other cephalosporins: Toxic epidermal necrolysis, abdominal pain, superinfection, renal dysfunction, toxic nephropathy, aplastic anemia, hemolytic anemia, hemorrhage, prothrombin time prolonged, BUN increased, creatinine increased, eosinophilia, pancytopenia, seizure

Dental Usual Dosage Orofacial infections: Oral: Adults: Dosage range: 250-500 mg every 8 hours

Dosage

Usual dosage range: Oral:

Children: 30 mg/kg/day divided twice daily up to a maximum of 2000 mg daily

Adults: 1000-2000 mg daily in 2 divided doses

Indication-specific dosing: Oral:

Pharyngitis, group A streptococci (IDSA guidelines): Children and Adults: 30 mg/kg once daily (maximum: 1000 mg daily) for 10 days (Shulman, 2012). **Note:** Recommended as an alternative agent in penicillin-allergic patients; however, avoid in patients with immediate type hypersensitivity to penicillin.

Orofacial infections: Adults: 250-500 mg every 8 hours

Prosthetic joint infection, chronic oral antimicrobial suppression, staphylococci (oxacillin-susceptible) (preferred) (unlabeled use): Adults: 500 mg every 12 hours (Osmon, 2013)

Dosage adjustment in renal impairment:

Cl_{cr} 10-25 mL/minute: Administer every 24 hours

Cl_{cr} <10 mL/minute: Administer every 36 hours

Dosage adjustment in hepatic impairment: No dosage adjustment provided in manufacturer's labeling.

Mechanism of Action Inhibits bacterial cell wall synthesis by binding to one or more of the penicillin-binding proteins (PBPs) which in turn inhibits the final transpeptidation step of peptidoglycan synthesis in bacterial cell walls, thus inhibiting cell wall biosynthesis. Bacteria eventually lyse due to ongoing activity of cell wall autolytic enzymes (autolysins and murein hydrolases) while cell wall assembly is arrested.

Contraindications Hypersensitivity to cefadroxil, any component of the formulation, or other cephalosporins

◀ **Warnings/Precautions** Modify dosage in patients with severe renal impairment. Use with caution in patients with a history of penicillin allergy, especially IgE-mediated reactions (eg, anaphylaxis, angioedema, urticaria). Prolonged use may result in fungal or bacterial superinfection, including *C. difficile*-associated diarrhea (CDAD) and pseudomembranous colitis; CDAD has been observed >2 months postantibiotic treatment.

Drug Interactions

Metabolism/Transport Effects None known.

Avoid Concomitant Use

Avoid concomitant use of Cefadroxil with any of the following: BCG

Increased Effect/Toxicity

Cefadroxil may increase the levels/effects of: Vitamin K Antagonists

The levels/effects of Cefadroxil may be increased by: Probenecid

Decreased Effect

Cefadroxil may decrease the levels/effects of: BCG; Sodium Picosulfate; Typhoid Vaccine

Ethanol/Nutrition/Herb Interactions Food: Concomitant administration with food, infant formula, or cow's milk does **not** significantly affect absorption.

Pharmacodynamics/Kinetics

Half-life Elimination 1-2 hours; Renal failure: 20-24 hours

Time to Peak Serum: 70-90 minutes

Pregnancy Risk Factor B

Pregnancy Considerations Adverse events were not observed in animal reproduction studies. Cefadroxil crosses the placenta. Limited data is available concerning the use of cefadroxil in pregnancy; however, adverse fetal effects were not noted in a small clinical trial.

Lactation Enters breast milk/use caution (AAP rates "compatible"; AAP 2001 update pending)

Breast-Feeding Considerations Very small amounts of cefadroxil are excreted in breast milk. The manufacturer recommends that caution be exercised when administering cefadroxil to nursing women. Nondose-related effects could include modification of bowel flora.

Dosage Forms

Capsule, oral: 500 mg

Powder for suspension, oral: 250 mg/5 mL (50 mL, 100 mL); 500 mg/5 mL (75 mL, 100 mL)

Tablet, oral: 1 g

References

American Dental Association Council on Scientific Affairs, "Combating Antibiotic Resistance," *J Am Dent Assoc*, 2004, 135(4):484-7.

Donowitz GR and Mandell GL, "Drug Therapy. Beta-Lactam Antibiotics (1)," *N Engl J Med*, 1988, 318(7):419-26.

Donowitz GR and Mandell GL, "Drug Therapy. Beta-Lactam Antibiotics (2)," *N Engl J Med*, 1988, 318(8):490-500.

Gustaferro CA and Steckelberg JM, "Cephalosporin Antimicrobial Agents and Related Compounds," *Mayo Clin Proc*, 1991, 66 (10):1064-73.

Wilson W, Taubert KA, Gewitz M, et al, "Prevention of Infective Endocarditis. Guidelines From the American Heart Association. A Guideline From the American Heart Association Rheumatic Fever, Endocarditis, and Kawasaki Disease Committee, Council on Cardiovascular Disease in the Young, and the Council on Clinical Cardiology, Council on Cardiovascular Surgery and Anesthesia, and the Quality of Care and Outcomes Research Interdisciplinary Working Group," *Circulation*, 2007, 115. Available at http://circ.ahajournals.org/cgi/reprint/CIRCULATIONAHA.106.183095v1; last accessed July 26, 2007.

CeFAZolin (sef A zoe lin)

Related Information

Antibiotic Prophylaxis *on page 1542*

Brand Names: Canada Cefazolin For Injection; Cefazolin For Injection, USP

Generic Availability (U.S.) Yes

Pharmacologic Category Antibiotic, Cephalosporin (First Generation)

Dental Use Alternative antibiotic for prevention of infective endocarditis when parenteral administration is needed. Individuals allergic to amoxicillin (penicillins) may receive cefazolin provided they have not had an immediate, local, or systemic IgE-mediated anaphylactic allergic reaction to penicillin. Alternate antibiotic for premedication in patients not allergic to penicillin who may be at potential increased risk of hematogenous total joint infection when parenteral administration is needed.

Use Treatment of respiratory tract, skin, genital, urinary tract, biliary tract, bone and joint infections, and septicemia due to susceptible gram-positive cocci (except *Enterococcus*); some gram-negative bacilli including *E. coli*, *Proteus*, and *Klebsiella* may be susceptible; surgical prophylaxis

Unlabeled Use Prophylaxis against infective endocarditis

Local Anesthetic/Vasoconstrictor Precautions No information available to require special precautions

Effects on Dental Treatment No significant effects or complications reported

Effects on Bleeding May potentiate the anticoagulant effects of vitamin K anticoagulants (ie, warfarin) due to alterations of gut flora.

Adverse Effects Frequency not defined.

Central nervous system: Fever, seizure

Dermatologic: Rash, pruritus, Stevens-Johnson syndrome

Gastrointestinal: Diarrhea, nausea, vomiting, abdominal cramps, anorexia, pseudomembranous colitis, oral candidiasis

Genitourinary: Vaginitis

Hepatic: Transaminases increased, hepatitis

Hematologic: Eosinophilia, neutropenia, leukopenia, thrombocytopenia, thrombocytosis

Local: Pain at injection site, phlebitis

Renal: BUN increased, serum creatinine increased, renal failure

Miscellaneous: Anaphylaxis

Reactions reported with other cephalosporins: Toxic epidermal necrolysis, abdominal pain, cholestasis, superinfection, toxic nephropathy, aplastic anemia, hemolytic anemia, hemorrhage, prothrombin time prolonged, pancytopenia

Dental Usual Dosage

Infective endocarditis prophylaxis (unlabeled use): I.M., I.V.:

Infants and Children: 50 mg/kg 30-60 minutes before procedure; maximum dose: 1000 mg

Adults: 1000 mg 30-60 minutes before procedure.

Note: Intramuscular injections should be avoided in patients who are receiving anticoagulant therapy. In these circumstances, orally administered regimens should be given whenever possible. Intravenously administered antibiotics should be used for patients who are unable to tolerate or absorb oral medications.

Note: American Heart Association (AHA) guidelines now recommend prophylaxis only in patients undergoing invasive procedures and in whom underlying cardiac conditions may predispose to a higher risk of adverse outcomes should infection occur. As of April 2007, routine prophylaxis for GI/GU procedures is no longer recommended by the AHA.

Prophylaxis in total joint replacement patient: I.M., I.V.: Adults: 1000 mg 1 hour prior to the procedure

Dosage

Usual dosage range: I.M., I.V.:

Children >1 month: 25-100 mg/kg/day divided every 6-8 hours; maximum: 6 **g** daily

Adults: 250-1500 mg every 6-12 (usually 8) hours, depending on severity of infection; maximum dose: 12 **g** daily

Indication-specific dosing:

Infants and Children: I.M., I.V.:

Community-acquired pneumonia (CAP) (IDSA/ PIDS, 2011), moderate-to-severe infection, *S. aureus* (methicillin-susceptible) (preferred): Infants >3 months and Children: 150 mg/kg/day divided every 8 hours

Prophylaxis against infective endocarditis (unlabeled use): 50 mg/kg 30-60 minutes before procedure; maximum dose: 1000 mg. Intramuscular injections should be avoided in patients who are receiving anticoagulant therapy. In these circumstances, orally administered regimens should be given whenever possible. Intravenously administered antibiotics should be used for patients who are unable to tolerate or absorb oral medications.

Note: American Heart Association (AHA) guidelines now recommend prophylaxis only in patients undergoing invasive procedures and in whom underlying cardiac conditions may predispose to a higher risk of adverse outcomes should infection occur. As of April 2007, routine prophylaxis for GI/ GU procedures is no longer recommended by the AHA.

Adults: I.M., I.V.:

Cholecystitis, mild-to-moderate: I.V.: 1000-2000 mg every 8 hours for 4-7 days (provided source controlled)

Endocarditis due to MSSA (without prosthesis) (unlabeled use): I.V.: 2000 mg every 8 hours; **Note:** Recommended for penicillin-allergic (nonanaphylactoid) patients (Baddour, 2005)

Group B streptococcus (neonatal prophylaxis): I.V.: 2000 mg once, then 1000 mg every 8 hours until delivery (CDC, 2010)

Intra-abdominal infection, complicated, community-acquired, mild-to-moderate (in combination with metronidazole): I.V.: 1000-2000 mg every 8 hours for 4-7 days (provided source controlled)

Prophylaxis against infective endocarditis (unlabeled use): 1000 mg 30-60 minutes before procedure. Intramuscular injections should be avoided in patients who are receiving anticoagulant therapy. In these circumstances, orally administered regimens should be given whenever possible. Intravenously administered antibiotics should be used for patients who are unable to tolerate or absorb oral medications.

Note: American Heart Association (AHA) guidelines now recommend prophylaxis only in patients undergoing invasive procedures and in whom underlying cardiac conditions may predispose to a higher risk of adverse outcomes should infection occur. As of April 2007, routine prophylaxis for GI/ GU procedures is no longer recommended by the AHA.

Moderate-to-severe infections: 500-1000 mg every 6-8 hours

Mild infection with gram-positive cocci: 250-500 mg every 8 hours

Perioperative prophylaxis: 1000-2000 mg within 60 minutes prior to surgery (may repeat in 2-5 hours intraoperatively); followed by 500-1000 mg every 6-8 hours for 24 hours postoperatively

Cardiothoracic surgery: 1000 mg (see **"Note"**) within 60 minutes prior to incision, followed by 1000 mg at sternotomy and 1000 mg after cardiopulmonary bypass; may continue 1000 mg every 6 hours for 24-48 hours postoperatively (Eagle, 2004)

Note: For patients weighing >60 kg, the Society of Thoracic Surgeons recommends a preoperative dose of 2000 mg administered within 60 minutes of skin incision. If the surgical incision remains open in the operating room, follow with 1000 mg every 3-4 hours unless cardiopulmonary bypass is to be discontinued within 4 hours then delay administration (Engelman, 2007).

Cholecystectomy: 1000-2000 mg every 8 hours, discontinue within 24 hours unless infection outside gallbladder suspected

Total joint replacement: 1000 mg 1 hour prior to the procedure

Pneumococcal pneumonia: 500 mg every 12 hours

Prosthetic joint infection, *Staphylococci* (oxacillin-susceptible): 1000-2000 mg every 8 hours for 2-6 weeks (in combination with rifampin) followed by oral antibiotic treatment and suppressive regimens (Osmon, 2013)

Severe infection: 1000-1500 mg every 6 hours

UTI (uncomplicated): 1000 mg every 12 hours

Dosage adjustment in renal impairment:

Cl_{cr} 35-54 mL/minute: Administer full dose in intervals of ≥8 hours

Cl_{cr} 11-34 mL/minute: Administer 50% of usual dose every 12 hours

Cl_{cr} ≤10 mL/minute: Administer 50% of usual dose every 18-24 hours

Intermittent hemodialysis (IHD) (administer after hemodialysis on dialysis days): Dialyzable (20% to 50%): 500-1000 mg every 24 hours **or** use 1000-2000 mg every 48-72 hours (Heintz, 2009); **Note:** Dosing dependent on the assumption of 3 times weekly, complete IHD sessions. Alternatively, may administer 15-20 mg/kg (maximum dose: 2000 mg) after dialysis without regularly scheduled dosing (Ahern, 2003; Sowinski, 2001).

Peritoneal dialysis (PD): 500 mg every 12 hours

Continuous renal replacement therapy (CRRT) (Heintz, 2009; Trotman, 2005): Drug clearance is highly dependent on the method of renal replacement, filter type, and flow rate. Appropriate dosing requires close monitoring of pharmacologic response, signs of adverse reactions due to drug accumulation, as well as drug concentrations in relation to target trough (if appropriate). The following are general recommendations only (based on dialysate flow/ultrafiltration rates of 1-2 L/hour and minimal residual renal function) and should not supersede clinical judgment:

CVVH: Loading dose of 2000 mg followed by 1000-2000 mg every 12 hours

CVVHD/CVVHDF: Loading dose of 2000 mg followed by either 1000 mg every 8 hours **or** 2000 mg every 12 hours. **Note:** Dosage of 1000 mg every 8 hours results in similar steady-state concentrations as 2000 mg every 12 hours and is more cost effective (Heintz, 2009).

Dosage adjustment in hepatic impairment: No dosage adjustment provided in manufacturer's labeling.

Mechanism of Action Inhibits bacterial cell wall synthesis by binding to one or more of the penicillin-binding proteins (PBPs) which in turn inhibits the final transpeptidation step of peptidoglycan synthesis in bacterial cell walls, thus inhibiting cell wall biosynthesis. Bacteria eventually lyse due to ongoing activity of cell wall autolytic enzymes (autolysins and murein hydrolases) while cell wall assembly is arrested.

Contraindications Hypersensitivity to cefazolin sodium, any component of the formulation, or other cephalosporins

Warnings/Precautions Modify dosage in patients with severe renal impairment. Use with caution in patients with a history of penicillin allergy, especially IgE-mediated reactions (eg, anaphylaxis, angioedema, urticaria). Prolonged use may result in fungal or bacterial superinfection, including *C. difficile*-associated diarrhea (CDAD) and pseudomembranous colitis; CDAD has been observed >2 months postantibiotic treatment. May be associated with increased INR, especially in nutritionally-deficient patients, prolonged treatment, hepatic or renal disease. Use with caution in patients with a history of seizure disorder; high levels, particularly in the presence of renal impairment, may increase risk of seizures.

Drug Interactions
Metabolism/Transport Effects None known.
Avoid Concomitant Use
Avoid concomitant use of CeFAZolin with any of the following: BCG
Increased Effect/Toxicity
CeFAZolin may increase the levels/effects of: Fosphenytoin; Phenytoin; Vitamin K Antagonists

The levels/effects of CeFAZolin may be increased by: Probenecid
Decreased Effect
CeFAZolin may decrease the levels/effects of: BCG; Sodium Picosulfate; Typhoid Vaccine
Dietary Considerations Some products may contain sodium.
Pharmacodynamics/Kinetics
Half-life Elimination 90-150 minutes; prolonged with renal impairment
Time to Peak Serum: I.M.: 0.5-2 hours
Pregnancy Risk Factor B
Pregnancy Considerations Adverse effects were not observed in animal reproduction studies. Cefazolin crosses the placenta. Adverse events have not been reported in the fetus following administration of cefazolin prior to caesarean section. Cefazolin is recommended for group B streptococcus prophylaxis in pregnant patients with a nonanaphylactic penicillin allergy. It is also one of the antibiotics recommended for prophylactic use prior to cesarean delivery and may be used in certain situations prior to vaginal delivery in women at high risk for endocarditis.

Due to pregnancy-induced physiologic changes, the pharmacokinetics of cefazolin are altered. The half-life is shorter, the AUC is smaller, and the clearance and volume of distribution are increased.
Lactation Enters breast milk/use caution (AAP rates "compatible"; AAP 2001 update pending)
Breast-Feeding Considerations Small amounts of cefazolin are excreted in breast milk. The manufacturer recommends that caution be exercised when administering cefazolin to nursing women. Nondose-related effects could include modification of bowel flora.

Dosage Forms
Infusion, premixed iso-osmotic dextrose solution: 1 g (50 mL)
Injection, powder for reconstitution: 500 mg, 1 g, 2 g, 10 g, 20 g, 100 g, 300 g

References
American Dental Association Council on Scientific Affairs, "Combating Antibiotic Resistance," *J Am Dent Assoc*, 2004, 135(4):484-7.
Donowitz GR and Mandell GL, "Drug Therapy. Beta-Lactam Antibiotics (1)," *N Engl J Med*, 1988, 318(7):419-26.
Donowitz GR and Mandell GL, "Drug Therapy. Beta-Lactam Antibiotics (2)," *N Engl J Med*, 1988, 318(8):490-500.
Gustaferro CA and Steckelberg JM, "Cephalosporin Antimicrobial Agents and Related Compounds," *Mayo Clin Proc*, 1991, 66 (10):1064-73.
Jevsevar DS and Abt E, "The New AAOS-ADA Clinical Practice Guideline on Prevention of Orthopaedic Implant Infection in Patients Undergoing Dental Procedures," *J Am Acad Orthop Surg*, 2013, 21 (3):195-7.
Wilson W, Taubert KA, Gewitz M, et al, "Prevention of Infective Endocarditis. Guidelines From the American Heart Association. A Guideline From the American Heart Association Rheumatic Fever, Endocarditis, and Kawasaki Disease Committee, Council on Cardiovascular Disease in the Young, and the Council on Clinical Cardiology, Council on Cardiovascular Surgery and Anesthesia, and the Quality of Care and Outcomes Research Interdisciplinary Working Group," *Circulation*, 2007, 115. Available at http://circ.-ahajournals.org/cgi/reprint/CIRCULATIONAHA.106.183095v1; last accessed July 26, 2007.

Cefdinir (SEF di ner)

Brand Names: U.S. Omnicef® [DSC]
Pharmacologic Category Antibiotic, Cephalosporin (Third Generation)
Use Treatment of community-acquired pneumonia, acute exacerbations of chronic bronchitis, acute bacterial otitis media, acute maxillary sinusitis, pharyngitis/tonsillitis, and uncomplicated skin and skin structure infections.
Local Anesthetic/Vasoconstrictor Precautions No information available to require special precautions
Effects on Dental Treatment No significant effects or complications reported
Effects on Bleeding No information available to require special precautions
Adverse Effects
>10%: Gastrointestinal: Diarrhea (8% to 15%)
1% to 10%:
  Central nervous system: Headache (2%)
  Dermatologic: Rash (≤3%)
  Endocrine & metabolic: Bicarbonate decreased (≤1%), hyperglycemia (≤1%), hyperphosphatemia (≤1%)
  Gastrointestinal: Nausea (≤3%), abdominal pain (≤1%), vomiting (≤1%)
  Genitourinary: Vaginal moniliasis (≤4%), urine leukocytes increased (≤2%), urine pH increased (≤1%), urine specific gravity increased (≤1%), vaginitis (≤1%)
  Hematologic: Lymphocytes increased (≤2%), eosinophils increased (1%), lymphocytes decreased (1%), platelets increased (≤1%), PMN changes (≤1%), WBC decreased/increased (≤1%)
  Hepatic: Alkaline phosphatase increased (≤1%), ALT increased (≤1%)
  Renal: Proteinuria (1% to 2%), microhematuria (≤1%), glycosuria (≤1%)
  Miscellaneous: GGT increased (≤1%), lactate dehydrogenase increased (≤1%)

Additional reactions reported with other cephalosporins: Agranulocytosis, angioedema, aplastic anemia, asterixis, encephalopathy, hemorrhage, interstitial nephritis, neuromuscular excitability, PT prolonged, seizure, superinfection, and toxic nephropathy

General Dosage Range Dosage adjustment recommended in patients with renal impairment
Oral:
Children 6 months to 12 years: 14 mg/kg/day in 1-2 divided doses (maximum: 600 mg/day)
Children >12 years and Adults: 600 mg/day in 1-2 divided doses

Mechanism of Action Inhibits bacterial cell wall synthesis by binding to one or more of the penicillin-binding proteins (PBPs) which in turn inhibits the final transpeptidation step of peptidoglycan synthesis in bacterial cell walls, thus inhibiting cell wall biosynthesis. Bacteria eventually lyse due to ongoing activity of cell wall autolytic enzymes (autolysins and murein hydrolases) while cell wall assembly is arrested.

Pharmacodynamics/Kinetics
Half-life Elimination ~100 minutes
Time to Peak 3 hours
Pregnancy Risk Factor B
Pregnancy Considerations Teratogenic events have not been observed in animal reproduction studies. An increase in most types of birth defects was not found following first trimester exposure to cephalosporins.

Cefditoren (sef de TOR en)

Related Information
Bacterial Infections *on page 1562*
Brand Names: U.S. Spectracef®
Generic Availability (U.S.) Yes
Pharmacologic Category Antibiotic, Cephalosporin (Third Generation)
Dental Use Bactericidal antibiotic for infections due to susceptible organisms
Use Treatment of acute bacterial exacerbation of chronic bronchitis or community-acquired pneumonia (due to susceptible organisms including *Haemophilus influenzae, Haemophilus parainfluenzae, Streptococcus pneumoniae*-penicillin susceptible only, *Moraxella catarrhalis*); pharyngitis or tonsillitis (*Streptococcus pyogenes*); and uncomplicated skin and skin-structure infections (*Staphylococcus aureus* - not MRSA, *Streptococcus pyogenes*)
Local Anesthetic/Vasoconstrictor Precautions No information available to require special precautions
Effects on Dental Treatment No significant effects or complications reported
Effects on Bleeding No information available to require special precautions
Adverse Effects
>10%: Gastrointestinal: Diarrhea (11% to 15%)
1% to 10%:
Central nervous system: Headache (2% to 3%)
Endocrine & metabolic: Glucose increased (1% to 2%)
Gastrointestinal: Nausea (4% to 6%), abdominal pain (2%), dyspepsia (1% to 2%), vomiting (1%)
Genitourinary: Vaginal moniliasis (3% to 6%)
Hematologic: Hematocrit decreased (2%)
Renal: Hematuria (3%), urinary white blood cells increased (2%)
Reactions reported with other cephalosporins: Anaphylaxis, aplastic anemia, cholestasis, hemorrhage, hemolytic anemia, renal dysfunction, reversible hyperactivity, serum sickness-like reaction, toxic nephropathy
Dental Usual Dosage Dental infections (unlabeled use): Children ≥12 years and Adults: Oral: 400 mg twice daily for 10 days

Dosage
Usual dosage range:
Children ≥12 years and Adults: Oral: 200-400 mg twice daily
Indication-specific dosing:
Children ≥12 years and Adults: Oral:
Acute bacterial exacerbation of chronic bronchitis: 400 mg twice daily for 10 days
Dental infections (unlabeled use): 400 mg twice daily for 10 days
Community-acquired pneumonia: 400 mg twice daily for 14 days
Pharyngitis, tonsillitis, uncomplicated skin and skin structure infections: 200 mg twice daily for 10 days
Dosage adjustment in renal impairment:
Cl_{cr} 30-49 mL/minute/1.73 m^2: Maximum dose: 200 mg twice daily
Cl_{cr} <30 mL/minute/1.73 m^2: Maximum dose: 200 mg once daily
End-stage renal disease: Appropriate dosing not established
Dosage adjustment in hepatic impairment:
Mild-to-moderate impairment: Adjustment not required
Severe impairment (Child-Pugh Class C): Specific guidelines not available
Mechanism of Action Inhibits bacterial cell wall synthesis by binding to one or more of the penicillin-binding proteins (PBPs) which in turn inhibits the final transpeptidation step of peptidoglycan synthesis in bacterial cell walls, thus inhibiting cell wall biosynthesis. Bacteria eventually lyse due to ongoing activity of cell wall autolytic enzymes (autolysins and murein hydrolases) while cell wall assembly is arrested.
Contraindications Hypersensitivity to cefditoren, any component of the formulation, other cephalosporins, or milk protein; carnitine deficiency
Warnings/Precautions Use with caution in patients with a history of penicillin allergy, especially IgE-mediated reactions (eg, anaphylaxis, urticaria). Prolonged use may result in fungal or bacterial superinfection, including *C. difficile*-associated diarrhea (CDAD) and pseudomembranous colitis; CDAD has been observed >2 months postantibiotic treatment. Caution in individuals with seizure disorders; high levels, particularly in the presence of renal impairment, may increase risk of seizures. Use caution in patients with renal or hepatic impairment; modify dosage in patients with severe renal impairment. Cefditoren causes renal excretion of carnitine; do not use in patients with carnitine deficiency; not for long-term therapy due to the possible development of carnitine deficiency over time. May prolong prothrombin time; use with caution in patients with a history of bleeding disorder. Cefditoren tablets contain sodium caseinate, which may cause hypersensitivity reactions in patients with milk protein hypersensitivity; this does not affect patients with lactose intolerance.
Drug Interactions
Metabolism/Transport Effects None known.
Avoid Concomitant Use There are no known interactions where it is recommended to avoid concomitant use.
Increased Effect/Toxicity
Cefditoren may increase the levels/effects of: Vitamin K Antagonists

The levels/effects of Cefditoren may be increased by: Probenecid

Decreased Effect

The levels/effects of Cefditoren may be decreased by: Antacids; H2-Antagonists; Proton Pump Inhibitors

Ethanol/Nutrition/Herb Interactions Food: Moderate- to high-fat meals increase bioavailability and maximum plasma concentration. Management: Take with meals. Maintain adequate hydration, unless instructed to restrict fluid intake.

Dietary Considerations Cefditoren should be taken with meals. Plasma carnitine levels are decreased during therapy (39% with 200 mg dosing, 63% with 400 mg dosing); normal concentrations return within 7-10 days after treatment is discontinued.

Pharmacodynamics/Kinetics

Half-life Elimination 1.6 ± 0.4 hours

Time to Peak 1.5-3 hours

Pregnancy Risk Factor B

Pregnancy Considerations Adverse events have not been observed in animal reproduction studies. An increase in most types of birth defects was not found following first trimester exposure to cephalosporins.

Lactation Excretion in breast milk unknown/use caution

Breast-Feeding Considerations It is not known whether cefditoren is excreted in human milk. The manufacturer recommends caution when using cefditoren during breast-feeding. If cefditoren reaches the breast milk, the limited oral absorption may minimize the effect on the nursing infant. Nondose-related effects could include modification of bowel flora.

Dosage Forms

Tablet, oral: 200 mg, 400 mg

Spectracef®: 200 mg, 400 mg

Cefepime (SEF e pim)

Brand Names: Canada Maxipime®

Pharmacologic Category Antibiotic, Cephalosporin (Fourth Generation)

Use Treatment of uncomplicated and complicated urinary tract infections, including pyelonephritis caused by *Escherichia coli, Klebsiella pneumoniae,* or *Proteus mirabilis*; monotherapy for febrile neutropenia; uncomplicated skin and skin structure infections caused by *Streptococcus pyogenes* or methicillin-susceptible staphylococci; moderate-to-severe pneumonia caused by *Streptococcus pneumoniae, Pseudomonas aeruginosa, Klebsiella pneumoniae,* or *Enterobacter* species; complicated intra-abdominal infections (in combination with metronidazole) caused by *E. coli, P. aeruginosa, K. pneumoniae, Enterobacter* species, or *Bacteroides fragilis* against methicillin-susceptible staphylococci, *Enterobacter* sp, and many other gram-negative bacilli.

Children 2 months to 16 years: Empiric therapy of febrile neutropenia patients, uncomplicated skin/soft tissue infections, pneumonia, and uncomplicated/complicated urinary tract infections, including pyelonephritis.

Unlabeled Use Brain abscess (postneurosurgical prevention); malignant otitis externa; prosthetic joint infection; septic lateral/cavernous sinus thrombosis

Local Anesthetic/Vasoconstrictor Precautions No information available to require special precautions

Effects on Dental Treatment No significant effects or complications reported

Effects on Bleeding No information available to require special precautions

Adverse Effects

>10%: Hematologic: Positive Coombs' test without hemolysis (16%)

1% to 10%:

Central nervous system: Fever (1%), headache (1%)

Dermatologic: Rash (1% to 4%), pruritus (1%)

Endocrine & metabolic: Hypophosphatemia (3%)

Gastrointestinal: Diarrhea (≤3%), nausea (≤2%), vomiting (≤1%)

Hematologic: Eosinophils (2%)

Hepatic: ALT increased (3%), AST increased (2%), PTT abnormal (2%), PT abnormal (1%)

Local: Inflammation, phlebitis, and pain (1%)

Reactions reported with other cephalosporins: Aplastic anemia, erythema multiforme, hemolytic anemia, hemorrhage, pancytopenia, PT prolonged, renal dysfunction, Stevens-Johnson syndrome, superinfection, toxic epidermal necrolysis, toxic nephropathy, vaginitis

General Dosage Range Dosage adjustment recommended in patients with renal impairment

I.M.:

Children ≥2 months: 50 mg/kg/dose every 12 hours

Adults: 500-1000 mg every 12 hours

I.V.:

Children ≥2 months: 50 mg/kg/dose every 8-12 hours

Adults: 1-2 g every 8-12 hours

Mechanism of Action Inhibits bacterial cell wall synthesis by binding to one or more of the penicillin-binding proteins (PBPs) which in turn inhibits the final transpeptidation step of peptidoglycan synthesis in bacterial cell walls, thus inhibiting cell wall biosynthesis. Bacteria eventually lyse due to ongoing activity of cell wall autolytic enzymes (autolysins and murein hydrolases) while cell wall assembly is arrested.

Pharmacodynamics/Kinetics

Half-life Elimination 2 hours

Time to Peak I.M.: 1-2 hours; I.V.: 0.5 hours

Pregnancy Risk Factor B

Pregnancy Considerations Adverse events were not observed in animal reproduction studies. Cefepime crosses the placenta.

Cefixime (sef IKS eem)

Related Information

Sexually-Transmitted Diseases *on page 1536*

Brand Names: U.S. Suprax®

Brand Names: Canada Suprax®

Pharmacologic Category Antibiotic, Cephalosporin (Third Generation)

Use Treatment of urinary tract infections, otitis media, respiratory infections due to susceptible organisms including *S. pneumoniae* and *S. pyogenes, H. influenzae,* and many Enterobacteriaceae; uncomplicated cervical/urethral gonorrhea due to *N. gonorrhoeae*

Note: Due to concerns of resistance, the CDC no longer recommends use of cefixime as a first-line regimen in the treatment of uncomplicated gonorrhea in the U.S.; ceftriaxone is the preferred cephalosporin (CDC, 2012).

Unlabeled Use Acute bacterial rhinosinusitis (ABRS) (pediatric) in combination with clindamycin

Local Anesthetic/Vasoconstrictor Precautions No information available to require special precautions

Effects on Dental Treatment No significant effects or complications reported

Effects on Bleeding No information available to require special precautions

Adverse Effects

>10%: Gastrointestinal: Diarrhea (16%)

2% to 10%: Gastrointestinal: Abdominal pain, nausea, dyspepsia, flatulence, loose stools

Reactions reported with other cephalosporins: Interstitial nephritis, aplastic anemia, hemolytic anemia, hemorrhage, pancytopenia, agranulocytosis, colitis, superinfection

General Dosage Range Dosage adjustment recommended in patients with renal impairment

Oral:

Children ≥6 months to 12 years and ≤50 kg: 8-20 mg/kg/day divided every 12-24 hours (maximum: 400 mg/day)

Children >12 years or >50 kg and Adults: 400 mg/day divided every 12-24 hours **or** 20-30 mg/kg/day in 2 divided doses

Mechanism of Action Inhibits bacterial cell wall synthesis by binding to one or more of the penicillin-binding proteins (PBPs); which in turn inhibits the final transpeptidation step of peptidoglycan synthesis in bacterial cell walls, thus inhibiting cell wall biosynthesis. Bacteria eventually lyse due to ongoing activity of cell wall autolytic enzymes (autolysins and murein hydrolases) while cell wall assembly is arrested.

Pharmacodynamics/Kinetics

Half-life Elimination Normal renal function: 3-4 hours; Renal failure: Up to 11.5 hours

Time to Peak Serum: 2-6 hours; delayed with food

Pregnancy Risk Factor B

Pregnancy Considerations Teratogenic effects were not observed in animal reproduction studies. Cefixime crosses the placenta and can be detected in the amniotic fluid. An increase in most types of birth defects was not found following first trimester exposure to cephalosporins. Cefixime may be used for the treatment of gonococcal infections in pregnant women in certain situations (refer to current guidelines).

Cefotaxime (sef oh TAKS eem)

Brand Names: U.S. Claforan®
Brand Names: Canada Cefotaxime Sodium For Injection; Claforan®
Pharmacologic Category Antibiotic, Cephalosporin (Third Generation)
Use Treatment of susceptible organisms in lower respiratory tract, skin and skin structure, bone and joint, urinary tract, intra-abdominal, gynecologic as well as bacteremia/septicemia, and documented or suspected central nervous system infections (eg, meningitis). Active against most gram-negative bacilli (not *Pseudomonas* spp) and gram-positive cocci (not enterococcus). Active against many penicillin-resistant pneumococci.
Unlabeled Use Acute bacterial rhinosinusitis (ABRS)
Local Anesthetic/Vasoconstrictor Precautions No information available to require special precautions
Effects on Dental Treatment No significant effects or complications reported
Effects on Bleeding No information available to require special precautions
Adverse Effects
1% to 10%:
Dermatologic: Pruritus, rash
Gastrointestinal: Colitis, diarrhea, nausea, vomiting
Local: Pain at injection site
Reactions reported with other cephalosporins: Aplastic anemia, hemorrhage, pancytopenia, renal dysfunction, seizure, superinfection, toxic nephropathy.

General Dosage Range Dosage adjustment recommended in patients with hepatic or renal impairment

I.M.:

Infants and Children 1 month to 12 years and <50 kg: 50-200 mg/kg/day in divided doses every 6-8 hours (maximum: 12 g/day)

Children ≥50 kg, Children >12 years, and Adults: 1-2 g every 4-12 hours **or** 0.5-1 g as a single dose

I.V.:

Infants and Children 1 month to 12 years and <50 kg: 50-200 mg/kg/day in divided doses every 6-8 hours (maximum: 12 g/day)

Children ≥50 kg, Children >12 years, and Adults: 1-2 g every 4-12 hours

Mechanism of Action Inhibits bacterial cell wall synthesis by binding to one or more of the penicillin-binding proteins (PBPs) which in turn inhibits the final transpeptidation step of peptidoglycan synthesis in bacterial cell walls, thus inhibiting cell wall biosynthesis. Bacteria eventually lyse due to ongoing activity of cell wall autolytic enzymes (autolysins and murein hydrolases) while cell wall assembly is arrested.

Pharmacodynamics/Kinetics

Half-life Elimination

Cefotaxime: Infants ≤1500 g: 4.6 hours; Infants >1500 g: 3.4 hours; Adults: 1-1.5 hours; prolonged with renal and/or hepatic impairment

Desacetylcefotaxime: 1.5-1.9 hours; prolonged with renal impairment

Time to Peak Serum: I.M.: Within 30 minutes

Pregnancy Risk Factor B

Pregnancy Considerations Teratogenic effects were not observed in animal reproduction studies. Cefotaxime crosses the human placenta and can be found in fetal tissue. An increase in most types of birth defects was not found following first trimester exposure to cephalosporins. During pregnancy, peak cefotaxime serum concentrations are decreased and the serum half-life is shorter. Cefotaxime is approved for use in women undergoing cesarean section (consult current guidelines for appropriate use).

CefoTEtan (SEF oh tee tan)

Generic Availability (U.S.) Yes
Pharmacologic Category Antibiotic, Cephalosporin (Second Generation)
Use Surgical prophylaxis; intra-abdominal infections and other mixed infections; respiratory tract, skin and skin structure, bone and joint, urinary tract and gynecologic infections as well as septicemia; active against gram-negative enteric bacilli including *E. coli*, *Klebsiella*, and *Proteus*; less active against staphylococci and streptococci than first generation cephalosporins, but active against anaerobes including *Bacteroides fragilis*
Local Anesthetic/Vasoconstrictor Precautions No information available to require special precautions
Effects on Dental Treatment No significant effects or complications reported
Effects on Bleeding May potentiate the anticoagulant effects of vitamin K anticoagulants (ie, warfarin) due to alterations of gut flora. Cefotetan may have additional hypoprothrombinemic activity.

Adverse Effects

1% to 10%:
Gastrointestinal: Diarrhea (1%)
Hepatic: Transaminases increased (1%)
Miscellaneous: Hypersensitivity reactions (1%)
Reactions reported with other cephalosporins: Seizure, Stevens-Johnson syndrome, toxic epidermal necrolysis, renal dysfunction, toxic nephropathy, cholestasis, aplastic anemia, hemolytic anemia, hemorrhage, pancytopenia, agranulocytosis, colitis, superinfection

Dosage

Usual dosage range:
Children (unlabeled use): I.M., I.V.: 20-40 mg/kg/dose every 12 hours (maximum: 6 g/day)
Adults: I.M., I.V.: 1-6 g/day in divided doses every 12 hours

Indication-specific dosing:
Children (unlabeled use):
Preoperative prophylaxis: I.M., I.V.: 40 mg/kg 30-60 minutes prior to surgery
Adolescents and Adults:
Pelvic inflammatory disease: I.V.: 2 g every 12 hours; used in combination with doxycycline
Adults:
Orbital cellulitis, odontogenic infections: I.V.: 2 g every 12 hours
Preoperative prophylaxis: I.M., I.V.: 1-2 g 30-60 minutes prior to surgery; when used for cesarean section, dose should be given as soon as umbilical cord is clamped
Susceptible infections: I.M., I.V.: 1-6 g/day in divided doses every 12 hours; usual dose: 1-2 g every 12 hours for 5-10 days; 1-2 g may be given every 24 hours for urinary tract infection; **Note:** Due to high rates of *B. fragilis* group resistance, not recommended for the treatment of community-acquired intra-abdominal infections (Solomkin, 2010)
Urinary tract infection: I.M., I.V.: 1-2 g may be given every 24 hours

Dosage adjustment in renal impairment:
Cl$_{cr}$ 10-30 mL/minute: Administer every 24 hours
Cl$_{cr}$ <10 mL/minute: Administer every 48 hours
Hemodialysis: Dialyzable (5% to 20%); administer 1/4 the usual dose every 24 hours on days between dialysis; administer 1/2 the usual dose on the day of dialysis.
Continuous arteriovenous or venovenous hemodiafiltration effects: Administer 750 mg every 12 hours
Dosage adjustment in hepatic impairment: No dosage adjustment provided in manufacturer's labeling.

Mechanism of Action Inhibits bacterial cell wall synthesis by binding to one or more of the penicillin-binding proteins (PBPs) which in turn inhibits the final transpeptidation step of peptidoglycan synthesis in bacterial cell walls, thus inhibiting cell wall biosynthesis. Bacteria eventually lyse due to ongoing activity of cell wall autolytic enzymes (autolysins and murein hydrolases) while cell wall assembly is arrested.

Contraindications Hypersensitivity to cefotetan, any component of the formulation, or other cephalosporins; previous cephalosporin-associated hemolytic anemia

Warnings/Precautions Modify dosage in patients with severe renal impairment. Although cefotetan contains the methyltetrazolethiol side chain, bleeding has not been a significant problem. Use with caution in patients with a history of penicillin allergy, especially IgE-mediated reactions (eg, anaphylaxis, urticaria). Cefotetan has been associated with a higher risk of hemolytic anemia relative to other cephalosporins (approximately threefold); monitor carefully during use and consider cephalosporin-associated immune anemia in patients who have received cefotetan within 2-3 weeks (either as treatment or prophylaxis). Prolonged use may result in fungal or bacterial superinfection, including *C. difficile*-associated diarrhea (CDAD) and pseudomembranous colitis; CDAD has been observed >2 months postantibiotic treatment. May be associated with increased INR, especially in nutritionally-deficient patients, prolonged treatment, hepatic or renal disease.

Drug Interactions

Metabolism/Transport Effects None known.

Avoid Concomitant Use
Avoid concomitant use of CefoTEtan with any of the following: BCG

Increased Effect/Toxicity
CefoTEtan may increase the levels/effects of: Alcohol (Ethyl); Aminoglycosides; Vitamin K Antagonists

The levels/effects of CefoTEtan may be increased by: Probenecid

Decreased Effect
CefoTEtan may decrease the levels/effects of: BCG; Sodium Picosulfate; Typhoid Vaccine

Ethanol/Nutrition/Herb Interactions Ethanol: Avoid ethanol (may cause a disulfiram-like reaction).

Dietary Considerations Some products may contain sodium.

Pharmacodynamics/Kinetics

Half-life Elimination 3-5 hours
Time to Peak Serum: I.M.: 1.5-3 hours

Pregnancy Risk Factor B

Pregnancy Considerations Adverse events have not been observed in animal reproduction studies. Cefotetan crosses the placenta and produces therapeutic concentrations in the amniotic fluid and cord serum. Cefotetan is one of the antibiotics recommended for prophylactic use prior to cesarean delivery.

Lactation Enters breast milk/use caution

Breast-Feeding Considerations Very small amounts of cefotetan are excreted in human milk. The manufacturer recommends caution when giving cefotetan to a breast-feeding mother. Nondose-related effects could include modification of bowel flora.

Dosage Forms

Injection, powder for reconstitution: 1 g, 2 g, 10 g

CefOXitin (se FOKS i tin)

Brand Names: U.S. Mefoxin®
Brand Names: Canada Cefoxitin For Injection
Generic Availability (U.S.) Yes: Excludes infusion
Pharmacologic Category Antibiotic, Cephalosporin (Second Generation)
Use Less active against staphylococci and streptococci than first generation cephalosporins, but active against anaerobes including *Bacteroides fragilis*; active against gram-negative enteric bacilli including *E. coli*, *Klebsiella*, and *Proteus*; used predominantly for respiratory tract, skin, bone and joint, urinary tract and gynecologic infections as well as septicemia; surgical prophylaxis; intra-abdominal infections and other mixed infections; indicated for bacterial *Eikenella corrodens* infections
Local Anesthetic/Vasoconstrictor Precautions No information available to require special precautions
Effects on Dental Treatment No significant effects or complications reported

Effects on Bleeding May potentiate the anticoagulant effects of vitamin K anticoagulants (ie, warfarin) due to alterations of gut flora.

Adverse Effects

1% to 10%: Gastrointestinal: Diarrhea

Reactions reported with other cephalosporins: Agranulocytosis, aplastic anemia, cholestasis, colitis, erythema multiforme, hemolytic anemia, hemorrhage, pancytopenia, renal dysfunction, serum-sickness reactions, seizure, Stevens-Johnson syndrome, superinfection, toxic nephropathy, vaginitis

Dosage

Usual dosage range:

Infants >3 months and Children: I.M., I.V.: 80-160 mg/kg/day in divided doses every 4-6 hours (maximum dose: 12 g/day)

Adults: I.M., I.V.: 1-2 g every 6-8 hours (maximum dose: 12 g/day)

Note: I.M. injection is painful

Indication-specific dosing:

Infants >3 months and Children:

Mild-to-moderate infection: I.M., I.V.: 80-100 mg/kg/day in divided doses every 4-6 hours

Perioperative prophylaxis: I.V.: 30-40 mg/kg 30-60 minutes prior to surgery followed by 30-40 mg/kg/dose every 6 hours for no more than 24 hours after surgery depending on the procedure

Severe infection: I.M., I.V.: 100-160 mg/kg/day in divided doses every 4-6 hours

Adolescents and Adults:

Perioperative prophylaxis: I.M., I.V.: 1-2 g 30-60 minutes prior to surgery (may repeat in 2-5 hours intraoperatively) followed by 1-2 g every 6-8 hours for no more than 24 hours after surgery depending on the procedure

Adults:

Amnionitis, endomyometritis: I.M., I.V.: 2 g every 6-8 hours

Aspiration pneumonia, empyema, orbital cellulitis, parapharyngeal space, human bites: I.M., I.V.: 2 g every 8 hours

Intra-abdominal infection, complicated, community acquired, mild-to-moderate: I.V.: 2 g every 6 hours for 4-7 days (provided source controlled)

Liver abscess: I.V.: 1 g every 4 hours

Mycobacterium species, not MTB or MAI: I.V.: 12 g/day with amikacin

Pelvic inflammatory disease:

Inpatients: I.V.: 2 g every 6 hours **plus** doxycycline 100 mg I.V. or 100 mg orally every 12 hours until improved, followed by doxycycline 100 mg orally twice daily to complete 14 days

Outpatients: I.M.: 2 g **plus** probenecid 1 g orally as a single dose, followed by doxycycline 100 mg orally twice daily for 14 days

Dosage adjustment in renal impairment:

Cl$_{cr}$ 30-50 mL/minute: Administer 1-2 g every 8-12 hours

Cl$_{cr}$ 10-29 mL/minute: Administer 1-2 g every 12-24 hours

Cl$_{cr}$ 5-9 mL/minute: Administer 0.5-1 g every 12-24 hours

Cl$_{cr}$ <5 mL/minute: Administer 0.5-1 g every 24-48 hours

Hemodialysis: Moderately dialyzable (20% to 50%); administer a loading dose of 1-2 g after each hemodialysis; maintenance dose as noted above based on Cl$_{cr}$

Continuous arteriovenous or venovenous hemodiafiltration effects: Dose as for Cl$_{cr}$ 10-50 mL/minute

Dosage adjustment in hepatic impairment: No dosage adjustment provided in manufacturer's labeling.

Mechanism of Action Inhibits bacterial cell wall synthesis by binding to one or more of the penicillin-binding proteins (PBPs) which in turn inhibits the final transpeptidation step of peptidoglycan synthesis in bacterial cell walls, thus inhibiting cell wall biosynthesis. Bacteria eventually lyse due to ongoing activity of cell wall autolytic enzymes (autolysins and murein hydrolases) while cell wall assembly is arrested.

Contraindications Hypersensitivity to cefoxitin, any component of the formulation, or other cephalosporins

Warnings/Precautions Modify dosage in patients with severe renal impairment. Prolonged use may result in superinfection. Use with caution in patients with a history of penicillin allergy, especially IgE-mediated reactions (eg, anaphylaxis, urticaria). Prolonged use may result in fungal or bacterial superinfection, including C. difficile-associated diarrhea (CDAD) and pseudomembranous colitis; CDAD has been observed >2 months postantibiotic treatment.

Drug Interactions

Metabolism/Transport Effects None known.

Avoid Concomitant Use

Avoid concomitant use of CefOXitin with any of the following: BCG

Increased Effect/Toxicity

CefOXitin may increase the levels/effects of: Aminoglycosides; Vitamin K Antagonists

The levels/effects of CefOXitin may be increased by: Probenecid

Decreased Effect

CefOXitin may decrease the levels/effects of: BCG; Sodium Picosulfate; Typhoid Vaccine

Dietary Considerations Some products may contain sodium.

Pharmacodynamics/Kinetics

Half-life Elimination 45-60 minutes; significantly prolonged with renal impairment

Time to Peak Serum: I.M.: 20-30 minutes

Pregnancy Risk Factor B

Pregnancy Considerations Adverse events have not been observed in animal reproduction studies. Cefoxitin crosses the placenta and reaches the cord serum and amniotic fluid.

Peak serum concentrations of cefoxitin during pregnancy may be similar to or decreased compared to nonpregnant values. Maternal half-life may be shorter at term. Pregnancy-induced hypertension increases trough concentrations in the immediate postpartum period. Cefoxitin is one of the antibiotics recommended for prophylactic use prior to cesarean delivery.

Lactation Enters breast milk/use caution (AAP rates "compatible"; AAP 2001 update pending)

Breast-Feeding Considerations Very small amounts of cefoxitin are excreted in breast milk. The manufacturer recommends that caution be exercised when administering cefoxitin to nursing women. Nondose-related effects could include modification of bowel flora. Cefoxitin pharmacokinetics may be altered immediately postpartum.

Dosage Forms

Infusion, premixed iso-osmotic dextrose solution: Mefoxin®: 1 g (50 mL); 2 g (50 mL)

Injection, powder for reconstitution: 1 g, 2 g, 10 g

Cefpodoxime (sef pode OKS eem)

Pharmacologic Category Antibiotic, Cephalosporin (Third Generation)

Use Treatment of susceptible acute, community-acquired pneumonia caused by *S. pneumoniae* or nonbeta-lactamase producing *H. influenzae*; acute uncomplicated gonorrhea caused by *N. gonorrhoeae*; uncomplicated skin and skin structure infections caused by *S. aureus* or *S. pyogenes*; acute otitis media caused by *S. pneumoniae*, *H. influenzae*, or *M. catarrhalis*; pharyngitis or tonsillitis; and uncomplicated urinary tract infections caused by *E. coli*, *Klebsiella*, and *Proteus*

Unlabeled Use Acute bacterial rhinosinusitis (ABRS) (pediatric) in combination with clindamycin

Local Anesthetic/Vasoconstrictor Precautions No information available to require special precautions

Effects on Dental Treatment No significant effects or complications reported

Effects on Bleeding No information available to require special precautions

Adverse Effects

>10%:
Dermatologic: Diaper rash (12%)
Gastrointestinal: Diarrhea in infants and toddlers (15%)
1% to 10%:
Central nervous system: Headache (1%)
Dermatologic: Rash (1%)
Gastrointestinal: Diarrhea (7%), nausea (4%), abdominal pain (2%), vomiting (1% to 2%)
Genitourinary: Vaginal infection (3%)
Reactions reported with other cephalosporins: Seizure, Stevens-Johnson syndrome, toxic epidermal necrolysis, erythema multiforme, urticaria, serum-sickness reactions, renal dysfunction, interstitial nephritis toxic nephropathy, cholestasis, aplastic anemia, hemolytic anemia, hemorrhage, pancytopenia, agranulocytosis, colitis, vaginitis, superinfection

General Dosage Range Dosage adjustment recommended in patients with renal impairment

Oral:
Children 2 months to 12 years: 10 mg/kg/day divided every 12 hours (maximum: 200 mg/dose)
Children ≥12 years and Adults: 100-400 mg every 12 hours **or** 200 mg as a single dose

Mechanism of Action Inhibits bacterial cell wall synthesis by binding to one or more of the penicillin-binding proteins (PBPs) which in turn inhibits the final transpeptidation step of peptidoglycan synthesis in bacterial cell walls, thus inhibiting cell wall biosynthesis. Bacteria eventually lyse due to ongoing activity of cell wall autolytic enzymes (autolysins and murein hydrolases) while cell wall assembly is arrested.

Pharmacodynamics/Kinetics

Half-life Elimination 2.2 hours; prolonged with renal impairment

Time to Peak Within 1 hour

Pregnancy Risk Factor B

Pregnancy Considerations Teratogenic events were not observed in animal reproduction studies. An increase in most types of birth defects was not found following first trimester exposure to cephalosporins.

Cefprozil (sef PROE zil)

Brand Names: Canada Apo-Cefprozil®; Auro-Cefprozil; Ava-Cefprozil; Cefzil®; RAN™-Cefprozil; Sandoz-Cefprozil

Generic Availability (U.S.) Yes

Pharmacologic Category Antibiotic, Cephalosporin (Second Generation)

Use Treatment of otitis media and infections involving the respiratory tract and skin and skin structure; active against methicillin-sensitive staphylococci, many streptococci, and various gram-negative bacilli including *E. coli*, some *Klebsiella*, *P. mirabilis*, *H. influenzae*, and *Moraxella*.

Local Anesthetic/Vasoconstrictor Precautions No information available to require special precautions

Effects on Dental Treatment No significant effects or complications reported

Effects on Bleeding No information available to require special precautions

Adverse Effects

1% to 10%:
Central nervous system: Dizziness (1%)
Dermatologic: Diaper rash (2%)
Gastrointestinal: Diarrhea (3%), nausea (4%), vomiting (1%), abdominal pain (1%)
Genitourinary: Vaginitis, genital pruritus (2%)
Hepatic: Transaminases increased (2%)
Miscellaneous: Superinfection
Reactions reported with other cephalosporins: Seizure, toxic epidermal necrolysis, renal dysfunction, interstitial nephritis, toxic nephropathy, aplastic anemia, hemolytic anemia, hemorrhage, pancytopenia, agranulocytosis, colitis, vaginitis, superinfection

Dosage

Usual dosage range:
Infants and Children >6 months to 12 years: Oral: 7.5-15 mg/kg/day divided every 12 hours
Children >12 years and Adults: Oral: 250-500 mg every 12 hours or 500 mg every 24 hours

Indication-specific dosing:
Infants and Children >6 months to 12 years: Oral:
Otitis media: 15 mg/kg every 12 hours for 10 days
Children 2-12 years: Oral:
Pharyngitis/tonsillitis: 7.5-15 mg/kg/day divided every 12 hours for 10 days (administer for >10 days if due to *S. pyogenes*; maximum: 1 g/day
Uncomplicated skin and skin structure infections: 20 mg/kg every 24 hours for 10 days; maximum: 1 g/day
Children >12 years and Adults: Oral:
Pharyngitis/tonsillitis: 500 mg every 24 hours for 10 days
Secondary bacterial infection of acute bronchitis or acute bacterial exacerbation of chronic bronchitis: 500 mg every 12 hours for 10 days
Uncomplicated skin and skin structure infections: 250 mg every 12 hours or 500 mg every 12-24 hours for 10 days

Dosage adjustment in renal impairment: Cl_{cr} <30 mL/minute: Reduce dose by 50%

Hemodialysis: Reduced by hemodialysis; administer dose after the completion of hemodialysis

Dosage adjustment in hepatic impairment: No dosage adjustment necessary.

Mechanism of Action Inhibits bacterial cell wall synthesis by binding to one or more of the penicillin-binding proteins (PBPs) which in turn inhibits the final transpeptidation step of peptidoglycan synthesis in bacterial cell walls, thus inhibiting cell wall biosynthesis. Bacteria eventually lyse due to ongoing activity of cell wall autolytic enzymes (autolysins and murein hydrolases) while cell wall assembly is arrested.

Contraindications Hypersensitivity to cefprozil, any component of the formulation, or other cephalosporins

Warnings/Precautions Modify dosage in patients with severe renal impairment. Use with caution in patients with a history of penicillin allergy, especially IgE-mediated reactions (eg, anaphylaxis, urticaria). Prolonged use may result in fungal or bacterial superinfection, including *C. difficile*-associated diarrhea (CDAD) and pseudomembranous colitis; CDAD has been observed >2 months postantibiotic treatment. Some products may contain phenylalanine.

Drug Interactions

Metabolism/Transport Effects None known.

Avoid Concomitant Use

Avoid concomitant use of Cefprozil with any of the following: BCG

Increased Effect/Toxicity

Cefprozil may increase the levels/effects of: Aminoglycosides; Vitamin K Antagonists

The levels/effects of Cefprozil may be increased by: Probenecid

Decreased Effect

Cefprozil may decrease the levels/effects of: BCG; Sodium Picosulfate; Typhoid Vaccine

Ethanol/Nutrition/Herb Interactions Food: Food delays cefprozil absorption.

Dietary Considerations May be taken with food. Oral suspension may contain phenylalanine; consult product labeling.

Pharmacodynamics/Kinetics

Half-life Elimination Normal renal function: 1.3 hours

Time to Peak Serum: Fasting: 1.5 hours

Pregnancy Risk Factor B

Pregnancy Considerations Adverse events were not observed in animal reproduction studies.

Lactation Enters breast milk/use caution (AAP rates "compatible"; AAP 2001 update pending)

Breast-Feeding Considerations Small amounts of cefprozil are excreted in breast milk. The manufacturer recommends that caution be exercised when administering cefprozil to nursing women. Nondose-related effects could include modification of bowel flora.

Dosage Forms

Powder for suspension, oral: 125 mg/5 mL (50 mL, 75 mL, 100 mL); 250 mg/5 mL (50 mL, 75 mL, 100 mL)

Tablet, oral: 250 mg, 500 mg

Ceftaroline Fosamil (sef TAR oh leen FOS a mil)

Brand Names: U.S. Teflaro™

Pharmacologic Category Antibiotic, Cephalosporin (Fifth Generation)

Use Treatment of acute bacterial skin and skin structure infections (ABSSSI) caused by susceptible isolates of *Staphylococcus aureus* (including methicillin-susceptible and -resistant isolates), *Streptococcus pyogenes, Streptococcus agalactiae, Escherichia coli, Klebsiella pneumoniae,* and *Klebsiella oxytoca,* and community-acquired pneumonia (CAP) caused by *Streptococcus pneumoniae* (including cases with concurrent bacteremia), *Staphylococcus aureus* (methicillin-susceptible isolates only), *Haemophilus influenzae, Klebsiella pneumoniae, Klebsiella oxytoca,* and *Escherichia coli*

Local Anesthetic/Vasoconstrictor Precautions No information available to require special precautions

Effects on Dental Treatment No significant effects or complications reported

Effects on Bleeding No information available to require special precautions

Adverse Effects

>10%: Hematologic: Positive Coombs' test without hemolysis (~11%)

2% to 10%:

Central nervous system: Headache (3% to 5%), insomnia (3% to 4%)

Dermatologic: Pruritus (3% to 4%), rash (3%)

Endocrine & metabolic: Hypokalemia (2%)

Gastrointestinal: Diarrhea (5%), nausea (4%), constipation (2%), vomiting (2%)

Hepatic: Transaminases increased (2%)

Local: Phlebitis (2%)

General Dosage Range Dosage adjustment recommended in patients with renal impairment.

I.V.: *Adults:* 600 mg every 12 hours

Mechanism of Action Inhibits bacterial cell wall synthesis by binding to penicillin-binding proteins (PBPs) 1 through 3. This action blocks the final transpeptidation step of peptidoglycan synthesis in bacterial cell walls and inhibits cell wall biosynthesis.Bacteria eventually lyse due to ongoing activity of cell wall autolytic enzymes (autolysis and murein hydrolases) while cell wall assembly is arrested. Ceftaroline has a strong affinity for PBP2a, a modified PBP in MRSA, and PBP2x in *S. pneumoniae*, contributing to its spectrum of activity against these bacteria.

Pharmacodynamics/Kinetics

Half-life Elimination Normal renal function: 2.4 hours; Moderate renal impairment (Cl$_{cr}$ 30-50 mL/minute): 4.5 hours

Time to Peak 1 hour

Pregnancy Risk Factor B

Pregnancy Considerations Skeletal abnormalities have been observed in some but not all animal studies using maternally toxic doses. There are no adequate and well-controlled studies in pregnant women.

CefTAZidime (SEF tay zi deem)

Brand Names: U.S. Fortaz®; Tazicef®

Brand Names: Canada Ceftazidime For Injection; Fortaz®

Pharmacologic Category Antibiotic, Cephalosporin (Third Generation)

Use Treatment of documented susceptible *Pseudomonas aeruginosa* infection and infections due to other susceptible aerobic gram-negative organisms; empiric therapy of a febrile, granulocytopenic patient

Unlabeled Use Bacterial endophthalmitis

Local Anesthetic/Vasoconstrictor Precautions No information available to require special precautions

Effects on Dental Treatment No significant effects or complications reported

Effects on Bleeding No information available to require special precautions

Adverse Effects

1% to 10%:

Gastrointestinal: Diarrhea (1%)

Local: Pain at injection site (1%)

Miscellaneous: Hypersensitivity reactions (2%)

Reactions reported with other cephalosporins: Seizure, urticaria, serum-sickness reactions, renal dysfunction, interstitial nephritis, toxic nephropathy, BUN increased, creatinine increased, cholestasis, aplastic anemia, hemolytic anemia, pancytopenia, agranulocytosis, colitis, prolonged PT, hemorrhage, superinfection

◀ **General Dosage Range** Dosage adjustment recommended in patients with renal impairment
I.M.: *Adults:* 500 mg to 2 g every 8-12 hours
I.V.:
Children 1 month to 12 years: 30-50 mg/kg every 8 hours (maximum: 6 g daily)
Children ≥12 years and Adults: 500 mg to 2 g every 8-12 hours (maximum: 6 g daily)

Mechanism of Action Inhibits bacterial cell wall synthesis by binding to one or more of the penicillin-binding proteins (PBPs) which in turn inhibits the final transpeptidation step of peptidoglycan synthesis in bacterial cell walls, thus inhibiting cell wall biosynthesis. Bacteria eventually lyse due to ongoing activity of cell wall autolytic enzymes (autolysins and murein hydrolases) while cell wall assembly is arrested.

Pharmacodynamics/Kinetics
Half-life Elimination 1-2 hours, prolonged with renal impairment; Neonates <23 days: 2.2-4.7 hours
Time to Peak Serum: I.M.: ~1 hour

Pregnancy Risk Factor B

Pregnancy Considerations Teratogenic effects were not observed in animal reproduction studies. Ceftazidime crosses the placenta and reaches the cord serum and amniotic fluid. An increase in most types of birth defects was not found following first trimester exposure to cephalosporins. Maternal peak serum concentration is unchanged in the first trimester. After the first trimester, serum concentrations decrease by approximately 50% of those in nonpregnant patients. Renal clearance is increased during pregnancy.

Ceftibuten (sef TYE byoo ten)

Related Information
Bacterial Infections *on page 1562*
Brand Names: U.S. Cedax®
Generic Availability (U.S.) No
Pharmacologic Category Antibiotic, Cephalosporin (Third Generation)
Use Treatment of acute exacerbations of chronic bronchitis, acute bacterial otitis media, and pharyngitis/tonsillitis
Local Anesthetic/Vasoconstrictor Precautions No information available to require special precautions
Effects on Dental Treatment No significant effects or complications reported
Effects on Bleeding No information available to require special precautions
Adverse Effects
1% to 10%:
Central nervous system: Headache (≤3%), dizziness (≤1%)
Gastrointestinal: Nausea (≤4%), diarrhea (3% to 4%), dyspepsia (≤2%), loose stools (≤2%), abdominal pain (1% to 2%), vomiting (1% to 2%)
Hematologic: Eosinophils increased (3%), hemoglobin decreased (1% to 2%), platelets increased (≤1%)
Hepatic: ALT increased (≤1%), bilirubin increased (≤1%)
Renal: BUN increased (2% to 4%)
Additional reactions reported with other cephalosporins: Allergic reaction, agranulocytosis, angioedema, aplastic anemia, anaphylaxis, asterixis, cholestasis, drug fever, encephalopathy, erythema multiforme, hemolytic anemia, hemorrhage, interstitial nephritis, neuromuscular excitability, neutropenia, pancytopenia, prolonged PT, renal dysfunction, seizure, superinfection, toxic nephropathy

Dosage
Usual dosage range:
Children 6 months to <12 years: Oral: 9 mg/kg/day for 10 days (maximum dose: 400 mg/day)
Children ≥12 years and Adults: Oral: 400 mg once daily for 10 days
Dosage adjustment in renal impairment:
Cl_{cr} ≥50 mL//minute: No adjustment needed
Cl_{cr} 30-49 mL//minute: Administer 4.5 mg/kg or 200 mg every 24 hours
Cl_{cr} 5-29 mL/minute: Administer 2.25 mg/kg or 100 mg every 24 hours.
Hemodialysis: Administer 400 mg or 9 mg/kg (maximum: 400 mg) after each hemodialysis session
Dosage adjustment in hepatic impairment: No dosage adjustment provided in manufacturer's labeling.
Mechanism of Action Inhibits bacterial cell wall synthesis by binding to one or more of the penicillin-binding proteins (PBPs) which in turn inhibits the final transpeptidation step of peptidoglycan synthesis in bacterial cell walls, thus inhibiting cell wall biosynthesis. Bacteria eventually lyse due to ongoing activity of cell wall autolytic enzymes (autolysins and murein hydrolases) while cell wall assembly is arrested.
Contraindications Hypersensitivity to ceftibuten, any component of the formulation, or other cephalosporins
Warnings/Precautions Modify dosage in patients with moderate-to-severe renal impairment. Prolonged use may result in fungal or bacterial superinfection, including *C. difficile*-associated diarrhea (CDAD) and pseudomembranous colitis; CDAD has been observed >2 months postantibiotic treatment. Use with caution in patients with a history of colitis and other gastrointestinal diseases. Use with caution in patients with a history of penicillin allergy, especially IgE-mediated reactions (eg, anaphylaxis, urticaria). Oral suspension formulation contains sucrose.
Drug Interactions
Metabolism/Transport Effects None known.
Avoid Concomitant Use
Avoid concomitant use of Ceftibuten with any of the following: BCG
Increased Effect/Toxicity
Ceftibuten may increase the levels/effects of: Aminoglycosides; Vitamin K Antagonists

The levels/effects of Ceftibuten may be increased by: Probenecid
Decreased Effect
Ceftibuten may decrease the levels/effects of: BCG; Sodium Picosulfate; Typhoid Vaccine

The levels/effects of Ceftibuten may be decreased by: Multivitamins/Minerals (with ADEK, Folate, Iron); Zinc Salts
Dietary Considerations
Capsule: Take without regard to food.
Suspension: Take 2 hours before or 1 hour after meals.
Pharmacodynamics/Kinetics
Half-life Elimination 2 hours; Cl_{cr} 30-49 mL/minute: 7 hours; Cl_{cr} 5-29 mL/minute: 13 hours; Cl_{cr} <5 mL/minute: 22 hours
Time to Peak 2-3 hours
Pregnancy Risk Factor B
Pregnancy Considerations Teratogenic effects were not observed in animal reproduction studies. An increase in most types of birth defects was not found following first trimester exposure to cephalosporins.
Lactation Excretion in breast milk unknown/use caution

Breast-Feeding Considerations Ceftibuten was not detectable in milk after a single 200 mg dose (limit of detection: 1 mcg/mL). It is not known if it would be detectable after a 400 mg dose or multiple doses. The manufacturer recommends that caution be exercised when administering ceftibuten to nursing women. If ceftibuten does reach the human milk, nondose-related effects could include modification of bowel flora.

Dosage Forms

Capsule, oral:
Cedax®: 400 mg

Powder for suspension, oral:
Cedax®: 90 mg/5 mL (60 mL, 90 mL, 120 mL); 180 mg/5 mL (30 mL, 60 mL)

CefTRIAXone (sef trye AKS one)

Related Information
Antibiotic Prophylaxis *on page 1542*
Sexually-Transmitted Diseases *on page 1536*
Brand Names: U.S. Rocephin®
Brand Names: Canada Ceftriaxone for Injection; Ceftriaxone Sodium for Injection BP; Rocephin®
Pharmacologic Category Antibiotic, Cephalosporin (Third Generation)
Use Treatment of lower respiratory tract infections, acute bacterial otitis media, skin and skin structure infections, bone and joint infections, intra-abdominal and urinary tract infections, pelvic inflammatory disease (PID), uncomplicated gonorrhea, bacterial septicemia, and meningitis; used in surgical prophylaxis
Unlabeled Use Treatment of chancroid, epididymitis, complicated gonococcal infections; sexually-transmitted diseases (STD); periorbital or buccal cellulitis; salmonellosis or shigellosis; atypical community-acquired pneumonia; acute bacterial rhinosinusitis (ABRS); epiglottitis, Lyme disease; used in chemoprophylaxis for high-risk contacts (close exposure to patients with invasive meningococcal disease); sexual assault; typhoid fever, Whipple's disease
Local Anesthetic/Vasoconstrictor Precautions No information available to require special precautions
Effects on Dental Treatment No significant effects or complications reported
Effects on Bleeding May potentiate the anticoagulant effects of vitamin K anticoagulants (ie, warfarin) due to alterations of gut flora.
Adverse Effects
>10%: Local: Induration (I.M. 5% to 17%), warmth (I.M.), tightness (I.M.)
1% to 10%:
Dermatologic: Rash (2%)
Gastrointestinal: Diarrhea (3%)
Hematologic: Eosinophilia (6%), thrombocytosis (5%), leukopenia (2%)
Hepatic: Transaminases increased (3%)
Local: Tenderness at injection site (I.V. 1%), pain
Renal: BUN increased (1%)
Reactions reported with other cephalosporins: Angioedema, allergic reaction, aplastic anemia, asterixis, cholestasis, encephalopathy, hemorrhage, hepatic dysfunction, hyperactivity (reversible), hypertonia, interstitial nephritis, LDH increased, neuromuscular excitability, pancytopenia, paresthesia, renal dysfunction, superinfection, toxic nephropathy

General Dosage Range Dosage adjustment recommended in patients with hepatic and renal impairment
I.M.:
Children: 50-100 mg/kg/day divided every 12-24 hours (maximum: 4 g/day) **or** 125 mg or 50 mg/kg as a single dose
Adults: 1-2 g every 12-24 hours **or** 125-250 mg as a single dose
I.V.:
Children: 50-100 mg/kg/day divided every 12-24 hours (maximum: 4 g/day)
Adults: 1-2 g every 12-24 hours
Mechanism of Action Inhibits bacterial cell wall synthesis by binding to one or more of the penicillin-binding proteins (PBPs) which in turn inhibits the final transpeptidation step of peptidoglycan synthesis in bacterial cell walls, thus inhibiting cell wall biosynthesis. Bacteria eventually lyse due to ongoing activity of cell wall autolytic enzymes (autolysins and murein hydrolases) while cell wall assembly is arrested.
Pharmacodynamics/Kinetics
Half-life Elimination Normal renal and hepatic function: 5-9 hours; Renal impairment (mild-to-severe): 12-16 hours
Time to Peak Serum: I.M.: 2-3 hours
Pregnancy Risk Factor B
Pregnancy Considerations Teratogenic effects have not been observed in animal reproduction studies. Ceftriaxone crosses the placenta and distributes to amniotic fluid. An increase in most types of birth defects was not found following first trimester exposure to cephalosporins. Pregnancy was found to influence the single dose pharmacokinetics of ceftriaxone when administered prior to delivery. The pharmacokinetics of ceftriaxone following multiple doses in the third trimester are similar to those of nonpregnant patients. Ceftriaxone is recommended for use in pregnant women for the treatment of gonococcal infections, Lyme disease, and may be used in certain situations prior to vaginal delivery in women at high risk for endocarditis (consult current guidelines).

Cefuroxime (se fyoor OKS eem)

Related Information
Bacterial Infections *on page 1562*
Brand Names: U.S. Ceftin®; Zinacef®
Brand Names: Canada Apo-Cefuroxime®; Auro-Cefuroxime; Ceftin®; Cefuroxime For Injection; Cefuroxime For Injection, USP; PRO-Cefuroxime; ratio-Cefuroxime
Generic Availability (U.S.) Yes
Pharmacologic Category Antibiotic, Cephalosporin (Second Generation)
Use Treatment of infections caused by staphylococci, group B streptococci, *H. influenzae* (type A and B), *E. coli, Enterobacter, Salmonella,* and *Klebsiella*; treatment of susceptible infections of the upper and lower respiratory tract, otitis media, urinary tract, uncomplicated skin and soft tissue, bone and joint, sepsis, uncomplicated gonorrhea, and early Lyme disease; surgical prophylaxis
Local Anesthetic/Vasoconstrictor Precautions No information available to require special precautions
Effects on Dental Treatment No significant effects or complications reported
Effects on Bleeding No information available to require special precautions

Adverse Effects
>10%: Gastrointestinal: Diarrhea (4% to 11%, duration-dependent)
1% to 10%:
Dermatologic: Diaper rash (3%)
Endocrine & metabolic: Alkaline phosphatase increased (2%), lactate dehydrogenase increased (1%)
Gastrointestinal: Nausea/vomiting (3% to 7%)
Genitourinary: Vaginitis (≤5%)
Hematologic: Eosinophilia (7%), hemoglobin and hematocrit decreased (10%)
Hepatic: Transaminases increased (2% to 4%)
Local: Thrombophlebitis (2%)
Reactions reported with other cephalosporins: Agranulocytosis, aplastic anemia, asterixis, encephalopathy, hemorrhage, neuromuscular excitability, serum-sickness reactions, superinfection, toxic nephropathy

Dosage Note: Cefuroxime axetil film-coated tablets and oral suspension are not bioequivalent and are not substitutable on a mg/mg basis

Usual dosage range:
Children 3 months to 12 years:
Oral: 20-30 mg/kg/day in 2 divided doses
I.M., I.V.: 75-150 mg/kg/day divided every 8 hours (maximum dose: 6 g/day)
Children ≥13 years and Adults:
Oral: 250-500 mg twice daily
I.M., I.V.: 750 mg to 1.5 g every 6-8 hours or 100-150 mg/kg/day in divided doses every 6-8 hours (maximum: 6 g/day)
Indication-specific dosing:
Children ≥3 months to 12 years:
Acute bacterial maxillary sinusitis, acute otitis media, and impetigo:
Oral: Suspension: 30 mg/kg/day in 2 divided doses for 10 days (maximum dose: 1 g/day); tablet: 250 mg twice daily for 10 days
I.M., I.V.: 75-150 mg/kg/day divided every 8 hours (maximum dose: 6 g/day)
Epiglottitis: Oral: 150 mg/kg/day in 3 divided doses for 7-10 days
Pharyngitis/tonsillitis:
Oral: Suspension: 20 mg/kg/day (maximum: 500 mg/day) in 2 divided doses for 10 days; tablet: 125 mg every 12 hours for 10 days
I.M., I.V.: 75-150 mg/kg day divided every 8 hours (maximum: 6 g/day)
Children ≥13 years and Adults (all oral doses listed are for tablet formulation):
Bronchitis (acute and exacerbations of chronic bronchitis):
Oral: 250-500 mg every 12 hours for 10 days
I.V.: 500-750 mg every 8 hours (complete therapy with oral dosing)
Cellulitis, orbital: I.V.: 1.5 g every 8 hours
Gonorrhea:
Disseminated: I.M., I.V.: 750 mg every 8 hours
Uncomplicated:
Oral: 1 g as a single dose
I.M.: 1.5 g as single dose (administer in 2 different sites with probenecid)
Lyme disease (early): Oral: 500 mg twice daily for 20 days
Pharyngitis/tonsillitis and sinusitis: Oral: 250 mg twice daily for 10 days
Pneumonia (uncomplicated): I.V.: 750 mg every 8 hours

Severe or complicated infections: I.M., I.V.: 1.5 g every 8 hours (up to 1.5 g every 6 hours in life-threatening infections)
Skin/skin structure infection (uncomplicated):
Oral: 250-500 mg every 12 hours for 10 days
I.M., I.V.: 750 mg every 8 hours
Surgical prophylaxis: I.V.: 1.5 g 30 minutes to 1 hour prior to procedure (if procedure is prolonged can give 750 mg every 8 hours I.M.)
Open heart: I.V.: 1.5 g every 12 hours to a total of 6 g
Urinary tract infection (uncomplicated):
Oral: 125-250 mg every 12 hours for 7-10 days
I.M., I.V.: 750 mg every 8 hours
Adults:
Cholecystitis, mild-to-moderate: I.V.: 1.5 g every 8 hours for 4-7 days (provided source controlled)
Intra-abdominal infection, complicated, community-acquired, mild-to-moderate (in combination with metronidazole): I.V.: 1.5 g every 8 hours for 4-7 days (provided source controlled)
Surgical prophylaxis:
Cholecystectomy: I.V.: 1.5 g every 8 hours, discontinue within 24 hours unless infection outside gallbladder suspected

Dosage adjustment in renal impairment:
Cl_{cr} 10-20 mL/minute: Administer every 12 hours
Cl_{cr} <10 mL/minute: Administer every 24 hours
Hemodialysis: Dialyzable (25%)
Peritoneal dialysis: Dose every 24 hours
Continuous renal replacement therapy (CRRT): 1 g every 12 hours
Dosage adjustment in hepatic impairment: No dosage adjustment provided in manufacturer's labeling.
Mechanism of Action Inhibits bacterial cell wall synthesis by binding to one or more of the penicillin-binding proteins (PBPs) which in turn inhibits the final transpeptidation step of peptidoglycan synthesis in bacterial cell walls, thus inhibiting cell wall biosynthesis. Bacteria eventually lyse due to ongoing activity of cell wall autolytic enzymes (autolysins and murein hydrolases) while cell wall assembly is arrested.
Contraindications Hypersensitivity to cefuroxime, any component of the formulation, or other cephalosporins
Warnings/Precautions Modify dosage in patients with severe renal impairment. Use with caution in patients with a history of penicillin allergy, especially IgE-mediated reactions (eg, anaphylaxis, urticaria). Prolonged use may result in fungal or bacterial superinfection, including *C. difficile*-associated diarrhea (CDAD) and pseudomembranous colitis; CDAD has been observed >2 months postantibiotic treatment. May be associated with increased INR, especially in nutritionally-deficient patients, prolonged treatment, hepatic or renal disease. Tablets and oral suspension are not bioequivalent (do not substitute on a mg-per-mg basis). Some products may contain phenylalanine.
Drug Interactions
Metabolism/Transport Effects None known.
Avoid Concomitant Use
Avoid concomitant use of Cefuroxime with any of the following: BCG
Increased Effect/Toxicity
Cefuroxime may increase the levels/effects of: Aminoglycosides; Vitamin K Antagonists

The levels/effects of Cefuroxime may be increased by: Probenecid

Decreased Effect

Cefuroxime may decrease the levels/effects of: BCG; Sodium Picosulfate; Typhoid Vaccine

The levels/effects of Cefuroxime may be decreased by: Antacids; H2-Antagonists

Ethanol/Nutrition/Herb Interactions Food: Bioavailability is increased with food; cefuroxime serum levels may be increased if taken with food or dairy products.

Dietary Considerations Some products may contain phenylalanine and/or sodium.

Oral suspension: May be taken with food.

Pharmacodynamics/Kinetics

Half-life Elimination Children 1-2 hours; Adults: 1-2 hours; prolonged with renal impairment

Time to Peak Serum: I.M.: ~15-60 minutes; I.V.: 2-3 minutes; Oral: Children: 3-4 hours; Adults: 2-3 hours

Pregnancy Risk Factor B

Pregnancy Considerations Adverse events were not observed in animal reproduction studies. Cefuroxime crosses the placenta and reaches the cord serum and amniotic fluid. Placental transfer is decreased in the presence of oligohydramnios. Several studies have failed to identify an increased teratogenic risk to the fetus following maternal cefuroxime use.

During pregnancy, mean plasma concentrations of cefuroxime are 50% lower, the AUC is 25% lower, and the plasma half-life is shorter than nonpregnant values. At term, plasma half-life is similar to nonpregnant values and peak maternal concentrations after I.M. administration are slightly decreased. Pregnancy does not alter the volume of distribution. Cefuroxime is one of the antibiotics recommended for prophylactic use prior to cesarean delivery.

Lactation Enters breast milk

Breast-Feeding Considerations Cefuroxime is excreted in breast milk. Manufacturer recommendations vary; caution is recommended if cefuroxime I.V. is given to a nursing woman and it is recommended to consider discontinuing nursing temporarily during treatment following oral cefuroxime. Nondose-related effects could include modification of bowel flora.

Dosage Forms

Infusion, premixed iso-osmotic solution:
Zinacef®: 750 mg (50 mL); 1.5 g (50 mL)

Injection, powder for reconstitution: 750 mg, 1.5 g, 7.5 g, 75 g
Zinacef®: 750 mg, 1.5 g

Powder for suspension, oral: 125 mg/5 mL (100 mL); 250 mg/5 mL (50 mL, 100 mL)
Ceftin®: 125 mg/5 mL (100 mL); 250 mg/5 mL (50 mL, 100 mL)

Tablet, oral: 250 mg, 500 mg
Ceftin®: 250 mg, 500 mg

Celecoxib (se le KOKS ib)

Related Information

Oral Pain *on page 1558*
Rheumatoid Arthritis, Osteoarthritis, and Osteoporosis *on page 1526*

Brand Names: U.S. CeleBREX®

Brand Names: Canada Celebrex®

Generic Availability (U.S.) No

Pharmacologic Category Nonsteroidal Anti-inflammatory Drug (NSAID), COX-2 Selective

Dental Use Management of acute dental pain

Use Relief of the signs and symptoms of osteoarthritis, ankylosing spondylitis, juvenile idiopathic arthritis (JIA), and rheumatoid arthritis; management of acute pain; treatment of primary dysmenorrhea

Local Anesthetic/Vasoconstrictor Precautions No information available to require special precautions

Effects on Dental Treatment Key adverse event(s) related to dental treatment: Stomatitis, abnormal taste, xerostomia (normal salivary flow resumes upon discontinuation), and tooth disorder.

Effects on Bleeding No effects on bleeding or platelet function have been reported. See Dental Comment.

Adverse Effects

≥2%

Cardiovascular: Peripheral edema

Central nervous system: Dizziness, fever, headache, insomnia

Dermatologic: Rash

Gastrointestinal: Abdominal pain, diarrhea, dyspepsia, flatulence, nausea, vomiting

Neuromuscular & skeletal: Arthralgia, back pain

Respiratory: Cough, nasopharyngitis, pharyngitis, rhinitis, sinusitis, upper respiratory tract infection

0.1% to 1.9%:

Cardiovascular: Angina, aortic valve incompetence, chest pain, coronary artery disorder, edema, facial edema, hypertension (aggravated), MI, palpitation, sinus bradycardia, tachycardia, ventricular hypertrophy

Central nervous system: Anxiety, depression, fatigue, hypoesthesia, migraine, nervousness, pain, somnolence, vertigo

Dermatologic: Alopecia, bruising, cellulitis, dermatitis, dry skin, photosensitivity, pruritus, rash (erythematous), rash (maculopapular), urticaria

Endocrine & metabolic: Hot flashes, hypercholesterolemia, hyperglycemia, hypokalemia, ovarian cyst, testosterone decreased

Gastrointestinal: Anorexia, appetite increased, constipation, diverticulitis, dysphagia, eructation, esophagitis, gastritis, gastroenteritis, gastroesophageal reflux, gastrointestinal ulcer, hemorrhoids, hiatal hernia, melena, stomatitis, tenesmus, weight gain, xerostomia

Genitourinary: Cystitis, dysuria, urinary frequency

Hematologic: Anemia, thrombocythemia

Hepatic: Alkaline phosphatase increased, transaminases increased

Neuromuscular & skeletal: Arthrosis, CPK increased, hypertonia, leg cramps, myalgia, paresthesia, synovitis, tendonitis

Ocular: Conjunctival hemorrhage, vitreous floaters

Otic: Deafness, labyrinthitis, tinnitus

Renal: Albuminuria, BUN increased, creatinine increased, hematuria, nonprotein nitrogen increased, renal calculi

Respiratory: Bronchitis, bronchospasm, dyspnea, epistaxis, laryngitis, pneumonia

Miscellaneous: Allergic reactions, allergy aggravated, cyst, diaphoresis, flu-like syndrome

Dental Usual Dosage Acute dental pain: Adults: Oral: 400 mg, followed by an additional 200 mg if needed on day 1; maintenance dose: 200 mg twice daily as needed

Dosage Note: Use the lowest effective dose for the shortest duration of time, consistent with individual patient treatment goals. Oral:

Children ≥2 years: Juvenile idiopathic arthritis (JIA):
≥10 kg to ≤25 kg: 50 mg twice daily
>25 kg: 100 mg twice daily

Adults:

Acute pain or primary dysmenorrhea: Initial dose: 400 mg, followed by an additional 200 mg if needed on day 1; maintenance dose: 200 mg twice daily as needed.

Canadian labeling: Recommended maximum dose for treatment of acute pain: 400 mg/day up to 7 days

Ankylosing spondylitis: 200 mg/day as a single dose or in divided doses twice daily; if no effect after 6 weeks, may increase to 400 mg/day. If no response following 6 weeks of treatment with 400 mg/day, consider discontinuation and alternative treatment.

Canadian labeling: Recommended maximum dose: 200 mg/day

Osteoarthritis: 200 mg/day as a single dose or in divided doses twice daily

Rheumatoid arthritis: 100-200 mg twice daily

Elderly: No specific adjustment based on age is recommended. However, the AUC in elderly patients may be increased by 50% as compared to younger subjects. Initiate at the lowest recommended dose in patients weighing <50 kg.

Dosing adjustment in poor CYP2C9 metabolizers (eg, CYP2C9*3/*3): Consider reducing initial dose by 50%; consider alternative treatment in patients with JIA who are poor CYP2C9 metabolizers.

Canadian labeling: Recommended maximum dose: 100 mg/day

Dosing adjustment in renal impairment:

Advanced renal disease: Use is not recommended; however, if celecoxib treatment cannot be avoided, monitor renal function closely

Severe renal insufficiency: Use is not recommended.

Canadian labeling: Cl_{cr} <30 mL/minute: Use is contraindicated.

Abnormal renal function tests (persistent or worsening): Discontinue use

Dosing adjustment in hepatic impairment:

Moderate hepatic impairment (Child-Pugh class B): Reduce dose by 50%

Severe hepatic impairment (Child-Pugh class C): Use is not recommended

Canadian labeling: Use is contraindicated.

Abnormal liver function tests (persistent or worsening): Discontinue use

Mechanism of Action Inhibits prostaglandin synthesis by decreasing the activity of the enzyme, cyclooxygenase-2 (COX-2), which results in decreased formation of prostaglandin precursors; has antipyretic, analgesic, and anti-inflammatory properties. Celecoxib does not inhibit cyclooxygenase-1 (COX-1) at therapeutic concentrations.

Contraindications Hypersensitivity to celecoxib, sulfonamides, aspirin, other NSAIDs, or any component of the formulation; perioperative pain in the setting of coronary artery bypass graft (CABG) surgery

Canadian labeling: Additional contraindications (not in U.S. labeling): Pregnancy (third trimester); women who are breast-feeding; severe, uncontrolled heart failure; active gastrointestinal ulcer (gastric, duodenal, peptic) or bleeding; inflammatory bowel disease; cerebrovascular bleeding; severe liver impairment or active hepatic disease; severe renal impairment (Cl_{cr} <30 mL/minute) or deteriorating renal disease; known hyperkalemia; use in children

Warnings/Precautions [U.S. Boxed Warning]: NSAIDs are associated with an increased risk of serious (and potentially fatal) adverse cardiovascular thrombotic events, including MI and stroke. Risk

may be increased with duration of use or pre-existing cardiovascular risk factors or disease. Carefully evaluate individual cardiovascular risk profiles prior to prescribing. New-onset or exacerbation of hypertension may occur (NSAIDS may impair response to thiazide or loop diuretics); may contribute to cardiovascular events; monitor blood pressure; use with caution in patients with hypertension. May cause sodium and fluid retention; use with caution in patients with edema, cerebrovascular disease, or ischemic heart disease. Avoid use in heart failure. Long-term cardiovascular risk in children has not been evaluated.

[U.S. Boxed Warning]: Celecoxib is contraindicated for treatment of perioperative pain in the setting of coronary artery bypass graft (CABG) surgery. Risk of MI and stroke may be increased with use following CABG surgery.

[U.S. Boxed Warning]: NSAIDs may increase risk of serious gastrointestinal ulceration, bleeding, and perforation (may be fatal). These events may occur at any time during therapy and without warning. Use caution with a history of GI disease (bleeding or ulcers), concurrent therapy with aspirin, anticoagulants and/or corticosteroids, smoking, use of alcohol, the elderly or debilitated patients. When used concomitantly with ≤325 mg of aspirin, a substantial increase in the risk of gastrointestinal complications (eg, ulcer) occurs; concomitant gastroprotective therapy (eg, proton pump inhibitors) is recommended (Bhatt, 2008).

Use the lowest effective dose for the shortest duration of time, consistent with individual patient goals, to reduce risk of cardiovascular or GI adverse events. Alternate therapies should be considered for patients at high risk.

NSAIDs may cause serious skin adverse events including exfoliative dermatitis, Stevens-Johnson syndrome (SJS), and toxic epidermal necrolysis (TEN); may occur without warning and in patients without prior known sulfa allergy. Anaphylactoid reactions may occur, even without prior exposure; patients with "aspirin triad" (bronchial asthma, aspirin intolerance, rhinitis) may be at increased risk. Do not use in patients who experience bronchospasm, asthma, rhinitis, or urticaria with NSAID or aspirin therapy. Use with caution in other forms of asthma.

Use with caution in patients with decreased hepatic (dosage adjustments are recommended for moderate hepatic impairment; not recommended for patients with severe hepatic impairment) or renal function. Transaminase elevations have been reported with use; closely monitor patients with any abnormal LFT. Severe hepatic reactions (eg, fulminant hepatitis, liver failure) have occurred with NSAID use, rarely; discontinue if signs or symptoms of liver disease develop, if systemic manifestations occur, or with persistent or worsening abnormal hepatic function tests. NSAID use may compromise existing renal function; dose-dependent decreases in prostaglandin synthesis may result from NSAID use, causing a reduction in renal blood flow which may cause renal decompensation (usually reversible). Patients with impaired renal function, dehydration, heart failure, liver dysfunction, those taking diuretics, ACE inhibitors, angiotensin II receptor blockers, and the elderly are at greater risk for renal toxicity. Rehydrate patient before starting therapy; monitor renal function closely. Not recommended for use in patients with advanced renal disease or severe renal insufficiency; discontinue use with persistent or worsening abnormal renal function tests. Long-term NSAID use may result in renal papillary necrosis. Should not be considered a treatment or replacement of corticosteroid-dependent diseases.

Anaphylactoid reactions may occur, even with no prior exposure to celecoxib. Use with caution in patients with known or suspected deficiency of cytochrome P450 isoenzyme 2C9; poor metabolizers may have higher plasma levels due to reduced metabolism; consider reduced initial doses. Alternate therapies should be considered in patients with JIA who are poor metabolizers of CYP2C9.

Anemia may occur with use; monitor hemoglobin or hematocrit in patients on long-term treatment. Celecoxib does not affect PT, PTT or platelet counts; does not inhibit platelet aggregation at approved doses.

When used for juvenile idiopathic arthritis (JIA), celecoxib is not FDA-approved in children <2 years of age or in children <10 kg. Use caution with systemic onset JIA (may be at risk for disseminated intravascular coagulation). Safety and efficacy have not been established for use in children for indications other than JIA.

Drug Interactions

Metabolism/Transport Effects Substrate of CYP2C9 (major), CYP3A4 (minor); **Note:** Assignment of Major/Minor substrate status based on clinically relevant drug interaction potential; **Inhibits** CYP2C8 (moderate), CYP2D6 (moderate)

Avoid Concomitant Use

Avoid concomitant use of Celecoxib with any of the following: Floctafenine; Ketorolac (Nasal); Ketorolac (Systemic); Nonsteroidal Anti-Inflammatory Agents; NSAID (COX-2 Inhibitor); Omacetaxine; Thioridazine

Increased Effect/Toxicity

Celecoxib may increase the levels/effects of: Agents with Antiplatelet Properties; Aliskiren; Aminoglycosides; Anticoagulants; ARIPiprazole; Bisphosphonate Derivatives; CycloSPORINE (Systemic); CYP2C8 Substrates; CYP2D6 Substrates; Deferasirox; Desmopressin; Digoxin; Eplerenone; Estrogen Derivatives; Fesoterodine; Haloperidol; Lithium; Methotrexate; Metoprolol; Nebivolol; NSAID (COX-2 Inhibitor); Omacetaxine; Porfimer; Potassium-Sparing Diuretics; PRALAtrexate; Prilocaine; Quinolone Antibiotics; Thioridazine; Thrombolytic Agents; Vancomycin; Vitamin K Antagonists

The levels/effects of Celecoxib may be increased by: ACE Inhibitors; Angiotensin II Receptor Blockers; Antidepressants (Tricyclic, Tertiary Amine); Aspirin; Corticosteroids (Systemic); CycloSPORINE (Systemic); CYP2C9 Inhibitors (Moderate); CYP2C9 Inhibitors (Strong); Floctafenine; Herbs (Anticoagulant/Antiplatelet Properties); Ketorolac (Nasal); Ketorolac (Systemic); Mifepristone; Nonsteroidal Anti-Inflammatory Agents; Probenecid; Propafenone; Selective Serotonin Reuptake Inhibitors; Sodium Phosphates; Treprostinil

Decreased Effect

Celecoxib may decrease the levels/effects of: ACE Inhibitors; Agents with Antiplatelet Properties; Aliskiren; Angiotensin II Receptor Blockers; Beta-Blockers; Codeine; Eplerenone; HydrALAZINE; Loop Diuretics; Potassium-Sparing Diuretics; Selective Serotonin Reuptake Inhibitors; Tamoxifen; Thiazide Diuretics; TraMADol

The levels/effects of Celecoxib may be decreased by: Bile Acid Sequestrants; CYP2C9 Inducers (Strong); Peginterferon Alfa-2b

Ethanol/Nutrition/Herb Interactions

Ethanol: Avoid ethanol (increased GI irritation).

Food: Peak concentrations are delayed and AUC is increased by 10% to 20% when taken with a high-fat meal.

Herb/Nutraceutical: Avoid concomitant use with herbs possessing anticoagulation/antiplatelet properties, including alfalfa, anise, bilberry, bladderwrack, bromelain, cat's claw, celery, chamomile, coleus, cordyceps, dong quai, evening primrose, fenugreek, feverfew, garlic, ginger, ginkgo biloba, ginseng (American, Panax, Siberian), grapeseed, green tea, guggul, horse chestnuts, horseradish, licorice, prickly ash, red clover, reishi, SAMe (S-adenosylmethionine), sweet clover, turmeric, white willow.

Dietary Considerations May be taken without regard to meals.

Pharmacodynamics/Kinetics

Half-life Elimination ~11 hours (fasted)

Time to Peak ~3 hours

Pregnancy Risk Factor C (prior to 30 weeks gestation)/D (≥30 weeks gestation)

Pregnancy Considerations Teratogenic effects have been observed in some animal studies; therefore, celecoxib is classified as pregnancy category C. Celecoxib is a NSAID that primarily inhibits COX-2 whereas other currently available NSAIDs are nonselective for COX-1 and COX-2. The effects of this selective inhibition to the fetus have not been well studied and limited information is available specific to celecoxib. NSAID exposure during the first trimester is not strongly associated with congenital malformations; however, cardiovascular anomalies and cleft palate have been observed following NSAID exposure in some studies. The use of a NSAID close to conception may be associated with an increased risk of miscarriage. Nonteratogenic effects have been observed following NSAID administration during the third trimester including: Myocardial degenerative changes, prenatal constriction of the ductus arteriosus, fetal tricuspid regurgitation, failure of the ductus arteriosus to close postnatally; renal dysfunction or failure, oligohydramnios; gastrointestinal bleeding or perforation, increased risk of necrotizing enterocolitis; intracranial bleeding (including intraventricular hemorrhage), platelet dysfunction with resultant bleeding; pulmonary hypertension. Because it may cause premature closure of the ductus arteriosus, the use of celecoxib is not recommended ≥30 weeks gestation. The chronic use of NSAIDs in women of reproductive age may be associated with infertility that is reversible upon discontinuation of the medication. A registry is available for pregnant women exposed to autoimmune medications including celecoxib. For additional information contact the Organization of Teratology Information Specialists, OTIS Autoimmune Diseases Study, at 877-311-8972.

Lactation Enters breast milk/use caution

Breast-Feeding Considerations Small amounts of celecoxib are found in breast milk. The manufacturer recommends that caution be exercised when administering celecoxib to nursing women.

Dosage Forms

Capsule, oral:

CeleBREX®: 50 mg, 100 mg, 200 mg, 400 mg

Dental Comment The product labeling for **all** prescription nonsteroidal anti-inflammatory agents (NSAIDs) now include boxed warnings regarding an increased risk of cardiovascular (CV) events and gastrointestinal (GI) bleeding associated with their use and a contraindication for use in patients who have recently undergone coronary artery bypass graft (CABG) surgery.

Medication guides are also now required for these products. Manufacturers of over-the-counter products are to include warnings about potential skin reactions, which are already included in prescription labeling.

The FDA encourages physicians to consider this information in risk-to-benefit evaluations while considering the use of the COX-2 selective celecoxib (CeleBREX®) in patients. Similar COX-2 selective drugs, including rofecoxib (Vioxx®) and valdecoxib (Bextra®), were pulled from the market due to increased risks of adverse CV events associated with their use. In addition, the FDA advises an evaluation of alternative therapy. If physicians determine that continued use is appropriate for individual patients, the lowest effective dose of celecoxib should be prescribed.

The association between selective COX-2 inhibitors and increased cardiovascular risk has been noted previously and prompted by publication of a meta-analysis entitled "Risk of Cardiovascular Events Associated With Selective COX-2 Inhibitors" in the August 22, 2001, edition of the *Journal of the American Medical Association (JAMA)*. The researchers re-evaluated four previously published trials, assessing cardiovascular events in patients receiving either celecoxib or rofecoxib. They found an association between the use of COX-2 inhibitors and cardiovascular events (including MI and ischemic stroke). The annualized MI rate was found to be significantly higher in patients receiving celecoxib or rofecoxib than in the control (placebo) group from a recent meta-analysis of primary prevention trials. Although cause and effect cannot be established (these trials were originally designed to assess GI effects, not cardiovascular ones), the authors believe the available data raise a cautionary flag concerning the risk of cardiovascular events with the use of COX-2 inhibitors.

Cross-reactivity, including bronchospasm, is a concern with aspirin and other NSAIDs, in aspirin-sensitive patients. The manufacturer suggests that celecoxib should not be administered to patients with this type of aspirin sensitivity and should be used with caution in patients with pre-existing asthma.

The manufacturer studied the effect of celecoxib on the anticoagulant effect of warfarin and found no alteration of anticoagulant effect, as determined by prothrombin time, in patients taking 2-5 mg daily. However, the manufacturer has issued a caution when using celecoxib with warfarin since those patients are at increased risk of bleeding complications.

References

Doyle G, Jayawardena S, Ashraf E, et al, "Efficacy and Tolerability of Nonprescription Ibuprofen Versus Celecoxib for Dental Pain," *J Clin Pharmacol*, 2002, 42(8):912-9.

Moore PA and Hersh EV, "Celecoxib and Rofecoxib. The Role of COX-2 Inhibitors in Dental Practice," *J Am Dent Assoc*, 2001, 132 (4):451-6.

Cellulose (Oxidized/Regenerated)

(SEL yoo lose, OKS i dyzed re JEN er aye ted)

Related Information

Antiplatelet and Anticoagulation Considerations in Dentistry *on page 1503*

Brand Names: U.S. Surgicel®; Surgicel® Fibrillar; Surgicel® NuKnit

Generic Availability (U.S.) No

Pharmacologic Category Hemostatic Agent

Dental Use To control bleeding created during a dental procedure

Use Hemostatic; temporary packing for the control of capillary, venous, or small arterial hemorrhage

Local Anesthetic/Vasoconstrictor Precautions No information available to require special precautions

Effects on Dental Treatment No significant effects or complications reported

Effects on Bleeding No information available to require special precautions

Adverse Effects Frequency not defined.

Central nervous system: Headache

Respiratory: Nasal burning or stinging, sneezing (rhinological procedures)

Miscellaneous: Encapsulation of fluid, foreign body reactions (with or without) infection

Dental Usual Dosage Control bleeding created during a dental procedure: Topical: Minimal amounts of the fabric strip are laid on the bleeding site or held firmly against the tissues until hemostasis occurs; remove excess material

Dosage Minimal amounts of the fabric strip are laid on the bleeding site or held firmly against the tissues until hemostasis occurs; remove excess material

Mechanism of Action Cellulose, oxidized regenerated is saturated with blood at the bleeding site and swells into a brownish or black gelatinous mass which aids in the formation of a clot. When used in small amounts, it is absorbed from the sites of implantation with little or no tissue reaction. In addition to providing hemostasis, oxidized regenerated cellulose also has been shown *in vitro* to have bactericidal properties.

Contraindications Hypersensitivity to any component of the formulation; implantation into bone defects; hemorrhage from large arteries; nonhemorrhagic oozing; use as an adhesion product

Warnings/Precautions Pain, numbness, or paralysis have been reported if used near a bony or neural space and left inside patient; use minimum amount necessary to achieve hemostasis. Remove as much of agent as possible after hemostasis is achieved. Do not leave in a contaminated or infected space. Always remove completely following hemostasis if applied in proximity to foramina in bone, areas of bony confine, the spinal cord or optic nerve and chasm; product may swell and exert unwanted pressure. The material should not be moistened before insertion since the hemostatic effect is greater when applied dry. The material should not be impregnated with anti-infective agents. Its hemostatic effect is not enhanced by the addition of thrombin.

Drug Interactions

Metabolism/Transport Effects None known.

Avoid Concomitant Use There are no known interactions where it is recommended to avoid concomitant use.

Increased Effect/Toxicity There are no known significant interactions involving an increase in effect.

Decreased Effect There are no known significant interactions involving a decrease in effect.

Pregnancy Considerations Has been evaluated for use in gynecologic surgeries (Sharma, 2003; Sharma, 2006).

Dosage Forms

Fabric, fibrous:

Surgicel® Fibrillar:

1" x 2" (10s)

2" x 4" (10s)

4" x 4" (10s)

Fabric, knitted:
Surgicel® NuKnit:
1" x 1" (24s)
1" x 3¹/₂" (10s)
3" x 4" (24s)
6" x 9" (10s)
Fabric, sheer weave:
Surgicel®:
¹/₂" x 2" (24s)
2" x 3" (24s)
2" x 14" (24s)
4" x 8" (24s)

Cephalexin (sef a LEKS in)

Related Information
Antibiotic Prophylaxis on page 1542
Bacterial Infections on page 1562
Related Sample Prescriptions
Bacterial Infections and Periodontal Diseases on page 1609
Infective Endocarditis (Prevention) on page 1604
Prosthetic Joint Late Infections (Prevention) on page 1605
Brand Names: U.S. Keflex®
Brand Names: Canada Apo-Cephalex®; Dom-Cephalexin; Keflex®; Novo-Lexin; Nu-Cephalex; PMS-Cephalexin
Generic Availability (U.S.) Yes
Pharmacologic Category Antibiotic, Cephalosporin (First Generation)
Dental Use Prophylaxis in total joint replacement patients undergoing dental procedures; alternative oral antibiotic for prevention of infective endocarditis in individuals allergic to penicillins or ampicillin
Note: Individuals allergic to amoxicillin (penicillins) may receive cephalexin provided they have not had an immediate, local, or systemic IgE-mediated anaphylactic allergic reaction to penicillin.
Use Treatment of susceptible bacterial infections including respiratory tract infections, otitis media, skin and skin structure infections, bone infections, and genitourinary tract infections, including acute prostatitis; alternative therapy for acute infective endocarditis prophylaxis
Unlabeled Use Chronic antimicrobial suppression of prosthetic joint infection
Local Anesthetic/Vasoconstrictor Precautions No information available to require special precautions
Effects on Dental Treatment No significant effects or complications reported (see Dental Comment)
Effects on Bleeding No information available to require special precautions
Adverse Effects Frequency not defined.
Central nervous system: Agitation, confusion, dizziness, fatigue, hallucinations, headache
Dermatologic: Angioedema, erythema multiforme (rare), rash, Stevens-Johnson syndrome (rare), toxic epidermal necrolysis (rare), urticaria
Gastrointestinal: Abdominal pain, diarrhea, dyspepsia, gastritis, nausea (rare), pseudomembranous colitis, vomiting (rare)
Genitourinary: Genital pruritus, genital moniliasis, vaginitis, vaginal discharge
Hematologic: Eosinophilia, hemolytic anemia, neutropenia, thrombocytopenia

Hepatic: ALT increased, AST increased, cholestatic jaundice (rare), transient hepatitis (rare)
Neuromuscular & skeletal: Arthralgia, arthritis, joint disorder
Renal: Interstitial nephritis (rare)
Miscellaneous: Allergic reactions, anaphylaxis
Dental Usual Dosage
Prophylaxis against infective endocarditis (dental, oral, or respiratory tract procedures): Oral:
Children >1 year: 50 mg/kg 30-60 minutes prior to procedure; maximum: 2 g
Children >15 years and Adults: 2 g 30-60 minutes prior to procedure
Note: American Heart Association (AHA) guidelines now recommend prophylaxis only in patients undergoing invasive procedures and in whom underlying cardiac conditions may predispose to a higher risk of adverse outcomes should infection occur.
Prophylaxis in total joint replacement patients undergoing dental procedures which produce bacteremia: Oral: Adults: 2 g 1 hour prior to procedure
Dosage
Usual dosage range:
Children >1 year: Oral: 25-100 mg/kg/day every 6-8 hours (maximum: 4 g/day)
Adults: Oral: 250-1000 mg every 6 hours; maximum: 4 g/day
Indication-specific dosing:
Infants >3 months and Children: Oral:
Community-acquired pneumonia (CAP) (IDSA/PIDS, 2011), S. aureus (methicillin-susceptible), mild infection or step-down therapy (preferred): 75-100 mg/kg/day in 3-4 divided doses
Children:
Furunculosis: 25-50 mg/kg/day in 4 divided doses
Impetigo: 25 mg/kg/day in 4 divided doses
Otitis media: 75-100 mg/kg/day in 4 divided doses
Prophylaxis against infective endocarditis (dental, oral, or respiratory tract procedures): 50 mg/kg 30-60 minutes prior to procedure (maximum: 2 g). **Note:** American Heart Association (AHA) guidelines now recommend prophylaxis only in patients undergoing invasive procedures and in whom underlying cardiac conditions may predispose to a higher risk of adverse outcomes should infection occur.
Severe infections: 50-100 mg/kg/day in divided doses every 6-8 hours
Skin abscess: 50 mg/kg/day in 4 divided doses (maximum: 4 g)
Skin and skin structure infections: Children >1 year: 25-50 mg/kg/day divided every 12 hours
Streptococcal pharyngitis: Children >1 year: 25-50 mg/kg/day divided every 12 hours. **Note:** Recommended by the Infectious Disease Society of America (IDSA) as an alternative agent for group A streptococcal pharyngitis in penicillin-allergic patients (avoid in patients with immediate-type hypersensitivity to penicillin) at a dose of 40 mg/kg/day divided twice daily (maximum: 1000 mg daily) for 10 days (Shulman, 2012).
Adolescents >15 years and Adults: Oral:
Cellulitis and mastitis: 500 mg every 6 hours
Furunculosis/skin abscess: 250 mg 4 times/day
Prophylaxis against infective endocarditis (dental, oral, or respiratory tract procedures): 2 g 30-60 minutes prior to procedure. **Note:** American Heart Association (AHA) guidelines now recommend prophylaxis only in patients undergoing invasive procedures and in whom underlying cardiac

conditions may predispose to a higher risk of adverse outcomes should infection occur.

Prophylaxis in total joint replacement patients undergoing dental procedures which produce bacteremia: 2 g 1 hour prior to procedure

Prosthetic joint infection, chronic oral antimicrobial suppression (unlabeled use): Oral:

Propionibacterium spp (alternative to penicillin or amoxicillin): 500 mg every 6-8 hours (Osmon, 2013)

Staphylococci, oxacillin-susceptible (preferred): 500 mg every 6-8 hours (Osmon, 2013)

Streptococci, beta-hemolytic (alternative to penicillin or amoxicillin): 500 mg every 6-8 hours (Osmon, 2013)

Skin and skin structure infections: 500 mg every 12 hours

Streptococcal pharyngitis: 500 mg every 12 hours.

Note: Recommended by the Infectious Disease Society of America (IDSA) as an alternative agent for group A streptococcal pharyngitis in penicillin-allergic patients (avoid in patients with immediate-type hypersensitivity to penicillin) with a duration of 10 days (Shulman, 2012).

Uncomplicated cystitis: 500 mg every 12 hours for 7-14 days

Dosage adjustment in renal impairment: Adults:
Cl_{cr} 10-50 mL/minute: 500 mg every 8-12 hours
Cl_{cr} <10: 250-500 mg every 12-24 hours
Hemodialysis: 250 mg every 12-24 hours; moderately dialyzable (20% to 50%); give dose after dialysis session

Dosage adjustment in hepatic impairment: No dosage adjustment provided in manufacturer's labeling.

Mechanism of Action Inhibits bacterial cell wall synthesis by binding to one or more of the penicillin-binding proteins (PBPs) which in turn inhibits the final transpeptidation step of peptidoglycan synthesis in bacterial cell walls, thus inhibiting cell wall biosynthesis. Bacteria eventually lyse due to ongoing activity of cell wall autolytic enzymes (autolysins and murein hydrolases) while cell wall assembly is arrested.

Contraindications Hypersensitivity to cephalexin, any component of the formulation, or other cephalosporins

Warnings/Precautions Modify dosage in patients with severe renal impairment. Use with caution in patients with a history of penicillin allergy, especially IgE-mediated reactions (eg, anaphylaxis, urticaria). Prolonged use may result in fungal or bacterial superinfection, including *C. difficile*-associated diarrhea (CDAD) and pseudomembranous colitis; CDAD has been observed >2 months postantibiotic treatment. May be associated with increased INR, especially in nutritionally-deficient patients, prolonged treatment, hepatic or renal disease.

Drug Interactions

Metabolism/Transport Effects None known.

Avoid Concomitant Use

Avoid concomitant use of Cephalexin with any of the following: BCG

Increased Effect/Toxicity

Cephalexin may increase the levels/effects of: MetFORMIN; Vitamin K Antagonists

The levels/effects of Cephalexin may be increased by: Probenecid

Decreased Effect

Cephalexin may decrease the levels/effects of: BCG; Sodium Picosulfate; Typhoid Vaccine

The levels/effects of Cephalexin may be decreased by: Multivitamins/Minerals (with ADEK, Folate, Iron); Zinc Salts

Ethanol/Nutrition/Herb Interactions Food: Peak antibiotic serum concentration is lowered and delayed, but total drug absorbed is not affected. Cephalexin serum levels may be decreased if taken with food.

Dietary Considerations Take without regard to food. If GI distress, take with food.

Pharmacodynamics/Kinetics

Half-life Elimination Adults: 0.5-1.2 hours; prolonged with renal impairment

Time to Peak Serum: ~1 hour

Pregnancy Risk Factor B

Pregnancy Considerations Adverse events were not observed in animal reproduction studies. Cephalexin crosses the placenta and produces therapeutic concentrations in the fetal circulation and amniotic fluid. An increased risk of teratogenic effects has not been observed following maternal use of cephalexin. Peak concentrations in pregnant patients are similar to those in nonpregnant patients. Prolonged labor may decrease oral absorption.

Lactation Enters breast milk/use caution

Breast-Feeding Considerations Small amounts of cephalexin are excreted in breast milk. The manufacturer recommends that caution be exercised when administering cephalexin to nursing women. Maximum milk concentration occurs ~4 hours after a single oral dose and gradually disappears by 8 hours after administration. Nondose-related effects could include modification of bowel flora.

Dosage Forms

Capsule, oral: 250 mg, 500 mg
Keflex®: 250 mg, 500 mg, 750 mg

Powder for suspension, oral: 125 mg/5 mL (100 mL, 200 mL); 250 mg/5 mL (100 mL, 200 mL)

Tablet, oral: 250 mg, 500 mg

Dental Comment Cephalexin is effective against anaerobic bacteria, but the sensitivity of alpha-hemolytic *Streptococcus* vary; approximately 10% of strains are resistant. Nearly 70% are intermediately sensitive. Patients allergic to penicillins can use a cephalosporin; the incidence of cross-reactivity between penicillins and cephalosporins is 1% when the allergic reaction to penicillin is delayed. If the patient has a history of immediate reaction to penicillin, the incidence of cross-reactivity is 20%; cephalosporins are contraindicated in these patients.

References

American Dental Association Council on Scientific Affairs, "Combating Antibiotic Resistance," *J Am Dent Assoc*, 2004, 135(4):484-7.

Jevsevar DS and Abt E, "The New AAOS-ADA Clinical Practice Guideline on Prevention of Orthopaedic Implant Infection in Patients Undergoing Dental Procedures," *J Am Acad Orthop Surg*, 2013, 21 (3):195-7.

Saxon A, Beall GN, Rohr AS, et al, "Immediate Hypersensitivity Reactions to Beta-Lactam Antibiotics," *Ann Intern Med*, 1987, 107 (2):204-15.

Wilson W, Taubert KA, Gewitz M, et al, "Prevention of Infective Endocarditis. Guidelines From the American Heart Association. A Guideline From the American Heart Association Rheumatic Fever, Endocarditis, and Kawasaki Disease Committee, Council on Cardiovascular Disease in the Young, and the Council on Clinical Cardiology, Council on Cardiovascular Surgery and Anesthesia, and the Quality of Care and Outcomes Research Interdisciplinary Working Group," *Circulation*, 2007, 115. Available at http://circ.-ahajournals.org/cgi/reprint/CIRCULATIONAHA.106.183095v1; last accessed July 26, 2007.

Wynn RL, Bergman SA, Meiller TF, et al, "Antibiotics in Treating Oral-Facial Infections of Odontogenic Origin: An Update," *Gen Dent*, 2001, 49(3):238-40, 242, 244 passim.

Certolizumab Pegol (cer to LIZ u mab PEG ol)

Related Information
Rheumatoid Arthritis, Osteoarthritis, and Osteoporosis on page 1526

Brand Names: U.S. Cimzia®

Brand Names: Canada Cimzia®

Pharmacologic Category Antirheumatic, Disease Modifying; Gastrointestinal Agent, Miscellaneous; Tumor Necrosis Factor (TNF) Blocking Agent

Use Treatment of moderately- to severely-active Crohn's disease in patients who have inadequate response to conventional therapy; moderately- to severely-active rheumatoid arthritis (as monotherapy or in combination with nonbiological disease-modifying antirheumatic drugs [DMARDS])

Local Anesthetic/Vasoconstrictor Precautions No information available to require special precautions

Effects on Dental Treatment Key adverse event(s) related to dental treatment: Aphthous ulcers reported in <1% of patients.

Effects on Bleeding No information available to require special precautions

Adverse Effects
>10%:
Gastrointestinal: Nausea (≤11%)
Respiratory: Upper respiratory infection (6% to 20%)
Miscellaneous: Infection (38%; serious: 3%)
1% to 10%:
Cardiovascular: Hypertension (≤5%)
Central nervous system: Headache (5%), fever (3%), fatigue (≤3%)
Dermatologic: Rash (≤9%)
Genitourinary: Urinary tract infection (≤8%)
Neuromuscular & skeletal: Arthralgia (6% to 7%), back pain (≤4%)
Respiratory: Cough (≤6%), nasopharyngitis (5%), bronchitis (≤3%), pharyngitis (≤3%)
Miscellaneous: Antibody formation (7% to 8%), positive ANA (≤4%)

General Dosage Range SubQ: Adults: Initial: 400 mg, repeat dose 2 and 4 weeks after initial dose; Maintenance: 400 mg every 4 weeks **or** 200 mg every other week

Mechanism of Action Certolizumab pegol is a pegylated humanized antibody Fab' fragment of tumor necrosis factor alpha (TNF-alpha) monoclonal antibody. Certolizumab pegol binds to and selectively neutralizes human TNF-alpha activity. (Elevated levels of TNF-alpha have a role in the inflammatory process associated with Crohn's disease and in joint destruction associated with rheumatoid arthritis.) Since it is not a complete antibody (lacks Fc region), it does not induce complement activation, antibody-dependent cell-mediated cytotoxicity, or apoptosis. Pegylation of certolizumab allows for delayed elimination and therefore an extended half-life.

Pharmacodynamics/Kinetics
Half-life Elimination ~14 days
Time to Peak Plasma: 54-171 hours

Pregnancy Risk Factor B

Pregnancy Considerations Adverse effects were not observed in animal reproduction studies. Certolizumab pegol was found to cross the human placenta. Serum concentrations in 12 infants of 10 mothers were ≥75% lower than the maternal serum at delivery (last maternal dose of 400 mg given 5-42 days prior to birth). Although placental transfer was low, infants may have a slower rate of elimination than adults. In one infant,

certolizumab pegol serum concentrations decreased from 1.02 to 0.84 mcg/mL over 4 weeks. Adverse events were not reported. The safety of administering live or live-attenuated vaccines to exposed infants is not known. Healthcare providers are encouraged to enroll women exposed to certolizumab pegol during pregnancy in the Cimzia® Pregnancy Registry (877-311-8972); patients may also enroll themselves.

Cetirizine (se TI ra zeen)

Brand Names: U.S. All Day Allergy [OTC]; ZyrTEC® Allergy [OTC]; ZyrTEC® Children's Allergy [OTC]; Zyr-TEC® Children's Hives Relief [OTC]

Brand Names: Canada Aller-Relief [OTC]; Apo-Cetirizine® [OTC]; Extra Strength Allergy Relief [OTC]; PMS-Cetirizine; Reactine [OTC]; Reactine™

Generic Availability (U.S.) Yes: Excludes liquid gel capsule

Pharmacologic Category Histamine H_1 Antagonist; Histamine H_1 Antagonist, Second Generation; Piperazine Derivative

Use Perennial and seasonal allergic rhinitis and other allergic symptoms including urticaria; chronic idiopathic urticaria

Local Anesthetic/Vasoconstrictor Precautions No information available to require special precautions

Effects on Dental Treatment Key adverse event(s) related to dental treatment: Xerostomia and increased salivation (normal salivary flow resumes upon discontinuation).

Effects on Bleeding No information available to require special precautions

Adverse Effects
>10%: Central nervous system: Headache (children 11% to 14%, placebo 12%), somnolence (adults 14%, children 2% to 4%)
2% to 10%:
Central nervous system: Insomnia (children 9%, adults <2%), fatigue (adults 6%), malaise (4%), dizziness (adults 2%)
Gastrointestinal: Abdominal pain (children 4% to 6%), dry mouth (adults 5%), diarrhea (children 2% to 3%), nausea (children 2% to 3%, placebo 2%), vomiting (children 2% to 3%)
Respiratory: Epistaxis (children 2% to 4%, placebo 3%), pharyngitis (children 3% to 6%, placebo 3%), bronchospasm (children 2% to 3%, placebo 2%)

Dosage Oral:
Children:
6-12 months: Chronic urticaria, perennial allergic rhinitis: 2.5 mg once daily
12 months to <2 years: Chronic urticaria, perennial allergic rhinitis: 2.5 mg once daily; may increase to 2.5 mg every 12 hours if needed
2-5 years: Chronic urticaria, perennial or seasonal allergic rhinitis: Initial: 2.5 mg once daily; may be increased to 2.5 mg every 12 hours **or** 5 mg once daily
Children ≥6 years and Adults: Chronic urticaria, perennial or seasonal allergic rhinitis: 5-10 mg once daily, depending upon symptom severity
Elderly: Initial: 5 mg once daily; may increase to 10 mg/day. **Note:** Manufacturer recommends 5 mg/day in patients ≥77 years of age.
Dosage adjustment in renal/hepatic impairment:
Children <6 years: Cetirizine use not recommended
Children 6-11 years: <2.5 mg once daily

Children ≥12 and Adults:
Cl$_{cr}$ 11-31 mL/minute, hemodialysis, or hepatic impairment: Administer 5 mg once daily
Cl$_{cr}$ <11 mL/minute, not on dialysis: Cetirizine use not recommended

Mechanism of Action Competes with histamine for H$_1$-receptor sites on effector cells in the gastrointestinal tract, blood vessels, and respiratory tract

Contraindications Hypersensitivity to cetirizine, hydroxyzine, or any component of the formulation

Warnings/Precautions Cetirizine should be used cautiously in patients with hepatic or renal dysfunction; dosage adjustment recommended. Use with caution in the elderly; may be more sensitive to adverse effects. May cause drowsiness; use caution performing tasks which require alertness (eg, operating machinery or driving). Effects may be potentiated when used with other sedative drugs or ethanol.

Drug Interactions
Metabolism/Transport Effects Substrate of CYP3A4 (minor), P-glycoprotein; **Note:** Assignment of Major/Minor substrate status based on clinically relevant drug interaction potential

Avoid Concomitant Use
Avoid concomitant use of Cetirizine with any of the following: Aclidinium; Azelastine (Nasal); Ipratropium (Oral Inhalation); Paraldehyde; Tiotropium

Increased Effect/Toxicity
Cetirizine may increase the levels/effects of: Alcohol (Ethyl); Anticholinergics; Azelastine (Nasal); Buprenorphine; CNS Depressants; Methotrimeprazine; Metyrosine; Mirtazapine; Paraldehyde; Pramipexole; ROPINIRole; Rotigotine; Selective Serotonin Reuptake Inhibitors; Tiotropium; Zolpidem

The levels/effects of Cetirizine may be increased by: Aclidinium; Droperidol; HydrOXYzine; Ipratropium (Oral Inhalation); Magnesium Sulfate; Methotrimeprazine; Perampanel; P-glycoprotein/ABCB1 Inhibitors; Pramlintide; Sodium Oxybate

Decreased Effect
Cetirizine may decrease the levels/effects of: Acetylcholinesterase Inhibitors (Central); Benzylpenicilloyl Polylysine; Betahistine; Hyaluronidase

The levels/effects of Cetirizine may be decreased by: Acetylcholinesterase Inhibitors (Central); Amphetamines; P-glycoprotein/ABCB1 Inducers

Ethanol/Nutrition/Herb Interactions Ethanol: May increase CNS depression; monitor for increased effects with coadministration. Caution patients about effects.

Dietary Considerations May be taken with or without food.

Pharmacodynamics/Kinetics
Onset of Action Suppression of skin wheal and flare: 0.7 hours (Simons, 1999)
Duration of Action Suppression of skin wheal and flare: ≥24 hours (Simons, 1999)
Half-life Elimination 8 hours
Time to Peak Serum: 1 hour

Pregnancy Considerations Maternal use of cetirizine has not been associated with an increased risk of major malformations. The use of antihistamines for the treatment of rhinitis during pregnancy is generally considered to be safe at recommended doses. Although safety data is limited, cetirizine may be a preferred second generation antihistamine for the treatment of rhinitis during pregnancy.

Breast-Feeding Considerations Cetirizine is excreted into breast milk.

Dosage Forms
Capsule, liquid gel, oral:
ZyrTEC® Allergy [OTC]: 10 mg
Solution, oral: 5 mg/5 mL (5 mL)
Syrup, oral: 5 mg/5 mL (5 mL, 118 mL, 120 mL, 473 mL, 480 mL)
ZyrTEC® Children's Allergy [OTC]: 5 mg/5 mL (118 mL)
ZyrTEC® Children's Hives Relief [OTC]: 5 mg/5 mL (118 mL)
Tablet, oral: 5 mg, 10 mg
All Day Allergy [OTC]: 10 mg
ZyrTEC® Allergy [OTC]: 10 mg
Tablet, chewable, oral: 5 mg, 10 mg
All Day Allergy [OTC]: 5 mg, 10 mg
ZyrTEC® Children's Allergy [OTC]: 5 mg, 10 mg

Cetirizine and Pseudoephedrine
(se TI ra zeen & soo doe e FED rin)

Related Information
Cetirizine *on page 281*
Pseudoephedrine *on page 1159*
Brand Names: U.S. ZyrTEC-D® Allergy & Congestion [OTC]
Brand Names: Canada Reactine® Allergy and Sinus
Pharmacologic Category Alpha/Beta Agonist; Decongestant; Histamine H$_1$ Antagonist; Histamine H$_1$ Antagonist, Second Generation; Piperazine Derivative
Use Treatment of symptoms of seasonal or perennial allergic rhinitis
Local Anesthetic/Vasoconstrictor Precautions Use with caution since pseudoephedrine is a sympathomimetic amine which could interact with epinephrine to cause a pressor response
Effects on Dental Treatment Key adverse event(s) related to dental treatment: Pseudoephedrine: Xerostomia (normal salivary flow resumes upon discontinuation).
Effects on Bleeding No information available to require special precautions
Adverse Effects Percentages reported with combination product. Additional adverse effects reported; also see individual agents.
1% to 10%:
Central nervous system: Insomnia (4%), fatigue (2%), somnolence (2%), dizziness (1%)
Gastrointestinal: Xerostomia (4%)
Respiratory: Pharyngitis (2%), epistaxis (1%)
General Dosage Range Dosage adjustment recommended in patients with hepatic or renal impairment
Oral: *Children ≥12 years:* 1 tablet twice daily (maximum: 2 tablets/day)
Mechanism of Action Cetirizine is an antihistamine; exhibits selective inhibition of H$_1$ receptors. Pseudoephedrine is a sympathomimetic and exerts a decongestant action on nasal mucosa.
Pharmacodynamics/Kinetics
Half-life Elimination Cetirizine: 7.9 hours; Pseudoephedrine: 6 hours
Time to Peak Cetirizine: 2.2 hours; Pseudoephedrine: 4.4 hours

Cetrorelix (set roe REL iks)

Brand Names: U.S. Cetrotide®
Brand Names: Canada Cetrotide®
Pharmacologic Category Gonadotropin Releasing Hormone Antagonist

Use Inhibits premature luteinizing hormone (LH) surges in women undergoing controlled ovarian stimulation

Local Anesthetic/Vasoconstrictor Precautions No information available to require special precautions

Effects on Dental Treatment No significant effects or complications reported

Effects on Bleeding No information available to require special precautions

Adverse Effects 1% to 10%:
Central nervous system: Headache (1%)
Endocrine & metabolic: Ovarian hyperstimulation syndrome, WHO grade II or III (4%)
Gastrointestinal: Nausea (1%)
Hepatic: ALT, AST, GGT, and alkaline phosphatase increased (1% to 2%)

General Dosage Range SubQ: *Adults (females):* 0.25 mg once daily **or** 3 mg as a single dose

Mechanism of Action Competes with naturally-occurring GnRH for binding on receptors of the pituitary. This delays luteinizing hormone surge, preventing ovulation until the follicles are of adequate size.

Pharmacodynamics/Kinetics
Onset of Action 0.25 mg dose: 2 hours; 3 mg dose: 1 hour
Duration of Action 3 mg dose (single dose): 4 days
Half-life Elimination 0.25 mg dose: 5 hours; 0.25 mg multiple doses: 20.6 hours; 3 mg dose: 62.8 hours
Time to Peak 0.25 mg dose: 1 hour; 3 mg dose: 1.5 hours

Pregnancy Risk Factor X

Pregnancy Considerations Adverse effects, including fetal resorption and implantation loss, have been observed in animal reproduction studies. Resorption resulting in fetal loss would be expected if used in a pregnant woman; use is contraindicated during pregnancy.

Cetuximab (se TUK see mab)

Brand Names: U.S. Erbitux®
Brand Names: Canada Erbitux®
Pharmacologic Category Antineoplastic Agent, Monoclonal Antibody; Epidermal Growth Factor Receptor (EGFR) Inhibitor

Use Treatment of *KRAS* mutation-negative (wild-type), EGFR-expressing metastatic colorectal cancer (in combination with FOLFIRI [irinotecan, fluorouracil, and leucovorin] as first-line treatment, in combination with irinotecan [in patients refractory to irinotecan-based chemotherapy], or as a single agent in patients who have failed oxaliplatin and irinotecan based chemotherapy or who are intolerant to irinotecan); treatment of squamous cell cancer of the head and neck (as a single agent for recurrent or metastatic disease after platinum-based chemotherapy failure; in combination with radiation therapy as initial treatment of locally or regionally advanced disease; in combination with platinum and fluorouracil-based chemotherapy as first-line treatment of locoregional or metastatic disease)

Note: Cetuximab is not indicated for the treatment of *KRAS* mutation-positive colorectal cancer.

Unlabeled Use Treatment of EGFR-expressing advanced nonsmall cell lung cancer (NSCLC); treatment of unresectable squamous cell skin cancer

Local Anesthetic/Vasoconstrictor Precautions No information available to require special precautions

Effects on Dental Treatment No significant effects or complications reported

Effects on Bleeding No information available to require special precautions

Adverse Effects Except where noted, percentages reported for studies with cetuximab monotherapy.
>10%:
Central nervous system: Fatigue (91%), pain (59%), sensory neuropathy (45%; grades 3/4: 1%), headache (38%), insomnia (27%), fever (25%), confusion (18%), anxiety (14%), chills/rigors (16%), depression (14%)
Dermatologic: Rash/desquamation (95%; grades 3/4: 16%), acneiform rash (all studies: 76% to 88%; grades 3/4: 1% to 17%; onset: ≤14 days), dry skin (57%), pruritus (47%), nail changes (31%)
Endocrine & metabolic: Hypomagnesemia (all studies: 55%; grades 3/4: 6% to 17%), dehydration (13%)
Gastrointestinal: Nausea (64%), abdominal pain (59%), constipation (53%), diarrhea (42%), vomiting (37% to 40%), stomatitis (32%), xerostomia (12%)
Neuromuscular & skeletal: Bone pain (15%), arthralgia (14%)
Respiratory: Dyspnea (48% to 49%), cough (30%)
Miscellaneous: Infection (all studies: 13% to 44%; grades 3/4: 11%), infusion reaction (all studies: 15% to 21%; grades 3/4: 2% to 5%; 90% of severe reactions occurred with first infusion)
1% to 10%:
Cardiovascular: Cardiopulmonary arrest (2%; with radiation therapy; 3% with platinum/fluorouracil-based chemotherapy)
Gastrointestinal: Taste disturbance (10%)
Renal: Renal failure (all studies: 1%)
Miscellaneous: Antibody formation (5%), sepsis (all studies: 1% to 4%)

General Dosage Range Dosage adjustment recommended in patients who develop toxicities
I.V.: *Adults:* Loading dose: 400 mg/m²; Maintenance: 250 mg/m² weekly

Mechanism of Action Recombinant human/mouse chimeric monoclonal antibody which binds specifically to the epidermal growth factor receptor (EGFR, HER1, c-ErbB-1) and competitively inhibits the binding of epidermal growth factor (EGF) and other ligands. Binding to the EGFR blocks phosphorylation and activation of receptor-associated kinases, resulting in inhibition of cell growth, induction of apoptosis, and decreased matrix metalloproteinase and vascular endothelial growth factor production. EGFR signal transduction results in *KRAS* wild-type activation; cells with *KRAS* mutations appear to be unaffected by EGFR inhibition.

Pharmacodynamics/Kinetics
Half-life Elimination ~112 hours (range: 63-230 hours)

Pregnancy Risk Factor C

Pregnancy Considerations In pregnant cynomolgus monkeys, cetuximab was detected in the amniotic fluid and in the serum of embryos. Although teratogenic effects were not observed in animal reproduction studies, increases in embryolethality and fetal loss were noted. It is not known whether cetuximab can cause fetal harm or affect reproductive capacity. Because cetuximab inhibits epidermal growth factor (EGF), a component of fetal development, adverse effects on pregnancy would be expected. Cetuximab should only be given to a pregnant woman if the potential benefit justifies the potential risk to the fetus.

Cetylpyridinium (SEE til peer i DI nee um)

Brand Names: U.S. Cepacol® [OTC]; DiabetAid Therapeutic Gingivitis Mouth Rinse [OTC] [DSC]
Generic Availability (U.S.) No
Pharmacologic Category Antiseptic, Oral Mouthwash
Dental Use Antiseptic to aid in the prevention and reduction of plaque and gingivitis, and to freshen breath
Use Antiseptic to aid in the prevention and reduction of plaque and gingivitis, and to freshen breath
Local Anesthetic/Vasoconstrictor Precautions No information available to require special precautions
Effects on Dental Treatment Key adverse event(s) related to dental treatment: Tooth and tongue staining and oral irritation.
Effects on Bleeding No information available to require special precautions
Adverse Effects Frequency not defined: Gastrointestinal: Tooth and tongue staining, oral irritation
Dental Usual Dosage Prevention and reduction of plaque and gingivitis, and to freshen breath: Children ≥6 years and Adults: Oral (OTC labeling): Rinse or gargle as directed; may be used before or after brushing (2 times/day)
Dosage Oral: Children ≥6 years and Adults: OTC labeling: Swish 20 mL thoroughly between teeth for 30 seconds then spit; use twice daily; may be used before or after brushing; do not swallow.
Contraindications Hypersensitivity to cetylpyridinium or any component of the formulation
Warnings/Precautions If an amount greater than used for rinsing is swallowed, seek professional assistance or contact a poison control center immediately. Stop use and consult a healthcare professional if symptoms or condition worsens or persists; if gingivitis, bleeding, redness persists for more than 2 weeks; if gums are painful and swollen; if pus from the gum line, loose teeth, or increased spacing between the teeth occurs. Avoid contact with eyes.
Drug Interactions
Metabolism/Transport Effects None known.
Avoid Concomitant Use There are no known interactions where it is recommended to avoid concomitant use.
Increased Effect/Toxicity There are no known significant interactions involving an increase in effect.
Decreased Effect There are no known significant interactions involving a decrease in effect.
Pregnancy Considerations
Cetylpyridinium chloride mouthwash (alcohol free) has been associated with a reduction in preterm births in pregnant women with periodontal disease (Jeffcoat, 2011).
Dosage Forms
Liquid, oral:
Cepacol® [OTC]: 0.05% (710 mL)

Cetylpyridinium and Benzocaine
(SEE til peer i DI nee um & BEN zoe kane)

Related Information
Benzocaine on page 176
Cetylpyridinium on page 284
Brand Names: Canada Cepacol®; Kank-A®
Pharmacologic Category Local Anesthetic
Dental Use Antiseptic/anesthetic for oral cavity
Use Symptomatic relief of sore throat

Local Anesthetic/Vasoconstrictor Precautions No information available to require special precautions
Effects on Dental Treatment No significant effects or complications reported
Effects on Bleeding No information available to require special precautions
Dosage Antiseptic/anesthetic: Oral: Dissolve in mouth as needed for sore throat
Drug Interactions
Metabolism/Transport Effects None known.
Avoid Concomitant Use There are no known interactions where it is recommended to avoid concomitant use.
Increased Effect/Toxicity
Cetylpyridinium and Benzocaine may increase the levels/effects of: Prilocaine
Decreased Effect There are no known significant interactions involving a decrease in effect.
Product Availability Not available in U.S.

Cevimeline (se vi ME leen)

Related Information
Dentin Hypersensitivity, Acid Erosion, High Caries Index, Management of Alveolar Osteitis, and Xerostomia on page 1582
Management of Patients Undergoing Cancer Therapy on page 1596
Brand Names: U.S. Evoxac®
Brand Names: Canada Evoxac®
Generic Availability (U.S.) Yes
Pharmacologic Category Cholinergic Agonist
Dental Use Treatment of symptoms of dry mouth in patients with Sjögren's syndrome
Use Treatment of symptoms of dry mouth in patients with Sjögren's syndrome
Local Anesthetic/Vasoconstrictor Precautions No information available to require special precautions
Effects on Dental Treatment Key adverse event(s) related to dental treatment: Excessive salivation, salivary gland pain, xerostomia (normal salivary flow resumes upon discontinuation), ulcerative stomatitis, and tooth disorder.
Effects on Bleeding No information available to require special precautions
Adverse Effects
>10%:
Gastrointestinal: Nausea (14%)
Respiratory: Sinusitis (12%), rhinitis (11%), upper respiratory infection (11%)
Miscellaneous: Diaphoresis increased (19%)
1% to 10%:
Cardiovascular: Chest pain, edema, palpitation, peripheral edema
Central nervous system: Fatigue (3%), insomnia (2%), depression, fever, hypoesthesia, migraine, vertigo
Dermatologic: Erythematous rash, pruritus, skin disorder
Endocrine & metabolic: Hot flashes (2%)
Gastrointestinal: Abdominal pain (8%), vomiting (5%), excessive salivation (2%), amylase increased, anorexia, constipation, eructation, flatulence, gastroesophageal reflux, salivary gland pain, sialoadenitis, toothache, ulcerative stomatitis, xerostomia
Genitourinary: Urinary tract infection (6%), cystitis, vaginitis
Hematologic: Anemia
Local: Abscess

Neuromuscular & skeletal: Back pain (5%), arthralgia (4%), skeletal pain (3%), weakness (1%), hypertonia, hyporeflexia, leg cramps, myalgia, tremor
Ocular: Abnormal vision, eye abnormality, eye infection, eye pain, xerophthalmia
Otic: Earache, otitis media
Respiratory: Coughing (6%), bronchitis (4%), epistaxis, pneumonia
Miscellaneous: Allergy, flu-like syndrome, fungal infection, hiccups, infection, moniliasis

Dental Usual Dosage Dry mouth (in Sjögren's syndrome): Adults: Oral: 30 mg 3 times/day
Dosage Oral:
Adults: 30 mg 3 times/day
Elderly: No specific dosage adjustment is recommended; however, use caution when initiating due to potential for increased sensitivity
Dosage adjustment in renal impairment: No dosage adjustment provided in the manufacturer's labeling.
Dosage adjustment in hepatic impairment: No dosage adjustment provided in the manufacturer's labeling.
Mechanism of Action Binds to muscarinic (cholinergic) receptors, causing an increase in secretion of exocrine glands (including salivary glands)
Contraindications Hypersensitivity to cevimeline or any component of the formulation; uncontrolled asthma; narrow-angle glaucoma; acute iritis; other conditions where miosis is undesirable
Warnings/Precautions May alter cardiac conduction and/or heart rate; use caution in patients with significant cardiovascular disease, including angina, myocardial infarction, or conduction disturbances. Cevimeline has the potential to increase bronchial smooth muscle tone, airway resistance, and bronchial secretions; use with caution in patients with controlled asthma, COPD, or chronic bronchitis. May cause decreased visual acuity (particularly at night and in patients with central lens changes) and impaired depth perception. Patients should be cautioned about driving at night or performing hazardous activities in reduced lighting. May cause a variety of parasympathomimetic effects, which may be particularly dangerous in elderly patients; excessive sweating may lead to dehydration in some patients.

Use with caution in patients with a history of biliary stones or nephrolithiasis; cevimeline may induce smooth muscle spasms, precipitating cholangitis, cholecystitis, biliary obstruction, renal colic, or ureteral reflux in susceptible patients. Patients with a known or suspected deficiency of CYP2D6 may be at higher risk of adverse effects.
Drug Interactions
Metabolism/Transport Effects Substrate of CYP2D6 (minor), CYP3A4 (minor); **Note:** Assignment of Major/Minor substrate status based on clinically relevant drug interaction potential
Avoid Concomitant Use There are no known interactions where it is recommended to avoid concomitant use.
Increased Effect/Toxicity
The levels/effects of Cevimeline may be increased by: Acetylcholinesterase Inhibitors; Beta-Blockers
Decreased Effect
The levels/effects of Cevimeline may be decreased by: Peginterferon Alfa-2b
Dietary Considerations Take with or without food.
Pharmacodynamics/Kinetics
Half-life Elimination 4-6 hours
Time to Peak 1.5-2 hours

Pregnancy Risk Factor C
Pregnancy Considerations Adverse effects were observed in animal reproduction studies.
Lactation Excretion in breast milk unknown/not recommended
Dosage Forms
Capsule, oral: 30 mg
Evoxac®: 30 mg

Charcoal, Activated (CHAR kole AK tiv ay ted)

Brand Names: U.S. Actidose® with Sorbitol [OTC]; Actidose®-Aqua [OTC]; Charcoal Plus® DS [OTC]; CharcoCaps® [OTC]; EZ-Char® [OTC]; Kerr Insta-Char® in Aqueous Base [OTC]; Kerr Insta-Char® in Sorbitol Base [OTC]; Requa® Activated Charcoal [OTC]
Brand Names: Canada Charac-25 [OTC]; Charac-50 [OTC]; Charactol-25 [OTC]; Charactol-50 [OTC]; Charcodote Susp [OTC]; Charcodote TFS [OTC]; Charcodote-Aqueous Sus; Premium Activated Charcoal [OTC]
Pharmacologic Category Antidote
Use
Suspension: Activated charcoal is a nonabsorbable adsorbent that may be considered in the management of poisonings when gastrointestinal decontamination of drugs or chemicals is indicated (eg, presentation to a treatment facility within 1 hour of ingestion). Activated charcoal is generally an effective adsorbent of drugs and chemicals with a molecular weight range of 100-1000 daltons. Multidose activated charcoal may be considered if a patient has ingested a life-threatening amount of carbamazepine, dapsone, phenobarbital, quinine, or theophylline (Vale, 1999).
Capsules, tablets: Digestive aid
Local Anesthetic/Vasoconstrictor Precautions No information available to require special precautions
Effects on Dental Treatment No significant effects or complications reported
Effects on Bleeding No information available to require special precautions
Adverse Effects Frequency not defined.
Gastrointestinal: Abdominal distention, appendicitis, bowel obstruction, constipation, vomiting
Ocular: Corneal abrasion (with direct contact)
Respiratory: Aspiration, respiratory failure
Miscellaneous: Fecal discoloration (black)
General Dosage Range Oral, NG:
Infants <1 year: Initial: 10-25 g; additional doses of 10-25 g can be given every 4 hours
Children 1-12 years: Initial: 25-50 g; additional doses of 10-25 g can be given every 4 hours
Children >12 years and Adults: Initial: 25-100 g; additional doses of 25-50 g can be given every 4 hours
Mechanism of Action Adsorbs toxic substances, thus inhibiting GI absorption
Pregnancy Considerations Activated charcoal is not absorbed systemically following oral administration. Systemic absorption would be required in order for activated charcoal to cross the placenta and reach the fetus. In general, medications used as antidotes should take into consideration the health and prognosis of the mother (Bailey, 2003).

Chloral Hydrate (KLOR al HYE drate)

Brand Names: U.S. Somnote® [DSC]
Brand Names: Canada PMS-Chloral Hydrate
Generic Availability (U.S.) No
Pharmacologic Category Hypnotic, Miscellaneous

Dental Use Short-term sedative/hypnotic for dental procedures

Use Short-term sedative and hypnotic (<2 weeks); sedative/hypnotic for diagnostic procedures; sedative prior to EEG evaluations

Local Anesthetic/Vasoconstrictor Precautions No information available to require special precautions

Effects on Dental Treatment No significant effects or complications reported

Effects on Bleeding No information available to require special precautions

Adverse Effects Frequency not defined.

Central nervous system: Ataxia, disorientation, sedation, excitement (paradoxical), dizziness, fever, headache, confusion, lightheadedness, nightmares, hallucinations, drowsiness, "hangover" effect

Dermatologic: Rash, urticaria

Gastrointestinal: Gastric irritation, nausea, vomiting, diarrhea, flatulence

Hematologic: Leukopenia, eosinophilia, acute intermittent porphyria

Miscellaneous: Physical and psychological dependence may occur with prolonged use of large doses

Dental Usual Dosage

Conscious sedation: Children: Oral: 50-75 mg/kg/dose 30-60 minutes prior to procedure; may repeat 30 minutes after initial dose if needed, to a total maximum dose of 120 mg/kg or 1 g total

Hypnotic: Adults: Oral: 500-1000 mg at bedtime or 30 minutes prior to procedure, not to exceed 2 g/24 hours

Sedation, anxiety: Oral:

Children: 5-15 mg/kg/dose every 8 hours (maximum: 500 mg/dose)

Adults: 250 mg 3 times/day

Dosage

Children:

Sedation or anxiety: Oral, rectal: 5-15 mg/kg/dose every 8 hours (maximum: 500 mg/dose)

Prior to EEG: Oral, rectal: 20-25 mg/kg/dose, 30-60 minutes prior to EEG; may repeat in 30 minutes to maximum of 100 mg/kg or 2 g total

Hypnotic: Oral, rectal: 20-40 mg/kg/dose up to a maximum of 50 mg/kg/24 hours or 1 g/dose or 2 g/24 hours

Conscious sedation: Oral: 50-75 mg/kg/dose 30-60 minutes prior to procedure; may repeat 30 minutes after initial dose if needed, to a total maximum dose of 120 mg/kg or 1 g total

Adults: Oral:

Sedation, anxiety: 250 mg 3 times/day

Hypnotic: 500-1000 mg at bedtime or 30 minutes prior to procedure, not to exceed 2 g/24 hours

Discontinuation: Withdraw gradually over 2 weeks if patient has been maintained on high doses for prolonged period of time. Do not stop drug abruptly; sudden withdrawal may result in delirium.

Dosing adjustment/comments in renal impairment: Cl$_{cr}$ <50 mL/minute: Avoid use

Hemodialysis: Dialyzable (50% to 100%); supplemental dose is not necessary

Dosing adjustment/comments in hepatic impairment: Avoid use in patients with severe hepatic impairment

Mechanism of Action Central nervous system depressant effects are due to its active metabolite trichloroethanol, mechanism unknown

Contraindications Hypersensitivity to chloral hydrate or any component of the formulation; hepatic or renal impairment; gastritis or ulcers; severe cardiac disease

Warnings/Precautions Hazardous agent - use appropriate precautions for handling and disposal (EPA, U-listed). Use with caution in patients with porphyria. Use with caution in neonates. Drug may accumulate with repeated use; prolonged use in neonates associated with hyperbilirubinemia. Tolerance to hypnotic effect develops, therefore, not recommended for use >2 weeks. Taper dosage to avoid withdrawal with prolonged use. Trichloroethanol (TCE), a metabolite of chloral hydrate, is a carcinogen in mice; there is no data in humans. Avoid use in older adults, potential risks exceed benefits; doses only 3 times the recommended dose are associated with overdosage potential; in addition, tolerance develops within 10 days of use (Beers Criteria). Recent interpretive guidelines from the Centers for Medicare and Medicaid Services (CMS) discourage the use of chloral hydrate in residents of long-term care facilities.

Drug Interactions

Metabolism/Transport Effects None known.

Avoid Concomitant Use

Avoid concomitant use of Chloral Hydrate with any of the following: Azelastine (Nasal); Furosemide; Paraldehyde; Sodium Oxybate

Increased Effect/Toxicity

Chloral Hydrate may increase the levels/effects of: Alcohol (Ethyl); Azelastine (Nasal); Buprenorphine; CNS Depressants; Highest Risk QTc-Prolonging Agents; Methotrimeprazine; Metyrosine; Mirtazapine; Moderate Risk QTc-Prolonging Agents; Paraldehyde; Pramipexole; ROPINIRole; Rotigotine; Selective Serotonin Reuptake Inhibitors; Sodium Oxybate; Vitamin K Antagonists; Zolpidem

The levels/effects of Chloral Hydrate may be increased by: Droperidol; Furosemide; HydrOXYzine; Magnesium Sulfate; Methotrimeprazine; Mifepristone; Perampanel

Decreased Effect

The levels/effects of Chloral Hydrate may be decreased by: Flumazenil

Ethanol/Nutrition/Herb Interactions

Ethanol: May increase CNS depression; monitor for increased effects with coadministration. Caution patients about effects.

Herb/Nutraceutical: Avoid valerian, St John's wort, kava kava, gotu kola (may increase CNS depression).

Pharmacodynamics/Kinetics

Onset of Action Time to sleep: 0.5-1 hour

Duration of Action 4-8 hours

Half-life Elimination Active metabolite: 8-11 hours

Pregnancy Risk Factor C

Pregnancy Considerations Animal reproduction studies have not been conducted. Chloral hydrate crosses the placenta and has been found in amniotic fluid and fetal blood.

Lactation Enters breast milk/not recommended

Controlled Substance C-IV

Chlorambucil (klor AM byoo sil)

Brand Names: U.S. Leukeran®

Brand Names: Canada Leukeran®

Pharmacologic Category Antineoplastic Agent, Alkylating Agent

Use Management of chronic lymphocytic leukemia (CLL), Hodgkin lymphoma, non-Hodgkin's lymphomas (NHL)

Canadian labeling: Additional uses (not in U.S. labeling): Management of Waldenström's macroglobulinemia

Unlabeled Use Treatment of nephrotic syndrome (steroid sensitive) in children; treatment of Waldenström's macroglobulinemia (unlabeled in U.S.)

Local Anesthetic/Vasoconstrictor Precautions No information available to require special precautions

Effects on Dental Treatment Key adverse event(s) related to dental treatment: Stomatitis.

Effects on Bleeding Thrombocytopenia has been reported to occur 1-2 weeks after a short course of therapy and persist for up to 4 weeks.

Adverse Effects Frequency not always defined.
Central nervous system: Agitation (rare), ataxia (rare), confusion (rare), drug fever, fever, focal/generalized seizure (rare), hallucinations (rare)
Dermatologic: Angioneurotic edema, erythema multiforme (rare), rash, skin hypersensitivity, Stevens-Johnson syndrome (rare), toxic epidermal necrolysis (rare), urticaria
Endocrine & metabolic: Amenorrhea, infertility, SIADH (rare)
Gastrointestinal: Diarrhea (infrequent), nausea (infrequent), oral ulceration (infrequent), vomiting (infrequent)
Genitourinary: Azoospermia, cystitis (sterile)
Hematologic: Neutropenia (onset: 3 weeks; recovery: 10 days after last dose), bone marrow failure (irreversible), bone marrow suppression, anemia, leukemia (secondary), leukopenia, lymphopenia, pancytopenia, thrombocytopenia
Hepatic: Hepatotoxicity, jaundice
Neuromuscular & skeletal: Flaccid paresis (rare), muscular twitching (rare), myoclonia (rare), peripheral neuropathy, tremor (rare)
Respiratory: Interstitial pneumonia, pulmonary fibrosis
Miscellaneous: Allergic reactions, malignancies (secondary)

General Dosage Range Dosage adjustment recommended in patients with hepatic impairment or who develop toxicities
Oral: *Adults:* 0.1-0.2 mg/kg/day for 3-6 weeks **or** 0.4 mg/kg intermittently, biweekly, or monthly (may increase by 0.1 mg/kg/dose)

Mechanism of Action Alkylating agent; interferes with DNA replication and RNA transcription by alkylation and cross-linking the strands of DNA

Pharmacodynamics/Kinetics
Half-life Elimination ~1.5 hours; Phenylacetic acid mustard: ~1.8 hours

Time to Peak Within 1 hour; Phenylacetic acid mustard: 1.2-2.6 hours

Pregnancy Risk Factor D

Pregnancy Considerations Animal reproduction studies have demonstrated teratogenicity. Chlorambucil crosses the human placenta. Following exposure during the first trimester, case reports have noted adverse renal effects (unilateral agenesis). Women of childbearing potential should avoid becoming pregnant while receiving treatment. **[U.S. Boxed Warning]: Affects human fertility; probably mutagenic and teratogenic as well;** chromosomal damage has been documented. Reversible and irreversible sterility (when administered to prepubertal and pubertal males), azoospermia (in adult males) and amenorrhea (in females) have been observed. Fibrosis, vasculitis and depletion of primordial follicles have been noted on autopsy of the ovaries.

Chloramphenicol (klor am FEN i kole)

Brand Names: Canada Chloromycetin®; Chloromycetin® Succinate; Diochloram®; Pentamycetin®
Pharmacologic Category Antibiotic, Miscellaneous
Use Treatment of serious infections due to organisms resistant to other less toxic antibiotics or when its penetrability into the site of infection is clinically superior to other antibiotics to which the organism is sensitive; useful in infections caused by *Bacteroides*, *H. influenzae*, *Neisseria meningitidis*, *Salmonella*, and *Rickettsia*; active against many vancomycin-resistant enterococci

Local Anesthetic/Vasoconstrictor Precautions No information available to require special precautions

Effects on Dental Treatment Key adverse event(s) related to dental treatment: Glossitis and stomatitis.

Effects on Bleeding Thrombocytopenia has been reported with short or long courses of therapy due to bone marrow suppression.

Adverse Effects Frequency not defined.
Central nervous system: Confusion, delirium, depression, fever, headache
Dermatologic: Angioedema, rash, urticaria
Gastrointestinal: Diarrhea, enterocolitis, glossitis, nausea, stomatitis, vomiting
Hematologic: Aplastic anemia, bone marrow suppression, granulocytopenia, hypoplastic anemia, pancytopenia, thrombocytopenia
Ocular: Optic neuritis
Miscellaneous: Anaphylaxis, hypersensitivity reactions, Gray syndrome

General Dosage Range I.V.: *Infants >30 days, Children, and Adults:* 50-100 mg/kg/day divided every 6 hours (maximum: 4 g/day)

Mechanism of Action Reversibly binds to 50S ribosomal subunits of susceptible organisms preventing amino acids from being transferred to growing peptide chains thus inhibiting protein synthesis

Pharmacodynamics/Kinetics
Half-life Elimination
Normal renal function:
Chloramphenicol: Adults: ~4 hours; Children 4-6 hours; Infants: Significantly prolonged
Chloramphenicol succinate: Adults: ~3 hours
End-stage renal disease: Chloramphenicol: 3-7 hours
Hepatic disease: Prolonged

Pregnancy Considerations Chloramphenicol crosses the placenta producing cord concentrations approaching maternal serum concentrations. An increased risk of teratogenic effects has not been identified for chloramphenicol and there have been no reports of fetal harm related to use of chloramphenicol in pregnancy. "Gray Syndrome" has occurred in premature infants and newborns receiving chloramphenicol. In most cases, chloramphenicol was started during the first 48 hours of life, but it has also occurred in older patients after high doses. Symptoms began after 3-4 days of therapy, starting with abdominal distention and continuing to progressive pallid cyanosis, vasomotor collapse, irregular respiration, and death within a few hours of symptom onset. Stopping therapy can reverse the process and allow complete recovery. There is one case report of an infant with gray baby syndrome after *in utero* exposure to a single maternal dose during labor, followed by a 10-fold overdose of chloramphenicol in the first day of life. The extent of the contribution of the single dose given during labor is unknown. The manufacturer recommends caution if used in a pregnant patient near term or during labor.

ChlordiazePOXIDE (klor dye az e POKS ide)

Pharmacologic Category Benzodiazepine

Use Management of anxiety disorder or for the short-term relief of symptoms of anxiety; withdrawal symptoms of acute alcoholism; preoperative apprehension and anxiety

Local Anesthetic/Vasoconstrictor Precautions No information available to require special precautions

Effects on Dental Treatment Key adverse event(s) related to dental treatment: Xerostomia (normal salivary flow resumes upon discontinuation).

Effects on Bleeding No information available to require special precautions

Adverse Effects

>10%:
Central nervous system: Drowsiness, fatigue, ataxia, lightheadedness, memory impairment, dysarthria, irritability
Dermatologic: Rash
Endocrine & metabolic: Libido decreased, menstrual disorders
Gastrointestinal: Xerostomia, salivation decreased, appetite increased or decreased, weight gain/loss
Genitourinary: Micturition difficulties

1% to 10%:
Cardiovascular: Hypotension
Central nervous system: Confusion, dizziness, disinhibition, akathisia
Dermatologic: Dermatitis
Endocrine & metabolic: Libido increased
Gastrointestinal: Salivation increased
Genitourinary: Sexual dysfunction, incontinence
Neuromuscular & skeletal: Rigidity, tremor, muscle cramps
Otic: Tinnitus
Respiratory: Nasal congestion

General Dosage Range Dosage adjustment recommended in patients with renal or hepatic impairment.

Oral:
Children ≥6 years: 10-30 mg/day in 2-4 divided doses
Adults: 15-100 mg/day in 3-4 divided doses
Elderly: 10-20 mg/day in 2-4 divided doses

Mechanism of Action Binds to stereospecific benzodiazepine receptors on the postsynaptic GABA neuron at several sites within the central nervous system, including the limbic system, reticular formation. Enhancement of the inhibitory effect of GABA on neuronal excitability results by increased neuronal membrane permeability to chloride ions. This shift in chloride ions results in hyperpolarization (a less excitable state) and stabilization.

Pharmacodynamics/Kinetics

Half-life Elimination 6.6-25 hours; End-stage renal disease: 5-30 hours; Cirrhosis: 30-63 hours

Time to Peak Serum: Within 2 hours

Pregnancy Considerations Adverse events were observed in some animal reproduction studies. Chlordiazepoxide crosses the human placenta and fetal serum concentrations are similar to those in the mother. Teratogenic effects have been observed with some

benzodiazepines (including chlordiazepoxide); however, additional studies are needed. The incidence of premature birth and low birth weights may be increased following maternal use of benzodiazepines; hypoglycemia and respiratory problems in the neonate may occur following exposure late in pregnancy. Neonatal withdrawal symptoms may occur within days to weeks after birth and "floppy infant syndrome" (which also includes withdrawal symptoms) has been reported with some benzodiazepines.

Controlled Substance C-IV

Chlorhexidine Gluconate
(klor HEKS i deen GLOO koe nate)

Related Information
Bacterial Infections *on page 1562*
Dentin Hypersensitivity, Acid Erosion, High Caries Index, Management of Alveolar Osteitis, and Xerostomia *on page 1582*
Management of Patients Undergoing Cancer Therapy *on page 1596*
Osteonecrosis of the Jaw *on page 1529*
Periodontal Diseases *on page 1570*
Ulcerative, Erosive, and Painful Oral Mucosal Disorders *on page 1578*

Related Sample Prescriptions
Antimicrobial Oral Rinses *on page 1613*

Brand Names: U.S. Avagard™ [OTC]; Bactoshield® CHG [OTC]; Betasept® [OTC]; ChloraPrep® Frepp® [OTC]; ChloraPrep® Sepp® [OTC]; ChloraPrep® [OTC]; Chlorascrub™ Maxi [OTC]; Chlorascrub™ [OTC]; Dyna-Hex® [OTC]; Hibiclens® [OTC]; Hibistat® [OTC]; Operand® Chlorhexidine Gluconate [OTC]; Peridex®; periochip®; PerioGard® [OTC]

Brand Names: Canada Hibidil® 1:2000; ORO-Clense; Peridex® Oral Rinse

Generic Availability (U.S.) Yes: Oral liquid

Pharmacologic Category Antibiotic, Oral Rinse; Antibiotic, Topical

Dental Use
Antibacterial dental rinse; chlorhexidine is active against gram-positive and gram-negative organisms, facultative anaerobes, aerobes, and yeast
Chip, for periodontal pocket insertion: Indicated as an adjunct to scaling and root planing procedures for reduction of pocket depth in patients with adult periodontitis; may be used as part of a periodontal maintenance program

Use Skin cleanser for line placement, skin wounds, preoperative skin preparation; germicidal hand rinse; antibacterial dental rinse. Chlorhexidine is active against gram-positive and gram-negative organisms, facultative anaerobes, aerobes, and yeast. Chip, for periodontal pocket insertion: Reduces pocket depth in patients with adult periodontitis

Orphan drug: Peridex®: Oral mucositis with cytoreductive therapy when used for patients undergoing bone marrow transplant

Local Anesthetic/Vasoconstrictor Precautions No information available to require special precautions

Effects on Dental Treatment Key adverse event(s) related to dental treatment: Increased tartar on teeth, altered taste perception, staining of oral surfaces (mucosa, teeth, dorsum of tongue), and oral/tongue irritation. Staining may be visible as soon as 1 week after therapy begins and is more pronounced when there is a heavy accumulation of unremoved plaque and when teeth fillings have rough surfaces. Stain does not have a clinically adverse effect but because removal may not be possible, patient with frontal restoration should be advised of the potential permanency of the stain.

Effects on Bleeding No information available to require special precautions

Adverse Effects

Oral:

>10%: Tartar on teeth increased, taste changes. Staining of oral surfaces (mucosa, teeth, dorsum of tongue) may be visible as soon as 1 week after therapy begins and is more pronounced when there is a heavy accumulation of unremoved plaque and when teeth fillings have rough surfaces. Stain does not have a clinically adverse effect but because removal may not be possible, patient with frontal restoration should be advised of the potential permanency of the stain.

1% to 10%: Gastrointestinal: Tongue irritation, oral irritation

Topical: Skin erythema and roughness, dryness, sensitization, allergic reactions

Dental Usual Dosage Adults:

Oral rinse (Peridex®, PerioGard®):

Floss and brush teeth, completely rinse toothpaste from mouth and swish 15 mL (one capful) undiluted oral rinse around in mouth for 30 seconds, then expectorate. Caution patient not to swallow the medicine and instruct not to eat for 2-3 hours after treatment (cap on bottle measures 15 mL).

Treatment of gingivitis: Oral prophylaxis: Swish for 30 seconds with 15 mL chlorhexidine, then expectorate; repeat twice daily (morning and evening). Patient should have a re-evaluation followed by a dental prophylaxis every 6 months.

Periodontal chip: One chip is inserted into a periodontal pocket with a probing pocket depth ≥5 mm. Up to 8 chips may be inserted in a single visit. Treatment is recommended every 3 months in pockets with a remaining depth ≥5 mm. If dislodgment occurs 7 days or more after placement, the subject is considered to have had the full course of treatment. If dislodgment occurs within 48 hours, a new chip should be inserted. The chip biodegrades completely and does not need to be removed. Patients should avoid dental floss at the site of periochip® insertion for 10 days after placement because flossing might dislodge the chip.

Insertion of periodontal chip: Pocket should be isolated and surrounding area dried prior to chip insertion. The chip should be grasped using forceps with the rounded edges away from the forceps. The chip should be inserted into the periodontal pocket to its maximum depth. It may be maneuvered into position using the tips of the forceps or a flat instrument.

Dosage Adults:

Oral rinse (Peridex®, PerioGard®):

Floss and brush teeth, completely rinse toothpaste from mouth and swish 15 mL (one capful) undiluted oral rinse around in mouth for 30 seconds, then expectorate. Caution patient not to swallow the medicine and instruct not to eat for 2-3 hours after treatment (cap on bottle measures 15 mL).

Treatment of gingivitis: Oral prophylaxis: Swish for 30 seconds with 15 mL chlorhexidine, then expectorate; repeat twice daily (morning and evening). Patient should have a re-evaluation followed by a dental prophylaxis every 6 months.

Periodontal chip: One chip is inserted into a periodontal pocket with a probing pocket depth ≥5 mm. Up to 8 chips may be inserted in a single visit. Treatment is recommended every 3 months in pockets with a remaining depth ≥5 mm. If dislodgment occurs 7 days or more after placement, the subject is considered to have had the full course of treatment. If dislodgment occurs within 48 hours, a new chip should be inserted. The chip biodegrades completely and does not need to be removed. Patients should avoid dental floss at the site of periochip® insertion for 10 days after placement because flossing might dislodge the chip.

Insertion of periodontal chip: Pocket should be isolated and surrounding area dried prior to chip insertion. The chip should be grasped using forceps with the rounded edges away from the forceps. The chip should be inserted into the periodontal pocket to its maximum depth. It may be maneuvered into position using the tips of the forceps or a flat instrument.

Cleanser:

Surgical scrub: Scrub 3 minutes and rinse thoroughly, wash for an additional 3 minutes

Hand sanitizer (Avagard™): Dispense 1 pumpful in palm of one hand; dip fingertips of opposite hand into solution and work it under nails. Spread remainder evenly over hand and just above elbow, covering all surfaces. Repeat on other hand. Dispense another pumpful in each hand and reapply to each hand up to the wrist. Allow to dry before gloving.

Hand wash: Wash for 15 seconds and rinse

Hand rinse: Rub 15 seconds and rinse

Mechanism of Action The bactericidal effect of chlorhexidine is a result of the binding of this cationic molecule to negatively charged bacterial cell walls and extramicrobial complexes. At low concentrations, this causes an alteration of bacterial cell osmotic equilibrium and leakage of potassium and phosphorous resulting in a bacteriostatic effect. At high concentrations of chlorhexidine, the cytoplasmic contents of the bacterial cell precipitate and result in cell death.

Contraindications Hypersensitivity to chlorhexidine gluconate or any component of the formulation

Warnings/Precautions

Oral: Staining of oral surfaces (mucosa, teeth, tooth restorations, dorsum of tongue) may occur; may be visible as soon as 1 week after therapy begins and is more pronounced when there is a heavy accumulation of unremoved plaque and when teeth fillings have rough surfaces. Stain does not have a clinically adverse effect, but because removal may not be possible, patient with frontal restoration should be advised of the potential permanency of the stain.

Topical: For topical use only. Avoid application over large surfaces or into open wounds. Keep out of eyes and ears. May stain fabric. There have been case reports of anaphylaxis following chlorhexidine disinfection. Not for preoperative preparation of face or head; avoid contact with meninges (do not use on lumbar puncture sites). Solutions may be flammable (contain isopropyl alcohol); avoid exposure to open flame and/or ignition source (eg, electrocautery) until completely dry; avoid application to hairy areas which may significantly delay drying time. Avoid use in children <2 months of age due to increased absorption and/or irritation.

Drug Interactions

Metabolism/Transport Effects None known.

Avoid Concomitant Use There are no known interactions where it is recommended to avoid concomitant use.

Increased Effect/Toxicity There are no known significant interactions involving an increase in effect.

◀ **Decreased Effect** There are no known significant interactions involving a decrease in effect.

Pharmacodynamics/Kinetics

Duration of Action Avagard™: Topical hand sanitizer: Duration of antimicrobial protection: 6 hours

Time to Peak Peridex®, PerioGard®: Plasma: Detectable levels not present after 12 hours

Pregnancy Risk Factor B/C (manufacturer specific)

Pregnancy Considerations Adverse events have not been observed in animal reproduction studies following use of the oral rinse; use of periodontal chip has not been studied. Chlorhexidine gluconate oral rinse is poorly absorbed from the gastrointestinal tract.

Lactation Excretion in breast milk unknown/use caution

Dosage Forms

Chip, for periodontal pocket insertion:
periochip®: 2.5 mg (20s)

Liquid, oral: 0.12% (15 mL, 473 mL, 475 mL, 480 mL)
Peridex®: 0.12% (118 mL, 473 mL, 1893 mL)
PerioGard® [OTC]: 0.12% (480 mL)

Liquid, topical:
Betasept® [OTC]: 4% (118 mL, 237 mL, 473 mL, 946 mL, 3840 mL)
Dyna-Hex® [OTC]: 2% (120 mL, 480 mL, 960 mL, 3840 mL); 4% (120 mL, 240 mL, 480 mL, 960 mL, 3840 mL)
Hibiclens® [OTC]: 4% (15 mL, 118 mL, 236 mL, 473 mL, 946 mL, 3840 mL)
Operand® Chlorhexidine Gluconate [OTC]: 4% (118 mL, 237 mL, 472 mL, 946 mL, 3785 mL)

Lotion, topical:
Avagard™ [OTC]: 1% (500 mL)

Solution, topical:
Bactoshield® CHG [OTC]: 2% (120 mL, 480 mL, 750 mL, 960 mL, 3840 mL); 4% (120 mL, 473 mL, 960 mL, 3840 mL)

Sponge, topical:
ChloraPrep® [OTC]: 2% (25s); 2% (25s); 2% (25s); 2% (25s); 2% (25s); 2% (25s); 2% (25s); 2% (25s)
ChloraPrep® Frepp® [OTC]: 2% (20s)
ChloraPrep® Sepp® [OTC]: 2% (200s)

Sponge/Brush, topical:
Bactoshield® CHG [OTC]: 4% (300s)

Swab, topical:
Chlorascrub™ [OTC]: 3.15% (100s)

Swabsticks, topical:
ChloraPrep® [OTC]: 2% (48s, 120s)
Chlorascrub™ [OTC]: 3.15% (50s)
Chlorascrub™ Maxi [OTC]: 3.15% (30s)

Wipe, topical:
Hibistat® [OTC]: 0.5% (50s)

References

Gonzales JR, Harnack L, Schmitt-Corsitto G, et al, "A Novel Approach to the Use of Subgingival Controlled-Release Chlorhexidine Delivery in Chronic Periodontitis: A Randomized Clinical Trial," *J Periodontol*, 2011, 82(8):1131-9.
Johnson BT, "Uses of Chlorhexidine in Dentistry," *Gen Dent*, 1995, 43 (2):126-32, 134-40.
Noiri Y, Okami Y, Narimatsu M, et al, "Effects of Chlorhexidine, Minocycline, and Metronidazole on Porphyromonas Gingivalis Strain 381 in Biofilms," *J Periodontol*, 2003, 74(11):1647-51.
Reddy MS, Jeffcoat MK, Geurs NC, et al, "Efficacy of Controlled-Release Subgingival Chlorhexidine to Enhance Periodontal Regeneration," *J Periodontol*, 2003, 74(4):411-9.
Soskolne WA, Proskin HM, and Stabholz A, "Probing Depth Changes Following 2 Years of Periodontal Maintenance Therapy Including Adjunctive Controlled Release of Chlorhexidine," *J Periodontol*, 2003, 74(4):420-7.

Chlorophyll (KLOR oh fil)

Brand Names: U.S. Nullo® [OTC]
Pharmacologic Category Gastrointestinal Agent, Miscellaneous

Use Control fecal odors in colostomy or ileostomy

Local Anesthetic/Vasoconstrictor Precautions No information available to require special precautions

Effects on Dental Treatment No significant effects or complications reported

Effects on Bleeding No information available to require special precautions

Adverse Effects Frequency not defined: Gastrointestinal: Diarrhea, green stools, abdominal cramping

General Dosage Range

Oral: *Children >12 years and Adults:* 100-200 mg/day in divided doses (maximum: 300 mg/day)

Ostomy: *Children >12 years and Adults:* Place 1-2 tablets in empty pouch each time it is reused or changed

Chloroprocaine (klor oh PROE kane)

Related Information
Oral Pain *on page 1558*

Brand Names: U.S. Nesacaine®; Nesacaine®-MPF
Brand Names: Canada Nesacaine®-CE
Pharmacologic Category Local Anesthetic

Use Infiltration anesthesia, peripheral nerve block, epidural anesthesia

Local Anesthetic/Vasoconstrictor Precautions No information available to require special precautions

Effects on Dental Treatment No significant effects or complications reported

Effects on Bleeding No information available to require special precautions

Adverse Effects Frequency not always defined.
Cardiovascular: Bradycardia, cardiac arrest, hypotension, ventricular arrhythmia
Central nervous system: Anxiety, dizziness, restlessness, tinnitus, unconsciousness
Dermatologic: Angioneurotic edema, erythema, pruritus, urticaria
Neuromuscular & skeletal: Chondrolysis (continuous intra-articular administration)
Ocular: Blurred vision
Respiratory: Respiratory arrest
Miscellaneous: Allergic reactions, anaphylactoid reactions

General Dosage Range

Caudal block: *Adults:* Preservative-free: 2% or 3%: 15-25 mL; may repeat at 40-60 minute intervals

Infiltration and peripheral nerve block:
Children >3 years: Infiltration: Concentrations of 0.5-1% (maximum without epinephrine: 11 mg/kg); Nerve block: Concentrations of 1% to 1.5% (maximum without epinephrine: 11 mg/kg)
Adults: Dosage varies greatly depending on indication

Lumbar epidural block: *Adults:* Preservative-free: 2% or 3%: 2-2.5 mL per segment; Usual total volume: 15-25 mL, may repeat with doses that are 2-6 mL less than total initial dose every 40-50 minutes

Mechanism of Action Chloroprocaine HCl is benzoic acid, 4-amino-2-chloro-2-(diethylamino) ethyl ester monohydrochloride. Chloroprocaine is an ester-type local anesthetic, which stabilizes the neuronal membranes and prevents initiation and transmission of nerve impulses thereby affecting local anesthetic actions. Local anesthetics including chloroprocaine, reversibly prevent generation and conduction of electrical impulses in neurons by decreasing the transient increase in permeability to sodium. The differential sensitivity generally depends on the size of the fiber; small fibers are more sensitive than larger fibers and require a longer period for recovery. Sensory pain fibers are usually blocked first, followed by fibers that transmit sensations of temperature, touch, and deep pressure. High concentrations block sympathetic somatic sensory and somatic motor fibers. The spread of anesthesia depends upon the distribution of the solution. This is primarily dependent on the volume of drug injected.

Pharmacodynamics/Kinetics

Onset of Action 6-12 minutes

Duration of Action 30-60 minutes

Half-life Elimination *In vitro,* plasma: Adults: 21 seconds; Neonates: 43 seconds

Pregnancy Risk Factor C

Pregnancy Considerations Animal reproduction studies have not been conducted. Local anesthetics rapidly cross the placenta and may cause varying degrees of maternal, fetal, and neonatal toxicity. Close maternal and fetal monitoring (heart rate and electronic fetal monitoring advised) are required during obstetrical use. Maternal hypotension has resulted from regional anesthesia. Positioning the patient on her left side and elevating the legs may help. Epidural, paracervical, or pudendal anesthesia may alter the forces of parturition through changes in uterine contractility or maternal expulsive efforts. The use of some local anesthetic drugs during labor and delivery may diminish muscle strength and tone for the first day or two of life. Administration as a paracervical block is not recommended with toxemia of pregnancy, fetal distress, or prematurity. Administration of a paracervical block early in pregnancy has resulted in maternal seizures and cardiovascular collapse. Fetal bradycardia and acidosis also have been reported. Fetal depression has occurred following unintended fetal intracranial injection while administering a paracervical and/or pudendal block.

Chloroquine (KLOR oh kwin)

Related Information

Clinical Risk Related to Drugs Prolonging QT Interval *on page 1510*

Brand Names: U.S. Aralen®

Brand Names: Canada Aralen®; Novo-Chloroquine

Pharmacologic Category Aminoquinoline (Antimalarial)

Use Suppression/chemoprophylaxis or treatment of acute malaria due to susceptible *Plasmodium malariae, P. vivax, P. ovale, P. falciparum*; extraintestinal amebiasis

Unlabeled Use Rheumatoid arthritis; discoid lupus erythematosus

Local Anesthetic/Vasoconstrictor Precautions Chloroquine is one of the drugs confirmed to prolong the QT interval and is accepted as having a risk of causing torsade de pointes. The risk of drug-induced torsade de pointes is extremely low when a single QT interval prolonging drug is prescribed. In terms of epinephrine, it is not known what effect vasoconstrictors in the local anesthetic regimen will have in patients with a known history of congenital prolonged QT interval or in patients taking any medication that prolongs the QT interval. Until more information is obtained, it is suggested that the clinician consult with the physician prior to the use of a vasoconstrictor in suspected patients, and that the vasoconstrictor (epinephrine, mepivacaine and levonordefrin [Carbocaine® 2% with Neo-Cobefrin®]) be used with caution.

Effects on Dental Treatment Key adverse event(s) related to dental treatment: Stomatitis.

Effects on Bleeding Thrombocytopenia has been reported.

Adverse Effects Frequency not defined.

Cardiovascular: Cardiomyopathy, ECG changes (rare; including prolonged QRS and QT_c intervals), hypotension (rare), torsade de pointes (rare)

Central nervous system: Agitation, anxiety, confusion, delirium, depression, hallucinations, headache, insomnia, personality changes, polyneuritis, psychosis,

Dermatologic: Alopecia, erythema multiforme (rare), exfoliative dermatitis (rare), hair bleaching, lichen planus eruptions, photosensitivity, pleomorphic skin eruptions, pruritus, skin/mucosal pigmentary changes (blue-black), Stevens-Johnson syndrome (rare), toxic epidermal necrolysis (rare), urticaria

Gastrointestinal: Abdominal cramps, anorexia, diarrhea, nausea, vomiting

Hematologic: Rare cases of agranulocytosis (reversible), aplastic anemia, neutropenia, pancytopenia, thrombocytopenia

Hepatic: Hepatitis, liver enzymes increased

Neuromuscular & skeletal: Depression of deep tendon reflexes, myopathy, neuromyopathy, proximal muscle atrophy

Ocular: Accommodation disturbances, blurred vision, corneal opacities (reversible), nyctalopia, retinopathy (including irreversible changes in some patients long-term or high-dose therapy), visual field defects

Otic: Hearing reduced (risk increased in patients with pre-existing auditory damage), nerve deafness, tinnitus

Miscellaneous: Anaphylaxis, angioedema

General Dosage Range Dosage adjustment recommended in patients with renal impairment

Oral: *Children and Adults:* Dosage varies greatly depending on indication

Mechanism of Action Binds to and inhibits DNA and RNA polymerase; interferes with metabolism and hemoglobin utilization by parasites; inhibits prostaglandin effects; chloroquine concentrates within parasite acid vesicles and raises internal pH resulting in inhibition of parasite growth; may involve aggregates of ferriprotoporphyrin IX acting as chloroquine receptors causing membrane damage; may also interfere with nucleoprotein synthesis

Pharmacodynamics/Kinetics

Duration of Action Small amounts may be present in urine months following discontinuation of therapy

Half-life Elimination 3-5 days

Time to Peak Serum: 1-2 hours

Pregnancy Considerations There are no adequate and well-controlled studies using chloroquine during pregnancy. However, based on clinical experience and because malaria infection in pregnant women may be more severe than in nonpregnant women, chloroquine prophylaxis may be considered in areas of chloroquine-sensitive *P. falciparum* malaria. Pregnant women should be advised not to travel to areas of *P. falciparum* resistance to chloroquine. Consult current CDC guidelines for the treatment of malaria during pregnancy.

Dental Comment Chloroquine is known to prolong the QT interval. The QT interval is measured as the time and distance between the Q point of the QRS complex and the end of the T wave in the ECG tracing. After adjustment for heart rate, the QT interval is defined as prolonged if it is more than 450 msec in men and 460 msec in women. A long QT syndrome was first described in the 1950s and 60s as a congenital syndrome involving QT interval prolongation and syncope and sudden death. Some of the congenital long QT syndromes were characterized by a peculiar electrocardiographic appearance of the QRS complex involving a premature atria beat followed by a pause, then a subsequent sinus beat showing marked QT prolongation and deformity. This type of cardiac arrhythmia was originally termed "torsade de pointes" (translated from the French as "twisting of the points"). Chloroquine is considered as having a risk of causing torsade de pointes. Since it is not known what effect vasoconstrictors in the local anesthetic regimen will have in patients with a known history of congenital prolonged QT interval or in patients taking any medication that prolongs the QT interval, a medical consult is suggested.

Chlorothiazide (klor oh THYE a zide)

Related Information
Cardiovascular Diseases *on page 1492*
Brand Names: U.S. Diuril®; Sodium Diuril®
Brand Names: Canada Diuril®
Pharmacologic Category Diuretic, Thiazide
Use Management of hypertension; adjunctive treatment of edema
Local Anesthetic/Vasoconstrictor Precautions No information available to require special precautions
Effects on Dental Treatment Key adverse event(s) related to dental treatment: Orthostatic hypotension.
Effects on Bleeding No information available to require special precautions
Adverse Effects Frequency not defined.
Cardiovascular: Hypotension, orthostatic hypotension, necrotizing angiitis
Central nervous system: Dizziness, fever, headache, restlessness, vertigo
Dermatologic: Alopecia, erythema multiforme, exfoliative dermatitis, photosensitivity, purpura, rash, Stevens-Johnson syndrome, toxic epidermal necrolysis, urticaria
Endocrine & metabolic: Cholesterol increased, hypercalcemia, hyperglycemia, hyperuricemia, hypochloremic alkalosis, hypokalemia, hyponatremia, hypomagnesemia, triglycerides increased
Gastrointestinal: Abdominal cramping, anorexia, constipation, diarrhea, gastric irritation, nausea, pancreatitis, sialadenitis, vomiting
Genitourinary: Impotence
Hematologic: Agranulocytosis, aplastic anemia, hemolytic anemia, leukopenia, thrombocytopenia
Hepatic: Jaundice
Neuromuscular & skeletal: Muscle spasm, paresthesia, weakness
Ocular: Blurred vision, xanthopsia
Renal: Glycosuria, hematuria (I.V.), interstitial nephritis, renal failure, renal dysfunction
Respiratory: Pneumonitis, pulmonary edema, respiratory distress
Miscellaneous: Anaphylactic reactions, systemic lupus erythematosus
General Dosage Range
I.V.: *Adults:* 250-1000 mg once or twice daily (maximum: 1000 mg daily)
Oral:
Children <6 months: 10-30 mg/kg/day in 2 divided doses (maximum: 375 mg daily)
Children ≥6 months: 10-20 mg/kg/day in 1-2 divided doses (maximum: 375 mg daily)

Adults: 250-2000 mg daily in 1-2 divided doses (maximum: 1000 mg daily [CHF])
Mechanism of Action Inhibits sodium and chloride reabsorption in the distal tubules causing increased excretion of sodium, chloride, and water resulting in diuresis. Loss of potassium, hydrogen ions, magnesium, phosphate, and bicarbonate also occurs.
Pharmacodynamics/Kinetics
Onset of Action Diuresis: Oral: Within 2 hours; I.V.: 15 minutes; Peak effect: Oral: ~4 hours; I.V.: 30 minutes
Duration of Action Diuretic action: Oral: ~6-12 hours
Half-life Elimination 45-120 minutes
Pregnancy Risk Factor C
Pregnancy Considerations Adverse events were not observed in animal reproduction studies; however, studies were not complete. Chlorothiazide crosses the placenta and is found in cord blood. Maternal use may cause may cause fetal or neonatal jaundice, thrombocytopenia, or other adverse events observed in adults. Use of thiazide diuretics during normal pregnancies is not appropriate; use may be considered when edema is due to pathologic causes (as in the nonpregnant patient); monitor.

Chlorpheniramine (klor fen IR a meen)

Related Information
Bacterial Infections *on page 1562*
Related Sample Prescriptions
Sinus Infection Treatment *on page 1611*
Brand Names: U.S. Aller-chlor® [OTC]; Allergy Relief [OTC]; Chlor Hist [OTC]; Chlor-Trimeton® Allergy [OTC]; Chlorphen [OTC]; Chlorphen-12™ [OTC]; ED Chlorped Jr [OTC]; Ed ChlorPed [OTC]; Ed-Chlortan [OTC]
Brand Names: Canada Chlor-Tripolon®; Novo-Pheniram
Generic Availability (U.S.) Yes
Pharmacologic Category Alkylamine Derivative; Histamine H_1 Antagonist; Histamine H_1 Antagonist, First Generation
Dental Use Treatment of histamine-induced allergic symptoms
Use Perennial and seasonal allergic rhinitis and other allergic symptoms including urticaria
Local Anesthetic/Vasoconstrictor Precautions No information available to require special precautions
Effects on Dental Treatment Key adverse event(s) related to dental treatment: Xerostomia (normal salivary flow resumes upon discontinuation). Chronic use of antihistamines will inhibit salivary flow, particularly in elderly patients; this may contribute to periodontal disease and oral discomfort.
Effects on Bleeding No information available to require special precautions
Adverse Effects
>10%:
Central nervous system: Slight to moderate drowsiness
Respiratory: Thickening of bronchial secretions
1% to 10%:
Central nervous system: Headache, excitability, fatigue, nervousness, dizziness
Gastrointestinal: Nausea, xerostomia, diarrhea, abdominal pain, appetite increase, weight gain
Genitourinary: Urinary retention

Neuromuscular & skeletal: Arthralgia, weakness

Ocular: Diplopia

Renal: Polyuria

Respiratory: Pharyngitis

Dosage Oral: **Chlorpheniramine maleate:**

Children: Immediate release:

2-5 years: 1 mg every 4-6 hours; do not exceed 6 mg/ 24 hours

6-11 years: 2 mg every 4-6 hours; do not exceed 12 mg/24 hours

Children ≥12 years and Adults:

Immediate release: 4 mg every 4-6 hours; do not exceed 24 mg/24 hours

Extended release: 12 mg every 12 hours; do not exceed 24 mg/24 hours

Mechanism of Action Competes with histamine for H_1-receptor sites on effector cells in the gastrointestinal tract, blood vessels, and respiratory tract

Contraindications Hypersensitivity to chlorpheniramine maleate or any component of the formulation; narrow-angle glaucoma; bladder neck obstruction; symptomatic prostate hypertrophy; during acute asthmatic attacks; stenosing peptic ulcer; pyloroduodenal obstruction. Avoid use in premature and term newborns due to possible association with SIDS.

Warnings/Precautions Causes sedation, caution must be used in performing tasks which require alertness (eg, operating machinery or driving). Sedative effects of CNS depressants or ethanol are potentiated. Use with caution in patients with urinary tract obstruction, symptomatic prostatic hyperplasia, thyroid dysfunction, increased intraocular pressure, and cardiovascular disease (including hypertension and ischemic heart disease). In the elderly, avoid use of this potent anticholinergic agent due to increased risk of confusion, dry mouth, constipation, and other anticholinergic effects; clearance decreases in patients of advanced age (Beers Criteria). Antihistamines may cause excitation in young children. Not for OTC use in children <2 years of age.

Drug Interactions

Metabolism/Transport Effects Substrate of CYP2D6 (major), CYP3A4 (minor); **Note:** Assignment of Major/Minor substrate status based on clinically relevant drug interaction potential; **Inhibits** CYP2D6 (weak)

Avoid Concomitant Use

Avoid concomitant use of Chlorpheniramine with any of the following: Aclidinium; Azelastine (Nasal); Ipratropium (Oral Inhalation); Paraldehyde; Tiotropium

Increased Effect/Toxicity

Chlorpheniramine may increase the levels/effects of: Alcohol (Ethyl); Anticholinergics; ARIPiprazole; Azelastine (Nasal); Buprenorphine; CNS Depressants; Methotrimeprazine; Metyrosine; Mirtazapine; Paraldehyde; Pramipexole; ROPINIRole; Rotigotine; Selective Serotonin Reuptake Inhibitors; Tiotropium; Zolpidem

The levels/effects of Chlorpheniramine may be increased by: Abiraterone Acetate; Aclidinium; CYP2D6 Inhibitors (Moderate); CYP2D6 Inhibitors (Strong); Darunavir; Droperidol; HydrOXYzine; Ipratropium (Oral Inhalation); Magnesium Sulfate; Methotrimeprazine; Perampanel; Pramlintide; Sodium Oxybate

Decreased Effect

Chlorpheniramine may decrease the levels/effects of: Acetylcholinesterase Inhibitors (Central); Benzylpenicilloyl Polylysine; Betahistine; Hyaluronidase

The levels/effects of Chlorpheniramine may be decreased by: Acetylcholinesterase Inhibitors (Central); Amphetamines; Peginterferon Alfa-2b

Ethanol/Nutrition/Herb Interactions Ethanol: May increase CNS depression; monitor for increased effects with coadministration. Caution patients about effects.

Dietary Considerations May be taken with food or water. Some products may contain phenylalanine.

Pharmacodynamics/Kinetics

Half-life Elimination Serum: Children: 10-13 hours; Adults: 14-24 hours (Paton, 1985)

Time to Peak 2-3 hours (Sharma, 2003)

Pregnancy Considerations Maternal chlorpheniramine use has generally not resulted in an increased risk of birth defects. Antihistamines are recommended for the treatment of rhinitis, urticaria, and pruritus with rash in pregnant women (although second generation antihistamines may be preferred). Antihistamines are not recommended for treatment of pruritus associated with intrahepatic cholestasis in pregnancy.

Breast-Feeding Considerations Information specific to the use of chlorpheniramine is limited. Antihistamines may decrease maternal serum prolactin concentrations when administered prior to the establishment of nursing.

Dosage Forms

Liquid, oral:

Ed ChlorPed [OTC]: 2 mg/mL (60 mL)

Syrup, oral:

Aller-chlor® [OTC]: 2 mg/5 mL (118 mL)

ED Chlorped Jr [OTC]: 2 mg/5 mL (473 mL)

Tablet, oral: 4 mg

Aller-chlor® [OTC]: 4 mg

Allergy Relief [OTC]: 4 mg

Chlor Hist [OTC]: 4 mg

Chlor-Trimeton® Allergy [OTC]: 4 mg

Chlorphen [OTC]: 4 mg

Ed-Chlortan [OTC]: 4 mg

Tablet, extended release, oral:

Chlorphen-12™ [OTC]: 12 mg

Chlorpheniramine and Acetaminophen

(klor fen IR a meen & a seet a MIN oh fen)

Related Information

Acetaminophen *on page 27*

Chlorpheniramine *on page 292*

Brand Names: U.S. Coricidin HBP® Cold and Flu [OTC]

Pharmacologic Category Alkylamine Derivative; Analgesic, Miscellaneous; Histamine H_1 Antagonist; Histamine H_1 Antagonist, First Generation

Use Symptomatic relief of congestion, headache, aches and pains of colds and flu

Local Anesthetic/Vasoconstrictor Precautions No information available to require special precautions

Effects on Dental Treatment Key adverse event(s) related to dental treatment: Chronic use of antihistamines will inhibit salivary flow, particularly in elderly patients; this may contribute to periodontal disease and oral discomfort. See Dental Comment.

Effects on Bleeding No information available to require special precautions

Adverse Effects See individual agents.

General Dosage Range Oral: *Adults:* 2 tablets every 4 hours

◀ **Dental Comment** Hepatotoxicity caused by acetaminophen is potentiated by chronic alcohol consumption. People who are taking acetaminophen, even at therapeutic doses, and consume alcohol are at risk of developing hepatotoxicity.

Acetaminophen may increase the levels and enhance the anticoagulant effects of vitamin K antagonists acenocoumarol and warfarin (Coumadin®). Studies have reported that acetaminophen has increased the INR in warfarin treated patients with daily acetaminophen doses as low as 2 g, particularly when taking acetaminophen for >1 week (Antlitz, 1968; Boeijinga, 1982; Gebauer, 2003; Hylek, 1998; Rubin, 1984). In addition, case reports of bleeding as a result of increased INR have been published (Bagheri, 1999; Bartle, 1991). There is no known mechanism of the interaction; furthermore, some studies have failed to demonstrate this interaction (Gadisseur, 2003; Kwan, 1995; van den Bemt, 2002). In terms of risk, the data suggest that acetaminophen and warfarin could interact in some clinically significant manner but that the benefits of concomitant use of acetaminophen for pain control in dental patients taking warfarin usually outweigh the risks. An appropriate monitoring plan should be in place to identify potential negative effects and dosage adjustments may be necessary in a minority of patients. The interaction may be more likely to occur with daily acetaminophen doses of >1.3 g for >1 week.

There are no reports of acetaminophen interacting with antiplatelet drugs such as aspirin, clopidogrel (Plavix®), or prasugrel (Effient™). Also, there are no reports of acetaminophen in combination with hydrocodone, codeine, or oxycodone interacting with warfarin (Coumadin®).

Chlorpheniramine and Phenylephrine
(klor fen IR a meen & fen il EF rin)

Related Information
Chlorpheniramine *on page 292*
Phenylephrine (Systemic) *on page 1087*
Brand Names: U.S. Ed ChlorPed D [OTC]; Ed-A-Hist™ [OTC]; LoHist [OTC]; Maxichlor PEH [OTC]; nasohist™ [OTC]; NoHist LQ [OTC]; NoHist [OTC] [DSC]; Sudafed PE® Sinus + Allergy [OTC]; Triaminic® Children's Cold & Allergy [OTC]; Virdec [OTC]
Pharmacologic Category Alkylamine Derivative; Alpha-Adrenergic Agonist; Decongestant; Histamine H₁ Antagonist; Histamine H₁ Antagonist, First Generation
Use Temporary relief of upper respiratory conditions such as nasal congestion, runny nose, and sneezing due to the common cold, hay fever, or allergic or vasomotor rhinitis
Local Anesthetic/Vasoconstrictor Precautions Use with caution since phenylephrine is a sympathomimetic amine which could interact with epinephrine to cause a pressor response
Effects on Dental Treatment Key adverse event(s) related to dental treatment:
Chlorpheniramine: Prolonged use will cause significant xerostomia (normal salivary flow resumes upon discontinuation).
Phenylephrine: Up to 10% of patients could experience tachycardia, palpitations, and xerostomia (prolonged use worsens); use vasoconstrictor with caution.
Effects on Bleeding No information available to require special precautions

Adverse Effects See individual agents.
General Dosage Range Oral: *Children ≥2 years and Adults:* Dosage varies greatly depending on product

Chlorpheniramine and Pseudoephedrine
(klor fen IR a meen & soo doe e FED rin)

Related Information
Chlorpheniramine *on page 292*
Pseudoephedrine *on page 1159*
Brand Names: U.S. Dicel® Chewable [OTC]; LoHist-D [OTC]; Maxichlor PSE [OTC]; Neutrahist Pediatric [OTC]; SudoGest™ Sinus & Allergy [OTC]
Brand Names: Canada Triaminic® Cold & Allergy
Pharmacologic Category Alkylamine Derivative; Alpha/Beta Agonist; Decongestant; Histamine H₁ Antagonist; Histamine H₁ Antagonist, First Generation
Use Relief of nasal congestion associated with the common cold, hay fever, allergic rhinitis, and other allergies
Local Anesthetic/Vasoconstrictor Precautions Use with caution since pseudoephedrine is a sympathomimetic amine which could interact with epinephrine to cause a pressor response
Effects on Dental Treatment Key adverse event(s) related to dental treatment:
Chlorpheniramine: Prolonged use will cause significant xerostomia (normal salivary flow resumes upon discontinuation).
Pseudoephedrine: Xerostomia (prolonged use worsens; normal salivary flow resumes upon discontinuation).
Effects on Bleeding No information available to require special precautions
Adverse Effects See individual agents.
General Dosage Range Oral: *Children ≥6 years and Adults:* Dosage varies greatly depending on product.
Mechanism of Action
Chlorpheniramine competes with histamine for H₁-receptor sites on effector cells in the gastrointestinal tract, blood vessels, and respiratory tract.
Pseudoephedrine is a sympathomimetic amine and isomer of ephedrine; acts as a decongestant in respiratory tract mucous membranes with less vasoconstrictor action than ephedrine in normotensive individuals.
Pregnancy Risk Factor C
Pregnancy Considerations Reproduction studies have not been conducted with this combination product. See individual agents.

Chlorpheniramine, Phenylephrine, and Dextromethorphan
(klor fen IR a meen, fen il EF rin, & deks troe meth OR fan)

Related Information
Chlorpheniramine *on page 292*
Dextromethorphan *on page 406*
Phenylephrine (Systemic) *on page 1087*
Brand Names: U.S. Cardec™ DM [OTC]; Corfen-DM [OTC]; De-Chlor DM [OTC]; Ed A-Hist DM [OTC]; EndaCof [OTC]; Father John's® Plus [OTC]; Maxichlor PEH DM [OTC] [DSC]; nasohist™ DM pediatric [OTC]; Neo DM [OTC]; NoHist DM [OTC]; PE-Hist-DM [OTC]; Virdec DM [OTC]

Pharmacologic Category Alkylamine Derivative; Alpha-Adrenergic Agonist; Antitussive; Decongestant; Histamine H₁ Antagonist; Histamine H₁ Antagonist, First Generation

Use Temporary relief of cough and upper respiratory symptoms associated with allergies or the common cold

Local Anesthetic/Vasoconstrictor Precautions
Chlorpheniramine, Dextromethorphan: No information available to require special precautions

Phenylephrine: Use with caution since phenylephrine is a sympathomimetic amine which could interact with epinephrine to cause a pressor response

Effects on Dental Treatment Key adverse event(s) related to dental treatment:

Chlorpheniramine: Prolonged use will cause significant xerostomia (normal salivary flow resumes upon discontinuation).

Dextromethorphan: No significant effects or complications reported

Phenylephrine: Up to 10% of patients could experience tachycardia, palpitations, and xerostomia (prolonged use worsens); use vasoconstrictor with caution.

Effects on Bleeding No information available to require special precautions

Adverse Effects See individual agents.

General Dosage Range Oral: *Children ≥2 years and Adults:* Dosage varies greatly depending on product

Chlorpheniramine, Pseudoephedrine, and Codeine
(klor fen IR a meen, soo doe e FED rin, & KOE deen)

Related Information
Chlorpheniramine *on page 292*
Codeine *on page 344*
Pseudoephedrine *on page 1159*

Brand Names: U.S. Phenylhistine DH [OTC]; Tricode® AR

Pharmacologic Category Alkylamine Derivative; Alpha/Beta Agonist; Analgesic, Opioid; Antitussive; Decongestant; Histamine H₁ Antagonist; Histamine H₁ Antagonist, First Generation

Use Temporary relief of cough associated with minor throat or bronchial irritation or nasal congestion due to common cold, allergic rhinitis, or sinusitis

Local Anesthetic/Vasoconstrictor Precautions
Use with caution since pseudoephedrine is a sympathomimetic amine which could interact with epinephrine to cause a pressor response

Effects on Dental Treatment Key adverse event(s) related to dental treatment:
Chlorpheniramine: Significant xerostomia with prolonged use (normal salivary flow resumes upon discontinuation).
Pseudoephedrine: Xerostomia (normal salivary flow resumes upon discontinuation).

Effects on Bleeding No information available to require special precautions

Adverse Effects See individual agents.

General Dosage Range Oral:
Children 6-11 years: 5 mL every 4 hours (maximum: 20 mL/24 hours)
Children ≥12 years and Adults: 10 mL every 4 hours (maximum: 40 mL/24 hours)
Controlled Substance C-V

ChlorproMAZINE (klor PROE ma zeen)

Related Information
Clinical Risk Related to Drugs Prolonging QT Interval *on page 1510*
Brand Names: Canada Chlorpromazine Hydrochloride Inj; Teva-Chlorpromazine
Pharmacologic Category Antimanic Agent; Antipsychotic Agent, Typical, Phenothiazine
Use Management of psychotic disorders (control of mania, treatment of schizophrenia); control of nausea and vomiting; relief of restlessness and apprehension before surgery; acute intermittent porphyria; adjunct in the treatment of tetanus; intractable hiccups; combativeness and/or explosive hyperexcitable behavior in children 1-12 years of age and in short-term treatment of hyperactive children
Unlabeled Use Behavioral symptoms associated with dementia (elderly); psychosis/agitation related to Alzheimer's dementia

Local Anesthetic/Vasoconstrictor Precautions
Most pharmacology textbooks state that in presence of phenothiazines, systemic doses of epinephrine paradoxically decrease the blood pressure. This is the so called "epinephrine reversal" phenomenon. This has never been observed when epinephrine is given by infiltration as part of the anesthesia procedure. Chlorpromazine is one of the drugs confirmed to prolong the QT interval and is accepted as having a risk of causing torsade de pointes. The risk of drug-induced torsade de pointes is extremely low when a single QT interval prolonging drug is prescribed. In terms of epinephrine, it is not known what effect vasoconstrictors in the local anesthetic regimen will have in patients with a known history of congenital prolonged QT interval or in patients taking any medication that prolongs the QT interval. Until more information is obtained, it is suggested that the clinician consult with the physician prior to the use of a vasoconstrictor in suspected patients, and that the vasoconstrictor (epinephrine, mepivacaine and levonordefrin [Carbocaine® 2% with Neo-Cobefrin®]) be used with caution.

Effects on Dental Treatment Key adverse event(s) related to dental treatment:
Xerostomia (normal salivary flow resumes upon discontinuation).
Significant hypotension may occur, especially when the drug is administered parenterally. Orthostatic hypotension is due to alpha-receptor blockade; elderly are at greater risk.
Tardive dyskinesia: Prevalence rate may be 40% in elderly; development of the syndrome and the irreversible nature are proportional to duration and total cumulative dose over time. Extrapyramidal reactions are more common in elderly with up to 50% developing these reactions after 60 years of age. Drug-induced Parkinson's syndrome occurs often; akathisia is the most common extrapyramidal reaction in elderly.
Increased confusion, memory loss, psychotic behavior, and agitation frequently occur as a consequence of anticholinergic effects. Antipsychotic-associated sedation in nonpsychotic patients is extremely unpleasant due to feelings of depersonalization, derealization, and dysphoria.

Effects on Bleeding No information available to require special precautions
Adverse Effects Frequency not defined.
Cardiovascular: Orthostatic hypotension, tachycardia, dizziness, nonspecific QT changes

◄ Central nervous system: Drowsiness, dystonias, akathisia, pseudoparkinsonism, tardive dyskinesia, neuroleptic malignant syndrome, seizure

Dermatologic: Photosensitivity, dermatitis, skin pigmentation (slate gray)

Endocrine & metabolic: Lactation, breast engorgement, false-positive pregnancy test, amenorrhea, gynecomastia, hyper- or hypoglycemia

Gastrointestinal: Xerostomia, constipation, nausea

Genitourinary: Urinary retention, ejaculatory disorder, impotence

Hematologic: Agranulocytosis, eosinophilia, leukopenia, hemolytic anemia, aplastic anemia, thrombocytopenic purpura

Hepatic: Jaundice

Ocular: Blurred vision, corneal and lenticular changes, epithelial keratopathy, pigmentary retinopathy

General Dosage Range

I.M., I.V.:

Children ≥6 months: 0.5-1 mg/kg every 6-8 hours (maximum: <5 years [<22.7 kg]: 40 mg/day; 5-12 years [22.7-45.5 kg]: 75 mg/day)

Adults: Initial: 25 mg; may repeat (25-50 mg) in 1-4 hours; Usual dose: 300-800 mg/day (maximum: 400 mg every 4-6 hours)

Oral:

Children ≥6 months: 0.5-1 mg/ kg every 4-6 hours as needed

Adults: Dosage varies greatly depending on indication

Mechanism of Action Chlorpromazine is an aliphatic phenothiazine antipsychotic which blocks postsynaptic mesolimbic dopaminergic receptors in the brain; exhibits a strong alpha-adrenergic blocking effect and depresses the release of hypothalamic and hypophyseal hormones; believed to depress the reticular activating system, thus affecting basal metabolism, body temperature, wakefulness, vasomotor tone, and emesis

Pharmacodynamics/Kinetics

Onset of Action I.M.: 15 minutes; Oral: 30-60 minutes

Half-life Elimination Biphasic: Initial: 2 hours; Terminal: 30 hours

Pregnancy Considerations Embryotoxicity was observed in animal reproduction studies. Jaundice or hyper-/hyporeflexia have been reported in newborn infants following maternal use of phenothiazines. Antipsychotic use during the third trimester of pregnancy has a risk for abnormal muscle movements (extrapyramidal symptoms [EPS]) and withdrawal symptoms in newborns following delivery. Symptoms in the newborn may include agitation, feeding disorder, hypertonia, hypotonia, respiratory distress, somnolence, and tremor; these effects may be self-limiting or require hospitalization.

Dental Comment Chlorpromazine is known to prolong the QT interval. The QT interval is measured as the time and distance between the Q point of the QRS complex and the end of the T wave in the ECG tracing. After adjustment for heart rate, the QT interval is defined as prolonged if it is more than 450 msec in men and 460 msec in women. A long QT syndrome was first described in the 1950s and 60s as a congenital syndrome involving QT interval prolongation and syncope and sudden death. Some of the congenital long QT syndromes were characterized by a peculiar electrocardiographic appearance of the QRS complex involving a premature atria beat followed by a pause, then a subsequent sinus beat showing marked QT prolongation and deformity. This type of cardiac arrhythmia was originally termed "torsade de pointes" (translated from the French as "twisting of the points"). Chlorpromazine is considered as having a risk of causing torsade de pointes. Since it is not known what effect vasoconstrictors in the local anesthetic regimen will have in patients with a known history of congenital prolonged QT interval or in patients taking any medication that prolongs the QT interval, a medical consult is suggested.

ChlorproPAMIDE (klor PROE pa mide)

Related Information
Endocrine Disorders and Pregnancy *on page 1517*

Brand Names: Canada Apo-Chlorpropamide®

Pharmacologic Category Antidiabetic Agent, Sulfonylurea

Use Management of blood sugar in type 2 diabetes mellitus (noninsulin dependent, NIDDM) as an adjunct to diet and exercise to lower blood glucose

Unlabeled Use Central (neurogenic) diabetes insipidus

Local Anesthetic/Vasoconstrictor Precautions No information available to require special precautions

Effects on Dental Treatment Chlorpropamide-dependent patients with diabetes (noninsulin dependent, Type 2) should be appointed for dental treatment in morning in order to minimize chance of stress-induced hypoglycemia.

Effects on Bleeding No information available to require special precautions

Adverse Effects Frequency not always defined.

Central nervous system: Dizziness, headache

Dermatologic: Pruritus (<3%), maculopapular eruptions (≤1%), urticaria (≤1%), erythema multiforme, exfoliative dermatitis, photosensitivity

Endocrine & metabolic: Disulfiram-like reactions, hypoglycemia, SIADH

Gastrointestinal: Nausea (<5%), anorexia (<2%), diarrhea (<2%), hunger (<2%), vomiting (<2%), proctocolitis (<1%), weight gain

Hematologic: Agranulocytosis, aplastic anemia, eosinophilia, hemolytic anemia, leukopenia, pancytopenia, porphyria cutanea tarda, thrombocytopenia

Hepatic: Cholestatic jaundice, hepatic porphyria, hepatitis, liver failure

General Dosage Range Oral:

Adults: Initial: 250 mg daily; Maintenance: 100-500 mg daily (maximum: 750 mg daily)

Elderly: Initial: 100-125 mg daily

Mechanism of Action Stimulates insulin release from the pancreatic beta cells; reduces glucose output from the liver; insulin sensitivity is increased at peripheral target sites

Pharmacodynamics/Kinetics

Onset of Action 1 hour; Peak effect: 3-6 hours

Duration of Action 24 hours

Half-life Elimination ~36 hours, prolonged in elderly or with renal impairment; End-stage renal disease: 50-200 hours

Time to Peak Serum: 2-4 hours

Pregnancy Risk Factor C

Pregnancy Considerations Animal reproduction studies have not been conducted; therefore, the manufacturer classifies chlorpropamide as pregnancy category C. Chlorpropamide crosses the placenta and measurable serum concentrations can be found in infants exposed *in utero*. Teratogenic effects have been associated with chlorpropamide use in some studies; however, it is unknown if this is related to the medication or uncontrolled diabetes. Nonteratogenic adverse effects (eg, severe neonatal hypoglycemia, increased perinatal mortality) have also been associated with maternal chlorpropamide use. Maternal hyperglycemia can be associated with adverse effects in the fetus, including macrosomia, neonatal hyperglycemia, and hyperbilirubinemia; the risk of congenital malformations is increased when the Hb A_{1c} is above the normal range. Diabetes can also be associated with adverse effects in the mother. Poorly-treated diabetes may cause end-organ damage that may in turn negatively affect obstetric outcomes. Physiologic glucose levels should be maintained prior to and during pregnancy to decrease the risk of adverse events in the mother and the fetus. Until additional safety and efficacy data are obtained, the use of oral agents is generally not recommended as routine management of GDM or type 2 diabetes mellitus during pregnancy. The manufacturer recommends if chlorpropamide is used during pregnancy, it should be discontinued at least 1 month before the expected delivery date. Insulin is the drug of choice for the control of diabetes mellitus during pregnancy.

Chlorthalidone (klor THAL i done)

Related Information
Cardiovascular Diseases *on page 1492*
Brand Names: U.S. Thalitone® [DSC]
Brand Names: Canada Apo-Chlorthalidone®
Pharmacologic Category Diuretic, Thiazide
Use Management of mild-to-moderate hypertension when used alone or in combination with other agents; treatment of edema associated with heart failure, renal dysfunction, hepatic cirrhosis, or corticosteroid and estrogen therapy.
Unlabeled Use Pediatric hypertension
Local Anesthetic/Vasoconstrictor Precautions No information available to require special precautions
Effects on Dental Treatment No significant effects or complications reported
Effects on Bleeding No information available to require special precautions
Adverse Effects Frequency not defined.
Dermatologic: Photosensitivity
Endocrine & metabolic: Hypokalemia
Gastrointestinal: Anorexia, dyspepsia
General Dosage Range Oral:
Adults: 25-100 mg/day (maximum: 200 mg/day)
Elderly: Initial: 12.5-25 mg once daily or every other day
Mechanism of Action Sulfonamide-derived diuretic that inhibits sodium and chloride reabsorption in the cortical-diluting segment of the ascending loop of Henle
Pharmacodynamics/Kinetics
Onset of Action Peak effect: 2-6 hours
Duration of Action 24-72 hours
Half-life Elimination 40-60 hours; may be prolonged with renal impairment; Anuria: 81 hours
Pregnancy Risk Factor B
Pregnancy Considerations Adverse events were not observed in animal reproduction studies. Chlorthalidone crosses the placenta and can be detected in cord blood and amniotic fluid. Maternal use may cause may cause fetal or neonatal jaundice, thrombocytopenia, or other adverse events observed in adults. Use of thiazide diuretics during normal pregnancies is not appropriate; use may be considered when edema is due to pathologic causes (as in the nonpregnant patient); monitor.

Chlorzoxazone (klor ZOKS a zone)

Related Information
Temporomandibular Dysfunction (TMD), Chronic Pain, and Fibromyalgia *on page 1590*
Brand Names: U.S. Lorzone™; Parafon Forte® DSC
Generic Availability (U.S.) Yes
Pharmacologic Category Skeletal Muscle Relaxant
Dental Use Treatment of muscle spasm and pain associated with acute temporomandibular joint pain (TMJ)
Use Symptomatic treatment of muscle spasm and pain associated with acute musculoskeletal conditions
Local Anesthetic/Vasoconstrictor Precautions No information available to require special precautions
Effects on Dental Treatment No significant effects or complications reported
Effects on Bleeding No information available to require special precautions
Adverse Effects Frequency not defined.
Central nervous system: Dizziness, drowsiness lightheadedness, paradoxical stimulation, malaise
Dermatologic: Rash (rare), petechiae (rare), ecchymoses (rare), angioedema (very rare)
Gastrointestinal: Diarrhea, GI bleeding (rare), nausea, vomiting
Genitourinary: Urine discoloration
Hepatic: Liver dysfunction
Miscellaneous: Anaphylaxis (very rare)
Dental Usual Dosage Treatment of muscle spasm and pain associated with acute TMJ pain: Oral:
Adults: Oral: 500 mg 3-4 times daily, may increase up to 750 mg 3-4 times daily. May consider dose reductions as symptoms improve.
Dosage Muscle spasm:
Adults: Oral: 500 mg 3-4 times daily, may increase up to 750 mg 3-4 times daily. May consider dose reductions as symptoms improve.
Elderly: In general, avoid use or use cautiously at lower doses. Refer to adult dosing.

Dosage adjustment in renal impairment: No dosage adjustment provided in manufacturer's labeling.
Dosage adjustment in hepatic impairment: No dosage adjustment provided in manufacturer's labeling.
Mechanism of Action Acts on the spinal cord and subcortical areas of the brain to inhibit polysynaptic reflex arcs involved in causing and maintaining skeletal muscle spasms
Contraindications Hypersensitivity to chlorzoxazone or any component of the formulation
Warnings/Precautions Rare, serious (including fatal) idiosyncratic and unpredictable hepatocellular toxicity has been reported with use. Discontinue immediately if early signs/symptoms of hepatic toxicity arise (eg. fever, rash, anorexia, nausea, vomiting, fatigue, right upper quadrant pain, dark urine or jaundice). Also discontinue if elevated liver enzymes develop. May cause drowsiness, dizziness, or lightheadedness; effects may be potentiated by ethanol or other CNS depressants. Caution patients about performing tasks which require mental alertness (eg. operating machinery or driving) This class of medication is poorly tolerated by the elderly due to anticholinergic effects, sedation, and weakness. Efficacy is questionable at dosages tolerated by elderly patients (Beers Criteria).

◄ **Drug Interactions**

Metabolism/Transport Effects Substrate of CYP1A2 (minor), CYP2A6 (minor), CYP2D6 (minor), CYP2E1 (minor), CYP3A4 (minor); **Note:** Assignment of Major/Minor substrate status based on clinically relevant drug interaction potential; **Inhibits** CYP2E1 (weak), CYP3A4 (weak)

Avoid Concomitant Use

Avoid concomitant use of Chlorzoxazone with any of the following: Azelastine (Nasal); Paraldehyde; Pimozide

Increased Effect/Toxicity

Chlorzoxazone may increase the levels/effects of: Alcohol (Ethyl); ARIPiprazole; Azelastine (Nasal); Buprenorphine; CNS Depressants; Lomitapide; Methotrimeprazine; Metyrosine; Mirtazapine; Paraldehyde; Pimozide; Pramipexole; ROPINIRole; Rotigotine; Selective Serotonin Reuptake Inhibitors; Zolpidem

The levels/effects of Chlorzoxazone may be increased by: Disulfiram; Droperidol; HydrOXYzine; Isoniazid; Magnesium Sulfate; Methotrimeprazine; Perampanel; Sodium Oxybate

Decreased Effect

The levels/effects of Chlorzoxazone may be decreased by: Peginterferon Alfa-2b

Ethanol/Nutrition/Herb Interactions Ethanol: May increase CNS depression; monitor for increased effects with coadministration. Caution patients about effects.

Pharmacodynamics/Kinetics

Onset of Action ~1 hour

Duration of Action Up to 6 hours (Desiraju, 1983)

Half-life Elimination

~1 hour (Desiraju, 1983)

Time to Peak 1-2 hours

Pregnancy Considerations Animal reproduction studies have not been conducted.

Lactation Excretion in breast milk unknown

Dosage Forms

Caplet, oral:
Parafon Forte® DSC: 500 mg

Tablet, oral: 500 mg
Lorzone™: 375 mg, 750 mg

Cholecalciferol (kole e kal SI fer ole)

Brand Names: U.S. Bio-D-Mulsion Forte® [OTC]; Bio-D-Mulsion® [OTC]; D-3 [OTC]; D3-50™ [OTC]; D3-5™ [OTC]; DDrops® Baby [OTC]; DDrops® Kids [OTC]; DDrops® [OTC]; Delta® D3 [OTC]; Enfamil® D-Vi-Sol™ [OTC]; Maximum D3® [OTC]; Vitamin D3 [OTC]

Brand Names: Canada D-Vi-Sol®

Pharmacologic Category Vitamin D Analog

Use Dietary supplement, treatment of vitamin D deficiency, or prophylaxis of deficiency

Unlabeled Use Osteoporosis prevention

Local Anesthetic/Vasoconstrictor Precautions No information available to require special precautions

Effects on Dental Treatment Key adverse event(s) related to dental treatment: Metallic taste and xerostomia (normal salivary flow resumes upon discontinuation).

Effects on Bleeding No information available to require special precautions

Adverse Effects Frequency not defined: Endocrine & metabolic: Hypervitaminosis D (signs and symptoms include hypercalcemia, resulting in headache, nausea, vomiting, lethargy, confusion, sluggishness, abdominal pain, bone pain, polyuria, polydipsia, weakness, cardiac arrhythmias [eg, QT shortening, sinus tachycardia], soft tissue calcification, calciuria, and nephrocalcinosis)

General Dosage Range Oral:

Children 0-12 months: Adequate intake: 400 units/day

Children 1 year to Adults ≤70 years: RDA: 600 units/day

Elderly >70 years: RDA: 800 units/day

Pharmacodynamics/Kinetics

Half-life Elimination 14 hours

Time to Peak 11 hours

Pregnancy Considerations Adverse events were observed in animals when high maternal doses of vitamin D were administered during pregnancy. Vitamin D crosses the placenta but the transfer to the fetus from the mother is low. Maternal supplementation has not been shown to affect pregnancy outcomes. Vitamin D requirements are the same in pregnant and nonpregnant females (IOM, 2011).

Cholestyramine Resin
(koe LES teer a meen REZ in)

Related Information

Cardiovascular Diseases *on page 1492*

Brand Names: U.S. Prevalite®; Questran®; Questran® Light

Brand Names: Canada Novo-Cholamine; Novo-Cholamine Light; Olestyr; PMS-Cholestyramine; Questran®; Questran® Light Sugar Free; ZYM-Cholestyramine-Light; ZYM-Cholestyramine-Regular

Pharmacologic Category Antilipemic Agent, Bile Acid Sequestrant

Use Adjunct in the management of primary hypercholesterolemia; pruritus associated with elevated levels of bile acids; regression of arteriosclerosis

Unlabeled Use Diarrhea associated with excess fecal bile acids (Westergaard, 2007); may be used to enhance elimination of digoxin when non-life-threatening toxicity occurs (Henderson, 1988)

Local Anesthetic/Vasoconstrictor Precautions No information available to require special precautions

Effects on Dental Treatment No significant effects or complications reported

Effects on Bleeding No information available to require special precautions

Adverse Effects Frequency not defined.

Cardiovascular: Edema, syncope

Central nervous system: Anxiety, dizziness, drowsiness, eructation, fatigue, headache, vertigo

Dermatologic: Bruising, rash, skin irritation, urticaria

Endocrine & metabolic: Hyperchloremic acidosis (children), libido increased

Gastrointestinal: Abdominal pain, anorexia, biliary colic, black stools, constipation, dental bleeding, dental caries, dental erosion, diarrhea, diverticulitis, duodenal ulcer bleeding, dysphagia, eructation, flatulence, gallbladder calcification, GI hemorrhage, intestinal obstruction (rare), hemorrhoidal bleeding, nausea, pancreatitis, perianal irritation, rectal bleeding, rectal pain, steatorrhea, taste disturbance, tongue irritation, tooth discoloration, ulcer, vomiting, weight gain/loss

Hepatic: Hypothrombinemia, liver function abnormalities, prothrombin time increased

Hematologic: Anemia, bleeding

Neuromuscular & skeletal: Arthritis, backache, joint/muscle/nerve pain, osteoporosis, paresthesia

Ocular: Night blindness (rare), uveitis

Otic: Tinnitus

Renal: Diuresis, dysuria, hematuria

Respiratory: Asthma, dyspnea, wheezing

Miscellaneous: Hiccups, swollen glands

General Dosage Range Oral: *Adults:* 4-24 g/day in 1-6 divided doses

Mechanism of Action Forms a nonabsorbable complex with bile acids in the intestine, releasing chloride ions in the process; inhibits enterohepatic reuptake of intestinal bile salts and thereby increases the fecal loss of bile salt-bound low density lipoprotein cholesterol

Pharmacodynamics/Kinetics

Onset of Action Peak effect: 21 days

Pregnancy Risk Factor C

Pregnancy Considerations Cholestyramine is not absorbed systemically, but may interfere with vitamin absorption; therefore, regular prenatal supplementation may not be adequate. There are no studies in pregnant women; use with caution.

Choline Magnesium Trisalicylate
(KOE leen mag NEE zhum trye sa LIS i late)

Related Information

Temporomandibular Dysfunction (TMD), Chronic Pain, and Fibromyalgia *on page 1590*

Generic Availability (U.S.) Yes

Pharmacologic Category Salicylate

Use Management of osteoarthritis, rheumatoid arthritis, and other arthritis; acute painful shoulder

Local Anesthetic/Vasoconstrictor Precautions No information available to require special precautions

Effects on Dental Treatment The dentist should be aware of the potential of abnormal coagulation. Caution should also be exercised in the use of NSAIDs in patients already on anticoagulant therapy with drugs such as warfarin (Coumadin®). See Effects on Bleeding.

Effects on Bleeding Nonacetylated salicylates, such as choline salicylate or magnesium salicylate, do not affect platelet aggregation and do not increase bleeding time. There have been rare reports of thrombocytopenia with salicylates.

Adverse Effects

<20%:

Gastrointestinal: Nausea, vomiting, diarrhea, heartburn, dyspepsia, epigastric pain, constipation

Otic: Tinnitus

<2%:

Central nervous system: Headache, lightheadedness, dizziness, drowsiness, lethargy

Otic: Hearing impairment

Dosage Oral (based on total salicylate content):

Children <37 kg: 50 mg/kg/day given in 2 divided doses; 2250 mg/day for heavier children

Adults: 500 mg to 1.5 g 2-3 times/day **or** 3 g at bedtime; usual maintenance dose: 1-4.5 g/day

Elderly: 750 mg 3 times/day

Dosage adjustment in renal impairment: Avoid use in severe renal impairment.

Dosage adjustment in hepatic impairment: No dosage adjustment provided in manufacturer's labeling; use with caution.

Mechanism of Action Weakly inhibits cyclooxygenase enzymes, which results in decreased formation of prostaglandin precursors; antipyretic, analgesic, and anti-inflammatory properties.

Other proposed mechanisms not fully elucidated (and possibly contributing to the anti-inflammatory effect to varying degrees) include inhibiting chemotaxis, altering lymphocyte activity, inhibiting neutrophil aggregation/activation, and decreasing proinflammatory cytokine levels.

Contraindications Hypersensitivity to salicylates, other nonacetylated salicylates, other NSAIDs, or any component of the formulation; bleeding disorders; pregnancy (3rd trimester)

Warnings/Precautions Salicylate salts may not inhibit platelet aggregation and, therefore, should not be substituted for aspirin in the prophylaxis of thrombosis. Use with caution in patients with impaired hepatic or renal function, dehydration, erosive gastritis, asthma, or peptic ulcer. Children and teenagers who have or are recovering from chickenpox or flu-like symptoms should not use this product. Changes in behavior (along with nausea and vomiting) may be an early sign of Reye's syndrome; patients should be instructed to contact their healthcare provider if these occur.

Elderly are a high-risk population for adverse effects from NSAIDs. As many as 60% of elderly can develop peptic ulceration and/or hemorrhage asymptomatically. Use lowest effective dose for shortest period possible. Tinnitus or impaired hearing may indicate toxicity. Tinnitus may be a difficult and unreliable indication of toxicity due to age-related hearing loss or eighth cranial nerve damage. CNS adverse effects may be observed in the elderly at lower doses than younger adults.

Drug Interactions

Metabolism/Transport Effects None known.

Avoid Concomitant Use

Avoid concomitant use of Choline Magnesium Trisalicylate with any of the following: Influenza Virus Vaccine (Live/Attenuated)

Increased Effect/Toxicity

Choline Magnesium Trisalicylate may increase the levels/effects of: Anticoagulants; Carbonic Anhydrase Inhibitors; Corticosteroids (Systemic); Divalproex; Drotrecogin Alfa (Activated); Hypoglycemic Agents; Methotrexate; PRALAtrexate; Salicylates; Thrombolytic Agents; Valproic Acid; Varicella Virus-Containing Vaccines; Vitamin K Antagonists

The levels/effects of Choline Magnesium Trisalicylate may be increased by: Agents with Antiplatelet Properties; Ammonium Chloride; Calcium Channel Blockers (Nondihydropyridine); Ginkgo Biloba; Herbs (Anticoagulant/Antiplatelet Properties); Influenza Virus Vaccine (Live/Attenuated); Loop Diuretics; Potassium Acid Phosphate; Treprostinil

Decreased Effect

Choline Magnesium Trisalicylate may decrease the levels/effects of: ACE Inhibitors; Hyaluronidase; Loop Diuretics; Probenecid

The levels/effects of Choline Magnesium Trisalicylate may be decreased by: Corticosteroids (Systemic)

Ethanol/Nutrition/Herb Interactions

Ethanol: Avoid ethanol (may enhance gastric mucosal irritation).

Food: May decrease the rate but not the extent of oral absorption.

Herb/Nutraceutical: Avoid cat's claw, dong quai, evening primrose, feverfew, garlic, ginger, ginkgo, red clover, horse chestnut, green tea, ginseng (all have additional antiplatelet activity). Limit curry powder, paprika, licorice, Benedictine liqueur, prunes, raisins, tea, and gherkins; may cause salicylate accumulation. These foods contain 6 mg salicylate/100 g.

Dietary Considerations Take with food or large volume of water or milk to minimize GI upset. Liquid may be mixed with fruit juice just before drinking. Hypermagnesemia resulting from magnesium salicylate; avoid or use with caution in renal insufficiency.

Pharmacodynamics/Kinetics
Onset of Action Peak effect: ~2 hours
Half-life Elimination Dose dependent: Low dose: 2-3 hours; High dose: 30 hours
Time to Peak Serum: ~2 hours
Pregnancy Risk Factor C/D (3rd trimester)
Pregnancy Considerations Animal reproduction studies have not been conducted. Due to the known effects of other salicylates (closure of ductus arteriosus), use during late pregnancy should be avoided.

Lactation Enters breast milk/use caution
Breast-Feeding Considerations Excreted in breast milk; peak levels occur 9-12 hours after dose. Use caution if used during breast-feeding.

Dosage Forms
Liquid, oral: 500 mg/5 mL (240 mL)

Chorionic Gonadotropin (Human)
(kor ee ON ik goe NAD oh troe pin, HYU man)

Related Information
Chorionic Gonadotropin (Recombinant) *on page 300*
Brand Names: U.S. Novarel®; Pregnyl®
Brand Names: Canada Chorionic Gonadotropin for Injection; Pregnyl®
Pharmacologic Category Gonadotropin; Ovulation Stimulator
Use Induces ovulation and pregnancy in anovulatory, infertile females; treatment of hypogonadotropic hypogonadism, prepubertal cryptorchidism; spermatogenesis induction with follitropin alfa
Local Anesthetic/Vasoconstrictor Precautions No information available to require special precautions
Effects on Dental Treatment No significant effects or complications reported
Effects on Bleeding No information available to require special precautions
Adverse Effects Frequency not always defined.
Cardiovascular: Edema
Central nervous system: Depression, fatigue, headache, irritability, restlessness
Endocrine & metabolic: Gynecomastia, precocious puberty
Local: Injection site reaction, pain at injection site
Miscellaneous: Hypersensitivity reaction (local or systemic)
General Dosage Range I.M.:
Children: Dosage varies greatly depending on indication
Adults (females): 5000-10,000 units 1 day following last dose of menotropins
Adults (males): 1000-2000 units 2-3 times/week
Mechanism of Action Luteinizing hormone obtained from the urine of pregnant women. Stimulates production of gonadal steroid hormones by causing production of androgen by the testes; as a substitute for luteinizing hormone (LH) to stimulate ovulation

Pharmacodynamics/Kinetics
Half-life Elimination Biphasic: Initial: 11 hours; Terminal: 23 hours
Pregnancy Risk Factor X
Pregnancy Considerations Teratogenic effects (forelimb, CNS) have been noted in animal studies at doses intended to induce superovulation (used in combination with gonadotropin). Testicular tumors in otherwise healthy men have been reported when treating secondary infertility.

Chorionic Gonadotropin (Recombinant)
(kor ee ON ik goe NAD oh troe pin ree KOM be nant)

Related Information
Chorionic Gonadotropin (Human) *on page 300*
Brand Names: U.S. Ovidrel®
Brand Names: Canada Ovidrel®
Pharmacologic Category Gonadotropin; Ovulation Stimulator
Use As part of an assisted reproductive technology (ART) program, induces ovulation in infertile females who have been pretreated with follicle stimulating hormones (FSH); induces ovulation and pregnancy in infertile females when the cause of infertility is functional
Local Anesthetic/Vasoconstrictor Precautions No information available to require special precautions
Effects on Dental Treatment No significant effects or complications reported
Effects on Bleeding No information available to require special precautions
Adverse Effects
2% to 10%:
Endocrine & metabolic: Ovarian cyst (3%), ovarian hyperstimulation (<2% to 3%)
Gastrointestinal: Abdominal pain (3% to 4%), nausea (3%), vomiting (3%)
Local: Injection site: Pain (8%), bruising (3% to 5%), reaction (<2% to 3%), inflammation (<2% to 2%)
Miscellaneous: Postoperative pain (5%)
<2%:
Cardiovascular: Cardiac arrhythmia, heart murmur
Central nervous system: Dizziness, emotional lability, fever, headache, insomnia, malaise
Dermatologic: Pruritus, rash
Endocrine & metabolic: Breast pain, hot flashes, hyperglycemia, intermenstrual bleeding, vaginal hemorrhage
Gastrointestinal: Abdominal enlargement, diarrhea, flatulence
Genitourinary: Cervical carcinoma, cervical lesion, dysuria, genital herpes, genital moniliasis, leukorrhea, urinary incontinence, urinary tract infection, vaginal discomfort, vaginal hemorrhage, vaginitis
Hematologic: Leukocytosis
Neuromuscular & skeletal: Back pain, paresthesia
Renal: Albuminuria
Respiratory: Cough, pharyngitis, upper respiratory tract infection
Miscellaneous: Ectopic pregnancy, hiccups
In addition, the following have been reported with menotropin therapy: Adnexal torsion, hemoperitoneum, mild-to-moderate ovarian enlargement, pulmonary and vascular complications. Ovarian neoplasms have also been reported (rare) with multiple drug regimens used for ovarian induction (relationship not established).

General Dosage Range SubQ: *Adults (females):* 250 mcg given 1 day following last dose of follicle stimulating agent

Mechanism of Action Luteinizing hormone analogue produced by recombinant DNA techniques; stimulates late follicular maturation and intitates rupture of the ovarian follicle once follicular development has occurred

Pharmacodynamics/Kinetics

Half-life Elimination Initial: 4 hours; Terminal: 29 hours

Time to Peak 12-24 hours

Pregnancy Risk Factor X

Pregnancy Considerations Intrauterine death and impaired birth were observed in animal studies. Ectopic pregnancy, premature labor, postpartum fever, and spontaneous abortion have been reported in clinical trials. Congenital abnormalities have also been observed, however, the incidence is similar during natural conception.

Ciclesonide (Oral Inhalation)
(sye KLES oh nide)

Related Information
Respiratory Diseases *on page 1514*

Brand Names: U.S. Alvesco®

Brand Names: Canada Alvesco®

Generic Availability (U.S.) No

Pharmacologic Category Corticosteroid, Inhalant (Oral)

Use Prophylactic management of bronchial asthma

Local Anesthetic/Vasoconstrictor Precautions No information available to require special precautions

Effects on Dental Treatment No significant effects or complications reported

Effects on Bleeding No information available to require special precautions

Adverse Effects
>10%:
Central nervous system: Headache (≤11%)
Respiratory: Nasopharyngitis (≤11%)
1% to 10%:
Cardiovascular: Facial edema (≥3%)
Central nervous system: Dizziness (≥3%), fatigue (≥3%), dysphonia (1%)
Dermatologic: Urticaria (≥3%)
Gastrointestinal: Gastroenteritis (≥3%), oral candidiasis (≥3%)
Neuromuscular & skeletal: Arthralgia (≥3%), musculoskeletal chest pain (≥3%), back pain (≥3%), extremity pain (≥3%)
Ocular: Conjunctivitis (≥3%)
Otic: Ear pain (2%)
Respiratory: Upper respiratory infection (≤9%), nasal congestion (≤6%), pharyngolaryngeal pain (≤5%), hoarseness (≥3%), pneumonia (≥3%), sinusitis (≥3%), paradoxical bronchospasm (2%)
Miscellaneous: Influenza (≥3%)

Dosage Oral inhalation (Alvesco®):
Asthma: **Note:** Titrate to the lowest effective dose once asthma stability is achieved:
U.S. labeling: Children ≥12 years and Adults:
Prior therapy with bronchodilators alone: Initial: 80 mcg twice daily (maximum dose: 320 mcg/day)
Prior therapy with inhaled corticosteroids: Initial: 80 mcg twice daily (maximum dose: 640 mcg/day)
Prior therapy with oral corticosteroids: Initial: 320 mcg twice daily (maximum dose: 640 mcg/day)

Canadian labeling:
Children 6-11 years: Initial: 100-200 mcg once daily; maintenance: 100-200 mcg/day (1-2 puffs once daily)
Children ≥12 years and Adults: Initial: 400 mcg once daily; maintenance: 100-800 mcg/day (1-2 puffs once daily; more severe asthma may require 400 mcg twice daily)
Note: Canadian Thoracic Society 2010 Asthma Management guidelines recommend dose titration in children 6-11 years who fail to achieve an adequate response in spite of adherence to therapy and/or lack of alternative factors (eg, environmental triggers) which might impair response. In children ≥12 years and adults, doses >200 mcg/day may provide minimal additional benefit while increasing risks for adverse events; add-on therapy should be considered prior to dose increases >200 mcg/day (Lougheed, 2010).
Global Strategy for Asthma Management and Prevention, 2011: Children >5 years and Adults:
"Low" dose: 80-160 mcg/day
"Medium" dose: >160-320 mcg/day
"High" dose: >320 mcg/day

Conversion from oral to orally-inhaled steroid: Initiation of oral inhalation therapy should begin in patients who have previously been stabilized on oral corticosteroids (OCS). A gradual dose reduction of OCS should begin ~7-10 days after starting inhaled therapy. U.S. labeling recommends reducing prednisone dose no more rapidly than ≤2.5 mg/day on a weekly basis. The Canadian labeling recommends decreasing the daily dose of prednisone by 1 mg (or equivalent of other OCS) every 7 days in closely monitored patients, and every 10 days in patients whom close monitoring is not possible. In the presence of withdrawal symptoms, resume previous OCS dose for 1 week before attempting further dose reductions.

Dosage adjustment in renal impairment: There are no dosage adjustments provided in the manufacturer labeling (has not been studied); however, dose adjustments may not be necessary as ≤20% of drug is eliminated renally.

Dosage adjustment in hepatic impairment: Dosage adjustments are not necessary.

Mechanism of Action Ciclesonide is a nonhalogenated, glucocorticoid prodrug that is hydrolyzed to the pharmacologically active metabolite des-ciclesonide following administration. Des-ciclesonide has a high affinity for the glucocorticoid receptor and exhibits anti-inflammatory activity. The mechanism of action for corticosteroids is believed to be a combination of three important properties – anti-inflammatory activity, immunosuppressive properties, and antiproliferative actions.

Contraindications Hypersensitivity to ciclesonide or any component of the formulation; primary treatment of acute asthma or status asthmaticus

Canadian labeling: Additional contraindications (not in U.S. labeling): Untreated fungal, bacterial, or tuberculosis infections of the respiratory tract; moderate-to-severe bronchiectasis

Warnings/Precautions May cause hypercorticism or suppression of hypothalamic-pituitary-adrenal (HPA) axis, particularly in younger children or in patients receiving high doses for prolonged periods. HPA axis suppression may lead to adrenal crisis. Withdrawal and discontinuation of a corticosteroid should be done slowly and carefully. Particular care is required when patients are transferred from systemic corticosteroids to inhaled ▶

products due to possible adrenal insufficiency or with-drawal from steroids, including an increase in allergic symptoms. Patients receiving >20 mg per day of pre-dnisone (or equivalent) may be most susceptible. Fatal-ities have occurred due to adrenal insufficiency in asthmatic patients during and after transfer from sys-temic corticosteroids to aerosol steroids; aerosol ste-roids do **not** provide the systemic steroid needed to treat patients having trauma, surgery, or infections.

Bronchospasm may occur with wheezing after inhala-tion; if this occurs stop steroid and treat with a fast-acting bronchodilator. Supplemental steroids (oral or parenteral) may be needed during stress or severe asthma attacks. Not to be used in status asthmaticus or for the relief of acute bronchospasm. Oropharyngeal thrush due to candida albicans infection may occur with use. Prolonged use of corticosteroids may also increase the incidence of secondary infection, mask acute infec-tion (including fungal infections), prolong or exacerbate viral infections, or limit response to vaccines. Exposure to chickenpox and measles should be avoided; cortico-steroids should not be used to treat ocular herpes simplex. Close observation is required in patients with latent tuberculosis and/or TB reactivity; restrict use in active TB (only in conjunction with antituberculosis treat-ment). Use in patients with TB is contraindicated in the Canadian labeling. Prolonged treatment with cortico-steroids has been associated with the development of Kaposi's sarcoma (case reports); if noted, discontinua-tion of therapy should be considered.

Use with caution in patients with cardiovascular disease, diabetes, severe hepatic impairment, thyroid disease, psychiatric disturbances, myasthenia gravis, glaucoma, cataracts, patients at risk for osteoporosis, and patients at risk for seizures. Use in renally-impaired patients has not been studied; however, ≤20% of drug is eliminated renally. Use with caution in elderly patients.

Orally inhaled corticosteroids may cause a reduction in growth velocity in pediatric patients (~1 cm per year [range: 0.3-1.8 cm per year] and related to dose and duration of exposure). To minimize the systemic effects of orally inhaled corticosteroids, each patient should be titrated to the lowest effective dose. Growth should be routinely monitored in pediatric patients.

Drug Interactions

Metabolism/Transport Effects Substrate of CYP3A4 (major); **Note:** Assignment of Major/Minor substrate status based on clinically relevant drug interaction potential

Avoid Concomitant Use

Avoid concomitant use of Ciclesonide (Oral Inhalation) with any of the following: Aldesleukin

Increased Effect/Toxicity

Ciclesonide (Oral Inhalation) may increase the levels/ effects of: Deferasirox

The levels/effects of Ciclesonide (Oral Inhalation) may be increased by: CYP3A4 Inhibitors (Moderate); Dasa-tinib; Ivacaftor; Mifepristone; Telaprevir

Decreased Effect

Ciclesonide (Oral Inhalation) may decrease the levels/ effects of: Aldesleukin; Corticorelin; Hyaluronidase; Telaprevir

Pharmacodynamics/Kinetics

Half-life Elimination ~6-7 hours (active metabolite)

Time to Peak ~1 hour (active metabolite)

Pregnancy Risk Factor C

Pregnancy Considerations Teratogenic effects were reported following subcutaneous administration of cicle-sonide in animal reproduction studies. Hypoadrenalism may occur in infants born to mothers receiving cortico-steroids during pregnancy. Inhaled corticosteroids are recommended for the treatment of asthma during preg-nancy (ACOG, 2008; NAEPP, 2005).

Lactation Excretion in breast milk unknown/use caution

Breast-Feeding Considerations Systemic corticoste-roids are excreted in human milk. It is not known if sufficient quantities of ciclesonide are absorbed follow-ing oral inhalation to produce detectable amounts in breast milk; however, oral absorption is limited (<1%). The use of inhaled corticosteroids is not considered a contraindication to breast-feeding (NAEPP, 2005).

Dosage Forms

Aerosol, for oral inhalation:

Alvesco®: 80 mcg/inhalation (6.1 g); 160 mcg/inhala-tion (6.1 g)

Dosage Forms: Canada

Aerosol for oral inhalation:

Alvesco®: 100 mcg/inhalation; 200 mcg/inhalation

Ciclesonide (Nasal) (sye KLES oh nide)

Brand Names: U.S. Omnaris®; Zetonna™

Brand Names: Canada Omnaris®

Pharmacologic Category Corticosteroid, Nasal

Use Management of seasonal and perennial allergic rhinitis

Unlabeled Use Adjunct to antibiotics in empiric treat-ment of acute bacterial rhinosinusitis (ABRS) (Chow, 2012)

Local Anesthetic/Vasoconstrictor Precautions No information available to require special precautions

Effects on Dental Treatment No significant effects or complications reported

Effects on Bleeding No information available to require special precautions

Adverse Effects

>10%:

Central nervous system: Headache (≤11%), fever (chil-dren 3%)

Respiratory: Epistaxis (≤11%), nasopharyngitis (≤11%)

1% to 10%:

Central nervous system: Dysphonia (1%)

Gastrointestinal: Nausea (≥2%)

Genitourinary: Urinary tract infection (≥2%)

Neuromuscular & skeletal: Back pain (≥2%), muscle strain (≥2%)

Respiratory: Upper respiratory infection (≤9%), nasal congestion (≤6%), sinusitis (≤6%), nasal discomfort (3% to 6%), pharyngolaryngeal pain (≤5%), hoarse-ness (≥3%), pneumonia (≥3%), bronchitis (≥2%), cough (≥2%), nasal septum disorder (≥2%), pharyng-itis (≥2%), paradoxical bronchospasm (2%)

Miscellaneous: Influenza (≥2%)

General Dosage Range Intranasal:

Omnaris®: *Children ≥6 years and Adults:* 2 sprays (50 mcg/spray) per nostril once daily (maximum: 200 mcg/day)

Zetonna™: *Children ≥12 years and Adults:* 1 spray (37 mcg/spray) per nostril once daily (maximum: 74 mcg/day)

Pharmacodynamics/Kinetics

Onset of Action 24-48 hours; further improvement observed over 1-2 weeks in seasonal allergic rhinitis or 5 weeks in perennial allergic rhinitis

Pregnancy Risk Factor C

Pregnancy Considerations Teratogenic effects were reported following subcutaneous administration of ciclesonide in animal reproduction studies. The extent of intranasal absorption of ciclesonide systemically is low but variable. Hypoadrenalism may occur in infants born to mothers receiving corticosteroids during pregnancy. Intranasal corticosteroids may be used in the treatment of rhinitis during pregnancy (Wallace, 2008).

Ciclopirox (sye kloe PEER oks)

Brand Names: U.S. Ciclodan®; Ciclodan® Kit; Loprox®; Pedipirox™ -4 Kit; Penlac®
Brand Names: Canada Apo-Ciclopirox®; Loprox®; Penlac®; Stieprox®; Taro-Ciclopirox
Pharmacologic Category Antifungal Agent, Topical
Use
Cream/suspension: Treatment of tinea pedis (athlete's foot), tinea cruris (jock itch), tinea corporis (ringworm), cutaneous candidiasis, and tinea versicolor (pityriasis)
Gel: Treatment of tinea pedis (athlete's foot), tinea corporis (ringworm); seborrheic dermatitis of the scalp
Lacquer (solution): Topical treatment of mild-to-moderate onychomycosis of the fingernails and toenails due to *Trichophyton rubrum* (not involving the lunula) and the immediately-adjacent skin
Shampoo: Treatment of seborrheic dermatitis of the scalp
Local Anesthetic/Vasoconstrictor Precautions No information available to require special precautions
Effects on Dental Treatment No significant effects or complications reported
Effects on Bleeding No information available to require special precautions
Adverse Effects
Cardiovascular: Ventricular tachycardia (shampoo)
Central nervous system: Headache
Dermatologic: Acne, alopecia, contact dermatitis, dry skin, erythema, facial edema, hair discoloration (rare; shampoo formulation in light-haired individuals), nail disorder (shape or color change with lacquer), pruritus, rash
Local: Burning sensation (gel: 7% to 34%; ≤1% with other forms), irritation, pain, or redness
Ocular: Eye pain
General Dosage Range Topical:
Cream/suspension: *Children >10 years and Adults:* Apply twice daily
Gel: *Children >16 years and Adults:* Apply twice daily
Lacquer: *Children ≥12 years and Adults:* Apply to adjacent skin and affected nails daily; remove with alcohol every 7 days
Shampoo: *Children >16 years and Adults:* Apply 5-10 mL to wet hair, lather, and leave in place ~3 minutes, rinse; repeat twice weekly (allow minimum of 3 days between applications)
Mechanism of Action Inhibiting transport of essential elements in the fungal cell disrupting the synthesis of DNA, RNA, and protein
Pharmacodynamics/Kinetics
Half-life Elimination Biologic: Cream, suspension: 1.7 hours; Elimination: Gel: 5.5 hours
Pregnancy Risk Factor B
Pregnancy Considerations Teratogenic effects were not observed in animal studies, however, there are no adequate and well-controlled studies in pregnant women. Use during pregnancy only if clearly needed.

Cidofovir (si DOF o veer)

Related Information
Systemic Viral Diseases *on page 1537*
Brand Names: U.S. Vistide®
Pharmacologic Category Antiviral Agent
Use Treatment of cytomegalovirus (CMV) retinitis in patients with acquired immunodeficiency syndrome (AIDS). **Note:** Should be administered with probenecid.
Local Anesthetic/Vasoconstrictor Precautions No information available to require special precautions
Effects on Dental Treatment Key adverse event(s) related to dental treatment: Stomatitis and abnormal taste.
Effects on Bleeding No reports of bleeding or thrombocytopenia with cidofovir alone.
Adverse Effects
>10%:
Central nervous system: Chills, fever, headache, pain
Dermatologic: Alopecia, rash
Gastrointestinal: Nausea, vomiting, diarrhea, anorexia
Hematologic: Anemia, neutropenia
Neuromuscular & skeletal: Weakness
Ocular: Intraocular pressure decreased, iritis, ocular hypotony, uveitis
Renal: Creatinine increased, proteinuria, renal toxicity
Respiratory: Cough, dyspnea
Miscellaneous: Infection, oral moniliasis, serum bicarbonate decreased
1% to 10%:
Renal: Fanconi syndrome
Respiratory: Pneumonia
Frequency not defined (limited to important or life-threatening reactions):
Cardiovascular: Cardiomyopathy, cardiovascular disorder, CHF, edema, orthostatic hypotension, shock, syncope, tachycardia
Central nervous system: Agitation, amnesia, anxiety, confusion, convulsion, dizziness, hallucinations, insomnia, malaise, vertigo
Dermatologic: Photosensitivity reaction, skin discoloration, urticaria
Endocrine & metabolic: Adrenal cortex insufficiency
Gastrointestinal: Abdominal pain, aphthous stomatitis, colitis, constipation, dysphagia, fecal incontinence, gastritis, GI hemorrhage, gingivitis, melena, proctitis, splenomegaly, stomatitis, tongue discoloration
Genitourinary: Urinary incontinence
Hematologic: Hypochromic anemia, leukocytosis, leukopenia, lymphadenopathy, lymphoma-like reaction, pancytopenia, thrombocytopenia, thrombocytopenic purpura
Hepatic: Hepatomegaly, hepatosplenomegaly, jaundice, liver function tests abnormal, liver damage, liver necrosis
Local: Injection site reaction
Neuromuscular & skeletal: Tremor
Ocular: Amblyopia, blindness, cataract, conjunctivitis, corneal lesion, diplopia, vision abnormal
Otic: Hearing loss
Miscellaneous: Allergic reaction, sepsis
General Dosage Range Dosage adjustment recommended in patients with renal impairment
I.V.: *Adults:* Induction: 5 mg/kg once weekly for 2 consecutive weeks; Maintenance: 5 mg/kg once every 2 weeks

◀ **Mechanism of Action** Cidofovir is converted to cidofovir diphosphate which is the active intracellular metabolite; cidofovir diphosphate suppresses CMV replication by selective inhibition of viral DNA synthesis. Incorporation of cidofovir into growing viral DNA chain results in reductions in the rate of viral DNA synthesis.

Pharmacodynamics/Kinetics

Half-life Elimination Plasma: ~2.6 hours

Pregnancy Risk Factor C

Pregnancy Considerations [U.S. Boxed Warning]: Possibly carcinogenic and teratogenic based on animal data. May cause hypospermia. Cidofovir was shown to be teratogenic and embryotoxic in animal studies, some at doses which also produced maternal toxicity. Reduced testes weight and hypospermia were also noted in animal studies. There are no adequate and well-controlled studies in pregnant women; use during pregnancy only if the potential benefit to the mother outweighs the possible risk to the fetus. Women of childbearing potential should use effective contraception during therapy and for 1 month following treatment. Males should use a barrier contraceptive during therapy and for 3 months following treatment.

Cilazapril (sye LAY za pril)

Brand Names: Canada Apo-Cilazapril®; CO Cilazapril; Inhibace®; Mylan-Cilazapril; Novo-Cilazapril; PHL-Cilazapril; PMS-Cilazapril

Pharmacologic Category Angiotensin-Converting Enzyme (ACE) Inhibitor

Use Management of hypertension; treatment of heart failure

Local Anesthetic/Vasoconstrictor Precautions No information available to require special precautions

Effects on Dental Treatment Key adverse event(s) related to dental treatment: Orthostatic hypotension.

Effects on Bleeding No information available to require special precautions

Adverse Effects 1% to 10%:

Cardiovascular: Palpitation (up to 1%), hypotension (symptomatic, up to 1% in HF patients), orthostatic hypotension (2%)

Central nervous system: Headache (3% to 5%), dizziness (3% to 8%), fatigue (2% to 3%)

Gastrointestinal: Nausea (1% to 3%)

Neuromuscular & skeletal: Weakness (≤2%)

Renal: Serum creatinine increased

Respiratory: Cough (2% in hypertension, up to 8% in HF patients)

General Dosage Range Dosage adjustment recommended in patients with hepatic or renal impairment

Oral:

Adults: Initial: 0.5-2.5 mg once daily (maximum: 5 mg/day [CHF]; 10 mg/day [HTN])

Elderly: Initial: 0.5-1.25 mg once daily (maximum: 2.5 mg/day [CHF]; 10 mg/day [HTN])

Mechanism of Action Cilazapril is a prodrug that is rapidly converted to cilazaprilat (active metabolite), a competitive inhibitor of angiotensin-converting enzyme (ACE); prevents conversion of angiotensin I to angiotensin II, a potent vasoconstrictor; results in lower levels of angiotensin II which causes an increase in plasma renin activity and a reduction in aldosterone secretion.

Pharmacodynamics/Kinetics

Onset of Action Antihypertensive: ~1-2 hour

Duration of Action Therapeutic effect: Up to 24 hours

Half-life Elimination Cilazaprilat: Terminal: 36-49 hours

Time to Peak 2-7 hours

Pregnancy Considerations [Canadian Boxed Warning]: Drugs that act on the renin-angiotensin system can cause injury and death to the developing fetus. Discontinue as soon as possible once pregnancy is detected. Teratogenic effects may occur following maternal use during pregnancy. Drugs that act on the renin-angiotensin system are associated with oligohydramnios. Oligohydramnios, due to decreased fetal renal function, may lead to fetal lung hypoplasia and skeletal malformations. Their use in pregnancy is also associated with anuria, hypotension, renal failure, skull hypoplasia, and death in the fetus/neonate. Infants exposed to an ACE inhibitor *in utero* should be monitored for hyperkalemia, hypotension, and oliguria.

Product Availability Not available in U.S.

Cilazapril and Hydrochlorothiazide
(sye LAY za pril & hye droe klor oh THYE a zide)

Related Information

Cilazapril *on page 304*

Hydrochlorothiazide *on page 687*

Brand Names: Canada Apo-Cilazapril®/Hctz; Inhibace® Plus; Novo-Cilazapril/HCTZ

Pharmacologic Category Angiotensin-Converting Enzyme (ACE) Inhibitor; Diuretic, Thiazide

Use Treatment of mild-to-moderate hypertension; not indicated for initial treatment of hypertension

Local Anesthetic/Vasoconstrictor Precautions No information available to require special precautions

Effects on Dental Treatment Key adverse event(s) related to dental treatment: Orthostatic hypotension.

Effects on Bleeding No information available to require special precautions

Adverse Effects 1% to 10%:

Cardiovascular: Palpitation (1%)

Central nervous system: Dizziness (4%), fatigue (3%), somnolence (1%)

Gastrointestinal: Nausea (1%)

Genitourinary: Polyuria (1%)

Hematologic: Transient neutropenia (1%)

Hepatic: Transaminases increased (≤1%)

Respiratory: Cough (3%)

General Dosage Range Dosage adjustment recommended in hepatic impairment.

Oral: Adults: Dose is individualized; range: Cilazapril 2.5-10 mg/hydrochlorothiazide 6.25-25 mg/day

Pregnancy Considerations [Canadian Boxed Warning]: Drugs that act on the renin-angiotensin system can cause injury and death to the developing fetus. Discontinue as soon as possible once pregnancy is detected. Use is contraindicated in pregnant women. See individual agents.

Product Availability Not available in U.S.

Cilostazol (sil OH sta zol)

Related Information

Antiplatelet and Anticoagulation Considerations in Dentistry *on page 1503*

Cardiovascular Diseases *on page 1492*

Brand Names: U.S. Pletal®

Pharmacologic Category Antiplatelet Agent; Phosphodiesterase-3 Enzyme Inhibitor

Use Symptomatic management of peripheral vascular disease, primarily intermittent claudication

Unlabeled Use Adjunct with aspirin and clopidogrel for prevention of stent thrombosis and restenosis after coronary stent placement; as an alternative agent to either aspirin or clopidogrel in a dual antiplatelet regimen when allergy or drug intolerance to either agent occurs in patients who have undergone elective PCI with bare metal or drug-eluting stent placement; secondary prevention of noncardioembolic ischemic stroke or transient ischemic attack (TIA)

Local Anesthetic/Vasoconstrictor Precautions No information available to require special precautions

Effects on Dental Treatment No significant effects or complications reported

Effects on Bleeding Cilostazol causes reversible inhibition of platelet aggregation. To restore platelet function, cilostazol should be discontinued for 96 hours (4 days). A medical consult is recommended to determine the benefit:risk of continuing or discontinuing cilostazol for invasive dental procedures.

Adverse Effects
>10%:
Central nervous system: Headache (27% to 34%)
Gastrointestinal: Abnormal stools (12% to 15%), diarrhea (12% to 19%)
Respiratory: Rhinitis (7% to 12%)
Miscellaneous: Infection (10% to 14%)
2% to 10%:
Cardiovascular: Peripheral edema (7% to 9%), palpitation (5% to 10%), tachycardia (4%)
Central nervous system: Dizziness (9% to 10%), vertigo (up to 3%)
Gastrointestinal: Dyspepsia (6%), nausea (6% to 7%), abdominal pain (4% to 5%), flatulence (2% to 3%)
Neuromuscular & skeletal: Back pain (6% to 7%), myalgia (2% to 3%)
Respiratory: Pharyngitis (7% to 10%), cough (3% to 4%)

General Dosage Range Dosage adjustment recommended in patients on concomitant therapy
Oral: *Adults:* 100 mg twice daily

Mechanism of Action Cilostazol and its metabolites are inhibitors of phosphodiesterase III. As a result, cyclic AMP is increased leading to reversible inhibition of platelet aggregation, vasodilation, and inhibition of vascular smooth muscle cell proliferation.

Pharmacodynamics/Kinetics
Onset of Action 2-4 weeks; may require up to 12 weeks
Half-life Elimination 11-13 hours
Pregnancy Risk Factor C
Pregnancy Considerations In animal studies, abnormalities of the skeletal, renal and cardiovascular system were increased. In addition, the incidence of stillbirth and decreased birth weights were increased.

Cimetidine (sye MET i deen)

Related Information
Gastrointestinal Disorders *on page 1512*
Brand Names: U.S. Tagamet HB 200® [OTC]
Brand Names: Canada Apo-Cimetidine®; Dom-Cimetidine; Mylan-Cimetidine; Novo-Cimetidine; Nu-Cimet; PMS-Cimetidine

Pharmacologic Category Histamine H_2 Antagonist
Use Short-term treatment of active duodenal ulcers and benign gastric ulcers; maintenance therapy of duodenal ulcer; treatment of gastric hypersecretory states; treatment of gastroesophageal reflux disease (GERD)

OTC labeling: Prevention or relief of heartburn, acid indigestion, or sour stomach
Unlabeled Use Part of a multidrug regimen for *H. pylori* eradication to reduce the risk of duodenal ulcer recurrence

Local Anesthetic/Vasoconstrictor Precautions No information available to require special precautions

Effects on Dental Treatment No significant effects or complications reported

Effects on Bleeding No information available to require special precautions

Adverse Effects
1% to 10%:
Central nervous system: Headache (2% to 4%), dizziness (1%), somnolence (1%), agitation
Endocrine & metabolic: Gynecomastia (<1% to 4%)
Gastrointestinal: Diarrhea (1%)
Frequency not defined:
Cardiovascular: AV block, bradycardia, hypotension, tachycardia, vasculitis
Central nervous system: Confusion, fever
Dermatologic: Alopecia, erythema multiforme, exfoliative dermatitis, Stevens-Johnson syndrome, toxic epidermal necrolysis, rash
Endocrine & metabolic: Edema of the breasts, sexual ability decreased
Gastrointestinal: Nausea, pancreatitis, vomiting
Hematologic: Agranulocytosis, aplastic anemia, hemolytic anemia (immune-based), neutropenia, pancytopenia, thrombocytopenia
Hepatic: ALT increased, AST increased, hepatic fibrosis (case report)
Neuromuscular & skeletal: Arthralgia, myalgia, polymyositis
Renal: Creatinine increased, interstitial nephritis
Miscellaneous: Anaphylaxis, pneumonia (causal relationship not established)

General Dosage Range Dosage adjustment recommended in patients with renal impairment
Oral:
Children <12 years: 20-40 mg/kg/day divided every 6 hours
Children ≥12 years: 20-40 mg/kg/day divided every 6 hours **or** 200 mg 1-2 times/day [OTC]
Adults: 300-600 mg 4 times/day **or** 400-800 mg 1-2 times/day **or** 200 mg 1-2 times/day [OTC]

Mechanism of Action Competitive inhibition of histamine at H_2 receptors of the gastric parietal cells resulting in reduced gastric acid secretion, gastric volume and hydrogen ion concentration reduced

Pharmacodynamics/Kinetics
Onset of Action 1 hour
Duration of Action 80% reduction in gastric acid secretion for 4-5 hours after 300 mg dose
Half-life Elimination Neonates: 3.6 hours; Children: 1.4 hours; Adults: 2 hours
Time to Peak Serum: Oral: 1-2 hours
Pregnancy Risk Factor B

Pregnancy Considerations Teratogenic effects were not observed in animal reproduction studies; therefore, cimetidine is classified as pregnancy category B. Cimetidine crosses the placenta. An increased risk of congenital malformations or adverse events in the newborn has generally not been observed following maternal use of cimetidine during pregnancy. Histamine H$_2$ antagonists have been evaluated for the treatment of gastroesophageal reflux disease (GERD), as well as gastric and duodenal ulcers during pregnancy. Although if needed, cimetidine is not the agent of choice. Histamine H$_2$ antagonists may be used for aspiration prophylaxis prior to cesarean delivery.

Cinacalcet (sin a KAL cet)

Brand Names: U.S. Sensipar®
Brand Names: Canada Sensipar®
Pharmacologic Category Calcimimetic
Use Treatment of secondary hyperparathyroidism in patients with chronic kidney disease (CKD) on dialysis; treatment of hypercalcemia in patients with parathyroid carcinoma; treatment of severe hypercalcemia in patients with primary hyperparathyroidism who are unable to undergo parathyroidectomy
Local Anesthetic/Vasoconstrictor Precautions No information available to require special precautions
Effects on Dental Treatment No significant effects or complications reported
Effects on Bleeding No information available to require special precautions
Adverse Effects
>10%:
Central nervous system: Fatigue (12% to 21%), headache (≤21%), depression (10% to 18%)
Endocrine & metabolic: Hypocalcemia (≤66%), dehydration (≤24%), hypercalcemia (12% to 21%)
Gastrointestinal: Nausea (31% to 66%), vomiting (27% to 52%), diarrhea (≤21%), anorexia (6% to 21%), constipation (10% to 18%)
Hematologic: Anemia (6% to 17%)
Neuromuscular & skeletal: Parasthesia (14% to 29%), fracture (12% to 21%), weakness (7% to 17%), arthralgia (6% to 17%), myalgia (≤15%), limb pain (10% to 12%)
Respiratory: Upper respiratory infection (10% to 12%)
1% to 10%:
Cardiovascular: Hypertension (≤7%)
Central nervous system: Dizziness (≤10%), seizure (1%)
Endocrine & metabolic: Testosterone decreased
Neuromuscular & skeletal: Chest pain (noncardiac; ≤6%)
General Dosage Range Dosage adjustment recommended in patients on concomitant therapy or who develop toxicities
Oral: *Adults:* Initial: 30 mg once or twice daily; Maintenance: Increase dose incrementally every 2-4 weeks to normalize calcium levels or maintain iPTH level (maximum: 360 mg/day [parathyroid cancer, primary hyperparathyroidism]; 180 mg/day [secondary hyperparathyroidism])
Mechanism of Action Increases the sensitivity of the calcium-sensing receptor on the parathyroid gland thereby, concomitantly lowering parathyroid hormone (PTH), serum calcium, and serum phosphorus levels, preventing progressive bone disease and adverse events associated with mineral metabolism disorders.

Pharmacodynamics/Kinetics
Half-life Elimination Terminal: 30-40 hours; moderate hepatic impairment: 65 hours; severe hepatic impairment: 84 hours
Time to Peak ~2-6 hours
Pregnancy Risk Factor C
Pregnancy Considerations In animal studies, there were no teratogenic effects observed, although decreased pup weights were noted. There are no adequate or well-controlled studies in pregnant women. Use in pregnancy only if potential benefit to mother justifies risk to the fetus. Women who become pregnant during cinacalcet treatment are encouraged to enroll in Amgen's Pregnancy Surveillance Program (1-800-772-6436).

Ciprofloxacin (Systemic) (sip roe FLOKS a sin)

Related Information
Periodontal Diseases *on page 1570*
Related Sample Prescriptions
Bacterial Infections and Periodontal Diseases *on page 1609*
Brand Names: U.S. Cipro®; Cipro® I.V.
Brand Names: Canada Apo-Ciproflox®; Auro-Ciprofloxacin; Ciprofloxacin Injection; Ciprofloxacin Intravenous Infusion; Cipro®; Cipro® XL; CO Ciprofloxacin; Dom-Ciprofloxacin; JAMP-Ciprofloxacin; Mar-Ciprofloxacin; Mint-Ciprofloxacin; Mylan-Ciprofloxacin; Novo-Ciprofloxacin; PHL-Ciprofloxacin; PMS-Ciprofloxacin; PRO-Ciprofloxacin; RAN™-Ciproflox; ratio-Ciprofloxacin; Riva-Ciprofloxacin; Sandoz-Ciprofloxacin; Taro-Ciprofloxacin
Generic Availability (U.S.) Yes: Excludes suspension
Pharmacologic Category Antibiotic, Quinolone
Dental Use Useful as a single agent or in combination with metronidazole in the treatment of periodontitis associated with the presence of *Actinobacillus actinomycetemcomitans* (AA), as well as enteric rods/pseudomonads
Use
Children: Complicated urinary tract infections and pyelonephritis due to *E. coli*. **Note:** Although effective, ciprofloxacin is not the drug of first choice in children.
Children and Adults: To reduce incidence or progression of disease following exposure to aerolized *Bacillus anthracis*.
Adults: Treatment of the following infections when caused by susceptible bacteria: Urinary tract infections; acute uncomplicated cystitis in females; chronic bacterial prostatitis; lower respiratory tract infections (including acute exacerbations of chronic bronchitis); acute sinusitis; skin and skin structure infections; bone and joint infections; complicated intra-abdominal infections (in combination with metronidazole); infectious diarrhea; typhoid fever due to *Salmonella typhi* (eradication of chronic typhoid carrier state has not been proven); uncomplicated cervical and urethra gonorrhea (due to *N. gonorrhoeae*); nosocomial pneumonia; empirical therapy for febrile neutropenic patients (in combination with piperacillin)
Note: As of April 2007, the CDC no longer recommends the use of fluoroquinolones for the treatment of gonococcal disease.

Unlabeled Use Acute pulmonary exacerbations in cystic fibrosis (children); cutaneous/gastrointestinal/oropharyngeal anthrax (treatment, children and adults); disseminated gonococcal infection (adults); chancroid (adults); epididymitis (adults); prophylaxis to *Neisseria meningitidis* following close contact with an infected person; empirical therapy (oral) for febrile neutropenia in low-risk cancer patients; HACEK group endocarditis; infectious diarrhea (children); periodontitis; chronic oral antimicrobial suppression of prosthetic joint infection

Local Anesthetic/Vasoconstrictor Precautions No information available to require special precautions

Effects on Dental Treatment No significant effects or complications reported

Effects on Bleeding No information available to require special precautions

Adverse Effects 1% to 10%:

Central nervous system: Neurologic events (children 2%, includes dizziness, insomnia, nervousness, somnolence); fever (children 2%); headache (I.V. administration); restlessness (I.V. administration)

Dermatologic: Rash (children 2%, adults 1%)

Gastrointestinal: Nausea (3%); diarrhea (children 5%, adults 2%); vomiting (children 5%, adults 1%); abdominal pain (children 3%, adults <1%); dyspepsia (children 3%)

Hepatic: ALT increased, AST increased (adults 1%)

Local: Injection site reactions (I.V. administration)

Respiratory: Rhinitis (children 3%)

Dental Usual Dosage Treatment of periodontitis: Adults: Oral: 500 mg every 12 hours for 8-10 days

Dosage Note: Extended release tablets and immediate release formulations are not interchangeable. Unless otherwise specified, oral dosing reflects the use of immediate release formulations.

Usual dosage ranges:

Children (see Warnings/Precautions):

Oral: See indication-specific dosing; maximum dose: 1500 mg daily

I.V.: See indication-specific dosing; maximum dose: 800 mg daily

Adults:

Oral: 250-750 mg every 12 hours

I.V.: 200-400 mg every 12 hours

Indication-specific dosing:

Infants >3 months and Children:

Community-acquired pneumonia (CAP) (IDSA/PIDS, 2011): *H. influenzae,* moderate-to-severe infection (alternative to ampicillin, ceftriaxone, or cefotaxime): I.V.: 30 mg/kg/day divided every 12 hours

Children:

Anthrax:

Inhalational (postexposure prophylaxis):

Oral: 15 mg/kg/dose every 12 hours for 60 days; maximum: 500 mg dose

I.V.: 10 mg/kg/dose every 12 hours for 60 days; do **not** exceed 400 mg dose (800 mg daily)

Cutaneous (treatment, CDC guidelines): Oral: 10-15 mg/kg every 12 hours for 60 days (maximum: 1000 mg daily); amoxicillin 80 mg/kg/day divided every 8 hours is an option for completion of treatment after clinical improvement. **Note:** In the presence of systemic involvement, extensive edema, lesions on head/neck, refer to I.V. dosing for treatment of inhalational/gastrointestinal/oropharyngeal anthrax.

Inhalational/gastrointestinal/oropharyngeal (treatment, CDC guidelines): I.V.: Initial: 10-15 mg/kg every 12 hours for 60 days (maximum: 500 mg dose); switch to oral therapy when clinically appropriate; refer to adult dosing for notes on combined therapy and duration

Cystic fibrosis (unlabeled use):

Oral: 40 mg/kg/day divided every 12 hours administered following 1 week of I.V. therapy has been reported in a clinical trial; total duration of therapy: 10-21 days (Rubio, 1997)

I.V.: 30 mg/kg/day divided every 8 hours for 1 week, followed by oral therapy, has been reported in a clinical trial (Rubio, 1997)

Shigella dysentery type 1 (unlabeled use): Oral: 30 mg/kg/day in 2 divided doses for 3 days (WHO, 2005)

Urinary tract infection (complicated) or pyelonephritis:

Oral: 20-40 mg/kg/day in 2 divided doses (every 12 hours) for 10-21 days; maximum: 1500 mg daily. **Note:** 30-40 mg/kg/day reserved for severe infections (Red Book, 2012)

I.V.: 6-10 mg/kg every 8 hours for 10-21 days (maximum: 400 mg dose)

Adults:

Anthrax:

Inhalational (postexposure prophylaxis):

Oral: 500 mg every 12 hours for 60 days

I.V.: 400 mg every 12 hours for 60 days

Cutaneous (treatment, CDC guidelines): Oral: Immediate release formulation: 500 mg every 12 hours for 60 days. **Note:** In the presence of systemic involvement, extensive edema, lesions on head/neck, refer to I.V. dosing for treatment of inhalational/gastrointestinal/oropharyngeal anthrax

Inhalational/gastrointestinal/oropharyngeal (treatment, CDC guidelines): I.V.: 400 mg every 12 hours. **Note:** Initial treatment should include two or more agents predicted to be effective (per CDC recommendations). Continue combined therapy for 60 days.

Bone/joint infections:

Oral: 500-750 mg twice daily for ≥4-6 weeks

I.V.: Mild-to-moderate: 400 mg every 12 hours for ≥4-6 weeks; Severe/complicated: 400 mg every 8 hours for ≥4-6 weeks

Chancroid (unlabeled use): Oral: 500 mg twice daily for 3 days (CDC, 2010)

Endocarditis due to HACEK organisms (AHA guidelines, unlabeled use): Note: Not first-line option; use only if intolerant of beta-lactam therapy:

Oral: 500 mg every 12 hours for 4 weeks

I.V.: 400 mg every 12 hours for 4 weeks

Epididymitis, chlamydial (unlabeled use): Oral: 500 mg single dose (Canadian STI Guidelines, 2008)

Febrile neutropenia: I.V.: 400 mg every 8 hours for 7-14 days (combination therapy with piperacillin generally recommended)

Gonococcal infections:

Urethral/cervical gonococcal infections: Oral: 250-500 mg as a single dose (CDC recommends concomitant doxycycline or azithromycin due to possible coinfection with *Chlamydia*); **Note:** As of April 2007, the CDC no longer recommends the use of fluoroquinolones for the treatment of uncomplicated gonococcal disease.

Disseminated gonococcal infection (CDC guidelines): Oral: 500 mg twice daily to complete 7 days of therapy (initial treatment with ceftriaxone 1 g I.M./I.V. daily for 24-48 hours after improvement begins); **Note:** As of April 2007, the CDC no longer recommends the use of fluoroquinolones for the treatment of more serious gonococcal disease, unless no other options exist and susceptibility can be confirmed via culture.

Granuloma inguinale (donovanosis) (unlabeled use): Oral: 750 mg twice daily for at least 3 weeks (and until lesions have healed) (CDC, 2010)

Infectious diarrhea: Oral:

Salmonella: 500 mg twice daily for 5-7 days

Shigella (including Shigella dysentery type 1) (unlabeled regimen): 500 mg twice daily for 3 days (IDSA, 2001)

Traveler's diarrhea (unlabeled regimen): Mild: 750 mg as a single dose (CDC, 2012; de la Cabada Bauch, 2011); Severe: 500 mg twice daily for 3 days (IDSA, 2001)

Vibrio cholerae (unlabeled regimen): 1 g as a single dose (CDC, 2011)

Intra-abdominal, complicated, community-acquired (in combination with metronidazole): Note: Avoid using in settings where *E. coli* susceptibility to fluoroquinolones is <90%:

Oral: 500 mg every 12 hours for 7-14 days

I.V.: 400 mg every 12 hours for 7-14 days; **Note:** 2010 IDSA guidelines recommend treatment duration of 4-7 days (provided source controlled)

Lower respiratory tract:

Oral: 500-750 mg twice daily for 7-14 days

I.V.: Mild-to-moderate: 400 mg every 12 hours for 7-14 days; Severe/complicated: 400 mg every 8 hours for 7-14 days

Meningococcal meningitis prophylaxis (unlabeled use): Oral: 500 mg as a single dose (CDC, 2005)

Nosocomial pneumonia: I.V.: 400 mg every 8 hours for 10-14 days

Periodontitis (unlabeled use): Oral: 500 mg every 12 hours for 8-10 days (Rams, 1992)

Prostatitis (chronic, bacterial):

Oral: 500 mg every 12 hours for 28 days

I.V.: 400 mg every 12 hours for 28 days

Sinusitis (acute):

Oral: 500 mg every 12 hours for 10 days

I.V.: 400 mg every 12 hours for 10 days

Skin/skin structure infections:

Oral: 500-750 mg twice daily for 7-14 days

I.V.: Mild-to-moderate: 400 mg every 12 hours for 7-14 days; Severe/complicated: 400 mg every 8 hours for 7-14 days

Typhoid fever: Oral: 500 mg every 12 hours for 10 days

Urinary tract infection:

Acute uncomplicated, cystitis:

Oral:

Immediate release formulation: 250 mg every 12 hours for 3 days

Extended release formulation (Cipro® XR): 500 mg every 24 hours for 3 days

I.V.: 200 mg every 12 hours for 7-14 days

Complicated (including pyelonephritis):

Oral:

Immediate release formulation: 500 mg every 12 hours for 7-14 days

Extended release formulation (Cipro® XR): 1000 mg every 24 hours for 7-14 days

I.V.: 400 mg every 12 hours for 7-14 days

Elderly: No adjustment needed in patients with normal renal function

Dosing adjustment in renal impairment: Adults:

Manufacturer's recommendations:

Oral, immediate release:

Cl_{cr} >50 mL/minute: No dosage adjustment necessary

Cl_{cr} 30-50 mL/minute: 250-500 mg every 12 hours

Cl_{cr} 5-29 mL/minute: 250-500 mg every 18 hours

ESRD on intermittent hemodialysis (IHD)/peritoneal dialysis (PD) (administer after dialysis on dialysis days): 250-500 mg every 24 hours

Oral, extended release:

Cl_{cr} ≥30 mL/minute: No dosage adjustment necessary

Cl_{cr} <30 mL/minute: 500 mg every 24 hours

ESRD on intermittent hemodialysis (IHD)/peritoneal dialysis (PD) (administer after dialysis on dialysis days): 500 mg every 24 hours

I.V.:

Cl_{cr} ≥30 mL/minute: No dosage adjustment necessary

Cl_{cr} 5-29 mL/minute: 200-400 mg every 18-24 hours

Alternate recommendations: Oral (immediate release), I.V.:

Cl_{cr} >50 mL/minute: No dosage adjustment necessary (Aronoff, 2007)

Cl_{cr} 10-50 mL/minute: Administer 50% to 75% of usual dose every 12 hours (Aronoff, 2007)

Cl_{cr} <10 mL/minute: Administer 50% of usual dose every 12 hours (Aronoff, 2007)

Intermittent hemodialysis (IHD) (administer after hemodialysis on dialysis days): Minimally dialyzable (<10%): Oral: 250-500 mg every 24 hours **or** I.V.: 200-400 mg every 24 hours (Heintz, 2009). **Note:** Dosing dependent on the assumption of 3 times weekly, complete IHD sessions.

Continuous renal replacement therapy (CRRT) (Heintz, 2009; Trotman, 2005): Drug clearance is highly dependent on the method of renal replacement, filter type, and flow rate. Appropriate dosing requires close monitoring of pharmacologic response, signs of adverse reactions due to drug accumulation, as well as drug concentrations in relation to target trough (if appropriate). The following are general recommendations only (based on dialysate flow/ultrafiltration rates of 1-2 L/hour and minimal residual renal function) and should not supersede clinical judgment:

CVVH/CVVHD/CVVHDF: I.V.: 200-400 mg every 12-24 hours

Mechanism of Action Inhibits DNA-gyrase in susceptible organisms; inhibits relaxation of supercoiled DNA and promotes breakage of double-stranded DNA

Contraindications Hypersensitivity to ciprofloxacin, any component of the formulation, or other quinolones; concurrent administration of tizanidine

Warnings/Precautions [U.S. Boxed Warning]: There have been reports of tendon inflammation and/or rupture with quinolone antibiotics in all ages; risk may be increased with concurrent corticosteroids, solid organ transplant recipients, and in patients >60 years of age. Rupture of the Achilles tendon sometimes requiring surgical repair has been reported most frequently; but other tendon sites (eg, rotator cuff, biceps) have also been reported. Strenuous physical activity, rheumatoid arthritis, and renal impairment may be an independent risk factor for tendonitis. Inflammation and rupture may occur bilaterally. Cases have been reported within the first 48 hours, during, and up to several months after discontinuation of therapy. Discontinue at first sign of tendon inflammation or pain. Use with caution in patients with rheumatoid arthritis; may increase risk of tendon rupture. Use with caution in patients with a history of tendon disorders.

CNS effects may occur (tremor, restlessness, confusion, and hallucinations, increased intracranial pressure [including pseudotumor cerebri] or seizures). Reactions may occur following the first dose. Use with caution in patients with known or suspected CNS disorder or consider discontinuation if CNS effects develop. Potential for seizures, although very rare, may be increased with concomitant NSAID therapy. Use with caution in individuals at risk of seizures (CNS disorders or concurrent therapy with medications which may lower seizure threshold; status epilepticus has occurred) or if clinically appropriate, consider alternative antimicrobial therapy. Discontinue if seizures occur.

Fluoroquinolones may prolong QT_c interval; avoid use in patients with a history of or at risk for QT_c prolongation, torsade de pointes, uncorrected hypokalemia, hypomagnesemia, cardiac disease (heart failure, myocardial infarction, bradycardia) or concurrent administration of other medications known to prolong the QT interval (including Class Ia and Class III antiarrhythmics, cisapride, erythromycin, antipsychotics, and tricyclic antidepressants). Hepatocellular, cholestatic, or mixed liver injury has been reported, including hepatic necrosis, life-threatening hepatic events, and fatalities. Acute liver injury can be rapid onset (range: 1-39 days), often associated with hypersensitivity. Most fatalities occurred in patients >55 years of age. Discontinue immediately if signs/symptoms of hepatitis (abdominal tenderness, dark urine, jaundice, pruritus) occur. Additionally, temporary increases in transaminases or alkaline phosphatase or cholestatic jaundice may occur (highest risk in patients with previous liver damage).

Prolonged use may result in fungal or bacterial superinfection, including C. difficile-associated diarrhea (CDAD) and pseudomembranous colitis; CDAD has been observed >2 months postantibiotic treatment. Rarely crystalluria has occurred; urine alkalinity may increase the risk. Ensure adequate hydration during therapy. Adverse effects, including those related to joints and/or surrounding tissues, are increased in pediatric patients and therefore, ciprofloxacin should not be considered as drug of choice in children (exception is anthrax treatment). Rare cases of peripheral neuropathy may occur.

Fluoroquinolones have been associated with the development of serious, and sometimes fatal, hypoglycemia, most often in elderly diabetics but also in patients without diabetes. This occurred most frequently with gatifloxacin (no longer available systemically), but may occur at a lower frequency with other quinolones.

Severe hypersensitivity reactions, including anaphylaxis, have occurred with quinolone therapy. Reactions may present as typical allergic symptoms after a single dose, or may manifest as severe idiosyncratic dermatologic, vascular, pulmonary, renal, hepatic, and/or hematologic events, usually after multiple doses. Prompt

discontinuation of drug should occur if skin rash or other symptoms arise. **[U.S. Boxed Warning]: Quinolones may exacerbate myasthenia gravis; avoid use (rare, potentially life-threatening weakness of respiratory muscles may occur).** Use caution in renal impairment. Avoid excessive sunlight and take precautions to limit exposure (eg, loose fitting clothing, sunscreen); may cause moderate-to-severe photosensitivity/phototoxicity reactions. Discontinue use if photosensitivity occurs. Since ciprofloxacin is ineffective in the treatment of syphilis and may mask symptoms, all patients should be tested for syphilis at the time of gonorrheal diagnosis and 3 months later. Hemolytic reactions may (rarely) occur with quinolone use in patients with latent or actual glucose-6-phosphate dehydrogenase (G6PD) deficiency.

Potentially significant interactions may exist, requiring dose or frequency adjustment, additional monitoring, and/or selection of alternative therapy. Serious and fatal reactions including seizures, status epilepticus, cardiac arrest and respiratory failure have been reported with concomitant administration of theophylline. If concurrent use is unavoidable, monitor serum theophylline levels and adjust theophylline dose as warranted.

Drug Interactions

Metabolism/Transport Effects Substrate of P-glycoprotein; **Inhibits** CYP1A2 (strong), CYP3A4 (weak)

Avoid Concomitant Use

Avoid concomitant use of Ciprofloxacin (Systemic) with any of the following: BCG; Pimozide; Pirfenidone; Pomalidomide; Strontium Ranelate; TIZANidine

Increased Effect/Toxicity

Ciprofloxacin (Systemic) may increase the levels/effects of: ARIPiprazole; Bendamustine; Caffeine; CloZAPine; Corticosteroids (Systemic); CYP1A2 Substrates; Erlotinib; Highest Risk QTc-Prolonging Agents; Lomitapide; Methotrexate; Moderate Risk QTc-Prolonging Agents; Pentoxifylline; Pimozide; Pirfenidone; Pomalidomide; Porfimer; Roflumilast; ROPINIRole; Ropivacaine; Sulfonylureas; Theophylline Derivatives; TIZANidine; Varenicline; Vitamin K Antagonists

The levels/effects of Ciprofloxacin (Systemic) may be increased by: Insulin; Mifepristone; Nonsteroidal Anti-Inflammatory Agents; P-glycoprotein/ABCB1 Inhibitors; Probenecid

Decreased Effect

Ciprofloxacin (Systemic) may decrease the levels/effects of: BCG; Didanosine; Fosphenytoin; Mycophenolate; Phenytoin; Sodium Picosulfate; Sulfonylureas; Typhoid Vaccine

The levels/effects of Ciprofloxacin (Systemic) may be decreased by: Antacids; Calcium Salts; Didanosine; Iron Salts; Lanthanum; Magnesium Salts; Multivitamins/Minerals (with ADEK, Folate, Iron); P-glycoprotein/ABCB1 Inducers; Quinapril; Sevelamer; Strontium Ranelate; Sucralfate; Zinc Salts

Ethanol/Nutrition/Herb Interactions

Food: Food decreases rate, but not extent, of absorption. Ciprofloxacin serum levels may be decreased if taken with divalent or trivalent cations. Ciprofloxacin may increase serum caffeine levels if taken concurrently. Rarely, crystalluria may occur. Enteral feedings may decrease plasma concentrations of ciprofloxacin probably by >30% inhibition of absorption. Management: May administer with food to minimize GI upset. Avoid or take ciprofloxacin 2 hours before or 6 hours after antacids, dairy products, or calcium-fortified juices alone or in a meal containing >800 mg calcium, oral multivitamins, or mineral supplements containing divalent and/or trivalent cations. Restrict caffeine intake if excessive cardiac or CNS stimulation occurs. Ensure adequate hydration during therapy. Ciprofloxacin should not be administered with enteral feedings. The feeding would need to be discontinued for 1-2 hours prior to and after ciprofloxacin administration. Nasogastric administration produces a greater loss of ciprofloxacin bioavailability than does nasoduodenal administration.

Herb/Nutraceutical: Dong quai and St John's wort may also cause photosensitization. Management: Avoid dong quai and St John's wort.

Dietary Considerations Food: Drug may cause GI upset; take without regard to meals (manufacturer prefers that immediate release tablet is taken 2 hours after meals). Extended release tablet may be taken with meals that contain dairy products (calcium content <800 mg), but not with dairy products alone.

Dairy products, calcium-fortified juices, oral multivitamins, and mineral supplements: Absorption of ciprofloxacin is decreased by divalent and trivalent cations. The manufacturer states that the usual dietary intake of calcium (including meals which include dairy products) has not been shown to interfere with ciprofloxacin absorption. Immediate release ciprofloxacin and Cipro® XR may be taken 2 hours before or 6 hours after any of these products.

Caffeine: Patients consuming regular large quantities of caffeinated beverages may need to restrict caffeine intake if excessive cardiac or CNS stimulation occurs.

Pharmacodynamics/Kinetics

Half-life Elimination Children: 2.5 hours; Adults: Normal renal function: 3-5 hours

Time to Peak Oral:
Immediate release tablet: 0.5-2 hours
Extended release tablet: Cipro® XR: 1-2.5 hours

Pregnancy Risk Factor C

Pregnancy Considerations Adverse events have been observed in some animal reproduction studies. Ciprofloxacin crosses the placenta and produces measurable concentrations in the amniotic fluid and cord serum (Ludlam, 1997). An increased risk of teratogenic effects has not been observed in animals or humans following ciprofloxacin use during pregnancy; however, because of concerns of cartilage damage in immature animals, ciprofloxacin should only be used during pregnancy if a safer option is not available. Ciprofloxacin is recommended for prophylaxis and treatment of pregnant women exposed to anthrax (CDC, 2001a; CDC, 2001b). Serum concentrations of ciprofloxacin may be lower during pregnancy than in nonpregnant patients (Giamarellou, 1989).

Lactation Enters breast milk/not recommended (AAP rates "compatible"; AAP 2001 update pending)

Breast-Feeding Considerations Ciprofloxacin is excreted in breast milk. Due to the potential for serious adverse reactions in the nursing infant, the manufacturer recommends a decision be made whether to discontinue nursing or to discontinue the drug, taking into account the importance of treatment to the mother. However, due to the low concentrations in human milk, minimal toxicity would be expected in the nursing infant and infant serum levels were undetectable in one report (Gardner, 1992). Nondose-related effects could include modification of bowel flora. There has been a single case report of perforated pseudomembranous colitis in a breast-feeding infant whose mother was taking ciprofloxacin (Harmon, 1992).

Dosage Forms

Infusion, premixed in D₅W: 200 mg (100 mL); 400 mg (200 mL)
Cipro® I.V.: 400 mg (200 mL)
Infusion, premixed in D₅W [preservative free]: 200 mg (100 mL); 400 mg (200 mL)
Injection, solution: 10 mg/mL (20 mL, 40 mL, 120 mL)
Injection, solution [preservative free]: 10 mg/mL (20 mL, 40 mL)
Microcapsules for suspension, oral:
Cipro®: 250 mg/5 mL (100 mL); 500 mg/5 mL (100 mL)
Tablet, oral: 100 mg, 250 mg, 500 mg, 750 mg
Cipro®: 250 mg, 500 mg
Tablet, extended release, oral: 500 mg, 1000 mg

Ciprofloxacin and Dexamethasone
(sip roe FLOKS a sin & deks a METH a sone)

Brand Names: U.S. Ciprodex®
Brand Names: Canada Ciprodex®
Pharmacologic Category Antibiotic, Otic; Antibiotic/Corticosteroid, Otic; Corticosteroid, Otic
Use Treatment of acute otitis media in pediatric patients with tympanostomy tubes or acute otitis externa in children and adults
Local Anesthetic/Vasoconstrictor Precautions No information available to require special precautions
Effects on Dental Treatment No significant effects or complications reported
Effects on Bleeding No information available to require special precautions
Adverse Effects 1% to 10%: Otic: Discomfort (3%), pain (<1% to 2%), pruritus (1%)
General Dosage Range Otic: *Children and Adults:* Instill 4 drops into affected ear(s) twice daily
Mechanism of Action Ciprofloxacin is a quinolone antibiotic; dexamethasone is a corticosteroid used to decrease inflammation accompanying bacterial infections
Pharmacodynamics/Kinetics
Time to Peak Plasma: Otic: Ciprofloxacin: 15 minutes to 2 hours
Pregnancy Risk Factor C
Pregnancy Considerations Animal reproduction studies have not been conducted with this combination. Refer to individual agents.

Ciprofloxacin and Hydrocortisone
(sip roe FLOKS a sin & hye droe KOR ti sone)

Brand Names: U.S. Cipro® HC
Brand Names: Canada Cipro® HC
Pharmacologic Category Antibiotic/Corticosteroid, Otic
Use Treatment of acute otitis externa, sometimes known as "swimmer's ear"
Local Anesthetic/Vasoconstrictor Precautions No information available to require special precautions
Effects on Dental Treatment No significant effects or complications reported
Effects on Bleeding No information available to require special precautions
Adverse Effects 1% to 10%: Central nervous system: Headache (1%)
General Dosage Range Otic: *Children >1 year and Adults:* 3 drops into affected ear(s) twice daily
Pregnancy Risk Factor C

Pregnancy Considerations Animal reproduction studies have not been conducted with this combination. Refer to individual agents.

Cisapride (SIS a pride)

Brand Names: U.S. Propulsid®

Pharmacologic Category Gastrointestinal Agent, Prokinetic

Use Treatment of nocturnal symptoms of gastroesophageal reflux disease (GERD); has demonstrated effectiveness for gastroparesis, refractory constipation, and nonulcer dyspepsia

Local Anesthetic/Vasoconstrictor Precautions Cisapride is one of the drugs confirmed to prolong the QT interval and is accepted as having a risk of causing torsade de pointes. The risk of drug-induced torsade de pointes is extremely low when a single QT interval prolonging drug is prescribed. In terms of epinephrine, it is not known what effect vasoconstrictors in the local anesthetic regimen will have in patients with a known history of congenital prolonged QT interval or in patients taking any medication that prolongs the QT interval. Until more information is obtained, it is suggested that the clinician consult with the physician prior to the use of a vasoconstrictor in suspected patients, and that the vasoconstrictor (epinephrine, mepivacaine and levonordefrin [Carbocaine® 2% with Neo-Cobefrin®]) be used with caution.

Effects on Dental Treatment Key adverse event(s) related to dental treatment: Xerostomia (normal salivary flow resumes upon discontinuation).

Effects on Bleeding No information available to require special precautions

Adverse Effects

>5%:

Central nervous system: Headache

Dermatologic: Rash

Gastrointestinal: Diarrhea, GI cramping, dyspepsia, flatulence, nausea, xerostomia

Respiratory: Rhinitis

<5%:

Cardiovascular: Tachycardia

Central nervous system: Extrapyramidal effects, somnolence, fatigue, seizure, insomnia, anxiety

Hematologic: Thrombocytopenia, increased LFTs, pancytopenia, leukopenia, granulocytopenia, aplastic anemia

Respiratory: Sinusitis, cough, upper respiratory tract infection, increased incidence of viral infection

General Dosage Range

Oral:

Children: 0.15-0.3 mg/kg 3-4 times/day (maximum: 10 mg/dose)

Adults: Initial: 5-10 mg 4 times/day, may increase to 20 mg 4 times/day if needed

Mechanism of Action Enhances the release of acetylcholine at the myenteric plexus. In vitro studies have shown cisapride to have serotonin-4 receptor agonistic properties which may increase gastrointestinal motility and cardiac rate; increases lower esophageal sphincter pressure and lower esophageal peristalsis; accelerates gastric emptying of both liquids and solids.

Pharmacodynamics/Kinetics

Onset of Action 0.5-1 hour

Half-life Elimination 6-12 hours

Pregnancy Risk Factor C

Pregnancy Considerations Adverse events were observed in animal reproduction studies.

Prescribing and Access Restrictions In U.S., available via limited-access protocol only. Call 877-795-4247 for more information.

Dental Comment Cisapride is known to prolong the QT interval. The QT interval is measured as the time and distance between the Q point of the QRS complex and the end of the T wave in the ECG tracing. After adjustment for heart rate, the QT interval is defined as prolonged if it is more than 450 msec in men and 460 msec in women. A long QT syndrome was first described in the 1950s and 60s as a congenital syndrome involving QT interval prolongation and syncope and sudden death. Some of the congenital long QT syndromes were characterized by a peculiar electrocardiographic appearance of the QRS complex involving a premature atria beat followed by a pause, then a subsequent sinus beat showing marked QT prolongation and deformity. This type of cardiac arrhythmia was originally termed "torsade de pointes" (translated from the French as "twisting of the points"). Cisapride is considered as having a risk of causing torsade de pointes. Since it is not known what effect vasoconstrictors in the local anesthetic regimen will have in patients with a known history of congenital prolonged QT interval or in patients taking any medication that prolongs the QT interval, a medical consult is suggested.

CISplatin (SIS pla tin)

Pharmacologic Category Antineoplastic Agent, Alkylating Agent; Antineoplastic Agent, Platinum Analog

Use Treatment of advanced bladder cancer, metastatic testicular cancer, and metastatic ovarian cancer

Unlabeled Use Treatment of breast cancer (metastatic), central nervous system tumors, cervical cancer, endometrial cancer, esophageal cancer, gastric cancer, germ cell tumors, gestational trophoblastic disease (refractory), head and neck cancer, hepatobiliary cancer, hepatoblastoma, Hodgkin lymphoma, malignant pleural mesothelioma, melanoma (metastatic), multiple myeloma, neuroblastoma, neuroendocrine tumors, non-Hodgkin lymphoma (NHL), nonsmall cell lung cancer (NSCLC), osteosarcoma, pancreatic cancer (advanced), prostate cancer, small cell lung cancer (SCLC), soft tissue sarcomas, and unknown primary cancers

Local Anesthetic/Vasoconstrictor Precautions No information available to require special precautions

Effects on Dental Treatment No significant effects or complications reported

Effects on Bleeding Cisplatin causes relatively less bone marrow suppression than many other antineoplastic agents. Thrombocytopenia may occur 18-23 days following treatment.

Adverse Effects

>10%:

Central nervous system: Neurotoxicity: Peripheral neuropathy is dose- and duration-dependent.

Gastrointestinal: Nausea and vomiting (76% to 100%)

Hematologic: Anemia (≤40%), leukopenia (25% to 30%; nadir: Day 18-23; recovery: By day 39; dose related), thrombocytopenia (25% to 30%; nadir: Day 18-23; recovery: By day 39; dose related)

Hepatic: Liver enzymes increased

Renal: Nephrotoxicity (28% to 36%; acute renal failure and chronic renal insufficiency)

Otic: Ototoxicity (children 40% to 60%; adults 10% to 31%; as tinnitus, high frequency hearing loss)

1% to 10%: Local: Tissue irritation

General Dosage Range Dosage adjustment recommended in patients with renal impairment

I.V.: *Adults:* 50-70 mg/m² every 3-4 weeks **or** 75-100 mg/m²/day every 3-4 weeks **or** 20 mg/m²/day for 5 days every 3 weeks

Mechanism of Action Inhibits DNA synthesis by the formation of DNA cross-links; denatures the double helix; covalently binds to DNA bases and disrupts DNA function; may also bind to proteins; the *cis*-isomer is 14 times more cytotoxic than the *trans*-isomer; both forms cross-link DNA but cis-platinum is less easily recognized by cell enzymes and, therefore, not repaired. Cisplatin can also bind two adjacent guanines on the same strand of DNA producing intrastrand cross-linking and breakage.

Pharmacodynamics/Kinetics

Half-life Elimination Initial: 14-49 minutes; Beta: 0.7-4.6 hours; Gamma: 24-127 hours (O'Dwyer, 2000)

Pregnancy Risk Factor D

Pregnancy Considerations Animal reproduction studies have demonstrated teratogenicity and embryotoxicity. Women of childbearing potential should be advised to avoid pregnancy. If used in pregnancy, or if patient becomes pregnant during treatment, the patient should be apprised of potential hazard to the fetus.

Citalopram (sye TAL oh pram)

Related Information

Clinical Risk Related to Drugs Prolonging QT Interval *on page 1510*

Escitalopram *on page 499*

Vasoconstrictor Interactions With Antidepressants *on page 1650*

Brand Names: U.S. CeleXA®

Brand Names: Canada Apo-Citalopram®; Auro-Citalopram; Ava-Citalopram; Celexa®; Citalopram-Odan; CO Citalopram; CTP 30; Dom-Citalopram; JAMP-Citalopram; Manda-Citalopram; Mint-Citalopram; Mylan-Citalopram; PHL-Citalopram; PMS-Citalopram; Q-Citalopram; RAN™-Citalo; ratio-Citalopram; Riva-Citalopram; Sandoz-Citalopram; Septa-Citalopram; Teva-Citalopram

Generic Availability (U.S.) Yes

Pharmacologic Category Antidepressant, Selective Serotonin Reuptake Inhibitor

Use Treatment of depression

Unlabeled Use Obsessive-compulsive disorder (OCD)

Local Anesthetic/Vasoconstrictor Precautions Although caution should be used in patients taking tricyclic antidepressants, no interactions have been reported with vasoconstrictors and citalopram, a non-tricyclic antidepressant which acts to increase serotonin; no precautions appear to be needed

Citalopram is one of the drugs confirmed to prolong the QT interval and is accepted as having a risk of causing torsade de pointes. The risk of drug-induced torsade de pointes is extremely low when a single QT interval prolonging drug is prescribed. In terms of epinephrine, it is not known what effect vasoconstrictors in the local anesthetic regimen will have in patients with a known history of congenital prolonged QT interval or in patients taking any medication that prolongs the QT interval. Until more information is obtained, it is suggested that the clinician consult with the physician prior to the use of a vasoconstrictor in suspected patients, and that the vasoconstrictor (epinephrine, mepivacaine and levonordefrin [Carbocaine® 2% with Neo-Cobefrin®]) be used with caution.

Effects on Dental Treatment Key adverse event(s) related to dental treatment: Xerostomia (normal salivary flow resumes upon discontinuation). Premarketing trials reported abnormal taste. See Effects on Bleeding and Dental Comment.

Effects on Bleeding Selective serotonin reuptake inhibitors, such as citalopram, may impair platelet aggregation due to platelet serotonin depletion, possibly increasing the risk of a bleeding complication. The risk of a bleeding complication can be increased by coadministration of other antiplatelet agents, such as NSAIDs and aspirin.

Adverse Effects

>10%:

Central nervous system: Somnolence (18%; dose related), insomnia (15%; dose related)

Gastrointestinal: Nausea (21%), xerostomia (20%)

Miscellaneous: Diaphoresis (11%; dose related)

1% to 10%:

Cardiovascular: QT prolongation (2%), hypotension (≥1%), orthostatic hypotension (≥1%), tachycardia (≥1%), bradycardia (1%)

Central nervous system: Fatigue (5%; dose related), anxiety (4%), agitation (3%), fever (2%), yawning (2%; dose related), amnesia (≥1%), apathy (≥1%), concentration impaired (≥1%), confusion (≥1%), depression (≥1%), migraine (≥1%), suicide attempt (≥1%)

Dermatologic: Rash (≥1%), pruritus (≥1%)

Endocrine & metabolic: Libido decreased (1% to 4%), dysmenorrhea (3%), amenorrhea (≥1%)

Gastrointestinal: Diarrhea (8%), dyspepsia (5%), anorexia (4%), vomiting (4%), abdominal pain (3%), appetite increased (≥1%), flatulence (≥1%), salivation increased (≥1%), taste perversion (≥1%), weight gain/loss (≥1%)

Genitourinary: Ejaculation disorder (6%), impotence (3%; dose related), polyuria (≥1%)

Neuromuscular & skeletal: Tremor (8%), arthralgia (2%), myalgia (2%), paresthesia (≥1%)

Ocular: Abnormal accommodation (≥1%)

Respiratory: Rhinitis (5%), upper respiratory tract infection (5%), sinusitis (3%), cough (≥1%)

Dosage Oral:

Children and Adolescents: Obsessive-compulsive disorder (unlabeled use): 10-40 mg daily (Mukaddes, 2003; Thomsen, 1997; Thomsen, 2001)

Adults <60 years: Depression: Initial: 20 mg once daily; increase the dose by 20 mg at an interval of ≥1 week to a maximum dose of 40 mg daily. **Note:** Doses >40 mg daily are not recommended due to the risk of QT prolongation; additional efficacy with doses >40 mg daily has not been demonstrated in clinical trials.

Poor metabolizers of CYP2C19 or concurrent use of moderate-to-strong CYP2C19 inhibitors (eg, cimetidine, omeprazole): Maximum dose: 20 mg daily

Elderly ≥60 years: Depression: Initial: 20 mg once daily; maximum dose in adults ≥60 years: 20 mg daily due to increased exposure and the risk of QT prolongation. Refer to adult dosing.

MAO inhibitor recommendations:

Switching to or from an MAO inhibitor intended to treat psychiatric disorders:

Allow 14 days to elapse between discontinuing an MAO inhibitor intended to treat psychiatric disorders and initiation of citalopram.

Allow 14 days to elapse between discontinuing citalopram and initiation of an MAO inhibitor intended to treat psychiatric disorders.

Use with other MAO inhibitors (linezolid or I.V. methylene blue):

Do not initiate citalopram in patients receiving linezolid or I.V. methylene blue; consider other interventions for psychiatric condition.

If urgent treatment with linezolid or I.V. methylene blue is required in a patient already receiving citalopram and potential benefits outweigh potential risks, discontinue citalopram promptly and administer linezolid or I.V. methylene blue. Monitor for serotonin syndrome for 2 weeks or until 24 hours after the last dose of linezolid or I.V. methylene blue, whichever comes first. May resume citalopram 24 hours after the last dose of linezolid or I.V. methylene blue.

Dosage adjustment in renal impairment:
Mild-to-moderate impairment: No dosage adjustment necessary.

Severe impairment: Cl_{cr} <20 mL/minute: No dosage adjustment provided in manufacturer's labeling (has not been studied); use caution.

Dosage adjustment in hepatic impairment: Initial: 20 mg once daily; maximum recommended dose: 20 mg daily due to decreased clearance and the risk of QT prolongation

Mechanism of Action A racemic bicyclic phthalane derivative, citalopram selectively inhibits serotonin reuptake in the presynaptic neurons and has minimal effects on norepinephrine or dopamine. Uptake inhibition of serotonin is primarily due to the S-enantiomer of citalopram. Displays little to no affinity for serotonin, dopamine, adrenergic, histamine, GABA, or muscarinic receptor subtypes.

Contraindications Hypersensitivity to citalopram or any component of the formulation; use of MAO inhibitors intended to treat psychiatric disorders (concurrently or within 14 days of discontinuing either citalopram or the MAO inhibitor); initiation of citalopram in a patient receiving linezolid or intravenous methylene blue; concomitant use with pimozide

Warnings/Precautions [U.S. Boxed Warning]: Antidepressants increase the risk of suicidal thinking and behavior in children, adolescents, and young adults (18-24 years of age) with major depressive disorder (MDD) and other psychiatric disorders; consider risk prior to prescribing. Short-term studies did not show an increased risk in patients >24 years of age and showed a decreased risk in patients ≥65 years. Closely monitor patients for clinical worsening, suicidality, or unusual changes in behavior, particularly during the initial 1-2 months of therapy or during periods of dosage adjustments (increases or decreases); the patient's family or caregiver should be instructed to closely observe the patient and communicate condition with healthcare provider. A medication guide concerning the use of antidepressants should be dispensed with each prescription. **Citalopram is not FDA approved for use in children.**

The possibility of a suicide attempt is inherent in major depression and may persist until remission occurs. Use caution in high-risk patients. Worsening depression and severe abrupt suicidality that are not part of the presenting symptoms may require discontinuation or modification of drug therapy. The patient's family or caregiver should be alerted to monitor patients for the emergence of suicidality and associated behaviors (such as agitation, irritability, hostility, impulsivity, and hypomania) and call healthcare provider.

May worsen psychosis in some patients or precipitate a shift to mania or hypomania in patients with bipolar disorder. Patients presenting with depressive symptoms should be screened for bipolar disorder. Monotherapy in patients with bipolar disorder should be avoided. **Citalopram is not FDA approved for the treatment of bipolar depression.**

Potentially life-threatening serotonin syndrome (SS) has occurred with serotonergic agents (eg, SSRIs, SNRIs), particularly when used in combination with other serotonergic agents (eg, triptans, TCAs, fentanyl, lithium, tramadol, buspirone, St John's wort, tryptophan) or agents that impair metabolism of serotonin (eg, MOA inhibitors intended to treat psychiatric disorders, other MAO inhibitors [ie, linezolid and intravenous methylene blue]). Discontinue treatment (and any concomitant serotonergic agent) immediately if signs/symptoms arise. May increase the risks associated with electroconvulsive therapy. Has a low potential to impair cognitive or motor performance; caution operating hazardous machinery or driving.

Citalopram causes dose-dependent QT_c prolongation; torsade de pointes, ventricular tachycardia, and sudden death have been reported. Use is not recommended in patients with congenital long QT syndrome, bradycardia, recent MI, uncompensated heart failure, hypokalemia, and/or hypomagnesemia, or patients receiving concomitant medications which prolong the QT interval; if use is essential and cannot be avoided in these patients, ECG monitoring is recommended. Discontinue therapy in any patient with persistent QT_c measurements >500 msec. Serum electrolytes, particularly potassium and magnesium, should be monitored prior to initiation and periodically during therapy in any patient at increased risk for significant electrolyte disturbances; hypokalemia and/or hypomagnesemia should be corrected prior to use. Due to the QT prolongation risk, doses >40 mg/day are not recommended. Additionally, the maximum daily dose should not exceed 20 mg/day in certain populations (eg, CYP2C19 poor metabolizers, patients with hepatic impairment, elderly patients). Potentially significant interactions may exist, requiring dose or frequency adjustment, additional monitoring, and/or selection of alternative therapy. Consult drug interactions database for more detailed information.

Use with caution in patients with a previous seizure disorder or condition predisposing to seizures such as brain damage or alcoholism. May cause or exacerbate sexual dysfunction. Upon discontinuation of citalopram therapy, gradually taper dose. If intolerable symptoms occur following a decrease in dosage or upon discontinuation of therapy, then resuming the previous dose with a more gradual taper should be considered. May cause hyponatremia/SIADH (elderly at increased risk); volume depletion and diuretics may increase risk. Monitor sodium closely with initiation or dosage adjustments in older adults (Beers Criteria). Citalopram is not FDA-approved for use in children; however, if used, monitor weight and growth regularly during therapy due to the potential for decreased appetite and weight loss with SSRI use.

Drug Interactions

Metabolism/Transport Effects Substrate of CYP2C19 (major), CYP2D6 (minor), CYP3A4 (major); **Note:** Assignment of Major/Minor substrate status based on clinically relevant drug interaction potential;

◀ **Inhibits** CYP1A2 (weak), CYP2B6 (weak), CYP2C19 (weak), CYP2D6 (weak)

Avoid Concomitant Use

Avoid concomitant use of Citalopram with any of the following: Conivaptan; Highest Risk QTc-Prolonging Agents; Iobenguane I 123; Ivabradine; Linezolid; MAO Inhibitors; Methylene Blue; Mifepristone; Moderate Risk QTc-Prolonging Agents; Pimozide; Tryptophan

Increased Effect/Toxicity

Citalopram may increase the levels/effects of: Agents with Antiplatelet Properties; Anticoagulants; Antidepressants (Serotonin Reuptake Inhibitor/Antagonist); Aspirin; BusPIRone; CarBAMazepine; CloZAPine; Collagenase (Systemic); Dabigatran Etexilate; Desmopressin; Dextromethorphan; Drotrecogin Alfa (Activated); Highest Risk QTc-Prolonging Agents; Hypoglycemic Agents; Ibritumomab; Methadone; Methylene Blue; Metoclopramide; Mexiletine; NSAID (COX-2 Inhibitor); NSAID (Nonselective); Pimozide; RisperiDONE; Rivaroxaban; Salicylates; Serotonin Modulators; Thrombolytic Agents; Tositumomab and Iodine I 131 Tositumomab; TraMADol; Tricyclic Antidepressants; Vitamin K Antagonists

The levels/effects of Citalopram may be increased by: Alcohol (Ethyl); Analgesics (Opioid); Antipsychotics; BusPIRone; Cimetidine; CNS Depressants; Cobicistat; Conivaptan; CYP2C19 Inhibitors (Moderate); CYP2C19 Inhibitors (Strong); CYP3A4 Inhibitors (Moderate); CYP3A4 Inhibitors (Strong); Dasatinib; Fluconazole; Glucosamine; Herbs (Anticoagulant/Antiplatelet Properties); Ivabradine; Ivacaftor; Linezolid; Lithium; Macrolide Antibiotics; MAO Inhibitors; Metoclopramide; Metyrosine; Mifepristone; Moderate Risk QTc-Prolonging Agents; Multivitamins/Minerals (with ADEK, Folate, Iron); Omega-3 Fatty Acids; Pentosan Polysulfate Sodium; Pentoxifylline; Prostacyclin Analogues; QTc-Prolonging Agents (Indeterminate Risk and Risk Modifying); Tipranavir; TraMADol; Tryptophan; Vitamin E

Decreased Effect

Citalopram may decrease the levels/effects of: Iobenguane I 123; Ioflupane I 123

The levels/effects of Citalopram may be decreased by: CarBAMazepine; CYP2C19 Inducers (Strong); CYP3A4 Inducers (Strong); Cyproheptadine; Deferasirox; NSAID (COX-2 Inhibitor); NSAID (Nonselective); Peginterferon Alfa-2b; Tocilizumab

Ethanol/Nutrition/Herb Interactions

Ethanol: May increase CNS depression; monitor for increased effects with coadministration. Caution patients about effects.

Herb/Nutraceutical: Avoid valerian, St John's wort, tryptophan, SAMe, kava kava, and gotu kola (may increase CNS depression).

Dietary Considerations May be taken without regard to food.

Pharmacodynamics/Kinetics

Onset of Action Depression: The onset of action is 1-4 weeks; however, individual response varies greatly and full response may not be seen until 8-12 weeks after initiation of treatment.

Half-life Elimination 24-48 hours (average: 35 hours); doubled with hepatic impairment and increased by 30% (following multiple doses) to 50% (following single dose) in elderly patients (≥60 years)

Time to Peak Serum: 1-6 hours, average within 4 hours

Pregnancy Risk Factor C

Pregnancy Considerations Adverse events have been observed in animal reproduction studies. Citalopram and its metabolites cross the human placenta. An increased risk of teratogenic effects, including cardiovascular defects, may be associated with maternal use of citalopram or other SSRIs; however, available information is conflicting. Nonteratogenic effects in the newborn following SSRI/SNRI exposure late in the third trimester include respiratory distress, cyanosis, apnea, seizures, temperature instability, feeding difficulty, vomiting, hypoglycemia, hypo- or hypertonia, hyper-reflexia, jitteriness, irritability, constant crying, and tremor. Symptoms may be due to the toxicity of the SSRIs/SNRIs or a discontinuation syndrome and may be consistent with serotonin syndrome associated with SSRI treatment. Persistent pulmonary hypertension of the newborn (PPHN) has also been reported with SSRI exposure. The long-term effects of *in utero* SSRI exposure on infant development and behavior are not known.

Due to pregnancy-induced physiologic changes, women who are pregnant may require adjusted doses of citalopram to achieve euthymia. The ACOG recommends that therapy with SSRIs or SNRIs during pregnancy be individualized; treatment of depression during pregnancy should incorporate the clinical expertise of the mental health clinician, obstetrician, primary healthcare provider, and pediatrician. According to the American Psychiatric Association (APA), the risks of medication treatment should be weighed against other treatment options and untreated depression. For women who discontinue antidepressant medications during pregnancy and who may be at high risk for postpartum depression, the medications can be restarted following delivery. Treatment algorithms have been developed by the ACOG and the APA for the management of depression in women prior to conception and during pregnancy.

Lactation Enters breast milk/consider risk:benefit

Breast-Feeding Considerations Citalopram and its metabolites are excreted in breast milk. According to the manufacturer, the decision to continue or discontinue breast-feeding during therapy should take into account the risk of exposure to the infant and the benefits of treatment to the mother. Excessive somnolence, decreased feeding, colic, irritability, restlessness, and weight loss have been reported in breast-fed infants. The long-term effects on development and behavior have not been studied; therefore, citalopram should be prescribed to a mother who is breast-feeding only when the benefits outweigh the potential risks. Maternal use of an SSRI during pregnancy may cause delayed milk secretion.

Dosage Forms

Solution, oral: 10 mg/5 mL (240 mL)

Tablet, oral: 10 mg, 20 mg, 40 mg

CeleXA®: 10 mg, 20 mg, 40 mg

Dental Comment Problems with SSRI-induced bruxism have been reported and may preclude their use; clinicians attempting to evaluate any patient with bruxism or involuntary muscle movement, who is simultaneously being treated with an SSRI drug, should be aware of the potential association.

Citalopram is known to prolong the QT interval. The QT interval is measured as the time and distance between the Q point of the QRS complex and the end of the T wave in the ECG tracing. After adjustment for heart rate, the QT interval is defined as prolonged if it is more than 450 msec in men and 460 msec in women. A long QT syndrome was first described in the 1950s and 60s as a congenital syndrome involving QT interval prolongation and syncope and sudden death. Some of the congenital long QT syndromes were characterized by a peculiar electrocardiographic appearance of the QRS complex involving a premature atria beat followed by a pause, then a subsequent sinus beat showing marked QT prolongation and deformity. This type of cardiac arrhythmia was originally termed "torsade de pointes" (translated from the French as "twisting of the points"). Citalopram is considered as having a risk of causing torsade de pointes. Since it is not known what effect vasoconstrictors in the local anesthetic regimen will have in patients with a known history of congenital prolonged QT interval or in patients taking any medication that prolongs the QT interval, a medical consult is suggested.

Citric Acid, Magnesium Carbonate, and Glucono-Delta-Lactone
(SI trik AS id, mag NEE see um KAR bo nate, and GLOO kon o DEL ta LAK tone)

Brand Names: U.S. Renacidin®
Pharmacologic Category Genitourinary Irrigant; Urinary Tract Product
Use Prevention of formation of calcifications of indwelling urinary tract catheters; treatment of renal and bladder calculi of the apatite or struvite type
Local Anesthetic/Vasoconstrictor Precautions No information available to require special precautions
Effects on Dental Treatment No significant effects or complications reported
Effects on Bleeding No information available to require special precautions
Adverse Effects
>10%:
  Central nervous system: Fever (20% to 40%)
  Genitourinary: Urothelial ulceration with or without edema (13%)
  Miscellaneous: Transient flank pain
1% to 10%:
  Endocrine & metabolic: Hypermagnesemia, hyperphosphatemia
  Genitourinary: Urinary tract infection, dysuria, hematuria, bladder irritability
  Neuromuscular & skeletal: Back pain
  Renal: Creatinine increased
General Dosage Range Irrigation: *Adults:* 30-60 mL into catheter 2-3 times/day **or** 30 mL into bladder, retained for 30-60 minutes then drained 4-6 times **or** 60-120 mL/hour
Mechanism of Action Magnesium from the irrigating solution is exchanged for calcium in the stone matrix. The magnesium stones are soluble and are able to dissolve in the acidic pH of the solution.
Pregnancy Risk Factor C
Pregnancy Considerations Reproduction studies have not been conducted.

Citric Acid, Sodium Citrate, and Potassium Citrate
(SIT rik AS id, SOW dee um SIT rate, & poe TASS ee um SIT rate)

Related Information
  Potassium Citrate *on page 1121*
Brand Names: U.S. Cytra-3; Tricitrates
Pharmacologic Category Alkalinizing Agent

Use Conditions where long-term maintenance of an alkaline urine is desirable as in control and dissolution of uric acid and cystine calculi of the urinary tract
Local Anesthetic/Vasoconstrictor Precautions No information available to require special precautions
Effects on Dental Treatment No significant effects or complications reported
Effects on Bleeding No information available to require special precautions
Adverse Effects Frequency not defined.
  Cardiovascular: Cardiac abnormalities
  Endocrine & metabolic: Metabolic alkalosis, calcium levels, hyperkalemia, hypernatremia
  Gastrointestinal: Diarrhea
  Neuromuscular & skeletal: Tetany
General Dosage Range Oral:
  Children: 5-15 mL after meals and at bedtime
  Adults: 15-30 mL after meals and at bedtime
Pregnancy Risk Factor Not established
Pregnancy Considerations Use caution with toxemia of pregnancy.

Cladribine (KLA dri been)

Pharmacologic Category Antineoplastic Agent, Antimetabolite; Antineoplastic Agent, Antimetabolite (Purine Analog)
Use Treatment of active hairy cell leukemia
Unlabeled Use Treatment of acute myeloid leukemia (AML), chronic lymphocytic leukemia (CLL), non-Hodgkin's lymphomas (mantle cell), Waldenström's macroglobulinemia, refractory Langerhans cell histiocytosis
Local Anesthetic/Vasoconstrictor Precautions No information available to require special precautions
Effects on Dental Treatment No significant effects or complications reported
Effects on Bleeding The major dose-limiting adverse effect of cladribine is bone marrow suppression including severe (grade 4) thrombocytopenia in ~12% of patients receiving repeated courses of therapy; recovery is usually by day 12.
Adverse Effects
>10%:
  Central nervous system: Fever (33% to 69%; ≥100°F: 67%; ≥104°F: 11%), fatigue (11% to 45%), headache (7% to 22%)
  Dermatologic: Rash (10% to 27%)
  Gastrointestinal: Nausea (22% to 28%), appetite decreased (8% to 17%), vomiting (9% to 13%)
  Hematologic: Neutropenia (grade 4: 70%; recovery: by week 5); anemia (1% to 37%; recovery: by week 8); myelosuppression (34%; prolonged), neutropenic fever (8% to 47%; severe: 32%), thrombocytopenia (grade 4: 12%; recovery: by day 12)
  Local: Injection site reactions (9% to 19%)
  Respiratory: Abnormal breath sounds (4% to 11%)
  Miscellaneous: Infection (month 1: 28% [serious: 6%]; month 2: 6%)
1% to 10%:
  Cardiovascular: Edema (2% to 6%), tachycardia (2% to 6%), thrombosis (2%)
  Central nervous system: Chills (2% to 9%), dizziness (6% to 9%), insomnia (3% to 7%), malaise (5% to 7%), pain (6%), anxiety (1%)
  Dermatologic: Purpura (10%), petechiae (2% to 8%), pruritus (2% to 6%), erythema (6%), hyperhidrosis (3%), bruising (1% to 2%)

Gastrointestinal: Diarrhea (7% to 10%), constipation (4% to 9%), abdominal pain (4% to 6%), flatulence (1%)

Local: Phlebitis (2%)

Neuromuscular & skeletal: Weakness (6% to 9%), myalgia (6% to 7%), arthralgia (3% to 5%), muscle weakness (1%)

Respiratory: Cough (7% to 10%), abnormal chest sounds (9%), dyspnea (5% to 7%), epistaxis (5%), rales (1%)

Miscellaneous: Diaphoresis (9%)

General Dosage Range Dosage adjustment recommended in patients with renal impairment

I.V.: *Adults:* Continuous infusion: 0.09 mg/kg/day for 7 days

Mechanism of Action A purine nucleoside analogue; prodrug which is activated via phosphorylation by deoxycytidine kinase to a 5'-triphosphate derivative (2-CaAMP). This active form incorporates into DNA to result in the breakage of DNA strand and shutdown of DNA synthesis and repair. This also results in a depletion of nicotinamide adenine dinucleotide and adenosine triphosphate (ATP). Cladribine is cell-cycle nonspecific.

Pharmacodynamics/Kinetics

Half-life Elimination After a 2-hour infusion (with normal renal function): 5.4 hours

Pregnancy Risk Factor D

Pregnancy Considerations Teratogenic effects and fetal mortality were observed in animal reproduction studies. May cause fetal harm if administered during pregnancy. Women of reproductive potential should use highly effective contraception during treatment.

Clarithromycin (kla RITH roe mye sin)

Related Information

Antibiotic Prophylaxis *on page 1542*

Bacterial Infections *on page 1562*

Clinical Risk Related to Drugs Prolonging QT Interval *on page 1510*

Gastrointestinal Disorders *on page 1512*

Brand Names: U.S. Biaxin®; Biaxin® XL

Brand Names: Canada Apo-Clarithromycin®; Ava-Clarithromycin; Biaxin®; Biaxin® XL; Dom-Clarithromycin; Mylan-Clarithromycin; PMS-Clarithromycin; RAN™-Clarithromycin; ratio-Clarithromycin; Riva-Clarithromycin; Sandoz-Clarithromycin

Generic Availability (U.S.) Yes

Pharmacologic Category Antibiotic, Macrolide

Dental Use Alternate oral antibiotic for prevention of infective endocarditis in individuals allergic to penicillins or ampicillin, when amoxicillin cannot be used; alternate antibiotic in the treatment of common orofacial infections caused by aerobic gram-positive cocci and susceptible anaerobes

Use

Children:

Acute maxillary sinusitis due to susceptible *H. influenzae, S. pneumoniae,* or *Moraxella catarrhalis*

Acute otitis media due to susceptible *H. influenzae, M. catarrhalis,* or *S. pneumoniae*

Community-acquired pneumonia due to susceptible *Mycoplasma pneumoniae, S. pneumoniae,* or *Chlamydia pneumoniae* (TWAR)

Disseminated mycobacterial infections due to *M. avium* or *M. intracellulare*

Pharyngitis/tonsillitis due to susceptible *S. pyogenes*

Prevention of disseminated mycobacterial infections due to MAC disease in patients with advanced HIV infection

Uncomplicated skin/skin structure infection due to susceptible *S. aureus, S. pyogenes,* or mycobacterial infections

Adults:

Pharyngitis/tonsillitis due to susceptible *S. pyogenes*

Acute maxillary sinusitis due to susceptible *H. influenzae, M. catarrhalis,* or *S. pneumoniae*

Acute exacerbation of chronic bronchitis due to susceptible *H. influenzae, H. parainfluenzae, M. catarrhalis,* or *S. pneumoniae*

Community-acquired pneumonia due to susceptible *H. influenzae, H. parainfluenzae, M. catarrhalis, Mycoplasma pneumoniae, S. pneumoniae,* or *Chlamydia pneumoniae* (TWAR)

Uncomplicated skin/skin structure infections due to susceptible *S. aureus, S. pyogenes*

Disseminated mycobacterial infections due to *M. avium* or *M. intracellulare*

Prevention of disseminated mycobacterial infections due to *M. avium* complex (MAC) disease (eg, patients with advanced HIV infection)

Duodenal ulcer disease due to *H. pylori* in regimens with other drugs including amoxicillin and lansoprazole or omeprazole, or in combination with omeprazole or ranitidine bismuth citrate (no longer marketed in the U.S.). **Note:** Regimens that contain clarithromycin as the single antimicrobial agent are more likely to be associated with the development of clarithromycin resistance.

Unlabeled Use Pertussis (CDC guidelines); alternate antibiotic for prophylaxis of infective endocarditis in patients who are allergic to penicillin and undergoing dental procedures (ACC/AHA guidelines)

Local Anesthetic/Vasoconstrictor Precautions Clarithromycin is one of the drugs confirmed to prolong the QT interval and is accepted as having a risk of causing torsade de pointes. In terms of epinephrine, it is not known what effect vasoconstrictors in the local anesthetic regimen will have in patients with a known history of congenital prolonged QT interval or in patients taking any medication that prolongs the QT interval. Until more information is obtained, it is suggested that the clinician consult with the physician prior to the use of a vasoconstrictor in suspected patients, and that the vasoconstrictor (epinephrine, mepivacaine and levonordefrin [Carbocaine® 2% with Neo-Cobefrin®]) be used with caution. See Dental Comment.

Effects on Dental Treatment Key adverse event(s) related to dental treatment: Abnormal taste.

Effects on Bleeding No information available to require special precautions

Adverse Effects 1% to 10%:

Central nervous system: Headache (2%)

Dermatologic: Rash (children 3%)

Gastrointestinal: Abnormal taste (adults 3% to 7%), diarrhea (adults 3% to 6%; children 6%), vomiting (children 6%), nausea (adults 3%), abdominal pain (adults 2%; children 3%), dyspepsia (adults 2%)

Hepatic: Prothrombin time increased (adults 1%)

Renal: BUN increased (4%)

Dental Usual Dosage Prophylaxis against infective endocarditis (unlabeled use): Oral:

Children: 15 mg/kg 30-60 minutes before procedure

Adults: 500 mg 30-60 minutes prior to procedure

Note: American Heart Association (AHA) guidelines now recommend prophylaxis only in patients undergoing invasive procedures and in whom underlying cardiac conditions may predispose to a higher risk of adverse outcomes should infection occur. As of April 2007, routine prophylaxis for GI/GU procedures is no longer recommended by the AHA.

Dosage

Usual dosage range:

Children ≥6 months: Oral: 7.5 mg/kg every 12 hours (maximum: 500 mg/dose) for 10 days

Adults: Oral: 250-500 mg every 12 hours **or** 1000 mg (two 500 mg extended release tablets) once daily for 7-14 days

Indication-specific dosing:

Children: Oral:

Community-acquired pneumonia (CAP) (IDSA/ PIDS, 2011): Infants >3 months and Children: **Note:** A beta-lactam antibiotic should be added if typical bacterial pneumonia cannot be ruled out.

Presumed atypical *(M. pneumoniae, C. pneumoniae, C. trachomatis)* infection, mild-to-severe atypical infection or step-down therapy (alternative to azithromycin): 7.5 mg/kg/dose (maximum: 1000 mg) every 12 hours

Mycobacterial infection (prevention and treatment):

Manufacturer's recommendation: 7.5 mg/kg/dose (maximum: 500 mg/dose) twice daily. **Note:** Safety of clarithromycin for MAC not studied in children <20 months.

HIV-exposed/-positive (unlabeled use; CDC, 2009):

Primary prophylaxis: 7.5 mg/kg/dose (maximum: 500 mg/dose) twice daily

Secondary prophylaxis: 7.5 mg/kg/dose (maximum: 500 mg/dose) twice daily, plus ethambutol, with or without rifabutin

Treatment: 7.5-15 mg/kg/dose (maximum: 500 mg/dose) twice daily plus ethambutol, plus rifabutin (for severe disease)

Pertussis (unlabeled use; CDC, 2005):

Children 1-5 months: 7.5 mg/kg/dose every 12 hours for 7 days

Children ≥6 months: 7.5 mg/kg/dose every 12 hours for 7 days (maximum: 1000 mg daily)

Pharyngitis, group A streptococci in penicillin-allergic patients (IDSA guidelines): 7.5 mg/kg/dose every 12 hours (maximum: 500 mg daily) for 10 days (Shulman, 2012)

Prophylaxis against infective endocarditis (unlabeled use): 15 mg/kg 30-60 minutes before procedure. **Note:** American Heart Association (AHA) guidelines now recommend prophylaxis only in patients undergoing invasive procedures and in whom underlying cardiac conditions may predispose to a higher risk of adverse outcomes should infection occur. As of April 2007, routine prophylaxis for GI/GU procedures is no longer recommended by the AHA.

Sinusitis, bronchitis, skin infections: 7.5 mg/kg/dose every 12 hours for 10 days

Adults: Oral:

Acute exacerbation of chronic bronchitis:

M. catarrhalis and *S. pneumoniae:* 250 mg every 12 hours for 7-14 days **or** 1000 mg (two 500 mg extended release tablets) once daily for 7 days

H. influenzae: 500 mg every 12 hours for 7-14 days **or** 1000 mg (two 500 mg extended release tablets) once daily for 7 days

H. parainfluenzae: 500 mg every 12 hours for 7 days **or** 1000 mg (two 500 mg extended release tablets) once daily for 7 days

Acute maxillary sinusitis: 500 mg every 12 hours **or** 1000 mg (two 500 mg extended release tablets) once daily for 14 days

Mycobacterial infection (prevention and treatment): 500 mg twice daily (use with other antimycobacterial drugs, eg, ethambutol or rifampin)

Peptic ulcer disease: Eradication of *Helicobacter pylori:* Dual or triple combination regimens with bismuth subsalicylate, amoxicillin, an H_2-receptor antagonist, or proton-pump inhibitor: 500 mg every 8-12 hours for 10-14 days

Pertussis (unlabeled use; CDC, 2005): 500 mg twice daily for 7 days

Pharyngitis, tonsillitis: 250 mg every 12 hours for 10 days. **Note:** Recommended by the Infectious Disease Society of America (IDSA) as an alternative agent for group A streptococcal pharyngitis in penicillin-allergic patients (Shulman, 2012).

Pneumonia:

C. pneumoniae, M. pneumoniae, and *S. pneumoniae:* 250 mg every 12 hours for 7-14 days **or** 1000 mg (two 500 mg extended release tablets) once daily for 7 days

H. influenzae: 250 mg every 12 hours for 7 days **or** 1000 mg (two 500 mg extended release tablets) once daily for 7 days

H. parainfluenzae and *M. catarrhalis:* 1000 mg (two 500 mg extended release tablets) once daily for 7 days

Prophylaxis against infective endocarditis (unlabeled use): 500 mg 30-60 minutes prior to procedure. **Note:** American Heart Association (AHA) guidelines now recommend prophylaxis only in patients undergoing invasive procedures and in whom underlying cardiac conditions may predispose to a higher risk of adverse outcomes should infection occur. As of April 2007, routine prophylaxis for GI/GU procedures is no longer recommended by the AHA.

Skin and skin structure infection, uncomplicated: 250 mg every 12 hours for 7-14 days

Elderly: Pharmacokinetics are similar to those in younger adults; may have age-related reductions in renal function; monitor and adjust dose if necessary

Dosing adjustment in renal impairment:

Cl_{cr} <30 mL/minute: Decrease clarithromycin dose by 50%

Hemodialysis: Administer after HD session is completed (Aronoff, 2007).

In combination with atazanavir or ritonavir:

Cl_{cr} 30-60 mL/minute: Decrease clarithromycin dose by 50%

Cl_{cr} <30 mL/minute: Decrease clarithromycin dose by 75%

Dosing adjustment in hepatic impairment: No dosing adjustment is needed as long as renal function is normal

Mechanism of Action Exerts its antibacterial action by binding to 50S ribosomal subunit resulting in inhibition of protein synthesis. The 14-OH metabolite of clarithromycin is twice as active as the parent compound against certain organisms.

Contraindications Hypersensitivity to clarithromycin, erythromycin, or any macrolide antibiotic; use with ergot derivatives, pimozide, cisapride, astemizole, terfenadine, colchicine (if patient has concomitant renal or hepatic impairment), lovastatin, simvastatin; history of cholestatic jaundice or hepatic dysfunction with prior clarithromycin use; history of QT prolongation or ventricular arrhythmia, including torsade de pointes

Warnings/Precautions Dosage adjustment required with severe renal impairment; decreased dosage or prolonged dosing interval may be appropriate. May cause hepatotoxicity (elevated liver function tests, hepatitis, jaundice, hepatic failure); use caution with preexisting hepatic disease or hepatotoxic medications. Use with caution in patients with myasthenia gravis. Colchicine toxicity (including fatalities) has been reported with concomitant use; concomitant use is contraindicated in patients with renal or hepatic impairment. Major inhibitor of CYP3A4; use caution with any agents with substantial metabolism through the CYP3A4 pathway; high potential for drug interactions exists. Prolonged use may result in fungal or bacterial superinfection, including *C. difficile*-associated diarrhea (CDAD) and pseudomembranous colitis; CDAD has been observed >2 months postantibiotic treatment. Decreased *H. pylori* eradication rates have been observed with short-term (≤7 days) combination therapy. The American College of Gastroenterology recommends 10-14 days of therapy (triple or quadruple) for eradication of *H. pylori* (Chey, 2007). Macrolides (including clarithromycin) have been associated with rare cardiac conduction alterations, and use is contraindicated in patients with a history of QT prolongation and ventricular arrhythmias, including torsade de pointes; avoid use in patients with uncorrected hypokalemia or hypomagnesemia, clinically significant bradycardia, and patients receiving Class IA (eg, quinidine, procainamide) or Class III (eg, amiodarone, dofetilide, sotalol) antiarrhythmic agents. Elderly patients may be at increased risk of torsade de pointes, particularly if concurrent renal/hepatic impairment. Severe acute reactions have (rarely) been reported, including anaphylaxis, Stevens-Johnson syndrome (SJS), toxic epidermal necrolysis (TEN), drug rash with eosinophilia and systemic symptoms (DRESS), and Henoch-Schönlein purpura (IgA vasculitis); discontinue therapy immediately and urgently initiate treatment. Use caution in patients with coronary artery disease. Avoid use of extended release tablets (Biaxin® XL) in patients with known stricture/narrowing of the GI tract.

Drug Interactions

Metabolism/Transport Effects Substrate of CYP3A4 (major); **Note:** Assignment of Major/Minor substrate status based on clinically relevant drug interaction potential; **Inhibits** CYP1A2 (weak), CYP3A4 (strong), P-glycoprotein

Avoid Concomitant Use

Avoid concomitant use of Clarithromycin with any of the following: Ado-Trastuzumab Emtansine; Alfuzosin; Apixaban; Avanafil; Axitinib; BCG; Bosutinib; Cabozantinib; Cisapride; Conivaptan; Crizotinib; Dihydroergotamine; Disopyramide; Dronedarone; Eplerenone; Ergotamine; Everolimus; Fluticasone (Oral Inhalation); Halofantrine; Highest Risk QTc-Prolonging Agents; Ivabradine; Lapatinib; Lomitapide; Lovastatin; Lurasidone; Mifepristone; Nilotinib; Nisoldipine; Pimozide; Pomalidomide; QuiNINE; Ranolazine; Red Yeast Rice; Regorafenib; RomiDEPsin; Salmeterol; Silodosin; Simvastatin; Tamsulosin; Terfenadine; Ticagrelor; Tolvaptan; Topotecan; Toremifene; VinCRIStine (Liposomal)

Increased Effect/Toxicity

Clarithromycin may increase the levels/effects of: Ado-Trastuzumab Emtansine; Alfentanil; Alfuzosin; Almotriptan; Alosetron; Antifungal Agents (Azole Derivatives, Systemic); Antineoplastic Agents (Vinca Alkaloids); Apixaban; ARIPiprazole; Avanafil; Axitinib; Bedaquiline; Benzodiazepines (metabolized by oxidation); Boceprevir; Bortezomib; Bosutinib; Brentuximab Vedotin; Brinzolamide; Budesonide (Nasal); Budesonide (Systemic, Oral Inhalation); BusPIRone; Cabozantinib; Calcium Channel Blockers; CarBAMazepine; Cardiac Glycosides; Cilostazol; Cisapride; CloZAPine; Cobicistat; Colchicine; Conivaptan; Corticosteroids (Orally Inhaled); Corticosteroids (Systemic); Crizotinib; CycloSPORINE (Systemic); CYP3A4 Inducers (Strong); CYP3A4 Substrates; Dabigatran Etexilate; Dienogest; Dihydroergotamine; Disopyramide; Dronedarone; Dutasteride; Eletriptan; Enzalutamide; Eplerenone; Ergot Derivatives; Ergotamine; Everolimus; FentaNYL; Fesoterodine; Fluticasone (Nasal); Fluticasone (Oral Inhalation); GlipiZIDE; GlyBURIDE; GuanFACINE; Halofantrine; Highest Risk QTc-Prolonging Agents; HMG-CoA Reductase Inhibitors; Iloperidone; Ivabradine; Ivacaftor; Ixabepilone; Lapatinib; Lomitapide; Lovastatin; Lumefantrine; Lurasidone; Maraviroc; MethylPREDNISolone; Mifepristone; Moderate Risk QTc-Prolonging Agents; Nilotinib; Nisoldipine; Ospemifene; Paricalcitol; Pazopanib; P-glycoprotein/ABCB1 Substrates; Pimecrolimus; Pimozide; Pomalidomide; Ponatinib; Propafenone; Protease Inhibitors; Prucalopride; QuiNIDine; QuiNINE; Ranolazine; Red Yeast Rice; Regorafenib; Repaglinide; Rifamycin Derivatives; Rivaroxaban; RomiDEPsin; Ruxolitinib; Salmeterol; Saxagliptin; Selective Serotonin Reuptake Inhibitors; Sildenafil; Silodosin; Simvastatin; Sirolimus; SORAfenib; Tacrolimus (Systemic); Tacrolimus (Topical); Tadalafil; Tamsulosin; Telaprevir; Temsirolimus; Terfenadine; Theophylline Derivatives; Ticagrelor; Tofacitinib; Tolterodine; Tolvaptan; Topotecan; Toremifene; Vardenafil; Vemurafenib; Vilazodone; VinCRIStine (Liposomal); Vitamin K Antagonists; Zidovudine; Zopiclone; Zuclopenthixol

The levels/effects of Clarithromycin may be increased by: Antifungal Agents (Azole Derivatives, Systemic); Boceprevir; Cobicistat; CYP3A4 Inducers (Strong); CYP3A4 Inhibitors (Moderate); CYP3A4 Inhibitors (Strong); Dasatinib; Ivabradine; Mifepristone; Protease Inhibitors; QTc-Prolonging Agents (Indeterminate Risk and Risk Modifying); Telaprevir

Decreased Effect

Clarithromycin may decrease the levels/effects of: BCG; Clopidogrel; Ifosfamide; Prasugrel; Sodium Picosulfate; Ticagrelor; Typhoid Vaccine; Zidovudine

The levels/effects of Clarithromycin may be decreased by: CYP3A4 Inducers (Strong); Deferasirox; Etravirine; Herbs (CYP3A4 Inducers); Protease Inhibitors; Tocilizumab

Ethanol/Nutrition/Herb Interactions

Food: Immediate release: Food delays rate, but not extent of absorption; Extended release: Food increases clarithromycin AUC by ~30% relative to fasting conditions.

Herb/Nutraceutical: St John's wort may decrease clarithromycin levels.

Dietary Considerations Clarithromycin immediate release tablets and oral suspension may be given with or without meals, and may be taken with milk. Extended release tablets should be taken with food.

Pharmacodynamics/Kinetics

Half-life Elimination Immediate release: Clarithromycin: 3-7 hours; 14-OH-clarithromycin: 5-9 hours

Time to Peak Immediate release: 2-3 hours; Extended release: 5-8 hours

Pregnancy Risk Factor C
Pregnancy Considerations Adverse fetal effects have been documented in some animal reproduction studies. Clarithromycin crosses the placenta. The manufacturer recommends that clarithromycin not be used in a pregnant woman unless there are no alternative therapies. An increased risk of teratogenic events has not been observed following maternal use of clarithromycin.
Lactation Excretion in breast milk unknown/use caution
Breast-Feeding Considerations It is not known if clarithromycin is excreted in human breast milk. The manufacturer recommends that caution be exercised when administering clarithromycin to breast-feeding women.

Other macrolides are considered compatible with breast-feeding and clarithromycin is used therapeutically in infants. Nondose-related effects could include modification of bowel flora.
Dosage Forms
Granules for suspension, oral: 125 mg/5 mL (50 mL, 100 mL); 250 mg/5 mL (50 mL, 100 mL)
Biaxin®: 125 mg/5 mL (50 mL, 100 mL); 250 mg/5 mL (50 mL, 100 mL)
Tablet, oral: 250 mg, 500 mg
Biaxin®: 250 mg, 500 mg
Tablet, extended release, oral: 500 mg
Biaxin® XL: 500 mg
Dental Comment The FDA issued a special alert in December 2005 stating that short-term therapy with clarithromycin in patients with stable coronary artery disease may cause significantly higher cardiovascular mortality. The use of 500 mg clarithromycin daily for 14 days in patients with the above condition resulted in significantly higher all-cause mortality compared to patients taking placebo. This information is provided to the dental practitioner on the possible association between short-term use of clarithromycin for infections and increases in mortality in patients with a history of stable coronary artery disease.

Clarithromycin is known to prolong the QT interval. The QT interval is measured as the time and distance between the Q point of the QRS complex and the end of the T wave in the ECG tracing. After adjustment for heart rate, the QT interval is defined as prolonged if it is more than 450 msec in men and 460 msec in women. A long QT syndrome was first described in the 1950s and 60s as a congenital syndrome involving QT interval prolongation and syncope and sudden death. Some of the congenital long QT syndromes were characterized by a peculiar electrocardiographic appearance of the QRS complex involving a premature atria beat followed by a pause, then a subsequent sinus beat showing marked QT prolongation and deformity. This type of cardiac arrhythmia was originally termed "torsade de pointes" (translated from the French as "twisting of the points"). Clarithromycin is considered as having a risk of causing torsade de pointes. Since it is not known what effect vasoconstrictors in the local anesthetic regimen will have in patients with a known history of congenital prolonged QT interval or in patients taking any medication that prolongs the QT interval, a medical consult is suggested.
References
ADA Division of Legal Affairs, "A Legal Perspective on Antibiotic Prophylaxis," *J Am Dent Assoc*, 2003, 134(9):1260.
American Dental Association Council on Scientific Affairs, "Combating Antibiotic Resistance," *J Am Dent Assoc*, 2004, 135(4):484-7.
Amsden GW, "Erythromycin, Clarithromycin, and Azithromycin: Are the Differences Real?" *Clin Ther*, 1996, 18(1):56-72.
Wilson W, Taubert KA, Gewitz M, et al, "Prevention of Infective Endocarditis. Guidelines From the American Heart Association. A Guideline From the American Heart Association Rheumatic Fever, Endocarditis, and Kawasaki Disease Committee, Council on Cardiovascular Disease in the Young, and the Council on Clinical Cardiology, Council on Cardiovascular Surgery and Anesthesia, and the Quality of Care and Outcomes Research Interdisciplinary Working Group," *Circulation*, 2007, 115. Available at http://circ.ahajournals.org/cgi/reprint/CIRCULATIONAHA.106.183095v1; last accessed July 26, 2007.
Wynn RL, Bergman SA, Meiller TF, et al, "Antibiotics in Treating Oral-Facial Infections of Odontogenic Origin: An Update," *Gen Dent*, 2001, 49(3):238-40, 242, 244 passim.

Clemastine (KLEM as teen)

Brand Names: U.S. Tavist® Allergy [OTC]
Pharmacologic Category Ethanolamine Derivative; Histamine H_1 Antagonist; Histamine H_1 Antagonist, First Generation
Use Perennial and seasonal allergic rhinitis and other allergic symptoms including urticaria
Local Anesthetic/Vasoconstrictor Precautions No information available to require special precautions
Effects on Dental Treatment Key adverse event(s) related to dental treatment: Xerostomia (normal salivary flow resumes upon discontinuation).
Effects on Bleeding No information available to require special precautions
Adverse Effects Frequency not defined.
Cardiovascular: Palpitation, hypotension, tachycardia
Central nervous system: Dyscoordination, sedation, somnolence slight to moderate, sleepiness, confusion, restlessness, nervousness, insomnia, irritability, fatigue, headache, dizziness increased
Dermatologic: Rash, photosensitivity
Gastrointestinal: Diarrhea, nausea, xerostomia, epigastric distress, vomiting, constipation
Genitourinary: Urinary frequency, difficult urination, urinary retention
Hematologic: Hemolytic anemia, thrombocytopenia, agranulocytosis
Ocular: Blurred vision
Otic: Tinnitus
Respiratory: Thickening of bronchial secretions
Miscellaneous: Anaphylaxis
General Dosage Range Oral:
Children <6 years: 0.05 mg/kg/day (base) **or** 0.335-0.67 mg/day (fumarate) in 2-3 divided doses (maximum: 1.34 mg/day [fumarate] or 1 mg/day [base])
Children 6-12 years: 0.67-1.34 mg fumarate (0.5-1 mg base) twice daily (maximum: 4.02 mg/day [3 mg base])
Children ≥12 years and Adults: 1.34-2.68 mg fumarate (1-2 mg base) 2-3 times/day (maximum: 8.04 mg/day [6 mg base])
Mechanism of Action Competes with histamine for H_1-receptor sites on effector cells in the gastrointestinal tract, blood vessels, and respiratory tract
Pharmacodynamics/Kinetics
Onset of Action Peak effect: Therapeutic: 5-7 hours
Duration of Action 8-12 hours; may persist for 24 hours
Half-life Elimination ~21 hours (range: 10-33 hours) (Sharma, 2003)
Time to Peak 2-4 hours
Pregnancy Risk Factor B

Pregnancy Considerations Maternal clemastine use has generally not resulted in an increased risk of birth defects. Antihistamines are recommended for the treatment of rhinitis, urticaria, and pruritus with rash in pregnant women (although second generation antihistamines may be preferred). Antihistamines are not recommended for treatment of pruritus associated with intrahepatic cholestasis in pregnancy.

Clevidipine (klev ID i peen)

Related Information
Calcium Channel Blockers and Gingival Hyperplasia *on page 1640*
Brand Names: U.S. Cleviprex®
Pharmacologic Category Calcium Channel Blocker; Calcium Channel Blocker, Dihydropyridine
Use Management of hypertension
Local Anesthetic/Vasoconstrictor Precautions No information available to require special precautions
Effects on Dental Treatment Key adverse event(s) related to dental treatment: Although other calcium channel blockers (eg, nifedipine, diltiazem) have been associated with gingival hyperplasia, there are no reports that clevidipine has caused this adverse effect.
Effects on Bleeding No information available to require special precautions
Adverse Effects
>10%:
Cardiovascular: Atrial fibrillation (21%)
Central nervous system: Fever (19%), insomnia (12%)
Gastrointestinal: Nausea (5% to 21%)
1% to 10%:
Central nervous system: Headache (6%)
Gastrointestinal: Vomiting (3%)
Hematologic: Postprocedural hemorrhage (3%)
Renal: Acute renal failure (9%)
Respiratory: Pneumonia (3%), respiratory failure (3%)
General Dosage Range I.V.: *Adults:* Initial: 1-2 mg/hour; Usual maintenance: 4-6 mg/hour; Maximum: 21 mg/hour (1000 mL/24 hours)
Mechanism of Action Dihydropyridine calcium channel blocker with potent arterial vasodilating activity. Inhibits calcium ion influx through the L-type calcium channels during depolarization in arterial smooth muscle, producing a decrease in mean arterial pressure (MAP) by reducing systemic vascular resistance.
Pharmacodynamics/Kinetics
Onset of Action 2-4 minutes after start of infusion
Duration of Action I.V.: 5-15 minutes
Half-life Elimination Biphasic: Initial: 1 minute (predominant); Terminal: 15 minutes
Pregnancy Risk Factor C
Pregnancy Considerations Adverse events were observed in animal reproduction studies. There are no adequate and well-controlled studies in pregnant women. Use only if potential benefit justifies potential risks.

Clidinium and Chlordiazepoxide
(kli DI nee um & klor dye az e POKS ide)

Related Information
ChlordiazePOXIDE *on page 288*
Brand Names: U.S. Librax®
Brand Names: Canada Apo-Chlorax®; Librax®
Pharmacologic Category Antispasmodic Agent, Gastrointestinal; Benzodiazepine

Use Adjunct treatment of peptic ulcer; treatment of irritable bowel syndrome
Local Anesthetic/Vasoconstrictor Precautions No information available to require special precautions
Effects on Dental Treatment Key adverse event(s) related to dental treatment: Xerostomia and changes in salivation (normal salivary flow resumes upon discontinuation).
Effects on Bleeding No information available to require special precautions
Adverse Effects 1% to 10%:
Central nervous system: Drowsiness, ataxia, confusion, anticholinergic side effects
Gastrointestinal: Dry mouth, constipation, nausea
General Dosage Range Oral: *Adults:* 1-2 capsules 3-4 times/day
Pregnancy Risk Factor D
Pregnancy Considerations An increased risk of congenital malformations has been associated with the use of minor tranquilizers during the 1st trimester. Because use of these drugs is rarely a matter of urgency, their use should be avoided during this period.

Clindamycin (Systemic) (klin da MYE sin)

Related Information
Antibiotic Prophylaxis *on page 1542*
Bacterial Infections *on page 1562*
Osteonecrosis of the Jaw *on page 1529*
Periodontal Diseases *on page 1570*
Related Sample Prescriptions
Bacterial Infections and Periodontal Diseases *on page 1609*
Infective Endocarditis (Prevention) *on page 1604*
Prosthetic Joint Late Infections (Prevention) *on page 1605*
Brand Names: U.S. Cleocin HCl®; Cleocin Pediatric®; Cleocin Phosphate®
Brand Names: Canada Apo-Clindamycin®; Ava-Clindamycin; Clindamycin Injection, USP; Clindamycine; Dalacin™ C; Mylan-Clindamycin; PMS-Clindamycin; Riva-Clindamycin; Teva-Clindamycin
Generic Availability (U.S.) Yes
Pharmacologic Category Antibiotic, Lincosamide
Dental Use Alternate oral antibiotic for prevention of infective endocarditis in individuals allergic to penicillins or ampicillin, when amoxicillin cannot be used; alternate I.M. or I.V. antibiotic for prevention of infective endocarditis in patients allergic to penicillins or ampicillin and unable to take oral medication; alternate oral antibiotic for prophylaxis for dental patients with total joint replacement who are allergic to penicillin; alternate I.V. antibiotic for prophylaxis for dental patients with total joint replacement who are allergic to penicillin and unable to take oral medications; alternate antibiotic in the treatment of common orofacial infections caused by aerobic gram-positive cocci and susceptible anaerobes; treatment of periodontal disease
Use Treatment of susceptible bacterial infections, mainly those caused by anaerobes, streptococci, pneumococci, and staphylococci; pelvic inflammatory disease (I.V.)
Unlabeled Use May be useful in PCP; alternate treatment for toxoplasmosis; bacterial vaginosis (oral); alternate treatment for MRSA infections; alternate antibiotic for prophylaxis of infective endocarditis in patients who are allergic to penicillin and undergoing surgical or dental procedures (ACC/AHA guidelines); group B

streptococcus (GBS) infection (maternal use for neonatal prophylaxis); treatment of severe or uncomplicated malaria; treatment of babesiosis; treatment of acute bacterial rhinosinusitis (ABRS) (pediatric) (in combination with a third-generation cephalosporin)

Local Anesthetic/Vasoconstrictor Precautions No information available to require special precautions

Effects on Dental Treatment No significant effects or complications reported

Effects on Bleeding No information available to require special precautions

Adverse Effects Frequency not defined.

Cardiovascular: Cardiac arrest (rare; I.V. administration), hypotension (rare; I.V. administration)

Dermatologic: Erythema multiforme (rare), exfoliative dermatitis (rare), pruritus, rash, Stevens-Johnson syndrome (rare), urticaria

Gastrointestinal: Abdominal pain, diarrhea, esophagitis, nausea, pseudomembranous colitis, vomiting

Genitourinary: Vaginitis

Hematologic: Agranulocytosis, eosinophilia (transient), neutropenia (transient), thrombocytopenia

Hepatic: Jaundice, liver function test abnormalities

Local: Induration/pain/sterile abscess (I.M.), thrombophlebitis (I.V.)

Neuromuscular & skeletal: Polyarthritis (rare)

Renal: Renal dysfunction (rare)

Miscellaneous: Anaphylactoid reactions (rare)

Dental Usual Dosage

Orofacial infection:

Children:

Oral: 10-20 mg/kg/day in 3-4 equally divided doses

I.V.: 15-25 mg/kg/day in 3-4 equally divided doses

Adults:

Oral: 150-450 mg/dose for 7 days; maximum dose: 1.8 g/day

I.V.: 600-900 mg every 8 hours

Treatment of periodontal disease: Oral: 300 mg every 8 hours for 8 days

Infective endocarditis prophylaxis:

Children:

Oral: 20 mg/kg 30-60 minutes before procedure

I.M., I.V.: 20 mg/kg 30-60 minutes before procedure.
Note: Intramuscular injections should be avoided in patients who are receiving anticoagulant therapy. In these circumstances, orally administered regimens should be given whenever possible. Intravenously administered antibiotics should be used for patients who are unable to tolerate or absorb oral medications.

Adults:

Oral: 600 mg 30-60 minutes before procedure

I.M., I.V.: 600 mg 30-60 minutes before procedure.
Note: Intramuscular injections should be avoided in patients who are receiving anticoagulant therapy. In these circumstances, orally administered regimens should be given whenever possible. Intravenously administered antibiotics should be used for patients who are unable to tolerate or absorb oral medications.

Prophylaxis in total joint replacement patients undergoing dental procedures which produce bacteremia:

Adults:

Oral: 600 mg 1 hour prior to procedure

I.V.: 600 mg 1 hour prior to procedure (for patients unable to take oral medication)

Dosage

Usual dosage ranges:

Infants and Children:

Oral: 8-40 mg/kg/day in 3-4 divided doses; Manufacturer's labeling: 8-20 mg/kg/day (as hydrochloride) or 8-25 mg/kg/day (as palmitate) in 3-4 divided doses; minimum dose of palmitate: 37.5 mg 3 times daily

I.M., I.V.: Manufacturer's labeling: 20-40 mg/kg/day in 3-4 divided doses

Adults:

Oral: 150-450 mg/dose every 6-8 hours; maximum dose: 1800 mg daily

I.M., I.V.: 1200-2700 mg daily in 2-4 divided doses; maximum dose: 4800 mg daily

Indication-specific dosing:

Infants >3 months and Children:

Community-acquired pneumonia (CAP) (IDSA/PIDS, 2011): Note: In children ≥5 years, a macrolide antibiotic should be added if atypical pneumonia cannot be ruled out.

Group A *Streptococcus:*

Moderate-to-severe infection (alternative to ampicillin/penicillin): I.V.: 40 mg/kg/day divided every 6-8 hours

Mild infection, step-down therapy (alternative to amoxicillin/penicillin): Oral: 40 mg/kg/day divided every 8 hours

Presumed bacterial (in addition to recommended antibiotic therapy), *S. pneumoniae* moderate-to-severe (MICs to penicillin ≤2.0 mcg/mL) (alternative to ampicillin/penicillin): I.V.: 40 mg/kg/day divided every 6-8 hours

S. pneumoniae:

Moderate-to-severe infection (MICs to penicillin ≥4.0 mcg/mL) (alternative to ceftriaxone): I.V.: 40 mg/kg/day divided every 6-8 hours

Mild infection, step-down therapy (MICs to penicillin ≥4.0 mcg/mL) (alternative to levofloxacin or linezolid): Oral: 30-40 mg/kg/day divided every 8 hours

S. aureus (methicillin-susceptible):

Moderate-to-severe infection (alternative to cefazolin or oxacillin): I.V.: 40 mg/kg/day divided every 6-8 hours

Mild infection, step-down therapy (alternative to cephalexin): Oral: 30-40 mg/kg/day divided every 6-8 hours

S. aureus (methicillin-resistant/clindamycin-susceptible):

Moderate-to-severe infection (preferred): I.V.: 40 mg/kg/day divided every 6-8 hours; recommended duration: 7-21 days (Liu, 2011)

Mild infection, step-down therapy (preferred): Oral: 30-40 mg/kg/day divided every 6-8 hours; recommended duration: 7-21 days (Liu, 2011)

Children:

Acute bacterial rhinosinusitis (unlabeled use): Oral: 30-40 mg/kg/day divided every 8 hours with concomitant cefixime or cefpodoxime for 10-14 days. **Note:** Recommended in patients with non-type I penicillin allergy, after failure of initial therapy or in patients at risk for antibiotic resistance (eg, daycare attendance, age <2 years, recent hospitalization, antibiotic use within the past month) (Chow, 2012).

Anthrax (unlabeled use): I.V.: 30 mg/kg/day divided every 6 hours

Babesiosis (unlabeled use): Oral: 20-40 mg/kg/day divided every 8 hours for 7-10 days *plus* quinine (*Medical Letter*, 2007)

Cellulitis due to MRSA (unlabeled use): Oral: 10-13 mg/kg/dose every 6-8 hours for 5-10 days (maximum: 40 mg/kg/day) (Liu, 2011)

Complicated skin/soft tissue infection due to MRSA (unlabeled use): Oral, I.V.: 10-13 mg/kg/dose every 6-8 hours for 7-14 days (maximum: 40 mg/kg/day) (Liu, 2011)

Healthcare-associated pneumonia (HAP) (methicillin-resistant/clindamycin-susceptible): Oral, I.V.: 30-40 mg/kg/day divided every 6-8 hours for 7-21 days (Liu, 2011)

Malaria, severe (unlabeled use): I.V.: Load: 10 mg/kg followed by 15 mg/kg/day divided every 8 hours *plus* I.V. quinidine gluconate; switch to oral therapy (clindamycin *plus* quinine) when able for total clindamycin treatment duration of 7 days (**Note:** Quinine duration is region specific, consult CDC for current recommendations) (CDC, 2009)

Malaria, uncomplicated treatment (unlabeled use): Oral: 20 mg/kg/day divided every 8 hours for 7 days *plus* quinine (CDC, 2009)

Osteomyelitis due to MRSA (unlabeled use): Oral, I.V.: 10-13 mg/kg/dose every 6-8 hours for a minimum of 4-6 weeks (maximum: 40 mg/kg/day) (Liu, 2011)

Pharyngitis, group A streptococci (IDSA recommendations): Oral:
Acute treatment in penicillin-allergic patients: 21 mg/kg/day divided every 8 hours (maximum: 300 mg per dose) for 10 days (Shulman, 2012).
Chronic carrier treatment: 20-30 mg/kg/day divided every 8 hours (maximum: 300 mg per dose) for 10 days (Shulman, 2012).

Prophylaxis against infective endocarditis (unlabeled use):
Oral: 20 mg/kg 30-60 minutes before procedure (Wilson, 2007)
I.M., I.V.: 20 mg/kg 30-60 minutes before procedure. Intramuscular injections should be avoided in patients who are receiving anticoagulant therapy. In these circumstances, orally administered regimens should be given whenever possible. Intravenously administered antibiotics should be used for patients who are unable to tolerate or absorb oral medications. (Wilson, 2007)
Note: American Heart Association (AHA) guidelines now recommend prophylaxis only in patients undergoing invasive procedures and in whom underlying cardiac conditions may predispose to a higher risk of adverse outcomes should infection occur. As of April 2007, routine prophylaxis for GI/GU procedures is no longer recommended by the AHA.

Septic arthritis due to MRSA (unlabeled use): Oral, I.V.: 10-13 mg/kg/dose every 6-8 hours for minimum of 3-4 weeks (maximum: 40 mg/kg/day) (Liu, 2011)

Toxoplasmosis (HIV-exposed/-positive; secondary prevention [unlabeled use]): Oral: 20-30 mg/kg/day divided every 6-8 hours (*plus* pyrimethamine and leucovorin calcium) (CDC, 2009)

Adults:
Amnionitis: I.V.: 450-900 mg every 8 hours
Anthrax (unlabeled use): I.V.: 900 mg every 8 hours with ciprofloxacin or doxycycline

Babesiosis (unlabeled use):
Oral: 600 mg 3 times daily for 7-10 days with quinine (Wormser, 2006; Vannier, 2012)
I.V.: 300-600 mg every 6 hours for 7-10 days with quinine (Wormser, 2006, Vannier, 2012)
Note: Relapsing infection may require at least 6 weeks of therapy (Vannier, 2012)

Bacterial vaginosis (unlabeled use): Oral: 300 mg twice daily for 7 days (CDC, 2010)

Bite wounds (canine): Oral: 300 mg 4 times daily with a fluoroquinolone

Cellulitis due to MRSA (unlabeled use): Oral: 300-450 mg 3 times daily for 5-10 days (Liu, 2011)

Complicated skin/soft tissue infection due to MRSA (unlabeled use): I.V., Oral: 600 mg 3 times daily for 7-14 days (Liu, 2011)

Gangrenous pyomyositis: I.V.: 900 mg every 8 hours with penicillin G

Group B streptococcus (neonatal prophylaxis) (unlabeled use): I.V.: 900 mg every 8 hours until delivery (CDC, 2010)

Malaria, severe (unlabeled use): I.V.: Load: 10 mg/kg followed by 15 mg/kg/day divided every 8 hours *plus* I.V. quinidine gluconate; switch to oral therapy (clindamycin *plus* quinine) when able for total clindamycin treatment duration of 7 days (**Note:** Quinine duration is region specific, consult CDC for current recommendations) (CDC, 2009)

Malaria, uncomplicated treatment (unlabeled use): Oral: 20 mg/kg/day divided every 8 hours for 7 days *plus* quinine (CDC, 2009)

Orofacial/parapharyngeal space infections:
Oral: 150-450 mg every 6 hours for 7 days, maximum 1800 mg daily
I.V.: 600-900 mg every 8 hours

Osteomyelitis due to MRSA (unlabeled use): I.V., Oral: 600 mg 3 times daily for a minimum of 8 weeks (some experts combine with rifampin) (Liu, 2011)

Pelvic inflammatory disease: I.V.: 900 mg every 8 hours with gentamicin (conventional or single daily dosing); 24 hours after clinical improvement may convert to oral doxycycline 100 mg twice daily **or** clindamycin 450 mg 4 times daily to complete 14 days of total therapy. Avoid doxycycline if tubo-ovarian abscess is present (CDC, 2010).

Pharyngitis, group A streptococci (IDSA recommendations):
Acute treatment in penicillin-allergic patients: 21 mg/kg/day divided every 8 hours (maximum: 300 mg per dose) for 10 days (Shulman, 2012)
Chronic carrier treatment: 20-30 mg/kg/day divided every 8 hours (maximum: 300 mg per dose) for 10 days (Shulman, 2012)

***Pneumocystis jirovecii* pneumonia (unlabeled use):**
I.V.: 600-900 mg every 6-8 hours with primaquine for 21 days (CDC, 2009)
Oral: 300-450 mg every 6-8 hours with primaquine for 21 days (CDC, 2009)

Pneumonia due to MRSA (unlabeled use): I.V., Oral: 600 mg 3 times daily for 7-21 days (Liu, 2011)

Prophylaxis against infective endocarditis (unlabeled use):
Oral: 600 mg 30-60 minutes before procedure (Wilson, 2007)

I.M., I.V.: 600 mg 30-60 minutes before procedure. Intramuscular injections should be avoided in patients who are receiving anticoagulant therapy. In these circumstances, orally administered regimens should be given whenever possible. Intravenously administered antibiotics should be used for patients who are unable to tolerate or absorb oral medications. (Wilson, 2007)

Note: American Heart Association (AHA) guidelines now recommend prophylaxis only in patients undergoing invasive procedures and in whom underlying cardiac conditions may predispose to a higher risk of adverse outcomes should infection occur. As of April 2007, routine prophylaxis for GI/GU procedures is no longer recommended by the AHA.

Prophylaxis in total joint replacement patients undergoing dental procedures which produce bacteremia (unlabeled use):
Oral: 600 mg 1 hour prior to procedure (ADA, 2003)
I.V.: 600 mg 1 hour prior to procedure (for patients unable to take oral medication) (ADA, 2003)

Prosthetic joint infection:
Chronic antimicrobial suppression, Staphylococci (oxacillin-susceptible) (alternative to cephalexin or cefadroxil) (unlabeled use): Oral: 300 mg every 6 hours (Osmon, 2013)
Propionibacterium acnes, treatment (alternative to penicillin G or ceftriaxone):
Oral: 300-450 mg every 6 hours for 4-6 weeks (Osmon, 2013)
I.V.: 600-900 mg every 8 hours for 4-6 weeks (Osmon, 2013)

Septic arthritis due to MRSA (unlabeled use): I.V., Oral: 600 mg 3 times daily for 3-4 weeks (Liu, 2011)
Toxic shock syndrome: I.V.: 900 mg every 8 hours with penicillin G or ceftriaxone
Toxoplasmosis (HIV-exposed/positive; secondary prevention [unlabeled use]): Oral: 600 mg every 8 hours (with pyrimethamine and leucovorin calcium) (CDC, 2009)

Dosing adjustment in renal impairment: No dosage adjustment required in renal impairment.
Poorly dialyzed; no supplemental dose or dosage adjustment necessary, including patients on intermittent hemodialysis, peritoneal dialysis, or continuous renal replacement therapy (eg, CVVHD).
Dosing adjustment in hepatic impairment: No adjustment required. Use caution with severe hepatic impairment.

Mechanism of Action Reversibly binds to 50S ribosomal subunits preventing peptide bond formation thus inhibiting bacterial protein synthesis; bacteriostatic or bactericidal depending on drug concentration, infection site, and organism

Contraindications Hypersensitivity to clindamycin, lincomycin, or any component of the formulation

Warnings/Precautions Dosage adjustment may be necessary in patients with severe hepatic dysfunction. **[U.S. Boxed Warning]: Can cause severe and possibly fatal colitis.** Prolonged use may result in fungal or bacterial superinfection, including *C. difficile*-associated diarrhea (CDAD) and pseudomembranous colitis; CDAD has been observed >2 months postantibiotic treatment. Use with caution in patients with a history of gastrointestinal disease. Discontinue drug if significant diarrhea, abdominal cramps, or passage of blood and mucus occurs. Some dosage forms contain benzyl alcohol or tartrazine. Use caution in atopic patients.

Not appropriate for use in the treatment of meningitis due to inadequate penetration into the CSF.

Drug Interactions
Metabolism/Transport Effects Substrate of CYP3A4 (minor); **Note:** Assignment of Major/Minor substrate status based on clinically relevant drug interaction potential
Avoid Concomitant Use
Avoid concomitant use of Clindamycin (Systemic) with any of the following: BCG; Erythromycin (Systemic)
Increased Effect/Toxicity
Clindamycin (Systemic) may increase the levels/effects of: Neuromuscular-Blocking Agents
Decreased Effect
Clindamycin (Systemic) may decrease the levels/effects of: BCG; Erythromycin (Systemic); Sodium Picosulfate; Typhoid Vaccine

The levels/effects of Clindamycin (Systemic) may be decreased by: Kaolin
Ethanol/Nutrition/Herb Interactions
Food: Peak concentrations may be delayed with food.
Herb/Nutraceutical: St John's wort may decrease clindamycin levels.
Dietary Considerations May be taken with food.
Pharmacodynamics/Kinetics
Half-life Elimination Neonates: Premature: 8.7 hours; Full-term: 3.6 hours; Children: ~2 hours; Adults: ~2-3 hours; Elderly 4 hours (range: 3.4-5.1 hours)
Time to Peak Serum: Oral: Within 60 minutes; I.M.: 1-3 hours
Pregnancy Risk Factor B
Pregnancy Considerations Adverse events were not observed in animal reproduction studies. Clindamycin crosses the placenta throughout pregnancy and at term, but use during pregnancy has not been shown to cause adverse fetal effects. Clindamycin pharmacokinetics are not affected by pregnancy. Clindamycin therapy is recommended in certain pregnant patients for prophylaxis of group B streptococcal disease in newborns, prophylaxis and treatment of *Toxoplasma gondii* encephalitis, or for the treatment of *Pneumocystis* pneumonia (PCP), bacterial vaginosis, or malaria.
Lactation Enters breast milk/not recommended (AAP rates "compatible"; AAP 2001 update pending)
Breast-Feeding Considerations Small amounts of clindamycin transfer to human milk. The manufacturer does not recommend the use of clindamycin during breast-feeding. Nondose-related effects could include modification of bowel flora. One case of bloody stools in an infant occurred after a mother received clindamycin while breast-feeding; however, a casual relationship was not confirmed.

Dosage Forms
Capsule, oral: 75 mg, 150 mg, 300 mg
Cleocin HCl®: 75 mg, 150 mg, 300 mg
Granules for solution, oral: 75 mg/5 mL (100 mL)
Cleocin Pediatric®: 75 mg/5 mL (100 mL)
Infusion, premixed in D₅W: 300 mg (50 mL); 600 mg (50 mL); 900 mg (50 mL)
Cleocin Phosphate®: 300 mg (50 mL); 600 mg (50 mL); 900 mg (50 mL)
Injection, solution: 150 mg/mL (2 mL, 4 mL, 6 mL, 60 mL)
Cleocin Phosphate®: 150 mg/mL (2 mL, 4 mL, 6 mL, 60 mL)
Dental Comment Clindamycin has not been shown to interfere with oral contraceptive activity; however, it reduces GI microflora, thus, oral contraceptive users should be advised to use additional methods of birth ▶

control. About 1% of clindamycin users develop pseudomembranous colitis. Symptoms may occur 2-9 days after initiation of therapy; however, it has never occurred with the 1-dose regimen of clindamycin used to prevent bacterial endocarditis.

References

ADA Division of Legal Affairs, "A Legal Perspective on Antibiotic Prophylaxis," *J Am Dent Assoc*, 2003, 134(9):1260.

American Dental Association Council on Scientific Affairs, "Combating Antibiotic Resistance," *J Am Dent Assoc*, 2004, 135(4):484-7.

Jevsevar DS and Abt E, "The New AAOS-ADA Clinical Practice Guideline on Prevention of Orthopaedic Implant Infection in Patients Undergoing Dental Procedures," *J Am Acad Orthop Surg*, 2013, 21 (3):195-7.

Sandor GK, Low DE, Judd PL, et al, "Antimicrobial Treatment Options in the Management of Odontogenic Infections," *J Can Dent Assoc*, 1998, 64(7):508-14.

Wilson W, Taubert KA, Gewitz M, et al, "Prevention of Infective Endocarditis. Guidelines From the American Heart Association. A Guideline From the American Heart Association Rheumatic Fever, Endocarditis, and Kawasaki Disease Committee, Council on Cardiovascular Disease in the Young, and the Council on Clinical Cardiology, Council on Cardiovascular Surgery and Anesthesia, and the Quality of Care and Outcomes Research Interdisciplinary Working Group," *Circulation*, 2007, 115. Available at http://circ.ahajournals.org/cgi/reprint/CIRCULATIONAHA.106.183095v1; last accessed July 26, 2007.

Clindamycin (Topical) (klin da MYE sin)

Brand Names: U.S. Cleocin T®; Cleocin®; Cleocin® Vaginal Ovule; Clindagel®; ClindaMax®; Clindesse®; Evoclin®

Brand Names: Canada Clinda-T; Clindasol™; Clindets; Dalacin® T; Dalacin® Vaginal; Taro-Clindamycin

Pharmacologic Category Antibiotic, Lincosamide; Topical Skin Product, Acne

Use Treatment of bacterial vaginosis (vaginal cream, vaginal suppository); topically in treatment of severe acne

Local Anesthetic/Vasoconstrictor Precautions No information available to require special precautions

Effects on Dental Treatment No significant effects or complications reported

Effects on Bleeding No information available to require special precautions

Adverse Effects

Topical:

>10%: Dermatologic: Dryness, burning, itching, scaliness, or peeling of skin (lotion, solution); erythema (foam, lotion, solution); oiliness (gel, lotion)

1% to 10%: Central nervous system: Headache (3%)

Vaginal:

>10%: Genitourinary: Vaginal moniliasis (≤14%), vulvovaginal pruritus

1% to 10%:

Central nervous system: Headache (7%)

Dermatologic: Pruritus (≤1%)

Gastrointestinal: Constipation (2%)

Genitourinary: Vulvovaginal disorder (3% to 7%), vulvovaginitis (4% to 6%), urinary tract infection (2%), vaginal pain (≤2%), trichomonal vaginitis (1%)

Neuromuscular & skeletal: Back pain (5%)

Miscellaneous: Fungal infection (1% to 2%)

General Dosage Range

Intravaginal: *Adults:* Insert 1 ovule or applicatorful once daily **or** 1 applicatorful as a single dose (Clindesse®)

Topical: *Children ≥12 years and Adults:* Apply once or twice daily

Mechanism of Action Reversibly binds to 50S ribosomal subunits preventing peptide bond formation thus inhibiting bacterial protein synthesis; bacteriostatic or bactericidal depending on drug concentration, infection site, and organism

Pharmacodynamics/Kinetics

Half-life Elimination Vaginal cream: 1.5-2.6 hours following repeated dosing; Vaginal suppository: 11 hours (range: 4-35 hours, limited by absorption rate)

Time to Peak Vaginal cream: ~10-14 hours (range: 4-24 hours); Vaginal suppository: ~5 hours (range: 1-10 hours)

Pregnancy Risk Factor B

Pregnancy Considerations Adverse effects were not observed in animal reproduction studies. Clindamycin has been shown to cross the placenta throughout pregnancy and at term following oral and parenteral dosing; use during pregnancy has not been shown to cause adverse fetal effects. Refer to the Clindamycin (Systemic) monograph for details. The amount of clindamycin available systemically is less following topical and vaginal application than with I.V. or oral administration. Oral clindamycin is recommended in certain pregnant patients for the treatment of bacterial vaginosis; however, vaginal therapy is not recommended for use in the second half of pregnancy.

Clindamycin and Benzoyl Peroxide
(klin da MYE sin & BEN zoe il peer OKS ide)

Related Information

Benzoyl Peroxide *on page 180*

Clindamycin (Topical) *on page 324*

Brand Names: U.S. Acanya®; BenzaClin®; Duac®

Brand Names: Canada BenzaClin®; Clindoxyl

Pharmacologic Category Acne Products; Topical Skin Product; Topical Skin Product, Acne

Use Topical treatment of acne vulgaris

Local Anesthetic/Vasoconstrictor Precautions No information available to require special precautions

Effects on Dental Treatment No significant effects or complications reported

Effects on Bleeding No information available to require special precautions

Adverse Effects

>10%: Dermatologic: Erythema (≤26%), scaling (≤18%), peeling (2% to 17%), dry skin (≤15%), itching (≤15%)

1% to 10%:

Dermatologic: Burning (≤8%), stinging (≤6%), pruritus (2%), sunburn (1%)

Local: Application site reaction (3%)

General Dosage Range Topical: *Children ≥12 years and Adults:* Apply once daily (Acanya®, Duac®) **or** twice daily (BenzaClin®) to affected areas

Mechanism of Action Clindamycin and benzoyl peroxide have activity against *Propionibacterium acnes in vitro*. This organism has been associated with acne vulgaris. Benzoyl peroxide releases free-radical oxygen which oxidizes bacterial proteins in the sebaceous follicles decreasing the number of anaerobic bacteria and decreasing irritating-type free fatty acids. Clindamycin reversibly binds to 50S ribosomal subunits preventing peptide bond formation thus inhibiting bacterial protein synthesis; bacteriostatic or bactericidal depending on drug concentration, infection site, and organism.

Pregnancy Risk Factor C

Pregnancy Considerations Animal reproduction studies have not been conducted; use during pregnancy only if clearly needed.

Clindamycin and Tretinoin
(klin da MYE sin & TRET i noyn)

Related Information
Clindamycin (Topical) *on page 324*
Tretinoin (Topical) *on page 1356*
Brand Names: U.S. Veltin™; Ziana®
Pharmacologic Category Acne Products; Retinoic Acid Derivative; Topical Skin Product; Topical Skin Product, Acne
Use Treatment of acne vulgaris
Local Anesthetic/Vasoconstrictor Precautions No information available to require special precautions
Effects on Dental Treatment No significant effects or complications reported
Effects on Bleeding No information available to require special precautions
General Dosage Range Topical: *Children ≥12 years and Adults:* Apply pea-size amount to entire face once daily at bedtime
Mechanism of Action Clindamycin reversibly binds to 50S ribosomal subunits preventing peptide chain elongation thus inhibiting bacterial protein synthesis. Clindamycin exhibits *in vitro* activity against *Propionibacterium acnes*, an organism associated with acne vulgaris. Topical tretinoin is believed to decrease follicular epithelial cells cohesiveness and increase follicular epithelial cell turnover resulting in decreased microcomedo formation and increased expulsion of comedones.
Pregnancy Risk Factor C
Pregnancy Considerations Teratogenic effects were not observed in topical animal studies. Refer to individual monographs.

CloBAZam (KLOE ba zam)

Brand Names: U.S. Onfi™
Brand Names: Canada Apo-Clobazam®; Clobazam-10; Dom-Clobazam; Frisium®; Novo-Clobazam; PMS-Clobazam
Pharmacologic Category Benzodiazepine
Use Adjunctive treatment of seizures associated with Lennox-Gastaut syndrome

Canadian labeling: Adjunctive treatment of epilepsy
Unlabeled Use Catamenial epilepsy; epilepsy (monotherapy)
Local Anesthetic/Vasoconstrictor Precautions No information available to require special precautions
Effects on Dental Treatment Key adverse event(s) related to dental treatment: Xerostomia (normal salivary flow resumes upon discontinuation). Paradoxical reactions (including excitation, agitation, hallucinations, and psychosis) are known to occur with benzodiazepines.
Effects on Bleeding No information available to require special precautions
Adverse Effects
>10%:
Central nervous system: Somnolence (22%), fever (13%), lethargy (10%)
Respiratory: Upper respiratory tract infection (12%)
1% to 10%:
Central nervous system: Aggressiveness (8%), irritability (7%), ataxia (5%), fatigue (5%), insomnia (5%), sedation (5%), psychomotor hyperactivity (4%)
Gastrointestinal: Salivation increased (9%), vomiting (7%), constipation (5%), appetite increased (3%), dysphagia (2%)
Genitourinary: Urinary tract infection (4%)

Neuromuscular & skeletal: Dysarthria (3%)
Respiratory: Cough (5%), pneumonia (4%), bronchitis (2%)
General Dosage Range Dosage adjustment recommended in patients with hepatic impairment or CYP2C19 poor metabolizers.
Oral: *Children ≥2 years and Adults:* Initial: 5-10 mg/day; Maintenance: Up to 40 mg/day
Mechanism of Action Clobazam is a 1,5 benzodiazepine which binds to stereospecific benzodiazepine receptors on the postsynaptic GABA neuron at several sites within the central nervous system, including the limbic system, reticular formation. Enhancement of the inhibitory effect of GABA on neuronal excitability results by increased neuronal membrane permeability to chloride ions. This shift in chloride ions results in hyperpolarization (a less excitable state) and stabilization.
Pharmacodynamics/Kinetics
Half-life Elimination 36-42 hours; N-desmethyl (active): 71-82 hours
Time to Peak 30 minutes to 4 hours
Pregnancy Considerations Clobazam was shown to be teratogenic in some animal studies. Clobazam crosses the placenta. Teratogenic effects have been observed with some benzodiazepines; however, additional studies are needed. Epilepsy itself, the number of medications, genetic factors, or a combination of these probably influence the teratogenicity of anticonvulsant therapy. The incidence of premature birth and low birth weights may be increased following maternal use of benzodiazepines; hypoglycemia and respiratory problems in the neonate may occur following exposure late in pregnancy. Neonatal withdrawal symptoms may occur within days to weeks after birth and "floppy infant syndrome" (which also includes withdrawal symptoms) has been reported with some benzodiazepines. An increased risk of fetal malformations may be associated with first trimester exposure. The Canadian labeling contraindicates use in the first trimester.

Patients exposed to clobazam during pregnancy are encouraged to enroll themselves into the AED Pregnancy Registry by calling 1-888-233-2334. Additional information is available at www.aedpregnancyregistry.org.
Product Availability Onfi™ oral suspension: FDA approved December 2012; anticipated availability is midyear to third quarter 2013.
Controlled Substance C-IV

Clobetasol (kloe BAY ta sol)

Related Information
Mild Lichen Planus *on page 1618*
Ulcerative, Erosive, and Painful Oral Mucosal Disorders *on page 1578*
Related Sample Prescriptions
Erosive Lichen Planus, Other Biopsy-Proven Desquamative Oral Diseases, and Major Aphthae *on page 1618*
Mild Lichen Planus *on page 1618*
Recurrent Aphthous Stomatitis *on page 1618*
Brand Names: U.S. Clobex®; Cormax®; Olux-E™; Olux®; Temovate E®; Temovate®
Brand Names: Canada Clobex®; Dermovate®; Mylan-Clobetasol Cream; Mylan-Clobetasol Ointment; Mylan-Clobetasol Scalp Application; Novo-Clobetasol; PMS-Clobetasol; ratio-Clobetasol; Taro-Clobetasol
Generic Availability (U.S.) Yes: Excludes spray

◀ **Pharmacologic Category** Corticosteroid, Topical

Dental Use Short-term relief of oral mucosal inflammation

Use Short-term relief of inflammation of moderate-to-severe corticosteroid-responsive dermatoses (very high potency topical corticosteroid)

Local Anesthetic/Vasoconstrictor Precautions No information available to require special precautions

Effects on Dental Treatment No significant effects or complications reported

Effects on Bleeding No information available to require special precautions

Adverse Effects Frequency not defined; may depend upon formulation used, length of application, surface area covered, and the use of occlusive dressings.

Central nervous system: Intracranial hypertension (systemic effect reported in children treated with topical corticosteroids)

Endocrine & metabolic: Adrenal suppression, Cushing's syndrome, hyperglycemia

Local: Application site: Burning, cracking/fissuring of the skin, dryness, erythema, folliculitis, irritation, numbness, pruritus, skin atrophy, stinging, telangiectasia

Renal: Glucosuria

Effects reported with other high-potency topical steroids: Acneiform eruptions, allergic contact dermatitis, hypertrichosis, hypopigmentation, maceration of the skin, miliaria, perioral dermatitis, secondary infection

Dental Usual Dosage Oral mucosal inflammation: Children ≥12 years and Adults: Cream: Apply twice daily for up to 2 weeks (maximum dose: 50 g/week); discontinue application when control is achieved; if no improvement is seen, reassessment of diagnosis may be necessary

Dosage Topical: Discontinue when control achieved; if improvement not seen within 2 weeks, reassessment of diagnosis may be necessary.

Children <12 years: Use is not recommended

Children ≥12 years and Adults:

Oral mucosal inflammation, dental (unlabeled use): Cream: Apply twice daily for up to 2 weeks (maximum dose: 50 g/week); discontinue application when control is achieved; if no improvement is seen, reassessment of diagnosis may be necessary

Steroid-responsive dermatoses:

Cream, emollient cream, gel, ointment: Apply twice daily for up to 2 weeks (maximum dose: 50 g/week)

Foam (Olux-E™): Apply to affected area twice daily for up to 2 weeks (maximum dose: 50 g/week); do not apply to face or intertriginous areas

Steroid-responsive dermatoses: Foam (Olux®), solution: Apply to affected scalp twice daily for up to 2 weeks (maximum dose: 50 g/week or 50 mL/week)

Mild-to-moderate plaque-type psoriasis of nonscalp areas: Foam (Olux®): Apply to affected area twice daily for up to 2 weeks (maximum dose: 50 g/week); do not apply to face or intertriginous areas

Children ≥16 years and Adults: Moderate-to-severe plaque-type psoriasis: Emollient cream, lotion: Apply twice daily for up to 2 weeks, has been used for up to 4 weeks when application is <10% of body surface area; use with caution (maximum dose: 50 g/week)

Children ≥18 years and Adults:

Moderate-to-severe plaque-type psoriasis: Spray: Apply by spraying directly onto affected area twice daily; should be gently rubbed into skin. Should be used for not longer than 4 weeks; treatment beyond 2 weeks should be limited to localized lesions which

have not improved sufficiently. Total dose should not exceed 50 g/week or 59 mL/week.

Scalp psoriasis: Shampoo: Apply thin film to dry scalp once daily; leave in place for 15 minutes, then add water, lather; rinse thoroughly

Steroid-responsive dermatoses: Lotion: Apply twice daily for up to 2 weeks (maximum dose: 50 g/week)

Mechanism of Action Stimulates the synthesis of enzymes needed to decrease inflammation, suppress mitotic activity, and cause vasoconstriction

Contraindications Hypersensitivity to clobetasol or any component of the formulation; viral, fungal, or tubercular skin lesions

Warnings/Precautions Systemic absorption of topical corticosteroids may cause hypothalamic-pituitary-adrenal (HPA) axis suppression (reversible) particularly in younger children. HPA axis suppression may lead to adrenal crisis. Risk is increased when used over large surface areas, for prolonged periods, or with occlusive dressings. Allergic contact dermatitis can occur, it is usually diagnosed by failure to heal rather than clinical exacerbation. Prolonged treatment with corticosteroids has been associated with the development of Kaposi's sarcoma (case reports); if noted, discontinuation of therapy should be considered. Adverse systemic effects including hyperglycemia, glycosuria, fluid and electrolyte changes, and HPA suppression may occur when used on large surface areas, for prolonged periods, or with an occlusive dressing. Use in children <12 years of age is not recommended. Do not use on the face, axillae, or groin.

Drug Interactions

Metabolism/Transport Effects None known.

Avoid Concomitant Use

Avoid concomitant use of Clobetasol with any of the following: Aldesleukin

Increased Effect/Toxicity

Clobetasol may increase the levels/effects of: Deferasirox

The levels/effects of Clobetasol may be increased by: Telaprevir

Decreased Effect

Clobetasol may decrease the levels/effects of: Aldesleukin; Corticorelin; Hyaluronidase; Telaprevir

Pregnancy Risk Factor C

Pregnancy Considerations Extensive use in pregnant women is not recommended. There are no adequate and well-controlled studies in pregnant women, however, teratogenic effects were observed in animal studies.

Lactation Excretion in breast milk unknown/use caution

Breast-Feeding Considerations It is not known if topical application will result in detectable quantities in breast milk.

Dosage Forms

Aerosol, foam, topical: 0.05% (50 g, 100 g)
  Olux-E™: 0.05% (50 g, 100 g)
  Olux®: 0.05% (50 g, 100 g)

Cream, topical: 0.05% (15 g, 30 g, 45 g, 60 g)
  Temovate E®: 0.05% (60 g)
  Temovate®: 0.05% (30 g, 60 g)

Gel, topical: 0.05% (15 g, 30 g, 60 g)
  Temovate®: 0.05% (60 g)

Lotion, topical: 0.05% (59 mL, 118 mL)
  Clobex®: 0.05% (30 mL, 59 mL, 118 mL)

Ointment, topical: 0.05% (15 g, 30 g, 45 g, 60 g)
  Temovate®: 0.05% (15 g, 30 g)

Shampoo, topical: 0.05% (118 mL)
  Clobex®: 0.05% (118 mL)

Solution, topical: 0.05% (25 mL, 50 mL)
Clobex®: 0.05% (59 mL, 125 mL)
Cormax®: 0.05% (50 mL)
Temovate®: 0.05% (50 mL)

Clocortolone (kloe KOR toe lone)

Brand Names: U.S. Cloderm®
Brand Names: Canada Cloderm®
Pharmacologic Category Corticosteroid, Topical
Use Inflammation of corticosteroid-responsive dermatoses (intermediate-potency topical corticosteroid)
Local Anesthetic/Vasoconstrictor Precautions No information available to require special precautions
Effects on Dental Treatment No significant effects or complications reported
Effects on Bleeding No information available to require special precautions
Adverse Effects 1% to 10%:
Dermatologic: Itching, erythema
Local: Burning, dryness, irritation, papular rash
General Dosage Range Topical: *Adults:* Apply sparingly to affected area 1-4 times/day
Mechanism of Action Stimulates the synthesis of enzymes needed to decrease inflammation, suppress mitotic activity, and cause vasoconstriction
Pregnancy Risk Factor C
Pregnancy Considerations Teratogenic effects have been observed in animals administered potent topical corticosteroids. Topical products are not recommended for extensive use, in large quantities, or for long periods of time in pregnant women.

Clodronate (KLOE droh nate)

Related Information
Osteonecrosis of the Jaw *on page 1529*
Brand Names: Canada Bonefos®; Clasteon®
Pharmacologic Category Bisphosphonate Derivative
Use Management of hypercalcemia of malignancy; management of osteolysis due to bone metastases of malignancy
Local Anesthetic/Vasoconstrictor Precautions No information available to require special precautions
Effects on Dental Treatment Osteonecrosis of the jaw (ONJ), generally associated with local infection and/or tooth extraction and often with delayed healing, has been reported in patients taking bisphosphonates. Symptoms included nonhealing extraction socket or an exposed jawbone. Most reported cases of bisphosphonate-associated osteonecrosis have been in cancer patients treated with intravenous bisphosphonates. However, some have occurred in patients with postmenopausal osteoporosis taking oral bisphosphonates. Dental surgery, particularly tooth extraction, may increase the risk for ONJ. Patients who develop ONJ while on bisphosphonate therapy should receive care by an oral surgeon. See Dental Comment.
Effects on Bleeding No information available to require special precautions
Adverse Effects
>10%: Hepatic: Transaminases increased (≤18%; >2 x ULN: 2%)
1% to 10%:
Endocrine & metabolic: Hypocalcemia (≤3%)
Gastrointestinal: GI disturbances (≤10%; includes anorexia, diarrhea, gastric pain, nausea, vomiting)

Renal: Serum creatinine increased (1%), BUN increased
General Dosage Range Dosage adjustment recommended in patients with renal impairment
I.V.: *Adults:* 1500 mg as single dose (Clasteon®) or 300 mg/day (Clasteon®, Bonefos®); Maximum therapy: 10 days (Clasteon®); 7 days (Bonefos®)
Oral: *Adults:* 1600-2400 mg/day in 1-2 divided doses (maximum: 3200 mg/day)
Mechanism of Action A bisphosphonate which lowers serum calcium by inhibition of bone resorption via actions on osteoclasts or on osteoclast precursors.
Pharmacodynamics/Kinetics
Onset of Action Calcium-lowering effects: I.V.: Within 48 hours
Duration of Action Calcium-lowering effects: 5 days to 3 weeks following discontinuation
Half-life Elimination Terminal: Oral: ~6 hours; I.V.: 13 hours (serum); prolonged in bone tissue
Time to Peak Plasma: Oral: 30 minutes
Pregnancy Considerations Bisphosphonates have been shown to cross the placenta and cause embryo/fetal effects in animals. Bisphosphonates are incorporated into the bone matrix and gradually released over time. Theoretically, there may be a risk of fetal harm when pregnancy follows the completion of therapy. There are no adequate and well-controlled studies in pregnant women; use is contraindicated during pregnancy.
Product Availability Not available in U.S.
Dental Comment A review of 2408 published cases of bisphosphonate-associated osteonecrosis of the jaw bone (BP-associated ONJ) was done by Filleul, 2010. BP therapy was associated with 89% of the cases to treat malignancies and 11% of the cases to treat nonmalignant conditions. Information on the specific bisphosphonate used was available for 1694 of the patients. Intravenous therapy (primarily zoledronic acid) was received by 88% of the patients and 12% received oral treatment (primarily alendronate). Of all the cases of BP-associated ONJ, 67% were preceded by tooth extraction and for 26% of patients, there was no predisposing factor identified.

A 2010 retrospective case review reported the prevalence of BP-associated ONJ in patients using alendronate-type drugs was 1 out of 952 patients or ~0.1% (Lo, 2010). Of the 8572 respondents, nine cases of ONJ were identified; five had developed ONJ spontaneously and four developed ONJ after tooth extraction. When extrapolated to patient-years of bisphosphonate exposure, this prevalence rate of 0.1% equates to a frequency of 28 cases per 100,000 person-years of oral bisphosphonate treatment. An Australian group (Mavrokokki, 2007), identified the frequency of BP-associated ONJ in osteoporotic patients, mainly taking weekly oral alendronate, was 1 in 8470 to 1 in 2260 (0.01% to 0.04%) patients. If extractions were carried out, the calculated frequency was 1 in 1130 to 1 in 296 (0.09% to 0.34%) patients. The median time to onset of ONJ in alendronate patients was 24 months.

According to the 2011 report by the American Dental Association (ADA), the incidence of BP-associated ONJ remains low and the benefits of using oral bisphosphonates significantly outweighs the risk of developing BP-associated ONJ for treatment and prevention of osteoporosis and cancer treatment (Hellstein, 2011). The full 47 page report can be accessed at http://www.ada.org/sections/professionalResources/pdfs/topics_AR-ONJ_report.pdf.

The ADA review of 2011 stated the incidence of oral BP-associated ONJ was one case for every 1000 individuals exposed to oral bisphosphonates (0.1%) (Hellstein, 2011).

Clofarabine (klo FARE a been)

Brand Names: U.S. Clolar®
Brand Names: Canada Clolar®
Pharmacologic Category Antineoplastic Agent, Antimetabolite (Purine Analog)
Use Treatment of acute lymphoblastic leukemia (ALL) in children (ages 1-21 years)
Unlabeled Use Treatment of relapsed/refractory acute lymphoblastic leukemia (ALL) in adults; treatment of acute myeloid leukemia (AML) in adults ≥60 years of age
Local Anesthetic/Vasoconstrictor Precautions No information available to require special precautions
Effects on Dental Treatment Key adverse event(s) related to dental treatment: Mucosal inflammation and gingival bleeding.
Effects on Bleeding Chemotherapy may result in significant myelosuppression, potentially including significant reduction in platelet counts and altered hemostasis. In patients who are under active treatment with these agents, medical consult is suggested.

Due to the thrombocytopenic effects of clofarabine, an increased risk of bleeding may be seen in patients receiving concomitant NSAIDs (including aspirin).
Adverse Effects
>10%:
Cardiovascular: Tachycardia (35%), hypotension (29%; grade 3: 11%; grade 4: 8%), flushing (19%), hypertension (13%), edema (12%)
Central nervous system: Headache (43%), fever (39%), chills (34%), fatigue (34%), anxiety (21%), pain (15%)
Dermatologic: Pruritus (43%), rash (38%), petechiae (26%), palmar-plantar erythrodysesthesia syndrome (16%), erythema (11%)
Gastrointestinal: Vomiting (78%; grades 3/4: 9%), nausea (73%; grades 3/4: 15%), diarrhea (56%), abdominal pain (8% to 35%), anorexia (30%), gingival bleeding (17%), mucosal inflammation (16%), oral candidiasis (11%)
Hematologic: Leukopenia (grades 3/4: 88%), anemia (83%; grades 3/4: 75%), lymphopenia (grades 3/4: 82%), thrombocytopenia (81%; grades 3/4: 80%), neutropenia (grades 3/4: 10% to 64%), febrile neutropenia (55%; grade 4: 3%)
Hepatic: ALT increased (81%; grades 3/4: 43% to 44%), AST increased (74%; grades 3/4: 36%), bilirubin increased (45%; grades 3/4: 13%)
Neuromuscular & skeletal: Limb pain (30%), myalgia (14%)
Renal: Creatinine increased (50%; grades 3/4: 8%), hematuria (13%)
Respiratory: Epistaxis (27%), dyspnea (13%), pleural effusion (12%)
Miscellaneous: Infection (83%; includes bacterial, fungal, and viral), sepsis/septic shock (17%), catheter-related infection (12%)
1% to 10%:
Cardiovascular: Pericardial effusion (8%)
Central nervous system: Irritability (10%), lethargy (10%), somnolence (10%), agitation (5%), mental status change (1% to 4%)
Dermatologic: Cellulitis (8%), pruritic rash (8%)

Gastrointestinal: Proctalgia (8%), clostridium colitis (7%), stomatitis (7%), oral mucosal petechiae (5%), cecitis (1% to 4%), pancreatitis (1% to 4%)
Hepatic: Jaundice (8%)
Neuromuscular & skeletal: Back pain (10%), bone pain (10%), weakness (10%), arthralgia (9%)
Respiratory: Pneumonia (10%), respiratory distress (10%), tachypnea (9%), upper respiratory tract infection (5%), pulmonary edema (1% to 4%)
Miscellaneous: Herpes simplex (10%), bacteremia (9%), candidiasis (7%), herpes zoster (7%), staphylococcus bacteremia (6%), tumor lysis syndrome (grade 3: 6%), capillary leak syndrome (4%), hypersensitivity (1% to 4%), SIRS (2%)
General Dosage Range Dosage adjustment recommended in patients with renal impairment or who develop toxicities.
I.V.: *Children >1 year and Adults ≤21 years:* 52 mg/m^2/day days 1 through 5; repeat every 2-6 weeks
Mechanism of Action Clofarabine, a purine (deoxyadenosine) nucleoside analog, is metabolized to clofarabine 5'-triphosphate. Clofarabine 5'-triphosphate decreases cell replication and repair as well as causing cell death. To decrease cell replication and repair, clofarabine 5'-triphosphate competes with deoxyadenosine triphosphate for the enzymes ribonucleotide reductase and DNA polymerase. Cell replication is decreased when clofarabine 5'-triphosphate inhibits ribonucleotide reductase from reacting with deoxyadenosine triphosphate to produce deoxynucleotide triphosphate which is needed for DNA synthesis. Cell replication is also decreased when clofarabine 5'-triphosphate competes with DNA polymerase for incorporation into the DNA chain; when done during the repair process, cell repair is affected. To cause cell death, clofarabine 5'-triphosphate alters the mitochondrial membrane by releasing proteins, an inducing factor and cytochrome C.
Pharmacodynamics/Kinetics
Half-life Elimination Children: ~5 hours; Children and Adults: 7 hours (Bonate, 2011); half-life may be increased in elderly and in patients with renal impairment (Bonate, 2011)
Pregnancy Risk Factor D
Pregnancy Considerations Teratogenic effects and resorptions were observed in animal reproduction studies. May cause fetal harm if administered to a pregnant woman. Women of childbearing potential should be advised to use effective contraception and avoid becoming pregnant during therapy.

ClomiPHENE (KLOE mi feen)

Brand Names: U.S. Clomid®; Serophene®
Brand Names: Canada Clomid®; Serophene®
Pharmacologic Category Ovulation Stimulator; Selective Estrogen Receptor Modulator (SERM)
Use Treatment of ovulatory dysfunction in patients desiring pregnancy
Local Anesthetic/Vasoconstrictor Precautions No information available to require special precautions
Effects on Dental Treatment No significant effects or complications reported
Effects on Bleeding No information available to require special precautions
Adverse Effects
>10%: Endocrine & metabolic: Ovarian enlargement (14%)

1% to 10%:
Central nervous system: Headache (1%)
Endocrine & metabolic: Hot flashes (10%), breast discomfort (2%), abnormal uterine bleeding (1%)
Gastrointestinal: Distention/bloating/discomfort (6%), nausea (2%), vomiting (2%)
Ocular: Visual symptoms (2%, includes blurred vision, diplopia, floaters, lights, phosphenes, photophobia, scotomata, waves)

General Dosage Range Oral: *Adults (females):* 50-100 mg daily for 5 days

Mechanism of Action Clomiphene is a racemic mixture consisting of zuclomiphene (~38%) and enclomiphene (~62%), each with distinct pharmacologic properties. Enclomiphene is much less potent in inducing ovulation; however, it is more rapidly absorbed and metabolized, allowing the more potent activity of zuclomiphene to predominate. Zuclomiphene acts at the level of the hypothalamus, occupying cell surface and intracellular estrogen receptors (ERs) for longer durations than estrogen. This interferes with receptor recycling, effectively depleting hypothalamic ERs and inhibiting normal estrogenic negative feedback. Impairment of the feedback signal results in increased pulsatile GnRH secretion from the hypothalamus and subsequent pituitary gonadotropin (FSH, LH) release, causing growth of the ovarian follicle, followed by follicular rupture.

Pharmacodynamics/Kinetics

Onset of Action Ovulation: 5-10 days following course of treatment

Duration of Action Effects are cumulative; ovulation may occur in the cycle following the last treatment

Half-life Elimination 5 days

Time to Peak ~6 hours

Pregnancy Risk Factor X

Pregnancy Considerations Embryofetal and structural malformations were observed in animal reproduction studies. The incidence of adverse fetal effects following maternal use of clomiphene for ovulation induction is similar to those seen in the general population. Clomiphene is not indicated for use in women who are already pregnant.

ClomiPRAMINE (kloe MI pra meen)

Related Information
Vasoconstrictor Interactions With Antidepressants *on page 1650*

Brand Names: U.S. Anafranil®

Brand Names: Canada Anafranil®; Apo-Clomipramine®; CO Clomipramine; Dom-Clomipramine; Novo-Clomipramine

Pharmacologic Category Antidepressant, Tricyclic (Tertiary Amine)

Use Treatment of obsessive-compulsive disorder (OCD)

Unlabeled Use Depression, panic attacks, chronic pain

Local Anesthetic/Vasoconstrictor Precautions Use with caution; epinephrine and levonordefrin have been shown to have an increased pressor response in combination with TCAs. Clomipramine is one of the drugs confirmed to prolong the QT interval and is accepted as having a risk of causing torsade de pointes. The risk of drug-induced torsade de pointes is extremely low when a single QT interval prolonging drug is prescribed. In terms of epinephrine, it is not known what effect vasoconstrictors in the local anesthetic regimen will have in patients with a known history of congenital prolonged QT interval or in patients taking any medication that prolongs the QT interval. Until more information is obtained, it is suggested that the clinician consult with the physician prior to the use of a vasoconstrictor in suspected patients, and that the vasoconstrictor (epinephrine, mepivacaine and levonordefrin [Carbocaine® 2% with Neo-Cobefrin®]) be used with caution.

Effects on Dental Treatment Key adverse event(s) related to dental treatment: Xerostomia and changes in salivation (normal salivary flow resumes upon discontinuation). Long-term treatment with TCAs, such as clomipramine, increases the risk of caries by reducing salivation and salivary buffer capacity.

Effects on Bleeding No information available to require special precautions

Adverse Effects Data shown for children reflects both children and adolescents studied in clinical trials.
>10%:
Central nervous system: Dizziness (54%), somnolence (54%), drowsiness, headache (52%; children 28%), fatigue (39%), insomnia (25%; children 11%), malaise, nervousness (18%; children 4%)
Endocrine & metabolic: Libido changes (21%), hot flushes (5%)
Gastrointestinal: Xerostomia (84%, children 63%) constipation (47%; children 22%), nausea (33%; children 9%), dyspepsia (22%; children 13%), weight gain (18%; children 2%), diarrhea (13%; children 7%), anorexia (12%; children 22%), abdominal pain (11%), appetite increased (11%)
Genitourinary: Ejaculation failure (42%), impotence (20%), micturition disorder (14%; children 4%)
Neuromuscular & skeletal: Tremor (54%), myoclonus (13%; children 2%), myalgia (13%)
Ocular: Abnormal vision (18%; children 7%)
Respiratory: Pharyngitis (14%), rhinitis (12%)
Miscellaneous: Diaphoresis increased (29%; children 9%)
1% to 10%:
Cardiovascular: Flushing (8%), orthostatic hypotension (6%), palpitation (4%), tachycardia (4%; children 2%), chest pain (4%), edema (2%)
Central nervous system: Anxiety (9%), memory impairment (9%), twitching (7%), depression (5%), concentration impaired (5%), fever (4%), hypertonia (4%), abnormal dreaming (3%), agitation (3%), confusion (3%), migraine (3%), pain (3%), psychosomatic disorder (3%), speech disorder (3%), yawning (3%), aggressiveness (children 2%), chills (2%), depersonalization (2%), emotional lability (2%), irritability (2%), panic reaction (1%)
Dermatologic: Rash (8%), pruritus (6%), purpura (3%), dermatitis (2%), acne (2%), dry skin (2%), urticaria (1%)
Endocrine & metabolic: Amenorrhea (1%), breast enlargement (2%), breast pain (1%), hot flashes (5%), lactation (nonpuerperal) (4%)
Gastrointestinal: Taste disturbance (8%), vomiting (7%), flatulence (6%), dental caries and teeth grinding (5%), dysphagia (2%), esophagitis (1%)
Genitourinary: UTI (2% to 6%), micturition frequency (5%), dysuria (2%), leucorrhea (2%), vaginitis (2%), urinary retention (2%)
Neuromuscular & skeletal: Paresthesia (9%), back pain (6%), arthralgia (3%), paresis (children 2%), weakness (1%)
Ocular: Lacrimation abnormal (3%), mydriasis (2%), conjunctivitis (1%)
Otic: Tinnitus (6%)
Respiratory: Sinusitis (6%), coughing (6%), bronchospasm (2%; children 7%), epistaxis (2%)

General Dosage Range Oral:

Children ≥10 years: Initial: 25 mg/day; Maintenance: Up to 3 mg/kg/day (maximum: 200 mg/day)

Adults: Initial: 25 mg/day; Maintenance: Up to 250 mg/day

Mechanism of Action Clomipramine appears to affect serotonin uptake while its active metabolite, desmethylclomipramine, affects norepinephrine uptake

Pharmacodynamics/Kinetics

Half-life Elimination Clomipramine: Mean: 32 hours (range: 19-37 hours); DMI: Mean: 69 hours (range: 54-77 hours)

Time to Peak 2-6 hours

Pregnancy Risk Factor C

Pregnancy Considerations Adverse events were observed in some animal reproduction studies. Withdrawal symptoms (including jitteriness, tremor, and seizures) have been observed in neonates whose mothers took clomipramine up to delivery.

Dental Comment Clomipramine is known to prolong the QT interval. The QT interval is measured as the time and distance between the Q point of the QRS complex and the end of the T wave in the ECG tracing. After adjustment for heart rate, the QT interval is defined as prolonged if it is more than 450 msec in men and 460 msec in women. A long QT syndrome was first described in the 1950s and 60s as a congenital syndrome involving QT interval prolongation and syncope and sudden death. Some of the congenital long QT syndromes were characterized by a peculiar electrocardiographic appearance of the QRS complex involving a premature atria beat followed by a pause, then a subsequent sinus beat showing marked QT prolongation and deformity. This type of cardiac arrhythmia was originally termed "torsade de pointes" (translated from the French as "twisting of the points"). Clomipramine is considered as having a risk of causing torsade de pointes. Since it is not known what effect vasoconstrictors in the local anesthetic regimen will have in patients with a known history of congenital prolonged QT interval or in patients taking any medication that prolongs the QT interval, a medical consult is suggested.

ClonazePAM (kloe NA ze pam)

Brand Names: U.S. KlonoPIN®

Brand Names: Canada Apo-Clonazepam®; Clonapam; Clonazepam-R; CO Clonazepam; Dom-Clonazepam; Dom-Clonazepam-R; Mylan-Clonazepam; Novo-Clonazepam; PHL-Clonazepam; PHL-Clonazepam-R; PMS-Clonazepam; PRO-Clonazepam; ratio-Clonazepam; Riva-Clonazepam; Rivotril®; Sandoz-Clonazepam; ZYM-Clonazepam

Generic Availability (U.S.) Yes

Pharmacologic Category Benzodiazepine

Dental Use Burning mouth syndrome

Use Alone or as an adjunct in the treatment of petit mal variant (Lennox-Gastaut), akinetic, and myoclonic seizures; petit mal (absence) seizures unresponsive to succimides; panic disorder with or without agoraphobia

Unlabeled Use Restless legs syndrome; neuralgia; multifocal tic disorder; parkinsonian dysarthria; bipolar disorder; adjunct therapy for schizophrenia; burning mouth syndrome; essential tremor

Local Anesthetic/Vasoconstrictor Precautions No information available to require special precautions

Effects on Dental Treatment Key adverse event(s) related to dental treatment: Xerostomia and changes in salivation (normal salivary flow resumes upon discontinuation), gum soreness, and coated tongue.

Effects on Bleeding No information available to require special precautions

Adverse Effects Reactions reported in patients with seizure and/or panic disorder. Frequency not always defined.

Cardiovascular: Edema (ankle or facial), palpitation

Central nervous system: Amnesia, ataxia (seizure disorder ~30%; panic disorder 5%), behavior problems (seizure disorder ~25%), coma, confusion, coordination impaired, depression, dizziness, drowsiness (seizure disorder ~50%), emotional lability, fatigue, fever, hallucinations, headache, hysteria, insomnia, intellectual ability reduced, memory disturbance, nervousness; paradoxical reactions (including aggressive behavior, agitation, anxiety, excitability, hostility, irritability, nervousness, nightmares, sleep disturbance, vivid dreams); psychosis, slurred speech, somnolence (panic disorder 37%), vertigo

Dermatologic: Hair loss, hirsutism, skin rash

Endocrine & metabolic: Dysmenorrhea, libido increased/decreased

Gastrointestinal: Abdominal pain, anorexia, appetite increased/decreased, coated tongue, constipation, dehydration, diarrhea, encopresis, gastritis, gum soreness, nausea, weight changes (loss/gain), xerostomia

Genitourinary: Colpitis, dysuria, ejaculation delayed, enuresis, impotence, micturition frequency, nocturia, urinary retention, urinary tract infection

Hematologic: Anemia, eosinophilia, leukopenia, thrombocytopenia

Hepatic: Alkaline phosphatase increased (transient), hepatomegaly, transaminases increased (transient)

Neuromuscular & skeletal: Choreiform movements, coordination abnormal, dysarthria, hypotonia, muscle pain, muscle weakness, myalgia, tremor

Ocular: Blurred vision, eye movements abnormal, diplopia, nystagmus

Respiratory: Bronchitis, chest congestion, cough, hypersecretions, pharyngitis, respiratory depression, respiratory tract infection, rhinitis, rhinorrhea, shortness of breath, sinusitis

Miscellaneous: Allergic reaction, aphonia, dysdiadochokinesis, "glassy-eyed" appearance, hemiparesis, flu-like syndrome, lymphadenopathy

<1% (Limited to important or life-threatening): Apathy, burning skin, chest pain, depersonalization, dyspnea, excessive dreaming, hyperactivity, hypoesthesia, hypotension postural, infection, migraine, organic disinhibition, pain, paresthesia, paresis, periorbital edema, polyuria, suicidal attempt, suicide ideation, thick tongue, twitching, visual disturbance, xerophthalmia

Dental Usual Dosage Burning mouth syndrome (unlabeled use): Adults: Oral: 0.25-3 mg/day in 2 divided doses, in morning and evening

Dosage

Children <10 years or <30 kg: Seizure disorders: Oral: Initial daily dose: 0.01-0.03 mg/kg/day (maximum: 0.05 mg/kg/day) given in 2-3 divided doses; increase by no more than 0.25-0.5 mg every third day until seizures are controlled or adverse effects seen

Usual maintenance dose: 0.1-0.2 mg/kg/day divided 3 times daily, not to exceed 0.2 mg/kg/day

Children >10 years or ≥30 kg, Adolescents, and Adults:
Seizure disorders: Oral:
Initial daily dose not to exceed 1.5 mg given in 3 divided doses; may increase by 0.5-1 mg every third day until seizures are controlled or adverse effects seen (maximum: 20 mg daily)
Usual maintenance dose: 2-8 mg daily in 1-2 divided doses (Brodie, 1997); do not exceed 20 mg daily
Adults:
Panic disorder: Oral: 0.25 mg twice daily; increase in increments of 0.125-0.25 mg twice daily every 3 days; target dose: 1 mg daily (maximum: 4 mg daily)
Discontinuation of treatment: To discontinue, treatment should be withdrawn gradually. Decrease dose by 0.125 mg twice daily every 3 days until medication is completely withdrawn.
Burning mouth syndrome (unlabeled use):
Oral: Initial: 0.25 at bedtime for 1 week; increase dose by ≤0.25 mg every week; maximum dose: 3 mg daily in 3 divided doses. **Note:** Use should be limited (Buchanan, 2008; Grushka, 1998).
Topical: May administer topically with 1 mg 3 times daily (after each meal). **Note:** Patient should be instructed to suck on the tablet, retain saliva in mouth near the pain sites without swallowing for 3 minutes, and then expectorate saliva (Gremeau-Richard, 2004).
Essential tremor (unlabeled use): Oral: Initial: 0.5 mg at bedtime; increase dose by 0.5 mg every 3-4 days; maximum dose: 6 mg daily (Biary, 1987; Thompson, 1984; Zesiewicz, 2005; Zesiewicz, 2011).
REM sleep behavior disorder (unlabeled use): 0.25-2 mg 30 minutes prior to bedtime (maximum: 4 mg 30 minutes prior to bedtime). **Note:** Use with caution in patients with dementia, gait disorders, or obstructive sleep apnea (Aurora, 2010).
Elderly: Initiate with low doses and observe closely

Dosage adjustment in renal impairment: No dosage adjustment provided in manufacturer's labeling; use with caution. Clonazepam metabolites may accumulate in patients with renal impairment.

Dosage adjustment in hepatic impairment: No dosage adjustment provided in manufacturer's labeling; use with caution.

Mechanism of Action The exact mechanism is unknown, but believed to be related to its ability to enhance the activity of GABA; suppresses the spike-and-wave discharge in absence seizures by depressing nerve transmission in the motor cortex

Contraindications Hypersensitivity to clonazepam or any component of the formulation (cross-sensitivity with other benzodiazepines may exist); significant liver disease; acute narrow-angle glaucoma

Warnings/Precautions Hazardous agent - use appropriate precautions for handling and disposal (NIOSH, 2012). Antiepileptics are associated with an increased risk of suicidal behavior/thoughts with use (regardless of indication); patients should be monitored for signs/symptoms of depression, suicidal tendencies, and other unusual behavior changes during therapy and instructed to inform their healthcare provider immediately if symptoms occur.

Use with caution in elderly or debilitated patients, patients with hepatic disease (including alcoholics), or renal impairment. Use with caution in patients with respiratory disease or impaired gag reflex or ability to protect the airway from secretions (salivation may be increased). Worsening of seizures may occur when added to patients with multiple seizure types.

Concurrent use with valproic acid may result in absence status. Monitoring of CBC and liver function tests has been recommended during prolonged therapy.

Causes CNS depression (dose related) resulting in sedation, dizziness, confusion, or ataxia which may impair physical and mental capabilities. Patients must be cautioned about performing tasks which require mental alertness (eg, operating machinery or driving). Use with caution in patients receiving other CNS depressants or psychoactive agents. Effects with other sedative drugs or ethanol may be potentiated. Benzodiazepines have been associated with falls and traumatic injury and should be used with extreme caution in patients who are at risk of these events.

Use caution in patients with depression, particularly if suicidal risk may be present. Use with caution in patients with a history of drug dependence. Benzodiazepines have been associated with dependence and acute withdrawal symptoms, including seizures, on discontinuation or reduction in dose. Acute withdrawal, including seizures, may be precipitated in patients after administration of flumazenil to patients receiving long-term benzodiazepine therapy.

Benzodiazepines have been associated with anterograde amnesia. Paradoxical reactions, including hyperactive or aggressive behavior, have been reported with benzodiazepines, particularly in adolescent/pediatric or psychiatric patients. Does not have analgesic, antidepressant, or antipsychotic properties.

In older adults, benzodiazepines increase the risk of impaired cognition, delirium, falls, fractures, and motor vehicle accidents. Due to increased sensitivity in this age group and slower metabolism of long-acting agents (such as clonazepam), avoid use for treatment of insomnia, agitation, or delirium (Beers Criteria).

Drug Interactions

Metabolism/Transport Effects Substrate of CYP3A4 (major); **Note:** Assignment of Major/Minor substrate status based on clinically relevant drug interaction potential

Avoid Concomitant Use

Avoid concomitant use of ClonazePAM with any of the following: Azelastine (Nasal); Conivaptan; OLANZapine; Paraldehyde; Sodium Oxybate

Increased Effect/Toxicity

ClonazePAM may increase the levels/effects of: Alcohol (Ethyl); Azelastine (Nasal); Buprenorphine; CloZApine; CNS Depressants; Fosphenytoin; Methotrimeprazine; Metyrosine; Mirtazapine; Paraldehyde; Phenytoin; Pramipexole; ROPINIRole; Rotigotine; Selective Serotonin Reuptake Inhibitors; Sodium Oxybate; Zolpidem

The levels/effects of ClonazePAM may be increased by: Antifungal Agents (Azole Derivatives, Systemic); Aprepitant; Calcium Channel Blockers (Nondihydropyridine); Cimetidine; Cobicistat; Conivaptan; Contraceptives (Estrogens); Contraceptives (Progestins); Cosyntropin; CYP3A4 Inhibitors (Moderate); CYP3A4 Inhibitors (Strong); Dasatinib; Droperidol; Fosaprepitant; Grapefruit Juice; HydrOXYzine; Isoniazid; Ivacaftor; Macrolide Antibiotics; Magnesium Sulfate; Methotrimeprazine; Mifepristone; OLANZapine; Perampanel; Proton Pump Inhibitors; Selective Serotonin Reuptake Inhibitors

◀ **Decreased Effect**

The levels/effects of ClonazePAM may be decreased by: CarBAMazepine; CYP3A4 Inducers (Strong); Deferasirox; Rifamycin Derivatives; St Johns Wort; Theophylline Derivatives; Tocilizumab; Yohimbine

Ethanol/Nutrition/Herb Interactions

Ethanol: May increase CNS depression; monitor for increased effects with coadministration. Caution patients about effects.

Food: Clonazepam serum concentration is unlikely to be increased by grapefruit juice because of clonazepam's high oral bioavailability.

Herb/Nutraceutical: St John's wort may decrease clonazepam levels. Avoid valerian, St John's wort, kava kava, gotu kola (may increase CNS depression).

Pharmacodynamics/Kinetics

Onset of Action ~20-40 minutes (Hanson, 1972)

Duration of Action Infants and young children: 6-8 hours (Hanson, 1972); Adults: ≤12 hours (Hanson, 1972)

Half-life Elimination Children: 22-33 hours (Walson, 1996); Adults: 17-60 hours (Walson, 1996)

Time to Peak Serum: 1-4 hours

Pregnancy Risk Factor D

Pregnancy Considerations Clonazepam was shown to be teratogenic in some animal studies. Clonazepam crosses the placenta. Teratogenic effects have been observed with some benzodiazepines; however, additional studies are needed. Epilepsy itself, the number of medications, genetic factors, or a combination of these probably influence the teratogenicity of anticonvulsant therapy. The incidence of premature birth and low birth weights may be increased following maternal use of benzodiazepines; hypoglycemia and respiratory problems in the neonate may occur following exposure late in pregnancy. Neonatal withdrawal symptoms may occur within days to weeks after birth and "floppy infant syndrome" (which also includes withdrawal symptoms) has been reported with some benzodiazepines, including clonazepam.

Patients exposed to clonazepam during pregnancy are encouraged to enroll themselves into the AED Pregnancy Registry by calling 1-888-233-2334. Additional information is available at www.aedpregnancyregistry.org.

Lactation Enters breast milk/not recommended

Breast-Feeding Considerations Clonazepam enters breast milk. Drowsiness, lethargy, or weight loss in nursing infants have been observed in case reports following maternal use of some benzodiazepines.

Controlled Substance C-IV

Dosage Forms

Tablet, oral: 0.5 mg, 1 mg, 2 mg

KlonoPIN®: 0.5 mg, 1 mg, 2 mg

Tablet, orally disintegrating, oral: 0.125 mg, 0.25 mg, 0.5 mg, 1 mg, 2 mg

References

Buchanan J and Zakrzewska J, "Burning Mouth Syndrome," *Clin Evid (online)*, March 14, 2008. Available at http://www.ncbi.nlm.nih.gov/pmc/articles/PMC2907957/pdf/2008-1301.pdf.

Minguez Serra MP, Salort Llorca C, Silvestre Donat FJ, "Pharmacological Treatment of Burning Mouth Syndrome: A Review and Update," *Med Oral Patol Oral Cir Bucal*, 2007, 12(4):E299-304.

CloNIDine (KLON i deen)

Related Information

Cardiovascular Diseases *on page 1492*

Brand Names: U.S. Catapres-TTS®-1; Catapres-TTS®-2; Catapres-TTS®-3; Catapres®; Duraclon®; Kapvay®

Brand Names: Canada Apo-Clonidine®; Catapres®; Dixarit®; Dom-Clonidine; Novo-Clonidine

Generic Availability (U.S.) Yes: Excludes extended release tablets

Pharmacologic Category Alpha$_2$-Adrenergic Agonist

Use

Oral:

Immediate release: Management of hypertension (monotherapy or as adjunctive therapy)

Extended release (Kapvay™): Treatment of attention-deficit/hyperactivity disorder (ADHD) (monotherapy or as adjunctive therapy)

Epidural (Duraclon®): For continuous epidural administration as adjunctive therapy with opioids for treatment of severe cancer pain in patients tolerant to or unresponsive to opioids alone; epidural clonidine is generally more effective for neuropathic pain and less effective (or possibly ineffective) for somatic or visceral pain

Transdermal patch: Management of hypertension (monotherapy or as adjunctive therapy)

Unlabeled Use Heroin or nicotine withdrawal; severe pain; dysmenorrhea; vasomotor symptoms associated with menopause; ethanol dependence; prophylaxis of migraines; glaucoma; diabetes-associated diarrhea; impulse control disorder, clozapine-induced sialorrhea; aid in the diagnosis of growth hormone deficiency; attention-deficit/hyperactivity disorder (ADHD) and associated insomnia in children; Tourette's syndrome in children; aggression associated with conduct disorder

Local Anesthetic/Vasoconstrictor Precautions No information available to require special precautions

Effects on Dental Treatment Key adverse event(s) related to dental treatment: Significant xerostomia (normal salivary flow resumes upon discontinuation), orthostatic hypotension, and abnormal taste.

Effects on Bleeding No information available to require special precautions

Adverse Effects Frequency not always defined.

Oral, Transdermal: Incidence of adverse events may be less with transdermal compared to oral due to the lower peak/trough ratio.

Cardiovascular: Bradycardia (≤4%), palpitation (1%), tachycardia (1%), arrhythmia, atrioventricular block, chest pain, CHF, ECG abnormalities, flushing, orthostatic hypotension, pallor, Raynaud's phenomenon, syncope

Central nervous system: Drowsiness (12% to 38%), headache (1% to 29%), fatigue (4% to 16%), dizziness (2% to 16%), sedation (3% to 10%), insomnia (≤6%), lethargy (3%), nervousness (1% to 3%), mental depression (1%), aggression, agitation, anxiety, behavioral changes, CVA, delirium, delusional perception, fever, hallucinations (visual and auditory), irritability, malaise, nightmares, restlessness, vivid dreams

Dermatologic: Transient localized skin reactions characterized by pruritus and erythema (transdermal 15% to 50%), contact dermatitis (transdermal 8% to 34%), vesiculation (transdermal 7%), allergic contact sensitization (transdermal 5%), hyperpigmentation (transdermal 5%), burning (transdermal 3%), edema (3%), excoriation (transdermal 3%) blanching (transdermal 1%), generalized macular rash (1%), papules (transdermal 1%), throbbing (transdermal 1%), alopecia, angioedema, hives, localized hypopigmentation (transdermal), rash, urticaria

Endocrine & metabolic: Sexual dysfunction (3%), gynecomastia (1%), creatine phosphokinase increased (transient; oral), hyperglycemia (transient; oral), libido decreased

Gastrointestinal: Xerostomia (≤40%), constipation (2% to 10%), anorexia (1%), taste perversion (1%), weight gain (<1%), abdominal pain (oral), diarrhea, nausea, parotid gland pain (oral), parotitis (oral), pseudo-obstruction (oral), throat pain, vomiting

Genitourinary: Erectile dysfunction (2% to 3%), nocturia (1%), dysuria, enuresis, urinary retention

Hematologic: Thrombocytopenia (oral)

Hepatic: Liver function test (mild transient abnormalities; ≤1%), hepatitis

Neuromuscular & skeletal: Weakness (10%), arthralgia (1%), myalgia (1%), leg cramps (<1%), numbness (localized, transdermal), pain in extremities, paresthesia, tremor

Ocular: Accommodation disorder, blurred vision, burning eyes, dry eyes, lacrimation decreased, lacrimation increased

Otic: Ear pain, otitis media

Renal: Pollakiuria

Respiratory: Asthma, epistaxis, nasal congestion, nasal dryness, nasopharyngitis, respiratory tract infection, rhinorrhea

Miscellaneous: Withdrawal syndrome (1%), flu-like syndrome, thirst

Epidural: Note: The following adverse events occurred more often than placebo in cancer patients with intractable pain being treated with concurrent epidural morphine.

>10%:

Cardiovascular: Hypotension (45%), orthostatic hypotension (32%)

Central nervous system: Confusion (13%), dizziness (13%)

Gastrointestinal: Xerostomia (13%)

1% to 10%:

Cardiovascular: Chest pain (5%)

Central nervous system: Hallucinations (5%)

Gastrointestinal: Nausea/vomiting (8%)

Otic: Tinnitus (5%)

Miscellaneous: Diaphoresis (5%)

Dosage Note: Dosing is expressed as the salt (clonidine hydrochloride) unless otherwise noted. Formulations of clonidine (immediate release versus extended release) are not interchangeable on a mg:mg basis due to different pharmacokinetic profiles.

Children:

Oral:

Hypertension (unlabeled use): Children ≥12 years: Immediate release: Initial: 0.2 mg/day in 2 divided doses; increase gradually, if needed, in 0.1 mg/day increments at weekly intervals; maximum: 2.4 mg/day (rarely required) (NHBPEP, Fourth Report)

Severe hypertension (unlabeled use): Children: Immediate release: 0.05-0.1 mg/dose; may repeat up to a maximum total dose of 0.8 mg (NHBPEP, Fourth Report)

Clonidine tolerance test (test of growth hormone release from pituitary) (unlabeled use):

0.15 mg/m² as a single dose (Lanes, 1982)

or

5 mcg/kg as a single dose; maximum dose: 250 mcg (Richmond, 2008)

ADHD: **Note:** May be used alone or as an adjunct to stimulants.

Immediate release (unlabeled indication; Pliszka, 2007):

Children ≤45 kg: Initial: 0.05 mg at bedtime; sequentially increase every 3-7 days by 0.05 mg increments as twice daily, then 3 times daily, then 4 times daily; maximum daily dose: 0.2 mg/day for patients weighing 27-40.5 kg; 0.3 mg/day for patients weighing 40.5-45 kg. When discontinuing therapy, taper gradually over 1-2 weeks.

Children >45 kg: Initial: 0.1 mg at bedtime; sequentially increase every 3-7 days by 0.1 mg increments as twice daily, then 3 times daily, then 4 times daily; maximum daily dose: 0.4 mg/day. When discontinuing therapy, taper gradually over 1-2 weeks.

Extended release (Kapvay™): Children ≥6 years: Initial: 0.1 mg at bedtime; increase in 0.1 mg/day increments every 7 days until desired response, doses should be administered twice daily (either split equally or with the higher split dosage given at bedtime); maximum: 0.4 mg/day. **Note:** Maintenance treatment for >5 weeks has not been evaluated. When discontinuing therapy, taper daily dose by ≤0.1 mg every 3-7 days.

Epidural infusion: Pain management: Reserved for cancer patients with severe intractable pain, unresponsive to other opioid analgesics: Initial: 0.5 mcg/kg/**hour**; adjust with caution, based on clinical effect

Adults:

Oral:

Hypertension: Immediate release: Initial dose: 0.1 mg twice daily (maximum recommended dose: 2.4 mg/day); usual dose range (JNC 7): 0.1-0.8 mg/day in 2 divided doses

Acute hypertension (urgency) (unlabeled use): Initial 0.1-0.2 mg; may be followed by additional doses of 0.1 mg every hour, if necessary, to a maximum total dose of 0.7 mg (Atkin, 1992; Jaker, 1989)

Unlabeled route of administration: Sublingual: Initial: 0.1-0.2 mg; followed by 0.05-0.1 mg every hour until blood pressure controlled or a cumulative dose of 0.7 mg is reached (Cunningham, 1994; Matuschka, 1999)

Nicotine withdrawal symptoms (unlabeled use): Initial: 0.1 mg twice daily; titrate by 0.1 mg/day every 7 days if needed; dosage range used in clinical trials: 0.15-0.75 mg/day; duration of therapy ranged from 3-10 weeks in clinical trials (Fiore, 2008)

Transdermal:

Hypertension: Initial: 0.1 mg/24 hour patch applied once every 7 days and increase by 0.1 mg at 1- to 2-week intervals (dosages >0.6 mg/24 hours do not improve efficacy); usual dose range (JNC 7): 0.1-0.3 mg/24 hour patch applied once every 7 days

Nicotine withdrawal symptoms (unlabeled use): Initial: 0.1 mg/24 hour patch applied once every 7 days and increase by 0.1 mg at 1-week intervals if necessary; dosage range used in clinical trials: 0.1-0.2 mg/24 hour patch applied once every 7 days; duration of therapy ranged from 3-10 weeks in clinical trials (Fiore, 2008)

Epidural infusion: Pain management: Reserved for cancer patients with severe intractable pain, unresponsive to other opioid analgesics: Starting dose: 30 mcg/hour; titrate as required for relief of pain or presence of side effects; experience with doses >40 mcg/hour is limited; should be considered an adjunct to opioid therapy

Conversion from oral to transdermal: **Note:** If transitioning from oral to transdermal therapy, overlap oral regimen for 1-2 days; transdermal route takes 2-3 days to achieve therapeutic effects. An example transition is below:

Day 1: Place Catapres-TTS® 1; administer 100% of oral dose.

Day 2: Administer 50% of oral dose.

Day 3: Administer 25% of oral dose.

Day 4: Patch remains, no further oral supplement necessary.

Conversion from transdermal to oral: After transdermal patch removal, therapeutic clonidine levels persist for ~8 hours and then slowly decrease over several days. Consider starting oral clonidine no sooner than 8 hours after patch removal.

Elderly: Oral: Immediate release: Hypertension: Initial: 0.1 mg once daily at bedtime, increase gradually as needed

Dosage adjustment in renal impairment:

Children: Oral (extended release), epidural: The manufacturer recommends dosage adjustment according to degree of renal impairment; however, no specific dosage adjustment provided (has not been studied).

Adults: Oral (immediate release), transdermal, epidural: The manufacturer recommends dosage adjustment according to degree of renal impairment; however, no specific dosage adjustment provided in manufacturer's labeling. Bradycardia, sedation, and hypotension may be more likely to occur in patients with renal failure; half-life significantly prolonged in patients with severe renal failure; consider use of lower initial doses and monitor closely.

Hemodialysis: Not dialyzable (0% to 5%); supplemental dose is not necessary. Oral antihypertensive drugs given preferentially at night may reduce the nocturnal surge of blood pressure and minimize the intradialytic hypotension that may occur when taken the morning before a dialysis session (K/DOQI, 2005).

Dosage adjustment in hepatic impairment: No dosage adjustment provided in manufacturer's labeling.

Mechanism of Action Stimulates alpha₂-adrenoceptors in the brain stem, thus activating an inhibitory neuron, resulting in reduced sympathetic outflow from the CNS, producing a decrease in peripheral resistance, renal vascular resistance, heart rate, and blood pressure; epidural clonidine may produce pain relief at spinal presynaptic and postjunctional alpha₂-adrenoceptors by preventing pain signal transmission; pain relief occurs only for the body regions innervated by the spinal segments where analgesic concentrations of clonidine exist. For the treatment of ADHD, the mechanism of action is unknown; it has been proposed that postsynaptic alpha₂-agonist stimulation regulates subcortical activity in the prefrontal cortex, the area of the brain responsible for emotions, attentions, and behaviors and causes reduced hyperactivity, impulsiveness, and distractibility.

Contraindications Hypersensitivity to clonidine hydrochloride or any component of the formulation

Epidural administration: Injection site infection; concurrent anticoagulant therapy; bleeding diathesis; administration above the C4 dermatome

Warnings/Precautions May cause CNS depression, which may impair physical or mental abilities; patients must be cautioned about performing tasks which require mental alertness (eg, operating machinery or driving). Sedating effects may be potentiated when used with other CNS-depressant drugs or ethanol. Use with caution in patients with severe coronary insufficiency; conduction disturbances; recent MI, CVA, or chronic renal insufficiency. May cause dose dependent reductions in heart rate; use with caution in patients with preexisting bradycardia or those predisposed to developing bradycardia. Caution in sinus node dysfunction. Use with caution in patients concurrently receiving agents known to reduce SA node function and/or AV nodal conduction (eg, digoxin, diltiazem, metoprolol, verapamil). May cause significant xerostomia. Clonidine may cause eye dryness in patients who wear contact lenses.

[U.S. Boxed Warning]: Must dilute concentrated epidural injectable (500 mcg/mL) solution prior to use. Epidural clonidine is not recommended for perioperative, obstetrical, or postpartum pain due to risk of hemodynamic instability. Clonidine injection should be administered via a continuous epidural infusion device. Monitor closely for catheter-related infection such as meningitis or epidural abscess. Epidural clonidine is not recommended for use in patients with severe cardiovascular disease or hemodynamic instability; may lead to cardiovascular instability (hypotension, bradycardia). Symptomatic hypotension may occur with use; in all patients, use epidural clonidine with caution due to the potential for severe hypotension especially in women and those of low body weight. Most hypotensive episodes occur within the first 4 days of initiation; however, episodes may occur throughout the duration of therapy.

Gradual withdrawal is needed (taper oral immediate release or epidural dose gradually over 2-4 days to avoid rebound hypertension) if drug needs to be stopped. Patients should be instructed about abrupt discontinuation (causes rapid increase in BP and symptoms of sympathetic overactivity). In patients on both a beta-blocker and clonidine where withdrawal of clonidine is necessary, withdraw the beta-blocker first and several days before clonidine withdrawal, then slowly decrease clonidine. In children and adolescents, extended release formulation (Kapvay™) should be tapered in decrements of no more than 0.1 mg every 3-7 days. Discontinue oral immediate release formulations within 4 hours of surgery then restart as soon as possible afterwards. Discontinue oral extended release formulations up to 28 hours prior to surgery, then restart the following day.

Oral formulations of clonidine (immediate release versus extended release) are not interchangeable on a mg:mg basis due to different pharmacokinetic profiles.

Transdermal patch may contain conducting metal (eg, aluminum); remove patch prior to MRI. Due to the potential for altered electrical conductivity, remove transdermal patch before cardioversion or defibrillation. Localized contact sensitization to the transdermal system has been reported; in these patients, allergic reactions (eg, generalized rash, urticaria, angioedema) have also occurred following subsequent substitution of oral therapy.

In the elderly, avoid use as first-line antihypertensive due to high risk of CNS adverse effects; may also cause orthostatic hypotension and bradycardia (Beers Criteria). In pediatric patients, epidural clonidine should be reserved for cancer patients with severe intractable pain, unresponsive to other analgesics or epidural or spinal opioids. Use oral formulations with caution in pediatric patients since children commonly have gastrointestinal illnesses with vomiting and are susceptible to hypertensive episodes due to abrupt inability to take oral medication.

Drug Interactions

Metabolism/Transport Effects None known.

Avoid Concomitant Use

Avoid concomitant use of CloNIDine with any of the following: Azelastine (Nasal); Iobenguane I 123; Paraldehyde

Increased Effect/Toxicity

CloNIDine may increase the levels/effects of: Alcohol (Ethyl); Amifostine; Antihypertensives; Azelastine (Nasal); Beta-Blockers; Buprenorphine; Calcium Channel Blockers (Nondihydropyridine); Cardiac Glycosides; CNS Depressants; Hypotensive Agents; Methotrimeprazine; Metyrosine; Paraldehyde; Pramipexole; RiTUXimab; ROPINIRole; Rotigotine; Selective Serotonin Reuptake Inhibitors; Zolpidem

The levels/effects of CloNIDine may be increased by: Alfuzosin; Beta-Blockers; Diazoxide; Droperidol; Herbs (Hypotensive Properties); HydrOXYzine; Magnesium Sulfate; MAO Inhibitors; Methotrimeprazine; Methylphenidate; Pentoxifylline; Perampanel; Phosphodiesterase 5 Inhibitors; Prostacyclin Analogues; Sodium Oxybate

Decreased Effect

CloNIDine may decrease the levels/effects of: Iobenguane I 123

The levels/effects of CloNIDine may be decreased by: Antidepressants (Alpha2-Antagonist); Herbs (Hypertensive Properties); Serotonin/Norepinephrine Reuptake Inhibitors; Tricyclic Antidepressants; Yohimbine

Ethanol/Nutrition/Herb Interactions

Ethanol: Avoid ethanol (may increase CNS depression). Herb/Nutraceutical: Avoid dong quai if using for hypertension (has estrogenic activity). Avoid ephedra, yohimbe, ginseng (may worsen hypertension). Avoid valerian, St John's wort, kava kava, gotu kola (may increase CNS depression).

Pharmacodynamics/Kinetics

Onset of Action Oral: Immediate release: 0.5-1 hour (maximum reduction in blood pressure: 2-4 hours); Transdermal: Initial application: 2-3 days

Duration of Action Oral: Immediate release: 6-10 hours

Half-life Elimination Adults: Normal renal function: 12-16 hours; Renal impairment: Up to 41 hours

Epidural administration: CSF half-life elimination: 0.8-1.8 hours

Transdermal: Half-life elimination (after patch removal): ~20 hours (due to skin depot effect; increase in plasma clonidine concentrations may occur after patch removal [MacGregor, 1985])

Time to Peak Plasma: Oral: Immediate release: 1-3 hours; Extended release: 7-8 hours

Pregnancy Risk Factor C

Pregnancy Considerations Adverse events have been observed in some animal reproduction studies. Clonidine crosses the placenta; concentrations in the umbilical cord plasma are similar to those in the maternal serum and concentrations in the amniotic fluid may

be 4 times those in the maternal serum. **[U.S. Boxed Warning]: Epidural clonidine is not recommended for obstetrical or postpartum pain** due to risk of hemodynamic instability.

Lactation Enters breast milk/not recommended

Breast-Feeding Considerations Enters breast milk with concentrations approximately twice maternal serum concentrations

Dosage Forms

Injection, solution [preservative free]: 100 mcg/mL (10 mL); 500 mcg/mL (10 mL)

Duraclon®: 100 mcg/mL (10 mL); 500 mcg/mL (10 mL)

Patch, transdermal: 0.1 mg/24 hours (4s); 0.2 mg/24 hours (4s); 0.3 mg/24 hours (4s)

Catapres-TTS®-1: 0.1 mg/24 hours (4s)

Catapres-TTS®-2: 0.2 mg/24 hours (4s)

Catapres-TTS®-3: 0.3 mg/24 hours (4s)

Tablet, oral: 0.1 mg, 0.2 mg, 0.3 mg

Catapres®: 0.1 mg, 0.2 mg, 0.3 mg

Tablet, extended release, oral:

Kapvay®: 0.1 mg, 0.2 mg, 0.1 mg AM dose, 0.2 mg PM dose

Clonidine and Chlorthalidone
(KLON i deen & klor THAL i done)

Related Information

Chlorthalidone *on page 297*

CloNIDine *on page 332*

Brand Names: U.S. Clorpres®

Pharmacologic Category Alpha$_2$-Adrenergic Agonist; Diuretic, Thiazide

Use Treatment of hypertension

Local Anesthetic/Vasoconstrictor Precautions No information available to require special precautions

Effects on Dental Treatment Key adverse event(s) related to dental treatment: Clonidine: Significant xerostomia (normal salivary flow resumes upon discontinuation), orthostatic hypotension, and abnormal taste.

Effects on Bleeding No information available to require special precautions

Adverse Effects Reactions which follow have been reported with the combination product; see individual drug agents for additional adverse reactions that may be expected from each agent.

>10%:

Central nervous system: Drowsiness (33%), dizziness (16%)

Gastrointestinal: Xerostomia (40%)

1% to 10%:

Central nervous system: Sedation (10%)

Gastrointestinal: Constipation (10%)

General Dosage Range Oral: *Adults:* One tablet (clonidine 0.1-0.3 mg/chlorthalidone 15 mg per tablet) 1-2 times daily (maximum: clonidine 0.6 mg; chlorthalidone 30 mg daily)

Pregnancy Risk Factor C

Pregnancy Considerations Refer to Clonidine monograph.

Clopidogrel (kloh PID oh grel)

Related Information

Antiplatelet and Anticoagulation Considerations in Dentistry *on page 1503*

Cardiovascular Diseases *on page 1492*

Brand Names: U.S. Plavix®

Brand Names: Canada Apo-Clopidogrel®; CO Clopidogrel; Dom-Clopidogrel; Mylan-Clopidogrel; Plavix®; PMS-Clopidogrel; RAN™-Clopidogrel; Sandoz-Clopidogrel; Teva-Clopidogrel

Generic Availability (U.S.) Yes

Pharmacologic Category Antiplatelet Agent; Antiplatelet Agent, Thienopyridine

Use Reduces rate of atherothrombotic events (myocardial infarction, stroke, vascular deaths) in patients with recent MI or stroke, or established peripheral arterial disease; reduces rate of atherothrombotic events in patients with unstable angina (UA) or non-ST-segment elevation MI (NSTEMI) managed medically or with percutaneous coronary intervention (PCI) (with or without stent) or CABG; reduces rate of death and atherothrombotic events in patients with ST-segment elevation MI (STEMI) managed medically

Canadian labeling: Additional use (not in U.S. labeling): Prevention of atherothrombotic and thromboembolic events, including stroke, in patients with atrial fibrillation with at least 1 risk factor for vascular events who are not suitable for treatment with an anticoagulant and are at a low risk for bleeding.

Unlabeled Use In patients with allergy or major gastrointestinal intolerance to aspirin, initial treatment of acute coronary syndromes (ACS) or prevention of coronary artery bypass graft closure (saphenous vein); stable coronary artery disease (in combination with aspirin); in patients having undergone peripheral artery percutaneous transluminal angioplasty; symptomatic carotid artery stenosis (including recent carotid endarterectomy)

Local Anesthetic/Vasoconstrictor Precautions No information available to require special precautions

Effects on Dental Treatment Aspirin in combination with clopidogrel (Plavix®), prasugrel (Effient®), or ticagrelor (Brilinta™) is the primary prevention strategy against stent thrombosis after placement of drug-eluting metal stents in coronary patients. Premature discontinuation of combination antiplatelet therapy (ie, dual antiplatelet therapy) strongly increases the risk of a catastrophic event of stent thrombosis leading to myocardial infarction and/or death, so says a science advisory issued in January 2007 from the American Heart Association in collaboration with the American Dental Association and other professional healthcare organizations. The advisory stresses a 12-month therapy of dual antiplatelet therapy after placement of a drug-eluting stent in order to prevent thrombosis at the stent site. Any elective surgery should be postponed for 1 year after stent implantation, and if surgery must be performed, consideration should be given to continuing the antiplatelet therapy during the perioperative period in high-risk patients with drug-eluting stents.

This advisory was issued from a science panel made up of representatives from the American Heart Association (AHA), the American College of Cardiology, the Society for Cardiovascular Angiography and Interventions, the American College of Surgeons, the American Dental Association (ADA), and the American College of Physicians (Grines, 2007).

Effects on Bleeding Clopidogrel irreversibly inhibits platelet aggregation which persists for the life of the platelet (7-10 days) and until new platelets are released. Clopidogrel should **not** be discontinued in patients with cardiac stents that have not completed their full course of dual antiplatelet therapy (eg, aspirin and clopidogrel [prasugrel or ticagrelor]); patient-specific situations need to be discussed with cardiologist. If normal platelet

function is desired, clopidogrel should be discontinued for at least 5 days. A medical consult is recommended to determine the benefit:risk of continuing or discontinuing clopidogrel therapy for invasive dental procedures.

Adverse Effects As with all drugs which may affect hemostasis, bleeding is associated with clopidogrel. Hemorrhage may occur at virtually any site. Risk is dependent on multiple variables, including the concurrent use of multiple agents which alter hemostasis and patient susceptibility.

3% to 10%:
Dermatologic: Rash (4%), pruritus (3%)
Hematologic: Bleeding (major 4%; minor 5%), purpura/ bruising (5%), epistaxis (3%)
1% to 3%:
Gastrointestinal: GI hemorrhage (2%)
Hematologic: Hematoma

Dosage Oral: Adults:

Recent MI, recent stroke, or established peripheral arterial disease (PAD): 75 mg once daily. **Note:** The ACCF/AHA guidelines for PAD recommend clopidogrel as an alternative to aspirin (Class Ib recommendation) or in conjunction with aspirin for those who are not at an increased risk of bleeding but are of high cardiovascular risk (Class IIb recommendation). These recommendations also pertain to those with intermittent claudication or critical limb ischemia, prior lower extremity revascularization, or prior amputation for lower extremity ischemia (Rooke, 2011).

Coronary artery disease (CAD), established: 75 mg once daily. **Note:** Established CAD defined as patients 1-year post ACS, with prior revascularization, coronary stenosis >50% by angiogram, and/or evidence for cardiac ischemia on diagnostic testing (includes patients after the first year post-ACS and/or with prior CABG surgery) (Guyatt, 2012).

Secondary prevention of cardioembolic stroke (patient not candidate for oral anticoagulation): 75 mg once daily (in combination with aspirin) (Guyatt, 2012)

Acute coronary syndrome (ACS):
Unstable angina, non-ST-segment elevation myocardial infarction (UA/NSTEMI): Initial: 300 mg loading dose, followed by 75 mg once daily for up to 12 months (in combination with aspirin indefinitely) (Jneid, 2012). The American College of Chest Physicians recommends combination aspirin dose of 75-100 mg (Guyatt, 2012).

ST-segment elevation myocardial infarction (STEMI): 75 mg once daily (in combination with aspirin 162-325 mg initially followed by 81-162 mg/day **or** 75-100 mg/day [Guyatt, 2012]). **Note:** CLARITY-TIMI 28 used a 300 mg loading dose (with thrombolysis) demonstrating an improvement in patency rate of the infarct related artery and reduction in ischemic complications. The duration of therapy was <28 days (usually until hospital discharge) unless nonprimary percutaneous coronary intervention (PCI) was performed (Sabatine, 2005).

Percutaneous coronary intervention (PCI) for acute coronary syndrome (eg, UA/NSTEMI or STEMI): Loading dose: 600 mg given as early as possible before or at the time of PCI, followed by 75 mg once daily (in combination with aspirin 81 mg/day). **Note:** If fibrinolytic administered within the previous 24 hours, administer 300 mg loading dose instead (Levine, 2011). The use of ticagrelor (instead of clopidogrel) in combination with aspirin has been suggested (Guyatt, 2012).

Higher versus standard maintenance dosing: May consider a maintenance dose of 150 mg once daily for 6 days, then 75 mg once daily thereafter in patients not at high risk for bleeding (CURRENT-OASIS 7 Investigators, 2010; Jneid, 2012); however, in another study, in patients with high on-treatment platelet reactivity, the use of 150 mg once daily for 6 months did not demonstrate a difference in 6-month incidence of death from cardiovascular causes, nonfatal MI, or stent thrombosis compared to standard dose therapy (Price, 2011).

Duration of clopidogrel (in combination with aspirin) after stent placement for ACS and non-ACS indications: **Premature interruption of therapy may result in stent thrombosis with subsequent fatal and nonfatal MI.** At least 12 months of clopidogrel is recommended for those with ACS receiving either stent type (bare metal [BMS] or drug eluting stent [DES]) or those receiving a DES for a non-ACS indication. Those receiving a BMS for a non-ACS indication (ie, elective PCI) should be given at least 1 month and ideally up to 12 months; if patient is at increased risk of bleeding, give for a minimum of 2 weeks. A duration >12 months, regardless of indication, may be considered in patients with DES placement (Jneid, 2012; Levine, 2011).

CYP2C19 poor metabolizers (ie, *CYP2C19*2* or *3 carriers): Although routine genetic testing is not recommended in patients treated with clopidogrel undergoing PCI, testing may be considered to identify poor metabolizers who would be at risk for poor outcomes while receiving clopidogrel; if identified, these patients may be considered for an alternative P2Y$_{12}$ inhibitor (Levine, 2011). An appropriate regimen for this patient population has not been established in clinical outcome trials. Although the manufacturer suggests a 600 mg loading dose, followed by 150 mg once daily, it does not appear that this dosing strategy improves outcomes for this patient population (Price, 2011).

Atrial fibrillation (in patients not candidates for warfarin and at a low risk of bleeding) (Canadian labeling; ACTIVE Investigators, 2009; unlabeled use in U.S.): 75 mg once daily (in combination with aspirin 75-100 mg once daily). **Note:** Combination may also be used as an alternative for patients with atrial fibrillation and mitral stenosis (Guyatt, 2012).

Carotid artery stenosis, symptomatic (including recent carotid endarterectomy) (unlabeled use): 75 mg once daily (Guyatt, 2012)

Peripheral artery percutaneous transluminal angioplasty (with or without stenting) or peripheral artery bypass graft surgery, postprocedure (unlabeled use): 75 mg once daily. **Note:** For below-knee bypass graft surgery with prosthetic grafts, combine with aspirin 75-100 mg/day (Guyatt, 2012).

Prevention of coronary artery bypass graft closure (saphenous vein) and postoperative adverse cardiovascular events (unlabeled use): Aspirin-allergic patients: 75 mg once daily (Hillis, 2011)

Dosing adjustment in renal impairment and elderly: None necessary

Dosing adjustment in hepatic impairment: Use with caution; experience is limited. **Note:** Inhibition of ADP-induced platelet aggregation and mean bleeding time prolongation were similar in patients with severe hepatic impairment compared to healthy subjects after repeated doses of 75 mg once daily for 10 days.

Mechanism of Action Clopidogrel requires *in vivo* biotransformation to an active thiol metabolite. The active metabolite irreversibly blocks the P2Y$_{12}$ component of ADP receptors on the platelet surface, which prevents activation of the GPIIb/IIIa receptor complex, thereby reducing platelet aggregation. Platelets blocked by clopidogrel are affected for the remainder of their lifespan (~7-10 days).

Contraindications Hypersensitivity to clopidogrel or any component of the formulation; active pathological bleeding such as peptic ulcer or intracranial hemorrhage

Canadian labeling: Additional contraindications (not in U.S. labeling): Significant liver impairment or cholestatic jaundice

Warnings/Precautions [U.S. Boxed Warning]: Patients with one or more copies of the variant *CYP2C19*2* and/or *CYP2C19*3* alleles (and potentially other reduced-function variants) may have reduced conversion of clopidogrel to its active thiol metabolite. Lower active metabolite exposure may result in reduced platelet inhibition and, thus, a higher rate of cardiovascular events following MI or stent thrombosis following PCI. Although evidence is insufficient to recommend routine genetic testing, tests are available to determine CYP2C19 genotype and may be used to determine therapeutic strategy; alternative treatment or treatment strategies may be considered if patient is identified as a CYP2C19 poor metabolizer. Genetic testing may be considered prior to initiating clopidogrel in patients at moderate or high risk for poor outcomes (eg, PCI in patients with extensive and/or very complex disease). The optimal dose for CYP2C19 poor metabolizers has yet to be determined. After initiation of clopidogrel, functional testing (eg, VerifyNow® P2Y12 assay) may also be done to determine clopidogrel responsiveness (Holmes, 2010).

Use with caution in patients who may be at risk of increased bleeding, including patients with PUD, trauma, or surgery. In patients with coronary stents, premature interruption of therapy may result in stent thrombosis with subsequent fatal and nonfatal MI. Duration of therapy, in general, is determined by the type of stent placed (bare metal or drug eluting) and whether an ACS event was ongoing at the time of placement. Consider discontinuing 5 days before elective surgery (except in patients with cardiac stents that have not completed their full course of dual antiplatelet therapy; patient-specific situations need to be discussed with cardiologist; AHA/ACC/SCAI/ACS/ADA Science Advisory provides recommendations). Discontinue at least 5 days before elective CABG; when urgent CABG is necessary, the ACCF/AHA CABG guidelines recommend discontinuation for at least 24 hours prior to surgery (Hillis, 2011).

Because of structural similarities, cross-reactivity is possible among the thienopyridines (clopidogrel, prasugrel, and ticlopidine); use with caution or avoid in patients with previous thienopyridine hypersensitivity. Use of clopidogrel is contraindicated in patients with hypersensitivity to clopidogrel, although desensitization may be considered for mild-to-moderate hypersensitivity.

Use caution in concurrent treatment with anticoagulants (eg, heparin, warfarin) or other antiplatelet drugs; bleeding risk is increased. Concurrent use with drugs known to inhibit CYP2C19 (eg, proton pump inhibitors) may reduce levels of active metabolite and subsequently reduce clinical efficacy and increase the risk of ▶

◀ cardiovascular events; if possible, avoid concurrent use of moderate-to-strong CYP2C19 inhibitors. In patients requiring antacid therapy, consider use of an acid-reducing agent lacking (eg, ranitidine/famotidine) or with less CYP2C19 inhibition. According to the manufacturer, avoid concurrent use of omeprazole (even when scheduled 12 hours apart) or esomeprazole; if a PPI is necessary, the use of an agent with comparatively less effect on the antiplatelet activity of clopidogrel is recommended. Of the PPIs, pantoprazole has the lowest degree of CYP2C19 inhibition *in vitro* (Li, 2004) and has been shown to have has less effect on conversion of clopidogrel to its active metabolite compared to omeprazole (Angiolillo, 2011). Although lansoprazole exhibits the most potent CYP2C19 inhibition *in vitro* (Li, 2004; Ogilvie, 2012), an *in vivo* study of extensive CYP2C19 metabolizers showed less reduction of the active metabolite of clopidogrel by lansoprazole/dexlansoprazole compared to esomeprazole/omeprazole (Frelinger, 2012). Avoidance of rabeprazole appears prudent due to potent *in vitro* CYP2C19 inhibition and lack of sufficient comparative *in vivo* studies with other PPIs. In contrast to these warnings, others have recommended the continued use of PPIs, regardless of the degree of inhibition, in patients with multiple risk factors for GI bleeding who are also receiving clopidogrel since no evidence has established clinically meaningful differences in outcome; however, a clinically-significant interaction cannot be excluded in those who are poor metabolizers of clopidogrel. Staggering PPIs with clopidogrel is not recommended until further evidence is available (Abraham, 2010). Concurrent use of aspirin and clopidogrel is not recommended for secondary prevention of ischemic stroke or TIA in patients unable to take oral anticoagulants due to hemorrhagic risk (Furie, 2011).

Use with caution in patients with severe liver or renal disease (experience is limited). Cases of TTP (usually occurring within the first 2 weeks of therapy), resulting in some fatalities, have been reported; urgent plasmapheresis is required. Use in patients with severe hepatic impairment or cholestatic jaundice is contraindicated in the Canadian labeling. Cases of TTP (usually occurring within the first 2 weeks of therapy), resulting in some fatalities, have been reported; urgent plasmapheresis is required. In patients with recent lacunar stroke (within 180 days), the use of clopidogrel in addition to aspirin did not significantly reduce the incidence of the primary outcome of stroke recurrence (any ischemic stroke or intracranial hemorrhage) compared to aspirin alone; the use of clopidogrel in addition to aspirin did however increase the risk of major hemorrhage and the rate of all-cause mortality (SPS3 Investigators, 2012).

Assess bleeding risk carefully prior to initiating therapy in patients with atrial fibrillation (Canadian labeling; not an approved use in U.S. labeling); in clinical trials, a significant increase in major bleeding events (including intracranial hemorrhage and fatal bleeding events) were observed in patients receiving clopidogrel plus aspirin versus aspirin alone. Vitamin K antagonist (VKA) therapy (in suitable patients) has demonstrated a greater benefit in stroke reduction than aspirin (with or without clopidogrel).

Drug Interactions

Metabolism/Transport Effects **Substrate** of CYP2C19 (major), CYP3A4 (minor); **Note:** Assignment of Major/Minor substrate status based on clinically relevant drug interaction potential; **Inhibits** CYP2B6 (moderate), CYP2C9 (weak)

Avoid Concomitant Use
Avoid concomitant use of Clopidogrel with any of the following: CYP2C19 Inhibitors (Moderate); CYP2C19 Inhibitors (Strong); Esomeprazole; Omeprazole

Increased Effect/Toxicity
Clopidogrel may increase the levels/effects of: Agents with Antiplatelet Properties; Anticoagulants; Collagenase (Systemic); CYP2B6 Substrates; Dabigatran Etexilate; Drotrecogin Alfa (Activated); Ibritumomab; Rivaroxaban; Salicylates; Thrombolytic Agents; Tositumomab and Iodine I 131 Tositumomab; Warfarin

The levels/effects of Clopidogrel may be increased by: Dasatinib; Glucosamine; Herbs (Anticoagulant/Antiplatelet Properties); Multivitamins/Minerals (with ADEK, Folate, Iron); Nonsteroidal Anti-Inflammatory Agents; Omega-3 Fatty Acids; Pentosan Polysulfate Sodium; Pentoxifylline; Prostacyclin Analogues; Rifamycin Derivatives; Tipranavir; Vitamin E

Decreased Effect
The levels/effects of Clopidogrel may be decreased by: Amiodarone; Calcium Channel Blockers; CYP2C19 Inhibitors (Moderate); CYP2C19 Inhibitors (Strong); Dexlansoprazole; Esomeprazole; Lansoprazole; Macrolide Antibiotics; Nonsteroidal Anti-Inflammatory Agents; Omeprazole; Pantoprazole; RABEprazole

Ethanol/Nutrition/Herb Interactions Herb/Nutraceutical: Avoid alfalfa, anise, bilberry, bladderwrack, bromelain, cat's claw, chamomile, coleus, cordyceps, dong quai, evening primrose oil, fenugreek, feverfew, garlic, ginger, ginkgo biloba, ginseng (American), ginseng (Panax), ginseng (Siberian), grape seed, green tea, guggul, horse chestnut seed, horseradish, licorice, prickly ash, red clover, reishi, SAMe (S-adenosylmethionine), sweet clover, turmeric, white willow (all have additional antiplatelet activity).

Dietary Considerations May be taken without regard to meals.

Pharmacodynamics/Kinetics

Onset of Action
Onset of action: Inhibition of platelet aggregation (IPA): Dose-dependent:
  300-600 mg loading dose: Detected within 2 hours
  50-100 mg/day: Detected by the second day of treatment
Peak effect: Time to maximal IPA: Dose-dependent:
  Note: Degree of IPA based on adenosine diphosphate (ADP) concentration used during light aggregometry:
  300-600 mg loading dose:
    ADP 5 micromole/L: 20% to 30% IPA at 6 hours post administration (Montelescot, 2006)
    ADP 20 micromole/L: 30% to 37% IPA at 6 hours post administration (Montelescot, 2006)
  50-100 mg/day: ADP 5 micromole/L: 50% to 60% IPA at 5-7 days (Herbert, 1993)

Half-life Elimination Parent drug: ~6 hours; Active metabolite: ~30 minutes

Time to Peak Serum: ~0.75 hours

Pregnancy Risk Factor B

Pregnancy Considerations Teratogenic effects were not observed in animal studies. Use during pregnancy only if clearly needed.

Lactation Excretion in breast milk unknown/not recommended

Dosage Forms

Tablet, oral: 75 mg, 300 mg
Plavix®: 75 mg, 300 mg

Dental Comment There is no scientific evidence to warrant the discontinuance of clopidogrel prior to dental surgery. Patients taking one clopidogrel tablet daily as an antithrombotic and who require dental surgery should be given special consideration in consultation with physician.

References

Grines CL, Bonow RO, Casey DE, et al, "AHA/ACC/SCAI/ACS/ADA Science Advisory, Prevention of Premature Discontinuation of Dual Antiplatelet Therapy in Patients With Coronary Artery Stents. A Science Advisory From the American Heart Association, American College of Cardiology, Society of Cardiovascular Angiography and Interventions, American College of Surgeons, and American Dental Association With Representation From The Amercian College Of Physicians," Circulation, 2007, 115(6):813-8. Available at http://www.acc.org/qualityandscience/clinical/pdfs/Final_Dual_Antiplatelet_Statement_010507.pdf.
Jeske AH, Suchko GD, ADA Council on Scientific Affairs and Division of Science, et al, "Lack of a Scientific Basis for Routine Discontinuation of Oral Anticoagulation Therapy Before Dental Treatment," J Am Dent Assoc, 2003, 134(11):1492-7.
Wynn RL, "Clopidogrel (Plavix): Dental Considerations of an Antiplatelet Drug," Gen Dent, 2001, 49(6):564-8.

Clorazepate (klor AZ e pate)

Brand Names: U.S. Tranxene® T-Tab®
Brand Names: Canada Apo-Clorazepate®; Novo-Clopate
Pharmacologic Category Benzodiazepine
Use Treatment of generalized anxiety disorder; management of ethanol withdrawal; adjunct anticonvulsant in management of partial seizures
Local Anesthetic/Vasoconstrictor Precautions No information available to require special precautions
Effects on Dental Treatment Key adverse event(s) related to dental treatment: Xerostomia (normal salivary flow resumes upon discontinuation). Many patients will experience drowsiness; orthostatic hypotension is possible. It is suggested that opioid analgesics not be given for pain control to patients taking clorazepate due to enhanced sedation.
Effects on Bleeding No information available to require special precautions
Adverse Effects Frequency not defined.
Cardiovascular: Hypotension
Central nervous system: Drowsiness, fatigue, ataxia, lightheadedness, memory impairment, insomnia, anxiety, headache, depression, slurred speech, confusion, nervousness, dizziness, irritability
Dermatologic: Rash
Endocrine & metabolic: Libido decreased
Gastrointestinal: Xerostomia, constipation, diarrhea, nausea, salivation decreased, vomiting, appetite increased or decreased
Hepatic: Jaundice, transaminase increased
Neuromuscular & skeletal: Dysarthria, tremor
Ocular: Blurred vision, diplopia
General Dosage Range Oral:
Children 9-12 years: Initial: 3.75-7.5 mg twice daily; Maintenance: Up to 60 mg/day in 2-3 divided doses
Children >12 years: Initial: Up to 7.5 mg 2-3 times/day; Maintenance: Up to 90 mg/day
Adults: Initial: 7.5-15 mg 2-4 times/day; Maintenance: Up to 90 mg/day
Elderly: Anxiety: 7.5 mg 1-2 times/day
Mechanism of Action Binds to stereospecific benzodiazepine receptors on the postsynaptic GABA neuron at several sites within the central nervous system, including the limbic system, reticular formation. Enhancement of the inhibitory effect of GABA on neuronal excitability results by increased neuronal membrane permeability to chloride ions. This shift in chloride ions results in hyperpolarization (a less excitable state) and stabilization.
Pharmacodynamics/Kinetics
Onset of Action 1-2 hours
Duration of Action Variable, 8-24 hours
Half-life Elimination Adults: Nordiazepam: 40-50 hours; Oxazepam: 6-8 hours
Time to Peak Serum: ~1 hour
Pregnancy Considerations Nordiazepam, the active metabolite of clorazepate, crosses the placenta and is measurable in cord blood and amniotic fluid. Teratogenic effects have been observed with some benzodiazepines (including clorazepate); however, additional studies are needed. The incidence of premature birth and low birth weights may be increased following maternal use of benzodiazepines; hypoglycemia and respiratory problems in the neonate may occur following exposure late in pregnancy. Neonatal withdrawal symptoms may occur within days to weeks after birth and "floppy infant syndrome" (which also includes withdrawal symptoms) has been reported with some benzodiazepines.

Patients exposed to clorazepate during pregnancy are encouraged to enroll themselves into the AED Pregnancy Registry by calling 1-888-233-2334. Additional information is available at www.aedpregnancyregistry.org.
Controlled Substance C-IV

Clotrimazole (Oral) (kloe TRIM a zole)

Related Information
Fungal Infections on page 1573
Related Sample Prescriptions
Fungal Infections Requiring Topical Therapy on page 1614
Generic Availability (U.S.) Yes
Pharmacologic Category Antifungal Agent, Oral Nonabsorbed
Dental Use Treatment of susceptible fungal infections, including oropharyngeal candidiasis; limited data suggest that clotrimazole troches may be effective for prophylaxis against oropharyngeal candidiasis in neutropenic patients
Use Treatment of susceptible fungal infections, including oropharyngeal candidiasis; limited data suggest that clotrimazole troches may be effective for prophylaxis against oropharyngeal candidiasis in neutropenic patients
Local Anesthetic/Vasoconstrictor Precautions No information available to require special precautions
Effects on Dental Treatment No significant effects or complications reported
Effects on Bleeding No information available to require special precautions
Adverse Effects
>10%: Hepatic: Abnormal liver function tests
Frequency not defined:
Dermatologic: Pruritus
Gastrointestinal: Nausea, vomiting
Dental Usual Dosage Oropharyngeal candidiasis: Children >3 years and Adults: Oral:
Prophylaxis: 10 mg troche dissolved 3 times/day for the duration of chemotherapy or until steroids are reduced to maintenance levels
Treatment: 10 mg troche dissolved slowly 5 times/day for 14 consecutive days

▶

◀ **Dosage** Oral: Children >3 years and Adults:
Prophylaxis: 10 mg troche dissolved 3 times/day for the duration of chemotherapy or until steroids are reduced to maintenance levels
Treatment: 10 mg troche dissolved slowly 5 times/day for 14 consecutive days

Mechanism of Action Binds to phospholipids in the fungal cell membrane altering cell wall permeability resulting in loss of essential intracellular elements

Contraindications Hypersensitivity to clotrimazole or any component of the formulation

Warnings/Precautions Clotrimazole should not be used for treatment of systemic fungal infection. Safety and effectiveness of clotrimazole lozenges (troches) in children <3 years of age have not been established.

Drug Interactions
Metabolism/Transport Effects Inhibits CYP1A2 (weak), CYP2A6 (weak), CYP2B6 (weak), CYP2C19 (weak), CYP2C8 (weak), CYP2C9 (weak), CYP2D6 (weak), CYP2E1 (weak), CYP3A4 (moderate)

Avoid Concomitant Use
Avoid concomitant use of Clotrimazole (Oral) with any of the following: Bosutinib; Ivabradine; Lomitapide; Pimozide; Tolvaptan

Increased Effect/Toxicity
Clotrimazole (Oral) may increase the levels/effects of: ARIPiprazole; Avanafil; Bosutinib; Budesonide (Systemic, Oral Inhalation); Colchicine; CYP3A4 Substrates; Eplerenone; Everolimus; FentaNYL; Halofantrine; Ivabradine; Ivacaftor; Lomitapide; Lurasidone; Pimecrolimus; Pimozide; Propafenone; Ranolazine; Salmeterol; Saxagliptin; Tacrolimus (Systemic); Tolvaptan; Vilazodone; Zuclopenthixol

Decreased Effect
Clotrimazole (Oral) may decrease the levels/effects of: Ifosfamide; Saccharomyces boulardii

Pregnancy Risk Factor C

Pregnancy Considerations In animal reproduction studies, adverse events were observed with oral administration of clotrimazole.

Lactation Excretion in breast milk unknown

Dosage Forms
Troche, oral: 10 mg

Clotrimazole (Topical) (kloe TRIM a zole)

Brand Names: U.S. Anti-Fungal™ [OTC]; Cruex® [OTC]; Gyne-Lotrimin® 3 [OTC]; Gyne-Lotrimin® 7 [OTC]; Lotrimin® AF Athlete's Foot [OTC]; Lotrimin® AF for Her [OTC]; Lotrimin® AF Jock Itch [OTC]

Brand Names: Canada Canesten® Topical; Canesten® Vaginal; Clotrimaderm; Trivagizole-3®

Generic Availability (U.S.) Yes

Pharmacologic Category Antifungal Agent, Topical; Antifungal Agent, Vaginal

Use Treatment of susceptible fungal infections, including dermatophytoses, superficial mycoses, and cutaneous candidiasis, as well as vulvovaginal candidiasis

Local Anesthetic/Vasoconstrictor Precautions No information available to require special precautions

Effects on Dental Treatment No significant effects or complications reported

Effects on Bleeding No information available to require special precautions

Adverse Effects Vaginal: 1% to 10%: Genitourinary: Vulvar/vaginal burning

Dental Usual Dosage Cutaneous candidiasis: Children >3 years and Adults: Topical (cream, solution): Apply twice daily; if no improvement occurs after 4 weeks of therapy, re-evaluate diagnosis.

Dosage
Children >3 years and Adults: Topical (cream, solution): Apply twice daily; if no improvement occurs after 4 weeks of therapy, re-evaluate diagnosis
Children >12 years and Adults:
Vaginal: Cream:
1%: Insert 1 applicatorful vaginal cream daily (preferably at bedtime) for 7 consecutive days
2%: Insert 1 applicatorful vaginal cream daily (preferably at bedtime) for 3 consecutive days
Topical (cream, solution): Apply to affected area twice daily (morning and evening) for 7 consecutive days

Mechanism of Action Binds to phospholipids in the fungal cell membrane altering cell wall permeability resulting in loss of essential intracellular elements

Contraindications Hypersensitivity to clotrimazole or any component of the formulation

Warnings/Precautions Avoid contact with eyes.

Drug Interactions
Metabolism/Transport Effects None known.
Avoid Concomitant Use There are no known interactions where it is recommended to avoid concomitant use.
Increased Effect/Toxicity There are no known significant interactions involving an increase in effect.
Decreased Effect There are no known significant interactions involving a decrease in effect.

Pharmacodynamics/Kinetics
Time to Peak Serum: Vaginal cream: ~24 hours

Pregnancy Risk Factor B

Pregnancy Considerations In animal reproduction studies, adverse events were not observed with vaginal administration of clotrimazole. Following topical and vaginal administration, clotrimazole is poorly absorbed systemically. Adverse events have not been reported following vaginal use during the second and third trimesters of pregnancy.

Lactation Excretion in breast milk unknown/use caution

Breast-Feeding Considerations Following topical and vaginal administration, clotrimazole is poorly absorbed systemically.

Dosage Forms
Cream, topical: 1% (15 g, 30 g, 45 g)
Anti-Fungal™ [OTC]: 1% (113 g)
Cruex® [OTC]: 1% (15 g)
Lotrimin® AF Athlete's Foot [OTC]: 1% (12 g)
Lotrimin® AF for Her [OTC]: 1% (24 g)
Lotrimin® AF Jock Itch [OTC]: 1% (12 g)
Cream, vaginal: 1% (45 g); 2% (21 g)
Gyne-Lotrimin® 7 [OTC]: 1% (45 g)
Gyne-Lotrimin® 3 [OTC]: 2% (21 g)
Solution, topical: 1% (10 mL, 30 mL)

Cloxacillin (kloks a SIL in)

Brand Names: Canada Apo-Cloxi®; Novo-Cloxin; Nu-Cloxi

Pharmacologic Category Antibiotic, Penicillin

Dental Use Treatment of susceptible orofacial infections (notably penicillinase-producing staphylococci)

Use Treatment of bacterial infections including endocarditis, pneumonia, bone and joint infections, skin and soft-tissue infections, and sepsis that are caused by susceptible strains of penicillinase-producing staphylococci. **Note:** Exhibits good activity against

Staphylococcus aureus; has activity against many strep-tococci, but is less active than penicillin and is generally not used in clinical practice to treat streptococcal infections.

Local Anesthetic/Vasoconstrictor Precautions No information available to require special precautions

Effects on Dental Treatment Key adverse event(s) related to dental treatment: Prolonged use of penicillins may lead to development of oral candidiasis.

Effects on Bleeding No information available to require special precautions

Adverse Effects Frequency not defined.

Cardiovascular: Hypotension

Central nervous system: Confusion, fever, lethargy, seizure (high doses and/or renal failure)

Dermatologic: Pruritus, rash, urticaria

Gastrointestinal: Abdominal pain, black or hairy tongue, diarrhea, flatulence, nausea, oral candidiasis, pseudo-membranous colitis, stomatitis, vomiting

Hematologic: Agranulocytosis, bone marrow depression, eosinophilia, granulocytopenia, hemolytic anemia, leukopenia, neutropenia, thrombocytopenia

Hepatic: Alkaline phosphatase increased, ALT increased, AST increased, hepatotoxicity

Local: Thrombophlebitis

Neuromuscular & skeletal: Arthralgia, myalgia, myoclonus

Renal: Hematuria, interstitial nephritis, proteinuria, renal insufficiency, renal tubular damage

Respiratory: Bronchospasm, laryngeal edema, laryngo-spasm, sneezing, wheezing

Miscellaneous: Anaphylaxis, angioedema, allergic reaction, serum sickness-like reaction

Dental Usual Dosage Susceptible orofacial infections: Children >20 kg and Adults: Oral: 250-500 mg every 6 hours

Dosage Note: Dose and duration of therapy can vary depending on infecting organism, severity of infection, and clinical response of patient. Treat severe staphylococcal infections for at least 14 days; endocarditis and osteomyelitis require an extended duration of therapy for 4-6 weeks. The intravenous route should be used for severe infections.

Usual dosage range (manufacturer's labeling):
Oral:
Children ≤20 kg: 25-50 mg/kg/day in divided doses every 6 hours
Children >20 kg and Adults: 250-500 mg every 6 hours (maximum adult dose: 6 g/day)
I.M., I.V.:
Children ≤20 kg: 25-50 mg/kg/day in divided doses every 6 hours; up to 200 mg/kg/day has been used in some studies for severe infections (Nunn, 2007; St. John, 1981)
Children >20 kg and Adults: 250-500 mg every 6 hours (maximum adult dose: 6 g/day)

Indication-specific dosing: Dosing recommendations of World Health Organization unless otherwise noted:
Arthritis (septic), methicillin-sensitive *Staphylococcus aureus* (MSSA) (unlabeled dosing):
Children 2 months to 5 years: I.M., I.V.: 25-50 mg/kg (maximum: 2 g) every 4-6 hours given with ceftriaxone until clinical improvement, **followed by** oral therapy: 12.5 mg/kg (maximum: 500 mg) every 6 hours; total duration of therapy 2-3 weeks

Children >5 years: I.M., I.V.: 25-50 mg/kg (maximum: 2 g) every 4-6 hours (maximum daily dose: 12 g/day) until clinical improvement, **followed by** oral therapy: 25 mg/kg (maximum: 500 mg) every 6 hours; total duration of therapy 2-3 weeks

Adults: I.M., I.V.: 2 g every 6 hours for 2-3 weeks; **Note:** Oral therapy of 1 g every 6 hours may be used to complete therapy if parenteral therapy is discontinued prior to 2-3 week duration

Endocarditis (MSSA) (unlabeled dosing): I.V.:
Children: 50 mg/kg (maximum: 2 g) every 4 hours for 6 weeks; give with gentamicin for initial 7 days
Adults:
Native valve: 2 g every 4 hours for 6 weeks; may give with gentamicin for initial 5 days (Choudri, 2000)
Prosthetic valve: 2 g every 4 hours for 6 weeks; give with gentamicin for 2 weeks and rifampin for 6 weeks (Choudri, 2000)
Uncomplicated endocarditis in I.V. drug users: 2 g every 4 hours for 4 weeks and gentamicin for initial 5 days **or** 2 g every 4 hours and gentamicin both given for 2 weeks total (Choudri, 2000)

Osteomyelitis (MSSA) (unlabeled dosing):
Children 2 months to 5 years: I.M., I.V.: 25-50 mg/kg (maximum: 2 g) every 4-6 hours given with ceftriaxone until clinical improvement, **followed by** oral therapy: 12.5 mg/kg (maximum: 500 mg) every 6 hours; total duration of therapy 3-4 weeks
Children >5 years: I.M., I.V.: 25-50 mg/kg (maximum: 2 g) every 4-6 hours (maximum daily dose: 12 g/day) until clinical improvement, **followed by** oral therapy: 25 mg/kg (maximum: 500 mg) every 6 hours; total duration of therapy 3-4 weeks
Adults: I.M., I.V.: 2 g every 6 hours for 4-6 weeks (preferred) **or** for a minimum of 14 days, **followed by** 1 g every 6 hours orally to complete 4-6 weeks of therapy

Pneumonia (MSSA) (unlabeled dosing):
Children 2 months to 5 years: Oral: 25-50 mg/kg (maximum: 2 g) every 6 hours for at least 3 weeks with gentamicin
Children >5 years: I.M., I.V.: 50 mg/kg (maximum: 2 g) every 6 hours for 10-14 days
Adults: I.M., I.V.: 1-2 g every 6 hours for 10-14 days

Dosage adjustment in renal impairment: No dosage adjustment necessary.

Dosage adjustment in hepatic impairment: No dosage adjustment provided in manufacturer's labeling.

Mechanism of Action Inhibits bacterial cell wall synthesis by binding to one or more of the penicillin-binding proteins (PBPs) which in turn inhibit the final transpeptidation step of peptidoglycan synthesis in bacterial cell walls, thus inhibiting cell wall biosynthesis. Bacteria eventually lyse due to ongoing activity of cell wall autolytic enzymes (autolysins and murein hydrolases) while cell wall assembly is arrested.

Contraindications Hypersensitivity to cloxacillin, other penicillins, cephalosporins, or any component of the formulation

Warnings/Precautions Serious and occasionally severe or fatal hypersensitivity (anaphylactoid) reactions have been reported in patients on penicillin therapy, especially with a history of beta-lactam hypersensitivity, history of sensitivity to multiple allergens, or previous IgE-mediated reactions (eg, anaphylaxis, angioedema, urticaria). Use with caution in renal impairment as the rate of elimination is decreased. Use with caution in asthmatic patients. Prolonged use may result in fungal or bacterial superinfection, including *C. difficile*-associated diarrhea (CDAD) and pseudomembranous colitis;

CDAD has been observed >2 months postantibiotic treatment. Use with caution in patients with a history of seizure disorders, particularly in the presence of renal impairment as increased serum levels may increase risk for seizures. Penicillin transport across the blood-brain barrier may be enhanced by inflamed meninges or during cardiopulmonary bypass increasing the risk of myoclonia, seizures, or reduced consciousness especially in patients with renal failure. Penicillin use has been associated with hematologic disorders (eg, agranulocytosis, neutropenia, thrombocytopenia) believed to be a hypersensitivity phenomena. Reactions are most often reversible upon discontinuing therapy. Renal clearance may be reduced in neonates; more frequent evaluation of clinical status and serum levels as well as more frequent dosage adjustments may be necessary with this patient population.

Drug Interactions

Metabolism/Transport Effects None known.

Avoid Concomitant Use

Avoid concomitant use of Cloxacillin with any of the following: BCG

Increased Effect/Toxicity

Cloxacillin may increase the levels/effects of: Methotrexate; Vitamin K Antagonists

The levels/effects of Cloxacillin may be increased by: Probenecid

Decreased Effect

Cloxacillin may decrease the levels/effects of: BCG; Mycophenolate; Sodium Picosulfate; Typhoid Vaccine; Vitamin K Antagonists

The levels/effects of Cloxacillin may be decreased by: Fusidic Acid; Tetracycline Derivatives

Ethanol/Nutrition/Herb Interactions Food: Food decreases cloxacillin absorption; serum levels are reduced by ~50%. Management: Administer with water on an empty stomach 1 hour before or 2 hours after meals.

Dietary Considerations Should be taken 1 hour before or 2 hours after meals with water.

Pharmacodynamics/Kinetics

Half-life Elimination 0.5-1.5 hours; prolonged with renal impairment and in neonates

Time to Peak Serum: ~1 hour

Pregnancy Considerations Cloxacillin crosses the placenta and distributes into fetal tissue. In general, penicillins as a class are considered safe for use during pregnancy.

Lactation Enters breast milk/use caution

Product Availability Not available in U.S.

Dosage Forms: Canada

Capsule, oral: 250 mg, 500 mg

Injection, powder for reconstitution: 250 mg, 500 mg, 1000 mg, 2000 mg

Powder for suspension, oral: 125 mg/5 mL

CloZAPine (KLOE za peen)

Brand Names: U.S. Clozaril®; FazaClo®

Brand Names: Canada Apo-Clozapine®; Clozaril®; Gen-Clozapine

Pharmacologic Category Antipsychotic Agent, Atypical

Use Treatment-refractory schizophrenia; to reduce risk of recurrent suicidal behavior in schizophrenia or schizoaffective disorder

Unlabeled Use Schizoaffective disorder, bipolar disorder, childhood psychosis, severe obsessive-compulsive disorder; psychosis/agitation related to Alzheimer's dementia

Local Anesthetic/Vasoconstrictor Precautions Most pharmacology textbooks state that in presence of phenothiazines, systemic doses of epinephrine paradoxically decrease the blood pressure. This is the so called "epinephrine reversal" phenomenon. This has never been observed when epinephrine is given by infiltration as part of the local anesthesia procedure.

Effects on Dental Treatment Key adverse event(s) related to dental treatment: Sialorrhea and xerostomia (normal salivary flow resumes upon discontinuation). Many patients may experience orthostatic hypotension with clozapine; precautions should be taken; do not use atropine-like drugs for xerostomia in patients taking clozapine due to significant potentiation.

Effects on Bleeding No information available to require special precautions

Adverse Effects

>10%:

Cardiovascular: Tachycardia (25%)

Central nervous system: Drowsiness (39% to 46%), dizziness (19% to 27%), insomnia (2% to 20%)

Gastrointestinal: Sialorrhea (31% to 48%), weight gain (4% to 31%), constipation (14% to 25%), nausea/vomiting (3% to 17%), abdominal discomfort/heartburn (4% to 14%)

1% to 10%:

Cardiovascular: Hypotension (9%), syncope (6%), hypertension (4%), angina (1%), ECG changes (1%)

Central nervous system: Headache (7%), agitation (4%), akinesia (4%), nightmares (4%), restlessness (4%), akathisia (3%), confusion (3%), seizure (3%), fatigue (2%), anxiety (1%), ataxia (1%), depression (1%), lethargy (1%), myoclonic jerks (1%), slurred speech (1%)

Dermatologic: Rash (2%)

Gastrointestinal: Xerostomia (6%), diarrhea (2%), anorexia (1%), throat discomfort (1%)

Genitourinary: Urinary abnormalities (eg, abnormal ejaculation, retention, urgency, incontinence; 1% to 2%)

Hematologic: Leukopenia (3%), agranulocytosis (1%), eosinophilia (1%)

Hepatic: Liver function tests abnormal (1%)

Neuromuscular & skeletal: Tremor (6%), hypokinesia (4%), rigidity (3%), hyperkinesia (1%), weakness (1%), pain (1%), spasm (1%)

Ocular: Visual disturbances (5%)

Respiratory: Dyspnea (1%), nasal congestion (1%)

Miscellaneous: Diaphoresis (6%), tongue numbness (1%)

General Dosage Range Dosage adjustment recommended in patients who develop toxicities

Oral: *Adults:* Initial: 12.5 mg once or twice daily; Maintenance: 12.5-900 mg/day (maximum: 900 mg/day)

Mechanism of Action Clozapine (dibenzodiazepine antipsychotic) exhibits weak antagonism of D_1, D_2, D_3, and D_5 dopamine receptor subtypes, but shows high affinity for D_4; in addition, it blocks the serotonin ($5\text{-}HT_2$), alpha-adrenergic, histamine H_1, and cholinergic receptors

Pharmacodynamics/Kinetics

Half-life Elimination Steady state: 12 hours (range: 4-66 hours)

Time to Peak 2.5 hours (range: 1-6 hours)

Pregnancy Risk Factor B

Pregnancy Considerations Teratogenic effects were not seen in animal studies. Clozapine crosses the placenta and can be detected in the fetal blood and amniotic fluid (Barnas, 1994). Antipsychotic use during the third trimester of pregnancy has a risk for abnormal muscle movements (extrapyramidal symptoms [EPS]) and withdrawal symptoms in newborns following delivery. Symptoms in the newborn may include agitation, feeding disorder, hypertonia, hypotonia, respiratory distress, somnolence, and tremor; these effects may be self-limiting or require hospitalization. Healthcare providers are encouraged to enroll women 18-45 years of age exposed to clozapine during pregnancy in the Atypical Antipsychotics Pregnancy Registry (1-866-961-2388 or http://www.womensmentalhealth. org/pregnancyregistry). Women with amenorrhea associated with use of other antipsychotic agents may return to normal menstruation when switching to clozapine therapy. Reliable contraceptive measures should be employed by women of childbearing potential switching to clozapine therapy.

Product Availability Versacloz™ oral suspension: FDA approved February 2013; anticipated availability currently unknown. Consult prescribing information for additional information.

Prescribing and Access Restrictions

U.S.: Clozaril® is deemed to have a REMS program (approval pending from FDA). As a requirement of the REMS program, access to this medication is restricted. Patient-specific registration is required to dispense clozapine. Information specific to each monitoring program is available from the individual manufacturers. If a patient is switched from one brand/manufacturer of clozapine to another, the patient must be entered into a new registry (must be completed by the prescriber and delivered to the dispensing pharmacy). Healthcare providers, including pharmacists dispensing clozapine, should verify the patient's hematological status and qualification to receive clozapine with all existing registries. The manufacturer of Clozaril® requests that healthcare providers submit all WBC/ANC values following discontinuation of therapy to the Clozaril National Registry for all nonrechallengable patients until WBC is ≥3500/mm³ and ANC is ≥2000/mm³.

Canada: Currently, there are multiple manufacturers that distribute clozapine and each manufacturer has its own registry and distribution system. Patients must be registered in a database that includes their location, prescribing physician, testing laboratory, and dispensing pharmacist before using clozapine. Information specific to each monitoring program is available from the individual manufacturers.

Coal Tar (KOLE tar)

Brand Names: U.S. Balnetar® [OTC]; Betatar Gel® [OTC]; Cutar® [OTC]; Denorex® Therapeutic Protection 2-in-1 Shampoo + Conditioner [OTC]; Denorex® Therapeutic Protection [OTC]; DHS® Tar [OTC]; DHS™ Tar Gel [OTC]; Exorex® Penetrating Emulsion #2 [OTC]; Exorex® Penetrating Emulsion [OTC]; ionil-T® Plus [OTC]; ionil-T® [OTC]; MG217® Medicated Tar Extra Strength [OTC]; MG217® Medicated Tar Intensive Strength [OTC]; MG217® Medicated Tar [OTC]; Neutrogena® T/Gel® Extra Strength [OTC]; Neutrogena® T/Gel® Stubborn Itch Control [OTC]; Neutrogena® T/Gel® [OTC]; Oxipor® VHC [OTC]; Pentrax® [OTC]; Scytera™ [OTC]; Tera-Gel™ [OTC]; Thera-Gel [OTC]; Zetar® [OTC]

Brand Names: Canada Doak Oil Forte [OTC]; Doak Oil [OTC]; Emorex Gel [OTC]; Neuotrogena T/Gel Therapeutic Shampoo [OTC]; Odans Liquor Carbonis Detergens [OTC]; Pentrax Gold Shampoo [OTC]; Pentrax Tar Shampoo [OTC]; Psoriasin [OTC]; T/Gel Therapeutic Shampoo Extra Strength [OTC]; Targel® [OTC]; Tersa Tar Shp [OTC]

Pharmacologic Category Topical Skin Product

Use Topically for controlling dandruff, seborrheic dermatitis, or psoriasis

Local Anesthetic/Vasoconstrictor Precautions No information available to require special precautions

Effects on Dental Treatment No significant effects or complications reported

Effects on Bleeding No information available to require special precautions

Adverse Effects Frequency not defined: Dermatologic: Dermatitis, folliculitis. irritation, photosensitivity

General Dosage Range Topical: *Adults:*
Bath: Add 60-90 mL (5-20%) or 15-25 mL (30%) to bath water, soak 5-20 minutes, use once daily to every 3 days
Scalp: Apply to lesions 3-12 hours before each shampoo
Shampoo: Rub into wet hair, rinse, repeat leaving on 5 minutes; apply twice weekly for 2 weeks then once weekly
Skin: Apply to affected areas 1-4 times/day, decrease to 2-3 times/week once condition controlled
Soap: Use on affected areas instead of regular soap

Pregnancy Considerations Limited application of coal tar during pregnancy for the treatment of psoriasis appears to be safe in pregnant women (Gelmetti, 2009; Landau, 2011).

Coal Tar and Salicylic Acid
(KOLE tar & sal i SIL ik AS id)

Related Information
Coal Tar *on page 343*
Salicylic Acid *on page 1219*

Brand Names: U.S. Tarsum® [OTC]; X-Seb T® Pearl [OTC]; X-Seb T® Plus [OTC]

Brand Names: Canada Sebcur/T®

Pharmacologic Category Topical Skin Product

Use Relief of symptoms of seborrheal dermatitis, dandruff, and psoriasis

Local Anesthetic/Vasoconstrictor Precautions No information available to require special precautions

Effects on Dental Treatment No significant effects or complications reported

Effects on Bleeding No information available to require special precautions

General Dosage Range Topical:
Gel: *Adults:* Apply to plaques, leave on up to 1 hour then rinse
Shampoo: *Adults:* Apply to wet hair, massage into scalp then rinse

Pregnancy Considerations The amount of coal tar and salicylic acid available systemically following topical application is unknown.

Cocaine (koe KANE)

Related Information
Management of the Chemically Dependent Patient *on page 1550*
Pharmacologic Category Local Anesthetic

Use Topical anesthesia (and vasoconstriction) for mucous membranes

Local Anesthetic/Vasoconstrictor Precautions Although plain local anesthetic is not contraindicated, vasoconstrictor is absolutely contraindicated in any patient under the influence of or within 2 hours of cocaine use

Effects on Dental Treatment Key adverse event(s) related to dental treatment: Loss of taste perception. See Dental Comment.

Effects on Bleeding No information available to require special precautions

Adverse Effects
>10%:
Central nervous system: CNS stimulation
Gastrointestinal: Loss of taste perception
Respiratory: Rhinitis, nasal congestion
Miscellaneous: Loss of smell
1% to 10%:
Cardiovascular: Heart rate decreased with low doses, tachycardia with moderate doses, hypertension, cardiomyopathy, cardiac arrhythmia, myocarditis, QRS prolongation, Raynaud's phenomenon, cerebral vasculitis, thrombosis, fibrillation (atrial), flutter (atrial), sinus bradycardia, CHF, pulmonary hypertension, sinus tachycardia, tachycardia (supraventricular), arrhythmia (ventricular), vasoconstriction
Central nervous system: Fever, nervousness, restlessness, euphoria, excitation, headache, psychosis, hallucinations, agitation, seizure, slurred speech, hyperthermia, dystonic reactions, cerebral vascular accident, vasculitis, clonic-tonic reactions, paranoia, sympathetic storm
Dermatologic: Skin infarction, pruritus, madarosis
Gastrointestinal: Nausea, anorexia, colonic ischemia, spontaneous bowel perforation
Genitourinary: Priapism, uterine rupture
Hematologic: Thrombocytopenia
Neuromuscular & skeletal: Chorea (extrapyramidal), paresthesia, tremor, fasciculations
Ocular: Mydriasis (peak effect at 45 minutes; may last up to 12 hours), sloughing of the corneal epithelium, ulceration of the cornea, iritis, mydriasis, chemosis
Renal: Myoglobinuria, necrotizing vasculitis
Respiratory: Tachypnea, nasal mucosa damage (when snorting), hyposmia, bronchiolitis obliterans organizing pneumonia
Miscellaneous: "Washed-out" syndrome

General Dosage Range Topical: *Adults:* Maximum total dose: 3 mg/kg **or** 200 mg (1% to 10% concentration)

Mechanism of Action Ester local anesthetic blocks both the initiation and conduction of nerve impulses by decreasing the neuronal membrane's permeability to sodium ions, which results in inhibition of depolarization with resultant blockade of conduction; interferes with the uptake of norepinephrine by adrenergic nerve terminals producing vasoconstriction

Pharmacodynamics/Kinetics
Onset of Action ~1 minute; Peak effect: ~5 minutes
Duration of Action Dose dependent: ≥30 minutes; cocaine metabolites may appear in urine of neonates up to 5 days after birth due to maternal cocaine use shortly before birth
Half-life Elimination 75 minutes
Pregnancy Risk Factor C
Pregnancy Considerations Animal reproduction studies have not been conducted with this product. Cocaine rapidly crosses the placenta in concentrations equal to those in the mother. Adverse events occur in the fetus (eg, congenital malformations, growth restriction), infant (neonatal abstinence syndrome), and mother (eg, preterm labor, placental abruption) following maternal abuse (Fajemirokun-Odudeyi, 2004).

Controlled Substance C-II

Dental Comment The cocaine user, regardless of how the cocaine was administered, presents a potential life-threatening situation in the dental operatory. A patient under the influence of cocaine could be compared to a car going 100 mph. Blood pressure is elevated, heart rate is likely increased, and the use of a local anesthetic with epinephrine may result in a medical emergency. Such patients can be identified by their jitteriness, irritability, talkativeness, tremors, and short, abrupt speech patterns. These same signs and symptoms may also be seen in a normal dental patient with preoperative dental anxiety; therefore, the dentist must be particularly alert to identify the potential cocaine abuser. If cocaine use is suspected, the patient should never be given a local anesthetic with vasoconstrictor, for fear of exacerbating the cocaine-induced sympathetic response. Life-threatening episodes of cardiac arrhythmias and hypertensive crises have been reported when local anesthetic with vasoconstrictor was administered to a patient under the influence of cocaine. No local anesthetic, used by any dentist, can interfere with, nor test positive by cocaine in any urine testing screen. Therefore, the dentist does not need to be concerned with any false drug-use accusations associated with dental anesthesia.

Codeine (KOE deen)

Related Information
Oral Pain *on page 1558*
Brand Names: Canada Codeine Contin®; PMS-Codeine; ratio-Codeine
Generic Availability (U.S.) Yes
Pharmacologic Category Analgesic, Opioid; Antitussive
Dental Use Treatment of postoperative pain
Use Management of mild-to-moderately-severe pain
Unlabeled Use Short-term relief of cough in select patients

Local Anesthetic/Vasoconstrictor Precautions No information available to require special precautions

Effects on Dental Treatment No significant effects or complications reported (see Dental Comment)

Effects on Bleeding No information available to require special precautions

Adverse Effects Frequency not defined.
Cardiovascular: Bradycardia, cardiac arrest, circulatory depression, flushing, hyper-/hypotension, palpitation, shock, syncope, tachycardia
Central nervous system: Abnormal dreams, agitation, anxiety, apprehension, chills, coordination impaired, depression, disorientation, dizziness, drowsiness, dysphoria, euphoria, faintness, fatigue, hallucinations, headache, insomnia, intracranial pressure increased, lightheadedness, nervousness, sedation, shakiness, somnolence, vertigo
Dermatologic: Pruritus, rash, urticaria
Gastrointestinal: Abdominal cramps/pain, anorexia, biliary tract spasm, constipation, diarrhea, nausea, pancreatitis, taste disturbance, vomiting, xerostomia
Genitourinary: Urinary hesitancy/retention
Neuromuscular & skeletal: Paresthesia, rigidity, tremor, weakness

Ocular: Blurred vision, diplopia, miosis, nystagmus, visual disturbances

Respiratory: Bronchospasm, dyspnea, laryngospasm, respiratory arrest, respiratory depression

Miscellaneous: Allergic reaction, diaphoresis

Dental Usual Dosage Postoperative pain: Adults: Oral (immediate release): 30 mg every 4-6 hours as needed; patients with prior opiate exposure may require higher initial doses. Usual range: 15-120 mg every 4-6 hours as needed

Dosage Oral:

Pain management (analgesic): **Note:** These are guidelines and do not represent the maximum doses that may be required in all patients. Doses should be titrated to pain relief/prevention.

Children (unlabeled use): Immediate release (tablet, oral solution): Initial: 0.5-1 mg/kg/dose every 4 hours as needed; maximum: 60 mg/dose (American Pain Society, 2008)

Adults:

Immediate release (tablet, oral solution): Initial: 15-60 mg every 4 hours as needed; maximum total daily dose: 360 mg/day; patients with prior opioid exposure may require higher initial doses. **Note:** The American Pain Society recommends an initial dose of 30-60 mg for adults with moderate pain (American Pain Society, 2008).

Controlled release: Codeine Contin® (Canadian availability; not available in U.S.): **Note:** Titrate at intervals of ≥48 hours until adequate analgesia has been achieved. Daily doses >600 mg/day should not be used; patients requiring higher doses should be switched to an opioid approved for use in severe pain. In patients who receive both Codeine Contin® and an immediate release or combination codeine product for breakthrough pain, the rescue dose of the immediate release codeine product should be ≤12.5% of the total daily Codeine Contin® dose.

Opioid-naive patients: Initial: 50 mg every 12 hours *Conversion from immediate release codeine preparations:* Immediate release codeine preparations contain ~75% codeine base. Therefore, patients who are switching from immediate release codeine preparations may be transferred to a ~25% lower total daily dose of Codeine Contin®, equally divided into 2 daily doses.

Conversion from a combination codeine product (eg, codeine with acetaminophen or aspirin): See table:

Number of 30 mg Codeine Combination Tablets Daily	Initial Dose of Codeine Contin®	Maintenance Dose of Codeine Contin®
≤6	50 mg every 12 h	100 mg every 12 h
7-9	100 mg every 12 h	150 mg every 12 h
10-12	150 mg every 12 h	200 mg every 12 h
>12	200 mg every 12 h	200-300 every 12 h (maximum: 300 mg every 12 h)

Conversion from another opioid analgesic: Using the patient's current opioid dose, calculate an equivalent daily dose of immediate release codeine. A ~25% lower dose of Codeine Contin® should then be initiated, equally divided into 2 daily doses.

Discontinuation of therapy: **Note:** Gradual dose reduction is recommended if clinically appropriate. Initially reduce the total daily dose by 50% and administer equally divided into 2 daily doses for 2 days followed by a 25% reduction every 2 days thereafter.

Treatment of cough (unlabeled use): Adults: Reported doses vary; range: 7.5-120 mg/day as a single dose or in divided doses (Bolser, 2006; Smith, 2010); **Note:** The American College of Chest Physicians does not recommend the routine use of codeine as an antitussive in patients with upper respiratory infections (Bolser, 2006).

Dosing adjustment in renal impairment:

Manufacturer's recommendations: Clearance may be reduced; active metabolites may accumulate. Initiate at lower doses or longer dosing intervals followed by careful titration.

Alternate recommendations: The following guidelines have been used by some clinicians (Aronoff, 2007):

Cl_{cr} 10-50 mL/minute: Administer 75% of dose

Cl_{cr} <10 mL/minute: Administer 50% of dose

Dosing adjustment in hepatic impairment: No dosage adjustment provided in manufacturer's labeling (has not been studied); however, initial lower doses or longer dosing intervals followed by careful titration are recommended.

Mechanism of Action Binds to opioid receptors in the CNS, causing inhibition of ascending pain pathways, altering the perception of and response to pain; causes cough suppression by direct central action in the medulla; produces generalized CNS depression

Contraindications Hypersensitivity to codeine or any component of the formulation; respiratory depression in the absence of resuscitative equipment; acute or severe bronchial asthma or hypercarbia; presence or suspicion of paralytic ileus

Canadian labeling: Additional contraindications (not in U.S. labeling): Hypersensitivity to other opioid analgesics; cor pulmonale; acute alcoholism; delirium tremens; severe CNS depression; convulsive disorders; increased cerebrospinal or intracranial pressure; head injury; suspected surgical abdomen; use with or within 14 days of MAO inhibitors.

Warnings/Precautions May cause dose-related respiratory depression. The risk is increased in elderly patients, debilitated patients, and patients with conditions associated with hypoxia, hypercapnia, or upper airway obstruction. Use with caution in patients with pre-existing respiratory compromise (hypoxia and/or hypercapnia), COPD or other obstructive pulmonary disease, and kyphoscoliosis or other skeletal disorder which may alter respiratory function; critical respiratory depression may occur, even at therapeutic dosages.

Use may cause or aggravate constipation; chronic use may result in obstructive bowel disease, particularly in those with underlying intestinal motility disorders. Avoid use in patients with gastrointestinal obstruction, particularly paralytic ileus. May cause hypotension; use with caution in patients with hypovolemia, cardiovascular disease (including acute MI), or drugs which may exaggerate hypotensive effects (including phenothiazines or general anesthetics). May cause CNS depression, which may impair physical or mental abilities; patients must be cautioned about performing tasks which require mental alertness (eg, operating machinery or driving).

Use with extreme caution in patients with head injury, intracranial lesions, or elevated intracranial pressure; exaggerated elevation of ICP may occur. Use with caution in patients with hypersensitivity reactions to other phenanthrene-derivative opioid agonists (hydrocodone, hydromorphone, levorphanol, oxycodone, oxymorphone), adrenal insufficiency (including Addison's disease), biliary tract dysfunction, CNS depression or coma, thyroid dysfunction, morbid obesity, prostatic hyperplasia and/or urinary stricture, or severe hepatic or renal impairment. Use may obscure diagnosis or clinical course of patients with acute abdominal conditions. May induce or aggravate seizures; use with caution in patients with seizure disorders.

Use with caution in patients with a history of drug abuse or acute alcoholism; potential for drug dependency exists. Tolerance, psychological and physical dependence may occur with prolonged use. Effects may be potentiated when used with other sedative drugs or ethanol. Concurrent use of agonist/antagonist analgesics may precipitate withdrawal symptoms and/or reduced analgesic efficacy in patients following prolonged therapy with mu opioid agonists. Abrupt discontinuation following prolonged use may also lead to withdrawal symptoms.

Use caution in patients with two or more copies of the variant CYP2D6*2 allele; may have extensive conversion to morphine and thus increased opioid-mediated effects.

Some preparations contain sulfites which may cause allergic reactions. Healthcare provider should be alert to the potential for abuse, misuse, and diversion.

Drug Interactions

Metabolism/Transport Effects Substrate of CYP2D6 (major); **Note:** Assignment of Major/Minor substrate status based on clinically relevant drug interaction potential

Avoid Concomitant Use

Avoid concomitant use of Codeine with any of the following: Azelastine (Nasal); Paraldehyde

Increased Effect/Toxicity

Codeine may increase the levels/effects of: Alcohol (Ethyl); Alvimopan; Azelastine (Nasal); CNS Depressants; Desmopressin; Metyrosine; Mirtazapine; Paraldehyde; Pramipexole; ROPINIRole; Rotigotine; Selective Serotonin Reuptake Inhibitors; Thiazide Diuretics; Zolpidem

The levels/effects of Codeine may be increased by: Amphetamines; Antipsychotic Agents (Phenothiazines); Droperidol; HydrOXYzine; Magnesium Sulfate; Perampanel; Sodium Oxybate; Somatostatin Analogs; Succinylcholine

Decreased Effect

Codeine may decrease the levels/effects of: Pegvisomant

The levels/effects of Codeine may be decreased by: Ammonium Chloride; CYP2D6 Inhibitors (Moderate); CYP2D6 Inhibitors (Strong); Mixed Agonist / Antagonist Opioids

Ethanol/Nutrition/Herb Interactions

Ethanol: May increase CNS depression; monitor for increased effects with coadministration. Caution patients about effects.

Herb/Nutraceutical: St John's wort may decrease codeine levels. Avoid valerian, St John's wort, kava kava, gotu kola (may increase CNS depression).

Pharmacodynamics/Kinetics

Onset of Action Oral: Immediate release: 0.5-1 hour; Peak effect: Oral: Immediate release: 1-1.5 hours

Duration of Action Immediate release: 4-6 hours

Half-life Elimination ~3 hours

Time to Peak Plasma: Immediate release: 1 hour; Controlled release (Canadian availability; not available in the U.S.): 3.3 hours

Pregnancy Risk Factor C

Pregnancy Considerations Adverse events have been observed in animal reproduction studies. Opioid analgesics cross the placenta. In humans, birth defects (including some heart defects) have been associated with maternal use of opioid analgesics, including codeine, during the first trimester of pregnancy (Broussard, 2011). Use of opioids during pregnancy may produce physical dependence in the neonate. Symptoms of opioid withdrawal may include excessive crying, diarrhea, fever, hyper-reflexia, irritability, respiratory rate increased, sneezing, tremors, vomiting, or yawning; respiratory depression may occur in the newborn if opioids are used prior to delivery.

Lactation Enters breast milk/use caution (AAP rates "compatible"; AAP 2001 update pending)

Breast-Feeding Considerations Codeine and its metabolite (morphine) are found in breast milk and can be detected in the serum of nursing infants. The relative dose to a nursing infant has been calculated to be ~1% of the weight-adjusted maternal dose. Higher levels of morphine may be found in the breast milk of lactating mothers who are "ultrarapid metabolizers" of codeine; patients with two or more copies of the variant CYP2D6*2 allele may have extensive conversion to morphine and thus increased opioid-mediated effects. In one case, excessively high serum concentrations of morphine were reported in a breast-fed infant following maternal use of acetaminophen with codeine. The mother was later found to be an "ultrarapid metabolizer" of codeine; symptoms in the infant included feeding difficulty and lethargy, followed by death. Caution should be used since most persons are not aware if they have the genotype resulting in "ultra-rapid metabolizer" status. When codeine is used in breast-feeding women, it is recommended to use the lowest dose for the shortest duration of time and observe the infant for increased sleepiness, difficulty in feeding or breathing, or limpness (FDA, 2007; Koren, 2006).

Controlled Substance C-II

Dosage Forms

Powder, for prescription compounding: USP: 100% (10 g, 25 g)

Solution, oral: 30 mg/5 mL (500 mL)

Tablet, oral: 15 mg, 30 mg, 60 mg

Dosage Forms: Canada

Tablet, controlled release:

Codeine Contin®: 50 mg, 100 mg, 150 mg, 200 mg

Dental Comment It is recommended that codeine not be used as the sole entity for analgesia because of moderate efficacy along with relatively high incidence of nausea, sedation, and constipation. In addition, codeine has some opioid addiction liability. Codeine in combination with acetaminophen or aspirin is recommended. Maximum effective analgesic dose of codeine is 60 mg (1 grain). Beyond 60 mg increases respiratory depression only.

Colchicine (KOL chi seen)

Brand Names: U.S. Colcrys®

Brand Names: Canada Jamp-Colchicine

Pharmacologic Category Antigout Agent

Use Prevention and treatment of acute gout flares; treatment of familial Mediterranean fever (FMF)

Unlabeled Use Primary biliary cirrhosis; pericarditis

Local Anesthetic/Vasoconstrictor Precautions No information available to require special precautions

Effects on Dental Treatment No significant effects or complications reported

Effects on Bleeding No information available to require special precautions

Adverse Effects

>10%: Gastrointestinal: Gastrointestinal disorders including abdominal pain, cramping, nausea, vomiting (up to 26%), diarrhea (up to 23%)

1% to 10%: Respiratory: Pharyngolaryngeal pain (3%)

General Dosage Range Dosage adjustment recommended in patients with renal impairment or on concomitant therapy

Oral:

Children 4-6 years: 0.3-1.8 mg/day in 1-2 divided doses

Children 6-12 years: 0.9-1.8 mg/day in 1-2 divided doses

Children 12-16 years: 1.2-2.4 mg/day in 1-2 divided doses

Children >16 years and Adults: 0.6-2.4 mg/day in 1-2 divided doses **or** Initial: 1.2 mg; repeat with 0.6 mg in 1 hour (maximum total therapy: 1.8 mg)

Mechanism of Action Disrupts cytoskeletal functions by inhibiting β-tubulin polymerization into microtubules, preventing activation, degranulation, and migration of neutrophils associated with mediating some gout symptoms. In familial Mediterranean fever, may interfere with intracellular assembly of the inflammasome complex present in neutrophils and monocytes that mediate activation of interleukin-1β.

Pharmacodynamics/Kinetics

Onset of Action Oral: Pain relief: ~18-24 hours

Half-life Elimination 27-31 hours (multiple oral doses; young, healthy volunteers)

Time to Peak Serum: Oral: 0.5-3 hours

Pregnancy Risk Factor C

Pregnancy Considerations Adverse events were observed in animal reproduction studies. Colchicine crosses the human placenta. Use during pregnancy in the treatment of familial Mediterranean fever has not shown an increase in miscarriage, stillbirth, or teratogenic effects (limited data).

Colchicine and Probenecid
(KOL chi seen & proe BEN e sid)

Related Information

Colchicine *on page 346*

Probenecid *on page 1142*

Pharmacologic Category Anti-inflammatory Agent; Antigout Agent; Uricosuric Agent

Use Treatment of chronic gouty arthritis when complicated by frequent, recurrent acute attacks of gout

Local Anesthetic/Vasoconstrictor Precautions No information available to require special precautions

Effects on Dental Treatment No significant effects or complications reported

Effects on Bleeding No information available to require special precautions

Adverse Effects See individual agents.

General Dosage Range Dosage adjustment recommended in patients with renal impairment

Oral: *Adults:* Initial: One tablet daily; Maintenance: 1 tablet twice daily

Pregnancy Considerations See individual agents.

Colesevelam (koh le SEV a lam)

Related Information

Cardiovascular Diseases *on page 1492*

Brand Names: U.S. Welchol®

Brand Names: Canada Lodalis™

Generic Availability (U.S.) No

Pharmacologic Category Antilipemic Agent, Bile Acid Sequestrant

Use Management of elevated LDL in primary hypercholesterolemia (Fredrickson type IIa) when used alone or in combination with an HMG-CoA reductase inhibitor; management of heterozygous familial hypercholesterolemia (heFH) in adolescent patients (males and postmenarcheal females 10-17 years of age) when used alone or in combination with an HMG-CoA reductase inhibitor, in patients who after an adequate trial of dietary therapy have LDL-C ≥190 mg/dL or LDL-C ≥160 mg/dL with positive family history of premature cardiovascular disease (CVD) or with two or more CVD risk factors; improve glycemic control in type 2 diabetes mellitus (noninsulin dependent, NIDDM) in conjunction with diet, exercise, and insulin or oral antidiabetic agents

Canadian labeling (Lodalis™): Adjunct to diet and lifestyle modifications in the management of primary hypercholesterolemia (Fredrickson type IIa) as monotherapy or in combination with an HMG-CoA reductase inhibitor

Local Anesthetic/Vasoconstrictor Precautions No information available to require special precautions

Effects on Dental Treatment No significant effects or complications reported

Effects on Bleeding No information available to require special precautions

Adverse Effects Actual frequency may be dependent upon indication. Unless otherwise noted, frequency of adverse effects is reported for adult patients.

>10%: Gastrointestinal: Constipation (9% to 11%)

1% to 10%:

Cardiovascular: Hypertension (3%)

Central nervous system: Headache (children 4% to 8%), fatigue (children 4%)

Endocrine & metabolic: Hypertriglyceridemia (4% to 5%), hypoglycemia (3%), CPK increased (children 2%)

Gastrointestinal: Dyspepsia (4% to 8%), nausea (3%), vomiting (children 2%)

Neuromuscular & skeletal: Weakness (4%), myalgia (2%)

Respiratory: Nasopharyngitis (children 5% to 6%), upper respiratory tract infection (children 5%), pharyngitis (3%), rhinitis (children 2%)

Miscellaneous: Flu-like syndrome (children 4%)

Dosage Oral:

Children 10-17 years (males and postmenarchal females): Dyslipidemia (heterozygous familial hypercholesterolemia):

Once-daily dosing: 3.75 g (oral suspension or 6 tablets)

Twice-daily dosing: 1.875 g (3 tablets)

Note: Due to large tablet size, oral suspension is recommended in pediatric patients.

Adults:

U.S. labeling: Dyslipidemia, type 2 diabetes (combination therapy with insulin or oral antidiabetic agents):
Once-daily dosing: 3.75 g (oral suspension or 6 tablets)
Twice-daily dosing: 1.875 g (3 tablets)

Canadian labeling: Dyslipidemia:
Combination therapy: 2.5-3.75 g (4-6 tablets) daily; maximum dose: 3.75 g (6 tablets) given once daily or 1.875 g (3 tablets) given twice daily
Monotherapy: Initial: 1.875 g (3 tablets) twice daily or 3.75 g (6 tablets) once daily; maximum dose: 4.375 g (7 tablets) daily

Elderly: Refer to adult dosing.

Dosage adjustment in renal impairment: No dosage adjustment necessary; not absorbed from the gastrointestinal tract.

Dosage adjustment in hepatic impairment: No dosage adjustment necessary; not absorbed from the gastrointestinal tract.

Mechanism of Action Cholesterol is the major precursor of bile acid. Colesevelam binds with bile acids in the intestine to form an insoluble complex that is eliminated in feces. This increased excretion of bile acids results in an increased oxidation of cholesterol to bile acid and a lowering of the serum cholesterol.

Contraindications History of bowel obstruction; serum triglyceride concentration >500 mg/dL; history of hypertriglyceridemia-induced pancreatitis

Canadian labeling: Hypersensitivity to colesevelam or any component of the formulation; bowel or biliary obstruction

Warnings/Precautions Use with caution in treating patients with serum triglyceride concentrations >300 mg/dL and in patients using insulin or sulfonylureas (may cause increased concentrations) or in patients susceptible to fat-soluble vitamin deficiencies. Discontinue if triglyceride concentrations exceed 500 mg/dL or hypertriglyceridemia-induced pancreatitis occurs. Use in patients with gastroparesis, other severe GI motility disorders, or a history of major GI tract surgery is not recommended due to constipating effects of colesevelam. Patients with dysphagia or swallowing disorders should use the oral suspension form of colesevelam due to large tablet size and risk for esophageal obstruction.

Minimal effects are seen on HDL-C and triglyceride levels. Secondary causes of hypercholesterolemia should be excluded before initiation. Colesevelam has not been studied in Fredrickson Type I, III, IV, or V dyslipidemias. Colesevelam is not indicated for the management of type 1 diabetes, particularly in the acute management (eg, DKA). It is also not indicated in type 2 diabetes mellitus as monotherapy and must be used as an adjunct to diet, exercise, and glycemic control with insulin or oral antidiabetic agents. Combination with dipeptidyl peptidase 4 inhibitors or thiazolidinediones has not been studied extensively.

Use with caution in patients susceptible to fat-soluble vitamin deficiencies. Absorption of fat soluble vitamins A, D, E, and K may be decreased; patients should take vitamins ≥4 hours before colesevelam. May decrease the absorption of many drugs; refer to Drug Interactions for further detail. Some products may contain phenylalanine.

Drug Interactions

Metabolism/Transport Effects None known.

Avoid Concomitant Use

Avoid concomitant use of Colesevelam with any of the following: Deferasirox

Increased Effect/Toxicity There are no known significant interactions involving an increase in effect.

Decreased Effect

Colesevelam may decrease the levels/effects of: Amiodarone; Antidiabetic Agents (Thiazolidinedione); AtorvaSTATin; Chenodiol; Contraceptives (Estrogens); Contraceptives (Progestins); Corticosteroids (Oral); CycloSPORINE (Systemic); Deferasirox; Ethinyl Estradiol; Ezetimibe; Glimepiride; GlipiZIDE; GlyBURIDE; Leflunomide; Lomitapide; Loop Diuretics; Methotrexate; Multivitamins/Minerals (with ADEK, Folate, Iron); Niacin; Nonsteroidal Anti-Inflammatory Agents; Norethindrone; Olmesartan; Phenytoin; Pravastatin; Propranolol; Raloxifene; Teriflunomide; Tetracycline Derivatives; Thiazide Diuretics; Thyroid Products; Ursodiol; Vancomycin; Vitamin D Analogs; Vitamin K Antagonists

Dietary Considerations Should be taken with meal(s) and a liquid. Follow dietary guidelines. Some products may contain phenylalanine.

Pharmacodynamics/Kinetics

Onset of Action

Lipid lowering: Therapeutic: ~2 weeks
Reduction of hemoglobin A_{1C} (Type II diabetes): 4-6 weeks initial onset; 12-18 weeks maximal effect

Pregnancy Risk Factor B

Pregnancy Considerations Adverse effects have not been observed in animal reproduction studies. Colesevelam is not absorbed systemically, but may interfere with vitamin absorption; therefore, regular supplementation may not be adequate.

Lactation Does not enter breast milk/use caution

Breast-Feeding Considerations Due to lack of systemic absorption, colesevelam is not expected to be excreted in breast milk; however, the tendency of colesevelam to interfere with the vitamin absorption may have an effect on the nursing infant.

Dosage Forms

Granules for suspension, oral:
Welchol®: 3.75 g/packet (30s)

Tablet, oral:
Welchol®: 625 mg

Dosage Forms: Canada

Tablet, oral:
Lodalis™: 625 mg

Colestipol (koe LES ti pole)

Related Information
Cardiovascular Diseases *on page 1492*

Brand Names: U.S. Colestid®; Colestid® Flavored

Brand Names: Canada Colestid®

Pharmacologic Category Antilipemic Agent, Bile Acid Sequestrant

Use Adjunct in management of primary hypercholesterolemia

Unlabeled Use Diarrhea associated with excess fecal bile acids (Westergaard, 2007); relief of pruritus associated with elevated levels of bile acids (Datta, 1963; Scaldaferri, 2011)

Local Anesthetic/Vasoconstrictor Precautions No information available to require special precautions

Effects on Dental Treatment No significant effects or complications reported

Effects on Bleeding Because colestipol can bind with and impair the absorption of dietary vitamin K, hypoprothrombinemia can occur

Adverse Effects Frequency not defined.

Cardiovascular: Angina, chest pain, edema of hands or feet, tachycardia

Central nervous system: Dizziness, fatigue, headache (including migraine and sinus), lightheadedness, insomnia

Dermatologic: Dermatitis, rash, urticaria

Gastrointestinal: Abdominal pain and cramping, anorexia, bloating, constipation, cholecystitis, cholelithiasis, diarrhea, dysphagia, esophageal obstruction, flatulence, indigestion, heartburn, hemorrhoids (bleeding), nausea, peptic ulceration, vomiting

Hepatic: Alkaline phosphatase increased, ALT increased, AST increased

Neuromuscular & skeletal: Arthritis, backache, joint/muscle pain, weakness

Respiratory: Dyspnea

General Dosage Range Oral: *Adults:* Granules: Initial: 5 g 1-2 times/day; Maintenance: 5-30 g/day once or in divided doses; Tablets: Initial: 2 g 1-2 times/day; Maintenance: 2-16 g/day once or in divided doses

Mechanism of Action Binds with bile acids to form an insoluble complex that is eliminated in feces; it thereby increases the fecal loss of bile acid-bound low density lipoprotein cholesterol

Pregnancy Considerations Colestipol is not absorbed systemically (<0.17%), but may interfere with vitamin absorption; therefore, regular prenatal supplementation may not be adequate. There are no studies in pregnant women; use with caution.

Colistimethate (koe lis ti METH ate)

Brand Names: U.S. Coly-Mycin® M

Brand Names: Canada Coly-Mycin® M

Pharmacologic Category Antibiotic, Miscellaneous

Use Treatment of acute or chronic infections due to sensitive strains of certain gram-negative bacilli (particularly *Pseudomonas aeruginosa*) which are resistant to other antibacterials or in patients allergic to other antibacterials

Unlabeled Use Used as nebulized inhalation in the prevention of *Pseudomonas aeruginosa* respiratory tract infections in immunocompromised patients; used as nebulized inhalation adjunct agent for the treatment of *P. aeruginosa* infections in patients with cystic fibrosis and other seriously ill or chronically ill patients; used as nebulized inhalation in the treatment of ventilator-associated pneumonia (VAP) due to multidrug-resistant *P. aeruginosa* or *Acinetobacter baumannii*

Local Anesthetic/Vasoconstrictor Precautions No information available to require special precautions

Effects on Dental Treatment No significant effects or complications reported

Effects on Bleeding No information available to require special precautions

Adverse Effects Frequency not defined.

Central nervous system: Dizziness, fever, headache, slurred speech, vertigo

Dermatologic: Pruritus, rash, urticaria

gastrointestinal: GI upset

Neuromuscular & skeletal: Paresthesia (extremities, oral); weakness (lower limb)

Renal: BUN increased, creatinine increased, nephrotoxicity, proteinuria, urine output decreased

Respiratory: Apnea, respiratory distress

General Dosage Range Dosage adjustment recommended in patients with renal impairment or who develop toxicities.

I.M., I.V.: *Children and Adults:* 2.5-5 mg/kg/day **colistin base** in 2-4 divided doses; maximum: 5 mg/kg/day

Mechanism of Action Colistimethate (or the sodium salt [colistimethate sodium]) is the inactive prodrug which is hydrolyzed to colistin, which acts as a cationic detergent and damages the bacterial cytoplasmic membrane causing leaking of intracellular substances and cell death

Pharmacodynamics/Kinetics

Half-life Elimination I.M., I.V.: 2-3 hours; Anuria: ≤2-3 days

Time to Peak I.V.: 10 minutes

Pregnancy Risk Factor C

Pregnancy Considerations Adverse events have been observed in animal reproduction studies; therefore, the manufacturer classifies colistimethate as pregnancy category C. Colistimethate crosses the placenta in humans. There are no adequate and well-controlled studies in pregnant women.

Collagen (Absorbable) (KOL la jen, ab SORB able)

Related Information

Antiplatelet and Anticoagulation Considerations in Dentistry *on page 1503*

Brand Names: U.S. CollaCote®; CollaPlug®; CollaTape®

Generic Availability (U.S.) Yes

Pharmacologic Category Hemostatic Agent

Dental Use Control of bleeding created during dental surgery

Use Hemostatic

Local Anesthetic/Vasoconstrictor Precautions No information available to require special precautions

Effects on Dental Treatment No significant effects or complications reported

Effects on Bleeding No information available to require special precautions

Adverse Effects No data reported.

Dental Usual Dosage Control of bleeding: Children and Adults: Topical: A sufficiently large dressing should be selected so as to completely cover the oral wound

Dosage Children and Adults: A sufficiently large dressing should be selected so as to completely cover the oral wound

Mechanism of Action The highly porous sponge structure absorbs blood and wound exudate. The collagen component causes aggregation of platelets which bind to collagen fibrils. The aggregated platelets degranulate, releasing coagulation factors that promote the formation of fibrin.

Contraindications No data reported

Warnings/Precautions Should not be used on infected or contaminated wounds

Drug Interactions

Metabolism/Transport Effects None known.

Avoid Concomitant Use There are no known interactions where it is recommended to avoid concomitant use.

Increased Effect/Toxicity There are no known significant interactions involving an increase in effect.

Decreased Effect There are no known significant interactions involving a decrease in effect.

Lactation Compatible

Dosage Forms
Wound dressing:
Generics:
3/8" x 3/4"
3/4" x 1 1/2"
1" x 3"
Brands:
CollaCote®, CollaPlug®, CollaTape®:
3/8" x 3/4"
3/4" x 1 1/2"
1" x 3"

Collagenase (Systemic) (KOL la je nase)

Brand Names: U.S. Xiaflex®
Pharmacologic Category Enzyme
Use Treatment of Dupuytren's contracture with a palpable cord
Adverse Effects
>10%:
Dermatologic: Bruising (70%), pruritus (15%)
Hematologic: Lymphadenopathy (13%)
Local: Injection site hemorrhage (38%), injection site reaction (24% to 35%; includes erythema, inflammation, irritation, pain, swelling, tenderness)
Miscellaneous: Antibody formation (≥86%), peripheral edema (primarily as swelling of injected hand: 73%), pain in extremity (35%), neutralizing antibodies (10% to 21% to AUX-I and AUX-II, respectively)
1% to 10%:
Dermatologic: laceration (9%), erythema (6%)
Miscellaneous: Lymph node pain (8%), axillary pain (6%)
General Dosage Range Intralesional: *Adults:* 0.58 mg per cord
Mechanism of Action Collagenase clostridium histolyticum contains two forms of microbial collagenase (Collagenase AUX-1 and Collagenase AUX-II) isolated and purified from the fermentation of *Clostridium histolyticum* bacteria; collagenase lyses collagen, leading to enzymatic disruption of contracted Dupuytren's cord (comprised primarily of collagen)
Pregnancy Risk Factor B
Pregnancy Considerations Adverse events were not observed in animal reproduction studies. Pharmacokinetic studies in humans did not show quantifiable systemic levels following intralesional injection into a Dupuytren's cord. IgE-anti-drug antibodies commonly develop in treated patients; effects to the fetus are unknown.

Collagenase (Topical) (KOL la je nase)

Brand Names: U.S. Santyl®
Brand Names: Canada Santyl®
Pharmacologic Category Enzyme, Topical Debridement
Use Promotes debridement of necrotic tissue in dermal ulcers and severe burns
Local Anesthetic/Vasoconstrictor Precautions No information available to require special precautions
Effects on Dental Treatment No significant effects or complications reported
Effects on Bleeding No information available to require special precautions
Adverse Effects Frequency not defined.
Local: Irritation, pain and burning may occur at site of application

General Dosage Range Topical: *Children and Adults:* Apply once daily
Mechanism of Action Collagenase is an enzyme derived from the fermentation of *Clostridium histolyticum* and differs from other proteolytic enzymes in that its enzymatic action has a high specificity for native and denatured collagen. Collagenase will not attack collagen in healthy tissue or newly formed granulation tissue. In addition, it does not act on fat, fibrin, keratin, or muscle.
Pregnancy Considerations It is not known if systemic absorption occurs following topical application.

Collagen Hemostat (KOL la jen HEE moe stat)

Related Information
Antiplatelet and Anticoagulation Considerations in Dentistry *on page 1503*
Brand Names: U.S. Avitene®; Avitene® Flour; Avitene® Ultrafoam™; EndoAvitene®; Helistat®; Helitene®; Instat™ MCH; SyringeAvitene™
Generic Availability (U.S.) No
Pharmacologic Category Hemostatic Agent
Dental Use Adjunct to hemostasis when control of bleeding by ligature is ineffective or impractical
Use Adjunct to hemostasis when control of bleeding by ligature is ineffective or impractical
Local Anesthetic/Vasoconstrictor Precautions No information available to require special precautions
Effects on Dental Treatment No significant effects or complications reported
Effects on Bleeding Used in surgical procedures as an adjunct to hemostasis when control of bleeding by ligature or conventional procedures is ineffective or impractical.
Adverse Effects Frequency not defined.
Miscellaneous: Adhesion formation, allergic reaction, edema, foreign body reaction, hematoma, inflammation, potentiation of infection
Dental Usual Dosage Hemostasis: Adults: Topical: Apply dry directly to source of bleeding; remove excess material after ~10-15 minutes
Dosage Apply dry directly to source of bleeding; remove excess material after ~10-15 minutes
Mechanism of Action Collagen hemostat is an absorbable topical hemostatic agent prepared from purified bovine corium collagen and shredded into fibrils. Physically, microfibrillar collagen hemostat yields a large surface area. Chemically, it is collagen with hydrochloric acid noncovalently bound to some of the available amino groups in the collagen molecules. When in contact with a bleeding surface, collagen hemostat attracts platelets which adhere to its fibrils and undergo the release phenomenon. This triggers aggregation of the platelets into thrombi in the interstices of the fibrous mass, initiating the formation of a physiologic platelet plug.
Contraindications Hypersensitivity to any component of the formulation; products of bovine origin; closure of skin incisions; contaminated wounds; application to bone surfaces to which prosthetic materials are attached with methylmethacrylate adhesives
Warnings/Precautions Pain, numbness, or paralysis have been reported if used near a bony or neural space and left inside patient; use minimum amount necessary to achieve hemostasis. Remove as much of agent as possible after hemostasis is achieved. Do not leave in a contaminated or infected space. Fragments of MCH may pass through filters of blood scavenging systems; avoid reintroduction of blood from operative sites treated

with MCH. Not intended to treat systemic coagulation disorders. Not for use when origin of bleeding is unknown.

Drug Interactions

Metabolism/Transport Effects None known.

Avoid Concomitant Use There are no known interactions where it is recommended to avoid concomitant use.

Increased Effect/Toxicity There are no known significant interactions involving an increase in effect.

Decreased Effect There are no known significant interactions involving a decrease in effect.

Pharmacodynamics/Kinetics

Onset of Action Hemostasis: 2-5 minutes

Dosage Forms

Powder, topical:
Avitene® Flour: (0.5 g, 1 g, 5 g)
Helitene®: (0.5 g, 1 g)
Instat™ MCH: (0.5 g, 1 g)
SyringeAvitene™: (1 g)

Sheet, topical:
Avitene®: (1s, 6s)
EndoAvitene®: (6s)

Sponge, topical:
Avitene® Ultrafoam™: (6s)
Helistat®: (10s, 18s)

Conivaptan (koe NYE vap tan)

Brand Names: U.S. Vaprisol®

Pharmacologic Category Vasopressin Antagonist

Use Treatment of euvolemic and hypervolemic hyponatremia in hospitalized patients

Local Anesthetic/Vasoconstrictor Precautions No information available to require special precautions

Effects on Dental Treatment Key adverse event(s) related to dental treatment: Dry mouth, oral candidiasis, orthostatic hypotension.

Effects on Bleeding No information available to require special precautions

Adverse Effects

>10%:
Cardiovascular: Orthostatic hypotension (6% to 14%)
Central nervous system: Fever (5% to 11%)
Endocrine & metabolic: Hypokalemia (10% to 22%)
Local: Injection site reactions including pain, erythema, phlebitis, swelling (63% to 73%)

1% to 10%:
Cardiovascular: Hypertension (6% to 8%), hypotension (5% to 8%), peripheral edema (3% to 8%), phlebitis (5%), atrial fibrillation (2% to 5%), ECG abnormality (≤5%)
Central nervous system: Headache (8% to 10%), insomnia (4% to 5%), confusion (≤5%), pain (2%)
Dermatologic: Pruritus (1% to 5%), erythema (3%)
Endocrine & metabolic: Hyponatremia (6% to 8%), hypomagnesemia (2% to 5%), hyper-/hypoglycemia (3%)
Gastrointestinal: Constipation (6% to 8%), vomiting (5% to 7%), diarrhea (≤7%), nausea (3% to 5%), dry mouth (4%), dehydration (2%), oral candidiasis (2%)
Genitourinary: Urinary tract infection (4% to 5%)
Hematologic: Anemia (5% to 6%)
Renal: Polyuria (5% to 6%), hematuria (2%)
Respiratory: Pneumonia (2% to 5%), pharyngolaryngeal pain (1% to 5%)
Miscellaneous: Thirst (3% to 6%)

General Dosage Range Dosage adjustment recommended in patients with hepatic impairment

I.V.: *Adults:* Loading dose: 20 mg bolus, followed by 20 mg as continuous infusion over 24 hours; Maintenance: 20-40 mg/day as a continuous infusion over 24 hours (maximum therapy: 4 days)

Mechanism of Action Conivaptan is an arginine vasopressin (AVP) receptor antagonist with affinity for AVP receptor subtypes V_{1A} and V_2. The antidiuretic action of AVP is mediated through activation of the V_2 receptor, which functions to regulate water and electrolyte balance at the level of the collecting ducts in the kidney. Serum levels of AVP are commonly elevated in euvolemic or hypervolemic hyponatremia, which results in the dilution of serum sodium and the relative hyponatremic state. Antagonism of the V_2 receptor by conivaptan promotes the excretion of free water (without loss of serum electrolytes) resulting in net fluid loss, increased urine output, decreased urine osmolality, and subsequent restoration of normal serum sodium concentrations.

Pharmacodynamics/Kinetics

Half-life Elimination ~5-8 hours

Pregnancy Risk Factor C

Pregnancy Considerations Animal studies indicate that conivaptan accumulates in the placenta (2.2-fold relative to maternal plasma); systemic exposure to fetus is likely. No teratogenic effects have been observed in animal studies; however, these studies have shown decreased neonatal viability and delayed growth and development at doses lower than those required for therapeutic efficacy. There are no adequate and well-controlled studies in pregnant women. Use only if benefit outweighs risk.

Copper (KOP er)

Pharmacologic Category Trace Element, Parenteral

Use Supplement to intravenous solutions given for total parenteral nutrition (TPN) to maintain copper serum levels and to prevent depletion of endogenous stores and subsequent deficiency symptoms

Local Anesthetic/Vasoconstrictor Precautions No information available to require special precautions

Effects on Dental Treatment No significant effects or complications reported

Effects on Bleeding No information available to require special precautions

Adverse Effects Note: Generally well tolerated; excessive copper levels may result in the following adverse effects:
Hepatic: Hepatic dysfunction (including hepatic necrosis)

General Dosage Range I.V. (as a parenteral nutrition component):
Infants and Children: 20 mcg/kg/day
Adults: 0.3-1.5 mg/day

Mechanism of Action Copper is an essential nutrient which serves as a cofactor for serum ceruloplasmin, an oxidase necessary for proper formation of the iron carrier protein, transferrin. It also helps maintain normal rates of red and white blood cell formation and helps prevent development of deficiency symptoms: Leukopenia, neutropenia, anemia, depressed ceruloplasmin levels, impaired transferring formation, secondary iron deficiency and osteoporosis.

Pregnancy Risk Factor C

◄ **Pregnancy Considerations** Animal reproduction studies have not been conducted. It is not known whether administration to a pregnant woman can cause fetal harm or can affect reproductive capacity.

Corticorelin (kor ti koe REL in)

Brand Names: U.S. Acthrel®

Pharmacologic Category Diagnostic Agent

Use Diagnostic test used in adrenocorticotropic hormone (ACTH)-dependent Cushing's syndrome to differentiate between pituitary and ectopic production of ACTH

Local Anesthetic/Vasoconstrictor Precautions No information available to require special precautions

Effects on Dental Treatment No significant effects or complications reported

Effects on Bleeding No information available to require special precautions

Adverse Effects

>10%: Cardiovascular: Flushing (face, neck and upper chest, 16%)

1% to 10%: Respiratory: Dyspnea (urge to inspire, 6%)

General Dosage Range I.V.: *Adults:* 1 mcg/kg

Mechanism of Action Corticorelin ovine, a peptide of ovine corticotropin-releasing hormone (oCRH) and an analogue of human CRH (hCRH), stimulates adrenocorticotropic hormone (ACTH) release from the anterior pituitary. ACTH stimulates the adrenal cortex to produce cortisol. Depending on the plasma ACTH and cortisol response following the corticorelin stimulation test, the results aid the clinician in the differentiation between the source of ACTH-dependent hypercortisolism (pituitary vs ectopic).

Pharmacodynamics/Kinetics

Onset of Action I.V.: Plasma ACTH level increases 2 minutes after injection; plasma cortisol level increases within 10 minutes after injection

Duration of Action I.V.: Plasma ACTH and cortisol levels remain elevated for up to 2 hours

Time to Peak Plasma: ACTH: 15-60 minutes; Cortisol: 30-120 minutes; both levels show a dose-dependent, biphasic response with a second lower peak 2-3 hours after injection; basal and peak response levels vary depending on AM or PM administration (baseline ACTH and cortisol levels are generally higher in the AM)

Pregnancy Risk Factor C

Pregnancy Considerations Animal reproduction studies have not been conducted.

Corticotropin (kor ti koe TROE pin)

Brand Names: U.S. H.P. Acthar®

Pharmacologic Category Corticosteroid, Systemic

Use Acute exacerbations of multiple sclerosis; infantile spasms; adjunctive therapy for exacerbations/acute episodes of rheumatic disorders (psoriatic arthritis, rheumatoid arthritis, juvenile idiopathic arthritis [JIA], ankylosing spondylitis); exacerbations or maintenance therapy for collagen diseases (systemic lupus erythematosus, systemic dermatomyositis); severe erythema multiforme; Stevens-Johnson syndrome; serum sickness; severe acute/chronic allergic and inflammatory ophthalmic disease (keratitis, iritis, iridocyclitis, diffuse posterior uveitis and choroiditis, optic neuritis, chorioretinitis, anterior segment inflammation); symptomatic sarcoidosis; to induce diuresis for remission of proteinuria in patients with nephrotic syndrome without idiopathic uremia or due to lupus erythematosus

Local Anesthetic/Vasoconstrictor Precautions No information available to require special precautions

Effects on Dental Treatment No significant effects or complications reported

Effects on Bleeding No information available to require special precautions

Adverse Effects

Adverse events associated with cortisol elevation; frequency not defined:

Cardiovascular: Blood pressure increased

Central nervous system: Behavioral changes, mood changes

Endocrine & metabolic: Fluid retention, glucose intolerance

Gastrointestinal: Appetite increased, weight gain

Adverse events associated with infantile spasm treatment:

>10%:

Cardiovascular: Hypertension (11%)

Central nervous system: Seizure (12%)

Miscellaneous: Infection (20%)

1% to 10%:

Cardiovascular: Cardiac hypertrophy (3%)

Central nervous system: Irritability (7%), pyrexia (5%)

Endocrine & metabolic: Cushingoid syndrome (3%)

Gastrointestinal: Appetite decreased (3%), diarrhea (3%), vomiting (3%), weight gain (1%)

Respiratory: Nasal congestion (1%)

General Dosage Range

I.M.:

Children <2 years: 75 units/m²/dose twice daily (infantile spasms) followed by gradual downward titration of dose

Children >2 years: 40-80 units every 24-72 hours

Adults: 80-120 units/day for 2-3 weeks (MS) **or** 40-80 units every 24-72 hours (indications other than MS)

SubQ:

Children >2 years: 40-80 units every 24-72 hours

Adults: 80-120 units/day for 2-3 weeks (MS) **or** 40-80 units every 24-72 hours (indications other than MS)

Mechanism of Action Stimulates the adrenal cortex to secrete adrenal steroids (including hydrocortisone, cortisone), androgenic substances, and a small amount of aldosterone

Pharmacodynamics/Kinetics

Half-life Elimination ACTH: 15 minutes

Pregnancy Considerations Embryocidal effects may be observed following corticotropin use during pregnancy. Endogenous ACTH levels are increased during pregnancy. Some studies have shown an association between first trimester systemic corticosteroid use and oral clefts; adverse events in the fetus/neonate have been noted in case reports following large doses of systemic corticosteroids during pregnancy.

Prescribing and Access Restrictions H.P. Acthar® Gel is only available through specialty pharmacy distribution and not through traditional distribution sources (eg, wholesalers, retail pharmacies). Hospitals wishing to acquire H.P. Acthar® Gel should contact CuraScript Specialty Distribution (1-877-599-7748).

After treatment is initiated, discharge or outpatient prescriptions should be submitted to the Acthar Support and Access Program (A.S.A.P.) in order to ensure an uninterrupted supply of the medication. The Acthar Referral/Prescription form is available online at http://www.acthar.com/files/Acthar-Prescription-Referral-Form.pdf.

Additional information is available for the A.S.A.P. at http://www.acthar.com/healthcare-professionals/physi-cian-patient-referrals or by calling 1-888-435-2284.

Cortisone (KOR ti sone)

Related Information
Respiratory Diseases *on page 1514*
Triamcinolone (Systemic) *on page 1357*
Pharmacologic Category Corticosteroid, Systemic
Use Management of adrenocortical insufficiency
Local Anesthetic/Vasoconstrictor Precautions No information available to require special precautions
Effects on Dental Treatment A compromised immune response may occur if patient has been taking systemic cortisone. The need for corticosteroid coverage in these patients should be considered before any dental treatment; consult with physician.
Effects on Bleeding Variable effects on anticoagulant therapy are observed with glucocorticoids, such as cortisone.
Adverse Effects
>10%:
Central nervous system: Insomnia, nervousness
Gastrointestinal: Increased appetite, indigestion
1% to 10%:
Dermatologic: Hirsutism
Endocrine & metabolic: Diabetes mellitus
Neuromuscular & skeletal: Arthralgia
Ocular: Cataracts, glaucoma
Respiratory: Epistaxis
General Dosage Range Oral:
Children: 0.5-10 mg/kg/day **or** 20-300 mg/m²/day divided every 6-8 hours
Adults: 25-300 mg /day divided every 12-24 hours
Mechanism of Action Decreases inflammation by suppression of migration of polymorphonuclear leukocytes and reversal of increased capillary permeability
Pharmacodynamics/Kinetics
Onset of Action Peak effect: Oral: ~2 hours; I.M.: 20-48 hours
Duration of Action 30-36 hours
Half-life Elimination 0.5-2 hours; End-stage renal disease: 3.5 hours
Pregnancy Considerations Adverse events have been observed with corticosteroids in animal reproduction studies. Cortisone is found in cord blood; endogenous maternal cortisol (active) is metabolized by placental enzymes to cortisone (inactive), regulating the amount of maternal glucocorticoids reaching the fetus. Some studies have shown an association between first trimester systemic corticosteroid use and oral clefts; adverse events in the fetus/neonate have been noted in case reports following large doses of systemic corticosteroids during pregnancy. Women exposed to cortisone during pregnancy for the treatment of an autoimmune disease may contact the OTIS Autoimmune Diseases Study at 877-311-8972.

Cosyntropin (koe sin TROE pin)

Brand Names: U.S. Cortrosyn™
Brand Names: Canada Cortrosyn™; Synacthen® Depot
Pharmacologic Category Corticosteroid, Systemic; Diagnostic Agent

Use Diagnostic test to differentiate primary adrenal from secondary (pituitary) adrenocortical insufficiency

Synacthen® Depot (Canadian availability): Additional indications: Treatment of various disease states (eg, collagen, dermatologic, endocrine, ocular, hemolytic). Consult manufacturer labeling for detailed list.
Local Anesthetic/Vasoconstrictor Precautions No information available to require special precautions
Effects on Dental Treatment No significant effects or complications reported
Effects on Bleeding No information available to require special precautions
Adverse Effects Frequency not defined. **Note:** Adverse events associated with other corticosteroids may be observed when Synacthen® Depot (Canadian availability) is used for therapeutic purposes. Refer to corticosteroid monographs for comprehensive lists.

Cardiovascular: Bradycardia, hypertension, peripheral edema, tachycardia
Dermatologic: Rash
Local: Whealing with redness at the injection site
Miscellaneous: Anaphylaxis, hypersensitivity reaction
General Dosage Range I.M., I.V.:
Children ≤2 years: 0.125 mg
Children >2 years and Adults: 0.25 mg
Mechanism of Action Stimulates the adrenal cortex to secrete adrenal steroids (including hydrocortisone, cortisone), androgenic substances, and a small amount of aldosterone
Pharmacodynamics/Kinetics
Duration of Action Synacthen® Depot (Canadian availability): I.M.: Plasma concentrations of 200-300 pg/mL maintained for 12 hours
Half-life Elimination Synacthen® Depot (Canadian availability): 7 minutes
Time to Peak Serum: I.M., I.V. push: ~1 hour; plasma cortisol levels rise in healthy individuals within 5 minutes
Pregnancy Risk Factor C
Pregnancy Considerations Animal reproduction studies have not been conducted.

Crizotinib (kriz OH ti nib)

Related Information
Clinical Risk Related to Drugs Prolonging QT Interval *on page 1510*
Brand Names: U.S. Xalkori®
Brand Names: Canada Xalkori™
Generic Availability (U.S.) No
Pharmacologic Category Antineoplastic Agent, Anaplastic Lymphoma Kinase Inhibitor; Antineoplastic Agent, Tyrosine Kinase Inhibitor
Use Treatment of locally advanced or metastatic non-small cell lung cancer (NSCLC) that is anaplastic lymphoma kinase (ALK) positive (as detected by an approved test)
Local Anesthetic/Vasoconstrictor Precautions Crizotinib is one of the drugs confirmed to prolong the QT interval and is accepted as having a risk of causing torsade de pointes. The risk of drug-induced torsade de pointes is extremely low when a single QT interval prolonging drug is prescribed. In terms of epinephrine, it is not known what effect vasoconstrictors in the local anesthetic regimen will have in patients with a known history of congenital prolonged QT interval or in patients taking any medication that prolongs the QT interval. Until more information is obtained, it is suggested that

the clinician consult with the physician prior to the use of a vasoconstrictor in suspected patients, and that the vasoconstrictor (epinephrine, mepivacaine, and levonordefrin [Carbocaine® 2% with Neo-Cobefrin®]) be used with caution.

Effects on Dental Treatment Key adverse event(s) related to dental treatment: Stomatitis and taste alteration have been reported

Effects on Bleeding No reports of bleeding or thrombocytopenia

Adverse Effects

>10%:
Cardiovascular: Edema (28%)
Central nervous system: Fatigue (20%), dizziness (16%)
Gastrointestinal: Nausea (53%), diarrhea (43%), vomiting (40%), constipation (27%), appetite decreased (19%), taste alteration (12%), esophageal disorder (11%; includes dyspepsia, dysphagia, epigastric burning/discomfort/pain, esophageal obstruction/pain/spasm/ulcer, esophagitis, gastroesophageal reflux, odynophagia, reflux esophagitis)
Hematologic: Lymphopenia (grades 3/4: 11%)
Hepatic: ALT increased (13%; grades 3/4: 5%)
Neuromuscular & skeletal: Neuropathy (13%; grades 3/4: <1%)
Ocular: Vision disorder (62%; onset: <2 weeks; includes blurred vision, diplopia, photophobia, photopsia, visual acuity decreased, visual brightness, visual field defect, visual impairment, vitreous floaters)

1% to 10%:
Cardiovascular: Bradycardia (5%), chest pain (1%)
Central nervous system: Headache (4%), insomnia (3%)
Dermatologic: Rash (10%)
Gastrointestinal: Abdominal pain (8%), stomatitis (6%)
Hematologic: Neutropenia (grades 3/4: 5%)
Hepatic: AST increased (9%; grades 3/4: 2%)
Neuromuscular & skeletal: Arthralgia (2%)
Renal: Renal cysts (1%)
Respiratory: Cough (4%), dyspnea (2%), pneumonitis (2%), upper respiratory infection (2%)

Dosage Oral: Adults: Nonsmall cell lung cancer, locally advanced or metastatic (ALK-positive): 250 mg twice daily, continue treatment until no longer clinically beneficial

Dosage adjustment for toxicity: Note: If dose reduction is necessary, reduce dose to 200 mg orally twice daily; if necessary, further reduce to 250 mg once daily
Hematologic toxicity (except lymphopenia, unless lymphopenia is associated with clinical events such as opportunistic infection):
Grade 3 toxicity (WBC 1000-2000/mm³, ANC 500-1000/mm³, platelets 25,000-50,000/mm³), grade 3 anemia: Withhold treatment until recovery to ≤grade 2, then resume at the same dose and schedule
Grade 4 toxicity (WBC <1000/mm³, ANC <500/mm³, platelets <25,000/mm³), grade 4 anemia: Withhold treatment until recovery to ≤grade 2, then resume at 200 mg twice daily
Recurrent grade 4 toxicity on 200 mg twice daily: Withhold treatment until recovery to ≤grade 2, then resume at 250 mg once daily
Recurrent grade 4 toxicity on 250 mg once daily: Permanently discontinue

Nonhematologic toxicities:
Grade 3 or 4 ALT or AST elevation (ALT or AST >5 x ULN) with ≤grade 1 total bilirubin elevation (total bilirubin ≤1.5 x ULN): Withhold treatment until recovery to ≤grade 1 (<2.5 X ULN) or baseline, then resume at 200 mg twice daily
Recurrent grade 3 or 4 ALT or AST elevation with ≤grade 1 total bilirubin elevation: Withhold treatment until recovery to ≤grade 1, then resume at 250 mg once daily
Recurrent grade 3 or 4 ALT or AST elevation on 250 mg once daily: Permanently discontinue
Grade 2, 3, or 4 ALT or AST elevation with concurrent grade 2, 3, or 4 total bilirubin elevation (>1.5 x ULN) in the absence of cholestasis or hemolysis: Permanently discontinue
Pneumonitis (any grade; not attributable to disease progression, infection, other pulmonary disease or radiation therapy): Permanently discontinue
Grade 3 QT_c prolongation (QT_c >500 msec without life-threatening signs or symptoms): Withhold treatment until recovery to ≤grade 1 (QT_c ≤470 msec), then resume at 200 mg twice daily
Recurrent grade 3 QT_c prolongation at 200 mg twice daily: Withhold treatment until recovery to ≤grade 1, then resume at 250 mg once daily
Recurrent grade 3 QT_c prolongation at 250 mg once daily: Permanently discontinue
Grade 4 QT_c prolongation: Permanently discontinue

Dosage adjustment in renal impairment:
Mild (Cl_{cr} 30-60 mL/minute) to moderate impairment (Cl_{cr} 60-90 mL/minute): No dosage adjustment required.
Severe impairment (Cl_{cr} <30 mL/minute): Data are insufficient to determine if dosage adjustment necessary; use with caution
End-stage renal disease (ESRD): Was not studied in patients with ESRD; use with caution

Dosage adjustment in hepatic impairment: Data are insufficient to determine if dosage adjustment necessary; however, crizotinib undergoes extensive hepatic metabolism and systemic exposure may be increased with impairment; use with caution

Mechanism of Action Tyrosine kinase receptor inhibitor, which inhibits anaplastic lymphoma kinase (ALK), Hepatocyte Growth Factor Receptor (HGFR, c-MET), and Recepteur d'Origine Nantais (RON). ALK gene abnormalities due to mutations or translocations may result in expression of oncogenic fusion proteins (eg, ALK fusion protein) which alter signaling and expression and result in increased cellular proliferation and survival in tumors which express these fusion proteins. Approximately 2% to 7% of patients with NSCLC have the abnormal echinoderm microtubule-associated protein-like 4, or EML4-ALK gene (which has a higher prevalence in never smokers or light smokers and in patients with adenocarcinoma). Crizotinib selectively inhibits ALK tyrosine kinase, which reduces proliferation of cells expressing the genetic alteration.

Contraindications There are no contraindications listed within the manufacturer's U.S. labeling.

Canadian labeling: Hypersensitivity to crizotinib or any component of the formulation; congenital long QT syndrome or with persistent Fridericia-corrected QT interval (QTcF) ≥500 msec

Warnings/Precautions Hazardous agent - use appropriate precautions for handling and disposal (meets NIOSH, 2012 criteria). Approved for use only in patients with locally advanced or metastatic nonsmall cell lung cancer (NSCLC) who test positive for the abnormal anaplastic lymphoma kinase (ALK) gene. The Vysis ALK break-apart FISH probe kit is approved to test for the gene abnormality.

Grade 3 or 4 ALT increases (usually asymptomatic and reversible) have been observed in clinical trials. May require dosage interruption and/or reduction; permanent discontinuation was necessary in some cases; concurrent ALT elevations >3 x ULN and total bilirubin elevations >2 x ULN (without alkaline phosphatase elevations) were observed rarely. Fatalities due to crizotinib-induced hepatotoxicity have also occurred (rare). Monitor liver function tests, including ALT and total bilirubin. Transaminase elevation onset was within 2 months of treatment initiation. Use with caution in patients with hepatic impairment (has not been studied); crizotinib is extensively metabolized in the liver and liver impairment is likely to increase crizotinib levels.

Severe, life-threatening, and potentially fatal pneumonitis has been associated with crizotinib. Onset was generally within 2 months of treatment initiation. Monitor for pulmonary symptoms which may indicate pneumonitis; exclude other potential causes (eg, disease progression, infection, other pulmonary disease, or radiation therapy). Permanently discontinue if treatment-related pneumonitis is confirmed.

QT$_c$ prolongation has been observed; consider periodic monitoring of ECG and electrolytes in patients with heart failure, bradyarrhythmias, electrolyte abnormalities, or who are taking medications known to prolong the QT interval. May require treatment interruption, dosage reduction, or discontinuation. Avoid use in patients with congenital long QT syndrome. Canadian labeling contraindicates use in patients with congenital long QT syndrome or persistent QTcF ≥500 msec.

Ocular toxicities (eg, blurred vision, diplopia, photophobia, photopsia, visual acuity decreased, visual brightness, visual field defect, visual impairment, and/or vitreous floaters) commonly occur. Onset is generally within 2 weeks of treatment initiation; consider ophthalmology exam, especially if photopsia or vitreous floaters occur. Severe or worsening vitreous floaters or photopsia could be a sign of retinal hole or impending detachment. Use with caution in patients with severe renal impairment; only one patient with severe renal impairment was studied in clinical trials and end stage renal disease was not studied. CYP3A4 inhibitors may increase crizotinib levels; avoid concomitant use with strong CYP3A4 inhibitors and use moderate CYP3A4 inhibitors with caution. CYP3A4 inducers may decrease crizotinib levels; avoid concomitant use with strong CYP3A4 inducers. Avoid concomitant use with CYP3A4 substrates.

Drug Interactions

Metabolism/Transport Effects Substrate of CYP3A4 (major), P-glycoprotein; **Note:** Assignment of Major/Minor substrate status based on clinically relevant drug interaction potential; **Inhibits** CYP2B6 (moderate), CYP3A4 (moderate), P-glycoprotein

Avoid Concomitant Use
Avoid concomitant use of Crizotinib with any of the following: Alfentanil; Bosutinib; CycloSPORINE (Systemic); CYP3A4 Inducers (Strong); CYP3A4 Inhibitors (Strong); Dihydroergotamine; Ergotamine; FentaNYL; Grapefruit Juice; Highest Risk QTc-Prolonging Agents; Ivabradine; Lomitapide; Mifepristone; Pimozide; Pomalidomide; QuiNIDine; Silodosin; Sirolimus; St Johns Wort; Tacrolimus (Systemic); Tolvaptan; Topotecan; VinCRIStine (Liposomal)

Increased Effect/Toxicity
Crizotinib may increase the levels/effects of: Alfentanil; ARIPiprazole; Avanafil; Bosutinib; Budesonide (Systemic, Oral Inhalation); Colchicine; CycloSPORINE (Systemic); CYP2B6 Substrates; CYP3A4 Substrates; Dabigatran Etexilate; Dihydroergotamine; Eplerenone; Ergotamine; Everolimus; FentaNYL; Highest Risk QTc-Prolonging Agents; Ivacaftor; Lomitapide; Lurasidone; Moderate Risk QTc-Prolonging Agents; P-glycoprotein/ABCB1 Substrates; Pimecrolimus; Pimozide; Pomalidomide; Prucalopride; QuiNIDine; Rivaroxaban; Salmeterol; Saxagliptin; Silodosin; Sirolimus; Tacrolimus (Systemic); Tolvaptan; Topotecan; Vilazodone; VinCRIStine (Liposomal); Vitamin K Antagonists

The levels/effects of Crizotinib may be increased by: CYP3A4 Inhibitors (Moderate); CYP3A4 Inhibitors (Strong); Dasatinib; Grapefruit Juice; Ivabradine; Ivacaftor; Mifepristone; P-glycoprotein/ABCB1 Inhibitors; QTc-Prolonging Agents (Indeterminate Risk and Risk Modifying)

Decreased Effect
Crizotinib may decrease the levels/effects of: Cardiac Glycosides; Ifosfamide; Vitamin K Antagonists

The levels/effects of Crizotinib may be decreased by: CYP3A4 Inducers (Strong); Deferasirox; P-glycoprotein/ABCB1 Inducers; St Johns Wort; Tocilizumab

Ethanol/Nutrition/Herb Interactions
Food: Grapefruit juice may increase serum crizotinib levels. Management: Avoid grapefruit and grapefruit juice.
Herb/Nutraceutical: St John's wort may decrease the serum concentration of crizotinib. Management: Avoid St John's wort.

Dietary Considerations May be taken with or without food. Avoid grapefruit and grapefruit juice.

Pharmacodynamics/Kinetics
Half-life Elimination Terminal: 42 hours
Time to Peak 4-6 hours

Pregnancy Risk Factor D
Pregnancy Considerations Embryotoxicity and fetal toxicity were observed in animal reproduction studies. Based on the mechanism of action, crizotinib may cause fetal harm if administered during pregnancy. Women of childbearing potential and men of reproductive potential should use adequate contraception methods during and for at least 90 days after treatment.

Lactation Excretion in breast milk unknown/not recommended
Breast-Feeding Considerations It is not known if crizotinib is excreted in breast milk. According to the manufacturer, the decision to discontinue crizotinib treatment or to discontinue breast-feeding should take into account the benefits of treatment to the mother.

Prescribing and Access Restrictions Available through specialty pharmacies. Further information may be obtained from the manufacturer, Pfizer, at 1-877-744-5675, or at http://www.pfizerpro.com
Dosage Forms
Capsule, oral:
Xalkori® 200 mg, 250 mg

Dental Comment Crizotinib is known to prolong the QT interval. The QT interval is measured as the time and distance between the Q point of the QRS complex and the end of the T wave in the ECG tracing. After adjustment for heart rate, the QT interval is defined as prolonged if it is more than 450 msec in men and 460 msec in women. A long QT syndrome was first described in the 1950s and 60s as a congenital syndrome involving QT interval prolongation and syncope and sudden death. Some of the congenital long QT syndromes were characterized by a peculiar electrocardiographic appearance of the QRS complex involving a premature atria beat followed by a pause, then a subsequent sinus beat showing marked QT prolongation and deformity. This type of cardiac arrhythmia was originally termed "torsade de pointes" (translated from the French as "twisting of the points"). Crizotinib is considered as having a risk of causing torsade de pointes. Since it is not known what effect vasoconstrictors in the local anesthetic regimen will have in patients with a known history of congenital prolonged QT interval or in patients taking any medication that prolongs the QT interval, a medical consult is suggested.

Crofelemer (kroe FEL e mer)

Brand Names: U.S. Fulyzaq™
Pharmacologic Category Antidiarrheal
Use Symptomatic relief of noninfectious diarrhea in patients with HIV/AIDS on antiretroviral therapy
Local Anesthetic/Vasoconstrictor Precautions No information available to require special precautions
Effects on Dental Treatment Key adverse event(s) related to dental treatment: Xerostomia and changes in salivation (normal salivary flow resumes upon discontinuation)
Effects on Bleeding No information available to require special precautions
Adverse Effects 1% to 10%:
Central nervous system: Anxiety (2%), depression (1% to 2%), dizziness (1% to 2%)
Dermatologic: Acne (1% to 2%), dermatitis (1% to 2%)
Gastrointestinal: Flatulence (3%), nausea (3%), abdominal distention (2%), giardiasis (2%), hemorrhoids (2%), abdominal pain (1% to 2%), constipation (1% to 2%), dyspepsia (1% to 2%), gastroenteritis (1% to 2%), xerostomia (1% to 2%)
Genitourinary: Urinary tract infection (2%), pollakiuria (1% to 2%)
Hematologic: Leukopenia (1% to 2%)
Hepatic: Hyperbilirubinemia (1% to 3%), ALT increased (2%), AST increased (1% to 2%)
Neuromuscular & skeletal: Arthralgia (3%), back pain (3%), musculoskeletal pain (2%), limb pain (1% to 2%)
Renal: Nephrolithiasis (1% to 2%)
Respiratory: Upper respiratory tract infection (6%), bronchitis (4%), cough (4%), nasopharyngitis (2%), sinusitis (1% to 2%)
Miscellaneous: Herpes zoster (1% to 2%), seasonal allergy (1% to 2%)
General Dosage Range Oral: *Adults:* 125 mg twice daily
Mechanism of Action Inhibits cyclic adenosine monophosphate (cAMP)-stimulated cystic fibrosis transmembrane conductance regulator (CFTR) chloride ion channel and calcium activated chloride ion channels at the enterocyte luminal membrane. This regulates fluid secretion and water loss (high volume) due to diarrhea, normalizing chloride ion and water flow in the GI tract.

Pregnancy Risk Factor C
Pregnancy Considerations Adverse events were observed in some animal reproduction studies; however, maternal toxicity was also present. Systemic absorption following oral administration is limited.
Product Availability Fulyzaq™: FDA approved December 2012; anticipated availability is early March 2013

Cromolyn (Systemic, Oral Inhalation) (KROE moe lin)

Related Information
Respiratory Diseases *on page 1514*
Brand Names: U.S. Gastrocrom®
Brand Names: Canada Nalcrom®; Nu-Cromolyn; PMS-Sodium Cromoglycate
Pharmacologic Category Mast Cell Stabilizer
Use
Inhalation: May be used as an adjunct in the prophylaxis of allergic disorders, including asthma; prevention of exercise-induced bronchospasm
Oral: Systemic mastocytosis
Unlabeled Use Oral: Food allergy, treatment of inflammatory bowel disease
Local Anesthetic/Vasoconstrictor Precautions No information available to require special precautions
Effects on Dental Treatment Key adverse event(s) related to dental treatment:
Inhalation: Unpleasant taste.
Systemic: Glossitis, stomatitis, and unpleasant taste.
Effects on Bleeding No information available to require special precautions
Adverse Effects Frequency not defined.
Cardiovascular: Angioedema, chest pain, edema, flushing, palpitation, premature ventricular contractions, tachycardia
Central nervous system: Anxiety, behavior changes, convulsions, depression, dizziness, fatigue, hallucinations, headache, irritability, insomnia, lethargy, migraine, nervousness, hypoesthesia, postprandial lightheadedness, psychosis
Dermatologic: Erythema, photosensitivity, pruritus, purpura, rash, urticaria
Gastrointestinal: Abdominal pain, constipation, diarrhea, dyspepsia, dysphagia, esophagospasm, flatulence, glossitis, nausea, stomatitis, vomiting
Genitourinary: Dysuria, urinary frequency
Hematologic: Neutropenia, pancytopenia, polycythemia
Hepatic: Liver function test abnormal
Local: Burning
Neuromuscular & skeletal: Arthralgia, leg stiffness, leg weakness, myalgia, paresthesia
Otic: Tinnitus
Respiratory: Dyspnea, pharyngitis
Miscellaneous: Lupus erythematosus
General Dosage Range
Inhalation: Nebulization: *Children ≥2 years and Adults:* Initial: 20 mg 4 times/day; Maintenance: 20 mg 3-4 times/day **or** 20 mg prior to exercise or allergen exposure
Oral:
Children 2-12 years: 100 mg 4 times/day (maximum: 40 mg/kg/day)
Children >12 years and Adults: 200 mg 4 times/day (maximum: 40 mg/kg/day)

Mechanism of Action Prevents the mast cell release of histamine, leukotrienes, and slow-reacting substance of anaphylaxis by inhibiting degranulation after contact with antigens

Pharmacodynamics/Kinetics

Onset of Action Response to treatment: Oral: May occur within 2-6 weeks

Half-life Elimination 80-90 minutes

Time to Peak Serum: Inhalation: ~15 minutes

Pregnancy Risk Factor B

Pregnancy Considerations Adverse events were not observed in animal reproduction studies. No data available on whether cromolyn crosses the placenta or clinical effects on the fetus. Available evidence suggests safe use during pregnancy.

Crotamiton (kroe TAM i tonn)

Brand Names: U.S. Eurax®

Brand Names: Canada Eurax Cream

Pharmacologic Category Scabicidal Agent

Use Treatment of scabies (*Sarcoptes scabiei*) and symptomatic treatment of pruritus

Local Anesthetic/Vasoconstrictor Precautions No information available to require special precautions

Effects on Dental Treatment No significant effects or complications reported

Effects on Bleeding No information available to require special precautions

Adverse Effects Frequency not defined. Topical:
Dermatologic: Contact dermatitis, pruritus, rash
Local: Local irritation
Miscellaneous: Allergic sensitivity reactions, warm sensation

General Dosage Range Topical: *Children and Adults:* Pruritus: Massage into affected areas as needed; Scabies: Apply a thin layer from the neck to the toes, repeat in 24 hours; take a cleansing bath 48 hours after final application, may repeat after 7-10 days

Mechanism of Action Crotamiton has scabicidal activity against *Sarcoptes scabiei*; mechanism of action unknown

Pregnancy Risk Factor C

Pregnancy Considerations Animal reproduction studies have not been conducted; use during pregnancy only if clearly needed.

Cyanocobalamin (sye an oh koe BAL a min)

Brand Names: U.S. Ener-B® [OTC]; Nascobal®; Twelve Resin-K [OTC]

Generic Availability (U.S.) Yes: Excludes nasal spray

Pharmacologic Category Vitamin, Water Soluble

Use Treatment of pernicious anemia; vitamin B_{12} deficiency due to dietary deficiencies or malabsorption diseases, inadequate secretion of intrinsic factor, and inadequate utilization of B_{12} (eg, during neoplastic treatment); increased B_{12} requirements due to pregnancy, thyrotoxicosis, hemorrhage, malignancy, liver or kidney disease

Local Anesthetic/Vasoconstrictor Precautions No information available to require special precautions

Effects on Dental Treatment No significant effects or complications reported

Effects on Bleeding No information available to require special precautions

Adverse Effects Frequency not defined.
Cardiovascular: CHF, peripheral vascular disorder, peripheral vascular thrombosis
Central nervous system: Anxiety, dizziness, headache, hypoesthesia, incoordination, pain, nervousness
Dermatologic: Itching, urticaria, exanthema (transient)
Gastrointestinal: Diarrhea, dyspepsia, glossitis, nausea, sore throat, vomiting
Hematologic: Polycythemia vera
Neuromuscular & skeletal: Abnormal gait, arthritis, back pain, myalgia, paresthesia, weakness
Respiratory: Dyspnea, pulmonary edema, rhinitis
Miscellaneous: Anaphylaxis (parenteral) and infection

Dosage

Adequate intake:
Children:
0-6 months: 0.4 mcg/day
7-12 months: 0.5 mcg/day

Recommended intake:
Children:
1-3 years: 0.9 mcg/day
4-8 years: 1.2 mcg/day
9-13 years: 1.8 mcg/day
Children >14 years and Adults: 2.4 mcg/day
Pregnancy: 2.6 mcg/day
Lactation: 2.8 mcg/day

Vitamin B_{12} deficiency:
I.M., deep SubQ:
Children (dosage not well established): 0.2 mcg/kg for 2 days, followed by 1000 mcg/day for 2-7 days, followed by 100 mcg/week for one month; for malabsorptive causes of B_{12} deficiency, monthly maintenance doses of 100 mcg have been recommended **or** as an alternative 100 mcg/day for 10-15 days, then once or twice weekly for several months
Adults: Initial: 30 mcg/day for 5-10 days; maintenance: 100-200 mcg/month
Intranasal: Adults (Nascobal®): 500 mcg in one nostril once weekly
Oral: Adults: 250 mcg/day

Pernicious anemia: I.M., deep SubQ (administer concomitantly with folic acid if needed, 1 mg/day for 1 month):
Children: 30-50 mcg/day for 2 or more weeks (to a total dose of 1000-5000 mcg), then follow with 100 mcg/month as maintenance dosage
Adults: 100 mcg/day for 6-7 days; if improvement, administer same dose on alternate days for 7 doses, then every 3-4 days for 2-3 weeks; once hematologic values have returned to normal, maintenance dosage: 100 mcg/month. **Note:** Alternative dosing of 1000 mcg/day for 5 days (followed by 500-1000 mcg/month) has been used.
Hematologic remission (without evidence of nervous system involvement): Adults:
Intranasal (Nascobal®): 500 mcg in one nostril once weekly
Oral: 1000-2000 mcg/day
I.M., SubQ: 100-1000 mcg/month

Dosage adjustment in renal impairment: No dosage adjustment provided in manufacturer's labeling. Use with caution; some formulations may also contain aluminum, which may accumulate in renal impairment.

Dosage adjustment in hepatic impairment: No dosage adjustment provided in manufacturer's labeling.

Mechanism of Action Coenzyme for various metabolic functions, including fat and carbohydrate metabolism and protein synthesis, used in cell replication and hematopoiesis

357

◄

Contraindications Hypersensitivity to cyanocobalamin, cobalt, or any component of the formulation

Warnings/Precautions I.M./SubQ routes are used to treat pernicious anemia; oral and intranasal administration are not indicated until hematologic remission and no signs of nervous system involvement. Treatment of severe vitamin B_{12} megaloblastic anemia may result in thrombocytosis and severe hypokalemia, sometimes fatal, due to intracellular potassium shift upon anemia resolution. Vitamin B_{12} deficiency masks signs of polycythemia vera; use caution in other conditions where folic acid or vitamin B_{12} administration alone might mask true diagnosis, despite hematologic response. Vitamin B_{12} deficiency for >3 months results in irreversible degenerative CNS lesions; neurologic manifestations will not be prevented with folic acid unless vitamin B_{12} is also given. Spinal cord degeneration might also occur when folic acid used as a substitute for vitamin B_{12} in anemia prevention. Use caution in Leber's disease patients; B_{12} treatment may result in rapid optic atrophy. Some parenteral products contain aluminum; use caution in patients with impaired renal function and neonates. Some products contain benzyl alcohol which has been associated with "gasping syndrome" in neonates. Avoid intravenous route; anaphylactic shock has occurred. Intradermal test dose of vitamin B_{12} is recommended for any patient suspected of cyanocobalamin sensitivity prior to intranasal or injectable administration. Efficacy of intranasal products in patients with nasal pathology or with other concomitant intranasal therapy has not been determined.

Drug Interactions

Metabolism/Transport Effects None known.

Avoid Concomitant Use There are no known interactions where it is recommended to avoid concomitant use.

Increased Effect/Toxicity There are no known significant interactions involving an increase in effect.

Decreased Effect

The levels/effects of Cyanocobalamin may be decreased by: Chloramphenicol; Colchicine

Ethanol/Nutrition/Herb Interactions Ethanol: Heavy consumption >2 weeks may impair vitamin B_{12} absorption.

Dietary Considerations Strict vegetarian diets (eg, without eggs or dairy products) may result in vitamin B_{12} deficiency.

Pregnancy Considerations Animal reproduction studies have not been conducted. Water soluble vitamins cross the placenta. Absorption of vitamin B_{12} may increase during pregnancy. Vitamin B_{12} requirements may be increased in pregnant women compared to nonpregnant women. Serum concentrations of vitamin B_{12} are higher in the neonate at birth than the mother (IOM, 1998).

Lactation Enters breast milk/compatible

Breast-Feeding Considerations Vitamin B_{12} is found in breast milk. Milk concentrations are similar to maternal serum concentrations and concentrations may be decreased in women who are vegetarians. Vitamin B_{12} requirements may be increased in nursing women compared to non-nursing women (IOM, 1998).

Dosage Forms

Injection, solution: 1000 mcg/mL (1 mL, 10 mL, 30 mL)

Lozenge, oral: 50 mcg (100s); 100 mcg (100s); 250 mcg (100s, 250s); 500 mcg (100s, 250s)

Lozenge, sublingual: 500 mcg (100s)

Solution, intranasal:

Nascobal®: 500 mcg/spray (2.3 mL)

Tablet, for buccal application/oral/sublingual:

Twelve Resin-K [OTC]: 1000 mcg

Tablet, oral: 50 mcg, 100 mcg, 250 mcg, 500 mcg, 1000 mcg

Ener-B® [OTC]: 100 mcg, 500 mcg, 1000 mcg

Tablet, sublingual: 1000 mcg, 2500 mcg, 5000 mcg

Tablet, timed release, oral: 1000 mcg

Ener-B® [OTC]: 1500 mcg

Cyclizine (SYE kli zeen)

Brand Names: U.S. Bonine® for Kids [OTC] [DSC]; Cyclivert® [OTC]; Marezine® [OTC]

Pharmacologic Category Histamine H_1 Antagonist; Histamine H_1 Antagonist, First Generation; Piperazine Derivative

Use Prevention and treatment of nausea, vomiting, and vertigo associated with motion sickness

Local Anesthetic/Vasoconstrictor Precautions No information available to require special precautions

Effects on Dental Treatment Key adverse event(s) related to dental treatment: Xerostomia (normal salivary flow resumes upon discontinuation).

Effects on Bleeding No information available to require special precautions

Adverse Effects

>10%:

Central nervous system: Drowsiness

Gastrointestinal: Xerostomia

1% to 10%:

Central nervous system: Headache

Dermatologic: Dermatitis

Gastrointestinal: Nausea

Genitourinary: Urinary retention

Ocular: Diplopia

Renal: Polyuria

General Dosage Range Oral:

Children 6-12 years: 25 mg up to 3 times/day (maximum: 75 mg/day)

Adults: 50 mg prior to departure; may repeat in 4-6 hours if needed (maximum: 200 mg/day)

Mechanism of Action Cyclizine is a piperazine derivative with properties of histamines. The precise mechanism of action in inhibiting the symptoms of motion sickness is not known. It may have effects directly on the labyrinthine apparatus and central actions on the labyrinthine apparatus and on the chemoreceptor trigger zone. Cyclizine exerts a central anticholinergic action.

Pharmacodynamics/Kinetics

Half-life Elimination Cyclizine: ~14 hours; Norcyclizine: ~24 hours; Norchlorcyclizine: ~6 days (Paton, 1985; Walker, 1996)

Pregnancy Considerations An increased risk of birth defects following maternal cyclizine use has generally not been observed. Although cyclizine has been evaluated for the treatment of nausea and vomiting in pregnancy, it is not currently recommended for this indication (consult current guidelines).

Cyclobenzaprine (sye kloe BEN za preen)

Related Information

Temporomandibular Dysfunction (TMD), Chronic Pain, and Fibromyalgia *on page 1590*

Brand Names: U.S. Amrix®; Fexmid® [DSC]; Flexeril®

Brand Names: Canada Apo-Cyclobenzaprine®; Auro-Cyclobenzaprine; Ava-Cyclobenzaprine; Dom-Cyclobenzaprine; JAMP-Cyclobenzaprine; Mylan-Cyclobenzaprine; Novo-Cycloprine; Nu-Cyclobenzaprine; PHL-Cyclobenzaprine; PMS-Cyclobenzaprine; Q-Cyclobenzaprine; ratio-Cyclobenzaprine; Riva-Cycloprine; ZYM-Cyclobenzaprine

Generic Availability (U.S.) Yes: Tablet

Pharmacologic Category Skeletal Muscle Relaxant

Dental Use Treatment of muscle spasm associated with acute temporomandibular joint pain (TMJ)

Use Treatment of muscle spasm associated with acute, painful musculoskeletal conditions

Unlabeled Use Treatment of muscle spasm associated with acute temporomandibular joint pain (TMJ)

Local Anesthetic/Vasoconstrictor Precautions No information available to require special precautions

Effects on Dental Treatment Key adverse event(s) related to dental treatment: Xerostomia and changes in salivation (normal salivary flow resumes upon discontinuation).

Effects on Bleeding No information available to require special precautions

Adverse Effects
>10%:
Central nervous system: Drowsiness (29% to 39%), dizziness (1% to 11%)
Gastrointestinal: Xerostomia (21% to 32%)
1% to 10%:
Central nervous system: Fatigue (1% to 6%), headache (1% to 5%), confusion (1% to 3%), irritability (1% to 3%), mental acuity decreased (1% to 3%), nervousness (1% to 3%), somnolence (1% to 2%)
Gastrointestinal: Dyspepsia (≤4%), abdominal pain (1% to 3%), constipation (1% to 3%), diarrhea (1% to 3%), gastric regurgitation (1% to 3%), nausea (1% to 3%), unpleasant taste (1% to 3%)
Neuromuscular & skeletal: Weakness (1% to 3%)
Ocular: Blurred vision (1% to 3%)
Respiratory: Pharyngitis (1% to 3%), upper respiratory infection (1% to 3%)

Dental Usual Dosage Treatment of muscle spasm associated with acute TMJ pain (**Note:** Do not use longer than 2-3 weeks): Oral:
Adults: Initial: 5 mg 3 times/day; may increase to 7.5-10 mg 3 times/day if needed
Elderly: 5 mg 3 times/day; plasma concentration and incidence of adverse effects are increased in the elderly; dose should be titrated slowly

Dosage Oral: Muscle spasm: **Note:** Do not use longer than 2-3 weeks
Capsule, extended release:
Adults: Usual: 15 mg once daily; some patients may require up to 30 mg once daily
Elderly: Use not recommended
Tablet, immediate release:
Children ≥15 years and Adults: Initial: 5 mg 3 times/day; may increase up to 10 mg 3 times/day if needed
Elderly: Initial: 5 mg; titrate dose slowly and consider less frequent dosing

Dosage adjustment in renal impairment: No dosage adjustment provided in manufacturer's labeling.

Dosage adjustment in hepatic impairment:
Capsule, extended release: Mild-to-severe impairment: Use not recommended.

Tablet, immediate release:
Mild impairment: Initial: 5 mg; use with caution; titrate slowly and consider less frequent dosing
Moderate-to-severe impairment: Use not recommended

Mechanism of Action Centrally-acting skeletal muscle relaxant pharmacologically related to tricyclic antidepressants; reduces tonic somatic motor activity influencing both alpha and gamma motor neurons

Contraindications Hypersensitivity to cyclobenzaprine or any component of the formulation; during or within 14 days of MAO inhibitors; hyperthyroidism; congestive heart failure; arrhythmias; heart block or conduction disturbances; acute recovery phase of MI

Warnings/Precautions May cause CNS depression, which may impair physical or mental abilities; patients must be cautioned about performing tasks which require mental alertness (eg, operating machinery or driving). Cyclobenzaprine shares the toxic potentials of the tricyclic antidepressants (including arrhythmias, tachycardia, and conduction time prolongation) and the usual precautions of tricyclic antidepressant therapy should be observed; use with caution in patients with urinary hesitancy or retention, angle-closure glaucoma or increased intraocular pressure, hepatic impairment, or in the elderly. Muscle relaxants are poorly tolerated by the elderly due to potent anticholinergic effects, sedation, and risk of fracture. Efficacy is questionable at dosages tolerated by elderly patients; avoid use (Beers Criteria). Extended release capsules not recommended for use in mild-to-severe hepatic impairment or in the elderly. Do not use concomitantly or within 14 days after MAO inhibitors; combination may cause hypertensive crisis, severe convulsions. Effects may be potentiated when used with other CNS depressants or ethanol.

Drug Interactions
Metabolism/Transport Effects Substrate of CYP1A2 (major), CYP2D6 (minor), CYP3A4 (minor); **Note:** Assignment of Major/Minor substrate status based on clinically relevant drug interaction potential

Avoid Concomitant Use
Avoid concomitant use of Cyclobenzaprine with any of the following: Aclidinium; Azelastine (Nasal); Ipratropium (Oral Inhalation); MAO Inhibitors; Paraldehyde; Tiotropium

Increased Effect/Toxicity
Cyclobenzaprine may increase the levels/effects of: Alcohol (Ethyl); Anticholinergics; Azelastine (Nasal); Buprenorphine; CNS Depressants; MAO Inhibitors; Metoclopramide; Metyrosine; Paraldehyde; Pramipexole; ROPINIRole; Rotigotine; Serotonin Modulators; Tiotropium; TraMADol; Zolpidem

The levels/effects of Cyclobenzaprine may be increased by: Abiraterone Acetate; Aclidinium; Antipsychotics; CYP1A2 Inhibitors (Moderate); CYP1A2 Inhibitors (Strong); Deferasirox; HydrOXYzine; Ipratropium (Oral Inhalation); Magnesium Sulfate; Perampanel; Pramlintide; Sodium Oxybate

Decreased Effect
Cyclobenzaprine may decrease the levels/effects of: Acetylcholinesterase Inhibitors (Central)

The levels/effects of Cyclobenzaprine may be decreased by: Acetylcholinesterase Inhibitors (Central); Peginterferon Alfa-2b

Ethanol/Nutrition/Herb Interactions
Ethanol: May increase CNS depression; monitor for increased effects with coadministration. Caution patients about effects.

◀ Food: Food increases bioavailability (peak plasma concentrations increased by 35% and area under the curve by 20%) of the extended release capsule.

Herb/Nutraceutical: Avoid valerian, kava kava, gotu kola (may increase CNS depression).

Pharmacodynamics/Kinetics

Half-life Elimination Range: 8-37 hours; Immediate release tablet: 18 hours; Extended release capsule: 32-33 hours

Time to Peak Extended release capsule: 7-8 hours

Pregnancy Risk Factor B

Pregnancy Considerations Teratogenic effects were not observed in animal studies. There are no adequate and well-controlled studies in pregnant women. Use during pregnancy only if clearly needed.

Lactation Excretion in breast milk unknown/use caution

Dosage Forms

Capsule, extended release, oral:
Amrix®: 15 mg, 30 mg

Tablet, oral: 5 mg, 7.5 mg, 10 mg
Flexeril®: 5 mg, 10 mg

Cyclopentolate (sye kloe PEN toe late)

Brand Names: U.S. AK-Pentolate™; Cyclogyl®

Brand Names: Canada AK Pentolate Oph Soln; Cyclogyl®; Diopentolate®; Minims Cyclopentolate; PMS-Cyclopentolate

Pharmacologic Category Anticholinergic Agent, Ophthalmic

Use Diagnostic procedures requiring mydriasis and cycloplegia

Local Anesthetic/Vasoconstrictor Precautions No information available to require special precautions

Effects on Dental Treatment No significant effects or complications reported

Effects on Bleeding No information available to require special precautions

Adverse Effects 1% to 10%:

Cardiovascular: Tachycardia

Central nervous system: Ataxia, hallucinations, hyperactivity, incoherent speech, psychosis, restlessness, seizure

Dermatologic: Burning sensation

Ocular: Intraocular pressure increased, loss of visual accommodation

Miscellaneous: Allergic reaction

General Dosage Range Ophthalmic:

Children: Instill 1 drop of 0.5%, 1%, or 2% in eye followed by 1 drop of 0.5% or 1% in 5 minutes, if necessary

Adults: Instill 1 drop of 1% followed by another drop in 5 minutes; 2% solution in heavily pigmented iris

Mechanism of Action Prevents the muscle of the ciliary body and the sphincter muscle of the iris from responding to cholinergic stimulation, causing mydriasis and cycloplegia

Pharmacodynamics/Kinetics

Onset of Action Peak effect: Cycloplegia: 25-75 minutes; Mydriasis: 30-60 minutes

Duration of Action ≤24 hours

Pregnancy Risk Factor C

Pregnancy Considerations Animal reproduction studies have not been conducted.

Cyclopentolate and Phenylephrine (sye kloe PEN toe late & fen il EF rin)

Related Information

Cyclopentolate *on page 360*

Brand Names: U.S. Cyclomydril®

Pharmacologic Category Ophthalmic Agent, Antiglaucoma

Use Induce mydriasis greater than that produced with cyclopentolate HCl alone

Local Anesthetic/Vasoconstrictor Precautions No information available to require special precautions

Effects on Dental Treatment No significant effects or complications reported

Effects on Bleeding No information available to require special precautions

Adverse Effects See individual agents.

General Dosage Range Ophthalmic: *Children and Adults:* Instill 1 drop into eyes every 5-10 minutes, for up to 3 doses

Pregnancy Risk Factor C

Pregnancy Considerations Animal reproduction studies have not been conducted with this combination.

Cyclophosphamide (sye kloe FOS fa mide)

Brand Names: Canada Procytox®

Generic Availability (U.S.) Yes

Pharmacologic Category Antineoplastic Agent, Alkylating Agent; Antirheumatic Miscellaneous; Immunosuppressant Agent

Dental Use Treatment of Wegener's granulomatosis, systemic lupus erythematosus

Use

Oncology-related uses: Treatment of Hodgkin lymphoma, non-Hodgkin lymphomas (including Burkitt's lymphoma), chronic lymphocytic leukemia (CLL), chronic myelocytic leukemia (CML), acute myelocytic leukemia (AML), acute lymphoblastic leukemia (ALL), mycosis fungoides, multiple myeloma, neuroblastoma, retinoblastoma; breast cancer; ovarian adenocarcinoma

Canadian labeling: Additional use (not in U.S. labeling): Treatment of lung cancer

Nononcology uses: Treatment of refractory nephrotic syndrome in children who are unresponsive or intolerant to corticosteroid therapy

Unlabeled Use

Oncology-related uses: Ewing's sarcoma, rhabdomyosarcoma, Wilms tumor, ovarian germ cell tumors, gestational trophoblastic tumors (high-risk), small cell lung cancer, testicular cancer, pheochromocytoma, hematopoietic stem cell transplant (HSCT) conditioning regimen

Nononcology uses: Severe rheumatoid disorders, granulomatosis with polyangiitis (GPA; Wegener's granulomatosis), myasthenia gravis, multiple sclerosis, lupus nephritis, autoimmune hemolytic anemia, idiopathic thrombocytic purpura (ITP), antibody-induced pure red cell aplasia

Local Anesthetic/Vasoconstrictor Precautions No information available to require special precautions

Effects on Dental Treatment Key adverse event(s) related to dental treatment: Mucositis and stomatitis.

Effects on Bleeding Hematologic toxicities including thrombocytopenia are among the important dose-limiting effects of cyclophosphamide. A medical consult is recommended.

Adverse Effects Frequency not defined.

Dermatologic: Alopecia (reversible; onset: 3-6 weeks after start of treatment)

Endocrine & metabolic: Amenorrhea, azoospermia, gonadal suppression, oligospermia, oogenesis impaired, sterility

Gastrointestinal: Abdominal pain, anorexia, diarrhea, mucositis, nausea/vomiting (dose-related), stomatitis

Genitourinary: Hemorrhagic cystitis

Hematologic: Anemia, leukopenia (dose-related; recovery: 7-10 days after cessation), myelosuppression, neutropenia, neutropenic fever, thrombocytopenia

Miscellaneous: Infection

Dosage Details concerning dosing in combination regimens should also be consulted. Antiemetics may be recommended (emetogenic potential varies by dose and combination therapy).

Children:

U.S. labeling:

Malignancy, solid tumor (single agent):

I.V.: 40-50 mg/kg in divided doses over 2-5 days **or** 10-15 mg/kg every 7-10 days **or** 3-5 mg/kg twice weekly

Oral: 1-5 mg/kg/day (initial and maintenance dosing)

Nephrotic syndrome, corticosteroid refractory or intolerant: Oral: 2.5-3 mg/kg/day every day for 60-90 days

Canadian labeling:

I.V.: Initial: 2-8 mg/kg (60-250 mg/m^2) in divided doses for 6 or more days; Maintenance: 10-15 mg/kg every 7-10 days or 30 mg/kg every 3-4 weeks or when bone marrow function recovers

Oral: Initial: 2-8 mg/kg (60-250 mg/m^2) in divided doses for 6 or more days; Maintenance: 2-5 mg/kg (50-150 mg/m^2) twice weekly

Indication specific and/or unlabeled uses/dosing:

Ewing's sarcoma (unlabeled use): I.V.: VAC/IE regimen: VAC: 1200 mg/m^2 (plus mesna) on day 1 of a 21-day treatment cycle (in combination with vincristine and doxorubicin [then dactinomycin when maximum doxorubicin dose reached]), alternates with IE (ifosfamide and etoposide) for a total of 17 cycles (Grier, 2003)

Hodgkin lymphoma (unlabeled dosing): I.V.: BEACOPP escalated regimen: 1200 mg/m^2 on day 0 of a 21-day treatment cycle (in combination with bleomycin, etoposide, doxorubicin, vincristine, prednisone, and procarbazine) for 4 cycles (Kelly, 2011)

Lupus nephritis (unlabeled use): I.V.: 500-1000 mg/m^2 every month for 6 months, then every 3 months for a total of 2.5-3 years (Austin, 1986; Gourley, 1996; Lehman, 2000)

Neuroblastoma (unlabeled dosing): I.V.: CE-CAdO regimen, courses 3 and 4: 300 mg/m^2 days 1-5 every 21 days for 2 cycles (Rubie, 1998) **or** 10 mg/kg days 1-5 every 21 days for 2 cycles (Rubie, 2001). **Note:** Decreased doses may be recommended for newborns or children <10 kg.

Transplant conditioning (unlabeled use): Myeloablative transplant: I.V.: 50 mg/kg/day for 4 days beginning 5 days before transplant (with or without antithymocyte globulin [equine]) (Champlin, 2007)

Adults:

U.S. labeling:

Single agent for solid tumors:

I.V.: 40-50 mg/kg in divided doses over 2-5 days **or** 10-15 mg/kg every 7-10 days **or** 3-5 mg/kg twice weekly

Oral: 1-5 mg/kg/day (initial and maintenance dosing)

Canadian labeling:

I.V.: Initial: 40-50 mg/kg (1500-1800 mg/m^2) administered as 10-20 mg/kg/day over 2-5 days; Maintenance: 10-15 mg/kg (350-550 mg/m^2) every 7-10 days **or** 3-5 mg/kg (110-185 mg/m^2) twice weekly

Oral: Initial 1-5 mg/kg/day (depending on tolerance); Maintenance: 1-5 mg/kg/day

Indication specific and/or unlabeled uses/dosing:

Acute lymphoblastic leukemia (unlabeled dosing): Multiple-agent regimens:

Hyper-CVAD regimen: I.V.: 300 mg/m^2 over 3 hours (with mesna) every 12 hours for 6 doses on days 1, 2, and 3 during odd-numbered cycles (cycles 1, 3, 5, 7) of an 8-cycle phase (Kantarjian, 2004)

Larson (CALGB8811) regimen: I.V.:

Adults <60 years: Induction phase: 1200 mg/m^2 on day 1 of a 4-week cycle; Early intensification phase: 1000 mg/m^2 on day 1 of a 4-week cycle (repeat once); Late intensification phase: 1000 mg/m^2 on day 29 of an 8-week cycle (Larson, 1995)

Adults ≥60 years: Induction phase: 800 mg/m^2 on day 1 of a 4-week cycle; Early intensification phase: 1000 mg/m^2 on day 1 of a 4-week cycle (repeat once); Late intensification phase: 1000 mg/m^2 on day 29 of an 8-week cycle (Larson, 1995)

Breast cancer (unlabeled dosing):

AC regimen: I.V.: 600 mg/m^2 on day 1 every 21 days (in combination with doxorubicin) for 4 cycles (Fisher, 1990)

CEF regimen: Oral: 75 mg/m^2/day days 1-14 every 28 days (in combination with epirubicin and fluorouracil) for 6 cycles (Levine, 1998)

CMF regimen: Oral: 100 mg/m^2/day days 1-14 every 28 days (in combination with methotrexate and fluorouracil) for 6 cycles (Levine, 1998) **or** I.V.: 600 mg/m^2 on day 1 every 21 days (in combination with methotrexate and fluorouracil); Goldhirsch, 1998)

Chronic lymphocytic leukemia (unlabeled dosing): I.V.: R-FC regimen: 250 mg/m^2/day for 3 days every 28 days (in combination with rituximab and fludarabine) for 6 cycles (Robak, 2010)

Ewing's sarcoma (unlabeled use): I.V.: VAC/IE regimen: VAC: 1200 mg/m^2 (plus mesna) on day 1 of a 21-day treatment cycle (in combination with vincristine and doxorubicin [then dactinomycin when maximum doxorubicin dose reached]), alternates with IE (ifosfamide and etoposide) for a total of 17 cycles (Grier, 2003)

Gestational trophoblastic tumors, high-risk (unlabeled use): I.V.: EMA/CO regimen: 600 mg/m^2 on day 8 of 2-week treatment cycle (in combination with etoposide, methotrexate, dactinomycin, and vincristine), continue for at least 2 treatment cycles after a normal hCG level (Escobar, 2003)

Granulomatosis with polyangiitis (GPA; Wegener's granulomatosis) (unlabeled use; in combination with glucocorticoids):

Low-dose: Oral: 1.5-2 mg/kg/day (Jayne, 2003; Stone, 2010) or 2 mg/kg/day until remission, followed by 1.5 mg/kg/day for 3 additional months (de Groot, 2009; Harper, 2012)

Pulse: I.V.: 15 mg/kg (maximum dose: 1200 mg) every 2 weeks for 3 doses, followed by maintenance pulses of either 15 mg/kg I.V. (maximum dose: 1200 mg) every 3 weeks or 2.5-5 mg/kg/day orally on days 1, 2, and 3 every 3 weeks for 3 months after remission achieved (de Groot, 2009; Harper, 2012)

Hodgkin lymphoma (unlabeled dosing): I.V.:

BEACOPP regimen: 650 mg/m² on day 1 every 3 weeks (in combination with bleomycin, etoposide, doxorubicin, vincristine, procarbazine, and prednisone) for 8 cycles (Diehl, 2003)

BEACOPP escalated regimen: 1200 mg/m² on day 1 every 3 weeks (in combination with bleomycin, etoposide, doxorubicin, vincristine, procarbazine, and prednisone) for 8 cycles (Diehl, 2003)

Multiple myeloma (unlabeled dosing): Oral: CyBorD regimen: 300 mg/m² on days 1, 8, 15, and 22 every 4 weeks (in combination with bortezomib and dexamethasone) for 4 cycles; may continue beyond 4 cycles (Khan, 2012)

Non-Hodgkin lymphoma (unlabeled dosing): I.V.:

R-CHOP regimen: 750 mg/m² on day 1 every 3 weeks (in combination with rituximab, doxorubicin, vincristine, and prednisone) for 8 cycles (Coiffier, 2002)

R-EPOCH (dose adjusted) regimen: 750 mg/m² on day 5 every 3 weeks (in combination with rituximab, etoposide, prednisone, vincristine, and doxorubicin) for 6-8 cycles (Garcia-Suarez, 2007)

CODOX-M/IVAC (Burkitt's lymphoma): Cycles 1 and 3 (CODOX-M): 800 mg/m² on day 1, followed by 200 mg/m² on days 2-5 (in combination with vincristine, doxorubicin, and methotrexate); CODOX-M alternates with IVAC (etoposide, ifosfamide, and cytarabine) for a total of 4 cycles (Magrath, 1996)

Lupus nephritis (unlabeled use): I.V.: 500 mg once every 2 weeks for 6 doses or 500-1000 mg/m² once every month for 6 doses (Hahn, 2012) or 500-1000 mg/m² every month every month for 6 months, then every 3 months for a total of at least 2.5 years (Austin, 1986; Gourley, 1996)

Transplant conditioning (unlabeled use): I.V.:

Nonmyeloablative transplant (allogeneic): 750 mg/m²/day for 3 days beginning 5 days prior to transplant (in combination with fludarabine) (Khouri, 2008)

Myeloablative transplant:

100 mg/kg (based on IBW, unless actual weight <95% of IBW) as a single dose 2 days prior to transplant (in combination with total body irradiation and etoposide) (Thompson, 2008)

50 mg/kg/day for 4 days beginning 5 days before transplant (with or without antithymocyte globulin [equine]) (Champlin, 2007)

50 mg/kg/day for 4 days beginning 5 days prior to transplant (in combination with busulfan) (Cassileth, 1993)

60 mg/kg/day for 2 days (in combination with busulfan and total body irradiation) (Anderson, 1996)

1800 mg/m²/day for 4 days beginning 7 days prior to transplant (in combination with etoposide and carmustine) (Reece, 1991)

Elderly: Refer to adult dosing. Adjust dosing for renal clearance.

Dosage adjustment for toxicity:

Hematologic toxicity: May require dose reduction or treatment interruption; Canadian labeling recommends reducing initial dose by 30% to 50% if bone marrow function compromised (due to prior radiation therapy, prior chemotherapy, or tumor infiltration)

Hemorrhagic cystitis, severe: Discontinue treatment.

Dosage adjustment in renal impairment:

U.S. labeling: No adjustment provided in the manufacturer's labeling (use with caution; elevated levels of metabolites may occur).

Canadian labeling:

Mild impairment: No dosage adjustment provided in manufacturer's labeling

Moderate impairment: Dose reduction may be necessary; manufacturer's labeling does not provide specific dosing recommendations

Severe impairment: Use is contraindicated.

The following adjustments have also been recommended:

Aronoff, 2007: Children and Adults:

Cl_{cr} ≥10 mL/minute: No dosage adjustment required.

Cl_{cr} <10 mL/minute: Administer 75% of normal dose.

Hemodialysis: Moderately dialyzable (20% to 50%); administer 50% of normal dose; administer after hemodialysis

Continuous ambulatory peritoneal dialysis (CAPD): Administer 75% of normal dose.

Continuous renal replacement therapy (CRRT): Administer 100% of normal dose.

Janus, 2010: Hemodialysis: Administer 75% of normal dose; administer after hemodialysis

Dosage adjustment in hepatic impairment: The pharmacokinetics of cyclophosphamide are not significantly altered in the presence of hepatic insufficiency.

U.S. labeling: No dosage adjustment provided in the manufacturer's labeling.

Canadian labeling:

Mild-to-moderate impairment: No dosage adjustment provided in the manufacturer's labeling.

Severe impairment: Use is contraindicated.

The following adjustments have been recommended (Floyd, 2006):

Serum bilirubin 3.1-5 mg/dL or transaminases >3 times ULN: Administer 75% of dose.

Serum bilirubin >5 mg/mL: Avoid use.

Mechanism of Action Cyclophosphamide is an alkylating agent that prevents cell division by cross-linking DNA strands and decreasing DNA synthesis. It is a cell cycle phase nonspecific agent. Cyclophosphamide also possesses potent immunosuppressive activity. Cyclophosphamide is a prodrug that must be metabolized to active metabolites in the liver.

Contraindications

U.S. labeling: Hypersensitivity to cyclophosphamide or any component of the formulation; severely depressed bone marrow function

Canadian labeling: Hypersensitivity to cyclophosphamide or its metabolites, urinary outflow obstructions, severe myelosuppression, severe renal or hepatic impairment, active infection (especially varicella zoster), severe immunosuppression

Warnings/Precautions Hazardous agent - use appropriate precautions for handling and disposal (NIOSH, 2012).

Cyclophosphamide is associated with the development of hemorrhagic cystitis; may rarely be severe and even fatal. Discontinue cyclophosphamide with severe hemorrhagic cystitis. Bladder injury is due to excretion of cyclophosphamide metabolites in the urine and appears to be dose- and treatment duration-dependent. Bladder fibrosis may also occur, either with or without cystitis. Increased hydration and frequent voiding is recommended to help prevent cystitis; some protocols utilize mesna to protect against hemorrhagic cystitis. Monitor urinalysis for hematuria. Severe or prolonged hemorrhagic cystitis may require medical or surgical treatment. Hematuria generally resolves within a few days after treatment is withheld, although it may persist. Cyclophosphamide may potentiate the cardiotoxicity of anthracyclines.

Cardiotoxicity has been reported, usually with high doses associated with transplant conditioning regimens, although may rarely occur with lower doses. Cardiac abnormalities do not appear to persist. Cardiotoxicities reported have included arrhythmia, congestive heart failure, heart block, hemorrhagic myocarditis, hemopericardium (secondary to hemorrhagic myocarditis and myocardial necrosis), pericarditis, and tachyarrhythmias. Cardiotoxicity is related to endothelial capillary damage; symptoms may be managed with diuretics, ACE inhibitors, beta blockers, or inotropics (Floyd, 2005). Use with caution in patients with pre-existing cardiovascular disease. For patients with multiple cardiac risk factors, considering monitoring during treatment (Floyd, 2005).

Pulmonary toxicities, including pneumonitis and acute respiratory distress syndrome, have been reported. Consider pulmonary function testing to assess the severity of pneumonitis (Morgan, 2011). Cyclophosphamide-induced pneumonitis is rare and may present as early (within 1-6 months) or late onset (several months to years); early onset has been reversible with discontinuation; late onset is associated with pleural thickening and may persist chronically (Malik, 1996).

Dose-related neutropenia is common; thrombocytopenia and anemia may also occur. Monitor for infections; immunosuppression and serious infections may occur; infections may require dose reduction, or interruption or discontinuation of treatment. Nausea and vomiting commonly occur; premedication with antiemetics is recommended. Stomatitis/mucositis may also occur. Anaphylactic reactions have been reported; cross-sensitivity with other alkylating agents may occur. May interfere with wound healing. Secondary malignancies (bladder cancer, myeloproliferative, and lymphoproliferative malignancies) have been reported with both single-agent and with combination chemotherapy regimens; onset may be delayed (up to several years after treatment); bladder malignancy usually occurs in patients previously experiencing hemorrhagic cystitis. May impair fertility; interferes with oogenesis and spermatogenesis; effect on fertility is generally dependent on dose and duration of treatment and may be irreversible. The age at treatment initiation and cumulative dose were determined to be risk factors for ovarian failure in cyclophosphamide use for the treatment of systemic lupus erythematosus (SLE) (Mok, 1998). Use with caution in patients with renal and hepatic impairment; dosage adjustment may be needed (use is contraindicated in severe impairment in the Canadian labeling).

Drug Interactions

Metabolism/Transport Effects Substrate of CYP2A6 (minor), CYP2B6 (major), CYP2C19 (minor), CYP2C9 (minor), CYP3A4 (minor); **Note:** Assignment of Major/Minor substrate status based on clinically relevant drug interaction potential; **Inhibits** CYP3A4 (weak); **Induces** CYP2B6 (weak/moderate), CYP2C9 (weak/moderate)

Avoid Concomitant Use

Avoid concomitant use of Cyclophosphamide with any of the following: BCG; Belimumab; CloZAPine; Etanercept; Natalizumab; Pimecrolimus; Pimozide; Tacrolimus (Topical); Tofacitinib; Vaccines (Live)

Increased Effect/Toxicity

Cyclophosphamide may increase the levels/effects of: ARIPiprazole; CloZAPine; Leflunomide; Lomitapide; Natalizumab; Pimozide; Succinylcholine; Tofacitinib; Vaccines (Live); Vitamin K Antagonists

The levels/effects of Cyclophosphamide may be increased by: Allopurinol; Belimumab; CYP2B6 Inhibitors (Moderate); CYP2B6 Inhibitors (Strong); Denosumab; Etanercept; Pentostatin; Pimecrolimus; Quazepam; Roflumilast; Tacrolimus (Topical); Trastuzumab

Decreased Effect

Cyclophosphamide may decrease the levels/effects of: BCG; Cardiac Glycosides; Coccidioidin Skin Test; Sipuleucel-T; Vaccines (Inactivated); Vaccines (Live); Vitamin K Antagonists

The levels/effects of Cyclophosphamide may be decreased by: CYP2B6 Inducers (Strong); Echinacea

Ethanol/Nutrition/Herb Interactions Herb/Nutraceutical: Avoid black cohosh, dong quai in estrogen-dependent tumors.

Dietary Considerations Tablets should be administered during or after meals.

Pharmacodynamics/Kinetics

Half-life Elimination 3-12 hours

Time to Peak Serum: Oral: ~1 hour; I.V.: Metabolites: 2-3 hours

Pregnancy Risk Factor D

Pregnancy Considerations Studies in pregnant women have demonstrated a risk to the fetus. Women of childbearing potential should avoid pregnancy while receiving cyclophosphamide treatment. Cyclophosphamide may also cause sterility in males and females (reversible in some cases). According to the National Comprehensive Cancer Network (NCCN) breast cancer guidelines (v.3.2012), chemotherapy, if indicated, may be administered to pregnant women with breast cancer as part of a combination chemotherapy regimen (common regimens administered during pregnancy include doxorubicin, cyclophosphamide, and fluorouracil); chemotherapy should not be administered during the first trimester, after 35 weeks gestation, or within 3 weeks of planned delivery.

Lactation Enters breast milk/not recommended

Breast-Feeding Considerations Due to the potential for adverse effects and tumorigenicity, the decision to discontinue cyclophosphamide or to discontinue breast-feeding should take into account the benefits of treatment to the mother.

Dosage Forms

Injection, powder for reconstitution: 500 mg, 1 g, 2 g

Tablet, oral: 25 mg, 50 mg

Dosage Forms: Canada

Injection, powder for reconstitution: 200 mg

CycloSERINE (sye kloe SER een)

Brand Names: U.S. Seromycin®
Pharmacologic Category Antibiotic, Miscellaneous; Antitubercular Agent
Use Adjunctive treatment in pulmonary or extrapulmonary tuberculosis
Local Anesthetic/Vasoconstrictor Precautions No information available to require special precautions
Effects on Dental Treatment No significant effects or complications reported
Effects on Bleeding No information available to require special precautions
Adverse Effects Frequency not defined.
Cardiovascular: Cardiac arrhythmia, heart failure
Central nervous system: Coma, confusion, dizziness, drowsiness, headache, paresis, psychosis, restlessness, seizures, vertigo
Dermatologic: Rash
Endocrine & metabolic: Vitamin B_{12} deficiency
Hematologic: Folate deficiency
Hepatic: Liver enzymes increased
Neuromuscular & skeletal: Dysarthria, hyperreflexia, paresthesia, tremor
Miscellaneous: Allergic manifestations
General Dosage Range Dosage adjustment recommended in patients with renal impairment
Oral:
Children: 10-20 mg/kg/day in 2 divided doses (maximum: 1000 mg/day)
Adults: Initial: 250 mg every 12 hours for 14 days; Maintenance: 500-1000 mg/day in 2 divided doses
Mechanism of Action Inhibits bacterial cell wall synthesis by competing with amino acid (D-alanine) for incorporation into the bacterial cell wall; bacteriostatic or bactericidal
Pharmacodynamics/Kinetics
Half-life Elimination Normal renal function: 10 hours
Time to Peak Serum: 4-8 hours
Pregnancy Risk Factor C
Pregnancy Considerations Teratogenic effects have not been observed in animal reproduction studies. Cycloserine crosses the placenta and can be detected in the fetal blood and amniotic fluid. The American Thoracic Society recommends use in pregnant women only if there are no alternatives (CDC, 2003).

CycloSPORINE (Systemic) (SYE kloe spor een)

Brand Names: U.S. Gengraf®; Neoral®; SandIMMUNE®
Brand Names: Canada Apo-Cyclosporine®; Neoral®; Rhoxal-cyclosporine; Sandimmune® I.V.; Sandoz-Cyclosporine
Generic Availability (U.S.) Yes: Excludes non-modified solution
Pharmacologic Category Calcineurin Inhibitor; Immunosuppressant Agent
Dental Use Used as an immunosuppressive agent
Use Prophylaxis of organ rejection in kidney, liver, and heart transplants, has been used with azathioprine and/or corticosteroids; severe, active rheumatoid arthritis (RA) not responsive to methotrexate alone; severe, recalcitrant plaque psoriasis in nonimmunocompromised adults unresponsive to or unable to tolerate other systemic therapy

Unlabeled Use Allogenic stem cell transplants for prevention and treatment of graft-versus-host disease; also used in some cases of severe autoimmune disease (eg, SLE) that are resistant to corticosteroids and other therapy; focal segmental glomerulosclerosis; severe ulcerative colitis
Local Anesthetic/Vasoconstrictor Precautions No information available to require special precautions
Effects on Dental Treatment Key adverse event(s) related to dental treatment: Mouth sores, swallowing difficulty, gingivitis, gum hyperplasia, xerostomia (normal salivary flow resumes upon discontinuation), abnormal taste, tongue disorder, tooth disorder, and gingival bleeding.
Effects on Bleeding No information available to require special precautions
Adverse Effects Adverse reactions reported with systemic use, including rheumatoid arthritis, psoriasis, and transplantation (kidney, liver, and heart). Percentages noted include the highest frequency regardless of indication/dosage. Frequencies may vary for specific conditions or formulation.

>10%:
Cardiovascular: Hypertension (8% to 53%), edema (5% to 14%)
Central nervous system: Headache (2% to 25%)
Dermatologic: Hirsutism (21% to 45%), hypertrichosis (5% to 19%)
Endocrine & metabolic: Triglycerides increased (15%), female reproductive disorder (9% to 11%)
Gastrointestinal: Nausea (23%), diarrhea (3% to 13%), gum hyperplasia (2% to 16%), abdominal discomfort (<1% to 15%), dyspepsia (2% to 12%)
Neuromuscular & skeletal: Tremor (7% to 55%), paresthesia (1% to 11%), leg cramps/muscle contractions (2% to 12%)
Renal: Renal dysfunction/nephropathy (10% to 38%), creatinine increased (16% to ≥50%)
Respiratory: Upper respiratory infection (1% to 14%)
Miscellaneous: Infection (3% to 25%)
Kidney, liver, and heart transplant only (≤2% unless otherwise noted):
Cardiovascular: Flushes (<1% to 4%), glomerular capillary thrombosis, MI
Central nervous system: Convulsions (1% to 5%), anxiety, confusion, fever, lethargy
Dermatologic: Acne (1% to 6%), brittle fingernails, hair breaking, pruritus
Endocrine & metabolic: Gynecomastia (<1% to 4%), hyperglycemia, hypomagnesemia
Gastrointestinal: Nausea (2% to 10%), vomiting (2% to 10%), diarrhea (3% to 8%), abdominal discomfort (<1% to 7%), cramps (0% to 4%), anorexia, constipation, gastritis, mouth sores, pancreatitis, swallowing difficulty, upper GI bleed, weight loss
Hematologic: Leukopenia (<1% to 6%), anemia, thrombocytopenia
Hepatic: Hepatotoxicity (<1% to 7%)
Neuromuscular & skeletal: Paresthesia (1% to 3%), joint pain, muscle pain, tingling, weakness
Ocular: Conjunctivitis, visual disturbance
Otic: Hearing loss, tinnitus
Renal: Hematuria
Respiratory: Sinusitis (<1% to 7%)
Miscellaneous: Lymphoma (<1% to 6%), allergic reactions, hiccups, night sweats

Rheumatoid arthritis only (1% to <3% unless otherwise noted):

Cardiovascular: Hypertension (8%), edema (5%), chest pain (4%), arrhythmia (2%), abnormal heart sounds, cardiac failure, MI, peripheral ischemia

Central nervous system: Dizziness (8%), pain (6%), insomnia (4%), depression (3%), migraine (2%), anxiety, hypoesthesia, emotional lability, impaired concentration, malaise, nervousness, paranoia, somnolence, vertigo

Dermatologic: Purpura (3%), abnormal pigmentation, angioedema, cellulitis, dermatitis, dry skin, eczema, folliculitis, nail disorder, pruritus, skin disorder, urticaria

Endocrine & metabolic: Menstrual disorder (3%), breast fibroadenosis, breast pain, diabetes mellitus, goiter, hot flashes, hyperkalemia, hyperuricemia, hypoglycemia, libido increased/decreased

Gastrointestinal: Vomiting (9%), flatulence (5%), gingivitis (4%), gum hyperplasia (2%), constipation, dry mouth, dysphagia, enanthema, eructation, esophagitis, gastric ulcer, gastritis, gastroenteritis, gingival bleeding, glossitis, peptic ulcer, salivary gland enlargement, taste perversion, tongue disorder, gum hyperplasia, weight loss/gain

Genitourinary: Leukorrhea (1%), abnormal urine, micturition urgency, nocturia, polyuria, pyelonephritis, urinary incontinence, uterine hemorrhage

Hematologic: Anemia, leukopenia

Hepatic: Bilirubinemia

Neuromuscular & skeletal: Paresthesia (8%), tremor (8%), leg cramps/muscle contractions (2%), arthralgia, bone fracture, joint dislocation, myalgia, neuropathy, stiffness, synovial cyst, tendon disorder, weakness

Ocular: Abnormal vision, cataract, conjunctivitis, eye pain

Otic: Tinnitus, deafness, vestibular disorder

Renal: BUN increased, hematuria, renal abscess

Respiratory: Cough (5%), dyspnea (5%), sinusitis (4%), abnormal chest sounds, bronchospasm, epistaxis

Miscellaneous: Infection (9%), abscess, allergy, bacterial infection, carcinoma, fungal infection, herpes simplex, herpes zoster, lymphadenopathy, moniliasis, diaphoresis increased, tonsillitis, viral infection

Psoriasis only (1% to <3% unless otherwise noted):

Cardiovascular: Chest pain, flushes

Central nervous system: Psychiatric events (4% to 5%), pain (3% to 4%), dizziness, fever, insomnia, nervousness, vertigo

Dermatologic: Hypertrichosis (5% to 7%), acne, dry skin, folliculitis, keratosis, pruritus, rash, skin malignancies

Endocrine & metabolic: Hot flashes

Gastrointestinal: Nausea (5% to 6%), diarrhea (5% to 6%), gum hyperplasia (4% to 6%), abdominal discomfort (3% to 6%), dyspepsia (2% to 3%), abdominal distention, appetite increased, constipation, gingival bleeding

Genitourinary: Micturition increased

Hematologic: Bleeding disorder, clotting disorder, platelet disorder, red blood cell disorder

Hepatic: Hyperbilirubinemia

Neuromuscular & skeletal: Paresthesia (5% to 7%), arthralgia (1% to 6%)

Ocular: Abnormal vision

Respiratory: Bronchospasm (5%), cough (5%), dyspnea (5%), rhinitis (5%), respiratory infection

Miscellaneous: Flu-like syndrome (8% to 10%)

Dental Usual Dosage Note: Neoral®/Gengraf® and Sandimmune® are not bioequivalent and cannot be used interchangeably.

Autoimmune diseases: Adults: 1-3 mg/kg/day

Dosage Neoral®/Gengraf® and Sandimmune® are not bioequivalent and cannot be used interchangeably.

Children: Transplant: Refer to adult dosing; children may require, and are able to tolerate, larger doses than adults.

Adults:

Newly-transplanted patients: Adjunct therapy with corticosteroids is recommended. Initial dose should be given 4-12 hours prior to transplant or may be given postoperatively; adjust initial dose to achieve desired plasma concentration

Oral: Dose is dependent upon type of transplant and formulation:

Cyclosporine (modified):

Renal: 9 ± 3 mg/kg/day, divided twice daily

Liver: 8 ± 4 mg/kg/day, divided twice daily

Heart: 7 ± 3 mg/kg/day, divided twice daily

Cyclosporine (non-modified): Initial doses of 10-14 mg/kg/day have been used for renal transplants (the manufacturer's labeling includes dosing from initial clinical trials of 15 mg/kg/day [range: 14-18 mg/kg/day]; however, this higher dosing level is rarely used any longer). Continue initial dose daily for 1-2 weeks; taper by 5% per week to a maintenance dose of 5-10 mg/kg/day; some renal transplant patients may be dosed as low as 3 mg/kg/day

Note: When using the non-modified formulation, cyclosporine levels may increase in liver transplant patients when the T-tube is closed; dose may need decreased

I.V.: Cyclosporine (non-modified): Manufacturer's labeling: Initial dose: 5-6 mg/kg/day or one-third of the oral dose as a single dose, infused over 2-6 hours; use should be limited to patients unable to take capsules or oral solution; patients should be switched to an oral dosage form as soon as possible

Note: Many transplant centers administer cyclosporine as "divided dose" infusions (in 2-3 doses/day) or as a continuous (24-hour) infusion; dosages range from 3-7.5 mg/kg/day. Specific institutional protocols should be consulted.

Conversion to cyclosporine (modified) from cyclosporine (non-modified): Start with daily dose previously used and adjust to obtain preconversion cyclosporine trough concentration. Plasma concentrations should be monitored every 4-7 days and dose adjusted as necessary, until desired trough level is obtained. When transferring patients with previously poor absorption of cyclosporine (non-modified), monitor trough levels at least twice weekly (especially if initial dose exceeds 10 mg/kg/day); high plasma levels are likely to occur.

Rheumatoid arthritis: Oral: Cyclosporine (modified): Initial dose: 2.5 mg/kg/day, divided twice daily; salicylates, NSAIDs, and oral glucocorticoids may be continued (refer to Drug Interactions); dose may be increased by 0.5-0.75 mg/kg/day if insufficient response is seen after 8 weeks of treatment; additional dosage increases may be made again at 12 weeks (maximum dose: 4 mg/kg/day). Discontinue if no benefit is seen by 16 weeks of therapy.

◄ **Note:** Increase the frequency of blood pressure monitoring after each alteration in dosage of cyclosporine. Cyclosporine dosage should be decreased by 25% to 50% in patients with no history of hypertension who develop sustained hypertension during therapy and, if hypertension persists, treatment with cyclosporine should be discontinued.

Psoriasis: Oral: Cyclosporine (modified): Initial dose: 2.5 mg/kg/day, divided twice daily; dose may be increased by 0.5 mg/kg/day if insufficient response is seen after 4 weeks of treatment. Additional dosage increases may be made every 2 weeks if needed (maximum dose: 4 mg/kg/day). Discontinue if no benefit is seen by 6 weeks of therapy. Once patients are adequately controlled, the dose should be decreased to the lowest effective dose. Doses lower than 2.5 mg/kg/day may be effective. Treatment longer than 1 year is not recommended.

Note: Increase the frequency of blood pressure monitoring after each alteration in dosage of cyclosporine. Cyclosporine dosage should be decreased by 25% to 50% in patients with no history of hypertension who develop sustained hypertension during therapy and, if hypertension persists, treatment with cyclosporine should be discontinued.

Focal segmental glomerulosclerosis (unlabeled use): Oral: Initial: 3.5-5 mg/kg/day divided every 12 hours (in combination with oral prednisone) (Braun, 2008; Cattran, 1999)

Lupus nephritis (unlabeled use): Oral: Initial: 4 mg/kg/day for 1 month (reduce dose if trough concentrations >200 ng/mL); reduce dose by 0.5 mg/kg every 2 weeks to a maintenance dose of 2.5-3 mg/kg/day (Moroni, 2006)

Severe ulcerative colitis (steroid-refractory) (unlabeled use):

I.V.: Cyclosporine (non-modified): 2-4 mg/kg/day, infused continuously over 24 hours. (Lichtiger, 1994; Van Assche, 2003). **Note:** Some studies suggest no therapeutic difference between low-dose (2 mg/kg) and high-dose (4 mg/kg) cyclosporine regimens (Van Assche, 2003).

Oral: Cyclosporine (modified): 2.3-3 mg/kg every 12 hours (De Saussure 2005; Weber 2006)

Note: Patients responsive to I.V. therapy should be switched to oral therapy when possible.

Dosage adjustment in renal impairment: For severe psoriasis:

Serum creatinine levels ≥25% above pretreatment levels: Take another sample within 2 weeks; if the level remains ≥25% above pretreatment levels, decrease dosage of cyclosporine (modified) by 25% to 50%. If two dosage adjustments do not reverse the increase in serum creatinine levels, treatment should be discontinued.

Serum creatinine levels ≥50% above pretreatment levels: Decrease cyclosporine dosage by 25% or 50%. If two dosage adjustments do not reverse the increase in serum creatinine levels, treatment should be discontinued.

Hemodialysis: Supplemental dose is not necessary.

Peritoneal dialysis: Supplemental dose is not necessary.

Dosage adjustment in hepatic impairment: Probably necessary; monitor levels closely

Mechanism of Action Inhibition of production and release of interleukin II and inhibits interleukin II-induced activation of resting T-lymphocytes.

Contraindications Hypersensitivity to cyclosporine or any component of the formulation. I.V. cyclosporine is contraindicated in hypersensitivity to polyoxyethylated castor oil (Cremophor® EL).

Rheumatoid arthritis and psoriasis: Abnormal renal function, uncontrolled hypertension, malignancies. Concomitant treatment with PUVA or UVB therapy, methotrexate, other immunosuppressive agents, coal tar, or radiation therapy are also contraindications for use in patients with psoriasis.

Warnings/Precautions Hazardous agent - use appropriate precautions for handling and disposal (NIOSH, 2012).

[U.S. Boxed Warning]: Increased risk of lymphomas and other malignancies (including fatal outcomes), particularly those of the skin; risk is related to intensity/duration of therapy and the use of more than one immunosuppressive agent; all patients should avoid excessive sun/UV light exposure. **[U.S. Boxed Warning]: May cause hypertension.** Use caution when changing dosage forms.

[U.S. Boxed Warning]: Renal impairment, including structural kidney damage has occurred (when used at high doses); monitor renal function closely. Elevations in serum creatinine and BUN generally respond to dosage reductions. Use caution with other potentially nephrotoxic drugs (eg, acyclovir, aminoglycoside antibiotics, amphotericin B, ciprofloxacin). Elevations in serum creatinine and BUN associated with nephrotoxicity generally respond to dosage reductions. In renal transplant patients with rapidly rising BUN and creatinine, carefully evaluate to differentiate between cyclosporine-associated nephrotoxicity and renal rejection episodes. In cases of severe rejection that fail to respond to pulse steroids and monoclonal antibodies, switching to an alternative immunosuppressant agent may be preferred to increasing cyclosporine to an excessive dosage.

[U.S. Boxed Warning]: Increased risk of infection with use; serious and fatal infections have been reported. Bacterial, viral, fungal, and protozoal infections (including opportunistic infections) have occurred. Polyoma virus infections, such as the JC virus and BK virus, may result in serious and sometimes fatal outcomes. The JC virus is associated with progressive multifocal leukoencephalopathy (PML), and PML has been reported in patients receiving cyclosporine. PML may be fatal and presents with hemiparesis, apathy, confusion, cognitive deficiencies, and ataxia; consider neurologic consultation as indicated. The BK virus is associated with nephropathy, and polyoma virus-associated nephropathy (PVAN) has been reported in patients receiving cyclosporine. PVAN is associated with serious adverse effects including renal dysfunction and renal graft loss. If PML or PVAN occur in transplant patients, consider reducing immunosuppression therapy as well as the risk that reduced immunosuppression poses to grafts.

Liver injury, including cholestasis, jaundice, hepatitis, and liver failure, has been reported. These events were mainly in patients with confounding factors including infections, coadministration with other potentially hepatotoxic medications, underlying conditions, and significant comorbidities. Fatalities have also been reported rarely, primarily in transplant patients. Increased hepatic enzymes and bilirubin have occurred (when used at high doses); improvement usually seen with dosage reduction.

Should be used initially with corticosteroids in transplant patients. Significant hyperkalemia (with or without hyperchloremic metabolic acidosis) and hyperuricemia have occurred with therapy. Syndromes of microangiopathic hemolytic anemia and thrombocytopenia have occurred and may result in graft failure; it is accompanied by platelet consumption within the graft. Syndrome may occur without graft rejection. Although management of the syndrome is unclear, discontinuation or reduction of cyclosporine, in addition to streptokinase and heparin administration or plasmapheresis, has been associated with syndrome resolution. However, resolution seems to be dependent upon early detection of the syndrome via indium 111 labeled platelet scans.

May cause seizures, particularly if used with high-dose corticosteroids. Encephalopathy has also been reported; predisposing factors include hypertension, hypomagnesemia, hypocholesterolemia, high-dose corticosteroids, high cyclosporine serum concentration, and graft-versus-host disease (GVHD). Encephalopathy may be more common in patients with liver transplant compared to kidney transplant. Other neurotoxic events, such as optic disc edema (including papilloedema and potential visual impairment), have been rarely reported primarily in transplant patients.

Potentially significant drug-drug/drug-food interactions may exist, requiring dose or frequency adjustment, additional monitoring, and/or selection of alternative therapy. **[U.S. Boxed Warning]: Cyclosporine (modified) has increased bioavailability as compared to cyclosporine (non-modified) and cannot be used interchangeably without close monitoring.** Monitor cyclosporine concentrations closely following the addition, modification, or deletion of other medications; live, attenuated vaccines may be less effective; use should be avoided. Make dose adjustments based on cyclosporine blood concentrations. **[U.S. Boxed Warning]: Adjustment of dose should only be made under the direct supervision of an experienced physician.** Anaphylaxis has been reported with I.V. use; reserve for patients who cannot take oral form. **[U.S. Boxed Warning]: Risk of skin cancer may be increased in transplant patients.** Due to the increased risk for nephrotoxicity in renal transplantation, avoid using standard doses of cyclosporine in combination with everolimus; reduced cyclosporine doses are recommended; monitor cyclosporine concentrations closely. Cyclosporine and everolimus combination therapy may increase the risk for proteinuria. Cyclosporine combined with either everolimus or sirolimus may increase the risk for thrombotic microangiopathy/thrombotic thrombocytopenic purpura/hemolytic uremic syndrome (TMA/TTP/HUS).

Patients with psoriasis should avoid excessive sun exposure; safety and efficacy in children <18 years of age have not been established. **[U.S. Boxed Warning]: Risk of skin cancer may be increased with a history of PUVA and possibly methotrexate or other immunosuppressants, UVB, coal tar, or radiation.**

Rheumatoid arthritis: Safety and efficacy for use in juvenile idiopathic arthritis (JIA) have not been established. If receiving other immunosuppressive agents, radiation or UV therapy, concurrent use of cyclosporine is not recommended.

Products may contain corn oil, ethanol, or propylene glycol; injection also contains Cremophor® EL (polyoxyethylated castor oil), which has been associated with rare anaphylactic reactions.

Drug Interactions
Metabolism/Transport Effects Substrate of CYP3A4 (major), P-glycoprotein; **Note:** Assignment of Major/Minor substrate status based on clinically relevant drug interaction potential; **Inhibits** CYP2C9 (weak), CYP3A4 (moderate), P-glycoprotein
Avoid Concomitant Use
Avoid concomitant use of CycloSPORINE (Systemic) with any of the following: Aliskiren; AtorvaSTATin; BCG; Bosentan; Bosutinib; Conivaptan; Crizotinib; Dronedarone; Enzalutamide; Eplerenone; Ivabradine; Lomitapide; Lovastatin; Mifepristone; Natalizumab; Pimecrolimus; Pimozide; Pitavastatin; Pomalidomide; Potassium-Sparing Diuretics; Silodosin; Simvastatin; Sitaxentan; Tacrolimus (Systemic); Tacrolimus (Topical); Tofacitinib; Tolvaptan; Topotecan; Vaccines (Live); VinCRIStine (Liposomal)
Increased Effect/Toxicity
CycloSPORINE (Systemic) may increase the levels/effects of: Aliskiren; Ambrisentan; ARIPiprazole; AtorvaSTATin; Avanafil; Boceprevir; Bosentan; Bosutinib; Budesonide (Systemic, Oral Inhalation); Calcium Channel Blockers (Dihydropyridine); Calcium Channel Blockers (Nondihydropyridine); Cardiac Glycosides; Caspofungin; Colchicine; CYP3A4 Substrates; Dabigatran Etexilate; Dexamethasone (Systemic); DOXOrubicin; Dronedarone; Etoposide; Etoposide Phosphate; Everolimus; Ezetimibe; FentaNYL; Fibric Acid Derivatives; Fluvastatin; Halofantrine; Imipenem; Ivabradine; Ivacaftor; Leflunomide; Lomitapide; Loop Diuretics; Lovastatin; Lurasidone; Methotrexate; MethylPREDNISolone; Minoxidil (Systemic); Minoxidil (Topical); Natalizumab; Nonsteroidal Anti-Inflammatory Agents; P-glycoprotein/ABCB1 Substrates; Pimozide; Pitavastatin; Pomalidomide; Pravastatin; PredniSONE; Propafenone; Protease Inhibitors; Prucalopride; Ranolazine; Repaglinide; Rivaroxaban; Rosuvastatin; Salmeterol; Saxagliptin; Silodosin; Simvastatin; Sirolimus; Sitaxentan; Tacrolimus (Systemic); Tacrolimus (Topical); Tofacitinib; Tolvaptan; Topotecan; Vaccines (Live); Vilazodone; VinCRIStine (Liposomal); Zuclopenthixol

The levels/effects of CycloSPORINE (Systemic) may be increased by: ACE Inhibitors; AcetaZOLAMIDE; Aminoglycosides; Amiodarone; Amphotericin B; Androgens; Angiotensin II Receptor Blockers; Antifungal Agents (Azole Derivatives, Systemic); Boceprevir; Bromocriptine; Calcium Channel Blockers (Nondihydropyridine); Carvedilol; Chloramphenicol; Conivaptan; Crizotinib; CYP3A4 Inhibitors (Moderate); CYP3A4 Inhibitors (Strong); Dasatinib; Denosumab; Dexamethasone (Systemic); Eplerenone; Ezetimibe; Fluconazole; GlyBURIDE; Grapefruit Juice; Imatinib; Imipenem; Ivacaftor; Macrolide Antibiotics; Melphalan; Methotrexate; MethylPREDNISolone; Metoclopramide; MetroNIDAZOLE (Systemic); Mifepristone; Nonsteroidal Anti-Inflammatory Agents; Norfloxacin; Omeprazole; P-glycoprotein/ABCB1 Inhibitors; Pimecrolimus; Potassium-Sparing Diuretics; Pravastatin; PrednisoLONE (Systemic); PredniSONE; Protease Inhibitors; Pyrazinamide; Quinupristin; Roflumilast; Sirolimus; Sulfonamide Derivatives; Tacrolimus (Systemic); Tacrolimus (Topical); Telaprevir; Temsirolimus; Trastuzumab
Decreased Effect
CycloSPORINE (Systemic) may decrease the levels/effects of: BCG; Coccidioidin Skin Test; GlyBURIDE; Ifosfamide; Mycophenolate; Sipuleucel-T; Vaccines (Inactivated); Vaccines (Live)

The levels/effects of CycloSPORINE (Systemic) may be decreased by: Adalimumab; Armodafinil; Ascorbic Acid; Barbiturates; Bosentan; CarBAMazepine; Colesevelam; CYP3A4 Inducers (Strong); Deferasirox; Dexamethasone (Systemic); Echinacea; Efavirenz; Enzalutamide; Fibric Acid Derivatives; Fosphenytoin; Griseofulvin; Imipenem; MethylPREDNISolone; Modafinil; Multivitamins/Minerals (with ADEK, Folate, Iron); Nafcillin; Orlistat; P-glycoprotein/ABCB1 Inducers; Phenytoin; PrednisoLONE (Systemic); PredniSONE; Rifamycin Derivatives; Somatostatin Analogs; St Johns Wort; Sulfinpyrazone [Off Market]; Sulfonamide Derivatives; Tocilizumab; Vitamin E

Ethanol/Nutrition/Herb Interactions
Food: Grapefruit juice increases cyclosporine serum concentrations. Management: Avoid grapefruit juice.
Herb/Nutraceutical: St John's wort may increase the metabolism of and decrease plasma levels of cyclosporine; organ rejection and graft loss have been reported. Cat's claw and echinacea have immunostimulant properties. Management: Avoid St John's wort, cat's claw, and echinacea.

Dietary Considerations Administer this medication consistently with relation to time of day and meals. Avoid grapefruit juice with oral cyclosporine use.

Pharmacodynamics/Kinetics
Half-life Elimination Oral: May be prolonged with hepatic impairment and shorter in pediatric patients due to the higher metabolism rate
Cyclosporine (non-modified): Biphasic: Alpha: 1.4 hours; Terminal: 19 hours (range: 10-27 hours)
Cyclosporine (modified): Biphasic: Terminal: 8.4 hours (range: 5-18 hours)
Time to Peak Serum: Oral:
Cyclosporine (non-modified): 2-6 hours; some patients have a second peak at 5-6 hours
Cyclosporine (modified): Renal transplant: 1.5-2 hours
Pregnancy Risk Factor C
Pregnancy Considerations Adverse events were not observed following the use of oral cyclosporine in animal reproduction studies (using doses that were not maternally toxic). In humans, cyclosporine crosses the placenta; maternal concentrations do not correlate with those found in the umbilical cord. Cyclosporine may be detected in the serum of newborns for several days after birth. Based on clinical use, premature births and low birth weight were consistently observed in pregnant transplant patients (additional pregnancy complications also present).

A pregnancy registry has been established for pregnant women taking immunosuppressants following any solid organ transplant (National Transplantation Pregnancy Registry, Temple University, 877-955-6877).

A pregnancy registry has also been established for pregnant women taking Neoral® for psoriasis or rheumatoid arthritis (Neoral® Pregnancy Registry for Psoriasis and Rheumatoid Arthritis, Thomas Jefferson University, 888-522-5581).

Lactation Enters breast milk/not recommended
Breast-Feeding Considerations Cyclosporine is excreted in breast milk. Breast feeding is not recommended by the manufacturer.

Dosage Forms
Capsule, oral: 100 mg
Gengraf®: 25 mg, 100 mg
Capsule, softgel, oral: 25 mg, 50 mg, 100 mg
Neoral®: 25 mg, 100 mg
SandIMMUNE®: 25 mg, 100 mg

Injection, solution: 50 mg/mL (5 mL)
SandIMMUNE®: 50 mg/mL (5 mL)
Solution, oral: 100 mg/mL (50 mL)
Gengraf®: 100 mg/mL (50 mL)
Neoral®: 100 mg/mL (50 mL)
SandIMMUNE®: 100 mg/mL (50 mL)

CycloSPORINE (Ophthalmic)
(SYE kloe spor een)

Brand Names: U.S. Restasis®
Brand Names: Canada Restasis®
Pharmacologic Category Calcineurin Inhibitor; Immunosuppressant Agent
Use Increase tear production when suppressed tear production is presumed to be due to keratoconjunctivitis sicca-associated ocular inflammation (in patients not already using topical anti-inflammatory drugs or punctal plugs)
Local Anesthetic/Vasoconstrictor Precautions No information available to require special precautions
Effects on Dental Treatment No significant effects or complications reported
Effects on Bleeding No information available to require special precautions
Adverse Effects
>10%: Ocular: Burning (17%)
1% to 5%: Ocular: Blurred vision, conjunctival hyperemia, discharge, epiphora, eye pain, foreign body sensation, pruritus, stinging, visual disturbance
General Dosage Range Ophthalmic: *Adolescents ≥16 years and Adults:* Instill 1 drop in each eye every 12 hours
Pregnancy Risk Factor C
Pregnancy Considerations Adverse events were not observed following the use of oral cyclosporine in animal reproduction studies when using doses that were approximately 300,000 times greater than a human ophthalmic dose (assuming complete absorption).

Cyproheptadine (si proe HEP ta deen)

Brand Names: Canada Euro-Cyproheptadine; PMS-Cyproheptadine
Pharmacologic Category Histamine H_1 Antagonist; Histamine H_1 Antagonist, First Generation; Piperidine Derivative
Use Perennial and seasonal allergic rhinitis and other allergic symptoms including urticaria
Unlabeled Use Migraine headache prophylaxis, pruritus, spasticity associated with spinal cord damage
Local Anesthetic/Vasoconstrictor Precautions No information available to require special precautions
Effects on Dental Treatment Key adverse event(s) related to dental treatment: Xerostomia (normal salivary flow resumes upon discontinuation)
Effects on Bleeding No information available to require special precautions
Adverse Effects Frequency not defined.
Cardiovascular: Extrasystoles, hypotension, palpitation, tachycardia
Central nervous system: Confusion, coordination disturbed, dizziness, excitation, euphoria, faintness, hallucinations, headache, hysteria, insomnia, irritability, nervousness, neuritis, restlessness, sedation, seizure, sleepiness, tremor, vertigo
Dermatologic: Angioedema, photosensitivity, rash, urticaria

Gastrointestinal: Abdominal pain, anorexia, appetite increased, constipation, diarrhea, nausea, vomiting, xerostomia

Genitourinary: Difficult urination, urinary frequency, urinary retention

Hematologic: Agranulocytosis, hemolytic anemia, leukopenia, thrombocytopenia

Hepatic: Cholestasis, hepatic failure, hepatitis, jaundice

Neuromuscular & skeletal: Paresthesia

Ocular: Blurred vision, diplopia

Otic: Labyrinthitis (acute), tinnitus

Respiratory: Bronchial secretions (thickening), nasal congestion, pharyngitis

Miscellaneous: Allergic reactions, anaphylactic shock, chills, diaphoresis, fatigue

General Dosage Range
Oral:
Children 2-6 years: 2 mg every 8-12 hours (not to exceed 12 mg/day)
Children 7-14 years: 4 mg every 8-12 hours (not to exceed 16 mg/day)
Adults: 4-20 mg/day divided every 8 hours (not to exceed 0.5 mg/kg/day)

Mechanism of Action A potent antihistamine and serotonin antagonist, competes with histamine for H_1-receptor sites on effector cells in the gastrointestinal tract, blood vessels, and respiratory tract

Pharmacodynamics/Kinetics
Half-life Elimination Metabolites: ~16 hours (Paton, 1985)
Time to Peak Plasma: 6-9 hours (Paton, 1985)
Pregnancy Risk Factor B
Pregnancy Considerations Adverse events have been observed in some animal reproduction studies. Maternal antihistamine use has generally not resulted in an increased risk of birth defects; however, information specific to cyproheptadine is limited. Antihistamines are recommended for the treatment of rhinitis, urticaria, and pruritus with rash in pregnant women (although second generation antihistamines may be preferred). Antihistamines are not recommended for treatment of pruritus associated with intrahepatic cholestasis in pregnancy.

Cysteamine (Systemic) (sis TEE a meen)

Brand Names: U.S. Cystagon®
Pharmacologic Category Anticystine Agent; Urinary Tract Product
Use Treatment of nephropathic cystinosis
Local Anesthetic/Vasoconstrictor Precautions No information available to require special precautions
Effects on Dental Treatment No significant effects or complications reported
Effects on Bleeding No information available to require special precautions
Adverse Effects
>5%:
Central nervous system: Fever (22%), lethargy (11%)
Dermatologic: Rash (7%)
Gastrointestinal: Vomiting (35%), anorexia (31%), diarrhea (16%)
<5%:
Cardiovascular: Hypertension
Central nervous system: Abnormal thinking, ataxia, confusion, depression, dizziness, emotional lability, encephalopathy, hallucinations, headache, impaired cognition, jitteriness, nervousness, nightmares, seizure, somnolence

Dermatologic: Urticaria
Endocrine & metabolic: Dehydration
Gastrointestinal: Abdominal pain, constipation, duodenal ulceration, duodenitis, dyspepsia, gastroenteritis, gastrointestinal bleeding, gastrointestinal ulcers, halitosis, nausea
Hematologic: Anemia, leukopenia
Hepatic: Abnormal LFTs
Neuromuscular & skeletal: Hyperkinesia, tremor
Otic: Hearing decreased

General Dosage Range Oral:
Children <12 years: Initial: 1/4 to 1/6 of maintenance dose; Maintenance: 1.3 g/m²/day **or** 60 mg/kg/day in 4 divided doses (maximum dose: 1.95 g/m²/day; 90 mg/kg/day)
Children ≥12 years and Adults >110 lb: Initial: 1/4 to 1/6 of maintenance dose; Maintenance: 2 g/day in 4 divided doses (maximum: 1.95 g/m²/day; 90 mg/kg/day)

Mechanism of Action Reacts with cystine within the lysosome to convert it to cysteine and to a cysteine-cysteamine mixed disulfide, both of which can then exit the lysosome in patients with cystinosis, an inherited defect of lysosomal transport

Pharmacodynamics/Kinetics
Onset of Action 1-1.8 hours
Duration of Action 6 hours
Time to Peak 1.4 hours
Pregnancy Risk Factor C
Pregnancy Considerations Use only when the potential benefits outweigh the potential hazards to the fetus; in animal studies, cysteamine is teratogenic and fetotoxic. There are no adequate and well-controlled studies in pregnant women.

Cysteamine (Ophthalmic) (sis TEE a meen)

Pharmacologic Category Anticystine Agent; Ophthalmic Agent
Use Treatment of corneal cystine crystal accumulation in patients with cystinosis
Adverse Effects ≥10%:
Central nervous system: Headache
Ocular: Photophobia, erythema, irritation, pain, visual field defects
General Dosage Range Ophthalmic: *Adults:* Instill 1 drop in each eye every hour while awake
Mechanism of Action Reacts with cystine within the lysosome to convert it to cysteine and to a cysteine-cysteamine mixed disulfide, both of which can then exit the lysosome to reduce corneal cystine crystal accumulation in patients with cystinosis, an inherited defect of lysosomal transport
Pregnancy Risk Factor C
Pregnancy Considerations Adverse events were observed following oral administration in animal reproduction studies. However, systemic exposure is expected to be negligible following ophthalmic administration.
Product Availability
Cystaran™: FDA approved October 2012; anticipated availability currently unknown.
Cystaran™ is an ophthalmic solution approved for the treatment of corneal cystine crystal accumulation in patients with cystinosis.

Cysteine (SIS te een)

Pharmacologic Category Nutritional Supplement

◀ **Use** Supplement to crystalline amino acid solutions, in particular the specialized pediatric formulas (eg, Aminosyn® PF, TrophAmine®) to meet the intravenous amino acid nutritional requirements of infants receiving parenteral nutrition (PN)

Local Anesthetic/Vasoconstrictor Precautions No information available to require special precautions

Effects on Dental Treatment No significant effects or complications reported

Effects on Bleeding No information available to require special precautions

Adverse Effects Frequency not defined.

Cardiovascular: Flushing

Central nervous system: Fever

Endocrine & metabolic: Metabolic acidosis

Gastrointestinal: Nausea

Local: Erythema, phlebitis, thrombosis, warm sensation

Renal: Azotemia, BUN increased

General Dosage Range I.V.: *Infants:* Added as a fixed ratio to crystalline amino acid solution: 40 mg cysteine per g of amino acids; dosage will vary with the daily amino acid dosage; weight-based doses of cysteine (~70-160 mg/kg/day) have also been added directly to the daily parenteral nutrition solution

Mechanism of Action Cysteine is a sulfur-containing amino acid synthesized from methionine via the transulfuration pathway. It is a precursor of the tripeptide glutathione and also of taurine. Newborn infants have a relative deficiency of the enzyme necessary to affect this conversion. Cysteine may be considered an essential amino acid in infants.

Pregnancy Considerations Cysteine is generally considered to be a nonessential amino acid in adults because it can be synthesized from methionine (an essential amino acid). The RDA for methionine + cysteine is increased in pregnant women (IOM, 2005).

Cytarabine (Conventional)
(sye TARE a been con VEN sha nal)

Brand Names: Canada Cytarabine Injection; Cytosar®

Pharmacologic Category Antineoplastic Agent, Antimetabolite; Antineoplastic Agent, Antimetabolite (Pyrimidine Analog)

Use Remission induction in acute myeloid leukemia (AML), treatment of acute lymphocytic leukemia (ALL) and chronic myelocytic leukemia (CML; blast phase); prophylaxis and treatment of meningeal leukemia

Unlabeled Use AML consolidation treatment, AML salvage treatment; acute promyelocytic leukemia (APL) consolidation treatment; treatment of primary central nervous system (CNS) lymphoma; treatment of chronic lymphocytic leukemia (CLL); treatment of relapsed or refractory Hodgkin lymphoma; treatment of non-Hodgkin's lymphomas (NHL)

Local Anesthetic/Vasoconstrictor Precautions No information available to require special precautions

Effects on Dental Treatment Key adverse event(s) related to dental treatment: Mucositis

Effects on Bleeding Hematologic effects depend on dose and schedule of treatment. Platelets are one of the primary cell lines affected. Patients will develop thrombocytopenia on approximately day 7 which resolves about day 21-28. A medical consult is recommended.

Adverse Effects

Frequent:

Central nervous system: Fever

Dermatologic: Rash

Gastrointestinal: Anal inflammation, anal ulceration, anorexia, diarrhea, mucositis, nausea, vomiting

Hematologic: Myelosuppression, neutropenia (onset: 1-7 days; nadir [biphasic]: 7-9 days and at 15-24 days; recovery [biphasic]: 9-12 days and at 24-34 days), thrombocytopenia (onset: 5 days; nadir: 12-15 days; recovery 15-25 days), anemia, bleeding, leukopenia, megaloblastosis, reticulocytes decreased

Hepatic: Hepatic dysfunction, transaminases increased (acute)

Local: Thrombophlebitis

Less frequent:

Cardiovascular: Chest pain, pericarditis

Central nervous system: Dizziness, headache, neural toxicity, neuritis

Dermatologic: Alopecia, pruritus, skin freckling, skin ulceration, urticaria

Gastrointestinal: Abdominal pain, bowel necrosis, esophageal ulceration, esophagitis, pancreatitis, sore throat

Genitourinary: Urinary retention

Hepatic: Jaundice

Local: Injection site cellulitis

Ocular: Conjunctivitis

Renal: Renal dysfunction

Respiratory: Dyspnea

Miscellaneous: Allergic edema, anaphylaxis, sepsis

Infrequent and/or case reports: Acute respiratory distress syndrome, amylase increased, angina, aseptic meningitis, cardiopulmonary arrest (acute), cerebral dysfunction, cytarabine syndrome (bone pain, chest pain, conjunctivitis, fever, maculopapular rash, malaise, myalgia); exanthematous pustulosis, hepatic sinusoidal obstruction syndrome (SOS; veno-occlusive disease), hyperuricemia, injection site inflammation (SubQ injection), injection site pain (SubQ injection), interstitial pneumonitis, lipase increased, paralysis (intrathecal and I.V. combination therapy), reversible posterior leukoencephalopathy syndrome (RPLS), rhabdomyolysis, toxic megacolon

Adverse events associated with high-dose cytarabine (CNS, gastrointestinal, ocular, and pulmonary toxicities are more common with high-dose regimens):

Cardiovascular: Cardiomegaly, cardiomyopathy (in combination with cyclophosphamide)

Central nervous system: Cerebellar toxicity, coma, neurotoxicity (up to 55% in patients with renal impairment), personality change, somnolence

Dermatologic: Alopecia (complete), desquamation, rash (severe)

Gastrointestinal: Gastrointestinal ulcer, pancreatitis, peritonitis, pneumatosis cystoides intestinalis

Hepatic: Hyperbilirubinemia, liver abscess, liver damage, necrotizing colitis

Neuromuscular & skeletal: Peripheral neuropathy (motor and sensory)

Ocular: Corneal toxicity, hemorrhagic conjunctivitis

Respiratory: Pulmonary edema, syndrome of sudden respiratory distress

Miscellaneous: Sepsis

Adverse events associated with intrathecal cytarabine administration:

Central nervous system: Accessory nerve paralysis, fever, necrotizing leukoencephalopathy (with concurrent cranial irradiation, I.T. methotrexate, and I.T. hydrocortisone), neurotoxicity, paraplegia

Gastrointestinal: Dysphagia, nausea, vomiting

Ocular: Blindness (with concurrent systemic chemotherapy and cranial irradiation), diplopia

Respiratory: Cough, hoarseness

Miscellaneous: Aphonia

General Dosage Range Dosage adjustment recommended in patients with hepatic or renal impairment

I.V.: *Children and Adults:* AML Induction: 100-200 mg/m^2/day for 7 days

Mechanism of Action Inhibits DNA synthesis. Cytosine gains entry into cells by a carrier process, and then must be converted to its active compound, aracytidine triphosphate. Cytosine is a pyrimidine analog and is incorporated into DNA; however, the primary action is inhibition of DNA polymerase resulting in decreased DNA synthesis and repair. The degree of cytotoxicity correlates linearly with incorporation into DNA; therefore, incorporation into the DNA is responsible for drug activity and toxicity. Cytarabine is specific for the S phase of the cell cycle (blocks progression from the G_1 to the S phase).

Pharmacodynamics/Kinetics

Half-life Elimination I.V.: Initial: 7-20 minutes; Terminal: 1-3 hours; I.T.: 2-6 hours

Time to Peak I.M., SubQ: 20-60 minutes

Pregnancy Risk Factor D

Pregnancy Considerations Teratogenic effects were demonstrated in animal studies; limb and ear defects have been noted in case reports of cytarabine exposure during the first trimester of pregnancy. The following have also been noted in the neonate: Pancytopenia, WBC depression, electrolyte abnormalities, prematurity, low birth weight, decreased hematocrit or platelets. Risk to the fetus is decreased if treatment can be avoided during the first trimester; however, women of childbearing potential should be advised of the potential risks.

Cytarabine (Liposomal)
(sye TARE a been lye po SO mal)

Brand Names: U.S. DepoCyt®

Brand Names: Canada DepoCyt®

Pharmacologic Category Antineoplastic Agent, Antimetabolite; Antineoplastic Agent, Antimetabolite (Pyrimidine Analog)

Use Treatment of lymphomatous meningitis

Local Anesthetic/Vasoconstrictor Precautions No information available to require special precautions

Effects on Dental Treatment No significant effects or complications reported

Effects on Bleeding Hematologic effects depend on dose and schedule of treatment. Platelets are one of the primary cell lines affected. Patients will develop thrombocytopenia on approximately day 7 which resolves about day 21-28. A medical consult is recommended.

Adverse Effects

>10%:

Cardiovascular: Peripheral edema (11%)

Central nervous system: Chemical arachnoiditis (without dexamethasone premedication: 100%; with dexamethasone premedication: 33% to 42%; grade 4: 19% to 30%; onset: ≤5 days); headache (56%), confusion (33%), fever (32%), fatigue (25%), seizure (20% to 22%), dizziness (18%), lethargy (16%), insomnia (14%), memory impairment (14%), pain (14%)

Endocrine & metabolic: Dehydration (13%)

Gastrointestinal: Nausea (46%), vomiting (44%), constipation (25%), diarrhea (12%), appetite decreased (11%)

Genitourinary: Urinary tract infection (14%)

Hematologic: Anemia (12%), thrombocytopenia (3% to 11%)

Neuromuscular & skeletal: Weakness (40%), back pain (24%), abnormal gait (23%), limb pain (15%), neck pain (14%), arthralgia (11%), neck stiffness (11%)

Ocular: Blurred vision (11%)

1% to 10%:

Cardiovascular: Tachycardia (9%), hypotension (8%), hypertension (6%), syncope (3%), edema (2%)

Central nervous system: Agitation (10%), hypoesthesia (10%), depression (8%), anxiety (7%), sensory neuropathy (3%)

Dermatologic: Pruritus (2%)

Endocrine & metabolic: Hypokalemia (7%), hyponatremia (7%), hyperglycemia (6%)

Gastrointestinal: Abdominal pain (9%), dysphagia (8%), anorexia (5%), hemorrhoids (3%), mucosal inflammation (3%)

Genitourinary: Incontinence (7%), urinary retention (5%)

Hematologic: Neutropenia (10%), contusion (2%)

Neuromuscular & skeletal: Muscle weakness (10%), tremor (9%), peripheral neuropathy (3% to 4%), abnormal reflexes (3%)

Otic: Hypoacusis (6%)

Respiratory: Dyspnea (10%), cough (7%), pneumonia (6%)

Miscellaneous: Diaphoresis (2%)

General Dosage Range Dosage adjustment recommended in patients who develop toxicities

I.T.: *Adults:* Induction: 50 mg every 14 days for a total of 2 doses (weeks 1 and 3); Consolidation: 50 mg every 14 days for 3 doses (weeks 5, 7, and 9), followed by 50 mg at week 13; Maintenance: 50 mg every 28 days for 4 doses (weeks 17, 21, 25, and 29)

Mechanism of Action Cytarabine liposomal is a sustained-release formulation of the active ingredient cytarabine, an antimetabolite which acts through inhibition of DNA synthesis and is cell cycle-specific for the S phase of cell division. Cytarabine is converted intracellularly to its active metabolite cytarabine-5'-triphosphate (ara-CTP). Ara-CTP also appears to be incorporated into DNA and RNA; however, the primary action is inhibition of DNA polymerase, resulting in decreased DNA synthesis and repair. The liposomal formulation allows for gradual release, resulting in prolonged exposure.

Pharmacodynamics/Kinetics

Half-life Elimination CSF: 6-82 hours

Time to Peak CSF: Intrathecal: <1 hour

Pregnancy Risk Factor D

Pregnancy Considerations Reproductive studies have not been conducted with cytarabine liposomal. Cytarabine, the active component, has been associated with fetal malformations when given as a component of systemic combination chemotherapy during the first trimester. Systemic exposure following intrathecal administration of cytarabine liposomal is negligible; however, women of childbearing potential should avoid becoming pregnant during treatment.

Dabigatran Etexilate (da BIG a tran ett EX ill ate)

Related Information

Antiplatelet and Anticoagulation Considerations in Dentistry *on page 1503*

Brand Names: U.S. Pradaxa®

Brand Names: Canada Pradaxa®

Pharmacologic Category Anticoagulant, Thrombin Inhibitor

Use Prevention of stroke and systemic embolism in patients with nonvalvular atrial fibrillation

2011 ACCF/AHA/HRS atrial fibrillation guidelines: Not recommended for patients with coexisting prosthetic heart valve or hemodynamically significant valve disease, severe renal failure (Cl_{cr} <15 mL/minute), or advanced liver disease (impaired baseline clotting function)

Canadian labeling: Additional uses (not in U.S. labeling): Postoperative thromboprophylaxis in patients who have undergone total hip or knee replacement procedures

Local Anesthetic/Vasoconstrictor Precautions No information available to require special precautions

Effects on Dental Treatment Dabigatran etexilate is converted *in vivo* to the active dabigatran, a specific, reversible, direct thrombin inhibitor. It causes bleeding by preventing thrombin-mediated effects, and by inhibiting thrombin-induced platelet aggregation.

Effects on Bleeding Dabigatran increases the risk of bleeding and can cause significant and sometimes fatal bleeding. Risk factors include the use of dabigatran etexilate with drugs that increase the risk of bleeding (eg, nonsteroidal anti-inflammatory drugs [NSAIDs]). A medical consult is recommended.

Adverse Effects Adverse reactions listed below are reflective of both the U.S. and Canadian product information. **Important:** No specific antidote exists for dabigatran reversal. Therapy for severe hemorrhage may include transfusions of fresh frozen plasma, packed red blood cells, or surgical intervention when appropriate (Wann, 2011). The use of a prothrombin complex concentrate (PCC) (Cofact®, not available in the U.S.) has been shown to be **ineffective** for dabigatran reversal (Eerenberg, 2011).

>10%:
Gastrointestinal: Dyspepsia (11%; includes abdominal discomfort/pain, epigastric discomfort)
Hematologic: Bleeding (8% to 33%; major: ≤6%)
1% to 10%:
Gastrointestinal: GI hemorrhage (≤6%), gastritis-like symptoms (eg, GERD, esophagitis, erosive gastritis, GI ulcer)
Hematologic: Anemia (1% to 4%), hematoma (1% to 2%), hemoglobin decreased (1% to 2%), hemorrhage (postprocedural or wound: 1% to 2%)
Hepatic: ALT increased (≥3 x ULN: 2% to 3%)
Renal: Hematuria (1%)
Miscellaneous: Wound secretion (5%), postprocedural discharge (1%)

General Dosage Range Dosage adjustment recommended in patients with renal impairment or patients on concomitant therapy.

Oral: *Adults:* 150 mg twice daily

Mechanism of Action Prodrug lacking anticoagulant activity that is converted *in vivo* to the active dabigatran, a specific, reversible, direct thrombin inhibitor that inhibits both free and fibrin-bound thrombin. Inhibits coagulation by preventing thrombin-mediated effects, including cleavage of fibrinogen to fibrin monomers, activation of factors V, VIII, XI, and XIII, and inhibition of thrombin-induced platelet aggregation.

Pharmacodynamics/Kinetics

Half-life Elimination 12-17 hours; Elderly: 14-17 hours; Mild-to-moderate renal impairment: 15-18 hours; Severe renal impairment: 28 hours (Stangier, 2010)

Time to Peak Plasma: Dabigatran: 1 hour; delayed 2 hours by food (no effect on bioavailability)

Pregnancy Risk Factor C

Pregnancy Considerations Adverse events were observed in some animal reproduction studies. Data are insufficient to evaluate the safety of direct thrombin inhibitors during pregnancy; use of oral agents during pregnancy should be avoided (Guyatt, 2012). Consider the risks of bleeding and stroke if used during pregnancy.

Dental Comment At recommended therapeutic doses, dabigatran etexilate prolongs the activated partial thromboplastin time (aPTT). With an oral dose of 150 mg twice daily, the median peak aPTT is approximately twice that of control values. Twelve hours after the last dose, the median aPTT is 1.5 x control. The INR test is relatively insensitive to the activity of dabigatran etexilate and may not be elevated in patients on dabigatran etexilate.

Dacarbazine (da KAR ba zeen)

Brand Names: Canada Dacarbazine for Injection

Pharmacologic Category Antineoplastic Agent, Alkylating Agent (Triazene)

Use Treatment of malignant melanoma, Hodgkin's disease

Unlabeled Use Treatment of soft-tissue sarcomas, islet cell tumors, pheochromocytoma, medullary carcinoma of the thyroid

Local Anesthetic/Vasoconstrictor Precautions No information available to require special precautions

Effects on Dental Treatment Key adverse event(s) related to dental treatment: Metallic taste.

Effects on Bleeding Hematopoietic suppression (including platelets) is the most common toxicity of dacarbazine. Risk of thrombocytopenia, which can be life-threatening, reaches a nadir at 7-10 days. A medical consult is recommended.

Adverse Effects Frequency not always defined.
Dermatologic: Alopecia
Gastrointestinal: Nausea and vomiting (>90%), anorexia
Hematologic: Myelosuppression (onset: 5-7 days; nadir: 7-10 days; recovery: 21-28 days), leukopenia, thrombocytopenia
Local: Pain on infusion

General Dosage Range Dosage adjustment recommended in patients with renal impairment

I.V.:
Children: 375 mg/m^2 on days 1 and 15, repeat every 28 days
Adults: 375 mg/m^2 days 1 and 15 every 4 weeks **or** 250 mg/m^2 days 1-5 every 3 weeks

Mechanism of Action Alkylating agent which is converted to the active alkylating metabolite MTIC [(methyl-triazene-1-yl)-imidazole-4-carboxamide] via the cytochrome P450 system. The cytotoxic effects of MTIC are manifested through alkylation (methylation) of DNA at the O^6, N^7 guanine positions which lead to DNA double strand breaks and apoptosis. Non-cell cycle specific.

Pharmacodynamics/Kinetics

Half-life Elimination Biphasic: Initial: 20-40 minutes; Terminal: 5 hours; Patients with renal and hepatic dysfunction: Initial: 55 minutes, Terminal: 7.2 hours

Pregnancy Risk Factor C

Pregnancy Considerations [U.S. Boxed Warning]: **This agent is carcinogenic and/or teratogenic when used in animals;** adverse effects have been observed in animal studies. There are no adequate and well-controlled trials in pregnant women; use in pregnancy only if the potential benefit outweighs the potential risk to the fetus.

DACTINomycin (dak ti noe MYE sin)

Brand Names: U.S. Cosmegen®
Brand Names: Canada Cosmegen®
Pharmacologic Category Antineoplastic Agent, Antibiotic
Use Treatment of Wilms' tumor, childhood rhabdomyosarcoma, Ewing's sarcoma, metastatic testicular tumors (nonseminomatous), gestational trophoblastic neoplasm; regional perfusion (palliative or adjunctive) of locally recurrent or locoregional solid tumors (sarcomas, carcinomas and adenocarcinomas)
Unlabeled Use Treatment of ovarian cancer (germ cell or stromal tumors), osteosarcoma, soft tissue sarcoma (other than rhabdomyosarcoma)
Local Anesthetic/Vasoconstrictor Precautions No information available to require special precautions
Effects on Dental Treatment Key adverse event(s) related to dental treatment: Stomatitis and mucositis
Effects on Bleeding Onset of thrombocytopenia, which can be severe, occurs at 7 days with the nadir at 14-21 days. A medical consult is recommended.
Adverse Effects Frequency not defined.
Central nervous system: Fatigue, fever, lethargy, malaise
Dermatologic: Acne, alopecia (reversible), cheilitis, erythema multiforme, increased pigmentation, sloughing, or erythema of previously irradiated skin; skin eruptions, Stevens-Johnson syndrome, toxic epidermal necrolysis
Endocrine & metabolic: Growth retardation, hyperuricemia, hypocalcemia
Gastrointestinal: Abdominal pain, anorexia, diarrhea, dysphagia, esophagitis, GI ulceration, mucositis, nausea, pharyngitis, proctitis, stomatitis, vomiting
Hematologic: Agranulocytosis, anemia, aplastic anemia, febrile neutropenia, leukopenia, myelosuppression (onset: 7 days, nadir: 14-21 days, recovery: 21-28 days), neutropenia, pancytopenia, reticulocytopenia, thrombocytopenia, thrombocytopenia (immune mediated)
Hepatic: Ascites, bilirubin increased, hepatic failure, hepatitis, hepatomegaly, hepatopathy thrombocytopenia syndrome, hepatotoxicity, liver function test abnormality, hepatic sinusoidal obstruction syndrome (SOS; veno-occlusive liver disease)
Local: Erythema, edema, epidermolysis, pain, tissue necrosis, and ulceration (following extravasation)
Neuromuscular & skeletal: Myalgia
Renal: Renal function abnormality
Respiratory: Pneumonitis
Miscellaneous: Anaphylactoid reaction, infection, sepsis (including neutropenic sepsis)
General Dosage Range
I.V.:
Children >6 months: 15 mcg/kg/day **or** 400-600 mcg/m²/day for 5 days every 3-6 weeks
Adults: 12-15 mcg/kg/day **or** 400-600 mcg/m²/day for 5 days every 3-6 weeks **or** 1000 mcg/m² on day 1 **or** 500 mcg/dose days 1 and 2

Regional perfusion: *Adults:* Lower extremity or pelvis: 50 mcg/kg; Upper extremity: 35 mcg/kg
Mechanism of Action Binds to the guanine portion of DNA intercalating between guanine and cytosine base pairs inhibiting DNA and RNA synthesis and protein synthesis
Pharmacodynamics/Kinetics
Half-life Elimination ~36 hours; Children: Range: 14-43 hours (Veal, 2005)
Pregnancy Risk Factor D
Pregnancy Considerations Animal reproduction studies have demonstrated teratogenic effects and fetal loss. Women of childbearing potential are advised not to become pregnant. Use only when potential benefit justifies potential risk to the fetus. **[U.S. Boxed Warning]: Avoid exposure during pregnancy.**

Dalfampridine (dal FAM pri deen)

Brand Names: U.S. Ampyra™
Brand Names: Canada Fampyra™
Pharmacologic Category Potassium Channel Blocker
Use Treatment to improve walking in patients with multiple sclerosis (MS)
Local Anesthetic/Vasoconstrictor Precautions No information available to require special precautions
Effects on Dental Treatment No significant effects or complications reported
Effects on Bleeding No information available to require special precautions
Adverse Effects
>10%: Genitourinary: Urinary tract infection (12%)
1% to 10%:
Central nervous system: Insomnia (9%), dizziness (7%), headache (7%), multiple sclerosis relapse (4%), seizures (up to 4%; dose-dependent)
Gastrointestinal: Nausea (7%), constipation (3%), dyspepsia (2%)
Neuromuscular & skeletal: Weakness (7%), back pain (5%), balance disorder (5%), paresthesia (4%)
Respiratory: Nasopharyngitis (4%), pharyngolaryngeal pain (2%)
General Dosage Range Oral: Extended release: *Adults:* 10 mg every 12 hours
Mechanism of Action Nonspecific potassium channel blocker which improves conduction in focally demyelinated axons by delaying repolarization and prolonging the duration of action potentials. Enhanced neuronal conduction is thought to strengthen skeletal muscle fiber twitch activity, thereby, improving peripheral motor neurologic function.
Pharmacodynamics/Kinetics
Half-life Elimination 5.2-6.5 hours; prolonged in severe renal impairment (~3 times longer)
Time to Peak Plasma: 3-4 hours
Pregnancy Risk Factor C
Pregnancy Considerations Adverse events have been observed in animal reproduction studies, including decreased growth and death.

Dalteparin (dal TE pa rin)

Related Information
Cardiovascular Diseases *on page 1492*
Brand Names: U.S. Fragmin®
Brand Names: Canada Fragmin®
Pharmacologic Category Low Molecular Weight Heparin

Use Prevention of deep vein thrombosis (DVT) which may lead to pulmonary embolism, in patients requiring abdominal surgery who are at risk for thromboembolism complications (eg, patients >40 years of age, obesity, patients with malignancy, history of DVT or pulmonary embolism, and surgical procedures requiring general anesthesia and lasting >30 minutes); prevention of DVT in patients undergoing hip-replacement surgery; patients immobile during an acute illness; prevention of ischemic complications in patients with unstable angina or non-Q-wave myocardial infarction on concurrent aspirin therapy; in patients with cancer, extended treatment (6 months) of acute symptomatic venous thromboembolism (DVT and/or PE) to reduce the recurrence of venous thromboembolism

Canadian labeling: Additional use (unlabeled use in U.S.): Treatment of acute DVT; prevention of venous thromboembolism (VTE) in patients at risk of VTE undergoing general surgery; anticoagulant in extracorporeal circuit during hemodialysis and hemofiltration

Unlabeled Use Active treatment of deep vein thrombosis (noncancer patients)

Local Anesthetic/Vasoconstrictor Precautions No information available to require special precautions

Effects on Dental Treatment Key adverse event(s) related to dental treatment: Bleeding is the major adverse effect of dalteparin. Adverse reactions reported were generally less than those seen with heparin. See Effects on Bleeding.

Effects on Bleeding The risk of bleeding and thrombocytopenia is high with low molecular weight heparin anticoagulants such as dalteparin. The use of NSAIDs and aspirin should be avoided. A medical consult is recommended.

Adverse Effects Note: As with all anticoagulants, bleeding is the major adverse effect of dalteparin. Hemorrhage may occur at virtually any site. Risk is dependent on multiple variables.

>10%: Hematologic: Bleeding (3% to 14%), thrombocytopenia (including heparin-induced thrombocytopenia, <1%; cancer clinical trials: ~11%)

1% to 10%:

Hematologic: Major bleeding (up to 6%), wound hematoma (up to 3%)

Hepatic: AST >3 times upper limit of normal (5% to 9%), ALT >3 times upper limit of normal (4% to 10%)

Local: Pain at injection site (up to 12%), injection site hematoma (up to 7%)

General Dosage Range SubQ: *Adults:* Prophylaxis: 2500-5000 units daily; Treatment: 120 units/kg every 12 hours (maximum: 10,000 units/dose) or ~150-200 units/kg (maximum: 18,000 units/dose) once daily

Mechanism of Action Low molecular weight heparin analog with a molecular weight of 4000-6000 daltons; the commercial product contains 3% to 15% heparin with a molecular weight <3000 daltons, 65% to 78% with a molecular weight of 3000-8000 daltons and 14% to 26% with a molecular weight >8000 daltons; while dalteparin has been shown to inhibit both factor Xa and factor IIa (thrombin), the antithrombotic effect of dalteparin is characterized by a higher ratio of antifactor Xa to antifactor IIa activity (ratio = 4)

Pharmacodynamics/Kinetics

Onset of Action Anti-Xa activity: Within 1-2 hours

Duration of Action >12 hours

Half-life Elimination Route dependent: Anti-Xa activity: 2-5 hours; prolonged in chronic renal insufficiency: 3.7-7.7 hours (following a single 5000 unit dose)

Time to Peak Serum: Anti-Xa activity: ~4 hours

Pregnancy Risk Factor B

Pregnancy Considerations Adverse effects were not observed in animal reproduction studies. Low molecular weight heparin (LMWH) does not cross the placenta; increased risks of fetal bleeding or teratogenic effects have not been reported.

LMWH is recommended over unfractionated heparin for the treatment of acute venous thromboembolism (VTE) in pregnant women. LMWH is also recommended over unfractionated heparin for VTE prophylaxis in pregnant women with certain risk factors. LMWH should be discontinued at least 24 hours prior to induction of labor or a planned cesarean delivery. For women undergoing cesarean section and who have additional risk factors for developing VTE, the prophylactic use of LMWH may be considered. For women who require long-term anticoagulation with warfarin and who are considering pregnancy, LMWH substitution should be done prior to conception when possible. When choosing therapy, fetal outcomes (ie, pregnancy loss, malformations), maternal outcomes (ie, VTE, hemorrhage), burden of therapy, and maternal preference should be considered (Guyatt, 2012). Multiple-dose vials contain benzyl alcohol (avoid in pregnant women due to association with gasping syndrome in premature infants; use of preservative-free formulation is recommended.

Danaparoid (da NAP a roid)

Brand Names: Canada Organan®

Pharmacologic Category Anticoagulant; Heparinoid

Use Prevention of postoperative deep vein thrombosis (DVT) following orthopedic or major abdominal and thoracic surgery; prevention of DVT in patients with confirmed diagnosis of non-hemorrhagic stroke; management of heparin-induced thrombocytopenia (HIT)

Local Anesthetic/Vasoconstrictor Precautions No information available to require special precautions

Effects on Dental Treatment Key adverse event(s) related to dental treatment: Bleeding is the major adverse effect of danaparoid. See Effects on Bleeding.

Effects on Bleeding As with all anticoagulants, bleeding is the major adverse effect of danaparoid. Hemorrhage may occur at virtually any site; risk is dependent on multiple variables including the intensity of anticoagulation and patient susceptibility. At the recommended doses, LMWHs do not significantly influence platelet aggregation or affect global clotting time (ie, PT or aPTT). Medical consult is suggested.

Adverse Effects As with all anticoagulants, bleeding is the major adverse effect of danaparoid. Hemorrhage may occur at virtually any site. Risk is dependent on multiple variables.

Frequency not always defined.

Cardiovascular: Arterial pressure decreased, atrial fibrillation, cerebral infarction, DVT, hypotension, peripheral edema

Central nervous system: Pain (5%), fever (2% to 5%), confusion, fatigue, insomnia, loss of consciousness, restlessness

Dermatologic: Rash (1%), bruising

Gastrointestinal: Nausea (3%), constipation (2%)

Genitourinary: Urinary retention (1%), urinary incontinence

Hematologic: Cerebral hemorrhage, hematoma, hemorrhage, spinal or epidural hematomas (may occur following neuraxial anesthesia or spinal puncture, resulting in paralysis), thrombocytopenia

Hepatic: Alkaline phosphatase increased, ALT increased (transient), AST increased (transient)

Local: Injection site hematoma (≤5%)

Neuromuscular & skeletal: Hemiparesis, involuntary muscle contractions, tremor

Renal: Hematuria

Respiratory: Apnea, asthma

Miscellaneous: Infection (2%), allergic reaction, sepsis

General Dosage Range Dosage adjustment recommended in patients with renal impairment

SubQ:

Children: 10 units/kg every 12 hours

Adults: Dosage varies greatly depending on indication

I.V.:

Children: Initial bolus: 30 units/kg; maintenance: 1.2-4 units/kg/hour

Adults: Dosage varies greatly depending on indication

Mechanism of Action Inhibits factor Xa and IIa (anti-Xa effects >20 times anti-IIa effects). Prevents fibrin formation in the coagulation pathway via thrombin generation inhibition.

Pharmacodynamics/Kinetics

Onset of Action Peak effect: SubQ: Maximum anti-factor Xa activities occur in 4-5 hours

Half-life Elimination Anti-Xa activity: ~25 hours (renal impairment: 29-35 hours); Thrombin generation inhibition activity: ~7 hours

Pregnancy Considerations Teratogenic effects have not been observed in animal reproduction studies. The manufacturer labeling states that incidental observations in pregnant women during the last trimesters, gave no indication that use during pregnancy results in fetal abnormalities or exacerbation of bleeding in the mother or infant during delivery. Use in pregnant women however is generally not recommended unless deemed medically necessary and alternative therapy is unavailable. Danaparoid does not cross the placenta and is the preferred anticoagulant in pregnant women with HIT (Guyatt, 2012).

Product Availability Not available in U.S.

Danazol (DA na zole)

Brand Names: Canada Cyclomen®

Pharmacologic Category Androgen

Use Treatment of endometriosis, fibrocystic breast disease, and hereditary angioedema

Local Anesthetic/Vasoconstrictor Precautions No information available to require special precautions

Effects on Dental Treatment No significant effects or complications reported

Effects on Bleeding Thrombocytopenia and thrombotic events have been reported.

Adverse Effects Frequency not defined.

Cardiovascular: Benign intracranial hypertension (rare), edema, flushing, hypertension, MI, palpitation, tachycardia

Central nervous system: Anxiety (rare), chills (rare), convulsions (rare), depression, dizziness, emotional lability, fainting, fatigue, fever (rare), Guillain-Barré syndrome (rare), headache, nervousness, sleep disorders

Dermatologic: Acne, alopecia, erythema multiforme (rare), mild hirsutism, maculopapular rash, papular rash, petechial rash, pruritus, purpuric rash, seborrhea, Stevens-Johnson syndrome (rare), photosensitivity (rare), urticaria, vesicular rash

Endocrine & metabolic: Amenorrhea (which may continue post therapy), breast size reduction, clitoris hypertrophy (rare), glucose intolerance/glucagon changes, HDL decreased, LDL increased, libido changes, nipple discharge (rare), menstrual disturbances (spotting, altered timing of cycle), semen abnormalities (changes in volume, viscosity, sperm count/motility), sex hormone-binding globulin changes, spermatogenesis reduction, thyroid binding globulin changes

Gastrointestinal: Appetite changes (rare), bleeding gums (rare), constipation, gastroenteritis, nausea, pancreatitis (rare), splenic peliosis (rare), vomiting, weight gain

Genitourinary: Vaginal dryness, vaginal irritation, pelvic pain (rare)

Hematologic: Eosinophilia, erythrocytosis (reversible), leukocytosis, leukopenia, platelet count increased, polycythemia, RBC increased, thrombocytopenia

Hepatic: Cholestatic jaundice, hepatic adenoma, jaundice, liver enzymes increased, malignant tumors (after prolonged use), peliosis hepatis

Neuromuscular & skeletal: Back pain, carpal tunnel syndrome (rare), CPK changes, extremity pain, joint lockup, joint pain, joint swelling, muscle cramps, neck pain, paresthesia, spasms, tremor, weakness

Ocular: Cataracts (rare), visual disturbances

Renal: Hematuria

Respiratory: Interstitial pneumonitis, nasal congestion (rare)

Miscellaneous: Diaphoresis, voice change (hoarseness, sore throat, instability, deepening of pitch)

General Dosage Range Oral:

Adults (females): 100-800 mg/day in 2 divided doses

Adults (females/males): Hereditary angioedema: Initial: 200 mg 2-3 times/day; after favorable response decrease dosage by 50% or less

Mechanism of Action Suppresses pituitary output of follicle-stimulating hormone and luteinizing hormone that causes regression and atrophy of normal and ectopic endometrial tissue; decreases rate of growth of abnormal breast tissue; reduces attacks associated with hereditary angioedema by increasing levels of C4 component of complement

Pharmacodynamics/Kinetics

Onset of Action Therapeutic: ~4 weeks

Half-life Elimination ~10 hours (variable; up to 24 hours following long-term use for endometriosis)

Time to Peak Serum: Within 2-8 hours (median 4 hours)

Pregnancy Risk Factor X

Pregnancy Considerations [U.S. Boxed Warning]: Pregnancy should be ruled out prior to treatment using a sensitive test (beta subunit test, if available). Nonhormonal contraception should be used during therapy. May cause androgenic effects to the female fetus; clitoral hypertrophy, labial fusion, urogenital sinus defect, vaginal atresia, and ambiguous genitalia have been reported. Therapy should be discontinued for 2 months prior to attempting pregnancy (Caballero, 2012).

Dantrolene (DAN troe leen)

Brand Names: U.S. Dantrium®; Revonto®

Brand Names: Canada Dantrium®

Pharmacologic Category Skeletal Muscle Relaxant

Use Treatment of spasticity associated with upper motor neuron disorders (eg, spinal cord injury, stroke, cerebral palsy, or multiple sclerosis); management of malignant hyperthermia (MH); prevention of malignant hyperthermia in susceptible individuals (preoperative/postoperative administration)

Note: Dantrolene prophylaxis is not recommended for most MH-susceptible patients, provided nontriggering anesthetics are used and an adequate supply of dantrolene is available.

Unlabeled Use Neuroleptic malignant syndrome (NMS)

Local Anesthetic/Vasoconstrictor Precautions No information available to require special precautions

Effects on Dental Treatment No significant effects or complications reported

Effects on Bleeding No information available to require special precautions

Adverse Effects Frequency not defined.

Cardiovascular: Blood pressure (altered), heart failure, tachycardia

Central nervous system: Chills, confusion, dizziness, drowsiness, fatigue, fever, headache, insomnia, light-headedness, malaise, mental depression, nervousness, seizure, speech disturbance

Dermatologic: Eczematoid eruption, hair growth (abnormal), pruritus, rash, urticaria

Gastrointestinal: Abdominal cramps, anorexia, constipation, diarrhea, dysphagia, gastric irritation, gastrointestinal hemorrhage, nausea, taste change, vomiting

Genitourinary: Crystalluria, difficult erection, difficult urination, nocturia, polyuria, urinary incontinence, urinary retention

Hematologic: Anemia, aplastic anemia, leukopenia, thrombocytopenia

Hepatic: Hepatitis

Local: Injection site reaction (pain, erythema, swelling), thrombophlebitis, tissue necrosis

Neuromuscular & skeletal: Back pain, muscle weakness, myalgia

Ocular: Blurred vision, diplopia, tearing (excessive)

Renal: Hematuria

Respiratory: Feeling of suffocation, pleural effusion (associated with pericarditis), pulmonary edema, respiratory depression

Miscellaneous: Anaphylaxis, diaphoresis, lymphocytic lymphoma, sialorrhea

General Dosage Range

I.V.: *Children and Adults:* 1-2.5 mg/kg; may repeat up to cumulative dose of 10 mg/kg **or** 2.5 mg/kg as a single dose

Oral:

Children: 4-8 mg/kg/day in 4 divided doses **or** 0.5-2 mg/kg/dose 1-4 times daily (maximum: 400 mg daily)

Adults: 4-8 mg/kg/day in 4 divided doses **or** 25-100 mg 1-4 times daily (maximum: 400 mg daily)

Mechanism of Action Acts directly on skeletal muscle by interfering with release of calcium ion from the sarcoplasmic reticulum; prevents or reduces the increase in myoplasmic calcium ion concentration that activates the acute catabolic processes associated with malignant hyperthermia

Pharmacodynamics/Kinetics

Half-life Elimination 4-8 hours

Pregnancy Risk Factor C

Pregnancy Considerations Adverse events were observed in animal reproduction studies. Dantrolene crosses the human placenta. Cord blood concentrations are similar to those in the maternal plasma at term and dantrolene can be detected in the newborn serum at delivery. Adverse events were not observed in the newborn following maternal doses of 100 mg/day administered orally prior to delivery (Shime, 1988). Uterine atony has been reported following dantrolene injection after delivery; however, this may be due in part to the mannitol contained in the I.V. preparation (Shin, 1995; Weingarten, 1987). Prophylactic use of dantrolene is not routinely recommended in pregnant women susceptible to MH prior to obstetric surgery, if use is needed, close monitoring of the mother and newborn is recommended (Krause, 2004; Norman, 1995).

Dapsone (Systemic) (DAP sone)

Related Information

HIV Infection and AIDS *on page 1520*

Generic Availability (U.S.) Yes

Pharmacologic Category Antibiotic, Miscellaneous

Dental Use Pemphigus vulgaris (oral), aphthous ulcers (severe), bullous systemic lupus erythematosus; all in consultation with patient's physician as significant monitoring required

Use Treatment of leprosy (due to susceptible strains of *Mycobacterium leprae*) and dermatitis herpetiformis

Unlabeled Use Prophylaxis of toxoplasmosis in severely-immunocompromised patients; alternative agent for *Pneumocystis jirovecii* pneumonia (PCP) prophylaxis (monotherapy) and treatment (in combination with trimethoprim); pemphigus vulgaris (oral), aphthous ulcers (severe), bullous systemic lupus erythematosus; all in consultation with patient's physician as significant monitoring required

Local Anesthetic/Vasoconstrictor Precautions No information available to require special precautions

Effects on Dental Treatment No significant effects or complications reported

Effects on Bleeding No information available to require special precautions

Adverse Effects Frequency not always defined.

>10%: Hematologic: Reticulocyte increase (2% to 12%), hemolysis (>10%; dose related; seen in patients with and without G6PD deficiency), hemoglobin decrease (>10%; 1-2 g/dL; almost all patients), methemoglobinemia (>10%), red cell life span shortened (>10%), Agranulocytosis, anemia, leukopenia, pure red cell aplasia (case report)

Cardiovascular: Tachycardia

Central nervous system: Fever, headache, insomnia, psychosis, vertigo

Dermatologic: Bullous and exfoliative dermatitis, erythema nodosum, exfoliative dermatitis, morbilliform and scarlatiniform reactions, phototoxicity, Stevens-Johnson syndrome, toxic epidural necrolysis, urticaria

Endocrine & metabolic: Hypoalbuminemia (without proteinuria), male infertility

Gastrointestinal: Abdominal pain, nausea, pancreatitis, vomiting

Hepatic: Cholestatic jaundice, hepatitis

Neuromuscular & skeletal: Drug-induced lupus erythematosus, lower motor neuron toxicity (prolonged therapy), peripheral neuropathy (rare, nonleprosy patients)

Ocular: Blurred vision

Otic: Tinnitus

Renal: Albuminuria, nephrotic syndrome, renal papillary necrosis

Respiratory: Interstitial pneumonitis, pulmonary eosinophilia

Miscellaneous: Infectious mononucleosis-like syndrome (rash, fever, lymphadenopathy, hepatic dysfunction)

Dental Usual Dosage Oral: Adults:

Aphthous ulcers, severe (unlabeled use): 50 mg once daily

Bullous systemic lupus erythematosus (unlabeled use): 100 mg once daily

Dosage Oral:

Aphthous ulcers, severe (unlabeled use): Adults: 50 mg once daily

Bullous systemic lupus erythematosus (unlabeled use): Adults: 100 mg once daily

Leprosy:

Children: 1-2 mg/kg/24 hours, up to a maximum of 100 mg/day, in combination with other antileprosy agents; duration of therapy is variable

Adults: 100 mg/day, in combination with other antileprosy agents; duration of therapy is variable

Dermatitis herpetiformis: Adults: Start at 50 mg/day, increase to 300 mg/day, or higher to achieve full control, reduce dosage to minimum level as soon as possible

Pneumocystis jirovecii pneumonia, alternative therapy (unlabeled use):

Prophylaxis (primary or secondary):

Infants and Children: 2 mg/kg/day once daily (maximum dose: 100 mg/day) or 4 mg/kg/dose once weekly (maximum dose: 200 mg) (CDC, 2009)

Adolescents and Adults: 100 mg/day once daily or divided in 2 doses as monotherapy **or** 50 mg daily in combination with weekly pyrimethamine and leucovorin (CDC, 2009)

Treatment:

Infants and Children: 2 mg/kg/day once daily (maximum dose: 100 mg/day) in combination with trimethoprim for 21 days

Adolescents and Adults: 100 mg/day once daily in combination with trimethoprim for 21 days

Dosing adjustment in renal impairment: No specific guidelines are available

Mechanism of Action Competitive antagonist of para-aminobenzoic acid (PABA) and prevents normal bacterial utilization of PABA for the synthesis of folic acid

Contraindications Hypersensitivity to dapsone or any component of the formulation

Warnings/Precautions Use with caution in patients with severe anemia, G6PD, methemoglobin reductase deficiency or hemoglobin M deficiency; hypersensitivity to other sulfonamides; aplastic anemia, agranulocytosis and other severe blood dyscrasias have resulted in death; monitor carefully; serious dermatologic reactions (including toxic epidermal necrolysis) are rare but potential occurrences; sulfone reactions may also occur as potentially fatal hypersensitivity reactions; these, but not leprosy reactional states, require drug discontinuation. Motor loss and muscle weakness have been reported with use. Prolonged use may result in fungal or bacterial superinfection, including *C. difficile*-associated diarrhea and pseudomembranous colitis.

Drug Interactions

Metabolism/Transport Effects Substrate of CYP2C19 (minor), CYP2C8 (minor), CYP2C9 (major), CYP2E1 (minor), CYP3A4 (major); **Note:** Assignment of Major/Minor substrate status based on clinically relevant drug interaction potential

Avoid Concomitant Use

Avoid concomitant use of Dapsone (Systemic) with any of the following: BCG; Conivaptan

Increased Effect/Toxicity

Dapsone (Systemic) may increase the levels/effects of: Antimalarial Agents; Prilocaine; Trimethoprim

The levels/effects of Dapsone (Systemic) may be increased by: Antimalarial Agents; Conivaptan; CYP2C9 Inhibitors (Moderate); CYP2C9 Inhibitors (Strong); CYP3A4 Inhibitors (Moderate); CYP3A4 Inhibitors (Strong); Dasatinib; Ivacaftor; Mifepristone; Probenecid; Trimethoprim

Decreased Effect

Dapsone (Systemic) may decrease the levels/effects of: BCG; Sodium Picosulfate; Typhoid Vaccine

The levels/effects of Dapsone (Systemic) may be decreased by: CYP2C9 Inducers (Strong); CYP3A4 Inducers (Strong); Deferasirox; Herbs (CYP3A4 Inducers); Peginterferon Alfa-2b; Rifamycin Derivatives; Tocilizumab

Ethanol/Nutrition/Herb Interactions Herb/Nutraceutical: St John's wort may decrease dapsone levels.

Dietary Considerations Do not give with antacids, alkaline foods, or drugs.

Pharmacodynamics/Kinetics

Half-life Elimination 30 hours (range: 10-50 hours)

Pregnancy Risk Factor C

Pregnancy Considerations Because of adverse events observed in some animal studies, dapsone is classified as pregnancy category C. Per the manufacturer, dapsone has not shown an increased risk of congenital anomalies when given during all trimesters of pregnancy. Several reports have described adverse effects in the newborn after *in utero* exposure to dapsone, including neonatal hemolytic disease, methemoglobinemia, and hyperbilirubinemia. Dapsone is an alternative for prophylaxis and treatment of *Pneumocystis jirovecii* pneumonia (PCP) in pregnant, HIV-infected patients. Dapsone is also recommended for pregnant women requiring maintenance therapy of either leprosy or dermatitis herpetiformis

Lactation Enters breast milk/not recommended (AAP rates "compatible"; AAP 2001 update pending)

Breast-Feeding Considerations Dapsone is excreted in breast milk and can be detected in the serum of nursing infants. Hemolytic anemia has been reported in a breast-fed infant. Breast-feeding is not recommended by the manufacturer due to the potential for carcinogenicity observed in animal studies and the potential for hemolysis in the neonate, especially if there is a family history of G6PD deficiency.

Dosage Forms

Tablet, oral: 25 mg, 100 mg

References

Fabbri P, Cardinali C, Giomi B, et al, "Cutaneous Lupus Erythematosus: Diagnosis and Management," *Am J Clin Dermatol*, 2003, 4 (7):449-65.

Werth VP, Fivenson D, Pandya AG, et al, "Multicenter Randomized, Double-Blind, Placebo, Controlled Clinical Trial of Dapsone as a Glucocorticoid-Sparing Agent in Maintenance-Phase Pemphigus Vulgaris," *Arch Dermatol*, 2008, 144(1):25-32.

Dapsone (Topical) (DAP sone)

Brand Names: U.S. Aczone®

Brand Names: Canada Aczone™

Pharmacologic Category Topical Skin Product, Acne

Use Topical treatment of acne vulgaris

Local Anesthetic/Vasoconstrictor Precautions No information available to require special precautions

Effects on Dental Treatment No significant effects or complications reported

◀ Effects on Bleeding No information available to require special precautions

Adverse Effects Frequency not always defined.

Cardiovascular: Facial edema

Central nervous system: Depression, psychosis, suicide attempt, tonic-clonic movement

Gastrointestinal: Abdominal pain, pancreatitis, vomiting

Local: Application site reactions including burning, dryness, erythema, oiliness/peeling, and pruritus were reported at an incidence similar to or less than placebo

Respiratory: Sinusitis (2%), pharyngitis

General Dosage Range Topical: *Children ≥12 years, Adolescents, and Adults:* Apply pea-sized amount (approximately) in thin layer to affected areas twice daily

Pregnancy Risk Factor C

Pregnancy Considerations Because of adverse events observed in some animal studies, dapsone is classified as pregnancy category C. Dapsone has not shown an increased risk of congenital anomalies when given orally during pregnancy; however, adverse effects in the newborn have been reported following *in utero* exposure. Refer to the Dapsone (Systemic) monograph for details. The amount of dapsone available systemically is less following topical application than with oral administration. During pregnancy, treatment for acne is often discontinued. If treatment is deemed necessary due to the risk of significant scarring or severe disease, dapsone is generally not the topical antibiotic of choice.

DAPTOmycin (DAP toe mye sin)

Brand Names: U.S. Cubicin®

Brand Names: Canada Cubicin®

Pharmacologic Category Antibiotic, Cyclic Lipopeptide

Use Treatment of complicated skin and skin structure infections caused by susceptible aerobic gram-positive organisms; *Staphylococcus aureus* bacteremia, including right-sided native valve infective endocarditis caused by MSSA or MRSA

Unlabeled Use Treatment of severe infections caused by MRSA or VRE; treatment of prosthetic joint infection caused by staphylococci (oxacillin-susceptible or -resistant) or *Enterococcus* (penicillin-susceptible or -resistant)

Local Anesthetic/Vasoconstrictor Precautions No information available to require special precautions

Effects on Dental Treatment No significant effects or complications reported

Effects on Bleeding No information available to require special precautions

Adverse Effects

>10%:

Gastrointestinal: Diarrhea (5% to 12%), vomiting (3% to 12%), constipation (6% to 11%)

Hematologic: Anemia (2% to 13%)

1% to 10%:

Cardiovascular: Peripheral edema (7%), chest pain (7%), hypertension (1% to 6%), hypotension (2% to 5%)

Central nervous system: Insomnia (5% to 9%), headache (5% to7%), fever (2% to 7%), dizziness (2% to 6%), anxiety (5%)

Dermatologic: Rash (4% to 7%), pruritus (3% to 6%), erythema (5%)

Endocrine & metabolic: Hypokalemia (9%), hyperkalemia (5%), hyperphosphatemia (3%)

Gastrointestinal: Nausea (6% to 10%), abdominal pain (6%), dyspepsia (1% to 4%), loose stool (4%), GI hemorrhage (2%)

Genitourinary: Urinary tract infection (2% to 7%)

Hematologic: INR increased (2%), eosinophilia (2%)

Hepatic: Transaminases increased (2% to 3%), alkaline phosphatase increased (2%)

Local: Injection site reaction (3% to 6%)

Neuromuscular & skeletal: CPK increased (3% to 9%), limb pain (2% to 9%), back pain (7%), weakness (5%), arthralgia (1% to 3%)

Renal: Renal failure (2% to 3%)

Respiratory: Pharyngolaryngeal pain (8%), pleural effusion (6%), cough (3%), pneumonia (3%), dyspnea (2% to 3%)

Miscellaneous: Osteomyelitis (6%), bacteremia (5%), diaphoresis (5%), sepsis (5%), infection (fungal, 2% to 3%)

General Dosage Range Dosage adjustment recommended in patients with renal impairment

I.V.: *Adults:* 4-6 mg/kg once daily

Mechanism of Action Daptomycin binds to components of the cell membrane of susceptible organisms and causes rapid depolarization, inhibiting intracellular synthesis of DNA, RNA, and protein. Daptomycin is bactericidal in a concentration-dependent manner.

Pharmacodynamics/Kinetics

Half-life Elimination 8-9 hours (up to 28 hours in renal impairment)

Pregnancy Risk Factor B

Pregnancy Considerations Adverse events were not observed in animal reproduction studies. Successful use of daptomycin during the second and third trimesters of pregnancy has been described; however, only limited information is available from case reports.

Darbepoetin Alfa (dar be POE e tin AL fa)

Brand Names: U.S. Aranesp®; Aranesp® SingleJect®

Brand Names: Canada Aranesp®

Pharmacologic Category Colony Stimulating Factor; Erythropoiesis-Stimulating Agent (ESA); Growth Factor; Recombinant Human Erythropoietin

Use Treatment of anemia due to concurrent myelosuppressive chemotherapy in patients with cancer (nonmyeloid malignancies) receiving chemotherapy (palliative intent) for a planned minimum of 2 additional months of chemotherapy; treatment of anemia due to chronic kidney disease (including patients on dialysis and not on dialysis)

Note: Darbepoetin is **not** indicated for use under the following conditions:

• Cancer patients receiving hormonal therapy, therapeutic biologic products, or radiation therapy unless also receiving concurrent myelosuppressive chemotherapy

• Cancer patients receiving myelosuppressive chemotherapy when the expected outcome is curative

• As a substitute for RBC transfusion in patients requiring immediate correction of anemia

Note: In clinical trials, darbepoetin has not demonstrated improved quality of life, fatigue, or well-being.

Unlabeled Use Treatment of symptomatic anemia in myelodysplastic syndrome (MDS)

Local Anesthetic/Vasoconstrictor Precautions No information available to require special precautions

Effects on Dental Treatment No significant effects or complications reported

Effects on Bleeding Erythropoiesis-stimulating agents have been associated with thromboembolic events.

Adverse Effects
>10%:
Cardiovascular: Hypertension (31%), peripheral edema (17%), edema (6% to 13%)
Gastrointestinal: Abdominal pain (10% to 13%)
Respiratory: Dyspnea (17%), cough (12%)
1% to 10%:
Cardiovascular: Angina, fluid overload, hypotension, MI, thromboembolic events
Central nervous system: Cerebrovascular disorder
Dermatologic: Rash/erythema
Local: AV graft thrombosis, vascular access complications
Respiratory: Pulmonary embolism

General Dosage Range
I.V.:
Children 1-18 years: 6.25-200 mcg/week
Adults: 0.45 mcg/kg once weekly **or** every 4 weeks **or** 0.75 mcg/kg once every 2 weeks **or** 6.25-200 mcg/week
SubQ:
Children 1-18 years: 6.25-200 mcg/week
Adults: 0.45-4.5 mcg/kg/week **or** 0.45 mcg/kg every 4 weeks **or** 0.75 mcg/kg once every 2 weeks **or** 500 mcg once every 3 weeks **or** 6.25-200 mcg/week

Mechanism of Action Induces erythropoiesis by stimulating the division and differentiation of committed erythroid progenitor cells; induces the release of reticulocytes from the bone marrow into the bloodstream, where they mature to erythrocytes. There is a dose response relationship with this effect. This results in an increase in reticulocyte counts followed by a rise in hematocrit and hemoglobin levels. When administered SubQ or I.V., darbepoetin's half-life is ~3 times that of epoetin alfa concentrations.

Pharmacodynamics/Kinetics
Onset of Action Increased hemoglobin levels not generally observed until 2-6 weeks after initiating treatment
Half-life Elimination Note: Darbepoetin half-life is approximately threefold longer than epoetin alfa following I.V. administration
CKD: Adults:
I.V.: 21 hours
SubQ: Nondialysis patients: 70 hours (range: 35-139 hours); Dialysis patients: 46 hours (range: 12-89 hours)
Cancer: Adults: SubQ: 74 hours (range: 24-144 hours); Children: 49 hours
Time to Peak SubQ:
CKD: Adults: 48 hours (range: 12-72 hours; independent of dialysis); Children: 36 hours (range: 10-58 hours)
Cancer: Adults: 71-90 hours (range: 28-123 hours); Children: 71 hours (range: 21-143 hours)

Pregnancy Risk Factor C
Pregnancy Considerations Darbepoetin has been shown to have adverse effects (reduced weights, early postimplantation loss) in animal studies. There are no adequate and well-controlled studies in pregnant women. Darbepoetin alfa should be used in a pregnant woman only if potential benefit justifies the potential risk to the fetus. Women who become pregnant during treatment with darbepoetin are encouraged to enroll in Amgen's Pregnancy Surveillance Program (1-800-772-6436).

Prescribing and Access Restrictions As a requirement of the REMS program, access to this medication is restricted. Healthcare providers and hospitals must be enrolled in the ESA APPRISE (Assisting Providers and Cancer Patients with Risk Information for the Safe use of ESAs) Oncology Program (866-284-8089; http://www.esa-apprise.com) to prescribe or dispense ESAs (ie, darbepoetin alfa, epoetin alfa) to patients with cancer.

Darifenacin (dar i FEN a sin)

Brand Names: U.S. Enablex®
Brand Names: Canada Enablex®
Pharmacologic Category Anticholinergic Agent
Use Management of symptoms of bladder overactivity (urge incontinence, urgency, and frequency)
Local Anesthetic/Vasoconstrictor Precautions No information available to require special precautions
Effects on Dental Treatment Key adverse event(s) related to dental treatment: Xerostomia (normal salivary flow resumes upon discontinuation). Prolonged xerostomia may contribute to discomfort and dental disease (eg, caries, periodontal disease, and oral candidiasis).
Effects on Bleeding No information available to require special precautions
Adverse Effects
>10%: Gastrointestinal: Xerostomia (19% to 35%), constipation (15% to 21%)
1% to 10%:
Cardiovascular: Hypertension (≥1%), peripheral edema (≥1%)
Central nervous system: Headache (7%), dizziness (<2%), pain (≥1%)
Dermatological: Dry skin (≥1%), pruritus (≥1%), rash (≥1%)
Gastrointestinal: Dyspepsia (3% to 8%), abdominal pain (2% to 4%), nausea (2% to 4%), vomiting (≥1%), weight gain (≥1%)
Genitourinary: Urinary tract infection (4% to 5%), vaginitis (≥1%), urinary retention (acute)
Neuromuscular & skeletal: Weakness (<3%), arthralgia (≥1%), back pain (≥1%)
Ocular: Dry eyes (2%), abnormal vision (≥1%)
Respiratory: Bronchitis (≥1%), pharyngitis (≥1%), rhinitis (≥1%), sinusitis (≥1%)
Miscellaneous: Flu-like syndrome (1% to 3%)
General Dosage Range Dosage adjustment recommended in patients with hepatic impairment or on concomitant therapy
Oral: *Adults:* Initial: 7.5 mg once daily; Maintenance: 7.5-15 mg once daily
Mechanism of Action Selective antagonist of the M3 muscarinic (cholinergic) receptor subtype. Blockade of the receptor limits bladder contractions, reducing the symptoms of bladder irritability/overactivity (urge incontinence, urgency and frequency).
Pharmacodynamics/Kinetics
Half-life Elimination ~13-19 hours
Time to Peak Plasma: ~7 hours
Pregnancy Risk Factor C
Pregnancy Considerations Teratogenic effects and developmental delay were observed in some animal studies. There are no adequate and well-controlled studies in pregnant women; should be used only if potential benefit outweighs possible risk to the fetus.

Darunavir (dar OO na veer)

Related Information
HIV Infection and AIDS *on page 1520*
Brand Names: U.S. Prezista®
Brand Names: Canada Prezista®

Pharmacologic Category Antiretroviral Agent, Protease Inhibitor

Use Treatment of HIV-1 infections in combination with ritonavir and other antiretroviral agents

Local Anesthetic/Vasoconstrictor Precautions No information available to require special precautions

Effects on Dental Treatment No significant effects or complications reported

Effects on Bleeding Increased bleeding has been noted with protease inhibitors, such as darunavir, in patients with hemophilia A or B. No other information is available to require special precautions in other patients.

Adverse Effects As a class, protease inhibitors potentially cause dyslipidemias which includes elevated cholesterol and triglycerides and a redistribution of body fat centrally to cause increased abdominal girth, buffalo hump, facial atrophy, and breast enlargement. These agents also cause hyperglycemia. Frequency of adverse events is reported for darunavir/ritonavir. See also Ritonavir monograph.

>10%:

Endocrine & metabolic: Hypercholesterolemia (children: grade 3: 1%; adults: grade 2: 16% to 25%; grade 3: 1% to 10%), LDL increased (children: grade 3: 3%; adults: grade 2: 14%; grade 3: 5% to 8%)

Gastrointestinal: Vomiting (children: 13% to 33%; adults 2% to 5%), nausea (4% to 25%), diarrhea (children: 11% to 19%; adults: 8% to 14%)

2% to 10%:

Central nervous system: Headache (children: 9%; adults: 3% to 6%), fatigue (children: 3%; adults: ≤2%)

Dermatologic: Rash (children: 5% to 10%; adults: 6% to 7%), pruritus (children: 8%)

Endocrine & metabolic: Hyperglycemia (grade 2: 7% to 10%; grade 3: ≤1%; grade 4: <1%), triglycerides increased (grade 2: 3% to 10%; grade 3: 1% to 7%; grade 4: ≤3%), diabetes mellitus (2%)

Gastrointestinal: Abdominal pain (children: 8% to 10%; adults: 5% to 6%), amylase increased (children: grade 3: 4%, grade 4: 1%; adults: grade 2: 5% to 6%, grade 3: 3% to 7%), appetite decreased (children: 8%), lipase increased (children: grade 3: 1%; adults: grade 2: 2% to 3%, grade 3; ≤2%; grade 4: <1%), abdominal distention (2%), anorexia (2%), dyspepsia (2%)

Hepatic: ALT increased (children: grade 3: 3%; grade 4: 1%; adults: grade 2: 7%, grade 3: 2% to 3%; grade 4: ≤1%), AST increased (children: grade 3: 1%; adults: grade 2: 6%; grade 3: 2% to 4%; grade 4: <1%), alkaline phosphatase (grade 2: ≤2%; grade 3: <1%)

Neuromuscular & skeletal: Weakness (≤3%)

General Dosage Range Dosage adjustment recommended in patients on concomitant therapy or who develop toxicities.

Oral:

Children ≥3 years

≥10 kg to <11 kg: Darunavir 350 mg once daily with ritonavir 64 mg once daily or Darunavir 200 mg twice daily with ritonavir 32 mg twice daily

≥11 kg to <12 kg: Darunavir 385 mg once daily with ritonavir 64 mg once daily or Darunavir 220 mg twice daily with ritonavir 32 mg twice daily

≥12 kg to <13 kg: Darunavir 420 mg once daily with ritonavir 80 mg once daily or Darunavir 240 mg twice daily with ritonavir 40 mg twice daily

≥13 kg to <14 kg: Darunavir 455 mg once daily with ritonavir 80 mg once daily or Darunavir 260 mg twice daily with ritonavir 40 mg twice daily

≥14 kg to <15 kg: Darunavir 490 mg once daily with ritonavir 96 mg once daily or Darunavir 280 mg twice daily with ritonavir 48 mg twice daily

≥15 kg to <30 kg: Darunavir 600 mg once daily with ritonavir 100 mg once daily or Darunavir 375 mg twice daily with ritonavir 48 mg twice daily

≥30 kg to <40 kg: Darunavir 675 mg once daily with ritonavir 100 mg once daily or Darunavir 450 mg twice daily with ritonavir 60 mg twice daily

≥40 kg: Darunavir 800 mg once daily with ritonavir 100 mg once daily or Darunavir: 600 mg twice daily with ritonavir 100 mg twice daily

Adults: Darunavir: 600 mg twice daily; Ritonavir: 100 mg twice daily or Darunavir: 800 mg once daily; Ritonavir: 100 mg once daily

Mechanism of Action Binds to the site of HIV-1 protease activity and inhibits cleavage of viral Gag-Pol polyprotein precursors into individual functional proteins required for infectious HIV. This results in the formation of immature, noninfectious viral particles.

Pharmacodynamics/Kinetics

Half-life Elimination ~15 hours

Pregnancy Risk Factor C

Pregnancy Considerations Teratogenic effects have not been observed in animal reproduction studies. Darunavir crosses the placenta. Safety and pharmacokinetic data are limited in pregnancy. Serum concentrations may be low with once-daily dosing; therefore, some experts recommend twice-daily dosing during pregnancy (studies are ongoing). The DHHS Perinatal HIV Guidelines consider darunavir to be an alternative protease inhibitor (PI) when combined with low-dose ritonavir boosting. A small increased risk of preterm birth has been associated with maternal use of protease inhibitor-based combination antiretroviral (ARV) therapy during pregnancy; however, the benefits of use generally outweigh this risk and PIs should not be withheld if otherwise recommended. Hyperglycemia, new onset of diabetes mellitus, or diabetic ketoacidosis have been reported with PIs; it is not clear if pregnancy increases this risk.

Regardless of CD4 count or HIV RNA copy number, all HIV-infected pregnant women should receive a combination antepartum ARV drug regimen; this includes women who require therapy for their own health, as well as women who do not yet require therapy for their own health. ARV therapy should be started as soon as possible if required for the woman's health. Although earlier initiation may be more effective in reducing the perinatal transmission of HIV), also consider maternal conditions (eg, nausea and vomiting) and the potential risks of first trimester fetal exposure for specific agents. Plasma HIV RNA levels should be assessed at ~34-36 weeks gestation in order to help determine mode of delivery. If ARV therapy must be interrupted for <24 hours during the peripartum period, stop then restart all medications simultaneously in order to decrease the chance of developing resistance. Long-term follow-up is recommended for all infants exposed to ARV medications.

Healthcare providers are encouraged to enroll pregnant women exposed to antiretroviral medications in the Antiretroviral Pregnancy Registry (1-800-258-4263 or www.APRegistry.com). Healthcare providers caring for HIV-infected women and their infants may contact the

National Perinatal HIV Hotline (888-448-8765) for clinical consultation (DHHS [perinatal], 2012).

Product Availability Prezista® 100 mg/mL oral suspension: FDA approved December 2011; availability expected in the second quarter of 2012

Dasatinib (da SA ti nib)

Related Information
Clinical Risk Related to Drugs Prolonging QT Interval *on page 1510*

Brand Names: U.S. Sprycel®

Brand Names: Canada Sprycel®

Pharmacologic Category Antineoplastic Agent, Tyrosine Kinase Inhibitor

Use Treatment of chronic myelogenous leukemia (CML) in chronic, accelerated or blast (myeloid or lymphoid) phase resistant or intolerant to prior therapy (including imatinib); treatment of newly-diagnosed Philadelphia chromosome-positive (Ph+) CML in chronic phase; treatment of Philadelphia chromosome-positive (Ph+) acute lymphoblastic leukemia (ALL) resistant or intolerant to prior therapy

Unlabeled Use Post-stem cell transplant (allogeneic) follow-up treatment of CML; treatment of gastrointestinal stromal tumor (GIST)

Local Anesthetic/Vasoconstrictor Precautions Dasatinib is one of the drugs confirmed to prolong the QT interval and is accepted as having a risk of causing torsade de pointes. The risk of drug-induced torsade de pointes is extremely low when a single QT interval prolonging drug is prescribed. In terms of epinephrine, it is not known what effect vasoconstrictors in the local anesthetic regimen will have in patients with a known history of congenital prolonged QT interval or in patients taking any medication that prolongs the QT interval. Until more information is obtained, it is suggested that the clinician consult with the physician prior to the use of a vasoconstrictor in suspected patients, and that the vasoconstrictor (epinephrine, mepivacaine and levonordefrin [Carbocaine® 2% with Neo-Cobefrin®]) be used with caution.

Effects on Dental Treatment Key adverse event(s) related to dental treatment: Mucositis/stomatitis, taste perversion.

Effects on Bleeding Bleeding was experienced in ≤9% of patients with ≤7% severe. Thrombocytopenia is prevalent. A medical consult is recommended.

Adverse Effects
≥10%:
Cardiovascular: Fluid retention (21% to 35%; grades 3/4: 1% to 8%), superficial edema (3% to 19%; grades 3/4: ≤1%)
Central nervous system: Headache (12% to 33%), fatigue (8% to 24%), fever (5% to 18%)
Dermatologic: Rash (11% to 21%; includes drug eruption, erythema, erythema multiforme, erythematous rash, erythrosis, exfoliative rash, follicular rash, heat rash, macular rash, maculopapular rash, milia, papular rash, pruritic rash, pustular rash, skin exfoliation, skin irritation, urticaria vesiculosa, vesicular rash)
Endocrine & metabolic: Hypophosphatemia (grades 3/4: 5% to 18%), hypokalemia (grades 3/4: ≤15%), hypocalcemia (grades 3/4: <1% to 12%)
Gastrointestinal: Diarrhea (18% to 31%; grades 3/4: ≤5%), nausea (9% to 24%), vomiting (5% to 16%), abdominal pain (3% to 12%)

Hematologic: Thrombocytopenia (grades 3/4: 19% to 85%), neutropenia (grades 3/4: 22% to 79%), anemia (grades 3/4: 11% to 74%), hemorrhage (6% to 26%; grades 3/4: 1% to 9%), neutropenic fever (grades 3/4: 1% to 12%)
Neuromuscular & skeletal: Musculoskeletal pain (≤19%), myalgia (3% to 13%), arthralgia (≤12%)
Respiratory: Pleural effusion (12% to 24%; grades 3/4: ≤11%), dyspnea (3% to 20%; grades 3/4: 2% to 3%)
Miscellaneous: Infection (9% to 12%, includes bacterial, fungal, viral)
1% to <10%:
Cardiovascular: Generalized edema (≤1%), pericardial effusion (≤3%; grades 3/4: ≤1%), CHF/cardiac dysfunction (≤4%; includes cardiac failure, cardiomyopathy, diastolic dysfunction, ejection fraction decreased, left ventricular dysfunction, ventricular failure); arrhythmia, chest pain, flushing, hypertension, palpitation
Central nervous system: CNS bleeding (≤3%; grades 3/4: ≤3%), chills, depression, dizziness, insomnia, pain, somnolence
Dermatologic: Acne, alopecia, dermatitis, dry skin, eczema, hyperhidrosis, pruritus, urticaria
Gastrointestinal: Gastrointestinal bleeding (2% to 9%; grades 3/4: 1% to 7%), abdominal distention, anorexia, colitis (including neutropenic colitis), constipation, dyspepsia, enterocolitis, gastritis, mucositis/stomatitis, oral soft tissue disorder, taste alteration, weight loss/gain
Hematologic: Contusion, pancytopenia
Hepatic: Bilirubin increased (grades 3/4: ≤6%), ALT increased (grades 3/4: ≤5%), AST increased (grades 3/4: ≤4%)
Neuromuscular & skeletal: Muscle inflammation (4%), muscle weakness, neuropathy, peripheral neuropathy, weakness
Ocular: Visual disorder (blurred vision, acuity reduced, visual disturbance), xerophthalmia
Otic: Tinnitus
Renal: Serum creatinine increased (grades 3/4: ≤8%)
Respiratory: Pulmonary edema (≤4%; grades 3/4: ≤3%), cough, lung infiltration, pneumonia (bacterial, viral or fungal), pneumonitis, pulmonary hypertension, upper respiratory tract infection/inflammation
Miscellaneous: Herpes virus infection

General Dosage Range Dosage adjustment recommended in patients on concomitant therapy or who develop toxicities
Oral: *Adults:* 100-180 mg once daily

Mechanism of Action BCR-ABL tyrosine kinase inhibitor; targets most imatinib-resistant BCR-ABL mutations (except the T315I and F317V mutants) by distinctly binding to active and inactive ABL-kinase. Kinase inhibition halts proliferation of leukemia cells. Also inhibits SRC family (including SRC, LKC, YES, FYN); c-KIT, EPHA2 and platelet derived growth factor receptor (PDGFRβ)

Pharmacodynamics/Kinetics
Half-life Elimination Terminal: 3-5 hours
Time to Peak 0.5-6 hours

Pregnancy Risk Factor D

Pregnancy Considerations Animal reproduction studies have demonstrated fetal abnormalities (skeletal malformations, reduced ossification, edema, microhepatia) and fetal death. May cause fetal harm if administered to a pregnant woman. Not recommended for use during pregnancy or if contemplating pregnancy. Effective contraception is recommended for men and women of childbearing potential. Pregnant women are advised to avoid contact with crushed or broken tablets.

Dental Comment Dasatinib is known to prolong the QT interval. The QT interval is measured as the time and distance between the Q point of the QRS complex and the end of the T wave in the ECG tracing. After adjustment for heart rate, the QT interval is defined as prolonged if it is more than 450 msec in men and 460 msec in women. A long QT syndrome was first described in the 1950s and 60s as a congenital syndrome involving QT interval prolongation and syncope and sudden death. Some of the congenital long QT syndromes were characterized by a peculiar electrocardiographic appearance of the QRS complex involving a premature atria beat followed by a pause, then a subsequent sinus beat showing marked QT prolongation and deformity. This type of cardiac arrhythmia was originally termed "torsade de pointes" (translated from the French as "twisting of the points"). Dasatinib is considered as having a risk of causing torsade de pointes. Since it is not known what effect vasoconstrictors in the local anesthetic regimen will have in patients with a known history of congenital prolonged QT interval or in patients taking any medication that prolongs the QT interval, a medical consult is suggested.

DAUNOrubicin (Conventional)
(daw noe ROO bi sin con VEN sha nal)

Brand Names: U.S. Cerubidine®
Brand Names: Canada Cerubidine®
Pharmacologic Category Antineoplastic Agent, Anthracycline
Use Treatment of acute lymphocytic leukemia (ALL) and acute myeloid leukemia (AML)
Local Anesthetic/Vasoconstrictor Precautions No information available to require special precautions
Effects on Dental Treatment Key adverse event(s) related to dental treatment: Stomatitis and discoloration of saliva.
Effects on Bleeding Thrombocytopenia occurs with the nadir in 10-14 days and recovery in 21-28 days. A medical consult is suggested.
Adverse Effects
>10%:
  Cardiovascular: Transient ECG abnormalities (supraventricular tachycardia, S-T wave changes, atrial or ventricular extrasystoles); generally asymptomatic and self-limiting. CHF, dose related, may be delayed for 7-8 years after treatment.
  Dermatologic: Alopecia (reversible), radiation recall
  Gastrointestinal: Mild nausea or vomiting, stomatitis
  Genitourinary: Discoloration of urine (red)
  Hematologic: Myelosuppression (onset: 7 days; nadir: 10-14 days; recovery: 21-28 days), primarily leukopenia; thrombocytopenia and anemia
1% to 10%:
  Dermatologic: Skin "flare" at injection site; discoloration of saliva, sweat, or tears
  Endocrine & metabolic: Hyperuricemia
  Gastrointestinal: Abdominal pain, GI ulceration, diarrhea
General Dosage Range Dosage adjustment recommended in patients with hepatic or renal impairment
I.V.:
  Children <2 years or BSA <0.5 m²: 1 mg/kg/dose per protocol with frequency dependent on regimen employed (maximum cumulative dose: 10 mg/kg)

Children ≥2 years and BSA ≥0.5 m²: 25 mg/m² on day 1 every week for 4 cycles **or** 30-60 mg/m²/day for 3 days (maximum cumulative dose: 300 mg/m²)
Adults <60 years: 30-60 mg/m²/day for 2-3 days (maximum cumulative dose: 550 mg/m²; 400 mg/m² with chest irradiation)
Adults ≥60 years: 30 mg/m²/day for 2-3 days (maximum cumulative dose: 550 mg/m²; 400 mg/m² with chest irradiation)
Mechanism of Action Inhibition of DNA and RNA synthesis by intercalation between DNA base pairs and by steric obstruction. Daunomycin intercalates at points of local uncoiling of the double helix. Although the exact mechanism is unclear, it appears that direct binding to DNA (intercalation) and inhibition of DNA repair (topoisomerase II inhibition) result in blockade of DNA and RNA synthesis and fragmentation of DNA.
Pharmacodynamics/Kinetics
Half-life Elimination Distribution: 2 minutes; Elimination: 14-20 hours; Terminal: 18.5 hours; Daunorubicinol plasma half-life: 24-48 hours
Pregnancy Risk Factor D
Pregnancy Considerations May cause fetal harm when administered to a pregnant woman. Animal studies have shown an increased incidence of fetal abnormalities.

DAUNOrubicin (Liposomal)
(daw noe ROO bi sin lye po SO mal)

Brand Names: U.S. DaunoXome®
Pharmacologic Category Antineoplastic Agent, Anthracycline
Use First-line treatment of advanced HIV-associated Kaposi's sarcoma (KS)
Local Anesthetic/Vasoconstrictor Precautions No information available to require special precautions
Effects on Dental Treatment Key adverse event(s) related to dental treatment: Stomatitis.
Effects on Bleeding Thrombocytopenia occurs with the nadir in 14 days and recovery in 21 days. A medical consult is recommended.
Adverse Effects
>10%:
  Cardiovascular: Edema (11%)
  Central nervous system: Fatigue (49%), fever (47%), headache (25%), neutropenic fever (17%)
  Gastrointestinal: Nausea (54%), diarrhea (38%), abdominal pain (23%), anorexia (23%), vomiting (23%)
  Hematologic: Myelosuppression (onset: 7 days; nadir: 14 days; recovery 21 days), neutropenia (up to 55%; grade 4: 15%), anemia (up to 55%; grade 4: 2%), thrombocytopenia (up to 12%; grade 4: 1%)
  Neuromuscular & skeletal: Rigors (19%), back pain (16%), neuropathy (13%)
  Respiratory: Cough (28%), dyspnea (26%), rhinitis (12%)
  Miscellaneous: Opportunistic infections (40%), allergic reactions (24%), diaphoresis (14%), infusion-related reactions (14%; includes back pain, flushing, chest tightness)
1% to 10%:
  Cardiovascular: Chest pain (10%), hypertension (≤5%), palpitation (≤5%), syncope (≤5%), tachycardia (≤5%), LVEF decreased (3%), CHF/cardiomyopathy

Central nervous system: Depression (10%), malaise (10%), dizziness (8%), insomnia (6%), abnormal thinking (≤5%), amnesia (≤5%), anxiety (≤5%), ataxia (≤5%), confusion (≤5%), emotional lability (≤5%), hallucination (≤5%), meningitis (≤5%), seizure (≤5%), somnolence (≤5%)

Dermatologic: Alopecia (8%), pruritus (7%), dry skin (≤5%), folliculitis (≤5%), seborrhea (≤5%)

Endocrine & metabolic: Dehydration (≤5%), hot flashes (≤5%)

Gastrointestinal: Stomatitis (10%), constipation (7%), tenesmus (5%), appetite increased (≤5%), dental caries (≤5%), dysphagia (≤5%), gastrointestinal hemorrhage (≤5%), gastritis (≤5%), gingival bleeding (≤5%), hemorrhoids (≤5%), melena (≤5%), splenomegaly (≤5%), taste perversion (≤5%), xerostomia (≤5%)

Genitourinary: Dysuria (≤5%), nocturia (≤5%), polyuria (≤5%)

Hepatic: Hepatomegaly (≤5%)

Local: Injection site inflammation (≤5%)

Neuromuscular & skeletal: Arthralgia (7%), myalgia (7%), gait abnormal (≤5%), hyperkinesia (≤5%), hypertonia (≤5%), tremor (≤5%)

Ocular: Abnormal vision (5%) conjunctivitis (≤5%), eye pain (≤5%)

Otic: Deafness (≤5%), earache (≤5%), tinnitus (≤5%)

Respiratory: Sinusitis (8%), hemoptysis (≤5%), pulmonary infiltrate (≤5%), sputum increased (≤5%)

Miscellaneous: Flu-like syndrome (5%), hiccups (≤5%), lymphadenopathy (≤5%), thirst (≤5%)

General Dosage Range Dosage adjustment recommended in patients with hepatic or renal impairment

I.V.: *Adults:* 40 mg/m^2 every 2 weeks

Mechanism of Action Liposomes have been shown to penetrate solid tumors more effectively, possibly because of their small size and longer circulation time. Once in tissues, daunorubicin is released. Daunorubicin inhibits DNA and RNA synthesis by intercalation between DNA base pairs and by steric obstruction; and intercalates at points of local uncoiling of the double helix. Although the exact mechanism is unclear, it appears that direct binding to DNA (intercalation) and inhibition of DNA repair (topoisomerase II inhibition) result in blockade of DNA and RNA synthesis and fragmentation of DNA.

Pharmacodynamics/Kinetics

Half-life Elimination Distribution: 4.4 hours; Terminal: 3-5 hours

Pregnancy Risk Factor D

Pregnancy Considerations Teratogenic effects and embryotoxicity were noted in animal studies. There are no adequate and well-controlled studies in pregnant women. Women of childbearing potential should avoid becoming pregnant while receiving treatment.

Decitabine (de SYE ta been)

Brand Names: U.S. Dacogen®

Pharmacologic Category Antineoplastic Agent, DNA Methylation Inhibitor

Use Treatment of myelodysplastic syndrome (MDS)

Unlabeled Use Treatment of acute myelogenous leukemia (AML), sickle cell anemia

Local Anesthetic/Vasoconstrictor Precautions No information available to require special precautions

Effects on Dental Treatment Key adverse event(s) related to dental treatment: Oral mucosal petechiae, stomatitis, gingival bleeding, tongue ulceration, oral candidiasis, lip ulceration, mucosal inflammation, gingival pain have been reported.

Effects on Bleeding Gingival bleeding and oral mucosal petechiae have been reported with decitabine therapy as well as a high incidence (27% to 89%) of thrombocytopenia. A medical consult is recommended.

Adverse Effects

>10%:

Cardiovascular: Peripheral edema (25% to 27%), pallor (23%), edema (5% to 18%), cardiac murmur (16%), hypotension (6% to 11%)

Central nervous system: Fever (6% to 53%), fatigue (46%), headache (23% to 28%), insomnia (14% to 28%), dizziness (18% to 21%), chills (16%), pain (5% to 13%), confusion (8% to 12%), lethargy (12%), anxiety (9% to 11%), hypoesthesia (11%)

Dermatologic: Petechiae (12% to 39%), bruising (9% to 22%), rash (11% to 19%), erythema (5% to 14%), cellulitis (9% to 12%), lesions (5% to 11%), pruritus (9% to 11%)

Endocrine & metabolic: Hyperglycemia (6% to 33%), hypoalbuminemia (7% to 24%), hypomagnesemia (5% to 24%), hypokalemia (12% to 22%), hyperkalemia (13%), hyponatremia (19%)

Gastrointestinal: Nausea (40% to 42%), constipation (30% to 35%), diarrhea (28% to 34%), vomiting (16% to 25%), anorexia/appetite decreased (8% to 23%), abdominal pain (5% to 14%), oral mucosal petechiae (13%), stomatitis (11% to 12%), dyspepsia (10% to 12%)

Hematologic: Neutropenia (38% to 90%; grades 3/4: 37% to 87%; recovery 28-50 days), thrombocytopenia (27% to 89%; grades 3/4: 24% to 85%), anemia (31% to 82%; grades 3/4: 22%), febrile neutropenia (20% to 29%; grades 3/4: 23%), leukopenia (6% to 28%; grades 3/4: 22%), lymphadenopathy (12%)

Hepatic: Hyperbilirubinemia (6% to 14%), alkaline phosphatase increased (11%)

Local: Tenderness (11%)

Neuromuscular & skeletal: Rigors (22%), arthralgia (17% to 20%), limb pain (18% to 19%), back pain (17% to 18%), weakness (15%)

Respiratory: Cough (27% to 40%), dyspnea (29%), pneumonia (20% to 22%), pharyngitis (16%), lung crackles (14%), epistaxis (13%)

5% to 10%:

Cardiovascular: Tachycardia (8%), chest pain/discomfort (6% to 7%), facial edema (6%), hypertension (6%), heart failure (5%)

Central nervous system: Depression (9%), malaise (5%)

Dermatologic: Alopecia (8%), dry skin (8%), urticaria (6%)

Endocrine & metabolic: Hyperuricemia (10%), LDH increased (8%), bicarbonate increased (6%), dehydration (6% to 8%), hypochloremia (6%), bicarbonate decreased (5%), hypoproteinemia (5%)

Gastrointestinal: Mucosal inflammation (9%), weight loss (9%), gingival bleeding (8%), hemorrhoids (8%), loose stools (7%), tongue ulceration (7%), dysphagia (5% to 6%), oral candidiasis (6%), toothache (6%), abdominal distension (5%), gastroesophageal reflux (5%), glossodynia (5%), lip ulceration (5%), oral pain (5%), tooth abscess (5%)

Genitourinary: Urinary tract infection (7%), dysuria (6%), polyuria (5%)

Hematologic: Bacteremia (5% to 8%), hematoma (5%), pancytopenia (5%), thrombocythemia (5%)

Hepatic: Ascites (10%), AST increased (10%), hypo-bilirubinemia (5%)

Local: Catheter infection (8%), catheter site erythema (5%), catheter site pain (5%), injection site swelling (5%)

Neuromuscular & skeletal: Myalgia (5% to 9%), falling (8%), chest wall pain (7%), muscle spasm (7%), bone pain (6%), musculoskeletal pain/discomfort (5% to 6%), crepitation (5%)

Ocular: Blurred vision (6%)

Otic: Ear pain (6%)

Respiratory: Breath sounds abnormal (5% to 10%), hypoxia (10%), upper respiratory tract infection (10%), pharyngolaryngeal pain (8%), rales (8%), pulmonary edema (6%), sinusitis (5% to 6%), pleural effusion (5%), postnasal drip (5%), sinus congestion (5%)

Miscellaneous: Candidal infection (10%), staphylococcal infection (7%), transfusion reaction (7%), night sweats (5%)

General Dosage Range Dosage adjustment recommended in patients who develop toxicities

I.V.: *Adults:* 15 mg/m^2 every 8 hours for 3 days every 6 weeks **or** 20 mg/m^2 daily for 5 days every 28 days

Mechanism of Action After phosphorylation, decitabine is incorporated into DNA and inhibits DNA methyltransferase causing hypomethylation and subsequent cell death (within the S-phase of the cell cycle).

Pharmacodynamics/Kinetics

Half-life Elimination ~30-35 minutes

Time to Peak At end of infusion

Pregnancy Risk Factor D

Pregnancy Considerations Teratogenic effects, decreased fetal weight, and increased fetal deaths were observed in animal studies. There are no adequate and well-controlled studies in pregnant women. Women of childbearing potential should be advised to avoid pregnancy during treatment and for 1 month after treatment. In addition, males should be advised to avoid fathering a child while on decitabine therapy and for 2 months after treatment.

Deferasirox (de FER a sir ox)

Brand Names: U.S. Exjade®

Brand Names: Canada Exjade®

Pharmacologic Category Chelating Agent

Use Treatment of chronic iron overload due to blood transfusions (transfusional hemosiderosis) or non-transfusion-dependent thalassemia syndromes

Local Anesthetic/Vasoconstrictor Precautions No information available to require special precautions

Effects on Dental Treatment No significant effects or complications reported

Effects on Bleeding Thrombocytopenia (<1%) has been reported.

Adverse Effects

>10%:

Central nervous system: Fever (19%), headache (16%)

Dermatologic: Rash (dose related; 2% to 11%)

Gastrointestinal: Abdominal pain (dose related; 21% to 28%), nausea (dose related; 2% to 23%), vomiting (dose related; 10% to 21%), diarrhea (dose related; 5% to 20%)

Renal: Serum creatinine increased (dose related; 2% to 38%), proteinuria (19%)

Respiratory: Cough (14%), nasopharyngitis (13%), pharyngolaryngeal pain (11%)

Miscellaneous: Influenza (11%)

1% to 10%:

Central nervous system: Fatigue (6%)

Dermatologic: Urticaria (4%)

Hepatic: ALT increased (1% to 8%), transaminitis (4%)

Neuromuscular & skeletal: Arthralgia (7%), back pain (6%)

Otic: Ear infection (5%)

Respiratory: Respiratory tract infection (10%), bronchitis (9%), pharyngitis (8%), acute tonsillitis (6%), rhinitis (6%)

General Dosage Range Dosage adjustment recommended in patients with renal or hepatic impairment or on concomitant therapy

Oral: *Children ≥2 years, Adolescents, and Adults:* Initial: 20 mg/kg once daily; Maintenance (usual): 20-30 mg/kg once daily (maximum: 40 mg/kg/day)

Mechanism of Action Selectively binds iron, forming a complex which is excreted primarily through the feces.

Pharmacodynamics/Kinetics

Half-life Elimination 8-16 hours

Time to Peak ~1.5-4 hours

Pregnancy Risk Factor C

Pregnancy Considerations Teratogenic effects were observed in animal reproduction studies. Use during pregnancy only if the potential benefit justifies the potential risk to the fetus.

Prescribing and Access Restrictions Deferasirox (Exjade®) is only available through a restricted distribution program called EPASS™ Complete Care. Prescribers must enroll patients in this program in order to obtain the medication. For patient enrollment, contact 1-888-90-EPASS (1-888-903-7277).

Deferiprone (de FER i prone)

Related Information

Clinical Risk Related to Drugs Prolonging QT Interval *on page 1510*

Brand Names: U.S. Ferriprox®

Pharmacologic Category Chelating Agent

Use Treatment of transfusional iron overload due to thalassemia syndromes with inadequate response to other chelation therapy

Local Anesthetic/Vasoconstrictor Precautions Deferiprone is one of the drugs confirmed to prolong the QT interval and is accepted as having a risk of causing torsade de pointes. The risk of drug-induced torsade de pointes is extremely low when a single QT interval prolonging drug is prescribed. In terms of epinephrine, it is not known what effect vasoconstrictors in the local anesthetic regimen will have in patients with a known history of congenital prolonged QT interval or in patients taking any medication that prolongs the QT interval. Until more information is obtained, it is suggested that the clinician consult with the physician prior to the use of a vasoconstrictor in suspected patients, and that the vasoconstrictor (epinephrine, mepivacaine and levonordefrin [Carbocaine® 2% with Neo-Cobefrin®]) be used with caution.

Effects on Dental Treatment No significant effects or complications reported

Effects on Bleeding No information available to require special precautions

Adverse Effects

>10%:

Gastrointestinal: Nausea (13%)

Genitourinary: Chromaturia (15%)

1% to 10%:

Central nervous system: Headache (3%)

Gastrointestinal: Abdominal pain/discomfort (10%), vomiting (10%), appetite increased (4%), diarrhea (3%), dyspepsia (2%), weight gain (2%), appetite decreased (1%)

Hematologic: Neutropenia (6% to 7%), agranulocytosis (2%)

Hepatic: ALT increased (8%), AST increased (1%)

Neuromuscular and skeletal: Arthralgia (10%), back pain (2%), limb pain (2%), arthropathy (1%)

General Dosage Range Oral: *Adults:* 25-33 mg/kg 3 times/day (maximum: 99 mg/kg/day)

Mechanism of Action Iron-chelating agent with affinity for ferric ion (iron III); binds to ferric ion and forms a 3:1 (deferiprone:iron) complex which is excreted in the urine. Has a lower affinity for other metals such as copper, aluminum, and zinc.

Pharmacodynamics/Kinetics

Half-life Elimination 1.9 hours

Time to Peak ~1-2 hours

Pregnancy Risk Factor D

Pregnancy Considerations Adverse effects were observed in animal reproduction studies. Although there is limited data in humans, deferiprone may cause fetal harm if administered during pregnancy. During treatment with deferiprone in women of reproductive potential, pregnancy should be avoided.

Dental Comment Deferiprone is known to prolong the QT interval. The QT interval is measured as the time and distance between the Q point of the QRS complex and the end of the T wave in the ECG tracing. After adjustment for heart rate, the QT interval is defined as prolonged if it is more than 450 msec in men and 460 msec in women. A long QT syndrome was first described in the 1950s and 60s as a congenital syndrome involving QT interval prolongation and syncope and sudden death. Some of the congenital long QT syndromes were characterized by a peculiar electrocardiographic appearance of the QRS complex involving a premature atria beat followed by a pause, then a subsequent sinus beat showing marked QT prolongation and deformity. This type of cardiac arrhythmia was originally termed "torsade de pointes" (translated from the French as "twisting of the points"). Deferiprone is considered as having a risk of causing torsade de pointes. Since it is not known what effect vasoconstrictors in the local anesthetic regimen will have in patients with a known history of congenital prolonged QT interval or in patients taking any medication that prolongs the QT interval, a medical consult is suggested.

Deferoxamine (de fer OKS a meen)

Brand Names: U.S. Desferal®

Brand Names: Canada Desferal®; PMS-Deferoxamine

Pharmacologic Category Antidote; Chelating Agent

Use Adjunct in the treatment of acute iron intoxication; treatment of chronic iron overload secondary to multiple transfusions

Canadian labeling (unlabeled use in the U.S.): Diagnosis of aluminum overload; treatment of chronic aluminum overload in patients with end-stage renal failure undergoing maintenance dialysis

Unlabeled Use Diagnosis or treatment of aluminum induced toxicity associated with chronic kidney disease (CKD)

Local Anesthetic/Vasoconstrictor Precautions No information available to require special precautions

Effects on Dental Treatment No significant effects or complications reported

Effects on Bleeding No information available to require special precautions

Adverse Effects Frequency not defined.

Cardiovascular: Flushing, hypotension, shock, tachycardia

Central nervous system: Dizziness, encephalopathy (aluminum toxicity/dialysis-related), fever, headache, seizure

Dermatologic: Angioedema, rash, urticaria

Endocrine & metabolic: Growth retardation (children), hyperparathyroidism (aggravated), hypocalcemia

Gastrointestinal: Abdominal discomfort, abdominal pain, diarrhea, nausea, vomiting

Genitourinary: Dysuria, urine discoloration (reddish color)

Hematologic: Leukopenia, thrombocytopenia

Hepatic: Hepatic dysfunction, transaminases increased

Local: Injection site: Burning, crust, edema, erythema, eschar, induration, infiltration, irritation, pain, pruritus, swelling, vesicles, wheal formation

Neuromuscular & skeletal: Arthralgia, metaphyseal dysplasia (children <3 years; dose related), muscle spasms, myalgia, neuropathy (peripheral, sensory, motor, or mixed), paresthesia

Ocular: Blurred vision, cataract, corneal opacities, dyschromatopsia, loss of vision, night blindness, optic neuritis, peripheral vision impaired, retinal pigment abnormalities, scotoma, visual acuity decreased, visual field defects

Otic: Hearing loss, tinnitus

Renal: Acute renal failure, renal tubular disorders, serum creatinine increased

Respiratory: Acute respiratory distress syndrome (dyspnea, cyanosis, and/or interstitial infiltrates), asthma

Miscellaneous: Anaphylaxis (with or without shock), hypersensitivity reaction, infections (*Yersinia*, mucormycosis)

General Dosage Range Dosage adjustment recommended in patients with renal impairment

I.M.: *Adults:* Initial: 1000 mg, followed by 500 mg every 4 hours for 2 doses; Maintenance: 500 mg every 4-12 hours **or** 500-1000 mg once daily (maximum: 6000 mg/day)

I.V.:

Children ≥3 years: 20-40 mg/kg/day 5-7 days per week; dose should not exceed 40 mg/kg/day until growth has ceased

Adults: Initial: 1000 mg, followed by 500 mg every 4 hours for 2 doses; Maintenance: 500 mg every 4-12 hours (maximum: 6000 mg/day) **or** 40-50 mg/kg/day (maximum: 60 mg/kg/day) 5-7 days per week

SubQ:

Children ≥3 years: 20-40 mg/kg/day (maximum: 1000-2000 mg/day)

Adults: 1000-2000 mg/day **or** 20-40 mg/kg/day

Mechanism of Action Complexes with trivalent ions (ferric ions) to form ferrioxamine, which is removed by the kidneys, slows accumulation of hepatic iron and retards or eliminates progression of hepatic fibrosis. Also known to inhibit DNA synthesis *in vitro*.

Pharmacodynamics/Kinetics

Half-life Elimination 14 hours (plasma half-life: 20-30 minutes)

Pregnancy Risk Factor C

Pregnancy Considerations Skeletal anomalies and delayed ossification were observed in some but not all animal reproduction studies. Toxic amounts of iron or deferoxamine have not been noted to cross the placenta. In case of acute iron toxicity, treatment during pregnancy should not be withheld.

Defibrotide (DE fib ro tide)

Pharmacologic Category Antiplatelet Agent; Thrombolytic Agent

Unlabeled Use Prevention of hepatic sinusoidal obstruction syndrome (SOS; formerly called veno-occlusive disease) in hematopoietic stem cell transplant (HSCT); treatment of hepatic SOS associated with HSCT

Local Anesthetic/Vasoconstrictor Precautions No information available to require special precautions

Effects on Dental Treatment Key adverse event(s) related to dental treatment: Increased bleeding with invasive procedures (see Effects on Bleeding)

Effects on Bleeding Defibrotide has antiplatelet and fibrinolytic properties; expect increased bleeding with invasive dental procedures; medical consult is recommended

Adverse Effects Frequency not defined.

Cardiovascular: Hypotension

Central nervous system: CNS hemorrhage, fever

Endocrine: Hot flashes

Gastrointestinal: Abdominal pain, cramping, diarrhea, diarrhea (hemorrhagic), gastrointestinal bleeding, hematemesis, mouth hemorrhage, nausea, vomiting

Hematologic: Hemorrhage/bleeding

Local: Thrombophlebitis

Renal: Hematuria, renal failure

Respiratory: Diffuse alveolar hemorrhage, epistaxis, pulmonary hemorrhage

Miscellaneous: Allergic reaction

Mechanism of Action Defibrotide binds to and protects vascular hepatic endothelial cells (especially small vessels) by enhancing fibrinolysis and suppressing coagulation. Effects are local, with no significant effect on systemic coagulation. Has antithrombotic, anti-inflammatory, antiplatelet, and anti-ischemic properties.

Prescribing and Access Restrictions Defibrotide is an investigational agent available for the treatment of hepatic SOS through an Expanded Access Treatment IND Protocol (protocol 2006-05). Information on access is available at http://www.gentium.com/vod/about-vod/access-to-defibrotide.

Degarelix (deg a REL ix)

Brand Names: U.S. Firmagon®

Brand Names: Canada Firmagon®

Pharmacologic Category Antineoplastic Agent, Gonadotropin-Releasing Hormone Antagonist; Gonadotropin Releasing Hormone Antagonist

Use Treatment of advanced prostate cancer

Local Anesthetic/Vasoconstrictor Precautions Degarelix may prolong QT interval; it is suggested that the clinician consult with the physician prior to use of vasoconstrictor in suspected patients; use vasoconstrictor (epinephrine, mepivacaine and levonordefrin [Carbocaine® 2% with Neo-Cobefrin®]) with caution.

Effects on Dental Treatment No significant effects or complications reported

Effects on Bleeding No information available to require special precautions

Adverse Effects

>10%:

Endocrine & metabolic: Hot flashes (26%)

Local: Injections site reactions (35%, grade 3: ≤2%; pain 28%, erythema 17%, swelling 6%, induration 4%, nodule 3%)

1% to 10%:

Cardiovascular: Hypertension (6%)

Central nervous system: Chills (5%), dizziness (1% to 5%), fever (1% to 5%), headache (1% to 5%), insomnia (1% to 5%), fatigue (3%)

Dermatologic: Hyperhydrosis

Endocrine & metabolic: Hypercholesterolemia (3%), gynecomastia, testicular atrophy

Gastrointestinal: Weight gain (9%), constipation (5%), nausea (1% to 5%), diarrhea

Genitourinary: Urinary tract infection (5%), erectile dysfunction

Hepatic: ALT increased (10%; grade 3: <1%), AST increased (5%; grade 3: <1%), GGT increased

Neuromuscular & skeletal: Back pain (6%), arthralgia (5%), weakness (1% to 5%)

Miscellaneous: Antidegarelix antibody formation (10%), night sweats (1% to 5%)

General Dosage Range SubQ: *Adults:* Loading dose: 240 mg; Maintenance dose: 80 mg every 28 days

Mechanism of Action Gonadotropin-releasing hormone (GnRH) antagonist which reversibly binds to GnRH receptors in the anterior pituitary gland, blocking the receptor and decreasing secretion of luteinizing hormone (LH) and follicle stimulation hormone (FSH), resulting in rapid androgen deprivation by decreasing testosterone production, thereby decreasing testosterone levels. Testosterone levels do not exhibit an initial surge, or flare, as is typical with GnRH agonists.

Pharmacodynamics/Kinetics

Onset of Action Rapid; ~96% of patients had testosterone levels ≤50 ng/dL within 3 days (Klotz, 2008)

Half-life Elimination Loading dose: SubQ: ~53 days

Time to Peak Plasma: Loading dose: SubQ: Within 2 days

Pregnancy Risk Factor X

Pregnancy Considerations Adverse events were observed in animal reproduction studies. Use is contraindicated in women who are or may become pregnant.

Dental Comment Degarelix is known to prolong the QT interval. The QT interval is measured as the time and distance between the Q point of the QRS complex and the end of the T wave in the ECG tracing. After adjustment for heart rate, the QT interval is defined as prolonged if it is more than 450 msec in men and 460 msec in women. A long QT syndrome was first described in the 1950s and 60s as a congenital syndrome involving QT interval prolongation and syncope and sudden death. Some of the congenital long QT syndromes were characterized by a peculiar electrocardiographic appearance of the QRS complex involving a premature atria beat followed by a pause, then a subsequent sinus beat showing marked QT prolongation and deformity. This type of cardiac arrhythmia was originally termed "torsade de pointes" (translated from the French as "twisting of the points"). Degarelix is considered as having a risk of causing torsade de pointes. Since it is not known what effect vasoconstrictors in the local anesthetic regimen will have in patients with a known history of congenital prolonged QT interval or in patients taking any medication that prolongs the QT interval, a medical consult is suggested.

Delavirdine (de la VIR deen)

Related Information
HIV Infection and AIDS *on page 1520*

Brand Names: U.S. Rescriptor®

Brand Names: Canada Rescriptor®

Pharmacologic Category Antiretroviral Agent, Reverse Transcriptase Inhibitor (Non-nucleoside)

Use Treatment of HIV-1 infection in combination with at least two additional antiretroviral agents

Local Anesthetic/Vasoconstrictor Precautions No information available to require special precautions

Effects on Dental Treatment No significant effects or complications reported

Effects on Bleeding No reports of bleeding or thrombocytopenia.

Adverse Effects
Frequency of adverse reactions reported from occurrence in clinical trials with delavirdine when used as part of combination antiretroviral therapy.

>10%:
Central nervous system: Headache (19% to 20%), depressive symptoms (10% to 15%), fever (4% to 12%)

Dermatologic: Rash (16% to 32%)

Gastrointestinal: Nausea (20% to 25%), vomiting (3% to 11%)

1% to 10%:
Central nervous system: Anxiety (6% to 8%)

Endocrine & metabolic: Transaminases increased (2% to 5%), amylase increased (3%), bilirubin increased (2%)

Gastrointestinal: Diarrhea, vomiting, abdominal pain (4% to 6%)

Hematologic: Prothrombin time increased (2%), hemoglobin decreased (1% to 3%)

Respiratory: Bronchitis (6% to 8%)

Frequency not defined (limited to important or life threatening): Abscess, adenopathy, alkaline phosphatase increased, allergic reaction, angioedema, anorexia, arrhythmia, bloody stool, bone pain, bruising, cardiac insufficiency, cardiac rate abnormal, cardiomyopathy, chest congestion, cognitive impairment, colitis, confusion, conjunctivitis, dermal leukocytoclastic vasculitis, desquamation, diverticulitis, dyspnea, emotional lability, eosinophilia, erythema multiforme, fecal incontinence, fungal dermatitis, gamma glutamyl transpeptidase increased, gastroenteritis, gastrointestinal bleeding, granulocytosis, gum hemorrhage, hallucination, hematuria, hepatomegaly, hyperglycemia, hyperkalemia, hypertension, hypertriglyceridemia, hyperuricemia, hypocalcemia, hyponatremia, hypophosphatemia, infection, jaundice, kidney pain, leukopenia, lipase increased, menstrual irregularities, moniliasis (oral/vaginal), orthostatic hypotension, pancreatitis, pancytopenia, paralysis, peripheral vascular disorder, pneumonia, purpura, redistribution of body fat, renal calculi, serum creatinine increased, spleen disorder, Stevens-Johnson syndrome, tetany, thrombocytopenia, urinary tract infection, vertigo

General Dosage Range Oral: *Children ≥16 years and Adults:* 400 mg 3 times/day

Mechanism of Action Delavirdine binds directly to reverse transcriptase, blocking RNA-dependent and DNA-dependent DNA polymerase activities

Pharmacodynamics/Kinetics
Half-life Elimination 5.8 hours (range: 2-11 hours)

Time to Peak Plasma: 1 hour

Pregnancy Risk Factor C

Pregnancy Considerations Adverse events were observed in some animal reproduction studies. Hypersensitivity reactions (including hepatic toxicity and rash) are more common in women on NNRTI therapy; it is not known if pregnancy increases this risk.

Regardless of CD4 count or HIV RNA copy number, all HIV-infected pregnant women should receive a combination antepartum antiretroviral (ARV) drug regimen; this includes women who require therapy for their own health, as well as women who do not yet require therapy for their own health. ARV therapy should be started as soon as possible if required for the woman's health. Although earlier initiation may be more effective in reducing the perinatal transmission of HIV), also consider maternal conditions (eg, nausea and vomiting) and the potential risks of first trimester fetal exposure for specific agents. Plasma HIV RNA levels should be assessed at ~34-36 weeks gestation in order to help determine mode of delivery. If ARV therapy must be interrupted for <24 hours during the peripartum period, stop then restart all medications simultaneously in order to decrease the chance of developing resistance. Long-term follow-up is recommended for all infants exposed to ARV medications.

Healthcare providers are encouraged to enroll pregnant women exposed to antiretroviral medications in the Antiretroviral Pregnancy Registry (1-800-258-4263 or www.APRegistry.com). Healthcare providers caring for HIV-infected women and their infants may contact the National Perinatal HIV Hotline (888-448-8765) for clinical consultation (DHHS [perinatal], 2012).

Delmopinol (del MOE pi nol)

Brand Names: U.S. Decapinol®

Generic Availability (U.S.) No

Pharmacologic Category Antibacterial, Oral Rinse

Dental Use Treatment of gingivitis; used to decrease the adhesion of oral plaque

Local Anesthetic/Vasoconstrictor Precautions No information available to require special precautions

Effects on Dental Treatment No significant effects or complications reported

Dental Usual Dosage Treatment of gingivitis; used to decrease the adhesion of oral plaque: Adults: Oral: Rinse mouth with 10 mL for 1 minute twice daily (after brushing and flossing)

Mechanism of Action Reduces adhesion of plaque-causing bacteria, reducing the formation of new plaque and promoting the removal of deposits with normal mechanical disruption (brushing and flossing). Ultimately causes a reduction in both plaque and gingivitis. Decapinol® is regulated as a medical device because the primary mode of action is to serve as a physical barrier without chemical activity.

Contraindications Hypersensitivity to delmopinol or any component of the formulation

Warnings/Precautions Not for ingestion, patients should be instructed not to swallow solution. May cause transient anesthetic effects, dry mouth, or changes in taste following use. Light staining may occur, which may be removed by brushing the teeth. Patients should be instructed to avoid eating or drinking for 30 minutes following use. Should be used as an adjunct to normal mechanical hygiene. Avoid use in pregnant women (lack of data). Not recommended for use in children <12 years of age.

Note: Preliminary monograph: A decision to market this product within the U.S. is pending. At the time of publication, it is not possible to determine when this product will be available in the U.S. market.

Pregnancy Risk Factor The manufacturer does not recommend use in pregnant women.

Lactation Excretion unknown/not recommended

References

Hase JC, Attstrom R, Edwardsson S, et al, "6-Month Use of 0.2% Delmopinol Hydrochloride in Comparison With 0.2% Chlorhexidine Digluconate and Placebo (I). Effect on Plaque Formation and Gingivitis," *J Clin Periodontol,* 1998, 25(9):746-53.

Klinge B, Matsson L, Attstrom R, et al, "Effect of Local Application of Delmopinol Hydrochloride on Developing and Early Established Supragingival Plaque in Humans," *J Clin Periodontol,* 1996, 23 (6):543-7.

Lang NP, Hase JC, Grassi M, et al, "Plaque Formation and Gingivitis After Supervised Mouthrinsing With 0.2% Delmopinol Hydrochloride, 0.2% Chlorhexidine Digluconate and Placebo for 6 Months," *Oral Dis,* 1998, 4(2):105-13.

Demeclocycline (dem e kloe SYE kleen)

Pharmacologic Category Antibiotic, Tetracycline Derivative

Use Treatment of susceptible bacterial infections (eg, acne, urinary tract infections, respiratory infections) caused by both gram-negative and gram-positive organisms

Note: Use of demeclocycline as an antibacterial agent is uncommon; alternative tetracycline agents (eg, doxycycline, minocycline, tetracycline) are generally preferred.

Unlabeled Use Treatment of chronic syndrome of inappropriate secretion of antidiuretic hormone (SIADH)

Local Anesthetic/Vasoconstrictor Precautions No information available to require special precautions

Effects on Dental Treatment Tetracyclines are not recommended for use during pregnancy or in children ≤8 years of age since they have been reported to cause enamel hypoplasia and permanent teeth discoloration. Tetracyclines should only be used in these patients if other agents are contraindicated or alternative antimicrobials will not eradicate the organism. Long-term use associated with oral candidiasis.

Effects on Bleeding No information available to require special precautions

Adverse Effects Frequency not defined.

Cardiovascular: Pericarditis

Central nervous system: Bulging fontanels (infants), dizziness, headache, pseudotumor cerebri (adults)

Dermatologic: Angioedema, anogenital inflammatory lesions (with monilial overgrowth), erythema multiforme, erythematous rash, exfoliative dermatitis (rare), maculopapular rash, photosensitivity, pigmentation of skin, Stevens-Johnson syndrome (rare), urticaria

Endocrine & metabolic: Microscopic discoloration of thyroid gland (brown/black), nephrogenic diabetes insipidus, thyroid dysfunction (rare)

Gastrointestinal: Anorexia, diarrhea, dysphagia, enterocolitis, esophageal ulcerations, glossitis, nausea, pancreatitis, vomiting

Genitourinary: Balanitis

Hematologic: Eosinophilia, neutropenia, hemolytic anemia, thrombocytopenia

Hepatic: Hepatitis (rare), hepatotoxicity (rare), liver enzymes increased, liver failure (rare)

Neuromuscular & skeletal: Myasthenic syndrome, polyarthralgia, tooth discoloration (children <8 years, rarely in adults)

Ocular: Visual disturbances

Otic: Tinnitus

Renal: Acute renal failure, BUN increased

Respiratory: Pulmonary infiltrates

Miscellaneous: Anaphylaxis, anaphylactoid purpura, fixed drug eruptions (rare), lupus-like syndrome, superinfection, systemic lupus erythematosus exacerbation

General Dosage Range Dosage adjustment recommended in patients with renal and hepatic impairment

Oral:

Children >8 years: 7-13 mg/kg/day (maximum: 600 mg/day) divided every 6-12 hours

Adults: 600 mg/day in 2 or 4 divided doses

Mechanism of Action Inhibits protein synthesis by binding with the 30S and possibly the 50S ribosomal subunit(s) of susceptible bacteria; may also cause alterations in the cytoplasmic membrane; inhibits the action of ADH in patients with chronic SIADH

Pharmacodynamics/Kinetics

Onset of Action SIADH: 2-5 days

Half-life Elimination 10-16 hours

Time to Peak Serum: ~4 hours

Pregnancy Risk Factor D

Pregnancy Considerations Tetracyclines, including demeclocycline, cross the placenta and accumulate in developing teeth and long tubular bones. Tetracyclines may discolor fetal teeth following maternal use during pregnancy; the specific teeth involved and the portion of the tooth affected depends on the timing and duration of exposure relative to tooth calcification. As a class, tetracyclines are generally considered second-line antibiotics in pregnant women and their use should be avoided (Gibbons, 1960; Mylonas, 2011).

Denileukin Diftitox (de ni LOO kin DIF ti toks)

Brand Names: U.S. ONTAK®

Pharmacologic Category Antineoplastic Agent, Miscellaneous

Use Treatment of persistent or recurrent cutaneous T-cell lymphoma (CTCL) whose malignant cells express the CD25 component of the IL-2 receptor

Unlabeled Use Treatment of relapsed or refractory peripheral T-cell lymphoma (PTCL)

Local Anesthetic/Vasoconstrictor Precautions No information available to require special precautions

Effects on Dental Treatment No significant effects or complications reported

Effects on Bleeding No information available to require special precautions

Adverse Effects

>10%:

Cardiovascular: Capillary leak syndrome (33%; serious: 11%), peripheral edema (20% to 26%), vasodilation (22%), hypotension (7% to 16%), chest pain (4% to 13%), tachycardia (12%), thrombosis-related events (7% to 11%)

Central nervous system: Fever (49% to 64%), fatigue (44% to 47%), headache (26% to 29%), dizziness (11% to 13%), pain (11% to 13%)

Dermatologic: Rash (20% to 24%), pruritus (16% to 18%)

Endocrine & metabolic: Hypoalbuminemia (14% to 17%)

Gastrointestinal: Nausea (47% to 60%), vomiting (13% to 35%), diarrhea (22%), anorexia (9% to 20%), taste disturbance (11% to 13%)

Hematologic: Lymphopenia (70%; 24% had lymphopenia at baseline)

Hepatic: ALT increased (84%), AST increased (84%)

Neuromuscular & skeletal: Rigors (42% to 47%), myalgia (18% to 20%), weakness (18%), back pain (16% to 18%), arthralgia (13% to 16%)

Respiratory: Cough (18% to 20%), upper respiratory infection (13%), dyspnea (11% to 13%)

Miscellaneous: Antibody formation (76% to 100%) neutralizing antibodies (45% to 97%), flu-like syndrome (≤85%), infusion reaction (71%; serious: 8%), infection (48%)

1% to 10%:

Cardiovascular: Arrhythmia (6%), hypertension (6%)

Hematologic: Leukopenia (grades 3/4: 3% to 6%), neutropenia (grades 3/4: 3%), thrombocytopenia (grades 3/4: 3%)

Local: Injection site reaction (8%)

Ocular: Visual changes (serious: 4%; includes loss of visual acuity)

Renal: Serum creatinine increased (3% to 10%), proteinuria/casts/hematuria (6%)

General Dosage Range Dosage adjustment recommended in patients who develop toxicities

I.V.: *Adults:* 9 or 18 mcg/kg/day days 1-5 every 21 days

Mechanism of Action Denileukin diftitox is a fusion protein (a combination of amino acid sequences from diphtheria toxin and interleukin-2) which selectively delivers the cytotoxic activity of diphtheria toxin to targeted cells. It interacts with the high-affinity IL-2 receptor on the surface of malignant cells to inhibit intracellular protein synthesis, rapidly leading to cell death.

Pharmacodynamics/Kinetics

Half-life Elimination Distribution: 2-5 minutes; Terminal: 70-80 minutes

Pregnancy Considerations Animal reproduction studies have not been conducted. Should be given to a pregnant woman only if clearly needed

---

Denosumab (den OH sue mab)

Related Information

Osteonecrosis of the Jaw *on page 1529*

Rheumatoid Arthritis, Osteoarthritis, and Osteoporosis *on page 1526*

Brand Names: U.S. Prolia™; Xgeva®

Brand Names: Canada Prolia®; Xgeva®

Generic Availability (U.S.) No

Pharmacologic Category Bone-Modifying Agent; Monoclonal Antibody

Use Treatment of osteoporosis in men and in postmenopausal women at high risk for fracture; treatment of bone loss in men receiving androgen deprivation therapy (ADT) for nonmetastatic prostate cancer; treatment of bone loss in women receiving aromatase inhibitor (AI) therapy for breast cancer; prevention of skeletal-related events (eg, fracture, spinal cord compression, bone pain requiring surgery/radiation therapy) in patients with bone metastases from solid tumors

Unlabeled Use Treatment of bone destruction caused by rheumatoid arthritis

Local Anesthetic/Vasoconstrictor Precautions No information available to require special precautions

Effects on Dental Treatment Cases of osteonecrosis of the jaw bone (ONJ) have been associated with denosumab exposure. ONJ presents clinically as exposed necrotic bone of at least 8 weeks duration with or without the presence of pain, infection, or previous trauma in a patient who has not received radiation to the jaws. Since ONJ is also associated with bisphosphonate exposure, and osteoclasts are the common targets of bisphosphonates and denosumab, osteoclastic

inhibition may play a central role in ONJ associated with these two classes of drugs. Patients developing ONJ while on denosumab therapy should receive care by an oral surgeon. See Warnings/Precautions and Dental Comment.

Effects on Bleeding No information available to require special precautions

Adverse Effects A postmarketing safety program for Prolia® is available to collect information on adverse events; more information is available at http://www.proliasafety.com. To report adverse events for either Prolia® or Xgeva®, prescribers may also call Amgen at 800-772-6436 or FDA at 800-332-1088.

Percentages noted with Prolia® (60 mg every 6 months) unless specified as Xgeva® (120 mg every 4 weeks):

>10%:

Central nervous system: Fatigue (Xgeva®: 45%), headache (Xgeva®: 13%)

Dermatologic: Dermatitis (4% to 11%), eczema (4% to 11%), rash (3% to 11%)

Endocrine & metabolic: Hypophosphatemia (Xgeva®: 32%; grade 3: 15%), hypocalcemia (2%; Xgeva®: 18%; grade 3: 3%)

Gastrointestinal: Nausea (Xgeva®: 31%), diarrhea (Xgeva®: 20%)

Neuromuscular & skeletal: Weakness (Xgeva®: 45%), arthralgia (7% to 14%), limb pain (10% to 12%), back pain (8% to 12%)

Respiratory: Dyspnea (Xgeva®: 21%), cough (Xgeva®: 15%)

1% to 10%:

Cardiovascular: Peripheral edema (5%), angina (3%)

Endocrine & metabolic: Hypercholesterolemia (7%)

Gastrointestinal: Flatulence (2%)

Neuromuscular & skeletal: Musculoskeletal pain (6%), sciatica (5%), bone pain (4%), myalgia (3%), osteonecrosis of the jaw (ONJ; ≤2%)

Ocular: Cataracts (≤5%)

Respiratory: Nasopharyngitis (7%), upper respiratory tract infection (5%)

Miscellaneous: New malignancies (3% to 5%), infections (nonfatal, serious; 4%)

Dosage SubQ: Adults:

Prevention of skeletal-related events in bone metastases from solid tumors (Xgeva®): 120 mg every 4 weeks

Treatment of androgen deprivation-induced bone loss in men with prostate cancer (Prolia®): 60 mg as a single dose, once every 6 months (Fizazi, 2011; Henry, 2011; Stopeck, 2010)

Treatment of aromatase inhibitor-induced bone loss in women with breast cancer (Prolia®): 60 mg as a single dose, once every 6 months (Smith, 2009)

Treatment of osteoporosis in men or postmenopausal women (Prolia®): 60 mg as a single dose, once every 6 months (Ellis, 2008)

Dosage adjustment in renal impairment: Cl$_{cr}$ <30 mL/minute (including dialysis-dependent): No adjustment necessary when administered every 6 months (Prolia®); once-monthly dosing has not been evaluated in patients with renal impairment (Xgeva®). Monitor patients with severe impairment (Cl$_{cr}$ <30 mL/minute or on dialysis) due to increased risk of hypocalcemia.

Dosage adjustment in hepatic impairment: No dosage adjustment provided in manufacturer's labeling (has not been studied).

Mechanism of Action Denosumab is a monoclonal antibody with affinity for nuclear factor-kappa ligand (RANKL). Osteoblasts secrete RANKL; RANKL activates osteoclast precursors and subsequent osteolysis which promotes release of bone-derived growth factors, such as insulin-like growth factor-1 (IGF1) and transforming growth factor-beta (TGF-beta), and increases serum calcium levels. Denosumab binds to RANKL, blocks the interaction between RANKL and RANK (a receptor located on osteoclast surfaces), and prevents osteoclast formation, leading to decreased bone resorption and increased bone mass in osteoporosis. In solid tumors with bony metastases, RANKL inhibition decreases osteoclast activity leading to decreased skeletal related events and tumor-induced bone destruction.

Contraindications

Prolia®: Hypersensitivity to denosumab or any component of the formulation; pre-existing hypocalcemia; pregnancy

Xgeva®: There are no contraindications listed in the manufacturer's labeling.

Warnings/Precautions Denosumab may cause or exacerbate hypocalcemia; severe symptomatic cases (including fatalities) have been reported. Monitor calcium levels; correct pre-existing hypocalcemia prior to therapy. Use caution in patients with a history of hypoparathyroidism, thyroid surgery, parathyroid surgery, malabsorption syndromes, excision of small intestine, severe renal impairment/dialysis or other conditions which would predispose the patient to hypocalcemia; monitor calcium, phosphorus, and magnesium closely during therapy. Ensure adequate calcium and vitamin D intake; supplement with calcium and vitamin D; magnesium supplementation may also be necessary. Incidence of infections may be increased, including serious skin infections, abdominal, urinary, ear, or periodontal infections. Endocarditis has also been reported following use. Patients should be advised to contact healthcare provider if signs or symptoms of severe infection or cellulitis develop. Use with caution in patients with impaired immune systems or using concomitant immunosuppressive therapy; may be at increased risk for serious infections. Evaluate the need for continued treatment with serious infection.

Atypical femur fractures have been reported in patients receiving denosumab. The fractures include subtrochanteric femur (bone just below the hip joint) and diaphyseal femur (long segment of the thigh bone). Some patients experience prodromal pain weeks or months before the fracture occurs. It is unclear if denosumab therapy is the cause for these fractures. Consider interrupting therapy in patients who develop an atypical femoral fracture. Osteonecrosis of the jaw (ONJ) has been reported in patients receiving denosumab. ONJ may manifest as jaw pain, osteomyelitis, osteitis, bone erosion, tooth/periodontal infection, toothache, gingival ulceration/erosion. Risk factors include invasive dental procedures (eg, tooth extraction, dental implants, boney surgery); a diagnosis of cancer, concomitant chemotherapy or corticosteroids, poor oral hygiene, ill-fitting dentures; and comorbid disorders (anemia, coagulopathy, infection, pre-existing dental disease). Patients should maintain good oral hygiene during treatment. A dental exam and preventative dentistry should be performed prior to therapy. The benefit/risk must be assessed by the treating physician and/or dentist/surgeon prior to any invasive dental procedure; avoid invasive procedures in patients with bone metastases receiving therapy for prevention of skeletal-related events. Patients developing ONJ while on denosumab therapy should receive care by a dentist or oral surgeon; extensive dental surgery to treat ONJ may exacerbate ONJ; evaluate individually and consider discontinuing if extensive dental surgery is necessary.

Postmenopausal osteoporosis: For use in women at high risk for fracture which is defined as a history of osteoporotic fracture or multiple risk factors for fracture. May also be used in women who failed or did not tolerate other therapies.

Bone metastases: Denosumab is not indicated for the prevention of skeletal-related events in patients with multiple myeloma. In trials with multiple myeloma patients, denosumab was noninferior to zoledronic acid in delaying time to first skeletal-related event and mortality was increased in a subset of the denosumab-treated group.

Denosumab therapy results in significant suppression of bone turnover; the long term effects of treatment are not known but may contribute to adverse outcomes such as ONJ, atypical fractures, or delayed fracture healing; monitor. Use with caution in patients with renal impairment (Cl_{cr} <30 mL/minute) or patients on dialysis; risk of hypocalcemia is increased. Dose adjustment is not needed when administered at 60 mg every 6 months (Prolia®); once-monthly dosing has not been evaluated in patients with renal impairment (Xgeva®). Dermatitis, eczema, and rash (which are not necessarily specific to the injection site) have been reported; consider discontinuing if severe symptoms occur. Packaging may contain natural latex rubber. May impair bone growth in children with open growth plates or inhibit eruption of dentition. Do not administer Prolia® and Xgeva® to the same patient for different indications.

Drug Interactions

Metabolism/Transport Effects None known.

Avoid Concomitant Use There are no known interactions where it is recommended to avoid concomitant use.

Increased Effect/Toxicity

Denosumab may increase the levels/effects of: Immunosuppressants

Decreased Effect There are no known significant interactions involving a decrease in effect.

Ethanol/Nutrition/Herb Interactions Ethanol: Avoid ethanol (may increase risk of osteoporosis).

Dietary Considerations Ensure adequate calcium and vitamin D intake to prevent or treat hypocalcemia. Calcium 1000 mg/day and vitamin D ≥400 units/day is recommended in product labeling (Prolia®).

Women and men >50 years of age should consume elemental calcium 1200-1500 mg/day and vitamin D 800-1000 units/day (National Osteoporosis Foundation Guidelines, 2010).

Pharmacodynamics/Kinetics

Onset of Action Decreases markers of bone resorption by ~85% within 3 days; maximal reductions observed within 1 month

Duration of Action Markers of bone resorption return to baseline within 12 months of discontinuing therapy

Half-life Elimination ~25-28 days

Time to Peak Serum: 10 days (range 3-21 days)

Pregnancy Risk Factor D (Xgeva®)/X (Prolia®)

Pregnancy Considerations Adverse events were observed in animal reproduction studies. Specifically, increased fetal loss, stillbirths, postnatal mortality, absent lymph nodes, abnormal bone growth, and decreased neonatal growth was observed in cynomolgus monkeys exposed to denosumab throughout pregnancy. Denosumab was measurable in the offspring at one month of age. Fetal exposure to monoclonal antibodies is expected to increase as pregnancy progresses. Women should be advised to avoid pregnancy during denosumab treatment. If a pregnant woman is exposed, patients or their prescribers may contact the Amgen Pregnancy Surveillance Program (800-772-6436). In addition, there is potential for a fetus to be exposed to denosumab when a pregnant woman has unprotected sex with a man treated with denosumab. It is unknown the extent that denosumab is present in seminal fluid; however, the risk of harm to the fetus is expected to be low. Men receiving denosumab who have pregnant partners should be counseled regarding this potential risk.

Lactation Excretion unknown/not recommended

Breast-Feeding Considerations According to the manufacturer, the decision to discontinue denosumab or discontinue breast-feeding should take into account the benefits of treatment to the mother. In some animal studies, mammary gland development was impaired following exposure to denosumab during pregnancy, resulting in impaired lactation postpartum.

Dosage Forms

Injection, solution [preservative free]:

Prolia™: 60 mg/mL (1 mL)

Xgeva®: 70 mg/mL (1.7 mL)

Dental Comment In head-to-head comparison trials of denosumab and zoledronate (a bisphosphonate) for the treatment of bone metastasis in patients with cancer, 20 cases of ONJ were detected out of a total of 1026 subjects (2.0%) exposed to denosumab. There were 14 cases of ONJ observed out of a total of 1020 subjects (1.4%) exposed to zoledronate (Kyrgidis, 2010). The case of a 60-year old male cancer patient who developed ONJ after treatment with denosumab has been published (Taylor, 2010). In that report, the patient participated in a trial for a phase 3 study of denosumab. The patient had never been prescribed a bisphosphonate medication before treatment with denosumab. Clinical and radiological features of the lesion were diagnostic of probable ONJ. After discontinuation of the denosumab, the patient was treated with antibiotics and chlorhexidine rinses for a week. The necrotic bone sequestered 12 months later, and 15 months after initial presentation, the mucosa had healed with no further symptoms. Another case reported the development of ONJ in a 65-year old women being treated for giant cell tumor with denosumab. Although the patient was medically compromised and on multiple medications, the authors proposed that a common thread in ONJ development is inhibition of osteoclastic activity, mediated in this case by denosumab.

References

Kyrgidis A and Toulis KA, "Denosumab-Related Osteonecrosis of the Jaws," *Osteoporos Int*, 2010, [epub ahead of print].

Taylor KH, Middlefell LS, and Mizen KD, "Osteonecrosis of the Jaws Induced by Anti-RANK Ligand Therapy," *Br J Oral Maxillofac Surg*, 2010, 48(3):221-3.

Desipramine (des IP ra meen)

Related Information

Vasoconstrictor Interactions With Antidepressants *on page 1650*

Brand Names: U.S. Norpramin®

Brand Names: Canada Dom-Desipramine; Novo-Desipramine; Nu-Desipramine; PMS-Desipramine

Pharmacologic Category Antidepressant, Tricyclic (Secondary Amine)

Use Treatment of depression

Unlabeled Use Analgesic adjunct in chronic pain; peripheral neuropathies (including diabetic neuropathy); attention-deficit/hyperactivity disorder (ADHD); depression in children ≤12 years of age

Local Anesthetic/Vasoconstrictor Precautions Use with caution; epinephrine and levonordefrin have been shown to have an increased pressor response in combination with TCAs. Desipramine is one of the drugs confirmed to prolong the QT interval and is accepted as having a risk of causing torsade de pointes. The risk of drug-induced torsade de pointes is extremely low when a single QT interval prolonging drug is prescribed. In terms of epinephrine, it is not known what effect vasoconstrictors in the local anesthetic regimen will have in patients with a known history of congenital prolonged QT interval or in patients taking any medication that prolongs the QT interval. Until more information is obtained, it is suggested that the clinician consult with the physician prior to the use of a vasoconstrictor in suspected patients, and that the vasoconstrictor (epinephrine, mepivacaine and levonordefrin [Carbocaine® 2% with Neo-Cobefrin®]) be used with caution.

Effects on Dental Treatment Key adverse event(s) related to dental treatment: Xerostomia and changes in salivation (normal salivary flow resumes upon discontinuation), unpleasant taste, stomatitis, and black tongue. Long-term treatment with TCAs increases the risk of caries by reducing salivation and salivary buffer capacity.

Effects on Bleeding Thrombocytopenia has been reported.

Adverse Effects Frequency not defined.

Cardiovascular: Arrhythmias, edema, flushing, heart block, hyper-/hypotension, MI, palpitation, stroke, tachycardia

Central nervous system: Agitation, anxiety, ataxia, confusion, delusions, disorientation, dizziness, drowsiness, EEG alterations, exacerbation of psychosis, extrapyramidal symptoms, fatigue, fever, hallucinations, headache, hypomania, incoordination, insomnia, neuroleptic malignant syndrome, nightmares, restlessness, seizure, suicidal thinking and behavior

Dermatologic: Alopecia, itching, petechiae, photosensitivity, skin rash, urticaria

Endocrine & metabolic: Breast enlargement, galactorrhea, gynecomastia, hyper-/hypoglycemia, impotence, libido changes, SIADH

Gastrointestinal: Abdominal cramps, anorexia, black tongue, constipation, diarrhea, epigastric distress, nausea, parotid edema, paralytic ileus, stomatitis, sublingual adenitis, unpleasant taste, vomiting, weight gain/loss, xerostomia

Genitourinary: Micturition delayed, nocturia, painful ejaculation, polyuria, testicular edema, urinary retention

Hematologic: Agranulocytosis, eosinophilia, purpura, thrombocytopenia

◄ Hepatic: Alkaline phosphatase increased, cholestatic jaundice, hepatitis, liver enzymes increased

Neuromuscular & skeletal: Falling, numbness, paresthesia of extremities, peripheral neuropathy, tingling, tremor, weakness

Ocular: Blurred vision, disturbances of accommodation, intraocular pressure increased, mydriasis

Otic: Tinnitus

Miscellaneous: Allergic reaction, diaphoresis (excessive), withdrawal symptoms

General Dosage Range Oral:
Adolescents: 25-100 mg/day in single or divided doses (maximum: 150 mg/day)
Adults: 100-200 mg/day in single or divided doses (maximum: 300 mg/day)
Elderly: 25-100 mg/day in single or divided doses (maximum: 150 mg/day)

Mechanism of Action Traditionally believed to increase the synaptic concentration of norepinephrine (and to a lesser extent, serotonin) in the central nervous system by inhibition of its reuptake by the presynaptic neuronal membrane. However, additional receptor effects have been found including desensitization of adenyl cyclase, down regulation of beta-adrenergic receptors, and down regulation of serotonin receptors.

Pharmacodynamics/Kinetics
Onset of Action Earliest therapeutic effects: 2-5 days; Maximum antidepressant effect: >2 weeks
Half-life Elimination Adults: 15-24 hours (Weiner, 1981)
Time to Peak Plasma: ~6 hours (Weiner, 1981)

Pregnancy Considerations Animal reproduction studies are inconclusive.

Dental Comment Desipramine is known to prolong the QT interval. The QT interval is measured as the time and distance between the Q point of the QRS complex and the end of the T wave in the ECG tracing. After adjustment for heart rate, the QT interval is defined as prolonged if it is more than 450 msec in men and 460 msec in women. A long QT syndrome was first described in the 1950s and 60s as a congenital syndrome involving QT interval prolongation and syncope and sudden death. Some of the congenital long QT syndromes were characterized by a peculiar electrocardiographic appearance of the QRS complex involving a premature atria beat followed by a pause, then a subsequent sinus beat showing marked QT prolongation and deformity. This type of cardiac arrhythmia was originally termed "torsade de pointes" (translated from the French as "twisting of the points"). Desipramine is considered as having a risk of causing torsade de pointes. Since it is not known what effect vasoconstrictors in the local anesthetic regimen will have in patients with a known history of congenital prolonged QT interval or in patients taking any medication that prolongs the QT interval, a medical consult is suggested.

Desirudin (des i ROO din)

Related Information
Cardiovascular Diseases *on page 1492*
Brand Names: U.S. Iprivask®
Pharmacologic Category Anticoagulant, Thrombin Inhibitor
Use Prophylaxis of deep vein thrombosis (DVT) in patients undergoing surgery for hip replacement
Local Anesthetic/Vasoconstrictor Precautions No information available to require special precautions

Effects on Dental Treatment No significant effects or complications reported

Effects on Bleeding As with all anticoagulants, bleeding is a potential adverse effect of desirudin during dental surgery; risk is dependent on multiple variables, including the intensity of anticoagulation and patient susceptibility. Medical consult is suggested. It is unlikely that ambulatory patients presenting for dental treatment will be taking intravenous anticoagulant therapy such as desirudin.

Adverse Effects As with all anticoagulants, bleeding is the major adverse effect. Hemorrhage may occur at any site.

2% to 10%:
Gastrointestinal: Nausea (2%)
Hematologic: Hematoma (6%), hemorrhage (major, <1% to 3%; may include cases of intracranial, retroperitoneal, intraocular, intraspinal, or prosthetic joint hemorrhage), anemia (3%)
Local: Injection site mass (4%), deep thrombophlebitis (2%)
Miscellaneous: Wound secretion (4%)

General Dosage Range Dosage adjustment recommended in patients with renal impairment
SubQ: *Adults:* 15 mg every 12 hours

Mechanism of Action Desirudin is a direct, highly selective thrombin inhibitor. Reversibly binds to the active thrombin site of free and clot-associated thrombin. Inhibits fibrin formation, activation of coagulation factors V, VII, and XIII, and thrombin-induced platelet aggregation resulting in a dose-dependent prolongation of the activated partial thromboplastin time (aPTT).

Pharmacodynamics/Kinetics
Half-life Elimination ~2 hours; Prolonged with renal impairment (Cl_{cr} <31 mL/minute/1.73 m^2: Up to 12 hours)
Time to Peak Plasma: 1-3 hours
Pregnancy Risk Factor C
Pregnancy Considerations Teratogenic effects were observed in some animal reproduction studies. Data are insufficient to evaluate the safety of thrombin inhibitors during pregnancy (Guyatt, 2012).

Desloratadine (des lor AT a deen)

Brand Names: U.S. Clarinex®
Brand Names: Canada Aerius®; Aerius® Kids; Desloratadine Allergy Control
Generic Availability (U.S.) Yes: Excludes syrup
Pharmacologic Category Histamine H_1 Antagonist; Histamine H_1 Antagonist, Second Generation; Piperidine Derivative
Use Relief of nasal and non-nasal symptoms of seasonal allergic rhinitis (SAR) and perennial allergic rhinitis (PAR); treatment of chronic idiopathic urticaria (CIU)
Local Anesthetic/Vasoconstrictor Precautions No information available to require special precautions
Effects on Dental Treatment Key adverse event(s) related to dental treatment: Xerostomia (normal salivary flow resumes upon discontinuation)
Effects on Bleeding No information available to require special precautions
Adverse Effects Note: Frequency reported in children, unless otherwise noted.
>10%:
Central nervous system: Fever (12% to 17%), headache (adults 14%), irritability (12%)
Gastrointestinal: Diarrhea (15% to 20%)

Respiratory: Upper respiratory tract infection (11% to 21%), cough (11%)

1% to 10%:

Central nervous system: Somnolence (children 9%; adults 2%), insomnia (5%), fatigue (adults 2% to 5%), dizziness (adults 4%), emotional lability (3%)

Dermatologic: Erythema (3%), maculopapular rash (3%)

Endocrine & metabolic: Dysmenorrhea (adults 2%)

Gastrointestinal: Vomiting (6%), anorexia (5%), nausea (children 3%; adults 5%), nausea (5%), appetite increased (3%), dyspepsia (adults 3%), xerostomia (adults 3%)

Genitourinary: Urinary tract infection (4%)

Neuromuscular & skeletal: Myalgia (adults 2% to 3%)

Otic: Otitis media (children 6%)

Respiratory: Bronchitis (6%), rhinorrhea (5%), pharyngitis (children 3% to 5%; adults 3% to 4%), epistaxis (3%)

Miscellaneous: Varicella infection (4%), parasitic infection (3%)

Dosage Oral:

Children:

6-11 months: 1 mg once daily

12 months to 5 years: 1.25 mg once daily

6-11 years: 2.5 mg once daily

Children ≥12 years and Adults: 5 mg once daily

Dosage adjustment in renal impairment:

Children: No dosage adjustment provided in manufacturer's labeling (has not been studied).

Adults: Mild-to-severe impairment: 5 mg every other day.

Dosage adjustment in hepatic impairment:

Children: No dosage adjustment provided in manufacturer's labeling (has not been studied).

Adults: Mild-to-severe impairment: 5 mg every other day.

Mechanism of Action Desloratadine, a major active metabolite of loratadine, is a long-acting tricyclic antihistamine with selective peripheral histamine H_1 receptor antagonistic activity.

Contraindications Hypersensitivity to desloratadine, loratadine, or any component of the formulation

Warnings/Precautions Hypersensitivity reactions (including anaphylaxis) have been reported with use; discontinue therapy immediately with signs/symptoms of hypersensitivity. Dose should be adjusted in patients with liver or renal impairment. Use with caution in patients known to be slow metabolizers of desloratadine (incidence of side effects may be increased). Some products may contain phenylalanine.

Drug Interactions

Metabolism/Transport Effects Substrate of P-glycoprotein

Avoid Concomitant Use

Avoid concomitant use of Desloratadine with any of the following: Aclidinium; Azelastine (Nasal); Ipratropium (Oral Inhalation); Paraldehyde; Tiotropium

Increased Effect/Toxicity

Desloratadine may increase the levels/effects of: Alcohol (Ethyl); Anticholinergics; Azelastine (Nasal); Buprenorphine; CNS Depressants; Methotrimeprazine; Metyrosine; Mirtazapine; Paraldehyde; Pramipexole; ROPINIRole; Rotigotine; Selective Serotonin Reuptake Inhibitors; Tiotropium; Zolpidem

The levels/effects of Desloratadine may be increased by: Aclidinium; Droperidol; HydrOXYzine; Ipratropium (Oral Inhalation); Magnesium Sulfate; Methotrimeprazine; Perampanel; P-glycoprotein/ABCB1 Inhibitors; Pramlintide; Sodium Oxybate

Decreased Effect

Desloratadine may decrease the levels/effects of: Acetylcholinesterase Inhibitors (Central); Benzylpenicilloyl Polylysine; Betahistine; Hyaluronidase

The levels/effects of Desloratadine may be decreased by: Acetylcholinesterase Inhibitors (Central); Amphetamines; P-glycoprotein/ABCB1 Inducers

Ethanol/Nutrition/Herb Interactions

Ethanol: May increase CNS depression; monitor for increased effects with coadministration. Caution patients about effects.

Food: Does not affect bioavailability.

Dietary Considerations May be taken with or without food. Some products may contain phenylalanine.

Pharmacodynamics/Kinetics

Onset of Action Within 1 hour

Duration of Action 24 hours

Half-life Elimination 27 hours

Time to Peak 3 hours

Pregnancy Risk Factor C

Pregnancy Considerations Adverse events have been observed in animal reproduction studies; therefore, the manufacturer classifies desloratadine as pregnancy category C. The use of antihistamines for the treatment of rhinitis during pregnancy is generally considered to be safe at recommended doses. Information related to the use of desloratadine during pregnancy is limited; therefore, other agents may be preferred. Desloratadine is the primary metabolite of loratadine; refer to the Loratadine monograph for additional information.

Lactation Enters breast milk/not recommended

Breast-Feeding Considerations Desloratadine is excreted into breast milk. According to the manufacturer, the decision to continue or discontinue breast-feeding during therapy should take into account the risk of exposure to the infant and the benefits of treatment to the mother.

Dosage Forms

Syrup, oral:

Clarinex®: 0.5 mg/mL (480 mL)

Tablet, oral: 5 mg

Clarinex®: 5 mg

Tablet, orally disintegrating, oral: 2.5 mg, 5 mg

Desloratadine and Pseudoephedrine

(des lor AT a deen & soo doe e FED rin)

Related Information

Desloratadine on page 392

Pseudoephedrine on page 1159

Brand Names: U.S. Clarinex-D® 12 Hour; Clarinex-D® 24 Hour [DSC]

Pharmacologic Category Alpha/Beta Agonist; Decongestant; Histamine H_1 Antagonist; Histamine H_1 Antagonist, Second Generation; Piperidine Derivative

Use Relief of nasal and non-nasal symptoms of seasonal allergic rhinitis

Local Anesthetic/Vasoconstrictor Precautions No information available to require special precautions

Effects on Dental Treatment Key adverse event(s) related to dental treatment: Pseudoephedrine: Xerostomia (normal salivary flow resumes upon discontinuation).

Effects on Bleeding No information available to require special precautions

Adverse Effects See also individual agents. Percentages as reported with the combination products: 1% to 10%:

Central nervous system: Insomnia (5% to 10%), headache (6% to 8%), fatigue (3% to 4%), somnolence (3%), dizziness (2% to 3%), hyperactivity (2%), nervousness (2%)

Gastrointestinal: Xerostomia (8%), anorexia (2%), nausea (2%)

Respiratory: Pharyngitis (3%)

General Dosage Range Dosage adjustment recommended in patients with renal impairment.

Oral: *Children ≥12 years and Adults:* 12-hour formulation: 1 tablet twice daily; 24-hour formulation: 1 tablet once daily

Mechanism of Action

Desloratadine, a major active metabolite of loratadine, is a long-acting tricyclic antihistamine with selective peripheral histamine H_1 receptor antagonistic activity.

Pseudoephedrine directly stimulates alpha-adrenergic receptors of respiratory mucosa causing vasoconstriction; directly stimulates beta-adrenergic receptors causing bronchial relaxation, increased heart rate and contractility.

Pharmacodynamics/Kinetics

Onset of Action Antihistaminic activity: 1 hour

Time to Peak Desloratadine: 4-7 hours; Pseudoephedrine: 6-9 hours

Pregnancy Risk Factor C

Pregnancy Considerations Reproduction studies have not been conducted with this combination. See individual agents.

Desmopressin (des moe PRES in)

Brand Names: U.S. DDAVP®; Stimate®

Brand Names: Canada Apo-Desmopressin®; DDAVP®; DDAVP® Melt; Minirin®; Novo-Desmopressin; Octostim®; PMS-Desmopressin

Pharmacologic Category Antihemophilic Agent; Hemostatic Agent; Vasopressin Analog, Synthetic

Use

Injection: Treatment of diabetes insipidus; maintenance of hemostasis and control of bleeding in hemophilia A with factor VIII coagulant activity levels >5% and mild-to-moderate classic von Willebrand's disease (type 1) with factor VIII coagulant activity levels >5%

Nasal solutions (DDAVP® Nasal Spray and DDAVP® Rhinal Tube): Treatment of central diabetes insipidus

Nasal spray (Stimate®): Maintenance of hemostasis and control of bleeding in hemophilia A with factor VIII coagulant activity levels >5% and mild-to-moderate classic von Willebrand's disease (type 1) with factor VIII coagulant activity levels >5%

Tablet: Treatment of central diabetes insipidus, temporary polyuria and polydipsia following pituitary surgery or head trauma, primary nocturnal enuresis

Unlabeled Use Uremic bleeding associated with acute or chronic renal failure; prevention of surgical bleeding in patients with uremia

Local Anesthetic/Vasoconstrictor Precautions No information available to require special precautions

Effects on Dental Treatment No significant effects or complications reported

Effects on Bleeding Rare reports of thrombotic events including thromboembolism have been associated with desmopressin, although no causality has been determined.

Adverse Effects Frequency may not be defined (may be dose or route related).

Cardiovascular: Blood pressure increased/decreased (I.V.), facial flushing

Central nervous system: Headache (2% to 5%), dizziness (intranasal; ≤3%), chills (intranasal; 2%)

Dermatologic: Rash

Endocrine & metabolic: Hyponatremia, water intoxication

Gastrointestinal: Abdominal pain (intranasal; 2%), gastrointestinal disorder (intranasal; ≤2%), nausea (intranasal; ≤2%), abdominal cramps, sore throat

Hepatic: Transient increases in liver transaminases (associated primarily with tablets)

Local: Injection: Burning pain, erythema, and swelling at the injection site

Neuromuscular & Skeletal: Weakness (intranasal; ≤2%)

Ocular: Conjunctivitis (intranasal; ≤2%), eye edema (intranasal; ≤2%), lacrimation disorder (intranasal; ≤2%)

Respiratory: Rhinitis (intranasal; 3% to 8%), epistaxis (intranasal; ≤3%), nostril pain (intranasal; ≤2%), cough, nasal congestion, upper respiratory infection

General Dosage Range

I.V.:

Infants and Children ≥3 months: 0.3 mcg/kg as a single dose, may repeat dose if needed

Adults: 2-4 mcg/day in 2 divided doses **or** one-tenth ($^1/_{10}$) of the intranasal maintenance dose **or** 0.3 mcg/kg as a single dose

Intranasal:

Infants 3-11 months: Initial: 5 mcg/day (0.05 mL/day) in 1-2 divided doses; Maintenance: 5-30 mcg/day (0.05-0.3 mL/day) in 1-2 divided doses

Children 12 months to 12 years: Initial: 5 mcg/day (0.05 mL/day) in 1-2 divided doses; Maintenance: 5-30 mcg/day (0.05-0.3 mL/day) in 1-2 divided doses **or** 150 mcg (1 spray of high concentration) as a single dose

Children >12 years and Adults <50 kg: 10-40 mcg/day (0.1-0.4 mL) in 1-3 divided doses **or** 150 mcg (1 spray of high concentration spray) as a single dose

Children >12 years and Adults ≥50 kg: 10-40 mcg/day in 1-3 divided doses **or** 300 mcg (1 spray each nostril of high concentration spray) as a single dose

Oral:

Children 4-5 years: Initial: 0.05 mg twice daily; Maintenance: 0.1-1.2 mg/day in 2-3 divided doses

Children ≥6 years: Initial: 0.05 mg twice daily **or** 0.2 mg at bedtime; Maintenance: 0.1-1.2 mg/day in 2-3 divided doses **or** 0.2-0.6 mg at bedtime

Adults: 0.2-0.6 mg at bedtime **or** 0.1-1.2 mg/day in 2-3 divided doses

SubQ: *Adults:* 2-4 mcg/day in 2 divided doses **or** one-tenth ($^1/_{10}$) of the intranasal maintenance dose

Mechanism of Action In a dose dependent manner, desmopressin increases cyclic adenosine monophosphate (cAMP) in renal tubular cells which increases water permeability resulting in decreased urine volume and increased urine osmolality; increases plasma levels of von Willebrand factor, factor VIII, and t-PA contributing to a shortened activated partial thromboplastin time (aPTT) and bleeding time.

Pharmacodynamics/Kinetics
Onset of Action
Intranasal: Antidiuretic: 15-30 minutes; Increased factor VIII and von Willebrand factor (vWF) activity (dose related): 30 minutes
Peak effect: Antidiuretic: 1 hour; Increased factor VIII and vWF activity: 1.5 hours
I.V. infusion: Increased factor VIII and vWF activity: 30 minutes (dose related)
Peak effect: 1.5-2 hours
Oral tablet: Antidiuretic: ~1 hour
Peak effect: 4-7 hours
Duration of Action Intranasal, I.V. infusion, Oral tablet: ~6-14 hours
Half-life Elimination Intranasal: ~3.5 hours; I.V. infusion: 3 hours; Oral tablet: 2-3 hours
Renal impairment: ≤9 hours
Pregnancy Risk Factor B
Pregnancy Considerations Adverse events were not observed in animal reproduction studies. There are no adequate and well-controlled studies in pregnant women. Anecdotal reports suggest congenital anomalies and low birth weight. However, causal relationship has not been established. Desmopressin has been used safely during pregnancy.

Desonide (DES oh nide)

Brand Names: U.S. Desonate®; DesOwen®; LoKara™; Verdeso®
Brand Names: Canada Desocort®; PMS-Desonide; Tridesilon; Verdeso™
Pharmacologic Category Corticosteroid, Topical
Use Treatment of inflammatory and pruritic manifestations of corticosteroid responsive dermatosis (low-to-medium potency corticosteroid); mild-to-moderate atopic dermatitis
Local Anesthetic/Vasoconstrictor Precautions No information available to require special precautions
Effects on Dental Treatment No significant effects or complications reported
Effects on Bleeding No information available to require special precautions
General Dosage Range Topical:
Children ≥3 months: Foam, gel: Apply 2 times/day sparingly
Adults: Apply 2-3 times/day sparingly
Mechanism of Action Stimulates the synthesis of enzymes needed to decrease inflammation, suppress mitotic activity, and cause vasoconstriction
Pregnancy Risk Factor C
Pregnancy Considerations Teratogenic events were not observed in rats or rabbits following topical administration of the cream in doses similar to the maximum human dose, based on body surface area. Teratogenic events have been reported following systemic use of corticosteroids.

Desoximetasone (des oks i MET a sone)

Brand Names: U.S. Topicort®
Brand Names: Canada Desoxicream; Topicort®; Topicort® Gel; Topicort® Mild; Topicort® Ointment
Generic Availability (U.S.) Yes
Pharmacologic Category Corticosteroid, Topical
Dental Use Short-term relief of inflammation of moderate-to-severe corticosteroid-responsive dermatosis (intermediate- to high-potency topical corticosteroid)
Use Relieves inflammation and pruritic symptoms of corticosteroid-responsive dermatosis
Local Anesthetic/Vasoconstrictor Precautions No information available to require special precautions
Effects on Dental Treatment No significant effects or complications reported
Effects on Bleeding No information available to require special precautions
Dosage Therapy should be discontinued when control is achieved; if no improvement is seen within 4 weeks, reassessment of diagnosis may be necessary.
Topical: Children and Adults: Apply a thin film to affected area twice daily
Mechanism of Action Desoximetasone topical corticosteroid is considered to be of intermediate- to high-potency. Corticosteroids inhibit the initial manifestations of the inflammatory process (ie, capillary dilation and edema, fibrin deposition, and migration and diapedesis of leukocytes into the inflamed site) as well as later sequelae (angiogenesis, fibroblast proliferation).
Contraindications Hypersensitivity to desoximetasone or any component of the formulation
Warnings/Precautions Systemic absorption of topical corticosteroids may cause hypercorticism or suppression of hypothalamic-pituitary-adrenal (HPA) axis, particularly in younger children or in patients receiving high doses for prolonged periods. HPA axis suppression may lead to adrenal crisis. Absorption of topical corticosteroids may cause manifestations of Cushing's syndrome, hyperglycemia, or glycosuria. Absorption is increased by the use of occlusive dressings, application to denuded skin, or application to large surface areas.

Prolonged treatment with corticosteroids has been associated with the development of Kaposi's sarcoma (case reports); discontinuation of therapy should be considered. Prolonged use may also result in fungal or bacterial superinfection; discontinue if dermatological infection persists despite appropriate antimicrobial therapy. Use appropriate antibacterial or antifungal agents to treat concomitant skin infections; discontinue desoximetasone treatment if infection does not resolve promptly. Allergic contact dermatitis can occur; it is usually diagnosed by failure to heal rather than clinical exacerbation.

Children may absorb proportionally larger amounts after topical application and may be more prone to systemic effects. HPA axis suppression, intracranial hypertension, and Cushing's syndrome have been reported in children receiving topical corticosteroids. Prolonged use may affect growth velocity; monitor growth in pediatric patients.
Drug Interactions
Metabolism/Transport Effects None known.
Avoid Concomitant Use
Avoid concomitant use of Desoximetasone with any of the following: Aldesleukin
Increased Effect/Toxicity
Desoximetasone may increase the levels/effects of: Deferasirox

The levels/effects of Desoximetasone may be increased by: Telaprevir
Decreased Effect
Desoximetasone may decrease the levels/effects of: Aldesleukin; Corticorelin; Hyaluronidase; Telaprevir
Pregnancy Risk Factor C

Pregnancy Considerations Corticosteroids were found to be teratogenic following topical application in animal reproduction studies. In general, the use of topical corticosteroids during pregnancy is not considered to have significant risk; however, intrauterine growth retardation in the infant has been reported (rare). The use of large amounts or for prolonged periods of time should be avoided (Reed, 1997).

Lactation Excretion in breast milk unknown/use caution

Breast-Feeding Considerations Systemic corticosteroids are excreted in human milk. It is not known if sufficient quantities of desoximetasone are absorbed following topical administration to produce detectable amounts in breast milk. Hypertension in the nursing infant has been reported following corticosteroid ointment applied to the nipples; use with caution (Reed, 1997).

Dosage Forms

Cream, topical: 0.05% (15 g, 60 g); 0.25% (15 g, 60 g, 100 g)

Topicort®: 0.05% (15 g, 60 g); 0.25% (15 g, 60 g)

Gel, topical: 0.05% (15 g, 60 g)

Topicort®: 0.05% (15 g, 60 g)

Ointment, topical: 0.05% (60 g); 0.25% (15 g, 60 g)

Topicort®: 0.25% (15 g, 60 g)

Desvenlafaxine (des ven la FAX een)

Related Information

Vasoconstrictor Interactions With Antidepressants *on page 1650*

Brand Names: U.S. Pristiq®

Brand Names: Canada Pristiq®

Pharmacologic Category Antidepressant, Serotonin/ Norepinephrine Reuptake Inhibitor

Use Treatment of major depressive disorder (acute and maintenance)

Local Anesthetic/Vasoconstrictor Precautions Part of the mechanism of desvenlafaxine is to block reuptake of norepinephrine along with dopamine. Because of the potential for norepinephrine elevation within CNS synapses, it is suggested that vasoconstrictor be administered with caution and to monitor vital signs in dental patients taking antidepressants that affect norepinephrine in this way. This is particularly important in patients taking desvenlafaxine, which has been noted to cause a sustained increase in blood pressure or heart rate. Dose-related increase in systolic and diastolic blood pressure have also been reported.

Effects on Dental Treatment Key adverse event(s) related to dental treatment: Significant xerostomia (normal salivary flow resumes upon discontinuation). See Effects on Bleeding.

Effects on Bleeding Platelet dysfunction (ie, impaired platelet aggregation) may occur during treatment with serotonin norepinephrine reuptake inhibitors (SNRIs), such as desvenlafaxine, due to platelet serotonin depletion, possibly increasing the risk of a bleeding complication. NSAIDs may increase this risk.

Adverse Effects Reported for 50-100 mg/day.

>10%:

Central nervous system: Dizziness (10% to 13%), insomnia (9% to 12%)

Dermatologic: Hyperhidrosis (10% to 11%)

Gastrointestinal: Nausea (22% to 26%), xerostomia (11% to 17%)

1% to 10%:

Cardiovascular: Orthostatic hypotension (elderly 8%), syncope (<2%), tachycardia (<2%), hypertension (dose related; ≤1% of patients taking 50-100 mg daily had sustained diastolic BP ≥90 mm Hg)

Central nervous system: Somnolence (≤9%), fatigue (7%), anxiety (3% to 5%), abnormal dreams (2% to 3%), vertigo (≤2%), feeling jittery (≤2%), depersonalization (<2%), seizures (<2%), attention disturbance (≤1%)

Dermatologic: Alopecia (<2%), angioedema (<2%), photosensitivity reaction (<2%), rash (<2%)

Endocrine & metabolic: Libido decreased (males 4% to 5%), cholesterol (increased by ≥50 mg/dL and ≥261 mg/dL: 3% to 4%), anorgasmia (females 1%; males ≤3%), prolactin increased (<2%), hot flushes (1%), low density lipoprotein cholesterol (increased by ≥50 mg/dL and ≥190 mg/dL: ≤1%), sexual dysfunction (males ≤1%)

Gastrointestinal: Constipation (9%), appetite decreased (5% to 8%), vomiting (≤4%), weight gain (<2%)

Genitourinary: Urinary retention (<2%), urinary hesitancy (≤1%)

Hepatic: Liver function tests abnormal (<2%)

Neuromuscular & skeletal: Tremor (≤3%), dystonia (<2%), stiffness (<2%), weakness (<2%)

Ocular: Blurred vision (3% to 4%), mydriasis (2%)

Otic: Tinnitus (≤2%)

Renal: Proteinuria (6% to 8%)

Miscellaneous: Ejaculation retarded (1% to 5%), erectile dysfunction (3% to 6%), bruxism (<2%), yawning (1%), ejaculation failure (≤1%)

General Dosage Range Dosage adjustment recommended in patients with hepatic or renal impairment

Oral: *Adults:* Initial: 50 mg once daily

Mechanism of Action Desvenlafaxine is a potent and selective serotonin and norepinephrine reuptake inhibitor.

Pharmacodynamics/Kinetics

Half-life Elimination ~10-11 hours; prolonged in renal failure and hepatic failure

Pregnancy Risk Factor C

Pregnancy Considerations Adverse events have been observed in some animal reproduction studies. Nonteratogenic effects in the newborn following SSRI/ SNRI exposure late in the third trimester include respiratory distress, cyanosis, apnea, seizures, temperature instability, feeding difficulty, vomiting, hypoglycemia, hyper- or hypotonia, hyper-reflexia, jitteriness, irritability, constant crying, and tremor. Symptoms may be due to the toxicity of the SNRIs/SSRIs or a discontinuation syndrome and may be consistent with serotonin syndrome associated with treatment. The long-term effects of *in utero* SNRI/SSRI exposure on infant development and behavior are not known.

The ACOG recommends that therapy with SSRIs or SNRIs during pregnancy be individualized; treatment of depression during pregnancy should incorporate the clinical expertise of the mental health clinician, obstetrician, primary healthcare provider, and pediatrician. According to the American Psychiatric Association (APA), the risks of medication treatment should be weighed against other treatment options and untreated depression. For women who discontinue antidepressant medications during pregnancy and who may be at high risk for postpartum depression, the medications can be restarted following delivery. Treatment algorithms have been developed by the ACOG and the APA for the management of depression in women prior to conception and during pregnancy.

Desvenlafaxine is the major active metabolite of venlafaxine; also refer to the Venlafaxine monograph.

Dexamethasone (Systemic)
(deks a METH a sone)

Related Information
Respiratory Diseases *on page 1514*
Ulcerative, Erosive, and Painful Oral Mucosal Disorders *on page 1578*
Related Sample Prescriptions
Erosive Lichen Planus, Other Biopsy-Proven Desquamative Oral Diseases, and Major Aphthae *on page 1618*
Mild Lichen Planus *on page 1618*
Recurrent Aphthous Stomatitis *on page 1618*
Brand Names: U.S. Baycadron™; Dexamethasone Intensol™; DexPak® 10 Day TaperPak®; DexPak® 13 Day TaperPak®; DexPak® 6 Day TaperPak®
Brand Names: Canada Apo-Dexamethasone®; Dexasone®; Dom-Dexamethasone; PHL-Dexamethasone; PMS-Dexamethasone; PRO-Dexamethasone; ratio-Dexamethasone
Generic Availability (U.S.) Yes: Excludes concentrated oral solution
Pharmacologic Category Anti-inflammatory Agent; Antiemetic; Corticosteroid, Systemic
Dental Use Treatment of a variety of oral diseases of allergic, inflammatory or autoimmune origin; aphthous stomatitis (systemic dexamethasone used topically); lichen planus (erosive) and other oral vesiculoerosive diseases
Use Primarily as an anti-inflammatory or immunosuppressant agent in the treatment of a variety of diseases including those of allergic, dermatologic, endocrine, hematologic, inflammatory, neoplastic, nervous system, renal, respiratory, rheumatic, and autoimmune origin; may be used in management of cerebral edema, chronic swelling, as a diagnostic agent, diagnosis of Cushing's syndrome, antiemetic
Unlabeled Use Dexamethasone suppression test as an indicator of depression and/or risk of suicide; prevention and treatment of acute mountain sickness and high altitude cerebral edema; accelerate fetal lung maturation in patients with preterm labor
Local Anesthetic/Vasoconstrictor Precautions No information available to require special precautions
Effects on Dental Treatment No significant effects or complications reported
Effects on Bleeding No information available to require special precautions
Adverse Effects Frequency not defined.
Cardiovascular: Arrhythmia, bradycardia, cardiac arrest, cardiomyopathy, CHF, circulatory collapse, edema, hypertension, myocardial rupture (post-MI), syncope, thromboembolism, vasculitis
Central nervous system: Depression, emotional instability, euphoria, headache, intracranial pressure increased, insomnia, malaise, mood swings, neuritis, personality changes, pseudotumor cerebri (usually following discontinuation), psychic disorders, seizure, vertigo
Dermatologic: Acne, allergic dermatitis, alopecia, angioedema, bruising, dry skin, erythema, fragile skin, hirsutism, hyper-/hypopigmentation, hypertrichosis, perianal pruritus (following I.V. injection), petechiae,

rash, skin atrophy, skin test reaction impaired, striae, urticaria, wound healing impaired
Endocrine & metabolic: Adrenal suppression, carbohydrate tolerance decreased, Cushing's syndrome, diabetes mellitus, glucose intolerance decreased, growth suppression (children), hyperglycemia, hypokalemic alkalosis, menstrual irregularities, negative nitrogen balance, pituitary-adrenal axis suppression, protein catabolism, sodium retention
Gastrointestinal: Abdominal distention, appetite increased, gastrointestinal hemorrhage, gastrointestinal perforation, nausea, pancreatitis, peptic ulcer, ulcerative esophagitis, weight gain
Genitourinary: Altered (increased or decreased) spermatogenesis
Hepatic: Hepatomegaly, transaminases increased
Local: Postinjection flare (intra-articular use), thrombophlebitis
Neuromuscular & skeletal: Arthropathy, aseptic necrosis (femoral and humoral heads), fractures, muscle mass loss, myopathy (particularly in conjunction with neuromuscular disease or neuromuscular-blocking agents), neuropathy, osteoporosis, parasthesia, tendon rupture, vertebral compression fractures, weakness
Ocular: Cataracts, exophthalmos, glaucoma, intraocular pressure increased
Renal: Glucosuria
Respiratory: Pulmonary edema
Miscellaneous: Abnormal fat deposition, anaphylactoid reaction, anaphylaxis, avascular necrosis, diaphoresis, hiccups, hypersensitivity, impaired wound healing, infections, Kaposi's sarcoma, moon face, secondary malignancy
Dental Usual Dosage
Erosive lichen planus and major aphthae: Oral: For 3 days, rinse with 15 mL 4 times/day and swallow; then for 3 days, rinse with 5 mL 4 times/day and swallow; then for 3 days, rinse with 5 mL 4 times/day and swallow every other time. Then for 3 days rinse with 5 mL 4 times/day and expectorate. Continue the rinse and expectorate mode for 2 minutes, but discontinue medication when mouth becomes completely comfortable.
Recurrent aphthous stomatitis: Rinse with 5 mL for 2 minutes 4 times/day and expectorate
Dosage Refer to individual protocols.
Children:
Antiemetic (prior to chemotherapy): Refer to individual protocols and emetogenic potential: I.V.: 10 mg/m^2/dose every 12-24 hours on days of chemotherapy for severely emetogenic chemotherapy courses
Anti-inflammatory immunosuppressant: Oral, I.M., I.V.: 0.08-0.3 mg/kg/day **or** 2.5-10 mg/m^2/day in divided doses every 6-12 hours
Extubation or airway edema: Oral, I.M., I.V.: 0.5-2 mg/kg/day in divided doses every 6 hours beginning 24 hours prior to extubation and continuing for 4-6 doses afterwards
Cerebral edema: I.V.: Loading dose: 1-2 mg/kg/dose as a single dose; maintenance: 1-1.5 mg/kg/day (maximum: 16 mg/day) in divided doses every 4-6 hours, taper off over 1-6 weeks
Croup (laryngotracheobronchitis): Oral, I.M., I.V.: 0.6 mg/kg once; usual maximum dose: 16 mg (doses as high as 20 mg have been used) (Bjornson, 2004; Hegenbarth, 2008; Rittichier, 2000); a single oral dose of 0.15 mg/kg has been shown effective in children with mild-to-moderate croup (Russell, 2004; Sparrow, 2006)

Bacterial meningitis: Infants and Children >6 weeks: I.V.: 0.15 mg/kg/dose every 6 hours for the first 2-4 days of antibiotic treatment; start dexamethasone 10-20 minutes before or with the first dose of antibiotic

Physiologic replacement: Oral, I.M., I.V.: 0.03-0.15 mg/kg/day **or** 0.6-0.75 mg/m²/day in divided doses every 6-12 hours

Acute mountain sickness (AMS)/high altitude cerebral edema (HACE) (unlabeled use): Oral, I.M., I.V.: 0.15 mg/kg/dose every 6 hours; consider using for high altitude pulmonary edema because of associated HACE with this condition (Luks, 2010; Pollard, 2001)

Adults:

Antiemetic:

Prophylaxis: Oral, I.V.: 10-20 mg 15-30 minutes before treatment on each treatment day

Continuous infusion regimen: Oral or I.V.: 10 mg every 12 hours on each treatment day

Mildly emetogenic therapy: Oral, I.M., I.V.: 4 mg every 4-6 hours

Delayed nausea/vomiting: Oral: 4-10 mg 1-2 times/ day for 2-4 days **or**

8 mg every 12 hours for 2 days; then

4 mg every 12 hours for 2 days **or**

20 mg 1 hour before chemotherapy; then

10 mg 12 hours after chemotherapy; then

8 mg every 12 hours for 4 doses; then

4 mg every 12 hours for 4 doses

Anti-inflammatory:

Oral, I.M., I.V. (injections should be given as sodium phosphate): 0.75-9 mg/day in divided doses every 6-12 hours

Intra-articular, intralesional, or soft tissue (as sodium phosphate): 0.4-6 mg/day

Multiple myeloma: Oral, I.V.: 40 mg/day, days 1 to 4, 9 to 12, and 17 to 20, repeated every 4 weeks (alone or as part of a regimen)

Cerebral edema: I.V. 10 mg stat, 4 mg I.M./I.V. every 6 hours until response is maximized, then switch to oral regimen, then taper off if appropriate; dosage may be reduced after 2-4 days and gradually discontinued over 5-7 days

Extubation or airway edema: Oral, I.M., I.V. (injections should be given as sodium phosphate): 0.5-2 mg/kg/ day in divided doses every 6 hours beginning 24 hours prior to extubation and continuing for 4-6 doses afterwards

Dexamethasone suppression test (depression/suicide indicator) (unlabeled use): Oral: 1 mg at 11 PM, draw blood at 8 AM the following day for plasma cortisol determination

Cushing's syndrome, diagnostic: Oral: 1 mg at 11 PM, draw blood at 8 AM; greater accuracy for Cushing's syndrome may be achieved by the following:

Dexamethasone 0.5 mg by mouth every 6 hours for 48 hours (with 24-hour urine collection for 17-hydroxycorticosteroid excretion)

Differentiation of Cushing's syndrome due to ACTH excess from Cushing's due to other causes: Oral: Dexamethasone 2 mg every 6 hours for 48 hours (with 24-hour urine collection for 17-hydroxycorticosteroid excretion)

Multiple sclerosis (acute exacerbation): 30 mg/day for 1 week, followed by 4-12 mg/day for 1 month

Physiological replacement: Oral, I.M., I.V. (should be given as sodium phosphate): 0.03-0.15 mg/kg/day **or** 0.6-0.75 mg/m²/day in divided doses every 6-12 hours

Treatment of shock:

Addisonian crisis/shock (ie, adrenal insufficiency/ responsive to steroid therapy): I.V. (given as sodium phosphate): 4-10 mg as a single dose, which may be repeated if necessary

Unresponsive shock (ie, unresponsive to steroid therapy): I.V. (given as sodium phosphate): 1-6 mg/kg as a single I.V. dose or up to 40 mg initially followed by repeat doses every 2-6 hours while shock persists

Acute mountain sickness (AMS)/high altitude cerebral edema (HACE) (unlabeled use):

Prevention: Oral: 2 mg every 6 hours **or** 4 mg every 12 hours starting on the day of ascent; may be discontinued after staying at the same elevation for 2-3 days or if descent is initiated; do not exceed a 10 day duration (Luks, 2010). **Note:** In situations of rapid ascent to altitudes >3500 meters (such as rescue or military operations), 4 mg every 6 hours may be considered (Luks, 2010).

Treatment: Oral, I.M., I.V.:

AMS: 4 mg every 6 hours (Luks, 2010)

HACE: Initial: 8 mg as a single dose; Maintenance: 4 mg every 6 hours until symptoms resolve (Luks, 2010)

Dosage adjustment in renal impairment: No dosage adjustment provided in manufacturer's labeling; use with caution.

Hemodialysis: Supplemental dose is not necessary

Peritoneal dialysis: Supplemental dose is not necessary

Dosage adjustment in hepatic impairment: No dosage adjustment provided in manufacturer's labeling.

Mechanism of Action Decreases inflammation by suppression of neutrophil migration, decreased production of inflammatory mediators, and reversal of increased capillary permeability; suppresses normal immune response. Dexamethasone's mechanism of antiemetic activity is unknown.

Contraindications Hypersensitivity to dexamethasone or any component of the formulation; systemic fungal infections, cerebral malaria

Warnings/Precautions Use with caution in patients with thyroid disease, hepatic impairment, renal impairment, cardiovascular disease, diabetes, glaucoma, cataracts, myasthenia gravis, patients at risk for osteoporosis, patients at risk for seizures, or GI diseases (diverticulitis, peptic ulcer, ulcerative colitis) due to perforation risk. Use caution following acute MI (corticosteroids have been associated with myocardial rupture). Because of the risk of adverse effects, systemic corticosteroids should be used cautiously in the elderly in the smallest possible effective dose for the shortest duration. May affect growth velocity; growth should be routinely monitored in pediatric patients. Withdraw therapy with gradual tapering of dose.

May cause hypercorticism or suppression of hypothalamic-pituitary-adrenal (HPA) axis, particularly in younger children or in patients receiving high doses for prolonged periods. HPA axis suppression may lead to adrenal crisis. Withdrawal and discontinuation of a corticosteroid should be done slowly and carefully. Particular care is required when patients are transferred from systemic corticosteroids to inhaled products due to possible adrenal insufficiency or withdrawal from steroids, including an increase in allergic symptoms. Patients receiving >20 mg per day of prednisone (or equivalent) may be most susceptible. Fatalities have occurred due to adrenal insufficiency in asthmatic patients during and after transfer from systemic corticosteroids to aerosol steroids; aerosol steroids do not provide the systemic steroid needed to treat patients having trauma, surgery, or infections. Dexamethasone does not provide adequate mineralocorticoid activity in adrenal insufficiency (may be employed as a single dose while cortisol assays are performed). The lowest possible dose should be used during treatment; discontinuation and/or dose reductions should be gradual.

Acute myopathy has been reported with high dose corticosteroids, usually in patients with neuromuscular transmission disorders; may involve ocular and/or respiratory muscles; monitor creatine kinase; recovery may be delayed. Corticosteroid use may cause psychiatric disturbances, including depression, euphoria, insomnia, mood swings, and personality changes. Pre-existing psychiatric conditions may be exacerbated by corticosteroid use. Prolonged use of corticosteroids may also increase the incidence of secondary infection, mask acute infection (including fungal infections), prolong or exacerbate viral infections, or limit response to vaccines. Exposure to chickenpox should be avoided; corticosteroids should not be used to treat ocular herpes simplex. Corticosteroids should not be used for cerebral malaria or viral hepatitis. Close observation is required in patients with latent tuberculosis and/or TB reactivity; restrict use in active TB (only in conjunction with anti-tuberculosis treatment). Prolonged treatment with corticosteroids has been associated with the development of Kaposi's sarcoma (case reports); if noted, discontinuation of therapy should be considered. High-dose corticosteroids should not be used to manage acute head injury.

Drug Interactions

Metabolism/Transport Effects Substrate of CYP3A4 (major), P-glycoprotein; **Note:** Assignment of Major/Minor substrate status based on clinically relevant drug interaction potential; **Inhibits** P-glycoprotein; **Induces** CYP2A6 (weak/moderate), CYP2B6 (weak/moderate), CYP2C9 (weak/moderate), CYP3A4 (strong), P-glycoprotein

Avoid Concomitant Use

Avoid concomitant use of Dexamethasone (Systemic) with any of the following: Aldesleukin; Apixaban; Axitinib; BCG; Bedaquiline; Bosutinib; Cabozantinib; Conivaptan; Crizotinib; Dabigatran Etexilate; Dronedarone; Enzalutamide; Everolimus; Ivacaftor; Lapatinib; Lurasidone; Mifepristone; Natalizumab; Nilotinib; Nisoldipine; Pazopanib; Perampanel; Pimecrolimus; Pomalidomide; Ponatinib; Praziquantel; Ranolazine; Regorafenib; Rilpivirine; Rivaroxaban; RomiDEPsin; SORAfenib; Tacrolimus (Topical); Ticagrelor; Tofacitinib; Tolvaptan; Toremifene; Vandetanib; VinCRIStine (Liposomal)

Increased Effect/Toxicity

Dexamethasone (Systemic) may increase the levels/ effects of: Acetylcholinesterase Inhibitors; Amphotericin B; CycloSPORINE (Systemic); Deferasirox; Ifosfamide; Leflunomide; Lenalidomide; Loop Diuretics; Natalizumab; NSAID (COX-2 Inhibitor); NSAID (Nonselective); Thalidomide; Thiazide Diuretics; Tofacitinib; Vaccines (Live); Warfarin

The levels/effects of Dexamethasone (Systemic) may be increased by: Antifungal Agents (Azole Derivatives, Systemic); Aprepitant; Asparaginase (E. coli); Asparaginase (Erwinia); Calcium Channel Blockers (Nondihydropyridine); Conivaptan; CycloSPORINE (Systemic); CYP3A4 Inhibitors (Moderate); CYP3A4 Inhibitors (Strong); Dasatinib; Denosumab; Estrogen Derivatives; Fluconazole; Fosaprepitant; Indacaterol; Ivacaftor; Macrolide Antibiotics; Mifepristone;

Neuromuscular-Blocking Agents (Nondepolarizing); P-glycoprotein/ABCB1 Inhibitors; Pimecrolimus; Quinolone Antibiotics; Roflumilast; Salicylates; Tacrolimus (Topical); Telaprevir; Trastuzumab

Decreased Effect

Dexamethasone (Systemic) may decrease the levels/ effects of: Aldesleukin; Antidiabetic Agents; Apixaban; ARIPiprazole; Axitinib; BCG; Bedaquiline; Boceprevir; Bosutinib; Brentuximab Vedotin; Cabozantinib; Calcitriol; Caspofungin; Cobicistat; Coccidioidin Skin Test; Corticorelin; Crizotinib; CycloSPORINE (Systemic); CYP3A4 Substrates; Dabigatran Etexilate; Dasatinib; Dronedarone; Elvitegravir; Enzalutamide; Everolimus; Exemestane; Gefitinib; GuanFACINE; Hyaluronidase; Imatinib; Isoniazid; Ivacaftor; Ixabepilone; Lapatinib; Lurasidone; Maraviroc; NIFEdipine; Nilotinib; Nisoldipine; Pazopanib; Perampanel; P-glycoprotein/ABCB1 Substrates; Pomalidomide; Ponatinib; Praziquantel; Ranolazine; Regorafenib; Rilpivirine; Rivaroxaban; RomiDEPsin; Salicylates; Sipuleucel-T; SORAfenib; SUNItinib; Tadalafil; Telaprevir; Ticagrelor; Tolvaptan; Toremifene; Uliprisal; Vaccines (Inactivated); Vandetanib; Vemurafenib; VinCRIStine (Liposomal); Zuclopenthixol

The levels/effects of Dexamethasone (Systemic) may be decreased by: Aminoglutethimide; Antacids; Barbiturates; Bile Acid Sequestrants; CYP3A4 Inducers (Strong); Echinacea; Herbs (CYP3A4 Inducers); Mifepristone; Mitotane; P-glycoprotein/ABCB1 Inducers; Primidone; Rifamycin Derivatives; Tocilizumab

Ethanol/Nutrition/Herb Interactions

Ethanol: Avoid ethanol (may enhance gastric mucosal irritation).

Food: Dexamethasone interferes with calcium absorption. Limit caffeine.

Herb/Nutraceutical: Avoid cat's claw, echinacea (have immunostimulant properties).

Dietary Considerations May be taken with meals to decrease GI upset. May need diet with increased potassium, pyridoxine, vitamin C, vitamin D, folate, calcium, and phosphorus.

Pharmacodynamics/Kinetics

Onset of Action Acetate: Prompt

Duration of Action Metabolic effect: 72 hours; acetate is a long-acting repository preparation

Half-life Elimination Normal renal function: 1.8-3.5 hours; Biological half-life: 36-54 hours

Time to Peak Serum: Oral: 1-2 hours; I.M.: ~8 hours

Pregnancy Risk Factor C

Pregnancy Considerations Adverse events have been observed with corticosteroids in animal reproduction studies. Dexamethasone crosses the placenta; and is partially metabolized to an inactive metabolite by placental enzymes. Due to its positive effect on stimulating fetal lung maturation, the injection is often used in patients with premature labor (24-34 weeks gestation). Some studies have shown an association between first trimester systemic corticosteroid use and oral clefts; adverse events in the fetus/neonate have been noted in case reports following large doses of systemic corticosteroids during pregnancy. Women exposed to dexamethasone during pregnancy for the treatment of an autoimmune disease may contact the OTIS Autoimmune Diseases Study at 877-311-8972.

Lactation Excretion in breast milk unknown/use caution

Breast-Feeding Considerations Corticosteroids are excreted in human milk; information specific to dexamethasone has not been located.

Dosage Forms
Elixir, oral: 0.5 mg/5 mL (237 mL)
Baycadron™: 0.5 mg/5 mL (237 mL)
Injection, solution: 4 mg/mL (1 mL, 5 mL, 30 mL); 10 mg/mL (1 mL, 10 mL)
Injection, solution [preservative free]: 10 mg/mL (1 mL)
Solution, oral: 0.5 mg/5 mL (240 mL, 500 mL)
Dexamethasone Intensol™: 1 mg/mL (30 mL)
Tablet, oral: 0.5 mg, 0.75 mg, 1 mg, 1.5 mg, 2 mg, 4 mg, 6 mg
DexPak® 6 Day TaperPak®: 1.5 mg
DexPak® 10 Day TaperPak®: 1.5 mg
DexPak® 13 Day TaperPak®: 1.5 mg

Dexchlorpheniramine (deks klor fen EER a meen)

Pharmacologic Category Alkylamine Derivative; Histamine H_1 Antagonist; Histamine H_1 Antagonist, First Generation
Use Perennial and seasonal allergic rhinitis and other allergic symptoms including urticaria
Local Anesthetic/Vasoconstrictor Precautions No information available to require special precautions
Effects on Dental Treatment Key adverse event(s) related to dental treatment: Significant xerostomia (normal salivary flow resumes upon discontinuation)
Effects on Bleeding No information available to require special precautions
Adverse Effects
>10%:
Central nervous system: Slight to moderate drowsiness
Respiratory: Thickening of bronchial secretions
1% to 10%:
Central nervous system: Headache, fatigue, nervousness, dizziness
Gastrointestinal: Appetite increase, weight gain, nausea, diarrhea, abdominal pain, xerostomia
Neuromuscular & skeletal: Arthralgia
Respiratory: Pharyngitis
General Dosage Range Oral:
Regular release:
Children 2-5 years: 0.5 mg every 4-6 hours
Children 6-11 years: 1 mg every 4-6 hours
Adults: 2 mg every 4-6 hours
Timed release:
Children 6-11 years: 4 mg at bedtime
Adults: 4-6 mg at bedtime **or** every 8-10 hours
Mechanism of Action Competes with histamine for H_1-receptor sites on effector cells in the gastrointestinal tract, blood vessels, and respiratory tract. Dexchlorpheniramine is the predominant active isomer of chlorpheniramine and is approximately twice as active as the racemic compound.
Pharmacodynamics/Kinetics
Half-life Elimination 20-30 hours (Moreno, 2010)
Time to Peak ~3 hours (Moreno, 2010)
Pregnancy Considerations Maternal antihistamine use has generally not resulted in an increased risk of birth defects; however, information specific to dexchlorpheniramine is limited. Dexchlorpheniramine is the *dextro*-isomer of chlorpheniramine; also refer to the chlorpheniramine monograph. Antihistamines are recommended for the treatment of rhinitis, urticaria, and pruritus with rash in pregnant women (although second generation antihistamines may be preferred). Antihistamines are not recommended for treatment of pruritus associated with intrahepatic cholestasis in pregnancy.

Dexlansoprazole (deks lan SOE pra zole)

Related Information
Gastrointestinal Disorders *on page 1512*
Brand Names: U.S. Dexilant™
Brand Names: Canada Dexilant™
Pharmacologic Category Proton Pump Inhibitor; Substituted Benzimidazole
Use Short-term (4 weeks) treatment of heartburn associated with nonerosive GERD; short-term (up to 8 weeks) treatment of all grades of erosive esophagitis (EE); to maintain healing of erosive esophagitis and relief of heartburn for up to 6 months
Local Anesthetic/Vasoconstrictor Precautions No information available to require special precautions
Effects on Dental Treatment Key adverse event(s) related to dental treatment: Xerostomia (normal salivary flow resumes upon discontinuation) and taste alteration has been reported in <2% of patients.
Effects on Bleeding No information available to require special precautions
Adverse Effects 2% to 10%:
Gastrointestinal: Diarrhea (5%), abdominal pain (4%), nausea (3%), flatulence (1% to 3%), vomiting (1% to 2%)
Respiratory: Upper respiratory tract infection (2% to 3%)
General Dosage Range Dosage adjustment recommended in patients with hepatic impairment
Oral: *Adults:* 30-60 mg once daily
Mechanism of Action Proton pump inhibitor; decreases acid secretion in gastric parietal cells through inhibition of (H+, K+)-ATPase enzyme system, blocking the final step in gastric acid production
Pharmacodynamics/Kinetics
Half-life Elimination ~1-2 hours
Time to Peak Serum: **Note:** Two distinct peaks secondary to dual release formulation:
Peak 1: 1-2 hours
Peak 2: 4-5 hours
Pregnancy Risk Factor B
Pregnancy Considerations Animal studies have not shown teratogenic effects to the fetus. However, there are no adequate and well-controlled studies in pregnant women; use during pregnancy only if clearly needed.

Dexmedetomidine (deks MED e toe mi deen)

Brand Names: U.S. Precedex®
Brand Names: Canada Precedex®
Pharmacologic Category Alpha$_2$-Adrenergic Agonist; Sedative
Use Sedation of initially intubated and mechanically ventilated patients during treatment in an intensive care setting; sedation prior to and/or during surgical or other procedures of nonintubated patients
Unlabeled Use Unlabeled uses include premedication prior to anesthesia induction with thiopental; relief of pain and reduction of opioid dose following laparoscopic tubal ligation; as an adjunct anesthetic in ophthalmic surgery; treatment of shivering; premedication to attenuate the cardiostimulatory and postanesthetic delirium of ketamine; use in children
Local Anesthetic/Vasoconstrictor Precautions No information available to require special precautions
Effects on Dental Treatment Key adverse event(s) related to dental treatment: Xerostomia and changes in salivation (normal salivary flow resumes upon discontinuation)

Effects on Bleeding No information available to require special precautions

Adverse Effects

>10%:
Cardiovascular: Hypotension (24% to 54%), bradycardia (5% to 14%)
Respiratory: Respiratory depression (37%; placebo 32%)

1% to 10%:
Cardiovascular: Atrial fibrillation (4% to 5%), hypovolemia (3%)
Endocrine & metabolic: Hypocalcemia (1%)
Gastrointestinal: Nausea (3% to 9%), xerostomia (3% to 4%)
Renal: Urine output decreased (1%)
Respiratory: Pleural effusion (2%), wheezing (≤1%)

General Dosage Range I.V.: *Adults:* Loading infusion: 0.5-1 mcg/kg; Maintenance infusion: 0.2-1 mcg/kg/**hour**

Mechanism of Action Selective alpha₂-adrenoceptor agonist with anesthetic and sedative properties thought to be due to activation of G-proteins by alpha₂ₐ-adrenoceptors in the brainstem resulting in inhibition of norepinephrine release; peripheral alpha₂ᵦ-adrenoceptors are activated at high doses or with rapid I.V. administration resulting in vasoconstriction.

Pharmacodynamics/Kinetics

Onset of Action I.V. Bolus: 5-10 minutes; Peak effect: 15-30 minutes

Duration of Action Dose dependent: 60-120 minutes

Half-life Elimination Distribution: ~6 minutes; Terminal: ~up to 3 hours (Venn, 2002); significantly prolonged in patients with severe hepatic impairment (Cunningham, 1999)

Pregnancy Risk Factor C

Pregnancy Considerations Teratogenic effects were not observed in animal studies. There are no adequate and well-controlled studies in pregnant women.

Dexmethylphenidate (dex meth il FEN i date)

Brand Names: U.S. Focalin XR®; Focalin®

Pharmacologic Category Central Nervous System Stimulant

Use Treatment of attention-deficit/hyperactivity disorder (ADHD)

Local Anesthetic/Vasoconstrictor Precautions No information available to require special precautions

Effects on Dental Treatment Key adverse event(s) related to dental treatment: Xerostomia (normal salivary flow resumes upon discontinuation).

Effects on Bleeding No information available to require special precautions

Adverse Effects Actual frequency may be dependent upon dose and/or formulation.

>10%:
Central nervous system: Headache (25% to 39%), insomnia (children 5% to 17%), restlessness (adults 12%), anxiety (5% to 11%)
Gastrointestinal: Appetite decreased (children 30%), xerostomia (adults 7% to 20%), abdominal pain (children 15%)

1% to 10%:
Central nervous system: Dizziness (adults 6%), fever (children 5%), irritability (children ≤5%), depression (children ≤3%), mood swings (children ≤3%)
Dermatologic: Pruritus (children ≤3%)

Gastrointestinal: Nausea (children 9%), dyspepsia (5% to 9%), vomiting (children 2% to 9%), anorexia (children 5% to 7%), pharyngolaryngeal pain (adults 4% to 7%)
Respiratory: Nasal congestion (children ≤5%)
Also refer to Methylphenidate for adverse effects seen with other methylphenidate products.

General Dosage Range Oral:

Extended release:
Children ≥6 years: Initial: 5 mg once daily; Maintenance: Up to 30 mg/day
Adults: Initial: 10 mg once daily; Maintenance: Up to 40 mg/day

Immediate release: *Children ≥6 years and Adults:* Initial: 2.5 mg twice daily; Maintenance: Up to 20 mg/day in 2 divided doses (at least 4 hours apart)

Mechanism of Action Dexmethylphenidate is the more active, *d-threo*-enantiomer of racemic methylphenidate. It is a CNS stimulant; blocks the reuptake of norepinephrine and dopamine, and increases their release into the extraneuronal space.

Pharmacodynamics/Kinetics

Onset of Action Extended release: ≥0.5 hours

Duration of Action Extended release: 12 hours

Half-life Elimination Immediate release: Adults: 2-4.5 hours; children: 2-3 hours

Time to Peak Fasting:
Immediate release: 1-1.5 hours
Extended release: First peak: 1.5 hours (range: 1-4 hours); Second peak: 6.5 hours (range: 4.5-7 hours)

Pregnancy Risk Factor C

Pregnancy Considerations Teratogenic effects were noted in animal studies. There are no adequate and well-controlled studies in pregnant women. Use only if the potential benefit to the mother outweighs the possible risks to the fetus.

Controlled Substance C-II

Dexpanthenol (deks PAN the nole)

Pharmacologic Category Gastrointestinal Agent, Stimulant; Topical Skin Product

Use Prophylactic use to minimize paralytic ileus; treatment of postoperative distention; topical to relieve itching and to aid healing of minor dermatoses

Local Anesthetic/Vasoconstrictor Precautions No information available to require special precautions

Effects on Dental Treatment No significant effects or complications reported

Effects on Bleeding No information available to require special precautions

Adverse Effects Frequency not defined.
Cardiovascular: Slight drop in blood pressure
Central nervous system: Agitation
Dermatologic: Dermatitis, irritation, itching, urticaria
Gastrointestinal: Diarrhea, hyperperistalsis, vomiting
Neuromuscular & skeletal: Paresthesia
Respiratory: Dyspnea
Miscellaneous: Allergic reactions

General Dosage Range I.M.: *Adults:* Initial: 250-500 mg; repeat in 2 hours, followed by doses every 6 hours if needed

Mechanism of Action A pantothenic acid B vitamin analog that is converted to coenzyme A internally; coenzyme A is essential to normal fatty acid synthesis, amino acid synthesis and acetylation of choline in the production of the neurotransmitter, acetylcholine

Pregnancy Risk Factor C

Pregnancy Considerations There are no adequate and well-controlled studies in pregnant women; use only if possible benefit outweighs potential risk to the fetus

Dexrazoxane (deks ray ZOKS ane)

Brand Names: U.S. Totect®; Zinecard®
Brand Names: Canada Zinecard®
Pharmacologic Category Antidote; Cardioprotectant
Use
Zinecard®: Reduction of the incidence and severity of cardiomyopathy associated with doxorubicin administration in women with metastatic breast cancer who have received a cumulative doxorubicin dose of 300 mg/m² and who would benefit from continuing therapy with doxorubicin. (Not recommended for use with initial doxorubicin therapy.)
Totect®: Treatment of anthracycline-induced extravasation.

Unlabeled Use Reduction of the incidence and severity of cardiomyopathy associated with doxorubicin administration (cumulative doses >300 mg/m²) in patients with malignancies other than metastatic breast cancer who would benefit from continuing therapy with doxorubicin; reduction of the incidence and severity of cardiomyopathy associated with continued epirubicin administration for advanced breast cancer; prevention of doxorubicin cardiomyopathy associated with acute lymphoblastic leukemia treatment in children

Local Anesthetic/Vasoconstrictor Precautions No information available to require special precautions

Effects on Dental Treatment No significant effects or complications reported

Effects on Bleeding Thrombocytopenia has been reported in patients who are under active treatment with dexrazoxane. A medical consult is suggested.

Adverse Effects Note: Most adverse reactions are thought to be attributed to chemotherapy, except for increased myelosuppression, pain at injection site, and phlebitis.

Prevention of doxorubicin cardiomyopathy (reactions listed are those which were greater in the dexrazoxane arm in a comparison of chemotherapy plus dexrazoxane vs chemotherapy alone):
Central nervous system: Fatigue/malaise, fever
Dermatologic: Alopecia, streaking/erythema
Gastrointestinal: Serum amylase increased
Hematologic: Granulocytopenia, leukopenia, myelosuppression, thrombocytopenia
Local: Extravasation, injection site pain, phlebitis
Neuromuscular & skeletal: Neurotoxicity
Miscellaneous: Infection, sepsis

Anthracycline extravasation:
Cardiovascular: Peripheral edema
Central nervous system: Depression, dizziness, fatigue, fever, headache, insomnia
Dermatologic: Alopecia
Endocrine & metabolic: Hypercalcemia, hyponatremia
Gastrointestinal: Abdominal pain, anorexia, constipation, diarrhea, nausea, vomiting
Hematologic: Anemia, leukopenia, neutropenia, neutropenic fever, thrombocytopenia
Hepatic: Alkaline phosphatase increased, ALT increased, AST increased, bilirubin increased, LDH increased

Local: Injection site pain/discomfort, phlebitis
Renal: Creatinine increased
Respiratory: Cough, dyspnea, pneumonia
Miscellaneous: Infection

General Dosage Range Dosage adjustment recommended in patients with renal impairment and hepatic impairment
I.V.: *Adults:* A 10:1 ratio of dexrazoxane:doxorubicin (dexrazoxane 500 mg/m²:doxorubicin 50 mg/m²) (prevention of cardiomyopathy) **or** 1000 mg/m² on days 1 and 2 (maximum dose: 2000 mg), followed by 500 mg/m² on day 3 (maximum dose: 1000 mg) (anthracycline-induced extravasation)

Mechanism of Action Derivative of ethylenediaminetetraacetic acid (EDTA); potent intracellular chelating agent. The mechanism of cardioprotectant activity is not fully understood. Appears to be converted intracellularly to a ring-opened chelating agent that interferes with iron-mediated oxygen free radical generation thought to be responsible, in part, for anthracycline-induced cardiomyopathy. In the management of anthracycline-induced extravasation, dexrazoxane may act by reversibly inhibiting topoisomerase II, protecting tissue from anthracycline cytotoxicity, thereby decreasing tissue damage.

Pharmacodynamics/Kinetics
Half-life Elimination 2-2.5 hours
Pregnancy Risk Factor D
Pregnancy Considerations Adverse events were observed in animal reproduction studies using doses less than the equivalent human dose (based on BSA).

Dextran (DEKS tran)

Brand Names: U.S. LMD®
Pharmacologic Category Plasma Volume Expander, Colloid
Use Blood volume expander used in treatment of shock or impending shock when blood or blood products are not available; also used as a priming fluid in pump oxygenators during cardiopulmonary bypass and for prophylaxis of venous thrombosis and pulmonary embolism in surgical procedures associated with a high risk of thromboembolic complications

Local Anesthetic/Vasoconstrictor Precautions No information available to require special precautions

Effects on Dental Treatment No significant effects or complications reported

Effects on Bleeding No information available to require special precautions

Adverse Effects Frequency not defined.
Cardiovascular: Cardiac arrest, hypotension, tightness of chest
Dermatologic: Urticaria
Gastrointestinal: Nausea, vomiting
Hematologic (all dose related): Bleeding time (prolonged), wound bleeding, wound hematoma
Hepatic: Liver function tests (abnormal)
Renal: Acute renal failure
Respiratory: Pulmonary edema (dose related), wheezing
Miscellaneous: Anaphylactoid reaction

General Dosage Range I.V.:
Dextran 40:
Children: Infuse 10 mL/kg as rapidly as possible (maximum: 20 mL/kg/day for the first 24 hours; 10 mL/kg/day thereafter); therapy should not be continued beyond 5 days

Adults: Infuse 500-1000 mL (~10 mL/kg) as rapidly as possible (maximum: 20 mL/kg/day for first 24 hours; 10 mL/kg/day thereafter); (5 days total therapy) **or** 50-100 g on the day of surgery, then 50 g (4 mL/minute) every 2-3 days during the period of risk

Mechanism of Action Produces plasma volume expansion by virtue of its highly colloidal starch structure.

Pharmacodynamics/Kinetics

Duration of Action Plasma expanding effect lasts 3-4 hours

Pregnancy Risk Factor C

Pregnancy Considerations Animal reproduction studies have not been conducted.

Dextroamphetamine (deks troe am FET a meen)

Brand Names: U.S. Dexedrine® Spansule®; ProCentra®

Brand Names: Canada Dexedrine®

Pharmacologic Category Central Nervous System Stimulant

Use Narcolepsy; attention-deficit/hyperactivity disorder (ADHD)

Local Anesthetic/Vasoconstrictor Precautions Use vasoconstrictor with caution in patients taking dextroamphetamine. Amphetamines enhance the sympathomimetic response of epinephrine and norepinephrine leading to potential hypertension and cardiotoxicity.

Effects on Dental Treatment Key adverse event(s) related to dental treatment: Xerostomia (normal salivary flow resumes upon discontinuation). Up to 10% of patients taking dextroamphetamines may present with hypertension. Monitor blood pressure prior to using local anesthetic with vasoconstrictors.

Effects on Bleeding No information available to require special precautions

Adverse Effects Frequency not defined.

Cardiovascular: Cardiomyopathy, hypertension, palpitation, tachycardia

Central nervous system: Aggression, dizziness, dyskinesia, dysphoria, euphoria, exacerbation of motor and phonic tics, headache, insomnia, mania, overstimulation, psychosis, restlessness, Tourette's syndrome

Dermatologic: Urticaria

Endocrine & metabolic: Libido changes

Gastrointestinal: Anorexia, constipation, diarrhea, unpleasant taste, weight loss, xerostomia

Genitourinary: Impotence

Neuromuscular & skeletal: Tremor

Ocular: Accommodation abnormalities, blurred vision

General Dosage Range Oral:

Children 3-5 years: Initial: 2.5 mg once daily; Maintenance: 0.1-0.5 mg/kg once daily (maximum: 40 mg/day)

Children 6-12 years: Initial: 5 mg once or twice daily; Maintenance: 5-20 mg (0.1-0.5 mg/kg) once daily (maximum: 40 mg [ADHD]; 60 mg [narcolepsy])

Children >12 years: Initial: 5-10 mg/day in 1-2 divided doses; Maximum: Up to 40 mg/day [ADHD] or 60 mg/day [narcolepsy]

Adults: Initial: 10 mg once daily; Maximum: Up to 60 mg/day

Mechanism of Action Amphetamines are noncatecholamine, sympathomimetic amines that promote release of catecholamines (primarily dopamine and norepinephrine) from their storage sites in the presynaptic nerve terminals. A less significant mechanism may

include their ability to block the reuptake of catecholamines by competitive inhibition.

Pharmacodynamics/Kinetics

Onset of Action 1-1.5 hours

Half-life Elimination Adults: 10-13 hours

Time to Peak Serum: Immediate release: ~3 hours; sustained release: ~8 hours

Pregnancy Risk Factor C

Pregnancy Considerations Adverse effects have been observed in animal reproduction studies. The majority of human data is based on illicit amphetamine/methamphetamine exposure and not from therapeutic maternal use (Golub, 2005). Use of amphetamines during pregnancy may lead to an increased risk of premature birth and low birth weight; newborns may experience symptoms of withdrawal. Behavioral problems may also occur later in childhood (LaGasse, 2012).

Controlled Substance C-II

Dextroamphetamine and Amphetamine (deks troe am FET a meen & am FET a meen)

Related Information

Dextroamphetamine *on page 403*

Brand Names: U.S. Adderall XR®; Adderall®

Brand Names: Canada Adderall XR®

Generic Availability (U.S.) Yes

Pharmacologic Category Central Nervous System Stimulant

Use Attention-deficit/hyperactivity disorder (ADHD); narcolepsy

Local Anesthetic/Vasoconstrictor Precautions Use vasoconstrictor with caution in patients taking dextroamphetamine. Amphetamines enhance the sympathomimetic response of epinephrine and norepinephrine leading to potential hypertension and cardiotoxicity.

Effects on Dental Treatment Key adverse event(s) related to dental treatment: Up to 6% of patients taking dextroamphetamines exhibit tachycardia. Modest increases in blood pressure have been seen (2-4 mm Hb). Consider monitoring blood pressure prior to using local anesthetic with a vasoconstrictor. Teeth clenching and tooth infection have been reported with use.

Effects on Bleeding No information available to require special precautions

Adverse Effects

As reported with Adderall XR®:

>10%:

Central nervous system: Insomnia (12% to 27%), headache (up to 26% in adults)

Gastrointestinal: Appetite decreased (22% to 36%), abdominal pain (11% to 14%), dry mouth (2% to 35%), weight loss (4% to 11%)

1% to 10%:

Cardiovascular: Tachycardia (up to 6% in adults), palpitation (2% to 4%)

Central nervous system: Emotional lability (2% to 9%), agitation (up to 8% in adults), anxiety (8%), dizziness (2% to 7%), nervousness (6%), fever (5%), somnolence (2% to 4%)

Dermatologic: Photosensitization (2% to 4%)

Endocrine & metabolic: Dysmenorrhea (2% to 4%), impotence (2% to 4%), libido decreased (2% to 4%)

Gastrointestinal: Nausea (2% to 8%), vomiting (2% to 7%), diarrhea (2% to 6%), constipation (2% to 4%), dyspepsia (2% to 4%)

Genitourinary: Urinary tract infection (5%)

Neuromuscular & skeletal: Twitching (2% to 4%), weakness (2% to 6%)

Respiratory: Dyspnea (2% to 4%)

Miscellaneous: Diaphoresis (2% to 4%), infection (2% to 4%), speech disorder (2% to 4%)

Dosage Oral: **Note:** Use lowest effective individualized dose; administer first dose as soon as awake

ADHD:

Children: <3 years: Not recommended

Children: 3-5 years (Adderall®): Initial 2.5 mg/day given every morning; increase daily dose in 2.5 mg increments at weekly intervals until optimal response is obtained (maximum dose: 40 mg/day given in 1-3 divided doses); use intervals of 4-6 hours between additional doses

Children: ≥6 years:

Adderall®: Initial: 5 mg 1-2 times/day; increase daily dose in 5 mg increments at weekly intervals until optimal response is obtained (usual maximum dose: 40 mg/day given in 1-3 divided doses); use intervals of 4-6 hours between additional doses

Adderall XR®: 5-10 mg once daily in the morning; if needed, may increase daily dose in 5-10 mg increments at weekly intervals (maximum dose: 30 mg/day)

Adolescents 13-17 years (Adderall XR®): 10 mg once daily in the morning; maybe increased to 20 mg/day after 1 week if symptoms are not controlled; higher doses (up to 60 mg/day) have been evaluated; however, there is not adequate evidence that higher doses afford additional benefit

Adults (Adderall XR®): Initial: 20 mg once daily in the morning; higher doses (up to 60 mg once daily) have been evaluated; however, there is not adequate evidence that higher doses afforded additional benefit

Narcolepsy (Adderall®):

Children: 6-12 years: Initial: 5 mg/day; increase daily dose in 5 mg at weekly intervals until optimal response is obtained (maximum dose: 60 mg/day given in 1-3 divided doses with intervals of 4-6 hours between doses)

Children >12 years and Adults: Initial: 10 mg/day; increase daily dose in 10 mg increments at weekly intervals until optimal response is obtained (maximum dose: 60 mg/day given in 1-3 divided doses with intervals of 4-6 hours between doses)

Mechanism of Action Amphetamines are noncatecholamine, sympathomimetic amines that promote release of catecholamines (primarily dopamine and norepinephrine) from their storage sites in the presynaptic nerve terminals. A less significant mechanism may include their ability to block the reuptake of catecholamines by competitive inhibition.

Contraindications Hypersensitivity to dextroamphetamine, amphetamine, or any component of the formulation; advanced arteriosclerosis; symptomatic cardiovascular disease; moderate-to-severe hypertension; hyperthyroidism; hypersensitivity or idiosyncrasy to the sympathomimetic amines; glaucoma; agitated states; patients with a history of drug abuse; with or within 14 days following MAO inhibitor (hypertensive crisis)

Warnings/Precautions [U.S. Boxed Warning]: Use has been associated with serious cardiovascular events including sudden death in patients with pre-existing structural cardiac abnormalities or other serious heart problems (sudden death in children and adolescents; sudden death, stroke and MI in adults. These products should be avoided in the patients with known serious structural cardiac abnormalities, cardiomyopathy, serious heart rhythm abnormalities, or other serious cardiac problems that could increase the risk of sudden death that these conditions alone carry. Patients should be carefully evaluated for cardiac disease prior to initiation of therapy. Use with caution in patients with hypertension and other cardiovascular conditions that might be exacerbated by increases in blood pressure or heart rate. Amphetamines may impair the ability to engage in potentially hazardous activities. May cause visual disturbances.

Use with caution in patients with psychiatric or seizure disorders. May exacerbate symptoms of behavior and thought disorder in psychotic patients. Stimulants may unmask tics in individuals with coexisting Tourette's syndrome. **[U.S. Boxed Warning]: Potential for drug dependency exists; prolonged use may lead to drug dependency.** Use is contraindicated in patients with history of ethanol or drug abuse. Prescriptions should be written for the smallest quantity consistent with good patient care to minimize possibility of overdose. Abrupt discontinuation following high doses or for prolonged periods may result in symptoms for withdrawal.

Use caution in the elderly due to CNS stimulant adverse effects. Safety and efficacy have not been established in children <3 years of age. Appetite suppression may occur; monitor weight during therapy, particularly in children. Use of stimulants has been associated with suppression of growth; monitor growth rate during treatment.

Drug Interactions

Metabolism/Transport Effects Refer to individual components.

Avoid Concomitant Use

Avoid concomitant use of Dextroamphetamine and Amphetamine with any of the following: Iobenguane I 123; MAO Inhibitors

Increased Effect/Toxicity

Dextroamphetamine and Amphetamine may increase the levels/effects of: Analgesics (Opioid); Sympathomimetics

The levels/effects of Dextroamphetamine and Amphetamine may be increased by: Alkalinizing Agents; Antacids; AtoMOXetine; Cannabinoids; Carbonic Anhydrase Inhibitors; MAO Inhibitors; Proton Pump Inhibitors; Tricyclic Antidepressants

Decreased Effect

Dextroamphetamine and Amphetamine may decrease the levels/effects of: Antihistamines; Ethosuximide; Iobenguane I 123; Ioflupane I 123; PHENobarbital; Phenytoin

The levels/effects of Dextroamphetamine and Amphetamine may be decreased by: Ammonium Chloride; Antipsychotics; Gastrointestinal Acidifying Agents; Lithium; Methenamine; Multivitamins/Minerals (with ADEK, Folate, Iron); Peginterferon Alfa-2b

Ethanol/Nutrition/Herb Interactions

Ethanol: Ethanol use may increase CNS depression. Potential for drug dependency may increase with prolonged use. Management: Avoid ethanol. Use is contraindicated for patients with history of ethanol or drug abuse.

Food: Dextroamphetamine serum levels may be altered if taken with acidic food, juices, or vitamin C. Management: Avoid caffeine. Take 30 minutes before meals.

Herb/Nutraceutical: Ephedra may cause hypertension or arrhythmias. Management: Avoid ephedra.

Pharmacodynamics/Kinetics

Onset of Action 30-60 minutes

Duration of Action 4-6 hours

Half-life Elimination

Children 6-12 years: d-amphetamine: 9 hours; l-amphetamine: 11 hours

Adolescents 13-17 years: d-amphetamine: 11 hours; l-amphetamine: 13-14 hours

Adults: d-amphetamine: 10 hours; l-amphetamine: 13 hours

Time to Peak T_{max}: Adderall®: 3 hours; Adderall XR®: 7 hours

Pregnancy Risk Factor C

Pregnancy Considerations Adverse effects have been observed in animal reproduction studies. The majority of human data is based on illicit amphetamine/methamphetamine exposure and not from therapeutic maternal use (Golub, 2005). Use of amphetamines during pregnancy may lead to an increased risk of premature birth and low birth weight; newborns may experience symptoms of withdrawal. Behavioral problems may also occur later in childhood (LaGasse, 2012).

Lactation Enters breast milk/not recommended

Breast-Feeding Considerations The majority of human data is based on illicit amphetamine/methamphetamine exposure and not from therapeutic maternal use (Golub, 2005). Amphetamines are excreted into breast milk and use may decrease milk production. Increased irritability, agitation, and crying have been reported in nursing infants (ACOG, 2011). A case report describes maternal use of amphetamine 20 mg/day throughout pregnancy and while breastfeeding. Milk concentrations were higher in breast milk than the maternal serum. The milk/plasma ratio ranged from 2.8-7.5 when measured on days 10 and 42 following delivery (Steiner, 1984). The manufacturer recommends that mothers taking dextroamphetamine/amphetamine refrain from nursing.

Controlled Substance C-II

Dosage Forms

Capsule, extended release, oral:

5 mg [dextroamphetamine sulfate 1.25 mg, dextroamphetamine saccharate 1.25 mg, amphetamine aspartate monohydrate 1.25 mg, amphetamine sulfate 1.25 mg]

10 mg [dextroamphetamine sulfate 2.5 mg, dextroamphetamine saccharate 2.5 mg, amphetamine aspartate monohydrate 2.5 mg, amphetamine sulfate 2.5 mg]

15 mg [dextroamphetamine sulfate 3.75 mg, dextroamphetamine saccharate 3.75 mg, amphetamine aspartate monohydrate 3.75 mg, amphetamine sulfate 3.75 mg]

20 mg [dextroamphetamine sulfate 5 mg, dextroamphetamine saccharate 5 mg, amphetamine aspartate monohydrate 5 mg, amphetamine sulfate 5 mg]

25 mg [dextroamphetamine sulfate 6.25 mg, dextroamphetamine saccharate 6.25 mg, amphetamine aspartate monohydrate 6.25 mg, amphetamine sulfate 6.25 mg]

30 mg [dextroamphetamine sulfate 7.5 mg, dextroamphetamine saccharate 7.5 mg, amphetamine aspartate monohydrate 7.5 mg, amphetamine sulfate 7.5 mg]

Adderall XR®:

5 mg [dextroamphetamine 1.25 mg, dextroamphetamine saccharate 1.25 mg, amphetamine aspartate monohydrate 1.25 mg, amphetamine sulfate 1.25 mg]

10 mg [dextroamphetamine sulfate 2.5 mg, dextroamphetamine saccharate 2.5 mg, amphetamine aspartate monohydrate 2.5 mg, amphetamine sulfate 2.5 mg]

15 mg [dextroamphetamine sulfate 3.75 mg, dextroamphetamine saccharate 3.75 mg, amphetamine aspartate monohydrate 3.75 mg, amphetamine sulfate 3.75 mg]

20 mg [dextroamphetamine sulfate 5 mg, dextroamphetamine saccharate 5 mg, amphetamine aspartate monohydrate 5 mg, amphetamine sulfate 5 mg]

25 mg [dextroamphetamine sulfate 6.25 mg, dextroamphetamine saccharate 6.25 mg, amphetamine aspartate monohydrate 6.25 mg, amphetamine sulfate 6.25 mg]

30 mg [dextroamphetamine sulfate 7.5 mg, dextroamphetamine saccharate 7.5 mg, amphetamine aspartate monohydrate 7.5 mg, amphetamine sulfate 7.5 mg]

Tablet, oral: 5 mg, 7.5 mg, 10 mg, 12.5 mg, 15 mg, 20 mg, 30 mg

5 mg [dextroamphetamine sulfate 1.25 mg, dextroamphetamine saccharate 1.25 mg, amphetamine aspartate monohydrate 1.25 mg, amphetamine sulfate 1.25 mg]

7.5 mg [dextroamphetamine sulfate 1.875 mg, dextroamphetamine saccharate 1.875 mg, amphetamine aspartate monohydrate 1.875 mg, amphetamine sulfate 1.875 mg]

10 mg [dextroamphetamine sulfate 2.5 mg, dextroamphetamine saccharate 2.5 mg, amphetamine aspartate monohydrate 2.5 mg, amphetamine sulfate 2.5 mg]

12.5 mg [dextroamphetamine sulfate 3.125 mg, dextroamphetamine saccharate 3.125 mg, amphetamine aspartate monohydrate 3.125 mg, amphetamine sulfate 3.125 mg]

15 mg [dextroamphetamine sulfate 3.75 mg, dextroamphetamine saccharate 3.75 mg, amphetamine aspartate monohydrate 3.75 mg, amphetamine sulfate 3.75 mg]

20 mg [dextroamphetamine sulfate 5 mg, dextroamphetamine saccharate 5 mg, amphetamine aspartate monohydrate 5 mg, amphetamine sulfate 5 mg]

30 mg [dextroamphetamine sulfate 7.5 mg, dextroamphetamine saccharate 7.5 mg, amphetamine aspartate monohydrate 7.5 mg, amphetamine sulfate 7.5 mg]

Adderall®:

5 mg [dextroamphetamine sulfate 1.25 mg, dextroamphetamine saccharate 1.25 mg, amphetamine aspartate monohydrate 1.25 mg, amphetamine sulfate 1.25 mg]

7.5 mg [dextroamphetamine sulfate 1.875 mg, dextroamphetamine saccharate 1.875 mg, amphetamine aspartate monohydrate 1.875 mg, amphetamine sulfate 1.875 mg]

10 mg [dextroamphetamine sulfate 2.5 mg, dextroamphetamine saccharate 2.5 mg, amphetamine aspartate monohydrate 2.5 mg, amphetamine sulfate 2.5 mg]

12.5 mg [dextroamphetamine sulfate 3.125 mg, dextroamphetamine saccharate 3.125 mg, amphetamine aspartate monohydrate 3.125 mg, amphetamine sulfate 3.125 mg]

◀ 15 mg [dextroamphetamine sulfate 3.75 mg, dextroamphetamine saccharate 3.75 mg, amphetamine aspartate monohydrate 3.75 mg, amphetamine sulfate 3.75 mg]

20 mg [dextroamphetamine sulfate 5 mg, dextroamphetamine saccharate 5 mg, amphetamine aspartate monohydrate 5 mg, amphetamine sulfate 5 mg]

30 mg [dextroamphetamine sulfate 7.5 mg, dextroamphetamine saccharate 7.5 mg, amphetamine aspartate monohydrate 7.5 mg, amphetamine sulfate 7.5 mg]

Dextromethorphan (deks troe meth OR fan)

Brand Names: U.S. Creo-Terpin® [OTC]; Creomulsion® Adult Formula [OTC]; Creomulsion® for Children [OTC]; Delsym® [OTC]; Father John's® [OTC]; Hold® DM [OTC]; Nycoff [OTC]; PediaCare® Children's Long-Acting Cough [OTC]; Robafen Cough [OTC]; Robitussin® Children's Cough Long-Acting [OTC]; Robitussin® Lingering Cold Long-Acting Cough [OTC]; Robitussin® Lingering Cold Long-Acting CoughGels® [OTC]; Scot-Tussin® Diabetes [OTC]; Silphen-DM [OTC]; Triaminic® Children's Cough Long Acting [OTC]; Vicks® 44® Cough Relief [OTC]; Vicks® DayQuil® Cough [OTC]; Vicks® Nature Fusion™ Cough [OTC]

Pharmacologic Category Antitussive; N-Methyl-D-Aspartate Receptor Antagonist

Use Symptomatic relief of coughs caused by the common cold or inhaled irritants

Unlabeled Use N-methyl-D-aspartate (NMDA) antagonist

Local Anesthetic/Vasoconstrictor Precautions No information available to require special precautions

Effects on Dental Treatment No significant effects or complications reported

Effects on Bleeding No information available to require special precautions

General Dosage Range Oral:
Extended release:
Children 4-6 years: 15 mg twice daily (maximum: 30 mg/day)
Children 6-12 years: 30 mg twice daily (maximum: 60 mg/day)
Children >12 years and Adults: 60 mg twice daily (maximum: 120 mg/day)
Immediate release:
Children 4-6 years: 2.5-7.5 mg every 4-8 hours (maximum: 30 mg/day)
Children 6-12 years: 5-10 mg every 4 hours **or** 15 mg every 6-8 hours (maximum: 60 mg/day)
Children >12 years and Adults: 10-20 mg every 4 hours **or** 30 mg every 6-8 hours (maximum: 120 mg/day)

Mechanism of Action Decreases the sensitivity of cough receptors and interrupts cough impulse transmission by depressing the medullary cough center through sigma receptor stimulation; structurally related to codeine

Pharmacodynamics/Kinetics
Onset of Action Antitussive: 15-30 minutes
Duration of Action ≤6 hours
Half-life Elimination Dextromethorphan: Extensive metabolizers: 2-4 hours; poor metabolizers: 24 hours
Time to Peak 2-3 hours

Pregnancy Considerations Maternal use of standard OTC doses of dextromethorphan when used as an antitussive during the first trimester of pregnancy has not been found to increase the risk of teratogenic effects. Dextromethorphan is metabolized in the liver via CYP2D6 and CYP3A enzymes. The activity of both enzymes is increased in the mother during pregnancy. In the fetus, CYP2D6 activity is low in the fetal liver and CYP3A4 activity is present by ~17 weeks gestation.

Dextromethorphan and Chlorpheniramine
(deks troe meth OR fan & klor fen IR a meen)

Related Information
Chlorpheniramine *on page 292*
Dextromethorphan *on page 406*

Brand Names: U.S. Coricidin® HBP Cough & Cold [OTC]; Dimetapp® Children's Long Acting Cough Plus Cold [OTC]; Robitussin® Children's Cough & Cold Long-Acting [OTC]; Scot-Tussin® DM Maximum Strength [OTC]; Triaminic® Children's Softchews® Cough & Runny Nose [OTC]

Pharmacologic Category Alkylamine Derivative; Antitussive; Histamine H_1 Antagonist; Histamine H_1 Antagonist, First Generation

Use Symptomatic relief of runny nose, sneezing, itchy/watery eyes, cough, and other upper respiratory symptoms associated with hay fever, common cold, or upper respiratory allergies

Local Anesthetic/Vasoconstrictor Precautions No information available to require special precautions

Effects on Dental Treatment Key adverse event(s) related to dental treatment: Chlorpheniramine: Prolonged use will cause significant xerostomia (normal salivary flow resumes upon discontinuation).

Effects on Bleeding No information available to require special precautions

Adverse Effects See individual agents.

General Dosage Range Oral:
Children 6-11 years: Dextromethorphan 10-15 mg and chlorpheniramine 2 mg every 4-6 hours as needed (maximum: 60 mg dextromethorphan and 10 mg chlorpheniramine/24 hours)
Children ≥12 years and Adults: Dextromethorphan 30 mg and chlorpheniramine 4 mg every 6 hours as needed (maximum: 120 mg dextromethorphan and 16 mg chlorpheniramine/24 hours)

Mechanism of Action
Chlorpheniramine maleate: Antihistamine with H_1-receptor activity
Dextromethorphan: A non-narcotic antitussive, increases cough threshold by its activity on the medulla oblongata

Pregnancy Considerations Reproduction studies have not been conducted with this combination. See individual agents.

Dextromethorphan and Phenylephrine
(deks troe meth OR fan & fen il EF rin)

Related Information
Dextromethorphan *on page 406*
Phenylephrine (Systemic) *on page 1087*

Brand Names: U.S. PediaCare® Children's Multi-Symptom Cold [OTC]; Safetussin® CD [OTC]; Sudafed PE® Children's Cold & Cough [OTC]; Triaminic® Day Time Cold & Cough [OTC]

Pharmacologic Category Antitussive; Decongestant

Use Temporary relief of symptoms of hay fever, the common cold, and upper respiratory allergies including sinus/nasal congestion, minor bronchial/throat irritation, and cough

Local Anesthetic/Vasoconstrictor Precautions

Use with caution since phenylephrine is a sympathomimetic amine which could interact with epinephrine to cause a pressor response

Effects on Dental Treatment No significant effects or complications reported

Effects on Bleeding No information available to require special precautions

Adverse Effects See individual agents.

General Dosage Range Oral:

Children ≥4-12 years: Dosage varies greatly depending on product

Children ≥12 years and Adults: Safetussin® CD: 10 mL every 6 hours as needed (maximum: 40 mL/24 hours)

Mechanism of Action See individual agents.

Dextromethorphan and Quinidine

(deks troe meth OR fan & KWIN i deen)

Related Information

Dextromethorphan *on page 406*
QuiNIDine *on page 1171*

Brand Names: U.S. Nuedexta™

Brand Names: Canada Nuedexta™

Pharmacologic Category N-Methyl-D-Aspartate Receptor Antagonist

Use Treatment of pseudobulbar affect (PBA)

Local Anesthetic/Vasoconstrictor Precautions See individual agents

Effects on Dental Treatment See individual agents

Effects on Bleeding See individual agents

Adverse Effects Also see individual agents.

>10%: Gastrointestinal: Diarrhea (13%)

1% to 10%:

Cardiovascular: Peripheral edema (5%)

Central nervous system: Dizziness (10%)

Gastrointestinal: Vomiting (5%), flatulence (3%)

Genitourinary: Urinary tract infection (4%)

Hepatic: GGT increased (3%)

Neuromuscular & skeletal: Weakness (5%)

Respiratory: Cough (5%)

Miscellaneous: Influenza (4%)

General Dosage Range

Oral: *Adults:* Initial: Once capsule once daily for 7 days; Maintenance: One capsule twice daily

Mechanism of Action Dextromethorphan may relieve the symptoms of PBA by binding to sigma-1 receptors in the brain which may be involved in behavior, however the exact mechanism of action is not known. Quinidine is used to block the rapid metabolism of dextromethorphan, thereby increasing serum concentrations. The dose of quinidine in this combination product provides serum concentrations 1% to 3% of those needed to treat cardiac arrhythmias.

Pharmacodynamics/Kinetics

Half-life Elimination Dextromethorphan: 13 hours in extensive metabolizers; Quinidine: 7 hours in extensive metabolizers

Time to Peak Dextromethorphan: 3-4 hours; Quinidine: 1-2 hours

Pregnancy Risk Factor C

Pregnancy Considerations Adverse events were observed in animal reproduction studies using this combination.

Dental Comment See individual agents

Dextrose (DEKS trose)

Brand Names: U.S. BD™ Glucose [OTC]; Dex4® [OTC]; Enfamil® Glucose [OTC]; GlucoBurst® [OTC]; Glutol™ [OTC]; Glutose 15™ [OTC]; Glutose 45™ [OTC]; Insta-Glucose® [OTC]; Similac® Glucose [OTC]

Pharmacologic Category Antidote, Hypoglycemia; Intravenous Nutritional Therapy

Use

Oral: Treatment of hypoglycemia

5% and 10% solutions: Peripheral infusion to provide calories and fluid replacement

25% (hypertonic) solution: Treatment of acute symptomatic episodes of hypoglycemia in infants and children to restore depressed blood glucose levels; adjunctive treatment of hyperkalemia when combined with insulin

50% (hypertonic) solution: Treatment of insulin-induced hypoglycemia (hyperinsulinemia or insulin shock) and adjunctive treatment of hyperkalemia in adolescents and adults

≥10% solutions: Infusion after admixture with amino acids for nutritional support

Local Anesthetic/Vasoconstrictor Precautions No information available to require special precautions

Effects on Dental Treatment No significant effects or complications reported

Effects on Bleeding No information available to require special precautions

Adverse Effects Frequency not defined. **Note:** Most adverse effects are associated with excessive dosage or rate of infusion.

Cardiovascular: Edema, dehydration, hyper-/hypovolemia, phlebitis, venous thrombosis

Central nervous system: Fever, hyperosmolar syndrome, mental confusion, unconsciousness

Endocrine & metabolic: Acidosis, hyperglycemia, hypokalemia, hypophosphatemia, hypomagnesemia

Genitourinary: Ketonuria, glycosuria, polyuria

Gastrointestinal: Diarrhea (oral), nausea, polydipsia

Local: Pain, tissue necrosis, vein irritation

Respiratory: Pulmonary edema, tachypnea

General Dosage Range

I.V.:

Infants ≤6 months: 0.25-1 g/kg/dose (maximum: 25 g/dose)

Children >6 months to 12 years: 0.5-1 g/kg/dose (maximum: 25 g/dose)

Adolescents and and Adults: 10-50 g/dose

Oral: *Children >2 years and and Adults:* 10-20 g as a single dose, may repeat if needed

Mechanism of Action Dextrose, a monosaccharide, is a source of calories and fluid for patients unable to obtain an adequate oral intake; may decrease body protein and nitrogen losses; promotes glycogen deposition in the liver. When used in the treatment of hyperkalemia (combined with insulin), dextrose stimulates the uptake of potassium by cells, especially in muscle tissue, lowering serum potassium.

Pharmacodynamics/Kinetics

Onset of Action

Treatment of hypoglycemia: Oral: 10 minutes

Treatment of hyperkalemia: Maximum effect: I.V.: 30 minutes

Time to Peak Oral: 40 minutes

Pregnancy Risk Factor C (injection, infusion)

◄ **Pregnancy Considerations** In patients who require parenteral nutrition for treatment of hyperemesis gravidarum, dextrose is part of the parenteral nutrition regimen (ASPEN, 2002).

Diatrizoate Meglumine
(dye a tri ZOE ate MEG loo meen)

Brand Names: U.S. Cystografin®; Cystografin® Dilute

Pharmacologic Category Iodinated Contrast Media; Radiological/Contrast Media, Ionic (High Osmolality)

Use

Solution for instillation: Retrograde cystourethrography; retrograde or ascending pyelography

Solution for injection: Arthrography, cerebral angiography, direct cholangiography, discography, drip infusion pyelography, excretory urography, peripheral arteriography, splenoportography, venography; contrast enhancement of computed tomographic head and body imaging

Local Anesthetic/Vasoconstrictor Precautions No information available to require special precautions

Effects on Dental Treatment No significant effects or complications reported

Effects on Bleeding No information available to require special precautions

Adverse Effects

<10%:

Cardiovascular: Flushing (49%)

Gastrointestinal: Taste perversion (11%)

Local: Injection site reaction (12%)

Renal: Nephrosis (excretory urography: 23%)

1% to 10%:

Cardiovascular: Edema, hypertension

Central nervous system: Dizziness (5%), agitation, chills, fever, headache

Dermatologic: Urticaria (1%)

Gastrointestinal: Nausea (6%), vomiting (3%)

Local: Extravasation

Neuromuscular & skeletal: Parasthesia (6%)

Renal: Hematuria (retrograde GU procedures), urinary tract infections (retrograde GU procedures)

Respiratory: Cough (2%), rhinitis (1%), sneezing

Miscellaneous: Allergic reaction, diaphoresis

Pregnancy Risk Factor C

Pregnancy Considerations Animal reproduction studies have not been conducted. Diatrizoate salts cross the placenta and may enter fetal circulation. Abnormal neonatal opacification of the small intestine and colon have been reported in the newborn 4-6 days after delivery. In general, iodinated contrast media agents are avoided during pregnancy unless essential for diagnosis.

Diatrizoate Meglumine and Diatrizoate Sodium
(dye a tri ZOE ate MEG loo meen & dye a tri ZOE ate SOW dee um)

Related Information

Diatrizoate Meglumine *on page 408*

Brand Names: U.S. Gastrografin®; MD-76®R; MD-Gastroview®

Pharmacologic Category Iodinated Contrast Media; Radiological/Contrast Media, Ionic (High Osmolality)

Use

Oral/rectal: Examination of GI tract; adjunct to contrast enhancement in computed tomography of the torso (in conjunction with a radiopaque contrast agent)

Injection: Angiocardiography, aortography, contrast enhancement of brain or body computed tomographic (CT), digital subtraction angiography, excretory urography, peripheral arteriography, selective coronary arteriography (with or without left ventriculography), selective renal arteriography, selective visceral arteriography

Unlabeled Use For use in evaluating adhesive small intestine obstruction (ASIO) in patients without signs of strangulation and peritonism

Local Anesthetic/Vasoconstrictor Precautions No information available to require special precautions

Effects on Dental Treatment No significant effects or complications reported

Effects on Bleeding No information available to require special precautions

Adverse Effects

Oral/rectal: Frequency not defined.

Cardiovascular: Tachyarrhythmia

Dermatologic: Erythema, urticaria

Gastrointestinal: Diarrhea, nausea, vomiting

Respiratory: Dyspnea, hypoxia

Miscellaneous: Anaphylaxis

Injection: Frequency not defined (specific procedure-related adverse events may also occur):

Cardiovascular: Arrhythmia, cardiovascular reactions (severe including cardiac arrest), chills, disseminated intravascular coagulation, edema, fever, flushing, hyper-/hypotension, pallor, transient ECG changes (with coronary angiography), ventricular fibrillation (with excretion urography or coronary angiography), warmth

Central nervous system: Dizziness, headache

Dermatologic: Facial petechiae, itching, pruritus, rash, urticaria

Gastrointestinal: Choking, nausea, retching, vomiting

Hematologic: Neutropenia

Local: Injection site reactions: Burning, numbness, partial collapse of vein, stinging, thrombophlebitis, tissue necrosis with extravasation, venospasm, venous pain

Neuromuscular & skeletal: Cramps, tremors, weakness

Ocular: Conjunctival petechiae, lacrimation

Renal: Acute renal failure

With aortography: Renal damage, including renal infarction, acute tubular necrosis with oliguria and anuria

Respiratory: Sneezing, wheezing

Miscellaneous: Allergic reactions, anaphylaxis with severe asthmatic reaction (with excretion urography), diaphoresis, nonimmunologic anaphylaxis (formerly known as anaphylactoid reaction)

General Dosage Range

Intra-arterial: Dosage varies greatly depending on indication.

I.V.: Dosage varies greatly depending on indication.

Oral:

Children <5 years: 30 mL, may dilute 1:1 (if <10 kg or debilitated, dilute 1:3 in water)

Children 5-10 years: 60 mL, may dilute 1:1 (if <10 kg or debilitated, dilute 1:3 in water)

Adults: 30-90 mL **or** 25-77 mL in 1000 mL tap water (administer 240 mL of solution)

Rectal:

Children <5 years: Dilute 1:5 in tap water

Children ≥5 years: Dilute 90 mL in 500 mL tap water

Adults: Dilute 240 mL in 1000 mL tap water

Pharmacodynamics/Kinetics
Half-life Elimination Injectable formulation: Initial: 10 minutes; Terminal: 100 minutes
Pregnancy Risk Factor B
Pregnancy Considerations Teratogenic effects were not observed in animal reproduction studies. Following I.V. administration, diatrizoate salts cross the placenta and may enter fetal circulation. In general, iodinated contrast media agents are avoided during pregnancy unless essential for diagnosis.

Diatrizoate Meglumine and Iodipamide Meglumine
(dye a tri ZOE ate MEG loo meen & eye oh DI pa mide MEG loo meen)

Related Information
Diatrizoate Meglumine *on page 408*
Iodipamide Meglumine *on page 756*
Brand Names: U.S. Sinografin®
Pharmacologic Category Iodinated Contrast Media; Radiological/Contrast Media, Ionic (Low Osmolality)
Use Hysterosalpingography
Local Anesthetic/Vasoconstrictor Precautions No information available to require special precautions
Effects on Dental Treatment No significant effects or complications reported
Effects on Bleeding No information available to require special precautions
Adverse Effects Frequency not defined.
Cardiovascular: Bradycardia (rare), cardiac arrest (rare), hypotension, syncope
Central nervous system: Chills, dizziness, fever
Gastrointestinal: Abdominal pain, abdominal tenderness, nausea, vomiting
Miscellaneous: Anaphylactoid reactions, hypersensitivity reactions (including sweating, flushing, pruritus, urticaria, rash, arthralgia, respiratory distress, and circulatory collapse)
General Dosage Range Intrauterine: *Adults:* Usual dose: 3-4 mL; Total dosage range: 1.5-10 mL
Pregnancy Considerations The procedure for which this product is indicated is contraindicated during or within 6 months of pregnancy. Diatrizoate meglumine crosses the placenta and enters the fetal circulation. Also refer to individual agents.

Diazepam (dye AZ e pam)

Related Information
Management of the Patient With Anxiety or Depression *on page 1594*
Temporomandibular Dysfunction (TMD), Chronic Pain, and Fibromyalgia *on page 1590*
Related Sample Prescriptions
Sedation (Prior to Dental Treatment) *on page 1621*
Brand Names: U.S. Diastat®; Diastat® AcuDial™; Diazepam Intensol™; Valium®
Brand Names: Canada Apo-Diazepam®; Bio-Diazepam; Diastat®; Diazemuls®; Diazepam Auto Injector; Diazepam Injection USP; Novo-Dipam; PMS-Diazepam; Valium®
Generic Availability (U.S.) Yes
Pharmacologic Category Benzodiazepine
Dental Use Oral medication for preoperative dental anxiety; sedative component in I.V. conscious sedation in oral surgery patients; skeletal muscle relaxant

Use Management of anxiety disorders, ethanol withdrawal symptoms; skeletal muscle relaxant; treatment of convulsive disorders; preoperative or preprocedural sedation and amnesia
Rectal gel: Management of selected, refractory epilepsy patients on stable regimens of antiepileptic drugs requiring intermittent use of diazepam to control episodes of increased seizure activity
Unlabeled Use Panic disorders; short-term treatment of spasticity in children with cerebral palsy; sedation for mechanically-ventilated patients in the intensive care unit
Local Anesthetic/Vasoconstrictor Precautions No information available to require special precautions
Effects on Dental Treatment Key adverse event(s) related to dental treatment: Xerostomia and changes in salivation (normal salivary flow resumes upon discontinuation).
Effects on Bleeding No information available to require special precautions
Adverse Effects Frequency not defined. Adverse reactions may vary by route of administration.
Cardiovascular: Hypotension, vasodilatation
Central nervous system: Amnesia, ataxia, confusion, depression, drowsiness, fatigue, headache, slurred speech, paradoxical reactions (eg, aggressiveness, agitation, anxiety, delusions, hallucinations, inappropriate behavior, increased muscle spasms, insomnia, irritability, psychoses, rage, restlessness, sleep disturbances, stimulation), vertigo
Dermatologic: Rash
Endocrine & metabolic: Libido changes
Gastrointestinal: Constipation, diarrhea, nausea, salivation changes (dry mouth or hypersalivation)
Genitourinary: Incontinence, urinary retention
Hepatic: Jaundice
Local: Phlebitis, pain with injection
Neuromuscular & skeletal: Dysarthria, tremor, weakness
Ocular: Blurred vision, diplopia
Respiratory: Apnea, asthma, respiratory rate decreased
Dental Usual Dosage
Anxiety/sedation/skeletal muscle relaxant: Adults:
Oral: 2-10 mg 2-4 times/day
I.M., I.V.: 2-10 mg, may repeat in 3-4 hours if needed
Anxiety: Elderly: Oral: Initial: 1-2 mg 1-2 times/day; increase gradually as needed, rarely need to use >10 mg/day (watch for hypotension and excessive sedation)
Skeletal muscle relaxant: Elderly: Oral: Initial: 2-5 mg 2-4 times/day
Dosage Oral absorption is more reliable than I.M.
Children:
Conscious sedation for procedures: Oral: 0.2-0.3 mg/kg (maximum: 10 mg) 45-60 minutes prior to procedure
Muscle spasm associated with tetanus: I.V., I.M.:
Infants >30 days and Children <5 years: 1-2 mg/dose every 3-4 hours as needed
Children ≥5 years: 5-10 mg/dose every 3-4 hours as needed
Sedation/muscle relaxant/anxiety:
Oral: 0.12-0.8 mg/kg/day in divided doses every 6-8 hours
I.M., I.V.: 0.04-0.3 mg/kg/dose every 2-4 hours to a maximum of 0.6 mg/kg within an 8-hour period if needed
Spasticity in cerebral palsy (unlabeled use): Oral: Dose should be individualized:
Children ≤5 years: <8.5 kg: 0.5-1 mg at bedtime; 8.5-15 kg: 1-2 mg at bedtime (Mathew, 2005)

Children 5-16 years: 1.25 mg 3 times daily to 5 mg 4 times daily (Engle, 1966)

Status epilepticus:

I.V.: Infants >30 days and Children: 0.1-0.3 mg/kg (maximum dose: 10 mg) given over ≤5 mg/minute; may repeat dose after 5-10 minutes (Hegenbarth, 2008)

Manufacturer's recommendations:

Infants >30 days and Children <5 years: 0.2-0.5 mg given slowly every 2-5 minutes (maximum total dose: 5 mg); repeat in 2-4 hours if needed

Children ≥5 years: 1 mg given slowly every 2-5 minutes (maximum total dose: 10 mg); repeat in 2-4 hours if needed

Rectal gel: 0.5 mg/kg, then 0.25 mg/kg in 10 minutes if needed (maximum dose: 20 mg) (Hegenbarth, 2008).

Anticonvulsant (acute treatment): Rectal gel:

Children <2 years: Safety and efficacy have not been studied

Children 2-5 years: 0.5 mg/kg (maximum dose: 20 mg)

Children 6-11 years: 0.3 mg/kg (maximum dose: 20 mg)

Children ≥12 years: 0.2 mg/kg (maximum dose: 20 mg)

Note: Dosage should be rounded upward to the next available dose, 2.5, 5, 7.5, 10, 12.5, 15, 17.5, and 20 mg/dose; dose may be repeated in 4-12 hours if needed; do not use for more than 5 episodes per month or more than one episode every 5 days

Adolescents: Conscious sedation for procedures:

Oral: 10 mg

I.V.: 5 mg, may repeat with 1/2 dose if needed

Adults:

Acute ethanol withdrawal: Oral: 10 mg 3-4 times during first 24 hours, then decrease to 5 mg 3-4 times/day as needed

Anticonvulsant (acute treatment): Rectal gel: 0.2 mg/kg

Note: Dosage should be rounded upward to the next available dose, 2.5, 5, 7.5, 10, 12.5, 15, 17.5, and 20 mg/dose; dose may be repeated in 4-12 hours if needed; do not use for more than 5 episodes per month or more than one episode every 5 days.

Anxiety (symptoms/disorders): Oral, I.M, I.V.: 2-10 mg 2-4 times/day if needed

Muscle spasm: I.V., I.M.: Initial: 5-10 mg; then 5-10 mg in 3-4 hours, if necessary. Larger doses may be required if associated with tetanus.

Sedation in the ICU patient: I.V.: Loading dose: 5-10 mg; Maintenance dose: 0.03-0.1 mg/kg every 30 minutes to 6 hours (Barr, 2013)

Skeletal muscle relaxant (adjunct therapy): Oral: 2-10 mg 3-4 times/day

Status epilepticus:

I.V.: 5-10 mg every 5-10 minutes given over ≤5 mg/minute; maximum dose: 30 mg

Rectal gel: Premonitory/Out-of-hospital treatment: 10 mg once; may repeat once if necessary (Kälviäinen, 2007)

Rapid tranquilization of agitated patient (administer every 30-60 minutes): Oral: 5-10 mg; average total dose for tranquilization: 20-60 mg

Elderly/debilitated patients:

Oral: 2-2.5 mg 1-2 times/day initially; increase gradually as needed and tolerated

Rectal gel: Due to the increased half-life in elderly and debilitated patients, consider reducing dose.

Dosing adjustment in renal impairment: No dose adjustment recommended; decrease dose if administered for prolonged periods.

I.V.: Risk of propylene glycol toxicity; monitor closely if using for prolonged periods or at high doses

Hemodialysis: Not dialyzable (0% to 5%); supplemental dose is not necessary

Dosing adjustment in hepatic impairment: Decrease maintenance dose by 50%; half-life significantly prolonged.

Mechanism of Action Binds to stereospecific benzodiazepine receptors on the postsynaptic GABA neuron at several sites within the central nervous system, including the limbic system, reticular formation. Enhancement of the inhibitory effect of GABA on neuronal excitability results by increased neuronal membrane permeability to chloride ions. This shift in chloride ions results in hyperpolarization (a less excitable state) and stabilization.

Contraindications Hypersensitivity to diazepam or any component of the formulation (cross-sensitivity with other benzodiazepines may exist); myasthenia gravis; severe respiratory insufficiency; severe hepatic insufficiency; sleep apnea syndrome; acute narrow-angle glaucoma; not for use in children <6 months of age (oral)

Warnings/Precautions Withdrawal has also been associated with an increase in the seizure frequency. Use with caution with drugs which may decrease diazepam metabolism. Use with caution in debilitated patients, obese patients, patients with hepatic disease (including alcoholics), or renal impairment. Active metabolites with extended half-lives may lead to delayed accumulation and adverse effects. Use with caution in patients with respiratory disease or impaired gag reflex.

Acute hypotension, muscle weakness, apnea, and cardiac arrest have occurred with parenteral administration. Acute effects may be more prevalent in patients receiving concurrent barbiturates, narcotics, or ethanol. Appropriate resuscitative equipment and qualified personnel should be available during administration and monitoring. Avoid use of the injection in patients with shock, coma, or acute ethanol intoxication. Intra-arterial injection or extravasation of the parenteral formulation should be avoided. Parenteral formulation contains propylene glycol, which has been associated with toxicity when administered in high dosages. Administration of rectal gel should only be performed by individuals trained to recognize characteristic seizure activity and monitor response.

Causes CNS depression (dose-related) resulting in sedation, dizziness, confusion, or ataxia which may impair physical and mental capabilities. Patients must be cautioned about performing tasks which require mental alertness (eg, operating machinery or driving). Use with caution in patients receiving other CNS depressants or psychoactive agents. Effects with other sedative drugs or ethanol may be potentiated. The dosage of narcotics should be reduced by approximately one-third when diazepam is added. Benzodiazepines have been associated with falls and traumatic injury and should be used with extreme caution in patients who are at risk of these events. Benzodiazepines with long half-lives may produce prolonged sedation and increase the risk of falls and fracture. In older adults, benzodiazepines increase the risk of impaired cognition, delirium, falls, fractures, and motor vehicle accidents. Due to increased sensitivity in this age group and slower metabolism of long-acting agents (such as diazepam), avoid use for treatment of insomnia, agitation, or delirium (Beers Criteria).

Use with caution in patients taking strong CYP3A4 inhibitors, moderate or strong CYP3A4 and CYP2C19 inducers and major CYP3A4 substrates.

Use caution in patients with depression or anxiety associated with depression, particularly if suicidal risk may be present. Use with caution in patients with a history of drug dependence. Benzodiazepines have been associated with dependence and acute withdrawal symptoms on discontinuation or reduction in dose. Acute withdrawal, including seizures, may be precipitated in patients after administration of flumazenil to patients receiving long-term benzodiazepine therapy.

Diazepam has been associated with anterograde amnesia. Psychiatric and paradoxical reactions, including hyperactive or aggressive behavior, have been reported with benzodiazepines, particularly in adolescent/pediatric or elderly patients. Does not have analgesic, antidepressant, or antipsychotic properties.

Rectal gel: Safety and efficacy have not been established in children <2 years of age.
Oral: Safety and efficacy have not been established in children <6 months of age.
Injection: Safety and efficacy have not been established in children <30 days of age. Solution for injection may contain sodium benzoate, benzyl alcohol, or benzoic acid. Large amounts have been associated with "gasping syndrome" in neonates.

Drug Interactions

Metabolism/Transport Effects Substrate of CYP1A2 (minor), CYP2B6 (minor), CYP2C19 (major), CYP2C9 (minor), CYP3A4 (major); **Note:** Assignment of Major/Minor substrate status based on clinically relevant drug interaction potential; **Inhibits** CYP2C19 (weak), CYP3A4 (weak)

Avoid Concomitant Use

Avoid concomitant use of Diazepam with any of the following: Azelastine (Nasal); Conivaptan; OLANZapine; Paraldehyde; Pimozide; Sodium Oxybate

Increased Effect/Toxicity

Diazepam may increase the levels/effects of: Alcohol (Ethyl); ARIPiprazole; Azelastine (Nasal); Buprenorphine; CloZAPine; CNS Depressants; Fosphenytoin; Lomitapide; Methotrimeprazine; Metyrosine; Mirtazapine; Paraldehyde; Phenytoin; Pimozide; Pramipexole; ROPINIRole; Rotigotine; Selective Serotonin Reuptake Inhibitors; Sodium Oxybate; Zolpidem

The levels/effects of Diazepam may be increased by: Antifungal Agents (Azole Derivatives, Systemic); Aprepitant; Calcium Channel Blockers (Nondihydropyridine); Cimetidine; Conivaptan; Contraceptives (Estrogens); Contraceptives (Progestins); Cosyntropin; CYP2C19 Inhibitors (Moderate); CYP2C19 Inhibitors (Strong); CYP3A4 Inhibitors (Moderate); CYP3A4 Inhibitors (Strong); Dasatinib; Disulfiram; Droperidol; Etravirine; Fosamprenavir; Fosaprepitant; Grapefruit Juice; HydrOXYzine; Isoniazid; Ivacaftor; Macrolide Antibiotics; Magnesium Sulfate; Methotrimeprazine; Mifepristone; OLANZapine; Perampanel; Proton Pump Inhibitors; Ritonavir; Saquinavir; Selective Serotonin Reuptake Inhibitors

Decreased Effect

The levels/effects of Diazepam may be decreased by: CarBAMazepine; CYP2C19 Inducers (Strong); CYP3A4 Inducers (Strong); Deferasirox; Etravirine; Rifamycin Derivatives; St Johns Wort; Theophylline Derivatives; Tocilizumab; Yohimbine

Ethanol/Nutrition/Herb Interactions

Ethanol: Ethanol may increase CNS depression. Potential for drug dependency exists. Management: Avoid ethanol.
Food: Diazepam serum concentrations may be decreased if taken with food. Grapefruit juice may increase diazepam serum concentrations. Management: Avoid concurrent use of grapefruit juice. Maintain adequate hydration, unless instructed to restrict fluid intake.
Herb/Nutraceutical: St John's wort may decrease diazepam levels. Yohimbe may decrease the effectiveness of diazepam. Kava kava, valerian, and gotu kola may increase CNS depression. Avoid St John's wort, yohimbe, kava kava, valerian, and gotu kola.

Pharmacodynamics/Kinetics

Onset of Action I.V.: Almost immediate; Oral: Rapid
Duration of Action I.V.: 20-30 minutes; Oral: Variable (dose and frequency dependent)
Half-life Elimination Parent drug: Adults: 20-50 hours; increased half-life in neonates, elderly, and those with severe hepatic disorders; Active major metabolite (desmethyldiazepam): 50-100 hours; may be prolonged in neonates
Time to Peak Oral: 15 minutes to 2 hours

Pregnancy Risk Factor D

Pregnancy Considerations Teratogenic effects have been reported in animal studies. In humans, diazepam and its metabolites (N-desmethyldiazepam, temazepam, and oxazepam) cross the placenta. Teratogenic effects have been observed with diazepam; however, additional studies are needed. The incidence of premature birth and low birth weights may be increased following maternal use of benzodiazepines; hypoglycemia and respiratory problems in the neonate may occur following exposure late in pregnancy. Neonatal withdrawal symptoms may occur within days to weeks after birth and "floppy infant syndrome" (which also includes withdrawal symptoms) has been reported with some benzodiazepines (including diazepam).

Lactation Enters breast milk/not recommended (AAP rates "of concern"; AAP 2001 update pending)

Breast-Feeding Considerations Diazepam and N-desmethyldiazepam can be found in breast milk; the oxazepam metabolite has also been detected in the urine of a nursing infant. Drowsiness, lethargy, or weight loss in nursing infants have been observed in case reports following maternal use of some benzodiazepines, including diazepam.

Controlled Substance C-IV

Dosage Forms

Gel, rectal: 10 mg (2 mL); 20 mg (4 mL); 5 mg/mL (0.5 mL)
Diastat®: 5 mg/mL (0.5 mL)
Diastat® AcuDial™: 10 mg (2 mL); 20 mg (4 mL)
Injection, solution: 5 mg/mL (2 mL, 10 mL)
Solution, oral: 5 mg/5 mL (5 mL, 500 mL)
Diazepam Intensol™: 5 mg/mL (30 mL)
Tablet, oral: 2 mg, 5 mg, 10 mg
Valium®: 2 mg, 5 mg, 10 mg

Diazoxide (dye az OKS ide)

Brand Names: U.S. Proglycem®
Brand Names: Canada Proglycem®
Pharmacologic Category Antidote, Hyperglycemia; Vasodilator, Direct-Acting
Use Hypoglycemia related to islet cell adenoma, carcinoma, hyperplasia, or adenomatosis; nesidioblastosis; leucine sensitivity; extrapancreatic malignancy
Local Anesthetic/Vasoconstrictor Precautions No information available to require special precautions
Effects on Dental Treatment No significant effects or complications reported
Effects on Bleeding No information available to require special precautions
Adverse Effects Frequency not defined.
Cardiovascular: Hypotension, palpitation, tachycardia
Central nervous system: Anxiety, dizziness, fever, headache, insomnia, malaise, polyneuritis
Dermatologic: Hirsutism, pruritus, purpura, rash, scalp hair loss
Endocrine & metabolic: Breast lump enlargement, diabetic ketoacidosis, fluid retention, galactorrhea, gout, hyperglycemia, hyperosmolar nonketotic coma, sodium retention
Gastrointestinal: Abdominal pain, anorexia, diarrhea, ileus, nausea, pancreatitis, pancreatic necrosis, taste loss (transient), vomiting
Hematologic: Bleeding (excessive), eosinophilia, hemoglobin/hematocrit decreased, neutropenia (transient), thrombocytopenia
Hepatic: Alkaline phosphatase increased, AST increased
Neuromuscular & skeletal: Weakness
Ocular: Blurred vision, cataracts (transient), diplopia, lacrimation, ring scotoma, subconjunctival hemorrhage
Renal: Albuminuria, azotemia, creatinine clearance decreased, glucosuria, hematuria, nephrotic syndrome (reversible), uric acid increased, urinary output decreased
Miscellaneous: Abnormal facial features (children with chronic use), IgG decreased, lymphadenopathy
General Dosage Range Oral:
Infants: 8-15 mg/kg/day in divided doses every 8-12 hours
Children and Adults: 3-8 mg/kg/day in divided doses every 8-12 hours
Mechanism of Action Activates potassium channels. Inhibits insulin release from the pancreas
Pharmacodynamics/Kinetics
Onset of Action Hyperglycemic: Oral: ~1 hour
Duration of Action Hyperglycemic: Oral: Normal renal function: 8 hours
Half-life Elimination Oral: Children: 9-24 hours; Adults: 24-36 hours
Pregnancy Risk Factor C
Pregnancy Considerations Adverse events have been observed in animal studies. Diazoxide crosses the human placenta. Altered carbohydrate metabolism, hyperbilirubinemia, or thrombocytopenia have been reported in the fetus or neonate. Alopecia and hypertrichosis lanuginosa have also been reported in infants following maternal use of diazoxide during the last 19-60 days of pregnancy.

Dibucaine (DYE byoo kane)

Brand Names: U.S. Nupercainal® [OTC]

Generic Availability (U.S.) Yes
Pharmacologic Category Local Anesthetic
Dental Use Amide derivative local anesthetic for minor skin conditions
Use Fast, temporary relief of pain and itching due to hemorrhoids, minor burns
Local Anesthetic/Vasoconstrictor Precautions No information available to require special precautions
Effects on Dental Treatment No significant effects or complications reported
Effects on Bleeding No information available to require special precautions
Adverse Effects 1% to 10%:
Dermatologic: Angioedema, contact dermatitis
Local: Burning
Dental Usual Dosage Local pain (local anesthetic): Children and Adults: Topical: Apply gently to the affected areas; no more than 30 g for adults or 7.5 g for children should be used in any 24-hour period
Dosage Children and Adults: Topical: Apply gently to the affected areas; no more than 30 g for adults or 7.5 g for children should be used in any 24-hour period
Mechanism of Action Local anesthetics bind selectively to the intracellular surface of sodium channels to block influx of sodium into the axon. As a result, depolarization necessary for action potential propagation and subsequent nerve function is prevented. The block at the sodium channel is reversible. When drug diffuses away from the axon, sodium channel function is restored and nerve propagation returns.
Contraindications Hypersensitivity to amide-type anesthetics, ophthalmic use
Warnings/Precautions When topical anesthetics are used prior to cosmetic or medical procedures, the lowest amount of anesthetic necessary for pain relief should be applied. High systemic levels and toxic effects (eg, methhemoglobinemia, irregular heart beats, respiratory depression, seizures, death) have been reported in patients who (without supervision of a trained professional) have applied topical anesthetics in large amounts (or to large areas of the skin), left these products on for prolonged periods of time, or have used wraps/dressings to cover the skin following application.
Drug Interactions
Metabolism/Transport Effects None known.
Avoid Concomitant Use There are no known interactions where it is recommended to avoid concomitant use.
Increased Effect/Toxicity There are no known significant interactions involving an increase in effect.
Decreased Effect There are no known significant interactions involving a decrease in effect.
Pharmacodynamics/Kinetics
Onset of Action ~15 minutes
Duration of Action 2-4 hours
Pregnancy Considerations Dibucaine is not absorbed systemically following topical administration on intact skin. Systemic absorption would be required in order for dibucaine to cross the placenta and reach the fetus.
Breast-Feeding Considerations No data reported; however, topical administration is probably compatible.
Dosage Forms
Ointment, topical: 1% [10 mg/g] (30 g, 454 g)
Nupercainal® [OTC]: 1% [10 mg/g] (30 g, 60 g)

Diclofenac (Systemic) (dye KLOE fen ak)

Related Information
Rheumatoid Arthritis, Osteoarthritis, and Osteoporosis on page 1526
Temporomandibular Dysfunction (TMD), Chronic Pain, and Fibromyalgia on page 1590

Brand Names: U.S. Cambia™; Cataflam®; Voltaren®-XR; Zipsor®

Brand Names: Canada Apo-Diclo Rapide®; Apo-Diclo®; Apo-Diclo® SR®; Ava-Diclofenac; Ava-Diclofenac SR; Cambia®; Cataflam®; Diclofenac ECT; Diclofenac Sodium; Diclofenac Sodium SR; Diclofenac SR; Dom-Diclofenac; Dom-Diclofenac SR; NTP-Diclofenac; NTP-Diclofenac SR; Nu-Diclo; Nu-Diclo-SR; PMS-Diclofenac; PMS-Diclofenac SR; PMS-Diclofenac-K; PRO-Diclo-Rapide; Sandoz-Diclofenac; Sandoz-Diclofenac Rapide; Sandoz-Diclofenac SR; Teva-Diclofenac; Teva-Diclofenac K; Teva-Diclofenac SR; Voltaren Rapide®; Voltaren SR®; Voltaren®

Generic Availability (U.S.) Yes: Excludes capsule, oral solution

Pharmacologic Category Nonsteroidal Anti-inflammatory Drug (NSAID); Nonsteroidal Anti-inflammatory Drug (NSAID), Oral

Dental Use Immediate-release tablets: Acute treatment of mild-to-moderate pain

Use
Capsule: Relief of mild-to-moderate acute pain
Immediate-release tablet: Relief of mild-to-moderate pain; primary dysmenorrhea; acute and chronic treatment of rheumatoid arthritis, osteoarthritis
Delayed-release tablet: Acute and chronic treatment of rheumatoid arthritis, osteoarthritis, ankylosing spondylitis
Extended-release tablet: Chronic treatment of osteoarthritis, rheumatoid arthritis
Oral solution: Treatment of acute migraine with or without aura
Suppository (CAN; not available in U.S.): Symptomatic treatment of rheumatoid arthritis and osteoarthritis (including degenerative joint disease of hip)

Unlabeled Use Juvenile idiopathic arthritis (JIA)

Local Anesthetic/Vasoconstrictor Precautions No information available to require special precautions

Effects on Dental Treatment The dentist should be aware of the potential of abnormal coagulation. Caution should also be exercised in the use of NSAIDs in patients already on anticoagulant therapy with drugs such as warfarin (Coumadin®). See Effects on Bleeding.

Effects on Bleeding Nonselective NSAIDs such as diclofenac (systemic) inhibit platelet aggregation and prolong bleeding time in some patients. Unlike aspirin, the NSAID effect on platelet function is quantitatively less, of shorter duration, and reversible. Normal platelet function should occur in ~5 elimination half-lives or in <10 hours after discontinuation of diclofenac (systemic). Concomitant use of other NSAIDs should be avoided.

Adverse Effects
Oral:
1% to 10%:
Cardiovascular: Edema
Central nervous system: Dizziness, headache
Dermatologic: Pruritus, rash
Endocrine & metabolic: Fluid retention

Gastrointestinal: Abdominal distension, abdominal pain, constipation, diarrhea, dyspepsia, flatulence, GI perforation, heartburn, nausea, peptic ulcer/GI bleed, vomiting
Hematologic: Anemia, bleeding time increased
Hepatic: Liver enzyme abnormalities (>3 x ULN; ≤4%)
Otic: Tinnitus
Renal: Renal function abnormal
Miscellaneous: Diaphoresis increased

Rectal suppository (CAN; not available in U.S.): Also refer to adverse reactions associated with oral formulations.

Dental Usual Dosage Pain: Adults: Oral: Starting dose: 50 mg 3 times/day; maximum dose: 150 mg/day

Dosage Adults:
Oral:
Analgesia:
Immediate release tablet: Starting dose: 50 mg 3 times/day (maximum dose: 150 mg/day); may administer 100 mg loading dose, followed by 50 mg every 8 hours (maximum dose day 1: 200 mg/day; maximum dose day 2 and thereafter: 150 mg/day)
Canadian labeling: Maximum loading dose day 1: 200 mg/day; maximum dose day 2 and up to 7 days: 150 mg/day (50 mg every 6-8 hours)
Immediate release capsule: 25 mg 4 times/day
Primary dysmenorrhea: Immediate release tablet: Starting dose: 50 mg 3 times/day (maximum dose: 150 mg/day); may administer 100 mg loading dose, followed by 50 mg every 8 hours (maximum dose day 1: 200 mg/day; maximum dose day 2 and thereafter: 150 mg/day)
Canadian labeling: Maximum loading dose day 1: 200 mg/day; maximum dose day 2 and up to 7 days: 150 mg/day (50 mg every 6-8 hours)
Rheumatoid arthritis: Immediate release tablet: 150-200 mg/day in 3-4 divided doses; Delayed release tablet: 150-200 mg/day in 2-4 divided doses; Extended release tablet: 100 mg/day (may increase dose to 200 mg/day in 2 divided doses)
Canadian labeling: 150 mg/day in 3 divided doses (75-150 mg/day of slow release tablet)
Osteoarthritis: Immediate or delayed release tablet: 100-150 mg/day in 2-3 divided doses; Extended release tablet: 100 mg/day
Canadian labeling: 150 mg/day in 3 divided doses (75-150 mg/day of slow release tablet)
Ankylosing spondylitis: Delayed release tablet: 100-125 mg/day in 4-5 divided doses
Migraine: Oral solution: 50 mg (one packet) as a single dose at the time of migraine onset; safety and efficacy of a second dose have not been established
Rectal suppository (not available in U.S.):
Osteoarthritis: Canadian labeling: Insert 50 mg or 100 mg suppository rectally as single dose to substitute for final (third) oral daily dose; maximum combined dose (rectal and oral): 150 mg/day
Rheumatoid arthritis: Canadian labeling: Insert 50 mg or 100 mg suppository rectally as single dose to substitute for final (third) oral daily dose (maximum combined dose [rectal and oral]: 150 mg/day)

Dosage adjustment in renal impairment: Not recommended in patients with advanced renal disease or significant renal impairment

Dosage adjustment in hepatic impairment: May require dosage adjustment; use oral solution only if benefits outweigh risks

Elderly: No specific dosing recommendations; elderly may demonstrate adverse effects at lower doses than younger adults, and >60% may develop asymptomatic peptic ulceration with or without hemorrhage; monitor renal function

Mechanism of Action Reversibly inhibits cyclooxygenase-1 and 2 (COX-1 and 2) enzymes, which results in decreased formation of prostaglandin precursors; has antipyretic, analgesic, and anti-inflammatory properties

Other proposed mechanisms not fully elucidated (and possibly contributing to the anti-inflammatory effect to varying degrees), include inhibiting chemotaxis, altering lymphocyte activity, inhibiting neutrophil aggregation/activation, and decreasing proinflammatory cytokine levels.

Contraindications Hypersensitivity to diclofenac or any component of the formulation; hypersensitivity to bovine protein (capsule formulation only); patients who exhibit asthma, urticaria, or other allergic-type reactions after taking aspirin or other NSAIDs; perioperative pain in the setting of coronary artery bypass graft (CABG) surgery

Canadian labeling: Additional contraindications (not in U.S. labeling): Uncontrolled heart failure, active gastric/duodenal/peptic ulcer; active GI bleed or perforation; regional ulcer, gastritis, or ulcerative colitis; cerebrovascular bleeding or other bleeding disorders; inflammatory bowel disease; severe hepatic impairment; active hepatic disease; severe renal impairment (Cl_{cr} <30 mL/minute) or deteriorating renal disease; known hyperkalemia; patients <16 years of age; breast-feeding; pregnancy (third trimester); use of diclofenac suppository if recent history of bleeding or inflammatory lesions of rectum/anus

Warnings/Precautions [U.S. Boxed Warning]: NSAIDs are associated with an increased risk of adverse cardiovascular thrombotic events, including MI and stroke. Risk may be increased with duration of use or pre-existing cardiovascular risk factors or disease. Carefully evaluate individual cardiovascular risk profiles prior to prescribing. May cause new-onset hypertension or worsening of existing hypertension. Monitor blood pressure closely. Use caution with fluid retention. Avoid use in heart failure. Concurrent administration of ibuprofen, and potentially other nonselective NSAIDs, may interfere with aspirin's cardioprotective effect. **[U.S. Boxed Warning]: Use is contraindicated for treatment of perioperative pain in the setting of coronary artery bypass graft (CABG) surgery.** Risk of MI and stroke may be increased with use following CABG surgery.

NSAID use may compromise existing renal function; dose-dependent decreases in prostaglandin synthesis may result from NSAID use, reducing renal blood flow which may cause renal decompensation. NSAID use may increase the risk for hyperkalemia. Patients with impaired renal function, dehydration, heart failure, liver dysfunction, those taking diuretics and ACEI, and the elderly are at greater risk of renal toxicity and hyperkalemia. Rehydrate patient before starting therapy; monitor renal function closely. Not recommended for use in patients with advanced renal disease. Long-term NSAID use may result in renal papillary necrosis while persistent urinary symptoms (eg, dysuria, bladder pain), cystitis, or hematuria may occur anytime after initiating NSAID therapy. Discontinue therapy with symptom onset and evaluate for origin.

[U.S. Boxed Warning]: NSAIDs may increase risk of gastrointestinal irritation, inflammation, ulceration, bleeding, and perforation. These events may occur at any time during therapy and without warning. Use caution with a history of GI disease (bleeding or ulcers), concurrent therapy with aspirin, anticoagulants and/or corticosteroids, smoking, use of alcohol, the elderly or debilitated patients. When used concomitantly with ≤325 mg of aspirin, a substantial increase in the risk of gastrointestinal complications (eg, ulcer) occurs; concomitant gastroprotective therapy (eg, proton pump inhibitors) is recommended (Bhatt, 2008).

Use the lowest effective dose for the shortest duration of time, consistent with individual patient goals, to reduce risk of cardiovascular or GI adverse events. Alternate therapies should be considered for patients at high risk.

NSAIDs may cause photosensitivity or serious skin adverse events including exfoliative dermatitis, Stevens-Johnson syndrome (SJS), and toxic epidermal necrolysis (TEN); discontinue use at first sign of skin rash or hypersensitivity. Anaphylactoid reactions may occur, even without prior exposure; patients with "aspirin triad" (bronchial asthma, aspirin intolerance, rhinitis) may be at increased risk. Do not use in patients who experience bronchospasm, asthma, rhinitis, or urticaria with NSAID or aspirin therapy. Use caution in other forms of asthma. Platelet adhesion and aggregation may be decreased; may prolong bleeding time; patients with coagulation disorders or who are receiving anticoagulants should be monitored closely. Anemia may occur; patients on long-term NSAID therapy should be monitored for anemia. Rarely, NSAID use may cause severe blood dyscrasias (eg, agranulocytosis, aplastic anemia, thrombocytopenia).

Use with caution in patients with impaired hepatic function. Closely monitor patients with any abnormal LFT. Diclofenac can cause transaminase elevations; initiate monitoring 4-8 weeks into therapy. Rarely, severe hepatic reactions (eg, fulminant hepatitis, liver failure) have occurred; discontinue all formulations if signs or symptoms of liver disease develop, or if systemic manifestations occur. Use with caution in hepatic porphyria (may trigger attack).

NSAIDS may cause drowsiness, dizziness, blurred vision, and other neurologic effects which may impair physical or mental abilities; patients must be cautioned about performing tasks which require mental alertness (eg, operating machinery or driving). Discontinue use with blurred or diminished vision and perform ophthalmologic exam. Monitor vision with long-term therapy. May increase the risk of aseptic meningitis, especially in patients with systemic lupus erythematosus (SLE) and mixed connective tissue disorders. In the elderly, avoid chronic use (unless alternative agents ineffective and patient can receive concomitant gastroprotective agent); nonselective oral NSAID use is associated with an increased risk of GI bleeding and peptic ulcer disease in older adults in high risk category (eg, >75 years or age or receiving concomitant oral/parenteral corticosteroids, anticoagulants, or antiplatelet agents) (Beers Criteria).

Withhold for at least 4-6 half-lives prior to surgical or dental procedures. Safety and efficacy have not been established in children.

Capsule: Contains gelatin; use is contraindicated in patients with history of hypersensitivity to bovine protein.

Oral solution: Only indicated for the acute treatment of migraine; not indicated for migraine prophylaxis or cluster headache. Not bioequivalent to other forms of diclofenac (even same dose); do not interchange products. Contains phenylalanine.

Drug Interactions

Metabolism/Transport Effects Substrate of CYP1A2 (minor), CYP2B6 (minor), CYP2C19 (minor), CYP2C8 (minor), CYP2C9 (minor), CYP2D6 (minor), CYP3A4 (minor); **Note:** Assignment of Major/Minor substrate status based on clinically relevant drug interaction potential; **Inhibits** CYP1A2 (weak), CYP2C9 (weak), CYP2E1 (weak), CYP3A4 (weak), UGT1A6

Avoid Concomitant Use

Avoid concomitant use of Diclofenac (Systemic) with any of the following: Floctafenine; Ketorolac (Nasal); Ketorolac (Systemic); NSAID (COX-2 Inhibitor); Omacetaxine; Pimozide

Increased Effect/Toxicity

Diclofenac (Systemic) may increase the levels/effects of: Agents with Antiplatelet Properties; Aliskiren; Aminoglycosides; Anticoagulants; ARIPiprazole; Bisphosphonate Derivatives; Collagenase (Systemic); CycloSPORINE (Systemic); Dabigatran Etexilate; Deferasirox; Deferiprone; Desmopressin; Digoxin; Drotrecogin Alfa (Activated); Eplerenone; Haloperidol; Ibritumomab; Lithium; Lomitapide; Methotrexate; Nonsteroidal Anti-Inflammatory Agents; NSAID (COX-2 Inhibitor); Omacetaxine; PEMEtrexed; Pimozide; Porfimer; Potassium-Sparing Diuretics; PRALAtrexate; Quinolone Antibiotics; Rivaroxaban; Salicylates; Thrombolytic Agents; Tositumomab and Iodine I 131 Tositumomab; Vancomycin; Vitamin K Antagonists

The levels/effects of Diclofenac (Systemic) may be increased by: ACE Inhibitors; Angiotensin II Receptor Blockers; Antidepressants (Tricyclic, Tertiary Amine); Corticosteroids (Systemic); CycloSPORINE (Systemic); CYP2C9 Inhibitors (Strong); Dasatinib; Floctafenine; Glucosamine; Herbs (Anticoagulant/Antiplatelet Properties); Ketorolac (Nasal); Ketorolac (Systemic); Multivitamins/Minerals (with ADEK, Folate, Iron); Nonsteroidal Anti-Inflammatory Agents; Omega-3 Fatty Acids; Pentosan Polysulfate Sodium; Pentoxifylline; Probenecid; Prostacyclin Analogues; Selective Serotonin Reuptake Inhibitors; Serotonin/Norepinephrine Reuptake Inhibitors; Sodium Phosphates; Tipranavir; Treprostinil; Vitamin E; Voriconazole

Decreased Effect

Diclofenac (Systemic) may decrease the levels/effects of: ACE Inhibitors; Agents with Antiplatelet Properties; Aliskiren; Angiotensin II Receptor Blockers; Beta-Blockers; Eplerenone; HydrALAZINE; Loop Diuretics; Potassium-Sparing Diuretics; Salicylates; Selective Serotonin Reuptake Inhibitors; Thiazide Diuretics

The levels/effects of Diclofenac (Systemic) may be decreased by: Bile Acid Sequestrants; CYP2C9 Inducers (Strong); Nonsteroidal Anti-Inflammatory Agents; Peginterferon Alfa-2b; Salicylates

Ethanol/Nutrition/Herb Interactions

Ethanol: Avoid ethanol (may enhance gastric mucosal irritation).

Herb/Nutraceutical: Avoid alfalfa, anise, bilberry, bladderwrack, bromelain, cat's claw, celery, chamomile, coleus, cordyceps, dong quai, evening primrose, fenugreek, feverfew, garlic, ginger, ginkgo biloba, grapeseed, green tea, ginseng (Siberian), guggul, horse chestnut, horseradish, licorice, prickly ash, red clover, reishi, SAMe (s-adenosylmethionine), sweet clover, turmeric, white willow (all have additional antiplatelet activity).

Dietary Considerations Oral formulations may be taken with food to decrease GI distress. Food may reduce effectiveness of oral solution. Some products may contain phenylalanine.

Diclofenac potassium = Cataflam®; potassium content: 5.8 mg (0.15 mEq) per 50 mg tablet

Pharmacodynamics/Kinetics

Onset of Action

Cataflam® (potassium salt) is more rapid than the sodium salt because it dissolves in the stomach instead of the duodenum

Suppository: more rapid onset, but slower rate of absorption when compared to enteric coated tablet

Half-life Elimination ~2 hours

Time to Peak Serum:

Cambia™: ~0.25 hours

Cataflam®: ~1 hour

Voltaren® XR ~5 hours

Zipsor®: ~0.5 hour

Suppository: ≤1 hour; **Note:** Suppository: C_{max}: Approximately two-thirds of that observed with enteric coated tablet (equivalent 50 mg dose)

Tablet, delayed release (diclofenac sodium): ~2 hours

Pregnancy Risk Factor C (oral)/D (≥30 weeks gestation [oral])

Pregnancy Considerations Adverse events were not observed in the initial animal reproduction studies; therefore, manufacturers classify most dosage forms of diclofenac as pregnancy category C (oral: Category D ≥30 weeks gestation). Diclofenac crosses the placenta and can be detected in fetal tissue and amniotic fluid. NSAID exposure during the first trimester is not strongly associated with congenital malformations; however, cardiovascular anomalies and cleft palate have been observed following NSAID exposure in some studies. The use of a NSAID close to conception may be associated with an increased risk of miscarriage. Nonteratogenic effects have been observed following NSAID administration during the third trimester including: Myocardial degenerative changes, prenatal constriction of the ductus arteriosus, fetal tricuspid regurgitation, failure of the ductus arteriosus to close postnatally; renal dysfunction or failure, oligohydramnios; gastrointestinal bleeding or perforation, increased risk of necrotizing enterocolitis; intracranial bleeding (including intraventricular hemorrhage), platelet dysfunction with resultant bleeding; pulmonary hypertension. Because they may cause premature closure of the ductus arteriosus, use of NSAIDs late in pregnancy should be avoided (use after 31 or 32 weeks gestation is not recommended by some clinicians). Product labeling for Zipsor® specifically notes that use at ≥30 weeks gestation should be avoided and, therefore, classifies diclofenac as pregnancy category D at this time. Use in the third trimester is contraindicated in the Canadian labeling. The chronic use of NSAIDs in women of reproductive age may be associated with infertility that is reversible upon discontinuation of the medication. A registry is available for pregnant women exposed to autoimmune medications including diclofenac. For additional information contact the Organization of Teratology ▶

◀ Information Specialists, OTIS Autoimmune Diseases Study, at 877-311-8972

Lactation Excreted in breast milk/not recommended

Breast-Feeding Considerations Low concentrations of diclofenac can be found in breast milk. Breast-feeding is not recommended by the manufacturer. Use while breast-feeding is contraindicated in Canadian labeling.

Dosage Forms

Capsule, liquid filled, oral:
Zipsor®: 25 mg

Powder for solution, oral:
Cambia™: 50 mg/packet (1s)

Tablet, oral: 50 mg
Cataflam®: 50 mg

Tablet, delayed release, enteric coated, oral: 25 mg, 50 mg, 75 mg

Tablet, extended release, oral: 100 mg
Voltaren®-XR: 100 mg

Dosage Forms: Canada
Suppository:
Voltaren®: 50 mg, 100mg

References

Kubitzek F, Ziegler G, Gold MS, et al, "Analgesic Efficacy of Low-Dose Diclofenac Versus Paracetamol and Placebo in Postoperative Dental Pain," *J Orofac Pain*, 2003, 17(3):237-44.

Diclofenac (Topical) (dye KLOE fen ak)

Brand Names: U.S. Flector®; Pennsaid®; Solaraze®; Voltaren® Gel

Brand Names: Canada Pennsaid®; Voltaren® Emul-gel™

Pharmacologic Category Nonsteroidal Anti-inflammatory Drug (NSAID); Nonsteroidal Anti-inflammatory Drug (NSAID), Topical

Use
Topical gel 1%: Relief of osteoarthritis pain in joints amenable to topical therapy (eg, ankle, elbow, foot, hand, knee, wrist)
Canadian labeling (not in U.S. labeling): Relief of pain associated with acute, localized joint/muscle injuries (eg, sports injuries, strains) in patients ≥16 years of age
Topical gel 3%: Actinic keratosis (AK) in conjunction with sun avoidance
Topical patch: Acute pain due to minor strains, sprains, and contusions
Topical solution: Relief of osteoarthritis pain of the knee

Local Anesthetic/Vasoconstrictor Precautions No information available to require special precautions

Effects on Dental Treatment No significant effects or complications reported

Effects on Bleeding No information available to require special precautions

Adverse Effects

Topical gel:
>10%: Local: Application site reactions (incidence increased with 3% gel): Pruritus (≤52%), rash (35% to 46%), contact dermatitis (4% to 33%), dry skin (≤27%), pain (15% to 26%), exfoliation (3% gel; 6% to 24%), paresthesia (≤20%)
1% to 10% (reported for 3% gel):
Cardiovascular: Chest pain, hypertension
Central nervous system: Headache, pain
Dermatologic: Pruritus, rash, skin ulcer
Endocrine & metabolic: Hypercholesterolemia, hyperglycemia
Gastrointestinal: Abdominal pain, diarrhea, dyspepsia
Hepatic: Liver enzymes increased
Local: Alopecia, edema, photosensitivity

Neuromuscular and skeletal: Arthralgia, arthrosis, back pain, CPK increased, hypokinesia, myalgia, neck pain, weakness
Ocular: Conjunctivitis
Renal: Hematuria
Respiratory: Asthma, dyspnea, pneumonia, sinusitis
Miscellaneous: Flu-like syndrome

Topical solution:
>10%: Dermatologic: Dry skin (application site 32%; nonapplication site 2%)
1% to 10%:
Cardiovascular: Edema (3%)
Dermatologic: Contact dermatitis (2% to 9%), rash (3%), bruising (2%), pruritus (application site 4%; nonapplication site 2%)
Gastrointestinal: Dyspepsia (8%), abdominal pain (6%), diarrhea (4%), flatulence (4%), nausea (4%), constipation (3%), halitosis (1%)
Neuromuscular & skeletal: Paresthesia (2%)
Respiratory: Sinusitis (1%)
Miscellaneous: Infection (3%)

Transdermal patch:
1% to 10%:
Central nervous system: Dizziness, hypoesthesia
Dermatologic: Dermatitis (2%), dermal allergic reaction
Gastrointestinal: Nausea (3%), dysgeusia (2%), abdominal pain, constipation, diarrhea, gastritis, vomiting, xerostomia
Local: Application site dryness, irritation, erythema, atrophy, discoloration, hyperhidrosis, and vesicles, edema, itching
Neuromuscular & skeletal: Hyperkinesia

General Dosage Range Topical: *Adults:*
1% gel: Apply 2-4 g to affected joint 4 times/day (maximum: 16 g/day single joint of lower extremity, 8 g/day single joint of upper extremity); Maximum total body dose of 1% gel should not exceed 32 g per day.
3% gel: Apply to lesion area twice daily
Patch: Apply 1 patch twice daily
Solution: Apply 40 drops to each affected knee 4 times/day

Pharmacodynamics/Kinetics

Half-life Elimination Patch: ~12 hours

Time to Peak Serum: Flector®: 10-20 hours; Pennsaid®: 5-17 hours; Solaraze® Gel: ~5 hours; Voltaren® Gel: 10-14 hours

Pregnancy Risk Factor B (topical gel 3%) / C (topical gel 1%, topical solution, topical patch) / D (topical solution ≥30 weeks gestation)

Pregnancy Considerations Adverse events have been observed in some animal studies; therefore, the pregnancy category is product dependent (B topical gel 3%; C topical gel 1% and topical patch). When administered orally, diclofenac crosses the placenta. The amount of diclofenac available systemically following topical application is less in comparison to oral doses. Because it may cause prenatal constriction of the ductus arteriosus, the use of diclofenac topical late in pregnancy should be avoided. Reversible constriction of the ductus arteriosus *in utero* has been observed following topical application of diclofenac. Additional adverse fetal and maternal effects have been observed following oral use of diclofenac. Refer to the Diclofenac (Systemic) monograph for details. A registry is available for pregnant women exposed to autoimmune medications including diclofenac. For additional information contact the Organization of Teratology Information Specialists, OTIS Autoimmune Diseases Study, at 877-311-8972.

Diclofenac and Misoprostol
(dye KLOE fen ak & mye soe PROST ole)

Related Information
Diclofenac (Systemic) *on page 413*
Misoprostol *on page 930*
Rheumatoid Arthritis, Osteoarthritis, and Osteoporosis *on page 1526*
Brand Names: U.S. Arthrotec®
Brand Names: Canada Arthrotec®
Pharmacologic Category Nonsteroidal Anti-inflammatory Drug (NSAID), Oral; Prostaglandin
Use Treatment of osteoarthritis and rheumatoid arthritis in patients at high risk for NSAID-induced gastric and duodenal ulceration
Local Anesthetic/Vasoconstrictor Precautions No information available to require special precautions
Effects on Dental Treatment The dentist should be aware of the potential of abnormal coagulation. Caution should also be exercised in the use of NSAIDs in patients already on anticoagulant therapy with drugs such as warfarin (Coumadin®). See Effects on Bleeding.
Effects on Bleeding Nonselective NSAIDs, such as diclofenac, inhibit platelet aggregation and prolong bleeding time in some patients. Unlike aspirin, the NSAID effect on platelet function is quantitatively less, of shorter duration, and reversible.
Adverse Effects Percentages reported with combination product. Also see individual agents.
>10%: Gastrointestinal: Abdominal pain (21%), diarrhea (19%), dyspepsia (14%), nausea (11%)
1% to 10%: Gastrointestinal: Flatulence (9%)
General Dosage Range Oral: *Adults:* Arthrotec® 50: One tablet 2-4 times/day; Arthrotec® 75: One tablet twice daily
Mechanism of Action See individual agents.
Pregnancy Risk Factor X
Pregnancy Considerations Teratogenic effects were not observed with this combination in animal reproduction studies; however, adverse fetal events have been observed following *in utero* exposure to both diclofenac and misoprostol in human pregnancy. **[U.S. Boxed Warning]: Not to be used to reduce NSAID-induced ulcers in women of childbearing potential unless woman is capable of complying with effective contraceptive measures.** Do not use in women of childbearing potential without a negative serum pregnancy test within 2 weeks prior to therapy; therapy is normally begun on the second or third day of next normal menstrual period. Use to prevent NSAID-induced ulcers is contraindicated in pregnant women. Written and verbal warnings concerning the hazards of misoprostol should be provided. Also refer to individual monographs for Diclofenac and Misoprostol for additional information.

Dicloxacillin (dye kloks a SIL in)

Related Information
Bacterial Infections *on page 1562*
Generic Availability (U.S.) Yes
Pharmacologic Category Antibiotic, Penicillin
Dental Use Treatment of susceptible orofacial infections (notably penicillinase-producing staphylococci)
Use Treatment of systemic infections such as pneumonia, skin and soft tissue infections, and osteomyelitis caused by penicillinase-producing staphylococci

Local Anesthetic/Vasoconstrictor Precautions No information available to require special precautions
Effects on Dental Treatment Key adverse event(s) related to dental treatment: Prolonged use of penicillins may lead to development of oral candidiasis.
Effects on Bleeding Thrombocytopenia has been reported.
Adverse Effects 1% to 10%: Gastrointestinal: Nausea, diarrhea, abdominal pain
Dental Usual Dosage Susceptible orofacial infections: Children >40 kg and Adults: 125-250 mg every 6 hours
Dosage
Usual dosage range:
Newborns: Use not recommended
Children <40 kg: Oral: 12.5-100 mg/kg/day divided every 6 hours
Children >40 kg: Oral: 125-250 mg every 6 hours
Adults: Oral: 125-1000 mg every 6 hours
Indication-specific dosing:
Children: Oral:
Furunculosis: 25-50 mg/kg/day divided every 6 hours
Osteomyelitis: 50-100 mg/kg/day in divided doses every 6 hours
Adults: Oral:
Erysipelas, furunculosis, mastitis, otitis externa, septic bursitis, skin abscess: 500 mg every 6 hours
Impetigo: 250 mg every 6 hours
Prosthetic joint infection: Chronic suppression therapy: Staphylococci (oxacillin-susceptible) (unlabeled regimen): 500 mg every 6-8 hours (Osmon, 2013)
***Staphylococcus aureus,* methicillin susceptible infection if no I.V. access:** 500-1000 mg every 6-8 hours

Dosage adjustment in renal impairment: No specific adjustment provided in manufacturer's labeling; a reduction in total dosage should be considered in renal impairment.
Hemodialysis: Not dialyzable (0% to 5%); supplemental dosage not necessary
Peritoneal dialysis: Supplemental dosage not necessary
Continuous arteriovenous or venovenous hemofiltration: Supplemental dosage not necessary
Dosage adjustment in hepatic impairment: No dosage adjustment provided in manufacturer's labeling.
Mechanism of Action Inhibits bacterial cell wall synthesis by binding to one or more of the penicillin-binding proteins (PBPs) which in turn inhibits the final transpeptidation step of peptidoglycan synthesis in bacterial cell walls, thus inhibiting cell wall biosynthesis. Bacteria eventually lyse due to ongoing activity of cell wall autolytic enzymes (autolysins and murein hydrolases) while cell wall assembly is arrested.
Contraindications Hypersensitivity to dicloxacillin, penicillin, or any component of the formulation
Warnings/Precautions Monitor PT if patient concurrently on warfarin. Use with caution in neonates; elimination of drug is slow. Serious and occasionally severe or fatal hypersensitivity (anaphylactoid) reactions have been reported in patients on penicillin therapy, especially with a history of beta-lactam hypersensitivity, history of sensitivity to multiple allergens, or previous IgE-mediated reactions (eg, anaphylaxis, angioedema, urticaria). Use with caution in asthmatic patients. Prolonged use may result in fungal or bacterial superinfection, including *C. difficile*-associated diarrhea and pseudomembranous colitis.

Drug Interactions

Metabolism/Transport Effects Induces CYP3A4 (weak/moderate)

Avoid Concomitant Use

Avoid concomitant use of Dicloxacillin with any of the following: Axitinib; BCG

Increased Effect/Toxicity

Dicloxacillin may increase the levels/effects of: Methotrexate; Vitamin K Antagonists

The levels/effects of Dicloxacillin may be increased by: Probenecid

Decreased Effect

Dicloxacillin may decrease the levels/effects of: ARIPiprazole; Axitinib; BCG; Mycophenolate; Saxagliptin; Sodium Picosulfate; Typhoid Vaccine; Vitamin K Antagonists

The levels/effects of Dicloxacillin may be decreased by: Fusidic Acid; Tetracycline Derivatives

Ethanol/Nutrition/Herb Interactions Food: Food decreases drug absorption rate and serum concentration. Management: Administer around-the-clock on an empty stomach with a large glass of water 1 hour before or 2 hours after meals.

Dietary Considerations Administer on an empty stomach 1 hour before or 2 hours after meals. Some products may contain sodium.

Pharmacodynamics/Kinetics

Half-life Elimination 0.6-0.8 hour; slightly prolonged with renal impairment

Time to Peak Serum: 0.5-2 hours

Pregnancy Risk Factor B

Pregnancy Considerations Adverse events have not been observed in animal studies; therefore, dicloxacillin is classified as pregnancy category B. Dicloxacillin crosses the placenta. Teratogenic effects have not been reported with dicloxacillin, but adequate and well-controlled studies of dicloxacillin have not been completed in pregnant women. Other penicillins are considered safe for use in pregnancy.

Lactation Excretion in breast milk unknown/use caution

Breast-Feeding Considerations It is not known if dicloxacillin crosses into human milk. The manufacturer recommends that caution be exercised when administering dicloxacillin to nursing women. Other penicillins distribute into human milk and are considered safe for use during breast-feeding. Nondose-related effects could include modification of bowel flora.

Dosage Forms

Capsule, oral: 250 mg, 500 mg

Dicyclomine (dye SYE kloe meen)

Brand Names: U.S. Bentyl®

Brand Names: Canada Bentylol®; Dicyclomine Hydrochloride Injection; Formulex®; Jamp-Dicyclomine; Protylol; Riva-Dicyclomine

Pharmacologic Category Anticholinergic Agent

Use Treatment of functional bowel/irritable bowel syndrome

Local Anesthetic/Vasoconstrictor Precautions No information available to require special precautions

Effects on Dental Treatment Key adverse event(s) related to dental treatment: Xerostomia and changes in salivation (normal salivary flow resumes upon discontinuation)

Effects on Bleeding No information available to require special precautions

Adverse Effects

>10%:

Central nervous system: Dizziness (40%)

Gastrointestinal: Xerostomia (33%), nausea (14%)

Ocular: Blurred vision (27%)

1% to 10%:

Central nervous system: Somnolence (9%), nervousness (6%)

Neuromuscular & skeletal: Weakness (7%)

General Dosage Range

I.M.: Adults: 10-20 mg 4 times daily

Oral: Adults: Initial: 20 mg 4 times daily; may increase to 40 mg 4 times daily

Mechanism of Action Blocks the action of acetylcholine at parasympathetic sites in smooth muscle, secretory glands and the CNS

Pharmacodynamics/Kinetics

Half-life Elimination Initial phase: ~1.8 hours; Terminal phase: Undetermined, but somewhat longer than the initial phase

Time to Peak Oral: 60-90 minutes

Pregnancy Risk Factor B

Pregnancy Considerations Teratogenic effects have not been observed in animal reproduction studies. In epidemiologic studies, birth defects were not observed in pregnant women taking doses up to 40 mg daily; information has not been located when used in pregnant women at recommended doses (80-160 mg daily). Use for the treatment of irritable bowel syndrome (IBS) is not recommended during pregnancy (Mahadevan, 2006).

Didanosine (dye DAN oh seen)

Related Information

HIV Infection and AIDS on page 1520

Brand Names: U.S. Videx®; Videx® EC

Brand Names: Canada Videx®; Videx® EC

Pharmacologic Category Antiretroviral Agent, Reverse Transcriptase Inhibitor (Nucleoside)

Use Treatment of HIV infection; always to be used in combination with at least two other antiretroviral agents

Local Anesthetic/Vasoconstrictor Precautions No information available to require special precautions

Effects on Dental Treatment Key adverse event(s) related to dental treatment: Xerostomia (normal salivary flow resumes upon discontinuation).

Effects on Bleeding Thrombocytopenia has been reported in <1% of patients treated.

Adverse Effects As reported in monotherapy studies; risk of toxicity may increase when combined with other agents.

>10%:

Gastrointestinal: Diarrhea (19% to 28%), amylase increased (15% to 17%), abdominal pain (7% to 13%)

Neuromuscular & skeletal: Peripheral neuropathy (17% to 20%)

1% to 10%:

Dermatologic: Rash/pruritus (7% to 9%)

Endocrine & metabolic: Uric acid increased (2% to 3%)

Gastrointestinal: Pancreatitis (1% to 7% dose dependent); patients >65 years of age had a higher frequency of pancreatitis than younger patients patients (10% vs 5% in younger patients)

Hepatic: AST increased (7% to 9%), ALT increased (6% to 9%), alkaline phosphatase increased (1% to 4%)

General Dosage Range Dosage adjustment recommended in patients with renal impairment

Oral:

Delayed release:

Children ≥6 years and 20 kg to <25 kg: 200 mg once daily

Children ≥6 years and 25 kg to <60 kg and Adults <60 kg: 250 mg once daily

Children and Adults ≥60 kg: 400 mg once daily

Pediatric powder for oral solution (Videx®):

Infants 2 weeks to 8 months: 100 mg/m² twice daily

Children >8 months to 18 years: 120 mg/m² twice daily

Adolescents and Adults <60 kg: 125 mg twice daily **or** 250 mg once daily

Adolescents and Adults ≥60 kg: 200 mg twice daily **or** 400 mg once daily

Mechanism of Action Didanosine, a purine nucleoside (adenosine) analog and the deamination product of dideoxyadenosine (ddA), inhibits HIV replication *in vitro* in both T cells and monocytes. Didanosine is converted within the cell to the mono-, di-, and triphosphates of ddA. These ddA triphosphates act as substrate and inhibitor of HIV reverse transcriptase substrate and inhibitor of HIV reverse transcriptase thereby blocking viral DNA synthesis and suppressing HIV replication.

Pharmacodynamics/Kinetics

Half-life Elimination

Children and Adolescents: 0.8 hour

Adults: Normal renal function: 1.5 hours; however, active metabolite, ddATP, has an intracellular half-life >12 hours *in vitro*; Renal impairment: 2.5-5 hours

Time to Peak Delayed release capsules: 2 hours; Powder for suspension: 0.25-1.5 hours

Pregnancy Risk Factor B

Pregnancy Considerations Adverse events have not been observed in animal reproduction studies. Didanosine has been shown to cross the placenta. Based on data from the Antiretroviral Pregnancy Registry, an increased rate of birth defects has been observed following maternal use of didanosine during pregnancy; no pattern of defects has been observed and clinical relevance is uncertain. Pharmacokinetics are not significantly altered during pregnancy; dose adjustments are not needed. Cases of lactic acidosis/hepatic steatosis syndrome related to mitochondrial toxicity have been reported in pregnant women with prolonged use of nucleoside analogues. It is not known if pregnancy itself potentiates this known side effect; however, women may be at increased risk of lactic acidosis and liver damage. In addition, these adverse events are similar to other rare but life-threatening syndromes which occur during pregnancy (eg, HELLP syndrome). Hepatic enzymes and electrolytes should be monitored in women receiving nucleoside analogues and clinicians should watch for early signs of the syndrome. In addition, mitochondrial dysfunction may develop in infants following *in utero* exposure. Due to the reports of lactic acidosis, maternal, and neonatal mortality, didanosine and stavudine should **not** be used in combination during pregnancy. The DHHS Perinatal HIV Guidelines recommend didanosine to be used only in special circumstances during pregnancy.

Regardless of CD4 count or HIV RNA copy number, all HIV-infected pregnant women should receive a combination antepartum antiretroviral (ARV) drug regimen; this includes women who require therapy for their own health, as well as women who do not yet require therapy for their own health. ARV therapy should be started as soon as possible if required for the woman's health. Although earlier initiation may be more effective in reducing the perinatal transmission of HIV), also consider maternal conditions (eg, nausea and vomiting) and the potential risks of first trimester fetal exposure for specific agents. Plasma HIV RNA levels should be assessed at ~34-36 weeks gestation in order to help determine mode of delivery. If ARV therapy must be interrupted for <24 hours during the peripartum period, stop then restart all medications simultaneously in order to decrease the chance of developing resistance. Long-term follow-up is recommended for all infants exposed to ARV medications.

Healthcare providers are encouraged to enroll pregnant women exposed to antiretroviral medications in the Antiretroviral Pregnancy Registry (1-800-258-4263 or www.APRegistry.com). Healthcare providers caring for HIV-infected women and their infants may contact the National Perinatal HIV Hotline (888-448-8765) for clinical consultation (DHHS [perinatal], 2012).

Dienogest (dye EN oh jest)

Brand Names: Canada Visanne®

Pharmacologic Category Antiandrogen

Use Management of pelvic pain associated with endometriosis

Local Anesthetic/Vasoconstrictor Precautions No information available to require special precautions

Effects on Dental Treatment No significant effects or complications reported

Effects on Bleeding No information available to require special precautions

Adverse Effects 1% to 10%:

Central nervous system: Headache (7%), depression (3%), sleep disturbance (2%), irritability (1%), migraine (1%), nervousness (1%)

Dermatologic: Acne (2%), alopecia (1%)

Endocrine & metabolic: Breast discomfort (5%), ovarian cyst (3%), libido decreased (2%)

Gastrointestinal: Nausea (4%), weight gain (4%), abdominal pain (2%)

Genitourinary: Vaginal bleeding (1%)

Neuromuscular & skeletal: Weakness (2%)

General Dosage Range Oral: *Adult females:* 2 mg once daily

Mechanism of Action Dienogest is a steroid with antiandrogen properties that lacks androgen, mineralcorticoid or glucocorticoid activity. Exhibits strong progestogenic effects although it binds uterine progesterone receptors with an affinity much lower (about one-tenth) than that of progesterone. Decreases estradiol production and thus suppresses estradiol's trophic effects on eutopic and ectopic endometrium. Inhibits cellular proliferation via direct antiproliferative, immunologic, and antiangiogenic effects.

Pharmacodynamics/Kinetics

Half-life Elimination ~9-10 hours

Time to Peak ~1.5 hours

◄ **Pregnancy Considerations** In animal studies, teratogenic effects were not observed; however, use of high dose dienogest during late pregnancy impaired fertility of female offspring. Based on limited data, inadvertent exposure in pregnancy has not shown adverse effects to the fetus, however use in known or suspected pregnancy is contraindicated. Rule out pregnancy prior to initiating therapy. Use of hormonal contraceptives is not recommended during dienogest therapy. Nonhormonal contraceptives should be employed during treatment. Ovulation is often inhibited during therapy although normal menstruation usually returns within 2 months of therapy discontinuation.

Product Availability Not available in the U.S.

Diethylene Triamine Penta-Acetic Acid
(dye ETH i leen TRYE a meen PEN ta a SEE tik AS id)

Brand Names: U.S. Ca-DTPA; Zn-DTPA
Pharmacologic Category Antidote
Use Treatment of known or suspected internal contamination with plutonium, americium, or curium
Local Anesthetic/Vasoconstrictor Precautions No information available to require special precautions
Effects on Dental Treatment Key adverse event(s) related to dental treatment: Metallic taste
Effects on Bleeding No information available to require special precautions
Adverse Effects Frequency not defined.
Cardiovascular: Chest pain
Central nervous system: Chills, fever, headache, lightheadedness
Dermatologic: Dermatitis, pruritus
Endocrine & metabolic: Magnesium depletion, manganese depletion, zinc depletion (calcium diethylene triamine penta-acetic acid [Ca-DTPA])
Gastrointestinal: Diarrhea, metallic taste, nausea, vomiting
Local: Injection site reactions
Neuromuscular & skeletal: Muscle cramps, pelvic pain
Respiratory: Cough and/or wheezing (nebulization in patients with asthma)
Miscellaneous: Allergic reaction
General Dosage Range
I.V.:
Children <12 years: Initial: Ca-DTPA: 14 mg/kg/day (maximum dose: 1 g/day); Maintenance: Zn-DTPA: 14 mg/kg/day (maximum: 1 g/day)
Children ≥12 years and Adults: Ca-DTPA: 1 g/day; Zn-DTPA: 1 g/day
Inhalation: *Children ≥12 years and Adults:* Ca-DTPA: 1 g/day; Zn-DTPA: 1 g/day
Mechanism of Action Calcium diethylene triamine penta-acetic acid (Ca-DTPA) and zinc diethylene triamine penta-acetic acid (Zn-DTPA) form chelates with some metal ions by exchanging calcium or zinc for a metal of greater binding capacity. The radioactive chelates are then excreted in the urine. Treatment is most effective when radiocontaminants are in circulation or interstitial fluids. Radiocontaminants eventually sequester in liver and bone; therefore, the efficacy of treatment decreases with time after the exposure.
Pharmacodynamics/Kinetics
Half-life Elimination Ca-DTPA, Zn-DTPA: May be increased by renal impairment
Pregnancy Risk Factor
C (calcium diethylene triamine penta-acetic acid [Ca-DTPA])
B (zinc diethylene triamine penta-acetic acid [Zn-DTPA])

Pregnancy Considerations Teratogenic effects have been reported with calcium diethylene triamine penta-acetic acid (Ca-DTPA) in animal studies. Multiple doses during pregnancy may increase adverse effects to the fetus due to zinc depletion. Reproduction studies with zinc diethylene triamine penta-acetic acid (Zn-DTPA) did not show teratogenic effects in animals; there are no well-controlled studies in pregnant women. Except in cases of high internal contamination, treatment should be initiated and maintained with Zn-DTPA during pregnancy.

Diethylpropion (dye eth il PROE pee on)

Brand Names: Canada Tenuate®; Tenuate® Dospan®
Pharmacologic Category Anorexiant; Central Nervous System Stimulant; Sympathomimetic
Use Short-term (few weeks) adjunct in the management of exogenous obesity

Pharmacotherapy for weight loss is recommended only for obese patients with a body mass index ≥30 kg/m², or ≥27 kg/m² in the presence of other risk factors such as hypertension, diabetes, and/or dyslipidemia or a high waist circumference; therapy should be used in conjunction with a comprehensive weight management program.

Local Anesthetic/Vasoconstrictor Precautions Use vasoconstrictor with caution in patients taking diethylpropion. Amphetamine-like drugs such as diethylpropion enhance the sympathomimetic response of epinephrine and norepinephrine leading to potential hypertension and cardiotoxicity.
Effects on Dental Treatment Key adverse event(s) related to dental treatment: Xerostomia and changes in salivation (normal salivary flow resumes upon discontinuation), and metallic taste (the use of local anesthetic without vasoconstrictor is recommended in these patients).
Effects on Bleeding No information available to require special precautions
Adverse Effects Frequency not defined.
Cardiovascular: Arrhythmia, ECG changes, hypertension, palpitation, precordial pain, pulmonary hypertension, tachycardia, valvulopathy
Central nervous system: Anxiety, CVA, depression, dizziness, drowsiness, dysphoria, euphoria, headache, insomnia, jitteriness, malaise, nervousness, overstimulation, psychosis, restlessness, seizure
Dermatologic: Alopecia, ecchymosis, erythema, rash, urticaria
Endocrine & metabolic: Libido changes, gynecomastia, menstrual irregularities
Gastrointestinal: Abdominal discomfort, constipation, diarrhea, nausea, unpleasant taste, vomiting, xerostomia
Genitourinary: Dysuria, impotence, polyuria
Hematologic: Bone marrow depression, agranulocytosis, leukopenia
Neuromuscular & skeletal: Dyskinesia, muscle pain, tremor
Ocular: Blurred vision, mydriasis
Respiratory: Dyspnea
Miscellaneous: Diaphoresis, tachyphylaxis
General Dosage Range Oral:
Controlled release: *Children >16 years and Adults:* 75 mg at midmorning
Immediate release: *Children >16 years and Adults:* 25 mg 3 times/day

Mechanism of Action Diethylpropion is a sympathomimetic amine with pharmacologic properties similar to the amphetamines. It is also structurally similar to bupropion. The mechanism of action in reducing appetite appears to be secondary to CNS effects, including stimulation of the hypothalamus to release norepinephrine

Pharmacodynamics/Kinetics

Half-life Elimination Aminoketone metabolites: ~4-6 hours

Pregnancy Risk Factor B

Pregnancy Considerations Teratogenic effects have not been observed in animal studies. Crosses the human placenta; spontaneous reports of congenital malformations have been reported, but an association with diethylpropion has not been established. Withdrawal symptoms may occur in the neonate following maternal use of diethylpropion.

Controlled Substance C-IV

Difenoxin and Atropine
(dye fen OKS in & A troe peen)

Related Information
Atropine on page 148

Brand Names: U.S. Motofen®

Pharmacologic Category Antidiarrheal

Use Treatment of diarrhea

Local Anesthetic/Vasoconstrictor Precautions No information available to require special precautions

Effects on Dental Treatment Key adverse event(s) related to dental treatment: Xerostomia (normal salivary flow resumes upon discontinuation)

Effects on Bleeding No information available to require special precautions

Adverse Effects 1% to 10%:
Central nervous system: Dizziness, drowsiness, lightheadedness, headache
Gastrointestinal: Nausea, vomiting, xerostomia, epigastric distress

General Dosage Range Oral: *Adults:* 2 tablets (each tablet contains difenoxin hydrochloride 1 mg and atropine sulfate 0.025 mg) initially, then 1 tablet after each loose stool (maximum: 8 tablets/day)

Pharmacodynamics/Kinetics

Time to Peak Plasma: Within 40-60 minutes

Pregnancy Risk Factor C

Pregnancy Considerations Adverse events were observed in some animal reproduction studies.

Controlled Substance C-IV

Diflorasone (dye FLOR a sone)

Brand Names: U.S. ApexiCon® E; ApexiCon™

Pharmacologic Category Corticosteroid, Topical

Use Relieves inflammation and pruritic symptoms of corticosteroid-responsive dermatosis (high to very high potency topical corticosteroid)

Local Anesthetic/Vasoconstrictor Precautions No information available to require special precautions

Effects on Dental Treatment No significant effects or complications reported

Effects on Bleeding No information available to require special precautions

General Dosage Range Topical: *Adults:* Cream: Apply 2-4 times/day; Ointment: Apply 1-3 times/day

Mechanism of Action Decreases inflammation by suppression of migration of polymorphonuclear leukocytes and reversal of increased capillary permeability

Pregnancy Risk Factor C

Pregnancy Considerations Teratogenic effects have been observed in animals administered potent topical corticosteroids. Topical products are not recommended for extensive use, in large quantities, or for long periods of time in pregnant women.

Diflunisal (dye FLOO ni sal)

Related Information
Oral Pain on page 1558
Rheumatoid Arthritis, Osteoarthritis, and Osteoporosis on page 1526
Temporomandibular Dysfunction (TMD), Chronic Pain, and Fibromyalgia on page 1590

Related Sample Prescriptions
Mild/Moderate Oral Pain on page 1606

Brand Names: Canada Apo-Diflunisal®; Novo-Diflunisal; Nu-Diflunisal

Generic Availability (U.S.) Yes

Pharmacologic Category Nonsteroidal Anti-inflammatory Drug (NSAID), Oral

Dental Use Treatment of postoperative pain

Use Management of inflammatory disorders usually including rheumatoid arthritis and osteoarthritis; can be used as an analgesic for treatment of mild-to-moderate pain

Local Anesthetic/Vasoconstrictor Precautions No information available to require special precautions

Effects on Dental Treatment The dentist should be aware of the potential of abnormal coagulation. Caution should also be exercised in the use of NSAIDs in patients already on anticoagulant therapy with drugs such as warfarin (Coumadin®). See Effects on Bleeding.

Effects on Bleeding As an inhibitor of prostaglandin synthetase, diflunisal has a dose-related effect on platelet function and bleeding time. In healthy volunteers, 250 mg twice daily for 8 days had no effect on platelet function, and 500 mg twice daily (the usual recommended dose) had a slight effect. However, at 1000 mg twice daily (which exceeds the maximum recommended dosage), diflunisal inhibited platelet function. In contrast with aspirin, these effects of diflunisal were reversible because diflunisal is a salicylic acid derivative.

Adverse Effects 1% to 10%:
Central nervous system: Headache (3% to 9%), dizziness (1% to 3%), insomnia (1% to 3%), somnolence (1% to 3%), fatigue (1% to 3%)
Dermatologic: Rash (3% to 9%)
Gastrointestinal: Nausea (3% to 9%), dyspepsia (3% to 9%), GI pain (3% to 9%), diarrhea (3% to 9%), constipation (1% to 3%), flatulence (1% to 3%), vomiting (1% to 3%), GI ulceration
Otic: Tinnitus (1% to 3%)

Dental Usual Dosage Mild-to-moderate pain: Adults: Oral: Initial: 500-1000 mg followed by 250-500 mg every 8-12 hours; maximum daily dose: 1.5 g

Dosage Adults: Oral:
Mild-to-moderate pain: Initial: 500-1000 mg followed by 250-500 mg every 8-12 hours; maximum daily dose: 1.5 g
Arthritis: 500-1000 mg/day in 2 divided doses; maximum daily dose: 1.5 g

Dosage adjustment in renal impairment: Use with caution; Cl$_{cr}$ <50 mL/minute: Administer 50% of normal dose (Aronoff, 1998)

Hemodialysis: No supplement required

CAPD: No supplement require

CAVH: Dose for GFR 10-50

Dosage adjustment in hepatic impairment: No dosage adjustment provided in manufacturer's labeling.

Mechanism of Action Reversibly inhibits cyclooxygenase-1 and 2 (COX-1 and 2) enzymes, which results in decreased formation of prostaglandin precursors; has antipyretic, analgesic, and anti-inflammatory properties.

Other proposed mechanisms not fully elucidated (and possibly contributing to the anti-inflammatory effect to varying degrees) include inhibiting chemotaxis, altering lymphocyte activity, inhibiting neutrophil aggregation/ activation, and decreasing proinflammatory cytokine levels.

Contraindications Hypersensitivity to diflunisal, aspirin, other NSAIDs, or any component of the formulation; perioperative pain in the setting of coronary artery bypass graft (CABG) surgery

Warnings/Precautions [U.S. Boxed Warning]: NSAIDs are associated with an increased risk of adverse cardiovascular thrombotic events, including MI and stroke. Risk may be increased with duration of use or pre-existing cardiovascular risk factors or disease. Carefully evaluate individual cardiovascular risk profiles prior to prescribing. May cause new-onset hypertension or worsening of existing hypertension. Use caution with fluid retention. Avoid use in heart failure. Concurrent administration of ibuprofen, and potentially other nonselective NSAIDs, may interfere with aspirin's cardioprotective effect. **[U.S. Boxed Warning]: Use is contraindicated for treatment of perioperative pain in the setting of coronary artery bypass graft (CABG) surgery.** Risk of MI and stroke may be increased with use following CABG surgery.

[U.S. Boxed Warning]: NSAIDs may increase risk of gastrointestinal irritation, inflammation, ulceration, bleeding, and perforation. Use caution with a history of GI disease (bleeding or ulcers), concurrent therapy with aspirin, anticoagulants and/or corticosteroids, smoking, use of alcohol, the elderly or debilitated patients. When used concomitantly with ≤325 mg of aspirin, a substantial increase in the risk of gastrointestinal complications (eg, ulcer) occurs; concomitant gastroprotective therapy (eg, proton pump inhibitors) is recommended (Bhatt, 2008).

In the elderly, avoid chronic use (unless alternative agents ineffective and patient can receive concomitant gastroprotective agent); nonselective oral NSAID use is associated with an increased risk of GI bleeding and peptic ulcer disease in older adults in high risk category (eg, >75 years or age or receiving concomitant oral/ parenteral corticosteroids, anticoagulants, or antiplatelet agents) (Beers Criteria).

Platelet adhesion and aggregation may be decreased; may prolong bleeding time; patients with coagulation disorders or who are receiving anticoagulants should be monitored closely. Anemia may occur; patients on long-term NSAID therapy should be monitored for anemia. Rarely, NSAID use may cause severe blood dyscrasias (eg, agranulocytosis, aplastic anemia, thrombocytopenia).

NSAID use may compromise existing renal function; dose-dependent decreases in prostaglandin synthesis may result from NSAID use, reducing renal blood flow which may cause renal decompensation. NSAID use may increase the risk for hyperkalemia. Patients with impaired renal function, dehydration, heart failure, liver dysfunction, those taking diuretics, and ACE inhibitors, and the elderly are at greater risk of renal toxicity and hyperkalemia. Rehydrate patient before starting therapy; monitor renal function closely. Not recommended for use in patients with advanced renal disease. Long-term NSAID use may result in renal papillary necrosis. Use with caution in patients with decreased hepatic function.

NSAIDS may cause drowsiness, dizziness, blurred vision and other neurologic effects which may impair physical or mental abilities; patients must be cautioned about performing tasks which require mental alertness (eg, operating machinery or driving). Discontinue use with blurred or diminished vision and perform ophthalmologic exam. Monitor vision with long-term therapy.

Use the lowest effective dose for the shortest duration of time, consistent with individual patient goals, to reduce risk of cardiovascular or GI adverse events.

NSAIDs may cause serious skin adverse events including exfoliative dermatitis, Stevens-Johnson syndrome (SJS), and toxic epidermal necrolysis (TEN); discontinue use at first sign of skin rash or hypersensitivity. Do not use in patients who experience bronchospasm, asthma, rhinitis, or urticaria with NSAID or aspirin therapy. Use caution in other forms of asthma.

A hypersensitivity syndrome has been reported; monitor for constitutional symptoms and cutaneous findings; other organ dysfunction may be involved.

Diflunisal is a derivative of acetylsalicylic acid and therefore may be associated with Reye's syndrome. Withhold for at least 4-6 half-lives prior to surgical or dental procedures.

Drug Interactions

Metabolism/Transport Effects None known.

Avoid Concomitant Use

Avoid concomitant use of Diflunisal with any of the following: Floctafenine; Ketorolac (Nasal); Ketorolac (Systemic); NSAID (COX-2 Inhibitor); Omacetaxine

Increased Effect/Toxicity

Diflunisal may increase the levels/effects of: Agents with Antiplatelet Properties; Aliskiren; Aminoglycosides; Anticoagulants; Bisphosphonate Derivatives; Collagenase (Systemic); CycloSPORINE (Systemic); Dabigatran Etexilate; Deferasirox; Desmopressin; Digoxin; Drotrecogin Alfa (Activated); Eplerenone; Haloperidol; Ibritumomab; Lithium; Methotrexate; Nonsteroidal Anti-Inflammatory Agents; NSAID (COX-2 Inhibitor); Omacetaxine; PEMEtrexed; Porfimer; Potassium-Sparing Diuretics; PRALAtrexate; Quinolone Antibiotics; Rivaroxaban; Salicylates; Thrombolytic Agents; Tositumomab and Iodine I 131 Tositumomab; Vancomycin; Vitamin K Antagonists

The levels/effects of Diflunisal may be increased by: ACE Inhibitors; Angiotensin II Receptor Blockers; Antidepressants (Tricyclic, Tertiary Amine); Corticosteroids (Systemic); CycloSPORINE (Systemic); Dasatinib; Floctafenine; Glucosamine; Herbs (Anticoagulant/Antiplatelet Properties); Ketorolac (Nasal); Ketorolac (Systemic); Multivitamins/Minerals (with ADEK, Folate, Iron); Nonsteroidal Anti-Inflammatory Agents; Omega-3 Fatty Acids; Pentosan Polysulfate Sodium;

Pentoxifylline; Probenecid; Prostacyclin Analogues; Selective Serotonin Reuptake Inhibitors; Serotonin/ Norepinephrine Reuptake Inhibitors; Sodium Phosphates; Tipranavir; Treprostinil; Vitamin E

Decreased Effect

Diflunisal may decrease the levels/effects of: ACE Inhibitors; Agents with Antiplatelet Properties; Aliskiren; Angiotensin II Receptor Blockers; Beta-Blockers; Eplerenone; HydrALAZINE; Loop Diuretics; Potassium-Sparing Diuretics; Salicylates; Selective Serotonin Reuptake Inhibitors; Thiazide Diuretics

The levels/effects of Diflunisal may be decreased by: Bile Acid Sequestrants; Nonsteroidal Anti-Inflammatory Agents; Salicylates

Ethanol/Nutrition/Herb Interactions

Ethanol: Avoid ethanol (may enhance gastric mucosal irritation).

Herb/Nutraceutical: Avoid alfalfa, anise, bilberry, bladderwrack, bromelain, cat's claw, celery, chamomile, coleus, cordyceps, dong quai, evening primrose, fenugreek, feverfew, garlic, ginger, ginkgo biloba, ginseng (American, Panax, Siberian), grapeseed, green tea, guggul, horse chestnut seed, horseradish, licorice, prickly ash, red clover, reishi, SAMe (S-adenosylmethionine), sweet clover, turmeric, white willow (all have additional antiplatelet activity).

Dietary Considerations Should be taken with food to decrease GI upset.

Pharmacodynamics/Kinetics

Onset of Action Analgesic: ~1 hour; maximal effect: 2-3 hours

Duration of Action 8-12 hours

Half-life Elimination 8-12 hours; prolonged with renal impairment

Time to Peak Serum: 2-3 hours

Pregnancy Risk Factor C

Pregnancy Considerations Adverse events were not observed in the initial animal reproduction studies; therefore, the manufacturer classifies diflunisal as pregnancy category C. NSAID exposure during the first trimester is not strongly associated with congenital malformations; however, cardiovascular anomalies and cleft palate have been observed following NSAID exposure in some studies. The use of a NSAID close to conception may be associated with an increased risk of miscarriage. Nonteratogenic effects have been observed following NSAID administration during the third trimester including: Myocardial degenerative changes, prenatal constriction of the ductus arteriosus, fetal tricuspid regurgitation, failure of the ductus arteriosus to close postnatally; renal dysfunction or failure, oligohydramnios; gastrointestinal bleeding or perforation, increased risk of necrotizing enterocolitis; intracranial bleeding (including intraventricular hemorrhage), platelet dysfunction with resultant bleeding; pulmonary hypertension. Because they may cause premature closure of the ductus arteriosus, use of NSAIDs late in pregnancy should be avoided (use after 31 or 32 weeks gestation is not recommended by some clinicians). The chronic use of NSAIDs in women of reproductive age may be associated with infertility that is reversible upon discontinuation of the medication.

Lactation Enters breast milk/not recommended

Breast-Feeding Considerations Diflunisal is excreted into breast milk at levels of 2% to 7% of those in maternal plasma. Breast-feeding is not recommended by the manufacturer.

Dosage Forms

Tablet, oral: 500 mg

Dental Comment The advantage of diflunisal as a pain reliever is its 12-hour duration of effect. In many cases, this long effect will ensure a full night sleep during the postoperative pain period.

References

Forbes JA, Calderazzo JP, Bowser MW, et al, "A 12-Hour Evaluation of the Analgesic Efficacy of Diflunisal, Aspirin, and Placebo in Postoperative Dental Pain," *J Clin Pharmacol*, 1982, 22(2-3):89-96.

Selcuk E, Gomel M, Bellibas SE, et al, "Comparison of the Analgesic Effects of Diflunisal and Paracetamol in the Treatment of Postoperative Dental Pain," *Int J Clin Pharmacol Res*, 1996, 16 (2-3):57-65.

Difluprednate (dye floo PRED nate)

Brand Names: U.S. Durezol®

Pharmacologic Category Corticosteroid, Ophthalmic

Use Treatment of inflammation and pain following ocular surgery; treatment of endogenous anterior uveitis

Local Anesthetic/Vasoconstrictor Precautions No information available to require special precautions

Effects on Dental Treatment No significant effects or complications reported

Effects on Bleeding No information available to require special precautions

Adverse Effects

Adverse reactions following ocular surgery:

5% to 15%: Ocular: Anterior chamber cells/flare, blepharitis, ciliary and conjunctival hyperemia, conjunctival/corneal edema, pain, photophobia, posterior capsule opacification

1% to 5%: Ocular: Inflammation, iritis, punctuate keratitis, visual acuity reduced

Adverse reactions associated with treatment of endogenous anterior uveitis:

5% to 10%:

Central nervous system: Headache

Ocular: Blurred vision, hyperemia (conjunctival and limbal), intraocular pressure increased, irritation, pain, punctate keratitis, uveitis

2% to 5%: Ocular: Anterior chamber flare, corneal edema, dry eye, iridocyclitis, photophobia, visual acuity decreased

General Dosage Range Ophthalmic: *Adults:* Instill 1 drop in affected eye(s) 2-4 times/day (ocular surgery) **or** 4 times/day for 14 days (uveitis); taper to discontinue

Mechanism of Action Corticosteroids inhibit the inflammatory response including edema, capillary dilation, leukocyte migration, and scar formation. Difluprednate penetrates cells readily to induce the production of lipocortins. These proteins modulate the activity of prostaglandins and leukotrienes.

Pregnancy Risk Factor C

Pregnancy Considerations Difluprednate was shown to be teratogenic in animal reproduction studies when administered subcutaneously. The amount of difluprednate absorbed systemically following ophthalmic administration is below the limit of quantification (<50 ng/mL).

Digoxin (di JOKS in)

Related Information

Cardiovascular Diseases *on page 1492*

Brand Names: U.S. Lanoxin®

Brand Names: Canada Apo-Digoxin®; Digoxin Injection CSD; Lanoxin®; Pediatric Digoxin CSD; PMS-Digoxin; Toloxin®

Generic Availability (U.S.) Yes

Pharmacologic Category Antiarrhythmic Agent, Miscellaneous; Cardiac Glycoside

Use Treatment of mild-to-moderate (or stage C as recommended by the ACCF/AHA) heart failure (HF); atrial fibrillation (rate-control)

Note: In treatment of atrial fibrillation (AF), use is not considered first-line unless AF coexistent with heart failure or in sedentary patients (Fuster, 2006).

Unlabeled Use Fetal tachycardia with or without hydrops; to slow ventricular rate in supraventricular tachyarrhythmias such as supraventricular tachycardia (SVT) excluding atrioventricular reciprocating tachycardia (AVRT)

Local Anesthetic/Vasoconstrictor Precautions Use vasoconstrictor with caution due to risk of cardiac arrhythmias with digoxin

Effects on Dental Treatment Sensitive gag reflex may cause difficulty in taking a dental impression.

Effects on Bleeding No information available to require special precautions

Adverse Effects Incidence not always reported.

Cardiovascular: Accelerated junctional rhythm, asystole, atrial tachycardia with or without block, AV dissociation, first-, second- (Wenckebach), or third-degree heart block, facial edema, PR prolongation, PVCs (especially bigeminy or trigeminy), ST segment depression, ventricular tachycardia or ventricular fibrillation

Central nervous system: Dizziness (6%), mental disturbances (5%), headache (4%), apathy, anxiety, confusion, delirium, depression, fever, hallucinations

Dermatologic: Rash (erythematous, maculopapular [most common], papular, scarlatiniform, vesicular or bullous), pruritus, urticaria, angioneurotic edema

Gastrointestinal: Nausea (4%), vomiting (2%), diarrhea (4%), abdominal pain, anorexia

Neuromuscular & skeletal: Weakness

Ocular: Visual disturbances (blurred or yellow vision)

Respiratory: Laryngeal edema

Dosage

Children: When changing from oral (tablets or liquid) or I.M. to I.V. therapy, dosage should be reduced by 20% to 25%. Refer to the following: See table.

Dosage Recommendations for Digoxin[1]

Age	Total Digitalizing Dose[2,3] (mcg/kg)		Daily Maintenance Dose[3,4] (mcg/kg)	
	Oral	I.V. or I.M.[5]	Oral	I.V. or I.M.[5]
Preterm infant	20-30	15-25	5-7.5	4-6
Full-term infant	25-35	20-30	6-10	5-8
1 mo - 2 y	35-60	30-50	10-15	7.5-12
2-5 y	30-40	25-35	7.5-10	6-9
5-10 y	20-35	15-30	5-10	4-8
>10 y	10-15	8-12	2.5-5	2-3

[1]Heart failure: A lower serum digoxin concentration may be adequate to treat heart failure (compared to cardiac arrhythmias); consider doses at the lower end of the recommended range for treatment of heart failure; a digitalizing dose (loading dose) may not be necessary when treating heart failure (Ross, 2001).

[2]Do not give full total digitalizing dose (TDD) at once. Give one-half of the total digitalizing dose (TDD) in the initial dose, then give one-quarter of the TDD in each of two subsequent doses at 6- to 8-hour intervals. Obtain ECG 6 hours after each dose to assess potential toxicity.

[3]Based on lean body weight and normal renal function for age. Decrease dose in patients with decreased renal function; digitalizing dose often not recommended in infants and children.

[4]Divided every 12 hours in infants and children <10 years of age. Given once daily to children >10 years of age and adults.

[5]I.M. not preferred due to severe injection site pain. If I.M. route is necessary, administer as deep injection followed by massage of injection site.

Adults:

Atrial fibrillation (rate control) in patients with heart failure: Loading dose: I.V.: 0.25 mg every 2 hours, up to 1.5 mg within 24 hours; for nonacute situations,

may administer 0.5 mg orally once daily for 2 days followed by oral maintenance dose. Maintenance dose: I.V., Oral: 0.125-0.375 mg once daily (Fuster, 2006)

Heart failure: Daily maintenance dose (**Note:** Loading dose not recommended): Oral: 0.125-0.25 mg once daily; higher daily doses (up to 0.5 mg/day) are rarely necessary. If patient is >70 years of age, has impaired renal function, or has a low lean body mass, low doses (eg, 0.125 mg daily or every other day) should be used (Hunt, 2009).

Supraventricular tachyarrhythmias (rate control):

Initial: Total digitalizing dose:

Oral: 0.75-1.5 mg

I.V., I.M.: 0.5-1 mg (**Note:** I.M. not preferred due to severe injection site pain.)

Give 1/2 (one-half) of the total digitalizing dose (TDD) as the initial dose, then give 1/4 (one-quarter) of the TDD in each of 2 subsequent doses at 6- to 8-hour intervals. Obtain ECG 6 hours after each dose to assess potential toxicity.

Daily maintenance dose:

Oral: 0.125-0.5 mg once daily

I.V., I.M.: 0.1-0.4 mg once daily (**Note:** I.M. not preferred due to severe injection site pain.)

Elderly: Dose is based on assessment of lean body mass and renal function. Elderly patients with low lean body mass may experience higher digoxin concentrations due to reduced volume of distribution (Cheng, 2010). Decrease dose in patients with decreased renal function.

Heart failure: If patient is >70 years, low doses (eg, 0.125 mg daily or every other day) should be used (Hunt, 2009).

Dosage adjustment in renal impairment:

Loading dose:

ESRD: If loading dose necessary, reduce dose by 50%

Acute renal failure: Based on expert opinion, if patient in acute renal failure requires ventricular rate control (eg, in atrial fibrillation), consider alternative therapy. If loading digoxin becomes necessary, patient volume of distribution may be increased and reduction in loading dose may not be necessary; however, maintenance dosing will require adjustment as long as renal failure persists.

Maintenance dose:

Cl_{cr} 10-50 mL/minute: Administer 25% to 75% of dose or every 36 hours

Cl_{cr} <10 mL/minute: Administer 10% to 25% of dose or every 48 hours

Hemodialysis: Not dialyzable

Dosage adjustment in hepatic impairment: No dosage adjustment provided in manufacturer's labeling.

Mechanism of Action

Heart failure: Inhibition of the sodium/potassium ATPase pump in myocardial cells results in a transient increase of intracellular sodium, which in turn promotes calcium influx via the sodium-calcium exchange pump leading to increased contractility.

Supraventricular arrhythmias: Direct suppression of the AV node conduction to increase effective refractory period and decrease conduction velocity - positive inotropic effect, enhanced vagal tone, and decreased ventricular rate to fast atrial arrhythmias. Atrial fibrillation may decrease sensitivity and increase tolerance to higher serum digoxin concentrations.

Contraindications Hypersensitivity to digoxin (rare) or other forms of digitalis, or any component of the formulation; ventricular fibrillation

Warnings/Precautions Watch for proarrhythmic effects (especially with digoxin toxicity). Withdrawal in clinically stable patients with HF may lead to recurrence of HF symptoms. During an episode of atrial fibrillation or flutter in patients with an accessory bypass tract (eg, Wolff-Parkinson-White syndrome), use has been associated with increased anterograde conduction down the accessory pathway leading to ventricular fibrillation; avoid use in such patients. Avoid use in patients with second- or third-degree heart block (except in patients with a functioning artificial pacemaker); incomplete AV block (eg, Stokes-Adams attack) may progress to complete block with digoxin administration. HF patients with preserved left ventricular function including patients with restrictive cardiomyopathy, constrictive pericarditis, and amyloid heart disease may be susceptible to digoxin toxicity; avoid use unless used to control ventricular response with atrial fibrillation. Digoxin should not be used in patients with low EF, sinus rhythm, and no HF symptoms since the risk of harm may be greater than clinical benefit. Avoid use in patients with hypertrophic cardiomyopathy (HCM) and outflow tract obstruction unless used to control ventricular response with atrial fibrillation; outflow obstruction may worsen due to the positive inotropic effects of digoxin.

Use with caution in patients with hyperthyroidism, hypothyroidism, recent acute MI (within 6 months), sinus nodal disease (eg, sick sinus syndrome). Reduce dose with renal impairment and when amiodarone, propafenone, quinidine, or verapamil are added to a patient on digoxin; use with caution in patients taking strong inducers or inhibitors of P-glycoprotein (eg, cyclosporine). Avoid rapid I.V. administration of calcium in digitalized patients; may produce serious arrhythmias.

Atrial arrhythmias associated with hypermetabolic states are very difficult to treat; treat underlying condition first; if digoxin is used, ensure digoxin toxicity does not occur. Patients with beri beri heart disease may fail to adequately respond to digoxin therapy; treat underlying thiamine deficiency concomitantly. Correct electrolyte disturbances, especially hypokalemia or hypomagnesemia, prior to use and throughout therapy; toxicity may occur despite therapeutic digoxin concentrations. Hypercalcemia may increase the risk of digoxin toxicity; maintain normocalcemia. It is not necessary to routinely reduce or hold digoxin therapy prior to elective electrical cardioversion for atrial fibrillation; however, exclusion of digoxin toxicity (eg, clinical and ECG signs) is necessary prior to cardioversion. If signs of digoxin excess exist, withhold digoxin and delay cardioversion until toxicity subsides; usually >24 hours. Use with caution in the elderly; decreases in renal clearance may result in toxic effects; in general, avoid doses >0.125 mg/day; in heart failure, higher doses may increase the risk of potential toxicity and have not been shown to provide additional benefit (Beers Criteria).

Drug Interactions

Metabolism/Transport Effects Substrate of CYP3A4 (minor), P-glycoprotein; **Note:** Assignment of Major/Minor substrate status based on clinically relevant drug interaction potential

Avoid Concomitant Use There are no known interactions where it is recommended to avoid concomitant use.

Increased Effect/Toxicity

Digoxin may increase the levels/effects of: Adenosine; Carvedilol; Colchicine; Dronedarone; Midodrine

The levels/effects of Digoxin may be increased by: Aminoquinolines (Antimalarial); Amiodarone; Antithyroid Agents; AtorvaSTATin; Beta-Blockers; Boceprevir; Calcium Channel Blockers (Nondihydropyridine); Calcium Polystyrene Sulfonate; Carvedilol; CloNIDine; Conivaptan; CycloSPORINE (Systemic); Dronedarone; Etravirine; Glycopyrrolate; Itraconazole; Lenalidomide; Loop Diuretics; Macrolide Antibiotics; Mifepristone; Milnacipran; Mirabegron; Multivitamins/Minerals (with ADEK, Folate, Iron); Nefazodone; Neuromuscular-Blocking Agents; NIFEdipine; Nonsteroidal Anti-Inflammatory Agents; Paricalcitol; P-glycoprotein/ABCB1 Inhibitors; Posaconazole; Potassium-Sparing Diuretics; Propafenone; Protease Inhibitors; QuiNIDine; QuiNINE; Ranolazine; Reserpine; SitaGLIPtin; Sodium Polystyrene Sulfonate; Spironolactone; Telaprevir; Telmisartan; Ticagrelor; Tolvaptan; Vitamin D Analogs

Decreased Effect

Digoxin may decrease the levels/effects of: Antineoplastic Agents (Anthracycline, Systemic)

The levels/effects of Digoxin may be decreased by: 5-ASA Derivatives; Acarbose; Aminoglycosides; Antineoplastic Agents; Antineoplastic Agents (Anthracycline, Systemic); Bile Acid Sequestrants; Kaolin; PenicillAMINE; P-glycoprotein/ABCB1 Inducers; Potassium-Sparing Diuretics; St Johns Wort; Sucralfate

Ethanol/Nutrition/Herb Interactions

Food: Digoxin peak serum concentrations may be decreased if taken with food. Meals containing increased fiber (bran) or foods high in pectin may decrease oral absorption of digoxin.

Herb/Nutraceutical: Avoid ephedra (risk of cardiac stimulation). Avoid natural licorice (causes sodium and water retention and increases potassium loss).

Dietary Considerations Maintain adequate amounts of potassium in diet to decrease risk of hypokalemia (hypokalemia may increase risk of digoxin toxicity).

Pharmacodynamics/Kinetics

Onset of Action

Heart rate control: Oral: 1-2 hours; I.V.: 5-60 minutes

Peak effect: Heart rate control: Oral: 2-8 hours; I.V.: 1-6 hours; **Note:** In patients with atrial fibrillation, median time to ventricular rate control in one study was 6 hours (range: 3-15 hours) (Siu, 2009)

Duration of Action Adults: 3-4 days

Half-life Elimination

Age, renal and cardiac function dependent:

Neonates: Premature: 61-170 hours; Full-term: 35-45 hours

Infants: 18-25 hours

Children: 18-36 hours

Adults: 36-48 hours

Adults, anephric: 3.5-5 days

Parent drug: 38 hours; Metabolites: Digoxigenin: 4 hours; Monodigitoxoside: 3-12 hours

Time to Peak Serum: Oral: 1-3 hours

Pregnancy Risk Factor C

Pregnancy Considerations Animal reproduction studies have not been conducted. Digoxin crosses the placenta and can be detected in the fetus. Digoxin is recommended as first-line in the treatment of fetal tachycardia determined to be SVT. In pregnant women with atrial fibrillation or SVT, use of digoxin is

◄ recommended (Class I recommendation; Blomström-Lundqvist, 2003; Fuster, 2006).

Lactation Enters breast milk/use caution (AAP rates "compatible"; AAP 2001 update pending)

Breast-Feeding Considerations Digoxin is excreted into breast milk and similar concentrations are found within mother's serum and milk. The manufacturer recommends that caution be used in nursing women.

Dosage Forms

Injection, solution: 250 mcg/mL (1 mL, 2 mL)
Lanoxin®: 100 mcg/mL (1 mL); 250 mcg/mL (2 mL)
Solution, oral: 50 mcg/mL (2.5 mL, 5 mL, 60 mL)
Tablet, oral: 125 mcg, 250 mcg
Lanoxin®: 125 mcg, 250 mcg

Dosage Forms: Canada

Tablet, oral:
Apo-Digoxin®: 62.5 mcg, 125 mcg, 250 mcg

Digoxin Immune Fab (di JOKS in i MYUN fab)

Brand Names: U.S. DigiFab®
Brand Names: Canada DigiFab®
Pharmacologic Category Antidote
Use Treatment of life-threatening or potentially life-threatening digoxin intoxication, including:
- acute digoxin ingestion (ie, >10 mg in adults; >0.1 mg/kg or >4 mg in children; ingestions resulting in serum concentrations >10 ng/mL)
- chronic ingestions leading to steady-state digoxin concentrations >6 ng/mL in adults or >4 ng/mL in children
- manifestations of digoxin toxicity due to overdose (eg, life-threatening ventricular arrhythmias, progressive bradycardia, second- or third-degree heart block not responsive to atropine, serum potassium >5.5 mEq/L in adults or >6 mEq/L in children)

Local Anesthetic/Vasoconstrictor Precautions No information available to require special precautions

Effects on Dental Treatment No significant effects or complications reported

Effects on Bleeding No information available to require special precautions

Adverse Effects Frequency not defined.

Cardiovascular: Heart failure exacerbation (due to withdrawal of digoxin), orthostatic hypotension, rapid ventricular response (patients with atrial fibrillation; due to withdrawal of digoxin)
Endocrine & metabolic: Hypokalemia
Local: Phlebitis
Miscellaneous: Allergic reactions, serum sickness

General Dosage Range I.V.:

Acute ingestion of known amount: *Children and Adults:* Digoxin Immune Fab Dose (vials) = Total body load (mg) / (0.5)

Based on steady-state digoxin concentration:

Infants and Children ≤20 kg: Digoxin Immune Fab Dose (mg) = [(serum digoxin concentration [ng/mL] x weight [kg]) / 100] x (digoxin immune Fab amount per vial [mg/vial])

Note: Digoxin immune Fab amount per vial: 40 mg/vial.

Children >20 kg and Adults: Digoxin Immune Fab Dose (vials) = (serum digoxin concentration [ng/mL] x weight [kg]) / 100

Amount ingested and blood level unknown:

Children ≤20 kg: Acute toxicity: 20 vials total in 2 divided doses; Chronic toxicity: 1 vial may be sufficient

Children >20 kg and Adults: Acute toxicity: 20 vials total in 2 divided doses; Chronic toxicity: 6 vials

Mechanism of Action Digoxin immune antigen-binding fragments (Fab) are specific antibodies for the treatment of digitalis intoxication in carefully selected patients; binds with molecules of digoxin or digitoxin and is then excreted by the kidneys and removed from the body

Pharmacodynamics/Kinetics

Onset of Action I.V.: Digitalis toxicity: Improvement may be seen in ≤30 minutes

Half-life Elimination 15-20 hours; prolonged with renal impairment

Pregnancy Risk Factor C

Pregnancy Considerations Animal reproduction studies have not been conducted. Safety and efficacy in pregnant women have not been established. Use during pregnancy only if clearly needed. In general, medications used as antidotes should take into consideration the health and prognosis of the mother (Bailey, 2003).

Dihydrocodeine, Aspirin, and Caffeine (dye hye droe KOE deen, AS pir in, & KAF een)

Related Information

Aspirin *on page 135*
Caffeine *on page 229*
Codeine *on page 344*
Oral Pain *on page 1558*

Brand Names: U.S. Synalgos®-DC
Generic Availability (U.S.) No
Pharmacologic Category Analgesic, Opioid
Dental Use Management of postoperative pain
Use Management of mild-to-moderate pain that requires relaxation

Local Anesthetic/Vasoconstrictor Precautions No information available to require special precautions

Effects on Dental Treatment Key adverse event(s) related to dental treatment: Dihydrocodeine: nausea, followed by sedation and constipation. Elderly are a high-risk population for adverse effects from nonsteroidal anti-inflammatory agents. As many as 60% of elderly patients with GI complications from NSAIDs can develop peptic ulceration and/or hemorrhage asymptomatically. Concomitant disease and drug use contribute to the risk of GI adverse effects. Use lowest effective dose for shortest period possible. Consider renal function decline with age.

Aspirin: As with all drugs which may affect hemostasis, bleeding is associated with aspirin. Hemorrhage may occur at virtually any site; risk is dependent on multiple variables including dosage, concurrent use of multiple agents which alter hemostasis, and patient susceptibility. Many adverse effects of aspirin are dose related, and are rare at low dosages. Other serious reactions are idiosyncratic, related to allergy or individual sensitivity (see Effects on Bleeding).

Effects on Bleeding Aspirin irreversibly inhibits platelet aggregation which can prolong bleeding. Upon discontinuation, normal platelet function returns only when new platelets are released (~7-10 days). However, in the case of dental surgery, there is no scientific evidence to support discontinuation of aspirin.

Adverse Effects

>10%:

Central nervous system: Lightheadedness, dizziness, drowsiness, sedation

Dermatologic: Pruritus, skin reactions

Gastrointestinal: Nausea, vomiting, constipation

1% to 10%:

Cardiovascular: Hypotension, palpitation, bradycardia, peripheral vasodilation

Central nervous system: Increased intracranial pressure

Endocrine & metabolic: Antidiuretic hormone release

Gastrointestinal: Biliary tract spasm

Genitourinary: Urinary tract spasm

Ocular: Miosis

Respiratory: Respiratory depression

Miscellaneous: Histamine release, physical and psychological dependence with prolonged use

Dental Usual Dosage Management of postoperative pain: Oral:

Adults: 1-2 capsules every 4-6 hours as needed for pain

Elderly: Initial dosing should be cautious (low end of adult dosing range)

Dosage

Adults: Oral: 1-2 capsules every 4-6 hours as needed for pain

Elderly: Initial dosing should be cautious (low end of adult dosing range)

Dosage adjustment in renal impairment: No dosage adjustment provided in manufacturer's labeling.

Dosage adjustment in hepatic impairment: No dosage adjustment provided in manufacturer's labeling.

Mechanism of Action Binds to opiate receptors in the CNS, causing inhibition of ascending pain pathways, altering the perception of and response to pain; causes cough suppression by direct central action in the medulla; produces generalized CNS depression

Contraindications Hypersensitivity to dihydrocodeine or any component of the formulation; pregnancy (prolonged use or high doses at term)

Warnings/Precautions May cause CNS depression, which may impair physical or mental abilities; patients must be cautioned about performing tasks which require mental alertness (eg, operating machinery or driving). Discontinue use if tinnitus or impaired hearing occurs. Use with caution in patients with hypersensitivity reactions to other phenanthrene-derivative opioid agonists (morphine, hydrocodone, hydromorphone, levorphanol, oxycodone, oxymorphone); patients with sensitivity to tartrazine dyes, nasal polyps, and asthma may have an increased risk of salicylate sensitivity; respiratory diseases including asthma, emphysema, COPD, adrenal insufficiency, biliary tract impairment, CNS depression, coma, head trauma, prostatic hyperplasia, urinary stricture, thyroid dysfunction bleeding disorders, GI disease, or severe liver or renal insufficiency; may obscure diagnosis or clinical course of patients with acute abdominal conditions; heavy ethanol use (>3 drinks/day) can increase bleeding risks; ASA should be avoided (if possible) in surgical patients for 1-2 weeks prior to surgery; some preparations contain sulfites which may cause allergic reactions; dextromethorphan has equivalent antitussive activity but has much lower toxicity in accidental overdose; tolerance of drug dependence may result from extended use

Drug Interactions

Metabolism/Transport Effects Refer to individual components.

Avoid Concomitant Use

Avoid concomitant use of Dihydrocodeine, Aspirin, and Caffeine with any of the following: Azelastine (Nasal); Floctafenine; Influenza Virus Vaccine (Live/Attenuated); Iobenguane I 123; Ketorolac (Nasal); Ketorolac (Systemic); Omacetaxine; Paraldehyde

Increased Effect/Toxicity

Dihydrocodeine, Aspirin, and Caffeine may increase the levels/effects of: Alcohol (Ethyl); Alendronate; Alvimopan; Anticoagulants; Azelastine (Nasal); Carbonic Anhydrase Inhibitors; CNS Depressants; Collagenase (Systemic); Corticosteroids (Systemic); Dabigatran Etexilate; Desmopressin; Divalproex; Drotrecogin Alfa (Activated); Formoterol; Heparin; Hypoglycemic Agents; Ibritumomab; Indacaterol; Methotrexate; Metyrosine; Mirtazapine; NSAID (COX-2 Inhibitor); Omacetaxine; Paraldehyde; PRALAtrexate; Pramipexole; Rivaroxaban; ROPINIRole; Rotigotine; Salicylates; Selective Serotonin Reuptake Inhibitors; Sympathomimetics; Thiazide Diuretics; Thrombolytic Agents; Ticagrelor; Tositumomab and Iodine I 131 Tositumomab; Valproic Acid; Varicella Virus-Containing Vaccines; Vitamin K Antagonists; Zolpidem

The levels/effects of Dihydrocodeine, Aspirin, and Caffeine may be increased by: Abiraterone Acetate; Agents with Antiplatelet Properties; Ammonium Chloride; Amphetamines; Antidepressants (Tricyclic, Tertiary Amine); Antipsychotic Agents (Phenothiazines); AtoMOXetine; Calcium Channel Blockers (Nondihydropyridine); CYP1A2 Inhibitors (Moderate); CYP1A2 Inhibitors (Strong); Dasatinib; Deferasirox; Droperidol; Floctafenine; Ginkgo Biloba; Glucosamine; Herbs (Anticoagulant/Antiplatelet Properties); HydrOXYzine; Influenza Virus Vaccine (Live/Attenuated); Ketorolac (Nasal); Ketorolac (Systemic); Linezolid; Loop Diuretics; Magnesium Sulfate; Multivitamins/Minerals (with ADEK, Folate, Iron); NSAID (Nonselective); Omega-3 Fatty Acids; Pentosan Polysulfate Sodium; Pentoxifylline; Perampanel; Potassium Acid Phosphate; Prostacyclin Analogues; Quinolone Antibiotics; Selective Serotonin Reuptake Inhibitors; Serotonin/Norepinephrine Reuptake Inhibitors; Sodium Oxybate; Succinylcholine; Tipranavir; Treprostinil; Vitamin E

Decreased Effect

Dihydrocodeine, Aspirin, and Caffeine may decrease the levels/effects of: ACE Inhibitors; Adenosine; Hyaluronidase; Iobenguane I 123; Loop Diuretics; Multivitamins/Minerals (with ADEK, Folate, Iron); NSAID (Nonselective); Pegvisomant; Probenecid; Regadenoson; Ticagrelor; Tiludronate

The levels/effects of Dihydrocodeine, Aspirin, and Caffeine may be decreased by: Ammonium Chloride; Corticosteroids (Systemic); Floctafenine; Ketorolac (Nasal); Ketorolac (Systemic); Mixed Agonist / Antagonist Opioids; NSAID (Nonselective); Peginterferon Alfa-2b; QuiNIDine; Teriflunomide

Ethanol/Nutrition/Herb Interactions Ethanol: May increase CNS depression; monitor for increased effects with coadministration. Caution patients about effects.

Pharmacodynamics/Kinetics

Onset of Action 10-30 minutes

Duration of Action 4-6 hours

Half-life Elimination Serum: 3.8 hours

Time to Peak Serum: 30-60 minutes

Pregnancy Considerations Animal reproduction studies have not been conducted with this combination. Birth defects, including some heart defects, have been associated with maternal use of opioid analgesics during the first trimester of pregnancy (Broussard, 2011). Use of opioids during pregnancy may produce physical dependence in the neonate (Rathmell, 1997). Dihydrocodeine is a semisynthetic analogue of codeine; it has been shown to cause respiratory depression in the fetus when administered to women during labor (Leppert, 2010; Myers, 1958; Sliom, 1970). Also refer to the aspirin and caffeine monographs for additional information.

Breast-Feeding Considerations Dihydrocodeine, aspirin, and caffeine are excreted in breast milk. Also refer to the aspirin and caffeine monographs for additional information.

Controlled Substance C-III

Dosage Forms

Capsule, oral:
Synalgos®-DC: Dihydrocodeine 16 mg, aspirin 356.4 mg, and caffeine 30 mg

Dental Comment There is no scientific evidence to warrant discontinuance of aspirin prior to dental surgery. Patients taking one aspirin tablet daily as an antithrombotic and who require dental surgery should be given special consideration in consultation with the physician before removal of the aspirin relative to prevention of postoperative bleeding.

Dihydrocodeine, Chlorpheniramine, and Phenylephrine
(dye hye droe KOE deen, klor fen IR a meen, & fen il EF rin)

Related Information

Chlorpheniramine on page 292
Codeine on page 344
Phenylephrine (Systemic) on page 1087

Brand Names: U.S. Coldcough PD; Novahistine DH; Tusscough DHC™

Pharmacologic Category Alkylamine Derivative; Alpha-Adrenergic Agonist; Analgesic, Opioid; Antitussive; Decongestant; Histamine H$_1$ Antagonist; Histamine H$_1$ Antagonist, First Generation

Use Symptomatic relief of cough and congestion associated with the upper respiratory tract

Local Anesthetic/Vasoconstrictor Precautions No information available to require special precautions

Effects on Dental Treatment Key adverse event(s) related to dental treatment:
Chlorpheniramine: Prolonged use will cause significant xerostomia (normal salivary flow resumes upon discontinuation).
Phenylephrine: Up to 10% of patients could experience tachycardia, palpitations, and xerostomia; use vasoconstrictor with caution.

Effects on Bleeding No information available to require special precautions

Adverse Effects See individual agents.

General Dosage Range

Oral:
Children 2-6 years: Novahistine DH: 1.25-2.5 mL every 4-6 hours as needed (maximum: 10 mL/day)
Children 6-12 years: Novahistine DH: 2.5-5 mL every 4-6 hours as needed (maximum: 20 mL/day)
Children >12 years and Adults: Novahistine DH: 5-10 mL every 4-6 hours as needed (maximum: 40 mL/day)

Mechanism of Action

Dihydrocodeine: Binds to opiate receptors in the CNS; suppresses cough in medullary center; produces generalized CNS depression

Chlorpheniramine: Competes with histamine for H$_1$-receptor sites on effector cells in the gastrointestinal tract, blood vessels, and respiratory tract

Phenylephrine: Potent, direct-acting alpha-adrenergic stimulator with weak beta-adrenergic activity; causes vasoconstriction of the arterioles of the nasal mucosa and conjunctiva

Controlled Substance C-III; C-V

Dihydroergotamine (dye hye droe er GOT a meen)

Brand Names: U.S. D.H.E. 45®; Migranal®
Brand Names: Canada Migranal®
Pharmacologic Category Antimigraine Agent; Ergot Derivative
Use Treatment of migraine headache with or without aura; injection also indicated for treatment of cluster headaches
Unlabeled Use Adjunct for DVT prophylaxis for hip surgery, for orthostatic hypotension, xerostomia secondary to antidepressant use, and pelvic congestion with pain

Local Anesthetic/Vasoconstrictor Precautions Use vasoconstrictor with caution in patients taking dihydroergotamine; this ergot alkaloid derivative directly stimulates vascular smooth muscle resulting in vasoconstriction of peripheral vasculature

Effects on Dental Treatment Key adverse event(s) related to dental treatment: Rhinitis and abnormal taste.

Effects on Bleeding No information available to require special precautions

Adverse Effects
>10%: Nasal spray: Respiratory: Rhinitis (26%)
1% to 10%: Nasal spray:
Central nervous system: Dizziness (4%), somnolence (3%)
Endocrine & metabolic: Hot flashes (1%)
Gastrointestinal: Nausea (10%), taste disturbance (8%), vomiting (4%), diarrhea (2%)
Local: Application site reaction (6%)
Neuromuscular & skeletal: Weakness (1%), stiffness (1%)
Respiratory: Pharyngitis (3%)

General Dosage Range
I.M., SubQ: Adults: 1 mg initially, may repeat hourly up to 3 mg total (maximum: 6 mg/week)
I.V.: Adults: 1 mg initially, may repeat hourly up to 2 mg total (maximum: 6 mg/week)
Intranasal: Adults: 1 spray (0.5 mg) in each nostril initially, may repeat after 15 minutes up to 4 sprays total (maximum: 6 sprays/24 hours; 8 sprays/week)

Mechanism of Action Ergot alkaloid alpha-adrenergic blocker directly stimulates vascular smooth muscle to vasoconstrict peripheral and cerebral vessels; also has effects on serotonin receptors

Pharmacodynamics/Kinetics
Onset of Action I.M.: 15-30 minutes
Duration of Action I.M.: 3-4 hours
Half-life Elimination ~9-10 hours
Time to Peak Serum: I.M.: 24 minutes; I.V.: 1-2 minutes; Intranasal: 30-60 minutes; SubQ 15-45 minutes

Pregnancy Risk Factor X
Pregnancy Considerations Dihydroergotamine is oxytocic and should not be used during pregnancy.

Diltiazem (dil TYE a zem)

Related Information

Calcium Channel Blockers and Gingival Hyperplasia *on page 1640*

Cardiovascular Diseases *on page 1492*

Brand Names: U.S. Cardizem®; Cardizem® CD; Cardizem® LA; Cartia XT®; Dilacor XR®; Dilt-CD; Dilt-XR; Diltia XT®; Diltzac; Matzim® LA; Taztia XT®; Tiazac®

Brand Names: Canada Apo-Diltiaz CD®; Apo-Diltiaz SR®; Apo-Diltiaz TZ®; Apo-Diltiaz®; Apo-Diltiaz® Injectable; Ava-Diltiazem; Cardizem® CD; CO Diltiazem CD; CO Diltiazem T; Diltiazem HCl ER®; Diltiazem Hydrochloride Injection; Diltiazem TZ; Diltiazem-CD; Nu-Diltiaz; Nu-Diltiaz-CD; PMS-Diltiazem CD; ratio-Diltiazem CD; Sandoz-Diltiazem CD; Sandoz-Diltiazem T; Teva-Diltiazem; Teva-Diltiazem CD; Teva-Diltiazem HCL ER Capsules; Tiazac®; Tiazac® XC

Generic Availability (U.S.) Yes

Pharmacologic Category Antianginal Agent; Antiarrhythmic Agent, Class IV; Calcium Channel Blocker; Calcium Channel Blocker, Nondihydropyridine

Use

Oral: Essential hypertension; chronic stable angina or angina from coronary artery spasm

Injection: Control of rapid ventricular rate in patients with atrial fibrillation or atrial flutter; conversion of paroxysmal supraventricular tachycardia (PSVT)

Unlabeled Use ACLS guidelines: Injection: Stable narrow-complex tachycardia uncontrolled or unconverted by adenosine or vagal maneuvers or if SVT is recurrent Hypertrophic cardiomyopathy; pediatric hypertension

Local Anesthetic/Vasoconstrictor Precautions No information available to require special precautions

Effects on Dental Treatment Key adverse event(s) related to dental treatment: Diltiazem has been reported to cause >10% incidence of gingival hyperplasia; usually disappears with discontinuation (consultation with physician is suggested).

Effects on Bleeding No information available to require special precautions

Adverse Effects Note: Frequencies represent ranges for various dosage forms. Patients with impaired ventricular function and/or conduction abnormalities may have higher incidence of adverse reactions.

>10%:
Cardiovascular: Edema (2% to 15%)
Central nervous system: Headache (5% to 12%)
2% to 10%:
Cardiovascular: AV block (first degree 2% to 8%), edema (lower limb 2% to 8%), pain (6%), bradycardia (2% to 6%), hypotension (<2% to 4%), vasodilation (2% to 3%), extrasystoles (2%), flushing (1% to 2%), palpitation (1% to 2%)
Central nervous system: Dizziness (3% to 10%), nervousness (2%)
Dermatologic: Rash (1% to 4%)
Endocrine & metabolic: Gout (1% to 2%)
Gastrointestinal: Dyspepsia (1% to 6%), constipation (<2% to 4%), vomiting (2%), diarrhea (1% to 2%)
Local: Injection site reactions: Burning, itching (4%)
Neuromuscular & skeletal: Weakness (1% to 4%), myalgia (2%)
Respiratory: Rhinitis (<2% to 10%), pharyngitis (2% to 6%), dyspnea (1% to 6%), bronchitis (1% to 4%), cough (≤3%), sinus congestion (1% to 2%)

Dosage

Children (unlabeled use): Minimal information available; some centers use the following: Oral: Hypertension: Immediate release tablets: Initial: 1.5-2 mg/kg/day divided in 3 doses/day (maximum dose 6 mg/kg/day up to 360 mg/day) (Flynn, 2000)

Adults:
Oral:
Angina:
Capsule, extended release:
Dilacor XR®, Dilt-XR, Diltia XT®: Initial: 120 mg once daily; titrate over 7-14 days; usual dose range: 120-320 mg/day: maximum: 480 mg/day
Cardizem® CD, Cartia XT®, Dilt-CD: Initial: 120-180 mg once daily; titrate over 7-14 days; usual dose range: 120-320 mg/day; maximum: 480 mg/day
Tiazac®, Taztia XT®: Initial: 120-180 mg once daily; titrate over 7-14 days; usual dose range: 120-320 mg/day; maximum: 540 mg/day
Tablet, extended release (Cardizem® LA, Matzim® LA, Tiazac® XC [CAN; not available in U.S.]): 180 mg once daily; may increase at 7- to 14-day intervals; usual dose range: 120-320 mg/day; maximum: 360 mg/day
Tablet, immediate release (Cardizem®): Usual starting dose: 30 mg 4 times/day; titrate dose gradually at 1- to 2-day intervals; usual dose range: 120-320 mg/day
Hypertension:
Capsule, extended release (once-daily dosing):
Cardizem® CD, Cartia XT®, Dilt-CD: Initial: 180-240 mg once daily; dose adjustment may be made after 14 days; usual dose range (JNC 7): 180-420 mg/day; maximum: 480 mg/day
Dilacor® XR, Diltia XT®, Dilt-XR: Initial: 180-240 mg once daily; dose adjustment may be made after 14 days; usual dose range (JNC 7): 180-420 mg/day; maximum: 540 mg/day
Tiazac®, Taztia XT®: Initial: 120-240 mg once daily; dose adjustment may be made after 14 days; usual dose range (JNC 7): 180-420 mg/day; maximum: 540 mg/day
Capsule, extended release (twice-daily dosing): Initial: 60-120 mg twice daily; dose adjustment may be made after 14 days; usual range: 240-360 mg/day
Note: Diltiazem is available as a generic intended for either once- or twice-daily dosing, depending on the formulation; verify appropriate extended release capsule formulation is administered.
Tablet, extended release (Cardizem® LA, Matzim® LA, Tiazac® XC [CAN; not available in U.S.]): Initial: 180-240 mg once daily; dose adjustment may be made after 14 days; usual dose range (JNC 7): 120-540 mg/day
Note: Elderly: Consider lower initial doses (eg, 120 mg once daily using extended release capsule) and titrate to response (Aronow, 2011)
I.V.: *Atrial fibrillation, atrial flutter, PSVT:*
Initial bolus dose: 0.25 mg/kg actual body weight over 2 minutes (average adult dose: 20 mg); ACLS guideline recommends 15-20 mg
Repeat bolus dose (may be administered after 15 minutes if the response is inadequate): 0.35 mg/kg actual body weight over 2 minutes (average adult dose: 25 mg); ACLS guideline recommends 20-25 mg

◀ Continuous infusion (infusions >24 hours or infusion rates >15 mg/hour are not recommended): Initial infusion rate of 10 mg/hour; rate may be increased in 5 mg/hour increments up to 15 mg/hour as needed; some patients may respond to an initial rate of 5 mg/hour.

If diltiazem injection is administered by continuous infusion for >24 hours, the possibility of decreased diltiazem clearance, prolonged elimination half-life, and increased diltiazem and/or diltiazem metabolite plasma concentrations should be considered.

Conversion from I.V. diltiazem to oral diltiazem:
Oral dose (mg/day) is approximately equal to [rate (mg/hour) x 3 + 3] x 10.
3 mg/hour = 120 mg/day
5 mg/hour = 180 mg/day
7 mg/hour = 240 mg/day
11 mg/hour = 360 mg/day

Dosing adjustment in renal impairment: Use with caution; no dosing adjustments recommended
Dialysis: Not removed by hemo- or peritoneal dialysis; supplemental dose is not necessary.

Dosing adjustment in hepatic impairment: Use with caution; no specific dosing recommendations available; extensively metabolized by the liver; half-life is increased in patients with cirrhosis

Mechanism of Action Nondihydropyridine calcium channel blocker which inhibits calcium ion from entering the "slow channels" or select voltage-sensitive areas of vascular smooth muscle and myocardium during depolarization, producing a relaxation of coronary vascular smooth muscle and coronary vasodilation; increases myocardial oxygen delivery in patients with vasospastic angina

Contraindications

Oral: Hypersensitivity to diltiazem or any component of the formulation; sick sinus syndrome (except in patients with a functioning artificial pacemaker); second- or third-degree AV block (except in patients with a functioning artificial pacemaker); severe hypotension (systolic <90 mm Hg); acute MI and pulmonary congestion

Intravenous (I.V.): Hypersensitivity to diltiazem or any component of the formulation; sick sinus syndrome (except in patients with a functioning artificial pacemaker); second- or third-degree AV block (except in patients with a functioning artificial pacemaker); severe hypotension (systolic <90 mm Hg); cardiogenic shock; administration concomitantly or within a few hours of the administration of I.V. beta-blockers; atrial fibrillation or flutter associated with accessory bypass tract (eg, Wolff-Parkinson-White syndrome); ventricular tachycardia (with wide-complex tachycardia, must determine whether origin is supraventricular or ventricular)

Canadian labeling: Additional contraindications (not in U.S. labeling): I.V. and Oral: Pregnancy; use in women of childbearing potential

Warnings/Precautions Can cause first-, second-, and third-degree AV block or sinus bradycardia and risk increases with agents known to slow cardiac conduction. The most common side effect is peripheral edema; occurs within 2-3 weeks of starting therapy. Symptomatic hypotension with or without syncope can rarely occur; blood pressure must be lowered at a rate appropriate for the patient's clinical condition. Use caution when using diltiazem together with a beta-blocker; may result in conduction disturbances, hypotension, and worsened LV function. Simultaneous administration of I.V. diltiazem and an I.V. beta-blocker or

administration within a few hours of each other may result in asystole and is contraindicated. Use with other agents known to either reduce SA node function and/or AV nodal conduction (eg, digoxin) or reduce sympathetic outflow (eg, clonidine) may increase the risk of serious bradycardia. Use caution in left ventricular dysfunction (may exacerbate condition). Avoid use of diltiazem in patients with heart failure and reduced ejection fraction (Hunt, 2009). Use with caution with hypertrophic obstructive cardiomyopathy; routine use is currently not recommended due to insufficient evidence (Maron, 2003). Use with caution in hepatic or renal dysfunction. Transient dermatologic reactions have been observed with use; if reaction persists, discontinue. May (rarely) progress to erythema multiforme or exfoliative dermatitis.

Drug Interactions

Metabolism/Transport Effects Substrate of CYP2C9 (minor), CYP2D6 (minor), CYP3A4 (major), P-glycoprotein; **Note:** Assignment of Major/Minor substrate status based on clinically relevant drug interaction potential; **Inhibits** CYP2C9 (weak), CYP2D6 (weak), CYP3A4 (moderate)

Avoid Concomitant Use

Avoid concomitant use of Diltiazem with any of the following: Bosutinib; Conivaptan; Dantrolene; Ivabradine; Lomitapide; Pimozide; Tolvaptan

Increased Effect/Toxicity

Diltiazem may increase the levels/effects of: Alfentanil; Amifostine; Amiodarone; Antihypertensives; Aprepitant; ARIPiprazole; AtorvaSTATin; Atosiban; Avanafil; Benzodiazepines (metabolized by oxidation); Beta-Blockers; Bosutinib; Budesonide (Systemic, Oral Inhalation); BusPIRone; Calcium Channel Blockers (Dihydropyridine); CarBAMazepine; Cardiac Glycosides; Colchicine; Corticosteroids (Systemic); CycloSPORINE (Systemic); CYP3A4 Substrates; Dronedarone; Eletriptan; Eplerenone; Everolimus; Fingolimod; Fosaprepitant; Fosphenytoin; Halofantrine; Hypotensive Agents; Ivabradine; Ivacaftor; Lithium; Lomitapide; Lovastatin; Lurasidone; Magnesium Salts; Midodrine; Neuromuscular-Blocking Agents (Nondepolarizing); Nitroprusside; Phenytoin; Pimecrolimus; Pimozide; Propafenone; QuiNIDine; Ranolazine; Red Yeast Rice; RiTUXimab; Rivaroxaban; Salicylates; Salmeterol; Saxagliptin; Simvastatin; Tacrolimus (Systemic); Tacrolimus (Topical); Tolvaptan; Vilazodone; Zuclopenthixol

The levels/effects of Diltiazem may be increased by: Alpha1-Blockers; Anilidopiperidine Opioids; Antifungal Agents (Azole Derivatives, Systemic); Aprepitant; AtorvaSTATin; Calcium Channel Blockers (Dihydropyridine); Cimetidine; CloNIDine; Conivaptan; CycloSPORINE (Systemic); CYP3A4 Inhibitors (Moderate); CYP3A4 Inhibitors (Strong); Dantrolene; Dasatinib; Diazoxide; Dronedarone; Fluconazole; Fosaprepitant; Grapefruit Juice; Herbs (Hypotensive Properties); Ivabradine; Ivacaftor; Lovastatin; Macrolide Antibiotics; Magnesium Salts; MAO Inhibitors; Mifepristone; Pentoxifylline; P-glycoprotein/ABCB1 Inhibitors; Phosphodiesterase 5 Inhibitors; Prostacyclin Analogues; Protease Inhibitors; Simvastatin

Decreased Effect

Diltiazem may decrease the levels/effects of: Clopidogrel; Ifosfamide

The levels/effects of Diltiazem may be decreased by: Barbiturates; Calcium Salts; CarBAMazepine; Colestipol; CYP3A4 Inducers (Strong); Deferasirox; Herbs (CYP3A4 Inducers); Herbs (Hypertensive Properties);

Methylphenidate; Nafcillin; Peginterferon Alfa-2b; P-glycoprotein/ABCB1 Inducers; Rifamycin Derivatives; Tocilizumab; Yohimbine

Ethanol/Nutrition/Herb Interactions

Ethanol: Ethanol may increase risk of hypotension or vasodilation. Management: Avoid ethanol.

Food: Diltiazem serum levels may be elevated if taken with food. Serum concentrations were not altered by grapefruit juice in small clinical trials.

Herb/Nutraceutical: St John's wort may decrease diltiazem levels. Some herbal medications may worsen hypertension (eg, licorice); others may increase the antihypertensive effect of diltiazem (eg, shepherd's purse). Management: Avoid St John's wort, bayberry, blue cohosh, cayenne, ephedra, ginger, ginseng (American), kola, licorice, and yohimbe. Avoid black cohosh, California poppy, coleus, golden seal, hawthorn, mistletoe, periwinkle, quinine, and shepherd's purse.

Pharmacodynamics/Kinetics

Onset of Action Oral: Immediate release tablet: 30-60 minutes; I.V.: 3 minutes

Duration of Action I.V.: Bolus: 1-3 hours; Continuous infusion (after discontinuation): 0.5-10 hours

Half-life Elimination Immediate release tablet: 3-4.5 hours, may be prolonged with renal impairment; Extended release tablet: 6-9 hours; Extended release capsules: 5-10 hours; I.V.: single dose: ~3.4 hours; continuous infusion: 4-5 hours

Time to Peak Serum: Immediate release tablet: 2-4 hours; Extended release tablet: 11-18 hours; Extended release capsule: 10-14 hours

Pregnancy Risk Factor C

Pregnancy Considerations Teratogenic and embryotoxic effects have been demonstrated in animal reproduction studies.

Lactation Enters breast milk/not recommended (AAP considers "compatible"; AAP 2001 update pending)

Breast-Feeding Considerations Diltiazem is excreted into breastmilk in concentrations similar to those in the maternal plasma.

Dosage Forms

Capsule, extended release, oral: 60 mg, 90 mg, 120 mg, 180 mg, 240 mg, 300 mg, 360 mg, 420 mg

Cardizem® CD: 120 mg, 180 mg, 240 mg, 300 mg, 360 mg

Cartia XT®: 120 mg, 180 mg, 240 mg, 300 mg

Dilacor XR®: 240 mg

Dilt-CD: 120 mg, 180 mg, 240 mg, 300 mg

Dilt-XR: 120 mg, 180 mg, 240 mg

Diltia XT®: 120 mg, 180 mg, 240 mg

Diltzac: 120 mg, 180 mg, 240 mg, 300 mg, 360 mg

Taztia XT®: 120 mg, 180 mg, 240 mg, 300 mg, 360 mg

Tiazac®: 120 mg, 180 mg, 240 mg, 300 mg, 360 mg, 420 mg

Injection, powder for reconstitution: 100 mg

Injection, solution: 5 mg/mL (5 mL, 10 mL, 25 mL)

Tablet, oral: 30 mg, 60 mg, 90 mg, 120 mg

Cardizem®: 30 mg, 60 mg, 90 mg, 120 mg

Tablet, extended release, oral:

Cardizem® LA: 120 mg, 180 mg, 240 mg, 300 mg, 360 mg, 420 mg

Matzim® LA: 180 mg, 240 mg, 300 mg, 360 mg, 420 mg

Dosage Forms: Canada

Tablet, extended release:

Tiazac® XC: 120 mg, 180 mg, 240 mg, 300 mg, 360 mg

DimenhyDRINATE (dye men HYE dri nate)

Brand Names: U.S. Dramamine® for kids [OTC]; Dramamine® [OTC]; Driminate [OTC]; TripTone® [OTC]

Brand Names: Canada Apo-Dimenhydrinate® [OTC]; Children's Motion Sickness Liquid [OTC]; Dimenhydrinate Injection; Dinate® [OTC]; Gravol IM; Gravol® [OTC]; Jamp-Dimenhydrinate [OTC]; Nauseatol [OTC]; Novo-Dimenate [OTC]; PMS-Dimenhydrinate [OTC]; Sandoz-Dimenhydrinate [OTC]; Travel Tabs [OTC]

Pharmacologic Category Ethanolamine Derivative; Histamine H_1 Antagonist; Histamine H_1 Antagonist, First Generation

Use Treatment and prevention of nausea, vertigo, and vomiting associated with motion sickness

Unlabeled Use Nausea and vomiting of pregnancy (NVP)

Local Anesthetic/Vasoconstrictor Precautions No information available to require special precautions

Effects on Dental Treatment Key adverse event(s) related to dental treatment: Significant xerostomia (normal salivary flow resumes upon discontinuation).

Effects on Bleeding No information available to require special precautions

Adverse Effects Frequency not defined.

Cardiovascular: Tachycardia

Central nervous system: Dizziness, drowsiness, excitation, headache, insomnia, lassitude, nervousness, restlessness

Dermatologic: Rash

Gastrointestinal: Anorexia, epigastric distress, nausea, xerostomia

Genitourinary: Dysuria

Ocular: Blurred vision

Respiratory: Thickening of bronchial secretions

General Dosage Range

Oral:

Children 2-5 years: 12.5-25 mg every 6-8 hours (maximum: 75 mg/day)

Children 6-12 years: 25-50 mg every 6-8 hours (maximum: 150 mg/day)

I.M.:

Children: 1.25 mg/kg or 37.5 mg/m² 4 times/day (maximum: 300 mg/day)

Adults: 50-100 mg every 4 hours

I.V.: *Adults:* 50-100 mg every 4 hours

Mechanism of Action Competes with histamine for H_1-receptor sites on effector cells in the gastrointestinal tract, blood vessels, and respiratory tract; blocks chemoreceptor trigger zone, diminishes vestibular stimulation, and depresses labyrinthine function through its central anticholinergic activity

Pregnancy Risk Factor B

Pregnancy Considerations Adverse events have not been observed in animal reproduction studies. The risk of fetal abnormalities was not increased following maternal use of dimenhydrinate during any trimester of pregnancy. Dimenhydrinate is recommended for the treatment of nausea and vomiting of pregnancy. Dimenhydrinate may have an oxytocic effect if used during labor.

Dimercaprol (dye mer KAP role)

Brand Names: U.S. BAL in Oil®
Pharmacologic Category Antidote

Use Antidote to gold, arsenic (except arsine), or acute mercury poisoning (except nonalkyl mercury); adjunct to edetate CALCIUM disodium in acute lead poisoning

Local Anesthetic/Vasoconstrictor Precautions No information available to require special precautions

Effects on Dental Treatment No significant effects or complications reported

Effects on Bleeding No information available to require special precautions

Adverse Effects
Frequency not always defined.
Cardiovascular: Chest pain, hypertension (dose related), tachycardia (dose related)
Central nervous system: Anxiety, fever (children ~30%), headache, nervousness
Dermatologic: Abscess
Gastrointestinal: Abdominal pain, burning sensation (lips, mouth, throat), nausea, salivation, throat irritation/pain, vomiting
Genitourinary: Burning sensation (penis)
Hematologic: Leukopenia (polymorphonuclear)
Local: Injection site pain
Neuromuscular & skeletal: Paresthesias (hand), weakness
Ocular: Blepharospasm, conjunctivitis, lacrimation
Renal: Acute renal insufficiency
Respiratory: Rhinorrhea, throat constriction
Miscellaneous: Diaphoresis

General Dosage Range I.M.: *Children and Adults:* Dosage varies greatly depending on indication

Mechanism of Action Sulfhydryl group combines with ions of various heavy metals to form relatively stable, nontoxic, soluble chelates which are excreted in urine

Pharmacodynamics/Kinetics
Time to Peak Serum: 0.5-1 hour

Pregnancy Risk Factor C

Pregnancy Considerations Animal reproduction studies have not been conducted. There are no adequate and well-controlled studies in pregnant women.

Lead poisoning: Lead is known to cross the placenta in amounts related to maternal plasma levels. Prenatal lead exposure may be associated with adverse events such as spontaneous abortion, preterm delivery, decreased birth weight, and impaired neurodevelopment. Some adverse outcomes may occur with maternal blood lead levels <10 mcg/dL. In addition, pregnant women exposed to lead may have an increased risk of gestational hypertension. Consider chelation therapy in pregnant women with confirmed blood lead levels ≥45 mcg/dL (pregnant women with blood lead levels ≥70 mcg/dL should be considered for chelation regardless of trimester); consultation with experts in lead poisoning and high-risk pregnancy is recommended. Encephalopathic pregnant women should be chelated regardless of trimester (CDC, 2010).

Dimethyl Fumarate (dye meth il FYOO ma rate)

Brand Names: U.S. Tecfidera™
Pharmacologic Category Fumaric Acid Derivative; Immunomodulator, Systemic
Use Treatment of relapsing forms of multiple sclerosis (MS)

Local Anesthetic/Vasoconstrictor Precautions No information available to require special precautions

Effects on Dental Treatment No significant effects or complications reported

Effects on Bleeding No information available to require special precautions

Adverse Effects
>10%:
Cardiovascular: Flushing (40%)
Gastrointestinal: Abdominal pain (18%), diarrhea (14%), nausea (12%)
Infection: Infection (60%; placebo: 58%)
1% to 10%:
Dermatologic: Pruritus (8%), skin rash (8%), erythema (5%)
Gastrointestinal: Vomiting (9%), dyspepsia (5%)
Genitourinary: Proteinuria (6%)
Hematologic: Lymphocytopenia (2% to 6%)
Hepatic: Increased serum AST (4%)

General Dosage Range Oral: *Adults:* Initial: 120 mg twice daily; Maintenance: 240 mg twice daily

Mechanism of Action DMF and its active metabolite, monomethyl fumarate (MMF), have been shown to activate the nuclear factor (erythyroid-derived 2)-like 2 (Nrf2) pathway, which is involved in cellular response to oxidative stress. The mechanism by which dimethyl fumarate (DMF) exerts a therapeutic effect in MS is unknown, although it is believed to result from its anti-inflammatory and cytoprotective properties via activation of the Nrf2 pathway (Fox, 2012; Gold, 2012).

Pharmacodynamics/Kinetics
Half-life Elimination MMF: ~1 hour
Time to Peak 2-2.5 hours

Pregnancy Risk Factor C

Pregnancy Considerations Adverse events were observed in animal reproduction studies.

Women exposed to dimethyl fumarate during pregnancy are encouraged to enroll in the Pregnancy Registry by calling 800-456-2255.

Dinoprostone (dye noe PROST one)

Brand Names: U.S. Cervidil®; Prepidil®; Prostin E₂®
Brand Names: Canada Cervidil®; Prepidil®; Prostin E₂®
Pharmacologic Category Abortifacient; Prostaglandin
Use
Endocervical gel (Prepidil®): Promote cervical ripening in patients at or near term in whom there is a medical or obstetrical indication for the induction of labor
Suppositories (Prostin E₂®): Terminate pregnancy from 12th through 20th week of gestation; evacuate uterus in cases of missed abortion or intrauterine fetal death up to 28 weeks of gestation; manage benign hydatidiform mole (nonmetastatic gestational trophoblastic disease)
Tablet (oral) (Prostin E₂®; Canadian availability): Elective induction of labor; when indications for induction of labor exist (eg, premature rupture of amniotic membranes, toxemia of pregnancy, Rh incompatibility, diabetes mellitus, hypertension, postmaturity, intrauterine death or fetal growth retardation)
Vaginal gel (Prostin E₂®; Canadian availability): Induction of labor in patients at or near term with singleton pregnancy, vertex presentation, and favorable induction features
Vaginal insert (Cervidil®): Initiation and/or continuation of cervical ripening in patients at or near term in whom there is a medical or obstetrical indication for the induction of labor

Local Anesthetic/Vasoconstrictor Precautions No information available to require special precautions

Effects on Dental Treatment No significant effects or complications reported

Effects on Bleeding No information available to require special precautions

Adverse Effects

Endocervical gel: 1% to 10%:
Central nervous system: Fever (1%)
Gastrointestinal: GI upset (6%)
Genitourinary: Abnormal uterine contractions (7%), warm feeling in vagina (2%)
Neuromuscular & skeletal: Back pain (3%)

Suppository: Frequency not defined:
Cardiovascular: Arrhythmia, chest pain, chest tightness, hypotension, syncope
Central nervous system: Chills, dizziness, fever, headache, shivering, tension
Dermatologic: Rash, skin discoloration
Endocrine & metabolic: Breast tenderness, endometritis, hot flashes
Gastrointestinal: Dehydration, diarrhea, nausea, vomiting
Genitourinary: Uterine rupture, urinary retention, vaginal pain, vaginismus, vaginitis, vulvitis
Neuromuscular & skeletal: Arthralgia, backache, joint inflammation/pain (new or exacerbated), leg cramps (nocturnal), muscle cramp/pain, myalgia, paresthesia, stiff neck, tremor, weakness
Ocular: Blurred vision, eye pain
Otic: Hearing impairment
Respiratory: Cough, dyspnea, laryngitis, pharyngitis, wheezing
Miscellaneous: Diaphoresis

Tablets (oral) (Canadian availability):
>10%: Gastrointestinal: Vomiting (with or without nausea/diarrhea): 21% to 50% (dose dependent)
1% to 10%: Genitourinary: Uterine hypertonus (3%)
<1%: Bronchospasm, chills, dizziness, dyspnea, fever, flushing, headache, hiccups, hyper-/hypotension, postpartum hemorrhage, rash, tachycardia
Frequency not defined:
Cardiovascular: Cardiac arrest
Central nervous system: Transient vasovagal symptoms
Genitourinary: Abnormal uterine contractions, placental abruption, rapid cervical dilation, uterine rupture
Neuromuscular & skeletal: Back pain
Respiratory: Asthma, pulmonary amniotic fluid embolism
Miscellaneous: Hypersensitivity reactions including anaphylaxis, anaphylactic shock, and nonimmunologic anaphylaxis (formerly known as anaphylactoid reaction)

Vaginal gel (Canadian availability):
1% to 10%: Genitourinary: Uterine hypercontractility (3%), failed induction (2%)
Frequency not defined:
Cardiovascular: Cardiac arrest
Central nervous system: Fever
Gastrointestinal: Diarrhea, nausea, vomiting
Genitourinary: Abnormal uterine contractions, uterine rupture, warm feeling in vagina
Neuromuscular & skeletal: Back pain
Miscellaneous: Hypersensitivity reactions including anaphylaxis, anaphylactic shock, and nonimmunologic anaphylaxis (formerly known as anaphylactoid reaction)

Vaginal insert: 1% to 10%: Genitourinary: Uterine hyperstimulation *without* fetal distress (2% to 5%), uterine hyperstimulation *with* fetal distress (3%)

General Dosage Range

Endocervical: *Children (females of reproductive age) and Adults (females):* 0.5 mg; may repeat every 6 hours if needed. Maximum cumulative dose: 1.5 mg/24 hours

Intravaginal: *Children (females of reproductive age) and Adults (females):* Insert: 10 mg; remove at onset of active labor or after 12 hours; Suppository: 20 mg every 3-5 hours until abortion occurs

Mechanism of Action Dinoprostone (prostaglandin E$_2$) is an endogenous hormone found in low concentrations in most tissues of the body. When administered as an abortifacient, it stimulates uterine contractions similar to those seen during natural labor. When administered for labor induction, it relaxes the smooth muscle of the cervix allowing dilation and passage of the fetus through the birth canal.

Pharmacodynamics/Kinetics

Onset of Action Uterine contractions: Vaginal suppository: Within 10 minutes

Duration of Action Vaginal insert: 0.3 mg/hour over 12 hours; Vaginal suppository: Up to 2-3 hours

Half-life Elimination 2.5-5 minutes

Time to Peak Endocervical gel: 30-45 minutes

Pregnancy Risk Factor C

Pregnancy Considerations Skeletal anomalies and embryotoxicity have been observed in animal reproduction studies. Although these effects would not be expected in humans when administered after the period of organogenesis, a sustained increase in uterine tone may have increased risks of adverse events to the fetus.

Fetal distress without corresponding maternal uterine hyperstimulation was observed in 3% to 4% of infants exposed to Cervidil® *in utero.* No adverse effects on physical or psychomotor function were observed in a 3 year follow-up study of exposed infants. Abnormal fetal heart rates were observed in 17% of infants exposed to Prepidil® gel *in utero.* Deceleration, intrauterine fetal sepsis, fetal depression and fetal acidosis have also been reported with administration of the endocervical gel. Still births, abnormal fetal heart rate and fetal distress have been reported with administration of Prostin E$_2$® vaginal gel and oral tablets (Canadian availability).

When used for termination of pregnancy, dinoprostone is not considered feticidal, but is used to terminate pregnancy due to its ability to stimulate uterine contractions; do not use if fetus has reached the stage of viability.

DiphenhydrAMINE (Systemic)
(dye fen HYE dra meen)

Related Information
Management of Patients Undergoing Cancer Therapy *on page 1596*
Ulcerative, Erosive, and Painful Oral Mucosal Disorders *on page 1578*
Viral Infections *on page 1575*

Related Sample Prescriptions
Recurrent Aphthous Stomatitis *on page 1618*

Brand Names: U.S. Aler-Cap [OTC]; Aler-Dryl [OTC]; Aler-Tab [OTC]; AllerMax® [OTC]; Altaryl [OTC]; Anti-Hist [OTC]; Banophen™ [OTC]; Benadryl® Allergy Quick Dissolve [OTC]; Benadryl® Allergy [OTC]; Benadryl® Children's Allergy FastMelt® [OTC]; Benadryl® Children's Allergy Perfect Measure™ [OTC]; Benadryl® Children's Allergy [OTC]; Benadryl®

Children's Dye Free Allergy [OTC]; Benadryl® Dye-Free Allergy [OTC]; Compoz® [OTC]; Diphen [OTC]; Diphenhist® [OTC]; Geri-Dryl; Histaprin [OTC]; Nytol® Quick Caps [OTC]; Nytol® Quick Gels [OTC]; Pedia-Care® Children's Allergy [OTC]; PediaCare® Children's NightTime Cough [OTC]; Q-dryl [OTC]; Quenalin [OTC]; Siladryl Allergy [OTC]; Silphen [OTC]; Simply Sleep® [OTC]; Sleep-ettes D [OTC]; Sleep-Tabs [OTC]; Sleepinal® [OTC]; Sominex® Maximum Strength [OTC]; Sominex® [OTC]; Theraflu® Thin Strips® Multi Symptom [OTC]; Twilite® [OTC]; Unisom® SleepGels® Maximum Strength [OTC]; Unisom® SleepMelts™ [OTC]; Vicks® ZzzQuil™ [OTC]

Brand Names: Canada Allerdryl®); Allernix; Benadryl®); Nytol®; Nytol® Extra Strength; PMS-Diphenhydramine; Simply Sleep®; Sominex®

Generic Availability (U.S.) Yes: Excludes orally-disintegrating tablet, strip

Pharmacologic Category Ethanolamine Derivative; Histamine H_1 Antagonist; Histamine H_1 Antagonist, First Generation

Dental Use Symptomatic relief of nasal mucosal congestion; symptomatic relief of oral erosions (systemic diphenhydramine used topically) including aphthous stomatitis

Use Symptomatic relief of allergic symptoms caused by histamine release including nasal allergies and allergic dermatosis; adjunct to epinephrine in the treatment of anaphylaxis; nighttime sleep aid; prevention or treatment of motion sickness; antitussive; management of Parkinsonian syndrome including drug-induced extrapyramidal symptoms

Local Anesthetic/Vasoconstrictor Precautions No information available to require special precautions

Effects on Dental Treatment Key adverse event(s) related to dental treatment: Xerostomia (normal salivary flow resumes upon discontinuation) and dry mucous membranes. Chronic use of antihistamines will inhibit salivary flow, particularly in elderly patients; may contribute to periodontal disease and oral discomfort. See Dental Comment.

Effects on Bleeding No information available to require special precautions

Adverse Effects Frequency not defined.

Cardiovascular: Chest tightness, extrasystoles, hypotension, palpitation, tachycardia

Central nervous system: Chills, confusion, convulsion, disturbed coordination, dizziness, euphoria, excitation, fatigue, headache, insomnia, irritability, nervousness, paradoxical excitement, restlessness, sedation, sleepiness, vertigo

Endocrine & metabolic: Menstrual irregularities (early menses)

Gastrointestinal: Anorexia, constipation, diarrhea, dry mucous membranes, epigastric distress, nausea, throat tightness, vomiting, xerostomia

Genitourinary: Difficult urination, urinary frequency, urinary retention

Hematologic: Agranulocytosis, hemolytic anemia, thrombocytopenia

Neuromuscular & skeletal: Neuritis, paresthesia, tremor

Ocular: Blurred vision, diplopia

Otic: Labyrinthitis (acute), tinnitus

Respiratory: Nasal stuffiness, thickening of bronchial secretions, wheezing

Miscellaneous: Anaphylactic shock, diaphoresis

Dental Usual Dosage

Symptomatic relief of nasal mucosal congestion: Adults: Oral: 25-50 mg every 6-8 hours

Symptomatic relief of oral erosions (used topically): Adults: Rinse with 5-10 mL every 2 hours and expectorate

Dosage Note: Dosages are expressed as the hydrochloride salt.

Children:

Allergic reactions or motion sickness: Oral, I.M., I.V.: 5 mg/kg/day or 150 mg/m²/day in divided doses every 6-8 hours, not to exceed 300 mg/day

Alternate dosing by age: Oral:

2 to <6 years: 6.25 mg every 4-6 hours; maximum: 37.5 mg/day

6 to <12 years: 12.5-25 mg every 4-6 hours; maximum: 150 mg/day

≥12 years: 25-50 mg every 4-6 hours; maximum: 300 mg/day

Night-time sleep aid: Oral: Children ≥12 years: 50 mg at bedtime

Antitussive: Oral:

2 to <6 years: 6.25 mg every 4 hours; maximum: 37.5 mg/day

6 to <12 years: 12.5 mg every 4 hours; maximum: 75 mg/day

≥12 years: 25 mg every 4 hours; maximum: 150 mg/day

Treatment of dystonic reactions: I.M., I.V.: 0.5-1 mg/kg/dose

Adults:

Allergic reactions or motion sickness: Oral: 25-50 mg every 6-8 hours

Antitussive: Oral: 25 mg every 4 hours; maximum: 150 mg/24 hours

Night-time sleep aid: Oral: 50 mg at bedtime

Allergic reactions or motion sickness: I.M., I.V.: 10-50 mg per dose; single doses up to 100 mg may be used if needed; not to exceed 400 mg/day

Dystonic reaction: I.M., I.V.: 50 mg in a single dose; may repeat in 20-30 minutes if necessary

Elderly: Initial: 25 mg 2-3 times/day increasing as needed

Mechanism of Action Competes with histamine for H_1-receptor sites on effector cells in the gastrointestinal tract, blood vessels, and respiratory tract; anticholinergic and sedative effects are also seen

Contraindications Hypersensitivity to diphenhydramine or any component of the formulation; acute asthma; neonates or premature infants; breast-feeding; use as a local anesthetic (injection)

Warnings/Precautions Causes sedation, caution must be used in performing tasks which require alertness (eg, operating machinery or driving). Sedative effects of CNS depressants or ethanol are potentiated. Antihistamines may cause excitation in young children. Use with caution in patients with angle-closure glaucoma, pyloroduodenal obstruction (including stenotic peptic ulcer), urinary tract obstruction (including bladder neck obstruction and symptomatic prostatic hyperplasia), asthma, hyperthyroidism, increased intraocular pressure, and cardiovascular disease (including hypertension and tachycardia). Some preparations contain soy protein; avoid use in patients with soy protein or peanut allergies. Some products may contain phenylalanine.

Oral products: In the elderly, avoid use of this potent anticholinergic agent due to increased risk of confusion, dry mouth, constipation, and other anticholinergic effects; clearance decreases in patients of advanced age; tolerance develops to hypnotic effects; when used for severe allergic reaction, use may be appropriate (Beers Criteria).

Self-medication (OTC use): Do not use with other products containing diphenhydramine, even ones used on the skin. Oral products are not for OTC use in children <6 years of age.

Drug Interactions

Metabolism/Transport Effects Inhibits CYP2D6 (moderate)

Avoid Concomitant Use

Avoid concomitant use of DiphenhydrAMINE (Systemic) with any of the following: Aclidinium; Azelastine (Nasal); Ipratropium (Oral Inhalation); Paraldehyde; Thioridazine; Tiotropium

Increased Effect/Toxicity

DiphenhydrAMINE (Systemic) may increase the levels/effects of: Alcohol (Ethyl); Anticholinergics; ARIPiprazole; Azelastine (Nasal); Buprenorphine; CNS Depressants; CYP2D6 Substrates; Fesoterodine; Highest Risk QTc-Prolonging Agents; Methotrimeprazine; Metoprolol; Metyrosine; Mirtazapine; Moderate Risk QTc-Prolonging Agents; Nebivolol; Paraldehyde; Pramipexole; ROPINIRole; Rotigotine; Selective Serotonin Reuptake Inhibitors; Thioridazine; Tiotropium; Zolpidem

The levels/effects of DiphenhydrAMINE (Systemic) may be increased by: Aclidinium; Droperidol; HydrOXYzine; Ipratropium (Oral Inhalation); Magnesium Sulfate; Methotrimeprazine; Mifepristone; Perampanel; Pramlintide; Propafenone; Sodium Oxybate

Decreased Effect

DiphenhydrAMINE (Systemic) may decrease the levels/effects of: Acetylcholinesterase Inhibitors (Central); Benzylpenicilloyl Polylysine; Betahistine; Codeine; Hyaluronidase; Tamoxifen; TraMADol

The levels/effects of DiphenhydrAMINE (Systemic) may be decreased by: Acetylcholinesterase Inhibitors (Central); Amphetamines

Ethanol/Nutrition/Herb Interactions

Ethanol: May increase CNS depression; monitor for increased effects with coadministration. Caution patients about effects.

Herb/Nutraceutical: Avoid valerian, St John's wort, kava kava, gotu kola (may increase CNS depression).

Dietary Considerations Some products may contain sodium and/or phenylalanine.

Pharmacodynamics/Kinetics

Duration of Action

Histamine-induced wheal suppression: ≤10 hours (Simons, 1990)

Histamine-induced flare suppression: ≤12 hours (Simons, 1990)

Half-life Elimination Children: 5 hours (range: 4-7 hours); Adults: 9 hours (range: 7-12 hours); Elderly: 13.5 hours (range: 9-18 hours) (Blyden, 1986; Simons, 1990)

Time to Peak Serum: ~2 hours (Blyden, 1986; Simons, 1990)

Pregnancy Risk Factor B

Pregnancy Considerations Adverse events have not been observed in animal reproduction studies. Diphenhydramine crosses the placenta. Maternal diphenhydramine use has generally not resulted in an increased risk of birth defects; however, adverse events (withdrawal symptoms, respiratory depression) have been reported in newborns exposed to diphenhydramine *in utero*. Antihistamines are recommended for the treatment of rhinitis, urticaria, and pruritus with rash in pregnant women (although second generation antihistamines may be preferred). Antihistamines are not recommended for treatment of pruritus associated with intrahepatic cholestasis in pregnancy.

Lactation Enters breast milk/contraindicated

Breast-Feeding Considerations Diphenhydramine is excreted into breast milk; drowsiness has been reported in a breast-feeding infant. Premature infants and newborns have a higher risk of intolerance to antihistamines. Breast-feeding is contraindicated by the manufacturer. Antihistamines may decrease maternal serum prolactin concentrations when administered prior to the establishment of nursing.

Dosage Forms

Caplet, oral:
Aler-Dryl [OTC]: 50 mg
AllerMax® [OTC]: 50 mg
Anti-Hist [OTC]: 25 mg
Compoz® [OTC]: 50 mg
Histaprin [OTC]: 25 mg
Nytol® Quick Caps [OTC]: 25 mg
Simply Sleep® [OTC]: 25 mg
Sleep-ettes D [OTC]: 50 mg
Sominex® Maximum Strength [OTC]: 50 mg
Twilite® [OTC]: 50 mg

Capsule, oral: 25 mg, 50 mg
Aler-Cap [OTC]: 25 mg
Banophen™ [OTC]: 25 mg
Benadryl® Allergy [OTC]: 25 mg
Diphen [OTC]: 25 mg
Diphenhist® [OTC]: 25 mg
Q-dryl [OTC]: 25 mg
Sleepinal® [OTC]: 50 mg

Capsule, liquid filled, oral:
Vicks® ZzzQuil™ [OTC]: 25 mg

Capsule, softgel, oral:
Benadryl® Dye-Free Allergy [OTC]: 25 mg
Compoz® [OTC]: 50 mg
Nytol® Quick Gels [OTC]: 50 mg
Unisom® SleepGels® Maximum Strength [OTC]: 50 mg

Captab, oral:
Diphenhist® [OTC]: 25 mg

Elixir, oral:
Altaryl [OTC]: 12.5 mg/5 mL (480 mL, 3840 mL)
Banophen™ [OTC]: 12.5 mg/5 mL (120 mL, 480 mL)

Injection, solution: 50 mg/mL (1 mL, 10 mL)

Injection, solution [preservative free]: 50 mg/mL (1 mL)

Liquid, oral:
AllerMax® [OTC]: 12.5 mg/5 mL (120 mL)
Benadryl® Children's Allergy [OTC]: 12.5 mg/5 mL (118 mL, 236 mL)
Benadryl® Children's Allergy Perfect Measure™ [OTC]: 12.5 mg/5 mL (5 mL)
Benadryl® Children's Dye Free Allergy [OTC]: 12.5 mg/5 mL (118 mL)
Siladryl Allergy [OTC]: 12.5 mg/5 mL (118 mL, 237 mL, 473 mL)
Vicks® ZzzQuil™ [OTC]: 50 mg/30 mL (177 mL, 354 mL)

Solution, oral: 12.5 mg/5 mL (5 mL, 10 mL, 20 mL)
Diphenhist® [OTC]: 12.5 mg/5 mL (118 mL, 473 mL)
Q-dryl [OTC]: 12.5 mg/5 mL (120 mL, 240 mL, 480 mL)

Strip, orally disintegrating, oral:
Benadryl® Allergy Quick Dissolve [OTC]: 25 mg (10s)
Theraflu® Thin Strips® Multi Symptom [OTC]: 25 mg (12s, 24s)

Syrup, oral:
PediaCare® Children's Allergy [OTC]: 12.5 mg/5 mL (118 mL)
PediaCare® Children's NightTime Cough [OTC]: 12.5 mg/5 mL (118 mL)
Quenalin [OTC]: 12.5 mg/5 mL (118 mL)
Silphen [OTC]: 12.5 mg/5 mL (118 mL, 237 mL, 473 mL)
Tablet, oral: 25 mg, 50 mg
Aler-Tab [OTC]: 25 mg
Banophen™ [OTC]: 25 mg
Benadryl® Allergy [OTC]: 25 mg
Geri-Dryl: 25 mg
Sleep-Tabs [OTC]: 25 mg
Sominex® [OTC]: 25 mg
Tablet, orally dissolving, oral:
Benadryl® Children's Allergy FastMelt® [OTC]: 12.5 mg
Unisom® SleepMelts™ [OTC]: 25 mg
Dental Comment 25-50 mg of diphenhydramine orally every 4-6 hours can be used to treat mild dermatologic manifestations of allergic reactions to penicillin and other antibiotics. Diphenhydramine is not recommended as local anesthetic for either infiltration route or nerve block since the vehicle has caused local necrosis upon injection. A 50:50 mixture of diphenhydramine liquid (12.5 mg/5 mL) in Kaopectate® or Maalox® is used as a local application for recurrent aphthous ulcers; swish 15 mL for 2 minutes 4 times/day.

DiphenhydrAMINE (Topical)
(dye fen HYE dra meen)

Brand Names: U.S. Banophen™ Anti-Itch [OTC]; Benadryl® Extra Strength Itch Stopping [OTC]; Benadryl® Itch Relief Extra Strength [OTC]; Benadryl® Itch Stopping Extra Strength [OTC]; Benadryl® Itch Stopping [OTC]; Dermamycin® [OTC]
Brand Names: Canada Benadryl® Cream; Benadryl® Itch Relief Stick; Benadryl® Spray
Generic Availability (U.S.) Yes: Excludes gel, liquid stick, spray
Pharmacologic Category Ethanolamine Derivative; Histamine H₁ Antagonist; Histamine H₁ Antagonist, First Generation; Topical Skin Product
Use Topically for relief of pain and itching associated with insect bites, minor cuts and burns, or rashes due to poison ivy, poison oak, and poison sumac
Local Anesthetic/Vasoconstrictor Precautions No information available to require special precautions
Effects on Dental Treatment No significant effects or complications reported
Effects on Bleeding No information available to require special precautions
Adverse Effects Frequency not defined.
Dermatologic: Photosensitivity, rash, urticaria
Dosage Topical: Relief of pain and itching: Children ≥2 years and Adults: Apply 1% or 2% to affected area up to 3-4 times/day
Contraindications Hypersensitivity to diphenhydramine or any component of the formulation; neonates or premature infants; breast-feeding
Warnings/Precautions Self-medication (OTC use): Topical products should not be used on large areas of the body, or on chicken pox or measles. Healthcare provider should be contacted if topical use is needed for >7 days. Topical products are not for OTC use in children <2 years of age. Do not use with other products containing diphenhydramine.

Drug Interactions
Metabolism/Transport Effects None known.
Avoid Concomitant Use
Avoid concomitant use of DiphenhydrAMINE (Topical) with any of the following: Aclidinium; Azelastine (Nasal); Ipratropium (Oral Inhalation); Paraldehyde; Tiotropium
Increased Effect/Toxicity
DiphenhydrAMINE (Topical) may increase the levels/ effects of: Alcohol (Ethyl); Anticholinergics; Azelastine (Nasal); Buprenorphine; CNS Depressants; Methotrimeprazine; Metyrosine; Mirtazapine; Paraldehyde; Pramipexole; ROPINIRole; Rotigotine; Selective Serotonin Reuptake Inhibitors; Tiotropium; Zolpidem

The levels/effects of DiphenhydrAMINE (Topical) may be increased by: Aclidinium; Droperidol; HydrOXYzine; Ipratropium (Oral Inhalation); Magnesium Sulfate; Methotrimeprazine; Perampanel; Pramlintide; Sodium Oxybate
Decreased Effect
DiphenhydrAMINE (Topical) may decrease the levels/ effects of: Acetylcholinesterase Inhibitors (Central); Benzylpenicilloyl Polylysine; Betahistine; Hyaluronidase

The levels/effects of DiphenhydrAMINE (Topical) may be decreased by: Acetylcholinesterase Inhibitors (Central); Amphetamines
Pregnancy Considerations When administered orally, diphenhydramine crosses the placenta. Diphenhydramine can also be measurable in the serum following topical administration to large areas of the body. Refer to the diphenhydramine (systemic) monograph.
Breast-Feeding Considerations When administered orally, diphenhydramine can be detected in breast milk. Diphenhydramine can also be measurable in the serum following topical administration to large areas of the body. Refer to the diphenhydramine (systemic) monograph.
Dosage Forms
Cream, topical: 2% (30 g)
Banophen™ Anti-Itch [OTC]: 2% (28.4 g)
Benadryl® Itch Stopping [OTC]: 1% (14.2 g, 28.3 g)
Benadryl® Itch Stopping Extra Strength [OTC]: 2% (14.2 g)
Dermamycin® [OTC]: 2% (28 g)
Gel, topical:
Benadryl® Extra Strength Itch Stopping [OTC]: 2% (120 mL)
Liquid, topical:
Benadryl® Itch Relief Extra Strength [OTC]: 2% (14 mL)
Benadryl® Itch Stopping Extra Strength [OTC]: 2% (59 mL)
Dermamycin® [OTC]: 2% (60 mL)

Diphenhydramine and Ibuprofen
(dye fen HYE dra meen & eye byoo PROE fen)

Brand Names: U.S. Advil® PM Caplets [OTC]; Advil® PM Liqui-Gels® [OTC]
Pharmacologic Category Analgesic, Miscellaneous; Ethanolamine Derivative; Histamine H₁ Antagonist; Histamine H₁ Antagonist, First Generation; Nonsteroidal Anti-inflammatory Drug (NSAID), Oral
Use Aid in the relief of insomnia accompanied by minor aches and pains
Local Anesthetic/Vasoconstrictor Precautions No information available to require special precautions

Effects on Dental Treatment Key adverse event(s) related to dental treatment: Diphenhydramine causes xerostomia (normal salivary flow resumes upon discontinuation) and dry mucous membranes. Chronic use of antihistamines will inhibit salivary flow, particularly in elderly patients; may contribute to periodontal disease and oral discomfort.

In a statement released on September 8, 2006, the FDA notified consumers and healthcare professionals that the administration of ibuprofen for pain relief to patients taking aspirin for cardioprotection may interfere with aspirin's cardiovascular benefits. The FDA states that ibuprofen can interfere with the antiplatelet effect of low-dose aspirin (81 mg/day). This could result in diminished effectiveness of aspirin as used for cardioprotection and stroke prevention. The FDA adds that although ibuprofen and aspirin can be taken together, it is recommended that consumers talk with their healthcare providers for additional information. For more information, including how to advise aspirin patients requiring ibuprofen for pain relief, see Effects on Bleeding and Dental Comment.

Effects on Bleeding Nonselective NSAIDs such as ibuprofen inhibit platelet aggregation and prolong bleeding time in some patients. Unlike aspirin, the NSAID effect on platelet function is quantitatively less, of shorter duration, and reversible. This may not be a significant issue here as the product is taken on an as-needed basis at bedtime. The patient may be instructed to avoid use the night before a dental procedure depending upon the time of the procedure.

Adverse Effects See individual agents.

General Dosage Range Oral: *Children ≥12 years, Adolescents, and Adults:* Diphenhydramine hydrochloride 50 mg/ibuprofen 400 mg at bedtime **or** diphenhydramine citrate 76 mg/ibuprofen 400 mg at bedtime

Dental Comment New information from the FDA states that ibuprofen can interfere with the antiplatelet effect of low-dose aspirin (81 mg/day), potentially rendering aspirin less effective when used for cardioprotection and stroke protection. In situations where these drugs could be used concomitantly, the FDA has provided the following information.

Patients who use immediate release aspirin (not enteric-coated aspirin) and take a single dose or chronic doses of ibuprofen 400 mg, should dose the ibuprofen at least **30 minutes or longer after aspirin ingestion or more than 8 hours before aspirin ingestion** to avoid attenuation of aspirin's effect.

At this time, recommendations about the timing of ibuprofen 400 mg in patients taking enteric-coated low-dose aspirin cannot be made based on available data. One study however, showed that the antiplatelet effect of enteric-coated low-dose aspirin was attenuated when ibuprofen 400 mg was dosed 2, 7, and 12 hours after aspirin (Catella-Lawson, 2001).

With occasional use of ibuprofen, there is likely to be minimal risk from any attenuation of the antiplatelet effect of low-dose aspirin, because of a long-lasting effect of aspirin on platelets.

Diphenhydramine and Phenylephrine
(dye fen HYE dra meen & fen il EF rin)

Related Information
DiphenhydrAMINE (Systemic) *on page 433*
Phenylephrine (Systemic) *on page 1087*

Brand Names: U.S. Aldex® CT; Benadryl-D® Allergy & Sinus [OTC]; Benadryl-D® Children's Allergy & Sinus [OTC]; Dimetapp® Children's Nighttime Cold & Congestion [OTC]; Triaminic® Children's Night Time Cold & Cough [OTC]

Pharmacologic Category Alpha-Adrenergic Agonist; Decongestant; Ethanolamine Derivative; Histamine H_1 Antagonist; Histamine H_1 Antagonist, First Generation

Use Temporary relief of symptoms of allergic rhinitis, sinusitis, and other upper respiratory conditions, including sinus/nasal congestion, sneezing, stuffy/runny nose, itchy/watery eyes, and cough

Local Anesthetic/Vasoconstrictor Precautions Use with caution since phenylephrine is a sympathomimetic amine which could interact with epinephrine or mepivacaine and levonordefrin (Carbocaine® 2% with Neo-Cobefrin®) to cause a pressor response.

Effects on Dental Treatment Key adverse event(s) related to dental treatment:
Diphenhydramine: Prolonged use will cause significant xerostomia (normal salivary flow resumes upon discontinuation).
Phenylephrine: Up to 10% of patients could experience tachycardia, palpitations, and xerostomia.

Effects on Bleeding No information available to require special precautions

Adverse Effects Frequency not defined.
Cardiovascular: Chest tightness, extrasystoles, hypotension, palpitation, tachycardia
Central nervous system: Chills, confusion, coordination impaired, dizziness, drowsiness, euphoria, excitation, fatigue, headache, insomnia, irritability, nervousness, neuritis, restlessness, sedation, seizure, vertigo
Dermatologic: Photosensitivity, rash, urticaria
Endocrine & metabolic: Early menses
Gastrointestinal: Anorexia, constipation, diarrhea, dry mucous membranes, epigastric distress, nausea, vomiting, xerostomia
Genitourinary: Dysuria, polyuria, urinary retention
Hematologic: Agranulocytosis, hemolytic anemia, thrombocytopenia
Neuromuscular & skeletal: Paresthesia, tremor
Ocular: Blurred vision, diplopia
Otic: Labyrinthitis, tinnitus
Respiratory: Bronchial secretions (thickening), nasal congestion, throat tightness, wheezing
Miscellaneous: Anaphylaxis, diaphoresis

General Dosage Range Oral:
Children 6-11 years: Aldex® CT: 1/2 to 1 tablet every 6 hours; OTC labeling: 5-10 mL every 4 hours as needed (maximum: 6 doses/24 hours)
Children ≥12 years and Adults: Aldex® CT: 1-2 tablets every 6 hours; OTC labeling: 10-20 mL every 4 hours as needed or 1 tablet every 4 hours as needed (maximum: 6 doses/24 hours)

Mechanism of Action
Diphenhydramine is an H_1-receptor antagonist.
Phenylephrine is a potent, direct-acting alpha-adrenergic stimulator.

Diphenoxylate and Atropine
(dye fen OKS i late & A troe peen)

Related Information
Atropine *on page 148*
Brand Names: U.S. Lomotil®
Brand Names: Canada Lomotil®
Pharmacologic Category Antidiarrheal
Use Treatment of diarrhea
Local Anesthetic/Vasoconstrictor Precautions No information available to require special precautions
Effects on Dental Treatment Key adverse event(s) related to dental treatment: Significant xerostomia (normal salivary flow resumes upon discontinuation).
Effects on Bleeding No information available to require special precautions
Adverse Effects Frequency not defined.
Cardiovascular: Tachycardia
Central nervous system: Confusion, depression, dizziness, drowsiness, euphoria, flushing, headache, hyperthermia, lethargy, malaise, restlessness, sedation
Dermatologic: Angioneurotic edema, dry skin, pruritus, urticaria
Gastrointestinal: Abdominal discomfort, anorexia, gum swelling, nausea, pancreatitis, paralytic ileus, toxic megacolon, vomiting, xerostomia
Genitourinary: Urinary retention
Neuromuscular & skeletal: Numbness
Miscellaneous: Anaphylaxis
General Dosage Range Oral:
Children 2-12 years: Initial: Diphenoxylate 0.3-0.4 mg/kg/day in 4 divided doses (maximum: 10 mg/day); Maintenance: Reduce as needed, may be as low as 25% of the initial daily dose
Adults: Initial: Diphenoxylate 5 mg 4 times/day (maximum: 20 mg/day); Maintenance: Reduce as needed, may be as low as 5 mg/day
Mechanism of Action Diphenoxylate inhibits excessive GI motility and GI propulsion; commercial preparations contain a subtherapeutic amount of atropine to discourage abuse
Pharmacodynamics/Kinetics
Onset of Action Diphenoxylate: Antidiarrheal: 45-60 minutes
Duration of Action Diphenoxylate: Antidiarrheal: 3-4 hours
Half-life Elimination Diphenoxylate: 2.5 hours; Diphenoxylic acid: 12-14 hours
Time to Peak Diphenoxylate: Serum: 2 hours
Pregnancy Risk Factor C
Pregnancy Considerations Teratogenic effects were not noted in animal studies; decreased maternal weight, fertility and litter sizes were observed. There are no adequate and well-controlled studies in pregnant women.
Controlled Substance C-V

Diphtheria and Tetanus Toxoids, Acellular Pertussis, and Poliovirus Vaccine
(dif THEER ee a & TET a nus TOKS oyds, ay CEL yoo lar per TUS sis & POE lee oh VYE rus vak SEEN)

Brand Names: U.S. Kinrix®
Brand Names: Canada Adacel®-Polio
Pharmacologic Category Vaccine, Inactivated (Bacterial); Vaccine, Inactivated (Viral)

Use Kinrix®: Active immunization against diphtheria, tetanus, pertussis, and poliomyelitis, used as the fifth dose in the DTaP series and the 4th dose in the IPV series

The Advisory Committee on Immunization Practices (ACIP) recommends routine vaccination for use as the fifth dose in the DTaP series and the fourth dose in the IPV series in children who received DTaP (Infanrix®) and/or DTaP-Hepatitis B-IPV (Pediarix®) as the first 3 doses and DTaP (Infanrix®) as the fourth dose. Whenever feasible, the same manufacturer should be used to provide the pertussis component; however, vaccination should not be deferred if a specific brand is not known or is not available.

Adacel®-Polio (Canadian availability): Active booster immunization against diphtheria, tetanus, pertussis, and poliomyelitis; alternative to fifth dose of DTaP-IPV; May be used for wound management when a tetanus toxoid-containing vaccine is needed for wound management [refer to current National Advisory Committee on Immunization (NACI) guidelines]

Local Anesthetic/Vasoconstrictor Precautions No information available to require special precautions
Effects on Dental Treatment No significant effects or complications reported
Effects on Bleeding No information available to require special precautions
Adverse Effects All serious adverse reactions must be reported to the U.S. Department of Health and Human Services (DHHS) Vaccine Adverse Event Reporting System (VAERS) 1-800-822-7967 or online at https://vaers.hhs.gov/esub/index. In Canada, adverse reactions may be reported to local provincial/territorial health agencies or to the Vaccine Safety Section at Public Health Agency of Canada (1-866-844-0018).
Adverse events reported within 4 days of vaccination: >10%:
Central nervous system: Drowsiness (19%, grade 3: 1%), fever (≥99.5°F: 16%, >100.4: 7%, >104: <1%)
Gastrointestinal: Loss of appetite (16%; grade 3: 1%)
Local: Injection site: Pain (57%; grade 3: 2%), redness (37%; ≤50 mm: 18%, ≥110 mm: 3%), arm circumference increase (36%, >20 mm: 7%, >30 mm: 2%), swelling (26%; ≥50 mm: 10%, ≥110 mm: 1%)
General Dosage Range I.M.: *Children 4-6 years:* 0.5 mL
Mechanism of Action Promotes active immunity to diphtheria, tetanus, pertussis, and poliovirus (types 1, 2 and 3) by inducing production of specific antibodies and antitoxins.
Pharmacodynamics/Kinetics
Onset of Action Immune response observed to all components ~1 month following vaccination
Pregnancy Risk Factor C
Pregnancy Considerations Reproduction studies have not been conducted; Kinrix® is not indicated for women of childbearing age. Adacel®-Polio is not recommended for use in pregnant women unless a definite risk of pertussis exists.

Diphtheria and Tetanus Toxoids, Acellular Pertussis, Hepatitis B (Recombinant), Poliovirus (Inactivated), and *Haemophilus influenzae* B Conjugate (Adsorbed) Vaccine

(dif THEER ee a & TET a nus TOKS oyds, ay CEL yoo lar per TUS sis, hep a TYE tis bee ree KOM be nant, POE lee oh VYE rus in ak ti VAY ted, & hem OF fi lus in floo EN za bee KON joo gate ad SORBED vak SEEN)

Brand Names: Canada Infanrix Hexa™

Pharmacologic Category Vaccine, Inactivated (Bacterial, Viral)

Use Active primary immunization against diphtheria, tetanus, pertussis, hepatitis B, poliomyelitis and disease caused by *Haemophilus influenzae* type b in infants and children 6 weeks to 2 years of age; booster immunization (at 18 months) in infants who previously received a full primary vaccination course of each component of the vaccine

Local Anesthetic/Vasoconstrictor Precautions No information available to require special precautions

Effects on Dental Treatment No significant effects or complications reported

Effects on Bleeding No information available to require special precautions

Adverse Effects All serious adverse reactions may be reported to local provincial/territorial health agencies or to the Vaccine Safety Section at Public Health Agency of Canada (1-866-844-0018).

Frequency not always defined.

>10%:
Central nervous system: Irritability (83%), sleeping increased (63%), fever ≥38°C (100.4°F) (56%), sleeping decreased (51%), crying abnormal (43%), fatigue, restlessness

Local: Injection Site: Redness (49%), pain (43%), swelling (36%)

Gastrointestinal: Loss of appetite (49%), diarrhea (36%), vomiting (25%)

1% to 10%:
Central nervous system: Fever >39.5°C (103.1°F), nervousness

Local: Injection site: Induration

General Dosage Range I.M.: *Children 6 weeks to 2 years:* Primary immunization: 0.5 mL every 8 weeks for a total of 3 doses; booster dose: 0.5 mL

Mechanism of Action Promotes active immunity to diphtheria, tetanus, pertussis, hepatitis B, poliovirus (types 1, 2, and 3), and *Haemophilus influenzae* type B by inducing production of specific antibodies and antitoxins.

Pharmacodynamics/Kinetics
Onset of Action Immune response observed to all components 1 month following the 3-dose series

Pregnancy Considerations Not indicated for use in pregnant women.

Product Availability Not available in U.S.

Diphtheria and Tetanus Toxoids, Acellular Pertussis, Poliovirus and *Haemophilus* b Conjugate Vaccine

(dif THEER ee a & TET a nus TOKS oyds ay CEL yoo lar per TUS sis POE lee oh VYE rus & hem OF fi lus bee KON joo gate vak SEEN)

Brand Names: U.S. Pentacel®

Brand Names: Canada Pediacel®; Pentacel®

Pharmacologic Category Vaccine, Inactivated (Bacterial); Vaccine, Inactivated (Viral)

Use Active immunization against diphtheria, tetanus, pertussis, poliomyelitis, and invasive disease caused by *H. influenzae* type b in children 6 weeks through 4 years of age

Advisory Committee on Immunization Practices (ACIP) recommends that Pentacel® (DTaP-IPV/Hib) may be used to provide the recommended DTaP, IPV, and Hib immunization in children <5 years of age. Whenever feasible, the same manufacturer should be used to provide the pertussis component; however, vaccination should not be deferred if a specific brand is not known or is not available. The Hib component in Pentacel® contains a tetanus toxoid conjugate. A Hib vaccine containing the PRP-OMP conjugate (PedvaxHIB®) may provide a more rapid seroconversion following the first dose and may be preferable to use in certain populations (eg, American Indian or Alaska Native children).

Local Anesthetic/Vasoconstrictor Precautions No information available to require special precautions

Effects on Dental Treatment No significant effects or complications reported

Effects on Bleeding No information available to require special precautions

Adverse Effects All serious adverse reactions must be reported to the U.S. Department of Health and Human Services (DHHS) Vaccine Adverse Event Reporting System (VAERS) 1-800-822-7967 or online at https://vaers.hhs.gov/esub/index. In Canada, adverse reactions may be reported to local provincial/territorial health agencies or to the Vaccine Safety Section at Public Health Agency of Canada (1-866-844-0018).

>10%:
Central nervous system: Fussiness/irritability (54% to 77%; >3 hours 4% to 5%), inconsolable crying (36% to 60%; >3 hours ≤2%), lethargy/decreased activity (24% to 46%; severe ≤3%), fever ≥38°C (6% to 16%)

Local: Injection site reactions: Tenderness (39% to 56%; severe 1% to 5%), arm circumference increase >5 mm (34%; >40 mm <1%), redness >5 mm (7% to 17%)

1% to 10%: Local: Injection site reaction: Swelling >5 mm (5% to 10%)

General Dosage Range I.M.: *Children 6 weeks to ≤4 years:* 0.5 mL

Pregnancy Risk Factor C

Pregnancy Considerations Animal reproduction studies have not been conducted for this combination product. This product is not indicated for use in women of childbearing age.

Diphtheria, Tetanus Toxoids, Acellular Pertussis, Hepatitis B (Recombinant), and Poliovirus (Inactivated) Vaccine

(dif THEER ee a, TET a nus TOKS oyds, ay CEL yoo lar per TUS sis, hep a TYE tis bee ree KOM be nant, & POE lee oh VYE rus in ak ti VAY ted vak SEEN)

Related Information
Hepatitis B Vaccine (Recombinant) *on page 682*
Poliovirus Vaccine (Inactivated) *on page 1110*
Tetanus Toxoid (Adsorbed) *on page 1305*

Brand Names: U.S. Pediarix®

Brand Names: Canada Pediarix®

◀ **Pharmacologic Category** Vaccine, Inactivated (Bacterial); Vaccine, Inactivated (Viral)

Use Combination vaccine for the active immunization against diphtheria, tetanus, pertussis, hepatitis B virus (all known subtypes), and poliomyelitis (caused by poliovirus types 1, 2, and 3)

The Advisory Committee on Immunization Practices (ACIP) recommends Pediarix® for the following:
- Primary vaccination for DTaP, Hep B, and IPV in children at 2, 4, and 6 months of age.
- To complete the primary vaccination series in children who have received DTaP (Infanrix®) and who are scheduled to receive the other components of the vaccine. Whenever feasible, the same manufacturer should be used to provide the pertussis component; however, vaccination should not be deferred if a specific brand is not known or is not available. HepB and IPV from different manufacturers are interchangeable.

Local Anesthetic/Vasoconstrictor Precautions No information available to require special precautions

Effects on Dental Treatment No significant effects or complications reported

Effects on Bleeding No information available to require special precautions

Adverse Effects All serious adverse reactions must be reported to the U.S. Department of Health and Human Services (DHHS) Vaccine Adverse Event Reporting System (VAERS) 1-800-822-7967 or online at https://vaers.hhs.gov/esub/index. In Canada, adverse reactions may be reported to local provincial/territorial health agencies or to the Vaccine Safety Section at Public Health Agency of Canada (1-866-844-0018).

Adverse events reported within 4 days of vaccination at 2-, 4-, and 6 months of age in patients given Pediarix® concomitantly with Hib conjugate vaccine and PCV7 vaccine.

>10%:
Central nervous system: Irritability/fussiness (61% to 65%; grade 3: 3% to 4%), drowsiness (41% to 57%), fever ≥100.4°F (28% to 39%)
Gastrointestinal: Loss of appetite (26% to 31%; grade 3: <1%)
Local: Injection site: Redness (25% to 40%; >20 mm: 1% to 3%), pain (31% to 36%; grade 3: 2% to 3%), swelling (17% to 29%; >20 mm: 2% to 3%)
1% to 10%: Central nervous system: Fever >103.1°F (≤1%)

Additional and postmarketing events: Anaphylactic/anaphylactoid reaction, angioedema, anorexia, apnea, arthus-type hypersensitivity reactions, brachial neuritis, bulging fontanelle, consciousness depressed, cough, cranial mononeuropathy, crying, cyanosis, demyelinating disease, diarrhea, dyspnea, encephalitis, erythema, fatigue, febrile convulsion, Guillain-Barré syndrome, hypersensitivity reaction, hypotonia, hypotonic-hyporesposnive episode, injection site reactions (cellulitis, induration, itching, nodule, warmth, vesicles), insomnia, lethargy, limb pain, limb swelling, liver function test abnormalities, nervousness, pallor, peripheral mononeuropathy, petechiae, rash, restlessness, screaming, seizure, SIDS, somnolence, upper respiratory tract infection, urticaria, vomiting

General Dosage Range I.M.: *Children 6 weeks to <7 years:* 0.5 mL/dose for a total of 3 doses

Mechanism of Action Promotes active immunity to diphtheria, tetanus, pertussis, hepatitis B and poliovirus (types 1, 2 and 3) by inducing production of specific antibodies and antitoxins.

Pharmacodynamics/Kinetics
Onset of Action Immune response observed to all components 1 month following the 3-dose series.

Pregnancy Risk Factor C

Pregnancy Considerations Reproduction studies have not been conducted; not indicated for women of childbearing age.

Dipivefrin (dye PI ve frin)

Brand Names: Canada Ophtho-Dipivefrin™; PMS-Dipivefrin; Propine®

Pharmacologic Category Alpha/Beta Agonist; Ophthalmic Agent, Antiglaucoma; Ophthalmic Agent, Vasoconstrictor

Use Reduces elevated intraocular pressure in chronic open-angle glaucoma; also used to treat ocular hypertension, low tension, and secondary glaucomas

Local Anesthetic/Vasoconstrictor Precautions No information available to require special precautions

Effects on Dental Treatment No significant effects or complications reported

Effects on Bleeding No information available to require special precautions

Adverse Effects 1% to 10%:
Central nervous system: Headache
Local: Burning, stinging
Ocular: Blepharoconjunctivitis, blurred vision, bulbar conjunctival follicles, cystoid macular edema, ocular congestion, ocular pain, mydriasis, photophobia

General Dosage Range Ophthalmic: *Adults:* Instill 1 drop every 12 hours

Mechanism of Action Dipivefrin is a prodrug of epinephrine which is the active agent that stimulates alpha- and/or beta-adrenergic receptors increasing aqueous humor outflow

Pharmacodynamics/Kinetics
Onset of Action
Ocular pressure: ~30 minutes
Mydriasis: ~30 minutes
Duration of Action
Ocular pressure effect: ≥12 hours
Mydriasis: Several hours

Pregnancy Risk Factor B

Pregnancy Considerations Adverse events have not been observed in animal reproduction studies when administered orally. Systemic adverse events (eg, arrhythmias, hypertension) have been reported following ophthalmic application; use is not recommended in pregnancy (Razeghinejad, 2011).

Dipyridamole (dye peer ID a mole)

Brand Names: U.S. Persantine®

Brand Names: Canada Apo-Dipyridamole FC®; Dipyridamole For Injection; Persantine®

Pharmacologic Category Antiplatelet Agent; Vasodilator

Use
Oral: Used with warfarin to decrease thrombosis in patients after artificial heart valve replacement
I.V.: Diagnostic agent in CAD

Unlabeled Use Stroke prevention (in combination with aspirin); **Note:** For this indication, the use of aspirin/extended release dipyridamole is recommended (Guyatt, 2012).

Local Anesthetic/Vasoconstrictor Precautions No information available to require special precautions

Effects on Dental Treatment No significant effects or complications reported

Effects on Bleeding Dipyridamole inhibits platelet aggregation and may increase the risk of bleeding.

Adverse Effects
Oral:
>10%: Dizziness (14%)
1% to 10%:
Central nervous system: Headache (2%)
Dermatologic: Rash (2%)
Gastrointestinal: Abdominal distress (6%)
Frequency not defined: Diarrhea, vomiting, flushing, pruritus, angina pectoris, liver dysfunction
I.V.:
>10%:
Cardiovascular: Exacerbation of angina pectoris (20%)
Central nervous system: Dizziness (12%), headache (12%)
1% to 10%:
Cardiovascular: Hypotension (5%), hypertension (2%), blood pressure lability (2%), ECG abnormalities (ST-T changes, extrasystoles; 5% to 8%), pain (3%), tachycardia (3%)
Central nervous system: Flushing (3%), fatigue (1%)
Gastrointestinal: Nausea (5%)
Neuromuscular & skeletal: Paresthesia (1%)
Respiratory: Dyspnea (3%)

General Dosage Range
I.V.: *Adults:* 0.14 mg/kg/minute for 4 minutes (maximum: 60 mg)
Oral: *Children ≥12 years and Adults:* 75-100 mg 4 times/day

Mechanism of Action Inhibits the activity of adenosine deaminase and phosphodiesterase, which causes an accumulation of adenosine, adenine nucleotides, and cyclic AMP; these mediators then inhibit platelet aggregation and may cause vasodilation; may also stimulate release of prostacyclin or PGD_2; causes coronary vasodilation

Pharmacodynamics/Kinetics
Half-life Elimination Terminal: 10-12 hours
Time to Peak Serum: 2-2.5 hours

Pregnancy Risk Factor B
Pregnancy Considerations Teratogenic effects were not observed in animal studies.

Disopyramide (dye soe PEER a mide)

Related Information
Clinical Risk Related to Drugs Prolonging QT Interval *on page 1510*

Brand Names: U.S. Norpace®; Norpace® CR
Brand Names: Canada Norpace®; Rythmodan®; Rythmodan®-LA

Pharmacologic Category Antiarrhythmic Agent, Class Ia

Use Life-threatening ventricular arrhythmias (eg, sustained ventricular tachycardia)

Unlabeled Use Alternative agent for the prevention of recurrent symptomatic focal atrial tachycardia (in combination with an AV nodal blocking agent), atrial fibrillation (especially vagally-induced), or atrial flutter (in combination with an AV nodal-blocking agent); obstructive hypertrophic cardiomyopathy (HCM) in combination with ventricular rate-controlling agents (eg, beta blockers or verapamil) to control symptoms of angina or dyspnea who are unresponsive to rate-controlling agents alone; atrial fibrillation in patients with HCM in combination with rate-controlling agents

Local Anesthetic/Vasoconstrictor Precautions Disopyramide is one of the drugs confirmed to prolong the QT interval and is accepted as having a risk of causing torsade de pointes. The risk of drug-induced torsade de pointes is extremely low when a single QT interval prolonging drug is prescribed. In terms of epinephrine, it is not known what effect vasoconstrictors in the local anesthetic regimen will have in patients with a known history of congenital prolonged QT interval or in patients taking any medication that prolongs the QT interval. Until more information is obtained, it is suggested that the clinician consult with the physician prior to the use of a vasoconstrictor in suspected patients, and that the vasoconstrictor (epinephrine, mepivacaine and levonordefrin [Carbocaine® 2% with Neo-Cobefrin®]) be used with caution.

Effects on Dental Treatment Key adverse event(s) related to dental treatment: Xerostomia (normal salivary flow resumes upon discontinuation).

Effects on Bleeding No information available to require special precautions

Adverse Effects The most common adverse effects are related to cholinergic blockade. The most serious adverse effects of disopyramide are hypotension and CHF.

>10%:
Gastrointestinal: Xerostomia (32%), constipation (11%)
Genitourinary: Urinary hesitancy (14% to 23%)
1% to 10%:
Cardiovascular: CHF, hypotension, cardiac conduction disturbance, edema, syncope, chest pain
Central nervous system: Fatigue, headache, malaise, dizziness, nervousness
Dermatologic: Rash, generalized dermatoses, pruritus
Endocrine & metabolic: Cholesterol increased, hypokalemia, triglycerides increased
Gastrointestinal: Dry throat, nausea, abdominal distension, flatulence, abdominal bloating, anorexia, diarrhea, vomiting, weight gain
Genitourinary: Urinary retention, urinary frequency, urinary urgency, impotence (1% to 3%)
Neuromuscular & skeletal: Muscle weakness, muscular pain
Ocular: Blurred vision, dry eyes
Respiratory: Dyspnea

General Dosage Range Dosage adjustment recommended in patients with hepatic or renal impairment
Oral:
Controlled release:
Adults <50 kg: 200 mg every 12 hours
Adults ≥50 kg: 300 mg every 12 hours
Immediate release:
Children <1 year: 10-30 mg/kg/day in 4 divided doses
Children 1-4 years: 10-20 mg/kg/day in 4 divided doses
Children 4-12 years: 10-15 mg/kg/day in 4 divided doses
Children 12-18 years: 6-15 mg/kg/day in 4 divided doses
Adults <50 kg: 100 mg every 6 hours
Adults ≥50 kg: 150 mg every 6 hours

◀ **Mechanism of Action** Class Ia antiarrhythmic: Decreases myocardial excitability and conduction velocity; reduces disparity in refractory between normal and infarcted myocardium; possesses anticholinergic, peripheral vasoconstrictive, and negative inotropic effects

Pharmacodynamics/Kinetics

Onset of Action 0.5-3.5 hours

Duration of Action Immediate release: 1.5-8.5 hours

Half-life Elimination Adults: 4-10 hours; prolonged with hepatic or renal impairment

Time to Peak Serum: Immediate release: Within 2 hours; Controlled release: 4-7 hours

Pregnancy Risk Factor C

Pregnancy Considerations Adverse events have been observed in animal reproduction studies. Disopyramide levels have been reported in human fetal blood. Disopyramide may stimulate contractions in pregnant women. In a case report, disopyramide use in the third trimester resulted in painful uterine contractions after the first dose and hemorrhage after the second dose (Abbi, 1999).

Dental Comment Disopyramide is known to prolong the QT interval. The QT interval is measured as the time and distance between the Q point of the QRS complex and the end of the T wave in the ECG tracing. After adjustment for heart rate, the QT interval is defined as prolonged if it is more than 450 msec in men and 460 msec in women. A long QT syndrome was first described in the 1950s and 60s as a congenital syndrome involving QT interval prolongation and syncope and sudden death. Some of the congenital long QT syndromes were characterized by a peculiar electrocardiographic appearance of the QRS complex involving a premature atria beat followed by a pause, then a subsequent sinus beat showing marked QT prolongation and deformity. This type of cardiac arrhythmia was originally termed "torsade de pointes" (translated from the French as "twisting of the points"). Disopyramide is considered as having a risk of causing torsade de pointes. Since it is not known what effect vasoconstrictors in the local anesthetic regimen will have in patients with a known history of congenital prolonged QT interval or in patients taking any medication that prolongs the QT interval, a medical consult is suggested.

Disulfiram (dye SUL fi ram)

Brand Names: U.S. Antabuse®

Pharmacologic Category Aldehyde Dehydrogenase Inhibitor

Use Management of chronic alcoholism

Local Anesthetic/Vasoconstrictor Precautions No information available to require special precautions

Effects on Dental Treatment No significant effects or complications reported

Effects on Bleeding No information available to require special precautions

Adverse Effects Frequency not defined.

Central nervous system: Drowsiness, headache, fatigue, polyneuritis, psychosis

Dermatologic: Rash, acneiform eruptions, allergic dermatitis

Gastrointestinal: Metallic or garlic-like aftertaste

Genitourinary: Impotence

Hepatic: Hepatitis (cholestatic and fulminant), hepatic failure (multiple case reports)

Neuromuscular & skeletal: Peripheral neuritis, peripheral neuropathy

Ocular: Optic neuritis

General Dosage Range Oral: *Adults:* Initial: 500 mg once daily; Maintenance: 125-500 mg once daily (maximum: 500 mg daily)

Mechanism of Action Disulfiram is a thiuram derivative which interferes with aldehyde dehydrogenase. When taken concomitantly with alcohol, there is an increase in serum acetaldehyde levels. High acetaldehyde causes uncomfortable symptoms including flushing, nausea, thirst, palpitations, chest pain, vertigo, and hypotension. This reaction is the basis for disulfiram use in postwithdrawal long-term care of alcoholism.

Pharmacodynamics/Kinetics

Onset of Action Full effect: 12 hours

Duration of Action ~1-2 weeks after last dose

DOBUTamine (doe BYOO ta meen)

Brand Names: Canada Dobutamine Injection, USP; Dobutrex®

Pharmacologic Category Adrenergic Agonist Agent

Use Short-term management of patients with cardiac decompensation

Unlabeled Use Positive inotropic agent for use in myocardial dysfunction related to sepsis; stress echocardiography

Local Anesthetic/Vasoconstrictor Precautions No information available to require special precautions

Effects on Dental Treatment No significant effects or complications reported

Effects on Bleeding No information available to require special precautions

Adverse Effects Incidence of adverse events is not always reported.

Cardiovascular: Increased heart rate, increased blood pressure, increased ventricular ectopic activity, hypotension, premature ventricular beats (5%, dose related), anginal pain (1% to 3%), nonspecific chest pain (1% to 3%), palpitation (1% to 3%)

Central nervous system: Fever (1% to 3%), headache (1% to 3%), paresthesia

Endocrine & metabolic: Slight decrease in serum potassium

Gastrointestinal: Nausea (1% to 3%)

Hematologic: Thrombocytopenia (isolated cases)

Local: Phlebitis, local inflammatory changes and pain from infiltration, cutaneous necrosis (isolated cases)

Neuromuscular & skeletal: Mild leg cramps

Respiratory: Dyspnea (1% to 3%)

General Dosage Range I.V.: *Children and Adults:* 2.5-20 mcg/kg/minute (maximum: 40 mcg/kg/minute)

Mechanism of Action Stimulates $beta_1$-adrenergic receptors, causing increased contractility and heart rate, with little effect on $beta_2$- or alpha-receptors

Pharmacodynamics/Kinetics

Onset of Action I.V.: 1-10 minutes; Peak effect: 10-20 minutes

Half-life Elimination 2 minutes

Pregnancy Risk Factor B

Pregnancy Considerations Adverse events have not been observed in animal reproduction studies.

DOCEtaxel (doe se TAKS el)

Brand Names: U.S. Docefrez™; Taxotere®

Brand Names: Canada Docetaxel for Injection; Taxotere®

Pharmacologic Category Antineoplastic Agent, Anti-microtubular; Antineoplastic Agent, Natural Source (Plant) Derivative; Antineoplastic Agent, Taxane Derivative

Use

U.S. labeling:

Docefrez™: Treatment of breast cancer (locally advanced/metastatic) after prior chemotherapy failure; treatment of nonsmall cell lung cancer (NSCLC) after failure of prior platinum-based chemotherapy; metastatic prostate cancer

Taxotere®: Treatment of breast cancer (locally advanced/metastatic or adjuvant treatment of operable node-positive); locally-advanced or metastatic nonsmall cell lung cancer (NSCLC); hormone refractory, metastatic prostate cancer; advanced gastric adenocarcinoma; locally-advanced squamous cell head and neck cancer

Canadian labeling: Treatment of breast cancer (locally advanced/metastatic or adjuvant treatment of operable node-positive); locally-advanced or metastatic nonsmall cell lung cancer (NSCLC); hormone refractory, metastatic prostate cancer; recurrent and/or metastatic squamous cell head and neck cancer; treatment of metastatic ovarian cancer following failure of first-line or subsequent chemotherapy

Unlabeled Use Treatment of bladder cancer (metastatic), ovarian cancer, cervical cancer (recurrent), esophageal cancer, small cell lung cancer (relapsed), soft tissue sarcoma, Ewing's sarcoma, osteosarcoma, and unknown-primary adenocarcinoma

Local Anesthetic/Vasoconstrictor Precautions No information available to require special precautions

Effects on Dental Treatment Key adverse event(s) related to dental treatment: Mucositis, stomatitis, and taste perversion.

Effects on Bleeding Thrombocytopenia (8% to 14%) and bleeding episodes have been reported. A medical consult is recommended.

Adverse Effects Percentages reported for docetaxel monotherapy; frequency may vary depending on diagnosis, dose, liver function, prior treatment, and premedication. The incidence of adverse events was usually higher in patients with elevated liver function tests.

>10%:

Cardiovascular: Fluid retention (13% to 60%; dose dependent)

Central nervous system: Neurosensory events (20% to 58%; including neuropathy), fever (31% to 35%), neuromotor events (16%)

Dermatologic: Alopecia (56% to 76%), cutaneous events (20% to 48%), nail disorder (11% to 41%)

Gastrointestinal: Stomatitis (19% to 53%; severe 1% to 8%), diarrhea (23% to 43%; severe: 5% to 6%), nausea (34% to 42%), vomiting (22% to 23%)

Hematologic: Neutropenia (84% to 99%; grade 4: 75% to 86%; nadir (median): 7 days, duration (severe neutropenia): 7 days; dose dependent), leukopenia (84% to 99%; grade 4: 32% to 44%), anemia (65% to 94%; dose dependent; grades 3/4: 8% to 9%), thrombocytopenia (8% to 14%; grade 4: 1%; dose dependent), febrile neutropenia (6% to 12%; dose dependent)

Hepatic: Transaminases increased (4% to 19%)

Neuromuscular & skeletal: Weakness (53% to 66%; severe 13% to 18%), myalgia (3% to 23%)

Respiratory: Pulmonary events (41%)

Miscellaneous: Infection (1% to 34%; dose dependent), hypersensitivity (1% to 21%; with premedication 15%)

1% to 10%:

Cardiovascular: Left ventricular ejection fraction decreased (prostate cancer: 10%; metastatic breast cancer: 8%), hypotension (3%)

Gastrointestinal: Taste perversion (6%)

Hepatic: Bilirubin increased (9%), alkaline phosphatase increased (4% to 7%)

Local: Infusion-site reactions (4%, including hyperpigmentation, inflammation, redness, dryness, phlebitis, extravasation, swelling of the vein)

Neuromuscular and skeletal: Arthralgia (3% to 9%)

Ocular: Epiphora associated with canalicular stenosis (≤77% with weekly administration; ≤1% with every 3-week administration)

General Dosage Range Dosage adjustment recommended in patients with hepatic impairment, on concomitant therapy, or who develop toxicities.

I.V.: *Adults:* 60-100 mg/m^2 every 3 weeks

Mechanism of Action Docetaxel promotes the assembly of microtubules from tubulin dimers, and inhibits the depolymerization of tubulin which stabilizes microtubules in the cell. This results in inhibition of DNA, RNA, and protein synthesis. Most activity occurs during the M phase of the cell cycle.

Pharmacodynamics/Kinetics

Half-life Elimination Terminal: ~11 hours

Pregnancy Risk Factor D

Pregnancy Considerations Adverse events have been observed in animal reproduction studies. An *ex vivo* human placenta perfusion model illustrated that docetaxel crossed the placenta at term. Placental transfer was low and affected by the presence of albumin; higher albumin concentrations resulted in lower docetaxel placental transfer (Berveiller, 2012). Women of childbearing potential should avoid becoming pregnant. A pregnancy registry is available for all cancers diagnosed during pregnancy at Cooper Health (877-635-4499).

Docosanol (doe KOE san ole)

Related Sample Prescriptions

Herpes Simplex (Recurrent) *on page 1616*

Brand Names: U.S. Abreva® [OTC]

Generic Availability (U.S.) No

Pharmacologic Category Antiviral Agent, Topical

Dental Use Treatment of herpes simplex of the face or lips

Use Treatment of herpes simplex of the face or lips

Local Anesthetic/Vasoconstrictor Precautions No information available to require special precautions

Effects on Dental Treatment No significant effects or complications reported (see Dental Comment)

Effects on Bleeding No information available to require special precautions

Adverse Effects Limited information; headache reported (frequency similar to placebo)

Dental Usual Dosage Herpes simplex (face/lips): Children ≥12 years and Adults: Topical: Apply 5 times/day to affected area of face or lips. Start at first sign of cold sore or fever blister and continue until healed.

Dosage Children ≥12 years and Adults: Topical: Apply 5 times/day to affected area of face or lips. Start at first sign of cold sore or fever blister and continue until healed.

Mechanism of Action Prevents viral entry and replication at the cellular level

Contraindications Hypersensitivity to docosanol or any component of the formulation

Warnings/Precautions For external use only. Do not apply to inside of mouth or around eyes. Not for use in children <12 years of age.

Drug Interactions

Metabolism/Transport Effects None known.

Avoid Concomitant Use There are no known interactions where it is recommended to avoid concomitant use.

Increased Effect/Toxicity There are no known significant interactions involving an increase in effect.

Decreased Effect There are no known significant interactions involving a decrease in effect.

Dosage Forms

Cream, topical:
Abreva® [OTC]: 10% (2 g)

Dental Comment Wash hands before and after applying cream. Begin treatment at first tingle of cold sore or fever blister. Rub into area gently, but completely. Do not apply directly to inside of mouth or around eyes. Contact healthcare provider if sore gets worse or does not heal within 10 days. Do not share this product with others, may spread infection. Notify healthcare professional if pregnant or breast-feeding.

Docusate (DOK yoo sate)

Brand Names: U.S. Colace® [OTC]; Correctol® [OTC]; Diocto [OTC]; Doc-Q-Lace [OTC]; Docu-Soft [OTC]; DocuSoft S™ [OTC]; Dok™ [OTC]; DSS® [OTC]; Dulcolax® Stool Softener [OTC]; Dulcolax® [OTC]; Enemeez® Plus [OTC]; Enemeez® [OTC]; Fleet® Pedia-Lax™ Liquid Stool Softener [OTC]; Fleet® Sof-Lax® [OTC]; Kao-Tin [OTC]; Kaopectate® Stool Softener [OTC]; Phillips'® Liquid-Gels® [OTC]; Phillips'® Stool Softener Laxative [OTC]; Silace [OTC]

Brand Names: Canada Apo-Docusate-Sodium®; Colace®; Colax-C®; Novo-Docusate Calcium; Novo-Docusate Sodium; PMS-Docusate Calcium; PMS-Docusate Sodium; Regulex®; Selax®; Soflax™

Pharmacologic Category Stool Softener

Use Stool softener in patients who should avoid straining during defecation and constipation associated with hard, dry stools; prophylaxis for straining (Valsalva) following myocardial infarction. A safe agent to be used in elderly; some evidence that doses <200 mg are ineffective; stool softeners are unnecessary if stool is well hydrated or "mushy" and soft; shown to be ineffective used long-term.

Unlabeled Use Ceruminolytic

Local Anesthetic/Vasoconstrictor Precautions No information available to require special precautions

Effects on Dental Treatment Key adverse event(s) related to dental treatment: Throat irritation.

Effects on Bleeding No information available to require special precautions

Adverse Effects 1% to 10%:
Gastrointestinal: Intestinal obstruction, diarrhea, abdominal cramping
Miscellaneous: Throat irritation

General Dosage Range

Oral:
Children <3 years: 10-40 mg/day in 1-4 divided doses
Children 3-6 years: 20-60 mg/day in 1-4 divided doses
Children 6-12 years: 40-150 mg/day in 1-4 divided doses

Adolescents and Adults: 50-500 mg/day in 1-4 divided doses

Rectal: *Older children and Adults:* Add 50-100 mg to enema fluid

Mechanism of Action Reduces surface tension of the oil-water interface of the stool resulting in enhanced incorporation of water and fat allowing for stool softening

Pharmacodynamics/Kinetics

Onset of Action 12-72 hours

Pregnancy Considerations Short-term use of docusate is generally considered safe during pregnancy (Mahadevan, 2006). Hypomagnesemia was reported in a newborn following chronic maternal overuse throughout pregnancy (Schindler, 1984).

Dofetilide (doe FET il ide)

Related Information

Clinical Risk Related to Drugs Prolonging QT Interval *on page 1510*

Brand Names: U.S. Tikosyn®

Brand Names: Canada Tikosyn®

Pharmacologic Category Antiarrhythmic Agent, Class III

Use Maintenance of normal sinus rhythm in patients with chronic atrial fibrillation/atrial flutter of longer than 1-week duration who have been converted to normal sinus rhythm; conversion of atrial fibrillation and atrial flutter to normal sinus rhythm

Unlabeled Use Alternative antiarrhythmic for the treatment of atrial fibrillation in patients with hypertrophic cardiomyopathy (HCM)

Local Anesthetic/Vasoconstrictor Precautions Dofetilide is one of the drugs confirmed to prolong the QT interval and is accepted as having a risk of causing torsade de pointes. The risk of drug-induced torsade de pointes is extremely low when a single QT interval prolonging drug is prescribed. In terms of epinephrine, it is not known what effect vasoconstrictors in the local anesthetic regimen will have in patients with a known history of congenital prolonged QT interval or in patients taking any medication that prolongs the QT interval. Until more information is obtained, it is suggested that the clinician consult with the physician prior to the use of a vasoconstrictor in suspected patients, and that the vasoconstrictor (epinephrine, mepivacaine and levonordefrin [Carbocaine® 2% with Neo-Cobefrin®]) be used with caution.

Effects on Dental Treatment No significant effects or complications reported

Effects on Bleeding No information available to require special precautions

Adverse Effects

Supraventricular arrhythmia patients:
>10%: Central nervous system: Headache (11%)
2% to 10%:
Central nervous system: Dizziness (8%), insomnia (4%)
Cardiovascular: Ventricular tachycardia (2.6% to 3.7%), chest pain (10%), torsade de pointes (3.3% in HF patients and 0.9% in patients with a recent MI; up to 10.5% in patients receiving doses in excess of those recommended). Torsade de pointes occurs most frequently within the first 3 days of therapy.
Dermatologic: Rash (3%)
Gastrointestinal: Nausea (5%), diarrhea (3%), abdominal pain (3%)
Neuromuscular & skeletal: Back pain (3%)

Respiratory: Respiratory tract infection (7%), dyspnea (6%)

Miscellaneous: Flu-like syndrome (4%)

<2%:

Central nervous system: CVA, facial paralysis, flaccid paralysis, migraine, paralysis

Cardiovascular: AV block (0.4% to 1.5%), bundle branch block (0.1% to 0.5%), heart block (0.1% to 0.5%), ventricular fibrillation (0% to 0.4%), bradycardia, cardiac arrest, edema, MI, sudden death, syncope

Dermatologic: Angioedema

Gastrointestinal: Liver damage

Neuromuscular & skeletal: Paresthesia

Respiratory: Cough

General Dosage Range Dosage adjustment recommended in patients with renal impairment

Oral: *Adults:* Initial: 500 mcg twice daily; Maintenance: 125-500 mcg twice daily **or** 125 mcg once daily

Mechanism of Action Vaughan Williams Class III antiarrhythmic activity. Blockade of the cardiac ion channel carrying the rapid component of the delayed rectifier potassium current. Dofetilide has no effect on sodium channels, adrenergic alpha-receptors, or adrenergic beta-receptors. It increases the monophasic action potential duration due to delayed repolarization. The increase in the QT interval is a function of prolongation of both effective and functional refractory periods in the His-Purkinje system and the ventricles. Changes in cardiac conduction velocity and sinus node function have not been observed in patients with or without structural heart disease. PR and QRS width remain the same in patients with pre-existing heart block and or sick sinus syndrome.

Pharmacodynamics/Kinetics

Half-life Elimination ~10 hours; prolonged with renal impairment

Time to Peak Serum: Fasting: 2-3 hours

Pregnancy Risk Factor C

Pregnancy Considerations Dofetilide has been shown to adversely affect *in utero* growth, organogenesis, and survival of rats and mice. There are no adequate and well-controlled studies in pregnant women. Dofetilide should be used with extreme caution in pregnant women and in women of childbearing age only when the benefit to the patient unequivocally justifies the potential risk to the fetus.

Prescribing and Access Restrictions As a requirement of the REMS program, access to this medication is restricted. Tikosyn® is only available to prescribers and hospitals that have confirmed their participation in a designated Tikosyn® Education Program. The program provides comprehensive education about the importance of in-hospital treatment initiation and individualized dosing.

T.I.P.S. is the Tikosyn® In Pharmacy System designated to allow retail pharmacies to stock and dispense Tikosyn® once they have been enrolled. A participating pharmacy must confirm receipt of the T.I.P.S. program materials and educate its pharmacy staff about the procedures required to fill an outpatient prescription for Tikosyn®. The T.I.P.S. enrollment form is available at www.tikosyn.com. Tikosyn® is only available from a special mail order pharmacy, and enrolled retail pharmacies. Pharmacists must verify that the hospital/prescriber is a confirmed participant before Tikosyn® is provided. For participant verification, the pharmacist may call 1-800-788-7353 or use the web site located at www.tikosynlist.com. Further details and directions on the program are provided at www.tikosyn.com.

Dofetilide therapy must be initiated/adjusted in a hospital setting with proper monitoring under the guidance of experienced personnel.

Dental Comment Dofetilide is known to prolong the QT interval. The QT interval is measured as the time and distance between the Q point of the QRS complex and the end of the T wave in the ECG tracing. After adjustment for heart rate, the QT interval is defined as prolonged if it is more than 450 msec in men and 460 msec in women. A long QT syndrome was first described in the 1950s and 60s as a congenital syndrome involving QT interval prolongation and syncope and sudden death. Some of the congenital long QT syndromes were characterized by a peculiar electrocardiographic appearance of the QRS complex involving a premature atria beat followed by a pause, then a subsequent sinus beat showing marked QT prolongation and deformity. This type of cardiac arrhythmia was originally termed "torsade de pointes" (translated from the French as "twisting of the points"). Dofetilide is considered as having a risk of causing torsade de pointes. Since it is not known what effect vasoconstrictors in the local anesthetic regimen will have in patients with a known history of congenital prolonged QT interval or in patients taking any medication that prolongs the QT interval, a medical consult is suggested.

Dolasetron (dol A se tron)

Related Information

Clinical Risk Related to Drugs Prolonging QT Interval *on page 1510*

Brand Names: U.S. Anzemet®

Brand Names: Canada Anzemet®

Pharmacologic Category Antiemetic; Selective 5-HT$_3$ Receptor Antagonist

Use

U.S. labeling:

Injection: Prevention and treatment of postoperative nausea and vomiting

Oral: Prevention of nausea and vomiting associated with emetogenic cancer chemotherapy (initial and repeat courses); prevention of postoperative nausea and vomiting

Canadian labeling: Oral: Prevention of nausea and vomiting associated with emetogenic cancer chemotherapy (initial and repeat courses)

Local Anesthetic/Vasoconstrictor Precautions Dolasetron is one of the drugs confirmed to prolong the QT interval and is accepted as having a risk of causing torsade de pointes. The risk of drug-induced torsade de pointes is extremely low when a single QT interval prolonging drug is prescribed. In terms of epinephrine, it is not known what effect vasoconstrictors in the local anesthetic regimen will have in patients with a known history of congenital prolonged QT interval or in patients taking any medication that prolongs the QT interval. Until more information is obtained, it is suggested that the clinician consult with the physician prior to the use of a vasoconstrictor in suspected patients, and that the vasoconstrictor (epinephrine, mepivacaine and levonordefrin [Carbocaine® 2% with Neo-Cobefrin®]) be used with caution.

Effects on Dental Treatment Key adverse event(s) related to dental treatment: Taste alterations.

Effects on Bleeding No information available to require special precautions

Adverse Effects Adverse events may vary according to indication

>10%:

Central nervous system: Headache (7% to 24%)

Gastrointestinal: Diarrhea (2% to 12%)

1% to 10%:

Cardiovascular: Bradycardia (4% to 5%), hypertension (≤3%), tachycardia (2% to 3%)

Central nervous system: Dizziness (1% to 6%), fatigue (3% to 6%), fever (4%), pain (≤2%), chills/shivering (1% to 2%)

Gastrointestinal: Dyspepsia (≤3%), abdominal pain (≤3%)

Hepatic: Abnormal hepatic function (4%)

Renal: Oliguria (3%)

General Dosage Range

I.V.:

Children 2-16 years: 0.35 mg/kg as a single dose (maximum: 12.5 mg)

Adults: 12.5 mg or 100 mg as a single dose

Oral:

Children 2-16 years: 1.2-1.8 mg/kg as a single dose (maximum: 100 mg/dose)

Adults: 100 mg as single dose

Mechanism of Action Selective serotonin receptor (5-HT$_3$) antagonist, blocking serotonin both peripherally (primary site of action) and centrally at the chemoreceptor trigger zone

Pharmacodynamics/Kinetics

Half-life Elimination Dolasetron: ≤10 minutes; hydrodolasetron: Adults: 6-8 hours; Children: 4-6 hours; Severe renal impairment: 11 hours; Severe hepatic impairment: 11 hours

Time to Peak Hydrodolasetron: I.V.: 0.6 hours; Oral: ~1 hour

Pregnancy Risk Factor B

Pregnancy Considerations Teratogenic effects were not observed in animal studies. There are no adequate and well-controlled studies in pregnant women.

Dental Comment Dolasetron is known to prolong the QT interval. The QT interval is measured as the time and distance between the Q point of the QRS complex and the end of the T wave in the ECG tracing. After adjustment for heart rate, the QT interval is defined as prolonged if it is more than 450 msec in men and 460 msec in women. A long QT syndrome was first described in the 1950s and 60s as a congenital syndrome involving QT interval prolongation and syncope and sudden death. Some of the congenital long QT syndromes were characterized by a peculiar electrocardiographic appearance of the QRS complex involving a premature atria beat followed by a pause, then a subsequent sinus beat showing marked QT prolongation and deformity. This type of cardiac arrhythmia was originally termed "torsade de pointes" (translated from the French as "twisting of the points"). Dolasetron is considered as having a risk of causing torsade de pointes. Since it is not known what effect vasoconstrictors in the local anesthetic regimen will have in patients with a known history of congenital prolonged QT interval or in patients taking any medication that prolongs the QT interval, a medical consult is suggested.

Donepezil (doh NEP e zil)

Brand Names: U.S. Aricept®; Aricept® ODT

Brand Names: Canada Aricept®; Aricept® RDT

Generic Availability (U.S.) Yes

Pharmacologic Category Acetylcholinesterase Inhibitor (Central)

Use Treatment of mild, moderate, or severe dementia of the Alzheimer's type

Unlabeled Use Behavioral syndromes in dementia; mild-to-moderate dementia associated with Parkinson's disease; Lewy body dementia

Local Anesthetic/Vasoconstrictor Precautions No information available to require special precautions

Effects on Dental Treatment No significant effects or complications reported

Effects on Bleeding No information available to require special precautions

Adverse Effects

>10%:

Central nervous system: Insomnia (2% to 14%)

Gastrointestinal: Nausea (3% to 19%; dose related), diarrhea (5% to 15%; dose related)

Miscellaneous: Accident (7% to 13%), infection (11%)

1% to 10%:

Cardiovascular: Hypertension (3%), chest pain (2%), hemorrhage (2%), syncope (2%), hypotension, atrial fibrillation, bradycardia, ECG abnormal, edema, heart failure, hot flashes, peripheral edema, vasodilation

Central nervous system: Headache (3% to 10%), pain (3% to 9%), fatigue (1% to 8%), dizziness (2% to 8%), abnormal dreams (3%), hostility (3%), nervousness (1% to 3%), hallucinations (3%), depression (2% to 3%), confusion (2%), emotional lability (2%), personality disorder (2%), fever (2%), somnolence (2%), abnormal crying, aggression, agitation, anxiety, aphasia, delusions, irritability, restlessness, seizure, vertigo

Dermatologic: Bruising (4% to 5%), eczema (3%), pruritus, rash, skin ulcer, urticaria

Endocrine & metabolic: Dehydration (1% to 2%), hyperlipemia (2%), libido increased

Gastrointestinal: Anorexia (2% to 8%), vomiting (3% to 9%; dose related), weight loss (3% to 5%; dose related), abdominal pain, bloating, constipation, dyspepsia, epigastric pain, fecal incontinence, gastroenteritis, GI bleeding, toothache

Genitourinary: Urinary frequency (2%), urinary incontinence (1% to 3%), cystitis, hematuria, glycosuria, nocturia, UTI

Hematologic: Contusion (≤2%), anemia

Hepatic: Alkaline phosphatase increased

Neuromuscular & skeletal: Muscle cramps (3% to 8%), back pain (3%), CPK increased (3%), arthritis (1% to 2%), ataxia, bone fracture, gait abnormal, lactate dehydrogenase increased, paresthesia, tremor, weakness (1% to 2%)

Ocular: Blurred vision, cataract, eye irritation

Respiratory: Bronchitis, cough increased, dyspnea, pharyngitis, pneumonia, sore throat

Miscellaneous: Diaphoresis, fungal infection, flu symptoms, wandering

Dosage Oral:

Adults: Alzheimer's dementia:

Mild-to-moderate: Initial: 5 mg once daily; may increase to 10 mg once daily after 4-6 weeks; effective dosage range in clinical studies: 5-10 mg/day

Moderate-to-severe: Initial: 5 mg once daily; may increase to 10 mg once daily after 4-6 weeks; may increase further to 23 mg once daily after ≥3 months; effective dosage range in clinical studies: 10-23 mg/day

Elderly: Refer to adult dosing. **Note:** The Canadian labeling recommends a maximum dose of 5 mg once daily in elderly women of low body weight.

Dosage adjustment in renal impairment: No adjustment provided in manufacturer's labeling. Limited data suggest severe renal impairment does not adversely affect donepezil clearance.

Dosage adjustment in hepatic impairment: No adjustment provided in manufacturer's labeling.

Mechanism of Action Alzheimer's disease is characterized by cholinergic deficiency in the cortex and basal forebrain, which contributes to cognitive deficits. Donepezil reversibly and noncompetitively inhibits centrally-active acetylcholinesterase, the enzyme responsible for hydrolysis of acetylcholine. This appears to result in increased concentrations of acetylcholine available for synaptic transmission in the central nervous system.

Contraindications Hypersensitivity to donepezil, piperidine derivatives, or any component of the formulation

Warnings/Precautions Cholinesterase inhibitors may have vagotonic effects which may cause bradycardia and/or heart block with or without a history of cardiac disease; syncopal episodes have been associated with donepezil. Alzheimer's treatment guidelines consider bradycardia to be a relative contraindication for use of centrally-active cholinesterase inhibitors. Use with caution with sick sinus syndrome or other supraventricular cardiac conduction abnormalities, COPD, or asthma. Use with caution in patients with a history of seizure disorder; cholinomimetics may potentially cause generalized seizures, although seizure activity may also result from Alzheimer's disease. Use with caution in patients at risk of ulcer disease (eg, previous history or NSAID use), or in patients with bladder outlet obstruction. May cause dose-related diarrhea, nausea, and/or vomiting, which usually resolves in 1-3 weeks. May cause anorexia and/or weight loss (dose-related). Patients weighing <55 kg may experience more nausea, vomiting, and weight loss than patients ≥55 kg. May exaggerate neuromuscular blockade effects of depolarizing neuromuscular-blocking agents (eg, succinylcholine). Potentially significant interactions may exist, requiring dose or frequency adjustment, additional monitoring, and/or selection of alternative therapy. Consult drug interactions database for more detailed information.

Drug Interactions

Metabolism/Transport Effects Substrate of CYP2D6 (minor), CYP3A4 (minor); **Note:** Assignment of Major/Minor substrate status based on clinically relevant drug interaction potential

Avoid Concomitant Use There are no known interactions where it is recommended to avoid concomitant use.

Increased Effect/Toxicity
Donepezil may increase the levels/effects of: Antipsychotics; Beta-Blockers; Cholinergic Agonists; Succinylcholine

The levels/effects of Donepezil may be increased by: Corticosteroids (Systemic)

Decreased Effect
Donepezil may decrease the levels/effects of: Anticholinergics; Neuromuscular-Blocking Agents (Nondepolarizing)

The levels/effects of Donepezil may be decreased by: Anticholinergics; Dipyridamole; Peginterferon Alfa-2b

Ethanol/Nutrition/Herb Interactions
Ethanol: Avoid ethanol (may increase CNS adverse events).

Herb/Nutraceutical: St John's wort may decrease donepezil levels. Ginkgo biloba may increase adverse effects/toxicity of acetylcholinesterase inhibitors.

Dietary Considerations May take with or without food.

Pharmacodynamics/Kinetics
Half-life Elimination 70 hours; time to steady-state: 15 days

Time to Peak Plasma: Tablet, 10 mg: 3 hours; Tablet, 23 mg: ~8 hours; **Note:** Peak plasma concentrations almost twofold higher for the 23 mg tablet compared to the 10 mg tablet

Pregnancy Risk Factor C

Pregnancy Considerations Teratogenic effects were not observed in animal reproduction studies. There are no adequate and well-controlled studies in pregnant women.

Lactation Excretion in breast milk unknown/not recommended

Dosage Forms
Tablet, oral: 5 mg, 10 mg
Aricept®: 5 mg, 10 mg, 23 mg
Tablet, orally disintegrating, oral: 5 mg, 10 mg
Aricept® ODT: 5 mg, 10 mg

Doripenem (dore i PEN em)

Brand Names: U.S. Doribax®
Brand Names: Canada Doribax®
Pharmacologic Category Antibiotic, Carbapenem
Use Treatment of complicated intra-abdominal infections and complicated urinary tract infections (including pyelonephritis) due to susceptible aerobic gram-positive, aerobic gram-negative (including *Pseudomonas aeruginosa*), and anaerobic bacteria

Canadian labeling: Additional use (not in U.S. labeling): Treatment of healthcare-associated pneumonia (including ventilator-associated pneumonia)

Unlabeled Use Treatment of intravascular catheter-related bloodstream infection due to extended-spectrum β-lactamase (ESBL)-producing *Escherichia coli* and *Klebsiella* spp

Local Anesthetic/Vasoconstrictor Precautions No information available to require special precautions

Effects on Dental Treatment Prolonged use of doripenem may lead to development of oral candidiasis.

Effects on Bleeding Thrombocytopenia has been reported through postmarketing surveillance

Adverse Effects
>10%:
Central nervous system: Headache (4% to 16%)
Gastrointestinal: Nausea (4% to 12%), diarrhea (6% to 11%)
1% to 10%:
Dermatologic: Rash (1% to 5%; includes allergic/bullous dermatitis, erythema, macular/papular eruptions, urticaria, and erythema multiforme), pruritus (≤3%)
Gastrointestinal: Oral candidiasis (1%)
Hematologic: Anemia (2% to 10%)
Hepatic: Transaminases increased (1% to 2%)
Local: Phlebitis (4% to 8%)
Renal: Renal impairment/failure (≤1%)
Miscellaneous: Vulvomycotic infection (1% to 2%)

General Dosage Range Dosage adjustment recommended in patients with renal impairment
I.V.: *Adults:* 500 mg every 8 hours

◀ **Mechanism of Action** Inhibits bacterial cell wall synthesis by binding to several of the penicillin-binding proteins (PBP-2, PBP-3, PBP-4), which in turn inhibits the final transpeptidation step of peptidoglycan synthesis in bacterial cell walls, thus inhibiting cell wall biosynthesis; bacteria eventually lyse due to ongoing activity of cell wall autolytic enzymes (autolysins and murein hydrolases) while cell wall assembly is arrested.

Pharmacodynamics/Kinetics
Half-life Elimination ~1 hour
Pregnancy Risk Factor B
Pregnancy Considerations Adverse events have not been observed in animal reproduction studies. Information related to use during pregnancy has not been located.

Dornase Alfa (DOOR nase AL fa)

Brand Names: U.S. Pulmozyme®
Brand Names: Canada Pulmozyme®
Pharmacologic Category Enzyme; Mucolytic Agent
Use Management of cystic fibrosis patients to reduce the frequency of respiratory infections that require parenteral antibiotics in patients with FVC ≥40% of predicted; in conjunction with standard therapies, to improve pulmonary function in patients with cystic fibrosis
Unlabeled Use Infected parapneumonic effusion (following alteplase administration)
Local Anesthetic/Vasoconstrictor Precautions No information available to require special precautions
Effects on Dental Treatment Key adverse event(s) related to dental treatment: Pharyngitis
Effects on Bleeding No information available to require special precautions
Adverse Effects Adverse events were similar in children using the PARI BABY™ nebulizer (facemask as opposed to mouthpiece) with the addition of cough (45% in children 3 months to <5 years; 30% in children 5 to ≤10 years).
>10%:
Cardiovascular: Chest pain (18% to 25%)
Central nervous system: Fever (32% in patients with FVC <40%)
Dermatologic: Rash (3% to 12%)
Respiratory: Pharyngitis (32% to 40%), rhinitis (30% in patients with FVC <40%); FVC decrease ≥10% of predicted (22% in patients with FVC <40%), dyspnea (17% in patients with FVC <40%)
Miscellaneous: Voice alteration (12% to 18%)
1% to 10%:
Gastrointestinal: Dyspepsia (≤3%)
Ocular: Conjunctivitis (1% to 5%)
Respiratory: Laryngitis (3% to 4%)
Miscellaneous: Dornase alfa serum antibodies (2% to 4%)
Postmarketing and/or case reports: Headache, urticaria
General Dosage Range Inhalation: *Children >5 years and Adults:* 2.5 mg once daily
Mechanism of Action The hallmark of cystic fibrosis lung disease is the presence of abundant, purulent airway secretions composed primarily of highly polymerized DNA. The principal source of this DNA is the nuclei of degenerating neutrophils, which is present in large concentrations in infected lung secretions. The presence of this DNA produces a viscous mucous that may contribute to the decreased mucociliary transport and persistent infections that are commonly seen in this population. Dornase alfa is a deoxyribonuclease (DNA) enzyme produced by recombinant gene technology.

Dornase selectively cleaves DNA, thus reducing mucous viscosity and as a result, airflow in the lung is improved and the risk of bacterial infection may be decreased.
Pharmacodynamics/Kinetics
Onset of Action Nebulization: Enzyme levels are measured in sputum in ~15 minutes
Duration of Action Rapidly declines
Pregnancy Risk Factor B
Pregnancy Considerations Teratogenic effects were not observed in animal reproduction studies.

Dorzolamide (dor ZOLE a mide)

Brand Names: U.S. Trusopt®
Brand Names: Canada Sandoz-Dorzolamide; Trusopt®
Pharmacologic Category Carbonic Anhydrase Inhibitor; Ophthalmic Agent, Antiglaucoma
Use Treatment of elevated intraocular pressure in patients with ocular hypertension or open-angle glaucoma
Local Anesthetic/Vasoconstrictor Precautions No information available to require special precautions
Effects on Dental Treatment No significant effects or complications reported
Effects on Bleeding No information available to require special precautions
Adverse Effects
>10%:
Gastrointestinal: Bitter taste following administration (25%)
Ocular: Burning, stinging or discomfort immediately following administration (33%); superficial punctate keratitis (10% to 15%); signs and symptoms of ocular allergic reaction (10%)
1% to 5%: Ocular: Blurred vision, conjunctivitis, dryness, lid reactions, photophobia, redness, tearing
General Dosage Range Ophthalmic: *Children and Adults:* Instill 1 drop into affected eye(s) 3 times/day
Mechanism of Action Reversible inhibition of the enzyme carbonic anhydrase resulting in reduction of hydrogen ion secretion at renal tubule and an increased renal excretion of sodium, potassium, bicarbonate, and water to decrease production of aqueous humor; also inhibits carbonic anhydrase in central nervous system to retard abnormal and excessive discharge from CNS neurons
Pharmacodynamics/Kinetics
Onset of Action Peak effect: 2 hours
Duration of Action 8-12 hours
Half-life Elimination Terminal RBC: 147 days; washes out of RBCs nonlinearly, resulting in a rapid decline of drug concentration initially, followed by a slower elimination phase with a half-life of about 4 months
Pregnancy Risk Factor C
Pregnancy Considerations Adverse events have been observed in animal reproduction studies following systemic administration. IOP is usually lower during pregnancy. If topical medications for the treatment of glaucoma in pregnant women cannot be discontinued because small increases in IOP cannot be tolerated, the minimum effective dose should be used in combination with punctual occlusion to decrease exposure to the fetus (Johnson, 2001).

Dorzolamide and Timolol
(dor ZOLE a mide & TYE moe lole)

Related Information
Dorzolamide *on page 448*
Timolol (Ophthalmic) *on page 1326*
Brand Names: U.S. Cosopt®; Cosopt® PF
Brand Names: Canada Apo-Dorzo-Timop; Cosopt®; Cosopt® Preservative Free; Sandoz-Dorzolamide/Timolol
Pharmacologic Category Beta-Adrenergic Blocker, Nonselective; Carbonic Anhydrase Inhibitor; Ophthalmic Agent, Antiglaucoma
Use Treatment of elevated intraocular pressure in patients with ocular hypertension or open-angle glaucoma
Local Anesthetic/Vasoconstrictor Precautions No information available to require special precautions
Effects on Dental Treatment Key adverse event(s) related to dental treatment: Taste perversion.
Effects on Bleeding No information available to require special precautions
Adverse Effects Percentages as reported with combination product. Also see individual agents.
>5%:
Gastrointestinal: Taste perversion (≤30%)
Ocular: Burning/stinging (≤30%), blurred vision (5% to 15%), conjunctival hyperemia (5% to 15%), itching (5% to 15%), superficial punctuate keratitis (5% to 15%)
1% to 5%:
Cardiovascular: Hypertension
Central nervous system: Dizziness, headache
Gastrointestinal: Abdominal pain, dyspepsia, nausea
Genitourinary: Urinary tract infection
Neuromuscular & skeletal: Back pain
Ocular: Blepharitis, cloudy vision, conjunctival discharge, conjunctival edema, conjunctival follicles, conjunctivitis, corneal erosion, corneal staining, cortical lens opacity, dryness, eye debris, eye/eyelid discharge, eye/eyelid pain, eyelid edema, eyelid erythema, eyelid exudate/scales, foreign body sensation, glaucomatous cupping, lens nucleus discoloration, lens opacity, post-subcapsular cataract, tearing, visual field defect, vitreous detachment
Respiratory: Bronchitis, cough, pharyngitis, sinusitis, upper respiratory infection
Miscellaneous: Flu
General Dosage Range Ophthalmic: *Children ≥2 years and Adults:* Instill 1 drop into affected eye(s) twice daily
Mechanism of Action
Dorzolamide: Inhibits carbonic anhydrase in the ciliary processes of the eye resulting decreased bicarbonate ion formation which decreases sodium and fluid transport, thus decreasing aqueous humor secretion and reduces intraocular pressure.
Timolol: Blocks both beta$_1$- and beta$_2$-adrenergic receptors, reduces intraocular pressure by reducing aqueous humor production or possibly outflow
Pregnancy Risk Factor C
Pregnancy Considerations There are no adequate and well-controlled studies in pregnant women with the combination product. Use only if benefit outweighs risk. See individual agents.

Doxapram (DOKS a pram)

Brand Names: U.S. Dopram®

Pharmacologic Category Respiratory Stimulant
Use Respiratory stimulant for respiratory depression secondary to anesthesia, mild-to-moderate drug-induced respiratory and CNS depression; acute hypercapnia secondary to COPD

Note: In general, the use of doxapram as a respiratory stimulant in adults is limited; alternate therapies are preferred.
Local Anesthetic/Vasoconstrictor Precautions No information available to require special precautions
Effects on Dental Treatment No significant effects or complications reported
Effects on Bleeding No information available to require special precautions
Adverse Effects Frequency not defined.
Cardiovascular: Arrhythmia, blood pressure increased, chest pain, chest tightness, flushing, heart rate changes, T waves lowered, ventricular tachycardia, ventricular fibrillation
Central nervous system: Apprehension, Babinski turns positive, disorientation, dizziness, hallucinations, headache, hyperactivity, pyrexia, seizure
Dermatologic: Burning sensation, pruritus
Gastrointestinal: Defecation urge, diarrhea, nausea, vomiting
Genitourinary: Spontaneous voiding, urinary retention
Hematologic: Hematocrit decreased, hemoglobin decreased, hemolysis, red blood cell count decreased
Local: Phlebitis
Neuromuscular & skeletal: Clonus, deep tendon reflexes increase, fasciculations, involuntary muscle movement, muscle spasm, paresthesia
Ocular: Pupillary dilatation
Renal: Albuminuria, BUN increased
Respiratory: Bronchospasm, cough, dyspnea, hiccups, hyperventilation, laryngospasm, rebound hypoventilation, tachypnea
Miscellaneous: Diaphoresis
General Dosage Range I.V.: *Children ≥12 years, Adolescents, and Adults:* Initial: 0.5-1 mg/kg as an intermittent injection every 5 minutes until response (maximum total dose: 2 mg/kg) **or** 1-5 mg/minute as an I.V. infusion until response; should not be continued >2 hours (maximum total dose: 4 mg/kg [3000 mg daily])
Mechanism of Action Stimulates respiration through action on peripheral carotid chemoreceptors; respiratory center in medulla is also directly stimulated as dosage is increased
Pharmacodynamics/Kinetics
Onset of Action Respiratory stimulation: Single I.V. injection: 20-40 seconds; Peak effect: Single I.V. injection: 1-2 minutes
Duration of Action Single I.V. injection: 5-12 minutes
Half-life Elimination Serum: Adults: Mean: 3.4 hours (range: 2.4-4.1 hours)
Pregnancy Risk Factor B
Pregnancy Considerations Adverse fetal effects have not been observed in animal reproduction studies.

Doxazosin (doks AY zoe sin)

Related Information
Cardiovascular Diseases *on page 1492*
Brand Names: U.S. Cardura®; Cardura® XL
Brand Names: Canada Alti-Doxazosin; Apo-Doxazosin®; Cardura-1™; Cardura-2™; Cardura-4™; Gen-Doxazosin; Mylan-Doxazosin; Novo-Doxazosin

◄ **Generic Availability (U.S.)** Yes: Excludes extended release tablet

Pharmacologic Category Alpha$_1$ Blocker

Use

Immediate release formulation: Treatment of hypertension as monotherapy or in conjunction with diuretics, ACE inhibitors, beta-blockers, or calcium antagonists; treatment of urinary outflow obstruction and/or obstructive and irritative symptoms associated with benign prostatic hyperplasia (BPH)

Extended release formulation: Treatment of urinary outflow obstruction and/or obstructive and irritative symptoms associated with BPH

Unlabeled Use Pediatric hypertension; facilitation of distal ureteral stone expulsion; erectile dysfunction in patients with concomitant BPH

Local Anesthetic/Vasoconstrictor Precautions No information available to require special precautions

Effects on Dental Treatment Key adverse event(s) related to dental treatment: Xerostomia (normal salivary flow resumes upon discontinuation) and orthostatic hypotension

Effects on Bleeding No information available to require special precautions

Adverse Effects Note: Type and frequency of adverse reactions reflect combined data from BPH and hypertension trials and immediate release and extended release products.

>10%: Central nervous system: Dizziness (5% to 19%), malaise (12%), fatigue (8% to 12%), headache (6% to 10%)

1% to 10%:

Cardiovascular: Edema (3% to 4%), hypotension (1% to 2%), orthostatic hypotension (dose related; 0.3% up to 2%), arrhythmia (1%), facial edema (1%), flushing (1%)

Central nervous system: Vertigo (2% to 4%), somnolence (1% to 5%), pain (2%), anxiety (1%), ataxia (1%), hypertonia (1%), insomnia (1%), movement disorder (1%)

Endocrine & metabolic: Sexual dysfunction (2%)

Gastrointestinal: Abdominal pain (2%), nausea (1% to 2%), dyspepsia (1%), xerostomia (1%)

Genitourinary: Polyuria (2%), impotence (1%), incontinence (1%), urinary tract infection (1%)

Neuromuscular & skeletal: Weakness (4% to 7%), arthritis (1%), muscle cramps (1%), muscle weakness (1%), myalgia (1%)

Ocular: Abnormal vision (2%)

Otic: Tinnitus (1%)

Respiratory: Respiratory tract infection (5%), rhinitis (3%), dyspnea (1% to 3%), epistaxis (1%)

Dosage Oral:

Children and Adolescents 1-17 years (unlabeled use): Hypertension: Immediate release: Initial: 1 mg once daily; maximum: 4 mg daily (NHBPEP, 2004)

Adults:

Immediate release: 1 mg once daily in morning or evening; may be increased to 2 mg once daily. Thereafter titrate upwards, if needed, every 1-2 weeks, balancing therapeutic benefit with doxazosin-induced postural hypotension.

BPH: Goal: 4-8 mg daily; maximum dose: 8 mg daily

Hypertension: Maximum dose: 16 mg daily

Distal ureteral stone expulsion (unlabeled use): 4 mg once daily in evening (Gurbuz, 2011; Resorlu, 2011). **Note:** Patients with stones >10 mm were excluded from studies.

Reinitiation of therapy: If therapy is discontinued for several days, restart at 1 mg dose and titrate as before

Extended release: BPH: 4 mg once daily with breakfast; titrate based on response and tolerability every 3-4 weeks to maximum recommended dose of 8 mg daily

Reinitiation of therapy: If therapy is discontinued for several days, restart at 4 mg dose and titrate as before.

Conversion to extended release from immediate release: Omit final evening dose of immediate release prior to starting morning dosing with extended release product; initiate extended release product using 4 mg once daily

Elderly: Hypertension: Consider lower initial doses (eg, immediate release: 0.5 mg once daily) and titrate to response (Aronow, 2011)

Dosage adjustment in renal impairment: No dosage adjustment provided in the manufacturer's labeling (limited data suggest renal impairment does not significantly alter pharmacokinetic parameters).

Dosage adjustment in hepatic impairment: Use with caution in mild-to-moderate hepatic dysfunction. Do not use with severe impairment.

Mechanism of Action

Hypertension: Competitively inhibits postsynaptic alpha$_1$-adrenergic receptors which results in vasodilation of veins and arterioles and a decrease in total peripheral resistance and blood pressure; ~50% as potent on a weight by weight basis as prazosin.

BPH: Competitively inhibits postsynaptic alpha$_1$-adrenergic receptors in prostatic stromal and bladder neck tissues. This reduces the sympathetic tone-induced urethral stricture causing BPH symptoms.

Contraindications Hypersensitivity to quinazolines (prazosin, terazosin), doxazosin, or any component of the formulation

Warnings/Precautions Can cause significant orthostatic hypotension and syncope, especially with first dose; anticipate a similar effect if therapy is interrupted for a few days, if dosage is rapidly increased, or if another antihypertensive drug (particularly vasodilators) or a PDE-5 inhibitor is introduced. Discontinue if symptoms of angina occur or worsen. Patients should be cautioned about performing hazardous tasks when starting new therapy or adjusting dosage upward. Priapism has been associated with use (rarely). Prostate cancer should be ruled out before starting for BPH. Use with caution in mild-to-moderate hepatic impairment; not recommended in severe dysfunction. Intraoperative floppy iris syndrome has been observed in cataract surgery patients who were on or were previously treated with alpha$_1$-blockers. Causality has not been established and there appears to be no benefit in discontinuing alpha-blocker therapy prior to surgery. In the elderly, avoid use as an antihypertensive due to high risk of orthostatic hypotension; alternative agents preferred due to a more favorable risk/benefit profile (Beers Criteria).

The extended release formulation consists of drug within a nondeformable matrix; following drug release/ absorption, the matrix/shell is expelled in the stool. The use of nondeformable products in patients with known stricture/narrowing of the GI tract has been associated with symptoms of obstruction. Use caution in patients with increased GI retention (eg, chronic constipation) as doxazosin exposure may be increased. Extended release formulation is not indicated for use in women or for the treatment of hypertension.

Drug Interactions

Metabolism/Transport Effects Substrate of CYP2C19 (minor), CYP2D6 (minor), CYP3A4 (major); **Note:** Assignment of Major/Minor substrate status based on clinically relevant drug interaction potential

Avoid Concomitant Use

Avoid concomitant use of Doxazosin with any of the following: Alpha1-Blockers; Conivaptan

Increased Effect/Toxicity

Doxazosin may increase the levels/effects of: Alpha1-Blockers; Amifostine; Antihypertensives; Calcium Channel Blockers; Hypotensive Agents; RiTUXimab

The levels/effects of Doxazosin may be increased by: Beta-Blockers; Conivaptan; CYP3A4 Inhibitors (Moderate); CYP3A4 Inhibitors (Strong); Dasatinib; Diazoxide; Herbs (Hypotensive Properties); Ivacaftor; MAO Inhibitors; Mifepristone; Pentoxifylline; Phosphodiesterase 5 Inhibitors; Prostacyclin Analogues

Decreased Effect

Doxazosin may decrease the levels/effects of: Alpha-/Beta-Agonists; Alpha1-Agonists

The levels/effects of Doxazosin may be decreased by: CYP3A4 Inducers (Strong); Deferasirox; Herbs (CYP3A4 Inducers); Herbs (Hypertensive Properties); Methylphenidate; Peginterferon Alfa-2b; Tocilizumab; Yohimbine

Ethanol/Nutrition/Herb Interactions Herb/Nutraceutical: Avoid dong quai if using for hypertension (has estrogenic activity). Avoid ephedra, yohimbe, ginseng (may worsen hypertension). Avoid saw palmetto when used for BPH (due to limited experience with this combination). Avoid garlic (may have increased antihypertensive effect).

Dietary Considerations Cardura® XL: Take with morning meal.

Pharmacodynamics/Kinetics

Duration of Action >24 hours

Half-life Elimination Immediate release: ~22 hours; Extended release: 15-19 hours

Time to Peak Serum: Immediate release: 2-3 hours; Extended release: 8-9 hours

Pregnancy Risk Factor C

Pregnancy Considerations Adverse events were observed in some animal reproduction studies. Delayed postnatal development was also noted. There are no adequate and well-controlled studies in pregnant women.

Lactation Excretion in breast milk unknown/use caution

Breast-Feeding Considerations The extended release formulation is not indicated for use in women.

Dosage Forms

Tablet, oral: 1 mg, 2 mg, 4 mg, 8 mg
  Cardura®: 1 mg, 2 mg, 4 mg, 8 mg

Tablet, extended release, oral:
  Cardura® XL: 4 mg, 8 mg

Doxepin (Systemic) (DOKS e pin)

Related Information

Management of the Patient With Anxiety or Depression *on page 1594*

Vasoconstrictor Interactions With Antidepressants *on page 1650*

Brand Names: U.S. Silenor®

Brand Names: Canada Apo-Doxepin®; Doxepine; Novo-Doxepin; Silenor®; Sinequan®; Zonalon

Generic Availability (U.S.) Yes: Excludes tablet

Pharmacologic Category Antidepressant, Tricyclic (Tertiary Amine)

Use Depression; treatment of insomnia (with difficulty of sleep maintenance)

Unlabeled Use Analgesic for certain chronic and neuropathic pain; anxiety

Local Anesthetic/Vasoconstrictor Precautions Doxepin is one of the drugs confirmed to prolong the QT interval and is accepted as having a risk of causing torsade de pointes. In terms of epinephrine, it is not known what effect vasoconstrictors in the local anesthetic regimen will have in patients with a known history of congenital prolonged QT interval or in patients taking any medication that prolongs the QT interval. Until more information is obtained, it is suggested that the clinician consult with the physician prior to the use of a vasoconstrictor in suspected patients, and that the vasoconstrictor (epinephrine, mepivacaine, and levonordefrin [Carbocaine® 2% with Neo-Cobefrin®]) be used with caution. See Dental Comment.

Effects on Dental Treatment Key adverse event(s) related to dental treatment: Xerostomia and changes in salivation (normal salivary flow resumes upon discontinuation)

Oral: Aphthous stomatitis, unpleasant taste, trouble with gums

Long-term treatment with TCAs increases the risk of caries by reducing salivation and salivary buffer capacity.

Effects on Bleeding No information available to require special precautions

Adverse Effects Actual frequency may be dependent on diagnosis.

Cardiovascular: Flushing, hypertension (<3%), hypotension, tachycardia

Central nervous system: Ataxia, chills, confusion, disorientation, dizziness, drowsiness, fatigue, hallucinations, headache, seizure, somnolence/sedation (6% to 9%)

Dermatologic: Alopecia, photosensitivity, pruritus, rash

Endocrine & metabolic: Blood sugar increased/decreased, breast enlargement, galactorrhea, gynecomastia, libido increased/decreased, SIADH

Gastrointestinal: Anorexia, aphthous stomatitis, constipation, diarrhea, gastroenteritis (≤2%), indigestion, nausea (2%), trouble with gums, unpleasant taste, vomiting, weight gain, xerostomia; lower esophageal sphincter tone decrease may cause GE reflux

Genitourinary: Testicular edema, urinary retention

Hematologic: Agranulocytosis, eosinophilia, leukopenia, purpura, thrombocytopenia, purpura

Hepatic: Jaundice

Neuromuscular & skeletal: Extrapyramidal symptoms, numbness, paresthesia, tardive dyskinesia, tremor, weakness

Ocular: Blurred vision

Otic: Tinnitus

Respiratory: Asthma exacerbation, nasopharyngitis/upper respiratory tract infection (≤4%)

Miscellaneous: Allergic reactions, diaphoresis (excessive)

◀ **Dosage** Oral:

Depression or anxiety (entire daily dose may be given at bedtime):

Adults: Initial: 25-150 mg/day at bedtime or in 2-3 divided doses; may gradually increase up to 300 mg/day; single dose should not exceed 150 mg; select patients may respond to 25-50 mg/day

Elderly: Initial: 10-25 mg at bedtime; increase by 10-25 mg every 3 days for inpatients and weekly for outpatients if tolerated. Rarely does the maximum dose required exceed 75 mg/day; a single bedtime dose is recommended.

Insomnia (Silenor®):

Adults: 3-6 mg once daily 30 minutes prior to bedtime; maximum dose: 6 mg/day

Elderly: 3 mg once daily; increase to 6 mg once daily if clinically needed

Dosage adjustment in renal impairment: No dosage adjustment provided in manufacturer's labeling.

Dosage adjustment in hepatic impairment: Use a lower dose and adjust gradually

Silenor®: Initial: 3 mg once daily

Mechanism of Action Increases the synaptic concentration of serotonin and norepinephrine in the central nervous system by inhibition of their reuptake by the presynaptic neuronal membrane; antagonizes the histamine (H_1) receptor for sleep maintenance

Contraindications Hypersensitivity to doxepin, drugs from similar chemical class, or any component of the formulation; narrow-angle glaucoma; urinary retention; use of MAO inhibitors within 14 days

Warnings/Precautions [U.S. Boxed Warning]: Antidepressants increase the risk of suicidal thinking and behavior in children, adolescents, and young adults (18-24 years of age) with major depressive disorder (MDD) and other psychiatric disorders; consider risk prior to prescribing. Short-term studies did not show an increased risk in patients >24 years of age and showed a decreased risk in patients ≥65 years. Closely monitor for clinical worsening, suicidality, or unusual changes in behavior; the patient's family or caregiver should be instructed to closely observe the patient and communicate condition with healthcare provider. A medication guide should be dispensed with each prescription. **Doxepin is approved for treatment of depression in adolescents.**

The possibility of a suicide attempt is inherent in major depression and may persist until remission occurs. Monitor for worsening of depression or suicidality, especially during initiation of therapy (generally first 1-2 months) or with dose increases or decreases. Use caution in high-risk patients. Worsening depression and severe abrupt suicidality that are not part of the presenting symptoms may require discontinuation or modification of drug therapy. The patient's family or caregiver should be alerted to monitor patients for the emergence of suicidality and associated behaviors (such as agitation, irritability, hostility, impulsivity, and hypomania) and call healthcare provider.

Risk of suicidal behavior may be increased regardless of doxepin dose; antidepressant doses of doxepin are 10- to 100-fold higher than doses for insomnia.

May worsen psychosis in some patients or precipitate a shift to mania or hypomania in patients with bipolar disorder. Patients presenting with depressive symptoms should be screened for bipolar disorder. Monotherapy in patients with bipolar disorder should be avoided.

Doxepin is not FDA approved for the treatment of bipolar depression.

Should only be used for insomnia after evaluation of potential causes of sleep disturbance. Failure of sleep disturbance to resolve after 7-10 days may indicate psychiatric or medical illness. An increased risk for hazardous sleep-related activities has been noted; discontinue use with any sleep-related episodes. The risks of sedative and anticholinergic effects are high relative to other antidepressant agents. Doxepin frequently causes sedation, which may result in impaired performance of tasks requiring alertness (eg, operating machinery or driving). Sedative effects may be additive with other CNS depressants and/or ethanol. Also use caution in patients with benign prostatic hyperplasia, xerostomia, visual problems, constipation, or history of bowel obstruction.

May cause orthostatic hypotension or conduction disturbances (risks are moderate relative to other antidepressants). Use with caution in patients with a history of cardiovascular disease (including previous MI, stroke, tachycardia, or conduction abnormalities). Use with caution in patients with respiratory compromise or sleep apnea; use is generally not recommended with severe sleep apnea. Consider discontinuation, when possible, prior to elective surgery. Therapy should not be abruptly discontinued in patients receiving high doses for prolonged periods.

Use caution in patients with a previous seizure disorder or condition predisposing to seizures such as brain damage, alcoholism, or concurrent therapy with other drugs which lower the seizure threshold. Use with caution in hyperthyroid patients or those receiving thyroid supplementation. Use with caution in patients with hepatic or renal dysfunction.

In the elderly, avoid doses >6 mg/day in this age group due to its potent anticholinergic and sedative properties, and potential to cause orthostatic hypotension; safety of doses ≤6 mg/day is comparable to placebo. In addition, may also cause or exacerbate syndrome of inappropriate antidiuretic hormone secretion or hyponatremia; monitor sodium closely with initiation or dosage adjustments in older adults (Beers Criteria).

Drug Interactions

Metabolism/Transport Effects Substrate of CYP1A2 (minor), CYP2C19 (minor), CYP2D6 (major), CYP3A4 (minor); **Note:** Assignment of Major/Minor substrate status based on clinically relevant drug interaction potential

Avoid Concomitant Use

Avoid concomitant use of Doxepin (Systemic) with any of the following: Aclidinium; Iobenguane I 123; Ipratropium (Oral Inhalation); Linezolid; MAO Inhibitors; Methylene Blue; Tiotropium

Increased Effect/Toxicity

Doxepin (Systemic) may increase the levels/effects of: Alpha-/Beta-Agonists (Direct-Acting); Alpha1-Agonists; Amphetamines; Anticholinergics; Aspirin; Beta2-Agonists; Desmopressin; Highest Risk QTc-Prolonging Agents; Methylene Blue; Metoclopramide; Moderate Risk QTc-Prolonging Agents; NSAID (COX-2 Inhibitor); NSAID (Nonselective); QuiNIDine; Serotonin Modulators; Sodium Phosphates; Sulfonylureas; Tiotropium; TraMADol; Vitamin K Antagonists; Yohimbine

The levels/effects of Doxepin (Systemic) may be increased by: Abiraterone Acetate; Aclidinium; Altretamine; Antipsychotics; BuPROPion; Cimetidine; Cinacalcet; Cobicistat; CYP2D6 Inhibitors (Moderate); CYP2D6 Inhibitors (Strong); Dexmethylphenidate; CYP2D6 Inhibitors (Strong); DULoxetine; Ipratropium (Oral Inhalation); Linezolid; Lithium; MAO Inhibitors; Methylphenidate; Metoclopramide; Metyrosine; Mifepristone; Pramlintide; Protease Inhibitors; QuiNIDine; Selective Serotonin Reuptake Inhibitors; Terbinafine (Systemic); Valproic Acid

Decreased Effect

Doxepin (Systemic) may decrease the levels/effects of: Acetylcholinesterase Inhibitors (Central); Alpha2-Agonists; Iobenguane I 123

The levels/effects of Doxepin (Systemic) may be decreased by: Acetylcholinesterase Inhibitors (Central); Barbiturates; CarBAMazepine; Peginterferon Alfa-2b; St Johns Wort

Ethanol/Nutrition/Herb Interactions

Ethanol: May increase CNS depression; monitor for increased effects with coadministration. Caution patients about effects.

Food: A high-fat meal increases the bioavailability of Silenor® and delays the peak plasma concentration by ~3 hours

Herb/Nutraceutical: Avoid valerian, St John's wort, SAMe, kava kava (may increase risk of serotonin syndrome and/or excessive sedation).

Pharmacodynamics/Kinetics

Onset of Action Peak effect: Antidepressant: Usually >2 weeks; Anxiolytic: May occur sooner

Half-life Elimination Adults: Doxepin: ~15 hours; N-desmethyldoxepin: 31 hours

Time to Peak Serum: Hypnotic: 3.5 hours

Pregnancy Risk Factor C

Pregnancy Considerations Decreased fetal body weight and fetal structural abnormalities were observed in animal reproduction studies at doses greater than the maximum recommended human dose. There are no adequate and well-controlled studies in pregnant women.

Lactation Enters breast milk/use caution (AAP rates "of concern"; AAP 2001 update pending)

Breast-Feeding Considerations Drowsiness and apnea have been reported in a nursing infant following maternal use of doxepin for depression.

Dosage Forms

Capsule, oral: 10 mg, 25 mg, 50 mg, 75 mg, 100 mg, 150 mg

Solution, oral: 10 mg/mL (118 mL, 120 mL)

Tablet, oral:

Silenor®: 3 mg, 6 mg

Dental Comment Doxepin is known to prolong the QT interval. The QT interval is measured as the time and distance between the Q point of the QRS complex and the end of the T wave in the ECG tracing. After adjustment for heart rate, the QT interval is defined as prolonged if it is more than 450 msec in men and 460 msec in women. A long QT syndrome was first described in the 1950s and 60s as a congenital syndrome involving QT interval prolongation and syncope and sudden death. Some of the congenital long QT syndromes were characterized by a peculiar electrocardiographic appearance of the QRS complex involving a premature atria beat followed by a pause, then a subsequent sinus beat showing marked QT prolongation and deformity. This type of cardiac arrhythmia was originally termed "torsade de pointes" (translated from

the French as "twisting of the points"). Doxepin is considered as having a risk of causing torsade de pointes. Since it is not known what effect vasoconstrictors in the local anesthetic regimen will have in patients with a known history of congenital prolonged QT interval or in patients taking any medication that prolongs the QT interval, a medical consult is suggested.

References

Jastak JT and Yagiela JA, "Vasoconstrictors and Local Anesthesia: A Review and Rationale for Use," *J Am Dent Assoc*, 1983, 107 (4):623-30.

Rundegren J, van Dijken J, Mörnstad H, et al, "Oral Conditions in Patients Receiving Long-Term Treatment With Cyclic Antidepressant Drugs," *Swed Dent J*, 1985, 9(2):55-64.

Yagiela JA, "Adverse Drug Interactions in Dental Practice: Interactions Associated With Vasoconstrictors. Part V of a Series," *J Am Dent Assoc*, 1999, 130(5):701-9.

Doxepin (Topical) (DOKS e pin)

Brand Names: U.S. Prudoxin™; Zonalon®

Brand Names: Canada Zonalon®

Generic Availability (U.S.) No

Pharmacologic Category Topical Skin Product

Dental Use Cream: Treatment of burning mouth syndrome and neuropathic pain

Use Short-term (<8 days) management of moderate pruritus in adults with atopic dermatitis or lichen simplex chronicus

Unlabeled Use Cream: Treatment of burning mouth syndrome and neuropathic pain

Local Anesthetic/Vasoconstrictor Precautions No information available to require special precautions

Effects on Dental Treatment Key adverse event(s) related to dental treatment: Xerostomia and changes in salivation (normal salivary flow resumes upon discontinuation)

Topical: Taste alteration

Long-term treatment with TCAs increases the risk of caries by reducing salivation and salivary buffer capacity.

Effects on Bleeding No information available to require special precautions

Adverse Effects

>10%:

Central nervous system: Drowsiness (22%)

Dermatologic: Stinging/burning (23%)

1% to 10%:

Cardiovascular: Edema: (1%)

Central nervous system: Dizziness (2%), emotional changes (2%)

Gastrointestinal: Xerostomia (10%), taste alteration (2%)

Dental Usual Dosage Treatment of burning mouth syndrome and neuropathic pain (unlabeled uses): Adults: Oral: Topical: Cream: Apply 3-4 times daily

Dosage

Oral: Topical: Burning mouth syndrome (unlabeled use): Cream: Apply 3-4 times daily

Topical: Pruritus: Adults and Elderly: Apply a thin film 4 times/day with at least 3- to 4-hour interval between applications; not recommended for use >8 days. **Note:** Low-dose (25-50 mg) oral administration has also been used to treat pruritus, but systemic effects are increased.

Contraindications Hypersensitivity to doxepin, drugs from similar chemical class, or any component of the formulation; narrow-angle glaucoma; urinary retention; use of MAO inhibitors within 14 days; use in a patient during acute recovery phase of MI

◄ **Warnings/Precautions** Cream formulation is for external use only (not for ophthalmic, vaginal, or oral use). Do not use occlusive dressings. Use for >8 days may increase risk of contact sensitization. Doxepin is significantly absorbed following topical administration; plasma levels may be similar to those achieved with oral administration. Systemic absorption may be significant. The risks of sedative and anticholinergic effects caused by doxepin are high relative to other antidepressant agents. Doxepin frequently causes sedation, which may result in impaired performance of tasks requiring alertness (eg, operating machinery or driving). Sedative effects may be additive with other CNS depressants and/or ethanol. Also use caution in patients with benign prostatic hyperplasia, xerostomia, visual problems, constipation, or history of bowel obstruction.

May cause orthostatic hypotension or conduction disturbances. Use with caution in patients with a history of cardiovascular disease (including previous MI, stroke, tachycardia, or conduction abnormalities). Consider discontinuation, when possible, prior to elective surgery. Use caution in patients with a previous seizure disorder or condition predisposing to seizures such as brain damage, alcoholism, or concurrent therapy with other drugs which lower the seizure threshold. Use with caution in hyperthyroid patients or those receiving thyroid supplementation. Use with caution in patients with hepatic or renal dysfunction.

Drug Interactions

Metabolism/Transport Effects Substrate of CYP1A2 (minor), CYP2C19 (minor), CYP2D6 (major), CYP3A4 (minor); **Note:** Assignment of Major/Minor substrate status based on clinically relevant drug interaction potential

Avoid Concomitant Use

Avoid concomitant use of Doxepin (Topical) with any of the following: Aclidinium; Iobenguane I 123; Ipratropium (Oral Inhalation); Linezolid; MAO Inhibitors; Methylene Blue; Tiotropium

Increased Effect/Toxicity

Doxepin (Topical) may increase the levels/effects of: Alpha-/Beta-Agonists (Direct-Acting); Alpha1-Agonists; Amphetamines; Anticholinergics; Aspirin; Beta2-Agonists; Desmopressin; Highest Risk QTc-Prolonging Agents; Methylene Blue; Metoclopramide; Moderate Risk QTc-Prolonging Agents; NSAID (COX-2 Inhibitor); NSAID (Nonselective); QuiNIDine; Serotonin Modulators; Sodium Phosphates; Sulfonylureas; Tiotropium; TraMADol; Vitamin K Antagonists; Yohimbine

The levels/effects of Doxepin (Topical) may be increased by: Abiraterone Acetate; Aclidinium; Altretamine; Antipsychotics; BuPROPion; Cimetidine; Cinacalcet; Cobicistat; CYP2D6 Inhibitors (Moderate); CYP2D6 Inhibitors (Strong); Dexmethylphenidate; Divalproex; DULoxetine; Ipratropium (Oral Inhalation); Linezolid; Lithium; MAO Inhibitors; Methylphenidate; Metoclopramide; Metyrosine; Mifepristone; Pramlintide; Protease Inhibitors; QuiNIDine; Selective Serotonin Reuptake Inhibitors; Terbinafine (Systemic); Valproic Acid

Decreased Effect

Doxepin (Topical) may decrease the levels/effects of: Acetylcholinesterase Inhibitors (Central); Alpha2-Agonists; Iobenguane I 123

The levels/effects of Doxepin (Topical) may be decreased by: Acetylcholinesterase Inhibitors (Central); Barbiturates; CarBAMazepine; Peginterferon Alfa-2b; St Johns Wort

Pregnancy Risk Factor B

Pregnancy Considerations Teratogenic effects were not observed in animal studies. Following topical application, plasma levels may be similar to those achieved with oral administration

Lactation Enters breast milk/not recommended (AAP rates "of concern"; AAP 2001 update pending)

Breast-Feeding Considerations Drowsiness and apnea have been reported in a nursing infant following maternal use of oral doxepin. Following topical application, plasma levels may be similar to those achieved with oral administration.

Dosage Forms

Cream, topical:
Prudoxin™: 5% (45 g)
Zonalon®: 5% (30 g, 45 g)

References

Buchanan J and Zakrzewska J, "Burning Mouth Syndrome," *Clin Evid* (online), March 14, 2008. Available at http://www.ncbi.nlm.nih.gov/pmc/articles/PMC2907957/pdf/2008-1301.pdf.

Mínguez Serra MP, Salort Llorca C, Silvestre Donat FJ, "Pharmacological Treatment of Burning Mouth Syndrome: A Review and Update," *Med Oral Patol Oral Cir Bucal*, 2007, 12(4):E299-304.

Doxercalciferol (doks er kal si fe FEER ole)

Brand Names: U.S. Hectorol®

Brand Names: Canada Hectorol®

Pharmacologic Category Vitamin D Analog

Use Treatment of secondary hyperparathyroidism in patients with chronic kidney disease

Local Anesthetic/Vasoconstrictor Precautions No information available to require special precautions

Effects on Dental Treatment No significant effects or complications reported

Effects on Bleeding No information available to require special precautions

Adverse Effects

Note: As reported in dialysis patients.

>10%:
Cardiovascular: Edema (34%)
Central nervous system: Headache (28%), malaise (28%), dizziness (12%)
Gastrointestinal: Nausea/vomiting (21%)
Respiratory: Dyspnea (12%)

1% to 10%:
Cardiovascular: Bradycardia (7%)
Central nervous system: Sleep disorder (3%)
Dermatologic: Pruritus (8%)
Endocrine & metabolic: Hypercalcemia (I.V. ~1%), hyperphosphatemia (I.V. 2% to 4%)
Gastrointestinal: Anorexia (5%), dyspepsia (5%), weight gain (5%)
Neuromuscular & skeletal: Arthralgia (5%)
Miscellaneous: Abscess (3%)

General Dosage Range

I.V.: *Adults:* Initial: 4 mcg 3 times/week after dialysis; Maintenance: Up to 18 mcg/week

Oral:
Adults (dialysis patients): Initial: 10 mcg 3 times/week at dialysis; Maintenance: Up to 60 mcg/week
Adults (predialysis patients): Initial: 1 mcg/day; Maintenance: Up to 3.5 mcg/day

Mechanism of Action Doxercalciferol is metabolized to the active form of vitamin D. The active form of vitamin D controls the intestinal absorption of dietary calcium, the tubular reabsorption of calcium by the kidneys, and in conjunction with PTH, the mobilization of calcium from the skeleton.

Pharmacodynamics/Kinetics
Half-life Elimination Active metabolite: 32-37 hours; up to 96 hours
Pregnancy Risk Factor B
Pregnancy Considerations Reproduction in animals (usual and high dose) do not reveal teratogenic or fetotoxic effects.

DOXOrubicin (doks oh ROO bi sin)

Related Information
DOXOrubicin (Liposomal) *on page 455*
Brand Names: U.S. Adriamycin®
Brand Names: Canada Adriamycin®; Doxorubicin Hydrochloride Injection
Pharmacologic Category Antineoplastic Agent, Anthracycline
Use Treatment of acute lymphocytic leukemia (ALL), acute myeloid leukemia (AML), Hodgkin's disease, malignant lymphoma, soft tissue and bone sarcomas, thyroid cancer, small cell lung cancer, breast cancer, gastric cancer, ovarian cancer, bladder cancer, neuroblastoma, and Wilms' tumor
Unlabeled Use Treatment of multiple myeloma, endometrial carcinoma, uterine sarcoma, head and neck cancer, liver cancer, kidney cancer
Local Anesthetic/Vasoconstrictor Precautions No information available to require special precautions
Effects on Dental Treatment Key adverse event(s) related to dental treatment: Stomatitis and mucositis.
Effects on Bleeding Severe myelosuppression with thrombocytopenia and anemia occur. Medical consult suggested.
Adverse Effects Frequency not defined.
Cardiovascular:
Acute cardiotoxicity: Atrioventricular block, bradycardia, bundle branch block, ECG abnormalities, extrasystoles (atrial or ventricular), sinus tachycardia, ST-T wave changes, supraventricular tachycardia, tachyarrhythmia, ventricular tachycardia
Delayed cardiotoxicity: LVEF decreased, CHF (manifestations include ascites, cardiomegaly, dyspnea, edema, gallop rhythm, hepatomegaly, oliguria, pleural effusion, pulmonary edema, tachycardia); myocarditis, pericarditis
Central nervous system: Malaise
Dermatologic: Alopecia, itching, photosensitivity, radiation recall, rash; discoloration of saliva, sweat, or tears
Endocrine & metabolic: Amenorrhea, dehydration, infertility (may be temporary), hyperuricemia
Gastrointestinal: Abdominal pain, anorexia, colon necrosis, diarrhea, GI ulceration, mucositis, nausea, vomiting
Genitourinary: Discoloration of urine
Hematologic: Leukopenia/neutropenia (75%; nadir: 10-14 days; recovery: by day 21); thrombocytopenia and anemia
Local: Skin "flare" at injection site, urticaria
Neuromuscular & skeletal: Weakness
General Dosage Range Dosage adjustment recommended in patients with hepatic impairment or who develop toxicities

I.V.: *Children and Adults:* Dosage varies greatly depending on indication
Mechanism of Action Inhibition of DNA and RNA synthesis by intercalation between DNA base pairs by inhibition of topoisomerase II and by steric obstruction. Doxorubicin intercalates at points of local uncoiling of the double helix. Although the exact mechanism is unclear, it appears that direct binding to DNA (intercalation) and inhibition of DNA repair (topoisomerase II inhibition) result in blockade of DNA and RNA synthesis and fragmentation of DNA. Doxorubicin is also a powerful iron chelator; the iron-doxorubicin complex can bind DNA and cell membranes and produce free radicals that immediately cleave the DNA and cell membranes.
Pharmacodynamics/Kinetics
Half-life Elimination
Distribution: 5-10 minutes
Elimination: Doxorubicin: 1-3 hours; Metabolites: 3-3.5 hours
Terminal: 17-48 hours
Male: 54 hours; Female: 35 hours
Pregnancy Risk Factor D
Pregnancy Considerations Teratogenicity and embryotoxicity were observed in animal studies. There are no adequate and well-controlled studies in pregnant women. Advise patients to avoid becoming pregnant (females) and to avoid causing pregnancy (males) during treatment. According to the National Comprehensive Cancer Network (NCCN) breast cancer guidelines, doxorubicin, if indicated, may be administered to pregnant women with breast cancer as part of a combination chemotherapy regimen, although chemotherapy should not be administered during the first trimester or after 35 weeks gestation.

DOXOrubicin (Liposomal)
(doks oh ROO bi sin lye po SO mal)

Related Information
DOXOrubicin *on page 455*
Brand Names: U.S. Doxil®
Brand Names: Canada Caelyx®; Myocet™
Pharmacologic Category Antineoplastic Agent, Anthracycline
Use
U.S. labeling: Treatment of ovarian cancer (progressive or recurrent after platinum-based treatment); multiple myeloma (in combination with bortezomib in patients who are bortezomib naïve and after failure of at least 1 prior therapy); AIDS-related Kaposi's sarcoma (after failure of or intolerance to prior systemic therapy)

Canadian labeling: Treatment of metastatic breast cancer (as monotherapy [Caelyx®] or in combination with cyclophosphamide [Myocet™]); advanced ovarian cancer (after failure of first-line treatment [Caelyx®]); AIDS-related Kaposi's sarcoma (after failure of or intolerance to prior systemic therapy [Caelyx®])

Unlabeled Use Treatment of metastatic breast cancer, Hodgkin lymphoma (salvage treatment), cutaneous T-cell lymphomas (mycosis fungoides and Sézary syndrome), advanced soft tissue sarcomas; advanced or recurrent uterine sarcoma
Local Anesthetic/Vasoconstrictor Precautions No information available to require special precautions
Effects on Dental Treatment Key adverse event(s) related to dental treatment: Xerostomia (normal salivary flow resumes upon discontinuation), mucositis, gingivitis, glossitis, mouth ulceration, taste perversion, and stomatitis.

◀ Effects on Bleeding Severe myelosuppression with thrombocytopenia and anemia occur. Medical consult suggested.

Adverse Effects

>10%:

Cardiovascular: Peripheral edema (≤11%)

Central nervous system: Fever (8% to 21%), headache (≤11%), pain (≤21%)

Dermatologic: Palmar-plantar erythrodysesthesia/ hand-foot syndrome (≤51% in ovarian cancer [grades 3/4: 24%]; 3% in Kaposi's sarcoma), rash (≤29% in ovarian cancer, ≤5% in Kaposi's sarcoma), alopecia (9% to 19%)

Gastrointestinal: Nausea (17% to 46%), stomatitis (5% to 41%), vomiting (8% to 33%), constipation (≤30%), diarrhea (5% to 21%), anorexia (≤20%), mucositis (≤14%), dyspepsia (≤12%), intestinal obstruction (≤11%)

Hematologic: Myelosuppression (onset: 7 days; nadir: 10-14 days; recovery: 21-28 days), thrombocytopenia (13% to 65%; grades 3/4: 1%), neutropenia (12% to 62%; grade 4: 4%), leukopenia (36%), anemia (6% to 74%; grade 4: <1%)

Neuromuscular & skeletal: Weakness (7% to 40%), back pain (≤12%)

Respiratory: Pharyngitis (≤16%), dyspnea (≤15%)

Miscellaneous: Infection (≤12%)

1% to 10%:

Cardiovascular: Cardiac arrest, chest pain, deep thrombophlebitis, edema, hypotension, pallor, tachycardia, vasodilation

Central nervous system: Agitation, anxiety, chills, confusion, depression, dizziness, emotional lability, insomnia, somnolence, vertigo

Dermatologic: Acne, bruising, dry skin (6%), exfoliative dermatitis, fungal dermatitis, furunculosis, maculopapular rash, pruritus, skin discoloration, vesiculobullous rash

Endocrine & metabolic: Dehydration, hypercalcemia, hyperglycemia, hypokalemia, hyponatremia

Gastrointestinal: Abdomen enlarged, anorexia, ascites, cachexia, dyspepsia, dysphagia, esophagitis, flatulence, gingivitis, glossitis, ileus, mouth ulceration, oral moniliasis, rectal bleeding, taste perversion, weight loss, xerostomia

Genitourinary: Cystitis, dysuria, leukorrhea, pelvic pain, polyuria, urinary incontinence, urinary tract infection, urinary urgency, vaginal bleeding, vaginal moniliasis

Hematologic: Hemolysis, prothrombin time increased

Hepatic: ALT increased, alkaline phosphatase increased, hyperbilirubinemia

Local: Thrombophlebitis

Neuromuscular & skeletal: Arthralgia, hypertonia, myalgia, neuralgia, neuritis (peripheral), neuropathy, paresthesia (≤10%), pathological fracture

Ocular: Conjunctivitis, dry eyes, retinitis

Otic: Ear pain

Renal: Albuminuria, hematuria

Respiratory: Apnea, cough (≤10%), epistaxis, pleural effusion, pneumonia, rhinitis, sinusitis

Miscellaneous: Allergic reaction; infusion-related reactions (7%; includes bronchospasm, chest tightness, chills, dyspnea, facial edema, flushing, headache, herpes simplex/zoster, hypotension, pruritus); moniliasis, diaphoresis

General Dosage Range Dosage adjustment recommended in patients with hepatic impairment or who develop toxicities

I.V.: *Adults:* 20-30 mg/m² every 3 weeks **or** 50 mg/m² every 4 weeks

Mechanism of Action Doxorubicin inhibits DNA and RNA synthesis by intercalating between DNA base pairs causing steric obstruction and inhibits topoisomerase-II at the point of DNA cleavage. Doxorubicin is also a powerful iron chelator. The iron-doxorubicin complex can bind DNA and cell membranes, producing free hydroxyl (OH) radicals that cleave DNA and cell membranes. Active throughout entire cell cycle. Doxorubicin liposomal is a pegylated formulation which protects the liposomes, and thereby increases blood circulation time.

Pharmacodynamics/Kinetics

Half-life Elimination Terminal: Distribution: 4.7-5.2 hours, Elimination: 44-55 hours

Pregnancy Risk Factor D

Pregnancy Considerations Adverse events were observed in animal reproduction studies at doses less than the equivalent human dose (based on BSA). May cause fetal harm if administered during pregnancy. Women of childbearing potential should avoid becoming pregnant during treatment.

Doxycycline (doks i SYE kleen)

Related Information

Periodontal Diseases *on page 1570*

Sexually-Transmitted Diseases *on page 1536*

Related Sample Prescriptions

Bacterial Infections and Periodontal Diseases *on page 1609*

Brand Names: U.S. Adoxa®; Alodox™; Doryx®; Doxy 100™; Monodox®; Ocudox™; Oracea®; Oraxyl™; Vibramycin®

Brand Names: Canada Apo-Doxy Tabs®; Apo-Doxy®; Dom-Doxycycline; Doxycin; Doxytab; Novo-Doxylin; Nu-Doxycycline; Periostat®; PHL-Doxycycline; PMS-Doxycycline; Vibra-Tabs®; Vibramycin®

Generic Availability (U.S.) Yes: Excludes capsule (variable release), powder for suspension, syrup

Pharmacologic Category Antibiotic, Tetracycline Derivative

Dental Use Treatment of periodontitis associated with presence of *Actinobacillus actinomycetemcomitans* (AA); adjunct to scaling and root planing to promote attachment level gain and to reduce pocket depth in adult periodontitis (systemic levels are subinhibitory against bacteria)

Use Principally in the treatment of infections caused by susceptible *Rickettsia*, *Chlamydia*, and *Mycoplasma*; alternative to mefloquine for malaria prophylaxis; treatment for syphilis, uncomplicated *Neisseria gonorrhoeae* (alternative agent), *Listeria*, *Actinomyces israelii*, and *Clostridium* infections in penicillin-allergic patients; used for community-acquired pneumonia and other common infections due to susceptible organisms; anthrax due to *Bacillus anthracis*, including inhalational anthrax (postexposure); treatment of infections caused by uncommon susceptible gram-negative and gram-positive organisms including *Borrelia recurrentis*, *Ureaplasma urealyticum*, *Haemophilus ducreyi*, *Yersinia pestis*, *Francisella tularensis*, *Vibrio cholerae*, *Campylobacter fetus*, *Brucella* spp, *Bartonella bacilliformis*, and *Klebsiella granulomatis*, Q fever, Lyme disease; treatment of inflammatory lesions associated with rosacea; intestinal amebiasis; severe acne

Unlabeled Use Sclerosing agent for pleural effusion (injection); vancomycin-resistant enterococci (VRE); alternate treatment for MRSA infections; treatment of periodontitis (refractory); localized juvenile periodontitis (LJP); treatment of acute bacterial rhinosinusitis (ABRS) (adults); oral phase treatment of prosthetic joint infection; chronic oral antimicrobial suppression of prosthetic joint infection

Local Anesthetic/Vasoconstrictor Precautions No information available to require special precautions

Effects on Dental Treatment Key adverse event(s) related to dental treatment: Glossitis and tooth discoloration (children). Opportunistic "superinfection" with *Candida albicans*; tetracyclines are not recommended for use during pregnancy or in children ≤8 years of age since they have been reported to cause enamel hypoplasia and permanent teeth discoloration. The use of tetracyclines should only be used in these patients if other agents are contraindicated or alternative antimicrobials will not eradicate the organism.

Effects on Bleeding Hemolytic anemia and thrombocytopenia have been reported

Adverse Effects Frequency not defined.

Cardiovascular: Intracranial hypertension, pericarditis

Dermatologic: Angioneurotic edema, erythema multiforme, exfoliative dermatitis (rare), photosensitivity, rash, skin hyperpigmentation, Stevens-Johnson syndrome, toxic epidermal necrolysis, urticaria

Endocrine & metabolic: Brown/black discoloration of thyroid gland (no dysfunction reported), hypoglycemia

Gastrointestinal: Anorexia, diarrhea, dysphagia, enterocolitis, esophagitis (rare), esophageal ulcerations (rare), glossitis, inflammatory lesions in anogenital region, nausea, oral (mucosal) pigmentation, pseudomembranous colitis, tooth discoloration (children), vomiting

Hematologic: Eosinophilia, hemolytic anemia, neutropenia, thrombocytopenia

Hepatic: Hepatotoxicity (rare)

Renal: BUN increased (dose related)

Miscellaneous: Anaphylactoid purpura, anaphylaxis, bulging fontanels (infants), serum sickness, SLE exacerbation

Note: Adverse effects in clinical trials occurring at a frequency more than 1% greater than placebo:

Periostat®: Diarrhea, dyspepsia, joint pain, menstrual cramp, nausea, dyspepsia, pain

Oracea®: Abdominal distention, abdominal pain, anxiety, AST increased, back pain, fungal infection, hyperglycemia, influenza, LDH increased, nasal congestion, nasopharyngitis, pain, sinus headache, sinusitis, xerostomia

Dental Usual Dosage

Adults: Oral: Treatment of periodontitis (refractory): 100-200 mg once daily for 21 days (Jolkovsky, 2006). **Note:** A specific formulation (Periostat® [available in Canada]) containing a subantimicrobial dosage is also available for use as an adjunct to scaling and root planing. In addition, doxycycline gel (Atridox™) is available for subgingival application (see Doxycycline Hyclate Periodontal Extended-Release Liquid monograph).

Dosage

Usual dosage range:

Children >8 years (≤45 kg): Oral, I.V.: 2-5 mg/kg/day in 1-2 divided doses, not to exceed 200 mg/day

Children >8 years (>45 kg) and Adults: Oral, I.V.: 100-200 mg/day in 1-2 divided doses

Indication-specific dosing:

Children:

Anthrax: Doxycycline should be used in children if antibiotic susceptibility testing, exhaustion of drug supplies, or allergic reaction preclude use of penicillin or ciprofloxacin. For treatment, the consensus recommendation does not include a loading dose for doxycycline.

Inhalational (postexposure prophylaxis) (ACIP, 2010): Oral, I.V. (use oral route when possible):

≤8 years: 2.2 mg/kg every 12 hours for 60 days

>8 years and ≤45 kg: 2.2 mg/kg every 12 hours for 60 days

>8 years and >45 kg: 100 mg every 12 hours for 60 days

Cutaneous (treatment): Oral: See dosing for "Inhalational (postexposure prophylaxis)"

Note: In the presence of systemic involvement, extensive edema, and/or lesions on head/neck, doxycycline should initially be administered I.V.

Inhalational/gastrointestinal/oropharyngeal (treatment): I.V.: Refer to dosing for inhalational anthrax (postexposure prophylaxis); switch to oral therapy when clinically appropriate

Note: Initial treatment should include two or more agents predicted to be effective (CDC, 2001). Agents suggested for use in conjunction with doxycycline or ciprofloxacin include rifampin, vancomycin, imipenem, penicillin, ampicillin, chloramphenicol, clindamycin, and clarithromycin. May switch to oral antimicrobial therapy when clinically appropriate. Continue combined therapy for 60 days

Community-acquired pneumonia (CAP) (IDSA/PIDS, 2011): Oral: Children >7 years: **Note:** A beta-lactam antibiotic should be added if typical bacterial pneumonia cannot be ruled out.

Presumed atypical, mild atypical (*M. pneumoniae, C. pneumoniae, C. trachomatis*) infection or step-down therapy (alternative to azithromycin): 2-4 mg/kg/day in 2 divided doses (maximum: 200 mg/day)

Cellulitis (purulent) due to community-acquired MRSA (unlabeled use): Oral: Children >8 years and ≤45 kg: 2 mg/kg/dose every 12 hours for 5-10 days (Liu, 2011)

Localized juvenile periodontitis (LJP) (unlabeled use): Oral: 50-100 mg/day

Q fever: Oral, I.V.: 2.2 mg/kg twice/day for 15-21 days (CDC, 2009). Some clinicians may recommend trimethoprim/sulfamethoxazole for children <8 years of age (Hartzell, 2008). **Note:** Use of tetracyclines should be avoided during tooth development (children ≤8 years of age) unless other drugs are unlikely to be effective or are contraindicated.

Tickborne rickettsial disease: Oral, I.V.: Children ≤8 years: 2.2 mg/kg (maximum dose: 100 mg) every 12 hours for 5-7 days; severe or complicated disease may require longer treatment; human granulocytotropic anaplasmosis (HGA) should be treated for 10-14 days. **Note:** The American Academy of Pediatrics Committee on Infectious Diseases identifies doxycycline as the drug of choice in children of any age.

Tularemia: I.V. (may transition to oral if clinically indicated) (Dennis, 2001):
Children <45 kg: 2.2 mg/kg every 12 hours for 14-21 days
Children ≥45 kg: 100 mg every 12 hours for 14-21 days
Children ≥8 years:
Lyme disease: Oral (Halperin, 2007; Wormser, 2006):
Prevention: 4 mg/kg (maximum: 200 mg) administered as a single dose; **Note:** Initiate within 72 hours of tick removal
Treatment (early lyme disease without neurologic manifestations): 1-2 mg/kg twice daily for 10-21 days (maximum: 100 mg/dose)
Treatment (meningitis and other early neurologic manifestations): 4-8 mg/kg/day in 2 divided doses for 10-28 days (maximum: 200 mg/dose)
Malaria chemoprophylaxis: Oral: 2.2 mg/kg/day (maximum: 100 mg/day). Start 1-2 days prior to travel to endemic area; continue daily during travel and for 4 weeks after leaving endemic area (CDC, 2012)
Malaria, severe, treatment (unlabeled use): Oral, I.V.:
<45 kg: 2.2 mg/kg (maximum dose: 100 mg) every 12 hours for 7 days with quinidine gluconate. **Note:** Quinidine gluconate duration is region specific; consult CDC for current recommendations (CDC, 2011).
≥45 kg: 100 mg every 12 hours for 7 days with quinidine gluconate. **Note:** Quinidine gluconate duration is region specific; consult CDC for current recommendations (CDC, 2011).
Malaria, uncomplicated, treatment (unlabeled use): Oral: 2.2 mg/kg (maximum dose: 100 mg) every 12 hours for 7 days with quinine sulfate. **Note:** Quinine sulfate duration is region specific; consult CDC for current recommendations (CDC, 2011).
Children >8 years (and >45 kg) and Adults:
Cellulitis (purulent) due to community-acquired MRSA (unlabeled use): Oral: 100 mg twice daily for 5-10 days (Liu, 2011)
Chlamydial infections, uncomplicated: Oral: 100 mg twice daily for 7 days
Tickborne rickettsial disease: Oral, I.V.: 100 mg twice daily for 5-7 days; severe or complicated disease may require longer treatment; human granulocytotropic anaplasmosis (HGA) should be treated for 10-14 days. **Note:** The American Academy of Pediatrics Committee on Infectious Diseases identifies doxycycline as the drug of choice in children of any age.
Adults:
Acute bacterial rhinosinusitis (unlabeled use): Oral: 200 mg/day in 1-2 divided doses for 5-7 days (Chow, 2012)
Anthrax:
Inhalational (postexposure prophylaxis): Oral, I.V. (use oral route when possible): 100 mg every 12 hours for 60 days (ACIP, 2010)
Cutaneous (treatment): Oral: 100 mg every 12 hours for 60 days. **Note:** In the presence of systemic involvement, extensive edema, lesions on head/neck, refer to I.V. dosing for treatment of inhalational/gastrointestinal/oropharyngeal anthrax
Inhalational/gastrointestinal/oropharyngeal (treatment): I.V.: Initial: 100 mg every 12 hours; switch to oral therapy when clinically appropriate; some recommend initial loading dose of 200 mg, followed by 100 mg every 8-12 hours (Franz, 1997). **Note:** Initial treatment should include two or more agents predicted to be effective (CDC, 2001). Agents suggested for use in conjunction with doxycycline or ciprofloxacin include rifampin, vancomycin, imipenem, penicillin, ampicillin, chloramphenicol, clindamycin, and clarithromycin. May switch to oral antimicrobial therapy when clinically appropriate. Continue combined therapy for 60 days
Brucellosis: Oral: 100 mg twice daily for 6 weeks with rifampin or streptomycin
Community-acquired pneumonia, bronchitis: Oral, I.V.: 100 mg twice daily (Ailani, 1999; Mandell, 2007)
Epididymitis: Oral: 100 mg twice daily for 10 days (in combination with ceftriaxone) (CDC, 2010)
Gonococcal infection, uncomplicated: Oral: **Note:** Azithromycin is preferred over doxycycline as the second antimicrobial in combination with ceftriaxone in uncomplicated infections due to a high prevalence of tetracycline resistance in isolates (CDC, 2012).
Cervix, rectum, urethra: 100 mg twice daily for 7 days in combination with ceftriaxone (preferred) or cefixime (only if ceftriaxone is not available and test-of-cure follow up in 7 days) (CDC, 2012).
Pharynx: 100 mg twice daily for 7 days in combination with ceftriaxone (CDC, 2012).
Alternatively, the manufacturer recommends a single-visit dose in nonanorectal infections in men: 300 mg initially, repeat dose in 1 hour (total dose: 600 mg)
Granuloma inguinale (donovanosis): Oral: 100 mg twice daily for at least 3 weeks (and until lesions have healed) (CDC, 2010)
Lyme disease: Oral (Halperin, 2007; Wormser, 2006):
Prevention: Initiate within 72 hours of tick removal: 200 mg administered as a single dose
Treatment (early lyme disease with neurologic manifestations): 100 mg twice daily for 10-21 days
Treatment (meningitis or other early neurologic manifestations): 100-200 mg twice daily for 14 days (range: 10-28 days)
Lymphogranuloma venereum: Oral: 100 mg twice daily for 21 days (CDC, 2010)
Malaria chemoprophylaxis: Oral: 100 mg/day. Start 1-2 days prior to travel to endemic area; continue daily during travel and for 4 weeks after leaving endemic area
Malaria, severe, treatment (unlabeled use): Oral, I.V.: 100 mg every 12 hours for 7 days with quinidine gluconate. **Note:** Quinidine gluconate duration is region specific; consult CDC for current recommendations (CDC, 2011).
Malaria, uncomplicated, treatment (unlabeled use): Oral: 100 mg twice daily for 7 days with quinine sulfate. **Note:** Quinine sulfate duration is region specific; consult CDC for current recommendations (CDC, 2011).
Nongonococcal urethritis: Oral: 100 mg twice daily for 7 days (CDC, 2010)
Pelvic inflammatory disease:
Treatment, inpatient: Oral, I.V.: 100 mg twice daily (in combination with cefoxitin or cefotetan); may transition to oral doxycycline (add clindamycin or metronidazole if tubo-ovarian abscess present) to complete 14 days of treatment (CDC, 2010)

Treatment, outpatient: Oral: 100 mg twice daily for 14 days (with or without metronidazole); preceded by a single I.M. dose of cefoxitin (plus oral probenecid) or ceftriaxone (CDC, 2010)

Periodontitis: Oral (Periostat®): 20 mg twice daily as an adjunct following scaling and root planing

Periodontitis, refractory (unlabeled use): Oral: 100-200 mg daily (Jolkovsky, 2006)

Proctitis: Oral: 100 mg twice daily for 7 days (in combination with ceftriaxone) (CDC, 2010)

Prosthetic joint infection (unlabeled use): Oral: Chronic oral antimicrobial suppression:

Propionibacterium spp (alternative to penicillin or amoxicillin): 100 mg twice daily (Osmon, 2013)

Staphylococci (oxacillin-resistant): 100 mg twice daily (Osmon, 2013)

Staphylococci (oxacillin-sensitive or –resistant) oral phase treatment (after completion of pathogen-specific I.V) following 1-stage exchange:

Total ankle, elbow, hip, or shoulder arthroplasty: 100 mg twice daily for 3 months; **Note:** Must be used in combination with rifampin (Osmon, 2013).

Total knee arthroplasty: 100 mg twice daily for 6 months; **Note:** Must be used in combination with rifampin (Osmon, 2013)

Q fever: Oral: 100 mg every 12 hours for 15-21 days (CDC, 2009)

Rosacea (Oracea®): Oral: 40 mg once daily in the morning

Sclerosing agent for pleural effusion (unlabeled use): Intrapleural: 500 mg as a single dose in 100 mL NS (Porcel, 2006); may require a repeat dose (Kvale, 2007)

Syphilis:

Primary/secondary syphilis: Oral: 100 mg twice daily for 14 days (CDC, 2010)

Latent syphilis: Oral: 100 mg twice daily for 28 days (CDC, 2010)

Tularemia: I.V. (may transition to oral if clinically appropriate): Initial: 100 mg every 12 hours for 14-21 days (Dennis, 2001)

Vibrio cholerae: Oral: 300 mg as a single dose (WHO, 2004)

***Yersinia pestis* (plague):** Oral, I.V.: 200 mg initially then 100 mg twice daily **or** 200 mg once daily for 10 days (Daya, 2005; Inglesby, 2000)

Dosage adjustment in renal impairment: No dosage adjustment necessary in renal impairment.

Poorly dialyzed; no supplemental dose or dosage adjustment necessary, including patients on intermittent hemodialysis, peritoneal dialysis, or continuous renal replacement therapy (eg, CVVHD).

Dosage adjustment in hepatic impairment: No dosage adjustment provided in manufacturer's labeling.

Mechanism of Action Inhibits protein synthesis by binding with the 30S and possibly the 50S ribosomal subunit(s) of susceptible bacteria; may also cause alterations in the cytoplasmic membrane

Periostat® capsules (proposed mechanism): Has been shown to inhibit collagenase activity *in vitro*. Also has been noted to reduce elevated collagenase activity in the gingival crevicular fluid of patients with periodontal disease. Systemic levels do not reach inhibitory concentrations against bacteria.

Contraindications Hypersensitivity to doxycycline, tetracycline or any component of the formulation

Warnings/Precautions Photosensitivity reaction may occur with this drug; avoid prolonged exposure to sunlight or tanning equipment. Antianabolic effects of tetracyclines can increase BUN (dose-related). Autoimmune syndromes have been reported. Hepatotoxicity rarely occurs; if symptomatic, conduct LFT and discontinue drug. Pseudotumor cerebri has been (rarely) reported with tetracycline use; usually resolves with discontinuation. Prolonged use may result in fungal or bacterial superinfection, including *C. difficile*-associated diarrhea (CDAD) and pseudomembranous colitis; CDAD has been observed >2 months postantibiotic treatment. May cause tissue hyperpigmentation, enamel hypoplasia, or permanent tooth discoloration; use of tetracyclines should be avoided during tooth development (children <8 years of age) unless other drugs are not likely to be effective or are contraindicated. However, recommended in treatment of anthrax exposure and tickborne rickettsial diseases. Do not use during pregnancy. In addition to affecting tooth development, tetracycline use has been associated with retardation of skeletal development and reduced bone growth.

Additional specific warnings: Oracea®: Should not be used for the treatment or prophylaxis of bacterial infections, since the lower dose of drug per capsule may be subefficacious and promote resistance. Syrup contains sodium metabisulfite. Effectiveness of products intended for use in periodontitis has not been established in patients with coexistent oral candidiasis; use with caution in patients with a history or predisposition to oral candidiasis.

Drug Interactions

Metabolism/Transport Effects Inhibits CYP3A4 (weak)

Avoid Concomitant Use

Avoid concomitant use of Doxycycline with any of the following: BCG; Pimozide; Retinoic Acid Derivatives; Strontium Ranelate

Increased Effect/Toxicity

Doxycycline may increase the levels/effects of: ARIPiprazole; Lomitapide; Mipomersen; Neuromuscular-Blocking Agents; Pimozide; Porfimer; Retinoic Acid Derivatives; Vitamin K Antagonists

Decreased Effect

Doxycycline may decrease the levels/effects of: BCG; Penicillins; Sodium Picosulfate; Typhoid Vaccine

The levels/effects of Doxycycline may be decreased by: Antacids; Barbiturates; Bile Acid Sequestrants; Bismuth; Bismuth Subsalicylate; Calcium Salts; CarBAMazepine; Fosphenytoin; Iron Salts; Lanthanum; Magnesium Salts; Multivitamins/Minerals (with ADEK, Folate, Iron); Phenytoin; Quinapril; Strontium Ranelate; Sucralfate

Ethanol/Nutrition/Herb Interactions

Ethanol: Chronic ethanol ingestion may reduce the serum concentration of doxycycline.

Food: Doxycycline serum levels may be slightly decreased if taken with food or milk. Administration with iron or calcium may decrease doxycycline absorption. May decrease absorption of calcium, iron, magnesium, zinc, and amino acids.

Herb/Nutraceutical: St John's wort may decrease doxycycline levels. Avoid dong quai, St John's wort (may also cause photosensitization).

◄ **Dietary Considerations**
Tetracyclines (in general): Take with food if gastric irritation occurs. While administration with food may decrease GI absorption of doxycycline by up to 20%, administration on an empty stomach is not recommended due to GI intolerance. Of currently available tetracyclines, doxycycline has the least affinity for calcium.
Oracea®: Take on an empty stomach 1 hour before or 2 hours after meals.
Some products may contain sodium.

Pharmacodynamics/Kinetics
Half-life Elimination 12-15 hours (usually increases to 22-24 hours with multiple doses); End-stage renal disease: 18-25 hours; Oracea®: 21 hours
Time to Peak Serum: 1.5-4 hours
Pregnancy Risk Factor D
Pregnancy Considerations Tetracyclines cross the placenta and accumulate in developing teeth and long tubular bones. Therapeutic doses of doxycycline during pregnancy are unlikely to produce substantial teratogenic risk, but data are insufficient to say that there is no risk. In general, reports of exposure have been limited to short durations of therapy in the first trimester. Tetracyclines may discolor fetal teeth following maternal use during pregnancy; the specific teeth involved and the portion of the tooth affected depends on the timing and duration of exposure relative to tooth calcification. As a class, tetracyclines are generally considered second-line antibiotics in pregnant women and their use should be avoided. Tetracycline medications should be used during pregnancy only when other medications are contraindicated or ineffective (Mylonas, 2011).
Lactation Enters breast milk/not recommended
Breast-Feeding Considerations Doxycycline is excreted in breast milk (Chung, 2002). According to the manufacturer, the decision to continue or discontinue breast-feeding during therapy should take into account the risk of exposure to the infant and the benefits of treatment to the mother. Although nursing is not specifically contraindicated, the effects of long-term exposure via breast milk are not known. Oral absorption of doxycycline is not markedly influenced by simultaneous ingestion of milk; therefore, oral absorption of doxycycline by the breast-feeding infant would not be expected to be diminished by the calcium in the maternal milk. Nondose-related effects could include modification of bowel flora.

Dosage Forms
Capsule, oral: 50 mg, 75 mg, 100 mg, 150 mg
Adoxa®: 150 mg
Monodox®: 75 mg, 100 mg
Ocudox™: 50 mg
Oracea®: 40 mg [30 mg (immediate release) and 10 mg (delayed release)]
Oraxyl™: 20 mg
Vibramycin®: 100 mg
Injection, powder for reconstitution: 100 mg
Doxy 100™: 100 mg
Powder for suspension, oral:
Vibramycin®: 25 mg/5 mL (60 mL)
Syrup, oral:
Vibramycin®: 50 mg/5 mL (473 mL)
Tablet, oral: 20 mg, 50 mg, 75 mg, 100 mg, 150 mg
Alodox™: 20 mg
Periostat®: 20 mg
Tablet, delayed release coated beads, oral: 75 mg, 100 mg, 150 mg
Tablet, delayed release coated pellets, oral:
Doryx®: 150 mg

References
Jolkovsky DL and Ciancio S, "Chemotherapeutic Agents," Newman MG, Takei HH, Klokkevold PR, et al, eds, *Clinical Periodontology*, 10th ed, St Louis, MO: Saunders/Elsevier, 2006, 802-3.

Doxycycline Hyclate Periodontal Extended-Release Liquid
(doks i SYE kleen HI klayt per ee oh DON tal ik STEN did ri LES LIK wid)

Related Information
Doxycycline *on page 456*
Periodontal Diseases *on page 1570*
Brand Names: U.S. Atridox®
Brand Names: Canada Atridox®
Generic Availability (U.S.) No
Pharmacologic Category Antibiotic, Tetracycline Derivative
Dental Use Treatment of chronic adult periodontitis for gain in clinical attachment, reduction in probing depth, and reduction in bleeding upon probing
Use Used exclusively in dental applications
Local Anesthetic/Vasoconstrictor Precautions No information available to require special precautions
Effects on Dental Treatment Key adverse event(s) related to dental treatment: Discoloration of teeth (in children), gum discomfort, toothache, periodontal abscess, tooth sensitivity, broken tooth, tooth mobility, endodontic abscess, and jaw pain

Mechanical oral hygiene procedures (ie, tooth brushing, flossing) should be avoided in any treated area for 7 days.
Effects reported in clinical trials were similar in incidence between doxycycline-containing product and vehicle alone; comparable to standard therapies including scaling and root planing or oral hygiene. Although there is no known relationship between doxycycline and hypertension, unspecified essential hypertension was noted in 1.6% of the doxycycline gel group, as compared to 0.2% in the vehicle group (allergic reactions to the vehicle were also reported in two patients).
Effects on Bleeding No information available to require special precautions
Adverse Effects
>10%: Discoloration of teeth in children
Doxycycline periodontal gel (Atridox®): The adverse effects reported in clinical trials were similar in incidence between doxycycline-containing product and vehicle alone. In addition, these effects were comparable to standard therapies including scaling and root planing or oral hygiene. Events associated with application reported with an incidence >1% included: gum discomfort (18%), toothache (14%), periodontal abscess (10%), tooth sensitivity (8%), broken tooth (5%), tooth mobility (2%), endodontic abscess (2%) and jaw pain (1%). Systemic adverse events included headache (27%), muscle aches (7%), diarrhea (3%), upset stomach (4%), and nausea (2%). Although there is no known relationship between doxycycline and hypertension, unspecified essential hypertension was noted in 1.6% of the doxycycline gel group, as compared to 0.2% in the vehicle group. Allergic reactions to the vehicle were also reported in two patients.
Dental Usual Dosage Oral, subgingival: Dose depends on size, shape and number of pockets treated. Application may be repeated four months after initial treatment. The delivery system consists of 2 separate syringes in a single pouch. Syringe A contains 450 mg of a bioabsorbable polymer gel; syringe B contains doxycycline

hyclate 50 mg. To prepare for instillation, couple syringe A to syringe B. Inject contents of syringe A (purple stripe) into syringe B, then push contents back into syringe A. Repeat this mixing cycle at a rate of one cycle per second for 100 cycles. If syringes are stored prior to use (a maximum of 3 days), repeat mixing cycle 10 times before use. After appropriate mixing, contents should be in syringe A. Holding syringes vertically, with syringe A at the bottom, pull back on the syringe A plunger, allowing contents to flow down barrel for several seconds. Uncouple syringes and attach enclosed blunt cannula to syringe A. Local anesthesia is not required for placement. Cannula tip may be bent to resemble periodontal probe and used to explore pocket. Express product from syringe until pocket is filled. To separate tip from formulation, turn tip towards the tooth and press against tooth surface to achieve separation. An appropriate dental instrument may be used to pack gel into the pocket. Pockets may be covered with either Coe-pak™ or Octyldent™ dental adhesive.

Dosage Adults: Subgingival application: Dose depends on size, shape and number of pockets treated. Contains 50 mg doxycycline hyclate per 500 mg of formulation in each final blended syringe product. Application may be repeated four months after initial treatment.

Atridox® subgingival controlled-release product: The delivery system consists of 2 separate syringes in a single pouch. Syringe A contains 450 mg of a bioabsorbable polymer gel; syringe B contains doxycycline hyclate 50 mg. To prepare for instillation, couple syringe A to syringe B. Inject contents of syringe A (purple stripe) into syringe B, then push contents back into syringe A. Repeat this mixing cycle at a rate of one cycle per second for 100 cycles. If syringes are stored prior to use (a maximum of 3 days), repeat mixing cycle 10 times before use. After appropriate mixing, contents should be in syringe A. Holding syringes vertically, with syringe A at the bottom, pull back on the syringe A plunger, allowing contents to flow down barrel for several seconds. Uncouple syringes and attach enclosed blunt cannula to syringe A. Local anesthesia is not required for placement. Cannula tip may be bent to resemble periodontal probe and used to explore pocket. Express product from syringe until pocket is filled. To separate tip from formulation, turn tip towards the tooth and press against tooth surface to achieve separation. An appropriate dental instrument may be used to pack gel into the pocket. Pockets may be covered with either Coe-Pak™ or Octyldent™ dental adhesive.

Mechanism of Action Inhibits protein synthesis by binding with the 30S and possibly the 50S ribosomal subunit(s) of susceptible bacteria; may also cause alterations in the cytoplasmic membrane

Doxycycline inhibits collagenase *in vitro* and has been shown to inhibit collagenase in the gingival crevicular fluid in adults with periodontitis

Contraindications Hypersensitivity to doxycycline, tetracycline or any component of the formulation; children <8 years of age

Warnings/Precautions Photosensitivity reaction may occur with this drug; avoid prolonged exposure to sunlight or tanning equipment. Prolonged use may result in fungal or bacterial superinfection, including *C. difficile*-associated diarrhea (CDAD) and pseudomembranous colitis; CDAD has been observed >2 months postantibiotic treatment. May cause tissue hyperpigmentation, enamel hypoplasia, or permanent tooth discoloration; use of tetracyclines should be avoided during tooth development (children <8 years of age) unless other

drugs are not likely to be effective or are contraindicated.

Additional specific warnings for doxycycline gel (Atridox®) for subgingival application: This product has not been evaluated or tested in immunocompromised patients, in patients with oral candidiasis, or in conditions characterized by severe periodontal defects with little remaining periodontium. May result in overgrowth of nonsusceptible organisms, including fungi. Effects of treatment >6 months have not been evaluated. Has not been evaluated for use in regeneration of alveolar bone

Drug Interactions

Metabolism/Transport Effects None known.

Avoid Concomitant Use There are no known interactions where it is recommended to avoid concomitant use.

Increased Effect/Toxicity There are no known significant interactions involving an increase in effect.

Decreased Effect There are no known significant interactions involving a decrease in effect.

Dietary Considerations May be taken with food, milk, or water.

Pregnancy Risk Factor D

Pregnancy Considerations Exposure to tetracyclines during the second or third trimester may cause permanent discoloration of the teeth. Most reports do not show an increase risk for teratogenicity with the exception of a potential small increased risk for cleft palate or esophageal atresia/stenosis. Serum concentrations following subgingival use are significantly less than with oral tablets.

Lactation Excretion in breast milk unknown/not recommended

Breast-Feeding Considerations Tetracyclines, including oral doxycycline, are excreted in breast milk and therefore, breast-feeding is not recommended by the manufacturer.

Doxycycline is less bound to the calcium in maternal milk which may lead to increased absorption compared to other tetracyclines. Only minimal amounts of oral doxycycline are excreted in human milk and the relative amount of tooth staining has been reported to be lower when compared to other tetracycline analogs. Nondose-related effects could include modification of bowel flora. Serum concentrations following subgingival use are significantly less than with oral tablets.

Dosage Forms

Liquid, subgingival:
Atridox®: 10% (6 units)

Doxylamine (dox IL a meen)

Brand Names: U.S. Aldex® AN
Brand Names: Canada Unisom®-2
Pharmacologic Category Ethanolamine Derivative; Histamine H_1 Antagonist; Histamine H_1 Antagonist, First Generation
Use Treatment of short-term insomnia
Unlabeled Use Nausea and vomiting of pregnancy (NVP)
Local Anesthetic/Vasoconstrictor Precautions No information available to require special precautions
Effects on Dental Treatment Key adverse event(s) related to dental treatment: Dry mucous membranes and significant xerostomia (normal salivary flow resumes upon discontinuation)
Effects on Bleeding No information available to require special precautions

▶

◀ **Adverse Effects** Frequency not defined.
Cardiovascular: Palpitation, tachycardia
Central nervous system: Dizziness, disorientation, drowsiness, headache, paradoxical CNS stimulation, vertigo
Gastrointestinal: Anorexia, dry mucous membranes, diarrhea, constipation, epigastric pain, xerostomia
Genitourinary: Dysuria, urinary retention
Ocular: Blurred vision, diplopia

General Dosage Range Oral: *Adults:* 1 tablet 30 minutes before bedtime

Mechanism of Action Doxylamine competes with histamine for H_1-receptor sites on effector cells; blocks chemoreceptor trigger zone, diminishes vestibular stimulation, and depresses labyrinthine function through its central anticholinergic activity.

Pharmacodynamics/Kinetics
Half-life Elimination 10-12 hours (Paton, 1985; Friedman, 1985); may be increased in the elderly (Friedman, 1989)
Time to Peak 2-4 hours (Paton, 1985; Friedman, 1985; Friedman, 1989)

Pregnancy Considerations Maternal use of doxylamine in combination with pyridoxine during pregnancy has not been shown to increase the baseline risk of major malformations. Doxylamine is recommended for the treatment of nausea and vomiting of pregnancy.

Dronabinol (droe NAB i nol)

Brand Names: U.S. Marinol®
Brand Names: Canada Marinol®
Pharmacologic Category Antiemetic; Appetite Stimulant
Use Chemotherapy-associated nausea and vomiting refractory to other antiemetic(s); AIDS-related anorexia
Unlabeled Use Cancer-related anorexia
Local Anesthetic/Vasoconstrictor Precautions No information available to require special precautions
Effects on Dental Treatment Key adverse event(s) related to dental treatment: Xerostomia (normal salivary flow resumes upon discontinuation) and orthostatic hypotension
Effects on Bleeding No information available to require special precautions
Adverse Effects Frequency not always specified.
>1%:
Cardiovascular: Palpitations, tachycardia, vasodilation/facial flushing
Central nervous system: Euphoria (8% to 24%, dose related), abnormal thinking (3% to 10%), dizziness (3% to 10%), paranoia (3% to 10%), somnolence (3% to 10%), amnesia, anxiety, ataxia, confusion, depersonalization, hallucination
Gastrointestinal: Abdominal pain (3% to 10%), nausea (3% to 10%), vomiting (3% to 10%)
Neuromuscular & skeletal: Weakness

General Dosage Range Oral:
Children: Initial: 5 mg/m² as a single dose; Maintenance: 5 mg/m²/dose every 2-4 hours for a total of 4-6 doses/day (maximum: 15 mg/m²/dose)
Adults: Initial: 5 mg/m² as a single dose; Maintenance: 5 mg/m²/dose every 2-4 hours for a total of 4-6 doses/day (maximum: 15 mg/m²/dose) **or** Initial: 2.5 mg twice daily; Maintenance: Titrate up to 20 mg/day in 2 divided doses

Mechanism of Action Unknown, may inhibit endorphins in the brain's emetic center, suppress prostaglandin synthesis, and/or inhibit medullary activity through an unspecified cortical action. Some pharmacologic effects appear to involve sympathimometic activity; tachyphylaxis to some effect (eg, tachycardia) may occur, but appetite-stimulating effects do not appear to wane over time. Antiemetic activity may be due to effect on cannabinoid receptors (CB1) within the central nervous system.

Pharmacodynamics/Kinetics
Onset of Action Within 1 hour; Peak effect: 2-4 hours
Duration of Action 24 hours (appetite stimulation)
Half-life Elimination Dronabinol: 25-36 hours (terminal); Dronabinol metabolites: 44-59 hours
Time to Peak Serum: 0.5-4 hours

Pregnancy Risk Factor C
Pregnancy Considerations Adverse events have been observed in animal reproduction studies.
Controlled Substance C-III

Dronedarone (droe NE da rone)

Related Information
Clinical Risk Related to Drugs Prolonging QT Interval *on page 1510*
Brand Names: U.S. Multaq®
Brand Names: Canada Multaq®
Pharmacologic Category Antiarrhythmic Agent, Class III
Use To reduce the risk of hospitalization for atrial fibrillation (AF) in patients in sinus rhythm with a history of paroxysmal or persistent AF
Unlabeled Use Alternative antiarrhythmic for the treatment of atrial fibrillation in patients with hypertrophic cardiomyopathy (HCM)
Local Anesthetic/Vasoconstrictor Precautions Dronedarone is one of the drugs confirmed to prolong the QT interval and is accepted as having a risk of causing torsade de pointes. The risk of drug-induced torsade de pointes is extremely low when a single QT interval prolonging drug is prescribed. In terms of epinephrine, it is not known what effect vasoconstrictors in the local anesthetic regimen will have in patients with a known history of congenital prolonged QT interval or in patients taking any medication that prolongs the QT interval. Until more information is obtained, it is suggested that the clinician consult with the physician prior to the use of a vasoconstrictor in suspected patients, and that the vasoconstrictor (epinephrine, mepivacaine and levonordefrin [Carbocaine® 2% with Neo-Cobefrin®]) be used with caution.
Effects on Dental Treatment No significant effects or complications reported (see Dental Comment)
Effects on Bleeding No information available to require special precautions
Adverse Effects
>10%:
Cardiovascular: QT_c (Bazett) prolongation (28% [placebo: 19%]; defined as >450 msec in males or >470 msec in females)
Renal: Serum creatinine increased ≥10% (51%; occurred 5 days after initiation)
1% to 10%:
Cardiovascular: Bradycardia (3%)
Dermatologic: Allergic dermatitis (≤5%), dermatitis (≤5%), eczema (≤5%), pruritus (≤5%), rash (≤5%; described as generalized, macular, maculopapular, erythematous)

Gastrointestinal: Diarrhea (9%), nausea (5%), abdominal pain (4%), dyspepsia (2%), vomiting (2%)

Neuromuscular & skeletal: Weakness (7%)

General Dosage Range Oral: *Adults:* 400 mg twice daily

Mechanism of Action A noniodinated antiarrhythmic agent structurally related to amiodarone exhibiting properties of all 4 antiarrhythmic classes. Dronedarone inhibits sodium (I_{Na}) and potassium (I_{Kr}, I_{KS}, I_{K1}, and I_{K-ACh}) channels resulting in prolongation of the action potential and refractory period in myocardial tissue without reverse-use dependent effects; decreases AV conduction and sinus node function through inhibition of calcium (I_{Ca-L}) channels and beta$_1$-receptor blocking activity. Similar to amiodarone, dronedarone also inhibits alpha$_1$-receptor mediated increases in blood pressure.

Pharmacodynamics/Kinetics

Half-life Elimination 13-19 hours

Time to Peak Plasma: 3-6 hours

Pregnancy Risk Factor X

Pregnancy Considerations Teratogenic effects were observed in animal studies. May cause fetal harm when administered to a pregnant woman, use is contraindicated.

Dental Comment Dronedarone is known to prolong the QT interval. The QT interval is measured as the time and distance between the Q point of the QRS complex and the end of the T wave in the ECG tracing. After adjustment for heart rate, the QT interval is defined as prolonged if it is more than 450 msec in men and 460 msec in women. A long QT syndrome was first described in the 1950s and 60s as a congenital syndrome involving QT interval prolongation and syncope and sudden death. Some of the congenital long QT syndromes were characterized by a peculiar electrocardiographic appearance of the QRS complex involving a premature atria beat followed by a pause, then a subsequent sinus beat showing marked QT prolongation and deformity. This type of cardiac arrhythmia was originally termed "torsade de pointes" (translated from the French as "twisting of the points"). Dronedarone is considered as having a risk of causing torsade de pointes. Since it is not known what effect vasoconstrictors in the local anesthetic regimen will have in patients with a known history of congenital prolonged QT interval or in patients taking any medication that prolongs the QT interval, a medical consult is suggested.

Droperidol (droe PER i dole)

Related Information

Clinical Risk Related to Drugs Prolonging QT Interval *on page 1510*

Brand Names: Canada Droperidol Injection, USP

Pharmacologic Category Antiemetic; Antipsychotic Agent, Typical

Use Prevention and/or treatment of nausea and vomiting from surgical and diagnostic procedures

Local Anesthetic/Vasoconstrictor Precautions Manufacturer's information states that droperidol may block vasopressor activity of epinephrine. This has not been observed during use of epinephrine as a vasoconstrictor in local anesthesia. Droperidol is one of the drugs confirmed to prolong the QT interval and is accepted as having a risk of causing torsade de pointes. The risk of drug-induced torsade de pointes is extremely low when a single QT interval prolonging drug is prescribed. In terms of epinephrine, it is not known what

effect vasoconstrictors in the local anesthetic regimen will have in patients with a known history of congenital prolonged QT interval or in patients taking any medication that prolongs the QT interval. Until more information is obtained, it is suggested that the clinician consult with the physician prior to the use of a vasoconstrictor in suspected patients, and that the vasoconstrictor (epinephrine, mepivacaine and levonordefrin [Carbocaine® 2% with Neo-Cobefrin®]) be used with caution.

Effects on Dental Treatment Key adverse event(s) related to dental treatment: Orthostatic hypotension

Effects on Bleeding No information available to require special precautions

Adverse Effects Frequency not defined.

Cardiovascular: Cardiac arrest, hypertension, hypotension (especially orthostatic), QT_c prolongation (dose dependent), tachycardia, torsade de pointes, ventricular tachycardia

Central nervous system: Anxiety, chills, depression (postoperative, transient), dizziness, drowsiness (postoperative) increased, dysphoria, extrapyramidal symptoms (akathisia, dystonia, oculogyric crisis), hallucinations (postoperative), hyperactivity, neuroleptic malignant syndrome (NMS) (rare), restlessness

Respiratory: Bronchospasm, laryngospasm

Miscellaneous: Anaphylaxis, shivering

General Dosage Range I.M., I.V.:

Children 2-12 years: Maximum: 0.1 mg/kg; additional doses may be repeated

Adults: Maximum initial dose: 2.5 mg; additional doses of 1.25 mg may be administered

Mechanism of Action Droperidol is a butyrophenone antipsychotic; antiemetic effect is a result of blockade of dopamine stimulation of the chemoreceptor trigger zone. Other effects include alpha-adrenergic blockade, peripheral vascular dilation, and reduction of the pressor effect of epinephrine resulting in hypotension and decreased peripheral vascular resistance; may also reduce pulmonary artery pressure

Pharmacodynamics/Kinetics

Onset of Action 3-10 minutes; Peak effect: Within 30 minutes

Duration of Action 2-4 hours, may extend to 12 hours

Half-life Elimination ~2.3 hours

Pregnancy Risk Factor C

Pregnancy Considerations While teratogenicity has not been demonstrated in animal studies, a slight increase in fetal mortality rate has been observed in some animal studies. Droperidol crosses the placenta. Use during pregnancy only if the potential benefits outweigh potential risks to the fetus.

Dental Comment Droperidol is known to prolong the QT interval. The QT interval is measured as the time and distance between the Q point of the QRS complex and the end of the T wave in the ECG tracing. After adjustment for heart rate, the QT interval is defined as prolonged if it is more than 450 msec in men and 460 msec in women. A long QT syndrome was first described in the 1950s and 60s as a congenital syndrome involving QT interval prolongation and syncope and sudden death. Some of the congenital long QT syndromes were characterized by a peculiar electrocardiographic appearance of the QRS complex involving a premature atria beat followed by a pause, then a subsequent sinus beat showing marked QT prolongation and deformity. This type of cardiac arrhythmia was originally termed "torsade de pointes" (translated from the French as "twisting of the points"). Droperidol is considered as having a risk of causing torsade de pointes. Since it is not known what effect

◀ vasoconstrictors in the local anesthetic regimen will have in patients with a known history of congenital prolonged QT interval or in patients taking any medication that prolongs the QT interval, a medical consult is suggested.

Drospirenone and Estradiol
(droh SPYE re none & es tra DYE ole)

Brand Names: U.S. Angeliq®
Brand Names: Canada Angeliq®
Pharmacologic Category Estrogen and Progestin Combination
Use Treatment of moderate-to-severe vasomotor symptoms associated with menopause; treatment of vulvar and vaginal atrophy associated with menopause
Local Anesthetic/Vasoconstrictor Precautions No information available to require special precautions
Effects on Bleeding No information available to require special precautions related to hemostasis in dental procedures.
Adverse Effects
>10%:
  Endocrine & metabolic: Breast pain (6% to 18%)
  Genitourinary: Genital tract bleeding (3% to 14%)
1% to 10%:
  Central nervous system: Emotional lability (1%), migraine (≤1%)
  Gastrointestinal: Abdominal/GI pain (4% to 7%)
  Genitourinary: Cervical polyp (≤1%)
General Dosage Range Oral: *Adults (females):* 1 tablet daily
Mechanism of Action
  Drospirenone is a synthetic progestin and spironolactone analog with antimineralocorticoid and antiandrogenic activity. Counteracts estrogen effects causing endometrial thinning.
  Estrogens are responsible for the development and maintenance of the female reproductive system and secondary sexual characteristics. Estradiol is the principal intracellular human estrogen and is more potent than estrone and estriol at the receptor level; it is the primary estrogen secreted prior to menopause. Following menopause, estrone and estrone sulfate are more highly produced. Estrogens modulate the pituitary secretion of gonadotropins, luteinizing hormone, and follicle-stimulating hormone through a negative feedback system; estrogen replacement reduces elevated levels of these hormones in postmenopausal women.
Pharmacodynamics/Kinetics
  Half-life Elimination Drospirenone: ~36-42 hours
  Time to Peak Plasma: Drospirenone: 1 hour; Estradiol: ~2 hours (range 0.3-10 hours)
Pregnancy Considerations Use is contraindicated during pregnancy

DULoxetine (doo LOX e teen)

Related Information
  Vasoconstrictor Interactions With Antidepressants *on page 1650*
Brand Names: U.S. Cymbalta®
Brand Names: Canada Cymbalta®
Pharmacologic Category Antidepressant, Serotonin/Norepinephrine Reuptake Inhibitor
Use Acute and maintenance treatment of major depressive disorder (MDD); treatment of generalized anxiety disorder (GAD); management of diabetic peripheral neuropathic pain (DPNP); management of fibromyalgia

(FM); chronic musculoskeletal pain (eg, chronic low back pain, osteoarthritis)
Unlabeled Use Treatment of stress incontinence
Local Anesthetic/Vasoconstrictor Precautions Although duloxetine is not a tricyclic antidepressant, it does block norepinephrine reuptake within the CNS synapses as part of its mechanism. It has been suggested that vasoconstrictors be administered with caution and to monitor vital signs in dental patients taking antidepressants that affect norepinephrine in this way.
Effects on Dental Treatment Key adverse event(s) related to dental treatment: Xerostomia and changes in salivation (normal salivary flow resumes upon discontinuation). See Effects on Bleeding.
Effects on Bleeding Platelet dysfunction (ie, impaired platelet aggregation) may occur during treatment with serotonin norepinephrine reuptake inhibitors (SNRIs) such as duloxetine due to platelet serotonin depletion, possibly increasing the risk of a bleeding complication. Concurrent NSAID use may increase this risk.
Adverse Effects
>10%:
  Central nervous system: Headache (13% to 14%), somnolence (10% to 12%; dose related), fatigue (10% to 11%)
  Gastrointestinal: Nausea (23% to 25%), xerostomia (11% to 15%; dose related)
1% to 10%:
  Cardiovascular: Palpitation (1% to 2%)
  Central nervous system: Dizziness (10%), insomnia (10%; dose related), agitation (3% to 5%), anxiety (3%), dreams abnormal (1% to 2%), yawning (1% to 2%), hypoesthesia (≥1%), lethargy (≥1%), vertigo (≥1%), chills (1%), sleep disorder (1%)
  Dermatologic: Hyperhydrosis (6% to 7%)
  Endocrine & metabolic: Libido decreased (2% to 4%), hot flushes (1% to 3%), orgasm abnormality (1% to 3%)
  Gastrointestinal: Constipation (10%; dose related), diarrhea (9% to 10%), appetite decreased (7% to 9%; dose related), abdominal pain (4% to 6%), vomiting (3% to 5%), dyspepsia (2%), weight loss (2%), flatulence (≥1%), taste abnormal (≥1%), weight gain (≥1%)
  Genitourinary: Erectile dysfunction (4% to 5%), ejaculation delayed (3%; dose related), ejaculatory dysfunction (2%)
  Hepatic: ALT >3x ULN (1%)
  Neuromuscular & skeletal: Muscle spasms (3%), tremor (2% to 3%; dose related), musculoskeletal pain (≥1%), paresthesia (≥1%), rigors (≥1%)
  Ocular: Blurred vision (1% to 3%)
  Respiratory: Nasopharyngitis (5%), cough (3%)
  Miscellaneous: Influenza (3%)
General Dosage Range Oral:
  Adults: 30-60 mg/day in 1-2 divided doses (maximum: 120 mg/day)
  Elderly: Initial: 20 mg 1-2 times/day
Mechanism of Action Duloxetine is a potent inhibitor of neuronal serotonin and norepinephrine reuptake and a weak inhibitor of dopamine reuptake. Duloxetine has no significant activity for muscarinic cholinergic, H_1-histaminergic, or alpha$_2$-adrenergic receptors. Duloxetine does not possess MAO-inhibitory activity.
Pharmacodynamics/Kinetics
  Half-life Elimination 12 hours (range: 8-17 hours)
  Time to Peak 6 hours; 10 hours when ingested with food
Pregnancy Risk Factor C

Pregnancy Considerations Adverse events were observed in animal reproduction studies. Nonteratogenic effects in the newborn following SSRI/SNRI exposure late in the third trimester include respiratory distress, cyanosis, apnea, seizures, temperature instability, feeding difficulty, vomiting, hypoglycemia, hyper- or hypotonia, hyper-reflexia, jitteriness, irritability, constant crying, and tremor. Symptoms may be due to the toxicity of the SNRIs/SSRIs or a discontinuation syndrome and may be consistent with serotonin syndrome associated with SSRI treatment. The long-term effects of *in utero* SNRI/SSRI exposure on infant development and behavior are not known.

The ACOG recommends that therapy with SSRIs or SNRIs during pregnancy be individualized; treatment of depression during pregnancy should incorporate the clinical expertise of the mental health clinician, obstetrician, primary healthcare provider, and pediatrician. According to the American Psychiatric Association (APA), the risks of medication treatment should be weighed against other treatment options and untreated depression. For women who discontinue antidepressant medications during pregnancy and who may be at high risk for postpartum depression, the medications can be restarted following delivery. Treatment algorithms have been developed by the ACOG and the APA for the management of depression in women prior to conception and during pregnancy.

Healthcare providers are encouraged to enroll women exposed to duloxetine during pregnancy in the Cymbalta® Pregnancy Registry (866-814-6975 or http://cymbaltapregnancyregistry.com).

Dutasteride (doo TAS teer ide)

Brand Names: U.S. Avodart®
Brand Names: Canada Avodart®
Pharmacologic Category 5 Alpha-Reductase Inhibitor
Use Treatment of symptomatic benign prostatic hyperplasia (BPH) as monotherapy or combination therapy with tamsulosin
Unlabeled Use Treatment of male pattern baldness
Local Anesthetic/Vasoconstrictor Precautions No information available to require special precautions
Effects on Dental Treatment No significant effects or complications reported
Effects on Bleeding No information available to require special precautions
Adverse Effects
1% to 10%: Endocrine & metabolic: Impotence (1% to 5%), libido decreased (≤3%), ejaculation disorders (≤1%), gynecomastia (including breast tenderness, breast enlargement; ≤1%)
Note: Frequency of adverse events (except gynecomastia) tends to decrease with continued use (>6 months).
General Dosage Range Oral: *Adults (males):* 0.5 mg once daily
Mechanism of Action Dutasteride is a 4-azo analog of testosterone and is a competitive, selective inhibitor of both reproductive tissues (type 2) and skin and hepatic (type 1) 5α-reductase. This results in inhibition of the conversion of testosterone to dihydrotestosterone and markedly suppresses serum dihydrotestosterone levels.
Pharmacodynamics/Kinetics
Half-life Elimination Terminal: ~5 weeks
Time to Peak 2-3 hours
Pregnancy Risk Factor X

Pregnancy Considerations Preclinical data (animal studies) suggests that the suppression of circulating levels of dihydrotestosterone may inhibit the development of the external genital organs and lead to feminization of a male fetus carried by a woman exposed to dutasteride. Pregnant woman and those who may become pregnant should not handle the capsules because dutasteride is absorbed through the skin. It is distributed into the semen.

Dutasteride and Tamsulosin
(doo TAS teer ide & tam SOO loe sin)

Related Information
Dutasteride *on page 465*
Tamsulosin *on page 1282*
Brand Names: U.S. Jalyn™
Pharmacologic Category 5 Alpha-Reductase Inhibitor; Alpha₁ Blocker
Use Treatment of symptomatic benign prostatic hyperplasia (BPH)
Local Anesthetic/Vasoconstrictor Precautions No information available to require special precautions
Effects on Dental Treatment Key adverse event(s) related to dental treatment: Tamsulosin: Orthostatic hypotension has been reported; monitor patient for dizziness while rising from dental chair.
Effects on Bleeding No information available to require special precautions
Adverse Effects Frequencies reported for when products used in combination. See individual monographs for additional adverse effects reported with each agent.
1% to 10%:
Central nervous system: Dizziness (2%)
Endocrine & metabolic: Libido decreased (5%), breast enlargement/tenderness (3%)
Genitourinary: Abnormal ejaculation (10%), impotence (8%)
General Dosage Range Oral: *Adults (males):* 1 capsule (0.5 mg dutasteride/0.4 mg tamsulosin) once daily
Mechanism of Action
Dutasteride is a 4-azo analog of testosterone and is a competitive, selective inhibitor of both reproductive tissues (type 2) and skin and hepatic (type 1) 5α-reductase. This results in inhibition of the conversion of testosterone to dihydrotestosterone and markedly suppresses serum dihydrotestosterone levels.

Tamsulosin is an antagonist of alpha₁ₐ-adrenoreceptors in the prostate. Smooth muscle tone in the prostate is mediated by alpha₁ₐ-adrenoreceptors; blocking them leads to relaxation of smooth muscle in the bladder neck and prostate, causing an improvement of urine flow and decreased symptoms of BPH. Approximately 75% of the alpha₁-receptors in the prostate are of the alpha₁ₐ-subtype.
Pregnancy Risk Factor X
Pregnancy Considerations Use contraindicated in pregnancy. Not indicated for use in women. See individual agents.

Dyclonine (DYE kloe neen)

Brand Names: U.S. Sucrets® Children's [OTC]; Sucrets® Maximum Strength [OTC]; Sucrets® Regular Strength [OTC]
Pharmacologic Category Local Anesthetic, Oral
Use Temporary relief of pain associated with oral mucosa ▶

Local Anesthetic/Vasoconstrictor Precautions No information available to require special precautions

Effects on Dental Treatment No significant effects or complications reported

Effects on Bleeding No information available to require special precautions

Adverse Effects
Local: Irritation, numbness, pain, stinging
Miscellaneous: Allergic reactions, cold/heat sensation

General Dosage Range Oral: Lozenge: *Children ≥2 years and Adults:* One lozenge every 2 hours as needed (maximum: 10 lozenges/day)

Dyphylline (DYE fi lin)

Brand Names: U.S. Lufyllin®

Pharmacologic Category Phosphodiesterase Enzyme Inhibitor, Nonselective

Use Bronchodilator in reversible airway obstruction due to asthma, chronic bronchitis, or emphysema

Local Anesthetic/Vasoconstrictor Precautions No information available to require special precautions

Effects on Dental Treatment Do not prescribe any erythromycin product to patients taking theophylline products. Erythromycin will delay the normal metabolic inactivation of theophyllines leading to increased blood levels; this has resulted in nausea, vomiting and CNS restlessness.

Effects on Bleeding No information available to require special precautions

Adverse Effects Frequency not defined. Reactions reported with other xanthine derivatives and may be dose related.
Cardiovascular: Circulatory failure, extrasystoles, flushing, hypotension, palpitation, tachycardia, ventricular arrhythmias
Central nervous system: Agitation, headache, hyperexcitability, insomnia, irritability, restlessness, seizure
Endocrine & metabolic: SIADH, hyperglycemia
Gastrointestinal: Diarrhea, epigastric pain, hematemesis, nausea, vomiting
Neuromuscular & skeletal: Muscle twitching
Renal: Albuminuria, diuresis, hematuria
Respiratory: Tachypnea

General Dosage Range Oral: *Adults:* Up to 15 mg/kg 4 times daily

Mechanism of Action Causes bronchodilatation, through phosphodiesterase inhibition which increases concentrations of cyclic adenine monophosphate (cAMP) and produces relaxation of bronchial smooth muscle.

Pharmacodynamics/Kinetics
Half-life Elimination ~2 hours (may be increased in renal impairment)
Time to Peak ~45 minutes
Pregnancy Risk Factor C
Pregnancy Considerations Animal reproduction studies have not been conducted.

Ecallantide (e KAL lan tide)

Brand Names: U.S. Kalbitor®

Pharmacologic Category Kallikrein Inhibitor

Use Treatment of acute attacks of hereditary angioedema (HAE)

Local Anesthetic/Vasoconstrictor Precautions No information available to require special precautions

Effects on Dental Treatment No significant effects or complications reported

Effects on Bleeding No information available to require special precautions

Adverse Effects
>10%:
Central nervous system: Headache (8% to 16%), fatigue (12%)
Gastrointestinal: Nausea (5% to 13%), diarrhea (4% to 11%)
1% to 10%:
Central nervous system: Fever (4% to 5%)
Dermatologic: Pruritus (5%), rash (3%), urticaria (2%)
Gastrointestinal: Vomiting (6%), upper abdominal pain (5%)
Local: Injection site reactions (3% to 7%; includes bruising, erythema, irritation, pain, pruritus, urticaria)
Respiratory: Upper respiratory infection (8%), nasopharyngitis (3% to 6%)
Miscellaneous: Antibody formation (5% to 7%), anaphylaxis (4%)

General Dosage Range SubQ: *Children ≥16 years and Adults:* 30 mg; may repeat once (maximum: 60 mg/24 hours)

Mechanism of Action Ecallantide is a recombinant protein which inhibits the conversion of high molecular weight kininogen to bradykinin by selectively and reversibly inhibiting plasma kallikrein. Unregulated bradykinin production is thought to contribute to the increased vascular permeability and angioedema observed in HAE.

Pharmacodynamics/Kinetics
Onset of Action 30 minutes to 4 hours
Half-life Elimination 1.5-2.5 hours
Time to Peak ~2-3 hours
Pregnancy Risk Factor C
Pregnancy Considerations Adverse effects were noted in animal studies. There are no adequate and well-controlled studies in pregnant women. Use during pregnancy only if the potential benefits justify the potential risk to the fetus.

Echothiophate Iodide
(ek oh THYE oh fate EYE oh dide)

Brand Names: U.S. Phospholine Iodide®

Pharmacologic Category Acetylcholinesterase Inhibitor; Ophthalmic Agent, Antiglaucoma; Ophthalmic Agent, Miotic

Use Used as miotic in treatment of chronic, open-angle glaucoma; may be useful in specific cases of angle-closure glaucoma (postiridectomy or where surgery refused/contraindicated); postcataract surgery-related glaucoma; accommodative esotropia

Local Anesthetic/Vasoconstrictor Precautions No information available to require special precautions

Effects on Dental Treatment No significant effects or complications reported

Effects on Bleeding No information available to require special precautions

Adverse Effects Frequency not defined.
Cardiovascular: Bradycardia, cardiac irregularities, flushing, hypotension
Gastrointestinal: Diarrhea, nausea, vomiting
Neurologic & skeletal: Muscle weakness

Ocular: Blurred vision, browache, burning eyes, ciliary redness, conjunctival redness/thickening, intraocular pressure increases (paradoxical), iris cysts, lacrimation, lid muscle twitching, miosis, myopia, latent iritis or uveitis activation, lens opacities, retinal detachment, stinging

Respiratory: Dyspnea

Miscellaneous: Diaphoresis, nasolacrimal canal obstruction

General Dosage Range Ophthalmic:

Children: Diagnosis: Instill 1 drop of (0.125%) into both eyes at bedtime for 2-3 weeks; Treatment: Instill 1 drop of 0.06% once daily **or** 0.125% every other day (maximum: 0.125% daily)

Adults: Initial: 1 drop (0.03%) twice daily; Maintenance: 1 dose daily or every other day

Mechanism of Action Long-acting inhibition of cholinesterase enhances activity of endogenous acetylcholine. Reduced degradation of acetylcholine leads to continuous stimulation of the ciliary muscle producing miosis; other effects include potentiation of accommodation and facilitation of aqueous humor outflow, with attendant reduction in intraocular pressure.

Pharmacodynamics/Kinetics

Onset of Action Miosis: 10-30 minutes; Intraocular pressure decrease: 4-8 hours

Peak effect: Intraocular pressure decrease: 24 hours

Duration of Action Miosis: 1-4 weeks

Pregnancy Risk Factor C

Pregnancy Considerations Animal reproduction studies have not been conducted. There are no adequate and well-controlled studies in pregnant women. Use only if clearly needed.

Econazole (e KONE a zole)

Pharmacologic Category Antifungal Agent, Topical

Use Topical treatment of tinea pedis (athlete's foot), tinea cruris (jock itch), tinea corporis (ringworm), tinea versicolor, and cutaneous candidiasis

Local Anesthetic/Vasoconstrictor Precautions No information available to require special precautions

Effects on Dental Treatment No significant effects or complications reported

Effects on Bleeding No information available to require special precautions

Adverse Effects 1% to 10%: Dermatologic: Burning (3%), erythema (3%), itching (3%), stinging (3%)

General Dosage Range Topical: *Children and Adults:* Apply sufficient quantity once or twice daily

Mechanism of Action Alters fungal cell wall membrane permeability; may interfere with RNA and protein synthesis, and lipid metabolism

Pregnancy Risk Factor C

Pregnancy Considerations Fetotoxic and embryotoxic events were observed in animal reproduction studies following oral administration.

Eculizumab (e kue LIZ oo mab)

Brand Names: U.S. Soliris®

Brand Names: Canada Soliris®

Pharmacologic Category Monoclonal Antibody; Monoclonal Antibody, Complement Inhibitor

Use Treatment of paroxysmal nocturnal hemoglobinuria (PNH) to reduce hemolysis; treatment of atypical hemolytic uremic syndrome (aHUS) to inhibit complement-mediated thrombotic microangiopathy

Note: Not indicated for the treatment of hemolytic uremic syndrome related to Shiga toxin *E. coli* (STEC-HUS)

Local Anesthetic/Vasoconstrictor Precautions No information available to require special precautions

Effects on Dental Treatment No significant effects or complications reported

Effects on Bleeding No information available to require special precautions

Adverse Effects

>10%:

Cardiovascular: Hypertension (aHUS: 35%), tachycardia (aHUS: children 21%), peripheral edema (11%)

Central nervous system: Headache (30% to 44%; serious: 2%), insomnia (14%), fatigue (11% to 12%), fever (2% to 11%; children 47%), vertigo (11%)

Gastrointestinal: Diarrhea (32%), vomiting (21% to 22%), nausea (16% to 19%), abdominal pain (11%)

Genitourinary: Urinary tract infection (16%)

Hematologic: Anemia (24%; serious: 2%), leukopenia (16%)

Neuromuscular & skeletal: Back pain (19%), limb pain (7% to 11%)

Respiratory: Respiratory tract infection (7% to 35%), cough (12% to 26%), nasopharyngitis (23%), nasal congestion (aHUS: children 21%), pharyngolaryngeal pain (14%)

1% to 10%:

Gastrointestinal: Constipation (7%)

Neuromuscular & skeletal: Myalgia (7%)

Respiratory: Sinusitis (7%)

Miscellaneous: Herpes infections (7%), flu-like syndrome (5%), viral infection (serious: 2%), meningococcal infection (≤1%)

General Dosage Range I.V.:

Children 5 kg to <10 kg: Induction: 300 mg weekly for 1 dose; Maintenance: 300 mg at week 2, then 300 mg every 3 weeks

Children 10 kg to <20 kg: Induction: 600 mg weekly for 1 dose; Maintenance: 300 mg at week 2, then 300 mg every 2 weeks

Children 20 kg to <30 kg: Induction: 600 mg weekly for 2 doses; Maintenance: 600 mg at week 3, then 600 mg every 2 weeks

Children 30 kg to <40 kg: Induction: 600 mg weekly for 2 doses; Maintenance: 900 mg at week 3, then 900 mg every 2 weeks

Children ≥40 kg: Induction: 900 mg weekly for 4 doses; Maintenance: 1200 mg at week 5, then 1200 mg every 2 weeks

Adults: aHUS: Induction: 900 mg weekly for 4 doses; Maintenance: 1200 mg at week 5, then 1200 mg every 2 weeks **or** PNH: Induction: 600 mg weekly for 4 doses; Maintenance: 900 mg at week 5, then 900 mg every 2 weeks

Mechanism of Action Terminal complement-mediated intravascular hemolysis is a key clinical feature of paroxysmal nocturnal hemoglobinuria (PNH); blocking the formation of membrane attack complex (MAC) results in stabilization of hemoglobin and a reduction in the need for RBC transfusions. Impairment of complement activity regulation leads to uncontrolled complement activation in atypical hemolytic uremic syndrome (aHUS). Eculizumab is a humanized monoclonal IgG antibody that binds to complement protein C5, preventing cleavage into C5a and C5b. Blocking the formation of C5b inhibits the subsequent formation of terminal complex C5b-9 or MAC.

◄ **Pharmacodynamics/Kinetics**
Onset of Action PNH: Reduced hemolysis: ≤1 week
Half-life Elimination PNH: ~11 days (range: ~8-15 days); aHUS: ~12 days (during plasma exchange the half-life is reduced to 1.26 hours)
Pregnancy Risk Factor C
Pregnancy Considerations Animal studies have demonstrated fetal abnormalities. Eculizumab is a recombinant IgG molecule with IgG2 and IgG4 sequences; human IgG is known to cross the placenta, however IgG2 may have reduced placental transfer compared to other IgG subclasses. There are no adequate and well-controlled studies in pregnant women. Pregnant women with PNH and their fetuses have high rates of morbidity and mortality during pregnancy and the postpartum period. Limited information is available related to use during pregnancy. Use during pregnancy only if clearly needed.
Prescribing and Access Restrictions Patients and providers must enroll with Soliris® OneSource™ (1-888-765-4747) program prior to treatment initiation.

Edetate CALCIUM Disodium
(ED e tate KAL see um dye SOW dee um)

Brand Names: U.S. Calcium Disodium Versenate®
Pharmacologic Category Chelating Agent
Use Treatment of symptomatic acute and chronic lead poisoning
Local Anesthetic/Vasoconstrictor Precautions No information available to require special precautions
Effects on Dental Treatment No significant effects or complications reported
Effects on Bleeding No information available to require special precautions
Adverse Effects Frequency not defined.
Cardiovascular: Arrhythmia, ECG changes, hypotension
Central nervous system: Chills, fatigue, fever, headache, malaise
Dermatologic: Cheilosis, dermatitis, rash
Endocrine & metabolic: Hypercalcemia, hypokalemia
Gastrointestinal: Anorexia, GI upset, nausea, thirst (excessive), vomiting
Hematologic: Anemia, bone marrow suppression (transient)
Hepatic: Alkaline phosphatase decreased, liver function test increased (mild)
Local: Pain at injection site (I.M. injection), thrombophlebitis (I.V. infusion when concentration >5 mg/mL)
Neuromuscular & skeletal: Arthralgia, myalgia, numbness, paresthesia, tremor
Ocular: Lacrimation
Renal: Glucosuria, microscopic hematuria, nephrosis, nephrotoxicity, proteinuria, renal tubular necrosis, urinary frequency/urgency
Respiratory: Nasal congestion, sneezing
Miscellaneous: Iron, magnesium, and/or zinc deficiency (with chronic therapy)
General Dosage Range Dosage adjustment recommended in patients with renal impairment
I.M., I.V.: *Children and Adults:* 1000-1500 mg/m^2/day (25-75 mg/kg/day)
Mechanism of Action Calcium is displaced by divalent and trivalent heavy metals, forming a nonionizing soluble complex that is excreted in urine
Pharmacodynamics/Kinetics
Onset of Action Chelation of lead: I.V.: 1 hour
Half-life Elimination 20-60 minutes
Pregnancy Risk Factor B

Pregnancy Considerations Adverse events were observed in some animal reproduction studies; there are no well controlled studies of edetate CALCIUM disodium in pregnant women. Lead is known to cross the placenta in amounts related to maternal plasma levels. Prenatal lead exposure may be associated with adverse events such as spontaneous abortion, preterm delivery, decreased birth weight, and impaired neurodevelopment. Some adverse outcomes may occur with maternal blood lead levels <10 mcg/dL. In addition, pregnant women exposed to lead may have an increased risk of gestational hypertension. Consider chelation therapy in pregnant women with confirmed blood lead levels ≥45 mcg/dL (pregnant women with blood lead levels ≥70 mcg/dL should be considered for chelation regardless of trimester); consultation with experts in lead poisoning and high-risk pregnancy is recommended. Encephalopathic pregnant women should be chelated regardless of trimester (CDC, 2010).

Edrophonium (ed roe FOE nee um)

Brand Names: U.S. Enlon®
Brand Names: Canada Enlon®; Tensilon®
Pharmacologic Category Acetylcholinesterase Inhibitor; Antidote; Diagnostic Agent
Use Diagnosis of myasthenia gravis; differentiation of cholinergic crises from myasthenia crises; reversal of nondepolarizing neuromuscular blockers
Local Anesthetic/Vasoconstrictor Precautions No information available to require special precautions
Effects on Dental Treatment No significant effects or complications reported
Effects on Bleeding No information available to require special precautions
Adverse Effects Frequency not defined.
Cardiovascular: Arrhythmias (especially bradycardia), AV block, carbon monoxide decreased, cardiac arrest, ECG changes (nonspecific), flushing, hypotension, nodal rhythm, syncope, tachycardia
Central nervous system: Convulsions, dizziness, drowsiness, dysarthria, dysphonia, headache, loss of consciousness
Dermatologic: Skin rash, thrombophlebitis (I.V.), urticaria
Gastrointestinal: Diarrhea, dysphagia, flatulence, hyperperistalsis, nausea, salivation, stomach cramps, vomiting
Genitourinary: Urinary urgency
Neuromuscular & skeletal: Arthralgias, fasciculations, muscle cramps, spasms, weakness
Ocular: Lacrimation, small pupils
Respiratory: Bronchiolar constriction, bronchospasm, dyspnea, bronchial secretions increased, laryngospasm, respiratory arrest, respiratory depression, respiratory muscle paralysis
Miscellaneous: Allergic reactions, anaphylaxis, diaphoresis increased
General Dosage Range
I.M.:
Infants: 0.5-1 mg
Children ≤34 kg: 1 mg
Children >34 kg: 5 mg
Adults: 10 mg, followed by 2 mg if no response

I.V.:
Infants: 0.1 mg, followed by 0.4 mg if no response (maximum total dose: 0.5 mg)

Children ≤34 kg: 0.04 mg/kg as single dose or followed by 0.16 mg/kg if no response **or** 1 mg, followed by 1mg every 30-45 seconds if no response (maximum total dose: 5 mg)

Children >34 kg: 0.04 mg/kg as single dose or followed by 0.16 mg/kg if no response **or** 2 mg, followed by 1 mg every 30-45 seconds if no response (maximum total dose: 10 mg)

Adults: 2 mg test dose, followed by 8 mg if no response **or** 1-10 mg as a single dose **or** 10 mg every 5-10 minutes up to 40 mg **or** 1 mg; may repeat after 1 minute

Mechanism of Action Inhibits destruction of acetylcholine by acetylcholinesterase. This facilitates transmission of impulses across myoneural junction and results in increased cholinergic responses such as miosis, increased tonus of intestinal and skeletal muscles, bronchial and ureteral constriction, bradycardia, and increased salivary and sweat gland secretions.

Pharmacodynamics/Kinetics
Onset of Action I.M.: 2-10 minutes; I.V.: 30-60 seconds
Duration of Action I.M.: 5-30 minutes: I.V.: 10 minutes
Half-life Elimination Adults: 1.2-2.4 hours; Anephric patients: 2.4-4.4 hours

---

Edrophonium and Atropine
(ed roe FOE nee um & A troe peen)

Related Information
Atropine *on page 148*
Edrophonium *on page 468*
Brand Names: U.S. Enlon-Plus®
Pharmacologic Category Acetylcholinesterase Inhibitor; Anticholinergic Agent; Antidote
Use Reversal of nondepolarizing neuromuscular blockers; adjunct treatment of respiratory depression caused by curare overdose
Local Anesthetic/Vasoconstrictor Precautions Bradyarrhythmias, tachycardia, and premature ventricular contractions have been reported; use vasoconstrictor with caution
Effects on Dental Treatment No significant effects or complications reported
Effects on Bleeding No information available to require special precautions
Adverse Effects See individual agents.
General Dosage Range I.V.: *Adults:* 0.05-0.1 mL/kg (0.5-1 mg/kg of edrophonium and 0.007-0.014 mg/kg of atropine)
Mechanism of Action
Edrophonium: Inhibits destruction of acetylcholine by acetylcholinesterase. This facilitates transmission of impulses across myoneural junction and results in increased cholinergic response.
Atropine: Minimizes or prevents the muscarinic cholinergic effects caused by edrophonium (eg, bradycardia, bronchocontriction, and increased secretions).
Pharmacodynamics/Kinetics
Onset of Action Edrophonium: Antagonism of nondepolarizing muscle relaxants: 3 minutes; Atropine: Heart rate: Immediate
Duration of Action Edrophonium: Antagonism of nondepolarizing muscle relaxants: 70 minutes; Atropine: Heart rate: 170 minutes

Half-life Elimination Edrophonium: Adults: 1.2-2.4 hours; Anephric patients: 2.4-4.4 hours
Time to Peak Edrophonium: Antagonism of nondepolarizing muscle relaxants: 1.2 minutes; Atropine: Heart rate: 2-16 minutes
Pregnancy Risk Factor C
Pregnancy Considerations See Atropine monograph.

Efavirenz (e FAV e renz)

Related Information
HIV Infection and AIDS *on page 1520*
Brand Names: U.S. Sustiva®
Brand Names: Canada Sustiva®
Pharmacologic Category Antiretroviral Agent, Reverse Transcriptase Inhibitor (Non-nucleoside)
Use Treatment of HIV-1 infections in combination with at least two other antiretroviral agents
Local Anesthetic/Vasoconstrictor Precautions No information available to require special precautions
Effects on Dental Treatment Key adverse event(s) related to dental treatment: Abnormal taste
Effects on Bleeding No information available to require special precautions related to hemostasis.
Adverse Effects Unless otherwise noted, frequency of adverse events is as reported in adults receiving combination antiretroviral therapy.
>10%:
Central nervous system: Dizziness (2% to 28%; children 16%), fever (children 21%), depression (≤19%; severe: 1% to 2%), insomnia (≤16%), anxiety (2% to 13%), pain (1% to 13%; children 14%), headache (2% to 8%; children 11%)
Dermatologic: Rash (5% to 26%, grade 3/4: <1%; children ≤46%, grade 3/4: 2% to 4%)
Endocrine & metabolic: HDL increased (25% to 35%), total cholesterol increased (20% to 40%), triglycerides increased (≥751 mg/dL: 6% to 11%)
Gastrointestinal: Diarrhea (3% to 14%; children: ≤39%), nausea (2% to 10%; children 12%), vomiting (3% to 6%; children 12%)
Respiratory: Cough (children 16%)
1% to 10%:
Central nervous system: Impaired concentration (≤8%), somnolence (≤7%), fatigue (≤8%), abnormal dreams (1% to 6%), nervousness (2% to 7%), hallucinations (1%)
Dermatologic: Pruritus (≤9%)
Endocrine & metabolic: Hyperglycemia (>250 mg/dL: 2% to 5%)
Gastrointestinal: Dyspepsia (≤4%), abdominal pain (2% to 3%), anorexia (≤ 2%), amylase increased (grade 3/4: ≤6%)
Hematologic: Neutropenia (grade 3/4: 2% to 10%)
Hepatic: Incidence higher with hepatitis B and/or C coinfection: ALT increased (grades 3/4: 2% to 8%), AST increased (grades 3/4: 5% to 8%)
General Dosage Range Dosage adjustment recommended in patients on concomitant therapy
Oral:
Children ≥3 years and 10 kg to <15 kg: 200 mg once daily
Children ≥3 years and 15 kg to <20 kg: 250 mg once daily
Children ≥3 years and 20 kg to <25 kg: 300 mg once daily
Children ≥3 years and 25 kg to <32.5 kg: 350 mg once daily

◄ *Children ≥3 years and 32.5 kg to <40 kg:* 400 mg once daily

Children ≥3 years and ≥40 kg and Adults: 600 mg once daily

Mechanism of Action As a non-nucleoside reverse transcriptase inhibitor, efavirenz has activity against HIV-1 by binding to reverse transcriptase. It consequently blocks the RNA-dependent and DNA-dependent DNA polymerase activities including HIV-1 replication. It does not require intracellular phosphorylation for antiviral activity.

Pharmacodynamics/Kinetics

Half-life Elimination Single dose: 52-76 hours; Multiple doses: 40-55 hours

Time to Peak 3-5 hours

Pregnancy Risk Factor D

Pregnancy Considerations Teratogenic effects have been observed in primates receiving efavirenz. Efavirenz crosses the placenta. Based on data from the Antiretroviral Pregnancy Registry, an increased risk of overall birth defects has not been observed following first trimester exposure to efavirenz; however, neural tube and other CNS defects have been reported. Due to the low number of first trimester exposures and the low incidence of neural tube defects in the general population, available data are insufficient to evaluate risk. Other antiretroviral agents should strongly be considered for use in women of childbearing potential who are planning to become pregnant or who are sexually active and not using effective contraception. Nonpregnant women of reproductive age should undergo pregnancy testing prior to initiation of efavirenz. Barrier contraception should be used in combination with other (hormonal) methods of contraception during therapy and for 12 weeks after efavirenz is discontinued. Neural tube defects would occur following exposure during the first 5-6 weeks of gestation (most pregnancies are not detected before 4-6 weeks gestation). For women who present in the first trimester already on an efavirenz-containing regimen and who have adequate viral suppression, efavirenz may be continued; changing regimens may lead to loss of viral control and increase the risk of perinatal transmission. Pharmacokinetic data from available studies do not suggest dose alterations are needed during pregnancy. Hypersensitivity reactions (including hepatic toxicity and rash) are more common in women on NNRTI therapy; it is not known if pregnancy increases this risk

Regardless of CD4 count or HIV RNA copy number, all HIV-infected pregnant women should receive a combination antepartum antiretroviral (ARV) drug regimen; this includes women who require therapy for their own health, as well as women who do not yet require therapy for their own health. ARV therapy should be started as soon as possible if required for the woman's health. Although earlier initiation may be more effective in reducing the perinatal transmission of HIV), also consider maternal conditions (eg, nausea and vomiting) and the potential risks of first trimester fetal exposure for specific agents. Plasma HIV RNA levels should be assessed at ~34-36 weeks gestation in order to help determine mode of delivery. If ARV therapy must be interrupted for <24 hours during the peripartum period, stop then restart all medications simultaneously in order to decrease the chance of developing resistance. Long-term follow-up is recommended for all infants exposed to ARV medications.

Healthcare providers are encouraged to enroll pregnant women exposed to antiretroviral medications in the Antiretroviral Pregnancy Registry (1-800-258-4263 or www.APRegistry.com). Healthcare providers caring for HIV-infected women and their infants may contact the National Perinatal HIV Hotline (888-448-8765) for clinical consultation (DHHS [perinatal], 2012).

Prescribing and Access Restrictions Efavirenz oral solution is available only through an expanded access (compassionate use) program. Enrollment information may be obtained by calling 877-372-7097.

Efavirenz, Emtricitabine, and Tenofovir
(e FAV e renz, em trye SYE ta been, & te NOE fo veer)

Related Information

Efavirenz *on page 469*
Emtricitabine *on page 473*
HIV Infection and AIDS *on page 1520*
Tenofovir *on page 1299*

Brand Names: U.S. Atripla®

Brand Names: Canada Atripla®

Pharmacologic Category Antiretroviral Agent, Reverse Transcriptase Inhibitor (Non-nucleoside); Antiretroviral Agent, Reverse Transcriptase Inhibitor (Nucleoside); Antiretroviral Agent, Reverse Transcriptase Inhibitor (Nucleotide)

Use Treatment of HIV infection

Local Anesthetic/Vasoconstrictor Precautions No information available to require special precautions

Effects on Dental Treatment Key adverse event(s) related to dental treatment: Efavirenz alone has caused xerostomia (normal salivary flow resumes upon discontinuation) and abnormal taste (see individual monograph). No significant effects or complications reported with combination drug.

Effects on Bleeding No information available to require special precautions related to hemostasis.

Adverse Effects The complete adverse reaction profile of combination therapy has not been established. **See individual agents.** The following adverse effects were noted in clinical trials with combination therapy:

>10%: Endocrine & metabolic: Hypercholesterolemia (22%)

1% to 10%:

Central nervous system: Depression (9%), fatigue (9%), dizziness (8%), headache (6%), anxiety (5%), insomnia (5%), somnolence (4%), abnormal dreams

Dermatologic: Rash (7%)

Endocrine & metabolic: Triglycerides increased (4%), hyperglycemia (2%)

Gastrointestinal: Nausea (9%), diarrhea (9%), serum amylase increased (8%), vomiting (2%)

Hematologic: Neutropenia (3%)

Hepatic: AST increased (3%), ALT increased (2%), alkaline phosphatase increased (1%)

Neuromuscular & skeletal: Creatine increased (9%)

Renal: Hematuria (3%)

Respiratory: Sinusitis (8%), upper respiratory infection (8%), nasopharyngitis (5%)

General Dosage Range Oral: *Children ≥12 years and ≥40 kg, Adolescents, and Adults:* 1 tablet (efavirenz 600 mg/emtricitabine 200 mg/tenofovir 300 mg) once daily

Mechanism of Action See individual agents.

Pregnancy Risk Factor D
Pregnancy Considerations See individual agents.

Eflornithine (ee FLOR ni theen)

Brand Names: U.S. Vaniqa®
Brand Names: Canada Vaniqa®
Pharmacologic Category Antiprotozoal; Topical Skin Product
Use Reduce unwanted hair from face and adjacent areas under the chin
Unlabeled Use Injection: Treatment of meningoencephalitic stage of *Trypanosoma brucei gambiense* infection (sleeping sickness). **Note:** Eflornithine has specific activity against *T.b. gambiense* in early and late stages (not effective for *T.b. rhodesiense*).
Local Anesthetic/Vasoconstrictor Precautions No information available to require special precautions
Effects on Dental Treatment No significant effects or complications reported
Effects on Bleeding No information available to require special precautions
Adverse Effects
Injection (Priotto, 2009):
>10%:
Cardiovascular: Arrhythmia (22%), hypertension (13%), chest pain (11%)
Central nervous system: Headache (46%), fever (43%), dizziness (17%)
Dermatologic: Pruritus (19%), rash (14%)
Gastrointestinal: Abdominal pain (30%), diarrhea (29%), nausea (20%), vomiting (20%), anorexia (14%)
Hematologic: Neutropenia (33%)
Local: Injection site reaction (11%)
Neuromuscular & skeletal: Myalgia/arthralgia (30%), weakness (20%)
Miscellaneous: Infection (2% to 16%)
1% to 10%:
Cardiovascular: Edema (4%), hypotension/shock (3%)
Central nervous system: Insomnia (10%), seizure (9%), anxiety (8%), coma (2%), amnesia (1%), ataxia (1%), confusion (1%), depression (1%), hallucination (1%), lethargy (1%)
Endocrine & metabolic: Dehydration (2%)
Gastrointestinal: Dysphagia (9%), xerostomia (5%), constipation (4%), taste disturbance (2%)
Genitourinary: Urinary frequency/urgency (4%), urinary incontinence (3%)
Hematologic: Anemia (9%), leukopenia (4%), thrombocytopenia (4%)
Local: Extravasation (8%)
Neuromuscular & skeletal: Peripheral neuropathy (1% to 4%), tremor (1%)
Otic: Inner ear disturbance (5%)
Renal: Bilirubin altered (5%), ALT altered (3%), creatinine altered (1%)
Respiratory: Cough (10%), epistaxis (2%), dyspnea (1%), respiratory distress (1%)
Miscellaneous: Hiccups (2%)

Topical:
>10%: Dermatologic: Acne (11% to 21%), pseudofolliculitis barbae (5% to 16%)
1% to 10%:
Central nervous system: Headache (4%), dizziness (1% to 2%)

Dermatologic: Stinging (4% to 8%), burning skin (4%), pruritus (3% to 4%), tingling skin (2% to 4%), dry skin (2% to 3%), rash (2% to 3%), erythema (1% to 3%), alopecia (1% to 2%), skin irritation (1% to 2%), folliculitis (≤1%), ingrown hair (≤1%)
Gastrointestinal: Dyspepsia (2% to 3%), anorexia (1%)
General Dosage Range
Topical: *Children and Adults:* Apply thin layer to affected areas twice daily
Mechanism of Action
Cream: Eflornithine inhibits the enzyme ornithine decarboxylase (ODC) which inhibits cell division and synthetic functions and thereby affects the rate of hair growth.
Injection: Eflornithine exerts antitumor and antiprotozoal effects through specific, irreversible ("suicide") inhibition of the enzyme ornithine decarboxylase (ODC). ODC is the rate-limiting enzyme in the biosynthesis of putrescine, spermine, and spermidine, the major polyamines in nucleated cells. Polyamines are necessary for the synthesis of DNA, RNA, and proteins and are, therefore, necessary for cell growth and differentiation. Although many microorganisms and higher plants are able to produce polyamines from alternate biochemical pathways, all mammalian cells depend on ornithine decarboxylase to produce polyamines. Eflornithine inhibits ODC and rapidly depletes animal cells of putrescine and spermidine; the concentration of spermine remains the same or may even increase. Rapidly dividing cells appear to be most susceptible to the effects of eflornithine.
Pharmacodynamics/Kinetics
Onset of Action Decreased hair growth: 4-8 weeks
Half-life Elimination I.V.: 3-3.5 hours; Topical: 8 hours
Pregnancy Risk Factor C
Pregnancy Considerations When administered topically, teratogenic effects were not observed in animal reproduction studies. Discontinuation or not initiating therapy should be considered since information related to topical use in pregnancy is limited.
Prescribing and Access Restrictions Injectable eflornithine is donated to World Health Organization (WHO) by the manufacturer. Further information may be found on WHO website at http://www.who.int/trypanosomiasis_african/diagnosis/en/index.html or by contacting the CDC Drug Service (404-639-3670).

Eletriptan (el e TRIP tan)

Related Information
Temporomandibular Dysfunction (TMD), Chronic Pain, and Fibromyalgia *on page 1590*
Brand Names: U.S. Relpax®
Brand Names: Canada Relpax®
Pharmacologic Category Antimigraine Agent; Serotonin 5-HT$_{1B, 1D}$ Receptor Agonist
Use Acute treatment of migraine, with or without aura
Local Anesthetic/Vasoconstrictor Precautions No information available to require special precautions
Effects on Dental Treatment Key adverse event(s) related to dental treatment: Xerostomia (normal salivary flow resumes upon discontinuation)
Effects on Bleeding No information available to require special precautions
Adverse Effects 1% to 10%:
Cardiovascular: Chest pain/tightness (1% to 4%; placebo 1%), palpitation

Central nervous system: Dizziness (3% to 7%; placebo 3%), somnolence (3% to 7%; placebo 4%), headache (3% to 4%; placebo 3%), chills, pain, vertigo

Gastrointestinal: Nausea (4% to 8%; placebo 5%), xerostomia (2% to 4%, placebo 2%), dysphagia (1% to 2%), abdominal pain/discomfort (1% to 2%; placebo 1%), dyspepsia (1% to 2%; placebo 1%)

Neuromuscular & skeletal: Weakness (4% to 10%), paresthesia (3% to 4%), back pain, hypertonia, hypoesthesia

Respiratory: Pharyngitis

Miscellaneous: Diaphoresis

General Dosage Range Oral: *Adults:* 20-40 mg as a single dose, may repeat (maximum: 80 mg/day)

Mechanism of Action Selective agonist for serotonin (5-HT$_{1B}$ and 5-HT$_{1D}$ receptors) in cranial arteries; causes vasoconstriction and reduces sterile inflammation associated with antidromic neuronal transmission correlating with relief of migraine

Pharmacodynamics/Kinetics

Half-life Elimination ~4 hours (Elderly: 4.4-5.7 hours); Metabolite: ~13 hours

Time to Peak Plasma: 1.5-2 hours

Pregnancy Risk Factor C

Pregnancy Considerations Teratogenic effects were observed in animal studies.

Eltrombopag (el TROM boe pag)

Brand Names: U.S. Promacta®
Brand Names: Canada Revolade™
Pharmacologic Category Colony Stimulating Factor; Thrombopoietic Agent
Use Treatment of thrombocytopenia in patients with chronic immune (idiopathic) thrombocytopenic purpura (ITP) at risk for bleeding who have had insufficient response to corticosteroids, immune globulin, or splenectomy; treatment of thrombocytopenia in patients with chronic hepatitis C in order to allow and maintain interferon-based therapy

Local Anesthetic/Vasoconstrictor Precautions No information available to require special precautions

Effects on Dental Treatment Key adverse event(s) related to dental treatment: Risk of bleeding in soft tissues upon discontinuation of therapy due to rebound thrombocytopenia; monitor for at least 4 weeks after discontinuation of treatment.

Effects on Bleeding Eltrombopag is used in the management of severe thrombocytopenia. Medical consultation is warranted.

Adverse Effects Adverse reactions and incidences reported are associated with ITP unless otherwise indicated.

>10%:

Central nervous system: Fever (chronic hepatitis C 30%), fatigue (4%; chronic hepatitis C 28%), headache (10%; chronic hepatitis C 21%), insomnia (chronic hepatitis C 16%), chills (chronic hepatitis C 14%)

Dermatologic: Pruritus (chronic hepatitis C 15%)

Gastrointestinal: Diarrhea (9%; chronic hepatitis C 19%), nausea (4% to 9%; chronic hepatitis C 19%), appetite decreased (chronic hepatitis C 18%)

Hematologic: Myelofibrosis (bone marrow biopsy): Grade ≤1: 93%; grade 2: 7%; grade 3: <3%) anemia (chronic hepatitis C 40%)

Hepatic: Liver function tests abnormal (11%)

Neuromuscular & skeletal: Weakness (chronic hepatitis C 16%), myalgia (5% to 12%)

Respiratory: Cough (chronic hepatitis C 15%)

Miscellaneous: Flu-like syndrome (3%; chronic hepatitis C 18%)

1% to 10%:

Cardiovascular: Peripheral edema (chronic hepatitis C 10%), thrombosis (chronic hepatitis C 3%)

Dermatologic: Alopecia (2%; chronic hepatitis C 10%), rash (3%)

Gastrointestinal: Vomiting (6%), xerostomia (2%)

Genitourinary: Urinary tract infection (5%)

Hematologic: Rebound thrombocytopenia (8%)

Hepatic: Ascites and encephalopathy (chronic hepatitis C 7%), hyperbilirubinemia (6% to 8%), ALT increased (5% to 6%), AST increased (4%), alkaline phosphatase increased (2%)

Neuromuscular & skeletal: Back pain (3%), paresthesia (3%), musculoskeletal pain (2%)

Ocular: Cataract (4% to 8%)

Respiratory: Upper respiratory infection (7%), oropharyngeal pain (4%), pharyngitis (4%)

General Dosage Range Dosage adjustment recommended in patients with hepatic impairment, of East-Asian ethnicity, or who develop toxicities

Oral: *Adults:* Initial: 25-50 mg once daily (maximum: 75 mg once daily for ITP; 100 mg once daily for chronic hepatitis C-associated thrombocytopenia)

Mechanism of Action Thrombopoietin (TPO) nonpeptide agonist which increases platelet counts by binding to and activating the human TPO receptor. Activates intracellular signal transduction pathways to increase proliferation and differentiation of marrow progenitor cells. Does not induce platelet aggregation or activation.

Pharmacodynamics/Kinetics

Onset of Action Platelet count increase: Within 1-2 weeks; Peak platelet count increase: 14-16 days

Duration of Action Platelets return to baseline: 1-2 weeks after last dose

Half-life Elimination ~21-32 hours in healthy individuals; ~26-35 hours in patients with ITP

Time to Peak 2-6 hours

Pregnancy Risk Factor C

Pregnancy Considerations Adverse effects were observed in animal reproduction studies. Use during pregnancy only if the potential benefit to the mother outweighs the potential risk to the fetus. A Promacta® pregnancy registry has been established to monitor outcomes of women exposed to eltrombopag during pregnancy (1-888-825-5249).

Elvitegravir, Cobicistat, Emtricitabine, and Tenofovir

(el vi TEG ra vir, koe BIK i stat, em trye SYE ta been, & te NOE fo veer)

Related Information
HIV Infection and AIDS *on page 1520*
Brand Names: U.S. Stribild™
Brand Names: Canada Stribild™
Pharmacologic Category Antiretroviral Agent, Integrase Inhibitor; Antiretroviral Agent, Reverse Transcriptase Inhibitor (Nucleoside); Antiretroviral Agent, Reverse Transcriptase Inhibitor (Nucleotide)
Use Treatment of human immunodeficiency virus type 1 (HIV-1) infection in antiretroviral treatment-naive adult patients

Local Anesthetic/Vasoconstrictor Precautions No information available to require special precautions

Effects on Dental Treatment No significant effects or complications reported

Effects on Bleeding No information available to require special precautions

Adverse Effects Percentages as reported for combination product.

>10%:
Gastrointestinal: Nausea (16%), diarrhea (12%)
Renal: Proteinuria (39%)

1% to 10%:
Central nervous system: Abnormal dreams (9%), headache (7%), fatigue (5%), dizziness (3%), insomnia (3%), somnolence (1%)
Dermatologic: Rash (3%)
Endocrine & metabolic: Cholesterol increased (grades 3/4: ≤1%), triglycerides increased (grades 3/4: ≤1%)
Gastrointestinal: Amylase increased (2%), flatulence (2%)
Hepatic: AST increased (2%)
Neuromuscular & skeletal: CPK increased (5%), fractures (1%)
Renal: Creatinine increased (7%), hematuria (3%)

General Dosage Range Oral: *Adults:* One tablet once daily

Mechanism of Action Integrase strand transfer inhibitor, CYP3A enzyme inhibitor plus nucleoside and nucleotide reverse transcriptase inhibitor combination; the viral cDNA strand produced by reverse transcriptase is processed and inserted into the human genome by the enzyme HIV-1 integrase. Elvitegravir inhibits the catalytic activity of integrase, thus preventing integration of the proviral gene into human DNA. Cobicistat inhibits enzymes of the CYP3A subfamily and enhances systemic exposure to elvitegravir. Emtricitabine is a cytosine analogue and tenofovir disoproxil fumarate (TDF) is an analog of adenosine 5'-monophosphate. Emtricitabine and tenofovir interfere with HIV viral RNA dependent DNA polymerase activities resulting in inhibition of viral replication.

Pharmacodynamics/Kinetics
Half-life Elimination Elvitegravir ~13 hours; cobicistat ~4 hours; emtricitabine ~10 hours; tenofovir ~17 hours
Time to Peak Plasma: ~3 hours (range: 2-4 hours)

Pregnancy Risk Factor B

Pregnancy Considerations Adverse events were not observed in animal reproduction studies following administration of the individual agents contained in this combination product. Also see individual agents. Healthcare providers are encouraged to enroll pregnant women exposed to antiretroviral medications in the Antiretroviral Pregnancy Registry (1-800-258-4263 or www.APRegistry.com). Healthcare providers caring for HIV-infected women and their infants may contact the National Perinatal HIV Hotline (888-448-8765) for clinical consultation (DHHS [perinatal], 2012).

Emedastine (em e DAS teen)

Brand Names: U.S. Emadine®
Pharmacologic Category Histamine H_1 Antagonist; Histamine H_1 Antagonist, Second Generation
Use Treatment of allergic conjunctivitis
Local Anesthetic/Vasoconstrictor Precautions No information available to require special precautions
Effects on Dental Treatment No significant effects or complications reported
Effects on Bleeding No information available to require special precautions

Adverse Effects
>10%: Central nervous system: Headache (11%)
1% to 10%:
Cardiovascular: Hyperemia
Central nervous system: Abnormal dreams
Dermatologic: Dermatitis, keratitis, pruritus
Gastrointestinal: Taste (unpleasant)
Neuromuscular & skeletal: Weakness
Ocular: Blurred vision, corneal infiltrates, corneal staining, dry eyes, transient burning or stinging
Respiratory: Rhinitis, sinusitis
Miscellaneous: Tearing

General Dosage Range Ophthalmic: *Children ≥3 years and Adults:* Instill 1 drop in affected eye up to 4 times/day

Mechanism of Action Selective histamine H_1-receptor antagonist for topical ophthalmic use

Pharmacodynamics/Kinetics
Half-life Elimination Oral: Plasma: 3-4 hours

Pregnancy Risk Factor B

Pregnancy Considerations Teratogenic events have not been observed in animal reproduction studies. Systemic absorption is limited following ocular administration.

Emtricitabine (em trye SYE ta been)

Related Information
HIV Infection and AIDS *on page 1520*
Brand Names: U.S. Emtriva®
Brand Names: Canada Emtriva®
Pharmacologic Category Antiretroviral Agent, Reverse Transcriptase Inhibitor (Nucleoside)
Use Treatment of HIV infection in combination with at least two other antiretroviral agents
Local Anesthetic/Vasoconstrictor Precautions No information available to require special precautions
Effects on Dental Treatment No significant effects or complications reported
Effects on Bleeding No information available to require special precautions related to hemostasis.

Adverse Effects Clinical trials were conducted in patients receiving other antiretroviral agents, and it is not possible to correlate frequency of adverse events with emtricitabine alone. The range of frequencies of adverse events is generally comparable to comparator groups, with the exception of hyperpigmentation, which occurred more frequently in patients receiving emtricitabine. Unless otherwise noted, percentages are as reported in adults.

>10%:
Central nervous system: Dizziness (4% to 25%), headache (6% to 22%), fever (children 18%), insomnia (5% to 16%), abnormal dreams (2% to 11%)
Dermatologic: Hyperpigmentation (children 32%; adults 2% to 4%; primarily of palms and/or soles but may include tongue, arms, lip and nails; generally mild and nonprogressive without associated local reactions such as pruritus or rash); rash (17% to 30%; includes pruritus, maculopapular rash, vesiculobullous rash, pustular rash, and allergic reaction)
Gastrointestinal: Diarrhea (children 20%; adults 9% to 23%), vomiting (children 23%; adults 9%), nausea (13% to 18%), abdominal pain (8% to 14%), gastroenteritis (children 11%)
Neuromuscular & skeletal: Weakness (12% to 16%), CPK increased (grades 3/4: 11% to 12%)
Otic: Otitis media (children 23%)

Respiratory: Cough (children 28%; adults 14%), rhinitis (children 20%; adults 12% to 18%), pneumonia (children 15%)

Miscellaneous: Infection (children 44%)

1% to 10%:

Central nervous system: Depression (6% to 9%), neuropathy/neuritis (4%)

Endocrine & metabolic: Serum triglycerides increased (grades 3/4: 4% to 10%), disordered glucose homeostasis (grades 3/4: 2% to 3%), serum amylase increased (grades 3/4: children 9%; adults 2% to 5%), serum lipase increased (grades 3/4: ≤1%)

Gastrointestinal: Dyspepsia (4% to 8%), serum amylase increased (grades 3/4: 8%)

Genitourinary: Hematuria (grades 3/4: 3%)

Hematologic: Anemia (children: 7%), neutropenia (grades 3/4: children 2%; adults 5%)

Hepatic: Transaminases increased (grades 3/4: 2% to 6%), alkaline phosphatase increased (>550 units/L: 1%), bilirubin increased (grades 3/4: 1%)

Neuromuscular & skeletal: Creatinine kinase increased (grades 3/4: 9%), myalgia (4% to 6%), paresthesia (5% to 6%), arthralgia (3% to 5%)

Respiratory: Upper respiratory tract infection (8%), sinusitis (8%), pharyngitis (5%)

General Dosage Range Dosage adjustment recommended in patients with renal impairment

Oral:

Capsule: *Children 3 months to 17 years and >33 kg and Adults:* 200 mg once daily

Solution:

Children <3 months: 3 mg/kg/day

Children 3 months to 17 years: 6 mg/kg once daily (maximum: 240 mg/day)

Adults: 240 mg once daily

Mechanism of Action Nucleoside reverse transcriptase inhibitor; emtricitabine is a cytosine analogue which is phosphorylated intracellularly to emtricitabine 5'-triphosphate which interferes with HIV viral RNA dependent DNA polymerase resulting in inhibition of viral replication.

Pharmacodynamics/Kinetics

Half-life Elimination Normal renal function: Adults: 10 hours; children: 5-18 hours

Time to Peak Plasma: 1-2 hours

Pregnancy Risk Factor B

Pregnancy Considerations Adverse events were not observed in animal studies. Emtricitabine crosses the placenta; no increased risk of overall birth defects has been observed according to data collected by the antiretroviral pregnancy registry. Cases of lactic acidosis/hepatic steatosis syndrome related to mitochondrial toxicity have been reported in pregnant women with prolonged use of nucleoside analogues. It is not known if pregnancy itself potentiates this known side effect; however, women may be at increased risk of lactic acidosis and liver damage. In addition, these adverse events are similar to other rare but life-threatening syndromes which occur during pregnancy (eg, HELLP syndrome). Hepatic enzymes and electrolytes should be monitored in women receiving nucleoside analogues and clinicians should watch for early signs of the syndrome. In addition, mitochondrial dysfunction may develop in infants following *in utero* exposure. A pharmacokinetic study shows a slight decrease in emtricitabine serum levels during the third trimester; however, there is no clear need to adjust the dose. The DHHS Perinatal HIV Guidelines consider emtricitabine to be an alternative NRTI in dual nucleoside combination regimens. The DHHS Perinatal HIV Guidelines consider emtricitabine plus tenofovir a recommended dual NRTI/NtRTI backbone for HIV/HBV coinfected pregnant women.

Regardless of CD4 count or HIV RNA copy number, all HIV-infected pregnant women should receive a combination antepartum antiretroviral (ARV) drug regimen; this includes women who require therapy for their own health, as well as women who do not yet require therapy for their own health. ARV therapy should be started as soon as possible if required for the woman's health. Although earlier initiation may be more effective in reducing the perinatal transmission of HIV, also consider maternal conditions (eg, nausea and vomiting) and the potential risks of first trimester fetal exposure for specific agents. Plasma HIV RNA levels should be assessed at ~34-36 weeks gestation in order to help determine mode of delivery. If ARV therapy must be interrupted for <24 hours during the peripartum period, stop then restart all medications simultaneously in order to decrease the chance of developing resistance. Long-term follow-up is recommended for all infants exposed to ARV medications.

Healthcare providers are encouraged to enroll pregnant women exposed to antiretroviral medications in the Antiretroviral Pregnancy Registry (1-800-258-4263 or www.APRegistry.com). Healthcare providers caring for HIV-infected women and their infants may contact the National Perinatal HIV Hotline (888-448-8765) for clinical consultation (DHHS [perinatal], 2012).

Emtricitabine and Tenofovir
(em trye SYE ta been & te NOE fo veer)

Related Information

Emtricitabine *on page 473*

HIV Infection and AIDS *on page 1520*

Tenofovir *on page 1299*

Brand Names: U.S. Truvada®

Brand Names: Canada Truvada®

Pharmacologic Category Antiretroviral Agent, Reverse Transcriptase Inhibitor (Nucleoside); Antiretroviral Agent, Reverse Transcriptase Inhibitor (Nucleotide)

Use

Treatment of HIV-1 infection in combination with other antiretroviral agents in adults and pediatric patients ≥12 years of age

Pre-exposure prophylaxis (PrEP) for prevention of HIV-1 infection in adults who are at high risk for acquiring HIV

High risk individuals include those with partners known to be HIV-1 infected or who engage in sexual activity within a high prevalence area or social network, and one or more of the following:

- Inconsistent or no condom use

- Diagnosis of sexually-transmitted infections

- Exchange of sex for commodities

- Use of illicit drugs or alcohol dependence

- Incarceration

- Partner of unknown HIV-1 status with any of the above risk factors

When prescribing PrEP healthcare providers **MUST:**

- Include PrEP as part of a comprehensive prevention strategy because PrEP alone is not always effective in preventing HIV-1 infection

- Counsel all uninfected patients to strictly adhere to the dosing schedule, because adherence was strongly correlated with effectiveness in clinical trials

- Confirm a negative HIV-1 test prior to starting PrEP; if a candidate has acute viral infection symptoms and unprotected exposure events <1 month prior, delay PrEP for at least 1 month and retest HIV-1 status or use an Food and Drug Administration (FDA) test approved for HIV-1 diagnosis, including acute or primary HIV-1 infection
- Retest for HIV-1 infection at least every 3 months while the patient receives PrEP

Unlabeled Use Treatment of hepatitis B in patients with antiviral-resistant HBV or coinfection with HIV

Local Anesthetic/Vasoconstrictor Precautions No information available to require special precautions

Effects on Dental Treatment No significant effects or complications reported

Effects on Bleeding No information available to require special precautions related to hemostasis.

Adverse Effects The adverse reaction profile of combination therapy has not been established. See individual agents.

General Dosage Range Dosage adjustment recommended in patients with renal impairment

Oral: *Children ≥12 (and >35 kg), Adolescents (≥35 kg), and Adults:* 1 tablet (emtricitabine 200 mg and tenofovir 300 mg) once daily

Mechanism of Action Nucleoside and nucleotide reverse transcriptase inhibitor combination; emtricitabine is a cytosine analogue while tenofovir disoproxil fumarate (TDF) is an analog of adenosine 5'-monophosphate. Each drug interferes with HIV viral RNA dependent DNA polymerase resulting in inhibition of viral replication.

Pregnancy Risk Factor B

Pregnancy Considerations Although approved for use in combination with safer sex practices for the prevention of HIV-1 infection in adults who are at high risk for acquiring HIV (preexposure prophylaxis [PrEP]), data on use in heterosexual HIV serodiscordant couples wishing to conceive are limited. In addition, preconception use of PrEP in the uninfected partner when the HIV-infected partner is receiving antiretroviral therapy has not been studied. Women of reproductive age should have a pregnancy test prior to starting PrEP and at regular intervals during therapy. In addition to pregnancy testing, uninfected women considering PrEP therapy should also undergo screening for HIV and other sexually transmitted diseases. Serodiscordant couples wishing to conceive should seek expert consultation to determine the safest approach for their specific situation. If HIV infection is documented during PrEP therapy, the antiretroviral agents should be discontinued in order to minimize drug resistance. If pregnancy is detected during therapy, the potential risks and benefits of continuing PrEP during pregnancy should be discussed (DHHS [perinatal], 2012; CDC, 2012). Refer to individual monographs for additional information.

Healthcare providers are encouraged to enroll pregnant women exposed to antiretroviral medications in the Antiretroviral Pregnancy Registry (1-800-258-4263 or www.APRegistry.com). Healthcare providers caring for HIV-infected women and their infants may contact the National Perinatal HIV Hotline (888-448-8765) for clinical consultation (DHHS [perinatal], 2012).

Emtricitabine, Rilpivirine, and Tenofovir
(em trye SYE ta been, ril pi VIR een, & te NOE fo veer)

Related Information
HIV Infection and AIDS *on page 1520*
Brand Names: U.S. Complera™
Brand Names: Canada Complera™
Pharmacologic Category Antiretroviral Agent, Reverse Transcriptase Inhibitor (Non-nucleoside); Antiretroviral Agent, Reverse Transcriptase Inhibitor (Nucleoside); Antiretroviral Agent, Reverse Transcriptase Inhibitor (Nucleotide)

Use Treatment of human immunodeficiency virus type 1 (HIV-1) infection in antiretroviral treatment-naive patients with HIV-1 RNA ≤100,000 copies/mL at the start of therapy

Local Anesthetic/Vasoconstrictor Precautions No information available to require special precautions

Effects on Dental Treatment No significant effects or complications reported

Effects on Bleeding No information available to require special precautions

Adverse Effects Observed in patients receiving the same doses of emtricitabine, rilpivirine and tenofovir as the combination product; also see individual agents.
>10%:
Endocrine & metabolic: Cholesterol increased [≥200-239 mg/dL: (13%)], LDL increased [≥130 and <159 mg/dL: (11%)]
Hepatic: ALT increased [≤2.5 x ULN: (16%)], AST increased [≤2.5 x ULN: (13%)]
2% to 10%:
Central nervous system: Depression, headache, insomnia
Endocrine & metabolic: Cholesterol increased (≥240-300 mg/dL), LDL increased (≥ 160 and ≤ 190 mg/dL)
Hepatic: ALT increased (≥2.5 and ≤5 x ULN; >5 x ULN), AST increased (>2.5 and ≤5 x ULN), bilirubin increased (≤2.5 x ULN)
Renal: Creatinine increased (≥1.1 and ≤1.3 x ULN)

General Dosage Range Oral: *Adults:* One tablet once daily

Mechanism of Action Non-nucleoside, nucleoside, and nucleotide reverse transcriptase inhibitor combination; rilpivirine binds to reverse transcriptase and does not require intracellular phosphorylation for antiviral activity; emtricitabine is a cytosine analogue while tenofovir disoproxil fumarate (TDF) is an analog of adenosine 5'-monophosphate. Each drug interferes with HIV viral RNA dependent DNA polymerase activities resulting in inhibition of viral replication.

Pregnancy Risk Factor B

Pregnancy Considerations See individual agents.

Enalapril (e NAL a pril)

Related Information
Cardiovascular Diseases *on page 1492*
Brand Names: U.S. Vasotec®
Brand Names: Canada Apo-Enalapril®; CO Enalapril; Mylan-Enalapril; Novo-Enalapril; PMS-Enalapril; PRO-Enalapril; RAN™-Enalapril; ratio-Enalapril; Riva-Enalapril; Sandoz-Enalapril; Sig-Enalapril; Taro-Enalapril; Teva-Enalapril; Vasotec®
Generic Availability (U.S.) Yes

◀ **Pharmacologic Category** Angiotensin-Converting Enzyme (ACE) Inhibitor

Use Treatment of hypertension; treatment of symptomatic heart failure; treatment of asymptomatic left ventricular dysfunction

Unlabeled Use To delay the progression of nephropathy and reduce risks of cardiovascular events in hypertensive patients with type 1 or 2 diabetes mellitus; hypertensive crisis, diabetic nephropathy, hypertension secondary to scleroderma renal crisis, diagnosis of aldosteronism, idiopathic edema, Bartter's syndrome, postmyocardial infarction for prevention of ventricular failure

Local Anesthetic/Vasoconstrictor Precautions No information available to require special precautions

Effects on Dental Treatment Key adverse event(s) related to dental treatment: Abnormal taste and orthostatic hypotension

Effects on Bleeding No information available to require special precautions

Adverse Effects Note: Frequency ranges include data from hypertension and heart failure trials. Higher rates of adverse reactions have generally been noted in patients with CHF. However, the frequency of adverse effects associated with placebo is also increased in this population.

1% to 10%:
Cardiovascular: Hypotension (1% to 7%), chest pain (2%), syncope (≤2%), orthostasis (2%), orthostatic hypotension (2%)
Central nervous system: Headache (2% to 5%), dizziness (4% to 8%), fatigue (2% to 3%)
Dermatologic: Rash (2%)
Gastrointestinal: Abnormal taste, abdominal pain, vomiting, nausea, diarrhea, anorexia, constipation
Neuromuscular & skeletal: Weakness
Renal: Serum creatinine increased (≤20%), worsening of renal function (in patients with bilateral renal artery stenosis or hypovolemia)
Respiratory (1% to 2%): Bronchitis, cough, dyspnea

Dosage Use lower listed initial dose in patients with hyponatremia, hypovolemia, severe congestive heart failure, decreased renal function, or in those receiving diuretics.

Oral:
Children 1 month to 17 years: Hypertension: Initial: 0.08 mg/kg/day (up to 5 mg) in 1-2 divided doses; adjust dosage based on patient response; doses >0.58 mg/kg (40 mg) have not been evaluated in pediatric patients
Infants and Children: Heart failure (unlabeled dosing): Initial: 0.1 mg/kg/day in 1-2 divided doses; increase as required over 2 weeks to maximum of 0.5 mg/kg/day. **Note:** Mean dose required for CHF improvement in 39 children (9 days to 17 years) was 0.36 mg/kg/day; select individuals have been treated with doses up to 0.94 mg/kg/day (Leversha, 1994).
Adults:
Asymptomatic left ventricular dysfunction: 2.5 mg twice daily, titrated as tolerated to 20 mg/day
Heart failure: Initial: 2.5 mg once or twice daily (usual range: 5-40 mg/day in 2 divided doses); titrate slowly at 1- to 2-week intervals. Target dose: 10-20 mg twice daily (ACC/AHA 2009 Heart Failure Guidelines)
Hypertension: 2.5-5 mg/day then increase as required, usually at 1- to 2-week intervals; usual dose range (JNC 7): 2.5-40 mg/day in 1-2 divided doses. **Note:** Initiate with 2.5 mg if patient is taking

a diuretic which cannot be discontinued. May add a diuretic if blood pressure cannot be controlled with enalapril alone.
Conversion from I.V. **enalaprilat** to oral **enalapril** therapy: If not concurrently receiving diuretics, initiate enalapril 5 mg once daily; if concurrently receiving diuretics and responding to enalaprilat 0.625 mg I.V. every 6 hours, initiate with enalapril 2.5 mg once daily; subsequent titration as needed.

Dosing adjustment in renal impairment: Note: Use in infants and children ≤16 years of age with GFR <30 mL/minute/1.73 m² is not recommended (no dosing data exists).
Manufacturer's recommendations:
Cl_{cr} >30 mL/minute: No dosage adjustment necessary
Cl_{cr} ≤30 mL/minute: Administer 2.5 mg day; titrated upward until blood pressure is controlled.
Heart failure patients with sodium <130 mEq/L or serum creatinine >1.6 mg/dL: Initiate dosage with 2.5 mg/day, increasing to twice daily as needed. Increase further in increments of 2.5 mg/dose at >4-day intervals to a maximum daily dose of 40 mg.
Intermittent hemodialysis (IHD): Moderately dialyzable (20% to 50%): Initial: 2.5 mg on dialysis days; adjust dose on nondialysis days depending on blood pressure response.
Conversion from I.V. **enalaprilat** to oral **enalapril** therapy:
Cl_{cr} >30 mL/minute: May initiate enalapril 5 mg once daily.
Cl_{cr} ≤30 mL/minute: May initiate enalapril 2.5 mg once daily.
Alternate recommendations (Aronoff, 2007):
Cl_{cr} >50 mL/minute: No dosage adjustment necessary
Cl_{cr} 10-50 mL/minute: Administer 75-100% of usual dose
Cl_{cr} <10 mL/minute: Administer 50% of usual dose
Peritoneal dialysis: Supplemental dose is not necessary, although some removal of drug occurs.

Dosing adjustment in hepatic impairment: Hydrolysis of enalapril to enalaprilat may be delayed and/or impaired in patients with severe hepatic impairment, but the pharmacodynamic effects of the drug do not appear to be significantly altered; no dosage adjustment.

Mechanism of Action Competitive inhibitor of angiotensin-converting enzyme (ACE); prevents conversion of angiotensin I to angiotensin II, a potent vasoconstrictor; results in lower levels of angiotensin II which causes an increase in plasma renin activity and a reduction in aldosterone secretion

Contraindications Hypersensitivity to enalapril or enalaprilat; angioedema related to previous treatment with an ACE inhibitor; patients with idiopathic or hereditary angioedema; concomitant use with aliskiren in patients with diabetes mellitus

Warnings/Precautions Anaphylactic reactions may occur rarely with ACE inhibitors. At any time during treatment (especially following first dose) angioedema may occur rarely with ACE inhibitors; it may involve the head and neck (potentially compromising airway) or the intestine (presenting with abdominal pain). African-Americans may be at an increased risk. Prolonged frequent monitoring may be required especially if tongue, glottis, or larynx are involved as they are associated with airway obstruction. Patients with a history of airway surgery may have a higher risk of airway obstruction. Aggressive early and appropriate management is critical. Use in patients with idiopathic or hereditary angioedema or previous angioedema associated with ACE inhibitor therapy is contraindicated. Severe anaphylactoid reactions may be seen during hemodialysis (eg, CVVHD) with high-flux dialysis membranes (eg, AN69), and rarely, during low density lipoprotein apheresis with dextran sulfate cellulose. Rare cases of anaphylactoid reactions have been reported in patients undergoing sensitization treatment with hymenoptera (bee, wasp) venom while receiving ACE inhibitors.

Symptomatic hypotension with or without syncope can occur with ACE inhibitors (usually with the first several doses); effects are most often observed in volume depleted patients; correct volume depletion prior to initiation; close monitoring of patient is required especially with initial dosing and dosing increases; blood pressure must be lowered at a rate appropriate for the patient's clinical condition. Initiation of therapy in patients with ischemic heart disease or cerebrovascular disease warrants close observation due to the potential consequences posed by falling blood pressure (eg, MI, stroke). Use with caution in hypertrophic cardiomyopathy with outflow tract obstruction, severe aortic stenosis, or before, during, or immediately after major surgery. **[U.S. Boxed Warning]: Drugs that act on the renin-angiotensin system can cause injury and death to the developing fetus. Discontinue as soon as possible once pregnancy is detected.**

Hyperkalemia may occur with ACE inhibitors; risk factors include renal dysfunction, diabetes mellitus, concomitant use of potassium-sparing diuretics, potassium supplements, and/or potassium-containing salts. Use cautiously, if at all, with these agents and monitor potassium closely. Cough may occur with ACE inhibitors. Other causes of cough should be considered (eg, pulmonary congestion in patients with heart failure) and excluded prior to discontinuation.

May be associated with deterioration of renal function and/or increases in serum creatinine, particularly in patients with low renal blood flow (eg, renal artery stenosis, heart failure) whose glomerular filtration rate (GFR) is dependent on efferent arteriolar vasoconstriction by angiotensin II; deterioration may result in oliguria, acute renal failure, and progressive azotemia. Small increases in serum creatinine may occur following initiation; consider discontinuation only in patients with progressive and/or significant deterioration in renal function. Use with caution in patients with unstented unilateral/bilateral renal artery stenosis. When unstented bilateral renal artery stenosis is present, use is generally avoided due to the elevated risk of deterioration in renal function unless possible benefits outweigh risks. Concomitant use of an angiotensin receptor blocker (ARB) or renin inhibitor (eg, aliskiren) is associated with an increased risk of hypotension, hyperkalemia, and renal dysfunction; concomitant use with aliskiren should be avoided in patients with GFR <60 mL/minute and is contraindicated in patients with diabetes mellitus (regardless of GFR).

Rare toxicities associated with ACE inhibitors include cholestatic jaundice (which may progress to fulminant hepatic necrosis), agranulocytosis, neutropenia or leukopenia with myeloid hypoplasia. Patients with collagen vascular diseases (especially with concomitant renal impairment) or renal impairment alone may be at increased risk for hematologic toxicity; periodically monitor CBC with differential in these patients.

Drug Interactions
Metabolism/Transport Effects None known.
Avoid Concomitant Use There are no known interactions where it is recommended to avoid concomitant use.
Increased Effect/Toxicity
Enalapril may increase the levels/effects of: Allopurinol; Amifostine; Antihypertensives; AzaTHIOprine; CycloSPORINE (Systemic); Ferric Gluconate; Gold Sodium Thiomalate; Hypotensive Agents; Iron Dextran Complex; Lithium; Nonsteroidal Anti-Inflammatory Agents; RiTUXimab; Sodium Phosphates

The levels/effects of Enalapril may be increased by: Alfuzosin; Aliskiren; Angiotensin II Receptor Blockers; Canagliflozin; Diazoxide; DPP-IV Inhibitors; Eplerenone; Everolimus; Herbs (Hypotensive Properties); Loop Diuretics; MAO Inhibitors; Pentoxifylline; Phosphodiesterase 5 Inhibitors; Potassium Salts; Potassium-Sparing Diuretics; Prostacyclin Analogues; Sirolimus; Temsirolimus; Thiazide Diuretics; TiZANidine; Tolvaptan; Trimethoprim
Decreased Effect
The levels/effects of Enalapril may be decreased by: Antacids; Aprotinin; Herbs (Hypertensive Properties); Icatibant; Lanthanum; Methylphenidate; Nonsteroidal Anti-Inflammatory Agents; Salicylates; Yohimbine
Ethanol/Nutrition/Herb Interactions
Food: Potassium supplements and/or potassium-containing salts may cause or worsen hyperkalemia. Management: Consult prescriber before consuming a potassium-rich diet, potassium supplements, or salt substitutes.
Herb/Nutraceutical: Some herbal medications may worsen hypertension (eg, licorice); others may increase the antihypertensive effect of enalapril (eg, shepherd's purse). Management: Avoid bayberry, blue cohosh, cayenne, ephedra, ginger, ginseng (American), kola, licorice, and yohimbe. Avoid black cohosh, California poppy, coleus, golden seal, hawthorn, mistletoe, periwinkle, quinine, and shepherd's purse.
Dietary Considerations Limit salt substitutes or potassium-rich diet.
Pharmacodynamics/Kinetics
Onset of Action ~1 hour; Peak effect: 4-6 hours
Duration of Action 12-24 hours
Half-life Elimination
Enalapril: Adults: Healthy: 2 hours; Congestive heart failure: 3.4-5.8 hours
Enalaprilat: Infants 6 weeks to 8 months of age: 6-10 hours (Lloyd, 1989); Adults: ~35 hours (Till, 1984; Ulm, 1982)
Time to Peak Serum: Oral: Enalapril: 0.5-1.5 hours; Enalaprilat (active metabolite): 3-4.5 hours
Pregnancy Risk Factor D
Pregnancy Considerations [U.S. Boxed Warning]: Drugs that act on the renin-angiotensin system can cause injury and death to the developing fetus. Discontinue as soon as possible once pregnancy is detected. Enalaprilat, the active metabolite of enalapril, crosses the placenta; teratogenic effects may occur following maternal use during pregnancy. Drugs that act on the renin-angiotensin system are associated with oligohydramnios. Oligohydramnios, due to decreased fetal renal function, may lead to fetal lung hypoplasia and skeletal malformations. The use of these drugs in pregnancy is also associated with anuria, hypotension, renal failure, skull hypoplasia, and death in the fetus/neonate. Chronic maternal hypertension itself is also associated with adverse events in the ▶

◄ fetus/infant. ACE inhibitors are not recommended during pregnancy to treat maternal hypertension or heart failure. Use of an ACE inhibitor should also be avoided in any woman of reproductive age. Women who are planning a pregnancy should be considered for other medication options if an ACE inhibitor is currently prescribed or the ACE inhibitor should be discontinued as soon as possible once pregnancy is detected. The exposed fetus should be monitored for fetal growth, amniotic fluid volume, and organ formation. Infants exposed to an ACE inhibitor *in utero* should be monitored for hyperkalemia, hypotension, and oliguria.

Lactation Enters breast milk/not recommended (AAP rates "compatible"; AAP 2001 update pending)

Breast-Feeding Considerations Enalapril and enalaprilat are excreted in breast milk. Breast-feeding is not recommended by the manufacturer.

Dosage Forms
Tablet, oral: 2.5 mg, 5 mg, 10 mg, 20 mg
Vasotec®: 2.5 mg, 5 mg, 10 mg, 20 mg

Enalapril and Hydrochlorothiazide
(e NAL a pril & hye droe klor oh THYE a zide)

Related Information
Enalapril *on page 475*
Hydrochlorothiazide *on page 687*
Brand Names: U.S. Vaseretic®
Brand Names: Canada Vaseretic®
Pharmacologic Category Angiotensin-Converting Enzyme (ACE) Inhibitor; Diuretic, Thiazide
Use Treatment of hypertension
Local Anesthetic/Vasoconstrictor Precautions No information available to require special precautions
Effects on Dental Treatment No significant effects or complications reported
Effects on Bleeding No information available to require special precautions
Adverse Effects See individual agents.
General Dosage Range Oral: *Adults:* Enalapril 5-10 mg and hydrochlorothiazide 12.5-25 mg once daily (maximum: 40 mg/day [enalapril]; 50 mg/day [hydrochlorothiazide])
Pregnancy Risk Factor D
Pregnancy Considerations [U.S. Boxed Warning]: Drugs that act on the renin-angiotensin system can cause injury and death to the developing fetus. Discontinue as soon as possible once pregnancy is detected. See individual agents.

Enalaprilat (en AL a pril at)

Brand Names: Canada Vasotec® I.V
Pharmacologic Category Angiotensin-Converting Enzyme (ACE) Inhibitor
Use Treatment of hypertension when oral therapy is not practical
Unlabeled Use Severe congestive heart failure in infants, acute cardiogenic pulmonary edema
Local Anesthetic/Vasoconstrictor Precautions No information available to require special precautions
Effects on Dental Treatment Key adverse event(s) related to dental treatment: Abnormal taste and orthostatic hypotension
Effects on Bleeding No information available to require special precautions

Adverse Effects Note: Since enalapril is converted to enalaprilat, adverse reactions associated with enalapril may also occur with enalaprilat (also refer to Enalapril monograph). Frequency ranges include data from hypertension and heart failure trials. Higher rates of adverse reactions have generally been noted in patients with CHF. However, the frequency of adverse effects associated with placebo is also increased in this population.

1% to 10%:
Cardiovascular: Hypotension (2% to 5%)
Central nervous system: Headache (3%)
Gastrointestinal: Nausea (1%)

General Dosage Range Dosage adjustment recommended in patients with renal impairment.
I.V.: *Adults:* 0.625-5 mg every 6 hours

Mechanism of Action Competitive inhibitor of angiotensin-converting enzyme (ACE); prevents conversion of angiotensin I to angiotensin II, a potent vasoconstrictor; results in lower levels of angiotensin II which causes an increase in plasma renin activity and a reduction in aldosterone secretion

Pharmacodynamics/Kinetics
Onset of Action I.V.: ≤15 minutes; Peak effect: I.V.: 1-4 hours
Duration of Action I.V.: ~6 hours
Half-life Elimination Infants 6 weeks to 8 months of age: 6-10 hours (Lloyd, 1989); Adults: ~35 hours (Till, 1984; Ulm, 1982)
Pregnancy Risk Factor C (1st trimester); D (2nd and 3rd trimesters)
Pregnancy Considerations [U.S. Boxed Warning]: Drugs that act on the renin-angiotensin system can cause injury and death to the developing fetus. Discontinue as soon as possible once pregnancy is detected. Enalaprilat, the active metabolite of enalapril, crosses the placenta; teratogenic effects may occur following maternal use during pregnancy. Drugs that act on the renin-angiotensin system are associated with oligohydramnios. Oligohydramnios, due to decreased fetal renal function, may lead to fetal lung hypoplasia and skeletal malformations. The use of these drugs in pregnancy is also associated with anuria, hypotension, renal failure, skull hypoplasia, and death in the fetus/neonate. Chronic maternal hypertension itself is also associated with adverse events in the fetus/infant. ACE inhibitors are not recommended during pregnancy to treat maternal hypertension or heart failure. Use of an ACE inhibitor should also be avoided in any woman of reproductive age. Women who are planning a pregnancy should be considered for other medication options if an ACE inhibitor is currently prescribed or the ACE inhibitor should be discontinued as soon as possible once pregnancy is detected. The exposed fetus should be monitored for fetal growth, amniotic fluid volume, and organ formation. Infants exposed to an ACE inhibitor *in utero* should be monitored for hyperkalemia, hypotension, and oliguria.

Enfuvirtide (en FYOO vir tide)

Related Information
HIV Infection and AIDS *on page 1520*
Brand Names: U.S. Fuzeon®
Brand Names: Canada Fuzeon®
Pharmacologic Category Antiretroviral Agent, Fusion Protein Inhibitor

Use Treatment of HIV-1 infection in combination with other antiretroviral agents in treatment-experienced patients with evidence of HIV-1 replication despite ongoing antiretroviral therapy

Local Anesthetic/Vasoconstrictor Precautions No information available to require special precautions

Effects on Dental Treatment Key adverse event(s) related to dental treatment: Xerostomia (normal salivary flow resumes upon discontinuation) and taste disturbance

Effects on Bleeding No information available to require special precautions related to hemostasis.

Adverse Effects

>10%:
Gastrointestinal: Diarrhea (32%), nausea (23%)
Local: Injection site infection (children 11%), injection site reactions (98%; may include pain, erythema, induration, pruritus, ecchymosis, nodule or cyst formation)

1% to 10%:
Dermatologic: Folliculitis (2%)
Gastrointestinal: Weight loss (7%), abdominal pain (4%), appetite decreased (3%), pancreatitis (3%), anorexia (2%), xerostomia (2%)
Hematologic: Eosinophilia (2% to 9%)
Hepatic: Transaminases increased (4%, grade 4: 1%)
Local: Injection site infection (adults 2%)
Neuromuscular & skeletal: CPK increased (3% to 7%), limb pain (3%), myalgia (3%)
Ocular: Conjunctivitis (2%)
Respiratory: Sinusitis (6%), cough (4%), bacterial pneumonia (3%)
Miscellaneous: Infections (4% to 6%), herpes simplex (4%), flu-like syndrome (2%)

General Dosage Range Dosage adjustment recommended in patients with renal impairment

SubQ:
Children 6-16 years: 2 mg/kg twice daily (maximum: 90 mg/dose)
Adolescents ≥16 years and Adults: 90 mg twice daily

Mechanism of Action Binds to the first heptad-repeat (HR1) in the gp41 subunit of the viral envelope glycoprotein. Inhibits the fusion of HIV-1 virus with CD4 cells by blocking the conformational change in gp41 required for membrane fusion and entry into CD4 cells

Pharmacodynamics/Kinetics

Half-life Elimination 3.8 hours

Time to Peak 4-8 hours

Pregnancy Risk Factor B

Pregnancy Considerations Teratogenic effects were not observed in animal studies. Limited data suggest that enfuvirtide does not cross the placenta. The DHHS Perinatal HIV Guidelines note that data are insufficient to recommend use during pregnancy.

Regardless of CD4 count or HIV RNA copy number, all HIV-infected pregnant women should receive a combination antepartum antiretroviral (ARV) drug regimen; this includes women who require therapy for their own health, as well as women who do not yet require therapy for their own health. ARV therapy should be started as soon as possible if required for the woman's health. Although earlier initiation may be more effective in reducing the perinatal transmission of HIV, also consider maternal conditions (eg, nausea and vomiting) and the potential risks of first trimester fetal exposure for specific agents. Plasma HIV RNA levels should be assessed at ~34-36 weeks gestation in order to help determine mode of delivery. If ARV therapy must be interrupted for <24 hours during the peripartum period, stop then restart all medications simultaneously in order to decrease the chance of developing resistance. Long-term follow-up is recommended for all infants exposed to ARV medications.

Healthcare providers are encouraged to enroll pregnant women exposed to antiretroviral medications in the Antiretroviral Pregnancy Registry (1-800-258-4263 or www.APRegistry.com). Healthcare providers caring for HIV-infected women and their infants may contact the National Perinatal HIV Hotline (888-448-8765) for clinical consultation (DHHS [perinatal], 2012).

Enoxaparin (ee noks a PA rin)

Related Information
Cardiovascular Diseases *on page 1492*

Brand Names: U.S. Lovenox®

Brand Names: Canada Enoxaparin Injection; Lovenox®; Lovenox® HP

Pharmacologic Category Low Molecular Weight Heparin

Use
Acute coronary syndromes: Unstable angina (UA), non-ST-elevation (NSTEMI), and ST-elevation myocardial infarction (STEMI)
DVT prophylaxis: Following hip or knee replacement surgery, abdominal surgery, or in medical patients with severely-restricted mobility during acute illness who are at risk for thromboembolic complications
Note: Patients at risk of thromboembolic complications who undergo abdominal surgery include those with one or more of the following risk factors: >40 years of age, obesity, general anesthesia lasting >30 minutes, malignancy, history of deep vein thrombosis or pulmonary embolism
DVT treatment (acute): Inpatient treatment (patients with or without pulmonary embolism) and outpatient treatment (patients without pulmonary embolism)

Unlabeled Use Prophylaxis and treatment of thromboembolism in children; anticoagulant bridge therapy during temporary interruption of vitamin K antagonist therapy in patients at high risk for thromboembolism; DVT prophylaxis following moderate-risk general surgery, major gynecologic surgery and following higher-risk general surgery for cancer; management of venous thromboembolism (VTE) during pregnancy; anticoagulant used during percutaneous coronary intervention (PCI)

Local Anesthetic/Vasoconstrictor Precautions No information available to require special precautions

Effects on Dental Treatment Key adverse event(s) related to dental treatment: Bleeding is the major adverse effect of enoxaparin. See Effects on Bleeding.

Effects on Bleeding As with all anticoagulants, bleeding is the major adverse effect of enoxaparin. Hemorrhage may occur at virtually any site. Routine coagulation tests, such as prothrombin time (PT) and aPTT, are relatively insensitive measures of enoxaparin injection activity and, therefore, unsuitable for monitoring. Moderate thrombocytopenia occurred at a rate of ~1%. Medical consult is suggested.

Adverse Effects As with all anticoagulants, bleeding is the major adverse effect of enoxaparin. Hemorrhage may occur at virtually any site. Risk is dependent on multiple variables. At the recommended doses, single injections of enoxaparin do not significantly influence platelet aggregation or affect global clotting time (ie, PT or aPTT).

◀ 1% to 10%:
Central nervous system: Fever (5% to 8%), confusion (2%), pain
Dermatologic: Bruising
Gastrointestinal: Nausea (3%), diarrhea (2%)
Hematologic: Hemorrhage (major, <1% to 4%; includes cases of intracranial, retroperitoneal, or intraocular hemorrhage; incidence varies with indication/population), thrombocytopenia (moderate 1%; severe 0.1% - see **"Note"** below), anemia (<2%)
Hepatic: ALT increased (6%), AST increased (6%)
Local: Injection site hematoma (9%), local reactions (irritation, pain, ecchymosis, erythema)
Renal: Hematuria (≤2%)
Note: Thrombocytopenia with thrombosis: Cases of heparin-induced thrombocytopenia (some complicated by organ infarction, limb ischemia, or death) have been reported.

General Dosage Range Dosage varies greatly depending on indication.

Mechanism of Action Standard heparin consists of components with molecular weights ranging from 4000-30,000 daltons with a mean of 16,000 daltons. Heparin acts as an anticoagulant by enhancing the inhibition rate of clotting proteases by antithrombin III impairing normal hemostasis and inhibition of factor Xa. Low molecular weight heparins have a small effect on the activated partial thromboplastin time and strongly inhibit factor Xa. Enoxaparin is derived from porcine heparin that undergoes benzylation followed by alkaline depolymerization. The average molecular weight of enoxaparin is 4500 daltons which is distributed as (≤20%) 2000 daltons (≥68%) 2000-8000 daltons, and (≤15%) >8000 daltons. Enoxaparin has a higher ratio of antifactor Xa to antifactor IIa activity than unfractionated heparin.

Pharmacodynamics/Kinetics
Onset of Action Peak effect: SubQ: Antifactor Xa and antithrombin (antifactor IIa): 3-5 hours
Duration of Action 40 mg dose: Antifactor Xa activity: ~12 hours
Half-life Elimination Plasma: 2-4 times longer than standard heparin, independent of dose; based on anti-Xa activity: 4.5-7 hours

Pregnancy Risk Factor B
Pregnancy Considerations Adverse events were not observed in animal reproduction studies. Low molecular weight heparin (LMWH) does not cross the placenta; increased risks of fetal bleeding or teratogenic effects have not been reported.

LMWH is recommended over unfractionated heparin for the treatment of acute venous thromboembolism (VTE) in pregnant women. LMWH is also recommended over unfractionated heparin for VTE prophylaxis in pregnant women with certain risk factors (eg, homozygous factor V Leiden, antiphospholipid antibody syndrome with ≥3 previous pregnancy losses). Prophylaxis is not routinely recommended for women undergoing assisted reproduction therapy; however, LMWH therapy is recommended for women who develop severe ovarian hyperstimulation syndrome. LMWH should be discontinued at least 24 hours prior to induction of labor or a planned cesarean delivery. For women undergoing cesarean section and who have additional risk factors for developing VTE, the prophylactic use of LMWH may be considered.

LMWH may also be used in women with mechanical heart valves (consult current ACCP guidelines for details). Women who require long-term anticoagulation with warfarin and who are considering pregnancy, LMWH substitution should be done prior to conception when possible. When choosing therapy, fetal outcomes (ie, pregnancy loss, malformations), maternal outcomes (ie, VTE, hemorrhage), burden of therapy, and maternal preference should be considered (Guyatt, 2012). Monitoring antifactor Xa levels is recommended.

Multiple-dose vials contain benzyl alcohol (avoid in pregnant women due to association with gasping syndrome in premature infants); use of preservative-free formulations is recommended.

Entacapone (en TA ka pone)

Brand Names: U.S. Comtan®
Brand Names: Canada Comtan®; Sandoz-Entacapone; Teva-Entacapone
Pharmacologic Category Anti-Parkinson's Agent, COMT Inhibitor
Use Adjunct to levodopa/carbidopa therapy in patients with idiopathic Parkinson's disease who experience "wearing-off" symptoms at the end of a dosing interval
Local Anesthetic/Vasoconstrictor Precautions No information available to require special precautions
Effects on Dental Treatment Key adverse event(s) related to dental treatment: Orthostatic hypotension and abnormal taste. Dopaminergic therapy in Parkinson's disease (ie, treatment with levodopa) is associated with orthostatic hypotension. Entacapone enhances levodopa bioavailability and may increase the occurrence of hypotension/syncope in the dental patient. The patient should be carefully assisted from the chair and observed for signs of orthostatic hypotension.
Effects on Bleeding No information available to require special precautions
Adverse Effects
>10%:
Gastrointestinal: Nausea (14%)
Neuromuscular & skeletal: Dyskinesia (25%), placebo (15%)
1% to 10%:
Cardiovascular: Orthostatic hypotension (4%), syncope (1%)
Central nervous system: Dizziness (8%), fatigue (6%), hallucinations (4%), anxiety (2%), somnolence (2%), agitation (1%)
Dermatologic: Purpura (2%)
Gastrointestinal: Diarrhea (10%), abdominal pain (8%), constipation (6%), vomiting (4%), dry mouth (3%), dyspepsia (2%), flatulence (2%), gastritis (1%), taste perversion (1%)
Genitourinary: Brown-orange urine discoloration (10%)
Neuromuscular & skeletal: Hyperkinesia (10%), hypokinesia (9%), back pain (4%), weakness (2%)
Respiratory: Dyspnea (3%)
Miscellaneous: Diaphoresis increased (2%), bacterial infection (1%)
General Dosage Range Oral: *Adults:* 200 mg with each dose of levodopa/carbidopa (maximum: 1600 mg/day)
Mechanism of Action Entacapone is a reversible and selective inhibitor of catechol-O-methyltransferase (COMT). When entacapone is taken with levodopa, the pharmacokinetics are altered, resulting in more sustained levodopa serum levels compared to levodopa taken alone. The resulting levels of levodopa provide for

increased concentrations available for absorption across the blood-brain barrier, thereby providing for increased CNS levels of dopamine, the active metabolite of levodopa.

Pharmacodynamics/Kinetics

Onset of Action Rapid; Peak effect: 1 hour

Half-life Elimination B phase: 0.4-0.7 hours; Y phase: 2.4 hours

Time to Peak Serum: 1 hour

Pregnancy Risk Factor C

Pregnancy Considerations Not recommended

Entecavir (en TE ka veer)

Related Information

HIV Infection and AIDS *on page 1520*

Systemic Viral Diseases *on page 1537*

Brand Names: U.S. Baraclude®

Brand Names: Canada Baraclude®

Pharmacologic Category Antiretroviral Agent, Reverse Transcriptase Inhibitor (Nucleoside)

Use Treatment of chronic hepatitis B virus (HBV) infection, with compensated or decompensated liver disease, in patients with evidence of active viral replication and either evidence of persistent transaminase elevations or histologically-active disease

Unlabeled Use HBV reinfection prophylaxis, post liver transplant; HIV/HBV coinfection

Local Anesthetic/Vasoconstrictor Precautions No information available to require special precautions

Effects on Dental Treatment No significant effects or complications reported

Effects on Bleeding No information available to require special precautions related to hemostasis.

Adverse Effects

>10%:

Cardiovascular: Peripheral edema (16% with decompensated liver disease)

Central nervous system: Pyrexia (14% with decompensated liver disease)

Hepatic: Ascites (15% with decompensated liver disease), ALT increased (>5 x ULN: 11% to 12%; post-treatment flare [lamivudine refractory]: >10 x ULN and >2 x baseline: 12%)

1% to 10%:

Central nervous system: Headache (2% to 4%), fatigue (1% to 3%), dizziness

Endocrine & metabolic: Hyperglycemia (2% to 3%), blood bicarbonate decreased (2% with decompensated liver disease)

Gastrointestinal: Lipase increased (7%), amylase increased (2% to 3%), diarrhea (≤1%), dyspepsia (≤1%), nausea

Hepatic: Hepatic encephalopathy (10% with decompensated liver disease), bilirubin increased (2% to 3%), ALT increased (>10 x ULN and >2 x baseline: 2%; post-treatment flare [nucleoside-naive]: >10 x ULN and >2 x baseline: 2% to 8%)

Renal: Hematuria (9%), glycosuria (4%), creatinine increased (1% to 2%)

Respiratory: Upper respiratory tract infection (10% with decompensated liver disease)

General Dosage Range Dosage adjustment recommended in patients with renal impairment.

Oral: *Adolescents ≥16 years and Adults:* 0.5-1 mg once daily

Mechanism of Action Entecavir is intracellularly phosphorylated to guanosine triphosphate which competes with natural substrates to effectively inhibit hepatitis B viral polymerase; enzyme inhibition blocks reverse transcriptase activity thereby reducing viral DNA synthesis.

Pharmacodynamics/Kinetics

Half-life Elimination Terminal: ~5-6 days; accumulation: ~24 hours

Time to Peak 0.5-1.5 hours

Pregnancy Risk Factor C

Pregnancy Considerations Teratogenic effects have been observed in animal studies. There are no adequate and well-controlled studies in pregnant women. Use only if benefit outweighs risk. Pregnant women taking entecavir should enroll in the pregnancy registry by calling 1-800-258-4263.

Enzalutamide (en za LOO ta mide)

Brand Names: U.S. Xtandi®

Pharmacologic Category Antiandrogen; Antineoplastic Agent, Antiandrogen

Use Treatment of metastatic, castration-resistant prostate cancer in patients previously treated with docetaxel

Local Anesthetic/Vasoconstrictor Precautions No information available to require special precautions

Effects on Dental Treatment No significant effects or complications reported

Effects on Bleeding Although significant myelosuppression with associated altered hemostasis has been reported for many chemotherapeutic agents, myelosuppression is not common with enzalutamide and no specific precautions appear to necessary.

Adverse Effects

>10%:

Cardiovascular: Peripheral edema (15%)

Central nervous system: Fatigue (51%), headache (12%)

Endocrine & metabolic: Hot flashes (20%)

Gastrointestinal: Diarrhea (22%)

Hematologic: Neutropenia (15%; grades 3/4: 1%)

Neuromuscular & skeletal: Back pain (26%), arthralgia (21%), musculoskeletal pain (15%)

Respiratory: Upper respiratory tract infection (11%)

1% to 10%:

Cardiovascular: Hypertension (6%)

Central nervous system: Dizziness (10%), insomnia (9%), anxiety (7%), hypoesthesia (4%), mental impairment (4%), hallucinations (2%)

Dermatologic: Dry skin (4%), pruritus (4%)

Genitourinary: Hematuria (7%), pollakiuria (5%)

Hepatic: Bilirubin increased (3%)

Neuromuscular & skeletal: Muscle weakness (10%), paresthesia (7%), falling (5%), fractures (4%), stiffness (3%)

Respiratory: Lower respiratory tract infection (9%), epistaxis (3%)

Miscellaneous: Infection (≤6%; including sepsis)

General Dosage Range Dosage adjustment recommended in patients on concomitant therapy or who develop toxicities.

Oral: *Adults:* 160 mg once daily

Mechanism of Action Enzalutamide is a pure androgen receptor signaling inhibitor; unlike other antiandrogen therapies, it has no known agonistic properties. It inhibits androgen receptor nuclear translocation, DNA binding, and coactivator mobilization, leading to cellular apoptosis and decreased prostate tumor volume.

Pharmacodynamics/Kinetics
Half-life Elimination 5.8 days (range: 2.8-10.2 days)
Time to Peak 1 hour (range: 0.5-3 hours)
Pregnancy Risk Factor X
Pregnancy Considerations Enzalutamide is an androgen receptor inhibitor. Although animal reproduction studies have not been conducted, it is expected to cause fetal harm based on its mechanism of action. Enzalutamide is not indicated for use in women and is specifically contraindicated for use in women who are or may become pregnant. Men using this medication should use a condom if having intercourse with a pregnant woman. A condom plus another effective method of birth control is recommended during therapy and for 3 months after treatment for men using this medication and who are having intercourse with a woman of reproductive potential.

EPHEDrine (Systemic) (e FED rin)

Pharmacologic Category Alpha/Beta Agonist
Use Treatment of nasal congestion, anesthesia-induced hypotension
Unlabeled Use Postoperative nausea and vomiting (PONV) refractory to traditional antiemetics; idiopathic orthostatic hypotension
Local Anesthetic/Vasoconstrictor Precautions Use vasoconstrictor with caution since ephedrine may enhance cardiostimulation and vasopressor effects of sympathomimetics such as epinephrine
Effects on Dental Treatment Key adverse event(s) related to dental treatment: Xerostomia (normal salivary flow resumes upon discontinuation)
Effects on Bleeding No information available to require special precautions
Adverse Effects Frequency not defined.
Cardiovascular: Arrhythmias, chest pain, elevation or depression of blood pressure, hypertension, palpitation, tachycardia, unusual pallor
Central nervous system: Agitation, anxiety, apprehension, CNS stimulating effects, dizziness, excitation, fear, headache hyperactivity, insomnia, irritability, nervousness, restlessness, tension
Gastrointestinal: Anorexia, GI upset, nausea, vomiting, xerostomia
Genitourinary: Painful urination
Neuromuscular & skeletal: Trembling, tremor (more common in the elderly), weakness
Respiratory: Dyspnea
Miscellaneous: Diaphoresis increased
General Dosage Range
I.V.:
Children: 0.2-0.3 mg/kg/dose every 4-6 hours
Adults: 5-25 mg/dose; repeat after 5-10 minutes as needed, then every 3-4 hours (maximum: 150 mg/day)
Oral: Children ≥12 years and Adults: 12.5-50 mg every 4 hours as needed (maximum: 150 mg/day)
Mechanism of Action Releases tissue stores of norepinephrine and thereby produces an alpha- and beta-adrenergic stimulation; longer-acting and less potent than epinephrine
Pharmacodynamics/Kinetics
Duration of Action Oral: 3-6 hours
Half-life Elimination 2.5-3.6 hours
Pregnancy Risk Factor C

Pregnancy Considerations Animal reproduction studies have not been conducted. Ephedrine crosses the placenta (Hughes, 1985). Ephedrine injection is used at delivery for the prevention and/or treatment of maternal hypotension associated with spinal anesthesia in women undergoing cesarean section (ASA, 2007).

Epinastine (ep i NAS teen)

Brand Names: U.S. Elestat®
Pharmacologic Category Histamine H_1 Antagonist; Histamine H_1 Antagonist, Second Generation
Use Treatment of allergic conjunctivitis
Local Anesthetic/Vasoconstrictor Precautions No information available to require special precautions
Effects on Dental Treatment No significant effects or complications reported
Effects on Bleeding No information available to require special precautions
Adverse Effects 1% to 10%:
Central nervous system: Headache (1% to 3%)
Ocular: Burning sensation, folliculosis, hyperemia, pruritus
Respiratory: Cough (1% to 3%), pharyngitis (1% to 3%), rhinitis (1% to 3%), sinusitis (1% to 3%)
Miscellaneous: Infection (10%; defined as cold symptoms and upper respiratory infection)
General Dosage Range Ophthalmic: Children ≥2 years and Adults: Instill 1 drop into each eye twice daily
Mechanism of Action Selective H_1-receptor antagonist; inhibits release of histamine from the mast cell; also has affinity for the H_2, alpha$_1$, alpha$_2$, and the 5-HT$_2$ receptors
Pharmacodynamics/Kinetics
Onset of Action 3-5 minutes
Duration of Action 8 hours
Half-life Elimination 12 hours
Pregnancy Risk Factor C
Pregnancy Considerations Teratogenic effects were not observed in animal studies. There are no adequate and well-controlled studies in pregnant women.

EPINEPHrine (Systemic, Oral Inhalation) (ep i NEF rin)

Brand Names: U.S. Adrenalin®; Asthmanefrin™ [OTC]; Auvi-Q™; EpiPen 2-Pak®; EpiPen Jr 2-Pak®; S2® [OTC]; Twinject® [DSC]
Brand Names: Canada Adrenalin®; Epi E-Z Pen®; EpiPen®; EpiPen® Jr; Twinject®
Generic Availability (U.S.) Yes: Solution for injection
Pharmacologic Category Alpha/Beta Agonist
Dental Use Emergency drug for treatment of anaphylactic reactions; used as vasoconstrictor to prolong local anesthesia
Use Treatment of bronchospasms, bronchial asthma, viral croup, anaphylactic reactions, cardiac arrest; added to local anesthetics to decrease systemic absorption of intraspinal and local anesthetics and increase duration of action; decrease superficial hemorrhage; induction and maintenance of mydriasis during intraocular surgery
Unlabeled Use ACLS guidelines: Ventricular fibrillation (VF) or pulseless ventricular tachycardia (VT) unresponsive to initial defibrillatory shocks; pulseless electrical activity; asystole; hypotension/shock unresponsive to volume resuscitation; symptomatic bradycardia unresponsive to atropine or pacing; inotropic support

Local Anesthetic/Vasoconstrictor Precautions No information available to require special precautions

Effects on Dental Treatment Key adverse event(s) related to dental treatment: Xerostomia (normal salivary flow resumes upon discontinuation) and dry throat.

Effects on Bleeding No information available to require special precautions

Adverse Effects Frequency not defined.

Cardiovascular: Angina, cardiac arrhythmia, chest pain, flushing, hypertension, pallor, palpitation, sudden death, tachycardia (parenteral), vasoconstriction, ventricular ectopy, ventricular fibrillation

Central nervous system: Anxiety (transient), apprehensiveness, cerebral hemorrhage, dizziness, headache, insomnia, lightheadedness, nervousness, restlessness

Gastrointestinal: Dry throat, loss of appetite, nausea, vomiting, xerostomia

Genitourinary: Acute urinary retention in patients with bladder outflow obstruction

Neuromuscular & skeletal: Tremor, weakness

Ocular: Allergic lid reaction, burning, corneal endothelial damage (intraocular use), eye pain, ocular irritation, precipitation of or exacerbation of narrow-angle glaucoma, transient stinging

Respiratory: Dyspnea, pulmonary edema

Miscellaneous: Diaphoresis

Dental Usual Dosage Hypersensitivity reaction: Self-administration following severe allergic reactions (eg, insect stings, food): **Note:** World Health Organization (WHO) and Anaphylaxis Canada recommend the availability of 1 dose for every 10-20 minutes of travel time to a medical emergency facility. More than 2 sequential doses should only be administered under direct medical supervision.

Children:

Auvi-Q™: I.M., SubQ:

Children 15-29 kg: 0.15 mg; if anaphylactic symptoms persist, dose may be repeated

Children ≥30 kg: 0.3 mg; if anaphylactic symptoms persist, dose may be repeated

EpiPen® Jr: I.M., SubQ: Children 15-29 kg: 0.15 mg; if anaphylactic symptoms persist, dose may be repeated in 5-15 minutes using an additional EpiPen® Jr

EpiPen®: I.M., SubQ: Children ≥30 kg: 0.3 mg; if anaphylactic symptoms persist, dose may be repeated in 5-15 minutes using an additional EpiPen®

Twinject®: I.M. SubQ:

Children 15-29 kg: 0.15 mg; if anaphylactic symptoms persist, dose may be repeated in 5-15 minutes using the same device after partial disassembly

Children ≥30 kg: 0.3 mg; if anaphylactic symptoms persist, dose may be repeated in 5-15 minutes using the same device after partial disassembly

Adults:

Auvi-Q™: I.M., SubQ: 0.3 mg; if anaphylactic symptoms persist, dose may be repeated

EpiPen®: I.M., SubQ: 0.3 mg; if anaphylactic symptoms persist, dose may be repeated in 5-15 minutes using an additional EpiPen®

Twinject®: I.M., SubQ: 0.3 mg; if anaphylactic symptoms persist, dose may be repeated in 5-15 minutes using the same device after partial disassembly

Dosage

Infants and Children:

Asystole/pulseless arrest, pulseless VT/VF (after failed defibrillation attempts) (PALS, 2010):

I.V., I.O.: 0.01 mg/kg (0.1 mL/kg of **1:10,000** [0.1 mg/mL] solution) (maximum single dose: 1 mg) every 3-5 minutes until return of spontaneous circulation

Endotracheal: 0.1 mg/kg (0.1 mL/kg of **1:1000** [1 mg/mL] solution) (maximum single dose: 2.5 mg) every 3-5 minutes until I.V./I.O. access established or return of spontaneous circulation. Flush with 5 mL of NS immediately after administration. May cause false-negative reading with exhaled CO_2 detectors; use second method to confirm tube placement if CO_2 is not detected (Neumar, 2010).

Postresuscitation infusion to maintain cardiac output or stabilize: I.V., I.O.: 0.1-1 mcg/kg/minute; doses <0.3 mcg/kg/minute generally produce beta-adrenergic effects and higher doses (>0.3 mcg/kg/minute) generally produce alpha-adrenergic vasoconstriction; titrate dosage to desired effect

Bradycardia (symptomatic; unresponsive to atropine or pacing):

I.V., I.O.: 0.01 mg/kg (0.1 mL/kg of **1:10,000** [0.1 mg/mL] solution) (maximum single dose: 1 mg) every 3-5 minutes as needed

Endotracheal: 0.1 mg/kg or (0.1 mL/kg of **1:1000** [1 mg/mL] solution) (maximum single dose: 2.5 mg) every 3-5 minutes as needed until I.V./I.O. access established. Flush with 5 mL of NS immediately after administration. May cause false-negative reading with exhaled CO_2 detectors; use second method to confirm tube placement if CO_2 is not detected (Neumar, 2010).

Continuous infusion: I.V., I.O.: 0.1-1 mcg/kg/minute; doses <0.3 mcg/kg/minute generally produce beta-adrenergic effects and higher doses (>0.3 mcg/kg/minute) generally produce alpha-adrenergic vasoconstriction; titrate dosage to desired effect

Bronchodilator:

SubQ: 0.01 mg/kg (0.01 mL/kg of **1:1000** [1 mg/mL] solution) (maximum single dose: 0.5 mg) every 20 minutes for 3 doses

Nebulization: S2® (racepinephrine, OTC labeling):

Children <4 years: Jet nebulizer: Croup: 0.05 mL/kg (maximum dose: 0.5 mL); dilute in 3 mL of NS. Administer over ~15 minutes; do not administer more frequently than every 2 hours

Children ≥4 years: Refer to adult dosing.

Inhalation: Children ≥4 years: Primatene® Mist: Refer to adult dosing.

Hypersensitivity reaction (eg, anaphylaxis): **Note:** SubQ administration results in slower absorption and is less reliable. I.M. administration in the anterolateral aspect of the middle third of the thigh is preferred in the setting of anaphylaxis (ACLS guidelines, 2010; Kemp, 2008).

I.M., SubQ: Larger I.M. or SubQ doses, use of I.V. route, or continuous I.V. infusion may be needed for severe anaphylactic reactions (Kemp, 2008; Lieberman, 2010). If clinician deems appropriate, the 5-minute interval between injections may be shortened to allow for more frequent administration (Lieberman, 2010).

Children <30 kg: 0.01 mg/kg (0.01 mL/kg of 1:**1000** [1 mg/mL] solution) (maximum single dose: 0.3 mg) every 5-10 minutes

Children ≥30 kg: 0.3-0.5 mg (0.3-0.5 mL of 1:**1000** [1 mg/mL] solution) every 5-10 minutes

Self-administration following severe allergic reactions (eg, insect stings, food): **Note:** World Health Organization (WHO) and Anaphylaxis Canada recommend the availability of 1 dose for every 10-20 minutes of travel time to a medical emergency facility. More than 2 sequential doses should only be administered under direct medical supervision.

Auvi-Q™: I.M., SubQ:

Children 15-29 kg: 0.15 mg; if anaphylactic symptoms persist, dose may be repeated

Children ≥30 kg: 0.3 mg; if anaphylactic symptoms persist, dose may be repeated

EpiPen® Jr: I.M., SubQ: Children 15-29 kg: 0.15 mg; if anaphylactic symptoms persist, dose may be repeated in 5-15 minutes using an additional EpiPen® Jr

EpiPen®: I.M., SubQ: Children ≥30 kg: 0.3 mg; if anaphylactic symptoms persist, dose may be repeated in 5-15 minutes using an additional EpiPen®

Twinject®: I.M. SubQ:

Children 15-29 kg: 0.15 mg; if anaphylactic symptoms persist, dose may be repeated in 5-15 minutes using the same device after partial disassembly

Children ≥30 kg: 0.3 mg; if anaphylactic symptoms persist, dose may be repeated in 5-15 minutes using the same device after partial disassembly

Alternate auto-injector dose: I.M. (Sicherer, 2007):

Children 10-25 kg: 0.15 mg

Children >25 kg: 0.3 mg

Hypotension/shock, fluid-resistant (unlabeled use): Continuous I.V. infusion: 0.1-1 mcg/kg/minute; doses up to 5 mcg/kg/minute may rarely be necessary (Hegenbarth, 2008)

Mydriasis during intraocular surgery, induction and maintenance: Intraocular: Must dilute 1:**1000** (1 mg/mL) solution to a concentration of 1:**100,000** to 1:**1,000,000** (10 **mcg**/mL to 1 **mcg**/mL) prior to intraocular use: May use as an irrigation solution as needed during the procedure or may administer intracamerally (ie, directly into the anterior chamber of the eye) with a bolus dose of 0.1 mL of a 1:**100,000** to 1:**400,000** (10 **mcg**/mL to 2.5 **mcg**/mL) dilution.

Adults:

Asystole/pulseless arrest, pulseless VT/VF (ACLS, 2010):

I.V., I.O.: 1 mg every 3-5 minutes until return of spontaneous circulation; if this approach fails, higher doses of epinephrine (up to 0.2 mg/kg) have been used for treatment of specific problems (eg, beta-blocker or calcium channel blocker overdose)

Endotracheal: 2-2.5 mg every 3-5 minutes until I.V./I.O. access established or return of spontaneous circulation; dilute in 5-10 mL NS or sterile water. **Note:** Absorption may be greater with sterile water (Naganobu, 2000). May cause false-negative reading with exhaled CO_2 detectors; use second method to confirm tube placement if CO_2 is not detected (Neumar, 2010).

Bradycardia (symptomatic; unresponsive to atropine or pacing): I.V. infusion: 2-10 mcg/minute **or** 0.1-0.5 mcg/kg/minute (7-35 mcg/minute in a 70 kg patient); titrate to desired effect (ACLS, 2010)

Bronchodilator:

SubQ: 0.3-0.5 mg (**1:1000** [1 mg/mL] solution) every 20 minutes for 3 doses

Nebulization: S2® (racepinephrine, OTC labeling):

Hand-bulb nebulizer: Add 0.5 mL (~10 drops) to nebulizer; 1-3 inhalations up to every 3 hours if needed

Jet nebulizer: Add 0.5 mL (~10 drops) to nebulizer and dilute with 3 mL of NS; administer over ~15 minutes every 3-4 hours as needed

Inhalation: Primatene® Mist (OTC labeling): One inhalation, wait at least 1 minute; if not relieved, may use once more. Do not use again for at least 3 hours.

Hypersensitivity reaction (eg, anaphylaxis):**Note:** SubQ administration results in slower absorption and is less reliable. I.M. administration in the anterolateral aspect of the middle third of the thigh is preferred in the setting of anaphylaxis (ACLS guidelines, 2010; Kemp, 2008).

I.M., SubQ: 0.2-0.5 mg (**1:1000** [1 mg/mL] solution) every 5-15 minutes in the absence of clinical improvement (ACLS, 2010; Kemp, 2008; Lieberman, 2010). If clinician deems appropriate, the 5-minute interval between injections may be shortened to allow for more frequent administration (Lieberman, 2010).

I.V.: 0.1 mg (**1:10,000** [0.1 mg/mL] solution) over 5 minutes; may infuse at 1-4 mcg/minute to prevent the need to repeat injections frequently **or** may initiate with an infusion at 5-15 mcg/minute (with crystalloid administration) (ACLS, 2010; Brown, 2004). In general, I.V. administration should only be done in patients who are profoundly hypotensive or are in cardiopulmonary arrest refractory to volume resuscitation and several epinephrine injections (Lieberman, 2010).

Self-administration following severe allergic reactions (eg, insect stings, food): **Note:** The World Health Organization (WHO) and Anaphylaxis Canada recommend the availability of one dose for every 10-20 minutes of travel time to a medical emergency facility. More than 2 sequential doses should only be administered under direct medical supervision.

Auvi-Q™: I.M., SubQ: 0.3 mg; if anaphylactic symptoms persist, dose may be repeated

EpiPen®: I.M., SubQ: 0.3 mg; if anaphylactic symptoms persist, dose may be repeated in 5-15 minutes using an additional EpiPen®

Twinject®: I.M., SubQ: 0.3 mg; if anaphylactic symptoms persist, dose may be repeated in 5-15 minutes using the same device after partial disassembly

Hypotension/shock, severe and fluid resistant (unlabeled use): I.V. infusion: Initial: 0.1-0.5 mcg/kg/minute (7-35 mcg/minute in a 70 kg patient); titrate to desired response (ACLS, 2010)

Mydriasis during intraocular surgery, induction and maintenance: Intraocular: Must dilute 1:**1000** (1 mg/mL) solution to a concentration of 1:**100,000** to 1:**1,000,000** (10 **mcg**/mL to 1 **mcg**/mL) prior to intraocular use: May use as an irrigation solution as needed during the procedure or may administer intracamerally (ie, directly into the anterior chamber of the eye) with a bolus dose of 0.1 mL of a 1:**100,000** to 1:**400,000** (10 **mcg**/mL to 2.5 **mcg**/mL) dilution.

Dosage adjustment in renal impairment: No dosage adjustment provided in manufacturer's labeling.

Dosage adjustment in hepatic impairment: No dosage adjustment provided in manufacturer's labeling.

Mechanism of Action Stimulates alpha-, beta$_1$-, and beta$_2$-adrenergic receptors resulting in relaxation of smooth muscle of the bronchial tree, cardiac stimulation (increasing myocardial oxygen consumption), and dilation of skeletal muscle vasculature; small doses can cause vasodilation via beta$_2$-vascular receptors; large doses may produce constriction of skeletal and vascular smooth muscle

Contraindications There are no absolute contraindications to the use of injectable epinephrine (including Auvi-Q™, EpiPen®, EpiPen® Jr, and Twinject®) in a life-threatening situation.

Oral inhalation: Concurrent use or within 2 weeks of MAO inhibitors

Injectable solution: There are no contraindications listed in the manufacturer's labeling.

Warnings/Precautions Use with caution in elderly patients, patients with diabetes mellitus, cardiovascular diseases (eg, coronary artery disease, hypertension), thyroid disease, cerebrovascular disease, Parkinson's disease, or patients taking tricyclic antidepressants. Some products contain sulfites as preservatives; the presence of sulfites in some products should not deter administration during a serious allergic or other emergency situation even if the patient is sulfite-sensitive. Accidental injection into digits, hands, or feet may result in local reactions, including injection site pallor, coldness and hypoesthesia or injury, resulting in bruising, bleeding, discoloration, erythema or skeletal injury; patient should seek immediate medical attention if this occurs. Rapid I.V. administration may cause death from cerebrovascular hemorrhage or cardiac arrhythmias; however, rapid I.V. administration during pulseless arrest is necessary. Prior to intraocular use, must dilute 1:**1000** (1 mg/mL) solution to a concentration of 1:**100,000** to 1:**1,000,000** (10 **mcg**/mL to 1 **mcg**/mL) prior to intraocular use. When used undiluted, has been associated with corneal endothelial damage.

Oral inhalation: Use with caution in patients with prostate enlargement or urinary retention; may cause temporary worsening of symptoms.

Self medication (OTC use): Oral inhalation: Prior to self-medication, patients should contact healthcare provider. The product should only be used in persons with a diagnosis of asthma. If symptoms are not relieved in 20 minutes or become worse do not continue to use the product - seek immediate medical assistance. The product should not be used more frequently or at higher doses than recommended unless directed by a healthcare provider. This product should not be used in patients who have required hospitalization for asthma or if a patient is taking prescription medication for asthma. Do not use if you have taken a MAO inhibitor (certain drugs used for depression, Parkinson's disease, or other conditions) within 2 weeks.

Drug Interactions

Metabolism/Transport Effects Substrate of COMT

Avoid Concomitant Use

Avoid concomitant use of EPINEPHrine (Systemic, Oral Inhalation) with any of the following: Ergot Derivatives; Iobenguane I 123; Lurasidone

Increased Effect/Toxicity

EPINEPHrine (Systemic, Oral Inhalation) may increase the levels/effects of: Bromocriptine; Lurasidone; Sympathomimetics

The levels/effects of EPINEPHrine (Systemic, Oral Inhalation) may be increased by: Antacids; AtoMOXetine; Beta-Blockers; Cannabinoids; Carbonic

Anhydrase Inhibitors; COMT Inhibitors; Ergot Derivatives; Hyaluronidase; Inhalational Anesthetics; MAO Inhibitors; Serotonin/Norepinephrine Reuptake Inhibitors; Tricyclic Antidepressants

Decreased Effect

EPINEPHrine (Systemic, Oral Inhalation) may decrease the levels/effects of: Benzylpenicilloyl Polylysine; Iobenguane I 123

The levels/effects of EPINEPHrine (Systemic, Oral Inhalation) may be decreased by: Alpha1-Blockers; Promethazine; Spironolactone

Ethanol/Nutrition/Herb Interactions Herb/Nutraceutical: Avoid ephedra, yohimbe (may cause CNS stimulation).

Pharmacodynamics/Kinetics

Onset of Action Bronchodilation: SubQ: ~5-10 minutes; Inhalation: ~1 minute

Pregnancy Risk Factor C

Pregnancy Considerations Teratogenic effects have been observed in animal reproduction studies. Epinephrine crosses the placenta and may cause fetal anoxia. Use during pregnancy when the potential benefit to the mother outweighs the possible risk to the fetus.

Lactation Excretion in breast milk unknown/use caution

Breast-Feeding Considerations It is not known if epinephrine is excreted in breast milk. The manufacturer recommends that caution be exercised when administering epinephrine to nursing women.

Dosage Forms

Injection, solution: 0.1 mg/mL (10 mL); 1 mg/mL (1 mL, 30 mL)

Adrenalin®: 1 mg/mL (1 mL, 30 mL)

Auvi-Q™: 0.15 mg/0.15 mL (0.76 mL); 0.3 mg/0.3 mL (0.76 mL)

EpiPen 2-Pak®: 0.3 mg/0.3 mL (2 mL)

EpiPen Jr 2-Pak®: 0.15 mg/0.3 mL (2 mL)

Injection, solution [preservative free]: 1 mg/mL (1 mL)

Solution, for oral inhalation [preservative free]:

Asthmanefrin™ [OTC]: Racepinephrine 2.25% (0.5 mL)

S2® [OTC]: Racepinephrine 2.25% (0.5 mL)

References

"2005 American Heart Association Guidelines for Cardiopulmonary Resuscitation and Emergency Cardiovascular Care," *Circulation*, 2005, 112(24 Suppl): 1-211.

National Asthma Education and Prevention Program, "Expert Panel Report 2: Guidelines for the Diagnosis and Management of Asthma," Bethesda, MD, National Institutes of Health, 1997. NIH publication 97-4051.

Stiell IG, Hebert PC, Wells GA, et al, "Vasopressin Versus Epinephrine for Inhospital Cardiac Arrest: A Randomised Controlled Trial," *Lancet*, 2001, 358(9276):105-9.

Wenzel V, Krismer AC, Arntz HR, et al, "A Comparison of Vasopressin and Epinephrine for Out-of-Hospital Cardiopulmonary Resuscitation. European Resuscitation Council Vasopressor during Cardiopulmonary Resuscitation Study Group," *N Engl J Med*, 2004, 350 (2):105-13.

Epinephrine and Chlorpheniramine

(ep i NEF rin & klor fen IR a meen)

Related Information

Chlorpheniramine *on page 292*

EPINEPHrine (Systemic, Oral Inhalation) *on page 482*

Brand Names: U.S. Ana-Kit®

Pharmacologic Category Antidote

Use Anaphylaxis emergency treatment of insect bites or stings by the sensitive patient that may occur within minutes of insect sting or exposure to an allergic substance

Local Anesthetic/Vasoconstrictor Precautions No information available to require special precautions

◄ **Effects on Dental Treatment** No significant effects or complications reported

Effects on Bleeding No information available to require special precautions

General Dosage Range

I.M., SubQ: Epinephrine (1:1000):
  Children *<2 years:* 0.05-0.1 mL
  Children *2-6 years:* 0.15 mL
  Children *6-12 years:* 0.2 mL
  Children *>12 years and Adults:* 0.3 mL

Oral: Chlorpheniramine (2 mg/tablet):
  Children *<6 years:* 1 tablet
  Children *6-12 years:* 2 tablets
  Children *>12 years and Adults:* 4 tablets

Pregnancy Considerations Refer to Epinephrine monograph.

Epinephrine (Racemic) and Aluminum Potassium Sulfate

(ep i NEF rin, ra SEE mik and a LOO mi num poe TASS ee um SUL fate)

Related Information
  EPINEPHrine (Systemic, Oral Inhalation) *on page 482*

Brand Names: U.S. Van R Gingibraid®

Generic Availability (U.S.) No

Pharmacologic Category Adrenergic Agonist Agent; Alpha/Beta Agonist; Astringent; Vasoconstrictor

Dental Use Gingival retraction

Use Gingival retraction

Local Anesthetic/Vasoconstrictor Precautions No information available to require special precautions

Effects on Dental Treatment Key adverse event(s) related to dental treatment: Tissue retraction around base of the tooth (therapeutic effect).

Effects on Bleeding No information available to require special precautions

Adverse Effects No data reported.

Dental Usual Dosage Gingival retraction: Adults: Pass the impregnated yarn around the neck of the tooth and place into gingival sulcus; normal tissue moisture, water, or gingival retraction solutions activate impregnated yarn. Limit use to one quadrant of the mouth at a time; recommended use is for 3-8 minutes in the mouth.

Mechanism of Action Epinephrine stimulates alpha₁ adrenergic receptors to cause vasoconstriction in blood vessels in gingiva; aluminum potassium sulfate, precipitates tissue and blood proteins

Contraindications Hypersensitivity to epinephrine or any component of the formulation; cardiovascular disease, hyperthyroidism, or diabetes; do not apply to areas of heavy or deep bleeding or over exposed bone

Warnings/Precautions Caution should be exercised whenever using gingival retraction cords with epinephrine since it delivers vasoconstrictor doses of racemic epinephrine to patients; the general medical history should be thoroughly evaluated before using in any patient

Dosage Forms

Yarn, saturated in solution of racemic epinephrine 8% and aluminum potassium sulfate 7% (Van R Gingibraid®):
  Type "0e": 0.20 ± 0.10 mg epinephrine/inch; Type "1e": 0.40 ± 0.20 mg epinephrine/inch; Type "2e": 0.60 ± 0.20 mg epinephrine/inch

---

Epirubicin (ep i ROO bi sin)

Brand Names: U.S. Ellence®

Brand Names: Canada Ellence®; Epirubicin for Injection; Epirubicin Hydrochloride Injection; Pharmorubicin®

Pharmacologic Category Antineoplastic Agent, Anthracycline

Use Adjuvant therapy component for primary breast cancer

Unlabeled Use Treatment of esophageal cancer, gastric cancer, soft tissue sarcoma, uterine sarcoma

Local Anesthetic/Vasoconstrictor Precautions No information available to require special precautions

Effects on Dental Treatment Key adverse event(s) related to dental treatment: Mucositis

Effects on Bleeding Causes severe myelosuppression, including severe thrombocytopenia (grades 3/4: <5%) and anemia. In patients who are under active treatment with this agent, medical consult is suggested.

Adverse Effects Percentages reported as part of combination chemotherapy regimens.
  >10%:
    Central nervous system: Lethargy (1% to 46%)
    Dermatologic: Alopecia (70% to 96%)
    Endocrine & metabolic: Amenorrhea (69% to 72%), hot flashes (5% to 39%)
    Gastrointestinal: Nausea/vomiting (83% to 92%; grades 3/4: 22% to 25%), mucositis (9% to 59%; grades 3/4: ≤9%), diarrhea (7% to 25%)
    Hematologic: Leukopenia (50% to 80%; grades 3/4: 2% to 59%), neutropenia (54% to 80%; grades 3/4: 11% to 67%; nadir: 10-14 days; recovery: by day 21), anemia (13% to 72%; grades 3/4: ≤6%), thrombocytopenia (5% to 49%; grades 3/4: ≤5%)
    Local: Injection site reactions (3% to 20%; grades 3/4: <1%)
    Ocular: Conjunctivitis (1% to 15%)
    Miscellaneous: Infection (15% to 22%; grades 3/4: ≤2%)
  1% to 10%:
    Cardiovascular: LVEF decreased (asymptomatic; delayed: 1% to 2%), HF (0.4% to 1.5%)
    Central nervous system: Fever (1% to 5%)
    Dermatologic: Rash (1% to 9%), skin changes (1% to 5%)
    Gastrointestinal: Anorexia (2% to 3%)
    Hematologic: Neutropenic fever (grades 3/4: ≤6%)

General Dosage Range Dosage adjustment recommended in patients with hepatic or renal impairment or who develop toxicities

I.V.: *Adults:* 100 mg/m² on day 1 every 3 weeks **or** 60 mg/m² on days 1 and 8 every 4 weeks

Mechanism of Action Epirubicin is an anthracycline antineoplastic agent; known to inhibit DNA and RNA synthesis by steric obstruction after intercalating between DNA base pairs; active throughout entire cell cycle. Intercalation triggers DNA cleavage by topoisomerase II, resulting in cytocidal activity. Also inhibits DNA helicase, and generates cytotoxic free radicals.

Pharmacodynamics/Kinetics

Half-life Elimination Triphasic; Mean terminal: 33 hours

Pregnancy Risk Factor D

Pregnancy Considerations Teratogenic effects and embryotoxicity were noted in animal studies. If a pregnant woman is treated with epirubicin, or if a woman becomes pregnant while receiving this drug, she should be informed of the potential hazard to the fetus. Limited information is available from retrospective studies of women who received epirubicin during the second or third (prior to week 35) trimester for the treatment of pregnancy-associated breast cancer; premature births and intrauterine growth retardation have been observed (Peccatori, 2009; Ring, 2005). Women of childbearing potential should be advised to use effective contraception and avoid becoming pregnant during treatment. Men undergoing treatment should use effective contraception. Epirubicin may cause irreversible amenorrhea in premenopausal women.

Eplerenone (e PLER en one)

Related Information
Cardiovascular Diseases *on page 1492*
Brand Names: U.S. Inspra™
Brand Names: Canada Inspra™
Pharmacologic Category Diuretic, Potassium-Sparing; Selective Aldosterone Blocker
Use
U.S. labeling: Treatment of hypertension (may be used alone or in combination with other antihypertensive agents); treatment of heart failure (HF) (LVEF ≤40%) following acute MI

Canadian labeling: Treatment of NYHA class II chronic heart failure (HF) with left ventricular systolic dysfunction; treatment of HF following acute MI
Local Anesthetic/Vasoconstrictor Precautions No information available to require special precautions
Effects on Dental Treatment No significant effects or complications reported
Effects on Bleeding No information available to require special precautions
Adverse Effects
>10%: Endocrine & metabolic: Hyperkalemia ([HF post-MI: K >5.5 mEq/L: 16%; K ≥6 mEq/L: 6%] [HTN: K >5.5 mEq/L at doses ≤200 mg: ≤1%; dose of 400 mg: 9%]), hypertriglyceridemia (1% to 15%, dose related)
1% to 10%:
Central nervous system: Dizziness (3%), fatigue (2%)
Endocrine & metabolic: Hyponatremia (2%, dose related), breast pain (males <1% to 1%), gynecomastia (males <1% to 1%), hypercholesterolemia (<1% to 1%)
Gastrointestinal: Diarrhea (2%), abdominal pain (1%)
Genitourinary: Abnormal vaginal bleeding (<1% to 2%)
Renal: Creatinine increased (HF post-MI: 6%), albuminuria (1%)
Respiratory: Cough (2%)
Miscellaneous: Flu-like syndrome (2%)
General Dosage Range Dosage adjustment recommended in patients on concomitant therapy or based on potassium concentrations
Oral: *Adults:* Initial: 25-50 mg once daily; Maintenance: 50 mg once or twice daily (maximum: 100 mg/day)
Mechanism of Action Aldosterone, a mineralocorticoid, increases blood pressure primarily by inducing sodium and water retention. Overexpression of aldosterone is thought to contribute to myocardial fibrosis (especially following myocardial infarction) and vascular fibrosis. Mineralocorticoid receptors are located in the kidney, heart, blood vessels, and brain. Eplerenone selectively blocks mineralocorticoid receptors reducing blood pressure in a dose-dependent manner and appears to prevent myocardial and vascular fibrosis.
Pharmacodynamics/Kinetics
Half-life Elimination 4-6 hours
Time to Peak Plasma: ~1.5 hours; may take up to 4 weeks for full antihypertensive effect

Pregnancy Risk Factor B
Pregnancy Considerations No teratogenic effects were seen in animal reproduction studies, however, there are no adequate and well-controlled studies in pregnant women. Use during pregnancy only if the potential benefit to the mother outweighs the possible risk to the fetus.

Epoetin Alfa (e POE e tin AL fa)

Brand Names: U.S. Epogen®; Procrit®
Brand Names: Canada Eprex®
Pharmacologic Category Colony Stimulating Factor; Erythropoiesis-Stimulating Agent (ESA); Growth Factor; Recombinant Human Erythropoietin
Use Treatment of anemia due to concurrent myelosuppressive chemotherapy in patients with cancer (non-myeloid malignancies) receiving chemotherapy (palliative intent) for a planned minimum of 2 additional months of chemotherapy; treatment of anemia due to chronic kidney disease (including patients on dialysis and not on dialysis) to decrease the need for RBC transfusion; treatment of anemia associated with HIV (zidovudine) therapy when endogenous erythropoietin levels ≤500 mUnits/mL; reduction of allogeneic RBC transfusion for elective, noncardiac, nonvascular surgery when perioperative hemoglobin is >10 to ≤13 g/dL and there is a high risk for blood loss

Note: Epoetin is **not** indicated for use under the following conditions:
  • Cancer patients receiving hormonal therapy, therapeutic biologic products, or radiation therapy unless also receiving concurrent myelosuppressive chemotherapy
  • Cancer patients receiving myelosuppressive chemotherapy when the expected outcome is curative
  • Surgery patients who are willing to donate autologous blood
  • Surgery patients undergoing cardiac or vascular surgery
  • As a substitute for RBC transfusion in patients requiring immediate correction of anemia

Note: In clinical trials (and one meta-analysis), epoetin has not demonstrated improved quality of life, fatigue, or well-being.
Unlabeled Use Treatment of symptomatic anemia in myelodysplastic syndrome (MDS)
Local Anesthetic/Vasoconstrictor Precautions No information available to require special precautions
Effects on Dental Treatment No significant effects or complications reported
Effects on Bleeding Although ESAs have been associated with thromboembolic events, there is no information available to require special precautions for dental procedures.
Adverse Effects
>10%:
Cardiovascular: Hypertension (3% to 28%)
Central nervous system: Fever (10% to 42%), headache (5% to 18%)
Dermatologic: Pruritus (12% to 21%), rash (2% to 19%)
Gastrointestinal: Nausea (35% to 56%), vomiting (12% to 28%)
Local: Injection site reaction (7% to 13%)
Neuromuscular & skeletal: Arthralgia (10% to 16%)
Respiratory: Cough (4% to 26%)

1% to 10%:
  Cardiovascular: Deep vein thrombosis, edema, thrombosis
  Central nervous system: Chills, depression, dizziness, insomnia
  Dermatologic: Urticaria
  Endocrine & metabolic: Hyperglycemia, hypokalemia
  Gastrointestinal: Dysphagia, stomatitis, weight loss
  Hematologic: Leukopenia
  Local: Clotted vascular access
  Neuromuscular & skeletal: Bone pain, muscle spasm, myalgia
  Respiratory: Pulmonary embolism, respiratory congestion, upper respiratory infection

General Dosage Range I.V., SubQ: Children and Adults: Dosage varies greatly depending on indication

Mechanism of Action Induces erythropoiesis by stimulating the division and differentiation of committed erythroid progenitor cells; induces the release of reticulocytes from the bone marrow into the bloodstream, where they mature to erythrocytes. There is a dose response relationship with this effect. This results in an increase in reticulocyte counts followed by a rise in hematocrit and hemoglobin levels.

Pharmacodynamics/Kinetics

Onset of Action Several days; Peak effect: Hemoglobin level: 2-6 weeks

Half-life Elimination Cancer: SubQ: 16-67 hours; Chronic kidney disease: I.V.: 4-13 hours

Time to Peak Serum: Chronic kidney disease: SubQ: 5-24 hours

Pregnancy Risk Factor C

Pregnancy Considerations Adverse events were observed in animal reproduction studies. In vitro studies suggest that recombinant erythropoietin does not cross the human placenta (Reisenberger, 1997). Polyhydramnios and intrauterine growth retardation have been reported with use in women with chronic kidney disease (adverse effects also associated with maternal disease). Hypospadias and pectus excavatum have been reported with first trimester exposure (case report).

Recombinant erythropoietin alfa has been evaluated as adjunctive treatment for severe pregnancy associated iron deficiency anemia (Breymann, 2001; Krafft, 2009) and has been used in pregnant women with iron-deficiency anemia associated with chronic kidney disease (CKD) (Furaz-Czerpak 2012; Josephson, 2007).

Amenorrheic premenopausal women should be cautioned that menstruation may resume following treatment with recombinant erythropoietin (Furaz-Czerpak, 2012). Multidose formulations containing benzyl alcohol are contraindicated for use in pregnant women; if treatment during pregnancy is needed, single dose preparations should be used.

Women who become pregnant during treatment with epoetin are encouraged to enroll in Amgen's Pregnancy Surveillance Program (1-800-772-6436).

Prescribing and Access Restrictions As a requirement of the REMS program, access to this medication is restricted. Healthcare providers and hospitals must be enrolled in the ESA APPRISE (Assisting Providers and Cancer Patients with Risk Information for the Safe use of ESAs) Oncology Program (866-284-8089; http://www.esa-apprise.com) to prescribe or dispense ESAs (ie, epoetin alfa, darbepoetin alfa) to patients with cancer.

Epoprostenol (e poe PROST en ole)

Brand Names: U.S. Flolan®; Veletri®

Brand Names: Canada Flolan®

Pharmacologic Category Prostacyclin; Prostaglandin; Vasodilator

Use Treatment of pulmonary arterial hypertension (PAH) (WHO Group I) in patients with NYHA Class III or IV symptoms to improve exercise capacity

Unlabeled Use Acute vasodilator testing in pulmonary arterial hypertension (PAH)

Inhalation: Intraoperative treatment of pulmonary hypertension in patients undergoing cardiac surgery with cardiopulmonary bypass; post-cardiothoracic surgery pulmonary hypertension, right ventricular dysfunction, or refractory hypoxemia

Local Anesthetic/Vasoconstrictor Precautions No information available to require special precautions

Effects on Dental Treatment No significant effects or complications reported. Epoprostenol is an inhibitor of platelet aggregation and may enhance the risk of bleeding with other antiplatelet agents (such as aspirin and/or NSAIDs).

Effects on Bleeding Epoprostenol is a potent inhibitor of platelet aggregation and increases the risk of hemorrhagic complications. A medical consult is suggested.

Adverse Effects Note: Adverse events reported during dose initiation and escalation include flushing (58%), headache (49%), nausea/vomiting (32%), hypotension (16%), anxiety/nervousness/agitation (11%), chest pain (11%); dizziness, abdominal pain, bradycardia, musculoskeletal pain, dyspnea, back pain, diaphoresis, dyspepsia, hypoesthesia/paresthesia, and tachycardia are also reported. Although some adverse reactions may be related to the underlying disease state, abdominal pain, anxiety/nervousness/agitation, arthralgia, bleeding, bradycardia, diarrhea, diaphoresis, flu-like syndrome, flushing, headache, hypotension, jaw pain, nausea, pain, pulmonary edema, rash, tachycardia, thrombocytopenia, and vomiting are clearly contributed to epoprostenol. The following adverse events have been reported during chronic administration for idiopathic or heritable PAH:

>10%:
  Cardiovascular: Tachycardia (35% to 43%), flushing (23% to 42%), hypotension (13%)
  Central nervous system: Dizziness (83%), headache (46% to 83%), chills/fever/sepsis/flu-like syndrome (25%), anxiety/nervousness/tremor (21%)
  Dermatologic: Skin ulcer (39%), eczema/rash/urticaria (25%)
  Gastrointestinal: Nausea/vomiting (41% to 67%), anorexia (66%), diarrhea (37% to 50%)
  Local: Injection site reactions: Infection (18%), pain (11%)
  Neuromuscular & skeletal: Pain/neck pain/arthralgia (84%), jaw pain (54% to 75%), arthritis (52%), myalgia (44%), musculoskeletal pain (35%), hypoesthesia/hyperesthesia/paresthesia (5% to 12%)

General Dosage Range I.V.: Adults: Initial: 1-2 ng/kg/minute; increase dose in increments of 1-2 ng/kg/minute every 15 minutes until response

Mechanism of Action Epoprostenol is also known as prostacyclin and PGI$_2$. It is a strong vasodilator of all vascular beds. In addition, it is a potent endogenous inhibitor of platelet aggregation. The reduction in platelet aggregation results from epoprostenol's activation of intracellular adenylate cyclase and the resultant increase in cyclic adenosine monophosphate concentrations within the platelets. Additionally, it is capable of decreasing thrombogenesis and platelet clumping in the lungs by inhibiting platelet aggregation.

Pharmacodynamics/Kinetics
Half-life Elimination ~6 minutes
Pregnancy Risk Factor B
Pregnancy Considerations Teratogenic effects were not reported in animal studies. There are no adequate and well-controlled studies in pregnant women. Women with IPAH are encouraged to avoid pregnancy.

Prescribing and Access Restrictions Orders for epoprostenol are distributed by two sources in the United States. Information on orders or reimbursement assistance may be obtained from either Accredo Health, Inc (1-800-935-6526) or TheraCom, Inc (1-877-356-5264).

Eprosartan (ep roe SAR tan)

Related Information
Cardiovascular Diseases *on page 1492*
Brand Names: U.S. Teveten®
Brand Names: Canada Teveten®
Generic Availability (U.S.) Yes
Pharmacologic Category Angiotensin II Receptor Blocker
Use Treatment of hypertension; may be used alone or in combination with other antihypertensives
Local Anesthetic/Vasoconstrictor Precautions No information available to require special precautions
Effects on Dental Treatment No significant effects or complications reported
Effects on Bleeding No information available to require special precautions
Adverse Effects 1% to 10%:
Central nervous system: Fatigue (2%), depression (1%)
Endocrine & metabolic: Hypertriglyceridemia (1%)
Gastrointestinal: Abdominal pain (2%)
Genitourinary: Urinary tract infection (1%)
Respiratory: Upper respiratory tract infection (8%), rhinitis (4%), pharyngitis (4%), cough (4%)
Miscellaneous: Viral infection (2%), injury (2%)
Dosage Adults: Oral: Dosage must be individualized; can administer once or twice daily with total daily doses of 400-800 mg. Usual starting dose is 600 mg once daily as monotherapy in patients who are euvolemic. Limited clinical experience with doses >800 mg.
Dosage adjustment in renal impairment: Moderate-to-severe impairment: No initial starting dosage adjustment is necessary; however, carefully monitor the patient. Maximum dose: 600 mg daily.
Hemodialysis: Poorly removed (Cl$_{HD}$ <1 L/hour)
Dosage adjustment in hepatic impairment: No starting dosage adjustment is necessary; however, carefully monitor the patient
Elderly: No starting dosage adjustment is necessary; however, carefully monitor the patient
Mechanism of Action Angiotensin II is formed from angiotensin I in a reaction catalyzed by angiotensin-converting enzyme (ACE, kininase II). Angiotensin II is the principal pressor agent of the renin-angiotensin system, with effects that include vasoconstriction, stimulation of synthesis and release of aldosterone, cardiac stimulation, and renal reabsorption of sodium. Eprosartan blocks the vasoconstrictor and aldosterone-secreting effects of angiotensin II by selectively blocking the binding of angiotensin II to the AT1 receptor in many tissues, such as vascular smooth muscle and the

adrenal gland. Its action is therefore independent of the pathways for angiotensin II synthesis. Blockade of the renin-angiotensin system with ACE inhibitors, which inhibit the biosynthesis of angiotensin II from angiotensin I, is widely used in the treatment of hypertension. ACE inhibitors also inhibit the degradation of bradykinin, a reaction also catalyzed by ACE. Because eprosartan does not inhibit ACE (kininase II), it does not affect the response to bradykinin. Whether this difference has clinical relevance is not yet known. Eprosartan does not bind to or block other hormone receptors or ion channels known to be important in cardiovascular regulation.

Contraindications Hypersensitivity to eprosartan or any component of the formulation; concomitant use with aliskiren in patients with diabetes mellitus

Warnings/Precautions [U.S. Boxed Warning]: Drugs that act on the renin-angiotensin system can cause injury and death to the developing fetus. Discontinue as soon as possible once pregnancy is detected. May cause hyperkalemia; avoid potassium supplementation unless specifically required by healthcare provider. Avoid use or use a smaller dose in patients who are volume depleted; correct depletion first. May be associated with deterioration of renal function and/or increases in serum creatinine, particularly in patients with low renal blood flow (eg, renal artery stenosis, heart failure) whose glomerular filtration rate (GFR) is dependent on efferent arteriolar vasoconstriction by angiotensin II. Use with caution in unstented unilateral/bilateral renal artery stenosis. When unstented bilateral renal artery stenosis is present, use is generally avoided due to the elevated risk of deterioration in renal function unless possible benefits outweigh risks. Use with caution in pre-existing renal insufficiency; significant aortic/mitral stenosis. Concomitant use of an angiotensin-converting enzyme (ACE) inhibitor or renin inhibitor (eg, aliskiren) is associated with an increased risk of hypotension, hyperkalemia, and renal dysfunction; concomitant use with aliskiren should be avoided in patients with GFR <60 mL/minute and is contraindicated in patients with diabetes mellitus (regardless of GFR).

Drug Interactions
Metabolism/Transport Effects Inhibits CYP2C9 (weak)
Avoid Concomitant Use There are no known interactions where it is recommended to avoid concomitant use.

Increased Effect/Toxicity
Eprosartan may increase the levels/effects of: ACE Inhibitors; Amifostine; Antihypertensives; CycloSPORINE (Systemic); Hypotensive Agents; Lithium; Nonsteroidal Anti-Inflammatory Agents; Potassium-Sparing Diuretics; RiTUXimab; Sodium Phosphates

The levels/effects of Eprosartan may be increased by: Alfuzosin; Aliskiren; Canagliflozin; Diazoxide; Eplerenone; Herbs (Hypotensive Properties); MAO Inhibitors; Pentoxifylline; Phosphodiesterase 5 Inhibitors; Potassium Salts; Prostacyclin Analogues; Tolvaptan; Trimethoprim

Decreased Effect
The levels/effects of Eprosartan may be decreased by: Herbs (Hypotensive Properties); Methylphenidate; Nonsteroidal Anti-Inflammatory Agents; Yohimbine

Ethanol/Nutrition/Herb Interactions Herb/Nutraceutical: Dong quai has estrogenic activity. Some herbal medications may worsen hypertension (eg, ephedra); garlic may have additional antihypertensive effects.

◄ Management: Avoid dong quai if using for hypertension. Avoid ephedra, yohimbe, ginseng, and garlic.

Pharmacodynamics/Kinetics
Half-life Elimination Terminal: 5-9 hours
Time to Peak Serum: Fasting: 1-2 hours
Pregnancy Risk Factor D
Pregnancy Considerations [U.S. Boxed Warning]: Drugs that act on the renin-angiotensin system can cause injury and death to the developing fetus. Discontinue as soon as possible once pregnancy is detected. The use of drugs which act on the renin-angiotensin system are associated with oligohydramnios. Oligohydramnios, due to decreased fetal renal function, may lead to fetal lung hypoplasia and skeletal malformations. Use is also associated with anuria, hypotension, renal failure, skull hypoplasia, and death in the fetus/neonate. The exposed fetus should be monitored for fetal growth, amniotic fluid volume, and organ formation. Infants exposed *in utero* should be monitored for hyperkalemia, hypotension, and oliguria.

Lactation Not recommended

Dosage Forms
Tablet, oral: 600 mg
Teveten®: 400 mg, 600 mg

Eprosartan and Hydrochlorothiazide
(ep roe SAR tan & hye droe klor oh THYE a zide)

Related Information
Eprosartan *on page 489*
Hydrochlorothiazide *on page 687*
Brand Names: U.S. Teveten® HCT
Brand Names: Canada Teveten® HCT; Teveten® Plus
Pharmacologic Category Angiotensin II Receptor Blocker; Diuretic, Thiazide
Use Treatment of hypertension (not indicated for initial treatment)
Local Anesthetic/Vasoconstrictor Precautions No information available to require special precautions
Effects on Dental Treatment No significant effects or complications reported
Effects on Bleeding No information available to require special precautions
Adverse Effects Percentages reported with combination product; other reactions have been reported (see individual agents for additional information).

1% to 10%:
Central nervous system: Dizziness (4%), headache (3%), fatigue (2%)
Hematologic: Neutrophil count decreased (1%)
Neuromuscular & skeletal: Back pain (3%)
Renal: BUN increased (1%)
General Dosage Range Oral: *Adults:* Eprosartan 600 mg and hydrochlorothiazide 12.5-25 mg once daily
Mechanism of Action Hydrochlorothiazide inhibits sodium reabsorption in the distal tubules causing increased excretion of sodium and water as well as potassium and hydrogen ions. **Eprosartan** blocks the vasoconstrictor and aldosterone-secreting effects of angiotensin II by selectively blocking the binding of angiotensin II to the AT1 receptor in many tissues, such as vascular smooth muscle and the adrenal gland.
Pregnancy Risk Factor D
Pregnancy Considerations [U.S. Boxed Warning]: Drugs that act on the renin-angiotensin system can cause injury and death to the developing fetus. Discontinue as soon as possible once pregnancy is detected. Also see individual agents.

Eptifibatide (ep TIF i ba tide)

Related Information
Cardiovascular Diseases *on page 1492*
Brand Names: U.S. Integrilin®
Brand Names: Canada Integrilin®
Pharmacologic Category Antiplatelet Agent, Glycoprotein IIb/IIIa Inhibitor
Use Treatment of patients with acute coronary syndrome (unstable angina/non-ST-segment elevation myocardial infarction [UA/NSTEMI]), including patients who are to be managed medically and those undergoing percutaneous coronary intervention (PCI including angioplasty, intracoronary stenting)
Unlabeled Use To support PCI during ST-elevation myocardial infarction (administered at the time of primary PCI); elective PCI for stable ischemic heart disease (in combination with unfractionated heparin)
Local Anesthetic/Vasoconstrictor Precautions No information available to require special precautions
Effects on Dental Treatment Key adverse event(s) related to dental treatment: Bleeding; patients weighing <70 kg may have an increased risk of major bleeding. See Effects on Bleeding.
Effects on Bleeding Bleeding is the most common complication. Eptifibatide inhibits platelet aggregation. Vascular and other trauma should be avoided. It is unlikely that dental work would be performed in patients undergoing treatment for acute coronary syndrome.
Adverse Effects Bleeding is the major drug-related adverse effect. Access site is often primary source of bleeding complications. Incidence of bleeding is also related to heparin intensity. Patients weighing <70 kg may have an increased risk of major bleeding.

>10%: Hematologic: Bleeding (major: 1% to 11%; minor: 3% to 14%; transfusion required: 2% to 13%)
1% to 10%:
Cardiovascular: Hypotension (up to 7%)
Hematologic: Thrombocytopenia (1% to 3%)
Local: Injection site reaction
General Dosage Range Dosage adjustment recommended in patients with renal impairment
I.V.: *Adults:* Bolus: 180 mcg/kg (maximum: 22.6 mg), repeat once for PCI; Infusion: 2 mcg/kg/minute (maximum: 15 mg/hour)
Mechanism of Action Eptifibatide is a cyclic heptapeptide which blocks the platelet glycoprotein IIb/IIIa receptor, the binding site for fibrinogen, von Willebrand factor, and other ligands. Inhibition of binding at this final common receptor reversibly blocks platelet aggregation and prevents thrombosis.
Pharmacodynamics/Kinetics
Onset of Action Within 1 hour
Duration of Action Platelet function restored ~4 hours following discontinuation
Half-life Elimination 2.5 hours
Pregnancy Risk Factor B
Pregnancy Considerations Teratogenic effects were not observed in animal studies.

Ergocalciferol (er goe kal SIF e role)

Brand Names: U.S. Calciferol™ [OTC]; Drisdol®; Drisdol® [OTC]
Brand Names: Canada Drisdol®; Ostoforte®
Pharmacologic Category Vitamin D Analog

Use Treatment of refractory rickets, hypophosphatemia, hypoparathyroidism; dietary supplement

Unlabeled Use Prevention and treatment of vitamin D deficiency in patients with chronic kidney disease (CKD); osteoporosis prevention

Local Anesthetic/Vasoconstrictor Precautions No information available to require special precautions

Effects on Dental Treatment Key adverse event(s) related to dental treatment: Metallic taste and xerostomia (normal salivary flow resumes upon discontinuation).

Effects on Bleeding No information available to require special precautions

Adverse Effects Frequency not defined: Endocrine & metabolic: Hypervitaminosis D (signs and symptoms include hypercalcemia, resulting in headache, nausea, vomiting, lethargy, confusion, sluggishness, abdominal pain, bone pain, polyuria, polydipsia, weakness, cardiac arrhythmias [eg, QT shortening, sinus tachycardia], soft tissue calcification, calciuria, and nephrocalcinosis)

General Dosage Range Oral:
Children 0-12 months: Adequate intake: 400 units/day
Children 1 year to Adults ≤70 years: RDA: 600 units/day
Elderly >70 years: RDA: 800 units/day

Mechanism of Action Stimulates calcium and phosphate absorption from the small intestine, promotes secretion of calcium from bone to blood; promotes renal tubule phosphate resorption

Pharmacodynamics/Kinetics
Onset of Action Peak effect: ~1 month following daily doses

Pregnancy Risk Factor C (manufacturer); A/C (dose exceeding RDA recommendation; per expert analysis)

Pregnancy Considerations Abnormalities have been observed in animal studies with maternal doses causing hypervitaminosis D. Doses larger than the RDA should be avoided during pregnancy.

Ergoloid Mesylates (ER goe loid MES i lates)

Brand Names: Canada Hydergine®
Pharmacologic Category Ergot Derivative
Use Treatment of cerebrovascular insufficiency in primary progressive dementia, Alzheimer's dementia, and senile onset

Local Anesthetic/Vasoconstrictor Precautions Although ergoloid mesylates are derivatives of the natural ergot alkaloids, they lack any vasoconstricting effects; there is no information available to require special precautions with vasoconstrictor

Effects on Dental Treatment Key adverse event(s) related to dental treatment: Orthostatic hypotension.

Effects on Bleeding No information available to require special precautions

Adverse Effects Adverse effects are minimal; most common include transient nausea, gastrointestinal disturbances and sublingual irritation with SL tablets; other common side effects include:

Cardiovascular: Bradycardia, orthostatic hypotension
Dermatologic: Flushing, skin rash
Ocular: Blurred vision
Respiratory: Nasal congestion

General Dosage Range Oral: *Adults:* Initial: 1 mg 3 times/day; Maintenance: 3-12 mg/day in 3 divided doses

Mechanism of Action Ergoloid mesylates do not have the vasoconstrictor effects of the natural ergot alkaloids; exact mechanism in dementia is unknown; originally classed as peripheral and cerebral vasodilator, now considered a "metabolic enhancer"; there is no specific evidence which clearly establishes the mechanism by which ergoloid mesylate preparations produce mental effects, nor is there conclusive evidence that the drug particularly affects cerebral arteriosclerosis or cerebrovascular insufficiency

Pharmacodynamics/Kinetics
Half-life Elimination Serum: 3.5 hours
Time to Peak Serum: ~1 hour

Ergonovine (er goe NOE veen)

Brand Names: Canada Ergonovine Maleate Injection
Pharmacologic Category Ergot Derivative
Use Prevention and treatment of postpartum and post-abortion hemorrhage caused by uterine atony

Unlabeled Use Diagnostically to identify Prinzmetal's angina

Local Anesthetic/Vasoconstrictor Precautions Use vasoconstrictor with caution in patients taking ergonovine; this ergot alkaloid derivative causes constriction of peripheral blood vessels

Effects on Dental Treatment No significant effects or complications reported

Effects on Bleeding Rare but significant events related to hemorrhage (cerebral hemorrhage, subarachnoid hemorrhage, and stroke) have occurred following injection of some agents in this class. However, there is no information related to special precautions associated with bleeding related to dental procedures.

Adverse Effects Frequency not defined.
Cardiovascular: Angina (transient), bradycardia, hypertension, MI, palpitation, shock, thrombophlebitis
Central nervous system: Dizziness, hallucination, headache, vertigo
Endocrine & metabolic: Water intoxication
Gastrointestinal: Abdominal pain, diarrhea, nausea, vomiting
Renal: Hematuria
Respiratory: Dyspnea
Miscellaneous: Allergic reactions, diaphoresis, ergotism

General Dosage Range I.M., I.V.: *Adults:* 0.2 mg, may repeat in 2-4 hours if needed, up to maximum of 5 total doses

Mechanism of Action Similar smooth muscle actions as seen with ergotamine; however, it affects primarily uterine smooth muscles producing sustained contractions and thereby shortens the third stage of labor.

Pharmacodynamics/Kinetics
Onset of Action I.M.: 2-3 minutes; I.V.: 1 minute
Duration of Action I.M.: Uterine effect: 3 hours; I.V.: ~45 minute

Pregnancy Considerations Ergonovine is used in the third stage of labor for the prevention or treatment of postpartum hemorrhage and should not be used prior to delivery of the placenta. Prior to administration, the placenta should be delivered and the possibility of twin pregnancy ruled out. Administration causes hyperstimulation of the uterus and may cause uterine tetany, decreased uteroplacental blood flow, uterine rupture, cervical and perineal lacerations, amniotic fluid embolism, and possible trauma to the infant.

Product Availability Not available in the U.S.

Ergotamine (er GOT a meen)

Brand Names: U.S. Ergomar®

Pharmacologic Category Antimigraine Agent; Ergot Derivative

Use Abort or prevent vascular headaches, such as migraine, migraine variants, or so-called "histaminic cephalalgia"

Local Anesthetic/Vasoconstrictor Precautions Use vasoconstrictor with caution in patients taking ergotamine; this ergot alkaloid derivative causes constriction of peripheral blood vessels

Effects on Dental Treatment No significant effects or complications reported

Effects on Bleeding No information available to require special precautions

Adverse Effects Frequency not defined.

Cardiovascular: Absence of pulse, bradycardia, cardiac valvular fibrosis, cyanosis, edema, ECG changes, gangrene, hypertension, ischemia, precordial distress and pain, tachycardia, vasospasm

Central nervous system: Vertigo

Dermatologic: Itching

Gastrointestinal: Nausea, vomiting

Genitourinary: Retroperitoneal fibrosis

Neuromuscular & skeletal: Muscle pain, numbness, paresthesia, weakness

Respiratory: Pleuropulmonary fibrosis

Miscellaneous: Cold extremities

General Dosage Range Sublingual: *Adults:* 1 tablet initially, then 1 tablet every 30 minutes if needed (maximum: 3 tablets/day; 5 tablets/week)

Mechanism of Action Has partial agonist and/or antagonist activity against tryptaminergic, dopaminergic and alpha-adrenergic receptors depending upon their site; is a highly active uterine stimulant; it causes constriction of peripheral and cranial blood vessels and produces depression of central vasomotor centers

Pharmacodynamics/Kinetics

Half-life Elimination 2 hours

Time to Peak Serum: Ergotamine: 0.5-3 hours

Pregnancy Risk Factor X

Pregnancy Considerations May cause prolonged constriction of the uterine vessels and/or increased myometrial tone leading to reduced placental blood flow. This has contributed to fetal growth retardation in animals.

Ergotamine and Caffeine
(er GOT a meen & KAF een)

Related Information

Caffeine *on page 229*

Ergotamine *on page 492*

Brand Names: U.S. Cafergot®; Migergot®

Brand Names: Canada Cafergor®

Pharmacologic Category Antimigraine Agent; Central Nervous System Stimulant; Ergot Derivative

Use Abort or prevent vascular headaches, such as migraine, migraine variants, or so-called "histaminic cephalalgia"

Local Anesthetic/Vasoconstrictor Precautions Use vasoconstrictor with caution in patients taking ergotamine; this ergot alkaloid derivative causes constriction of peripheral blood vessels

Effects on Dental Treatment No significant effects or complications reported

Effects on Bleeding No information available to require special precautions

Adverse Effects Frequency not defined.

Cardiovascular: Absence of pulse, bradycardia, cardiac valvular fibrosis, cyanosis, edema, ECG changes, gangrene, hypertension, ischemia, precordial distress and pain, tachycardia, vasospasm

Central nervous system: Vertigo

Dermatologic: Itching

Gastrointestinal: Anal or rectal ulcer (with overuse of suppository), nausea, vomiting

Genitourinary: Retroperitoneal fibrosis

Neuromuscular & skeletal: Muscle pain, numbness, paresthesia, weakness

Respiratory: Pleuropulmonary fibrosis

Miscellaneous: Cold extremities

General Dosage Range

Oral: *Adults:* 2 tablets initially, then 1 tablet every 30 minutes as needed (maximum: 6 tablets/attack; 10 tablets/week)

Rectal: *Adults:* 1 suppository initially; may repeat after 1 hour if needed (maximum: 2 doses/attack; 5 doses/week)

Mechanism of Action Has partial agonist and/or antagonist activity against tryptaminergic, dopaminergic and alpha-adrenergic receptors depending upon their site; is a highly active uterine stimulant; it causes constriction of peripheral and cranial blood vessels and produces depression of central vasomotor centers

Pharmacodynamics/Kinetics

Half-life Elimination 2 hours

Time to Peak Serum: Ergotamine: 0.5-3 hours

Pregnancy Risk Factor X

Pregnancy Considerations May cause prolonged constriction of the uterine vessels and/or increased myometrial tone leading to reduced placental blood flow. This has contributed to fetal growth retardation in animals.

Eribulin (er i BUE lin)

Brand Names: U.S. Halaven™

Brand Names: Canada Halaven™

Pharmacologic Category Antineoplastic Agent, Antimicrotubular

Use Treatment of metastatic breast cancer in patients who have received at least 2 prior chemotherapy regimens

Local Anesthetic/Vasoconstrictor Precautions No information available to require special precautions

Effects on Dental Treatment Key adverse event(s) related to dental treatment: Xerostomia (normal salivary flow resumes upon discontinuation), stomatitis, mucosal inflammation, or taste alteration.

Effects on Bleeding Anemia is a primary adverse effect. A medical consult is suggested.

Adverse Effects

>10%:

Central nervous system: Central nervous system: Fatigue (54%), fever (21%), headache (19%)

Dermatologic: Alopecia (45%)

Gastrointestinal: Nausea (35%), stomatitis (5% to 18%), constipation (25%), weight loss (21%), anorexia (20%), diarrhea (18%), vomiting (18%)

Hematologic: Neutropenia (82%; grades 3: 28%; grade 4: 29%; nadir: 13 days; recovery: 8 days), anemia (58%; grades 3/4: 2%)

Hepatic: ALT increased (18%)

Neuromuscular & skeletal: Weakness (54%), peripheral neuropathy (35%; grades 3/4: ≤8%), arthralgia/myalgia (22%), back pain (16%), bone pain (12%), limb pain (11%)
Respiratory: Dyspnea (16%), cough (14%)
1% to 10%:
Cardiovascular: Peripheral edema
Central nervous system: Depression, dizziness, insomnia
Dermatologic: Rash
Endocrine & metabolic: Hypokalemia
Gastrointestinal: Mucosal inflammation (9%), abdominal pain, dyspepsia, taste alteration, xerostomia
Genitourinary: Urinary tract infection (10%)
Hematologic: Neutropenic fever (5%), thrombocytopenia (grades 3/4: 1%)
Neuromuscular & skeletal: Muscle spasm
Ocular: Lacrimation increased
Respiratory: Upper respiratory infection

General Dosage Range Dosage adjustment recommended in patients with renal or hepatic impairment or who develop toxicities
I.V.: *Adults:* 1.4 mg/m^2/dose days 1 and 8 every 3 weeks

Mechanism of Action Eribulin is a non-taxane microtubule inhibitor which is a halichondrin B analog. It inhibits the growth phase of the microtubule by inhibiting formation of mitotic spindles causing mitotic blockage and arresting the cell cycle at the G$_2$/M phase; suppresses microtubule polymerization yet does not affect depolymerization.

Pharmacodynamics/Kinetics
Half-life Elimination ~40 hours
Pregnancy Risk Factor D
Pregnancy Considerations Teratogenicity and fetal loss were observed in animal studies. There are no adequate and well-controlled studies in pregnant women. Based on its mechanism of action, eribulin would be expected to cause fetal harm if administered during pregnancy.

Erlotinib (er LOE tye nib)

Brand Names: U.S. Tarceva®
Brand Names: Canada Tarceva®
Pharmacologic Category Antineoplastic Agent, Tyrosine Kinase Inhibitor; Epidermal Growth Factor Receptor (EGFR) Inhibitor
Use Treatment of locally advanced or metastatic nonsmall cell lung cancer (NSCLC) refractory to at least 1 prior chemotherapy regimen (as monotherapy); maintenance treatment of locally advanced or metastatic NCSLC which has not progressed after 4-6 cycles of first line platinum-based chemotherapy; locally advanced, unresectable or metastatic pancreatic cancer (first-line therapy in combination with gemcitabine)

Canadian labeling: First-line treatment of locally advanced or metastatic nonsmall cell lung cancer (NSCLC) with known EGFR mutation (as monotherapy); treatment of locally advanced or metastatic NSCLC refractory to at least 1 prior chemotherapy regimen and positive or unknown EGFR status (as monotherapy); maintenance treatment of locally advanced or metastatic NCSLC which has not progressed after 4 cycles of first line platinum-based chemotherapy
Unlabeled Use First-line treatment of NSCLC with known EGFR mutation (unlabeled in U.S.)
Local Anesthetic/Vasoconstrictor Precautions No information available to require special precautions

Effects on Dental Treatment Key adverse event(s) related to dental treatment: Xerostomia (normal salivary flow resumes upon discontinuation), mucositis, abnormal taste, and stomatitis
Effects on Bleeding In treatment of pancreatic carcinoma, has been noted to cause microangiopathic hemolytic anemia with thrombocytopenia

Adverse Effects
Adverse reactions reported with monotherapy:
>10%:
Cardiovascular: Chest pain (≤17%)
Central nervous system: Fatigue (9% to 52%), pyrexia (≤11%)
Dermatologic: Rash (49% to 75%; grade 3: 5% to 13%; grade 4: <1%; median onset: 8 days), dry skin (4% to 17%), paronychia (4% to 16%), alopecia (14% to 15%), pruritus (7% to 13%), acne (6% to 12%)
Gastrointestinal: Diarrhea (20% to 57%; grade 3: 2% to 6%; grade 4: <1%; median onset: 12 days), anorexia (9% to 52%), nausea (23% to 33%), appetite decreased (≤28%), vomiting (13% to 23%), stomatitis (11% to 17%), mucosal inflammation (≤17%), abdominal pain (3% to 11%), constipation (≤8%)
Genitourinary: Urinary tract infection (≤4%)
Hematologic: Anemia (≤11%; grade 4: 1%)
Neuromuscular & skeletal: Weakness (≤53%), back pain (≤16%)
Ocular: Conjunctivitis (12%), keratoconjunctivitis sicca (12%)
Respiratory: Dyspnea (41%), cough (33% to 45%)
Miscellaneous: Infection (4% to 24%)
1% to 10%:
Cardiovascular: Peripheral edema (≤5%)
Central nervous system: Pain (≤9%), headache (≤7%), anxiety (≤5%), dizziness (≤4%), dysphonia (≤4%), insomnia (≤4%), neurotoxicity (≤4%)
Dermatologic: Folliculitis (≤8%), nail disorder (≤7%), exfoliative rash (5%), hypertrichosis (5%), skin fissures (5%), dermatitis acneiform (4% to 5%), erythema (≤5%), dermatitis (4%), erythematous rash (≤4%), palmar-plantar erythrodysesthesia (≤4%)
Gastrointestinal: Dyspepsia (≤5%), weight loss (4% to 5%), xerostomia (≤3%), taste disturbance (≤1%)
Hematologic: Lymphopenia (≤4%; grade 3: 1%), leukopenia (≤3%), thrombocytopenia (≤1%)
Hepatic: Hyperbilirubinemia (7%; grade 3: ≤1%), ALT increased (grade 2: 2% to 4%; grade 3: 1% to 3%), GGT increased (≤4%)
Neuromuscular & skeletal: Arthralgia (≤10%), musculoskeletal pain (≤9%), bone pain (≤4%), muscle spasms (≤4%), musculoskeletal chest pain (≤4%), paresthesia (≤4%)
Otic: Tinnitus (≤1%)
Renal: Renal failure (≤1%), serum creatinine increased (≤1%)
Respiratory: Nasopharyngitis (≤7%), epistaxis (≤4%), pulmonary embolus (≤4%), respiratory tract infection (≤4%), pneumonitis/pulmonary infiltrate (3%), pulmonary fibrosis (3%)

Adverse reactions reported with combination (erlotinib plus gemcitabine) therapy:
>10%:
Cardiovascular: Edema (37%), thrombotic events (grades 3/4: 11%)
Central nervous system: Fatigue (73% to 79%), fever (36%), depression (19%), dizziness (15%), headache (15%), anxiety (13%)
Dermatologic: Rash (69%), alopecia (14%)

Gastrointestinal: Nausea (60%), anorexia (52%), diarrhea (48%), abdominal pain (46%), vomiting (42%), weight loss (39%), stomatitis (22%), dyspepsia (17%), flatulence (13%)

Hepatic: ALT increased (grade 2: 31%, grade 3: 13%, grade 4: <1%), AST increased (grade 2: 24%, grade 3: 10%, grade 4 <1%), hyperbilirubinemia (grade 2: 17%, grade 3: 10%, grade 4: <1%)

Neuromuscular & skeletal: Bone pain (25%), myalgia (21%), neuropathy (13%), rigors (12%)

Respiratory: Dyspnea (24%), cough (16%)

Miscellaneous: Infection (39%)

1% to 10%:

Cardiovascular: Arrhythmia (<5%), syncope (<5%), deep venous thrombosis (4%), cerebrovascular accident (2%; including cerebral hemorrhage), MI/myocardial ischemia (2%)

Gastrointestinal: Ileus (<5%), pancreatitis (<5%)

Hematologic: Hemolytic anemia (<5%), microangiopathic hemolytic anemia with thrombocytopenia (1%)

Renal: Renal insufficiency (<5%)

Respiratory: Interstitial lung disease-like events (<3%)

General Dosage Range Dosage adjustment recommended in patients with hepatic impairment, on concomitant therapy, who smoke, or who develop toxicities

Oral: *Adults:* 100-150 mg/day

Mechanism of Action The mechanism of erlotinib's antitumor action is not fully characterized. It is known to inhibit overall epidermal growth factor receptor (HER1/EGFR) - tyrosine kinase. Active competitive inhibition of adenosine triphosphate inhibits downstream signal transduction of ligand dependent HER1/EGFR activation.

Pharmacodynamics/Kinetics

Half-life Elimination 24-36 hours

Time to Peak Plasma: 1-7 hours

Pregnancy Risk Factor D

Pregnancy Considerations Animal reproduction studies have demonstrated fetal harm and abortion. Women of childbearing potential should be advised to avoid pregnancy; adequate contraception is recommended during treatment and for at least 2 weeks after treatment has been completed.

Ertapenem (er ta PEN em)

Brand Names: U.S. INVanz®

Brand Names: Canada Invanz®

Pharmacologic Category Antibiotic, Carbapenem

Use Treatment of the following moderate-to-severe infections: Complicated intra-abdominal infections, complicated skin and skin structure infections (including diabetic foot infections without osteomyelitis, animal and human bites), complicated UTI (including pyelonephritis), acute pelvic infections (including postpartum endomyometritis, septic abortion, postsurgical gynecologic infections), and community-acquired pneumonia. Prophylaxis of surgical site infection following elective colorectal surgery. Antibacterial coverage includes aerobic gram-positive organisms, aerobic gram-negative organisms, and anaerobic organisms.

Note: Methicillin-resistant *Staphylococcus aureus*, *Enterococcus* spp, penicillin-resistant strains of *Streptococcus pneumoniae*, *Acinetobacter*, and *Pseudomonas aeruginosa*, are **resistant** to ertapenem while most extended-spectrum β-lactamase (ESBL)-producing bacteria remain sensitive to ertapenem.

Unlabeled Use Treatment of intravenous catheter-related bloodstream infection; treatment of prosthetic joint infection

Local Anesthetic/Vasoconstrictor Precautions No information available to require special precautions

Effects on Dental Treatment Key adverse event(s) related to dental treatment: Oral candidiasis

Effects on Bleeding No information available to require special precautions

Adverse Effects

>10%: Gastrointestinal: Diarrhea (2% to 12%)

1% to 10%:

Cardiovascular: Edema (3%), chest pain (1% to 2%), hypertension (1% to 2%), hypotension (1% to 2%), tachycardia (1% to 2%)

Central nervous system: Headache (4% to 7%); altered mental status (eg, agitation, confusion, disorientation, mental acuity decreased, somnolence, stupor) (3% to 5%); fever (2% to 5%), insomnia (3%), dizziness (2%), hypothermia (infants, children, and adolescents <2%), fatigue (1%), anxiety (1%)

Dermatologic: Diaper rash (infants and children 5%), rash (2% to 3%), pruritus (1% to 2%), erythema (1% to 2%), genital rash (infants, children, and adolescents <2%), skin lesions (infants, children, and adolescents <2%)

Endocrine & metabolic: Hypokalemia (2%), hyperglycemia (1% to 2%), hyperkalemia (≤1%)

Gastrointestinal: Vomiting (2% to 10%), nausea (6% to 9%), abdominal pain (4% to 5%), constipation (2% to 4%), acid regurgitation (1% to 2%), appetite decreased (infants, children, and adolescents <2%), dyspepsia (1%), oral candidiasis (≤1%)

Genitourinary: Urine WBCs increased (2% to 3%), urine RBCs increased (1% to 3%), vaginitis (1% to 3%)

Hematologic: Thrombocytosis (4% to 7%), hematocrit/hemoglobin decreased (3% to 5%), eosinophils increased (1% to 2%), leukopenia (1% to 2%), neutrophils decreased (1% to 2%), thrombocytopenia (1%), prothrombin time increased (≤1%)

Hepatic: Hepatic enzyme increased (7% to 9%), alkaline phosphatase increase (4% to 7%), albumin decreased (1% to 2%), bilirubin (total) increased (1% to 2%)

Local: Infused vein complications (5% to 7%), phlebitis/thrombophlebitis (2%), extravasation (1% to 2%)

Neuromuscular & skeletal: Arthralgia (infants, children, and adolescents <2%), weakness (1%), leg pain (≤1%)

Otic: Otitis media (infants, children, and adolescents <2%)

Renal: Serum creatinine increased (1%)

Respiratory: Cough (1% to 4%), dyspnea (1% to 3%), nasopharyngitis (infants, children, and adolescents <2%), rhinitis (infants, children, and adolescents <2%), rhinorrhea (infants, children, and adolescents <2%), upper respiratory tract infection (infants, children, and adolescents <2%), wheezing (infants, children, and adolescents <2%), pharyngitis (1%), rales/rhonchi (1%), respiratory distress (≤1%)

Miscellaneous: Herpes simplex (infants, children, and adolescents <2%)

General Dosage Range Dosage adjustment recommended in patients with renal impairment

I.M., I.V.:

Children 3 months to 12 years: 15 mg/kg twice daily (maximum: 1 g daily)

Adolescents ≥13 years and Adults: 1 g once daily or as single dose

Mechanism of Action Inhibits bacterial cell synthesis by binding to one or more of the penicillin-binding proteins; which in turn inhibits the final transpeptidation step of peptidoglycan synthesis in bacterial cell walls, thus inhibiting cell wall biosynthesis. Bacteria eventually lyse due to ongoing activity of cell wall autolytic enzymes (autolysins and murein hydrolases) while cell wall assembly is arrested.

Pharmacodynamics/Kinetics

Half-life Elimination
Children 3 months to 12 years: ~2.5 hours
Children ≥13 years and Adults: ~4 hours

Time to Peak I.M.: ~2.3 hours

Pregnancy Risk Factor B

Pregnancy Considerations Teratogenic effects were not observed in animal reproduction studies. Ertapenem is approved for the treatment of postpartum endomyometritis, septic abortion, and postsurgical infections. Information related to use during pregnancy has not been located.

Erythromycin (Systemic) (er ith roe MYE sin)

Related Information
Bacterial Infections *on page 1562*
Clinical Risk Related to Drugs Prolonging QT Interval *on page 1510*

Related Sample Prescriptions
Bacterial Infections and Periodontal Diseases *on page 1609*

Brand Names: U.S. E.E.S.®; Ery-Tab®; EryPed®; Erythro-RX; Erythrocin®; Erythrocin® Lactobionate-I.V.; PCE®

Brand Names: Canada Apo-Erythro Base®; Apo-Erythro E-C®; Apo-Erythro-ES®; Apo-Erythro-S®; EES®; Erybid™; Eryc®; Novo-Rythro Estolate; Novo-Rythro Ethylsuccinate; Nu-Erythromycin-S; PCE®

Generic Availability (U.S.) Yes: Capsule, tablet (as base, ethylsuccinate, and stearate)

Pharmacologic Category Antibiotic, Macrolide

Dental Use Alternative to penicillin VK for treatment of orofacial infections

Use Treatment of susceptible bacterial infections including *S. pyogenes,* some *S. pneumoniae,* some *S. aureus, M. pneumoniae, Legionella pneumophila,* diphtheria, pertussis, *Chlamydia,* erythrasma, *N. gonorrhoeae, E. histolytica,* syphilis and nongonococcal urethritis, and *Campylobacter* gastroenteritis; used in conjunction with neomycin for decontaminating the bowel

Unlabeled Use Management of gastroparesis, chancroid; preoperative gut sterilization

Local Anesthetic/Vasoconstrictor Precautions Erythromycin is one of the drugs confirmed to prolong the QT interval and is accepted as having a risk of causing torsade de pointes. In terms of epinephrine, it is not known what effect vasoconstrictors in the local anesthetic regimen will have in patients with a known history of congenital prolonged QT interval or in patients taking any medication that prolongs the QT interval. Until more information is obtained, it is suggested that the clinician consult with the physician prior to the use of a vasoconstrictor in suspected patients, and that the vasoconstrictor (epinephrine, mepivacaine and levonordefrin [Carbocaine® 2% with Neo-Cobefrin®]) be used with caution. See Dental Comment.

Effects on Dental Treatment Key adverse event(s) related to dental treatment: Oral candidiasis.

Effects on Bleeding No information available to require special precautions

Adverse Effects Frequency not defined. Incidence may vary with formulation.

Cardiovascular: QT_c prolongation, torsade de pointes, ventricular arrhythmia, ventricular tachycardia

Central nervous system: Seizure

Dermatologic: Erythema multiforme, pruritus, rash, Stevens-Johnson syndrome, toxic epidermal necrolysis

Gastrointestinal: Abdominal pain, anorexia, diarrhea, infantile hypertrophic pyloric stenosis, nausea, oral candidiasis, pancreatitis, pseudomembranous colitis, vomiting

Hepatic: Cholestatic jaundice (most common with estolate), hepatitis, liver function tests abnormal

Local: Phlebitis at the injection site, thrombophlebitis

Neuromuscular & skeletal: Weakness

Otic: Hearing loss

Miscellaneous: Allergic reactions, anaphylaxis, hypersensitivity reactions, interstitial nephritis, urticaria

Dental Usual Dosage Treatment of orofacial infections:
Adults: Oral:
Base: 250-500 mg every 6-12 hours
Ethylsuccinate: 400-800 mg every 6-12 hours

Dosage Note: Due to differences in absorption, 400 mg erythromycin ethylsuccinate produces the same serum levels as 250 mg erythromycin base or stearate.

Usual dosage range:
Infants and Children:
Oral:
Base: 30-50 mg/kg/day in 2-4 divided doses; maximum: 2 g daily
Ethylsuccinate: 30-50 mg/kg/day in 2-4 divided doses; maximum: 3.2 g daily
Stearate: 30-50 mg/kg/day in 2-4 divided doses; maximum: 2 g daily
I.V.: Lactobionate: 15-50 mg/kg/day divided every 6 hours, not to exceed 4 g daily
Adults:
Oral:
Base: 250-500 mg every 6-12 hours; maximum: 4 g daily
Ethylsuccinate: 400-800 mg every 6-12 hours; maximum: 4 g daily
I.V.: Lactobionate: 15-20 mg/kg/day divided every 6 hours or 500 mg to 1 g every 6 hours, or given as a continuous infusion over 24 hours; maximum: 4 g daily

Indication-specific dosing:
Infants and Children:
Bartonella sp infections (bacillary angiomatosis **[BA], peliosis hepatis [PH]) (unlabeled use):** Oral: 40 mg/kg/day (ethylsuccinate) in 4 divided doses (maximum: 2 g daily) for 3 months (BA) or 4 months (PH)
Chlamydial infection *(C. trachomatis):* Children <45 kg: Oral: 50 mg/kg/day (base or ethylsuccinate) in 4 divided doses for 14 days (CDC, 2010)
Community-acquired pneumonia (CAP) (IDSA/PIDS, 2011): Infants >3 months and Children: **Note:** A beta-lactam antibiotic should be added if typical bacterial pneumonia cannot be ruled out.
Presumed atypical *(M. pneumoniae, C. pneumoniae, C. trachomatis)* infection, mild atypical infection or step-down therapy (alternative to azithromycin): Oral: 10 mg/kg/dose every 6 hours
Moderate-to-severe atypical infection (alternative to azithromycin): I.V.: 5 mg/kg/dose every 6 hours

Mild/moderate infection: Oral: 30-50 mg/kg/day in divided doses every 6-12 hours

Pertussis: Oral: 40-50 mg/kg/day in 4 divided doses for 14 days; maximum 2 g daily (not preferred agent for infants <1 month due to IHPS)

Pharyngitis, tonsillitis (streptococcal): Oral: 20 mg (base)/kg/day or 40 mg (ethylsuccinate)/kg/day in 2 divided doses for 10 days. **Note:** No longer preferred therapy due to increased organism resistance.

Preop bowel preparation: Oral: 20 mg (base)/kg at 1, 2, and 11 PM on the day before surgery combined with mechanical cleansing of the large intestine and oral neomycin

Severe infection: I.V.: 15-50 mg/kg/day; maximum: 4 g daily

Adults:

Bartonella sp infections (bacillary angiomatosis **[BA], peliosis hepatis [PH]) (unlabeled use):** Oral: 500 mg (base) 4 times daily for 3 months (BA) or 4 months (PH)

Chancroid (unlabeled use): Oral: 500 mg (base) 3 times daily for 7 days; **Note:** Not a preferred agent; isolates with intermediate resistance have been documented (CDC, 2010)

Gastroparesis (unlabeled use):
I.V.: 3 mg/kg administered over 45 minutes every 8 hours (Camilleri, 2013)
Oral: Patients refractory/intolerant to other prokinetic agents (eg, metoclopramide, domperidone): 250-500 mg (base) 3 times daily before meals. Limit duration of therapy, tachyphylaxis may occur after 4 weeks (Camilleri, 2013).

Granuloma inguinale (donovanosis) (unlabeled use): Oral: 500 mg (base) 4 times daily for 21 days (CDC, 2010)

Legionnaires' disease: Oral: 1.6-4 g (ethylsuccinate) daily or 1-4 g (base) daily in divided doses for 21 days. **Note:** No longer preferred therapy and only used in nonhospitalized patients.

Lymphogranuloma venereum: Oral: 500 mg (base) 4 times daily for 21 days; **Note:** Preferred therapy for pregnant or lactating women (CDC, 2010)

Nongonococcal urethritis (including coinfection with *C. trachomatis*): Oral: 500 mg (base) 4 times daily for 7 days or 800 mg (ethylsuccinate) 4 times daily for 7 days. **Note:** May use 250 mg (base) or 400 mg (ethylsuccinate) 4 times daily for 14 days if gastrointestinal intolerance.

Pertussis: Oral: 500 mg (base) every 6 hours for 14 days

Preop bowel preparation: Oral: 1 g erythromycin base at 1, 2, and 11 PM on the day before surgery combined with mechanical cleansing of the large intestine and oral neomycin

Dosage adjustment in renal impairment: Dialysis: Slightly dialyzable (5% to 20%); no supplemental dosage necessary in hemo- or peritoneal dialysis or in continuous arteriovenous or venovenous hemofiltration

Dosage adjustment in hepatic impairment: No dosage adjustment provided in manufacturer's labeling; use with caution.

Mechanism of Action Inhibits RNA-dependent protein synthesis at the chain elongation step; binds to the 50S ribosomal subunit resulting in blockage of transpeptidation

Contraindications Hypersensitivity to erythromycin, any macrolide antibiotics, or any component of the formulation

Concomitant use with pimozide, cisapride, ergotamine or dihydroergotamine, terfenadine, astemizole, lovastatin, or simvastatin

Warnings/Precautions Use caution with hepatic impairment with or without jaundice has occurred, it may be accompanied by malaise, nausea, vomiting, abdominal colic, and fever; discontinue use if these occur. Use caution with other medication relying on CYP3A4 metabolism; high potential for drug interactions exists. Prolonged use may result in fungal or bacterial superinfection, including *C. difficile*-associated diarrhea (CDAD) and pseudomembranous colitis; CDAD has been observed >2 months postantibiotic treatment. Use in infants has been associated with infantile hypertrophic pyloric stenosis (IHPS). Macrolides have been associated with rare QT$_c$ prolongation and ventricular arrhythmias, including torsade de pointes; avoid use in patients with prolonged QT interval, uncorrected hypokalemia or hypomagnesemia, clinically significant bradycardia, or concurrent use of Class IA (eg, quinidine, procainamide) or Class III (eg, amiodarone, dofetilide, sotalol) antiarrhythmic agents. Avoid concurrent use with strong CYP3A inhibitors; may increase the risk of sudden cardiac death (Ray, 2004). Use caution in elderly patients, as risk of adverse events may be increased. Use caution in myasthenia gravis patients; erythromycin may aggravate muscular weakness.

Drug Interactions

Metabolism/Transport Effects Substrate of CYP2B6 (minor), CYP3A4 (major), P-glycoprotein; **Note:** Assignment of Major/Minor substrate status based on clinically relevant drug interaction potential; **Inhibits** CYP3A4 (moderate), P-glycoprotein

Avoid Concomitant Use

Avoid concomitant use of Erythromycin (Systemic) with any of the following: BCG; Bosutinib; Cisapride; Conivaptan; Disopyramide; Highest Risk QTc-Prolonging Agents; Ivabradine; Lincosamide Antibiotics; Lomitapide; Lovastatin; Mifepristone; Pimozide; Pomalidomide; QuiNINE; Silodosin; Simvastatin; Terfenadine; Tolvaptan; Topotecan

Increased Effect/Toxicity

Erythromycin (Systemic) may increase the levels/ effects of: Alfentanil; Antifungal Agents (Azole Derivatives, Systemic); Antineoplastic Agents (Vinca Alkaloids); ARIPiprazole; Avanafil; Benzodiazepines (metabolized by oxidation); Bosutinib; Budesonide (Systemic, Oral Inhalation); BusPIRone; Calcium Channel Blockers; CarBAMazepine; Cardiac Glycosides; Cilostazol; Cisapride; CloZAPine; Colchicine; Corticosteroids (Systemic); CycloSPORINE (Systemic); CYP3A4 Substrates; Dabigatran Etexilate; Disopyramide; Eletriptan; Eplerenone; Ergot Derivatives; Everolimus; FentaNYL; Fexofenadine; Highest Risk QTc-Prolonging Agents; HMG-CoA Reductase Inhibitors; Ivacaftor; Lomitapide; Lovastatin; Lurasidone; Moderate Risk QTc-Prolonging Agents; P-glycoprotein/ABCB1 Substrates; Pimecrolimus; Pimozide; Pomalidomide; QuiNIDine; QuiNINE; Repaglinide; Rifamycin Derivatives; Rivaroxaban; Salmeterol; Saxagliptin; Selective Serotonin Reuptake Inhibitors; Sildenafil; Silodosin; Simvastatin; Sirolimus; Tacrolimus (Systemic); Tacrolimus (Topical); Telaprevir; Temsirolimus; Terfenadine; Theophylline Derivatives; Tolvaptan; Topotecan; Vardenafil; Vitamin K Antagonists; Zopiclone

The levels/effects of Erythromycin (Systemic) may be increased by: Antifungal Agents (Azole Derivatives, Systemic); Conivaptan; CYP3A4 Inhibitors (Moderate); CYP3A4 Inhibitors (Strong); Dasatinib; Ivabradine;

Ivacaftor; Mifepristone; P-glycoprotein/ABCB1 Inhibitors; QTc-Prolonging Agents (Indeterminate Risk and Risk Modifying); Telaprevir

Decreased Effect

Erythromycin (Systemic) may decrease the levels/ effects of: BCG; Clopidogrel; Ifosfamide; Sodium Picosulfate; Typhoid Vaccine; Zafirlukast

The levels/effects of Erythromycin (Systemic) may be decreased by: CYP3A4 Inducers (Strong); Deferasirox; Etravirine; Herbs (CYP3A4 Inducers); Lincosamide Antibiotics; P-glycoprotein/ABCB1 Inducers; Tocilizumab

Ethanol/Nutrition/Herb Interactions

Ethanol: Ethanol may decrease absorption of erythromycin or enhance effects of ethanol. Management: Avoid ethanol.

Food: Erythromycin serum levels may be altered if taken with food (formulation-dependent). GI upset, including diarrhea, is common. Management: May be taken with food to decrease GI upset, otherwise take around-the-clock with a full glass of water. Do not give with milk or acidic beverages (eg, soda, juice).

Herb/Nutraceutical: St John's wort may decrease erythromycin levels. Management: Avoid St John's wort.

Dietary Considerations Drug may cause GI upset; may take with food. Some products may contain sodium.

Pharmacodynamics/Kinetics

Half-life Elimination Peak: 1.5-2 hours; End-stage renal disease: 5-6 hours

Time to Peak Serum: Base: 4 hours; Ethylsuccinate: 0.5-2.5 hours; delayed with food due to differences in absorption

Pregnancy Risk Factor B

Pregnancy Considerations Adverse events were not observed in animal reproduction studies. Erythromycin crosses the placenta and low concentrations are found in the fetal serum. Most reports do not identify an increase in risk for congenital abnormalities due to prenatal exposure to erythromycin. Cardiovascular anomalies following exposure in early pregnancy have been reported in some observational studies. Most studies also do not support a link between prenatal exposure to erythromycin and pyloric stenosis in the neonate. In general, serum concentrations of erythromycin are lower in pregnant women. Erythromycin therapy in patients with preterm, premature rupture of membranes is associated with a range of health benefits to the neonate and no long-term adverse events to the child have been observed. However, maternal use of erythromycin in women with preterm labor, intact membranes, and no documented infection does not improve neonatal health and may have adverse effects in childhood (use is not recommended). In patients with acute infections during pregnancy, erythromycin may be given if an antibiotic is required and appropriate based on bacterial sensitivity. Erythromycin is the antibiotic of choice for preterm premature rupture of membranes (with membrane rupture prior to 34 weeks gestation), the treatment of granuloma inguinale and lymphogranuloma venereum in pregnancy, and the treatment of or long-term suppression of *Bartonella* infection in HIV-infected pregnant patients. Erythromycin may be appropriate as an alternative agent for the treatment of chlamydial infections in pregnant women (consult current guidelines).

Lactation Enters breast milk/use caution (AAP considers "compatible"; AAP 2001 update pending)

Breast-Feeding Considerations Erythromycin is excreted in breast milk; therefore, the manufacturer recommends that caution be exercised when administering erythromycin to breast-feeding women.

Due to the low concentrations in human milk, minimal toxicity would be expected in the nursing infant. One case report and a cohort study raise the possibility for a connection with pyloric stenosis in neonates exposed to erythromycin via breast milk and an alternative antibiotic may be preferred for breast-feeding mothers of infants in this age group. Nondose-related effects could include modification of bowel flora.

Dosage Forms

Capsule, delayed release, enteric coated pellets, oral: 250 mg

Granules for suspension, oral:

E.E.S.®: Erythromycin activity 200 mg/5 mL (100 mL, 200 mL)

Injection, powder for reconstitution:

Erythrocin® Lactobionate-I.V.: Erythromycin activity 500 mg

Powder, for prescription compounding:

Erythro-RX: USP: 100% (50 g)

Powder for suspension, oral:

EryPed®: Erythromycin activity 200 mg/5 mL (100 mL); Erythromycin activity 400 mg/5 mL (100 mL)

Tablet, oral: 250 mg, Erythromycin activity 400 mg, 500 mg

E.E.S.®: Erythromycin activity 400 mg

Erythrocin®: Erythromycin activity 250 mg, Erythromycin activity 500 mg

Tablet, delayed release, enteric coated, oral:

Ery-Tab®: 250 mg, 333 mg, 500 mg

Tablet, polymer coated particles, oral:

PCE®: 333 mg, 500 mg

Dental Comment Erythromycin is known to prolong the QT interval. The QT interval is measured as the time and distance between the Q point of the QRS complex and the end of the T wave in the ECG tracing. After adjustment for heart rate, the QT interval is defined as prolonged if it is more than 450 msec in men and 460 msec in women. A long QT syndrome was first described in the 1950s and 60s as a congenital syndrome involving QT interval prolongation and syncope and sudden death. Some of the congenital long QT syndromes were characterized by a peculiar electrocardiographic appearance of the QRS complex involving a premature atria beat followed by a pause, then a subsequent sinus beat showing marked QT prolongation and deformity. This type of cardiac arrhythmia was originally termed "torsade de pointes" (translated from the French as "twisting of the points"). Erythromycin is considered as having a risk of causing torsade de pointes. Since it is not known what effect vasoconstrictors in the local anesthetic regimen will have in patients with a known history of congenital prolonged QT interval or in patients taking any medication that prolongs the QT interval, a medical consult is suggested.

Many patients cannot tolerate erythromycin because of abdominal pain and nausea; the mechanism of this adverse effect appears to be the motilin agonistic properties of erythromycin in the GI tract. For these patients, clindamycin is indicated as the alternative antibiotic for treatment of orofacial infections.

HMG-CoA reductase inhibitors, also known as the statins, effectively decrease the hepatic cholesterol biosynthesis resulting in the reduction of blood LDL-cholesterol concentrations. The AUC of atorvastatin (Lipitor®) was increased 33% by erythromycin administration. Combination of erythromycin and lovastatin (Mevacor®) has been associated with rhabdomyolysis (Ayanian, et al). The mechanism of erythromycin is inhibiting the CYP3A4 metabolism of atorvastatin, lovastatin, and cerivastatin. Simvastatin (Zocor®) would likely be affected in a similar manner by the coadministration of erythromycin. Clarithromycin (Biaxin®) may exert a similar effect as erythromycin on atorvastatin, lovastatin, cerivastatin, and simvastatin.

References

American Dental Association Council on Scientific Affairs, "Combating Antibiotic Resistance," *J Am Dent Assoc*, 2004, 135(4):484-7.

Wynn RL and Bergman SA, "Antibiotics and Their Use in the Treatment of Orofacial Infections, Part I and Part II," *Gen Dent*, 1994, 42 (5):398-402, 498-502.

Wynn RL, "Current Concepts of the Erythromycins," *Gen Dent*, 1991, 39(6):408, 410-1.

Erythromycin and Benzoyl Peroxide
(er ith roe MYE sin & BEN zoe il per OKS ide)

Related Information

Benzoyl Peroxide *on page 180*

Brand Names: U.S. Benzamycin®; Benzamycin® Pak

Brand Names: Canada Benzamycin®

Pharmacologic Category Acne Products; Topical Skin Product, Acne

Use Topical control of acne vulgaris

Local Anesthetic/Vasoconstrictor Precautions No information available to require special precautions

Effects on Dental Treatment No significant effects or complications reported

Effects on Bleeding No information available to require special precautions

Adverse Effects

1% to 10%:

Dermatologic: Dry skin (3% to 8%), urticaria (3%), pruritus (2% to 3%), burning (1% to 3%), erythema (1% to 3%), stinging (1% to 3%), photosensitivity (1%), oiliness, peeling, skin discoloration, skin tenderness, swelling

Ocular: Blepharitis (≤2%)

General Dosage Range Topical: *Adolescents ≥12 years and Adults:* Apply twice daily

Pregnancy Risk Factor C

Pregnancy Considerations Animal reproduction studies have not been conducted with this combination. Refer to individual monographs.

Erythromycin and Sulfisoxazole
(er ith roe MYE sin & sul fi SOKS a zole)

Related Information

Erythromycin (Systemic) *on page 495*

Brand Names: U.S. E.S.P.®

Brand Names: Canada Pediazole®

Pharmacologic Category Antibiotic, Macrolide; Antibiotic, Macrolide Combination; Antibiotic, Sulfonamide Derivative

Use Treatment of otitis media caused by susceptible strains of *Haemophilus influenzae*

Local Anesthetic/Vasoconstrictor Precautions No information available to require special precautions

Effects on Dental Treatment Key adverse event(s) related to dental treatment: Oral candidiasis.

Effects on Bleeding No information available to require special precautions

Adverse Effects Frequency not defined. Adverse events specific to this combination have not been identified.

Cardiovascular: Allergic myocarditis, arteritis, cyanosis, edema (including periorbital), flushing, intracranial hypertension, palpitations, periarteritis nodosa, syncope, tachycardia, torsade de pointes, vasculitis, ventricular arrhythmia

Central nervous system: Anxiety, ataxia, depression, disorientation, dizziness, drowsiness, fatigue, fever, hallucinations, headache, insomnia, psychosis, seizure, vertigo

Dermatologic: Angioedema, erythema multiforme, exfoliative dermatitis, photosensitivity, pruritus, purpura, rash, Stevens-Johnson syndrome, toxic epidermal necrolysis, urticaria

Endocrine & metabolic: Goiter (rare), hypoglycemia (rare)

Gastrointestinal: Abdominal pain, anorexia, diarrhea, flatulence, gastrointestinal hemorrhage, glossitis, hypertrophic pyloric stenosis, melena, nausea, oral candidiasis, pancreatitis, pseudomembranous colitis, salivary gland swelling, stomatitis, vomiting

Genitourinary: Urinary retention

Hematologic: Agranulocytosis, anemia, aplastic anemia, clotting disorders (including hypoprothrombinemia, hypofibrinogenemia, sulfhemoglobinemia, methemoglobinemia), eosinophilia, hemolytic anemia, leukopenia, thrombocytopenia

Hepatic: Hepatotoxicity (including hepatitis, hepatic necrosis, and cholestatic jaundice), liver enzymes increased

Neuromuscular & skeletal: Paresthesia, peripheral neuritis, rigors, weakness

Otic: Hearing loss (reversible), tinnitus

Renal: Acute renal failure, blood urea nitrogen increased, crystalluria, diuresis (rare), hematuria, nephritis, serum creatinine increased, toxic nephrosis (with oliguria and anuria)

Respiratory: Cough, dyspnea, pneumonitis, pulmonary infiltrates

Miscellaneous: Anaphylaxis, hypersensitivity reactions, serum sickness, systemic lupus erythematosus (SLE)

General Dosage Range Oral: *Infants ≥2 months and Children:* Erythromycin 50 mg/kg/day and sulfisoxazole 150 mg/kg/day in divided doses every 6-8 hours (maximum: Erythromycin 2 g/day or sulfisoxazole 6 g/day)

Mechanism of Action Erythromycin inhibits bacterial protein synthesis; sulfisoxazole competitively inhibits bacterial synthesis of folic acid from para-aminobenzoic acid

Pharmacodynamics/Kinetics

Half-life Elimination Sulfisoxazole: 5-8 hours

Time to Peak Sulfisoxazole: 1-4 hours

Pregnancy Risk Factor C

Pregnancy Considerations Animal reproduction studies have not been conducted with this combination; therefore, the manufacturer classifies erythromycin/sulfisoxazole as pregnancy category C. Erythromycin and sulfisoxazole cross the placenta. Sulfisoxazole is contraindicated in late pregnancy because sulfonamides may cause kernicterus in the newborn. Neonatal healthcare providers should be informed if maternal sulfonamide therapy is used near the time of delivery. See individual agents.

Escitalopram (es sye TAL oh pram)

Related Information

Citalopram *on page 312*

Clinical Risk Related to Drugs Prolonging QT Interval *on page 1510*

Vasoconstrictor Interactions With Antidepressants *on page 1650*

Brand Names: U.S. Lexapro®

Brand Names: Canada Cipralex®

Generic Availability (U.S.) Yes

Pharmacologic Category Antidepressant, Selective Serotonin Reuptake Inhibitor

Use Treatment of major depressive disorder; generalized anxiety disorders (GAD)

Canadian labeling: Additional use (not in U.S. labeling): Treatment of obsessive-compulsive disorder (OCD)

Unlabeled Use Treatment of mild dementia-associated agitation in nonpsychotic patients; treatment of vasomotor symptoms associated with menopause

Local Anesthetic/Vasoconstrictor Precautions Although caution should be used in patients taking tricyclic antidepressants, no interactions have been reported with vasoconstrictors and escitalopram, a nontricyclic antidepressant which acts to increase serotonin; no precautions appear to be needed

Escitalopram is one of the drugs confirmed to prolong the QT interval and is accepted as having a risk of causing torsade de pointes. The risk of drug-induced torsade de pointes is extremely low when a single QT interval prolonging drug is prescribed. In terms of epinephrine, it is not known what effect vasoconstrictors in the local anesthetic regimen will have in patients with a known history of congenital prolonged QT interval or in patients taking any medication that prolongs the QT interval. Until more information is obtained, it is suggested that the clinician consult with the physician prior to the use of a vasoconstrictor in suspected patients, and that the vasoconstrictor (epinephrine, mepivacaine, and levonordefrin [Carbocaine® 2% with Neo-Cobefrin®]) be used with caution.

Effects on Dental Treatment Key adverse event(s) related to dental treatment: Xerostomia (normal salivary flow resumes upon discontinuation) and toothache. See Effects on Bleeding.

Effects on Bleeding Selective serotonin reuptake inhibitors such as escitalopram may impair platelet aggregation due to platelet serotonin depletion, possibly increasing the risk of a bleeding complication. The risk of a bleeding complication can be increased by coadministration of other antiplatelet agents such as NSAIDs and aspirin.

Adverse Effects

>10%:

Central nervous system: Headache (24%), somnolence (4% to 13%), insomnia (7% to 12%)

Gastrointestinal: Diarrhea (6% to 14%), nausea (15% to 18%)

Genitourinary: Ejaculation disorder (9% to 14%)

1% to 10%:

Central nervous system: Fatigue (2% to 8%), dizziness (4% to 7%), abnormal dreaming (3%), lethargy (3%), yawning (2%)

Endocrine & metabolic: Libido decreased (3% to 7%), anorgasmia (2% to 6%), menstrual disorder (2%)

Gastrointestinal: Xerostomia (4% to 9%), constipation (3% to 6%), indigestion (2% to 6%), appetite decreased (3%), vomiting (3%), abdominal pain (2%), flatulence (2%), toothache (2%)

Genitourinary: Impotence (2% to 3%), urinary tract infection (children ≥2%)

Neuromuscular & skeletal: Neck/shoulder pain (3%), back pain (children ≥2%), paresthesia (2%)

Respiratory: Rhinitis (5%), sinusitis (3%), nasal congestion (children ≥2%)

Miscellaneous: Diaphoresis (3% to 8%), flu-like syndrome (5%)

Dosage Oral:

U.S. labeling:

Children ≥12 years: Major depressive disorder: Initial: 10 mg once daily; dose may be increased to a maximum of 20 mg once daily after at least 3 weeks

Adults: Major depressive disorder, generalized anxiety disorder: Initial: 10 mg once daily; dose may be increased to a maximum of 20 mg once daily after at least 1 week

Elderly: 10 mg once daily

Canadian labeling:

Adults: Major depressive disorder, generalized anxiety disorder (GAD), obsessive compulsive disorder (OCD): Initial: 10 mg once daily (may consider 5 mg once daily where sensitivity is a concern); dose may be increased as tolerated to a maximum of 20 mg once daily. Patients with GAD or OCD who require extended therapy should be maintained at the lowest effective dose and assessed periodically to determine the need for continued therapy. **Note:** Initiate treatment in poor CYP2C19 metabolizers at a dose of 5 mg once daily; may increase dose to a maximum of 10 mg once daily.

Elderly: Initial: 5 mg once daily; dose may be increased as tolerated to a maximum of 10 mg once daily

Unlabeled use: Adults: Vasomotor symptoms associated with menopause: Initial: 10 mg once daily, increase to 20 mg once daily after 4 weeks if symptoms not adequately controlled (Carpenter, 2012; Freeman, 2011).

MAO inhibitor recommendations: *U.S. labeling:*

Switching to or from an MAO inhibitor intended to treat psychiatric disorders:

Allow 14 days to elapse between discontinuing an MAO inhibitor intended to treat psychiatric disorders and initiation of escitalopram.

Allow 14 days to elapse between discontinuing escitalopram and initiation of an MAO inhibitor intended to treat psychiatric disorders.

Use with other MAO inhibitors (linezolid or I.V. methylene blue):

Do not initiate escitalopram in patients receiving linezolid or I.V. methylene blue; consider other interventions for psychiatric condition.

If urgent treatment with linezolid or I.V. methylene blue is required in a patient already receiving escitalopram and potential benefits outweigh potential risks, discontinue escitalopram promptly and administer linezolid or I.V. methylene blue. Monitor for serotonin syndrome for 2 weeks or until 24 hours after the last dose of linezolid or I.V. methylene blue, whichever comes first. May resume escitalopram 24 hours after the last dose of linezolid or I.V. methylene blue.

Dosage adjustment with concomitant medications: *Canadian labeling:* Escitalopram dose should not exceed 10 mg once daily in patients taking omeprazole or cimetidine.

Dosage adjustment in renal impairment:
Mild-to-moderate impairment: No dosage adjustment is necessary
Severe impairment: Cl_{cr} <20 mL/minute (U.S. labeling) or Cl_{cr} <30 mL/minute (Canadian labeling): Use with caution.

Dosage adjustment in hepatic impairment:
U.S. labeling: 10 mg once daily
Canadian labeling:
Mild or moderate impairment (Child-Pugh class A or B): Initial: 5 mg once daily; dose may be increased as tolerated to 10 mg once daily (maximum dose)
Severe Impairment (Child-Pugh class C): No dosage adjustment provided in manufacturer's labeling; has not been studied. Use with caution.

Mechanism of Action Escitalopram is the S-enantiomer of the racemic derivative citalopram, which selectively inhibits the reuptake of serotonin with little to no effect on norepinephrine or dopamine reuptake. It has no or very low affinity for $5\text{-}HT_{1-7}$, alpha- and beta-adrenergic, D_{1-5}, H_{1-3}, M_{1-5}, and benzodiazepine receptors. Escitalopram does not bind to or has low affinity for Na^+, K^+, Cl^-, and Ca^{++} ion channels.

Contraindications Hypersensitivity to escitalopram, citalopram, or any component of the formulation; use of MAO inhibitors intended to treat psychiatric disorders (concurrently or within 14 days of discontinuing either escitalopram or the MAO inhibitor); initiation of escitalopram in a patient receiving linezolid or intravenous methylene blue

Canadian labeling: Additional contraindications (not in U.S. labeling): Known QT-interval prolongation or congenital long QT syndrome

Warnings/Precautions [U.S. Boxed Warning]: Antidepressants increase the risk of suicidal thinking and behavior in children, adolescents, and young adults (18-24 years of age) with major depressive disorder (MDD) and other psychiatric disorders; consider risk prior to prescribing. Short-term studies did not show an increased risk in patients >24 years of age and showed a decreased risk in patients ≥65 years. Closely monitor patients for clinical worsening, suicidality, or unusual changes in behavior, particularly during the initial 1-2 months of therapy or during periods of dosage adjustments (increases or decreases); the patient's family or caregiver should be instructed to closely observe the patient and communicate condition with healthcare provider. A medication guide concerning the use of antidepressants should be dispensed with each prescription. **Escitalopram is not FDA approved for use in children <12 years of age.**

The possibility of a suicide attempt is inherent in major depression and may persist until remission occurs. Use caution in high-risk patients. Worsening depression and severe abrupt suicidality that are not part of the presenting symptoms may require discontinuation or modification of drug therapy. The patient's family or caregiver should be alerted to monitor patients for the emergence of suicidality and associated behaviors (such as agitation, irritability, hostility, impulsivity, and hypomania) and call healthcare provider.

May worsen psychosis in some patients or precipitate a shift to mania or hypomania in patients with bipolar disorder. Patients presenting with depressive symptoms should be screened for bipolar disorder. Monotherapy in patients with bipolar disorder should be avoided. Escitalopram is not FDA approved for the treatment of bipolar depression. Escitalopram is not FDA approved for the treatment of bipolar depression.

Potentially life-threatening serotonin syndrome (SS) has occurred with serotonergic agents (eg, SSRIs, SNRIs), particularly when used in combination with other serotonergic agents (eg, triptans, TCAs, fentanyl, lithium, tramadol, buspirone, St John's wort, tryptophan) or agents that impair metabolism of serotonin (eg, MOA inhibitors intended to treat psychiatric disorders, other MAO inhibitors [ie, linezolid and intravenous methylene blue]). Discontinue treatment (and any concomitant serotonergic agent) immediately if signs/symptoms arise. May increase the risks associated with electroconvulsive therapy. Has a low potential to impair cognitive or motor performance; caution operating hazardous machinery or driving.

Use with caution in patients with a recent history of MI or unstable heart disease. Use has been associated with dose-dependent QT-interval prolongation with doses of 10 mg and 30 mg/day in healthy subjects (mean change from baseline: 4.3 msec and 10.7 msec, respectively); prolongation of QT interval and ventricular arrhythmia (including torsade de pointes) have been reported, particularly in females with pre-existing QT prolongation or other risk factors (eg, hypokalemia, other cardiac disease).

Use caution with a previous seizure disorder or condition predisposing to seizures such as brain damage, alcoholism, or concurrent therapy with other drugs which lower the seizure threshold. May cause hyponatremia/SIADH (elderly at increased risk); volume depletion (diuretics may increase risk) may occur. Use caution in patients with metabolic disease. May cause or exacerbate sexual dysfunction. Use caution in elderly patients; may cause or exacerbate syndrome of inappropriate antidiuretic hormone secretion or hyponatremia; monitor sodium closely with initiation or dosage adjustments in older adults (Beers Criteria). Bioavailability and half-life are increased by 50% in the elderly. Use caution with severe renal impairment or liver impairment; concomitant CNS depressants. Use with caution in patients who are hemodynamically unstable. UPotentially significant interactions may exist, requiring dose or frequency adjustment, additional monitoring, and/or selection of alternative therapy. Consult drug interactions database for more detailed information.

Upon discontinuation of escitalopram therapy, gradually taper dose. If intolerable symptoms occur following a decrease in dosage or upon discontinuation of therapy, then resuming the previous dose with a more gradual taper should be considered.

Drug Interactions

Metabolism/Transport Effects Substrate of CYP2C19 (major), CYP3A4 (major); **Note:** Assignment of Major/Minor substrate status based on clinically relevant drug interaction potential; **Inhibits** CYP2D6 (weak)

Avoid Concomitant Use

Avoid concomitant use of Escitalopram with any of the following: Conivaptan; Highest Risk QTc-Prolonging Agents; Iobenguane I 123; Ivabradine; Linezolid; MAO Inhibitors; Methylene Blue; Mifepristone; Moderate Risk QTc-Prolonging Agents; Pimozide; Tryptophan

Increased Effect/Toxicity

Escitalopram may increase the levels/effects of:
Agents with Antiplatelet Properties; Anticoagulants; Antidepressants (Serotonin Reuptake Inhibitor/Antagonist); Aspirin; BusPIRone; CarBAMazepine; CloZAPine; Collagenase (Systemic); Dabigatran Etexilate; Desmopressin; Dextromethorphan; Drotrecogin Alfa (Activated); Highest Risk QTc-Prolonging Agents; Hypoglycemic Agents; Ibritumomab; Methadone; Methylene Blue; Metoclopramide; Mexiletine; NSAID (COX-2 Inhibitor); NSAID (Nonselective); Pimozide; RisperiDONE; Rivaroxaban; Salicylates; Serotonin Modulators; Thrombolytic Agents; Tositumomab and Iodine I 131 Tositumomab; TraMADol; Tricyclic Antidepressants; Vitamin K Antagonists

The levels/effects of Escitalopram may be increased by: Alcohol (Ethyl); Analgesics (Opioid); Antipsychotics; BusPIRone; Cimetidine; CNS Depressants; Cobicistat; Conivaptan; CYP2C19 Inhibitors (Moderate); CYP2C19 Inhibitors (Strong); CYP3A4 Inhibitors (Moderate); CYP3A4 Inhibitors (Strong); Dasatinib; Glucosamine; Herbs (Anticoagulant/Antiplatelet Properties); Ivabradine; Ivacaftor; Linezolid; Lithium; Macrolide Antibiotics; MAO Inhibitors; Metoclopramide; Metyrosine; Mifepristone; Moderate Risk QTc-Prolonging Agents; Multivitamins/Minerals (with ADEK, Folate, Iron); Omega-3 Fatty Acids; Omeprazole; Pentosan Polysulfate Sodium; Pentoxifylline; Prostacyclin Analogues; QTc-Prolonging Agents (Indeterminate Risk and Risk Modifying); Tipranavir; TraMADol; Tryptophan; Vitamin E

Decreased Effect

Escitalopram may decrease the levels/effects of: Iobenguane I 123; Ioflupane I 123

The levels/effects of Escitalopram may be decreased by: Boceprevir; CarBAMazepine; CYP2C19 Inducers (Strong); CYP3A4 Inducers (Strong); Cyproheptadine; Deferasirox; NSAID (COX-2 Inhibitor); NSAID (Nonselective); Telaprevir; Tocilizumab

Ethanol/Nutrition/Herb Interactions

Ethanol: May increase CNS depression; monitor for increased effects with coadministration. Caution patients about effects.

Herb/Nutraceutical: Avoid valerian, St John's wort, tryptophan, SAMe, kava kava, and gotu kola (may increase CNS depression and/or increase risk of serotonin syndrome).

Dietary Considerations May be taken with or without food.

Pharmacodynamics/Kinetics

Onset of Action Depression: The onset of action is within a week; however, individual response varies greatly and full response may not be seen until 8-12 weeks after initiation of treatment.

Half-life Elimination ~27-32 hours (increased ~50% in the elderly and doubled in patients with hepatic impairment)

Time to Peak Escitalopram: ~5 hours

Pregnancy Risk Factor C

Pregnancy Considerations Adverse events have been observed in animal reproduction studies. Escitalopram crosses the placenta and is distributed into the amniotic fluid. An increased risk of teratogenic effects, including cardiovascular defects, may be associated with maternal use of escitalopram or other SSRIs; however, available information is conflicting. Nonteratogenic effects in the newborn following SSRI/SNRI exposure late in the third trimester include respiratory distress, cyanosis, apnea, seizures, temperature instability, feeding difficulty, vomiting, hypoglycemia, hypo- or hypertonia, hyper-reflexia, jitteriness, irritability, constant crying, and tremor. Symptoms may be due to the toxicity of the SSRIs/SNRIs or a discontinuation syndrome and may be consistent with serotonin syndrome associated with SSRI treatment. Persistent pulmonary hypertension of the newborn (PPHN) has also been reported with SSRI exposure. The long-term effects of *in utero* SSRI exposure on infant development and behavior are not known. Escitalopram is the S-enantiomer of the racemic derivative citalopram; also refer to the Citalopram monograph.

Due to pregnancy-induced physiologic changes, some pharmacokinetic parameters of escitalopram may be altered. The ACOG recommends that therapy with SSRIs or SNRIs during pregnancy be individualized; treatment of depression during pregnancy should incorporate the clinical expertise of the mental health clinician, obstetrician, primary healthcare provider, and pediatrician. According to the American Psychiatric Association (APA), the risks of medication treatment should be weighed against other treatment options and untreated depression. For women who discontinue antidepressant medications during pregnancy and who may be at high risk for postpartum depression, the medications can be restarted following delivery. Treatment algorithms have been developed by the ACOG and the APA for the management of depression in women prior to conception and during pregnancy.

Lactation Enters breast milk/consider risk:benefit

Breast-Feeding Considerations Escitalopram and its metabolite are excreted into breast milk. Limited data is available concerning the effects escitalopram may have in the nursing infant and the long-term effects on development and behavior have not been studied. Adverse effects have been reported in nursing infants exposed to some SSRIs. According to the manufacturer, the decision to continue or discontinue breast-feeding during therapy should take into account the risk of exposure to the infant and the benefits of treatment to the mother. Maternal use of an SSRI during pregnancy may cause delayed milk secretion. Escitalopram is the S-enantiomer of the racemic derivative citalopram; also refer to the Citalopram monograph.

Dosage Forms

Solution, oral: 1 mg/mL (240 mL)
  Lexapro®: 1 mg/mL (240 mL)

Tablet, oral: 5 mg, 10 mg, 20 mg
  Lexapro®: 5 mg, 10 mg, 20 mg

Dosage Forms: Canada

Tablet:
  Cipralex®: 10 mg, 20 mg

Dental Comment Escitalopram is known to prolong the QT interval. The QT interval is measured as the time and distance between the Q point of the QRS complex and the end of the T wave in the ECG tracing. After adjustment for heart rate, the QT interval is defined as prolonged if it is more than 450 msec in men and 460 msec in women. A long QT syndrome was first described in the 1950s and 60s as a congenital syndrome involving QT interval prolongation and syncope and sudden death. Some of the congenital long QT syndromes were characterized by a peculiar electrocardiographic appearance of the QRS complex involving a premature atria beat followed by a pause, then a subsequent sinus beat showing marked QT prolongation and deformity. This type of cardiac arrhythmia was originally termed "torsade de pointes" (translated from the French as "twisting of the points"). Escitalopram is considered as having a risk of causing torsade de pointes. Since it is not known what effect vasoconstrictors in the local anesthetic regimen will have in patients with a known history of congenital prolonged QT interval or in patients taking any medication that prolongs the QT interval, a medical consult is suggested.

Esmolol (ES moe lol)

Brand Names: U.S. Brevibloc
Brand Names: Canada Brevibloc®; Brevibloc® Premixed
Pharmacologic Category Antiarrhythmic Agent, Class II; Beta-Blocker, Beta-1 Selective
Use Treatment of supraventricular tachycardia (SVT) and atrial fibrillation/flutter (control ventricular rate); treatment of intraoperative and postoperative tachycardia and/or hypertension; treatment of noncompensatory sinus tachycardia
Unlabeled Use
Children: SVT and postoperative hypertension
Adults: Arrhythmia/rate control during acute coronary syndrome (eg, acute myocardial infarction, unstable angina), aortic dissection, intubation, thyroid storm, pheochromocytoma, electroconvulsive therapy
Local Anesthetic/Vasoconstrictor Precautions No information available to require special precautions
Effects on Dental Treatment Esmolol is a cardioselective beta-blocker. Local anesthetic with vasoconstrictor can be safely used in patients medicated with esmolol. Nonselective beta-blockers (ie, propranolol, nadolol) enhance the pressor response to epinephrine, resulting in hypertension and bradycardia; this has not been reported for esmolol. Many nonsteroidal anti-inflammatory drugs, such as ibuprofen and indomethacin, can reduce the hypotensive effect of beta-blockers after 3 or more weeks of therapy with the NSAID. Short-term NSAID use (ie, 3 days) requires no special precautions in patients taking beta-blockers.
Effects on Bleeding No information available to require special precautions
Adverse Effects
>10%: Cardiovascular: Blood pressure decreased (20% to 50%), asymptomatic hypotension (dose related: 25%), symptomatic hypotension (dose related: 12%)
1% to 10%:
Cardiovascular: Peripheral ischemia (1%)
Central nervous system: Dizziness (3%), somnolence (3%), confusion (2%), headache (2%), agitation (2%)
Gastrointestinal: Nausea (7%), vomiting (1%)
Local: Infusion site reaction (8%; including irritation, inflammation, and severe reactions associated with extravasation [eg, thrombophlebitis, necrosis, and blistering])
General Dosage Range I.V.: *Adults:* Bolus: 0.5 **mg**/kg or 1 mg/kg; Infusion: 50-200 mcg/kg/minute (maximum: 300 mcg/kg/minute)
Mechanism of Action Class II antiarrhythmic: Competitively blocks response to $beta_1$-adrenergic stimulation with little or no effect of $beta_2$-receptors except at high doses, no intrinsic sympathomimetic activity, no membrane stabilizing activity
Pharmacodynamics/Kinetics
Onset of Action Beta-blockade: I.V.: 2-10 minutes (quickest when loading doses are administered)
Duration of Action Hemodynamic effects: 10-30 minutes; prolonged following higher cumulative doses, extended duration of use

Half-life Elimination Adults: Esmolol: 9 minutes; Acid metabolite: 3.7 hours; elimination of metabolite decreases with end-stage renal disease
Pregnancy Risk Factor C
Pregnancy Considerations Adverse events were observed in some animal reproduction studies. Esmolol has been shown to decrease fetal heart rate. Adverse fetal/neonatal events have also been observed with the chronic use of beta-blockers during pregnancy. Esmolol is a short-acting beta-blocker and not indicated for the chronic treatment of hypertension. Esmolol may be considered for the acute management of atrial fibrillation in pregnant women (Fuster, 2006). Esmolol has been evaluated for use during intubation as an agent to offset the exaggerated pressor response observed in pregnant women with hypertension undergoing surgery (Bansal, 2002).

Esomeprazole (es oh ME pray zol)

Related Information
Gastrointestinal Disorders *on page 1512*
Omeprazole *on page 1009*
Brand Names: U.S. NexIUM®; NexIUM® I.V.
Brand Names: Canada Apo-Esomeprazole®; Mylan-Esomeprazole; Nexium®
Generic Availability (U.S.) No
Pharmacologic Category Proton Pump Inhibitor; Substituted Benzimidazole
Use
Oral: Short-term (4-8 weeks) treatment of erosive esophagitis; maintaining symptom resolution and healing of erosive esophagitis; treatment of symptomatic gastroesophageal reflux disease (GERD); as part of a multidrug regimen for *Helicobacter pylori* eradication in patients with duodenal ulcer disease (active or history of within the past 5 years); prevention of gastric ulcers in patients at risk (age ≥60 years and/or history of gastric ulcer) associated with continuous NSAID therapy; long-term treatment of pathological hypersecretory conditions including Zollinger-Ellison syndrome
Canadian labeling: Additional use (not in U.S. labeling): Oral: Treatment of nonerosive reflux disease (NERD); treatment of NSAID-induced gastric ulcers

I.V.: Short-term (≤10 days) treatment of gastroesophageal reflux disease (GERD) when oral therapy is not possible or appropriate
Unlabeled Use I.V.: Prevention of recurrent peptic ulcer bleeding postendoscopy
Local Anesthetic/Vasoconstrictor Precautions No information available to require special precautions
Effects on Dental Treatment Key adverse event(s) related to dental treatment: Xerostomia (normal salivary flow resumes upon discontinuation)
Effects on Bleeding No information available to require special precautions
Adverse Effects Unless otherwise specified, percentages represent adverse reactions identified in clinical trials evaluating the oral formulation.
>10%: Central nervous system: Headache (I.V. 11%; oral 2% to 8%)
1% to 10%:
Central nervous system: Dizziness (I.V. 3%; oral <1%), somnolence (adults <1%; children 2%)
Dermatologic: Pruritus (I.V. 1%; oral <1%)

Gastrointestinal: Flatulence (I.V. 10%; oral ≤5%), diarrhea (I.V. 4%; oral 2% to <7%), abdominal pain (I.V. 6%; oral 1% to ≤6%), nausea (I.V. 6%; oral 2% to ≤6%), xerostomia (I.V. 4%; oral 3%), constipation (I.V. 3%; oral 2%)

Local: Injection site reaction (I.V. 2%)

Dosage

Oral:

Children 1 month to <1 year: Erosive esophagitis (healing): **Note:** Safety and efficacy of doses >1.33 mg/kg/day and/or therapy beyond 6 weeks have not been established.

3-5 kg: 2.5 mg once daily for up to 6 weeks

>5-7.5 kg: 5 mg once daily for up to 6 weeks

>7.5 kg: 10 mg once daily for up to 6 weeks

Children 1-11 years: **Note:** Safety and efficacy of doses >1 mg/kg/day and/or therapy beyond 8 weeks have not been established.

Symptomatic GERD: 10 mg once daily for up to 8 weeks

Erosive esophagitis (healing):

<20 kg: 10 mg once daily for 8 weeks

≥20 kg: 10-20 mg once daily for 8 weeks

Nonerosive reflux disease (NERD) (Canadian labeling): 10 mg once daily for up to 8 weeks

Adolescents 12-17 years:

GERD: 20-40 mg once daily for up to 8 weeks

NERD (Canadian labeling): 20 mg once daily for 2-4 weeks; lack of symptom control after 4 weeks warrants further evaluation

Adults:

Erosive esophagitis (healing): Initial: 20-40 mg once daily for 4-8 weeks; if incomplete healing, may continue for an additional 4-8 weeks; maintenance: 20 mg once daily (controlled studies did not extend beyond 6 months)

NERD (Canadian labeling): Initial: 20 mg once daily for 2-4 weeks; lack of symptom control after 4 weeks warrants further evaluation; maintenance (in patients with successful initial therapy): 20 mg once daily as needed

Symptomatic GERD: 20 mg once daily for 4 weeks; may continue an additional 4 weeks if symptoms persist

Helicobacter pylori eradication:

Manufacturer labeling: 40 mg once daily administered with amoxicillin 1000 mg *and* clarithromycin 500 mg twice daily for 10 days

American College of Gastroenterology guidelines (Chey, 2007):

Nonpenicillin allergy: 40 mg once daily administered with amoxicillin 1000 mg *and* clarithromycin 500 mg twice daily for 10-14 days

Penicillin allergy: 40 mg once daily administered with clarithromycin 500 mg *and* metronidazole 500 mg twice daily for 10-14 days **or** 40 mg once daily administered with bismuth subsalicylate 525 mg *and* metronidazole 250 mg *plus* tetracycline 500 mg 4 times daily for 10-14 days

Canadian labeling: 20 mg twice daily for 7 days; requires combination therapy

Prevention of NSAID-induced gastric ulcers:

U.S. labeling: 20-40 mg once daily for up to 6 months

Canadian labeling: 20 mg once daily for up to 6 months

Note: 40 mg daily did not show additional benefit over 20 mg daily in clinical trials.

Treatment of NSAID-induced gastric ulcers (Canadian labeling; unlabeled in U.S.): 20 mg once daily for 4-8 weeks (Goldstein, 2007)

Pathological hypersecretory conditions (Zollinger-Ellison syndrome): 40 mg twice daily; adjust regimen to individual patient needs; doses up to 240 mg daily have been administered

I.V.:

Treatment of GERD (short-term): **Note:** Indicated only in cases where oral therapy is inappropriate or not possible; safety/efficacy ≥10 days has not been established.

Children 1 month to <1 year: 0.5 mg/kg once daily

Children 1-17 years: <55 kg: 10 mg once daily; ≥55 kg: 20 mg once daily

Adults: 20 mg or 40 mg once daily

Prevention of recurrent peptic ulcer bleeding postendoscopy (unlabeled use; Sung, 2009): Adults: 80 mg over 30 minutes, followed by 8 mg/hour infusion for 72 hours, then 40 mg *orally* once daily for 27 additional days

Elderly: No dosage adjustment needed.

Dosage adjustment in renal impairment: No dosage adjustment necessary

Dosage adjustment in hepatic impairment:

Safety and efficacy not established in children with hepatic impairment.

Mild-to-moderate impairment (Child-Pugh class A or B): No dosage adjustment necessary

Severe impairment (Child-Pugh class C): Dose should not exceed 20 mg daily

Mechanism of Action Proton pump inhibitor suppresses gastric acid secretion by inhibition of the H^+/K^+-ATPase in the gastric parietal cell. Esomeprazole is the S-isomer of omeprazole.

Contraindications Hypersensitivity to esomeprazole, other substituted benzimidazole proton pump inhibitors, or any component of the formulation

Warnings/Precautions Use of proton pump inhibitors (PPIs) may increase the risk of gastrointestinal infections (eg, *Salmonella, Campylobacter*). Relief of symptoms does not preclude the presence of a gastric malignancy. Atrophic gastritis (by biopsy) has been noted with long-term omeprazole therapy; this may also occur with esomeprazole. No reports of enterochromaffin-like (ECL) cell carcinoids, dysplasia, or neoplasia have occurred. Use of PPIs may increase risk of CDAD, especially in hospitalized patients; consider CDAD diagnosis in patients with persistent diarrhea that does not improve. Use the lowest dose and shortest duration of PPI therapy appropriate for the condition being treated. Severe liver dysfunction may require dosage reductions. Safety and efficacy of I.V. therapy >10 days have not been established; transition from I.V. to oral therapy as soon possible. Bioavailability may be increased in Asian populations, the elderly, and patients with hepatic dysfunction. Decreased *H. pylori* eradication rates have been observed with short-term (≤7 days) combination therapy. The American College of Gastroenterology recommends 10-14 days of therapy (triple or quadruple) for eradication of *H. pylori* (Chey, 2007).

PPIs may diminish the therapeutic effect of clopidogrel, thought to be due to reduced formation of the active metabolite of clopidogrel. The manufacturer of clopidogrel recommends either avoidance of both omeprazole (even when scheduled 12 hours apart) and esomeprazole or use of a PPI with comparatively less effect on the active metabolite of clopidogrel (eg, pantoprazole). In contrast to these warnings, others have recommended the continued use of PPIs, regardless of the degree of inhibition, in patients with a history of GI bleeding or multiple risk factors for GI bleeding who are also receiving clopidogrel since no evidence has established clinically meaningful differences in outcome; however, a clinically-significant interaction cannot be excluded in those who are poor metabolizers of clopidogrel (Abraham, 2010; Levine, 2011). Additionally, concomitant use of esomeprazole with other drugs may require cautious use, may not be recommended, or may require dosage adjustments.

Increased incidence of osteoporosis-related bone fractures of the hip, spine, or wrist may occur with PPI therapy. Patients on high-dose or long-term therapy should be monitored. Use the lowest effective dose for the shortest duration of time, use vitamin D and calcium supplementation, and follow appropriate guidelines to reduce risk of fractures in patients at risk.

Hypomagnesemia, reported rarely, usually with prolonged PPI use of >3 months (most cases >1 year of therapy); may be symptomatic or asymptomatic; severe cases may cause tetany, seizures, and cardiac arrhythmias. Consider obtaining serum magnesium concentrations prior to beginning long-term therapy, especially if taking concomitant digoxin, diuretics, or other drugs known to cause hypomagnesemia; and periodically thereafter. Hypomagnesemia may be corrected by magnesium supplementation, although discontinuation of esomeprazole may be necessary; magnesium levels typically return to normal within 1 week of stopping. Serum chromogranin A levels may be increased if assessed while patient on esomeprazole; may lead to diagnostic errors related to neuroendocrine tumors.

Drug Interactions

Metabolism/Transport Effects Substrate of CYP2C19 (major), CYP3A4 (minor); **Note:** Assignment of Major/Minor substrate status based on clinically relevant drug interaction potential; **Inhibits** CYP2C19 (moderate)

Avoid Concomitant Use

Avoid concomitant use of Esomeprazole with any of the following: Clopidogrel; Dasatinib; Delavirdine; Erlotinib; Nelfinavir; Ponatinib; Posaconazole; Rifampin; Rilpivirine; Risedronate; St Johns Wort

Increased Effect/Toxicity

Esomeprazole may increase the levels/effects of: Amphetamines; Benzodiazepines (metabolized by oxidation); Cilostazol; Citalopram; CYP2C19 Substrates; Dexmethylphenidate; Methotrexate; Methylphenidate; Raltegravir; Risedronate; Saquinavir; Tacrolimus (Systemic); Vitamin K Antagonists

The levels/effects of Esomeprazole may be increased by: Fluconazole; Ketoconazole (Systemic)

Decreased Effect

Esomeprazole may decrease the levels/effects of: Atazanavir; Bisphosphonate Derivatives; Bosutinib; Cefditoren; Clopidogrel; Dabigatran Etexilate; Dasatinib; Delavirdine; Erlotinib; Gefitinib; Indinavir; Iron Salts; Itraconazole; Ketoconazole (Systemic); Mesalamine; Multivitamins/Minerals (with ADEK, Folate, Iron); Mycophenolate; Nelfinavir; Nilotinib; Ponatinib; Posaconazole; Rilpivirine; Risedronate; Vismodegib

The levels/effects of Esomeprazole may be decreased by: CYP2C19 Inducers (Strong); Rifampin; St Johns Wort; Tipranavir

Ethanol/Nutrition/Herb Interactions

Food: Absorption is decreased by 43% to 53% when taken with food. Management: Take at least 1 hour before meals at the same time each day, best if before breakfast.

Herb/Nutraceutical: St John's wort may decrease the efficacy of esomeprazole. Management: Avoid St John's wort.

Dietary Considerations Take at least 1 hour before meals; best if taken before breakfast.

Pharmacodynamics/Kinetics

Half-life Elimination ~1-1.5 hours

Time to Peak Oral: 1.5-2 hours

Pregnancy Risk Factor B

Pregnancy Considerations Teratogenic effects were not observed in animal studies. However, there are no adequate and well-controlled studies in pregnant women. Congenital abnormalities have been reported sporadically following omeprazole use during pregnancy.

Lactation Excretion in breast milk unknown/not recommended

Breast-Feeding Considerations Esomeprazole excretion into breast milk has not been studied. However, omeprazole is excreted in breast milk, and therefore considered likely that esomeprazole is similarly excreted; breast-feeding is not recommended.

Dosage Forms

Capsule, delayed release, oral:
NexIUM®: 20 mg, 40 mg

Granules for suspension, delayed release, oral:
NexIUM®: 10 mg/packet (30s); 20 mg/packet (30s); 40 mg/packet (30s)

Injection, powder for reconstitution:
NexIUM® I.V.: 20 mg, 40 mg

Dosage Forms: Canada Note: Strength expressed as base.

Granules, for oral suspension, delayed release, as magnesium:
Nexium®: 10 mg/packet (28s)

Tablet, extended release, as magnesium:
Nexium®: 20 mg, 40 mg

Estazolam (es TA zoe lam)

Pharmacologic Category Benzodiazepine

Use Short-term management of insomnia

Local Anesthetic/Vasoconstrictor Precautions No information available to require special precautions

Effects on Dental Treatment Key adverse event(s) related to dental treatment: Significant xerostomia (normal salivary flow resumes upon discontinuation)

Effects on Bleeding No information available to require special precautions

Adverse Effects

>10%: Central nervous system: Somnolence (42%)

1% to 10%:
Central nervous system: Hypokinesia (8%), dizziness (7%), abnormal coordination (4%), hangover effect (3%), abnormal thoughts (2%), confusion (2%), anxiety (≥1%)

Dermatologic: Pruritus (1%)

Gastrointestinal: Constipation (≥1%), xerostomia (≥1%)

Neuromuscular & skeletal: Lower extremity pain (3%), stiffness (1%)

General Dosage Range Oral: *Adults:* 0.5-2 mg at bedtime

Mechanism of Action Binds to stereospecific benzo-diazepine receptors on the postsynaptic GABA neuron at several sites within the central nervous system, including the limbic system, reticular formation. Enhancement of the inhibitory effect of GABA on neuronal excitability results by increased neuronal membrane permeability to chloride ions. This shift in chloride ions results in hyperpolarization (a less excitable state) and stabilization.

Pharmacodynamics/Kinetics

Duration of Action Variable

Half-life Elimination 10-24 hours (no significant changes in elderly)

Time to Peak Serum: 0.5-6 hours

Pregnancy Risk Factor X

Pregnancy Considerations Although information specific to estazolam has not been located, all benzodiazepines are assumed to cross the placenta. Teratogenic effects have been observed with some benzodiazepines; however, additional studies are needed. The incidence of premature birth and low birth weights may be increased following maternal use of benzodiazepines; hypoglycemia and respiratory problems in the neonate may occur following exposure late in pregnancy. Neonatal withdrawal symptoms may occur within days to weeks after birth and "floppy infant syndrome" (which also includes withdrawal symptoms) has been reported with some benzodiazepines. The use of estazolam is contraindicated in pregnant women.

Controlled Substance C-IV

Estradiol (Systemic) (es tra DYE ole)

Related Information

Endocrine Disorders and Pregnancy *on page 1517*
Rheumatoid Arthritis, Osteoarthritis, and Osteoporosis *on page 1526*

Brand Names: U.S. Alora®; Climara®; Delestrogen®; Depo®-Estradiol; Divigel®; Elestrin®; Estrace®; Estra-sorb®; EstroGel®; Evamist®; Femring®; Femtrace®; Menostar®; Minivelle™; Vivelle-Dot®

Brand Names: Canada Climara®; Depo®-Estradiol; Estraderm®; Estradot®; EstroGel®; Menostar®; Oesclim®; Sandoz-Estradiol Derm 100; Sandoz-Estradiol Derm 50; Sandoz-Estradiol Derm 75

Pharmacologic Category Estrogen Derivative

Use Treatment of moderate-to-severe vasomotor symptoms associated with menopause; treatment of moderate-to-severe vulvar and vaginal atrophy associated with menopause; hypoestrogenism (due to hypogonadism, castration, or primary ovarian failure); advanced prostatic cancer (palliation); metastatic breast cancer (palliation) in men and postmenopausal women; postmenopausal osteoporosis (prophylaxis)

Local Anesthetic/Vasoconstrictor Precautions No information available to require special precautions

Effects on Dental Treatment No significant effects or complications reported

Effects on Bleeding No information available to require special precautions

Adverse Effects Frequency not defined. Some adverse reactions observed with estrogen and/or progestin combination therapy.

Cardiovascular: Chest pain, DVT, edema, hypertension, MI, stroke, syncope, TIA, vasodilation, venous thromboembolism

Central nervous system: Anxiety, dementia, dizziness, epilepsy exacerbation, headache, insomnia, irritability, mental depression, migraine, mood disturbances, nervousness

Dermatologic: Angioedema, chloasma, dermatitis, erythema multiforme, erythema nodosum, hemorrhagic eruption, hirsutism, loss of scalp hair, melasma, rash, pruritus, urticaria

Endocrine & metabolic: Breast cancer, breast enlargement, breast pain, breast tenderness, carbohydrate intolerance, fibrocystic breast changes, fluid retention, galactorrhea, hot flashes, hypocalcemia, libido changes, nipple discharge, nipple pain

Gastrointestinal: Abdominal cramps, abdominal pain, bloating, cholecystitis, cholelithiasis, constipation, diarrhea, dyspepsia, flatulence, gallbladder disease, gastritis, nausea, pancreatitis, vomiting, weight gain/loss

Genitourinary: Alterations in frequency and flow of bleeding patterns, breakthrough bleeding, cervical ectropion changes, cervical secretion changes, cystitis, dysmenorrhea, endometrial cancer, endometrial hyperplasia, genital eruption, menorrhagia, metrorrhagia, ovarian cancer, ovarian cyst, Pap smear suspicious, spotting, uterine leiomyomata size increased, leukorrhea, uterine cancer, uterine enlargement, uterine pain, urinary incontinence, urogenital pruritus, vaginal candidiasis, vaginal discharge, vaginal moniliasis, vaginitis

Hematologic: Aggravation of porphyria

Hepatic: Cholestatic jaundice, hepatic hemangioma enlargement

Local: Thrombophlebitis

Gel, spray: Application site reaction

Transdermal patches: Erythema, irritation

Neuromuscular & skeletal: Arthralgia, back pain, chorea, leg cramps, myalgia, muscle cramps, skeletal pain, weakness

Ocular: Blindness, contact lens intolerance, corneal curvature steepening, retinal vascular thrombosis

Respiratory: Asthma exacerbation, pulmonary thromboembolism

Miscellaneous: Anaphylactoid/anaphylactic reactions, hypersensitivity reactions

General Dosage Range

I.M.:

Cypionate:

Adults (females): Hypoestrogenism: 1.5-2 mg monthly

Adults (females): Menopause: 1-5 mg every 3-4 weeks

Valerate:

Adults (females): Menopause: 10-20 mg every 4 weeks

Adults (males): Prostate cancer: 30 mg or more every 1-2 weeks

Oral:

Adults (females):

Estrace®: Breast cancer: 10 mg 3 times/day; Hypoestrogenism: 1-2 mg/day; Menopause: 0.5-2 mg/day

Femtrace®: Menopause: 0.45-1.8 mg/day

Adults (males): Estrace®: Prostate cancer: 1-2 mg 3 times/day; Breast cancer: 10 mg 3 times/day

Intravaginal: *Adults (females):* (Femring®): 0.05-0.1 mg, leave in place for 3 months

Topical: *Adults (females):*

Emulsion (Estrasorb®): 3.48 g applied once daily in the morning

Gel: 1.25 g/day (EstroGel®) or 0.87-1.7 g/day (Elestrin®) or 0.25-1 g/day (Divigel®) applied at the same time each day

Spray (Evamist®): 1 spray (1.53 mg) per day; dosing range: 1-3 sprays/day

Transdermal: *Adults (females):*

Alora®, Estraderm®, Minivelle™, Vivelle-Dot®: Apply twice weekly continuously or cyclically (3 weeks on, 1 week off)

Climara®: Apply once weekly continuously or cyclically (3 weeks on, 1 week off)

Menostar®: Apply once weekly continuously

Mechanism of Action Estrogens are responsible for the development and maintenance of the female reproductive system and secondary sexual characteristics. Estradiol is the principle intracellular human estrogen and is more potent than estrone and estriol at the receptor level; it is the primary estrogen secreted prior to menopause. Following menopause, estrone and estrone sulfate are more highly produced. Estrogens modulate the pituitary secretion of gonadotropins, luteinizing hormone, and follicle-stimulating hormone through a negative feedback system; estrogen replacement reduces elevated levels of these hormones in postmenopausal women.

Pharmacodynamics/Kinetics

Half-life Elimination Femtrace®: 21-26 hours

Time to Peak Plasma: Oral: Femtrace®: 0.4-0.75 hours

Pregnancy Risk Factor X

Pregnancy Considerations In general, the use of estrogen and progestin as in combination hormonal contraceptives has not been associated with teratogenic effects when inadvertently taken early in pregnancy. These products are contraindicated for use during pregnancy.

Estradiol and Dienogest
(es tra DYE ole & dye EN oh jest)

Related Information

Dienogest *on page 419*

Estradiol (Systemic) *on page 505*

Brand Names: U.S. Natazia®

Pharmacologic Category Contraceptive; Estrogen and Progestin Combination

Use Prevention of pregnancy; treatment of heavy menstrual bleeding

Unlabeled Use Pain associated with endometriosis; dysmenorrhea

Local Anesthetic/Vasoconstrictor Precautions No information available to require special precautions

Effects on Dental Treatment No significant effects or complications reported

Effects on Bleeding No information available to require special precautions

Adverse Effects

>10%: Central nervous system: Headache (13%, including migraine)

1% to 10%:

Central nervous system: Mood changes (3%, including depression)

Dermatologic: Acne (4%)

Endocrine & metabolic: Metrorrhagia and irregular menstruation (7% to 8%), breast pain/discomfort/tenderness (7%)

Gastrointestinal: Nausea or vomiting (7%), weight gain (3%)

The following reactions have been associated with oral contraceptive use; frequency not defined:

Cardiovascular: Arterial thromboembolism, cerebral hemorrhage, cerebral thrombosis, DVT, edema, hypertension, mesenteric thrombosis, MI, varicose vein aggravation, venous thrombosis (with or without embolism)

Dermatologic: Chloasma, melasma, rash

Endocrine & metabolic: Amenorrhea, breakthrough bleeding, breast changes (enlargement, pain, secretion, tenderness), fluid retention, infertility (temporary), lactation decreased (with use immediately postpartum), menstrual flow changes, ruptured ovarian cyst, spotting

Gastrointestinal: Abdominal bloating, abdominal cramps, abdominal pain, appetite changes, gallbladder disease, nausea, weight changes, vomiting

Genitourinary: Cervical ectropion, cervical secretion, uterine leiomyoma, vaginal candidiasis, vaginitis

Hematologic: Folate decreased, porphyria exacerbation

Hepatic: Cholestatic jaundice, focal nodular hyperplasia of the liver, hepatic adenomas, liver tumors (benign)

Local: Thrombophlebitis

Neuromuscular & skeletal: Chorea exacerbation

Ocular: Contact lens intolerance, corneal curvature changes (steepening), retinal thrombosis

Respiratory: Pulmonary embolism

Miscellaneous: Anaphylactic/anaphylactoid reactions (including angioedema, circulatory collapse, respiratory collapse, urticaria), SLE exacerbation

General Dosage Range Oral: *Children and Adults (females, postmenarche):* 1 tablet daily

Mechanism of Action Combination hormonal contraceptives inhibit ovulation and may also cause changes in the cervical mucus, rendering it unfavorable for sperm penetration even if ovulation occurs. The four-phasic formulation provides the estrogen in decreasing concentrations and the progestin in increasing concentrations over the 28-day cycle.

Pharmacodynamics/Kinetics

Half-life Elimination Estradiol: ~14 hours; Dienogest: ~11 hours

Time to Peak Estradiol: ~6 hours; Dienogest: ~1 hour

Pregnancy Considerations Pregnancy should be ruled out prior to treatment and discontinued if pregnancy occurs. In general, the use of combination hormonal contraceptives when inadvertently taken early in pregnancy has not been associated with teratogenic effects. Hormonal contraceptives may be less effective in obese patients. An increase in oral contraceptive failure was noted in women with a BMI >27.3 kg/m². Similar findings were noted in patients weighing ≥90 kg (198 lb) using the contraceptive patch. This product was not studied in women with a BMI >30 kg/m².

Due to increased risk of venous thromboembolism (VTE) postpartum, combination hormonal contraceptives should not be started in any woman <21 days following delivery. Women without risk factors for VTE and who are not breast-feeding may start combination hormonal contraceptives during 21-42 days postpartum. After 42 days postpartum, restrictions for use are not related to postpartum status and should be based on other medical conditions (CDC, 2011). The manufacturer states that combination hormonal contraceptives should not be started until ≥4 weeks after delivery in women who choose not to breastfeed, or ≥4 weeks after a second trimester abortion or miscarriage

Estradiol and Levonorgestrel
(es tra DYE ole & LEE voe nor jes trel)

Related Information
Endocrine Disorders and Pregnancy *on page 1517*
Brand Names: U.S. ClimaraPro®
Pharmacologic Category Estrogen and Progestin Combination
Use Women with an intact uterus: Treatment of moderate-to-severe vasomotor symptoms associated with menopause; prevention of postmenopausal osteoporosis
Local Anesthetic/Vasoconstrictor Precautions No information available to require special precautions
Effects on Dental Treatment No significant effects or complications reported
Effects on Bleeding No information available to require special precautions related to hemostasis in dental procedures.
Adverse Effects Percentages reported as greater in ClimaraPro™ when compared to estradiol alone:

>10%:
Central nervous system: Depression (12%)
Endocrine & metabolic: Breast pain (40%)
Genitourinary: Vaginal bleeding (78%)
Local: Application site reaction (86%)
Neuromuscular & skeletal: Back pain (13%)
Respiratory: Upper respiratory tract infection (28%)
1% to 10%: Cardiovascular: Edema (8%)
Other adverse events reported with **estrogen and/or estrogen/progestin** therapy: Abdominal cramps, acne, abnormal uterine bleeding, aggravation of porphyria, amenorrhea, anaphylactoid reactions, anaphylaxis, angioedema, antifactor Xa decreased, antithrombin III decreased, appetite changes, bloating, breast enlargement, breast tenderness, carbohydrate tolerance decreased, cerebral embolism, cerebral thrombosis, chloasma, cholestatic jaundice, cholecystitis, cholelithiasis, chorea, contact lens intolerance, corneal curvature steepening, cystitis-like syndrome, dizziness; factors VII, VIII, IX, X, XII, VII-X complex, and II-VII-X complex increased; endometrial hyperplasia, erythema multiforme, erythema nodosum, galactorrhea, hemorrhagic eruption, fatigue, fibrinogen increased, glucose tolerance impaired, HDL-cholesterol increased, hirsutism, hypertension, gallbladder disease, insomnia, LDL-cholesterol decreased, libido changes, melasma, migraine, nervousness, optic neuritis, pancreatitis, platelet aggregability and platelet count increased, premenstrual-like syndrome, PT and PTT accelerated, pulmonary embolism, pyrexia, retinal thrombosis, scalp hair loss, size of uterine leiomyomata increased, somnolence, thrombophlebitis, thyroid-binding globulin increased, total thyroid hormone (T_4) increased, triglycerides increased, urticaria, vaginal candidiasis, vomiting, weight gain/loss
General Dosage Range Transdermal: *Adults (females):* Apply 1 patch (estradiol 0.045 mg/levonorgestrel 0.015 mg) weekly
Mechanism of Action Estrogens are responsible for the development and maintenance of the female reproductive system and secondary sexual characteristics.

Estradiol is the principle intracellular human estrogen and is more potent than estrone and estriol at the receptor level; it is the primary estrogen secreted prior to menopause. Following menopause, estrone and estrone sulfate are more highly produced. Estrogens modulate the pituitary secretion of gonadotropins, luteinizing hormone, and follicle-stimulating hormone through a negative feedback system; estrogen replacement reduces elevated levels of these hormones in postmenopausal women.

Levonorgestrel inhibits gonadotropin production; when used in this combination, it counteracts the proliferative effects of estradiol on the endometrium.
Pharmacodynamics/Kinetics
Half-life Elimination Estradiol: 3 ± 0.67 hours; Levonorgestrel: 28 ± 6.4 hours
Time to Peak Serum: Topical: Estradiol (mean): 2-2.5 days; Levonorgestrel: 2.5 days
Pregnancy Considerations Use of this combination is contraindicated during pregnancy. Estrogens are not indicated for use during pregnancy or immediately postpartum. Increased risk of fetal reproductive tract disorders and other birth defects have been observed with diethylstilbestrol (DES). Epidemiologic studies have not shown an increased risk of birth defects when levonorgestrel is used prior to pregnancy or inadvertently during early pregnancy, although rare reports of congenital anomalies have been reported. This product is intended to be used only in postmenopausal women.

Estradiol and Norethindrone
(es tra DYE ole & nor eth IN drone)

Related Information
Estradiol (Systemic) *on page 505*
Norethindrone *on page 990*
Brand Names: U.S. Activella®; CombiPatch®; Mimvey™
Brand Names: Canada Estalis-Sequi®; Estalis®
Pharmacologic Category Estrogen and Progestin Combination
Use Women with an intact uterus:
Tablet: Treatment of moderate-to-severe vasomotor symptoms associated with menopause; treatment of vulvar and vaginal atrophy; prophylaxis for postmenopausal osteoporosis
Transdermal patch: Treatment of moderate-to-severe vasomotor symptoms associated with menopause; treatment of vulvar and vaginal atrophy; treatment of hypoestrogenism due to hypogonadism, castration, or primary ovarian failure
Local Anesthetic/Vasoconstrictor Precautions No information available to require special precautions
Effects on Dental Treatment No significant effects or complications reported
Effects on Bleeding No information available to require special precautions related to hemostasis in dental procedures.
Adverse Effects Frequency not defined.
Cardiovascular: Altered blood pressure, cardiovascular accident, edema, MI, stroke, venous thromboembolism, thrombophlebitis
Central nervous system: Dementia, dizziness, emotional lability, fatigue, headache, insomnia, irritability, mental depression, migraine, mood changes, nervousness, seizure

Dermatologic: Chloasma, erythema multiforme, erythema nodosum, hemorrhagic eruption, hirsutism, itching, loss of scalp hair, melasma, pruritus, seborrhea, skin rash

Endocrine & metabolic: Breast cancer, breast enlargement, breast tenderness, breast pain, fibrocystic breast changes, galactorrhea, hypocalcemia, libido changes, nipple discharge, triglycerides increased

Gastrointestinal: Abdominal pain, bloating, changes in appetite, cramps, flatulence, gallbladder disease, gastroenteritis, nausea, pancreatitis, vomiting, weight gain/loss

Genitourinary: Alterations in frequency and flow of menses, changes in cervical secretions, cystitis-like syndrome, endometrial cancer, endometrial hyperplasia, endometrial thickening, endometriosis exacerbation, genital moniliasis, ovarian cancer, ovarian cyst, postmenopausal bleeding, premenstrual-like syndrome, size of uterine leiomyomata increased, uterine fibroid, vaginal candidiasis, vaginal hemorrhage, vaginitis

Hematologic: Aggravation of porphyria

Hepatic: Cholestatic jaundice

Local: Application site reaction (transdermal patch)

Neuromuscular & skeletal: Arthralgia, back pain, chorea, extremity pain, leg cramps, myalgia, weakness

Ocular: Contact lens intolerance, corneal curvature steepening, retinal vascular thrombosis

Respiratory: Asthma exacerbation, nasopharyngitis, pharyngitis, pulmonary thromboembolism, rhinitis, sinusitis, upper respiratory tract infection

Miscellaneous: Allergic reactions, carbohydrate intolerance, flu-like syndrome, viral infection

General Dosage Range

Oral: *Adults (females):* 1 tablet daily

Transdermal: *Adults (females):* Apply 1 patch twice weekly

Pharmacodynamics/Kinetics

Half-life Elimination Activella®: Estradiol: 12-14 hours; Norethindrone: 8-11 hours

Time to Peak Activella®: Estradiol: 5-8 hours

Pregnancy Considerations Not for use prior to menopause; use during pregnancy is contraindicated.

Estradiol and Norgestimate
(es tra DYE ole & nor JES ti mate)

Related Information

Estradiol (Systemic) *on page 505*

Rheumatoid Arthritis, Osteoarthritis, and Osteoporosis *on page 1526*

Brand Names: U.S. Prefest™

Pharmacologic Category Estrogen and Progestin Combination

Use Women with an intact uterus: Treatment of moderate-to-severe vasomotor symptoms associated with menopause; treatment of atrophic vaginitis; prevention of osteoporosis

Local Anesthetic/Vasoconstrictor Precautions No information available to require special precautions

Effects on Dental Treatment No significant effects or complications reported

Effects on Bleeding No information available to require special precautions related to hemostasis in dental procedures.

Adverse Effects

>10%:

Central nervous system: Headache (23%)

Endocrine & metabolic: Breast pain (16%)

Gastrointestinal: Abdominal pain (12%)

Neuromuscular & skeletal: Back pain (12%)

Respiratory: Upper respiratory tract infection (21%)

Miscellaneous: Flu-like syndrome (11%)

1% to 10%:

Central nervous system: Fatigue (6%), pain (6%), depression (5%), dizziness (5%)

Endocrine & metabolic: Vaginal bleeding (9%), dysmenorrhea (8%), vaginitis (7%)

Gastrointestinal: Nausea (6%), flatulence (5%)

Neuromuscular & skeletal: Arthralgia (9%), myalgia (5%)

Respiratory: Sinusitis (8%), pharyngitis (7%), cough (5%)

Miscellaneous: Viral infection (6%)

Additional adverse effects associated with **estrogens and progestins**; frequency not defined:

Cardiovascular: Edema, hypertension, MI, stroke, venous thrombosis

Central nervous system: Anxiety, epilepsy exacerbation, insomnia, irritability, migraine, mood disturbances, nervousness, pyrexia, somnolence

Dermatologic: Acne, chloasma, erythema multiforme, erythema nodosum, hemorrhagic eruptions, hirsutism, itching, melasma, pruritus, rash, scalp hair loss, urticaria

Endocrine & metabolic: Amenorrhea, breast cancer, breast discharge, breast enlargement, Breast tenderness, carbohydrate tolerance decreased, endometrial cancer, endometrial hyperplasia, fibrocystic breast changes, galactorrhea, hypocalcemia, libido changes, ovarian cancer, triglycerides increased

Gastrointestinal: Abdominal cramps, appetite changes, bloating, gallbladder disease, pancreatitis, vomiting, weight gain/loss

Genitourinary: Abnormal withdrawal bleeding/flow, breakthrough bleeding, cervical secretion changes, cystitis syndrome, uterine leiomyomata size increased, vaginal candidiasis, vaginal bleeding/spotting

Hematologic: Anemia, porphyria

Hepatic: Cholestatic jaundice

Local: Thrombophlebitis

Neuromuscular & skeletal: Chorea

Ocular: Contact lens intolerance, corneal curvature steepening, neuro-ocular lesions

Respiratory: Asthma exacerbation, pulmonary embolism

Miscellaneous: Anaphylaxis

General Dosage Range Oral: *Adults (females):* 1 tablet of estradiol 1 mg once daily for 3 days, followed by 1 tablet of estradiol 1 mg and norgestimate 0.09 mg once daily for 3 days; repeat sequence continuously

Mechanism of Action Estrogens are responsible for the development and maintenance of the female reproductive system and secondary sexual characteristics. Estradiol is the principle intracellular human estrogen and is more potent than estrone and estriol at the receptor level; it is the primary estrogen secreted prior to menopause. Following menopause, estrone and estrone sulfate are more highly produced. Estrogens modulate the pituitary secretion of gonadotropins, luteinizing hormone, and follicle-stimulating hormone through a negative feedback system; estrogen replacement reduces elevated levels of these hormones in postmenopausal women.

Progestins inhibit gonadotropin production which then prevents follicular maturation and ovulation. In women with adequate estrogen, progestins transform a proliferative endometrium into a secretory endometrium; when administered with estradiol, reduces the incidence of endometrial hyperplasia and risk of adenocarcinoma.

Pharmacodynamics/Kinetics
Half-life Elimination Norgestimate: 17-deacetylnorgestimate: 37 hours
Pregnancy Risk Factor X
Pregnancy Considerations Estrogens are not indicated for use during pregnancy or immediately postpartum. Increased risk of fetal reproductive tract disorders and other birth defects have been observed with diethylstilbestrol (DES); do not use during pregnancy. Progestins are associated with fetal genital abnormalities when used during the first trimester; not recommended for use during pregnancy.

Estramustine (es tra MUS teen)

Brand Names: U.S. Emcyt®
Brand Names: Canada Emcyt®
Pharmacologic Category Antineoplastic Agent, Alkylating Agent; Antineoplastic Agent, Hormone; Antineoplastic Agent, Hormone (Estrogen/Nitrogen Mustard)
Use Palliative treatment of progressive or metastatic prostate cancer
Local Anesthetic/Vasoconstrictor Precautions No information available to require special precautions
Effects on Dental Treatment No significant effects or complications reported
Effects on Bleeding Thrombocytopenia has been reported in a small number of patients
Adverse Effects
>10%:
Cardiovascular: Edema (20%)
Endocrine & metabolic: Gynecomastia (75%), breast tenderness (71%), libido decreased
Gastrointestinal: Nausea (16%), diarrhea (13%), gastrointestinal upset (12%)
Hepatic: LDH increased (2% to 33%), AST increased (2% to 33%)
Respiratory: Dyspnea (12%)
1% to 10%:
Cardiovascular: CHF (3%), MI (3%), cerebrovascular accident (2%), chest pain (1%), flushing (1%)
Central nervous system: Lethargy (4%), insomnia (3%), emotional lability (2%), anxiety (1%), headache (1%)
Dermatologic: Bruising (3%), dry skin (2%), pruritus (2%), hair thinning (1%), rash (1%), skin peeling (1%)
Gastrointestinal: Anorexia (4%), flatulence (2%), burning throat (1%), gastrointestinal bleeding (1%), thirst (1%), vomiting (1%)
Hematologic: Leukopenia (4%), thrombocytopenia (1%)
Hepatic: Bilirubin increased (1% to 2%)
Local: Thrombophlebitis (3%)
Neuromuscular & skeletal: Leg cramps (9%)
Ocular: Tearing (1%)
Respiratory: Pulmonary embolism (2%), upper respiratory discharge (1%), hoarseness (1%)
General Dosage Range Oral: *Adults (males):* 14 mg/kg/day (range: 10-16 mg/kg/day) in 3 or 4 divided doses
Mechanism of Action Combines the effects of estradiol and nitrogen mustard. It appears to bind to microtubule proteins, preventing normal tubulin function. The antitumor effect may be due solely to an estrogenic effect. Estramustine causes a marked decrease in plasma testosterone and an increase in estrogen levels.
Pharmacodynamics/Kinetics
Half-life Elimination Terminal: 15-24 hours
Time to Peak Serum: 2-3 hours
Pregnancy Considerations Estramustine is not indicated for use in women. Men who were impotent on estrogen therapy have regained potency while taking estramustine; effective contraception should be used for male patients with partners of childbearing potential.

Estrogens (Conjugated A/Synthetic)
(ES troe jenz, KON joo gate ed, aye, sin THET ik)

Related Information
Endocrine Disorders and Pregnancy *on page 1517*
Brand Names: U.S. Cenestin®
Brand Names: Canada Cenestin
Pharmacologic Category Estrogen Derivative
Use Treatment of moderate-to-severe vasomotor symptoms of menopause; treatment of vulvar and vaginal atrophy
Local Anesthetic/Vasoconstrictor Precautions No information available to require special precautions
Effects on Dental Treatment No significant effects or complications reported
Effects on Bleeding No information available to require special precautions related to hemostasis in dental procedures.
Adverse Effects
>10%:
Central nervous system: Headache (11% to 68%), dizziness (11%), pain (11%)
Endocrine & metabolic: Breast pain (29%), endometrial thickening (19%), metrorrhagia (14%)
Gastrointestinal: Abdominal pain (9% to 28%), nausea (9% to 18%)
Neuromuscular & skeletal: Paresthesia (8% to 33%), back pain (14%)
Respiratory: Upper respiratory tract infection (13%)
Miscellaneous: Infection (2% to 14%)
1% to 10%:
Central nervous system: Anxiety (6%), fever (1%)
Gastrointestinal: Dyspepsia (10%), vomiting (7%), constipation (6%), diarrhea (6%), weight gain (6%)
Genitourinary: Vaginitis (8%)
Neuromuscular & skeletal: Leg cramps (10%), hypertonia (6%)
Respiratory: Rhinitis (6% to 8%), cough (6%)

In addition, the following have been reported with estrogen and/or progestin therapy:
Cardiovascular: Edema, hypertension, MI, stroke, venous thromboembolism
Central nervous system: Epilepsy exacerbation, irritability, mental depression, migraine, mood disturbances, nervousness
Dermatologic: Angioedema, chloasma, erythema multiforme, erythema nodosum, hemorrhagic eruption, hirsutism, melasma, pruritus, rash, scalp hair loss, urticaria
Endocrine & metabolic: Breast cancer, breast enlargement, breast tenderness, glucose tolerance impaired, HDL-cholesterol increased, hyper-/hypocalcemia, LDL-cholesterol decreased, libido changes, serum triglycerides/phospholipids increased, thyroid-binding globulin increased, total thyroid hormone (T_4) increased

Gastrointestinal: Abdominal cramps, bloating, chole-cystitis, cholelithiasis, gallbladder disease, pancrea-titis, weight gain/loss

Genitourinary: Alterations in frequency and flow of menses, cervical secretion changes, endometrial cancer, endometrial hyperplasia, uterine leiomyomata size increased, vaginal candidiasis

Hematologic: Aggravation of porphyria, antithrombin III and antifactor Xa decreased, fibrinogen levels increased, platelet aggregability and platelet count increased; prothrombin and factors VII, VIII, IX, X increased

Hepatic: Cholestatic jaundice, hepatic hemangiomas enlarged

Neuromuscular & skeletal: Arthralgias, chorea, leg cramps

Local: Thrombophlebitis

Ocular: Contact lens intolerance, retinal vascular thrombosis, corneal curvature steepening

Respiratory: Asthma exacerbation, pulmonary thromboembolism

Miscellaneous: Anaphylactoid/anaphylactic reactions, carbohydrate intolerance

General Dosage Range Oral: *Adults (females):* 0.3-1.25 mg once daily

Mechanism of Action Conjugated A/synthetic estrogens contain a mixture of 9 synthetic estrogen substances, including sodium estrone sulfate, sodium equilin sulfate, sodium 17 alpha-dihydroequilin, sodium 17 alpha-estradiol and sodium 17 beta-dihydroequilin. Estrogens are responsible for the development and maintenance of the female reproductive system and secondary sexual characteristics. Estradiol is the principle intracellular human estrogen and is more potent than estrone and estriol at the receptor level; it is the primary estrogen secreted prior to menopause. Following menopause, estrone and estrone sulfate are more highly produced. Estrogens modulate the pituitary secretion of gonadotropins, luteinizing hormone, and follicle-stimulating hormone through a negative feedback system; estrogen replacement reduces elevated levels of these hormones in postmenopausal women.

Pregnancy Considerations Use during pregnancy is contraindicated.

Estrogens (Conjugated B/Synthetic)
(ES troe jenz, KON joo gate ed, bee, sin THET ik)

Brand Names: U.S. Enjuvia™

Pharmacologic Category Estrogen Derivative

Use Treatment of moderate-to-severe vasomotor symptoms of menopause; treatment of vulvar and vaginal atrophy associated with menopause; treatment of moderate-to-severe vaginal dryness and pain with intercourse associated with menopause

Local Anesthetic/Vasoconstrictor Precautions No information available to require special precautions

Effects on Dental Treatment No significant effects or complications reported

Effects on Bleeding No information available to require special precautions related to hemostasis in dental procedures.

Adverse Effects

>10%:

Central nervous system: Headache (15% to 25%), pain (10% to 19%)

Endocrine & metabolic: Breast pain (up to 14%)

Gastrointestinal: Abdominal pain (4% to 15%), nausea (7% to 12%)

1% to 10%:

Central nervous system: Dizziness (1% to 7%)

Endocrine & metabolic: Dysmenorrhea (1% to 8%)

Gastrointestinal: Flatulence (4% to 7%)

Genitourinary: Vaginitis (2% to 7%)

Neuromuscular & skeletal: Paresthesia (up to 6%)

Respiratory: Bronchitis (up to 7%), rhinitis (4% to 7%), sinusitis (3% to 7%)

Miscellaneous: Flu-like syndrome (4% to 7%)

In addition, the following have been reported with estrogen and/or progestin therapy:

Cardiovascular: Edema, hypertension, MI, stroke, venous thromboembolism

Central nervous system: Epilepsy exacerbation, irritability, mental depression, migraine, mood disturbances, nervousness

Dermatologic: Angioedema, chloasma, erythema multiforme, erythema nodosum, hemorrhagic eruption, hirsutism, loss of scalp hair, melasma, pruritus, rash, urticaria

Endocrine & metabolic: Breast cancer, breast enlargement, breast tenderness, HDL-cholesterol increased, hyper-/hypocalcemia, impaired glucose tolerance, LDL-cholesterol decreased, libido (changes in), serum triglycerides/phospholipids increased, thyroid-binding globulin increased, total thyroid hormone (T_4) increased

Gastrointestinal: Abdominal cramps, bloating, cholecystitis, cholelithiasis, gallbladder disease, pancreatitis, weight gain/loss

Genitourinary: Alterations in frequency and flow of menses, changes in cervical secretions, endometrial cancer, endometrial hyperplasia, increased size of uterine leiomyomata, vaginal candidiasis

Hematologic: Aggravation of porphyria; antithrombin III and antifactor Xa decreased; fibrinogen levels increased; platelet aggregability and platelet count increased; prothrombin and factors VII, VIII, IX, X increased

Hepatic: Cholestatic jaundice, hepatic hemangiomas enlarged

Local: Thrombophlebitis

Neuromuscular & skeletal: Arthralgias, chorea, leg cramps

Ocular: Contact lens intolerance, corneal curvature steepening, retinal vascular thrombosis

Respiratory: Asthma exacerbation, pulmonary thromboembolism

Miscellaneous: Anaphylactoid/anaphylactic reactions, carbohydrate intolerance

General Dosage Range Oral: *Adults (females):* 0.3-1.25 mg once daily

Mechanism of Action Conjugated B/synthetic estrogens contain a mixture of 10 synthetic estrogen substances, including sodium estrone sulfate, sodium equilin sulfate, sodium 17-alpha-dihydroequilin, sodium 17-alpha-estradiol, and sodium 17-beta-dihydroequilin. Estrogens are responsible for the development and maintenance of the female reproductive system and secondary sexual characteristics. Estradiol is the principle intracellular human estrogen and is more potent than estrone and estriol at the receptor level; it is the primary estrogen secreted prior to menopause. Following menopause, estrone and estrone sulfate are more highly produced. Estrogens modulate the pituitary secretion of gonadotropins, luteinizing hormone, and follicle-stimulating hormone through a negative feedback system; estrogen replacement reduces elevated levels of these hormones in postmenopausal women.

Pharmacodynamics/Kinetics
Half-life Elimination Conjugated estrone: 8-20 hours; conjugated equilin: 5-17 hours
Pregnancy Considerations Use during pregnancy is contraindicated.

Estrogens (Conjugated/Equine, Systemic) (ES troe jenz KON joo gate ed, EE kwine)

Related Information
Endocrine Disorders and Pregnancy on page 1517
Brand Names: U.S. Premarin®
Brand Names: Canada C.E.S.®; Congest; PMS-Conjugated Estrogens C.S.D.; Premarin®
Generic Availability (U.S.) No
Pharmacologic Category Estrogen Derivative
Use Treatment of moderate-to-severe vasomotor symptoms associated with menopause; treatment of vulvar and vaginal atrophy due to menopause; hypoestrogenism (due to hypogonadism, castration, or primary ovarian failure); prostatic cancer (palliation); breast cancer (palliation); postmenopausal osteoporosis (prophylaxis); abnormal uterine bleeding
Unlabeled Use Uremic bleeding
Local Anesthetic/Vasoconstrictor Precautions No information available to require special precautions
Effects on Dental Treatment No significant effects or complications reported
Effects on Bleeding No information available to require special precautions
Adverse Effects Note: Percentages reported in postmenopausal women following oral use.
>10%:
Central nervous system: Headache (26% to 32%; placebo 28%), pain (17% to 20%; placebo 18%)
Endocrine & metabolic: Breast pain (7% to 12%; placebo 9%)
Gastrointestinal: Abdominal pain (15% to 17%), diarrhea (6% to 7%; placebo 6%)
Genitourinary: Vaginal hemorrhage (2% to 14%)
Neuromuscular & skeletal: Back pain (13% to 14%), arthralgia (7% to 14%; placebo 12%)
Respiratory: Pharyngitis (10% to 12%; placebo 11%), sinusitis: (6% to 11%; placebo 7%)
1% to 10%:
Central nervous system: Depression (5% to 8%), dizziness (4% to 6%), nervousness (2% to 5%)
Dermatologic: Pruritus (4% to 5%)
Gastrointestinal: Flatulence (6% to 7%)
Genitourinary: Vaginitis (5% to 7%), leukorrhea (4% to 7%), vaginal moniliasis (5% to 6%)
Neuromuscular & skeletal: Weakness (7% to 8%), leg cramps (3% to 7%)
Respiratory: Cough increased (4% to 7%)
Additional adverse reactions reported with injection; frequency not defined: Local: injection site: Edema, pain, phlebitis
Dosage Adults:
Males: Androgen-dependent prostate cancer palliation: Oral: 1.25-2.5 mg 3 times/day

Females:
Prevention of postmenopausal osteoporosis: Oral:
U.S. labeling: Initial: 0.3 mg/day cyclically* or daily, depending on medical assessment of patient. Dose may be adjusted based on bone mineral density and clinical response. The lowest effective dose should be used.
Canadian labeling: 0.625 mg once daily

Moderate-to-severe vasomotor symptoms associated with menopause: Oral: Initial: 0.3 mg/day, cyclically* or daily, depending on medical assessment of patient. Adjust dose based on patient's response. The lowest dose that will control symptoms should be used.
Vulvar and vaginal atrophy: Oral: Initial: 0.3 mg/day; the lowest dose that will control symptoms should be used. May be given cyclically* or daily, depending on medical assessment of patient. Adjust dose based on patient's response.
Abnormal uterine bleeding: Acute/heavy bleeding:
Oral (unlabeled route): 10-20 mg/day in 4 divided doses has been used in place of I.M./I.V. doses (ACOG, 2000)
I.M., I.V.: 25 mg, may repeat in 6-12 hours if needed (manufacturer's labeling) **or** 25 mg I.V. repeated every 4 hours for 24 hours (ACOG, 2000). Patients who do not respond to 1-2 doses should be re-evaluated (ACOG, 2000).
Note: Treatment should be followed by a low-dose oral contraceptive; medroxyprogesterone acetate along with or following estrogen therapy can also be given
Female hypogonadism: Oral: 0.3-0.625 mg/day given cyclically*; dose may be titrated in 6- to 12-month intervals; progestin treatment should be added to maintain bone mineral density once skeletal maturity is achieved.
Female castration, primary ovarian failure: Oral: 1.25 mg/day given cyclically*; adjust according to severity of symptoms and patient response. For maintenance, adjust to the lowest effective dose.
*Cyclic administration: Either 3 weeks on, 1 week off or 25 days on, 5 days off

Males and Females:
Breast cancer palliation, metastatic disease in selected patients: Oral: 10 mg 3 times/day for at least 3 months
Uremic bleeding (unlabeled use): I.V.: 0.6 mg/kg/day for 5 days (Livio, 1986)

Elderly: Refer to adult dosing; a higher incidence of stroke and invasive breast cancer was observed in women >75 years in a WHI substudy.

Dosage adjustment in renal impairment: No dosage adjustment provided in manufacturer's labeling (has not been studied). Use with caution; may increase risk of fluid retention.
Dosage adjustment in hepatic impairment: Use is contraindicated with hepatic dysfunction or disease.
Mechanism of Action Conjugated estrogens contain a mixture of estrone sulfate, equilin sulfate, 17 alpha-dihydroequilin, 17 alpha-estradiol and 17 beta-dihydroequilin. Estrogens are responsible for the development and maintenance of the female reproductive system and secondary sexual characteristics. Estradiol is the principle intracellular human estrogen and is more potent than estrone and estriol at the receptor level; it is the primary estrogen secreted prior to menopause. Following menopause, estrone and estrone sulfate are more highly produced. Estrogens modulate the pituitary secretion of gonadotropins, luteinizing hormone, and follicle-stimulating hormone through a negative feedback system; estrogen replacement reduces elevated levels of these hormones in postmenopausal women.
Contraindications Angioedema or anaphylactic reaction to estrogens or any component of the formulation; undiagnosed abnormal vaginal bleeding; history of or current thrombophlebitis or venous thromboembolic

disorders (including DVT, PE); active or history of arterial thromboembolic disease (eg, stroke, MI); carcinoma of the breast (except in appropriately selected patients being treated for metastatic disease); estrogen-dependent tumor; hepatic dysfunction or disease; known protein C, protein S, antithrombin deficiency or other known thrombophilic disorders; pregnancy

Canadian labeling: Additional contraindications (not in U.S. labeling): Endometrial hyperplasia; partial or complete vision loss due to ophthalmic vascular disease; migraine with aura

Warnings/Precautions Hazardous agent - use appropriate precautions for handling and disposal (NIOSH, 2012). Anaphylaxis requiring emergency medical management has been reported within minutes to hours of taking conjugated estrogen (CE) tablets. Angioedema involving the face, feet, hands, larynx, and tongue has also been reported. Exogenous estrogens may exacerbate symptoms in women with hereditary angioedema.

[U.S. Boxed Warning]: Based on data from the Women's Health Initiative (WHI) studies, an increased risk of invasive breast cancer was observed in postmenopausal women using conjugated estrogens (CE) in combination with medroxyprogesterone acetate (MPA). This risk may be associated with duration of use and declines once combined therapy is discontinued (Chlebowski, 2009). The risk of invasive breast cancer was decreased in postmenopausal women with a hysterectomy using CE only, regardless of weight. However, the risk was not significantly decreased in women at high risk for breast cancer (family history of breast cancer, personal history of benign breast disease) (Anderson, 2012). An increase in abnormal mammogram findings has also been reported with estrogen alone or in combination with progestin therapy. Estrogen use may lead to severe hypercalcemia in patients with breast cancer and bone metastases; discontinue estrogen if hypercalcemia occurs. **[U.S. Boxed Warning]: The use of unopposed estrogen in women with an intact uterus is associated with an increased risk of endometrial cancer. The addition of a progestin to estrogen therapy may decrease the risk of endometrial hyperplasia, a precursor to endometrial cancer. Adequate diagnostic measures, including endometrial sampling if indicated, should be performed to rule out malignancy in postmenopausal women with undiagnosed abnormal vaginal bleeding.** Estrogens may exacerbate endometriosis. Malignant transformation of residual endometrial implants has been reported posthysterectomy with unopposed estrogen therapy. Consider adding a progestin in women with residual endometriosis posthysterectomy. Postmenopausal estrogen therapy and combined estrogen/progesterone therapy may increase the risk of ovarian cancer; however, the absolute risk to an individual woman is small. Although results from various studies are not consistent, risk does not appear to be significantly associated with the duration, route, or dose of therapy. In one study, the risk decreased after 2 years following discontinuation of therapy (Mørch, 2009). Although the risk of ovarian cancer is rare, women who are at an increased risk (eg, family history) should be counseled about the association (NAMS, 2012).

[U.S. Boxed Warning]: Estrogens with or without progestin should not be used to prevent cardiovascular disease. Using data from the Women's Health Initiative (WHI) studies, an increased risk of deep vein thrombosis (DVT) and stroke has been reported with CE

and an increased risk of DVT, stroke, pulmonary emboli (PE) and myocardial infarction (MI) has been reported with CE with MPA in postmenopausal women. Additional risk factors include diabetes mellitus, hypercholesterolemia, hypertension, SLE, obesity, tobacco use, and/or history of venous thromboembolism (VTE). Adverse cardiovascular events have also been reported in males taking estrogens for prostate cancer. Risk factors should be managed appropriately; discontinue use if adverse cardiovascular events occur or are suspected. Women with inherited thrombophilias (eg, protein C or S deficiency) may have increased risk of venous thromboembolism (DeSancho, 2010; van Vlijmen, 2011). Use is contraindicated in women with protein C, protein S, antithrombin deficiency, or other known thrombophilic disorders.

[U.S. Boxed Warning]: Estrogens with or without progestin should not be used to prevent dementia. In the Women's Health Initiative Memory Study (WHIMS), an increased incidence of dementia was observed in women ≥65 years of age taking CE alone or in combination with MPA.

Estrogen compounds are generally associated with lipid effects such as increased HDL-cholesterol and decreased LDL-cholesterol. Triglycerides may also be increased; discontinue if pancreatitis occurs. Use with caution in patients with familial defects of lipoprotein metabolism. Estrogens may increase thyroid-binding globulin (TBG) levels leading to increased circulating total thyroid hormone levels. Women on thyroid replacement therapy may require higher doses of thyroid hormone while receiving estrogens. Use caution in patients with hypoparathyroidism; estrogen-induced hypocalcemia may occur. May have adverse effects on glucose tolerance; use caution in women with diabetes. Use caution in patients with asthma, epilepsy, hepatic hemangiomas, porphyria, or SLE; may exacerbate disease. Use with caution in patients with diseases which may be exacerbated by fluid retention, including cardiac or renal dysfunction. Use of postmenopausal estrogen may be associated with an increased risk of gallbladder disease requiring surgery. Use caution with migraine; may exacerbate disease. Canadian labeling contraindicates use in migraine with aura. Estrogens may cause retinal vascular thrombosis; discontinue if migraine, loss of vision, proptosis, diplopia, or other visual disturbances occur; discontinue permanently if papilledema or retinal vascular lesions are observed on examination.

Estrogens are poorly metabolized in patients with hepatic dysfunction. Use caution with a history of cholestatic jaundice associated with prior estrogen use or pregnancy. Discontinue if jaundice develops or if acute or chronic hepatic disturbances occur. Use is contraindicated with hepatic disease.

Whenever possible, estrogens should be discontinued at least 4-6 weeks prior to elective surgery associated with an increased risk of thromboembolism or during periods of prolonged immobilization. Avoid use of oral estrogen (with or without progestins) in the elderly due to potential of increased risk of breast and endometrial cancers, and lack of proven cardioprotection and cognitive protection (Beers Criteria). Prior to puberty, estrogens may cause premature closure of the epiphyses, premature breast development in girls or gynecomastia in boys. Vaginal bleeding and vaginal cornification may also be induced in girls. The use of estrogens and/or progestins may change the results of some laboratory tests (eg, coagulation factors, lipids, glucose tolerance, binding proteins). The dose, route, and the specific estrogen/progestin influences these changes. In addition, personal risk factors (eg, cardiovascular disease, smoking, diabetes, age) also contribute to adverse events; use of specific products may be contraindicated in women with certain risk factors.

[U.S. Boxed Warning]: Estrogens with or without progestin should be used for the shortest duration possible at the lowest effective dose consistent with treatment goals. Before prescribing estrogen therapy to postmenopausal women, the risks and benefits must be weighed for each patient. Women should be informed of these risks and benefits, as well as possible effects of progestin when added to estrogen therapy. Patients should be reevaluated as clinically appropriate to determine if treatment is still necessary. Available data related to treatment risks are from Women's Health Initiative (WHI) studies, which evaluated oral CE 0.625 mg with or without MPA 2.5 mg relative to placebo in postmenopausal women. Other combinations and dosage forms of estrogens and progestins were not studied. **Outcomes reported from clinical trials using CE with or without MPA should be assumed to be similar for other doses and other dosage forms of estrogens and progestins until comparable data becomes available.**

Vulvar and vaginal atrophy use: Moderate-to-severe symptoms of vulvar and vaginal atrophy include vaginal dryness, dyspareunia, and atrophic vaginitis. When used solely for the treatment of vulvar and vaginal atrophy, topical vaginal products should be considered (NAMS, 2007).

Osteoporosis use: For use only in women at significant risk of osteoporosis and for who other nonestrogen medications are not considered appropriate.

Drug Interactions

Metabolism/Transport Effects Substrate of CYP1A2 (major), CYP2A6 (minor), CYP2B6 (minor), CYP2C19 (minor), CYP2C9 (minor), CYP2D6 (minor), CYP2E1 (minor), CYP3A4 (major); **Note:** Assignment of Major/Minor substrate status based on clinically relevant drug interaction potential; **Inhibits** CYP1A2 (weak); **Induces** CYP3A4 (weak/moderate)

Avoid Concomitant Use

Avoid concomitant use of Estrogens (Conjugated/Equine, Systemic) with any of the following: Anastrozole; Axitinib; Ospemifene

Increased Effect/Toxicity

Estrogens (Conjugated/Equine, Systemic) may increase the levels/effects of: Corticosteroids (Systemic); Ospemifene; ROPINIRole; Tipranavir

The levels/effects of Estrogens (Conjugated/Equine, Systemic) may be increased by: Ascorbic Acid; Herbs (Estrogenic Properties); NSAID (COX-2 Inhibitor)

Decreased Effect

Estrogens (Conjugated/Equine, Systemic) may decrease the levels/effects of: Anastrozole; ARIPiprazole; Axitinib; Chenodiol; Hyaluronidase; Ospemifene; Saxagliptin; Somatropin; Thyroid Products; Ursodiol

The levels/effects of Estrogens (Conjugated/Equine, Systemic) may be decreased by: CYP1A2 Inducers (Strong); CYP3A4 Inducers (Strong); Cyproterone; Deferasirox; Herbs (CYP3A4 Inducers); Peginterferon Alfa-2b; Tipranavir; Tocilizumab

Ethanol/Nutrition/Herb Interactions

Ethanol: Avoid ethanol (routine use increases estrogen plasma concentrations and risk of breast cancer). Ethanol may also increase the risk of osteoporosis.
Food: Folic acid absorption may be decreased.
Herb/Nutraceutical: St John's wort may decrease levels. Herbs with estrogenic properties may enhance the adverse/toxic effect of estrogen derivatives; examples include alfalfa, black cohosh, bloodroot, hops, kudzu, licorice, red clover, saw palmetto, soybean, thyme, wild yam, yucca.

Dietary Considerations Ensure adequate calcium and vitamin D intake when used for the prevention of osteoporosis. Powder for reconstitution for injection (25 mg) contains lactose 200 mg.

Pharmacodynamics/Kinetics

Half-life Elimination Total estrone: 27 hours

Time to Peak Total estrone: 7 hours

Pregnancy Considerations Estrogens are not indicated for use during pregnancy or immediately postpartum. In general, the use of estrogen and progestin as in combination hormonal contraceptives have not been associated with teratogenic effects when inadvertently taken early in pregnancy. These products are contraindicated for use during pregnancy.

Lactation Enters breast milk/use caution

Breast-Feeding Considerations Estrogen has been shown to decrease the quantity and quality of human milk. Use only if clearly needed. Monitor the growth of the infant closely.

Dosage Forms

Injection, powder for reconstitution:
Premarin®: 25 mg
Tablet, oral:
Premarin®: 0.3 mg, 0.45 mg, 0.625 mg, 0.9 mg, 1.25 mg

Estrogens (Conjugated/Equine) and Medroxyprogesterone

(ES troe jenz KON joo gate ed/EE kwine & me DROKS ee proe JES te rone)

Related Information

Endocrine Disorders and Pregnancy *on page 1517*
Estrogens (Conjugated/Equine, Systemic) *on page 511*
MedroxyPROGESTERone *on page 861*

Brand Names: U.S. Premphase®; Prempro®

Brand Names: Canada Premphase®; Premplus®; Prempro®

Pharmacologic Category Estrogen and Progestin Combination

Use Women with an intact uterus: Treatment of moderate-to-severe vasomotor symptoms associated with menopause; treatment of moderate-to-severe vulvar and vaginal atrophy due to menopause; postmenopausal osteoporosis (prophylaxis)

Local Anesthetic/Vasoconstrictor Precautions No information available to require special precautions

Effects on Dental Treatment No significant effects or complications reported

Effects on Bleeding No information available to require special precautions related to hemostasis in dental procedures

Adverse Effects

>10%:
Central nervous system: Headache (15% to 19%)
Endocrine & metabolic: Breast pain (13% to 36%), dysmenorrhea (3% to 13%)
Gastrointestinal: Abdominal pain (7% to 17%)

1% to 10%:
Cardiovascular: Edema (≤4%), peripheral edema (2% to 3%), hypertension (2%), vasodilation (≤2%), chest pain (1%), palpitation (≤1%)
Central nervous system: Depression (7% to 8%), pain (5%), emotional lability (3%), dizziness (2% to 3%), migraine (2% to 3%), nervousness (1% to 3%), anxiety (2%), insomnia (1% to 2%)
Dermatologic: Pruritus (2% to 6%), rash (2%), acne (≤2%), alopecia (≤2%), skin discoloration (1% to 2%), dry skin (≤1%)
Endocrine & metabolic: Leukorrhea (3% to 8%), breast enlargement (2% to 5%), breakthrough bleeding (1% to 4%), breast cancer (≤1%), breast engorgement (≤1%), glucose tolerance decreased (≤1%), menorrhagia (≤1%)
Gastrointestinal: Nausea (6% to 8%), flatulence (4% to 8%), diarrhea (≤6%), weight gain (3%), constipation (2%), appetite increased (≤2%), eructation (≤1%)
Genitourinary: Pelvic pain (2% to 5%), vaginal hemorrhage (≤5%), vaginitis (2% to 4%), monilial vaginitis (1% to 4%), uterine spasm (1% to 4%), cervical changes (1% to 3%), Pap smear suspicious (≤2%), incontinence (≤1%)
Neuromuscular & skeletal: Weakness (3% to 6%), back pain (2% to 7%), leg cramps (2% to 4%), hypertonia (1% to 2%)
Respiratory: Pharyngitis (>5%), sinusitis (>5%)
Miscellaneous: Moniliasis (≤2%), diaphoresis (≤1%), flu-like syndrome (≤1%), infection (≤1%)

General Dosage Range Oral: *Adults (females):* Prempro®: Conjugated estrogen 0.3-0.625 mg/mPA 1.5-5 mg once daily **or** Premphase®: One 0.625 mg tablet daily on days 1 through 14 and 1 conjugated estrogen 0.625 mg/mPA 5 mg tablet daily on days 15 through 28

Mechanism of Action

Conjugated estrogens contain a mixture of estrone sulfate, equilin sulfate, 17 alpha-dihydroequilin, 17 alpha-estradiol, and 17 beta-dihydroequilin. Estrogens are responsible for the development and maintenance of the female reproductive system and secondary sexual characteristics. Estradiol is the principle intracellular human estrogen and is more potent than estrone and estriol at the receptor level; it is the primary estrogen secreted prior to menopause. Following menopause, estrone and estrone sulfate are more highly produced. Estrogens modulate the pituitary secretion of gonadotropins, luteinizing hormone, and follicle-stimulating hormone through a negative feedback system; estrogen replacement reduces elevated levels of these hormones in postmenopausal women.

MPA inhibits gonadotropin production which then prevents follicular maturation and ovulation. In women with adequate estrogen, MPA transforms a proliferative endometrium into a secretory endometrium; when administered with conjugated estrogens, reduces the incidence of endometrial hyperplasia and risk of adenocarcinoma.

Pregnancy Considerations See individual agents; use of this combination is contraindicated during pregnancy

---

Estrogens (Esterified) (ES troe jenz, es TER i fied)

Related Information
Endocrine Disorders and Pregnancy *on page 1517*
Brand Names: U.S. Menest®
Brand Names: Canada Estragyn; Estratab®; Menest®

Pharmacologic Category Estrogen Derivative

Use Treatment of moderate-to-severe vasomotor symptoms associated with menopause; treatment of moderate-to-severe vulvar and vaginal atrophy associated with menopause; hypoestrogenism (due to hypogonadism, castration, or primary ovarian failure); advanced prostatic cancer (palliation), metastatic breast cancer (palliation) in men and postmenopausal women

Local Anesthetic/Vasoconstrictor Precautions No information available to require special precautions

Effects on Dental Treatment No significant effects or complications reported

Effects on Bleeding No information available to require special precautions related to hemostasis in dental procedures.

Adverse Effects Frequency not defined.
Cardiovascular: Edema, hypertension, MI, stroke, venous thromboembolism
Central nervous system: Dementia exacerbation, dizziness, epilepsy exacerbation, headache, irritability, mental depression, migraine, mood disturbances, nervousness
Dermatologic: Angioedema, chloasma, erythema multiforme, erythema nodosum, hemorrhagic eruption, hirsutism, pruritus, loss of scalp hair, melasma, rash, urticaria
Endocrine & metabolic: Breast cancer, breast enlargement, breast tenderness, carbohydrate intolerance, fibrocystic breast changes, galactorrhea, hypocalcemia, libido (changes in), nipple discharge, premenstrual like syndrome
Gastrointestinal: Abdominal cramps, bloating, gallbladder disease, nausea, pancreatitis, vomiting, weight gain/loss
Genitourinary: Alterations in frequency and flow of menstrual patterns, breakthrough bleeding, changes in cervical secretions, cervical ectropion changes, cystitis-like syndrome, dysmenorrhea, endometrial hyperplasia, endometrial cancer, increased size of uterine leiomyomata, ovarian cancer, vaginal candidiasis, vaginitis
Hematologic: Aggravation of porphyria
Hepatic: Cholestatic jaundice, hemangioma enlargement
Local: Thrombophlebitis
Neuromuscular & skeletal: Arthralgia, chorea, leg cramps
Ocular: Contact lens intolerance, corneal curvature steepening, retinal vascular thrombosis
Respiratory: Asthma exacerbation, pulmonary embolism
Miscellaneous: Anaphylactoid/anaphylactic reactions

General Dosage Range
Oral:
Adults (females): Hypogonadism: 2.5-7.5 mg/day for 20 days followed by a 10-day rest, repeat until response; Castration or ovarian failure: 1.25 mg/day, cyclically; Menopause 0.3-1.25 mg/day given cyclically; Breast cancer: 10 mg 3 times/day
Adults (males): Breast cancer: 10 mg 3 times/day; Prostate cancer: 1.25-2.5 mg 3 times/day

Mechanism of Action Esterified estrogens contain a mixture of estrogenic substances; the principle component is estrone. Preparations contain 75% to 85% sodium estrone sulfate and 6% to 15% sodium equilin sulfate such that the total is not <90%. Estrogens are responsible for the development and maintenance of the female reproductive system and secondary sexual characteristics. Estradiol is the principle intracellular human estrogen and is more potent than estrone and estriol at the receptor level; it is the primary estrogen secreted prior to menopause. In males and following menopause in females, estrone and estrone sulfate are more highly produced. Estrogens modulate the pituitary secretion of gonadotropins, luteinizing hormone, and follicle-stimulating hormone through a negative feedback system; estrogen replacement reduces elevated levels of these hormones.

Pregnancy Considerations In general, the use of estrogen and progestin as in combination hormonal contraceptives have not been associated with teratogenic effects when inadvertently taken early in pregnancy. This product is contraindicated for use during pregnancy.

Estrogens (Esterified) and Methyltestosterone
(ES troe jenz es TER i fied & meth il tes TOS te rone)

Related Information
Endocrine Disorders and Pregnancy *on page 1517*
Estrogens (Esterified) *on page 514*
MethylTESTOSTERone *on page 906*

Brand Names: U.S. Covaryx®; Covaryx® H.S.; EEMT™; EEMT™ HS

Pharmacologic Category Estrogen and Androgen Combination

Use Treatment of moderate-to-severe vasomotor symptoms associated with menopause not improved by estrogens alone

Local Anesthetic/Vasoconstrictor Precautions No information available to require special precautions

Effects on Dental Treatment No significant effects or complications reported

Effects on Bleeding No information available to require special precautions related to hemostasis in dental procedures.

Adverse Effects Refer to the Estrogens (Esterified) and the Testosterone monographs.

General Dosage Range Oral: *Adults (females):* Usual dosage range (based on esterified estrogen component): 0.625-1.25 mg every day for 3 weeks and then discontinued for 1 week off

Mechanism of Action
Conjugated estrogens: Activate estrogen receptors (DNA protein complex) located in estrogen-responsive tissues. Once activated, regulate transcription of certain genes leading to observed effects.
Testosterone: Increases synthesis of DNA, RNA, and various proteins in target tissues

Pregnancy Risk Factor X

Pregnancy Considerations [U.S. Boxed Warning]: Estrogens should not be used during pregnancy. This product is specifically contraindicated during pregnancy. Refer to the Estrogens (Esterified) monograph and the Testosterone monograph for additional information.

Estropipate (ES troe pih pate)

Related Information
Endocrine Disorders and Pregnancy *on page 1517*
Brand Names: Canada Ogen®
Pharmacologic Category Estrogen Derivative
Use Treatment of moderate-to-severe vasomotor symptoms associated with menopause; treatment of vulvar and vaginal atrophy; hypoestrogenism (due to hypogonadism, castration, or primary ovarian failure); osteoporosis (prophylaxis)

Local Anesthetic/Vasoconstrictor Precautions No information available to require special precautions

Effects on Dental Treatment No significant effects or complications reported

Effects on Bleeding No information available to require special precautions related to hemostasis in dental procedures.

Adverse Effects Frequency not defined.
Cardiovascular: Edema, hypertension, venous thromboembolism
Central nervous system: Dizziness, headache, mental depression, migraine
Dermatologic: Chloasma, erythema multiforme, erythema nodosum, hemorrhagic eruption, hirsutism, loss of scalp hair, melasma
Endocrine & metabolic: Breast enlargement, breast tenderness, libido (changes in), increased thyroid-binding globulin, increased total thyroid hormone (T_4), increased serum triglycerides/phospholipids, increased HDL-cholesterol, decreased LDL-cholesterol, impaired glucose tolerance, hypercalcemia
Gastrointestinal: Abdominal cramps, bloating, cholecystitis, cholelithiasis, gallbladder disease, nausea, pancreatitis, vomiting, weight gain/loss
Genitourinary: Alterations in frequency and flow of menses, changes in cervical secretions, endometrial cancer, increased size of uterine leiomyomata, vaginal candidiasis
Hematologic: Antithrombin III decreased; antifactor Xa decreased; fibrinogen levels increased; platelet aggregability increased; platelet count increased; porphyria aggravation; prothrombin and factors VII, VIII, IX, X increased
Hepatic: Cholestatic jaundice
Neuromuscular & skeletal: Chorea
Ocular: Ocular: Contact lens intolerance, corneal curvature steepening
Respiratory: Pulmonary thromboembolism
Miscellaneous: Carbohydrate intolerance

General Dosage Range Dosage adjustment recommended in patients with hepatic impairment
Oral: *Adults (females):* 0.75-6 mg once daily or cyclically [menopause] **or** 1.5-9 mg for the first 3 weeks, followed by a rest period of 8-10 days [hypoestrogenism] **or** 0.75 mg for 25 days of a 31 day cycle [osteoporosis]

Mechanism of Action Estrogens are responsible for the development and maintenance of the female reproductive system and secondary sexual characteristics. Estradiol is the principle intracellular human estrogen and is more potent than estrone and estriol at the receptor level; it is the primary estrogen secreted prior to menopause. In males and following menopause in females, estrone and estrone sulfate are more highly produced. Estrogens modulate the pituitary secretion of gonadotropins, luteinizing hormone, and follicle-stimulating hormone through a negative feedback system; estrogen replacement reduces elevated levels of these hormones. Estropipate is prepared from purified crystalline estrone that has been solubilized as the sulfate and stabilized with piperazine.

Pregnancy Considerations This product is contraindicated for use during pregnancy.

Eszopiclone (es zoe PIK lone)

Brand Names: U.S. Lunesta®
Generic Availability (U.S.) No
Pharmacologic Category Hypnotic, Miscellaneous

Use Treatment of insomnia (with difficulty of sleep onset and/or sleep maintenance)

Local Anesthetic/Vasoconstrictor Precautions No information available to require special precautions

Effects on Dental Treatment Key adverse event(s) related to dental treatment: Unpleasant taste and xerostomia (normal salivary flow resumes upon discontinuation).

Effects on Bleeding No information available to require special precautions

Adverse Effects

>10%:

Central nervous system: Headache (15% to 21%)

Gastrointestinal: Unpleasant taste (8% to 34%)

1% to 10%:

Cardiovascular: Cardiovascular: Chest pain (≥1%), peripheral edema (≥1%)

Central nervous system: Somnolence (8% to 10%), dizziness (5% to 7%), pain (4% to 5%), nervousness (up to 5%), depression (1% to 4%), confusion (up to 3%), hallucinations (1% to 3%), anxiety (1% to 3%), abnormal dreams (1% to 3%), migraine

Dermatologic: Rash (3% to 4%), pruritus (1% to 4%)

Endocrine & metabolic: Libido decreased (up to 3%), dysmenorrhea (up to 3%), gynecomastia (males up to 3%)

Gastrointestinal: Xerostomia (3% to 7%), dyspepsia (2% to 6%), nausea (4% to 5%), diarrhea (2% to 4%), vomiting (up to 3%)

Genitourinary: Urinary tract infection (up to 3%)

Neuromuscular & skeletal: Neuralgia (up to 3%)

Miscellaneous: Infection (5% to 10%), viral infection (3%), accidental injury (up to 3%)

Dosage Oral:

Adults: Insomnia: Initial: 2 mg immediately before bedtime (maximum dose: 3 mg)

Concurrent use with strong CYP3A4 inhibitor: 1 mg immediately before bedtime; if needed, dose may be increased to 2 mg

Elderly:

Difficulty **falling** asleep: Initial: 1 mg immediately before bedtime; maximum dose: 2 mg

Difficulty **staying** asleep: 2 mg immediately before bedtime

Dosage adjustment in renal impairment: No dosage adjustment required

Dosage adjustment in hepatic impairment:

Mild-to-moderate impairment: Use with caution; no dosage adjustment required.

Severe impairment: Initial dose: 1 mg; use with caution; systemic exposure is doubled in severe impairment.

Mechanism of Action May interact with GABA-receptor complexes at binding domains located close to or allosterically coupled to benzodiazepine receptors.

Contraindications Hypersensitivity to eszopiclone or any component of the formulation.

Warnings/Precautions Symptomatic treatment of insomnia should be initiated only after careful evaluation of potential causes of sleep disturbance. Failure of sleep disturbance to resolve after 7-10 days may indicate psychiatric and/or medical illness. Administer only when the patient is able to stay in bed a full night (7-8 hours) before being active again. Tolerance did not develop over 6 months of use. May cause CNS depression impairing physical and mental capabilities; patients must be cautioned about performing tasks which require mental alertness (operating machinery or driving). Use with caution in patients with depression; the minimum dose that will effectively treat the individual patient

should be used. Prescriptions should be written for the smallest quantity consistent with good patient care. Use caution in patients with a history of drug dependence. Use with caution in patients receiving other CNS depressants or psychoactive medications; dose adjustments may be necessary. Effects with other sedative drugs or ethanol may be potentiated, including risk of sleep-related behaviors. Use with alcohol is not recommended. Hypnotics/sedatives have been associated with abnormal thinking and behavior changes including decreased inhibition, aggression, bizarre behavior, agitation, hallucinations, and depersonalization. These changes may occur unpredictably and may indicate previously unrecognized psychiatric disorders; evaluate appropriately. An increased risk for hazardous sleep-related activities such as sleep-driving, cooking and eating food, and making phone calls while asleep has also been noted; amnesia may also occur. Discontinue treatment in patients who report any sleep-related episodes. Use caution in patients with respiratory compromise; hepatic dysfunction (dose adjustment recommended with severe impairment); or those taking strong CYP3A4 inhibitors (dose adjustment may be necessary). Because of the rapid onset of action, administer immediately prior to bedtime or after the patient has gone to bed and is having difficulty falling asleep. Abrupt discontinuance may lead to withdrawal symptoms. Hypersensitivity reactions including anaphylaxis as well as angioedema have been reported, in some cases following initial dosing. Patients who develop severe reactions should not be rechallenged.

Use with caution in the elderly; dosage adjustment recommended. Closely monitor elderly or debilitated patients for impaired cognitive and/or motor performance, confusion, and potential for falling. Avoid chronic use (>90 days) in older adults; adverse events, including delirium, falls, fractures, have been observed with non-benzodiazepine hypnotic use in the elderly similar to events observed with benzodiazepines. Data suggests improvements in sleep duration and latency are minimal (Beers Criteria).

Drug Interactions

Metabolism/Transport Effects Substrate of CYP2E1 (minor), CYP3A4 (major); **Note:** Assignment of Major/Minor substrate status based on clinically relevant drug interaction potential

Avoid Concomitant Use

Avoid concomitant use of Eszopiclone with any of the following: Azelastine (Nasal); Conivaptan; Paraldehyde; Sodium Oxybate

Increased Effect/Toxicity

Eszopiclone may increase the levels/effects of: Alcohol (Ethyl); Azelastine (Nasal); Buprenorphine; CNS Depressants; Methotrimeprazine; Metyrosine; Mirtazapine; Paraldehyde; Pramipexole; ROPINIRole; Rotigotine; Selective Serotonin Reuptake Inhibitors; Sodium Oxybate; Zolpidem

The levels/effects of Eszopiclone may be increased by: Antifungal Agents (Azole Derivatives, Systemic); Conivaptan; CYP3A4 Inhibitors (Moderate); CYP3A4 Inhibitors (Strong); Dasatinib; Droperidol; HydrOXYzine; Ivacaftor; Magnesium Sulfate; Methotrimeprazine; Mifepristone; Perampanel

Decreased Effect

The levels/effects of Eszopiclone may be decreased by: CYP3A4 Inducers (Strong); Deferasirox; Flumazenil; Herbs (CYP3A4 Inducers); Tocilizumab

Ethanol/Nutrition/Herb Interactions

Ethanol: Ethanol may increase CNS depression. Management: Avoid ethanol.

Food: Onset of action may be reduced if taken with or immediately after a heavy meal. Management: Take immediately prior to bedtime, not with or immediately after a heavy or high-fat meal.

Herb/Nutraceutical: Some herbal medications may increase CNS depression. Management: Avoid valerian, St John's wort, kava kava, and gotu kola.

Dietary Considerations Avoid taking after a heavy meal; may delay onset.

Pharmacodynamics/Kinetics

Half-life Elimination ~6 hours; Elderly (≥65 years): ~9 hours

Time to Peak ~1 hour

Pregnancy Risk Factor C

Pregnancy Considerations Adverse effects were observed in animal reproduction studies. Eszopiclone is the S-enantiomer of the racemic derivative zopiclone. There is limited data on the use of eszopiclone during pregnancy.

Lactation Excretion in breast milk unknown

Breast-Feeding Considerations Eszopiclone is the S-enantiomer of the racemic derivative zopiclone; zopiclone is excreted in human milk. There is limited data on the use of eszopiclone during breast-feeding.

Controlled Substance C-IV

Dosage Forms

Tablet, oral:

Lunesta®: 1 mg, 2 mg, 3 mg

Etanercept (et a NER sept)

Related Information

Rheumatoid Arthritis, Osteoarthritis, and Osteoporosis on page 1526

Brand Names: U.S. Enbrel®; Enbrel® SureClick®

Brand Names: Canada Enbrel®

Generic Availability (U.S.) No

Pharmacologic Category Antirheumatic, Disease Modifying; Tumor Necrosis Factor (TNF) Blocking Agent

Use Treatment of moderately- to severely-active rheumatoid arthritis (RA); moderately- to severely-active polyarticular juvenile idiopathic arthritis (JIA); psoriatic arthritis; active ankylosing spondylitis (AS); moderate-to-severe chronic plaque psoriasis

Local Anesthetic/Vasoconstrictor Precautions No information available to require special precautions

Effects on Dental Treatment No significant effects or complications reported

Effects on Bleeding No information available to require special precautions

Adverse Effects

>10%:

Central nervous system: Headache (17% to 19%)

Dermatologic: Rash (3% to 13%)

Gastrointestinal: Abdominal pain (5%; children 19%), diarrhea (3% to 16%), vomiting (3%; children 13%)

Local: Injection site reaction (14% to 43%; bleeding, bruising, erythema, itching, pain, or swelling)

Respiratory: Respiratory tract infection (21% to 54%; upper: 38% to 65%), rhinitis (12%)

Miscellaneous: Infection (50% to 81%; children 62%), positive antidouble-stranded DNA antibodies (15% by RIA, 3% by *Crithidia luciliae* assay), positive ANA (11%)

≥3% to 10%:

Central nervous system: Dizziness (7%), fever (2% to 3%)

Dermatologic: Pruritus (2% to 5%)

Gastrointestinal: Nausea (children 9%), dyspepsia (4%)

Neuromuscular & skeletal: Weakness (5%)

Respiratory: Pharyngitis (7%), cough (6%), respiratory disorder (5%), sinusitis (3%)

Dosage SubQ:

Children 2-17 years: Juvenile idiopathic arthritis:

Once-weekly dosing: 0.8 mg/kg (maximum: 50 mg/dose) once weekly

Twice-weekly dosing: 0.4 mg/kg (maximum: 25 mg/dose) twice weekly (individual doses should be separated by 72-96 hours)

Adults:

Rheumatoid arthritis, psoriatic arthritis, ankylosing spondylitis:

Once-weekly dosing: 50 mg once weekly

Twice weekly dosing: 25 mg given twice weekly (individual doses should be separated by 72-96 hours)

Plaque psoriasis:

Initial: 50 mg twice weekly, 72-96 hours apart; maintain initial dose for 3 months (starting doses of 25 or 50 mg once weekly have also been used successfully)

Maintenance dose: 50 mg once weekly

Elderly: Refer to adult dosing. Although greater sensitivity of some elderly patients cannot be ruled out, no overall differences in safety or effectiveness were observed.

Dosage adjustment in renal impairment: No dosage adjustment provided in manufacturer's labeling (has not been studied).

Dosage adjustment in hepatic impairment: No dosage adjustment provided in manufacturer's labeling (has not been studied).

Mechanism of Action Etanercept is a recombinant DNA-derived protein composed of tumor necrosis factor receptor (TNFR) linked to the Fc portion of human IgG1. Etanercept binds tumor necrosis factor (TNF) and blocks its interaction with cell surface receptors. TNF plays an important role in the inflammatory processes and the resulting joint pathology of rheumatoid arthritis (RA), polyarticular-course juvenile idiopathic arthritis (JIA), ankylosing spondylitis (AS), and plaque psoriasis.

Contraindications Hypersensitivity to etanercept or any component of the formulation; patients with sepsis (mortality may be increased)

Warnings/Precautions [U.S. Boxed Warning]: Patients receiving etanercept are at increased risk for serious infections which may result in hospitalization and/or fatality; infections usually developed in patients receiving concomitant immunosuppressive agents (eg, methotrexate or corticosteroids) and may present as disseminated (rather than local) disease. Active tuberculosis (or reactivation of latent tuberculosis), invasive fungal (including aspergillosis, blastomycosis, candidiasis, coccidioidomycosis, histoplasmosis, and pneumocystosis) and bacterial, viral or other opportunistic infections (including legionellosis and listeriosis) have been reported in patients receiving TNF-blocking agents, including etanercept. Monitor closely for signs/symptoms of infection. Discontinue for serious infection or sepsis. Consider risks versus benefits prior to use in patients with a history of chronic or

recurrent infection. Consider empiric antifungal therapy in patients who are at risk for invasive fungal infection and develop severe systemic illness. Caution should be exercised when considering use in the elderly or in patients with conditions that predispose them to infections (eg, diabetes) or residence/travel from areas of endemic mycoses (blastomycosis, coccidioidomycosis, histoplasmosis), or with latent or localized infections. Do not initiate etanercept therapy with clinically important active infection. Patients who develop a new infection while undergoing treatment should be monitored closely. **[U.S. Boxed Warning]: Tuberculosis (disseminated or extrapulmonary) has been reported in patients receiving etanercept; both reactivation of latent infection and new infections have been reported.** Patients should be evaluated for tuberculosis risk factors and for latent tuberculosis infection with a tuberculin skin test prior to starting therapy. Treatment of latent tuberculosis should be initiated before etanercept therapy; consider antituberculosis treatment if adequate course of treatment cannot be confirmed in patients with a history of latent or active tuberculosis or with risk factors despite negative skin test. Some patients who tested negative prior to therapy have developed active infection; monitor for signs and symptoms of tuberculosis in all patients. Rare reactivation of hepatitis B virus (HBV) has occurred in chronic virus carriers; use with caution; evaluate prior to initiation and during treatment. Patients should be brought up to date with all immunizations before initiating therapy. Live vaccines should not be given concurrently with etanercept. Patients with a significant exposure to varicella virus should temporarily discontinue etanercept. Treatment with varicella zoster immune globulin should be considered.

[U.S. Boxed Warning]: Lymphoma and other malignancies have been reported in children and adolescent patients receiving TNF-blocking agents, including etanercept. Half of the malignancies reported in children were lymphomas (Hodgkin's and non-Hodgkin's) while other cases varied and included malignancies not typically observed in this population. The impact of etanercept on the development and course of malignancy is not fully defined. Compared to the general population, an increased risk of lymphoma has been noted in clinical trials; however, rheumatoid arthritis alone has been previously associated with an increased rate of lymphoma. Lymphomas and other malignancies were also observed (at rates higher than expected for the general population) in adult patients receiving etanercept. Etanercept is not recommended for use in patients with Wegener's granulomatosis who are receiving immunosuppressive therapy. Hepatosplenic T-cell lymphoma (HSTCL), a rare T-cell lymphoma, has also been associated with TNF-blocking agents, primarily reported in adolescent and young adult males with Crohn's disease or ulcerative colitis. Treatment may result in the formation of autoimmune antibodies; cases of autoimmune disease have not been described. Non-neutralizing antibodies to etanercept may also be formed. Rarely, a reversible lupus-like syndrome has occurred.

Allergic reactions may occur; if an anaphylactic reaction or other serious allergic reaction occurs, administration should be discontinued immediately and appropriate therapy initiated. Use with caution in patients with pre-existing or recent onset CNS demyelinating disorders; rare cases of new onset or exacerbation of CNS demyelinating disorders have occurred; may present with

mental status changes and some may be associated with permanent disability. Optic neuritis, transverse myelitis, multiple sclerosis, and new onset or exacerbation of seizures have been reported. Use with caution in patients with heart failure or decreased left ventricular function; worsening and new-onset heart failure has been reported. Use caution in patients with a history of significant hematologic abnormalities; has been associated with pancytopenia and aplastic anemia (rare). Discontinue if significant hematologic abnormalities are confirmed. Use with caution in patients with moderate to severe alcoholic hepatitis. Compared to placebo, the mortality rate in patients treated with etanercept was similar at one month but significantly higher after 6 months

Due to a higher incidence of serious infections, concomitant use with anakinra is not recommended. Some dosage forms may contain dry natural rubber (latex). Some dosage forms may contain benzyl alcohol which has been associated with "gasping syndrome" in neonates.

Drug Interactions

Metabolism/Transport Effects None known.

Avoid Concomitant Use

Avoid concomitant use of Etanercept with any of the following: Abatacept; Anakinra; BCG; Belimumab; Canakinumab; Certolizumab Pegol; Cyclophosphamide; Natalizumab; Pimecrolimus; Rilonacept; Tacrolimus (Topical); Tocilizumab; Tofacitinib; Vaccines (Live)

Increased Effect/Toxicity

Etanercept may increase the levels/effects of: Abatacept; Anakinra; Belimumab; Canakinumab; Certolizumab Pegol; Cyclophosphamide; Leflunomide; Natalizumab; Rilonacept; Tofacitinib; Vaccines (Live)

The levels/effects of Etanercept may be increased by: Denosumab; Pimecrolimus; Roflumilast; Tacrolimus (Topical); Tocilizumab; Trastuzumab

Decreased Effect

Etanercept may decrease the levels/effects of: BCG; Coccidioidin Skin Test; Sipuleucel-T; Vaccines (Inactivated); Vaccines (Live)

The levels/effects of Etanercept may be decreased by: Echinacea

Ethanol/Nutrition/Herb Interactions Herb/Nutraceutical: Echinacea may decrease the therapeutic effects of etanercept (avoid concurrent use).

Pharmacodynamics/Kinetics

Onset of Action ~2-3 weeks; RA: 1-2 weeks

Half-life Elimination RA: SubQ: 72-132 hour

Time to Peak RA: SubQ: 35-103 hours

Pregnancy Risk Factor B

Pregnancy Considerations Developmental toxicity studies performed in animals have revealed no evidence of harm to the fetus. There are no studies in pregnant women; this drug should be used during pregnancy only if clearly needed. A pregnancy registry has been established to monitor outcomes of women exposed to etanercept during pregnancy (877-311-8972).

Lactation Excretion in breast milk unknown/not recommended

Breast-Feeding Considerations It is not known whether etanercept is excreted in human milk. Because many drugs and immunoglobulins are excreted in human milk and the potential for serious adverse reactions exists, a decision should be made whether to discontinue nursing or to discontinue the drug, taking into account the importance of the drug to the mother.

Dosage Forms

Injection, powder for reconstitution [preservative free]:

Enbrel®: 25 mg

Injection, solution [preservative free]:

Enbrel®: 50 mg/mL (0.51 mL, 0.98 mL)

Enbrel® SureClick®: 50 mg/mL (0.98 mL)

Ethacrynic Acid (eth a KRIN ik AS id)

Brand Names: U.S. Edecrin®; Sodium Edecrin®

Brand Names: Canada Edecrin®; Sodium Edecrin®

Pharmacologic Category Diuretic, Loop

Use Management of edema associated with congestive heart failure; hepatic cirrhosis or renal disease; short-term management of ascites due to malignancy, idiopathic edema, and lymphedema

Local Anesthetic/Vasoconstrictor Precautions No information available to require special precautions

Effects on Dental Treatment No significant effects or complications reported

Effects on Bleeding No information available to require special precautions

Adverse Effects Frequency not defined.

Central nervous system: Headache, fatigue, apprehension, confusion, fever, chills, encephalopathy (patients with pre-existing liver disease); vertigo

Dermatologic: Skin rash, Henoch-Schönlein purpura (IgA vasculitis) (in patient with rheumatic heart disease)

Endocrine & metabolic: Hyponatremia, hyperglycemia, variations in phosphorus, CO_2 content, bicarbonate, and calcium; reversible hyperuricemia, gout, hyperglycemia, hypoglycemia (occurred in two uremic patients who received doses above those recommended)

Gastrointestinal: Anorexia, malaise, abdominal discomfort or pain, dysphagia, nausea, vomiting, diarrhea, gastrointestinal bleeding, acute pancreatitis (rare)

Genitourinary: Hematuria

Hepatic: Jaundice, abnormal liver function tests

Hematology: Agranulocytosis, severe neutropenia, thrombocytopenia

Local: Thrombophlebitis (with intravenous use), local irritation and pain

Ocular: Blurred vision

Otic: Tinnitus, temporary or permanent deafness

Renal: Serum creatinine increased

General Dosage Range

I.V.: *Adults:* 0.5-1 mg/kg/dose (maximum: 100 mg/dose)

Oral:

Children: 1-3 mg/kg/day

Adults: 50-400 mg/day in 1-2 divided doses

Elderly: Initial: 25-50 mg/day

Mechanism of Action Inhibits reabsorption of sodium and chloride in the ascending loop of Henle and distal renal tubule, interfering with the chloride-binding cotransport system, thus causing increased excretion of water, sodium, chloride, magnesium, and calcium

Pharmacodynamics/Kinetics

Onset of Action Diuresis: Oral: ~30 minutes; I.V.: 5 minutes; Peak effect: Oral: 2 hours; I.V.: 30 minutes

Duration of Action Oral: 12 hours; I.V.: 2 hours

Half-life Elimination Normal renal function: 2-4 hours

Pregnancy Risk Factor B

Pregnancy Considerations No data available. Generally, use of diuretics during pregnancy is avoided due to risk of decreased placental perfusion.

Ethambutol (e THAM byoo tole)

Brand Names: U.S. Myambutol®

Brand Names: Canada Etibi®

Pharmacologic Category Antitubercular Agent

Use Treatment of pulmonary tuberculosis in conjunction with other antituberculosis agents

Unlabeled Use Other mycobacterial diseases in conjunction with other antimycobacterial agents

Local Anesthetic/Vasoconstrictor Precautions No information available to require special precautions

Effects on Dental Treatment No significant effects or complications reported

Effects on Bleeding No information available to require special precautions

Adverse Effects Frequency not defined.

Cardiovascular: Myocarditis, pericarditis

Central nervous system: Confusion, disorientation, dizziness, fever, hallucinations, headache, malaise

Dermatologic: Dermatitis, erythema multiforme, exfoliative dermatitis, pruritus, rash

Endocrine & metabolic: Acute gout or hyperuricemia

Gastrointestinal: Abdominal pain, anorexia, GI upset, nausea, vomiting

Hematologic: Eosinophilia, leukopenia, lymphadenopathy, neutropenia, thrombocytopenia

Hepatic: Hepatitis, hepatotoxicity (possibly related to concurrent therapy), LFTs abnormal

Neuromuscular & skeletal: Arthralgia, peripheral neuritis

Ocular: Optic neuritis; symptoms may include decreased acuity, scotoma, color blindness, or visual defects (usually reversible with discontinuation, irreversible blindness has been described)

Renal: Nephritis

Respiratory: Infiltrates (with or without eosinophilia), pneumonitis

Miscellaneous: Anaphylaxis, anaphylactoid reaction; hypersensitivity syndrome (cutaneous reactions, eosinophilia, and organ-specific inflammation)

General Dosage Range Dosage adjustment recommended in patients with renal impairment

Oral:

Children: 15-20 mg/kg/day (maximum: 1 g/day) **or** 50 mg/kg twice weekly (maximum: 2.5 g/dose)

Adults: Daily therapy: 1.5-2.5 g/kg/day (maximum dose: 1.5-2.5 g); 3 times/week DOT: 25-30 mg/kg/dose (maximum dose: 2.4 g/dose); Twice weekly DOT: 50 mg/kg/dose (maximum dose: 4 g/dose)

Mechanism of Action Inhibits arabinosyl transferase resulting in impaired mycobacterial cell wall synthesis

Pharmacodynamics/Kinetics

Half-life Elimination 2.5-3.6 hours; End-stage renal disease: 7-15 hours

Time to Peak Serum: 2-4 hours

Pregnancy Risk Factor C

Pregnancy Considerations Teratogenic effects have been seen in animals. There are no adequate and well-controlled studies in pregnant women; there have been reports of ophthalmic abnormalities in infants born to women receiving ethambutol as a component of antituberculous therapy. Use only during pregnancy if benefits outweigh risks.

Ethanolamine Oleate (ETH a nol a meen OH lee ate)

Brand Names: U.S. Ethamolin®

Pharmacologic Category Sclerosing Agent

◄ **Use Orphan drug:** Sclerosing agent used for bleeding esophageal varices

Local Anesthetic/Vasoconstrictor Precautions No information available to require special precautions

Effects on Dental Treatment No significant effects or complications reported

Effects on Bleeding No information available to require special precautions

Adverse Effects 1% to 10%:

Central nervous system: Pyrexia (1.8%)

Gastrointestinal: Esophageal ulcer (2%), esophageal stricture (1.3%)

Respiratory: Pleural effusion (2%), pneumonia (1.2%)

Miscellaneous: Retrosternal pain (1.6%)

General Dosage Range Injection: *Adults:* 1.5-5 mL per varix (maximum: 20 mL total)

Mechanism of Action Derived from oleic acid and similar in physical properties to sodium morrhuate; however, the exact mechanism of the hemostatic effect used in endoscopic injection sclerotherapy is not known. Intravenously injected ethanolamine oleate produces a sterile inflammatory response resulting in fibrosis and occlusion of the vein; a dose-related extravascular inflammatory reaction occurs when the drug diffuses through the venous wall. Autopsy results indicate that variceal obliteration occurs secondary to mural necrosis and fibrosis. Thrombosis appears to be a transient reaction.

Pregnancy Risk Factor C

Pregnancy Considerations Animal reproduction studies have not been conducted.

Ethinyl Estradiol and Desogestrel

(ETH in il es tra DYE ole & des oh JES trel)

Brand Names: U.S. Apri®; Azurette™; Caziant®; Cyclessa®; Desogen®; Emoquette™; Kariva®; Mircette®; Ortho-Cept®; Reclipsen®; Velivet™; Viorele

Brand Names: Canada Cyclessa®; Linessa®; Marvelon®; Ortho-Cept®

Generic Availability (U.S.) Yes

Pharmacologic Category Contraceptive; Estrogen and Progestin Combination

Use Prevention of pregnancy

Unlabeled Use Treatment of hypermenorrhea (menorrhagia); pain associated with endometriosis; dysmenorrhea; dysfunctional uterine bleeding

Local Anesthetic/Vasoconstrictor Precautions No information available to require special precautions

Effects on Dental Treatment When prescribing antibiotics, patient must be warned to use additional methods of birth control if on oral contraceptives.

Effects on Bleeding No information available to require special precautions

Adverse Effects The following reactions have been associated with oral contraceptive use:

Increased risk or evidence of association with use:

Cardiovascular: Arterial thromboembolism, cerebral hemorrhage, cerebral thrombosis, hypertension, mesenteric thrombosis, MI, venous thrombosis (with or without embolism)

Gastrointestinal: Gallbladder disease

Hepatic: Hepatic adenomas, liver tumors (benign)

Local: Thrombophlebitis

Ocular: Retinal thrombosis

Respiratory: Pulmonary embolism

Adverse reactions considered drug related:

Cardiovascular: Edema, varicose vein aggravation

Central nervous system: Depression, migraine, mood changes

Dermatologic: Chloasma, melasma, rash (allergic)

Endocrine & metabolic: Amenorrhea, breakthrough bleeding, breast changes (enlargement, pain, secretion, tenderness), fluid retention, infertility (temporary), lactation decreased (with use immediately postpartum), menstrual flow changes, spotting

Gastrointestinal: Abdominal bloating, abdominal cramps, abdominal pain, appetite changes, nausea, weight changes, vomiting

Genitourinary: Cervical ectropion, cervical secretion, vaginal candidiasis, vaginitis

Hematologic: Folate decreased, porphyria exacerbation

Hepatic: Cholestatic jaundice

Neuromuscular & skeletal: Chorea exacerbation

Ocular: Contact lens intolerance, corneal curvature changes (steepening)

Miscellaneous: Anaphylactic/anaphylactoid reactions (including angioedema, circulatory collapse, respiratory collapse, urticaria), SLE exacerbation

Adverse reactions in which association is not confirmed or denied: Acne, Budd-Chiari syndrome, cataracts, colitis, cystitis-like syndrome, dizziness, dysmenorrhea, erythema multiforme, erythema nodosum, headache, hemolytic uremic syndrome, hemorrhagic eruption, hirsutism, libido changes, nervousness, optic neuritis (with or without partial or complete loss of vision), pancreatitis, premenstrual syndrome, renal function impaired, scalp hair loss

Dosage Oral: Adults: Females: Contraception:

Schedule 1 (Sunday starter): Dose begins on first Sunday after onset of menstruation; if the menstrual period starts on Sunday, take first tablet that very same day. **With a Sunday start, an additional method of contraception should be used until after the first 7 days of consecutive administration.**

For 21-tablet package: Dosage is 1 tablet daily for 21 consecutive days, followed by 7 days off of the medication; a new course begins on the 8th day after the last tablet is taken.

For 28-tablet package: Dosage is 1 tablet daily without interruption.

Schedule 2 (Day 1 starter): Dose starts on first day of menstrual cycle taking 1 tablet daily.

For 21-tablet package: Dosage is 1 tablet daily for 21 consecutive days, followed by 7 days off of the medication; a new course begins on the 8th day after the last tablet is taken.

For 28-tablet package: Dosage is 1 tablet daily without interruption.

If all doses have been taken on schedule and one menstrual period is missed, continue dosing cycle. If two consecutive menstrual periods are missed, pregnancy test is required before new dosing cycle is started.

Missed doses **monophasic formulations** (refer to package insert for complete information):

One dose missed: Take as soon as remembered or take 2 tablets next day

Two consecutive doses missed in the first 2 weeks: Take 2 tablets as soon as remembered or 2 tablets next 2 days. **An additional method of contraception should be used for 7 days after missed dose.**

Two consecutive doses missed in week 3 or three consecutive doses missed at any time:

Schedule 1 (Sunday starter): Continue to take 1 tablet daily until Sunday, then discard the rest of the pack, and a new pack is started that same day.

Schedule 2 (Day 1 starter): Current pack should be discarded, and a new pack started that same day. **An additional method of contraception should be used for 7 days after missed dose.**

Missed doses **biphasic/triphasic formulations** (refer to package insert for complete information):

One dose missed: Take as soon as remembered or take 2 tablets next day.

Two consecutive doses missed in week 1 or week 2 of the pack: Take 2 tablets as soon as remembered and 2 tablets the next day. Resume taking 1 tablet daily until the pack is empty. **An additional method of contraception should be used for 7 days after a missed dose.**

Two consecutive doses missed in week 3 of the pack; **an additional method of contraception must be used for 7 days after a missed dose:**

Schedule 1 (Sunday starter): Take 1 tablet every day until Sunday. Discard the remaining pack and start a new pack of pills on the same day.

Schedule 2 (Day 1 starter): Discard the remaining pack and start a new pack the same day.

Three or more consecutive doses missed; **an additional method of contraception must be used for 7 days after a missed dose:**

Schedule 1 (Sunday starter): Take 1 tablet every day until Sunday; on Sunday, discard the pack and start a new pack.

Schedule 2 (Day 1 starter): Discard the remaining pack and begin new pack of tablets starting on the same day.

Dosage adjustment in renal impairment: Specific guidelines not available; use with caution and monitor blood pressure closely. Consider other forms of contraception.

Dosage adjustment in hepatic impairment: Contraindicated in patients with hepatic impairment

Mechanism of Action Combination hormonal contraceptives inhibit ovulation via a negative feedback mechanism on the hypothalamus, which alters the normal pattern of gonadotropin secretion of a follicle-stimulating hormone (FSH) and luteinizing hormone by the anterior pituitary. The follicular phase FSH and midcycle surge of gonadotropins are inhibited. In addition, combination hormonal contraceptives produce alterations in the genital tract, including changes in the cervical mucus, rendering it unfavorable for sperm penetration even if ovulation occurs. Changes in the endometrium may also occur, producing an unfavorable environment for nidation. Combination hormonal contraceptive drugs may alter the tubal transport of the ova through the fallopian tubes. Progestational agents may also alter sperm fertility.

Contraindications Hypersensitivity to ethinyl estradiol, etonogestrel, desogestrel, or any component of the formulation; breast cancer or other estrogen- or progestin-dependent neoplasms (current or a history of), hepatic tumors or disease, pregnancy, undiagnosed abnormal uterine bleeding, cholestatic jaundice of pregnancy, jaundice with prior combination hormonal contraceptive use

Use is also contraindicated in women at high risk of arterial or venous thrombotic diseases including: Cerebrovascular disease, coronary artery disease, diabetes mellitus with vascular disease, DVT or PE (current or history of), headaches with focal neurological symptoms, hypertension (uncontrolled), valvular heart disease with complications, major surgery with prolonged immobilization

Warnings/Precautions Hazardous agent - use appropriate precautions for handling and disposal (NIOSH, 2012). Combination hormonal contraceptives do not protect against HIV infection or other sexually-transmitted diseases. **[U.S. Boxed Warning]: The risk of cardiovascular side effects is increased in women who smoke cigarettes; risk increases with age (especially women >35 years of age) and the number of cigarettes smoked; women who use combination hormonal contraceptives should be strongly advised not to smoke. Should not be used in patients >35 years of age who smoke.** Use with caution in patients with risk factors for coronary artery disease (eg, hypertension, hypercholesterolemia, morbid obesity, diabetes, or women who smoke); may lead to increased risk of myocardial infarction. May have a dose-related risk of vascular disease and hypertension; women with hypertension should be encouraged to use another form of contraception. May increase the risk of thromboembolism; discontinue use of combination hormonal contraceptives if an arterial or venous thrombotic event occurs. Women with inherited thrombophilias (eg, protein C or S deficiency) may have increased risk of venous thromboembolism (DeSancho, 2010; van Vlijmen, 2011). Whenever possible, combination hormonal contraceptives should be discontinued at least 4 weeks prior to and for 2 weeks following elective surgery associated with an increased risk of thromboembolism or during periods of prolonged immobilization. Women with hypertension or renal disease should be encouraged to use another form of contraception.

The use of combination hormonal contraceptives has been associated with a slight increase in frequency of breast cancer; however, studies are not consistent. Use is contraindicated in women with (or history of) breast cancer. Combination hormonal contraceptives may cause glucose intolerance or affect serum triglyceride and lipoprotein levels. May have a dose-related risk of gallbladder disease. Estrogens may increase thyroid-binding globulin (TBG) levels leading to increased circulating total thyroid hormone levels. Women on thyroid replacement therapy may require higher doses of thyroid hormone while receiving estrogens. Estrogens may cause retinal vascular thrombosis; discontinue if migraine, loss of vision, proptosis, diplopia or other visual disturbances occur; discontinue permanently if papilledema or retinal vascular lesions are observed on examination. Use caution in conditions that may be aggravated by fluid retention, depression, or history of migraine. Extremely rare adenomas and focal nodular hyperplasia resulting in fatal intra-abdominal hemorrhage have been reported in association with long-term oral contraceptive use. Presentation of an abdominal mass, acute abdominal pain, or intra-abdominal bleeding warrants further evaluation to rule out source. Combination hormonal contraceptives may be poorly metabolized in women with hepatic impairment. Discontinue if jaundice develops during therapy or if liver function becomes abnormal. Risk of cholestasis may be increased with previous cholestatic jaundice of pregnancy or jaundice with prior oral contraceptive use. Presentation of irregular, unresolving vaginal bleeding warrants further evaluation including endometrial sampling, if indicated, to rule out malignancy. Not for use prior to menarche.

The minimum dosage combination of estrogen/progestin that will effectively treat the individual patient should be used. New patients should be started on products containing ≤0.035 mg of estrogen per tablet. The use of estrogens and/or progestins may change the results of some laboratory tests (eg, coagulation factors, lipids, glucose tolerance, binding proteins). The dose, route, and the specific estrogen/progestin influences these changes. In addition, personal risk factors (eg, cardiovascular disease, smoking, diabetes, age) also contribute to adverse events; use of specific products may be contraindicated in women with certain risk factors.

Drug Interactions

Avoid Concomitant Use

Avoid concomitant use of Ethinyl Estradiol and Desogestrel with any of the following: Anastrozole; Griseofulvin; Ospemifene; Pimozide; Pirfenidone

Increased Effect/Toxicity

Ethinyl Estradiol and Desogestrel may increase the levels/effects of: ARIPiprazole; Benzodiazepines (metabolized by oxidation); Corticosteroids (Systemic); CYP1A2 Substrates; Lomitapide; Ospemifene; Pimozide; Pirfenidone; ROPINIRole; Selegiline; Theophylline Derivatives; Tipranavir; TiZANidine; Tranexamic Acid; Voriconazole

The levels/effects of Ethinyl Estradiol and Desogestrel may be increased by: Ascorbic Acid; Atazanavir; Boceprevir; Cobicistat; Herbs (Estrogenic Properties); Herbs (Progestogenic Properties); Mifepristone; NSAID (COX-2 Inhibitor); Voriconazole

Decreased Effect

Ethinyl Estradiol and Desogestrel may decrease the levels/effects of: Anastrozole; Chenodiol; Hyaluronidase; LamoTRIgine; Ospemifene; Thyroid Products; Ursodiol; Vitamin K Antagonists

The levels/effects of Ethinyl Estradiol and Desogestrel may be decreased by: Acitretin; Aminoglutethimide; Aprepitant; Armodafinil; Artemether; Barbiturates; Bexarotene (Systemic); Bile Acid Sequestrants; Boceprevir; Bosentan; CarBAMazepine; ClOBAZam; Cobicistat; Colesevelam; CYP3A4 Inducers (Strong); Deferasirox; Elvitegravir; Exenatide; Felbamate; Fosaprepitant; Fosphenytoin; Griseofulvin; LamoTRIgine; Mifepristone; Modafinil; Mycophenolate; Nafcillin; Nevirapine; OXcarbazepine; Perampanel; Phenytoin; Protease Inhibitors; Prucalopride; Retinoic Acid Derivatives; Rifamycin Derivatives; Rufinamide; St Johns Wort; Telaprevir; Tipranavir; Tocilizumab; Topiramate

Ethanol/Nutrition/Herb Interactions

Food: CNS effects of caffeine may be enhanced if combination hormonal contraceptives are used concurrently with caffeine. Grapefruit juice increases ethinyl estradiol concentrations and would be expected to increase progesterone serum levels as well; clinical implications are unclear.

Herb/Nutraceutical: St John's wort may decrease levels. Herbs with estrogenic properties may enhance the adverse/toxic effect of estrogen derivatives; examples include alfalfa, black cohosh, bloodroot, hops, kudzu, licorice, red clover, saw palmetto, soybean, thyme, wild yam, yucca. Herbs with progestogenic properties may enhance the adverse/toxic effect of progestins; examples include bloodroot, chasteberry, damiana, oregano, yucca.

Dietary Considerations
Should be taken at same time each day.

Pharmacodynamics/Kinetics

Half-life Elimination Etonogestrel: ~38 hours; Ethinyl estradiol: ~26 hours

Pregnancy Risk Factor X

Pregnancy Considerations
Pregnancy should be ruled out prior to treatment and discontinued if pregnancy occurs. In general, the use of combination hormonal contraceptives when inadvertently taken early in pregnancy has not been associated with teratogenic effects. Hormonal contraceptives may be less effective in obese patients. An increase in oral contraceptive failure was noted in women with a BMI >27.3 kg/m^2. Similar findings were noted in patients weighing ≥90 kg (198 lb) using the contraceptive patch.

Due to increased risk of venous thromboembolism (VTE) postpartum, combination hormonal contraceptives should not be started in any woman <21 days following delivery. Women without risk factors for VTE and who are not breast-feeding may start combination hormonal contraceptives during 21-42 days postpartum. After 42 days postpartum, restrictions for use are not related to postpartum status and should be based on other medical conditions (CDC, 2011).

Lactation Enters breast milk/not recommended

Breast-Feeding Considerations Jaundice and breast enlargement in the nursing infant have been reported following the use of combination hormonal contraceptives. May decrease the quality and quantity of breast milk; a nonhormonal form of contraception is recommended (per manufacturer). The theoretical concerns about decreased milk production are greatest early in the postpartum period when milk production is being established. Postpartum risk status for VTE should be considered when initiating combination hormonal contraceptives after delivery. Combined hormonal contraceptives should not be started <21 days postpartum due to increased risk of VTE. Risk of VTE is still elevated in breast-feeding women until ~42 days postpartum and is greater in women with additional risk factors. After 42 days postpartum, restrictions for use are not related to postpartum VTE risk and should be based on other medical conditions (CDC, 2011).

Dosage Forms

Tablet, oral [low dose formulation]:

Azurette™:
  Day 1-21: Ethinyl estradiol 0.02 mg and desogestrel 0.15 mg [21 white tablets]
  Day 22-23: 2 inactive green tablets
  Day 24-28: Ethinyl estradiol 0.01 mg [5 blue tablets] (28s)

Kariva®:
  Day 1-21: Ethinyl estradiol 0.02 mg and desogestrel 0.15 mg [21 white tablets]
  Day 22-23: 2 inactive light green tablets
  Day 24-28: Ethinyl estradiol 0.01 mg [5 light blue tablets] (28s)

Mircette®, Viorele:
  Day 1-21: Ethinyl estradiol 0.02 mg and desogestrel 0.15 mg [21 white tablets]
  Day 22-23: 2 inactive green tablets
  Day 24-28: Ethinyl estradiol 0.01 mg [5 yellow tablets] (28s)

Tablet, oral [monophasic formulation]:

Apri® 28: Ethinyl estradiol 0.03 mg and desogestrel 0.15 mg [21 rose tablets and 7 white inactive tablets] (28s)

Desogen®, Reclipsen®: Ethinyl estradiol 0.03 mg and desogestrel 0.15 mg [21 white tablets and 7 green inactive tablets] (28s)

Emoquette™: Ethinyl estradiol 0.03 mg and desogestrel 0.15 mg [21 white tablets and 7 light green inactive tablets] (28s)

Ortho-Cept® 28: Ethinyl estradiol 0.03 mg and desogestrel 0.15 mg [21 light orange tablets and 7 green inactive tablets] (28s)

Tablet, oral [triphasic formulation]:
Caziant®:
Day 1-7: Ethinyl estradiol 0.025 mg and desogestrel 0.1 mg [7 white tablets]
Day 8-14: Ethinyl estradiol 0.025 mg and desogestrel 0.125 mg [7 light blue tablets]
Day 15-21: Ethinyl estradiol 0.025 mg and desogestrel 0.15 mg [7 blue tablets]
Day 22-28: 7 green inactive tablets (28s)
Cyclessa®:
Day 1-7: Ethinyl estradiol 0.025 mg and desogestrel 0.1 mg [7 light yellow tablets]
Day 8-14: Ethinyl estradiol 0.025 mg and desogestrel 0.125 mg [7 orange tablets]
Day 15-21: Ethinyl estradiol 0.025 mg and desogestrel 0.15 mg [7 red tablets]
Day 22-28: 7 green inactive tablets (28s)
Velivet™:
Day 1-7: Ethinyl estradiol 0.025 mg and desogestrel 0.1 mg [7 beige tablets]
Day 8-14: Ethinyl estradiol 0.025 mg and desogestrel 0.125 mg [7 orange tablets]
Day 15-21: Ethinyl estradiol 0.025 mg and desogestrel 0.15 mg [7 pink tablets]
Day 22-28: 7 white inactive tablets (28s)

Ethinyl Estradiol and Drospirenone
(ETH in il es tra DYE ole & droh SPYE re none)

Related Information
Endocrine Disorders and Pregnancy *on page 1517*
Brand Names: U.S. Gianvi™; Loryna™; Ocella™; Syeda™; Vestura™; Yasmin®; Yaz®; Zarah®
Brand Names: Canada Yasmin®; Yaz®
Generic Availability (U.S.) Yes
Pharmacologic Category Contraceptive; Estrogen and Progestin Combination
Use Prevention of pregnancy; treatment of premenstrual dysphoric disorder (PMDD); treatment of acne
Unlabeled Use Treatment of hypermenorrhea (menorrhagia); pain associated with endometriosis; dysmenorrhea; dysfunctional uterine bleeding
Local Anesthetic/Vasoconstrictor Precautions No information available to require special precautions
Effects on Dental Treatment When prescribing antibiotics, patient must be warned to use additional methods of birth control if on oral contraceptives.
Effects on Bleeding No information available to require special precautions
Adverse Effects The following reactions have been associated with oral contraceptive use:
Increased risk or evidence of association with use:
Cardiovascular: Arterial thromboembolism, cerebral hemorrhage, cerebral thrombosis, hypertension, mesenteric thrombosis, MI
Gastrointestinal: Gallbladder disease
Hepatic: Hepatic adenomas, liver tumors (benign)
Local: Thrombophlebitis
Ocular: Retinal thrombosis
Respiratory: Pulmonary embolism
Adverse reactions considered drug related:
Cardiovascular: Edema, varicose vein aggravation
Central nervous system: Depression, migraine
Dermatologic: Melasma, rash (allergic)
Endocrine & metabolic: Amenorrhea, breakthrough bleeding, breast changes (enlargement, pain, secretion, tenderness), carbohydrate tolerance decreased, infertility (temporary), lactation decreased (with use immediately postpartum), menstrual flow changes, spotting

Gastrointestinal: Abdominal bloating, abdominal cramps, nausea, weight changes, vomiting
Genitourinary: Cervical ectropion, cervical secretion/erosion, vaginal candidiasis
Hematologic: Folate decreased, porphyria exacerbation
Hepatic: Cholestatic jaundice
Neuromuscular & skeletal: Chorea exacerbation
Ocular: Contact lens intolerance, corneal curvature changes (steepening)
Miscellaneous: Anaphylactic/anaphylactoid reactions (including angioedema, circulatory collapse, respiratory collapse, urticaria), SLE exacerbation
Adverse reactions in which association is not confirmed or denied: Acne, appetite changes, Budd-Chiari syndrome, cataracts, colitis, cystitis-like syndrome, dizziness, dysmenorrhea, erythema multiforme, erythema nodosum, headache, hemolytic uremic syndrome, hemorrhagic eruption, hirsutism, libido changes, nervousness, optic neuritis (with or without partial or complete loss of vision), pancreatitis, premenstrual syndrome, porphyria, renal function impaired, scalp hair loss, vaginitis

Dosage Oral:
Children ≥14 years and Adults: Females: Acne (Yaz®): Refer to dosing for contraception
Adults: Females: Contraception (Yasmin®, Yaz®), PMDD (Yaz®): Dosage is 1 tablet daily for 28 consecutive days. Dosing may be started on the first day of menstrual period (Day 1 starter) or on the first Sunday after the onset of the menstrual period (Sunday starter). **An additional method of contraception should be used until after the first 7 days of consecutive administration.**
Day 1 starter: Dose starts on first day of menstrual cycle taking 1 tablet daily.
Sunday starter: Dose begins on first Sunday after onset of menstruation; if the menstrual period starts on Sunday, take first tablet that very same day.
Switching from a different contraceptive:
Oral contraceptive: Start on the same day that a new pack of the previous oral contraceptive would have been taken
Transdermal patch, vaginal ring, injection: Start on the day the next dose would have been due
IUD or implant: Start on the day of removal
Use after childbirth (in women who are not breast-feeding) or after second trimester abortion: Therapy may be started ≥4 weeks postpartum. Pregnancy should be ruled out prior to treatment if menstrual periods have not restarted and an additional method of contraception (nonhormonal) should be used until after the first 7 days of consecutive administration.

Missed doses:
If all doses have been taken on schedule and one menstrual period is missed, continue dosing cycle. If two consecutive menstrual periods are missed, pregnancy test is required before new dosing cycle is started.
If doses have been missed during the first 3 weeks and the menstrual period is missed, pregnancy should be ruled out prior to continuing treatment.
Missed doses (monophasic formulations) (refer to package insert for complete information):
One dose missed: Take as soon as remembered or take 2 tablets next day

Two consecutive doses missed in the first 2 weeks: Take 2 tablets as soon as remembered or 2 tablets next 2 days. **An additional method of contraception should be used for 7 days after missed dose.**

Two consecutive doses missed in week 3 or three consecutive doses missed at any time: **An additional method of contraception must be used for 7 days after a missed dose.**

Day 1 starter: Current pack should be discarded, and a new pack should be started that same day.

Sunday starter: Continue dose of 1 tablet daily until Sunday, then discard the rest of the pack, and a new pack should be started that same day.

Any number of doses missed in week 4: Continue taking one pill each day until pack is empty; no back-up method of contraception is needed

Dosage adjustment in renal impairment: Contraindicated in patients with renal dysfunction

Dosage adjustment in hepatic impairment: Contraindicated in patients with hepatic dysfunction

Mechanism of Action Combination oral contraceptives inhibit ovulation via a negative feedback mechanism on the hypothalamus, which alters the normal pattern of gonadotropin secretion of a follicle-stimulating hormone (FSH) and luteinizing hormone by the anterior pituitary. The follicular phase FSH and midcycle surge of gonadotropins are inhibited. In addition, oral contraceptives produce alterations in the genital tract, including changes in the cervical mucus, rendering it unfavorable for sperm penetration even if ovulation occurs. Changes in the endometrium may also occur, producing an unfavorable environment for nidation. Oral contraceptive drugs may alter the tubal transport of the ova through the fallopian tubes. Progestational agents may also alter sperm fertility. Drospirenone is a spironolactone analogue with antimineralocorticoid and antiandrogenic activity.

Contraindications Adrenal insufficiency, breast cancer or other estrogen- or progestin-dependent neoplasms (current or a history of), hepatic tumors or disease, pregnancy, renal impairment, undiagnosed abnormal uterine bleeding. Use is also contraindicated in women at high risk of arterial or venous thrombotic diseases including: Cerebrovascular disease, coronary artery disease, diabetes mellitus with vascular disease, DVT or PE (current or history of), hypercoagulopathies (inherited or acquired), headaches with focal neurological symptoms, hypertension (uncontrolled), migraine headaches if >35 years of age, thrombogenic valvular or rhythm diseases of the heart (eg, subacute bacterial endocarditis with valvular disease or atrial fibrillation), women >35 years of age who smoke.

Warnings/Precautions Hazardous agent - use appropriate precautions for handling and disposal (NIOSH, 2012). Oral contraceptives do not protect against HIV infection or other sexually-transmitted diseases.**[U.S. Boxed Warning]: The risk of cardiovascular side effects is increased in women who smoke cigarettes; risk increases with age (especially women >35 years of age) and the number of cigarettes smoked; women who use combination hormonal contraceptives should be strongly advised not to smoke. Use is contraindicated in patients >35 years of age who smoke.** Oral contraceptives may lead to increased risk of stroke or myocardial infarction, use with caution in patients with risk factors for cardiovascular disease (eg, hypertension, hypercholesterolemia, morbid obesity, diabetes, or women who smoke). Contraceptives may increase the risk of thromboembolism;

discontinue if an arterial or venous thrombotic event occurs. Risk may be greater with contraceptives containing drospirenone. Women with inherited thrombophilias (eg, protein C or S deficiency) may have increased risk of venous thromboembolism (DeSancho, 2010; van Vlijmen, 2011). Use is contraindicated in women with hypercoagulopathies (inherited or acquired). Whenever possible, combination hormonal contraceptives should be discontinued at least 4 weeks prior to and for 2 weeks following elective surgery associated with an increased risk of thromboembolism or during periods of prolonged immobilization. Oral contraceptives may have a dose-related risk of vascular disease, hypertension, and gallbladder disease. Women with hypertension should be encouraged to use another form of contraception. The use of combination hormonal contraceptives has been associated with a slight increase in frequency of breast cancer; however, studies are not consistent. Use is contraindicated in women with (or history of) breast cancer.

May have adverse effects on glucose tolerance; use caution in women with diabetes. Estrogens may cause retinal vascular thrombosis; discontinue if migraine, loss of vision, proptosis, diplopia or other visual disturbances occur; discontinue permanently if papilledema or retinal vascular lesions are observed on examination. Use with caution in patients with conditions that may be aggravated by fluid retention, depression, or patients with history of migraine. Evaluate new, recurrent, severe or persistent headaches. Not for use prior to menarche. Estrogens may induce or exacerbate symptoms in women with hereditary angioedema. Use caution with a history of chloasma gravidarum; women with a tendency to chloasma should avoid sun and ultraviolet radiation exposure during therapy. Extremely rare adenomas and focal nodular hyperplasia resulting in fatal intra-abdominal hemorrhage have been reported in association with long-term oral contraceptive use. Presentation of an abdominal mass, acute abdominal pain, or intra-abdominal bleeding warrants further evaluation to rule out source. Combination hormonal contraceptives may be poorly metabolized in women with hepatic impairment. Discontinue if jaundice develops during therapy or if liver function becomes abnormal. Risk of cholestasis may be increased with previous cholestatic jaundice of pregnancy or jaundice with prior oral contraceptive use. Combination hormonal contraceptives may affect serum triglyceride and lipoprotein levels. Use with caution in patients with familial defects of lipoprotein metabolism; consider an alternate form of contraception in women with uncontrolled dyslipidemias. Estrogens may increase thyroid-binding globulin (TBG) levels leading to increased circulating total thyroid hormone levels. Women on thyroid replacement therapy may require higher doses of thyroid hormone while receiving estrogens. The use of estrogens and/or progestins may change the results of some laboratory tests (eg, coagulation factors, lipids, glucose tolerance, binding proteins). Drospirenone can also cause an increase in plasma renin activity and plasma aldosterone. The dose, route, and the specific estrogen/progestin influences these changes. In addition, personal risk factors (eg, cardiovascular disease, smoking, diabetes, age) also contribute to adverse events; use of specific products may be contraindicated in women with certain risk factors.

The minimum dosage combination of estrogen/progestin that will effectively treat the individual patient should be used. Unscheduled bleeding/spotting may especially occur within the first 3 months of use. Development of irregular, unresolving vaginal bleeding following previously regular cycles warrants further evaluation including endometrial sampling, if indicated, to rule out malignancy.

Acne use: For use only in females ≥14 years who have reached menarche, who also desire combination hormonal contraceptive therapy, are unresponsive to topical treatments, and have no contraindications to combination hormonal contraceptive use.

PMDD use: For use only in females who desire combination hormonal contraceptive therapy; use for more than 3 menstrual cycles has not been evaluated. Has not been evaluated for the treatment of premenstrual syndrome

Drospirenone has antimineralocorticoid activity that may lead to hyperkalemia in patients with renal insufficiency, hepatic dysfunction, or adrenal insufficiency. Use caution with medications that may increase serum potassium.

Drug Interactions
Avoid Concomitant Use
Avoid concomitant use of Ethinyl Estradiol and Drospirenone with any of the following: Anastrozole; Boceprevir; CycloSPORINE (Systemic); Griseofulvin; Ospemifene; Pimozide; Pirfenidone; Tacrolimus (Systemic)

Increased Effect/Toxicity
Ethinyl Estradiol and Drospirenone may increase the levels/effects of: ACE Inhibitors; Amifostine; Ammonium Chloride; Antihypertensives; ARIPiprazole; Benzodiazepines (metabolized by oxidation); Cardiac Glycosides; Corticosteroids (Systemic); CycloSPORINE (Systemic); CYP1A2 Substrates; Hypotensive Agents; Lomitapide; Ospemifene; Pimozide; Pirfenidone; Potassium-Sparing Diuretics; RiTUXimab; ROPINIRole; Selegiline; Sodium Phosphates; Tacrolimus (Systemic); Theophylline Derivatives; Tipranavir; TiZANidine; Tranexamic Acid; Voriconazole

The levels/effects of Ethinyl Estradiol and Drospirenone may be increased by: Alfuzosin; Angiotensin II Receptor Blockers; Ascorbic Acid; Atazanavir; Boceprevir; Canagliflozin; Cobicistat; Diazoxide; Eplerenone; Herbs (Estrogenic Properties); Herbs (Hypotensive Properties); Herbs (Progestogenic Properties); MAO Inhibitors; Mifepristone; Nonsteroidal Anti-Inflammatory Agents; NSAID (COX-2 Inhibitor); Pentoxifylline; Phosphodiesterase 5 Inhibitors; Potassium Salts; Prostacyclin Analogues; Tolvaptan; Voriconazole

Decreased Effect
Ethinyl Estradiol and Drospirenone may decrease the levels/effects of: Anastrozole; Cardiac Glycosides; Chenodiol; Hyaluronidase; LamoTRIgine; Ospemifene; QuiNIDine; Thyroid Products; Ursodiol; Vitamin K Antagonists

The levels/effects of Ethinyl Estradiol and Drospirenone may be decreased by: Acitretin; Aminoglutethimide; Aprepitant; Armodafinil; Artemether; Barbiturates; Bexarotene (Systemic); Bile Acid Sequestrants; Boceprevir; Bosentan; CarBAMazepine; CloBAZam; Cobicistat; Colesevelam; CYP3A4 Inducers (Strong); Deferasirox; Elvitegravir; Exenatide; Felbamate; Fosaprepitant; Fosphenytoin; Griseofulvin; Herbs (Hypertensive Properties); LamoTRIgine; Methylphenidate; Mifepristone; Modafinil; Mycophenolate; Nafcillin; Nevirapine; Nonsteroidal Anti-Inflammatory Agents; OXcarbazepine; Perampanel; Phenytoin; Protease Inhibitors; Prucalopride; Retinoic Acid Derivatives; Rifamycin Derivatives; Rufinamide; St Johns Wort; Telaprevir; Tipranavir; Tocilizumab; Topiramate; Yohimbine

Ethanol/Nutrition/Herb Interactions
Food: CNS effects of caffeine may be enhanced if oral contraceptives are used concurrently with caffeine. Grapefruit juice increases ethinyl estradiol plasma concentrations; clinical implications are unclear.

Herb/Nutraceutical: St John's wort may decrease levels. Herbs with estrogenic properties may enhance the adverse/toxic effect of estrogen derivatives; examples include alfalfa, black cohosh, bloodroot, hops, kudzu, licorice, red clover, saw palmetto, soybean, thyme, wild yam, yucca. Herbs with progestogenic properties may enhance the adverse/toxic effect of progestins; examples include bloodroot, chasteberry, damiana, oregano, yucca.

Dietary Considerations
Should be taken at the same time each day; may be taken with or without a meal

Pharmacodynamics/Kinetics
Half-life Elimination Terminal: Drospirenone: ~30 hours; Ethinyl estradiol: ~24 hours

Time to Peak 1-3 hours

Pregnancy Risk Factor X

Pregnancy Considerations In general, the use of oral contraceptives when inadvertently taken early in pregnancy have not been associated with teratogenic effects. Esophageal atresia was reported in one infant with a single-cycle exposure to ethinyl estradiol and drospirenone *in utero* (association not known). Pregnancy should be ruled out prior to treatment and discontinued if pregnancy occurs. Hormonal contraceptives may be less effective in obese patients. An increase in oral contraceptive failure was noted in women with a BMI >27.3 kg/m^2. Similar findings were noted in patients weighing ≥90 kg (198 lb) using the contraceptive patch.

Due to increased risk of venous thromboembolism (VTE) postpartum, combination hormonal contraceptives should not be started in any woman <21 days following delivery. Women without risk factors for VTE and who are not breast-feeding may start combination hormonal contraceptives during 21-42 days postpartum. After 42 days postpartum, restrictions for use are not related to postpartum status and should be based on other medical conditions (CDC, 2011). The manufacturer states that combination hormonal contraceptives should not be started until ≥4 weeks after delivery in women who choose not to breast-feed, or ≥4 weeks after a second trimester abortion or miscarriage.

Lactation Enters breast milk/not recommended

Breast-Feeding Considerations The amount of drospirenone excreted in breast milk is ~0.02%, resulting in a maximum of ~3 mcg/day drospirenone to the infant. Jaundice and breast enlargement in the nursing infant have been reported following the use of other oral contraceptives. In addition, may decrease the quality and quantity of breast milk. Other forms of contraception are recommended while breast-feeding (per manufacturer). The theoretical concerns about decreased milk production are greatest early in the postpartum period when milk production is being established. Postpartum risk status for VTE should be considered when initiating combination hormonal contraceptives after delivery. Combined hormonal contraceptives should not be started <21 days postpartum due to increased risk of VTE. Risk of VTE is still elevated in breast-feeding women until ~42 days postpartum and is greater in women with additional risk factors. After 42 days postpartum, restrictions for use are not related to postpartum VTE risk and should be based on other medical conditions (CDC, 2011).

Dosage Forms

Tablet, oral: Ethinyl estradiol 0.03 mg and drospirenone 3 mg [21 active tablets and 7 inactive tablets] (28s)

Gianvi™: Ethinyl estradiol 0.03 mg and drospirenone 3 mg [24 light pink active tablets and 4 white inactive tablets] (28s)

Loryna™: Ethinyl estradiol 0.02 mg and drospirenone 3 mg [24 peach active tablets and 4 white inactive tablets] (28s)

Ocella™, Syeda™, Yasmin®: Ethinyl estradiol 0.03 mg and drospirenone 3 mg [21 yellow active tablets and 7 white inactive tablets] (28s)

Vestura™: Ethinyl estradiol 0.02 mg and drospirenone 3 mg [24 pink active tablets and 4 peach inactive tablets] (28s)

Yaz®: Ethinyl estradiol 0.02 mg and drospirenone 3 mg [24 light pink active tablets and 4 white inactive tablets] (28s)

Zarah®: Ethinyl estradiol 0.03 mg and drospirenone 3 mg [21 blue active tablets and 7 peach inactive tablets] (28s)

Ethinyl Estradiol and Ethynodiol Diacetate

(ETH in il es tra DYE ole & e thye noe DYE ole dye AS e tate)

Brand Names: U.S. Kelnor™; Zovia®

Brand Names: Canada Demulen® 30

Generic Availability (U.S.) Yes

Pharmacologic Category Contraceptive; Estrogen and Progestin Combination

Use Prevention of pregnancy

Unlabeled Use Treatment of hypermenorrhea (menorrhagia); pain associated with endometriosis; dysmenorrhea; dysfunctional uterine bleeding

Local Anesthetic/Vasoconstrictor Precautions No information available to require special precautions

Effects on Dental Treatment When prescribing antibiotics, patient must be warned to use additional methods of birth control if on oral contraceptives.

Effects on Bleeding No information available to require special precautions

Adverse Effects Frequency not defined.

Cardiovascular: Arterial thromboembolism, cerebral hemorrhage, cerebral thrombosis, edema, hypertension, mesenteric thrombosis, MI

Central nervous system: Depression, dizziness, headache, migraine, nervousness, premenstrual syndrome, stroke

Dermatologic: Acne, erythema multiforme, erythema nodosum, hirsutism, loss of scalp hair, melasma (may persist), rash (allergic)

Endocrine & metabolic: Amenorrhea, breakthrough bleeding, breast enlargement, breast secretion, breast tenderness, carbohydrate intolerance, lactation decreased (postpartum), glucose tolerance decreased, libido changes, menstrual flow changes, sex hormone-binding globulins (SHBG) increased, spotting, temporary infertility (following discontinuation), thyroid-binding globulin increased, triglycerides increased

Gastrointestinal: Abdominal cramps, appetite changes, bloating, cholestasis, colitis, gallbladder disease, jaundice, nausea, vomiting, weight gain/loss

Genitourinary: Cervical erosion changes, cervical secretion changes, cystitis-like syndrome, vaginal candidiasis, vaginitis

Hematologic: Antithrombin III decreased, folate levels decreased, hemolytic uremic syndrome, norepinephrine induced platelet aggregability increased, porphyria, prothrombin increased; factors VII, VIII, IX, and X increased

Hepatic: Benign liver tumors, Budd-Chiari syndrome, cholestatic jaundice, hepatic adenomas

Local: Thrombophlebitis

Ocular: Cataracts, change in corneal curvature (steepening), contact lens intolerance, optic neuritis, retinal thrombosis

Renal: Impaired renal function

Respiratory: Pulmonary thromboembolism

Miscellaneous: Hemorrhagic eruption

Dosage Oral: Adults: Females: Contraception:

Schedule 1 (Sunday starter): Dose begins on first Sunday after onset of menstruation; if the menstrual period starts on Sunday, take first tablet that very same day. **With a Sunday start, an additional method of contraception should be used until after the first 7 days of consecutive administration.**

For 21-tablet package: 1 tablet/day for 21 consecutive days, followed by 7 days off of the medication; a new course begins on the 8th day after the last tablet is taken.

For 28-tablet package: 1 tablet/day without interruption.

Schedule 2 (Day 1 starter): Dose starts on first day of menstrual cycle taking 1 tablet daily.

For 21-tablet package: 1 tablet/day for 21 consecutive days, followed by 7 days off of the medication; a new course begins on the 8th day after the last tablet is taken.

For 28-tablet package: 1 tablet/day without interruption.

If all doses have been taken on schedule and one menstrual period is missed, continue dosing cycle. If two consecutive menstrual periods are missed, pregnancy test is required before new dosing cycle is started.

Missed doses **monophasic formulations** (refer to package insert for complete information):

One dose missed: Take as soon as remembered or take 2 tablets next day

Two consecutive doses missed in the first 2 weeks: Take 2 tablets as soon as remembered or 2 tablets next 2 days. **An additional method of contraception should be used for 7 days after missed dose.**

Two consecutive doses missed in week 3 or three consecutive doses missed at any time: **An additional method of contraception should be used for 7 days after missed dose:**

Schedule 1 (Sunday starter): Continue dose of 1 tablet daily until Sunday, then discard the rest of the pack, and a new pack should be started that same day.

Schedule 2 (Day 1 starter): Current package should be discarded, and a new pack should be started that same day.

Dosage adjustment in renal impairment: Specific guidelines not available; use with caution and monitor blood pressure closely. Consider other forms of contraception.

Dosage adjustment in hepatic impairment: Contraindicated in patients with hepatic impairment

Mechanism of Action Combination hormonal contraceptives inhibit ovulation via a negative feedback mechanism on the hypothalamus, which alters the normal pattern of gonadotropin secretion of a follicle-stimulating hormone (FSH) and luteinizing hormone by the anterior pituitary. The follicular phase FSH and midcycle surge of gonadotropins are inhibited. In addition, combination hormonal contraceptives produce alterations in the genital tract, including changes in the cervical mucus, rendering it unfavorable for sperm penetration even if ovulation occurs. Changes in the endometrium may also occur, producing an unfavorable environment for nidation. Combination hormonal contraceptive drugs may alter the tubal transport of the ova through the fallopian tubes. Progestational agents may also alter sperm fertility.

Contraindications Breast cancer or other estrogen- or progestin-dependent neoplasms (current or a history of), hepatic tumors or disease, cholestatic jaundice of pregnancy, jaundice with prior combination hormonal contraceptive use, pregnancy, undiagnosed abnormal uterine bleeding

Use is also contraindicated in women at high risk of arterial or venous thrombotic diseases including: Cerebrovascular disease, coronary artery disease, DVT or PE (current or history of)

Warnings/Precautions Hazardous agent - use appropriate precautions for handling and disposal (NIOSH, 2012). Combination hormonal contraceptives do not protect against HIV infection or other sexually-transmitted diseases. **[U.S. Boxed Warning]: The risk of cardiovascular side effects is increased in women who smoke cigarettes; risk increases with age (especially women >35 years of age) and the number of cigarettes smoked; women who use combination hormonal contraceptives should be strongly advised not to smoke. Should not be used in patients >35 years of age who smoke.** Use with caution in patients with risk factors for coronary artery disease (eg, hypertension, hypercholesterolemia, morbid obesity, diabetes, or women who smoke); may lead to increased risk of myocardial infarction. May have a dose-related risk of vascular disease and hypertension; women with hypertension should be encouraged to use a nonhormonal form of contraception. May increase the risk of thromboembolism; discontinue use of combination hormonal contraceptives if an arterial or venous thrombotic event occurs. Women with inherited thrombophilias (eg, protein C or S deficiency) may have increased risk of venous thromboembolism (DeSancho, 2010; van Vlijmen, 2011). Whenever possible, combination hormonal contraceptives should be discontinued at least 4 weeks prior to and for 2 weeks following elective surgery associated with an increased risk of thromboembolism or during periods of prolonged immobilization.

Combination hormonal contraceptives may have a dose-related risk of gallbladder disease. Women with renal disease should be encouraged to use a nonhormonal form of contraception. The use of combination hormonal contraceptives has been associated with a slight increase in frequency of breast cancer; however, studies are not consistent. Use is contraindicated in women with (or history of) breast cancer. Combination hormonal contraceptives may cause glucose intolerance or affect serum triglyceride and lipoprotein levels. Estrogens may increase thyroid-binding globulin (TBG) levels leading to increased circulating total thyroid hormone levels. Women on thyroid replacement therapy may require higher doses of thyroid hormone while receiving estrogens. Estrogens may cause retinal vascular thrombosis; discontinue if migraine, loss of vision, proptosis, diplopia or other visual disturbances occur; discontinue permanently if papilledema or retinal vascular lesions are observed on examination. Use caution with conditions that may be aggravated by fluid retention, depression, or history of migraine. Not for use prior to menarche. Presentation of irregular, unresolving vaginal bleeding warrants further evaluation including endometrial sampling, if indicated, to rule out malignancy. Extremely rare adenomas and focal nodular hyperplasia resulting in fatal intra-abdominal hemorrhage have been reported in association with long-term oral contraceptive use. Presentation of an abdominal mass, acute abdominal pain, or intra-abdominal bleeding warrants further evaluation to rule out source. Combination hormonal contraceptives may be poorly metabolized in women with hepatic impairment. Discontinue if jaundice develops during therapy or if liver function becomes abnormal. Risk of cholestasis may be increased with previous cholestatic jaundice of pregnancy or jaundice with prior oral contraceptive use. The use of estrogens and/or progestins may change the results of some laboratory tests (eg, coagulation factors, lipids, glucose tolerance, binding proteins). The dose, route, and the specific estrogen/progestin influences these changes. In addition, personal risk factors (eg, cardiovascular disease, smoking, diabetes, age) also contribute to adverse events; use of specific products may be contraindicated in women with certain risk factors.

The minimum dosage combination of estrogen/progestin that will effectively treat the individual patient should be used. New patients should be started on products containing ≤0.035 mg of estrogen per tablet.

Drug Interactions

Avoid Concomitant Use

Avoid concomitant use of Ethinyl Estradiol and Ethynodiol Diacetate with any of the following: Anastrozole; Griseofulvin; Ospemifene; Pimozide; Pirfenidone

Increased Effect/Toxicity

Ethinyl Estradiol and Ethynodiol Diacetate may increase the levels/effects of: ARIPiprazole; Benzodiazepines (metabolized by oxidation); Corticosteroids (Systemic); CYP1A2 Substrates; Lomitapide; Ospemifene; Pimozide; Pirfenidone; ROPINIRole; Selegiline; Theophylline Derivatives; Tipranavir; TiZANidine; Tranexamic Acid; Voriconazole

The levels/effects of Ethinyl Estradiol and Ethynodiol Diacetate may be increased by: Ascorbic Acid; Atazanavir; Boceprevir; Cobicistat; Herbs (Estrogenic Properties); Herbs (Progestogenic Properties); Mifepristone; NSAID (COX-2 Inhibitor); Voriconazole

Decreased Effect

Ethinyl Estradiol and Ethynodiol Diacetate may decrease the levels/effects of: Anastrozole; Chenodiol; Hyaluronidase; LamoTRIgine; Ospemifene; Thyroid Products; Ursodiol; Vitamin K Antagonists

The levels/effects of Ethinyl Estradiol and Ethynodiol Diacetate may be decreased by: Acitretin; Aminoglutethimide; Aprepitant; Armodafinil; Artemether; Barbiturates; Bexarotene (Systemic); Bile Acid Sequestrants; Boceprevir; Bosentan; CarBAMazepine; CloBAZam; Cobicistat; Colesevelam; CYP3A4 Inducers (Strong); Deferasirox; Elvitegravir; Exenatide; Felbamate; Fosaprepitant; Fosphenytoin; Griseofulvin; LamoTRIgine; Mifepristone; Modafinil; Mycophenolate; Nafcillin; Nevirapine; OXcarbazepine; Perampanel; Phenytoin; Protease Inhibitors; Prucalopride; Retinoic ▶

527

Acid Derivatives; Rifamycin Derivatives; Rufinamide; St Johns Wort; Telaprevir; Tipranavir; Tocilizumab; Topiramate

Ethanol/Nutrition/Herb Interactions

Food: CNS effects of caffeine may be enhanced if combination hormonal contraceptives are used concurrently with caffeine. Grapefruit juice increases ethinyl estradiol concentrations and would be expected to increase progesterone serum levels as well; clinical implications are unclear.

Herb/Nutraceutical: St John's wort may decrease levels. Herbs with estrogenic properties may enhance the adverse/toxic effect of estrogen derivatives; examples include alfalfa, black cohosh, bloodroot, hops, kudzu, licorice, red clover, saw palmetto, soybean, thyme, wild yam, yucca. Herbs with progestogenic properties may enhance the adverse/toxic effect of progestins; examples include bloodroot, chasteberry, damiana, oregano, yucca.

Dietary Considerations Should be taken with food at same time each day.

Pharmacodynamics/Kinetics

Half-life Elimination Ethynodiol diacetate (converted to norethindrone) Terminal: 5-14 hours

Pregnancy Risk Factor X

Pregnancy Considerations Pregnancy should be ruled out prior to treatment and discontinued if pregnancy occurs. In general, the use of combination hormonal contraceptives when inadvertently taken early in pregnancy have not been associated with teratogenic effects. Hormonal contraceptives may be less effective in obese patients. An increase in oral contraceptive failure was noted in women with a BMI >27.3 kg/m^2. Similar findings were noted in patients weighing ≥90 kg (198 lb) using the contraceptive patch.

Due to increased risk of venous thromboembolism (VTE) postpartum, combination hormonal contraceptives should not be started in any woman <21 days following delivery. Women without risk factors for VTE and who are not breast-feeding may start combination hormonal contraceptives during 21-42 days postpartum. After 42 days postpartum, restrictions for use are not related to postpartum status and should be based on other medical conditions (CDC, 2011).

Lactation Enters breast milk/not recommended

Breast-Feeding Considerations Jaundice and breast enlargement in the nursing infant have been reported following the use of combination hormonal contraceptives. May decrease the quality and quantity of breast milk; a nonhormonal form of contraception is recommended (per manufacturer). Postpartum risk status for VTE should be considered when initiating combination hormonal contraceptives after delivery. Combined hormonal contraceptives should not be started <21 days postpartum due to increased risk of VTE. Risk of VTE is still elevated in breast-feeding women until ~42 days postpartum and is greater in women with additional risk factors. After 42 days postpartum, restrictions for use are not related to postpartum VTE risk and should be based on other medical conditions (CDC, 2011).

Dosage Forms

Tablet, oral [monophasic formulation]:

Kelnor™ 1/35: Ethinyl estradiol 0.035 mg and ethynodiol diacetate 1 mg [21 light yellow tablets and 7 white inactive tablets] (28s)

Zovia® 1/35-28: Ethinyl estradiol 0.035 mg and ethynodiol diacetate 1 mg [21 light pink tablets and 7 white inactive tablets] (28s)

Zovia® 1/50-28: Ethinyl estradiol 0.05 mg and ethynodiol diacetate 1 mg [21 pink tablets and 7 white inactive tablets] (28s)

Ethinyl Estradiol and Etonogestrel

(ETH in il es tra DYE ole & et oh noe JES trel)

Related Information

Endocrine Disorders and Pregnancy *on page 1517*

Etonogestrel *on page 557*

Brand Names: U.S. NuvaRing®

Brand Names: Canada NuvaRing®

Generic Availability (U.S.) No

Pharmacologic Category Contraceptive; Estrogen and Progestin Combination

Use Prevention of pregnancy

Unlabeled Use Treatment of hypermenorrhea (menorrhagia); pain associated with endometriosis; dysmenorrhea; dysfunctional uterine bleeding

Local Anesthetic/Vasoconstrictor Precautions No information available to require special precautions

Effects on Dental Treatment When prescribing antibiotics, patient must be warned to use additional methods of birth control if on oral contraceptives.

Effects on Bleeding No information available to require special precautions

Adverse Effects

The most common adverse reactions associated with NuvaRing® (5% to 14%): Headache, nausea, sinusitis, upper respiratory tract infection, vaginal secretion, vaginitis, and weight gain. The following reactions have been associated with combination hormonal contraceptive use:

Increased risk or evidence of association with use:

Cardiovascular: Arterial thromboembolism, cerebral hemorrhage, cerebral thrombosis, hypertension, mesenteric thrombosis, MI, venous thrombosis (with or without embolism)

Gastrointestinal: Gallbladder disease

Hepatic: Hepatic adenomas, liver tumors (benign)

Local: Thrombophlebitis

Ocular: Retinal thrombosis

Respiratory: Pulmonary embolism

Adverse reactions considered drug related:

Cardiovascular: Edema, varicose vein aggravation

Central nervous system: Depression, migraine, mood changes

Dermatologic: Chloasma, melasma, rash (allergic)

Endocrine & metabolic: Amenorrhea, breakthrough bleeding, breast changes (enlargement, pain, secretion, tenderness), fluid retention, infertility (temporary), lactation decreased (with use immediately postpartum), menstrual flow changes, spotting

Gastrointestinal: Abdominal bloating, abdominal cramps, abdominal pain, appetite changes, nausea, weight changes, vomiting

Genitourinary: Cervical ectropion, cervical secretion, vaginal candidiasis, vaginitis

Hematologic: Folate decreased, porphyria exacerbation

Hepatic: Cholestatic jaundice

Neuromuscular & skeletal: Chorea exacerbation

Ocular: Contact lens intolerance, corneal curvature changes (steepening)

Miscellaneous: Anaphylactic/anaphylactoid reactions (including angioedema, circulatory collapse, respiratory collapse, urticaria), SLE exacerbation

Adverse reactions in which association is not confirmed or denied: Acne, Budd-Chiari syndrome, cataracts, colitis, cystitis-like syndrome, dizziness, dysmenorrhea, erythema multiforme, erythema nodosum, headache, hemolytic uremic syndrome, hemorrhagic eruption, hirsutism, libido changes, nervousness, optic neuritis (with or without partial or complete loss of vision), pancreatitis, premenstrual syndrome, renal function impaired, scalp hair loss

Dosage Vaginal: Adults: Females: Contraception: One ring, inserted vaginally and left in place for 3 consecutive weeks, then removed for 1 week. A new ring is inserted 7 days after the last was removed (even if bleeding is not complete) and should be inserted at approximately the same time of day the ring was removed the previous week.

Initial treatment should begin as follows (pregnancy should always be ruled out first):

No hormonal contraceptive use in the past month: Insert ring on the first day of menstrual cycle ("Day 1"). May also insert on days 2-5 even if bleeding is not complete, however, **a spermicide or barrier method of contraception should be used for the following 7 days.***

Switching from combination oral contraceptive: Ring can be inserted on any day within 7 days after the last **active** tablet in the cycle was taken and no later than the first day a new cycle of tablets would begin. Additional forms of contraception are not needed.

Switching from progestin-only contraceptive: **A spermicide or barrier method of contraception should be used for the following 7 days with any of the following.***

If previously using a progestin-only mini-pill, insert the ring on any day of the month; do not skip days between the last pill and insertion of the ring.

If previously using an implant, insert the ring on the same day of implant removal.

If previously using a progestin-containing IUD, insert the ring on day of IUD removal.

If previously using a progestin injection, insert the ring on the day the next injection would be given.

Following complete 1st trimester abortion: Insert ring within the first 5 days of abortion. If not inserted within 5 days, follow instructions for "No hormonal contraceptive use within the past month" and instruct patient to use a nonhormonal contraceptive in the interim.

Following delivery or 2nd trimester abortion: Insert ring 4 weeks postpartum (in women who are not breastfeeding) or following 2nd trimester abortion. **A spermicide or barrier method of contraception should be used for the following 7 days.***

If the ring is accidentally removed from the vagina at anytime during the 3-week period of use, it may be rinsed with cool or lukewarm water (not hot) and reinserted as soon as possible. If the ring is not reinserted within 3 hours, contraceptive effectiveness will be decreased. **A spermicide or barrier method of contraception should be used until the ring has been in place for 7 consecutive days.***

If the ring has been removed for longer than 1 week, pregnancy must be ruled out prior to restarting therapy. **A spermicide or barrier method of contraception should be used for the following 7 days.***

If the ring has been left in place for >3 weeks, a new ring should be inserted following a 1-week (ring-free) interval. Protection continues during week 4, however, if the ring is left in place >4 weeks, pregnancy must be ruled out prior to insertion and **a spermicide or barrier method of contraception should be used for the following 7 days.***

Disconnected ring: In the event the ring disconnects at the weld joint, discard and replace with a new ring.

***Note:** Diaphragms may interfere with proper ring placement, and therefore, are not recommended for use as an additional form of contraception.

Dosage adjustment in renal impairment: Specific guidelines not available; use with caution and monitor blood pressure closely. Consider other forms of contraception.

Dosage adjustment in hepatic impairment: Contraindicated in patients with hepatic impairment

Mechanism of Action Combination hormonal contraceptives inhibit ovulation via a negative feedback mechanism on the hypothalamus, which alters the normal pattern of gonadotropin secretion of a follicle-stimulating hormone (FSH) and luteinizing hormone by the anterior pituitary. The follicular phase FSH and midcycle surge of gonadotropins are inhibited. In addition, combination hormonal contraceptives produce alterations in the genital tract, including changes in the cervical mucus, rendering it unfavorable for sperm penetration even if ovulation occurs. Changes in the endometrium may also occur, producing an unfavorable environment for nidation. Combination hormonal contraceptive drugs may alter the tubal transport of the ova through the fallopian tubes. Progestational agents may also alter sperm fertility.

Contraindications Hypersensitivity to ethinyl estradiol, etonogestrel, or any component of the formulation; breast cancer or other estrogen- or progestin-dependent neoplasms (current or a history of), hepatic tumors or disease, pregnancy, undiagnosed abnormal uterine bleeding, cholestatic jaundice of pregnancy, jaundice with prior combination hormonal contraceptive use

Use is also contraindicated in women at high risk of arterial or venous thrombotic diseases including: Cerebrovascular disease, coronary artery disease, diabetes mellitus with vascular disease, DVT or PE (current or history of), headaches with focal neurological symptoms, hypertension (uncontrolled), valvular heart disease with thrombogenic complications, women >35 years of age who smoke, major surgery with prolonged immobilization.

Warnings/Precautions Hazardous agent - use appropriate precautions for handling and disposal (NIOSH, 2012). Combination hormonal contraceptive agents do not protect against HIV infection or other sexually-transmitted diseases.**[U.S. Boxed Warning]: The risk of cardiovascular side effects is increased in women who smoke cigarettes; risk increases with age (especially women >35 years of age) and the number of cigarettes smoked; women who use combination hormonal contraceptives should be strongly advised not to smoke. Use is contraindicated in patients >35 years of age who smoke.** May lead to increased risk of myocardial infarction, use with caution in patients with risk factors for coronary artery disease (eg, hypertension, hypercholesterolemia, morbid obesity, diabetes, or women who smoke). May increase the risk of thromboembolism; discontinue use of combination hormonal contraceptives if an arterial or venous thrombotic event occurs. Women with inherited thrombophilias (eg, protein C or S deficiency) may have increased risk of venous thromboembolism (DeSancho, 2010; van Vlijmen, 2011). Whenever possible, combination hormonal contraceptives should be discontinued at least 4 weeks prior to and for 2 weeks following elective surgery associated with an increased risk of thromboembolism or during periods of prolonged immobilization. May have a dose-related risk of vascular disease, hypertension, and gallbladder disease. Women with hypertension or renal disease should be encouraged to use another form of contraception. The use of combination hormonal contraceptives has been associated with a slight increase in frequency of breast cancer; however, studies are not consistent. Use is contraindicated in women with (or history of) breast cancer.

Combination hormonal contraceptives may affect serum triglyceride and lipoprotein levels. May have adverse effects on glucose tolerance; use caution in women with diabetes. Estrogens may cause retinal vascular thrombosis; discontinue if migraine, loss of vision, proptosis, diplopia or other visual disturbances occur; discontinue permanently if papilledema or retinal vascular lesions are observed on examination. Use caution with conditions that may be aggravated by fluid retention, depression, or history of migraine. Extremely rare adenomas and focal nodular hyperplasia resulting in fatal intra-abdominal hemorrhage have been reported in association with long-term oral contraceptive use. Presentation of an abdominal mass, acute abdominal pain, or intra-abdominal bleeding warrants further evaluation to rule out source. Combination hormonal contraceptives may be poorly metabolized in women with hepatic impairment. Discontinue if jaundice develops during therapy or if liver function becomes abnormal. Risk of cholestasis may be increased with previous cholestatic jaundice of pregnancy or jaundice with prior oral contraceptive use. Estrogens may increase thyroid-binding globulin (TBG) levels leading to increased circulating total thyroid hormone levels. Women on thyroid replacement therapy may require higher doses of thyroid hormone while receiving estrogens. Presentation of irregular, unresolving vaginal bleeding warrants further evaluation including endometrial sampling, if indicated, to rule out malignancy. Not for use prior to menarche. The use of estrogens and/or progestins may change the results of some laboratory tests (eg, coagulation factors, lipids, glucose tolerance, binding proteins). The dose, route, and the specific estrogen/progestin influences these changes. In addition, personal risk factors (eg, cardiovascular disease, smoking, diabetes, age) also contribute to adverse events; use of specific products may be contraindicated in women with certain risk factors.

Vaginally-administered combination hormonal contraceptive agents may have a similar adverse effects associated with oral contraceptive products. In order to reduce some of the possible risks, the minimum dosage combination of estrogen/progestin that will effectively treat the individual patient should be used. May not be appropriate for use in women with conditions that make the vagina susceptible to irritation or ulceration. Ensure proper vaginal placement of the ring to avoid inadvertent urinary bladder insertion.

Drug Interactions

Metabolism/Transport Effects Refer to individual components.

Avoid Concomitant Use

Avoid concomitant use of Ethinyl Estradiol and Etonogestrel with any of the following: Anastrozole; Griseofulvin; Ospemifene; Pimozide; Pirfenidone

Increased Effect/Toxicity

Ethinyl Estradiol and Etonogestrel may increase the levels/effects of: ARIPiprazole; Benzodiazepines (metabolized by oxidation); Corticosteroids (Systemic); CYP1A2 Substrates; Lomitapide; Ospemifene; Pimozide; Pirfenidone; ROPINIRole; Selegiline; Theophylline Derivatives; Tipranavir; TiZANidine; Tranexamic Acid; Voriconazole

The levels/effects of Ethinyl Estradiol and Etonogestrel may be increased by: Ascorbic Acid; Atazanavir; Boceprevir; Cobicistat; Herbs (Estrogenic Properties); Herbs (Progestogenic Properties); Mifepristone; NSAID (COX-2 Inhibitor); Voriconazole

Decreased Effect

Ethinyl Estradiol and Etonogestrel may decrease the levels/effects of: Anastrozole; Chenodiol; Hyaluronidase; LamoTRIgine; Ospemifene; Thyroid Products; Ursodiol; Vitamin K Antagonists

The levels/effects of Ethinyl Estradiol and Etonogestrel may be decreased by: Acitretin; Aminoglutethimide; Aprepitant; Armodafinil; Artemether; Barbiturates; Bexarotene (Systemic); Bile Acid Sequestrants; Boceprevir; Bosentan; CarBAMazepine; CloBAZam; Cobicistat; Colesevelam; CYP3A4 Inducers (Strong); Deferasirox; Efavirenz; Elvitegravir; Exenatide; Felbamate; Fosaprepitant; Fosphenytoin; Griseofulvin; LamoTRIgine; Mifepristone; Modafinil; Mycophenolate; Nafcillin; Nevirapine; OXcarbazepine; Perampanel; Phenytoin; Protease Inhibitors; Prucalopride; Retinoic Acid Derivatives; Rifamycin Derivatives; Rufinamide; St Johns Wort; Telaprevir; Tipranavir; Tocilizumab; Topiramate

Ethanol/Nutrition/Herb Interactions

Food: CNS effects of caffeine may be enhanced if combination hormonal contraceptives are used concurrently with caffeine. Grapefruit juice increases ethinyl estradiol concentrations and would be expected to increase progesterone serum levels as well; clinical implications are unclear.

Herb/Nutraceutical: St John's wort may decrease levels. Herbs with estrogenic properties may enhance the adverse/toxic effect of estrogen derivatives; examples include alfalfa, black cohosh, bloodroot, hops, kudzu, licorice, red clover, saw palmetto, soybean, thyme, wild yam, yucca. Herbs with progestogenic properties may enhance the adverse/toxic effect of progestins; examples include bloodroot, chasteberry, damiana, oregano, yucca.

Pharmacodynamics/Kinetics

Duration of Action Serum levels (contraceptive effectiveness) decrease after 3 weeks of continuous use

Half-life Elimination Ethinyl estradiol: 45 hours; Etonogestrel: 29 hours

Time to Peak Vaginal: Ethinyl estradiol: 60 hours; Etonogestrel: 200 hours

Pregnancy Risk Factor X

Pregnancy Considerations Pregnancy should be ruled out prior to treatment and discontinued if pregnancy occurs. In general, the use of combination hormonal contraceptives, when inadvertently used early in pregnancy, have not been associated with teratogenic effects. Hormonal contraceptives may be less effective in obese patients. An increase in oral contraceptive failure was noted in women with a BMI >27.3 kg/m^2. Similar findings were noted in patients weighing ≥90 kg (198 lb) using the contraceptive patch. In a study using the vaginal ring, ethinyl estradiol serum concentrations were decreased in obese women (BMI 30-39.9 kg/m^2; n=19) in comparison to women of normal weight (BMI

19-24.9 kg/m^2; n=18; p= 0.004); etonogestrel concentrations did not differ significantly. Bleeding and spotting were more frequent in the obese women. The study was not powered to evaluate contraceptive effectiveness (Westhoff, 2012).

Due to increased risk of venous thromboembolism (VTE) postpartum, combination hormonal contraceptives should not be started in any woman <21 days following delivery. Women without risk factors for VTE and who are not breast-feeding may start combination hormonal contraceptives during 21-42 days postpartum. After 42 days postpartum, restrictions for use are not related to postpartum status and should be based on other medical conditions (CDC, 2011). The manufacturer states that combination hormonal contraceptives should not be started until ≥4 weeks after delivery in women who choose not to breastfeed, or ≥4 weeks after a second trimester abortion or miscarriage.

Lactation Enters breast milk/not recommended

Breast-Feeding Considerations Jaundice and breast enlargement in the nursing infant have been reported following the use of combination hormonal contraceptives. May decrease the quality and quantity of breast milk; alternative form of contraception is recommended (per manufacturer). The theoretical concerns about decreased milk production are greatest early in the postpartum period when milk production is being established. Postpartum risk status for VTE should be considered when initiating combination hormonal contraceptives after delivery. Combined hormonal contraceptives should not be started <21 days postpartum due to increased risk of VTE. Risk of VTE is still elevated in breast-feeding women until ~42 days postpartum and is greater in women with additional risk factors. After 42 days postpartum, restrictions for use are not related to postpartum VTE risk and should be based on other medical conditions (CDC, 2011).

Dosage Forms

Ring, vaginal:

NuvaRing®: Ethinyl estradiol 0.015 mg/day and etonogestrel 0.12 mg/day (3s) [3-week duration]

Ethinyl Estradiol and Levonorgestrel

(ETH in il es tra DYE ole & LEE voe nor jes trel)

Related Information

Levonorgestrel on page 813

Brand Names: U.S. Altavera™; Amethia™; Amethia™ Lo; Amethyst™; Aviane™; camrese™; Chateal™; Enpresse®; Falmina™; Introvale™; Jolessa™; Kurvelo™; Lessina®; Levonest™; Levora®; LoSeasonique®; Lutera®; Lybrel®; Marlissa; Myzilra™; Nordette® 28 [DSC]; Orsythia™; Portia®; Quasense®; Seasonale® [DSC]; Seasonique®; Sronyx®; Trivora®

Brand Names: Canada Alesse®; Aviane®; Min-Ovral®; Seasonale®; Triphasil®; Triquilar®

Generic Availability (U.S.) Yes

Pharmacologic Category Contraceptive; Estrogen and Progestin Combination

Use Prevention of pregnancy; postcoital contraception

Unlabeled Use Treatment of hypermenorrhea (menorrhagia); pain associated with endometriosis; dysmenorrhea; dysfunctional uterine bleeding

Local Anesthetic/Vasoconstrictor Precautions No information available to require special precautions

Effects on Dental Treatment When prescribing antibiotics, patient must be warned to use additional methods of birth control if on oral contraceptives.

Effects on Bleeding No information available to require special precautions

Adverse Effects The following reactions have been associated with oral contraceptive use:

Increased risk or evidence of association with use:

Cardiovascular: Arterial thromboembolism, cerebral hemorrhage, cerebral thrombosis, hypertension, mesenteric thrombosis, MI, venous thrombosis (with or without embolism)

Gastrointestinal: Gallbladder disease

Hepatic: Hepatic adenomas, liver tumors (benign)

Local: Thrombophlebitis

Ocular: Retinal thrombosis

Respiratory: Pulmonary embolism

Adverse reactions considered drug related:

Cardiovascular: Edema, varicose vein aggravation

Central nervous system: Depression, migraine, mood changes

Dermatologic: Chloasma, melasma, rash (allergic)

Endocrine & metabolic: Amenorrhea, breakthrough bleeding, breast changes (enlargement, pain, secretion, tenderness), carbohydrate tolerance decreased, fluid retention, infertility (temporary), lactation decreased (with use immediately postpartum), menstrual flow changes, spotting

Gastrointestinal: Abdominal bloating, abdominal cramps, abdominal pain, appetite changes, nausea, weight changes, vomiting

Genitourinary: Cervical ectropion, cervical secretion/erosion, endocervical hyperplasia, fibroid enlargement, vaginal candidiasis, vaginitis

Hematologic: Folate decreased, porphyria exacerbation

Hepatic: Cholestatic jaundice, focal nodular hyperplasia

Neuromuscular & skeletal: Chorea exacerbation

Ocular: Contact lens intolerance, corneal curvature changes (steepening)

Respiratory: Rhinitis

Miscellaneous: Anaphylactic/anaphylactoid reactions (including angioedema, circulatory collapse, respiratory collapse, urticaria), SLE exacerbation

Adverse reactions in which association is not confirmed or denied: Acne, auditory disturbances, Budd-Chiari syndrome, cataracts, cervical smear abnormal, colitis, cystitis-like syndrome, dizziness, dysmenorrhea, erythema multiforme, erythema nodosum, headache, hemolytic uremic syndrome, hemorrhagic eruption, hirsutism, libido changes, nervousness, optic neuritis (with or without partial or complete loss of vision), pancreatitis, premenstrual syndrome, renal function impaired, scalp hair loss

Dosage Oral: Adults: Females:

Contraception, 28-day cycle:

Schedule 1 (Sunday starter): Dose begins on first Sunday after onset of menstruation; if the menstrual period starts on Sunday, take first tablet that very same day. With a Sunday start, an additional method of contraception should be used until after the first 7 days of consecutive administration:

For 21-tablet package: 1 tablet/day for 21 consecutive days, followed by 7 days off of the medication; a new course begins on the 8th day after the last tablet is taken

For 28-tablet package: 1 tablet/day without interruption

Schedule 2 (Day 1 starter): Dose starts on first day of menstrual cycle taking 1 tablet/day:

For 21-tablet package: 1 tablet/day for 21 consecutive days, followed by 7 days off of the medication; a new course begins on the 8th day after the last tablet is taken

For 28-tablet package: 1 tablet/day without interruption

If all doses have been taken on schedule and one menstrual period is missed, continue dosing cycle. If two consecutive menstrual periods are missed, pregnancy test is required before new dosing cycle is started.

Missed doses **monophasic formulations** (refer to package insert for complete information):

One dose missed: Take as soon as remembered or take 2 tablets next day

Two consecutive doses missed in the first 2 weeks: Take 2 tablets as soon as remembered or 2 tablets next 2 days. An additional method of contraception should be used for 7 days after missed dose.

Two consecutive doses missed in week 3 or three consecutive doses missed at any time: An additional method of contraception must be used for 7 days after a missed dose:

Schedule 1 (Sunday starter): Continue dose of 1 tablet daily until Sunday, then discard the rest of the pack, and a new pack should be started that same day.

Schedule 2 (Day 1 starter): Current pack should be discarded, and a new pack should be started that same day.

Missed doses **biphasic/triphasic formulations** (refer to package insert for complete information):

One dose missed: Take as soon as remembered or take 2 tablets next day.

Two consecutive doses missed in week 1 or week 2 of the pack: Take 2 tablets as soon as remembered and 2 tablets the next day. Resume taking 1 tablet daily until the pack is empty. An additional method of contraception should be used for 7 days after a missed dose.

Two consecutive doses missed in week 3 of the pack: An additional method of contraception must be used for 7 days after a missed dose.

Schedule 1 (Sunday starter): Take 1 tablet every day until Sunday. Discard the remaining pack and start a new pack of pills on the same day.

Schedule 2 (Day 1 starter): Discard the remaining pack and start a new pack the same day.

Three or more consecutive doses missed: An additional method of contraception must be used for 7 days after a missed dose.

Schedule 1 (Sunday starter): Take 1 tablet every day until Sunday; on Sunday, discard the pack and start a new pack.

Schedule 2 (Day 1 starter): Discard the remaining pack and begin new pack of tablets starting on the same day.

Contraception, 91-day cycle (extended cycle regimen): Dose begins on first Sunday after onset of menstruation; if the menstrual period starts on Sunday, take first tablet that very same day. An additional method of contraception should be used until after the first 7 days of consecutive administration:

Seasonale®: One active tablet/day for 84 consecutive days, followed by 1 inactive tablet/day for 7 days; if all doses have been taken on schedule and one menstrual period is missed, pregnancy should be ruled out prior to continuing therapy.

Seasonique®, LoSeasonique®: One active tablet/day for 84 consecutive days, followed by 1 low dose estrogen tablet/day for 7 days; if all doses have been taken on schedule and one menstrual period is missed, pregnancy should be ruled out prior to continuing therapy.

Missed doses:

One dose missed: Take as soon as remembered or take 2 tablets the next day

Two consecutive doses missed: Take 2 tablets as soon as remembered or 2 tablets the next 2 days. An additional nonhormonal method of contraception should be used for 7 consecutive days after the missed dose.

Three or more consecutive doses missed: Do not take the missed doses; continue taking 1 tablet/day until pack is complete. Bleeding may occur during the following week. An additional nonhormonal method of contraception should be used for 7 consecutive days after the missed dose.

Any number of pills during week 13: Throw away the missed pills and keep taking scheduled pills until the pack is finished. A back-up method of contraception is not needed

Contraception, continuous use (extended cycle regimen): Lybrel®: Take one tablet daily, at the same time each day, without a tablet-free interval. Therapy should be initiated as follows:

No previous contraception: Begin on the first day of menstrual cycle. Back-up contraception is not needed.

Previously taking a 21-day or 28-day combination hormonal contraceptive: Begin on day 1 of the withdrawal bleed (at the latest, 7 days after the last active tablet). Back-up contraception is not needed.

Previously using a progestin-only pill: Begin the day after taking a progestin only pill. Back-up contraception is needed for the first 7 days of therapy.

Previously using contraceptive implant: Begin the day of implant removal. Back-up contraception is needed for the first 7 days of therapy.

Previously using contraceptive injection: Begin when the next injection is due. Back-up contraception is needed for the first 7 days of therapy.

Missed doses:

One dose missed: Take as soon as remembered then take the next tablet at the regular time (2 tablets in 1 day). An additional nonhormonal method of contraception should also be used for 7 consecutive days.

Two consecutive doses missed: If remembered the day of the second missed tablet, take 2 tablets as soon as remembered, then 1 tablet the next day. If remembered the day after the second tablet is missed, take 2 tablets the day remembered, then 2 tablets the next day. An additional nonhormonal method of contraception should also be used for 7 consecutive days.

Three or more consecutive doses missed: Take 1 tablet daily and contact healthcare provider; do not take the missed pills. An additional nonhormonal method of contraception should also be used for 7 consecutive days.

Dosage adjustment in renal impairment: Specific guidelines not available; use with caution and monitor blood pressure closely. Consider other forms of contraception.

Dosage adjustment in hepatic impairment: Contraindicated in patients with hepatic impairment

Mechanism of Action Combination hormonal contraceptives inhibit ovulation via a negative feedback mechanism on the hypothalamus, which alters the normal pattern of gonadotropin secretion of a follicle-stimulating hormone (FSH) and luteinizing hormone by the anterior pituitary. The follicular phase FSH and midcycle surge of gonadotropins are inhibited. In addition, combination hormonal contraceptives produce alterations in the genital tract, including changes in the cervical mucus, rendering it unfavorable for sperm penetration even if ovulation occurs. Changes in the endometrium may also occur, producing an unfavorable environment for nidation. Combination hormonal contraceptive drugs may alter the tubal transport of the ova through the fallopian tubes. Progestational agents may also alter sperm fertility.

Contraindications Breast cancer or other estrogen- or progestin-dependent neoplasms (current or a history of), hepatic tumors or disease, pregnancy, undiagnosed abnormal uterine bleeding

Use is also contraindicated in women at high risk of arterial or venous thrombotic diseases including: Cerebrovascular disease, coronary artery disease, diabetes mellitus with vascular disease, DVT or PE (current or history of), hypercoagulopathies (inherited or acquired), headaches with focal neurological symptoms, hypertension (uncontrolled), migraine headaches if >35 years of age, thrombogenic valvular or rhythm diseases of the heart (eg, subacute bacterial endocarditis with valvular disease or atrial fibrillation), women >35 years of age who smoke.

Canadian-labeling: Additional contraindication: Ocular lesions due to ophthalmic vascular disease including partial or complete loss of vision or defect in visual fields; severe dyslipoproteinemia; hereditary or acquired predisposition for venous or arterial thrombosis

Warnings/Precautions Hazardous agent - use appropriate precautions for handling and disposal (NIOSH, 2012). Combination hormonal contraceptives do not protect against HIV infection or other sexually-transmitted diseases. **[U.S. Boxed Warning]: The risk of cardiovascular side effects is increased in women who smoke cigarettes; risk increases with age (especially women >35 years of age) and the number of cigarettes smoked; women who use combination hormonal contraceptives should be strongly advised not to smoke. Use is contraindicated in patients >35 years of age who smoke.** Use with caution in patients with risk factors for coronary artery disease (eg, hypertension, hypercholesterolemia, morbid obesity, diabetes, or women who smoke); may lead to increased risk of myocardial infarction. May have a dose-related risk of vascular disease and hypertension; women with hypertension should be encouraged to use a nonhormonal form of contraception. May increase the risk of thromboembolism; discontinue use of combination hormonal contraceptives if an arterial or venous thrombotic event occurs. Women with inherited thrombophilias (eg, protein C or S deficiency) may have increased risk of venous thromboembolism (DeSancho, 2010; van Vlijmen, 2011). Use is contraindicated in women with hypercoagulopathies (inherited or acquired). Whenever possible, combination hormonal contraceptives should be discontinued at least 4 weeks prior to and for 2 weeks following elective surgery associated with an increased risk of thromboembolism or during periods of prolonged immobilization. Combination hormonal contraceptives may have a dose-related risk of gallbladder disease and may worsen existing gallbladder disease. Women with renal disease should be encouraged to use another form of contraception. May have adverse effects on glucose tolerance; use caution in women with diabetes.

Combination hormonal contraceptives may affect serum triglyceride and lipoprotein levels. Triglycerides may also be increased; use with caution in patients with familial defects of lipoprotein metabolism. The use of combination hormonal contraceptives has been associated with a slight increase in frequency of breast cancer; however, studies are not consistent. Use is contraindicated in women with (or history of) breast cancer. Use caution with conditions that may be aggravated by fluid retention, depression, or history of migraine. Evaluate new, recurrent, severe or persistent headaches. Use with migraine headaches with or without aura if >35 years of age is contraindicated. Not for use prior to menarche. Estrogens may cause retinal vascular thrombosis; discontinue if migraine, loss of vision, proptosis, diplopia or other visual disturbances occur; discontinue permanently if papilledema or retinal vascular lesions are observed on examination. Risk of chloasma may be increased with history of chloasma gravidarum. Women with history of chloasma should avoid exposure to sun or ultraviolet radiation during therapy. May induce or exacerbate symptoms of hereditary angioedema.

Presentation of irregular, unresolving vaginal bleeding warrants further evaluation including endometrial sampling, if indicated, to rule out malignancy; evaluate hypothalamic-pituitary-function in women with persistent (≥6 months) amenorrhea (especially associated with breast secretion) following discontinuation of therapy. Discontinue use with the onset of sudden enlargement, pain, or tenderness of fibroids (leiomyomata). Extremely rare adenomas and focal nodular hyperplasia resulting in fatal intra-abdominal hemorrhage have been reported in association with long-term oral contraceptive use. Presentation of an abdominal mass, acute abdominal pain, or intra-abdominal bleeding warrants further evaluation to rule out source. Combination hormonal contraceptives may be poorly metabolized in women with hepatic impairment. Discontinue if jaundice develops during therapy or if liver function becomes abnormal. Risk of cholestasis may be increased with previous cholestatic jaundice of pregnancy or jaundice with prior oral contraceptive use. Estrogens may increase thyroid-binding globulin (TBG) levels leading to increased circulating total thyroid hormone levels. Women on thyroid replacement therapy may require higher doses of thyroid hormone while receiving estrogens. The use of estrogens and/or progestins may change the results of some laboratory tests (eg, coagulation factors, lipids, glucose tolerance, binding proteins). The dose, route, and the specific estrogen/progestin influences these changes. In addition, personal risk factors (eg, cardiovascular disease, smoking, diabetes, age) also contribute to adverse events; use of specific products may be contraindicated in women with certain risk factors. Some products may contain tartrazine, which may cause allergic reactions in certain individuals.

The minimum dosage combination of estrogen/progestin that will effectively treat the individual patient should be used. New patients should be started on products containing ≤0.035 mg of estrogen per tablet. Extended cycle regimen contraceptives provide more hormonal exposure per year than conventional monthly contraceptives.

◀ **Drug Interactions**

Metabolism/Transport Effects Refer to individual components.

Avoid Concomitant Use

Avoid concomitant use of Ethinyl Estradiol and Levonorgestrel with any of the following: Anastrozole; Griseofulvin; Ospemifene; Pimozide; Pirfenidone

Increased Effect/Toxicity

Ethinyl Estradiol and Levonorgestrel may increase the levels/effects of: ARIPiprazole; Benzodiazepines (metabolized by oxidation); Corticosteroids (Systemic); CYP1A2 Substrates; Lomitapide; Ospemifene; Pimozide; Pirfenidone; ROPINIRole; Selegiline; Theophylline Derivatives; Tipranavir; TiZANidine; Tranexamic Acid; Voriconazole

The levels/effects of Ethinyl Estradiol and Levonorgestrel may be increased by: Ascorbic Acid; Atazanavir; Boceprevir; Cobicistat; Herbs (Estrogenic Properties); Herbs (Progestogenic Properties); Mifepristone; NSAID (COX-2 Inhibitor); Voriconazole

Decreased Effect

Ethinyl Estradiol and Levonorgestrel may decrease the levels/effects of: Anastrozole; Chenodiol; Hyaluronidase; LamoTRIgine; Ospemifene; Thyroid Products; Ursodiol; Vitamin K Antagonists

The levels/effects of Ethinyl Estradiol and Levonorgestrel may be decreased by: Acitretin; Aminoglutethimide; Aprepitant; Armodafinil; Artemether; Barbiturates; Bexarotene (Systemic); Bile Acid Sequestrants; Boceprevir; Bosentan; CarBAMazepine; CloBAZam; Cobicistat; Colesevelam; CYP3A4 Inducers (Strong); Deferasirox; Elvitegravir; Exenatide; Felbamate; Fosaprepitant; Fosphenytoin; Griseofulvin; LamoTRIgine; Mifepristone; Modafinil; Mycophenolate; Nafcillin; Nevirapine; OXcarbazepine; Perampanel; Phenytoin; Protease Inhibitors; Prucalopride; Retinoic Acid Derivatives; Rifamycin Derivatives; Rufinamide; St Johns Wort; Telaprevir; Tipranavir; Tocilizumab; Topiramate

Ethanol/Nutrition/Herb Interactions

Food: CNS effects of caffeine may be enhanced if combination hormonal contraceptives are used concurrently with caffeine. Grapefruit juice increases ethinyl estradiol plasma concentrations and would be expected to increase progesterone serum levels as well; clinical implications are unclear.

Herb/Nutraceutical: St John's wort may decrease levels. Herbs with estrogenic properties may enhance the adverse/toxic effect of estrogen derivatives; examples include alfalfa, black cohosh, bloodroot, hops, kudzu, licorice, red clover, saw palmetto, soybean, thyme, wild yam, yucca. Herbs with progestogenic properties may enhance the adverse/toxic effect of progestins; examples include bloodroot, chasteberry, damiana, oregano, yucca. Impaired folate metabolism and reduced serum levels of cyanocobalamin have been reported with oral contraceptive use; increased dietary intake or supplementation may be necessary.

Dietary Considerations Should be taken at the same time each day.

Pharmacodynamics/Kinetics

Half-life Elimination Ethinyl estradiol: 12-23 hours; Levonorgestrel: 22-49 hours

Pregnancy Risk Factor X

Pregnancy Considerations Pregnancy should be ruled out prior to treatment and discontinued if pregnancy occurs. In general, the use of combination hormonal contraceptives when inadvertently taken early in pregnancy have not been associated with teratogenic effects. Hormonal contraceptives may be less effective in obese patients. An increase in oral contraceptive failure was noted in women with a BMI >27.3 kg/m^2. Similar findings were noted in patients weighing ≥90 kg (198 lb) using the contraceptive patch.

Due to increased risk of venous thromboembolism (VTE) postpartum, combination hormonal contraceptives should not be started in any woman <21 days following delivery. Women without risk factors for VTE and who are not breast-feeding may start combination hormonal contraceptives during 21-42 days postpartum. After 42 days postpartum, restrictions for use are not related to postpartum status and should be based on other medical conditions (CDC, 2011).

Lactation Enters breast milk/not recommended

Breast-Feeding Considerations Jaundice and breast enlargement in the nursing infant have been reported following the use of combination hormonal contraceptives. May decrease the quality and quantity of breast milk; alternative form of contraception is recommended (per manufacturer). The theoretical concerns about decreased milk production are greatest early in the postpartum period when milk production is being established. Postpartum risk status for VTE should be considered when initiating combination hormonal contraceptives after delivery. Combined hormonal contraceptives should not be started <21 days postpartum due to increased risk of VTE. Risk of VTE is still elevated in breast-feeding women until ~42 days postpartum and is greater in women with additional risk factors. After 42 days postpartum, restrictions for use are not related to postpartum VTE risk and should be based on other medical conditions (CDC, 2011).

Product Availability Quartette™: FDA approved March 2013; anticipated availability currently unknown. Consult prescribing information for additional information.

Dosage Forms

Tablet, oral [low-dose formulation]: Ethinyl estradiol 0.02 mg and levonorgestrel 0.1 mg [21 tablets and 7 inactive tablets] (28s)

Aviane™: Ethinyl estradiol 0.02 mg and levonorgestrel 0.1 mg [21 orange tablets and 7 light green inactive tablets] (28s)

Falmina™: Ethinyl estradiol 0.02 mg and levonorgestrel 0.1 mg [21 orange tablets and 7 white inactive tablets] (28s)

Lessina®: Ethinyl estradiol 0.02 mg and levonorgestrel 0.1 mg [21 pink tablets and 7 white inactive tablets] (28s)

Lutera®, Sronyx®: Ethinyl estradiol 0.02 mg and levonorgestrel 0.1 mg [21 white tablets and 7 peach inactive tablets] (28s)

Orsythia™: Ethinyl estradiol 0.02 mg and levonorgestrel 0.1 mg [21 pink tablets and 7 light green inactive tablets] (28s)

Tablet, oral [monophasic formulation]: Ethinyl estradiol 0.03 mg and levonorgestrel 0.15 mg [21 tablets and 7 inactive tablets] (28s)

Altavera™: Ethinyl estradiol 0.03 mg and levonorgestrel 0.15 mg [21 peach tablets and 7 white inactive tablets] (28s)

Chateal™: Ethinyl estradiol 0.03 mg and levonorgestrel 0.15 mg [21 white tablets and 7 green inactive tablets] (28s)

Kurvelo™: Ethinyl estradiol 0.03 mg and levonorgestrel 0.15 mg [21 light orange tablets and 7 pink inactive tablets] (28s)

Levora®: Ethinyl estradiol 0.03 mg and levonorgestrel 0.15 mg [21 white tablets and 7 peach inactive tablets] (28s)

Marlissa: Ethinyl estradiol 0.03 mg and levonorgestrel 0.15 mg [21 light orange tablets and 7 pink inactive tablets] (28s)

Portia® 28: Ethinyl estradiol 0.03 mg and levonorgestrel 0.15 mg [21 pink tablets and 7 white inactive tablets] (28s)

Tablet, oral [extended cycle regimen]: Ethinyl estradiol 0.02 mg and levonorgestrel 0.1 mg [84 tablets] and ethinyl estradiol 0.01 mg [7 tablets] (91s)

Amethia™:Ethinyl estradiol 0.03 mg and levonorgestrel 0.15 mg [84 white tablets] and ethinyl estradiol 0.01 mg [7 light blue tablets] (91s)

Amethia™ Lo: Ethinyl estradiol 0.02 mg and levonorgestrel 0.1 mg [84 white tablets] and ethinyl estradiol 0.01 mg [7 blue tablets] (91s)

camrese™: Ethinyl estradiol 0.03 mg and levonorgestrel 0.15 mg [84 light blue-green tablets] and ethinyl estradiol 0.01 mg [7 yellow tablets] (91s)

Introvale™: Ethinyl estradiol 0.03 mg and levonorgestrel 0.15 mg [84 peach tablets and 7 white inactive tablets] (91s)

Jolessa™: Ethinyl estradiol 0.03 mg and levonorgestrel 0.15 mg [84 pink tablets and 7 white inactive tablets] (91s)

LoSeasonique®: Ethinyl estradiol 0.02 mg and levonorgestrel 0.1 mg [84 orange tablets] and ethinyl estradiol 0.01 mg [7 yellow tablets] (91s)

Quasense®: Ethinyl estradiol 0.03 mg and levonorgestrel 0.15 mg] [84 white tablets and 7 peach inactive tablets] (91s)

Seasonique®: Ethinyl estradiol 0.03 mg and levonorgestrel 0.15 mg [84 light blue-green tablets] and ethinyl estradiol 0.01 mg [7 yellow tablets] (91s)

Tablet, oral [noncyclic regimen]:
Amethyst™: Ethinyl estradiol 0.02 mg and levonorgestrel 0.09 mg [28 white tablets] (28s)
Lybrel®: Ethinyl estradiol 0.02 mg and levonorgestrel 0.09 mg [28 yellow tablets] (28s)

Tablet, oral [triphasic formulation]:
Enpresse®:
Day 1-6: Ethinyl estradiol 0.03 mg and levonorgestrel 0.05 mg [6 pink tablets]
Day 7-11: Ethinyl estradiol 0.04 mg and levonorgestrel 0.075 mg [5 white tablets]
Day 12-21: Ethinyl estradiol 0.03 mg and levonorgestrel 0.125 mg [10 orange tablets]
Day 22-28: 7 light green inactive tablets (28s)
Levonest™:
Day 1-6: Ethinyl estradiol 0.03 mg and levonorgestrel 0.05 mg [6 yellow tablets]
Day 7-11: Ethinyl estradiol 0.04 mg and levonorgestrel 0.075 mg [5 green tablets]
Day 12-21: Ethinyl estradiol 0.03 mg and levonorgestrel 0.125 mg [10 light brown tablets]
Day 22-28: 7 white inactive tablets (28s)
Myzilra™:
Day 1-6: Ethinyl estradiol 0.03 mg and levonorgestrel 0.05 mg [6 beige tablets]
Day 7-11: Ethinyl estradiol 0.04 mg and levonorgestrel 0.075 mg [5 white tablets]
Day 12-21: Ethinyl estradiol 0.03 mg and levonorgestrel 0.125 mg [10 light yellow tablets]
Day 22-28: 7 light green inactive tablets (28s)

Trivora®:
Day 1-6: Ethinyl estradiol 0.03 mg and levonorgestrel 0.05 mg [6 blue tablets]
Day 7-11: Ethinyl estradiol 0.04 mg and levonorgestrel 0.075 mg [5 white tablets]
Day 12-21: Ethinyl estradiol 0.03 mg and levonorgestrel 0.125 mg [10 pink tablets]
Day 22-28: 7 peach inactive tablets (28s)

Ethinyl Estradiol and Norelgestromin
(ETH in il es tra DYE ole & nor el JES troe min)

Brand Names: U.S. Ortho Evra®
Brand Names: Canada Evra®
Pharmacologic Category Contraceptive; Estrogen and Progestin Combination
Use Prevention of pregnancy
Local Anesthetic/Vasoconstrictor Precautions No information available to require special precautions
Effects on Dental Treatment When prescribing antibiotics, patient must be warned to use additional methods of birth control if on oral contraceptives.
Effects on Bleeding No information available to require special precautions
Adverse Effects The following reactions have been reported with the contraceptive patch. Adverse reactions associated with oral combination hormonal contraceptive agents are also likely to appear with the topical contraceptive patch (frequency difficult to anticipate). See individual oral contraceptive monographs for additional information.

>10%:
Central nervous system: Headache (21%)
Endocrine & metabolic: Breast symptoms (22%; including discomfort, engorgement, pain)
Gastrointestinal: Nausea (17%)
Miscellaneous: Application site disorder (17%)
1% to 10%:
Cardiovascular: Blood pressure increased (<2.5%)
Central nervous system: Anxiety/mood disorders (6%), dizziness (3%), fatigue (3%), migraine (3%), insomnia (<2.5%), malaise (<2.5%)
Dermatologic: Acne (3%), pruritus (3%), chloasma (<2.5%), contact dermatitis (<2.5%), erythema (<2.5%), skin irritation (<2.5%)
Endocrine & metabolic: Dysmenorrhea (8%), menstrual disorders (6%), weight gain (3%), fluid retention (<2.5%), galactorrhea (<2.5%), libido changes (<2.5%)
Gastrointestinal: Abdominal pain (8%), vomiting (5%), diarrhea (4%), vaginal yeast infection (4%), abdominal distension (<2.5%)
Genitourinary: Vaginal bleeding (6%), genital discharge (<2.5%), uterine spasm (<2.5%), vaginal discharge (<2.5%), vulvovaginal dryness (<2.5%)
Hepatic: Cholecystitis (<2.5%), lipid disorders (<2.5%)
Neuromuscular & skeletal: Muscle spasms (<2.5%)
Respiratory: Pulmonary embolism (<2.5%)
Miscellaneous: Premenstrual syndrome (<2.5%)
Dosage Topical: Adults: Females:
Contraception: Apply one patch each week for 3 weeks (21 total days); followed by one week that is patch-free. Each patch should be applied on the same day each week ("patch change day") and only one patch should be worn at a time. No more than 7 days should pass during the patch-free interval.

Schedule 1 (Sunday starter): Dose begins on first Sunday after onset of menstruation; if the menstrual period starts on Sunday, apply one patch that very same day. **With a Sunday start, an additional method of contraception (nonhormonal) must be used until after the first 7 days of consecutive administration.** Each patch change will then occur on Sunday.

Schedule 2 (Day 1 starter): Dose starts on first day of menstrual cycle, applying one patch during the first 24 hours of menstrual cycle. No back-up method of contraception is needed as long as the patch is applied on the first day of cycle. Each patch change will then occur on that same day of the week.

Additional dosing considerations:

No bleeding during patch-free week/missed menstrual period: If patch has been applied as directed, continue treatment on usual "patch change day". If used correctly, no bleeding during patch-free week does not necessarily indicate pregnancy. However, if no withdrawal bleeding occurs for 2 consecutive cycles, pregnancy should be ruled out. If patch has not been applied as directed, and one menstrual period is missed, pregnancy should be ruled out prior to continuing treatment.

If a patch becomes partially or completely detached for <24 hours: Try to reapply to same place, or replace with a new patch immediately. Do not reapply if patch is no longer sticky, if it is sticking to itself or another surface, or if it has material sticking to it.

If a patch becomes partially or completely detached for >24 hours (or time period is unknown): Apply a new patch and use this day of the week as the new "patch change day" from this point on. **An additional method of contraception (nonhormonal) must be used until after the first 7 days of consecutive administration.**

Switching from oral contraceptives or vaginal ring: Complete current cycle and apply the first patch on the day the next pill cycle would be started or ring would be inserted. If there is no menstrual bleeding within 7 days of taking the last active tablet, the patient can initiate the first patch application; however, pregnancy must be ruled out. If patch is applied later than 7 days after the last active pill or removal of the vaginal ring, **an additional method of contraception (nonhormonal) should be used until after the first 7 days of consecutive administration**

Use after childbirth: Therapy should not be started <4 weeks after childbirth. Pregnancy should be ruled out prior to treatment if menstrual periods have not restarted. **An additional method of contraception (nonhormonal) should be used until after the first 7 days of consecutive administration.**

Use after abortion or miscarriage: Therapy may be started immediately if abortion/miscarriage occurs within the first trimester. If therapy is not started within 5 days, follow instructions for first time use. An additional method of contraception (nonhormonal) should be used until after the first 7 days of consecutive administration. If abortion/miscarriage occurs during the second trimester, therapy should not be started for at least 4 weeks. Follow directions for use after childbirth.

Dosage adjustment in renal impairment: Specific guidelines not available; use with caution and monitor blood pressure closely. Consider other forms of contraception.

Dosage adjustment in hepatic impairment: Contraindicated in patients with hepatic impairment

Mechanism of Action Combination hormonal contraceptives inhibit ovulation via a negative feedback mechanism on the hypothalamus, which alters the normal pattern of gonadotropin secretion of a follicle-stimulating hormone (FSH) and luteinizing hormone by the anterior pituitary. The follicular phase FSH and midcycle surge of gonadotropins are inhibited. In addition, combination hormonal contraceptives produce alterations in the genital tract, including changes in the cervical mucus, rendering it unfavorable for sperm penetration even if ovulation occurs. Changes in the endometrium may also occur, producing an unfavorable environment for nidation. Combination hormonal contraceptive drugs may alter the tubal transport of the ova through the fallopian tubes. Progestational agents may also alter sperm fertility.

Contraindications Hypersensitivity to ethinyl estradiol, norelgestromin, or any component of the formulation; breast cancer or other estrogen- or progestin-dependent neoplasms (current or a history of), hepatic tumors or disease, pregnancy, undiagnosed abnormal uterine bleeding, cholestatic jaundice of pregnancy, jaundice with prior combination hormonal contraceptive use

Use is also contraindicated in women at high risk of arterial or venous thrombotic diseases including: Cerebrovascular disease, coronary artery disease, diabetes mellitus with vascular disease, DVT or PE (current or history of), headaches with focal neurological symptoms, persistent blood pressure values of ≥160/100 mm Hg, valvular heart disease with complications, major surgery with prolonged immobilization

Warnings/Precautions Hazardous agent - use appropriate precautions for handling and disposal (NIOSH, 2012). Combination hormonal contraceptives do not protect against HIV infection or other sexually-transmitted diseases. **[U.S. Boxed Warning]: The risk of cardiovascular side effects is increased in women who smoke cigarettes; risk increases with age (especially women >35 years of age) and the number of cigarettes smoked; women who use combination hormonal contraceptives should be strongly advised not to smoke. Should not be used in patients >35 years of age who smoke.** Combination hormonal contraceptives may lead to increased risk of myocardial infarction, use with caution in patients with risk factors for coronary artery disease. All combination hormonal contraceptives may increase the risk of thromboembolism; discontinue use of combination hormonal contraceptives if an arterial or venous thrombotic event occurs. **[U.S. Boxed Warning]: The risk of venous thromboembolism (VTE) may be further increased with use of the contraceptive patch due to increased estrogen exposure in comparison to oral contraceptives.** Women with inherited thrombophilias (eg, protein C or S deficiency) may have increased risk of venous thromboembolism (DeSancho, 2010; van Vlijmen, 2011). Whenever possible, combination hormonal contraceptives should be discontinued at least 4 weeks prior to and for 2 weeks following elective surgery associated with an increased risk of thromboembolism or during periods of prolonged immobilization. Combination hormonal contraceptives may have a dose-related risk of vascular disease, hypertension, and gallbladder disease. Women with hypertension or renal disease should be encouraged to use a nonhormonal form of contraception. The use of combination hormonal contraceptives has been associated with a slight increase in frequency of breast cancer; however, studies are not consistent. Use is contraindicated in women with (or history of) breast cancer.

Combination hormonal contraceptives may cause glucose intolerance or affect serum triglyceride and lipoprotein levels. Estrogens may cause retinal vascular thrombosis; discontinue if migraine, loss of vision, proptosis, diplopia or other visual disturbances occur; discontinue permanently if papilledema or retinal vascular lesions are observed on examination. Use caution with conditions that may be aggravated by fluid retention, depression, or history of migraine. Presentation of irregular, unresolving vaginal bleeding warrants further evaluation including endometrial sampling, if indicated, to rule out malignancy. Extremely rare adenomas and focal nodular hyperplasia resulting in fatal intra-abdominal hemorrhage have been reported in association with long-term oral contraceptive use. Combination hormonal contraceptives may be poorly metabolized in women with hepatic impairment. Discontinue if jaundice develops during therapy or if liver function becomes abnormal. Risk of cholestasis may be increased with previous cholestatic jaundice of pregnancy or jaundice with prior oral contraceptive use. Estrogens may increase thyroid-binding globulin (TBG) levels leading to increased circulating total thyroid hormone levels. Women on thyroid replacement therapy may require higher doses of thyroid hormone while receiving estrogens. The minimum dosage combination of estrogen/progestin that will effectively treat the individual patient should be used. Not for use prior to menarche.

The use of estrogens and/or progestins may change the results of some laboratory tests (eg, coagulation factors, lipids, glucose tolerance, binding proteins). The dose, route, and the specific estrogen/progestin influences these changes. In addition, personal risk factors (eg, cardiovascular disease, smoking, diabetes, age) also contribute to adverse events; use of specific products may be contraindicated in women with certain risk factors. The combination hormonal contraceptive patch may have adverse effects similar to those associated with oral contraceptive products. Risk of complications increases with other risk factors such as hypertension, hyperlipidemias, obesity and diabetes. The topical patch may be less effective in patients weighing ≥90 kg (198 lb) and an increased incidence of pregnancy has been reported in this population; consider another form of contraception.

Drug Interactions
Metabolism/Transport Effects Refer to individual components.
Avoid Concomitant Use
Avoid concomitant use of Ethinyl Estradiol and Norelgestromin with any of the following: Anastrozole; Griseofulvin; Ospemifene; Pimozide; Pirfenidone
Increased Effect/Toxicity
Ethinyl Estradiol and Norelgestromin may increase the levels/effects of: ARIPiprazole; Benzodiazepines (metabolized by oxidation); Corticosteroids (Systemic); CYP1A2 Substrates; Lomitapide; Ospemifene; Pimozide; Pirfenidone; ROPINIRole; Selegiline; Theophylline Derivatives; Tipranavir; TiZANidine; Tranexamic Acid; Voriconazole

The levels/effects of Ethinyl Estradiol and Norelgestromin may be increased by: Ascorbic Acid; Atazanavir; Boceprevir; Cobicistat; Herbs (Estrogenic Properties); Herbs (Progestogenic Properties); Mifepristone; NSAID (COX-2 Inhibitor); Voriconazole

Decreased Effect
Ethinyl Estradiol and Norelgestromin may decrease the levels/effects of: Anastrozole; Chenodiol; Hyaluronidase; LamoTRIgine; Ospemifene; Thyroid Products; Ursodiol; Vitamin K Antagonists

The levels/effects of Ethinyl Estradiol and Norelgestromin may be decreased by: Acitretin; Aminoglutethimide; Aprepitant; Armodafinil; Artemether; Barbiturates; Bexarotene (Systemic); Bile Acid Sequestrants; Boceprevir; Bosentan; CarBAMazepine; CloBAZam; Cobicistat; Colesevelam; CYP3A4 Inducers (Strong); Deferasirox; Elvitegravir; Exenatide; Felbamate; Fosaprepitant; Fosphenytoin; Griseofulvin; LamoTRIgine; Mifepristone; Modafinil; Mycophenolate; Nafcillin; Nevirapine; OXcarbazepine; Perampanel; Phenytoin; Protease Inhibitors; Prucalopride; Retinoic Acid Derivatives; Rifamycin Derivatives; Rufinamide; St Johns Wort; Telaprevir; Tipranavir; Tocilizumab; Topiramate

Ethanol/Nutrition/Herb Interactions
Food: CNS effects of caffeine may be enhanced if combination hormonal contraceptives are used concurrently with caffeine. Grapefruit juice increases ethinyl estradiol concentrations and would be expected to increase progesterone serum levels as well; clinical implications are unclear.
Herb/Nutraceutical: St John's wort may decrease levels. Herbs with estrogenic properties may enhance the adverse/toxic effect of estrogen derivatives; examples include alfalfa, black cohosh, bloodroot, hops, kudzu, licorice, red clover, saw palmetto, soybean, thyme, wild yam, yucca. Herbs with progestogenic properties may enhance the adverse/toxic effect of progestins; examples include bloodroot, chasteberry, damiana, oregano, yucca.
Pharmacodynamics/Kinetics
Half-life Elimination Topical: Ethinyl estradiol: ~17 hours; Norelgestromin: ~28 hours
Pregnancy Risk Factor X
Pregnancy Considerations Pregnancy should be ruled out prior to treatment and discontinued if pregnancy occurs. In general, the use of combination hormonal contraceptives when inadvertently taken early in pregnancy have not been associated with teratogenic effects. The topical patch may be less effective in patients weighing ≥90 kg (198 lb) and an increased incidence of pregnancy has been reported in this population; consider another form of contraception.

Due to increased risk of venous thromboembolism (VTE) postpartum, combination hormonal contraceptives should not be started in any woman <21 days following delivery. Women without risk factors for VTE and who are not breast-feeding may start combination hormonal contraceptives during 21-42 days postpartum. After 42 days postpartum, restrictions for use are not related to postpartum status and should be based on other medical conditions (CDC, 2011). The manufacturer states that combination hormonal contraceptives should not be started until ≥4 weeks after delivery in women who choose not to breastfeed, or ≥4 weeks after a second trimester abortion or miscarriage.
Lactation Enters breast milk/not recommended
Breast-Feeding Considerations Jaundice and breast enlargement in the nursing infant have been reported following the use of combination hormonal contraceptives. May decrease the quality and quantity of breast milk; a nonhormonal form of contraception is recommended (per manufacturer). The theoretical concerns about decreased milk production are greatest early in

the postpartum period when milk production is being established. Postpartum risk status for VTE should be considered when initiating combination hormonal contraceptives after delivery. Combined hormonal contraceptives should not be started <21 days postpartum due to increased risk of VTE. Risk of VTE is still elevated in breast-feeding women until ~42 days postpartum and is greater in women with additional risk factors. After 42 days postpartum, restrictions for use are not related to postpartum VTE risk and should be based on other medical conditions (CDC, 2011).

Dosage Forms
Patch, transdermal:
Ortho Evra®: Ethinyl estradiol 0.75 mg and norelgestromin 6 mg [releases ethinyl estradiol 20 mcg and norelgestromin 150 mcg per day] (1s, 3s)
Dosage Forms: Canada
Patch, transdermal:
Evra®: Ethinyl estradiol 0.6 mg and norelgestromin 6 mg (1s, 3s)

Ethinyl Estradiol and Norethindrone
(ETH in il es tra DYE ole & nor eth IN drone)

Related Information
Endocrine Disorders and Pregnancy *on page 1517*
Norethindrone *on page 990*
Rheumatoid Arthritis, Osteoarthritis, and Osteoporosis *on page 1526*
Brand Names: U.S. Alyacen 1/35; Alyacen 7/7/7; Aranelle®; Balziva™; Brevicon®; Briellyn; Cyclafem™ 1/35; Cyclafem™ 7/7/7; Dasetta™ 1/35; Dasetta™ 7/7/7; Estrostep® Fe; Femcon® Fe; femhrt®; femhrt® Lo; Generess™ Fe; Gildess® FE 1.5/30; Gildess® FE 1/20; Jevantique™ [DSC]; Jinteli™; Junel® 1.5/30; Junel® 1/20; Junel® Fe 1.5/30; Junel® Fe 1/20; Leena®; Lo Loestrin™ Fe; Loestrin® 21 1.5/30; Loestrin® 21 1/20; Loestrin® 24 Fe; Loestrin® Fe 1.5/30; Loestrin® Fe 1/20; Microgestin® 1.5/30; Microgestin® 1/20; Microgestin® Fe 1.5/30; Microgestin® Fe 1/20; Modicon®; Necon® 0.5/35; Necon® 1/35; Necon® 10/11; Necon® 7/7/7; Norinyl® 1+35; Nortrel® 0.5/35; Nortrel® 1/35; Nortrel® 7/7/7; Ortho-Novum® 1/35; Ortho-Novum® 7/7/7; Ovcon® 35; Ovcon® 50 [DSC]; Tilia™ Fe; Tri-Legest™ Fe; Tri-Norinyl®; Wera™; Wymzya™ Fe; Zenchent Fe™; Zenchent®; Zeosa™
Brand Names: Canada Brevicon® 0.5/35; Brevicon® 1/35; FemHRT®; Loestrin™ 1.5/30; Minestrin™ 1/20; Ortho® 0.5/35; Ortho® 1/35; Ortho® 7/7/7; Select™ 1/35; Synphasic®
Generic Availability (U.S.) Yes
Pharmacologic Category Contraceptive; Estrogen and Progestin Combination
Use Prevention of pregnancy; treatment of acne; moderate-to-severe vasomotor symptoms associated with menopause; prevention of osteoporosis (in women at significant risk only)
Unlabeled Use Treatment of hypermenorrhea (menorrhagia); pain associated with endometriosis, dysmenorrhea; dysfunctional uterine bleeding
Local Anesthetic/Vasoconstrictor Precautions No information available to require special precautions
Effects on Dental Treatment When prescribing antibiotics, patient must be warned to use additional methods of birth control if on oral contraceptives.
Effects on Bleeding No information available to require special precautions

Adverse Effects The following reactions have been associated with oral contraceptive use:
Increased risk or evidence of association with use:
Cardiovascular: Arterial thromboembolism, cerebral hemorrhage, cerebral thrombosis, hypertension, mesenteric thrombosis, MI, venous thrombosis (with or without embolism)
Gastrointestinal: Gallbladder disease
Hepatic: Hepatic adenomas, liver tumors (benign)
Local: Thrombophlebitis
Ocular: Retinal thrombosis
Renal: Impaired renal function
Respiratory: Pulmonary embolism
Adverse reactions considered drug related:
Cardiovascular: Edema, varicose vein aggravation
Central nervous system: Depression, migraine, mood changes
Dermatologic: Chloasma, melasma, rash (allergic)
Endocrine & metabolic: Amenorrhea, breakthrough bleeding, breast changes (enlargement, pain, secretion, tenderness), fluid retention, infertility (temporary), lactation decreased (with use immediately postpartum), menstrual flow changes, spotting
Gastrointestinal: Abdominal bloating, abdominal cramps, abdominal pain, appetite changes, nausea, weight changes, vomiting
Genitourinary: Cervical ectropion, cervical secretion, vaginal candidiasis, vaginitis
Hematologic: Folate decreased, porphyria exacerbation
Hepatic: Cholestatic jaundice
Neuromuscular & skeletal: Chorea exacerbation
Ocular: Contact lens intolerance, corneal curvature changes (steepening)
Miscellaneous: Anaphylactic/anaphylactoid reactions (including angioedema, circulatory collapse, respiratory collapse, urticaria), SLE exacerbation
Adverse reactions in which association is not confirmed or denied: Acne, Budd-Chiari syndrome, cataracts, colitis, cystitis-like syndrome, dizziness, dysmenorrhea, erythema multiforme, erythema nodosum, headache, hemolytic uremic syndrome, hemorrhagic eruption, hirsutism, libido changes, nervousness, optic neuritis (with or without partial or complete loss of vision), pancreatitis, premenstrual syndrome, renal function impaired, scalp hair loss

The following have been associated with femhrt® and in general, are similar to placebo. Also refer to adverse reactions observed with oral contraceptives for additional reactions observed with estrogen/progestin therapy:
>10%: Central nervous system: Headache (15% to 18%)
1% to 10%:
Central nervous system: Depression (4% to 6%), nervousness (2% to 5%)
Endocrine & metabolic: Breast pain (8% to 9%)
Gastrointestinal: Abdominal pain (8% to 10%), nausea/vomiting (5% to 7%), diarrhea (4% to 6%), dyspepsia (3% to 5%)
Genitourinary: Urinary tract infection (4% to 6%), vaginitis (5%)
Respiratory: Sinusitis (8% to 9%)
Dosage Oral:
Adolescents ≥15 years and Adults: Females: Acne: Estrostep® Fe: Refer to dosing for contraception

Adults: Females:

Moderate-to-severe vasomotor symptoms associated with menopause: Initial: femhrt® 0.5/2.5: 1 tablet daily; patient should be re-evaluated at 3- to 6-month intervals to determine if treatment is still necessary; patient should be maintained at the lowest effective dose

Prevention of osteoporosis: Initial: femhrt® 0.5/2.5: 1 tablet daily; patient should be maintained on the lowest effective dose

Contraception:

Schedule 1 (Sunday starter): Dose begins on first Sunday after onset of menstruation; if the menstrual period starts on Sunday, take first tablet that very same day. This schedule is not preferred for Lo Loestrin™ Fe. With a Sunday start, an additional method of contraception should be used until after the first 7 days of consecutive administration (all products).

For 21-tablet package: Dosage is 1 tablet daily for 21 consecutive days, followed by 7 days off of the medication; a new course begins on the 8th day after the last tablet is taken.

For 28-tablet package: Dosage is 1 tablet daily without interruption.

Schedule 2 (Day 1 starter): Dose starts on first day of menstrual cycle taking 1 tablet daily.

For 21-tablet package: Dosage is 1 tablet daily for 21 consecutive days, followed by 7 days off of the medication; a new course begins on the 8th day after the last tablet is taken.

For 28-tablet package: Dosage is 1 tablet daily without interruption.

If all doses have been taken on schedule and one menstrual period is missed, continue dosing cycle. If two consecutive menstrual periods are missed, pregnancy test is required before new dosing cycle is started.

Missed doses **monophasic formulations** (refer to package insert for complete information):

One dose missed: Take as soon as remembered. Take the next tablet at your regular time. You may take 2 tablets in 1 day.

Two consecutive doses missed in the first 2 weeks: Take 2 tablets as soon as remembered and 2 tablets the next day. An additional method of contraception should be used for 7 days after missed dose.

Two consecutive doses missed in week 3 (all products) or in week 4 (Lo Loestrin™ Fe), or three consecutive doses missed at any time (all products): An additional method of contraception must be used for 7 days after a missed dose.

Schedule 1 (Sunday starter): Continue dose of 1 tablet daily until Sunday, then discard the rest of the pack, and a new pack should be started that same day.

Schedule 2 (Day 1 starter): Current pack should be discarded, and a new pack should be started that same day.

Missed doses **biphasic/triphasic formulations** (refer to package insert for complete information):

One dose missed: Take the next tablet at your regular time. You may take 2 tablets in 1 day.

Two consecutive doses missed in week 1 or week 2 of the pack: Take 2 tablets as soon as remembered and 2 tablets the next day. Resume taking 1 tablet daily until the pack is empty. An additional method of contraception should be used for 7 days after a missed dose.

Two consecutive doses missed in week 3 of the pack: An additional method of contraception must be used for 7 days after a missed dose.

Schedule 1 (Sunday Starter): Take 1 tablet every day until Sunday. Discard the remaining pack and start a new pack of pills on the same day.

Schedule 2 (Day 1 starter): Discard the remaining pack and start a new pack the same day.

Three or more consecutive doses missed: An additional method of contraception must be used for 7 days after a missed dose.

Schedule 1 (Sunday Starter): Take 1 tablet every day until Sunday; on Sunday, discard the pack and start a new pack.

Schedule 2 (Day 1 Starter): Discard the remaining pack and begin new pack of tablets starting on the same day.

Switching from a different contraceptive:

Oral contraceptive: Start on the same day that a new pack of the previous oral contraceptive would have been taken.

Transdermal patch, vaginal ring, injection: Start on the day the next dose would have been due.

IUD or implant: Start on the day of removal. A backup method of contraception may be required following IUD removal.

Use after childbirth (in women who are not breast-feeding) or after second trimester abortion: Therapy may be started ≥4 weeks postpartum. Pregnancy should be ruled out prior to treatment if menstrual periods have not restarted and an additional method of contraception (nonhormonal) should be used until after the first 7 days of consecutive administration.

Dosage adjustment in renal impairment: Specific guidelines not available; use with caution and monitor blood pressure closely. Consider other forms of contraception.

Dosage adjustment in hepatic impairment: Contraindicated in patients with hepatic impairment.

Mechanism of Action Combination oral contraceptives inhibit ovulation via a negative feedback mechanism on the hypothalamus, which alters the normal pattern of gonadotropin secretion of a follicle-stimulating hormone (FSH) and luteinizing hormone by the anterior pituitary. The follicular phase FSH and midcycle surge of gonadotropins are inhibited. In addition, combination hormonal contraceptives produce alterations in the genital tract, including changes in the cervical mucus, rendering it unfavorable for sperm penetration even if ovulation occurs. Changes in the endometrium may also occur, producing an unfavorable environment for nidation. Combination hormonal contraceptive drugs may alter the tubal transport of the ova through the fallopian tubes. Progestational agents may also alter sperm fertility.

In postmenopausal women, exogenous estrogen is used to replace decreased endogenous production. The addition of progestin reduces the incidence of endometrial hyperplasia and risk of endometrial cancer in women with an intact uterus.

Contraindications Angioedema, anaphylactic reaction, or hypersensitivity to ethinyl estradiol, norethindrone, norethindrone acetate, or any component of the formulation; breast cancer or other estrogen- or progestin-dependent neoplasms (current or a history of), hepatic tumors or disease, pregnancy, undiagnosed abnormal uterine bleeding

Use is also contraindicated in women at high risk of arterial or venous thrombotic diseases including: Cerebrovascular disease, coronary artery disease, diabetes mellitus with vascular disease, DVT or PE (current or history of), hypercoagulopathies (inherited or acquired), headaches with focal neurological symptoms, hypertension (uncontrolled), migraine headaches if >35 years of age, thrombogenic valvular or rhythm diseases of the heart (eg, subacute bacterial endocarditis with valvular disease or atrial fibrillation), women >35 years of age who smoke.

Warnings/Precautions Hazardous agent - use appropriate precautions for handling and disposal (NIOSH, 2012).

[U.S. Boxed Warning]: Based on data from the Women's Health Initiative (WHI) studies, an increased risk of invasive breast cancer was observed in postmenopausal women using conjugated estrogens (CE) in combination with medroxyprogesterone acetate (MPA). This risk may be associated with duration of use and declines once combined therapy is discontinued (Chlebowski, 2009). The risk of invasive breast cancer was decreased in postmenopausal women with a hysterectomy using CE only, regardless of weight. However, the risk was not significantly decreased in women at high risk for breast cancer (family history of breast cancer, personal history of benign breast disease) (Anderson, 2012). An increase in abnormal mammogram findings has also been reported with estrogen alone or in combination with progestin therapy. Estrogen use may lead to severe hypercalcemia in patients with breast cancer and bone metastases; discontinue estrogen if hypercalcemia occurs. The use of combination hormonal contraceptives has been associated with a slight increase in frequency of breast cancer, however studies are not consistent. Use is contraindicated in patients with known or suspected breast cancer.

[U.S. Boxed Warning]: The use of unopposed estrogen in women with an intact uterus is associated with an increased risk of endometrial cancer. The addition of a progestin to estrogen therapy may decrease the risk of endometrial hyperplasia, a precursor to endometrial cancer. Adequate diagnostic measures, including endometrial sampling if indicated, should be performed to rule out malignancy in postmenopausal women with undiagnosed abnormal vaginal bleeding. Estrogens may exacerbate endometriosis. Malignant transformation of residual endometrial implants has been reported posthysterectomy with unopposed estrogen therapy. Consider adding a progestin in women with residual endometriosis posthysterectomy. Postmenopausal estrogen therapy and combined estrogen/progesterone therapy may increase the risk of ovarian cancer; however, the absolute risk to an individual woman is small. Although results from various studies are not consistent, risk does not appear to be significantly associated with the duration, route, or dose of therapy. In one study, the risk decreased after 2 years following discontinuation of therapy (Mørch, 2009). Although the risk of ovarian cancer is rare, women who are at an increased risk (eg, family history) should be counseled about the association (NAMS, 2012).

[U.S. Boxed Warning]: Estrogens with or without progestin should not be used to prevent cardiovascular disease. Using data from the Women's Health Initiative (WHI) studies, an increased risk of deep vein thrombosis (DVT) and stroke has been reported with CE and an increased risk of DVT, stroke, pulmonary emboli (PE) and myocardial infarction (MI) has been reported with CE with MPA in postmenopausal women.

Additional risk factors include diabetes mellitus, hypercholesterolemia, hypertension, SLE, obesity, tobacco use, and/or history of venous thromboembolism (VTE). Risk factors should be managed appropriately; discontinue use if adverse cardiovascular events occur or are suspected. **[U.S. Boxed Warning]: The risk of cardiovascular side effects is increased in women who smoke cigarettes; risk increases with age (especially women >35 years of age) and the number of cigarettes smoked; women who use combination hormonal contraceptives should be strongly advised not to smoke. Use is contraindicated in patients >35 years of age who smoke.** When used for contraception, use with caution in patients with risk factors for cardiovascular disease. May have a dose-related risk of vascular disease and hypertension; women with hypertension should be encouraged to use another form of contraception. Monitor women with well-controlled hypertension and discontinue if blood pressure rises significantly. Use is contraindicated with uncontrolled hypertension. Combination hormonal contraceptives may affect serum triglyceride and lipoprotein levels. Estrogen compounds are generally associated with lipid effects such as increased HDL-cholesterol and decreased LDL-cholesterol. Progestins may be associated with decreased HDL-cholesterol. Triglycerides may also be increased; use with caution in patients with familial defects of lipoprotein metabolism. Women with inherited thrombophilias (eg, protein C or S deficiency) may have increased risk of venous thromboembolism (DeSancho, 2010; van Vlijmen, 2011). Use is contraindicated in women with hypercoagulopathies (inherited or acquired).

[U.S. Boxed Warning]: Estrogens with or without progestin should not be used to prevent dementia. In the Women's Health Initiative Memory Study (WHIMS), an increased incidence of dementia was observed in women ≥65 years of age taking CE alone or in combination with MPA.

Steroid hormones may be poorly metabolized in patients with hepatic dysfunction. Use caution with a history of cholestatic jaundice associated with prior estrogen use or pregnancy. Discontinue if jaundice develops or if acute or chronic hepatic disturbances occur. Use is contraindicated with hepatic disease. Estrogens may cause retinal vascular thrombosis; discontinue if migraine, loss of vision, proptosis, diplopia or other visual disturbances occur; discontinue permanently if papilledema or retinal vascular lesions are observed on examination. May have adverse effects on glucose tolerance; use caution in women with diabetes. Use caution with a history of chloasma gravidarum; women with a tendency to chloasma should avoid sun and ultraviolet radiation exposure during therapy. Use with caution in patients with diseases which may be exacerbated by fluid retention, including cardiac or renal dysfunction. Women with renal disease should be encouraged to use a nonhormonal form of contraception. Use with caution in patients with gallbladder disease. May have a dose-related risk of gallbladder disease. Use of postmenopausal estrogen may be associated with an increased risk of gallbladder disease requiring surgery. Exogenous estrogens may exacerbate angioedema symptoms in women with hereditary angioedema. Use caution in patients with asthma, depression, epilepsy, hepatic hemangioma, severe hypocalcemia, porphyria, or SLE. Use with caution in patients with a history of migraine. Evaluate new, recurrent, severe, or persistent headaches. Use of combination oral contraceptives is contraindicated in women with headaches with focal neurological symptoms or migraine headaches if >35 years of age. Estrogens may increase thyroid-binding globulin (TBG) levels leading to increased circulating total thyroid hormone levels. Women on thyroid replacement therapy may require higher doses of thyroid hormone while receiving estrogens.

Whenever possible, should be discontinued at least 4-6 weeks prior to and for 2 weeks following elective surgery associated with an increased risk of thromboembolism or during periods of prolonged immobilization.

Unscheduled bleeding/spotting may occur within the first 3 months of combination oral contraceptive use. Presentation of irregular, unresolving vaginal bleeding following previously regular cycles warrants further evaluation including endometrial sampling, if indicated, to rule out malignancy. Extremely rare adenomas and focal nodular hyperplasia resulting in fatal intra-abdominal hemorrhage have been reported in association with long-term oral contraceptive use. Presentation of an abdominal mass, acute abdominal pain, or intra-abdominal bleeding warrants further evaluation to rule out source. The minimum dosage combination of estrogen/progestin that will effectively treat the individual patient should be used. New patients should be started on products containing ≤0.035 mg of estrogen per tablet. Combination hormonal contraceptives are not for use prior to menarche. Safety and efficacy of some products (eg, Generess Fe, Lo Loestrin™ Fe) have not been established in women with a BMI >35 kg/m^2. Combination hormonal contraceptives do not protect against HIV infection or other sexually-transmitted diseases. When used for acne, use only in females ≥15 years of age, who also desire combination hormonal contraceptive therapy, are unresponsive to topical treatments, have no contraindications to combination hormonal contraceptive use, and plan to stay on therapy for ≥6 months.

[U.S. Boxed Warning]: Estrogens with or without progestin should be used for the shortest duration possible at the lowest effective dose consistent with treatment goals. Before prescribing estrogen therapy to postmenopausal women, the risks and benefits must be weighed for each patient. Women should be informed of these risks and benefits, as well as possible effects of progestin when added to estrogen therapy. Patients should be reevaluated as clinically appropriate to determine if treatment is still necessary. Available data related to treatment risks are from Women's Health Initiative (WHI) studies, which evaluated oral CE 0.625 mg with or without MPA 2.5 mg relative to placebo in postmenopausal women. Other combinations and dosage forms of estrogens and progestins were not studied. Outcomes reported from clinical trials using CE with or without MPA should be assumed to be similar for other doses and other dosage forms of estrogens and progestins until comparable data becomes available. When used for menopause, use only in women at significant risk of osteoporosis and for who other non-estrogen medications are not considered appropriate.

The use of estrogens and/or progestins may change the results of some laboratory tests (eg, coagulation factors, lipids, glucose tolerance, binding proteins). The dose, route, and the specific estrogen/progestin influences these changes. In addition, personal risk factors (eg, cardiovascular disease, smoking, diabetes, age) also contribute to adverse events; use of specific products may be contraindicated in women with certain risk factors. Some products may contain tartrazine, which may cause allergic reactions in certain individuals.

Drug Interactions

Metabolism/Transport Effects Refer to individual components.

Avoid Concomitant Use
Avoid concomitant use of Ethinyl Estradiol and Norethindrone with any of the following: Anastrozole; Griseofulvin; Ospemifene; Pimozide; Pirfenidone

Increased Effect/Toxicity
Ethinyl Estradiol and Norethindrone may increase the levels/effects of: ARIPiprazole; Benzodiazepines (metabolized by oxidation); Corticosteroids (Systemic); CYP1A2 Substrates; Lomitapide; Ospemifene; Pimozide; Pirfenidone; ROPINIRole; Selegiline; Theophylline Derivatives; Tipranavir; TiZANidine; Tranexamic Acid; Voriconazole

The levels/effects of Ethinyl Estradiol and Norethindrone may be increased by: Ascorbic Acid; Atazanavir; Boceprevir; Cobicistat; Herbs (Estrogenic Properties); Herbs (Progestogenic Properties); Mifepristone; NSAID (COX-2 Inhibitor); Voriconazole

Decreased Effect
Ethinyl Estradiol and Norethindrone may decrease the levels/effects of: Anastrozole; Chenodiol; Hyaluronidase; LamoTRIgine; Ospemifene; Thyroid Products; Ursodiol; Vitamin K Antagonists

The levels/effects of Ethinyl Estradiol and Norethindrone may be decreased by: Acitretin; Aminoglutethimide; Aprepitant; Armodafinil; Artemether; Barbiturates; Bexarotene (Systemic); Bile Acid Sequestrants; Boceprevir; Bosentan; CarBAMazepine; CloBAZam; Cobicistat; Colesevelam; CYP3A4 Inducers (Strong); Darunavir; Deferasirox; Elvitegravir; Exenatide; Felbamate; Fosaprepitant; Fosphenytoin; Griseofulvin; LamoTRIgine; Mifepristone; Modafinil; Mycophenolate; Nafcillin; Nevirapine; OXcarbazepine; Perampanel; Phenytoin; Protease Inhibitors; Prucalopride; Retinoic Acid Derivatives; Rifamycin Derivatives; Rufinamide; St Johns Wort; Telaprevir; Tipranavir; Tocilizumab; Topiramate

Ethanol/Nutrition/Herb Interactions

Ethanol: Routine use increases estrogen level and risk of breast cancer; avoid ethanol. Ethanol may also increase the risk of osteoporosis.

Food: CNS effects of caffeine may be enhanced if combination hormonal contraceptives are used concurrently with caffeine. Grapefruit juice increases ethinyl estradiol concentrations and would be expected to increase progesterone serum levels as well; clinical implications are unclear. Norethindrone absorption is increased by 27% following administration with food.

Herb/Nutraceutical: St John's wort may decrease levels. Herbs with estrogenic properties may enhance the adverse/toxic effect of estrogen derivatives; examples include alfalfa, black cohosh, bloodroot, hops, kudzu, licorice, red clover, saw palmetto, soybean, thyme, wild yam, yucca. Herbs with progestogenic properties may enhance the adverse/toxic effect of progestins; examples include bloodroot, chasteberry, damiana, oregano, yucca.

Dietary Considerations Should be taken at same time each day. May be taken without regard to meals. Ensure adequate calcium and vitamin D intake when used for the prevention of osteoporosis.

Pharmacodynamics/Kinetics

Half-life Elimination Ethinyl estradiol: 19-24 hours

◀ **Pregnancy Risk Factor** X

Pregnancy Considerations Pregnancy should be ruled out prior to treatment and discontinued if pregnancy occurs. In general, the use of combination hormonal contraceptives when inadvertently taken early in pregnancy have not been associated with teratogenic effects. Hormonal contraceptives may be less effective in obese patients. An increase in oral contraceptive failure was noted in women with a BMI >27.3 kg/m^2. Similar findings were noted in patients weighing ≥90 kg (198 lb) using the contraceptive patch.

Due to increased risk of venous thromboembolism (VTE) postpartum, combination hormonal contraceptives should not be started in any woman <21 days following delivery. Women without risk factors for VTE and who are not breast-feeding may start combination hormonal contraceptives during 21-42 days postpartum. After 42 days postpartum, restrictions for use are not related to postpartum status and should be based on other medical conditions (CDC, 2011). May be started immediately following first trimester abortion or miscarriage.

Lactation Enters breast milk/not recommended

Breast-Feeding Considerations Jaundice and breast enlargement in the nursing infant have been reported following the use of combination hormonal contraceptives. May decrease the quality and quantity of breast milk; alternative form of contraception is recommended (per manufacturer). The theoretical concerns about decreased milk production are greatest early in the postpartum period when milk production is being established. Postpartum risk status for VTE should be considered when initiating combination hormonal contraceptives after delivery. Combined hormonal contraceptives should not be started <21 days postpartum due to increased risk of VTE. Risk of VTE is still elevated in breast-feeding women until ~42 days postpartum and is greater in women with additional risk factors. After 42 days postpartum, restrictions for use are not related to postpartum VTE risk and should be based on other medical conditions (CDC, 2011).

Dosage Forms

Tablet, oral:
femhrt® 1/5: Ethinyl estradiol 0.005 mg and norethindrone acetate 1 mg [white tablets] (28s, 90s)

femhrt® Lo 0.5/2.5: Ethinyl estradiol 0.0025 mg and norethindrone acetate 0.5 mg [white tablets] (28s)

Tablet, oral [monophasic formulation]:
Alyacen 1/35: Ethinyl estradiol 0.035 mg and norethindrone 1 mg [21 peach tablets and 7 light green inactive tablets] (28s)

Balziva™: Ethinyl estradiol 0.035 mg and norethindrone 0.4 mg [21 light peach tablets and 7 white inactive tablets] (28s)

Brevicon®: Ethinyl estradiol 0.035 mg and norethindrone 0.5 mg [21 blue tablets and 7 orange inactive tablets] (28s)

Briellyn: Ethinyl estradiol 0.035 mg and norethindrone 0.4 mg [21 light peach tablets and 7 white-off-white inactive tablets] (28s)

Cyclafem™ 1/35: Ethinyl estradiol 0.035 mg and norethindrone 1 mg [21 pink tablets and 7 light green inactive tablets] (28s)

Dasetta™ 1/35: Ethinyl estradiol 0.035 mg and norethindrone 1 mg [21 orange tablets and 7 white inactive tablets] (28s)

Gildess® FE 1/20: Ethinyl estradiol 0.02 mg and norethindrone acetate 1 mg [21 white tablets] and ferrous fumarate 75 mg [7 white-speckled brown tablets] (28s)

Gildess® FE 1.5/30: Ethinyl estradiol 0.03 mg and norethindrone acetate 1.5 mg [21 light green tablets] and ferrous fumarate 75 mg [7 white-speckled brown tablets] (28s)

Junel® 1/20: Ethinyl estradiol 0.02 mg and norethindrone acetate 1 mg [yellow tablets] (21s)

Junel® 1.5/30, Loestrin® 21 1.5/30: Ethinyl estradiol 0.03 mg and norethindrone acetate 1.5 mg [pink tablets] (21s)

Junel® Fe 1/20: Ethinyl estradiol 0.02 mg and norethindrone acetate 1 mg [21 yellow tablets] and ferrous fumarate 75 mg [7 brown tablets] (28s)

Junel® Fe 1.5/30, Loestrin® Fe 21 1.5/30: Ethinyl estradiol 0.03 mg and norethindrone acetate 1.5 mg [21 pink tablets] and ferrous fumarate 75 mg [7 brown tablets] (28s)

Loestrin® 21 1/20: Ethinyl estradiol 0.02 mg and norethindrone acetate 1 mg [light yellow tablets] (21s)

Lo Loestrin™ Fe: Ethinyl estradiol 0.01 mg and norethindrone acetate 1mg [24 blue tablets] and ethinyl estradiol 0.01 mg [2 white tablets] and ferrous fumarate 75 mg [2 brown tablets] (28s)

Loestrin® 24 Fe: Ethinyl estradiol 0.02 mg and norethindrone acetate 1 mg [24 white tablets] and ferrous fumarate 75 mg [4 brown tablets] (28s)

Loestrin® Fe 1/20: Ethinyl estradiol 0.02 mg and norethindrone acetate 1 mg [21 light yellow tablets] and ferrous fumarate 75 mg [7 brown tablets] (28s)

Loestrin® Fe 1.5/30: Ethinyl estradiol 0.03 mg and norethindrone acetate 1.5 mg [21 pink tablets] and ferrous fumarate 75 mg [7 brown tablets] (28s)

Microgestin® 1/20: Ethinyl estradiol 0.02 mg and norethindrone acetate 1 mg [white tablets] (21s)

Microgestin® 1.5/30: Ethinyl estradiol 0.03 mg and norethindrone acetate 1.5 mg [green tablets] (21s)

Microgestin® Fe 1/20: Ethinyl estradiol 0.02 mg and norethindrone acetate 1 mg [21 white tablets] and ferrous fumarate 75 mg [7 brown tablets] (28s)

Microgestin® Fe 1.5/30: Ethinyl estradiol 0.03 mg and norethindrone acetate 1.5 mg [21 green tablets] and ferrous fumarate 75 mg [7 brown tablets] (28s)

Modicon®: Ethinyl estradiol 0.035 mg and norethindrone 0.5 mg [21 white tablets and 7 green inactive tablets] (28s)

Necon® 0.5/35, Nortrel® 0.5/35: Ethinyl estradiol 0.035 mg and norethindrone 0.5 mg [21 light yellow tablets and 7 white inactive tablets] (28s)

Necon® 1/35: Ethinyl estradiol 0.035 mg and norethindrone 1 mg [21 dark yellow tablets and 7 white inactive tablets] (28s)

Norinyl® 1+35: Ethinyl estradiol 0.035 mg and norethindrone 1 mg [21 yellow-green tablets and 7 orange inactive tablets] (28s)

Nortrel® 1/35:
Ethinyl estradiol 0.035 mg and norethindrone 1 mg [yellow tablets] (21s)

Ethinyl estradiol 0.035 mg and norethindrone 1 mg [21 yellow tablets and 7 white inactive tablets] (28s)

Ortho-Novum® 1/35: Ethinyl estradiol 0.035 mg and norethindrone 1 mg [21 peach tablets and 7 green inactive tablets] (28s)

Ovcon® 35: Ethinyl estradiol 0.035 mg and norethindrone 0.4 mg [21 light peach tablets and 7 green inactive tablets] (28s)

Wera™: Ethinyl estradiol 0.035 mg and norethindrone 0.5 mg [21 light peach tablets and 7 white inactive tablets] (28s)

Zenchent®: Ethinyl estradiol 0.035 mg and norethindrone 0.4 mg [21 orange tablets and 7 white inactive tablets] (28s)

Tablet, chewable, oral [monophasic formulation]:
Ethinyl estradiol 0.035 mg and norethindrone 0.4 mg [21 tablets] and ferrous fumarate 75 mg [7 tablets] (28s)

Femcon® Fe, Wymzya™ Fe: Ethinyl estradiol 0.035 mg and norethindrone 0.4 mg [21 white tablets] and ferrous fumarate 75 mg [7 brown tablets] (28s)

Generess™ Fe: Ethinyl estradiol 0.025 mg and norethindrone 0.8 mg [24 light green tablets] and ferrous fumarate 75 mg [4 brown tablets] (28s)

Zenchent Fe™, Zeosa™: Ethinyl estradiol 0.035 mg and norethindrone 0.4 mg [21 light yellow tablets] and ferrous fumarate 75 mg [7 brown tablets] (28s)

Tablet, oral [biphasic formulation]:
Necon® 10/11:
Day 1-10: Ethinyl estradiol 0.035 mg and norethindrone 0.5 mg [10 light yellow tablets]
Day 11-21: Ethinyl estradiol 0.035 mg and norethindrone 1 mg [11 dark yellow tablets]
Day 22-28: 7 white inactive tablets (28s)

Tablet, oral [triphasic formulation]:
Alyacen 7/7/7:
Day 1-7: Ethinyl estradiol 0.035 mg and norethindrone 0.5 mg [7 white-off-white tablets]
Day 8-14: Ethinyl estradiol 0.035 mg and norethindrone 0.75 mg [7 light peach tablets]
Day 15-21: Ethinyl estradiol 0.035 mg and norethindrone 1 mg [7 peach tablets]
Day 22-28: 7 light green inactive tablets (28s)
Aranelle®:
Day 1-7: Ethinyl estradiol 0.035 mg and norethindrone 0.5 mg [7 light yellow tablets]
Day 8-16: Ethinyl estradiol 0.035 mg and norethindrone 1 mg [9 white tablets]
Day 17-21: Ethinyl estradiol 0.035 mg and norethindrone 0.5 mg [5 light yellow tablets]
Day 22-28: 7 peach inactive tablets (28s)
Cyclafem™ 7/7/7:
Day 1-7: Ethinyl estradiol 0.035 mg and norethindrone 0.5 mg [7 white tablets]
Day 8-14: Ethinyl estradiol 0.035 mg and norethindrone 0.75 mg [7 light pink tablets]
Day 15-21: Ethinyl estradiol 0.035 mg and norethindrone 1 mg [7 pink tablets]
Day 22-28: 7 light green inactive tablets (28s)
Dasetta™ 7/7/7:
Day 1-7: Ethinyl estradiol 0.035 mg and norethindrone 0.5 mg [7 light peach tablets]
Day 8-14: Ethinyl estradiol 0.035 mg and norethindrone 0.75 mg [7 peach tablets]
Day 15-21: Ethinyl estradiol 0.035 mg and norethindrone 1 mg [7 orange tablets]
Day 22-28: 7 white inactive tablets (28s)
Estrostep® Fe, Tilia™ Fe:
Day 1-5: Ethinyl estradiol 0.02 mg and norethindrone acetate 1 mg [5 white triangular tablets]
Day 6-12: Ethinyl estradiol 0.03 mg and norethindrone acetate 1 mg [7 white square tablets]
Day 13-21: Ethinyl estradiol 0.035 mg and norethindrone acetate 1 mg [9 white round tablets]
Day 22-28: Ferrous fumarate 75 mg [7 brown tablets] (28s)

Leena®:
Day 1-7: Ethinyl estradiol 0.035 mg and norethindrone 0.5 mg [7 light blue tablets]
Day 8-16: Ethinyl estradiol 0.035 mg and norethindrone 1 mg [9 light yellow-green tablets]
Day 17-21: Ethinyl estradiol 0.035 mg and norethindrone 0.5 mg [5 light blue tablets]
Day 22-28: 7 orange inactive tablets (28s)
Necon® 7/7/7, Ortho-Novum® 7/7/7:
Day 1-7: Ethinyl estradiol 0.035 mg and norethindrone 0.5 mg [7 white tablets]
Day 8-14: Ethinyl estradiol 0.035 mg and norethindrone 0.75 mg [7 light peach tablets]
Day 15-21: Ethinyl estradiol 0.035 mg and norethindrone 1 mg [7 peach tablets]
Day 22-28: 7 green inactive tablets (28s)
Nortrel® 7/7/7:
Day 1-7: Ethinyl estradiol 0.035 mg and norethindrone 0.5 mg [7 light yellow tablets]
Day 8-14: Ethinyl estradiol 0.035 mg and norethindrone 0.75 mg [7 blue tablets]
Day 15-21: Ethinyl estradiol 0.035 mg and norethindrone 1 mg [7 peach tablets]
Day 22-28: 7 white inactive tablets (28s)
Tri-Legest™ Fe:
Day 1-5: Ethinyl estradiol 0.02 mg and norethindrone acetate 1 mg [5 light pink tablets]
Day 6-12: Ethinyl estradiol 0.03 mg and norethindrone acetate 1 mg [7 light yellow tablets]
Day 13-21: Ethinyl estradiol 0.035 mg and norethindrone acetate 1 mg [9 light blue tablets]
Day 22-28: Ferrous fumarate 75 mg [7 brown tablets] (28s)
Tri-Norinyl®:
Day 1-7: Ethinyl estradiol 0.035 mg and norethindrone 0.5 mg [7 blue tablets]
Day 8-16: Ethinyl estradiol 0.035 mg and norethindrone 1 mg [9 yellow-green tablets]
Day 17-21: Ethinyl estradiol 0.035 mg and norethindrone 0.5 mg [5 blue tablets]
Day 22-28: 7 orange inactive tablets (28s)

Ethinyl Estradiol and Norgestimate
(ETH in il es tra DYE ole & nor JES ti mate)

Related Information
Endocrine Disorders and Pregnancy *on page 1517*
Brand Names: U.S. Estarylla™; MonoNessa®; Ortho Tri-Cyclen®; Ortho Tri-Cyclen® Lo; Ortho-Cyclen®; Previfem®; Sprintec®; Tri-Estarylla™; Tri-Previfem®; Tri-Sprintec®; TriNessa®
Brand Names: Canada Cyclen®; Tri-Cyclen®; Tri-Cyclen® Lo
Generic Availability (U.S.) Yes
Pharmacologic Category Contraceptive; Estrogen and Progestin Combination
Use Prevention of pregnancy; treatment of acne
Unlabeled Use Treatment of hypermenorrhea (menorrhagia); pain associated with endometriosis; dysmenorrhea; dysfunctional uterine bleeding
Local Anesthetic/Vasoconstrictor Precautions No information available to require special precautions
Effects on Dental Treatment When prescribing antibiotics, patient must be warned to use additional methods of birth control if on oral contraceptives.
Effects on Bleeding No information available to require special precautions

Adverse Effects The following reactions have been associated with oral contraceptive use:

Increased risk or evidence of association with use:

Cardiovascular: Arterial thromboembolism, cerebral hemorrhage, cerebral thrombosis, hypertension, mesenteric thrombosis, MI, venous thrombosis (with or without embolism)

Gastrointestinal: Gallbladder disease

Hepatic: Hepatic adenomas, liver tumors (benign)

Local: Thrombophlebitis

Ocular: Retinal thrombosis

Respiratory: Pulmonary embolism

Adverse reactions considered drug related:

Cardiovascular: Edema, varicose vein aggravation

Central nervous system: Depression, migraine, mood changes

Dermatologic: Chloasma, melasma, rash (allergic)

Endocrine & metabolic: Amenorrhea, breakthrough bleeding, breast changes (enlargement, pain, secretion, tenderness), fluid retention, infertility (temporary), lactation decreased (with use immediately postpartum), menstrual flow changes, spotting

Gastrointestinal: Abdominal bloating, abdominal cramps, abdominal pain, appetite changes, nausea, weight changes, vomiting

Genitourinary: Cervical ectropion, cervical secretion, vaginal candidiasis, vaginitis

Hematologic: Folate decreased, porphyria exacerbation

Hepatic: Cholestatic jaundice

Neuromuscular & skeletal: Chorea exacerbation

Ocular: Contact lens intolerance, corneal curvature changes (steepening)

Miscellaneous: Anaphylactic/anaphylactoid reactions (including angioedema, circulatory collapse, respiratory collapse, urticaria), SLE exacerbation

Adverse reactions in which association is not confirmed or denied: Acne, Budd-Chiari syndrome, cataracts, colitis, cystitis-like syndrome, dizziness, dysmenorrhea, erythema multiforme, erythema nodosum, headache, hemolytic uremic syndrome, hemorrhagic eruption, hirsutism, libido changes, nervousness, optic neuritis (with or without partial or complete loss of vision), pancreatitis, premenstrual syndrome, renal function impaired, scalp hair loss

Dosage Oral:

Children ≥15 years and Adults: Females: Acne (Ortho Tri-Cyclen®): Refer to dosing for contraception

Adults: Females:

Contraception:

Schedule 1 (Sunday starter): Dose begins on first Sunday after onset of menstruation; if the menstrual period starts on Sunday, take first tablet that very same day. **With a Sunday start, an additional method of contraception should be used until after the first 7 days of consecutive administration.**

For 21-tablet package: Dosage is 1 tablet daily for 21 consecutive days, followed by 7 days off of the medication; a new course begins on the 8th day after the last tablet is taken.

For 28-tablet package: Dosage is 1 tablet daily without interruption.

Schedule 2 (Day 1 starter): Dose starts on first day of menstrual cycle taking 1 tablet daily.

For 21-tablet package: Dosage is 1 tablet daily for 21 consecutive days, followed by 7 days off of the medication; a new course begins on the 8th day after the last tablet is taken.

For 28-tablet package: Dosage is 1 tablet daily without interruption.

If all doses have been taken on schedule and one menstrual period is missed, continue dosing cycle. If two consecutive menstrual periods are missed, pregnancy test is required before new dosing cycle is started.

Missed doses **monophasic formulations** (refer to package insert for complete information):

One dose missed: Take as soon as remembered or take 2 tablets next day

Two consecutive doses missed in the first 2 weeks: Take 2 tablets as soon as remembered or 2 tablets next 2 days. **An additional method of contraception should be used for 7 days after missed dose.**

Two consecutive doses missed in week 3 or three consecutive doses missed at any time: **An additional method of contraception must be used for 7 days after a missed dose:**

Schedule 1 (Sunday starter): Continue dose of 1 tablet daily until Sunday, then discard the rest of the pack, and a new pack should be started that same day.

Schedule 2 (Day 1 starter): Current pack should be discarded, and a new pack should be started that same day.

Missed doses **biphasic/triphasic formulations** (refer to package insert for complete information):

One dose missed: Take as soon as remembered or take 2 tablets next day.

Two consecutive doses missed in week 1 or week 2 of the pack: Take 2 tablets as soon as remembered and 2 tablets the next day. Resume taking 1 tablet daily until the pack is empty. **An additional method of contraception must be used for 7 days after a missed dose.**

Two consecutive doses missed in week 3 of the pack. **An additional method of contraception must be used for 7 days after a missed dose.**

Schedule 1 (Sunday starter): Take 1 tablet every day until Sunday. Discard the remaining pack and start a new pack of pills on the same day.

Schedule 2 (Day 1 starter): Discard the remaining pack and start a new pack the same day.

Three or more consecutive doses missed. **An additional method of contraception must be used for 7 days after a missed dose.**

Schedule 1 (Sunday starter): Take 1 tablet every day until Sunday; on Sunday, discard the pack and start a new pack.

Schedule 2 (Day 1 starter): Discard the remaining pack and begin new pack of tablets starting on the same day.

Dosage adjustment in renal impairment: Specific guidelines not available; use with caution and monitor blood pressure closely. Consider other forms of contraception.

Dosage adjustment in hepatic impairment: Contraindicated in patients with hepatic impairment.

Mechanism of Action Combination hormonal contraceptives inhibit ovulation via a negative feedback mechanism on the hypothalamus, which alters the normal pattern of gonadotropin secretion of a follicle-stimulating hormone (FSH) and luteinizing hormone by the anterior pituitary. The follicular phase FSH and midcycle surge of gonadotropins are inhibited. In addition, combination hormonal contraceptives produce alterations in the genital tract, including changes in the cervical mucus, rendering it unfavorable for sperm penetration even if ovulation occurs. Changes in the endometrium may also occur, producing an unfavorable environment for nidation. Combination hormonal contraceptive drugs may alter the tubal transport of the ova through the fallopian tubes. Progestational agents may also alter sperm fertility.

Contraindications Hypersensitivity to ethinyl estradiol, norgestimate, or any component of the formulation; breast cancer or other estrogen- or progestin-dependent neoplasms (current or a history of), hepatic tumors or disease, pregnancy, undiagnosed abnormal uterine bleeding, cholestatic jaundice of pregnancy, jaundice with prior combination hormonal contraceptive use

Use is also contraindicated in women at high risk of arterial or venous thrombotic diseases including: Cerebrovascular disease, coronary artery disease, diabetes mellitus with vascular disease, DVT or PE (current or history of), headaches with focal neurological symptoms, hypertension (uncontrolled), valvular heart disease with complications, major surgery with prolonged immobilization

Warnings/Precautions Hazardous agent - use appropriate precautions for handling and disposal (NIOSH, 2012). Combination hormonal contraceptives do not protect against HIV infection or other sexually-transmitted diseases. **[U.S. Boxed Warning]: The risk of cardiovascular side effects is increased in women who smoke cigarettes; risk increases with age (especially women >35 years of age) and the number of cigarettes smoked; women who use combination hormonal contraceptives should be strongly advised not to smoke. Should not be used in patients >35 years of age who smoke.** Combination hormonal contraceptives may lead to increased risk of myocardial infarction, use with caution in patients with risk factors for coronary artery disease (eg, hypertension, hypercholesterolemia, morbid obesity, diabetes, or women who smoke). May increase the risk of thromboembolism; discontinue use of combination hormonal contraceptives if an arterial or venous thrombotic event occurs. Women with inherited thrombophilias (eg, protein C or S deficiency) may have increased risk of venous thromboembolism (DeSancho, 2010; van Vlijmen, 2011). Whenever possible, combination hormonal contraceptives should be discontinued at least 4 weeks prior to and for 2 weeks following elective surgery associated with an increased risk of thromboembolism or during periods of prolonged immobilization. Combination hormonal contraceptives may have a dose-related risk of vascular disease, hypertension, and gallbladder disease. Women with hypertension or renal disease should be encouraged to use a nonhormonal form of contraception. The use of combination hormonal contraceptives has been associated with a slight increase in frequency of breast cancer; however, studies are not consistent. Use is contraindicated in women with (or history of) breast cancer.

Combination hormonal contraceptives may cause glucose intolerance or affect serum triglyceride and lipoprotein levels. Estrogens may increase thyroid-binding globulin (TBG) levels leading to increased circulating total thyroid hormone levels. Women on thyroid replacement therapy may require higher doses of thyroid hormone while receiving estrogens. Estrogens may cause retinal vascular thrombosis; discontinue if migraine, loss of vision, proptosis, diplopia or other visual disturbances occur; discontinue permanently if papilledema or retinal vascular lesions are observed on examination. Extremely rare adenomas and focal

nodular hyperplasia resulting in fatal intra-abdominal hemorrhage have been reported in association with long-term oral contraceptive use. Presentation of an abdominal mass, acute abdominal pain, or intra-abdominal bleeding warrants further evaluation to rule out source. Combination hormonal contraceptives may be poorly metabolized in women with hepatic impairment. Discontinue if jaundice develops during therapy or if liver function becomes abnormal. Risk of cholestasis may be increased with previous cholestatic jaundice of pregnancy or jaundice with prior oral contraceptive use. Presentation of irregular, unresolving vaginal bleeding warrants further evaluation including endometrial sampling, if indicated, to rule out malignancy. Use caution with conditions that may be aggravated by fluid retention, depression, or history of migraine. Not for use prior to menarche.

The use of estrogens and/or progestins may change the results of some laboratory tests (eg, coagulation factors, lipids, glucose tolerance, binding proteins). The dose, route, and the specific estrogen/progestin influences these changes. In addition, personal risk factors (eg, cardiovascular disease, smoking, diabetes, age) also contribute to adverse events; use of specific products may be contraindicated in women with certain risk factors.

The minimum dosage combination of estrogen/progestin that will effectively treat the individual patient should be used. New patients should be started on products containing ≤0.035 mg of estrogen per tablet.

Acne: For use only in females ≥15 years of age, who also desire combination hormonal contraceptive therapy, are unresponsive to topical treatments, and have no contraindications to combination hormonal contraceptive use.

Drug Interactions
Avoid Concomitant Use
Avoid concomitant use of Ethinyl Estradiol and Norgestimate with any of the following: Anastrozole; Griseofulvin; Ospemifene; Pimozide; Pirfenidone

Increased Effect/Toxicity
Ethinyl Estradiol and Norgestimate may increase the levels/effects of: ARIPiprazole; Benzodiazepines (metabolized by oxidation); Corticosteroids (Systemic); CYP1A2 Substrates; Lomitapide; Ospemifene; Pimozide; Pirfenidone; ROPINIRole; Selegiline; Theophylline Derivatives; Tipranavir; TiZANidine; Tranexamic Acid; Voriconazole

The levels/effects of Ethinyl Estradiol and Norgestimate may be increased by: Ascorbic Acid; Atazanavir; Boceprevir; Cobicistat; Herbs (Estrogenic Properties); Herbs (Progestogenic Properties); Mifepristone; NSAID (COX-2 Inhibitor); Voriconazole

Decreased Effect
Ethinyl Estradiol and Norgestimate may decrease the levels/effects of: Anastrozole; Chenodiol; Hyaluronidase; LamoTRIgine; Ospemifene; Thyroid Products; Ursodiol; Vitamin K Antagonists

The levels/effects of Ethinyl Estradiol and Norgestimate may be decreased by: Acitretin; Aminoglutethimide; Aprepitant; Armodafinil; Artemether; Barbiturates; Bexarotene (Systemic); Bile Acid Sequestrants; Boceprevir; Bosentan; CarBAMazepine; CloBAZam; Cobicistat; Colesevelam; CYP3A4 Inducers (Strong); Deferasirox; Efavirenz; Elvitegravir; Exenatide; Felbamate; Fosaprepitant; Fosphenytoin; Griseofulvin; LamoTRIgine; Mifepristone; Modafinil;

Mycophenolate; Nafcillin; Nevirapine; OXcarbazepine; Perampanel; Phenytoin; Protease Inhibitors; Prucalopride; Retinoic Acid Derivatives; Rifamycin Derivatives; Rufinamide; St Johns Wort; Telaprevir; Tipranavir; Tocilizumab; Topiramate

Ethanol/Nutrition/Herb Interactions

Food: CNS effects of caffeine may be enhanced if combination hormonal contraceptives are used concurrently with caffeine. Grapefruit juice increases ethinyl estradiol concentrations and would be expected to increase progesterone serum levels as well; clinical implications are unclear.

Herb/Nutraceutical: St John's wort may decrease levels. Herbs with estrogenic properties may enhance the adverse/toxic effect of estrogen derivatives; examples include alfalfa, black cohosh, bloodroot, hops, kudzu, licorice, red clover, saw palmetto, soybean, thyme, wild yam, yucca. Herbs with progestogenic properties may enhance the adverse/toxic effect of progestins; examples include bloodroot, chasteberry, damiana, oregano, yucca.

Dietary Considerations Should be taken at same time each day.

Pharmacodynamics/Kinetics

Half-life Elimination EE: 10-16 hours; NGMN: 18-25 hours; NG: 38-45 hours

Time to Peak EE and NGM: ~2 hours

Pregnancy Risk Factor X

Pregnancy Considerations Pregnancy should be ruled out prior to treatment and discontinued if pregnancy occurs. In general, the use of combination hormonal contraceptives when inadvertently taken early in pregnancy have not been associated with teratogenic effects. Hormonal contraceptives may be less effective in obese patients. An increase in oral contraceptive failure was noted in women with a BMI >27.3 kg/m^2. Similar findings were noted in patients weighing ≥90 kg (198 lb) using the contraceptive patch.

Due to increased risk of venous thromboembolism (VTE) postpartum, combination hormonal contraceptives should not be started in any woman <21 days following delivery. Women without risk factors for VTE and who are not breast-feeding may start combination hormonal contraceptives during 21-42 days postpartum. After 42 days postpartum, restrictions for use are not related to postpartum status and should be based on other medical conditions (CDC, 2011).

Lactation Enters breast milk/not recommended

Breast-Feeding Considerations Jaundice and breast enlargement in the nursing infant have been reported following the use of combination hormonal contraceptives. May decrease the quality and quantity of breast milk; a nonhormonal form of contraception is recommended (per manufacturer). The theoretical concerns about decreased milk production are greatest early in the postpartum period when milk production is being established. Postpartum risk status for VTE should be considered when initiating combination hormonal contraceptives after delivery. Combined hormonal contraceptives should not be started <21 days postpartum due to increased risk of VTE. Risk of VTE is still elevated in breast-feeding women until ~42 days postpartum and is greater in women with additional risk factors. After 42 days postpartum, restrictions for use are not related to postpartum VTE risk and should be based on other medical conditions (CDC, 2011).

Dosage Forms

Tablet, oral [monophasic formulation]:

Estarylla™: Ethinyl estradiol 0.035 mg and norgestimate 0.25 mg [21 blue tablets and 7 green inactive tablets] (28s)

MonoNessa®, Ortho-Cyclen®: Ethinyl estradiol 0.035 mg and norgestimate 0.25 mg [21 blue tablets and 7 dark green inactive tablets] (28s)

Previfem®: Ethinyl estradiol 0.035 mg and norgestimate 0.25 mg [21 blue tablets and 7 light green inactive tablets] (28s)

Sprintec®: Ethinyl estradiol 0.035 mg and norgestimate 0.25 mg [21 blue tablets and 7 white inactive tablets] (28s)

Tablet, oral [triphasic formulation]:

Ortho Tri-Cyclen®, TriNessa®:
Day 1-7: Ethinyl estradiol 0.035 mg and norgestimate 0.18 mg [7 white tablets]
Day 8-14: Ethinyl estradiol 0.035 mg and norgestimate 0.215 mg [7 light blue tablets]
Day 15-21: Ethinyl estradiol 0.035 mg and norgestimate 0.25 mg [7 blue tablets]
Day 22-28: 7 dark green inactive tablets (28s)

Tri-Estarylla™
Day 1-7: Ethinyl estradiol 0.035 mg and norgestimate 0.18 mg [7 white tablets]
Day 8-14: Ethinyl estradiol 0.035 mg and norgestimate 0.215 mg [7 light blue tablets]
Day 15-21: Ethinyl estradiol 0.035 mg and norgestimate 0.25 mg [7 blue tablets]
Day 22-28: 7 green inactive tablets (28s)

Tri-Previfem®::
Day 1-7: Ethinyl estradiol 0.035 mg and norgestimate 0.18 mg [7 white tablets]
Day 8-14: Ethinyl estradiol 0.035 mg and norgestimate 0.215 mg [7 light blue tablets]
Day 15-21: Ethinyl estradiol 0.035 mg and norgestimate 0.25 mg [7 blue tablets]
Day 22-28: 7 light green inactive tablets (28s)

Tri-Sprintec®:
Day 1-7: Ethinyl estradiol 0.035 mg and norgestimate 0.18 mg [7 gray tablets]
Day 8-14: Ethinyl estradiol 0.035 mg and norgestimate 0.215 mg [7 light blue tablets]
Day 15-21: Ethinyl estradiol 0.035 mg and norgestimate 0.25 mg [7 blue tablets]
Day 22-28: 7 white inactive tablets (28s)

Ortho Tri-Cyclen® Lo:
Day 1-7: Ethinyl estradiol 0.025 mg and norgestimate 0.18 mg [7 white tablets]
Day 8-14: Ethinyl estradiol 0.025 mg and norgestimate 0.215 mg [7 light blue tablets]
Day 15-21: Ethinyl estradiol 0.025 mg and norgestimate 0.25 mg [7 dark blue tablets]
Day 22-28: 7 dark green inactive tablets (28s)

Ethinyl Estradiol and Norgestrel
(ETH in il es tra DYE ole & nor JES trel)

Brand Names: U.S. Cryselle® 28; Lo/Ovral®-28; Low-Ogestrel®; Ogestrel®

Brand Names: Canada Lo-Femenal 21; Ovral®

Generic Availability (U.S.) Yes

Pharmacologic Category Contraceptive; Estrogen and Progestin Combination

Use Prevention of pregnancy; postcoital contraceptive or "morning after" pill

Unlabeled Use Treatment of hypermenorrhea (menorrhagia); pain associated with endometriosis; dysmenorrhea; dysfunctional uterine bleeding

Local Anesthetic/Vasoconstrictor Precautions No information available to require special precautions

Effects on Dental Treatment When prescribing antibiotics, patient must be warned to use additional methods of birth control if on oral contraceptives.

Effects on Bleeding No information available to require special precautions

Adverse Effects Frequency not defined.

Cardiovascular: Arterial thromboembolism, cerebral hemorrhage, cerebral thrombosis, edema, hypertension, mesenteric thrombosis, MI

Central nervous system: Depression, dizziness, headache, migraine, nervousness, premenstrual syndrome, stroke

Dermatologic: Acne, erythema multiforme, erythema nodosum, hirsutism, loss of scalp hair, melasma (may persist), rash (allergic)

Endocrine & metabolic: Amenorrhea, breakthrough bleeding, breast enlargement, breast secretion, breast tenderness, carbohydrate intolerance, lactation decreased (postpartum), glucose tolerance decreased, libido changes, menstrual flow changes, sex hormone-binding globulins (SHBG) increased, spotting, temporary infertility (following discontinuation), thyroid-binding globulin increased, triglycerides increased

Gastrointestinal: Abdominal cramps, appetite changes, bloating, cholestasis, colitis, gallbladder disease, jaundice, nausea, vomiting, weight gain/loss

Genitourinary: Cervical erosion changes, cervical secretion changes, cystitis-like syndrome, vaginal candidiasis, vaginitis

Hematologic: Antithrombin III decreased, folate levels decreased, hemolytic uremic syndrome, norepinephrine induced platelet aggregability increased, porphyria, prothrombin increased; factors VII, VIII, IX, and X

Hepatic: Benign liver tumors, Budd-Chiari syndrome, cholestatic jaundice, hepatic adenomas

Local: Thrombophlebitis

Ocular: Cataracts, change in corneal curvature (steepening), contact lens intolerance, optic neuritis, retinal thrombosis

Renal: Impaired renal function

Respiratory: Pulmonary thromboembolism

Miscellaneous: Hemorrhagic eruption

Dosage Oral: Adults: Females:

Contraception:

Schedule 1 (Sunday starter): Dose begins on first Sunday after onset of menstruation; if the menstrual period starts on Sunday, take first tablet that very same day. **With a Sunday start, an additional method of contraception should be used until after the first 7 days of consecutive administration.**

For 21-tablet package: Dosage is 1 tablet daily for 21 consecutive days, followed by 7 days off of the medication; a new course begins on the 8th day after the last tablet is taken.

For 28-tablet package: Dosage is 1 tablet daily without interruption.

Schedule 2 (Day 1 starter): Dose starts on first day of menstrual cycle taking 1 tablet daily.

For 21-tablet package: Dosage is 1 tablet daily for 21 consecutive days, followed by 7 days off of the medication; a new course begins on the 8th day after the last tablet is taken.

For 28-tablet package: Dosage is 1 tablet daily without interruption.

If all doses have been taken on schedule and one menstrual period is missed, continue dosing cycle. If two consecutive menstrual periods are missed, pregnancy test is required before new dosing cycle is started.

Missed doses **monophasic formulations** (refer to package insert for complete information):

One dose missed: Take as soon as remembered or take 2 tablets next day

Two consecutive doses missed in the first 2 weeks: Take 2 tablets as soon as remembered or 2 tablets next 2 days. **An additional method of contraception should be used for 7 days after missed dose.**

Two consecutive doses missed in week 3 or three consecutive doses missed at any time:

Schedule 1 (Sunday starter): Continue to take 1 tablet daily until Sunday, then discard the rest of the pack, and a new pack is started that same day.

Schedule 2 (Day 1 starter): Current pack should be discarded, and a new pack started that same day. **An additional method of contraception should be used for 7 days after missed dose.**

Postcoital contraception:

Ethinyl estradiol 0.03 mg and norgestrel 0.3 mg formulation: 4 tablets within 72 hours of unprotected intercourse and 4 tablets 12 hours after first dose

Ethinyl estradiol 0.05 mg and norgestrel 0.5 mg formulation: 2 tablets within 72 hours of unprotected intercourse and 2 tablets 12 hours after first dose

Dosage adjustment in renal impairment: Specific guidelines not available; use with caution and monitor blood pressure closely. Consider other forms of contraception.

Dosage adjustment in hepatic impairment: Contraindicated in patients with hepatic impairment.

Mechanism of Action Combination hormonal contraceptives inhibit ovulation via a negative feedback mechanism on the hypothalamus, which alters the normal pattern of gonadotropin secretion of a follicle-stimulating hormone (FSH) and luteinizing hormone by the anterior pituitary. The follicular phase FSH and midcycle surge of gonadotropins are inhibited. In addition, combination hormonal contraceptives produce alterations in the genital tract, including changes in the cervical mucus, rendering it unfavorable for sperm penetration even if ovulation occurs. Changes in the endometrium may also occur, producing an unfavorable environment for nidation. Combination hormonal contraceptive drugs may alter the tubal transport of the ova through the fallopian tubes. Progestational agents may also alter sperm fertility.

Contraindications Hypersensitivity to ethinyl estradiol, norgestrel, or any component of the formulation; breast cancer or other estrogen- or progestin-dependent neoplasms (current or a history of), hepatic tumors or disease, pregnancy, undiagnosed abnormal uterine bleeding, cholestatic jaundice of pregnancy, jaundice with prior combination hormonal contraceptive use

Use is also contraindicated in women at high risk of arterial or venous thrombotic diseases including: Cerebrovascular disease, coronary artery disease, diabetes mellitus with vascular disease, DVT or PE (current or history of), hypercoagulopathies (inherited or acquired), headaches with focal neurological symptoms, hypertension (uncontrolled), thrombogenic valvular or rhythm diseases of the heart, major surgery with prolonged immobilization

Warnings/Precautions Hazardous agent - use appropriate precautions for handling and disposal (NIOSH, 2012). Combination hormonal contraceptives do not protect against HIV infection or other sexually-transmitted diseases. **[U.S. Boxed Warning]: The risk of cardiovascular side effects is increased in women who smoke cigarettes; risk increases with age (especially women >35 years of age) and the number of cigarettes smoked; women who use combination hormonal contraceptives should be strongly advised not to smoke. Should not be used in patients >35 years of age who smoke.** Combination hormonal contraceptives may lead to increased risk of myocardial infarction, use with caution in patients with risk factors for coronary artery disease (eg, hypertension, hypercholesterolemia, morbid obesity, diabetes, or women who smoke). May increase the risk of thromboembolism; discontinue use of combination hormonal contraceptives if an arterial or venous thrombotic event occurs. Women with inherited thrombophilias (eg, protein C or S deficiency) may have increased risk of venous thromboembolism (DeSancho, 2010; van Vlijmen, 2011). Whenever possible, combination hormonal contraceptives should be discontinued at least 4 weeks prior to and for 2 weeks following elective surgery associated with an increased risk of thromboembolism or during periods of prolonged immobilization. Combination hormonal contraceptives may have a dose-related risk of vascular disease, hypertension, and gallbladder disease. Women with hypertension or renal disease should be encouraged to use another form of contraception. The use of combination hormonal contraceptives has been associated with a slight increase in frequency of breast cancer; however, studies are not consistent. Use is contraindicated in women with (or history of) breast cancer.

Combination hormonal contraceptives may cause glucose intolerance or affect serum triglyceride and lipoprotein levels. Estrogens may increase thyroid-binding globulin (TBG) levels leading to increased circulating total thyroid hormone levels. Women on thyroid replacement therapy may require higher doses of thyroid hormone while receiving estrogens. Estrogens may cause retinal vascular thrombosis; discontinue if migraine, loss of vision, proptosis, diplopia or other visual disturbances occur; discontinue permanently if papilledema or retinal vascular lesions are observed on examination. Use caution with conditions that may be aggravated by fluid retention, depression, or history of migraine. Extremely rare adenomas and focal nodular hyperplasia resulting in fatal intra-abdominal hemorrhage have been reported in association with long-term oral contraceptive use. Presentation of an abdominal mass, acute abdominal pain, or intra-abdominal bleeding warrants further evaluation to rule out source. Combination hormonal contraceptives may be poorly metabolized in women with hepatic impairment. Discontinue if jaundice develops during therapy or if liver function becomes abnormal. Risk of cholestasis may be increased with previous cholestatic jaundice of pregnancy or jaundice with prior oral contraceptive use. The use of estrogens and/or progestins may change the results of some laboratory tests (eg, coagulation factors, lipids, glucose tolerance, binding proteins). The dose, route, and the specific estrogen/progestin influences these changes. In addition, personal risk factors (eg, cardiovascular disease, smoking, diabetes, age) also contribute to adverse events; use of specific products may be contraindicated in women with certain risk factors.

Not for use prior to menarche. Presentation of irregular, unresolving vaginal bleeding warrants further evaluation including endometrial sampling, if indicated, to rule out malignancy.

The minimum dosage combination of estrogen/progestin that will effectively treat the individual patient should be used. New patients should be started on products containing ≤0.035 mg of estrogen per tablet.

Drug Interactions

Avoid Concomitant Use

Avoid concomitant use of Ethinyl Estradiol and Norgestrel with any of the following: Anastrozole; Griseofulvin; Ospemifene; Pimozide; Pirfenidone

Increased Effect/Toxicity

Ethinyl Estradiol and Norgestrel may increase the levels/effects of: ARIPiprazole; Benzodiazepines (metabolized by oxidation); Corticosteroids (Systemic); CYP1A2 Substrates; Lomitapide; Ospemifene; Pimozide; Pirfenidone; ROPINIRole; Selegiline; Theophylline Derivatives; Tipranavir; TiZANidine; Tranexamic Acid; Voriconazole

The levels/effects of Ethinyl Estradiol and Norgestrel may be increased by: Ascorbic Acid; Atazanavir; Boceprevir; Cobicistat; Herbs (Estrogenic Properties); Herbs (Progestogenic Properties); Mifepristone; NSAID (COX-2 Inhibitor); Voriconazole

Decreased Effect

Ethinyl Estradiol and Norgestrel may decrease the levels/effects of: Anastrozole; Chenodiol; Hyaluronidase; LamoTRIgine; Ospemifene; Thyroid Products; Ursodiol; Vitamin K Antagonists

The levels/effects of Ethinyl Estradiol and Norgestrel may be decreased by: Acitretin; Aminoglutethimide; Aprepitant; Armodafinil; Artemether; Barbiturates; Bexarotene (Systemic); Bile Acid Sequestrants; Boceprevir; Bosentan; CarBAMazepine; CloBAZam; Cobicistat; Colesevelam; CYP3A4 Inducers (Strong); Deferasirox; Elvitegravir; Exenatide; Felbamate; Fosaprepitant; Fosphenytoin; Griseofulvin; LamoTRIgine; Mifepristone; Modafinil; Mycophenolate; Nafcillin; Nevirapine; OXcarbazepine; Perampanel; Phenytoin; Protease Inhibitors; Prucalopride; Retinoic Acid Derivatives; Rifamycin Derivatives; Rufinamide; St Johns Wort; Telaprevir; Tipranavir; Tocilizumab; Topiramate

Ethanol/Nutrition/Herb Interactions

Food: CNS effects of caffeine may be enhanced if combination hormonal contraceptives are used concurrently with caffeine. Grapefruit juice increases ethinyl estradiol concentrations and would be expected to increase progesterone serum levels as well; clinical implications are unclear.

Herb/Nutraceutical: St John's wort may decrease levels. Herbs with estrogenic properties may enhance the adverse/toxic effect of estrogen derivatives; examples include alfalfa, black cohosh, bloodroot, hops, kudzu, licorice, red clover, saw palmetto, soybean, thyme, wild yam, yucca. Herbs with progestogenic properties may enhance the adverse/toxic effect of progestins; examples include bloodroot, chasteberry, damiana, oregano, yucca.

Dietary Considerations Should be taken at same time each day.

Pregnancy Risk Factor X

Pregnancy Considerations Pregnancy should be ruled out prior to treatment and discontinued if pregnancy occurs. In general, the use of combination hormonal contraceptives when inadvertently taken early in pregnancy have not been associated with teratogenic effects. Hormonal contraceptives may be less effective in obese patients. An increase in oral contraceptive failure was noted in women with a BMI >27.3 kg/m². Similar findings were noted in patients weighing ≥90 kg (198 lb) using the contraceptive patch.

Due to increased risk of venous thromboembolism (VTE) postpartum, combination hormonal contraceptives should not be started in any woman <21 days following delivery. Women without risk factors for VTE and who are not breast-feeding may start combination hormonal contraceptives during 21-42 days postpartum. After 42 days postpartum, restrictions for use are not related to postpartum status and should be based on other medical conditions (CDC, 2011).

Lactation Enters breast milk/not recommended

Breast-Feeding Considerations Jaundice and breast enlargement in the nursing infant have been reported following the use of combination hormonal contraceptives. May decrease the quality and quantity of breast milk; a nonhormonal form of contraception is recommended (per manufacturer). The theoretical concerns about decreased milk production are greatest early in the postpartum period when milk production is being established. Postpartum risk status for VTE should be considered when initiating combination hormonal contraceptives after delivery. Combined hormonal contraceptives should not be started <21 days postpartum due to increased risk of VTE. Risk of VTE is still elevated in breast-feeding women until ~42 days postpartum and is greater in women with additional risk factors. After 42 days postpartum, restrictions for use are not related to postpartum VTE risk and should be based on other medical conditions (CDC, 2011).

Dosage Forms

Tablet, oral [monophasic formulation]: Ethinyl estradiol 0.03 mg and norgestrel 0.3 mg [21 tablets and 7 inactive tablets] (28s)

Cryselle® 28: Ethinyl estradiol 0.03 mg and norgestrel 0.3 mg [21 white tablets and 7 light green inactive tablets] (28s)

Low-Ogestrel®: Ethinyl estradiol 0.03 mg and norgestrel 0.3 mg [21 white tablets and 7 peach inactive tablets] (28s)

Lo/Ovral®-28: Ethinyl estradiol 0.03 mg and norgestrel 0.3 mg [21 white tablets and 7 pink inactive tablets] (28s)

Ogestrel®: Ethinyl estradiol 0.05 mg and norgestrel 0.5 mg [21 white tablets and 7 peach inactive tablets] (28s)

Ethinyl Estradiol, Drospirenone, and Levomefolate

(ETH in il es tra DYE ole, droh SPYE re none, & lee voe me FOE late)

Brand Names: U.S. Beyaz™; Safyral™

Pharmacologic Category Contraceptive; Estrogen and Progestin Combination

Use Prevention of pregnancy; treatment of premenstrual dysphoric disorder (PMDD); treatment of acne; folate supplementation

Unlabeled Use Treatment of hypermenorrhea (menorrhagia); pain associated with endometriosis; dysmenorrhea; dysfunctional uterine bleeding

Local Anesthetic/Vasoconstrictor Precautions No information available to require special precautions

Effects on Dental Treatment When prescribing antibiotics, patient must be warned to use additional methods of birth control if on oral contraceptives.

Effects on Bleeding No information available to require special precautions

Adverse Effects Note: Percentages reported with Beyaz™

>10%:

Central nervous system: Headache/migraine (6% to 13%)

Endocrine & metabolic: Menstrual irregularities (4% to 25%, including menorrhagia, metrorrhagia, spotting, vaginal hemorrhage), breast pain/tenderness (3% to 11%)

Gastrointestinal: Nausea/vomiting (4% to 16%)

1% to 10%:

Central nervous system: Fatigue (4%), irritability (3%), affect lability (2%)

Endocrine & metabolic: Libido decreased (3%)

Gastrointestinal: Weight gain (3%)

Frequency not defined: Cervical dysplasia, cervix carcinoma stage 0

For additional adverse events and postmarketing reports, refer to the Ethinyl Estradiol and Drospirenone (Yasmin®, Yaz®) monograph.

Dosage Oral:

Children ≥14 years and Adults: Females: Acne (Beyaz™): Refer to dosing for contraception

Adults: Females: PMDD (Beyaz™): Refer to dosing for contraception

Adults: Females: Contraception (Beyaz™, Safyral™): Dosage is 1 tablet daily

Beyaz™: One pink tablet daily for 24 consecutive days, then one light orange tablet daily on days 25-28

Safyral™: One orange tablet daily for 21 consecutive days, then one light orange tablet daily on days 22-28

Dose should be taken at the same time each day, either after the evening meal or at bedtime. Dosing may be started on the first day of menstrual period (Day 1 starter) or on the first Sunday after the onset of the menstrual period (Sunday starter).

Day 1 starter: Dose starts on first day of menstrual cycle taking 1 tablet daily. If first dose is taken later than the first day of the menstrual cycle, **an additional method of contraception should be used until after the first 7 days of consecutive administration.**

Sunday starter: Dose begins on first Sunday after onset of menstruation; if the menstrual period starts on Sunday, take first tablet that very same day. **With a Sunday start, an additional method of contraception should be used until after the first 7 days of consecutive administration.**

Switching from a different contraceptive:

Oral contraceptive: Start on the same day that a new pack of the previous oral contraceptive would have been taken

Transdermal patch, vaginal ring, injection: Start on the day the next dose would have been due

IUD or implant: Start on the day of removal

Use after childbirth (in women who are not breast-feeding) or after second trimester abortion: Therapy may be started ≥4 weeks postpartum. Pregnancy should be ruled out prior to treatment if menstrual periods have not restarted and an additional method of contraception (nonhormonal) should be used until after the first 7 days of consecutive administration.

Missed doses:

If all doses have been taken on schedule and one menstrual period is missed, continue dosing cycle. If two consecutive menstrual periods are missed, rule out pregnancy and discontinue if pregnancy is confirmed.

If doses have been missed during the first 3 weeks or if active tablets (pink tablets) were started later than as directed and the menstrual period is missed, pregnancy should be ruled out prior to continuing treatment.

Missed doses (monophasic formulations) (refer to package insert for complete information):

One dose missed: Take as soon as remembered or take 2 tablets next day

Two consecutive doses missed in the first 2 weeks: Take 2 tablets as soon as remembered or 2 tablets next 2 days. **An additional method of contraception should be used for 7 days after missed dose.**

Two consecutive doses missed in week 3 or three consecutive doses missed at any time: **An additional method of contraception must be used for 7 days after a missed dose.**

Day 1 starter: Current pack should be discarded, and a new pack should be started that same day.

Sunday starter: Continue dose of 1 tablet daily until Sunday, then discard the rest of the pack, and a new pack should be started that same day.

Any number of doses missed in week 4: Throw away the pills that were missed. Continue taking one pill each day until pack is empty; no back-up method of contraception is needed

Dosage adjustment in renal impairment: Contraindicated in patients with renal dysfunction

Dosage adjustment in hepatic impairment: Contraindicated in patients with hepatic disease. Exposure to drospirenone is ~3 times higher with moderate liver impairment; information not available for severe impairment.

Mechanism of Action Combination oral contraceptives inhibit ovulation via a negative feedback mechanism on the hypothalamus, which alters the normal pattern of gonadotropin secretion of a follicle-stimulating hormone (FSH) and luteinizing hormone by the anterior pituitary. The follicular phase FSH and midcycle surge of gonadotropins are inhibited. In addition, oral contraceptives produce alterations in the genital tract, including changes in the cervical mucus, rendering it unfavorable for sperm penetration even if ovulation occurs. Changes in the endometrium may also occur, producing an unfavorable environment for nidation. Oral contraceptive drugs may alter the tubal transport of the ova through the fallopian tubes. Progestational agents may also alter sperm fertility. Drospirenone is a spironolactone analogue with antimineralocorticoid and antiandrogenic activity.

Contraindications Adrenal insufficiency, breast cancer or other estrogen- or progestin-dependent neoplasms (current or a history of), hepatic tumors or disease, pregnancy, renal impairment, undiagnosed abnormal uterine bleeding. Use is also contraindicated in women at high risk of arterial or venous thrombotic diseases including: Cerebrovascular disease, coronary artery disease, diabetes mellitus with vascular disease, DVT or PE (current or history of), hypercoagulopathies (inherited or acquired), headaches with focal neurological symptoms, hypertension (uncontrolled), migraine headaches if >35 years of age, thrombogenic valvular or rhythm diseases of the heart (eg, subacute bacterial endocarditis with valvular disease or atrial fibrillation), women >35 years of age who smoke.

Warnings/Precautions Hazardous agent - use appropriate precautions for handling and disposal (NIOSH, 2012). **[U.S. Boxed Warning]: The risk of cardiovascular side effects is increased in women who smoke cigarettes; risk increases with age (especially women >35 years of age) and the number of cigarettes smoked; women who use combination hormonal contraceptives should be strongly advised not to smoke. Use is contraindicated in patients >35 years of age who smoke.** Use with caution in patients with risk factors for coronary artery disease (eg, hypertension, hypercholesterolemia, morbid obesity, diabetes, or women who smoke); may lead to increased risk of myocardial infarction or stroke. May have a dose-related risk of vascular disease and hypertension; women with hypertension should be encouraged to use another form of contraception. Monitor women with well-controlled hypertension and discontinue if blood pressure rises significantly. Use is contraindicated with uncontrolled hypertension or hypertension with vascular disease. Contraceptives may increase the risk of thromboembolism. Discontinue if an arterial or deep venous thrombotic event occurs. Risk may be greater with contraceptives containing drospirenone. Women with inherited thrombophilias (eg, protein C or S deficiency) may have increased risk of venous thromboembolism (DeSancho, 2010; van Vlijmen, 2011). Use is contraindicated in women with hypercoagulopathies (inherited or acquired). Estrogens may induce or exacerbate symptoms of angioedema in women with hereditary angioedema.

Steroid hormones are poorly metabolized in patients with hepatic dysfunction. Discontinue if jaundice develops or if acute or chronic hepatic disturbances occur. Use is contraindicated with hepatic disease. Cholestasis may occur in women with a history of pregnancy related or previous oral contraceptive related cholestasis. Drospirenone has antimineralocorticoid activity that may lead to hyperkalemia in patients with renal insufficiency, hepatic dysfunction, or adrenal insufficiency; use caution with medications that may increase serum potassium. Combination hormonal contraceptives may affect serum triglyceride and lipoprotein levels. Estrogen compounds are generally associated with lipid effects such as increased HDL-cholesterol and decreased LDL-cholesterol. Progestins may be associated with decreased HDL-cholesterol. Triglycerides may also be increased; use with caution in patients with familial defects of lipoprotein metabolism. Combination hormonal contraceptives may have adverse effects on glucose tolerance; use caution in women with diabetes. Use may have a dose-related risk of gallbladder disease. Estrogens may increase thyroid-binding globulin (TBG) levels leading to increased circulating total thyroid hormone levels. Women on thyroid replacement therapy may require higher doses of thyroid hormone while receiving estrogens.

The use of combination hormonal contraceptives has been associated with a slight increase in frequency of breast cancer; however, studies are not consistent. Use is contraindicated in women with breast cancer (current or history of). Extremely rare adenomas and focal nodular hyperplasia resulting in fatal intra-abdominal hemorrhage have been reported in association with long-term oral contraceptive use. Presentation of an abdominal mass, acute abdominal pain, or intra-abdominal bleeding warrants further evaluation to rule out source.

Estrogens may cause retinal vascular thrombosis; discontinue if migraine, loss of vision, proptosis, diplopia or other visual disturbances occur; discontinue permanently if papilledema or retinal vascular lesions are observed on examination. Use with caution in patients with a history of migraine. Evaluate new, recurrent, severe, or persistent headaches. Use is contraindicated in women with headaches with focal neurological symptoms or migraine headaches if >35 years of age. Use with caution in patients with diseases which may be exacerbated by fluid retention, including asthma, epilepsy, diabetes or renal dysfunction; use with caution in patients with depression. Use caution with a history of chloasma gravidarum; women with a tendency to chloasma should avoid sun and ultraviolet radiation exposure during therapy.

Unscheduled bleeding/spotting may occur within the first 3 months of use. Presentation of irregular, unresolving vaginal bleeding following previously regular cycles warrants further evaluation including endometrial sampling, if indicated, to rule out malignancy. Inform patients that oral contraceptives do not protect against HIV infection or other sexually-transmitted diseases. The minimum dosage combination of estrogen/progestin that will effectively treat the individual patient should be used. Not for use prior to menarche. Whenever possible, should be discontinued at least 4 weeks prior to and for 2 weeks following elective surgery associated with an increased risk of thromboembolism or during periods of prolonged immobilization. The use of estrogens and/or progestins may change the results of some laboratory tests (eg, coagulation factors, lipids, glucose tolerance, binding proteins). Drospirenone also can caused an increase in plasma renin activity and plasma aldosterone. Folates may mask vitamin B12 deficiency. The dose, route, and the specific estrogen/progestin influences these changes. In addition, personal risk factors (eg, cardiovascular disease, smoking, diabetes, age) also contribute to adverse events; use of specific products may be contraindicated in women with certain risk factors.

Acne use: For use only in females ≥14 years of age who have reached menarche, who also desire combination hormonal contraceptive therapy.

PMDD use: For use only in females who desire combination hormonal contraceptive therapy; use for more than 3 menstrual cycles has not been evaluated. Has not been evaluated for the treatment of premenstrual syndrome.

Drug Interactions

Avoid Concomitant Use

Avoid concomitant use of Ethinyl Estradiol, Drospirenone, and Levomefolate with any of the following: Anastrozole; Boceprevir; CycloSPORINE (Systemic); Griseofulvin; Ospemifene; Pimozide; Pirfenidone; Raltitrexed; Tacrolimus (Systemic)

Increased Effect/Toxicity

Ethinyl Estradiol, Drospirenone, and Levomefolate may increase the levels/effects of: ACE Inhibitors; Amifostine; Ammonium Chloride; Antihypertensives; ARIPiprazole; Benzodiazepines (metabolized by oxidation); Cardiac Glycosides; Corticosteroids (Systemic); CycloSPORINE (Systemic); CYP1A2 Substrates; Hypotensive Agents; Lomitapide; Ospemifene; Pimozide; Pirfenidone; Potassium-Sparing Diuretics; RiTUXimab; ROPINIRole; Selegiline; Sodium Phosphates; Tacrolimus (Systemic); Theophylline Derivatives; Tipranavir; TiZANidine; Tranexamic Acid; Voriconazole

The levels/effects of Ethinyl Estradiol, Drospirenone, and Levomefolate may be increased by: Alfuzosin; Angiotensin II Receptor Blockers; Ascorbic Acid; Atazanavir; Boceprevir; Canagliflozin; Cobicistat; Diazoxide; Eplerenone; Herbs (Estrogenic Properties); Herbs (Hypotensive Properties); Herbs (Progestogenic Properties); MAO Inhibitors; Mifepristone; Nonsteroidal Anti-Inflammatory Agents; NSAID (COX-2 Inhibitor); Pentoxifylline; Phosphodiesterase 5 Inhibitors; Potassium Salts; Prostacyclin Analogues; Tolvaptan; Voriconazole

Decreased Effect

Ethinyl Estradiol, Drospirenone, and Levomefolate may decrease the levels/effects of: Anastrozole; Cardiac Glycosides; Chenodiol; Fosphenytoin; Hyaluronidase; LamoTRIgine; Ospemifene; PHENobarbital; Phenytoin; Primidone; QuiNIDine; Raltitrexed; Thyroid Products; Ursodiol; Vitamin K Antagonists

The levels/effects of Ethinyl Estradiol, Drospirenone, and Levomefolate may be decreased by: Acitretin; Aminoglutethimide; Aprepitant; Armodafinil; Artemether; Barbiturates; Bexarotene (Systemic); Bile Acid Sequestrants; Boceprevir; Bosentan; CarBAMazepine; CloBAZam; Cobicistat; Colesevelam; CYP3A4 Inducers (Strong); Deferasirox; Elvitegravir; Exenatide; Felbamate; Fosaprepitant; Fosphenytoin; Griseofulvin; Herbs (Hypertensive Properties); LamoTRIgine; Methylphenidate; Mifepristone; Modafinil; Mycophenolate; Nafcillin; Nevirapine; Nonsteroidal Anti-Inflammatory Agents; OXcarbazepine; Perampanel; Phenytoin; Protease Inhibitors; Prucalopride; Retinoic Acid Derivatives; Rifamycin Derivatives; Rufinamide; St Johns Wort; Telaprevir; Tipranavir; Tocilizumab; Topiramate; Yohimbine

Ethanol/Nutrition/Herb Interactions

Food: CNS effects of caffeine may be enhanced if oral contraceptives are used concurrently with caffeine. Grapefruit juice increases ethinyl estradiol plasma concentrations; clinical implications are unclear. Food decreases the maximum plasma concentrations of drospirenone and ethinyl estradiol by ~40%.

Herb/Nutraceutical: St John's wort may decrease levels. Herbs with estrogenic properties may enhance the adverse/toxic effect of estrogen derivatives; examples include alfalfa, black cohosh, bloodroot, hops, kudzu, licorice, red clover, saw palmetto, soybean, thyme, wild yam, yucca. Herbs with progestogenic properties may enhance the adverse/toxic effect of progestins; examples include bloodroot, chasteberry, damiana, oregano, yucca.

Dietary Considerations

Should be taken at the same time each day; may be taken with or without a meal. Consider other sources of folic acid and ensure supplementation continues once therapy is discontinued. The RDA for folate in women 14–50 years of age is 400 mcg/day of dietary folate equivalents. The USPSTF recommends that all women of reproductive potential should take a supplement containing folic acid 400-800 mcg/day in order to decrease the risk of neural tube defects.

Pharmacodynamics/Kinetics

Half-life Elimination Terminal: Drospirenone: ~31 hours; Ethinyl estradiol: ~24 hours; levomefolate calcium: ~4-5 hours

Time to Peak Drospirenone, ethinyl estradiol: 1-2 hours; Levomefolate calcium: 0.5-1.5 hours

Pregnancy Considerations In general, the use of oral contraceptives when inadvertently taken early in pregnancy have not been associated with teratogenic effects. The addition of levomefolate in this product is intended to decrease the risk of neural tube defects if pregnancy inadvertently occurs during therapy or shortly after discontinuation. Hormonal contraceptives may be less effective in obese patients. An increase in oral contraceptive failure was noted in women with a BMI >27.3 kg/m^2. Similar findings were noted in patients weighing ≥90 kg (198 lb) using the contraceptive patch.

Due to increased risk of venous thromboembolism (VTE) postpartum, combination hormonal contraceptives should not be started in any woman <21 days following delivery. Women without risk factors for VTE and who are not breast-feeding may start combination hormonal contraceptives during 21-42 days postpartum. After 42 days postpartum, restrictions for use are not related to postpartum status and should be based on other medical conditions (CDC, 2011). The manufacturer states that combination hormonal contraceptives should not be started until ≥4 weeks after delivery in women who choose not to breastfeed, or ≥4 weeks after a second trimester abortion or miscarriage.

Lactation Enters breast milk/not recommended

Breast-Feeding Considerations The amount of drospirenone excreted in breast milk is ~0.02%, resulting in a maximum of ~3 mcg/day drospirenone to the infant. Jaundice and breast enlargement in the nursing infant have been reported following the use of other oral contraceptives. In addition, may decrease the quality and quantity of breast milk. Other forms of contraception are recommended while breast-feeding (per manufacturer). The theoretical concerns about decreased milk production are greatest early in the postpartum period when milk production is being established. Postpartum risk status for VTE should be considered when initiating combination hormonal contraceptives after delivery. Combined hormonal contraceptives should not be started <21 days postpartum due to increased risk of VTE. Risk of VTE is still elevated in breast-feeding women until ~42 days postpartum and is greater in women with additional risk factors. After 42 days postpartum, restrictions for use not related to postpartum VTE risk and should be based on other medical conditions (CDC, 2011).

Dosage Forms

Tablet, oral:

Beyaz™: Ethinyl estradiol 0.02 mg, drospirenone 3 mg, and levomefolate calcium 0.451 mg [24 pink tablets] and levomefolate calcium 0.451 mg [4 light orange tablets] (28s)

Safyral™: Ethinyl estradiol 0.03 mg, drospirenone 3 mg, and levomefolate calcium 0.451 mg [21 orange tablets] and levomefolate calcium 0.451 mg [7 light orange tablets] (28s)

Ethionamide (e thye on AM ide)

Brand Names: U.S. Trecator®
Brand Names: Canada Trecator®
Pharmacologic Category Antitubercular Agent
Use Treatment of tuberculosis and other mycobacterial diseases, in conjunction with other antituberculosis agents, when first-line agents have failed or resistance has been demonstrated

Local Anesthetic/Vasoconstrictor Precautions No information available to require special precautions

Effects on Dental Treatment Key adverse event(s) related to dental treatment: Postural hypotension, metallic taste, and stomatitis.

Effects on Bleeding No information available to require special precautions

Adverse Effects Frequency not defined.
Cardiovascular: Orthostatic hypotension
Central nervous system: Depression, dizziness, drowsiness, headache, psychiatric disturbances, restlessness, seizure
Dermatologic: Acne, alopecia, photosensitivity, purpura, rash
Endocrine & metabolic: Gynecomastia, hypoglycemia, hypothyroidism or goiter, menstrual irregularities, pellagra-like syndrome
Gastrointestinal: Abdominal pain, anorexia, diarrhea, excessive salivation, metallic taste, nausea, stomatitis, vomiting, weight loss
Genitourinary: Impotence
Hematologic: Leukopenia, thrombocytopenia
Hepatic: Bilirubin increased, hepatitis, jaundice, liver function tests increased
Neuromuscular & skeletal: Arthralgia, peripheral neuritis
Ocular: Blurred vision, diplopia, optic neuritis
Respiratory: Olfactory disturbances
Miscellaneous: Hypersensitivity reaction

General Dosage Range Dosage adjustment recommended in patients with renal impairment
Oral:
Children: 15-20 mg/kg/day in 2-3 divided doses (maximum: 1 g/day)
Adults: 250-750 mg/day in 1-4 divided doses (maximum: 1 g/day)

Mechanism of Action Inhibits peptide synthesis; bacteriostatic

Pharmacodynamics/Kinetics
Half-life Elimination 2 hours
Time to Peak Serum: 1 hour
Pregnancy Risk Factor C
Pregnancy Considerations Ethionamide crosses the placenta; teratogenic effects were observed in animal studies. Use during pregnancy is not recommended.

Ethosuximide (eth oh SUKS i mide)

Brand Names: U.S. Zarontin®
Brand Names: Canada Zarontin®
Pharmacologic Category Anticonvulsant, Succinimide
Use Management of absence (petit mal) seizures

Local Anesthetic/Vasoconstrictor Precautions No information available to require special precautions

Effects on Dental Treatment No significant effects or complications reported

Effects on Bleeding No information available to require special precautions

Adverse Effects Frequency not defined.
Central nervous system: Aggressiveness, ataxia, concentration impaired, dizziness, drowsiness, euphoria, fatigue, headache, hyperactivity, irritability, lethargy, mental depression (with cases of overt suicidal intentions), night terrors, paranoid psychosis, sleep disturbance
Dermatologic: Hirsutism, pruritus, rash, Stevens-Johnson syndrome, urticaria
Endocrine & metabolic: Libido increased
Gastrointestinal: Abdominal pain, anorexia, cramps, diarrhea, epigastric pain, gastric upset, gum hypertrophy, nausea, tongue swelling, vomiting, weight loss
Genitourinary: Hematuria (microscopic), vaginal bleeding
Hematologic: Agranulocytosis, eosinophilia, leukopenia, pancytopenia
Ocular: Myopia

Miscellaneous: Allergic reaction, drug rash with eosinophilia and systemic symptoms (DRESS), hiccups, systemic lupus erythematosus

General Dosage Range Oral:
Children 3-6 years: Initial: 250 mg/day; Maintenance: 20 mg/kg/day (maximum: 1.5 g/day in divided doses)
Children ≥6 years: Initial: 500 mg/day; Maintenance: 20 mg/kg/day (maximum: 1.5 g/day in divided doses)
Adults: Initial: 500 mg/day (maximum: 1.5 g/day in divided doses)

Mechanism of Action Increases the seizure threshold and suppresses paroxysmal spike-and-wave pattern in absence seizures; depresses nerve transmission in the motor cortex

Pharmacodynamics/Kinetics
Half-life Elimination Serum: Children: 30 hours; Adults: 50-60 hours
Time to Peak Serum: Capsule: ~2-4 hours; Syrup: <2-4 hours

Pregnancy Considerations Ethosuximide crosses the placenta. Cases of birth defects have been reported in infants. Epilepsy itself, the number of medications, genetic factors, or a combination of these probably influence the teratogenicity of anticonvulsant therapy.

Patients exposed to ethosuximide during pregnancy are encouraged to enroll themselves into the NAAED Pregnancy Registry by calling 1-888-233-2334. Additional information is available at www.aedpregnancyregistry.org.

Ethotoin (ETH oh toyn)

Brand Names: U.S. Peganone®
Pharmacologic Category Anticonvulsant, Hydantoin
Use Generalized tonic-clonic or complex-partial seizures
Local Anesthetic/Vasoconstrictor Precautions No information available to require special precautions
Effects on Dental Treatment No significant effects or complications reported
Effects on Bleeding No information available to require special precautions
Adverse Effects Frequency not defined.
Cardiovascular: Chest pain
Central nervous system: Ataxia, dizziness, fatigue, fever, headache, insomnia
Dermatologic: Skin rash, Stevens-Johnson syndrome
Gastrointestinal: Diarrhea, gingival hyperplasia, nausea, vomiting
Hematologic: Blood dyscrasias
Neuromuscular & skeletal: Numbness
Ocular: Diplopia, nystagmus
Miscellaneous: Lymphadenopathy, systemic lupus erythematosus (SLE)-like syndrome
General Dosage Range Oral:
Children ≥1 year: Maximum initial dose: 750 mg/day; usual maintenance dose: 0.5-1 g/day; maximum dose: 3 g/day
Adults: Initial dose: ≤1 g/day; usual maintenance dose: 2-3 g/day
Mechanism of Action Stabilizes the seizure threshold and prevents the spread of seizure activity
Pharmacodynamics/Kinetics
Half-life Elimination 3-9 hours
Pregnancy Risk Factor D
Pregnancy Considerations Maternal ingestion of antiepileptic agents has been associated with neonatal coagulation defects/bleeding usually within 24 hours of birth. Congenital malformations (including a pattern of

malformations termed the "fetal hydantoin syndrome" or "fetal anticonvulsant syndrome") have been reported with the use of other hydantoin derivatives, however, case reports using ethotoin during pregnancy are few. Epilepsy itself, the number of medications, genetic factors, or a combination of these probably influence the teratogenicity of anticonvulsant therapy.

Patients exposed to ethotoin during pregnancy are encouraged to enroll themselves into the AED Pregnancy Registry by calling 1-888-233-2334. Additional information is available at www.aedpregnancyregistry.org.

Ethyl Chloride (ETH il KLOR ide)

Brand Names: U.S. Gebauer's Ethyl Chloride®
Pharmacologic Category Local Anesthetic
Use Local anesthetic in minor operative procedures; control pain associated with injections, starting I.V. lines, and venipuncture; relieve pain caused by minor sport injury, bruises, myofascial and visceral pain syndromes
Local Anesthetic/Vasoconstrictor Precautions No information available to require special precautions
Effects on Dental Treatment Key adverse event(s) related to dental treatment: Mucous membrane irritation. See Dental Comment.
Effects on Bleeding No information available to require special precautions
Adverse Effects Frequency not defined.
Dermatologic: Mucous membrane irritation, freezing may alter skin pigment, sensitization (rare)
General Dosage Range Topical: *Adults:* Dosage varies greatly depending on indication
Pharmacodynamics/Kinetics
Duration of Action A few seconds to 1 minute
Pregnancy Considerations Skin absorption may occur; the amount of ethyl chloride available systemically is unknown.
Dental Comment Spray for a few seconds until the tissue becomes white; avoid prolonged spraying of skin beyond this point and avoid frosting of the skin

Etidronate (e ti DROE nate)

Related Information
Osteonecrosis of the Jaw *on page 1529*
Brand Names: U.S. Didronel® [DSC]
Brand Names: Canada Co-Etidronate; Mylan-Etidronate
Pharmacologic Category Bisphosphonate Derivative
Use Symptomatic treatment of Paget's disease; prevention and treatment of heterotopic ossification due to spinal cord injury or after total hip replacement
Local Anesthetic/Vasoconstrictor Precautions No information available to require special precautions
Effects on Dental Treatment Key adverse event(s) related to dental treatment: Abnormal taste.
Osteonecrosis of the jaw (ONJ), generally associated with local infection and/or tooth extraction and often with delayed healing, has been reported in patients taking bisphosphonates. Symptoms included nonhealing extraction socket or an exposed jawbone. Most reported cases of bisphosphonate-associated osteonecrosis have been in cancer patients treated with intravenous bisphosphonates. However, some have occurred in patients with postmenopausal osteoporosis taking oral bisphosphonates. Dental surgery, particularly tooth extraction, may increase the risk for

ONJ. Patients who develop ONJ while on bisphosphonate therapy should receive care by an oral surgeon. See Dental Comment.

Effects on Bleeding No information available to require special precautions

Adverse Effects Frequency not defined.
Gastrointestinal: Diarrhea, nausea
Neuromuscular & skeletal: Bone pain

General Dosage Range Oral: *Adults:* 5-20 mg/kg/day

Mechanism of Action Decreases bone resorption by inhibiting osteocystic osteolysis; decreases mineral release and matrix or collagen breakdown in bone

Pharmacodynamics/Kinetics
Onset of Action 1-3 months
Duration of Action Can persist for 12 months without continuous therapy
Half-life Elimination 1-6 hours

Pregnancy Risk Factor C

Pregnancy Considerations Teratogenic effects have been reported in some but not all animal studies. There are no adequate and well-controlled studies in pregnant women. Bisphosphonates are incorporated into the bone matrix and gradually released over time. Theoretically, there may be a risk of fetal harm when pregnancy follows the completion of therapy. Based on limited case reports with pamidronate, serum calcium levels in the newborn may be altered if administered during pregnancy.

Dental Comment A review of 2408 published cases of bisphosphonate-associated osteonecrosis of the jaw bone (BP-associated ONJ) was done by Filleul, 2010. BP therapy was associated with 89% of the cases to treat malignancies and 11% of the cases to treat nonmalignant conditions. Information on the specific bisphosphonate used was available for 1694 of the patients. Intravenous therapy (primarily zoledronic acid) was received by 88% of the patients and 12% received oral treatment (primarily alendronate). Of all the cases of BP-associated ONJ, 67% were preceded by tooth extraction and for 26% of patients, there was no predisposing factor identified.

A 2010 retrospective case review reported the prevalence of BP-associated ONJ in patients using alendronate-type drugs was one out of 952 patients or ~0.1% (Lo, 2010). Of the 8572 respondents, nine cases of ONJ were identified; five had developed ONJ spontaneously and four developed ONJ after tooth extraction. When extrapolated to patient-years of bisphosphonate exposure, this prevalence rate of 0.1% equates to a frequency of 28 cases per 100,000 person-years of oral bisphosphonate treatment. An Australian group (Mavrokokki, 2007), identified the frequency of BP-associated ONJ in osteoporotic patients, mainly taking weekly oral alendronate, was 1 in 8470 to 1 in 2260 (0.01% to 0.04%) patients. If extractions are carried out, the calculated frequency was 1 in 1130 to 1 in 296 (0.09% to 0.34%) patients. The median time to onset of ONJ in alendronate patients was 24 months.

According to the 2011 report by the American Dental Association (ADA), the incidence of BP-associated ONJ remains low and the benefits of using oral bisphosphonates significantly outweighs the risk of developing BP-associated ONJ for treatment and prevention of osteoporosis and cancer treatment (Hellstein, 2011). The full 47 page report can be accessed at http://www.ada.org/sections/professionalResources/pdfs/topics_ARONJ_report.pdf.

The ADA review of 2011 stated the incidence of oral BP-associated ONJ was one case for every 1000 individuals exposed to oral bisphosphonates (0.1%) (Hellstein, 2011).

Etidronate and Calcium Carbonate
(e ti DROE nate & KAL see um KAR bun ate)

Related Information
Calcium Carbonate *on page 233*
Etidronate *on page 553*
Brand Names: Canada CO Etidrocal; Didrocal®; Mylan-Eti-Cal Carepac; Novo-Etidronatecal
Pharmacologic Category Bisphosphonate Derivative; Calcium Salt
Use Treatment and prevention of postmenopausal osteoporosis; prevention of corticosteroid-induced osteoporosis
Local Anesthetic/Vasoconstrictor Precautions No information available to require special precautions
Effects on Dental Treatment Osteonecrosis of the jaw (ONJ), generally associated with local infection and/or tooth extraction and often with delayed healing, has been reported in patients taking bisphosphonates. Symptoms included nonhealing extraction socket or an exposed jawbone. Most reported cases of bisphosphonate-associated osteonecrosis have been in cancer patients treated with intravenous bisphosphonates. However, some have occurred in patients with postmenopausal osteoporosis taking oral bisphosphonates. Dental surgery, particularly tooth extraction, may increase the risk for ONJ. Patients who develop ONJ while on bisphosphonate therapy should receive care by an oral surgeon. See Dental Comment.
Effects on Bleeding No information available to require special precautions
Adverse Effects >10%:
Central nervous system: Dizziness (16%), headache (13%)
Gastrointestinal: Diarrhea (37%), nausea (18%), flatulence (17%), constipation (13%), dyspepsia (12%), vomiting (11%)
General Dosage Range Oral: *Adults:* Etidronate disodium 400 mg once daily for 14 days, followed by calcium carbonate 1250 mg (500 mg elemental calcium) once daily for 76 days
Mechanism of Action See individual agents.
Pregnancy Considerations Etidronate: Teratogenic effects have been reported in some but not all animal studies. There are no adequate and well-controlled studies in pregnant women. Bisphosphonates are incorporated into the bone matrix and gradually released over time. Theoretically, there may be a risk of fetal harm when pregnancy follows the completion of therapy. Based on limited case reports with pamidronate, serum calcium levels in the newborn may be altered if administered during pregnancy.
Product Availability Not available in U.S.
Dental Comment See Etidronate monograph.

Etodolac (ee toe DOE lak)

Related Information
Oral Pain *on page 1558*
Rheumatoid Arthritis, Osteoarthritis, and Osteoporosis *on page 1526*
Temporomandibular Dysfunction (TMD), Chronic Pain, and Fibromyalgia *on page 1590*
Brand Names: Canada Apo-Etodolac®; Utradol™

Generic Availability (U.S.) Yes

Pharmacologic Category Nonsteroidal Anti-inflammatory Drug (NSAID), Oral

Dental Use Management of postoperative pain

Use Acute and long-term use in the management of signs and symptoms of osteoarthritis; rheumatoid arthritis and juvenile idiopathic arthritis (JIA); management of acute pain

Local Anesthetic/Vasoconstrictor Precautions No information available to require special precautions

Effects on Dental Treatment The dentist should be aware of the potential of abnormal coagulation. Caution should also be exercised in the use of NSAIDs in patients already on anticoagulant therapy with drugs such as warfarin (Coumadin®). See Effects on Bleeding.

Effects on Bleeding Nonselective NSAIDs such as etodolac inhibit platelet aggregation and prolong bleeding time in some patients. Unlike aspirin, the NSAID effect on platelet function is quantitatively less, of shorter duration, and reversible.

Adverse Effects 1% to 10%:
Central nervous system: Dizziness (3% to 9%), chills/fever (1% to 3%), depression (1% to 3%), nervousness (1% to 3%)
Dermatologic: Rash (1% to 3%), pruritus (1% to 3%)
Gastrointestinal: Dyspepsia (10%), abdominal cramps (3% to 9%), diarrhea (3% to 9%), flatulence (3% to 9%), nausea (3% to 9%), vomiting (1% to 3%), constipation (1% to 3%), melena (1% to 3%), gastritis (1% to 3%)
Genitourinary: Dysuria (1% to 3%)
Neuromuscular & skeletal: Weakness (3% to 9%)
Ocular: Blurred vision (1% to 3%)
Otic: Tinnitus (1% to 3%)
Renal: Polyuria (1% to 3%)

Dental Usual Dosage Acute pain: Adults: Oral: Immediate release formulation: 200-400 mg every 6-8 hours, as needed, not to exceed total daily doses of 1000 mg

Dosage Note: For chronic conditions, response is usually observed within 2 weeks.
Children 6-16 years: Oral: Juvenile idiopathic arthritis (JIA): Extended release formulation:
20-30 kg: 400 mg once daily
31-45 kg: 600 mg once daily
46-60 kg: 800 mg once daily
>60 kg: 1000 mg once daily
Adults: Oral:
Acute pain: Immediate release formulation: 200-400 mg every 6-8 hours, as needed, not to exceed total daily doses of 1000 mg
Rheumatoid arthritis, osteoarthritis:
Immediate release formulation: 400 mg 2 times/day or 300 mg 2-3 times/day or 500 mg 2 times/day (doses >1000 mg/day have not been evaluated)
Extended release formulation: 400-1000 mg once daily
Elderly: Refer to adult dosing; in patients ≥65 years, no dosage adjustment required based on pharmacokinetics. The elderly are more sensitive to antiprostaglandin effects and may need dosage adjustments.

Dosage adjustment in renal impairment:
Mild-to-moderate: No adjustment required
Severe: Use not recommended; use with caution
Hemodialysis: Not removed

Dosage adjustment in hepatic impairment: No adjustment required.

Mechanism of Action Reversibly inhibits cyclooxygenase-1 and 2 (COX-1 and 2) enzymes, which results in decreased formation of prostaglandin precursors; has antipyretic, analgesic, and anti-inflammatory properties

Other proposed mechanisms not fully elucidated (and possibly contributing to the anti-inflammatory effect to varying degrees), include inhibiting chemotaxis, altering lymphocyte activity, inhibiting neutrophil aggregation/activation, and decreasing proinflammatory cytokine levels.

Contraindications Hypersensitivity to etodolac, aspirin, other NSAIDs, or any component of the formulation; perioperative pain in the setting of coronary artery bypass graft (CABG) surgery

Warnings/Precautions [U.S. Boxed Warning]: NSAIDs are associated with an increased risk of adverse cardiovascular thrombotic events, including MI and stroke. Risk may be increased with duration of use or pre-existing cardiovascular risk factors or disease. Carefully evaluate individual cardiovascular risk profiles prior to prescribing. May cause new-onset hypertension or worsening of existing hypertension. Use caution with fluid retention. Avoid use in heart failure. Concurrent administration of ibuprofen, and potentially other nonselective NSAIDs, may interfere with aspirin's cardioprotective effect. **[U.S. Boxed Warning]: Use is contraindicated for treatment of perioperative pain in the setting of coronary artery bypass graft (CABG) surgery.** Risk of MI and stroke may be increased with use following CABG surgery.

[U.S. Boxed Warning]: NSAIDs may increase risk of gastrointestinal irritation, inflammation, ulceration, bleeding, and perforation. These events may occur at any time during therapy and without warning. Use caution with a history of GI disease (bleeding or ulcers), concurrent therapy with aspirin, anticoagulants and/or corticosteroids, smoking, use of alcohol, the elderly or debilitated patients. When used concomitantly with ≤325 mg of aspirin, a substantial increase in the risk of gastrointestinal complications (eg, ulcer) occurs; concomitant gastroprotective therapy (eg, proton pump inhibitors) is recommended (Bhatt, 2008).

Platelet adhesion and aggregation may be decreased; may prolong bleeding time; patients with coagulation disorders or who are receiving anticoagulants should be monitored closely. Anemia may occur; patients on long-term NSAID therapy should be monitored for anemia. Rarely, NSAID use may cause severe blood dyscrasias (eg, agranulocytosis, aplastic anemia, thrombocytopenia).

NSAID use may compromise existing renal function; dose-dependent decreases in prostaglandin synthesis may result from NSAID use, reducing renal blood flow which may cause renal decompensation. NSAID use may increase the risk for hyperkalemia. Patients with impaired renal function, dehydration, heart failure, liver dysfunction, those taking diuretics and ACE inhibitors, and the elderly are at greater risk for renal toxicity and hyperkalemia. Rehydrate patient before starting therapy; monitor renal function closely. Not recommended for use in patients with advanced renal disease. Long-term NSAID use may result in renal papillary necrosis.

Use the lowest effective dose for the shortest duration of time, consistent with individual patient goals, to reduce risk of cardiovascular or GI adverse events. Alternate therapies should be considered for patients at high risk.

NSAIDs may cause serious skin adverse events including exfoliative dermatitis, Stevens-Johnson syndrome (SJS), and toxic epidermal necrolysis (TEN); discontinue use at first sign of skin rash or hypersensitivity. Anaphylactoid reactions may occur, even without prior exposure; patients with "aspirin triad" (bronchial asthma, aspirin intolerance, rhinitis) may be at increased risk. Do not use in patients who experience bronchospasm, asthma, rhinitis, or urticaria with NSAID or aspirin therapy. Use caution in other forms of asthma.

Use with caution in patients with decreased hepatic function. Closely monitor patients with any abnormal LFT. Severe hepatic reactions (eg, fulminant hepatitis, liver failure) have occurred with NSAID use, rarely; discontinue if signs or symptoms of liver disease develop, or if systemic manifestations occur.

NSAIDS may cause drowsiness, dizziness, blurred vision and other neurologic effects which may impair physical or mental abilities; patients must be cautioned about performing tasks which require mental alertness (eg, operating machinery or driving). Discontinue use with blurred or diminished vision and perform ophthalmologic exam. Monitor vision with long-term therapy. In the elderly, avoid chronic use (unless alternative agents ineffective and patient can receive concomitant gastroprotective agent); nonselective oral NSAID use is associated with an increased risk of GI bleeding and peptic ulcer disease in older adults in high risk category (eg, >75 years or age or receiving concomitant oral/parenteral corticosteroids, anticoagulants, or antiplatelet agents) (Beers Criteria).

Withhold for at least 4-6 half-lives prior to surgical or dental procedures.

Use of extended release product consisting of a nondeformable matrix should be avoided in patients with stricture/narrowing of the GI tract; symptoms of obstruction have been associated with nondeformable products.

Drug Interactions

Metabolism/Transport Effects None known.

Avoid Concomitant Use

Avoid concomitant use of Etodolac with any of the following: Floctafenine; Ketorolac (Nasal); Ketorolac (Systemic); NSAID (COX-2 Inhibitor); Omacetaxine

Increased Effect/Toxicity

Etodolac may increase the levels/effects of: Agents with Antiplatelet Properties; Aliskiren; Aminoglycosides; Anticoagulants; Bisphosphonate Derivatives; Collagenase (Systemic); CycloSPORINE (Systemic); Dabigatran Etexilate; Deferasirox; Desmopressin; Digoxin; Drotrecogin Alfa (Activated); Eplerenone; Haloperidol; Ibritumomab; Lithium; Methotrexate; Nonsteroidal Anti-Inflammatory Agents; NSAID (COX-2 Inhibitor); Omacetaxine; PEMEtrexed; Porfimer; Potassium-Sparing Diuretics; PRALAtrexate; Quinolone Antibiotics; Rivaroxaban; Salicylates; Thrombolytic Agents; Tositumomab and Iodine I 131 Tositumomab; Vancomycin; Vitamin K Antagonists

The levels/effects of Etodolac may be increased by: ACE Inhibitors; Angiotensin II Receptor Blockers; Antidepressants (Tricyclic, Tertiary Amine); Corticosteroids (Systemic); CycloSPORINE (Systemic); Dasatinib; Floctafenine; Glucosamine; Herbs (Anticoagulant/Antiplatelet Properties); Ketorolac (Nasal); Ketorolac (Systemic); Multivitamins/Minerals (with ADEK, Folate, Iron); Nonsteroidal Anti-Inflammatory Agents; Omega-3 Fatty Acids; Pentosan Polysulfate Sodium;

Pentoxifylline; Probenecid; Prostacyclin Analogues; Selective Serotonin Reuptake Inhibitors; Serotonin/ Norepinephrine Reuptake Inhibitors; Sodium Phosphates; Tipranavir; Treprostinil; Vitamin E

Decreased Effect

Etodolac may decrease the levels/effects of: ACE Inhibitors; Agents with Antiplatelet Properties; Aliskiren; Angiotensin II Receptor Blockers; Beta-Blockers; Eplerenone; HydrALAZINE; Loop Diuretics; Potassium-Sparing Diuretics; Salicylates; Selective Serotonin Reuptake Inhibitors; Thiazide Diuretics

The levels/effects of Etodolac may be decreased by: Bile Acid Sequestrants; Nonsteroidal Anti-Inflammatory Agents; Salicylates

Ethanol/Nutrition/Herb Interactions

Ethanol: Avoid ethanol (may enhance gastric mucosal irritation).

Food: Etodolac peak serum levels may be decreased if taken with food.

Herb/Nutraceutical: Avoid alfalfa, anise, bilberry, bladderwrack, bromelain, cat's claw, celery, chamomile, coleus, cordyceps, dong quai, evening primrose, fenugreek, feverfew, garlic, ginger, ginkgo biloba, ginseng (American, Panax, Siberian), grapeseed, green tea, guggul, horse chestnut seed, horseradish, licorice, prickly ash, red clover, reishi, SAMe (S-adenosylmethionine), sweet clover, turmeric, white willow (all have additional antiplatelet activity).

Dietary Considerations May be taken with food to decrease GI upset.

Pharmacodynamics/Kinetics

Onset of Action Analgesic: 2-4 hours; Maximum anti-inflammatory effect: A few days

Half-life Elimination Terminal: Adults: 5-8 hours; Extended release: Children (6-16 years): 12 hours

Time to Peak Immediate release: Adults: 1-2 hours; Extended release: 5-7 hours, increased 1.4-3.8 hours with food

Pregnancy Risk Factor C

Pregnancy Considerations Adverse events were not observed in the initial animal reproduction studies; therefore, the manufacturer classifies etodolac as pregnancy category C. NSAID exposure during the first trimester is not strongly associated with congenital malformations; however, cardiovascular anomalies and cleft palate have been observed following NSAID exposure in some studies. The use of an NSAID close to conception may be associated with an increased risk of miscarriage. Nonteratogenic effects have been observed following NSAID administration during the third trimester including: Myocardial degenerative changes, prenatal constriction of the ductus arteriosus, fetal tricuspid regurgitation, failure of the ductus arteriosus to close postnatally; renal dysfunction or failure, oligohydramnios; gastrointestinal bleeding or perforation, increased risk of necrotizing enterocolitis; intracranial bleeding (including intraventricular hemorrhage), platelet dysfunction with resultant bleeding; pulmonary hypertension. Because they may cause premature closure of the ductus arteriosus, use of NSAIDs late in pregnancy should be avoided (use after 31 or 32 weeks gestation is not recommended by some clinicians). The chronic use of NSAIDs in women of reproductive age may be associated with infertility that is reversible upon discontinuation of the medication.

Lactation Excretion in breast milk unknown/not recommended

Breast-Feeding Considerations It is not known if etodolac is excreted into breast milk. Use of etodolac while breast-feeding is not recommended by the manufacturer.

Dosage Forms
Capsule, oral: 200 mg, 300 mg
Tablet, oral: 400 mg, 500 mg
Tablet, extended release, oral: 400 mg, 500 mg, 600 mg

Etomidate (e TOM i date)

Brand Names: U.S. Amidate®
Brand Names: Canada Amidate®
Pharmacologic Category General Anesthetic
Use Induction and maintenance of general anesthesia
Unlabeled Use Sedation for diagnosis of seizure foci; procedural sedation
Local Anesthetic/Vasoconstrictor Precautions No information available to require special precautions
Effects on Dental Treatment Key adverse event(s) related to dental treatment: Hiccups.
Effects on Bleeding No information available to require special precautions
Adverse Effects
>10%:
Endocrine & metabolic: Adrenal suppression
Gastrointestinal: Nausea, vomiting on emergence from anesthesia
Local: Pain at injection site (30% to 80%)
Neuromuscular & skeletal: Myoclonus (33%), transient skeletal movements, uncontrolled eye movements
1% to 10%: Hiccups
General Dosage Range I.V.: *Children >10 years and Adults:* Induction: 0.2-0.6 mg/kg; Maintenance: 5-20 mcg/kg/minute
Mechanism of Action Ultrashort-acting nonbarbiturate hypnotic (benzimidazole) used for the induction of anesthesia; chemically, it is a carboxylated imidazole which produces a rapid induction of anesthesia with minimal cardiovascular effects; produces EEG burst suppression at high doses
Pharmacodynamics/Kinetics
Onset of Action 30-60 seconds; Peak effect: 1 minute
Duration of Action 3-5 minutes; terminated by redistribution
Half-life Elimination Terminal: 2.6 hours
Pregnancy Risk Factor C
Pregnancy Considerations Adverse events have been observed in animal reproduction studies.

Etonogestrel (e toe noe JES trel)

Brand Names: U.S. Implanon®; Nexplanon®
Pharmacologic Category Contraceptive; Progestin
Use Prevention of pregnancy; for use in women who request long-acting (up to 3 years) contraception
Local Anesthetic/Vasoconstrictor Precautions No information available to require special precautions
Effects on Dental Treatment Key adverse event(s) related to dental treatment: Until more is known about the mechanism of interaction, use caution in prescribing antibiotics to female patients taking progestin-only contraceptives.
Effects on Bleeding No information available to require special precautions

Adverse Effects
>10%:
Central nervous system: Headache (25%)
Dermatologic: Acne (14%)
Endocrine & metabolic: Infrequent menstrual bleeding (<3 episodes/90 days: 34%), amenorrhea (no bleeding in 90 days: 22%), prolonged menstrual bleeding (lasting >14 days: 18%), breast pain (13%), menstrual bleeding irregularities requiring discontinuation (11%)
Gastrointestinal: Weight gain (14%), abdominal pain (11%)
Genitourinary: Vaginitis (15%)
Respiratory: Pharyngitis (11%)
1% to 10%:
Central nervous system: Dizziness (7%), emotional lability (7%), depression (6%), nervousness (6%), pain (6%)
Endocrine & metabolic: Dysmenorrhea (7%), frequent menstrual bleeding (>5 episodes/90 days: 7%)
Gastrointestinal: Nausea (6%)
Genitourinary: Leukorrhea (10%)
Local: Implant site reactions (9%), insertion site pain (3% to 5%)
Neuromuscular & skeletal: Back pain (7%)
Miscellaneous: Flu-like syndrome (8%), hypersensitivity reactions (5%)
General Dosage Range Subdermal: *Adults (females, postmenarche):* Implant 1 rod for up to 3 years
Mechanism of Action Etonogestrel is the active metabolite of desogestrel. It prevents pregnancy by suppressing ovulation, increasing the viscosity of cervical mucous, and inhibiting endometrial proliferation.
Pharmacodynamics/Kinetics
Onset of Action Serum levels sufficient to inhibit ovulation: ≤8 hours of implant
Duration of Action Implant: Each rod maintains etonogestrel levels sufficient to inhibit ovulation for 3 years
Half-life Elimination ~25 hours
Pregnancy Considerations Teratogenic effects were not observed in animal studies. Not for use during pregnancy; rule out pregnancy prior to insertion. Remove implant if pregnancy is detected during use. Ovulation may return within 1 week of implant removal; alternate forms of contraception may be required. In a multicenter clinical trial, 11 out of 46 women no longer using contraception became pregnant between 1 and 18 weeks following removal of the implant. Do not insert <21 days postpartum. Women weighing >130% of their ideal body weight were not included in clinical studies. With oral combination hormonal contraceptives, an increase in contraceptive failure was noted in women with a BMI >27.3. Similar findings were noted in patients weighing ≥90 kg (198 lb) using the contraceptive patch.
Prescribing and Access Restrictions Only healthcare providers who have undergone training in the insertion and removal procedures will be able to order Implanon® or Nexplanon®. Materials related to the insertion and removal of Implanon® or Nexplanon® are available from the manufacturer (877-467-5266).

Etoposide (e toe POE side)

Brand Names: U.S. Toposar®
Brand Names: Canada Etoposide Injection USP; Vepesid™

Pharmacologic Category Antineoplastic Agent, Podophyllotoxin Derivative; Antineoplastic Agent, Topoisomerase II Inhibitor

Use Treatment of refractory testicular tumors (injectable formulation); treatment of small cell lung cancer (SCLC)

Canadian labeling: Treatment of small cell lung cancer (SCLC; first- and second-line); treatment of nonsmall cell lung cancer (NSCLC); treatment of non-Hodgkin lymphomas (first-line); treatment of testicular cancer (first-line [injectable formulation] and refractory)

Unlabeled Use Treatment of acute lymphocytic leukemia (ALL), refractory acute myeloid leukemia (AML), recurrent or metastatic breast cancer, central nervous system tumors, Ewing's sarcoma, gestational trophoblastic disease, Hodgkin lymphoma, merkel cell cancer, refractory multiple myeloma, neuroblastoma, neuroendocrine tumors (adrenal gland and carcinoid tumors), non-Hodgkin lymphomas, nonsmall cell lung cancer (NSCLC), osteosarcoma, ovarian cancer (refractory), prostate cancer, retinoblastoma, metastatic soft tissue sarcoma, thymic malignancies (locally advanced or metastatic), unknown-primary adenocarcinoma, Wilms' tumor; conditioning regimen for hematopoietic cell transplantation

Local Anesthetic/Vasoconstrictor Precautions No information available to require special precautions

Effects on Dental Treatment Key adverse event(s) related to dental treatment: Mucositis (especially at high doses) and stomatitis.

Effects on Bleeding Myelosuppression is dose related. When thrombocytopenia occurs, platelet nadirs develop 9-16 days after drug administration. Bone marrow recovery is usually complete by day 20, and no cumulative toxicity has been reported.

Adverse Effects Note: The following may occur with higher doses used in stem cell transplantation: Alopecia, ethanol intoxication, hepatitis, hypotension (infusion-related), metabolic acidosis, mucositis, nausea and vomiting (severe), secondary malignancy, skin lesions (resembling Stevens-Johnson syndrome).

>10%:
Dermatologic: Alopecia (8% to 66%)
Gastrointestinal: Nausea/vomiting (31% to 43%), anorexia (10% to 13%), diarrhea (1% to 13%)
Hematologic: Leukopenia (60% to 91%; grade 4: 3% to 17%; nadir: 7-14 days; recovery: by day 20), thrombocytopenia (22% to 41%; grades 3/4: 1% to 20%; nadir 9-16 days; recovery: by day 20), anemia (≤33%)

1% to 10%:
Cardiovascular: Hypotension (1% to 2%; due to rapid infusion)
Gastrointestinal: Stomatitis (1% to 6%), abdominal pain (up to 2%)
Hepatic: Hepatic toxicity (up to 3%)
Neuromuscular & skeletal: Peripheral neuropathy (1% to 2%)
Miscellaneous: Anaphylactic-like reaction (I.V. infusion 1% to 2%; oral capsules <1%; including chills, fever, tachycardia, bronchospasm, dyspnea)

General Dosage Range Dosage adjustment recommended in patients with hepatic impairment, renal impairment, or who develop toxicities.
I.V., oral: *Adults:* Dosage varies greatly depending on indication

Mechanism of Action Etoposide has been shown to delay transit of cells through the S phase and arrest cells in late S or early G_2 phase. The drug may inhibit mitochondrial transport at the NADH dehydrogenase

level or inhibit uptake of nucleosides into HeLa cells. It is a topoisomerase II inhibitor and appears to cause DNA strand breaks. Etoposide does not inhibit microtubular assembly.

Pharmacodynamics/Kinetics
Half-life Elimination Terminal: I.V.: 4-11 hours; Children: Normal renal/hepatic function: 6-8 hours

Pregnancy Risk Factor D

Pregnancy Considerations Animal reproduction studies have demonstrated teratogenicity and fetal loss. There are no adequate and well-controlled studies in pregnant women. Women of childbearing potential should be advised to avoid pregnancy.

Etoposide Phosphate (e toe POE side FOS fate)

Related Information
Etoposide *on page 557*
Brand Names: U.S. Etopophos®
Pharmacologic Category Antineoplastic Agent, Podophyllotoxin Derivative; Antineoplastic Agent, Topoisomerase II Inhibitor

Use Treatment of refractory testicular tumors; treatment of small cell lung cancer

Local Anesthetic/Vasoconstrictor Precautions No information available to require special precautions

Effects on Dental Treatment Key adverse event(s) related to dental treatment: Mucositis (especially at high doses), stomatitis, and taste perversion.

Effects on Bleeding Myelosuppression is dose related. When thrombocytopenia occurs, platelet nadirs develop 10-15 days after drug administration. Bone marrow recovery is usually complete by day 21, and no cumulative toxicity has been reported.

Adverse Effects Note: Also see adverse reactions for **etoposide;** etoposide phosphate is converted to etoposide, adverse reactions experienced with etoposide would also be expected with etoposide phosphate.

>10%:
Central nervous system: Chills/fever (24%)
Dermatologic: Alopecia (33% to 44%)
Gastrointestinal: Nausea/vomiting (37%), anorexia (16%), mucositis (11%)
Hematologic: Leukopenia (91%; grade 4: 17%; nadir: day 15-22; recovery: usually by day 21), neutropenia (88%; grade 4: 37%; nadir: day 12-19; recovery: usually by day 21), anemia (72%; grades 3/4: 19%), thrombocytopenia (23%; grade 4: 9%; nadir: day 10-15; recovery: usually by day 21)
Neuromuscular & skeletal: Weakness/malaise (39%)

1% to 10%:
Cardiovascular: Hypotension (1% to 5%), hypertension (3%), facial flushing (2%)
Central nervous system: Dizziness (5%)
Dermatologic: Skin rash (3%)
Gastrointestinal: Constipation (8%), abdominal pain (7%), diarrhea (6%), taste perversion (6%)
Local: Extravasation/phlebitis (5%; including swelling, pain, cellulitis, necrosis, and/or skin necrosis at site of infiltration)
Miscellaneous: Anaphylactic-type reactions (3%; including chills, diaphoresis, fever, rigor, tachycardia, bronchospasm, dyspnea, pruritus)

General Dosage Range Dosage adjustment recommended in patients with hepatic or renal impairment
I.V.: *Adults:* Dosage varies greatly depending on indication

Mechanism of Action Etoposide phosphate is converted *in vivo* to the active moiety, etoposide, by dephosphorylation. Etoposide inhibits mitotic activity; inhibits cells from entering prophase; inhibits DNA synthesis. Initially thought to be mitotic inhibitors similar to podophyllotoxin, but actually have no effect on microtubule assembly. However, later shown to induce DNA strand breakage and inhibition of topoisomerase II (an enzyme which breaks and repairs DNA); etoposide acts in late S or early G2 phases.

Pharmacodynamics/Kinetics

Half-life Elimination Terminal: 4-11 hours; Children: Normal renal/hepatic function: 6-8 hours

Pregnancy Risk Factor D

Pregnancy Considerations Animal studies have demonstrated teratogenicity and fetal loss. There are no adequate and well-controlled studies in pregnant women. Women of childbearing potential should be advised to avoid pregnancy.

Etravirine (et ra VIR een)

Related Information

HIV Infection and AIDS *on page 1520*

Brand Names: U.S. Intelence®

Brand Names: Canada Intelence®

Pharmacologic Category Antiretroviral Agent, Reverse Transcriptase Inhibitor (Non-nucleoside)

Use Treatment of HIV-1 infection in combination with at least two additional antiretroviral agents in treatment-experienced patients exhibiting viral replication with documented non-nucleoside reverse transcriptase inhibitor (NNRTI) resistance

Local Anesthetic/Vasoconstrictor Precautions No information available to require special precautions

Effects on Dental Treatment Key adverse event(s) related to dental treatment: Stomatitis has been reported.

Effects on Bleeding No information available to require special precautions related to hemostasis.

Adverse Effects

>10%:

Dermatologic: Rash (≥grade 2: 10% to 15%)

Endocrine & metabolic: Cholesterol (total) increased (≤300 mg/dL: 20%; >300 mg/dL: 8%), hyperglycemia (≤250 mg/dL: 15%; 251-500 mg/dL: 4%), LDL increased (≤190 mg/dL: 13%)

Gastrointestinal: Nausea

2% to 10%:

Endocrine & metabolic: Triglycerides increased (≤750 mg/dL: 9%; >750 mg/dL: 4% to 6%)

Gastrointestinal: Diarrhea (children and adolescents ≥2%), amylase increased (>5 x ULN: 2%)

Hepatic: ALT increased (≤5 x ULN: 6%; >5 x ULN: 3%), AST increased (≤5 x ULN: 6%; >5 x ULN: 3%)

Neuromuscular & skeletal: Peripheral neuropathy (≥ grade 2: 4%)

Renal: Creatinine increased (≤1.8 x ULN: 6%; >1.8 x ULN: 2%)

General Dosage Range Oral:

Children ≥6 years and ≥16 kg to <20 kg: 100 mg twice daily

Children ≥6 years and ≥20 kg to <25 kg: 125 mg twice daily

Children ≥6 years and ≥25 kg to <30 kg: 150 mg twice daily

Children ≥6 years and ≥30 kg and Adults: 200 mg twice daily

Mechanism of Action As a non-nucleoside reverse transcriptase inhibitor, etravirine has activity against HIV-1 by binding to reverse transcriptase. It consequently blocks the RNA-dependent and DNA-dependent DNA polymerase activities, including HIV-1 replication. It does not require intracellular phosphorylation for antiviral activity.

Pharmacodynamics/Kinetics

Half-life Elimination 41 hours (± 20 hours)

Time to Peak 2.5-4 hours

Pregnancy Risk Factor B

Pregnancy Considerations Adverse events have not been noted in animal reproduction studies. Etravirine crosses the placenta. Based on limited data, dose adjustments are not needed in pregnant women. However, because available data in pregnant women are insufficient, the DHHS Perinatal HIV Guidelines do not recommend use in antiretroviral-naive women unless other alternatives are not available. Hypersensitivity reactions (including hepatic toxicity and rash) are more common in women on NNRTI therapy; it is not known if pregnancy increases this risk.

Regardless of CD4 count or HIV RNA copy number, all HIV-infected pregnant women should receive a combination antepartum antiretroviral (ARV) drug regimen; this includes women who require therapy for their own health, as well as women who do not yet require therapy for their own health. ARV therapy should be started as soon as possible if required for the woman's health. Although earlier initiation may be more effective in reducing the perinatal transmission of HIV, also consider maternal conditions (eg, nausea and vomiting) and the potential risks of first trimester fetal exposure for specific agents. Plasma HIV RNA levels should be assessed at ~34-36 weeks gestation in order to help determine mode of delivery. If ARV therapy must be interrupted for <24 hours during the peripartum period, stop then restart all medications simultaneously in order to decrease the chance of developing resistance. Long-term follow-up is recommended for all infants exposed to ARV medications.

Healthcare providers are encouraged to enroll pregnant women exposed to antiretroviral medications in the Antiretroviral Pregnancy Registry (1-800-258-4263 or www.APRegistry.com). Healthcare providers caring for HIV-infected women and their infants may contact the National Perinatal HIV Hotline (888-448-8765) for clinical consultation (DHHS [perinatal], 2012).

Everolimus (e ver OH li mus)

Brand Names: U.S. Afinitor®; Afinitor® Disperz; Zortress®

Brand Names: Canada Afinitor®

Pharmacologic Category Antineoplastic Agent, mTOR Kinase Inhibitor; Immunosuppressant Agent; mTOR Kinase Inhibitor

Use

Afinitor®: Treatment of advanced hormone receptor-positive, HER2-negative breast cancer in postmenopausal women (in combination with exemestane and after letrozole or anastrozole failure); treatment of advanced renal cell cancer (RCC), after sunitinib or sorafenib failure; treatment of renal angiomyolipoma with tuberous sclerosis complex (TSC) not requiring immediate surgery; treatment of subependymal giant cell astrocytoma (SEGA) associated with TSC which requires intervention, but cannot be curatively resected; treatment of advanced, metastatic or unresectable pancreatic neuroendocrine tumors (PNET)

Afinitor® Disperz: Treatment of subependymal giant cell astrocytoma (SEGA) associated with TSC which requires intervention, but cannot be curatively resected

Zortress®: Prophylaxis of organ rejection in renal transplantation patients at low-moderate immunologic risk (in combination with basiliximab, cyclosporine, and corticosteroids); prophylaxis of organ rejection in liver transplantation (in combination with tacrolimus and corticosteroids)

Unlabeled Use Treatment of relapsed or refractory Waldenström's macroglobulinemia (WM); treatment of progressive advanced carcinoid tumors

Local Anesthetic/Vasoconstrictor Precautions No information available to require special precautions

Effects on Dental Treatment Key adverse event(s) related to dental treatment: High incidence of mouth ulcers, mucositis, and stomatitis; xerostomia and taste alterations have been observed (normal salivary flow resumes upon discontinuation)

Effects on Bleeding No information available to require special precautions

Adverse Effects

>10%:

Cardiovascular: Peripheral edema (4% to 45%), hypertension (4% to 30%; hypertensive crisis: 1%)

Central nervous system: Fatigue (7% to 45%), fever (13% to 32%), headache (18% to 30%), seizure (5% to 29%), behavioral changes (anxiety/aggression/behavioral disturbance; SEGA: 21%), insomnia (6% to 17%), dizziness (7% to 14%)

Dermatologic: Skin rash (18% to 59%), cellulitis (SEGA: 29%), acneiform eruption (3% to 25%), nail disease (including onychoclasis, 4% to 22%), acne vulgaris (3% to 22%), pruritus (13% to 21%), xeroderma (9% to 18%), contact dermatitis (14%), excoriation (14%)

Endocrine & metabolic: Hypercholesterolemia (17% to 85%), hyperglycemia (12% to 75%; grades 3/4: <1% to 17%), hypertriglyceridemia (73%), decreased serum bicarbonate (≤56%), hypophosphatemia (9% to 49%), hypocalcemia (17% to 37%), decreased serum albumin (≤33%), diabetes mellitus ([new onset] <10%; liver transplant: 32%), hypoglycemia (≤32%), hypokalemia (12% to 29%), hyperlipidemia (renal, liver transplant: 21% to 24%), hyperkalemia (renal transplant: 18%), amenorrhea (≤17%), hyponatremia (≤16%), lipid metabolism disorder (renal transplant: 15%), hypomagnesemia (renal transplant: 14%)

Gastrointestinal: Stomatitis (oncology uses: 44% to 86%; grade 3: 4% to 9%; grade 4: <1%; renal transplant: 8%), diarrhea (14% to 50%; grade 3: ≤5%; grade 4: <1%), constipation (10% to 38%), abdominal pain (3% to 36%), nausea (8% to 32%; grade 3: ≤2%; grade 4: <1%), decreased appetite (6% to 30%), anorexia (1% to 30%), vomiting (15% to 29%; grade 3: ≤2%; grade 4: <1%), weight loss (9% to 28%), dysgeusia (1% to 22%), gastroenteritis (1% to 18%), xerostomia (8% to 11%)

Genitourinary: Urinary tract infection (5% to 22%), hematuria (renal transplant: 12%), dysuria (renal transplant: 11%)

Hematologic & oncologic: Anemia (26% to 92%; grades 3/4: ≤15%; grade 4: <1%), prolonged partial thromboplastin time (SEGA: 72%), leukopenia

(oncology uses: 26% to 58%; renal, liver transplant: 3% to 12%), lymphocytopenia (20% to 54%; grades 3/4: ≤18%), thrombocytopenia (oncology uses: 19% to 54%; grade 3: ≤3%; renal transplant: <10%), neutropenia (≤46%; grades 3/4: ≤9%)

Hepatic: Increased serum AST (23% to 89%; grade 3: ≤4%; grade 4: <1%), increased serum alkaline phosphatase (oncology uses: 32% to 74%; renal, liver transplant: <10%), increased serum ALT (18% to 51%; grade 3: ≤4%; grade 4: 1%)

Infection: Infection (13% to 62%; grade 3: 4% to 7%; grade 4: 1% to 3%)

Musculoskeletal: Weakness (13% to 33%), arthralgia (≤20%), back pain (11% to 15%), limb pain (8% to 14%)

Otic: Otitis (6% to 36%)

Renal: Increased serum creatinine (11% to 50%)

Respiratory: Upper respiratory tract infection (11% to 82%), sinusitis (3% to 39%), cough (7% to 30%), dyspnea (20% to 24%; grade 3: 2% to 6%; grade 4: ≤1%), epistaxis (≤22%), pneumonitis (including alveolitis, interstitial lung disease, lung infiltrate, pulmonary alveolar hemorrhage, pulmonary toxicity, 1% to 19%; grade 3: 3% to 4%; grade 4: <1%), nasal congestion (14%), rhinitis (14%), pharyngitis (4% to 11%)

Miscellaneous: Wound healing impairment (liver transplant: 11%; oncology uses: <1%)

1% to 10%:

Cardiovascular: Chest pain (5%), tachycardia (3%), cardiac failure (1%), angina pectoris, atrial fibrillation, chest discomfort, deep vein thrombosis, edema (generalized), hypotension, palpitations, syncope, venous thromboembolism

Central nervous system: Depression (5%), migraine (5%), paresthesia (5%), chills (4%), agitation, drowsiness, hallucination, hemiparesis, hypoesthesia, lethargy, malaise, neuralgia

Dermatologic: Eczema (10%), alopecia (≤10%), palmar-plantar erythrodysesthesia ([hand-foot syndrome] 5%), papule (5%), erythema (4%), pityriasis rosea (4%), skin lesion (4%), hirsutism, hyperhidrosis, hypertrichosis

Endocrine & metabolic: Hypermenorrhea (6% to 10%), menstrual disease (6% to 10%), dysmenorrhea (6%), irregular menses (6%), exacerbation of diabetes mellitus (2%), cushingoid appearance, cyanocobalamin deficiency, dehydration, gout, hypercalcemia, hyperparathyroidism, hyperphosphatemia, hyperuricemia, iron deficiency, ovarian cyst, scrotal edema

Gastrointestinal: Gastritis (7%), hemorrhoids (5%), dyspepsia (4%), dysphagia (4%), ageusia (1%), abdominal distention, epigastric distress, flatulence, gastroesophageal reflux disease, gingival hyperplasia, hematemesis, intestinal obstruction, oral herpes

Genitourinary: Vaginal hemorrhage (8%), bladder spasm, erectile dysfunction, pollakiuria, pyuria, urinary retention, urinary urgency

Hematologic & oncologic: Neoplasm (liver transplant: 4%), hemorrhage (3%), leukocytosis, lymphadenopathy, pancytopenia (renal, liver transplant)

Hepatic: Increased serum bilirubin (3% to 10%; grades 3/4: ≤1%), abnormal hepatic function tests (liver transplant: 7%), ascites (liver transplant: 4%), increased serum transaminases

Hypersensitivity: Hypersensitivity (including anaphylaxis, dyspnea, flushing, chest pain, angioedema, 3%)

Infection: BK virus infection, candidiasis, herpes infection, sepsis

Musculoskeletal: Muscle spasm (≤10%), tremor (8% to 9%), jaw pain (3%), joint swelling, musculoskeletal pain, myalgia, osteonecrosis, osteopenia, osteoporosis, spondylitis

Ophthalmic: Eyelid edema (4%), ocular hyperemia (4%), conjunctivitis (2%), blurred vision, cataract

Renal: Renal failure (3%), hydronephrosis, increased blood urea nitrogen, interstitial nephritis, polyuria, proteinuria, renal artery thrombosis, renal insufficiency

Respiratory: Pleural effusion (5% to 7%), nasopharyngitis (6%), pneumonia (6%), bronchitis (4%), pharyngolaryngeal pain (4%), rhinorrhea (3%), atelectasis, lower respiratory tract infection, oropharyngeal pain, pulmonary edema, pulmonary embolism, sinus congestion, wheezing

Miscellaneous: Night sweats, peritonitis, postoperative wound complication (including incisional hernia)

General Dosage Range Dosage adjustment recommended in patients with hepatic impairment, on concomitant therapy, or who develop toxicities

Oral: *Children ≥1 year and Adults:* Dosage varies greatly depending on indication

Mechanism of Action Everolimus is a macrolide immunosuppressant and an m-TOR inhibitor which has antiproliferative and antiangiogenic properties, and also reduces lipoma volume in patients with angiomyolipoma. Reduces protein synthesis and cell proliferation by binding to the FK binding protein-12 (FKBP-12), an intracellular protein, to form a complex that inhibits activation of mTOR (mammalian target of rapamycin) serine-threonine kinase activity. Also reduces angiogenesis by inhibiting vascular endothelial growth factor (VEGF) and hypoxia-inducible factor (HIF-1) expression. Angiomyolipomas may occur due to unregulated mTOR activity in TSC-associated renal angiomyolipoma (Budde, 2012); everolimus reduces lipoma volume (Bissler, 2012).

Pharmacodynamics/Kinetics

Half-life Elimination ~30 hours

Time to Peak 1-2 hours

Pregnancy Risk Factor D (Afinitor®) / C (Zortress®)

Pregnancy Considerations Embryotoxicity, fetotoxicity, malformations, and growth retardation were observed in animal reproduction studies with exposures lower than expected with human doses. Based on the mechanism of action, may cause fetal harm if administered during pregnancy. Women of childbearing potential should be advised to avoid pregnancy. Women of childbearing potential should use highly effective birth control during treatment, and continue for 8 weeks after everolimus discontinuation.

Product Availability Afinitor Disperz (tablets for oral suspension): FDA approved August 2012; anticipated availability in November 2012. Consult prescribing information for additional information.

Exemestane (ex e MES tane)

Brand Names: U.S. Aromasin®

Brand Names: Canada Aromasin®; CO Exemestane

Pharmacologic Category Antineoplastic Agent, Aromatase Inactivator

Use Treatment of advanced breast cancer in postmenopausal women whose disease has progressed following tamoxifen therapy; adjuvant treatment of postmenopausal estrogen receptor-positive early breast cancer following 2-3 years of tamoxifen (for a total of 5 years of adjuvant therapy)

Unlabeled Use Risk reduction for invasive breast cancer in postmenopausal women; treatment of endometrial cancer; treatment of uterine sarcoma

Local Anesthetic/Vasoconstrictor Precautions No information available to require special precautions

Effects on Dental Treatment No significant effects or complications reported

Effects on Bleeding No information available to require special precautions

Adverse Effects

>10%:

Cardiovascular: Hypertension (5% to 15%)

Central nervous system: Fatigue (8% to 22%), insomnia (11% to 14%), pain (13%), headache (7% to 13%), depression (6% to 13%)

Dermatological: Hyperhidrosis (4% to 18%), alopecia (15%)

Endocrine & metabolic: Hot flashes (13% to 33%)

Gastrointestinal: Nausea (9% to 18%), abdominal pain (6% to 11%)

Hepatic: Alkaline phosphatase increased (14% to 15%)

Neuromuscular & skeletal: Arthralgia (15% to 29%)

1% to 10%:

Cardiovascular: Edema (6% to 7%); cardiac ischemic events (2%: MI, angina, myocardial ischemia); chest pain

Central nervous system: Dizziness (8% to 10%), anxiety (4% to 10%), fever (5%), confusion, hypoesthesia

Dermatologic: Dermatitis (8%), itching, rash

Endocrine & metabolic: Weight gain (8%)

Gastrointestinal: Diarrhea (4% to 10%), vomiting (7%), anorexia (6%), constipation (5%), appetite increased (3%), dyspepsia

Genitourinary: Urinary tract infection (2% to 5%)

Hepatic: Bilirubin increased (5% to 7%)

Neuromuscular & skeletal: Back pain (9%), limb pain (9%), myalgia (6%), osteoarthritis (6%), weakness (6%), osteoporosis (5%), pathological fracture (4%), paresthesia (3%), carpal tunnel syndrome (2%), cramps (2%)

Ocular: Visual disturbances (5%)

Renal: Creatinine increased (6%)

Respiratory: Dyspnea (10%), cough (6%), bronchitis, pharyngitis, rhinitis, sinusitis, upper respiratory infection

Miscellaneous: Flu-like syndrome (6%), lymphedema, infection

A dose-dependent decrease in sex hormone-binding globulin has been observed with daily doses of ≥2.5 mg. Serum luteinizing hormone and follicle-stimulating hormone levels have increased with this medicine.

General Dosage Range Dosage adjustment recommended in patients on concomitant therapy

Oral: *Adults (postmenopausal females):* 25 mg once daily

Mechanism of Action Exemestane is an irreversible, steroidal aromatase inactivator. It is structurally related to androstenedione, and is converted to an intermediate that irreversibly blocks the active site of the aromatase enzyme, leading to inactivation ("suicide inhibition") and thus preventing conversion of androgens to estrogens in peripheral tissues. In postmenopausal breast cancers where growth is estrogen-dependent, this medicine will lower circulating estrogens.

Pharmacodynamics/Kinetics

Half-life Elimination 24 hours

Time to Peak Women with breast cancer: 1.2 hours

◀ **Pregnancy Risk Factor** X

Pregnancy Considerations According to the manufacturer, the decision to continue or discontinue breastfeeding during therapy should take into account the risk of exposure to the infant and the benefits of treatment to the mother. Not indicated for use in premenopausal women.

Exenatide (ex EN a tide)

Brand Names: U.S. Bydureon™; Byetta®
Brand Names: Canada Byetta®
Pharmacologic Category Antidiabetic Agent, Glucagon-Like Peptide-1 (GLP-1) Receptor Agonist
Use Treatment of type 2 diabetes mellitus (noninsulin dependent, NIDDM) to improve glycemic control
Local Anesthetic/Vasoconstrictor Precautions No information available to require special precautions
Effects on Dental Treatment No significant effects or complications reported
Effects on Bleeding No information available to require special precautions
Adverse Effects
>10%:
Endocrine & metabolic: Hypoglycemia (monotherapy 2% to 5%; combination therapy with sulfonylurea 14% to 36%, with metformin ≤4%, with thiazolidinedione 11%)
Gastrointestinal: Nausea (monotherapy 8% to 11%; combination therapy 13% to 44%; dose-dependent), vomiting (monotherapy 4%; combination therapy 11% to 13%), diarrhea (monotherapy <2% to 11%; combination therapy 6% to 20%), constipation (monotherapy 9%; combination therapy 6% to 10%)
Local: Injection site nodule (Bydureon™ 6% to 77%), injection site reactions (2% to 18%; includes erythema, hematoma, pruritus)
Miscellaneous: Anti-exenatide antibodies (low titers 38% to 49%, high titers 6% to 12%)
1% to 10%:
Central nervous system: Nervousness (9%), dizziness (monotherapy <2%; combination therapy 9%), headache (5% to 9%), fatigue (3% to 6%)
Dermatologic: Hyperhidrosis (3%)
Gastrointestinal: Viral gastroenteritis (6% to 9%), dyspepsia (monotherapy 3% to 7%; combination therapy 5% to 7%), GERD (3% to 7%), appetite decreased (1% to 5%)
Neuromuscular & skeletal: Weakness (4%)
General Dosage Range SubQ: *Adults:*
Immediate release: Initial: 5 mcg twice daily; Maintenance: 5-10 mcg twice daily
Extended release: 2 mg once weekly
Mechanism of Action Exenatide is an analog of the hormone incretin (glucagon-like peptide 1 or GLP-1) which increases glucose-dependent insulin secretion, decreases inappropriate glucagon secretion, increases B-cell growth/replication, slows gastric emptying, and decreases food intake. Exenatide administration results in decreases in hemoglobin A_{1c} by approximately 0.5% to 1% (immediate release) or 1.5% to 1.9% (extended release).
Pharmacodynamics/Kinetics
Half-life Elimination
Immediate release (daily) formulation: 2.4 hours
Extended release (weekly) formulation: ~2 weeks

Time to Peak SubQ:
Immediate release (daily) formulation: 2.1 hours
Extended release (weekly) formulation: Triphasic: Phase 1: 2-5 hours; Phase 2: ~2 weeks; Phase 3: ~7 weeks
Pregnancy Risk Factor C
Pregnancy Considerations Due to adverse events observed in some animal studies, exenatide is classified as pregnancy category C. Based on *in vitro* data, exenatide has a low potential to cross the placenta. Maternal hyperglycemia can be associated with adverse effects in the fetus, including macrosomia, neonatal hyperglycemia, and hyperbilirubinemia; the risk of congenital malformations is increased when the Hb A_{1c} is above the normal range. Diabetes can also be associated with adverse effects in the mother. Poorly-treated diabetes may cause end-organ damage that may in turn negatively affect obstetric outcomes. Physiologic glucose levels should be maintained prior to and during pregnancy to decrease the risk of adverse events in the mother and the fetus. Until additional safety and efficacy data are obtained, the use of exenatide is generally not recommended in the routine management of diabetes mellitus during pregnancy. Insulin is the drug of choice for the control of diabetes mellitus during pregnancy. A registry has been established for women exposed to exenatide during pregnancy (1-800-633-9081).

Ezetimibe (ez ET i mibe)

Related Information
Cardiovascular Diseases *on page 1492*
Brand Names: U.S. Zetia®
Brand Names: Canada Ezetrol®
Generic Availability (U.S.) No
Pharmacologic Category Antilipemic Agent, 2-Azetidinone
Use Use in combination with dietary therapy for the treatment of primary hypercholesterolemia (as monotherapy or in combination with HMG-CoA reductase inhibitors); homozygous sitosterolemia; homozygous familial hypercholesterolemia (in combination with atorvastatin or simvastatin); mixed hyperlipidemia (in combination with fenofibrate)
Local Anesthetic/Vasoconstrictor Precautions No information available to require special precautions
Effects on Dental Treatment No significant effects or complications reported
Effects on Bleeding No information available to require special precautions
Adverse Effects 1% to 10%:
Central nervous system: Fatigue (2%)
Gastrointestinal: Diarrhea (4%)
Hepatic: Transaminases increased (with HMG-CoA reductase inhibitors) (≥3 x ULN, 1%)
Neuromuscular & skeletal: Arthralgia (3%), pain in extremity (3%)
Respiratory: Upper respiratory tract infection (4%), sinusitis (3%)
Miscellaneous: Influenza (2%)
Dosage Oral:
Children ≥10 years and Adults: 10 mg/day
Elderly: Refer to adult dosing

Dosage adjustment in renal impairment: AUC increased with severe impairment (Cl_{cr} <30 mL/minute); no dosing adjustment necessary
Dosage adjustment in hepatic impairment: AUC increased with hepatic impairment

Mild impairment (Child-Pugh class A): No dosing adjustment necessary

Moderate-to-severe impairment (Child-Pugh class B or C): Use of ezetimibe not recommended

Mechanism of Action Inhibits absorption of cholesterol at the brush border of the small intestine via the sterol transporter, Niemann-Pick C1-Like1 (NPC1L1). This leads to a decreased delivery of cholesterol to the liver, reduction of hepatic cholesterol stores and an increased clearance of cholesterol from the blood; decreases total C, LDL-cholesterol (LDL-C), ApoB, and triglycerides (TG) while increasing HDL-cholesterol (HDL-C).

Contraindications Hypersensitivity to ezetimibe or any component of the formulation; concomitant use with an HMG-CoA reductase inhibitor in patients with active hepatic disease, unexplained persistent elevations in serum transaminases; pregnancy; breast-feeding

Warnings/Precautions Secondary causes of hyperlipidemia should be ruled out prior to therapy. Use caution with severe renal (Cl_{cr} <30 mL/minute); if using concurrent simvastatin in patients with moderate-to-severe renal impairment, the manufacturer of ezetimibe recommends that simvastatin doses exceeding 20 mg be used with caution and close monitoring for adverse events (eg, myopathy). Use caution with mild hepatic impairment (Child-Pugh class A); not recommended for use with moderate or severe hepatic impairment (Child-Pugh classes B and C). Concurrent use of ezetimibe and fibric acid derivatives may increase the risk of cholelithiasis.

Drug Interactions

Metabolism/Transport Effects Substrate of SLCO1B1

Avoid Concomitant Use There are no known interactions where it is recommended to avoid concomitant use.

Increased Effect/Toxicity

Ezetimibe may increase the levels/effects of: Cyclo-SPORINE (Systemic)

The levels/effects of Ezetimibe may be increased by: CycloSPORINE (Systemic); Eltrombopag; Fibric Acid Derivatives

Decreased Effect

The levels/effects of Ezetimibe may be decreased by: Bile Acid Sequestrants

Ethanol/Nutrition/Herb Interactions Food: Ezetimibe did not cause meaningful reductions in fat-soluble vitamin concentrations during a 2-week clinical trial. Effects of long-term therapy have not been evaluated.

Dietary Considerations May be taken without regard to meals. Before initiation of therapy, patients should be placed on a standard cholesterol-lowering diet for 6 weeks and the diet should be continued during drug therapy.

Pharmacodynamics/Kinetics

Half-life Elimination 22 hours (ezetimibe and metabolite)

Time to Peak Plasma: 4-12 hours

Pregnancy Risk Factor C

Pregnancy Considerations Safety and efficacy have not been established; use during pregnancy only if the potential benefit to the mother outweighs the possible risk to the fetus.

Lactation Excretion in breast milk unknown/not recommended

Dosage Forms

Tablet, oral:

Zetia®: 10 mg

Ezetimibe and Simvastatin
(ez ET i mibe & SIM va stat in)

Related Information

Ezetimibe *on page 562*

Simvastatin *on page 1236*

Brand Names: U.S. Vytorin®

Pharmacologic Category Antilipemic Agent, 2-Azetidinone; Antilipemic Agent, HMG-CoA Reductase Inhibitor

Use Used in combination with dietary modification for the treatment of primary hypercholesterolemia and homozygous familial hypercholesterolemia

Local Anesthetic/Vasoconstrictor Precautions No information available to require special precautions

Effects on Dental Treatment No significant effects or complications reported

Effects on Bleeding No information available to require special precautions

Adverse Effects Percentages refer to combination Vytorin®. Also see individual agents.

1% to 10%:

Central nervous system: Headache (6%)

Gastrointestinal: Diarrhea (3%)

Hepatic: ALT increased (4%)

Neuromuscular & skeletal: Myalgia (4%), pain in extremity (2%)

Respiratory: Upper respiratory infection (4%)

Miscellaneous: Influenza (2%)

General Dosage Range Dosage adjustment recommended in patients with renal impairment or on concomitant therapy

Oral: *Adults:* Ezetimibe 10 mg and simvastatin 10-40 mg once daily

Mechanism of Action

Ezetimibe: Inhibits absorption of cholesterol at the brush border of the small intestine, leading to a decreased delivery of cholesterol to the liver. Ezetimibe inhibits the enzyme Niemann-Pick C1-Like1 (NPC1L1), a sterol transporter.

Simvastatin: A methylated derivative of lovastatin that acts by competitively inhibiting 3-hydroxy-3-methylglutaryl-coenzyme A (HMG-CoA) reductase, the enzyme that catalyzes the rate-limiting step in cholesterol biosynthesis.

Pregnancy Risk Factor X

Pregnancy Considerations Use is contraindicated in pregnant women. See individual agents.

Ezogabine (e ZOG a been)

Related Information

Clinical Risk Related to Drugs Prolonging QT Interval *on page 1510*

Brand Names: U.S. Potiga™

Pharmacologic Category Anticonvulsant, Neuronal Potassium Channel Opener

Use Adjuvant treatment of partial-onset seizures

Local Anesthetic/Vasoconstrictor Precautions Ezogabine is one of the drugs confirmed to prolong the QT interval and is accepted as having a risk of causing torsade de pointes. The risk of drug-induced torsade de pointes is extremely low when a single QT interval prolonging drug is prescribed. In terms of epinephrine, it is not known what effect vasoconstrictors in the local anesthetic regimen will have in patients with a known history of congenital prolonged QT interval or in patients taking any medication that prolongs the QT interval. Until more information is obtained, it is suggested that the clinician consult with the physician prior to the use of a vasoconstrictor in suspected patients, and that the vasoconstrictor (epinephrine, mepivacaine and levonordefrin [Carbocaine® 2% with Neo-Cobefrin®]) be used with caution.

Effects on Dental Treatment Key adverse event(s) related to dental treatment: Xerostomia and changes in salivation (normal salivary flow resumes upon discontinuation)

Effects on Bleeding No information available to require special precautions

Adverse Effects

>10%: Central nervous system: Dizziness (dose related; 23%), somnolence (dose related; 22%), fatigue (15%)

2% to 10%:

Central nervous system: Confusion (dose related; 9%), vertigo (8%), coordination impaired (dose related; 7%), attention disturbance (6%), memory impairment (dose related; 6%), aphasia (dose related; 4%), balance disorder (dose related; 4%), anxiety (3%), amnesia (2%), disorientation (2%)

Gastrointestinal: Nausea (7%), constipation (dose related; 3%), weight gain (dose related; 3%), dysphagia (2%)

Ocular: Diplopia (7%), blurred vision (dose related; 5%)

Neuromuscular & skeletal: Tremor (dose related; 8%), weakness (5%), abnormal gait (dose related; 4%), dysarthria (4%), paresthesia (3%)

Renal: Chromaturia (dose related; 2%), dysuria (dose related; 2%), hematuria (2%), urinary hesitation (2%)

Miscellaneous: Influenza infection (3%)

General Dosage Range Dosage adjustment recommended in patients with renal impairment or hepatic impairment.

Oral:

Adults: Initial: 100 mg 3 times/day; Maintenance: 200-400 mg 3 times/day (maximum: 1200 mg/day)

Elderly: Initial: 50 mg 3 times/day; Maintenance: 250 mg 3 times/day (maximum: 750 mg/day)

Mechanism of Action Ezogabine binds the KCNQ (Kv7.2-7.5) voltage-gated potassium channels, thereby stabilizing the channels in the open formation and enhancing the M-current. As a result, neuronal excitability is regulated and epileptiform activity is suppressed. In addition, ezogabine may also exert therapeutic effects through augmentation of GABA-mediated currents.

Pharmacodynamics/Kinetics

Half-life Elimination Ezogabine and NAMR: 7-11 hours; increased by ~30% in elderly patients

Time to Peak Plasma: 0.5-2 hours; delayed by 0.75 hours when administered with high-fat food

Pregnancy Risk Factor C

Pregnancy Considerations Adverse events were observed in animal reproduction studies. Patients exposed to ezogabine during pregnancy are encouraged to enroll themselves into the North American Antiepileptic Drug (NAAED) Pregnancy Registry by calling 1-888-233-2334. Additional information is available at www.aedpregnancyregistry.org.

Controlled Substance C-V

Dental Comment Ezogabine is known to prolong the QT interval. The QT interval is measured as the time and distance between the Q point of the QRS complex and the end of the T wave in the ECG tracing. After adjustment for heart rate, the QT interval is defined as prolonged if it is more than 450 msec in men and 460 msec in women. A long QT syndrome was first described in the 1950s and 60s as a congenital syndrome involving QT interval prolongation and syncope and sudden death. Some of the congenital long QT syndromes were characterized by a peculiar electrocardiographic appearance of the QRS complex involving a premature atria beat followed by a pause, then a subsequent sinus beat showing marked QT prolongation and deformity. This type of cardiac arrhythmia was originally termed "torsade de pointes" (translated from the French as "twisting of the points"). Ezogabine is considered as having a risk of causing torsade de pointes. Since it is not known what effect vasoconstrictors in the local anesthetic regimen will have in patients with a known history of congenital prolonged QT interval or in patients taking any medication that prolongs the QT interval, a medical consult is suggested.

Factor VIIa (Recombinant)

(FAK ter SEV en aye ree KOM be nant)

Brand Names: U.S. NovoSeven® RT

Brand Names: Canada Niastase®; Niastase® RT

Pharmacologic Category Antihemophilic Agent

Use Treatment of bleeding episodes and prevention of bleeding in surgical interventions in patients with either hemophilia A or B with inhibitors to factor VIII or factor IX, acquired hemophilia, or congenital factor VII deficiency

Unlabeled Use Warfarin-related intracerebral hemorrhage; treatment of refractory bleeding after cardiac surgery in nonhemophiliac patients

Local Anesthetic/Vasoconstrictor Precautions No information available to require special precautions

Effects on Dental Treatment No significant effects or complications reported

Effects on Bleeding Serious thromboembolic events are associated with use. Medical consult recommended.

Adverse Effects 1% to 10%:

Cardiovascular: Hypertension (2%), bradycardia (1%), edema (1%), hypotension (1%)

Central nervous system: Fever (4%), headache (1%), pain (1%)

Dermatologic: Pruritus (1%), purpura (1%), rash (1%)

Gastrointestinal: Vomiting (1%)

Hematologic: Plasma fibrinogen decreased (2%), disseminated intravascular coagulation (1%), fibrinolysis increased (1%), prothrombin decreased (1%)

Local: Injection site reaction (1%)

Neuromuscular & skeletal: Arthrosis (1%)

Renal: Abnormal renal function (1%)

Respiratory: Pneumonia (1%)

Miscellaneous: Allergic reactions (1%)

General Dosage Range I.V.: *Children and Adults:* Dosage varies greatly depending on indication

Mechanism of Action Recombinant factor VIIa, a vitamin K-dependent glycoprotein, promotes hemostasis by activating the extrinsic pathway of the coagulation cascade. It replaces deficient activated coagulation factor VII, which complexes with tissue factor and may activate coagulation factor X to Xa and factor IX to IXa. When complexed with other factors, coagulation factor Xa converts prothrombin to thrombin, a key step in the formation of a fibrin-platelet hemostatic plug.

Pharmacodynamics/Kinetics

Half-life Elimination 2.3 hours (range: 1.7-2.7)

Pregnancy Risk Factor C

Pregnancy Considerations Adverse events were observed in animal reproduction studies.

Factor IX Complex (Human)
(FAK ter nyne KOM pleks HYU man)

Brand Names: U.S. Bebulin® VH; Profilnine® SD

Pharmacologic Category Antihemophilic Agent; Blood Product Derivative; Prothrombin Complex Concentrate (PCC)

Use Prevention and control of bleeding in patients with factor IX deficiency (hemophilia B or Christmas disease)

Unlabeled Use Emergent correction of warfarin-induced coagulopathy (with clinically significant bleeding); **Note:** Products contain low or nontherapeutic levels of factor VII component; use of fresh frozen plasma (FFP) should be considered

Local Anesthetic/Vasoconstrictor Precautions No information available to require special precautions

Effects on Dental Treatment No significant effects or complications reported

Effects on Bleeding Associated with disseminated intravascular coagulation and thromboembolism

Adverse Effects Frequency not defined.

Cardiovascular: Flushing, thrombosis (sometimes fatal)

Central nervous system: Chills, fever, headache, lethargy, somnolence

Dermatologic: Rash, urticaria

Gastrointestinal: Nausea, vomiting

Hematologic: DIC

Neuromuscular & skeletal: Paresthesia

Respiratory: Dyspnea

Miscellaneous: Anaphylactic shock, clotting factor antibodies (development of), heparin-induced thrombocytopenia (with products containing heparin)

General Dosage Range I.V.: *Children and Adults:* Dosage varies greatly depending on indication

Mechanism of Action Replaces deficient clotting factor including factor X; hemophilia B, or Christmas disease, is an X-linked recessively inherited disorder of blood coagulation characterized by insufficient or abnormal synthesis of the clotting protein factor IX. Factor IX is a vitamin K-dependent coagulation factor which is synthesized in the liver. Factor IX is activated by factor XIa in the intrinsic coagulation pathway. Activated factor IX (IXa), in combination with factor VII:C, activates factor X to Xa, resulting ultimately in the conversion of prothrombin to thrombin and the formation of a fibrin clot. The infusion of exogenous factor IX to replace the deficiency present in hemophilia B temporarily restores hemostasis.

Pharmacodynamics/Kinetics

Half-life Elimination IX component: ~24 hours

Pregnancy Risk Factor C

Pregnancy Considerations Animal reproduction studies have not been conducted. There are no adequate and well-controlled studies in pregnant women.

Factor IX (Human) (FAK ter nyne HYU man)

Brand Names: U.S. AlphaNine® SD; Mononine®

Brand Names: Canada Immunine® VH

Pharmacologic Category Antihemophilic Agent; Blood Product Derivative

Use Prevention and control of bleeding in patients with hemophilia B (congenital factor IX deficiency or Christmas disease)

NOTE: Contains **nondetectable levels of factors II, VII, and X**. Therefore, **NOT INDICATED** for replacement therapy of any other clotting factor besides factor IX or for reversal of anticoagulation due to either vitamin K

antagonists or other anticoagulants (eg, dabigatran), for hemophilia A patients with factor VIII inhibitors, or for patients in a hemorrhagic state caused by reduced production of liver-dependent coagulation factors (eg, hepatitis, cirrhosis).

Local Anesthetic/Vasoconstrictor Precautions No information available to require special precautions

Effects on Dental Treatment No significant effects or complications reported

Effects on Bleeding Associated with disseminated intravascular coagulation and thromboembolism

Adverse Effects Frequency not defined.

Cardiovascular: Cyanosis, flushing, hypotension, chest tightness, thrombosis

Central nervous system: Chills, dizziness, drowsiness, fever (including transient fever following rapid administration), headache, lethargy, lightheadedness, somnolence

Dermatologic: Angioedema, photosensitivity reaction, rash, urticaria

Gastrointestinal: Abnormal taste, diarrhea, nausea, vomiting

Hematologic: Disseminated intravascular coagulation (DIC)

Hepatic: Alkaline phosphatase increased, ALT increased, AST increased

Local: Injection site reactions: Cellulitis, discomfort, pain, phlebitis, stinging

Neuromuscular & skeletal: Neck tightness, paresthesia, rigors

Ocular: Visual disturbance

Respiratory: Allergic rhinitis, asthma, cough, dyspnea, hypoxia, laryngeal edema, lung disorder

Miscellaneous: Allergic reaction, anaphylaxis, burning sensation in jaw/skull, factor IX inhibitor development, hypersensitivity reaction

General Dosage Range I.V.: *Infants, Children, Adolescents, and Adults:* Dosage varies greatly depending on indication

Mechanism of Action Replaces deficient clotting factor IX. Hemophilia B, or Christmas disease, is an X-linked inherited disorder of blood coagulation characterized by insufficient or abnormal synthesis of the clotting protein factor IX. Factor IX is a vitamin K-dependent coagulation factor which is synthesized in the liver. Factor IX is activated by factor XIa in the intrinsic coagulation pathway. Activated factor IX (IXa), in combination with factor VII:C activates factor X to Xa, resulting ultimately in the conversion of prothrombin to thrombin and the formation of a fibrin clot. The infusion of exogenous factor IX to replace the deficiency present in hemophilia B temporarily restores hemostasis.

Pharmacodynamics/Kinetics

Half-life Elimination IX component: ~21-25 hours

Pregnancy Risk Factor C

Pregnancy Considerations Animal reproduction studies have not been conducted. Safety and efficacy in pregnant women have not been established. Use during pregnancy only if clearly needed. Parvovirus B19 or hepatitis A, which may be present in plasma-derived products, may affect a pregnant woman more seriously than a nonpregnant woman.

Factor IX (Recombinant)
(FAK ter nyne ree KOM be nant)

Brand Names: U.S. BeneFix®

Brand Names: Canada BeneFix®

Pharmacologic Category Antihemophilic Agent

Use Prevention and control of bleeding in patients with hemophilia B (congenital factor IX deficiency or Christmas disease); perioperative management in patients with hemophilia B

NOTE: Contains **only factor IX.** Therefore, **NOT INDICATED** for replacement therapy of any other clotting factor besides factor IX or for reversal of anticoagulation due to either vitamin K antagonists or other anticoagulants (eg, dabigatran), for hemophilia A patients with factor VIII inhibitors, or for patients in a hemorrhagic state caused by reduced production of liver-dependent coagulation factors (eg, hepatitis, cirrhosis).

Local Anesthetic/Vasoconstrictor Precautions No information available to require special precautions

Effects on Dental Treatment No significant effects or complications reported

Effects on Bleeding Associated with disseminated intravascular coagulation and thromboembolism

Adverse Effects
>10%: Central nervous system: Headache (11%)
1% to 10%:
Cardiovascular: Flushing (3%), chest tightness (2%)
Central nervous system: Dizziness (8%), fever (3%; including transient fever following rapid administration), drowsiness (2%), chills (2%)
Dermatologic: Rash (2% to 6%), urticaria (3% to 5%)
Gastrointestinal: Nausea (6%), abnormal taste (5%), vomiting (2%)
Local: Injection reaction (2% to 8%; including cellulitis, pain, phlebitis)
Ocular: Blurred vision (2%)
Renal: Renal infarct (2%)
Respiratory: Dyspnea (3%), cough (2%), hypoxia (2%)
Miscellaneous: Factor IX inhibitor development (2% to 3%), shaking (2%)

General Dosage Range I.V.: *Infants, Children, Adolescents, and Adults:* Dosage varies greatly depending on indication

Mechanism of Action Replaces deficient clotting factor IX. Hemophilia B, or Christmas disease, is an X-linked inherited disorder of blood coagulation characterized by insufficient or abnormal synthesis of the clotting protein factor IX. Factor IX is a vitamin K-dependent coagulation factor which is synthesized in the liver. Factor IX is activated by factor XIa in the intrinsic coagulation pathway. Activated factor IX (IXa) in combination with factor VII:C activates factor X to Xa, resulting ultimately in the conversion of prothrombin to thrombin and the formation of a fibrin clot. The infusion of exogenous factor IX to replace the deficiency present in hemophilia B temporarily restores hemostasis.

Pharmacodynamics/Kinetics
Half-life Elimination Adolescents ≥16 years and adults: 11-36 hours; children: 14-28 hours

Pregnancy Risk Factor C

Pregnancy Considerations Animal reproduction studies have not been conducted. Safety and efficacy in pregnant women have not been established. Use during pregnancy only if clearly needed.

Factor XIII Concentrate (Human)
(FAK ter THIR teen KON cen trate HYU man)

Brand Names: U.S. Corifact®
Pharmacologic Category Antihemophilic Agent; Blood Product Derivative
Use Prophylaxis against bleeding episodes and management of perioperative surgical bleeding in patients with congenital factor XIII deficiency

Local Anesthetic/Vasoconstrictor Precautions No information available to require special precautions

Effects on Dental Treatment No significant effects or complications reported

Effects on Bleeding Thrombosis and thromboembolism reported. Consider medical consult.

Adverse Effects >1%:
Central nervous system: Chills, fever, headache
Dermatologic: Bruising, erythema, pruritus, rash
Hematologic: Hematoma, thrombin-antithrombin levels increased
Hepatic: LDH increased
Neuromuscular & skeletal: Arthralgia, joint inflammation
Respiratory: Epistaxis
Miscellaneous: Hypersensitivity

General Dosage Range I.V.: *Infants, Children, Adolescents, and Adults:* Initial: 40 units/kg; Maintenance: Varies depending on desired factor XIII trough levels; Usual: 40 units/kg every 28 days

Mechanism of Action Factor XIII (FXIII) is an endogenous plasma glycoprotein found in platelets, monocytes and macrophages that is converted to activated factor XIII (FXIIIa) in the presence of calcium ions. Once activated, FXIIIa cross-links fibrin and cross-links plasmin inhibitor to protect and strengthen the hemostatic platelet plug.

Pharmacodynamics/Kinetics
Duration of Action Plasma levels of FXIII: ~28 days; FXIII activity maintained at ≥5% in ≥97% of patients and ≥10% in ≥85% of patients
Half-life Elimination Children (<16): 5.7 days; Adults: 7.1 days
Time to Peak 1.7 hours postinfusion
Pregnancy Risk Factor C
Pregnancy Considerations Use in pregnant women only when benefit exceeds potential risk to the fetus. Thromboembolic events have been reported with use of factor XIII; pregnant women may be at increased risk due to hypercoagulable state.

Famciclovir (fam SYE kloe veer)

Related Information
Systemic Viral Diseases *on page 1537*
Viral Infections *on page 1575*
Related Sample Prescriptions
Herpes Simplex (Recurrent) *on page 1616*
Shingles (Varicella-Zoster Virus) *on page 1616*
Brand Names: U.S. Famvir®
Brand Names: Canada Apo-Famciclovir®; Ava-Famciclovir; CO Famciclovir; Famvir®; PMS-Famciclovir; Sandoz-Famciclovir
Generic Availability (U.S.) Yes
Pharmacologic Category Antiviral Agent
Dental Use Management of acute herpes zoster (shingles); treatment of recurrent herpes labialis in immunocompetent patients
Use Treatment of acute herpes zoster (shingles) in immunocompetent patients; treatment and suppression of recurrent episodes of genital herpes in immunocompetent patients; treatment of herpes labialis (cold sores) in immunocompetent patients; treatment of recurrent orolabial/genital (mucocutaneous) herpes simplex in HIV-infected patients

Local Anesthetic/Vasoconstrictor Precautions No information available to require special precautions
Effects on Dental Treatment No significant effects or complications reported

Effects on Bleeding No information available to require special precautions

Adverse Effects Note: Frequencies vary with dose and duration.

>10%:
Central nervous system: Headache (9% to 39%)
Gastrointestinal: Nausea (2% to 13%)
1% to 10%:
Central nervous system: Fatigue (1% to 5%), migraine (1% to 3%)
Dermatologic: Pruritus (≤4%), rash (≤3%)
Endocrine & metabolic: Dysmenorrhea (≤8%)
Gastrointestinal: Diarrhea (2% to 9%), abdominal pain (≤8%), vomiting (1% to 5%), flatulence (≤5%)
Hematologic: Neutropenia (3%)
Hepatic: Transaminases increased (2% to 3%), bilirubin increased (2%)
Neuromuscular & skeletal: Paresthesia (≤3%)

Dosage Adults: Oral:
Immunocompetent patients:
Acute herpes zoster: 500 mg every 8 hours for 7 days (**Note:** Initiate therapy as soon as possible after diagnosis and within 72 hours of rash onset)
Genital herpes simplex virus (HSV) infection:
Initial episode: 250 mg 3 times/day for 7-10 days (CDC, 2010)
Recurrence: 1000 mg twice daily for 1 day (**Note:** Initiate therapy as soon as possible and within 6 hours of symptoms/lesions onset)
Alternatively, the following regimens are also recommended: 125 mg twice daily for 5 days or 500 mg as a single dose, followed by 250 mg twice daily for 2 days (CDC, 2010). **Note:** Canadian labeling recommends 125 mg twice daily for 5 days.
Suppressive therapy: 250 mg twice daily for up to 1 year; **Note:** Duration not established, but efficacy/safety have been demonstrated for 1 year (CDC, 2010)
Recurrent herpes labialis (cold sores): 1500 mg as a single dose; initiate therapy at first sign or symptom such as tingling, burning, or itching (initiated within 1 hour in clinical studies)
HIV patients (**Note:** Initiate therapy as soon as possible and within 48 hours of symptoms/lesions onset):
Recurrent orolabial/genital (mucocutaneous) HSV infection: 500 mg twice daily for 7 days or 5-10 days (CDC, 2010).
Prevention of HSV reactivation: 500 mg twice daily (CDC, 2010)

Dosing adjustment in renal impairment:
Herpes zoster:
Cl_{cr} ≥60 mL/minute: No dosage adjustment necessary
Cl_{cr} 40-59 mL/minute: Administer 500 mg every 12 hours
Cl_{cr} 20-39 mL/minute: Administer 500 mg every 24 hours
Cl_{cr} <20 mL/minute: Administer 250 mg every 24 hours
Hemodialysis: Administer 250 mg after each dialysis session.
Recurrent genital herpes: Treatment:
U.S. labeling (single-day regimen):
Cl_{cr} ≥60 mL/minute: No dosage adjustment necessary
Cl_{cr} 40-59 mL/minute: Administer 500 mg every 12 hours for 1 day
Cl_{cr} 20-39 mL/minute: Administer 500 mg as a single dose

Cl_{cr} <20 mL/minute: Administer 250 mg as a single dose
Hemodialysis: Administer 250 mg as a single dose after a dialysis session.
Canadian labeling:
Cl_{cr} >20 mL/minute/1.73 m^2: No dosage adjustment necessary
Cl_{cr} <20 mL/minute/1.73 m^2: Administer 125 mg every 24 hours
Hemodialysis: Administer 125 mg after each dialysis session.
Recurrent genital herpes: Suppression:
Cl_{cr} ≥40 mL/minute: No dosage adjustment necessary
Cl_{cr} 20-39 mL/minute: Administer 125 mg every 12 hours
Cl_{cr} <20 mL/minute: Administer 125 mg every 24 hours
Hemodialysis: Administer 125 mg after each dialysis session.
Recurrent herpes labialis: Treatment (single-dose regimen):
Cl_{cr} ≥60 mL/minute: No dosage adjustment necessary
Cl_{cr} 40-59 mL/minute: Administer 750 mg as a single dose
Cl_{cr} 20-39 mL/minute: Administer 500 mg as a single dose
Cl_{cr} <20 mL/minute: Administer 250 mg as a single dose
Hemodialysis: Administer 250 mg as a single dose after a dialysis session.
Recurrent orolabial/genital (mucocutaneous) herpes in HIV-infected patients:
Cl_{cr} ≥40 mL/minute: No dosage adjustment necessary
Cl_{cr} 20-39 mL/minute: Administer 500 mg every 24 hours
Cl_{cr} <20 mL/minute: Administer 250 mg every 24 hours
Hemodialysis: Administer 250 mg after each dialysis session.

Dosage adjustment in hepatic impairment:
Mild-to-moderate impairment: No dosage adjustment is necessary
Severe impairment: No dosage adjustment provided in manufacturer's labeling; has not been studied. However, a 44% decrease in the C_{max} of penciclovir (active metabolite) was noted in patients with mild-to-moderate impairment; impaired conversion of famciclovir to penciclovir may affect efficacy.

Mechanism of Action Famciclovir undergoes rapid biotransformation to the active compound, penciclovir (prodrug), which is phosphorylated by viral thymidine kinase in HSV-1, HSV-2, and VZV-infected cells to a monophosphate form; this is then converted to penciclovir triphosphate and competes with deoxyguanosine triphosphate to inhibit HSV-2 polymerase, therefore, herpes viral DNA synthesis/replication is selectively inhibited.

Contraindications Hypersensitivity to famciclovir, penciclovir, or any component of the formulation

Warnings/Precautions Has not been established for use in immunocompromised patients (except HIV-infected patients with orolabial or genital herpes, patients with ophthalmic or disseminated zoster or with initial episode of genital herpes, and in Black and African American patients with recurrent episodes of genital herpes. Acute renal failure has been reported with use of inappropriate high doses in patients with underlying renal disease. Dosage adjustment is required in patients with renal insufficiency. Tablets contain lactose; do not use with galactose intolerance, severe lactase deficiency, or glucose-galactose malabsorption syndromes.

Drug Interactions
Metabolism/Transport Effects None known.
Avoid Concomitant Use
Avoid concomitant use of Famciclovir with any of the following: Zoster Vaccine
Increased Effect/Toxicity There are no known significant interactions involving an increase in effect.
Decreased Effect
Famciclovir may decrease the levels/effects of: Zoster Vaccine
Ethanol/Nutrition/Herb Interactions Food: Rate of absorption and/or conversion to penciclovir and peak concentration are reduced with food, but bioavailability is not affected.
Dietary Considerations May be taken without regard to meals.
Pharmacodynamics/Kinetics
Half-life Elimination Penciclovir: 2-4 hours; Prolonged in renal impairment: Cl_{cr} 20-39 mL/minute: 5-8 hours, Cl_{cr} <20 mL/minute: 3-24 hours
Time to Peak Penciclovir: ~1 hour
Pregnancy Risk Factor B
Pregnancy Considerations Teratogenic effects were not observed in animal reproduction studies. Data in pregnant women is limited. A registry has been established for women exposed to famciclovir during pregnancy (888-669-6682).
Lactation Excretion in breast milk unknown/not recommended
Breast-Feeding Considerations There is no specific data describing the excretion of famciclovir in breast milk. Breast-feeding is not recommended by the manufacturer unless the potential benefits outweigh any possible risk. If herpes lesions are on breast, breast-feeding should be avoided in order to avoid transmission to infant.
Dosage Forms
Tablet, oral: 125 mg, 250 mg, 500 mg
Famvir®: 125 mg, 250 mg, 500 mg

Famotidine (fa MOE ti deen)

Related Information
Gastrointestinal Disorders on page 1512
Brand Names: U.S. Heartburn Relief Maximum Strength [OTC]; Heartburn Relief [OTC]; Pepcid®; Pepcid® AC Maximum Strength [OTC]; Pepcid® AC [OTC]
Brand Names: Canada Acid Control; Apo-Famotidine®; Apo-Famotidine® Injectable; Famotidine Omega; Mylan-Famotidine; Novo-Famotidine; Nu-Famotidine; Pepcid®; Pepcid® AC; Pepcid® I.V.; Ulcidine
Generic Availability (U.S.) Yes: Infusion, Injection, oral suspension, tablet
Pharmacologic Category Histamine H_2 Antagonist
Use Maintenance therapy and treatment of duodenal ulcer; treatment of gastroesophageal reflux disease (GERD), active benign gastric ulcer; pathological hypersecretory conditions
OTC labeling: Relief of heartburn, acid indigestion, and sour stomach
Unlabeled Use Part of a multidrug regimen for H. pylori eradication to reduce the risk of duodenal ulcer recurrence; stress ulcer prophylaxis in critically-ill patients; symptomatic relief in gastritis
Local Anesthetic/Vasoconstrictor Precautions No information available to require special precautions
Effects on Dental Treatment No significant effects or complications reported

Effects on Bleeding No information available to require special precautions
Adverse Effects Note: Agitation and vomiting have been reported in up to 14% of pediatric patients <1 year of age.
1% to 10%:
Central nervous system: Headache (5%), dizziness (1%)
Gastrointestinal: Diarrhea (2%), constipation (1%), necrotizing enterocolitis (VLBW neonates; Guillet, 2006)
Dosage
Children: Treatment duration and dose should be individualized
Peptic ulcer: 1-16 years:
Oral: 0.5 mg/kg/day at bedtime or divided twice daily (maximum dose: 40 mg/day); doses of up to 1 mg/kg/day have been used in clinical studies
I.V.: 0.25 mg/kg every 12 hours (maximum dose: 40 mg/day); doses of up to 0.5 mg/kg have been used in clinical studies
GERD: Oral:
<3 months: 0.5 mg/kg once daily
3-12 months: 0.5 mg/kg twice daily
1-16 years: 1 mg/kg/day divided twice daily (maximum dose: 40 mg twice daily); doses of up to 2 mg/kg/day have been used in clinical studies

Children ≥12 years and Adults: Heartburn, indigestion, sour stomach: OTC labeling: Oral: 10-20 mg every 12 hours; dose may be taken 15-60 minutes before eating foods known to cause heartburn

Adults:
Duodenal ulcer: Oral: Acute therapy: 40 mg/day at bedtime (or 20 mg twice daily) for 4-8 weeks; maintenance therapy: 20 mg/day at bedtime
Helicobacter pylori eradication (unlabeled use): Oral: 40 mg once daily; requires combination therapy with antibiotics
Gastric ulcer: Oral: Acute therapy: 40 mg/day at bedtime
GERD: Oral: 20 mg twice daily for 6 weeks
Hypersecretory conditions: Oral: Initial: 20 mg every 6 hours, may increase in increments up to 160 mg every 6 hours
Esophagitis and accompanying symptoms due to GERD: Oral: 20 mg or 40 mg twice daily for up to 12 weeks
Stress ulcer prophylaxis, ICU patients (unlabeled use): Oral, I.V., or nasogastric (NG) tube: 20 mg twice daily (ASHP, 1999; Baghaie, 1995); **Note:** Intended for patients with associated risk factors (eg, coagulopathy, mechanical ventilation for >48 hours, severe sepsis); discontinue use once risk factors have resolved. The Surviving Sepsis Campaign guidelines suggest the use of proton pump inhibitors rather than H_2 antagonist therapy (Dellinger, 2013).
Patients unable to take oral medication: I.V.: 20 mg every 12 hours

Dosing adjustment in renal impairment:
Cl_{cr} <50 mL/minute: Manufacturer recommendation: Administer 50% of dose **or** increase the dosing interval to every 36-48 hours (to limit potential CNS adverse effects).
Stress ulcer prophylaxis (ASHP, 1999): Adults: Cl_{cr} <30 mL/minute: Oral, I.V., or nasogastric (NG) tube: 20 mg once daily

Mechanism of Action Competitive inhibition of histamine at H_2 receptors of the gastric parietal cells, which inhibits gastric acid secretion

Contraindications Hypersensitivity to famotidine, other H_2 antagonists, or any component of the formulation

Warnings/Precautions Modify dose in patients with moderate-to-severe renal impairment. Prolonged QT interval has been reported in patients with renal dysfunction. The FDA has received reports of torsade de pointes occurring with famotidine (Poluzzi, 2009). Relief of symptoms does not preclude the presence of a gastric malignancy. Reversible confusional states, usually clearing within 3-4 days after discontinuation, have been linked to use. Increased age (>50 years) and renal or hepatic impairment are thought to be associated. Multidose vials for injection contain benzyl alcohol.

OTC labeling: When used for self-medication, patients should be instructed not to use if they have difficulty swallowing, are vomiting blood, or have bloody or black stools. Not for use with other acid reducers.

Drug Interactions

Metabolism/Transport Effects None known.

Avoid Concomitant Use

Avoid concomitant use of Famotidine with any of the following: Dasatinib; Delavirdine; Ponatinib; Risedronate

Increased Effect/Toxicity

Famotidine may increase the levels/effects of: Dexmethylphenidate; Highest Risk QTc-Prolonging Agents; Methylphenidate; Moderate Risk QTc-Prolonging Agents; Risedronate; Saquinavir; Varenicline

The levels/effects of Famotidine may be increased by: Mifepristone

Decreased Effect

Famotidine may decrease the levels/effects of: Atazanavir; Bosutinib; Cefditoren; Cefpodoxime; Cefuroxime; Dasatinib; Delavirdine; Erlotinib; Fosamprenavir; Gefitinib; Indinavir; Iron Salts; Itraconazole; Ketoconazole (Systemic); Mesalamine; Multivitamins/Minerals (with ADEK, Folate, Iron); Nelfinavir; Nilotinib; Ponatinib; Posaconazole; Rilpivirine; Vismodegib

Ethanol/Nutrition/Herb Interactions

Ethanol: Avoid ethanol (may cause gastric mucosal irritation).

Food: Famotidine bioavailability may be increased if taken with food.

Dietary Considerations May be taken without regard to meals.

Pharmacodynamics/Kinetics

Onset of Action Antisecretory effect: Oral: Within 1 hour; I.V.: Within 30 minutes

Peak effect: Antisecretory effect: Oral: Within 1-3 hours (dose-dependent)

Duration of Action Antisecretory effect: I.V., Oral: 10-12 hours

Half-life Elimination

Infants: 0-3 months: ~8-10.5 hours; >3-12 months: ~4.5 hours

Children: 3.4 hours

Adults: 2.5-3.5 hours; prolonged with renal impairment; Oliguria: >20 hours

Time to Peak Serum: Oral: ~1-3 hours

Pregnancy Risk Factor B

Pregnancy Considerations Adverse events have not been observed in animal reproduction studies; therefore, famotidine is classified as pregnancy category B. Famotidine crosses the placenta. An increased risk of congenital malformations or adverse events in the newborn has generally not been observed following maternal use of famotidine during pregnancy. Histamine H_2 antagonists have been evaluated for the treatment of gastroesophageal reflux disease (GERD), as well as gastric and duodenal ulcers, during pregnancy. Although if needed, famotidine is not the agent of choice. Histamine H_2 antagonists may be used for aspiration prophylaxis prior to cesarean delivery.

Lactation Enters breast milk/not recommended

Breast-Feeding Considerations Famotidine is excreted into breast milk with peak concentrations occurring ~6 hours after the maternal dose. According to the manufacturer, the decision to continue or discontinue breast-feeding during therapy should take into account the risk of exposure to the infant and the benefits of treatment to the mother.

Dosage Forms

Infusion, premixed in NS [preservative free]: 20 mg (50 mL)

Injection, solution: 10 mg/mL (4 mL, 20 mL, 50 mL)

Injection, solution [preservative free]: 10 mg/mL (2 mL)

Powder for suspension, oral: 40 mg/5 mL (50 mL)
Pepcid®: 40 mg/5 mL (50 mL)

Tablet, oral: 10 mg, 20 mg, 40 mg
Heartburn Relief [OTC]: 10 mg
Heartburn Relief Maximum Strength [OTC]: 20 mg
Pepcid®: 20 mg, 40 mg
Pepcid® AC [OTC]: 10 mg
Pepcid® AC Maximum Strength [OTC]: 20 mg

Tablet, chewable, oral:
Pepcid® AC Maximum Strength [OTC]: 20 mg

Famotidine, Calcium Carbonate, and Magnesium Hydroxide

(fa MOE ti deen, KAL see um KAR bun ate, & mag NEE zhum hye DROKS ide)

Related Information

Calcium Carbonate *on page 233*
Famotidine *on page 568*
Magnesium Hydroxide *on page 852*

Brand Names: U.S. Pepcid® Complete® [OTC]; Tums® Dual Action [OTC]

Brand Names: Canada Pepcid® Complete® [OTC]

Pharmacologic Category Antacid; Histamine H_2 Antagonist

Use Relief of heartburn due to acid indigestion

Local Anesthetic/Vasoconstrictor Precautions No information available to require special precautions

Effects on Dental Treatment No significant effects or complications reported

Effects on Bleeding No information available to require special precautions

Adverse Effects See individual agents.

General Dosage Range Oral: *Children ≥12 years and Adults:* 1 tablet (famotidine 10 mg/calcium carbonate 800 mg/magnesium hydroxide 165 mg) as needed (maximum: 2 tablets/day)

Mechanism of Action
Famotidine: H_2 antagonist
Calcium carbonate: Antacid
Magnesium hydroxide: Antacid

Pregnancy Considerations See individual agents.

Fat Emulsion (fat e MUL shun)

Brand Names: U.S. Intralipid®; Liposyn® III
Brand Names: Canada Intralipid®; Liposyn® II

Pharmacologic Category Caloric Agent

Use Source of calories and essential fatty acids for patients requiring parenteral nutrition of extended duration; prevention and treatment of essential fatty acid deficiency (EFAD)

Unlabeled Use Treatment of local anesthetic-induced cardiac arrest unresponsive to conventional resuscitation

Local Anesthetic/Vasoconstrictor Precautions No information available to require special precautions

Effects on Dental Treatment No significant effects or complications reported

Effects on Bleeding No information available to require special precautions

Adverse Effects <1%: Allergic reactions, back pain, brown pigment deposition in the reticuloendothelial system ("intravenous fat pigment"), chest pain, cholestasis, cyanosis, diaphoresis, dizziness, dyspnea, eye pressure, fever, flushing, headache, hepatomegaly, hypercoagulability, hyperlipidemia, infusion site irritation, jaundice, leukopenia, liver function tests increased, nausea, pancreatitis, overloading syndrome (focal seizures, fever, leukocytosis, hepatomegaly, splenomegaly, shock), sleepiness, thrombocytopenia, vomiting

General Dosage Range I.V.:

Infants: Initial: 1-2 g/kg/day; Maintenance: Up to 3 g/kg/day

Children: 1-2 g/kg/day; Maintenance: Up to 2-3 g/kg/day **or** 8% to 10% of caloric intake given 2-3 times weekly

Adolescents and Adults: Initial: 1 g/kg/day; Maintenance: Up to 2.5 g/kg/day **or** 8% to 10% of caloric intake given 2-3 times weekly

Mechanism of Action Fat emulsion is metabolized and utilized as an energy source; provides the essential fatty acids, linoleic acid, and alpha linolenic acid necessary for normal structure and function of cell membranes; in local anesthetic toxicity, lipid emulsion probably extracts lipophilic local anesthesia from cardiac muscle

In local anesthetic toxicity, exogenous lipids provide an alternative source of binding of lipid-soluble local anesthetics (Rowlingson, 2008), commonly known as the "lipid sink" effect. This is more relevant to bupivacaine, levobupivacaine, and ropivacaine than mepivacaine and prilocaine. High lipid partition constant and large volumes of distribution are good predictors of success when using lipid therapy (French, 2011). Lipid administration may also affect the heart in a metabolically advantageous way by improving fatty acid transport (Weinberg, 2008).

Pharmacodynamics/Kinetics

Half-life Elimination 0.5-1 hour

Pregnancy Risk Factor C

Pregnancy Considerations Reproductive studies have not been conducted. Indications for fat emulsion therapy in pregnant women are the same as in nonpregnant women. The ASPEN guidelines for parenteral and enteral nutrition state that intravenous fat emulsion may be used safely in pregnant women to provide calories and prevent essential fatty acid deficiency (ASPEN Guidelines, 2002).

Febuxostat (feb UX oh stat)

Brand Names: U.S. Uloric®
Brand Names: Canada Uloric®
Pharmacologic Category Antigout Agent; Xanthine Oxidase Inhibitor
Use Chronic management of hyperuricemia in patients with gout

Local Anesthetic/Vasoconstrictor Precautions No information available to require special precautions

Effects on Dental Treatment Key adverse event(s) related to dental treatment: Xerostomia (normal salivary flow resumes upon discontinuation) and taste alteration has been reported in <1% of patients.

Effects on Bleeding No information available to require special precautions

Adverse Effects 1% to 10%:
Dermatologic: Rash (1% to 2%)
Gastrointestinal: Nausea (1%)
Hepatic: Liver function abnormalities (5% to 7%)
Neuromuscular & skeletal: Arthralgia (1%)

General Dosage Range Oral: *Adults:* 40-80 mg once daily

Mechanism of Action Selectively inhibits xanthine oxidase, the enzyme responsible for the conversion of hypoxanthine to xanthine to uric acid thereby decreasing uric acid. At therapeutic concentration does not inhibit other enzymes involved in purine and pyrimidine synthesis.

Pharmacodynamics/Kinetics

Half-life Elimination ~5-8 hours

Time to Peak Plasma: 1-1.5 hours

Pregnancy Risk Factor C

Pregnancy Considerations Animal studies have demonstrated increased neonatal mortality and reduction in weight gain, but not teratogenic effects. There are no adequate and well-controlled studies in pregnant women. Use during pregnancy only if potential benefit to the mother outweighs potential risk to the fetus.

Felbamate (FEL ba mate)

Brand Names: U.S. Felbatol®
Pharmacologic Category Anticonvulsant, Miscellaneous
Use Monotherapy or adjunctive therapy in the treatment of partial seizures (with and without generalization); adjunctive therapy in the treatment of partial and generalized seizures associated with Lennox-Gastaut syndrome; not indicated for use as first-line treatment

Local Anesthetic/Vasoconstrictor Precautions No information available to require special precautions

Effects on Dental Treatment Key adverse event(s) related to dental treatment: Xerostomia (normal salivary flow resumes upon discontinuation) and abnormal taste.

Effects on Bleeding Associated with marked increase in aplastic anemia and may present with signs of infection, bleeding, or anemia; therefore, incidents of abnormal bleeding should be reported to prescribing physician. Incidence of thrombocytopenia is ≤1%.

Adverse Effects
>10%:
Central nervous system: Somnolence (children 48%; adults 19%), headache (children 7%; adults 7% to 37%), fever (children 23%; adults 3%), dizziness (18%), insomnia (9% to 18%), fatigue (7% to 17%), nervousness (children 16%; adults 7%)
Dermatologic: Purpura (children 13%)
Gastrointestinal: Anorexia (children 55%; adults 19%), vomiting (children 39%; adults 9% to 17%), nausea (children 7%; adults 34%), dyspepsia (9% to 12%), constipation (7% to 11%)
Respiratory: Upper respiratory infection (children 45%; adults 5% to 9%)
1% to 10%:
Cardiovascular: Chest pain (3%), facial edema (3%), palpitation (≥1%), tachycardia (≥1%)

Central nervous system: Abnormal thinking (children 7%), ataxia (children 7%; adults 4%), emotional lability (children 7%), anxiety (5%), depression (5%), stupor (3%), malaise (≥1%), agitation (≥1%), psychological disturbances (≥1%), aggressive reaction (≥1%), euphoria (≤1%), hallucination (≤1%), migraine (≤1%), suicide attempt (≤1%)

Dermatologic: Skin rash (children 10%; adults 3% to 4%), acne (3%), pruritus (≥1%), bullous eruption (≤1%), urticaria (≤1%)

Endocrine and metabolic: Hypophosphatemia (≤1% to 3%), intramenstrual bleeding (3%), hypokalemia (≤1%), hyponatremia (≤1%)

Gastrointestinal: Hiccup (children 10%), weight loss (children 7%; adults 3%), taste perversion (6%), abdominal pain (5%), diarrhea (5%), xerostomia (3%), weight gain (≥1%), appetite increased (≤1%), esophagitis (≤1%)

Genitourinary: Urinary tract infection (3%)

Hematologic: Leukopenia (children 7%; adults ≤1%), granulocytopenia (≤1%), leukocytosis (≤1%), lymphadenopathy (≤1%), thrombocytopenia (≤1%)

Hepatic: Liver function tests increased (1% to 5%), alkaline phosphatase increased (≤1%)

Neuromuscular & skeletal: Abnormal gait (children 10%; adults 5%), pain (children 7%), tremor (6%), paresthesia (4%), myalgia (3%), weakness (≥1%), dystonia (≤1%)

Ocular: Miosis (children 7%), diplopia (3% to 6%), abnormal vision (5%)

Otic: Otitis media (children 10%; adults 3%)

Respiratory: Pharyngitis (children 10%; adults 3%), cough (children 7%), rhinitis (7%), sinusitis (4%)

Miscellaneous: Flu-like syndrome (≥1%), LDH increased (≤1%)

General Dosage Range Dosage adjustment recommended in patients with renal impairment or on concomitant therapy

Oral:
Children 2-14 years: Initial: 15 mg/kg/day in divided doses 3 or 4 times/day; Maintenance: Up to 45 mg/kg/day in divided doses 3 or 4 times/day (maximum: 3600 mg/day)

Children >14 years and Adults: Initial: 1200 mg/day in divided doses 3 or 4 times/day; Maintenance: Up to 3600 mg/day in divided doses 3 or 4 times/day.

Mechanism of Action Mechanism of action is unknown but has properties in common with other marketed anticonvulsants; has weak inhibitory effects on GABA-receptor binding, benzodiazepine receptor binding, and is devoid of activity at the MK-801 receptor binding site of the NMDA receptor-ionophore complex.

Pharmacodynamics/Kinetics
Half-life Elimination 20-23 hours (average); prolonged by 9-15 hours in renal impairment
Time to Peak Serum: 3-5 hours
Pregnancy Risk Factor C

Pregnancy Considerations Adverse events were not observed in animal reproduction studies. Postmarketing case reports in humans include fetal death, genital malformation, anencephaly, encephalocele, and placental disorder.

Patients exposed to felbamate during pregnancy are encouraged to enroll themselves into the North American Antiepileptic Drug (AED) Pregnancy Registry by calling 1-888-233-2334. Additional information is available at www.aedpregnancyregistry.org.

Prescribing and Access Restrictions A patient "informed consent" form should be completed and signed by the patient and physician. Copies are available from MEDA Pharmaceuticals by calling 800-526-3840.

Felodipine (fe LOE di peen)

Related Information
Calcium Channel Blockers and Gingival Hyperplasia *on page 1640*
Cardiovascular Diseases *on page 1492*
Brand Names: Canada Plendil®; Renedil®; Sandoz-Felodipine
Pharmacologic Category Calcium Channel Blocker; Calcium Channel Blocker, Dihydropyridine
Use Treatment of hypertension
Unlabeled Use Pediatric hypertension
Local Anesthetic/Vasoconstrictor Precautions No information available to require special precautions
Effects on Dental Treatment Key adverse event(s) related to dental treatment: Gingival hyperplasia (fewer reports than other CCBs, resolves upon discontinuation, consultation with physician is suggested).
Effects on Bleeding No information available to require special precautions
Adverse Effects
>10%: Central nervous system: Headache (11% to 15%)
2% to 10%: Cardiovascular: Peripheral edema (2% to 17%), tachycardia (0.4% to 2.5%), flushing (4% to 7%)
General Dosage Range Dosage adjustment recommended in patients with hepatic impairment
Oral:
Adults: Initial: 2.5-10 mg once daily; Maintenance: 2.5-20 mg once daily (maximum: 20 mg/day)
Elderly: Initial: 2.5 mg/day
Mechanism of Action Inhibits calcium ions from entering the "slow channels" or select voltage-sensitive areas of vascular smooth muscle and myocardium during depolarization, producing a relaxation of coronary vascular smooth muscle and coronary vasodilation; increases myocardial oxygen delivery in patients with vasospastic angina
Pharmacodynamics/Kinetics
Onset of Action Antihypertensive: 2-5 hours
Duration of Action Antihypertensive effect: 24 hours
Half-life Elimination Immediate release: 11-16 hours
Pregnancy Risk Factor C
Pregnancy Considerations Adverse events were observed in animal reproduction studies.

Fenofibrate (fen oh FYE brate)

Related Information
Cardiovascular Diseases *on page 1492*
Brand Names: U.S. Antara®; Fenoglide®; Lipofen®; Lofibra®; TriCor®; Triglide®
Brand Names: Canada Apo-Feno-Micro®; Apo-Feno-Super®; Apo-Fenofibrate®; Ava-Fenofibrate Micro; Dom-Fenofibrate Micro; Feno-Micro-200; Fenofibrate Micro; Fenofibrate-S; Fenomax; Lipidil EZ®; Lipidil Micro®; Lipidil Supra®; Mylan-Fenofibrate Micro; Novo-Fenofibrate Micronized; PHL-Fenofibrate Micro; PMS-Fenofibrate Micro; PRO-Feno-Super; Q-Fenofibrate Micro; ratio-Fenofibrate MC; Riva-Fenofibrate Micro; Sandoz-Fenofibrate E; Sandoz-Fenofibrate S; Teva-Fenofibrate S

◀ **Generic Availability (U.S.)** Yes: Micronized capsule, tablet

Pharmacologic Category Antilipemic Agent, Fibric Acid

Use Adjunct to dietary therapy for the treatment of adults with elevations of serum triglyceride levels (Fredrickson types IV and V hyperlipidemia); adjunct to dietary therapy for the reduction of low density lipoprotein cholesterol (LDL-C), total cholesterol (total-C), triglycerides, and apolipoprotein B (apo B), and to increase high density lipoprotein cholesterol (HDL-C) in adult patients with primary hypercholesterolemia or mixed dyslipidemia (Fredrickson types IIa and IIb hyperlipidemia)

Unlabeled Use Adjunctive therapy for the treatment of hyperuricemia in patients with gout

Local Anesthetic/Vasoconstrictor Precautions No information available to require special precautions

Effects on Dental Treatment Key adverse event(s) related to dental treatment: Dry mouth and tooth disorder.

Effects on Bleeding Thrombocytopenia has been reported through postmarketing surveillance.

Adverse Effects

>10%: Hepatic: Liver function tests increased (dose related; 3% to 13%; ALT/AST increased >3 x ULN: 5% to 13%)

1% to 10%:

Central nervous system: Headache (3%)

Dermatologic: Urticaria (1%)

Gastrointestinal: Abdominal pain (5%), constipation (2%), nausea (2%)

Neuromuscular & skeletal: Back pain (3%), CPK increased (3%)

Respiratory: Respiratory disorder (6%), rhinitis (2%)

Dosage Oral: **Note:** At least 2-3 months of therapy is required to determine efficacy.

Adults:

Hypertriglyceridemia: Initial:

Antara® (micronized): 43-130 mg once daily; maximum dose: 130 mg once daily

Fenoglide®: 40-120 mg once daily; maximum dose: 120 mg once daily

Fenomax™ [CAN; not available in U.S.]: 160 mg once daily; maximum dose: 200 mg once daily

Lipidil EZ® [CAN; not available in U.S.]: 145 mg once daily; maximum dose: 145 mg once daily

Lipidil Micro® [CAN; not available in U.S.]: 200 mg once daily; maximum dose: 200 mg once daily

Lipidil Supra® [CAN; not available in U.S.]: 160 mg once daily; maximum dose: 200 mg once daily

Lipofen®: 50-150 mg once daily; maximum dose: 150 mg once daily

Lofibra® (micronized): 67-200 mg once daily; maximum dose: 200 mg once daily

Lofibra® (tablets): 54-160 mg once daily; maximum dose: 160 mg once daily

TriCor®: 48-145 mg once daily; maximum dose: 145 mg once daily

Triglide®: 50-160 mg once daily; maximum dose: 160 mg once daily

Hypercholesterolemia or mixed hyperlipidemia:

Antara® (micronized): 130 mg once daily

Fenoglide®: 120 mg once daily

Fenomax™ [CAN; not available in U.S.]: 160 mg once daily; maximum dose: 200 mg once daily

Lipidil EZ® [CAN; not available in U.S.]: 145 mg once daily; maximum dose: 145 mg once daily

Lipidil Micro® [CAN; not available in U.S.]: 200 mg once daily; maximum dose: 200 mg once daily

Lipidil Supra® [CAN; not available in U.S.]: 160 mg once daily; maximum dose: 200 mg once daily

Lipofen®: 150 mg once daily

Lofibra® (micronized): 200 mg once daily

Lofibra® (tablets): 160 mg once daily

TriCor®: 145 mg once daily

Triglide®: 160 mg once daily

Elderly: Initial:

Antara® (micronized): 43 mg once daily

Fenoglide®: Adjust dosage based on creatinine clearance

Lipidil EZ® [CAN; not available in U.S.]: 48 mg once daily

Lipidil Micro® [CAN; not available in U.S.]: Adjust dosage based on creatinine clearance

Lipidil Supra® [CAN; not available in U.S.]: Adjust dosage based on creatinine clearance

Lipofen®: Adjust dosage based on creatinine clearance

Lofibra® (micronized): 67 mg once daily

Lofibra® (tablets): 54 mg once daily

TriCor®: Adjust dosage based on creatinine clearance

Triglide®: Adjust dosage based on creatinine clearance

Dosage adjustment in renal impairment: Monitor renal function and lipid panel before adjusting. **Note:** Use in severe renal impairment (including patients on dialysis) is contraindicated (see specific product labeling):

Antara® (micronized):

Cl_{cr} ≥50 mL/minute: No dosage adjustment necessary.

Cl_{cr} <50 mL/minute: Initiate at 43 mg once daily (contraindicated in severe impairment)

Fenoglide®:

Cl_{cr} >80 mL/minute or eGFR ≥60 mL/minute/1.73 m^2: No dosage adjustment necessary.

Cl_{cr} 31-80 mL/minute or eGFR 30-59 mL/minute/1.73 m^2: Initiate at 40 mg once daily

Cl_{cr} ≤30 mL/minute or eGFR <30 mL/minute/1.73 m^2: Use is contraindicated.

Fenomax™ [CAN; not available in U.S.]:

Cl_{cr} ≥20-100 mL/minute: Initiate at 100 mg once daily

Cl_{cr} <20 mL/minute: Use is contraindicated.

Lipidil EZ® [CAN; not available in U.S.]: **Note:** Interrupt treatment in patients with an increase in creatinine concentrations >50% the upper limit of normal (ULN).

Cl_{cr} ≥20-50 mL/minute: Initiate at 48 mg once daily

Cl_{cr} <20 mL/minute: Use is contraindicated.

Lipidil Micro® [CAN; not available in U.S.]: **Note:** Interrupt treatment in patients with an increase in creatinine concentrations >50% the upper limit of normal (ULN).

Cl_{cr} ≥20-85 mL/minute (women) or ≥20-95 mL/minute (men): Initiate therapy with Lipidil EZ® formulation with a dose of 48 mg once daily.

Cl_{cr} <20 mL/minute: Use is contraindicated.

Lipidil Supra® [CAN; not available in U.S.]: **Note:** Interrupt treatment in patients with an increase in creatinine concentrations >50% the upper limit of normal (ULN).

Cl_{cr} ≥20-100 mL/minute: Initiate at 100 mg once daily

Cl_{cr} <20 mL/minute: Use is contraindicated.

Lipofen®:

Cl_{cr} >80 mL/minute: No dosage adjustment necessary.

Cl_{cr} 31-80 mL/minute: Initiate at 50 mg once daily

Cl_{cr} ≤30 mL/minute: Use is contraindicated.

Lofibra® (micronized):

Cl_{cr} >80 mL/minute: No dosage adjustment necessary.

Cl_{cr} 31-80 mL/minute: Initiate at 67 mg once daily

Cl_{cr} ≤30 mL/minute: Use is contraindicated.

Lofibra® (tablets):

Cl_{cr} >80 mL/minute: No dosage adjustment necessary.

Cl_{cr} 31-80 mL/minute: Initiate at 54 mg once daily

Cl_{cr} ≤30 mL/minute: Use is contraindicated.

TriCor®:

Cl_{cr} >80 mL/minute: No dosage adjustment necessary.

Cl_{cr} 31-80 mL/minute: Initiate at 48 mg once daily

Cl_{cr} ≤30 mL/minute: Use is contraindicated.

Triglide®:

Cl_{cr} >80 mL/minute: No dosage adjustment necessary.

Cl_{cr} 31-80 mL/minute: Initiate at 50 mg once daily

Cl_{cr} ≤30 mL/minute: Use is contraindicated.

Dosage adjustment in hepatic impairment: Use is contraindicated.

Mechanism of Action Fenofibric acid, an agonist for the nuclear transcription factor peroxisome proliferator-activated receptor-alpha (PPAR-alpha), downregulates apoprotein C-III (an inhibitor of lipoprotein lipase) and upregulates the synthesis of apolipoprotein A-I, fatty acid transport protein, and lipoprotein lipase resulting in an increase in VLDL catabolism, fatty acid oxidation, and elimination of triglyceride-rich particles; as a result of a decrease in VLDL levels, total plasma triglycerides are reduced by 30% to 60%; modest increase in HDL occurs in some hypertriglyceridemic patients.

Contraindications Hypersensitivity to fenofibrate or any component of the formulation; hepatic dysfunction including primary biliary cirrhosis and unexplained persistent liver function abnormalities; severe renal impairment (including patients on dialysis); pre-existing gallbladder disease; breast-feeding (Fenoglide®, Lipofen®, TriCor®, and Triglide®)

Canadian labeling: Additional contraindications (not in U.S. labeling): Pregnancy; breast-feeding; known photoallergy or phototoxic reaction during treatment with fibrates or ketoprofen

Lipidil EZ®; Lipidil Micro®; Lipidil Supra®: Additional contraindications: Allergy to soya lecithin or peanut or arachis oil; chronic or acute pancreatitis; patients <18 years of age; coadministration with HMG-CoA reductase inhibitors in patients with a predisposition for myopathy.

Warnings/Precautions Secondary causes of hyperlipidemia should be ruled out prior to therapy. Hepatic transaminases can become significantly elevated (dose-related); hepatocellular, chronic active, and cholestatic hepatitis have been reported. Regular monitoring of liver function tests is required. Use with caution in patients with mild-to-moderate renal impairment; dosage adjustment may be required. Contraindicated with severe renal impairment including those receiving dialysis. Increases in serum creatinine (>2 mg/dL) have been observed with use; clinical significance unknown. Fenofibrate has been shown to increase creatinine production (unknown mechanism) resulting in an equal increase of creatinuria thereby demonstrating that the increase does not reflect a reduction in creatinine clearance (Hottelart, 2002). Monitor renal function in patients with renal impairment and consider monitoring patients with increased risk for developing renal impairment. May cause cholelithiasis. Use with caution in patient taking oral anticoagulants (eg, warfarin); adjustments in anticoagulation therapy may be required. Use caution with HMG-CoA reductase inhibitors or colchicine (may lead to myopathy, myositis, rhabdomyolysis). No incremental benefit of combination therapy on cardiovascular morbidity and mortality over statin monotherapy has been established. In patients with type 2 diabetes mellitus, neither fenofibrate monotherapy nor the addition of fenofibrate to simvastatin compared to placebo has been shown to reduce cardiovascular disease morbidity and mortality in patients with type 2 diabetes. In combination with HMG-CoA reductase inhibitors, fenofibrate is generally regarded as safer than gemfibrozil due to limited pharmacokinetic interaction with statins. Therapy should be withdrawn if an adequate response is not obtained after 2-3 months of therapy at the maximal daily dose. In patients with severe hypertriglyceridemia, the occurrence of pancreatitis may represent a failure of efficacy, a direct effect of the drug, or obstruction of the common bile duct due to biliary tract stone or sludge formation. A paradoxical, severe, and reversible decrease in HDL-C (as low as 2 mg/dL) with a simultaneous decrease in apolipoprotein A1 has been reported within 2 weeks to years after initiation of fibrate therapy; clinical significance unknown. Monitor HDL-C within a few months of initiation of therapy and discontinue if HDL-C becomes severely depressed; do not restart therapy. The occurrence of pancreatitis may represent a failure of efficacy in patients with severely elevated triglycerides. May cause mild-to-moderate decreases in hemoglobin, hematocrit, and WBC upon initiation of therapy which usually stabilizes with long-term therapy. Agranulocytosis and thrombocytopenia have been reported (rare). Periodic monitoring of blood counts is recommended during the first year of therapy.

Rare hypersensitivity reactions may occur. Use has been associated with pulmonary embolism (PE) and deep vein thrombosis (DVT). Use with caution in patients with risk factors for VTE. Dose adjustment may be required for elderly patients.

Some products may contain soya lecithin or peanut or arachis oil; use is contraindicated in patients with a soya lecithin allergy or a peanut or arachis allergy for applicable formulations.

Drug Interactions

Metabolism/Transport Effects **Substrate** of CYP3A4 (minor); **Note:** Assignment of Major/Minor substrate status based on clinically relevant drug interaction potential; **Inhibits** CYP2A6 (weak), CYP2C8 (weak), CYP2C9 (weak)

Avoid Concomitant Use There are no known interactions where it is recommended to avoid concomitant use.

Increased Effect/Toxicity

Fenofibrate may increase the levels/effects of: Colchicine; Ezetimibe; HMG-CoA Reductase Inhibitors; Sulfonylureas; Vitamin K Antagonists; Warfarin

The levels/effects of Fenofibrate may be increased by: CycloSPORINE (Systemic); Tacrolimus (Systemic)

Decreased Effect

Fenofibrate may decrease the levels/effects of: Chenodiol; CycloSPORINE (Systemic); Ursodiol

The levels/effects of Fenofibrate may be decreased by: Bile Acid Sequestrants

Dietary Considerations

Fenoglide®, Lofibra® (capsules [micronized] and tablets), Lipofen®: Take with meals.

Antara®, TriCor®, Triglide®: May be taken with or without food.

Canadian products [not available in U.S.]:
Fenomax™, Lipidil Micro®, Lipidil Supra®: Take with meals.
Lipidil EZ®: May be taken with or without food.

Pharmacodynamics/Kinetics

Half-life Elimination Half-life elimination: Fenofibric acid: Mean: 20 hours (range: 10-35 hours); half-life prolonged in patients with renal impairment

Time to Peak 2-8 hours

Pregnancy Risk Factor C

Pregnancy Considerations Maternal toxicity was observed in pregnant rats at doses approximately equivalent to the human dose; adverse events were not observed in reproduction studies done in rabbits. Reports of using fenofibrate during pregnancy are limited (Goldberg, 2012; Sunman, 2012; Whitten, 2011). Other agents are generally preferred if treatment for hypertriglyceridemia during pregnancy (Berglund, 2012) or treatment of lipid disorders in women of reproductive age (NCEP, 2001) is required. Use during pregnancy is specifically contraindicated in Canadian product labeling; some products recommend using effective birth control when treating women of reproductive age and discontinuing therapy several months prior to conception if planning a pregnancy.

Lactation Excretion in breast milk unknown/not recommended

Breast-Feeding Considerations It is not known if fenofibrate is excreted into breast milk. Some products are specifically contraindicated in nursing women. According to the manufacturers, the decision to continue or discontinue breast-feeding during therapy should take into account the risk of exposure to the infant and the benefits of treatment to the mother.

Dosage Forms

Capsule, oral: 43 mg, 67 mg, 130 mg, 134 mg, 200 mg
Antara®: 43 mg, 130 mg
Lipofen®: 50 mg, 150 mg
Lofibra®: 67 mg, 134 mg, 200 mg
Tablet, oral: 48 mg, 54 mg, 145 mg, 160 mg
Fenoglide®: 40 mg, 120 mg
Lofibra®: 54 mg, 160 mg
TriCor®: 48 mg, 145 mg
Triglide®: 50 mg, 160 mg

Fenofibric Acid (fen oh FYE brik AS id)

Related Information
Cardiovascular Diseases *on page 1492*

Brand Names: U.S. Fibricor®; TriLipix®

Generic Availability (U.S.) Yes

Pharmacologic Category Antilipemic Agent, Fibric Acid

Use Adjunct to dietary therapy for the treatment of severely elevated serum triglyceride levels; adjunct to dietary therapy for the reduction of low density lipoprotein cholesterol (LDL-C), total cholesterol (total-C), triglycerides, and apolipoprotein B (apo B) and to increase high density lipoprotein cholesterol (HDL-C) in patients with primary hypercholesterolemia or mixed dyslipidemia

TriLipix™ is also indicated as adjunct to dietary therapy concomitantly with a statin to reduce triglyceride levels and increase HDL-C levels in patients with mixed dyslipidemia and coronary heart disease (CHD) or at risk for CHD

Local Anesthetic/Vasoconstrictor Precautions No information available to require special precautions

Effects on Dental Treatment No significant effects or complications reported

Effects on Bleeding Thrombocytopenia has been reported through postmarketing surveillance.

Adverse Effects Adverse reactions and frequency reported as observed during monotherapy and concurrent administration with a statin (HMG-CoA reductase inhibitor).

>10%: Central nervous system: Headache (12% to 13%)

1% to 10%:
Central nervous system: Dizziness (3% to 4%), pain (1% to 4%), fatigue (2% to 3%)
Gastrointestinal: Nausea (4% to 6%), dyspepsia (3% to 5%), diarrhea (3% to 4%), constipation (3%)
Hepatic: ALT increased (monotherapy: 1%; coadministered with statin: 3%)
Neuromuscular & skeletal: Back pain (4% to 6%), pain in extremities (3% to 5%), arthralgia (4%), myalgia (3% to 4%), muscle spasm (2% to 3%)
Respiratory: Nasopharyngitis (4% to 5%), upper respiratory infection (4% to 5%), sinusitis (3% to 4%)

Additional adverse reactions when fenofibric acid coadministered with a statin (frequency not defined): AST increased, bronchitis, cough, CPK increased, hepatic enzymes increased, hypertension, influenza, insomnia, musculoskeletal pain, pharyngolaryngeal pain, urinary tract infection

Dosage Oral:

Adults:
Mixed dyslipidemia (coadministered with a statin): TriLipix™: 135 mg once daily (maximum: 135 mg/day)
Hypertriglyceridemia:
Fibricor®: Initial: 35-105 mg once daily; Maintenance: Individualize according to patient response (maximum: 105 mg/day)
TriLipix™: Initial: 45-135 mg once daily; Maintenance: Individualize according to patient response (maximum: 135 mg/day)
Primary hypercholesterolemia or mixed dyslipidemia:
Fibricor®: 105 mg once daily (maximum: 105 mg/day)
TriLipix™: 135 mg once daily (maximum: 135 mg/day)
Elderly: Dosage based on renal function

Dosage adjustment in renal impairment:
Normal renal function:
Fibricor®: Cl_{cr} >80 mL/minute: No dosage adjustment necessary
TriLipix™: eGFR ≥60 mL/minute/1.73 m^2: No dosage adjustment necessary.
Mild-to-moderate renal impairment
Fibricor®: Cl_{cr} 30-80 mL/minute: Initial: 35 mg once daily
TriLipix™: eGFR 30-59 mL/minute/1.73 m^2: Initial: 45 mg once daily
Severe renal impairment (with or without dialysis):
Fibricor®: Cl_{cr} <30 mL/minute: Use is contraindicated.
TriLipix™: eGFR <30 mL/minute/1.73 m^2: Use is contraindicated.

Dosage adjustment in hepatic impairment: Use is contraindicated in active liver disease, including primary biliary cirrhosis and unexplained persistent liver function abnormalities.

Mechanism of Action Fenofibric acid, an agonist for the nuclear transcription factor peroxisome proliferator-activated receptor-alpha (PPAR-alpha), downregulates apoprotein C-III (an inhibitor of lipoprotein lipase) and upregulates the synthesis of apolipoprotein A-I, fatty acid transport protein, and lipoprotein lipase resulting in an increase in VLDL catabolism, fatty acid oxidation, and elimination of triglyceride-rich particles; as a result of a decrease in VLDL levels, total plasma triglycerides are reduced by 30% to 60%; modest increased in HDL occurs in some hypertriglyceridemia patients.

Contraindications Hypersensitivity to fenofibric acid, fenofibrate, or any component of the formulation; hepatic dysfunction including primary biliary cirrhosis and unexplained persistent liver function abnormalities; severe renal impairment (including patients on dialysis); pre-existing gallbladder disease; breast-feeding

Warnings/Precautions Secondary causes of hyperlipidemia should be ruled out prior to therapy. Has been associated with rare myositis or rhabdomyolysis; patients should be monitored closely. Risk increased in the elderly, patients with diabetes mellitus, renal failure, or hypothyroidism. Patients should be instructed to report unexplained muscle pain, tenderness, weakness, or brown urine. Hepatic transaminases can become significantly elevated (dose-related); hepatocellular, chronic active, and cholestatic hepatitis have been reported. Regular monitoring of liver function tests is required. Use with caution in patients with mild-to-moderate renal impairment; dosage adjustment required. Contraindicated with severe renal impairment including those receiving dialysis. Reversible increases in serum creatinine (>2 mg/dL) have been observed with use; no adverse effects on clinical outcomes (ie, adverse renal or cardiovascular outcomes) seen in one analysis (Bonds, 2012). Fenofibrate has been shown to increase creatinine production (unknown mechanism) resulting in an equal increase of creatinuria demonstrating that the increase does not reflect a reduction in creatinine clearance (Hottelart, 2002). Monitor renal function in patients with renal impairment and consider monitoring patients with increased risk for developing renal impairment. May cause cholelithiasis discontinue if gallstones found upon gallbladder studies. A paradoxical, severe, and reversible decrease in HDL cholesterol (as low as 2 mg/dL) with a simultaneous decrease in apolipoprotein A1 may occur within 2 weeks to years after initiation. Monitor HDL-C within a few months of initiation of therapy and discontinue if HDL-C becomes severely depressed; do not restart therapy. Use caution with oral anticoagulants; adjustments in therapy may be required.

Use caution with HMG-CoA reductase inhibitors or colchicine (may lead to myopathy, rhabdomyolysis). No incremental benefit of combination therapy on cardiovascular morbidity and mortality over HMG-CoA reductase inhibitor monotherapy has been established. In patients with type 2 diabetes mellitus, neither fenofibrate monotherapy nor the addition of fenofibrate to simvastatin compared to placebo has been shown to reduce cardiovascular disease morbidity and mortality in patients with type 2 diabetes. In combination with HMG-CoA reductase inhibitors, fenofibric acid derivatives are generally regarded as safer than gemfibrozil due to limited pharmacokinetic interaction. Therapy should be withdrawn if an adequate response is not obtained after 2-3 months of therapy at the maximal daily dose. The occurrence of pancreatitis may represent a failure of efficacy in patients with severely elevated triglycerides. May cause mild-to-moderate decreases in hemoglobin, hematocrit, and WBC upon initiation of therapy, which usually stabilizes with long-term therapy. Rare hypersensitivity reactions may occur. Use has been associated with pulmonary embolism (PE) and deep vein thrombosis (DVT). Use with caution in patients with risk factors for VTE. Dose adjustment is required for renal impairment and elderly patients.

Drug Interactions

Metabolism/Transport Effects Inhibits CYP2A6 (weak), CYP2C8 (weak), CYP2C9 (moderate)

Avoid Concomitant Use There are no known interactions where it is recommended to avoid concomitant use.

Increased Effect/Toxicity

Fenofibric Acid may increase the levels/effects of: Carvedilol; Colchicine; CYP2C9 Substrates; Ezetimibe; HMG-CoA Reductase Inhibitors; Sulfonylureas; Vitamin K Antagonists; Warfarin

The levels/effects of Fenofibric Acid may be increased by: CycloSPORINE (Systemic); Tacrolimus (Systemic)

Decreased Effect

Fenofibric Acid may decrease the levels/effects of: Chenodiol; CycloSPORINE (Systemic); Ursodiol

The levels/effects of Fenofibric Acid may be decreased by: Bile Acid Sequestrants

Dietary Considerations May be taken with or without food. Patients should follow appropriate lipid-lowering diet.

Pharmacodynamics/Kinetics

Half-life Elimination ~20 hours

Time to Peak Fibricor®: ~2.5 hours; TriLipix™: 4-5 hours

Pregnancy Risk Factor C

Pregnancy Considerations Adverse events were observed in animal reproduction studies. When treatment is required during pregnancy, other agents are preferred (NCEP, 2002).

Lactation Excretion in breast milk unknown/contraindicated

Breast-Feeding Considerations It is not known if fenofibric acid is excreted in breast milk. Due to the potential for serious adverse reactions in the nursing infant, use is contraindicated in nursing women.

Dosage Forms

Capsule, delayed release, oral:
TriLipix®: 45 mg, 135 mg

Tablet, oral: 35 mg, 105 mg
Fibricor®: 35 mg, 105 mg

Fenoldopam (fe NOL doe pam)

Brand Names: U.S. Corlopam®

Pharmacologic Category Dopamine Agonist

Use Treatment of severe hypertension (up to 48 hours in adults), including in patients with renal compromise; short-term (up to 4 hours) blood pressure reduction in pediatric patients

Local Anesthetic/Vasoconstrictor Precautions No information available to require special precautions

Effects on Dental Treatment Key adverse event(s) related to dental treatment: Xerostomia and changes in salivation (normal salivary flow resumes upon discontinuation).

Effects on Bleeding No information available to require special precautions

Adverse Effects

≥5%:
Cardiovascular: Cutaneous flushing, hypotension
Central nervous system: Headache
Gastrointestinal: Nausea

◄ <5%:
Cardiovascular: Angina, bradycardia, chest pain, extrasystoles, heart failure, MI, orthostatic hypotension, palpitation, ST-T abnormalities, T-wave inversion, tachycardia
Central nervous system: Anxiety, dizziness, fever, insomnia
Endocrine & metabolic: Hyperglycemia, hypokalemia, LDH increased
Gastrointestinal: Abdominal pain/fullness, constipation, diarrhea, vomiting
Genitourinary: Urinary tract infection
Hematologic: Bleeding, leukocytosis
Hepatic: Transaminases increased
Local: Injection site reactions
Neuromuscular & skeletal: Back pain, limb cramps
Ocular: Intraocular pressure increased
Renal: BUN increased, creatinine increased, oliguria
Respiratory: Dyspnea, nasal congestion
Miscellaneous: Diaphoresis

General Dosage Range I.V.:
Children: Initial: 0.2 mcg/kg/minute, may increase to 0.3-0.5 mcg/kg/minute every 20-30 minutes (maximum: 0.8 mcg/kg/minute)
Adults: Initial: 0.03-0.1 mcg/kg/minute, may increase in increments of 0.05-0.1 mcg/kg/minute every 15 minutes (maximum: 1.6 mcg/kg/minute)

Mechanism of Action A selective postsynaptic dopamine agonist (D_1-receptors) which exerts hypotensive effects by decreasing peripheral vasculature resistance with increased renal blood flow, diuresis, and natriuresis; 6 times as potent as dopamine in producing renal vasodilatation; has minimal adrenergic effects

Pharmacodynamics/Kinetics
Onset of Action I.V.: 10 minutes
Duration of Action I.V.: 1 hour
Half-life Elimination I.V.: Children: 3-5 minutes; Adults: ~5 minutes

Pregnancy Risk Factor B

Pregnancy Considerations Fetal harm was not observed in animal studies; however, safety and efficacy have not been established for use during pregnancy. Use during pregnancy only if clearly needed.

Fenoprofen (fen oh PROE fen)

Related Information
Rheumatoid Arthritis, Osteoarthritis, and Osteoporosis *on page 1526*
Temporomandibular Dysfunction (TMD), Chronic Pain, and Fibromyalgia *on page 1590*
Brand Names: U.S. Nalfon®
Brand Names: Canada Nalfon®
Generic Availability (U.S.) Yes: Tablet
Pharmacologic Category Nonsteroidal Anti-inflammatory Drug (NSAID), Oral
Use Symptomatic treatment of acute and chronic rheumatoid arthritis and osteoarthritis; relief of mild-to-moderate pain
Unlabeled Use Migraine prophylaxis
Local Anesthetic/Vasoconstrictor Precautions No information available to require special precautions
Effects on Dental Treatment The dentist should be aware of the potential of abnormal coagulation. Caution should also be exercised in the use of NSAIDs in patients already on anticoagulant therapy with drugs such as warfarin (Coumadin®). See Effects on Bleeding.

Effects on Bleeding Nonselective NSAIDs such as fenoprofen inhibit platelet aggregation and prolong bleeding time in some patients. Unlike aspirin, the NSAID effect on platelet function is quantitatively less, of shorter duration, and reversible.

Adverse Effects 1% to 10%:
Cardiovascular: Peripheral edema (5%), palpitation (3%)
Central nervous system: Headache (9%), somnolence (9%), dizziness (7%), nervousness (6%), fatigue (2%), confusion (1%)
Dermatologic: Itching (4%), rash (4%)
Gastrointestinal: Dyspepsia (10%), nausea (8%), constipation (7%), vomiting (3%), abdominal pain (2%)
Neuromuscular & skeletal: Weakness (5%), tremor (2%)
Ocular: Blurred vision (2%)
Otic: Tinnitus (5%), hearing decreased (2%)
Respiratory: Dyspnea (3%), nasopharyngitis (1%)
Miscellaneous: Diaphoresis (5%)

Dosage Adults: Oral:
Rheumatoid arthritis, osteoarthritis: 300-600 mg 3-4 times/day; maximum dose: 3.2 g/day
Mild-to-moderate pain: 200 mg every 4-6 hours as needed; maximum dose: 3.2 g/day

Dosage adjustment in renal impairment: Not recommended in patients with advanced renal disease
Dosage adjustment in hepatic impairment: No dosage adjustment provided in manufacturer's labeling.
Mechanism of Action Reversibly inhibits cyclooxygenase-1 and 2 (COX-1 and 2) enzymes, which results in decreased formation of prostaglandin precursors; has antipyretic, analgesic, and anti-inflammatory properties

Other proposed mechanisms not fully elucidated (and possibly contributing to the anti-inflammatory effect to varying degrees), include inhibiting chemotaxis, altering lymphocyte activity, inhibiting neutrophil aggregation/activation, and decreasing proinflammatory cytokine levels.

Contraindications Hypersensitivity to fenoprofen, aspirin, or other NSAIDs, or any component of the formulation; perioperative pain in the setting of coronary artery bypass graft (CABG) surgery; significant renal dysfunction

Warnings/Precautions [U.S. Boxed Warning]: NSAIDs are associated with an increased risk of adverse cardiovascular thrombotic events, including MI and stroke. Risk may be increased with duration of use or pre-existing cardiovascular risk factors or disease. Carefully evaluate individual cardiovascular risk profiles prior to prescribing. May cause new-onset hypertension or worsening of existing hypertension. Use caution with fluid retention. Avoid use in heart failure. Concurrent administration of ibuprofen, and potentially other nonselective NSAIDs, may interfere with aspirin's cardioprotective effect. **[U.S. Boxed Warning]: Use is contraindicated for treatment of perioperative pain in the setting of coronary artery bypass graft (CABG) surgery.** Risk of MI and stroke may be increased with use following CABG surgery.

NSAID use may compromise existing renal function; dose-dependent decreases in prostaglandin synthesis may result from NSAID use, reducing renal blood flow which may cause renal decompensation. NSAID use may increase the risk for hyperkalemia. Patients with impaired renal function, dehydration, heart failure, liver dysfunction, those taking diuretics, and ACE inhibitors, and the elderly are at greater risk of renal toxicity and hyperkalemia. Rehydrate patient before starting therapy; monitor renal function closely. Not recommended for use in patients with advanced renal disease. Long-term NSAID use may result in renal papillary necrosis.

[U.S. Boxed Warning]: NSAIDs may increase risk of gastrointestinal irritation, inflammation, ulceration, bleeding, and perforation. These events may occur at any time during therapy and without warning. Use caution with a history of GI disease (bleeding or ulcers), concurrent therapy with aspirin, anticoagulants and/or corticosteroids, smoking, use of alcohol, the elderly or debilitated patients. When used concomitantly with ≤325 mg of aspirin, a substantial increase in the risk of gastrointestinal complications (eg, ulcer) occurs; concomitant gastroprotective therapy (eg, proton pump inhibitors) is recommended (Bhatt, 2008).

Platelet adhesion and aggregation may be decreased; may prolong bleeding time; patients with coagulation disorders or who are receiving anticoagulants should be monitored closely. Anemia may occur; patients on long-term NSAID therapy should be monitored for anemia. Rarely, NSAID use has been associated with potentially severe blood dyscrasias (eg, agranulocytosis, thrombocytopenia, aplastic anemia).

Use the lowest effective dose for the shortest duration of time, consistent with individual patient goals, to reduce risk of cardiovascular or GI adverse events. Alternate therapies should be considered for patients at high risk.

NSAIDs may cause serious skin adverse events including exfoliative dermatitis, Stevens-Johnson syndrome (SJS), and toxic epidermal necrolysis (TEN); discontinue use at first sign of skin rash or hypersensitivity. Anaphylactoid reactions may occur, even without prior exposure; patients with "aspirin triad" (bronchial asthma, aspirin intolerance, rhinitis) may be at increased risk. Do not use in patients who experience bronchospasm, asthma, rhinitis, or urticaria with NSAID or aspirin therapy. Use caution in other forms of asthma.

Use with caution in patients with decreased hepatic function. Closely monitor patients with any abnormal LFT. Severe hepatic reactions (eg, fulminant hepatitis, liver failure) have occurred with NSAID use, rarely; discontinue if signs or symptoms of liver disease develop, or if systemic manifestations occur.

NSAIDS may cause drowsiness, dizziness, blurred vision and other neurologic effects which may impair physical or mental abilities; patients must be cautioned about performing tasks which require mental alertness (eg, operating machinery or driving). Discontinue use with blurred or diminished vision and perform ophthalmologic exam. Monitor vision with long-term therapy.

In the elderly, avoid chronic use (unless alternative agents ineffective and patient can receive concomitant gastroprotective agent); nonselective oral NSAID use is associated with an increased risk of GI bleeding and peptic ulcer disease in older adults in high risk category (eg, >75 years or age or receiving concomitant oral/parenteral corticosteroids, anticoagulants, or antiplatelet agents) (Beers Criteria).

Withhold for at least 4-6 half-lives prior to surgical or dental procedures.

Drug Interactions

Metabolism/Transport Effects None known.

Avoid Concomitant Use

Avoid concomitant use of Fenoprofen with any of the following: Floctafenine; Ketorolac (Nasal); Ketorolac (Systemic); NSAID (COX-2 Inhibitor); Omacetaxine

Increased Effect/Toxicity

Fenoprofen may increase the levels/effects of: Agents with Antiplatelet Properties; Aliskiren; Aminoglycosides; Anticoagulants; Bisphosphonate Derivatives; Collagenase (Systemic); CycloSPORINE (Systemic); Dabigatran Etexilate; Deferasirox; Desmopressin; Digoxin; Drotrecogin Alfa (Activated); Eplerenone; Haloperidol; Ibritumomab; Lithium; Methotrexate; Nonsteroidal Anti-Inflammatory Agents; NSAID (COX-2 Inhibitor); Omacetaxine; PEMEtrexed; Porfimer; Potassium-Sparing Diuretics; PRALAtrexate; Quinolone Antibiotics; Rivaroxaban; Salicylates; Thrombolytic Agents; Tositumomab and Iodine I 131 Tositumomab; Vancomycin; Vitamin K Antagonists

The levels/effects of Fenoprofen may be increased by: ACE Inhibitors; Angiotensin II Receptor Blockers; Antidepressants (Tricyclic, Tertiary Amine); Corticosteroids (Systemic); CycloSPORINE (Systemic); Floctafenine; Glucosamine; Herbs (Anticoagulant/Antiplatelet Properties); Ketorolac (Nasal); Ketorolac (Systemic); Multivitamins/Minerals (with ADEK, Folate, Iron); Nonsteroidal Anti-Inflammatory Agents; Omega-3 Fatty Acids; Pentosan Polysulfate Sodium; Pentoxifylline; Probenecid; Prostacyclin Analogues; Selective Serotonin Reuptake Inhibitors; Serotonin/Norepinephrine Reuptake Inhibitors; Sodium Phosphates; Tipranavir; Treprostinil; Vitamin E

Decreased Effect

Fenoprofen may decrease the levels/effects of: ACE Inhibitors; Agents with Antiplatelet Properties; Aliskiren; Angiotensin II Receptor Blockers; Beta-Blockers; Eplerenone; HydrALAZINE; Loop Diuretics; Potassium-Sparing Diuretics; Salicylates; Selective Serotonin Reuptake Inhibitors; Thiazide Diuretics

The levels/effects of Fenoprofen may be decreased by: Bile Acid Sequestrants; Nonsteroidal Anti-Inflammatory Agents; Salicylates

Ethanol/Nutrition/Herb Interactions

Ethanol: Avoid ethanol (may enhance gastric mucosal irritation).

Food: Fenoprofen peak serum levels may be decreased if taken with food; total amount absorbed is not affected.

Herb/Nutraceutical: Avoid alfalfa, anise, bilberry, bladderwrack, bromelain, cat's claw, celery, chamomile, coleus, cordyceps, dong quai, evening primrose, fenugreek, feverfew, garlic, ginger, ginkgo biloba, ginseng (American, Panax, Siberian), grapeseed, green tea, guggul, horse chestnut seed, horseradish, licorice, prickly ash, red clover, reishi, SAMe (S-adenosylmethionine), sweet clover, turmeric, white willow (all have additional antiplatelet activity).

Dietary Considerations May be taken with food to decrease GI distress.

Pharmacodynamics/Kinetics

Onset of Action A few days; full benefit: up to 2-3 weeks

Half-life Elimination 2.5-3 hours

Time to Peak Serum: ~2 hours

Pregnancy Risk Factor C

Pregnancy Considerations Adverse events were not observed in the initial animal reproduction studies; therefore, the manufacturer classifies fenoprofen as pregnancy category C. NSAID exposure during the first trimester is not strongly associated with congenital malformations; however, cardiovascular anomalies and cleft palate have been observed following NSAID exposure in some studies. The use of an NSAID close to conception may be associated with an increased risk of miscarriage. Nonteratogenic effects have been observed following NSAID administration during the third trimester including: Myocardial degenerative changes, prenatal constriction of the ductus arteriosus, fetal tricuspid regurgitation, failure of the ductus arteriosus to close postnatally; renal dysfunction or failure, oligohydramnios; gastrointestinal bleeding or perforation, increased risk of necrotizing enterocolitis; intracranial bleeding (including intraventricular hemorrhage), platelet dysfunction with resultant bleeding; pulmonary hypertension. Because they may cause premature closure of the ductus arteriosus, use of NSAIDs late in pregnancy should be avoided (use after 31 or 32 weeks gestation is not recommended by some clinicians). The chronic use of NSAIDs in women of reproductive age may be associated with infertility that is reversible upon discontinuation of the medication.

Lactation Enters breast milk/not recommended

Breast-Feeding Considerations Very low levels of fenoprofen are found in breast milk. Breast-feeding is not recommended by the manufacturer.

Dosage Forms
Capsule, oral:
Nalfon®: 200 mg, 400 mg
Tablet, oral: 600 mg

FentaNYL (FEN ta nil)

Brand Names: U.S. Abstral®; Actiq®; Duragesic®; Fentora®; Lazanda®; Onsolis®; Subsys®
Brand Names: Canada Abstral™; Actiq®; Apo-Fentanyl® Matrix; Duragesic®; Duragesic® MAT; Fentanyl Citrate Injection, USP; Novo-Fentanyl; Onsolis®; PMS-Fentanyl MTX; RAN™-Fentanyl Matrix Patch; RAN™-Fentanyl Transdermal System; ratio-Fentanyl; Sandoz Fentanyl Patch; Teva-Fentanyl
Generic Availability (U.S.) Yes: Injection, lozenge, patch
Pharmacologic Category Analgesic, Opioid; Anilidopiperidine Opioid; General Anesthetic
Dental Use Adjunct in preoperative intravenous conscious sedation in patients undergoing dental surgery
Use
Injection: Relief of pain, preoperative medication, adjunct to general or regional anesthesia
Transdermal patch (eg, Duragesic®): Management of persistent moderate-to-severe chronic pain in opioid-tolerant patients when around-the-clock analgesia is needed for an extended period of time
Transmucosal lozenge (eg, Actiq®), buccal tablet (Fentora®), buccal film (Onsolis®), nasal spray (Lazanda®), sublingual tablet (Abstral®), sublingual spray (Subsys®): Management of breakthrough cancer pain in opioid-tolerant patients
Note: "Opioid-tolerant" patients are defined as patients who are taking at least:
Oral morphine 60 mg/day, **or**
Transdermal fentanyl 25 mcg/hour, **or**
Oral oxycodone 30 mg/day, **or**
Oral hydromorphone 8 mg/day, **or**
Oral oxymorphone 25 mg/day, **or**
Equianalgesic dose of another opioid for at least 1 week

Local Anesthetic/Vasoconstrictor Precautions No information available to require special precautions

Effects on Dental Treatment Key adverse event(s) related to dental treatment: Xerostomia, changes in salivation (normal salivary flow resumes upon discontinuation), and orthostatic hypotension. Actiq® may contribute to dental caries due to sugar content of oral lozenge; advise patients to maintain good oral hygiene. See Dental Comment.

Effects on Bleeding No information available to require special precautions

Adverse Effects
>10%:
Cardiovascular: Bradycardia, edema
Central nervous system: CNS depression, confusion, dizziness, drowsiness, fatigue, headache, sedation
Endocrine & metabolic: Dehydration
Gastrointestinal: Constipation, nausea, vomiting, xerostomia
Local: Application-site reaction erythema
Neuromuscular & skeletal: Chest wall rigidity (high dose I.V.), muscle rigidity, weakness
Ocular: Miosis
Respiratory: Dyspnea, respiratory depression
Miscellaneous: Diaphoresis

1% to 10%:
Cardiovascular: Cardiac arrhythmia, cardiorespiratory arrest, chest pain, DVT, flushing, hyper-/hypotension, orthostatic hypotension, pallor, palpitation, peripheral edema, sinus tachycardia, syncope, tachycardia, vasodilation
Central nervous system: Abnormal dreams, abnormal thinking, agitation, amnesia, anxiety, attention disturbance, chills, depression, disorientation, dysphoria, euphoria, fever, hallucinations, hypoesthesia, insomnia, irritability, lethargy, malaise, mental status change, migraine, nervousness, paranoid reaction, restlessness, somnolence, stupor, vertigo
Dermatologic: Alopecia, bruising, cellulitis, decubitus ulcer, erythema, hyperhidrosis, papules, pruritus, rash
Endocrine & metabolic: Breast pain, dehydration, hot flashes, hyper-/hypocalcemia, hyper-/hypoglycemia, hypoalbuminemia, hypokalemia, hypomagnesemia, hyponatremia
Gastrointestinal: Abdominal distension, abdominal pain, abnormal taste, anorexia, appetite decreased, biliary tract spasm, diarrhea, dyspepsia, dysphagia (buccal tablet/film/sublingual spray), flatulence, gastritis, gastroenteritis, gastroesophageal reflux, GI hemorrhage, gingival pain (buccal tablet), gingivitis (lozenge), glossitis (lozenge), hematemesis, ileus, intestinal obstruction (buccal film), periodontal abscess (lozenge/buccal tablet), proctalgia, stomatitis (lozenge/buccal tablet/sublingual tablet/sublingual spray), tongue disorder (sublingual tablet), ulceration (gingival, lip, mouth; transmucosal use/nasal spray), weight loss
Genitourinary: Dysuria, erectile dysfunction, urinary incontinence, urinary retention, urinary tract infection, vaginitis, vaginal hemorrhage
Hematologic: Anemia, leukopenia, neutropenia, thrombocytopenia
Hepatic: Alkaline phosphatase increased, ascites, AST increased, jaundice
Local: Application site pain, application site irritation
Neuromuscular & skeletal: Abnormal coordination, abnormal gait, arthralgia, back pain, limb pain, myalgia, neuropathy, paresthesia, rigors, tremor
Ocular: Blurred vision, diplopia, dry eye, swelling, ptosis, strabismus
Renal: Renal failure

Respiratory: Apnea, asthma, bronchitis, cough, dyspnea (exertional), epistaxis, hemoptysis, hypoventilation, hypoxia, laryngitis, nasal congestion (nasal spray), nasal discomfort (nasal spray), nasopharyngitis, pharyngolaryngeal pain, pharyngitis, pneumonia, postnasal drip (nasal spray), pulmonary embolism (nasal spray), rhinitis, rhinorrhea (nasal spray), sinusitis, upper respiratory infection, wheezing

Miscellaneous: Flu-like syndrome, hiccups, hypersensitivity, lymphadenopathy, night sweats, parosmia, speech disorder, withdrawal syndrome

Dental Usual Dosage Surgery: Adults:

Premedication: I.M., slow I.V.: 25-100 mcg/dose 30-60 minutes prior to surgery

Adjunct to regional anesthesia. Slow I.V.: 25-100 mcg/dose over 1-2 minutes. **Note:** An I.V. should be in place with regional anesthesia so the I.M. route is rarely used but still maintained as an option in the package labeling.

Dosage Note: Ranges listed may not represent the maximum doses that may be required in all patients. Doses and dosage intervals should be titrated to pain relief/prevention. Monitor vital signs routinely. Single I.M. doses have duration of 1-2 hours, single I.V. doses last 0.5-1 hour.

Minor procedures/analgesia (unlabeled use): I.V.:

Children 1-12 years: 0.5-2 mcg/kg/dose given 3 minutes prior to procedure; may repeat every 1-2 hours

Children >12 years: 0.5-2 mcg/kg/dose (maximum: 50 mcg/dose) given 3 minutes prior to procedure; may repeat in 5 minutes if necessary; if more than 2 doses are needed, repeat with a maximum of 25 mcg/dose up to 5 times

Surgery:

Children ≥2 years: Adjunct to anesthesia (induction and maintenance): Slow I.V.: 2-3 mcg/kg/dose every 1-2 hours as needed

Adults:

Premedication: I.M., slow I.V.: 50-100 mcg/dose 30-60 minutes prior to surgery

Adjunct to regional anesthesia: Slow I.V.: 25-100 mcg/dose over 1-2 minutes. **Note:** An I.V. should be in place with regional anesthesia so the I.M. route is rarely used but still maintained as an option in the package labeling.

Adjunct to general anesthesia: Slow I.V.:

Low dose: 0.5-2 mcg/kg/dose depending on the indication

Moderate dose: Initial: 2-20 mcg/kg/dose; Maintenance (bolus or infusion): 1-2 mcg/kg/**hour**. Discontinuing fentanyl infusion 30-60 minutes prior to the end of surgery will usually allow adequate ventilation upon emergence from anesthesia. For "fast-tracking" and early extubation following major surgery, total fentanyl doses are limited to 10-15 mcg/kg.

High dose: 20-50 mcg/kg/dose; **Note:** High-dose fentanyl as an adjunct to general anesthesia is rarely used, but is still described in the manufacturer's label.

Pain management:

Children (unlabeled use): I.V.: 0.5-2 mcg/kg/dose given every 1-2 hours as needed; continuous infusion: 0.5-2 mcg/kg/**hour**; titrate to desired effects

Patient-controlled analgesia (PCA) (unlabeled use; American Pain Society, 2008): Children <50 kg: **Note:** Opiate-naive: Consider lower end of dosing range:

Usual concentration: 10 mcg/mL

Demand dose: 0.5-1 mcg/kg/dose

Lockout interval: 6-8 minutes

Usual basal rate: 0-0.5 mcg/kg/**hour**

Adults:

I.V. (unlabeled use): Bolus at start of infusion: 1-2 mcg/kg **or** 25-100 mcg/dose; continuous infusion rate: 1-2 mcg/kg/**hour or** 25-200 mcg/hour

Severe pain: I.M, I.V. (unlabeled): 50-100 mcg/dose every 1-2 hours as needed; patients with prior opiate exposure may tolerate higher initial doses

Patient-controlled analgesia (PCA) (unlabeled use): I.V.:

Usual concentration: 10 mcg/mL

Demand dose: Usual: 20 mcg; range: 10-50 mcg

Lockout interval: 5-8 minutes

Usual basal rate: ≤50 mcg/hour

Critically-ill patients (unlabeled dose): Slow I.V.: 25-35 mcg (based on ~70 kg patient) **or** 0.35-0.5 mcg/kg every 30-60 minutes as needed (Barr, 2013). **Note:** More frequent dosing may be needed (eg, mechanically-ventilated patients).

Continuous infusion: 50-700 mcg/hour (based on ~70 kg patient) **or** 0.7-10 mcg/kg/**hour** (Barr, 2013)

Intrathecal (I.T.) (unlabeled use; American Pain Society, 2008): **Must be preservative-free.** Doses must be adjusted for age, injection site, and patient's medical condition and degree of opioid tolerance.

Single dose: 5-25 mcg/dose; may provide adequate relief for up to 6 hours

Continuous infusion: Not recommended in acute pain management due to risk of excessive accumulation. For chronic cancer pain, infusion of very small doses may be practical (American Pain Society, 2008).

Epidural (unlabeled use; American Pain Society, 2008): **Must be preservative-free.** Doses must be adjusted for age, injection site, and patient's medical condition and degree of opioid tolerance

Single dose: 25-100 mcg/dose; may provide adequate relief for up to 8 hours

Continuous infusion: 25-100 mcg/hour

Breakthrough cancer pain: For patients who are tolerant to and currently receiving opioid therapy for persistent cancer pain; dosing should be individually titrated to provide adequate analgesia with minimal side effects. Dose titration should be done if patient requires more than 1 dose/breakthrough pain episode for several consecutive episodes. Patients experiencing >4 breakthrough pain episodes/day should have the dose of their long-term opioid re-evaluated.

Children ≥16 years and Adults: Transmucosal: Lozenge (Actiq®): Initial dose: 200 mcg; the second dose may be started 15 minutes after completion of the first dose if pain unrelieved. A maximum of 1 additional dose can be given per pain episode; must wait at least 4 hours before treating another episode. Consumption should be limited to ≤4 units/day. Additional requirements suggest need for improved baseline therapy.

Adults: Transmucosal:

Buccal film (Onsolis®): Initial dose: 200 mcg for all patients **Note:** Patients previously using another transmucosal product should be initiated at doses of 200 mcg; do **not** switch patients using any other fentanyl product on a mcg-per-mcg basis.

Dose titration: If titration required, increase dose in 200 mcg increments once per episode using multiples of the 200 mcg film; do not redose within a single episode of breakthrough pain and separate single doses by ≥2 hours. During titration, do not exceed 4 simultaneous applications of the 200 mcg films (800 mcg). If >800 mcg required, treat next episode with one 1200 mcg film (maximum dose: 1200 mcg). Once maintenance dose is determined, all other unused films should be disposed of and that strength (using a single film) should be used. During any pain episode, if adequate relief is not achieved after 30 minutes following buccal film application, a rescue medication (as determined by healthcare provider) may be used.

Maintenance: Determined dose applied as a single film once per episode and separated by ≥2 hours (dose range: 200-1200 mcg); limit to 4 applications/day. Consider increasing the around-the-clock opioid therapy in patients experiencing >4 breakthrough pain episodes/day.

Buccal tablet (Fentora®): Initial dose: 100 mcg; a second 100 mcg dose, if needed, may be started 30 minutes after the start of the first dose. **Note:** For patients previously using the transmucosal lozenge (Actiq®), the initial dose should be selected using the conversions listed below (maximum: 2 doses per breakthrough pain episode every 4 hours).

Dose titration, if required, should be done using multiples of the 100 mcg tablets. Patient can use two 100 mcg tablets (one on each side of mouth). If that dose is not successful, can use four 100 mcg tablets (two on each side of mouth). If titration requires >400 mcg/dose, then use 200 mcg tablets. **Note:** Buccal tablet may be administered sublingually once an effective maintenance dose has been established.

Conversion from lozenge to buccal tablet (Fentora®):

Lozenge dose 200-400 mcg, then buccal tablet 100 mcg

Lozenge dose 600-800 mcg, then buccal tablet 200 mcg

Lozenge dose 1200-1600 mcg, then buccal tablet 400 mcg

Note: Four 100 mcg buccal tablets deliver approximately 12% and 13% higher values of C_{max} and AUC, respectively, compared to one 400 mcg buccal tablet. To prevent confusion, patient should only have one strength available at a time. Using more than four buccal tablets at a time has not been studied.

Nasal spray (Lazanda®):

Initial dose: 100 mcg (one 100 mcg spray in one nostril) for all patients. **Note:** Patients previously using another fentanyl product should be initiated at a dose of 100 mcg; do not convert patients from other fentanyl products to Lazanda® on a mcg-per-mcg basis.

Dose titration: If pain is relieved within 30 minutes, that same dose should be used to treat subsequent episodes. If pain is unrelieved, may increase to a higher dose using the recommended titration steps. **Must wait at least 2 hours before treating another episode with nasal spray.** Dose titration steps: If no relief with 100 mcg dose, increase to 200 mcg dose per episode (one 100 mcg spray in each nostril); if no relief with 200 mcg dose, increase to 400 mcg per episode (one 400 mcg spray); if no relief with 400 mcg dose, increase to 800 mcg dose per episode (one 400 mcg spray in each nostril). **Note:** Single doses >800 mcg have not been evaluated. There are no data supporting the use of a combination of dose strengths.

Maintenance dose: Once maintenance dose for breakthrough pain episode has been determined, use that dose for subsequent episodes. For pain that is not relieved after 30 minutes of Lazanda® administration or if a separate breakthrough pain episode occurs within the 2 hour window before the next Lazanda® dose is permitted, a rescue medication may be used. Limit Lazanda® use to ≤4 episodes of breakthrough pain per day. If response to maintenance dose changes (increase in adverse reactions or alterations in pain relief), dose readjustment may be necessary. If patient is experiencing >4 breakthrough pain episodes/day, consider increasing the around-the-clock, long-acting opioid therapy; if long-acting opioid therapy dose is altered, re-evaluate and retitrate Lazanda® dose as needed.

Sublingual spray (Subsys®):

Initial dose: 100 mcg for all patients. If pain is unrelieved, 1 additional 100 mcg dose may be given 30 minutes after administration of the first dose. A maximum of 2 doses can be given per breakthrough pain episode; must wait at least 4 hours before treating another episode. **Note:** Patients must remain on around-the-clock opioids during use. Patients previously using other fentanyl products should be initiated at a dose of 100 mcg; do not convert patients from any other fentanyl product (transmucosal, transdermal, or parenteral) to Subsys® on a mcg-per-mcg basis.

Dose titration: If pain is relieved within 30 minutes, that same dose should be used to treat subsequent episodes and no titration is necessary. If pain is unrelieved, may increase to a higher dose using the recommended titration steps. Goal is to determine the dose that provides adequate analgesia (with tolerable side effects) using a single dose per breakthrough pain episode. For each breakthrough pain episode, if pain unrelieved after 30 minutes only 1 additional dose using the same strength may be given (maximum: 2 doses per breakthrough pain episode). **Must wait at least 4 hours before treating another episode with Subsys®.**

Dose titration steps: If no relief with 100 mcg dose, increase to 200 mcg dose per episode (one 200 mcg unit); if no relief with 200 mcg dose, increase to 400 mcg per episode (one 400 mcg unit); if no relief with 400 mcg dose, increase to 600 mcg dose per episode (one 600 mcg unit); if no relief with 600 mcg dose, increase to 800 mcg dose per episode (one 800 mcg unit); if no relief with 800 mcg dose, increase to 1200 mcg dose per episode (two 600 mcg units); if no relief with 1200 mcg dose, increase to 1600 mcg per episode (two 800 mcg units).

Maintenance dose: Once maintenance dose for breakthrough pain episode has been determined, use that dose for subsequent episodes. If occasional episodes of unrelieved breakthrough pain occur following 30 minutes of Subsys® administration, 1 additional dose using the same strength may be administered (maximum: 2 doses per breakthrough pain episode); patient must wait 4 hours before treating another breakthrough pain episode with Subsys®. Once maintenance dose is determined, limit Susbsys™ use to ≤4 episodes of breakthrough pain per day. If response to maintenance dose changes (increase in adverse reactions or alterations in pain relief), dose readjustment may be necessary. If patient is experiencing >4 breakthrough pain episodes/day, consider increasing the around-the-clock, long-acting opioid therapy.

Sublingual tablet (Abstral®):

Initial dose:

U.S. labeling: 100 mcg for all patients; if pain is unrelieved, a second dose may be given 30 minutes after administration of the first dose. A maximum of 2 doses can be given per breakthrough pain episode; must wait at least 2 hours before treating another episode.

Canadian labeling: 100 mcg for all patients; if pain is unrelieved 30 minutes after administration of Abstral™, an alternative rescue medication (other than Abstral™) may be given. Administer only 1 dose of Abstral™ per breakthrough pain episode; must wait at least 2 hours before treating another episode.

Note: Patients previously using another fentanyl product should be initiated at a dose of 100 mcg; do not convert patients from other fentanyl products to Abstral® on a mcg-per-mcg basis.

Dose titration: If titration required, increase in 100 mcg increments (up to 400 mcg) over consecutive breakthrough episodes. If titration requires >400 mcg/dose, increase in increments of 200 mcg, starting with 600 mcg dose. During titration, patients may use multiples of 100 mcg and/or 200 mcg tablets for any single dose; do not exceed 4 tablets at one time; safety and efficacy of doses >800 mcg have not been evaluated.

Maintenance dose: Once maintenance dose for breakthrough pain episode has been determined, use only 1 tablet in the appropriate strength per episode; if pain is unrelieved with maintenance dose:

U.S. labeling recommendations: A second dose may be given after 30 minutes; maximum of 2 doses/episode of breakthrough pain; separate treatment of subsequent episodes by ≥2 hours; limit treatment to ≤4 breakthrough episodes/day.

Canadian labeling recommendations: Administer alternative rescue medication after 30 minutes; maximum of 1 Abstral™ dose/episode of breakthrough pain; separate treatment of subsequent episodes by ≥2 hours; limit treatment to ≤4 breakthrough episodes/day.

Consider increasing the around-the-clock long-acting opioid therapy in patients experiencing >4 breakthrough pain episodes/day; if long-acting opioid therapy dose altered, re-evaluate and retitrate Abstral® dose as needed.

Elderly >65 years: Transmucosal lozenge (eg, Actiq®): In clinical trials, patients who were >65 years of age were titrated to a mean dose that was 200 mcg less than that of younger patients.

Chronic pain management: Children ≥2 years and Adults (opioid-tolerant patients): Transdermal patch (Duragesic®):

Initial: To convert patients from oral or parenteral opioids to transdermal patch, a 24-hour analgesic requirement should be calculated (based on prior opiate use). Using the tables, the appropriate initial dose can be determined. The initial fentanyl dosage may be approximated from the 24-hour morphine dosage equivalent and titrated to minimize adverse effects and provide analgesia. With the initial application, the absorption of transdermal fentanyl requires several hours to reach plateau; therefore transdermal fentanyl is inappropriate for management of acute pain. Change patch every 72 hours.

Conversion from continuous infusion of fentanyl: In patients who have adequate pain relief with a fentanyl infusion, fentanyl may be converted to transdermal dosing at a rate equivalent to the intravenous rate. A two-step taper of the infusion to be completed over 12 hours has been recommended (Kornick, 2001) after the patch is applied. The infusion is decreased to 50% of the original rate six hours after the application of the first patch, and subsequently discontinued twelve hours after application.

Titration: Short-acting agents may be required until analgesic efficacy is established and/or as supplements for "breakthrough" pain. The amount of supplemental doses should be closely monitored. Appropriate dosage increases may be based on daily supplemental dosage using the ratio of 45 mg/24 hours of oral morphine to a 12.5 mcg/hour increase in fentanyl dosage.

Frequency of adjustment: The dosage should not be titrated more frequently than every 3 days after the initial dose or every 6 days thereafter. Patients should wear a consistent fentanyl dosage through two applications (6 days) before dosage increase based on supplemental opiate dosages can be estimated. **Note:** Upon discontinuation, ~17 hours are required for a 50% decrease in fentanyl levels.

Frequency of application: The majority of patients may be controlled on every 72-hour administration; however, a small number of patients require every 48-hour administration.

Dose conversion guidelines for transdermal fentanyl (see tables).

Note: U.S. and Canadian dose conversion guidelines differ. Consult appropriate table.

U.S. Labeling: Dose Conversion Guidelines: Recommended Initial Duragesic® Dose Based Upon Daily Oral Morphine Dose[1,2]

Oral 24-Hour Morphine (mg/day)	Duragesic® Dose[3] (mcg/h)
60-134	25
135-224	50
225-314	75
315-404	100
405-494	125
495-584	150
585-674	175
675-764	200
765-854	225
855-944	250
945-1034	275
1035-1124	300

[1]The table should NOT be used to convert from transdermal fentanyl (Duragesic®) to other opioid analgesics. Rather, following removal of the patch, titrate the dose of the new opioid until adequate analgesia is achieved.

[2]Recommendations are based on U.S. product labeling for Duragesic®.

[3]Pediatric patients initiating therapy on a 25 mcg/hour Duragesic® system should be opioid-tolerant and receiving at least 60 mg oral morphine equivalents per day.

U.S. Labeling: Dose Conversion Guidelines[1,2]

Current Analgesic	Daily Dosage (mg/day)			
Morphine (I.M./I.V.)	10-22	23-37	38-52	53-67
Oxycodone (oral)	30-67	67.5-112	112.5-157	157.5-202
Codeine (oral)	150-447	-	-	-
Hydromorphone (oral)	8-17	17.1-28	28.1-39	39.1-51
Hydromorphone (I.V.)	1.5-3.4	3.5-5.6	5.7-7.9	8-10
Meperidine (I.M.)	75-165	166-278	279-390	391-503
Methadone (oral)	20-44	45-74	75-104	105-134
Fentanyl transdermal recommended dose (mcg/h)	25 mcg/h	50 mcg/h	75 mcg/h	100 mcg/h

[1]The table should NOT be used to convert from transdermal fentanyl (Duragesic®) to other opioid analgesics. Rather, following removal of the patch, titrate the dose of the new opioid until adequate analgesia is achieved.

[2]Recommendations are based on U.S. product labeling for Duragesic®.

Transdermal patch (Duragesic® MAT [Canada; not available in U.S.]): Adults:

Canadian Labeling: Dose Conversion Guidelines (Adults): Recommended Initial Duragesic® MAT Dose Based Upon Daily Oral Morphine Dose[1,2]

Oral 24-Hour Morphine (Current Dose in mg/day)	Duragesic® MAT Dose (Initial Dose in mcg/h)
45-59	12
60-134	25
135-179	37
180-224	50
225-269	62
270-314	75
315-359	87
360-404	100
405-494	125
495-584	150
585-674	175
675-764	200
765-854	225
855-944	250
945-1034	275
1035-1124	300

[1]The table should NOT be used to convert from transdermal fentanyl (Duragesic® MAT) to other opioid analgesics. Rather, following removal of the patch, titrate the dose of the new opioid until adequate analgesia is achieved.

[2]Recommendations are based on Canadian product labeling for Duragesic® MAT.

Note: The 12 mcg/hour dose included in this table is to be used for incremental dose adjustment and is generally not recommended for initial dosing, except for patients in whom lower starting doses are deemed clinically appropriate.

Canadian Labeling: Dose Conversion Guidelines (Adults)[1,2]

Current Analgesic	Daily Dosage (mg/day)						
Morphine[3] (I.M./I.V.)	20-44	45-60	61-75	76-90	n/a[4]	n/a[4]	n/a[4]
Oxycodone (oral)	30-66	67-90	91-112	113-134	135-157	158-179	180-202
Codeine (oral)	150-447	448-597	598-747	748-897	898-1047	1048-1197	1198-1347
Hydromorphone (oral)	8-16	17-22	23-28	29-33	34-39	40-45	46-51
Hydromorphone (I.V.)	4-8.4	8.5-11.4	11.5-14.4	14.5-16.5	16.6-19.5	19.6-22.5	22.6-25.5
Fentanyl transdermal recommended dose (mcg/h)	25 mcg/h	37 mcg/h	50 mcg/h	62 mcg/h	75 mcg/h	87 mcg/h	100 mcg/h

[1]The table should NOT be used to convert from transdermal fentanyl (Duragesic® MAT) to other opioid analgesics. Rather, following removal of the patch, titrate the dose of the new opioid until adequate analgesia is achieved.

[2]Recommendations are based on Canadian product labeling for Duragesic® MAT.

[3]Morphine dose conversion based upon I.M to oral dose ratio of 1:3.

[4]Insufficient data available to provide specific dosing recommendations. Use caution; adjust dose conservatively.

Dosage adjustment in renal impairment:
Injection: No dosage adjustment provided in manufacturer's labeling; use with caution.
Transdermal (patch): Degree of impairment (ie, Cl$_{cr}$) not defined in manufacturer's labeling.
Mild-to-moderate impairment: Initial: Reduce dose by 50%.
Severe impairment: Use not recommended.
Transmucosal (buccal film/tablet, sublingual spray/tablet, lozenge) and nasal spray: Although fentanyl pharmacokinetics may be altered in renal disease, fentanyl can be used successfully in the management of breakthrough cancer pain. Doses should be titrated to reach clinical effect with careful monitoring of patients with severe renal disease.

Dosage adjustment in hepatic impairment:
Injection: No dosage adjustment provided in manufacturer's labeling; use with caution.
Transdermal (patch):
Mild-to-moderate impairment: Initial: Reduce dose by 50%.
Severe impairment: Use not recommended.
Transmucosal (buccal film/tablet, sublingual spray/tablet, lozenge) and nasal spray: Although fentanyl pharmacokinetics may be altered in hepatic disease, fentanyl can be used successfully in the management of breakthrough cancer pain. Doses should be titrated to reach clinical effect with careful monitoring of patients with severe hepatic disease.

Mechanism of Action Binds with stereospecific receptors at many sites within the CNS, increases pain threshold, alters pain reception, inhibits ascending pain pathways

Contraindications Hypersensitivity to fentanyl or any component of the formulation

Additional contraindications for transdermal patches (eg, Duragesic®): Severe respiratory disease or depression including acute asthma (unless patient is mechanically ventilated); paralytic ileus; patients requiring short-term therapy, management of acute or intermittent pain, postoperative or mild pain, and in patients who are **not** opioid tolerant

Additional contraindications for transmucosal buccal tablets (Fentora®), buccal films (Onsolis™), lozenges (eg, Actiq®), sublingual tablets (Abstral®), sublingual spray (Subsys®), nasal spray (Lazanda®): Contraindicated in the management of acute or postoperative pain (including headache, migraine, or dental pain), and in patients who are **not** opioid tolerant. Abstral® and Onsolis™ also are contraindicated for acute pain management in the emergency room.

Canadian labeling: Additional contraindication (not in U.S. labeling): Sublingual tablets (Abstral™): Severe respiratory depression or severe obstructive lung disease

Warnings/Precautions An opioid-containing analgesic regimen should be tailored to each patient's needs and based upon the type of pain being treated (acute versus chronic), the route of administration, degree of tolerance for opioids (naive versus chronic user), age, weight, and medical condition. The optimal analgesic dose varies widely among patients. Doses should be titrated to pain relief/prevention. May cause CNS depression, which may impair physical or mental abilities; patients must be cautioned about performing tasks which require mental alertness (eg, operating machinery or driving). When using with other CNS depressants, reduce dose

of one or both agents. Fentanyl shares the toxic potentials of opiate agonists, and precautions of opiate agonist therapy should be observed; use with caution in patients with bradycardia or bradyarrhythmias; rapid I.V. infusion may result in skeletal muscle and chest wall rigidity leading to respiratory distress and/or apnea, bronchoconstriction, laryngospasm; inject slowly over 3-5 minutes. **[U.S. Boxed Warning]: Healthcare provider should be alert to problems of abuse, misuse, and diversion.** Tolerance or drug dependence may result from extended use. The elderly may be particularly susceptible to the CNS depressant and constipating effects of narcotics. Use extreme caution in patients with COPD or other chronic respiratory conditions. Use caution with head injuries, morbid obesity, renal impairment, or hepatic dysfunction. **[U.S. Boxed Warning]: Use with strong or moderate CYP3A4 inhibitors may result in increased effects and potentially fatal respiratory depression.** Use is not recommended with MAO inhibitors or within 14 days of MAO inhibitor use; severe and unpredictable adverse effects may result. Concurrent use of agonist/antagonist analgesics may precipitate withdrawal symptoms and/or reduced analgesic efficacy in patients following prolonged therapy with mu opioid agonists. Abrupt discontinuation following prolonged use may also lead to withdrawal symptoms.

Pediatric patients: **[U.S. Boxed Warning]: Buccal film, buccal tablet, nasal spray, sublingual tablet, sublingual spray, transdermal patch, and lozenge preparations contain an amount of medication that can be fatal to children. Keep all used and unused products out of the reach of children at all times and discard products properly.** Patients and caregivers should be counseled on the dangers to children including the risk of exposure to partially-consumed products.

[U.S. Boxed Warning] Abstral®, Actiq®, Duragesic®, Fentora®, Lazanda®, Onsolis®, Subsys®: May cause potentially life-threatening hypoventilation, respiratory depression, and/or death; Abstral®, Actiq®, Duragesic®, Fentora®, Lazanda®, Onsolis®, or Subsys® should only be prescribed for opioid-tolerant patients. Risk of respiratory depression increased in elderly patients, debilitated patients, and patients with conditions associated with hypoxia or hypercapnia; usually occurs after administration of initial dose in nontolerant patients or when given with other drugs that depress respiratory function.

Transmucosal (buccal film/tablet, sublingual spray/tablet, lozenge) and nasal spray: **[U.S. Boxed Warning]: Transmucosal and nasal fentanyl formulations are contraindicated in the management of acute or postoperative pain and in opioid nontolerant patients.** Should be used only for the care of opioid-tolerant cancer patients with breakthrough pain and is intended for use by specialists who are knowledgeable in treating cancer pain. **[U.S. Boxed Warning]: Substantial differences exist in the pharmacokinetic profile of fentanyl products. Do not convert patients on a mcg-per-mcg basis from one fentanyl product to another fentanyl product; the substitution of one fentanyl product for another fentanyl product may result in a fatal overdose. [U.S. Boxed Warning]: Available only through the TIRF REMS ACCESS program, a restricted distribution program with outpatients, prescribers who prescribe to outpatients, pharmacies (inpatient and outpatient), and distributor-required enrollment.** Avoid use of topical nasal decongestants (eg, oxymetazoline) during episodes of rhinitis when using fentanyl nasal spray; response to fentanyl may be delayed or reduced. Avoid use of sublingual spray in cancer patients with grade 2 or higher mucositis (fentanyl exposure increased); use with caution in patients with grade 1 mucositis, and closely monitor for respiratory and CNS depression.

Transdermal patch: **[U.S. Boxed Warning]: Transdermal patch is contraindicated in the management of short-term analgesia, or in the management of postoperative pain, and in patients who are opioid nontolerant. Should only be prescribed by healthcare professionals who are knowledgeable in the use of potent opioids in the management of chronic pain. Monitor closely for respiratory depression during use, particularly during first two applications after initiation of therapy or after dose increases. [U.S. Boxed Warning]: Avoid exposure of application site and surrounding area to direct external heat sources. Patients who experience fever or increase in core body temperature should be monitored closely.** Serum fentanyl concentrations may increase by approximately one-third for patients with a body temperature of 40°C (104°F) secondary to a temperature-dependent increase in fentanyl release from the patch and increased skin permeability.**[U.S. Boxed Warning]: Accidental exposure may lead to severe respiratory depression, including death, in children and adults; proper procedures for handling and disposal of patches should be followed.** Avoid unclothed/unwashed application site exposure, inadvertent person-to-person patch transfer (eg, while hugging), incidental exposure (eg, sharing same bed, sitting on patch), intentional exposure (eg, chewing), or accidental exposure by caregivers when applying/removing patch. Should be applied only to intact skin. Use of a patch that has been cut, damaged, or altered in any way may result in overdosage. Patients who experience adverse reactions should be monitored for at least 24 hours after removal of the patch. May contain conducting metal (eg, aluminum); remove patch prior to MRI.

Drug Interactions

Metabolism/Transport Effects Substrate of CYP3A4 (major); **Note:** Assignment of Major/Minor substrate status based on clinically relevant drug interaction potential; **Inhibits** CYP3A4 (weak)

Avoid Concomitant Use

Avoid concomitant use of FentaNYL with any of the following: Azelastine (Nasal); Crizotinib; Enzalutamide; MAO Inhibitors; Mifepristone; Paraldehyde; Pimozide

Increased Effect/Toxicity

FentaNYL may increase the levels/effects of: Alcohol (Ethyl); Alvimopan; ARIPiprazole; Azelastine (Nasal); Beta-Blockers; Calcium Channel Blockers (Nondihydropyridine); CNS Depressants; Desmopressin; Lomitapide; MAO Inhibitors; Metyrosine; Mirtazapine; Paraldehyde; Pimozide; Pramipexole; ROPINIRole; Rotigotine; Selective Serotonin Reuptake Inhibitors; Thiazide Diuretics; Zolpidem

The levels/effects of FentaNYL may be increased by: Amphetamines; Antipsychotic Agents (Phenothiazines); Crizotinib; CYP3A4 Inhibitors (Moderate); CYP3A4 Inhibitors (Strong); Dasatinib; Droperidol; HydrOXYzine; Ivacaftor; Magnesium Sulfate; MAO Inhibitors; Mifepristone; Perampanel; Sodium Oxybate; Succinylcholine

Decreased Effect

FentaNYL may decrease the levels/effects of: Ioflupane I 123; Pegvisomant

The levels/effects of FentaNYL may be decreased by: Alpha-/Beta-Agonists (Indirect-Acting); Alpha1-Agonists; Ammonium Chloride; Enzalutamide; Mixed Agonist / Antagonist Opioids; Rifamycin Derivatives

Ethanol/Nutrition/Herb Interactions

Ethanol: Ethanol may increase CNS depression. Management: Monitor for increased effects with coadministration. Caution patients about effects.

Food: Fentanyl concentrations may be increased by grapefruit juice. Management: Avoid concurrent intake of large quantities (>1 quart/day) of grapefruit juice.

Herb/Nutraceutical: St John's wort may decrease fentanyl levels; gotu kola, valerian, and kava kava may increase CNS depression. Management: Avoid St John's wort, gotu kola, valerian, and kava kava.

Dietary Considerations Transmucosal lozenge contains 2 g sugar per unit.

Pharmacodynamics/Kinetics

Onset of Action Analgesic: I.M.: 7-8 minutes; I.V.: Almost immediate; Transdermal (initial placement): 6 hours; Transmucosal: 5-15 minutes

Duration of Action I.M.: 1-2 hours; I.V.: 0.5-1 hour; Transdermal (removal of patch/no replacement): Related to blood level; some effects may last 72-96 hours due to extended half-life and absorption from the skin, fentanyl concentrations decrease by ~50% in 20-27 hours; Transmucosal: Related to blood level; respiratory depressant effect may last longer than analgesic effect

Half-life Elimination

I.V.: 2-4 hours; when administered as a continuous infusion, the half-life prolongs with infusion duration due to the large volume of distribution (Sessler, 2008)

Transdermal patch: 20-27 hours (apparent half-life is influenced by continued fentanyl absorption from skin)

Transmucosal products: 3-14 hours (dose dependent); Nasal spray: 15-25 hours (based on a multiple-dose pharmacokinetic study when doses are administered in the same nostril and separated by a 1-, 2-, or 4-hour time lapse)

Time to Peak

Buccal film: 0.75-4 hours (median: 1 hour)

Buccal tablet: 20-240 minutes (median: 47 minutes)

Lozenge: 20-480 minutes (median: 20-40 minutes)

Nasal spray: Median: 15-21 minutes

Sublingual spray: 10-120 minutes (median: 90 minutes)

Sublingual tablet: 15-240 minutes (median: 30-60 minutes)

Transdermal patch: 20-72 hours; steady state serum concentrations are reached after two sequential 72-hour applications

Pregnancy Risk Factor C

Pregnancy Considerations Adverse events were observed in animal reproduction studies. Fentanyl crosses the placenta and the injectable formulation has been used safely during labor (Gomar, 2000). Chronic use during pregnancy has shown detectable serum concentrations in the newborn with transient respiratory depression, behavioral changes, or seizures in the newborn infant characteristic of neonatal abstinence syndrome; transient neonatal muscular rigidity has also been observed. Transdermal patch, transmucosal lozenge, nasal spray (Lazanda®), sublingual tablet, sublingual spray (Subsys®), buccal tablet (Fentora®), and buccal film (Onsolis®) are not recommended for analgesia during labor and delivery.

Lactation Enters breast milk/not recommended (AAP rates "compatible"; AAP 2001 update pending)

Breast-Feeding Considerations Fentanyl is excreted in low concentrations into breast milk. Breast-feeding is considered acceptable following single doses to the mother; however, limited information is available when used long-term (Spigset, 2000). **Note:** Transdermal patch, transmucosal lozenge, sublingual tablet, sublingual spray (Subsys®), buccal tablet (Fentora®), and buccal film (Onsolis®) are not recommended in nursing women due to potential for sedation and/or respiratory depression. Symptoms of opioid withdrawal may occur in infants following the cessation of breast-feeding.

Controlled Substance C-II

Prescribing and Access Restrictions As a requirement of the REMS program, access is restricted.

Transmucosal immediate-release fentanyl products (eg, sublingual tablets and spray, oral lozenges, buccal tablets and soluble film, nasal spray) are only available through the Transmucosal Immediate-Release Fentanyl (TIRF) REMS ACCESS program. Enrollment in the program is required for outpatients, prescribers for outpatient use, pharmacies (inpatient and outpatient), and distributors. Enrollment is not required for inpatient administration (eg, hospitals, hospices, long-term care facilities), inpatients, and prescribers who prescribe to inpatients. Further information is available at 1-866-822-1483 or at www.TIRFREMSaccess.com

Note: Effective December, 2011, individual REMs programs for TIRF products were combined into a single access program (TIRF REMS Access). Prescribers and pharmacies that were enrolled in at least one individual REMS program for these products will automatically be transitioned to the single access program.

Dosage Forms

Film, for buccal application:
Onsolis®: 200 mcg (30s); 400 mcg (30s); 600 mcg (30s); 800 mcg (30s); 1200 mcg (30s)

Injection, solution [preservative free]: 0.05 mg/mL (2 mL, 5 mL, 10 mL, 20 mL, 30 mL, 50 mL)

Liquid, sublingual, [spray]:
Subsys®: 100 mcg (30s); 200 mcg (30s); 400 mcg (30s); 600 mcg (30s); 800 mcg (30s)

Lozenge, oral: 200 mcg (30s); 400 mcg (30s); 600 mcg (30s); 800 mcg (30s); 1200 mcg (30s); 1600 mcg (30s)
Actiq®: 200 mcg (30s); 400 mcg (30s); 600 mcg (30s); 800 mcg (30s); 1200 mcg (30s); 1600 mcg (30s)

Patch, transdermal: 12 [delivers 12.5 mcg/hr] (5s); 25 [delivers 25 mcg/hr] (5s); 50 [delivers 50 mcg/hr] (5s); 75 [delivers 75 mcg/hr] (5s); 100 [delivers 100 mcg/hr] (5s)
Duragesic®: 12 [delivers 12.5 mcg/hr] (5s); 25 [delivers 25 mcg/hr] (5s); 50 [delivers 50 mcg/hr] (5s); 75 [delivers 75 mcg/hr] (5s); 100 [delivers 100 mcg/hr] (5s)

Powder, for prescription compounding: USP: 100% (1 g)

Solution, intranasal, as citrate [spray]:
Lazanda®: 100 mcg/spray (5 mL); 400 mcg/spray (5 mL) [delivers 8 metered sprays]

Tablet, for buccal application:
Fentora®: 100 mcg (28s); 200 mcg (28s); 400 mcg (28s); 600 mcg (28s); 800 mcg (28s)

Tablet, sublingual:
Abstral®: 100 mcg (12s, 32s); 200 mcg (12s, 32s); 300 mcg (12s, 32s); 400 mcg (12s, 32s); 600 mcg (32s); 800 mcg (32s)

Dosage Forms: Canada
Patch, transdermal, as base: 12 mcg/hr (5s); 25 mcg/hr (5s); 50 mcg/hr (5s); 75 mcg/hr (5s); 100 mcg/hr (5s)
Duragesic® MAT: 12 mcg/hr (5s); 25 mcg/hr (5s); 50 mcg/hr (5s); 75 mcg/hr (5s); 100 mcg/hr (5s)

Dental Comment Transdermal fentanyl should not be used as a pain reliever in dentistry due to danger of hypoventilation

Actiq® is a solid formulation of fentanyl with a high sugar content of 2 g hydrated dextrates per unit. Frequent use of Actiq® could result in significant dental problems including risk of dental decay. Dry mouth caused by fentanyl could add to the risk of caries. Oral adverse reactions reported in clinical trials have included tooth caries, gum hemorrhage, mouth ulcerations, oral moniliasis, dry mouth, and cheilitis.

Sedation: There is a subsequent slow release from muscle and fat which results in a terminal half-life that is beyond that of morphine. Fentanyl does not induce the release of histamine; therefore, fentanyl is preferable in patients with a predisposition to bronchospasm. Fentanyl is a good choice for use in cardiac patients because it lacks direct myocardial depression. The incidence of nausea is less than that reported with morphine or meperidine. The clinician should wait 2 to 3 minutes between doses to allow time for observation of the clinical effects of each administered dose.

References
Dionne RA, Yagiela JA, Moore PA, et al, "Comparing Efficacy and Safety of Four Intravenous Sedation Regimens in Dental Outpatients," *Am Dent Assoc*, 2001, 132(6):740-51.

Ferric Gluconate (FER ik GLOO koe nate)

Brand Names: U.S. Ferrlecit®; Nulecit™ [DSC]

Brand Names: Canada Ferrlecit®

Pharmacologic Category Iron Salt

Use Treatment of iron-deficiency anemia in patients undergoing hemodialysis in conjunction with erythropoietin therapy

Unlabeled Use Cancer-/chemotherapy-associated anemia

Local Anesthetic/Vasoconstrictor Precautions No information available to require special precautions

Effects on Dental Treatment Key adverse event(s) related to dental treatment: Xerostomia (normal salivary flow resumes upon discontinuation). Do not prescribe tetracyclines simultaneously with iron since GI tract absorption of both tetracycline and iron may be inhibited.

Effects on Bleeding No information available to require special precautions

Adverse Effects Percentages reported in adults unless otherwise noted:

>10%:
Cardiovascular: Hypotension (children 35%; adults 29%), hypertension (children 23%; adults 13%), tachycardia (children 17%; adults 5%)
Central nervous system: Headache (children 24%; adults 7%), dizziness (13%)
Gastrointestinal: Vomiting (adults ≤35%; children 11%), nausea (adults ≤35%; children 9%), diarrhea (adults ≤35%; children 8%)
Hematologic: Erythrocytes abnormal (11% [changes in morphology, color, or number])
Local: Injection site reaction (33%)
Neuromuscular & skeletal: Cramps (25%)
Respiratory: Dyspnea (11%)
1% to 10%:
Cardiovascular: Chest pain (10%), syncope (6%), edema (5%), angina pectoris, bradycardia, hypervolemia, MI, peripheral edema, vasodilation

Central nervous system: Pain (10%), fever (children 9%; adults 5%), fatigue (6%), agitation, chills, consciousness decreased, lightheadedness, malaise, rigors, somnolence

Dermatologic: Pruritus (6%), rash

Endocrine & metabolic: Hyperkalemia (6%), hypoglycemia, hypokalemia

Gastrointestinal: Abdominal pain (children 9%; adults 6%), anorexia, dyspepsia, eructation, flatulence, GI disorder, melena, rectal disorder

Genitourinary: Menorrhagia, UTI

Hematologic: Thrombosis (children 6%), anemia, leukocytosis, lymphadenopathy

Neuromuscular & skeletal: Leg cramps (10%), weakness (7%), paresthesias (6%), arm pain, arthralgia, back pain, leg edema, myalgia

Ocular: Arcus senilis, conjunctivitis, diplopia, puffy eyelids, redness of eyes, rolling of eyes, watery eyes

Otic: Deafness

Respiratory: Pharyngitis (children 9%), cough (6%), rhinitis (children 6%), upper respiratory infections (6%), pneumonia, pulmonary edema

Miscellaneous: Abscess, carcinoma, diaphoresis, flu-like symptoms, infection, sepsis

General Dosage Range I.V.:

Children ≥6 years: 1.5 mg/kg of elemental iron per dialysis session (maximum: 125 mg/dose)

Adults: 125 mg of elemental iron per dialysis session

Mechanism of Action Supplies a source to elemental iron necessary to the function of hemoglobin, myoglobin and specific enzyme systems; allows transport of oxygen via hemoglobin

Pharmacodynamics/Kinetics

Half-life Elimination Bound iron: 1 hour

Pregnancy Risk Factor B

Pregnancy Considerations Adverse events were not observed in animal reproduction studies. It is recommended that pregnant women meet the dietary requirements of iron with diet and/or supplements in order to prevent adverse events associated with iron deficiency anemia in pregnancy. Treatment of iron deficiency anemia in pregnant women is the same as in nonpregnant women and in most cases, oral iron preparations may be used. Except in severe cases of maternal anemia, the fetus achieves normal iron stores regardless of maternal concentrations.

Ferric Hexacyanoferrate
(FER ik hex a SYE an oh fer ate)

Brand Names: U.S. Radiogardase®

Pharmacologic Category Antidote

Use Treatment of known or suspected internal contamination with radioactive cesium and/or radioactive or nonradioactive thallium

Local Anesthetic/Vasoconstrictor Precautions No information available to require special precautions

Effects on Dental Treatment No significant effects or complications reported

Effects on Bleeding No information available to require special precautions

Adverse Effects

>10%: Gastrointestinal: Constipation (24%)

1% to 10%: Endocrine & metabolic: Hypokalemia (7%)

Frequency not defined: Gastrointestinal: Gastric distress, fecal discoloration (blue)

General Dosage Range Oral:

Children 2-12 years: 1 g 3 times/day

Children >12 years and Adults: 1-3 g 3 times/day

Mechanism of Action Binds to cesium and thallium isotopes in the gastrointestinal tract following their ingestion or excretion in the bile; reduces their gastrointestinal reabsorption (enterohepatic circulation)

Pharmacodynamics/Kinetics

Half-life Elimination

Cesium-137: Effective: Adults: 80 days, decreased by 69% with ferric hexacyanoferrate; adolescents: 62 days, decreased by 46% with ferric hexacyanoferrate; children: 42 days, decreased by 43% with ferric hexacyanoferrate

Nonradioactive thallium: Biological: 8-10 days; with ferric hexacyanoferrate: 3 days

Pregnancy Risk Factor C

Pregnancy Considerations Ferric hexacyanoferrate is not absorbed from the gastrointestinal tract and reproduction studies have not been conducted. Cesium-137 crosses the placenta; in one case, reported levels were equal in the mother and the neonate. Thallium also crosses the placenta; fetal death, failure to thrive, and alopecia in the neonate have been reported. Toxicity from exposure to thallium or radioactive cesium is expected to be greater than the risk of toxicity to ferric hexacyanoferrate. Oligospermia or azoospermia has been reported following whole body radiation in doses >1 Gy of cesium-137.

Ferric Subsulfate (FER ik sub SULL fate)

Brand Names: U.S. AstrinGyn®

Pharmacologic Category Hemostatic Agent

Use Hemostatic in minor surgical procedures

Local Anesthetic/Vasoconstrictor Precautions No information available to require special precautions

Effects on Dental Treatment No significant effects or complications reported

Effects on Bleeding Effective hemostatic agent when applied topically

Adverse Effects Dermatologic: Hyperpigmentation (application site)

General Dosage Range Topical: *Adults:* Apply evenly to wound.

Mechanism of Action Causes agglutination of surface proteins resulting in hemostasis

Pharmacodynamics/Kinetics

Onset of Action Hemostasis: ≤20 seconds

Pregnancy Considerations Ferric subsulfate is used as a hemostatic agent following cervical biopsies (Manca, 1997; Tam, 2005). May cause vaginal pain if leakage of solution occurs (Tam, 2005). A case report also describes use following a miscarriage; fertility was not impaired and a successful pregnancy occurred 7 months later (Disu, 2007).

Ferrous Fumarate (FER us FYOO ma rate)

Brand Names: U.S. Femiron® [OTC]; Ferretts® [OTC]; Ferro-Sequels® [OTC]; Ferrocite™ [OTC]; Hemocyte® [OTC]; Ircon® [OTC]

Brand Names: Canada Palafer®

Pharmacologic Category Iron Salt

Use Prevention and treatment of iron-deficiency anemias

Local Anesthetic/Vasoconstrictor Precautions No information available to require special precautions

Effects on Dental Treatment Key adverse event(s) related to dental treatment: Staining of teeth. Do not prescribe tetracyclines simultaneously with iron since GI tract absorption of both tetracycline and iron may be inhibited.

Effects on Bleeding No information available to require special precautions

Adverse Effects

>10%: Gastrointestinal: Constipation, dark stools, nausea, stomach cramping, vomiting

1% to 10%:

Gastrointestinal: Diarrhea, heartburn, staining of teeth

Genitourinary: Discoloration of urine

General Dosage Range Oral:

Children: 1-6 mg elemental iron/kg/day in 1-3 divided doses

Adults: 60 mg elemental iron 2-4 times/day

Mechanism of Action Replaces iron found in hemoglobin, myoglobin, and enzymes; allows the transportation of oxygen via hemoglobin

Pharmacodynamics/Kinetics

Onset of Action Hematologic response: Oral, parenteral iron salts: ~3-10 days

Peak effect: Reticulocytosis: 5-10 days; hemoglobin values increase within 2-4 weeks

Pregnancy Considerations It is recommended that pregnant women meet the dietary requirements of iron with diet and/or supplements in order to prevent adverse events associated with iron deficiency anemia in pregnancy. Treatment of iron deficiency anemia in pregnant women is the same as in nonpregnant women and in most cases, oral iron preparations may be used. Except in severe cases of maternal anemia, the fetus achieves normal iron stores regardless of maternal concentrations.

Ferrous Gluconate (FER us GLOO koe nate)

Brand Names: U.S. Ferate [OTC]; Fergon® [OTC]

Brand Names: Canada Apo-Ferrous Gluconate®; Novo-Ferrogluc

Pharmacologic Category Iron Salt

Use Prevention and treatment of iron-deficiency anemias

Local Anesthetic/Vasoconstrictor Precautions No information available to require special precautions

Effects on Dental Treatment Key adverse event(s) related to dental treatment: Staining of teeth. Do not prescribe tetracyclines simultaneously with iron since GI tract absorption of both tetracycline and iron may be inhibited.

Effects on Bleeding No information available to require special precautions

Adverse Effects

>10%: Gastrointestinal: Constipation, dark stools, nausea, stomach cramping, vomiting

1% to 10%:

Gastrointestinal: Diarrhea, heartburn, staining of teeth

Genitourinary: Discoloration of urine

General Dosage Range Oral:

Children: 1-6 mg Fe/kg/day in 1-3 divided doses

Adults: 60 mg 1-4 times/day

Mechanism of Action Replaces iron found in hemoglobin, myoglobin, and enzymes; allows the transportation of oxygen via hemoglobin

Pharmacodynamics/Kinetics

Onset of Action Hematologic response: Oral: 3-10 days; peak reticulocytosis occurs in 5-10 days, and hemoglobin values increase in ~2-4 weeks

Pregnancy Considerations It is recommended that pregnant women meet the dietary requirements of iron with diet and/or supplements in order to prevent adverse events associated with iron deficiency anemia in pregnancy. Treatment of iron deficiency anemia in pregnant women is the same as in nonpregnant women and in

most cases, oral iron preparations may be used. Except in severe cases of maternal anemia, the fetus achieves normal iron stores regardless of maternal concentrations.

Ferrous Sulfate (FER us SUL fate)

Brand Names: U.S. Feosol® [OTC]; Fer-In-Sol® [OTC]; Fer-iron [OTC]; MyKidz Iron 10™ [OTC]; Slow FE® [OTC]; Slow Release [OTC]

Brand Names: Canada Apo-Ferrous Sulfate®; Fer-In-Sol®; Ferodan™

Pharmacologic Category Iron Salt

Use Prevention and treatment of iron-deficiency anemias

Local Anesthetic/Vasoconstrictor Precautions No information available to require special precautions

Effects on Dental Treatment Do not prescribe tetracyclines simultaneously with iron since GI tract absorption of both tetracycline and iron may be inhibited. Liquid preparations may temporarily stain the teeth.

Effects on Bleeding No information available to require special precautions

Adverse Effects

>10%: Gastrointestinal: Constipation, dark stools, epigastric pain, GI irritation, nausea, stomach cramping, vomiting

1% to 10%:

Gastrointestinal: Diarrhea, heartburn

Genitourinary: Discoloration of urine

Miscellaneous: Liquid preparations may temporarily stain the teeth

General Dosage Range Oral:

Extended release: *Adults:* 250 mg 1-2 times/day

Immediate release:

Children: 1-6 mg Fe/kg/day in 1-3 divided doses (maximum: 15 mg/day [prophylaxis dosing])

Adults: 300 mg 1-4 times/day

Mechanism of Action Replaces iron, found in hemoglobin, myoglobin, and other enzymes; allows the transportation of oxygen via hemoglobin

Pharmacodynamics/Kinetics

Onset of Action Hematologic response: Oral: ~3-10 days

Peak effect: Reticulocytosis: 5-10 days; hemoglobin increases within 2-4 weeks

Pregnancy Considerations It is recommended that pregnant women meet the dietary requirements of iron with diet and/or supplements in order to prevent adverse events associated with iron deficiency anemia in pregnancy. Treatment of iron deficiency anemia in pregnant women is the same as in nonpregnant women and in most cases, oral iron preparations may be used. Except in severe cases of maternal anemia, the fetus achieves normal iron stores regardless of maternal concentrations.

Ferumoxytol (fer ue MOX i tol)

Brand Names: U.S. Feraheme®

Brand Names: Canada Feraheme®

Pharmacologic Category Iron Salt

Use Treatment of iron-deficiency anemia in chronic kidney disease

Local Anesthetic/Vasoconstrictor Precautions No information available to require special precautions

Effects on Dental Treatment No significant effects or complications reported

Effects on Bleeding No information available to require special precautions

Adverse Effects 1% to 10%:
Cardiovascular: Hypotension (≤3%), edema (2%), peripheral edema (2%), chest pain (1%), hypertension (1%)
Central nervous system: Dizziness (3%), headache (2%), fever (1%)
Dermatologic: Pruritus (1%), rash (1%)
Gastrointestinal: Diarrhea (4%), nausea (3%), constipation (2%), vomiting (2%), abdominal pain (1%)
Neuromuscular & skeletal: Back pain (1%), muscle spasms (1%)
Respiratory: Cough (1%), dyspnea (1%)
Miscellaneous: Hypersensitivity reactions (≤4%; serious reactions: <1%)

General Dosage Range I.V.: *Adults:* 510 mg (17 mL) as a single dose; repeat once 3-8 days later

Mechanism of Action Superparamagnetic iron oxide coated with a low molecular weight semisynthetic carbohydrate; iron-carbohydrate complex enters the reticuloendothelial system macrophages of the liver, spleen, and bone marrow where the iron is released from the complex. The released iron is either transported into storage pools or is transported via plasma transferrin for incorporation into hemoglobin.

Pharmacodynamics/Kinetics
Half-life Elimination ~15 hours; ferumoxytol is not removed by hemodialysis
Pregnancy Risk Factor C
Pregnancy Considerations Fetal malformations and decreased fetal weights were observed in animal studies at maternally toxic doses. There are no adequate and well-controlled studies in pregnant women. Use in pregnancy only if potential benefit justifies potential risk to fetus. It is recommended that pregnant women meet the dietary requirements of iron with diet and/or supplements in order to prevent adverse events associated with iron-deficiency anemia in pregnancy. Treatment of iron-deficiency anemia in pregnant women is the same as in nonpregnant women and in most cases, oral iron preparations may be used. Except in severe cases of maternal anemia, the fetus achieves normal iron stores regardless of maternal concentrations.

Fesoterodine (fes oh TER oh deen)

Brand Names: U.S. Toviaz®
Pharmacologic Category Anticholinergic Agent
Use Treatment of patients with an overactive bladder with symptoms of urinary frequency, urgency, or urge incontinence.
Local Anesthetic/Vasoconstrictor Precautions No information available to require special precautions
Effects on Dental Treatment Key adverse event(s) related to dental treatment: Prolonged use will cause significant xerostomia (normal salivary flow resumes upon discontinuation).
Effects on Bleeding No information available to require special precautions
Adverse Effects
>10%: Gastrointestinal: Xerostomia (19% to 35%; dose related)
1% to 10%:
Central nervous system: Insomnia (1%)
Dermatological: Rash (1%)
Gastrointestinal: Constipation (4% to 6%), dyspepsia (2%), nausea (1% to 2%), abdominal pain (1%)
Genitourinary: Urinary tract infection (3% to 4%), dysuria (1% to 2%), urinary retention (1%)
Hepatic: ALT increased (1%), GGT increased (1%)

Neuromuscular & skeletal: Back pain (1% to 2%)
Ocular: Dry eyes (1% to 4%)
Respiratory: Upper respiratory tract infection (2% to 3%), cough (1% to 2%), dry throat (1% to 2%)
Miscellaneous: Peripheral edema (1%)
General Dosage Range Dosage adjustment recommended in patients with renal impairment or on concomitant therapy
Oral: *Adults:* 4-8 mg once daily
Mechanism of Action Fesoterodine acts as a prodrug and is converted to an active metabolite, 5-hydroxymethyl tolterodine (5-HMT); 5-HMT is responsible for fesoterodine's antimuscarinic activity and acts as a competitive antagonist of muscarinic receptors.

Urinary bladder contractions are mediated by muscarinic receptors; fesoterodine inhibits the receptors in the bladder preventing symptoms of urgency and frequency.
Pharmacodynamics/Kinetics
Half-life Elimination ~7 hours
Time to Peak Plasma: 5-HMT: ~5 hours; C_{max} higher in poor CYP2D6 metabolizers
Pregnancy Risk Factor C
Pregnancy Considerations Teratogenic effects were observed in some animal reproduction studies.

Fexofenadine (feks oh FEN a deen)

Brand Names: U.S. Allegra®; Allegra® Allergy 12 Hour [OTC]; Allegra® Allergy 24 Hour [OTC]; Allegra® Children's Allergy ODT [OTC]; Allegra® Children's Allergy [OTC]
Brand Names: Canada Allegra®
Generic Availability (U.S.) Yes: Excludes orally disintegrating tablet and suspension
Pharmacologic Category Histamine H_1 Antagonist; Histamine H_1 Antagonist, Second Generation; Piperidine Derivative
Use Relief of symptoms associated with seasonal allergic rhinitis; treatment of chronic idiopathic urticaria
OTC labeling: Relief of symptoms associated with allergic rhinitis
Local Anesthetic/Vasoconstrictor Precautions No information available to require special precautions
Effects on Dental Treatment No significant effects or complications reported
Effects on Bleeding No information available to require special precautions
Adverse Effects
>10%:
Central nervous system: Headache (5% to 11%)
Gastrointestinal: Vomiting (children 6 months to 5 years: 4% to 12%)
1% to 10%:
Central nervous system: Fatigue (1% to 3%), somnolence (1% to 3%), dizziness (2%), fever (2%), pain (2%), drowsiness (1%)
Endocrine & metabolic: Dysmenorrhea (2%)
Gastrointestinal: Diarrhea (3% to 4%), nausea (2%), dyspepsia (1% to 2%)
Neuromuscular & skeletal: Myalgia (3%), back pain (2% to 3%), pain in extremities (2%)
Otic: Otitis media (2% to 4%)
Respiratory: Upper respiratory tract infection (3% to 4%), cough (2% to 4%), rhinorrhea (1% to 2%)
Miscellaneous: Viral infection (3%)
Dosage Oral:
Chronic idiopathic urticaria: Children 6 months to <2 years: 15 mg twice daily

Chronic idiopathic urticaria, seasonal allergic rhinitis:
Children 2-11 years: 30 mg twice daily
Children ≥12 years and Adults: 60 mg twice daily **or** 180 mg once daily
Elderly: Starting dose: Use caution; adjust dose for renal impairment
Allergic rhinitis (OTC labeling):
Children 2-11 years: 30 mg twice daily
Children ≥12 years and Adults: 60 mg twice daily **or** 180 mg once daily

Dosage adjustment in renal impairment: Cl_{cr} <80 mL/minute:
Children 6 months to <2 years: Initial: 15 mg once daily
Children 2-11 years: Initial: 30 mg once daily
Children ≥12 years and Adults: Initial: 60 mg once daily
Hemodialysis: Not effectively removed by hemodialysis
Dosage adjustment in hepatic impairment: No dosage adjustment provided in manufacturer's labeling; however, need for adjustment not likely since undergoes minimal hepatic metabolism.

Mechanism of Action Fexofenadine is an active metabolite of terfenadine and like terfenadine it competes with histamine for H_1-receptor sites on effector cells in the gastrointestinal tract, blood vessels and respiratory tract; it appears that fexofenadine does not cross the blood-brain barrier to any appreciable degree, resulting in a reduced potential for sedation

Contraindications Hypersensitivity to fexofenadine or any component of the formulation

Warnings/Precautions Use with caution in patients with renal impairment; dosage adjustment recommended. Safety and efficacy in children <6 months of age have not been established; orally disintegrating tablet not recommended for use in children <6 years of age. Orally disintegrating tablet contains phenylalanine.

Drug Interactions
Metabolism/Transport Effects Substrate of CYP3A4 (minor), P-glycoprotein, SLCO1B1; **Note:** Assignment of Major/Minor substrate status based on clinically relevant drug interaction potential; **Inhibits** CYP2D6 (weak)

Avoid Concomitant Use
Avoid concomitant use of Fexofenadine with any of the following: Aclidinium; Azelastine (Nasal); Ipratropium (Oral Inhalation); Paraldehyde; Tiotropium

Increased Effect/Toxicity
Fexofenadine may increase the levels/effects of: Alcohol (Ethyl); Anticholinergics; ARIPiprazole; Azelastine (Nasal); Buprenorphine; CNS Depressants; Methotrimeprazine; Metyrosine; Mirtazapine; Paraldehyde; Pramipexole; ROPINIRole; Rotigotine; Selective Serotonin Reuptake Inhibitors; Tiotropium; Zolpidem

The levels/effects of Fexofenadine may be increased by: Aclidinium; Droperidol; Eltrombopag; Erythromycin (Systemic); HydrOXYzine; Ipratropium (Oral Inhalation); Itraconazole; Ketoconazole (Systemic); Magnesium Sulfate; Methotrimeprazine; Perampanel; P-glycoprotein/ABCB1 Inhibitors; Pramlintide; Sodium Oxybate; Verapamil

Decreased Effect
Fexofenadine may decrease the levels/effects of: Acetylcholinesterase Inhibitors (Central); Benzylpenicilloyl Polylysine; Betahistine; Hyaluronidase

The levels/effects of Fexofenadine may be decreased by: Acetylcholinesterase Inhibitors (Central); Amphetamines; Antacids; Grapefruit Juice; P-glycoprotein/ABCB1 Inducers; Rifampin

Ethanol/Nutrition/Herb Interactions
Ethanol: Ethanol may increase CNS depression. Management: Avoid ethanol.
Food: Fruit juice (apple, grapefruit, orange) may decrease bioavailability of fexofenadine by ~36%. Management: Administer with water only, avoid fruit juice.
Herb/Nutraceutical: St John's wort may decrease fexofenadine levels.

Dietary Considerations Some products may contain phenylalanine and/or sodium. Take suspension and tablets with water only; do not administer with fruit juices.

Pharmacodynamics/Kinetics
Onset of Action 60 minutes
Duration of Action Antihistaminic effect: ≥12 hours
Half-life Elimination 14.4 hours (31% to 72% longer in renal impairment)
Time to Peak Serum: ODT: 2 hours (4 hours with high-fat meal); Tablet: ~2.6 hours; Suspension: ~1 hour
Pregnancy Risk Factor C
Pregnancy Considerations Adverse events have been observed in animal reproduction studies; therefore, the manufacturer classifies fexofenadine as pregnancy category C. The use of antihistamines for the treatment of rhinitis during pregnancy is generally considered to be safe at recommended doses. Information related to the use of fexofenadine during pregnancy is limited; therefore, other agents are preferred.
Lactation Excretion in breast milk unknown/use caution (AAP rates "compatible"; AAP 2001 update pending)
Breast-Feeding Considerations It is not known if fexofenadine is excreted in breast milk. The manufacturer recommends that caution be exercised when administering fexofenadine to nursing women.

Dosage Forms
Suspension, oral:
Allegra®: 6 mg/mL (300 mL)
Allegra® Children's Allergy [OTC]: 6 mg/mL (120 mL)
Tablet, oral: 30 mg, 60 mg, 180 mg
Allegra® Allergy 12 Hour [OTC]: 60 mg
Allegra® Allergy 24 Hour [OTC]: 180 mg
Allegra® Children's Allergy [OTC]: 30 mg
Tablet, orally disintegrating, oral:
Allegra® Children's Allergy ODT [OTC]: 30 mg

Fexofenadine and Pseudoephedrine
(feks oh FEN a deen & soo doe e FED rin)

Related Information
Fexofenadine *on page 588*
Pseudoephedrine *on page 1159*
Brand Names: U.S. Allegra-D® 12 Hour; Allegra-D® 24 Hour
Brand Names: Canada Allegra-D®
Pharmacologic Category Alpha/Beta Agonist; Decongestant; Histamine H_1 Antagonist; Histamine H_1 Antagonist, Second Generation; Piperidine Derivative
Use Relief of symptoms associated with seasonal allergic rhinitis in adults and children ≥12 years of age
Local Anesthetic/Vasoconstrictor Precautions Use with caution since pseudoephedrine is a sympathomimetic amine which could interact with epinephrine to cause a pressor response

589

Effects on Dental Treatment Key adverse event(s) related to dental treatment: Pseudoephedrine: Xerostomia (normal salivary flow resumes upon discontinuation).

Effects on Bleeding No information available to require special precautions

Adverse Effects See individual agents.

General Dosage Range Dosage adjustment recommended in patients with renal impairment

Oral: *Children ≥12 years and Adults:* 1 tablet (fexofenadine 60 mg/pseudoephedrine 120 mg) twice daily **or** 1 tablet (fexofenadine 180 mg/pseudoephedrine 240 mg) once daily

Pregnancy Risk Factor C

Pregnancy Considerations Animal studies using this combination showed reduced fetal weight, delayed ossification, and decreased survival. Also refer to individual monographs.

Fibrinogen Concentrate (Human)
(fi BRIN o gin KON suhn trate HYU man)

Brand Names: U.S. RiaSTAP®

Pharmacologic Category Blood Product Derivative

Use Treatment of acute bleeding episodes in patients with congenital fibrinogen deficiency (afibrinogenemia and hypofibrinogenemia)

Local Anesthetic/Vasoconstrictor Precautions No information available to require special precautions

Effects on Dental Treatment No significant effects or complications reported

Effects on Bleeding Serious thromboembolism and thrombosis have been reported.

General Dosage Range I.V.: *Children and Adults:* When baseline fibrinogen level is known: Dose (mg/kg) = [Target level (mg/dL) - measured level (mg/dL)] **divided by** 1.7 (mg/dL per mg/kg body weight) **or** when baseline fibrinogen level is not known: 70 mg/kg

Mechanism of Action Fibrinogen (coagulation factor I), a protein found in normal plasma, is required to clot blood. Fibrinogen concentrate made from pooled human plasma replaces this protein which is missing or reduced in patients with a congenital fibrinogen deficiency.

Pharmacodynamics/Kinetics

Half-life Elimination 61-97 hours (range 56-117 hours); may be decreased in children <16 years of age

Pregnancy Risk Factor C

Pregnancy Considerations Animal reproduction studies have not been conducted. Increased pregnancy loss is associated with untreated congenital fibrinogen disorders.

Fibrin Sealant (FI brin SEEL ent)

Related Information

Antiplatelet and Anticoagulation Considerations in Dentistry *on page 1503*

Brand Names: U.S. Artiss; Evicel™; TachoSil®; Tisseel

Brand Names: Canada Tisseel

Pharmacologic Category Blood Product Derivative; Hemostatic Agent

Use

Artiss: Aid in adhering autologous skin grafts in burn patients or tissue flaps during facial rhytidectomy surgery (facelift) (not indicated for hemostasis)

Evicel™: Adjunct to hemostasis in surgery when control of bleeding by conventional surgical techniques is ineffective or impractical

TachoSil®: Adjunct to hemostasis in cardiovascular surgery when control of bleeding by conventional surgical technique is ineffective or impractical

Tisseel: Adjunct to hemostasis in cardiopulmonary bypass surgery (including fully heparinized patients) and splenic injury (due to blunt or penetrating trauma to the abdomen) when the control of bleeding by conventional surgical techniques is ineffective or impractical; adjunctive sealant for closure of colostomies

Local Anesthetic/Vasoconstrictor Precautions No information available to require special precautions

Effects on Dental Treatment No significant effects or complications reported

Effects on Bleeding No information available to require special precautions

Adverse Effects May be related to aprotinin contained in some products. Frequency may vary by product.

1% to 10%:

Cardiovascular: Bradycardia (≤10%)

Central nervous system: Fever (6%)

Dermatologic: Pruritus (≤1%)

Hematologic: Hematoma/seroma (Artiss: Facial rhytidectomy: 1% to 4%)

Local: Skin graft failure (Artiss: 3%)

General Dosage Range Topical: *Children >6 months and Adults:* Dosage varies greatly depending on product

Mechanism of Action Formation of a biodegradable adhesive is done by duplicating the last step of the coagulation cascade, the formation of fibrin from fibrinogen. Fibrinogen is the main component of the sealant solution. The solution also contains thrombin, which transforms fibrinogen from the sealer protein solution into fibrin, and fibrinolysis inhibitor (aprotinin), which prevents the premature degradation of fibrin. When mixed as directed, a viscous solution forms that sets into an elastic coagulum.

Pharmacodynamics/Kinetics

Onset of Action Artiss: Full adherence achieved: ~2 hours

Time to hemostasis: Evicel™: 4-10 minutes; TachoSil®: 6 minutes; Tisseel: 5 minutes

Pregnancy Risk Factor C

Pregnancy Considerations Animal reproduction studies have not been conducted.

Product Availability Evarrest™ (fibrin sealant patch): FDA approved December 2012; limited distribution to select facilities expected in mid-December 2012 with full availability expected by the end of 2013. Consult prescribing information for additional information.

Fidaxomicin (fye DAX oh mye sin)

Brand Names: U.S. Dificid™

Brand Names: Canada Dificid™

Pharmacologic Category Antibiotic, Macrolide

Use Treatment of *Clostridium difficile*-associated diarrhea (CDAD)

Local Anesthetic/Vasoconstrictor Precautions No information available to require special precautions

Effects on Dental Treatment No significant effects or complications reported

Effects on Bleeding No information available to require special precautions

Adverse Effects

>10%: Gastrointestinal: Nausea (11%)

2% to 10%:

Gastrointestinal: Gastrointestinal hemorrhage (4%), abdominal pain, vomiting

Hematologic: Anemia (2%), neutropenia (2%)

General Dosage Range No dosage adjustment recommended in patients with hepatic or renal impairment.

Oral: *Adults:* 200 mg twice daily

Mechanism of Action Inhibits RNA polymerase sigma subunit resulting in inhibition of protein synthesis and cell death in susceptible organisms including *C. difficile*; bactericidal

Pregnancy Risk Factor B

Pregnancy Considerations Adverse events were not observed in animal reproduction studies. Due to the limited oral absorption of fidaxomicin, exposure to the fetus is expected to be low. There are no adequate and well-controlled studies in pregnant women.

Filgrastim (fil GRA stim)

Brand Names: U.S. Neupogen®

Brand Names: Canada Neupogen®

Pharmacologic Category Colony Stimulating Factor

Use

Cancer patients (nonmyeloid malignancies) receiving myelosuppressive chemotherapy to decrease the incidence of infection (febrile neutropenia) in regimens associated with a high incidence of neutropenia with fever

Acute myelogenous leukemia (AML) following induction or consolidation chemotherapy to shorten time to neutrophil recovery and reduce the duration of fever

Cancer patients (nonmyeloid malignancies) receiving bone marrow transplant to shorten the duration of neutropenia and neutropenia-related events (eg, neutropenic fever)

Peripheral stem cell transplantation to mobilize hematopoietic progenitor cells for apheresis collection

Severe chronic neutropenia (SCN; chronic administration) to reduce the incidence and duration of neutropenic complications (fever, infections, oropharyngeal ulcers) in symptomatic patients with congenital, cyclic, or idiopathic neutropenia

Unlabeled Use Treatment of anemia in myelodysplastic syndrome (in combination with epoetin); mobilization of hematopoietic stem cells (HSC) for collection and subsequent autologous transplantation (in combination with plerixafor) in patients with non-Hodgkin's lymphoma (NHL) and multiple myeloma (MM); treatment of neutropenia in HIV-infected patients receiving zidovudine; hepatitis C treatment-associated neutropenia

Local Anesthetic/Vasoconstrictor Precautions No information available to require special precautions

Effects on Dental Treatment No significant effects or complications reported

Effects on Bleeding No information available to require special precautions. Medical consultation may be considered to confirm adequate platelet counts.

Adverse Effects

>10%:

Central nervous system: Fever (12%)

Dermatologic: Petechiae (≤17%), rash (≤12%)

Endocrine & metabolic: LDH increased, uric acid increased

Gastrointestinal: Splenomegaly (severe chronic neutropenia: 30%; rare in other patients)

Hepatic: Alkaline phosphatase increased (21%)

Neuromuscular & skeletal: Bone/skeletal pain (22% to 33%; dose related), commonly in the lower back, posterior iliac crest, and sternum

Respiratory: Epistaxis (9% to 15%)

1% to 10%:

Cardiovascular: Hyper-/hypotension (4%), myocardial infarction/arrhythmias (3%)

Central nervous system: Headache (7%)

Gastrointestinal: Nausea (10%), vomiting (7%), peritonitis (≤2%)

Hematologic: Leukocytosis (2%)

Miscellaneous: Transfusion reaction (≤10%)

General Dosage Range

I.V.: *Children and Adults:* 5-10 mcg/kg/day

SubQ: *Children and Adults:* 5-10 mcg/kg/day **or** 6 mcg/kg twice daily

Mechanism of Action Stimulates the production, maturation, and activation of neutrophils; filgrastim activates neutrophils to increase both their migration and cytotoxicity.

Pharmacodynamics/Kinetics

Onset of Action ~24 hours; plateaus in 3-5 days

Duration of Action Neutrophil counts generally return to baseline within 4 days

Half-life Elimination 1.8-3.5 hours

Time to Peak Serum: SubQ: 2-8 hours

Pregnancy Risk Factor C

Pregnancy Considerations Animal studies have demonstrated adverse effects and fetal loss. Filgrastim has been shown to cross the placenta in humans. There are no adequate and well-controlled studies in pregnant women. Use only if potential benefit to mother justifies risk to the fetus. Women who become pregnant during filgrastim treatment are encouraged to enroll in Amgen's Pregnancy Surveillance Program (1-800-772-6436).

Product Availability

Tbo-filgrastim: FDA approved August 2012; availability anticipated November 2013.

Tbo-filgrastim is a short-acting recombinant form of G-CSF (biologically similar to Neupogen®), indicated to reduce the duration of severe neutropenia in patients with nonmyeloid malignancies.

Finasteride (fi NAS teer ide)

Brand Names: U.S. Propecia®; Proscar®

Brand Names: Canada Apo-Finasteride; CO Finasteride; JAMP-Finasteride; Mint-Finasteride; Mylan-Finasteride; PMS-Finasteride; Propecia®; Proscar®; ratio-Finasteride; Sandoz-Finasteride; Teva-Finasteride

Pharmacologic Category 5 Alpha-Reductase Inhibitor

Use

Propecia®: Treatment of male pattern hair loss in **men only**. Safety and efficacy were demonstrated in men between 18-41 years of age.

Proscar®: Treatment of symptomatic benign prostatic hyperplasia (BPH); can be used in combination with an alpha-blocker, doxazosin

Unlabeled Use Treatment of female hirsutism

Local Anesthetic/Vasoconstrictor Precautions No information available to require special precautions

Effects on Dental Treatment No significant effects or complications reported

Effects on Bleeding No information available to require special precautions

Adverse Effects Note: "Combination therapy" refers to finasteride and doxazosin.

>10%:

Endocrine & metabolic: Impotence (5% to 19%; combination therapy 23%), libido decreased (2% to 10%; combination therapy 12%)

Neuromuscular & skeletal: Weakness (5%; combination therapy 17%)

1% to 10%:

Cardiovascular: Orthostatic hypotension (9%; combination therapy 18%), edema (1%; combination therapy 3%)

Central nervous system: Dizziness (7%; combination therapy 23%), somnolence (2%; combination therapy 3%)

Dermatologic: Rash (1%)

Genitourinary: Ejaculation disturbances (<1% to 7%; combination therapy 14%), decreased volume of ejaculate (2% to 4%)

Endocrine & metabolic: Gynecomastia (1% to 2%), breast tenderness (≤1%)

Respiratory: Dyspnea (1%; combination therapy 2%), rhinitis (1%; combination therapy 2%)

General Dosage Range Oral: *Adults:* 1 mg or 5 mg once daily

Mechanism of Action Finasteride is a competitive inhibitor of both tissue and hepatic 5-alpha reductase. This results in inhibition of the conversion of testosterone to dihydrotestosterone and markedly suppresses serum dihydrotestosterone levels

Pharmacodynamics/Kinetics

Onset of Action BPH: 6 months; Male pattern hair loss: ≥3 months of daily use.

Duration of Action

After a single oral dose as small as 0.5 mg: 65% depression of plasma dihydrotestosterone levels persists 5-7 days

After 6 months of treatment with 5 mg/day: Circulating dihydrotestosterone levels are reduced to castrate levels without significant effects on circulating testosterone; levels return to normal within 14 days of discontinuation of treatment

Half-life Elimination 6 hours (range: 3-16 hours); Elderly: 8 hours (range: 6-15 hours)

Time to Peak Serum: 1-2 hours

Pregnancy Risk Factor X

Pregnancy Considerations Abnormalities of external male genitalia were reported in animal reproduction studies. Use is not indicated in women. Pregnant women are advised to avoid contact with crushed or broken tablets and the semen from a male partner exposed to finasteride.

Fingolimod (fin GOL i mod)

Brand Names: U.S. Gilenya®

Brand Names: Canada Gilenya®

Pharmacologic Category Sphingosine 1-Phosphate (S1P) Receptor Modulator

Use Treatment of relapsing forms of multiple sclerosis (MS) to reduce the frequency of clinical exacerbations and delay disability progression

Local Anesthetic/Vasoconstrictor Precautions No information available to require special precautions

Effects on Dental Treatment Key adverse event(s) related to dental treatment: Increased blood pressure may occur with fingolimod; assess and plan treatment according to patient's blood pressure. Fingolimod causes immune suppression; medical consult needed prior to dental surgery.

Effects on Bleeding No information available to require special precautions

Adverse Effects

>10%:

Central nervous system: Headache (25%)

Gastrointestinal: Diarrhea (12%)

Hepatic: ALT increased (14%), AST increased (14%)

Neuromuscular & skeletal: Back pain (12%)

Miscellaneous: Flu-like syndrome (13%)

1% to 10%:

Cardiovascular: Hypertension (6%), bradycardia (4%)

Central nervous system: Depression (8%), dizziness (7%), migraine (5%)

Dermatologic: Alopecia (4%), eczema (3%), pruritus (3%)

Endocrine & metabolic: Triglycerides increased (3%)

Gastrointestinal: Gastroenteritis (5%), weight loss (5%)

Hematologic: Lymphopenia (4%), leukopenia (3%)

Hepatic: GGT increased (5%)

Neuromuscular & skeletal: Paresthesia (5%), weakness (3%)

Ocular: Blurred vision (4%), eye pain (3%)

Respiratory: Cough (10%), bronchitis (8%), dyspnea (8%), sinusitis (7%)

Miscellaneous: Herpes infection (9%), tinea infection (4%)

General Dosage Range Oral: *Adults:* 0.5 mg once daily

Mechanism of Action Fingolimod-phosphate, active metabolite of fingolimod, binds to sphingosine 1-phosphate receptors 1, 3, 4, and 5. The amount of lymphocytes available to the central nervous system are decreased which reduces central inflammation.

Pharmacodynamics/Kinetics

Half-life Elimination 6-9 days

Time to Peak Plasma: 12-16 hours

Pregnancy Risk Factor C

Pregnancy Considerations Teratogenic and adverse effects have been observed in animal reproduction studies. Elimination of fingolimod takes approximately 2 months; to avoid potential fetal harm, women of childbearing potential should avoid pregnancy during and for 2 months after discontinuing treatment. Healthcare providers are encouraged to enroll pregnant women, or pregnant women may enroll themselves, in the Gilenya™ Pregnancy Registry (1-877-598-7237 or www.gilenyapregnancyregistry.com).

Flavocoxid (fla vo KOKS id)

Brand Names: U.S. Limbrel 250™; Limbrel 500™; Limbrel™ [DSC]

Pharmacologic Category Anti-inflammatory Agent; Nutritional Supplement

Use Clinical dietary management of the metabolic processes of osteoarthritis

Local Anesthetic/Vasoconstrictor Precautions No information available to require special precautions

Effects on Dental Treatment No significant effects or complications reported. May enhance risk of bleeding associated with NSAIDs.

Effects on Bleeding No information available to require special precautions

Adverse Effects ≥2%:
Cardiovascular: Hypertension, varicose veins
Dermatologic: Psoriasis
Gastrointestinal: Occult stools (statistically similar to placebo)
Neuromuscular & skeletal: Fluid on the knee
General Dosage Range Oral: *Adults:* 250-500 mg every 12 hours
Mechanism of Action Exerts anti-inflammatory properties through nonspecific inhibition of cyclooxygenase (COX) and lipoxygenase (5-LOX) pathways; may also possess general analgesic and antioxidant/anticytokine properties
Pharmacodynamics/Kinetics
Onset of Action 1-2 hours
Pregnancy Considerations Flavocoxid has not been studied in pregnant women; use during pregnancy is not recommended.

FlavoxATE (fla VOKS ate)

Brand Names: Canada Apo-Flavoxate®; Urispas®
Pharmacologic Category Antispasmodic Agent, Urinary
Use Antispasmodic to provide symptomatic relief of dysuria, nocturia, suprapubic pain, urgency, and incontinence in patients with cystitis, urethritis, urethrocystitis, urethrotrigonitis, and prostatitis
Local Anesthetic/Vasoconstrictor Precautions No information available to require special precautions
Effects on Dental Treatment Key adverse event(s) related to dental treatment: Xerostomia and changes in salivation (normal salivary flow resumes upon discontinuation), and dry throat.
Effects on Bleeding No information available to require special precautions
Adverse Effects Frequency not defined.
Cardiovascular: Palpitations, tachycardia
Central nervous system: Confusion (especially in the elderly), drowsiness, headache, hyperpyrexia, nervousness, vertigo
Dermatologic: Rash, urticaria
Gastrointestinal: Nausea, vomiting, xerostomia
Genitourinary: Dysuria
Hematologic: Eosinophilia, leukopenia
Ocular: Blurred vision, intraocular pressure increased, ocular accommodation disorder
General Dosage Range Oral: *Children >12 years and Adults:* 100-200 mg 3-4 times daily
Mechanism of Action Synthetic antispasmotic with similar actions to that of propantheline; it exerts a direct relaxant effect on smooth muscles via phosphodiesterase inhibition, providing relief to a variety of smooth muscle spasms; it is especially useful for the treatment of bladder spasticity, whereby it produces an increase in urinary capacity
Pharmacodynamics/Kinetics
Onset of Action 55 minutes
Pregnancy Risk Factor B
Pregnancy Considerations Adverse events have not been observed in animal reproduction studies.

Flecainide (fle KAY nide)

Related Information
Clinical Risk Related to Drugs Prolonging QT Interval *on page 1510*
Brand Names: U.S. Tambocor™
Brand Names: Canada Apo-Flecainide®; Tambocor™

Pharmacologic Category Antiarrhythmic Agent, Class Ic
Use Prevention and suppression of documented life-threatening ventricular arrhythmias (eg, sustained ventricular tachycardia); controlling symptomatic, disabling supraventricular tachycardias in patients without structural heart disease in whom other agents fail
Local Anesthetic/Vasoconstrictor Precautions Flecainide is one of the drugs confirmed to prolong the QT interval and is accepted as having a risk of causing torsade de pointes. The risk of drug-induced torsade de pointes is extremely low when a single QT interval prolonging drug is prescribed. In terms of epinephrine, it is not known what effect vasoconstrictors in the local anesthetic regimen will have in patients with a known history of congenital prolonged QT interval or in patients taking any medication that prolongs the QT interval. Until more information is obtained, it is suggested that the clinician consult with the physician prior to the use of a vasoconstrictor in suspected patients, and that the vasoconstrictor (epinephrine, mepivacaine and levonordefrin [Carbocaine® 2% with Neo-Cobefrin®]) be used with caution.
Effects on Dental Treatment No significant effects or complications reported
Effects on Bleeding No information available to require special precautions
Adverse Effects
>10%:
Central nervous system: Dizziness (19% to 30%)
Ocular: Visual disturbances (16%)
Respiratory: Dyspnea (~10%)
1% to 10%:
Cardiovascular: Palpitation (6%), chest pain (5%), edema (3.5%), tachycardia (1% to 3%), proarrhythmic (4% to 12%), sinus node dysfunction (1.2%)
Central nervous system: Headache (4% to 10%), fatigue (8%), nervousness (5%) additional symptoms occurring at a frequency between 1% and 3%: fever, malaise, hypoesthesia, paresis, ataxia, vertigo, syncope, somnolence, tinnitus, anxiety, insomnia, depression
Dermatologic: Rash (1% to 3%)
Gastrointestinal: Nausea (9%), constipation (1%), abdominal pain (3%), anorexia (1% to 3%), diarrhea (0.7% to 3%)
Neuromuscular & skeletal: Tremor (5%), weakness (5%), paresthesia (1%)
Ocular: Diplopia (1% to 3%), blurred vision
General Dosage Range Dosage adjustment recommended in patients with renal impairment
Oral:
Children: Initial: 3 mg/kg/day **or** 50-100 mg/m^2/day in 3 divided doses; Maintenance: 3-6 mg/kg/day **or** 100-150 mg/m^2/day in 3 divided doses (maximum: 11 mg/kg/day; 200 mg/m^2/day)
Adults: Initial: 50-100 mg every 12 hours; Maintenance: 100-400 mg/day in 2 divided doses (maximum: 400 mg/day)
Mechanism of Action Class Ic antiarrhythmic; slows conduction in cardiac tissue by altering transport of ions across cell membranes; causes slight prolongation of refractory periods; decreases the rate of rise of the action potential without affecting its duration; increases electrical stimulation threshold of ventricle, His-Purkinje system; possesses local anesthetic and moderate negative inotropic effects

Pharmacodynamics/Kinetics

Half-life Elimination Infants: 11-12 hours; Children: 8 hours; Adults: 7-22 hours, increased with congestive heart failure or renal dysfunction; End-stage renal disease: 19-26 hours

Time to Peak Serum: ~1.5-3 hours

Pregnancy Risk Factor C

Pregnancy Considerations Adverse events have been observed in some animal reproduction studies.

Dental Comment Flecainide is known to prolong the QT interval. The QT interval is measured as the time and distance between the Q point of the QRS complex and the end of the T wave in the ECG tracing. After adjustment for heart rate, the QT interval is defined as prolonged if it is more than 450 msec in men and 460 msec in women. A long QT syndrome was first described in the 1950s and 60s as a congenital syndrome involving QT interval prolongation and syncope and sudden death. Some of the congenital long QT syndromes were characterized by a peculiar electrocardiographic appearance of the QRS complex involving a premature atria beat followed by a pause, then a subsequent sinus beat showing marked QT prolongation and deformity. This type of cardiac arrhythmia was originally termed "torsade de pointes" (translated from the French as "twisting of the points"). Flecainide is considered as having a risk of causing torsade de pointes. Since it is not known what effect vasoconstrictors in the local anesthetic regimen will have in patients with a known history of congenital prolonged QT interval or in patients taking any medication that prolongs the QT interval, a medical consult is suggested.

Floctafenine (flok ta FEN een)

Related Information

Rheumatoid Arthritis, Osteoarthritis, and Osteoporosis *on page 1526*

Brand Names: Canada Apo-Floctafenine®

Pharmacologic Category Nonsteroidal Anti-inflammatory Drug (NSAID), Oral

Use Short-term management of acute, mild-to-moderate pain

Local Anesthetic/Vasoconstrictor Precautions No information available to require special precautions

Effects on Dental Treatment Key adverse event(s) related to dental treatment: Xerostomia and changes in salivation (normal salivary flow resumes upon discontinuation), bitter taste. See Effects on Bleeding.

Effects on Bleeding Nonselective NSAIDs are known to reversibly decrease platelet aggregation via mechanisms different than observed with aspirin. Platelet function is restored as the drug is eliminated from the body. Dental professionals should be aware that recommendations differ between dental and general medical surgery. NSAIDs should be avoided (if possible) in general medical surgery patients for 3-5 half-lives of the drug (usually 1-3 days) prior to surgery to reduce the risk of excessive bleeding. However, there is no scientific evidence to warrant discontinuance of NSAIDs prior to dental surgery. In medically complicated patients or extensive oral surgery, the decision to interrupt therapy must be based on the risk to benefit in an individual patient and a medical consult is suggested. Routine interruption of NSAID therapy for most dental procedures is not warranted. If therapy is continued without interruption, the clinician should anticipate the potential for slower clotting times.

Adverse Effects Frequency not defined.

Cardiovascular: Edema, flushing, tachycardia

Central nervous system: Depression, dizziness, drowsiness, fatigue, headache, insomnia, irritability, malaise, nervousness, vertigo

Dermatologic: Angioedema, pruritus, rash, urticaria

Endocrine & metabolic: Fluid retention, hyperkalemia

Gastrointestinal: Abdominal pain, bitter taste, constipation, diarrhea, dyspepsia, flatulence, gastrointestinal bleeding, gastrointestinal ulcer, gross bleeding with perforation, heartburn, nausea, vomiting, xerostomia

Hematologic: Agranulocytosis, aplastic anemia, bleeding, leukopenia, neutropenia, thrombocytopenia

Hepatic: Hepatotoxicity, liver enzymes increased

Ocular: Blurred and/or diminished vision

Otic: Tinnitus

Renal: Burning micturition, cystitis, dysuria, hematuria, interstitial nephritis, polyuria, reversible acute renal insufficiency with or without oliguria/anuria, strong smelling urine, urethritis

Respiratory: Asthmatic-type dyspnea

Miscellaneous: Anaphylaxis, diaphoresis, thirst

General Dosage Range Dosage adjustment recommended in patients with renal impairment

Oral: *Adults:* 200-400 mg every 6-8 hours as needed (maximum: 1200 mg/day)

Mechanism of Action Reversibly inhibits cyclooxygenase-1 and 2 (COX-1 and 2) enzymes, which results in decreased formation of prostaglandin precursors; has antipyretic, analgesic, and anti-inflammatory properties

Other proposed mechanisms not fully elucidated (and possibly contributing to the anti-inflammatory effect to varying degrees), include inhibiting chemotaxis, altering lymphocyte activity, inhibiting neutrophil aggregation/activation, and decreasing proinflammatory cytokine levels.

Pharmacodynamics/Kinetics

Duration of Action 6-8 hours

Half-life Elimination Initial phase (distribution): 1 hour; second phase (elimination): 8 hours

Time to Peak 1-2 hours

Pregnancy Considerations Floctafenic acid (active metabolite) crosses the placenta; therefore, the benefits of use must be weighed against risk to mother and fetus. In late pregnancy, NSAIDs may cause premature closure of the ductus arteriosus.

Product Availability Not available in U.S.

Floxuridine (floks YOOR i deen)

Brand Names: Canada FUDR®

Pharmacologic Category Antineoplastic Agent, Antimetabolite; Antineoplastic Agent, Antimetabolite (Pyrimidine Analog)

Use Management of hepatic metastases of colorectal and gastric cancers

Local Anesthetic/Vasoconstrictor Precautions No information available to require special precautions

Effects on Dental Treatment Key adverse event(s) related to dental treatment: Stomatitis.

Effects on Bleeding Thrombocytopenia and anemia can occur.

Adverse Effects

>10%:

Gastrointestinal: Stomatitis, diarrhea; may be dose limiting

Hematologic: Myelosuppression, may be dose limiting; leukopenia, thrombocytopenia, anemia
  Onset: 4-7 days
  Nadir: 5-9 days
  Recovery: 21 days
1% to 10%:
  Dermatologic: Alopecia, photosensitivity, hyperpigmentation of the skin, localized erythema, dermatitis
  Gastrointestinal: Anorexia
  Hepatic: Biliary sclerosis, cholecystitis, jaundice
General Dosage Range Dosage adjustment recommended in patients with hepatic impairment
  Intra-arterial: *Adults:* 0.1-0.6 mg/kg/day
Mechanism of Action Mechanism of action and pharmacokinetics are very similar to fluorouracil; floxuridine is the deoxyribonucleotide of fluorouracil. Floxuridine is a fluorinated pyrimidine antagonist which inhibits DNA and RNA synthesis and methylation of deoxyuridylic acid to thymidylic acid.
Pregnancy Risk Factor D
Pregnancy Considerations Teratogenic effects have been observed in animal reproduction studies. Medications that inhibit DNA synthesis are known to be teratogenic in humans. Women of childbearing potential should avoid pregnancy.

Fluconazole (floo KOE na zole)

Related Information
Clinical Risk Related to Drugs Prolonging QT Interval *on page 1510*
Fungal Infections *on page 1573*
Related Sample Prescriptions
Fungal Infections Requiring Systemic Therapy *on page 1614*
Brand Names: U.S. Diflucan®
Brand Names: Canada Apo-Fluconazole®; CanesOral®; CO Fluconazole; Diflucan®; Dom-Fluconazole; Fluconazole Injection; Fluconazole Omega; Monicure; Mylan-Fluconazole; Novo-Fluconazole; PHL-Fluconazole; PMS-Fluconazole; PRO-Fluconazole; Riva-Fluconazole; Taro-Fluconazole; ZYM-Fluconazole
Generic Availability (U.S.) Yes
Pharmacologic Category Antifungal Agent, Oral; Antifungal Agent, Parenteral
Dental Use Treatment of susceptible fungal infections in the oral cavity including candidiasis, oral thrush, and chronic mucocutaneous candidiasis treatment of esophageal and oropharyngeal candidiasis caused by *Candida* species; treatment of severe, chronic mucocutaneous candidiasis caused by *Candida* species
Use Treatment of candidiasis (esophageal, oropharyngeal, peritoneal, urinary tract, vaginal); systemic candida infections (eg, candidemia, disseminated candidiasis, and pneumonia); cryptococcal meningitis; antifungal prophylaxis in allogeneic bone marrow transplant recipients
Unlabeled Use Cryptococcal pneumonia; candidal intertrigo
Local Anesthetic/Vasoconstrictor Precautions Fluconazole is one of the drugs confirmed to prolong the QT interval and is accepted as having a risk of causing torsade de pointes. The risk of drug-induced torsade de pointes is extremely low when a single QT interval prolonging drug is prescribed. In terms of epinephrine, it is not known what effect vasoconstrictors in the local anesthetic regimen will have in patients with a known history of congenital prolonged QT interval or in patients taking any medication that prolongs the QT interval. Until more information is obtained, it is suggested that the clinician consult with the physician prior to the use of a vasoconstrictor in suspected patients, and that the vasoconstrictor (epinephrine, mepivacaine and levonordefrin [Carbocaine® 2% with Neo-Cobefrin®]) be used with caution.
Effects on Dental Treatment Key adverse event(s) related to dental treatment: Abnormal taste.
Effects on Bleeding No information available to require special precautions
Adverse Effects Frequency not always defined.
  Cardiovascular: Angioedema (rare)
  Central nervous system: Headache (2% to 13%), dizziness (1%)
  Dermatologic: Rash (2%)
  Gastrointestinal: Nausea (2% to 7%), abdominal pain (2% to 6%), vomiting (2% to 5%), diarrhea (2% to 3%), dysgeusia (1%), dyspepsia (1%)
  Hepatic: Alkaline phosphatase increased, ALT increased, AST increased, hepatic failure (rare), hepatitis, jaundice
  Miscellaneous: Anaphylactic reactions (rare)
Dental Usual Dosage Candidiasis: Adults:
  Usual dosage range: 200-400 mg/day; duration and dosage depends on severity of infection
  Oropharyngeal (long-term suppression): 200 mg/day; chronic therapy is recommended in immunocompromised patients with history of oropharyngeal candidiasis (OPC)
Dosage The daily dose of fluconazole is the same for oral and I.V. administration
Usual dosage ranges: Oral, I.V:
  Children: Loading dose: 6-12 mg/kg/dose; maintenance: 3-12 mg/kg/dose once daily; duration and dosage depend on location and severity of infection
  Adults: 150 mg once **or** Loading dose: 200-800 mg; maintenance: 200-800 mg once daily; duration and dosage depend on location and severity of infection

Indication-specific dosing:
Children:
  Candidiasis: Oral, I.V.:
    Esophageal:
      Manufacturer's recommendation: Loading dose: 6 mg/kg/dose; maintenance: 3-12 mg/kg/dose once daily for 21 days and for at least 2 weeks following resolution of symptoms (maximum: 600 mg/day)
      HIV-exposed/-infected: Loading dose: 6 mg/kg/dose once on day 1; maintenance: 3-6 mg/kg/dose once daily for 4-21 days (maximum: 400 mg/day) (CDC, 2009)
      Relapse suppression (HIV-exposed/-infected): 3-6 mg/kg/dose once daily (maximum: 200 mg/day) (CDC, 2009)
      Invasive disease (alternative therapy): 5-6 mg/kg/dose every 12 hours for ≥28 days (maximum: 600 mg/day) (CDC, 2009)
    Oropharyngeal:
      Manufacturer's recommendation: Loading dose: 6 mg/kg/dose; maintenance: 3 mg/kg/dose once daily for ≥2 weeks (maximum: 600 mg/day)
      HIV-exposed/-infected: 3-6 mg/kg/dose once daily for 7-14 days (maximum: 400 mg/day) (CDC, 2009)

Coccidiodomycosis: Oral, I.V.: *Meningeal infection, or in a stable patient with diffuse pulmonary or disseminated disease* (HIV-exposed/-infected):
Treatment: 5-6 mg/kg/dose twice daily (maximum daily dose: 800 mg/**day**) (CDC, 2009), followed by chronic suppressive therapy (see below)
Relapse suppression: 6 mg/kg/dose once daily (maximum daily dose: 400 mg/**day**) (CDC, 2009)

Cryptococcosis: Oral, I.V.:
Manufacturer's recommendation: Meningitis: 12 mg/kg/dose for 1 dose, then 6-12 mg/kg/day for 10-12 weeks following negative CSF culture
HIV-exposed/-infected:
CNS disease (alternative therapy in patients intolerant of amphotericin B): Induction: 12 mg/kg/dose for 1 dose, then 6-12 mg/kg/day (maximum: 800 mg/day) for ≥2 weeks (in combination with flucytosine) (CDC, 2009)
Consolidation: 10-12 mg/kg/day for 8 weeks (Perfect, 2010) **or** 12 mg/kg/dose for 1 dose, then 6-12 mg/kg/day (maximum: 800 mg/day) for 8 weeks (CDC, 2009)
Maintenance (suppression): 6 mg/kg/day (maximum: 200 mg/day) (CDC, 2009; Perfect, 2010)
Non-CNS disease, disseminated (including severe pulmonary disease) (alternative therapy; unlabeled use): Induction: 12 mg/kg/dose for 1 dose, then 6-12 mg/kg/day (maximum: 600 mg/day) (CDC, 2009)
Non-CNS disease, localized (including isolated pulmonary disease) (unlabeled use): 12 mg/kg/dose for 1 dose, then 6-12 mg/kg/day (maximum: 600 mg/day). **Note:** Duration depends upon infection site and severity (CDC, 2009). For patients with pulmonary disease (not delineated by severity), the IDSA recommends a duration of 6-12 months (Perfect, 2010).

Adults:

Blastomycosis (unlabeled use): Oral: *CNS disease:* Consolidation: 800 mg daily for ≥12 months and until resolution of CSF abnormalities (Chapman, 2008)

Candidiasis: Oral, I.V.:
Candidemia (neutropenic and non-neutropenic): Loading dose: 800 mg (12 mg/kg) on day 1, then 400 mg daily (6 mg/kg/day) for 14 days after first negative blood culture and resolution of signs/symptoms. **Note:** Not recommended for patients with recent azole exposure, critical illness, or if *C. krusei* or *C. glabrata* are suspected (Pappas, 2009).
Chronic, disseminated: 400 mg daily (6 mg/kg/day) until calcification or lesion resolution (Pappas, 2009)
CNS candidiasis (alternative therapy): 400-800 mg daily (6-12 mg/kg/day) until CSF/radiological abnormalities resolved. **Note:** Recommended as alternative therapy in patients intolerant of amphotericin B (Pappas, 2009).
Endocarditis, prosthetic valve (unlabeled use): 400-800 mg daily (6-12 mg/kg/day) for 6 weeks after valve replacement (as step-down in stable, culture-negative patients); long-term suppression in absence of valve replacement: 400-800 mg daily (Pappas, 2009)
Endophthalmitis (unlabeled use): 400-800 mg daily (6-12 mg/kg/day) for 4-6 weeks until examination indicates resolution (Pappas, 2009)
Esophageal:
Manufacturer's recommendation: Loading dose: 200 mg on day 1, then maintenance dose of 100-400 mg daily for 21 days and for at least 2 weeks following resolution of symptoms

Alternative dosing: 200-400 mg daily for 14-21 days; suppressive therapy of 100-200 mg 3 times weekly may be used for recurrent infections (Pappas, 2009)
Intertrigo (unlabeled use): 50 mg daily or 150 mg once weekly (Coldiron, 1991; Nozickova, 1998; Stengel, 1994)
Oropharyngeal:
Manufacturer's recommendation: Loading dose: 200 mg on day 1; maintenance dose 100 mg daily for ≥2 weeks. **Note:** Therapy with 100 mg daily is associated with resistance development (Rex, 1995).
Alternative dosing: 100-200 mg daily for 7-14 days for uncomplicated, moderate-to-severe disease; chronic therapy of 100 mg 3 times weekly is recommended in immunocompromised patients with history of oropharyngeal candidiasis (OPC) (Pappas, 2009)
Osteoarticular: 400 mg daily for 6-12 months (osteomyelitis) or 6 weeks (septic arthritis) (Pappas, 2009)
Pacemaker (or ICD, VAD) infection (unlabeled use): 400-800 mg daily (6-12 mg/kg/day) for 4- 6 weeks after device removal (as step-down in stable, culture-negative patients); long-term suppression when VAD cannot be removed: 400-800 mg daily (Pappas, 2009)
Pericarditis or myocarditis: 400-800 mg daily for several months (Pappas, 2009)
Peritonitis: 50-200 mg/day. **Note:** Some clinicians do not recommend using <200 mg daily (Chen, 2004).
Prophylaxis:
Bone marrow transplant: 400 mg once daily. Patients anticipated to have severe granulocytopenia should start therapy several days prior to the anticipated onset of neutropenia and continue for 7 days after the neutrophil count is >1000 mm³.
High-risk ICU patients in units with high incidence of invasive candidiasis: 400 mg once daily (Pappas, 2009)
Neutropenic patients: 400 mg once daily for duration of neutropenia (Pappas, 2009)
Peritoneal dialysis associated infection (concurrently treated with antibiotics), prevention of secondary fungal infection: 200 mg every 48 hours (Restrepo, 2010)
Solid organ transplant: 200-400 mg once daily for at least 7-14 days (Pappas, 2009)
Thrombophlebitis, suppurative (unlabeled use): 400-800 mg daily (6-12 mg/kg/day) and as step-down in stable patients for ≥ 2 weeks (Pappas, 2009)
Urinary tract:
Cystitis:
Manufacturer's recommendation: UTI: 50-200 mg once daily
Asymptomatic, patient undergoing urologic procedure: 200-400 mg once daily several days before and after the procedure (Pappas, 2009)
Symptomatic: 200 mg once daily for 2 weeks (Pappas, 2009)
Fungus balls: 200-400 mg once daily (Pappas, 2009)
Pyelonephritis: 200-400 mg once daily for 2 weeks (Pappas, 2009)
Vaginal:
Uncomplicated: Manufacturer's recommendation: 150 mg as a single oral dose
Complicated: 150 mg every 72 hours for 3 doses (Pappas, 2009)

Recurrent: 150 mg once daily for 10-14 days, followed by 150 mg once weekly for 6 months (Pappas, 2009), or fluconazole (oral) 100 mg, 150 mg, or 200 mg every third day for a total of 3 doses (day 1, 4, and 7), then 100 mg, 150 mg, or 200 mg dose weekly for 6 months (CDC, 2010)

Coccidioidomycosis, treatment: Oral, I.V.:

HIV-infected (unlabeled use):

Meningitis: 400-800 mg once daily continued indefinitely (CDC, 2009)

Pneumonia, focal, mild or positive serology alone: 400 mg once daily continued indefinitely (CDC, 2009)

Pneumonia, diffuse or severe extrathoracic disseminated disease (after clinical improvement noted with amphotericin B): 400 mg once daily (CDC, 2009)

Non-HIV infected (unlabeled use):

Disseminated, extrapulmonary: 400 mg once daily (some experts use 2000 mg daily [Galgiani, 2005])

Meningitis: 400 mg once daily (some experts use initial doses of 800-1000 mg daily), lifelong duration (Galgiani, 2005)

Pneumonia, acute, uncomplicated: 200-400 mg daily for 3-6 months (Catanzaro, 1995; Galgiani, 2000)

Pneumonia, chronic progressive, fibrocavitary: 200-400 mg daily for 12 months (Catanzaro, 1995; Galgiani, 2000)

Pneumonia, diffuse: Consolidation after amphotericin B induction: 400 mg daily for 12 months (lifelong in chronically immunosuppressed) (Galgiani, 2005)

Coccidioidomycosis, prophylaxis: Oral:

HIV-infected, positive serology, CD4+ count <250 cells/microL (unlabeled use): 400 mg once daily (CDC, 2009)

Solid organ transplant (unlabeled use): **Note:** Prophylaxis regimens in this setting have not been established; the following regimen has been proposed for transplant recipients who maintain residence in a *Coccidioides* spp endemic area.

Previous history >12 months prior to transplant: 200 mg once daily for 6-12 months (Vikram, 2009; Vucicevic, 2011)

Previous history ≤12 months prior to transplant: 400 mg once daily, lifelong treatment (Vikram, 2009; Vucicevic, 2011)

Positive serology before or at transplant: 400 mg once daily, lifelong treatment; if serology is negative at 12 months, consider a dose reduction to 200 mg daily (Vikram, 2009; Vucicevic, 2011)

No history (at risk for *de novo* post-transplant disease): some clinicians treat with 200 mg daily for 6-12 months (Vucicevic, 2011)

Cryptococcosis: Oral, I.V.:

Meningitis: Manufacturer's recommendation: 400 mg for 1 dose, then 200-400 mg once daily for 10-12 weeks following negative CSF culture

HIV-infected:

Meningitis (in patients amphotericin B resistant or intolerant): Induction: 400-800 mg once daily for 4-6 weeks with concomitant flucytosine (CDC, 2009) **or** 800-1200 mg once daily with concomitant flucytosine for 6 weeks (Perfect, 2010)

Consolidation: 400 mg once daily for 8 weeks (CDC, 2009)

Maintenance (suppression): 200 mg once daily lifelong or until CD4+ count >200 (CDC, 2009)

Pulmonary (immunocompetent) (unlabeled use): 400 mg once daily for 6-12 months (Perfect, 2010)

Dosage adjustment in renal impairment:

Manufacturer's recommendation: **Note:** Renal function estimated using the Cockcroft-Gault formula

No adjustment for vaginal candidiasis single-dose therapy

For multiple dosing in adults, administer loading dose of 50-400 mg, then adjust daily doses as follows (dosage reduction in children should parallel adult recommendations): Cl_{cr} ≤50 mL/minute (no dialysis): Administer 50% of recommended dose daily

Intermittent hemodialysis (IHD): Dialyzable (50%): May administer 100% of daily dose (according to indication) after each dialysis session. Alternatively, doses of 200-400 mg every 48-72 hours **or** 100- 200 mg every 24 hours have been recommended. **Note:** Dosing dependent on the assumption of 3 times/week, complete IHD sessions (Heintz, 2009).

Continuous renal replacement therapy (CRRT) (Heintz, 2009; Trotman, 2005): Drug clearance is highly dependent on the method of renal replacement, filter type, and flow rate. Appropriate dosing requires close monitoring of pharmacologic response, signs of adverse reactions due to drug accumulation, as well as drug concentrations in relation to target trough (if appropriate). The following are general recommendations only (based on dialysate flow/ultrafiltration rates of 1-2 L/hour and minimal residual renal function) and should not supersede clinical judgment:

CVVH: Loading dose of 400-800 mg followed by 200-400 mg every 24 hours

CVVHD/CVVHDF: Loading dose of 400-800 mg followed by 400-800 mg every 24 hours (CVVHD or CVVHDF) **or** 800 mg every 24 hours (CVVHDF)

Note: Higher maintenance doses of 400 mg every 24 hours (CVVH), 800 mg every 24 hours (CVVHD), and 500-600 mg every 12 hours (CVVHDF) may be considered when treating resistant organisms and/or when employing combined ultrafiltration and dialysis flow rates of ≥2 L/hour for CVVHD/CVVHDF (Heintz, 2009; Trotman, 2005).

Dosage adjustment in hepatic impairment: No dosage adjustment provided in manufacturer's labeling; use with caution.

Mechanism of Action Interferes with fungal cytochrome P450 activity (lanosterol 14-α-demethylase), decreasing ergosterol synthesis (principal sterol in fungal cell membrane) and inhibiting cell membrane formation

Contraindications Hypersensitivity to fluconazole or any component of the formulation (cross-reaction with other azole antifungal agents may occur, but has not been established; use caution); coadministration of CYP3A4 substrates which may lead to QT_c prolongation (eg, cisapride, pimozide, or quinidine)

Warnings/Precautions Should be used with caution in patients with renal and hepatic dysfunction or previous hepatotoxicity from other azole derivatives. Patients who develop abnormal liver function tests during fluconazole therapy should be monitored closely and discontinued if symptoms consistent with liver disease develop. Rare exfoliative skin disorders have been observed; monitor closely if rash develops and discontinue if lesions progress. Cases of QT_c prolongation and torsade de pointes associated with fluconazole use have been reported (usually high dose or in combination with agents known to prolong the QT interval); use caution in patients with concomitant medications or conditions which are arrhythmogenic. Use caution in patients treated with medications having a narrow therapeutic window and which are metabolized via CYP2C9 or CYP3A4 (monitor). Use with erythromycin should be avoided (may increase risk of cardiotoxicity). May occasionally cause dizziness or seizures; use caution driving or operating machines. Powder for oral suspension contains sucrose; use caution with fructose intolerance, sucrose-isomaltase deficiency, or glucose-galactose malabsorption.

Drug Interactions

Metabolism/Transport Effects Inhibits CYP1A2 (weak), CYP2C19 (strong), CYP2C9 (strong), CYP3A4 (moderate)

Avoid Concomitant Use

Avoid concomitant use of Fluconazole with any of the following: Bosutinib; Cisapride; Clopidogrel; Conivaptan; Dofetilide; Ivabradine; Lomitapide; Ospemifene; Pimozide; Ranolazine; Tolvaptan; Voriconazole

Increased Effect/Toxicity

Fluconazole may increase the levels/effects of: Alfentanil; Aprepitant; ARIPiprazole; AtorvaSTATin; Avanafil; Benzodiazepines (metabolized by oxidation); Bosentan; Bosutinib; Budesonide (Systemic, Oral Inhalation); BusPIRone; Busulfan; Calcium Channel Blockers; CarBAMazepine; Carvedilol; Cilostazol; Cinacalcet; Cisapride; Citalopram; Colchicine; Conivaptan; Corticosteroids (Systemic); CycloSPORINE (Systemic); CYP2C19 Substrates; CYP2C9 Substrates; CYP3A4 Substrates; Diclofenac (Systemic); DOCEtaxel; Dofetilide; Eletriptan; Eplerenone; Erlotinib; Eszopiclone; Etravirine; Everolimus; FentaNYL; Fluvastatin; Fosaprepitant; Fosphenytoin; Gefitinib; Halofantrine; Highest Risk QTc-Prolonging Agents; Imatinib; Irbesartan; Irinotecan; Ivabradine; Ivacaftor; Lomitapide; Losartan; Lovastatin; Lurasidone; Macrolide Antibiotics; Methadone; Moderate Risk QTc-Prolonging Agents; Nevirapine; Ospemifene; Phenytoin; Pimecrolimus; Pimozide; Propafenone; Proton Pump Inhibitors; QuiNIDine; Ramelteon; Ranolazine; Red Yeast Rice; Repaglinide; Rifamycin Derivatives; Salmeterol; Saxagliptin; Sildenafil; Simvastatin; Sirolimus; Solifenacin; Sulfonylureas; SUNItinib; Tacrolimus (Systemic); Tacrolimus (Topical); Tadalafil; Temsirolimus; Tipranavir; Tofacitinib; Tolterodine; Tolvaptan; Vardenafil; Vilazodone; Vitamin K Antagonists; Voriconazole; Zidovudine; Ziprasidone; Zolpidem; Zuclopenthixol

The levels/effects of Fluconazole may be increased by: Etravirine; Grapefruit Juice; Macrolide Antibiotics; Mifepristone

Decreased Effect

Fluconazole may decrease the levels/effects of: Amphotericin B; Clopidogrel; Ifosfamide; Saccharomyces boulardii

The levels/effects of Fluconazole may be decreased by: Didanosine; Etravirine; Rifamycin Derivatives

Dietary Considerations Take without regard to meals.

Pharmacodynamics/Kinetics

Half-life Elimination Normal renal function: ~30 hours (range: 20-50 hours); Elderly: ~46 hours

Time to Peak Oral: 1-2 hours

Pregnancy Risk Factor C (single dose for vaginal candidiasis)/D (all other indications)

Pregnancy Considerations Adverse events have been observed in some animal reproduction studies. When used in high doses, fluconazole is teratogenic in animal studies. Following exposure during the first trimester, case reports have noted similar malformations in humans when used in higher doses (400 mg/day) over extended periods of time (Aleck, 1997).

Abnormalities reported include abnormal facies, abnormal calvarial development, arthrogryposis, brachycephaly, cleft palate, congenital heart disease, femoral bowing, thin ribs and long bones. Use of lower doses (150 mg as a single dose) does not suggest an increase risk to the fetus. Most azole antifungals, including fluconazole, are recommended to be avoided during pregnancy (Pappas, 2009).

Lactation Enters breast milk/use caution (AAP rates "compatible"; AAP 2001 update pending)

Breast-Feeding Considerations Fluconazole is excreted in breast milk. The manufacturer recommends that caution be exercised when administering fluconazole to nursing women. Fluconazole is found in breast milk at concentrations similar to maternal plasma.

Dosage Forms

Infusion, premixed iso-osmotic dextrose solution: 200 mg (100 mL); 400 mg (200 mL)

Infusion, premixed iso-osmotic sodium chloride solution: 100 mg (50 mL); 200 mg (100 mL); 400 mg (200 mL)

Infusion, premixed iso-osmotic sodium chloride solution [preservative free]: 200 mg (100 mL); 400 mg (200 mL)

Powder for suspension, oral: 10 mg/mL (35 mL); 40 mg/mL (35 mL)

Diflucan®: 10 mg/mL (35 mL); 40 mg/mL (35 mL)

Tablet, oral: 50 mg, 100 mg, 150 mg, 200 mg

Diflucan®: 50 mg, 100 mg, 150 mg, 200 mg

Dental Comment Fluconazole is known to prolong the QT interval. The QT interval is measured as the time and distance between the Q point of the QRS complex and the end of the T wave in the ECG tracing. After adjustment for heart rate, the QT interval is defined as prolonged if it is more than 450 msec in men and 460 msec in women. A long QT syndrome was first described in the 1950s and 60s as a congenital syndrome involving QT interval prolongation and syncope and sudden death. Some of the congenital long QT syndromes were characterized by a peculiar electrocardiographic appearance of the QRS complex involving a premature atria beat followed by a pause, then a subsequent sinus beat showing marked QT prolongation and deformity. This type of cardiac arrhythmia was originally termed "torsade de pointes" (translated from the French as "twisting of the points"). Fluconazole is considered as having a risk of causing torsade de pointes. Since it is not known what effect vasoconstrictors in the local anesthetic regimen will have in patients with a known history of congenital prolonged QT interval or in patients taking any medication that prolongs the QT interval, a medical consult is suggested.

Flucytosine (floo SYE toe seen)

Brand Names: U.S. Ancobon®

Pharmacologic Category Antifungal Agent, Oral

Use Adjunctive treatment of systemic fungal infections (eg, septicemia, endocarditis, UTI, meningitis, or pulmonary) caused by susceptible strains of *Candida* or *Cryptococcus*

Local Anesthetic/Vasoconstrictor Precautions No information available to require special precautions

Effects on Dental Treatment No significant effects or complications reported

Effects on Bleeding No information available to require special precautions

Adverse Effects Frequency not defined.

Cardiovascular: Cardiac arrest, myocardial toxicity, ventricular dysfunction, chest pain

Central nervous system: Ataxia, confusion, fatigue, hallucinations, headache, parkinsonism, psychosis, pyrexia, sedation, seizure, vertigo

Dermatologic: Rash, photosensitivity, pruritus, toxic epidermal necrolysis, urticaria

Endocrine & metabolic: Hypoglycemia, hypokalemia

Gastrointestinal: Abdominal pain, anorexia, diarrhea, duodenal ulcer, enterocolitis, hemorrhage, nausea, ulcerative colitis, vomiting, xerostomia

Hematologic: Agranulocytosis, anemia, aplastic anemia, bone marrow aplasia, eosinophilia, leukopenia, pancytopenia, thrombocytopenia

Hepatic: Acute hepatic injury, bilirubin increased, hepatic dysfunction, jaundice, liver enzymes increased

Neuromuscular & skeletal: Paresthesia, peripheral neuropathy, weakness

Otic: Hearing loss

Renal: Azotemia, BUN increased, crystalluria, renal failure, serum creatinine increased

Respiratory: Dyspnea, respiratory arrest

Miscellaneous: Allergic reaction

General Dosage Range Dosage adjustment recommended in patients with renal impairment

Oral: *Adults:* 50-150 mg/kg daily in 3 or 4 divided doses

Mechanism of Action Penetrates fungal cells and is converted to fluorouracil which competes with uracil interfering with fungal RNA and protein synthesis

Pharmacodynamics/Kinetics

Half-life Elimination Normal renal function: 2-5 hours; Anuria: 85 hours (range: 30-250); End stage renal disease: 75-200 hours

Time to Peak Serum: ~1-2 hours

Pregnancy Risk Factor C

Pregnancy Considerations Adverse events have been observed in some animal reproduction studies. Flucytosine is metabolized to fluorouracil which may cause adverse events if administered during pregnancy; refer to the Fluorouracil (Systemic) monograph for additional information.

Fludarabine (floo DARE a been)

Brand Names: U.S. Fludara®

Brand Names: Canada Fludara®

Pharmacologic Category Antineoplastic Agent, Antimetabolite (Purine Analog)

Use Treatment of progressive or refractory B-cell chronic lymphocytic leukemia (CLL)

Canadian labeling: Second-line treatment of chronic lymphocytic leukemia (CLL); second-line treatment of low-grade, refractory non-Hodgkin lymphoma (NHL)

Unlabeled Use Treatment of non-Hodgkin lymphomas (NHL); acute myeloid leukemia (AML), either refractory or in poor risk patients; relapsed acute lymphocytic leukemia (ALL) or AML in pediatric patients; Waldenström's macroglobulinemia (WM); reduced-intensity conditioning regimens prior to allogeneic hematopoietic stem cell transplantation (generally administered in combination with busulfan or cyclophosphamide and antithymocyte globulin or lymphocyte immune globulin, or in combination with melphalan and alemtuzumab)

Local Anesthetic/Vasoconstrictor Precautions No information available to require special precautions

Effects on Dental Treatment Key adverse event(s) related to dental treatment: Stomatitis.

Effects on Bleeding Thrombocytopenia (nadir: 16 days) and anemia reported in the majority of patients.

Adverse Effects

>10%:

Cardiovascular: Edema (8% to 19%)

Central nervous system: Fever (60% to 69%), fatigue (10% to 38%), pain (20% to 22%), chills (11% to 19%)

Dermatologic: Rash (15%)

Gastrointestinal: Nausea/vomiting (31% to 36%), anorexia (7% to 34%), diarrhea (13% to 15%), gastrointestinal bleeding (3% to 13%)

Genitourinary: Urinary tract infection (2% to 15%)

Hematologic: Myelosuppression (nadir: 10-14 days; recovery: 5-7 weeks; dose-limiting toxicity), anemia (60%), neutropenia (grade 4: 59%; nadir: ~13 days), thrombocytopenia (55%; nadir: ~16 days)

Neuromuscular & skeletal: Weakness (9% to 65%), myalgia (4% to 16%), paresthesia (4% to 12%)

Ocular: Visual disturbance (3% to 15%)

Respiratory: Cough (10% to 44%), pneumonia (16% to 22%), dyspnea (9% to 22%), upper respiratory infection (2% to 16%)

Miscellaneous: Infection (33% to 44%), diaphoresis (1% to 13%)

1% to 10%:

Cardiovascular: Angina (≤6%), arrhythmia (≤3%), cerebrovascular accident (≤3%), heart failure (≤3%), MI (≤3%), supraventricular tachycardia (≤3%), deep vein thrombosis (1% to 3%), phlebitis (1% to 3%), aneurysm (≤1%), transient ischemic attack (≤1%)

Central nervous system: Malaise (6% to 8%), headache (≤3%), sleep disorder (1% to 3%), cerebellar syndrome (≤1%), depression (≤1%), mentation impaired (≤1%)

Dermatologic: Alopecia (≤3%), pruritus (1% to 3%), seborrhea (≤1%)

Endocrine & metabolic: Hyperglycemia (1% to 6%), dehydration (≤1%)

Gastrointestinal: Stomatitis (≤9%), esophagitis (≤3%), constipation (1% to 3%), mucositis (≤2%), dysphagia (≤1%)

Genitourinary: Dysuria (3% to 4%), hesitancy (≤3%)

Hematologic: Hemorrhage (≤1%)

Hepatic: Cholelithiasis (≤3%), liver function tests abnormal (1% to 3%), liver failure (≤1%)

Neuromuscular & skeletal: Osteoporosis (≤2%), arthralgia (≤1%)

Otic: Hearing loss (2% to 6%)

Renal: Hematuria (2% to 3%), renal failure (≤1%), renal function test abnormal (≤1%), proteinuria (≤1%)

Respiratory: Pharyngitis (≤9%), allergic pneumonitis (≤6%), hemoptysis (1% to 6%), sinusitis (≤5%), bronchitis (≤1%), epistaxis (≤1%), hypoxia (≤1%)

Miscellaneous: Anaphylaxis (≤1%), tumor lysis syndrome (≤1%)

General Dosage Range Dosage adjustment recommended in patients with renal impairment or who develop toxicities.

I.V.: *Adults:* 25 mg/m^2/day for 5 days every 28 days

Mechanism of Action Fludarabine inhibits DNA synthesis by inhibition of DNA polymerase and ribonucleotide reductase; also inhibits DNA primase and DNA ligase I

Pharmacodynamics/Kinetics

Half-life Elimination 2-fluoro-ara-A: ~20 hours

Time to Peak Oral: 1-2 hours

Pregnancy Risk Factor D

◀ **Pregnancy Considerations** Teratogenic effects were observed in animal studies. Based on the mechanism of action, fludarabine has the potential to cause fetal harm if administered during pregnancy. There are no adequate and well-controlled studies in pregnant women. Effective contraception is recommended during and for 6 months after treatment for women and men with female partners of reproductive potential.

Fludrocortisone (floo droe KOR ti sone)

Brand Names: Canada Florinef®
Generic Availability (U.S.) Yes
Pharmacologic Category Corticosteroid, Systemic

Use Partial replacement therapy for primary and secondary adrenocortical insufficiency in Addison's disease; treatment of salt-losing adrenogenital syndrome (or congenital adrenal hyperplasia)

Unlabeled Use Treatment of idiopathic orthostatic hypotension in conjunction with increased sodium intake

Local Anesthetic/Vasoconstrictor Precautions No information available to require special precautions

Effects on Dental Treatment No significant effects or complications reported

Effects on Bleeding No information available to require special precautions

Adverse Effects Frequency not defined.

Cardiovascular: Cardiac enlargement, CHF, edema, hypertension

Central nervous system: Delirium, depression, emotional instability, euphoria, hallucinations, headache, insomnia, intracranial pressure increased, malaise, mood swings, nervousness, personality changes, pseudotumor cerebri, psychiatric disorders, psychoses, seizure, vertigo

Dermatologic: Acne, bruising, erythema, hirsutism, hives, hyperpigmentation, maculopapular rash, petechiae, purpura, rash, skin test reaction impaired, striae, subcutaneous fat atrophy, thin fragile skin, urticaria, wound healing (impaired)

Endocrine & metabolic: Cushing's syndrome, diabetes mellitus, glucose intolerance, growth suppression, hyperglycemia, hypokalemia, hypokalemic alkalosis, menstrual irregularities, negative nitrogen balance, pituitary-adrenal axis suppression

Gastrointestinal: Abdominal distention, esophagitis ulceration, pancreatitis, peptic ulcer

Neuromuscular & skeletal: Fractures, necrosis (femoral and humeral heads), muscle mass loss, muscle weakness, myopathy, osteoporosis, vertebral compression fractures

Ocular: Cataracts, exophthalmos, glaucoma, increased intraocular pressure

Renal: Glycosuria

Miscellaneous: Anaphylaxis (generalized), diaphoresis

Dosage Oral:

Infants, Children, and Adolescents: Congenital adrenal hyperplasia due to 21-hydroxylase deficiency (Endocrine Society guidelines): 0.05-0.2 mg daily in 1-2 divided doses in combination with sodium chloride supplementation (Speiser, 2010).

Adults:

Addison's disease: Initial: 0.1 mg daily; if transient hypertension develops, reduce dose to 0.05 mg daily; maintenance dosage range: 0.1 mg 3 times weekly to 0.2 mg daily. Preferred administration with cortisone (10-37.5 mg daily) or hydrocortisone (10-30 mg daily).

Salt-losing adrenogenital syndrome (or congenital adrenal hyperplasia): 0.1-0.2 mg daily

The Endocrine Society recommends a maintenance dose range of 0.05-0.2 mg once daily (in combination with hydrocortisone) for patients with congenital adrenal hyperplasia due to 21-hydroxylase deficiency (Speiser, 2010).

Orthostatic hypotension (unlabeled use; Kearney, 2009; Lahrmann, 2006; Lanier, 2011): Initial: 0.1 mg daily in conjunction with a high-salt diet and adequate fluid intake; may be increased in increments of 0.1 mg per week; maximum dose: 1 mg daily. **Note:** Doses exceeding 0.3 mg daily may not be beneficial and predispose patient to unwanted side effects (eg, hypertension, hypokalemia).

Dosage adjustment in renal impairment: No dosage adjustment provided in manufacturer's labeling; use with caution.

Dosage adjustment in hepatic impairment: No dosage adjustment provided in manufacturer's labeling.

Mechanism of Action Very potent mineralocorticoid with high glucocorticoid activity; used primarily for its mineralocorticoid effects. Promotes increased reabsorption of sodium and loss of potassium from renal distal tubules.

Contraindications Hypersensitivity to fludrocortisone, hypersensitivity to other corticosteroids, or any component of the formulation; systemic fungal infections

Warnings/Precautions May cause hypercorticism or suppression of hypothalamic-pituitary-adrenal (HPA) axis, particularly in younger children or in patients receiving high doses for prolonged periods. HPA axis suppression may lead to adrenal crisis. Withdrawal and discontinuation of a corticosteroid should be done slowly and carefully. Fludrocortisone is primarily a mineralocorticoid agonist, but may also inhibit the HPA axis. Prolonged use may increase risk of infection, mask acute infection, prolong or exacerbate viral infections, or limit response to vaccinations. Exposure to chickenpox should be avoided. Corticosteroids should not be used to treat ocular herpes simplex, cerebral malaria, or viral hepatitis. Close observation is required in patients with latent tuberculosis (TB) and/or TB reactivity. Restrict use in active TB (only in conjunction with antituberculosis treatment). Prolonged treatment with corticosteroids has been associated with the development of Kaposi's sarcoma (case reports); if noted, discontinuation of therapy should be considered. Acute myopathy has been reported with high-dose corticosteroids, usually in patients with neuromuscular transmission disorders; may involve ocular and/or respiratory muscles; monitor creatine kinase; recovery may be delayed.

Corticosteroid use may cause psychiatric disturbances, including depression, euphoria, insomnia, mood swings, and personality changes. Pre-existing psychiatric conditions may be exacerbated by corticosteroid use. Use with caution in patients with HF; use may be associated with fluid retention, edema, weight gain and hypertension. Use with caution in patients with sodium retention and potassium loss, diabetes mellitus, GI diseases (diverticulitis, peptic ulcer, ulcerative colitis), hepatic impairment, myasthenia gravis, post- myocardial infarction, osteoporosis, and/or renal impairment. Use with caution in patients with cataracts and/or glaucoma; increased intraocular pressure, open-angle glaucoma, and cataracts have occurred with prolonged use. Consider routine eye exams in chronic users. Use with caution in patients with a history of seizure disorder; seizures have been reported with adrenal crisis.

Changes in thyroid status may necessitate dosage adjustments; metabolic clearance of corticosteroids increases in hyperthyroid patients and decreases in hypothyroid ones. Use with caution in the elderly. May affect growth velocity in pediatric patients. Withdraw therapy with gradual tapering of dose.

Drug Interactions

Metabolism/Transport Effects None known.

Avoid Concomitant Use

Avoid concomitant use of Fludrocortisone with any of the following: Aldesleukin; BCG; Mifepristone; Natalizumab; Pimecrolimus; Tacrolimus (Topical); Tofacitinib

Increased Effect/Toxicity

Fludrocortisone may increase the levels/effects of: Acetylcholinesterase Inhibitors; Amphotericin B; Deferasirox; Leflunomide; Loop Diuretics; Natalizumab; NSAID (COX-2 Inhibitor); NSAID (Nonselective); Thiazide Diuretics; Tofacitinib; Vaccines (Live); Warfarin

The levels/effects of Fludrocortisone may be increased by: Antifungal Agents (Azole Derivatives, Systemic); Aprepitant; Calcium Channel Blockers (Nondihydropyridine); Denosumab; Estrogen Derivatives; Fluconazole; Fosaprepitant; Indacaterol; Macrolide Antibiotics; Mifepristone; Neuromuscular-Blocking Agents (Nondepolarizing); Pimecrolimus; Quinolone Antibiotics; Roflumilast; Salicylates; Tacrolimus (Topical); Telaprevir; Trastuzumab

Decreased Effect

Fludrocortisone may decrease the levels/effects of: Aldesleukin; Antidiabetic Agents; BCG; Calcitriol; Coccidioidin Skin Test; Corticorelin; Hyaluronidase; Isoniazid; Salicylates; Sipuleucel-T; Telaprevir; Vaccines (Inactivated)

The levels/effects of Fludrocortisone may be decreased by: Aminoglutethimide; Antacids; Barbiturates; Bile Acid Sequestrants; Echinacea; Mifepristone; Mitotane; Primidone; Rifamycin Derivatives

Dietary Considerations Systemic use of mineralocorticoids/corticosteroids may require a diet with increased potassium, vitamins A, B_6, C, D, folate, calcium, zinc, and phosphorus, and decreased sodium. With fludrocortisone, a decrease in dietary sodium is often not required as the increased retention of sodium is usually the desired therapeutic effect.

Pharmacodynamics/Kinetics

Half-life Elimination Plasma: ~3.5 hours; Biological: 18-36 hours

Pregnancy Risk Factor C

Pregnancy Considerations Animal reproduction studies have not been conducted with fludrocortisone; adverse events have been observed with corticosteroids in animal reproduction studies. Some studies have shown an association between first trimester systemic corticosteroid use and oral clefts; adverse events in the fetus/neonate have been noted in case reports following large doses of systemic corticosteroids during pregnancy. Monitor for hypoadrenalism in infants exposed to fludrocortisone during pregnancy.

Lactation Excretion in breast milk unknown/use caution

Breast-Feeding Considerations Corticosteroids are excreted in human milk; information specific to fludrocortisone has not been located.

Dosage Forms

Tablet, oral: 0.1 mg

Flumazenil (FLOO may ze nil)

Brand Names: U.S. Romazicon® [DSC]

Brand Names: Canada Anexate®; Flumazenil Injection; Flumazenil Injection, USP; Romazicon®

Generic Availability (U.S.) Yes

Pharmacologic Category Antidote

Use Benzodiazepine antagonist; reverses sedative effects of benzodiazepines used in conscious sedation and general anesthesia; treatment of benzodiazepine overdose

Local Anesthetic/Vasoconstrictor Precautions No information available to require special precautions

Effects on Dental Treatment Key adverse event(s) related to dental treatment: Xerostomia (normal salivary flow resumes upon discontinuation).

Effects on Bleeding No information available to require special precautions

Adverse Effects

>10%: Gastrointestinal: Vomiting (11%)

1% to 10%:

Cardiovascular: Palpitation (3% to 9%), flushing (1% to 3%), vasodilation (1% to 3%)

Central nervous system: Ataxia (10%), dizziness (10%), vertigo (10%), agitation (3% to 9%), anxiety (3% to 9%), insomnia (3% to 9%), nervousness (3% to 9%), abnormal crying (1% to 3%), depersonalization (1% to 3%), depression (1% to 3%), dysphoria (1% to 3%), emotional lability (1% to 3%), euphoria (1% to 3%), fatigue (1% to 3%), headache (1% to 3%), malaise (1% to 3%), paranoia (1% to 3%)

Endocrine & metabolic: Hot flashes (1% to 3%)

Gastrointestinal: Xerostomia (3% to 9%), nausea (1% to 3%)

Local: Pain at injection site (3% to 9%), injection site reaction (1% to 3%), rash (1% to 3%), skin abnormality (1% to 3%), thrombophlebitis (1% to 3%)

Neuromuscular & skeletal: Hypoesthesia (1% to 3%), paresthesia (1% to 3%), weakness (1% to 3%), tremor

Ocular: Blurred vision (3% to 9%), abnormal vision (1% to 3%), lacrimation (1% to 3%)

Respiratory: Dyspnea (3% to 9%), hyperventilation (3% to 9%)

Miscellaneous: Diaphoresis (1% to 3%)

Dosage

I.V.:

Children ≥1 year: Reversal of conscious sedation:

Initial dose: 0.01 mg/kg over 15 seconds (maximum: 0.2 mg)

Repeat doses (maximum: 4 doses): If desired level of consciousness is not obtained, 0.01 mg/kg (maximum: 0.2 mg) repeated at 1-minute intervals

Maximum total cumulative dose: 1 mg or 0.05 mg/kg (whichever is lower)

Mean total dose: 0.65 mg (range: 0.08-1 mg)

Adults:

Reversal of conscious sedation and general anesthesia:

Initial dose: 0.2 mg over 15 seconds

Repeat doses (maximum: 4 doses): If desired level of consciousness is not obtained, 0.2 mg may be repeated at 1-minute intervals.

Maximum total cumulative dose: 1 mg (usual total dose: 0.6-1 mg). In the event of resedation: Repeat doses may be given at 20-minute intervals as needed at 0.2 mg per minute to a maximum of 1 mg total dose and 3 mg in 1 hour.

Suspected benzodiazepine overdose:

Initial dose: 0.2 mg over 30 seconds; if the desired level of consciousness is not obtained 30 seconds after the dose, 0.3 mg can be given over 30 seconds

◀ Repeat doses: 0.5 mg over 30 seconds repeated at 1-minute intervals

Maximum total cumulative dose: 3 mg (usual total dose: 1-3 mg). Patients with a partial response at 3 mg may require (rare) additional titration up to a total dose of 5 mg (although doses >3 mg do not reliably produce additional effects). If a patient has not responded 5 minutes after cumulative dose of 5 mg, the major cause of sedation is not likely due to benzodiazepines. In the event of resedation, repeat doses may be given at 20-minute intervals if needed, at 0.5 mg per minute to a maximum of 1 mg total dose and 3 mg in 1 hour.

Elderly: No differences in safety or efficacy have been reported; however, increased sensitivity may occur in some elderly patients.

Dosing in renal impairment: No dosage adjustment provided in manufacturer's labeling; however, pharmacokinetics are not significantly affected by renal failure (Cl$_{cr}$ <10 mL/minute) or hemodialysis.

Dosing in hepatic impairment: Initial reversal: No dosage adjustment necessary. Repeat doses: Reduce dose or frequency.

Mechanism of Action Competitively inhibits the activity at the benzodiazepine receptor site on the GABA/benzodiazepine receptor complex. Flumazenil does not antagonize the CNS effect of drugs affecting GABA-ergic neurons by means other than the benzodiazepine receptor (ethanol, barbiturates, general anesthetics) and does not reverse the effects of opioids

Contraindications Hypersensitivity to flumazenil, benzodiazepines, or any component of the formulation; patients given benzodiazepines for control of potentially life-threatening conditions (eg, control of intracranial pressure or status epilepticus); patients who are showing signs of serious cyclic-antidepressant overdosage

Warnings/Precautions [U.S. Boxed Warning]: Benzodiazepine reversal may result in seizures; seizures may occur more frequently in patients on benzodiazepines for long-term sedation or following tricyclic antidepressant overdose. Dose should be individualized and practitioners should be prepared to manage seizures. Seizures may also develop in patients with concurrent major sedative-hypnotic drug withdrawal, recent therapy with repeated doses of parenteral benzodiazepines, myoclonic jerking or seizure activity prior to flumazenil administration. Use with caution in patients relying on a benzodiazepine for seizure control. May cause CNS depression, which may impair physical or mental abilities; patients must be cautioned about performing tasks which require mental alertness (eg, operating machinery or driving) for 24 hours after discharge.

Flumazenil may not reliably reverse respiratory depression/hypoventilation. Flumazenil is not a substitute for evaluation of oxygenation; establishing an airway and assisting ventilation, as necessary, is always the initial step in overdose management. Resedation occurs more frequently in patients where a large single dose or cumulative dose of a benzodiazepine is administered along with a neuromuscular-blocking agent and multiple anesthetic agents. Flumazenil should be used with caution in the intensive care unit because of increased risk of unrecognized benzodiazepine dependence in such settings. Should not be used to diagnose benzodiazepine-induced sedation. Reverse neuromuscular blockade before considering use. Flumazenil does not antagonize the CNS effects of other GABA agonists (such as ethanol, barbiturates, or general anesthetics);

nor does it reverse narcotics. Flumazenil does not consistently reverse amnesia; patient may not recall verbal instructions after procedure.

Use with caution in patients with a history of panic disorder; may provoke panic attacks. Use caution in drug and ethanol-dependent patients; these patients may also be dependent on benzodiazepines. Not recommended for treatment of benzodiazepine dependence. Use with caution in patients with a head injury; may alter cerebral blood flow or precipitate convulsions in patients receiving benzodiazepines. Use caution in patients with mixed drug overdoses; toxic effects of other drugs taken may emerge once benzodiazepine effects are reversed. Use caution in hepatic dysfunction; repeated doses of the drug should be reduced in frequency or amount.

Drug Interactions

Metabolism/Transport Effects None known.

Avoid Concomitant Use There are no known interactions where it is recommended to avoid concomitant use.

Increased Effect/Toxicity There are no known significant interactions involving an increase in effect.

Decreased Effect

Flumazenil may decrease the levels/effects of: Hypnotics (Nonbenzodiazepine)

Dietary Considerations Avoid alcohol for the first 24 hours after administration or as long as the effects of benzodiazepines exist.

Pharmacodynamics/Kinetics

Onset of Action 1-2 minutes; 80% response within 3 minutes; Peak effect: 6-10 minutes

Duration of Action Resedation occurs after ~1 hour (range: 19-50 minutes); duration related to dose given and benzodiazepine plasma concentrations; reversal effects of flumazenil may wear off before effects of benzodiazepine

Half-life Elimination Adults: Alpha: 4-11 minutes; Terminal: 40-80 minutes; Moderate hepatic dysfunction: 1.3 hours; Severe hepatic impairment: 2.4 hours

Pregnancy Risk Factor C

Pregnancy Considerations Teratogenic effects were not seen in animal reproduction studies. Embryocidal effects were seen at large doses. Use during labor and delivery is not recommended. In general, medications used as antidotes should take into consideration the health and prognosis of the mother (Bailey, 2003).

Lactation Excretion in breast milk unknown/use caution

Breast-Feeding Considerations It is not known if flumazenil is excreted in breast milk. The manufacturer recommends that caution be used if administering to breast-feeding women.

Dosage Forms

Injection, solution: 0.1 mg/mL (5 mL, 10 mL)

Dental Comment Sedation: Patients should be monitored for at least 1 hour following administration of flumazenil to ensure full recovery. Flumazenil should only be used in an emergency situation and not as a means of hastening recovery from conscious sedation. When used to hasten recovery, emergence can be sudden and unpleasant. Flumazenil should be used with caution in patients routinely taking benzodiazepines for other therapeutic uses, withdrawal symptoms will be induced.

Flunarizine (floo NAR i zeen)

Brand Names: Canada Novo-Flunarizine
Pharmacologic Category Calcium Channel Blocker

Use Prophylaxis of migraine (with and without aura)

Local Anesthetic/Vasoconstrictor Precautions No information available to require special precautions

Effects on Dental Treatment Key adverse event(s) related to dental treatment: Xerostomia and changes in salivation (normal salivary flow resumes upon discontinuation).

Effects on Bleeding No information available to require special precautions

Adverse Effects Frequency not defined.

Central nervous system: Anxiety, depression, dizziness, drowsiness, fatigue, insomnia, sedation, vertigo

Dermatologic: Rash

Endocrine & metabolic: Galactorrhea, menstrual irregularities, prolactin levels increased

Gastrointestinal: Appetite increased, epigastric pain, heartburn, nausea, vomiting, weight gain, xerostomia

Neuromuscular & skeletal: Extrapyramidal symptoms, muscle ache, weakness

General Dosage Range Oral: *Adults <65 years:* 10 mg once daily

Mechanism of Action Flunarizine is a selective calcium channel blocker that prevents cellular calcium overload by reducing transmembrane calcium influx; also has antihistamine properties. Has greater effect on decreasing the frequency of migraine attacks than on decreasing the severity or duration of attacks.

Pharmacodynamics/Kinetics

Half-life Elimination ~19 days

Time to Peak 2-4 hours

Pregnancy Considerations Teratogenic events have not been observed in animal reproduction studies.

Product Availability Not available in U.S.

Flunisolide (Nasal) (floo NISS oh lide)

Brand Names: Canada Apo-Flunisolide®; Nasalide®; Rhinalar®

Pharmacologic Category Corticosteroid, Nasal

Use Seasonal or perennial rhinitis

Unlabeled Use Adjunct to antibiotics in empiric treatment of acute bacterial rhinosinusitis (ABRS) (Chow, 2012)

Local Anesthetic/Vasoconstrictor Precautions No information available to require special precautions

Effects on Dental Treatment Key adverse event(s) related to dental treatment: *Candida* infections of the nose, atrophic rhinitis, sneezing, nasal congestion, nasal dryness and burning, increased susceptibility to infections, dry throat, epistaxis

Effects on Bleeding No information available to require special precautions

Adverse Effects

>10%: Respiratory: Nasal congestion (15%), nasal burning/stinging (13%)

1% to 10%:

Respiratory: Nasal dryness, nasal irritation, rhinitis, sneezing

Miscellaneous: Loss of smell

General Dosage Range Intranasal:

Children 6-14 years: 1-2 sprays 2-3 times/day (maximum: 4 sprays/day in each nostril)

Children ≥15 years and Adults: 2 sprays twice daily (maximum: 8 sprays/day in each nostril)

Mechanism of Action Decreases inflammation by suppression of migration of polymorphonuclear leukocytes and reversal of increased capillary permeability; does not depress hypothalamus

Pregnancy Risk Factor C

Pregnancy Considerations Teratogenic effects were observed in animal studies. A decrease in fetal growth has not been observed with inhaled corticosteroid use during pregnancy. Inhaled corticosteroids are recommended for the treatment of allergic rhinitis during pregnancy.

Flunisolide (Oral Inhalation) (floo NISS oh lide)

Related Information

Respiratory Diseases *on page 1514*

Brand Names: U.S. Aerospan™

Pharmacologic Category Corticosteroid, Inhalant (Oral)

Use Maintenance treatment and prophylactic therapy for asthma; to reduce or eliminate the need for oral corticosteroids in steroid-dependent asthma patients

Local Anesthetic/Vasoconstrictor Precautions No information available to require special precautions

Effects on Dental Treatment Key adverse event(s) related to dental treatment: *Candida* infections of the pharynx, sore throat, bitter taste, palpitations, dizziness, headache, nervousness, GI irritation, sneezing, coughing, upper respiratory tract infection, bronchitis, increased susceptibility to infections, xerostomia (normal salivary flow resumes upon discontinuation), dry throat, loss of taste, and diaphoresis.

Effects on Bleeding No information available to require special precautions

Adverse Effects

>10%:

Central nervous system: Headache (9% to 14%)

Respiratory: Pharyngitis (17% to 18%), rhinitis (4% to 16%)

1% to 10%:

Cardiovascular: Chest pain (1% to 3%), edema (1% to 3%)

Central nervous system: Fever (1% to 7%), pain (2% to 5%), dizziness (1% to 3%), insomnia (1% to 3%), migraine (1% to 3%)

Dermatologic: Rash (2% to 4%), erythema multiforme (1% to 3%)

Endocrine & metabolic: Dysmenorrhea (1% to 3%)

Gastrointestinal: Vomiting (≤5%), dyspepsia (2% to 4%), abdominal pain (1% to 3%), diarrhea (1% to 3%), gastroenteritis (1% to 3%), nausea (1% to 3%), oral moniliasis (1% to 3%), taste perversion (1% to 3%)

Genitourinary: Urinary tract infection (1% to 4%), vaginitis (1% to 3%)

Neuromuscular & skeletal: Back pain (1% to 3%), myalgia (1% to 3%), neck pain (1% to 3%)

Ocular: Conjunctivitis (1% to 3%)

Otic: Ear pain (1% to 3)

Respiratory: Sinusitis (4% to 9%), cough increased (2% to 9%), bronchitis (1% to 3%), laryngitis (1% to 3%), epistaxis (≤3%)

Miscellaneous: Allergic reaction (4% to 5%), bacterial infection (1% to 4%), infection (1% to 3%), voice alteration (1% to 3%)

General Dosage Range Oral inhalation:

Children 6-11 years: 80 mcg twice daily (maximum: 160 mcg twice daily)

Children ≥12 years, Adolescents, and Adults: 160 mcg twice daily (maximum: 320 mcg twice daily)

Mechanism of Action Decreases airway inflammation by suppression of endogenous inflammatory mediators (kinins, histamine, liposomal enzymes, prostaglandins). Inhibits inflammatory cell migration and reverses increased capillary permeability to decrease access of inflammatory cells to the site of inflammation; does not depress hypothalamus.

Pharmacodynamics/Kinetics

Half-life Elimination 1.3-1.7 hours

Time to Peak Within 5-10 minutes

Pregnancy Risk Factor C

Pregnancy Considerations Teratogenic and fetotoxic effects were observed in animal studies. A decrease in fetal growth has not been observed with inhaled corticosteroid use during pregnancy. Inhaled corticosteroids are recommended for the treatment of asthma (most information available using budesonide) during pregnancy.

Product Availability Aerospan®: FDA approved September 2012; availability anticipated for Fall of 2013.

Fluocinolone (Topical) (floo oh SIN oh lone)

Brand Names: U.S. Capex®; Derma-Smoothe/FS®

Brand Names: Canada Capex®; Derma-Smoothe/FS®; Synalar®

Generic Availability (U.S.) Yes: Excludes shampoo

Pharmacologic Category Corticosteroid, Topical

Dental Use Relief of inflammatory and pruritic manifestations (low, medium, high potency topical corticosteroid)

Use Relief of susceptible inflammatory dermatosis (low, medium corticosteroid); dermatitis or psoriasis of the scalp; atopic dermatitis in adults and children ≥3 months of age

Local Anesthetic/Vasoconstrictor Precautions No information available to require special precautions

Effects on Dental Treatment No significant effects or complications reported

Effects on Bleeding No information available to require special precautions

Adverse Effects Frequency not defined.

Cardiovascular: Intracranial hypertension (rare)

Central nervous system: Telangiectasia

Dermatologic: Acneiform eruptions, allergic contact dermatitis, atopic dermatitis (secondary), burning, dryness, erythema, folliculitis, irritation, itching, hypertrichosis, hypopigmentation, keratosis pilaris, miliaria, papules, perioral dermatitis, pustules, shiny skin, skin atrophy, striae

Endocrine & metabolic: Cushing's syndrome, HPA axis suppression

Otic: Ear infection

Miscellaneous: Herpes simplex, secondary infection

Dental Usual Dosage Inflammatory and pruritic manifestations: Adults: Topical: Apply to oral lesion 4 times/day, after meals and at bedtime

Dosage Topical:

Atopic dermatitis (Derma-Smoothe/FS® body oil):

Children ≥3 months: Moisten skin; apply a thin film to affected area twice daily; do not use for longer than 4 weeks

Adults: Apply a thin film to affected area 3 times/day

Corticosteroid-responsive dermatoses: Children and Adults: Cream, ointment, solution: Apply a thin layer to affected area 2-4 times/day; may use occlusive dressings to manage psoriasis or recalcitrant conditions

Inflammatory and pruritic manifestations (dental use): Adults: Apply to oral lesion 4 times/day, after meals and at bedtime

Scalp psoriasis (Derma-Smoothe/FS® scalp oil): Adults: Massage thoroughly into wet or dampened hair/scalp; cover with shower cap. Leave on overnight (or for at least 4 hours). Remove by washing hair with shampoo and rinsing thoroughly.

Seborrheic dermatitis of the scalp (Capex®): Adults: Apply no more than 1 ounce to scalp once daily; work into lather and allow to remain on scalp for ~5 minutes. Remove from hair and scalp by rinsing thoroughly with water.

Mechanism of Action A synthetic fluorinated corticosteroid of low-to-moderate potency. The mechanism of action for all topical corticosteroids is not well defined, however, is believed to be a combination of anti-inflammatory, antipruritic, and vasoconstrictive properties.

Contraindications Hypersensitivity to fluocinolone or any component of the formulation; TB of skin, herpes (including varicella)

Warnings/Precautions Adverse systemic effects may occur when used on large areas of the body, denuded areas, for prolonged periods of time, or with an occlusive dressing. Infants and children may be more susceptible to systemic toxicity from equivalent doses due to larger skin surface to body mass ratio. Infants and small children may be more susceptible to adrenal axis suppression from topical corticosteroid therapy. Allergic contact dermatitis can occur, it is usually diagnosed by failure to heal rather than clinical exacerbation.

Topical: Not for oral, ophthalmic, or intravaginal use; do not apply to the face, axillae, groin, or diaper area unless directed by hea lthcare provider. Safety and efficacy of Derma-Smoothe/FS® body oil have not been established in children <3 months of age. Derma-Smoothe/FS® and contains peanut oil; use caution in peanut-sensitive individuals.

Drug Interactions

Metabolism/Transport Effects None known.

Avoid Concomitant Use

Avoid concomitant use of Fluocinolone (Topical) with any of the following: Aldesleukin

Increased Effect/Toxicity

Fluocinolone (Topical) may increase the levels/effects of: Deferasirox

The levels/effects of Fluocinolone (Topical) may be increased by: Telaprevir

Decreased Effect

Fluocinolone (Topical) may decrease the levels/effects of: Aldesleukin; Corticorelin; Hyaluronidase; Telaprevir

Pregnancy Risk Factor C

Pregnancy Considerations Adverse events have been observed with corticosteroids in animal reproduction studies. In general, the use of topical corticosteroids during pregnancy is not considered to have significant risk; however, intrauterine growth retardation in the infant has been reported (rare). The use of large amounts or for prolonged periods of time should be avoided.

Lactation Excretion in breast milk unknown/use caution

Breast-Feeding Considerations Systemic corticosteroids are excreted in human milk. It is not known if sufficient quantities of fluocinolone are absorbed following topical administration to produce detectable amounts in breast milk. Hypertension in the nursing infant has been reported following corticosteroid ointment applied to the nipples. Use with caution.

Dosage Forms
Cream, topical: 0.01% (15 g, 60 g); 0.025% (15 g, 60 g)
Oil, topical: 0.01% (118 mL)
Derma-Smoothe/FS®: 0.01% (120 mL)
Ointment, topical: 0.025% (15 g, 60 g)
Shampoo, topical:
Capex®: 0.01% (120 mL)
Solution, topical: 0.01% (60 mL)

Fluocinolone, Hydroquinone, and Tretinoin
(floo oh SIN oh lone, HYE droe kwin one, & TRET i noyn)

Related Information
Fluocinolone (Topical) on page 604
Hydroquinone on page 702
Tretinoin (Topical) on page 1356
Brand Names: U.S. Tri-Luma®
Pharmacologic Category Corticosteroid, Topical; Depigmenting Agent; Retinoic Acid Derivative
Use Short-term treatment of moderate-to-severe melasma of the face
Local Anesthetic/Vasoconstrictor Precautions No information available to require special precautions
Effects on Dental Treatment Key adverse event(s) related to dental treatment: Xerostomia (normal salivary flow resumes upon discontinuation).
Effects on Bleeding No information available to require special precautions
Adverse Effects
>10%:
Dermatologic: Erythema (41%), desquamation (38%), burning (18%), dry skin (14%), pruritus (11%)
1% to 10%:
Cardiovascular: Telangiectasia (3%)
Central nervous system: Hyperesthesia (2%)
Dermatologic: Acne (5%), pigmentation change (2%), irritation (2%), papules (1%), rash (1%), rosacea (1%), vesicles (1%)
Gastrointestinal: Xerostomia (1%)
Neuromuscular & skeletal: Paresthesia (3%)
General Dosage Range Topical: *Adults:* Apply a thin film once daily to affected areas.
Mechanism of Action Not clearly defined. Hydroquinone may interrupt melanin synthesis (tyrosine-tyrosinase pathway); reduces hyperpigmentation.
Pregnancy Risk Factor C
Pregnancy Considerations There are no adequate and well-controlled studies in pregnant women. Tretinoin appears to have a low risk of teratogenicity when used topically since it is rapidly metabolized by the skin; however, there are rare reports of fetal defects. Risk may be greatest in 1st trimester. Use topically only if benefit to mother outweighs potential risk to fetus. In general, the use of topical corticosteroids during pregnancy is not considered to have significant risk, however, intrauterine growth retardation in the infant has been reported (rare). The use of large amounts or for prolonged periods of time should be avoided. Consider delaying treatment until after delivery.

Fluocinonide (floo oh SIN oh nide)

Related Information
Ulcerative, Erosive, and Painful Oral Mucosal Disorders on page 1578
Related Sample Prescriptions
Mild Lichen Planus on page 1618
Recurrent Aphthous Stomatitis on page 1618
Brand Names: U.S. Vanos®
Brand Names: Canada Lidemol®; Lidex®; Lyderm®; Tiamol®; Topactin; Topsyn®
Generic Availability (U.S.) Yes
Pharmacologic Category Corticosteroid, Topical
Dental Use Relief of inflammatory and pruritic manifestations (high potency topical corticosteroid)
Use Anti-inflammatory, antipruritic; treatment of plaque-type psoriasis (up to 10% of body surface area) [high-potency topical corticosteroid]
Local Anesthetic/Vasoconstrictor Precautions No information available to require special precautions
Effects on Dental Treatment No significant effects or complications reported
Effects on Bleeding No information available to require special precautions
Adverse Effects Frequency not defined.
Cardiovascular: Intracranial hypertension
Dermatologic: Acne, allergic dermatitis, contact dermatitis, dry skin, folliculitis, hypertrichosis, hypopigmentation, maceration of the skin, miliaria, perioral dermatitis, pruritus, skin atrophy, striae, telangiectasia
Endocrine & metabolic: Cushing's syndrome, growth retardation, HPA axis suppression, hyperglycemia
Local: Burning, irritation
Renal: Glycosuria
Miscellaneous: Secondary infection
Dental Usual Dosage Pruritus and inflammation: Children and Adults: Topical (0.05% cream): Apply thin layer to affected area 2-4 times/day depending on the severity of the condition. Therapy should be discontinued when control is achieved; if no improvement is seen, reassessment of diagnosis may be necessary.
Dosage
Children and Adults: Pruritus and inflammation: Topical (0.05% cream): Apply thin layer to affected area 2-4 times/day depending on the severity of the condition. Therapy should be discontinued when control is achieved; if no improvement is seen, reassessment of diagnosis may be necessary.
Children ≥12 years and Adults: Plaque-type psoriasis (Vanos™): Topical (0.1% cream): Apply a thin layer once or twice daily to affected areas (limited to <10% of body surface area). **Note:** Not recommended for use >2 consecutive weeks or >60 g/week total exposure. Discontinue when control is achieved.
Mechanism of Action Fluorinated topical corticosteroid considered to be of high potency. The mechanism of action for all topical corticosteroids is not well defined, however, is felt to be a combination of three important properties: anti-inflammatory activity, immunosuppressive properties, and antiproliferative actions.
Contraindications Hypersensitivity to fluocinonide or any component of the formulation; viral, fungal, or tubercular skin lesions, herpes simplex

Warnings/Precautions Systemic absorption of topical corticosteroids may cause hypercorticism or suppression of hypothalamic-pituitary-adrenal (HPA) axis, particularly in younger children or in patients receiving high doses for prolonged periods. HPA axis suppression may lead to adrenal crisis. Absorption of topical corticosteroids may cause manifestations of Cushing's syndrome, hyperglycemia, or glycosuria. Absorption is increased by the use of occlusive dressings, application to denuded skin, or application to large surface areas.

Allergic contact dermatitis can occur, it is usually diagnosed by failure to heal rather than clinical exacerbation. Prolonged treatment with corticosteroids has been associated with the development of Kaposi's sarcoma (case reports); if noted, discontinuation of therapy should be considered. Lower-strength cream (0.05%) may be used cautiously on face or opposing skin surfaces that may rub or touch (eg, skin folds of the groin, axilla, and breasts); higher-strength (0.1%) should not be used on the face, groin, or axillae. Use of the 0.1% cream for >2 weeks or in patients <12 years of age is not recommended. Children may absorb proportionally larger amounts after topical application and may be more prone to systemic effects. HPA axis suppression, intracranial hypertension, and Cushing's syndrome have been reported in children receiving topical corticosteroids. Prolonged use may affect growth velocity; growth should be routinely monitored in pediatric patients.

Drug Interactions

Metabolism/Transport Effects None known.

Avoid Concomitant Use

Avoid concomitant use of Fluocinonide with any of the following: Aldesleukin

Increased Effect/Toxicity

Fluocinonide may increase the levels/effects of: Deferasirox

The levels/effects of Fluocinonide may be increased by: Telaprevir

Decreased Effect

Fluocinonide may decrease the levels/effects of: Aldesleukin; Corticorelin; Hyaluronidase; Telaprevir

Pregnancy Risk Factor C

Pregnancy Considerations Teratogenic effects have been observed in animals administered potent topical corticosteroids. Topical products are not recommended for extensive use, in large quantities, or for long periods of time in pregnant women.

Lactation Excretion unknown/not recommended

Breast-Feeding Considerations It is not known if topical application will result in detectable quantities in breast milk.

Dosage Forms

Cream, topical:
Vanos®: 0.1% (30 g, 60 g, 120 g)
Cream, anhydrous, emollient, topical: 0.05% (15 g, 30 g, 60 g, 120 g)
Cream, aqueous, emollient, topical: 0.05% (15 g, 30 g, 60 g)
Gel, topical: 0.05% (15 g, 30 g, 60 g)
Ointment, topical: 0.05% (15 g, 30 g, 60 g)
Solution, topical: 0.05% (20 mL, 60 mL)

Fluoride (FLOR ide)

Related Information

Dentin Hypersensitivity, Acid Erosion, High Caries Index, Management of Alveolar Osteitis, and Xerostomia *on page 1582*

Brand Names: U.S. Act® Kids [OTC]; Act® Restoring™ [OTC]; Act® Total Care™ [OTC]; Act® [OTC]; CaviRinse™; Clinpro™ 5000; ControlRx™; ControlRx™ Multi; Denta 5000 Plus™; DentaGel™; Epiflur™; Fluor-A-Day®; Fluorabon™; Fluorinse®; Fluoritab; Flura-Drops®; Gel-Kam® Rinse; Gel-Kam® [OTC]; Just For Kids™ [OTC]; Lozi-Flur™; NeutraCare®; NeutraGard® Advanced; Omni Gel™ [OTC]; OrthoWash™; PerioMed™; Phos-Flur®; Phos-Flur® Rinse [OTC]; Previ-Dent®; PreviDent® 5000 Booster; PreviDent® 5000 Dry Mouth; PreviDent® 5000 Plus®; PreviDent® 5000 Sensitive; StanGard® Perio; Stop®

Brand Names: Canada Fluor-A-Day

Generic Availability (U.S.) Yes: Excludes lozenge, gel drops

Pharmacologic Category Nutritional Supplement

Dental Use Prevention of dental caries

Use Prevention of dental caries

Local Anesthetic/Vasoconstrictor Precautions No information available to require special precautions

Effects on Dental Treatment Key adverse event(s) related to dental treatment: Products containing stannous fluoride may stain teeth. See Dental Comment.

Effects on Bleeding No information available to require special precautions

Dosage Oral:

The recommended daily dose of oral fluoride supplement (mg), based on fluoride ion content (ppm) in drinking water (2.2 mg of sodium fluoride is equivalent to 1 mg of fluoride ion): See table.

Fluoride Ion

Fluoride Content of Drinking Water	Daily Dose, Oral (mg)
<0.3 ppm	
Birth - 6 mo	None
6 mo - 3 y	0.25
3-6 y	0.5
6-16 y	1
0.3-0.6 ppm	
Birth - 6 mo	None
6 mo - 3 y	None
3-6 y	0.25
6-16 y	0.5

Adapted from Recommended Dosage Schedule of The American Dental Association, The American Academy of Pediatric Dentistry, and The American Academy of Pediatrics.

Cream: Children ≥6 years and Adults: Brush teeth with cream once daily regardless of fluoride content of drinking water

Dental rinse or gel:
Children 6-12 years: 5-10 mL rinse or apply to teeth and spit daily after brushing
Adults: 10 mL rinse or apply to teeth and spit daily after brushing

PreviDent® rinse: Children >6 years and Adults: Once weekly, rinse 10 mL vigorously around and between teeth for 1 minute, then spit; this should be done preferably at bedtime, after thoroughly brushing teeth; for maximum benefit, do not eat, drink, or rinse mouth for at least 30 minutes after treatment; do not swallow

Fluorinse®: Children >6 years and Adults: Once weekly, vigorously swish 5-10 mL in mouth for 1 minute, then spit

Lozenge (Lozi-Flur™): Adults: One lozenge daily regardless of fluoride content of drinking water

Mechanism of Action Promotes remineralization of decalcified enamel; inhibits the cariogenic microbial process in dental plaque; increases tooth resistance to acid dissolution

Contraindications Hypersensitivity to fluoride, tartrazine, or any component of the formulation; when fluoride content of drinking water exceeds 0.7 ppm; low sodium or sodium-free diets; do not use 1 mg tablets in children <3 years of age or when drinking water fluoride content is ≥0.3 ppm; do not use 1 mg/5 mL rinse (as supplement) in children <6 years of age

Warnings/Precautions Prolonged ingestion with excessive doses may result in dental fluorosis and osseous changes; do **not** exceed recommended dosage. Some products contain tartrazine.

Drug Interactions

Metabolism/Transport Effects None known.

Avoid Concomitant Use There are no known interactions where it is recommended to avoid concomitant use.

Increased Effect/Toxicity There are no known significant interactions involving an increase in effect.

Decreased Effect There are no known significant interactions involving a decrease in effect.

Dietary Considerations Do not administer with milk; do **not** allow eating or drinking for 30 minutes after use.

Pregnancy Risk Factor B

Pregnancy Considerations Adverse events have not been observed in animal reproduction studies; epidemiological studies in areas with high levels of fluorinated water have not shown an increase in adverse effects. Heavy exposure *in utero* may be linked to skeletal fluorosis seen later in childhood.

Breast-Feeding Considerations Low concentrations of fluoride can be found in breast milk and the amount is not significantly affected by supplementation or concentrations in drinking water (IOM, 1997).

Dosage Forms

Cream, oral: 1.1% (51 g)
Denta 5000 Plus™: 1.1% (51 g)
PreviDent® 5000 Plus®: 1.1% (51 g)

Gel, oral:
PreviDent® 5000 Booster: 1.1% (100 mL, 106 mL)
PreviDent® 5000 Dry Mouth: 1.1% (100 mL)
PreviDent® 5000 Sensitive: 1.1% (100 mL)

Gel, topical: 1.1% (56 g)
DentaGel™: 1.1% (56 g)
Gel-Kam® [OTC]: 0.4% (129 g)
Just For Kids™ [OTC]: 0.4% (122 g)
NeutraCare®: 1.1% (60 g)
NeutraGard® Advanced: 1.1% (60 g)
Omni Gel™ [OTC]: 0.4% (122 g); 0.4% (122 g)
Phos-Flur®: 1.1% (51 g)
PreviDent®: 1.1% (56 g)
Stop®: 0.4% (120 g)

Liquid, oral:
Fluoritab: 0.125 mg/drop

Lozenge, oral:
Lozi-Flur™: 2.21 mg (90s)

Paste, oral:
Clinpro™ 5000: 1.1% (113 g)
ControlRx™: 1.1% (57 g)
ControlRx™ Multi: 1.1% (57 g)

Solution, oral: 1.1 mg/mL (50 mL); 0.2% (473 mL); 0.63% (300 mL)
Act® [OTC]: 0.05% (532 mL)
Act® Kids [OTC]: 0.05% (500 mL, 532 mL)
Act® Restoring™ [OTC]: 0.02% (1000 mL); 0.05% (532 mL)
Act® Total Care™ [OTC]: 0.02% (1000 mL); 0.05% (88 mL, 532 mL)
CaviRinse™: 0.2% (240 mL)
Fluor-A-Day®: 0.278 mg/drop (30 mL)
Fluorabon™: 0.55 mg/0.6 mL (60 mL)
Fluorinse®: 0.2% (480 mL)
Flura-Drops®: 0.55 mg/drop (24 mL)
Gel-Kam® Rinse: 0.63% (300 mL)
OrthoWash™: 0.044% (480 mL)
PerioMed™: 0.63% (284 mL)
Phos-Flur® Rinse [OTC]: 0.044% (473 mL, 500 mL)
PreviDent®: 0.2% (473 mL)
StanGard® Perio: 0.63% (284 mL)

Tablet, chewable, oral: 0.55 mg, 1.1 mg, 2.2 mg
Epiflur™: 0.55 mg, 1.1 mg, 2.2 mg
Fluor-A-Day®: 0.55 mg, 1.1 mg, 2.2 mg
Fluoritab: 1.1 mg, 2.2 mg

Dental Comment Neutral pH fluoride preparations are preferred in patients with oral mucositis to reduce tissue irritation; long-term use of acidulated fluorides has been associated with enamel demineralization and damage to porcelain crowns

References

Wynn RL, "Fluoride: After 50 Years, a Clearer Picture of Its Mechanism," *Gen Dent*, 2002, 50(2):118-22, 124, 126.

Fluorometholone (flure oh METH oh lone)

Brand Names: U.S. Flarex®; FML Forte®; FML®
Brand Names: Canada Flarex®; FML Forte®; FML®; PMS-Fluorometholone

Pharmacologic Category Corticosteroid, Ophthalmic

Use Treatment of steroid-responsive inflammatory conditions of the eye

Local Anesthetic/Vasoconstrictor Precautions No information available to require special precautions

Effects on Dental Treatment No significant effects or complications reported

Effects on Bleeding No information available to require special precautions

Adverse Effects

Frequency not defined:

Gastrointestinal: Taste perversion

Ocular: Blurred vision, burning, cataract formation, delayed wound healing, glaucoma, glaucoma with optic nerve damage, intraocular pressure increased, irritation, secondary ocular infection (bacterial, fungal, viral), stinging, visual acuity and field defects

Miscellaneous: Allergic reaction, systemic hypercorticoidism (rare)

Effects reported with other corticosteroids: Anterior uveitis, bleb formation increased, conjunctival hyperemia, conjunctivitis, corneal ulcers, keratitis, loss of accommodation, mydriasis, perforation of the globe, ptosis

General Dosage Range Ophthalmic:

Ointment: *Children ≥2 years, Adolescents, and Adults:* Apply small amount (~1/2" ribbon) every 4 hours (initial: 24-48 hours) **or** 1-3 times daily

Suspension:
Children ≥2 years, Adolescents, and Adults (FML®, FML® Forte): Instill 1 drop every 4 hours (initial: 24-48 hours) **or** 1 drop 2-4 times daily
Adults (Flarex®): Instill 2 drops (initial: 24-48 hours) **or** 1-2 drops 2-4 times daily

Mechanism of Action Corticosteroids inhibit the inflammatory response including edema, capillary dilation, leukocyte migration, and scar formation. Fluorometholone penetrates cells readily to induce the production of lipocortins. These proteins modulate the activity of prostaglandins and leukotrienes.

Pregnancy Risk Factor C

Pregnancy Considerations Teratogenic effects were observed in animal reproduction studies following use of ophthalmic fluorometholone. The extent of systemic absorption following topical application of the ophthalmic drops is not known.

Fluorouracil (Systemic) (flure oh YOOR a sil)

Related Information
Capecitabine *on page 239*
Brand Names: U.S. Adrucil®
Pharmacologic Category Antineoplastic Agent, Antimetabolite; Antineoplastic Agent, Antimetabolite (Pyrimidine Analog)
Use Treatment of breast cancer, colon cancer, rectal cancer, pancreatic cancer, and stomach (gastric) cancer
Unlabeled Use Treatment of anal cancer, bladder cancer, cervical cancer, esophageal cancer, head and neck cancer, hepatobiliary cancers, neuroendocrine tumors, penile cancer (metastatic), thymic cancers, and unknown primary cancer
Local Anesthetic/Vasoconstrictor Precautions No information available to require special precautions
Effects on Dental Treatment Key adverse event(s) related to dental treatment: Stomatitis.
Effects on Bleeding Thrombocytopenia and anemia can occur during systemic therapy.
Adverse Effects Toxicity depends on duration of treatment and/or rate of administration
Cardiovascular: Angina, arrhythmia, heart failure, MI, myocardial ischemia, vasospasm, ventricular ectopy
Central nervous system: Acute cerebellar syndrome, confusion, disorientation, euphoria, headache, nystagmus, stroke
Dermatologic: Alopecia, dermatitis, dry skin, fissuring, nail changes (nail loss), palmar-plantar erythrodysesthesia syndrome, pruritic maculopapular rash, photosensitivity, Stevens-Johnson syndrome, toxic epidermal necrolysis, vein pigmentation
Gastrointestinal: Anorexia, bleeding, diarrhea, esophagopharyngitis, mesenteric ischemia (acute), nausea, sloughing, stomatitis, ulceration, vomiting
Hematologic: Agranulocytosis, anemia, leukopenia (nadir: days 9-14; recovery by day 30), pancytopenia, thrombocytopenia
Local: Thrombophlebitis
Ocular: Lacrimation, lacrimal duct stenosis, photophobia, visual changes
Respiratory: Epistaxis
Miscellaneous: Anaphylaxis, generalized allergic reactions
General Dosage Range Dosage adjustment recommended in patients with hepatic or renal impairment or who develop toxicities
I.V.: *Adults:* Dosage varies greatly depending on indication

Mechanism of Action A pyrimidine analog antimetabolite that interferes with DNA and RNA synthesis; after activation, F-UMP (an active metabolite) is incorporated into RNA to replace uracil and inhibit cell growth; the active metabolite F-dUMP, inhibits thymidylate synthetase, depleting thymidine triphosphate (a necessary component of DNA synthesis).

Pharmacodynamics/Kinetics
Half-life Elimination 16 minutes (range: 8-20 minutes); two metabolites, F-dUMP and F-UMP, have prolonged half-lives depending on the type of tissue
Pregnancy Risk Factor D
Pregnancy Considerations Adverse effects (increased resorptions, embryolethality, and teratogenicity) have been observed in animal reproduction studies. Based on the mechanism of action, fluorouracil may cause fetal harm if administered during pregnancy (according to the manufacturer's labeling). The National Comprehensive Cancer Network (NCCN) breast cancer guidelines (v.3.2012) state that chemotherapy, if indicated, may be administered to pregnant women with breast cancer as part of a combination chemotherapy regimen (common regimens administered during pregnancy include doxorubicin, cyclophosphamide, and fluorouracil); chemotherapy should not be administered during the first trimester, after 35 weeks gestation, or within 3 weeks of planned delivery.

FLUoxetine (floo OKS e teen)

Related Information
Clinical Risk Related to Drugs Prolonging QT Interval *on page 1510*
Management of the Patient With Anxiety or Depression *on page 1594*
Vasoconstrictor Interactions With Antidepressants *on page 1650*
Brand Names: U.S. PROzac®; PROzac® Weekly™; Sarafem®
Brand Names: Canada Apo-Fluoxetine®; Ava-Fluoxetine; CO Fluoxetine; Dom-Fluoxetine; Fluoxetine Capsules BP; FXT 40; Gen-Fluoxetine; JAMP-Fluoxetine; Mint-Fluoxetine; Mylan-Fluoxetine; Novo-Fluoxetine; Nu-Fluoxetine; PHL-Fluoxetine; PMS-Fluoxetine; PRO-Fluoxetine; Prozac®; Q-Fluoxetine; ratio-Fluoxetine; Riva-Fluoxetine; Sandoz-Fluoxetine; Teva-Fluoxetine; ZYM-Fluoxetine
Generic Availability (U.S.) Yes
Pharmacologic Category Antidepressant, Selective Serotonin Reuptake Inhibitor
Use Treatment of major depressive disorder (MDD); treatment of binge-eating and vomiting in patients with moderate-to-severe bulimia nervosa; obsessive-compulsive disorder (OCD); premenstrual dysphoric disorder (PMDD); panic disorder with or without agoraphobia; in combination with olanzapine for treatment-resistant or bipolar I depression
Unlabeled Use Selective mutism; treatment of mild dementia-associated agitation in nonpsychotic patients; post-traumatic stress disorder (PTSD); social anxiety disorder; fibromyalgia; Raynaud's phenomenon; treatment of paraphilia/hypersexuality
Local Anesthetic/Vasoconstrictor Precautions Although caution should be used in patients taking tricyclic antidepressants, no interactions have been reported with vasoconstrictors and fluoxetine, a nontricyclic antidepressant which acts to increase serotonin; no precautions appear to be needed. Fluoxetine is one of the drugs confirmed to prolong the QT interval and is

accepted as having a risk of causing torsade de pointes. The risk of drug-induced torsade de pointes is extremely low when a single QT interval prolonging drug is prescribed. In terms of epinephrine, it is not known what effect vasoconstrictors in the local anesthetic regimen will have in patients with a known history of congenital prolonged QT interval or in patients taking any medication that prolongs the QT interval. Until more information is obtained, it is suggested that the clinician consult with the physician prior to the use of a vasoconstrictor in suspected patients, and that the vasoconstrictor (epinephrine, mepivacaine and levonordefrin [Carbocaine® 2% with Neo-Cobefrin®]) be used with caution.

Effects on Dental Treatment Key adverse event(s) related to dental treatment: Xerostomia (normal salivary flow resumes upon discontinuation) and taste perversion. Problems with SSRI-induced bruxism have been reported and may preclude their use. Clinicians attempting to evaluate any patient with bruxism or involuntary muscle movement, who is simultaneously being treated with an SSRI drug, should be aware of this potential association. See Effects on Bleeding.

Effects on Bleeding Selective serotonin reuptake inhibitors such as fluoxetine may impair platelet aggregation due to platelet serotonin depletion, possibly increasing the risk of a bleeding complication. The risk of a bleeding complication can be increased by coadministration of other antiplatelet agents such as NSAIDs and aspirin.

Adverse Effects Percentages listed for adverse effects as reported in placebo-controlled trials and were generally similar in adults and children; actual frequency may be dependent upon diagnosis and in some cases the range presented may be lower than or equal to placebo for a particular disorder.

>10%:
Central nervous system: Insomnia (10% to 33%), headache (21%), somnolence (5% to 17%), anxiety (6% to 15%), nervousness (8% to 14%)
Endocrine & metabolic: Libido decreased (1% to 11%)
Gastrointestinal: Nausea (12% to 29%), diarrhea (8% to 18%), anorexia (4% to 17%), xerostomia (4% to 12%)
Neuromuscular & skeletal: Weakness (7% to 21%), tremor (3% to 13%)
Respiratory: Pharyngitis (3% to 11%), yawn (≤11%)
1% to 10%:
Cardiovascular: Vasodilation (1% to 5%), chest pain, hemorrhage, hypertension, palpitation
Central nervous system: Dizziness (9%), abnormal dreams (1% to 5%), abnormal thinking (2%), agitation, amnesia, chills, confusion, emotional lability, sleep disorder
Dermatologic: Rash (2% to 6%), pruritus (4%)
Endocrine & metabolic: Ejaculation abnormal (≤7%), impotence (≤7%), menorrhagia (≥2%)
Gastrointestinal: Dyspepsia (6% to 10%), constipation (5%), flatulence (3%), vomiting (3%), thirst (≥2%), weight loss (2%), appetite increased, taste perversion, weight gain
Genitourinary: Urinary frequency
Neuromuscular & skeletal: Hyperkinesia (≥2%)
Ocular: Vision abnormal (2%)
Otic: Ear pain, tinnitus
Respiratory: Sinusitis (1% to 6%)
Miscellaneous: Flu-like syndrome (3% to 10%), diaphoresis (2% to 8%), epistaxis (≥2%)

Dosage Oral: **Note:** Upon discontinuation of fluoxetine therapy, gradually taper dose. If intolerable symptoms occur following a dose reduction, consider resuming the previously prescribed dose and/or decrease dose at a more gradual rate.

Children:
Depression: 8-18 years: 10-20 mg/day; lower-weight children can be started at 10 mg/day, may increase to 20 mg/day after 1 week if needed
Obsessive-compulsive disorder: 7-17 years: Initial: 10 mg/day; may increase after 2 weeks if inadequate clinical response to 20 mg/day; further increases may be considered after several weeks to recommended range of 20-30 mg/day (lower weight children) or 20-60 mg/day (adolescents and higher weight children)
Selective mutism (unlabeled use): 5-18 years: Initial: 5-10 mg/day; titrate upwards as needed (usual maximum dose: 60 mg/day)

Adults: 20 mg/day in the morning; may increase after several weeks by 20 mg/day increments; maximum: 80 mg/day; doses >20 mg may be given once daily or divided twice daily. **Note:** Lower doses of 5-10 mg/day have been used for initial treatment.
Indication-specific dosing:
Bulimia nervosa: 60 mg/day
Depression: Initial: 20 mg/day; may increase after several weeks if inadequate response (maximum: 80 mg/day). Patients maintained on Prozac® 20 mg/day may be changed to Prozac® Weekly™ 90 mg/week, starting dose 7 days after the last 20 mg/day dose
Depression associated with bipolar disorder (in combination with olanzapine): Initial: 20 mg in the evening; adjust as tolerated to usual range of 20-50 mg/day. See **"Note"** below.
Fibromyalgia (unlabeled use): Range: 20-80 mg/day (Arnold, 2002)
Obsessive-compulsive disorder: Initial: 20 mg/day; may increase after several weeks if inadequate response; recommended range: 20-60 mg/day (maximum: 80 mg/day)
Panic disorder: Initial: 10 mg/day; after 1 week, increase to 20 mg/day; may increase after several weeks; doses >60 mg/day have not been evaluated
Post-traumatic stress disorder (PTSD) (unlabeled use): 20-40 mg/day
Premenstrual dysphoric disorder (Sarafem®): 20 mg/day continuously, **or** 20 mg/day starting 14 days prior to menstruation and through first full day of menses (repeat with each cycle)
Raynaud's phenomena (unlabeled use): 20 mg/day (Coleiro, 2001)
Social anxiety disorder (unlabeled use): Target dose: 40 mg/day; range 30-60 mg/day (Davidson, 2004)
Treatment-resistant depression (in combination with olanzapine): Initial: 20 mg in the evening; adjust as tolerated to usual range of 20-50 mg/day. See **"Note"**
Note: When using individual components of fluoxetine with olanzapine rather than fixed dose combination product (Symbyax®), approximate dosage correspondence is as follows:
Olanzapine 2.5 mg + fluoxetine 20 mg = Symbyax® 3/25
Olanzapine 5 mg + fluoxetine 20 mg = Symbyax® 6/25
Olanzapine 12.5 mg + fluoxetine 20 mg = Symbyax® 12/25

Olanzapine 5 mg + fluoxetine 50 mg = Symbyax® 6/50

Olanzapine 12.5 mg + fluoxetine 50 mg = Symbyax® 12/50

Elderly: Depression: Some patients may require an initial dose of 10 mg/day with dosage increases of 10 and 20 mg every several weeks as tolerated; should not be taken at night unless patient experiences sedation

MAO inhibitor recommendations:

Switching to or from an MAO inhibitor intended to treat psychiatric disorders:

Allow 14 days to elapse between discontinuing an MAO inhibitor intended to treat psychiatric disorders and initiation of fluoxetine.

Allow 5 weeks to elapse between discontinuing fluoxetine and initiation of an MAO inhibitor intended to treat psychiatric disorders.

Use with other MAO inhibitors (linezolid or I.V. methylene blue):

Do not initiate fluoxetine in patients receiving linezolid or I.V. methylene blue; consider other interventions for psychiatric condition.

If urgent treatment with linezolid or I.V. methylene blue is required in a patient already receiving fluoxetine and potential benefits outweigh potential risks, discontinue fluoxetine promptly and administer linezolid or I.V. methylene blue. Monitor for serotonin syndrome for 5 weeks or until 24 hours after the last dose of linezolid or I.V. methylene blue, whichever comes first. May resume fluoxetine 24 hours after the last dose of linezolid or I.V. methylene blue.

Dosing adjustment in renal impairment:

Single dose studies: Pharmacokinetics of fluoxetine and norfluoxetine were similar among subjects with all levels of impaired renal function, including anephric patients on chronic hemodialysis

Chronic administration: Additional accumulation of fluoxetine or norfluoxetine may occur in patients with severely impaired renal function

Hemodialysis: Not removed by hemodialysis; use of lower dose or less frequent dosing is not usually necessary.

Dosing adjustment in hepatic impairment: Elimination half-life of fluoxetine is prolonged in patients with hepatic impairment; a lower or less frequent dose of fluoxetine should be used in these patients

Cirrhosis patients: Administer a lower dose or less frequent dosing interval

Compensated cirrhosis without ascites: Administer 50% of normal dose

Mechanism of Action Inhibits CNS neuron serotonin reuptake; minimal or no effect on reuptake of norepinephrine or dopamine; does not significantly bind to alpha-adrenergic, histamine, or cholinergic receptors

Contraindications Hypersensitivity to fluoxetine or any component of the formulation; use of MAO inhibitors intended to treat psychiatric disorders (concurrently, within 5 weeks of discontinuing fluoxetine, or within 2 weeks of discontinuing the MAO inhibitor); initiation of fluoxetine in a patient receiving linezolid or intravenous methylene blue; use with pimozide or thioridazine (**Note:** Thioridazine should not be initiated until 5 weeks after the discontinuation of fluoxetine)

Warnings/Precautions [U.S. Boxed Warning]: Antidepressants increase the risk of suicidal thinking and behavior in children, adolescents, and young adults (18-24 years of age) with major depressive disorder (MDD) and other psychiatric disorders; consider risk prior to prescribing. Short-term studies did not show an increased risk in patients >24 years of age and showed a decreased risk in patients ≥65 years. Closely monitor patients for clinical worsening, suicidality, or unusual changes in behavior, particularly during the initial 1-2 months of therapy or during periods of dosage adjustments (increases or decreases); the patient's family or caregiver should be instructed to closely observe the patient and communicate condition with healthcare provider. A medication guide concerning the use of antidepressants should be dispensed with each prescription. **Fluoxetine is FDA approved for the treatment of OCD in children ≥7 years of age and MDD in children ≥8 years of age.**

The possibility of a suicide attempt is inherent in major depression and may persist until remission occurs. Use caution in high-risk patients. Worsening depression and severe abrupt suicidality that are not part of the presenting symptoms may require discontinuation or modification of drug therapy. The patient's family or caregiver should be alerted to monitor patients for the emergence of suicidality and associated behaviors (such as agitation, irritability, hostility, impulsivity, and hypomania) and call healthcare provider.

May worsen psychosis in some patients or precipitate a shift to mania or hypomania in patients with bipolar disorder. Patients presenting with depressive symptoms should be screened for bipolar disorder. Monotherapy in patients with bipolar disorder should be avoided. **Fluoxetine monotherapy is not FDA approved for the treatment of bipolar depression.** May cause insomnia, anxiety, nervousness, or anorexia. Use with caution in patients where weight loss is undesirable. May impair cognitive or motor performance; caution operating hazardous machinery or driving.

Potentially life-threatening serotonin syndrome (SS) has occurred with serotonergic agents (eg, SSRIs, SNRIs), particularly when used in combination with other serotonergic agents (eg, triptans, TCAs, fentanyl, lithium, tramadol, buspirone, St John's wort, tryptophan) or agents that impair metabolism of serotonin (eg, MOA inhibitors intended to treat psychiatric disorders, other MAO inhibitors [ie, linezolid and intravenous methylene blue]). Discontinue treatment (and any concomitant serotonergic agent) immediately if signs/symptoms arise. Fluoxetine use has been associated with occurrences of significant rash and allergic events, including vasculitis, lupus-like syndrome, laryngospasm, anaphylactoid reactions, and pulmonary inflammatory disease. Discontinue if underlying cause of rash cannot be identified.

Use caution in patients with a previous seizure disorder or condition predisposing to seizures such as brain damage, alcoholism, or concurrent therapy with other drugs which lower the seizure threshold. Use with caution in patients with hepatic or severe renal dysfunction and in elderly patients. Use caution in elderly patients; may cause or exacerbate syndrome of inappropriate antidiuretic hormone secretion or hyponatremia; monitor sodium closely with initiation or dosage adjustments in older adults (Beers Criteria). May also cause agitation, sleep disturbances, and excessive CNS stimulation. May cause hyponatremia/SIADH (elderly at increased risk); volume depletion (diuretics may increase risk). May increase the risks associated with electroconvulsive treatment. Use caution with history of MI or unstable heart disease; use in these patients is limited. May alter glycemic control in patients with diabetes. Due to the long half-life of fluoxetine and its metabolites, the effects and interactions noted may persist for prolonged periods following discontinuation. May cause or exacerbate sexual dysfunction. May cause mydriasis; use caution in patients at risk of acute narrow-angle glaucoma or with increased intraocular pressure. Discontinuation symptoms (eg, dysphoric mood, irritability, agitation, confusion, anxiety, insomnia, hypomania) may occur upon abrupt discontinuation. Taper dose when discontinuing therapy. Potentially significant interactions may exist, requiring dose or frequency adjustment, additional monitoring, and/or selection of alternative therapy. Consult drug interactions database for more detailed information.

Drug Interactions

Metabolism/Transport Effects Substrate of CYP1A2 (minor), CYP2B6 (minor), CYP2C19 (minor), CYP2C9 (major), CYP2D6 (major), CYP2E1 (minor), CYP3A4 (minor); **Note:** Assignment of Major/Minor substrate status based on clinically relevant drug interaction potential; **Inhibits** CYP1A2 (moderate), CYP2B6 (weak), CYP2C19 (moderate), CYP2C9 (weak), CYP2D6 (strong)

Avoid Concomitant Use

Avoid concomitant use of FLUoxetine with any of the following: Clopidogrel; Iobenguane I 123; Linezolid; MAO Inhibitors; Methylene Blue; Pimozide; Pirfenidone; Tamoxifen; Thioridazine; Tryptophan

Increased Effect/Toxicity

FLUoxetine may increase the levels/effects of: Agents with Antiplatelet Properties; Anticoagulants; Antidepressants (Serotonin Reuptake Inhibitor/Antagonist); ARIPiprazole; Aspirin; AtoMOXetine; Benzodiazepines (metabolized by oxidation); Beta-Blockers; BusPIRone; CarBAMazepine; CloZAPine; Collagenase (Systemic); CYP1A2 Substrates; CYP2C19 Substrates; CYP2D6 Substrates; Dabigatran Etexilate; Desmopressin; Dextromethorphan; Drotrecogin Alfa (Activated); Fesoterodine; Fosphenytoin; Galantamine; Haloperidol; Highest Risk QTc-Prolonging Agents; Hypoglycemic Agents; Ibritumomab; Methadone; Methylene Blue; Metoclopramide; Metoprolol; Mexiletine; Moderate Risk QTc-Prolonging Agents; NIFEdipine; NiMODipine; NSAID (COX-2 Inhibitor); NSAID (Nonselective); Phenytoin; Pimozide; Pirfenidone; Propafenone; QuiNIDine; RisperiDONE; Rivaroxaban; Salicylates; Serotonin Modulators; Tetrabenazine; Thioridazine; Thrombolytic Agents; Tositumomab and Iodine I 131 Tositumomab; TraMADol; Tricyclic Antidepressants; Vitamin K Antagonists

The levels/effects of FLUoxetine may be increased by: Abiraterone Acetate; Alcohol (Ethyl); Analgesics (Opioid); Antipsychotics; ARIPiprazole; BusPIRone; Cimetidine; CNS Depressants; Cobicistat; CYP2C9 Inhibitors (Moderate); CYP2C9 Inhibitors (Strong); CYP2D6 Inhibitors (Moderate); CYP2D6 Inhibitors (Strong); Darunavir; Dasatinib; Glucosamine; Herbs (Anticoagulant/Antiplatelet Properties); Linezolid; Lithium; Macrolide Antibiotics; MAO Inhibitors; Metoclopramide; Metyrosine; Mifepristone; Multivitamins/Minerals (with ADEK, Folate, Iron); Omega-3 Fatty Acids; Pentosan Polysulfate Sodium; Pentoxifylline; Prostacyclin Analogues; Tipranavir; TraMADol; Tryptophan; Vitamin E

Decreased Effect

FLUoxetine may decrease the levels/effects of: Clopidogrel; Iobenguane I 123; Ioflupane I 123; Tamoxifen

The levels/effects of FLUoxetine may be decreased by: CarBAMazepine; CYP2C9 Inducers (Strong); Cyproheptadine; NSAID (COX-2 Inhibitor); NSAID (Nonselective); Peginterferon Alfa-2b

Ethanol/Nutrition/Herb Interactions

Ethanol: May increase CNS depression; monitor for increased effects with coadministration. Caution patients about effects.

Herb/Nutraceutical: Avoid valerian, St John's wort, tryptophan, kava kava, gotu kola (may increase CNS depression and/or risk of serotonin syndrome).

Dietary Considerations May be taken without regard to meals.

Pharmacodynamics/Kinetics

Onset of Action Depression: The onset of action is within a week; however, individual response varies greatly and full response may not be seen until 8-12 weeks after initiation of treatment.

Half-life Elimination Adults: Parent drug: 1-3 days (acute), 4-6 days (chronic), 7.6 days (cirrhosis); Metabolite (norfluoxetine): 9.3 days (range: 4-16 days), 12 days (cirrhosis)

Time to Peak Serum: 6-8 hours

Pregnancy Risk Factor C

Pregnancy Considerations Adverse events have been observed in animal reproduction studies. Fluoxetine and its metabolite cross the human placenta. An increased risk of teratogenic effects, including cardiovascular defects, may be associated with maternal use of fluoxetine or other SSRIs; however, available information is conflicting. Nonteratogenic effects in the newborn following SSRI/SNRI exposure late in the third trimester include respiratory distress, cyanosis, apnea, seizures, temperature instability, feeding difficulty, vomiting, hypoglycemia, hypo- or hypertonia, hyper-reflexia, jitteriness, irritability, constant crying, and tremor. Symptoms may be due to the toxicity of the SSRIs/SNRIs or a discontinuation syndrome and may be consistent with serotonin syndrome associated with SSRI treatment. Persistent pulmonary hypertension of the newborn (PPHN) has also been reported with SSRI exposure. The long-term effects of *in utero* SSRI exposure on infant development and behavior are not known.

Due to pregnancy-induced physiologic changes, women who are pregnant may require dose adjustments of fluoxetine to achieve euthymia. The ACOG recommends that therapy with SSRIs or SNRIs during pregnancy be individualized; treatment of depression during pregnancy should incorporate the clinical expertise of the mental health clinician, obstetrician, primary healthcare provider, and pediatrician. According to the American Psychiatric Association (APA), the risks of medication treatment should be weighed against other treatment options and untreated depression. For women who discontinue antidepressant medications during pregnancy and who may be at high risk for postpartum depression, the medications can be restarted following delivery. Treatment algorithms have been developed by the ACOG and the APA for the management of depression in women prior to conception and during pregnancy.

Lactation Enters breast milk/not recommended (AAP rates "of concern"; AAP 2001 update pending)

Breast-Feeding Considerations Fluoxetine and its metabolite are excreted into breast milk and can be detected in the serum of breast-feeding infants. Concentrations in breast milk are variable. In comparison to other SSRIs, fluoxetine concentrations in breast milk are higher and adverse events have been observed in

◀ nursing infants. Maternal use of an SSRI during pregnancy may cause delayed milk secretion. Breast-feeding is not recommended by the manufacturer. Long-term effects on development and behavior have not been studied.

Dosage Forms

Capsule, oral: 10 mg, 20 mg, 40 mg
PROzac®: 10 mg, 20 mg, 40 mg
Capsule, delayed release, enteric coated pellets, oral: 90 mg
PROzac® Weekly™: 90 mg
Solution, oral: 20 mg/5 mL (5 mL, 120 mL)
Tablet, oral: 10 mg, 20 mg, 60 mg
Sarafem®: 10 mg, 15 mg, 20 mg

Dental Comment Fluoxetine is known to prolong the QT interval. The QT interval is measured as the time and distance between the Q point of the QRS complex and the end of the T wave in the ECG tracing. After adjustment for heart rate, the QT interval is defined as prolonged if it is more than 450 msec in men and 460 msec in women. A long QT syndrome was first described in the 1950s and 60s as a congenital syndrome involving QT interval prolongation and syncope and sudden death. Some of the congenital long QT syndromes were characterized by a peculiar electrocardiographic appearance of the QRS complex involving a premature atria beat followed by a pause, then a subsequent sinus beat showing marked QT prolongation and deformity. This type of cardiac arrhythmia was originally termed "torsade de pointes" (translated from the French as "twisting of the points"). Fluoxetine is considered as having a risk of causing torsade de pointes. Since it is not known what effect vasoconstrictors in the local anesthetic regimen will have in patients with a known history of congenital prolonged QT interval or in patients taking any medication that prolongs the QT interval, a medical consult is suggested.

References

Friedlander AH and Mahler ME, "Major Depressive Disorder. Psychopathology, Medical Management, and Dental Implications," *J Am Dent Assoc*, 2001, 132(5):629-38.
Gerber PE and Lynd LD, "Selective Serotonin Reuptake Inhibitor-induced Movement Disorders," *Ann Pharmacother*, 1998, 32 (6):692-8.
Wynn RL, "New Antidepressant Medications," *Gen Dent*, 1997, 45 (1):24-8.

Fluoxymesterone (floo oks i MES te rone)

Brand Names: U.S. Androxy™
Pharmacologic Category Androgen
Use Replacement therapy in the treatment of delayed male puberty; male hypogonadism (primary or hypogonadotropic); inoperable metastatic female breast cancer

Local Anesthetic/Vasoconstrictor Precautions No information available to require special precautions
Effects on Dental Treatment No significant effects or complications reported
Effects on Bleeding No information available to require special precautions
Adverse Effects Frequency not defined.
Male: Gynecomastia, oligospermia (at higher doses), priapism, prostatic carcinoma, prostatic hypertrophy, testicular atrophy
Female: Menstrual irregularities (including amenorrhea), virilism (including deepening of the voice, clitoris hypertrophy)
Cardiovascular: Edema
Central nervous system: Anxiety, depression, headache
Dermatologic: Acne, hirsutism, "male pattern" baldness

Endocrine & metabolic: Electrolyte abnormalities (sodium, chloride, calcium, potassium, and inorganic phosphate retention), hypercholesterolemia, libido changes (increased or decreased), water retention
Gastrointestinal: GI irritation, nausea, vomiting
Genitourinary: Prostatic hyperplasia
Hematologic: Clotting factor suppression, polycythemia
Hepatic: Cholestatic jaundice, hepatic coma (rare), hepatic dysfunction, hepatocellular neoplasms (rare), liver function tests abnormal, peliosis hepatitis (rare)
Neuromuscular & skeletal: Paresthesia
Miscellaneous: Hypersensitivity, nonimmunologic anaphylaxis (formerly known as anaphylactoid reaction)

General Dosage Range Oral:
Adults (females): 10-40 mg daily in divided doses
Adults (males): 2.5-20 mg daily
Mechanism of Action Synthetic derivative of testosterone; responsible for the normal growth and development of male sex hormones, male sex organs, and maintenance of secondary sex characteristics; large doses suppress endogenous testosterone release
Pharmacodynamics/Kinetics
Half-life Elimination 10 hours (range: 10-100 minutes)
Pregnancy Risk Factor X
Pregnancy Considerations Use is contraindicated in women who are or may become pregnant. May cause androgenic effects to the female fetus; clitoral hypertrophy, labial fusion, urogenital sinus defect, vaginal atresia, and ambiguous genitalia have been reported.
Controlled Substance C-III

FluPHENAZine (floo FEN a zeen)

Brand Names: Canada Apo-Fluphenazine Decanoate®; Apo-Fluphenazine®; Modecate®; Modecate® Concentrate; PMS-Fluphenazine Decanoate
Pharmacologic Category Antipsychotic Agent, Typical, Phenothiazine
Use Management of manifestations of psychotic disorders and schizophrenia; depot formulation may offer improved outcome in individuals with psychosis who are nonadherent with oral antipsychotics
Unlabeled Use Psychosis/agitation related to Alzheimer's dementia
Local Anesthetic/Vasoconstrictor Precautions Most pharmacology textbooks state that in the presence of phenothiazines, systemic doses of epinephrine paradoxically decrease the blood pressure. This is the so called "epinephrine reversal" phenomenon. This has never been observed when epinephrine is given by infiltration as part of the anesthesia procedure.
Effects on Dental Treatment Key adverse event(s) related to dental treatment: Xerostomia and increased salivation (normal salivary flow resumes upon discontinuation). Orthostatic hypotension and nasal congestion are possible and since the drug is a dopamine antagonist, extrapyramidal symptoms of the TMJ are a possibility.
Effects on Bleeding No information available to require special precautions
Adverse Effects Frequency not defined.
Cardiovascular: Hyper-/hypotension, tachycardia, fluctuations in blood pressure, arrhythmia, edema

Central nervous system: Parkinsonian symptoms, akathisia, dystonias, tardive dyskinesia, dizziness, hyperreflexia, headache, cerebral edema, drowsiness, lethargy, restlessness, excitement, bizarre dreams, EEG changes, depression, seizure, NMS, altered central temperature regulation

Dermatologic: Dermatitis, eczema, erythema, itching, photosensitivity, rash, seborrhea, skin pigmentation, urticaria

Endocrine & metabolic: Menstrual cycle changes, breast pain, amenorrhea, galactorrhea, gynecomastia, libido changes, prolactin increased, SIADH

Gastrointestinal: Weight gain, appetite loss, salivation, xerostomia, constipation, paralytic ileus, laryngeal edema

Genitourinary: Ejaculatory disturbances, impotence, polyuria, bladder paralysis, enuresis

Hematologic: Agranulocytosis, leukopenia, thrombocytopenia, nonthrombocytopenic purpura, eosinophilia, pancytopenia

Hepatic: Cholestatic jaundice, hepatotoxicity

Neuromuscular & skeletal: Trembling of fingers, SLE, facial hemispasm

Ocular: Pigmentary retinopathy, cornea and lens changes, blurred vision, glaucoma

Respiratory: Nasal congestion, asthma

General Dosage Range
I.M. (hydrochloride): *Adults:* Initial: 1.25 mg as a single dose; Maintenance: 2.5-10 mg/day in divided doses every 6-8 hours
I.M., SubQ (Depot): *Adults:* Initial: 6.25-25 mg every 2-4 weeks (maximum: 100 mg)
Oral: *Adults:* 1-20 mg/day in divided doses every 6-8 hours (maximum: 40 mg/day)

Mechanism of Action Fluphenazine is a piperazine phenothiazine antipsychotic which blocks postsynaptic mesolimbic dopaminergic D_1 and D_2 receptors in the brain; depresses the release of hypothalamic and hypophyseal hormones; believed to depress the reticular activating system, thus affecting basal metabolism, body temperature, wakefulness, vasomotor tone, and emesis

Pharmacodynamics/Kinetics
Onset of Action Decanoate: 24-72 hours; Peak effect: Neuroleptic: Decanoate: 48-96 hours
Duration of Action Hydrochloride salt: 6-8 hours; Decanoate: ~4 weeks
Half-life Elimination Derivative dependent: Hydrochloride: ~14-16.4 hours; Decanoate: ~14 days
Time to Peak Serum: Hydrochloride: Oral: 2 hours; Decanoate: 8-10 hours

Pregnancy Considerations Jaundice or hyper-/hyporeflexia have been reported in newborn infants following maternal use of phenothiazines. Antipsychotic use during the third trimester of pregnancy has a risk for abnormal muscle movements (extrapyramidal symptoms [EPS]) and withdrawal symptoms in newborns following delivery. Symptoms in the newborn may include agitation, feeding disorder, hypertonia, hypotonia, respiratory distress, somnolence, and tremor; these effects may be self-limiting or require hospitalization.

Flurandrenolide (flure an DREN oh lide)

Brand Names: U.S. Cordran®; Cordran® SP
Brand Names: Canada Cordran®
Pharmacologic Category Corticosteroid, Topical

Use Treatment of pruritic and inflammatory corticosteroid-responsive dermatoses (medium potency topical corticosteroid)
Local Anesthetic/Vasoconstrictor Precautions No information available to require special precautions
Effects on Dental Treatment No significant effects or complications reported
Effects on Bleeding No information available to require special precautions
Adverse Effects Frequency not defined.
Dermatologic: Acne, acneiform eruptions, allergic contact dermatitis, dry skin, folliculitis, hypopigmentation, hypertrichosis, itching, maceration of the skin, miliaria, perioral dermatitis, skin atrophy, striae
Local: Burning, irritation
Miscellaneous: Secondary infection
General Dosage Range Topical:
Children: Cream, tape: Apply 1-2 times per day; Lotion: Apply 2-3 times per day
Adults: Cream, lotion: Apply 2-3 times per day; Tape: Apply 1-2 times per day
Mechanism of Action Decreases inflammation by suppression of migration of polymorphonuclear leukocytes and reversal of increased capillary permeability
Pregnancy Risk Factor C
Pregnancy Considerations Some corticosteroids were found to be teratogenic following topical application in animal reproduction studies. Topical products are not recommended for extensive use, in large quantities, or for long periods of time in pregnant women.

Flurazepam (flure AZ e pam)

Brand Names: Canada Apo-Flurazepam®; Dalmane®; Som Pam
Generic Availability (U.S.) Yes
Pharmacologic Category Hypnotic, Benzodiazepine
Use Short-term treatment of insomnia
Local Anesthetic/Vasoconstrictor Precautions No information available to require special precautions
Effects on Dental Treatment Key adverse event(s) related to dental treatment: Xerostomia and changes in salivation (normal salivary flow resumes upon discontinuation), and bitter taste.
Effects on Bleeding No information available to require special precautions
Adverse Effects Frequency not defined.
Cardiovascular: Chest pain, flushing, hypotension, palpitation
Central nervous system: Apprehension, ataxia, confusion, depression, dizziness, drowsiness, euphoria, faintness, falling, hallucinations, hangover effect, headache, irritability, lightheadedness, memory impairment, nervousness, paradoxical reactions, restlessness, slurred speech, staggering, talkativeness
Dermatologic: Pruritus, rash
Gastrointestinal: Appetite increased/decreased, bitter taste, constipation, diarrhea, GI pain, heartburn, nausea, salivation increased/excessive, upset stomach, vomiting, weight gain/loss, xerostomia
Hematologic: Granulocytopenia, leukopenia
Hepatic: Alkaline phosphatase increased, ALT increased, AST increased, cholestatic jaundice, total bilirubin increased
Neuromuscular & skeletal: Body/joint pain, dysarthria, reflex slowing, weakness
Ocular: Blurred vision, burning eyes, difficulty focusing
Respiratory: Apnea, dyspnea
Miscellaneous: Diaphoresis, drug dependence

Postmarketing and/or case reports: Anaphylaxis, angioedema, complex sleep-related behavior (sleep-driving, cooking or eating food, making phone calls)

Dosage Oral: Insomnia:

Children:

<15 years: Dose not established

≥15 years: 15 mg at bedtime

Adults: 15-30 mg at bedtime

Elderly: 15 mg at bedtime; avoid use if possible

Dosage adjustment in renal impairment: No dosage adjustment provided in manufacturer's labeling; use with caution.

Dosage adjustment in hepatic impairment: No dosage adjustment provided in manufacturer's labeling; use with caution.

Mechanism of Action Binds to stereospecific benzodiazepine receptors on the postsynaptic GABA neuron at several sites within the central nervous system, including the limbic system, reticular formation. Enhancement of the inhibitory effect of GABA on neuronal excitability results by increased neuronal membrane permeability to chloride ions. This shift in chloride ions results in hyperpolarization (a less excitable state) and stabilization.

Contraindications Hypersensitivity to flurazepam or any component of the formulation (cross-sensitivity with other benzodiazepines may exist); narrow-angle glaucoma; pregnancy

Warnings/Precautions Use with caution in elderly or debilitated patients, patients with hepatic disease (including alcoholics), or renal impairment. Use with caution in patients with respiratory disease or impaired gag reflex. Avoid use in patients with sleep apnea.

Causes CNS depression (dose related); patients must be cautioned about performing tasks which require mental alertness (eg, operating machinery or driving). Use with caution in patients receiving other CNS depressants or psychoactive agents. Benzodiazepines have been associated with falls and traumatic injury and should be used with extreme caution in patients who are at risk of these events. In older adults, benzodiazepines increase the risk of impaired cognition, delirium, falls, fractures, and motor vehicle accidents. Due to increased sensitivity in this age group and slower metabolism of long-acting agents (such as flurazepam), avoid use for treatment of insomnia, agitation, or delirium (Beers Criteria).

Use caution in patients with depression, particularly if suicidal risk may be present. Use with caution in patients with a history of drug dependence. Benzodiazepines have been associated with dependence and acute withdrawal symptoms on discontinuation or reduction in dose (may occur after as little as 10 days of use).

As a hypnotic, should be used only after evaluation of potential causes of sleep disturbance. Failure of sleep disturbance to resolve after 7-10 days may indicate psychiatric or medical illness. A worsening of insomnia or the emergence of new abnormalities of thought or behavior may represent unrecognized psychiatric or medical illness and requires immediate and careful evaluation. Postmarketing studies have indicated that the use of hypnotic/sedative agents for sleep has been associated with hypersensitivity reactions including anaphylaxis as well as angioedema. An increased risk for hazardous sleep-related activities such as sleep-driving; cooking and eating food, and making phone calls while asleep have also been noted.

Benzodiazepines have been associated with anterograde amnesia. Paradoxical reactions have been reported, particularly in adolescent/pediatric or psychiatric patients. Does not have analgesic, antidepressant, or antipsychotic properties.

Drug Interactions

Metabolism/Transport Effects Substrate of CYP3A4 (major); **Note:** Assignment of Major/Minor substrate status based on clinically relevant drug interaction potential; **Inhibits** CYP2E1 (weak)

Avoid Concomitant Use

Avoid concomitant use of Flurazepam with any of the following: Azelastine (Nasal); Conivaptan; OLANZapine; Paraldehyde; Sodium Oxybate

Increased Effect/Toxicity

Flurazepam may increase the levels/effects of: Alcohol (Ethyl); Azelastine (Nasal); Buprenorphine; CloZAPine; CNS Depressants; Methotrimeprazine; Metyrosine; Mirtazapine; Paraldehyde; Phenytoin; Pramipexole; ROPINIRole; Rotigotine; Selective Serotonin Reuptake Inhibitors; Sodium Oxybate; Zolpidem

The levels/effects of Flurazepam may be increased by: Antifungal Agents (Azole Derivatives, Systemic); Aprepitant; Calcium Channel Blockers (Nondihydropyridine); Cimetidine; Conivaptan; Contraceptives (Estrogens); Contraceptives (Progestins); CYP3A4 Inhibitors (Moderate); CYP3A4 Inhibitors (Strong); Dasatinib; Droperidol; Fosamprenavir; Fosaprepitant; Grapefruit Juice; HydrOXYzine; Isoniazid; Ivacaftor; Macrolide Antibiotics; Magnesium Sulfate; Methotrimeprazine; Mifepristone; OLANZapine; Perampanel; Proton Pump Inhibitors; Ritonavir; Saquinavir; Selective Serotonin Reuptake Inhibitors

Decreased Effect

The levels/effects of Flurazepam may be decreased by: CarBAMazepine; CYP3A4 Inducers (Strong); Deferasirox; Rifamycin Derivatives; St Johns Wort; Theophylline Derivatives; Tocilizumab; Yohimbine

Ethanol/Nutrition/Herb Interactions

Ethanol: May increase CNS depression; monitor for increased effects with coadministration. Caution patients about effects.

Food: Serum levels and response to flurazepam may be increased by grapefruit juice, but unlikely because of flurazepam's high oral bioavailability.

Herb/Nutraceutical: Avoid valerian, St John's wort, kava kava, gotu kola (may increase CNS depression).

Pharmacodynamics/Kinetics

Onset of Action Hypnotic: 15-20 minutes; Peak effect: 3-6 hours

Duration of Action 7-8 hours

Half-life Elimination

Flurazepam: 2.3 hours

N-desalkylflurazepam:

Adults: Single dose: 74-90 hours; Multiple doses: 111-113 hours

Elderly (61-85 years): Single dose: 120-160 hours; Multiple doses: 126-158 hours

Time to Peak N-desalkylflurazepam: 10.6 hours (range: 7.6-13.6 hours); N-hydroxyethylflurazepam: ~1 hour

Pregnancy Considerations Although information specific to flurazepam has not been located, all benzodiazepines are assumed to cross the placenta. Teratogenic effects have been observed with some benzodiazepines; however, additional studies are needed. The incidence of premature birth and low birth weights may be increased following maternal use of benzodiazepines; hypoglycemia and respiratory problems in the neonate may occur following exposure late in pregnancy. Neonatal withdrawal symptoms may occur within days to weeks after birth and "floppy infant syndrome" (which also includes withdrawal symptoms) has been reported with some benzodiazepines. Neonatal depression has been observed, specifically following exposure to flurazepam when used maternally for 10 consecutive days prior to delivery. Serum levels of N-desalkylflurazepam were measurable in the infant during the first 4 days of life. Use of flurazepam during pregnancy is contraindicated.

Lactation Excretion in breast milk unknown

Breast-Feeding Considerations Drowsiness, lethargy, or weight loss in nursing infants have been observed in case reports following maternal use of some benzodiazepines.

Controlled Substance C-IV

Dosage Forms

Capsule, oral: 15 mg, 30 mg

Flurbiprofen (Systemic) (flure BI proe fen)

Related Information

Rheumatoid Arthritis, Osteoarthritis, and Osteoporosis *on page 1526*

Temporomandibular Dysfunction (TMD), Chronic Pain, and Fibromyalgia *on page 1590*

Brand Names: Canada Alti-Flurbiprofen; Ansaid®; Apo-Flurbiprofen®; Froben-SR®; Froben®; Novo-Flurprofen; Nu-Flurprofen

Generic Availability (U.S.) Yes

Pharmacologic Category Nonsteroidal Anti-inflammatory Drug (NSAID), Oral

Dental Use Management of postoperative pain

Use Treatment of rheumatoid arthritis and osteoarthritis

Unlabeled Use Management of postoperative pain

Local Anesthetic/Vasoconstrictor Precautions No information available to require special precautions

Effects on Dental Treatment The dentist should be aware of the potential of abnormal coagulation. Caution should also be exercised in the use of NSAIDs in patients already on anticoagulant therapy with drugs such as warfarin (Coumadin®). See Effects on Bleeding.

Effects on Bleeding Nonselective NSAIDs such as flurbiprofen inhibit platelet aggregation and prolong bleeding time in some patients. Unlike aspirin, the NSAID effect on platelet function is quantitatively less, of shorter duration, and reversible.

Adverse Effects >1%:

Cardiovascular: Edema

Central nervous system: Amnesia, anxiety, depression, dizziness, headache, insomnia, malaise, nervousness, somnolence, vertigo

Dermatologic: Rash

Gastrointestinal: Abdominal pain, constipation, diarrhea, dyspepsia, flatulence, GI bleeding, nausea, vomiting, weight changes

Hepatic: Liver enzymes increased

Neuromuscular & skeletal: Reflexes increased, tremor, weakness

Ocular: Vision changes

Otic: Tinnitus

Respiratory: Rhinitis

Dental Usual Dosage Management of postoperative pain: Adults: Oral: 100 mg every 12 hours

Dosage Oral:

Rheumatoid arthritis and osteoarthritis: 200-300 mg/day in 2, 3, or 4 divided doses; do not administer more than 100 mg for any single dose; maximum: 300 mg/day

Dental: Management of postoperative pain (unlabeled use): 100 mg every 12 hours

Dosage adjustment in renal impairment: Not recommended in patients with advanced renal disease.

Dosage adjustment in hepatic impairment: No dosage adjustment provided in manufacturer's labeling; patients with hepatic insufficiency may require reduced doses due to extensive hepatic metabolism.

Mechanism of Action Reversibly inhibits cyclooxygenase-1 and 2 (COX-1 and 2) enzymes, which results in decreased formation of prostaglandin precursors; has antipyretic, analgesic, and anti-inflammatory properties

Other proposed mechanisms not fully elucidated (and possibly contributing to the anti-inflammatory effect to varying degrees), include inhibiting chemotaxis, altering lymphocyte activity, inhibiting neutrophil aggregation/activation, and decreasing proinflammatory cytokine levels.

Contraindications Hypersensitivity to flurbiprofen, aspirin, other NSAIDs, or any component of the formulation; perioperative pain in the setting of coronary artery bypass (CABG) surgery

Warnings/Precautions [U.S. Boxed Warning]: NSAIDs are associated with an increased risk of adverse cardiovascular thrombotic events, including MI and stroke. Risk may be increased with duration of use or pre-existing cardiovascular risk factors or disease. Carefully evaluate individual cardiovascular risk profiles prior to prescribing. May cause new-onset hypertension or worsening of existing hypertension. Use caution with fluid retention. Avoid use in heart failure. Concurrent administration of ibuprofen, and potentially other nonselective NSAIDs, may interfere with aspirin's cardioprotective effect. **[U.S. Boxed Warning]: Use is contraindicated for treatment of perioperative pain in the setting of coronary artery bypass graft (CABG) surgery.** Risk of MI and stroke may be increased with use following CABG surgery.

Platelet adhesion and aggregation may be decreased; may prolong bleeding time; patients with coagulation disorders or who are receiving anticoagulants should be monitored closely. Anemia may occur; patients on long-term NSAID therapy should be monitored for anemia. NSAID use may compromise existing renal function; dose-dependent decreases in prostaglandin synthesis may result from NSAID use, reducing renal blood flow which may cause renal decompensation. Patients with impaired renal function, dehydration, heart failure, liver dysfunction, those taking diuretics, and ACE inhibitors, and the elderly are at greater risk of renal toxicity. Rehydrate patient before starting therapy; monitor renal function closely. Not recommended for use in patients with advanced renal disease. Long-term NSAID use may result in renal papillary necrosis.

[U.S. Boxed Warning]: NSAIDs may increase risk of gastrointestinal irritation, inflammation, ulceration, bleeding, and perforation. These events may occur at any time during therapy and without warning. Use caution with a history of GI disease (bleeding or ulcers), concurrent therapy with aspirin, anticoagulants and/or corticosteroids, smoking, use of alcohol, the elderly, or debilitated patients. When used concomitantly with

◄ ≤325 mg of aspirin, a substantial increase in the risk of gastrointestinal complications (eg, ulcer) occurs; concomitant gastroprotective therapy (eg, proton pump inhibitors) is recommended (Bhatt, 2008).

Use the lowest effective dose for the shortest duration of time, consistent with individual patient goals, to reduce risk of cardiovascular or GI adverse events. Alternate therapies should be considered for patients at high risk.

NSAIDs may cause serious skin adverse events including exfoliative dermatitis, Stevens-Johnson syndrome (SJS), and toxic epidermal necrolysis (TEN); discontinue use at first sign of skin rash or hypersensitivity. Anaphylactoid reactions may occur, even without prior exposure; patients with "aspirin triad" (bronchial asthma, aspirin intolerance, rhinitis) may be at increased risk. Do not use in patients who experience bronchospasm, asthma, rhinitis, or urticaria with NSAID or aspirin therapy. Use caution in other forms of asthma.

Use with caution in patients with decreased hepatic function. Closely monitor patients with any abnormal LFT. Severe hepatic reactions (eg, fulminant hepatitis, liver failure) have occurred with NSAID use, rarely; discontinue if signs or symptoms of liver disease develop, or if systemic manifestations occur.

The elderly are at increased risk for adverse effects (especially peptic ulceration, CNS effects, renal toxicity) from NSAIDs even at low doses.

Withhold for at least 4-6 half-lives prior to surgical or dental procedures. Safety and efficacy have not been established in children.

Drug Interactions

Metabolism/Transport Effects Substrate of CYP2C9 (minor); **Note:** Assignment of Major/Minor substrate status based on clinically relevant drug interaction potential; **Inhibits** CYP2C9 (weak)

Avoid Concomitant Use

Avoid concomitant use of Flurbiprofen (Systemic) with any of the following: Floctafenine; Ketorolac (Nasal); Ketorolac (Systemic); NSAID (COX-2 Inhibitor); Omacetaxine

Increased Effect/Toxicity

Flurbiprofen (Systemic) may increase the levels/effects of: Agents with Antiplatelet Properties; Aliskiren; Aminoglycosides; Anticoagulants; Bisphosphonate Derivatives; Collagenase (Systemic); CycloSPORINE (Systemic); Dabigatran Etexilate; Deferasirox; Desmopressin; Digoxin; Drotrecogin Alfa (Activated); Eplerenone; Haloperidol; Ibritumomab; Lithium; Methotrexate; Nonsteroidal Anti-Inflammatory Agents; NSAID (COX-2 Inhibitor); Omacetaxine; PEMEtrexed; Porfimer; Potassium-Sparing Diuretics; PRALAtrexate; Quinolone Antibiotics; Rivaroxaban; Salicylates; Thrombolytic Agents; Tositumomab and Iodine I 131 Tositumomab; Vancomycin; Vitamin K Antagonists

The levels/effects of Flurbiprofen (Systemic) may be increased by: ACE Inhibitors; Angiotensin II Receptor Blockers; Antidepressants (Tricyclic, Tertiary Amine); Corticosteroids (Systemic); CycloSPORINE (Systemic); Dasatinib; Floctafenine; Glucosamine; Herbs (Anticoagulant/Antiplatelet Properties); Ketorolac (Nasal); Ketorolac (Systemic); Multivitamins/Minerals (with ADEK, Folate, Iron); Nonsteroidal Anti-Inflammatory Agents; Omega-3 Fatty Acids; Pentosan Polysulfate Sodium; Pentoxifylline; Probenecid; Prostacyclin Analogues; Selective Serotonin Reuptake Inhibitors; Serotonin/Norepinephrine Reuptake Inhibitors; Sodium Phosphates; Tipranavir; Treprostinil; Vitamin E

Decreased Effect

Flurbiprofen (Systemic) may decrease the levels/effects of: ACE Inhibitors; Agents with Antiplatelet Properties; Aliskiren; Angiotensin II Receptor Blockers; Beta-Blockers; Eplerenone; HydrALAZINE; Loop Diuretics; Potassium-Sparing Diuretics; Salicylates; Selective Serotonin Reuptake Inhibitors; Thiazide Diuretics

The levels/effects of Flurbiprofen (Systemic) may be decreased by: Bile Acid Sequestrants; Nonsteroidal Anti-Inflammatory Agents; Salicylates

Ethanol/Nutrition/Herb Interactions

Ethanol: Avoid ethanol (may enhance gastric mucosal irritation).

Food: Food may decrease the rate but not the extent of absorption.

Herb/Nutraceutical: Avoid alfalfa, anise, bilberry, bladderwrack, bromelain, cat's claw, celery, chamomile, coleus, cordyceps, dong quai, evening primrose, fenugreek, feverfew, garlic, ginger, ginkgo biloba, ginseng (American, Panax, Siberian), grapeseed, green tea, guggul, horse chestnut seed, horseradish, licorice, prickly ash, red clover, reishi, SAMe (S-adenosylmethionine), sweet clover, turmeric, white willow (all have additional antiplatelet activity).

Dietary Considerations May be taken with food, milk, or antacid to decrease GI effects.

Pharmacodynamics/Kinetics

Onset of Action ~1-2 hours

Half-life Elimination 5.7 hours

Time to Peak 1.5 hours

Pregnancy Risk Factor C

Pregnancy Considerations Adverse events were not observed in the initial animal reproduction studies; therefore, the manufacturer classifies flurbiprofen as pregnancy category C. NSAID exposure during the first trimester is not strongly associated with congenital malformations; however, cardiovascular anomalies and cleft palate have been observed following NSAID exposure in some studies. The use of an NSAID close to conception may be associated with an increased risk of miscarriage. Nonteratogenic effects have been observed following NSAID administration during the third trimester including myocardial degenerative changes, prenatal constriction of the ductus arteriosus, fetal tricuspid regurgitation, failure of the ductus arteriosus to close postnatally; renal dysfunction or failure, oligohydramnios; gastrointestinal bleeding or perforation, increased risk of necrotizing enterocolitis; intracranial bleeding (including intraventricular hemorrhage), platelet dysfunction with resultant bleeding; pulmonary hypertension. Because they may cause premature closure of the ductus arteriosus, use of NSAIDs late in pregnancy should be avoided (use after 31 or 32 weeks gestation is not recommended by some clinicians). The chronic use of NSAIDs in women of reproductive age may be associated with infertility that is reversible upon discontinuation of the medication.

Lactation Enters breast milk/not recommended

Breast-Feeding Considerations Low levels of flurbiprofen are found in breast milk. Breast-feeding is not recommended by the manufacturer. The pharmacokinetics of flurbiprofen immediately postpartum are similar to healthy volunteers.

Dosage Forms

Tablet, oral: 50 mg, 100 mg

References

Bragger U, Muhle T, Fourmousis I, et al, "Effect of the NSAID Flurbiprofen on Remodeling After Periodontal Surgery," *J Periodontal Res*, 1997, 32(7):575-82.

Cooper SA and Kupperman A, "The Analgesic Efficacy of Flurbiprofen Compared to Acetaminophen With Codeine," *J Clin Dent*, 1991, 2 (3):70-4.

Dionne RA, "Suppression of Dental Pain by the Preoperative Administration of Flurbiprofen," *Am J Med*, 1986, 80(3A):41-9.

Dionne RA, Snyder J, and Hargreaves KM, "Analgesic Efficacy of Flurbiprofen in Comparison With Acetaminophen, Acetaminophen Plus Codeine, and Placebo After Impacted Third Molar Removal," *J Oral Maxillofac Surg*, 1994, 52(9):919-24.

Doroschak AM, Bowles WR, and Hargreaves KM, "Evaluation of the Combination of Flurbiprofen and Tramadol for Management of Endodontic Pain," *J Endod*, 1999, 25(10):660-3.

Jeffcoat MK, Reddy MS, Haigh S, et al, "A Comparison of Topical Ketorolac, Systemic Flurbiprofen, and Placebo for the Inhibition of Bone Loss in Adult Periodontitis," *J Periodontol*, 1995, 66(5):329-38.

Jeffcoat MK, Reddy MS, Wang IC, et al, "The Effect of Systemic Flurbiprofen on Bone Supporting Dental Implants," *J Am Dent Assoc*, 1995, 126(3):305-11.

Flutamide (FLOO ta mide)

Brand Names: Canada Apo-Flutamide®; Euflex®; Eulexin®; Novo-Flutamide; PMS-Flutamide; Teva-Flutamide

Pharmacologic Category Antineoplastic Agent, Antiandrogen

Use Treatment of metastatic prostatic carcinoma in combination therapy with LHRH agonist analogues

Unlabeled Use Female hirsutism

Local Anesthetic/Vasoconstrictor Precautions No information available to require special precautions

Effects on Dental Treatment No significant effects or complications reported

Effects on Bleeding Hemolytic anemia has been reported.

Adverse Effects

>10%:

Endocrine & metabolic: Gynecomastia, hot flashes, breast tenderness, galactorrhea (9% to 42%), impotence, libido decreased, tumor flare

Gastrointestinal: Nausea, vomiting (11% to 12%)

Hepatic: AST increased (transient; mild), LDH increased (transient; mild)

1% to 10%:

Cardiovascular: Hypertension (1%), edema

Central nervous system: Drowsiness, confusion, depression, anxiety, nervousness, headache, dizziness, insomnia

Dermatologic: Ecchymosis, photosensitivity, pruritus

Gastrointestinal: Anorexia, appetite increased, constipation, indigestion, upset stomach (4% to 6%); diarrhea

Hematologic: Anemia (6%), leukopenia (3%), thrombocytopenia (1%)

Neuromuscular & skeletal: Weakness (1%)

Miscellaneous: Herpes zoster

General Dosage Range Oral: *Adults:* 250 mg 3 times/day

Mechanism of Action Nonsteroidal antiandrogen that inhibits androgen uptake or inhibits binding of androgen in target tissues

Pharmacodynamics/Kinetics

Half-life Elimination 5-6 hours (2-hydroxyflutamide)

Pregnancy Risk Factor D

Pregnancy Considerations

Adverse events have been observed in animal reproduction studies. When used for the treatment of hirsutism, adequate contraception is recommended throughout therapy and for 3 months after therapy is complete (Falsetti, 2000).

Fluticasone (Oral Inhalation) (floo TIK a sone)

Related Information

Respiratory Diseases *on page 1514*

Brand Names: U.S. Flovent® Diskus®; Flovent® HFA

Brand Names: Canada Flovent® Diskus®; Flovent® HFA

Generic Availability (U.S.) No

Pharmacologic Category Corticosteroid, Inhalant (Oral)

Use Maintenance treatment of asthma as prophylactic therapy; also indicated for patients requiring oral corticosteroid therapy for asthma to assist in total discontinuation or reduction of total oral dose

Local Anesthetic/Vasoconstrictor Precautions No information available to require special precautions

Effects on Dental Treatment Localized infections with *Candida albicans* or *Aspergillus niger* have occurred frequently in the mouth and pharynx with repetitive use of oral inhaler of corticosteroids. These infections may require treatment with appropriate antifungal therapy or discontinuance of treatment with corticosteroid inhaler.

Effects on Bleeding No information available to require special precautions

Adverse Effects

>10%:

Central nervous system: Malaise/fatigue (16%), headache (2% to 14%)

Gastrointestinal: Oral candidiasis (≤31%)

Neuromuscular & skeletal: Arthralgia/articular rheumatism (17%), musculoskeletal pain (2% to 12%)

Respiratory: Sinusitis/sinus infection (≤33%), upper respiratory tract infection (≤31%), throat irritation (3% to 22%), nasal congestion/blockage (16%), rhinitis (≤13%)

1% to 10%:

Central nervous system: Pain (10%), fever (1% to 7%)

Dermatologic: Rash (8%), pruritus (6%)

Gastrointestinal: Nausea/vomiting (1% to 9%), gastrointestinal infection (including viral; 1% to 5%), gastrointestinal discomfort/pain (1% to 4%)

Neuromuscular & skeletal: Muscle injury (≤5%)

Respiratory: Hoarseness/dysphonia (2% to 9%), cough (1% to 9%), viral respiratory infection (1% to 9%), bronchitis (≤8%), upper respiratory tract inflammation (≤5%)

Miscellaneous: Viral infection (≤5%)

Dosage Inhalation, oral: Asthma: **Note:** Titrate to lowest effective dose once asthma stability achieved.

Flovent® HFA:

U.S. labeling:

Children 4-11 years: Initial: 88 mcg twice daily; maximum: 88 mcg twice daily

Children ≥12 years and Adults: Dosing based on previous asthma therapy: **Note:** May increase dose after 2 weeks of therapy in patients who are not adequately controlled.

Bronchodilator alone: Initial: 88 mcg twice daily; maximum: 440 mcg twice daily

Inhaled corticosteroids: Initial: 88-220 mcg twice daily (initial dose >88 mcg twice daily may be considered in patients previously requiring higher doses of inhaled corticosteroids); maximum: 440 mcg twice daily

Oral corticosteroids (OCS): Initial: 440 mcg twice daily; maximum: 880 mcg twice daily

NIH Asthma Guidelines (NIH, 2007) (administer in divided doses twice daily):
"Low" dose:
0-4 years: 176 mcg/day
5-11 years: 88-176 mcg/day
≥12 years: 88-264 mcg/day
"Medium" dose:
0-4 years: >176-352 mcg/day
5-11 years: >176-352 mcg/day
≥12 years: >264-440 mcg/day
"High" dose:
0-4 years: >352 mcg/day
5-11 years: >352 mcg/day
≥12 years: >440 mcg/day

Canadian labeling:
Children 1-3 years: 100 mcg twice daily
Children 4-15 years: 100 mcg twice daily. **Note:** Canadian labeling recommends Flovent® HFA be administered as a minimum of 2 inhalations twice daily; therefore, patients requiring lower or higher dosages than 100 mg twice daily should use Flovent® Diskus®.
Children ≥16 years and Adults: **Note:** May increase dose after ~1 week of therapy in patients who are not adequately controlled.
Mild asthma: 100-250 mcg twice daily
Moderate asthma: 250-500 mcg twice daily
Severe asthma: 500 mcg twice daily; may increase up to 1000 mcg twice daily in very severe patients (eg, patients using oral corticosteroids [OCS])

Flovent® Diskus®:
U.S. labeling:
Children 4-11 years: Initial: 50 mcg twice daily; may increase to maximum dose of 100 mcg twice daily in patients not adequately controlled after 2 weeks of therapy. Initial dose >50 mcg twice daily may be considered in patients with poorer asthma control or those previously requiring high ranges of inhaled corticosteroids
Children ≥12 years and Adults: **Note:** May increase dose after 2 weeks of therapy in patients who are not adequately controlled.
Dosing based on previous asthma therapy:
Bronchodilator alone: Initial: 100 mcg twice daily; maximum: 500 mcg twice daily
Inhaled corticosteroids: Initial: 100-250 mcg twice daily; maximum: 500 mcg twice daily; initial dose >100 mcg twice daily may be considered in patients with poorer asthma control or those previously requiring high ranges of inhaled corticosteroids
Oral corticosteroids (OCS): Initial: 500-1000 mcg twice daily; maximum: 1000 mcg twice daily
NIH Asthma Guidelines (NIH, 2007) (administer in divided doses twice daily):
"Low" dose:
5-11 years: 100-200 mcg/day
≥12 years: 100-300 mcg/day
"Medium" dose:
5-11 years: >200-400 mcg/day
≥12 years: >300-500 mcg/day
"High" dose:
5-11 years: >400 mcg/day
≥12 years: >500 mcg/day

Canadian labeling:
Children 4-16 years: Initial: 50-100 mcg twice daily; may increase up to 200 mcg twice daily after ~1 week of therapy in patients not adequately controlled

Children ≥16 years and Adults: **Note:** May increase dose after ~1 week of therapy in patients who are not adequately controlled.
Mild asthma: 100-250 mcg twice daily
Moderate asthma: 250-500 mcg twice daily
Severe asthma: 500 mcg twice daily; may increase up to 1000 mcg twice daily in very severe patients (eg, patients using oral corticosteroids [OCS])

Conversion from oral systemic corticosteroids to orally inhaled corticosteroids: When converting from oral corticosteroids (OCS) to orally inhaled corticosteroids, initiate oral inhalation therapy in patients whose asthma is previously stabilized on OCS. Gradual OCS dose reductions should begin ~7 days after starting inhaled therapy. U.S. labeling recommends reducing prednisone dose no more rapidly than 2.5-5 mg/day (or equivalent of other OCS) weekly in children ≥12 years but does not provide a recommendation for children <12 years. A similar approach to OCS dose reduction would however seem advisable. The Canadian labeling recommends decreasing the daily dose of prednisone by 1 mg (or equivalent of other OCS) no more rapidly than weekly (adults) or every 8 days (children) if closely monitored or every 10 days (adults) and 20 days (children) if not closely monitored. If adrenal insufficiency occurs, resume OCS therapy; initiate a more gradual withdrawal. When transitioning from systemic to inhaled corticosteroids, supplemental systemic corticosteroid therapy may be necessary during periods of stress or during severe asthma attacks.

Elderly: Refer to adult dosing.

Dosage adjustment in renal impairment: No dosage adjustment provided in manufacturer's labeling (has not been studied).

Dosage adjustment in hepatic impairment: No dosage adjustment provided in manufacturer's labeling (has not been studied); however, fluticasone is primarily cleared in the liver and plasma levels may be increased in patients with hepatic impairment. Use with caution; monitor.

Mechanism of Action Fluticasone belongs to a group of corticosteroids which utilizes a fluorocarbothioate ester linkage at the 17 carbon position; extremely potent vasoconstrictive and anti-inflammatory activity. The effectiveness of inhaled fluticasone is due to its direct local effect.

Contraindications Hypersensitivity to fluticasone or any component of the formulation; severe hypersensitivity to milk proteins or lactose (Flovent® Diskus®); primary treatment of status asthmaticus or other acute episodes of asthma requiring intensive measures

Canadian labeling: Additional contraindications (not in U.S. labeling): Moderate-to-severe bronchiectasis; untreated fungal, bacterial or tubercular infections of the respiratory tract

Warnings/Precautions May cause hypercorticism or suppression of hypothalamic-pituitary-adrenal (HPA) axis, particularly in younger children or in patients receiving high doses for prolonged periods. HPA axis suppression may lead to adrenal crisis. Withdrawal and discontinuation of a corticosteroid should be done slowly and carefully. Particular care is required when patients are transferred from systemic corticosteroids to inhaled products due to possible adrenal insufficiency or withdrawal from steroids, including an increase in allergic symptoms. Patients receiving ≥20 mg per day of prednisone (or equivalent) may be most susceptible. Fatalities have occurred due to adrenal insufficiency in asthmatic patients during and after transfer from systemic corticosteroids to aerosol steroids; aerosol steroids do **not** provide the systemic steroid needed to treat patients having trauma, surgery, or infections.

Bronchospasm may occur with wheezing after inhalation; if this occurs, stop steroid and treat with a fast-acting bronchodilator. Supplemental steroids (oral or parenteral) may be needed during stress or severe asthma attacks. Corticosteroid use may cause psychiatric disturbances, including depression, euphoria, insomnia, mood swings, and personality changes. Pre-existing psychiatric conditions may be exacerbated by corticosteroid use. Prolonged use of corticosteroids may also increase the incidence of secondary infection, mask acute infection (including fungal infections), prolong or exacerbate viral infections, or limit response to vaccines. Avoid use in patients with ocular herpes or untreated viral, fungal, parasitic or bacterial systemic infections (Canadian labeling contraindicates use with untreated respiratory infections). Exposure to chickenpox should be avoided. Close observation is required in patients with latent tuberculosis and/or TB reactivity; restrict use in active TB (only in conjunction with anti-tuberculosis treatment). Rare cases of vasculitis (Churg-Strauss syndrome) or other eosinophilic conditions can occur. Prolonged treatment with corticosteroids has been associated with the development of Kaposi's sarcoma (case reports); if noted, discontinuation of therapy should be considered.

Use with caution in patients with thyroid disease, hepatic impairment, renal impairment, cardiovascular disease, diabetes, glaucoma, cataracts, myasthenia gravis, patients at risk for osteoporosis, patients at risk for seizures, or GI diseases (diverticulitis, peptic ulcer, ulcerative colitis) due to perforation risk. Use caution following acute MI (corticosteroids have been associated with myocardial rupture). Because of the risk of adverse effects, systemic corticosteroids should be used cautiously in the elderly in the smallest possible effective dose for the shortest duration.

Orally-inhaled corticosteroids may cause a reduction in growth velocity in pediatric patients (~1 centimeter per year [range: 0.3-1.8 cm per year] and related to dose and duration of exposure). To minimize the systemic effects of orally-inhaled corticosteroids, each patient should be titrated to the lowest effective dose. Growth should be routinely monitored in pediatric patients.

Use with strong CYP3A4 inhibitors is not recommended (see Drug Interactions). Not to be used in status asthmaticus or for the relief of acute bronchospasm. Flovent® Diskus® contains lactose; very rare anaphylactic reactions have been reported in patients with severe milk protein allergy. There have been reports of systemic corticosteroid withdrawal symptoms (eg, joint/muscle pain, lassitude, depression) when withdrawing oral inhalation therapy. Local yeast infections (eg, oral pharyngeal candidiasis) may occur.

Drug Interactions

Metabolism/Transport Effects Substrate of CYP3A4 (major); **Note:** Assignment of Major/Minor substrate status based on clinically relevant drug interaction potential

Avoid Concomitant Use

Avoid concomitant use of Fluticasone (Oral Inhalation) with any of the following: Aldesleukin; BCG; Cobicistat; CYP3A4 Inhibitors (Strong); Natalizumab; Pimecrolimus; Tacrolimus (Topical); Tofacitinib

Increased Effect/Toxicity

Fluticasone (Oral Inhalation) may increase the levels/effects of: Amphotericin B; Deferasirox; Leflunomide; Loop Diuretics; Natalizumab; Thiazide Diuretics; Tofacitinib

The levels/effects of Fluticasone (Oral Inhalation) may be increased by: Cobicistat; CYP3A4 Inhibitors (Moderate); CYP3A4 Inhibitors (Strong); Dasatinib; Denosumab; Ivacaftor; Mifepristone; Pimecrolimus; Tacrolimus (Topical); Telaprevir; Trastuzumab

Decreased Effect

Fluticasone (Oral Inhalation) may decrease the levels/effects of: Aldesleukin; Antidiabetic Agents; BCG; Coccidioidin Skin Test; Corticorelin; Hyaluronidase; Sipuleucel-T; Telaprevir; Vaccines (Inactivated)

The levels/effects of Fluticasone (Oral Inhalation) may be decreased by: Echinacea

Ethanol/Nutrition/Herb Interactions Herb/Nutraceutical: In theory, St John's wort may decrease serum levels of fluticasone by inducing CYP3A4 isoenzymes.

Dietary Considerations Flovent® Diskus® contains lactose; very rare anaphylactic reactions have been reported in patients with severe milk protein allergy.

Pharmacodynamics/Kinetics

Onset of Action Maximal benefit may take 1-2 weeks or longer

Half-life Elimination ~11-12 hours (Thorsson, 2001)

Pregnancy Risk Factor C

Pregnancy Considerations Adverse events have been observed with systemic corticosteroids in animal reproduction studies. A decrease in fetal growth has not been observed with inhaled corticosteroid use during pregnancy. Inhaled corticosteroids are recommended for the treatment of asthma (most information available using budesonide) during pregnancy.

Lactation Excretion in breast milk unknown/use caution

Breast-Feeding Considerations Systemic corticosteroids are excreted in human milk. It is not known if sufficient quantities of fluticasone are absorbed following inhalation to produce detectable amounts in breast milk. The use of inhaled corticosteroids is not considered a contraindication to breast feeding.

Dosage Forms

Aerosol, for oral inhalation:
Flovent® HFA: 44 mcg/inhalation (10.6 g); 110 mcg/inhalation (12 g); 220 mcg/inhalation (12 g)

Powder, for oral inhalation:
Flovent® Diskus®: 50 mcg (60s); 100 mcg (60s); 250 mcg (60s)

Dosage Forms: Canada

Aerosol, for oral inhalation:
Flovent® HFA: 50 mcg/inhalation (120 actuations); 125 mcg/inhalation (60 or 120 actuations); 250 mcg/inhalation (60 or 120 actuations)

Powder, for oral inhalation
Flovent® Diskus®: 50 mcg (60s); 100 mcg (60s); 250 mcg (60s); 500 mcg (60s)

Fluticasone (Nasal) (floo TIK a sone)

Brand Names: U.S. Flonase®; Veramyst®

Brand Names: Canada Apo-Fluticasone®; Avamys®; Flonase®; ratio-Fluticasone

Pharmacologic Category Corticosteroid, Nasal

Use

Flonase®: Management of seasonal and perennial allergic rhinitis and nonallergic rhinitis

Veramyst®, Avamys® [CAN]: Management of seasonal and perennial allergic rhinitis

Unlabeled Use Adjunct to antibiotics in empiric treatment of acute bacterial rhinosinusitis (ABRS) (Chow, 2012)

Local Anesthetic/Vasoconstrictor Precautions No information available to require special precautions

Effects on Dental Treatment No significant effects or complications reported

Effects on Bleeding No information available to require special precautions

Adverse Effects

>10%: Central nervous system: Headache (7% to 16%)

1% to 10%:

Central nervous system: Dizziness (1% to 3%), fever (1% to 5%)

Gastrointestinal: Nausea/vomiting (3% to 5%), abdominal pain (1% to 3%), diarrhea (1% to 3%)

Neuromuscular & skeletal: Back pain (1%)

Respiratory: Pharyngitis (6% to 8%), epistaxis (4% to 7%), asthma symptoms (3% to 7%), cough (3% to 4%), pharyngolaryngeal pain (2% to 4%), blood in nasal mucous (1% to 3%), bronchitis (1% to 3%), runny nose (1% to 3%), nasal ulcer (1%)

Miscellaneous: Aches and pains (1% to 3%), flu-like syndrome (1% to 3%)

General Dosage Range Intranasal:

Propionate (Flonase®):

Children ≥4 years: Initial: 1 spray (50 mcg/spray) per nostril once daily (100 mcg/day); Maintenance: 1-2 sprays per nostril once daily (100-200 mcg/day); (maximum: 2 sprays in each nostril [200 mcg]/day)

Adults: Initial: 2 sprays (50 mcg/spray) per nostril once daily (200 mcg/day); Maintenance: 1-2 sprays per nostril once daily (100-200 mcg/day)

Furoate (Veramyst®):

Children 2-11 years: Initial: 1 spray (27.5 mcg/spray) per nostril once daily (55 mcg/day); Maintenance 1-2 sprays per nostril once daily (55-110 mcg/day) (maximum: 2 sprays in each nostril [110 mcg]/day)

Children ≥12 years and Adults: Initial: 2 sprays (27.5 mcg/spray) per nostril once (110 mcg/day); Maintenance 1-2 sprays per nostril once daily (55-110 mcg/day) (maximum: 2 sprays in each nostril [110 mcg]/day)

Mechanism of Action Fluticasone belongs to a group of corticosteroids which utilizes a fluorocarbothioate ester linkage at the 17 carbon position; extremely potent vasoconstrictive and anti-inflammatory activity

Pharmacodynamics/Kinetics

Onset of Action Maximal benefit may take several days

Pregnancy Risk Factor C

Pregnancy Considerations Adverse events have been observed with systemic corticosteroids in animal reproduction studies; teratogenic effects were not observed following administration of fluticasone furoate via inhalation to pregnant rats or rabbits. A decrease in fetal growth has not been observed with inhaled corticosteroid use during pregnancy. Inhaled corticosteroids are recommended for the treatment of allergic rhinitis during pregnancy.

Fluticasone and Salmeterol

(floo TIK a sone & sal ME te role)

Related Information

Fluticasone (Oral Inhalation) on page 617

Salmeterol on page 1221

Brand Names: U.S. Advair Diskus®; Advair® HFA

Brand Names: Canada Advair Diskus®; Advair®

Generic Availability (U.S.) No

Pharmacologic Category Beta$_2$ Agonist; Beta$_2$-Adrenergic Agonist, Long-Acting; Corticosteroid, Inhalant (Oral)

Use Maintenance treatment of asthma; maintenance treatment of COPD

Local Anesthetic/Vasoconstrictor Precautions No information available to require special precautions

Effects on Dental Treatment Localized infections with Candida albicans or Aspergillus niger have occurred frequently in the mouth and pharynx with repetitive use of oral inhaler of corticosteroids. These infections may require treatment with appropriate antifungal therapy or discontinuance of treatment with corticosteroid inhaler.

Effects on Bleeding No information available to require special precautions

Adverse Effects Percentages reported in patients with asthma; also see individual agents:

>10%:

Central nervous system: Headache (12% to 21%)

Respiratory: Upper respiratory tract infection (16% to 27%), pharyngitis (9% to 13%)

>3% to 10%:

Central nervous system: Dizziness (1% to 4%)

Endocrine & metabolic: Menstruation symptoms (3% to 5%)

Gastrointestinal: Nausea/vomiting (3% to 6%), diarrhea (2% to 4%), pain/discomfort (1% to 4%), oral candidiasis (1% to 4%), gastrointestinal infections (including viral, ≤4%)

Neuromuscular & skeletal: Musculoskeletal pain (2% to 7%), muscle pain (≤4%)

Respiratory: Throat irritation (7% to 9%), bronchitis (2% to 8%), upper respiratory tract inflammation (4% to 7%), lower respiratory tract infections/pneumonia (1% to 7%; COPD diagnosis and age >65 years increase risk), cough (3% to 6%), sinusitis (4% to 5%), hoarseness/dysphonia (1% to 5%), viral respiratory tract infection (3% to 5%)

1% to 3%:

Cardiovascular: Arrhythmia, chest symptoms, fluid retention, MI, palpitation, syncope, tachycardia

Central nervous system: Compressed nerve syndromes, hypnagogic effects, migraine, pain, sleep disorders, tremor

Dermatologic: Dermatitis, dermatosis, eczema, hives, skin flakiness, urticaria, viral skin infection

Endocrine & metabolic: Hypothyroidism

Gastrointestinal: Constipation, dental discomfort/pain, gastrointestinal infection, hemorrhoids, oral discomfort/pain, oral erythema/rash, oral ulcerations, unusual taste, weight gain

Genitourinary: Urinary tract infection

Hematologic: Contusions/hematomas

Hepatic: Abnormal liver function tests

Neuromuscular & skeletal: Arthralgia, articular rheumatism, bone/cartilage disorders, bone pain, cramps, fractures, muscle injuries (≤3%), muscle spasm, muscle stiffness, tightness/rigidity

Ocular: Conjunctivitis, edema, eye redness, keratitis, xerophthalmia

Respiratory: Blood in nasal mucosa, congestion, ear/nose/throat infection, epistaxis, laryngitis, lower respiratory hemorrhage, nasal irritation, rhinitis, rhinorrhea/postnasal drip, sneezing

Miscellaneous: Allergies/allergic reactions, bacterial infection, burns, candidiasis (≤3%), diaphoresis, sweat/sebum disorders, viral infection, wounds and lacerations

Dosage Oral inhalation: **Note:** Do not use to transfer patients from systemic corticosteroid therapy.

COPD: Adults:

Advair Diskus®: Fluticasone 250 mcg/salmeterol 50 mcg twice daily, 12 hours apart. **Note:** This is the maximum dose.

Advair Diskus® [Canadian labeling; not in approved U.S. labeling]: Fluticasone 250 mcg/salmeterol 50 mcg **or** fluticasone 500 mcg/salmeterol 50 mcg twice daily, 12 hours apart.

Maximum dose: Fluticasone 500 mcg/salmeterol 50 mcg per inhalation (2 inhalations/day)

Asthma:

Children 4-11 years: Advair Diskus®: Fluticasone 100 mcg/salmeterol 50 mcg twice daily, 12 hours apart. **Note:** This is the maximum dose.

Children ≥12 years and Adults:

Advair Diskus®: One inhalation twice daily, morning and evening, 12 hours apart

Maximum dose: Fluticasone 500 mcg/salmeterol 50 mcg per inhalation (2 inhalations/day)

Advair® HFA: Two inhalations twice daily, morning and evening, 12 hours apart

Maximum dose: Fluticasone 230 mcg/salmeterol 21 mcg per inhalation (4 inhalations/day)

Advair® 125 or Advair® 250 [Canadian labeling; not in approved U.S. labeling]: Two inhalations twice daily, morning and evening, 12 hours apart

Maximum dose: Fluticasone 250 mcg/salmeterol 25 mcg per inhalation (4 inhalations/day)

Note: Initial dose prescribed should be based upon previous dose of inhaled-steroid asthma therapy. Dose should be increased after 2 weeks if adequate response is not achieved. Patients should be titrated to lowest effective dose once stable. Each suggestion below specifies the product strength to use; remember to **use 1 inhalation for Diskus® and 2 inhalations for HFA.**

Patients not currently on inhaled corticosteroids:

Advair Diskus®: Fluticasone 100 mcg/salmeterol 50 mcg **or** fluticasone 250 mcg/salmeterol 50 mcg

Advair® HFA: Fluticasone 45 mcg/salmeterol 21 mcg **or** fluticasone 115 mcg/salmeterol 21 mcg

Patients currently using inhaled beclomethasone dipropionate:

≤160 mcg/day: Fluticasone 100 mcg/salmeterol 50 mcg **or** Advair® HFA: Fluticasone 45 mcg/salmeterol 21 mcg

320 mcg/day: Fluticasone 250 mcg/salmeterol 50 mcg **or** Advair® HFA: Fluticasone 115 mcg/salmeterol 21 mcg

640 mcg/day: Fluticasone 500 mcg/salmeterol 50 mcg **or** Advair® HFA: Fluticasone 230 mcg/salmeterol 21 mcg

Patients currently using inhaled budesonide:

≤400 mcg/day: Fluticasone 100 mcg/salmeterol 50 mcg **or** Advair® HFA: Fluticasone 45 mcg/salmeterol 21 mcg

800-1200 mcg/day: Fluticasone 250 mcg/salmeterol 50 mcg **or** Advair® HFA: Fluticasone 115 mcg/salmeterol 21 mcg

1600 mcg/day: Fluticasone 500 mcg/salmeterol 50 mcg **or** Advair® HFA: Fluticasone 230 mcg/salmeterol 21 mcg

Patients currently using inhaled flunisolide CFC aerosol:

≤1000 mcg/day: Fluticasone 100 mcg/salmeterol 50 mcg **or** Advair® HFA: Fluticasone 45 mcg/salmeterol 21 mcg

1250-2000 mcg/day: Fluticasone 250 mcg/salmeterol 50 mcg **or** Advair® HFA: Fluticasone 115 mcg/salmeterol 21 mcg

Patients currently using inhaled flunisolide HFA inhalation aerosol:

≤320 mcg/day: Fluticasone 100 mcg/salmeterol 50 mcg **or** Advair® HFA: Fluticasone 45 mcg/salmeterol 21 mcg

640 mcg/day: Fluticasone 250 mcg/salmeterol 50 mcg **or** Advair® HFA: Fluticasone 115 mcg/salmeterol 21 mcg

Patients currently using inhaled fluticasone HFA aerosol:

≤176 mcg/day: Fluticasone 100 mcg/salmeterol 50 mcg **or** Advair® HFA: Fluticasone 45 mcg/salmeterol 21 mcg

440 mcg/day: Fluticasone 250 mcg/salmeterol 50 mcg **or** Advair® HFA: Fluticasone 115 mcg/salmeterol 21 mcg

660-880 mcg/day: Fluticasone 500 mcg/salmeterol 50 mcg **or** Advair® HFA: Fluticasone 230 mcg/salmeterol 21 mcg

Patients currently using inhaled fluticasone propionate powder:

≤200 mcg/day: Fluticasone 100 mcg/salmeterol 50 mcg **or** Advair® HFA: Fluticasone 45 mcg/salmeterol 21 mcg

500 mcg/day: Fluticasone 250 mcg/salmeterol 50 mcg **or** Advair® HFA: Fluticasone 115 mcg/salmeterol 21 mcg

1000 mcg/day: Fluticasone 500 mcg/salmeterol 50 mcg **or** Advair® HFA: Fluticasone 230 mcg/salmeterol 21 mcg

Patients currently using inhaled mometasone furoate powder:

220 mcg/day: Fluticasone 100 mcg/salmeterol 50 mcg **or** Advair® HFA: Fluticasone 45 mcg/salmeterol 21 mcg

440 mcg/day: Fluticasone 250 mcg/salmeterol 50 mcg **or** Advair® HFA: Fluticasone 115 mcg/salmeterol 21 mcg

880 mcg/day: Fluticasone 500 mcg/salmeterol 50 mcg **or** Advair® HFA: Fluticasone 230 mcg/salmeterol 21 mcg

Patients currently using inhaled triamcinolone acetonide:

≤1000 mcg/day: Fluticasone 100 mcg/salmeterol 50 mcg **or** Advair® HFA: Fluticasone 45 mcg/salmeterol 21 mcg

1100-1600 mcg/day: Fluticasone 250 mcg/salmeterol 50 mcg **or** Advair® HFA: Fluticasone 115 mcg/salmeterol 21 mcg

Elderly: No differences in safety or effectiveness have been seen in studies of patients ≥65 years of age. However, increased sensitivity may be seen in the elderly. Use with caution in patients with concomitant cardiovascular disease.

▶

Dosage adjustment in renal impairment: No dosage adjustment provided in manufacturer's labeling (has not been studied). However, fluticasone and salmeterol are predominately eliminated by hepatic metabolism.

Dosage adjustment in hepatic impairment: No dosage adjustment required; manufacturer suggests close monitoring of patients with hepatic impairment.

Mechanism of Action Combination of fluticasone (corticosteroid) and salmeterol (long-acting beta₂-agonist) designed to improve pulmonary function and control over what is produced by either agent when used alone. Because fluticasone and salmeterol act locally in the lung, plasma levels do not predict therapeutic effect.

Fluticasone: The mechanism of action for all topical corticosteroids is believed to be a combination of three important properties: Anti-inflammatory activity, immunosuppressive properties, and antiproliferative actions. Fluticasone has extremely potent vasoconstrictive and anti-inflammatory activity.

Salmeterol: Relaxes bronchial smooth muscle by selective action on beta₂-receptors with little effect on heart rate

Contraindications Hypersensitivity to fluticasone, salmeterol, or any component of the formulation; status asthmaticus; acute episodes of asthma or COPD; severe hypersensitivity to milk proteins (Advair Diskus®)

Warnings/Precautions See individual agents.

Drug Interactions

Metabolism/Transport Effects Refer to individual components.

Avoid Concomitant Use

Avoid concomitant use of Fluticasone and Salmeterol with any of the following: Aldesleukin; BCG; Cobicistat; CYP3A4 Inhibitors (Strong); Natalizumab; Pimecrolimus; Tacrolimus (Topical); Tofacitinib

Increased Effect/Toxicity

Fluticasone and Salmeterol may increase the levels/effects of: Amphotericin B; Deferasirox; Leflunomide; Loop Diuretics; Natalizumab; Thiazide Diuretics; Tofacitinib

The levels/effects of Fluticasone and Salmeterol may be increased by: Cobicistat; CYP3A4 Inhibitors (Moderate); CYP3A4 Inhibitors (Strong); Dasatinib; Denosumab; Ivacaftor; Mifepristone; Pimecrolimus; Tacrolimus (Topical); Telaprevir; Trastuzumab

Decreased Effect

Fluticasone and Salmeterol may decrease the levels/effects of: Aldesleukin; Antidiabetic Agents; BCG; Coccidioidin Skin Test; Corticorelin; Hyaluronidase; Sipuleucel-T; Telaprevir; Vaccines (Inactivated)

The levels/effects of Fluticasone and Salmeterol may be decreased by: Echinacea

Dietary Considerations Advair Diskus® powder for oral inhalation contains lactose; very rare anaphylactic reactions have been reported in patients with severe milk protein allergy.

Pregnancy Risk Factor C

Pregnancy Considerations See individual agents.

Lactation

Fluticasone: Excretion in breast milk unknown/use caution

Salmeterol: Enters breast milk/use caution

Dosage Forms

Aerosol, for oral inhalation:

Advair® HFA:

45/21: Fluticasone propionate 45 mcg and salmeterol 21 mcg (8 g, 12 g) [chlorofluorocarbon free]

115/21: Fluticasone propionate 115 mcg and salmeterol 21 mcg (8 g, 12 g) [chlorofluorocarbon free]

230/21: Fluticasone propionate 230 mcg and salmeterol 21 mcg (8 g, 12 g) [chlorofluorocarbon free]

Powder, for oral inhalation:

Advair Diskus®:

100/50: Fluticasone propionate 100 mcg and salmeterol 50 mcg (14s, 60s)

250/50: Fluticasone propionate 250 mcg and salmeterol 50 mcg (60s)

500/50: Fluticasone propionate 500 mcg and salmeterol 50 mcg (60s)

Dosage Forms: Canada

Aerosol, for oral inhalation:

Advair®: 125/25: Fluticasone propionate 125 mcg and salmeterol 25 mcg (12 g); 250/25: Fluticasone propionate 250 mcg and salmeterol 25 mcg (12 g)

Fluvastatin (FLOO va sta tin)

Related Information

Cardiovascular Diseases *on page 1492*

Brand Names: U.S. Lescol®; Lescol® XL

Brand Names: Canada Lescol®; Lescol® XL; Teva-Fluvastatin

Pharmacologic Category Antilipemic Agent, HMG-CoA Reductase Inhibitor

Use To be used as a component of multiple risk factor intervention in patients at risk for atherosclerosis vascular disease due to hypercholesterolemia

Adjunct to dietary therapy to reduce elevated total cholesterol (total-C), LDL-C, triglyceride, and apolipoprotein B (apo-B) levels and to increase HDL-C in primary hypercholesterolemia and mixed dyslipidemia (Fredrickson types IIa and IIb); to slow the progression of coronary atherosclerosis in patients with coronary heart disease; reduce risk of coronary revascularization procedures in patients with coronary heart disease

Local Anesthetic/Vasoconstrictor Precautions No information available to require special precautions

Effects on Dental Treatment No significant effects or complications reported

Effects on Bleeding No information available to require special precautions

Adverse Effects As reported with fluvastatin capsules; in general, adverse reactions reported with fluvastatin extended release tablet were similar, but the incidence was less.

1% to 10%:

Central nervous system: Headache (9%), fatigue (3%), insomnia (3%)

Gastrointestinal: Dyspepsia (8%), diarrhea (5%), abdominal pain (5%), nausea (3%)

Genitourinary: Urinary tract infection (2%)

Neuromuscular & skeletal: Myalgia (5%)

Respiratory: Sinusitis (3%), bronchitis (2%)

General Dosage Range Oral:

Extended release: *Adolescents 10-16 years (females 1 year postmenarche) and Adults:* 80 mg once daily

Immediate release:
Adolescents 10-16 years (females 1 year postmenarche): Initial: 20 mg once daily; Maintenance: Up to 80 mg/day in 2 divided doses
Adults: Initial: 20-40 mg once daily; Maintenance: Up to 80 mg/day in 2 divided doses

Mechanism of Action Acts by competitively inhibiting 3-hydroxy-3-methylglutaryl-coenzyme A (HMG-CoA) reductase, the enzyme that catalyzes the reduction of HMG-CoA to mevalonate; this is an early rate-limiting step in cholesterol biosynthesis. HDL is increased while total, LDL, and VLDL cholesterols; apolipoprotein B; and plasma triglycerides are decreased.

Pharmacodynamics/Kinetics

Onset of Action Peak effect: Maximal LDL-C reductions achieved within 4 weeks

Half-life Elimination Capsule: <3 hours; Extended release tablet: 9 hours

Time to Peak Capsule: 1 hour; Extended release tablet: 3 hours

Pregnancy Risk Factor X

Pregnancy Considerations Adverse events were not observed in animal reproduction studies. There are reports of congenital anomalies following maternal use of HMG-CoA reductase inhibitors in pregnancy; however, maternal disease, differences in specific agents used, and the low rates of exposure limit the interpretation of the available data (Godfrey, 2012; Lecarpentier, 2012). Cholesterol biosynthesis may be important in fetal development; serum cholesterol and triglycerides increase normally during pregnancy. The discontinuation of lipid lowering medications temporarily during pregnancy is not expected to have significant impact on the long term outcomes of primary hypercholesterolemia treatment.

Use of fluvastatin is contraindicated in pregnancy. HMG-CoA reductase inhibitors should be discontinued prior to pregnancy (ADA, 2013). If treatment of dyslipidemias is needed in pregnant women or in women of reproductive age, other agents are preferred (Berglund, 2012; NCEP, 2002). The manufacturer recommends administration to women of childbearing potential only when conception is highly unlikely and patients have been informed of potential hazards.

FluvoxaMINE (floo VOKS a meen)

Related Information
Management of the Patient With Anxiety or Depression *on page 1594*
Vasoconstrictor Interactions With Antidepressants *on page 1650*

Brand Names: U.S. Luvox® CR
Brand Names: Canada Alti-Fluvoxamine; Apo-Fluvoxamine®; Luvox®; Novo-Fluvoxamine; Nu-Fluvoxamine; PMS-Fluvoxamine; Rhoxal-fluvoxamine; Riva-Fluvox; Sandoz-Fluvoxamine

Generic Availability (U.S.) Yes
Pharmacologic Category Antidepressant, Selective Serotonin Reuptake Inhibitor
Use Treatment of obsessive-compulsive disorder (OCD)
Unlabeled Use Treatment of major depression; panic disorder; anxiety disorders in children; treatment of mild dementia-associated agitation in nonpsychotic patients; post-traumatic stress disorder (PTSD); social anxiety disorder (SAD); patients; treatment of paraphilia/hypersexuality

---

Local Anesthetic/Vasoconstrictor Precautions
Although caution should be used in patients taking tricyclic antidepressants, no interactions have been reported with vasoconstrictors and fluvoxamine, a non-tricyclic antidepressant which acts to increase serotonin; no precautions appear to be needed

Effects on Dental Treatment Key adverse event(s) related to dental treatment: Xerostomia (normal salivary flow resumes upon discontinuation) and abnormal taste. Problems with SSRI-induced bruxism have been reported and may preclude their use; clinicians attempting to evaluate any patient with bruxism or involuntary muscle movement, who is simultaneously being treated with an SSRI drug, should be aware of the potential association. See Effects on Bleeding and Dental Comment.

Effects on Bleeding Selective serotonin reuptake inhibitors such as fluvoxamine may impair platelet aggregation due to platelet serotonin depletion, possibly increasing the risk of a bleeding complication. The risk of a bleeding complication can be increased by coadministration of other antiplatelet agents such as NSAIDs and aspirin.

Adverse Effects Frequency varies by dosage form and indication. Adverse reactions reported as a composite of all indications.
>10%:
Central nervous system: Headache (22% to 35%), insomnia (21% to 35%), somnolence (22% to 27%), dizziness (11% to 15%), nervousness (10% to 12%)
Gastrointestinal: Nausea (34% to 40%), diarrhea (11% to 18%), xerostomia (10% to 14%), anorexia (6% to 14%)
Genitourinary: Ejaculation abnormal (8% to 11%)
Neuromuscular & skeletal: Weakness (14% to 26%)
1% to 10%:
Cardiovascular: Chest pain (3%), palpitation (3%), vasodilation (2% to 3%), hypertension (1% to 2%), edema (≤1%), hypotension (≤1%), syncope (≤1%), tachycardia (≤1%)
Central nervous system: Pain (10%), anxiety (5% to 8%), abnormal dreams (3%), abnormal thinking (3%), agitation (2% to 3%), apathy (≥1% to 3%), chills (2%), CNS stimulation (2%), depression (2%), neurosis (2%), amnesia, malaise, manic reaction, psychotic reaction
Dermatologic: Bruising (4%), acne (2%)
Endocrine & metabolic: Libido decreased (2% to 10%; incidence higher in males), anorgasmia (2% to 5%), sexual function abnormal (2% to 4%), menorrhagia (2%)
Gastrointestinal: Dyspepsia (8% to 10%), constipation (4% to 10%), vomiting (4% to 6%), abdominal pain (5%), flatulence (4%), taste perversion (2% to 3%), toothache and dental caries (2% to 3%), dysphagia (2%), gingivitis (2%), weight loss (≤1% to 2%), weight gain
Genitourinary: Polyuria (2% to 3%), impotence (2%), urinary tract infection (2%), urinary retention (1%)
Hepatic: Liver function tests abnormal (≥1% to 2%)
Neuromuscular & skeletal: Tremor (5% to 8%), myalgia (5%), paresthesia (3%), hypertonia (2%), twitching (2%), hyper-/hypokinesia, myoclonus
Ocular: Amblyopia (2% to 3%)
Respiratory: Upper respiratory infection (9%), pharyngitis (6%), yawn (2% to 5%), laryngitis (3%), bronchitis (2%), dyspnea (2%), epistaxis (2%), cough increased, sinusitis
Miscellaneous: Diaphoresis (6% to 7%), flu-like syndrome (3%), viral infection (2%)

◄ **Dosage** Oral:

Obsessive-compulsive disorder:

Children 8-17 years: Immediate release: Initial: 25 mg once daily at bedtime; may be increased in 25 mg increments at 4- to 7-day intervals, as tolerated, to maximum therapeutic benefit; usual dose range: 50-200 mg/day. **Note:** When total daily dose exceeds 50 mg, the dose should be given in 2 divided doses with larger portion administered at bedtime.

Maximum: Children: 8-11 years: 200 mg/day, adolescents: 300 mg/day; lower doses may be effective in female versus male patients

Adults:

Immediate release: Initial: 50 mg once daily at bedtime; may be increased in 50 mg increments at 4- to 7-day intervals, as tolerated; usual dose range: 100-300 mg/day; maximum dose: 300 mg/day. **Note:** When total daily dose exceeds 100 mg, the dose should be given in 2 divided doses with larger portion administered at bedtime.

Extended release: Initial: 100 mg once daily at bedtime; may be increased in 50 mg increments at intervals of at least 1 week; usual dosage range: 100-300 mg/day; maximum dose: 300 mg/day

Social anxiety disorder (unlabeled use): Adults: Extended release: Initial: 100 mg once daily at bedtime; may be increased in 50 mg increments at intervals of at least 1 week; usual dosage range: 100-300 mg/day; maximum dose: 300 mg/day (Davidson, 2004; Stein, 2003; Westenberg, 2004)

Post-traumatic stress disorder (PTSD) (unlabeled use): Adults: Immediate release: 75 mg twice daily (Spivak, 2006)

Elderly: Reduce dose, titrate slowly

MAO inhibitor recommendations:

Switching to or from an MAO inhibitor intended to treat psychiatric disorders:

Allow 14 days to elapse between discontinuing an MAO inhibitor intended to treat psychiatric disorders and initiation of fluvoxamine.

Allow 14 days to elapse between discontinuing fluvoxamine and initiation of an MAO inhibitor intended to treat psychiatric disorders.

Use with other MAO inhibitors (linezolid or I.V. methylene blue):

Do not initiate fluvoxamine in patients receiving linezolid or I.V. methylene blue; consider other interventions for psychiatric condition.

If urgent treatment with linezolid or I.V. methylene blue is required in a patient already receiving fluvoxamine and potential benefits outweigh potential risks, discontinue fluvoxamine promptly and administer linezolid or I.V. methylene blue. Monitor for serotonin syndrome for 2 weeks or until 24 hours after the last dose of linezolid or I.V. methylene blue, whichever comes first. May resume fluvoxamine 24 hours after the last dose of linezolid or I.V. methylene blue.

Dosage adjustment in renal impairment: No dosage adjustment provided in manufacturer's labeling. Limited data suggest fluvoxamine does not accumulate in patients with renal impairment.

Dosage adjustment in hepatic impairment: No dosage adjustment provided in manufacturer's labeling. Limited data suggest fluvoxamine clearance is reduced in patients with hepatic impairment. Reduced initial dose and slow titration may be required.

Mechanism of Action Inhibits CNS neuron serotonin uptake; minimal or no effect on reuptake of norepinephrine or dopamine; does not significantly bind to alpha-adrenergic, histamine or cholinergic receptors

Contraindications Concurrent use with alosetron, pimozide, ramelteon, thioridazine, or tizanidine; use of MAO inhibitors intended to treat psychiatric disorders (concurrently or within 14 days of discontinuing either fluvoxamine or the MAO inhibitor); initiation of fluvoxamine in a patient receiving linezolid or intravenous methylene blue

Warnings/Precautions [U.S. Boxed Warning]: Antidepressants increase the risk of suicidal thinking and behavior in children, adolescents, and young adults (18-24 years of age) with major depressive disorder (MDD) and other psychiatric disorders; consider risk prior to prescribing. Short-term studies did not show an increased risk in patients >24 years of age and showed a decreased risk in patients ≥65 years. Closely monitor patients for clinical worsening, suicidality, or unusual changes in behavior, particularly during the initial 1-2 months of therapy or during periods of dosage adjustments (increases or decreases); the patient's family or caregiver should be instructed to closely observe the patient and communicate condition with healthcare provider. A medication guide concerning the use of antidepressants should be dispensed with each prescription. **Fluvoxamine is FDA approved for the treatment of OCD in children ≥8 years of age; extended release capsules are not FDA approved for use in children.**

The possibility of a suicide attempt is inherent in major depression and may persist until remission occurs. Use caution in high-risk patients. Worsening depression and severe abrupt suicidality that are not part of the presenting symptoms may require discontinuation or modification of drug therapy. The patient's family or caregiver should be alerted to monitor patients for the emergence of suicidality and associated behaviors (such as agitation, irritability, hostility, impulsivity, and hypomania) and call healthcare provider.

May worsen psychosis in some patients or precipitate a shift to mania or hypomania in patients with bipolar disorder. Patients presenting with depressive symptoms should be screened for bipolar disorder. Monotherapy in patients with bipolar disorder should be avoided. **Fluvoxamine is not FDA approved for the treatment of bipolar depression.**

Potentially life-threatening serotonin syndrome (SS) has occurred with serotonergic agents (eg, SSRIs, SNRIs), particularly when used in combination with other serotonergic agents (eg, triptans, TCAs, fentanyl, lithium, tramadol, buspirone, St John's wort, tryptophan) or agents that impair metabolism of serotonin (eg, MOA inhibitors intended to treat psychiatric disorders, other MAO inhibitors [ie, linezolid and intravenous methylene blue]). Discontinue treatment (and any concomitant serotonergic agent) immediately if signs/symptoms arise. Fluvoxamine has a low potential to impair cognitive or motor performance; caution operating hazardous machinery or driving. Use caution in patients with a previous seizure disorder or condition predisposing to seizures such as brain damage, alcoholism, or concurrent therapy with other drugs which lower the seizure threshold. Potentially significant interactions may exist, requiring dose or frequency adjustment, additional monitoring, and/or selection of alternative therapy. Consult drug interactions database for more detailed information. Fluvoxamine levels may be lower in patients who smoke.

May increase the risks associated with electroconvulsive therapy. Use with caution in patients with hepatic dysfunction and in elderly patients. May cause hyponatremia/SIADH (elderly at increased risk); volume depletion (diuretics may increase risk). Use with caution in patients at risk of bleeding or receiving concurrent anticoagulant therapy, although not consistently noted, fluvoxamine may cause impairment in platelet function. May cause or exacerbate sexual dysfunction. Use caution in elderly patients; monitor sodium closely with initiation or dosage adjustments in older adults (Beers Criteria).

Drug Interactions

Metabolism/Transport Effects Substrate of CYP1A2 (major), CYP2D6 (major); **Note:** Assignment of Major/Minor substrate status based on clinically relevant drug interaction potential; **Inhibits** CYP1A2 (strong), CYP2B6 (weak), CYP2C19 (strong), CYP2C9 (weak), CYP2D6 (weak), CYP3A4 (weak)

Avoid Concomitant Use

Avoid concomitant use of FluvoxaMINE with any of the following: Alosetron; Clopidogrel; Iobenguane I 123; Linezolid; MAO Inhibitors; Methylene Blue; Pimozide; Pirfenidone; Pomalidomide; Ramelteon; Thioridazine; TiZANidine; Tryptophan

Increased Effect/Toxicity

FluvoxaMINE may increase the levels/effects of: Agents with Antiplatelet Properties; Alosetron; Anticoagulants; Antidepressants (Serotonin Reuptake Inhibitor/Antagonist); Asenapine; Aspirin; Bendamustine; Benzodiazepines (metabolized by oxidation); Bromazepam; BusPIRone; CarBAMazepine; CloZAPine; Collagenase (Systemic); CYP1A2 Substrates; CYP2C19 Substrates; Dabigatran Etexilate; Desmopressin; Drotrecogin Alfa (Activated); DULoxetine; Erlotinib; Fosphenytoin; Haloperidol; Hypoglycemic Agents; Ibritumomab; Lomitapide; Methadone; Methylene Blue; Metoclopramide; Mexiletine; NSAID (COX-2 Inhibitor); NSAID (Nonselective); OLANZapine; Phenytoin; Pimozide; Pirfenidone; Pomalidomide; Propafenone; Propranolol; QuiNIDine; Ramelteon; Rivaroxaban; Roflumilast; Ropivacaine; Salicylates; Serotonin Modulators; Theophylline Derivatives; Thioridazine; Thrombolytic Agents; TiZANidine; Tositumomab and Iodine I 131 Tositumomab; TraMADol; Tricyclic Antidepressants; Vitamin K Antagonists; Zolpidem

The levels/effects of FluvoxaMINE may be increased by: Abiraterone Acetate; Alcohol (Ethyl); Analgesics (Opioid); Antipsychotics; BusPIRone; Cimetidine; CNS Depressants; Cobicistat; CYP1A2 Inhibitors (Moderate); CYP1A2 Inhibitors (Strong); CYP2D6 Inhibitors (Moderate); CYP2D6 Inhibitors (Strong); Darunavir; Dasatinib; Deferasirox; DULoxetine; Glucosamine; Grapefruit Juice; Herbs (Anticoagulant/Antiplatelet Properties); Linezolid; Lithium; MAO Inhibitors; Metoclopramide; Metyrosine; Multivitamins/Minerals (with ADEK, Folate, Iron); Omega-3 Fatty Acids; Pentosan Polysulfate Sodium; Pentoxifylline; Prostacyclin Analogues; Tipranavir; TraMADol; Tryptophan; Vitamin E

Decreased Effect

FluvoxaMINE may decrease the levels/effects of: Clopidogrel; Iobenguane I 123; Ioflupane I 123

The levels/effects of FluvoxaMINE may be decreased by: CarBAMazepine; CYP1A2 Inducers (Strong); Cyproheptadine; Cyproterone; NSAID (COX-2 Inhibitor); NSAID (Nonselective); Peginterferon Alfa-2b

Ethanol/Nutrition/Herb Interactions

Ethanol: May increase CNS depression; monitor for increased effects with coadministration. Caution patients about effects.

Herb/Nutraceutical: Avoid valerian, St John's wort, tryptophan, SAMe, kava kava (may increase risk of serotonin syndrome and/or excessive sedation). Avoid alfalfa, anise, bilberry, bladderwrack, bromelain, cat's claw, celery, chamomile, coleus, cordyceps, dong quai, evening primrose, fenugreek, feverfew, garlic, ginger, ginkgo biloba, ginseng (American), ginseng (Panax), ginseng (Siberian), grape seed, green tea, guggul, horse chestnuts, horseradish, licorice, prickly ash, red clover, reishi, SAMe (S-adenosylmethionine), sweet clover, turmeric, white willow (all have additional antiplatelet activity). Bioavailability of melatonin may be increased by fluvoxamine.

Dietary Considerations May be taken with or without food.

Pharmacodynamics/Kinetics

Onset of Action Depression: The onset of action is within a week; however, individual response varies greatly and full response may not be seen until 8-12 weeks after initiation of treatment.

Half-life Elimination 15-16 hours; 17-26 hours in the elderly

Time to Peak Plasma: 3-8 hours

Pregnancy Risk Factor C

Pregnancy Considerations Adverse events have been observed in animal reproduction studies. Fluvoxamine crosses the human placenta. An increased risk of teratogenic effects, including cardiovascular defects, may be associated with maternal use of fluvoxamine or other SSRIs; however, available information is conflicting. Nonteratogenic effects in the newborn following SSRI/SNRI exposure late in the third trimester include respiratory distress, cyanosis, apnea, seizures, temperature instability, feeding difficulty, vomiting, hypoglycemia, hypo- or hypertonia, hyper-reflexia, jitteriness, irritability, constant crying, and tremor. Symptoms may be due to the toxicity of the SSRIs/SNRIs or a discontinuation syndrome and may be consistent with serotonin syndrome associated with SSRI treatment. Persistent pulmonary hypertension of the newborn (PPHN) has also been reported with SSRI exposure. The long-term effects of *in utero* SSRI exposure on infant development and behavior are not known.

The ACOG recommends that therapy with SSRIs or SNRIs during pregnancy be individualized; treatment of depression during pregnancy should incorporate the clinical expertise of the mental health clinician, obstetrician, primary healthcare provider, and pediatrician. According to the American Psychiatric Association (APA), the risks of medication treatment should be weighed against other treatment options and untreated depression. For women who discontinue antidepressant medications during pregnancy and who may be at high risk for postpartum depression, the medications can be restarted following delivery. Treatment algorithms have been developed by the ACOG and the APA for the management of depression in women prior to conception and during pregnancy.

Lactation Enters breast milk/consider risk:benefit (AAP rates "of concern"; AAP 2001 update pending)

Breast-Feeding Considerations Fluvoxamine is excreted in breast milk. Based on case reports, the dose the infant receives is relatively small and adverse events have not been observed. Adverse events have been reported in nursing infants exposed to some SSRIs. According to the manufacturer, the decision to continue or discontinue breast-feeding during therapy should take into account the risk of exposure to the infant and the benefits of treatment to the mother.

The long-term effects on development and behavior have not been studied; therefore, fluvoxamine should be prescribed to a mother who is breast-feeding only when the benefits outweigh the potential risks. Maternal use of an SSRI during pregnancy may cause delayed milk secretion.

Dosage Forms

Capsule, extended release, oral: 100 mg, 150 mg
Luvox® CR: 100 mg, 150 mg

Tablet, oral: 25 mg, 50 mg, 100 mg

Dental Comment Problems with SSRI-induced bruxism have been reported and may preclude their use. Clinicians attempting to evaluate any patient with bruxism or involuntary muscle movement, who is simultaneously being treated with an SSRI drug, should be aware of the potential association.

References

Friedlander AH and Mahler ME, "Major Depressive Disorder. Psychopathology, Medical Management, and Dental Implications," *J Am Dent Assoc*, 2001, 132(5):629-38.
Gerber PE and Lynd LD, "Selective Serotonin Reuptake Inhibitor-induced Movement Disorders," *Ann Pharmacother*, 1998, 32 (6):692-8.
Wynn RL, "New Antidepressant Medications," *Gen Dent*, 1997, 45 (1):24-8.

Folic Acid (FOE lik AS id)

Brand Names: U.S. Folacin-800 [OTC]

Brand Names: Canada Apo-Folic®

Generic Availability (U.S.) Yes

Pharmacologic Category Vitamin, Water Soluble

Use Treatment of megaloblastic and macrocytic anemias due to folate deficiency; dietary supplement to prevent neural tube defects

Unlabeled Use Adjunctive cofactor therapy in methanol toxicity (alternative to leucovorin calcium)

Local Anesthetic/Vasoconstrictor Precautions No information available to require special precautions

Effects on Dental Treatment No significant effects or complications reported

Effects on Bleeding No information available to require special precautions

Adverse Effects Frequency not defined.
Cardiovascular: Flushing (slight)
Central nervous system: Malaise (general)
Dermatologic: Erythema, pruritus, rash
Respiratory: Bronchospasm
Miscellaneous: Allergic reaction

Dosage

Oral, I.M., I.V., SubQ: Anemia:
Infants: 0.1 mg/day
Children <4 years: Up to 0.3 mg/day
Children >4 years and Adults: 0.4 mg/day
Pregnant and lactating women: 0.8 mg/day

Oral:

Adequate intake (AI) (IOM, 1998): Expressed as folate equivalents: Infants:
1-6 months: 65 mcg/day
7-12 months: 80 mcg/day

Recommended daily allowance (RDA) (IOM, 1998): Expressed as dietary folate equivalents:
Children:
1-3 years: 150 mcg/day
4-8 years: 200 mcg/day
9-13 years: 300 mcg/day
Children ≥14 years and Adults: 400 mcg/day
Pregnancy: 600 mcg/day
Lactation: 500 mcg/day
Elderly: Vitamin B_{12} deficiency must be ruled out before initiating folate therapy due to frequency of combined nutritional deficiencies: RDA requirements (1999): 400 mcg/day (0.4 mg) minimum
Prevention of neural tube defects:
Females of childbearing potential: 400-800 mcg/day (USPSTF, 2009)
Females at high risk or with family history of neural tube defects: 4 mg/day (ACOG, 2003)

Mechanism of Action Folic acid is necessary for formation of a number of coenzymes in many metabolic systems, particularly for purine and pyrimidine synthesis; required for nucleoprotein synthesis and maintenance in erythropoiesis; stimulates WBC and platelet production in folate deficiency anemia. Folic acid enhances the metabolism of formic acid, the toxic metabolite of methanol, to nontoxic metabolites (unlabeled use).

Contraindications Hypersensitivity to folic acid or any component of the formulation

Warnings/Precautions Not appropriate for monotherapy with pernicious, aplastic, or normocytic anemias when anemia is present with vitamin B_{12} deficiency. Doses >0.1 mg/day may obscure pernicious anemia with continuing irreversible nerve damage progression. Resistance to treatment may occur with depressed hematopoiesis, alcoholism, and deficiencies of other vitamins. Injection contains benzyl alcohol (1.5%) as preservative (use care in administration to neonates).

Drug Interactions

Metabolism/Transport Effects None known.

Avoid Concomitant Use

Avoid concomitant use of Folic Acid with any of the following: Raltitrexed

Increased Effect/Toxicity There are no known significant interactions involving an increase in effect.

Decreased Effect

Folic Acid may decrease the levels/effects of: Fosphenytoin; PHENobarbital; Phenytoin; Primidone; Raltitrexed

The levels/effects of Folic Acid may be decreased by: Green Tea

Dietary Considerations As of January 1998, the FDA has required manufacturers of enriched flour, bread, corn meal, pasta, rice, and other grain products to add folic acid to their products. The intent is to help decrease the risk of neural tube defects by increasing folic acid intake. Other foods which contain folic acid include dark green leafy vegetables, citrus fruits and juices, and lentils.

Pharmacodynamics/Kinetics

Onset of Action Peak effect: Oral: 0.5-1 hour

Pregnancy Risk Factor A

Pregnancy Considerations Water soluble vitamins cross the placenta. Folate requirements increase during pregnancy. Folate supplementation during the periconceptual period decreases the risk of neural tube defects. Folate supplementation (doses larger than the RDA) is recommended for women who may become pregnant (IOM, 1998).

Lactation Enters breast milk/compatible

Breast-Feeding Considerations Folate is found in breast milk; concentrations are not affected by dietary intake unless the mother has a severe deficiency (IOM, 1998).

Dosage Forms
Injection, solution: 5 mg/mL (10 mL)
Tablet, oral: 0.4 mg, 0.8 mg, 1 mg
Folacin-800 [OTC]: 0.8 mg

Folic Acid, Cyanocobalamin, and Pyridoxine
(FOE lik AS id, sye an oh koe BAL a min, & peer i DOKS een)

Related Information
Cyanocobalamin *on page 357*
Folic Acid *on page 626*
Pyridoxine *on page 1163*

Brand Names: U.S. FaBB; Folastin; Folbee®; Folbic™; Folcaps™; Folgard RX®; Folgard® [OTC] [DSC]; Folplex 2.2; Foltabs™ 800 [OTC]; Foltx® [DSC]; Homocysteine Guard [OTC]; Lev-Tov [OTC]; Tri-B® [OTC]; Tricardio B; Virt-Vite Forte; Vita-Respa®

Pharmacologic Category Vitamin

Use Nutritional supplement in end-stage renal failure, dialysis, hyperhomocysteinemia, homocystinuria, malabsorption syndromes, dietary deficiencies

Local Anesthetic/Vasoconstrictor Precautions No information available to require special precautions

Effects on Dental Treatment No significant effects or complications reported

Effects on Bleeding No information available to require special precautions

Adverse Effects See individual agents.

General Dosage Range Oral: *Adults:* 1 tablet (folic acid 0.4-2.5 mg/cyanocobalamin 115-2000 mcg/pyridoxine 10-25 mg) daily

Pregnancy Considerations See individual agents.

Follitropin Alfa (foe li TRO pin AL fa)

Brand Names: U.S. Gonal-f®; Gonal-f® RFF; Gonal-f® RFF Pen

Brand Names: Canada Gonal-f®; Gonal-f® Pen

Pharmacologic Category Gonadotropin; Ovulation Stimulator

Use
Gonal-f®: Induction of ovulation in anovulatory infertile patients in whom the cause of infertility is functional and not caused by primary ovarian failure; development of multiple follicles with Assisted Reproductive Technology (ART); induction of spermatogenesis in men with primary and secondary hypogonadotropic hypogonadism in whom the cause of infertility is not due to primary testicular failure.

Gonal-f® RFF: Induction of ovulation in oligo-anovulatory infertile patients in whom the cause of infertility is functional and not caused by primary ovarian failure; development of multiple follicles with ART

Local Anesthetic/Vasoconstrictor Precautions No information available to require special precautions

Effects on Dental Treatment Key adverse event(s) related to dental treatment: Stomatitis and toothache.

Effects on Bleeding No information available to require special precautions

Adverse Effects Percentage may vary by indication, product formulation
>10%:
Central nervous system: Headache

Dermatologic: Acne (males)
Endocrine & metabolic: Breast pain (males), ovarian cyst
Gastrointestinal: Abdomen enlarged, abdominal pain, nausea
Miscellaneous: Upper respiratory infection
1% to 10%:
Cardiovascular: Chest pain, hypotension, palpitation
Central nervous system: Anxiety, dizziness, emotional lability, fatigue, fever, malaise, migraine, nervousness, pain, somnolence
Dermatologic: Acne (females), pruritus
Endocrine & metabolic: Breast pain (females), cervix lesion, dysmenorrhea, gynecomastia, hot flashes, intermenstrual bleeding, menstrual disorder, ovarian disorder, ovarian hyperstimulation
Gastrointestinal: Anorexia, constipation, diarrhea, dyspepsia, flatulence, stomatitis (ulcerative), toothache, vomiting, weight gain
Genitourinary: Cystitis, leukorrhea, micturition frequency, pelvic pain, urinary tract infection, uterine hemorrhage, vaginal hemorrhage
Local: Injection site bruising, edema, inflammation, pain, reaction
Neuromuscular & skeletal: Back pain, myalgia, paresthesia
Respiratory: Asthma, cough, dyspnea, pharyngitis, rhinitis, sinusitis
Miscellaneous: Flu-like syndrome, infection, moniliasis, thirst increased

General Dosage Range SubQ:
Adults (females): Initial: 75-225 units/day; Maximum: Up to 300-450 units/day
Adults (males): Gonal-f®: Initial: 150 units 3 times/week; Maximum: Up to 300 units 3 times/week

Mechanism of Action Follitropin alfa is a human FSH preparation of recombinant DNA origin. Follitropins stimulate ovarian follicular growth in women who do not have primary ovarian failure, and stimulate spermatogenesis in men with hypogonadotrophic hypogonadism. FSH is required for normal follicular growth, maturation, gonadal steroid production, and spermatogenesis.

Pharmacodynamics/Kinetics
Onset of Action Peak effect:
Spermatogenesis, median: 6.8-12.4 months (range: 2.7-18.1 months)
Follicle development: Within cycle
Half-life Elimination
I.M.: 50 hours in healthy female volunteers
SubQ: 24 hours in healthy female volunteers; 32 hours with *in vitro* fertilization/embryo transfer patients; 32-41 hours in healthy male volunteers
Time to Peak In healthy volunteers:
Females: SubQ: 8-16 hours; I.M.: 25 hours
Males: SubQ: 11-20 hours
Pregnancy Risk Factor X
Pregnancy Considerations Ectopic pregnancy, congenital abnormalities, spontaneous abortion, and multiple births have been reported. The incidence of congenital abnormality may be slightly higher after ART than with spontaneous conception; higher incidence may be related to parenteral characteristics (maternal age, sperm characteristics). Follitropin Alfa is used for the induction of ovulation; use is contraindicated in women who are already pregnant.

Follitropin Beta (foe li TRO pin BAY ta)

Brand Names: U.S. Follistim® AQ; Follistim® AQ Cartridge

◄ **Brand Names: Canada** Puregon®

Pharmacologic Category Gonadotropin; Ovulation Stimulator

Use

Females: Induction of ovulation and pregnancy in anovulatory infertile patients in whom the cause of infertility is functional and not caused by primary ovarian failure; induction of pregnancy in normal ovulatory women undergoing Assisted Reproductive Technology (ART) (eg, *in vitro* fertilization [IVF], intracytoplasmic sperm injection [ICSI])

Males: Induction of spermatogenesis in men with primary and secondary hypogonadotropic hypogonadism in whom the cause of infertility is not due to primary testicular failure.

Local Anesthetic/Vasoconstrictor Precautions No information available to require special precautions

Effects on Dental Treatment No significant effects or complications reported

Effects on Bleeding No information available to require special precautions

Adverse Effects Frequency may vary based on indication.

Central nervous system: Headache (7%), fatigue (2%)

Dermatologic: Acne (7%), rash (3%)

Endocrine & metabolic: Pelvic discomfort (8%), ovarian hyperstimulation (6% to 8%), pelvic pain (6%), gynecomastia (3%), ovarian cyst (3%)

Gastrointestinal: Nausea (4%), abdominal pain/discomfort (2% to 3%)

Local: Injection site pain (7%), injection site reaction (7%)

Postmarketing and/or case reports: Abdominal distension, breast tenderness, constipation, diarrhea, metrorrhagia, miscarriage, ovarian enlargement, ovarian neoplasm, ovarian torsion, thromboembolism, vaginal hemorrhage

General Dosage Range

I.M., SubQ: *Adults (females):* Initial: 75-225 units/day; Maintenance: Up to 175-600 units/day

SubQ: *Adults (males):* 450 units/week

Mechanism of Action Follitropin beta is a human FSH preparation of recombinant DNA origin. Follitropins stimulate ovarian follicular growth in women who do not have primary ovarian failure and stimulate spermatogenesis in men with hypogonadotrophic hypogonadism. FSH is required for normal follicular growth, maturation, gonadal steroid production, and spermatogenesis.

Pharmacodynamics/Kinetics

Onset of Action Peak effect: Females: Follicle development: Within cycle

Half-life Elimination Females: I.M.: 44 hours (single dose), 27-30 hours (multiple doses); SubQ: 33 hours (single dose)

Time to Peak Females: SubQ: 13 hours

Pregnancy Risk Factor X

Pregnancy Considerations

Ectopic pregnancies, congenital abnormalities, and multiple births have been reported. The incidence of congenital abnormality may be slightly higher after ART than with spontaneous conception; higher incidence may be related to parenteral characteristics (maternal age, sperm characteristics). Follitropin Beta is used for the induction of ovulation; use is contraindicated in women who are already pregnant.

Fomepizole (foe ME pi zole)

Brand Names: U.S. Antizol®

Brand Names: Canada Antizol®

Pharmacologic Category Antidote

Use Treatment of methanol or ethylene glycol poisoning alone or in combination with hemodialysis

Unlabeled Use Pediatric administration; treatment of propylene glycol toxicity

Local Anesthetic/Vasoconstrictor Precautions No information available to require special precautions

Effects on Dental Treatment Key adverse event(s) related to dental treatment: Bad/metallic taste.

Effects on Bleeding No information available to require special precautions

Adverse Effects

>10%:

Central nervous system: Headache (14%)

Gastrointestinal: Nausea (11%)

1% to 10% (≤3% unless otherwise noted):

Cardiovascular: Bradycardia, facial flush, hypotension, shock, tachycardia

Central nervous system: Dizziness (6%), drowsiness increased (6%), agitation, anxiety, fever, lightheadedness, seizure, vertigo

Dermatologic: Rash

Gastrointestinal: Bad/metallic taste (6%), abdominal pain, appetite decreased, diarrhea, heartburn, vomiting

Hematologic: Anemia, disseminated intravascular coagulation (DIC), eosinophilia, lymphangitis

Hepatic: Liver function tests increased

Local: Application site reaction, injection site inflammation, pain during injection, phlebitis

Neuromuscular & skeletal: Backache

Ocular: Nystagmus, transient blurred vision, visual disturbances

Renal: Anuria

Respiratory: Abnormal smell, hiccups, pharyngitis

Miscellaneous: Multiorgan failure, speech disturbances

General Dosage Range Dosage adjustment recommended in patients with renal impairment

I.V.: *Adults:* Loading dose of 15 mg/kg, followed by 10 mg/kg every 12 hours for 4 doses, then 15 mg/kg every 12 hours

Mechanism of Action Fomepizole competitively inhibits alcohol dehydrogenase, an enzyme which catalyzes the metabolism of ethanol, ethylene glycol, and methanol to their toxic metabolites. Ethylene glycol is metabolized to glycoaldehyde, then oxidized to glycolate, glyoxylate, and oxalate. Glycolate and oxalate are responsible for metabolic acidosis and renal damage. Methanol is metabolized to formaldehyde, then oxidized to formic acid. Formic acid is responsible for metabolic acidosis and visual disturbances.

Pharmacodynamics/Kinetics

Onset of Action Peak effect: Maximum: 1.5-2 hours

Half-life Elimination Has not been calculated; varies with dose

Pregnancy Risk Factor C

Pregnancy Considerations Animal reproduction studies have not been conducted. In general, medications used as antidotes should take into consideration the health and prognosis of the mother (Bailey, 2003).

Fondaparinux (fon da PARE i nuks)

Brand Names: U.S. Arixtra®

Brand Names: Canada Arixtra®

Pharmacologic Category Factor Xa Inhibitor

Use Prophylaxis of deep vein thrombosis (DVT) in patients undergoing surgery for hip replacement, knee replacement, hip fracture (including extended prophylaxis following hip fracture surgery), or abdominal surgery (in patients at risk for thromboembolic complications); treatment of acute pulmonary embolism (PE); treatment of acute DVT without PE

Canadian labeling: Additional uses (not approved in U.S.): Unstable angina or non-ST segment elevation myocardial infarction (UA/NSTEMI) for the prevention of death and subsequent MI; ST segment elevation MI (STEMI) for the prevention of death and myocardial reinfarction

Unlabeled Use Prophylaxis of DVT in patients with a history of heparin-induced thrombocytopenia (HIT); treatment of acute thrombosis (unrelated to HIT) in patients with a past history of HIT; acute symptomatic superficial vein thrombosis (≥5 cm in length) of the legs

Local Anesthetic/Vasoconstrictor Precautions No information available to require special precautions

Effects on Dental Treatment Key adverse event(s) related to dental treatment: Hemorrhage may occur at any site. See Effects on Bleeding.

Effects on Bleeding Dose related bleeding is the most common adverse event. Bleeding from the gums is reported (3%). Moderate thrombocytopenia occurs in 3% of patients and severe thrombocytopenia in 0.2%. Medical consult recommended.

Adverse Effects As with all anticoagulants, bleeding is the major adverse effect. Hemorrhage may occur at any site. Risk appears increased by a number of factors including renal dysfunction, age (>75 years), and weight (<50 kg).

>10%:
Central nervous system: Fever (4% to 14%)
Gastrointestinal: Nausea (11%)
Hematologic: Anemia (20%)

1% to 10%:
Cardiovascular: Edema (9%), hypotension (4%), thrombosis PCI catheter (without heparin 1%)
Central nervous system: Insomnia (5%), dizziness (4%), headache (2% to 5%), confusion (3%), pain (2%)
Dermatologic: Rash (8%), purpura (4%), bullous eruption (3%)
Endocrine & metabolic: Hypokalemia (1% to 4%)
Gastrointestinal: Constipation (5% to 9%), nausea (3%), vomiting (6%), diarrhea (3%), dyspepsia (2%)
Genitourinary: Urinary tract infection (4%), urinary retention (3%)
Hematologic: Moderate thrombocytopenia (50,000-100,000/mm^3: 3%), major bleeding (1% to 3%), minor bleeding (2% to 4%), hematoma (3%); risk of major bleeding increased as high as 5% in patients receiving initial dose <6 hours following surgery
Hepatic: ALT increased (≤3%), AST increased (≤2%)
Local: Injection site reaction (bleeding, rash, pruritus)
Miscellaneous: Wound drainage increased (5%)

General Dosage Range SubQ:
Adults <50 kg: Treatment: 5 mg once daily
Adults 50-100 kg: Prophylaxis: 2.5 mg once daily; Treatment: 7.5 mg once daily
Adults >100 kg: Prophylaxis: 2.5 mg once daily; Treatment: 10 mg once daily

Mechanism of Action Fondaparinux is a synthetic pentasaccharide that causes an antithrombin III-mediated selective inhibition of factor Xa. Neutralization of factor Xa interrupts the blood coagulation cascade and inhibits thrombin formation and thrombus development.

Pharmacodynamics/Kinetics
Half-life Elimination 17-21 hours; prolonged with renal impairment
Time to Peak SubQ: 2-3 hours
Pregnancy Risk Factor B
Pregnancy Considerations Adverse events were not observed in animal reproduction studies. Based on case reports, small amounts of fondaparinux have been detected in the umbilical cord following multiple doses during pregnancy (Dempfle, 2004). Use of fondaparinux in pregnancy should be limited to those women who have severe allergic reactions to heparin, including heparin-induced thrombocytopenia, and who cannot receive danaparoid (Guyatt, 2012).

Formoterol (for MOH te rol)

Related Information
Respiratory Diseases *on page 1514*
Brand Names: U.S. Foradil® Aerolizer®; Perforomist®
Brand Names: Canada Foradil®; Oxeze® Turbuhaler®
Pharmacologic Category Beta$_2$ Agonist; Beta$_2$-Adrenergic Agonist, Long-Acting
Use U.S. labeling: Treatment of asthma (only as concomitant therapy with an inhaled corticosteroid) in patients with reversible obstructive airway disease, including patients with symptoms of nocturnal asthma (Foradil® Aerolizer®); maintenance treatment of bronchoconstriction in patients with COPD (Foradil® Aerolizer®, Perforomist®); prevention of exercise-induced bronchospasm when administered on an as-needed basis (monotherapy may be indicated in patients without persistent asthma) (Foradil® Aerolizer®)

Canadian labeling: Treatment of asthma (only as concomitant therapy with an inhaled corticosteroid) in patients with reversible obstructive airway disease, including patients with symptoms of nocturnal asthma (Foradil®, Oxeze® Turbuhaler®); maintenance treatment of COPD (Foradil®); prevention of exercise-induced bronchospasm when administered on an as-needed basis (monotherapy may be indicated in patients without persistent asthma) (Oxeze® Turbuhaler®)

Local Anesthetic/Vasoconstrictor Precautions No information available to require special precautions
Effects on Dental Treatment Key adverse event(s) related to dental treatment: Xerostomia (normal salivary flow resumes upon discontinuation).
Effects on Bleeding No information available to require special precautions
Adverse Effects
1% to 10%:
Cardiovascular: Chest pain (2% to 3%), palpitation
Central nervous system: Anxiety (2%), dizziness (2%), fever (2%), insomnia (2%), dysphonia (1%), headache
Dermatologic: Pruritus (2%), rash (1%)
Gastrointestinal: Diarrhea (5%), nausea (5%), xerostomia (1% to 3%), vomiting (2%), abdominal pain, dyspepsia, gastroenteritis
Neuromuscular & skeletal: Muscle cramps (2%), tremor

Respiratory: Infection (3% to 7%), asthma exacerbation (age 5-12 years: 5% to 6%; age >12 years: <4%), bronchitis (5%), pharyngitis (3% to 4%), sinusitis (3%), dyspnea (2%), tonsillitis (1%)

General Dosage Range Inhalation:

Powder for inhalation: *Children ≥5 years, Adolescents, and Adults:* 12 mcg every 12 hours (maximum: 24 mcg daily) **or** 12 mcg inhaled prior to exercise

Solution for nebulization: *Adults:* 20 mcg twice daily (maximum: 40 mcg daily)

Mechanism of Action Relaxes bronchial smooth muscle by selective action on beta$_2$ receptors with little effect on heart rate. Formoterol has a long-acting effect.

Pharmacodynamics/Kinetics

Onset of Action Powder for inhalation: Within 3 minutes

Peak effect: Powder for inhalation: 80% of peak effect within 15 minutes; Solution for nebulization: 2 hours

Duration of Action Improvement in FEV$_1$ observed for 12 hours in most patients

Half-life Elimination Powder: ~10-14 hours; Nebulized solution: ~7 hours

Time to Peak Maximum improvement in FEV$_1$ in 1-3 hours

Pregnancy Risk Factor C

Pregnancy Considerations When given orally to rats throughout organogenesis, formoterol caused delayed ossification and decreased fetal weight, but no malformations. There were no adverse events when given to pregnant rats in late pregnancy. Doses used were ≥70 times the recommended daily inhalation dose in humans. There are no adequate and well-controlled studies in pregnant women. Use only if benefit outweighs risk to the fetus. Beta-agonists interfere with uterine contractility so use during labor only if benefit outweighs risk to the fetus.

Fosamprenavir (FOS am pren a veer)

Related Information

HIV Infection and AIDS *on page 1520*

Brand Names: U.S. Lexiva®

Brand Names: Canada Telzir®

Pharmacologic Category Antiretroviral Agent, Protease Inhibitor

Use Treatment of HIV infections in combination with at least two other antiretroviral agents

Local Anesthetic/Vasoconstrictor Precautions No information available to require special precautions

Effects on Dental Treatment No significant effects or complications reported

Effects on Bleeding No information available to require special precautions

Adverse Effects

>10%:

Dermatologic: Rash (≤19%; onset: ~11 days; duration: ~13 days)

Endocrine & metabolic: Hypertriglyceridemia (>750 mg/dL: ≤11%)

Gastrointestinal: Diarrhea (moderate-to-severe; 5% to 13%)

1% to 10%:

Central nervous system: Headache (moderate-to-severe; 2% to 4%), fatigue (moderate-to-severe; 2% to 4%)

Dermatologic: Pruritus (7% to 8%)

Endocrine & metabolic: Hyperglycemia (>251 mg/dL: ≤2%)

Gastrointestinal: Serum lipase increased (>2 times ULN: 5% to 8%), nausea (moderate-to-severe; 3% to 7%), vomiting (moderate-to-severe; 2% to 6%), abdominal pain (moderate-to-severe; ≤2%)

Hematologic: Neutropenia (<750 cells/mm^3: 3%)

Hepatic: Transaminases increased (>5 times ULN: 4% to 8%)

Frequency not defined: Diabetes mellitus, fat redistribution, and immune reconstitution syndrome have been associated with protease inhibitor therapy. Spontaneous bleeding has been reported in patients with hemophilia A or B following treatment with protease inhibitors. Acute hemolytic anemia has been reported in association with amprenavir use.

General Dosage Range Dosage adjustment recommended in patients with hepatic impairment or on concomitant therapy

Oral:

Infants ≥4 weeks (PI-naive patients) or Infants ≥6 months (PI-experienced patients): Ritonavir-boosted regimen:

<11 kg: 45 mg/kg/dose twice daily (plus ritonavir); maximum: 700 mg/dose

11 to <15 kg: 30 mg/kg/dose twice daily (plus ritonavir); maximum: 700 mg/dose

15 to <20 kg: 23 mg/kg/dose twice daily (plus ritonavir); maximum: 700 mg/dose

≥20 kg: 18 mg/kg/dose twice daily (plus ritonavir); maximum: 700 mg/dose

Children ≥2 years (PI-naive patients): Unboosted regimen:

<47 kg: 30 mg/kg/dose twice daily; maximum: 1400 mg/dose

≥47 kg: 1400 mg twice daily

Adults:

Ritonavir-boosted regimen: 700 mg twice daily **or** 1400 mg once daily

Unboosted regimen: 1400 mg twice daily

Mechanism of Action Fosamprenavir is rapidly and almost completely converted to amprenavir by cellular phosphatases *in vivo*. Amprenavir binds to the site of HIV-1 protease activity and inhibits cleavage of viral Gag-Pol polyprotein precursors into individual functional proteins required for infectious HIV. This results in the formation of immature, noninfectious viral particles.

Pharmacodynamics/Kinetics

Half-life Elimination ~7.7 hours (amprenavir)

Time to Peak 1.5-4 hours (median: 2.5 hours)

Pregnancy Risk Factor C

Pregnancy Considerations Adverse events were observed in some animal reproduction studies. It is not known if fosamprenavir crosses the human placenta. A small increased risk of preterm birth has been associated with maternal use of protease inhibitor-based combination antiretroviral (ARV) therapy during pregnancy; however, the benefits of use generally outweigh this risk and protease inhibitors (PIs) should not be withheld if otherwise recommended. Hyperglycemia, new onset of diabetes mellitus, or diabetic ketoacidosis have been reported with PIs; it is not clear if pregnancy increases this risk. The DHHS Perinatal HIV Guidelines note there are insufficient data to recommend use during pregnancy; however, if used, they recommend that fosamprenavir be given with low-dose ritonavir boosting.

Regardless of CD4 count or HIV RNA copy number, all HIV-infected pregnant women should receive a combination antepartum ARV drug regimen; this includes women who require therapy for their own health, as well as women who do not yet require therapy for their own health. ARV therapy should be started as soon as possible if required for the woman's health. Although earlier initiation may be more effective in reducing the perinatal transmission of HIV, also consider maternal conditions (eg, nausea and vomiting) and the potential risks of first trimester fetal exposure for specific agents. Plasma HIV RNA levels should be assessed at ~34-36 weeks gestation in order to help determine mode of delivery. If ARV therapy must be interrupted for <24 hours during the peripartum period, stop then restart all medications simultaneously in order to decrease the chance of developing resistance. Long-term follow-up is recommended for all infants exposed to ARV medications.

Healthcare providers are encouraged to enroll pregnant women exposed to antiretroviral medications in the Antiretroviral Pregnancy Registry (1-800-258-4263 or www.APRegistry.com). Healthcare providers caring for HIV-infected women and their infants may contact the National Perinatal HIV Hotline (888-448-8765) for clinical consultation (DHHS [perinatal], 2012).

Fosaprepitant (fos a PRE pi tant)

Brand Names: U.S. Emend® for Injection
Brand Names: Canada Emend® IV
Pharmacologic Category Antiemetic; Substance P/ Neurokinin 1 Receptor Antagonist
Use Prevention of acute and delayed nausea and vomiting associated with moderately- and highly-emetogenic chemotherapy (in combination with other antiemetics)
Local Anesthetic/Vasoconstrictor Precautions No information available to require special precautions
Effects on Dental Treatment Key adverse event(s) related to dental treatment: Stomatitis, taste disturbances, xerostomia (normal salivary flow resumes upon discontinuation).
Effects on Bleeding No information available to require special precautions
Adverse Effects Adverse reactions reported with aprepitant and fosaprepitant (as part of a combination chemotherapy regimen) occurring at a higher frequency than standard antiemetic therapy:
1% to 10%:
 Central nervous system: Fatigue (1% to 3%), headache (1% to 3%)
 Gastrointestinal: Anorexia (2%), constipation 2%), dyspepsia (2%), diarrhea (1%), eructation (1%)
 Hepatic: ALT increased (1% to 3%), AST increased (1%)
 Local: Injection site reactions (3%; includes erythema, induration, pain, pruritus, or thrombophlebitis)
 Neuromuscular & skeletal: Weakness (3%)
 Miscellaneous: Hiccups (5%)
General Dosage Range I.V.: *Adults:* 150 mg as a single dose
Mechanism of Action Fosaprepitant is a prodrug of aprepitant, a substance P/neurokinin 1 (NK1) receptor antagonist. It is rapidly converted to aprepitant which prevents acute and delayed vomiting by inhibiting the substance P/neurokinin 1 (NK1) receptor; augments the antiemetic activity of the 5-HT$_3$ receptor antagonist and corticosteroid activity and inhibits chemotherapy-induced emesis.
Pharmacodynamics/Kinetics
 Half-life Elimination Fosaprepitant: ~2 minutes; Aprepitant: ~9-13 hours
 Time to Peak Fosaprepitant is converted to aprepitant within 30 minutes after the end of infusion

Pregnancy Risk Factor B
Pregnancy Considerations Teratogenic effects were not observed in animal reproduction studies for aprepitant. Use during pregnancy only if clearly needed. Efficacy of hormonal contraceptive may be reduced; alternative or additional methods of contraception should be used both during treatment with fosaprepitant or aprepitant and for at least 1 month following the last fosaprepitant/aprepitant dose.

Foscarnet (fos KAR net)

Related Information
Systemic Viral Diseases *on page 1537*
Brand Names: U.S. Foscavir®
Brand Names: Canada Foscavir®
Generic Availability (U.S.) Yes
Pharmacologic Category Antiviral Agent
Dental Use Treatment of acyclovir-resistant mucocutaneous herpes simplex virus (HSV) infections in immunocompromised persons (eg, with advanced AIDS); treatment of CMV retinitis in persons with HIV
Use Treatment of acyclovir-resistant mucocutaneous herpes simplex virus (HSV) infections in immunocompromised persons (eg, with advanced AIDS); treatment of CMV retinitis in persons with HIV
Unlabeled Use Other CMV infections (eg, colitis, esophagitis, neurological disease); CMV prophylaxis for cancer patients receiving alemtuzumab therapy or allogeneic stem cell transplant
Local Anesthetic/Vasoconstrictor Precautions Foscarnet is one of the drugs confirmed to prolong the QT interval and is accepted as having a risk of causing torsade de pointes. In terms of epinephrine, it is not known what effect vasoconstrictors in the local anesthetic regimen will have in patients with a known history of congenital prolonged QT interval or in patients taking any medication that prolongs the QT interval. Until more information is obtained, it is suggested that the clinician consult with the physician prior to the use of a vasoconstrictor in suspected patients, and that the vasoconstrictor (epinephrine, mepivacaine and levonordefrin [Carbocaine® 2% with Neo-Cobefrin®]) be used with caution. See Dental Comment.
Effects on Dental Treatment Key adverse event(s) related to dental treatment: Xerostomia (normal salivary flow resumes upon discontinuation), taste perversion, and ulcerative stomatitis.
Effects on Bleeding No information available to require special precautions
Adverse Effects
>10%:
 Central nervous system: Fever (65%), headache (26%)
 Endocrine & metabolic: Hypokalemia (16% to 48%), hypocalcemia (15% to 30%), hypomagnesemia (15% to 30%), hypophosphatemia (8% to 26%)
 Gastrointestinal: Nausea (47%), diarrhea (30%), vomiting (26%)
 Hematologic: Anemia (33%), granulocytopenia (17%)
 Renal: Abnormal renal function/decreased creatinine clearance (12%; without adequate hydration: 33%)
1% to 10%:
 Cardiovascular: Chest pain (1% to 5%), edema (1% to 5%), facial edema (1% to 5%), flushing (1% to 5%), hyper-/hypotension (1% to 5%), palpitation (1% to 5%), ECG changes (1% to 5%)

Central nervous system: Seizures (8% to 10%), anxiety (≥5%), confusion (≥5%), depression (≥5%), dizziness (≥5%), fatigue (≥5%), hypoesthesia (≥5%), malaise (≥5%), pain (≥5%), aggressiveness (1% to 5%), agitation (1% to 5%), amnesia (1% to 5%), aphasia (1% to 5%), ataxia (1% to 5%), coordination abnormal (1% to 5%), dementia (1% to 5%), EEG abnormal (1% to 5%), hallucination (1% to 5%), insomnia (1% to 5%), meningitis (1% to 5%), nervousness (1% to 5%), somnolence (1% to 5%), stupor (1% to 5%)

Dermatologic: Rash (≥5%), erythematous rash (1% to 5%), maculopapular rash (1% to 5%), pruritus (1% to 5%), seborrhea (1% to 5%), skin discoloration (1% to 5%), skin ulceration (1% to 5%)

Endocrine & metabolic: Hyperphosphatemia (6%), acidosis (1% to 5%), hyponatremia (1% to 5%)

Gastrointestinal: Abdominal pain (≥5%), anorexia (≥5%), cachexia (1% to 5%), constipation (1% to 5%), dyspepsia (1% to 5%), dysphagia (1% to 5%), flatulence (1% to 5%), melena (1% to 5%), pancreatitis (1% to 5%), rectal hemorrhage (1% to 5%), taste perversion (1% to 5%), ulcerative stomatitis (1% to 5%), weight loss (1% to 5%), xerostomia (1% to 5%)

Genitourinary: Dysuria (1% to 5%), nocturia (1% to 5%), urinary retention (1% to 5%), urinary tract infection (1% to 5%)

Hematologic: Bone marrow suppression (10%), leukopenia (≥5%), lymphadenopathy (1% to 5%), thrombocytopenia (1% to 5%), thrombosis (1% to 5%)

Hepatic: Alkaline phosphatase increased (1% to 5%), ALT increased (1% to 5%), AST increased (1% to 5%), hepatic function abnormal (1% to 5%), LDH increased (1% to 5%)

Local: Abscess (1% to 5%), injection site pain/inflammation (1% to 5%)

Neuromuscular & skeletal: Paresthesia (≥5%), involuntary muscle contractions (≥5%), rigors (≥5%), neuropathy (peripheral; ≥5%), weakness (≥5%), arthralgia (1% to 5%), back pain (1% to 5%), leg cramps (1% to 5%), myalgia (1% to 5%), tremor (1% to 5%)

Ocular: Vision abnormalities (≥5%), conjunctivitis (1% to 5%), eye pain (1% to 5%)

Renal: Acute renal failure (1% to 5%), albuminuria (1% to 5%), BUN increased (1% to 5%), polyuria (1% to 5%)

Respiratory: Cough (≥5%), dyspnea (≥5%), bronchospasm (1% to 5%), hemoptysis (1% to 5%), pharyngitis (1% to 5%), pneumonia (1% to 5%), pneumothorax (1% to 5%), pulmonary infiltrates (1% to 5%), respiratory failure (1% to 5%), rhinitis (1% to 5%), sinusitis (1% to 5%), stridor (1% to 5%)

Miscellaneous: Diaphoresis (≥5%), sepsis (≥5%), flu-like syndrome (1% to 5%), infection (includes bacterial and fungal; 1% to 5%), malignancies (lymphoma/sarcoma 1% to 5%), thirst (1% to 5%)

Dental Usual Dosage Herpes simplex infections (acyclovir-resistant): Induction: I.V.: 40 mg/kg/dose every 8-12 hours for 14-21 days

Dosage

CMV retinitis: I.V.:

Induction treatment: 60 mg/kg/dose every 8 hours **or** 90 mg/kg every 12 hours for 14-21 days

Maintenance therapy: 90-120 mg/kg/day as a single daily infusion

Herpes simplex infections (acyclovir-resistant): Induction: I.V.: 40 mg/kg/dose every 8-12 hours for 14-21 days

Therapy of CMV infection in cancer patients (unlabeled use): I.V.:

Prophylaxis: 60 mg/kg every 8-12 hours for 7 days, followed by 90-120 mg/kg daily until day 100 after HSCT

Pre-emptive treatment: 60 mg/kg every 12 hours for 14 days; if CMV still detectable, continue with 90 mg/kg daily for 5 days/week for 2 additional weeks

Treatment: 90 mg/kg every 12 hours for 2 weeks, followed by 120 mg/kg daily for ≥2 weeks

Dosage adjustment in renal impairment: Induction and maintenance dosing schedules based on creatinine clearance (mL/minute/kg): See tables.

Induction Dosing of Foscarnet in Patients With Abnormal Renal Function

Cl_{cr} (mL/min/kg)	HSV Equivalent to 40 mg/kg q12h	HSV Equivalent to 40 mg/kg q8h	CMV Equivalent to 60 mg/kg q8h	CMV Equivalent to 90 mg/kg q12h
<0.4	Not recommended	Not recommended	Not recommended	Not recommended
≥0.4-0.5	20 mg/kg every 24 hours	35 mg/kg every 24 hours	50 mg/kg every 24 hours	50 mg/kg every 24 hours
>0.5-0.6	25 mg/kg every 24 hours	40 mg/kg every 24 hours	60 mg/kg every 24 hours	60 mg/kg every 24 hours
>0.6-0.8	35 mg/kg every 24 hours	25 mg/kg every 12 hours	40 mg/kg every 12 hours	80 mg/kg every 24 hours
>0.8-1.0	20 mg/kg every 12 hours	35 mg/kg every 12 hours	50 mg/kg every 12 hours	50 mg/kg every 12 hours
>1.0-1.4	30 mg/kg every 12 hours	30 mg/kg every 8 hours	45 mg/kg every 8 hours	70 mg/kg every 12 hours
>1.4	40 mg/kg every 12 hours	40 mg/kg every 8 hours	60 mg/kg every 8 hours	90 mg/kg every 12 hours

Maintenance Dosing of Foscarnet in Patients With Abnormal Renal Function

Cl_{cr} (mL/min/kg)	CMV Equivalent to 90 mg/kg q24h	CMV Equivalent to 120 mg/kg q24h
<0.4	Not recommended	Not recommended
≥0.4-0.5	50 mg/kg every 48 hours	65 mg/kg every 48 hours
>0.5-0.6	60 mg/kg every 48 hours	80 mg/kg every 48 hours
>0.6-0.8	80 mg/kg every 48 hours	105 mg/kg every 48 hours
>0.8-1.0	50 mg/kg every 24 hours	65 mg/kg every 24 hours
>1.0-1.4	70 mg/kg every 24 hours	90 mg/kg every 24 hours
>1.4	90 mg/kg every 24 hours	120 mg/kg every 24 hours

Hemodialysis:

Foscarnet is highly removed by hemodialysis (up to ~38% in 2.5 hours HD with high-flux membrane)

Doses of 50 mg/kg/dose posthemodialysis have been found to produce similar serum concentrations as doses of 90 mg/kg twice daily in patients with normal renal function

Doses of 60-90 mg/kg/dose loading dose (posthemodialysis) followed by 45-60 mg/kg/dose posthemodialysis (3 times/week) with the monitoring of weekly plasma concentrations to maintain peak plasma concentrations in the range of 400-800 µMolar have been recommended by some clinicians

Continuous arteriovenous or venovenous hemodiafiltration effects: Dose as for Cl_{cr} 10-50 mL/minute

Dosage adjustment in hepatic impairment: No dosage adjustment provided in manufacturer's labeling.

Mechanism of Action Pyrophosphate analogue which acts as a noncompetitive inhibitor of many viral RNA and DNA polymerases as well as HIV reverse transcriptase. Similar to ganciclovir, foscarnet is a virostatic agent. Foscarnet does not require activation by thymidine kinase.

Contraindications Hypersensitivity to foscarnet or any component of the formulation

Warnings/Precautions [U.S. Boxed Warning]: Indicated only for immunocompromised patients with CMV retinitis and mucocutaneous acyclovir-resistant HSV infection. [U.S. Boxed Warning]: Renal impairment occurs to some degree in the majority of patients treated with foscarnet; renal impairment may occur at any time and is usually reversible within 1 week following dose adjustment or discontinuation of therapy, however, several patients have died with renal failure within 4 weeks of stopping foscarnet; therefore, renal function should be closely monitored. To reduce the risk of nephrotoxicity and the potential to administer a relative overdose, always calculate the creatine clearance even if serum creatinine is within the normal range. Adequate hydration may reduce the risk of nephrotoxicity; the manufacturer makes specific recommendations regarding this.

Imbalance of serum electrolytes or minerals occurs in at least 15% of patients (hypocalcemia, low ionized calcium, hyper/hypophosphatemia, hypomagnesemia, or hypokalemia). Correct electrolytes before initiating therapy. Use caution when administering other medications that cause electrolyte imbalances. Patients who experience signs or symptoms of an electrolyte imbalance should be assessed immediately. **[U.S. Boxed Warning]: Seizures related to plasma electrolyte/mineral imbalance may occur;** incidence has been reported in up to 10% of HIV patients. Risk factors for seizures include impaired baseline renal function, low total serum calcium, and underlying CNS conditions. May cause anemia and granulocytopenia. May cause genital/vascular tissue irritation/ulceration; adequately hydrate and administer only into vein with adequate blood flow to minimize risk. Foscarnet is deposited in teeth and bone of young, growing animals; it has adversely affected tooth enamel development in rats.

Drug Interactions

Metabolism/Transport Effects None known.

Avoid Concomitant Use There are no known interactions where it is recommended to avoid concomitant use.

Increased Effect/Toxicity

Foscarnet may increase the levels/effects of: Highest Risk QTc-Prolonging Agents; Moderate Risk QTc-Prolonging Agents

The levels/effects of Foscarnet may be increased by: Mifepristone

Decreased Effect There are no known significant interactions involving a decrease in effect.

Pharmacodynamics/Kinetics

Half-life Elimination Elimination: ~3-4 hours; terminal: ~88 hours (due to bone deposition)

Pregnancy Risk Factor C

Pregnancy Considerations Associated with an increase in skeletal anomalies in animal studies at approximately the equivalent of 13% to 33% of the maximal daily human dose. There are no adequate and well controlled studies in pregnant women. A single case report of use during the third trimester with normal infant outcome was observed. Monitoring of amniotic fluid volumes by ultrasound is recommended weekly after 20 weeks of gestation to detect oligohydramnios.

Lactation Excretion in breast milk unknown/contraindicated

Breast-Feeding Considerations The CDC recommends **not** to breast-feed if diagnosed with HIV to avoid postnatal transmission of the virus.

Dosage Forms

Injection, solution [preservative free]: 24 mg/mL (250 mL, 500 mL)

Foscavir®: 24 mg/mL (250 mL)

Dental Comment Foscarnet is known to prolong the QT interval. The QT interval is measured as the time and distance between the Q point of the QRS complex and the end of the T wave in the ECG tracing. After adjustment for heart rate, the QT interval is defined as prolonged if it is more than 450 msec in men and 460 msec in women. A long QT syndrome was first described in the 1950s and 60s as a congenital syndrome involving QT interval prolongation and syncope and sudden death. Some of the congenital long QT syndromes were characterized by a peculiar electrocardiographic appearance of the QRS complex involving a premature atria beat followed by a pause, then a subsequent sinus beat showing marked QT prolongation and deformity. This type of cardiac arrhythmia was originally termed "torsade de pointes" (translated from the French as "twisting of the points"). Foscarnet is considered as having a risk of causing torsade de pointes. Since it is not known what effect vasoconstrictors in the local anesthetic regimen will have in patients with a known history of congenital prolonged QT interval or in patients taking any medication that prolongs the QT interval, a medical consult is suggested.

Fosfomycin (fos foe MYE sin)

Brand Names: U.S. Monurol®

Brand Names: Canada Monurol®

Pharmacologic Category Antibiotic, Miscellaneous

Use Single oral dose in the treatment of uncomplicated urinary tract infections in women due to susceptible strains of *E. coli* and *Enterococcus faecalis*

Unlabeled Use Multiple doses have been investigated for complicated urinary tract infections in men

Local Anesthetic/Vasoconstrictor Precautions No information available to require special precautions

Effects on Dental Treatment No significant effects or complications reported

Effects on Bleeding No information available to require special precautions

Adverse Effects 1% to 10%:

Central nervous system: Headache (4% to 10%), pain (2%), dizziness (1% to 2%)

Dermatologic: Rash (1%)

Endocrine and metabolic: Dysmenorrhea (3%)

Gastrointestinal: Diarrhea (9% to 10%), nausea (4% to 5%), abdominal pain (2%), dyspepsia (1% to 2%)

Genitourinary: Vaginitis (6% to 8%)

Neuromuscular & skeletal: Back pain (3%), weakness (1% to 2%)

Respiratory: Rhinitis (5%), pharyngitis (3%)

General Dosage Range Oral: *Adults (females):* 3 g once

Mechanism of Action As a phosphoric acid derivative, fosfomycin inhibits bacterial wall synthesis (bactericidal) by inactivating the enzyme, pyruvyl transferase, which is critical in the synthesis of cell walls by bacteria

Pharmacodynamics/Kinetics
Half-life Elimination 4-8 hours; Cl_{cr} <54 mL/minute: 50 hours
Time to Peak Serum: 2 hours; within 4 hours with high-fat meal
Pregnancy Risk Factor B
Pregnancy Considerations Fosfomycin crosses the placenta. Because teratogenicity was not observed in animals, fosfomycin is classified pregnancy category B. There have been several human studies using single dose therapy with fosfomycin for the treatment of asymptomatic bacteriuria during pregnancy. In these studies, fosfomycin was well-tolerated and adverse fetal effects were not observed.

Fosinopril (foe SIN oh pril)

Related Information
Cardiovascular Diseases *on page 1492*
Brand Names: Canada Apo-Fosinopril®; Jamp-Fosinopril; Monopril®; Mylan-Fosinopril; PMS-Fosinopril; RAN™-Fosinopril; Riva-Fosinopril; Teva-Fosinopril
Generic Availability (U.S.) Yes
Pharmacologic Category Angiotensin-Converting Enzyme (ACE) Inhibitor
Use Treatment of hypertension, either alone or in combination with other antihypertensive agents; treatment of heart failure (HF)
Local Anesthetic/Vasoconstrictor Precautions No information available to require special precautions
Effects on Dental Treatment Key adverse event(s) related to dental treatment: Orthostatic hypotension.
Effects on Bleeding No information available to require special precautions
Adverse Effects Note: Frequency ranges include data from hypertension and heart failure trials. Higher rates of adverse reactions have generally been noted in patients with CHF. However, the frequency of adverse effects associated with placebo is also increased in this population.

>10%: Central nervous system: Dizziness (2% to 12%)
1% to 10%:
Cardiovascular: Orthostatic hypotension (1% to 2%), palpitation (1%)
Central nervous system: Dizziness (1% to 2%; up to 12% in CHF patients), headache (3%), fatigue (1% to 2%)
Endocrine & metabolic: Hyperkalemia (2.6%)
Gastrointestinal: Diarrhea (2%), nausea/vomiting (1.2% to 2.2%)
Hepatic: Transaminases increased
Neuromuscular & skeletal: Musculoskeletal pain (<1% to 3%), noncardiac chest pain (<1% to 2%), weakness (1%)
Renal: Serum creatinine increased, renal function worsening (in patients with bilateral renal artery stenosis or hypovolemia)
Respiratory: Cough (2% to 10%)
Miscellaneous: Upper respiratory infection (2%)
>1% but ≤ frequency in patients receiving placebo: Sexual dysfunction, fever, flu-like syndrome, dyspnea, rash, headache, insomnia
Other events reported with ACE inhibitors: Neutropenia, agranulocytosis, eosinophilic pneumonitis, cardiac arrest, pancytopenia, hemolytic anemia, anemia, aplastic anemia, thrombocytopenia, acute renal failure, hepatic failure, jaundice, symptomatic hyponatremia, bullous pemphigus, exfoliative dermatitis, Stevens-Johnson syndrome. In addition, a syndrome which may include fever, myalgia, arthralgia, interstitial nephritis, vasculitis, rash, eosinophilia and positive ANA, and elevated ESR has been reported for other ACE inhibitors.

Dosage Oral:
Children ≥6 years and >50 kg: Hypertension: Initial: 5-10 mg once daily (maximum: 40 mg/day)
Adults:
Heart failure: Initial: 10 mg/day (5 mg if renal dysfunction present) and increase, as needed, to a maximum of 40 mg once daily over several weeks; usual dose: 20-40 mg/day. If hypotension, orthostasis, or azotemia occur during titration, consider decreasing concomitant diuretic dose, if any.
Hypertension: Initial: 10 mg/day; most patients are maintained on 20-40 mg/day (maximum: 80 mg/day). May need to divide the dose into two if trough effect is inadequate; discontinue the diuretic, if possible 2-3 days before initiation of therapy; resume diuretic therapy carefully, if needed.
Dosing adjustment/comments in renal impairment: None needed since hepatobiliary elimination compensates adequately diminished renal elimination.
Hemodialysis: Moderately dializable (20% to 50%)
Mechanism of Action Competitive inhibitor of angiotensin-converting enzyme (ACE); prevents conversion of angiotensin I to angiotensin II, a potent vasoconstrictor; results in lower levels of angiotensin II which causes an increase in plasma renin activity and a reduction in aldosterone secretion; a CNS mechanism may also be involved in hypotensive effect as angiotensin II increases adrenergic outflow from CNS; vasoactive kallikreins may be decreased in conversion to active hormones by ACE inhibitors, thus reducing blood pressure
Contraindications Hypersensitivity to fosinopril, any other ACE inhibitor, or any component of the formulation; angioedema related to previous treatment with an ACE inhibitor; concomitant use with aliskiren in patients with diabetes mellitus
Warnings/Precautions Anaphylactic reactions may occur rarely with ACE inhibitors. At any time during treatment (especially following first dose), angioedema may occur rarely with ACE inhibitors; it may involve the head and neck (potentially compromising airway) or the intestine (presenting with abdominal pain). African-Americans may be at an increased risk and patients with idiopathic or hereditary angioedema may be at an increased risk. Prolonged frequent monitoring may be required especially if tongue, glottis, or larynx are involved as they are associated with airway obstruction. Patients with a history of airway surgery may have a higher risk of airway obstruction. Aggressive early and appropriate management is critical. Use in patients with previous angioedema associated with ACE inhibitor therapy is contraindicated. Severe anaphylactoid reactions may be seen during hemodialysis (eg, CVVHD) with high-flux dialysis membranes (eg, AN69), and rarely, during low density lipoprotein apheresis with dextran sulfate cellulose. Rare cases of anaphylactoid reactions have been reported in patients undergoing sensitization treatment with hymenoptera (bee, wasp) venom while receiving ACE inhibitors.

Symptomatic hypotension with or without syncope can occur with ACE inhibitors (usually with the first several doses); effects are most often observed in volume-depleted patients; correct volume depletion prior to initiation; close monitoring of patient is required especially with initial dosing and dosing increases; blood pressure must be lowered at a rate appropriate for the patient's clinical condition. Initiation of therapy in patients with ischemic heart disease or cerebrovascular disease warrants close observation due to the potential consequences posed by falling blood pressure (eg, MI, stroke). Use with caution in hypertrophic cardiomyopathy with outflow tract obstruction, severe aortic stenosis, or before, during, or immediately after major surgery. **[U.S. Boxed Warning]: Based on human data, ACEIs can cause injury and death to the developing fetus when used in the second and third trimesters. ACEIs should be discontinued as soon as possible once pregnancy is detected.**

Hyperkalemia may occur with ACE inhibitors; risk factors include renal dysfunction, diabetes mellitus, concomitant use of potassium-sparing diuretics, potassium supplements, and/or potassium-containing salts. Use cautiously, if at all, with these agents and monitor potassium closely. Cough may occur with ACE inhibitors. Other causes of cough should be considered (eg, pulmonary congestion in patients with heart failure) and excluded prior to discontinuation.

May be associated with deterioration of renal function and/or increases in serum creatinine, particularly in patients with low renal blood flow (eg, renal artery stenosis, heart failure) whose glomerular filtration rate (GFR) is dependent on efferent arteriolar vasoconstriction by angiotensin II; deterioration may result in oliguria, acute renal failure, and progressive azotemia. Small increases in serum creatinine may occur following initiation; consider discontinuation only in patients with progressive and/or significant deterioration in renal function. Use with caution in patients with unstented unilateral/bilateral renal artery stenosis. When unstented bilateral renal artery stenosis is present, use is generally avoided due to the elevated risk of deterioration in renal function unless possible benefits outweigh risks. Concomitant use of an angiotensin receptor blocker (ARB) or renin inhibitor (eg, aliskiren) is associated with an increased risk of hypotension, hyperkalemia, and renal dysfunction; concomitant use with aliskiren should be avoided in patients with GFR <60 mL/minute and is contraindicated in patients with diabetes mellitus (regardless of GFR).

Rare toxicities associated with ACE inhibitors include cholestatic jaundice (which may progress to fulminant hepatic necrosis), agranulocytosis, neutropenia or leukopenia with myeloid hypoplasia. Patients with collagen vascular diseases (especially with concomitant renal impairment) or renal impairment alone may be at increased risk for hematologic toxicity; periodically monitor CBC with differential in these patients.

Drug Interactions
Metabolism/Transport Effects None known.
Avoid Concomitant Use There are no known interactions where it is recommended to avoid concomitant use.
Increased Effect/Toxicity
Fosinopril may increase the levels/effects of: Allopurinol; Amifostine; Antihypertensives; AzaTHIOprine; CycloSPORINE (Systemic); Ferric Gluconate; Gold Sodium Thiomalate; Hypotensive Agents; Iron Dextran Complex; Lithium; Nonsteroidal Anti-Inflammatory Agents; RiTUXimab; Sodium Phosphates

The levels/effects of Fosinopril may be increased by: Alfuzosin; Aliskiren; Angiotensin II Receptor Blockers; Canagliflozin; Diazoxide; DPP-IV Inhibitors; Eplerenone; Everolimus; Herbs (Hypotensive Properties);

Loop Diuretics; MAO Inhibitors; Pentoxifylline; Phosphodiesterase 5 Inhibitors; Potassium Salts; Potassium-Sparing Diuretics; Prostacyclin Analogues; Sirolimus; Temsirolimus; Thiazide Diuretics; TiZANidine; Tolvaptan; Trimethoprim
Decreased Effect
The levels/effects of Fosinopril may be decreased by: Antacids; Aprotinin; Herbs (Hypertensive Properties); Icatibant; Lanthanum; Methylphenidate; Nonsteroidal Anti-Inflammatory Agents; Salicylates; Yohimbine
Ethanol/Nutrition/Herb Interactions
Food: Potassium supplements and/or potassium-containing salts may cause or worsen hyperkalemia. Management: Consult prescriber before consuming a potassium-rich diet, potassium supplements, or salt substitutes.
Herb/Nutraceutical: Some herbal medications may worsen hypertension (eg, licorice); others may increase the antihypertensive effect of fosinopril (eg, shepherd's purse). Management: Avoid bayberry, blue cohosh, cayenne, ephedra, ginger, ginseng (American), kola, licorice, and yohimbe. Avoid black cohosh, california poppy, coleus, golden seal, hawthorn, mistletoe, periwinkle, quinine, and shepherd's purse.
Dietary Considerations Should not take a potassium salt supplement without the advice of healthcare provider.
Pharmacodynamics/Kinetics
Onset of Action 1 hour
Duration of Action 24 hours
Half-life Elimination Serum (fosinoprilat): 12 hours
Time to Peak Serum: ~3 hours
Pregnancy Risk Factor C (1st trimester); D (2nd and 3rd trimesters)
Pregnancy Considerations Due to adverse events observed in some animal studies, fosinopril is considered pregnancy category C during the first trimester. Based on human data, fosinopril is considered pregnancy category D if used during the second and third trimesters (per the manufacturer; however, one study suggests that fetal injury may occur at anytime during pregnancy). First trimester exposure to ACE inhibitors may cause major congenital malformations. An increased risk of cardiovascular and/or central nervous system malformations was observed in one study; however, an increased risk of teratogenic events was not observed in other studies. Second and third trimester use of an ACE inhibitor is associated with oligohydramnios. Oligohydramnios due to decreased fetal renal function may lead to fetal limb contractures, craniofacial deformation, and hypoplastic lung development. The use of ACE inhibitors during the second and third trimesters is also associated with anuria, hypotension, renal failure (reversible or irreversible), skull hypoplasia, and death in the fetus/neonate. Chronic maternal hypertension itself is also associated with adverse events in the fetus/infant. ACE inhibitors are not recommended during pregnancy to treat maternal hypertension or heart failure. Those who are planning a pregnancy should be considered for other medication options if an ACE inhibitor is currently prescribed or the ACE inhibitor should be discontinued as soon as possible once pregnancy is detected. The exposed fetus should be monitored for fetal growth, amniotic fluid volume, and organ formation. Infants exposed to an ACE inhibitor *in utero*, especially during the second and third trimester, should be monitored for hyperkalemia, hypotension, and oliguria.

◀ **[U.S. Boxed Warning]:** Based on human data, ACE inhibitors can cause injury and death to the developing fetus when used in the second and third trimesters. ACE inhibitors should be discontinued as soon as possible once pregnancy is detected.

Lactation Enters breast milk/not recommended

Breast-Feeding Considerations Fosinoprilat is excreted in breast milk. Breast-feeding is not recommended by the manufacturer.

Dosage Forms
Tablet, oral: 10 mg, 20 mg, 40 mg

Fosinopril and Hydrochlorothiazide
(foe SIN oh pril & hye droe klor oh THYE a zide)

Related Information
Fosinopril on page 634
Hydrochlorothiazide on page 687

Brand Names: U.S. Monopril-HCT® [DSC]
Brand Names: Canada Monopril-HCT®
Pharmacologic Category Angiotensin-Converting Enzyme (ACE) Inhibitor; Diuretic, Thiazide
Use Treatment of hypertension; not indicated for first-line treatment

Local Anesthetic/Vasoconstrictor Precautions No information available to require special precautions
Effects on Dental Treatment No significant effects or complications reported
Effects on Bleeding No information available to require special precautions
Adverse Effects Reactions reported with combination product. Also see individual agents.
2% to 10%:
Central nervous system: Headache (7%, less than placebo), fatigue (4%), dizziness (3%), orthostatic hypotension (2%)
Neuromuscular & skeletal: Musculoskeletal pain (2%)
Respiratory: Cough (6%), upper respiratory infection (2%, less than placebo)

General Dosage Range Oral: *Adults:* Fosinopril 10-80 mg and hydrochlorothiazide 12.5-50 mg once daily

Mechanism of Action Fosinopril is a competitive inhibitor of angiotensin-converting enzyme (ACE); prevents conversion of angiotensin I to angiotensin II, a potent vasoconstrictor; results in lower levels of angiotensin II which causes an increase in plasma renin activity and a reduction in aldosterone secretion; a CNS mechanism may also be involved in hypotensive effect as angiotensin II increases adrenergic outflow from CNS; vasoactive kallikreins may be decreased in conversion to active hormones by ACE inhibitors, thus reducing blood pressure. Hydrochlorothiazide inhibits sodium reabsorption in the distal tubules causing increased excretion of sodium and water as well as potassium and hydrogen ions.

Pregnancy Risk Factor C (1st trimester); D (2nd and 3rd trimester)

Pregnancy Considerations [U.S. Boxed Warning]: Based on human data, ACEIs can cause injury and death to the developing fetus when used in the second and third trimesters. ACEIs should be discontinued as soon as possible once pregnancy is detected. See individual agents.

Fosphenytoin (FOS fen i toyn)

Related Information
Phenytoin on page 1088

Brand Names: Canada Cerebyx®
Pharmacologic Category Anticonvulsant, Hydantoin
Use Used for the control of generalized convulsive status epilepticus and prevention and treatment of seizures occurring during neurosurgery; indicated for short-term parenteral administration when other means of phenytoin administration are unavailable, inappropriate, or deemed less advantageous (the safety and effectiveness of fosphenytoin use for more than 5 days has not been systematically evaluated)

Local Anesthetic/Vasoconstrictor Precautions No information available to require special precautions
Effects on Dental Treatment Key adverse event(s) related to dental treatment: Tongue disorder and dry mouth.
Effects on Bleeding No information available to require special precautions
Adverse Effects The more important adverse clinical events caused by the I.V. use of fosphenytoin or phenytoin are cardiovascular collapse and/or central nervous system depression. Hypotension can occur when either drug is administered rapidly by the I.V. route.

The adverse clinical events most commonly observed with the use of fosphenytoin in clinical trials were nystagmus, dizziness, pruritus, paresthesia, headache, somnolence, and ataxia. Paresthesia and pruritus were seen more often following fosphenytoin (versus phenytoin) administration and occurred more often with I.V. fosphenytoin than with I.M. administration. These events were dose and rate related (adult doses ≥15 mg/kg at a rate of 150 mg PE/minute) and occurred in up to 64% of patients. These sensations, generally described as itching, burning, or tingling are usually not at the infusion site. The location of the discomfort varied with the groin mentioned most frequently. The paresthesia and pruritus were transient events that occurred within several minutes of the start of infusion and generally resolved within 10 minutes after completion of infusion.

Transient pruritus, tinnitus, nystagmus, somnolence, and ataxia occurred 2-3 times more often at adult doses ≥15 mg/kg and rates ≥150 mg PE/minute.

Also refer to phenytoin monograph for additional adverse reactions.

I.V. and I.M. administration (as reported in clinical trials):
1% to 10%:
Cardiovascular: Facial edema, hypertension
Central nervous system: Chills, fever, intracranial hypertension, nervousness
Endocrine & metabolic: Hypokalemia
Neuromuscular & skeletal: Hyperreflexia, myasthenia

I.V. administration (maximum dose/rate):
>10%:
Central nervous system: Paresthesia (4% to 64%), nystagmus (44%), dizziness (31%), somnolence (20%), ataxia (11%)
Dermatologic: Pruritus (49% to 64%)
1% to 10%:
Cardiovascular: Hypotension (7%), vasodilation (6%), tachycardia (2%)

Central nervous system: Stupor (7%), extrapyramidal syndrome (4%), incoordination (4%), agitation (3%), tremor (3%), brain edema (2%), headache (2%), hypoesthesia (2%), vertigo (2%)

Gastrointestinal: Nausea (9%), tongue disorder (4%), xerostomia (4%), taste perversion (3%), vomiting (2%)

Neuromuscular & skeletal: Pelvic pain (4%), back pain (2%), dysarthria (2%), weakness (2%)

Ocular: Diplopia (3%), amblyopia (2%)

Otic: Tinnitus (9%), deafness (2%)

I.M. administration (substitute for oral phenytoin):
>10%: Central nervous system: Nystagmus (15%)
1% to 10%:
Central nervous system: Tremor (10%), headache (9%), ataxia (8%), incoordination (8%), somnolence (7%), dizziness (5%), paresthesia (4%), reflexes decreased (3%)
Dermatologic: Bruising (7%), pruritus (3%)
Gastrointestinal: Nausea (5%), vomiting (3%)
Neuromuscular & skeletal: Weakness (4%)

General Dosage Range

I.M.: *Adults:* Loading: 10-20 mg PE/kg; Maintenance: 4-6 mg PE/kg/day

I.V.: *Adults:* Loading: 10-20 mg PE/kg; Maintenance: 4-6 mg PE/kg/day

Mechanism of Action Diphosphate ester salt of phenytoin which acts as a water soluble prodrug of phenytoin; after administration, plasma esterases convert fosphenytoin to phosphate, formaldehyde, and phenytoin as the active moiety; phenytoin works by stabilizing neuronal membranes and decreasing seizure activity by increasing efflux or decreasing influx of sodium ions across cell membranes in the motor cortex during generation of nerve impulses

Pharmacodynamics/Kinetics

Half-life Elimination Fosphenytoin: Conversion half-life: 15 minutes; Phenytoin: Variable (mean: 12-29 hours); kinetics of phenytoin are saturable

Time to Peak Conversion to phenytoin: Following I.V. administration (maximum rate of administration): 15 minutes; following I.M. administration, peak phenytoin levels are reached in 3 hours; therapeutic phenytoin concentrations may be achieved as early as 5-20 minutes following I.M. (gluteal) administration (Pryor, 2001)

Pregnancy Risk Factor D

Pregnancy Considerations Fosphenytoin is the prodrug of phenytoin. Refer to Phenytoin monograph for additional information.

Fospropofol (fos PROE po fole)

Brand Names: U.S. Lusedra™ [DSC]

Generic Availability (U.S.) No

Pharmacologic Category Sedative

Use Monitored anesthesia care (MAC) sedation in patients undergoing diagnostic or therapeutic procedures

Local Anesthetic/Vasoconstrictor Precautions No information available to require special precautions

Effects on Dental Treatment No significant effects or complications reported

Effects on Bleeding No information available to require special precautions

Adverse Effects

>10%:
Dermatologic: Pruritus (see **"Note"** below; 8% to 28%)
Neuromuscular & skeletal: Paresthesia (see **"Note"** below; 52% to 74%)
Respiratory: Hypoxemia (1% to 11%)
1% to 10%:
Cardiovascular: Hypotension (2% to 7%)
Central nervous system: Headache (1% to 2%)
Gastrointestinal: Nausea (≤4%), vomiting (≤3%)
Miscellaneous: Procedural pain (≤2%)

Note: Paresthesias (including perineal discomfort or burning sensation) and pruritus (including genital, perineal, and generalized pruritus) are mostly limited to the first 5 minutes of administration and usually described as mild-moderate in intensity. No pretreatments are helpful in reducing the incidence of these adverse effects.

Dosage Monitored anesthesia care (MAC) sedation: I.V.:
Note: Onset of effect is delayed as compared to propofol-emulsion due to need for conversion to active component. If <60 kg, base dosing on 60 kg; however, lower doses may be used to achieve lower levels of sedation. If >90 kg, base dosing on 90 kg.

Healthy adults <65 years or with mild systemic disease (ASA-PS1 or -PS2): *Standard dosing regimen:* Initial: 6.5 mg/kg (maximum initial dose: 577.5 mg or 16.5 mL), followed by supplemental doses of 1.6 mg/kg (maximum supplemental dose: 140 mg or 4 mL) no more frequently than every 4 minutes as needed to achieve desired level of sedation.

Elderly patients ≥65 years or patients with severe systemic disease (ASA-PS3 or -PS4): *Modified dosing regimen:* Initial: 4.9 mg/kg (maximum initial dose: 437.5 mg or 12.5 mL), followed by supplemental doses of 1.2 mg/kg (maximum supplemental dose: 105 mg or 3 mL) no more frequently than every 4 minutes as needed to achieve desired level of sedation.

Dosage adjustment in renal impairment: No dosage adjustment recommended. Use with caution in patients with severe renal impairment (Cl_{cr} <30 mL/minute); limited safety and efficacy data available in these patients.

Dosage adjustment in hepatic impairment: No dosage adjustment recommended. Use with caution in patients with hepatic impairment; has not been adequately studied in this population.

Mechanism of Action Fospropofol disodium is a prodrug of propofol. Propofol interacts with the $GABA_A$ receptor, which is the presumed mechanism of action whereby it produces a sedative/hypnotic effect. Propofol is an alkyl-phenolic compound with intravenous general anesthetic properties.

Contraindications There are no contraindications in the manufacturer's FDA approved labeling.

Note: Applicable contraindications to propofol include: Hypersensitivity to propofol; when general anesthesia or sedation is contraindicated

Warnings/Precautions The major cardiovascular effect is hypotension; use with caution in patients who are hemodynamically unstable, hypovolemic, have abnormally low vascular tone (eg, sepsis) or compromised myocardial function (eg, heart failure). The **onset of action will be delayed** due to need for conversion to the active metabolite, propofol. If supplemental doses are administered before full effect occurs, the risk of dose-stacking may be elevated resulting in deeper sedation than intended.

◀ Use requires careful patient monitoring; should only be administered by persons trained in the administration of general anesthesia and not involved in the conduct of the diagnostic or therapeutic procedure. Sedated patients should be continuously monitored, and facilities for maintenance of a patent airway, providing artificial ventilation, administering supplemental oxygen, and instituting cardiovascular resuscitation must be immediately available. Patients should be continuously monitored during sedation and through the recovery process for early signs of hypotension, apnea, airway obstruction, and/or oxygen desaturation. Use to induce moderate (conscious) sedation in patients warrants monitoring equivalent to that seen with general anesthesia. May cause loss of spontaneous respiration and/or hypoxemia; supplemental oxygen is recommended for all patients receiving fospropofol; monitor patient closely. The risk of these effects may be increased with the concomitant use of opioids and/or other sedatives. May cause patients to become unresponsive or minimally responsive to vigorous tactile or painful stimuli.

Use lower doses in patients ≥65 years and/or ASA-PS 3/4 patients to reduce the incidence of unwanted cardiorespiratory and neurologic depressive events. Use with caution in patients with hepatic impairment or severe renal impairment (Cl_cr <30 mL/minute). Use with caution in patients with respiratory disease; risk of cardiorespiratory depression may be increased. Use with caution in patients with a history of epilepsy or seizures; seizure may occur during recovery phase.

Concomitant use of opioids/sedative-hypnotics may lead to increased sedative or respiratory depressant effects of fospropofol, more pronounced decreases in systolic, diastolic, and mean arterial pressures, heart rate, and cardiac output. Fospropofol lacks analgesic properties; pain management requires specific use of analgesic agents. Fospropofol should only be used in pregnancy if clearly needed. Not recommended for use in obstetrics, including cesarean section deliveries. Safety and efficacy have not been established in patients <18 years of age.

Drug Interactions

Metabolism/Transport Effects Substrate of CYP1A2 (minor), CYP2B6 (major), CYP2C9 (minor), CYP3A4 (minor); **Note:** Assignment of Major/Minor substrate status based on clinically relevant drug interaction potential; **Inhibits** CYP1A2 (weak), CYP2C9 (weak), CYP2E1 (weak), CYP3A4 (weak)

Avoid Concomitant Use

Avoid concomitant use of Fospropofol with any of the following: Pimozide

Increased Effect/Toxicity

Fospropofol may increase the levels/effects of: ARIPiprazole; Lomitapide; Pimozide; Ropivacaine

The levels/effects of Fospropofol may be increased by: Alfentanil; CYP2B6 Inhibitors (Moderate); CYP2B6 Inhibitors (Strong); Quazepam

Decreased Effect There are no known significant interactions involving a decrease in effect.

Pharmacodynamics/Kinetics

Onset of Action Bolus (dose dependent): Attainment of adequate sedation was achieved between 2-28 minutes (median: 8 minutes)

Duration of Action Duration of sedation: Time to fully alert: ≤1 hour (median: 5 minutes)

Half-life Elimination
Fospropofol: 0.8-0.96 hours
Propofol: 0.85-1.41 hours
Time to Peak Propofol (from fospropofol): Median: 12 minutes
Pregnancy Risk Factor B
Pregnancy Considerations Adverse events were not observed in animal reproduction studies; however, fospropofol should only be used in pregnancy if clearly needed. Fospropofol is not recommended for obstetrics, including cesarean section deliveries. It is not known if fospropofol crosses the placenta. However, propofol crosses the placenta, and therefore, may be associated with neonatal CNS and respiratory depression.
Lactation Propofol (the active metabolite of fospropofol) enters breast milk/not recommended
Controlled Substance C-IV
References

Cohen LB, "Clinical Trial: a dose-response study of fospropofol disodium for moderate sedation during colonoscopy," *Aliment Pharmacol Ther*, 2008, 27(7):597-608.
Silvestri GA, Vincent BD, Wahidi MM, et al, "A Phase 3, Randomized, Double-blind, Study to Assess the Efficacy and Safety of Fospropofol Disodium Injection for Moderate Sedation in Patients Undergoing Flexible Bronchoscopy," *Chest*, 2009, 135(1):41-7.

Frovatriptan (froe va TRIP tan)

Related Information
Temporomandibular Dysfunction (TMD), Chronic Pain, and Fibromyalgia *on page 1590*
Brand Names: U.S. Frova®
Brand Names: Canada Frova®
Generic Availability (U.S.) No
Pharmacologic Category Antimigraine Agent; Serotonin 5-HT_{1B, 1D} Receptor Agonist
Use Acute treatment of migraine with or without aura
Unlabeled Use Short-term prevention of menstrually-associated migraines (MAMs)
Local Anesthetic/Vasoconstrictor Precautions No information available to require special precautions
Effects on Dental Treatment No significant effects or complications reported
Effects on Bleeding No information available to require special precautions
Adverse Effects 1% to 10%:
Cardiovascular: Flushing (4%), chest pain (2%), palpitation (1%)
Central nervous system: Dizziness (8%), fatigue (5%), headache (4%), hot or cold sensation (3%), somnolence (≥2%), anxiety (1%), dysesthesia (1%), hypoesthesia (1%), insomnia (1%), pain (1%)
Gastrointestinal: Xerostomia (3%), nausea (≥2%), dyspepsia (2%), abdominal pain (1%), diarrhea (1%), vomiting (1%)
Neuromuscular & skeletal: Paresthesia (4%), skeletal pain (3%)
Ocular: Vision abnormal (1%)
Otic: Tinnitus (1%)
Respiratory: Rhinitis (1%), sinusitis (1%)
Miscellaneous: Diaphoresis (1%)
Dosage Oral: Adults: Migraine:
U.S. labeling: 2.5 mg; if headache recurs, a second dose may be given if first dose provided relief and at least 2 hours have elapsed since the first dose (maximum daily dose: 7.5 mg)
Canadian labeling: 2.5 mg; if headache recurs, a second dose may be given if first dose provided relief and at least 4 hours have elapsed since the first dose (maximum daily dose: 5 mg)

Note: The safety of treating more than 4 migraines/month has not been established.

Dosage adjustment in renal impairment: No adjustment necessary

Dosage adjustment in hepatic impairment: No adjustment necessary in mild-to-moderate hepatic impairment; use with caution in severe impairment (has not been studied in severe impairment).
Canadian labeling (not in U.S. labeling): Use is contraindicated in severe hepatic impairment.

Mechanism of Action Selective agonist for serotonin (5-HT$_{1B}$ and 5-HT$_{1D}$ receptors) in cranial arteries; causes vasoconstriction and reduces sterile inflammation associated with antidromic neuronal transmission correlating with relief of migraine.

Contraindications Hypersensitivity to frovatriptan or any component of the formulation; patients with ischemic heart disease or signs or symptoms of ischemic heart disease (including Prinzmetal's angina, angina pectoris, myocardial infarction, silent myocardial ischemia); cerebrovascular syndromes (including strokes, transient ischemic attacks); peripheral vascular syndromes (including ischemic bowel disease); uncontrolled hypertension; use within 24 hours of ergotamine derivatives; use within 24 hours of another 5-HT$_1$ agonist; management of hemiplegic or basilar migraine

Canadian labeling: Additional contraindications (not in U.S. labeling): Cardiac arrhythmias, valvular heart disease, congenital heart disease, atherosclerotic disease; management of ophthalmoplegic migraine; severe hepatic impairment

Warnings/Precautions Not intended for migraine prophylaxis, or treatment of cluster headaches, hemiplegic or basilar migraines. Rule out underlying neurologic disease in patients with atypical headache, migraine (with no prior history of migraine) or inadequate clinical response to initial dosing. Cardiac events (coronary artery vasospasm, transient ischemia, MI, ventricular tachycardia/fibrillation, cardiac arrest, and death), cerebral/subarachnoid hemorrhage, stroke, peripheral vascular ischemia, and colonic ischemia have been reported with 5-HT$_1$ agonist administration. Patients who experience sensations of chest pain/pressure/tightness or symptoms suggestive of angina following dosing should be evaluated for coronary artery disease or Prinzmetal's angina before receiving additional doses; if dosing is resumed and similar symptoms recur, monitor with ECG. May cause vasospastic reactions resulting in colonic, peripheral, or coronary ischemia. Do not give to patients with risk factors for CAD until a cardiovascular evaluation has been performed; if evaluation is satisfactory, the healthcare provider should administer the first dose (consider ECG monitoring) and cardiovascular status should be periodically evaluated. Significant elevation in blood pressure, including hypertensive crisis, has also been reported on rare occasions in patients using other 5-HT$_{1D}$ agonists with and without a history of hypertension. May lower seizure threshold, use caution in epilepsy or structural brain lesions. Symptoms of agitation, confusion, hallucinations, hyper-reflexia, myoclonus, shivering, and tachycardia (serotonin syndrome) may occur with concomitant proserotonergic drugs (ie, SSRIs/SNRIs or triptans) or agents which reduce frovatriptan's metabolism. Concurrent use of serotonin precursors (eg, tryptophan) is not recommended. If concomitant administration with SSRIs is warranted, monitor closely, especially at initiation and with dose increases. Safety and efficacy in pediatric patients have not been established.

Drug Interactions
Metabolism/Transport Effects Substrate of CYP1A2 (minor); **Note:** Assignment of Major/Minor substrate status based on clinically relevant drug interaction potential

Avoid Concomitant Use
Avoid concomitant use of Frovatriptan with any of the following: Ergot Derivatives

Increased Effect/Toxicity
Frovatriptan may increase the levels/effects of: Ergot Derivatives; Metoclopramide; Serotonin Modulators

The levels/effects of Frovatriptan may be increased by: Antipsychotics; Ergot Derivatives

Decreased Effect There are no known significant interactions involving a decrease in effect.

Ethanol/Nutrition/Herb Interactions Food: Food does not affect frovatriptan bioavailability.

Pharmacodynamics/Kinetics
Half-life Elimination ~26 hours
Time to Peak 2-4 hours

Pregnancy Risk Factor C

Pregnancy Considerations There are no adequate and well-controlled studies using frovatriptan in pregnant women. Use only if potential benefit to the mother outweighs the potential risk to the fetus.

Lactation Excretion in breast milk unknown/use caution

Breast-Feeding Considerations It is not known if frovatriptan is excreted in breast milk. The manufacturer recommends that caution be exercised when administering frovatriptan to nursing women.

Dosage Forms
Tablet, oral:
Frova®: 2.5 mg

Fructose, Dextrose, and Phosphoric Acid (FRUK tose, DEKS trose, & foss FOR ik AS id)

Related Information
Dextrose on page 407
Brand Names: U.S. Emetrol® [OTC]; Formula EM [OTC]; Kalmz [OTC]; Nausea Relief [OTC]; Nausetrol® [OTC]

Pharmacologic Category Antiemetic

Use Relief of nausea associated with upset stomach that occurs with intestinal or stomach flu, and food indiscretions

Local Anesthetic/Vasoconstrictor Precautions No information available to require special precautions

Effects on Dental Treatment No significant effects or complications reported

Effects on Bleeding No information available to require special precautions

General Dosage Range Oral:
Children ≥2-12 years: 5-10 mL every 15 minutes as needed; do not take for more than 1 hour (5 doses)
Children ≥12 years and Adults: 15-30 mL every 15 minutes as needed; do not take for more than 1 hour (5 doses)

Fulvestrant (fool VES trant)

Brand Names: U.S. Faslodex®
Brand Names: Canada Faslodex®
Pharmacologic Category Antineoplastic Agent, Estrogen Receptor Antagonist

Use Treatment of hormone receptor positive metastatic breast cancer in postmenopausal women with disease progression following antiestrogen therapy

Local Anesthetic/Vasoconstrictor Precautions No information available to require special precautions

Effects on Dental Treatment No significant effects or complications reported

Effects on Bleeding No information available to require special precautions

Adverse Effects Adverse reactions reported with 500 mg dose.

>10%:

Endocrine & metabolic: Hot flushes (7% to 13%)

Hepatic: Alkaline phosphatase increased (>15%; grades 3/4: 1% to 2%), transaminases increased (>15%; grades 3/4: 1% to 2%)

Local: Injection site pain (12% to 14%)

Neuromuscular & skeletal: Joint disorders (14% to 19%)

1% to 10%:

Cardiovascular: Ischemic disorder (1%)

Central nervous system: Fatigue (8%), headache (8%)

Gastrointestinal: Nausea (10%), anorexia (6%), vomiting (6%), constipation (5%), weight gain (≤1%)

Genitourinary: Urinary tract infection (2% to 4%)

Neuromuscular & skeletal: Bone pain (9%), arthralgia (8%), back pain (8%), extremity pain (7%), musculoskeletal pain (6%), weakness (6%)

Respiratory: Cough (5%), dyspnea (4%)

General Dosage Range Dosage adjustment recommended in patients with hepatic impairment

I.M.: *Adults (postmenopausal women):* Initial: 500 mg on days 1, 15, and 29; Maintenance: 500 mg once monthly

Mechanism of Action Estrogen receptor antagonist; competitively binds to estrogen receptors on tumors and other tissue targets, producing a nuclear complex that causes a dose-related down-regulation of estrogen receptors and inhibits tumor growth.

Pharmacodynamics/Kinetics

Duration of Action I.M.: Steady state concentrations reached within first month, when administered with additional dose given 2 weeks following the initial dose; plasma levels maintained for at least 1 month

Half-life Elimination 250 mg: ~40 days

Pregnancy Risk Factor D

Pregnancy Considerations Fetal loss and abnormalities were observed in animal studies. Approved for use only in postmenopausal women. If used prior to confirmed menopause, women of reproductive potential should be advised not to become pregnant.

Furosemide (fyoor OH se mide)

Related Information

Cardiovascular Diseases *on page 1492*

Brand Names: U.S. Lasix®

Brand Names: Canada Apo-Furosemide®; AVA-Furosemide; Bio-Furosemide; Dom-Furosemide; Furosemide Injection Sandoz Standard; Furosemide Injection, USP; Furosemide Special; Furosemide Special Injection; Lasix®; Lasix® Special; Novo-Semide; NTP-Furosemide; Nu-Furosemide; PMS-Furosemide; Teva-Furosemide

Generic Availability (U.S.) Yes

Pharmacologic Category Diuretic, Loop

Use Management of edema associated with heart failure and hepatic or renal disease; acute pulmonary edema; treatment of hypertension (alone or in combination with other antihypertensives)

Canadian labeling: Additional use: Furosemide Special Injection and Lasix® Special (products not available in the U.S.): Adjunctive treatment of oliguria in patients with severe renal impairment

Local Anesthetic/Vasoconstrictor Precautions No information available to require special precautions

Effects on Dental Treatment No significant effects or complications reported

Effects on Bleeding No information available to require special precautions

Adverse Effects Frequency not defined.

Cardiovascular: Acute hypotension, chronic aortitis, necrotizing angiitis, orthostatic hypotension, vasculitis

Central nervous system: Dizziness, fever, headache, hepatic encephalopathy, lightheadedness, restlessness, vertigo

Dermatologic: Bullous pemphigoid, cutaneous vasculitis, drug rash with eosinophilia and systemic symptoms (DRESS), erythema multiforme, exanthematous pustulosis (generalized), exfoliative dermatitis, photosensitivity, pruritus, purpura, rash, Stevens-Johnson syndrome, toxic epidermal necrolysis, urticaria

Endocrine & metabolic: Cholesterol and triglycerides increased, glucose tolerance test altered, gout, hyperglycemia, hyperuricemia, hypocalcemia, hypochloremia, hypokalemia, hypomagnesemia, hyponatremia, metabolic alkalosis

Gastrointestinal: Anorexia, constipation, cramping, diarrhea, nausea, oral and gastric irritation, pancreatitis, vomiting

Genitourinary: Urinary bladder spasm, urinary frequency

Hematological: Agranulocytosis (rare), anemia, aplastic anemia (rare), eosinophilia, hemolytic anemia, leukopenia, thrombocytopenia

Hepatic: Intrahepatic cholestatic jaundice, ischemic hepatitis, liver enzymes increased

Local: Injection site pain (following I.M. injection), thrombophlebitis

Neuromuscular & skeletal: Muscle spasm, paresthesia, weakness

Ocular: Blurred vision, xanthopsia

Otic: Hearing impairment (reversible or permanent with rapid I.V. or I.M. administration), tinnitus

Renal: Allergic interstitial nephritis, fall in glomerular filtration rate and renal blood flow (due to overdiuresis), glycosuria, transient rise in BUN

Miscellaneous: Anaphylaxis (rare), exacerbate or activate systemic lupus erythematosus

Dosage

Infants and Children: Edema, heart failure:

Oral: Initial: 2 mg/kg/dose increased in increments of 1-2 mg/kg/dose with each succeeding dose at intervals of 6-8 hours until a satisfactory response is achieved; maximum dose: 6 mg/kg/dose

I.M., I.V.: Initial: 1 mg/kg/dose; if response not adequate, may increase dose in increments of 1 mg/kg/dose and administer not sooner than 2 hours after previous dose, until a satisfactory response is achieved; may administer maintenance dose at intervals of every 6-12 hours; maximum dose: 6 mg/kg/dose

Children 1-17 years: Hypertension, resistant (unlabeled; AAP, 2004): Oral: Initial: 0.5-2 mg/kg/dose once or twice daily; maximum dose: 6 mg/kg/dose

Adults:

Edema, heart failure:

Oral: Initial: 20-80 mg/dose; if response is not adequate, may repeat the same dose or increase dose in increments of 20-40 mg/dose at intervals of 6-8 hours; may be titrated up to 600 mg/day with severe edematous states; usual maintenance dose interval is once or twice daily. **Note:** Dosing frequency may be adjusted based on patient-specific diuretic needs.

I.M., I.V.: Initial: 20-40 mg/dose; if response is not adequate, may repeat the same dose or increase dose in increments of 20 mg/dose and administer 1-2 hours after previous dose (maximum dose: 200 mg/dose). Individually determined dose should then be given once or twice daily although some patients may initially require dosing as frequent as every 6 hours. **Note:** ACC/AHA 2009 guidelines for heart failure recommend a maximum single dose of 160-200 mg.

Continuous I.V. infusion (Howard, 2001; Hunt, 2009): Initial: I.V. bolus dose 20-40 mg over 1-2 minutes, followed by continuous I.V. infusion doses of 10-40 mg/hour. If urine output is <1 mL/kg/hour, double as necessary to a maximum of 80-160 mg/hour. The risk associated with higher infusion rates (80-160 mg/hour) must be weighed against alternative strategies. **Note:** ACC/AHA 2009 guidelines for heart failure recommend 40 mg I.V. load, then 10-40 mg/hour infusion.

Acute pulmonary edema: I.V.: 40 mg over 1-2 minutes. If response not adequate within 1 hour, may increase dose to 80 mg. **Note:** ACC/AHA 2009 guidelines for heart failure recommend a maximum single dose of 160-200 mg.

Hypertension, resistant (Chobanian, 2003; JNC 7): Oral: 20-80 mg/day in 2 divided doses

Refractory heart failure: Oral, I.V.: Doses up to 8 g/day have been used.

Elderly: Oral, I.M., I.V.: Initial: 20 mg/day; increase slowly to desired response.

Dosing adjustment/comments in renal impairment: Acute renal failure: High doses (up to 1-3 g/day - oral/ I.V.) have been used to initiate desired response; avoid use in oliguric states.

Dialysis: Not removed by hemo- or peritoneal dialysis; supplemental dose is not necessary.

Dosing adjustment/comments in hepatic disease: Diminished natriuretic effect with increased sensitivity to hypokalemia and volume depletion in cirrhosis; monitor effects, particularly with high doses.

Mechanism of Action Inhibits reabsorption of sodium and chloride in the ascending loop of Henle and distal renal tubule, interfering with the chloride-binding cotransport system, thus causing increased excretion of water, sodium, chloride, magnesium, and calcium

Contraindications Hypersensitivity to furosemide or any component of the formulation; anuria

Canadian labeling: Additional contraindications (not in U.S. labeling): Hypersensitivity to sulfonamide-derived drugs; complete renal shutdown; hepatic coma and precoma; uncorrected states of electrolyte depletion, hypovolemia, or hypotension; jaundiced newborn infants or infants with disease(s) capable of causing hyperbilirubinemia and possibly kernicterus; breastfeeding. **Note:** Manufacturer labeling for Lasix® Special and Furosemide Special Injection also includes: GFR <5 mL/minute or GFR >20 mL/minute; hepatic cirrhosis; renal failure accompanied by hepatic coma and precoma; renal failure due to poisoning with nephrotoxic or hepatotoxic substances.

Warnings/Precautions [U.S. Boxed Warning]: If given in excessive amounts, furosemide, similar to other loop diuretics, can lead to profound diuresis, resulting in fluid and electrolyte depletion; close medical supervision and dose evaluation are required. Watch for and correct electrolyte disturbances; adjust dose to avoid dehydration. When electrolyte depletion is present, therapy should not be initiated unless serum electrolytes, especially potassium, are normalized. In cirrhosis, avoid electrolyte and acid/base imbalances that might lead to hepatic encephalopathy; correct electrolyte and acid/base imbalances prior to initiation when hepatic coma is present. Coadministration of antihypertensives may increase the risk of hypotension.

Monitor fluid status and renal function in an attempt to prevent oliguria, azotemia, and reversible increases in BUN and creatinine; close medical supervision of aggressive diuresis is required. May increase risk of contrast-induced nephropathy. Rapid I.V. administration, renal impairment, excessive doses, hypoproteinemia, and concurrent use of other ototoxins is associated with ototoxicity. Asymptomatic hyperuricemia has been reported with use; rarely, gout may precipitate. Photosensitization may occur.

Use with caution in patients with prediabetes or diabetes mellitus; may see a change in glucose control. Use with caution in patients with systemic lupus erythematosus (SLE); may cause SLE exacerbation or activation. Use with caution in patients with prostatic hyperplasia/urinary stricture; may cause urinary retention. May lead to nephrocalcinosis or nephrolithiasis in premature infants or in children <4 years of age with chronic use. May prevent closure of patent ductus arteriosus in premature infants. Chemical similarities are present among sulfonamides, sulfonylureas, carbonic anhydrase inhibitors, thiazides, and loop diuretics (except ethacrynic acid). A risk of cross-reaction exists in patients with allergy to any of these compounds; avoid use when previous reaction has been severe. Discontinue if signs of hypersensitivity are noted.

Drug Interactions

Metabolism/Transport Effects None known.

Avoid Concomitant Use

Avoid concomitant use of Furosemide with any of the following: Chloral Hydrate; Ethacrynic Acid

Increased Effect/Toxicity

Furosemide may increase the levels/effects of: ACE Inhibitors; Allopurinol; Amifostine; Aminoglycosides; Antihypertensives; Cardiac Glycosides; Chloral Hydrate; CISplatin; Dofetilide; Ethacrynic Acid; Hypotensive Agents; Lithium; Methotrexate; Neuromuscular-Blocking Agents; RisperiDONE; RiTUXimab; Salicylates; Sodium Phosphates; Topiramate

The levels/effects of Furosemide may be increased by: Alfuzosin; Beta2-Agonists; Corticosteroids (Orally Inhaled); Corticosteroids (Systemic); CycloSPORINE (Systemic); Diazoxide; Herbs (Hypotensive Properties); Licorice; MAO Inhibitors; Methotrexate; Pentoxifylline; Phosphodiesterase 5 Inhibitors; Probenecid; Prostacyclin Analogues

Decreased Effect

Furosemide may decrease the levels/effects of: Hypoglycemic Agents; Lithium; Neuromuscular-Blocking Agents

◀ *The levels/effects of Furosemide may be decreased by:* Aliskiren; Bile Acid Sequestrants; Fosphenytoin; Herbs (Hypertensive Properties); Methotrexate; Methylphenidate; Nonsteroidal Anti-Inflammatory Agents; Phenytoin; Probenecid; Salicylates; Sucralfate; Yohimbine

Ethanol/Nutrition/Herb Interactions
Food: Furosemide serum levels may be decreased if taken with food.

Herb/Nutraceutical: Avoid bayberry, blue cohosh, cayenne, ephedra, ginger, ginseng (American), kola, licorice (may worsen hypertension). Avoid black cohosh, California poppy, coleus, golden seal, hawthorn, mistletoe, periwinkle, quinine, shepherd's purse (may increase antihypertensive effect). Licorice may also cause or worsen hypokalemia.

Dietary Considerations
May cause potassium loss; potassium supplement or dietary changes may be required.

Pharmacodynamics/Kinetics
Onset of Action Diuresis: Oral, S.L.: 30-60 minutes; I.M.: 30 minutes; I.V.: ~5 minutes

Symptomatic improvement with acute pulmonary edema: Within 15-20 minutes; occurs prior to diuretic effect

Peak effect: Oral: 1-2 hours

Duration of Action Oral, S.L.: 6-8 hours; I.V.: 2 hours

Half-life Elimination Normal renal function: 0.5-2 hours; End-stage renal disease: 9 hours

Pregnancy Risk Factor C
Pregnancy Considerations Animal studies have demonstrated maternal death, fetal toxicity, and fetal loss. There are no adequate and well-controlled studies in pregnant women. Crosses the placenta. Increased fetal urine production, electrolyte disturbances reported. Generally, use of diuretics during pregnancy is avoided due to risk of decreased placental perfusion. Monitor fetal growth if used during pregnancy; may increase birth weight.

Lactation Enters breast milk/use caution

Breast-Feeding Considerations Crosses into breast milk; may suppress lactation

Dosage Forms
Injection, solution [preservative free]: 10 mg/mL (2 mL, 4 mL, 10 mL)

Solution, oral: 40 mg/5 mL (5 mL, 500 mL); 10 mg/mL (4 mL, 60 mL, 120 mL)

Tablet, oral: 20 mg, 40 mg, 80 mg
Lasix®: 20 mg, 40 mg, 80 mg

Dosage Forms: Canada
Injection, solution [preservative free]:
Furosemide Special Injection: 10 mg/mL (25 mL)
Tablet, oral:
Lasix® Special: 500 mg [scored]

Fusidic Acid and Hydrocortisone
(fyoo SI dik AS id & hye droe KOR ti sone)

Brand Names: Canada Fucidin H
Pharmacologic Category Antibiotic, Topical; Corticosteroid, Topical

Use Treatment of mild- to moderately-severe atopic dermatitis caused by susceptible organisms

Local Anesthetic/Vasoconstrictor Precautions No information available to require special precautions

Effects on Dental Treatment No significant effects or complications reported

Effects on Bleeding No information available to require special precautions

Adverse Effects
Dermatologic: Dermatitis exacerbation (2%), acne rosacea, atrophy of subcutaneous tissues, burning, dryness, hypertrichosis, itching, pigmentation changes, secondary infection, skin atrophy, striae, telangiectasia
Local: Irritation (2%)
Miscellaneous: Hypersensitivity

General Dosage Range Topical: *Children ≥3 years and Adults:* Apply 3 times/day

Mechanism of Action See individual agents.
Pregnancy Considerations See individual agents.
Product Availability Not available in U.S.

Gabapentin (GA ba pen tin)

Related Information
Temporomandibular Dysfunction (TMD), Chronic Pain, and Fibromyalgia *on page 1590*

Brand Names: U.S. Gralise™; Neurontin®
Brand Names: Canada Apo-Gabapentin®; Auro-Gabapentin; CO Gabapentin; Dom-Gabapentin; GD-Gabapentin; JAMP-Gabapentin; Mylan-Gabapentin; Neurontin®; PHL-Gabapentin; PMS-Gabapentin; PRO-Gabapentin; RAN™-Gabapentin; ratio-Gabapentin; Riva-Gabapentin; Teva-Gabapentin

Generic Availability (U.S.) Yes
Pharmacologic Category Anticonvulsant, Miscellaneous; GABA Analog
Dental Use Neuropathic pain (consult with physician)
Use Adjunct for treatment of partial seizures with and without secondary generalized seizures in patients >12 years of age with epilepsy; adjunct for treatment of partial seizures in pediatric patients 3-12 years of age; management of postherpetic neuralgia (PHN) in adults
Unlabeled Use Neuropathic pain, diabetic peripheral neuropathy, fibromyalgia, postoperative pain (adjunct), restless legs syndrome (RLS), vasomotor symptoms

Local Anesthetic/Vasoconstrictor Precautions No information available to require special precautions

Effects on Dental Treatment Key adverse event(s) related to dental treatment: Xerostomia (normal salivary flow resumes upon discontinuation), dry throat, and dental abnormalities.

Effects on Bleeding No information available to require special precautions

Adverse Effects As reported for immediate release (IR) formulations in patients >12 years of age, unless otherwise noted in children (3-12 years) or with use of extended release (ER) formulation

>10%:
Central nervous system: Dizziness (IR: 17% to 28%; children 3%; ER: 11%), somnolence (IR: 19% to 21%; children 8%; ER: 5%), ataxia (3% to 13%), fatigue (11%; children 3%)
Miscellaneous: Viral infection (children 11%)

1% to 10%:
Cardiovascular: Peripheral edema (IR: 2% to 8%; ER: 4%), vasodilatation (1%)
Central nervous system: Fever (children 10%), hostility (children 5% to 8%), emotional lability (children 4% to 6%), headache (IR: 3%; ER: 4%), abnormal thinking (2% to 3%; children 2%), amnesia (2%), depression (2%), nervousness (2%), abnormal coordination (1% to 2%), pain (ER: 1% to 2%), hyperesthesia (1%), lethargy (ER: 1%), twitching (1%), vertigo (ER: 1%)
Dermatologic: Pruritus (1%), rash (1%)
Endocrine & metabolic: Hyperglycemia (1%)

Gastrointestinal: Diarrhea (IR: 6%; ER: 3%), nausea/vomiting (3% to 4%; children 8%), abdominal pain (3%), xerostomia (IR: 2% to 5%; ER: 3%), constipation (IR: 1% to 4%; ER: 1%), weight gain (IR: adults and children 2% to 3%; ER: 2%), dyspepsia (IR: 2%; ER: 1%), flatulence (2%), dry throat (2%), dental abnormalities (2%), appetite stimulation (1%)

Genitourinary: Impotence (2%), urinary tract infection (ER: 2%)

Hematologic: Decreased WBC (1%), leukopenia (1%)

Neuromuscular & skeletal: Tremor (7%), weakness (6%), hyperkinesia (children 3% to 5%), abnormal gait (2%), back pain (IR: 2%; ER: 2%), dysarthria (2%), limb pain (ER: 2%), myalgia (2%), fracture (1%)

Ocular: Nystagmus (8%), diplopia (1% to 6%), blurred vision (3% to 4%), conjunctivitis (1%)

Otic: Otitis media (1%)

Respiratory: Rhinitis (4%), bronchitis (children 3%), nasopharyngitis (ER: 3%), respiratory infection (children 3%), pharyngitis (1% to 3%), cough (2%)

Miscellaneous: Infection (5%)

Dental Usual Dosage

Pain (unlabeled use): Children >12 years and Adults: Oral: 300-1800 mg/day given in 3 divided doses has been the most common dosage range

Postherpetic neuralgia or neuropathic pain: Adults: Oral: Day 1: 300 mg, Day 2: 300 mg twice daily, Day 3: 300 mg 3 times/day; dose may be titrated as needed for pain relief (range: 1800-3600 mg/day, daily doses >1800 mg do not generally show greater benefit)

Dosage Oral:

Children: Immediate release: Anticonvulsant:

3-12 years: Initial: 10-15 mg/kg/day in 3 divided doses; titrate to effective dose over ~3 days; dosages of up to 50 mg/kg/day have been tolerated in clinical studies

3-4 years: Usual dose: 40 mg/kg/day in 3 divided doses

≥5-12 years: Usual dose: 25-35 mg/kg/day in 3 divided doses

See **"Note"** in adult dosing.

Children >12 years and Adults: Immediate release: Anticonvulsant: Initial: 300 mg 3 times/day; if necessary the dose may be increased up to 1800 mg/day; Maintenance: 900-1800 mg/day administered in 3 divided doses; doses of up to 2400 mg/day have been tolerated in long-term clinical studies; up to 3600 mg/day has been tolerated in short-term studies.

Note: If gabapentin is discontinued or if another anticonvulsant is added to therapy, it should be done slowly over a minimum of 1 week

Adults:

Immediate release:

Diabetic neuropathy (unlabeled use): 900-3600 mg/day (Bril, 2011)

Neuropathic pain (unlabeled use): 300-3600 mg/day (Attal, 2010; Dworkin, 2010)

Neuropathic pain, critically-ill patients (unlabeled use): Initial: 100 mg 3 times daily in combination with I.V. opioids; Maintenance: 300-1200 mg 3 times daily; maximum dose: 3600 mg daily (Barr, 2013)

Postherpetic neuralgia: Day 1: 300 mg, Day 2: 300 mg twice daily, Day 3: 300 mg 3 times/day; dose may be titrated as needed for pain relief (range: 1800-3600 mg/day in divided doses, daily doses >1800 mg do not generally show greater benefit)

Postoperative pain (adjunct) (unlabeled use): Usual dose: 300-1200 mg given the night before or 1-2 hours prior to surgery (Dauri, 2009)

Restless legs syndrome (RLS) (unlabeled use): Initial: 300 mg once daily 2 hours before bedtime. Doses ≥600 mg/day have been given in 2 divided doses (late afternoon and 2 hours before bedtime). Dose may be titrated every 2 weeks until symptom relief achieved (range: 300-1800 mg/day). Suggested maintenance dosing schedule: One-third of total daily dose given at 12 pm, remaining two-thirds total daily dose given at 8 pm. (Garcia-Borreguero, 2002; Happe, 2003; Saletu, 2010; Vignatelli, 2006)

Vasomotor symptoms associated with menopause (unlabeled use): Day 1: 300 mg at bedtime, Day 2: 300 mg twice daily, followed by 300 mg 3 times/day for 4 weeks and then tapered off (Butt, 2008)

Extended release (Gralise™): Postherpetic neuralgia: Day 1: 300 mg, Day 2: 600 mg, Days 3-6: 900 mg once daily, Days 7-10: 1200 mg once daily, Days 11-14: 1500 mg once daily, Days ≥15: 1800 mg once daily

Elderly: Studies in elderly patients have shown a decrease in clearance as age increases. This is most likely due to age-related decreases in renal function; dose reductions may be needed.

Dosing adjustment in renal impairment: Children ≥12 years and Adults: **Note:** Renal function may be estimated using the Cockcroft-Gault formula for dosage adjustment purposes.

Immediate release:

Cl_{cr} ≥60 mL/minute: 300-1200 mg 3 times/day

Cl_{cr} >30-59 mL/minute: 200-700 mg twice daily

Cl_{cr} >15-29 mL/minute: 200-700 mg once daily

Cl_{cr} 15 mL/minute: 100-300 mg once daily

Cl_{cr} <15 mL/minute: Reduce daily dose in proportion to creatinine clearance based on dose for creatinine clearance of 15 mL/minute (eg, reduce dose by one-half [range: 50-150 mg/day] for Cl_{cr} 7.5 mL/minute)

ESRD requiring hemodialysis: Dose for Cl_{cr} <15 mL/minute plus single supplemental dose of 125-350 mg (given after each 4 hours of hemodialysis)

Extended release: **Note:** Follow initial dose titration schedule if treatment-naive.

Cl_{cr} ≥60 mL/minute: 1800 mg once daily

Cl_{cr} >30-59 mL/minute: 600-1800 mg once daily; dependent on tolerability and clinical response

Cl_{cr} <30 mL/minute: Use is not recommended.

ESRD requiring hemodialysis: Use is not recommended.

Dosing adjustment in hepatic impairment: There are no dosage adjustments provided in the manufacturer's labeling; however, gabapentin is not hepatically metabolized.

Mechanism of Action Gabapentin is structurally related to GABA. However, it does not bind to GABA_A or GABA_B receptors, and it does not appear to influence synthesis or uptake of GABA. High affinity gabapentin binding sites have been located throughout the brain; these sites correspond to the presence of voltage-gated calcium channels specifically possessing the alpha-2-delta-1 subunit. This channel appears to be located presynaptically, and may modulate the release of excitatory neurotransmitters which participate in epileptogenesis and nociception.

Contraindications Hypersensitivity to gabapentin or any component of the formulation

Warnings/Precautions Antiepileptics are associated with an increased risk of suicidal behavior/thoughts with use (regardless of indication); patients should be monitored for signs/symptoms of depression, suicidal tendencies, and other unusual behavior changes during therapy and instructed to inform their healthcare provider immediately if symptoms occur. Avoid abrupt withdrawal, may precipitate seizures; Gralise™ should be withdrawn over ≥1 week. Use cautiously in patients with severe renal dysfunction; male rat studies demonstrated an association with pancreatic adenocarcinoma (clinical implication unknown). May cause CNS depression, which may impair physical or mental abilities. Patients must be cautioned about performing tasks which require mental alertness (eg, operating machinery or driving). Effects with other sedative drugs or ethanol may be potentiated. Pediatric patients (3-12 years of age) have shown increased incidence of CNS-related adverse effects, including emotional lability, hostility, thought disorder, and hyperkinesia. Gabapentin immediate release and extended release (Gralise™) products are not interchangeable with each other **or** with gabapentin enacarbil (Horizant™). The safety and efficacy of extended release gabapentin (Gralise™) has not been studied in patients with epilepsy. Potentially serious, sometimes fatal multiorgan hypersensitivity (also known as drug reaction with eosinophilia and systemic symptoms [DRESS]) has been reported with some antiepileptic drugs, including gabapentin; may affect lymphatic, hepatic, renal, cardiac, and/or hematologic systems; fever, rash, and eosinophilia may also be present. Discontinue immediately if suspected.

Drug Interactions

Metabolism/Transport Effects None known.

Avoid Concomitant Use

Avoid concomitant use of Gabapentin with any of the following: Azelastine (Nasal); Paraldehyde

Increased Effect/Toxicity

Gabapentin may increase the levels/effects of: Alcohol (Ethyl); Azelastine (Nasal); Buprenorphine; CNS Depressants; Methotrimeprazine; Metyrosine; Mirtazapine; Paraldehyde; Pramipexole; ROPINIRole; Rotigotine; Selective Serotonin Reuptake Inhibitors; Zolpidem

The levels/effects of Gabapentin may be increased by: Droperidol; HydrOXYzine; Magnesium Sulfate; Methotrimeprazine; Perampanel; Sodium Oxybate

Decreased Effect

The levels/effects of Gabapentin may be decreased by: Antacids; Ketorolac (Nasal); Ketorolac (Systemic); Mefloquine

Ethanol/Nutrition/Herb Interactions

Ethanol: May increase CNS depression; monitor for increased effects with coadministration. Caution patients about effects.

Food: Tablet, solution (immediate release): No significant effect on rate or extent of absorption; tablet (extended release): Increases rate and extent of absorption.

Herb/Nutraceutical: Avoid evening primrose (seizure threshold decreased). Avoid valerian, St John's wort, kava kava, gotu kola (may increase CNS depression).

Dietary Considerations Immediate release tablet and solution may be taken without regard to meals; extended release tablet should be taken with food.

Pharmacodynamics/Kinetics

Half-life Elimination 5-7 hours; anuria 132 hours; during dialysis 3.8 hours

Time to Peak Immediate release: 2-4 hours; extended release: 8 hours

Pregnancy Risk Factor C

Pregnancy Considerations Adverse events have been observed in animal reproduction studies. Gabapentin crosses the placenta. In a small study (n=6), the umbilical/maternal plasma concentration ratio was ~1.74. Neonatal concentrations declined quickly after delivery and at 24 hours of life were ~27% of the cord blood concentrations at birth (gabapentin neonatal half-life ~14 hours) (Ohman, 2005). Outcome data following maternal use of gabapentin during pregnancy is limited (Holmes, 2012).

Patients exposed to gabapentin during pregnancy are encouraged to enroll in the North American Antiepileptic Drug (NAAED) Pregnancy Registry by calling 1-888-233-2334. Additional information is available at www.aedpregnancyregistry.org.

Lactation Enters breast milk/use caution

Breast-Feeding Considerations Gabapentin is excreted in human breast milk. Per the manufacturer, a nursed infant could be exposed to ~1 mg/kg/day of gabapentin; the effect on the child is not known. Use in breast-feeding women only if the benefits to the mother outweigh the potential risk to the infant.

In a small study of breast-feeding women (n=6), the estimated exposure of gabapentin to the nursing infants was ~1% to 4% of the weight-adjusted maternal dose (sampling occurred from 12-97 days after delivery and maternal doses ranged from 600-2100 mg daily). Gabapentin was detected in the serum of 2 nursing infants 2-3 weeks after delivery and in 1 infant after 3 months of breast-feeding. Serum concentrations were <12% of the maternal plasma concentrations and <5% of those measured in the umbilical cord. Adverse events were not reported in the breast-fed infants (Ohman, 2005).

Dosage Forms

Capsule, oral: 100 mg, 300 mg, 400 mg
  Neurontin®: 100 mg, 300 mg, 400 mg
Solution, oral: 250 mg/5 mL (470 mL, 473 mL)
  Neurontin®: 250 mg/5 mL (470 mL)
Tablet, oral: 600 mg, 800 mg
  Gralise™: 300 mg, 600 mg, 300 mg (9s) [white tablets; contains soybean lecithin] and 600 mg (69s) [beige tablets]
  Neurontin®: 600 mg, 800 mg

References

Laird MA and Gidal BE, "Use of Gabapentin in the Treatment of Neuropathic Pain," *Ann Pharmacother*, 2000, 34(6):802-7.
Rose MA and Kam PCA, "Gabapentin: Pharmacology and Its Use in Pain Management," *Anaesthesia*, 2002, 57:451-62.
Rosenberg JM, Harrell C, Ristic H, et al, "The Effect of Gabapentin on Neuropathic Pain," *Clin J Pain*, 1997, 13(3):251-5.
Rowbotham M, Harden N, Stacey B, et al, "Gabapentin for the Treatment of Postherpetic Neuralgia: A Randomized Controlled Trial," *JAMA*, 1998, 280(21):1837-42.

Gabapentin Enacarbil (gab a PEN tin en a KAR bil)

Brand Names: U.S. Horizant™

Pharmacologic Category Anticonvulsant, Miscellaneous

Use Treatment of moderate-to-severe restless leg syndrome (RLS); management of postherpetic neuralgia (PHN)

Local Anesthetic/Vasoconstrictor Precautions No information available to require special precautions

Effects on Dental Treatment Key adverse event(s) related to dental treatment: Xerostomia (normal salivary flow resumes upon discontinuation).

Effects on Bleeding No information available to require special precautions

Adverse Effects Percentages reported are for restless leg syndrome (RLS) 600 mg daily and postherpetic neuralgia (PHN) 1200 mg daily.

>10%: Central nervous system: Sedation/somnolence (PHN 10%; RLS 20%), dizziness (13% to 17%), headache (10% to 12%)

1% to 10%:

Cardiovascular: Peripheral edema (PHN 6%; RLS <1%)

Central nervous system: Fatigue (6%), irritability (≤4%), insomnia (PHN 3%), balance disorder (<2%), depression (<2%), disorientation (<2%), lethargy (<2%), drunk feeling (<2%), vertigo (<2%)

Gastrointestinal: Nausea (6% to 8%), flatulence (≤3%), xerostomia (≤3%), weight gain (2% to 3%), appetite increased (≤2%)

Ocular: Blurred vision (≤2%)

General Dosage Range Dosage adjustment recommended in patients with renal impairment.

Oral: *Adults:* 600 mg once daily (RLS) **or** 600 mg once daily for 3 days, then 600 mg twice daily (PHN)

Mechanism of Action Gabapentin enacarbil is a prodrug of gabapentin. Gabapentin is structurally related to GABA. However, it does not bind to GABA$_A$ or GABA$_B$ receptors, and it does not appear to influence synthesis or uptake of GABA. High affinity gabapentin binding sites have been located throughout the brain; these sites correspond to the presence of voltage-gated calcium channels specifically possessing the alpha-2-delta-1 subunit. This channel appears to be located presynaptically, and may modulate the release of excitatory neurotransmitters. These effects on RLS are unknown.

Pharmacodynamics/Kinetics

Half-life Elimination Prodrug hydrolyzed primarily in the intestines to gabapentin (active metabolite)

Time to Peak 5-6 hours

Pregnancy Risk Factor C

Pregnancy Considerations Adverse events were observed in animal reproduction studies. Gabapentin enacarbil is the prodrug of gabapentin; bioavailability following gabapentin enacarbil is increased in comparison to gabapentin (Backonja, 2011). Refer to Gabapentin monograph for information related to gabapentin exposure during pregnancy.

Gadopentetate Dimeglumine
(gad oh PEN te tate dye MEG loo meen)

Brand Names: U.S. Magnevist®
Brand Names: Canada Magnevist®

Pharmacologic Category Diagnostic Agent; Gadolinium-Containing Contrast Agent; Radiological/Contrast Media, Ionic (High Osmolality); Radiological/Contrast Media, Paramagnetic Agent

Use Contrast medium for magnetic resonance imaging (MRI) to visualize CNS lesions with abnormal vascularity in the brain, spine and associated tissues, extracranial/extraspinal lesions with abnormal vascularity in the head and neck, and body lesions with abnormal vascularity (excluding the heart)

Unlabeled Use Contrast medium for magnetic resonance angiography (MRA)

Local Anesthetic/Vasoconstrictor Precautions No information available to require special precautions

Effects on Dental Treatment No significant effects or complications reported

Effects on Bleeding No information available to require special precautions

Adverse Effects 1% to 10%:

Central nervous system: Headache (5%), dizziness (1%)

Gastrointestinal: Nausea (3%)

Local: Injection site coldness/localized coldness (2%)

General Dosage Range I.V.: *Children ≥2 years and Adults:* 0.1 mmol/kg (0.2 mL/kg)

Mechanism of Action Exposure to an external magnetic field induces a large local magnetic field in gadopentetate exposed tissues. This local magnetism disrupts water protons in the vicinity, resulting in a change in proton density and spin characteristics, which can be detected by the imaging device.

Pharmacodynamics/Kinetics

Half-life Elimination 1.6 ± 0.13 hours

Pregnancy Risk Factor C

Pregnancy Considerations Adverse events were observed in some animal reproduction studies. Gadopentetate dimeglumine crosses the placenta in humans (Marcos, 1997). Gadolinium-based agents should not routinely be administered to pregnant women (Expert Panel on MR Safety, 2013; Wang, 2012).

Gadoteridol (gad oh TER i dol)

Brand Names: U.S. ProHance®; ProHance® Multipack™

Pharmacologic Category Diagnostic Agent; Gadolinium-Containing Contrast Agent; Radiological/Contrast Media, Nonionic (Low Osmolality); Radiological/Contrast Media, Paramagnetic Agent

Use Contrast medium for magnetic resonance imaging (MRI) to visualize CNS lesions with abnormal vascularity in the brain, spine, and associated tissues and to visualize extracranial/extraspinal tissues in the head and neck

Unlabeled Use Contrast medium for magnetic resonance angiography (MRA)

Local Anesthetic/Vasoconstrictor Precautions No information available to require special precautions

Effects on Dental Treatment No significant effects or complications reported

Effects on Bleeding No information available to require special precautions

Adverse Effects 1% to 10%: Gastrointestinal: Nausea (1%), taste perversion (1%)

General Dosage Range I.V.:

Children ≥2 years: 0.1 mmol/kg (0.2 mL/kg)

Adults: 0.1 mmol/kg (0.2 mL/kg); may repeat 0.2 mmol/kg (0.4 mL/kg) once if needed [CNS imaging]

Mechanism of Action Gadoteridol is a gadolinium-containing paramagnetic agent. Exposure to an external magnetic field induces a large local magnetic field in exposed tissues. This local magnetism disrupts water protons in the vicinity, resulting in a change in proton density and spin characteristics, which can be detected by the imaging device.

Pharmacodynamics/Kinetics

Half-life Elimination 1.57 ± 0.08 hours

Pregnancy Risk Factor C

Pregnancy Considerations Adverse events were observed in animal reproduction studies. Gadolinium-based contrast agents cross the placenta in humans. Gadolinium-based agents should not routinely be administered to pregnant women (Expert Panel on MR Safety, 2013; Wang, 2012).

Galantamine (ga LAN ta meen)

Brand Names: U.S. Razadyne®; Razadyne® ER
Brand Names: Canada Mylan-Galantamine ER; PAT-Galantamine ER; Reminyl®; Reminyl® ER
Pharmacologic Category Acetylcholinesterase Inhibitor (Central)
Use Treatment of mild-to-moderate dementia of Alzheimer's disease
Unlabeled Use Severe dementia associated with Alzheimer's disease; mild-to-moderate dementia associated with Parkinson's disease; Lewy body dementia
Local Anesthetic/Vasoconstrictor Precautions No information available to require special precautions
Effects on Dental Treatment No significant effects or complications reported
Effects on Bleeding No information available to require special precautions
Adverse Effects
>10%: Gastrointestinal: Nausea (13% to 24%), vomiting (6% to 13%), diarrhea (6% to 12%)
1% to 10%:
  Cardiovascular: Bradycardia (2% to 3%), hypertension (≥2%), peripheral edema (≥2%), syncope (0.4% to 2.2%: dose related), chest pain (≥1% to 2%)
  Central nervous system: Dizziness (9%), headache (8%), depression (7%), fatigue (5%), insomnia (5%), somnolence (4%), agitation (≥2%), anxiety (≥2%), confusion (≥2%), hallucination (≥2%), fever (≥1%), malaise (≥1%)
  Dermatologic: Purpura (≥2%)
  Gastrointestinal: Anorexia (7% to 9%), weight loss (5% to 7%), abdominal pain (5%), dyspepsia (5%), constipation (≥2%), flatulence (≥1%)
  Genitourinary: Urinary tract infection (8%), hematuria (<1% to 3%), incontinence (≥1% to 2%)
  Hematologic: Anemia (3%)
  Neuromuscular & skeletal: Tremor (3%), back pain (≥2%), fall (≥2%), weakness (≥1% to 2%)
  Respiratory: Rhinitis (4%), bronchitis (≥2%), cough (≥2%), upper respiratory tract infection (≥2%)
General Dosage Range Dosage adjustment recommended in patients with hepatic or renal impairment
Oral:
  Extended-release: *Adults:* Initial: 8 mg once daily; Maintenance: 16-24 mg once daily
  Immediate release: *Adults:* Initial: 4 mg twice daily; Maintenance: 16-24 mg/day in 2 divided doses
Mechanism of Action Centrally-acting cholinesterase inhibitor (competitive and reversible). It elevates acetylcholine in cerebral cortex by slowing the degradation of acetylcholine. Modulates nicotinic acetylcholine receptor to increase acetylcholine from surviving presynaptic nerve terminals. May increase glutamate and serotonin levels.
Pharmacodynamics/Kinetics
  Duration of Action 3 hours; maximum inhibition of erythrocyte acetylcholinesterase ~40% at 1 hour post 8 mg oral dose; levels return to baseline at 30 hours
  Half-life Elimination ~7 hours
  Time to Peak Immediate release: 1 hour (2.5 hours with food); extended release: 4.5-5 hours
Pregnancy Risk Factor B
Pregnancy Considerations Adverse events have been observed in animal reproduction studies.

Gallium Nitrate (GAL ee um NYE trate)

Brand Names: U.S. Ganite™
Pharmacologic Category Calcium-Lowering Agent
Use Treatment of symptomatic cancer-related hypercalcemia (refractory to adequate hydration)
Local Anesthetic/Vasoconstrictor Precautions No information available to require special precautions
Effects on Dental Treatment No significant effects or complications reported
Effects on Bleeding Anemia has been reported with very high doses. Medical consult recommended.
Adverse Effects Frequency not always defined.
  Cardiovascular: Edema (lower extremity), hypotension, tachycardia
  Central nervous system: Coma, confusion, dreams, encephalopathy, fever, hallucinations, hypothermia, lethargy
  Dermatologic: Rash
  Endocrine & metabolic: Hypophosphatemia (≤79%), serum bicarbonate decreased (40% to 50%), hypocalcemia (38%), respiratory alkalosis (mild)
  Gastrointestinal: Constipation, diarrhea, nausea, vomiting
  Hematologic: Anemia, leukopenia
  Neuromuscular & skeletal: Paresthesia, positive Cvostek's sign
  Ocular: Optic neuritis (<1%), blindness (case report)
  Otic: Auditory acuity decreased (<1%), tinnitus (<1%), hearing decreased
  Renal: BUN increased (13%), creatinine increased (13%), acute renal failure
  Respiratory: Dyspnea, pleural effusion, pulmonary infiltrates, rales, rhonchi
General Dosage Range I.V.: *Adults:* 100-200 mg/m²/day
Mechanism of Action Inhibits calcium resorption from bone by inhibiting osteoclast activity. Gallium nitrate appears to be effective in parathyroid hormone-related protein (PTHrP) and non-PTHrP-associated hypercalcemia.
Pharmacodynamics/Kinetics
  Onset of Action Onset of calcium lowering: Calcium begins to decrease within 24-48 hours; normocalcemia achieved within 5-9 days
  Duration of Action Normocalcemia: 7-10 days
  Half-life Elimination Continuous infusion: 105 hours
Pregnancy Risk Factor C
Pregnancy Considerations Reproduction studies have not been conducted. Gallium nitrate should be used in pregnant women only if clearly needed.

Galsulfase (gal SUL fase)

Brand Names: U.S. Naglazyme®
Pharmacologic Category Enzyme
Use Replacement therapy in mucopolysaccharidosis VI (MPS VI; Maroteaux-Lamy Syndrome) for improvement of walking and stair-climbing capacity
Local Anesthetic/Vasoconstrictor Precautions No information available to require special precautions
Effects on Dental Treatment No significant effects or complications reported
Effects on Bleeding No information available to require special precautions

Adverse Effects Note: Percentages reported are from a placebo-controlled study (39 patients, 19 on galsulfase); also included are adverse effects noted during other clinical studies.

Cardiovascular: Chest pain (16%), hypertension (11%)

Central nervous system: Pain (32%), chills (21%), malaise (11%), fever, headache

Dermatologic: Rash (21%), angioedema, pruritus, urticaria

Gastrointestinal: Abdominal pain (47%), gastroenteritis (11%), nausea, vomiting

Neuromuscular & skeletal: Arthralgia (42%), areflexia (11%)

Ocular: Conjunctivitis (21%), corneal opacification increased (11%)

Otic: Ear pain (42%), hearing impairment (11%)

Respiratory: Dyspnea (21%), pharyngitis (11%), nasal congestion (11%), apnea, laryngeal edema, respiratory distress

Miscellaneous: Antigalsulfase antibodies (98%), infusion reactions (56%), umbilical hernia (11%)

General Dosage Range I.V.: *Children >5 years and Adults:* 1 mg/kg once weekly

Mechanism of Action Galsulfase is a recombinant form of N-acetylgalactosamine 4-sulfatase, produced in Chinese hamster cells. A deficiency of this enzyme leads to accumulation of the glycosaminoglycan dermatan sulfate in various tissues, causing progressive disease which includes decreased growth, skeletal deformities, upper airway obstruction, clouding of the cornea, heart disease, and coarse facial features. Replacement of this enzyme has been shown to improve mobility and physical function (measured by walking and stair-climbing).

Pharmacodynamics/Kinetics

Half-life Elimination Week 1: Median 9 minutes (range: 6-21 minutes); Week 24: Median 26 minutes (range: 8-40 minutes)

Pregnancy Risk Factor B

Pregnancy Considerations Fetal harm was not reported in animal studies. There are no studies in pregnant women. Pregnant women are encouraged to enroll in the Clinical Surveillance Program.

Ganciclovir (Systemic) (gan SYE kloe veer)

Related Information

Systemic Viral Diseases *on page 1537*

ValGANciclovir *on page 1377*

Brand Names: U.S. Cytovene®-IV

Brand Names: Canada Cytovene®

Generic Availability (U.S.) Yes

Pharmacologic Category Antiviral Agent

Use Treatment of CMV retinitis in immunocompromised individuals, including patients with acquired immunodeficiency syndrome; prophylaxis of CMV infection in transplant patients

Unlabeled Use CMV retinitis: May be given in combination with foscarnet in patients who relapse after monotherapy with either drug

Local Anesthetic/Vasoconstrictor Precautions No information available to require special precautions

Effects on Dental Treatment No significant effects or complications reported

Effects on Bleeding Anemia (15% to 25%), thrombocytopenia (57% in bone marrow transplant patients; less common in other populations [8%]), and unusual bleeding are frequently reported.

Adverse Effects

>10%:

Central nervous system: Fever (48%)

Gastrointestinal: Diarrhea (44%), anorexia (14%), vomiting (13%)

Hematologic: Thrombocytopenia (57%), leukopenia (41%), anemia (16% to 26%), neutropenia with ANC <500/mm^3 (12% to 14%)

Ocular: Retinal detachment (11%; relationship to ganciclovir not established)

Renal: Serum creatinine increased (2% to 14%)

Miscellaneous: Sepsis (15%), diaphoresis (12%)

1% to 10%:

Central nervous system: Chills (10%), neuropathy (9%)

Dermatologic: Pruritus (5%)

<1%, postmarketing, and/or case reports (limited to important or life-threatening): Allergic reaction (including anaphylaxis), alopecia, arrhythmia, bronchospasm, cardiac arrest, cataracts, cholestasis, coma, dyspnea, edema, encephalopathy, exfoliative dermatitis, extrapyramidal symptoms, hepatitis, hepatic failure, pancreatitis, pancytopenia, pulmonary fibrosis, psychosis, rhabdomyolysis, seizure, alopecia, urticaria, eosinophilia, hemorrhage, Stevens-Johnson syndrome, torsade de pointes, renal failure, SIADH, visual loss

Dosage

CMV CNS infection in HIV-exposed/-infected patients (unlabeled use; CDC, 2009): Infants, Children, and Adults: I.V.: 5 mg/kg/dose every 12 hours plus foscarnet until symptoms improve followed by chronic suppression

CMV retinitis:

Children and Adults: I.V. (slow infusion):

Induction therapy: 5 mg/kg/dose every 12 hours for 14-21 days followed by maintenance therapy

Maintenance therapy: 5 mg/kg/day as a single daily dose for 7 days/week or 6 mg/kg/day for 5 days/week

Prevention (secondary) of CMV disease in HIV-exposed/-infected patients (unlabeled use; CDC, 2009): Infants, Children, and Adults: I.V.: 5 mg/kg/dose daily

Prevention (secondary) of CMV disease in transplant patients: Children and Adults: I.V. (slow infusion): 5 mg/kg/dose every 12 hours for 7-14 days; duration of maintenance therapy is dependent on clinical condition and degree of immunosuppression

Varicella zoster: Progressive outer retinal necrosis in HIV-exposed/-infected patients (unlabeled use; CDC, 2009): Infants, Children, and Adults: I.V.: 5 mg/kg/dose every 12 hours plus systemic foscarnet and intravitreal ganciclovir or intravitreal foscarnet

Elderly: Refer to adult dosing; in general, dose selection should be cautious, reflecting greater frequency of organ impairment

Dosage adjustment in renal impairment:

I.V. (Induction):

Cl$_{cr}$ 50-69 mL/minute: Administer 2.5 mg/kg/dose every 12 hours

Cl$_{cr}$ 25-49 mL/minute: Administer 2.5 mg/kg/dose every 24 hours

Cl$_{cr}$ 10-24 mL/minute: Administer 1.25 mg/kg/dose every 24 hours

Cl$_{cr}$ <10 mL/minute: Administer 1.25 mg/kg/dose 3 times/week following hemodialysis

◄ I.V. (Maintenance):
Cl$_{cr}$ 50-69 mL/minute: Administer 2.5 mg/kg/dose every 24 hours
Cl$_{cr}$ 25-49 mL/minute: Administer 1.25 mg/kg/dose every 24 hours
Cl$_{cr}$ 10-24 mL/minute: Administer 0.625 mg/kg/dose every 24 hours
Cl$_{cr}$ <10 mL/minute: Administer 0.625 mg/kg/dose 3 times/week following hemodialysis

Intermittent hemodialysis (IHD) (administer after hemodialysis on dialysis days): Dializable (50%): CMV Infection: I.V.: Induction: 1.25 mg/kg every 48-72 hours; Maintenance: 0.625 mg/kg every 48-72 hours. **Note:** Dosing dependent on the assumption of 3 times/week, complete IHD sessions.

Peritoneal dialysis (PD): Dose as for Cl$_{cr}$ <10 mL/minute.

Continuous renal replacement therapy (CRRT) (Heintz, 2009; Trotman, 2005): Drug clearance is highly dependent on the method of renal replacement, filter type, and flow rate. Appropriate dosing requires close monitoring of pharmacologic response, signs of adverse reactions due to drug accumulation, as well as drug concentrations in relation to target trough (if appropriate). The following are general recommendations only (based on dialysate flow/ultrafiltration rates of 1-2 L/hour and minimal residual renal function) and should not supersede clinical judgment: CMV Infection:

CVVH: I.V.: Induction: 2.5 mg/kg every 24 hours; Maintenance: 1.25 mg/kg every 24 hours
CVVHD/CVVHDF: I.V.: Induction: 2.5 mg/kg every 12 hours; Maintenance: 2.5 mg/kg every 24 hours

Dosage adjustment in hepatic impairment: No dosage adjustment provided in manufacturer's labeling.

Mechanism of Action Ganciclovir is phosphorylated to a substrate which competitively inhibits the binding of deoxyguanosine triphosphate to DNA polymerase resulting in inhibition of viral DNA synthesis

Contraindications Hypersensitivity to ganciclovir, acyclovir, or any component of the formulation

Warnings/Precautions Hazardous agent - use appropriate precautions for handling and disposal (NIOSH, 2012). **[U.S. Boxed Warning]: Granulocytopenia (neutropenia), anemia, and thrombocytopenia may occur.** Dosage adjustment or interruption of ganciclovir therapy may be necessary in patients with neutropenia and/or thrombocytopenia and patients with impaired renal function. **[U.S. Boxed Warning]: Animal studies have demonstrated carcinogenic and teratogenic effects, and inhibition of spermatogenesis;** contraceptive precautions for female and male patients need to be followed during and for at least 90 days after therapy with the drug; take care to administer only into veins with good blood flow. **[U.S. Boxed Warning]: Indicated only for treatment of CMV retinitis in the immunocompromised patient and CMV prevention in transplant patients at risk.**

Drug Interactions
Metabolism/Transport Effects None known.
Avoid Concomitant Use
Avoid concomitant use of Ganciclovir (Systemic) with any of the following: Imipenem
Increased Effect/Toxicity
Ganciclovir (Systemic) may increase the levels/effects of: Imipenem; Mycophenolate; Reverse Transcriptase Inhibitors (Nucleoside); Tenofovir

The levels/effects of Ganciclovir (Systemic) may be increased by: Mycophenolate; Probenecid; Tenofovir

Decreased Effect There are no known significant interactions involving a decrease in effect.
Dietary Considerations Some products may contain sodium.
Pharmacodynamics/Kinetics
Half-life Elimination 1.7-5.8 hours; prolonged with renal impairment; End-stage renal disease: 5-28 hours
Pregnancy Risk Factor C
Pregnancy Considerations [U.S. Boxed Warning]: Animal studies have demonstrated carcinogenic and teratogenic effects, and inhibition of spermatogenesis. Female patients should use effective contraception during therapy; male patients should use a barrier contraceptive during and for at least 90 days after therapy.
Lactation Excretion in breast milk unknown/not recommended
Breast-Feeding Considerations Due to the carcinogenic and teratogenic effects observed in animal studies, the possibility of adverse events in a nursing infant is considered likely. Therefore, nursing should be discontinued during therapy. In addition, the CDC recommends **not** to breast-feed if diagnosed with HIV to avoid postnatal transmission of the virus.
Dosage Forms
Injection, powder for reconstitution: 500 mg
Cytovene®-IV: 500 mg

Ganirelix (ga ni REL ix)

Brand Names: Canada Orgalutran®
Pharmacologic Category Gonadotropin Releasing Hormone Antagonist
Use Inhibits premature luteinizing hormone (LH) surges in women undergoing controlled ovarian hyperstimulation
Local Anesthetic/Vasoconstrictor Precautions No information available to require special precautions
Effects on Dental Treatment No significant effects or complications reported
Effects on Bleeding No information available to require special precautions
Adverse Effects 1% to 10%:
Central nervous system: Headache (3%)
Endocrine & metabolic: Ovarian hyperstimulation syndrome (2%)
Gastrointestinal: Abdominal pain (1%), nausea (1%)
Genitourinary: Pelvic pain (5%), vaginal bleeding (2%)
Local: Injection site reaction (1%)
General Dosage Range SubQ: *Adults:* 250 mcg/day
Mechanism of Action Competitively blocks the gonadotropin-release hormone receptors on the pituitary gonadotroph and transduction pathway. This suppresses gonadotropin secretion and luteinizing hormone secretion preventing ovulation until the follicles are of adequate size.
Pharmacodynamics/Kinetics
Duration of Action <48 hours
Half-life Elimination Single dose: 12.8 hours; Multiple dosing: 16.2 hours
Time to Peak 1.1 hours
Pregnancy Risk Factor X
Pregnancy Considerations Fetal resorption occurred in pregnant rats and rabbits. These effects are results of hormonal alterations and could result in fetal loss in humans. The drug should not be used in pregnant women.

Gatifloxacin (gat i FLOKS a sin)

Related Information
Bacterial Infections *on page 1562*
Brand Names: U.S. Zymaxid™
Brand Names: Canada Zymar™
Generic Availability (U.S.) No
Pharmacologic Category Antibiotic, Ophthalmic; Antibiotic, Quinolone
Use Treatment of bacterial conjunctivitis
Local Anesthetic/Vasoconstrictor Precautions No information available to require special precautions
Effects on Dental Treatment Key adverse event(s) related to dental treatment: Taste disturbance.
Effects on Bleeding No information available to require special precautions
Adverse Effects 1% to 10%:
Cardiovascular: Edema
Dermatologic: Contact dermatitis, erythema
Gastrointestinal: Taste disturbance
Ocular: Conjunctival irritation, discharge, dry eye, edema, irritation, keratitis, lacrimation increased, pain, papillary conjunctivitis, visual acuity decreased
Respiratory: Rhinorrhea
Dosage Ophthalmic: Children ≥1 year and Adults: Bacterial conjunctivitis:
Zymar™:
Days 1 and 2: Instill 1 drop into affected eye(s) every 2 hours while awake (maximum: 8 times/day)
Days 3-7: Instill 1 drop into affected eye(s) 4 times/day while awake
Zymaxid™:
Day 1: Instill 1 drop into affected eye(s) every 2 hours while awake (maximum: 8 times/day)
Days 2-7: Instill 1 drop into affected eye(s) 2-4 times/day while awake

Dosage adjustment in renal impairment: No dosage adjustment provided in manufacturer's labeling. However, dosage adjustment unlikely due to low systemic absorption.
Dosage adjustment in hepatic impairment: No dosage adjustment provided in manufacturer's labeling. However, dosage adjustment unlikely due to low systemic absorption.
Mechanism of Action Gatifloxacin is a DNA gyrase inhibitor, and also inhibits topoisomerase IV. DNA gyrase (topoisomerase II) is an essential bacterial enzyme that maintains the superhelical structure of DNA. DNA gyrase is required for DNA replication and transcription, DNA repair, recombination, and transposition; inhibition is bactericidal.
Contraindications
Zymaxid™: There are no contraindications listed in the manufacturer's labeling.
Zymar™: Hypersensitivity to gatifloxacin, other quinolones, or any component of the formulation
Warnings/Precautions Severe hypersensitivity reactions, including anaphylaxis, have occurred with systemic quinolone therapy. Reactions may present as typical allergic symptoms after a single dose, or may manifest as severe idiosyncratic dermatologic, vascular, pulmonary, renal, hepatic, and/or hematologic events, usually after multiple doses. Prompt discontinuation of drug should occur if skin rash or other symptoms arise. Prolonged use may result in fungal or bacterial superinfection. For topical ophthalmic use only. Do not inject ophthalmic solution subconjunctivally or introduce directly into the anterior chamber of the eye. Contact lenses should not be worn during treatment of ophthalmic infections.
Drug Interactions
Metabolism/Transport Effects None known.
Avoid Concomitant Use There are no known interactions where it is recommended to avoid concomitant use.
Increased Effect/Toxicity There are no known significant interactions involving an increase in effect.
Decreased Effect
Gatifloxacin may decrease the levels/effects of: Sodium Picosulfate
Pregnancy Risk Factor C
Pregnancy Considerations Gatifloxacin has been shown to be fetotoxic in animal studies. Quinolone exposure during human pregnancy has been reported with other agents (refer to Ciprofloxacin (Systemic), Ofloxacin (Systemic), and Norfloxacin monographs). Following ophthalmic administration, serum concentrations of gatifloxacin are below the limits of quantification (<5 ng/mL). Systemic absorption would be required in order for gatifloxacin to cross the placenta.
Lactation Excretion in breast milk unknown/use caution
Breast-Feeding Considerations Other quinolones are known to be excreted in breast milk. The manufacturer recommends using caution if gatifloxacin is administered while nursing.
Dosage Forms
Solution, ophthalmic:
Zymaxid™: 0.5% (2.5 mL)
Dosage Forms: Canada
Solution, ophthalmic [drops]:
Zymar™: 0.3% (1 mL, 2.5 mL, 5 mL)

Gefitinib (ge FI tye nib)

Brand Names: U.S. Iressa®
Brand Names: Canada IRESSA®
Pharmacologic Category Antineoplastic Agent, Tyrosine Kinase Inhibitor
Use Treatment of locally advanced or metastatic non-small cell lung cancer (NSCLC) after failure of platinum-based and docetaxel therapies. Treatment is limited to patients who are benefiting or have benefited from treatment with gefitinib.
Note: Due to the lack of improved survival data from clinical trials of gefitinib, and in response to positive survival data with another EGFR inhibitor, according to the U.S. labeling, physicians are advised to use treatment options other than gefitinib in patients with advanced nonsmall cell lung cancer following one or two prior chemotherapy regimens when they are refractory/intolerant to their most recent regimen.

Canada labeling: First-line treatment of locally advanced or metastatic NSCLC with activating mutations of EGFR-TK
Unlabeled Use First-line treatment of NSCLC with known EGFR mutation
Local Anesthetic/Vasoconstrictor Precautions No information available to require special precautions
Effects on Dental Treatment Key adverse event(s) related to dental treatment: Mouth ulceration.
Effects on Bleeding Bleeding has been reported in <1% of patients, but can be serious.
Adverse Effects
>10%:
Dermatologic: Rash (43% to 54%), acne (25% to 33%), dry skin (13% to 26%), paronychia (14%)

649

Gastrointestinal: Diarrhea (48% to 67%; grade 3: 1%), nausea (13% to 18%), vomiting (9% to 12%)

1% to 10%:
Cardiovascular: Peripheral edema (2%)
Dermatologic: Pruritus (8% to 9%)
Gastrointestinal: Anorexia (7% to 10%), weight loss (3% to 5%), mouth ulceration (1%)
Neuromuscular & skeletal: Weakness (4% to 6%)
Ocular: Amblyopia (2%), conjunctivitis (1%)
Respiratory: Dyspnea (2%), interstitial lung disease (1% to 2%; includes alveolitis, interstitial pneumonia, pneumonitis)

General Dosage Range Dosage adjustment recommended in patients on concomitant therapy or who develop toxicities.

Oral: *Adults:* 250 mg once daily

Mechanism of Action Gefitinib is a tyrosine kinase inhibitor (TKI) which inhibits numerous tyrosine kinases associated with transmembrane cell surface receptors found on both normal and cancer cells, including the tyrosine kinase associated with the epidermal growth factor receptor, EGFR. Tyrosine kinase activity appears to be vitally important to cell proliferation and survival.

Pharmacodynamics/Kinetics

Half-life Elimination Oral: 41 hours

Time to Peak Plasma: Oral: 3-7 hours

Pregnancy Risk Factor D

Pregnancy Considerations Animal studies have demonstrated fetal harm; there are no well-controlled studies in pregnant women. The risk of fetal harm should be carefully weighed. Women of childbearing potential should be advised to avoid pregnancy.

Prescribing and Access Restrictions As of September 15, 2005, distribution of gefitinib (IRESSA®) is limited to patients enrolled in the IRESSA® Access Program. Under this program, access to gefitinib will be limited to the following groups:

Patients who are currently receiving and benefiting from gefitinib

Patients who have previously received and benefited from gefitinib

Previously-enrolled patients or new patients in non-Investigational New Drug (IND) clinical trials involving gefitinib if these protocols were approved by an IRB prior to June 17, 2005

New patients may also receive gefitinib if the manufacturer (AstraZeneca) decides to make it available under IND, and the patients meet the criteria for enrollment under the IND

Additional information on the IRESSA® Access Program, including enrollment forms, may be obtained by calling AstraZeneca at 1-800-601-8933 or via the web at www.Iressa-access.com

---

Gelatin (Absorbable) (JEL a tin, ab SORB a ble)

Related Information
Antiplatelet and Anticoagulation Considerations in Dentistry *on page 1503*

Brand Names: U.S. Gelfilm®; Gelfoam®

Generic Availability (U.S.) No

Pharmacologic Category Hemostatic Agent

Dental Use Adjunct to provide hemostasis in oral and dental surgery

Use Adjunct to provide hemostasis in surgical procedures; adjunct in neuro, thoracic, or ocular surgeries to promote tissue repair and/or prevent adhesions (Gelfilm®)

Local Anesthetic/Vasoconstrictor Precautions No information available to require special precautions

Effects on Dental Treatment Key adverse event(s) related to dental treatment: Local infection and abscess formation.

Effects on Bleeding Used as adjunct to enhance hemostasis.

Adverse Effects
Frequency not defined:
Central nervous system: Fever
Local: Abscess and infection formation
Miscellaneous: Foreign body reactions, encapsulation of fluid and hematoma

Adverse events reported when used in various surgical procedures (Gelfoam®):
Cardiopulmonary bypass surgery: Atrial fibrillation (13%), wound infection (6%), heart failure (4%), atrial flutter (2%), peripheral vascular disorder (2%), pneumothorax (2%), respiratory arrest (2%), respiratory failure (2%), ventricular tachycardia (2%), fever (1%), heart block (1%)
Implant in brain: Compression of brain and spinal cord, giant-cell granuloma
Laminectomy operations: Arachnoiditis, bladder and bowel dysfunction, cauda equine syndrome, headaches, impotence, meningitis, pain, paresthesias, spinal stenosis
Nasal surgery: Toxic shock syndrome
Tendon repair: Fibrosis, fixation of tendon prolonged
Tympanoplasty: Failure of absorption, hearing loss

Dosage Children and Adults:
Hemostasis (Gelfoam®): **Note:** Use minimum amount of product necessary to produce hemostasis; once hemostasis attained, excess product should be removed.
Dental sponge: Insert rolled sponge (dry or wet) into cavity or socket; apply light finger pressure for 1-2 minutes
Sponge: Apply appropriate size (dry or wet) with moderate pressure directly to bleeding site until bleeding stops; if first application does not stop bleeding, additional applications may be used with a new sponge
Powder: Apply paste to bleeding surface; remove excess paste when bleeding has stopped. Consult manufacturer's labeling for additional information.
Neurosurgery, thoracic, or ocular surgery (Gelfilm®): Use as directed per manufacturer's labeling.

Mechanism of Action Arrests bleeding by forming artificial clot and producing mechanical matrix which facilitates clotting

Contraindications
Gelfilm®: There are no contraindications listed in the manufacturer's labeling.
Gelfoam®: Hypersensitivity to porcine collagen; intravascular placement (embolus risk); closure of skin incisions (interferes with healing)

Warnings/Precautions Do not sterilize by heat; do not use in the presence of infection

Drug Interactions

Metabolism/Transport Effects None known.

Avoid Concomitant Use There are no known interactions where it is recommended to avoid concomitant use.

Increased Effect/Toxicity There are no known significant interactions involving an increase in effect.

Decreased Effect There are no known significant interactions involving a decrease in effect.

Pregnancy Considerations When administered topically, gelatin is completely absorbed; however, the amount of gelatin available systemically following topical application is unknown.

Dosage Forms
Film, ophthalmic:
Gelfilm®: (6s)
Film, topical:
Gelfilm®: (1s)
Powder, topical:
Gelfoam®: (1 g)
Sponge, oral topical:
Gelfoam®: (12s)
Sponge, topical:
Gelfoam®: (4s, 6s, 12s)

Gemcitabine (jem SITE a been)

Brand Names: U.S. Gemzar®
Brand Names: Canada Gemcitabine For Injection; Gemcitabine For Injection, USP; Gemcitabine Sun For Injection; Gemzar®
Pharmacologic Category Antineoplastic Agent, Antimetabolite; Antineoplastic Agent, Antimetabolite (Pyrimidine Analog)
Use Treatment of metastatic breast cancer; inoperable locally-advanced or metastatic nonsmall cell lung cancer (NSCLC); locally advanced or metastatic pancreatic cancer; advanced, relapsed ovarian cancer
Unlabeled Use Treatment of biliary tract cancers (advanced), bladder cancer, cervical cancer (recurrent or persistent), Ewing's sarcoma (refractory), head and neck cancer (nasopharyngeal), Hodgkin lymphoma (relapsed), non-Hodgkin lymphomas (refractory), malignant pleural mesothelioma, osteosarcoma (refractory), renal cell cancer (metastatic), small cell lung cancer (refractory or relapsed), soft tissue sarcoma (advanced), testicular cancer (refractory germ cell tumors), thymic malignancies, uterine sarcoma, and unknown-primary adenocarcinoma
Local Anesthetic/Vasoconstrictor Precautions No information available to require special precautions
Effects on Dental Treatment Key adverse event(s) related to dental treatment: Stomatitis.
Effects on Bleeding Bleeding occurs in 2% to 17% of patients. Anemia (68% to 73%) and thrombocytopenia (24% to 36%) frequently occur. Medical consult is recommended.
Adverse Effects Frequency of adverse reactions reported for single-agent use of gemcitabine only.
>10%:
Cardiovascular: Peripheral edema (20%), edema (13%)
Central nervous system: Fever (38% to 41%), somnolence (11%)
Dermatologic: Rash (28% to 30%), alopecia (15% to 16%), pruritus (13%)
Gastrointestinal: Nausea/vomiting (69% to 71%; grade 3: 10% to 13%; grade 4: 1% to 2%), diarrhea (19% to 30%), stomatitis (10% to 11%)
Hematologic: Anemia (68% to 73%; grade 4: 1% to 2%), leukopenia (62% to 64%; grade 4: ≤1%), neutropenia (61% to 63%; grade 4: 6% to 7%), thrombocytopenia (24% to 36%; grade 4: ≤1%), hemorrhage (4% to 17%; grades 3: ≤2%; grade 4: <1%); myelosuppression is the dose-limiting toxicity

Hepatic: AST increased (67% to 78%; grade 3: 6% to 12%; grade 4: 2% to 5%), alkaline phosphatase increased (55% to 77%; grade 3: 7% to 16%; grade 4: 2% to 4%), ALT increased (68% to 72%; grade 3: 8% to 10%; grade 4: 1% to 2%), bilirubin increased (13% to 26%; grade 3: 2% to 6%; grade 4: ≤2%)
Renal: Proteinuria (32% to 45%; grades 3/4: <1%), hematuria (23% to 35%; grades 3/4: <1%), BUN increased (15% to 16%)
Respiratory: Dyspnea (10% to 23%)
Miscellaneous: Flu-like syndrome (19%), infection (10% to 16%; grade 3: 1% to 2%; grade 4: <1%)
1% to 10%:
Local: Injection site reactions (4%)
Neuromuscular & skeletal: Paresthesia (10%)
Renal: Creatinine increased (6% to 8%)
Respiratory: Bronchospasm (<2%)
General Dosage Range Dosage adjustment recommended in patients with hepatic impairment or who develop toxicities
I.V.: *Adults:* Dosage varies greatly depending on indication
Mechanism of Action A pyrimidine antimetabolite that inhibits DNA synthesis by inhibition of DNA polymerase and ribonucleotide reductase, cell cycle-specific for the S-phase of the cycle (also blocks cellular progression at G1/S-phase). Gemcitabine is phosphorylated intracellularly by deoxycytidine kinase to gemcitabine monophosphate, which is further phosphorylated to active metabolites gemcitabine diphosphate and gemcitabine triphosphate. Gemcitabine diphosphate inhibits DNA synthesis by inhibiting ribonucleotide reductase; gemcitabine triphosphate incorporates into DNA and inhibits DNA polymerase.
Pharmacodynamics/Kinetics
Half-life Elimination
Gemcitabine: Infusion time ≤70 minutes: 42-94 minutes; infusion time 3-4 hours: 4-10.5 hours (affected by age and gender)
Metabolite (gemcitabine triphosphate), terminal phase: 1.7-19.4 hours
Time to Peak 30 minutes after completion of infusion
Pregnancy Risk Factor D
Pregnancy Considerations Embryotoxicity and fetal malformations (cleft palate, incomplete ossification, fused pulmonary artery, absence of gallbladder) have been reported in animal studies. There are no adequate and well-controlled studies in pregnant women. If patient becomes pregnant, she should be informed of risks. May cause fetal harm if administered during pregnancy; adverse effects in reproduction are anticipated based on the mechanism of action.

Gemfibrozil (jem FI broe zil)

Related Information
Cardiovascular Diseases *on page 1492*
Brand Names: U.S. Lopid®
Brand Names: Canada Apo-Gemfibrozil®; Gen-Gemfibrozil; GMD-Gemfibrozil; Lopid®; Mylan-Gemfibrozil; Novo-Gemfibrozil; Nu-Gemfibrozil; PMS-Gemfibrozil
Generic Availability (U.S.) Yes
Pharmacologic Category Antilipemic Agent, Fibric Acid
Use Treatment of hypertriglyceridemia in Fredrickson types IV and V hyperlipidemia for patients who are at greater risk for pancreatitis and who have not responded to dietary intervention; to reduce the risk of CHD development in Fredrickson type IIb patients without a history

or symptoms of existing CHD who have not responded to dietary and other interventions (including pharmacologic treatment) and who have decreased HDL, increased LDL, and increased triglycerides

Local Anesthetic/Vasoconstrictor Precautions No information available to require special precautions

Effects on Dental Treatment No significant effects or complications reported

Effects on Bleeding Anemia has been reported in <1% of patients.

Adverse Effects

>10%: Gastrointestinal: Dyspepsia (20%)

1% to 10%:
Cardiovascular: Atrial fibrillation (1%)
Central nervous system: Fatigue (4%), vertigo (2%)
Dermatologic: Eczema (2%), rash (2%)
Gastrointestinal: Abdominal pain (10%), nausea/vomiting (3%)

Reports where causal relationship has not been established: Alopecia, anaphylaxis, cataracts, colitis, confusion, decreased fertility (male), drug-induced lupus-like syndrome, extrasystoles, hepatoma, intracranial hemorrhage, pancreatitis, peripheral vascular disease, photosensitivity, positive ANA, renal dysfunction, retinal edema, seizure, syncope, thrombocytopenia, vasculitis, weight loss

Dosage Adults: Oral: 600 mg twice daily; administer 30 minutes before breakfast and dinner

Dosage adjustment in renal impairment:
Mild-to-moderate impairment: Use caution; deterioration of renal function has been reported in patients with baseline serum creatinine >2 mg/dL
Severe impairment: Use is contraindicated
Hemodialysis: Not removed by hemodialysis; supplemental dose is not necessary

Dosage adjustment in hepatic impairment: Use is contraindicated

Mechanism of Action The exact mechanism of action of gemfibrozil is unknown, however, several theories exist regarding the VLDL effect; it can inhibit lipolysis and decrease subsequent hepatic fatty acid uptake as well as inhibit hepatic secretion of VLDL; together these actions decrease serum VLDL levels; increases HDL-cholesterol; the mechanism behind HDL elevation is currently unknown

Contraindications Hypersensitivity to gemfibrozil or any component of the formulation; hepatic or severe renal dysfunction; primary biliary cirrhosis; pre-existing gallbladder disease; concurrent use with repaglinide

Warnings/Precautions Secondary causes of hyperlipidemia should be ruled out prior to therapy. Possible increased risk of malignancy and cholelithiasis. Anemia, leukopenia, thrombocytopenia, and bone marrow hypoplasia have rarely been reported. Periodic monitoring recommended during the first year of therapy. Elevations in serum transaminases can be seen. Discontinue if lipid response not seen. Be careful in patient selection; this is not a first- or second-line choice. Other agents may be more suitable. Adjustments in warfarin therapy may be required with concurrent use. Has been associated with rare myositis or rhabdomyolysis; patients should be monitored closely. Patients should be instructed to report unexplained muscle pain, tenderness, weakness, or brown urine. Use caution when combining gemfibrozil with HMG-CoA reductase inhibitors (may lead to myopathy, rhabdomyolysis). Use with caution in patients with mild-to-moderate renal impairment; contraindicated in patients with severe impairment. Renal function deterioration has been seen when used in patients with a serum creatinine >2 mg/dL.

Drug Interactions

Metabolism/Transport Effects Substrate of CYP3A4 (minor); **Note:** Assignment of Major/Minor substrate status based on clinically relevant drug interaction potential; **Inhibits** CYP1A2 (moderate), CYP2C19 (strong), CYP2C8 (strong), CYP2C9 (strong)

Avoid Concomitant Use
Avoid concomitant use of Gemfibrozil with any of the following: AtorvaSTATin; Bexarotene (Systemic); Clopidogrel; Enzalutamide; Fluvastatin; Lovastatin; Pirfenidone; Pitavastatin; Pravastatin; Repaglinide; Rosuvastatin; Simvastatin

Increased Effect/Toxicity
Gemfibrozil may increase the levels/effects of: Antidiabetic Agents (Thiazolidinedione); AtorvaSTATin; Bexarotene (Systemic); Carvedilol; Citalopram; Colchicine; CYP1A2 Substrates; CYP2C19 Substrates; CYP2C8 Substrates; CYP2C9 Substrates; Diclofenac (Systemic); Enzalutamide; Ezetimibe; Fluvastatin; Lovastatin; Ospemifene; Pirfenidone; Pitavastatin; Pravastatin; Repaglinide; Rosuvastatin; Simvastatin; Sulfonylureas; Treprostinil; Vitamin K Antagonists

The levels/effects of Gemfibrozil may be increased by: CycloSPORINE (Systemic)

Decreased Effect
Gemfibrozil may decrease the levels/effects of: Chenodiol; Clopidogrel; CycloSPORINE (Systemic); Ursodiol

The levels/effects of Gemfibrozil may be decreased by: Bile Acid Sequestrants

Ethanol/Nutrition/Herb Interactions
Ethanol: Avoid ethanol to decrease triglycerides.
Food: When given after meals, the AUC of gemfibrozil is decreased.

Dietary Considerations Before initiation of therapy, patients should be placed on a standard cholesterol-lowering diet for 3-6 months and the diet should be continued during drug therapy. Should be taken 30 minutes prior to breakfast and dinner

Pharmacodynamics/Kinetics

Onset of Action May require several days

Half-life Elimination 1.5 hours

Time to Peak Serum: 1-2 hours

Pregnancy Risk Factor C

Pregnancy Considerations Adverse events were observed in animal reproduction studies. There are no adequate and well-controlled studies in pregnant women. Use only if benefits outweigh the risks.

Lactation Excretion in breast milk unknown/not recommended

Breast-Feeding Considerations It is not known if gemfibrozil is excreted in breast milk. Due to the potential for serious adverse reactions in the nursing infant, a decision should be made whether to discontinue nursing or to discontinue the drug, taking into account the importance of treatment to the mother.

Dosage Forms

Tablet, oral: 600 mg
Lopid®: 600 mg

Gemifloxacin (je mi FLOKS a sin)

Related Information
Bacterial Infections *on page 1562*
Clinical Risk Related to Drugs Prolonging QT Interval *on page 1510*

Brand Names: U.S. Factive®
Brand Names: Canada Factive®
Generic Availability (U.S.) No
Pharmacologic Category Antibiotic, Quinolone; Respiratory Fluoroquinolone
Use Treatment of acute exacerbation of chronic bronchitis; treatment of community-acquired pneumonia (CAP), including pneumonia caused by multidrug-resistant strains of *S. pneumoniae* (MDRSP)
Unlabeled Use Acute sinusitis

Local Anesthetic/Vasoconstrictor Precautions
Gemifloxacin is one of the drugs confirmed to prolong the QT interval and is accepted as having a risk of causing torsade de pointes. The risk of drug-induced torsade de pointes is extremely low when a single QT interval prolonging drug is prescribed. In terms of epinephrine, it is not known what effect vasoconstrictors in the local anesthetic regimen will have in patients with a known history of congenital prolonged QT interval or in patients taking any medication that prolongs the QT interval. Until more information is obtained, it is suggested that the clinician consult with the physician prior to the use of a vasoconstrictor in suspected patients, and that the vasoconstrictor (epinephrine, mepivacaine and levonordefrin [Carbocaine® 2% with Neo-Cobefrin®]) be used with caution.

Effects on Dental Treatment No significant effects or complications reported

Effects on Bleeding No information available to require special precautions

Adverse Effects 1% to 10%:
Central nervous system: Headache (4%), dizziness (2%)
Dermatologic: Rash (4%)
Gastrointestinal: Diarrhea (5%), nausea (4%), abdominal pain (2%), vomiting (2%)
Hepatic: Transaminases increased (1% to 4%)

Important adverse effects reported with other agents in this drug class include (not reported for gemifloxacin): Allergic reactions, CNS stimulation, hepatitis, jaundice, peripheral neuropathy, pneumonitis (eosinophilic); seizure; sensorimotor-axonal neuropathy (paresthesia, hypoesthesias, dysesthesias, weakness); severe dermatologic reactions (toxic epidermal necrolysis, Stevens-Johnson syndrome); torsade de pointes, vasculitis

Dosage
Usual dosage range:
Adults: Oral: 320 mg once daily
Indication-specific dosing:
Adults: Oral:
Acute exacerbations of chronic bronchitis: 320 mg once daily for 5 days
Community-acquired pneumonia (mild-to-moderate): 320 mg once daily for 5 or 7 days (decision to use 5- or 7-day regimen should be guided by initial sputum culture; 7 days are recommended for MDRSP, *Klebsiella*, or *M. catarrhalis* infection)
Sinusitis (unlabeled use): 320 mg once daily for 10 days
Elderly: Refer to adult dosing.

Dosage adjustment in renal impairment:
Cl_{cr} >40 mL/minute: No adjustment required
Cl_{cr} ≤40 mL/minute (or patients on hemodialysis/CAPD): 160 mg once daily (administer dose following hemodialysis)
Dosage adjustment in hepatic impairment: No adjustment required

Mechanism of Action Gemifloxacin is a DNA gyrase inhibitor and also inhibits topoisomerase IV. DNA gyrase (topoisomerase IV) is an essential bacterial enzyme that maintains the superhelical structure of DNA. DNA gyrase is required for DNA replication and transcription, DNA repair, recombination, and transposition; bactericidal

Contraindications Hypersensitivity to gemifloxacin, other fluoroquinolones, or any component of the formulation

Warnings/Precautions [U.S. Boxed Warning]: There have been reports of tendon inflammation and/or rupture with quinolone antibiotics; risk may be increased with concurrent corticosteroids, organ transplant recipients, and in patients >60 years of age. Rupture of the Achilles tendon sometimes requiring surgical repair has been reported most frequently; but other tendon sites (eg, rotator cuff, biceps) have also been reported. Strenuous physical activity, rheumatoid arthritis, and renal impairment may be an independent risk factor for tendonitis. Discontinue at first sign of tendon inflammation or pain. May occur even after discontinuation of therapy. Use with caution in patients with rheumatoid arthritis; may increase risk of tendon rupture. Fluoroquinolones may prolong QT_c interval; avoid use of gemifloxacin in patients with a history of QT_c prolongation, uncorrected hypokalemia, hypomagnesemia, or concurrent administration of other medications known to prolong the QT interval (including Class Ia and Class III antiarrhythmics, cisapride, erythromycin, antipsychotics, and tricyclic antidepressants). Use with caution in patients with significant bradycardia or acute myocardial ischemia. CNS effects may occur (tremor, restlessness, confusion, and very rarely hallucinations, increased intracranial pressure [including pseudotumor cerebri] or seizures). Use with caution in patients with known or suspected CNS disorder. Potential for seizures, although very rare, may be increased with concomitant NSAID therapy. Use with caution in individuals at risk of seizures. Use caution in renal dysfunction; dosage adjustment required for Cl_{cr} ≤40 mL/minute.

Fluoroquinolones have been associated with the development of serious, and sometimes fatal, hypoglycemia, most often in elderly diabetics, but also in patients without diabetes. This occurred most frequently with gatifloxacin (no longer available systemically) but may occur at a lower frequency with other quinolones.

Severe hypersensitivity reactions, including anaphylaxis, have occurred with quinolone therapy. Reactions may present as typical allergic symptoms after a single dose, or may manifest as severe idiosyncratic dermatologic, vascular, pulmonary, renal, hepatic, and/or hematologic events, usually after multiple doses. May cause maculopapular rash, usually 8-10 days after treatment initiation; risk factors may include age <40 years, female gender (including postmenopausal women on HRT), and treatment duration >7 days. Prompt discontinuation of drug should occur if skin rash or other symptoms arise. **[U.S. Boxed Warning]: Quinolones may exacerbate myasthenia gravis; avoid use (rare, potentially life-threatening weakness of respiratory muscles may occur).** Avoid excessive sunlight and ▶

◀ take precautions to limit exposure (eg, loose fitting clothing, sunscreen); may cause moderate-to-severe phototoxicity reactions. Discontinue use if photosensitivity occurs. Prolonged use may result in fungal or bacterial superinfection, including *C. difficile*-associated diarrhea (CDAD) and pseudomembranous colitis; CDAD has been observed >2 months postantibiotic treatment. Peripheral neuropathy has been linked to the use of quinolones; these cases were rare. Hemolytic reactions may (rarely) occur with quinolone use in patients with latent or actual G6PD deficiency.

Drug Interactions
Metabolism/Transport Effects None known.
Avoid Concomitant Use
Avoid concomitant use of Gemifloxacin with any of the following: BCG; Highest Risk QTc-Prolonging Agents; Ivabradine; Mifepristone; Strontium Ranelate
Increased Effect/Toxicity
Gemifloxacin may increase the levels/effects of: Corticosteroids (Systemic); Highest Risk QTc-Prolonging Agents; Moderate Risk QTc-Prolonging Agents; Porfimer; Sulfonylureas; Varenicline; Vitamin K Antagonists

The levels/effects of Gemifloxacin may be increased by: Insulin; Ivabradine; Mifepristone; Nonsteroidal Anti-Inflammatory Agents; Probenecid; QTc-Prolonging Agents (Indeterminate Risk and Risk Modifying)
Decreased Effect
Gemifloxacin may decrease the levels/effects of: BCG; Didanosine; Mycophenolate; Sodium Picosulfate; Sulfonylureas; Typhoid Vaccine

The levels/effects of Gemifloxacin may be decreased by: Antacids; Calcium Salts; Didanosine; Iron Salts; Magnesium Salts; Multivitamins/Minerals (with ADEK, Folate, Iron); Quinapril; Sevelamer; Strontium Ranelate; Sucralfate; Zinc Salts

Ethanol/Nutrition/Herb Interactions Herb/Nutraceutical: Avoid dong quai, St John's wort (may also cause photosensitization).

Dietary Considerations May take tablets with or without food, milk, or calcium supplements. Gemifloxacin should be taken 3 hours before or 2 hours after supplements (including multivitamins) containing iron, zinc, or magnesium.

Pharmacodynamics/Kinetics
Half-life Elimination 7 hours (range 4-12 hours)
Time to Peak Plasma: 0.5-2 hours
Pregnancy Risk Factor C
Pregnancy Considerations Adverse events have been observed in some animal studies; therefore, the manufacturer classifies gemifloxacin as pregnancy category C. Quinolone exposure during human pregnancy has been reported with other agents (see Ciprofloxacin [Systemic], Ofloxacin [Systemic], and Norfloxacin monographs). To date, no specific teratogenic effect or increased pregnancy risk has been identified; however, because of concerns of cartilage damage in immature animals exposed to quinolones and the limited gemifloxacin specific data, gemifloxacin should only be used during pregnancy if a safer option is not available.

Lactation Excretion in breast milk unknown/not recommended
Breast-Feeding Considerations It is not known if gemifloxacin is excreted in breast milk. Breast-feeding is not recommended by the manufacturer. Nondose-related effects could include modification of bowel flora.

Dosage Forms
Tablet, oral:
Factive®: 320 mg
Dental Comment Gemifloxacin is known to prolong the QT interval. The QT interval is measured as the time and distance between the Q point of the QRS complex and the end of the T wave in the ECG tracing. After adjustment for heart rate, the QT interval is defined as prolonged if it is more than 450 msec in men and 460 msec in women. A long QT syndrome was first described in the 1950s and 60s as a congenital syndrome involving QT interval prolongation and syncope and sudden death. Some of the congenital long QT syndromes were characterized by a peculiar electrocardiographic appearance of the QRS complex involving a premature atria beat followed by a pause, then a subsequent sinus beat showing marked QT prolongation and deformity. This type of cardiac arrhythmia was originally termed "torsade de pointes" (translated from the French as "twisting of the points"). Gemifloxacin is considered as having a risk of causing torsade de pointes. Since it is not known what effect vasoconstrictors in the local anesthetic regimen will have in patients with a known history of congenital prolonged QT interval or in patients taking any medication that prolongs the QT interval, a medical consult is suggested.

Gemtuzumab Ozogamicin
(gem TOO zoo mab oh zog a MY sin)

Pharmacologic Category Antineoplastic Agent, Monoclonal Antibody
Use Due to safety concerns, as well as lack of clinical benefit demonstrated in a post-approval clinical trial, gemtuzumab was withdrawn from the U.S. commercial market in 2010.
Unlabeled Use Treatment of relapsed or refractory CD33-positive acute myeloid leukemia (AML); salvage therapy for acute promyelocytic leukemia (APL)
Effects on Bleeding Bleeding reported in 13% of patients with gum hemorrhage reported in 9%. Bone marrow suppression with anemia and thrombocytopenia are common. Recovery of platelets may be delayed. Medical consult recommended.
Adverse Effects Frequency not defined.
Cardiovascular: Cerebral hemorrhage, hyper-/hypotension, peripheral edema, tachycardia
Central nervous system: Anxiety, chills, depression, dizziness, fever, headache, insomnia, intracranial hemorrhage, pain
Dermatologic: Bruising, petechiae, pruritus, rash
Endocrine & metabolic: Hyperglycemia, hypocalcemia, hypokalemia, hypomagnesemia, hypophosphatemia
Gastrointestinal: Abdominal pain, anorexia, diarrhea, dyspepsia, gingival hemorrhage, melena, mucositis, nausea, stomatitis, vomiting
Genitourinary: Vaginal bleeding, vaginal hemorrhage
Hematologic: Anemia, disseminated intravascular coagulation (DIC), hemorrhage, leukopenia, lymphopenia, neutropenia (median recovery 40-51 days), neutropenic fever, thrombocytopenia (median recovery 36-51 days)
Hepatic: Alkaline phosphatase increased, ALT increased, ascites, AST increased, hyperbilirubinemia, LDH increased, prothrombin time increased, PTT increased, sinusoidal obstruction syndrome (SOS; veno-occlusive disease; higher frequency in patients with prior history of or subsequent hematopoietic stem cell transplant)
Local: Local reaction

Neuromuscular & skeletal: Arthralgia, back pain, myalgia, weakness

Renal: Creatinine increased, hematuria

Respiratory: Cough, dyspnea, epistaxis, hypoxia, pharyngitis, pneumonia, rhinitis

Miscellaneous: Cutaneous herpes simplex, infection, infusion reaction, sepsis

Mechanism of Action Antibody to CD33 antigen, which is expressed on leukemic blasts in 80% of AML patients. Binds to the CD33 antigen, resulting in internalization of the antibody-antigen complex. Following internalization, the calicheamicin derivative is released inside the myeloid cell. The calicheamicin derivative binds to DNA resulting in double strand breaks and cell death. Pluripotent stem cells and nonhematopoietic cells are not affected.

Pharmacodynamics/Kinetics

Half-life Elimination Total calicheamicin: Initial: 41-45 hours, Repeat dose: 60-64 hours; Unconjugated: 100-143 hours (no change noted in repeat dosing)

Pregnancy Considerations Animal studies have demonstrated teratogenic effects, fetal loss, and maternal toxicity. There are no adequate and well-controlled studies in pregnant women. May cause fetal harm when administered to a pregnant woman. Women of childbearing potential should avoid becoming pregnant while receiving treatment.

Product Availability No longer commercially available in the U.S. market for new patients. Available in Canada through a special access program.

Prescribing and Access Restrictions As of June 2010, gemtuzumab has been withdrawn from the U.S. market and is no longer commercially available to new patients; gemtuzumab is only available in the U.S. under an Investigational New Drug (IND) protocol.

In Canada, gemtuzumab is available through a special access program (access information is available from Health Canada).

Gentamicin (Systemic) (jen ta MYE sin)

Brand Names: Canada Gentamicin Injection, USP

Pharmacologic Category Antibiotic, Aminoglycoside

Use Treatment of susceptible bacterial infections, normally gram-negative organisms, including *Pseudomonas*, *Proteus*, *Serratia*, and gram-positive *Staphylococcus*; treatment of bone infections, respiratory tract infections, skin and soft tissue infections, as well as abdominal and urinary tract infections, and septicemia; treatment of infective endocarditis

Local Anesthetic/Vasoconstrictor Precautions No information available to require special precautions

Effects on Dental Treatment No significant effects or complications reported

Effects on Bleeding No information available to require special precautions

Adverse Effects Frequency not defined.

Cardiovascular: Edema, hyper/hypotension

Central nervous system: Ataxia, confusion, depression, dizziness, drowsiness, encephalopathy, fever, headache, lethargy, pseudomotor cerebri, seizures, vertigo

Dermatologic: Alopecia, erythema, itching, purpura, rash, urticaria

Endocrine & metabolic: Hypocalcemia, hypokalemia, hypomagnesemia, hyponatremia

Gastrointestinal: Anorexia, appetite decreased, *C. difficile*-associated diarrhea, enterocolitis, nausea, salivation increased, splenomegaly, stomatitis, vomiting, weight loss

Hematologic: Agranulocytosis, anemia, eosinophilia, granulocytopenia, leukopenia, reticulocytes increased/decreased, thrombocytopenia

Hepatic: Hepatomegaly, LFTs increased

Local: Injection site reactions, pain at injection site, phlebitis/thrombophlebitis

Neuromuscular & skeletal: Arthralgia, gait instability, muscle cramps, muscle twitching, muscle weakness, myasthenia gravis-like syndrome, numbness, paresthesia, peripheral neuropathy, tremor, weakness

Ocular: Visual disturbances

Otic: Hearing impairment, hearing loss (associated with persistently increased serum concentrations; early toxicity usually affects high-pitched sound), tinnitus

Renal: BUN increased, casts (hyaline, granular) in urine, creatinine clearance decreased, distal tubular dysfunction, Fanconi-like syndrome (high dose, prolonged course) (infants and adults), oliguria, renal failure (high trough serum concentrations), polyuria, proteinuria, serum creatinine increased, tubular necrosis, urine specific gravity decreased

Respiratory: Dyspnea, laryngeal edema, pulmonary fibrosis, respiratory depression

Miscellaneous: Allergic reaction, anaphylaxis, anaphylactoid reactions

General Dosage Range Dosage adjustment recommended for the I.M. and I.V. routes in patients with renal impairment

I.M., I.V.:

Children <5 years: 2.5 mg/kg/dose every 8 hours

Children ≥5 years: 2-2.5 mg/kg/dose every 8 hours

Adults: 1-2.5 mg/kg/dose every 8-12 hours **or** 4-7 mg/kg once daily

Intrathecal: *Adults:* 4-8 mg/day

Mechanism of Action Interferes with bacterial protein synthesis by binding to 30S and 50S ribosomal subunits resulting in a defective bacterial cell membrane

Pharmacodynamics/Kinetics

Half-life Elimination

Infants: <1 week: 3-11.5 hours; 1 week to 6 months: 3-3.5 hours

Adults: 1.5-3 hours; End-stage renal disease: 36-70 hours

Time to Peak Serum: I.M.: 30-90 minutes; I.V.: 30 minutes after 30-minute infusion

Pregnancy Risk Factor D

Pregnancy Considerations Gentamicin crosses the placenta and produces detectable serum levels in the fetus. Renal toxicity has been described in two case reports following first trimester exposure. There are several reports of total irreversible bilateral congenital deafness in children whose mothers received streptomycin during pregnancy; therefore, the manufacturer classifies gentamicin as pregnancy category D. Although ototoxicity has not been reported following maternal use of gentamicin, a potential for harm exists. **[U.S. Boxed Warning]: Aminoglycosides may cause fetal harm if administered to a pregnant woman.**

Due to pregnancy induced physiologic changes, some pharmacokinetic parameters of gentamicin may be altered. Pregnant women have an average-to-larger volume of distribution which may result in lower serum peak levels than for the same dose in nonpregnant women. Serum half-life is also shorter.

Gentian Violet (JEN shun VYE oh let)

Pharmacologic Category Antibiotic, Topical; Antifungal Agent, Topical

Use Treatment of cutaneous or mucocutaneous infections caused by *Candida albicans* and other superficial skin infections; external treatment of minor abrasions or cuts

Local Anesthetic/Vasoconstrictor Precautions No information available to require special precautions

Effects on Dental Treatment Key adverse event(s) related to dental treatment: Ulceration of mucous membranes.

Effects on Bleeding No information available to require special precautions

Adverse Effects Frequency not defined.

Dermatologic: Necrotic skin reactions, staining, vesicle formation

Gastrointestinal: Esophagitis, gastrointestinal irritation, ulceration of mucous membranes

Genitourinary: Hemorrhagic cystitis

Local: Burning, irritation

Ocular: Keratoconjunctivitis

Respiratory: Epistaxis, laryngitis, laryngeal obstruction, tracheitis

Miscellaneous: Allergic contact dermatitis, sensitivity reactions

General Dosage Range Topical: *Children and Adults:* Apply 0.5% to 2% to affected area once or twice daily

Mechanism of Action Topical antiseptic/germicide effective against some vegetative gram-positive bacteria, particularly *Staphylococcus* sp, and some yeast; it is much less effective against gram-negative bacteria and is ineffective against acid-fast bacteria

Glatiramer Acetate (gla TIR a mer AS e tate)

Brand Names: U.S. Copaxone®
Brand Names: Canada Copaxone®
Pharmacologic Category Biological, Miscellaneous
Use Management of relapsing-remitting type multiple sclerosis, including patients with a first clinical episode with MRI features consistent with multiple sclerosis

Local Anesthetic/Vasoconstrictor Precautions No information available to require special precautions

Effects on Dental Treatment Key adverse event(s) related to dental treatment: Ulcerative stomatitis, salivary gland enlargement, and oral moniliasis.

Effects on Bleeding No information available to require special precautions

Adverse Effects
>10%:
Cardiovascular: Vasodilation (20%), chest pain (13%)
Central nervous system: Pain (20%), anxiety (13%)
Dermatologic: Rash (19%)
Gastrointestinal: Nausea (15%)
Local: Injection site reactions: Inflammation (49%), erythema (43%), pain (40%), pruritus (27%), mass (27%)
Neuromuscular & skeletal: Weakness (22%), back pain (12%)
Respiratory: Dyspnea (14%)
Miscellaneous: Infection (30%), flu-like syndrome (14%), diaphoresis (15%)
1% to 10%:
Cardiovascular: Edema (8%; includes peripheral and facial), palpitation (7%), tachycardia (5%), syncope (3%), hypertension (1%)
Central nervous system: Fever (6%), migraine (4%), chills (3%), nervousness (2%), speech disorder (2%), abnormal dreams (1%), emotional lability (1%), stupor (1%)

Dermatologic: Bruising (8%), pruritus (5%), erythema (4%), urticaria (3%), skin nodule (2%), eczema (1%), pustular rash (1%)
Endocrine & metabolic: Amenorrhea (1%), impotence (1%), menorrhagia (1%)
Gastrointestinal: Vomiting (7%), gastroenteritis (6%), weight gain (3%), dysphagia (2%), dental caries (1%)
Genitourinary: Urinary urgency (5%), vaginal moniliasis (4%)
Local: Injection site reactions: Hemorrhage (5%), hypersensitivity (4%), fibrosis (2%), lipoatrophy (2%), abscess (1%), edema (1%)
Neuromuscular & skeletal: Neck pain (8%), tremor (4%)
Ocular: Diplopia (3%), visual field defect (1%)
Respiratory: Rhinitis (7%), bronchitis (6%), cough (6%), laryngismus (5%), hyperventilation (1%)
Miscellaneous: Lymphadenopathy (7%), hypersensitivity (3%)
General Dosage Range SubQ: *Adults:* 20 mg daily
Mechanism of Action Glatiramer is a mixture of random polymers of four amino acids; L-alanine, L-glutamic acid, L-lysine, and L-tyrosine, the resulting mixture is antigenically similar to myelin basic protein, which is an important component of the myelin sheath of nerves; glatiramer is thought to induce and activate T-lymphocyte suppressor cells specific for a myelin antigen; it is also proposed that glatiramer interferes with the antigen-presenting function of certain immune cells opposing pathogenic T-cell function
Pregnancy Risk Factor B
Pregnancy Considerations Adverse events were not observed in animal studies. There are no adequate and well-controlled studies in pregnant women. Use in pregnancy only if clearly necessary.

Gliclazide (GLYE kla zide)

Brand Names: Canada Apo-Gliclazide®; AVA-Gliclazide; Diamicron®; Diamicron® MR; Gliclazide MR; Gliclazide-80; Mylan-Gliclazide; Novo-Gliclazide; PMS-Gliclazide
Pharmacologic Category Antidiabetic Agent, Sulfonylurea
Use Management of type 2 diabetes mellitus (noninsulin dependent, NIDDM)

Local Anesthetic/Vasoconstrictor Precautions No information available to require special precautions

Effects on Dental Treatment Gliclazide-dependent patients with diabetes (noninsulin dependent, type 2) should be appointed for dental treatment in morning in order to minimize chance of stress-induced hypoglycemia.

Effects on Bleeding No information available to require special precautions

Adverse Effects
>10%: Endocrine & metabolic: Hypoglycemia (11% to 12%)
1% to 10%:
Cardiovascular: Hypertension (3% to 4%), angina (2%), peripheral edema (1%)
Central nervous system: Headache (4% to 5%), dizziness (2%), depression (1% to 2%), insomnia (1% to 2%)
Dermatologic: Skin disorder (2%), dermatitis (1% to 2%), rash (1%; includes maculopapular, morbilliform), pruritus (≤1%)
Endocrine & metabolic: Hyperglycemia (2%), hyperlipidemia (1%), lipid metabolism disorder (1%)

Gastrointestinal: Diarrhea (2% to 3%), constipation (1% to 2%), gastroenteritis (1% to 2%), abdominal pain (1%), gastritis (1%), nausea (1%)

Genitourinary: Urinary tract infection (3%)

Neuromuscular & skeletal: Back pain (4% to 5%), arthralgia (3% to 4%), weakness (2% to 3%), arthrosis (2%), myalgia (2%), arthritis (1% to 2%), neuralgia (1%), tendonitis (1%)

Ocular: Conjunctivitis (1%)

Otic: Otitis media (1%)

Respiratory: Bronchitis (4% to 5%), rhinitis (4% to 5%), pharyngitis (4%), upper respiratory infection (3% to 4%), cough (2%), pneumonia (1% to 2%), sinusitis (1% to 2%)

Miscellaneous: Viral infection (6% to 8%)

Dosage Oral: Adults:

Type 2 diabetes: **Note:** There is no fixed-dosage regimen for the management of diabetes mellitus with gliclazide. Dose must be individualized based on frequent determinations of blood glucose during dose titration and throughout maintenance.

Immediate release tablet: Recommended initial: 80 mg twice daily; titrate based on blood glucose levels. Usual dosage range: 80-320 mg/day (maximum dose: 320 mg/day); dosage of ≥160 mg should be divided into 2 equal parts for twice-daily administration

Modified release tablet: Initial: 30 mg once daily; titrate in 30 mg increments every 2 weeks based on blood glucose levels. Maximum dose: 120 mg once daily

Maturity-onset diabetes: May consider conversion from insulin to gliclazide therapy in patients receiving <40 units/day insulin. Prior to conversion, discontinue insulin for 48-72 hours with close monitoring (≥3 times/day) of urine for glucose and ketones. Patients with ketonuria and glycosuria 12-24 hours after discontinuing insulin should not be converted to gliclazide therapy and should remain on insulin therapy.

Elderly: Refer to adult dosing.

Dosage adjustment in renal impairment:

Mild-to-moderate impairment: Initial dosage adjustments are not required; however, as gliclazide is primarily excreted in the urine, dose reductions may be necessary.

Severe impairment: Use is contraindicated.

Dosage adjustment in hepatic impairment:

Mild-to-moderate impairment: Initial dosage adjustments are not required; dose reductions may be necessary; however, as gliclazide is primarily excreted in the urine.

Severe impairment: Use is contraindicated.

Mechanism of Action Stimulates insulin release from the pancreatic beta cells; reduces insulin uptake and glucose output by the liver; insulin sensitivity is increased at peripheral target sites. Reduces microthrombosis by decreasing platelet aggregation and adhesion, and by restoring fibrinolysis with an increase in tissue plasminogen activator (t-PA) activity. Antioxidant effects include a decrease in plasma levels of peroxidized lipids and increased erythrocyte superoxide dismutase activity.

Contraindications Hypersensitivity to gliclazide, other sulfonylureas or sulfonamides, or any component of the formulation; unstable and/or type 1 diabetes mellitus (insulin dependent, IDDM); diabetic ketoacidosis; diabetic pre-coma and coma; severe renal or hepatic impairment; stress conditions (eg, serious infection, trauma, surgery); concurrent use with miconazole (systemic or oromucosal gel); pregnancy; breast-feeding

Warnings/Precautions All sulfonylurea drugs are capable of producing severe hypoglycemia. The incidence of hypoglycemia is least with gliclazide compared to other sulfonylureas (eg, glimepiride or glyburide) (Canadian Diabetes Association [CDA], 2008). Hypoglycemia is more likely to occur when caloric intake is deficient, after severe or prolonged exercise, when ethanol is ingested, or when more than one glucose-lowering drug is used. Hypoglycemia is also more likely in elderly patients, malnourished patients or in patients with endocrine disorders, severe vascular disease or impaired renal or hepatic function. Hypoglycemic effects (eg, dizziness, weakness) may impair physical or mental abilities; patients must be cautioned about performing tasks which require mental alertness (eg, operating machinery or driving).

Loss of efficacy may be observed following prolonged use as a result of the progression of type 2 diabetes mellitus which results in continued beta cell destruction. In patients who were previously responding to sulfonylurea therapy, consider additional factors which may be contributing to decreased efficacy (eg, inappropriate dose, nonadherence to diet and exercise regimen). If no contributing factors can be identified, consider discontinuing use of the sulfonylurea due to secondary failure of treatment. Additional antidiabetic therapy (eg, insulin) will be required. Diabetes self-management education (DSME) is essential to maximize the effectiveness of therapy.

Chemical similarities are present among sulfonamides, sulfonylureas, carbonic anhydrase inhibitors, thiazides, and loop diuretics (except ethacrynic acid). Use in patients with sulfonamide allergy is contraindicated in the product labeling due to the risk of cross-reaction that exists in patients with an allergy to any of these compounds especially when the previous reaction has been severe. Use with caution in hepatic or renal impairment as metabolism and/or excretion may be impaired; dose reductions may be necessary. Discontinue use if cholestatic jaundice occurs during therapy. Use in severe hepatic or renal impairment or during periods of stress (eg, trauma, infection, surgery) is contraindicated. Patients with glucose-6-phosphate dehydrogenase (G6PD) deficiency may be at an increased risk of sulfonylurea-induced hemolytic anemia; however, cases have also been described in patients without G6PD deficiency during postmarketing surveillance. Use with caution and consider a nonsulfonylurea alternative in patients with G6PD deficiency

U.S. product labeling of sulfonylureas states oral hypoglycemic drugs may be associated with an increased cardiovascular mortality as compared to treatment with diet alone or diet plus insulin. Data to support this association are limited, and several studies, including a large prospective trial (UKPDS), have not supported an association. Formulation may contain lactose; avoid use in patients with galactose intolerance, glucose-galactose malabsorption or Lapp lactose deficiency.

Drug Interactions

Metabolism/Transport Effects Substrate of CYP2C9 (major); **Note:** Assignment of Major/Minor substrate status based on clinically relevant drug interaction potential

Avoid Concomitant Use There are no known interactions where it is recommended to avoid concomitant use.

Increased Effect/Toxicity

Gliclazide may increase the levels/effects of: Alcohol (Ethyl); Hypoglycemic Agents; Porfimer; Vitamin K Antagonists

The levels/effects of Gliclazide may be increased by: Beta-Blockers; Chloramphenicol; Cimetidine; Cyclic Antidepressants; CYP2C9 Inhibitors (Moderate); CYP2C9 Inhibitors (Strong); Fibric Acid Derivatives; Fluconazole; GLP-1 Agonists; Herbs (Hypoglycemic Properties); MAO Inhibitors; Mifepristone; Pegvisomant; Probenecid; Quinolone Antibiotics; Ranitidine; Salicylates; Selective Serotonin Reuptake Inhibitors; Sulfonamide Derivatives; Vitamin K Antagonists; Voriconazole

Decreased Effect

The levels/effects of Gliclazide may be decreased by: Corticosteroids (Orally Inhaled); Corticosteroids (Systemic); CYP2C9 Inducers (Strong); Loop Diuretics; Luteinizing Hormone-Releasing Hormone Analogs; Peginterferon Alfa-2b; Quinolone Antibiotics; Rifampin; Somatropin; Thiazide Diuretics

Ethanol/Nutrition/Herb Interactions

Ethanol: Avoid ethanol (may cause hypoglycemia and/or rare disulfiram reactions).

Herb/Nutraceutical: Avoid chromium, garlic, gymnema (may cause hypoglycemia).

Dietary Considerations Should be taken with meals. Individualized medical nutrition therapy (MNT) based on CDA recommendations is an integral part of therapy.

Pharmacodynamics/Kinetics

Duration of Action Modified release tablet: 24 hours

Half-life Elimination Immediate release tablet: 10 hours; Modified release tablet: 16 hours (range: 12-20 hours)

Time to Peak Immediate release tablet: 4-6 hours; Modified release tablet: ~6 hours

Pregnancy Considerations Use during pregnancy is contraindicated. Maternal hyperglycemia can be associated with adverse effects in the fetus, including macrosomia, neonatal hyperglycemia, and hyperbilirubinemia; the risk of congenital malformations is increased when the Hb A_{1c} is above the normal range. Diabetes can also be associated with adverse effects in the mother. Poorly-treated diabetes may cause end-organ damage that may in turn negatively affect obstetric outcomes. Physiologic glucose levels should be maintained prior to and during pregnancy to decrease the risk of adverse events in the mother and the fetus. Insulin is the drug of choice for the control of diabetes mellitus during pregnancy.

Lactation Excretion in breast milk unknown/contraindicated

Breast-Feeding Considerations Potential for neonatal hypoglycemia in a nursing infant contraindicates use.

Product Availability Not available in U.S.

Dosage Forms: Canada

Tablet, oral:
Diamicron®: 80 mg

Tablet, modified release, oral:
Diamicron® MR: 30 mg, 60 mg

Glimepiride (GLYE me pye ride)

Related Information
Endocrine Disorders and Pregnancy *on page 1517*

Brand Names: U.S. Amaryl®

Brand Names: Canada Amaryl®; Apo-Glimepiride®; Novo-Glimepiride; PMS-Glimepiride; ratio-Glimepiride; Sandoz-Glimepiride

Generic Availability (U.S.) Yes

Pharmacologic Category Antidiabetic Agent, Sulfonylurea

Use Management of type 2 diabetes mellitus (noninsulin dependent, NIDDM) as an adjunct to diet and exercise to lower blood glucose; may be used in combination with metformin or insulin in patients whose hyperglycemia cannot be controlled by diet and exercise in conjunction with a single oral hypoglycemic agent

Local Anesthetic/Vasoconstrictor Precautions No information available to require special precautions

Effects on Dental Treatment Glimepiride-dependent patients with diabetes (noninsulin dependent, type 2) should be appointed for dental treatment in morning in order to minimize chance of stress-induced hypoglycemia.

Effects on Bleeding No information available to require special precautions

Adverse Effects
>10%: Endocrine & metabolic: Hypoglycemia (4% to 20%)

1% to 10%:
Central nervous system: Dizziness (2%), headache
Gastrointestinal: Nausea (5%)
Hepatic: ALT increased (2%)
Miscellaneous: Flu-like syndrome (5%)

Dosage Oral:
Adults: Initial: 1-2 mg once daily, administered with breakfast or the first main meal; based on response, may increase dose by 1-2 mg every 1-2 weeks up to maximum of 8 mg daily. If inadequate response to maximal dose, combination therapy with other agents (eg, metformin, insulin) may be considered. Combination therapy is individualized based on glycemic response.

Conversion from therapy with long half-life agents: Observe patient carefully for 1-2 weeks when converting from a longer half-life agent (eg, chlorpropamide) to glimepiride due to overlapping hypoglycemic effects.

Elderly: Initial: 1 mg once daily; dose titration and maintenance dosing should be conservative to avoid hypoglycemia

Dosing adjustment/comments in renal impairment:
U.S. labeling: Initial: 1 mg once daily; titrate carefully based on fasting blood glucose levels
Canadian labeling:
Mild-to-moderate impairment: Initial: 1 mg once daily; titrate carefully based on fasting blood glucose levels
Severe impairment: Use is contraindicated

Dosing adjustment in hepatic impairment:
U.S. labeling: No dosage adjustment provided in manufacturer's labeling (has not been studied).
Canadian labeling:
Mild-to-moderate impairment: No dosage adjustment provided in manufacturer's labeling (has not been studied).
Severe impairment: Use is contraindicated.

Mechanism of Action Stimulates insulin release from the pancreatic beta cells; reduces glucose output from the liver; insulin sensitivity is increased at peripheral target sites

Contraindications Hypersensitivity to glimepiride, any component of the formulation, or sulfonamides; diabetic ketoacidosis (with or without coma)

Canadian labeling: Additional contraindications (not in U.S. labeling): Pregnancy; breast-feeding; severe renal or hepatic impairment

Warnings/Precautions All sulfonylurea drugs are capable of producing severe hypoglycemia. Hypoglycemia is more likely to occur when caloric intake is deficient, after severe or prolonged exercise, when ethanol is ingested, or when more than one glucose-lowering drug is used. It is also more likely in elderly patients, malnourished patients and in patients with impaired renal or hepatic function; use with caution.

Loss of efficacy may be observed following prolonged use as a result of the progression of type 2 diabetes mellitus which results in continued beta cell destruction. In patients who were previously responding to sulfonylurea therapy, consider additional factors which may be contributing to decreased efficacy (eg, inappropriate dose, nonadherence to diet and exercise regimen). If no contributing factors can be identified, consider discontinuing use of the sulfonylurea due to secondary failure of treatment. Additional antidiabetic therapy (eg, insulin) will be required. It may be necessary to discontinue therapy and administer insulin if the patient is exposed to stress (fever, trauma, infection, surgery).

Chemical similarities are present among sulfonamides, sulfonylureas, carbonic anhydrase inhibitors, thiazides, and loop diuretics (except ethacrynic acid). Use in patients with sulfonamide allergy is not specifically contraindicated in product labeling, however, a risk of cross-reaction exists in patients with allergy to any of these compounds; avoid use when previous reaction has been severe. Patients with G6PD deficiency may be at an increased risk of sulfonylurea-induced hemolytic anemia; however, cases have also been described in patients without G6PD deficiency during postmarketing surveillance. Use with caution and consider a nonsulfonylurea alternative in patients with G6PD deficiency.

Product labeling states oral hypoglycemic drugs may be associated with an increased cardiovascular mortality as compared to treatment with diet alone or diet plus insulin. Data to support this association are limited, and several studies, including a large prospective trial (UKPDS) have not supported an association.

Drug Interactions

Metabolism/Transport Effects Substrate of CYP2C9 (major); **Note:** Assignment of Major/Minor substrate status based on clinically relevant drug interaction potential

Avoid Concomitant Use There are no known interactions where it is recommended to avoid concomitant use.

Increased Effect/Toxicity

Glimepiride may increase the levels/effects of: Alcohol (Ethyl); Hypoglycemic Agents; Porfimer; Vitamin K Antagonists

The levels/effects of Glimepiride may be increased by: Beta-Blockers; Chloramphenicol; Cimetidine; Cyclic Antidepressants; CYP2C9 Inhibitors (Moderate); CYP2C9 Inhibitors (Strong); Fibric Acid Derivatives; Fluconazole; GLP-1 Agonists; Herbs (Hypoglycemic Properties); MAO Inhibitors; Mifepristone; Pegvisomant; Probenecid; Quinolone Antibiotics; Ranitidine; Salicylates; Selective Serotonin Reuptake Inhibitors; Sulfonamide Derivatives; Vitamin K Antagonists; Voriconazole

Decreased Effect

The levels/effects of Glimepiride may be decreased by: Colesevelam; Corticosteroids (Orally Inhaled); Corticosteroids (Systemic); CYP2C9 Inducers (Strong); Loop Diuretics; Luteinizing Hormone-Releasing Hormone Analogs; Peginterferon Alfa-2b; Quinolone Antibiotics; Rifampin; Somatropin; Thiazide Diuretics

Ethanol/Nutrition/Herb Interactions

Ethanol: Caution with ethanol (may cause hypoglycemia).

Herb/Nutraceutical: Caution with chromium, garlic, gymnema (may cause hypoglycemia).

Dietary Considerations Take with breakfast or the first main meal of the day. Individualized medical nutrition therapy (MNT) based on ADA recommendations is an integral part of therapy.

Pharmacodynamics/Kinetics

Onset of Action Peak effect: Blood glucose reductions: 2-3 hours

Duration of Action 24 hours

Half-life Elimination 5-9 hours

Time to Peak 2-3 hours

Pregnancy Risk Factor C

Pregnancy Considerations Adverse events have been observed in animal studies; therefore, glimepiride is classified as pregnancy category C. Severe hypoglycemia lasting 4-10 days has been noted in infants born to mothers taking a sulfonylurea at the time of delivery. The manufacturer recommends that patients be switched to insulin during pregnancy. Maternal hyperglycemia can be associated with adverse effects in the fetus, including macrosomia, neonatal hyperglycemia, and hyperbilirubinemia; the risk of congenital malformations is increased when the Hb A_{1c} is above the normal range. Diabetes can also be associated with adverse effects in the mother. Poorly-treated diabetes may cause end-organ damage that may in turn negatively affect obstetric outcomes. Physiologic glucose levels should be maintained prior to and during pregnancy to decrease the risk of adverse events in the mother and the fetus. Until additional safety and efficacy data are obtained, the use of oral agents is generally not recommended as routine management of GDM or type 2 diabetes mellitus during pregnancy. Insulin is the drug of choice for the control of diabetes mellitus during pregnancy.

Lactation Excretion in breast milk unknown/not recommended

Breast-Feeding Considerations It is not known if glimepiride is excreted in breast milk. Breast-feeding is not recommended by the manufacturer. Potentially, hypoglycemia may occur in a nursing infant exposed to a sulfonylurea via breast milk.

Dosage Forms

Tablet, oral: 1 mg, 2 mg, 4 mg
Amaryl®: 1 mg, 2 mg, 4 mg

GlipiZIDE (GLIP i zide)

Related Information

Endocrine Disorders and Pregnancy *on page 1517*

Brand Names: U.S. Glucotrol XL®; Glucotrol®

Generic Availability (U.S.) Yes

Pharmacologic Category Antidiabetic Agent, Sulfonylurea

▶

Use Management of type 2 diabetes mellitus (noninsulin dependent, NIDDM) as an adjunct to diet and exercise to lower blood glucose; may be used in combination with metformin or insulin in patients whose hyperglycemia cannot be controlled by diet and exercise in conjunction with a single oral hypoglycemic agent

Local Anesthetic/Vasoconstrictor Precautions No information available to require special precautions

Effects on Dental Treatment Glipizide-dependent patients with diabetes (noninsulin dependent, type 2) should be appointed for dental treatment in morning in order to minimize chance of stress-induced hypoglycemia.

Effects on Bleeding No information available to require special precautions

Adverse Effects Frequency not always defined.
Cardiovascular: Syncope (<3%)
Central nervous system: Dizziness (2% to 7%), nervousness (4%), anxiety (<3%), depression (<3%), hypoesthesia (<3%), insomnia (<3%), pain (<3%), drowsiness (2%), headache (2%)
Dermatologic: Pruritus (1% to <3%), eczema (1%), erythema (1%), maculopapular eruptions (1%), morbilliform eruptions (1%), rash (1%), urticaria (1%)
Endocrine & metabolic: Hypoglycemia (<3%)
Gastrointestinal: Diarrhea (1% to 5%), flatulence (3%), constipation (1% to <3%), nausea (1% to <3%), dyspepsia (<3%), vomiting (<3%), abdominal pain (1%)
Hepatic: Alkaline phosphatase increased, AST increased, LDH increased
Neuromuscular & skeletal: Tremor (4%), arthralgia (<3%), leg cramps (<3%), myalgia (<3%), paresthesia (<3%)
Ocular: Blurred vision (<3%)
Renal: Blood urea nitrogen increased, creatinine increased
Respiratory: Rhinitis (<3%)
Miscellaneous: Diaphoresis (<3%)

Dosage Oral: Adults:
Immediate release tablet: Initial: 5 mg once daily; titrate in 2.5-5 mg increments no more frequently than every few days based on blood glucose response; if once-daily dose is ineffective, may divide the dose; doses >15 mg/day should be administered in divided doses. Maximum recommended once-daily dose: 15 mg; maximum recommended total daily dose: 40 mg (some clinicians recommend a maximum total daily dose of 20 mg [Defronzo, 1999]).
Extended release tablet (Glucotrol XL®): Initial: 5 mg once daily; usual dose: 5-10 mg once daily; maximum recommended dose: 20 mg/day; dosage adjustments based on blood glucose monitoring should be made no more frequently than every 7 days
When transferring from immediate release to extended release glipizide: May switch the total daily dose of immediate release to the nearest equivalent daily dose of the extended release tablet and administer once daily; alternatively, may initiate extended release at 5 mg once daily and titrate accordingly.
When transferring from insulin to glipizide immediate release or extended release tablet:
Current insulin requirement ≤20 units: Discontinue insulin and initiate glipizide at usual dose
Current insulin requirement >20 units: Decrease insulin by 50% and initiate glipizide at usual dose; gradually decrease insulin dose based on patient response

Conversion from therapy with long half-life agents: Observe patient carefully for 1-2 weeks when converting from a longer half-life agent (eg, chlorpropamide) to glipizide due to overlapping hypoglycemic effects.

Elderly:
Immediate release tablet: Initial: 2.5 mg once daily; consider titrating by 2.5-5 mg/day at 1- to 2-week intervals
Extended release tablet: Initial and maintenance dosing should be on the lower end of the recommended range.

Dosing adjustment in renal impairment: No dosage adjustment provided in manufacturer's labeling although caution is recommended.
The following guidelines have been used by some clinicians (Aronoff, 2007): GFR ≤50 mL/minute: Decrease dose by 50%

Dosing adjustment in hepatic impairment:
Immediate release tablet: Initial: 2.5 mg once daily
Extended release tablet: There are no dosage adjustments provided in manufacturer's labeling; however, drug undergoes hepatic metabolism and use of a lower initial and maintenance dose should be considered.

Mechanism of Action Stimulates insulin release from the pancreatic beta cells; reduces glucose output from the liver; insulin sensitivity is increased at peripheral target sites

Contraindications Hypersensitivity to glipizide or any component of the formulation; type 1 diabetes mellitus (insulin dependent, IDDM); diabetic ketoacidosis (with or without coma)

Warnings/Precautions All sulfonylurea drugs are capable of producing severe hypoglycemia. Hypoglycemia is more likely to occur when caloric intake is deficient, after severe or prolonged exercise, when ethanol is ingested, or when more than one glucose-lowering drug is used. It is also more likely in elderly patients, malnourished patients and in patients with impaired renal or hepatic function; use with caution. Autonomic neuropathy, advanced age, and concomitant use of beta-blockers or other sympatholytic agents may impair the patient's ability to recognize the signs and symptoms of hypoglycemia; use with caution.

Use with caution in patients with hepatic or renal impairment. It may be necessary to discontinue therapy and administer insulin if the patient is exposed to stress (fever, trauma, infection, surgery). Loss of efficacy may be observed following prolonged use as a result of the progression of type 2 diabetes mellitus which results in continued beta cell destruction. In patients who were previously responding to sulfonylurea therapy, consider additional factors which may be contributing to decreased efficacy (eg, inappropriate dose, nonadherence to diet and exercise regimen). If no contributing factors can be identified, consider discontinuing use of the sulfonylurea due to secondary failure of treatment. Additional antidiabetic therapy (eg, insulin) will be required.

Chemical similarities are present among sulfonamides, sulfonylureas, carbonic anhydrase inhibitors, thiazides, and loop diuretics (except ethacrynic acid). Use in patients with sulfonamide allergy is not specifically contraindicated in product labeling; however, a risk of cross-reaction exists in patients with allergy to any of these compounds; avoid use when previous reaction has been severe. Patients with G6PD deficiency may be at an increased risk of sulfonylurea-induced hemolytic anemia; however, cases have also been described in patients without G6PD deficiency during postmarketing surveillance. Use with caution and consider a nonsulfonylurea alternative in patients with G6PD deficiency.

Product labeling states oral hypoglycemic drugs may be associated with an increased cardiovascular mortality as compared to treatment with diet alone or diet plus insulin. Data to support this association are limited, and several studies, including a large prospective trial (UKPDS) have not supported an association. Avoid use of extended release tablets (Glucotrol XL®) in patients with known stricture/narrowing of the GI tract.

Drug Interactions

Metabolism/Transport Effects Substrate of CYP2C9 (major); **Note:** Assignment of Major/Minor substrate status based on clinically relevant drug interaction potential

Avoid Concomitant Use There are no known interactions where it is recommended to avoid concomitant use.

Increased Effect/Toxicity

GlipiZIDE may increase the levels/effects of: Alcohol (Ethyl); Hypoglycemic Agents; Porfimer; Vitamin K Antagonists

The levels/effects of GlipiZIDE may be increased by: Beta-Blockers; Chloramphenicol; Cimetidine; Clarithromycin; Cyclic Antidepressants; CYP2C9 Inhibitors (Moderate); CYP2C9 Inhibitors (Strong); Fibric Acid Derivatives; Fluconazole; GLP-1 Agonists; Herbs (Hypoglycemic Properties); MAO Inhibitors; Mifepristone; Pegvisomant; Posaconazole; Probenecid; Quinolone Antibiotics; Ranitidine; Salicylates; Selective Serotonin Reuptake Inhibitors; Sulfonamide Derivatives; Vitamin K Antagonists; Voriconazole

Decreased Effect

The levels/effects of GlipiZIDE may be decreased by: Colesevelam; Corticosteroids (Orally Inhaled); Corticosteroids (Systemic); CYP2C9 Inducers (Strong); Loop Diuretics; Luteinizing Hormone-Releasing Hormone Analogs; Peginterferon Alfa-2b; Quinolone Antibiotics; Rifampin; Somatropin; Thiazide Diuretics

Ethanol/Nutrition/Herb Interactions

Ethanol: Caution with ethanol (may cause hypoglycemia or rare disulfiram reaction).

Food: A delayed release of insulin may occur if glipizide is taken with food. Immediate release tablets should be administered 30 minutes before meals to avoid erratic absorption.

Herb/Nutraceutical: Herbs with hypoglycemic properties may enhance the hypoglycemic effect of glipizide. This includes alfalfa, aloe, bilberry, bitter melon, burdock, celery, damiana, fenugreek, garcinia, garlic, ginger, ginseng (American), gymnema, marshmallow, stinging nettle

Dietary Considerations Take immediate release tablets 30 minutes before meals (preferably before breakfast if once-daily dosing); extended release tablets should be taken with breakfast. Individualized medical nutrition therapy (MNT) based on ADA recommendations is an integral part of therapy.

Pharmacodynamics/Kinetics

Duration of Action 12-24 hours

Half-life Elimination 2-5 hours

Time to Peak 1-3 hours; extended release tablets: 6-12 hours

Pregnancy Risk Factor C

Pregnancy Considerations Adverse events have been observed in animal studies; therefore, glipizide is classified as pregnancy category C. Glipizide crosses the placenta. Severe hypoglycemia lasting 4-10 days has been noted in infants born to mothers taking a sulfonylurea at the time of delivery. Maternal hyperglycemia can be associated with adverse effects in the fetus, including macrosomia, neonatal hyperglycemia, and hyperbilirubinemia; the risk of congenital malformations is increased when the Hb A_{1c} is above the normal range. Diabetes can also be associated with adverse effects in the mother. Poorly-treated diabetes may cause end-organ damage that may in turn negatively affect obstetric outcomes. Physiologic glucose levels should be maintained prior to and during pregnancy to decrease the risk of adverse events in the mother and the fetus. Until additional safety and efficacy data are obtained, the use of oral agents is generally not recommended as routine management of GDM or type 2 diabetes mellitus during pregnancy. The manufacturer recommends if glipizide is used during pregnancy it should be discontinued at least 1 month before the expected delivery date. Insulin is the drug of choice for the control of diabetes mellitus during pregnancy.

Lactation Excretion in breast milk unknown/not recommended

Breast-Feeding Considerations Data from initial studies note that glipizide was not detected in breast milk. Breast-feeding is not recommended by the manufacturer. Potentially, hypoglycemia may occur in a nursing infant exposed to a sulfonylurea via breast milk.

Dosage Forms

Tablet, oral: 5 mg, 10 mg

Glucotrol®: 5 mg, 10 mg

Tablet, extended release, oral: 2.5 mg, 5 mg, 10 mg

Glucotrol XL®: 2.5 mg, 5 mg, 10 mg

Glipizide and Metformin
(GLIP i zide & met FOR min)

Related Information

GlipiZIDE on page 659

MetFORMIN on page 882

Brand Names: U.S. Metaglip™

Generic Availability (U.S.) Yes

Pharmacologic Category Antidiabetic Agent, Biguanide; Antidiabetic Agent, Sulfonylurea

Use Indicated as an adjunct to diet and exercise to improve glycemic control in adults with type 2 diabetes mellitus (noninsulin dependent, NIDDM)

Local Anesthetic/Vasoconstrictor Precautions No information available to require special precautions

Effects on Dental Treatment Key adverse event(s) related to dental treatment: Upper respiratory tract infection (8% to 10%). Dependent patients with diabetes (noninsulin dependent, type 2) should be appointed for dental treatment in the morning in order to minimize chance of stress-induced hypoglycemia.

Effects on Bleeding No information available to require special precautions

Adverse Effects Also see individual agents.

>10%:

Central nervous system: Headache (13%)

Endocrine & metabolic: Hypoglycemia (8% to 13%)

Gastrointestinal: Diarrhea (2% to 18%)

1% to 10%:

Cardiovascular: Hypertension (3% to 4%)

Central nervous system: Dizziness (2% to 5%)

Gastrointestinal: Nausea/vomiting (<1% to 8%), abdominal pain (6%)

Neuromuscular & skeletal: Musculoskeletal pain (8%)

Renal: Urinary tract infection (1%)

Respiratory: Upper respiratory tract infection (8% to 10%)

Dosage Oral: Type 2 diabetes:

Adults:

Patients inadequately controlled on diet and exercise alone: Initial dose: Glipizide 2.5 mg/metformin 250 mg once daily with a meal. In patients with fasting plasma glucose (FPG) 280-320 mg/dL, initiate therapy with glipizide 2.5 mg/metformin 500 mg twice daily.

Note: Increase dose by 1 tablet/day every 2 weeks (maximum daily dose: Glipizide 10 mg/metformin 2000 mg in divided doses)

Patients inadequately controlled on a sulfonylurea and/or metformin: Initial dose: Glipizide 2.5 mg/metformin 500 mg or glipizide 5 mg/metformin 500 mg twice daily with morning and evening meals; starting dose should not exceed current daily dose of glipizide (or sulfonylurea equivalent) and/or metformin.

Note: Increase dose in increments of no more than glipizide 5 mg/metformin 500 mg (maximum daily dose: Glipizide 20 mg/metformin 2000 mg)

Elderly: Conservative doses are recommended in the elderly due to potentially decreased renal function; **do not titrate to maximum dose**; should not be used in patients ≥80 years unless renal function is verified as normal

Dosage adjustment in renal impairment: Contraindicated in the presence of renal disease or renal dysfunction (serum creatinine ≥1.5 mg/dL [males], ≥1.4 mg/dL [females], or abnormal creatinine clearance)

Dosage adjustment in hepatic impairment: Avoid use in patients with impaired liver function

Mechanism of Action The combination of glipizide and metformin is used to improve glycemic control in patients with type 2 diabetes mellitus (noninsulin dependent, NIDDM) by using two different, but complementary, mechanisms of action:

Glipizide: Stimulates insulin release from the pancreatic beta cells; reduces glucose output from the liver; insulin sensitivity is increased at peripheral target sites

Metformin: Decreases hepatic glucose production, decreasing intestinal absorption of glucose and improves insulin sensitivity (increases peripheral glucose uptake and utilization)

Contraindications Hypersensitivity to glipizide, metformin, or any component of the formulation; renal disease or renal dysfunction (serum creatinine ≥1.5 mg/dL in males or ≥1.4 mg/dL in females, or abnormal creatinine clearance which may also result from conditions such as cardiovascular collapse, acute myocardial infarction, and septicemia); acute or chronic metabolic acidosis with or without coma (including diabetic ketoacidosis)

Note: Temporarily discontinue in patients undergoing radiologic studies in which intravascular iodinated contrast materials are utilized.

Warnings/Precautions Age, hepatic and renal impairment are independent risk factors for hypoglycemia. Use with caution in patients with hepatic impairment, malnourished or debilitated conditions, or adrenal or pituitary insufficiency. Use caution in patients with renal impairment. Use caution in the elderly and patients taking beta-blockers; signs and symptoms of hypoglycemia may be masked. Instruct patients to avoid excessive acute or chronic ethanol use; ethanol may potentiate metformin's effect on lactate metabolism and increase risk of hypoglycemia.

[U.S. Boxed Warning]: Lactic acidosis is a rare, but potentially severe consequence of therapy with metformin. Withhold therapy in hypoxemia, dehydration, or sepsis. The risk of lactic acidosis is increased in any patient with CHF requiring pharmacologic management. This risk is particularly high during acute or unstable CHF because of the risk of hypoperfusion and hypoxemia. Metformin is substantially excreted by the kidney. The risk of accumulation and lactic acidosis increases with the degree of impairment of renal function. Patients with renal function below the limit of normal for their age should not receive metformin. In elderly patients, renal function should be monitored regularly; should not be used in any patient ≥80 years of age unless normal renal function is confirmed. Use of concomitant medications that may affect renal function (ie, affect tubular secretion) may also affect metformin disposition. Metformin should be withheld in patients with dehydration and/or prerenal azotemia. Therapy should be suspended for any surgical procedures (resume only after oral intake resumed and normal renal function is verified). Intravascular iodinated contrast media used for radiologic studies are associated with alteration of renal function and may increase risk of lactic acidosis. Discontinue Metaglip™ at the time of or prior to the procedure and withhold for 48 hours subsequent to the procedure; reinstitute only after renal function has been re-evaluated and found to be normal.

It may be necessary to discontinue therapy and administer insulin if the patient is exposed to stress (fever, trauma, infection, surgery). Loss of efficacy may be observed following prolonged use as a result of the progression of type 2 diabetes mellitus which results in continued beta cell destruction. In patients who were previously responding to sulfonylurea therapy, consider additional factors which may be contributing to decreased efficacy (eg, inappropriate dose, nonadherence to diet and exercise regimen). If no contributing factors can be identified, consider discontinuing use of the sulfonylurea due to secondary failure of treatment. Additional antidiabetic therapy (eg, insulin) will be required.

Chemical similarities are present among sulfonamides, sulfonylureas, carbonic anhydrase inhibitors, thiazides, and loop diuretics (except ethacrynic acid). Use in patients with sulfonamide allergy is not specifically contraindicated in product labeling, however, a risk of cross-reaction exists in patients with allergy to any of these compounds; avoid use when previous reaction has been severe. Patients with G6PD deficiency may be at an increased risk of sulfonylurea-induced hemolytic anemia; however, cases have also been described in patients without G6PD deficiency during postmarketing surveillance. Use with caution and consider a nonsulfonylurea alternative in patients with G6PD deficiency.

Product labeling states oral hypoglycemic drugs may be associated with an increased cardiovascular mortality as compared to treatment with diet alone or diet plus insulin. Data to support this association are limited, and several studies, including a large prospective trial (UKPDS), have not supported an association.

Drug Interactions

Metabolism/Transport Effects Refer to individual components.

Avoid Concomitant Use There are no known interactions where it is recommended to avoid concomitant use.

Increased Effect/Toxicity

Glipizide and Metformin may increase the levels/effects of: Alcohol (Ethyl); Dalfampridine; Dofetilide; Hypoglycemic Agents; Porfimer; Vitamin K Antagonists

The levels/effects of Glipizide and Metformin may be increased by: Beta-Blockers; Carbonic Anhydrase Inhibitors; Cephalexin; Chloramphenicol; Cimetidine; Clarithromycin; Cyclic Antidepressants; CYP2C9 Inhibitors (Moderate); CYP2C9 Inhibitors (Strong); Dalfampridine; Fibric Acid Derivatives; Fluconazole; GLP-1 Agonists; Glycopyrrolate; Herbs (Hypoglycemic Properties); Iodinated Contrast Agents; LamoTRIgine; MAO Inhibitors; Mifepristone; Pegvisomant; Posaconazole; Probenecid; Quinolone Antibiotics; Ranitidine; Salicylates; Selective Serotonin Reuptake Inhibitors; Sulfonamide Derivatives; Trimethoprim; Vitamin K Antagonists; Voriconazole

Decreased Effect

Glipizide and Metformin may decrease the levels/effects of: Trospium

The levels/effects of Glipizide and Metformin may be decreased by: Colesevelam; Corticosteroids (Orally Inhaled); Corticosteroids (Systemic); CYP2C9 Inducers (Strong); Loop Diuretics; Luteinizing Hormone-Releasing Hormone Analogs; Peginterferon Alfa-2b; Quinolone Antibiotics; Rifampin; Somatropin; Thiazide Diuretics

Ethanol/Nutrition/Herb Interactions See individual agents.

Dietary Considerations May cause GI upset; should be taken with food to decrease GI upset. Individualized medical nutrition therapy (MNT) based on ADA recommendations is an integral part of therapy. Monitor for signs and symptoms of vitamin B_{12} and folic acid deficiency; supplementation may be required.

Pregnancy Risk Factor C

Pregnancy Considerations Animal reproduction studies were not conducted with this combination; therefore, glipizide/metformin is classified as pregnancy category C. Refer to individual agents.

Lactation

Glipizide: Excretion in breast milk unknown/not recommended

Metformin: Enters breast milk/not recommended

Breast-Feeding Considerations Refer to individual agents.

Dosage Forms

Tablet, oral: 2.5/250: Glipizide 2.5 mg and metformin 250 mg; 2.5/500: Glipizide 2.5 mg and metformin 500 mg; 5/500: Glipizide 5 mg and metformin 500 mg

Metaglip™: 2.5/500: Glipizide 2.5 mg and metformin 500 mg; 5/500: Glipizide 5 mg and metformin 500 mg

---

Glucagon (GLOO ka gon)

Brand Names: U.S. GlucaGen®; GlucaGen® Diagnostic Kit; GlucaGen® HypoKit®; Glucagon Emergency Kit

Brand Names: Canada GlucaGen®; GlucaGen® HypoKit®

Pharmacologic Category Antidote; Antidote, Hypoglycemia; Diagnostic Agent

Use Management of hypoglycemia; diagnostic aid in radiologic examinations to temporarily inhibit GI tract movement

Unlabeled Use Beta-blocker- or calcium channel blocker-induced myocardial depression (with or without hypotension) unresponsive to standard measures; suspected or documented hypoglycemia secondary to insulin or sulfonylurea overdose (as adjunct to dextrose)

Local Anesthetic/Vasoconstrictor Precautions No information available to require special precautions

Effects on Dental Treatment No significant effects or complications reported

Effects on Bleeding No information available to require special precautions

Adverse Effects Frequency not defined.

Cardiovascular: Hypotension (up to 2 hours after GI procedures), hypertension, tachycardia

Gastrointestinal: Nausea, vomiting (high incidence with rapid administration of high doses)

Miscellaneous: Hypersensitivity reactions, anaphylaxis

General Dosage Range

I.M.:

Children <20 kg: 0.5 mg **or** 20-30 mcg/kg/dose, may repeat

Children ≥20 kg: 1 mg, may repeat

Adults: 1 mg, may repeat **or** 1-2 mg prior to gastrointestinal procedure

I.V.:

Children <20 kg: 0.5 mg or 20-30 mcg/kg/dose, may repeat

Children ≥20 kg: 1 mg, may repeat

Adults: 1 mg, may repeat in 20 minutes **or** 0.25-2 mg 10 minutes prior to gastrointestinal procedure

SubQ:

Children <20 kg: 0.5 mg **or** 20-30 mcg/kg/dose, may repeat

Children ≥20 kg and Adults: 1 mg, may repeat

Mechanism of Action Stimulates adenylate cyclase to produce increased cyclic AMP, which promotes hepatic glycogenolysis and gluconeogenesis, causing a raise in blood glucose levels

Pharmacodynamics/Kinetics

Onset of Action Peak effect: Blood glucose levels: Parenteral: I.V.: 5-20 minutes; I.M.: 30 minutes; SubQ: 30-45 minutes

Duration of Action Glucose elevation: SubQ: 60-90 minutes; I.V.: 30 minutes

Half-life Elimination Plasma: 8-18 minutes

Pregnancy Risk Factor B

Pregnancy Considerations Adverse events have not been observed in animal reproduction studies.

Glucose Polymers (GLOO kose POL i merz)

Brand Names: U.S. Polycose® [OTC]

Pharmacologic Category Nutritional Supplement

Use Supplies calories for those persons not able to meet the caloric requirement with usual dietary intake

Local Anesthetic/Vasoconstrictor Precautions No information available to require special precautions

Effects on Dental Treatment No significant effects or complications reported

Effects on Bleeding No information available to require special precautions

General Dosage Range Oral: *Adults:* Add to foods, beverages, or water as needed

Glutamine (GLOO ta meen)

Brand Names: U.S. Enterex® Glutapak-10® [OTC]; NutreStore™; Resource® GlutaSolve® [OTC]; Sympt-X G.I. [OTC]; Sympt-X [OTC]

Pharmacologic Category Amino Acid; Gastrointestinal Agent, Miscellaneous

Use

NutreStore™: Treatment of short bowel syndrome (SBS) when used in combination with specialized nutritional support and growth hormone therapy

OTC products: Medical food used to promote GI tract healing and nutritional supplementation with GI disorders, HIV/AIDS, cancer, and other critical illnesses

Local Anesthetic/Vasoconstrictor Precautions No information available to require special precautions

Effects on Dental Treatment No significant effects or complications reported

Effects on Bleeding No information available to require special precautions

Adverse Effects Frequency not defined.

Cardiovascular: Facial edema, peripheral edema

Central nervous system: Dizziness, fever, headache, pain

Dermatologic: Pruritus, rash

Gastrointestinal: Abdominal pain, flatulence, nausea, pancreatitis, tenesmus, vomiting

Neuromuscular & skeletal: Arthralgia, back pain, hypoesthesia

Otic: Ear or hearing symptoms

Respiratory: Rhinitis

Miscellaneous: Flu-like syndrome, infection, sepsis

General Dosage Range Oral: *Adults:* 5-30 g/day in 3 divided doses **or** 5 g 6 times/day

Mechanism of Action Glutamine regulates gastrointestinal cell growth, function, and regeneration. Considered a "conditionally essential" amino acid during metabolic stress and injury.

Pharmacodynamics/Kinetics

Half-life Elimination I.V.: 1 hour

Pregnancy Risk Factor C

Pregnancy Considerations Reproduction studies have not been conducted.

GlyBURIDE (GLYE byoor ide)

Related Information

Endocrine Disorders and Pregnancy *on page 1517*

Brand Names: U.S. DiaBeta®; Glynase® PresTab®

Brand Names: Canada Apo-Glyburide®; DiaBeta®; Dom-Glyburide; Euglucon®; Med-Glybe; Mylan-Glybe; Novo-Glyburide; Nu-Glyburide; PMS-Glyburide; PRO-Glyburide; ratio-Glyburide; Riva-Glyburide; Sandoz-Glyburide; Teva-Glyburide

Generic Availability (U.S.) Yes

Pharmacologic Category Antidiabetic Agent, Sulfonylurea

Use Adjunct to diet and exercise for the management of type 2 diabetes mellitus (noninsulin dependent, NIDDM)

Unlabeled Use Alternative to insulin in women for the treatment of gestational diabetes mellitus (GDM) (11-33 weeks gestation)

Local Anesthetic/Vasoconstrictor Precautions No information available to require special precautions

Effects on Dental Treatment Glyburide-dependent patients with diabetes (noninsulin dependent, type 2) should be appointed for dental treatment in morning in order to minimize chance of stress-induced hypoglycemia.

Effects on Bleeding No information available to require special precautions

Adverse Effects Frequency not defined.

Cardiovascular: Vasculitis

Central nervous system: Dizziness, headache

Dermatologic: Angioedema, erythema, maculopapular eruptions, morbilliform eruptions, photosensitivity reaction, pruritus, purpura, rash, urticaria

Endocrine & metabolic: Disulfiram-like reaction, hypoglycemia, hyponatremia (SIADH reported with other sulfonylureas)

Gastrointestinal: Anorexia, constipation, diarrhea, epigastric fullness, heartburn, nausea

Genitourinary: Nocturia

Hematologic: Agranulocytosis, aplastic anemia, hemolytic anemia, leukopenia, pancytopenia, porphyria cutanea tarda, thrombocytopenia

Hepatic: Cholestatic jaundice, hepatitis, liver failure, transaminase increased

Neuromuscular & skeletal: Arthralgia, myalgia, paresthesia

Ocular: Blurred vision

Renal: Diuretic effect (minor)

Miscellaneous: Allergic reaction

Dosage Oral: Micronized glyburide tablets are **not** bioequivalent to conventional glyburide tablets; retitration should occur if patients are being transferred to a different glyburide formulation (eg, micronized-to-conventional or vice versa) or from other hypoglycemic agents.

DiaβBeta®: Adults:

Initial: 2.5-5 mg/day, administered with breakfast or the first main meal of the day. In patients who are more sensitive to hypoglycemic drugs, start at 1.25 mg/day.

Increase in increments of no more than 2.5 mg/day at weekly intervals based on the patient's blood glucose response

Maintenance: 1.25-20 mg/day given as single or divided doses. Some patients (especially those receiving >10 mg/day) may have a more satisfactory response with twice-daily dosing. Maximum: 20 mg/day

Elderly: Initial: 1.25-2.5 mg/day, increase by 1.25-2.5 mg/day every 1-3 weeks

Micronized tablets (Glynase® PresTab®): Adults:

Initial: 1.5-3 mg/day, administered with breakfast or the first main meal of the day in patients who are more sensitive to hypoglycemic drugs, start at 0.75 mg/day. Increase in increments of no more than 1.5 mg/day in weekly intervals based on the patient's blood glucose response.

Maintenance: 0.75-12 mg/day given as a single dose or in divided doses. Some patients (especially those receiving >6 mg/day) may have a more satisfactory response with twice-daily dosing. Maximum: 12 mg/day

Management of noninsulin-dependent diabetes mellitus in patients previously maintained on insulin: Initial dosage dependent upon previous insulin dosage, see table.

Dose Conversion: Insulin to Glyburide

Previous Daily Insulin Dosage (units/day)	Initial Glyburide Dosage Conventional Formulation (mg/day)	Initial Glyburide Dosage Micronized Formulation (mg/day)	Insulin Dosage Change (after glyburide started)
<20	2.5-5	1.5-3	Discontinue
20-40	5	3	Discontinue
>40	5 (increase in increments of 1.25-2.5 mg every 2-10 days)	3 (increase in increments of 0.75-1.5 mg every 2-10 days)	Reduce insulin dosage by 50% (gradually taper off insulin as glyburide dosage increased)

Dosing adjustment/comments in renal impairment: Cl_{cr} <50 mL/minute: **Not recommended**

Dosing adjustment in hepatic impairment: Use conservative initial and maintenance doses and avoid use in severe disease

Mechanism of Action Stimulates insulin release from the pancreatic beta cells; reduces glucose output from the liver; insulin sensitivity is increased at peripheral target sites

Contraindications Hypersensitivity to glyburide or any component of the formulation; type 1 diabetes mellitus (insulin dependent, IDDM), diabetic ketoacidosis; concomitant use with bosentan

Warnings/Precautions All sulfonylurea drugs are capable of producing severe hypoglycemia. Hypoglycemia is more likely to occur when caloric intake is deficient, after severe or prolonged exercise, when ethanol is ingested, or when more than one glucose-lowering drug is used. It is also more likely in elderly patients, malnourished patients and in patients with impaired renal or hepatic function; use with caution.

It may be necessary to discontinue therapy and administer insulin if the patient is exposed to stress (fever, trauma, infection, surgery). Loss of efficacy may be observed following prolonged use as a result of the progression of type 2 diabetes mellitus which results in continued beta cell destruction. In patients who were previously responding to sulfonylurea therapy, consider additional factors which may be contributing to decreased efficacy (eg, inappropriate dose, nonadherence to diet and exercise regimen). If no contributing factors can be identified, consider discontinuing use of the sulfonylurea due to secondary failure of treatment. Additional antidiabetic therapy (eg, insulin) will be required.

Elderly: Avoid use in older adults due to increased risk of prolonged hypoglycemia (Beers Criteria). Rapid and prolonged hypoglycemia (>12 hours) despite hypertonic glucose injections have been reported; age and hepatic and renal impairment are independent risk factors for hypoglycemia; dosage titration should be made at weekly intervals.

Chemical similarities are present among sulfonamides, sulfonylureas, carbonic anhydrase inhibitors, thiazides, and loop diuretics (except ethacrynic acid). Use in patients with sulfonamide allergy is not specifically contraindicated in product labeling, however, a risk of cross-reaction exists in patients with allergy to any of these compounds; avoid use when previous reaction has been severe.

Product labeling states oral hypoglycemic drugs may be associated with an increased cardiovascular mortality as compared to treatment with diet alone or diet plus insulin. Data to support this association are limited, and several studies, including a large prospective trial (UKPDS) have not supported an association.

Patients with G6PD deficiency may be at an increased risk of sulfonylurea-induced hemolytic anemia; however, cases have also been described in patients without G6PD deficiency during postmarketing surveillance. Use with caution and consider a nonsulfonylurea alternative in patients with G6PD deficiency.

Micronized glyburide tablets are **not** bioequivalent to *conventional* glyburide tablets; retitration should occur if patients are being transferred to a different glyburide formulation (eg, micronized-to-conventional or vice versa) or from other hypoglycemic agents.

Drug Interactions

Metabolism/Transport Effects Substrate of CYP2C9 (major); **Note:** Assignment of Major/Minor substrate status based on clinically relevant drug interaction potential; **Inhibits** CYP2C8 (weak), CYP3A4 (weak)

Avoid Concomitant Use

Avoid concomitant use of GlyBURIDE with any of the following: Bosentan; Pimozide

Increased Effect/Toxicity

GlyBURIDE may increase the levels/effects of: Alcohol (Ethyl); ARIPiprazole; Bosentan; CycloSPORINE (Systemic); Hypoglycemic Agents; Lomitapide; Pimozide; Porfimer; Vitamin K Antagonists

The levels/effects of GlyBURIDE may be increased by: Beta-Blockers; Chloramphenicol; Cimetidine; Clarithromycin; Cyclic Antidepressants; CYP2C9 Inhibitors (Moderate); CYP2C9 Inhibitors (Strong); Fibric Acid Derivatives; Fluconazole; GLP-1 Agonists; Herbs (Hypoglycemic Properties); MAO Inhibitors; Mifepristone; Pegvisomant; Probenecid; Quinolone Antibiotics; Ranitidine; Salicylates; Selective Serotonin Reuptake Inhibitors; Sulfonamide Derivatives; Vitamin K Antagonists; Voriconazole

Decreased Effect

GlyBURIDE may decrease the levels/effects of: Bosentan

The levels/effects of GlyBURIDE may be decreased by: Bosentan; Colesevelam; Corticosteroids (Orally Inhaled); Corticosteroids (Systemic); CycloSPORINE (Systemic); CYP2C9 Inducers (Strong); Loop Diuretics; Luteinizing Hormone-Releasing Hormone Analogs; Peginterferon Alfa-2b; Quinolone Antibiotics; Rifampin; Somatropin; Thiazide Diuretics

Ethanol/Nutrition/Herb Interactions

Ethanol: Caution with ethanol (may cause hypoglycemia).

Herb/Nutraceutical: Herbs with hypoglycemic properties may enhance the hypoglycemic effect of glyburide. This includes alfalfa, aloe, bilberry, bitter melon, burdock, celery, damiana, fenugreek, garcinia, garlic, ginger, ginseng (American), gymnema, marshmallow, stinging nettle

Dietary Considerations Should be taken with meals at the same time each day (twice-daily dosing may be beneficial if conventional glyburide doses are >10 mg or micronized glyburide doses are >6 mg).

Individualized medical nutrition therapy (MNT) based on ADA recommendations is an integral part of therapy.

Pharmacodynamics/Kinetics

Onset of Action Serum insulin levels begin to increase 15-60 minutes after a single dose

Duration of Action ≤24 hours

Half-life Elimination Diaβeta®: 10 hours; Glynase® PresTab®: ~4 hours; may be prolonged with renal or hepatic impairment

Time to Peak Serum: Adults: 2-4 hours

Pregnancy Risk Factor B/C (manufacturer dependent)

Pregnancy Considerations Reproduction studies differ by manufacturer labeling. Because adverse events were not observed in animal reproduction studies, one manufacturer classifies glyburide as pregnancy category B. Because adverse events were noted in animal studies during the period of lactation, another manufacturer classifies glyburide as pregnancy category C.

Glyburide was not found to significantly cross the placenta *in vitro* and was not found in the cord serum infants of mothers taking glyburide for gestational diabetes mellitus (GDM). Nonteratogenic effects such as hypoglycemia in the neonate have been associated with maternal glyburide use. Maternal hyperglycemia can be associated with adverse effects in the fetus, including macrosomia, neonatal hyperglycemia, and hyperbilirubinemia; the risk of congenital malformations is increased when the Hb A_{1c} is above the normal range. Diabetes can also be associated with adverse effects in the mother. Poorly-treated diabetes may cause end-organ damage that may in turn negatively affect obstetric outcomes. Physiologic glucose levels should be maintained prior to and during pregnancy to decrease the risk of adverse events in the mother and the fetus. The manufacturer recommends that if glyburide is used during pregnancy, it should be discontinued at least 2 weeks before the expected delivery date. Although studies have shown positive outcomes using glyburide for the treatment of GDM, use may not be appropriate for all women. Until additional safety and efficacy data are obtained, the use of oral agents is generally not recommended as routine management of type 2 diabetes mellitus during pregnancy. Insulin is considered the drug of choice for the control of diabetes mellitus during pregnancy.

Lactation Does not enter breast milk/use caution

Breast-Feeding Considerations Data from initial studies note that glyburide was not detected in breast milk. Breast-feeding is not recommended by the manufacturer. Potentially, hypoglycemia may occur in a nursing infant exposed to a sulfonylurea via breast milk.

Dosage Forms

Tablet, oral: 1.25 mg, 1.5 mg, 2.5 mg, 3 mg, 5 mg, 6 mg

DiaBeta®: 1.25 mg, 2.5 mg, 5 mg

Glynase® PresTab®: 1.5 mg, 3 mg, 6 mg

Glyburide and Metformin
(GLYE byoor ide & met FOR min)

Related Information

GlyBURIDE *on page 664*
MetFORMIN *on page 882*

Brand Names: U.S. Glucovance®

Generic Availability (U.S.) Yes

Pharmacologic Category Antidiabetic Agent, Biguanide; Antidiabetic Agent, Sulfonylurea

Use Adjunct to diet and exercise for the management of type 2 diabetes mellitus (noninsulin dependent, NIDDM)

Local Anesthetic/Vasoconstrictor Precautions No information available to require special precautions

Effects on Dental Treatment Glyburide-dependent patients with diabetes (noninsulin dependent, type 2) should be appointed for dental treatment in morning in order to minimize chance of stress-induced hypoglycemia. Metformin-dependent patients with diabetes (noninsulin dependent, type 2) should be appointed for dental treatment in morning in order to minimize chance of stress-induced hypoglycemia.

Effects on Bleeding No information available to require special precautions

Adverse Effects (Also refer to individual agents)
>10%:
Endocrine & metabolic: Hypoglycemia (11% to 38%, effects higher when increased doses were used as initial therapy)
Gastrointestinal: Diarrhea (17%)
Respiratory: Upper respiratory infection (17%)
1% to 10%:
Central nervous system: Headache (9%), dizziness (6%)
Gastrointestinal: Nausea (8%), vomiting (8%), abdominal pain (7%) (combined GI effects increased to 38% in patients taking high doses as initial therapy)

Dosage Note: Dose must be individualized. Dosages expressed as glyburide/metformin components.
Adults: Oral:
Initial therapy (no prior treatment with sulfonylurea or metformin): 1.25 mg/250 mg once daily with a meal; patients with Hb A_{1c} >9% or fasting plasma glucose (FPG) >200 mg/dL may start with 1.25 mg/250 mg twice daily with meals. **Note:** Doses of 5 mg/500 mg should not be used as initial therapy, due to risk of hypoglycemia.
Dosage may be increased in increments of 1.25 mg/250 mg, at intervals of not less than 2 weeks; maximum daily dose: 10 mg/2000 mg (limited experience with higher doses)
Previously treated with a sulfonylurea or metformin alone: Initial: 2.5 mg/500 mg or 5 mg/500 mg twice daily with meals; increase in increments no greater than 5 mg/500 mg; maximum daily dose: 20 mg/2000 mg
When switching patients previously on a sulfonylurea and metformin together, do not exceed the daily dose of glyburide (or glyburide equivalent) or metformin.
Note: May combine with a thiazolidinedione in patients with an inadequate response to glyburide/metformin therapy (risk of hypoglycemia may be increased). When adding thiazolidinedione, continue glyburide and metformin at current dose and initiate thiazolidinedione at recommended starting dose.

Elderly: Oral: Conservative doses are recommended in the elderly due to potentially decreased renal function; **do not titrate to maximum dose**; should not be used in patients ≥80 years of age unless renal function is verified as normal

Dosage adjustment in renal impairment: Use is contraindicated in patients with serum creatinine ≥1.5 mg/dL in males, or ≥1.4 mg/dL in females or abnormal creatinine clearance.

Dosage adjustment in hepatic impairment: No dosage adjustment provided in manufacturer's labeling (has not been studied).

Mechanism of Action The combination of glyburide and metformin is used to improve glycemic control in patients with type 2 diabetes mellitus by using two different, but complementary, mechanisms of action:

Glyburide: Stimulates insulin release from the pancreatic beta cells; reduces glucose output from the liver; insulin sensitivity is increased at peripheral target sites

Metformin: Decreases hepatic glucose production, decreasing intestinal absorption of glucose and improves insulin sensitivity (increases peripheral glucose uptake and utilization)

Contraindications Hypersensitivity to glyburide, metformin, or any component of the formulation; renal disease or renal dysfunction (serum creatinine ≥1.5 mg/dL in males or ≥1.4 mg/dL in females, or abnormal creatinine clearance) which may also result from conditions such as cardiovascular collapse, acute myocardial infarction, and septicemia; acute or chronic metabolic acidosis with or without coma (including diabetic ketoacidosis)

Note: Temporarily discontinue in patients undergoing radiologic studies in which intravascular iodinated contrast materials are utilized. Temporarily discontinue for surgical procedures.

Warnings/Precautions Age, hepatic and renal impairment are independent risk factors for hypoglycemia. Use with caution in patients with hepatic impairment, malnourished or debilitated conditions, or adrenal or pituitary insufficiency. Use caution in patients with renal impairment. Use with caution in the elderly. Instruct patients to avoid excessive acute or chronic ethanol use; ethanol may potentiate metformin's effect on lactate metabolism.

[U.S. Boxed Warning]: Lactic acidosis is a rare, but potentially fatal and severe consequence of therapy with metformin. Withhold therapy in hypoxemia, dehydration, or sepsis. The risk of lactic acidosis is increased in any patient with acutely decompensated HF requiring pharmacologic management. This risk is particularly high during acute or unstable acutely decompensated HF because of the risk of hypoperfusion and hypoxemia. Metformin is substantially excreted by the kidney. The risk of accumulation and lactic acidosis increases with the degree of renal impairment. Patients with renal function below the limit of normal for their age should not receive metformin. In elderly patients, renal function should be monitored regularly; should not be used in any patient ≥80 years of age unless normal renal function is confirmed. Use of concomitant medications that may affect renal function (ie, affect tubular secretion) may also affect metformin disposition. Metformin should be withheld in patients with dehydration and/or prerenal azotemia. Therapy should be suspended for any surgical procedures requiring food or fluid restriction (resume only after normal intake resumed and normal renal function is verified). Intravascular iodinated contrast media used for radiologic studies are associated with alteration of renal function and may increase risk of lactic acidosis. Discontinue Glucovance® at the time of or prior to the procedure and withhold for 48 hours subsequent to the procedure; reinstitute only after renal function has been re-evaluated and found to be normal.

Chemical similarities are present among sulfonamides, sulfonylureas, carbonic anhydrase inhibitors, thiazides, and loop diuretics (except ethacrynic acid). Use in patients with sulfonamide allergy is not specifically contraindicated in product labeling, however a risk of cross-reaction exists in patients with allergy to any of these compounds; avoid use when previous reaction has been severe. Patients with G6PD deficiency may be at an increased risk of sulfonylurea-induced hemolytic anemia; however, cases have also been described in patients without G6PD deficiency during postmarketing surveillance. Use with caution and consider a nonsulfonylurea alternative in patients with G6PD deficiency

Loss of efficacy may be observed following prolonged use as a result of the progression of type 2 diabetes mellitus which results in continued beta cell destruction. In patients who were previously responding to sulfonylurea therapy, consider additional factors which may be contributing to decreased efficacy (eg, inappropriate dose, nonadherence to diet and exercise regimen). If no contributing factors can be identified, consider discontinuing use of the sulfonylurea due to secondary failure of treatment. Additional antidiabetic therapy (eg, insulin) will be required. Product labeling states oral hypoglycemic drugs may be associated with an increased cardiovascular mortality as compared to treatment with diet alone or diet plus insulin. Data to support this association are limited, and several studies, including a large prospective trial (UKPDS), have not supported an association. Metformin does not appear to share this risk. Concurrent use with a thiazolidinedione may increase risk of hypoglycemia and/or weight gain; liver function tests should be monitored periodically with concurrent use.

Drug Interactions

Metabolism/Transport Effects Refer to individual components.

Avoid Concomitant Use

Avoid concomitant use of Glyburide and Metformin with any of the following: Bosentan; Pimozide

Increased Effect/Toxicity

Glyburide and Metformin may increase the levels/effects of: Alcohol (Ethyl); ARIPiprazole; Bosentan; CycloSPORINE (Systemic); Dalfampridine; Dofetilide; Hypoglycemic Agents; Lomitapide; Pimozide; Porfimer; Vitamin K Antagonists

The levels/effects of Glyburide and Metformin may be increased by: Beta-Blockers; Carbonic Anhydrase Inhibitors; Cephalexin; Chloramphenicol; Cimetidine; Clarithromycin; Cyclic Antidepressants; CYP2C9 Inhibitors (Moderate); CYP2C9 Inhibitors (Strong); Dalfampridine; Fibric Acid Derivatives; Fluconazole; GLP-1 Agonists; Glycopyrrolate; Herbs (Hypoglycemic Properties); Iodinated Contrast Agents; LamoTRIgine; MAO Inhibitors; Mifepristone; Pegvisomant; Probenecid; Quinolone Antibiotics; Ranitidine; Salicylates; Selective Serotonin Reuptake Inhibitors; Sulfonamide Derivatives; Trimethoprim; Vitamin K Antagonists; Voriconazole

Decreased Effect

Glyburide and Metformin may decrease the levels/effects of: Bosentan; Trospium

The levels/effects of Glyburide and Metformin may be decreased by: Bosentan; Colesevelam; Corticosteroids (Orally Inhaled); Corticosteroids (Systemic); CycloSPORINE (Systemic); CYP2C9 Inducers (Strong); Loop Diuretics; Luteinizing Hormone-Releasing Hormone Analogs; Peginterferon Alfa-2b; Quinolone Antibiotics; Rifampin; Somatropin; Thiazide Diuretics

▶

Ethanol/Nutrition/Herb Interactions

Ethanol: May cause hypoglycemia; incidence of lactic acidosis may be increased; a disulfiram-like reaction characterized by flushing, headache, nausea, vomiting, sweating, or tachycardia has been reported with sulfonylureas; avoid or limit use.

Food: Metformin decreases absorption of vitamin B_{12}. Metformin decreases absorption of folic acid.

Dietary Considerations May cause GI upset; take with food to decrease GI upset. Dietary modification based on ADA recommendations is a part of therapy. Individualized medical nutrition therapy (MNT) based on ADA recommendations is an integral part of therapy. Monitor for signs and symptoms of vitamin B_{12} and folic acid deficiency; supplementation may be required.

Pharmacodynamics/Kinetics

Time to Peak Glucovance®: 2.75 hours when taken with food

Pregnancy Risk Factor B

Pregnancy Considerations Animal reproduction studies were not conducted with this combination. Adverse events were not observed in animal studies of the individual agents; therefore, glyburide/metformin is classified as pregnancy category B. Refer to individual agents.

Lactation Excretion in breast milk unknown/not recommended

Breast-Feeding Considerations Refer to individual agents.

Dosage Forms

Tablet: Glyburide 1.25 mg and metformin 250 mg; glyburide 2.5 mg and metformin 500 mg; glyburide 5 mg and metformin 500 mg

Glucovance®: 2.5 mg/500 mg: Glyburide 2.5 mg and metformin 500 mg; 5 mg/500 mg: Glyburide 5 mg and metformin 500 mg

Glycerin (GLIS er in)

Related Information

Dentifrices: No Sodium Lauryl Sulfate (SLS) *on page 1643*

Brand Names: U.S. Fleet® Glycerin Suppositories [OTC]; Fleet® Liquid Glycerin [OTC]; Fleet® Pedia-Lax™ Glycerin Suppositories [OTC]; Fleet® Pedia-Lax™ Liquid Glycerin Suppositories [OTC]; Orajel® Dry Mouth [OTC]; Sani-Supp® [OTC]

Pharmacologic Category Laxative, Osmotic

Use Constipation; relief of dry mouth

Local Anesthetic/Vasoconstrictor Precautions No information available to require special precautions

Effects on Dental Treatment No significant effects or complications reported

Effects on Bleeding No information available to require special precautions

Adverse Effects Frequency not defined: Rectal: Gastrointestinal: Cramping pain, rectal irritation, tenesmus

General Dosage Range

Oral: *Children ≥2 years, Adolescents, and Adults:* Apply a one-inch strip directly to tongue and oral cavity as needed

Rectal:

Children 2 to <6 years: One pediatric suppository once daily as needed **or** as directed

Children ≥6 years, Adolescents, and Adults: One adult suppository once daily as needed **or** as directed

Mechanism of Action Osmotic dehydrating agent which increases osmotic pressure; draws fluid into colon and thus stimulates evacuation

Pharmacodynamics/Kinetics

Onset of Action Constipation: Suppository: 15-30 minutes

Pregnancy Considerations Glycerin suppositories are generally considered safe to use during pregnancy (Cullen, 2007; Wald, 2003).

Glycopyrrolate (glye koe PYE roe late)

Brand Names: U.S. Cuvposa™; Robinul®; Robinul® Forte

Brand Names: Canada Glycopyrrolate Injection, USP; Seebri® Breezhaler®

Pharmacologic Category Anticholinergic Agent

Use Inhibit salivation and excessive secretions of the respiratory tract preoperatively; control of upper airway secretions; intraoperatively to counteract drug-induced or vagal mediated bradyarrhythmias; adjunct in treatment of peptic ulcer (indication listed in product labeling but currently has no place in management of peptic ulcer disease)

Cuvposa™: Reduce chronic, severe drooling in those with neurologic conditions (eg, cerebral palsy) associated with drooling

Seebri® Breezhaler® (Canadian availability; not available in U.S.): Maintenance treatment of chronic obstructive pulmonary disease (COPD) including chronic bronchitis and emphysema

Unlabeled Use Adjunct with acetylcholinesterase inhibitors (eg, neostigmine, edrophonium, pyridostigmine) to antagonize cholinergic effects

Local Anesthetic/Vasoconstrictor Precautions No information available to require special precautions

Effects on Dental Treatment Key adverse event(s) related to dental treatment: Significant xerostomia (normal salivary flow resumes upon discontinuation).

Effects on Bleeding No information available to require special precautions

Adverse Effects

>10% (as reported with Cuvposa™):

Cardiovascular: Flushing (30%)

Central nervous system: Headache (15%)

Gastrointestinal: Vomiting (40%), xerostomia (40%), constipation (35%)

Genitourinary: Urinary retention (15%)

Respiratory: Nasal congestion (30%), sinusitis (15%), upper respiratory tract infection (15%)

<10% (frequency not always defined):

Cardiovascular: Pallor (≤2%), arrhythmias, cardiac arrest, heart block, hyper-/hypotension, malignant hyperthermia, palpitation, QT_c-interval prolongation, tachycardia

Central nervous system: Aggressiveness (≤2%), agitation (≤2%), crying (abnormal; ≤2%), irritability (≤2%), mood changes (≤2%), pain (≤2%), restlessness (≤2%), confusion, dizziness, drowsiness, excitement, insomnia, nervousness, seizure

Dermatologic: Dry skin (≤2%), pruritus (≤2%), rash (≤2%), urticaria

Endocrine & metabolic: Dehydration (≤2%), lactation suppression

Gastrointestinal: Abdominal distention (≤2%), abdominal pain (≤2%), flatulence (≤2%), retching (≤2%), bloated feeling, intestinal obstruction, loss of taste, nausea, pseudo-obstruction

Genitourinary: Urinary tract infection (≤2%), impotence, urinary hesitancy

Local: Injection site reactions (edema, erythema, pain)

Neuromuscular & skeletal: Weakness
Ocular: Nystagmus (≤2%), blurred vision, cycloplegia, mydriasis, ocular tension increased, photophobia, sensitivity to light increased
Respiratory: Bronchial secretion (thickening; ≤2%), nasal dryness (≤2%), pneumonia (≤2%), respiratory depression
Miscellaneous: Anaphylactoid reactions, diaphoresis decreased, hypersensitivity reactions

As reported with Seebri® Breezhaler® (Canadian availability; not available in U.S.): 1% to 10%:
Central nervous system: Headache (elderly: 2%)
Gastrointestinal: Xerostomia (2% to 3%), gastroenteritis (1% to 3%), dyspepsia (1%), vomiting (1%)
Genitourinary: Urinary tract infection (elderly: 3%), dysuria (1%)
Neuromuscular & skeletal: Musculoskeletal pain (2%)
Respiratory: Nasopharyngitis (9%), rhinitis (2%)

General Dosage Range
I.M.:
Children <2 years: 4-9 mcg/kg once **or** 4-10 mcg/kg every 3-4 hours (maximum: 0.2 mg/dose; 0.8 mg/day)
Children ≥2 years: 4 mcg/kg once **or** 4-10 mcg/kg every 3-4 hours (maximum: 0.2 mg/dose; 0.8 mg/day)
Adults: 4 mcg/kg once **or** 0.1-0.2 mg 3-4 times/day
I.V.:
Children: 4-10 mcg/kg every 3-4 hours (maximum: 0.2 mg/dose; 0.8 mg/day) **or** 4 mcg/kg (maximum: 0.1 mg); repeat as needed
Adults: 0.1-0.2 mg 3-4 times/day **or** 0.1 mg repeated as needed
Oral: *Children 3-16 years:* 0.02-0.1 mg/kg/dose 3 times/day (maximum: 3 mg/dose)

Mechanism of Action Blocks the action of acetylcholine at parasympathetic sites in smooth muscle, secretory glands, and the CNS; indirectly reduces the rate of salivation by preventing the stimulation of acetylcholine receptors

In COPD, competitively and reversibly inhibits the action of acetylcholine at muscarinic receptor subtypes 1-3 (greater affinity for subtypes 1 and 3) in bronchial smooth muscle thereby causing bronchodilation

Pharmacodynamics/Kinetics
Onset of Action Oral: 50 minutes; I.M.: 15-30 minutes; I.V.: ~1 minute
Peak effect: Oral: ~1 hour; I.M.: 30-45 minutes
Duration of Action Vagal effect: 2-3 hours; Inhibition of salivation: Up to 7 hours; Anticholinergic: Oral: 8-12 hours
Half-life Elimination Infants: 22-130 minutes; Children 19-99 minutes; Adults: ~60-75 minutes; Oral solution: Adults: 3 hours; Oral powder for inhalation: 13-22 hours (Sechaud, 2012)
Time to Peak Plasma: Oral powder for inhalation: 5 minutes

Pregnancy Risk Factor B (injection) / C (oral solution)
Pregnancy Considerations Teratogenic effects were not observed in animal studies. Small amounts of glycopyrrolate cross the human placenta.

Gold Sodium Thiomalate
(gold SOW dee um thye oh MAL ate)

Brand Names: U.S. Myochrysine® [DSC]
Brand Names: Canada Myochrysine®
Pharmacologic Category Gold Compound

Use Adjunctive treatment of active rheumatoid arthritis
Local Anesthetic/Vasoconstrictor Precautions No information available to require special precautions
Effects on Dental Treatment Key adverse event(s) related to dental treatment: Stomatitis, gingivitis, and glossitis.
Effects on Bleeding No information available to require special precautions
Adverse Effects Frequency not defined.
Cardiovascular: Bradycardia, syncope
Central nervous system: Confusion, fever, Guillain-Barré syndrome, hallucinations, seizure
Dermatologic: Alopecia, angioedema, dermatitis, nail shedding, pruritus, rash, urticaria
Gastrointestinal: Anorexia, abdominal cramps, diarrhea, dysphagia, enterocolitis (ulcerative), gingivitis, glossitis, nausea, stomatitis, taste disturbance (metallic), thick tongue, vomiting
Hematologic: Agranulocytosis, aplastic anemia, eosinophilia, leukopenia, purpura, thrombocytopenia
Hepatic: Cholestasis, hepatitis, hepatotoxicity, jaundice
Neuromuscular & skeletal: Arthralgia, peripheral neuropathy
Ocular: Conjunctivitis, corneal ulcers, gold deposits in ocular tissues, iritis
Respiratory: Dyspnea, gold bronchitis, interstitial pneumonitis, pulmonary fibrosis
Renal: Glomerulitis, hematuria, nephrotic syndrome, proteinuria
Miscellaneous: Anaphylactoid reaction, anaphylaxis, nitritoid reaction
General Dosage Range Dosage adjustment recommended in patients with renal impairment or who develop toxicities
I.M.:
Children: Test dose (recommended): 10 mg first week; Initial dosing: 1 mg/kg/week (maximum: 50 mg/injection); Maintenance: 1 mg/kg/dose (maximum: 50 mg/injection)
Adults: Test dose: 10 mg first week; Initial dosing: 25 mg second week, then 25-50 mg/week until 1 g cumulative dose has been given; Maintenance: 25-50 mg every other week for 2-20 weeks, then every 3-4 weeks
Mechanism of Action Unknown, may decrease prostaglandin synthesis or may alter cellular mechanisms by inhibiting sulfhydryl systems
Pharmacodynamics/Kinetics
Onset of Action Delayed; may require up to 3 months
Half-life Elimination 5 days; may be prolonged with multiple doses
Time to Peak Serum: 4-6 hours
Pregnancy Risk Factor C
Pregnancy Considerations Adverse events were observed in animal reproduction studies

Golimumab (goe LIM ue mab)

Related Information
Rheumatoid Arthritis, Osteoarthritis, and Osteoporosis *on page 1526*
Brand Names: U.S. Simponi®
Brand Names: Canada Simponi®
Pharmacologic Category Antipsoriatic Agent; Antirheumatic, Disease Modifying; Monoclonal Antibody; Tumor Necrosis Factor (TNF) Blocking Agent
Use Treatment of active rheumatoid arthritis (moderate-to-severe), active psoriatic arthritis, and active ankylosing spondylitis

◀ Local Anesthetic/Vasoconstrictor Precautions No information available to require special precautions

Effects on Dental Treatment No significant effects or complications reported

Effects on Bleeding No information available to require special precautions

Adverse Effects
>10%:
Respiratory: Upper respiratory tract infection (16%; includes laryngitis, nasopharyngitis, pharyngitis, and rhinitis)
Miscellaneous: Infection (28%)
1% to 10%:
Cardiovascular: Hypertension (3%)
Central nervous system: Dizziness (2%), fever (1%)
Gastrointestinal: Constipation (1%)
Hepatic: ALT increased (4%), AST increased (3%)
Local: Injection site reactions (6%)
Neuromuscular & skeletal: Paresthesia (2%)
Respiratory: Bronchitis (2%), sinusitis (2%)
Miscellaneous: Viral infection (5%; includes herpes and influenza), antibody formation (4%), fungal infection (superficial; 2%)

General Dosage Range SubQ: *Adults:* 50 mg once per month

Mechanism of Action Human monoclonal antibody that binds to human tumor necrosis factor alpha (TNFα), thereby interfering with endogenous TNFα activity. Biological activities of TNFα include the induction of proinflammatory cytokines (interleukin [IL]-6, IL-8, Granulocyte-colony stimulating factor, granulocyte-macrophage colony stimulating factor), expression of adhesion molecules (E-selectin, vascular cell adhesion molecule [VCAM]-1, intercellular adhesion molecule [ICAM]-1) necessary for leukocyte infiltration, activation of neutrophils and eosinophils.

Pharmacodynamics/Kinetics
Half-life Elimination ~2 weeks
Time to Peak SubQ: 2-6 days
Pregnancy Risk Factor B
Pregnancy Considerations Adverse events were not observed in animal reproduction studies. Golimumab crosses the placenta. Based on data from other TNF-blockers, antibodies may be present in the newborn serum for up to 6 months and infants exposed to golimumab *in utero* may be at risk of increased infection. Administration of live vaccines to newborns is not recommended until 6 months after the last maternal dose. Canadian labeling recommends that women of childbearing potential use reliable contraception during and for at least 6 months after discontinuation of golimumab therapy.

Gonadorelin (goe nad oh RELL in)

Brand Names: Canada Lutrepulse™
Pharmacologic Category Gonadotropin
Use Induction of ovulation in females with hypothalamic amenorrhea

Local Anesthetic/Vasoconstrictor Precautions No information available to require special precautions

Effects on Dental Treatment No significant effects or complications reported

Effects on Bleeding No information available to require special precautions

Adverse Effects Local: Injection site irritation, superficial thrombophlebitis

General Dosage Range I.V., SubQ: *Adults:* 1-20 mcg every 90 minutes

Mechanism of Action Stimulates the release of luteinizing hormone (LH) from the anterior pituitary gland

Pharmacodynamics/Kinetics
Onset of Action Response to therapy usually observed within 2-3 weeks
Half-life Elimination Terminal: ~10-40 minutes; increased in patients with renal impairment

Pregnancy Considerations The risk of fetal harm appears remote if gonadorelin is used during pregnancy. Clinical studies of pregnant women have not demonstrated an increased risk of fetal abnormalities during the first trimester. Follow-up reports of infants born to exposed mothers revealed no adverse effects or complications attributed to gonadorelin therapy. Based on its indicated use, gonadorelin treatment is continued for 2 weeks following ovulation to maintain the corpus luteum; initiation of treatment is not appropriate if pregnancy has been established.

Product Availability Not available in U.S.

Goserelin (GOE se rel in)

Brand Names: U.S. Zoladex®
Brand Names: Canada Zoladex®; Zoladex® LA
Pharmacologic Category Antineoplastic Agent, Gonadotropin-Releasing Hormone Agonist; Gonadotropin Releasing Hormone Agonist
Use Treatment of locally confined prostate cancer; palliative treatment of advanced prostate cancer; palliative treatment of advanced breast cancer in pre- and perimenopausal women; treatment of endometriosis, including pain relief and reduction of endometriotic lesions; endometrial thinning agent as part of treatment for dysfunctional uterine bleeding

Local Anesthetic/Vasoconstrictor Precautions No information available to require special precautions

Effects on Dental Treatment Key adverse event(s) related to dental treatment: Xerostomia (normal salivary flow resumes upon discontinuation) and taste disturbances.

Effects on Bleeding No information available to require special precautions

Adverse Effects Percentages reported with the 1-month implant:
>10%:
Cardiovascular: Peripheral edema (female 21%)
Central nervous system: Headache (female 32% to 75%; male 1% to 5%), emotional lability (female 60%), depression (female 54%; male 1% to 5%), pain (female 17%; male 8%), insomnia (female 11%; male 5%)
Dermatologic: Acne (female 42%), seborrhea (female 26%)
Endocrine & metabolic: Hot flashes (female 57% to 96%; male 62%), libido decreased (female 48% to 61%), sexual dysfunction (male 21%), breast atrophy (female 33%), breast enlargement (female 18%), erections decreased (18%), libido increased (female 12%)
Gastrointestinal: Nausea (female 8% to 11%; male 5%), abdominal pain (female 7% to 10%)
Genitourinary: Vaginitis (75%), pelvic symptoms (female 9% to 18%), dyspareunia (female 14%), lower urinary symptoms (male 13%)
Neuromuscular & skeletal: Bone mineral density decreased (female 23%; ~4% decrease from baseline in 6 months; postmarketing reports in males), weakness (female 11%)

Miscellaneous: Diaphoresis (female 16% to 45%; male 6%), tumor flare (female: 23%), infection (female 13%)

1% to 10%:

Cardiovascular: Arrhythmia, cerebrovascular accident, chest pain, edema, heart failure, hypertension, MI, palpitation, peripheral vascular disorder, tachycardia

Central nervous system: Abnormal thinking, anxiety, chills, dizziness, fever, lethargy, malaise, migraine, nervousness, somnolence

Dermatologic: Alopecia, bruising, dry skin, hair disorder, hirsutism, pruritus, rash, skin discoloration

Endocrine & metabolic: Breast pain, breast swelling/tenderness, dysmenorrhea, gout, hyperglycemia

Gastrointestinal: Anorexia, appetite increased, constipation, diarrhea, dyspepsia, flatulence, ulcer, vomiting, weight gain/loss, xerostomia

Genitourinary: Urinary frequency, urinary obstruction, urinary tract infection, vaginal hemorrhage, vulvovaginitis

Hematologic: Anemia, hemorrhage

Local: Application site reaction

Neuromuscular & skeletal: Arthralgia, back pain, hypertonia, joint disorder, leg cramps, myalgia, paresthesia

Ocular: Amblyopia, dry eyes

Renal: Renal insufficiency

Respiratory: Bronchitis, COPD, cough, epistaxis, pharyngitis, rhinitis, sinusitis, upper respiratory tract infection

Miscellaneous: Allergic reaction, flu-like syndrome, voice alteration

General Dosage Range SubQ: *Adults:* 3.6 mg every 28 days **or** 10.8 mg every 12 weeks

Mechanism of Action Goserelin (a gonadotropin-releasing hormone [GnRH] analog) causes an initial increase in luteinizing hormone (LH) and follicle stimulating hormone (FSH), chronic administration of goserelin results in a sustained suppression of pituitary gonadotropins. Serum testosterone falls to levels comparable to surgical castration. The exact mechanism of this effect is unknown, but may be related to changes in the control of LH or down-regulation of LH receptors.

Pharmacodynamics/Kinetics

Onset of Action

Females: Estradiol suppression reaches postmenopausal levels within 3 weeks and FSH and LH are suppressed to follicular phase levels within 4 weeks of initiation.

Males: Testosterone suppression reaches castrate levels within 2-4 weeks after initiation.

Duration of Action

Females: Estradiol, LH and FSH generally return to baseline levels within 12 weeks following the last monthly implant.

Males: Testosterone levels maintained at castrate levels throughout the duration of therapy.

Half-life Elimination SubQ: Male: ~4 hours, Female: ~2 hours; Renal impairment: Male: 12 hours

Time to Peak SubQ: Male: 12-15 days, Female: 8-22 days

Pregnancy Risk Factor X (endometriosis, endometrial thinning); D (advanced breast cancer)

Pregnancy Considerations Goserelin has been found to be teratogenic and increases pregnancy loss in animal studies. Goserelin induces hormonal changes which increase the risk for fetal loss and use is contraindicated in pregnancy unless being used for palliative treatment of advanced breast cancer.

Breast cancer: If used for the palliative treatment of breast cancer during pregnancy, the potential for increased fetal loss should be discussed with the patient.

Endometriosis, endometrial thinning: Women of childbearing potential should not receive therapy until pregnancy has been excluded. Nonhormonal contraception is recommended for premenopausal women during therapy and for 12 weeks after therapy is discontinued. Although ovulation is usually inhibited and menstruation may stop, pregnancy prevention is not ensured during goserelin therapy. Changes in reproductive function may occur following chronic administration.

Granisetron (gra NI se tron)

Related Information

Clinical Risk Related to Drugs Prolonging QT Interval *on page 1510*

Brand Names: U.S. Granisol™; Sancuso®

Brand Names: Canada Granisetron Hydrochloride Injection; Kytril®

Pharmacologic Category Antiemetic; Selective 5-HT$_3$ Receptor Antagonist

Use Prophylaxis of nausea and vomiting associated with emetogenic chemotherapy and radiation therapy; prophylaxis and treatment of postoperative nausea and vomiting (PONV)

Unlabeled Use Breakthrough treatment of nausea and vomiting associated with chemotherapy

Local Anesthetic/Vasoconstrictor Precautions Granisetron is one of the drugs confirmed to prolong the QT interval and is accepted as having a risk of causing torsade de pointes. The risk of drug-induced torsade de pointes is extremely low when a single QT interval prolonging drug is prescribed. In terms of epinephrine, it is not known what effect vasoconstrictors in the local anesthetic regimen will have in patients with a known history of congenital prolonged QT interval or in patients taking any medication that prolongs the QT interval. Until more information is obtained, it is suggested that the clinician consult with the physician prior to the use of a vasoconstrictor in suspected patients, and that the vasoconstrictor (epinephrine, mepivacaine and levonordefrin [Carbocaine® 2% with Neo-Cobefrin®]) be used with caution.

Effects on Dental Treatment No significant effects or complications reported

Effects on Bleeding No information available to require special precautions

Adverse Effects

>10%:

Central nervous system: Headache (3% to 21%; transdermal patch: 1%)

Gastrointestinal: Constipation (3% to 18%)

Neuromuscular & skeletal: Weakness (5% to 18%)

1% to 10%:

Cardiovascular: QT$_c$ prolongation (1% to 3%), hypertension (1% to 2%)

Central nervous system: Pain (10%), fever (3% to 9%), dizziness (4% to 5%), insomnia (<2% to 5%), somnolence (1% to 4%), anxiety (2%), agitation (<2%), CNS stimulation (<2%)

Dermatologic: Rash (1%)

Gastrointestinal: Diarrhea (3% to 9%), abdominal pain (4% to 6%), dyspepsia (3% to 6%), taste perversion (2%)

Hepatic: Liver enzymes increased (5% to 6%)

Renal: Oliguria (2%)

Respiratory: Cough (2%)
Miscellaneous: Infection (3%)

General Dosage Range

I.V.:

Children ≥2 years: 10 mcg/kg/dose (maximum: 1 mg/dose) as a single dose or every 12 hours

Adults: 10 mcg/kg/dose (maximum: 1 mg/dose) as a single dose or every 12 hours **or** 1 mg as a single dose

Oral: *Adults:* 2 mg/day in 1-2 divided dose

Transdermal: *Adults:* 1 patch prior to chemotherapy; Maximum duration: Patch may be worn up to 7 days

Mechanism of Action Selective 5-HT$_3$-receptor antagonist, blocking serotonin, both peripherally on vagal nerve terminals and centrally in the chemoreceptor trigger zone

Pharmacodynamics/Kinetics

Duration of Action Oral, I.V.: Generally up to 24 hours

Half-life Elimination Oral: 6 hours; I.V.: 9 hours

Time to Peak Transdermal patch: Maximum systemic concentrations: ~48 hours after application (range: 24-168 hours)

Pregnancy Risk Factor B

Pregnancy Considerations There are no adequate or well-controlled studies in pregnant women. Teratogenic effects were not observed in animal studies. Injection (1 mg/mL strength) contains benzyl alcohol which may cross the placenta. Use only if benefit exceeds the risk.

Dental Comment Granisetron is known to prolong the QT interval. The QT interval is measured as the time and distance between the Q point of the QRS complex and the end of the T wave in the ECG tracing. After adjustment for heart rate, the QT interval is defined as prolonged if it is more than 450 msec in men and 460 msec in women. A long QT syndrome was first described in the 1950s and 60s as a congenital syndrome involving QT interval prolongation and syncope and sudden death. Some of the congenital long QT syndromes were characterized by a peculiar electrocardiographic appearance of the QRS complex involving a premature atria beat followed by a pause, then a subsequent sinus beat showing marked QT prolongation and deformity. This type of cardiac arrhythmia was originally termed "torsade de pointes" (translated from the French as "twisting of the points"). Granisetron is considered as having a risk of causing torsade de pointes. Since it is not known what effect vasoconstrictors in the local anesthetic regimen will have in patients with a known history of congenital prolonged QT interval or in patients taking any medication that prolongs the QT interval, a medical consult is suggested.

Grass Pollen Allergen Extract

(GRAS POL uhn al er juhn EK strakt)

Brand Names: Canada Oralair™

Pharmacologic Category Allergen-Specific Immunotherapy

Use Treatment of allergic rhinitis with or without conjunctivitis due to moderate to severe seasonal grass pollen. For use only in patients with clinical symptoms ≥2 pollen seasons and who are not tolerant or responsive to conventional therapy. **Note:** Patients should have a positive skin test and a positive titer of IgE specific to *Poaceae* grass pollen.

Local Anesthetic/Vasoconstrictor Precautions No information available to require special precautions

Effects on Dental Treatment Key adverse event(s) related to dental treatment: Oral pruritus, throat irritation, cough, nasopharyngitis, and mouth edema

Effects on Bleeding No information available to require special precautions

Adverse Effects

>10%:

Central nervous system: Headache (adults 14%)

Gastrointestinal: Oral pruritus (29% to 43%), throat irritation (9% to 26%), mouth edema (5% to 13%)

Ocular: Ocular pruritus (1% to 13%)

Otic: Ear pruritus (adults 3% to 12%, children 4%)

Respiratory: Cough (11% to 25%), nasopharyngitis (8% to 14%)

1% to 10%:

Cardiovascular: Facial edema (adults ≤4%), chest discomfort (1% to 2%), hypertension (adults 1%)

Central nervous system: Dysphonia (3%), anxiety (1%), dizziness (children 1%)

Dermatologic: Atopic dermatitis (children 4%), cheilitis (children 1%), excoriation (adults 1%)

Gastrointestinal: Dyspepsia (adults 3% to 5%, children 1%), lip edema (3% to 5%), oral discomfort (adults 1% to 4%), tongue edema (1% to 4%), abdominal pain (1% to 3%), glossodynia (adults 1% to 3%), oral hypoesthesia (adults 1% to 3%), gastroenteritis (adults 2%), nausea (children 2%), oral mucosal blistering (children 2%), stomatitis (2%), dry throat (adults 1% to 2%), glossitis (1% to 2%), vomiting (1% to 2%), dysphagia (adults 1%), oral pain (adults 1%), stomach discomfort (adults 1%), toothache (1%), xerostomia (adults 1%)

Neuromuscular & skeletal: Oral paresthesia (adults 3% to 4%), neck pain (adults 1%), weakness (children 1%)

Ocular: Conjunctivitis (adults 6%), chalazion (adults ≤1%)

Respiratory: Nasal congestion (children 9%), asthma (children 7%), rhinitis (7%), tonsillitis (children 7%, adults 2%), pharyngolaryngeal pain (3% to 6%), pharyngolaryngeal edema (adults 4%), upper respiratory tract infection (4%), pharyngolaryngeal discomfort (adults 3%), bronchitis (children 2%), larynx irritation (children 2%), pharyngeal hypoesthesia (adults 2%), pneumonia (children 2%), oropharyngeal edema (adults ≤2%), throat tightness (1% to 2%), upper respiratory tract congestion (1%), viral respiratory tract infection (children 1%)

Miscellaneous: Viral infection (adults 1% to 3%), lymphadenopathy (adults ≤2%), flu-like syndrome (children 1%), infectious mononucleosis (children 1%)

General Dosage Range Sublingual: *Children >5 years, Adolescents, and Adults ≤50 years:* Initial: Day 1: 100 IR once; Day 2: 200 IR once; Day 3: 300 IR once; Maintenance: 300 IR once daily

Mechanism of Action

While the exact mechanism has not been fully elucidated, specific immunotherapy (SIT) may act by inducing a switch from T helper 2 cell response (Th2) to T helper 1 cell (Th1) response resulting in decreased interleukin-4 (IL-4) and interleukin-5 (IL-5) and increased interleukin-10 (IL-10), production of IgG-blocking antibodies that compete with IgE antibodies for allergen binding, proliferation of regulatory T lymphocytes and cytokines, and decreases in mast cells, eosinophils, and early- and late-phase allergic responses (Leith, 2006).

Pregnancy Considerations Adverse events have not been observed in animal reproduction studies.

Product Availability Not available in the U.S.

Griseofulvin (gri see oh FUL vin)

Brand Names: U.S. Grifulvin V®; Gris-PEG®
Pharmacologic Category Antifungal Agent, Oral
Use Treatment of tinea infections of the skin, hair, and nails caused by susceptible species of *Microsporum*, *Epidermophyton*, or *Trichophyton*
Local Anesthetic/Vasoconstrictor Precautions No information available to require special precautions
Effects on Dental Treatment Key adverse event(s) related to dental treatment: May cause soreness or irritation of mouth or tongue. May cause oral thrush.
Effects on Bleeding No information available to require special precautions
Adverse Effects Frequency not defined.
Central nervous system: Dizziness, fatigue, headache, insomnia, mental confusion
Dermatologic: Angioneurotic edema (rare), erythema multiforme-like drug reaction, photosensitivity, rash (most common), urticaria (most common)
Gastrointestinal: Diarrhea, epigastric distress, GI bleeding, nausea, vomiting
Hematologic: Granulocytopenia, leukopenia (rare)
Hepatic: Hepatotoxicity
Neuromuscular & skeletal: Paresthesia (rare)
Renal: Nephrosis, proteinuria (rare)
Miscellaneous: Drug-induced lupus-like syndrome (rare), oral thrush
Postmarketing and/or case reports: Bilirubin increased, liver transaminases increased, Stevens-Johnson syndrome, toxic epidermal necrolysis
General Dosage Range Oral:
Microsize:
Children >2 years: 10-20 mg/kg/day in single or divided doses (maximum: 1000 mg daily)
Adults: 500-1000 mg daily in single or divided doses
Ultramicrosize:
Children >2 years: 5-15 mg/kg/day in single dose or 2 divided doses (maximum: 750 mg daily)
Adults: 375 mg daily in single or divided doses or up to 750 mg daily in divided doses
Mechanism of Action Inhibits fungal cell mitosis at metaphase; binds to human keratin making it resistant to fungal invasion
Pharmacodynamics/Kinetics
Half-life Elimination 9-24 hours
Time to Peak Serum: 4 hours
Pregnancy Considerations Teratogenic effects have been observed in animal reproduction studies. Griseofulvin crosses the placenta. Because adverse events have also been observed in humans (two cases of conjoined twins), use during pregnancy is contraindicated. Effective contraception should be used during therapy and for 1 month after therapy is discontinued in women of reproductive potential. Men should avoid fathering a child for at least 6 months after therapy.

GuaiFENesin (gwye FEN e sin)

Brand Names: U.S. Allfen [OTC] [DSC]; Bidex®-400 [OTC]; Diabetic Siltussin DAS-Na [OTC]; Diabetic Tussin® EX [OTC]; Fenesin IR [OTC]; Geri-Tussin [OTC]; Humibid® Maximum Strength [OTC]; Iophen NR [OTC]; Liquituss GG [OTC]; Mucinex® Kid's Mini-Melts™ [OTC]; Mucinex® Kid's [OTC]; Mucinex® Maximum Strength [OTC]; Mucinex® [OTC]; Mucus Relief [OTC]; Organ-I NR [OTC]; Q-Tussin [OTC]; Refenesen™ 400 [OTC]; Refenesen™ [OTC]; Robafen [OTC]; Scot-Tussin® Expectorant [OTC]; Siltussin SA [OTC]; Vicks®

Casero™ Chest Congestion Relief [OTC]; Vicks® DayQuil® Mucus Control [OTC]; Xpect™ [OTC]
Brand Names: Canada Balminil Expectorant; Benylin® E Extra Strength; Koffex Expectorant; Robitussin®
Pharmacologic Category Expectorant
Use Help loosen phlegm and thin bronchial secretions to make coughs more productive
Local Anesthetic/Vasoconstrictor Precautions No information available to require special precautions
Effects on Dental Treatment No significant effects or complications reported
Effects on Bleeding No information available to require special precautions
Adverse Effects Frequency not defined.
Central nervous system: Dizziness, drowsiness, headache
Dermatologic: Rash
Endocrine & metabolic: Uric acid levels decreased
Gastrointestinal: Nausea, stomach pain, vomiting
General Dosage Range Oral:
Extended release: *Children ≥12 years and Adults:* 600-1200 mg every 12 hours (maximum: 2.4 g/day)
Immediate release:
Children 6 months to 2 years: 25-50 mg every 4 hours (maximum: 300 mg/day)
Children 2-5 years: 50-100 mg every 4 hours (maximum: 600 mg/day)
Children 6-11 years: 100-200 mg every 4 hours (maximum: 1.2 g/day)
Children ≥12 years and Adults: 200-400 mg every 4 hours (maximum: 2.4 g/day)
Mechanism of Action Thought to act as an expectorant by irritating the gastric mucosa and stimulating respiratory tract secretions, thereby increasing respiratory fluid volumes and decreasing mucous viscosity
Pharmacodynamics/Kinetics
Half-life Elimination ~1 hour
Pregnancy Considerations Based on the limited available data, an increased risk of adverse birth outcomes has not been observed following maternal use of guaifenesin in pregnancy. Alcohol may be present in some liquid formulations of guaifenesin. If consumed in sufficient quantities during pregnancy, fetal alcohol syndrome may result. Guaifenesin has been investigated as an agent to improve cervical mucus and improve fertility.

Guaifenesin and Codeine
(gwye FEN e sin & KOE deen)

Related Information
Codeine *on page 344*
GuaiFENesin *on page 673*
Brand Names: U.S. Allfen CD; Allfen CDX; Codar® GF; Dex-Tuss; Guaiatussin AC; Iophen C-NR; M-Clear; M-Clear WC; Mar-Cof® CG; Robafen AC
Pharmacologic Category Antitussive; Cough Preparation; Expectorant
Use Temporary control of cough due to minor throat and bronchial irritation
Local Anesthetic/Vasoconstrictor Precautions No information available to require special precautions
Effects on Dental Treatment Key adverse event(s) related to dental treatment: Xerostomia (normal salivary flow resumes upon discontinuation).
Effects on Bleeding No information available to require special precautions

◄ **Adverse Effects** Frequency not defined; also see individual agents.

Cardiovascular: Bradycardia, circulatory depression, flushing, orthostatic hypotension, palpitation, syncope, tachycardia

Central nervous system: Convulsions, CNS depression, disorientation, dizziness, dysphoria, euphoria, faintness, hallucinations (transient), headache, lightheadedness, sedation

Dermatologic: Angioneurotic edema, pruritus, urticaria

Gastrointestinal: Biliary tract spasm, colonic motility increase (with chronic ulcerative colitis), constipation, nausea, stomach pain, toxic dilation (with acute ulcerative colitis), vomiting

Genitourinary: Oliguria, urinary retention

Neuromuscular & skeletal: Weakness

Ocular: Visual disturbances

Respiratory: Laryngeal edema, respiratory depression

Miscellaneous: Anaphylaxis, diaphoresis

General Dosage Range Oral: *Children ≥6 years and Adults:* Dosage varies greatly depending on product

Mechanism of Action

Guaifenesin may act as an expectorant by irritating the gastric mucosa and stimulating respiratory tract secretions, thereby increasing respiratory fluid volumes and decreasing phlegm viscosity

Codeine is an antitussive that controls cough by depressing the medullary cough center

Pregnancy Considerations See individual agents.

Controlled Substance Capsule: C-V; Liquid products: C-V; Tablet: C-III

Guaifenesin and Dextromethorphan
(gwye FEN e sin & deks troe meth OR fan)

Related Information

Dextromethorphan *on page 406*

GuaiFENesin *on page 673*

Brand Names: U.S. Cheracol® D [OTC]; Cheracol® Plus [OTC]; Coricidin HBP® Chest Congestion and Cough [OTC]; Diabetic Siltussin-DM DAS-Na Maximum Strength [OTC]; Diabetic Siltussin-DM DAS-Na [OTC]; Diabetic Tussin® DM Maximum Strength [OTC]; Diabetic Tussin® DM [OTC]; Double Tussin DM [OTC]; Fenesin DM IR [OTC]; Guaicon DMS [OTC]; Iophen DM-NR [OTC]; Kolephrin® GG/DM [OTC]; Mucinex® DM Maximum Strength [OTC]; Mucinex® DM [OTC]; Mucinex® Kid's Cough Mini-Melts™ [OTC]; Mucinex® Kid's Cough [OTC]; Q-Tussin DM [OTC]; Refenesen™ DM [OTC]; Robafen DM Clear [OTC]; Robafen DM [OTC]; Robitussin® Peak Cold Cough + Chest Congestion DM [OTC]; Robitussin® Peak Cold Maximum Strength Cough + Chest Congestion DM [OTC]; Robitussin® Peak Cold Sugar-Free Cough + Chest Congestion DM [OTC]; Safe Tussin® DM [OTC]; Scot-Tussin® Senior [OTC]; Silexin [OTC]; Siltussin DM DAS [OTC]; Siltussin DM [OTC]; Vicks® 44E [OTC]; Vicks® DayQuil® Mucus Control DM [OTC]; Vicks® Nature Fusion™ Cough & Chest Congestion [OTC]; Vicks® Pediatric Formula 44E [OTC]

Brand Names: Canada Balminil DM E; Benylin® DM-E

Pharmacologic Category Antitussive; Cough Preparation; Expectorant

Use Temporary control of cough due to minor throat and bronchial irritation

Local Anesthetic/Vasoconstrictor Precautions No information available to require special precautions

Effects on Dental Treatment No significant effects or complications reported

Effects on Bleeding No information available to require special precautions

Adverse Effects See individual agents.

General Dosage Range Oral:

Children 2-6 years: Guaifenesin 50-100 mg and dextromethorphan 2.5-5 mg every 4 hours (maximum: Guaifenesin 600 mg/day; Dextromethorphan 30 mg/day)

Children 6-12 years: Guaifenesin 100-200 mg and dextromethorphan 5-10 mg every 4 hours (maximum: Guaifenesin 1200 mg/day; Dextromethorphan 60 mg/day)

Children ≥12 years and Adults: Guaifenesin 200-400 mg and dextromethorphan 10-20 mg every 4 hours (maximum: Guaifenesin 2400 mg/day; Dextromethorphan 120 mg/day)

Mechanism of Action

Guaifenesin is thought to act as an expectorant by irritating the gastric mucosa and stimulating respiratory tract secretions, thereby increasing respiratory fluid volumes and decreasing phlegm viscosity

Dextromethorphan is a chemical relative of morphine lacking narcotic properties except in overdose; controls cough by depressing the medullary cough center

Pregnancy Considerations See individual agents.

Guaifenesin and Phenylephrine
(gwye FEN e sin & fen il EF rin)

Related Information

GuaiFENesin *on page 673*

Phenylephrine (Systemic) *on page 1087*

Brand Names: U.S. Ambi 10PEH/400GFN [OTC]; Fenesin PE IR; J-Max [OTC]; Liquibid® D-R [OTC]; Liquibid® PD-R [OTC]; Medent®-PEI [OTC]; Mucinex® Cold [OTC]; Mucus Relief Sinus [OTC]; Nu-COPD [OTC]; OneTab™ Congestion & Cold [OTC]; Refenesen™ PE [OTC]; Rescon GG [OTC]; Sudafed PE® Non-Drying Sinus [OTC]; Triaminic® Children's Chest & Nasal Congestion [OTC]

Pharmacologic Category Decongestant; Expectorant

Use Temporary relief of nasal congestion, sinusitis, rhinitis, and hay fever; temporary relief of cough associated with upper respiratory tract conditions, especially when associated with dry, nonproductive cough

Local Anesthetic/Vasoconstrictor Precautions Use with caution since phenylephrine is a sympathomimetic amine which could interact with epinephrine to cause a pressor response

Effects on Dental Treatment Key adverse event(s) related to dental treatment:

Guaifenesin: No significant effects or complications reported

Phenylephrine: Up to 10% of patients could experience tachycardia, palpitations, and xerostomia (normal salivary flow resumes upon discontinuation); use vasoconstrictor with caution

Effects on Bleeding No information available to require special precautions

Adverse Effects See individual agents.

General Dosage Range Oral: *Children >2 years and Adults:* Dosage varies greatly depending on product

Mechanism of Action See individual agents.

Pregnancy Considerations See individual agents.

Guaifenesin and Pseudoephedrine
(gwye FEN e sin & soo doe e FED rin)

Related Information
GuaiFENesin *on page 673*
Pseudoephedrine *on page 1159*
Brand Names: U.S. Ambifed-G [OTC]; Congestac® [OTC]; ExeFen-IR; Maxifed [OTC]; Maxifed-G [OTC] [DSC]; Mucinex® D Maximum Strength [OTC]; Mucinex® D [OTC]; Refenesen Plus [OTC]; SudaTex-G [OTC]
Brand Names: Canada Contac® Cold-Chest Congestion, Non Drowsy, Regular Strength; Entex® LA; Novahistex® Expectorant with Decongestant
Pharmacologic Category Alpha/Beta Agonist; Expectorant
Use Temporary relief of nasal congestion and to help loosen phlegm and thin bronchial secretions in the treatment of cough
Local Anesthetic/Vasoconstrictor Precautions Use with caution since pseudoephedrine is a sympathomimetic amine which could interact with epinephrine to cause a pressor response
Effects on Dental Treatment Key adverse event(s) related to dental treatment:
Guaifenesin: No significant effects or complications reported
Pseudoephedrine: Xerostomia (normal salivary flow resumes upon discontinuation).
Effects on Bleeding No information available to require special precautions
Adverse Effects See individual agents.
General Dosage Range Oral: *Children >2 years and Adults:* Dosage varies greatly depending on product
Pregnancy Considerations See individual agents.

Guaifenesin, Dextromethorphan, and Phenylephrine
(gwye FEN e sin, deks troe meth OR fan, & fen il EF rin)

Related Information
Dextromethorphan *on page 406*
GuaiFENesin *on page 673*
Phenylephrine (Systemic) *on page 1087*
Brand Names: U.S. Maxiphen DM [DSC]; Maxiphen DMX; Mucinex® Children's Multi-Symptom Cold [OTC]; Robafen CF Cough & Cold [OTC]; Robitussin® Children's Cough & Cold CF [OTC]; Robitussin® Peak Cold Maximum Strength Multi-Symptom Cold [OTC]; Robitussin® Peak Cold Multi-Symptom Cold [OTC]; SINUtuss® DM [DSC]; Tusicof® [OTC]; Tusso™-DMR [DSC]
Pharmacologic Category Antitussive; Decongestant
Use Symptomatic relief of dry nonproductive coughs and upper respiratory symptoms associated with hay fever, colds, or the flu
Local Anesthetic/Vasoconstrictor Precautions Use with caution since phenylephrine is a sympathomimetic amine which could interact with epinephrine to cause a pressor response
Effects on Dental Treatment Key adverse event(s) related to dental treatment:
Dextromethorphan: No significant effects or complications reported
Guaifenesin: No significant effects or complications reported
Phenylephrine: Up to 10% of patients could experience tachycardia, palpitations, and xerostomia (normal

salivary flow resumes upon discontinuation); use vasoconstrictor with caution
Effects on Bleeding No information available to require special precautions
Adverse Effects Reactions which follow have been reported with the combination product; see individual drug monographs for additional adverse reactions that may be expected from each agent.
Cardiovascular: Cardiovascular collapse, palpitation, tachycardia
Central nervous system: Anxiety, CNS depression, convulsions, dizziness, drowsiness, excitability increased, fear, hallucinations, headache, insomnia, irritability increased, lightheadedness, nervousness
Gastrointestinal: Nausea, vomiting
Neuromuscular & skeletal: Tremor, weakness
Respiratory: Respiratory difficulties
General Dosage Range Oral: *Children >4 years and Adults:* Dosage varies greatly depending on product
Mechanism of Action See individual agents.
Pregnancy Considerations See individual agents.

Guaifenesin, Pseudoephedrine, and Codeine
(gwye FEN e sin, soo doe e FED rin, & KOE deen)

Related Information
Codeine *on page 344*
GuaiFENesin *on page 673*
Pseudoephedrine *on page 1159*
Brand Names: U.S. Cheratussin® DAC; Mytussin® DAC; Tricode® GF
Brand Names: Canada Benylin® 3.3 mg-D-E; Calmylin with Codeine
Pharmacologic Category Antitussive/Decongestant/Expectorant
Use Temporarily relieves nasal congestion and controls cough associated with upper respiratory infections and related conditions (common cold, sinusitis, bronchitis, influenza)
Local Anesthetic/Vasoconstrictor Precautions Use with caution since pseudoephedrine is a sympathomimetic amine which could interact with epinephrine to cause a pressor response
Effects on Dental Treatment Key adverse event(s) related to dental treatment:
Codeine: Xerostomia (normal salivary flow resumes upon discontinuation).
Guaifenesin: No significant effects or complications reported
Pseudoephedrine: Xerostomia (normal salivary flow resumes upon discontinuation).
Effects on Bleeding No information available to require special precautions
Adverse Effects See individual agents.
General Dosage Range Oral:
Children 6-12 years: 5 mL every 4 hours (maximum: 20 mL/24 hours)
Children >12 years and Adults: 10 mL every 4 hours (maximum: 40 mL/24 hours)
Pregnancy Risk Factor C
Pregnancy Considerations Reproduction studies have not been conducted with this combination. See individual agents.
Controlled Substance C-V

Guaifenesin, Pseudoephedrine, and Dextromethorphan
(gwye FEN e sin, soo doe e FED rin, & deks troe meth OR fan)

Related Information

Dextromethorphan *on page 406*

GuaiFENesin *on page 673*

Pseudoephedrine *on page 1159*

Brand Names: U.S. Ambifed DM; Ambifed-G DM; ExeFen-DMX; Maxifed DM [DSC]; Maxifed DMX

Brand Names: Canada Balminil DM + Decongestant + Expectorant; Benylin® DM-D-E

Pharmacologic Category Antitussive/Decongestant/Expectorant

Use Temporarily relieves nasal congestion and controls cough due to minor throat and bronchial irritation; helps loosen phlegm and thin bronchial secretions to make coughs more productive

Local Anesthetic/Vasoconstrictor Precautions Use with caution since pseudoephedrine is a sympathomimetic amine which could interact with epinephrine to cause a pressor response

Effects on Dental Treatment Key adverse event(s) related to dental treatment:

Dextromethorphan: No significant effects or complications reported

Guaifenesin: No significant effects or complications reported

Pseudoephedrine: Xerostomia (normal salivary flow resumes upon discontinuation).

Effects on Bleeding No information available to require special precautions

Adverse Effects See individual agents.

General Dosage Range Oral: *Children ≥6 years and Adults:* Dosage varies greatly depending on product

Mechanism of Action See individual agents.

Pregnancy Considerations See individual agents.

GuanFACINE (GWAHN fa seen)

Related Information

Cardiovascular Diseases *on page 1492*

Brand Names: U.S. Intuniv®; Tenex®

Pharmacologic Category Alpha$_2$-Adrenergic Agonist

Use

Tablet, immediate release: Management of hypertension

Tablet, extended release: Treatment of attention-deficit/hyperactivity disorder (ADHD) as monotherapy or adjunctive therapy to stimulants

Unlabeled Use Tic disorder; Tourette's syndrome

Local Anesthetic/Vasoconstrictor Precautions No information available to require special precautions

Effects on Dental Treatment Key adverse event(s) related to dental treatment: Xerostomia and changes in salivation (normal salivary flow resumes upon discontinuation).

Effects on Bleeding No information available to require special precautions

Adverse Effects

>10%:

Central nervous system: Somnolence (5% to 45%; dose-related), dizziness (2% to 15%; dose-related), headache (3% to 26%), fatigue (2% to 15%)

Gastrointestinal: Xerostomia (4% to 54%; dose-related), constipation (≤16%; dose-related), abdominal pain (≤11%; dose-related)

1% to 10%:

Cardiovascular: Hypotension (≤10%; dose-related), hypertension (2% to 5%), syncope (1% to 5%), AV block (<2%), bradycardia (<2%), chest pain (<2%), orthostasis (<2%), pallor (<2%), sinus arrhythmias (<2%)

Central nervous system: Insomnia (2% to 12%), fever (8%; Biederman, 2008), irritability (6%), lethargy (2% to 6%)

Gastrointestinal: Vomiting (9%), nausea (≤7%), weight gain (≤7%), appetite decreased (2% to 5%), diarrhea (2% to 5%), stomach discomfort (2% to 5%), dyspepsia (<2%)

Genitourinary: Impotence (≤7%), enuresis (<2%), urinary frequency (<2%)

Hepatic: ALT increased (<2%)

Neuromuscular & skeletal: Weakness (≤7%)

Respiratory: Asthma (<2%)

General Dosage Range Oral:

Immediate release: *Children ≥12 years and Adults:* 0.5-2 mg once daily

Extended release: *Children ≥6 years and Adolescents:* 1-4 mg once daily

Mechanism of Action Guanfacine is a selective alpha$_{2A}$-adrenoreceptor agonist which reduces sympathetic nerve impulses, resulting in reduced sympathetic outflow and a subsequent decrease in vasomotor tone and heart rate. In addition, guanfacine preferentially binds postsynaptic alpha$_{2A}$-adrenoreceptors in the prefrontal cortex and has been theorized to improve delay-related firing of prefrontal cortex neurons. As a result, underlying working memory and behavioral inhibition are affected; thereby improving symptoms associated with ADHD. Guanfacine is not a CNS stimulant.

Pharmacodynamics/Kinetics

Duration of Action Antihypertensive effect: 24 hours following single dose

Half-life Elimination

Immediate release: ~17 hours (range: 10-30 hours)

Extended release: 16 hours

Time to Peak Serum:

Immediate release: 2.6 hours (range: 1-4 hours)

Extended release: ~5 hours

Pregnancy Risk Factor B

Pregnancy Considerations Animal studies indicate decreased fetal survival when administered at higher doses than recommended in humans. There are no adequate and well-controlled studies in pregnant women. Use during pregnancy only if the benefits justify the risk to the fetus.

Guanidine (GWAHN i deen)

Pharmacologic Category Cholinergic Agonist

Use Reduction of the symptoms of muscle weakness associated with the myasthenic syndrome of Eaton-Lambert, not for myasthenia gravis

Local Anesthetic/Vasoconstrictor Precautions No information available to require special precautions

Effects on Dental Treatment No significant effects or complications reported

Effects on Bleeding No information available to require special precautions

Adverse Effects Frequency not defined.

Cardiovascular: Atrial fibrillation, flushing, hypotension, palpitation, tachycardia

Central nervous system: Ataxia, confusion, emotional lability, fever, hallucination, irritability, jitteriness, light-headedness, mood changes, nervousness, psychotic state

Dermatologic: Bruising, dry skin, folliculitis, petechiae, purpura, rash, skin eruptions

Gastrointestinal: Abdominal cramps, anorexia, diarrhea, gastric irritation, nausea, sore throat, xerostomia

Hematologic: Anemia, bone-marrow suppression, leukopenia, thrombocytopenia

Hepatic: Abnormal liver function tests

Neuromuscular & skeletal: Paresthesia, trembling, tremor

Renal: Creatinine increased, interstitial nephritis (acute or chronic), renal tubular necrosis, uremia

Miscellaneous: Cold extremities, diaphoresis

General Dosage Range Oral: *Adults:* Initial: 10-15 mg/kg/day in 3-4 divided doses; Maintenance: Up to 35 mg/kg/day

Pregnancy Considerations Animal reproduction studies have not been conducted.

Haemophilus b Conjugate Vaccine
(he MOF fi lus bee KON joo gate vak SEEN)

Brand Names: U.S. ActHIB®; Hiberix®; PedvaxHIB®
Brand Names: Canada ActHIB®; PedvaxHIB®
Pharmacologic Category Vaccine, Inactivated (Bacterial)
Use Routine immunization of children against invasive disease caused by *H. influenzae* type b

The Advisory Committee on Immunization Practices (ACIP) recommends routine vaccination of all children through age 59 months. Efficacy data are not available for use in older children and adults with chronic conditions associated with an increased risk of Hib disease. However, a single dose may also be considered for older children, adolescents, and adults who did not receive the childhood series and who have a chronic condition associated with an increased risk of Hib disease (eg, splenectomy, sickle cell disease, leukemia, HIV infection).

Local Anesthetic/Vasoconstrictor Precautions No information available to require special precautions
Effects on Dental Treatment No significant effects or complications reported
Effects on Bleeding No information available to require special precautions
Adverse Effects All serious adverse reactions must be reported to the U.S. Department of Health and Human Services (DHHS) Vaccine Adverse Event Reporting System (VAERS) 1-800-822-7967 or online at https://vaers.hhs.gov/esub/index. In Canada, adverse reactions may be reported to local provincial/territorial health agencies or to the Vaccine Safety Section at Public Health Agency of Canada (1-866-844-0018).

Frequency not defined:
Central nervous system: Crying (unusual, high pitched, prolonged), fever, fussiness, irritability, pain, restlessness, sleepiness
Dermatologic: Rash
Gastrointestinal: Anorexia, diarrhea, vomiting
Local: Injection site: Erythema, induration, pain, soreness, swelling
Otic: Otitis media
Respiratory: Upper respiratory tract infection
General Dosage Range I.M.: *Children:* 0.5 mL (number of doses determined by age at first dose)

Mechanism of Action Stimulates production of anti-capsular antibodies and provides active immunity to *Haemophilus influenzae* type b
Pharmacodynamics/Kinetics
Onset of Action Serum antibody response: 1-2 weeks
Duration of Action Immunity: 1.5 years
Pregnancy Risk Factor C
Pregnancy Considerations Reproduction studies have not been conducted.

Halcinonide (hal SIN oh nide)

Brand Names: U.S. Halog®
Pharmacologic Category Corticosteroid, Topical
Use Relief of inflammatory and pruritic effects of corticosteroid-responsive dermatoses [high potency topical corticosteroid]
Local Anesthetic/Vasoconstrictor Precautions No information available to require special precautions
Effects on Dental Treatment No significant effects or complications reported
Effects on Bleeding No information available to require special precautions
Adverse Effects Note: Frequency not defined. Adverse reactions reported with topical corticosteroids; may occur more frequently with occlusive dressing.
Cardiovascular: Intracranial hypertension (children)
Dermatologic: Acneiform eruptions, allergic contact dermatitis, dry skin, folliculitis, hypertrichosis, hypopigmentation, itching, miliaria, perioral dermatitis, skin atrophy, skin maceration, striae
Endocrine & metabolic: Cushing's syndrome, growth retardation (children), HPA axis suppression, hyperglycemia
Local: Burning, irritation
Renal: Glucosuria
Miscellaneous: Secondary infection
General Dosage Range Topical: *Children and Adults:* Apply sparingly 2-3 times daily
Mechanism of Action Decreases inflammation by suppression of migration of polymorphonuclear leukocytes and reversal of increased capillary permeability
Pregnancy Risk Factor C
Pregnancy Considerations Teratogenic effects have been observed in animals administered potent topical corticosteroids. Topical products are not recommended for extensive use, in large quantities, or for long periods of time in pregnant women (Reed, 1997).

Halobetasol (hal oh BAY ta sol)

Brand Names: U.S. Halonate™; Ultravate®
Brand Names: Canada Ultravate®
Generic Availability (U.S.) Yes
Pharmacologic Category Corticosteroid, Topical
Use Relief of inflammatory and pruritic manifestations of corticosteroid-response dermatoses [super high potency topical corticosteroid]
Local Anesthetic/Vasoconstrictor Precautions No information available to require special precautions
Effects on Dental Treatment No significant effects or complications reported
Effects on Bleeding No information available to require special precautions
Adverse Effects Frequency not always defined.
Central nervous system: Intracranial hypertension (systemic effect reported in children treated with topical corticosteroids)

▶

◀ Dermatologic: Itching (4%), acneiform eruptions, allergic contact dermatitis, dry skin, erythema, folliculitis, hypertrichosis, hypopigmentation, leukoderma, miliaria, perioral dermatitis, pruritus, pustulation, rash, skin atrophy, skin infection (secondary), striae, telangiectasia, vesicles, urticaria

Endocrine: Glycosuria, HPA axis suppression, metabolic effects (hyperglycemia, hypokalemia)

Local: Burning (2% to 4%), stinging (2% to 4%)

Neuromuscular & skeletal: Paresthesia

Dosage Topical: Children ≥12 years and Adults: Steroid-responsive dermatoses: Apply sparingly to skin once or twice daily, rub in gently and completely; treatment should not exceed 2 consecutive weeks and total dosage should not exceed 50 g/week. Therapy should be discontinued when control is achieved; if no improvement is seen, reassessment of diagnosis may be necessary.

Mechanism of Action Corticosteroids inhibit the initial manifestations of the inflammatory process (ie, capillary dilation and edema, fibrin deposition, and migration and diapedesis of leukocytes into the inflamed site) as well as later sequelae (angiogenesis, fibroblast proliferation)

Contraindications Hypersensitivity to halobetasol or any component of the formulation

Warnings/Precautions Topical corticosteroids may be absorbed percutaneously. Absorption of topical corticosteroids may cause manifestations of Cushing's syndrome, hyperglycemia, or glycosuria. Absorption is increased by the use of occlusive dressings, application to denuded skin, or application to large surface areas. May cause hypercorticism or suppression of hypothalamic-pituitary-adrenal (HPA) axis, particularly in younger children or in patients receiving high doses for prolonged periods. HPA axis suppression may lead to adrenal crisis. Children may absorb proportionally larger amounts of corticosteroids after topical application and may be more prone to systemic effects. HPA axis suppression, intracranial hypertension, and Cushing's syndrome have been reported in children receiving topical corticosteroids. Prolonged use may affect growth velocity; growth should be routinely monitored in pediatric patients.

Allergic contact dermatitis can occur, it is usually diagnosed by failure to heal rather than clinical exacerbation. Discontinue therapy if irritation develops. Use appropriate antibacterial or antifungal agents to treat concomitant skin infections; discontinue halobetasol treatment if infection does not resolve promptly. Prolonged treatment with corticosteroids has been associated with the development of Kaposi's sarcoma (case reports); if noted, discontinuation of therapy should be considered. Not for ophthalmic use. Topical halobetasol should not be used for the treatment of rosacea or perioral dermatitis. Not recommended for application to the face, groin, or axillae.

Drug Interactions

Metabolism/Transport Effects None known.

Avoid Concomitant Use

Avoid concomitant use of Halobetasol with any of the following: Aldesleukin

Increased Effect/Toxicity

Halobetasol may increase the levels/effects of: Deferasirox

The levels/effects of Halobetasol may be increased by: Telaprevir

Decreased Effect

Halobetasol may decrease the levels/effects of: Aldesleukin; Corticorelin; Hyaluronidase; Telaprevir

Pregnancy Risk Factor C

Pregnancy Considerations Teratogenic effects have been observed in animal reproduction studies. Topical products are not recommended for extensive use, in large quantities, or for long periods of time in pregnant women (Reed, 1997).

Lactation Excretion in breast milk unknown/use caution

Breast-Feeding Considerations Systemically administered corticosteroids appear in human milk and may cause adverse effects in a nursing infant. It is not known if the systemic absorption of topical halobetasol results in detectable quantities in human milk. Use with caution while breast-feeding; do not apply to nipples (Reed, 1997).

Dosage Forms

Cream, topical: 0.05% (15 g, 50 g)
  Ultravate®: 0.05% (50 g)
Ointment, topical: 0.05% (15 g, 50 g)
  Halonate™: 0.05% (50 g)
  Ultravate®: 0.05% (50 g)

Haloperidol (ha loe PER i dole)

Related Information

Clinical Risk Related to Drugs Prolonging QT Interval *on page 1510*

Brand Names: U.S. Haldol®; Haldol® Decanoate

Brand Names: Canada Apo-Haloperidol LA®; Apo-Haloperidol®; Haloperidol Injection, USP; Haloperidol Long Acting; Haloperidol-LA; Haloperidol-LA Omega; Novo-Peridol; PMS-Haloperidol; PMS-Haloperidol LA

Pharmacologic Category Antipsychotic Agent, Typical

Use Management of schizophrenia; control of tics and vocal utterances of Tourette's disorder in children and adults; severe behavioral problems in children

Unlabeled Use Treatment of nonschizophrenia psychosis; may be used for the emergency sedation of severely-agitated or delirious patients; treatment of ICU delirium; adjunctive treatment of ethanol dependence; postoperative nausea and vomiting (alternative therapy); psychosis/agitation related to Alzheimer's dementia

Local Anesthetic/Vasoconstrictor Precautions Manufacturer's information states that haloperidol may block vasopressor activity of epinephrine. This has not been observed during use of epinephrine as a vasoconstrictor in local anesthesia. Haloperidol is one of the drugs confirmed to prolong the QT interval and is accepted as having a risk of causing torsade de pointes. The risk of drug-induced torsade de pointes is extremely low when a single QT interval prolonging drug is prescribed. In terms of epinephrine, it is not known what effect vasoconstrictors in the local anesthetic regimen will have in patients with a known history of congenital prolonged QT interval or in patients taking any medication that prolongs the QT interval. Until more information is obtained, it is suggested that the clinician consult with the physician prior to the use of a vasoconstrictor in suspected patients, and that the vasoconstrictor (epinephrine, mepivacaine and levonordefrin [Carbocaine® 2% with Neo-Cobefrin®]) be used with caution.

Effects on Dental Treatment Key adverse event(s) related to dental treatment: Xerostomia (normal salivary flow resumes upon discontinuation). Orthostatic hypotension, and nasal congestion are possible; since the drug is a dopamine antagonist, extrapyramidal symptoms of the TMJ are a possibility.

Effects on Bleeding No information available to require special precautions

Adverse Effects Frequency not defined.

Cardiovascular: Abnormal T waves with prolonged ventricular repolarization, arrhythmia, hyper-/hypotension, QT prolongation, sudden death, tachycardia, torsade de pointes

Central nervous system: Agitation, akathisia, altered central temperature regulation, anxiety, confusion, depression, drowsiness, dystonic reactions, euphoria, extrapyramidal reactions, headache, insomnia, lethargy, neuroleptic malignant syndrome (NMS), pseudoparkinsonian signs and symptoms, restlessness, seizure, tardive dyskinesia, tardive dystonia, vertigo

Dermatologic: Alopecia, contact dermatitis, hyperpigmentation, photosensitivity (rare), pruritus, rash

Endocrine & metabolic: Amenorrhea, breast engorgement, galactorrhea, gynecomastia, hyper-/hypoglycemia, hyponatremia, lactation, mastalgia, menstrual irregularities, sexual dysfunction

Gastrointestinal: Anorexia, constipation, diarrhea, dyspepsia, hypersalivation, nausea, vomiting, xerostomia

Genitourinary: Priapism, urinary retention

Hematologic: Agranulocytosis (rare), leukopenia, leukocytosis, neutropenia, anemia, lymphomonocytosis

Hepatic: Cholestatic jaundice, obstructive jaundice

Ocular: Blurred vision

Respiratory: Bronchospasm, laryngospasm

Miscellaneous: Diaphoresis, heat stroke

General Dosage Range

I.M.:

Decanoate: *Adults:* Initial: 10-20 times daily oral dose at 4-week intervals; Maintenance: 10-15 times initial oral dose

Lactate:

Children 6-12 years: 1-3 mg/dose every 4-8 hours (maximum: 0.15 mg/kg/day)

Adults: 2-5 mg every 4-8 hours as needed

Oral:

Children 3-12 years (15-40 kg): Initial: 0.5 mg/day in 2-3 divided doses; Maintenance: 0.05-0.15 mg/kg/day in 2-3 divided doses

Adults: Initial: 0.5-5 mg 2-3 times/day; Maintenance: Up to 30 mg/day in 2-3 divided doses

Mechanism of Action Haloperidol is a butyrophenone antipsychotic which blocks postsynaptic mesolimbic dopaminergic D_1 and D_2 receptors in the brain; depresses the release of hypothalamic and hypophyseal hormones; believed to depress the reticular activating system thus affecting basal metabolism, body temperature, wakefulness, vasomotor tone, and emesis

Pharmacodynamics/Kinetics

Onset of Action Sedation: I.M., I.V.: 30-60 minutes

Duration of Action Decanoate: ~3 weeks

Half-life Elimination 18 hours; Decanoate: 21 days

Time to Peak Oral: 2-6 hours; I.M.: 20 minutes; decanoate: 7 days

Pregnancy Risk Factor C

Pregnancy Considerations Adverse events were observed in animal studies. Haloperidol crosses the placenta. There are case reports of limb malformations following first trimester exposure in humans. Antipsychotic use during the third trimester of pregnancy has a risk for abnormal muscle movements (extrapyramidal symptoms [EPS]) and withdrawal symptoms in newborns following delivery. Symptoms in the newborn may include agitation, feeding disorder, hypertonia, hypotonia, respiratory distress, somnolence, and tremor; these effects may be self-limiting or require hospitalization.

Dental Comment Haloperidol is known to prolong the QT interval. The QT interval is measured as the time and distance between the Q point of the QRS complex and the end of the T wave in the ECG tracing. After adjustment for heart rate, the QT interval is defined as prolonged if it is more than 450 msec in men and 460 msec in women. A long QT syndrome was first described in the 1950s and 60s as a congenital syndrome involving QT interval prolongation and syncope and sudden death. Some of the congenital long QT syndromes were characterized by a peculiar electrocardiographic appearance of the QRS complex involving a premature atria beat followed by a pause, then a subsequent sinus beat showing marked QT prolongation and deformity. This type of cardiac arrhythmia was originally termed "torsade de pointes" (translated from the French as "twisting of the points"). Haloperidol is considered as having a risk of causing torsade de pointes. Since it is not known what effect vasoconstrictors in the local anesthetic regimen will have in patients with a known history of congenital prolonged QT interval or in patients taking any medication that prolongs the QT interval, a medical consult is suggested.

Hemin (HEE min)

Brand Names: U.S. Panhematin®

Pharmacologic Category Blood Modifiers; Blood Product Derivative

Use Treatment of recurrent attacks of acute intermittent porphyria (AIP)

Local Anesthetic/Vasoconstrictor Precautions No information available to require special precautions

Effects on Dental Treatment No significant effects or complications reported

Effects on Bleeding No information available to require special precautions

Adverse Effects Frequency not defined.

Central nervous system: Pyrexia

Hematologic: Leukocytosis

Local: Phlebitis

General Dosage Range I.V.: *Children ≥16 years and Adults:* 1-4 mg/kg/day divided every 12 hours (maximum: 6 mg/kg/24 hours)

Mechanism of Action Inhibits the hepatic and/or marrow synthesis of ALA synthase, the enzyme that regulates the porphyrin/heme pathway

Pregnancy Risk Factor C

Pregnancy Considerations Animal reproduction studies have not been conducted. There are no adequate and well-controlled studies in pregnant women. Use during pregnancy only if the potential benefit out weighs the potential risk to the fetus.

Heparin (HEP a rin)

Related Information

Cardiovascular Diseases *on page 1492*

Brand Names: U.S. Hep-Lock; HepFlush®-10

Brand Names: Canada Hepalean®; Hepalean® Leo; Hepalean®-LOK

Pharmacologic Category Anticoagulant

Use Prophylaxis and treatment of thromboembolic disorders; as an anticoagulant for extracorporeal and dialysis procedures

Note: Heparin lock flush solution is intended only to maintain patency of I.V. devices and is **not** to be used for systemic anticoagulant therapy.

◀ **Unlabeled Use** ST-elevation myocardial infarction (STEMI) as an adjunct to thrombolysis; unstable angina/non-STEMI (UA/NSTEMI); anticoagulant used during percutaneous coronary intervention (PCI)

Local Anesthetic/Vasoconstrictor Precautions No information available to require special precautions

Effects on Dental Treatment Key adverse event(s) related to dental treatment: Bleeding from the gums. See Effects on Bleeding.

Effects on Bleeding The most serious adverse effect is bleeding, including bleeding from the gums. Medical consult is recommended.

Adverse Effects Note: Thrombocytopenia has been reported to occur at an incidence between 0% and 30%. It is often of no clinical significance. However, immunologically mediated heparin-induced thrombocytopenia (HIT) has been estimated to occur in 1% to 2% of patients, and is marked by a progressive fall in platelet counts and, in some cases, thromboembolic complications (skin necrosis, pulmonary embolism, gangrene of the extremities, stroke, or MI).

Frequency not defined.
Cardiovascular: Allergic vasospastic reaction (possibly related to thrombosis), chest pain, hemorrhagic shock, shock, thrombosis
Central nervous system: Chills, fever, headache
Dermatologic: Alopecia (delayed, transient), bruising (unexplained), cutaneous necrosis, dysesthesia pedis, erythematous plaques (case reports), eczema, urticaria, purpura
Endocrine & metabolic: Adrenal hemorrhage, hyperkalemia (suppression of aldosterone synthesis), ovarian hemorrhage, rebound hyperlipidemia on discontinuation
Gastrointestinal: Constipation, hematemesis, nausea, tarry stools, vomiting
Genitourinary: Frequent or persistent erection
Hematologic: Bleeding from gums, epistaxis, hemorrhage, ovarian hemorrhage, retroperitoneal hemorrhage, thrombocytopenia (see **"Note"**)
Hepatic: Liver enzymes increased
Local: Irritation, erythema, pain, hematoma, and ulceration have been rarely reported with deep SubQ injections; I.M. injection (not recommended) is associated with a high incidence of these effects
Neuromuscular & skeletal: Peripheral neuropathy, osteoporosis (chronic therapy effect)
Ocular: Conjunctivitis (allergic reaction), lacrimation
Renal: Hematuria
Respiratory: Asthma, bronchospasm (case reports), hemoptysis, pulmonary hemorrhage, rhinitis
Miscellaneous: Allergic reactions, anaphylactoid reactions, heparin resistance, hypersensitivity (including chills, fever, and urticaria)

General Dosage Range
I.V.:
  Children: Bolus: 50-100 units/kg; Initial infusion: 15-25 units/kg/hour; Maintenance: Increase dose by 2-4 units/kg/hour every 6-8 hours as needed **or** 50-100 units/kg every 4 hours intermittently
  Adults: Bolus: 60-80 units/kg; Infusion: 10-30 units/kg/hour **or** 10,000 units (initially), then 50-70 units/kg (5000-10,000 units) every 4-6 hours intermittently
  SubQ: *Adults:* Thromboprophylaxis: 5000 units every 8-12 hours; Treatment: 17,500 units every 12 hours

Mechanism of Action Potentiates the action of antithrombin III and thereby inactivates thrombin (as well as activated coagulation factors IX, X, XI, XII, and plasmin) and prevents the conversion of fibrinogen to fibrin;

heparin also stimulates release of lipoprotein lipase (lipoprotein lipase hydrolyzes triglycerides to glycerol and free fatty acids)

Pharmacodynamics/Kinetics
Onset of Action Anticoagulation: I.V.: Immediate; SubQ: ~20-30 minutes

Half-life Elimination
Dose-dependent: I.V. bolus: 25 units/kg: 30 minutes; 100 units/kg: 60 minutes; 400 units/kg: 150 minutes (Hirsh, 2008)
Mean: 1.5 hours; Range: 1-2 hours; affected by obesity, renal function, malignancy, presence of pulmonary embolism, and infections
Note: At therapeutic doses, elimination occurs rapidly via nonrenal mechanisms. With very high doses, renal elimination may play more of a role; however, dosage adjustment remains unnecessary for patients with renal impairment (Hirsh, 2008).

Pregnancy Risk Factor C

Pregnancy Considerations Increased resorptions were observed in some animal reproduction studies. Heparin does not cross the placenta. Heparin may be used for the prevention and treatment of thromboembolism in pregnant women; however the use of low molecular weight heparin (LMWH) is preferred. Twice-daily heparin should be discontinued prior to induction of labor or a planned cesarean delivery. In pregnant women with mechanical heart valves, adjusted-dose LMWH or adjusted-dose heparin may be used throughout pregnancy or until week 13 of gestation when therapy can be changed to warfarin. LMWH or heparin should be resumed close to delivery. In women who are at a very high risk for thromboembolism (older generation prosthesis in mitral position or history of thromboembolism), warfarin can be used throughout pregnancy and replaced with LMWH or heparin near term; the use of low-dose aspirin is also recommended. When choosing therapy, fetal outcomes (ie, pregnancy loss, malformations), maternal outcomes (ie, VTE, hemorrhage), burden of therapy, and maternal preference should be considered (Guyatt, 2012).

Some products contain benzyl alcohol as a preservative; their use in pregnant women is contraindicated by some manufacturers; use of a preservative free formulation is recommended.

Hepatitis A and Hepatitis B Recombinant Vaccine
(hep a TYE tis aye & hep a TYE tis bee ree KOM be nant vak SEEN)

Related Information
Systemic Viral Diseases *on page 1537*
Brand Names: U.S. Twinrix®
Brand Names: Canada Twinrix®; Twinrix® Junior
Pharmacologic Category Vaccine, Inactivated (Viral)
Use Active immunization against disease caused by hepatitis A virus and hepatitis B virus (all known subtypes) in populations desiring protection against or at high risk of exposure to these viruses.

Populations include travelers or people living in or relocating to areas of intermediate/high endemicity for **both** HAV and HBV and are at increased risk of HBV infection due to behavioral or occupational factors; patients with chronic liver disease; laboratory workers who handle live HAV and HBV; healthcare workers, police, and other personnel who render first-aid or medical assistance; workers who come in contact with sewage; employees of day care centers and correctional facilities; patients/staff of hemodialysis units; men who have sex with men; patients frequently receiving blood products; military personnel; users of injectable illicit drugs; close household contacts of patients with hepatitis A and hepatitis B infection; residents of drug and alcohol treatment centers

Local Anesthetic/Vasoconstrictor Precautions No information available to require special precautions

Effects on Dental Treatment Key adverse event(s) related to dental treatment: Flu-like syndrome and upper respiratory tract infection.

Effects on Bleeding No information available to require special precautions

Adverse Effects In the U.S., all serious adverse reactions must be reported to the U.S. Department of Health and Human Services (DHHS) Vaccine Adverse Event Reporting System (VAERS) 1-800-822-7967 or online at https://vaers.hhs.gov/esub/index.

Incidence of adverse effects of the combination product were similar to those occurring after administration of hepatitis A vaccine and hepatitis B vaccine alone. (Incidence reported is not versus placebo.)

Adults:
>10%:
Central nervous system: Headache (13% to 22%), fatigue (11% to 14%)
Local: Injection site reaction: Soreness (35% to 41%), redness (8% to 11%)
1% to 10%:
Central nervous system: Fever (2% to 4%)
Gastrointestinal: Diarrhea (4% to 6%), nausea (2% to 4%), vomiting (≤1%)
Local: Injection site reaction: Swelling (4% to 6%), induration
Respiratory: Upper respiratory tract infection

Children (as reported in Canadian labeling):
>10%: Local: Injection site pain/redness
1% to 10%:
Central nervous system: Fever (≥37.5°C), drowsiness, fatigue, headache, irritability, malaise
Gastrointestinal: Appetite decreased, diarrhea, nausea, vomiting
Local: Injection site edema

General Dosage Range I.M.: *Adults:* 3 doses (1 mL each) given on a 0-, 1-, and 6-month schedule

Mechanism of Action
Hepatitis A vaccine, an inactivated virus vaccine, offers active immunization against hepatitis A virus infection at an effective immune response rate in up to 99% of subjects.
Recombinant hepatitis B vaccine is a noninfectious subunit viral vaccine. The vaccine is derived from hepatitis B surface antigen (HB$_s$Ag) produced through recombinant DNA techniques from yeast cells. The portion of the hepatitis B gene which codes for HB$_s$Ag is cloned into yeast which is then cultured to produce hepatitis B vaccine.

In immunocompetent people, Twinrix® provides active immunization against hepatitis A virus infection (at an effective immune response rate >99% of subjects) and against hepatitis B virus infection (at an effective immune response rate of 93% to 97%) 30 days after completion of the 3-dose series. This is comparable to using hepatitis A vaccine and hepatitis B vaccine concomitantly.

Pharmacodynamics/Kinetics
Onset of Action Seroconversion for antibodies against HAV and HBV were detected 1 month after completion of the 3-dose series.
Duration of Action Patients remained seropositive for at least 4 years during clinical studies.
Pregnancy Risk Factor C
Pregnancy Considerations Reproduction studies have not been conducted with this combination. Healthcare providers are encouraged to call the manufacturer of Twinrix® to register any patients who may have received this vaccine during pregnancy (888-452-9622).

Hepatitis A Vaccine (hep a TYE tis aye vak SEEN)

Related Information
Systemic Viral Diseases *on page 1537*
Brand Names: U.S. Havrix®; VAQTA®
Brand Names: Canada Avaxim®; Avaxim®-Pediatric; HAVRIX®; VAQTA®
Pharmacologic Category Vaccine, Inactivated (Viral)
Use
Active immunization against disease caused by hepatitis A virus (HAV)
The Advisory Committee on Immunization Practices (ACIP) recommends routine vaccination for (CDC, 2006):
- All children ≥12 months of age
- All unvaccinated adults requesting protection from HAV infection
- All unvaccinated adults at risk for HAV infection, such as:
  Behavioral risks: Men who have sex with men; injection and non-injection illicit drug users
  Occupational risks: Persons who work with HAV-infected primates or with HAV in a research laboratory setting
  Medical risks: Persons with chronic liver disease; patients who receive clotting-factor concentrates
- Other risks: International travelers to regions with high or intermediate levels of endemic HAV infection (a list of countries is available at http://wwwnc.cdc.gov/travel/page/diseases.htm)
- Unvaccinated persons who anticipate close personal contact with international adoptee from a country of intermediate to high endemicity of HAV, during their first 60 days of arrival into the United States (eg, household contacts, babysitters)

Local Anesthetic/Vasoconstrictor Precautions No information available to require special precautions
Effects on Dental Treatment No significant effects or complications reported
Effects on Bleeding No information available to require special precautions
Adverse Effects All serious adverse reactions must be reported to the U.S. Department of Health and Human Services (DHHS) Vaccine Adverse Event Reporting System (VAERS) at 1-800-822-7967 or online at https://vaers.hhs.gov/esub/index.
Frequency dependent upon age, product used, and concomitant vaccine administration. In general, headache and injection site reactions were less common in younger children.
>10%:
Central nervous system: Drowsiness, fever ≥100.4°F (1-5 days post vaccination), fever >98.6°C (1-14 days post vaccination), headache, irritability
Gastrointestinal: Appetite decreased

Local: Injection site: Erythema, pain, soreness, swelling, tenderness, warmth

1% to 10%:

Central nervous system: Chills, fatigue, fever ≥102°F (1-5 days postvaccination), insomnia, malaise

Dermatologic: Rash

Endocrine & metabolic: Menstrual disorder

Gastrointestinal: Abdominal pain, anorexia, constipation, diarrhea, gastroenteritis, nausea, vomiting

Local: Injection site bruising, induration

Neuromuscular & skeletal: Arm pain, back pain, myalgia, stiffness, weakness/fatigue

Ocular: Conjunctivitis

Otic: Otitis media

Respiratory: Asthma, cough, nasopharyngitis, nasal congestion, pharyngitis, rhinorrhea, rhinitis, upper respiratory tract infection

Miscellaneous: Crying

General Dosage Range I.M.:

Children 12 months to 18 years: 0.5 mL

Adults: 1 mL

Mechanism of Action As an inactivated virus vaccine, hepatitis A vaccine offers active immunization against hepatitis A virus infection at an effective immune response rate in up to 99% of subjects

Pharmacodynamics/Kinetics

Onset of Action Protection: 2-4 weeks after a single dose; 2 weeks after vaccine administration, 54% to 62% of patients develop neutralizing antibodies; this percentage increases to 94% to 100% at 1 month postvaccination (CDC, 2006)

Duration of Action Neutralizing antibodies have persisted for up to 8 years; based on kinetic models, antibodies may be present ≥14-20 years in children and ≥25 years in adults who receive the complete vaccination series (CDC, 2006; Van Damme, 2003).

Pregnancy Risk Factor C

Pregnancy Considerations Reproduction studies have not been conducted. The safety of vaccination during pregnancy has not been determined, however, the theoretical risk to the infant is expected to be low. Inactivated vaccines have not been shown to cause increased risks to the fetus (CDC, 2011).

Hepatitis B Immune Globulin (Human)

(hep a TYE tis bee i MYUN GLOB yoo lin YU man)

Related Information

Systemic Viral Diseases *on page 1537*

Brand Names: U.S. HepaGam B®; HyperHEP B™ S/D; Nabi-HB®

Brand Names: Canada HepaGam B®; HyperHEP B™ S/D

Pharmacologic Category Blood Product Derivative; Immune Globulin

Use

Passive prophylactic immunity to hepatitis B following: Acute exposure to blood containing hepatitis B surface antigen (HB_sAg); perinatal exposure of infants born to HB_sAg-positive mothers; sexual exposure to HB_sAg-positive persons; household exposure to persons with acute HBV infection

Prevention of hepatitis B virus recurrence after liver transplantation in HB_sAg-positive transplant patients

Note: Hepatitis B immune globulin is not indicated for treatment of active hepatitis B infection and is ineffective in the treatment of chronic active hepatitis B infection.

Local Anesthetic/Vasoconstrictor Precautions No information available to require special precautions

Effects on Dental Treatment No significant effects or complications reported

Effects on Bleeding No information available to require special precautions

Adverse Effects Reported with postexposure prophylaxis; frequency not defined. Adverse events reported in liver transplant patients included tremor and hypotension, were associated with a single infusion during the first week of treatment, and did not recur with additional infusions.

Central nervous system: Dizziness, fainting, headache, lightheadedness, malaise

Dermatologic: Angioedema, bruising, urticaria

Gastrointestinal: Nausea, vomiting

Hematologic: WBC decreased

Hepatic: Alkaline phosphatase increased, AST increased

Local: Ache, erythema, pain, and/or tenderness at injection site

Neuromuscular & skeletal: Arthralgia, joint stiffness, myalgia

Renal: Creatinine increased

Respiratory: Cold symptoms

Miscellaneous: Anaphylaxis, flu-like syndrome

General Dosage Range

I.M.:

Newborns and Infants <12 months: 0.5 mL/dose

Children ≥12 months and Adults: 0.06 mL/kg/dose

I.V.: *Adults:* 20,000 units/dose daily for 8 days, then every 2 weeks for 6 doses, then once monthly

Mechanism of Action Hepatitis B immune globulin (HBIG) is a nonpyrogenic sterile solution containing immunoglobulin G (IgG) specific to hepatitis B surface antigen (HB_sAg). HBIG differs from immune globulin in the amount of anti-HB_s. Immune globulin is prepared from plasma that is not preselected for anti-HB_s content. HBIG is prepared from plasma preselected for high titer anti-HB_s. In the U.S., HBIG has an anti-HB_s high titer >1:100,000 by IRA.

Pharmacodynamics/Kinetics

Duration of Action Postexposure prophylaxis: 3-6 months

Half-life Elimination 17-25 days

Time to Peak Serum: I.M.: 2-10 days

Pregnancy Risk Factor C

Pregnancy Considerations Animal reproduction studies have not been conducted. Use of HBIG is not contraindicated in pregnant women and may be used for postexposure prophylaxis when indicated (CDC, 2001). In addition, use of HBIG has been evaluated to reduce maternal to fetal transmission of hepatis B virus during pregnancy (ACOG, 2007)

Hepatitis B Vaccine (Recombinant)

(hep a TYE tis bee vak SEEN ree KOM be nant)

Related Information

Systemic Viral Diseases *on page 1537*

Brand Names: U.S. Engerix-B®; Recombivax HB®

Brand Names: Canada Engerix-B®; Recombivax HB®

Pharmacologic Category Vaccine, Inactivated (Viral)

Use Immunization against infection caused by all known subtypes of hepatitis B virus (HBV)

The Advisory Committee on Immunization Practices (ACIP) recommends routine vaccination for the following (CDC, 2005; CDC, 2006; CDC, 2011):
- All infants at birth
- All infants and children (post-birth dose; refer to recommended vaccination schedule)
- All unvaccinated adults requesting protection from HBV infection
- All unvaccinated adults at risk for HBV infection such as those with:
  Behavioral risks: Sexually-active persons with >1 partner in a 6-month period; persons seeking evaluation or treatment for a sexually-transmitted disease; men who have sex with men; injection drug users
  Occupational risks: Healthcare and public safety workers with reasonably anticipated risk for exposure to blood or blood contaminated body fluids
  Medical risks: Persons with end-stage renal disease (including predialysis, hemodialysis, peritoneal dialysis, and home dialysis); persons with HIV infection; persons with chronic liver disease. Adults (19 through 59 years of age) with diabetes mellitus type 1 or type 2 should be vaccinated as soon as possible following diagnosis. Adults ≥60 years with diabetes mellitus may also be vaccinated at the discretion of their treating clinician.
  Other risks: Household contacts and sex partners of persons with chronic HBV infection; residents and staff of facilities for developmentally disabled persons; international travelers to regions with high or intermediate levels of endemic HBV infection

In addition, the ACIP recommends vaccination for any persons who are wounded in bombings or similar mass casualty events who have penetrating injuries or non-intact skin exposure, or who have contact with mucous membranes (exception - superficial contact with intact skin), and who cannot confirm receipt of a hepatitis B vaccination (CDC, 2008).

Local Anesthetic/Vasoconstrictor Precautions No information available to require special precautions

Effects on Dental Treatment No significant effects or complications reported

Effects on Bleeding No information available to require special precautions

Adverse Effects All serious adverse reactions must be reported to the U.S. Department of Health and Human Services (DHHS) Vaccine Adverse Event Reporting System (VAERS) at 1-800-822-7967 or online at https://vaers.hhs.gov/esub/index.
Frequency not defined. The most common adverse effects reported with both products included injection site reactions (>10%).
Cardiovascular: Flushing, hypotension
Central nervous system: Agitation, chills, dizziness, fatigue, fever (≥37.5°C/100°F), headache, insomnia, irritability, lightheadedness, malaise, somnolence, vertigo
Dermatologic: Angioedema, petechiae, pruritus, rash, urticaria
Gastrointestinal: Abdominal pain, anorexia, appetite decreased, constipation, cramps, diarrhea, dyspepsia, nausea, vomiting
Genitourinary: Dysuria
Local: Injection site reactions: Ecchymosis, erythema, induration, pain, nodule formation, soreness, swelling, tenderness, warmth
Neuromuscular & skeletal: Achiness, arthralgia, back pain, myalgia, neck pain, neck stiffness, paresthesia, shoulder pain, tingling, weakness

Otic: Earache
Respiratory: Cough, pharyngitis, rhinitis, upper respiratory tract infection
Miscellaneous: Diaphoresis, lymphadenopathy, flu-like syndrome

General Dosage Range Dosage adjustment recommended in patients with renal impairment.
I.M.:
Birth to 19 years: 0.5 mL
Adults ≥20 years: 1 mL

Mechanism of Action Recombinant hepatitis B vaccine is a noninfectious subunit viral vaccine, which confers active immunity via formation of antihepatitis B antibodies. The vaccine is derived from hepatitis B surface antigen (HB_sAg) produced through recombinant DNA techniques from yeast cells. The portion of the hepatitis B gene which codes for HB_sAg is cloned into yeast which is then cultured to produce hepatitis B vaccine.

Pharmacodynamics/Kinetics
Duration of Action Following a 3-dose series in children, up to 50% of patients will have low or undetectable anti-HB antibody 5-15 years postvaccination. However, anamnestic increases in anti-HB have been shown up to 23 years later suggesting a lifelong immune memory response.

Pregnancy Risk Factor C
Pregnancy Considerations Animal reproduction studies have not been conducted. The ACIP recommends HB_sAg testing for all pregnant women. Based on limited data, there is no apparent risk to the fetus when the hepatitis B vaccine is administered during pregnancy. Pregnancy itself is not a contraindication to vaccination; vaccination should be considered if otherwise indicated (CDC, 2006).

Dental Comment Immunization is recommended for dentists, oral surgeons, dental hygienists, dental nurses, and dental students

Hetastarch (HET a starch)

Brand Names: U.S. Hespan®; Hextend®
Brand Names: Canada Hextend®
Pharmacologic Category Plasma Volume Expander, Colloid
Use Blood volume expander used in treatment of hypovolemia; adjunct in leukapheresis to improve harvesting and increase the yield of granulocytes by centrifugation (Hespan®)
Unlabeled Use Priming fluid in pump oxygenators during cardiopulmonary bypass; plasma volume expansion during cardiopulmonary bypass

Local Anesthetic/Vasoconstrictor Precautions No information available to require special precautions

Effects on Dental Treatment No significant effects or complications reported

Effects on Bleeding Large volumes of isotonic solutions containing 6% hetastarch may transiently alter the coagulation mechanism due to hemodilution. This may prolong bleeding. Medical consult recommended.

Adverse Effects Frequency not defined.
Cardiovascular: Bradycardia, circulatory overload, heart failure, peripheral edema, tachycardia
Central nervous system: Chills, fever, headache, intracranial bleeding
Dermatologic: Itching, pruritus (dose dependent; may be delayed), rash

Endocrine & metabolic: Amylase levels increased (transient), metabolic acidosis, parotid gland enlargement

Gastrointestinal: Vomiting

Hematologic: Anemia, bleeding, bleeding time prolonged, clotting time prolonged, dilutional coagulopathy, disseminated intravascular coagulopathy (rare), factor VIII:C plasma levels decreased, hemolysis (rare), plasma aggregation decreased, PT prolonged, PTT prolonged, thrombocytopenia, von Willebrand factor decreased, wound hemorrhage

Hepatic: Bilirubin increased (indirect)

Neuromuscular & skeletal: Myalgia

Respiratory: Bronchospasm, pulmonary edema (noncardiac)

Miscellaneous: Anaphylactoid reactions, flu-like syndrome (mild), hypersensitivity

Postmarketing and/or case reports: Hypotension, urticaria

General Dosage Range Dosage adjustment recommended in patients with renal impairment

I.V.: *Adults:* 500-1500 mL/day **or** 20 mL/kg/day (up to 1500 mL/day)

Leukapheresis: *Adults:* 250-700 mL

Mechanism of Action Produces plasma volume expansion by virtue of its highly colloidal starch structure

Pharmacodynamics/Kinetics

Onset of Action Volume expansion: I.V.: ~30 minutes

Duration of Action 6-36 hours

Pregnancy Risk Factor C

Pregnancy Considerations Adverse events have been observed in some animal reproduction studies.

Hexachlorophene (heks a KLOR oh feen)

Brand Names: U.S. pHisoHex®

Brand Names: Canada pHisoHex®

Pharmacologic Category Antibiotic, Topical

Use Surgical scrub and as a bacteriostatic skin cleanser; control an outbreak of gram-positive infection when other procedures have been unsuccessful

Local Anesthetic/Vasoconstrictor Precautions No information available to require special precautions

Effects on Dental Treatment No significant effects or complications reported

Effects on Bleeding No information available to require special precautions

General Dosage Range Topical: *Children and Adults:* Apply 5 mL cleanser and water to area to be cleansed

Mechanism of Action Bacteriostatic polychlorinated biphenyl which inhibits membrane-bound enzymes and disrupts the cell membrane

Pharmacodynamics/Kinetics

Half-life Elimination Infants: 6.1-44.2 hours

Pregnancy Risk Factor C

Pregnancy Considerations Adverse events have been observed in animal reproduction studies. Hexachlorophene is absorbed systemically when applied topically. Following use as an antiseptic for vaginal exams during labor, hexachlorophene is detectable in the maternal serum and cord blood (Strickland, 1983). Vaginal use as a pack or tampon and application to mucous membranes is contraindicated.

Hexylresorcinol (heks il re ZOR si nole)

Brand Names: U.S. Sucrets® Original [OTC]

Pharmacologic Category Antiseptic, Topical; Local Anesthetic

Use Minor antiseptic and local anesthetic for sore throat; topical antiseptic for minor cuts or abrasions

Local Anesthetic/Vasoconstrictor Precautions No information available to require special precautions

Effects on Dental Treatment No significant effects or complications reported

Effects on Bleeding No information available to require special precautions

General Dosage Range Oral: *Children ≥6 years and Adults:* Up to 10 lozenges/day

---

Histrelin (his TREL in)

Brand Names: U.S. Supprelin® LA; Vantas®

Brand Names: Canada Vantas®

Pharmacologic Category Gonadotropin Releasing Hormone Agonist

Use Palliative treatment of advanced prostate cancer; treatment of children with central precocious puberty (CPP)

Local Anesthetic/Vasoconstrictor Precautions No information available to require special precautions

Effects on Dental Treatment No significant effects or complications reported

Effects on Bleeding Anemia reported in <2% of patients

Adverse Effects

CPP:

>10%: Local: Insertion site reaction (51%; includes bruising, discomfort, itching, pain, protrusion of implant area, soreness, swelling, tingling)

>2% to 10%:

Endocrine & metabolic: Metrorrhagia (4%)

Local: Keloid scar (6%), scar (6%), suture-related complication (6%), pain at the application site (4%), post procedural pain (4%)

Prostate cancer:

>10%:

Endocrine & metabolic: Hot flashes (66%)

Local: Implant site reaction (6% to 14%; includes bruising, erythema, pain, soreness, swelling, tenderness)

2% to 10%:

Central nervous system: Fatigue (10%), headache (3%), insomnia (3%)

Endocrine & metabolic: Gynecomastia (4%), sexual dysfunction (4%), libido decreased (2%)

Gastrointestinal: Constipation (4%), weight gain (2%)

Genitourinary: Expected pharmacological consequence of testosterone suppression: Testicular atrophy (5%)

Renal: Renal impairment (5%)

General Dosage Range SubQ: *Children ≥2 years and Adults:* 50 mg implant, inserted every 12 months

Mechanism of Action Potent inhibitor of gonadotropin secretion; continuous administration results in, after an initiation phase, the suppression of luteinizing hormone (LH), follicle-stimulating hormone (FSH), and a subsequent decrease in testosterone and dihydrotestosterone (males) and estrone and estradiol (premenopausal females). Testosterone levels are reduced to castrate levels in males (treated for prostate cancer) within 2-4 weeks. Additionally, in patients with CPP, linear growth velocity is slowed (improves chance of attaining predicted adult height).

Pharmacodynamics/Kinetics

Onset of Action Prostate cancer: Chemical castration: Within 2-4 weeks; CPP: Progression of sexual development stops and growth is decreased within 1 month

Duration of Action 1 year

Half-life Elimination Adults: Terminal: ~4 hours

Time to Peak Adults: 12 hours

Pregnancy Risk Factor X

Pregnancy Considerations Fetal harm and an increase in fetal mortalities have been noted in animal studies. Histrelin is contraindicated for use during pregnancy or in women who may become pregnant.

Homatropine (hoe MA troe peen)

Brand Names: U.S. Homatropaire; Isopto® Homatropine

Pharmacologic Category Anticholinergic Agent, Ophthalmic; Ophthalmic Agent, Mydriatic

Use Producing cycloplegia and mydriasis for refraction; treatment of acute inflammatory conditions of the uveal tract; optical aid in axial lens opacities

Local Anesthetic/Vasoconstrictor Precautions No information available to require special precautions

Effects on Dental Treatment Key adverse event(s) related to dental treatment: Nasal congestion.

Effects on Bleeding No information available to require special precautions

Adverse Effects Frequency not defined.

Gastrointestinal: Xerostomia

Local: Burning, irritation, stinging

Ocular: Blurred vision, eczematoid dermatitis, edema, exudate, follicular conjunctivitis, intraocular pressure increased, photophobia, vascular congestion

Miscellaneous: Thirst

General Dosage Range Ophthalmic:

Children >3 months: Instill 1-2 drops (2% solution) 2-6 times daily **or** 1-2 drops (2% solution) into eye(s); repeat every 10-15 minutes if necessary; maximum: 5 doses

Adults: Instill 1-2 drops (2% or 5% solution) into eye(s) 2-6 times daily **or** 1-2 drops (2% or 5% solution) into eye(s); repeat every 10-15 minutes if necessary; maximum 5 doses

Mechanism of Action Blocks response of iris sphincter muscle and the accommodative muscle of the ciliary body to cholinergic stimulation resulting in dilation (mydriasis) and paralysis of accommodation (cycloplegia)

Pregnancy Risk Factor C

Pregnancy Considerations Animal reproduction studies have not been conducted.

Hyaluronate and Derivatives
(hye al yoor ON ate & dah RIV ah tives)

Brand Names: U.S. Amvisc®; Amvisc® Plus; Bionect®; Euflexxa®; Hyalgan®; Hylase® Wound; Juvéderm® Ultra; Juvéderm® Ultra Plus; Juvéderm® Ultra Plus XC; Juvéderm® Ultra XC; Orthovisc®; Perlane®; Provisc®; Restylane®; Supartz®; Synvisc-One®; Synvisc®

Brand Names: Canada Cystistat®; Durolane®; OrthoVisc®; Suplasyn®

Pharmacologic Category Antirheumatic Miscellaneous; Ophthalmic Agent, Viscoelastic; Skin and Mucous Membrane Agent, Miscellaneous

Use

Intra-articular injection: Treatment of pain in osteoarthritis in knee in patients who have failed nonpharmacologic treatment and simple analgesics (Euflexxa®, Hyalgan®, OrthoVisc®, Supartz®, Synvisc®, Synvisc-One®)

Intradermal: Correction of moderate-to-severe facial wrinkles or folds (Juvederm® [all formulations], Perlane®, Restylane®)

Ophthalmic: Surgical aid in cataract extraction (Amvisc®, Amvisc® Plus, Provisc®); intraocular lens implantation (Amvisc®, Amvisc® Plus, Provisc®); corneal transplant (Amvisc®, Amvisc® Plus); glaucoma filtration (Amvisc®, Amvisc® Plus); and retinal attachment surgery (Amvisc®, Amvisc® Plus)

Submucosal: Lip augmentation (Restylane®)

Topical cream, gel: Management of skin ulcers and wounds (Bionect®, Hylase® Wound)

Unlabeled Use Treatment of refractory interstitial cystitis

Local Anesthetic/Vasoconstrictor Precautions No information available to require special precautions

Effects on Dental Treatment No significant effects or complications reported

Effects on Bleeding No information available to require special precautions

Adverse Effects Frequencies and/or type of local reaction may vary by formulation and site of application/injection.

>10%:

Local: Injection site (intradermal): Erythema (75% to 93%), tenderness (61% to 92%), swelling (81% to 91%), pain (47% to 90%), firmness (86% to 89%), bruising (52% to 87%), lumps/bumps (56% to 83%), skin discoloration (33% to 78%), pruritus (25% to 36%)

Neuromuscular & skeletal: Arthralgia (intra-articular 25%)

1% to 10%:

Cardiovascular: Blood pressure increased (4%)

Central nervous system: Fatigue (1%)

Gastrointestinal: Nausea (≤2%)

Local: Injection site (intra-articular): Pain (3%)

Neuromuscular & skeletal: Back pain (intra-articular <1% to 7%), joint effusion (intra-articular 2% to 6%), tendonitis (intra-articular 2%), arthrosis (intra-articular 1%), limb pain (intra-articular 1%), parasthesia (intra-articular 1%)

Miscellaneous: Infection (intra-articular 1%)

Frequency not defined: Ocular (intraocular): Postoperative inflammatory reactions (iritis, hypopyon), corneal edema, corneal decompensation, postoperative increase in IOP (transient)

General Dosage Range

Intra-articular: *Adults:* 16-30 mg once weekly for 3-5 doses (total injections: 3-5) **or** 48 mg once

Intradermal: *Adults:* Inject as required for cosmetic effect (maximum: 20 mL/60 kg/year [Juvederm® all formulations] or maximum: 6 mL/treatment [Perlane®, Restylane®])

Ophthalmic: *Adults:* Depends upon procedure (slowly introduce a sufficient quantity into eye)

Submucosal: *Adults ≥21 years:* Maximum 1.5 mL per lip (upper or lower) per treatment session (Restylane®)

Topical: *Adults:* Apply to affected area 1-3 times daily

Mechanism of Action Sodium hyaluronate is a biological polysaccharide which is distributed widely in the extracellular matrix of connective tissue in man (vitreous and aqueous humor of the eye, synovial fluid, skin, and umbilical cord). Sodium hyaluronate and its derivatives form a viscoelastic solution in water (at physiological pH and ionic strength) which makes it suitable for aqueous and vitreous humor in ophthalmic surgery, and functions as a tissue and/or joint lubricant which plays an important role in modulating the interactions between adjacent tissues. Intradermal injection may decrease the depth of facial wrinkles. In the topical management of wounds and ulcers, sodium hyaluronate protects the skin against friction and abrasion.

Pregnancy Considerations Adverse events were not observed in animal reproduction studies. Safety for use in pregnant women has not been established.

Hyaluronidase (hye al yoor ON i dase)

Brand Names: U.S. Amphadase™; Hylenex; Vitrase®
Pharmacologic Category Enzyme
Use Increase the dispersion and absorption of other injected drugs; increase rate of absorption of parenteral fluids given by subcutaneous administration (hypodermoclysis)
Unlabeled Use Management of drug extravasations; local anesthetic adjuvant in bupivacaine-lidocaine mixture for retrobulbar/peribulbar block
Local Anesthetic/Vasoconstrictor Precautions No information available to require special precautions
Effects on Dental Treatment No significant effects or complications reported
Effects on Bleeding No information available to require special precautions
Adverse Effects Frequency not defined.
Cardiovascular: Edema
Local: Injection site reactions
General Dosage Range
Intradermal: *Children and Adults:* 0.02 mL (3 units) of a 150 units/mL solution
SubQ:
Premature Infants: Volume of a single clysis/day should not exceed 25 mL/kg; rate of administration should not exceed 2 mL/minute
Children <3 years: Volume of a single clysis should not exceed 200 mL **or** 75 units over each scapula followed by injection of contrast medium at the same site
Children ≥3 years and Adults: Rate and volume of a single clysis should not exceed those used for infusion of I.V. fluids **or** 75 units over each scapula followed by injection of contrast medium at the same site
Mechanism of Action Modifies the permeability of connective tissue through hydrolysis of hyaluronic acid, one of the chief components of tissue cement which offers resistance to diffusion of liquids through tissues; hyaluronidase increases both the distribution and absorption of locally injected substances.
Pharmacodynamics/Kinetics
Onset of Action SubQ: Immediate
Duration of Action 24-48 hours
Pregnancy Risk Factor C
Pregnancy Considerations There are no adequate or well-controlled studies in pregnant women; use only if clearly needed. Administration during labor did not cause any increase in blood loss or differences in cervical trauma. It is not known whether it affects the fetus if used during labor.

HydrALAZINE (hye DRAL a zeen)

Related Information
Cardiovascular Diseases *on page 1492*
Brand Names: Canada Apo-Hydralazine®; Apresoline®; Novo-Hylazin; Nu-Hydral
Pharmacologic Category Vasodilator
Use Management of moderate-to-severe hypertension
Unlabeled Use Heart failure; hypertension secondary to pre-eclampsia/eclampsia
Local Anesthetic/Vasoconstrictor Precautions No information available to require special precautions
Effects on Dental Treatment No significant effects or complications reported
Effects on Bleeding No information available to require special precautions
Adverse Effects Frequency not defined.
Cardiovascular: Angina pectoris, flushing, orthostatic hypotension, palpitations, paradoxical hypertension, peripheral edema, tachycardia, vascular collapse
Central nervous system: Anxiety, chills, depression, disorientation, dizziness, fever, headache, increased intracranial pressure (I.V.; in patient with pre-existing increased intracranial pressure), psychotic reaction
Dermatologic: Pruritus, rash, urticaria
Gastrointestinal: Anorexia, constipation, diarrhea, nausea, paralytic ileus, vomiting
Genitourinary: Dysuria, impotence
Hematologic: Agranulocytosis, eosinophilia, erythrocyte count reduced, hemoglobin decreased, hemolytic anemia, leukopenia, thrombocytopenia (rare)
Neuromuscular & skeletal: Muscle cramps, peripheral neuritis, rheumatoid arthritis, tremor, weakness
Ocular: Conjunctivitis, lacrimation
Respiratory: Dyspnea, nasal congestion
Miscellaneous: Diaphoresis, drug-induced lupus-like syndrome (dose related; fever, arthralgia, splenomegaly, lymphadenopathy, asthenia, myalgia, malaise, pleuritic chest pain, edema, positive ANA, positive LE cells, maculopapular facial rash, positive direct Coombs' test, pericarditis, pericardial tamponade)
General Dosage Range Dosage adjustment recommended in patients with renal impairment
I.M., I.V.:
Children: 0.1-0.2 mg/kg/dose (not to exceed 20 mg) every 4-6 hours as needed (maximum: 3.5 mg/kg/day in 4-6 divided doses)
Adults: Initial: 10-20 mg/dose every 4-6 hours as needed; Maintenance: Up to 40 mg/dose every 4-6 hours **or** Eclampsia/pre-eclampsia: 5 mg/dose then 5-10 mg every 20-30 minutes as needed
Oral:
Children: Initial: 0.75-1 mg/kg/day in 2-4 divided doses; Maintenance: Up to 7.5 mg/kg/day in 2-4 divided doses (maximum: 200 mg/day)
Adults: Initial: 10-25 mg 3-4 times/day; Maintenance: 25-300 mg/day (target dose: 225-300 mg/day for CHF) in 2-4 divided doses (maximum: 300 mg/day)
Elderly: Initial: 10 mg 2-3 times/day, increase by 10-25 mg/day every 2-5 days; Target dose: 225-300 mg/day for CHF
Mechanism of Action Direct vasodilation of arterioles (with little effect on veins) with decreased systemic resistance
Pharmacodynamics/Kinetics
Onset of Action Oral: 20-30 minutes; I.V.: 5-20 minutes

Duration of Action Oral: Up to 8 hours; I.V.: 1-4 hours; **Note:** May vary depending on acetylator status of patient

Half-life Elimination Normal renal function: 2-8 hours; End-stage renal disease: 7-16 hours

Pregnancy Risk Factor C

Pregnancy Considerations Teratogenic effects were observed in animal studies at 20-30 times the maximum daily human dose. Hydralazine crosses the placenta. Hydralazine is recommended for use in the management of hypertension associated with pre-eclampsia.

Hydrochlorothiazide (hye droe klor oh THYE a zide)

Related Information
Cardiovascular Diseases *on page 1492*

Brand Names: U.S. Microzide®

Brand Names: Canada Apo-Hydro®; Bio-Hydrochlorothiazide; Dom-Hydrochlorothiazide; Novo-Hydrazide; Nu-Hydro; PMS-Hydrochlorothiazide

Generic Availability (U.S.) Yes

Pharmacologic Category Diuretic, Thiazide

Use Management of mild-to-moderate hypertension; treatment of edema in heart failure and nephrotic syndrome

Unlabeled Use Treatment of lithium-induced diabetes insipidus

Local Anesthetic/Vasoconstrictor Precautions No information available to require special precautions

Effects on Dental Treatment Key adverse event(s) related to dental treatment: Orthostatic hypotension and hypotension.

Effects on Bleeding No information available to require special precautions

Adverse Effects Frequency not defined; with capsule formulation, adverse events were observed at doses ≥25 mg in adults:

Cardiovascular: Hypotension, orthostatic hypotension

Central nervous system: Dizziness, fever, headache, vertigo

Dermatologic: Alopecia, erythema multiforme, exfoliative dermatitis, photosensitivity, purpura, rash, Stevens-Johnson syndrome, toxic epidermal necrolysis, urticaria

Endocrine & metabolic: Hyperglycemia, hypokalemia, hyperuricemia

Gastrointestinal: Anorexia, constipation, cramping, diarrhea, epigastric distress, gastric irritation, nausea, pancreatitis, sialadenitis, vomiting

Genitourinary: Glycosuria, impotence

Hematologic: Agranulocytosis, aplastic anemia, hemolytic anemia, leukopenia, thrombocytopenia

Hepatic: Jaundice

Neuromuscular & skeletal: Muscle spasm, paresthesia, restlessness, weakness

Ocular: Blurred vision (transient), xanthopsia

Renal: Interstitial nephritis, renal dysfunction, renal failure

Respiratory: Respiratory distress, pneumonitis, pulmonary edema

Miscellaneous: Anaphylactic reactions, necrotizing angiitis

Dosage Oral (effect of drug may be decreased when used every day):

Children (in pediatric patients, chlorothiazide may be preferred over hydrochlorothiazide as there are more dosage formulations [eg, suspension] available):

Edema, hypertension:

<6 months: 1-3 mg/kg/day in 2 divided doses

>6 months to 2 years: 1-3 mg/kg/day in 2 divided doses; maximum: 37.5 mg/day

>2-17 years: Initial: 1 mg/kg/day; maximum: 3 mg/kg/day (50 mg/day)

Adults:

Edema: 25-100 mg/day in 1-2 doses; maximum: 200 mg/day

Hypertension: 12.5-50 mg/day; minimal increase in response and more electrolyte disturbances are seen with doses >50 mg/day

Elderly: 12.5-25 mg once daily

Dosage adjustment in renal impairment: Cl_{cr} <10 mL/minute: Avoid use. Usually ineffective with GFR <30 mL/minute. Effective at lower GFR in combination with a loop diuretic.

Note: ACC/AHA 2009 Heart Failure guidelines suggest that thiazides lose their efficacy when Cl_{cr} <40 mL/minute.

Dosage adjustment in hepatic impairment: No dosage adjustment provided in manufacturer's labeling. Use with caution and monitor for precipitation of hepatic coma.

Mechanism of Action Inhibits sodium reabsorption in the distal tubules causing increased excretion of sodium and water as well as potassium and hydrogen ions

Contraindications Hypersensitivity to hydrochlorothiazide or any component of the formulation, thiazides, or sulfonamide-derived drugs; anuria

Warnings/Precautions Hypersensitivity reactions may occur with hydrochlorothiazide. Risk is increased in patients with a history of allergy or bronchial asthma. Avoid in severe renal disease (ineffective as a diuretic). Electrolyte disturbances (hypokalemia, hypochloremic alkalosis, hyponatremia) can occur. Use with caution in severe hepatic dysfunction; hepatic encephalopathy can be caused by electrolyte disturbances. Gout may be precipitated in certain patients with a history of gout, a familial predisposition to gout, or chronic renal failure. Thiazide diuretics reduce calcium excretion; pathologic changes in the parathyroid glands with hypercalcemia and hypophosphatemia have been observed with prolonged use. Use with caution in patients with prediabetes and diabetes; may alter glucose control. May cause SLE exacerbation or activation. Use with caution in patients with moderate or high cholesterol concentrations. Photosensitization may occur. Correct hypokalemia before initiating therapy. Thiazide diuretics may decrease renal calcium excretion; consider avoiding use in patients with hypercalcemia. May cause acute transient myopia and acute angle-closure glaucoma, typically occurring within hours to weeks following initiation; discontinue therapy immediately in patients with acute decreases in visual acuity or ocular pain. Risk factors may include a history of sulfonamide or penicillin allergy.

Chemical similarities are present among sulfonamides, sulfonylureas, carbonic anhydrase inhibitors, thiazides, and loop diuretics (except ethacrynic acid). Use in patients with sulfonamide allergy is specifically contraindicated in product labeling, however, a risk of cross-reaction exists in patients with allergy to any of these compounds; avoid use when previous reaction has been severe. Discontinue if signs of hypersensitivity are noted.

Drug Interactions

Metabolism/Transport Effects None known.

Avoid Concomitant Use

Avoid concomitant use of Hydrochlorothiazide with any of the following: Dofetilide

Increased Effect/Toxicity

Hydrochlorothiazide may increase the levels/effects of: ACE Inhibitors; Allopurinol; Amifostine; Antihypertensives; Benazepril; Calcium Salts; CarBAMazepine; Dofetilide; Hypotensive Agents; Lithium; Multivitamins/Minerals (with ADEK, Folate, Iron); OXcarbazepine; Porfimer; RiTUXimab; Sodium Phosphates; Topiramate; Toremifene; Valsartan; Vitamin D Analogs

The levels/effects of Hydrochlorothiazide may be increased by: Alcohol (Ethyl); Alfuzosin; Analgesics (Opioid); Barbiturates; Beta2-Agonists; Corticosteroids (Orally Inhaled); Corticosteroids (Systemic); Herbs (Hypotensive Properties); Licorice; MAO Inhibitors; Pentoxifylline; Phosphodiesterase 5 Inhibitors; Prostacyclin Analogues; Valsartan

Decreased Effect

Hydrochlorothiazide may decrease the levels/effects of: Antidiabetic Agents

The levels/effects of Hydrochlorothiazide may be decreased by: Benazepril; Bile Acid Sequestrants; Herbs (Hypertensive Properties); Methylphenidate; Nonsteroidal Anti-Inflammatory Agents; Yohimbine

Ethanol/Nutrition/Herb Interactions

Food: Hydrochlorothiazide peak serum levels may be decreased if taken with food. This product may deplete potassium, sodium, and magnesium.

Herb/Nutraceutical: Avoid herbs with *hypertensive* properties (bayberry, blue cohosh, cayenne, ephedra, ginger, ginseng [American], kola, licorice); may diminish the antihypertensive effect of hydrochlorothiazide. Avoid herbs with *hypotensive* properties (black cohosh, California poppy, coleus, golden seal, hawthorn, mistletoe, periwinkle, quinine, shepherd's purse); may enhance the hypotensive effect of hydrochlorothiazide.

Dietary Considerations May be taken with food or milk.

Pharmacodynamics/Kinetics

Onset of Action Diuresis: ~2 hours; Peak effect: 4-6 hours

Duration of Action 6-12 hours

Half-life Elimination 5.6-14.8 hours

Time to Peak 1-2.5 hours

Pregnancy Risk Factor B

Pregnancy Considerations Adverse events were not observed in animal reproduction studies. Thiazide diuretics cross the placenta and are found in cord blood. Maternal use may cause fetal or neonatal jaundice, thrombocytopenia, or other adverse events observed in adults. Use of thiazide diuretics during normal pregnancies is not appropriate; use may be considered when edema is due to pathologic causes (as in the nonpregnant patient); monitor.

Lactation Enters breast milk/not recommended (AAP rates "compatible"; AAP 2001 update pending)

Breast-Feeding Considerations Thiazide diuretics are found in breast milk. Following a single oral maternal dose of hydrochlorothiazide 50 mg, the mean breast milk concentration was 80 ng/mL (samples collected over 24 hours) and hydrochlorothiazide was not detected in the blood of the breast feeding infant (limit of detection 20 ng/mL). Peak plasma concentrations reported in adults following hydrochlorothiazide 12.5-100 mg are 70-490 ng/mL.

Dosage Forms

Capsule, oral: 12.5 mg

Microzide®: 12.5 mg

Tablet, oral: 12.5 mg, 25 mg, 50 mg

Hydrochlorothiazide and Spironolactone

(hye droe klor oh THYE a zide & speer on oh LAK tone)

Related Information

Hydrochlorothiazide *on page 687*

Spironolactone *on page 1254*

Brand Names: U.S. Aldactazide®

Brand Names: Canada Aldactazide 25®; Aldactazide 50®; Novo-Spirozine

Pharmacologic Category Diuretic, Thiazide; Selective Aldosterone Blocker

Use Management of mild-to-moderate hypertension; treatment of edema in congestive heart failure and nephrotic syndrome, and cirrhosis of the liver accompanied by edema and/or ascites

Local Anesthetic/Vasoconstrictor Precautions No information available to require special precautions

Effects on Dental Treatment No significant effects or complications reported

Effects on Bleeding No information available to require special precautions

Adverse Effects See individual agents.

General Dosage Range Oral: *Adults:* 12.5-50 mg hydrochlorothiazide and 12.5-50 mg spironolactone/day in 1-2 divided doses

Pregnancy Risk Factor C

Pregnancy Considerations See individual agents.

Hydrochlorothiazide and Triamterene

(hye droe klor oh THYE a zide & trye AM ter een)

Related Information

Hydrochlorothiazide *on page 687*

Triamterene *on page 1360*

Brand Names: U.S. Dyazide®; Maxzide®; Maxzide®-25

Brand Names: Canada Apo-Triazide®; Nu-Triazide; Pro-Triazide; Riva-Zide; Teva-Triamterene HCTZ

Generic Availability (U.S.) Yes

Pharmacologic Category Diuretic, Potassium-Sparing; Diuretic, Thiazide

Use Treatment of hypertension or edema (not recommended for initial treatment) when hypokalemia has developed on hydrochlorothiazide alone or when the development of hypokalemia must be avoided

Local Anesthetic/Vasoconstrictor Precautions No information available to require special precautions

Effects on Dental Treatment No significant effects or complications reported

Effects on Bleeding No information available to require special precautions

Adverse Effects Also see individual agents. Frequency not defined.

Cardiovascular: Angina, arrhythmia, orthostatic hypotension, tachycardia

Central nervous system: Anxiety, dizziness, depression, fatigue, headache, insomnia, restlessness, vertigo

Dermatologic: Photosensitivity, purpura, rash, subacute cutaneous lupus erythematosus-like reactions, urticaria

Endocrine & metabolic: Acidosis, diabetes mellitus, hypercalcemia, hyperglycemia, hyper-/hypokalemia, hyperuricemia, hypochloremia, hypomagnesemia, hyponatremia

Gastrointestinal: Abdominal pain, anorexia, burning of tongue, constipation, diarrhea, loss of appetite, nausea, pancreatitis, sialadenitis, stomach cramps, taste alteration, tongue discoloration (bright orange), upset stomach, vomiting, xerostomia

Genitourinary: Impotence

Hematologic: Aplastic anemia, agranulocytosis, hemolytic anemia, leukopenia, thrombocytopenia, megaloblastic anemia

Hepatic: Jaundice, liver function tests (abnormal)

Neuromuscular & skeletal: Muscle cramping, parasthesia, weakness

Ocular: Blurred vision (transient), xanthopsia

Renal: Acute renal failure, BUN increased, glycosuria, interstitial nephritis, necrotizing vasculitis, renal stone formation, serum creatinine increased, urinary sediment abnormal, urine discoloration

Respiratory: Allergic pneumonitis, dyspnea, pulmonary edema, respiratory distress

Miscellaneous: Anaphylaxis, systemic lupus erythematosus (SLE) exacerbation

Dosage Oral: Adults:
Hydrochlorothiazide 25 mg and triamterene 37.5 mg: 1-2 tablets/capsules once daily

Hydrochlorothiazide 50 mg and triamterene 75 mg: 1/2-1 tablet daily

Dosage adjustment in renal impairment: Efficacy of hydrochlorothiazide is limited in patients with Cl_{cr} <30 mL/minute, contraindicated in patients with anuria, acute and chronic renal insufficiency, or significant renal impairment.

Dosage adjustment in hepatic impairment: No dosage adjustment provided in manufacturer's labeling; use with caution. Use with caution and monitor for precipitation of hepatic coma.

Mechanism of Action

Based on **triamterene** component: Blocks epithelial sodium channels in the late distal convoluted tubule (DCT) and collecting duct which inhibits sodium reabsorption from the lumen. This effectively reduces intracellular sodium, decreasing the function of Na+/K+ ATPase, leading to potassium retention and decreased calcium, magnesium, and hydrogen excretion. As sodium uptake capacity in the DCT/collecting duct is limited, the natriuretic, diuretic, and antihypertensive effects are generally considered weak.

Based on **hydrochlorothiazide** component: Inhibits sodium reabsorption in the distal tubules causing increased excretion of sodium and water as well as potassium and hydrogen ions

Contraindications Hypersensitivity to hydrochlorothiazide, triamterene, any component of the formulation, or sulfonamide-derived drugs; anuria; acute and chronic renal insufficiency or significant renal impairment; patients receiving other potassium-sparing diuretics, potassium-containing salt substitutes, or potassium supplements (except in severe cases of hypokalemia); preexisting hyperkalemia

Warnings/Precautions See individual agents.

Drug Interactions

Metabolism/Transport Effects None known.

Avoid Concomitant Use

Avoid concomitant use of Hydrochlorothiazide and Triamterene with any of the following: CycloSPORINE (Systemic); Dofetilide; Tacrolimus (Systemic)

Increased Effect/Toxicity

Hydrochlorothiazide and Triamterene may increase the levels/effects of: ACE Inhibitors; Allopurinol; Amifostine; Ammonium Chloride; Antihypertensives; Benazepril; Calcium Salts; CarBAMazepine; Cardiac

Glycosides; CycloSPORINE (Systemic); Dofetilide; Hypotensive Agents; Lithium; Multivitamins/Minerals (with ADEK, Folate, Iron); OXcarbazepine; Porfimer; RiTUXimab; Sodium Phosphates; Tacrolimus (Systemic); Topiramate; Toremifene; Valsartan; Vitamin D Analogs

The levels/effects of Hydrochlorothiazide and Triamterene may be increased by: Alcohol (Ethyl); Alfuzosin; Analgesics (Opioid); Angiotensin II Receptor Blockers; Barbiturates; Beta2-Agonists; Canagliflozin; Corticosteroids (Orally Inhaled); Corticosteroids (Systemic); Drospirenone; Eplerenone; Herbs (Hypotensive Properties); Indomethacin; Licorice; MAO Inhibitors; Nonsteroidal Anti-Inflammatory Agents; Pentoxifylline; Phosphodiesterase 5 Inhibitors; Potassium Salts; Prostacyclin Analogues; Tolvaptan; Valsartan

Decreased Effect

Hydrochlorothiazide and Triamterene may decrease the levels/effects of: Antidiabetic Agents; Cardiac Glycosides; QuiNIDine

The levels/effects of Hydrochlorothiazide and Triamterene may be decreased by: Benazepril; Bile Acid Sequestrants; Herbs (Hypertensive Properties); Methylphenidate; Nonsteroidal Anti-Inflammatory Agents; Yohimbine

Ethanol/Nutrition/Herb Interactions Food: Avoid food with high potassium content and potassium-containing salt substitutes.

Dietary Considerations Should be taken after meals.

Pregnancy Risk Factor C

Pregnancy Considerations See individual agents.

Lactation Enters breast milk/not recommended

Breast-Feeding Considerations See individual agents.

Dosage Forms

Capsule: Hydrochlorothiazide 25 mg and triamterene 37.5 mg; hydrochlorothiazide 25 mg and triamterene 50 mg

Dyazide®: Hydrochlorothiazide 25 mg and triamterene 37.5 mg

Tablet: Hydrochlorothiazide 25 mg and triamterene 37.5 mg; hydrochlorothiazide 50 mg and triamterene 75 mg

Maxzide®: Hydrochlorothiazide 50 mg and triamterene 75 mg [scored]

Maxzide®-25: Hydrochlorothiazide 25 mg and triamterene 37.5 mg [scored]

Hydrocodone and Acetaminophen
(hye droe KOE done & a seet a MIN oh fen)

Related Information
Acetaminophen on page 27
Oral Pain on page 1558

Related Sample Prescriptions
Moderate/Moderately Severe Oral Pain on page 1606

Brand Names: U.S. hycet®; Lorcet® 10/650; Lorcet® Plus; Lortab®; Margesic® H; Maxidone®; Norco®; Stagesic™; Vicodin ES®; Vicodin HP®; Vicodin®; Xodol® 10/300; Xodol® 5/300; Xodol® 7.5/300; Zamicet™; Zolvit®; Zydone®

Generic Availability (U.S.) Yes: Oral solution, tablet

Pharmacologic Category Analgesic Combination (Opioid)

Dental Use Treatment of postoperative pain

Use Relief of moderate-to-severe pain

Local Anesthetic/Vasoconstrictor Precautions No information available to require special precautions

◄ **Effects on Dental Treatment** Key adverse event(s) related to dental treatment: Xerostomia (normal salivary flow resumes upon discontinuation). See Dental Comment.

Effects on Bleeding No information available to require special precautions

Adverse Effects Frequency not defined.

Cardiovascular: Bradycardia, cardiac arrest, circulatory collapse, coma, hypotension

Central nervous system: Anxiety, dizziness, drowsiness, dysphoria, euphoria, fear, lethargy, lightheadedness, malaise, mental clouding, mental impairment, mood changes, physiological dependence, sedation, somnolence, stupor

Dermatologic: Pruritus, rash

Endocrine & metabolic: Hypoglycemic coma

Gastrointestinal: Abdominal pain, constipation, gastric distress, heartburn, nausea, peptic ulcer, vomiting, xerostomia

Genitourinary: Ureteral spasm, urinary retention, vesical sphincter spasm

Hematologic: Agranulocytosis, bleeding time prolonged, hemolytic anemia, iron deficiency anemia, occult blood loss, thrombocytopenia

Hepatic: Hepatic necrosis, hepatitis

Neuromuscular & skeletal: Skeletal muscle rigidity

Otic: Hearing impairment or loss (chronic overdose)

Renal: Renal toxicity, renal tubular necrosis

Respiratory: Acute airway obstruction, apnea, dyspnea, respiratory depression (dose related)

Miscellaneous: Allergic reactions, clamminess, diaphoresis

Dental Usual Dosage Postoperative pain: Oral:

Children and Adults ≥50 kg: Average starting dose in opioid naive patients: Hydrocodone 5-10 mg 4 times/day; the dosage of acetaminophen should be limited to ≤4 g/day (and possibly less in patients with hepatic impairment or ethanol use).

Dosage ranges (based on specific product labeling): Hydrocodone 2.5-10 mg every 4-6 hours; maximum: 60 mg hydrocodone/day (maximum dose of hydrocodone may be limited by the acetaminophen content of specific product)

Elderly: Doses should be titrated to appropriate analgesic effect; 2.5-5 mg of the hydrocodone component every 4-6 hours. Do not exceed 4 g/day of acetaminophen.

Dosage Oral (doses should be titrated to appropriate analgesic effect): Analgesic:

Children 2-13 years or <50 kg: Hydrocodone 0.1-0.2 mg/kg/dose every 4-6 hours; do not exceed 6 doses/day or the maximum recommended dose of acetaminophen

Children and Adults ≥50 kg: Average starting dose in opioid naive patients: Hydrocodone 5-10 mg 4 times/day; the dosage of acetaminophen should be limited to ≤4 g/day (and possibly less in patients with hepatic impairment or ethanol use).

Dosage ranges (based on specific product labeling): Hydrocodone 2.5-10 mg every 4-6 hours (maximum dose of hydrocodone may be limited by the acetaminophen content of specific product)

Elderly: Doses should be titrated to appropriate analgesic effect; 2.5-5 mg of the hydrocodone component every 4-6 hours. Do not exceed 4 g/day of acetaminophen.

Dosage adjustment in renal impairment: No dosage adjustment provided in manufacturer's labeling; use with caution.

Dosage adjustment in hepatic impairment: Use with caution. Limited, low-dose therapy usually well tolerated in hepatic disease/cirrhosis; however, cases of hepatotoxicity at daily acetaminophen dosages <4 g/day have been reported. Avoid chronic use in hepatic impairment.

Mechanism of Action Hydrocodone, as with other narcotic (opiate) analgesics, blocks pain perception in the cerebral cortex by binding to specific receptor molecules (opiate receptors) within the neuronal membranes of synapses. This binding results in a decreased synaptic chemical transmission throughout the CNS thus inhibiting the flow of pain sensations into the higher centers. Mu and kappa are the two subtypes of the opiate receptor which hydrocodone binds to cause analgesia.

Acetaminophen inhibits the synthesis of prostaglandins in the CNS and peripherally blocks pain impulse generation; produces antipyresis from inhibition of hypothalamic heat-regulating center.

Contraindications Hypersensitivity to hydrocodone, acetaminophen, or any component of the formulation; CNS depression; severe respiratory depression

Warnings/Precautions Use with caution in patients with hypersensitivity reactions to other phenanthrene derivative opioid agonists (morphine, hydromorphone, levorphanol, oxycodone, oxymorphone); tolerance or drug dependence may result from extended use. Concurrent use of agonist/antagonist analgesics may precipitate withdrawal symptoms and/or reduced analgesic efficacy in patients following prolonged therapy with mu opioid agonists. Abrupt discontinuation following prolonged use may also lead to withdrawal symptoms.

Respiratory depressant effects may be increased with head injuries. Use caution with acute abdominal conditions; clinical course may be obscured. Use caution with adrenal insufficiency, biliary tract impairment, morbidly obese patients, toxic psychosis, thyroid dysfunction, prostatic hyperplasia, respiratory disease, hepatic or renal disease, and in the debilitated or elderly. Causes sedation; caution must be used in performing tasks which require alertness (eg, operating machinery or driving). Effects may be potentiated when used with other sedative drugs or ethanol. May cause hypotension.

Due to the role of CYP2D6 in the metabolism of hydrocodone to hydromorphone (an active metabolite with higher binding affinity to mu-opioid receptors compared to hydrocodone), patients with genetic variations of CYP2D6, including "poor metabolizers" or "extensive metabolizers," may have decreased or increased hydromorphone formation, respectively. Variable effects in positive and negative opioid effects have been reported in these patients; however, limited data exists to determine if clinically significant differences of analgesia and toxicity can be predicted based on CYP2D6 phenotype (Hutchinson, 2004; Otton, 1993; Zhou, 2009).

[U.S. Boxed Warning]: Acetaminophen may cause severe hepatotoxicity, potentially requiring liver transplant or resulting in death; hepatotoxicity is usually associated with excessive acetaminophen intake (>4 g/day). Risk is increased with alcohol use, pre-existing liver disease, and intake of more than one source of acetaminophen-containing medications. Chronic daily dosing in adults has also resulted in liver damage in some patients. Hypersensitivity and anaphylactic reactions have been reported with acetaminophen use; discontinue immediately if symptoms of allergic or hypersensitivity reactions occur. Use caution in patients with known G6PD deficiency.

Drug Interactions

Metabolism/Transport Effects Refer to individual components.

Avoid Concomitant Use

Avoid concomitant use of Hydrocodone and Acetaminophen with any of the following: Azelastine (Nasal); Paraldehyde; Pimozide

Increased Effect/Toxicity

Hydrocodone and Acetaminophen may increase the levels/effects of: Alcohol (Ethyl); Alvimopan; ARIPiprazole; Azelastine (Nasal); Busulfan; CNS Depressants; Dasatinib; Desmopressin; Imatinib; Lomitapide; Metyrosine; Mipomersen; Mirtazapine; Paraldehyde; Pimozide; Pramipexole; Prilocaine; ROPINIRole; Rotigotine; Selective Serotonin Reuptake Inhibitors; SORAfenib; Thiazide Diuretics; Vitamin K Antagonists; Zolpidem

The levels/effects of Hydrocodone and Acetaminophen may be increased by: Amphetamines; Antipsychotic Agents (Phenothiazines); Dasatinib; Droperidol; HydrOXYzine; Imatinib; Isoniazid; Magnesium Sulfate; MAO Inhibitors; Metyrapone; Perampanel; Probenecid; Sodium Oxybate; SORAfenib; Succinylcholine

Decreased Effect

Hydrocodone and Acetaminophen may decrease the levels/effects of: Pegvisomant

The levels/effects of Hydrocodone and Acetaminophen may be decreased by: Ammonium Chloride; Anticonvulsants (Hydantoin); Barbiturates; CarBAMazepine; Cholestyramine Resin; Mixed Agonist / Antagonist Opioids; Peginterferon Alfa-2b; QuiNIDine

Ethanol/Nutrition/Herb Interactions

Ethanol: Consuming ≥3 alcoholic drinks/day may increase the risk of liver damage. Ethanol may also increase CNS depression; monitor for increased effects with coadministration. Caution patients about effects.

Herb/Nutraceutical: Avoid valerian, St John's wort, SAMe, kava kava (may increase risk of excessive sedation).

Pharmacodynamics/Kinetics

Onset of Action Hydrocodone: Narcotic analgesic: 10-20 minutes

Duration of Action Hydrocodone: 4-8 hours

Half-life Elimination Hydrocodone: 3.3-4.4 hours

Pregnancy Risk Factor C

Pregnancy Considerations Hydrocodone is teratogenic in animal reproduction studies. In humans, birth defects, including some heart defects, have been associated with maternal use of opioid analgesics, including hydrocodone, during the first trimester of pregnancy (Broussard, 2011). Use of opioids during pregnancy may produce physical dependence in the neonate. Symptoms of opioid withdrawal may include excessive crying, diarrhea, fever, hyper-reflexia, irritability, respiratory rate increased, sneezing, tremors, vomiting, or yawning; respiratory depression may occur in the newborn if opioids are used prior to delivery. Also refer to acetaminophen monograph.

Lactation Enters breast milk/not recommended

Breast-Feeding Considerations Acetaminophen and hydrocodone are excreted in breast milk. In one study (n=30), the calculated dose of hydrocodone to a nursing infant was 0.2% to 9% (mean: 2.4%) of the weight-adjusted maternal dose. Hydromorphone was also measurable in 12 cases; the total opioid dose to a nursing infant was calculated to be 0.1% to 9.9% (mean: 1.5%) of the weight-adjusted maternal dose. Concentrations may be increased in women who are extensive metabolizers of CYP2D6. Caution should be used since most persons are not aware of their CYP2D6 genotype status. When hydrocodone is used in breast-feeding women, it is recommended to use the lowest dose for the shortest duration of time and observe the infant for adverse events. Some clinicians recommend limiting the dose to hydrocodone bitartrate 30 mg/day (Sauberan, 2011). The manufacturers recommend discontinuing the medication or to discontinue nursing during therapy. Also refer to acetaminophen monograph.

Controlled Substance C-III

Dosage Forms

Capsule, oral: Hydrocodone 5 mg and acetaminophen 500 mg

Margesic® H, Stagesic™: Hydrocodone 5 mg and acetaminophen 500 mg

Elixir, oral:

Lortab®: Hydrocodone 7.5 mg and acetaminophen 500 mg per 15 mL

Solution, oral: Hydrocodone 7.5 mg and acetaminophen 325 mg per 15 mL; hydrocodone 7.5 mg and acetaminophen 500 mg per 15 mL; hydrocodone 10 mg and acetaminophen 325 mg per 15 mL

hycet®: Hydrocodone 7.5 mg and acetaminophen 325 mg per 15 mL

Zamicet™: Hydrocodone 10 mg and acetaminophen 325 mg per 15 mL

Zolvit®: Hydrocodone 10 mg and acetaminophen 300 mg per 15 mL (480 mL)

Tablet, oral:

Generics:

Hydrocodone 2.5 mg and acetaminophen 500 mg

Hydrocodone 5 mg and acetaminophen 300 mg

Hydrocodone 5 mg and acetaminophen 325 mg

Hydrocodone 5 mg and acetaminophen 500 mg

Hydrocodone 7.5 mg and acetaminophen 300 mg

Hydrocodone 7.5 mg and acetaminophen 325 mg

Hydrocodone 7.5 mg and acetaminophen 500 mg

Hydrocodone 7.5 mg and acetaminophen 650 mg

Hydrocodone 7.5 mg and acetaminophen 750 mg

Hydrocodone 10 mg and acetaminophen 300 mg

Hydrocodone 10 mg and acetaminophen 325 mg

Hydrocodone 10 mg and acetaminophen 500 mg

Hydrocodone 10 mg and acetaminophen 650 mg

Hydrocodone 10 mg and acetaminophen 660 mg

Hydrocodone 10 mg and acetaminophen 750 mg

Brands:

Lorcet® 10/650: Hydrocodone 10 mg and acetaminophen 650 mg

Lorcet® Plus: Hydrocodone 7.5 mg and acetaminophen 650 mg

Lortab®: 5/500: Hydrocodone 5 mg and acetaminophen 500 mg; 7.5/500: Hydrocodone 7.5 mg and acetaminophen 500 mg; 10/500: Hydrocodone 10 mg and acetaminophen 500 mg

Maxidone®: Hydrocodone 10 mg and acetaminophen 750 mg

Norco®: Hydrocodone 5 mg and acetaminophen 325 mg; hydrocodone 7.5 mg and acetaminophen 325 mg; hydrocodone 10 mg and acetaminophen 325 mg

Vicodin®: Hydrocodone 5 mg and acetaminophen 300 mg

Vicodin ES®: Hydrocodone 7.5 mg and acetaminophen 300 mg

Vicodin HP®: Hydrocodone 10 mg and acetaminophen 300 mg

Xodol®: 5/300: Hydrocodone 5 mg and acetaminophen 300 mg; 7.5/300: Hydrocodone 7.5 mg and acetaminophen 300 mg; 10/300: Hydrocodone 10 mg and acetaminophen 300 mg

Zydone®: Hydrocodone 5 mg and acetaminophen 400 mg; hydrocodone 7.5 mg and acetaminophen 400 mg; hydrocodone 10 mg and acetaminophen 400 mg

Dental Comment Neither hydrocodone nor acetaminophen elicit anti-inflammatory effects. Because of addiction liability of opiate analgesics, the use of hydrocodone should be limited to 2-3 days postoperatively for treatment of dental pain. Nausea is the most common adverse effect seen after use in dental patients; sedation and constipation are second. Nausea elicited by opioid analgesics is centrally mediated and the presence or absence of food will not affect the degree nor incidence of nausea.

Hepatotoxicity caused by acetaminophen is potentiated by chronic alcohol consumption. People who are taking acetaminophen, even at therapeutic doses, and consume alcohol are at risk of developing hepatotoxicity.

Acetaminophen may increase the levels and enhance the anticoagulant effects of vitamin K antagonists acenocoumarol and warfarin (Coumadin®). Studies have reported that acetaminophen has increased the INR in warfarin treated patients with daily acetaminophen doses as low as 2 g, particularly when taking acetaminophen for >1 week (Antlitz, 1968; Boeijinga, 1982; Gebauer, 2003; Hylek, 1998; Rubin, 1984). In addition, case reports of bleeding as a result of increased INR have been published (Bagheri, 1999; Bartle, 1991). There is no known mechanism of the interaction; furthermore, some studies have failed to demonstrate this interaction (Gadisseur, 2003; Kwan, 1995; van den Bemt, 2002). In terms of risk, the data suggest that acetaminophen and warfarin could interact in some clinically significant manner but that the benefits of concomitant use of acetaminophen for pain control in dental patients taking warfarin usually outweigh the risks. An appropriate monitoring plan should be in place to identify potential negative effects and dosage adjustments may be necessary in a minority of patients. The interaction may be more likely to occur with daily acetaminophen doses of >1.3 g for >1 week.

There are no reports of acetaminophen interacting with antiplatelet drugs such as aspirin, clopidogrel (Plavix®), or prasugrel (Effient™). Also, there are no reports of acetaminophen in combination with hydrocodone, codeine, or oxycodone interacting with warfarin (Coumadin®).

References

Antlitz AM, Mead JA Jr, and Tolentino MA, "Potentiation of Oral Anticoagulant Therapy by Acetaminophen," *Curr Ther Res Clin Exp*, 1968, 10(10):501-7.

Bagheri H, Bernhard NB, and Montastruc JL, "Potentiation of the Acenocoumarol Anticoagulant Effect by Acetaminophen," *Ann Pharmacother*, 1999, 33(4):506.

Bartle WR and Blakely LA, "Potentiation of Warfarin Anticoagulation by Acetaminophen," *JAMA*, 1991, 265(10):1260.

Boeijinga JJ, Boerstra EE, Ris P, et al, "Interaction Between Paracetamol and Coumarin Anticoagulants," *Lancet*, 1982, 1(8270):506.

Gadisseur AP, Van Der Meer FJ, and Rosendaal FR, "Sustained Intake of Paracetamol (Acetaminophen) During Oral Anticoagulant Therapy With Coumarins Does Not Cause Clinically Important INR Changes: A Randomized Double-Blind Clinical Trial," *J Thromb Haemost*, 2003, 1(4):714-7.

Gebauer MG, Nyfort-Hansen K, Henschke PJ, et al, "Warfarin and Acetaminophen Interaction," *Pharmacotherapy*, 2003, 23(1):109-12.

Hylek EM, Heiman H, Skates SJ, et al, "Acetaminophen and Other Risk factors for excessive warfarin anticoagulation," *JAMA*, 1998, 279(9):657-62.

Kwan D, Bartle WR, and Walker SE, "The Effects of Acetaminophen on Pharmacokinetics and Pharmacodynamics of Warfarin," *J Clin Pharmacol*, 1999, 39(1):68-75.

Kwan D, Bartle WR, and Walker SE, "The Effects of Acute and Chronic Acetaminophen Dosing on the Pharmacodynamics and Pharmacokinetics of (R)- and (S)-Warfarin," *Clin Pharmacol Ther*, 1995, 57:212.

Rubin RN, Mentzer RL, and Budzynski AZ, "Potentiation of Anticoagulant Effect of Warfarin by Acetaminophen (Tylenol®)," *Clin Res*, 1984, 32:698a.

van den Bemt PM, Geven LM, Kuitert NA, et al, "The Potential Interaction Between Oral Anticoagulants and Acetaminophen in Everyday Practice," *Pharm World Sci*, 2002, 24(5):201-4.

Hydrocodone and Chlorpheniramine

(hye droe KOE done & klor fen IR a meen)

Related Information

Chlorpheniramine *on page 292*

Brand Names: U.S. TussiCaps®; Tussionex® Pennkinetic®

Pharmacologic Category Alkylamine Derivative; Analgesic, Opioid; Antitussive; Histamine H_1 Antagonist; Histamine H_1 Antagonist, First Generation

Use Symptomatic relief of cough and upper respiratory symptoms associated with cold and allergy

Local Anesthetic/Vasoconstrictor Precautions No information available to require special precautions

Effects on Dental Treatment Key adverse event(s) related to dental treatment: Prolonged use will cause significant xerostomia (normal salivary flow resumes upon discontinuation).

Effects on Bleeding No information available to require special precautions

Adverse Effects Also refer to Chlorpheniramine monograph. Frequency not defined.

Cardiovascular: Chest tightness

Central nervous system: Anxiety, dizziness, drowsiness, dysphoria, euphoria, fear, lethargy, mental impairment, mood changes, sedation

Dermatologic: Pruritus, rash

Gastrointestinal: Constipation, nausea, vomiting

Genitourinary: Ureteral spasm, urinary retention, vesicle sphincter spasm

Respiratory: Dryness of pharynx, respiratory depression

Miscellaneous: Psychological dependence

General Dosage Range Oral:

Children 6-12 years: TussiCaps® 5 mg/4 mg: 1 capsule every 12 hours (maximum: 2 capsules/24 hours); Tussionex®: 2.5 mL every 12 hours (maximum: 5 mL/24 hours)

Children >12 years and Adults: TussiCaps® 10 mg/8 mg: 1 capsule every 12 hours (maximum: 2 capsules/24 hours); Tussionex®: 5 mL every 12 hours (maximum: 10 mL/24 hours)

Mechanism of Action

Hydrocodone binds to opiate receptors in the CNS, altering the perception of and response to pain; suppresses cough in medullary center; produces generalized CNS depression

Chlorpheniramine competes with histamine for H_1-receptor sites on effector cells in the gastrointestinal tract, blood vessels, and respiratory tract

Pharmacodynamics/Kinetics

Duration of Action Hydrocodone: 4-8 hours

Half-life Elimination Hydrocodone: 3.3-4.4 hours

Pregnancy Risk Factor C

Pregnancy Considerations Hydrocodone is teratogenic in animal reproduction studies. In humans, birth defects, including some heart defects, have been associated with maternal use of opioid analgesics, including hydrocodone, during the first trimester of pregnancy (Broussard, 2011). Use of opioids during pregnancy may produce physical dependence in the neonate. Symptoms of opioid withdrawal may include excessive crying, diarrhea, fever, hyper-reflexia, irritability, respiratory rate increased, sneezing, tremors, vomiting, or yawning; respiratory depression may occur in the newborn if opioids are used prior to delivery. Also refer to the chlorpheniramine monograph.

Product Availability Vituz (hydrocodone bitartrate 5 mg and chlorpheniramine maleate 4 mg) oral solution: FDA approved February 2013; anticipated availability currently unknown. Refer to prescribing information for additional information.

Controlled Substance C-III

Hydrocodone and Homatropine
(hye droe KOE done & hoe MA troe peen)

Related Information
Homatropine *on page 685*
Brand Names: U.S. Hydromet®; Tussigon®
Pharmacologic Category Antitussive
Use Symptomatic relief of cough

Local Anesthetic/Vasoconstrictor Precautions No information available to require special precautions

Effects on Dental Treatment Key adverse event(s) related to dental treatment: Xerostomia (normal salivary flow resumes upon discontinuation).

Effects on Bleeding No information available to require special precautions

Adverse Effects Frequency not defined.
Central nervous system: Anxiety, dizziness, drowsiness, dysphoria, fear, lethargy, mental clouding, mental impairment, mood changes, sedation
Dermatologic: Pruritus, rash
Gastrointestinal: Constipation, nausea, vomiting, xerostomia
Genitourinary: Urinary retention, urinary tract spasm
Respiratory: Respiratory depression
Miscellaneous: Physical and psychological dependence with prolonged use

General Dosage Range Oral:
Children 6-11 years: 1/2 tablet or 2.5 mL every 4-6 hours as needed (maximum: 3 tablets or 15 mL/24 hours)
Children ≥12 years and Adults: 1 tablet or 5 mL every 4-6 hours as needed (maximum: 6 tablets/24 hours or 30 mL/24 hours)

Mechanism of Action
Hydrocodone binds to opiate receptors in the CNS, altering the perception of and response to pain; suppresses cough in medullary center; produces generalized CNS depression.
Homatropine is an anticholinergic agent, present in a subtherapeutic amount to discourage deliberate overdose.

Pharmacodynamics/Kinetics
Onset of Action Hydrocodone: Narcotic analgesic: 10-20 minutes
Duration of Action Hydrocodone: 4-8 hours
Half-life Elimination Hydrocodone: 3.3-4.4 hours

Pregnancy Risk Factor C
Pregnancy Considerations Animal reproduction studies have not been conducted with this combination. Birth defects, including some heart defects, have been associated with maternal use of opioid analgesics, including hydrocodone, during the first trimester of pregnancy (Broussard, 2011). Use of opioids during pregnancy may produce physical dependence in the neonate. Symptoms of opioid withdrawal may include excessive crying, diarrhea, fever, hyper-reflexia, irritability, respiratory rate increased, sneezing, tremors, vomiting, or

yawning; respiratory depression may occur in the newborn if opioids are used prior to delivery.
Controlled Substance C-III

Hydrocodone and Ibuprofen
(hye droe KOE done & eye byoo PROE fen)

Related Information
Ibuprofen *on page 711*
Oral Pain *on page 1558*
Related Sample Prescriptions
Moderate/Moderately Severe Oral Pain *on page 1606*
Brand Names: U.S. Ibudone®; Reprexain™; Vicoprofen®
Brand Names: Canada Vicoprofen®
Generic Availability (U.S.) Yes
Pharmacologic Category Analgesic Combination (Opioid); Nonsteroidal Anti-inflammatory Drug (NSAID), Oral

Dental Use Short-term management (generally <10 days) of moderate-to-severe acute postoperative dental pain where an anti-inflammatory effect is desired

Use Short-term (generally <10 days) management of moderate-to-severe acute pain; is not indicated for treatment of such conditions as osteoarthritis or rheumatoid arthritis

Local Anesthetic/Vasoconstrictor Precautions No information available to require special precautions

Effects on Dental Treatment Key adverse event(s) related to dental treatment: Xerostomia (normal salivary flow resumes upon discontinuation). See Effects on Bleeding.

Effects on Bleeding Nonselective NSAIDs such as ibuprofen inhibit platelet aggregation and prolong bleeding time in some patients. Unlike aspirin, the NSAID effect on platelet function is quantitatively less, of shorter duration, and reversible.

Adverse Effects
>10%:
Central nervous system: Headache (27%), somnolence (22%), dizziness (14%)
Gastrointestinal: Constipation (22%), nausea (21%), dyspepsia (12%)
1% to 10%:
Cardiovascular: Edema (3% to 9%), palpitation (<3%), vasodilation (<3%)
Central nervous system: Anxiety (3% to 9%), insomnia (3% to 9%), nervousness (3% to 9%), confusion (<3%), fever (<3%), thought abnormalities (<3%)
Dermatologic: Itching (3% to 9%)
Gastrointestinal: Abdominal pain (3% to 9%), diarrhea (3% to 9%), flatulence (3% to 9%), vomiting (3% to 9%), xerostomia (3% to 9%), gastritis (<3%), melena (<3%), mouth ulcers (<3%)
Genitourinary: Polyuria (<3%)
Neuromuscular & skeletal: Hypertonia (<3%), paresthesia (<3%)
Otic: Tinnitus (<3%)
Respiratory: Dyspnea (<3%), pharyngitis (<3%), rhinitis (<3%)
Miscellaneous: Diaphoresis (3% to 9%), infection (3% to 9%), flu-like syndrome (<3%), hiccups (<3%)

Dental Usual Dosage Moderate-to-severe acute postoperative dental pain: Adults: Oral: 1-2 tablets every 4-6 hours as needed for pain; maximum: 5 tablets/day

Dosage Oral:

Adults: 1 tablet every 4-6 hours as needed for pain; maximum: 5 tablets/day. **Note:** Short-term use is recommended (<10 days).

Elderly: Use with caution; consider reduced doses. Refer to dosing in individual monographs.

Mechanism of Action

Hydrocodone: Binds to opiate receptors in the CNS, altering the perception of and response to pain; suppresses cough in medullary center; produces generalized CNS depression

Ibuprofen: Reversibly inhibits cyclooxygenase-1 and 2 (COX-1 and 2) enzymes, which result in decreased formation of prostaglandin precursors; has antipyretic, analgesic, and anti-inflammatory properties

Contraindications Hypersensitivity to hydrocodone, ibuprofen, or any component of the formulation; patients who have experienced asthma, urticaria, or allergic-type reactions to aspirin or other NSAIDs; perioperative pain in the setting of coronary artery bypass graft (CABG) surgery

Warnings/Precautions [U.S. Boxed Warning]: NSAIDs are associated with an increased risk of adverse cardiovascular thrombotic events, including MI and stroke. Risk may be increased with duration of use or pre-existing cardiovascular risk factors or disease. May cause new-onset hypertension or worsening of existing hypertension. Use caution with fluid retention. Avoid use in heart failure. **[U.S. Boxed Warning]: Use of NSAIDs is contraindicated for treatment of perioperative pain in the setting of coronary artery bypass graft (CABG) surgery.** Risk of MI and stroke may be increased with use following CABG surgery. **[U.S. Boxed Warning]: NSAIDs may increase risk of gastrointestinal irritation, inflammation, ulceration, bleeding, and perforation.** When used concomitantly with ≤325 mg of aspirin, a substantial increase in the risk of gastrointestinal complications (eg, ulcer) occurs; concomitant gastroprotective therapy (eg, proton pump inhibitors) is recommended (Bhatt, 2008).

May increase the risk of aseptic meningitis, especially in patients with systemic lupus erythematosus (SLE) and mixed connective tissue disorders. Platelet adhesion and aggregation may be decreased; may prolong bleeding time; patients with coagulation disorders or who are receiving anticoagulants should be monitored closely. Anemia may occur; patients on long-term NSAID therapy should be monitored for anemia. Rarely, NSAID use may cause severe blood dyscrasias (eg, agranulocytosis, aplastic anemia, thrombocytopenia).

NSAIDS may cause drowsiness, dizziness, blurred vision and other neurologic effects which may impair physical or mental abilities; patients must be cautioned about performing tasks which require mental alertness (eg, operating machinery or driving). Discontinue use with blurred or diminished vision and perform ophthalmologic exam. Monitor vision with long-term therapy.

NSAID use may compromise existing renal function; dose-dependent decreases in prostaglandin synthesis may result from NSAID use, reducing renal blood flow which may cause renal decompensation. NSAID use may increase the risk for hyperkalemia. Patients with impaired renal function, dehydration, heart failure, liver dysfunction, those taking diuretics, and ACE inhibitors, and the elderly are at greater risk of renal toxicity and hyperkalemia. Rehydrate patient before starting therapy; monitor renal function closely. Not recommended for use in patients with advanced renal disease. Long-term NSAID use may result in renal papillary necrosis. NSAIDs may cause serious skin adverse events; discontinue use at first sign of skin rash or hypersensitivity. Anaphylactoid reactions may occur, even without prior exposure. Do not use in patients who experience bronchospasm, asthma, rhinitis, or urticaria with NSAID or aspirin therapy. Use caution in other forms of asthma. The elderly are at increased risk for adverse effects (especially peptic ulceration, CNS effects, renal toxicity) from NSAIDs even at low doses. Withhold for at least 4-6 half-lives prior to surgical or dental procedures.

Hydrocodone: May cause CNS depression. Effects may be potentiated when used with other sedative drugs or ethanol. May cause hypotension. Use with caution in patients with pre-existing respiratory compromise, and kyphoscoliosis or other skeletal disorder which may alter respiratory function. Use with caution in patients with hypersensitivity reactions to other phenanthrene derivative opioid agonists (codeine, hydrocodone, hydromorphone, levorphanol, oxycodone, oxymorphone). Use with extreme caution in patients with head injury, intracranial lesions, or elevated intracranial pressure. May obscure diagnosis or clinical course of patients with acute abdominal conditions. Use with caution in patients with severe hepatic dysfunction. Use with caution in patients with biliary tract dysfunction; acute pancreatitis may cause constriction of sphincter of Oddi. Use with caution in patients with adrenal insufficiency, thyroid dysfunction, seizure disorder, morbid obesity, toxic psychosis, prostatic hyperplasia and/or urinary stricture, severe hepatic dysfunction, or with a potential for or a history of drug abuse or acute alcoholism. May suppress cough reflex. Tolerance, psychological and physical dependence may occur with prolonged use. Concurrent use of agonist/antagonist analgesics may precipitate withdrawal symptoms and/or reduced analgesic efficacy in patients following prolonged therapy with mu opioid agonists. Abrupt discontinuation following prolonged use may also lead to withdrawal symptoms.

Due to the role of CYP2D6 in the metabolism of hydrocodone to hydromorphone (an active metabolite with higher binding affinity to mu-opioid receptors compared to hydrocodone), patients with genetic variations of CYP2D6, including "poor metabolizers" or "extensive metabolizers," may have decreased or increased hydromorphone formation, respectively. Variable effects in positive and negative opioid effects have been reported in these patients; however, limited data exists to determine if clinically significant differences of analgesia and toxicity can be predicted based on CYP2D6 phenotype (Hutchinson, 2004; Otton, 1993; Zhou, 2009).

Safety and efficacy in children <16 years have not been established.

Drug Interactions

Metabolism/Transport Effects Refer to individual components.

Avoid Concomitant Use

Avoid concomitant use of Hydrocodone and Ibuprofen with any of the following: Azelastine (Nasal); Floctafenine; Ketorolac (Nasal); Ketorolac (Systemic); NSAID (COX-2 Inhibitor); Omacetaxine; Paraldehyde

Increased Effect/Toxicity

Hydrocodone and Ibuprofen may increase the levels/ effects of: Agents with Antiplatelet Properties; Alcohol (Ethyl); Aliskiren; Alvimopan; Aminoglycosides; Anticoagulants; Azelastine (Nasal); Bisphosphonate Derivatives; CNS Depressants; Collagenase (Systemic); CycloSPORINE (Systemic); Dabigatran Etexilate;

Deferasirox; Desmopressin; Digoxin; Drotrecogin Alfa (Activated); Eplerenone; Haloperidol; Ibritumomab; Lithium; Methotrexate; Metyrosine; Mirtazapine; Nonsteroidal Anti-Inflammatory Agents; NSAID (COX-2 Inhibitor); Omacetaxine; Paraldehyde; PEMEtrexed; Porfimer; Potassium-Sparing Diuretics; PRALAtrexate; Pramipexole; Quinolone Antibiotics; Rivaroxaban; ROPINIRole; Rotigotine; Salicylates; Selective Serotonin Reuptake Inhibitors; Thiazide Diuretics; Thrombolytic Agents; Tositumomab and Iodine I 131 Tositumomab; Vancomycin; Vitamin K Antagonists; Zolpidem

The levels/effects of Hydrocodone and Ibuprofen may be increased by: ACE Inhibitors; Amphetamines; Angiotensin II Receptor Blockers; Antidepressants (Tricyclic, Tertiary Amine); Antipsychotic Agents (Phenothiazines); Corticosteroids (Systemic); CycloSPORINE (Systemic); Dasatinib; Droperidol; Floctafenine; Glucosamine; Herbs (Anticoagulant/Antiplatelet Properties); HydrOXYzine; Ketorolac (Nasal); Ketorolac (Systemic); Magnesium Sulfate; MAO Inhibitors; Multivitamins/Minerals (with ADEK, Folate, Iron); Nonsteroidal Anti-Inflammatory Agents; Omega-3 Fatty Acids; Pentosan Polysulfate Sodium; Pentoxifylline; Perampanel; Probenecid; Prostacyclin Analogues; Selective Serotonin Reuptake Inhibitors; Serotonin/Norepinephrine Reuptake Inhibitors; Sodium Oxybate; Sodium Phosphates; Succinylcholine; Tipranavir; Treprostinil; Vitamin E; Voriconazole

Decreased Effect
Hydrocodone and Ibuprofen may decrease the levels/ effects of: ACE Inhibitors; Agents with Antiplatelet Properties; Aliskiren; Angiotensin II Receptor Blockers; Beta-Blockers; Eplerenone; HydrALAZINE; Imatinib; Loop Diuretics; Pegvisomant; Potassium-Sparing Diuretics; Salicylates; Selective Serotonin Reuptake Inhibitors

The levels/effects of Hydrocodone and Ibuprofen may be decreased by: Ammonium Chloride; Bile Acid Sequestrants; Mixed Agonist / Antagonist Opioids; Nonsteroidal Anti-Inflammatory Agents; QuiNIDine; Salicylates

Ethanol/Nutrition/Herb Interactions
Based on **hydrocodone** component: Ethanol: May increase CNS depression; monitor for increased effects with coadministration. Caution patients about effects.

Based on **ibuprofen** component:
Ethanol: Avoid ethanol (may enhance gastric mucosal irritation).
Food: Ibuprofen peak serum levels may be decreased if taken with food.
Herb/Nutraceutical: Avoid alfalfa, anise, bilberry, bladderwrack, bromelain, cat's claw, celery, chamomile, coleus, cordyceps, dong quai, evening primrose, fenugreek, feverfew, garlic, ginger, ginkgo biloba, ginseng (American, Panax, Siberian), grapeseed, green tea, guggul, horse chestnut seed, horseradish, licorice, prickly ash, red clover, reishi, SAMe (S-adenosylmethionine), sweet clover, turmeric, white willow (all have additional antiplatelet activity).

Pharmacodynamics/Kinetics
Onset of Action Hydrocodone: Narcotic analgesic: 10-20 minutes
Duration of Action Hydrocodone: 4-8 hours
Half-life Elimination Hydrocodone: 4.5 hours
Time to Peak Hydrocodone: 1.7 hours
Pregnancy Risk Factor C

Pregnancy Considerations Adverse events were observed in animal reproduction studies. In humans, birth defects, including some heart defects, have been associated with maternal use of opioid analgesics, including hydrocodone, during the first trimester of pregnancy (Broussard, 2011). Use of opioids during pregnancy may produce physical dependence in the neonate. Symptoms of opioid withdrawal may include excessive crying, diarrhea, fever, hyper-reflexia, irritability, respiratory rate increased, sneezing, tremors, vomiting, or yawning; respiratory depression may occur in the newborn if opioids are used prior to delivery. As with other NSAID-containing products, this agent should be avoided in late pregnancy because it may cause premature closure of the ductus arteriosus. Also refer to the ibuprofen monograph.

Lactation Enters breast milk/not recommended
Breast-Feeding Considerations Hydrocodone and ibuprofen are excreted in breast milk. In one study, the calculated dose of hydrocodone to a nursing infant was 0.2% to 9% (mean: 2.4%) of the weight-adjusted maternal dose. Hydromorphone was also measurable in 12 cases; the total opioid dose to a nursing infant was calculated to be 0.1% to 9.9% (mean: 1.5%) of the weight-adjusted maternal dose. Concentrations may be increased in women who are extensive metabolizers of CYP2D6. Caution should be used since most persons are not aware of their CYP2D6 genotype status. When hydrocodone is used in breast-feeding women, it is recommended to use the lowest dose for the shortest duration of time and observe the infant for adverse events. Some clinicians recommend limiting the dose to hydrocodone bitartrate 30 mg/day (Sauberan, 2011). The manufacturers recommend discontinuing the medication or to discontinue nursing during therapy. Also refer to the ibuprofen monograph.

Controlled Substance C-III
Dosage Forms
Tablet: Hydrocodone 2.5 mg and ibuprofen 200 mg; Hydrocodone 5 mg and ibuprofen 200 mg; Hydrocodone 7.5 mg and ibuprofen 200 mg
Ibudone®: 5/200: Hydrocodone 5 mg and ibuprofen 200 mg; 10/200: Hydrocodone 10 mg and ibuprofen 200 mg
Reprexain™: 2.5/200: Hydrocodone 2.5 mg and ibuprofen 200 mg; 5/200: Hydrocodone 5 mg and ibuprofen 200 mg; 10/200: Hydrocodone 10 mg and ibuprofen 200 mg
Vicoprofen®: 7.5/200: Hydrocodone 7.5 mg and ibuprofen 200 mg

References
Sunshine A, Olson NZ, O'Neill E, et al, "Analgesic Efficacy of a Hydrocodone With Ibuprofen Combination Compared With Ibuprofen Alone for the Treatment of Acute Postoperative Pain," *J Clin Pharmacol*, 1997, 37(10):908-15.

Hydrocodone and Phenyltoloxamine
(hye droe KOE done & fen il to LOKS a meen)

Brand Names: Canada Tussionex®
Pharmacologic Category Alkylamine Derivative; Analgesic, Opioid; Antitussive; Histamine H_1 Antagonist; Histamine H_1 Antagonist, First Generation
Use Symptomatic relief of cough and upper respiratory symptoms associated with cold and allergy that does not respond to non-narcotic antitussives
Local Anesthetic/Vasoconstrictor Precautions No information available to require special precautions
Effects on Dental Treatment No significant effects or complications reported

Effects on Bleeding No information available to require special precautions

Adverse Effects Frequency not defined.

Cardiovascular: Tachycardia

Central nervous system: Drowsiness, hallucinations, seizures

Dermatologic: Facial pruritus

Gastrointestinal: Constipation, nausea

Respiratory: Dyspnea, respiratory depression

Miscellaneous: Allergic reactions, psychological dependence

General Dosage Range Oral:

Children ≥6 years: Hydrocodone 5 mg/phenyltoloxamine 10 mg (5 mL) every 12 hours (maximum dose: hydrocodone 10 mg/phenyltoloxamine 20 mg [10 mL] every 24 hours)

Adults: Hydrocodone 5 mg/phenyltoloxamine 10 mg (5 mL suspension or 1 tablet) every 8-12 hours (maximum dose: hydrocodone 10 mg/phenyltoloxamine 20 mg [10 mL suspension or 2 tablets] every 24 hours)

Mechanism of Action

Hydrocodone binds to opiate receptors in the CNS, altering the perception of and response to pain; suppresses cough in medullary center; produces generalized CNS depression.

Phenyltoloxamine competes with histamine for H_1-receptor sites on effector cells. May potentiate the antitussive effects of hydrocodone; sedative effects are also seen.

Pharmacodynamics/Kinetics

Duration of Action Antitussive effects: ≥8 hours

Half-life Elimination Hydrocodone: ~4 hours (Tussionex® Pennkinetic® U.S. prescribing information, 2008).

Pregnancy Considerations Birth defects, including some heart defects, have been associated with maternal use of opioid analgesics, including hydrocodone, during the first trimester of pregnancy (Broussard, 2011). Use of opioids during pregnancy may produce physical dependence in the neonate. Symptoms of opioid withdrawal may include excessive crying, diarrhea, fever, hyper-reflexia, irritability, respiratory rate increased, sneezing, tremors, vomiting, or yawning; respiratory depression may occur in the newborn if opioids are used prior to delivery.

Product Availability Tussionex® represents a different product in Canada than it does in the U.S. In Canada, Tussionex® contains hydrocodone and phenyltoloxamine while in the U.S. Tussionex® (Pennkinetic®) contains hydrocodone and chlorpheniramine.

Controlled Substance CDSA I

Hydrocodone and Pseudoephedrine
(hye droe KOE done & soo doe e FED rin)

Related Information

Pseudoephedrine *on page 1159*

Brand Names: U.S. Rezira™

Pharmacologic Category Antitussive/Decongestant

Use Symptomatic relief of cough and nasal congestion associated with common cold

Local Anesthetic/Vasoconstrictor Precautions Use with caution since pseudoephedrine is a sympathomimetic amine which could interact with epinephrine to cause a pressor response

Effects on Dental Treatment Key adverse event(s) related to dental treatment: Pseudoephedrine: Xerostomia (normal salivary flow resumes upon discontinuation).

Effects on Bleeding No information available to require special precautions

Adverse Effects See individual agents.

General Dosage Range Oral: *Adults:* 5 mL every 4-6 hours as needed (maximum: 20 mL/24 hours)

Mechanism of Action

Hydrocodone binds to opiate receptors in the CNS, altering the perception of and response to pain; suppresses cough in medullary center; produces generalized CNS depression.

Pseudoephedrine directly stimulates alpha-adrenergic receptors of respiratory mucosa causing vasoconstriction; directly stimulates beta-adrenergic receptors causing bronchial relaxation, increased heart rate and contractility.

Pharmacodynamics/Kinetics

Onset of Action Hydrocodone: Narcotic analgesic: 10-20 minutes

Duration of Action Hydrocodone: 4-8 hours

Half-life Elimination Hydrocodone: 3.3-4.4 hours

Pregnancy Risk Factor C

Pregnancy Considerations Animal reproduction studies have not been conducted with this combination. In humans, birth defects, including some heart defects, have been associated with maternal use of opioid analgesics, including hydrocodone, during the first trimester of pregnancy (Broussard, 2011). Use of opioids during pregnancy may produce physical dependence in the neonate. Symptoms of opioid withdrawal may include excessive crying, diarrhea, fever, hyper-reflexia, irritability, respiratory rate increased, sneezing, tremors, vomiting, or yawning; respiratory depression may occur in the newborn if opioids are used prior to delivery. Also refer to pseudoephedrine monograph.

Controlled Substance C-III

Hydrocodone, Chlorpheniramine, and Pseudoephedrine
(hye droe KOE done, klor fen IR a meen, & soo doe e FED rin)

Related Information

Chlorpheniramine *on page 292*

Pseudoephedrine *on page 1159*

Brand Names: U.S. Zutripro™

Pharmacologic Category Alpha/Beta Agonist; Analgesic, Opioid; Antitussive; Decongestant; Histamine H_1 Antagonist; Histamine H_1 Antagonist, First Generation

Use Temporary relief of cough and nasal congestion due to colds or upper respiratory allergies

Local Anesthetic/Vasoconstrictor Precautions Use with caution since pseudoephedrine is a sympathomimetic amine which could interact with epinephrine to cause a pressor response

Effects on Dental Treatment Key adverse event(s) related to dental treatment: Pseudoephedrine and chlorpheniramine: Xerostomia (normal salivary flow resumes upon discontinuation).

Effects on Bleeding No information available to require special precautions

Adverse Effects Also refer to the Chlorpheniramine and Pseudoephedrine individual monographs. Frequency not defined.

Cardiovascular: Bradycardia, hyper-/hypotension, orthostatic hypotension, palpitation, syncope, tachycardia

Central nervous system: Agitation, anxiety, confusion, dizziness, dysphoria, euphoria, fear, headache, insomnia, irritability, lethargy, lightheadedness, mental impairment, mood changes, nervousness, restlessness, sedation, somnolence, vertigo

Dermatologic: Erythema, hyperhidrosis, rash, pruritus, urticaria

Endocrine: Gynecomastia, hypoglycemia, lactation decreased, libido increased, menstrual irregularities

Gastrointestinal: Abdominal distension, abdominal pain, appetite changes, constipation, dyspepsia, epigastric distress, nausea, pancreatitis (acute), vomiting, xerostomia

Genitourinary: Dysuria, glycosuria, ureteral spasm, urinary frequency, urinary hesitancy, urinary retention

Neuromuscular & skeletal: Facial dyskinesia, tremor

Ocular: Hypermetropia, lacrimation increased, mydriasis, photophobia, visual disturbances

Otic: Labyrinthitis, tinnitus

Respiratory: Dyspnea, respiratory dryness, laryngismus, wheezing

Miscellaneous: Psychological dependence

General Dosage Range Oral: *Adults:* 5 mL every 4-6 hours as needed (maximum: 4 doses/24 hours)

Mechanism of Action

Pseudoephedrine: Directly stimulates alpha-adrenergic receptors of respiratory mucosa causing vasoconstriction; directly stimulates beta-adrenergic receptors causing bronchial relaxation

Hydrocodone: Binds to opiate receptors in the CNS; suppresses cough in medullary center; produces generalized CNS depression

Chlorpheniramine: Competes with histamine for H_1-receptor sites on effector cells in the gastrointestinal tract, blood vessels, and respiratory tract

Pharmacodynamics/Kinetics

Onset of Action Hydrocodone: Narcotic analgesic: 10-20 minutes

Duration of Action Hydrocodone: 4-8 hours

Half-life Elimination Hydrocodone: 3.3-4.4 hours

Time to Peak Hydrocodone: 1.4 hours

Pregnancy Risk Factor C

Pregnancy Considerations Animal reproduction studies have not been conducted with this combination product. In humans, birth defects, including some heart defects, have been associated with maternal use of opioid analgesics, including hydrocodone, during the first trimester of pregnancy (Broussard, 2011). Use of opioids during pregnancy may produce physical dependence in the neonate. Symptoms of opioid withdrawal may include excessive crying, diarrhea, fever, hyper-reflexia, irritability, respiratory rate increased, sneezing, tremors, vomiting, or yawning; respiratory depression may occur in the newborn if opioids are used prior to delivery. Also refer to the chlorpheniramine and pseudoephedrine monographs.

Controlled Substance C-III

Hydrocortisone (Systemic)
(hye droe KOR ti sone)

Related Information

Respiratory Diseases *on page 1514*

Brand Names: U.S. A-Hydrocort®; Cortef®; Solu-CORTEF®

Brand Names: Canada Cortef®; Solu-Cortef®

Generic Availability (U.S.) Yes: Tablet

Pharmacologic Category Corticosteroid, Systemic

Dental Use Treatment of a variety of oral diseases of allergic, inflammatory, or autoimmune origin

Use Management of adrenocortical insufficiency; anti-inflammatory or immunosuppressive

Unlabeled Use Management of septic shock when blood pressure is poorly responsive to fluid resuscitation and vasopressor therapy; treatment of thyroid storm

Local Anesthetic/Vasoconstrictor Precautions No information available to require special precautions

Effects on Dental Treatment No significant effects or complications reported

Effects on Bleeding No information available to require special precautions

Adverse Effects Frequency not defined.

Cardiovascular: Arrhythmias, bradycardia, cardiac arrest, cardiomegaly, circulatory collapse, congestive heart failure, edema, fat embolism, hypertension, hypertrophic cardiomyopathy (premature infants), myocardial rupture (post MI), syncope, tachycardia, thromboembolism, vasculitis

Central nervous system: Delirium, depression, emotional instability, euphoria, hallucinations, headache, insomnia, intracranial pressure increased, malaise, mood swings, nervousness, neuritis, neuropathy, personality changes, pseudotumor cerebri, psychic disorders, psychoses, seizure, vertigo

Dermatologic: Acne, allergic dermatitis, alopecia, bruising, burning/tingling, dry scaly skin, edema, erythema, hirsutism, hyper-/hypopigmentation, impaired wound healing, petechiae, rash, skin atrophy, skin test reaction impaired, sterile abscess, striae, urticaria

Endocrine & metabolic: Adrenal suppression, alkalosis, amenorrhea, carbohydrate intolerance increased, Cushing's syndrome, diabetes mellitus, glucose intolerance, growth suppression, hyperglycemia, hyperlipidemia, hypokalemia, hypokalemic alkalosis, menstrual irregularities, negative nitrogen balance, pituitary-adrenal axis suppression, potassium loss, protein catabolism, sodium and water retention, sperm motility increased/decreased, spermatogenesis increased/decreased

Gastrointestinal: Abdominal distention, appetite increased, bowel dysfunction (intrathecal administration), indigestion, nausea, pancreatitis, peptic ulcer, gastrointestinal perforation, ulcerative esophagitis, vomiting, weight gain

Genitourinary: Bladder dysfunction (intrathecal administration)

Hematologic: Leukocytosis (transient)

Hepatic: Hepatomegaly, transaminases increased

Local: Atrophy (at injection site), postinjection flare (intra-articular use), thrombophlebitis

Neuromuscular & skeletal: Arthralgia, necrosis (femoral and humoral heads), Charcot-like arthropathy, fractures, muscle mass loss, muscle weakness, myopathy, osteoporosis, tendon rupture, vertebral compression fractures

Ocular: Cataracts, exophthalmoses, glaucoma, intraocular pressure increased

Miscellaneous: Abnormal fat deposits, anaphylaxis, avascular necrosis, diaphoresis, hiccups, hypersensitivity reactions, infection, secondary malignancy

Dosage Dose should be based on severity of disease and patient response

Adrenal insufficiency (acute): I.M., I.V.:

Infants and Young Children: 1-2 mg/kg/dose bolus, then 25-150 mg/day in divided doses every 6-8 hours

Older Children: 1-2 mg/kg bolus then 150-250 mg/day in divided doses every 6-8 hours

Adults: 100 mg I.V. bolus, then 300 mg/day in divided doses every 8 hours or as a continuous infusion for 48 hours; once patient is stable change to oral, 50 mg every 8 hours for 6 doses, then taper to 30-50 mg/day in divided doses

Adrenal insufficiency (chronic), physiologic replacement (unlabeled dosing): Adults: Oral: 15-25 mg/day in 2-3 divided doses. **Note:** Studies suggest administering one-half to two-thirds of the daily dose in the morning in order to mimic the physiological cortisol secretion pattern. If the twice-daily regimen is utilized, the second dose should be administered 6-8 hours following the first dose (Arlt, 2003).

Anti-inflammatory or immunosuppressive:

Infants and Children:

Oral: 2.5-10 mg/kg/day **or** 75-300 mg/m²/day every 6-8 hours

I.M., I.V.: 1-5 mg/kg/day **or** 30-150 mg/m²/day divided every 12-24 hours

Adolescents and Adults: Oral, I.M., I.V.: 15-240 mg every 12 hours

Congenital adrenal hyperplasia (unlabeled dosing): Oral: **Note:** Doses must be individualized by monitoring growth, bone age, and hormonal levels.

Children: 10-15 mg/m²/day in 3 divided doses; higher initial doses may be required to achieve initial target hormone serum concentrations in infancy (Speiser, 2010)

Adolescents and Adults: 15-25 mg/day in 2-3 divided doses (Speiser, 2010)

Physiologic replacement: Children: Oral: 8-10 mg/m²/day divided every 8 hours; up to 12 mg/m²/day in some patients (Ahmet, 2011; Gupta, 2008; Maguire, 2007)

Status asthmaticus: Children and Adults: I.V.: 1-2 mg/kg/dose every 6 hours for 24 hours, then maintenance of 0.5-1 mg/kg every 6 hours

Stress dosing (surgery) in patients known to be adrenally-suppressed or on chronic systemic steroids: I.V.: Adults:

Minor stress (ie, inguinal herniorrhaphy): 25 mg/day for 1 day

Moderate stress (ie, joint replacement, cholecystectomy): 50-75 mg/day (25 mg every 8-12 hours) for 1-2 days

Major stress (pancreatoduodenectomy, esophagogastrectomy, cardiac surgery): 100-150 mg/day (50 mg every 8-12 hours) for 2-3 days

Septic shock (unlabeled use): I.V.:

Children: Initial: 1-2 mg/kg/day (intermittent or as continuous infusion); may titrate up to 50 mg/kg/day for shock reversal (Brierley, 2009); alternative dosing suggests 50 mg/m²/day (Dellinger, 2008). **Note:** Use recommended only in catecholamine-resistant shock and suspected or proven adrenal insufficiency.

Adults: 50 mg every 6 hours (Annane, 2002; Marik, 2008); not to exceed 300 mg/day (Dellinger, 2008). Practice guidelines also recommend alternative dosing of 100 mg bolus, followed by continuous infusion of 10 mg/hour (240 mg/day). Taper slowly (for total of 11 days) and do not stop abruptly. **Note:** Fludrocortisone is optional with use of hydrocortisone.

Thyroid storm (unlabeled use): I.V.: 300 mg loading dose, followed by 100 mg every 8 hours (Bahn, 2011)

Dosage adjustment in renal impairment: No dosage adjustment provided in manufacturer's labeling; use with caution.

Dosage adjustment in hepatic impairment: No dosage adjustment provided in manufacturer's labeling.

Mechanism of Action Decreases inflammation by suppression of migration of polymorphonuclear leukocytes and reversal of increased capillary permeability

Contraindications Hypersensitivity to hydrocortisone or any component of the formulation; serious infections, except septic shock or tuberculous meningitis; viral, fungal, or tubercular skin lesions; I.M. administration contraindicated in idiopathic thrombocytopenia purpura; intrathecal administration of injection

Warnings/Precautions Use with caution in patients with thyroid disease, hepatic impairment, renal impairment, heart failure, hypertension, diabetes, glaucoma, cataracts, myasthenia gravis, patients at risk for osteoporosis, patients at risk for seizures, or GI diseases (diverticulitis, peptic ulcer, ulcerative colitis) due to perforation risk. Use caution following acute MI (corticosteroids have been associated with myocardial rupture). Because of the risk of adverse effects, systemic corticosteroids should be used cautiously in the elderly in the smallest possible effective dose for the shortest duration. May affect growth velocity; growth should be routinely monitored in pediatric patients. Withdraw therapy with gradual tapering of dose.

May cause hypercorticism or suppression of hypothalamic-pituitary-adrenal (HPA) axis, particularly in younger children or in patients receiving high doses for prolonged periods. HPA axis suppression may lead to adrenal crisis. Withdrawal and discontinuation of a corticosteroid should be done slowly and carefully. Particular care is required when patients are transferred from systemic corticosteroids to inhaled products due to possible adrenal insufficiency or withdrawal from steroids, including an increase in allergic symptoms. Patients receiving >20 mg per day of prednisone (or equivalent) may be most susceptible. Fatalities have occurred due to adrenal insufficiency in asthmatic patients during and after transfer from systemic corticosteroids to aerosol steroids; aerosol steroids do not provide the systemic steroid needed to treat patients having trauma, surgery, or infections.

Acute myopathy has been reported with high dose corticosteroids, usually in patients with neuromuscular transmission disorders; may involve ocular and/or respiratory muscles; monitor creatine kinase; recovery may be delayed. Corticosteroid use may cause psychiatric disturbances, including depression, euphoria, insomnia, mood swings, and personality changes. Pre-existing psychiatric conditions may be exacerbated by corticosteroid use. Prolonged use of corticosteroids may also increase the incidence of secondary infection, mask acute infection (including fungal infections), prolong or exacerbate viral infections, or limit response to vaccines. Exposure to chickenpox should be avoided; corticosteroids should not be used to treat ocular herpes simplex. Corticosteroids should not be used for cerebral malaria or viral hepatitis. Oral steroid treatment is not recommended for the treatment of acute optic neuritis. Close observation is required in patients with latent tuberculosis and/or TB reactivity; restrict use in active TB (only in conjunction with antituberculosis treatment). Prolonged treatment with corticosteroids has been associated with the development of Kaposi's sarcoma (case reports); if noted, discontinuation of therapy should be considered. High-dose corticosteroids should not be used to manage acute head injury. Some dosage forms contain benzyl alcohol which has been associated with "gasping syndrome" in neonates.

Drug Interactions

Metabolism/Transport Effects Substrate of CYP3A4 (minor), P-glycoprotein; **Note:** Assignment of Major/Minor substrate status based on clinically relevant drug interaction potential; **Induces** CYP3A4 (weak/moderate)

Avoid Concomitant Use

Avoid concomitant use of Hydrocortisone (Systemic) with any of the following: Aldesleukin; Axitinib; BCG; Mifepristone; Natalizumab; Pimecrolimus; Tacrolimus (Topical); Tofacitinib

Increased Effect/Toxicity

Hydrocortisone (Systemic) may increase the levels/ effects of: Acetylcholinesterase Inhibitors; Amphotericin B; Deferasirox; Leflunomide; Loop Diuretics; Natalizumab; NSAID (COX-2 Inhibitor); NSAID (Nonselective); Thiazide Diuretics; Tofacitinib; Vaccines (Live); Warfarin

The levels/effects of Hydrocortisone (Systemic) may be increased by: Antifungal Agents (Azole Derivatives, Systemic); Aprepitant; Calcium Channel Blockers (Nondihydropyridine); Denosumab; Estrogen Derivatives; Fluconazole; Fosaprepitant; Indacaterol; Macrolide Antibiotics; Mifepristone; Neuromuscular-Blocking Agents (Nondepolarizing); P-glycoprotein/ABCB1 Inhibitors; Pimecrolimus; Quinolone Antibiotics; Roflumilast; Salicylates; Tacrolimus (Topical); Telaprevir; Trastuzumab

Decreased Effect

Hydrocortisone (Systemic) may decrease the levels/ effects of: Aldesleukin; Antidiabetic Agents; ARIPiprazole; Axitinib; BCG; Calcitriol; Coccidioidin Skin Test; Corticorelin; Hyaluronidase; Isoniazid; Salicylates; Sipuleucel-T; Telaprevir; Vaccines (Inactivated)

The levels/effects of Hydrocortisone (Systemic) may be decreased by: Aminoglutethimide; Antacids; Barbiturates; Bile Acid Sequestrants; Echinacea; Mifepristone; Mitotane; P-glycoprotein/ABCB1 Inducers; Primidone; Rifamycin Derivatives

Ethanol/Nutrition/Herb Interactions

Ethanol: Avoid ethanol (may enhance gastric mucosal irritation).

Food: Hydrocortisone interferes with calcium absorption.

Herb/Nutraceutical: St John's wort may decrease hydrocortisone levels. Avoid cat's claw, echinacea (have immunostimulant properties).

Dietary Considerations Systemic use of corticosteroids may require a diet with increased potassium, vitamins A, B_6, C, D, folate, calcium, zinc, phosphorus, and decreased sodium. Some products may contain sodium.

Pharmacodynamics/Kinetics

Onset of Action Hydrocortisone sodium succinate (water soluble): Rapid

Half-life Elimination Biologic: 8-12 hours

Pregnancy Risk Factor C

Pregnancy Considerations Adverse events have been observed with corticosteroids in animal reproduction studies. Hydrocortisone crosses the placenta. Some studies have shown an association between first trimester systemic corticosteroid use and oral clefts; adverse events in the fetus/neonate have been noted in case reports following large doses of systemic corticosteroids during pregnancy.

Lactation Enters breast milk/use caution

Breast-Feeding Considerations Corticosteroids are excreted in breast milk and endogenous hydrocortisone is also found in human milk; the effect of maternal hydrocortisone intake is not known.

Dosage Forms

Injection, powder for reconstitution:
A-Hydrocort®: 100 mg
Solu-CORTEF®: 100 mg

Injection, powder for reconstitution [preservative free]:
Solu-CORTEF®: 100 mg, 250 mg, 500 mg, 1000 mg
Tablet, oral: 5 mg, 10 mg, 20 mg
Cortef®: 5 mg, 10 mg, 20 mg

Hydrocortisone (Topical) (hye droe KOR ti sone)

Brand Names: U.S. Ala-Cort; Ala-Scalp; Anu-med HC; Anucort-HC™; Anusol-HC®; Aquanil HC® [OTC]; Beta-HC® [OTC]; Caldecort® [OTC]; Colocort®; Cortaid® Advanced [OTC]; Cortaid® Intensive Therapy [OTC]; Cortaid® Maximum Strength [OTC]; Cortenema®; CortiCool® [OTC]; Cortifoam®; Cortizone-10® Hydratensive Healing [OTC]; Cortizone-10® Hydratensive Soothing [OTC]; Cortizone-10® Intensive Healing Eczema [OTC]; Cortizone-10® Maximum Strength Cooling Relief [OTC]; Cortizone-10® Maximum Strength Easy Relief [OTC]; Cortizone-10® Maximum Strength Intensive Healing Formula [OTC]; Cortizone-10® Maximum Strength [OTC]; Cortizone-10® Plus Maximum Strength [OTC]; Dermarest® Eczema Medicated [OTC]; Hemril® -30; Hydrocortisone Plus [OTC]; Hydro-SKIN® [OTC]; Locoid Lipocream®; Locoid®; Pandel®; Pediaderm™ HC; Preparation H® Hydrocortisone [OTC]; Procto-Pak™; Proctocort®; ProctoCream®-HC; Proctosol-HC®; Proctozone-HC 2.5%™; Recort [OTC]; Scalpana [OTC]; Texacort™; U-Cort®; Westcort®

Brand Names: Canada Aquacort®; Cortamed®; Cortenema®; Cortifoam™; Emo-Cort®; Hycort™; Hyderm; HydroVal®; Locoid®; Prevex® HC; Sarna® HC; Westcort®

Generic Availability (U.S.) Yes: Excludes foam (acetate), cream (probutate), gel (base), liquid (base), lotion (base), lotion (butyrate), solution (base)

Pharmacologic Category Corticosteroid, Rectal; Corticosteroid, Topical

Use Relief of inflammation of corticosteroid-responsive dermatoses (low and medium potency topical corticosteroid); adjunctive treatment of ulcerative colitis; mild-to-moderate atopic dermatitis; inflamed hemorrhoids, postirradiation (factitial) proctitis, and other inflammatory conditions of anorectum and pruritus ani

Local Anesthetic/Vasoconstrictor Precautions No information available to require special precautions

Effects on Dental Treatment No significant effects or complications reported

Effects on Bleeding No information available to require special precautions

Adverse Effects Frequency not defined. Local adverse events presented. Adverse events similar to those observed with systemic absorption are also observed, especially following rectal use. Refer to the Hydrocortisone (Systemic) monograph for details.

Cream, ointment: Acneiform eruptions, burning, dryness, folliculitis, hypertrichosis, hypopigmentation, irritation, itching, maceration of skin, miliaria, perioral dermatitis, secondary infection, skin atrophy, striae

Enema: Burning, pain, rectal bleeding

Suppositories: Allergic contact dermatitis, burning, dryness, folliculitis, hypopigmentation, itching, secondary infection

Dental Usual Dosage Treatment of a variety of oral diseases of allergic, inflammatory, or autoimmune origin: Children >2 years and Adults: Topical: Apply to affected area 2-4 times/day

Dosage
Topical:
Children 3 months to 18 years: Atopic dermatitis: Hydrocortisone butyrate (Locoid Lipocream®): Apply thin film to affected area twice daily
Children and Adults: Dermatosis: Apply thin film to affected area 2-4 times/day. Products labeled for OTC use (self-medication) should not be used in children <2 years of age.
Children ≥12 years and Adults: External anal and genital itching: (OTC labeling): Apply to clean dry skin up to 3-4 times/day
Adults: Dermatosis:
Hydrocortisone probutate (Pandel®): Apply thin film to affected area 1-2 times/day
Hydrocortisone valerate (Westcort®): Apply thin film to affected area 2-3 times/day
Rectal: Adults:
Hemorrhoids: Suppository: One suppository (30 mg) twice daily for 2 weeks. For severe cases of proctitis, 1 suppository 3 times/day or 2 suppositories twice daily may be needed. For factitial proctitis, duration of treatment may be up to 6-8 weeks.
Ulcerative colitis:
Foam: One applicatorful (80 mg) 1-2 times/day for 2-3 weeks, and then every other day thereafter; use lowest dose to maintain clinical response; taper dose to discontinue long-term therapy
Suspension: One enema (100 mg) every night for 21 days or until remission (clinical improvement may precede improvement of mucosal integrity); 2-3 months of therapy may be required; taper dose to discontinue long-term therapy
Mechanism of Action Decreases inflammation by suppression of migration of polymorphonuclear leukocytes and reversal of increased capillary permeability
Contraindications Hypersensitivity to any component of the formulation.

Rectal enema: Systemic fungal infections; ileocolostomy during the immediate or early postoperative period

Cortifoam® is also contraindicated with obstruction, abscess, perforation, peritonitis, fresh intestinal anastomoses, extensive fistulas and sinus tracts (other enemas are labeled to be used with caution).

Warnings/Precautions May cause hypercorticism or suppression of hypothalamic-pituitary-adrenal (HPA) axis, particularly in younger children or in patients receiving high doses for prolonged periods. HPA axis suppression may lead to adrenal crisis. Withdrawal and discontinuation of a corticosteroid should be done slowly and carefully. Children may absorb proportionally larger amounts after topical application and may be more prone to systemic effects. HPA axis suppression, intracranial hypertension, and Cushing's syndrome have been reported in children receiving topical corticosteroids. Prolonged use may affect growth velocity; growth should be routinely monitored in pediatric patients. Rare cases of anaphylactoid reactions have been observed in patients receiving corticosteroids.

Prolonged use of corticosteroids may increase the incidence of secondary infection, mask acute infection (including fungal infections), prolong or exacerbate viral infections, or limit response to vaccines. Exposure to chickenpox should be avoided. Close observation is required in patients with latent tuberculosis and/or TB reactivity; restrict use in active TB (only in conjunction with antituberculosis treatment). Prolonged treatment with corticosteroids has been also associated with the development of Kaposi's sarcoma (case reports); if noted, discontinuation of therapy should be considered. Prolonged use of corticosteroids may produce cataracts or glaucoma and may enhance the establishment of secondary ocular infections Use caution with ocular herpes simplex.

Acute myopathy has been reported with high-dose corticosteroids, usually in patients with neuromuscular transmission disorders; may involve ocular and/or respiratory muscles; monitor creatine kinase; recovery may be delayed. Corticosteroid use may cause psychiatric disturbances, including depression, euphoria, insomnia, mood swings, and personality changes. Pre-existing psychiatric conditions may be exacerbated by corticosteroid use.

Use with caution in patients with hypertension, GI diseases (diverticulitis, peptic ulcer), hepatic impairment (including cirrhosis), osteoporosis, myasthenia gravis, osteoporosis, renal impairment, or thyroid disease. In patients with severe ulcerative colitis, it may be hazardous to delay surgery while waiting for response to treatment.

Topical corticosteroids may be absorbed percutaneously. Absorption is increased by the use of occlusive dressings, application to denuded skin, or application to large surface areas. Avoid use of topical preparations with occlusive dressings or on weeping or exudative lesions. Topical use has been associated with local sensitization (redness, irritation); discontinue if sensitization is noted. Because of the risk of adverse effects associated with systemic absorption, topical corticosteroids should be used cautiously in the elderly in the smallest possible effective dose for the shortest duration.

Rectal enema: Damage to the rectal wall may occur from improper or careless insertion of the enema tip.

Self-medication (OTC use): Contact healthcare provider if condition worsens, symptoms persist for >7 days, or rectal bleeding occurs. Consult with healthcare provider prior to use if needed for diaper rash.
Drug Interactions
Metabolism/Transport Effects Substrate of CYP3A4 (minor); **Note:** Assignment of Major/Minor substrate status based on clinically relevant drug interaction potential
Avoid Concomitant Use
Avoid concomitant use of Hydrocortisone (Topical) with any of the following: Aldesleukin
Increased Effect/Toxicity
Hydrocortisone (Topical) may increase the levels/effects of: Deferasirox

The levels/effects of Hydrocortisone (Topical) may be increased by: Telaprevir
Decreased Effect
Hydrocortisone (Topical) may decrease the levels/effects of: Aldesleukin; Corticorelin; Hyaluronidase; Telaprevir
Pregnancy Risk Factor C
Pregnancy Considerations Adverse events have been observed with corticosteroids in animal reproduction studies. Topical products are not recommended for extensive use, in large quantities, or for long periods of time in pregnant women (Reed, 1997).
Lactation Enters breast milk/use caution

Breast-Feeding Considerations Systemically administered corticosteroids are excreted in breast milk and endogenous hydrocortisone is also found in human milk. It is not known if systemic absorption following topical administration results in detectable quantities in human milk. Use with caution while breast-feeding; do not apply to nipples (Reed, 1997).

Dosage Forms

Aerosol, foam, rectal:
Cortifoam®: 10% (15 g)

Cream, topical: 0.1% (15 g, 45 g); 0.2% (15 g, 45 g, 60 g); 0.5% (0.9 g, 15 g, 28.4 g, 30 g, 60 g); 1% (0.9 g, 1 g, 1.5 g, 15 g, 20 g, 28.35 g, 28.4 g, 30 g, 114 g, 120 g, 454 g); 2% (43 g); 2.5% (20 g, 28 g, 28.35 g, 30 g, 454 g)
Ala-Cort: 1% (28.4 g, 85.2 g)
Anusol-HC®: 2.5% (30 g)
Caldecort® [OTC]: 1% (28.4 g)
Cortaid® Advanced [OTC]: 1% (42 g)
Cortaid® Intensive Therapy [OTC]: 1% (37 g, 56 g)
Cortaid® Maximum Strength [OTC]: 1% (14 g, 28 g, 37 g, 56 g)
Cortizone-10® Maximum Strength [OTC]: 1% (15 g, 28 g, 56 g)
Cortizone-10® Maximum Strength Intensive Healing Formula [OTC]: 1% (28 g, 56 g)
Cortizone-10® Plus Maximum Strength [OTC]: 1% (28 g, 56 g)
Hydrocortisone Plus [OTC]: 1% (28.4 g)
HydroSKIN® [OTC]: 1% (28 g)
Locoid Lipocream®: 0.1% (45 g, 60 g)
Pandel®: 0.1% (15 g, 45 g, 80 g)
Preparation H® Hydrocortisone [OTC]: 1% (26 g)
Procto-Pak™: 1% (28.4 g)
Proctocort®: 1% (28.35 g)
ProctoCream®-HC: 2.5% (30 g)
Proctosol-HC®: 2.5% (28.35 g)
Proctozone-HC 2.5%™: 2.5% (30 g)
Recort [OTC]: 1% (30 g)
U-Cort®: 1% (28 g)

Gel, topical:
CortiCool® [OTC]: 1% (0.9 g, 42.5 g)
Cortizone-10® Maximum Strength Cooling Relief [OTC]: 1% (28 g)

Liquid, topical:
Cortizone-10® Maximum Strength Easy Relief [OTC]: 1% (36 mL)
Scalpana [OTC]: 1% (85.5 mL)

Lotion, topical: 1% (114 g, 118 mL, 120 mL); 2.5% (59 mL, 60 mL, 118 mL)
Ala-Scalp: 2% (29.6 mL)
Aquanil HC® [OTC]: 1% (120 mL)
Beta-HC® [OTC]: 1% (60 mL)
Cortaid® Intensive Therapy [OTC]: 1% (98 g)
Cortizone-10® Hydratensive Healing [OTC]: 1% (113 g)
Cortizone-10® Hydratensive Soothing [OTC]: 1% (113 g)
Cortizone-10® Intensive Healing Eczema [OTC]: 1% (99 g)
Dermarest® Eczema Medicated [OTC]: 1% (118 mL)
HydroSKIN® [OTC]: 1% (118 mL)
Locoid®: 0.1% (60 mL)
Pediaderm™ HC: 2% (29.6 mL)

Ointment, topical: 0.1% (15 g, 45 g); 0.2% (15 g, 45 g, 60 g); 0.5% (30 g); 1% (25 g, 28.4 g, 30 g, 110 g, 430 g, 454 g); 2.5% (20 g, 28.35 g, 30 g, 454 g)
Cortaid® Maximum Strength [OTC]: 1% (28 g, 37 g)
Cortizone-10® Maximum Strength [OTC]: 1% (28 g, 56 g)
Locoid®: 0.1% (15 g, 45 g)
Westcort®: 0.2% (45 g, 60 g)

Powder, for prescription compounding: USP: 100% (10 g, 25 g, 50 g, 100 g, 1000 g)

Solution, topical: 0.1% (20 mL, 60 mL)
Cortaid® Intensive Therapy [OTC]: 1% (59 mL)
Locoid®: 0.1% (20 mL, 60 mL)
Texacort™: 2.5% (30 mL)

Suppository, rectal: 25 mg (12s, 24s, 1000s); 30 mg (12s)
Anu-med HC: 25 mg (12s)
Anucort-HC™: 25 mg (12s, 24s, 100s)
Anusol-HC®: 25 mg (12s, 24s)
Hemril® -30: 30 mg (12s, 24s)
Proctocort®: 30 mg (12s, 24s)

Suspension, rectal: 100 mg/60 mL (60 mL)
Colocort®: 100 mg/60 mL (60 mL)
Cortenema®: 100 mg/60 mL (60 mL)

HYDROmorphone (hye droe MOR fone)

Related Information
Oral Pain on page 1558
Oxymorphone on page 1037

Brand Names: U.S. Dilaudid-HP®; Dilaudid®; Exalgo®

Brand Names: Canada Dilaudid-HP®; Dilaudid®; Hydromorph Contin®; Hydromorphone HP; Hydromorphone HP® 10; Hydromorphone HP® 20; Hydromorphone HP® 50; Hydromorphone HP® Forte; Hydromorphone Hydrochloride Injection, USP; Jurnista™; PMS-Hydromorphone; Teva-Hydromorphone

Pharmacologic Category Analgesic, Opioid

Use Management of moderate-to-severe pain

Exalgo®: Management of moderate-to-severe pain in opioid-tolerant patients (requiring around-the-clock analgesia for an extended period of time)

Local Anesthetic/Vasoconstrictor Precautions No information available to require special precautions

Effects on Dental Treatment Key adverse event(s) related to dental treatment: Xerostomia (normal salivary flow resumes upon discontinuation).

Effects on Bleeding No information available to require special precautions

Adverse Effects Frequency not defined.

Cardiovascular: Bradycardia, extrasystoles, flushing of face, hyper-/hypotension, palpitation, peripheral edema, peripheral vasodilation, syncope, tachycardia

Central nervous system: Abnormal dreams, abnormal feelings, agitation, aggression, apprehension, attention disturbances, chills, coordination impaired, CNS depression, confusion, cognitive disorder, crying, dizziness, drowsiness, dysphoria, encephalopathy, euphoria, fatigue, hallucinations, headache, hyper-reflexia, hypo/hyperesthesia, hypothermia, increased intracranial pressure, insomnia, lightheadedness, listlessness, malaise, memory impairment, mental depression, mood alterations, nervousness, panic attacks, paranoia, psychomotor hyperactivity, restlessness, sedation, seizure, somnolence, suicide ideation, vertigo

Dermatologic: Hyperhidrosis, pruritus, rash, urticaria

Endocrine & metabolic: Amylase decreased, dehydration, erectile dysfunction, fluid retention, hyperuricemia, hypogonadism, hypokalemia, libido decreased, sexual dysfunction, testosterone decreased

Gastrointestinal: Abdominal distention, anal fissure, anorexia, appetite decreased/increased, bezoar (Exalgo®), biliary tract spasm, constipation, diarrhea, diverticulum, diverticulitis, duodenitis, dysgeusia, dysphagia, eructation, flatulence, gastric emptying impaired, gastrointestinal motility disorder (Exalgo®), gastroenteritis, hematochezia, ileus, intestinal obstruction (Exalgo®), large intestine perforation (Exalgo®), nausea, painful defecation, paralytic ileus, stomach cramps, taste perversion, vomiting, weight loss, xerostomia

Genitourinary: Dysuria, micturition disorder, ureteral spasm, urinary frequency, urinary hesitation, urinary retention, urinary tract spasm, urination decreased

Hepatic: LFTs increased

Local: Pain at injection site (I.M.), wheal/flare over vein (I.V.)

Neuromuscular & skeletal: Arthralgia, dysarthria, dyskinesia, muscle rigidity, muscle spasms, myalgia, myoclonus, paresthesia, trembling, tremor, uncoordinated muscle movements, weakness

Ocular: Blurred vision, diplopia, dry eyes, miosis, nystagmus

Otic: Tinnitus

Respiratory: Apnea, bronchospasm, dyspnea, hyperventilation, hypoxia, laryngospasm, oxygen saturation decreased, respiratory depression/distress, rhinorrhea

Miscellaneous: Antidiuretic effects, balance disorder, diaphoresis, difficulty walking, histamine release, physical and psychological dependence

General Dosage Range Dosage adjustment recommended in patients with hepatic or renal impairment

I.M., SubQ: *Children >50 kg and Adults:* 0.8-1 mg every 3-4 hours

I.V.: *Children >50 kg and Adults:* 0.2-0.6 mg every 2-3 hours as needed

Oral:

Children >50 kg: 2-4 mg every 4 hours as needed

Adults: 2-4 mg every 4 hours as needed; Extended release: 8-64 mg every 24 hours

Elderly: Initiation at the low end of dosage range is recommended

Rectal: *Children >50 kg and Adults:* 3 mg every 6-8 hours as needed

Mechanism of Action Binds to opioid receptors in the CNS, causing inhibition of ascending pain pathways, altering the perception of and response to pain; causes cough supression by direct central action in the medulla; produces generalized CNS depression

Pharmacodynamics/Kinetics

Onset of Action Analgesic:

Immediate release formulations:

Oral: 15-30 minutes; Peak effect: 30-60 minutes

I.V.: 5 minutes; Peak effect: 10-20 minutes

Extended release tablet: 6 hours; Peak effect: ~9 hours (Angst, 2001)

Duration of Action

Immediate release formulations: Oral, I.V.: 3-4 hours

Extended release tablet: ~13 hours (Angst, 2001)

Half-life Elimination

Immediate release formulations: 2-3 hours

Extended release tablets: Apparent half-life: ~11 hours (range: 8-15 hours)

Time to Peak Plasma:

Immediate release tablet: ≤1 hour

Extended release tablet: 12-16 hours

Pregnancy Risk Factor C

Pregnancy Considerations Hydromorphone was teratogenic in some, but not all, animal studies; however, maternal toxicity was also reported. Hydromorphone crosses the placenta. Chronic opioid use during pregnancy may lead to a withdrawal syndrome in the neonate. Symptoms include irritability, hyperactivity, loss of sleep pattern, abnormal crying, tremor, vomiting, diarrhea, weight loss, or failure to gain weight.

Controlled Substance C-II

Prescribing and Access Restrictions Exalgo®: As a requirement of the REMS program, healthcare providers who prescribe Exalgo® need to receive training on the proper use and potential risks of Exalgo®. For training, please refer to http://www.exalgorems.com. Prescribers will need retraining every 2 years or following any significant changes to the Exalgo® REMS program.

Hydroquinone (HYE droe kwin one)

Brand Names: U.S. Aclaro PD®; Aclaro®; Alphaquin HP®; Eldopaque Forte®; Eldopaque® [OTC]; Eldoquin Forte®; Eldoquin® [OTC]; EpiQuin® Micro; Esoterica® Daytime [OTC]; Esoterica® Nighttime [OTC]; Lustra-AF®; Lustra-Ultra™; Lustra®; Melpaque HP®; Melquin HP®; Melquin-3®; NeoStrata® HQ Skin Lightening [OTC]; Nuquin HP®; Palmer's® Skin Success® Eventone® Fade Cream [OTC]; Palmer's® Skin Success® Eventone® Fade Milk [OTC]; Palmer's® Skin Success® Eventone® Ultra Fade Serum [OTC]

Brand Names: Canada Eldopaque®; Eldoquin®; Glyquin® XM; Lustra®; NeoStrata® HQ; Solaquin Forte®; Solaquin®; Ultraquin™

Pharmacologic Category Depigmenting Agent

Use Gradual bleaching of hyperpigmented skin conditions

Local Anesthetic/Vasoconstrictor Precautions No information available to require special precautions

Effects on Dental Treatment No significant effects or complications reported

Effects on Bleeding No information available to require special precautions

Adverse Effects Frequency not defined.

Dermatologic: Dermatitis, dryness, erythema, stinging, inflammatory reaction, sensitization

Local: Irritation

General Dosage Range Topical: *Children >12 years and Adults:* Apply thin layer and rub in twice daily

Mechanism of Action Produces reversible depigmentation of the skin by suppression of melanocyte metabolic processes, in particular the inhibition of the enzymatic oxidation of tyrosine to DOPA (3,4-dihydroxyphenylalanine); sun exposure reverses this effect and will cause repigmentation.

Pharmacodynamics/Kinetics

Onset of Action Onset of depigmentation produced by hydroquinone varies among individuals

Duration of Action Onset and duration of depigmentation produced by hydroquinone varies among individuals

Pregnancy Risk Factor C

Pregnancy Considerations Animal reproduction studies have not been conducted with topical administration; the amount of systemic absorption is unknown.

Hydroxocobalamin (hye droks oh koe BAL a min)

Brand Names: U.S. Cyanokit®

Brand Names: Canada Cyanokit®

Pharmacologic Category Antidote; Vitamin, Water Soluble

Use

I.M. injection: Treatment of pernicious anemia; treatment of vitamin B_{12} deficiency due to dietary deficiencies or malabsorption diseases, inadequate secretion of intrinsic factor, competition for vitamin B_{12} by intestinal parasites/bacteria, or inadequate utilization of B_{12} (eg, during neoplastic treatment)

I.V. infusion (Cyanokit®): Treatment of cyanide poisoning (known or suspected)

Local Anesthetic/Vasoconstrictor Precautions No information available to require special precautions

Effects on Dental Treatment No significant effects or complications reported

Effects on Bleeding No information available to require special precautions

Adverse Effects

I.M. injection: Frequency not defined:

Dermatologic: Exanthema (transient), itching

Gastrointestinal: Diarrhea (mild, transient)

Local: Injection site pain

Miscellaneous: Anaphylaxis, feeling of swelling of the entire body

I.V. infusion (Cyanokit®):

>10%:

Cardiovascular: Blood pressure increased (18% to 28%)

Central nervous system: Headache (6% to 33%)

Dermatologic: Erythema (94% to 100%; may last up to 2 weeks), rash (predominantly acneiform; 20% to 44%; can appear 7-28 days after administration and usually resolves within a few weeks)

Gastrointestinal: Nausea (6% to 11%)

Genitourinary: Chromaturia (100%; may last up to 5 weeks after administration)

Hematologic: Lymphocytes decreased (8% to 17%)

Local: Infusion site reaction (6% to 39%)

Frequency not defined:

Cardiovascular: Chest discomfort, hot flashes, peripheral edema

Central nervous system: Dizziness, memory impairment, restlessness

Dermatologic: Pruritus, urticaria

Gastrointestinal: Abdominal discomfort, diarrhea, dyspepsia, dysphagia, hematochezia, vomiting

Ocular: Irritation, redness, swelling

Respiratory: Dry throat, dyspnea, throat tightness

Miscellaneous: Allergic reaction (including anaphylaxis)

General Dosage Range

I.M.:

Children: Initial: 100 mcg once daily for ≥2 weeks (total dose: 1-5 **mg**); maintenance: 30-50 mcg once per month

Adults: Initial: 30 mcg once daily for 5-10 days; maintenance: 100-200 mcg once per month **or** 1000 mcg once

I.V.: *Adults:* 5 **g** as a single infusion; may repeat if needed (maximum: 10 **g** cumulative dose)

Mechanism of Action Hydroxocobalamin (vitamin B_{12a}) is a precursor to cyanocobalamin (vitamin B_{12}). Cyanocobalamin acts as a coenzyme for various metabolic functions, including fat and carbohydrate metabolism and protein synthesis, used in cell replication and hematopoiesis. In the presence of cyanide, each hydroxocobalamin molecule can bind one cyanide ion by displacing it for the hydroxo ligand linked to the trivalent cobalt ion, forming cyanocobalamin, which is then excreted in the urine.

Pharmacodynamics/Kinetics

Half-life Elimination 26-31 hours

Pregnancy Risk Factor C

Pregnancy Considerations Animal studies are insufficient to determine the effect, if any, on pregnancy or fetal development. There are no adequate and well-controlled studies in pregnant women. Data on the use of hydroxocobalamin in pregnancy for the treatment of cyanide poisoning and cobalamin defects are limited. In general, medications used as antidotes should take into consideration the health and prognosis of the mother (Bailey, 2003).

Hydroxyamphetamine and Tropicamide (hye droks ee am FET a meen & troe PIK a mide)

Related Information

Tropicamide *on page 1369*

Brand Names: U.S. Paremyd®

Pharmacologic Category Adrenergic Agonist Agent, Ophthalmic

Use Short-term pupil dilation for diagnostic procedures and exams

Local Anesthetic/Vasoconstrictor Precautions No information available to require special precautions

Effects on Dental Treatment No significant effects or complications reported

Effects on Bleeding No information available to require special precautions

Adverse Effects Frequency not defined (as reported with Paremyd® or similar medications):

Cardiovascular: Hypotension, MI, pallor, tachycardia, ventricular fibrillation

Central nervous system: Behavioral disturbances, headache, psychotic reactions

Gastrointestinal: Dry mouth, nausea, vomiting

Neuromuscular & skeletal: Muscle rigidity

Ocular: Blurred vision, intraocular pressure increased, photophobia, transient stinging

Miscellaneous: Allergic reaction, cardiorespiratory collapse, vasomotor collapse

General Dosage Range Ophthalmic: *Adults:* Instill 1-2 drops into conjunctival sac(s)

Mechanism of Action Hydroxyamphetamine hydrobromide is an indirect acting sympathomimetic agent which causes the release of norepinephrine from adrenergic nerve terminals, resulting in mydriasis. Tropicamide is a parasympatholytic agent which produces mydriasis and paralysis by blocking the sphincter muscle in the iris and the ciliary muscle.

Pharmacodynamics/Kinetics

Onset of Action 15 minutes

Duration of Action 3 hours; complete recovery usually occurs in 6-8 hours, but may take up to 24 hours

Time to Peak 60 minutes

Pregnancy Risk Factor C

Pregnancy Considerations Animal reproduction studies have not been conducted.

Hydroxychloroquine (hye droks ee KLOR oh kwin)

Related Information

Rheumatoid Arthritis, Osteoarthritis, and Osteoporosis *on page 1526*

Brand Names: U.S. Plaquenil®

◄ **Brand Names: Canada** Apo-Hydroxyquine®; Gen-Hydroxychloroquine; Mylan-Hydroxychloroquine; Pla-quenil®; PRO-Hydroxyquine

Pharmacologic Category Aminoquinoline (Antimalarial)

Use Suppression and treatment of acute attacks of malaria; treatment of systemic lupus erythematosus (SLE) and rheumatoid arthritis

Unlabeled Use Porphyria cutanea tarda, polymorphous light eruptions

Local Anesthetic/Vasoconstrictor Precautions No information available to require special precautions

Effects on Dental Treatment No significant effects or complications reported

Effects on Bleeding Hematologic adverse effects such as anemia, aplastic anemia, and thrombocytopenia are rare.

Adverse Effects Frequency not defined.

Cardiovascular: Cardiomyopathy (rare, relationship to hydroxychloroquine unclear)

Central nervous system: Ataxia, dizziness, emotional changes, headache, irritability, lassitude, nervousness, nightmares, psychosis, seizure, vertigo

Dermatologic: Alopecia, angioedema, bleaching of hair, pigmentation changes (skin and mucosal; black-blue color), rash (acute generalized exanthematous pustulosis, erythema annulare centrifugum, exfoliative dermatitis, lichenoid, maculopapular, morbilliform, purpuric, Stevens-Johnson syndrome, urticarial), urticaria

Gastrointestinal: Abdominal cramping, anorexia, diarrhea, nausea, vomiting, weight loss

Hematologic: Agranulocytosis, aplastic anemia, hemolysis (in patients with glucose-6-phosphate deficiency), leukopenia, thrombocytopenia

Hepatic: Abnormal liver function/hepatic failure (isolated cases)

Neuromuscular & skeletal: Myopathy, palsy, or neuromyopathy leading to progressive weakness and atrophy of proximal muscle groups (may be associated with mild sensory changes, loss of deep tendon reflexes, and abnormal nerve conduction)

Ocular: Abnormal color vision, abnormal retinal pigmentation, atrophy, attenuation of retinal arterioles, corneal changes/deposits (visual disturbances, blurred vision, photophobia [reversible on discontinuation]), decreased visual acuity, disturbance in accommodation, keratopathy, macular edema, nystagmus, optic disc pallor/atrophy, pigmentary retinopathy, retinopathy (early changes reversible [may progress despite discontinuation if advanced]), scotoma

Otic: Deafness, tinnitus

Miscellaneous: Exacerbation of porphyria and nonlight sensitive psoriasis

Respiratory: Bronchospasm, respiratory failure (myopathy-related)

General Dosage Range Oral:

Children: 13 mg/kg for 1-2 doses, followed by 6.5 mg/kg for 3 doses or once weekly

Adults: Initial: 400-800 mg/day divided 1-2 times/day; Maintenance: 200-400 mg/day **or** 800 mg for 1-2 doses, followed by 400 mg for 3 doses or once weekly

Mechanism of Action Interferes with digestive vacuole function within sensitive malarial parasites by increasing the pH and interfering with lysosomal degradation of hemoglobin; inhibits locomotion of neutrophils and chemotaxis of eosinophils; impairs complement-dependent antigen-antibody reactions

Pharmacodynamics/Kinetics

Onset of Action Rheumatic disease: May require 4-6 weeks to respond

Half-life Elimination 32-50 days

Time to Peak Rheumatic disease: Several months

Pregnancy Considerations Malaria infection in pregnant women may be more severe than in nonpregnant women. Therefore, pregnant women and women who are likely to become pregnant are advised to avoid travel to malaria-risk areas. Hydroxychloroquine is recommended as an alternative treatment of pregnant women for uncomplicated malaria in chloroquine-sensitive regions. Women exposed to hydroxychloroquine for the treatment of rheumatoid arthritis or systemic lupus erythematosus during pregnancy may be enrolled in the Organization of Teratology Information Specialists (OTIS) Autoimmune Diseases Study pregnancy registry (877-311-8972).

Hydroxyprogesterone Caproate
(hye droks ee proe JES te rone CAP ro ate)

Brand Names: U.S. Makena™

Pharmacologic Category Progestin

Use To reduce the risk of preterm birth in women with singleton pregnancies who have a history of spontaneous preterm birth (delivery <37 weeks gestation) with previous singleton pregnancies

Local Anesthetic/Vasoconstrictor Precautions No information available to require special precautions

Effects on Dental Treatment No significant effects or complications reported

Effects on Bleeding No information available to require special precautions

Adverse Effects

>10%:
Dermatologic: Urticaria (12%)
Local: Injection site: Pain (35%), swelling (17%)
1% to 10%:
Dermatologic: Pruritus (8%)
Gastrointestinal: Nausea (6%), diarrhea (2%)
Local: Injection site pruritus (6%), nodule (5%)

General Dosage Range I.M.: *Pregnant females:* 250 mg every 7 days

Pharmacodynamics/Kinetics

Half-life Elimination Nonpregnant females: ~8 days; Pregnant females (singleton pregnancies): 16 days (range: 11-21 days) (Caritis, 2012)

Time to Peak Serum: I.M.: Nonpregnant females: 3-7 days; Pregnant females (singleton pregnancies): 1-4 days (Caritis, 2012)

Pregnancy Risk Factor B

Pregnancy Considerations Teratogenic events were not observed in animal reproduction studies; embryolethality was observed in some species. Teratogenic effects were not observed in human studies following second or third trimester exposure; first trimester data not available.

Maternal serum concentrations of hydroxyprogesterone caproate are widely variable and may be decreased in women with increased BMI. Hydroxyprogesterone is metabolized by the placenta and reaches the fetal circulation. In one study, the cord:maternal concentration ratio averaged 0.2. Hydroxyprogesterone caproate was detected in cord blood when delivery occurred ≥44 days after the last injection (Cartitis, 2012; Hemauer, 2008).

Prescribing and Access Restrictions The Makena Care Connection™ is a comprehensive program for patients and healthcare providers which provides administrative support (including insurance benefit investigation and prescription fulfillment); financial and co-pay assistance for eligible patients; and treatment support (including educational information, home health care service and scheduled treatment reminders). The Makena Care Connection™ is available by calling 1-800-847-3418, Monday-Friday, 8 AM to 9 PM EST.

Hydroxypropyl Cellulose
(hye droks ee PROE pil SEL yoo lose)

Related Information
Hydroxypropyl Methylcellulose *on page 705*

Brand Names: U.S. Lacrisert®

Brand Names: Canada Lacrisert®

Pharmacologic Category Ophthalmic Agent, Miscellaneous

Use Dry eyes (moderate-to-severe)

Local Anesthetic/Vasoconstrictor Precautions No information available to require special precautions

Effects on Dental Treatment No significant effects or complications reported

Effects on Bleeding No information available to require special precautions

Adverse Effects Frequency not defined: Ocular: Local irritation, blurred vision, edema of the eyelids

General Dosage Range Ophthalmic: *Adults:* Apply once daily

Pregnancy Considerations Hydroxypropyl cellulose is physiologically inert and is not metabolized. It was not absorbed following oral administration in animal studies. Systemic absorption would be required in order for hydroxypropyl cellulose to cross the placenta and reach the fetus.

Hydroxypropyl Methylcellulose
(hye droks ee PROE pil meth il SEL yoo lose)

Related Information
Hydroxypropyl Cellulose *on page 705*

Brand Names: U.S. Cellugel®; GenTeal® Mild [OTC]; GenTeal® [OTC]; Gonak™; Goniosoft™ [OTC]; Isopto® Tears [OTC]; Natural Balance Tears [OTC]; Nature's Tears [OTC]; Tears Again® MC Gel Drops™ [OTC]

Brand Names: Canada Genteal®; Isopto® Tears

Pharmacologic Category Diagnostic Agent, Ophthalmic; Lubricant, Ocular

Use Relief of burning and minor irritation due to dry eyes; diagnostic agent in gonioscopic examination

Local Anesthetic/Vasoconstrictor Precautions No information available to require special precautions

Effects on Dental Treatment No significant effects or complications reported

Effects on Bleeding No information available to require special precautions

General Dosage Range Ophthalmic: *Adults:* Instill 1-2 drops in affected eye(s) as needed

Hydroxyurea (hye droks ee yoor EE a)

Brand Names: U.S. Droxia®; Hydrea®

Brand Names: Canada Apo-Hydroxyurea®; Gen-Hydroxyurea; Hydrea®; Mylan-Hydroxyurea

Pharmacologic Category Antineoplastic Agent, Antimetabolite

Use Treatment of melanoma, refractory chronic myelocytic leukemia (CML); recurrent, metastatic, or inoperable ovarian cancer; management (with concomitant radiation therapy) of squamous cell head and neck cancer (excluding lip cancer); management of sickle cell patients who have had at least three painful crises in the previous 12 months (to reduce frequency of these crises and the need for blood transfusions)

Unlabeled Use Treatment of essential thrombocythemia, polycythemia vera, hypereosinophilic syndrome; management of hyperleukocytosis due to acute myeloid leukemia (AML); treatment of AML in poor-risk patients; treatment of meningiomas

Local Anesthetic/Vasoconstrictor Precautions No information available to require special precautions

Effects on Dental Treatment No significant effects or complications reported

Effects on Bleeding Can cause life-threatening anemia and thrombocytopenia. Usually resolves within 14 days of discontinuation. Used to treat thrombocytosis. Medical consult recommended.

Adverse Effects Frequency not defined.

Cardiovascular: Edema

Central nervous system: Chills, disorientation, dizziness, drowsiness (dose-related), fever, hallucinations, headache, malaise, seizure

Dermatologic: Alopecia, cutaneous vasculitic toxicities, dermatomyositis-like skin changes, facial erythema, gangrene, hyperpigmentation, maculopapular rash, nail atrophy, nail discoloration, peripheral erythema, scaling, skin atrophy, skin cancer, skin ulcer, vasculitis ulcerations, violet papules

Endocrine & metabolic: Hyperuricemia

Gastrointestinal: Anorexia, constipation, diarrhea, gastrointestinal irritation and mucositis, (potentiated with radiation therapy), nausea, pancreatitis, stomatitis, vomiting

Genitourinary: Dysuria

Hematologic: Myelosuppression (anemia, leukopenia/neutropenia [common], thrombocytopenia; hematologic recovery: within 2 weeks); macrocytosis, megaloblastic erythropoiesis, secondary leukemias (long-term use)

Hepatic: Hepatic enzymes increased, hepatotoxicity

Neuromuscular & skeletal: Peripheral neuropathy, weakness

Renal: BUN increased, creatinine increased, renal tubular dysfunction

Respiratory: Acute diffuse pulmonary infiltrates (rare), dyspnea, pulmonary fibrosis (rare)

General Dosage Range Dosage adjustment recommended in patients with renal impairment or who develop toxicities.

Oral: *Adults:* 15-35 mg/kg/day **or** 500-3000 mg/day as single or divided dose **or** 80 mg/kg as a single dose every third day

Mechanism of Action Antimetabolite which selectively inhibits ribonucleoside diphosphate reductase, preventing the conversion of ribonucleotides to deoxyribonucleotides, halting the cell cycle at the G1/S phase and therefore has radiation sensitizing activity by maintaining cells in the G_1 phase and interfering with DNA repair. In sickle cell anemia, hydroxyurea increases red blood cell (RBC) hemoglobin F levels, RBC water content, deformability of sickled cells, and alters adhesion of RBCs to endothelium.

Pharmacodynamics/Kinetics

Onset of Action Sickle cell anemia: Fetal hemoglobin increase: 4-12 weeks

Half-life Elimination 1.9-3.9 hours (Gwilt, 1998); Children: Sickle cell anemia: 1.7 hours (range: 0.7-3 hours) (Ware, 2011)

Time to Peak 1-4 hours

Pregnancy Risk Factor D

Pregnancy Considerations Animal reproduction studies have demonstrated teratogenicity and embryotoxicity at doses lower than the usual human dose (based on BSA). Hydroxyurea may cause fetal harm if administered during pregnancy. Women of childbearing potential should be advised to avoid becoming pregnant during treatment and should use effective contraception.

HydrOXYzine (hye DROKS i zeen)

Related Information
Management of the Patient With Anxiety or Depression *on page 1594*

Related Sample Prescriptions
Sedation (Prior to Dental Treatment) *on page 1621*

Brand Names: U.S. Vistaril®

Brand Names: Canada Apo-Hydroxyzine®; Atarax®; Hydroxyzine Hydrochloride Injection, USP; Novo-Hydroxyzin; Nu-Hydroxyzine; PMS-Hydroxyzine; Riva-Hydroxyzine

Generic Availability (U.S.) Yes

Pharmacologic Category Antiemetic; Histamine H_1 Antagonist; Histamine H_1 Antagonist, First Generation; Piperazine Derivative

Dental Use Treatment of anxiety, as a preoperative sedative in pediatric dentistry

Use Treatment of anxiety/agitation (including adjunctive therapy in alcoholism); adjunct to pre- and postoperative analgesia and anesthesia; antipruritic; antiemetic

Local Anesthetic/Vasoconstrictor Precautions No information available to require special precautions

Effects on Dental Treatment Key adverse event(s) related to dental treatment: Xerostomia (normal salivary flow resumes upon discontinuation).

Effects on Bleeding No information available to require special precautions

Adverse Effects Frequency not defined.

Central nervous system: Dizziness, drowsiness, fatigue, hallucination, headache, nervousness, seizure

Dermatologic: Pruritus, rash, urticaria

Gastrointestinal: Xerostomia

Neuromuscular & skeletal: Involuntary movements, paresthesia, tremor

Ocular: Blurred vision

Respiratory: Respiratory depression (at higher than recommended doses)

Miscellaneous: Allergic reaction

Dental Usual Dosage
Anxiety: Adults: Oral: 50-100 mg 4 times/day

Preoperative sedation:

Children:

Oral: 0.6 mg/kg/dose

I.M.: 0.5-1 mg/kg/dose

Adults:

Oral: 50-100 mg

I.M.: 25-100 mg

Dosage
Note: Adjust dose based on patient response.

Children:

Preoperative sedation:

Oral: 0.6 mg/kg/dose

I.M.: 1.1 mg/kg/dose

Pruritus, anxiety: Oral:

<6 years: 50 mg daily in divided doses

≥6 years: 50-100 mg daily in divided doses

Antiemetic: I.M.: 1.1 mg/kg/dose

Adults:

Antiemetic: I.M.: 25-100 mg/dose

Anxiety:

Oral: 50-100 mg 4 times/day

I.M.: Initial: 50-100 mg, then every 4-6 hours as needed

Preoperative sedation:

Oral: 50-100 mg

I.M.: 25-100 mg

Pruritus: Oral: 25 mg 3-4 times/day

Elderly: Initiate dosing using the lower end of the recommended dosage range due to an increased potential for anticholinergic side effects. Refer to adult dosing.

Dosing adjustment in renal impairment: No dosage adjustment provided in the manufacturer's labeling; however, the following guidelines have been used by some clinicians (Aronoff, 2007): Adults:

GFR >50 mL/minute: No adjustment recommended.

GFR ≤50 mL/minute: Administer 50% of normal dose.

Continuous renal replacement therapy (CRRT), hemodialysis, peritoneal dialysis: Administer 50% of the normal dose.

Dosing interval in hepatic impairment: Change dosing interval to every 24 hours in patients with primary biliary cirrhosis (Simons F, 1989).

Mechanism of Action Competes with histamine for H_1-receptor sites on effector cells in the gastrointestinal tract, blood vessels, and respiratory tract. Possesses skeletal muscle relaxing, bronchodilator, antihistamine, antiemetic, and analgesic properties.

Contraindications Hypersensitivity to hydroxyzine or any component of the formulation; early pregnancy; SubQ, intra-arterial, or I.V. injection

Warnings/Precautions Causes sedation, caution must be used in performing tasks which require alertness (eg, operating machinery or driving). Sedative effects of CNS depressants or ethanol are potentiated. SubQ, I.V., and intra-arterial administration are contraindicated since tissue damage, intravascular hemolysis, thrombosis, and digital gangrene can occur. Use with caution with narrow-angle glaucoma, prostatic hyperplasia, bladder neck obstruction, asthma, or COPD. In the elderly, avoid use of this potent anticholinergic agent due to increased risk of confusion, dry mouth, constipation, and other anticholinergic effects; clearance decreases in patients of advanced age (Beers Criteria).

Drug Interactions

Metabolism/Transport Effects Inhibits CYP2D6 (weak)

Avoid Concomitant Use

Avoid concomitant use of HydrOXYzine with any of the following: Aclidinium; Azelastine (Nasal); Ipratropium (Oral Inhalation); Paraldehyde; Tiotropium

Increased Effect/Toxicity

HydrOXYzine may increase the levels/effects of: Alcohol (Ethyl); Anticholinergics; ARIPiprazole; Azelastine (Nasal); Barbiturates; Buprenorphine; CNS Depressants; Meperidine; Methotrimeprazine; Metyrosine; Mirtazapine; Paraldehyde; Pramipexole; ROPINIRole; Rotigotine; Selective Serotonin Reuptake Inhibitors; Tiotropium; Zolpidem

The levels/effects of HydrOXYzine may be increased by: Aclidinium; Droperidol; Ipratropium (Oral Inhalation); Magnesium Sulfate; Methotrimeprazine; Perampanel; Pramlintide; Sodium Oxybate

Decreased Effect

HydrOXYzine may decrease the levels/effects of: Acetylcholinesterase Inhibitors (Central); Benzylpenicilloyl Polylysine; Betahistine; Hyaluronidase

The levels/effects of HydrOXYzine may be decreased by: Acetylcholinesterase Inhibitors (Central); Amphetamines

Ethanol/Nutrition/Herb Interactions

Ethanol: May increase CNS depression; monitor for increased effects with coadministration. Caution patients about effects.

Herb/Nutraceutical: Avoid valerian, St John's wort, kava kava, gotu kola (may increase CNS depression).

Pharmacodynamics/Kinetics

Onset of Action Oral: 15-30 minutes; Injection: Rapid

Duration of Action Decreased histamine-induced wheal and flare areas: 2 to ≥36 hours; Suppression of pruritus: 1-12 hours (Simons, 1984)

Half-life Elimination Adults: ~20 hours (Simons, 1984); Elderly: ~29 hours (Simons K, 1989); Hepatic dysfunction: ~37 hours (Simons F, 1989)

Time to Peak Oral administration: Serum: ~2 hours; Peak suppression of antihistamine-induced wheal and flare: 4-12 hours (Simons, 1984)

Pregnancy Considerations Adverse events were observed in animal reproduction studies. Hydroxyzine crosses the placenta. Maternal hydroxyzine use has generally not resulted in an increased risk of birth defects. Use of hydroxyzine early in pregnancy is contraindicated but hydroxyzine is approved for pre- and postpartum adjunctive therapy to reduce narcotic dosage, treat anxiety, and control emesis. Antihistamines are recommended for the treatment pruritus with rash in pregnant women (although second generation antihistamines may be preferred). Antihistamines are not recommended for treatment of pruritus associated with intrahepatic cholestasis in pregnancy. Possible withdrawal symptoms have been observed in neonates following chronic maternal use of hydroxyzine during pregnancy.

Lactation Excretion in breast milk unknown/not recommended

Breast-Feeding Considerations It is not known if hydroxyzine is excreted in breast milk. Breast-feeding is not recommended by the manufacturer. Antihistamines may decrease maternal serum prolactin concentrations when administered prior to the establishment of nursing.

Dosage Forms

Capsule, oral: 25 mg, 50 mg, 100 mg
Vistaril®: 25 mg, 50 mg

Injection, solution: 25 mg/mL (1 mL); 50 mg/mL (1 mL, 2 mL, 10 mL)

Solution, oral: 10 mg/5 mL (473 mL)

Syrup, oral: 10 mg/5 mL (118 mL, 473 mL)

Tablet, oral: 10 mg, 25 mg, 50 mg

Hyoscyamine (hye oh SYE a meen)

Brand Names: U.S. Anaspaz®; ED-SPAZ; HyoMax®-SR; HyoMax®-SL; HyoMax™-DT; HyoMax™-FT; Hyosyne; Levbid®; Levsin®; Levsin®/SL; NuLev®; Oscimin; Symax® DuoTab; Symax® FasTab; Symax® SL; Symax® SR

Brand Names: Canada Levsin®

Pharmacologic Category Anticholinergic Agent

Use

Oral: Adjunctive therapy for peptic ulcers, irritable bowel, neurogenic bladder/bowel; treatment of infant colic, GI tract disorders caused by spasm; to reduce rigidity, tremors, sialorrhea, and hyperhidrosis associated with parkinsonism; as a drying agent in acute rhinitis

Injection: Preoperative antimuscarinic to reduce secretions and block cardiac vagal inhibitory reflexes; to improve radiologic visibility of the kidneys; symptomatic relief of biliary and renal colic; reduce GI motility to facilitate diagnostic procedures (ie, endoscopy, hypotonic duodenography); reduce pain and hypersecretion in pancreatitis, certain cases of partial heart block associated with vagal activity; reversal of neuromuscular blockade

Local Anesthetic/Vasoconstrictor Precautions No information available to require special precautions

Effects on Dental Treatment Key adverse event(s) related to dental treatment: Xerostomia (normal salivary flow resumes upon discontinuation).

Effects on Bleeding No information available to require special precautions

Adverse Effects Frequency not defined.

Cardiovascular: Palpitation, tachycardia

Central nervous system: Ataxia, dizziness, drowsiness, headache, insomnia, mental confusion/excitement, nervousness, speech disorder

Dermatologic: Urticaria

Endocrine & metabolic: Lactation suppression

Gastrointestinal: Bloating, constipation, dry mouth, loss of taste, nausea, vomiting

Genitourinary: Impotence, urinary hesitancy, urinary retention

Neuromuscular & skeletal: Weakness

Ocular: Blurred vision, cycloplegia, increased ocular tension, mydriasis

Miscellaneous: Allergic reactions, sweating decreased

General Dosage Range

I.M., SubQ: *Adults:* 0.25-0.5 mg 4 times/day as needed

I.V.:

Children ≥2 years: 5 mcg/kg given 30-60 minutes prior to induction of anesthesia

Adults: 0.125-0.5 mg 4 times/day as needed **or** 0.25-0.5 mg or 5 mcg/kg as a single dose **or** 0.2 mg for every 1 mg neostigmine

Oral:

Regular release:

Children <2 years and 3.4 kg: 4 drops every 4 hours as needed (maximum: 24 drops/day)

Children <2 years and 5 kg: 5 drops every 4 hours as needed (maximum: 30 drops/day)

Children <2 years and 7 kg: 6 drops every 4 hours as needed (maximum: 36 drops/day)

Children <2 years and 10 kg: 8 drops every 4 hours as needed (maximum: 48 drops/day)

Children ≥2 years and 10 kg: 0.031-0.033 mg every 4 hours as needed (maximum: 0.75 mg/day)

Children ≥2 years and 20 kg: 0.0625 mg every 4 hours as needed (maximum: 0.75 mg/day)

Children ≥2 years and 40 kg: 0.0938 mg every 4 hours as needed (maximum: 0.75 mg/day)

Children ≥2 years and 50 kg: 0.125 mg every 4 hours as needed (maximum: 0.75 mg/day)

Adults: 0.125-0.25 mg every 4 hours or as needed (maximum: 1.5 mg/day)

Timed release: *Adults:* 0.375-0.75 mg every 12 hours (maximum: 1.5 mg/day)

S.L.:
Children ≥2 years and 10 kg: 0.031-0.033 mg every 4 hours as needed (maximum: 0.75 mg/day)
Children ≥2 years and 20 kg: 0.0625 mg every 4 hours as needed (maximum: 0.75 mg/day)
Children ≥2 years and 40 kg: 0.0938 mg every 4 hours as needed (maximum: 0.75 mg/day)
Children ≥2 years and 50 kg: 0.125 mg every 4 hours as needed (maximum: 0.75 mg/day)
Adults: 0.125-0.25 mg every 4 hours or as needed (maximum: 1.5 mg/day)

Mechanism of Action Blocks the action of acetylcholine at parasympathetic sites in smooth muscle, secretory glands, and the CNS; increases cardiac output, dries secretions, antagonizes histamine and serotonin

Pharmacodynamics/Kinetics
Onset of Action 2-3 minutes
Duration of Action 4-6 hours
Half-life Elimination 3-5 hours
Pregnancy Risk Factor C
Pregnancy Considerations Crosses the placenta, effects to the fetus not known; use during pregnancy only if clearly needed.

Hyoscyamine, Atropine, Scopolamine, and Phenobarbital

(hye oh SYE a meen, A troe peen, skoe POL a meen, & fee noe BAR bi tal)

Related Information
Atropine on page 148
Hyoscyamine on page 707
PHENobarbital on page 1080
Scopolamine (Systemic) on page 1226
Brand Names: U.S. Donnatal Extentabs®; Donnatal®; Hyonatol
Pharmacologic Category Anticholinergic Agent; Antispasmodic Agent, Gastrointestinal
Use Adjunct in treatment of irritable bowel syndrome, acute enterocolitis, duodenal ulcer
Local Anesthetic/Vasoconstrictor Precautions No information available to require special precautions
Effects on Dental Treatment Key adverse event(s) related to dental treatment: Xerostomia (normal salivary flow resumes upon discontinuation).
Effects on Bleeding No information available to require special precautions
Adverse Effects Frequency not defined.
Cardiovascular: Palpitation, tachycardia
Central nervous system: Dizziness, drowsiness, excitement, headache, insomnia, nervousness
Dermatologic: Urticaria
Endocrine & metabolic: Lactation suppressed
Gastrointestinal: Bloating, constipation, nausea, taste loss, vomiting, xerostomia
Genitourinary: Impotence, urinary hesitancy, urinary retention
Neuromuscular & skeletal: Musculoskeletal pain, weakness
Ocular: Blurred vision, cycloplegia, mydriasis, ocular tension increased
Miscellaneous: Allergic reaction (may be severe), anaphylaxis, sweating decreased
General Dosage Range Oral:
Extended release: Adults: 1 tablet every 8-12 hours
Immediate release:
Children ≥2 years:
9.1 kg: 1 mL every 4 hours **or** 1.5 mL every 6 hours
13.6 kg: 1.5 mL every 4 hours **or** 2 mL every 6 hours

22.7 kg: 2.5 mL every 4 hours **or** 3.75 mL every 6 hours
34 kg: 3.75 mL every 4 hours **or** 5 mL every 6 hours
45.4 kg: 5 mL every 4 hours **or** 7.5 mL every 6 hours
Adults: 1-2 tablets **or** 5-10 mL of elixir 3-4 times/day

Mechanism of Action Anticholinergic agents (hyoscyamine, atropine, and scopolamine) inhibit the muscarinic actions of acetylcholine at the postganglionic parasympathetic neuroeffector sites including smooth muscle, secretory glands, and CNS sites; specific anticholinergic responses are dose-related.

Pregnancy Risk Factor C
Pregnancy Considerations Reproduction studies with this combination have not been done; refer to individual monographs.

Ibandronate (eye BAN droh nate)

Related Information
Osteonecrosis of the Jaw on page 1529
Rheumatoid Arthritis, Osteoarthritis, and Osteoporosis on page 1526
Brand Names: U.S. Boniva®
Generic Availability (U.S.) Yes: Tablet
Pharmacologic Category Bisphosphonate Derivative
Use Treatment and prevention of osteoporosis in postmenopausal females
Unlabeled Use Hypercalcemia of malignancy; reduce bone pain and skeletal complications from metastatic bone disease due to breast cancer
Local Anesthetic/Vasoconstrictor Precautions No information available to require special precautions
Effects on Dental Treatment Key adverse event(s) related to dental treatment: Tooth disorder.
Osteonecrosis of the jaw (ONJ), generally associated with local infection and/or tooth extraction and often with delayed healing, has been reported in patients taking bisphosphonates. Symptoms included nonhealing extraction socket or an exposed jawbone. Most reported cases of bisphosphonate-associated osteonecrosis have been in cancer patients treated with intravenous bisphosphonates. However, some have occurred in patients with postmenopausal osteoporosis taking oral bisphosphonates. Dental surgery, particularly tooth extraction, may increase the risk for ONJ. Patients who develop ONJ while on bisphosphonate therapy should receive care by an oral surgeon. See Dental Comment.
Effects on Bleeding No information available to require special precautions
Adverse Effects Percentages vary based on frequency of administration (daily vs monthly). Unless specified, percentages are reported with oral use.
>10%:
Gastrointestinal: Dyspepsia (6% to 12%)
Neuromuscular & skeletal: Back pain (4% to 14%)
1% to 10%:
Cardiovascular: Hypertension (6% to 7%)
Central nervous system: Headache (3% to 7%), dizziness (1% to 4%), insomnia (1% to 2%)
Dermatologic: Rash (1% to 2%)
Endocrine & metabolic: Hypercholesterolemia (5%)
Gastrointestinal: Abdominal pain (5% to 8%), diarrhea (4% to 7%), nausea (5%), constipation (3% to 4%), vomiting (3%)
Genitourinary: Urinary tract infection (2% to 6%)
Hepatic: Alkaline phosphatase decreased (frequency not defined)
Local: Injection site reaction (<2%)

Neuromuscular & skeletal: Pain in extremity (1% to 8%), arthralgia (4% to 6%), myalgia (1% to 6%), joint disorder (4%), osteonecrosis of the jaw (4%), weakness (4%), osteoarthritis (localized; 1% to 3%), muscle cramp (2%)

Respiratory: Bronchitis (3% to 10%), pneumonia (6%), pharyngitis/nasopharyngitis (3% to 4%), upper respiratory infection (2%)

Miscellaneous: Acute phase reaction (I.V. 10%; oral 3% to 9%), infection (4%), flu-like syndrome (1% to 4%), allergic reaction (3%)

Dosage

Oral: Postmenopausal osteoporosis (prevention and treatment): 150 mg once a month; **Note:** Patients should receive supplemental calcium and vitamin D if dietary intake is inadequate

I.V.:

Postmenopausal osteoporosis (treatment): 3 mg every 3 months; **Note:** Patients should receive supplemental calcium and vitamin D if dietary intake is inadequate

Hypercalcemia of malignancy (unlabeled use): 2-6 mg over 1-2 hours (Pecherstorfer, 2003; Ralston, 1997)

Metastatic bone disease due to breast cancer (unlabeled use): 6 mg every 3-4 weeks (Diel, 2004)

Dosage adjustment in renal impairment:

Osteoporosis: Oral, I.V.:

Cl_{cr} ≥30 mL/minute: No dosage adjustment necessary.

Cl_{cr} <30 mL/minute: Use not recommended.

Oncologic uses (unlabeled): I.V.: Cl_{cr} <30 mL/minute: 2 mg every 3-4 weeks (von Moos, 2005)

Dosage adjustment in hepatic impairment: No dosage adjustment necessary.

Mechanism of Action A bisphosphonate which inhibits bone resorption via actions on osteoclasts or on osteoclast precursors; decreases the rate of bone resorption, leading to an indirect increase in bone mineral density.

Contraindications Hypersensitivity to ibandronate or any component of the formulation; hypocalcemia; oral tablets are also contraindicated in patients unable to stand or sit upright for at least 60 minutes and in patients with abnormalities of the esophagus which delay esophageal emptying, such as stricture or achalasia

Warnings/Precautions Hypocalcemia must be corrected before therapy initiation. Ensure adequate calcium and vitamin D intake. Osteonecrosis of the jaw (ONJ) has been reported in patients receiving bisphosphonates. Risk factors include invasive dental procedures (eg, tooth extraction, dental implants, boney surgery); a diagnosis of cancer, with concomitant chemotherapy or corticosteroids; poor oral hygiene, ill-fitting dentures; and comorbid disorders (anemia, coagulopathy, infection, pre-existing dental disease). Most reported cases occurred after I.V. bisphosphonate therapy; however, cases have been reported following oral therapy. A dental exam and preventative dentistry should be performed prior to placing patients with risk factors on chronic bisphosphonate therapy. The manufacturer's labeling states that discontinuing bisphosphonates in patients requiring invasive dental procedures may reduce the risk of ONJ. However, other experts suggest that there is no evidence that discontinuing therapy reduces the risk of developing ONJ (Assael, 2009). The benefit/risk must be assessed by the treating physician and/or dentist/surgeon prior to any invasive dental procedure. Patients developing ONJ while on bisphosphonates should receive care by an oral surgeon.

Atypical femur fractures have been reported in patients receiving bisphosphonates for treatment/prevention of osteoporosis. The fractures include subtrochanteric femur (bone just below the hip joint) and diaphyseal femur (long segment of the thigh bone). Some patients experience prodromal pain weeks or months before the fracture occurs. It is unclear if bisphosphonate therapy is the cause for these fractures, although the majority have been reported in patients taking bisphosphonates. Patients receiving long-term (>3-5 years) therapy may be at an increased risk. Discontinue bisphosphonate therapy in patients who develop a femoral shaft fracture.

Infrequently, severe (and occasionally debilitating) bone, joint, and/or muscle pain have been reported during bisphosphonate treatment. The onset of pain ranged from a single day to several months. Consider discontinuing therapy in patients who experience severe symptoms; symptoms usually resolve upon discontinuation. Some patients experienced recurrence when rechallenged with same drug or another bisphosphonate; avoid use in patients with a history of these symptoms in association with bisphosphonate therapy.

Oral bisphosphonates may cause dysphagia, esophagitis, esophageal or gastric ulcer; risk may increase in patients unable to comply with dosing instructions; discontinue use if new or worsening symptoms develop. Intravenous bisphosphonates may cause transient decreases in serum calcium and have also been associated with renal toxicity.

Use not recommended with severe renal impairment (Cl_{cr} <30 mL/minute).

Drug Interactions

Metabolism/Transport Effects None known.

Avoid Concomitant Use There are no known interactions where it is recommended to avoid concomitant use.

Increased Effect/Toxicity

Ibandronate may increase the levels/effects of: Deferasirox; Phosphate Supplements; SUNItinib

The levels/effects of Ibandronate may be increased by: Aminoglycosides; Nonsteroidal Anti-Inflammatory Agents

Decreased Effect

The levels/effects of Ibandronate may be decreased by: Antacids; Calcium Salts; Iron Salts; Magnesium Salts; Multivitamins/Minerals (with ADEK, Folate, Iron); Proton Pump Inhibitors

Ethanol/Nutrition/Herb Interactions

Ethanol: Ethanol may increase risk of osteoporosis. Management: Avoid ethanol.

Food: May reduce absorption; mean oral bioavailability is decreased up to 90% when given with food. Management: Take with a full glass (6-8 oz) of plain water, at least 60 minutes prior to any food, beverages, or medications. Mineral water with a high calcium content should be avoided. Wait at least 60 minutes after taking ibandronate before taking anything else.

Dietary Considerations Ensure adequate calcium and vitamin D intake; women and men >50 years of age should consume 1200-1500 mg/day of elemental calcium and 800-1000 units/day of vitamin D. Ibandronate tablet should be taken with a full glass (6-8 oz) of plain water, at least 60 minutes prior to any food, beverages, or medications. Mineral water with a high calcium content should be avoided.

Pharmacodynamics/Kinetics
Half-life Elimination
Oral: 150 mg dose: Terminal: 37-157 hours
I.V.: Terminal: ~5-25 hours
Time to Peak Oral: 0.5-2 hours
Pregnancy Risk Factor C
Pregnancy Considerations Adverse effects were demonstrated in animal reproduction studies. Bisphosphonates are incorporated into the bone matrix and are gradually released over time. Theoretically, there may be a risk of fetal harm when pregnancy follows the completion of therapy. Based on limited case reports with pamidronate, serum calcium levels in the newborn may be altered if administered during pregnancy.
Lactation Excretion in breast milk unknown/use caution
Dosage Forms
Injection, solution:
Boniva®: 1 mg/mL (3 mL)
Tablet, oral: 150 mg
Boniva®: 150 mg
Dental Comment A review of 2408 published cases of bisphosphonate-associated osteonecrosis of the jaw bone (BP-associated ONJ) was done by Filleul, 2010. BP therapy was associated with 89% of the cases to treat malignancies and 11% of the cases to treat non-malignant conditions. Information on the specific bisphosphonate used was available for 1694 of the patients. Intravenous therapy (primarily zoledronic acid) was received by 88% of the patients and 12% received oral treatment (primarily alendronate). Of all the cases of BP-associated ONJ, 67% were preceded by tooth extraction and for 26% of patients, there was no predisposing factor identified.

A 2010 retrospective case review reported the prevalence of BP-associated ONJ in patients using alendronate-type drugs was one out of 952 patients or ~0.1% (Lo, 2010). Of the 8572 respondents, nine cases of ONJ were identified; five had developed ONJ spontaneously and four developed ONJ after tooth extraction. When extrapolated to patient-years of bisphosphonate exposure, this prevalence rate of 0.1% equates to a frequency of 28 cases per 100,000 person-years of oral bisphosphonate treatment. An Australian group (Mavrokokki, 2007), identified the frequency of BP-associated ONJ in osteoporotic patients, mainly taking weekly oral alendronate, was 1 in 8470 to 1 in 2260 (0.01% to 0.04%) patients. If extractions were carried out, the calculated frequency was 1 in 1130 to 1 in 296 (0.09% to 0.34%) patients. The median time to onset of ONJ in alendronate patients was 24 months.

According to the 2011 report by the American Dental Association (ADA), the incidence of BP-associated ONJ remains low and the benefits of using oral bisphosphonates significantly outweighs the risk of developing BP-associated ONJ for treatment and prevention of osteoporosis and cancer treatment (Hellstein, 2011). The full 47 page report can be accessed at http://www.ada.org/sections/professionalResources/pdfs/topics_ARONJ_report.pdf.

The ADA review of 2011 stated the incidence of oral BP-associated ONJ was one case for every 1000 individuals exposed to oral bisphosphonates (0.1%) (Hellstein, 2011).

References
Durie BG, Katz M, and Crowley J, "Osteonecrosis of the Jaw and Bisphosphonates," *N Engl J Med*, 2005, 353(1):99-102.
Filleul O, Crompot E, and Saussez S, "Bisphosphonate-Induced Osteonecrosis of the Jaw: A Review of 2,400 Patient Cases," *J Cancer Res Clin Oncol*, 2010, 136(8):1117-24.

Hellstein JW, Adler RA, Edwards B, et al, "Managing the Care of Patients Receiving Antiresorptive Therapy for Prevention and Treatment of Osteoporosis: Executive Summary of Recommendations From the American Dental Association Council on Scientific Affairs," *J Am Dent Assoc*, 2011, 142(11):1243-51.
Hellstein JW, Adler RA, Edwards B, et al, "Managing the Care of Patients Receiving Antiresorptive Therapy for Prevention and Treatment of Osteoporosis: Recommendations From the American Dental Association Council on Scientific Affairs," 2011, Available at http://www.ada.org/sections/professionalResources/pdfs/topics_ARONJ_report.pdf. Accessed February 2013.
Lo JC, O'Ryan FS, Gordon NP, et al, "Prevalence of Osteonecrosis of the Jaw in Patients With Oral Bisphosphonate Exposure," *J Oral Maxillofac Surg*, 2010, 68(2):243-53.
Marx RE, Sawatari Y, Fortin M, et al, "Bisphosphonate-Induced Exposed Bone (Osteonecrosis/Osteopetrosis) of the Jaws: Risk Factors, Recognition, Prevention, and Treatment," *J Oral Maxillofac Surg*, 2005, 63(11):1567-75.
Mavrokokki T, Cheng A, Stein B, et al, "Nature and Frequency of Bisphosphonate-Associated Osteonecrosis of the Jaws in Australia," *J Oral Maxillofac Surg*, 2007, 65(3):415-23.
Ruggiero SL, Dodson TB, Assael LA, et al, "American Association of Oral and Maxillofacial Surgeons Position Paper on Bisphosphonate-Related Osteonecrosis of the Jaws-2009 Update," *J Oral Maxillofac Surg*, 2009, 67(5 Suppl):2-12.
Ruggiero S, Gralow J, Marx RE, et al, "Practical Guidelines for the Prevention, Diagnosis, and Treatment of Osteonecrosis of the Jaw in Patients With Cancer," *J Clin Oncol*, 2006, 2(1):7-14.

Ibritumomab (ib ri TYOO mo mab)

Brand Names: U.S. Zevalin®
Brand Names: Canada Zevalin®
Pharmacologic Category Antineoplastic Agent, Monoclonal Antibody; Radiopharmaceutical
Use Treatment of relapsed or refractory low-grade or follicular B-cell non-Hodgkin's lymphoma (NHL); treatment of follicular NHL in patients (previously untreated) who achieve a response (partial or complete) to first-line chemotherapy
Local Anesthetic/Vasoconstrictor Precautions No information available to require special precautions
Effects on Dental Treatment Key adverse event(s) related to dental treatment: Hypotension, cough, throat irritation, rhinitis.
Effects on Bleeding Chemotherapy may result in significant myelosuppression, potentially including significant reduction in platelet counts and altered hemostasis. In patients who are under active treatment with these agents, medical consult is suggested.
Adverse Effects
>10%:
Central nervous system: Fatigue (33%)
Gastrointestinal: Nausea (18%), abdominal pain (17%), diarrhea (11%)
Hematologic: Thrombocytopenia (62% to 95%; grades 3/4: 51% to 63%; nadir: 49-53 days; median duration: 24 days; median time to recovery: 13 days), neutropenia (45% to 77%; grades 3/4: 41% to 60%; nadir: 61-62 days; median duration: 22 days; median time to recovery: 12 days), anemia (22% to 61%; grades 3/4: 5% to 17%; nadir: 68-69 days; median duration: 24 days), leukopenia (43%; grades 3/4: 36%), lymphopenia (26%; grades 3/4: 18%)
Neuromuscular & skeletal: Weakness (15%)
Respiratory: Nasopharyngitis (19%), cough (11%)
Miscellaneous: Infection (29%; serious 1% to 3%)
1% to 10%:
Cardiovascular: Hypertension (7%)
Central nervous system: Fever (10%), dizziness (7%)
Dermatologic: Petechiae (8%), bruising (7%), pruritus (7%), rash (7%)
Gastrointestinal: Anorexia (8%)
Genitourinary: Urinary tract infection (7%)
Hematologic: Secondary malignancies (1% to 6%; includes acute myelogenous leukemia and myelodysplastic syndrome), prolonged cytopenia (severe: 5%)

Neuromuscular & skeletal: Myalgia (9%)
Respiratory: Bronchitis (8%), rhinitis (8%), pharyngo-laryngeal pain (7%), sinusitis (7%), epistaxis (5%)
Miscellaneous: Flu-like syndrome (8%), night sweats (8%), HAMA antibody formation (1% to 3%), biodistribution altered (1%)

General Dosage Range I.V.: *Adults:* Day 7, 8, or 9: 0.3-0.4 mCi/kg (11.1-14.8 MBq/kg) actual body weight (maximum: 32 mCi [1184 MBq])

Mechanism of Action Ibritumomab is a monoclonal antibody directed against the CD20 antigen found on pre-B and mature B lymphocytes (normal and malignant). Ibritumomab binding induces apoptosis in B lymphocytes *in vitro*. It is combined with the chelator tiuxetan, which acts as a specific chelation site for Yttrium-90 (Y-90). The monoclonal antibody acts as a delivery system to direct the radioactive isotope to the targeted cells, however, binding has been observed in lymphoid cells throughout the body and in lymphoid nodules in organs such as the large and small intestines. Beta-emission induces cellular damage through the formation of free radicals (in both target cells and surrounding cells).

Pharmacodynamics/Kinetics
Duration of Action B cell recovery begins in ~12 weeks; generally in normal range within 9 months
Half-life Elimination Y-90 ibritumomab: 30 hours; Yttrium-90 decays with a physical half-life of 64 hours
Pregnancy Risk Factor D
Pregnancy Considerations Animal reproduction studies have not been conducted. Based on the radioactivity, Y-90 ibritumomab may cause fetal harm if administered during pregnancy. IgG molecules are known to cross the placenta. Women of childbearing potential should avoid becoming pregnant during treatment with ibritumomab. Both males and females should use effective contraception for at least 12 months following treatment. The effect on future fertility is unknown.

Ibuprofen (eye byoo PROE fen)

Related Information
Antiplatelet and Anticoagulation Considerations in Dentistry *on page 1503*
Oral Pain *on page 1558*
Rheumatoid Arthritis, Osteoarthritis, and Osteoporosis *on page 1526*
Temporomandibular Dysfunction (TMD), Chronic Pain, and Fibromyalgia *on page 1590*
Related Sample Prescriptions
Mild/Moderate Oral Pain *on page 1606*
Moderate/Moderately Severe Oral Pain *on page 1606*
Brand Names: U.S. Addaprin [OTC]; Advil® Children's [OTC]; Advil® Infants' [OTC]; Advil® Migraine [OTC]; Advil® [OTC]; Caldolor®; I-Prin [OTC]; Ibu-200 [OTC]; Ibu®; Midol® Cramps & Body Aches [OTC]; Motrin® Children's [OTC]; Motrin® IB [OTC]; Motrin® Infants' [OTC]; Motrin® Junior [OTC]; NeoProfen®; Proprinal® [OTC]; TopCare® Junior Strength [OTC]; Ultraprin [OTC]
Brand Names: Canada Advil®; Advil® Children's; Apo-Ibuprofen®; Motrin® (Children's); Motrin® IB; Novo-Profen; Nu-Ibuprofen
Generic Availability (U.S.) Yes: Caplet, liquid-filled capsule, softgel capsule, suspension, tablet
Pharmacologic Category Nonsteroidal Anti-inflammatory Drug (NSAID), Oral; Nonsteroidal Anti-inflammatory Drug (NSAID), Parenteral
Dental Use Management of pain and swelling

Use
Oral: Inflammatory diseases and rheumatoid disorders including juvenile idiopathic arthritis (JIA), mild-to-moderate pain, fever, dysmenorrhea, osteoarthritis
Ibuprofen injection (Caldolor®): Management of mild-to-moderate pain; management moderate-to-severe pain when used concurrently with an opioid analgesic; reduction of fever
Ibuprofen lysine injection (NeoProfen®): To induce closure of a clinically-significant patent ductus arteriosus (PDA) in premature infants weighing between 500-1500 g and who are ≤32 weeks gestational age (GA) when usual treatments are ineffective
Unlabeled Use Ankylosing spondylitis, cystic fibrosis, gout, acute migraine headache, migraine prophylaxis, pericarditis
Local Anesthetic/Vasoconstrictor Precautions No information available to require special precautions
Effects on Dental Treatment In a statement released on September 8, 2006, the FDA notified consumers and healthcare professionals that the administration of ibuprofen for pain relief to patients taking aspirin for cardioprotection may interfere with aspirin's cardiovascular benefits. The FDA states that ibuprofen can interfere with the antiplatelet effect of low-dose aspirin (81 mg/day). This could result in diminished effectiveness of aspirin as used for cardioprotection and stroke prevention. The FDA adds that although ibuprofen and aspirin can be taken together, it is recommended that consumers talk with their healthcare providers for additional information. For more information, including how to advise aspirin patients requiring ibuprofen for pain relief, see Effects on Bleeding and Dental Comment.
Effects on Bleeding Nonselective NSAIDs such as ibuprofen inhibit platelet aggregation and prolong bleeding time in some patients. Unlike aspirin, the NSAID effect on platelet function is quantitatively less, of shorter duration, and reversible.
Adverse Effects
Oral:
1% to 10%:
Cardiovascular: Edema (1% to 3%)
Central nervous system: Dizziness (3% to 9%), headache (1% to 3%), nervousness (1% to 3%)
Dermatologic: Rash (3% to 9%), itching (1% to 3%)
Endocrine & metabolic: Fluid retention (1% to 3%)
Gastrointestinal: Epigastric pain (3% to 9%), heartburn (3% to 9%), nausea (3% to 9%), abdominal pain/cramps/distress (1% to 3%), appetite decreased (1% to 3%), constipation (1% to 3%), diarrhea (1% to 3%), dyspepsia (1% to 3%), flatulence (1% to 3%), vomiting (1% to 3%)
Otic: Tinnitus (3% to 9%)

Injection: Ibuprofen (Caldolor®):
Cardiovascular: Edema, hypertension
Central nervous system: Dizziness, headache
Dermatologic: Pruritus
Endocrine & metabolic: Hypernatremia, hypokalemia
Gastrointestinal: Abdominal pain, dyspepsia, flatulence, nausea, vomiting
Genitourinary: Urinary retention
Hematologic: Anemia, hemorrhage, neutropenia
Renal: BUN increased
Respiratory: Cough

Injection: Ibuprofen lysine (NeoProfen®):
>10%:
Cardiovascular: Intraventricular hemorrhage (29%; grade 3/4: 15%)
Dermatologic: Skin irritation (16%)

Endocrine & metabolic: Hypocalcemia (12%), hypogly-cemia (12%)

Gastrointestinal: GI disorders, non NEC (22%)

Hematologic: Anemia (32%)

Respiratory: Apnea (28%), respiratory infection (19%)

Miscellaneous: Sepsis (43%)

1% to 10%:

Cardiovascular: Edema (4%)

Endocrine & metabolic: Adrenal insufficiency (7%), hypernatremia (7%)

Genitourinary: Urinary tract infection (9%)

Renal: Urea increased (7%), renal impairment (6%), creatinine increased (3%), urine output decreased (3%; small decrease reported on days 2-6 with compensatory increase in output on day 9), renal failure (1%)

Respiratory: Respiratory failure (10%), atelecta-sis (4%)

Frequency not defined: Abdominal distension, choles-tasis, feeding problems, gastritis, GI reflux, heart fail-ure, hyperglycemia, hypotension, ileus, infection, inguinal hernia, injection site reaction, jaundice, neu-tropenia, seizure, tachycardia, thrombocytopenia

Dental Usual Dosage

Analgesic/pain/fever/dysmenorrhea: Oral:

Children: 4-10 mg/kg/dose every 6-8 hours

Adults: 200-400 mg/dose every 4-6 hours (maximum daily dose: 1.2 g, unless directed by physician; under physician supervision daily doses ≤2.4 g may be used)

OTC labeling (analgesic, antipyretic): **Note:** Treatment for >10 days is not recommended unless directed by healthcare provider. Oral:

Children 6 months to 11 years: See table; use of weight to select dose is preferred; doses may be repeated every 6-8 hours (maximum: 4 doses/day)

Children ≥12 years and Adults: 200 mg every 4-6 hours as needed (maximum: 1200 mg/24 hours)

Ibuprofen Dosing

Weight (lb)	Age	Dosage (mg)
12-17	6-11 mo	50
18-23	12-23 mo	75
24-35	2-3 y	100
36-47	4-5 y	150
48-59	6-8 y	200
60-71	9-10 y	250
72-95	11 y	300

Dosage

I.V.:

Neonates: Ibuprofen lysine (NeoProfen®): Infants between 500-1500 g and ≤32 weeks GA: Patent ductus arteriosus: Initial dose: Ibuprofen 10 mg/kg, followed by two doses of 5 mg/kg at 24 and 48 hours. Dose should be based on birth weight.

Adults (Caldolor®): **Note**: Patients should be well hydrated prior to administration

Analgesic: 400-800 mg every 6 hours as needed (maximum: 3.2 g/day)

Antipyretic: Initial: 400 mg, then every 4-6 hours or 100-200 mg every 4 hours as needed (maximum: 3.2 g/day)

Oral:

Children:

Antipyretic: 6 months to 12 years: Temperature <102.5°F (39°C): 5 mg/kg/dose; temperature >102.5°F: 10 mg/kg/dose given every 6-8 hours (maximum daily dose: 40 mg/kg/day)

Juvenile idiopathic arthritis (JIA): 30-50 mg/kg/24 hours divided every 8 hours; start at lower end of dosing range and titrate upward (maximum: 2.4 g/day)

Analgesic: 4-10 mg/kg/dose every 6-8 hours

Cystic fibrosis (unlabeled use): Chronic (>4 years) twice daily dosing adjusted to maintain serum con-centration of 50-100 mcg/mL has been associated with slowing of disease progression in younger patients with mild lung disease

OTC labeling (analgesic, antipyretic): **Note:** Treatment for >10 days is not recommended unless directed by healthcare provider.

Children 6 months to 11 years: Use of weight to select dose is preferred; doses may be repeated every 6-8 hours (maximum: 4 doses/day)

Children ≥12 years: 200 mg every 4-6 hours as needed (maximum: 1200 mg/24 hours)

Adults:

Inflammatory disease: 400-800 mg/dose 3-4 times/day (maximum dose: 3.2 g/day)

Analgesia/pain/fever/dysmenorrhea: 200-400 mg/dose every 4-6 hours (maximum daily dose: 1.2 g, unless directed by physician; under physician supervision daily doses ≤2.4 g may be used)

OTC labeling (analgesic, antipyretic): 200 mg every 4-6 hours as needed (maximum: 1200 mg/24 hours); treatment for >10 days is not recommended unless directed by healthcare provider.

Migraine: 400 mg at onset of symptoms (maximum: 400 mg/24 hours unless directed by healthcare provider)

Pericarditis (unlabeled use): 400-800 mg 3-4 times daily (maximum dose: 3.2 g daily) (Imazio, 2009); with pericarditis postmyocardial infarction, the ACCF/AHA prefers the use of aspirin (O'Gara, 2013).

Dosing adjustment/comments in renal impairment: If anuria or oliguria evident, hold dose until renal function returns to normal

Dosing adjustment/comments in severe hepatic impairment: Avoid use

Mechanism of Action Reversibly inhibits cyclooxyge-nase-1 and 2 (COX-1 and 2) enzymes, which results in decreased formation of prostaglandin precursors; has antipyretic, analgesic, and anti-inflammatory properties

Other proposed mechanisms not fully elucidated (and possibly contributing to the anti-inflammatory effect to varying degrees), include inhibiting chemotaxis, altering lymphocyte activity, inhibiting neutrophil aggregation/activation, and decreasing proinflammatory cytokine levels.

Contraindications Hypersensitivity to ibuprofen; his-tory of asthma, urticaria, or allergic-type reaction to aspirin or other NSAIDs; aspirin triad (eg, bronchial asthma, aspirin intolerance, rhinitis); perioperative pain in the setting of coronary artery bypass graft (CABG) surgery

Ibuprofen lysine (NeoProfen®): Preterm infants with untreated proven or suspected infection; congenital heart disease where patency of the PDA is necessary for pulmonary or systemic blood flow; bleeding (especially with active intracranial hemorrhage or GI bleed); thrombocytopenia; coagulation defects; proven or suspected necrotizing enterocolitis (NEC); significant renal dysfunction

Warnings/Precautions [U.S. Boxed Warning]: NSAIDs are associated with an increased risk of adverse cardiovascular thrombotic events, including fatal MI and stroke. Risk may be increased with duration of use or pre-existing cardiovascular risk factors or disease. Carefully evaluate individual cardiovascular risk profiles prior to prescribing. May cause new-onset hypertension or worsening of existing hypertension. Response to ACE inhibitors, thiazides, or loop diuretics may be impaired with concurrent use of NSAIDs. Use caution with fluid retention. Avoid use in heart failure. Concurrent administration of ibuprofen, and potentially other nonselective NSAIDs, may interfere with aspirin's cardioprotective effect. **[U.S. Boxed Warning]: Use is contraindicated for treatment of perioperative pain in the setting of coronary artery bypass graft (CABG) surgery.** Risk of MI and stroke may be increased with use following CABG surgery.

May increase the risk of aseptic meningitis, especially in patients with systemic lupus erythematosus (SLE) and mixed connective tissue disorders. Platelet adhesion and aggregation may be decreased; may prolong bleeding time; patients with coagulation disorders or who are receiving anticoagulants should be monitored closely. Anemia may occur; patients on long-term NSAID therapy should be monitored for anemia. Rarely, NSAID use may cause severe blood dyscrasias (eg, agranulocytosis, aplastic anemia, thrombocytopenia).

NSAID use may compromise existing renal function; dose-dependent decreases in prostaglandin synthesis may result from NSAID use, reducing renal blood flow which may cause renal decompensation. NSAID use may increase the risk for hyperkalemia. Patients with impaired renal function, dehydration, heart failure, liver dysfunction, those taking diuretics, and ACE inhibitors, and the elderly are at greater risk of renal toxicity and hyperkalemia. Rehydrate patient before starting therapy; monitor renal function closely. Not recommended for use in patients with advanced renal disease. Long-term NSAID use may result in renal papillary necrosis.

NSAIDs may increase risk of gastrointestinal irritation, inflammation, ulceration, bleeding, and perforation. These events can be fatal and may occur at any time during therapy and without warning. Use caution with a history of GI disease (bleeding or ulcers), concurrent therapy with aspirin, anticoagulants and/or corticosteroids, smoking, use of ethanol, the elderly or debilitated patients. When used concomitantly with aspirin, a substantial increase in the risk of gastrointestinal complications (eg, ulcer) occurs; concomitant gastroprotective therapy (eg, proton pump inhibitors) is recommended (Bhatt, 2008).

Use the lowest effective dose for the shortest duration of time, consistent with individual patient goals, to reduce risk of cardiovascular or GI adverse events. Alternate therapies should be considered for patients at high risk.

NSAIDs may cause serious skin adverse events including exfoliative dermatitis, Stevens-Johnson Syndrome (SJS) and toxic epidermal necrolysis (TEN); discontinue use at first sign of skin rash or hypersensitivity.

Anaphylactoid reactions may occur, even without prior exposure; patients with "aspirin triad" (bronchial asthma, aspirin intolerance, rhinitis) may be at increased risk. Do not use in patients who experience bronchospasm, asthma, rhinitis, or urticaria with NSAID or aspirin therapy. Use caution in other forms of asthma.

NSAIDS may cause drowsiness, dizziness, blurred vision and other neurologic effects which may impair physical or mental abilities; patients must be cautioned about performing tasks which require mental alertness (eg, operating machinery or driving). Monitor vision with long-term therapy. Blurred/diminished vision, scotomata, and changes in color vision have been reported. Discontinue use with altered vision and perform ophthalmologic exam.

Use with caution in patients with decreased hepatic function. Closely monitor patients with any abnormal LFT. Severe hepatic reactions (eg, fulminant hepatitis, liver failure) have occurred with NSAID use, rarely; discontinue if signs or symptoms of liver disease develop, or if systemic manifestations occur.

In the elderly, avoid chronic use (unless alternative agents ineffective and patient can receive concomitant gastroprotective agent); nonselective oral NSAID use is associated with an increased risk of GI bleeding and peptic ulcer disease in older adults in high risk category (eg, >75 years or age or receiving concomitant oral/parenteral corticosteroids, anticoagulants, or antiplatelet agents) (Beers Criteria).

Withhold for at least 4-6 half-lives prior to surgical or dental procedures. Some products may contain phenylalanine. Ibuprofen injection (Caldolor®) must be diluted prior to administration; hemolysis can occur if not diluted.

Ibuprofen lysine injection (NeoProfen®): Hold second or third doses if urinary output is <0.6 mL/kg/hour. May alter signs of infection. May inhibit platelet aggregation; monitor for signs of bleeding. May displace bilirubin; use caution when total bilirubin is elevated. Long-term evaluations of neurodevelopment, growth, or diseases associated with prematurity following treatment have not been conducted. A second course of treatment, alternative pharmacologic therapy or surgery may be needed if the ductus arteriosus fails to close or reopens following the initial course of therapy.

Self medication (OTC use): Prior to self-medication, patients should contact healthcare provider if they have had recurring stomach pain or upset, ulcers, bleeding problems, high blood pressure, heart or kidney disease, other serious medical problems, are currently taking a diuretic, aspirin, anticoagulant, or are ≥60 years of age. If patients are using for migraines, they should also contact healthcare provider if they have not had a migraine diagnosis by healthcare provider, a headache that is different from usual migraine, worst headache of life, fever and neck stiffness, headache from head injury or coughing, first headache at ≥50 years of age, daily headache, or migraine requiring bed rest. Recommended dosages should not be exceeded, due to an increased risk of GI bleeding. Stop use and consult a healthcare provider if symptoms get worse, newly appear, fever lasts for >3 days or pain lasts >3 days (children) and >10 days (adults). Do not give for >10 days unless instructed by healthcare provider. Consuming ≥3 alcoholic beverages/day or taking longer than recommended may increase the risk of GI bleeding.

Drug Interactions

Metabolism/Transport Effects Substrate of CYP2C19 (minor), CYP2C9 (minor); **Note:** Assignment of Major/Minor substrate status based on clinically relevant drug interaction potential; **Inhibits** CYP2C9 (weak)

Avoid Concomitant Use

Avoid concomitant use of Ibuprofen with any of the following: Floctafenine; Ketorolac (Nasal); Ketorolac (Systemic); NSAID (COX-2 Inhibitor); Omacetaxine

Increased Effect/Toxicity

Ibuprofen may increase the levels/effects of: Agents with Antiplatelet Properties; Aliskiren; Aminoglycosides; Anticoagulants; Bisphosphonate Derivatives; Collagenase (Systemic); CycloSPORINE (Systemic); Dabigatran Etexilate; Deferasirox; Desmopressin; Digoxin; Drotrecogin Alfa (Activated); Eplerenone; Haloperidol; Ibritumomab; Lithium; Methotrexate; Nonsteroidal Anti-Inflammatory Agents; NSAID (COX-2 Inhibitor); Omacetaxine; PEMEtrexed; Porfimer; Potassium-Sparing Diuretics; PRALAtrexate; Quinolone Antibiotics; Rivaroxaban; Salicylates; Thrombolytic Agents; Tositumomab and Iodine I 131 Tositumomab; Vancomycin; Vitamin K Antagonists

The levels/effects of Ibuprofen may be increased by: ACE Inhibitors; Angiotensin II Receptor Blockers; Antidepressants (Tricyclic, Tertiary Amine); Corticosteroids (Systemic); CycloSPORINE (Systemic); Dasatinib; Floctafenine; Glucosamine; Herbs (Anticoagulant/Antiplatelet Properties); Ketorolac (Nasal); Ketorolac (Systemic); Multivitamins/Minerals (with ADEK, Folate, Iron); Nonsteroidal Anti-Inflammatory Agents; Omega-3 Fatty Acids; Pentosan Polysulfate Sodium; Pentoxifylline; Probenecid; Prostacyclin Analogues; Selective Serotonin Reuptake Inhibitors; Serotonin/Norepinephrine Reuptake Inhibitors; Sodium Phosphates; Tipranavir; Treprostinil; Vitamin E; Voriconazole

Decreased Effect

Ibuprofen may decrease the levels/effects of: ACE Inhibitors; Agents with Antiplatelet Properties; Aliskiren; Angiotensin II Receptor Blockers; Beta-Blockers; Eplerenone; HydrALAZINE; Imatinib; Loop Diuretics; Potassium-Sparing Diuretics; Salicylates; Selective Serotonin Reuptake Inhibitors; Thiazide Diuretics

The levels/effects of Ibuprofen may be decreased by: Bile Acid Sequestrants; Nonsteroidal Anti-Inflammatory Agents; Salicylates

Ethanol/Nutrition/Herb Interactions

Ethanol: Avoid ethanol (may enhance gastric mucosal irritation).

Food: Ibuprofen peak serum levels may be decreased if taken with food.

Herb/Nutraceutical: Avoid alfalfa, anise, bilberry, bladderwrack, bromelain, cat's claw, celery, chamomile, coleus, cordyceps, dong quai, evening primrose, fenugreek, feverfew, garlic, ginger, ginkgo biloba, ginseng (American, Panax, Siberian), grapeseed, green tea, guggul, horse chestnut seed, horseradish, licorice, prickly ash, red clover, reishi, SAMe (S-adenosylmethionine), sweet clover, turmeric, white willow (all have additional antiplatelet activity).

Dietary Considerations Should be taken with food. Some products may contain phenylalanine and/or potassium.

Pharmacodynamics/Kinetics

Onset of Action Oral: Analgesic: 30-60 minutes; Anti-inflammatory: ≤7 days

Duration of Action Oral: 4-6 hours

Half-life Elimination

Premature infants (highly variable between studies):
Day 3: 35-51 hours
Day 5: 20-33 hours
Children 3 months to 10 years: 1.6 ± 0.7 hours
Adults: 2-4 hours; End-stage renal disease: Unchanged

Time to Peak Oral: ~1-2 hours

Pregnancy Risk Factor C/D ≥30 weeks gestation

Pregnancy Considerations Adverse events were not observed in the initial animal reproduction studies; therefore, the manufacturer classifies ibuprofen as pregnancy category C (category D: ≥30 weeks gestation). NSAID exposure during the first trimester is not strongly associated with congenital malformations; however, cardiovascular anomalies and cleft palate have been observed following NSAID exposure in some studies. The use of a NSAID close to conception may be associated with an increased risk of miscarriage. Non-teratogenic effects have been observed following NSAID administration during the third trimester including: Myocardial degenerative changes, prenatal constriction of the ductus arteriosus, fetal tricuspid regurgitation, failure of the ductus arteriosus to close postnatally; renal dysfunction or failure, oligohydramnios; gastrointestinal bleeding or perforation, increased risk of necrotizing enterocolitis; intracranial bleeding (including intraventricular hemorrhage), platelet dysfunction with resultant bleeding; pulmonary hypertension. Because they may cause premature closure of the ductus arteriosus, use of NSAIDs late in pregnancy should be avoided (use after 31 or 32 weeks gestation is not recommended by some clinicians). Product labeling for Caldolor® specifically notes that use at ≥30 weeks gestation should be avoided and therefore classifies ibuprofen as pregnancy category D at this time. The chronic use of NSAIDs in women of reproductive age may be associated with infertility that is reversible upon discontinuation of the medication. A registry is available for pregnant women exposed to autoimmune medications including ibuprofen. For additional information contact the Organization of Teratology Information Specialists, OTIS Autoimmune Diseases Study, at 877-311-8972.

Lactation Enters breast milk/not recommended (AAP rates "compatible"; AAP 2001 update pending)

Breast-Feeding Considerations Based on limited data, only very small amounts of ibuprofen are excreted into breast milk. Adverse events have not been reported in nursing infants. Because there is a potential for adverse events to occur in nursing infants, the manufacturer does not recommend the use of ibuprofen while breast-feeding. Use with caution in nursing women with hypertensive disorders of pregnancy or pre-existing renal disease.

Dosage Forms

Caplet, oral: 200 mg
Advil® [OTC]: 200 mg
Motrin® IB [OTC]: 200 mg
Motrin® Junior [OTC]: 100 mg

Capsule, liquid filled, oral: 200 mg
Advil® [OTC]: 200 mg
Advil® Migraine [OTC]: 200 mg

Gelcap, oral:
Advil® [OTC]: 200 mg

Injection, solution:
Caldolor®: 100 mg/mL (4 mL, 8 mL)

Injection, solution [preservative free]:
NeoProfen®: 17.1 mg/mL (2 mL)

Suspension, oral: 100 mg/5 mL (5 mL, 10 mL, 120 mL, 240 mL, 480 mL); 40 mg/mL (15 mL)
Advil® Children's [OTC]: 100 mg/5 mL (120 mL)
Advil® Infants' [OTC]: 40 mg/mL (15 mL)
Motrin® Children's [OTC]: 100 mg/5 mL (60 mL, 120 mL)
Motrin® Infants' [OTC]: 40 mg/mL (15 mL)
Tablet, oral: 200 mg, 400 mg, 600 mg, 800 mg
Addaprin [OTC]: 200 mg
Advil® [OTC]: 200 mg
I-Prin [OTC]: 200 mg
Ibu-200 [OTC]: 200 mg
Ibu®: 400 mg, 600 mg, 800 mg
Midol® Cramps & Body Aches [OTC]: 200 mg
Motrin® IB [OTC]: 200 mg
Proprinal® [OTC]: 200 mg
Ultraprin [OTC]: 200 mg
Tablet, chewable, oral:
Motrin® Junior [OTC]: 100 mg
TopCare® Junior Strength [OTC]: 100 mg

Dental Comment Preoperative use of ibuprofen at a dose of 400-600 mg every 6 hours 24 hours before the appointment decreases postoperative edema and hastens healing time.

New information from the FDA states that ibuprofen can interfere with the antiplatelet effect of low-dose aspirin (81 mg/day), potentially rendering aspirin less effective when used for cardioprotection and stroke protection. In situations where these drugs could be used concomitantly, the FDA has provided the following information.

Patients who use immediate release aspirin (not enteric-coated aspirin) and take a single dose or chronic doses of ibuprofen 400 mg, should dose the ibuprofen at least **30 minutes or longer after aspirin ingestion or more than 8 hours before aspirin ingestion** to avoid attenuation of aspirin's effect.

At this time, recommendations about the timing of ibuprofen 400 mg in patients taking enteric-coated low-dose aspirin cannot be made based on available data. One study however, showed that the antiplatelet effect of enteric-coated low-dose aspirin was attenuated when ibuprofen 400 mg was dosed 2, 7, and 12 hours after aspirin (Catella-Lawson, 2001).

With occasional use of ibuprofen, there is likely to be minimal risk from any attenuation of the antiplatelet effect of low-dose aspirin, because of a long-lasting effect of aspirin on platelets.

Other over-the-counter (OTC) NSAIDs (ie, naproxen sodium and ketoprofen) should be viewed as having the potential to interfere with the antiplatelet effect of low-dose aspirin until proven otherwise. However, the FDA is unaware of any studies that have looked at the same type of interference by ketoprofen with low-dose aspirin. One study of naproxen and low-dose aspirin has suggested that naproxen may interfere with aspirin's antiplatelet activity when they are coadministered (Steinhubl, 2005). However, naproxen 500 mg administered 2 hours before or after aspirin 100 mg, did not interfere with aspirin's antiplatelet effect. The FDA stated that there is no data looking at doses of naproxen <500 mg. Naproxen OTC strength is 220 mg tablets.

Ibuprofen, prescription dose of 800 mg 3 times daily, significantly diminishes the antiplatelet effects of low-dose aspirin (baby) in healthy volunteers. Diclofenac (Systemic), 50 mg 3 times daily, did not interfere with the antiplatelet effects of low-dose aspirin (baby) in healthy volunteers. Ibuprofen, and possibly other

nonselective NSAIDs, may reduce the cardioprotective effects of aspirin. It seems prudent to avoid regular, frequent use of ibuprofen in patients receiving aspirin for its cardioprotective effects. Alternative analgesics (eg, acetaminophen) or prescription diclofenac in place of prescription ibuprofen may be a safer choice.

References

Ahmad N, Grad HA, Haas DA, et al, "The Efficacy of Nonopioid Analgesics for Postoperative Dental Pain: A Meta-Analysis," *Anesth Prog*, 1997, 44(4):119-26.
Beaver WT, "Review of the Analgesic Efficacy of Ibuprofen," *Int J Clin Pract*, 2003, (Suppl 135):13-7.
Catella-Lawson F, Reilly MP, Kapoor SC, et al. "Cyclooxygenase Inhibitors and the Antiplatelet Effects of Aspirin," *N Engl J Med*, 2001, 345(25):1809-17.
Dionne RA and Berthold CW, "Therapeutic Uses of Nonsteroidal Anti-inflammatory Drugs in Dentistry," *Crit Rev Oral Biol Med*, 2001, 12(4):315-30.
Dionne R, "Additive Analgesia Without Opioid Side Effects," *Compend Contin Educ Dent*, 2000, 21(7):572-4, 576-7.
Dionne R, "Relative Efficacy of Selective COX-2 Inhibitors Compared With Over-The-Counter Ibuprofen," *Int J Clin Pract Suppl*, 2003, (135):18-22.
Doyle G, Jayawardena S, Ashraf E, et al, "Efficacy and Tolerability of Nonprescription Ibuprofen Versus Celecoxib for Dental Pain," *J Clin Pharmacol*, 2002, 42(8):912-9.
Gobetti JP, "Controlling Dental Pain," *J Am Dent Assoc*, 1992, 123(6):47-52.
Hersh EV, Levin LM, Cooper SA, et al, "Ibuprofen Liquigel for Oral Surgery Pain," *Clin Ther*, 2000, 22(11):1306-18.
Olson NZ, Otero AM, Marrero I, et al, "Onset of Analgesia for Liquigel Ibuprofen 400 mg, Acetaminophen 1000 mg, Ketoprofen 25 mg, and Placebo in the Treatment of Postoperative Dental Pain," *J Clin Pharmacol*, 2001, 41(11):1238-47.
Pearlman B, Boyatzis S, Daly C, et al, "The Analgesic Efficacy of Ibuprofen in Periodontal Surgery: A Multicentre Study," *Aust Dent J*, 1997, 42(5):328-34.
Nguyen AM, Graham DY, Gage T, et al, "Nonsteroidal Anti-inflammatory Drug Use in Dentistry: Gastrointestinal Implications," *Gen Dent*, 1999, 47(6):590-6.
Schuijt MP, Huntjens-Fleuren HW, de Metz M, et al, "The Interaction of Ibuprofen and Diclofenac With Aspirin in Healthy Volunteers," *Br J Pharmacol*, 2009, 157(6):931-4.
Steinhubl SR, "The Use of Anti-Inflammatory Analgesics in the Patient With Cardiovascular Disease: What a Pain," *J Am Coll Cardiol*, 2005, 45(8):1302-3.
Wynn RL, "Update on Nonprescription Pain Relievers for Dental Pain," *Gen Dent*, 2004, 52(2):94-8.

Ibuprofen and Famotidine
(eye byoo PROE fen & fa MOE ti deen)

Brand Names: U.S. Duexis®

Pharmacologic Category Histamine H_2 Antagonist; Nonsteroidal Anti-inflammatory Drug (NSAID), Oral

Use Reduction of the risk of NSAID-associated gastric ulcers in patients who require an NSAID for the treatment of rheumatoid arthritis or osteoarthritis

Local Anesthetic/Vasoconstrictor Precautions No information available to require special precautions

Effects on Dental Treatment See individual agents

Effects on Bleeding See individual agents

Adverse Effects Percentages as reported for combination product. Also see individual agents.

1% to 10%:
Cardiovascular: Hypertension (3%), peripheral edema (2%)
Central nervous system: Headache (3%)
Gastrointestinal: Nausea (6%), diarrhea (5%), dyspepsia (5%), constipation (4%), abdominal pain/discomfort (2% to 3%), GERD (2%), vomiting (2%)
Genitourinary: Urinary tract infection (2%)
Hematologic: Anemia (2%)
Neuromuscular & skeletal: Back pain (2%), arthralgia (1%)
Respiratory: Upper respiratory tract infection (4%), bronchitis (2%), cough (2%), nasopharyngitis (2%), pharyngolaryngeal pain (2%), sinusitis (2%)
Miscellaneous: Influenza (2%)

General Dosage Range Oral: *Adults:* One tablet (800 mg ibuprofen/26.6 mg famotidine) 3 times daily

Mechanism of Action

Ibuprofen: Reversibly inhibits cyclooxygenase-1 and 2 (COX-1 and 2) enzymes, which results in in decreased formation of prostaglandin precursors; has antipyretic, analgesic, and anti-inflammatory properties

Famotidine: Competitive inhibition of histamine at H_2 receptors of the gastric parietal cells, which inhibits gastric acid secretion

Pregnancy Risk Factor C

Pregnancy Considerations Reproduction studies have not been conducted with this combination. Use is contraindicated in late stages of pregnancy ($\geq$30 weeks gestation). See individual agents.

Dental Comment See individual agents

Ibutilide (i BYOO ti lide)

Related Information

Clinical Risk Related to Drugs Prolonging QT Interval *on page 1510*

Brand Names: U.S. Corvert®

Pharmacologic Category Antiarrhythmic Agent, Class III

Use Acute termination of atrial fibrillation or flutter of recent onset; the effectiveness of ibutilide has not been determined in patients with arrhythmias >90 days in duration

Local Anesthetic/Vasoconstrictor Precautions Ibutilide is one of the drugs confirmed to prolong the QT interval and is accepted as having a risk of causing torsade de pointes. The risk of drug-induced torsade de pointes is extremely low when a single QT interval prolonging drug is prescribed. In terms of epinephrine, it is not known what effect vasoconstrictors in the local anesthetic regimen will have in patients with a known history of congenital prolonged QT interval or in patients taking any medication that prolongs the QT interval. Until more information is obtained, it is suggested that the clinician consult with the physician prior to the use of a vasoconstrictor in suspected patients, and that the vasoconstrictor (epinephrine, mepivacaine and levonordefrin [Carbocaine® 2% with Neo-Cobefrin®]) be used with caution.

Effects on Dental Treatment No significant effects or complications reported

Effects on Bleeding No information available to require special precautions

Adverse Effects 1% to 10%:

Cardiovascular: Ventricular extrasystoles (5.1%), nonsustained monomorphic ventricular tachycardia (4.9%), nonsustained polymorphic ventricular tachycardia (2.7%), tachycardia/supraventricular tachycardia (2.7%), hypotension (2%), bundle branch block (1.9%), sustained polymorphic ventricular tachycardia (eg, torsade de pointes) (1.7%, often requiring cardioversion), AV block (1.5%), bradycardia (1.2%), QT segment prolongation, hypertension (1.2%), palpitation (1%)

Central nervous system: Headache (3.6%)

Gastrointestinal: Nausea (>1%)

General Dosage Range I.V.:

Adults <60 kg: 0.01 mg/kg; may repeat once

Adults ≥60 kg: 1 mg; may repeat once

Mechanism of Action Exact mechanism of action is unknown; prolongs the action potential in cardiac tissue

Pharmacodynamics/Kinetics

Onset of Action ~90 minutes after start of infusion ($\frac{1}{2}$ of conversions to sinus rhythm occur during infusion)

Half-life Elimination 2-12 hours (average: 6 hours)

Pregnancy Risk Factor C

Pregnancy Considerations Teratogenic and embryocidal in rats; avoid use in pregnancy

Dental Comment Ibutilide is known to prolong the QT interval. The QT interval is measured as the time and distance between the Q point of the QRS complex and the end of the T wave in the ECG tracing. After adjustment for heart rate, the QT interval is defined as prolonged if it is more than 450 msec in men and 460 msec in women. A long QT syndrome was first described in the 1950s and 60s as a congenital syndrome involving QT interval prolongation and syncope and sudden death. Some of the congenital long QT syndromes were characterized by a peculiar electrocardiographic appearance of the QRS complex involving a premature atria beat followed by a pause, then a subsequent sinus beat showing marked QT prolongation and deformity. This type of cardiac arrhythmia was originally termed "torsade de pointes" (translated from the French as "twisting of the points"). Ibutilide is considered as having a risk of causing torsade de pointes. Since it is not known what effect vasoconstrictors in the local anesthetic regimen will have in patients with a known history of congenital prolonged QT interval or in patients taking any medication that prolongs the QT interval, a medical consult is suggested.

Icatibant (eye KAT i bant)

Brand Names: U.S. Firazyr®

Pharmacologic Category Selective Bradykinin B2 Receptor Antagonist

Use Treatment of acute attacks of hereditary angioedema (HAE)

Local Anesthetic/Vasoconstrictor Precautions No information available to require special precautions

Effects on Dental Treatment No significant effects or complications reported

Effects on Bleeding No information available to require special precautions

Adverse Effects

>10%: Local: Injection site reaction (97%)

1% to 10%:

Central nervous system: Pyrexia (4%), dizziness (3%)

Hepatic: Transaminase increased (4%)

General Dosage Range SubQ: *Adults:* 30 mg/dose; maximum: 3 doses/24 hours

Mechanism of Action Icatibant is a selective competitive antagonist for the bradykinin B_2 receptor. Patients with HAE have an absence or dysfunction of C1-esterase-inhibitor which leads to the production of bradykinin. The presence of bradykinin may cause symptoms of localized swelling, inflammation, and pain. Icatibant inhibits bradykinin from binding at the B_2 receptor, thereby treating the symptoms associated with acute attack.

Pharmacodynamics/Kinetics

Onset of Action Median time to 50% decrease of symptoms: ~2 hours

Duration of Action Inhibits symptoms caused by bradykinin for ~6 hours

Half-life Elimination 1-1.8 hours

Time to Peak 0.75 hours

Pregnancy Risk Factor C

Pregnancy Considerations Adverse events were observed in animal reproduction studies with doses close to or less than the recommended human dose.

Icodextrin (eye KOE dex trin)

Brand Names: U.S. Extraneal
Pharmacologic Category Adhesiolytic; Peritoneal Dialysate, Osmotic
Use
Adept®: Reduction of postsurgical adhesions in gynecologic laparoscopic procedures
Extraneal®: Daily exchange for the long dwell (8- to 16-hour) during continuous ambulatory peritoneal dialysis (CAPD) or automated peritoneal dialysis (APD) for the management of end-stage renal disease (ESRD); improvement of long-dwell ultrafiltration and clearance of creatinine and urea nitrogen (compared to 4.25% dextrose) in patients with high/average or greater transport characteristics as measured by peritoneal equilibration test (PET)
Local Anesthetic/Vasoconstrictor Precautions No information available to require special precautions
Effects on Dental Treatment No significant effects or complications reported
Effects on Bleeding No information available to require special precautions
Adverse Effects
CAPD or APD (Extraneal®):
>10%:
Cardiovascular: Hypertension (13%)
Respiratory: Upper respiratory infection (15%)
Miscellaneous: Peritonitis (26% vs 25% in controls)
5% to 10%:
Cardiovascular: Edema (up to 6%), chest pain (5%), hypervolemia, hypotension
Central nervous system: Headache (9%), dizziness
Dermatological: Rash (10%), pruritus, skin disorder
Endocrine & metabolic: Hyperglycemia (5%), hyperphosphatemia, hypokalemia, hypoproteinemia
Gastrointestinal: Abdominal pain (8%), nausea (7%), dyspepsia (5%), diarrhea, vomiting
Hematologic: Anemia
Neuromuscular & skeletal: Arthralgia, pain, weakness
Respiratory: Cough increased (7%), dyspnea
Miscellaneous: Accidental injury (6%), flu syndrome (7%), infection
<5%:
Cardiovascular: Orthostatic hypotension, CHF
Central nervous system: Confusion
Dermatologic: Exfoliative dermatitis, erythema multiforme, eczema, maculopapular rash, vesicobullous rash
Endocrine & metabolic: Hypercalcemia, hypochloremia, hypoglycemia, hyponatremia, alkaline phosphatase increased
Gastrointestinal: Abdominal enlargement, cramps
Hepatic: ALT increased, AST increased
Local: Infusion pain
Miscellaneous: Cloudy effluent

Laparoscopic surgery (Adept®):
>10%:
Central nervous system: Headache (35%)
Endocrine & metabolic: Dysmenorrhea (13%)
Gastrointestinal: Nausea (6% to 17%), constipation (11%)
1% to 10%:
Central nervous system: Pyrexia (6%), insomnia (5%)
Gastrointestinal: Flatulence (8%), abdominal pain (7%), abdominal distention (6%), vomiting (6%), diarrhea (1%)

Genitourinary: Dysuria (7%), urinary tract infection (7%); labial, vulvar, or vaginal swelling (6%); vaginal bleeding (6%)
Neuromuscular & skeletal: Arthralgia (9%), back pain (8%)
Respiratory: Nasopharyngitis (7%), cough (4%)
General Dosage Range Intraperitoneal: *Adults:*
CAPD or APD (Extraneal®): Given as a single daily exchange in CAPD or APD; dwell time of 8-16 hours is suggested
Laparoscopic gynecologic surgery (Adept®): Irrigate with at least 100 mL every 30 minutes during surgery; aspirate remaining fluid after surgery is completed, then instill 1 L into the cavity
Mechanism of Action When used for dialysis, icodextrin exerts osmotic pressure across small intercellular pores resulting in transcapillary ultrafiltration throughout the dwell while providing electrolytes and lactate for the maintenance of both the electrolyte and acid-base balance. When used for laparoscopic surgery, the colloidal osmotic action allows the fluid to be retained in the peritoneal cavity for 3-4 days, physically providing a temporary separation of peritoneal surfaces and minimizing adhesion formation.
Pharmacodynamics/Kinetics
Time to Peak Plasma: 13 hours
Pregnancy Risk Factor C
Pregnancy Considerations Complete reproduction studies have not been conducted.

Icosapent Ethyl (eye KOE sa pent ETH il)

Brand Names: U.S. Vascepa™
Pharmacologic Category Antilipemic Agent, Omega-3 Fatty Acids
Use Adjunct to dietary therapy in the treatment of hypertriglyceridemia (≥500 mg/dL)
Local Anesthetic/Vasoconstrictor Precautions No information available to require special precautions
Effects on Dental Treatment Key adverse event(s) related to dental treatment: Oropharyngeal pain (rare)
Effects on Bleeding Prolongation of bleeding time has been observed in some clinical studies of omega-3 fatty acids including eicospentaenoic acid. Bleeding time may be prolonged in patients taking icosapent ethyl; may be more pronounced if used concomitantly with warfarin or antiplatelet agents.
Adverse Effects 1% to 10%: Neuromuscular & skeletal: Arthralgia (2%)
General Dosage Range Oral: *Adults:* 2 g twice daily
Mechanism of Action Icosapent ethyl, the ethyl ester of eicosapentaenoic acid (EPA), is an omega-3 fatty acid which aids in decreasing hepatic very low-density lipoprotein triglycerides (VLDL-TG) synthesis/secretion and increasing triglyceride clearance from VLDL particles. The mechanism has not been completely defined. Possible mechanisms include inhibition of acyl CoA: 1,2 diacylglycerol acyltransferase, increased hepatic beta-oxidation, a reduction in the hepatic synthesis of triglycerides, or an increase in plasma lipoprotein lipase activity.
Pharmacodynamics/Kinetics
Half-life Elimination EPA: ~89 hours
Time to Peak EPA: ~5 hours
Pregnancy Risk Factor C

◄ **Pregnancy Considerations** Adverse events were observed in animal reproduction studies. Maternal dietary consumption of omega-3-fatty acids (containing eicosapentaenoic acid [EPA] and docosahexaenoic acid [DHA]) influences fetal concentrations (Coletta, 2010; Miles, 2011). Information specific to the therapeutic use of this product in pregnancy has not been located; however, the use of omega-3-fatty acids to manage elevated triglycerides in pregnancy has been described in case reports (Goldberg, 2012; Papadakis, 2011).

IDArubicin (eye da ROO bi sin)

Brand Names: U.S. Idamycin PFS®
Brand Names: Canada Idamycin®
Pharmacologic Category Antineoplastic Agent, Anthracycline; Antineoplastic Agent, Antibiotic
Use Treatment of acute myeloid leukemia (AML)
Unlabeled Use Acute lymphocytic leukemia (ALL)
Local Anesthetic/Vasoconstrictor Precautions No information available to require special precautions
Effects on Dental Treatment Key adverse event(s) related to dental treatment: Stomatitis.
Effects on Bleeding Platelet counts reach a nadir by day 10-15 and recover by day 21-28. Bleeding during periods of thrombocytopenia may occur.
Adverse Effects
>10%:
  Cardiovascular: Transient ECG abnormalities (supraventricular tachycardia, S-T wave changes, atrial or ventricular extrasystoles); generally asymptomatic and self-limiting. CHF, dose related. The relative cardiotoxicity of idarubicin compared to doxorubicin is unclear. Some investigators report no increase in cardiac toxicity for adults at cumulative oral idarubicin doses up to 540 mg/m²; other reports suggest a maximum cumulative intravenous dose of 150 mg/m².
  Central nervous system: Headache
  Dermatologic: Alopecia (25% to 30%), radiation recall, skin rash (11%), urticaria
  Gastrointestinal: Nausea, vomiting (30% to 60%); diarrhea (9% to 22%); stomatitis (11%); GI hemorrhage (30%)
  Genitourinary: Discoloration of urine (darker yellow)
  Hematologic: Myelosuppression (nadir: 10-15 days; recovery: 21-28 days), primarily leukopenia; thrombocytopenia and anemia. Effects are generally less severe with oral dosing.
  Hepatic: Bilirubin and transaminases increased (44%)
1% to 10%:
  Central nervous system: Seizure
  Neuromuscular & skeletal: Peripheral neuropathy
General Dosage Range Dosage adjustment recommended in patients with hepatic or renal impairment
I.V.: *Adults:* Induction: 12 mg/m²/day for 3 days; Consolidation: 10-12 mg/m²/day for 2 days
Mechanism of Action Similar to doxorubicin and daunorubicin; inhibition of DNA and RNA synthesis by intercalation between DNA base pairs
Pharmacodynamics/Kinetics
  Half-life Elimination Oral: 14-35 hours; I.V.: 12-27 hours
  Time to Peak Serum: 1-5 hours
Pregnancy Risk Factor D

Pregnancy Considerations Adverse events were observed in animal studies. Fetal fatality was noted in a case report following use in a pregnant woman during the second trimester. The manufacturer recommends that women of childbearing potential avoid pregnancy.

Idursulfase (eye dur SUL fase)

Brand Names: U.S. Elaprase®
Brand Names: Canada Elaprase®
Pharmacologic Category Enzyme
Use Replacement therapy in mucopolysaccharidosis II (MPS II, Hunter syndrome) for improvement of walking capacity
Local Anesthetic/Vasoconstrictor Precautions No information available to require special precautions
Effects on Dental Treatment No significant effects or complications reported
Effects on Bleeding No information available to require special precautions
Adverse Effects >10%:
  Cardiovascular: Hypertension (25%), atrial abnormality (13%)
  Central nervous system: Pyrexia (63%), headache (59%), malaise (22%), anxiety (13%), irritability (13%)
  Dermatologic: Pruritus (28%), urticaria (16%), pruritic rash (13%), skin disorder (13%)
  Gastrointestinal: Dyspepsia (13%)
  Local: Abscess (16%), infusion site edema (13%)
  Neuromuscular & skeletal: Arthralgia (31%), limb pain (28%), chest wall musculoskeletal pain (16%), musculoskeletal dysfunction (16%)
  Ocular: Visual disturbance (22%)
  Respiratory: Wheezing (19%)
  Miscellaneous: Antibody development (51%), infusion reactions (15%), superficial injury (13%)
General Dosage Range I.V.: *Children ≥5 years and Adults:* 0.5 mg/kg once weekly
Mechanism of Action Idursulfase is a recombinant form of iduronate-2-sulfatase, an enzyme needed to hydrolyze the mucopolysaccharides dermatan sulfate and heparan sulfate in various cells. Accumulation of these polysaccharides can lead to various manifestations of disease, including physical changes, CNS involvement, cardiac, respiratory, and mobility dysfunction. Replacement of this enzyme has been shown to improve walking capacity in patients with a deficiency.
Pharmacodynamics/Kinetics
  Half-life Elimination Half-life elimination: 44-48 minutes
Pregnancy Risk Factor C
Pregnancy Considerations Animal reproduction studies have not been conducted.

Ifosfamide (eye FOSS fa mide)

Brand Names: U.S. Ifex
Brand Names: Canada Ifex
Pharmacologic Category Antineoplastic Agent, Alkylating Agent; Antineoplastic Agent, Alkylating Agent (Nitrogen Mustard)
Use
U.S. labeling: Treatment (third-line) of germ cell testicular cancer (in combination with other chemotherapy drugs and with concurrent mesna)

Canadian labeling (not approved indications in the U.S.): Treatment of soft tissue sarcoma, pancreatic cancer (relapsed or refractory), cervical cancer (advanced or recurrent; as monotherapy or in combination with cisplatin and bleomycin)

Unlabeled Use Treatment of bladder cancer (metastatic), cervical cancer (recurrent or metastatic), head and neck cancers (recurrent or metastatic), ovarian cancer, small cell lung cancer (relapsed), Hodgkin lymphoma (relapsed or refractory), non-Hodgkin lymphomas, thymomas and thymic cancers (advanced), sarcomas (Ewing's sarcoma, osteosarcoma, and soft tissue sarcoma)

Local Anesthetic/Vasoconstrictor Precautions No information available to require special precautions

Effects on Dental Treatment No significant effects or complications reported

Effects on Bleeding Thrombocytopenia occurs in ~20% of patients (grade 3/4: 8%). Medical consult recommended.

Adverse Effects
>10%:
Central nervous system: CNS toxicity or encephalopathy (12% to 15%)
Dermatologic: Alopecia (83% to 90%; 100% with combination therapy)
Endocrine & metabolic: Metabolic acidosis (31%)
Gastrointestinal: Nausea/vomiting (47% to 58%)
Hematologic: Leukopenia (50% to ≤100%; grade 4: ≤50%; nadir: 8-14 days), anemia (38%), thrombocytopenia (20%; grades 3/4: ≤8%)
Renal: Hematuria (6% to 92%; reduced with mesna; grade 2 [gross hematuria]: 8% to 12%)
1% to 10%:
Central nervous system: Fever (1%)
Gastrointestinal: Anorexia (1%)
Hematologic: Neutropenic fever (1%)
Hepatic: Bilirubin increased (2% to 3%), liver dysfunction (2% to 3%), transaminases increased (2% to 3%)
Local: Phlebitis (2% to 3%)
Renal: Renal impairment (6%)
Miscellaneous: Infection (8% to 10%)

General Dosage Range Dosage adjustment recommended in patients with hepatic or renal impairment or who develop toxicities.
I.V.: *Adults:* 1200 mg/m^2/day for 5 days every 21 days

Mechanism of Action Causes cross-linking of strands of DNA by binding with nucleic acids and other intracellular structures; inhibits protein synthesis and DNA synthesis

Pharmacodynamics/Kinetics
Half-life Elimination
Increased in the elderly
High dose (3800-5000 mg/m^2): ~15 hours
Lower dose (1600-2400 mg/m^2): ~7 hours

Pregnancy Risk Factor D

Pregnancy Considerations Embryotoxic and teratogenic effects have been observed in animal reproduction studies. Fetal growth retardation and neonatal anemia have been reported with exposure to ifosfamide-containing regimens during human pregnancy. Male and female fertility may be affected (dose and duration dependent). Ifosfamide interferes with oogenesis and spermatogenesis; amenorrhea, azoospermia, and sterility have been reported and may be irreversible. Avoid pregnancy during treatment; male patients should not father a child for at least 6 months after completion of therapy.

Iloperidone (eye loe PER i done)

Related Information
Clinical Risk Related to Drugs Prolonging QT Interval *on page 1510*
Brand Names: U.S. Fanapt®
Generic Availability (U.S.) No
Pharmacologic Category Antipsychotic Agent, Atypical
Use Acute treatment of schizophrenia

Local Anesthetic/Vasoconstrictor Precautions Iloperidone is one of the drugs confirmed to prolong the QT interval and is accepted as having a risk of causing torsade de pointes. The risk of drug-induced torsade de pointes is extremely low when a single QT interval prolonging drug is prescribed. In terms of epinephrine, it is not known what effect vasoconstrictors in the local anesthetic regimen will have in patients with a known history of congenital prolonged QT interval or in patients taking any medication that prolongs the QT interval. Until more information is obtained, it is suggested that the clinician consult with the physician prior to the use of a vasoconstrictor in suspected patients, and that the vasoconstrictor (epinephrine, mepivacaine and levonordefrin [Carbocaine® 2% with Neo-Cobefrin®]) be used with caution.

Effects on Dental Treatment Key adverse event(s) related to dental treatment: Xerostomia and changes in salivation (normal salivary flow resumes upon discontinuation), orthostatic hypotension

Effects on Bleeding No information available to require special precautions

Adverse Effects
>10%:
Cardiovascular: Tachycardia (3% to 12%; dose related)
Central nervous system: Dizziness (10% to 20%; dose related), somnolence (9% to 15%)
1% to 10%:
Cardiovascular: Orthostatic hypotension (3% to 5%), hypotension (<1% to 3%; dose related), palpitations (≥1%)
Central nervous system: Fatigue (4% to 6%), extrapyramidal symptoms (4% to 5%), tremor (3%), lethargy (1% to 3%), akathisia (2%), aggression (≥1%), delusion (≥1%), restlessness (≥1%)
Dermatologic: Rash (2% to 3%)
Gastrointestinal: Nausea (≤10%), xerostomia (8% to 10%), weight gain (1% to 9%; dose related), diarrhea (5% to 7%), abdominal discomfort (≤3%; dose related), weight loss (≥1%)
Genitourinary: Ejaculation failure (2%), erectile dysfunction (≥1%), urinary incontinence (≥1%)
Neuromuscular & skeletal: Arthralgia (3%), stiffness (1% to 3%; dose related), dyskinesia (<2%), muscle spasm (≥1%), myalgia (≥1%)
Ocular: Blurred vision (≤3%), conjunctivitis (≥1%)
Respiratory: Nasal congestion (5% to 8%), nasopharyngitis (≤4%), upper respiratory tract infection (2% to 3%), dyspnea (2%)

Dosage Oral: Adults: Schizophrenia: Initial: 1 mg twice daily; titrate to the recommended dosage range with dosage adjustments not to exceed 2 mg twice daily (4 mg daily) every 24 hours; recommended dosage range: 6-12 mg twice daily (maximum: 24 mg daily)

◀ **Note:** Titrate dose to effect (to avoid orthostatic hypotensive effects); treatment >6 weeks has not been evaluated; when reinitiating treatment after discontinuation (>3 days), the initial titration schedule should be followed.

Dosage adjustment in patients receiving strong CYP2D6 inhibitors (eg, paroxetine, fluoxetine, quinidine): Decrease iloperidone dose by 50%; when the CYP2D6 inhibitor is discontinued, return to previous dose.

Dosage adjustment in patients receiving strong CYP3A4 inhibitors (eg, ketoconazole, clarithromycin): Decrease iloperidone dose by 50%; when the CYP3A4 inhibitor is discontinued, return to previous dose.

Dosage adjustment in poor metabolizers of CYP2D6: Decrease iloperidone dose by 50%.

Dosage adjustment in renal impairment: No dosage adjustment provided in manufacturer's labeling; however, pharmacokinetics of iloperidone do not appear to be altered by renal impairment due to extensive hepatic metabolism.

Dosage adjustment in hepatic impairment: Use is not recommended in patients with hepatic impairment (has not been studied).

Mechanism of Action Iloperidone is a piperidinyl-benzisoxazole atypical antipsychotic with mixed $D_2/5-HT_2$ antagonist activity. It exhibits high affinity for $5-HT_{2A}$, D_2, and D_3 receptors, low to moderate affinity for D_1, D_4, H_1, $5-HT_{1A}$, $5-HT_6$, $5-HT_7$, and $NE_{\alpha 1}$ receptors, and no affinity for muscarinic receptors. The addition of serotonin antagonism to dopamine antagonism (classic neuroleptic mechanism) is thought to improve negative symptoms of psychoses and reduce the incidence of extrapyramidal side effects. Iloperidone's low affinity for histamine H_1 receptors may decrease the risk for weight gain and somnolence while its affinity for $NE_{\alpha 1/\alpha 2C}$ may provide antidepressant and anxiolytic activity and improved cognitive function.

Contraindications Hypersensitivity to iloperidone or any component of the formulation

Warnings/Precautions [U.S. Boxed Warning]: Elderly patients with dementia-related psychosis treated with antipsychotics are at an increased risk of death compared to placebo. Most deaths appeared to be either cardiovascular (eg, heart failure, sudden death) or infectious (eg, pneumonia) in nature. In addition, an increased incidence of cerebrovascular effects (eg, transient ischemic attack, cerebrovascular accidents) has been reported in studies of placebo-controlled trials of antipsychotics in elderly patients with dementia-related psychosis. Iloperidone is not approved for the treatment of dementia-related psychosis.

May be sedating; use with caution in disorders where CNS depression is a feature. Caution in patients with predisposition to seizures. Use is not recommended in patients with hepatic impairment. Esophageal dysmotility and aspiration have been associated with antipsychotic use; use with caution in patients at risk of aspiration pneumonia (ie, Alzheimer's disease). Use is associated with increased prolactin levels; clinical significance of hyperprolactinemia in patients with breast cancer or other prolactin-dependent tumors is unknown. May alter temperature regulation. Leukopenia, neutropenia, and agranulocytosis (sometimes fatal) have been reported in clinical trials and postmarketing reports; presence of risk factors (eg, pre-existing low WBC or history of drug-induced leuko-/neutropenia) should prompt periodic blood count assessment and discontinuation at first signs of blood dyscrasias.

May alter cardiac conduction and prolong the QT_c interval; life-threatening arrhythmias have occurred with therapeutic doses of antipsychotics. Risks may be increased by conditions or concomitant medications which cause bradycardia, hypokalemia, and/or hypomagnesemia. Avoid use in combination with QT_c-prolonging drugs and in patients with congenital long QT syndrome, history of cardiac arrhythmia, recent MI, or uncompensated heart failure. Discontinue treatment in patients found to have persistent QT_c intervals >500 msec. Further cardiac evaluation is warranted in patients with symptoms of dizziness, palpitations, or syncope. May cause orthostatic hypotension; use with caution in patients at risk of this effect (eg, concurrent medication use which may predispose to hypotension/bradycardia or presence of hypovolemia) or in those who would not tolerate transient hypotensive episodes. Use with caution in patients with cardiovascular diseases (eg, heart failure, history of myocardial infarction or ischemia, cerebrovascular disease, conduction abnormalities).

May cause anticholinergic effects (confusion, agitation, constipation, xerostomia, blurred vision, urinary retention); therefore, use with caution in patients with decreased gastrointestinal motility, urinary retention, BPH, xerostomia, or visual problems (including narrow-angle glaucoma). May cause extrapyramidal symptoms (EPS), including pseudoparkinsonism, acute dystonic reactions, akathisia, and tardive dyskinesia. Risk of dystonia (and probably other EPS) may be greater with increased doses, use of conventional antipsychotics, males, and younger patients. Risk of neuroleptic malignant syndrome (NMS) may be increased in patients with Parkinson's disease or Lewy body dementia. May cause hyperglycemia; in some cases may be extreme and associated with ketoacidosis, hyperosmolar coma, or death. Use with caution in patients with diabetes or other disorders of glucose regulation; monitor for worsening of glucose control. Dyslipidemia has been reported with atypical antipsychotics; risk profile may differ between agents. In clinical trials, changes in triglyceride and total cholesterol levels observed with iloperidone were similar to those observed with placebo or were clinically insignificant. Small reductions in cholesterol and triglycerides have been observed in longer term iloperidone trials.

Significant weight gain has been observed with antipsychotic therapy; incidence varies with product. Monitor waist circumference and BMI. Rare cases of priapism have been reported.

Use in elderly patients with dementia is associated with an increased risk of mortality and cerebrovascular accidents; avoid antipsychotic use for behavioral problems associated with dementia unless alternative nonpharmacologic therapies have failed and patient may harm self or others. In addition, use may cause or exacerbate syndrome of inappropriate antidiuretic hormone secretion or hyponatremia; monitor sodium closely with initiation or dosage adjustments in older adults (Beers Criteria).

Dosage adjustments are recommended for iloperidone when given concomitantly with strong CYP2D6 or CYP3A4 inhibitors or in poor metabolizers of CYP2D6. The possibility of a suicide attempt is inherent in psychotic illness; use caution in high-risk patients during initiation of therapy. Prescriptions should be written for the smallest quantity consistent with good patient care. Continued use for >6 weeks has not been evaluated.

Drug Interactions
Metabolism/Transport Effects Substrate of CYP2D6 (major), CYP3A4 (minor); **Note:** Assignment of Major/Minor substrate status based on clinically relevant drug interaction potential; **Inhibits** CYP3A4 (moderate)

Avoid Concomitant Use
Avoid concomitant use of Iloperidone with any of the following: Azelastine (Nasal); Bosutinib; Highest Risk QTc-Prolonging Agents; Ivabradine; Lomitapide; Metoclopramide; Mifepristone; Moderate Risk QTc-Prolonging Agents; Paraldehyde; Tolvaptan

Increased Effect/Toxicity
Iloperidone may increase the levels/effects of: Alcohol (Ethyl); ARIPiprazole; Avanafil; Azelastine (Nasal); Bosutinib; Budesonide (Systemic, Oral Inhalation); Buprenorphine; CNS Depressants; Colchicine; CYP3A4 Substrates; Eplerenone; Everolimus; FentaNYL; Highest Risk QTc-Prolonging Agents; Ivacaftor; Lomitapide; Lurasidone; Methotrimeprazine; Methylphenidate; Paraldehyde; Pimecrolimus; Salmeterol; Saxagliptin; Serotonin Modulators; Tolvaptan; Zolpidem

The levels/effects of Iloperidone may be increased by: Abiraterone Acetate; Acetylcholinesterase Inhibitors (Central); CYP2D6 Inhibitors (Moderate); CYP2D6 Inhibitors (Strong); CYP3A4 Inhibitors (Strong); HydrOXYzine; Ivabradine; Lithium formulations; Magnesium Sulfate; MAO Inhibitors; Methotrimeprazine; Methylphenidate; Metoclopramide; Metyrosine; Mifepristone; Moderate Risk QTc-Prolonging Agents; Perampanel; QTc-Prolonging Agents (Indeterminate Risk and Risk Modifying); Sodium Oxybate; Tetrabenazine

Decreased Effect
Iloperidone may decrease the levels/effects of: Amphetamines; Anti-Parkinson's Agents (Dopamine Agonist); Ifosfamide; Quinagolide

The levels/effects of Iloperidone may be decreased by: CYP2D6 Inhibitors (Strong); Lithium formulations; Peginterferon Alfa-2b

Ethanol/Nutrition/Herb Interactions
Ethanol: May increase CNS depression; monitor for increased effects with coadministration. Caution patients about effects.
Herb/Nutraceutical: Avoid St John's wort (may decrease serum levels of iloperidone). Avoid kava kava, gotu kola, valerian, St John's wort (may increase CNS depression).

Dietary Considerations May be given with or without food.

Pharmacodynamics/Kinetics
Half-life Elimination
Extensive metabolizers: Iloperidone: 18 hours; P88: 26 hours; P95: 23 hours
Poor metabolizers: Iloperidone: 33 hours; P88: 37 hours; P95: 31 hours
Time to Peak Plasma: 2-4 hours
Pregnancy Risk Factor C
Pregnancy Considerations Animal studies have shown an increased risk of developmental toxicity and fetal mortality. Antipsychotic use during the third trimester of pregnancy has a risk for abnormal muscle movements (extrapyramidal symptoms [EPS]) and withdrawal symptoms in newborns following delivery. Symptoms in the newborn may include agitation, feeding disorder, hypertonia, hypotonia, respiratory distress, somnolence, and tremor; these effects may be self-limiting or require hospitalization.

Lactation Excretion in breast milk unknown/not recommended
Dosage Forms
Tablet, oral:
Fanapt®: 1 mg, 2 mg, 4 mg, 6 mg, 8 mg, 10 mg, 12 mg, 1 mg (2s), 2 mg (2s), 4 mg (2s), and 6 mg (2s)

Dental Comment Iloperidone is known to prolong the QT interval. The QT interval is measured as the time and distance between the Q point of the QRS complex and the end of the T wave in the ECG tracing. After adjustment for heart rate, the QT interval is defined as prolonged if it is more than 450 msec in men and 460 msec in women. A long QT syndrome was first described in the 1950s and 60s as a congenital syndrome involving QT interval prolongation and syncope and sudden death. Some of the congenital long QT syndromes were characterized by a peculiar electrocardiographic appearance of the QRS complex involving a premature atria beat followed by a pause, then a subsequent sinus beat showing marked QT prolongation and deformity. This type of cardiac arrhythmia was originally termed "torsade de pointes" (translated from the French as "twisting of the points"). Iloperidone is considered as having a risk of causing torsade de pointes. Since it is not known what effect vasoconstrictors in the local anesthetic regimen will have in patients with a known history of congenital prolonged QT interval or in patients taking any medication that prolongs the QT interval, a medical consult is suggested.

Iloprost (EYE loe prost)

Brand Names: U.S. Ventavis®
Pharmacologic Category Prostacyclin; Prostaglandin; Vasodilator
Use Treatment of pulmonary arterial hypertension (PAH) (WHO Group I) in patients with NYHA Class III or IV symptoms to improve exercise tolerance, symptoms, and diminish clinical deterioration
Unlabeled Use WHO group III and IV pulmonary arterial hypertension (PAH)
Local Anesthetic/Vasoconstrictor Precautions No information available to require special precautions
Effects on Dental Treatment Key adverse event(s) related to dental treatment: Jaw pain (reported in >10% of patients).
Effects on Bleeding No information available to require special precautions
Adverse Effects
>10%:
Cardiovascular: Flushing (27%), hypotension (11%)
Central nervous system: Headache (30%)
Gastrointestinal: Nausea (13%)
Neuromuscular & skeletal: Trismus (12%), jaw pain (12%)
Respiratory: Cough increased (39%)
Miscellaneous: Flu-like syndrome (14%)
1% to 10%:
Cardiovascular: Syncope (8%), palpitation (7%)
Central nervous system: Insomnia (8%)
Gastrointestinal: Vomiting (7%), tongue pain (4%)
Hepatic: Alkaline phosphatase increased (6%), GGT increased (6%)
Neuromuscular & skeletal: Back pain (7%), muscle cramps (6%)
Respiratory: Hemoptysis (5%), pneumonia (4%)

◄ **General Dosage Range** Dosage adjustment recommended in patients with hepatic impairment.

Inhalation: *Adults:* Initial: 2.5 mcg/dose; Maintenance: 2.5-5 mcg/dose 6-9 times/day (maximum: 45 mcg/day)

Mechanism of Action Acutely, iloprost dilates systemic and pulmonary arterial vascular beds. With longer-term use, alters pulmonary vascular resistance and suppresses vascular smooth muscle proliferation. In addition, it is a mild endogenous inhibitor of platelet aggregation when aerosolized (Beghetti, 2002).

Pharmacodynamics/Kinetics

Duration of Action 30-60 minutes

Half-life Elimination 20-30 minutes (effect), 7-9 minutes (elimination)

Time to Peak Serum: Within 5 minutes after inhalation

Pregnancy Risk Factor C

Pregnancy Considerations Iloprost was shown to be embryolethal or teratogenic in some, but not all, animal studies. There are no adequate or well-controlled studies in pregnant women; use only if clearly needed. Women with pulmonary hypertension are urged to avoid pregnancy.

Imatinib (eye MAT eh nib)

Brand Names: U.S. Gleevec®

Brand Names: Canada Gleevec®

Pharmacologic Category Antineoplastic Agent, Tyrosine Kinase Inhibitor

Use Treatment of:

Gastrointestinal stromal tumors (GIST) kit-positive (CD117), including unresectable and/or metastatic malignant and adjuvant treatment following complete resection

Philadelphia chromosome-positive (Ph+) chronic myeloid leukemia (CML) in chronic phase (newly-diagnosed) in children and adults

Ph+ CML in blast crisis, accelerated phase, or chronic phase after failure of interferon therapy

Ph+ acute lymphoblastic leukemia (ALL) (relapsed or refractory)

Ph+ ALL (newly diagnosed; in combination with chemotherapy) in children

Aggressive systemic mastocytosis (ASM) without D816V c-Kit mutation (or c-Kit mutation status unknown)

Dermatofibrosarcoma protuberans (DFSP) (unresectable, recurrent and/or metastatic)

Hypereosinophilic syndrome (HES) and/or chronic eosinophilic leukemia (CEL)

Myelodysplastic/myeloproliferative disease (MDS/MPD) associated with platelet-derived growth factor receptor (PDGFR) gene rearrangements

Canadian labeling (not an approved indication in the U.S.): Ph+ ALL induction therapy (newly diagnosed; as a single agent)

Unlabeled Use Treatment of desmoid tumors or chordoma (soft tissue sarcomas); post-stem cell transplant (allogeneic) follow-up treatment for recurrence in CML; treatment of advanced or metastatic melanoma (C-KIT mutated tumors)

Local Anesthetic/Vasoconstrictor Precautions No information available to require special precautions

Effects on Dental Treatment Key adverse event(s) related to dental treatment: Mouth ulceration and taste disturbance.

Effects on Bleeding Bleeding was reported in 12% to 53% of patients. Cytopenias including thrombocytopenia (grade 4 severe: <33%) and anemia (25% to 80%; grade 4: <11%) have been reported. Medical consult is recommended.

Adverse Effects Note: Adverse reactions listed as a composite of data across many trials, except where noted for a specific indication.

>10%:

Cardiovascular: Edema/fluid retention (11% to 86%; grades 3/4: 3% to 13%; includes aggravated edema, anasarca, ascites, pericardial effusion, peripheral edema, pulmonary edema, and superficial edema); facial edema (≤17%), chest pain (7% to 11%), hypotension (Ph+ ALL [pediatric] grades 3/4: 11%)

Central nervous system: Fatigue (29% to 75%), pain (≤47%), fever (6% to 41%), headache (8% to 37%), dizziness (5% to 19%), insomnia (10% to 15%), depression (≤15%), anxiety (8% to 12%), chills (≤11%)

Dermatologic: Rash (9% to 50%; grades 3/4: 1% to 9%), dermatitis (GIST ≤39%), pruritus (8% to 26%), alopecia (GIST 10% to 15%)

Endocrine & metabolic: LDH increased (GIST ≤60%), hypokalemia (6% to 13%; Ph+ ALL [pediatric] grades 3/4: 34%), hypoproteinemia (≤32%), albumin decreased (≤21%; grade 3: ≤4%)

Gastrointestinal: Nausea (42% to 73%; Ph+ ALL [pediatric] grades 3/4: 16%), diarrhea (25% to 59%; Ph+ ALL [pediatric] grades 3/4: 9%), vomiting (11% to 58%), abdominal pain (3% to 57%), anorexia (≤36%), weight gain (5% to 32%), dyspepsia (11% to 27%), flatulence (≤25%), abdominal distension (≤19%), stomatitis/mucositis (≤10% to 16%), constipation (9% to 16%), taste disturbance (≤13%)

Hematologic: Anemia (25% to 80%; grade 3: 1% to 42%; grade 4: ≤11%), leukopenia (GIST 5% to 47%; grades 3/4: 2%), hemorrhage (3% to 53%; grades 3/4: ≤19%), neutropenia (12% to 16%, grade 3: 7% to 27%; grade 4: 3% to 48%), thrombocytopenia (grade 3: 1% to 31%; grade 4: <1% to 33%)

Hepatic: Transaminases and/or bilirubin increased (Ph+ ALL [pediatric] grades 3/4: 57%), AST increased (≤38%; grade 3: 2% to 5%; grade 4: ≤3%), ALT increased (≤34%; grade 3: 2% to 7%; grade 4: <3%), alkaline phosphatase increased (≤17%; grade 3: ≤6%; grade 4: <1%), bilirubin increased (≤13%; grade 3: 1% to 4%; grade 4: ≤3%)

Neuromuscular & skeletal: Muscle cramps (16% to 62%), arthralgia (≤40%), musculoskeletal pain (children 21%; adults 38% to 49%), myalgia (9% to 32%), joint pain (11% to 31%), weakness (≤21%), rigors (10% to 12%), paresthesia (≤12%), bone pain (≤11%)

Ocular: Periorbital edema (29% to ≤74%), lacrimation increased (DFSP 25%; GIST ≤18%), blurred vision (≤11%)

Renal: Serum creatinine increased (≤44%; grade 3: ≤3%; DFSP: grade 4: 8%)

Respiratory: Nasopharyngitis (1% to 31%), cough (11% to 27%), dyspnea (≤21%), upper respiratory tract infection (3% to 21%), pharyngolaryngeal pain (≤18%), rhinitis (DFSP 17%), pharyngitis (CML 10% to 15%), pneumonia (CML 4% to 13%), sinusitis (4% to 11%)

Miscellaneous: Infection (Ph+ ALL [pediatric] grades 3/4: 53%; GIST ≤28%), night sweats (CML 13% to 17%), flu-like syndrome (1% to 14%), diaphoresis (GIST ≤13%)

1% to 10%:
Cardiovascular: Pleural effusion (Ph+ ALL [pediatric] grades 3/4: 7%), palpitation (≤5%), flushing
Central nervous system: CNS/cerebral hemorrhage (≤9%), depression (≤8%), hypoesthesia
Dermatologic: Photosensitivity reaction (4% to 7%), dry skin (≤7%), erythema
Endocrine & metabolic: Hyperglycemia (≤10%), hypocalcemia (GIST ≤6%)
Gastrointestinal: Appetite decreased (10%), weight loss (≤10%), gastrointestinal hemorrhage (2% to 8%), gastritis, gastroesophageal reflux, xerostomia
Hematologic: Lymphopenia (GIST ≤10%; grades 3/4: 1% to 2%), neutropenic fever, pancytopenia
Neuromuscular & skeletal: Back pain (GIST ≤7%), limb pain (GIST ≤7%), peripheral neuropathy, joint swelling
Ocular: Conjunctivitis (5% to 8%), conjunctival hemorrhage, dry eyes
Respiratory: Hypoxia (9%), pneumonitis (Ph+ ALL [pediatric] grades 3/4: 8%), epistaxis

General Dosage Range Dosage adjustment recommended in patients with hepatic or renal impairment, on concomitant therapy, and/or who develop toxicities

Oral:
Children ≥1 year and Adolescents: 340 mg/m^2/day in 1-2 divided doses (maximum: 600 mg daily)
Adults: 100-800 mg daily in 1-2 divided doses

Mechanism of Action Inhibits Bcr-Abl tyrosine kinase, the constitutive abnormal gene product of the Philadelphia chromosome in chronic myeloid leukemia (CML). Inhibition of this enzyme blocks proliferation and induces apoptosis in Bcr-Abl positive cell lines as well as in fresh leukemic cells in Philadelphia chromosome positive CML. Also inhibits tyrosine kinase for platelet-derived growth factor (PDGF), stem cell factor (SCF), c-Kit, and cellular events mediated by PDGF and SCF.

Pharmacodynamics/Kinetics
Half-life Elimination Adults: Parent drug: ~18 hours; N-desmethyl metabolite: ~40 hours; Children: Parent drug: ~15 hours

Time to Peak 2-4 hours

Pregnancy Risk Factor D

Pregnancy Considerations Animal reproduction studies have demonstrated teratogenic effects and fetal loss. Women of childbearing potential are advised not to become pregnant (female patients and female partners of male patients); highly effective contraception is recommended. Case reports of pregnancies while on therapy (both males and females) include reports of spontaneous abortion, minor abnormalities (hypospadias, pyloric stenosis, and small intestine rotation) at or shortly after birth, and other congenital abnormalities including skeletal malformations, hypoplastic lungs, exomphalos, kidney abnormalities, hydrocephalus, cerebellar hypoplasia, and cardiac defects.

Retrospective case reports of women with CML in complete hematologic response (CHR) with cytogenic response (partial or complete) who interrupted imatinib therapy due to pregnancy, demonstrated a loss of response in some patients while off treatment. At 18 months after treatment reinitiation following delivery, CHR was again achieved in all patients and cytogenic response was achieved in some patients. Cytogenetic response rates may not be at as high as compared to patients with 18 months of uninterrupted therapy (Ault, 2006; Pye, 2008).

Imiglucerase (i mi GLOO ser ace)

Brand Names: U.S. Cerezyme®
Brand Names: Canada Cerezyme®
Pharmacologic Category Enzyme
Use Long-term enzyme replacement therapy for patients with type 1 Gaucher disease
Local Anesthetic/Vasoconstrictor Precautions No information available to require special precautions
Effects on Dental Treatment No significant effects or complications reported
Effects on Bleeding No information available to require special precautions
Adverse Effects 1% to 10%:
Cardiovascular: Tachycardia (<2%)
Central nervous system: Chills (<2%), dizziness (<2%), fatigue (<2%), fever (<2%), headache (<2%)
Dermatologic: Pruritus (<2%), rash (<2%)
Gastrointestinal: Abdominal discomfort (<2%), diarrhea (<2%), nausea (<2%), vomiting (<2%)
Neuromuscular & skeletal: Backache (<2%)
Miscellaneous: Hypersensitivity reaction (7%; symptoms may include pruritus, flushing, urticaria, angioedema, chest discomfort, dyspnea, coughing, cyanosis, hypotension)
General Dosage Range I.V.: *Children ≥2 years and Adults:* 2.5 units/kg 3 times weekly to 60 units/kg every 2 weeks.
Mechanism of Action Imiglucerase is an analogue of glucocerebrosidase; it is produced by recombinant DNA technology using mammalian cell culture. Glucocerebrosidase is an enzyme deficient in Gaucher's disease. It is needed to catalyze the hydrolysis of glucocerebroside to glucose and ceramide.
Pharmacodynamics/Kinetics
Half-life Elimination 3.6-10.4 minutes
Pregnancy Risk Factor C
Pregnancy Considerations Animal reproduction studies have not been conducted; however, imiglucerase has been used safely during pregnancy based on available data (Sherer, 2003; Zimran, 2009). Doses of imiglucerase should be based on prepregnancy weight and adjusted as clinically indicated (Granovsky, 2011).

Imipenem and Cilastatin
(i mi PEN em & sye la STAT in)

Brand Names: U.S. Primaxin® I.V.
Brand Names: Canada Imipenem and Cilastatin for Injection; Primaxin® I.V. Infusion; RAN™-Imipenem-Cilastatin
Pharmacologic Category Antibiotic, Carbapenem
Use Treatment of lower respiratory tract, urinary tract, intra-abdominal, gynecologic, bone and joint, skin and skin structure, endocarditis (caused by *Staphylococcus aureus*) and polymicrobic infections as well as bacterial septicemia. Antibacterial activity includes gram-positive bacteria (methicillin-sensitive *S. aureus* and *Streptococcus* spp), resistant gram-negative bacilli (including extended spectrum beta-lactamase-producing *Escherichia coli* and *Klebsiella* spp, *Enterobacter* spp, and *Pseudomonas aeruginosa*), and anaerobes.
Unlabeled Use Hepatic abscess; neutropenic fever; melioidosis
Local Anesthetic/Vasoconstrictor Precautions No information available to require special precautions
Effects on Dental Treatment No significant effects or complications reported

Effects on Bleeding No information available to require special precautions

Adverse Effects

1% to 10%:

Cardiovascular: Tachycardia (infants 2%; adults <1%)

Central nervous system: Seizure (infants 6%; adults <1%)

Dermatologic: Rash (≤1%, children 2%)

Gastrointestinal: Nausea (1% to 2%), diarrhea (children 3% to 4%; adults 1% to 2%), vomiting (≤2%)

Genitourinary: Oliguria/anuria (infants 2%; adults <1%)

Local: Phlebitis/thrombophlebitis (3%)

General Dosage Range Dosage adjustment recommended in patients with renal impairment

I.V.:

Children >3 months: 15-25 mg/kg every 6 hours (maximum: 4 g/day)

Adults 30 to <70 kg: 125 mg every 12 hours up to 1000 mg every 8 hours

Adults ≥70 kg: 250-1000 mg every 6-8 hours (maximum: 50 mg/kg/day; 4 g/day)

Mechanism of Action Inhibits bacterial cell wall synthesis by binding to one or more of the penicillin-binding proteins (PBPs); which in turn inhibits the final transpeptidation step of peptidoglycan synthesis in bacterial cell walls, thus inhibiting cell wall biosynthesis. Bacteria eventually lyse due to ongoing activity of cell wall autolytic enzymes (autolysins and murein hydrolases) while cell wall assembly is arrested. Cilastatin prevents renal metabolism of imipenem by competitive inhibition of dehydropeptidase along the brush border of the renal tubules.

Pharmacodynamics/Kinetics

Half-life Elimination I.V.: Both drugs: 60 minutes; prolonged with renal impairment

Pregnancy Risk Factor C

Pregnancy Considerations Teratogenic events have not been observed in animal reproduction studies. Due to pregnancy induced physiologic changes, some pharmacokinetic parameters of imipenem/cilastatin may be altered. Pregnant women have a larger volume of distribution resulting in lower serum peak levels than for the same dose in nonpregnant women. Clearance is also increased.

Imipramine (im IP ra meen)

Related Information

Vasoconstrictor Interactions With Antidepressants *on page 1650*

Brand Names: U.S. Tofranil-PM®; Tofranil®

Brand Names: Canada Apo-Imipramine®; Novo-Pramine; Tofranil®

Pharmacologic Category Antidepressant, Tricyclic (Tertiary Amine)

Use Treatment of depression; treatment of nocturnal enuresis in children

Unlabeled Use Analgesic for certain chronic and neuropathic pain (including diabetic neuropathy); panic disorder; attention-deficit/hyperactivity disorder (ADHD); post-traumatic stress disorder (PTSD)

Local Anesthetic/Vasoconstrictor Precautions Use with caution; epinephrine and levonordefrin have been shown to have an increased pressor response in combination with TCAs. Imipramine is one of the drugs confirmed to prolong the QT interval and is accepted as having a risk of causing torsade de pointes. The risk of drug-induced torsade de pointes is extremely low when a single QT interval prolonging drug is prescribed. In terms of epinephrine, it is not known what effect vasoconstrictors in the local anesthetic regimen will have in patients with a known history of congenital prolonged QT interval or in patients taking any medication that prolongs the QT interval. Until more information is obtained, it is suggested that the clinician consult with the physician prior to the use of a vasoconstrictor in suspected patients, and that the vasoconstrictor (epinephrine, mepivacaine and levonordefrin [Carbocaine® 2% with Neo-Cobefrin®]) be used with caution.

Effects on Dental Treatment Key adverse event(s) related to dental treatment: Xerostomia and changes in salivation (normal salivary flow resumes upon discontinuation). Long-term treatment with TCAs, such as imipramine, increases the risk of caries by reducing salivation and salivary buffer capacity. In a study by Rundergren, et al, pathological alterations were observed in the oral mucosa of 72% of 58 patients; 55% had new carious lesions after taking TCAs for a median of 5 ¹/₂ years. Current research is investigating the use of the salivary stimulant pilocarpine to overcome the xerostomia from imipramine.

Effects on Bleeding No information available to require special precautions

Adverse Effects Reported for tricyclic antidepressants in general. Frequency not defined.

Cardiovascular: Arrhythmia, CHF, ECG changes, heart block, hypertension, MI, orthostatic hypotension, palpitation, stroke, tachycardia

Central nervous system: Agitation, anxiety, confusion, delusions, disorientation, dizziness, drowsiness, fatigue, hallucination, headache, hypomania, insomnia, nightmares, psychosis, restlessness, seizure

Dermatologic: Alopecia, itching, petechiae, photosensitivity, purpura, rash, urticaria

Endocrine & metabolic: Breast enlargement, galactorrhea, gynecomastia, increase or decrease in blood sugar, increase or decrease in libido, SIADH

Gastrointestinal: Abdominal cramps, anorexia, black tongue, constipation, diarrhea, epigastric disorders, ileus, nausea, stomatitis, taste disturbance, vomiting, weight gain/loss, xerostomia

Genitourinary: Impotence, testicular swelling, urinary retention

Hematologic: Agranulocytosis, eosinophilia, thrombocytopenia

Hepatic: Cholestatic jaundice, transaminases increased

Neuromuscular & skeletal: Ataxia, extrapyramidal symptoms, incoordination, numbness, paresthesia, peripheral neuropathy, tingling, tremor, weakness

Ocular: Blurred vision, disturbances of accommodation, mydriasis

Otic: Tinnitus

Miscellaneous: Diaphoresis, falling, hypersensitivity (eg, drug fever, edema)

General Dosage Range Oral:

Children ≥6-12 years: Initial: 25 mg at bedtime, may increase to 50 mg at bedtime if no response (maximum: 2.5 mg/kg/day; 50 mg/day)

Children >12 years: Initial: 25 mg at bedtime, may increase to 75 mg at bedtime if not response (maximum: 75 mg/day) **or** 30-40 mg/day, increase gradually, to a maximum of 100 mg/day in single or divided doses

Adults: Initial: 75-150 mg/day, increase gradually to a maximum of 200 mg/day (outpatients) or 300 mg/day (inpatients) in divided doses or a single dose at bedtime

Elderly: Initial: 25-50 mg at bedtime (maximum: 100 mg/day)

Mechanism of Action Traditionally believed to increase the synaptic concentration of serotonin and/or norepinephrine in the central nervous system by inhibition of their reuptake by the presynaptic neuronal membrane. However, additional receptor effects have been found including desensitization of adenyl cyclase, down regulation of beta-adrenergic receptors, and down regulation of serotonin receptors.

Pharmacodynamics/Kinetics

Onset of Action Peak antidepressant effect: Usually after ≥2 weeks

Half-life Elimination 6-18 hours

Pregnancy Considerations Animal reproduction studies are inconclusive. Congenital abnormalities have been reported in humans; however, a casual relationship has not been established. Due to pregnancy-induced physiologic changes, women who are pregnant may require dose adjustments late in pregnancy to achieve euthymia.

Dental Comment Imipramine is known to prolong the QT interval. The QT interval is measured as the time and distance between the Q point of the QRS complex and the end of the T wave in the ECG tracing. After adjustment for heart rate, the QT interval is defined as prolonged if it is more than 450 msec in men and 460 msec in women. A long QT syndrome was first described in the 1950s and 60s as a congenital syndrome involving QT interval prolongation and syncope and sudden death. Some of the congenital long QT syndromes were characterized by a peculiar electrocardiographic appearance of the QRS complex involving a premature atria beat followed by a pause, then a subsequent sinus beat showing marked QT prolongation and deformity. This type of cardiac arrhythmia was originally termed "torsade de pointes" (translated from the French as "twisting of the points"). Imipramine is considered as having a risk of causing torsade de pointes. Since it is not known what effect vasoconstrictors in the local anesthetic regimen will have in patients with a known history of congenital prolonged QT interval or in patients taking any medication that prolongs the QT interval, a medical consult is suggested.

Imiquimod (i mi KWI mod)

Related Information

Systemic Viral Diseases *on page 1537*
Viral Infections *on page 1575*

Brand Names: U.S. Aldara®; Zyclara®

Brand Names: Canada Aldara®; Vyloma™; Zyclara®

Generic Availability (U.S.) Yes

Pharmacologic Category Skin and Mucous Membrane Agent; Topical Skin Product

Use

Aldara®: Treatment of external genital and perianal warts/condyloma acuminata; nonhyperkeratotic, nonhypertrophic actinic keratosis on face or scalp; superficial basal cell carcinoma (sBCC) with a maximum tumor diameter of 2 cm located on the trunk (excluding anogenital skin), neck, or extremities (excluding hands or feet)

Vyloma™ (Canadian availability; not available in the U.S.): Treatment of external genital and perianal warts/condyloma acuminata

Zyclara®:
U.S. labeling: Treatment of external genital and perianal warts/condyloma acuminata (3.75% formulation); treatment of clinically typical visible or palpable, actinic keratoses on face or scalp (2.5% or 3.75% formulation)
Canadian labeling: Treatment of clinically typical visible or palpable, actinic keratoses on face or scalp

Unlabeled Use Treatment of common warts

Local Anesthetic/Vasoconstrictor Precautions No information available to require special precautions

Effects on Dental Treatment No significant effects or complications reported

Effects on Bleeding No information available to require special precautions

Adverse Effects Note: Frequency may depend on indication/formulation.

>10%:
Local: Application site reactions are common. Frequency of reactions vary, and are related to the degree of inflammation associated with the treated disease, number of weekly applications, and individual sensitivity.
Burning, edema, erosion/ulceration, erythema, excoriation, flaking, induration, itching, scabbing/crusting, scaling/dryness, vesicles, weeping/exudate
Respiratory: Upper respiratory infection
Miscellaneous: Fungal infection

1% to 10%:
Cardiovascular: Chest pain
Central nervous system: Anxiety, dizziness, fatigue, fever, headache, pain
Dermatologic: Alopecia, cheilitis, eczema, seborrhoeic keratosis
Endocrine & metabolic: Blood glucose increased
Gastrointestinal: Anorexia, diarrhea, dyspepsia, nausea, vomiting
Genitourinary: Urinary tract infection
Local: Bleeding, hypopigmentation, infection, irritation, pain, papule, paresthesia, pruritus, rash, scar, sensitivity, soreness, stinging, tenderness
Neuromuscular & skeletal: Arthralgia, back pain, myalgia, rigors
Respiratory: Coughing, pharyngitis, rhinitis, sinusitis
Miscellaneous: Herpes simplex, influenza-like syndrome, lymphadenopathy, squamous cell carcinoma, tinea cruris

Dosage Topical: **Note:** Imiquimod treatment should not be prolonged beyond recommended period due to missed doses or rest periods.
U.S. labeling:
Actinic keratosis: Adults: **Note:** Prescribed course of therapy should be completed even if all lesions appear to be gone. Safety and efficacy of repeated use in a previously treated area has not been established.
Aldara®: Treatment should be limited to areas ≤25 cm², apply 2 times/week for 16 weeks to a treatment area on face or scalp (but not both concurrently); no more than 1 packet should be applied at each application and no more than 36 packets applied per 16 weeks; apply prior to bedtime and leave on skin for ~8 hours. Remove with mild soap and water.

Zyclara® 2.5%, 3.75%: Treatment consists of 2 cycles (14 days each) separated by 1 rest period (14 days) with no treatment. Apply up to 2 packets or 2 full actuations of pump daily at bedtime to affected area on either face or balding scalp (but not both concurrently); leave on skin for ~8 hours. Remove with mild soap and water. Patient should not receive more than 56 packets or 2 x 7.5 g pumps or 1 x 15 g pump per 2 cycles of treatment.

External genital and/or perianal warts/condyloma acuminata: Children ≥12 years and Adults:

Aldara®: Apply a thin layer 3 times/week prior to bedtime and leave on skin for 6-10 hours. Remove with mild soap and water. Examples of 3 times/week application schedules are: Monday, Wednesday, Friday; or Tuesday, Thursday, Saturday. Continue treatment until there is total clearance of the warts or a maximum duration of therapy of 16 weeks.

Zyclara® 3.75%: Apply a thin layer using up to 1 packet or 1 full actuation of pump once daily prior to bedtime and leave on skin for ~8 hours. Remove with mild soap and water. Continue treatment until there is total clearance of the warts or a maximum duration of therapy of 8 weeks. Patient should not receive more than 56 packets or 2 x 7.5 g pumps or 1 x 15 g pump per course of treatment.

Superficial basal cell carcinoma: Adults: Aldara®: Apply once daily prior to bedtime, 5 days/week for 6 weeks. No more than 36 packets should be used during the 6-week treatment period. Tumor treatment area should not exceed 3 cm (maximum of 2 cm tumor diameter plus a 1 cm margin of skin around the tumor). The diameter of cream droplet applied should range from 4 mm to 7 mm for tumor areas of 0.5 cm to 2 cm, respectively. Leave on skin for ~8 hours. Remove with mild soap and water. Safety and efficacy of repeated use in a previously treated area have not been established.

Canadian labeling:

Actinic keratosis: Adults: **Note:** Prescribed course of therapy should be completed even if all lesions appear to be gone; safety and efficacy of repeated use in a previously treated area have not been established.

Aldara®: Treatment should be limited to areas ≤25 cm^2; apply 2 times/week for 16 weeks to a treatment area on face or scalp (but not both concurrently); no more than 1 packet should be applied at each application; apply prior to bedtime and leave on skin for ~8 hours. Remove with mild soap and water.

Zyclara®: Treatment should be limited to an area <200 cm^2 on the face or scalp and consists of 2 cycles (14 days each) separated by 1 rest period (14 days) with no treatment. Apply up to 2 packets or 2 full actuations of pump once daily at bedtime to affected area on either face or balding scalp (but not both concurrently). Leave on skin for ~8 hours. Remove with mild soap and water. Patient should not receive more than 56 packets or 2 x 7.5 g pumps or 1 x 15 g pump per 2 cycles of treatment.

External genital and/or perianal warts/condyloma acuminata: Adults:

Aldara®: Apply a thin layer 3 times/week prior to bedtime and leave on skin for 6-10 hours. Remove with mild soap and water. Examples of 3 times/week application schedules are: Monday, Wednesday, Friday; or Tuesday, Thursday, Saturday. Continue treatment until there is total clearance of the warts or a maximum duration of therapy of 16 weeks.

Vyloma™: Apply a thin layer once daily prior to bedtime and leave on skin for ~8 hours. Remove with mild soap and water. Continue treatment until there is total clearance of the warts or maximum duration of therapy of 8 weeks.

Superficial basal cell carcinoma: Adults: Aldara®: Apply once daily prior to bedtime, 5 days/week for 6 weeks. Tumor treatment area should not exceed 3 cm (maximum of 2 cm tumor diameter plus a 1 cm margin of skin around the tumor). The diameter of cream droplet applied should range from 4 mm to 7 mm for tumor areas of 0.5 cm to 2 cm, respectively. Leave on skin for ~8 hours. Remove with mild soap and water. Safety and efficacy of repeated use in a previously treated area have not been established.

Unlabeled uses: Common warts (5% cream): Apply once daily prior to bedtime for 5 days/week for up to 16 weeks (Hengge, 2000) or apply twice daily for up to 24 weeks (Grussendorf-Conen, 2002)

Dosing adjustment for toxicity:

Local skin reactions (eg, erythema, edema, scabbing, etc): Temporarily interrupt treatment for up to several days for severe or intolerable reactions; may consider resuming therapy once reaction subsides.

Systemic/flu-like reactions (eg, malaise, fever, rigors, etc): Consider temporary interruption of therapy.

Vulvar swelling: Interrupt or discontinue therapy for severe vulvar swelling.

Dosing adjustment in renal impairment: No dosage adjustment provided in manufacturer's labeling.

Dosing adjustment in hepatic impairment: No dosage adjustment provided in manufacturer's labeling.

Mechanism of Action Precise mechanism of action is unknown; Toll-like receptor 7 agonist that induces cytokines, including interferon-alpha and others

Contraindications U.S. labeling: There are no contraindications listed within the approved manufacturer's labeling.

Canadian labeling: Hypersensitivity to imiquimod or any component of the formulation

Warnings/Precautions Imiquimod is not intended for oral, nasal, intravaginal, or ophthalmic use. Topical imiquimod administration is not recommended until tissue is healed from any previous drug or surgical treatment. Treatment should not be prolonged beyond recommended period due to missed doses or rest periods. Imiquimod has the potential to exacerbate inflammatory conditions of the skin (including chronic graft-versus-host disease). Intense inflammatory reactions may occur, and may be accompanied by systemic symptoms (fever, malaise, myalgia); interruption of therapy should be considered. Severe inflammation of female external genitalia following topical application may lead to severe vulvar swelling and urinary retention; interruption or discontinuation of therapy may be necessary.

May increase sunburn susceptibility; in an animal study, topical imiquimod administration and concurrent ultraviolet radiation decreased the median time to skin tumor formation. Patients should protect themselves from the sun and artificial forms of sunlight. Safety and efficacy have not been established for immunosuppressed patients, or for basal cell nevus syndrome or xeroderma pigmentosum. Following 2 randomized, double-blind, placebo-controlled trials, efficacy of imiquimod was not established for molluscum contagiosum in children 2-12 years of age. Use with caution in patients with pre-existing autoimmune disorders (onset or exacerbation of disease has been reported rarely with imiquimod).

Basal cell carcinoma: Use in basal cell carcinoma should be limited to superficial carcinomas with a maximum diameter of 2 cm. Safety and efficacy in treatment of sBCC lesions of the face, head, and anogenital area, or other subtypes of basal cell carcinoma (including nodular and morpheaform), have not been established.

Actinic keratosis: Safety and efficacy of repeated use of Aldara® or Zyclara® in a previously treated area have not been established. Prescribed course of therapy should be completed even if all lesions appear to be gone.

Genital warts: Safety and efficacy of Zyclara® 2.75% in the treatment of external genital warts have not been established. Imiquimod has not been evaluated for the treatment of urethral, intravaginal, cervical, rectal, or intra-anal human papilloma viral disease and is not recommended for these conditions.

Drug Interactions

Metabolism/Transport Effects Substrate of CYP1A2 (minor), CYP3A4 (minor); **Note:** Assignment of Major/Minor substrate status based on clinically relevant drug interaction potential

Avoid Concomitant Use

Avoid concomitant use of Imiquimod with any of the following: BCG; Natalizumab; Pimecrolimus; Tacrolimus (Topical); Tofacitinib; Vaccines (Live)

Increased Effect/Toxicity

Imiquimod may increase the levels/effects of: Leflunomide; Natalizumab; Tofacitinib; Vaccines (Live)

The levels/effects of Imiquimod may be increased by: Denosumab; Pimecrolimus; Roflumilast; Tacrolimus (Topical); Trastuzumab

Decreased Effect

Imiquimod may decrease the levels/effects of: BCG; Coccidioidin Skin Test; Sipuleucel-T; Vaccines (Inactivated); Vaccines (Live)

The levels/effects of Imiquimod may be decreased by: Echinacea

Pharmacodynamics/Kinetics

Time to Peak 9-12 hours

Pregnancy Risk Factor C

Pregnancy Considerations Teratogenic effects were noted in some animal studies following oral administration. Safety and efficacy have not been established in pregnant women.

Lactation Excretion in breast milk unknown/use caution

Breast-Feeding Considerations It is not known if imiquimod is excreted in breast milk. The manufacturer recommends that caution be exercised when administering imiquimod to nursing women.

Dosage Forms

Cream, topical: 5% (24s)
Aldara®: 5% (12s)
Zyclara®: 2.5% (7.5 g); 3.75% (7.5 g, 28s)

Dosage Forms: Canada

Cream, topical:
Vyloma™: 3.75% (28s)

Dental Comment Imiquimod cream 5% has been used for actinic cheilitis or keratosis. Imiquimod 2.5% and 3.75% cream is FDA approved to treat actinic keratosis. Adverse events of erosion/ulcerations have been reported with topical use. Imiquimod use in the treatment of oral papilloma virus remains inadequately studied.

Immune Globulin (i MYUN GLOB yoo lin)

Related Information

Systemic Viral Diseases *on page 1537*

Brand Names: U.S. Bivigam™; Carimune® NF; Flebogamma® DIF; GamaSTAN™ S/D; Gammagard S/D®; Gammagard® Liquid; Gammaked™; Gammaplex®; Gamunex®-C; Hizentra®; Octagam®; Privigen®

Brand Names: Canada Gamastan S/D; Gamimune® N; Gammagard Liquid; Gammagard S/D; Gamunex®; Hizentra®; IGIVnex®; Privigen®

Generic Availability (U.S.) No

Pharmacologic Category Blood Product Derivative; Immune Globulin

Use

Treatment of primary humoral immunodeficiency syndromes (congenital agammaglobulinemia, severe combined immunodeficiency syndromes [SCIDS], common variable immunodeficiency, X-linked immunodeficiency, Wiskott-Aldrich syndrome) (Bivigam™, Carimune® NF, Flebogamma® DIF, Gammagard® Liquid, Gammagard S/D®, Gammaked™, Gammaplex®, Gamunex®-C, Hizentra®, Octagam®, Privigen®)

Treatment of acute and chronic immune (idiopathic) thrombocytopenic purpura (ITP) (Carimune® NF, Gammagard S/D®, Gammaked™, Gammaplex® [chronic only], Gamunex®-C, Privigen® [chronic only])

Treatment of chronic inflammatory demyelinating polyneuropathy (CIDP) (Gammaked™, Gamunex®-C)

Treatment of multifocal motor neuropathy (MMN) (Gammagard® Liquid)

Prevention of coronary artery aneurysms associated with Kawasaki syndrome (in combination with aspirin) (Gammagard S/D®)

Prevention of bacterial infection in patients with hypogammaglobulinemia and/or recurrent bacterial infections with B-cell chronic lymphocytic leukemia (CLL) (Gammagard S/D®)

Prevention of serious infection in immunoglobulin deficiency (select agammaglobulinemias) (GamaSTAN™ S/D)

Provision of passive immunity in the following susceptible individuals (GamaSTAN™ S/D):

Hepatitis A: Pre-exposure prophylaxis; postexposure: within 14 days and/or prior to manifestation of disease

Measles: For use within 6 days of exposure in an unvaccinated person, who has not previously had measles

Rubella: Postexposure prophylaxis (within 72 hours) to reduce the risk of infection and fetal damage in exposed pregnant women who will not consider therapeutic abortion

Varicella: For immunosuppressed patients when varicella zoster immune globulin is not available

Unlabeled Use Acquired hypogammaglobulinemia secondary to malignancy; Guillain-Barré syndrome; hematopoietic stem cell transplantation (HSCT), to prevent bacterial infections among allogeneic recipients with severe hypogammaglobulinemia (IgG <400 mg/dL) at <100 days post transplant (CDC guidelines); HIV-associated thrombocytopenia; multiple sclerosis (relapsing, remitting when other therapies cannot be used); Lambert-Eaton myasthenic syndrome (LEMS); myasthenia gravis; refractory dermatomyositis/polymyositis

Local Anesthetic/Vasoconstrictor Precautions No information available to require special precautions

727

◄ **Effects on Dental Treatment** No significant effects or complications reported

Effects on Bleeding No information available to require special precautions

Adverse Effects Frequency not always defined.

Cardiovascular: Chest tightness (7%), hypertension (5% to 6%), angioedema, edema, flushing of the face, hypotension, palpitation, tachycardia

Central nervous system: Headache (16% to 48%), fever (6% to 16%), chills (3% to 6%), dizziness (1% to 6%), malaise (1%), anxiety, aseptic meningitis syndrome, drowsiness, fatigue, irritability, lethargy, lightheadedness, migraine, pain

Dermatologic: Bruising, contact dermatitis, eczema, erythema, hyperhidrosis, petechiae, pruritus, purpura, rash, urticaria

Endocrine & metabolic: Hyperglycemia (neuromuscular disease: 1%) dehydration

Gastrointestinal: Nausea (3% to 18%), anorexia (neuromuscular disease: 1%), abdominal cramps, abdominal pain, diarrhea, discomfort, dyspepsia, gastroenteritis, sore throat, toothache, vomiting

Hematologic: Anemia, autoimmune hemolytic anemia, hematocrit decreased, hematoma, hemolysis (mild), hemorrhage, thrombocytopenia

Hepatic: Bilirubin increased, LDH increased, liver function test increased

Local: Muscle stiffness at I.M. site; pain, swelling, redness or irritation at the infusion site

Neuromuscular & skeletal: Muscle spasm (MMN 7%), weakness (1%; MMN: 7%), arthralgia (1%), back or hip pain, leg cramps, muscle cramps, myalgia, neck pain, rigors

Ocular: Conjunctivitis

Otic: Ear pain

Renal: Acute renal failure, acute tubular necrosis, anuria, BUN increased, creatinine increased, oliguria, proximal tubular nephropathy, osmotic nephrosis

Respiratory: Oropharyngeal pain (7%), asthma aggravated, bronchitis, cough, dyspnea, epistaxis, nasal congestion, pharyngeal pain, pharyngitis, rhinitis, rhinorrhea, sinus headache, sinusitis, upper respiratory infection, wheezing

Miscellaneous: Anaphylaxis, diaphoresis, flu-like syndrome, hypersensitivity reactions, infusion reaction, thermal burn

Dosage Note: Some clinicians may administer IVIG formulations FDA approved only for intravenous administration as a subcutaneous infusion based on clinical judgment and patient tolerability. Also, some clinicians dose IVIG on ideal body weight or an adjusted ideal body weight in morbidly obese patients (Siegel, 2010).

Children and Adults:

B-cell chronic lymphocytic leukemia (CLL) (Gammagard S/D®): I.V.: 400 mg/kg every 3-4 weeks

Chronic inflammatory demyelinating polyneuropathy (CIDP) (Gammaked™, Gamunex-C®): I.V.: Loading dose: 2000 mg/kg (given in divided doses over 2-4 consecutive days); Maintenance: 1000 mg/kg every 3 weeks. Alternatively, administer 500 mg/kg/day for 2 consecutive days every 3 weeks.

Hepatitis A (GamaSTAN™ S/D): I.M.:

Pre-exposure prophylaxis upon travel into endemic areas (hepatitis A vaccine preferred):

0.02 **mL**/kg for anticipated risk of exposure <3 months

0.06 **mL**/kg for anticipated risk of exposure ≥3 months; repeat every 4-6 months.

Postexposure prophylaxis: 0.02 **mL**/kg given within 14 days of exposure and/or prior to manifestation of disease; not needed if at least 1 dose of hepatitis A vaccine was given at ≥1 month before exposure

Immunoglobulin deficiency (GamaSTAN™ S/D): I.M.: 0.66 **mL**/kg (minimum dose should be 100 mg/kg) every 3-4 weeks. Administer a double dose at onset of therapy; some patients may require more frequent injections.

Immune (idiopathic) thrombocytopenic purpura (ITP):

Carimune® NF: I.V.: Initial: 400 mg/kg/day for 2-5 days; Maintenance: 400 mg/kg as needed to maintain platelet count ≥30,000/mm³ and/or to control significant bleeding; may increase dose if needed (range: 800-1000 mg/kg)

Gammagard S/D®: I.V.: 1000 mg/kg; up to 3 additional doses may be given based on patient response and/or platelet count. **Note:** Additional doses should be given on alternate days.

Gammaked™, Gamunex-C®: I.V.: 1000 mg/kg/day for 2 consecutive days (second dose may be withheld if adequate platelet response in 24 hours) **or** 400 mg/kg once daily for 5 consecutive days

Privigen®: I.V.: 1000 mg/kg/day for 2 consecutive days

Kawasaki syndrome: I.V.:

Gammagard S/D®: 1000 mg/kg as a single dose **or** 400 mg/kg/day for 4 consecutive days. Begin within 7 days of onset of fever.

AHA guidelines (2004): 2000 mg/kg as a single dose within 10 days of disease onset

Note: Must be used in combination with aspirin: 80-100 mg/kg/day orally, divided every 6 hours for up to 14 days (until fever resolves for at least 48 hours); then decrease dose to 3-5 mg/kg/day once daily. In patients without coronary artery abnormalities, give lower dose for 6-8 weeks. In patients with coronary artery abnormalities, low-dose aspirin should be continued indefinitely.

Measles:

GamaSTAN™ S/D: I.M.:

Immunocompetent: 0.25 **mL**/kg given within 6 days of exposure followed by live attenuated measles vaccine in 5-6 months when indicated (CDC, 1998)

Immunocompromised children: 0.5 **mL**/kg (maximum dose: 15 **mL**) immediately following exposure

Gammaked™, Gamunex-C®, Octagam®: I.V.:

Prophylaxis in patients with primary humoral immunodeficiency (**ONLY** if routine dose is <400 mg/kg): ≥400 mg/kg immediately before expected exposure

Treatment in patients with primary immunodeficiency: 400 mg/kg administered as soon as possible after exposure

Hizentra®: SubQ infusion: Measles exposure in patients with primary humoral immunodeficiency: Weekly dose: ≥200 mg/kg for 2 consecutive weeks for patients at risk of measles exposure (eg, during an outbreak; travel to endemic area). In patients who have been exposed to measles, administer the minimum dose as soon as possible following exposure.

Primary humoral immunodeficiency disorders:

I.V. infusion dosing:

Bivigam™: I.V.: 300-800 mg/kg every 3-4 weeks; dose adjusted based on monitored trough serum IgG concentrations and clinical response

Carimune® NF: I.V.: 400-800 mg/kg every 3-4 weeks

Flebogamma® DIF, Gammagard® Liquid, Gammagard S/D®, Gammaked™, Gamunex-C®, Octagam®: I.V.: 300-600 mg/kg every 3-4 weeks; dose adjusted based on monitored trough serum IgG concentrations and clinical response

Privigen®: I.V.: 200-800 mg/kg every 3-4 weeks; dose adjusted based on monitored trough serum IgG concentrations and clinical response

Switching to weekly subcutaneous infusion dosing:
Gammagard® Liquid, Gammaked™, Gamunex-C®: SubQ infusion: Begin 1 week after last I.V. dose. Use the following equation to calculate initial dose: Initial weekly dose (g) = [1.37 x IGIV dose (g)] divided by [I.V. dose interval (weeks)]
Note: For subsequent dose adjustments, refer to product labeling.

Hizentra®: SubQ infusion: Begin 1 week after last I.V. dose. **Note:** Patient should have received an I.V. immune globulin routinely for at least 3 months before switching to SubQ. Use the following equation to calculate initial dose:
Initial weekly dose (g) = [1.53 x IGIV dose (g)] divided by [I.V. dose interval (weeks)]
Note: For subsequent dose adjustments, refer to product labeling.

Rubella (GamaSTAN™ S/D): I.M.: Prophylaxis during pregnancy: 0.55 **mL**/kg within 72 hours of exposure (CDC, 1998)

Varicella (GamaSTAN™ S/D): I.M.: Prophylaxis: 0.6-1.2 **mL**/kg (varicella zoster immune globulin preferred) within 72 hours of exposure

Adults:
Immune (idiopathic) thrombocytopenic purpura (ITP) (Gammaplex®): I.V.: 1000 mg/kg/day for 2 consecutive days
Multifocal motor neuropathy (MMN) (Gammagard® liquid): I.V.: 500-2400 mg/kg/month based upon response
Primary humoral immunodeficiency disorders: *I.V. infusion dosing* (Gammaplex®): I.V.: 300-800 mg/kg every 3-4 weeks; dose adjusted based on monitored trough serum IgG concentrations and clinical response

Unlabeled uses: I.V.:
Acquired hypogammaglobulinemia secondary to malignancy (unlabeled use): Adults: 400 mg/kg/dose every 3 weeks; reevaluate every 4-6 months (Anderson, 2007)
Guillain-Barré syndrome (unlabeled use): Children and Adults: Various regimens have been used, including: 400 mg/kg/day for 5 days (Hughes, 2003)
or
400 mg/kg/day for 6 days (Patwa, 2012)
or
2000 mg/kg in divided doses administered over 2-5 days (Feasby, 2007)
Hematopoietic stem cell transplantation with hypogammaglobulinemia (CDC guidelines, 2000; unlabeled use):
Children: 400 mg/kg per month; increase dose or frequency to maintain IgG levels >400 mg/dL
Adolescents and Adults: 500 mg/kg/week
HIV-associated thrombocytopenia (unlabeled use): Adults: 1000 mg/kg/day for 2 days (Anderson, 2007)
Lambert-Eaton myasthenic syndrome (LEMS) (unlabeled use): Adults: 1000 mg/kg/day for 2 days (Bain, 1996; Patwa, 2012)
Multiple sclerosis (relapsing-remitting, when other therapies cannot be used) (unlabeled use): Children and Adults: 1000 mg/kg per month, with or without an induction of 400 mg/kg/day for 5 days (Feasby, 2007)
Myasthenia gravis (severe exacerbation) (unlabeled use): Children and Adults: 2000 mg/kg per treatment course over 2-5 days (Feasby, 2007; Patwa, 2012)

Refractory dermatomyositis/polymyositis (unlabeled uses): Children and Adults: 2000 mg/kg per treatment course administered over 2-5 days (Feasby, 2007)

Dosage adjustment in renal impairment:
I.V.: Use with caution due to risk of immune globulin-induced renal dysfunction; the rate of infusion and concentration of solution should be minimized.
I.M., SubQ infusion: No dosage adjustment provided in the manufacturer's labeling; risk of immune globulin-induced renal dysfunction has not been identified with I.M. and SubQ infusion administration.

Dosage adjustment in hepatic impairment: I.M., I.V., SubQ infusion: No dosage adjustment provided in manufacturer's labeling.

Mechanism of Action Replacement therapy for primary and secondary immunodeficiencies, and IgG antibodies against bacteria, viral, parasitic and mycoplasma antigens; interference with F_c receptors on the cells of the reticuloendothelial system for autoimmune cytopenias and ITP; provides passive immunity by increasing the antibody titer and antigen-antibody reaction potential

Contraindications Hypersensitivity to immune globulin or any component of the formulation; IgA deficiency (with antibodies against IgA and history of hypersensitivity); hyperprolinemia (Hizentra®, Privigen®); isolated IgA deficiency (GamaSTAN™ S/D); severe thrombocytopenia or coagulation disorders where I.M. injections are contraindicated (GamaSTAN™ S/D)

Warnings/Precautions [U.S. Boxed Warning]: I.V. administration only: Acute renal dysfunction (increased serum creatinine, oliguria, acute renal failure, osmotic nephrosis) can rarely occur and has been associated with fatalities; usually within 7 days of use (more likely with products stabilized with sucrose). Use with caution in the elderly, patients with renal disease, diabetes mellitus, volume depletion, sepsis, paraproteinemia, and nephrotoxic medications due to risk of renal dysfunction. In patients at risk of renal dysfunction, the rate of infusion and concentration of solution should be minimized. Discontinue if renal function deteriorates. High-dose regimens (1 g/kg for 1-2 days) are not recommended for individuals with fluid overload or where fluid volume may be of concern. Hypersensitivity and anaphylactic reactions can occur; a severe fall in blood pressure may rarely occur with anaphylactic reaction; immediate treatment (including epinephrine 1:1000) should be available. Product of human plasma; may potentially contain infectious agents which could transmit disease. Screening of donors, as well as testing and/or inactivation or removal of certain viruses, reduces the risk. Infections thought to be transmitted by this product should be reported to the manufacturer. Aseptic meningitis may occur with high doses (≥1-2 g/kg [product-dependent]) and/or rapid infusion; syndrome usually appears within several hours to 2 days following treatment; usually resolves within several days after product is discontinued; patients with a migraine history may be at higher risk for AMS. Increased risk of hypersensitivity, especially in patients with anti-IgA antibodies; use is contraindicated in patients with IgA deficiency (with antibodies against IgA and history of hypersensitivity) or isolated IgA deficiency (GamaSTAN™ S/D). Increased risk of hematoma formation when administered subcutaneously for the treatment of ITP.

Intravenous immune globulin has been associated with antiglobulin hemolysis; monitor for signs of hemolytic anemia. Risk factors include high doses (≥2 g/kg) and non-O blood type. In chronic ITP, assess risk versus benefit of high-dose regimen in patients with increased risk of thrombosis, hemolysis, acute kidney injury, or volume overload.

Patients should be adequately hydrated prior to initiation of therapy. Hyperproteinemia, increased serum viscosity and hyponatremia may occur; distinguish hyponatremia from pseudohyponatremia to prevent volume depletion, a further increase in serum viscosity, and a higher risk of thrombotic events. There is clinical evidence of a possible association between thrombotic events and administration of intravenous immune globulin and subcutaneous immune globulin. Use caution in patients with a history of thrombotic events or a history of atherosclerosis or cardiovascular disease, advanced age, impaired cardiac output, or patients with known/ suspected hyperviscosity. Consider a baseline assessment of blood viscosity in patients at risk for hyperviscosity such as those with cryoglobulins, fasting chylomicronemia/severe hypertriglyceridemia, or monoclonal gammopathies. In patients at risk of thrombotic events, the rate of infusion should be minimized. Patients should be monitored for adverse events during and after the infusion. Stop administration with signs of infusion reaction (fever, chills, nausea, vomiting, and rarely shock). Risk may be increased with initial treatment, when switching brands of immune globulin, and with treatment interruptions of >8 weeks. Monitor for transfusion-related acute lung injury (TRALI); noncardiogenic pulmonary edema has been reported with intravenous immune globulin use. TRALI is characterized by severe respiratory distress, pulmonary edema, hypoxemia, and fever (in the presence of normal left ventricular function) and usually occurs within 1-6 hours after infusion. Response to live vaccinations may be impaired. Some clinicians may administer intravenous immune globulin products as a subcutaneous infusion based on patient tolerability and clinical judgment. SubQ infusion should begin 1 week after the last I.V. dose; dose should be individualized based on clinical response and serum IgG trough concentrations; consider premedicating with acetaminophen and diphenhydramine.

Some products may contain maltose, which may result in falsely-elevated blood glucose readings; maltose-containing products are contraindicated in patients with an allergy to corn. Some products may contain polysorbate 80, sodium, and/or sucrose. Some products may contain sorbitol; do not use in patients with fructose intolerance. Hizentra® and Privigen® contain the stabilizer L-proline and are contraindicated in patients with hyperprolinemia. Packaging of some products may contain natural latex/natural rubber; skin testing should not be performed with GamaSTAN™ S/D as local irritation can occur and be misinterpreted as a positive reaction.

Drug Interactions

Metabolism/Transport Effects None known.

Avoid Concomitant Use There are no known interactions where it is recommended to avoid concomitant use.

Increased Effect/Toxicity There are no known significant interactions involving an increase in effect.

Decreased Effect

Immune Globulin may decrease the levels/effects of: Vaccines (Live)

Dietary Considerations Some products may contain sodium.

Pharmacodynamics/Kinetics

Onset of Action I.V.: Provides immediate antibody levels

Duration of Action I.M., I.V.: Immune effects: 3-4 weeks (variable)

Half-life Elimination I.M.: ~23 days; I.V.: IgG (variable among patients): Healthy subjects: 14-24 days; Patients with congenital humoral immunodeficiencies: 26-40 days; hypermetabolism associated with fever and infection have coincided with a shortened half-life

Time to Peak

Plasma: SubQ: Gammagard® Liquid: 2.9 days; Hizentra®: 2.9 days

Serum: I.M.: ~48 hours

Pregnancy Risk Factor C

Pregnancy Considerations Reproduction studies have not been conducted. Immune globulins cross the placenta in increased amounts after 30 weeks gestation. Intravenous immune globulin has been recommended for use in fetal-neonatal alloimmune thrombocytopenia and pregnancy-associated ITP. May also be used in postexposure prophylaxis for rubella (within 72 hours) to reduce the risk of infection and fetal damage in exposed pregnant women who will not consider therapeutic abortion.

Lactation Excretion in breast milk unknown/use caution

Product Availability Bivigam™: FDA approved December 2012; anticipated availability is currently undetermined. Consult prescribing information for additional information.

Dosage Forms

Injection, powder for reconstitution [preservative free]:

Carimune® NF: 3 g, 6 g, 12 g

Gammagard S/D®: 5 g, 10 g

Injection, solution [preservative free]:

Bivigam™: 10% [100 mg/mL] (50 mL, 100 mL)

Flebogamma® DIF: 5% [50 mg/mL] (10 mL, 50 mL, 100 mL, 200 mL, 400 mL); 10% [100 mg/mL] (100 mL, 200 mL)

GamaSTAN™ S/D: 15% to 18% [150 to 180 mg/mL] (2 mL, 10 mL)

Gammagard® Liquid: 10% [100 mg/mL] (10 mL, 25 mL, 50 mL, 100 mL, 200 mL, 300 mL)

Gammaked™: 10% [100 mg/mL] (10 mL, 25 mL, 50 mL, 100 mL, 200 mL)

Gammaplex®: 5% [50 mg/mL] (50 mL, 100 mL, 200 mL)

Gamunex®-C: 10% [100 mg/mL] (10 mL, 25 mL, 50 mL, 100 mL, 200 mL)

Hizentra®: 20% [200 mg/mL] (5 mL, 10 mL, 20 mL)

Octagam®: 5% [50 mg/mL] (20 mL, 50 mL, 100 mL, 200 mL)

Privigen®: 10% [100 mg/mL] (50 mL, 100 mL, 200 mL)

IncobotulinumtoxinA
(in kuh BOT yoo lin num TOKS in aye)

Brand Names: U.S. Xeomin®

Brand Names: Canada Xeomin Cosmetic™; Xeomin®

Generic Availability (U.S.) No

Pharmacologic Category Neuromuscular Blocker Agent, Toxin; Ophthalmic Agent, Toxin

Use

U.S. labeling: Treatment of blepharospasm in patients previously treated with onabotulinumtoxinA (Botox®); treatment of cervical dystonia in botulinum toxin-naïve and previously treated patients; temporary improvement in the appearance of moderate-to-severe glabellar lines associated with corrugator and/or procerus muscle activity

Canadian labeling:

Xeomin®: Treatment of hypertonicity disorders of the seventh nerve (eg, blepharospasm, hemifacial spasm); treatment of poststroke spasticity of upper limb(s); treatment of cervical dystonia (spasmodic torticollis)

Xeomin Cosmetic™: Temporary improvement in the appearance of moderate-to-severe glabellar lines

Local Anesthetic/Vasoconstrictor Precautions No information available to require special precautions

Effects on Dental Treatment Key adverse event(s) related to dental treatment: Xerostomia (normal salivary flow resumes upon discontinuation).

Effects on Bleeding No information available to require special precautions

Adverse Effects

>10%:

Gastrointestinal: Dysphagia (cervical dystonia 13% to 18%), xerostomia (blepharospasm 16%)

Neuromuscular & skeletal: Muscular weakness (cervical dystonia 7% to 11%), neck pain (cervical dystonia 7% to 15%)

Ocular: Eyelid ptosis (blepharospasm 19%; reduction of glabellar lines <1%), dry eye (blepharospasm 16%), vision impaired (blepharospasm 12%)

1% to 10%:

Central nervous system: Headache (blepharospasm 7%; reduction of glabellar lines 5%, poststroke spasticity [Canadian labeling] 1%)

Gastrointestinal: Diarrhea (blepharospasm 8%)

Local: Injection site pain (cervical dystonia 4% to 9%)

Neuromuscular & skeletal: Pain (cervical dystonia 4% to 7%)

Respiratory: Dyspnea (blepharospasm 5%), nasopharyngitis (blepharospasm 5%), respiratory tract infection (blepharospasm 5%)

Miscellaneous: Neutralizing antibody formation (1%)

<1%, postmarketing and/or case reports: Any indication: Abdominal distension, abnormal dreams, allergic dermatitis, allergic reactions, alopecia, anaphylaxis, asthma, aspiration pneumonia, blurred vision, cardiovascular insufficiency, circulatory collapse, colitis, conjunctivitis, corneal perforation, cough, diaphoresis, diplopia, dysarthria, dysphonia, edema, erythema, eye edema, eye pain, eyelid ecchymosis, eyelid edema, fatigue, herpes zoster, hypersensitivity, injection site inflammation, injection site reaction, lymphadenopathy, madarosis, muscle spasm, myalgia, nausea, paresthesia, peripheral edema, pruritus, rash, reduced blinking leading to corneal ulceration, respiratory failure, serum sickness, soft tissue edema, somnolence, tremor, trismus, urinary incontinence, urticaria, vomiting, weakness

Dosage I.M.: Adults:

Blepharospasm:

U.S. labeling: Initial: Total dose should be the same as previously administered onabotulinumtoxinA dose. If prior onabotulinumtoxinA dose is not known: 1.25-2.5 units/injection site (maximum initial dose: 35 units/eye or 70 units/both eyes). Number and location of injection sites based on disease severity and previous dose/response to onabotulinumtoxinA (in clinical trials, a mean number of 6 injections per eye were administered). Cumulative dose should not exceed 35 units/eye or 70 units/both eyes administered no more frequently than every 3 months.

Canadian labeling: Initial: 1.25-2.5 units/injection site (maximum initial dose: 25 units/eye). Dose may be increased up to twice the previous dose if the response from the initial dose lasted ≤2 months; maximum dose per site: 5 units. Cumulative dose should not exceed 35 units/eye or 70 units/both eyes administered no more frequently than every 3 months.

Cervical dystonia:

U.S. labeling: Initial total dose: 120 units (in clinical trials, similar efficacy was noted with initial total doses of 120 and 240 units and between treatment experienced and treatment naïve patients). Dose and number of injection sites should be individualized based on prior treatment, response, duration of effect, adverse events, number/location of muscle(s) to be treated and disease severity. In clinical trials most patients received a total of 2-10 injections into treated muscles. Administer no more frequently than every 3 months

Canadian labeling: Usual total dose: 200 units (maximum: 300 units; maximum dose per injection site: 50 units); administer no more frequently than every 3 months

Reduction of glabellar lines: Inject 4 units into each of the 5 sites (2 injections in each corrugator muscle and 1 injection in the procerus muscle) for a total dose of 20 units per treatment session. Administer no more frequently than every 3 months.

Spasticity of upper limb (poststroke): Canadian labeling (not in U.S. labeling): Individualize dose based on patient size, extent, and location of muscle involvement, degree of spasticity, local muscle weakness, and response to prior treatment. In clinical trials, total doses up to 400 units were administered as separate injections typically divided among selected muscles; may repeat therapy at ≥3 months with appropriate dosage based upon the clinical condition of patient at time of retreatment.

Suggested guidelines for the treatment of stroke-related upper limb spasticity: Note: The lowest recommended starting dose should be used. Dosage and number of injection sites should be individualized. Multiple injections may minimize adverse effects. Dose listed is total dose administered to site:

Biceps: 80 units

Brachialis: 50 units

Brachioradialis: 60 units

Flexor carpi radialis: 50 units

Flexor carpi ulnaris: 40 units

Flexor digitorum profundus: 40 units

Flexor digitorum superficialis: 40 units

Adductor pollicis: 10 units

Flexor pollicis brevis: 10 units

Flexor pollicis longus: 20 units

Pronator quadratus 25 units

Pronator teres: 40 units

Elderly: Initiate therapy at lowest recommended dose and titrate upward cautiously.

Dosage adjustment in renal impairment: There are no dosage adjustments provided in manufacturer's labeling.

◀ **Dosage adjustment in hepatic impairment:** There are no dosage adjustments provided in manufacturer's labeling.

Mechanism of Action IncobotulinumtoxinA is a neurotoxin produced from *Clostridium botulinum* that inhibits acetylcholine release from peripheral cholinergic nerve endings. Inhibition occurs sequentially via binding and internalization of the neurotoxin into presynaptic cholinergic nerve terminals, translocation to the nerve terminal cytosol, and enzymatic cleavage of SNAP25, a protein necessary for acetylcholine release. Inhibition of acetylcholine release at the neuromuscular junction produces a state of denervation. Muscle inactivation persists until new fibrils grow from the nerve and form junction plates on new areas of the muscle-cell walls.

Contraindications Hypersensitivity to botulinum toxin, or any component of the formulation; infection at the proposed injection site(s)

Canadian labeling: Additional contraindications (not in U.S. labeling): Generalized disorders of muscle activity (eg, myasthenia gravis, Lambert-Eaton syndrome)

Warnings/Precautions [U.S. Boxed Warning]: Distant spread of botulinum toxin beyond the site of injection has been reported; dysphagia and breathing difficulties have occurred and may be life threatening; other symptoms reported include blurred vision, diplopia, dysarthria, dysphonia, generalized muscle weakness, ptosis, and urinary incontinence which may develop within hours or weeks following injection. The risk is likely greatest in children treated for the unapproved use of spasticity. Systemic effects have occurred following use in approved and unapproved uses, including low doses. Use caution in patients with underlying conditions which may predispose them to these symptoms. Immediate medical attention required if respiratory, speech, or swallowing difficulties appear. Higher doses, more frequent administration, or young age at disease onset may result in neutralizing antibody formation and loss of efficacy. Use caution in patients with bleeding disorders and/or receiving anticoagulation therapy. May impair ability to drive and/or operate machinery; if loss of strength, muscle weakness, or impaired vision occurs, patients should avoid driving or engaging in other hazardous activities.

Product contains albumin and may carry a remote risk of virus transmission. Use caution if there is excessive weakness or atrophy at the proposed injection site(s); use is contraindicated if infection is present at injection site. Have appropriate support in case of anaphylactic reaction. Use with caution in patients with neuromuscular diseases (such as myasthenia gravis or Lambert-Eaton syndrome [contraindicated in Canadian labeling]), neuropathic disorders (such as amyotrophic lateral sclerosis), patients taking aminoglycosides, neuromuscular-blocking agents, or other drugs that interfere with neuromuscular transmission and patients with pre-existing cardiovascular disease (rare reports of arrhythmia and MI). Long-term effects of chronic therapy are unknown. Botulinum products (abobotulinumtoxinA, incobotulinumtoxinA, onabotulinumtoxinA, rimabotulinumtoxinB) are not interchangeable; potency units are specific to each preparation and cannot be compared or converted to any other botulinum product.

Cervical dystonia: Dysphagia is common and may occur within hours to weeks and persist for several months after administration. If severe, alternative feeding methods may be required. Risk factors include smaller neck muscle mass or bilateral injections into the sternocleidomastoid muscle. Use extreme caution in patients with

pre-existing respiratory disease; may weaken accessory muscles that are necessary for these patients to maintain adequate ventilation. Risk of aspiration resulting from severe dysphagia is increased in patients with decreased respiratory function.

Ocular disease: Blepharospasm: Reduced blinking from injection of the orbicularis muscle can lead to corneal exposure and ulceration. Careful testing of corneal sensation, avoidance of lower lid injections to prevent ectropion, and treatment of epithelial defects are necessary. Soft contact lenses, application of protective drops or ointment, or covering the affected eye may help. Gentle pressure at injection site may limit bruising of eyelid. Use caution in patients with angle-closure glaucoma.

Pharmacodynamics/Kinetics
Onset of Action Improvement: ~4-7 days
Duration of Action ~3-4 months
Pregnancy Risk Factor C
Pregnancy Considerations Decreased fetal body weight, delayed ossification, maternal toxicity, abortions, and fetal malformations were observed in animal reproduction studies. Use during pregnancy only if benefits outweigh potential risks to fetus.

Lactation Excretion in breast milk unknown/use caution

Dosage Forms
Injection, powder for reconstitution:
  Xeomin®: 50 units, 100 units

Dosage Forms: Canada
Injection, powder for reconstitution:
  Xeomin Cosmetic™: 100 units

Indacaterol (in da KA ter ol)

Related Information
  Respiratory Diseases *on page 1514*
Brand Names: U.S. Arcapta™ Neohaler™
Brand Names: Canada Onbrez® Breezhaler®
Pharmacologic Category Beta$_2$ Agonist; Beta$_2$-Adrenergic Agonist, Long-Acting
Use Long-term maintenance treatment of airflow obstruction in chronic obstructive pulmonary disease (COPD) including chronic bronchitis and/or emphysema
Local Anesthetic/Vasoconstrictor Precautions No information available to require special precautions
Effects on Dental Treatment Key adverse event(s) related to dental treatment: oropharyngeal pain has been reported
Effects on Bleeding No information available to require special precautions
Adverse Effects
  >10%: Respiratory: Cough (post inhalation 7% to 24%)
  1% to 10%:
    Central nervous system: Headache (5%)
    Gastrointestinal: Nausea (2%)
    Respiratory: Nasopharyngitis (5%), oropharyngeal pain (2%)
General Dosage Range Inhalation: *Adults:* One inhalation once daily
Mechanism of Action Relaxes bronchial smooth muscle by selective action on beta$_2$-receptors with little effect on heart rate; acts locally in the lung.
Pharmacodynamics/Kinetics
  Onset of Action 5 minutes; Peak effect: 1-4 hours
  Duration of Action 24 hours
  Half-life Elimination 40-56 hours
  Time to Peak Serum: ~15 minutes
Pregnancy Risk Factor C

Pregnancy Considerations Adverse events were not observed in animal reproduction studies. Beta agonists may interfere with uterine contractility if administered during labor.

Indapamide (in DAP a mide)

Related Information
Cardiovascular Diseases *on page 1492*
Brand Names: Canada Apo-Indapamide®; Dom-Indapamide; Indapamide Hemihydrate; JAMP-Indapamide; Lozide®; Mylan-Indapamide; Novo-Indapamide; Nu-Indapamide; PHL-Indapamide; PMS-Indapamide; PRO-Indapamide; Riva-Indapamide
Pharmacologic Category Diuretic, Thiazide-Related
Use Management of mild-to-moderate hypertension; treatment of edema in heart failure
Unlabeled Use Nephrotic syndrome (Tanaka, 2005)
Local Anesthetic/Vasoconstrictor Precautions Indapamide is one of the drugs confirmed to prolong the QT interval and is accepted as having a risk of causing torsade de pointes. The risk of drug-induced torsade de pointes is extremely low when a single QT interval prolonging drug is prescribed. In terms of epinephrine, it is not known what effect vasoconstrictors in the local anesthetic regimen will have in patients with a known history of congenital prolonged QT interval or in patients taking any medication that prolongs the QT interval. Until more information is obtained, it is suggested that the clinician consult with the physician prior to the use of a vasoconstrictor in suspected patients, and that the vasoconstrictor (epinephrine, mepivacaine and levonordefrin [Carbocaine® 2% with Neo-Cobefrin®]) be used with caution.
Effects on Dental Treatment Key adverse event(s) related to dental treatment: Orthostatic hypotension, palpitations, flushing, xerostomia (normal salivary flow resumes upon discontinuation), and rhinorrhea.
Effects on Bleeding No information available to require special precautions
Adverse Effects
≥5%:
Central nervous system: Agitation, anxiety, dizziness, fatigue, headache, irritability, lethargy, malaise, nervousness (dose dependent), pain, tension, tiredness
Endocrine & metabolic: Hypokalemia (<3.5 mEq/L: 20% to 72%, dose dependent)
Neuromuscular & skeletal: Back pain, muscle cramps/spasm, paresthesia, weakness
Respiratory: Rhinitis
Miscellaneous: Infection
≥1% to <5%:
Cardiovascular: Arrhythmia, chest pain, flushing, orthostatic hypotension, palpitation, peripheral edema, PVC, vasculitis
Central nervous system: Depression, drowsiness, insomnia, lightheadedness, vertigo
Dermatologic: Hives, pruritus, rash
Endocrine & metabolic: Hyperglycemia, hyperuricemia, hypochloremia, hyponatremia, libido decreased
Gastrointestinal: Abdominal pain, anorexia, constipation, cramping, diarrhea, dyspepsia, gastric irritation, nausea, vomiting, weight loss, xerostomia
Genitourinary: Nocturia, polyuria
Neuromuscular & skeletal: Hypertonia
Ocular: Blurred vision, conjunctivitis

Renal: BUN increased, creatinine increased, glycosuria
Respiratory: Cough, pharyngitis, rhinorrhea, sinusitis
Miscellaneous: Flu-like syndrome
General Dosage Range Oral: *Adults:* 1.25-5 mg once daily
Mechanism of Action Diuretic effect is localized at the proximal segment of the distal tubule of the nephron; it does not appear to have significant effect on glomerular filtration rate nor renal blood flow; like other diuretics, it enhances sodium, chloride, and water excretion by interfering with the transport of sodium ions across the renal tubular epithelium
Pharmacodynamics/Kinetics
Half-life Elimination Biphasic: 14 and 25 hours
Time to Peak 2 hours
Pregnancy Risk Factor B
Pregnancy Considerations Adverse events were not observed in animal reproduction studies. Diuretics cross the placenta and are found in cord blood. Maternal use may cause may cause fetal or neonatal jaundice, thrombocytopenia, or other adverse events observed in adults. Use of diuretics during normal pregnancies is not appropriate; use may be considered when edema is due to pathologic causes (as in the nonpregnant patient); monitor.
Dental Comment Indapamide is known to prolong the QT interval. The QT interval is measured as the time and distance between the Q point of the QRS complex and the end of the T wave in the ECG tracing. After adjustment for heart rate, the QT interval is defined as prolonged if it is more than 450 msec in men and 460 msec in women. A long QT syndrome was first described in the 1950s and 60s as a congenital syndrome involving QT interval prolongation and syncope and sudden death. Some of the congenital long QT syndromes were characterized by a peculiar electrocardiographic appearance of the QRS complex involving a premature atria beat followed by a pause, then a subsequent sinus beat showing marked QT prolongation and deformity. This type of cardiac arrhythmia was originally termed "torsade de pointes" (translated from the French as "twisting of the points"). Indapamide is considered as having a risk of causing torsade de pointes. Since it is not known what effect vasoconstrictors in the local anesthetic regimen will have in patients with a known history of congenital prolonged QT interval or in patients taking any medication that prolongs the QT interval, a medical consult is suggested.

Indinavir (in DIN a veer)

Related Information
HIV Infection and AIDS *on page 1520*
Brand Names: U.S. Crixivan®
Brand Names: Canada Crixivan®
Pharmacologic Category Antiretroviral Agent, Protease Inhibitor
Use Treatment of HIV infection; should always be used as part of a multidrug regimen (at least three antiretroviral agents)
Local Anesthetic/Vasoconstrictor Precautions No information available to require special precautions
Effects on Dental Treatment Key adverse event(s) related to dental treatment: Abnormal taste.
Effects on Bleeding Spontaneous bleeding has been reported in patients with hemophilia and concurrent HIV infection. Medical consult recommended.

Adverse Effects

>10%:

Gastrointestinal: Abdominal pain (17%), nausea (12%)

Hepatic: Hyperbilirubinemia (14%; dose dependent)

Renal: Nephrolithiasis/urolithiasis, including flank pain with/without hematuria (29%, pediatric patients; 12% adult patients; dose dependent)

1% to 10%:

Central nervous system: Headache (5%), dizziness (3%), somnolence (2%), fever (2%), malaise (2%), fatigue (2%)

Dermatologic: Pruritus (4%), rash (1%)

Endocrine & metabolic: Hyperglycemia (1%)

Gastrointestinal: Vomiting (8%), diarrhea (3%), taste perversion (3%), acid reflux (3%), anorexia (3%), appetite increased (2%), dyspepsia (2%), serum amylase increased (2%)

Hematologic: Neutropenia (2%), anemia (1%), thrombocytopenia (1%)

Hepatic: Transaminases increased (4% to 5%), jaundice (2%)

Neuromuscular & skeletal: Back pain (8%), weakness (2%)

Renal: Dysuria (2%)

Respiratory: Cough (2%)

General Dosage Range Dosage adjustment recommended in patients with hepatic impairment or on concomitant therapy

Oral: *Adults:* 800 mg every 8 hours; Boosted regimen: 800 mg every 12 hours

Mechanism of Action Binds to the site of HIV-1 protease activity and inhibits cleavage of viral Gag-Pol polyprotein precursors into individual functional proteins required for infectious HIV. This results in the formation of immature, noninfectious viral particles.

Pharmacodynamics/Kinetics

Half-life Elimination 1.8 ± 0.4 hour; hepatic insufficiency: 2.8 ± 0.5 hour

Time to Peak 0.8 ± 0.3 hour

Pregnancy Risk Factor C

Pregnancy Considerations Adverse events were observed in some animal reproduction studies. Placental passage in humans is minimal. No increased risk of overall birth defects was observed according to data collected by the antiretroviral pregnancy registry. A small increased risk of preterm birth has been associated with maternal use of protease inhibitor-based combination antiretroviral (ARV) therapy during pregnancy; however, the benefits of use generally outweigh this risk and protease inhibitors (PIs) should not be withheld if otherwise recommended. Hyperglycemia, new onset of diabetes mellitus, or diabetic ketoacidosis have been reported with PIs; it is not clear if pregnancy increases this risk. Hyperbilirubinemia may occur in neonates following *in utero* exposure to indinavir. Until optimal dosing during pregnancy has been established, the manufacturer does not recommend indinavir use in pregnant patients. The DHHS Perinatal HIV Guidelines consider indinavir an agent to be used in special circumstances when preferred and alternative agents cannot be used; however, if needed, indinavir must be used in combination with low-dose ritonavir during pregnancy (with ritonavir boosting, 82% of pregnant women reached target trough concentrations).

Regardless of CD4 count or HIV RNA copy number, all HIV-infected pregnant women should receive a combination antepartum ARV drug regimen; this includes women who require therapy for their own health, as well as women who do not yet require therapy for their own health. ARV therapy should be started as soon as possible if required for the woman's health. Although earlier initiation may be more effective in reducing the perinatal transmission of HIV, also consider maternal conditions (eg, nausea and vomiting) and the potential risks of first trimester fetal exposure for specific agents. Plasma HIV RNA levels should be assessed at ~34-36 weeks gestation in order to help determine mode of delivery. If ARV therapy must be interrupted for <24 hours during the peripartum period, stop then restart all medications simultaneously in order to decrease the chance of developing resistance. Long-term follow-up is recommended for all infants exposed to ARV medications.

Healthcare providers are encouraged to enroll pregnant women exposed to antiretroviral medications in the Antiretroviral Pregnancy Registry (1-800-258-4263 or www.APRegistry.com). Healthcare providers caring for HIV-infected women and their infants may contact the National Perinatal HIV Hotline (888-448-8765) for clinical consultation (DHHS [perinatal], 2012).

Indium 111 Oxyquinoline
(IN dee um won e LEV en oks i KWIN oh leen)

Pharmacologic Category Radiopharmaceutical

Use Radiolabeling autologous leukocytes as an adjunct to detect inflammatory processes (eg, abscess or other infection) when localization or diagnosis by other methods (eg, ultrasound or computed tomography) fails or is ambiguous

Local Anesthetic/Vasoconstrictor Precautions No information available to require special precautions

Effects on Dental Treatment No significant effects or complications reported

Effects on Bleeding No information available to require special precautions

Adverse Effects Frequency not defined.

Central nervous system: Fever

Dermatologic: Urticaria

Miscellaneous: Hypersensitivity reactions

Mechanism of Action Creates radiolabeled autologous leukocytes to allow for detection of inflammatory processes such as abscesses or other infections.

Pharmacodynamics/Kinetics

Half-life Elimination Indium In-111: Physical half-life: 67.2 hours

Pregnancy Risk Factor C

Pregnancy Considerations Animal reproductive studies have not been conducted. In a related compound, indium nitrate adverse events were observed in animal reproductive studies. Elective examinations in women of reproductive potential should be conducted within 10 days of the onset of menses.

Indocyanine Green (in doe SYE a neen green)

Brand Names: U.S. IC-Green™

Pharmacologic Category Diagnostic Agent

Use Determining hepatic function, cardiac output, and liver blood flow; ophthalmic angiography

Local Anesthetic/Vasoconstrictor Precautions No information available to require special precautions

Effects on Dental Treatment No significant effects or complications reported

Effects on Bleeding No information available to require special precautions

Adverse Effects Frequency not defined.
Central nervous system: Headache
Dermatologic: Pruritus, urticaria
Gastrointestinal: Feces discoloration (green)
Miscellaneous: Anaphylactoid reactions, diaphoresis
General Dosage Range
Cardiac catheter:
Infants: 1.25 mg (maximum total dose: 2 mg/kg)
Children: 2.5 mg (maximum total dose: 2 mg/kg)
Adults: 5 mg (maximum total dose: 2 mg/kg)
I.V.: *Adults:* Hepatic function: 0.5 mg/kg; Ophthalmic angiography: ≤40 mg bolus
Pharmacodynamics/Kinetics
Half-life Elimination 2.5-3 minutes
Pregnancy Risk Factor C
Pregnancy Considerations Reproduction studies have not been done.

Indomethacin (in doe METH a sin)

Related Information
Rheumatoid Arthritis, Osteoarthritis, and Osteoporosis *on page 1526*
Temporomandibular Dysfunction (TMD), Chronic Pain, and Fibromyalgia *on page 1590*
Brand Names: U.S. Indocin®; Indocin® I.V.
Brand Names: Canada Apo-Indomethacin®; Indocid® P.D.A.; Novo-Methacin; Nu-Indo; Pro-Indo; ratio-Indomethacin; Sandoz-Indomethacin
Generic Availability (U.S.) Yes: Excludes oral suspension, suppository
Pharmacologic Category Nonsteroidal Anti-inflammatory Drug (NSAID), Oral; Nonsteroidal Anti-inflammatory Drug (NSAID), Parenteral
Use Acute gouty arthritis, acute bursitis/tendonitis, moderate-to-severe osteoarthritis, rheumatoid arthritis, ankylosing spondylitis; I.V. form used as alternative to surgery for closure of patent ductus arteriosus in neonates
Unlabeled Use Management of preterm labor; prevention of pancreatitis post-endoscopic retrograde cholangiopancreatography (ERCP)
Local Anesthetic/Vasoconstrictor Precautions No information available to require special precautions
Effects on Dental Treatment The dentist should be aware of the potential of abnormal coagulation. Caution should also be exercised in the use of NSAIDs in patients already on anticoagulant therapy with drugs such as warfarin (Coumadin®). See Effects on Bleeding.
Effects on Bleeding Nonselective NSAIDs such as indomethacin inhibit platelet aggregation and prolong bleeding time in some patients. Unlike aspirin, the NSAID effect on platelet function is quantitatively less, of shorter duration, and reversible.
Adverse Effects
>10%: Central nervous system: Headache (12%)
1% to 10%:
Central nervous system: Dizziness (3% to 9%), depression (<3%), fatigue (<3%), malaise (<3%), somnolence (<3%), vertigo (<3%)
Gastrointestinal: Dyspepsia (3% to 9%), epigastric pain (3% to 9%), heartburn (3% to 9%), indigestion (3% to 9%), nausea (3% to 9%), abdominal pain/cramps/distress (<3%), constipation (<3%), diarrhea (<3%), rectal irritation (suppository), tenesmus (suppository), vomiting
Otic: Tinnitus (<3%)

Dosage
Patent ductus arteriosus:
Neonates: I.V.: Initial: 0.2 mg/kg, followed by 2 doses depending on postnatal age (PNA):
PNA **at time of first dose** <48 hours: 0.1 mg/kg at 12- to 24-hour intervals
PNA **at time of first dose** 2-7 days: 0.2 mg/kg at 12- to 24-hour intervals
PNA **at time of first dose** >7 days: 0.25 mg/kg at 12- to 24-hour intervals
In general, may use 12-hour dosing interval if urine output >1 mL/kg/hour after prior dose; use 24-hour dosing interval if urine output is <1 mL/kg/hour but >0.6 mL/kg/hour; doses should be withheld if patient has oliguria (urine output <0.6 mL/kg/hour) or anuria
Inflammatory/rheumatoid disorders: **Note:** Use lowest effective dose.
Children ≥2 years: Oral: 1-2 mg/kg/day in 2-4 divided doses; maximum dose: 4 mg/kg/day; not to exceed 150-200 mg/day
Children >14 years and Adults: Oral, rectal: 25-50 mg/dose 2-3 times/day; maximum dose: 200 mg/day; extended release capsule should be given on a 1-2 times/day schedule (maximum dose for extended release: 150 mg/day). In patients with arthritis and persistent night pain and/or morning stiffness may give the larger portion (up to 100 mg) of the total daily dose at bedtime.
Bursitis/tendonitis: Oral, rectal: Adults: Initial dose: 75-150 mg/day in 3-4 divided doses **or** 1-2 divided doses for extended release; usual treatment is 7-14 days
Acute gouty arthritis: Oral, rectal: Adults: 50 mg 3 times daily until pain is tolerable then reduce dose; usual treatment <3-5 days
Prevention of pancreatitis post-endoscopic retrograde cholangiopancreatography (ERCP) (unlabeled use): Rectal: Adults: 100 mg immediately after ERCP (Elmunzer, 2012)

Elderly: Refer to adult dosing. Use lowest recommended dose and frequency in elderly to initiate therapy for indications listed in adult dosing.

Dosage adjustment in renal impairment: No dosage adjustment provided in the manufacturer's labeling; not recommended in patients with advanced renal disease.
Dosage adjustment in hepatic impairment: No dosage adjustment provided in the manufacturer's labeling; use with caution.
Mechanism of Action Reversibly inhibits cyclooxygenase-1 and 2 (COX-1 and 2) enzymes, which results in decreased formation of prostaglandin precursors; has antipyretic, analgesic, and anti-inflammatory properties

Other proposed mechanisms not fully elucidated (and possibly contributing to the anti-inflammatory effect to varying degrees), include inhibiting chemotaxis, altering lymphocyte activity, inhibiting neutrophil aggregation/activation, and decreasing proinflammatory cytokine levels.
Contraindications Hypersensitivity to indomethacin, aspirin, other NSAIDs, or any component of the formulation; perioperative pain in the setting of coronary artery bypass graft (CABG) surgery; patients with a history of proctitis or recent rectal bleeding (suppositories)

◀ Neonates: Necrotizing enterocolitis; impaired renal function; active bleeding (including intracranial hemorrhage and gastrointestinal bleeding), thrombocytopenia, coagulation defects; untreated infection; congenital heart disease where patent ductus arteriosus is necessary

Warnings/Precautions [U.S. Boxed Warning]: NSAIDs are associated with an increased risk of adverse cardiovascular thrombotic events, including MI and stroke. Risk may be increased with duration of use or pre-existing cardiovascular risk factors or disease. May cause new-onset hypertension or worsening of existing hypertension. Use caution with fluid retention. Avoid use in heart failure. Concurrent administration of ibuprofen, and potentially other nonselective NSAIDs, may interfere with aspirin's cardioprotective effect. **[U.S. Boxed Warning]: Use is contraindicated for treatment of perioperative pain in the setting of coronary artery bypass graft (CABG) surgery.** Risk of MI and stroke may be increased with use following CABG surgery.

Platelet adhesion and aggregation may be decreased; may prolong bleeding time; patients with coagulation disorders or who are receiving anticoagulants should be monitored closely. Anemia may occur; patients on long-term NSAID therapy should be monitored for anemia. Rarely, NSAID use may cause severe blood dyscrasias (eg, agranulocytosis, aplastic anemia, thrombocytopenia).

NSAID use may compromise existing renal function; dose-dependent decreases in prostaglandin synthesis may result from NSAID use, reducing renal blood flow which may cause renal decompensation. NSAID use may increase the risk for hyperkalemia. Patients with impaired renal function, dehydration, heart failure, liver dysfunction, those taking diuretics, and ACE inhibitors are at greater risk of renal toxicity and hyperkalemia. Rehydrate patient before starting therapy; monitor renal function closely. Not recommended for use in patients with advanced renal disease. Long-term NSAID use may result in renal papillary necrosis.

[U.S. Boxed Warning]: NSAIDs may increase risk of gastrointestinal irritation, inflammation, ulceration, bleeding, and perforation. Use caution with a history of GI disease (bleeding or ulcers), concurrent therapy with aspirin, anticoagulants and/or corticosteroids, smoking, use of alcohol, the elderly or debilitated patients. When used concomitantly with ≤325 mg of aspirin, a substantial increase in the risk of gastrointestinal complications (eg, ulcer) occurs; concomitant gastroprotective therapy (eg, proton pump inhibitors) is recommended (Bhatt, 2008).

Use the lowest effective dose for the shortest duration of time, consistent with individual patient goals, to reduce risk of cardiovascular or GI adverse events. Alternate therapies should be considered for patients at high risk.

NSAIDS may cause drowsiness, dizziness, blurred vision and other neurologic effects which may impair physical or mental abilities; patients must be cautioned about performing tasks which require mental alertness (eg, operating machinery or driving). Discontinue use with blurred or diminished vision and perform ophthalmologic exam. Monitor vision with long-term therapy.

NSAIDs may cause serious skin adverse events including exfoliative dermatitis, Stevens-Johnson syndrome (SJS) and toxic epidermal necrolysis (TEN); discontinue use at first sign of skin rash or hypersensitivity.

Anaphylactoid reactions may occur, even without prior exposure; patients with "aspirin triad" (bronchial asthma, aspirin intolerance, rhinitis) may be at increased risk. Do not use in patients who experience bronchospasm, asthma, rhinitis, or urticaria with NSAID or aspirin therapy. Use caution in other forms of asthma.

Use with caution in patients with decreased hepatic function. Closely monitor patients with any abnormal LFT. Severe hepatic reactions (eg, fulminant hepatitis, liver failure) have occurred with NSAID use, rarely; discontinue if signs or symptoms of liver disease develop, or if systemic manifestations occur. The elderly are at increased risk for adverse effects (especially peptic ulceration, CNS effects, renal toxicity) from NSAIDs even at low doses. Prolonged use may cause corneal deposits and retinal disturbances; discontinue if visual changes are observed. Use caution with depression, epilepsy, or Parkinson's disease.

Withhold for at least 4-6 half-lives prior to surgical or dental procedures.

Elderly: Nonselective oral NSAID use is associated with an increased risk of GI bleeding and peptic ulcer disease in older adults in high risk category (eg, >75 years or age or receiving concomitant oral/parenteral corticosteroids, anticoagulants, or antiplatelet agents). Risk of adverse events may be higher with indomethacin compared to other NSAIDs; avoid use in this age group (Beers Criteria).

Oral: Safety and efficacy have not been established in children <14 years of age. Hepatotoxicity has been reported in younger children treated for juvenile idiopathic arthritis (JIA). Closely monitor if use is needed in children ≥2 years of age.

Drug Interactions

Metabolism/Transport Effects Substrate of CYP2C19 (minor), CYP2C9 (minor); **Note:** Assignment of Major/Minor substrate status based on clinically relevant drug interaction potential; **Inhibits** CYP2C19 (weak), CYP2C9 (weak)

Avoid Concomitant Use

Avoid concomitant use of Indomethacin with any of the following: Floctafenine; Ketorolac (Nasal); Ketorolac (Systemic); NSAID (COX-2 Inhibitor); Omacetaxine

Increased Effect/Toxicity

Indomethacin may increase the levels/effects of: Agents with Antiplatelet Properties; Aliskiren; Aminoglycosides; Anticoagulants; Bisphosphonate Derivatives; Collagenase (Systemic); CycloSPORINE (Systemic); Dabigatran Etexilate; Deferasirox; Desmopressin; Digoxin; Drotrecogin Alfa (Activated); Eplerenone; Haloperidol; Ibritumomab; Lithium; Methotrexate; Nonsteroidal Anti-Inflammatory Agents; NSAID (COX-2 Inhibitor); Omacetaxine; PEMEtrexed; Porfimer; Potassium-Sparing Diuretics; PRALAtrexate; Quinolone Antibiotics; Rivaroxaban; Salicylates; Thrombolytic Agents; Tiludronate; Tositumomab and Iodine I 131 Tositumomab; Triamterene; Vancomycin; Vitamin K Antagonists

The levels/effects of Indomethacin may be increased by: ACE Inhibitors; Angiotensin II Receptor Blockers; Antidepressants (Tricyclic, Tertiary Amine); Corticosteroids (Systemic); CycloSPORINE (Systemic); Dasatinib; Floctafenine; Glucosamine; Herbs (Anticoagulant/Antiplatelet Properties); Ketorolac (Nasal); Ketorolac (Systemic); Multivitamins/Minerals (with ADEK, Folate, Iron); Nonsteroidal Anti-Inflammatory Agents; Omega-3 Fatty Acids; Pentosan Polysulfate Sodium;

Pentoxifylline; Probenecid; Prostacyclin Analogues; Selective Serotonin Reuptake Inhibitors; Serotonin/Norepinephrine Reuptake Inhibitors; Sodium Phosphates; Tipranavir; Treprostinil; Vitamin E

Decreased Effect

Indomethacin may decrease the levels/effects of: ACE Inhibitors; Agents with Antiplatelet Properties; Aliskiren; Angiotensin II Receptor Blockers; Beta-Blockers; Eplerenone; HydrALAZINE; Loop Diuretics; Potassium-Sparing Diuretics; Salicylates; Selective Serotonin Reuptake Inhibitors; Thiazide Diuretics

The levels/effects of Indomethacin may be decreased by: Bile Acid Sequestrants; Nonsteroidal Anti-Inflammatory Agents; Salicylates

Ethanol/Nutrition/Herb Interactions

Ethanol: Avoid ethanol (may enhance gastric mucosal irritation).

Food: Food may decrease the rate but not the extent of absorption. Indomethacin peak serum levels may be delayed if taken with food.

Herb/Nutraceutical: Avoid alfalfa, anise, bilberry, bladderwrack, bromelain, cat's claw, celery, chamomile, coleus, cordyceps, dong quai, evening primrose, fenugreek, feverfew, garlic, ginger, ginkgo biloba, ginseng (American, Panax, Siberian), grapeseed, green tea, guggul, horse chestnut seed, horseradish, licorice, prickly ash, red clover, reishi, SAMe (S-adenosylmethionine), sweet clover, turmeric, white willow (all have additional antiplatelet activity).

Dietary Considerations May cause GI upset; take with food or milk to minimize

Pharmacodynamics/Kinetics

Onset of Action ~30 minutes

Duration of Action 4-6 hours

Half-life Elimination 4.5 hours; prolonged with neonates

Time to Peak Oral: Immediate release: 2 hours

Pregnancy Risk Factor C

Pregnancy Considerations Adverse events have been observed in animal reproduction studies; therefore, the manufacturer classifies indomethacin as pregnancy category C. Indomethacin crosses the placenta and can be detected in fetal plasma and amniotic fluid. Indomethacin exposure during the first trimester is not strongly associated with congenital malformations; however, cardiovascular anomalies and cleft palate have been observed following NSAID exposure in some studies. The use of an NSAID close to conception may be associated with an increased risk of miscarriage. Nonteratogenic effects have been observed following NSAID administration during the third trimester, including myocardial degenerative changes, prenatal constriction of the ductus arteriosus, failure of the ductus arteriosus to close postnatally, and fetal tricuspid regurgitation; renal dysfunction or failure, oligohydramnios; gastrointestinal bleeding or perforation, increased risk of necrotizing enterocolitis; intracranial bleeding (including intraventricular hemorrhage), platelet dysfunction with resultant bleeding; and pulmonary hypertension. The risk of fetal ductal constriction following maternal use of indomethacin is increased with gestational age and duration of therapy. Because they may cause premature closure of the ductus arteriosus, use of NSAIDs late in pregnancy should be avoided (use after 31 or 32 weeks gestation is not recommended by some clinicians). Indomethacin has been used in the management of preterm labor. Indomethacin should be used with caution in pregnant women with hypertension. The chronic use of NSAIDs in women of reproductive age may be

associated with infertility that is reversible upon discontinuation of the medication.

Lactation Enters breast milk/not recommended (AAP rates "compatible"; AAP 2001 update pending)

Breast-Feeding Considerations Indomethacin is excreted into breast milk and low amounts have been measured in the plasma of nursing infants. Seizures in a nursing infant were observed in one case report, although adverse events have not been noted in other cases. Breast-feeding is not recommended by the manufacturer. (The therapeutic use of indomethacin is contraindicated in neonates with significant renal failure.) Hypertensive crisis and psychiatric side effects have been noted in case reports following use of indomethacin for analgesia in postpartum women. Use with caution in nursing women with hypertensive disorders of pregnancy or pre-existing renal disease.

Dosage Forms

Capsule, oral: 25 mg, 50 mg

Capsule, extended release, oral: 75 mg

Injection, powder for reconstitution: 1 mg
Indocin® I.V.: 1 mg

Suppository, rectal:
Indocin®: 50 mg (30s)

Suspension, oral:
Indocin®: 25 mg/5 mL (237 mL)

InFLIXimab (in FLIKS e mab)

Related Information

Rheumatoid Arthritis, Osteoarthritis, and Osteoporosis on page 1526

Brand Names: U.S. Remicade®

Brand Names: Canada Remicade®

Pharmacologic Category Antirheumatic, Disease Modifying; Gastrointestinal Agent, Miscellaneous; Immunosuppressant Agent; Monoclonal Antibody; Tumor Necrosis Factor (TNF) Blocking Agent

Use

Treatment of moderately- to severely-active rheumatoid arthritis (with methotrexate) (to reduce signs/symptoms of active arthritis and inhibit progression of structural damage and improve physical function)

Treatment of moderately- to severely-active Crohn's disease with inadequate response to conventional therapy (to reduce signs/symptoms and induce and maintain clinical remission) or to reduce the number of draining enterocutaneous and rectovaginal fistulas and maintain fistula closure

Treatment of psoriatic arthritis (to reduce signs/symptoms of active arthritis and inhibit progression of structural damage and improve physical function)

Treatment of chronic severe (extensive and/or disabling) plaque psoriasis as an alternative to other systemic therapy

Treatment of active ankylosing spondylitis (to reduce signs/symptoms)

Treatment of moderately- to severely-active ulcerative colitis with inadequate response to conventional therapy (to reduce signs/symptoms and induce and maintain clinical remission, mucosal healing and eliminate corticosteroid use)

Local Anesthetic/Vasoconstrictor Precautions No information available to require special precautions

Effects on Dental Treatment No significant effects or complications reported

Effects on Bleeding Has been associated with thrombocytopenia, anemia, and hemolytic anemia, but incidence may vary with indication.

Adverse Effects Although profile is similar, frequency of adverse effects may vary with disease state. Except where noted, percentages reported in adults with rheumatoid arthritis:

>10%:

Central nervous system: Headache (18%)

Gastrointestinal: Nausea (21%), diarrhea (12%), abdominal pain (12%, Crohn's 26%)

Hepatic: ALT increased (risk increased with concomitant methotrexate)

Respiratory: Upper respiratory tract infection (32%), sinusitis (14%), cough (12%), pharyngitis (12%)

Miscellaneous: Development of antinuclear antibodies (~50%), infection (36%), infusion reactions (20%; severe <1%), development of antibodies to double-stranded DNA (20%), development of new abscess (Crohn's patients with fistulizing disease: 15%), anti-infliximab antibodies (variable; ~10% to 15% [range: 6% to 61%]; Mayer, 2006)

5% to 10%:

Cardiovascular: Hypertension (7%)

Central nervous system: Fatigue (9%), pain (8%), fever (7%)

Dermatologic: Rash (1% to 10%), pruritus (7%)

Gastrointestinal: Dyspepsia (10%)

Genitourinary: Urinary tract infection (8%)

Neuromuscular & skeletal: Arthralgia (1% to 8%), back pain (8%)

Respiratory: Bronchitis (10%), rhinitis (8%), dyspnea (6%)

Miscellaneous: Moniliasis (5%)

The following adverse events were reported in children with Crohn's disease and were found more frequently in children than adults:

>10%:

Hepatic: Liver enzymes increased (18%; ≥5 times ULN: 1%)

Hematologic: Anemia (11%)

Miscellaneous: Infections (56%; more common with every 8-week versus every 12-week infusions)

1% to 10%:

Central nervous system: Flushing (9%)

Gastrointestinal: Blood in stool (10%)

Hematologic: Leukopenia (9%), neutropenia (7%)

Neuromuscular & skeletal: Bone fracture (7%)

Respiratory: Respiratory tract allergic reaction (6%)

Miscellaneous: Viral infection (8%), bacterial infection (6%), antibodies to infliximab (3%)

General Dosage Range Dosage adjustment is required in heart failure patients.

I.V.:

Children ≥6 years and Adolescents: Initial: 5 mg/kg at 0, 2, and 6 weeks; Maintenance: 5 mg/kg every 8 weeks

Adults: Initial: 3-10 mg/kg at 0, 2, and 6 weeks; Maintenance: 3-10 mg/kg every 8 weeks **or** 5 mg/kg every 6 weeks

Mechanism of Action Infliximab is a chimeric monoclonal antibody that binds to human tumor necrosis factor alpha (TNFα), thereby interfering with endogenous TNFα activity. Elevated TNFα levels have been found in involved tissues/fluids of patients with rheumatoid arthritis, ankylosing spondylitis, psoriatic arthritis, plaque psoriasis, Crohn's disease and ulcerative colitis. Biological activities of TNFα include the induction of proinflammatory cytokines (interleukins), enhancement of leukocyte migration, activation of neutrophils and eosinophils, and the induction of acute phase reactants and tissue degrading enzymes. Animal models have shown TNFα expression causes polyarthritis, and

infliximab can prevent disease as well as allow diseased joints to heal.

Pharmacodynamics/Kinetics

Onset of Action Crohn's disease: ~2 weeks

Half-life Elimination 7-12 days

Pregnancy Risk Factor B

Pregnancy Considerations Animal reproduction studies have not been conducted. Infliximab crosses the placenta and can be detected in the serum of infants for up to 6 months following *in utero* exposure. The safety of administering live or live-attenuated vaccines to exposed infants is not known. A Rheumatoid Arthritis and Pregnancy Registry has been established for women exposed to infliximab during pregnancy (Organization of Teratology Information Services, 877-311-8972).

Influenza Virus Vaccine (H5N1)
(in floo EN za VYE rus vak SEEN H5N1)

Pharmacologic Category Vaccine, Inactivated (Viral)

Use Active immunization of adults at increased risk of exposure to the H5N1 viral subtype of influenza

Local Anesthetic/Vasoconstrictor Precautions No information available to require special precautions

Effects on Dental Treatment No significant effects or complications reported

Effects on Bleeding No information available to require special precautions

Adverse Effects All serious adverse reactions must be reported to the U.S. Department of Health and Human Services (DHHS) Vaccine Adverse Event Reporting System (VAERS) 1-800-822-7967 or online at https://vaers.hhs.gov/esub/index.

>10%:

Central nervous system: Headache (3% to 36%), malaise (22%)

Local: Pain (74%), tenderness (70%), erythema/redness (20%), induration/swelling (15%)

Neuromuscular & skeletal: Myalgia (16%)

1% to 10%:

Central nervous system: Fever (up to 7%)

Gastrointestinal: Nausea (10%), diarrhea (6%)

Respiratory: Nasopharyngitis (2%), upper respiratory infection (2%), nasal congestion (1%)

Additional reactions observed with other influenza vaccine formulations: Allergic reaction, anaphylaxis, angioedema, asthma, encephalopathy, facial paralysis, hives, GBS, neuropathy, optic neuritis, vasculitis

General Dosage Range I.M.: *Adults 18-64 years:* 1 mL, followed by second 1 mL dose given 28 days later

Mechanism of Action A monovalent, split virus (inactivated) preparation of the H5N1 avian strain of influenza virus (A/Vietnam/1203/2004) which promotes active immunity to avian influenza.

Pharmacodynamics/Kinetics

Onset of Action Fourfold increase in antibody titers occurred in up to 58% of patients 28 days after second dose.

Pregnancy Risk Factor C

Pregnancy Considerations Reproduction studies have not been conducted. Vaccine should be given only if clearly needed. Inactivated viral vaccines have not been shown to cause increased risks to the fetus (CDC, 2011).

Prescribing and Access Restrictions Commercial distribution is not planned. The vaccine will be included as part of the U.S. Strategic National Stockpile. It will be distributed by public health officials if needed.

Influenza Virus Vaccine (Inactivated)
(in floo EN za VYE rus vak SEEN, in ak ti VAY ted)

Related Information
Systemic Viral Diseases *on page 1537*
Brand Names: U.S. Afluria®; Fluarix®; Flucelvax®; FluLaval®; Fluvirin®; Fluzone®; Fluzone® High-Dose; Fluzone® Intradermal
Brand Names: Canada Agriflu™; Fluad™; Fluviral®; Influvac®; Intanza®; Vaxigrip®
Pharmacologic Category Vaccine, Inactivated (Viral)
Use Provide active immunity to influenza virus strains contained in the vaccine

The Advisory Committee on Immunization Practices (ACIP) recommends annual vaccination with the seasonal inactivated influenza vaccine (IIV) (injection) for all persons ≥6 months of age.

When vaccine supply is limited, target groups for vaccination (those at higher risk of complications from influenza infection and their close contacts) include the following:
• Persons ≥50 years of age
• Residents of nursing homes and other chronic-care facilities that house persons of any age with chronic medical conditions
• Adults and children with chronic disorders of the pulmonary or cardiovascular systems (except hypertension), including asthma
• Adults and children who have chronic metabolic diseases (including diabetes mellitus), hepatic disease, renal dysfunction, hematologic disorders, or immunosuppression (including immunosuppression caused by medications or HIV)
• Adults and children with cognitive or neurologic/neuromuscular conditions (including conditions such as spinal cord injuries or seizure disorders) which may compromise respiratory function, the handling of respiratory secretions, or that can increase the risk of aspiration
• Children and adolescents (6 months to 18 years of age) who are receiving long-term aspirin therapy, and therefore, may be at risk for developing Reye's syndrome after influenza
• Women who are or will be pregnant during the influenza season
• Children 6-59 months of age
• Healthcare personnel
• Household contacts and caregivers of children <5 years (particularly children <6 months) and adults ≥50 years
• Household contacts and caregivers of persons with medical conditions which put them at high risk of complications from influenza infection
• American Indians/Alaska Natives
• Morbidly obese (BMI ≥40)

The Advisory Committee on Immunization Practices (ACIP) states that healthy, nonpregnant persons aged 2-49 years may receive vaccination with either the seasonal live, attenuated influenza vaccine (LAIV) (nasal spray) or the seasonal trivalent inactivated influenza vaccine (IIV) (injection).

Local Anesthetic/Vasoconstrictor Precautions No information available to require special precautions

Effects on Dental Treatment No significant effects or complications reported

Effects on Bleeding No information available to require special precautions

Adverse Effects All serious adverse reactions must be reported to the U.S. Department of Health and Human Services (DHHS) Vaccine Adverse Event Reporting System (VAERS) 1-800-822-7967 or online at https://vaers.hhs.gov/esub/index. In Canada, adverse reactions may be reported to local provincial/territorial health agencies or to the Vaccine Safety Section at Public Health Agency of Canada (1-866-844-0018).

Frequency not defined. Adverse reactions in adults ≥65 years of age may be greater using the high-dose vaccine, but are typically mild and transient.
Cardiovascular: Chest tightness, facial edema
Central nervous system: Chills, drowsiness, fatigue, fever, headache, irritability, malaise, migraine, shivering
Endocrine & metabolic: Dysmenorrhea
Gastrointestinal: Appetite decreased, diarrhea, nausea, sore throat, upper abdominal pain, vomiting
Local: Injection site reactions (including bruising, erythema, induration, inflammation, pain, soreness [≤64%; may last up to 2 days], pruritus, swelling, tenderness)
Neuromuscular & skeletal: Arthralgia, back pain, myalgia (may start within 6-12 hours and last 1-2 days; incidence generally equal to placebo in adults; occurs more frequently than placebo in children)
Ocular: Red eyes
Otic: Earache
Respiratory: Cough, nasal congestion, nasopharyngitis, pharyngolaryngeal pain, rhinitis, upper respiratory tract infection, wheezing
Miscellaneous: Diaphoresis

General Dosage Range
I.M.:
Children 6-35 months: 0.25 mL/dose (1 or 2 doses per season)
Children 3-9 years: 0.5 mL/dose (1 or 2 doses per season)
Children ≥9 years and Adults: 0.5 mL/dose (1 dose per season)
Intradermal: *Adults:* 18-64 years: 0.1 mL/dose (1 dose per season)

Mechanism of Action Promotes immunity to seasonal influenza virus by inducing specific antibody production. Each year the formulation is standardized according to the U.S. Public Health Service. Preparations from previous seasons must not be used.

Pharmacodynamics/Kinetics
Onset of Action Protective antibody titers achieved ~3 weeks after vaccination
Duration of Action Protective antibody titers persist approximately ≥6 months. Elderly: Protective antibody titers may fall ≤4 months after vaccination.

Pregnancy Risk Factor B/C (manufacturer specific)
Pregnancy Considerations Reproduction studies have not been conducted with all products. When conducted, adverse events were not observed in animal studies. Inactivated influenza vaccine has not been shown to cause fetal harm and has been shown to be safe and effective when given to pregnant women. Following maternal immunization with the influenza virus vaccine, vaccine specific antibodies are observed in the newborn.

Pregnant women are at an increased risk of complications from influenza infection (Rasmussen, 2008). Influenza vaccination with the inactivated influenza vaccine (IIV) is recommended for all women who are or will become pregnant during the influenza season and who do not otherwise have contraindications to the ►

vaccine. Pregnant women should observe the same precautions as nonpregnant women to reduce the risk of exposure to influenza and other respiratory infections. When vaccine supply is limited, focus on delivering the vaccine should be given to women who are pregnant or will be pregnant during the flu season, as well as mothers of newborns and contacts or caregivers of children <5 years of age (CDC, 2010). Most available studies show a decrease in influenza-related illnesses in pregnant women as well as children <6 months of age following maternal vaccination during pregnancy, thereby supporting current recommendations that all pregnant women should be vaccinated (Zaman, 2008).

Healthcare providers are encouraged to refer women exposed to the influenza vaccine during pregnancy to the *Vaccines and Medications in Pregnancy Surveillance System* (VAMPSS) by contacting The Organization of Teratology Information Specialists (OTIS) at (877) 311-8972. Women exposed to Flulaval® or Fluarix® during pregnancy may also contact the GlaxoSmithKline registry at 888-452-9622. Healthcare providers may enroll women exposed to Fluzone® Intradermal during pregnancy in the Sanofi Pasteur vaccination registry at 800-822-2463.

Product Availability
Fluarix® Quadrivalent:

Fluarix® Quadrivalent: FDA approved December 2012; availability expected during the 2013-2014 influenza season.

Fluarix® Quadrivalent is an inactivated influenza virus vaccine approved for patients ≥3 years of age. Seasonal quadrivalent influenza vaccines contain two subtype A strains and two subtype B strains; trivalent influenza vaccines contain two subtype A strains and one subtype B strain.

Influenza Virus Vaccine (Live/Attenuated)
(in floo EN za VYE rus vak SEEN live ah TEN yoo aye ted)

Brand Names: U.S. FluMist®
Brand Names: Canada FluMist®
Pharmacologic Category Vaccine, Live (Viral)
Use Provide active immunity to influenza virus strains contained in the vaccine

The Advisory Committee on Immunization Practices (ACIP) states that healthy, nonpregnant persons aged 2-49 years may receive vaccination with either the seasonal live, attenuated influenza vaccine (LAIV) (nasal spray) or the seasonal trivalent inactivated influenza vaccine (TIV) (injection).

Local Anesthetic/Vasoconstrictor Precautions No information available to require special precautions

Effects on Dental Treatment No significant effects or complications reported

Effects on Bleeding No information available to require special precautions

Adverse Effects All serious adverse reactions must be reported to the U.S. Department of Health and Human Services (DHHS) Vaccine Adverse Event Reporting System (VAERS) 1-800-822-7967 or online at https://vaers.hhs.gov/esub/index. In Canada, adverse reactions may be reported to local provincial/territorial health agencies or to the Vaccine Safety Section at Public Health Agency of Canada (1-866-844-0018).

Frequency of events reported within 10 days.

>10%:

Central nervous system: Headache (children 3% to 9%; adults 40%), irritability (children 12% to 21%), lethargy (children 7% to 14%)

Gastrointestinal: Appetite decreased (children 13% to 21%), abdominal pain (children 2% to 12%)

Neuromuscular & skeletal: Tiredness/weakness (adults 26%), muscle aches (children 2% to 6%; adults 17%)

Respiratory: Cough (adults 14%), nasal congestion/runny nose (children 51% to 58%; adults 9% to 44%), sore throat (children 5% to 11%; adults 28%)

1% to 10%:

Central nervous system: Chills (children 2% to 4%, adults 9%), fever (100°F to 101°F: children 6% to 9%; >101°F: children 1% to 4%)

Otic: Otitis media (children 3%)

Respiratory: Sinusitis (adults 4%), sneezing (children 2%), wheezing (children 6-23 months 6%; children 24-59 months 2%)

General Dosage Range Intranasal:

Children 2-8 years: 0.2 mL/dose (1 or 2 doses per season)

Children ≥9 years and Adults ≤49 years: 0.2 mL/dose (1 dose per season)

Mechanism of Action Promotes immunity to seasonal influenza virus by inducing specific antibody production. Each year the formulation is standardized according to the U.S. Public Health Service. Preparations from previous seasons must not be used.

Pharmacodynamics/Kinetics

Onset of Action Protective antibody titers achieved ~3 weeks after vaccination

Duration of Action Protective antibody titers persist approximately ≥6 months. Elderly: Protective antibody titers may fall ≤4 months after vaccination.

Pregnancy Risk Factor B

Pregnancy Considerations Adverse events were not observed in animal reproduction studies. LAIV is not recommended for use during pregnancy. Influenza vaccination with the trivalent inactivated vaccine (TIV) is recommended for all women who are or will become pregnant during the influenza season and who do not otherwise have contraindications to the vaccine.

Healthy pregnant women do not need to avoid contact with persons vaccinated with LAIV and pregnant healthcare providers may administer the LAIV. The nasal vaccine contains the same strains of influenza A and B found in the injection. Information specific to the use of LAIV in pregnancy has not been located. Refer to the Influenza Virus Vaccine (Inactivated) monograph for additional information.

Healthcare providers are encouraged to refer women exposed to the influenza vaccine during pregnancy to the Vaccines and Medications in Pregnancy Surveillance System (VAMPSS) by contacting The Organization of Teratology Information Specialists (OTIS) at (877) 311-8972.

Product Availability

FluMist® Quadrivalent Vaccine: FDA approved February 2012; availability anticipated for the 2013-2014 flu season. Consult prescribing information for additional information.

Seasonal quadrivalent influenza vaccines contain two subtype A strains and two subtype B strains; trivalent influenza vaccines contain two subtype A strains and one subtype B strain.

Influenza Virus Vaccine (Recombinant)
(in floo EN za VYE rus vak SEEN ree KOM be nant)

Brand Names: U.S. Flublok®
Pharmacologic Category Vaccine, Recombinant
Use Provide active immunity to influenza virus strains contained in the vaccine
Local Anesthetic/Vasoconstrictor Precautions No information available to require special precautions
Effects on Dental Treatment No significant effects or complications reported
Effects on Bleeding No information available to require special precautions
Adverse Effects All serious adverse reactions must be reported to the U.S. Department of Health and Human Services (DHHS) Vaccine Adverse Event Reporting System (VAERS) 1-800-822-7967 or online at https://vaers.hhs.gov/esub/index. In Canada, adverse reactions may be reported to local provincial/territorial health agencies or to the Vaccine Safety Section at Public Health Agency of Canada (1-866-844-0018).

>10%:
Central nervous system: Fatigue (15%)
Local: Injection site reactions: Pain (37%)
Neuromuscular & skeletal: Muscle pain (11%)
1% to 10%:
Central nervous system: Headache (1% to 2%)
Gastrointestinal: Nausea (6%)
Local: Injection site reactions: Redness (4%), Swelling (3%)
Respiratory: Cough (1% to 2%), nasal congestion (1% to 2%), nasopharyngitis (1% to 2%), pharyngolaryngeal pain (1% to 2%), rhinorrhea (1% to 2%), upper respiratory tract infection (1% to 2%)
General Dosage Range
I.M.: *Adults 18-49 years:* 0.5 mL/dose (1 per season)
Mechanism of Action Promotes immunity to seasonal influenza virus by inducing specific antibody production. Each year the formulation is standardized according to the U.S. Public Health Service. Preparations from previous seasons must not be used.
Pregnancy Risk Factor B
Pregnancy Considerations Adverse events were not observed in animal reproduction studies.

Pregnant women are at an increased risk of complications from influenza infection (Rasmussen, 2008). Inactivated influenza vaccination is recommended for all women who are or will become pregnant during the influenza season and who do not otherwise have contraindications to the vaccine. Information related to Flublok® in pregnancy is not yet available. Pregnant women should observe the same precautions as nonpregnant women to reduce the risk of exposure to influenza and other respiratory infections. When vaccine supply is limited, focus on delivering the vaccine should be given to women who are pregnant or will be pregnant during the flu season, as well as mothers of newborns and contacts or caregivers of children <5 years of age (CDC, 2010).

Healthcare providers are encouraged to refer women exposed to the influenza vaccine during pregnancy to the *Vaccines and Medications in Pregnancy Surveillance System* (VAMPSS) by contacting The Organization of Teratology Information Specialists (OTIS) at (877) 311-8972. Women exposed to Flublok® during pregnancy may also be enrolled in the Protein Sciences Corporation registry (888-855-7871).

Ingenol Mebutate (IN je nol MEB u tate)

Brand Names: U.S. Picato®
Pharmacologic Category Topical Skin Product
Use Topical treatment of actinic keratosis
Local Anesthetic/Vasoconstrictor Precautions No information available to require special precautions
Effects on Dental Treatment No significant effects or complications reported
Effects on Bleeding No information available to require special precautions
Adverse Effects
>10%: Dermatologic: Erythema (92% to 94%), flaking/scaling (85% to 90%), crusting (74% to 80%), swelling (64% to 79%), vesiculation/pustulation (44% to 56%), erosion/ulceration (26% to 32%), application site pain (2% to 15%)
1% to 10%:
Central nervous system: Headache (2%)
Dermatologic: Application site pruritus (8%), application site irritation (4%), application site infection (3%)
Ocular: Periorbital edema (3%)
Respiratory: Nasopharyngitis (2%)
General Dosage Range Topical: *Adults:* Apply once daily for 2 days (0.05%) or 3 days (0.015%)
Mechanism of Action Ingenol mebutate appears to induce primary necrosis of actinic keratosis with a subsequent neutrophil-mediated inflammatory response with antibody-dependent cytotoxicity of residual disease cells; killing residual disease cells may prevent future relapse.
Pregnancy Risk Factor C
Pregnancy Considerations Adverse events were observed in some animal reproduction studies following I.V. administration of ingenol mebutate. Absorption is limited in humans following topical application.

Inosine Pranobex (EYE no seen PRA no becks)

Brand Names: Canada Imunovir®
Pharmacologic Category Antiviral Agent; Immunomodulator, Systemic
Use Treatment of slowly progressive subacute sclerosing panencephalitis (SSPE); may delay neurologic deterioration and prolong life expectancy
Local Anesthetic/Vasoconstrictor Precautions No information available to require special precautions
Effects on Dental Treatment No significant effects or complications reported
Effects on Bleeding No information available to require special precautions
Adverse Effects Frequency not defined.
Central nervous system: Dizziness, fatigue, headache, insomnia, nervousness
Dermatologic: Itching, rash
Endocrine & metabolic: Hyperuricemia
Gastrointestinal: Constipation, diarrhea, stomach upset
Genitourinary: Urine output increased
Neuromuscular & skeletal: Joint ache
General Dosage Range Oral: *Children, Adolescents, and Adults:* Subacute sclerosing panencephalitis: 50 mg/kg/day in 3 or 4 equally divided doses (maximum: 3 g daily)
Mechanism of Action Exact mechanism has not been fully elucidated; may possess antiviral and immunomodulating effects by potentiating T-lymphocyte and macrophage cell function and by influencing cytokine production (Milano, 1991; Petrova, 2010; Wybran, 1978).

Pharmacodynamics/Kinetics
Half-life Elimination ~50 minutes (Campoli-Richards, 1986)
Time to Peak 1 hour (Campoli-Richards, 1986)
Pregnancy Considerations Adverse effects to the fetus were not observed in animal reproduction studies. Due to the altered immune status of pregnant women, SSPE may be exacerbated during pregnancy and may progress rapidly. Because this condition is rare, use of inosine pranobex in pregnant women is limited to case reports (Cole, 2007)
Product Availability Not available in the U.S.

Insulin Aspart (IN soo lin AS part)

Related Information
Endocrine Disorders and Pregnancy on page 1517
Insulin Regular on page 748
Brand Names: U.S. NovoLOG®; NovoLOG® FlexPen®; NovoLOG® Penfill®
Brand Names: Canada NovoRapid®
Pharmacologic Category Insulin, Rapid-Acting
Use Treatment of type 1 diabetes mellitus (insulin dependent, IDDM) and type 2 diabetes mellitus (non-insulin dependent, NIDDM) to improve glycemic control
Unlabeled Use Gestational diabetes mellitus (GDM); mild-to-moderate diabetic ketoacidosis (DKA); mild-to-moderate hyperosmolar hyperglycemic state (HHS)
Local Anesthetic/Vasoconstrictor Precautions No information available to require special precautions
Effects on Dental Treatment Patients with type 1 diabetes (insulin dependent) should be appointed for dental treatment in the morning in order to minimize chance of stress-induced hypoglycemia.
Effects on Bleeding No information available to require special precautions
General Dosage Range SubQ: *Children ≥2 years, Adolescents, and Adults:* Daily doses are expressed as the **total units/kg/day of all insulin formulations combined.** Diabetes mellitus, type 1: Initial: 0.2-0.6 units/kg/day in divided doses; usual maintenance: 0.5-1 units/kg/day in divided doses.
Mechanism of Action Insulin acts via specific membrane-bound receptors on target tissues to regulate metabolism of carbohydrate, protein, and fats. Target organs for insulin include the liver, skeletal muscle, and adipose tissue.

Within the liver, insulin stimulates hepatic glycogen synthesis. Insulin promotes hepatic synthesis of fatty acids, which are released into the circulation as lipoproteins. Skeletal muscle effects of insulin include increased protein synthesis and increased glycogen synthesis. Within adipose tissue, insulin stimulates the processing of circulating lipoproteins to provide free fatty acids, facilitating triglyceride synthesis and storage by adipocytes; it also directly inhibits the hydrolysis of triglycerides. In addition, insulin stimulates the cellular uptake of amino acids and increases cellular permeability to several ions, including potassium, magnesium, and phosphate. By activating sodium-potassium ATPases, insulin promotes the intracellular movement of potassium.

Normally secreted by the pancreas, insulin products are manufactured for pharmacologic use through recombinant DNA technology using either *E. coli* or *Saccharomyces cerevisiae*. Insulins are categorized based on the onset, peak, and duration of effect (eg, rapid-, short-, intermediate-, and long-acting insulin). Insulin aspart is a rapid-acting insulin analog.

Pharmacodynamics/Kinetics
Onset of Action 0.2-0.3 hours; Peak effect: 1-3 hours
Duration of Action 3-5 hours
Half-life Elimination SubQ: 81 minutes
Time to Peak Plasma: 40-50 minutes
Pregnancy Risk Factor B
Pregnancy Considerations Adverse events have not been observed in animal reproduction studies. Maternal hyperglycemia can be associated with adverse effects in the fetus, including macrosomia, neonatal hyperglycemia, and hyperbilirubinemia; the risk of congenital malformations is increased when the Hb A_{1c} is >1% above the normal range.

Insulin requirements tend to fall during the first trimester of pregnancy and increase in the later trimesters, peaking at 28-32 weeks of gestation. Following delivery, insulin requirements decrease rapidly. Diabetes can also be associated with adverse effects in the mother. Poorly-treated diabetes may cause end-organ damage that may in turn negatively affect obstetric outcomes. Physiologic glucose levels should be maintained prior to and during pregnancy to decrease the risk of adverse events in the fetus and the mother. Insulin is the drug of choice for the control of diabetes mellitus during pregnancy. Insulin aspart has been demonstrated to be as safe and effective as regular human insulin when used during pregnancy and may have advantages over regular insulin during pregnancy.

Insulin Aspart Protamine and Insulin Aspart (IN soo lin AS part PROE ta meen & IN soo lin AS part)

Related Information
Insulin Regular on page 748
Brand Names: U.S. NovoLOG® Mix 70/30; NovoLOG® Mix 70/30 FlexPen®
Brand Names: Canada NovoMix® 30
Pharmacologic Category Insulin, Combination
Use Treatment of type 1 diabetes mellitus (insulin dependent, IDDM) and type 2 diabetes mellitus (non-insulin dependent, NIDDM) to improve glycemic control
Local Anesthetic/Vasoconstrictor Precautions No information available to require special precautions
Effects on Dental Treatment Patients with type 1 diabetes (insulin dependent) should be appointed for dental treatment in the morning in order to minimize chance of stress-induced hypoglycemia.
Effects on Bleeding No information available to require special precautions
Adverse Effects Frequency not defined.
Cardiovascular: Palpitation, pallor, peripheral edema, tachycardia
Central nervous system: Fatigue, headache, hypothermia, loss of consciousness, mental confusion
Dermatologic: Pruritus, rash, redness, urticaria
Endocrine & metabolic: Hypoglycemia, hypokalemia
Gastrointestinal: Hunger, nausea, numbness of mouth, weight gain
Local: Injection site reaction (including edema, itching, pain or warmth, stinging), lipoatrophy, lipodystrophy
Neuromuscular & skeletal: Muscle weakness, paresthesia, tremor
Ocular: Transient presbyopia or blurred vision
Miscellaneous: Anaphylaxis, antibodies to insulin (no change in efficacy), diaphoresis, local allergy, systemic allergic symptoms

General Dosage Range SubQ: *Adults:* Diabetes mellitus, type 1 or 2: **Not** intended for initial therapy; basal insulin requirements should be established **first** to direct dosing of combination insulin products.

Mechanism of Action Insulin aspart protamine and insulin aspart is an intermediate-acting combination insulin product with a more rapid onset and similar duration of action as compared to that of insulin NPH and insulin regular combination products. Insulin acts via specific membrane-bound receptors on target tissues to regulate metabolism of carbohydrate, protein, and fats. Target organs for insulin include the liver, skeletal muscle, and adipose tissue.

Within the liver, insulin stimulates hepatic glycogen synthesis. Insulin promotes hepatic synthesis of fatty acids, which are released into the circulation as lipoproteins. Skeletal muscle effects of insulin include increased protein synthesis and increased glycogen synthesis. Within adipose tissue, insulin stimulates the processing of circulating lipoproteins to provide free fatty acids, facilitating triglyceride synthesis and storage by adipocytes; also directly inhibits the hydrolysis of triglycerides. In addition, insulin stimulates the cellular uptake of amino acids and increases cellular permeability to several ions, including potassium, magnesium, and phosphate. By activating sodium-potassium ATPases, insulin promotes the intracellular movement of potassium.

Normally secreted by the pancreas, insulin products are manufactured for pharmacologic use through recombinant DNA technology using either *E. coli* or *Saccharomyces cerevisiae*. Insulins are categorized based on the onset, peak, and duration of effect (eg, rapid-, short-, intermediate-, and long-acting insulin).

Pharmacodynamics/Kinetics
Onset of Action 10-20 minutes; Peak effect: 1-4 hours
Duration of Action 18-24 hours
Half-life Elimination ~8-9 hours
Time to Peak 1-1.5 hours
Pregnancy Risk Factor B
Pregnancy Considerations Biphasic insulin aspart (insulin aspart protamine suspension 70% [intermediate acting] and insulin aspart solution 30% [rapid acting]) was found to be comparable to biphasic human insulin (Insulin NPH suspension 70% [intermediate acting] and insulin regular solution 30% [short acting]) in a pilot study of women with gestational diabetes mellitus. All pregnancies have a background risk of adverse outcome; this risk is increased in pregnancies complicated by hyperglycemia and may be decreased with good metabolic control. Most available information for use of insulin aspart in pregnancy is from studies using the rapid action solution. Refer to Insulin Aspart monograph for additional information.

Insulin Detemir (IN soo lin DE te mir)

Related Information
Endocrine Disorders and Pregnancy *on page 1517*
Insulin Regular *on page 748*
Brand Names: U.S. Levemir®; Levemir® FlexPen®
Brand Names: Canada Levemir®
Pharmacologic Category Insulin, Intermediate- to Long-Acting
Use Treatment of type 1 diabetes mellitus (insulin dependent, IDDM) and type 2 diabetes mellitus (non-insulin dependent, NIDDM) to improve glycemic control
Local Anesthetic/Vasoconstrictor Precautions No information available to require special precautions

Effects on Dental Treatment Patients with type 1 diabetes (insulin dependent) should be appointed for dental treatment in the morning in order to minimize chance of stress-induced hypoglycemia.
Effects on Bleeding No information available to require special precautions
Adverse Effects Primarily symptoms of hypoglycemia
Cardiovascular: Pallor, palpitation, tachycardia
Central nervous system: Fatigue, headache, hypothermia, loss of consciousness, mental confusion
Dermatologic: Redness, urticaria
Endocrine & metabolic: Hypoglycemia, hypokalemia
Gastrointestinal: Hunger, nausea, numbness of mouth
Local: Atrophy or hypertrophy of SubQ fat tissue; edema, itching, pain or warmth at injection site; stinging
Neuromuscular & skeletal: Muscle weakness, paresthesia, tremor
Ocular: Transient presbyopia or blurred vision
Miscellaneous: Anaphylaxis, diaphoresis, local and/or systemic hypersensitivity reactions
General Dosage Range SubQ:
Children ≥2 years, Adolescents, and Adults: Diabetes mellitus, type 1: Initial dose: Approximately one-third of the total daily insulin requirement administered in 1-2 divided doses.
Adults: Diabetes mellitus, type 2: Initial: 10 units **or** 0.1-0.2 units/kg in 1-2 divided doses
Mechanism of Action Insulin acts via specific membrane-bound receptors on target tissues to regulate metabolism of carbohydrate, protein, and fats. Target organs for insulin include the liver, skeletal muscle, and adipose tissue.

Within the liver, insulin stimulates hepatic glycogen synthesis. Insulin promotes hepatic synthesis of fatty acids, which are released into the circulation as lipoproteins. Skeletal muscle effects of insulin include increased protein synthesis and increased glycogen synthesis. Within adipose tissue, insulin stimulates the processing of circulating lipoproteins to provide free fatty acids, facilitating triglyceride synthesis and storage by adipocytes; also directly inhibits the hydrolysis of triglycerides. In addition, insulin stimulates the cellular uptake of amino acids and increases cellular permeability to several ions, including potassium, magnesium, and phosphate. By activating sodium-potassium ATPases, insulin promotes the intracellular movement of potassium.

Normally secreted by the pancreas, insulin products are manufactured for pharmacologic use through recombinant DNA technology using either *E. coli* or *Saccharomyces cerevisiae*. Insulins are categorized based on the onset, peak, and duration of effect (eg, rapid-, short-, intermediate-, and long-acting insulin). Insulin detemir is an intermediate- to long-acting insulin analog.
Pharmacodynamics/Kinetics
Onset of Action 3-4 hours; Peak effect: 3-9 hours (Plank, 2005)
Duration of Action Dose dependent: 6-23 hours; **Note:** Duration is dose-dependent. At lower dosages (0.1-0.2 units/kg), mean duration is variable (5.7-12.1 hours). At 0.4 units/kg, the mean duration was 19.9 hours. At high dosages (≥0.8 units/kg) the duration is longer and less variable (mean of 22-23 hours) (Plank, 2005).
Half-life Elimination 5-7 hours (dose-dependent)
Time to Peak Plasma: 6-8 hours
Pregnancy Risk Factor B

Pregnancy Considerations Dose-related adverse events were observed in animal reproduction studies. Limited information is available related to the use of insulin detemir in pregnancy. Maternal hyperglycemia can be associated with adverse effects in the fetus, including macrosomia, neonatal hyperglycemia, and hyperbilirubinemia; the risk of congenital malformations is increased when the Hb A_{1c} is >1% above the normal range. Insulin requirements tend to fall during the first trimester of pregnancy and increase in the later trimesters, peaking at 28-32 weeks of gestation. Following delivery, insulin requirements decrease rapidly. Diabetes can also be associated with adverse effects in the mother. Poorly treated diabetes may cause end-organ damage that may in turn negatively affect obstetric outcomes. Physiologic glucose levels should be maintained prior to and during pregnancy to decrease the risk of adverse events in the fetus and the mother. Insulin is the drug of choice for the control of diabetes mellitus during pregnancy.

Insulin Glargine (IN soo lin GLAR jeen)

Related Information
Endocrine Disorders and Pregnancy *on page 1517*
Insulin Regular *on page 748*
Brand Names: U.S. Lantus®; Lantus® Solostar®
Brand Names: Canada Lantus®; Lantus® OptiSet®
Pharmacologic Category Insulin, Long-Acting
Use Treatment of type 1 diabetes mellitus (insulin dependent, IDDM) and type 2 diabetes mellitus (non-insulin dependent, NIDDM) to improve glycemic control
Local Anesthetic/Vasoconstrictor Precautions No information available to require special precautions
Effects on Dental Treatment Patients with type 1 diabetes (insulin dependent) should be appointed for dental treatment in the morning in order to minimize chance of stress-induced hypoglycemia.
Effects on Bleeding No information available to require special precautions
Adverse Effects Primarily symptoms of hypoglycemia
Cardiovascular: Pallor, palpitation, tachycardia
Central nervous system: Fatigue, headache, hypothermia, loss of consciousness, mental confusion
Dermatologic: Redness, urticaria
Endocrine & metabolic: Hypoglycemia, hypokalemia
Gastrointestinal: Hunger, nausea, numbness of mouth
Local: Atrophy or hypertrophy of SubQ fat tissue; edema, itching, pain or warmth at injection site; stinging
Neuromuscular & skeletal: Muscle weakness, paresthesia, tremor
Ocular: Transient presbyopia or blurred vision
Miscellaneous: Anaphylaxis, diaphoresis, local and/or systemic hypersensitivity reactions
General Dosage Range SubQ:
Children ≥6 years, Adolescents, and Adults: Diabetes mellitus, type 1: Initial dose: Approximately one-third of the total daily insulin requirement administered once daily
Adults: Diabetes mellitus, type 2: Initial: 10 units or 0.2 units/kg once daily
Mechanism of Action Insulin acts via specific membrane-bound receptors on target tissues to regulate metabolism of carbohydrate, protein, and fats. Target organs for insulin include the liver, skeletal muscle, and adipose tissue.

Within the liver, insulin stimulates hepatic glycogen synthesis. Insulin promotes hepatic synthesis of fatty acids, which are released into the circulation as lipoproteins. Skeletal muscle effects of insulin include increased protein synthesis and increased glycogen synthesis. Within adipose tissue, insulin stimulates the processing of circulating lipoproteins to provide free fatty acids, facilitating triglyceride synthesis and storage by adipocytes; also directly inhibits the hydrolysis of triglycerides. In addition, insulin stimulates the cellular uptake of amino acids and increases cellular permeability to several ions, including potassium, magnesium, and phosphate. By activating sodium-potassium ATPases, insulin promotes the intracellular movement of potassium.

Normally secreted by the pancreas, insulin products are manufactured for pharmacologic use through recombinant DNA technology using either *E. coli* or *Saccharomyces cerevisiae*. Insulins are categorized based on the onset, peak, and duration of effect (eg, rapid-, short-, intermediate-, and long-acting insulin). Insulin glargine is a long-acting insulin analog.

Pharmacodynamics/Kinetics
Onset of Action 3-4 hours; Peak effect: No pronounced peak
Duration of Action Generally 24 hours or longer; reported range: 10.8 to >24 hours (up to 32 hours documented in some studies)
Time to Peak Plasma: No pronounced peak
Pregnancy Risk Factor C
Pregnancy Considerations Adverse events have been shown in some animal studies. Maternal hyperglycemia can be associated with adverse effects in the fetus, including macrosomia, neonatal hyperglycemia, and hyperbilirubinemia; the risk of congenital malformations is increased when Hb A_{1c} is >1% above the normal range.

Insulin requirements tend to fall during the first trimester of pregnancy and increase in the later trimesters, peaking at 28-32 weeks of gestation. Following delivery, insulin requirements decrease rapidly. Diabetes can also be associated with adverse effects in the mother. Poorly-treated diabetes may cause end-organ damage that may in turn negatively affect obstetric outcomes. Physiologic glucose levels should be maintained prior to and during pregnancy to decrease the risk of adverse events in the fetus and the mother. Insulin is the drug of choice for the control of diabetes mellitus during pregnancy. When compared to NPH insulin, insulin glargine has not been found to increase the risk of adverse events during pregnancy.

Insulin Glulisine (IN soo lin gloo LIS een)

Related Information
Endocrine Disorders and Pregnancy *on page 1517*
Insulin Regular *on page 748*
Brand Names: U.S. Apidra®; Apidra® SoloStar®
Brand Names: Canada Apidra®
Pharmacologic Category Insulin, Rapid-Acting
Use Treatment of type 1 diabetes mellitus (insulin dependent, IDDM) and type 2 diabetes mellitus (non-insulin dependent, NIDDM) to improve glycemic control
Local Anesthetic/Vasoconstrictor Precautions No information available to require special precautions
Effects on Dental Treatment Patients with type 1 diabetes (insulin dependent) should be appointed for dental treatment in the morning in order to minimize chance of stress-induced hypoglycemia.

Effects on Bleeding No information available to require special precautions

Adverse Effects Primarily symptoms of hypoglycemia
Cardiovascular: Pallor, palpitation, tachycardia
Central nervous system: Fatigue, headache, hypothermia, loss of consciousness, mental confusion
Dermatologic: Redness, urticaria
Endocrine & metabolic: Hypoglycemia, hypokalemia
Gastrointestinal: Hunger, nausea, numbness of mouth
Local: Atrophy or hypertrophy of SubQ fat tissue; edema, itching, pain or warmth at injection site; stinging
Neuromuscular & skeletal: Muscle weakness, paresthesia, tremor
Ocular: Transient presbyopia or blurred vision
Miscellaneous: Anaphylaxis, diaphoresis, local and/or systemic hypersensitivity reactions

General Dosage Range SubQ: *Children ≥4 years, Adolescents and Adults:* Diabetes mellitus, type 1:
Note: Multiple daily doses or continuous subcutaneous infusions guided by blood glucose monitoring are the standard of diabetes care. Combinations of insulin formulations are commonly used. The daily doses presented below are expressed as the **total units/kg/day of all insulin formulations combined.**
Initial: 0.2-0.6 units/kg/day in divided doses; usual maintenance: 0.5-1 units/kg/day in divided doses.

Mechanism of Action Insulin acts via specific membrane-bound receptors on target tissues to regulate metabolism of carbohydrate, protein, and fats. Target organs for insulin include the liver, skeletal muscle, and adipose tissue.

Within the liver, insulin stimulates hepatic glycogen synthesis. Insulin promotes hepatic synthesis of fatty acids, which are released into the circulation as lipoproteins. Skeletal muscle effects of insulin include increased protein synthesis and increased glycogen synthesis. Within adipose tissue, insulin stimulates the processing of circulating lipoproteins to provide free fatty acids, facilitating triglyceride synthesis and storage by adipocytes; also directly inhibits the hydrolysis of triglycerides. In addition, insulin stimulates the cellular uptake of amino acids and increases cellular permeability to several ions, including potassium, magnesium, and phosphate. By activating sodium-potassium ATPases, insulin promotes the intracellular movement of potassium.

Normally secreted by the pancreas, insulin products are manufactured for pharmacologic use through recombinant DNA technology using either *E. coli* or *Saccharomyces cerevisiae*. Insulins are categorized based on the onset, peak, and duration of effect (eg, rapid-, short-, intermediate-, and long-acting insulin). Insulin glulisine is a rapid-acting insulin analog.

Pharmacodynamics/Kinetics
Onset of Action 0.2-0.5 hours; Peak effect: 1.6-2.8 hours
Duration of Action 3-4 hours
Half-life Elimination
I.V.: 13 minutes
SubQ: 42 minutes
Time to Peak Plasma: 0.6-2 hours
Pregnancy Risk Factor C
Pregnancy Considerations Adverse events were observed in some animal reproduction studies. Maternal hyperglycemia can be associated with adverse effects in the fetus, including macrosomia, neonatal hyperglycemia, and hyperbilirubinemia; the risk of congenital malformations is increased when the Hb A_{1c} is >1% above the normal range.

Insulin requirements tend to fall during the first trimester of pregnancy and increase in the later trimesters, peaking at 28-32 weeks of gestation. Following delivery, insulin requirements decrease rapidly. Diabetes can also be associated with adverse effects in the mother. Poorly-treated diabetes may cause end-organ damage that may in turn negatively affect obstetric outcomes. Physiologic glucose levels should be maintained prior to and during pregnancy to decrease the risk of adverse events in the fetus and mother. Insulin is the drug of choice for the control of diabetes mellitus during pregnancy. Due to lack of clinical studies with insulin glulisine in pregnant women, the manufacturer recommends use during pregnancy only if the potential benefit to the mother justifies any potential risk to the fetus.

Insulin Lispro (IN soo lin LYE sproe)

Related Information
Endocrine Disorders and Pregnancy *on page 1517*
Insulin Regular *on page 748*
Brand Names: U.S. HumaLOG®; HumaLOG® KwikPen™
Brand Names: Canada Humalog®
Pharmacologic Category Insulin, Rapid-Acting
Use Treatment of type 1 diabetes mellitus (insulin dependent, IDDM) and type 2 diabetes mellitus (non-insulin dependent, NIDDM) to improve glycemic control
Unlabeled Use Gestational diabetes mellitus (GDM); mild-to-moderate diabetic ketoacidosis (DKA); mild-to-moderate hyperosmolar hyperglycemic state (HHS)
Local Anesthetic/Vasoconstrictor Precautions No information available to require special precautions
Effects on Dental Treatment Patients with type 1 diabetes (insulin dependent) should be appointed for dental treatment in the morning in order to minimize chance of stress-induced hypoglycemia.
Effects on Bleeding No information available to require special precautions

Adverse Effects Primarily symptoms of hypoglycemia
Cardiovascular: Pallor, palpitation, tachycardia
Central nervous system: Fatigue, headache, hypothermia, loss of consciousness, mental confusion
Dermatologic: Redness, urticaria
Endocrine & metabolic: Hypoglycemia, hypokalemia
Gastrointestinal: Hunger, nausea, numbness of mouth
Local: Atrophy or hypertrophy of SubQ fat tissue; edema, itching, pain or warmth at injection site; stinging
Neuromuscular & skeletal: Muscle weakness, paresthesia, tremor
Ocular: Transient presbyopia or blurred vision
Miscellaneous: Anaphylaxis, diaphoresis, local and/or systemic hypersensitivity reactions

General Dosage Range SubQ: *Children ≥3 years, Adolescents and Adults:* Daily doses are expressed as the **total units/kg/day of all insulin formulations combined.** Diabetes mellitus, type 1: Initial: 0.2-0.6 units/kg/day in divided doses; usual maintenance: 0.5-1 units/kg/day in divided doses.

Mechanism of Action Insulin acts via specific membrane-bound receptors on target tissues to regulate metabolism of carbohydrate, protein, and fats. Target organs for insulin include the liver, skeletal muscle, and adipose tissue.

Within the liver, insulin stimulates hepatic glycogen synthesis. Insulin promotes hepatic synthesis of fatty acids, which are released into the circulation as lipoproteins. Skeletal muscle effects of insulin include increased protein synthesis and increased glycogen synthesis. Within adipose tissue, insulin stimulates the processing of circulating lipoproteins to provide free fatty acids, facilitating triglyceride synthesis and storage by adipocytes; also directly inhibits the hydrolysis of triglycerides. In addition, insulin stimulates the cellular uptake of amino acids and increases cellular permeability to several ions, including potassium, magnesium, and phosphate. By activating sodium-potassium ATPases, insulin promotes the intracellular movement of potassium.

Normally secreted by the pancreas, insulin products are manufactured for pharmacologic use through recombinant DNA technology using either *E. coli* or *Saccharomyces cerevisiae*. Insulins are categorized based on the onset, peak, and duration of effect (eg, rapid-, short-, intermediate-, and long-acting insulin). Insulin lispro is a rapid-acting insulin analog.

Pharmacodynamics/Kinetics
Onset of Action 0.25-0.5 hours; Peak effect: 0.5-2.5 hours
Duration of Action ≤5 hours
Half-life Elimination
I.V.: ~0.5-1 hour (dose-dependent)
SubQ: 1 hour
Time to Peak Plasma: 0.5-1.5 hours
Pregnancy Risk Factor B
Pregnancy Considerations Adverse events have not been observed in animal reproduction studies. Insulin lispro has not been shown to cross the placenta at standard clinical doses. Although congenital anomalies have been noted in case reports, when compared to regular insulin, insulin lispro has not been found to increase the risk of adverse events to the fetus in larger studies. Maternal hyperglycemia can be associated with adverse effects in the fetus, including macrosomia, neonatal hyperglycemia, and hyperbilirubinemia; the risk of congenital malformations is increased when Hb A_{1c} is >1% above the normal range.

Insulin requirements tend to fall during the first trimester of pregnancy and increase in the later trimesters, peaking at 28-32 weeks of gestation. Following delivery, insulin requirements decrease rapidly. Diabetes can also be associated with adverse effects in the mother. Poorly-treated diabetes may cause end-organ damage that may in turn negatively affect obstetric outcomes. Physiologic glucose levels should be maintained prior to and during pregnancy to decrease the risk of adverse events in the fetus and mother. Insulin is the drug of choice for the control of diabetes mellitus during pregnancy. The use of insulin lispro has been shown to be as effective as regular insulin to treat diabetes in pregnancy and may have advantages over regular insulin during pregnancy.

Insulin Lispro Protamine and Insulin Lispro
(IN soo lin LYE sproe PROE ta meen & IN soo lin LYE sproe)

Related Information
Insulin Regular *on page 748*
Brand Names: U.S. HumaLOG® Mix 50/50™; HumaLOG® Mix 50/50™ KwikPen™; HumaLOG® Mix 75/25™; HumaLOG® Mix 75/25™ KwikPen™
Brand Names: Canada Humalog® Mix 25
Pharmacologic Category Insulin, Combination
Use Treatment of type 1 diabetes mellitus (insulin dependent, IDDM) and type 2 diabetes mellitus (non-insulin dependent, NIDDM) to improve glycemic control

Local Anesthetic/Vasoconstrictor Precautions No information available to require special precautions
Effects on Dental Treatment Patients with type 1 diabetes (insulin-dependent) should be appointed for dental treatment in the morning in order to minimize chance of stress-induced hypoglycemia.
Effects on Bleeding No information available to require special precautions
Adverse Effects Primarily symptoms of hypoglycemia
Cardiovascular: Pallor, palpitation, tachycardia
Central nervous system: Fatigue, headache, hypothermia, loss of consciousness, mental confusion
Dermatologic: Redness, urticaria
Endocrine & metabolic: Hypoglycemia, hypokalemia
Gastrointestinal: Hunger, nausea, numbness of mouth
Local: Atrophy or hypertrophy of SubQ fat tissue; edema, itching, pain or warmth at injection site; stinging
Neuromuscular & skeletal: Muscle weakness, paresthesia, tremor
Ocular: Transient presbyopia or blurred vision
Miscellaneous: Anaphylaxis, diaphoresis, local and/or systemic hypersensitivity reactions
General Dosage Range SubQ: *Adults:* Diabetes mellitus, type 1 or 2: **Not** intended for initial therapy; basal insulin requirements should be established **first** to direct dosing of combination insulin products.
Mechanism of Action Insulin acts via specific membrane-bound receptors on target tissues to regulate metabolism of carbohydrate, protein, and fats. Target organs for insulin include the liver, skeletal muscle, and adipose tissue.

Within the liver, insulin stimulates hepatic glycogen synthesis. Insulin promotes hepatic synthesis of fatty acids, which are released into the circulation as lipoproteins. Skeletal muscle effects of insulin include increased protein synthesis and increased glycogen synthesis. Within adipose tissue, insulin stimulates the processing of circulating lipoproteins to provide free fatty acids, facilitating triglyceride synthesis and storage by adipocytes; also directly inhibits the hydrolysis of triglycerides. In addition, insulin stimulates the cellular uptake of amino acids and increases cellular permeability to several ions, including potassium, magnesium, and phosphate. By activating sodium-potassium ATPases, insulin promotes the intracellular movement of potassium.

Normally secreted by the pancreas, insulin products are manufactured for pharmacologic use through recombinant DNA technology using either *E. coli* or *Saccharomyces cerevisiae*. Insulins are categorized based on the onset, peak, and duration of effect (eg, rapid-, short-, intermediate-, and long-acting insulin). Insulin lispro protamine and insulin lispro is an intermediate-acting combination product with a more rapid onset and similar duration of action as compared to that of insulin NPH and insulin regular combination products.

Pharmacodynamics/Kinetics
Onset of Action 0.25-0.5 hours
Peak effect: Humalog® Mix 50/50™: 0.8-4.8 hours; Humalog® Mix 75/25™: 1-6.5 hours
Duration of Action 14-24 hours
Time to Peak Plasma: Humalog® Mix 50/50™: 0.75-13.5 hours; Humalog® Mix 75/25™: 0.5-4 hours
Pregnancy Risk Factor B
Pregnancy Considerations Adverse events have not been observed in animal reproduction studies. Insulin lispro has not been shown to cross the placenta at standard clinical doses. Although congenital anomalies have been noted in case reports, when compared to

regular insulin, insulin lispro has not been found to increase the risk of adverse events to the fetus in larger studies. Maternal hyperglycemia can be associated with adverse effects in the fetus, including macrosomia, neonatal hyperglycemia, and hyperbilirubinemia; the risk of congenital malformations is increased when Hb A_{1c} is >1% above the normal range.

Insulin requirements tend to fall during the first trimester of pregnancy and increase in the later trimesters, peaking at 28-32 weeks of gestation. Following delivery, insulin requirements decrease rapidly. Diabetes can also be associated with adverse effects in the mother. Poorly-treated diabetes may cause end-organ damage that may in turn negatively affect obstetric outcomes. Physiologic glucose levels should be maintained prior to and during pregnancy to decrease the risk of adverse events in the fetus and mother. Insulin is the drug of choice for the control of diabetes mellitus during pregnancy. The use of insulin lispro has been shown to be as effective as regular insulin to treat diabetes in pregnancy and may have advantages over regular insulin during pregnancy.

Insulin NPH (IN soo lin N P H)

Related Information
Endocrine Disorders and Pregnancy *on page 1517*
Insulin Regular *on page 748*
Brand Names: U.S. HumuLIN® N; NovoLIN® N
Brand Names: Canada Humulin® N; Novolin® ge NPH
Pharmacologic Category Insulin, Intermediate-Acting
Use Treatment of type 1 diabetes mellitus (insulin dependent, IDDM) and type 2 diabetes mellitus (non-insulin dependent, NIDDM) to improve glycemic control
Unlabeled Use Gestational diabetes mellitus (GDM)
Local Anesthetic/Vasoconstrictor Precautions No information available to require special precautions
Effects on Dental Treatment Patients with type 1 diabetes (insulin dependent) should be appointed for dental treatment in the morning in order to minimize chance of stress-induced hypoglycemia.
Effects on Bleeding No information available to require special precautions
Adverse Effects Primarily symptoms of hypoglycemia
Cardiovascular: Pallor, palpitation, tachycardia
Central nervous system: Fatigue, headache, hypothermia, loss of consciousness, mental confusion
Dermatologic: Redness, urticaria
Endocrine & metabolic: Hypoglycemia, hypokalemia
Gastrointestinal: Hunger, nausea, numbness of mouth
Local: Atrophy or hypertrophy of SubQ fat tissue; edema, itching, pain or warmth at injection site; stinging
Neuromuscular & skeletal: Muscle weakness, paresthesia, tremor
Ocular: Transient presbyopia or blurred vision
Miscellaneous: Anaphylaxis, diaphoresis, local and/or systemic hypersensitivity reactions
General Dosage Range SubQ:
Children ≥2 years, Adolescents, and Adults: Daily doses are expressed as the **total units/kg/day of all insulin formulations combined.** Diabetes mellitus, type 1: Initial: 0.2-0.6 units/kg/day in divided doses; usual maintenance: 0.5-1 units/kg/day in divided doses.
Adults: Diabetes mellitus, type 2: Initial: 0.2 units/kg/day or 10 units/day in divided doses before meals.

Mechanism of Action Insulin acts via specific membrane-bound receptors on target tissues to regulate metabolism of carbohydrate, protein, and fats. Target organs for insulin include the liver, skeletal muscle, and adipose tissue.

Within the liver, insulin stimulates hepatic glycogen synthesis. Insulin promotes hepatic synthesis of fatty acids, which are released into the circulation as lipoproteins. Skeletal muscle effects of insulin include increased protein synthesis and increased glycogen synthesis. Within adipose tissue, insulin stimulates the processing of circulating lipoproteins to provide free fatty acids, facilitating triglyceride synthesis and storage by adipocytes; also directly inhibits the hydrolysis of triglycerides. In addition, insulin stimulates the cellular uptake of amino acids and increases cellular permeability to several ions, including potassium, magnesium, and phosphate. By activating sodium-potassium ATPases, insulin promotes the intracellular movement of potassium.

Normally secreted by the pancreas, insulin products are manufactured for pharmacologic use through recombinant DNA technology using either *E. coli* or *Saccharomyces cerevisiae*. Insulins are categorized based on the onset, peak, and duration of effect (eg, rapid-, short-, intermediate-, and long-acting insulin). Insulin NPH, an isophane suspension of human insulin, is an intermediate-acting insulin.
Pharmacodynamics/Kinetics
Onset of Action 1-2 hours; Peak effect: 4-12 hours
Duration of Action 14-24 hours
Time to Peak Plasma: 6-10 hours
Pregnancy Considerations Maternal hyperglycemia can be associated with adverse effects in the fetus, including macrosomia, neonatal hyperglycemia, and hyperbilirubinemia; the risk of congenital malformations is increased when the Hb A_{1c} is >1% above the normal range. Insulin requirements tend to fall during the first trimester of pregnancy and increase in the later trimesters, peaking at 28-32 weeks of gestation. Following delivery, insulin requirements decrease rapidly. Diabetes can also be associated with adverse effects in the mother. Poorly-treated diabetes may cause end-organ damage that may in turn negatively affect obstetric outcomes. Physiologic glucose levels should be maintained prior to and during pregnancy to decrease the risk of adverse events in the fetus and mother. Insulin is the drug of choice for the control of diabetes mellitus during pregnancy.

Insulin NPH and Insulin Regular
(IN soo lin N P H & IN soo lin REG yoo ler)

Related Information
Insulin Regular *on page 748*
Brand Names: U.S. HumuLIN® 70/30; NovoLIN® 70/30
Brand Names: Canada Humulin® 20/80; Humulin® 70/30; Novolin® ge 30/70; Novolin® ge 40/60; Novolin® ge 50/50
Pharmacologic Category Insulin, Combination
Use Treatment of type 1 diabetes mellitus (insulin dependent, IDDM) and type 2 diabetes mellitus (non-insulin dependent, NIDDM) to improve glycemic control
Unlabeled Use Gestational diabetes mellitus (GDM)
Local Anesthetic/Vasoconstrictor Precautions No information available to require special precautions

◄ **Effects on Dental Treatment** Patients with type 1 diabetes (insulin dependent) should be appointed for dental treatment in the morning in order to minimize chance of stress-induced hypoglycemia.

Effects on Bleeding No information available to require special precautions

Adverse Effects Primarily symptoms of hypoglycemia

Cardiovascular: Pallor, palpitation, tachycardia

Central nervous system: Fatigue, headache, hypothermia, loss of consciousness, mental confusion

Dermatologic: Redness, urticaria

Endocrine & metabolic: Hypoglycemia, hypokalemia

Gastrointestinal: Hunger, nausea, numbness of mouth

Local: Atrophy or hypertrophy of SubQ fat tissue; edema, itching, pain or warmth at injection site; stinging

Neuromuscular & skeletal: Muscle weakness, paresthesia, tremor

Ocular: Transient presbyopia or blurred vision

Miscellaneous: Anaphylaxis, diaphoresis, local and/or systemic hypersensitivity reactions

General Dosage Range SubQ:

Children, Adolescents, and Adults: Daily doses are expressed as the **total units/kg/day of all insulin formulations combined.** Diabetes mellitus, type 1: Initial: 0.2-0.6 units/kg/day in divided doses; usual maintenance: 0.5-1 units/kg/day in divided doses.

Adults: Diabetes mellitus, type 2: **Not** intended for initial therapy; basal insulin requirements should be established **first** to direct dosing of combination insulin products.

Mechanism of Action Insulin acts via specific membrane-bound receptors on target tissues to regulate metabolism of carbohydrate, protein, and fats. Target organs for insulin include the liver, skeletal muscle, and adipose tissue.

Within the liver, insulin stimulates hepatic glycogen synthesis. Insulin promotes hepatic synthesis of fatty acids, which are released into the circulation as lipoproteins. Skeletal muscle effects of insulin include increased protein synthesis and increased glycogen synthesis. Within adipose tissue, insulin stimulates the processing of circulating lipoproteins to provide free fatty acids, facilitating triglyceride synthesis and storage by adipocytes; also directly inhibits the hydrolysis of triglycerides. In addition, insulin stimulates the cellular uptake of amino acids and increases cellular permeability to several ions, including potassium, magnesium, and phosphate. By activating sodium-potassium ATPases, insulin promotes the intracellular movement of potassium.

Normally secreted by the pancreas, insulin products are manufactured for pharmacologic use through recombinant DNA technology using either *E. coli* or *Saccharomyces cerevisiae*. Insulins are categorized based on the onset, peak, and duration of effect (eg, rapid-, short-, intermediate-, and long-acting insulin). Insulin NPH and insulin regular is an intermediate-acting combination insulin product with a more rapid onset than that of insulin NPH alone.

Pharmacodynamics/Kinetics

Onset of Action 0.5 hours; Peak effect: 2-12 hours

Duration of Action 18-24 hours

Time to Peak Based on individual components:

Insulin regular: 0.8-2 hours

Insulin NPH: 6-10 hours

Pregnancy Considerations See individual agents.

Insulin Regular (IN soo lin REG yoo ler)

Related Information

Endocrine Disorders and Pregnancy *on page 1517*

Insulin Aspart *on page 742*

Insulin Aspart Protamine and Insulin Aspart *on page 742*

Insulin Detemir *on page 743*

Insulin Glargine *on page 744*

Insulin Glulisine *on page 744*

Insulin Lispro *on page 745*

Insulin Lispro Protamine and Insulin Lispro *on page 746*

Insulin NPH *on page 747*

Insulin NPH and Insulin Regular *on page 747*

Brand Names: U.S. HumuLIN® R; HumuLIN® R U-500; NovoLIN® R

Brand Names: Canada Humulin® R; Novolin® ge Toronto

Pharmacologic Category Insulin, Short-Acting

Use Treatment of type 1 diabetes mellitus (insulin dependent, IDDM) and type 2 diabetes mellitus (non-insulin dependent, NIDDM) to improve glycemic control

Unlabeled Use Hyperkalemia; gestational diabetes mellitus (GDM), diabetic ketoacidosis (DKA); hyperosmolar hyperglycemic state (HHS); adjunct of parenteral nutrition

Local Anesthetic/Vasoconstrictor Precautions No information available to require special precautions

Effects on Dental Treatment Patients with type 1 diabetes (insulin dependent) should be appointed for dental treatment in the morning in order to minimize chance of stress-induced hypoglycemia.

Effects on Bleeding No information available to require special precautions

Adverse Effects Primarily symptoms of hypoglycemia

Cardiovascular: Pallor, palpitation, tachycardia

Central nervous system: Fatigue, headache, hypothermia, loss of consciousness, mental confusion

Dermatologic: Redness, urticaria

Endocrine & metabolic: Hypoglycemia, hypokalemia

Gastrointestinal: Hunger, nausea, numbness of mouth

Local: Atrophy or hypertrophy of SubQ fat tissue; edema, itching, pain or warmth at injection site; stinging

Neuromuscular & skeletal: Muscle weakness, paresthesia, tremor

Ocular: Transient presbyopia or blurred vision

Miscellaneous: Anaphylaxis, diaphoresis, local and/or systemic hypersensitivity reactions

General Dosage Range Dosage adjustment recommended in patients with renal impairment

I.V., SubQ: *Children and Adults:*

Diabetes mellitus, type 1: Initial: 0.5-1 unit/kg/day in divided doses; Usual maintenance: 0.5-1.2 units/kg/day in divided doses. **Note:** Generally, 50% to 75% of the total daily dose (TDD) is given as an intermediate- or long-acting form of insulin (1-2 daily injections) and the remaining portion is then divided and administered before or at mealtime (depending on the formulation) as a rapid-acting or short-acting form of insulin.

Diabetes mellitus, type 2: Initial basal insulin dose: 0.2 units/kg or 10 units/day given as an intermediate- or long-acting insulin at bedtime or long-acting insulin given in the morning

Mechanism of Action Insulin acts via specific membrane-bound receptors on target tissues to regulate metabolism of carbohydrate, protein, and fats. Target organs for insulin include the liver, skeletal muscle, and adipose tissue.

Within the liver, insulin stimulates hepatic glycogen synthesis. Insulin promotes hepatic synthesis of fatty acids, which are released into the circulation as lipoproteins. Skeletal muscle effects of insulin include increased protein synthesis and increased glycogen synthesis. Within adipose tissue, insulin stimulates the processing of circulating lipoproteins to provide free fatty acids, facilitating triglyceride synthesis and storage by adipocytes; also directly inhibits the hydrolysis of triglycerides. In addition, insulin stimulates the cellular uptake of amino acids and increases cellular permeability to several ions, including potassium, magnesium, and phosphate. By activating sodium-potassium ATPases, insulin promotes the intracellular movement of potassium.

Normally secreted by the pancreas, insulin products are manufactured for pharmacologic use through recombinant DNA technology using either *E. coli* or *Saccharomyces cerevisiae*. Insulins are categorized based on the onset, peak, and duration of effect (eg, rapid-, short-, intermediate-, and long-acting insulin).

Pharmacodynamics/Kinetics

Onset of Action SubQ: 0.5 hours; Peak effect: SubQ: 2.5-5 hours

Duration of Action SubQ:
U-100: 4-12 hours (may increase with dose)
U-500: Up to 24 hours

Half-life Elimination I.V.: ~0.5-1 hour (dose-dependent); SubQ: 1.5 hours

Time to Peak Plasma: SubQ: 0.8-2 hours

Pregnancy Risk Factor B

Pregnancy Considerations Minimal amounts of endogenous insulin cross the placenta. Exogenous insulin bound to anti-insulin antibodies has been detected in cord blood. Maternal hyperglycemia can be associated with adverse effects in the fetus, including macrosomia, neonatal hyperglycemia, and hyperbilirubinemia; the risk of congenital malformations is increased when the Hb A_{1c} is >1% above the normal range. Insulin requirements tend to fall during the first trimester of pregnancy and increase in the later trimesters, peaking at 28-32 weeks of gestation. Following delivery, insulin requirements decrease rapidly. Diabetes can also be associated with adverse effects in the mother. Poorly treated diabetes may cause end-organ damage that may in turn negatively affect obstetric outcomes. Physiologic glucose levels should be maintained prior to and during pregnancy to decrease the risk of adverse events in the fetus and the mother. Insulin is the drug of choice for the control of diabetes mellitus during pregnancy.

Interferon Alfa-2b (in ter FEER on AL fa too bee)

Related Information
Systemic Viral Diseases *on page 1537*
Brand Names: U.S. Intron® A
Brand Names: Canada Intron® A
Generic Availability (U.S.) No
Pharmacologic Category Interferon
Use
Patients ≥1 year of age: Chronic hepatitis B
Patients ≥3 years of age: Chronic hepatitis C (in combination with ribavirin)

Patients ≥18 years of age: Condyloma acuminata, chronic hepatitis B, chronic hepatitis C, hairy cell leukemia, malignant melanoma (high-risk of recurrence), AIDS-related Kaposi's sarcoma, follicular non-Hodgkin lymphoma

Unlabeled Use Treatment of cutaneous ulcerations of Behçet's disease, neuroendocrine tumors (including carcinoid syndrome and islet cell tumor), cutaneous T-cell lymphoma, desmoid tumor, hepatitis D, chronic myelogenous leukemia (CML), non-Hodgkin lymphomas (other than follicular lymphoma, see approved use), multiple myeloma, renal cell carcinoma, West Nile virus

Local Anesthetic/Vasoconstrictor Precautions No information available to require special precautions

Effects on Dental Treatment Key adverse event(s) related to dental treatment: Xerostomia (normal salivary flow resumes upon discontinuation), metallic taste, taste alteration, and gingivitis.

Effects on Bleeding Hematologic toxicity associated with dose and disease being treated. Thrombocytopenia may be as high as 15%. Medical consult recommended.

Adverse Effects Note: In a majority of patients, a flu-like syndrome (fever, chills, tachycardia, malaise, myalgia, headache), occurs within 1-2 hours of administration; may last up to 24 hours and may be dose limiting.

>10%:
Cardiovascular: Chest pain (≤28%)
Central nervous system: Fatigue (8% to 96%), fever (34% to 94%; more common in children), headache (21% to 62%), chills (≤54%), depression (3% to 40%; grades 3/4: 2%), somnolence (≤33%), dizziness (≤24%), irritability (≤22%), pain (≤18%), amnesia (≤14%), concentration impaired (≤14%), malaise (≤14%), confusion (≤12%), insomnia (≤12%)
Dermatologic: Alopecia (≤38%), rash (≤25%), pruritus (≤11%)
Endocrine & metabolic: Amenorrhea (≤12%)
Gastrointestinal: Anorexia (1% to 69%), nausea, (17% to 66%), diarrhea (2% to 45%), xerostomia (≤28%), vomiting (children 27%; adults 7% to 10%), taste alteration (≤24%), abdominal pain (1% to 23%), constipation (≤14%), gingivitis (≤14%), weight loss (<1% to 13%)
Hematologic: Neutropenia (≤92%; grade 4: 1% to 4%), leukopenia (≤68%), anemia (≤32%), thrombocytopenia (≤15%)
Hepatic: AST increased (≤63%; grades 3/4: 14%), ALT increased (≤15%), pain (upper right quadrant: up to 15%); alkaline phosphatase increased (≤13%)
Local: Injection site reaction (≤20%)
Neuromuscular & skeletal: Myalgia (28% to 75%), weakness (≤63%), rigors (≤42%), paresthesia (1% to 21%), skeletal pain (≤21%), arthralgia (≤19%), back pain (≤19%)
Renal: BUN increased (≤12%)
Respiratory: Dyspnea (≤34%), cough (≤31%), pharyngitis (≤31%), sinusitis (≤21%)
Miscellaneous: Flu-like syndrome (≤79%), diaphoresis (1% to 21%), moniliasis (≤17%)
5% to 10%:
Cardiovascular: Edema (≤10%), hypertension (≤9%)
Central nervous system: Hypoesthesia (≤10%), anxiety (≤9%), vertigo (≤8%), agitation (≤7%)
Dermatologic: Dry skin (≤10%), dermatitis (≤8%), purpura (≤5%)
Endocrine & metabolic: Libido decreased (≤5%)
Gastrointestinal: Loose stools (≤10%), dyspepsia (≤8%)

Genitourinary: Urinary tract infection (≤5%)

Renal: Polyuria (≤10%), serum creatinine increased (≤6%)

Respiratory: Bronchitis (≤10%), nasal congestion (≤10%), epistaxis (≤7%)

Miscellaneous: Infection (≤7%), herpes virus infections (≤5%)

Dosage Details concerning dosing in combination regimens should also be consulted. Consider premedication with acetaminophen prior to administration to reduce the incidence of some adverse reactions. Not all dosage forms and strengths are appropriate for all indications; refer to product labeling for details.

Children 1-17 years: **Note:** The following dosing may also be used in **infants** in the setting of HIV-exposure/-infection (CDC, 2009).

Chronic hepatitis B (including HIV coinfection): SubQ: 3 million units/m^2 3 times weekly for 1 week, followed by 6 million units/m^2 3 times weekly (maximum: 10 million units per dose); total duration of therapy 16-24 weeks (treat for 24 weeks in HIV-exposure/-infection)

Chronic hepatitis C with HIV coinfection: I.M., SubQ: 3-5 million units/m^2 3 times weekly (maximum: 3 million units per dose) with ribavirin for 48 weeks, regardless of HCV genotype (CDC, 2009)

Adults:

Hairy cell leukemia: I.M., SubQ: 2 million units/m^2 3 times weekly for up to 6 months (may continue treatment with sustained treatment response); discontinue for disease progression or failure to respond after 6 months

Lymphoma (follicular): SubQ: 5 million units 3 times weekly for up to 18 months

Malignant melanoma: Induction: 20 million units/m^2 I.V. for 5 consecutive days per week for 4 weeks, followed by maintenance dosing of 10 million units/m^2 SubQ 3 times weekly for 48 weeks

AIDS-related Kaposi's sarcoma: I.M., SubQ: 30 million units/m^2 3 times weekly; continue until disease progression or until maximal response has been achieved after 16 weeks

Chronic hepatitis B: I.M., SubQ: 5 million units daily or 10 million units 3 times weekly for 16 weeks

Chronic hepatitis C: I.M., SubQ: 3 million units 3 times weekly. In patients with normalization of ALT at 16 weeks, continue treatment (if tolerated) for 18-24 months; consider discontinuation if normalization does not occur at 16 weeks. **Note:** May be used in combination therapy with ribavirin in previously untreated patients or in patients who relapse following alpha interferon therapy.

Condyloma acuminata: Intralesionally: 1 million units/lesion (maximum: 5 lesions per treatment) 3 times weekly (on alternate days) for 3 weeks; may administer a second course at 12-16 weeks

Dosage adjustment for toxicity:

Neuropsychiatric disorders (during treatment):

Clinical depression or other psychiatric problem: Monitor closely during and for 6 months after treatment.

Severe depression or other psychiatric disorder: Discontinue treatment.

Persistent or worsening psychiatric symptoms, suicidal ideation, aggression towards others: Discontinue treatment and follow with appropriate psychiatric intervention.

Hypersensitivity reaction (acute, serious), ophthalmic disorders (new or worsening), thyroid abnormality development (which cannot be normalized with medication), signs or symptoms of liver failure: Discontinue treatment.

Hematologic toxicity (also refer to indication specified adjustments below): ANC <500/mm^3 or platelets <25,000/mm^3: Discontinue treatment.

Liver function abnormality, pulmonary infiltrate development, evidence of pulmonary function impairment, or autoimmune disorder development, triglycerides >1000 mg/dL: Monitor closely and discontinue if appropriate.

Manufacturer-recommended adjustments, listed according to indication:

Lymphoma (follicular):

Neutrophils >1000/mm^3 to <1500/mm^3: Reduce dose by 50%; may re-escalate to starting dose when neutrophils return to >1500/mm^3

Severe toxicity (neutrophils <1000/mm^3 or platelets <50,000/mm^3): Temporarily withhold.

AST >5 times ULN or serum creatinine >2 mg/dL: Permanently discontinue.

Hairy cell leukemia:

Platelet count <50,000/mm^3: Do not administer intramuscularly (administer SubQ instead).

Severe toxicity: Reduce dose by 50% or temporarily withhold and resume with 50% dose reduction; permanently discontinue if persistent or recurrent severe toxicity is noted.

Chronic hepatitis B:

WBC <1500/mm^3, granulocytes <750/mm^3, or platelet count <50,000/mm^3, or other laboratory abnormality or severe adverse reaction: Reduce dose by 50%; may re-escalate to starting dose upon resolution of hematologic toxicity. Discontinue for persistent intolerance.

WBC <1000/mm^3, granulocytes <500/mm^3, or platelet count <25,000/mm^3: Permanently discontinue.

Chronic hepatitis C: Severe toxicity: Reduce dose by 50% or temporarily withhold until subsides; permanently discontinue for persistent toxicities after dosage reduction.

AIDS-related Kaposi sarcoma: Severe toxicity: Reduce dose by 50% or temporarily withhold; may resume at reduced dose with toxicity resolution; permanently discontinue for persistent/recurrent toxicities.

Malignant melanoma (induction and maintenance):

Severe toxicity, including neutrophils >250/mm^3 to <500/mm^3 or ALT/AST >5-10 times ULN: Temporarily withhold; resume with a 50% dose reduction when adverse reaction abates.

Neutrophils <250/mm^3, ALT/AST >10 times ULN, or severe/persistent adverse reactions: Permanently discontinue.

Dosage adjustment in renal impairment: Combination therapy with ribavirin (hepatitis C) should not be used in patients with reduced renal function (Cl$_{cr}$ <50 mL/minute).

Dosage adjustment in hepatic impairment: No dosage adjustment provided in manufacturer's labeling.

Mechanism of Action Binds to a specific receptor on the cell wall to initiate intracellular activity; multiple effects can be detected including induction of gene transcription. Inhibits cellular growth, alters the state of cellular differentiation, interferes with oncogene expression, alters cell surface antigen expression, increases phagocytic activity of macrophages, and augments cytotoxicity of lymphocytes for target cells

Contraindications Hypersensitivity to interferon alfa or any component of the formulation; decompensated liver disease; autoimmune hepatitis

Combination therapy with interferon alfa-2b and ribavirin is also contraindicated in pregnancy, males with pregnant partners; hemoglobinopathies (eg, thalassemia major, sickle-cell anemia); renal dysfunction (Cl$_{cr}$ <50 mL/minute)

Warnings/Precautions [U.S. Boxed Warning]: May cause or aggravate fatal or life-threatening autoimmune disorders, neuropsychiatric symptoms (including depression and/or suicidal thoughts/ behaviors), ischemic, and/or infectious disorders; monitor closely with clinical and lab evaluations (periodic); discontinue treatment for severe persistent or worsening symptoms; some cases may resolve with discontinuation.

Neuropsychiatric disorders: May cause neuropsychiatric events, including depression, psychosis, mania, suicidal behavior/ideation, homicidal ideation; may occur in patients with or without previous psychiatric symptoms. Careful neuropsychiatric monitoring is recommended during and for 6 months after treatment in patients who develop psychiatric disorders (including clinical depression). New or exacerbated neuropsychiatric or substance abuse disorders are best managed with early intervention. Use with caution in patients with a history of psychiatric disorders. Drug screening and periodic health evaluation (including monitoring of psychiatric symptoms) is recommended if initiating treatment in patients with coexisting psychiatric condition or substance abuse disorders. Suicidal ideation or attempts may occur more frequently in pediatric patients when compared to adults. Higher doses in elderly patients, or diseases other than hairy cell leukemia, may result in increased CNS toxicity.

Hepatic disease: May cause hepatotoxicity; monitor closely if abnormal liver function tests develop. A transient increase in ALT (≥2 times baseline) may occur in patients treated with interferon alfa-2b for chronic hepatitis B. Therapy generally may continue; monitor. Worsening and potentially fatal liver disease, including jaundice, hepatic encephalopathy, and hepatic failure have been reported in patients receiving interferon alfa for chronic hepatitis B and C with decompensated liver disease, autoimmune hepatitis, history of autoimmune disease, and immunosuppressed transplant recipients; avoid use in these patients. Chronic hepatitis B or C patients with a history of autoimmune disease or who are immunosuppressed transplant recipients should not receive interferon alfa-2b. Discontinue treatment (if appropriate) in any patient developing signs or symptoms of liver failure.

Bone marrow suppression: Causes bone marrow suppression, including potentially severe cytopenias, and very rarely, aplastic anemia. Discontinue treatment for severe neutropenia (ANC <500/mm^3) or thrombocytopenia (platelets <25,000/mm^3). Hemolytic anemia (hemoglobin <10 g/dL) was observed when combined with ribavirin; anemia occurred within 1-2 weeks of initiation of therapy. Use caution in patients with preexisting myelosuppression and in patients with concomitant medications which cause myelosuppression.

Autoimmune disorders: Avoid use in patients with history of autoimmune disorders; development of autoimmune disorders (thrombocytopenia, vasculitis, Raynaud's disease, rheumatoid arthritis, lupus erythematosus and rhabdomyolysis) has been associated with use. Monitor closely; consider discontinuing. Worsening of psoriasis and sarcoidosis (and the development of new sarcoidosis) have been reported; use caution.

Cardiovascular disease/coagulation disorders: Use caution and monitor closely in patients with cardiovascular disease (ischemic or thromboembolic), arrhythmias, hypertension, and in patients with a history of MI or prior therapy with cardiotoxic drugs. Patients with pre-existing cardiac disease and/or advanced cancer should have baseline and periodic ECGs. May cause hypotension (during administration or delayed), arrhythmia, tachycardia, cardiomyopathy (~2% in AIDS-related Kaposi's Sarcoma patients) and/or MI. Hemorrhagic cerebrovascular events have been observed with therapy. Use caution in patients with coagulation disorders.

Endocrine disorders: Thyroid disorders (possibly reversible) have been reported; use caution in patients with pre-existing thyroid disease. TSH levels should be within normal limits prior to initiating interferon. Discontinue interferon use in patients who cannot maintain normal ranges with thyroid medication. Diabetes mellitus has been reported; discontinue if cannot effectively manage with medication. Use with caution in patients with a history of diabetes mellitus, particularly if prone to DKA. Hypertriglyceridemia has been reported; discontinue if persistent and severe, and/or combined with symptoms of pancreatitis.

Pulmonary disease: Dyspnea, pulmonary infiltrates, pulmonary hypertension, interstitial pneumonitis, pneumonia, bronchiolitis obliterans, and sarcoidosis may be induced or aggravated by treatment, sometimes resulting in respiratory failure or fatality. Has been reported more in patients being treated for chronic hepatitis C, although has also occurred with use for oncology indications. Patients with fever, cough, dyspnea or other respiratory symptoms should be evaluated with a chest x-ray; monitor closely and consider discontinuing treatment with evidence of impaired pulmonary function. Use with caution in patients with a history of pulmonary disease.

Ophthalmic disorders: Decreased or loss of vision, macular edema, optic neuritis, retinal hemorrhages, cotton wool spots, papilledema, retinal detachment (serous), and retinal artery or vein thrombosis have occurred (or been aggravated) in patients receiving alpha interferons. Use caution in patients with pre-existing eye disorders; monitor closely; a complete eye exam should be done promptly in patients who develop ocular symptoms; discontinue with new or worsening ophthalmic disorders.

Commonly associated with fever and flu-like symptoms; rule out other causes/infection with persistent fever; use with caution in patients with debilitating conditions. Acute hypersensitivity reactions have been reported. Do not treat patients with visceral AIDS-related Kaposi's sarcoma associated with rapidly-progressing or life-threatening disease. Some formulations contain albumin, which may carry a remote risk of viral transmission. Due to differences in dosage, patients should not change brands of interferons without the concurrence of their healthcare provider. Combination therapy with ribavirin is associated with birth defects and/or fetal mortality and hemolytic anemia. Do not use combination therapy with ribavirin in patients with renal dysfunction (Cl$_{cr}$ <50 mL/minute).

Drug Interactions

Metabolism/Transport Effects Inhibits CYP1A2 (weak)

Avoid Concomitant Use

Avoid concomitant use of Interferon Alfa-2b with any of the following: CloZAPine; Telbivudine

Increased Effect/Toxicity

Interferon Alfa-2b may increase the levels/effects of: Aldesleukin; CloZAPine; Methadone; Ribavirin; Telbivudine; Theophylline Derivatives; Zidovudine

Decreased Effect There are no known significant interactions involving a decrease in effect.

Pharmacodynamics/Kinetics

Half-life Elimination I.V.: ~2 hours; I.M., SubQ: ~2-3 hours

Time to Peak Serum: I.M., SubQ: ~3-12 hours; I.V.: By the end of a 30-minute infusion

Pregnancy Risk Factor C / X in combination with ribavirin

Pregnancy Considerations Animal reproduction studies have demonstrated abortifacient effects. Disruption of the normal menstrual cycle was also observed in animal studies; therefore, the manufacturer recommends that reliable contraception is used in women of childbearing potential. Alfa interferon is endogenous to normal amniotic fluid. *In vitro* administration studies have reported that when administered to the mother, it does not cross the placenta. Case reports of use in pregnant women are limited. The Perinatal HIV Guidelines Working Group does not recommend that interferon-alfa be used during pregnancy. Interferon alfa-2b monotherapy should only be used in pregnancy when the potential benefit to the mother justifies the possible risk to the fetus. Combination therapy with ribavirin is contraindicated in pregnancy (refer to Ribavirin monograph); two forms of contraception should be used during combination therapy and patients should have monthly pregnancy tests. A pregnancy registry has been established for women inadvertently exposed to ribavirin while pregnant (800-593-2214).

Lactation Enters breast milk/not recommended (AAP rates "compatible"; AAP 2001 update pending)

Breast-Feeding Considerations Breast milk samples obtained from a lactating mother prior to and after administration of interferon alfa-2b showed that interferon alfa is present in breast milk and administration of the medication did not significantly affect endogenous levels. Breast-feeding is not linked to the spread of hepatitis C virus; however, if nipples are cracked or bleeding, breast-feeding is not recommended. Mothers coinfected with HIV are discouraged from breast-feeding to decrease potential transmission of HIV.

Dosage Forms

Injection, powder for reconstitution [preservative free]:

Intron® A: 10 million units, 18 million units, 50 million units

Injection, solution:

Intron® A: 6 million units/mL (3 mL); 10 million units/mL (2.5 mL); 3 million units/0.2 mL (1.2 mL); 5 million units/0.2 mL (1.2 mL); 10 million units/0.2 mL (1.2 mL)

Interferon Alfa-2b and Ribavirin

(in ter FEER on AL fa too bee & rye ba VYE rin)

Related Information

Interferon Alfa-2b *on page 749*

Ribavirin *on page 1190*

Systemic Viral Diseases *on page 1537*

Brand Names: U.S. Rebetron®

Pharmacologic Category Antiviral Agent; Interferon

Use Combination therapy for the treatment of chronic hepatitis C in patients with compensated liver disease previously untreated with alpha interferon or who have relapsed after alpha interferon therapy

Local Anesthetic/Vasoconstrictor Precautions No information available to require special precautions

Effects on Dental Treatment Key adverse event(s) related to dental treatment: Xerostomia (normal salivary flow resumes upon discontinuation), metallic taste, and taste perversion.

Effects on Bleeding No information available to require special precautions

Adverse Effects Note: Adverse reactions listed are specific to combination regimen in previously untreated hepatitis patients. See individual agents for additional adverse reactions reported with each agent during therapy for other diseases.

>10%:

Central nervous system: Fatigue (children 61%; adults 68%), headache (63%), insomnia (children 14%; adults 39%), fever (children 61%; adults 37%), depression (children 13%; adults 32% to 36%), irritability (children 10%; adults 23% to 32%), dizziness (17% to 23%), emotional lability (children 16%; adults 7% to 11%), impaired concentration (5% to 14%)

Dermatologic: Alopecia (23% to 32%), pruritus (children 12%; adults 19% to 21%), rash (17% to 28%)

Gastrointestinal: Nausea (33% to 46%), anorexia (children 51%; adults 25% to 27%), dyspepsia (children <1%; adults 14% to 16%), vomiting (children 42%; adults 9% to 11%)

Hematologic: Leukopenia, neutropenia (usually recovers within 4 weeks of treatment discontinuation), anemia

Hepatic: Hyperbilirubinemia (27%; only 0.9% to 2% >3.0-6 mg/dL)

Local: Injection site inflammation (13%)

Neuromuscular & skeletal: Myalgia (children 32%; adults 61% to 64%), rigors (40%), arthralgia (children 15%; adults 30% to 33%), musculoskeletal pain (20% to 28%)

Respiratory: Dyspnea (children 5%; adults 18% to 19%)

Miscellaneous: Flu-like syndrome (children 31%; adults 14% to 18%)

1% to 10%:

Cardiovascular: Chest pain (5% to 9%)

Central nervous system: Nervousness (3% to 4%)

Endocrine & metabolic: Thyroid abnormalities (hyper- or hypothyroidism), serum uric acid increased, hyperglycemia

Gastrointestinal: Taste perversion (children <1%; adults 7% to 8%)

Hematologic: Hemolytic anemia (10%), thrombocytopenia, anemia

Local: Injection site reaction (7%)

Neuromuscular & skeletal: Weakness (5% to 9%)

Respiratory: Sinusitis (children <1%; adults 9% to 10%)

General Dosage Range

Oral (Rebetol®):

Children <3 years: Dosage not established

Children 3-5 years or ≤25 kg: 15 mg/kg/day in 2 divided doses

Children >5 years and 26-36 kg: 200 mg twice daily

Children >5 years and 37-49 kg: 200 mg in the morning and 400 mg in the evening

Children >5 years and 50-61 kg: 400 mg twice daily

Children >5 years and >61-75 kg: 400 mg in the morning and 600 mg in the evening

Children >5 years and >75 kg: 600 mg twice daily

Adults ≤75 kg: 400 mg in the morning and 600 mg in the evening

Adults >75 kg: 600 mg twice daily

SubQ (Intron® A):

Children <3 years: Dosage not established

Children ≥3 years and 25-61 kg: 3 million int. units/m^2 3 times/week

Children ≥3 years and >61 kg: 3 million int. units 3 times/week

Adults: 3 million int. units 3 times/week

Mechanism of Action

Interferon Alfa-2b: Alpha interferons are a family of proteins, produced by nucleated cells, that have antiviral, antiproliferative, and immune-regulating activity. There are 16 known subtypes of alpha interferons. Interferons interact with cells through high affinity cell surface receptors. Following activation, multiple effects can be detected including induction of gene transcription. Inhibits cellular growth, alters the state of cellular differentiation, interferes with oncogene expression, alters cell surface antigen expression, increases phagocytic activity of macrophages, and augments cytotoxicity of lymphocytes for target cells

Ribavirin: Inhibits replication of RNA and DNA viruses; inhibits influenza virus RNA polymerase activity and inhibits the initiation and elongation of RNA fragments resulting in inhibition of viral protein synthesis

Pregnancy Risk Factor X

Pregnancy Considerations Abortifacient and teratogenic effects have been reported with ribavirin. Negative pregnancy test is required before initiation and monthly thereafter. Avoid pregnancy in female patients and female partners of patients during therapy by using two effective forms of contraception; continue contraceptive measures for at least 6 months after completion of therapy. If patient or female partner becomes pregnant during treatment, she should be counseled about potential risks of exposure. Pregnancies that occur during use, or within 6 months after treatment, should be reported to the manufacturer (800-593-2214).

Interferon Alfa-n3 (in ter FEER on AL fa en three)

Related Information

Systemic Viral Diseases *on page 1537*

Brand Names: U.S. Alferon® N

Brand Names: Canada Alferon® N

Pharmacologic Category Interferon

Use Patients ≥18 years of age: Intralesional treatment of refractory or recurring genital or venereal warts (condylomata acuminata)

Local Anesthetic/Vasoconstrictor Precautions No information available to require special precautions

Effects on Dental Treatment Key adverse event(s) related to dental treatment: Xerostomia (normal salivary flow resumes upon discontinuation), metallic taste, tongue hyperesthesia, abnormal taste, thirst, rhinitis, pharyngitis, nosebleed, increased diaphoresis, taste disturbance, and gingivitis.

Effects on Bleeding No information available to require special precautions

Adverse Effects Note: Adverse reaction incidence noted below is specific to intralesional administration in patients with condylomata acuminata. Flu-like reactions, consisting of headache, fever, and/or myalgia, was reported in 30% of patients, and abated with repeated dosing.

>10%:

Central nervous system: Fever (40%), headache (31%), chills (14%), fatigue (14%)

Hematologic: Decreased WBC (11%)

Neuromuscular & skeletal: Myalgia (45%)

Miscellaneous: Flu-like syndrome (30%)

1% to 10%:

Central nervous system: Malaise (9%), dizziness (9%), depression (2%), insomnia (2%), thirst (1%)

Dermatologic: Pruritus (2%)

Gastrointestinal: Nausea (45), vomiting (3%), dyspepsia (3%), diarrhea (2%), tongue hyperesthesia (1%), taste disturbance (1%)

Genitourinary: Groin lymph node swelling (1%)

Neuromuscular & skeletal: Arthralgia (5%), back pain (4%), cramps (1%), paresthesia (1%)

Ocular: Visual disturbance (1%)

Respiratory: Rhinitis (2%), pharyngitis (1%), nosebleed (1%)

Miscellaneous: Diaphoresis increased (2%), vasovagal reaction (2%)

General Dosage Range Intralesional: *Adults:* Inject 250,000 units (0.05 mL) in each wart twice weekly (maximum: 8 weeks)

Mechanism of Action Interferons interact with cells through high affinity cell surface receptors. Following activation, multiple effects can be detected including induction of gene transcription. Inhibits cellular growth, alters the state of cellular differentiation, interferes with oncogene expression, alters cell surface antigen expression, increases phagocytic activity of macrophages, and augments cytotoxicity of lymphocytes for target cells

Pregnancy Risk Factor C

Pregnancy Considerations Safety and efficacy for use during pregnancy have not been established. Interferon alpha has been shown to decrease serum estradiol and progesterone levels in humans. Menstrual irregularities and abortion have been reported in animals. Effective contraception is recommended during treatment.

Interferon Beta-1a (in ter FEER on BAY ta won aye)

Brand Names: U.S. Avonex®; Avonex® Pen™; Rebif®; Rebif® Rebidose®; Rebif® Rebidose® Titration Pack; Rebif® Titration Pack

Brand Names: Canada Avonex®; Rebif®

Pharmacologic Category Interferon

Use Treatment of relapsing forms of multiple sclerosis (MS)

Canadian labeling: Additional uses (not in U.S. labeling): Avonex®: To decrease the number and volume of active brain lesions, decrease overall disease burden, and delay onset of clinically definite MS in patients who have experienced a single demyelinating event.

Local Anesthetic/Vasoconstrictor Precautions No information available to require special precautions

Effects on Dental Treatment Key adverse event(s) related to dental treatment: Xerostomia and changes in salivation (normal salivary flow resumes upon discontinuation), and toothache.

Effects on Bleeding Thrombocytopenia has been reported in 2% to 8% of patients. Medical consult recommended.

Adverse Effects Note: Adverse reactions reported as a composite of both commercially-available products. Spectrum and incidence of reactions is generally similar between products, but consult individual product labels for specific incidence.

>10%:
Central nervous system: Headache (58% to 70%), fatigue (33% to 41%), fever (20% to 28%), pain (23%), chills (19%), depression (18% to 25%), dizziness (14%)
Gastrointestinal: Nausea (23%), abdominal pain (8% to 22%)
Genitourinary: Urinary tract infection (17%)
Hematologic: Leukopenia (28% to 36%)
Hepatic: ALT increased (20% to 27%), AST increased (10% to 17%)
Local: Injection site reaction (3% to 92%)
Neuromuscular & skeletal: Myalgia (25% to 29%), back pain (23% to 25%), weakness (24%), skeletal pain (10% to 15%), rigors (6% to 13%)
Ocular: Vision abnormal (7% to 13%)
Respiratory: Sinusitis (14%), upper respiratory tract infection (14%)
Miscellaneous: Flu-like syndrome (49% to 59%), neutralizing antibodies (significance not known; Avonex® 5%; Rebif® 24%), lymphadenopathy (11% to 12%)

1% to 10%:
Cardiovascular: Chest pain (5% to 6%), vasodilation (2%)
Central nervous system: Migraine (5%), somnolence (4% to 5%), malaise (4% to 5%), seizure (1% to 5%)
Dermatologic: Erythematous rash (5% to 7%), maculopapular rash (4% to 5%), alopecia (4%), urticaria
Endocrine & metabolic: Thyroid disorder (4% to 6%)
Gastrointestinal: Xerostomia (1% to 5%), toothache (3%)
Genitourinary: Micturition frequency (2% to 7%), urinary incontinence (2% to 4%)
Hematologic: Thrombocytopenia (2% to 8%), anemia (3% to 5%)
Hepatic: Bilirubinemia (2% to 3%)
Local: Injection site pain (8%), injection site bruising (6%), injection site necrosis (1% to 3%), injection site inflammation
Neuromuscular & skeletal: Arthralgia (9%), hypertonia (6% to 7%), coordination abnormal (4% to 5%)
Ocular: Eye disorder (4%), xerophthalmia (1% to 3%)
Respiratory: Bronchitis (8%)
Miscellaneous: Infection (7%)

General Dosage Range Dosage adjustment recommended in patients who develop toxicities

I.M.: *Adults:* Initial: 30 mcg once weekly **or** 7.5 mcg (week 1) then titrate in increments of 7.5 mcg once weekly (weeks 2-4) to 30 mcg once weekly

SubQ: *Adults:* Initial: 4.4 or 8.8 mcg 3 times weekly for 2 weeks; Titration: 11 or 22 mcg 3 times weekly for 2 weeks; Maintenance: 22 or 44 mcg 3 times weekly

Mechanism of Action Interferon beta differs from naturally occurring human protein by a single amino acid substitution and the lack of carbohydrate side chains; alters the expression and response to surface antigens and can enhance immune cell activities. Properties of interferon beta that modify biologic responses are mediated by cell surface receptor interactions; mechanism in the treatment of MS is unknown.

Pharmacodynamics/Kinetics
Onset of Action Avonex®: 12 hours (based on biological response markers)
Duration of Action Avonex®: 4 days (based on biological response markers)
Half-life Elimination Avonex®: 10 hours; Rebif®: 69 hours
Time to Peak Serum: Avonex® (I.M.): ~15 hours (range: 6-36 hours); Rebif® (SubQ): 16 hours

Pregnancy Risk Factor C

Pregnancy Considerations Adverse events were observed in animal reproduction studies. Preliminary data from the Avonex® pregnancy registry (published in abstract) do not show an increased risk of adverse fetal events when exposure occurs during pregnancy (Richman, 2012; Tomczyk, 2013); however, other studies have reported conflicting results. Until additional information is available, consideration should be given to discontinuing treatment if a woman becomes pregnant, or 1 month prior to becoming pregnant in women with mild disease (Coyle, 2012; Houtchens, 2012; Lu, 2013).

Interferon Beta-1b (in ter FEER on BAY ta won bee)

Brand Names: U.S. Betaseron®; Extavia®
Brand Names: Canada Betaseron®; Extavia®
Pharmacologic Category Interferon
Use Treatment of relapsing forms of multiple sclerosis (MS); treatment of first clinical episode with MRI features consistent with MS

Canadian labeling: Additional use (not in U.S. labeling): Treatment of secondary-progressive MS

Local Anesthetic/Vasoconstrictor Precautions No information available to require special precautions

Effects on Dental Treatment No significant effects or complications reported

Effects on Bleeding Thrombocytopenia has been reported. Medical consult recommended.

Adverse Effects Note: Flu-like syndrome (including at least two of the following - headache, fever, chills, malaise, diaphoresis, and myalgia) are reported in the majority of patients (60%) and decrease over time (average duration ~1 week).

>10%:
Cardiovascular: Peripheral edema (15%), chest pain (11%)
Central nervous system: Headache (57%), fever (36%), pain (51%), chills (25%), dizziness (24%), insomnia (24%)
Dermatologic: Rash (24%), skin disorder (12%)
Endocrine & metabolic: Metrorrhagia (11%)
Gastrointestinal: Nausea (27%), diarrhea (19%), abdominal pain (19%), constipation (20%), dyspepsia (14%)
Genitourinary: Urinary urgency (13%)

Hematologic: Lymphopenia (88%), neutropenia (14%), leukopenia (14%)

Local: Injection site reaction (85%), inflammation (53%), pain (18%)

Neuromuscular & skeletal: Weakness (61%), myalgia (27%), hypertonia (50%), myasthenia (46%), arthralgia (31%), incoordination (21%)

Miscellaneous: Flu-like syndrome (decreases over treatment course; 60%), neutralizing antibodies (≤45%; significance not known)

1% to 10%:

Cardiovascular: Palpitation (4%), vasodilation (8%), hypertension (7%), tachycardia (4%), peripheral vascular disorder (6%)

Central nervous system: Anxiety (10%), malaise (8%), nervousness (7%)

Dermatologic: Alopecia (4%)

Endocrine & metabolic: Menorrhagia (8%), dysmenorrhea (7%)

Gastrointestinal: Weight gain (7%)

Genitourinary: Impotence (9%), pelvic pain (6%), cystitis (8%), urinary frequency (7%), prostatic disorder (3%)

Hematologic: Lymphadenopathy (8%)

Hepatic: ALT increased >5x baseline (10%), AST increased >5x baseline (3%)

Local: Injection site necrosis (4% to 5%), edema (3%), mass (2%)

Neuromuscular & skeletal: Leg cramps (4%)

Respiratory: Dyspnea (7%)

Miscellaneous: Diaphoresis (8%), hypersensitivity (3%)

General Dosage Range SubQ: *Adults:* 0.0625-0.25 mg (2-8 million units) every other day

Mechanism of Action Interferon beta-1b differs from naturally occurring human protein by a single amino acid substitution and the lack of carbohydrate side chains; mechanism in the treatment of MS is unknown; however, immunomodulatory effects attributed to interferon beta-1b include enhancement of suppressor T cell activity, reduction of proinflammatory cytokines, down-regulation of antigen presentation, and reduced trafficking of lymphocytes into the central nervous system. Improves MRI lesions, decreases relapse rate, and disease severity in patients with secondary progressive MS.

Pharmacodynamics/Kinetics
Half-life Elimination 8 minutes to 4.3 hours
Time to Peak 1-8 hours
Pregnancy Risk Factor C

Pregnancy Considerations A dose-related abortifacient activity was reported in Rhesus monkeys. There are no adequate and well-controlled studies in pregnant women. Treatment should be discontinued if a woman becomes pregnant, or plans to become pregnant during therapy.

Interferon Gamma-1b
(in ter FEER on GAM ah won bee)

Brand Names: U.S. Actimmune®
Brand Names: Canada Actimmune®
Pharmacologic Category Interferon

Use Reduce frequency and severity of serious infections associated with chronic granulomatous disease; delay time to disease progression in patients with severe, malignant osteopetrosis

Local Anesthetic/Vasoconstrictor Precautions No information available to require special precautions

Effects on Dental Treatment No significant effects or complications reported

Effects on Bleeding Dose related (>100 mcg/m^2 administered 3 times weekly) thrombocytopenia has been reported. Medical consult recommended.

Adverse Effects Based on 50 mcg/m^2 dose administered 3 times weekly for chronic granulomatous disease >10%:

Central nervous system: Fever (52%), headache (33%), chills (14%), fatigue (14%)

Dermatologic: Rash (17%)

Gastrointestinal: Diarrhea (14%), vomiting (13%)

Local: Injection site erythema or tenderness (14%)

1% to 10%:

Central nervous system: Depression (3%)

Gastrointestinal: Nausea (10%), abdominal pain (8%)

Neuromuscular & skeletal: Myalgia (6%), arthralgia (2%), back pain (2%)

Additional adverse reactions noted at doses >100 mcg/m^2 administered 3 times weekly: ALT increased, AST increased, autoantibodies increased, bronchospasm, chest discomfort, confusion, dermatomyositis exacerbation, disorientation, DVT, gait disturbance, GI bleeding, hallucinations, heart block, heart failure, hepatic insufficiency, hyperglycemia, hypertriglyceridemia, hyponatremia, hypotension, interstitial pneumonitis, lupus-like syndrome, MI, neutropenia, pancreatitis (may be fatal), Parkinsonian symptoms, PE, proteinuria, renal insufficiency (reversible), seizure, syncope, tachyarrhythmia, tachypnea, thrombocytopenia, TIA

General Dosage Range Dosage adjustment recommended in patients who develop toxicities

SubQ: *Children and Adults:*

BSA ≤0.5 m^2: 1.5 mcg/kg/dose 3 times/week

BSA >0.5 m^2: 50 mcg/m^2 (1 million units/m^2) 3 times/week

Mechanism of Action Interferon gamma participates in immunoregulation by enhancing the oxidative metabolism of macrophages; it also enhances antibody dependent cellular cytotoxicity, activates natural killer cells and has a role in the expression of Fc receptors and histocompatibility antigens. The exact mechanism of action for the treatment of chronic granulomatous disease or osteopetrosis has not been defined.

Pharmacodynamics/Kinetics
Half-life Elimination I.V.: 38 minutes; I.M.: ~3 hours, SubQ: ~6 hours
Time to Peak Plasma: I.M.: 4 hours (1.5 ng/mL); SubQ: 7 hours (0.6 ng/mL)
Pregnancy Risk Factor C

Pregnancy Considerations Teratogenic effects were not observed in animal studies. A dose-related abortifacient activity was reported in Rhesus monkeys. Safety and efficacy in pregnant women has not been established.

Iodine (EYE oh dyne)

Related Information
Trace Elements *on page 1345*
Brand Names: U.S. Iodex® [OTC]; Iodoflex™ [OTC]; Iodosorb® [OTC]
Pharmacologic Category Antiseptic, Topical

Use Used topically as an antiseptic in the management of minor, superficial skin wounds and has been used to disinfect the skin preoperatively

Local Anesthetic/Vasoconstrictor Precautions No information available to require special precautions

Effects on Dental Treatment No significant effects or complications reported

◄ **Effects on Bleeding** No information available to require special precautions

Adverse Effects

Reactions reported following topical application: Frequency not defined:

Endocrine & metabolic: TSH increased

Local: Eczema, edema, irritation, pain, redness

Miscellaneous: Allergic reaction

Reactions reported more likely observed following large doses or chronic iodine intoxication; frequency not defined:

Central nervous system: Fever, headache

Dermatologic: Skin rash, angioedema, urticaria, acne

Endocrine & metabolic: Hypothyroidism

Gastrointestinal: Metallic taste, diarrhea

Hematologic: Eosinophilia, hemorrhage (mucosal)

Neuromuscular & skeletal: Arthralgia

Ocular: Swelling of eyelids

Respiratory: Pulmonary edema

Miscellaneous: Ioderma, lymph node enlargement

General Dosage Range Topical: *Adults:* Antiseptic: Apply to affected area 1-3 times/day; Ulcer/wound cleansing: Apply to clean wound 3 times/week (maximum: 50 g/application; 150 g/week)

Mechanism of Action Iodine is required for thyroid hormone synthesis. Iodine is also known to be a powerful broad spectrum germicidal agent effective against a wide range of bacteria, viruses, fungi, protozoa, and spores. Iodosorb® and Iodoflex™ contain iodine in hydrophilic beads of cadexomer which allows a slow release of iodine into the wound and absorption of fluid, bacteria, and other substances from the wound

Pregnancy Considerations An adequate amount of iodine intake is essential for thyroid function. Iodine crosses the placenta and requirements are increased during pregnancy. Iodine deficiency in pregnancy can lead to neurologic damage in the newborn; an extreme form, cretinism, is characterized by gross mental retardation, short stature, deaf mutism, and spasticity. Large amounts of iodine during pregnancy can cause fetal goiter or hyperthyroidism. Transient hypothyroidism in the newborn has also been reported following topical or vaginal use prior to delivery.

Iodipamide Meglumine
(eye oh DI pa mide MEG loo meen)

Brand Names: U.S. Cholografin® Meglumine

Pharmacologic Category Iodinated Contrast Media; Radiological/Contrast Media, Ionic (High Osmolality)

Use Contrast medium for intravenous cholangiography and cholecystography

Local Anesthetic/Vasoconstrictor Precautions No information available to require special precautions

Effects on Dental Treatment No significant effects or complications reported

Effects on Bleeding No information available to require special precautions

Adverse Effects Frequency not defined.

Cardiovascular: Cardiac reactions (rare), cyanosis (rare), hypotension (rare)

Ocular: Edema of eyelids (rare)

Renal: Renal failure, renal function tests altered

Respiratory: Laryngospasm (rare), respiratory difficulties (rare)

Miscellaneous: Anaphylactoid reaction (rare); hypersensitivity reactions; infusion reactions (generally mild and transient; associated with rapid infusion rates; includes restlessness, sensations of warmth, sneezing,

perspiration, salivation, flushing, pressure in the upper abdomen, dizziness, nausea, vomiting, chills, fever, headache, pallor, tremors)

General Dosage Range I.V.:

Infants and Children: 0.3-0.6 mL/kg (maximum: 20 mL)

Adults: 20 mL

Pregnancy Considerations Reproduction studies have not been conducted. In general, iodinated contrast media agents are avoided during pregnancy unless essential for diagnosis.

Iodixanol (EYE oh dix an ole)

Brand Names: U.S. Visipaque™

Brand Names: Canada Visipaque™

Pharmacologic Category Iodinated Contrast Media; Radiological/Contrast Media, Nonionic (Iso-Osmolality)

Use

Intra-arterial: Digital subtraction angiography, angiocardiography, peripheral arteriography, visceral arteriography, cerebral arteriography

Intravenous: Contrast enhanced computed tomography imaging, excretory urography, and peripheral venography

Local Anesthetic/Vasoconstrictor Precautions No information available to require special precautions

Effects on Dental Treatment Key adverse event(s) related to dental treatment: Taste perversion.

Effects on Bleeding No information available to require special precautions

Adverse Effects

>10%: Local: Injection site reactions (discomfort/pain/warmth 30%)

1% to 10%:

Cardiovascular: Angina/chest pain (2%)

Central nervous system: Headache/migraine (3%), vertigo (2%)

Dermatologic: Nonurticarial rash/erythema (2%), pruritus (2%)

Gastrointestinal: Taste perversion (4%), nausea (3%)

Neuromuscular & skeletal: Paresthesia (1%)

Respiratory: Parosoma (1%)

General Dosage Range

I.V.:

Children >1-12 years: Iodixanol 270 mg iodine/mL: 1-2 mL/kg (maximum: 2 mL/kg)

Children >12 years and Adults: Iodixanol 270 mg and 320 mg iodine/mL: Concentration and dose vary based on study type; refer to product labeling (maximum total dose: 80 g iodine)

Intra-arterial:

Children >1-12 years: Iodixanol 320 mg iodine/mL: 1-2 mL/kg (maximum: 4 mL/kg)

Children >12 years and Adults: Iodixanol 320 mg iodine/mL: Dose individualized based on injection site and study type; refer to product labeling (maximum total dose: 80 g iodine)

Mechanism of Action Opacifies vessels in the path of flow permitting radiographic imaging of internal structures.

Pharmacodynamics/Kinetics

Half-life Elimination Children: 2-4 hours; Adults: 2 hours

Time to Peak Immediate; peak enhancement at 15-120 seconds; optimum renal contrast at 5-15 minutes; brain contrast at up to 1 hour

Pregnancy Risk Factor B

Pregnancy Considerations Fetal harm was not observed in animal studies. There are no adequate and well-controlled studies in pregnant women. In general, iodinated contrast media agents are avoided during pregnancy unless essential for diagnosis.

Iodoquinol (eye oh doe KWIN ole)

Brand Names: U.S. Yodoxin®
Brand Names: Canada Diodoquin®
Pharmacologic Category Amebicide
Use Treatment of intestinal amebiasis due to trophozoite and cyst forms of *Entamoeba histolytica*
Unlabeled Use *Blastocystis hominis* infections, *Balantidium coli* infections, *Dientamoeba fragilis* infections
Local Anesthetic/Vasoconstrictor Precautions No information available to require special precautions
Effects on Dental Treatment No significant effects or complications reported
Effects on Bleeding No information available to require special precautions
Adverse Effects Frequency not defined.
Central nervous system: Chills, fever, headache, vertigo
Dermatologic: Pruritus, rash, skin eruptions, urticaria
Endocrine & metabolic: Thyroid gland enlargement
Gastrointestinal: Abdominal cramps, anal itching, diarrhea, nausea, vomiting
Neuromuscular & skeletal: Peripheral neuropathy
Ocular: Optic atrophy, optic neuritis
General Dosage Range Oral:
Children: 30-40 mg/kg daily in 3 divided doses (maximum: 1.95 g daily)
Adults: 650 mg 3 times daily (maximum: 1.95 g daily)
Mechanism of Action Contact amebicide that works in the lumen of the intestine by an unknown mechanism
Pregnancy Considerations There is very limited data on the use of iodoquinol during pregnancy and safety has not been established. Adverse effects have occurred in children exposed to topical iodoquinol.

Iodoquinol and Hydrocortisone
(eye oh doe KWIN ole & hye droe KOR ti sone)

Related Information
Hydrocortisone (Topical) *on page 699*
Iodoquinol *on page 757*
Related Sample Prescriptions
Angular Cheilitis *on page 1614*
Brand Names: U.S. Alcortin® A; Dermazene®
Generic Availability (U.S.) Yes: Cream
Pharmacologic Category Antifungal Agent, Topical; Corticosteroid, Topical
Dental Use Reported to be useful in the treatment of angular cheilitis
Use Treatment of eczema (including impetiginized, nuchal, and nummular); acne urticaria; anogenital pruritus, atopic and contact dermatitis; chronic infectious dermatitis; chronic eczematoid otitis externa; folliculitis, intertrigo; lichen simplex chronicus; moniliasis; mycotic dermatoses; neurodermatitis (localized or systemic); pyoderma, stasis dermatitis
Local Anesthetic/Vasoconstrictor Precautions No information available to require special precautions
Effects on Dental Treatment No significant effects or complications reported
Effects on Bleeding No information available to require special precautions

Adverse Effects See individual agents.
Dental Usual Dosage Angular cheilitis: Adults: Topical: Apply 3-4 times daily
Dosage Topical: Children ≥12 years and Adults: Apply 3-4 times daily
Contraindications Hypersensitivity to iodoquinol, hydrocortisone, or any component of the formulation
Warnings/Precautions
Based on **iodoquinol** component: Optic neuritis, optic atrophy, and peripheral neuropathy have occurred following prolonged use; avoid long-term therapy

Based on **hydrocortisone** component:
Use with caution in patients with hyperthyroidism, cirrhosis, nonspecific ulcerative colitis, hypertension, osteoporosis, thromboembolic tendencies, CHF, convulsive disorders, myasthenia gravis, thrombophlebitis, peptic ulcer, diabetes
Acute adrenal insufficiency may occur with abrupt withdrawal (depending on degree of systemic absorption) after long-term therapy or with stress; young pediatric patients may be more susceptible to adrenal axis suppression from topical therapy
Drug Interactions
Metabolism/Transport Effects Refer to individual components.
Avoid Concomitant Use
Avoid concomitant use of Iodoquinol and Hydrocortisone with any of the following: Aldesleukin
Increased Effect/Toxicity
Iodoquinol and Hydrocortisone may increase the levels/effects of: Deferasirox

The levels/effects of Iodoquinol and Hydrocortisone may be increased by: Telaprevir
Decreased Effect
Iodoquinol and Hydrocortisone may decrease the levels/effects of: Aldesleukin; Corticorelin; Hyaluronidase; Telaprevir
Pregnancy Risk Factor C
Pregnancy Considerations Animal reproduction studies have not been conducted with this combination. Refer to individual monographs.
Lactation Excretion in breast milk unknown/use caution
Breast-Feeding Considerations See individual agents.
Dosage Forms
Cream, topical: Iodoquinol 1% and hydrocortisone 1% (30 g)
Dermazene®: Iodoquinol 1% and hydrocortisone 1% (30 g)
Gel, topical:
Alcortin® A: Iodoquinol 1% and hydrocortisone 2% (2 g)

Iohexol (eye oh HEX ole)

Brand Names: U.S. Omnipaque™ 140 [DSC]; Omnipaque™ 180; Omnipaque™ 240; Omnipaque™ 300; Omnipaque™ 350
Brand Names: Canada Omnipaque™
Pharmacologic Category Iodinated Contrast Media; Radiological/Contrast Media, Nonionic (Low Osmolality)
Use
Intrathecal: Myelography; contrast enhancement for computerized tomography
Intravascular: Angiocardiography, aortography, digital subtraction angiography, peripheral arteriography, excretory urography; contrast enhancement for computed tomographic imaging

Oral/body cavity: Arthrography, GI tract examination, hysterosalpingography, pancreatography, cholangiopancreatography, herniography, cystourethrography; enhanced computed tomography of the abdomen

Local Anesthetic/Vasoconstrictor Precautions No information available to require special precautions

Effects on Dental Treatment No significant effects or complications reported

Effects on Bleeding No information available to require special precautions

Adverse Effects Frequency not defined; **Note:** Children have a lower frequency of reactions than adults.

Cardiovascular: Asystole, arrhythmia, bradycardia, cardiopulmonary collapse, edema, heart failure, hypertension (in patients with phenochromocytoma after intra-arterial injection), hypotension, syncope, transient ischemic attacks, vasovagal attacks, venous thrombosis, ventricular fibrillation, ventricular tachycardia

Central nervous system: Anxiety, confusion, dizziness, headache, loss of consciousness, seizure, vertigo

Dermatologic: Pruritus, rash, urticaria

Endocrine & metabolic: Thyrotoxicosis exacerbation

Gastrointestinal: Cramping, diarrhea, nausea, salivary gland swelling, vomiting

Local: Burning sensation, pain at injection site, thrombophlebitis

Neuromuscular & skeletal: Parasthesia, polyarthropathy, tremor

Ocular: Vision abnormalities

Renal: Contrast-associated nephropathy, creatinine increased, renal dysfunction

Respiratory: Bronchospasm, cough, dyspnea, pulmonary edema, rhinitis, sneezing

Miscellaneous: Anaphylactoid reaction, diaphoresis, hypersensitivity reactions

Mechanism of Action Opacification of vessels and anatomical structures in the path of flow of the contrast media which allows for radiographic visualization

Pharmacodynamics/Kinetics

Duration of Action

CNS: ~30 minutes following intrathecal administration, 60 minutes following intravenous administration

Serum: 15-120 seconds

Pregnancy Risk Factor B

Pregnancy Considerations Fetal harm was not observed in animal studies. In general, iodinated contrast media agents are avoided during pregnancy unless essential for diagnosis.

Iopamidol (eye oh PA mi dole)

Brand Names: U.S. Isovue Multipack®; Isovue-M®; Isovue® 200; Isovue® 250; Isovue® 300; Isovue® 370

Pharmacologic Category Iodinated Contrast Media; Radiological/Contrast Media, Nonionic (Low Osmolality)

Use

Intrathecal (Isovue-M®): Myelography contrast enhancement of computed tomographic cisternography and ventriculography; thoracolumbar myelography

Intravascular (Isovue®, Isovue Multipack®): Angiography (eg, coronary, cerebral, peripheral arteriogram), pediatric angiocardiography, excretory urography; contrast enhancement of computed tomographic imaging (in adults and children); evaluation of certain malignancies; image enhancement of non-neoplastic lesions

Local Anesthetic/Vasoconstrictor Precautions No information available to require special precautions

Effects on Dental Treatment No significant effects or complications reported

Effects on Bleeding No information available to require special precautions

Adverse Effects

>10%: Central nervous system: Headache (1% to 16%)

≥1% to 10%:

Cardiovascular: Angina pectoris (3%), flushing (2%), bradycardia (1%), hypertension (1%), hypotension (1%), arrhythmias, circulatory collapse, MI, tachycardia, ventricular fibrillation

Central nervous system: Hot flashes (3%), pain (3%), chills, faintness, fever, vasovagal reaction

Dermatologic: Hives (1%), pruritus, rash, urticaria

Gastrointestinal: Nausea (1% to 7%), vomiting (1% to 4%), anorexia, taste alterations

Genitourinary: Urinary retention

Local: Burning sensation (1%), thrombophlebitis

Neuromuscular & skeletal: Muscle pain (1% to 2%)

Ocular: Visual disturbances

Respiratory: Dyspnea, nasal congestion, pulmonary edema

Miscellaneous: Diaphoresis

Mechanism of Action Opacification of vessels and anatomical structures in the path of flow of the contrast media which allows for radiographic visualization

Pharmacodynamics/Kinetics

Half-life Elimination 2 hours; prolonged in renal impairment

Pregnancy Risk Factor B

Pregnancy Considerations Fetal harm was not observed in animal studies. Diagnostic iodinated contrast agents have been shown to cross the placenta. There are no adequate or well-controlled studies in pregnant women. In general, iodinated contrast media agents are avoided during pregnancy unless essential for diagnosis.

Iopromide (eye oh PROE mide)

Brand Names: U.S. Ultravist®

Brand Names: Canada Ultravist®

Pharmacologic Category Iodinated Contrast Media; Radiological/Contrast Media, Nonionic (Low Osmolality)

Use Enhance imaging in cerebral arteriography and peripheral arteriography; coronary arteriography and left ventriculography; visceral angiography and aortography; contrast-enhanced computed tomographic imaging of the head and body, excretory urography, intra-arterial digital subtraction angiography, peripheral venography

Local Anesthetic/Vasoconstrictor Precautions No information available to require special precautions

Effects on Dental Treatment Key adverse event(s) related to dental treatment: Abnormal taste.

Effects on Bleeding No information available to require special precautions

Adverse Effects

1% to 10%:

Cardiovascular: Vasodilatation (4%), chest pain (3%), hypertension (1%)

Central nervous system: Headache (6%), pain (2%), dizziness (1%)

Gastrointestinal: Nausea (4%), vomiting (2%), abnormal taste (1%)

Genitourinary: Urinary urgency (3%)

Local: Injection site hematoma (3%), injection site pain (1%)

Neuromuscular & skeletal: Back pain (3%)

Ocular: Abnormal vision (2%)

Mechanism of Action Iopromide opacifies vessels in its path of flow, permitting radiographic visualization of internal structures.

Pharmacodynamics/Kinetics

Half-life Elimination Main elimination phase: 2 hours, terminal phase: 6.2 hours

Time to Peak

Intravascular: Contrast enhancement: 15-120 seconds after bolus injection

Intravenous: Contrast enhancement: Kidneys: 5-15 minutes

Pregnancy Risk Factor B

Pregnancy Considerations Animal studies do not show evidence of direct fetal harm. Embryolethality was observed, but may be related to maternal toxicity. Safety has not been established in pregnant women. Use during pregnancy only if clearly needed.

Iothalamate Meglumine
(eye oh thal A mate MEG loo meen)

Brand Names: U.S. Conray®; Conray® 30; Conray® 43; Cysto-Conray™ II

Brand Names: Canada Conray® 30; Conray® 43; Conray® 60; Cysto-Conray™ II

Pharmacologic Category Iodinated Contrast Media; Radiological/Contrast Media, Ionic (High Osmolality)

Use

Solution for injection: Arthrography, cerebral angiography, cranial computerized angiotomography, digital subtraction angiography, direct cholangiography, endoscopic retrograde cholangiopancreatography, excretory urography, peripheral arteriography, urography, venography; contrast enhancement of computed tomographic images

Solution for instillation: Retrograde cystography and cystourethrography

Local Anesthetic/Vasoconstrictor Precautions No information available to require special precautions

Effects on Dental Treatment No significant effects or complications reported

Effects on Bleeding No information available to require special precautions

Pregnancy Risk Factor B/C (product dependent)

Pregnancy Considerations In general, iodinated contrast media agents are avoided during pregnancy unless essential for diagnosis.

Ioversol (EYE oh ver sole)

Brand Names: U.S. Optiray® 240; Optiray® 300; Optiray® 320; Optiray® 350

Brand Names: Canada Optiray® 240; Optiray® 300; Optiray® 320; Optiray® 350

Pharmacologic Category Iodinated Contrast Media; Radiological/Contrast Media, Nonionic (Low Osmolality)

Use Arteriography, angiography, angiocardiography, ventriculography, excretory urography, and venography procedures; contrast enhanced tomographic imaging

Local Anesthetic/Vasoconstrictor Precautions No information available to require special precautions

Effects on Dental Treatment No significant effects or complications reported

Effects on Bleeding No information available to require special precautions

Adverse Effects

>10%: Central nervous system: Headache (16%)

1% to 10%:

Cardiovascular: Angina pectoris (3%), flushing (2%), bradycardia (1%), hypotension (1%), arrhythmias, hypertension (in patients with phenochromocytoma after intra-arterial injection), myocardial ischemia, tachycardia, venous thrombosis, ventricular fibrillation, ventricular tachycardia

Central nervous system: Hot flashes (3%), chills, fever, transient ischemic attack

Dermatologic: Hives (1%), pruritus, rash, urticaria

Gastrointestinal: Nausea (7%), vomiting (4%), anorexia, taste alterations

Genitourinary: Urinary retention

Local: Burning sensation (1%)

Neuromuscular & skeletal: Back pain (2%), leg pain (1%), neck pain (1%), back spasm, paresthesia

Ocular: Vision abnormalities

Renal: Contrast-associated nephropathy, creatinine increased, renal dysfunction

Respiratory: Bronchospasm, cough, dyspnea, pulmonary edema, rhinitis, sneezing

Miscellaneous: Diaphoresis, hypersensitivity reactions

General Dosage Range Dosage varies greatly depending on product.

Mechanism of Action Opacification of vessels and anatomical structures in the path of flow of the contrast media which allows for radiographic visualization.

Pharmacodynamics/Kinetics

Half-life Elimination ~2 hours

Pregnancy Risk Factor B

Pregnancy Considerations Fetal harm was not observed in animal studies. In general, iodinated contrast media agents are avoided during pregnancy unless essential for diagnosis.

Ioxaglate Meglumine and Ioxaglate Sodium
(eye ox AG late MEG loo meen & eye ox AG late SOW dee um)

Brand Names: U.S. Hexabrix™

Pharmacologic Category Iodinated Contrast Media; Radiological/Contrast Media, Ionic (Low Osmolality)

Use Angiocardiography, arteriography, aortography, arthrography, angiography, hysterosalpingography, venography, and urography procedures; contrast enhancement of computed tomographic imaging

Local Anesthetic/Vasoconstrictor Precautions No information available to require special precautions

Effects on Dental Treatment No significant effects or complications reported

Effects on Bleeding No information available to require special precautions

Pregnancy Risk Factor B

Pregnancy Considerations Animal reproduction studies did not show fetal harm. In general, iodinated contrast media agents are avoided during pregnancy unless essential for diagnosis.

Ipilimumab (ip i LIM u mab)

Brand Names: U.S. Yervoy®

Brand Names: Canada Yervoy®

Pharmacologic Category Antineoplastic Agent, Monoclonal Antibody; Monoclonal Antibody

Use Treatment of unresectable or metastatic melanoma

Local Anesthetic/Vasoconstrictor Precautions No information available to require special precautions

Effects on Dental Treatment No significant effects or complications reported

Effects on Bleeding No information available to require special precautions

Adverse Effects

>10%:

Central nervous system: Fatigue (41% to 42%; grades 3-5: 7%), headache (15%), fever (12%)

Dermatologic: Pruritus (24% to 31%), rash (19% to 29%; grades 3-5: 2%), dermatitis (grade 2: 12%; grades 3-5: 2% to 3% [includes Stevens-Johnson syndrome, toxic epidermal necrolysis, dermal ulceration, necrotic, bullous or hemorrhagic dermatitis])

Gastrointestinal: Nausea (35%), diarrhea (32% to 33%; grades 3-5: 5%), appetite decreased (27%), vomiting (24%), constipation (21%), abdominal pain (15%)

Hematologic: Anemia (12%)

Respiratory: Cough (16%), dyspnea (15%)

1% to 10%:

Dermatologic: Urticaria (2%), vitiligo (2%)

Endocrine & metabolic: Hypopituitarism (grade 2: 2%; grades 3-5: 4%), hypophysitis (2%), adrenal insufficiency (≤2%), hypothyroidism (≤2%)

Gastrointestinal: Colitis (8%; grades 3-5: 5%), enterocolitis (grade 2: 5%; grades 3-5: 7%), intestinal perforation (1%)

Hematologic: Eosinophilia (grades 3-5: 1%)

Hepatic: Hepatotoxicity (grade 2: 3%; grades 3-5: 1% to 2%), ALT increased (2%)

Renal: Nephritis (grades 3-5: 1%)

Miscellaneous: Antibody formation (1%)

General Dosage Range Dosage adjustment recommended in patients who develop toxicities.

I.V.: *Adults:* 3 mg/kg every 3 weeks

Mechanism of Action Ipilimumab is a recombinant human IgG1 immunoglobulin monoclonal antibody which binds to the cytotoxic T-lymphocyte associated antigen 4 (CTLA-4). CTLA-4 is a down-regulator of T-cell activation pathways. Blocking CTLA-4 allows for enhanced T-cell activation and proliferation. In melanoma, ipilimumab may indirectly mediate T-cell immune responses against tumors.

Pharmacodynamics/Kinetics

Half-life Elimination Terminal: 15.4 days

Pregnancy Risk Factor C

Pregnancy Considerations Adverse effects were observed in animal reproduction studies. Ipilimumab is an IgG1 immunoglobulin and human IgG1 is known to cross the placenta, therefore, ipilimumab may be expected to reach the fetus.

Ipratropium (Oral Inhalation)

(i pra TROE pee um)

Related Information

Respiratory Diseases *on page 1514*

Brand Names: U.S. Atrovent® HFA

Brand Names: Canada Atrovent® HFA; Gen-Ipratropium; Mylan-Ipratropium Sterinebs; Novo-Ipramide; Nu-Ipratropium; PMS-Ipratropium; Teva-Ipratropium Sterinebs

Pharmacologic Category Anticholinergic Agent

Use Anticholinergic bronchodilator used in bronchospasm associated with COPD, bronchitis, and emphysema

Local Anesthetic/Vasoconstrictor Precautions No information available to require special precautions

Effects on Dental Treatment Key adverse event(s) related to dental treatment: Xerostomia and changes in salivation (normal salivary flow resumes upon discontinuation), and dry mucous membranes.

Effects on Bleeding No information available to require special precautions

Adverse Effects

>10%: Respiratory: Bronchitis (10% to 23%), COPD exacerbation (8% to 23%), sinusitis (1% to 11%)

1% to 10%:

Central nervous system: Headache (6% to 7%), dizziness (3%)

Gastrointestinal: Dyspepsia (1% to 5%), nausea (4%), xerostomia (2% to 4%), taste perversion (1%)

Genitourinary: Urinary tract infection (2% to 10%)

Neuromuscular & skeletal: Back pain (2% to 7%)

Respiratory: Dyspnea (7% to 8%), cough (>3%), rhinitis (>3%), upper respiratory infection (>3%)

Miscellaneous: Flu-like syndrome (4% to 8%)

General Dosage Range

Inhalation: *Children >12 years and Adults:* 2 inhalations 4 times/day (maximum: 12 inhalations/day)

Nebulization: *Children >12 years and Adults:* 500 mcg every 6-8 hours

Mechanism of Action Blocks the action of acetylcholine at parasympathetic sites in bronchial smooth muscle causing bronchodilation; local application to nasal mucosa inhibits serous and seromucous gland secretions.

Pharmacodynamics/Kinetics

Onset of Action Bronchodilation: Within 15 minutes; Peak effect: 1-2 hours

Duration of Action 2-5 hours

Half-life Elimination 2 hours

Pregnancy Risk Factor B

Pregnancy Considerations Teratogenic effects were not observed in animal studies. Inhaled ipratropium is recommended for use as additional therapy for pregnant women with severe asthma exacerbations.

Ipratropium (Nasal) (i pra TROE pee um)

Brand Names: U.S. Atrovent®

Brand Names: Canada Alti-Ipratropium; Apo-Ipravent®; Atrovent®; Mylan-Ipratropium Solution

Pharmacologic Category Anticholinergic Agent

Use Symptomatic relief of rhinorrhea associated with the common cold and allergic and nonallergic rhinitis

Local Anesthetic/Vasoconstrictor Precautions No information available to require special precautions

Effects on Dental Treatment No significant effects or complications reported

Effects on Bleeding No information available to require special precautions

Adverse Effects 1% to 10%:

Central nervous system: Headache (4% to 10%)

Gastrointestinal: Taste perversion (≤4%), xerostomia (1% to 4%), diarrhea (2%), nausea (2%)

Respiratory: Upper respiratory tract infection (5% to 10%), epistaxis (6% to 9%), pharyngitis (≤8%), nasal dryness (<1% to 5%), nasal irritation (2%), nasal congestion (1%)

General Dosage Range Intranasal:

0.03% solution: *Children ≥6 years and Adults:* 2 sprays in each nostril 2-3 times/day

0.06% solution: *Children ≥5 years and Adults:* 2 sprays in each nostril 3-4 times/day

Mechanism of Action Local application to nasal mucosa inhibits serous and seromucous gland secretions.

Pharmacodynamics/Kinetics

Half-life Elimination 1.6 hours

Pregnancy Risk Factor B

Pregnancy Considerations Teratogenic effects were not observed in animal studies.

Ipratropium and Albuterol
(i pra TROE pee um & al BYOO ter ole)

Related Information
Albuterol on page 54
Ipratropium (Oral Inhalation) on page 760

Brand Names: U.S. Combivent®; Combivent® Respimat®; DuoNeb®

Brand Names: Canada CO Ipra-Sal; Combivent UDV; Gen-Combo Sterinebs; ratio-Ipra Sal UDV; Teva-Combo Sterinebs

Generic Availability (U.S.) Yes: Solution for nebulization

Pharmacologic Category Anticholinergic Agent; Beta$_2$-Adrenergic Agonist

Use Treatment of COPD in those patients who are currently on a regular bronchodilator who continue to have bronchospasms and require a second bronchodilator

Local Anesthetic/Vasoconstrictor Precautions No information available to require special precautions

Effects on Dental Treatment Key adverse event(s) related to dental treatment: Xerostomia (normal salivary flow resumes upon discontinuation), dry mucous membrane, and unusual taste.

Effects on Bleeding No information available to require special precautions

Adverse Effects Percentages reported with combination product (not versus placebo). Also see individual agents.

>10%: Respiratory: Bronchitis (2% to 12%), upper respiratory tract infection (3% to 11%)

1% to 10%:
Cardiovascular: Chest pain (≤3%), angina (<2%), arrhythmia (<2%), edema (<2%), hypertension (<2%), palpitation (<2%), tachycardia (<2%)
Central nervous system: Headache (3% to 6%), pain (1% to 3%), dizziness (<2%), fatigue (<2%), insomnia (<2%), nervousness (<2%)
Dermatologic: Pruritus (<2%), rash (<2%)
Endocrine & metabolic: Hypokalemia (<2%)
Gastrointestinal: Diarrhea (≤2%), dyspepsia (≤2%), nausea (1% to 2%), constipation (<2%), dry throat (<2%), sputum increased (<2%), taste perversion (<2%), vomiting (<2%), xerostomia (<2%)
Genitourinary: Urinary tract infection (≤2%), dysuria (<2%)
Neuromuscular & skeletal: Arthralgia (<2%), muscle spasms (<2%), myalgia (<2%), paresthesia (<2%), tremor (<2%), weakness (<2%), leg cramps (1%)
Ocular: Eye pain (<2%)
Respiratory: Lung disease (6%), dyspnea (2% to 5%), cough (3% to 7%), pharyngitis (2% to 4%), bronchospasm (<2%), pharyngolaryngeal pain (<2%), wheezing (<2%), respiratory disorder (3%), sinusitis (2%), pneumonia (1%), rhinitis (1%)
Miscellaneous: Dysphonia (<2%), flu-like syndrome (1%)

Dosage COPD: Inhalation: Adults:
Aerosol for inhalation:
Combivent®: Two inhalations 4 times daily (maximum: 12 inhalations/24 hours)
Combivent® Respimat®: One inhalation 4 times daily (maximum: 6 inhalations/24 hours)
Solution for nebulization: Initial: 3 mL every 6 hours (maximum: 3 mL every 4 hours)

Dosage adjustment in renal impairment: No dosage adjustment provided in manufacturer's labeling (has not been studied); use with caution.

Dosage adjustment in hepatic impairment: No dosage adjustment provided in manufacturer's labeling (has not been studied); use with caution.

Mechanism of Action See individual agents.

Contraindications Hypersensitivity to ipratropium, albuterol, atropine (and its derivatives) or any component of the formulation

Combivent® aerosol inhaler: Additional contraindication: Hypersensitivity to soya lecithin or related food products (eg, soybean and peanut)

Warnings/Precautions See individual agents. Combivent® aerosol inhaler contains soya lecithin; use is contraindicated in patients with allergy to soya lecithin or related food products (eg, soybean and peanut).

Drug Interactions

Metabolism/Transport Effects None known.

Avoid Concomitant Use
Avoid concomitant use of Ipratropium and Albuterol with any of the following: Aclidinium; Anticholinergics; Potassium Chloride; Tiotropium

Increased Effect/Toxicity
Ipratropium and Albuterol may increase the levels/effects of: AbobotulinumtoxinA; Anticholinergics; Cannabinoids; Mirabegron; OnabotulinumtoxinA; Potassium Chloride; RimabotulinumtoxinB; Tiotropium; Topiramate

The levels/effects of Ipratropium and Albuterol may be increased by: Aclidinium; Pramlintide

Decreased Effect
Ipratropium and Albuterol may decrease the levels/effects of: Acetylcholinesterase Inhibitors (Central); Secretin

The levels/effects of Ipratropium and Albuterol may be decreased by: Acetylcholinesterase Inhibitors (Central)

Dietary Considerations The Combivent® aerosol dosage form contains soya lecithin. Do not use in patients allergic to soya lecithin or related food products such as soybean and peanut.

Pregnancy Risk Factor C

Pregnancy Considerations Animal reproduction studies have not been conducted with this combination. See individual agents.

Breast-Feeding Considerations See individual agents.

Dosage Forms

Aerosol, for oral inhalation:
Combivent®: Ipratropium bromide 18 mcg and albuterol (base) 90 mcg per inhalation (14.7 g) [200 metered actuations]

Solution, for nebulization: Ipratropium 0.5 mg and albuterol (base) 2.5 mg per 3 mL (30s, 60s)
DuoNeb®: Ipratropium 0.5 mg and albuterol (base) 2.5 mg per 3 mL (30s, 60s)
Solution, for oral inhalation [spray]:
Combivent® Respimat®: Ipratropium bromide 20 mcg and albuterol (base) 100 mcg per inhalation (4 g) [120 metered actuations]

Ipratropium and Fenoterol
(i pra TROE pee um & fen oh TER ole)

Related Information
Ipratropium (Oral Inhalation) *on page 760*
Brand Names: Canada Duovent® UDV
Pharmacologic Category Anticholinergic Agent; Beta$_2$-Adrenergic Agonist
Use Treatment of bronchospasm associated with acute severe exacerbation of COPD or bronchial asthma
Local Anesthetic/Vasoconstrictor Precautions No information available to require special precautions
Effects on Dental Treatment Key adverse event(s) related to dental treatment: Xerostomia (normal salivary flow resumes upon discontinuation).
Effects on Bleeding No information available to require special precautions
Adverse Effects Frequency not defined.
Cardiovascular: Arrhythmias, atrial fibrillation, cardiac arrest, hyper-/hypotension, myocardial ischemia, palpitation, QT$_c$ prolongation, SVT, tachycardia
Central nervous system: Dizziness, headache, nervousness, psychological alterations
Gastrointestinal: Constipation, diarrhea, nausea, vomiting, xerostomia
Genitourinary: Urinary retention
Endocrine & metabolic: Hyperglycemia, hypokalemia
Neuromuscular & skeletal: Muscle cramps, myalgia, tremor, weakness
Ophthalmic: Accommodation disturbance, acute angle closure glaucoma, eye pain, intraocular pressure increased, mydriasis
Respiratory: Bronchospasm (inhalation induced), cough, pharyngitis, throat irritation
Miscellaneous: Allergic reactions (anaphylaxis, angioedema, bronchospasm, laryngospasm, oropharyngeal edema, skin rash, urticaria); diaphoresis
General Dosage Range Nebulization: *Children ≥12 years and Adults:* Usual dose: 4 mL; may repeat every 6 hours as needed
Mechanism of Action
Ipratropium: Blocks the action of acetylcholine at parasympathetic sites in bronchial smooth muscle causing bronchodilation
Fenoterol: Relaxes bronchial smooth muscle by action on beta$_2$-receptors
Pharmacodynamics/Kinetics
Onset of Action
Ipratropium: Bronchodilation: Within 15 minutes
Peak effect: 1-2 hours
Fenoterol: Bronchodilation: 5 minutes
Peak effect: 30-60 minutes
Duration of Action
Ipratropium: 6-8 hours
Fenoterol: 4-6 hours; In combination with ipratropium: 6-8 hours

Pregnancy Considerations Reproduction studies have not been conducted with this combination. Use with caution prior to delivery due to tocolytic effect of fenoterol.
Product Availability Not available in U.S.

Irbesartan (ir be SAR tan)

Related Information
Cardiovascular Diseases *on page 1492*
Brand Names: U.S. Avapro®
Brand Names: Canada Avapro®; CO Irbesartan; PMS-Irbesartan; ratio-Irbesartan; Sandoz-Irbesartan; Teva-Irbesartan
Generic Availability (U.S.) Yes
Pharmacologic Category Angiotensin II Receptor Blocker
Use Treatment of hypertension alone or in combination with other antihypertensives; treatment of diabetic nephropathy in patients with type 2 diabetes mellitus (noninsulin dependent, NIDDM) and hypertension
Unlabeled Use To slow the rate of progression of aortic-root dilation in pediatric patients with Marfan's syndrome
Local Anesthetic/Vasoconstrictor Precautions No information available to require special precautions
Effects on Dental Treatment Key adverse event(s) related to dental treatment: Orthostatic hypotension.
Effects on Bleeding No information available to require special precautions
Adverse Effects Unless otherwise indicated, percentage of incidence is reported for patients with hypertension.
>10%: Endocrine & metabolic: Hyperkalemia (19%, diabetic nephropathy; rarely seen in HTN)
1% to 10%:
Cardiovascular: Orthostatic hypotension (5%, diabetic nephropathy)
Central nervous system: Fatigue (4%), dizziness (10%, diabetic nephropathy)
Gastrointestinal: Diarrhea (3%), dyspepsia (2%)
Respiratory: Upper respiratory infection (9%), cough (2.8% versus 2.7% in placebo)
Dosage Oral:
Hypertension:
Children:
<6 years: Safety and efficacy have not been established.
≥6-12 years: Initial: 75 mg once daily; may be titrated to a maximum of 150 mg once daily
Children ≥13 years and Adults: 150 mg once daily; patients may be titrated to 300 mg once daily
Note: Starting dose in volume-depleted patients should be 75 mg
Aortic-root dilation with Marfan's syndrome (unlabeled use): Children 14 months to 16 years: Initial: 1.4 mg/kg/day; can be increased to a maximum of 2 mg/kg/day (not to exceed adult maximum of 300 mg/day)
Nephropathy in patients with type 2 diabetes and hypertension: Adults: Target dose: 300 mg once daily

Dosage adjustment in renal impairment: No dosage adjustment necessary with mild to severe impairment unless the patient is also volume depleted.
Dosage adjustment in hepatic impairment: No dosage adjustment necessary.

Mechanism of Action Irbesartan is an angiotensin receptor antagonist. Angiotensin II acts as a vasoconstrictor. In addition to causing direct vasoconstriction, angiotensin II also stimulates the release of aldosterone. Once aldosterone is released, sodium as well as water are reabsorbed. The end result is an elevation in blood pressure. Irbesartan binds to the AT1 angiotensin II receptor. This binding prevents angiotensin II from binding to the receptor thereby blocking the vasoconstriction and the aldosterone secreting effects of angiotensin II.

Contraindications Hypersensitivity to irbesartan or any component of the formulation; concomitant use with aliskiren in patients with diabetes mellitus

Warnings/Precautions [U.S. Boxed Warning]: Drugs that act on the renin-angiotensin system can cause injury and death to the developing fetus. Discontinue as soon as possible once pregnancy is detected. May cause hyperkalemia; avoid potassium supplementation unless specifically required by healthcare provider. May be associated with deterioration of renal function and/or increases in serum creatinine, particularly in patients with low renal blood flow (eg, renal artery stenosis, heart failure) whose glomerular filtration rate (GFR) is dependent on efferent arteriolar vasoconstriction by angiotensin II. Avoid use or use a much smaller dose in patients who are intravascularly volume-depleted; use caution in patients with unstented unilateral or bilateral renal artery stenosis. When unstented bilateral renal artery stenosis is present, use is generally avoided due to the elevated risk of deterioration in renal function unless possible benefits outweigh risks. AUCs of irbesartan (not the active metabolite) are about 50% greater in patients with Cl_{cr} <30 mL/minute and are doubled in hemodialysis patients. Concomitant use of an angiotensin-converting enzyme (ACE) inhibitor or renin inhibitor (eg, aliskiren) is associated with an increased risk of hypotension, hyperkalemia, and renal dysfunction; concomitant use with aliskiren should be avoided in patients with GFR <60 mL/minute and is contraindicated in patients with diabetes mellitus (regardless of GFR).

Drug Interactions

Metabolism/Transport Effects Substrate of CYP2C9 (minor); **Note:** Assignment of Major/Minor substrate status based on clinically relevant drug interaction potential; **Inhibits** CYP2C8 (moderate), CYP2C9 (moderate), CYP2D6 (weak), CYP3A4 (weak)

Avoid Concomitant Use
Avoid concomitant use of Irbesartan with any of the following: Pimozide

Increased Effect/Toxicity
Irbesartan may increase the levels/effects of: ACE Inhibitors; Amifostine; Antihypertensives; ARIPiprazole; Carvedilol; CycloSPORINE (Systemic); CYP2C8 Substrates; CYP2C9 Substrates; Hypotensive Agents; Lithium; Lomitapide; Nonsteroidal Anti-Inflammatory Agents; Pimozide; Potassium-Sparing Diuretics; RiTUXimab; Sodium Phosphates

The levels/effects of Irbesartan may be increased by: Alfuzosin; Aliskiren; Canagliflozin; Diazoxide; Eplerenone; Fluconazole; Herbs (Hypotensive Properties); MAO Inhibitors; Pentoxifylline; Phosphodiesterase 5 Inhibitors; Potassium Salts; Prostacyclin Analogues; Tolvaptan; Trimethoprim

Decreased Effect
The levels/effects of Irbesartan may be decreased by: Herbs (Hypertensive Properties); Methylphenidate; Nonsteroidal Anti-Inflammatory Agents; Rifamycin Derivatives; Yohimbine

Ethanol/Nutrition/Herb Interactions Herb/Nutraceutical: Dong quai has estrogenic activity. Some herbal medications may worsen hypertension (eg, ephedra); garlic may have additional antihypertensive effects. Management: Avoid dong quai if using for hypertension. Avoid ephedra, yohimbe, ginseng, and garlic.

Dietary Considerations May be taken with or without food.

Pharmacodynamics/Kinetics
Onset of Action Peak levels in 1-2 hours
Duration of Action >24 hours
Half-life Elimination Terminal: 11-15 hours
Time to Peak Serum: 1.5-2 hours

Pregnancy Risk Factor D

Pregnancy Considerations [U.S. Boxed Warning]: Drugs that act on the renin-angiotensin system can cause injury and death to the developing fetus. Discontinue as soon as possible once pregnancy is detected. The use of drugs which act on the renin-angiotensin system are associated with oligohydramnios. Oligohydramnios, due to decreased fetal renal function, may lead to fetal lung hypoplasia and skeletal malformations. Use is also associated with anuria, hypotension, renal failure, skull hypoplasia, and death in the fetus/neonate. The exposed fetus should be monitored for fetal growth, amniotic fluid volume, and organ formation. Infants exposed *in utero* should be monitored for hyperkalemia, hypotension, and oliguria.

Lactation Excretion in breast milk unknown/contraindicated

Dosage Forms
Tablet, oral: 75 mg, 150 mg, 300 mg
Avapro®: 75 mg, 150 mg, 300 mg

Irbesartan and Hydrochlorothiazide
(ir be SAR tan & hye droe klor oh THYE a zide)

Related Information
Hydrochlorothiazide *on page 687*
Irbesartan *on page 762*
Brand Names: U.S. Avalide®
Brand Names: Canada Avalide®; CO Irbesartan HCT; Irbesartan-HCTZ; PMS-Irbesartan HCTZ; Ran™-Irbesartan HCTZ; ratio-Irbesartan HCTZ; Sandoz-Irbesartan HCT; Teva-Irbesartan HCTZ

Pharmacologic Category Angiotensin II Receptor Blocker; Diuretic, Thiazide

Use Combination therapy for the management of hypertension; may be used as initial therapy in patients likely to need multiple drugs to achieve blood pressure goals

Local Anesthetic/Vasoconstrictor Precautions No information available to require special precautions

Effects on Dental Treatment No significant effects or complications reported

Effects on Bleeding No information available to require special precautions

Adverse Effects Reactions/percentages reported with combination product; also see individual agents.
1% to 10%:
Cardiovascular: Edema (3%), chest pain (2%), tachycardia (1%)
Central nervous system: Dizziness (8%; orthostatic: 1%), fatigue (6%)

Gastrointestinal: Nausea/vomiting (3%), abdominal pain (2%), dyspepsia (2%)

Genitourinary: Urination abnormal (2%)

Neuromuscular & skeletal: Musculoskeletal pain (6%)

Renal: BUN increased (2%), creatinine increased (1%)

Miscellaneous: Flu-like syndrome (3%)

General Dosage Range Oral: *Adults:* Irbesartan 150-300 mg and hydrochlorothiazide 12.5-25 mg once daily

Mechanism of Action

Irbesartan: Irbesartan is an angiotensin receptor antagonist. Angiotensin II acts as a vasoconstrictor. In addition to causing direct vasoconstriction, angiotensin II also stimulates the release of aldosterone. Once aldosterone is released, sodium as well as water are reabsorbed. The end result is an elevation in blood pressure. Irbesartan binds to the AT1 angiotensin II receptor. This binding prevents angiotensin II from binding to the receptor thereby blocking the vasoconstriction and the aldosterone secreting effects of angiotensin II.

Hydrochlorothiazide: Inhibits sodium reabsorption in the distal tubules causing increased excretion of sodium and water as well as potassium and hydrogen ions

Pregnancy Risk Factor D

Pregnancy Considerations [U.S. Boxed Warning]: Drugs that act on the renin-angiotensin system can cause injury and death to the developing fetus. Discontinue as soon as possible once pregnancy is detected. Also see individual agents.

Irinotecan (eye rye no TEE kan)

Brand Names: U.S. Camptosar®

Brand Names: Canada Camptosar®; Irinotecan Hydrochloride Trihydrate

Pharmacologic Category Antineoplastic Agent, Camptothecin; Antineoplastic Agent, Natural Source (Plant) Derivative; Antineoplastic Agent, Topoisomerase I Inhibitor

Use Treatment of metastatic carcinoma of the colon or rectum

Unlabeled Use Treatment of cervical cancer (recurrent or metastatic), central nervous system tumors (recurrent glioblastoma), esophageal cancer, Ewing's sarcoma (recurrent or progressive), gastric cancer (metastatic or locally advanced), nonsmall cell lung cancer (advanced), ovarian cancer (recurrent), pancreatic cancer (advanced), small cell lung cancer (extensive stage)

Local Anesthetic/Vasoconstrictor Precautions No information available to require special precautions

Effects on Dental Treatment Key adverse event(s) related to dental treatment: Increased salivation, mucositis, and stomatitis.

Effects on Bleeding Hematologic adverse effects include anemia (60% to 97%) and thrombocytopenia (96%; grades 3/4: 1% to 4%). Bleeding and hemorrhage have been noted in 1% to 5% of patients. Medical consult recommended.

Adverse Effects Frequency of adverse reactions reported for single-agent use of irinotecan only.

>10%:

Cardiovascular: Vasodilation (9% to 11%)

Central nervous system: Cholinergic toxicity (47% - includes rhinitis, increased salivation, miosis, lacrimation, diaphoresis, flushing and intestinal hyperperistalsis); fever (44% to 45%), pain (23% to 24%),

dizziness (15% to 21%), insomnia (19%), headache (17%), chills (14%)

Dermatologic: Alopecia (46% to 72%), rash (13% to 14%)

Endocrine & metabolic: Dehydration (15%)

Gastrointestinal: Diarrhea, late (83% to 88%; grade 3/4: 14% to 31%), diarrhea, early (43% to 51%; grade 3/4: 7% to 22%), nausea (70% to 86%), abdominal pain (57% to 68%), vomiting (62% to 67%), cramps (57%), anorexia (44% to 55%), constipation (30% to 32%), mucositis (30%), weight loss (30%), flatulence (12%), stomatitis (12%)

Hematologic: Anemia (60% to 97%; grades 3/4: 5% to 7%), leukopenia (63% to 96%, grades 3/4: 14% to 28%), thrombocytopenia (96%, grades 3/4: 1% to 4%), neutropenia (30% to 96%; grades 3/4: 14% to 31%)

Hepatic: Bilirubin increased (84%), alkaline phosphatase increased (13%)

Neuromuscular & skeletal: Weakness (69% to 76%), back pain (14%)

Respiratory: Dyspnea (22%), cough (17% to 20%), rhinitis (16%)

Miscellaneous: Diaphoresis (16%), infection (14%)

1% to 10%:

Cardiovascular: Edema (10%), hypotension (6%), thromboembolic events (5%)

Central nervous system: Somnolence (9%), confusion (3%)

Gastrointestinal: Abdominal fullness (10%), dyspepsia (10%)

Hematologic: Neutropenic fever (grades 3/4: 2% to 6%), hemorrhage (grades 3/4: 1% to 5%), neutropenic infection (grades 3/4: 1% to 2%)

Hepatic: AST increased (10%), ascites and/or jaundice (grades 3/4: 9%)

Respiratory: Pneumonia (4%)

Note: In limited pediatric experience, dehydration (often associated with severe hypokalemia and hyponatremia) was among the most significant grade 3/4 adverse events, with a frequency up to 29%. In addition, grade 3/4 infection was reported in 24%.

General Dosage Range Dosage adjustment recommended in patients with hepatic impairment or who develop toxicities

I.V.: *Adults:* Dosage varies greatly depending on indication

Mechanism of Action Irinotecan and its active metabolite (SN-38) bind reversibly to topoisomerase I-DNA complex preventing religation of the cleaved DNA strand. This results in the accumulation of cleavable complexes and double-strand DNA breaks. As mammalian cells cannot efficiently repair these breaks, cell death consistent with S-phase cell cycle specificity occurs, leading to termination of cellular replication.

Pharmacodynamics/Kinetics

Half-life Elimination Irinotecan: 6-12 hours; SN-38: ~10-20 hours

Time to Peak SN-38: Following 90-minute infusion: ~1 hour

Pregnancy Risk Factor D

Pregnancy Considerations Teratogenic effects were noted in animal studies. There are no adequate and well-controlled studies in pregnant women. Women of childbearing potential should avoid becoming pregnant while receiving treatment.

Iron Dextran Complex
(EYE ern DEKS tran KOM pleks)

Brand Names: U.S. Dexferrum®; INFeD®
Brand Names: Canada Dexiron™; Infufer®
Pharmacologic Category Iron Salt
Use Treatment of iron deficiency in patients in whom oral administration is infeasible or ineffective
Unlabeled Use Cancer-/chemotherapy-associated anemia
Local Anesthetic/Vasoconstrictor Precautions No information available to require special precautions
Effects on Dental Treatment Key adverse event(s) related to dental treatment: Metallic taste.
Effects on Bleeding No information available to require special precautions
Adverse Effects Frequency not defined. **Note:** Adverse event risk is reported to be higher with the high-molecular-weight iron dextran formulation.

Cardiovascular: Arrhythmia, bradycardia, cardiac arrest, chest pain, chest tightness, cyanosis, flushing, hyper-/hypotension, shock, syncope, tachycardia

Central nervous system: Chills, disorientation, dizziness, fever, headache, malaise, seizure, unconsciousness, unresponsiveness

Dermatologic: Pruritus, purpura, rash, urticaria

Gastrointestinal: Abdominal pain, diarrhea, nausea, taste alteration, vomiting

Genitourinary: Discoloration of urine

Hematologic: Leukocytosis, lymphadenopathy

Local: Injection site reactions (cellulitis, inflammation, pain, phlebitis, soreness, swelling), muscle atrophy/fibrosis (with I.M. injection), skin/tissue staining (at the site of I.M. injection), sterile abscess

Neuromuscular & skeletal: Arthralgia, arthritis/arthritis exacerbation, back pain, myalgia, paresthesia, weakness

Respiratory: Bronchospasm, dyspnea, respiratory arrest, wheezing

Renal: Hematuria

Miscellaneous: Anaphylactic reactions (sudden respiratory difficulty, cardiovascular collapse), diaphoresis

General Dosage Range Note: A 0.5 mL test dose (0.25 mL in infants) should be given prior to starting iron dextran therapy.

I.M., I.V.:

Children <5 kg and >4 months: Replacement iron (mg) = blood loss (mL) x Hct; **Note:** Total dose should be divided daily at not more than 25 mg/day

Children 5-15 kg and >4 months: Total Dose (mL) = 0.0442 (desired Hgb [usually 12 g/dL] - observed Hgb) x W (in kg) + (0.26 x W [in kg]) **or** replacement iron (mg) = blood loss (mL) x hematocrit; **Note:** Total dose should be divided daily at not more than 50 mg/day (5-10 kg) or 100 mg/day (10-15 kg)

Children >15 kg: Total Dose (mL) = 0.0442 (desired Hgb [usually 14.8 g/dL] - observed Hgb) x LBW + (0.26 x LBW) **or** replacement iron (mg) = blood loss (mL) x Hct; **Note:** Total dose should be divided daily at not more than 100 mg/day

Adults: Total Dose (mL) = 0.0442 (desired Hgb [usually 14.8 g/dL] - observed Hgb) x LBW + (0.26 x LBW) **or** replacement iron (mg) = blood loss (mL) x Hct; **Note:** Total dose should be divided daily at not more than 100 mg/day

Mechanism of Action The released iron, from the plasma, eventually replenishes the depleted iron stores in the bone marrow where it is incorporated into hemoglobin

Pharmacodynamics/Kinetics
Onset of Action I.V.: Serum ferritin peak: 7-9 days after dose
Pregnancy Risk Factor C
Pregnancy Considerations Adverse events have been observed in animal reproduction studies. It is not known if iron dextran (as iron dextran) crosses the placenta. It is recommended that pregnant women meet the dietary requirements of iron with diet and/or supplements in order to prevent adverse events associated with iron deficiency anemia in pregnancy. Treatment of iron deficiency anemia in pregnant women is the same as in nonpregnant women and in most cases, oral iron preparations may be used. Except in severe cases of maternal anemia, the fetus achieves normal iron stores regardless of maternal concentrations.

Iron Sucrose (EYE ern SOO krose)

Brand Names: U.S. Venofer®
Brand Names: Canada Venofer®
Pharmacologic Category Iron Salt
Use Treatment of iron-deficiency anemia in chronic kidney disease (CKD), including nondialysis-dependent and dialysis-dependent patients
Unlabeled Use Cancer-/chemotherapy-associated anemia
Local Anesthetic/Vasoconstrictor Precautions No information available to require special precautions
Effects on Dental Treatment Key adverse event(s) related to dental treatment: Taste perversion.
Effects on Bleeding No information available to require special precautions
Adverse Effects Events and incidences are associated with use in adults unless otherwise specified.

>10%:

Cardiovascular: Hypotension (2% to 3%; children 2%; 39% in hemodialysis patients; may be related to total dose or rate of administration)

Central nervous system: Headache (3% to 13%; children 6%)

Gastrointestinal: Nausea (5% to 15%; children 3%)

Neuromuscular & skeletal: Muscle cramps (1% to 3%; 29% in hemodialysis patients)

Respiratory: Nasopharyngitis (2% to 16%), pharyngitis (2% to 16%), sinusitis (2% to 16%), upper respiratory infection (2% to 16%; children 4%)

1% to 10%:

Cardiovascular: Hypertension (7% to 8%; children 2%), peripheral edema (3% to 7%), chest pain (1% to 6%), arteriovenous fistula thrombosis (children 2%), heart failure (>1%)

Central nervous system: Dizziness (1% to 7%; children 4%), fever (1% to 3%; children 4%)

Dermatologic: Pruritus (2% to 4%)

Endocrine & metabolic: Hypoglycemia (≤4%), fluid overload (1% to 3%), gout (≤3%), hyperglycemia (≤3%)

Gastrointestinal: Vomiting (5% to 9%; children 4%), diarrhea (5% to 8%), taste perversion (≤8%), peritonitis (children 4%), abdominal pain (1% to 4%)

Local: Injection site reaction (≤6%)

Neuromuscular & skeletal: Extremity pain (3% to 6%), arthralgia (1% to 4%), myalgia (≤4%), weakness (1% to 3%), back pain (1% to 2%)

Ocular: Conjunctivitis (≤3%)

Otic: Ear pain (≤2%)
Respiratory: Dyspnea (1% to 6%), cough (1% to 3%; children 4%), nasal congestion (≤1%)
Miscellaneous: Graft complication (≤10%), sepsis (>1%)

General Dosage Range I.V.:
Children ≥2 years and Adolescents: Maintenance therapy: 0.5 mg/kg/dose (maximum: 100 mg) every 2 weeks for 6 doses **or** every 4 weeks for 3 doses
Adults: 100 mg during consecutive dialysis sessions for 10 doses (total cumulative dose: 1000 mg) **or** 200 mg on 5 different occasions within a 14-day period (total cumulative dose: 1000 mg) **or** two 300 mg infusions administered 14 days apart, followed by a single 400 mg infusion 14 days later (total cumulative dose: 1000 mg)

Mechanism of Action Iron sucrose is dissociated by the reticuloendothelial system into iron and sucrose. The released iron increases serum iron concentrations and is incorporated into hemoglobin.

Pharmacodynamics/Kinetics
Half-life Elimination Healthy adults: 6 hours; Nondialysis-dependent adolescents: 8 hours

Pregnancy Risk Factor B

Pregnancy Considerations Teratogenic effects were not observed in animal studies. There are no adequate and well-controlled studies in pregnant women. Based on limited data, iron sucrose may be effective for the treatment of iron-deficiency anemia in pregnancy. It is recommended that pregnant women meet the dietary requirements of iron with diet and/or supplements in order to prevent adverse events associated with iron deficiency anemia in pregnancy. Treatment of iron deficiency anemia in pregnant women is the same as in nonpregnant women and in most cases, oral iron preparations may be used. Except in severe cases of maternal anemia, the fetus achieves normal iron stores regardless of maternal concentrations.

Isocarboxazid (eye soe kar BOKS a zid)

Related Information
Vasoconstrictor Interactions With Antidepressants *on page 1650*

Brand Names: U.S. Marplan®

Pharmacologic Category Antidepressant, Monoamine Oxidase Inhibitor

Use Treatment of depression

Local Anesthetic/Vasoconstrictor Precautions Attempts should be made to avoid use of vasoconstrictor due to possibility of hypertensive episodes with monoamine oxidase inhibitors

Effects on Dental Treatment Key adverse event(s) related to dental treatment: Orthostatic hypotension, xerostomia (normal salivary flow resumes upon discontinuation).

Effects on Bleeding No information available to require special precautions

Adverse Effects
>10%: Central nervous system: Dizziness (29%), headache (15%)
1% to 10%:
Cardiovascular: Orthostatic hypotension (4%), palpitation (2%), syncope (2%)
Central nervous system: Sleep disturbance (5%), drowsiness (4%), anxiety (2%), chills (2%), forgetfulness (2%), hyperactivity (2%), lethargy (2%), sedation (2%)

Gastrointestinal: Xerostomia (9%), constipation (7%), nausea (6%), diarrhea (2%)
Genitourinary: Urinary frequency (2%), impotence (2%), urinary hesitancy (1%)
Neuromuscular & skeletal: Tremor (4%), myoclonus (2%), paresthesia (2%)
Miscellaneous: Diaphoresis (2%), heavy feeling (2%)

General Dosage Range Oral: *Adults:* Initial: 10 mg 2 times/day; may increase to a maximum of 60 mg/day divided in 2-4 doses

Mechanism of Action Thought to act by increasing endogenous concentrations of epinephrine, norepinephrine, dopamine, and serotonin through inhibition of the enzyme (monoamine oxidase) responsible for the breakdown of these neurotransmitters

Pregnancy Risk Factor C

Pregnancy Considerations Animal reproduction studies have not been conducted.

Isoniazid (eye soe NYE a zid)

Brand Names: Canada Isotamine®; PMS-Isoniazid

Pharmacologic Category Antitubercular Agent

Use Treatment of susceptible tuberculosis infections; treatment of latent tuberculosis infection (LTBI)

Local Anesthetic/Vasoconstrictor Precautions No information available to require special precautions

Effects on Dental Treatment Key adverse event(s) related to dental treatment: Xerostomia (normal salivary flow resumes upon discontinuation).

Effects on Bleeding Anemia and thrombocytopenia have been reported.

Adverse Effects Frequency not defined.
Cardiovascular: Hypertension, palpitation, tachycardia, vasculitis
Central nervous system: Depression, dizziness, encephalopathy, fever, lethargy, memory impairment, psychosis, seizure, slurred speech, toxic encephalopathy
Dermatologic: Flushing, rash (morbilliform, maculopapular, pruritic, or exfoliative)
Endocrine & metabolic: Gynecomastia, hyperglycemia, metabolic acidosis, pellagra, pyridoxine deficiency
Gastrointestinal: Anorexia, epigastric distress, nausea, stomach pain, vomiting
Hematologic: Agranulocytosis, anemia (sideroblastic, hemolytic, or aplastic), eosinophilia, thrombocytopenia
Hepatic: LFTs mildly increased (10% to 20%), hyperbilirubinemia, bilirubinuria, jaundice, hepatic dysfunction, hepatitis (may involve progressive liver damage; risk increases with age; 2.3% in patients >50 years)
Neuromuscular & skeletal: Arthralgia, hyper-reflexia, paresthesia, peripheral neuropathy (dose-related incidence, 10% to 20% incidence with 10 mg/kg/day), weakness
Ocular: Blurred vision, loss of vision, optic neuritis and atrophy
Miscellaneous: Lupus-like syndrome, lymphadenopathy, rheumatic syndrome

General Dosage Range Oral, I.M.:
Children: 10-20 mg/kg/day once daily (maximum: 300 mg/day) **or** 20-40 mg/kg 2-3 times/week (maximum: 900 mg/dose)
Adults: 300 mg (5 mg/kg) once daily **or** 900 mg (15 mg/kg) 2-3 times/week

Mechanism of Action Unknown, but may include the inhibition of mycolic acid synthesis resulting in disruption of the bacterial cell wall

Pharmacodynamics/Kinetics
Half-life Elimination Fast acetylators: 30-100 minutes; Slow acetylators: 2-5 hours; may be prolonged with hepatic or severe renal impairment
Time to Peak Serum: 1-2 hours
Pregnancy Risk Factor C
Pregnancy Considerations Isoniazid was found to be embryocidal in animal studies; teratogenic effects were not noted. Isoniazid crosses the human placenta. Due to the risk of tuberculosis to the fetus, treatment is recommended when the probability of maternal disease is moderate to high. The CDC recommends isoniazid as part of the initial treatment regimen (CDC, 2003). Pyridoxine supplementation is recommended (25 mg/day).

Isoproterenol (eye soe proe TER e nole)

Brand Names: U.S. Isuprel®
Pharmacologic Category Beta$_1$- & Beta$_2$-Adrenergic Agonist Agent
Use Manufacturer's labeled indications (see **"Note"**): Mild or transient episodes of heart block that do not require electric shock or pacemaker therapy; serious episodes of heart block and Adams-Stokes attacks (except when caused by ventricular tachycardia or fibrillation); cardiac arrest until electric shock or pacemaker therapy is available; bronchospasm during anesthesia; adjunct to fluid and electrolyte replacement therapy and other drugs and procedures in the treatment of hypovolemic or septic shock and low cardiac output states (eg, decompensated heart failure, cardiogenic shock)

Note: The use of isoproterenol in advanced cardiac life support (ACLS) has largely been supplanted by the use of other adrenergic agents (eg, epinephrine and dopamine). The use of isoproterenol for bronchospasm during anesthesia and cardiogenic, hypovolemic, or septic shock is no longer recommended. See *Unlabeled Use* for more appropriate, yet unlabeled, uses.
Unlabeled Use Pharmacologic overdrive pacing for refractory torsade de pointes; pharmacologic provocation during tilt table testing for syncope; temporary control of bradycardia in denervated heart transplant patients unresponsive to atropine; ventricular arrhythmias due to AV nodal block; beta-blocker overdose; electrical storm associated with Brugada syndrome
Local Anesthetic/Vasoconstrictor Precautions Isoproterenol is selective for beta-adrenergic receptors and not alpha-receptors; therefore, there is no precaution in the use of vasoconstrictor such as epinephrine
Effects on Dental Treatment Key adverse event(s) related to dental treatment: Xerostomia and changes in salivation (normal salivary flow resumes upon discontinuation).
Effects on Bleeding No information available to require special precautions
Adverse Effects Frequency not defined.
Cardiovascular: Angina, flushing, hyper-/hypotension, pallor, palpitation, paradoxical bradycardia (with tilt table testing), premature ventricular beats, Stokes-Adams attacks, tachyarrhythmia, ventricular arrhythmia
Central nervous system: Dizziness, headache, nervousness, restlessness, Stokes-Adams seizure
Endocrine & metabolic: Hypokalemia, serum glucose increased
Gastrointestinal: Nausea, vomiting
Neuromuscular & skeletal: Tremor, weakness
Ocular: Blurred vision

Respiratory: Dyspnea, pulmonary edema
Miscellaneous: Diaphoresis
General Dosage Range Continuous I.V. infusion:
Children: 0.05-2 mcg/**kg**/minute; titrate to patient response
Adults: 2-10 mcg/minute; titrate to patient response
Mechanism of Action Stimulates beta$_1$- and beta$_2$-receptors resulting in relaxation of bronchial, GI, and uterine smooth muscle, increased heart rate and contractility, vasodilation of peripheral vasculature
Pharmacodynamics/Kinetics
Onset of Action I.V.: Immediate
Duration of Action I.V.: 10-15 minutes
Half-life Elimination 2.5-5 minutes
Pregnancy Risk Factor C
Pregnancy Considerations Animal reproduction studies have not been conducted. Adequate studies have not been conducted in pregnant women; use during pregnancy when the potential benefit to the mother outweighs the possible risk to the fetus.

Isosorbide Dinitrate
(eye soe SOR bide dye NYE trate)

Related Information
Cardiovascular Diseases *on page 1492*
Isosorbide Mononitrate *on page 769*
Brand Names: U.S. Dilatrate®-SR; IsoDitrate® ER; Isordil® Titradose™
Brand Names: Canada ISDN; Isosorbide; Novo-Sorbide; PMS-Isosorbide
Pharmacologic Category Antianginal Agent; Vasodilator
Use Prevention and treatment of angina pectoris

Note: Due to slower onset of action, not the drug of choice to abort an acute anginal episode.
Unlabeled Use Patients with heart failure (HF) who do not tolerate an ACE inhibitor or an angiotensin receptor blocker (ARB); African-American (self-identified) patients with HF remaining symptomatic despite optimal standard therapy; esophageal spastic disorders
Local Anesthetic/Vasoconstrictor Precautions No information available to require special precautions
Effects on Dental Treatment Key adverse event(s) related to dental treatment: Xerostomia and changes in salivation (normal salivary flow resumes upon discontinuation).
Effects on Bleeding No information available to require special precautions
Adverse Effects Frequency not defined.
Cardiovascular: Crescendo angina (uncommon), hypotension, orthostatic hypotension, rebound hypertension (uncommon), syncope (uncommon)
Central nervous system: Headache (most common), lightheadedness (related to blood pressure changes)
Hematologic: Methemoglobinemia (rare, overdose)
General Dosage Range
Oral:
Immediate release: *Adults:* 5-40 mg 2-3 times/day
Sustained release: *Adults:* 40-160 mg/day in divided doses
Sublingual: *Adults:* 2.5-5 mg every 5-10 minutes for maximum of 3 doses in 15-30 minutes **or** 2.5-5 mg 15 minutes prior to activities which may provoke an anginal episode

◀ **Mechanism of Action** Stimulation of intracellular cyclic-GMP results in vascular smooth muscle relaxation of both arterial and venous vasculature with more prominent effects on the veins. Primarily reduces cardiac oxygen demand by decreasing preload (left ventricular end-diastolic pressure); may modestly reduce afterload. Additionally, coronary artery dilation improves collateral flow to ischemic regions.

Pharmacodynamics/Kinetics

Onset of Action Sublingual tablet: ~3 minutes; Oral tablet and capsule (includes extended-release formulations): ~1 hour

Duration of Action Sublingual tablet: 1-2 hours; Oral tablet and capsule (includes extended-release formulations): Up to 8 hours

Half-life Elimination Parent drug: ~1 hour; Metabolites (5-mononitrate: 5 hours; 2-mononitrate: 2 hours)

Pregnancy Risk Factor C

Pregnancy Considerations Increased fetal mortality has been observed in animal studies using isosorbide dinitrate at doses much higher than those used in humans. There are no adequate and well-controlled studies in pregnant women.

Isosorbide Dinitrate and Hydralazine
(eye soe SOR bide dye NYE trate & hye DRAL a zeen)

Related Information

HydrALAZINE *on page 686*

Isosorbide Dinitrate *on page 767*

Brand Names: U.S. BiDil®

Generic Availability (U.S.) No

Pharmacologic Category Vasodilator

Use Treatment of heart failure, adjunct to standard therapy, in self-identified African-Americans

Local Anesthetic/Vasoconstrictor Precautions No information available to require special precautions

Effects on Dental Treatment No significant effects or complications reported

Effects on Bleeding No information available to require special precautions

Adverse Effects The following events were reported in the A-HeFT Study using the combination isosorbide dinitrate/hydralazine product. See individual drug monographs for additional information.

>10%:

Cardiovascular: Chest pain (16%)

Central nervous system: Headache (50%), dizziness (32%)

Neuromuscular & skeletal: Weakness (14%)

1% to 10%:

Cardiovascular: Hypotension (8%), palpitation (4%), ventricular tachycardia (4%), tachycardia (2%)

Central nervous system: Malaise (1%), somnolence (1%)

Dermatologic: Alopecia (1%), angioedema (1%)

Endocrine & metabolic: Hyperglycemia (4%), hyperlipidemia (3%), hypercholesterolemia (1%)

Gastrointestinal: Nausea (10%), vomiting (4%)

Hepatic: Cholecystitis (1%)

Neuromuscular & skeletal: Paresthesia (4%), arthralgia (1%), myalgia (1%), tendon disorder (1%)

Ocular: Amblyopia (3%)

Respiratory: Bronchitis (8%), sinusitis (4%), rhinitis (4%)

Miscellaneous: Allergic reaction (1%), diaphoresis (1%)

Dosage Oral: Adults: Initial: 1 tablet 3 times/day; may titrate to a maximum dose of 2 tablets 3 times/day

Dosage adjustment for toxicity: If patient experiences intolerable side effects, dose may be reduced to as little as one-half tablet 3 times/day; dose should be titrated upward as soon as tolerated.

Dosage adjustment in renal impairment: No dosage adjustment provided in manufacturer's labeling (has not been studied).

Dosage adjustment in hepatic impairment: No dosage adjustment provided in manufacturer's labeling (has not been studied).

Mechanism of Action

Hydralazine: Direct vasodilation of arterioles (with little effect on veins) resulting in decreased systemic resistance

Isosorbide Dinitrate: Stimulation of intracellular cyclic-GMP results in vascular smooth muscle relaxation of both arterial and venous vasculature with more prominent effects on the veins. Primarily reduces cardiac oxygen demand by decreasing preload (left ventricular end-diastolic pressure); may modestly reduce afterload. Additionally, coronary artery dilation improves collateral flow to ischemic regions.

Contraindications Hypersensitivity to organic nitrates; concurrent use with phosphodiesterase-5 inhibitors (sildenafil, tadalafil, or vardenafil)

Warnings/Precautions See individual agents.

Drug Interactions

Metabolism/Transport Effects Refer to individual components.

Avoid Concomitant Use

Avoid concomitant use of Isosorbide Dinitrate and Hydralazine with any of the following: Conivaptan; Phosphodiesterase 5 Inhibitors; Pimozide

Increased Effect/Toxicity

Isosorbide Dinitrate and Hydralazine may increase the levels/effects of: Amifostine; Antihypertensives; ARIPiprazole; Hypotensive Agents; Lomitapide; Pimozide; Prilocaine; RiTUXimab; Rosiglitazone

The levels/effects of Isosorbide Dinitrate and Hydralazine may be increased by: Alfuzosin; Conivaptan; CYP3A4 Inhibitors (Moderate); CYP3A4 Inhibitors (Strong); Dasatinib; Diazoxide; Herbs (Hypotensive Properties); Ivacaftor; MAO Inhibitors; Mifepristone; Pentoxifylline; Phosphodiesterase 5 Inhibitors; Prostacyclin Analogues

Decreased Effect

The levels/effects of Isosorbide Dinitrate and Hydralazine may be decreased by: CYP3A4 Inducers (Strong); Deferasirox; Herbs (CYP3A4 Inducers); Herbs (Hypertensive Properties); Methylphenidate; Nonsteroidal Anti-Inflammatory Agents; Tocilizumab; Yohimbine

Pharmacodynamics/Kinetics

Half-life Elimination Hydralazine: 4 hours; Isosorbide dinitrate: 2 hours

Time to Peak 1 hour (both agents)

Pregnancy Risk Factor C

Pregnancy Considerations See individual agents.

Lactation See individual agents.

Breast-Feeding Considerations See individual agents.

Dosage Forms

Tablet:

BiDil®: Isosorbide dinitrate 20 mg and hydralazine 37.5 mg

Isosorbide Mononitrate
(eye soe SOR bide mon oh NYE trate)

Related Information
Cardiovascular Diseases *on page 1492*
Isosorbide Dinitrate *on page 767*
Brand Names: U.S. Imdur®; Monoket® [DSC]
Brand Names: Canada Apo-ISMN®; Imdur®; PMS-ISMN; PRO-ISMN
Generic Availability (U.S.) Yes
Pharmacologic Category Antianginal Agent; Vasodilator
Use Prevention of angina pectoris
Local Anesthetic/Vasoconstrictor Precautions No information available to require special precautions
Effects on Dental Treatment No significant effects or complications reported
Effects on Bleeding No information available to require special precautions
Adverse Effects
>10%: Central nervous system: Headache (13% to 35%)
1% to 10%:
Cardiovascular: Angina (≤2%), flushing (≤2%)
Central nervous system: Dizziness (≤4%), fatigue (≤4%), pain (≤4%), emotional lability (≤2%)
Dermatologic: Pruritus (≤2%), rash (≤2%)
Gastrointestinal: Nausea (≤3%), abdominal pain (≤2%), diarrhea (≤2%)
Respiratory: Upper respiratory infection (≤4%), cough increased (≤2%)
Miscellaneous: Allergic reaction (≤2%)
Dosage Oral:
Adults:
Regular release tablet: Initial: 5-20 mg twice daily with the 2 doses given 7 hours apart (eg, 8 AM and 3 PM) to decrease tolerance development; patients initiating therapy with 5 mg twice daily (eg, small stature) should be titrated up to 10 mg twice daily in first 2-3 days.
Extended release tablet: Initial: 30-60 mg given once daily in the morning; titrate upward as needed, giving at least 3 days between increases; maximum daily single dose: 240 mg
Elderly: Start with lowest recommended adult dose.

Dosing adjustment in renal impairment: Dose adjustment not necessary
Hemodialysis: Dose supplementation is not necessary.
Peritoneal dialysis: Dose supplementation is not necessary.
Dosing adjustment in hepatic impairment: Dose adjustment not necessary

Note: Tolerance to nitrate effects develops with chronic exposure. Dose escalation does not overcome this effect. Tolerance can only be overcome by short periods of nitrate absence from the body. Short periods of nitrate withdrawal may help minimize tolerance. Recommended twice daily dosage regimens incorporate this interval. Administer sustained release tablet once daily in the morning.
Mechanism of Action Nitroglycerin and other nitrates form free radical nitric oxide. In smooth muscle, nitric oxide activates guanylate cyclase which increases guanosine 3'5' monophosphate (cGMP) leading to dephosphorylation of myosin light chains and smooth muscle relaxation. Produces a vasodilator effect on the peripheral veins and arteries with more prominent effects on the veins. Primarily reduces cardiac oxygen demand by decreasing preload (left ventricular end-diastolic pressure); may modestly reduce afterload; dilates coronary arteries and improves collateral flow to ischemic regions.
Contraindications Hypersensitivity to isosorbide mononitrate or any component of the formulation; hypersensitivity to organic nitrates; concurrent use with phosphodiesterase-5 (PDE-5) inhibitors (sildenafil, tadalafil, or vardenafil)
Warnings/Precautions Avoid use in hypertrophic cardiomyopathy with outflow tract obstruction; nitrates may reduce preload, exacerbating obstruction and cause hypotension or syncope and/or worsening of heart failure (Gersh, 2011). Use with caution in volume depletion, moderate hypotension, and extreme caution with inferior wall MI and suspected right ventricular infarctions. Nitrates may precipitate or aggravate increased intracranial pressure and subsequently may worsen clinical outcomes in patients with neurologic injury (eg, intracranial hemorrhage, traumatic brain injury). Postural hypotension, transient episodes of weakness, dizziness, or syncope may occur even with small doses; ethanol accentuates these effects; tolerance and cross-tolerance to nitrate antianginal and hemodynamic effects may occur during prolonged isosorbide mononitrate therapy; (minimized by using the smallest effective dose, by alternating coronary vasodilators or offering drug-free intervals of as little as 12 hours). Excessive doses may result in severe headache, blurred vision, or xerostomia; increased anginal symptoms may be a result of dosage increases. Avoid concurrent use with PDE-5 inhibitors (eg, sildenafil, tadalafil, vardenafil). When nitrate administration becomes medically necessary, may administer nitrates only if 24 hours have elapsed after use of sildenafil or vardenafil (48 hours after tadalafil use) (O'Connor, 2010).
Drug Interactions
Metabolism/Transport Effects Substrate of CYP3A4 (major); **Note:** Assignment of Major/Minor substrate status based on clinically relevant drug interaction potential
Avoid Concomitant Use
Avoid concomitant use of Isosorbide Mononitrate with any of the following: Conivaptan; Phosphodiesterase 5 Inhibitors
Increased Effect/Toxicity
Isosorbide Mononitrate may increase the levels/effects of: Hypotensive Agents; Prilocaine; Rosiglitazone

The levels/effects of Isosorbide Mononitrate may be increased by: Conivaptan; CYP3A4 Inhibitors (Moderate); CYP3A4 Inhibitors (Strong); Dasatinib; Ivacaftor; Mifepristone; Phosphodiesterase 5 Inhibitors
Decreased Effect
The levels/effects of Isosorbide Mononitrate may be decreased by: CYP3A4 Inducers (Strong); Deferasirox; Herbs (CYP3A4 Inducers); Tocilizumab
Ethanol/Nutrition/Herb Interactions Ethanol: Caution with ethanol (may increase risk of hypotension).
Pharmacodynamics/Kinetics
Onset of Action 30-60 minutes
Duration of Action Immediate release: ≥6 hours (Thadani, 1987); Extended release: ≥12-24 hours (Anderson, 2007)
Half-life Elimination Mononitrate: ~5-6 hours
Pregnancy Risk Factor B/C (manufacturer dependent)

▶

Pregnancy Considerations Teratogenic effects were not observed in animal reproduction studies. Adverse events in the offspring were observed with use later in pregnancy at doses that were also maternally toxic.

Lactation Excretion in breast milk unknown/use caution

Dosage Forms
Tablet, oral: 10 mg, 20 mg
Tablet, extended release, oral: 30 mg, 60 mg, 120 mg
Imdur®: 30 mg, 60 mg, 120 mg

ISOtretinoin (eye soe TRET i noyn)

Brand Names: U.S. Absorica™; Amnesteem®; Claravis™; Myorisan™; Sotret®; Zenatane™
Brand Names: Canada Accutane®; Clarus™
Pharmacologic Category Acne Products; Antineoplastic Agent, Miscellaneous; Retinoic Acid Derivative
Use Treatment of severe recalcitrant nodular acne unresponsive to conventional therapy
Unlabeled Use Management of moderate degrees of treatment-resistant acne, management of acne that produces physical or psychological scarring; treatment of cutaneous T-cell lymphomas (mycosis fungoides and Sézary syndrome); prevention of squamous cell skin cancers (in high-risk patients); treatment of high-risk neuroblastoma in children
Local Anesthetic/Vasoconstrictor Precautions No information available to require special precautions
Effects on Dental Treatment Key adverse event(s) related to dental treatment: Xerostomia and changes in salivation (normal salivary flow resumes upon discontinuation).
Effects on Bleeding No information available to require special precautions
Adverse Effects Frequency not always defined.
Cardiovascular: Chest pain, edema, flushing, palpitation, stroke, syncope, tachycardia, vascular thrombotic disease
Central nervous system: Aggressive behavior, depression, dizziness, drowsiness, emotional instability, fatigue, headache, insomnia, lethargy, malaise, nervousness, paresthesia, pseudotumor cerebri, psychosis, seizure, stroke, suicidal ideation, suicide attempts, suicide, violent behavior
Dermatologic: Abnormal wound healing acne fulminans, alopecia, bruising, cheilitis, cutaneous allergic reactions, dry nose, dry skin, eczema, eruptive xanthomas, facial erythema, fragility of skin, hair abnormalities, hirsutism, hyperpigmentation, hypopigmentation, increased sunburn susceptibility, nail dystrophy, paronychia, peeling of palms, peeling of soles, photoallergic reactions, photosensitizing reactions, pruritus, purpura, rash
Endocrine & metabolic: Triglycerides increased (25%), abnormal menses, blood glucose increased, cholesterol increased, HDL decreased, hyperuricemia
Gastrointestinal: Bleeding and inflammation of the gums, colitis, esophagitis, esophageal ulceration, inflammatory bowel disease, nausea, nonspecific gastrointestinal symptoms, pancreatitis, weight loss, xerostomia
Genitourinary: Nonspecific urogenital findings
Hematologic: Agranulocytosis (rare), anemia, neutropenia, pyogenic granuloma, thrombocytopenia
Hepatic: Alkaline phosphatase increased, ALT increased, AST increased, GGTP increased, hepatitis, LDH increased

Neuromuscular & skeletal: Back pain (29% in pediatric patients), arthralgia, arthritis, bone abnormalities, bone mineral density decreased, calcification of tendons and ligaments, CPK increased, myalgia, premature epiphyseal closure, skeletal hyperostosis, tendonitis, weakness
Ocular: Conjunctivitis (4%), blepharitis (1%), chalazion (1%), hordeolum (1%), cataracts, color vision disorder, corneal opacities, eyelid inflammation, keratitis, night vision decreased, optic neuritis, photophobia, visual disturbances
Otic: Hearing impairment, tinnitus
Renal: Glomerulonephritis, hematuria, proteinuria, pyuria, vasculitis
Respiratory: Bronchospasms, epistaxis, respiratory infection, voice alteration, Wegener's granulomatosis
Miscellaneous: Allergic reactions, anaphylactic reactions, disseminated herpes simplex, diaphoresis, infection, lymphadenopathy
General Dosage Range Dosage adjustments recommended in patients with hepatic impairment
Oral:
Children 12-17 years: 0.5-1 mg/kg/day in 2 divided doses
Adults: 0.5-2 mg/kg/day in 2 divided doses
Mechanism of Action Reduces sebaceous gland size and reduces sebum production in acne treatment; in neuroblastoma, decreases cell proliferation and induces differentiation
Pharmacodynamics/Kinetics
Half-life Elimination Terminal: Parent drug: 21 hours; Metabolite: 21-24 hours
Time to Peak Serum: 3-5 hours
Pregnancy Risk Factor X
Pregnancy Considerations Major fetal abnormalities (both internal and external), spontaneous abortion and premature births have been reported. **[U.S. Boxed Warnings]: Birth defects (facial, eye, ear, skull, central nervous system, cardiovascular, thymus and parathyroid gland abnormalities) have been noted following isotretinoin exposure during pregnancy and the risk for severe birth defects is high, with any dose or even with short treatment duration. Low IQ scores have also been reported. The risk for spontaneous abortion and premature births is increased. Because of the high likelihood of teratogenic effects, all patients (male and female), prescribers, wholesalers, and dispensing pharmacists must register and be active in the iPLEDGE™ risk evaluation and mitigation strategy (REMS) program; do not prescribe isotretinoin for women who are or who are likely to become pregnant while using the drug. If pregnancy occurs during therapy, isotretinoin should be discontinued immediately and the patient referred to an obstetrician-gynecologist specializing in reproductive toxicity.** This medication is contraindicated in females of childbearing potential unless they are able to comply with the guidelines of the iPLEDGE™ pregnancy prevention program. Females of childbearing potential should not become pregnant during therapy or for 1 month following discontinuation of isotretinoin. Upon discontinuation of treatment, females of childbearing potential should have a pregnancy test after their last dose and again one month after their last dose. Two forms of contraception should be continued during this time. Any pregnancies should be reported to the iPLEDGE™ program (www.ipledgeprogram.com or 866-495-0654).

Prescribing and Access Restrictions As a requirement of the REMS program, access to this medication is restricted. All patients (male and female), prescribers, wholesalers, and dispensing pharmacists must register and be active in the iPLEDGE™ risk management program, designed to eliminate fetal exposures to isotretinoin. This program covers all isotretinoin products (brand and generic). The iPLEDGE™ program requires that all patients meet qualification criteria and monthly program requirements (eg, pregnancy testing). Healthcare providers can only prescribe a maximum 30-day supply at each monthly visit and must counsel patients on the iPLEDGE™ program requirements and confirm counseling via the iPLEDGE™ automated system. Registration, activation, and additional information are provided at www.ipledgeprogram.com or by calling 866-495-0654.

Isoxsuprine (eye SOKS syoo preen)

Pharmacologic Category Vasodilator
Use Treatment of peripheral vascular diseases, such as arteriosclerosis obliterans, thromboangiitis obliterans (Buerger's disease), and Raynaud's disease; relief of symptoms associated with cerebrovascular insufficiency

Note: More appropriate therapies (medical or surgical) should be considered; efficacy of isoxsuprine in the treatment of these conditions has not been well established.
Local Anesthetic/Vasoconstrictor Precautions No information available to require special precautions
Effects on Dental Treatment May enhance effects of other vasodilators.
Effects on Bleeding No information available to require special precautions
Adverse Effects Frequency not defined.
Cardiovascular: Chest pain, hypotension, tachycardia
Central nervous system: Dizziness
Dermatologic: Rash
Gastrointestinal: Abdominal distress, nausea, vomiting
General Dosage Range Oral:
Adults: 10-20 mg 3-4 times/day
Elderly: Start with lower dose due to potential hypotension.
Mechanism of Action In studies on normal human subjects, isoxsuprine increases muscle blood flow, but skin blood flow is usually unaffected. Rather than increasing muscle blood flow by beta-receptor stimulation, isoxsuprine probably has a direct action on vascular smooth muscle. The generally accepted mechanism of action of isoxsuprine on the uterus is beta-adrenergic stimulation. Isoxsuprine was shown to inhibit prostaglandin synthetase at high serum concentrations, with low concentrations there was an increase in the P-G synthesis.
Pharmacodynamics/Kinetics
Time to Peak Time to peak, serum: ~1 hour; serum concentrations maintained for at least 3 hours
Pregnancy Considerations Isoxsuprine crosses the placenta. Adverse effects (eg, hypocalcemia, hypoglycemia, hypotension, and ileus) requiring treatment have been observed in infants born to mothers who received isoxsuprine during pregnancy. Maternal and fetal tachycardia have occurred with use and pulmonary edema has been reported with maternal use of beta stimulants (Brazy, 1979; Brazy, 1981). Although isoxsuprine has been evaluated for the treatment of premature labor, use for this indication is not currently recommended (ACOG, 2012).

Isradipine (iz RA di peen)

Related Information
Calcium Channel Blockers and Gingival Hyperplasia *on page 1640*
Cardiovascular Diseases *on page 1492*
Brand Names: U.S. DynaCirc CR® [DSC]
Pharmacologic Category Calcium Channel Blocker; Calcium Channel Blocker, Dihydropyridine
Use Treatment of hypertension
Unlabeled Use Pediatric hypertension
Local Anesthetic/Vasoconstrictor Precautions Isradipine is one of the drugs confirmed to prolong the QT interval and is accepted as having a risk of causing torsade de pointes. The risk of drug-induced torsade de pointes is extremely low when a single QT interval prolonging drug is prescribed. In terms of epinephrine, it is not known what effect vasoconstrictors in the local anesthetic regimen will have in patients with a known history of congenital prolonged QT interval or in patients taking any medication that prolongs the QT interval. Until more information is obtained, it is suggested that the clinician consult with the physician prior to the use of a vasoconstrictor in suspected patients, and that the vasoconstrictor (epinephrine, mepivacaine and levonordefrin [Carbocaine® 2% with Neo-Cobefrin®]) be used with caution.
Effects on Dental Treatment Unlike other calcium channel blockers, information is sparse as to whether isradipine causes gingival hyperplasia. Consultation with physician is suggested if hyperplasia is observed in patients taking isradipine.
Effects on Bleeding No information available to require special precautions
Adverse Effects Percentages reported with capsule formulation.
>10%: Central nervous system: Headache (dose related 2% to 22%)
1% to 10%:
    Cardiovascular: Edema (dose related 1% to 9%), palpitation (dose related 1% to 5%), flushing (dose related 1% to 5%), tachycardia (1% to 3%), chest pain (2% to 3%)
    Central nervous system: Dizziness (2% to 8%), fatigue (dose related 1% to 9%)
    Dermatologic: Rash (2%)
    Gastrointestinal: Nausea (1% to 5%), abdominal discomfort (≤3%), vomiting (≤1%), diarrhea (≤3%)
    Neuromuscular & skeletal: Weakness (≤1%)
    Renal: Urinary frequency (1% to 3%)
    Respiratory: Dyspnea (1% to 3%)
General Dosage Range Dosage adjustment recommended in patients with hepatic or renal impairment
Oral: *Adults:*
    Capsule: Initial: 2.5 mg twice daily; Usual range: 2.5-10 mg/day
    Controlled release tablet: Initial: 5 mg once daily; Maintenance: 5-20 mg once daily (maximum: 20 mg/day)
Mechanism of Action Inhibits calcium ion from entering the "slow channels" or select voltage-sensitive areas of vascular smooth muscle and myocardium during depolarization, producing a relaxation of coronary vascular smooth muscle and coronary vasodilation; increases myocardial oxygen delivery in patients with vasospastic angina
Pharmacodynamics/Kinetics
Onset of Action Immediate release: 2-3 hours
Duration of Action Immediate release: >12 hours

Half-life Elimination Terminal: 8 hours
Time to Peak Serum: 1-1.5 hours
Pregnancy Risk Factor C
Pregnancy Considerations Teratogenic effects were not observed in animal studies. Israpidine crosses the human placenta. There are no adequate and well-controlled studies in pregnant women.

Dental Comment Isradipine is known to prolong the QT interval. The QT interval is measured as the time and distance between the Q point of the QRS complex and the end of the T wave in the ECG tracing. After adjustment for heart rate, the QT interval is defined as prolonged if it is more than 450 msec in men and 460 msec in women. A long QT syndrome was first described in the 1950s and 60s as a congenital syndrome involving QT interval prolongation and syncope and sudden death. Some of the congenital long QT syndromes were characterized by a peculiar electrocardiographic appearance of the QRS complex involving a premature atria beat followed by a pause, then a subsequent sinus beat showing marked QT prolongation and deformity. This type of cardiac arrhythmia was originally termed "torsade de pointes" (translated from the French as "twisting of the points"). Isradipine is considered as having a risk of causing torsade de pointes. Since it is not known what effect vasoconstrictors in the local anesthetic regimen will have in patients with a known history of congenital prolonged QT interval or in patients taking any medication that prolongs the QT interval, a medical consult is suggested.

Itraconazole (i tra KOE na zole)

Related Information
Fungal Infections *on page 1573*
Brand Names: U.S. Onmel™; Sporanox®
Brand Names: Canada Sporanox®
Generic Availability (U.S.) Yes: Capsule
Pharmacologic Category Antifungal Agent, Oral
Dental Use Treatment of susceptible fungal infections in immunocompromised and immunocompetent patients including blastomycosis and histoplasmosis; has activity against *Aspergillus, Candida, Coccidioides, Cryptococcus, Sporothrix,* and chromomycosis. Useful in superficial mycoses including dermatophytoses (eg, tinea capitis), pityriasis versicolor, sebopsoriasis, vaginal and chronic mucocutaneous candidiases; systemic mycoses including candidiasis, meningeal and disseminated cryptococcal infections, paracoccidioidomycosis, coccidioidomycoses; miscellaneous mycoses such as sporotrichosis, chromomycosis, leishmaniasis, fungal keratitis, alternariosis, zygomycosis.
Use
Oral capsules: Treatment of susceptible fungal infections in immunocompromised and immunocompetent patients including blastomycosis and histoplasmosis; indicated for aspergillosis (in patients intolerant/refractory to amphotericin B), and onychomycosis of the toenail and fingernail (in nonimmunocompromised patients)
Oral solution: Treatment of oral and esophageal candidiasis

Canadian labeling: Oral capsules: Additional indications (not in U.S. labeling): Treatment of oral and esophageal candidiasis; treatment of cutaneous and lymphatic sporotrichosis, chromomycosis, or paracoccidioidomycosis in immunocompetent and immunosuppressed patients; treatment of onychomycosis in immunosuppressed patients; treatment of dermatomycoses due to tinea pedis, tinea cruris, tinea corporis and of pityriasis versicolor in immunocompetent and immunocompromised patients in whom oral therapy is appropriate

Local Anesthetic/Vasoconstrictor Precautions No information available to require special precautions
Effects on Dental Treatment No significant effects or complications reported
Effects on Bleeding No information available to require special precautions
Adverse Effects
>10%: Gastrointestinal: Nausea (3% to 11%), diarrhea (3% to 11%)
1% to 10%:
Cardiovascular: Edema (4%), hypertension (3%), chest pain (3%)
Central nervous system: Headache (4% to 10%), fever (2% to 7%), dizziness (2% to 4%), anxiety (3%), depression (2% to 3%), fatigue (2% to 3%), pain (2% to 3%), malaise (1% to 3%), dreams abnormal (2%)
Dermatologic: Rash (3% to 9%), pruritus (≤5%)
Endocrine & metabolic: Hypertriglyceridemia (≤3%), hypokalemia (2%)
Gastrointestinal: Vomiting (5% to 7%), abdominal pain (2% to 6%), dyspepsia (≤4%), flatulence (≤4%), gingivitis (3%), stomatitis (ulcerative) (≤3%), constipation (2% to 3%), appetite increased (2%), gastritis (2%), gastroenteritis (2%)
Hepatic: LFTs abnormal (≤4%)
Neuromuscular & skeletal: Bursitis (3%), myalgia (≤3%), tremor (2%), weakness (≤2%)
Renal: Cystitis (3%), urinary tract infection (3%)
Respiratory: Rhinitis (5% to 9%), upper respiratory tract infection (8%), sinusitis (2% to 7%), cough (4%), dyspnea (2%), pharyngitis (≤2%), pneumonia (2%), sputum increased (2%)
Miscellaneous: Diaphoresis increased (3%), herpes zoster (2%)
Dental Usual Dosage Oropharyngeal candidiasis: Adults: Oral solution: 200 mg once daily for 1-2 weeks; in patients unresponsive or refractory to fluconazole: 100 mg twice daily (clinical response expected in 1-2 weeks)
Dosage
Children: Oral: Manufacturer labeling states that a small number of patients 3-16 years of age have been treated with 100 mg/day for systemic fungal infections with no serious adverse effects reported. A dose of 5 mg/kg once daily was used in a pharmacokinetic study using the oral solution in patients 6 months to 12 years; duration of study was 2 weeks.

Indication-specific dosing:
Infants and Children (HIV-exposed/-positive; unlabeled use; CDC, 2009a): **Note:** Doses >200 mg daily should be administered in 2 divided doses.
Candidiasis:
Oropharyngeal: Oral solution: 2.5 mg/kg/dose twice daily (maximum: 200 mg daily [400 mg daily if fluconazole-refractory]) for 7-14 days
Esophageal: Oral solution: 5 mg/kg/day once daily or divided twice daily for 4-21 days
Coccidioidomycosis:
Treatment: Oral: 5-10 mg/kg/dose twice daily for 3 days, followed by 2-5 mg/kg/dose orally twice daily (maximum: 400 mg daily)
Relapse prevention: Oral: 2-5 mg/kg/dose twice daily (maximum: 400 mg daily)

Cryptococcus: *Relapse prevention:* Oral solution: 5 mg/kg/dose once daily (maximum: 200 mg daily)

Histoplasmosis:

Treatment of mild disseminated disease: Oral solution: 2-5 mg/kg/dose 3 times daily for 3 days (9 doses), followed by twice daily for 12 months (maximum: 200 mg per dose)

Consolidation treatment for moderate-severe to severe disseminated disease, including CNS infection (following appropriate induction therapy): 2-5 mg/kg/dose 3 times daily for 3 days, followed by 2-5 mg/kg/dose (maximum: 200 mg per dose) twice daily for 12 months for non-CNS-disseminated disease or for ≥12 months for CNS infection

Relapse prevention: Oral solution: 5 mg/kg/dose twice daily (maximum: 400 mg/day)

Adults: **Note:** Doses >200 mg daily should be administered in 2 divided doses.

Aspergillosis: 200-400 mg daily. **Note:** For life-threatening infections, administer a loading dose of 200 mg 3 times daily (total: 600 mg daily) for the first 3 days of therapy. Continue treatment for at least 3 months and until clinical and laboratory evidence suggest that infection has resolved.

Aspergillosis, invasive (salvage therapy): Duration of therapy should be a minimum of 6-12 weeks or throughout period of immunosuppression: Oral: 200-400 mg daily; **Note:** 2008 IDSA guidelines recommend 600 mg/day for 3 days, followed by 400 mg daily (Walsh, 2008)

Appropriate use: Itraconazole should **NOT** be used for voriconazole-refractory aspergillosis since the same antifungal and/or resistance mechanism(s) may be shared by both agents. Itraconazole oral solution and capsule formulations are not bioequivalent or interchangeable. Due to variable bioavailability of oral preparations, therapeutic drug monitoring is advisable (Walsh, 2008).

Aspergillosis, allergic (ABPA, sinusitis): 200 mg/day; may be used in conjunction with corticosteroids (Walsh, 2008)

Blastomycosis: Initial: 200 mg once daily; if no clinical improvement or evidence of progressive infection, may increase dose in increments of 100 mg up to maximum of 400 mg daily. **Note:** For life-threatening infections, administer a loading dose of 200 mg 3 times daily (total 600 mg/day) for the first 3 days of therapy. Continue treatment for at least 3 months and until clinical and laboratory evidence suggest that infection has resolved.

Alternative dosing (Chapman, 2008): 200 mg 3 times daily for 3 days, then 200 mg twice daily for 6-12 months; in moderately-severe to severe infection, therapy should be initiated with ~2 weeks of amphotericin B.

Candidiasis:

Esophageal:

Oral solution: 100-200 mg once daily for a minimum of 3 weeks; continue dosing for 2 weeks after resolution of symptoms

Oral capsules: Canadian labeling (not in U.S. labeling): 100 mg once daily for 4 weeks; increase dose to 200 mg once daily in patients with AIDS and neutropenic patients

Oropharyngeal:

Oral solution: 200 mg once daily for 1-2 weeks; in patients unresponsive or refractory to fluconazole: 100 mg twice daily (clinical response expected in 2-4 weeks)

Oral capsules: Canadian labeling (not in U.S. labeling): 100 mg once daily for 2 weeks; increase dose to 200 mg once daily in patients with AIDS and neutropenic patients

Chromomycosis: Canadian labeling (not in U.S. labeling): 200 mg once daily for 6 months (when due to *Fonsecaea pedrosoli*) or 100 mg once daily for 3 months (when due to *Cladosporium carrioni*)

Coccidioidomycosis (nonprogressive, nondisseminated disease): 200 mg twice daily or 3 times/day (Galgiani, 2005)

Histoplasmosis: Manufacturer labeling: Initial: 200 mg once daily; if no clinical improvement or evidence of progressive infection, may increase dose in increments of 100 mg up to maximum of 400 mg daily. **Note:** For life-threatening infections, administer a loading dose of 200 mg 3 times daily (total: 600 mg daily) for the first 3 days of therapy. Continue treatment for at least 3 months and until clinical and laboratory evidence suggest that infection has resolved.

Alternative dosing (Wheat, 2007): 200 mg 3 times daily for 3 days, then 200 mg twice daily (or once daily in mild-moderate disease) for 6-12 weeks in mild-moderate disease or ≥12 months in progressive disseminated or chronic cavitary pulmonary histoplasmosis; in moderately-severe to severe infection, therapy should be initiated with ~2 weeks of a lipid formation of amphotericin B.

Long-term suppression therapy: 200 mg daily (CDC, 2009b)

Meningitis:

Coccidioides: 400-600 mg/day (Galgiani, 2005)

Coccidioides, HIV-positive (unlabeled use): 200 mg 3 times/day for 3 days, then 200 mg twice daily; maintenance: 200 mg twice daily life-long (CDC, 2009b)

Appropriate use: Fluconazole is preferred for meningeal infections (CDC, 2009b; Galgiani, 2005)

Onychomycosis: 200 mg once daily for 12 consecutive weeks; alternative "pulse-dosing" may be considering for fingernail involvement only: 200 mg twice daily for 1 week; repeat 1-week course after 3-week off-time

Onychomycosis (toenails with or without fingernail involvement): Canadian labeling (not in U.S. labeling): "Pulse-dosing": 200 mg twice daily for 1 week; repeat 1-week course twice with 3-week off-time between each course

Paracoccidioidomycosis: Canadian labeling (not in U.S. labeling): 100 mg once daily for 6 months

Penicilliosis, HIV-positive (unlabeled use): 400 mg daily for 8 weeks (mild disease) or 10 weeks (severe infections). In severely-ill patients, initiate therapy with 2 weeks of amphotericin B. Maintenance: 200 mg daily (CDC, 2009b)

Pityriasis versicolor: Canadian labeling (not in U.S. labeling): 200 mg once daily for 7 days

Pneumonia:

Coccidioides: Mild-to-moderate: 200 mg twice daily

Coccidioides, HIV-positive (focal pneumonia): 200 mg 3 times/day for 3 days, then 200 mg twice daily (CDC, 2009b)

Sporotrichosis:

Lymphocutaneous: 100-200 mg daily for 3-6 months (Kauffman, 2007)

Canadian labeling (not in U.S. labeling): 100 mg once daily for 3 months

Osteoarticular and pulmonary: 200 mg twice daily for ≥1 years (may use amphotericin B initially for stabilization) (Kauffman, 2007)

Tinea corporis or tinea cruris: Canadian labeling (not in U.S. labeling): 100 mg once daily for 14 consecutive days or 200 mg once daily for 7 consecutive days. **Note:** Equivalency between regimens not established.

Tinea pedis: Canadian labeling (not in U.S. labeling): 100 mg once daily for 28 consecutive days or 200 mg twice daily for 7 consecutive days. **Note:** Equivalency between regimens not established. Patients with chronic resistant infection may benefit from lower dose and extended treatment time (100 mg once daily for 28 days).

Dosing adjustment in renal impairment: The manufacturer's labeling states to use with caution in patients with renal impairment. Limited data suggests that no dosage adjustments are required in renal impairment; wide variations observed in plasma concentrations versus time profiles in patients with uremia, or receiving hemodialysis or continuous ambulatory peritoneal dialysis (Boelaert, 1988).

Dosing adjustment in hepatic impairment: No dosage adjustment provided in manufacturer's labeling; however, use caution and monitor closely for signs/symptoms of toxicity.

Mechanism of Action Interferes with cytochrome P450 activity, decreasing ergosterol synthesis (principal sterol in fungal cell membrane) and inhibiting cell membrane formation

Contraindications Hypersensitivity to itraconazole (use caution in patients with a history of hypersensitivity to other azoles), any component of the formulation; concurrent administration with cisapride, dofetilide, ergot derivatives, felodipine, levomethadyl, lovastatin, methadone, midazolam (oral), nisoldipine, pimozide, quinidine, simvastatin, or triazolam; treatment of onychomycosis (or other non-life-threatening indications) in patients with evidence of ventricular dysfunction, heart failure (HF) or a history of HF; treatment of onychomycosis in patients who are pregnant or intend on becoming pregnant

Canadian labeling: Oral capsule: Additional contraindications (not in U.S. labeling): Concurrent administration with eletriptan; treatment of dermatomycosis (tinea pedis, tinea cruris, tinea corporis) and of pityriasis versicolor in patients who are pregnant or intend on becoming pregnant

Warnings/Precautions [U.S. Boxed Warning]: Negative inotropic effects have been observed following intravenous administration. Discontinue or reassess use if signs or symptoms of HF (heart failure) occur during treatment. [U.S. Boxed Warning]: Use is contraindicated for treatment of onychomycosis in patients with ventricular dysfunction or a history of HF. HF has been reported, particularly in patients receiving a total daily oral dose of 400 mg. Use with caution in patients with risk factors for HF (COPD, renal failure, edematous disorders, ischemic or valvular disease). Discontinue if signs or symptoms of HF or neuropathy occur during treatment. Due to potential toxicity, the manufacturer recommends confirmation of diagnosis testing of nail specimens prior to treatment of onychomycosis.

[U.S. Boxed Warning]: Serious cardiovascular adverse events including, QT prolongation, ventricular tachycardia, torsade de pointes, cardiac arrest and/or sudden death have been observed due to itraconazole-induced increased serum concentrations of the following: cisapride, dofetilide, ergot alkaloids (dihydroergotamine, ergonovine, ergotamine, methylergonovine), felodipine, levomethadyl, lovastatin, methadone, midazolam (oral), nisoldipine, pimozide, simvastatin, quinidine, or triazolam; concurrent use contraindicated.

Calcium channel blockers (CCBs) may cause additive negative inotropic effects when used concurrently with itraconazole. Itraconazole may also inhibit the metabolism of CCBs. Use caution with concurrent use of itraconazole and CCBs due to an increased risk of HF. Concurrent use of itraconazole and nisoldipine is contraindicated.

Use with caution in patients with renal impairment. Rare cases of serious hepatotoxicity (including liver failure and death) have been reported (including some cases occurring within the first week of therapy); hepatotoxicity was reported in some patients without pre-existing liver disease or risk factors. Use with caution in patients with pre-existing hepatic impairment; monitor liver function closely and dosage adjustment may be warranted. Not recommended for use in patients with active liver disease, elevated liver enzymes, or prior hepatotoxic reactions to other drugs unless the expected benefit exceeds the risk of hepatotoxicity. Transient or permanent hearing loss has been reported. Quinidine (a contraindicated drug) was used concurrently in several of these cases. Hearing loss usually resolves after discontinuation, but may persist in some patients.

Large differences in itraconazole pharmacokinetic parameters have been observed in cystic fibrosis patients receiving the solution; if a patient with cystic fibrosis does not respond to therapy, alternate therapies should be considered. Due to differences in bioavailability, oral capsules and oral solution cannot be used interchangeably. Only the oral solution has proven efficacy for oral and esophageal candidiasis. Initiation of treatment with oral solution is not recommended in patients at immediate risk for systemic candidiasis (eg, patients with severe neutropenia).

Drug Interactions

Metabolism/Transport Effects Substrate of CYP3A4 (major); **Note:** Assignment of Major/Minor substrate status based on clinically relevant drug interaction potential; **Inhibits** CYP3A4 (strong), P-glycoprotein

Avoid Concomitant Use

Avoid concomitant use of Itraconazole with any of the following: Ado-Trastuzumab Emtansine; Alfuzosin; Aliskiren; Apixaban; Avanafil; Axitinib; Bosutinib; Cabozantinib; Cisapride; Conivaptan; Crizotinib; CYP3A4 Inducers (Strong); Dihydroergotamine; Dofetilide; Dronedarone; Eletriptan; Eplerenone; Ergoloid Mesylates; Ergonovine; Ergotamine; Everolimus; Felodipine; Fluticasone (Oral Inhalation); Halofantrine; Ivabradine; Lapatinib; Lomitapide; Lovastatin; Lurasidone; Methadone; Methylergonovine; Midazolam; Nevirapine; Nilotinib; Nisoldipine; Pimozide; Pomalidomide; QuiNIDine; Ranolazine; Red Yeast Rice; Regorafenib; Rivaroxaban; RomiDEPsin; Salmeterol; Silodosin; Simvastatin; Tamsulosin; Ticagrelor; Tolvaptan; Topotecan; Toremifene; VinCRIStine (Liposomal)

Increased Effect/Toxicity

Itraconazole may increase the levels/effects of: Ado-Trastuzumab Emtansine; Alfentanil; Alfuzosin; Aliskiren; Almotriptan; Alosetron; Apixaban; Aprepitant; ARIPiprazole; AtorvaSTATin; Avanafil; Axitinib; Bedaquiline; Benzodiazepines (metabolized by oxidation); Boceprevir; Bortezomib; Bosentan; Bosutinib; Brentuximab Vedotin; Brinzolamide; Budesonide (Nasal); Budesonide (Systemic, Oral Inhalation); BusPIRone; Busulfan; Cabozantinib; Calcium Channel Blockers; CarBAMazepine; Cardiac Glycosides; Cilostazol; Cisapride; Cobicistat; Colchicine; Conivaptan; Corticosteroids (Orally Inhaled); Corticosteroids (Systemic); Crizotinib; CycloSPORINE (Systemic); CYP3A4 Substrates; Dabigatran Etexilate; Darunavir; Dienogest; Dihydroergotamine; DOCEtaxel; Dofetilide; Dronedarone; Dutasteride; Eletriptan; Elvitegravir; Enzalutamide; Eplerenone; Ergoloid Mesylates; Ergonovine; Ergotamine; Erlotinib; Eszopiclone; Etravirine; Everolimus; Felodipine; FentaNYL; Fesoterodine; Fexofenadine; Fluticasone (Nasal); Fluticasone (Oral Inhalation); Fosamprenavir; Fosaprepitant; Fosphenytoin; Gefitinib; GuanFACINE; Halofantrine; Highest Risk QTc-Prolonging Agents; Iloperidone; Imatinib; Indinavir; Irinotecan; Ivabradine; Ivacaftor; Ixabepilone; Lapatinib; Lomitapide; Losartan; Lovastatin; Lumefantrine; Lurasidone; Macrolide Antibiotics; Maraviroc; Methadone; Methylergonovine; MethylPREDNISolone; Midazolam; Mifepristone; Moderate Risk QTc-Prolonging Agents; Nilotinib; Nisoldipine; Ospemifene; Paliperidone; Paricalcitol; Pazopanib; P-glycoprotein/ABCB1 Substrates; Phenytoin; Pimecrolimus; Pimozide; Pomalidomide; Ponatinib; Pravastatin; Propafenone; Prucalopride; QuiNIDine; Ramelteon; Ranolazine; Red Yeast Rice; Regorafenib; Repaglinide; Rifamycin Derivatives; Rivaroxaban; RomiDEPsin; Rosuvastatin; Ruxolitinib; Salmeterol; Saquinavir; Saxagliptin; Sildenafil; Silodosin; Simvastatin; Sirolimus; Solifenacin; SORAfenib; SUNItinib; Tacrolimus (Systemic); Tacrolimus (Topical); Tadalafil; Tamsulosin; Telaprevir; Temsirolimus; Ticagrelor; Tofacitinib; Tolterodine; Tolvaptan; Topotecan; Toremifene; Vardenafil; Vemurafenib; Vilazodone; VinBLAStine; VinCRIStine; VinCRIStine (Liposomal); Vinorelbine; Vitamin K Antagonists; Ziprasidone; Zolpidem; Zuclopenthixol

The levels/effects of Itraconazole may be increased by: Boceprevir; Cobicistat; Darunavir; Etravirine; Fosamprenavir; Grapefruit Juice; Indinavir; Lopinavir; Macrolide Antibiotics; Ritonavir; Saquinavir; Telaprevir; Tipranavir

Decreased Effect

Itraconazole may decrease the levels/effects of: Amphotericin B; Ifosfamide; Prasugrel; Saccharomyces boulardii; Ticagrelor

The levels/effects of Itraconazole may be decreased by: Antacids; CYP3A4 Inducers (Strong); Deferasirox; Didanosine; Efavirenz; Etravirine; Fosphenytoin; H2-Antagonists; Herbs (CYP3A4 Inducers); Isoniazid; Nevirapine; Phenytoin; Proton Pump Inhibitors; Rifamycin Derivatives; Sucralfate; Tocilizumab

Ethanol/Nutrition/Herb Interactions

Food:

Capsules: Absorption enhanced by food and possibly by gastric acidity. Cola drinks have been shown to increase the absorption of the capsules in patients with achlorhydria or those taking H_2-receptor antagonists or other gastric acid suppressors. Grapefruit/grapefruit juice may increase serum levels. Management: Take capsules immediately after meals. Avoid grapefruit juice.

Solution: Food decreases the bioavailability and increases the time to peak concentration. Management: Take solution on an empty stomach 1 hour before or 2 hours after meals.

Herb/Nutraceutical: St John's wort may decrease itraconazole levels.

Dietary Considerations

Capsule: Take with food.

Solution: Take without food, if possible.

Pharmacodynamics/Kinetics

Half-life Elimination Oral: Single dose: ~21 hours; steady state: 64 hours; Cirrhosis (single dose): 37 hours (range 20-54 hours)

Time to Peak Plasma: Capsules: 3-5 hours; Oral solution: 2-3 hours

Pregnancy Risk Factor C

Pregnancy Considerations Dose related adverse events were observed in animal reproduction studies. Use is contraindicated for the treatment of onychomycosis during pregnancy. If used for the treatment of onychomycosis in women of reproductive potential, effective contraception should be used during treatment and for 2 months following treatment. Therapy should begin on the second or third day following menses. Congenital abnormalities have been reported during postmarketing surveillance, but a causal relationship has not been established.

Lactation Enters breast milk/not recommended

Product Availability Onmel™ 200 mg tablets: FDA approved November 2012; availability anticipated January 2013. Onmel™ is indicated for the treatment of onychomycosis of the toenail; consult prescribing information for additional information.

Dosage Forms

Capsule, oral: 100 mg
Sporanox®: 100 mg

Solution, oral:
Sporanox®: 10 mg/mL (150 mL)

Tablet, oral:
Onmel™: 200 mg

Ivacaftor (eye va KAF tor)

Brand Names: U.S. Kalydeco™

Brand Names: Canada Kalydeco™

Pharmacologic Category Cystic Fibrosis Transmembrane Conductance Regulator Potentiator

Use Treatment of cystic fibrosis (CF) in patients who have a G551D mutation in the cystic fibrosis transmembrane conductance regulator (CFTR) gene

Note: Not effective in patients with CF who are homozygous for the F508del mutation in the CTFR gene

Local Anesthetic/Vasoconstrictor Precautions No information available to require special precautions

Effects on Dental Treatment Key adverse event(s) related to dental treatment: Oropharyngeal pain has been reported

Effects on Bleeding No information available to require special precautions

Adverse Effects

>10%:

Central nervous system: Headache (4% to 24%)

Dermatologic: Rash (10% to 13%)

Gastrointestinal: Abdominal pain (16%), diarrhea (13%), nausea (10% to 12%)

Respiratory: Oropharyngeal pain (22%), upper respiratory tract infection (16% to 22%), nasal congestion (16% to 20%), nasopharyngitis (15%)

1% to 10%:

Central nervous system: Dizziness (5% to 9%)

Dermatologic: Acne (4% to 7%)

Endocrine & metabolic: Hyperglycemia (4% to 7%)

Hepatic: Transaminases increased (4% to 7%; >5 x ULN: 3%)

Neuromuscular & skeletal: Arthralgia (4% to 7%), musculoskeletal chest pain (4% to 7%), myalgia (4% to 7%)

Respiratory: Pharyngeal erythema (4% to 7%), pleuritic chest pain (4% to 7%), rhinitis (4% to 7%), sinus congestion (4% to 7%), wheezing (4% to 7%)

Miscellaneous: Bacteria in sputum (4% to 7%)

General Dosage Range Dosage adjustment recommended in patients with hepatic impairment or on concomitant therapy.

Oral: *Children ≥6 years and Adults:* 150 mg every 12 hours

Mechanism of Action Potentiates epithelial cell chloride ion transport of defective (G551D mutant) cell-surface CFTR protein thereby improving the regulation of salt and water absorption and secretion in various tissues (eg, lung, gastrointestinal tract).

Pharmacodynamics/Kinetics

Onset of Action FEV$_1$ increased, sweat chloride decreased within ~2 weeks

Half-life Elimination ~12 hours

Time to Peak ~4 hours

Pregnancy Risk Factor B

Pregnancy Considerations Adverse events were not observed in animal reproduction studies.

Ivermectin (Systemic) (eye ver MEK tin)

Brand Names: U.S. Stromectol®

Pharmacologic Category Anthelmintic

Use Treatment of the following infections: Strongyloidiasis of the intestinal tract due to the nematode parasite *Strongyloides stercoralis*. Onchocerciasis due to the immature form of the nematode parasite *Onchocerca volvulus*

Unlabeled Use Treatment of other parasitic infections, including *Ancylostoma braziliense, Ascaris lumbricoides, Sarcoptes scabiei, Gnathostoma spinigerum, Mansonella ozzardi, Mansonella streptocerca, Pediculus humanus capitis, Pediculus humanus corporis, Phthirus pubis, Trichuris trichiura, Wucheria bancrofti*

Local Anesthetic/Vasoconstrictor Precautions No information available to require special precautions

Effects on Dental Treatment No significant effects or complications reported

Effects on Bleeding No information available to require special precautions

Adverse Effects

>10%: Miscellaneous: Mazzotti-type reaction (with onchocerciasis): Pruritus (28%), fever (23%), skin involvement (23%; including edema/urticarial rash), lymph node tenderness (1% to 14%), lymph node enlargement (3% to 13%), arthralgia/synovitis (9%)

1% to 10%:

Cardiovascular: Tachycardia (4%), peripheral edema (3%), facial edema (1%), orthostatic hypotension (1%)

Central nervous system: Dizziness (3%)

Dermatologic: Pruritus (3%)

Gastrointestinal: Diarrhea (2%), nausea (2%)

Hematologic: Eosinophilia (3%), leukocytes decreased (3%), hemoglobin increased (1%)

Hepatic: ALT increased (2%), AST increased (2%)

General Dosage Range Oral: *Children ≥15 kg and Adults:* 150-200 mcg/kg as a single dose

Mechanism of Action Ivermectin is a semisynthetic anthelminthic agent; it binds selectively and with strong affinity to glutamate-gated chloride ion channels which occur in invertebrate nerve and muscle cells. This leads to increased permeability of cell membranes to chloride ions then hyperpolarization of the nerve or muscle cell, and death of the parasite.

Pharmacodynamics/Kinetics

Onset of Action

Peak effect in treatment of onchocerciasis: 3-6 months

Peak effect in treatment of strongyloides: 3 months

Half-life Elimination ~18 hours

Time to Peak ~4 hours

Pregnancy Risk Factor C

Pregnancy Considerations Teratogenic effects have been observed in animal reproduction studies; therefore, the manufacturer classifies ivermectin as pregnancy category C. Ivermectin is not recommended for use in pregnancy. Although studies during pregnancy are limited, several mass treatment programs have not identified an increased risk of adverse fetal, neonatal, or maternal outcomes following ivermectin use in the first and second trimesters.

Ivermectin (Topical) (eye ver MEK tin)

Brand Names: U.S. Sklice™

Pharmacologic Category Antiparasitic Agent, Topical; Pediculocide

Use Topical treatment of head lice (*Pediculus capitis*) infestation

Local Anesthetic/Vasoconstrictor Precautions No information available to require special precautions

Effects on Dental Treatment No significant effects or complications reported

Effects on Bleeding No information available to require special precautions

General Dosage Range Topical: *Children ≥6 months and Adults:* Apply sufficient amount (up to 1 tube) to completely cover dry scalp and hair; for single-dose use only

Mechanism of Action Ivermectin is a semisynthetic anthelminthic agent; it binds selectively and with strong affinity to glutamate-gated chloride ion channels which occur in invertebrate nerve and muscle cells. This leads to increased permeability of cell membranes to chloride ions then hyperpolarization of the nerve or muscle cell, and death of the parasite.

Pregnancy Risk Factor C

Pregnancy Considerations Teratogenic effects have been observed in animal reproduction studies following oral administration. Refer to the Ivermectin (Systemic) monograph for additional information. Systemic absorption is less following topical application than with oral administration.

Ixabepilone (ix ab EP i lone)

Brand Names: U.S. Ixempra®

Pharmacologic Category Antineoplastic Agent, Antimicrotubular; Antineoplastic Agent, Epothilone B Analog

Use Treatment of metastatic or locally-advanced breast cancer (refractory or resistant)

Unlabeled Use Treatment (second-line) of endometrial cancer

Local Anesthetic/Vasoconstrictor Precautions No information available to require special precautions

Effects on Dental Treatment Key adverse event(s) related to dental treatment: Stomatitis, mucositis, and taste perversion.

Effects on Bleeding Anemia and thrombocytopenia (grades 3/4: 2% to 5%) are dose-limiting toxicities. Medical consult recommended.

Adverse Effects Percentages reported with mono-therapy:

>10%:

Central nervous system: Headache (11%)

Dermatologic: Alopecia (48%)

Gastrointestinal: Nausea (42%), vomiting (29%), mucositis/stomatitis (29%), diarrhea (22%), anorexia (19%), constipation (16%), abdominal pain (13%)

Hematologic: Leukopenia (grade 3: 36%; grade 4: 13%), neutropenia (grade 3: 31%; grade 4: 23%)

Neuromuscular & skeletal: Peripheral neuropathy (63%; grades 3/4: 14%; grade 3/4 median onset: cycle 4), sensory neuropathy (62%; grades 3/4: 14%), weakness (56%), myalgia/arthralgia (49%), musculoskeletal pain (20%)

1% to 10%:

Cardiovascular: Edema (9%), chest pain (5%)

Central nervous system: Fever (8%), pain (8%), dizziness (7%), insomnia (5%)

Dermatologic: Nail disorder (9%), rash (9%), palmar-plantar erythrodysesthesia/hand-and-foot syndrome (8%), pruritus (6%), skin exfoliation (2%), hyperpigmentation (2%)

Endocrine & metabolic: Hot flush (6%), dehydration (2%)

Gastrointestinal: Gastroesophageal reflux disease (6%), taste perversion (6%), weight loss (6%)

Hematologic: Anemia (grade 3: 6%; grade 4: 2%), neutropenic fever (3%; grade 3: 3%), thrombocytopenia (grade 3: 5%; grade 4: 2%)

Neuromuscular & skeletal: Motor neuropathy (10%; grade 3: 1%)

Ocular: Lacrimation increased (4%)

Respiratory: Dyspnea (9%), upper respiratory tract infection (6%), cough (2%)

Miscellaneous: Hypersensitivity (5%; grade 3: 1%), infection (5%)

General Dosage Range Dosage adjustment recommended in patients with hepatic impairment or who develop toxicities

I.V.: *Adults:* 40 mg/m^2 every 3 weeks (maximum dose: 88 mg)

Mechanism of Action Epothilone B analog; binds to the beta-tubulin subunit of the microtubule, stabilizing microtubular promoting tubulin polymerization and stabilizing microtubular function, thus arresting the cell cycle (at the G2/M phase) and inducing apoptosis. Activity in taxane-resistant cells has been demonstrated.

Pharmacodynamics/Kinetics

Half-life Elimination ~52 hours

Time to Peak At the end of infusion (3 hours)

Pregnancy Risk Factor D

Pregnancy Considerations In animal studies, ixabepilone caused maternal toxicity and embryo/fetal toxicity at doses ~1/10 the human dose. There are no adequate and well-controlled studies in pregnant women. Women of childbearing potential should be advised to use effective contraception during treatment.

Japanese Encephalitis Virus Vaccine (Inactivated)

(jap a NEESE en sef a LYE tis VYE rus vak SEEN, in ak ti VAY ted)

Brand Names: U.S. Ixiaro®

Brand Names: Canada Ixiaro®

Pharmacologic Category Vaccine, Inactivated (Viral)

Use Active immunization against Japanese encephalitis Japanese encephalitis vaccine is not recommended for all persons traveling to or residing in Asia. The Advisory Committee on Immunization Practices (ACIP) recommends vaccination for:

- Persons spending ≥1 month in endemic areas during transmission season
- Research laboratory workers who may be exposed to the Japanese encephalitis virus

Vaccination may also be considered for the following:

- Travelers to areas with an ongoing outbreak
- Travelers spending <30 days in endemic areas during the transmission season and planning to go outside of urban areas and have an increased risk of exposure. For example, high-risk activities include extensive outdoor activity in rural areas especially at night; extensive outdoor activities such as camping, hiking, etc; staying in accommodations without air conditioning, screens or bed nets.
- Travelers to endemic areas who are unsure of specific destination, activities, or duration of travel

Local Anesthetic/Vasoconstrictor Precautions No information available to require special precautions

Effects on Dental Treatment No significant effects or complications reported

Effects on Bleeding No information available to require special precautions

Adverse Effects Report allergic or unusual adverse reactions to the Vaccine Adverse Event Reporting System (VAERS) 1-800-822-7967 or online at https://vaers.hhs.gov/esub/index. In Canada, adverse reactions may be reported to local provincial/territorial health agencies or to the Vaccine Safety Section at Public Health Agency of Canada (1-866-844-0018).

Percentage of adverse reactions reported over days 0-56. In general, incidence was similar to placebo.

>10%:

Central nervous system: Headache (28%), fatigue (11%)

Local: Injection site reaction: Tenderness (36%), pain (33%)

Neuromuscular & skeletal: Myalgia (16%)

Miscellaneous: Flu-like syndrome (12%)

1% to 10%:

Central nervous system: Pyrexia (3%)

Dermatologic: Rash (1%)

Gastrointestinal: Nausea (7%), diarrhea (2%), vomiting (1%)

Local: Injection site reaction: Erythema (10%), induration (8%), edema (4%), pruritus (4%)

Neuromuscular & skeletal: Back pain (1%)

Respiratory: Nasopharyngitis (5%), pharyngolaryngeal pain (2%), upper respiratory tract infection (2%), cough (1%), rhinitis (1%)

General Dosage Range

I.M.: *Adults ≥17 years:* 0.5 mL/dose on days 0 and 28

Pregnancy Risk Factor B

◀ **Pregnancy Considerations** Adverse events were not observed in animal reproduction studies. Risks of vaccine administration should be carefully considered and in general, pregnant women should only be vaccinated if they are at high risk for exposure. Infection from Japanese encephalitis during the first or second trimesters of pregnancy may increase risk of miscarriage. Intrauterine transmission of the Japanese encephalitis virus has been reported. To report inadvertent use of Ixiaro® during pregnancy, contact Novartis Vaccines (800-244-7668).

Pregnancy Considerations Hearing impairment in the offspring was observed following maternal use of kanamycin in animal studies; teratogenic events were not reported. Kanamycin crosses the placenta and produces detectable serum levels in the fetus. Because of several reports of total irreversible bilateral congenital deafness in children whose mothers received another aminoglycoside (streptomycin) during pregnancy, kanamycin has been classified by the manufacturer as pregnancy risk category D. There is also one case report of hearing impairment in a child with prenatal exposure to kanamycin.

Kanamycin (kan a MYE sin)

Pharmacologic Category Antibiotic, Aminoglycoside
Use Treatment of serious infections caused by susceptible strains of *E. coli*, *Proteus* species, *Enterobacter aerogenes*, *Klebsiella pneumoniae*, *Serratia marcescens*, and *Acinetobacter* species; second-line treatment of *Mycobacterium tuberculosis*
Local Anesthetic/Vasoconstrictor Precautions No information available to require special precautions
Effects on Dental Treatment Key adverse event(s) related to dental treatment: Salivation increased.
Effects on Bleeding No information available to require special precautions
Adverse Effects Frequency not defined.
Cardiovascular: Edema
Central nervous system: Neurotoxicity, drowsiness, headache, pseudomotor cerebri
Dermatologic: Skin itching, redness, rash, photosensitivity, erythema
Gastrointestinal: Nausea, vomiting, diarrhea, malabsorption syndrome (with prolonged and high-dose therapy of hepatic coma), anorexia, weight loss, salivation increased, enterocolitis
Hematologic: Granulocytopenia, agranulocytosis, thrombocytopenia
Local: Burning, stinging
Neuromuscular & skeletal: Weakness, tremor, muscle cramps
Otic: Ototoxicity (auditory), ototoxicity (vestibular)
Renal: Nephrotoxicity
Respiratory: Dyspnea
General Dosage Range Dosage adjustment of I.M. and I.V. route recommended in patients with renal impairment
I.M., I.V.:
Children: 15 mg/kg/day divided every 8-12 hours
Adults: 5-7.5 mg/kg every 8-12 hours
Elderly: 5-7.5 mg/kg every 12-24 hours
Inhalation, aerosol: Adults: 250 mg 2-4 times/day
Intraperitoneal: Adults: 500 mg
Irrigation: Adults: 0.25% (maximum: 1.5 g/day)
Mechanism of Action Interferes with protein synthesis in bacterial cell by binding to ribosomal subunit
Pharmacodynamics/Kinetics
Half-life Elimination 2-4 hours; Anuria: 80 hours; End-stage renal disease: 40-96 hours
Time to Peak Serum: I.M.: 1-2 hours (decreased in burn patients)
Pregnancy Risk Factor D

Ketamine (KEET a meen)

Brand Names: U.S. Ketalar®
Brand Names: Canada Ketalar®; Ketamine Hydrochloride Injection, USP
Pharmacologic Category General Anesthetic
Use Induction and maintenance of general anesthesia
Unlabeled Use Analgesia, sedation
Local Anesthetic/Vasoconstrictor Precautions No information available to require special precautions
Effects on Dental Treatment Key adverse event(s) related to dental treatment: Increased salivation.
Effects on Bleeding No information available to require special precautions
Adverse Effects Frequency not always defined.
Cardiovascular: Arrhythmia, bradycardia/tachycardia, hyper-/hypotension
Central nervous system: Intracranial pressure increased
Dermatologic: Erythema (transient), morbilliform rash (transient)
Gastrointestinal: Anorexia, nausea, salivation increased, vomiting
Local: Pain at the injection site, exanthema at the injection site
Neuromuscular & skeletal: Skeletal muscle tone enhanced (tonic-clonic movements)
Ocular: Diplopia, intraocular pressure increased, nystagmus
Respiratory: Airway obstruction, apnea, bronchial secretions increased, respiratory depression, laryngospasm
Miscellaneous: Anaphylaxis, dependence with prolonged use, emergence reactions (~12%; includes confusion, delirium, dreamlike state, excitement, hallucinations, irrational behavior, vivid imagery)
General Dosage Range
I.M.: Children ≥16 years and Adults: 2-6 mg/kg
I.V.: Children ≥16 years and Adults: 0.2-2 mg/kg **or** 0.1-0.5 mg/minute as a continuous infusion
Mechanism of Action Produces a cataleptic-like state in which the patient is dissociated from the surrounding environment by direct action on the cortex and limbic system. Ketamine is a noncompetitive NMDA receptor antagonist that blocks glutamate. Low (subanesthetic) doses produce analgesia, and modulate central sensitization, hyperalgesia and opioid tolerance. Reduces polysynaptic spinal reflexes.
Pharmacodynamics/Kinetics
Onset of Action
I.V.: Anesthetic effect: 30 seconds
I.M.: Anesthetic effect: 3-4 minutes
Duration of Action Anesthetic effect: I.V.: 5-10 minutes; I.M.: 12-25 minutes
Half-life Elimination Alpha: 10-15 minutes; Beta: 2.5 hours

Pregnancy Considerations Adverse events have not been observed in animal reproduction studies. Ketamine crosses the placenta and can be detected in fetal tissue. Ketamine produces dose dependent increases in uterine contractions; effects may vary by trimester. The plasma clearance of ketamine is reduced during pregnancy. Dose related neonatal depression and decreased APGAR scores have been reported with large doses administered at delivery (Ghoneim, 1977; Little, 1972; White, 1982).

Controlled Substance C-III

Ketoconazole (Systemic) (kee toe KOE na zole)

Related Information
Fungal Infections *on page 1573*
Related Sample Prescriptions
Fungal Infections Requiring Systemic Therapy *on page 1614*
Brand Names: Canada Apo-Ketoconazole®; Novo-Ketoconazole
Generic Availability (U.S.) Yes
Pharmacologic Category Antifungal Agent, Oral
Dental Use Treatment of susceptible fungal infections in the oral cavity including candidiasis, oral thrush, and chronic mucocutaneous candidiasis
Use Treatment of susceptible fungal infections, including candidiasis, oral thrush, blastomycosis, histoplasmosis, paracoccidioidomycosis, coccidioidomycosis, chromomycosis, candiduria, chronic mucocutaneous candidiasis, as well as certain recalcitrant cutaneous dermatophytes
Unlabeled Use Treatment of prostate cancer (androgen synthesis inhibitor)
Local Anesthetic/Vasoconstrictor Precautions No information available to require special precautions
Effects on Dental Treatment No significant effects or complications reported
Effects on Bleeding No information available to require special precautions
Adverse Effects 1% to 10%:
Dermatologic: Pruritus (2%)
Gastrointestinal: Nausea/vomiting (3% to 10%), abdominal pain (1%)
Dental Usual Dosage Oral fungal infections: Oral:
Children ≥2 years: 3.3-6.6 mg/kg/day as a single dose for 1-2 weeks for candidiasis, for at least 4 weeks in recalcitrant dermatophyte infections, and for up to 6 months for other systemic mycoses
Adults: 200-400 mg/day as a single daily dose for durations as stated above
Dosage Oral:
Fungal infections:
Children ≥2 years: 3.3-6.6 mg/kg/day as a single dose for 1-2 weeks for candidiasis, for at least 4 weeks in recalcitrant dermatophyte infections, and for up to 6 months for other systemic mycoses
Adults: 200-400 mg/day as a single daily dose for durations as stated above
Prostate cancer (unlabeled use): Adults: 400 mg 3 times/day

Dosing adjustment in renal impairment: Hemodialysis: Not dialyzable (0% to 5%)
Dosing adjustment in hepatic impairment: Dose reductions should be considered in patients with severe liver disease

Mechanism of Action Alters the permeability of the cell wall by blocking fungal cytochrome P450; inhibits biosynthesis of triglycerides and phospholipids by fungi; inhibits several fungal enzymes that results in a build-up of toxic concentrations of hydrogen peroxide; also inhibits androgen synthesis
Contraindications Hypersensitivity to ketoconazole or any component of the formulation; CNS fungal infections (due to poor CNS penetration); coadministration with ergot derivatives, cisapride, or triazolam is contraindicated due to risk of potentially fatal cardiac arrhythmias
Warnings/Precautions [U.S. Boxed Warning]: Ketoconazole has been associated with hepatotoxicity, including some fatalities; use with caution in patients with impaired hepatic function and perform periodic liver function tests. **[U.S. Boxed Warning]: Concomitant use with cisapride is contraindicated due to the occurrence of ventricular arrhythmias.** High doses of ketoconazole may depress adrenocortical function.
Drug Interactions
Metabolism/Transport Effects Substrate of CYP3A4 (major); **Note:** Assignment of Major/Minor substrate status based on clinically relevant drug interaction potential; **Inhibits** CYP1A2 (strong), CYP2A6 (moderate); CYP2B6 (weak), CYP2C19 (moderate), CYP2C8 (weak), CYP2C9 (strong), CYP2D6 (moderate), CYP3A4 (strong), P-glycoprotein
Avoid Concomitant Use
Avoid concomitant use of Ketoconazole (Systemic) with any of the following: Ado-Trastuzumab Emtansine; Alfuzosin; Apixaban; Avanafil; Axitinib; Bosutinib; Cabozantinib; Cisapride; Clopidogrel; Conivaptan; Crizotinib; Dihydroergotamine; Dofetilide; Domperidone; Dronedarone; Eletriptan; Eplerenone; Ergoloid Mesylates; Ergonovine; Ergotamine; Everolimus; Fluticasone (Oral Inhalation); Halofantrine; Ivabradine; Lapatinib; Lomitapide; Lovastatin; Lurasidone; Methylergonovine; Midazolam; Nevirapine; Nilotinib; Nisoldipine; Pimozide; Pirfenidone; Pomalidomide; QuiNIDine; Ranolazine; Red Yeast Rice; Regorafenib; Rivaroxaban; RomiDEPsin; Salmeterol; Silodosin; Simvastatin; Tamsulosin; Thioridazine; Ticagrelor; Tipranavir; Tolvaptan; Topotecan; Toremifene; VinCRIStine (Liposomal)
Increased Effect/Toxicity
Ketoconazole (Systemic) may increase the levels/effects of: Ado-Trastuzumab Emtansine; Alfentanil; Alfuzosin; Aliskiren; Almotriptan; Alosetron; Apixaban; Aprepitant; ARIPiprazole; AtorvaSTATin; Avanafil; Axitinib; Bedaquiline; Bendamustine; Benzodiazepines (metabolized by oxidation); Boceprevir; Bortezomib; Bosentan; Bosutinib; Brentuximab Vedotin; Brinzolamide; Budesonide (Nasal); Budesonide (Systemic, Oral Inhalation); BusPIRone; Busulfan; Cabozantinib; Calcium Channel Blockers; CarBAMazepine; Carvedilol; Cilostazol; Cinacalcet; Cisapride; Citalopram; Cobicistat; Colchicine; Conivaptan; Corticosteroids (Orally Inhaled); Corticosteroids (Systemic); Crizotinib; CycloSPORINE (Systemic); CYP1A2 Substrates; CYP2A6 Substrates; CYP2C19 Substrates; CYP2C9 Substrates; CYP2D6 Substrates; CYP3A4 Substrates; Dabigatran Etexilate; Darunavir; Diclofenac (Systemic); Dienogest; Dihydroergotamine; DOCEtaxel; Dofetilide; Domperidone; Dronedarone; Dutasteride; Eletriptan; Elvitegravir; Enzalutamide; Eplerenone; Ergoloid Mesylates; Ergonovine; Ergotamine; Erlotinib; Eszopiclone; Etravirine; Everolimus; FentaNYL; Fesoterodine; Fexofenadine; Fingolimod; Fluticasone (Nasal); Fluticasone (Oral Inhalation); Fosamprenavir; ▶

◀ Fosaprepitant; Fosphenytoin; Gefitinib; GuanFACINE; Halofantrine; Highest Risk QTc-Prolonging Agents; Iloperidone; Imatinib; Indinavir; Irinotecan; Ivabradine; Ivacaftor; Ixabepilone; Lapatinib; Lomitapide; Lopinavir; Losartan; Lovastatin; Lumefantrine; Lurasidone; Macrolide Antibiotics; Maraviroc; Methadone; Methylergonovine; MethylPREDNISolone; Metoprolol; Midazolam; Mifepristone; Mirabegron; Moderate Risk QTc-Prolonging Agents; Nebivolol; Nilotinib; Nisoldipine; Ospemifene; Paricalcitol; Pazopanib; P-glycoprotein/ABCB1 Substrates; Phenytoin; Pimecrolimus; Pimozide; Pirfenidone; Pomalidomide; Ponatinib; Praziquantel; Propafenone; Proton Pump Inhibitors; Prucalopride; QuiNIDine; Ramelteon; Ranolazine; Red Yeast Rice; Regorafenib; Repaglinide; Rifamycin Derivatives; Rilpivirine; Rivaroxaban; RomiDEPsin; Ruxolitinib; Salmeterol; Saquinavir; Saxagliptin; Sildenafil; Silodosin; Simvastatin; Sirolimus; Solifenacin; SORAfenib; SUNItinib; Tacrolimus (Systemic); Tacrolimus (Topical); Tadalafil; Tamsulosin; Telaprevir; Temsirolimus; Thioridazine; Ticagrelor; Tofacitinib; Tolterodine; Tolvaptan; Topotecan; Toremifene; Vardenafil; Vemurafenib; Vilazodone; VinCRIStine (Liposomal); Vitamin K Antagonists; Ziprasidone; Zolpidem; Zuclopenthixol

The levels/effects of Ketoconazole (Systemic) may be increased by: AtorvaSTATin; Boceprevir; Cobicistat; Darunavir; Domperidone; Etravirine; Fosamprenavir; Grapefruit Juice; Indinavir; Lopinavir; Macrolide Antibiotics; Ritonavir; Saquinavir; Telaprevir; Tipranavir

Decreased Effect

Ketoconazole (Systemic) may decrease the levels/effects of: Amphotericin B; Clopidogrel; Codeine; Ifosfamide; Prasugrel; Saccharomyces boulardii; Tamoxifen; Ticagrelor; TraMADol

The levels/effects of Ketoconazole (Systemic) may be decreased by: Antacids; CYP3A4 Inducers (Strong); Deferasirox; Didanosine; Etravirine; Fosphenytoin; H2-Antagonists; Herbs (CYP3A4 Inducers); Isoniazid; Nevirapine; Phenytoin; Proton Pump Inhibitors; Rifamycin Derivatives; Rilpivirine; Sucralfate; Tocilizumab

Ethanol/Nutrition/Herb Interactions
Food: Ketoconazole peak serum levels may be prolonged if taken with food.
Herb/Nutraceutical: St John's wort may decrease ketoconazole levels.

Dietary Considerations May be taken with food or milk to decrease GI adverse effects.

Pharmacodynamics/Kinetics
Half-life Elimination Biphasic: Initial: 2 hours; Terminal: 8 hours
Time to Peak Serum: 1-2 hours

Pregnancy Risk Factor C

Pregnancy Considerations Adverse effects were noted in animal reproduction studies.

Lactation Enters breast milk/not recommended

Breast-Feeding Considerations In a case report, ketoconazole in concentrations of ≤0.22 mcg/mL were detected in the breast milk of a woman 1 month postpartum. She had been taking oral ketoconazole 200 mg/day for 5 days at the time of sampling. The maximum milk concentration occurred 3.25 hours after the dose and concentrations were undetectable 24 hours after the dose. Based on the highest milk concentration, the estimated dose to the nursing infant was 1.4% of the maternal dose. Breast-feeding is not recommended by the manufacturer.

Dosage Forms
Tablet, oral: 200 mg

Ketoconazole (Topical) (kee toe KOE na zole)

Related Information
Fungal Infections *on page 1573*
Related Sample Prescriptions
Fungal Infections Requiring Topical Therapy *on page 1614*

Brand Names: U.S. Extina®; Nizoral®; Nizoral® A-D [OTC]; Xolegel®

Brand Names: Canada Ketoderm®; Xolegel®

Generic Availability (U.S.) Yes: Aerosol, cream, shampoo

Pharmacologic Category Antifungal Agent, Topical

Dental Use Treatment of susceptible fungal infections in the oral cavity including candidiasis, oral thrush, and chronic mucocutaneous candidiasis

Use
Cream: Treatment of tinea corporis, tinea cruris, tinea versicolor, cutaneous candidiasis, seborrheic dermatitis
Foam, gel: Treatment of seborrheic dermatitis
Shampoo: Treatment of dandruff, seborrheic dermatitis, tinea versicolor

Unlabeled Use Cream: Treatment of susceptible fungal infections in the oral cavity including candidiasis, oral thrush, and chronic mucocutaneous candidiasis

Local Anesthetic/Vasoconstrictor Precautions No information available to require special precautions

Effects on Dental Treatment No significant effects or complications reported

Effects on Bleeding No information available to require special precautions

Adverse Effects Frequency not always defined.
Topical cream/gel: Stinging (~5%), local burning (4%), acne, allergic reaction, contact dermatitis (possibly related to sulfites or propylene glycol), discharge, dizziness, dryness, erythema, facial swelling, headache, impetigo, keratoconjunctivitis sicca, nail discoloration, ocular irritation/swelling, pain, paresthesia, pruritus, pustules, pyogenic granuloma, severe irritation
Topical foam: Application site burning (10%), application site reaction (6%), contact sensitization, dryness, erythema, pruritus, rash
Shampoo: Application site reaction (≤3%), dry skin (≤3%), pruritus (≤3%), abnormal hair texture (<1%), hair loss increased (<1%), irritation (<1%), scalp pustules (<1%), alopecia, anaphylaxis, angioedema, burning sensation, contact dermatitis, hair discoloration, hypersensitivity, itching, oiliness/dryness of hair, rash, urticaria

Dental Usual Dosage Cream: Apply locally as directed with a thin coat to inner surface of denture and affected areas after meals

Dosage
Shampoo:
Seborrheic dermatitis (ketoconazole 1%): Children ≥12 years and Adults: Apply twice weekly for up to 8 weeks with at least 3 days between each shampoo
Tinea versicolor (ketoconazole 2%): Adults: Apply to damp skin, lather, leave on 5 minutes, and rinse (one application should be sufficient)

Topical:
Tinea infections: Adults: Cream: Rub gently into the affected area once daily. Duration of treatment: Tinea corporis, cruris: 2 weeks; tinea pedis: 6 weeks

Seborrheic dermatitis: Children ≥12 years and Adults: Cream: Rub gently into the affected area twice daily for 4 weeks or until clinical response is noted
Foam: Apply to affected area twice daily for 4 weeks
Gel: Rub gently into the affected area once daily for 2 weeks

Susceptible fungal infections in the oral cavity (candidiasis, oral thrush, and chronic mucocutaneous candidiasis) (unlabeled use): Adults: Cream: Apply locally as directed with a thin coat to inner surface of denture and affected areas after meals

Mechanism of Action Alters the permeability of the cell wall by blocking fungal cytochrome P450; inhibits biosynthesis of triglycerides and phospholipids by fungi; inhibits several fungal enzymes that results in a build-up of toxic concentrations of hydrogen peroxide; also inhibits androgen synthesis

Contraindications Hypersensitivity to ketoconazole or any component of the formulation

Warnings/Precautions Cases of hypersensitivity reactions (including rare cases of anaphylaxis) have been reported. Formulations may contain sulfites. Avoid exposure of gel to open flames or smoking during or immediately after application. Foam formulation contains alcohol and propane/butane; do not expose to open flame or smoking during or immediately after application; do not puncture or incinerate container. Use of shampoo may remove curl from permanently wavy hair, cause hair discoloration, and changes in hair texture; avoid contact with eyes. Discontinue use if irritation occurs.

Drug Interactions

Metabolism/Transport Effects None known.

Avoid Concomitant Use There are no known interactions where it is recommended to avoid concomitant use.

Increased Effect/Toxicity There are no known significant interactions involving an increase in effect.

Decreased Effect There are no known significant interactions involving a decrease in effect.

Pregnancy Risk Factor C

Pregnancy Considerations Adverse effects were noted in animal reproduction studies with oral ketoconazole. Ketoconazole is not detectable in the plasma following chronic use of the shampoo.

Lactation Excretion in breast milk unknown/use caution

Breast-Feeding Considerations Ketoconazole has been detected in breast milk following oral dosing. Although it is not detected in the plasma following chronic use of the shampoo, and concentrations in the plasma following application of the gel are <250 times those observed with oral dosing, the manufacturers recommend that caution be used when administering to a nursing woman.

Dosage Forms

Aerosol, foam, topical: 2% (50 g, 100 g)
Extina®: 2% (50 g, 100 g)

Cream, topical: 2% (15 g, 30 g, 60 g)

Gel, topical:
Xolegel®: 2% (45 g)

Shampoo, topical: 2% (120 mL)
Nizoral®: 2% (120 mL)
Nizoral® A-D [OTC]: 1% (120 mL, 210 mL)

Ketoprofen (kee toe PROE fen)

Related Information
Oral Pain on page 1558
Rheumatoid Arthritis, Osteoarthritis, and Osteoporosis on page 1526
Temporomandibular Dysfunction (TMD), Chronic Pain, and Fibromyalgia on page 1590

Brand Names: Canada Apo-Keto SR®; Apo-Keto-E®; Apo-Keto®; Ketoprofen SR; Ketoprofen-E; Nu-Ketoprofen; Nu-Ketoprofen-E; PMS-Ketoprofen; PMS-Ketoprofen-E

Generic Availability (U.S.) Yes

Pharmacologic Category Nonsteroidal Anti-inflammatory Drug (NSAID), Oral

Dental Use Management of pain and swelling

Use Acute and long-term treatment of rheumatoid arthritis and osteoarthritis; primary dysmenorrhea; mild-to-moderate pain

Unlabeled Use Migraine prophylaxis

Local Anesthetic/Vasoconstrictor Precautions No information available to require special precautions

Effects on Dental Treatment Key adverse event(s) related to dental treatment: Stomatitis.

According to the FDA, the over-the-counter NSAID ketoprofen should be viewed as having the potential to interfere with the antiplatelet effect of low-dose aspirin until proven otherwise. This statement was provided in the same warning from the FDA that ibuprofen can interfere with the antiplatelet effect of low-dose aspirin (81 mg/day), potentially rendering aspirin less effective when used for cardioprotection and stroke protection. In situations where these drugs could be used concomitantly, the FDA has provided the following information: Patients who use immediate release aspirin (not enteric-coated aspirin) and take single doses of ibuprofen 400 mg, should dose the ibuprofen at least 30 minutes or longer after aspirin ingestion or more than 8 hours before aspirin ingestion to avoid attenuation of aspirin's effect. Similar recommendations may hold for concomitant ketoprofen and aspirin use. See Effects on Bleeding.

At this time, recommendations about the timing of ibuprofen 400 mg or other NSAIDs (such as ketoprofen) in patients taking enteric-coated low-dose aspirin cannot be made based on available data.

Effects on Bleeding Nonselective NSAIDs such as ketoprofen inhibit platelet aggregation and prolong bleeding time in some patients. Unlike aspirin, the NSAID effect on platelet function is quantitatively less, of shorter duration, and reversible.

Adverse Effects
>10%:
Gastrointestinal: Dyspepsia (11%)
Hepatic: Liver function test abnormal (≤15%)
1% to 10%:
Cardiovascular: Peripheral edema (2%)
Central nervous system: Headache (3% to 9%), depression, dizziness (>1%), dreams, insomnia, malaise, nervousness, somnolence
Dermatologic: Rash (>1%)
Gastrointestinal: Abdominal pain (3% to 9%), constipation (3% to 9%), diarrhea (3% to 9%), flatulence (3% to 9%), nausea (3% to 9%), gastrointestinal bleeding (>2%), peptic ulcer (>2%), anorexia (>1%), stomatitis (>1%), vomiting (>1%)

Genitourinary: Urinary tract irritation (>1%)

Ocular: Visual disturbances (>1%)

Otic: Tinnitus (>1%)

Renal: Renal dysfunction (3% to 9%)

Dental Usual Dosage Mild-to-moderate pain: Children ≥16 years and Adults: Oral: Capsule: 25-50 mg every 6-8 hours up to a maximum of 300 mg/day

Dosage Note: The extended release formulation is not recommended for the treatment of acute pain. Oral: Adults:

Rheumatoid arthritis, osteoarthritis (lower doses may be used in small patients or in the elderly, or debilitated):

Regular release: 50 mg 4 times/day **or** 75 mg 3 times/day; up to a maximum of 300 mg/day

Extended release: 200 mg once daily

Dysmenorrhea, mild-to-moderate pain: Regular release: 25-50 mg every 6-8 hours up to a maximum of 300 mg/day

Elderly: Initial dose should be decreased in patients >75 years; use caution when dosage changes are made

Dosage adjustment in renal impairment: In general, NSAIDs are not recommended for use in patients with advanced renal disease, but the manufacturer of ketoprofen does provide some guidelines for adjustment in renal dysfunction:

Mild impairment: Maximum dose: 150 mg/day

Severe impairment: Cl$_{cr}$ <25 mL/minute: Maximum dose: 100 mg/day

Dosage adjustment in hepatic impairment and serum albumin <3.5 g/dL: Maximum dose: 100 mg/day

Mechanism of Action Reversibly inhibits cyclooxygenase-1 and 2 (COX-1 and 2) enzymes, which results in decreased formation of prostaglandin precursors; has antipyretic, analgesic, and anti-inflammatory properties

Other proposed mechanisms not fully elucidated (and possibly contributing to the anti-inflammatory effect to varying degrees), include inhibiting chemotaxis, altering lymphocyte activity, inhibiting neutrophil aggregation/activation, and decreasing proinflammatory cytokine levels.

Contraindications Hypersensitivity to ketoprofen, aspirin, other NSAIDs, or any component of the formulation; perioperative pain in the setting of coronary artery bypass graft (CABG) surgery

Warnings/Precautions [U.S. Boxed Warning]: NSAIDs are associated with an increased risk of adverse cardiovascular thrombotic events, including MI and stroke Risk may be increased with duration of use or pre-existing cardiovascular risk factors or disease. Carefully evaluate individual cardiovascular risk profiles prior to prescribing. May cause new-onset hypertension or worsening of existing hypertension. Use caution with fluid retention. Avoid use in heart failure. Concurrent administration of ibuprofen, and potentially other nonselective NSAIDs, may interfere with aspirin's cardioprotective effect. **[U.S. Boxed Warning]: Use is contraindicated for treatment of perioperative pain in the setting of coronary artery bypass graft (CABG) surgery.** Risk of MI and stroke may be increased with use following CABG surgery.

NSAID use may compromise existing renal function; dose-dependent decreases in prostaglandin synthesis may result from NSAID use, reducing renal blood flow which may cause renal decompensation. NSAID use may increase the risk for hyperkalemia. Patients with impaired renal function, dehydration, heart failure, liver dysfunction, those taking diuretics, and ACE inhibitors, and the elderly are at greater risk of renal toxicity and hyperkalemia. Rehydrate patient before starting therapy; monitor renal function closely. Not recommended for use in patients with advanced renal disease. Long-term NSAID use may result in renal papillary necrosis.

[U.S. Boxed Warning]: NSAIDs may increase risk of gastrointestinal irritation, inflammation, ulceration, bleeding, and perforation. These events may occur at any time during therapy and without warning. Use caution with a history of GI disease (bleeding or ulcers), concurrent therapy with aspirin, anticoagulants and/or corticosteroids, smoking, use of alcohol, the elderly or debilitated patients. When used concomitantly with ≤325 mg of aspirin, a substantial increase in the risk of gastrointestinal complications (eg, ulcer) occurs; concomitant gastroprotective therapy (eg, proton pump inhibitors) is recommended (Bhatt, 2008). Platelet adhesion and aggregation may be decreased; may prolong bleeding time; patients with coagulation disorders or who are receiving anticoagulants should be monitored closely. Anemia may occur; patients on long-term NSAID therapy should be monitored for anemia. Rarely, NSAID use may cause severe blood dyscrasias (eg, agranulocytosis, aplastic anemia, thrombocytopenia).

In the elderly, avoid chronic use (unless alternative agents ineffective and patient can receive concomitant gastroprotective agent); nonselective oral NSAID use is associated with an increased risk of GI bleeding and peptic ulcer disease in older adults in high risk category (eg, >75 years or age or receiving concomitant oral/parenteral corticosteroids, anticoagulants, or antiplatelet agents) (Beers Criteria).

Use the lowest effective dose for the shortest duration of time, consistent with individual patient goals, to reduce risk of cardiovascular or GI adverse events. Alternate therapies should be considered for patients at high risk.

NSAIDS may cause drowsiness, dizziness, blurred vision and other neurologic effects which may impair physical or mental abilities; patients must be cautioned about performing tasks which require mental alertness (eg, operating machinery or driving). Discontinue use with blurred or diminished vision and perform ophthalmologic exam. Monitor vision with long-term therapy.

NSAIDs may cause serious skin adverse events including exfoliative dermatitis, Stevens-Johnson syndrome (SJS), and toxic epidermal necrolysis (TEN); discontinue use at first sign of skin rash or hypersensitivity. Anaphylactoid reactions may occur, even without prior exposure; patients with "aspirin triad" (bronchial asthma, aspirin intolerance, rhinitis) may be at increased risk. Do not use in patients who experience bronchospasm, asthma, rhinitis, or urticaria with NSAID or aspirin therapy. Use caution in other forms of asthma.

Use with caution in patients with decreased hepatic function. Closely monitor patients with any abnormal LFT. Severe hepatic reactions (eg, fulminant hepatitis, liver failure) have occurred with NSAID use, rarely; discontinue if signs or symptoms of liver disease develop, or if systemic manifestations occur. The elderly are at increased risk for adverse effects (especially peptic ulceration, CNS effects, renal toxicity) from NSAIDs, even at low doses.

Withhold for at least 4-6 half-lives prior to surgical or dental procedures. Safety and efficacy have not been established in pediatric patients.

Drug Interactions

Metabolism/Transport Effects Inhibits CYP2C9 (weak)

Avoid Concomitant Use

Avoid concomitant use of Ketoprofen with any of the following: Floctafenine; Ketorolac (Nasal); Ketorolac (Systemic); NSAID (COX-2 Inhibitor); Omacetaxine

Increased Effect/Toxicity

Ketoprofen may increase the levels/effects of: Agents with Antiplatelet Properties; Aliskiren; Aminoglycosides; Anticoagulants; Bisphosphonate Derivatives; Collagenase (Systemic); CycloSPORINE (Systemic); Dabigatran Etexilate; Deferasirox; Desmopressin; Digoxin; Drotrecogin Alfa (Activated); Eplerenone; Haloperidol; Ibritumomab; Lithium; Methotrexate; Nonsteroidal Anti-Inflammatory Agents; NSAID (COX-2 Inhibitor); Omacetaxine; PEMEtrexed; Porfimer; Potassium-Sparing Diuretics; PRALAtrexate; Quinolone Antibiotics; Rivaroxaban; Salicylates; Thrombolytic Agents; Tositumomab and Iodine I 131 Tositumomab; Vancomycin; Vitamin K Antagonists

The levels/effects of Ketoprofen may be increased by: ACE Inhibitors; Angiotensin II Receptor Blockers; Antidepressants (Tricyclic, Tertiary Amine); Corticosteroids (Systemic); CycloSPORINE (Systemic); Dasatinib; Floctafenine; Glucosamine; Herbs (Anticoagulant/Antiplatelet Properties); Ketorolac (Nasal); Ketorolac (Systemic); Multivitamins/Minerals (with ADEK, Folate, Iron); Nonsteroidal Anti-Inflammatory Agents; Omega-3 Fatty Acids; Pentosan Polysulfate Sodium; Pentoxifylline; Probenecid; Prostacyclin Analogues; Selective Serotonin Reuptake Inhibitors; Serotonin/ Norepinephrine Reuptake Inhibitors; Sodium Phosphates; Tipranavir; Treprostinil; Vitamin E

Decreased Effect

Ketoprofen may decrease the levels/effects of: ACE Inhibitors; Agents with Antiplatelet Properties; Aliskiren; Angiotensin II Receptor Blockers; Beta-Blockers; Eplerenone; HydrALAZINE; Loop Diuretics; Potassium-Sparing Diuretics; Salicylates; Selective Serotonin Reuptake Inhibitors; Thiazide Diuretics

The levels/effects of Ketoprofen may be decreased by: Bile Acid Sequestrants; Nonsteroidal Anti-Inflammatory Agents; Salicylates

Ethanol/Nutrition/Herb Interactions

Ethanol: Avoid ethanol (due to GI irritation).

Food: Food slows rate of absorption resulting in delayed and reduced peak serum concentrations; total bioavailability is not affected by food.

Herb/Nutraceutical: Avoid alfalfa, anise, bilberry, bladderwrack, bromelain, cat's claw, celery, chamomile, coleus, cordyceps, dong quai, evening primrose, fenugreek, feverfew, garlic, ginger, ginkgo biloba, ginseng (American, Panax, Siberian), grapeseed, green tea, guggul, horse chestnut seed, horseradish, licorice, prickly ash, red clover, reishi, SAMe (S-adenosylmethionine), sweet clover, turmeric, and white willow (all have additional antiplatelet activity).

Dietary Considerations In order to minimize gastrointestinal effects, ketoprofen can be prescribed to be taken with food or milk.

Pharmacodynamics/Kinetics

Onset of Action Regular release: <30 minutes

Duration of Action Regular release: Up to 6 hours

Half-life Elimination

Regular release: 2-4 hours; Renal impairment: Mild: 3 hours; moderate-to-severe: 5-9 hours

Extended release: ~3-7.5 hours

Time to Peak Regular release: 0.5-2 hours; Extended release: 6-7 hours

Pregnancy Risk Factor C

Pregnancy Considerations Adverse events were not observed in the initial animal reproduction studies; therefore, the manufacturer classifies ketoprofen as pregnancy category C. Ketoprofen crosses the placenta. NSAID exposure during the first trimester is not strongly associated with congenital malformations; however, cardiovascular anomalies and cleft palate have been observed following NSAID exposure in some studies. The use of an NSAID close to conception may be associated with an increased risk of miscarriage. Nonteratogenic effects have been observed following NSAID administration during the third trimester including myocardial degenerative changes, prenatal constriction of the ductus arteriosus, fetal tricuspid regurgitation, failure of the ductus arteriosus to close postnatally; renal dysfunction or failure, oligohydramnios; gastrointestinal bleeding or perforation, increased risk of necrotizing enterocolitis; intracranial bleeding (including intraventricular hemorrhage), platelet dysfunction with resultant bleeding; pulmonary hypertension. Because they may cause premature closure of the ductus arteriosus, use of NSAIDs late in pregnancy should be avoided (use after 31or 32 weeks gestation is not recommended by some clinicians). The chronic use of NSAIDs in women of reproductive age may be associated with infertility that is reversible upon discontinuation of the medication.

Lactation Enters breast milk

Breast-Feeding Considerations Small amounts of ketoprofen are found in breast milk. Breast-feeding is not recommended by the manufacturer.

Dosage Forms

Capsule, oral: 50 mg, 75 mg

Capsule, extended release, oral: 200 mg

References

Brooks PM and Day RO, "Nonsteroidal Anti-inflammatory Drugs - Differences and Similarities," *N Engl J Med*, 1991, 324(24):1716-25.

Cooper SA, "Ketoprofen in Oral Surgery Pain: A Review," *J Clin Pharmacol*, 1988, 28(12 Suppl):S40-6.

Hersh EV, "The Efficacy and Safety of Ketoprofen in Postsurgical Dental Pain," *Compendium*, 1991, 12(4):234.

Ketorolac (Systemic) (KEE toe role ak)

Related Information

Oral Pain *on page 1558*

Rheumatoid Arthritis, Osteoarthritis, and Osteoporosis *on page 1526*

Temporomandibular Dysfunction (TMD), Chronic Pain, and Fibromyalgia *on page 1590*

Brand Names: Canada Apo-Ketorolac Injectable®; Apo-Ketorolac® Tablet; Ketorolac Tromethamine Injection, USP; Novo-Ketorolac; Nu-Ketorolac; Toradol®; Toradol® IM

Generic Availability (U.S.) Yes

Pharmacologic Category Nonsteroidal Anti-inflammatory Drug (NSAID), Oral; Nonsteroidal Anti-inflammatory Drug (NSAID), Parenteral

Dental Use Short-term (≤5 days) management of moderate-to-severe acute pain requiring analgesia at the opioid level

Use Short-term (≤5 days) management of moderate-to-severe acute pain requiring analgesia at the opioid level

Local Anesthetic/Vasoconstrictor Precautions No information available to require special precautions

Effects on Dental Treatment Key adverse event(s) related to dental treatment: Xerostomia (normal salivary flow resumes upon discontinuation) and stomatitis.

NSAID formulations are known to reversibly decrease platelet aggregation via mechanisms different than observed with aspirin. The dentist should be aware of the potential of abnormal coagulation. Caution should also be exercised in the use of NSAIDs in patients already on anticoagulant therapy with drugs such as warfarin (Coumadin®). See Dental Comment.

Effects on Bleeding Nonselective NSAIDs such as ketorolac inhibit platelet aggregation and prolong bleeding time in some patients. Unlike aspirin, the NSAID effect on platelet function is quantitatively less, of shorter duration, and reversible.

Adverse Effects

Frequencies noted for parenteral administration:
>10%:
Central nervous system: Headache (17%)
Gastrointestinal: Gastrointestinal pain (13%), dyspepsia (12%), nausea (12%)
>1% to 10%:
Cardiovascular: Edema (4%), hypertension
Central nervous system: Dizziness (7%), drowsiness (6%)
Dermatologic: Pruritus, purpura, rash
Gastrointestinal: Diarrhea (7%), constipation, flatulence, GI bleeding, GI fullness, GI perforation, GI ulcer, heartburn, stomatitis, vomiting
Hematologic: Anemia, bleeding time increased
Hepatic: Liver enzymes increased
Local: Injection site pain (2%)
Otic: Tinnitus
Renal: Renal function abnormal
Miscellaneous: Diaphoresis

Dental Usual Dosage

Short-term (≤5 days) management of moderate-to-severe acute pain requiring analgesia at the opioid level (**Note:** The maximum combined duration of treatment (for parenteral and oral) is 5 days; do not increase dose or frequency; supplement with low-dose opioids if needed for breakthrough pain). For patients <50 kg and/or ≥65 years, see Elderly dosing.
Adults:
I.M.: 60 mg as a single dose or 30 mg every 6 hours (maximum daily dose: 120 mg)
I.V.: 30 mg as a single dose or 30 mg every 6 hours (maximum daily dose: 120 mg)
Oral: 20 mg, followed by 10 mg every 4-6 hours; do not exceed 40 mg/day; oral dosing is intended to be a continuation of I.M. or I.V. therapy only

Dosage adjustments in elderly (≥65 years), renal insufficiency, or low body weight (<50 kg): Note: These groups have an increased incidence of GI bleeding, ulceration, and perforation. The maximum combined duration of treatment (for parenteral and oral) is 5 days.
I.M.: 30 mg as a single dose or 15 mg every 6 hours (maximum daily dose: 60 mg)
I.V.: 15 mg as a single dose or 15 mg every 6 hours (maximum daily dose: 60 mg)
Oral: 10 mg, followed by 10 mg every 4-6 hours; do not exceed 40 mg/day; oral dosing is intended to be a continuation of I.M. or I.V. therapy only

Dosage

Children ≥16 years and Adults (pain relief usually begins within 10 minutes with parenteral forms): **Note:** The maximum combined duration of treatment (for parenteral and oral) is 5 days; do not increase dose or frequency; supplement with low-dose opioids if needed for breakthrough pain. For patients <50 kg and/or ≥65 years, see Elderly dosing.

I.M.: 60 mg as a single dose or 30 mg every 6 hours (maximum daily dose: 120 mg)
I.V.: 30 mg as a single dose or 30 mg every 6 hours (maximum daily dose: 120 mg)
Critically-ill patients: Adults: I.M., I.V.: 30 mg once, followed by 15-30 mg every 6 hours for up to 5 days (maximum daily dose: 120 mg) (Barr, 2013).
Children ≥17 years and Adults: Oral: 20 mg, followed by 10 mg every 4-6 hours; do not exceed 40 mg/day; oral dosing is intended to be a continuation of I.M. or I.V. therapy only
Note: The maximum combined duration of treatment (for parenteral and oral) is 5 days; do not increase dose or frequency; supplement with low-dose opioids if needed for breakthrough pain. Therapy should not be initiated with oral formulation. For patients <50 kg and/or ≥65 years, see Elderly dosing.

Dosage adjustments in elderly (≥65 years), renal insufficiency, or low body weight (<50 kg): Note: These groups have an increased incidence of GI bleeding, ulceration, and perforation. The maximum combined duration of treatment (for parenteral and oral) is 5 days.
I.M.: 30 mg as a single dose or 15 mg every 6 hours (maximum daily dose: 60 mg)
I.V.: 15 mg as a single dose or 15 mg every 6 hours (maximum daily dose: 60 mg)
Oral: 10 mg, followed by 10 mg every 4-6 hours; do not exceed 40 mg/day; oral dosing is intended to be a continuation of I.M. or I.V. therapy only

Dosage adjustment in renal impairment: Contraindicated in patients with advanced renal impairment. Patients with moderately-elevated serum creatinine should use half the recommended dose, not to exceed 60 mg/day I.M./I.V.

Dosage adjustment in hepatic impairment: Use with caution, may cause elevation of liver enzymes; discontinue if clinical signs and symptoms of liver disease develop

Mechanism of Action Reversibly inhibits cyclooxygenase-1 and 2 (COX-1 and 2) enzymes, which results in decreased formation of prostaglandin precursors; has antipyretic, analgesic, and anti-inflammatory properties

Other proposed mechanisms not fully elucidated (and possibly contributing to the anti-inflammatory effect to varying degrees), include inhibiting chemotaxis, altering lymphocyte activity, inhibiting neutrophil aggregation/activation, and decreasing proinflammatory cytokine levels.

Contraindications Hypersensitivity to ketorolac, aspirin, other NSAIDs, or any component of the formulation; active or history of peptic ulcer disease; recent or history of GI bleeding or perforation; patients with advanced renal disease or risk of renal failure (due to volume depletion); prophylaxis before major surgery; suspected or confirmed cerebrovascular bleeding; hemorrhagic diathesis, incomplete hemostasis, or high risk of bleeding; concurrent ASA or other NSAIDs; concomitant probenecid or pentoxifylline; epidural or intrathecal administration; perioperative pain in the setting of coronary artery bypass graft (CABG) surgery; labor and delivery; breast-feeding

Warnings/Precautions [U.S. Boxed Warning]: May inhibit platelet function; contraindicated in patients with cerebrovascular bleeding (suspected or confirmed), hemorrhagic diathesis, incomplete hemostasis and patients at high risk for bleeding. Effects on platelet adhesion and aggregation may prolong bleeding time. Anemia may occur; patients on long-term

NSAID therapy should be monitored for anemia. Rarely, NSAID use has been associated with potentially severe blood dyscrasias (eg, agranulocytosis, thrombocytopenia, aplastic anemia).

[U.S. Boxed Warning]: NSAIDs are associated with an increased risk of adverse cardiovascular thrombotic events, including MI and stroke. Risk may be increased with duration of use or pre-existing cardiovascular risk factors or disease. Carefully evaluate individual cardiovascular risk profiles prior to prescribing. May cause new-onset hypertension or worsening of existing hypertension. Use caution with fluid retention. Avoid use in heart failure. Concurrent administration of ibuprofen, and potentially other nonselective NSAIDs, may interfere with aspirin's cardioprotective effect. **[U.S. Boxed Warning]: Use is contraindicated as prophylactic analgesic before any major surgery and is contraindicated for treatment of perioperative pain in the setting of coronary artery bypass graft (CABG) surgery.** Risk of MI and stroke may be increased with use following CABG surgery. Wound bleeding and postoperative hematomas have been associated with ketorolac use in the perioperative setting. Withhold for at least 4-6 half-lives prior to surgical or dental procedures.

[U.S. Boxed Warning]: Ketorolac is contraindicated in patients with advanced renal impairment and in patients at risk for renal failure due to volume depletion. NSAID use may compromise existing renal function; dose-dependent decreases in prostaglandin synthesis may result from NSAID use, reducing renal blood flow which may cause renal decompensation. NSAID use may increase the risk for hyperkalemia. Patients with impaired renal function, dehydration, heart failure, liver dysfunction, those taking diuretics and ACE inhibitors, and the elderly are at greater risk of renal toxicity. Use with caution in patients with impaired renal function or history of kidney disease; dosage adjustment is required in patients with moderate elevation in serum creatinine. Monitor renal function closely. Acute renal failure, interstitial nephritis, and nephrotic syndrome have been reported with ketorolac use; papillary necrosis and renal injury have been reported with the use of NSAIDs. Use of NSAIDs can compromise existing renal function. Rehydrate patient before starting therapy.

[U.S. Boxed Warning]: NSAIDs may increase risk of gastrointestinal irritation, inflammation, ulceration, bleeding, and perforation. These events may occur at any time during therapy and without warning. Use caution with a history of GI disease (bleeding, ulcers, inflammatory bowel disease), concurrent therapy with aspirin, anticoagulants and/or corticosteroids, smoking, use of alcohol, the elderly, or debilitated patients. When used concomitantly with ≤325 mg of aspirin, a substantial increase in the risk of gastrointestinal complications (eg, ulcer) occurs; concomitant gastroprotective therapy (eg, proton pump inhibitors) is recommended (Bhatt, 2008).

NSAIDs may cause serious skin adverse events including exfoliative dermatitis, Stevens-Johnson syndrome (SJS), and toxic epidermal necrolysis (TEN); discontinue use at first sign of skin rash or hypersensitivity. Hypersensitivity or anaphylactoid reactions may occur, even without prior exposure; patients with "aspirin triad" (bronchial asthma, aspirin intolerance, rhinitis) may be at increased risk. Do not use in patients who experience bronchospasm, asthma, rhinitis, or urticaria with NSAID or aspirin therapy. **[U.S. Boxed Warning]: Ketorolac injection is contraindicated in patients with prior hypersensitivity reaction to aspirin or NSAIDs.** Use caution in other forms of asthma.

Use with caution in patients with hepatic impairment or a history of liver disease. Closely monitor patients with any abnormal LFT. Rarely, severe hepatic reactions (eg, fulminant hepatitis, hepatic necrosis, liver failure) have occurred with NSAID use; discontinue if signs or symptoms of liver disease develop, or if systemic manifestations occur.

[U.S. Boxed Warning]: Dosage adjustment is required for patients ≥65 years of age. Avoid use in older adults; use is associated with an increased risk of GI bleeding and peptic ulcer disease in older adults in high risk category (eg, >75 years or age or receiving concomitant oral/parenteral corticosteroids, anticoagulants, or antiplatelet agents) (Beers Criteria). **[U.S. Boxed Warning]: Dosage adjustment is required for patients weighing <50 kg (<110 pounds). [U.S. Boxed Warning]: May inhibit uterine contractions and affect fetal circulation; inhibits prostaglandin synthesis in neonates; use is contraindicated in labor and delivery and breast-feeding women.** Avoid use in late pregnancy. **[U.S. Boxed Warning]: Concurrent use of ketorolac with aspirin or other NSAIDs is contraindicated due to the increased risk of adverse reactions.**

[U.S. Boxed Warning]: Contraindicated for epidural or intrathecal administration. [U.S. Boxed Warning]: Systemic ketorolac is indicated for short term (≤5 days) use in adults for treatment of moderately severe acute pain requiring opioid-level analgesia. Low doses of narcotics may be needed for breakthrough pain. **[U.S. Boxed Warning]: Oral therapy is only indicated for use as continuation treatment, following parenteral ketorolac and is not indicated for minor or chronic painful conditions. The maximum daily oral dose is 40 mg (adults); doses above 40 mg/day do not improve efficacy but may increase the risk of serious adverse effects.** The combined therapy duration (oral and parenteral) should not exceed 5 days. Use the lowest effective dose for the shortest duration of time, consistent with individual patient goals, to reduce risk of cardiovascular or GI adverse events. Alternate therapies should be considered for patients at high risk. **[U.S. Boxed Warning]: Oral ketorolac is not indicated for use in children.**

NSAIDS may cause drowsiness, dizziness, blurred vision and other neurologic effects which may impair physical or mental abilities; patients must be cautioned about performing tasks which require mental alertness (eg, operating machinery or driving). Discontinue use with blurred or diminished vision and perform ophthalmologic exam. Monitor vision with long-term therapy.

Drug Interactions

Metabolism/Transport Effects None known.

Avoid Concomitant Use

Avoid concomitant use of Ketorolac (Systemic) with any of the following: Aspirin; Floctafenine; Ketorolac (Nasal); Nonsteroidal Anti-Inflammatory Agents; NSAID (COX-2 Inhibitor); Omacetaxine; Pentoxifylline; Probenecid

Increased Effect/Toxicity

Ketorolac (Systemic) may increase the levels/effects of: Agents with Antiplatelet Properties; Aliskiren; Aminoglycosides; Anticoagulants; Aspirin; Bisphosphonate Derivatives; Collagenase (Systemic); CycloSPORINE (Systemic); Dabigatran Etexilate; ▶

Deferasirox; Desmopressin; Digoxin; Drotrecogin Alfa (Activated); Eplerenone; Haloperidol; Ibritumomab; Lithium; Methotrexate; Neuromuscular-Blocking Agents (Nondepolarizing); Nonsteroidal Anti-Inflammatory Agents; NSAID (COX-2 Inhibitor); Omacetaxine; PEMEtrexed; Pentoxifylline; Porfimer; Potassium-Sparing Diuretics; PRALAtrexate; Quinolone Antibiotics; Rivaroxaban; Salicylates; Thrombolytic Agents; Tositumomab and Iodine I 131 Tositumomab; Vancomycin; Vitamin K Antagonists

The levels/effects of Ketorolac (Systemic) may be increased by: ACE Inhibitors; Angiotensin II Receptor Blockers; Antidepressants (Tricyclic, Tertiary Amine); Corticosteroids (Systemic); CycloSPORINE (Systemic); Dasatinib; Floctafenine; Glucosamine; Herbs (Anticoagulant/Antiplatelet Properties); Ketorolac (Nasal); Multivitamins/Minerals (with ADEK, Folate, Iron); Omega-3 Fatty Acids; Pentosan Polysulfate Sodium; Probenecid; Prostacyclin Analogues; Selective Serotonin Reuptake Inhibitors; Serotonin/Norepinephrine Reuptake Inhibitors; Sodium Phosphates; Tipranavir; Treprostinil; Vitamin E

Decreased Effect

Ketorolac (Systemic) may decrease the levels/effects of: ACE Inhibitors; Agents with Antiplatelet Properties; Aliskiren; Angiotensin II Receptor Blockers; Anticonvulsants; Aspirin; Beta-Blockers; Eplerenone; HydrALAZINE; Loop Diuretics; Potassium-Sparing Diuretics; Salicylates; Selective Serotonin Reuptake Inhibitors; Thiazide Diuretics

The levels/effects of Ketorolac (Systemic) may be decreased by: Bile Acid Sequestrants; Salicylates

Ethanol/Nutrition/Herb Interactions

Ethanol: Avoid ethanol (may enhance gastric mucosal irritation).

Food: Oral: High-fat meals may delay time to peak (by ~1 hour) and decrease peak concentrations.

Herb/Nutraceutical: Avoid alfalfa, anise, bilberry, bladderwrack, bromelain, cat's claw, celery, chamomile, coleus, cordyceps, dong quai, evening primrose, fenugreek, feverfew, garlic, ginger, ginkgo biloba, ginseng (American, Panax, Siberian), grapeseed, green tea, guggul, horse chestnut seed, horseradish, licorice, prickly ash, red clover, reishi, SAMe (S-adenosylmethionine), sweet clover, turmeric, and white willow (all have additional antiplatelet activity).

Dietary Considerations Administer tablet with food or milk to decrease gastrointestinal distress.

Pharmacodynamics/Kinetics

Onset of Action Analgesic: I.M.: ~10 minutes; Peak effect: Analgesic: 2-3 hours

Duration of Action Analgesic: 6-8 hours

Half-life Elimination 2-6 hours; increased 30% to 50% in elderly; up to 19 hours in renal impairment

Time to Peak Serum: I.M.: 30-60 minutes

Pregnancy Risk Factor C

Pregnancy Considerations Adverse events were not observed in the initial animal reproduction studies; therefore, the manufacturer classifies ketorolac as pregnancy category C. Ketorolac crosses the placenta. NSAID exposure during the first trimester is not strongly associated with congenital malformations; however, cardiovascular anomalies and cleft palate have been observed following NSAID exposure in some studies. The use of an NSAID close to conception may be associated with an increased risk of miscarriage. Nonteratogenic effects have been observed following NSAID administration during the third trimester including myocardial degenerative changes, prenatal constriction

of the ductus arteriosus, fetal tricuspid regurgitation, failure of the ductus arteriosus to close postnatally; renal dysfunction or failure, oligohydramnios; gastrointestinal bleeding or perforation, increased risk of necrotizing enterocolitis; intracranial bleeding (including intraventricular hemorrhage), platelet dysfunction with resultant bleeding; pulmonary hypertension. Because they may cause premature closure of the ductus arteriosus, use of NSAIDs late in pregnancy should be avoided (use after 31 or 32 weeks gestation is not recommended by some clinicians). **[U.S. Boxed Warning]: Ketorolac is contraindicated during labor and delivery (may inhibit uterine contractions and adversely affect fetal circulation).** The chronic use of NSAIDs in women of reproductive age may be associated with infertility that is reversible upon discontinuation of the medication.

Lactation Enters breast milk/contraindicated (per manufacturer's labeling)

Breast-Feeding Considerations Low concentrations of ketorolac are found in breast milk (milk concentrations were <1% of the weight-adjusted maternal dose in one study). **[U.S. Boxed Warning]: Inhibition of prostaglandin synthesis may adversely affect neonates; use of systemic ketorolac is contraindicated in breast-feeding women.** The manufacturer of the ophthalmic product recommends that caution be used if administered to a breast-feeding woman. The maternal pharmacokinetics of ketorolac were not found to change immediately postpartum.

Dosage Forms

Injection, solution: 15 mg/mL (1 mL, 2 mL); 30 mg/mL (1 mL, 2 mL, 10 mL)

Tablet, oral: 10 mg

Dental Comment According to the manufacturer, ketorolac has been used inappropriately by physicians in the past. The drug had been prescribed to NSAID-sensitive patients, patients with GI bleeding, and for long-term use; a warning has been issued regarding increased incidence and severity of GI complications with increasing doses and duration of use. Labeling now includes the statement that ketorolac inhibits platelet function and is indicated for up to 5 days use only.

References

Balevi B, "Ketorolac Versus Ibuprofen: A Simple Cost-Efficacy Comparison for Dental Use," *J Can Dent Assoc*, 1994, 60(1):31-2.

Forbes JA, Butterworth GA, Burchfield WH, et al, "Evaluation of Ketorolac, Aspirin, and an Acetaminophen-Codeine Combination in Postoperative Oral Surgery Pain," *Pharmacotherapy*, 1990, 10(6 Pt 2):77S-93S.

Forbes JA, Kehm CJ, Grodin CD, et al, "Evaluation of Ketorolac, Ibuprofen, Acetaminophen, and an Acetaminophen-Codeine Combination in Postoperative Oral Surgery Pain," *Pharmacotherapy*, 1990, 10(6 Pt 2):94S-105S.

Fricke JR Jr, Angelocci D, Fox K, et al, "Comparison of the Efficacy and Safety of Ketorolac and Meperidine in the Relief of Dental Pain," *J Clin Pharmacol*, 1992, 32(4):376-84.

Fricke J, Halladay SC, Bynum L, et al, "Pain Relief After Dental Impaction Surgery Using Ketorolac, Hydrocodone Plus Acetaminophen, or Placebo," *Clin Ther*, 1993, 15(3):500-9.

Pendeville PE, Van Boven MJ, Contreras V, et al, "Ketorolac Tromethamine for Postoperative Analgesia in Oral Surgery," *Acta Anaesthesiol Belg*, 1995, 46(1):25-30.

Walton GM, Rood JP, Snowdon AT, et al, "Ketorolac and Diclofenac for Postoperative Pain Relief Following Oral Surgery," *Br J Oral Maxillofac Surg*, 1993, 31(3):158-60.

Ketorolac (Nasal) (KEE toe role ak)

Brand Names: U.S. Sprix®

Pharmacologic Category Nonsteroidal Anti-inflammatory Drug (NSAID), Nasal

Use Short-term (≤5 days) management of moderate-to-moderately-severe acute pain requiring analgesia at the opioid level

Local Anesthetic/Vasoconstrictor Precautions No information available to require special precautions

Effects on Dental Treatment Key adverse event(s) related to dental treatment: Nasal discomfort, rhinalgia, throat irritation; also see Ketorolac (Systemic)

Effects on Bleeding Nonselective NSAIDs such as ketorolac inhibit platelet aggregation and prolong bleeding time in some patients (<1% with intranasal use). Unlike aspirin, the NSAID effect on platelet function is quantitatively less, of shorter duration, and reversible.

Adverse Effects Events reported with intranasal use; refer to Ketorolac (Systemic) monograph for other potential ketorolac-related adverse events.

>10%: Respiratory: Nasal discomfort (15%), rhinalgia (13%)

>1% to 10%:
Cardiovascular: Bradycardia (2%), hypertension (2%)
Dermatologic: Rash (3%)
Gastrointestinal: Throat irritation (4%)
Genitourinary: Urine output decreased (2%)
Hepatic: ALT/AST increased (2%)
Ocular: Lacrimation increased (5%)
Respiratory: Rhinitis (2%)
Renal: Oliguria (3%)

General Dosage Range Dosage adjustment recommended in patients with renal impairment.

Intranasal:
Adults <65 years and ≥50 kg: one spray (15.75 mg) in each nostril (total dose: 31.5 mg) every 6-8 hours; maximum dose: 4 doses (126 mg)/day
Adults <50 kg and/or Elderly ≥65 years: One spray (15.75 mg) in 1 nostril (total dose: 15.75 mg) every 6-8 hours; maximum dose: 4 doses (63 mg)/day

Mechanism of Action Reversibly inhibits cyclooxygenase-1 and 2 (COX-1 and 2) enzymes, which results in decreased formation of prostaglandin precursors; has antipyretic, analgesic, and anti-inflammatory properties

Other proposed mechanisms not fully elucidated (and possibly contributing to the anti-inflammatory effect to varying degrees), include inhibiting chemotaxis, altering lymphocyte activity, inhibiting neutrophil aggregation/activation, and decreasing proinflammatory cytokine levels.

Pharmacodynamics/Kinetics

Onset of Action Analgesia: Within 20 minutes

Half-life Elimination
~5-6 hours (similar to I.M. administration); prolonged ~35% in elderly; up to 19 hours in renal impairment

Time to Peak 0.5-0.75 hours

Pregnancy Risk Factor C/D ≥30 weeks gestation

Pregnancy Considerations Adverse events were not observed in the initial animal reproduction studies; therefore, the manufacturer classifies ketorolac (nasal) as pregnancy category C (category D: ≥30 weeks gestation).When administered I.M., ketorolac crosses the placenta. The amount of ketorolac available systemically following intranasal administration is 60% to 70% in comparison to I.M. doses. Adverse fetal effects have been observed following maternal use of NSAIDs. Maternal use ≥30 weeks gestation increases the risk of premature closure of the ductus arteriosus. When used during labor and delivery, ketorolac may cause adverse effects on the fetal circulation, inhibit uterine contractions and increase the risk of uterine hemorrhage. Use during labor and delivery is contraindicated. Refer to the Ketorolac (Systemic) monograph for details.

Ketotifen (Systemic) (kee toe TYE fen)

Related Information
Respiratory Diseases *on page 1514*

Brand Names: Canada APO-Ketotifen®; Novo-Ketotifen; Nu-Ketotifen®; PMS-Ketotifen; Zaditen®

Pharmacologic Category Histamine H$_1$ Antagonist; Histamine H$_1$ Antagonist, Second Generation; Mast Cell Stabilizer; Piperidine Derivative

Use Adjunctive therapy in the chronic treatment of pediatric patients ≥6 months of age with mild, atopic asthma

Local Anesthetic/Vasoconstrictor Precautions No information available to require special precautions

Effects on Dental Treatment No significant effects or complications reported

Effects on Bleeding No information available to require special precautions

Adverse Effects 1% to 10%:
Central nervous system: Sedation (8%; less than placebo), headache (1%), sleep disturbance (1%)
Dermatologic: Rash (4%), urticaria (1%)
Gastrointestinal: Weight gain (5%), abdominal pain (1%), appetite increased (1%)
Respiratory: Respiratory infection (4%), epistaxis (1%)
Miscellaneous: Flu (3%), puffy eyelid (1%)

General Dosage Range Oral:
Children 6 months to 3 years: Initial: 0.05 mg/kg once daily or in 2 divided doses for 5 days; Maintenance: 0.05 mg/kg twice daily (maximum dose: 1 mg twice daily)
Children >3 years: Initial: 1 mg once daily or in 2 divided doses for 5 days; Maintenance: 1 mg twice daily

Mechanism of Action Exhibits noncompetitive H$_1$-receptor antagonist and mast cell stabilizer properties. Efficacy in asthma likely results from a combination of anti-inflammatory and antihistaminergic actions including interference with chemokine-induced migration of eosinophils into inflamed airways, inhibition of airway hyper-reactivity due to platelet activating factor (PAF), antagonism of leukotriene-induced bronchoconstriction.

Pharmacodynamics/Kinetics

Half-life Elimination ~9-9.5 hours

Time to Peak Plasma: 2-4 hours

Pregnancy Considerations Adverse fetal effects were found in some but not all animal studies. Safety in human pregnancy has not been established.

Product Availability Not available in the U.S.

Ketotifen (Ophthalmic) (kee toe TYE fen)

Brand Names: U.S. Alaway™ [OTC]; Claritin™ Eye [OTC]; Zaditor® [OTC]; ZyrTEC® Itchy Eye [OTC]

Brand Names: Canada Zaditor®

Pharmacologic Category Histamine H$_1$ Antagonist; Histamine H$_1$ Antagonist, Second Generation; Mast Cell Stabilizer; Piperidine Derivative

Use Temporary relief of eye itching due to allergic conjunctivitis

Local Anesthetic/Vasoconstrictor Precautions No information available to require special precautions

Effects on Dental Treatment Key adverse event(s) related to dental treatment: Pharyngitis.

Effects on Bleeding No information available to require special precautions

Adverse Effects 1% to 10%:

Ocular: Allergic reactions, burning or stinging, conjunctivitis, discharge, dry eyes, eye pain, eyelid disorder, itching, keratitis, lacrimation disorder, mydriasis, photophobia, rash

Respiratory: Pharyngitis

Miscellaneous: Flu syndrome

General Dosage Range Ophthalmic: *Children ≥3 years and Adults:* Instill 1 drop into the affected eye(s) twice daily, every 8-12 hours

Mechanism of Action Exhibits noncompetitive H_1-receptor antagonist and mast cell stabilizer properties. Efficacy in conjunctivitis likely results from a combination of anti-inflammatory and antihistaminergic actions including interference with chemokine-induced migration of eosinophils into inflamed conjunctiva.

Pharmacodynamics/Kinetics

Onset of Action Minutes

Duration of Action 8-12 hours

Pregnancy Risk Factor C

Pregnancy Considerations Topical ocular administration has not been studied.

Labetalol (la BET a lole)

Related Information

Cardiovascular Diseases *on page 1492*

Brand Names: U.S. Trandate®

Brand Names: Canada Apo-Labetalol®; Labetalol Hydrochloride Injection, USP; Normodyne®; Trandate®

Pharmacologic Category Beta-Blocker With Alpha-Blocking Activity

Use Treatment of mild-to-severe hypertension; I.V. for severe hypertension (eg, hypertensive emergencies)

Unlabeled Use Pediatric hypertension; management of pre-eclampsia; severe hypertension in pregnancy; hypertension during acute ischemic stroke

Local Anesthetic/Vasoconstrictor Precautions

Use with caution; epinephrine has interacted with non-selective beta-blockers to result in initial hypertensive episode followed by bradycardia

Effects on Dental Treatment Key adverse event(s) related to dental treatment: Taste disorder.

Many nonsteroidal anti-inflammatory drugs, such as ibuprofen and indomethacin, can reduce the hypotensive effect of beta-blockers after 3 or more weeks of therapy with the NSAID. Short-term NSAID use (ie, 3 days) requires no special precautions in patients taking beta-blockers.

Effects on Bleeding No information available to require special precautions

Adverse Effects

>10%:

Cardiovascular: Orthostatic hypotension (I.V. use; ≤58%)

Central nervous system: Dizziness (1% to 20%), fatigue (1% to 11%)

Gastrointestinal: Nausea (≤19%)

1% to 10%:

Cardiovascular: Hypotension (1% to 5%), edema (≤2%), flushing (1%), ventricular arrhythmia (I.V. use; 1%)

Central nervous system: Somnolence (3%), headache (2%), vertigo (1% to 2%)

Dermatologic: Scalp tingling (≤7%), pruritus (1%), rash (1%)

Gastrointestinal: Dyspepsia (≤4%), vomiting (≤3%), taste disturbance (1%)

Genitourinary: Ejaculatory failure (≤5%), impotence (1% to 4%)

Hepatic: Transaminases increased (4%)

Neuromuscular & skeletal: Paresthesia (≤5%), weakness (1%)

Ocular: Vision abnormal (1%)

Renal: BUN increased (≤8%)

Respiratory: Nasal congestion (1% to 6%), dyspnea (2%)

Miscellaneous: Diaphoresis (≤4%)

Other adverse reactions noted with beta-adrenergic blocking agents include mental depression, catatonia, disorientation, short-term memory loss, emotional lability, clouded sensorium, intensification of pre-existing AV block, laryngospasm, respiratory distress, agranulocytosis, thrombocytopenic purpura, nonthrombocytopenic purpura, mesenteric artery thrombosis, and ischemic colitis.

General Dosage Range

I.V.:

Children: 0.3-1 mg/kg/dose intermittently **or** 0.4-1 mg/kg/hour infusion (maximum: 3 mg/kg/hour)

Adults: Bolus: 20 mg, may give 40-80 mg at 10-minute intervals; Infusion: 2 mg/minute (maximum: 300 mg total cumulative dose)

Oral: *Adults:* Initial: 100 mg twice daily; Maintenance: 200-800 mg/day in 2 divided doses (maximum: 2.4 g/day)

Mechanism of Action Blocks alpha-, $beta_1$-, and $beta_2$-adrenergic receptor sites; elevated renins are reduced. The ratios of alpha- to beta-blockade differ depending on the route of administration: 1:3 (oral) and 1:7 (I.V.).

Pharmacodynamics/Kinetics

Onset of Action Oral: 20 minutes to 2 hours; I.V.: 2-5 minutes; Peak effect: Oral: 1-4 hours; I.V.: 5-15 minutes

Duration of Action Blood pressure response:

Oral: 8-12 hours (dose dependent)

I.V.: 2-18 hours (dose dependent; based on single and multiple sequential doses of 0.25-0.5 mg/kg with cumulative dosing up to 3.25 mg/kg)

Half-life Elimination Oral: 6-8 hours; I.V.: ~5.5 hours

Time to Peak Plasma: Oral: 1-2 hours

Pregnancy Risk Factor C

Pregnancy Considerations Because adverse events were observed in some animal reproduction studies, labetalol is classified as pregnancy category C. Labetalol crosses the placenta and can be detected in cord blood and infant serum after delivery. It has been shown to decrease maternal blood pressure without significantly effecting placental blood flow. In a cohort study, an increased risk of cardiovascular defects was observed following maternal use of beta-blockers during pregnancy. Intrauterine growth restriction (IUGR), small placentas, as well as fetal/neonatal bradycardia, hypoglycemia, and/or respiratory depression have been observed following *in utero* exposure to beta-blockers as a class. Adequate facilities for monitoring infants at birth should be available. Untreated chronic maternal hypertension and pre-eclampsia are also associated with adverse events in the fetus, infant, and mother. The pharmacokinetics of labetalol are not significantly changed during the third trimester of pregnancy. Labetalol is considered an appropriate agent for the treatment of hypertension in pregnancy; intravenous labetalol is also used for the management of pre-eclampsia.

Lacosamide (la KOE sa mide)

Brand Names: U.S. Vimpat®
Brand Names: Canada Vimpat®
Pharmacologic Category Anticonvulsant, Miscellaneous
Use Adjunctive therapy in the treatment of partial-onset seizures
Local Anesthetic/Vasoconstrictor Precautions Lacosamide may prolong PR interval resulting in cardiac conduction problems; it is not known what effect vasoconstrictors will have in patients taking medications that could prolong PR interval. It is suggested that the clinician consult with the physician prior to use of vasoconstrictor in suspected patients; use vasoconstrictor with caution.
Effects on Dental Treatment No significant effects or complications reported
Effects on Bleeding No information available to require special precautions
Adverse Effects
>10%:
Central nervous system: Dizziness (31%), headache (13%)
Gastrointestinal: Nausea (11%)
Ocular: Diplopia (11%)
1% to 10%:
Cardiovascular: Syncope (adults 1%; dose-related: >400 mg/day)
Central nervous system: Fatigue (9%), ataxia (8%), somnolence (7%), coordination impaired (4%), vertigo (4%), depression (2%), memory impairment (2%)
Dermatologic: Pruritus (2%)
Gastrointestinal: Vomiting (9%), diarrhea (4%)
Hepatic: ALT increased (1%)
Local: Contusion (3%), skin laceration (3%), injection site pain/discomfort (3%), irritation (1%)
Neuromuscular & skeletal: Tremor (7%), gait instability (2%), weakness (2%)
Ocular: Blurred vision (8%), nystagmus (5%)
General Dosage Range Dosage adjustment recommended in patients with hepatic or renal impairment
Oral: Adolescents ≥17 years and Adults: Initial: 50 mg twice daily; Maintenance dose: 200-400 mg daily
Mechanism of Action In vitro studies have shown that lacosamide stabilizes hyperexcitable neuronal membranes and inhibits repetitive neuronal firing by enhancing the slow inactivation of sodium channels (with no effects on fast inactivation of sodium channels).
Pharmacodynamics/Kinetics
Half-life Elimination ~13 hours
Time to Peak Oral: 1-4 hours
Pregnancy Risk Factor C
Pregnancy Considerations Adverse events were observed in animal reproduction studies. Available information related to use in pregnancy is limited; if inadvertent exposure occurs during pregnancy, close monitoring of the mother and fetus/newborn is recommended (Hoeltzenbein, 2011). Two registries are available for women exposed to lacosamide during pregnancy:
Pregnant women may contact the North American Antiepileptic Drug (AED) Pregnancy Registry (888-233-2334 or http://www.aedpregnancyregistry.org)
The healthcare provider or patient may contact the UCB AED Pregnancy Registry (888-537-7734)
Controlled Substance C-V

Lactase (LAK tase)

Brand Names: U.S. Lac-Dose® [OTC]; Lactaid® Fast Act [OTC]; Lactaid® Original [OTC]; Lactose Intolerance [OTC]; Lactrase® [OTC]
Brand Names: Canada Dairyaid®
Pharmacologic Category Enzyme
Use Help digest lactose in milk for patients with lactose intolerance
Local Anesthetic/Vasoconstrictor Precautions No information available to require special precautions
Effects on Dental Treatment No significant effects or complications reported
Effects on Bleeding No information available to require special precautions
General Dosage Range Oral: Adults: 1-2 capsules with meals or 5-15 drops or 1-2 capsules/quart of milk or 1-3 tablets with meals

Lactic Acid (LAK tik AS id)

Pharmacologic Category Topical Skin Product
Use Lubricate and moisturize the skin counteracting dryness and itching
Local Anesthetic/Vasoconstrictor Precautions No information available to require special precautions
Effects on Dental Treatment No significant effects or complications reported
Effects on Bleeding No information available to require special precautions
Adverse Effects Frequency not defined: Dermatologic: Burning, mild stinging, peeling
General Dosage Range Topical: Adults: Apply twice daily

Lactic Acid and Ammonium Hydroxide
(LAK tik AS id & a MOE nee um hye DROKS ide)

Related Information
Lactic Acid on page 789
Brand Names: U.S. AmLactin® [OTC]; Geri-Hydrolac™ [OTC]; Geri-Hydrolac™-12 [OTC]; Lac-Hydrin®; Lac-Hydrin® Five [OTC]; LAClotion™
Pharmacologic Category Topical Skin Product
Use Treatment of moderate-to-severe xerosis and ichthyosis vulgaris
Local Anesthetic/Vasoconstrictor Precautions No information available to require special precautions
Effects on Dental Treatment No significant effects or complications reported
Effects on Bleeding No information available to require special precautions
Adverse Effects
>10%: Dermatologic: Burning/stinging (3% to 15%), rash (2% to 15%; includes erythema and irritation)
1% to 10%: Dermatologic: Itching (5%), dry skin (2%)
General Dosage Range Topical:
Cream: Children ≥2 years and Adults: Apply twice daily to affected area
Lotion: Children and Adults: Apply twice daily to affected area
Mechanism of Action Exact mechanism of action unknown; lactic acid is a normal component in blood and tissues. When applied topically to the skin, acts as a humectant.
Pregnancy Risk Factor B

◄ **Pregnancy Considerations** Lactic acid is a normal component in blood and tissues. Topical application in animals has not shown fetal harm.

Lactobacillus (lak toe ba SIL us)

Related Information
Ulcerative, Erosive, and Painful Oral Mucosal Disorders *on page 1578*

Brand Names: U.S. Bacid® [OTC]; Culturelle® [OTC]; Dofus [OTC]; Flora-Q™ [OTC]; Floranex™ [OTC]; Kala® [OTC]; Lactinex™ [OTC]; Lacto-Bifidus [OTC]; Lacto-Key [OTC]; Lacto-Pectin [OTC]; Lacto-TriBlend [OTC]; Megadophilus® [OTC]; MoreDophilus® [OTC]; RisaQuad®-2 [OTC]; RisaQuad™ [OTC]; Superdophilus® [OTC]; VSL #3® [OTC]; VSL #3®-DS

Brand Names: Canada Bacid®; Fermalac

Generic Availability (U.S.) Yes

Pharmacologic Category Dietary Supplement; Probiotic

Dental Use Treatment of uncomplicated diarrhea, particularly that caused by antibiotic therapy; re-establish normal physiologic and bacterial flora of the intestinal tract

Use Promote normal bacterial flora of the intestinal tract

Local Anesthetic/Vasoconstrictor Precautions No information available to require special precautions

Effects on Dental Treatment No significant effects or complications reported

Effects on Bleeding No information available to require special precautions

Adverse Effects Gastrointestinal: Bloating (intestinal), flatulence

Dosage Dietary supplement: Oral: Dosing varies by manufacturer; consult product labeling

Children (Culturelle®): 1 capsule daily
Adults:
Bacid®: 2 caplets/day
Culturelle®: 1 capsule daily; may increase to twice daily
Flora-Q™: 1 capsule/day
Lacto-Key 100 or 600: 1-2 capsules/day
Lactinex™: 1 packet or 4 tablets 3-4 times/day
VSL #3®: 1-8 sachets or 2-32 capsules/day
VSL #3®-DS: 1-4 packets/day

Dosage adjustment in renal impairment: No dosage adjustment provided in manufacturer's labeling.

Dosage adjustment in hepatic impairment: No dosage adjustment provided in manufacturer's labeling.

Mechanism of Action Helps re-establish normal intestinal flora; suppresses the growth of potentially pathogenic microorganisms by producing lactic acid which favors the establishment of an aciduric flora.

Contraindications Hypersensitivity to any component of the formulation

Warnings/Precautions *Lactobacillus* species have been studied for various gastrointestinal disorders including diarrhea, inflammatory bowel disease, gastrointestinal infection. Effectiveness may be dependent upon actual species used; studies are ongoing. Currently, there are no FDA-approved disease-prevention or therapeutic indications for these products.

Drug Interactions

Metabolism/Transport Effects None known.

Avoid Concomitant Use There are no known interactions where it is recommended to avoid concomitant use.

Increased Effect/Toxicity There are no known significant interactions involving an increase in effect.

Decreased Effect There are no known significant interactions involving a decrease in effect.

Dietary Considerations Some products may contain potassium and/or sodium.

Dosage Forms

Capsule:
Culturelle® [OTC]: *L. rhamnosus* GG 10 billion colony-forming units
Dofus [OTC]: *L. acidophilus* and *L. bifidus* 10:1 ratio
Flora-Q™ [OTC]: *L. acidophilus* and *L. paracasei* ≥8 billion colony-forming units
Lacto-Key [OTC]:
  100: *L. acidophilus* 1 billion colony-forming units
  600: *L. acidophilus* 6 billion colony-forming units
Lacto-Bifidus [OTC]:
  100: *L. bifidus* 1 billion colony-forming units
  600: *L. bifidus* 6 billion colony-forming units
Lacto-Pectin [OTC]: *L. acidophilus* and *L. casei* ≥5 billion colony-forming units
Lacto-TriBlend [OTC]:
  100: *L. acidophilus*, *L. bifidus*, and *L. bulgaricus* 1 billion colony-forming units
  600: *L. acidophilus*, *L. bifidus*, and *L. bulgaricus* 6 billion colony-forming units
Megadophilus® [OTC], Superdophilus® [OTC]: *L. acidophilus* 2 billion units
RisaQuad™ [OTC]: *L. acidophilus* and *L. paracasei* 8 billion colony-forming units
VSL #3® [OTC]: *L. acidophilus*, *L. plantarum*, *L. paracasei*, *L. bulgaricus* 112 billion live cells

Capsule, double strength:
RisaQuad®-2 [OTC]: *L. acidophilus* and *L. paracasei* 16 billion colony-forming units

Capsule, softgel: *L. acidophilus* 100 active units

Caplet:
Bacid® [OTC]: *L. acidophilus 80%* and *L. bulgaricus 10%*

Granules:
Floranex™ [OTC], Lactinex™ [OTC]: *L. acidophilus* and *L. bulgaricus* 100 million live cells per 1 g packet (12s)

Powder:
Lacto-TriBlend [OTC]: *L. acidophilus*, *L. bifidus*, and *L. bulgaricus* 10 billion colony-forming units per ¼ teaspoon
Megadophilus® [OTC], Superdophilus® [OTC]: *L. acidophilus* 2 billion units per half-teaspoon
MoreDophilus® [OTC]: *L. acidophilus* 12.4 billion units per teaspoon
VSL #3® [OTC]: *L. acidophilus*, *L. plantarum*, *L. paracasei*, *L. bulgaricus* 450 billion live cells
VSL #3®-DS: *L. acidophilus*, *L. plantarum*, *L. paracasei*, *L. bulgaricus* 900 billion live cells

Tablet:
Kala® [OTC]: *L. acidophilus* 200 million units

Tablet, chewable: *L. reuteri* 100 million organisms
Floranex™ [OTC]: *L. acidophilus* and *L. bulgaricus* 1 million colony-forming units
Lactinex™ [OTC]: *L. acidophilus* and *L. bulgaricus* 1 million live cells

Wafer: *L. acidophilus* 90 mg and *L. bifidus* 25 mg (100s)

Lactulose (LAK tyoo lose)

Brand Names: U.S. Constulose; Enulose; Generlac; Kristalose®

Brand Names: Canada Acilac; Apo-Lactulose®; Lax-ilose; PMS-Lactulose

Pharmacologic Category Ammonium Detoxicant; Laxative, Osmotic

Use Prevention and treatment of portal-systemic ence-phalopathy (including hepatic precoma and coma); treatment of constipation

Local Anesthetic/Vasoconstrictor Precautions No information available to require special precautions

Effects on Dental Treatment No significant effects or complications reported

Effects on Bleeding No information available to require special precautions

Adverse Effects Frequency not defined.

Endocrine & metabolic: Dehydration, hypernatremia, hypokalemia

Gastrointestinal: Abdominal discomfort, abdominal dis-tention, belching, cramping, diarrhea (excessive dose), flatulence, nausea, vomiting

General Dosage Range

Oral:

Infants: 1.7-6.7 g/day (2.5-10 mL/day) in divided doses

Older Children and Adolescents: 26.7-60 g/day (40-90 mL/day) in divided doses

Adults: PSE: 20-30 g (30-45 mL) every hour initially, then 3-4 times/day; Constipation: 10-40 g (15-60 mL) daily

Rectal: *Adults:* Constipation: 200 g (300 mL); may repeat every 4-6 hours

Mechanism of Action The bacterial degradation of lactulose resulting in an acidic pH inhibits the diffusion of NH_3 into the blood by causing the conversion of NH_3 to NH_4+; also enhances the diffusion of NH_3 from the blood into the gut where conversion to NH_4+ occurs; produces an osmotic effect in the colon with resultant distention promoting peristalsis; reduces blood ammo-nia concentration to reduce the degree of portal sys-temic encephalopathy

Pharmacodynamics/Kinetics

Onset of Action

Constipation: Up to 24-48 hours to produce a normal bowel movement

Encephalopathy: At least 24-48 hours

Pregnancy Risk Factor B

Pregnancy Considerations Adverse events have not been observed in animal reproduction studies.

LamiVUDine (la MI vyoo deen)

Related Information

HIV Infection and AIDS *on page 1520*

Systemic Viral Diseases *on page 1537*

Brand Names: U.S. Epivir-HBV®; Epivir®

Brand Names: Canada 3TC®; Apo-Lamivudine®; Apo-Lamivudine® HBV; Heptovir®

Pharmacologic Category Antiretroviral Agent, Reverse Transcriptase Inhibitor (Nucleoside)

Use

Epivir®: Treatment of HIV infection when antiretroviral therapy is warranted; should always be used as part of a multidrug regimen (at least three antiretroviral agents)

Epivir-HBV®: Treatment of chronic hepatitis B associ-ated with evidence of hepatitis B viral replication and active liver inflammation. Resistance develops rapidly in hepatitis B; consider use only if other anti-HBV antiviral agents with more favorable resistance pat-terns cannot be used.

Unlabeled Use Postexposure prophylaxis for HIV expo-sure as part of a multidrug regimen

Local Anesthetic/Vasoconstrictor Precautions No information available to require special precautions

Effects on Dental Treatment No significant effects or complications reported

Effects on Bleeding No information available to require special precautions relative to hemostasis.

Adverse Effects Incidence data include patients on combination therapy with other antiretroviral agents.

>10%:

Central nervous system: Headache (21% to 35%), fatigue (24% to 27%), insomnia (11%)

Gastrointestinal: Nausea (15% to 33%), diarrhea (14% to 18%), pancreatitis (range: 0.3% to 18%; higher percentage in pediatric patients), abdominal pain (9% to 16%), vomiting (13% to 15%)

Hematologic: Neutropenia (7% to 15%)

Hepatic: Transaminases increased (2% to 11%)

Neuromuscular & skeletal: Myalgia (8% to 14%), neu-ropathy (12%), musculoskeletal pain (12%)

Respiratory: Nasal signs and symptoms (20%), cough (18%), sore throat (13%)

Miscellaneous: Infections (25%; includes ear, nose, and throat)

1% to 10%:

Central nervous system: Dizziness (10%), depression (9%), fever (7% to 10%), chills (7% to 10%)

Dermatologic: Rash (5% to 9%)

Gastrointestinal: Anorexia (10%), lipase increased (10%), abdominal cramps (6%), dyspepsia (5%), amylase increased (<1% to 4%), heartburn

Hematologic: Thrombocytopenia (1% to 4%), hemo-globinemia (2% to 3%)

Neuromuscular & skeletal: Creatine phosphokinase increased (9%), arthralgia (5% to 7%)

General Dosage Range Dosage adjustment recom-mended in patients with renal impairment

Oral:

Infants 1-3 months: HIV (DHHS [pediatric], 2010): 4 mg/kg/dose twice daily

Children 3 months to 2 years: HIV: 4 mg/kg/dose twice daily (maximum: 150 mg/dose twice daily)

Children 2-16 years and >16 years and <50 kg: Hep-atitis B: 3 mg/kg/dose once daily (maximum: 100 mg/day); HIV: 4 mg/kg/dose twice daily (maxi-mum: 150 mg/dose twice daily)

Children >16 years and ≥50 kg: Hepatitis B: 3 mg/kg/dose once daily (maximum: 100 mg/day); HIV: 150 mg twice daily **or** 300 mg once daily

Adults <50 kg: Hepatitis B: 100 mg/day; HIV (DHHS [pediatric], 2010): 4 mg/kg/dose twice daily (maxi-mum: 150 mg/dose twice daily)

Adults ≥50 kg: Hepatitis B: 100 mg/day; HIV: 150 mg twice daily **or** 300 mg once daily

Mechanism of Action Lamivudine is a cytosine ana-log. After lamivudine is triphosphorylated, the principle mode of action is inhibition of HIV reverse transcription via viral DNA chain termination; inhibits RNA- and DNA-dependent DNA polymerase activities of reverse tran-scriptase. The monophosphate form of lamivudine is incorporated into the viral DNA by hepatitis B virus polymerase, resulting in DNA chain termination.

Pharmacodynamics/Kinetics

Half-life Elimination Children: 2 hours; Adults: 5-7 hours

Time to Peak Fed: 3.2 hours; Fasted: 0.9 hours

Pregnancy Risk Factor C

◄ **Pregnancy Considerations** Adverse events were observed in some animal reproduction studies. Lamivudine crosses the human placenta. No increased risk of overall birth defects has been observed following first trimester exposure according to data collected by the antiretroviral pregnancy registry. The pharmacokinetics of lamivudine during pregnancy are not significantly altered and dosage adjustment is not required. Cases of lactic acidosis/hepatic steatosis syndrome related to mitochondrial toxicity have been reported in pregnant women with prolonged use of nucleoside analogues. It is not known if pregnancy itself potentiates this known side effect; however, women may be at increased risk of lactic acidosis and liver damage. In addition, these adverse events are similar to other rare but life-threatening syndromes which occur during pregnancy (eg, HELLP syndrome). Hepatic enzymes and electrolytes should be monitored in women receiving nucleoside analogues and clinicians should watch for early signs of the syndrome. In addition, mitochondrial dysfunction may develop in infants following in utero exposure The DHHS Perinatal HIV Guidelines recommend lamivudine for use during pregnancy; the combination of lamivudine with zidovudine is the recommended dual combination NRTI in pregnancy. The DHHS Perinatal HIV Guidelines consider lamivudine plus tenofovir a recommended dual NRTI/NtRTI backbone for HIV/HBV coinfected pregnant women. Use caution with hepatitis B coinfection; hepatitis B flare may occur if lamivudine is discontinued postpartum.

Regardless of CD4 count or HIV RNA copy number, all HIV-infected pregnant women should receive a combination antepartum antiretroviral (ARV) drug regimen; this includes women who require therapy for their own health, as well as women who do not yet require therapy for their own health. ARV therapy should be started as soon as possible if required for the woman's health. Although earlier initiation may be more effective in reducing the perinatal transmission of HIV), also consider maternal conditions (eg, nausea and vomiting) and the potential risks of first trimester fetal exposure for specific agents. Plasma HIV RNA levels should be assessed at ~34-36 weeks gestation in order to help determine mode of delivery. If ARV therapy must be interrupted for <24 hours during the peripartum period, stop then restart all medications simultaneously in order to decrease the chance of developing resistance. Long-term follow-up is recommended for all infants exposed to ARV medications.

Healthcare providers are encouraged to enroll pregnant women exposed to antiretroviral medications in the Antiretroviral Pregnancy Registry (1-800-258-4263 or www.APRegistry.com). Healthcare providers caring for HIV-infected women and their infants may contact the National Perinatal HIV Hotline (888-448-8765) for clinical consultation (DHHS [perinatal], 2012).

Lamivudine and Zidovudine
(la MI vyoo deen & zye DOE vyoo deen)

Related Information
HIV Infection and AIDS *on page 1520*
LamiVUDine *on page 791*
Zidovudine *on page 1419*
Brand Names: U.S. Combivir®
Brand Names: Canada Combivir®; Teva-Lamivudine/Zidovudine
Pharmacologic Category Antiretroviral Agent, Reverse Transcriptase Inhibitor (Nucleoside)

Use Treatment of HIV infection when therapy is warranted based on clinical and/or immunological evidence of disease progression
Local Anesthetic/Vasoconstrictor Precautions No information available to require special precautions
Effects on Dental Treatment No significant effects or complications reported
Effects on Bleeding No information available to require special precautions relative to hemostasis.
Adverse Effects See individual agents.
General Dosage Range Oral: *Adolescents ≥30 kg and Adults:* 1 tablet (lamivudine 150 mg/zidovudine 300 mg) twice daily
Mechanism of Action The combination of zidovudine and lamivudine is believed to act synergistically to inhibit reverse transcriptase via DNA chain termination after incorporation of the nucleoside analogue as well as to delay the emergence of mutations conferring resistance
Pregnancy Risk Factor C
Pregnancy Considerations See individual agents.

LamoTRIgine (la MOE tri jeen)

Brand Names: U.S. LaMICtal®; LaMICtal® ODT™; LaMICtal® XR™
Brand Names: Canada Apo-Lamotrigine®; Auro-Lamotrigine; Lamictal®; Mylan-Lamotrigine; PMS-Lamotrigine; ratio-Lamotrigine; Teva-Lamotrigine
Pharmacologic Category Anticonvulsant, Miscellaneous
Use
U.S. labeling:
  Immediate release: Adjunctive therapy in the treatment of generalized seizures of Lennox-Gastaut syndrome, primary generalized tonic-clonic seizures, and partial seizures; conversion to monotherapy in patients with partial seizures who are receiving treatment with a single antiepileptic drug (AED) (specifically carbamazepine, phenytoin, phenobarbital, primidone, or valproic acid); maintenance treatment of bipolar I disorder
  Extended release: Adjunctive therapy for primary generalized tonic-clonic seizures and partial seizures (with or without secondary generalization); conversion to monotherapy in patients with partial seizures who are receiving treatment with a single antiepileptic drug AED
Canadian labeling: Immediate release: Adjunctive therapy for epilepsy uncontrolled by conventional therapy; monotherapy of epilepsy following withdrawal of concurrent antiepileptic agents; adjunctive therapy for Lennox-Gastaut syndrome
Local Anesthetic/Vasoconstrictor Precautions No information available to require special precautions
Effects on Dental Treatment Key adverse event(s) related to dental treatment: Xerostomia (normal salivary flow resumes upon discontinuation).
Effects on Bleeding Thrombocytopenia and anemia have been reported in <1% of patients.
Adverse Effects Percentages reported in adults on monotherapy for epilepsy or bipolar disorder.
>10%: Gastrointestinal: Nausea (7% to 14%)
1% to 10%:
  Cardiovascular: Chest pain (5%), peripheral edema (2% to 5%), edema (1% to 5%)

Central nervous system: Insomnia (5% to 10%), somnolence (9%), fatigue (8%), coordination impaired (7%), dizziness (7%), anxiety (5%), pain (5%), ataxia (2% to 5%), irritability (2% to 5%), suicidal ideation (2% to 5%), agitation (1% to 5%), amnesia (1% to 5%), depression (1% to 5%), dream abnormality (1% to 5%), emotional lability (1% to 5%), fever (1% to 5%), hypoesthesia (1% to 5%), migraine (1% to 5%), thought abnormality (1% to 5%), confusion (1%)
Dermatologic: Rash (nonserious: 7%), dermatitis (2% to 5%), dry skin (2% to 5%)
Endocrine & metabolic: Dysmenorrhea (5%), libido increased (2% to 5%)
Gastrointestinal: Vomiting (5% to 9%), dyspepsia (7%), abdominal pain (6%), xerostomia (2% to 6%), constipation (5%), weight loss (5%), anorexia (2% to 5%), peptic ulcer (2% to 5%), rectal hemorrhage (2% to 5%), flatulence (1% to 5%), weight gain (1% to 5%)
Genitourinary: Urinary frequency (1% to 5%)
Neuromuscular & skeletal: Back pain (8%), weakness (2% to 5%), arthralgia (1% to 5%), myalgia (1% to 5%), neck pain (1% to 5%), paresthesia (1%)
Ocular: Nystagmus (2% to 5%), vision abnormal (2% to 5%), amblyopia (1%)
Respiratory: Rhinitis (7%), cough (5%), pharyngitis (5%), bronchitis (2% to 5%), dyspnea (2% to 5%), epistaxis (2% to 5%), sinusitis (1% to 5%)
Miscellaneous: Infection (5%), diaphoresis (2% to 5%), reflexes increased/decreased (2% to 5%), dyspraxia (1% to 5%)
General Dosage Range Dosage adjustment recommended in patients with hepatic or renal impairment or on concomitant therapy
Oral:
Immediate release formulation:
Children 2-12 years: Dosage varies greatly depending on indication
Children >12 years and Adults: Dosage varies greatly depending on indication
Extended release formulation: *Children ≥13 years and Adults:* Dosage varies greatly depending on indication
Mechanism of Action A triazine derivative which inhibits release of glutamate (an excitatory amino acid) and inhibits voltage-sensitive sodium channels, which stabilizes neuronal membranes. Lamotrigine has weak inhibitory effect on the 5-HT$_3$ receptor; *in vitro* inhibits dihydrofolate reductase.
Pharmacodynamics/Kinetics
Half-life Elimination Immediate release: Adults: 25-33 hours, Elderly: 25-43 hours; Extended release: Similar to immediate release
Concomitant valproic acid therapy: 48-70 hours
Concomitant phenytoin, phenobarbital, primidone, or carbamazepine therapy: 13-14 hours
Chronic renal failure: 43 hours
Hemodialysis: 13 hours during dialysis; 57 hours between dialysis (~20% of a dose is eliminated in a 4-hour dialysis session)
Hepatic impairment:
Mild: 26-66 hours
Moderate: 28-116 hours
Severe without ascites: 56-78 hours
Severe with ascites: 52-148 hours
Time to Peak Plasma: Immediate release: 1-1.5 hours; Extended release: 4-11 hours (dependent on adjunct therapy)
Pregnancy Risk Factor C

Pregnancy Considerations Lamotrigine has been found to decrease folate concentrations in animal studies. Teratogenic effects in animals were not observed. Lamotrigine crosses the human placenta and can be measured in the plasma of exposed newborns. Preliminary data from the North American Antiepileptic Drug Pregnancy Registry (NAAED) suggest an increased incidence of cleft lip and/or cleft palate following first trimester exposure. Healthcare providers may enroll patients in the Lamotrigine Pregnancy Registry by calling (800) 336-2176. Patients may enroll themselves in the NAAED registry by calling (888) 233-2334. Additional information is available at www.aedpregnancyregistry.org. Dose of lamotrigine may need adjustment during pregnancy to maintain clinical response; lamotrigine serum levels may decrease during pregnancy and return to prepartum levels following delivery. Monitor frequently during pregnancy, following delivery, and when adding or discontinuing combination hormonal contraceptives.

Lanolin, Cetyl Alcohol, Glycerin, Petrolatum, and Mineral Oil
(LAN oh lin, SEE til AL koe hol, GLIS er in, pe troe LAY tum, & MIN er al oyl)

Related Information
Glycerin *on page 668*
Brand Names: U.S. Lubriderm® Fragrance Free [OTC]; Lubriderm® [OTC]
Pharmacologic Category Topical Skin Product
Use Treatment of dry skin
Local Anesthetic/Vasoconstrictor Precautions No information available to require special precautions
Effects on Dental Treatment No significant effects or complications reported
Effects on Bleeding No information available to require special precautions
Adverse Effects 1% to 10%: Local irritation
General Dosage Range Topical: *Adults:* Apply to skin as necessary

Lanreotide (lan REE oh tide)

Brand Names: U.S. Somatuline® Depot
Brand Names: Canada Somatuline® Autogel®
Pharmacologic Category Somatostatin Analog
Use Long-term treatment of acromegaly in patients who are not candidates for or are unresponsive to surgery and/or radiotherapy
Local Anesthetic/Vasoconstrictor Precautions No information available to require special precautions
Effects on Dental Treatment No significant effects or complications reported
Effects on Bleeding No information available to require special precautions
Adverse Effects
>10%:
Cardiovascular: Bradycardia (5% to 18%)
Gastrointestinal: Diarrhea (26% to 65%; dose related), abdominal pain (7% to 19%; dose related), flatulence (≤14%; dose related), nausea (11%), weight loss (5% to 11%)
Hematologic: Anemia (3% to 14%)
Hepatic: Cholelithiasis/gall bladder sludge (2% to 20%)
Local: Injection site reaction (6% to 22%; induration 5%; pain 4%; mass 2%)

◀ 1% to 10%:
Cardiovascular: Hypertension (5%), sinus bradycardia (3%)
Central nervous system: Headache (7%)
Endocrine & metabolic: Hyper-/hypoglycemia/diabetes (7%)
Gastrointestinal: Constipation (8%), vomiting (7%), loose stools (6%)
Neuromuscular & skeletal: Arthralgia (7%)

General Dosage Range Dosage adjustment recommended in patients with hepatic or renal impairment
SubQ: *Adults:* Initial: 90 mg once every 4 weeks for 3 months; Maintenance: 60-120 mg every 4 weeks **or** 120 mg every 6-8 weeks

Mechanism of Action Synthetic octapeptide analogue of somatostatin which is a peptide inhibitor of multiple endocrine, neuroendocrine, and exocrine mechanisms. Displays a greater affinity for somatostatin type 2 (SSTR2) and type 5 (SSTR5) receptors found in pituitary gland, pancreas, and growth hormone (GH) secreting neoplasms of pituitary gland and a lesser affinity for somatostatin receptors 1, 3, and 4. Reduces GH secretion and also reduces the levels of insulin-like growth factor 1.

Pharmacodynamics/Kinetics
Half-life Elimination 23-36 days
Time to Peak Mean: 7-12 hours
Pregnancy Risk Factor C
Pregnancy Considerations Animal studies have demonstrated embryocidal and teratogenic effects, as well as transitory growth retardation. Very little data exists from clinical trials and/or postmarketing reports of lanreotide in pregnancy. There are no adequate and well-controlled studies in pregnant women. Use in pregnancy only if benefits outweigh potential risks to fetus.

Lansoprazole (lan SOE pra zole)

Related Information
Gastrointestinal Disorders *on page 1512*
Brand Names: U.S. First®-Lansoprazole; Prevacid®; Prevacid® 24 HR [OTC]; Prevacid® SoluTab™
Brand Names: Canada Apo-Lansoprazole®; Mylan-Lansoprazole; Prevacid®; Prevacid® FasTab; Teva-Lansoprazole
Generic Availability (U.S.) Yes: Capsule
Pharmacologic Category Proton Pump Inhibitor; Substituted Benzimidazole
Use Short-term (4 weeks) treatment of active duodenal ulcers; maintenance treatment of healed duodenal ulcers; as part of a multidrug regimen for *H. pylori* eradication to reduce the risk of duodenal ulcer recurrence; short-term (up to 8 weeks) treatment of active benign gastric ulcer; treatment of NSAID-associated gastric ulcer; to reduce the risk of NSAID-associated gastric ulcer in patients with a history of gastric ulcer who require an NSAID; short-term treatment of symptomatic GERD; short-term (up to 8 weeks) treatment for all grades of erosive esophagitis; to maintain healing of erosive esophagitis; long-term treatment of pathological hypersecretory conditions, including Zollinger-Ellison syndrome

OTC labeling: Relief of frequent heartburn (≥2 days/week)

Local Anesthetic/Vasoconstrictor Precautions No information available to require special precautions
Effects on Dental Treatment No significant effects or complications reported

Effects on Bleeding No information available to require special precautions
Adverse Effects 1% to 10%:
Central nervous system: Headache (children 1-11 years 3%, 12-17 years 7%), dizziness (children 12-17 years 3%; adults <1%)
Gastrointestinal: Diarrhea (1% to 5%; 60 mg/day: 7%), abdominal pain (children 12-17 years 5%; adults 2%), constipation (children 1-11 years 5%; adults 1%), nausea (children 12-17 years 3%; adults 1%)

Dosage Oral:
Children 1-11 years: GERD, erosive esophagitis:
≤30 kg: 15 mg once daily for up to 12 weeks
>30 kg: 30 mg once daily for up to 12 weeks
Note: Doses were increased in some pediatric patients if still symptomatic after 2 or more weeks of treatment (maximum dose: 30 mg twice daily)
Children 12-17 years:
Nonerosive GERD: 15 mg once daily for up to 8 weeks
Erosive esophagitis: 30 mg once daily for up to 8 weeks
Adults:
Duodenal ulcer: Short-term treatment: 15 mg once daily for 4 weeks; maintenance therapy: 15 mg once daily
Gastric ulcer: Short-term treatment: 30 mg once daily for up to 8 weeks
NSAID-associated gastric ulcer (healing): 30 mg once daily for 8 weeks; controlled studies did not extend past 8 weeks of therapy
NSAID-associated gastric ulcer (to reduce risk): 15 mg once daily for up to 12 weeks; controlled studies did not extend past 12 weeks of therapy
Symptomatic GERD: Short-term treatment: 15 mg once daily for up to 8 weeks
Erosive esophagitis: Short-term treatment: 30 mg once daily for up to 8 weeks; continued treatment for an additional 8 weeks may be considered for recurrence or for patients who do not heal after the first 8 weeks of therapy; maintenance therapy: 15 mg once daily
Hypersecretory conditions: Initial: 60 mg once daily; adjust dose based upon patient response and to reduce acid secretion to <10 mEq/hour (5 mEq/hour in patients with prior gastric surgery); doses of 90 mg twice daily have been used; administer doses >120 mg/day in divided doses
Helicobacter pylori eradication:
Manufacturer labeling: 30 mg 3 times daily administered with amoxicillin 1000 mg 3 times daily for 14 days **or** 30 mg twice daily administered with amoxicillin 1000 mg *and* clarithromycin 500 mg twice daily for 10-14 days
American College of Gastroenterology guidelines (Chey, 2007):
Nonpenicillin allergy: 30 mg twice daily administered with amoxicillin 1000 mg *and* clarithromycin 500 mg twice daily for 10-14 days
Penicillin allergy: 30 mg twice daily administered with clarithromycin 500 mg *and* metronidazole 500 mg twice daily for 10-14 days **or** 30 mg once or twice daily administered with bismuth subsalicylate 525 mg *and* metronidazole 250 mg *plus* tetracycline 500 mg 4 times daily for 10-14 days
Heartburn: OTC labeling: 15 mg once daily for 14 days; may repeat 14 days of therapy every 4 months. Do not take for >14 days or more often than every 4 months, unless instructed by healthcare provider.

Dosage adjustment in renal impairment: No dosage adjustment necessary.

Dosage adjustment in hepatic impairment: Bioavailability increased in hepatic impairment. Consider dose reduction in severe impairment.

Mechanism of Action Decreases acid secretion in gastric parietal cells through inhibition of (H+, K+)-ATPase enzyme system, blocking the final step in gastric acid production.

Contraindications Hypersensitivity to lansoprazole or any component of the formulation

Warnings/Precautions Use of proton pump inhibitors (PPIs) may increase the risk of gastrointestinal infections (eg, *Salmonella, Campylobacter*). Relief of symptoms does not preclude the presence of a gastric malignancy. Atrophic gastritis (by biopsy) has been noted with long-term omeprazole therapy; this may also occur with lansoprazole. No reports of enterochromaffin-like (ECL) cell carcinoids, dysplasia, or neoplasia have occurred. Use of proton pump inhibitors (PPIs) may increase risk of CDAD, especially in hospitalized patients; consider CDAD diagnosis in patients with persistent diarrhea that does not improve. Use the lowest dose and shortest duration of PPI therapy appropriate for the condition being treated. Severe liver dysfunction may require dosage reductions. Decreased *H. pylori* eradication rates have been observed with short-term (≤7 days) combination therapy. The American College of Gastroenterology recommends 10-14 days of therapy (triple or quadruple) for eradication of *H. pylori* (Chey, 2007).

PPIs may diminish the therapeutic effect of clopidogrel thought to be due to reduced formation of the active metabolite of clopidogrel. The manufacturer of clopidogrel recommends either avoidance of both omeprazole (even when scheduled 12 hours apart) and esomeprazole or use of a PPI with comparatively less effect on the active metabolite of clopidogrel (eg, pantoprazole). Although lansoprazole exhibits the most potent CYP2C19 inhibition *in vitro* (Li, 2004; Ogilvie, 2011), an *in vivo* study of extensive CYP2C19 metabolizers showed less reduction of the active metabolite of clopidogrel by lansoprazole/dexlansoprazole compared to esomeprazole/omeprazole (Frelinger, 2012). The manufacturer of lansoprazole states that no dosage adjustment is necessary for clopidogrel when used concurrently. In contrast to these warnings, others have recommended the continued use of PPIs, regardless of the degree of inhibition, in patients with a history of GI bleeding or multiple risk factors for GI bleeding who are also receiving clopidogrel since no evidence has established clinically meaningful differences in outcome; however, a clinically-significant interaction cannot be excluded in those who are poor metabolizers of clopidogrel (Abraham, 2010; Levine, 2011). Additionally, concomitant use of lansoprazole with some drugs may require cautious use, may not be recommended, or may require dosage adjustments.

Increased incidence of osteoporosis-related bone fractures of the hip, spine, or wrist may occur with PPI therapy. Patients on high-dose or long-term therapy should be monitored. Use the lowest effective dose for the shortest duration of time, use vitamin D and calcium supplementation, and follow appropriate guidelines to reduce risk of fractures in patients at risk. Lansoprazole has been shown to be ineffective for the treatment of symptomatic GERD in children 1 month to <1 year.

Hypomagnesemia, reported rarely, usually with prolonged PPI use of >3 months (most cases >1 year of therapy); may be symptomatic or asymptomatic; severe cases may cause tetany, seizures, and cardiac arrhythmias. Consider obtaining serum magnesium concentrations prior to beginning long-term therapy, especially if taking concomitant digoxin, diuretics, or other drugs known to cause hypomagnesemia; and periodically thereafter. Hypomagnesemia may be corrected by magnesium supplementation, although discontinuation of lansoprazole may be necessary; magnesium levels typically return to normal within 1 week of stopping.

When used for self-medication, patients should be instructed not to use if they have difficulty swallowing, are vomiting blood, or have bloody or black stools. Prior to use, patients should contact healthcare provider if they have liver disease, heartburn for >3 months, heartburn with dizziness, lightheadedness, or sweating, MI symptoms, frequent chest pain, frequent wheezing (especially with heartburn), unexplained weight loss, nausea/vomiting, stomach pain, or are taking antifungals, atazanavir, digoxin, tacrolimus, theophylline, or warfarin. Patients should stop use and consult a healthcare provider if heartburn continues or worsens, or if they need to take for >14 days or more often than every 4 months. Patients should be informed that it may take 1-4 days for full effect to be seen; should not be used for immediate relief.

Drug Interactions

Metabolism/Transport Effects Substrate of CYP2C19 (major), CYP2C9 (minor), CYP3A4 (major); **Note:** Assignment of Major/Minor substrate status based on clinically relevant drug interaction potential; **Inhibits** CYP2C19 (weak), CYP2C9 (weak), CYP2D6 (weak), CYP3A4 (weak); **Induces** CYP1A2 (weak/moderate)

Avoid Concomitant Use

Avoid concomitant use of Lansoprazole with any of the following: Dasatinib; Delavirdine; Erlotinib; Nelfinavir; Pimozide; Ponatinib; Posaconazole; Rilpivirine; Risedronate

Increased Effect/Toxicity

Lansoprazole may increase the levels/effects of: Amphetamines; ARIPiprazole; Dexmethylphenidate; Imatinib; Lomitapide; Methotrexate; Methylphenidate; Pimozide; Raltegravir; Risedronate; Saquinavir; Tacrolimus (Systemic); Vitamin K Antagonists; Voriconazole

The levels/effects of Lansoprazole may be increased by: Fluconazole; Ketoconazole (Systemic); Voriconazole

Decreased Effect

Lansoprazole may decrease the levels/effects of: Atazanavir; Bisphosphonate Derivatives; Bosutinib; Cefditoren; Clopidogrel; Dabigatran Etexilate; Dasatinib; Delavirdine; Erlotinib; Gefitinib; Indinavir; Iron Salts; Itraconazole; Ketoconazole (Systemic); Mesalamine; Multivitamins/Minerals (with ADEK, Folate, Iron); Mycophenolate; Nelfinavir; Nilotinib; Ponatinib; Posaconazole; Rilpivirine; Risedronate; Vismodegib

The levels/effects of Lansoprazole may be decreased by: CYP2C19 Inducers (Strong); CYP3A4 Inducers (Strong); Deferasirox; Herbs (CYP3A4 Inducers); Tipranavir; Tocilizumab

Ethanol/Nutrition/Herb Interactions

Ethanol: Avoid ethanol (may cause gastric mucosal irritation).

Food: Lansoprazole serum concentrations may be decreased if taken with food.

Herb/Nutraceutical: Avoid St John's wort (may decrease the levels/effect of lansoprazole).

Dietary Considerations Should be taken before eating; best if taken before breakfast. Some products may contain phenylalanine.

Pharmacodynamics/Kinetics

Onset of Action Gastric acid suppression: Oral: 1-3 hours

Duration of Action Gastric acid suppression: Oral: >1 day

Half-life Elimination 1.5 ± 1 hours; Elderly: 2-3 hours; Hepatic impairment: 3-7 hours

Time to Peak Plasma: 1.7 hours

Pregnancy Risk Factor B

Pregnancy Considerations Animal studies have not shown teratogenic effects to the fetus. However, there are no adequate and well-controlled studies in pregnant women; use during pregnancy only if clearly needed.

Lactation Excretion in breast milk unknown/not recommended

Dosage Forms

Capsule, delayed release, oral: 15 mg, 30 mg
Prevacid®: 15 mg, 30 mg
Prevacid® 24 HR [OTC]: 15 mg

Powder for suspension, oral:
First®-Lansoprazole: 3 mg/mL (90 mL, 150 mL, 300 mL)

Tablet, delayed release, orally disintegrating, oral:
Prevacid® SoluTab™: 15 mg, 30 mg

Lansoprazole, Amoxicillin, and Clarithromycin
(lan SOE pra zole, a moks i SIL in, & kla RITH roe mye sin)

Related Information
Amoxicillin *on page 96*
Clarithromycin *on page 316*
Gastrointestinal Disorders *on page 1512*
Lansoprazole *on page 794*
Brand Names: U.S. Prevpac®
Brand Names: Canada Hp-PAC®
Pharmacologic Category Antibiotic, Macrolide Combination; Antibiotic, Penicillin; Gastrointestinal Agent, Miscellaneous; Proton Pump Inhibitor; Substituted Benzimidazole
Use Eradication of *H. pylori* to reduce the risk of recurrent duodenal ulcer
Local Anesthetic/Vasoconstrictor Precautions No information available to require special precautions
Effects on Dental Treatment Key adverse event(s) related to dental treatment: Taste perversion.
Effects on Bleeding No information available to require special precautions
Adverse Effects Note: Frequencies noted refer to experience with combination therapy. Also see individual agents.
3% to 10%:
Central nervous system: Headache (6%)
Gastrointestinal: Diarrhea (7%), taste perversion (5%)
General Dosage Range Oral: *Adults:* Lansoprazole 30 mg, amoxicillin 1 g, and clarithromycin 500 mg taken together twice daily
Pregnancy Risk Factor C
Pregnancy Considerations Adverse events were observed in animal reproduction studies using clarithromycin. See individual agents.

Lanthanum (LAN tha num)

Brand Names: U.S. Fosrenol®

Brand Names: Canada Fosrenol®
Pharmacologic Category Phosphate Binder
Use Reduction of serum phosphate in patients with stage 5 chronic kidney disease (end-stage renal disease [ESRD]; kidney failure: GFR <15 mL/minute/1.73 m^2 or dialysis)
Local Anesthetic/Vasoconstrictor Precautions No information available to require special precautions
Effects on Dental Treatment No significant effects or complications reported
Effects on Bleeding No information available to require special precautions
Adverse Effects Reported in short-term (4-6 weeks) trials at frequency > placebo:
>10%: Gastrointestinal: Nausea (11%)
1% to 10%: Gastrointestinal: Vomiting (9%), abdominal pain (5%)
General Dosage Range Oral: *Adults:* Initial: 1500 mg/day in divided doses; Usual range: 1500-3000 mg/day
Mechanism of Action Disassociates in the upper gastrointestinal tract to lanthanum ions (La^{3+}) which bind to dietary phosphate resulting in insoluble lanthanum phosphate complexes and a net decrease in serum phosphate and calcium levels.
Pharmacodynamics/Kinetics
Half-life Elimination Plasma: 53 hours; Bone: 2-3.6 years
Pregnancy Risk Factor C
Pregnancy Considerations Teratogenic effects were observed in some, but not all, animal studies. The effect on absorption of vitamins and nutrients has not been studied. Lanthanum is not recommended for use during pregnancy.

Lapatinib (la PA ti nib)

Related Information
Clinical Risk Related to Drugs Prolonging QT Interval *on page 1510*
Brand Names: U.S. Tykerb®
Brand Names: Canada Tykerb®
Pharmacologic Category Antineoplastic Agent, Anti-HER2; Antineoplastic Agent, Tyrosine Kinase Inhibitor; Epidermal Growth Factor Receptor (EGFR) Inhibitor
Use Treatment of HER2 overexpressing advanced or metastatic breast cancer (in combination with capecitabine) in patients who have received prior therapy (with an anthracycline, a taxane, and trastuzumab) and HER2 overexpressing hormone receptor positive metastatic breast cancer in postmenopausal women where hormone therapy is indicated (in combination with letrozole)
Unlabeled Use Treatment (in combination with trastuzumab) of HER2 overexpressing metastatic breast cancer which had progressed on prior trastuzumab containing therapy; treatment of HER2 overexpressing metastatic breast cancer with brain metastases
Local Anesthetic/Vasoconstrictor Precautions Lapatinib is one of the drugs confirmed to prolong the QT interval and is accepted as having a risk of causing torsade de pointes. The risk of drug-induced torsade de pointes is extremely low when a single QT interval prolonging drug is prescribed. In terms of epinephrine, it is not known what effect vasoconstrictors in the local anesthetic regimen will have in patients with a known history of congenital prolonged QT interval or in patients taking any medication that prolongs the QT interval. Until more information is obtained, it is suggested that the clinician consult with the physician prior to the use of

a vasoconstrictor in suspected patients, and that the vasoconstrictor (epinephrine, mepivacaine and levonordefrin [Carbocaine® 2% with Neo-Cobefrin®]) be used with caution.

Effects on Dental Treatment Key adverse event(s) related to dental treatment: Stomatitis.

Effects on Bleeding Anemia and thrombocytopenia have been reported. Medical consult recommended.

Adverse Effects Percentages reported for combination therapy.

>10%:

Central nervous system: Fatigue (10% to 20%), headache (≤14%)

Dermatologic: Palmar-plantar erythrodysesthesia (hand-and-foot syndrome) (with capecitabine: 53%; grade 3: 12%), rash (28% to 44%), dry skin (10% to 13%), alopecia (≤13%), pruritus (≤12%), nail disorder (≤11%)

Gastrointestinal: Diarrhea (64% to 65%; grade 3: 9% to 13%; grade 4: ≤1%), nausea (31% to 44%), vomiting (17% to 26%), abdominal pain (≤15%), mucosal inflammation (≤15%), stomatitis (≤14%), anorexia (≤11%), dyspepsia (≤11%)

Hematologic: Anemia (with capecitabine: 56%; grade 3: <1%), neutropenia (with capecitabine: 22%; grade 3: 3%; grade 4: <1%), thrombocytopenia (with capecitabine: 18%; grade 3: <1%)

Hepatic: AST increased (49% to 53%; grade 3: 2% to 6%; grade 4: <1%), ALT increased (37% to 46%; grade 3: 2% to 5%; grade 4<1%) total bilirubin increased (22% to 45%; grade 3: ≤4%; grade 4: <1%)

Neuromuscular & skeletal: Limb pain (≤12%), weakness (≤12%), back pain (≤11%)

Respiratory:Dyspnea (≤12%), epistaxis (≤11%)

1% to 10%:

Cardiovascular: LVEF decreased (grades 1/2: 2% to 4%; grades 3/4: <1%)

Central nervous system: Insomnia (≤10%)

General Dosage Range Dosage adjustment recommended in patients with hepatic impairment, on concomitant therapy, or who develop toxicities

Oral: *Adults:* 1250-1500 mg once daily

Mechanism of Action Tyrosine kinase (dual kinase) inhibitor; inhibits EGFR (ErbB1) and HER2 (ErbB2) by reversibly binding to tyrosine kinase, blocking phosphorylation and activation of downstream second messengers (Erk1/2 and Akt), regulating cellular proliferation and survival in ErbB- and ErbB2-expressing tumors. Combination therapy with lapatinib and endocrine therapy may overcome endocrine resistance occurring in HER2+ and hormone receptor positive disease.

Pharmacodynamics/Kinetics

Half-life Elimination ~24 hours

Time to Peak ~4 hours (Burris, 2009)

Pregnancy Risk Factor D

Pregnancy Considerations Increased pup deaths were demonstrated in animal reproduction studies. Lapatinib may cause fetal harm if administered during pregnancy. Women of childbearing potential should be advised to avoid pregnancy during treatment.

Prescribing and Access Restrictions Lapatinib is available **only** at specialty pharmacies through a restricted-access program, Tykerb® CARES. Information is available at www.tykerbcares.com or 1-866-489-5372.

Dental Comment Lapatinib is known to prolong the QT interval. The QT interval is measured as the time and distance between the Q point of the QRS complex and the end of the T wave in the ECG tracing. After adjustment for heart rate, the QT interval is defined as prolonged if it is more than 450 msec in men and 460 msec in women. A long QT syndrome was first described in the 1950s and 60s as a congenital syndrome involving QT interval prolongation and syncope and sudden death. Some of the congenital long QT syndromes were characterized by a peculiar electrocardiographic appearance of the QRS complex involving a premature atria beat followed by a pause, then a subsequent sinus beat showing marked QT prolongation and deformity. This type of cardiac arrhythmia was originally termed "torsade de pointes" (translated from the French as "twisting of the points"). Lapatinib is considered as having a risk of causing torsade de pointes. Since it is not known what effect vasoconstrictors in the local anesthetic regimen will have in patients with a known history of congenital prolonged QT interval or in patients taking any medication that prolongs the QT interval, a medical consult is suggested.

Laronidase (lair OH ni days)

Brand Names: U.S. Aldurazyme®

Brand Names: Canada Aldurazyme®

Pharmacologic Category Enzyme

Use Treatment of Hurler and Hurler-Scheie forms of mucopolysaccharidosis I (MPS I); treatment of Scheie form of MPS I in patients with moderate-to-severe symptoms

Local Anesthetic/Vasoconstrictor Precautions No information available to require special precautions

Effects on Dental Treatment No significant effects or complications reported

Effects on Bleeding Thrombocytopenia has been reported.

Adverse Effects Note: Unless otherwise noted, frequency of adverse reactions is reported for patients ≥6 years of age.

>10%:

Cardiovascular: Flushing (11% to 23%), poor venous access (14%)

Central nervous system: Fever 11% (children 6 months to 5 years: 30%), chills (children 6 months to 5 years: 20%)

Dermatologic: Rash (13% to 36%; children 6 months to 5 years: ≥5%)

Local: Injection site reaction (18%)

Neuromuscular & skeletal: Hyper-reflexia (14%), paresthesia (14%)

Otic: Otitis media (children 6 months to 5 years: 20%)

Respiratory: Upper respiratory tract infection (32%)

Miscellaneous: Antibody development to laronidase (97%); infusion reactions (32% to 49%; may be severe; children 6 months to 5 years: 35%)

1% to 10%:

Cardiovascular: Hypertension (children 6 months to 5 years: 10%), tachycardia (children 6 months to 5 years: 10%), chest pain (9%), edema (9%), facial edema (9%), hypotension (9%), pallor (children 6 months to 5 years: ≥5%)

Central nervous system: Headache (9%)

Dermatologic: Pruritus (4%), urticaria (4%), hyperhidrosis

Gastrointestinal: Abdominal pain/discomfort (9%), diarrhea (7%), vomiting (4%)

Hematologic: Thrombocytopenia (9%)

Hepatic: Bilirubinemia (9%)

Local: Abscess (9%), injection site pain (9%)

Neuromuscular & skeletal: Tremor (children 6 months to 5 years: ≥5%), arthralgia (4%), back pain, musculoskeletal pain

Ocular: Corneal opacity (9%)

Respiratory: Oxygen saturation decreased (children 6 months to 5 years: 10%), crepitations (children 6 months to 5 years: ≥5%), respiratory distress (children 6 months to 5 years: ≥5%), wheezing (children 6 months to 5 years: ≥5%), bronchospasm, cough, dyspnea

Miscellaneous: Feeling warm/cold (7%), allergic reaction (severe/serious 1%)

General Dosage Range I.V.: *Children ≥6 months and Adults:* 0.58 mg/kg once weekly

Mechanism of Action Laronidase is a recombinant (replacement) form of α-L-iduronidase derived from Chinese hamster cells. α-L-iduronidase is an enzyme needed to break down endogenous glycosaminoglycans (GAGs) within lysosomes. A deficiency of α-L-iduronidase leads to an accumulation of GAGs, causing cellular, tissue, and organ dysfunction as seen in MPS I. Improved pulmonary function and walking capacity have been demonstrated with the administration of laronidase to patients with Hurler, Hurler-Scheie, or Scheie (with moderate-to-severe symptoms) forms of MPS.

Pharmacodynamics/Kinetics

Half-life Elimination 1.5-3.6 hours

Pregnancy Risk Factor B

Pregnancy Considerations Teratogenic effects were not observed in animal reproduction studies. Patients are encouraged to enroll in the MPS I registry (800-745-4447 or www.MPSIregistry.com).

Latanoprost (la TA noe prost)

Brand Names: U.S. Xalatan®

Brand Names: Canada Apo-Latanoprost®; CO Latanoprost; GD-Latanoprost; Xalatan®

Generic Availability (U.S.) Yes

Pharmacologic Category Ophthalmic Agent, Antiglaucoma; Prostaglandin, Ophthalmic

Use Reduction of elevated intraocular pressure in patients with open-angle glaucoma or ocular hypertension

Local Anesthetic/Vasoconstrictor Precautions No information available to require special precautions

Effects on Dental Treatment No significant effects or complications reported

Effects on Bleeding No information available to require special precautions

Adverse Effects

>5% to 15%: Ocular: Blurred vision, burning and stinging, conjunctival hyperemia, foreign body sensation, itching, increased pigmentation of the iris, punctate epithelial keratopathy

1% to 5%:

Cardiovascular: Angina pectoris (1% to 2%), chest pain (1% to 2%)

Dermatologic: Allergic skin reaction (1% to 2%), rash (1% to 2%)

Neuromuscular & skeletal: Arthralgia (1% to 2%), back pain (1% to 2%), myalgia (1% to 2%)

Ocular: Dry eye (1% to 4%), excessive tearing (1% to 4%), eye pain (1% to 4%), lid crusting (1% to 4%), lid edema (1% to 4%), lid erythema (1% to 4%), lid discomfort/pain (1% to 4%), photophobia (1% to 4%)

Respiratory: Cold (4%), flu (4%), upper respiratory tract infection (4%)

Miscellaneous: Flu-like syndrome (4%)

Dosage Adults: Ophthalmic: 1 drop (1.5 mcg) in the affected eye(s) once daily in the evening; do not exceed the once daily dosage because it has been shown that more frequent administration may decrease the IOP lowering effect

Note: A medication delivery device (Xal-Ease™) is available for use with Xalatan®.

Dosage adjustment in renal impairment: No dosage adjustment provided in manufacturer's labeling. However, dosage adjustment unlikely due to low systemic absorption.

Dosage adjustment in hepatic impairment: No dosage adjustment provided in manufacturer's labeling. However, dosage adjustment unlikely due to low systemic absorption.

Mechanism of Action Latanoprost is a prostaglandin F_2-alpha analog believed to reduce intraocular pressure by increasing the outflow of the aqueous humor

Contraindications Hypersensitivity to latanoprost, benzalkonium chloride, or any component of the formulation

Warnings/Precautions May permanently change/increase brown pigmentation of the iris, the eyelid skin, and eyelashes. In addition, may increase the length and/or number of eyelashes (may vary between eyes); changes occur slowly and may not be noticeable for months or years. Long-term consequences and potential injury to eye are not known. Use with caution in patients with intraocular inflammation, aphakic patients, pseudophakic patients with a torn posterior lens capsule, or patients with risk factors for macular edema. Safety and efficacy have not been determined for use in patients with angle-closure-, inflammatory-, or neovascular glaucoma.

There have been reports of bacterial keratitis associated with the use of multiple-dose containers of topical ophthalmic products. Contains benzalkonium chloride which may be absorbed by contact lenses; remove contacts prior to administration and wait 15 minutes before reinserting.

Drug Interactions

Metabolism/Transport Effects None known.

Avoid Concomitant Use There are no known interactions where it is recommended to avoid concomitant use.

Increased Effect/Toxicity

Latanoprost may increase the levels/effects of: Bimatoprost

Decreased Effect

The levels/effects of Latanoprost may be decreased by: NSAID (Ophthalmic)

Pharmacodynamics/Kinetics

Onset of Action 3-4 hours; Peak effect: Maximum: 8-12 hours

Half-life Elimination 17 minutes

Pregnancy Risk Factor C

Pregnancy Considerations Adverse events were observed in animal reproduction studies at maternally toxic doses.

Lactation Excretion in breast milk unknown/use caution

Dosage Forms

Solution, ophthalmic: 0.005% (2.5 mL)

Xalatan®: 0.005% (2.5 mL)

Latanoprost and Timolol
(la TA noe prost & TIM oh lol)

Related Information
Latanoprost *on page 798*
Timolol (Ophthalmic) *on page 1326*
Brand Names: Canada Xalacom™
Pharmacologic Category Beta-Blocker, Nonselective; Ophthalmic Agent, Antiglaucoma; Prostaglandin, Ophthalmic
Use Reduction of intraocular pressure (IOP) in patients with open-angle glaucoma or ocular hypertension who are insufficiently responsive to topical beta-blockers, prostaglandin analogues, or other IOP-reducing agents and in whom combination therapy is appropriate
Local Anesthetic/Vasoconstrictor Precautions No information available to require special precautions
Effects on Dental Treatment No significant effects or complications reported
Effects on Bleeding No information available to require special precautions
Adverse Effects Percentages as reported with combination product. Also see individual agents.
>10%: Ocular: Eyelash alterations (including darkening, lengthening, thickening) (≤37%), iris pigmentation increased (≤20%), eye irritation (12%)
1% to 10%:
Cardiovascular: Hypertension (≤4%), chest pain (1%)
Central nervous system: Depression (2%), headache (2%)
Dermatologic: Skin disorder (2%), rash (1%)
Endocrine & metabolic: Hypercholesterolemia (2%), diabetes mellitus (1%)
Neuromuscular & skeletal: Arthritis (2%), back pain (1%)
Ocular: Hyperemia (7%), vision abnormal (7%), visual field defect (5%), blepharitis (3%), cataract (3%), conjunctivitis (3%), corneal disorder (3%), eye pain (2%), photophobia (2%), refraction errors (2%), skin disorder (2%), conjunctival disorder (1%), keratitis (1%), meibomianitis (1%)
Respiratory: Upper respiratory infection (6%), sinusitis (2%), bronchitis (1%)
Miscellaneous: Flu-like symptoms (3%), infection (1%)
General Dosage Range Ophthalmic: *Adults:* Instill 1 drop once daily
Mechanism of Action
Latanoprost: A prostaglandin F$_2$-alpha analog believed to reduce intraocular pressure by increasing the outflow of the aqueous humor
Timolol: Blocks both beta$_1$- and beta$_2$-adrenergic receptors, reduces intraocular pressure by reducing aqueous humor production or possibly outflow; reduces blood pressure by blocking adrenergic receptors and decreasing sympathetic outflow, produces a negative chronotropic and inotropic activity through an unknown mechanism
Pregnancy Considerations Reproductive studies have not been conducted with this combination. See individual agents.
Product Availability Not available in U.S.

Leflunomide (le FLOO noh mide)

Related Information
Rheumatoid Arthritis, Osteoarthritis, and Osteoporosis *on page 1526*
Brand Names: U.S. Arava®

Brand Names: Canada Apo-Leflunomide®; Arava®; Mylan-Leflunomide; Novo-Leflunomide; PHL-Leflunomide; PMS-Leflunomide; Sandoz-Leflunomide
Pharmacologic Category Antirheumatic, Disease Modifying
Use Treatment of active rheumatoid arthritis; indicated to reduce signs and symptoms, and to inhibit structural damage and improve physical function
Unlabeled Use Treatment of cytomegalovirus (CMV) disease in transplant recipients resistant to standard antivirals; prevention of acute and chronic rejection in recipients of solid organ transplants
Local Anesthetic/Vasoconstrictor Precautions No information available to require special precautions
Effects on Dental Treatment Key adverse event(s) related to dental treatment: Xerostomia (normal salivary flow resumes upon discontinuation), stomatitis, oral candidiasis, abnormal taste, tooth disorder, enlarged salivary gland, esophagitis, and gingivitis.
Effects on Bleeding There have been rare reports of thrombocytopenia.
Adverse Effects
>10%:
Gastrointestinal: Diarrhea (17%)
Respiratory: Respiratory tract infection (4% to 15%)
1% to 10%:
Cardiovascular: Hypertension (10%), chest pain (2%), edema (peripheral), palpitation, tachycardia, varicose vein, vasculitis, vasodilation
Central nervous system: Headache (7%), dizziness (4%), pain (2%), anxiety, depression, fever, insomnia, malaise, migraine, sleep disorder, vertigo
Dermatologic: Alopecia (10%), rash (10%), pruritus (4%), dry skin (2%), eczema (2%), acne, bruising, dermatitis, hair discoloration, hematoma, nail disorder, skin disorder/discoloration, skin ulcer, subcutaneous nodule
Endocrine & metabolic: Hypokalemia (1%), diabetes mellitus, hyperglycemia, hyperlipidemia, hyperthyroidism, menstrual disorder
Gastrointestinal: Nausea (9%), abdominal pain (5% to 6%), dyspepsia (5%), weight loss (4%), anorexia (3%), gastroenteritis (3%), mouth ulceration (3%), vomiting (3%), candidiasis (oral), colitis, constipation, esophagitis, flatulence, gastritis, gingivitis, melena, salivary gland enlarged, stomatitis, taste disturbance, xerostomia
Genitourinary: Urinary tract infection (5%), albuminuria, cystitis, dysuria, prostate disorder, urinary frequency, vaginal candidiasis
Hematologic: Anemia
Hepatic: Abnormal LFTs (5%), cholelithiasis
Local: Abscess
Neuromuscular & skeletal: Back pain (5%), joint disorder (4%), tenosynovitis (3%), weakness (3%), paresthesia (2%), synovitis (2%), arthralgia (1%), leg cramps (1%), arthrosis, bone necrosis, bone pain, bursitis, CPK increased, myalgia, neck pain, neuralgia, neuritis, pelvic pain, tendon rupture
Ocular: Blurred vision, cataract, conjunctivitis, eye disorder
Renal: Hematuria
Respiratory: Bronchitis (7%), cough (3%), pharyngitis (3%), pneumonia (2%), rhinitis (2%), sinusitis (2%), asthma, dyspnea, epistaxis
Miscellaneous: Accidental injury (5%), allergic reactions (2%), flu-like syndrome (2%), cyst, diaphoresis, hernia, herpes infection

◀ **General Dosage Range** Dosage adjustment recommended in patients who develop toxicities
Oral: *Adults:* Initial: 100 mg/day for 3 days; Maintenance range: 10-20 mg/day
Mechanism of Action Leflunomide is an immunodulatory agent that inhibits pyrimidine synthesis, resulting in antiproliferative and anti-inflammatory effects. Leflunomide is a prodrug; the active metabolite is responsible for activity. For CMV, may interfere with virion assembly.
Pharmacodynamics/Kinetics
Half-life Elimination M1: Mean: 14-15 days; enterohepatic recycling appears to contribute to the long half-life of this agent, since activated charcoal and cholestyramine substantially reduce plasma half-life
Time to Peak M1: 6-12 hours
Pregnancy Risk Factor X
Pregnancy Considerations Has been associated with teratogenic and embryolethal effects in animal models at low doses. Leflunomide is contraindicated in pregnant women or women of childbearing potential who are not using reliable contraception. Pregnancy must be excluded prior to initiating treatment. **[U.S. Boxed Warning]: Women of childbearing potential should not receive therapy until pregnancy has been excluded,** they have been counseled concerning fetal risk, and reliable contraceptive measures have been confirmed. Following treatment, pregnancy should be avoided until undetectable serum concentrations (<0.02 mg/L) are verified. This may be accomplished by the use of an enhanced drug elimination procedure using cholestyramine. Serum concentrations <0.02 mg/L should be verified by two separate tests performed at least 14 days apart. If serum concentrations are >0.02 mg/L, additional cholestyramine treatment should be considered. Pregnant women exposed to leflunomide should be registered with the pregnancy registry (877-311-8972). It is not known if males taking leflunomide may contribute to fetal toxicity. Males taking leflunomide who wish to father a child should consider discontinuing therapy and using the cholestyramine procedure to eliminate the medication.

Lenalidomide (le na LID oh mide)

Brand Names: U.S. Revlimid®
Brand Names: Canada Revlimid®
Pharmacologic Category Angiogenesis Inhibitor; Antineoplastic Agent; Immunomodulator, Systemic
Use Treatment of low- or intermediate-1-risk myelodysplastic syndrome (MDS) in patients with deletion 5q (del 5q) cytogenetic abnormality (with or without other cytogenetic abnormalities) with transfusion-dependent anemia; treatment of multiple myeloma (in combination with dexamethasone) in patients who have received at least one prior therapy
Unlabeled Use Treatment of non-Hodgkin's lymphomas; systemic light chain amyloidosis; lower-risk myelodysplastic syndrome (MDS) in transfusion-dependent patients without deletion 5q (del 5q); maintenance treatment for multiple myeloma (after response to primary treatment or following autologous stem cell transplant)
Local Anesthetic/Vasoconstrictor Precautions No information available to require special precautions
Effects on Dental Treatment Key adverse event(s) related to dental treatment: Xerostomia (normal salivary flow resumes upon discontinuation), taste perversion.
Effects on Bleeding Associated with significant thrombocytopenia and anemia. Medical consult recommended.

Adverse Effects
>10%:
Cardiovascular: Peripheral edema (8% to 26%)
Central nervous system: Fatigue (31% to 44%), fever (21% to 28%), dizziness (20% to 23%), headache (20%)
Dermatologic: Pruritus (8% to 42%), rash (21% to 36%; grades 3/4: 7%), dry skin (9% to 14%)
Endocrine & metabolic: Hypokalemia (11% to 14%)
Gastrointestinal: Diarrhea (39% to 49%), constipation (24% to 41%), nausea (24% to 26%), weight loss (20%), anorexia (10% to 16%), taste perversion (6% to 15%), vomiting (10% to 12%), abdominal pain (8% to 12%)
Genitourinary: Urinary tract infection (9% to 11%)
Hematologic: Thrombocytopenia (22% to 62%; grades 3/4: 12% to 50%; MDS: onset: 28 days [range 8-290 days]; recovery: 22 days [range: 5-224 days]), neutropenia (42% to 59%; grades 3/4: 33% to 53%; MDS: onset: 42 days [range 14-411 days]; recovery: 17 days [range: 2-170 days]), anemia (12% to 31%; grades 3/4: 6% to 10%)
Neuromuscular & skeletal: Muscle cramp (18% to 33%), weakness (15%), arthralgia (22%), back pain (21% to 26%), tremor (21%), bone pain (14%), limb pain (11% to 12%)
Ocular: Blurred vision (17%)
Respiratory: Upper respiratory infection (15% to 25%), nasopharyngitis (18% to 23%), cough (≤20%), dyspnea (7% to 24%), pharyngitis (14% to 16%), epistaxis (15%), pneumonia (9% to 14%), bronchitis (6% to 11%)
1% to 10%:
Cardiovascular: Edema (10%), deep vein thrombosis (≤9%; grades 3/4: ≤8%), hypertension (6% to 8%), hypotension (7%), chest pain (5% to 8%), palpitation (5%), atrial fibrillation (grades 3/4: ≤4%), syncope (grade 3/4: 1% to 3%), cerebrovascular accident (2%), tachycardia (grades 3/4: 2%), angina pectoris (≥1%), bradycardia (≥1%), cerebral ischemia (≥1%), MI (≥1%), heart failure (1%)
Central nervous system: Insomnia (10%), hypoesthesia (7% to 10%), lethargy (7%), pain (7%), depression (5%), hallucinations (≥1%), malaise (≥1%), mood swings (≥1%)
Dermatologic: Bruising (5% to 8%), cellulitis (5%), erythema (5%), exanthem (≥1%), hirsutism (≥1%), hyperpigmentation (≥1%)
Endocrine & metabolic: Hypothyroidism (7%), hypomagnesemia (6% to 7%), hypocalcemia (9%), dehydration (7%), hypophosphatemia (grades 3/4: 3%), loss of libido (≥1%)
Gastrointestinal: Appetite decreased (7%), xerostomia (7%), loose stools (6%), glossodynia (≥1%), GI hemorrhage (≥1%)
Genitourinary: Dysuria (7%), erectile dysfunction (≥1%)
Hematologic: Leukopenia (8%; grade 3/4: 4% to 5%), febrile neutropenia (5%; grades 3/4: 2% to 4%), granulocytopenia (grades 3/4: 2%), lymphopenia (5%; grade 3: 3%), pancytopenia (grades 3/4: 2%), autoimmune hemolytic anemia (≥1%)
Hepatic: ALT increased (8%), liver function tests abnormal (≥1%)
Neuromuscular & skeletal: Myalgia (9%), neuropathy (5% to 7%), rigors (6%)
Ocular: Cataract (grades 3/4: 1% to 2%), blindness (≥1%), ocular hypertension (≥1%)

Respiratory: Sinusitis (7% to 8%), rhinitis (7%), pulmonary embolism (≤4%; grades 3/4: 2% to 4%), respiratory distress (grades 3/4: 1% to 2%), hoarseness (≥1%), hypoxia (grades 3/4: 1%), pleural effusion (grades 3/4: 1%), pneumonitis (grades 3/4: 1%), pulmonary hypertension (grades 3/4: 1%)

Miscellaneous: Diaphoresis (7% to 10%), night sweats (8%), sepsis (grades 3/4: 3%)

General Dosage Range Dosage adjustment recommended in patients with renal impairment or who develop toxicities

Oral: *Adults:* 10 once daily **or** 25 mg once daily for 21 of 28 days

Mechanism of Action Immunomodulatory, antiangiogenic, and antineoplastic characteristics via multiple mechanisms. Selectively inhibits secretion of proinflammatory cytokines (potent inhibitor of tumor necrosis factor-alpha secretion); enhances cell-mediated immunity by stimulating proliferation of anti-CD3 stimulated T cells (resulting in increased IL-2 and interferon gamma secretion); inhibits trophic signals to angiogenic factors in cells. Inhibits the growth of myeloma cells by inducing cell cycle arrest and cell death.

Pharmacodynamics/Kinetics

Half-life Elimination 3-5 hours; Moderate-to-severe renal impairment: Increased threefold; Hemodialysis patients: Increased ~4.5-fold

Time to Peak MDS or myeloma patients: 0.5-6 hours

Pregnancy Risk Factor X

Pregnancy Considerations [U.S. Boxed Warning]: Lenalidomide is an analogue of thalidomide (a human teratogen) and could potentially cause birth defects in humans; do not use during pregnancy (contraindication); avoid pregnancy while taking lenalidomide. Obtain 2 negative pregnancy tests prior to initiation of treatment; 2 forms of contraception (or abstain from heterosexual intercourse) must be used at least 4 weeks prior to, during, and for 4 weeks after lenalidomide treatment (and during treatment interruptions). Distribution is restricted; physicians, pharmacies, and patients must be registered with the Revlimid REMS™ program. Animal reproduction studies with lenalidomide in nonhuman primates have demonstrated malformations similar to those observed in humans with thalidomide.

Women of childbearing potential should be treated only if they are able to comply with the conditions of the Revlimid REMS™ program. Women of reproductive potential must avoid pregnancy 4 weeks prior to therapy, during therapy, during therapy interruptions, and for ≥4 weeks after therapy is discontinued. Two forms of effective contraception or total abstinence from heterosexual intercourse must be used by females who are not infertile or who have not had a hysterectomy. A negative pregnancy test (sensitivity of at least 50 mIU/mL) 10-14 days prior to therapy, within 24 hours prior to beginning therapy, weekly during the first 4 weeks, and every 4 weeks (every 2 weeks for women with irregular menstrual cycles) thereafter is required for women of childbearing potential. Lenalidomide must be immediately discontinued for a missed period, abnormal pregnancy test or abnormal menstrual bleeding; refer patient to a reproductive toxicity specialist if pregnancy occurs during treatment.

Lenalidomide is also present in the semen of males. Males (including those vasectomized) should use a latex or synthetic condom during any sexual contact with women of childbearing age during treatment, during treatment interruptions, and for 4 weeks after discontinuation. Male patients should not donate sperm during, and for 4 weeks after treatment, and during therapy interruptions.

The parent or legal guardian for patients between 12 and 18 years of age must agree to ensure compliance with the required guidelines. Any suspected fetal exposure should be reported to the FDA via the MedWatch program (1-800-FDA-1088) and to Celgene Corporation (1-888-423-5436).

Prescribing and Access Restrictions As a requirement of the REMS program, access to this medication is restricted. Lenalidomide is approved for marketing in the U.S. only under a Food and Drug Administration (FDA) approved, restricted distribution program called Revlimid REMS™ (www.celgeneriskmanagment.com or 1-888-423-5436). Prescriptions must be filled within 7 days (for females of reproductive potential) or within 30 days (for all other patients) after authorization number obtained. Subsequent prescriptions may be filled only if fewer than 7 days of therapy remain on the previous prescription. A new prescription is required for further dispensing (a telephone prescription may not be accepted.) Pregnancy testing is required for females of childbearing potential. In Canada, distribution is restricted through RevAid® (www.RevAid.ca or 1-888-738-2431).

Lepirudin (leh puh ROO din)

Related Information

Cardiovascular Diseases *on page 1492*

Brand Names: U.S. Refludan® [DSC]

Brand Names: Canada Refludan®

Pharmacologic Category Anticoagulant, Thrombin Inhibitor

Use Indicated for anticoagulation in patients with heparin-induced thrombocytopenia (HIT) and associated thromboembolic disease in order to prevent further thromboembolic complications

Local Anesthetic/Vasoconstrictor Precautions No information available to require special precautions

Effects on Dental Treatment Key adverse event(s) related to dental treatment: Bleeding is the major adverse effect of lepirudin. See Effects on Bleeding.

Effects on Bleeding The most serious adverse reaction associated with lepirudin therapy is bleeding. Bleeding from puncture sites and wounds was reported in 1% of patients. Hemorrhagic mouth bleeding has been reported. Lepirudin is used as an anticoagulant in patients with heparin-induced thrombocytopenia. Medical consult recommended.

Adverse Effects As with all anticoagulants, bleeding is the most common adverse event associated with lepirudin. Hemorrhage may occur at virtually any site. Risk is dependent on multiple variables.

HIT patients:

>10%: Hematologic: Anemia (12%), bleeding from puncture sites (11%), hematoma (11%)

1% to 10%:

Cardiovascular: Heart failure (3%), pericardial effusion (1%), ventricular fibrillation (1%)

Central nervous system: Fever (7%)

Dermatologic: Maculopapular rash (4%), eczema (3%)

Gastrointestinal: GI bleeding/rectal bleeding (5%)

Genitourinary: Vaginal bleeding (2%)

Hepatic: Transaminases increased (6%)

Renal: Hematuria (4%)

Respiratory: Epistaxis (4%)

Non-HIT populations (including those receiving thrombolytics and/or contrast media):

1% to 10%: Respiratory: Bronchospasm/stridor/dyspnea/cough

General Dosage Range Dosage adjustment recommended in patients with renal impairment

I.V.: *Adults:* Bolus: 0.2-0.4 mg/kg; Infusion: 0.1-0.15 mg/kg/hour (maximum: 0.21 mg/kg/hour)

Mechanism of Action Lepirudin is a highly specific direct inhibitor of thrombin; lepirudin is a recombinant hirudin derived from yeast cells

Pharmacodynamics/Kinetics

Half-life Elimination Initial: ~10 minutes: Terminal: Healthy volunteers: 1.3 hours; Significant renal impairment (Cl_{cr} <15 mL/minute and on hemodialysis): ≤2 days

Pregnancy Risk Factor B

Pregnancy Considerations Adverse events were not observed in animal reproduction studies. Data are insufficient to evaluate the safety of thrombin inhibitors during pregnancy. Use of parenteral thrombin inhibitors in pregnancy should be limited to those women who have severe allergic reactions to heparin, including heparin induced thrombocytopenia, and who cannot receive danaparoid (Guyatt, 2012).

Product Availability Not available in the U.S.

Letrozole (LET roe zole)

Brand Names: U.S. Femara®

Brand Names: Canada Femara®; JAMP-Letrozole; Letrozole Tablets, USP; MED-Letrozole; Myl-Letrozole; PMS-Letrozole; Sandoz-Letrozole

Pharmacologic Category Antineoplastic Agent, Aromatase Inhibitor

Use For use in postmenopausal women in the adjuvant treatment of hormone receptor positive early breast cancer, extended adjuvant treatment of early breast cancer after 5 years of tamoxifen, advanced breast cancer with disease progression following antiestrogen therapy, hormone receptor positive or hormone receptor unknown, locally-advanced, or first-line (or second-line) treatment of advanced or metastatic breast cancer

Unlabeled Use Treatment of ovarian (epithelial) cancer, endometrial cancer

Local Anesthetic/Vasoconstrictor Precautions No information available to require special precautions

Effects on Dental Treatment No significant effects or complications reported

Effects on Bleeding Thrombocytopenia has been reported but relationship to letrozole is unclear.

Adverse Effects

>10%:

Cardiovascular: Edema (7% to 18%)

Central nervous system: Headache (4% to 20%), dizziness (3% to 14%), fatigue (8% to 13%)

Endocrine & metabolic: Hypercholesterolemia (3% to 52%), hot flashes (6% to 50%)

Gastrointestinal: Nausea (9% to 17%), weight gain (2% to 13%), constipation (2% to 11%)

Neuromuscular & skeletal: Weakness (4% to 34%), arthralgia (8% to 25%), arthritis (7% to 25%), bone pain (5% to 22%), back pain (5% to 18%), bone mineral density decreased/osteoporosis (5% to 15%), bone fracture (10% to 14%)

Respiratory: Dyspnea (6% to 18%), cough (6% to 13%)

Miscellaneous: Diaphoresis (≤24%), night sweats (15%)

1% to 10%:

Cardiovascular: Chest pain (6% to 8%), hypertension (5% to 8%), chest wall pain (6%), peripheral edema (5%); cerebrovascular accident including hemorrhagic stroke, thrombotic stroke (2% to 3%); thromboembolic event including venous thrombosis, thrombophlebitis, portal vein thrombosis, pulmonary embolism (2% to 3%); MI (1% to 2%), angina (1% to 2%), transient ischemic attack

Central nervous system: Insomnia (6% to 7%), pain (5%), anxiety (<5%), depression (<5%), vertigo (<5%), somnolence (3%)

Dermatologic: Rash (5%), alopecia (3% to 5%), pruritus (1%)

Endocrine & metabolic: Breast pain (2% to 7%), hypercalcemia (<5%)

Gastrointestinal: Diarrhea (5% to 8%), vomiting (3% to 7%), weight loss (6% to 7%), abdominal pain (6%), anorexia (1% to 5%), dyspepsia (3%)

Genitourinary: Urinary tract infection (6%), vaginal bleeding (5%), vaginal dryness (5%), vaginal hemorrhage (5%), vaginal irritation (5%)

Neuromuscular & skeletal: Limb pain (4% to 10%), myalgia (7% to 9%)

Ocular: Cataract (2%)

Renal: Renal disorder (5%)

Respiratory: Pleural effusion (<5%)

Miscellaneous: Infection (7%), influenza (6%), viral infection (6%), secondary malignancy (2% to 4%)

General Dosage Range Dosage adjustment recommended in patients with hepatic impairment

Oral: *Adults (postmenopausal females):* 2.5 mg once daily

Mechanism of Action Nonsteroidal competitive inhibitor of the aromatase enzyme system which binds to the heme group of aromatase, a cytochrome P450 enzyme which catalyzes conversion of androgens to estrogens (specifically, androstenedione to estrone and testosterone to estradiol). This leads to inhibition of the enzyme and a significant reduction in plasma estrogen (estrone, estradiol and estrone sulfate) levels. Does not affect synthesis of adrenal or thyroid hormones, aldosterone, or androgens.

Pharmacodynamics/Kinetics

Half-life Elimination Terminal: ~2 days

Time to Peak Steady state, plasma: 2-6 weeks

Pregnancy Risk Factor X

Pregnancy Considerations Letrozole may cause fetal harm when administered to pregnant women. Animal studies have demonstrated embryotoxicity and fetotoxicity. There are no adequate and well-controlled studies in pregnant women. If used in pregnancy, or if patient becomes pregnant during treatment, the patient should be apprised of potential hazard to the fetus. Letrozole is FDA indicated for postmenopausal women only (no clinical benefit for breast cancer has been demonstrated in premenopausal women). Women who are perimenopausal or recently postmenopausal should use adequate contraception until postmenopausal status is fully established.

Leucovorin Calcium (loo koe VOR in KAL see um)

Brand Names: Canada Lederle Leucovorin

Pharmacologic Category Antidote; Chemotherapy Modulating Agent; Rescue Agent (Chemotherapy); Vitamin, Water Soluble

Use Antidote for folic acid antagonists (methotrexate, trimethoprim, pyrimethamine) and rescue therapy following high-dose methotrexate; in combination with fluorouracil in the treatment of colon cancer; treatment of megaloblastic anemias when folate is deficient as in infancy, sprue, pregnancy, and nutritional deficiency when oral folate therapy is not possible

Unlabeled Use Adjunctive cofactor therapy in methanol toxicity; prevention of pyrimethamine hematologic toxicity in HIV-positive patients

Local Anesthetic/Vasoconstrictor Precautions No information available to require special precautions

Effects on Dental Treatment No significant effects or complications reported

Effects on Bleeding No information available to require special precautions

Adverse Effects Frequency not defined. Toxicities (especially gastrointestinal toxicity) of fluorouracil is higher when used in combination with leucovorin.
Dermatologic: Rash, pruritus, erythema, urticaria
Hematologic: Thrombocytosis
Respiratory: Wheezing
Miscellaneous: Allergic reactions, anaphylactoid reactions

General Dosage Range
I.M.: *Children and Adults:* ≤1 mg/day [folate deficient megaloblastic anemia] **or** 15 mg (~10 mg/m^2) every 6 hours for 10 doses [methotrexate rescue dose]
I.V.:
Children: 15 mg (~10 mg/m^2) every 6 hours for 10 doses
Adults: Initial: 15 mg (~10 mg/m^2) every 6 hours for 10 doses [methotrexate rescue dose] **or** 200 mg/m^2 **or** 20 mg/m^2 as a single dose [colorectal cancer]
Oral: *Children and Adults:* 5-15 mg/day [weak folic acid antagonist overdose] **or** 15 mg (~10 mg/m^2) every 6 hours for 10 doses [methotrexate rescue dose]

Mechanism of Action A reduced form of folic acid, leucovorin supplies the necessary cofactor blocked by methotrexate. Leucovorin actively competes with methotrexate for transport sites, displaces methotrexate from intracellular binding sites, and restores active folate stores required for DNA/RNA synthesis. Stabilizes the binding of 5-dUMP and thymidylate synthetase, enhancing the activity of fluorouracil. When administered with pyrimethamine for the treatment of opportunistic infections, leucovorin reduces the risk for hematologic toxicity.

Methanol toxicity treatment: Formic acid (methanol's toxic metabolite) is normally metabolized to carbon dioxide and water by 10-formyltetrahydrofolate dehydrogenase after being bound to tetrahydrofolate. Administering a source of tetrahydrofolate may aid the body in eliminating formic acid.

Pharmacodynamics/Kinetics
Half-life Elimination ~4-8 hours
Time to Peak Oral: ~2 hours; I.V.: Total folates: 10 minutes; 5MTHF: ~1 hour
Pregnancy Risk Factor C
Pregnancy Considerations Animal reproduction studies have not been conducted. Leucovorin is a biologically active form of folic acid. Adequate amounts of folic acid are recommended during pregnancy. Refer to Folic Acid monograph.

Leuprolide (loo PROE lide)

Brand Names: U.S. Eligard®; Lupron Depot-Ped®; Lupron Depot®

Brand Names: Canada Eligard®; Lupron®; Lupron® Depot®
Pharmacologic Category Antineoplastic Agent, Gonadotropin-Releasing Hormone Agonist; Gonadotropin Releasing Hormone Agonist
Use Palliative treatment of advanced prostate cancer; management of endometriosis; treatment of anemia caused by uterine leiomyomata (fibroids); central precocious puberty
Unlabeled Use Treatment of breast cancer; infertility; treatment of paraphilia/hypersexuality
Local Anesthetic/Vasoconstrictor Precautions No information available to require special precautions
Effects on Dental Treatment Key adverse event(s) related to dental treatment: Gum hemorrhage, gingivitis, dry mucous membranes, and dysphagia.
Effects on Bleeding Decreased and increased platelet count has been reported.
Adverse Effects
Children (percentages based on 1-month and 3-month pediatric formulations combined):
>10%: Local: Injection site pain (≤20%)
2% to 10%:
Cardiovascular: Vasodilation (2%)
Central nervous system: Emotional lability (5%), mood altered (5%), headache (3% to 5%), pain (3%)
Dermatologic: Acne (3%), rash (3% including erythema multiforme), seborrhea (3%)
Gastrointestinal: Weight gain (≤7%)
Genitourinary: Vaginal bleeding (3%), vaginal discharge (3%), vaginitis (3%)
Local: Injection site reaction (≤9%)

Adults: Note: For prostate cancer treatment, an initial rise in serum testosterone concentrations may cause "tumor flare" or worsening of symptoms, including bone pain, neuropathy, hematuria, or ureteral or bladder outlet obstruction during the first 2 weeks. Similarly, an initial increase in estradiol levels, with a temporary worsening of symptoms, may occur in women treated with leuprolide.
Delayed release formulations:
>10%:
Cardiovascular: Edema (≤14%)
Central nervous system: Headache (≤65%), pain (<2% to 33%), depression (≤31%), insomnia (≤31%), fatigue (≤17%), dizziness/vertigo (≤16%)
Dermatologic: Skin reaction (≤12%)
Endocrine & metabolic: Hot flashes (25% to 98%), testicular atrophy (≤20%), hyperlipidemia (≤12%), libido decreased (≤11%)
Gastrointestinal: Nausea/vomiting (≤25%), bowel function altered (≤14%), weight gain/loss (≤13%)
Genitourinary: Vaginitis (11% to 28%), urinary disorder (13% to 15%)
Local: Injection site burning/stinging (transient: ≤35%)
Neuromuscular & skeletal: Weakness (≤18%), joint disorder (≤12%)
Miscellaneous: Flu-like syndrome (≤12%)
1% to 10% (limited to important or life-threatening):
Cardiovascular: Angina (<5%), arrhythmia (<5%), atrial fibrillation (<5%), bradycardia (<5%), CHF (<5%), deep thrombophlebitis (<5%), hyper-/hypotension (<5%), palpitation (<5%), syncope (<5%), tachycardia (<5%)
Central nervous system: Nervousness (≤8%), anxiety (≤6%), confusion (<5%), delusions (<5%), dementia (<5%), fever (<5%), seizure (<5%)

Dermatologic: Acne (≤10%), alopecia (≤5%), bruising (≤5%), cellulitis (<5%), pruritus (≤3%), rash (≤2%), hirsutism (<2%)

Endocrine & metabolic: Dehydration (≤8%), gynecomastia (≤7%), breast tenderness/pain (≤6%), bicarbonate decreased (≥5%), hyper-/hypocholesterolemia (≥5%), hyperglycemia (≥5%), hyperphosphatemia (≥5%), hyperuricemia (≥5%), hypoalbuminemia (≥5%), hypoproteinemia (≥5%), lactation (<5%), testicular pain (≤4%), menstrual disorder (≤2%)

Gastrointestinal: Dysphagia (<5%), gastrointestinal hemorrhage (<5%), intestinal obstruction (<5%), ulcer (<5%), constipation (≤3%), gastroenteritis/colitis (≤3%), diarrhea (≤2%)

Genitourinary: Prostatic acid phosphatase increased/decreased (≥5%), urine specific gravity increased/decreased (≥5%), impotence (≤5%), balanitis (<5%), incontinence (<5%), penile/testis disorder (<5%), urinary tract infection (<5%), nocturia (≤4%), polyuria (2% to 4%), dysuria (≤2%), bladder spasm (<2%), erectile dysfunction (<2%), hematuria (<2%), urinary retention (<2%), urinary urgency (<2%)

Hematologic: Eosinophilia (≥5%), leukopenia (≥5%), platelets increased (≥5%), anemia

Hepatic: Liver function tests abnormal (≥5%), partial thromboplastin time increased (≥5%), prothrombin time increased (≥5%), hepatomegaly (<5%)

Local: Injection site pain (2% to 5%), injection site erythema (1% to 3%)

Neuromuscular & skeletal: Myalgia (≤8%), paresthesia (≤8%), neuropathy (<5%), paralysis (<5%), pathologic fracture (<5%), bone pain (<2%), arthralgia (≤1%)

Renal: BUN increased (≥5%), creatinine increased (≥5%)

Respiratory: Emphysema (<5%), epistaxis (<5%), hemoptysis (<5%), pleural effusion (<5%), pulmonary edema (<5%), dyspnea (≤2%), cough (≤1%)

Miscellaneous: Diaphoresis (<5%), allergic reaction (<5%), infection (5%), lymphadenopathy (<5%)

Immediate release formulation:
>10%:

Cardiovascular: ECG changes/ischemia (19%), peripheral edema (12%)

Central nervous system: Pain (13%)

Endocrine & metabolic: Hot flashes (55%)

1% to 10% (limited to important or life-threatening):

Cardiovascular: Hypertension (8%), murmur (3%), thrombosis/phlebitis (2%), CHF (1%), angina, arrhythmia, MI, syncope

Central nervous system: Headache (7%), insomnia (7%), dizziness/lightheadedness (5%), anxiety, depression, fatigue, fever, nervousness

Dermatologic: Dermatitis (5%), alopecia, bruising, itching, lesions, pigmentation

Endocrine & metabolic: Gynecomastia/breast tenderness/pain (7%), testicular size decreased (7%), diabetes, hypercalcemia, hypoglycemia, libido decreased, thyroid enlarged

Gastrointestinal: Constipation (7%), anorexia (6%), nausea/vomiting (5%), diarrhea, dysphagia, gastrointestinal bleeding, peptic ulcer, rectal polyps

Genitourinary: Urinary frequency/urgency (6%), impotence (4%), urinary tract infection (3%), bladder spasm, dysuria, incontinence, testicular pain, urinary obstruction

Hematologic: Anemia (5%)

Local: Injection site reaction

Neuromuscular & skeletal: Weakness (10%), bone pain (5%), peripheral neuropathy

Ocular: Blurred vision

Renal: Hematuria (6%), BUN increased, creatinine increased

Respiratory: Dyspnea (2%), cough, pneumonia, pulmonary embolus, pulmonary fibrosis

Miscellaneous: Infection, inflammation

General Dosage Range I.M., SubQ: *Children and Adults:* Dosage varies greatly depending on indication

Mechanism of Action Leuprolide, is an agonist of luteinizing hormone-releasing hormone (LHRH). Acting as a potent inhibitor of gonadotropin secretion; continuous administration results in suppression of ovarian and testicular steroidogenesis due to decreased levels of LH and FSH with subsequent decrease in testosterone (male) and estrogen (female) levels. In males, testosterone levels are reduced to below castrate levels. Leuprolide may also have a direct inhibitory effect on the testes, and act by a different mechanism not directly related to reduction in serum testosterone.

Pharmacodynamics/Kinetics

Onset of Action Following transient increase, testosterone suppression occurs in ~2-4 weeks of continued therapy

Pregnancy Risk Factor X

Pregnancy Considerations Pregnancy must be excluded prior to the start of treatment. Although leuprolide usually inhibits ovulation and stops menstruation, contraception is not ensured and a nonhormonal contraceptive should be used. Fetal abnormalities and increased fetal mortality have been noted in animal studies.

Leuprolide and Norethindrone
(loo PROE lide & nor eth IN drone)

Pharmacologic Category Gonadotropin Releasing Hormone Agonist; Progestin

Use Management of initial and recurrent painful symptoms of endometriosis

Local Anesthetic/Vasoconstrictor Precautions No information available to require special precautions

Effects on Dental Treatment No significant effects or complications reported

Effects on Bleeding No information available to require special precautions

Adverse Effects
>10%:

Central nervous system: Headache (46% to 51%), depression (27% to 34%), pain (21% to 29%), insomnia (13% to 15%), dizziness (7% to 11%), nervousness (4% to 11%)

Dermatologic: Dermatological reaction (9% to 11%)

Endocrine & metabolic: Hot flash (57% to 87%), decreased HDL cholesterol (41% to 44%), androgen-like effect (5% to 18%), breast changes (8% to 13%), increased LDL cholesterol (7% to 11%)

Gastrointestinal: Nausea and vomiting (13% to 29%), constipation/diarrhea (10% to 15%), weight gain (4% to 13%)

Genitourinary: Vaginitis (8% to 15%), irregular menses (5%)

Musculoskeletal: Weakness (11% to 18%)

1% to 10%:

Cardiovascular: Edema (7% to 9%)

Central nervous system: Memory impairment (2% to 4%)

Endocrine & metabolic: Increased serum triglycerides (9% to 10%), decreased libido (4% to 7%), increased gamma-glutamyl transferase (1%)

Gastrointestinal: Dyspepsia (4% to 7%), change in appetite (6%)

Hepatic: Increased serum ALT (2%; ≥2 x ULN)

Local: Injection site reaction (3% to 9%)

Musculoskeletal: Leg cramps (3% to 9%)

General Dosage Range I.M./Oral: *Adults: Females:* Leuprolide acetate 11.25 mg I.M. once every 3 months and norethindrone acetate 5 mg orally once daily (maximum initial therapy duration: 6 months; may repeat treatment once for a maximum cumulative therapy duration: 12 months)

Mechanism of Action Leuprolide administration inhibits the production of estrogen through negative feedback of pituitary gonadotropins. This in turn decreases endometrial implants and symptoms of endometriosis such as pain. Norethindrone is used to decrease adverse events observed with the hypoestrogenic state caused by leuprolide and possibly mitigate bone mineral density loss (Surrey, 2010).

Pregnancy Risk Factor X

Pregnancy Considerations Adverse events were observed with leuprolide in animal reproduction studies. Pregnancy must be excluded prior to the start of treatment. Although leuprolide usually inhibits ovulation and stops menstruation, contraception is not ensured and a nonhormonal contraceptive should be used. Use in pregnant women or women who may be planning a pregnancy during therapy is contraindicated.

Fertility suppression observed with other leuprolide formulations is reversible following discontinuation of therapy. This formulation is indicated to treat pain associated with endometriosis; in infertile women with endometriosis, it does not necessarily improve the ability to conceive (ACOG, 2010; ASRM, 2012).

Product Availability Lupaneta Pack: FDA approved December 2012: anticipated availability is early third quarter of 2013. Refer to prescribing information for additional information.

Levalbuterol (leve al BYOO ter ole)

Related Information
Respiratory Diseases *on page 1514*
Brand Names: U.S. Xopenex HFA™; Xopenex®
Brand Names: Canada Xopenex®
Pharmacologic Category Beta₂ Agonist
Use Treatment or prevention of bronchospasm in children and adults with reversible obstructive airway disease

Local Anesthetic/Vasoconstrictor Precautions No information available to require special precautions

Effects on Dental Treatment No significant effects or complications reported

Effects on Bleeding No information available to require special precautions

Adverse Effects

>10%:
Endocrine & metabolic: Serum glucose increased, serum potassium decreased
Neuromuscular & skeletal: Tremor (≤7%)
Respiratory: Rhinitis (3% to 11%)
Miscellaneous: Viral infection (7% to 12%)

>2% to 10%:
Central nervous system: Headache (8% to 12%), nervousness (3% to 10%), dizziness (1% to 3%), anxiety (≤3%), migraine (≤3%), weakness (3%)
Cardiovascular: Tachycardia (~3%)
Dermatologic: Rash (≤8%)

Gastrointestinal: Diarrhea (2% to 6%), dyspepsia (1% to 3%)

Neuromuscular & skeletal: Leg cramps (≤3%)

Respiratory: Asthma (9%), pharyngitis (3% to 10%), cough (1% to 4%), sinusitis (1% to 4%), nasal edema (1% to 3%)

Miscellaneous: Flu-like syndrome (1% to 4%), accidental injury (≤3%)

Note: Immediate hypersensitivity reactions have occurred (including angioedema, oropharyngeal edema, urticaria, and anaphylaxis).

General Dosage Range

Inhalation (metered-dose inhaler): *Children ≥4 years and Adults:* 1-2 puffs every 4-6 hours

Nebulization (solution):

Children ≤4 years: 0.31-1.25 mg every 4-6 hours as needed

Children 5-11 years: 0.31-0.63 mg 3 times/day

Children ≥12 years and Adults: 0.63-1.25 mg every 8 hours as needed

Elderly: Initial: 0.63 mg

Mechanism of Action Relaxes bronchial smooth muscle by action on beta₂-receptors with little effect on heart rate

Pharmacodynamics/Kinetics

Onset of Action Measured as a 15% increase in FEV_1:
Aerosol: 5.5-10.2 minutes; Peak effect: ~77 minutes
Nebulization: 10-17 minutes; Peak effect: 1.5 hours

Duration of Action Measured as a 15% increase in FEV_1:
Aerosol: 3-4 hours (up to 6 hours in some patients)
Nebulization: 5-6 hours (up to 8 hours in some patients)

Half-life Elimination 3.3-4 hours

Time to Peak
Aerosol: Children: 0.8 hours, Adults: 0.5 hours
Nebulization: Children: 0.3-0.6 hours, Adults: 0.2 hours

Pregnancy Risk Factor C

Pregnancy Considerations Teratogenic effects were not observed in animal studies; however, racemic albuterol was teratogenic in some species. There are no adequate and well-controlled studies in pregnant women. This drug should be used during pregnancy only if benefit exceeds risk. Use caution if needed for bronchospasm during labor and delivery; has potential to interfere with uterine contractions.

LevETIRAcetam (lee va tye RA se tam)

Brand Names: U.S. Keppra XR®; Keppra®
Brand Names: Canada Apo-Levetiracetam®; Ava-Levetiracetam; CO Levetiracetam; Dom-Levetiracetam; Keppra®; PHL-Levetiracetam; PMS-Levetiracetam; PRO-Levetiracetam

Pharmacologic Category Anticonvulsant, Miscellaneous

Use Adjunctive therapy in the treatment of partial onset, myoclonic, and/or primary generalized tonic-clonic seizures

Local Anesthetic/Vasoconstrictor Precautions No information available to require special precautions

Effects on Dental Treatment No significant effects or complications reported

Effects on Bleeding No information available to require special precautions

Adverse Effects

>10%:

Central nervous system: Behavioral symptoms (agitation, aggression, anger, anxiety, apathy, depersonalization, depression, emotional lability, hostility, hyperkinesias, irritability, nervousness, neurosis and personality disorder: adults 5% to 13%; children 5% to 38%), somnolence (8% to 23%), headache (14%), hostility (2% to 12%)

Gastrointestinal: Vomiting (15%), anorexia (3% to 13%)

Neuromuscular & skeletal: Weakness (9% to 15%)

Respiratory: Pharyngitis (6% to 14%), rhinitis (4% to 13%), cough (2% to 11%)

Miscellaneous: Accidental injury (17%), infection (2% to 13%)

1% to 10%:

Cardiovascular: Facial edema (2%)

Central nervous system: Fatigue (10%), nervousness (4% to 10%), dizziness (5% to 9%), personality disorder (8%), pain (6% to 7%), agitation (4%), irritability (6% to 7%), emotional lability (2% to 6%), mood swings (5%), depression (3% to 5%), vertigo (3% to 5%), ataxia (3%), amnesia (2%), anxiety (2%), confusion (2%)

Dermatologic: Bruising (4%), pruritus (2%), rash (2%), skin discoloration (2%)

Endocrine & metabolic: Dehydration (2%)

Gastrointestinal: Diarrhea (8%), nausea (5%), gastroenteritis (4%), constipation (3%)

Genitourinary: Urine abnormality (2%)

Hematologic: Leukocytes decreased (2% to 3%)

Neuromuscular & skeletal: Neck pain (2% to 8%), paresthesia (2%), reflexes increased (2%)

Ocular: Conjunctivitis (3%), diplopia (2%), amblyopia (2%)

Otic: Ear pain (2%)

Renal: Albuminuria (4%)

Respiratory: Influenza (5%), asthma (2%), sinusitis (2%)

Miscellaneous: Flu-like syndrome (3% to 8%), viral infection (2%)

General Dosage Range Dosage adjustment recommended in patients with renal impairment

Oral:

Immediate release:

Children 1 to <6 months: Initial: 7 mg/kg twice daily; Maintenance: 7-21 mg/kg/dose twice daily (maximum: 42 mg/kg/day)

Children 6 months to <4 years: Initial: 10 mg/kg twice daily; Maintenance: 10-25 mg/kg twice daily (maximum: 50 mg/kg/day)

Children 4 to <16 years: Initial: 10 mg/kg twice daily; Maintenance: 10-30 mg/kg twice daily (maximum: 60 mg/kg/day or 3000 mg/day)

Children ≥12 years: Initial: 500 mg twice daily; Maintenance: 500-1500 mg twice daily (maximum: 3000 mg/day)

Adults: Initial: 500 mg twice daily; Maintenance: 500-1500 mg twice daily (maximum: 3000 mg/day)

Extended release: Children ≥16 years and Adults: Initial: 1000 mg once daily; Maintenance: 1000-3000 mg once daily (maximum: 3000 mg/day)

I.V.: Children ≥16 years and Adults: Initial: 500 mg twice daily; Maintenance: 500-1500 mg twice daily (maximum: 3000 mg/day)

Mechanism of Action The precise mechanism by which levetiracetam exerts its antiepileptic effect is unknown. However, several studies have suggested the mechanism may involve one or more of the following central pharmacologic effects: inhibition of voltage-dependent N-type calcium channels; facilitation of GABA-ergic inhibitory transmission through displacement of negative modulators; reduction of delayed rectifier potassium current; and/or binding to synaptic proteins which modulate neurotransmitter release.

Pharmacodynamics/Kinetics

Onset of Action Peak effect: Oral: 1 hour

Half-life Elimination ~6-8 hours; extended release tablet: ~7 hours; half-life increased in renal dysfunction

Time to Peak Oral: Immediate release: ~1 hour; Extended release: ~4 hours

Pregnancy Risk Factor C

Pregnancy Considerations Developmental toxicities were observed in animal reproduction studies. Levetiracetam crosses the placenta and can be detected in the neonate at birth. Concentrations in the umbical cord at delivery are similar to those in the maternal plasma. Serum concentrations of levetiracetam may decrease as pregnancy progresses; monitor carefully throughout pregnancy and postpartum (Tomson, 2007).

Two registries are available for women exposed to levetiracetam during pregnancy: Pregnant women may enroll themselves into the North American Antiepileptic Drug (AED) Pregnancy Registry (888-233-2334 or http://www.mgh.harvard.edu/aed/). The patient or healthcare provider may contact the UCB AED Pregnancy Registry (888-537-7734).

The North American AED registry has published data collected from pregnant women taking levetiracetam monotherapy from 1997-2011 (n=450). Eleven major malformations were diagnosed within 12 weeks of birth. The relative risk of major malformations was not increased in comparison to women with epilepsy not taking AEDs (n=442; RR 2.2, 95% CI 0.8-6.4) or in comparison to women using lamotrigine monotherapy (n=1562; RR 1.2, 95% CI 0.6-2.5) (Hernández-Díaz, 2012).

Levobunolol (lee voe BYOO noe lole)

Brand Names: U.S. Betagan®

Brand Names: Canada Apo-Levobunolol®; Betagan®; Novo-Levobunolol; PMS-Levobunolol; Ratio-Levobunolol; Sandoz-Levobunolol

Pharmacologic Category Beta-Adrenergic Blocker, Nonselective; Ophthalmic Agent, Antiglaucoma

Use To lower intraocular pressure in chronic open-angle glaucoma or ocular hypertension

Local Anesthetic/Vasoconstrictor Precautions No information available to require special precautions

Effects on Dental Treatment Key adverse event(s) related to dental treatment: Levobunolol is a nonselective beta-blocker and may enhance the pressor response to epinephrine, resulting in hypertension and bradycardia. Many nonsteroidal anti-inflammatory drugs, such as ibuprofen and indomethacin, can reduce the hypotensive effect of beta-blockers after 3 or more weeks of therapy with the NSAID. Short-term NSAID use (ie, 3 days) requires no special precautions in patients taking beta-blockers.

Effects on Bleeding No information available to require special precautions

Adverse Effects Frequency not always defined.

Cardiovascular: Arrhythmia, bradycardia, cardiac arrest cerebral ischemia, cerebrovascular accident, chest pain, congestive heart failure, heart block, hypotension, palpitation, syncope

Central nervous system: Ataxia (transient), confusion, depression, dizziness, headache, lethargy

Dermatologic: Alopecia, erythema, pruritus, rash, Stevens-Johnson syndrome, urticaria

Endocrine & metabolic: Hypoglycemia masked

Gastrointestinal: Diarrhea, nausea

Genitourinary: Impotence

Neuromuscular & skeletal: Myasthenia gravis exacerbation, paresthesia, weakness

Ocular: Stinging/burning (up to 33%), blepharoconjunctivitis (5%), blepharoptosis, conjunctivitis, corneal sensitivity decreased, diplopia, iridocyclitis, keratitis, ptosis, visual disturbances

Respiratory: Bronchospasm, dyspnea, nasal congestion, respiratory failure

Miscellaneous: Hypersensitivity

General Dosage Range Ophthalmic: *Adults:* Instill 1 drop in the affected eye(s) 1-2 times daily

Mechanism of Action A nonselective beta-adrenergic blocking agent that lowers intraocular pressure by reducing aqueous humor production and possibly increases the outflow of aqueous humor

Pharmacodynamics/Kinetics

Onset of Action Within 1 hour; Peak effect: 2-6 hours

Duration of Action Up to 24 hours

Pregnancy Risk Factor C

Pregnancy Considerations Adverse events have been observed in some animal reproduction studies. If ophthalmic agents are needed for the treatment of glaucoma during pregnancy, the minimum effective dose should be used in combination with punctual occlusion to decrease potential exposure to the fetus (Johnson, 2001; Samples, 1988)

Levocabastine (Nasal) (LEE voe kab as teen)

Brand Names: Canada Livostin®

Pharmacologic Category Histamine H₁ Antagonist; Histamine H₁ Antagonist, Second Generation; Piperidine Derivative

Use Symptomatic treatment of allergic rhinitis

Local Anesthetic/Vasoconstrictor Precautions No information available to require special precautions

Effects on Dental Treatment Key adverse event(s) related to dental treatment: Xerostomia (normal salivary flow resumes upon discontinuation)

Effects on Bleeding No information available to require special precautions

Adverse Effects Note: Most adverse reactions are transient; incidence often similar to placebo.

1% to 10%:
Central nervous system: Somnolence (4%), headache (3%), fatigue (1%)
Gastrointestinal: Xerostomia (3%)
Respiratory: Nasal irritation (5%), epistaxis (1%)

General Dosage Range Intranasal: *Children ≥12 years and Adults ≤65 years:* 2 sprays in each nostril 2-4 times/day

Mechanism of Action Potent, selective histamine H₁-receptor antagonist

Pharmacodynamics/Kinetics

Onset of Action 10 minutes

Half-life Elimination 33 hours

Pregnancy Considerations Adverse events were observed in some animal reproduction studies when using oral doses much larger than the equivalent maximum human nasal dose.

Product Availability Not available in U.S.

Levocabastine (Ophthalmic)
(LEE voe kab as teen)

Brand Names: Canada Livostin® Eye Drops

Pharmacologic Category Histamine H₁ Antagonist; Histamine H₁ Antagonist, Second Generation; Piperidine Derivative

Use Treatment of seasonal allergic conjunctivitis

Local Anesthetic/Vasoconstrictor Precautions No information available to require special precautions

Effects on Dental Treatment No significant effects or complications reported

Effects on Bleeding No information available to require special precautions

Adverse Effects
>10%: Ocular: Irritation (16%; similar to placebo)
1% to 10%:
Central nervous system: Fatigue (2%)
Respiratory: Epistaxis (1%)

General Dosage Range Ophthalmic: *Children ≥12 years and Adults ≤65 years:* Instill 1 drop in affected eye(s) 2-4 times/day

Mechanism of Action Potent, selective histamine H₁-receptor antagonist for topical ophthalmic use

Pharmacodynamics/Kinetics

Onset of Action 10-15 minutes

Half-life Elimination 33 hours

Pregnancy Considerations Adverse events were observed in animal reproduction studies when using doses much larger than the equivalent maximum human ophthalmic dose.

Product Availability Not available in U.S.

LevOCARNitine (lee voe KAR ni teen)

Brand Names: U.S. Carnitine-300 [OTC]; Carnitor®; Carnitor® SF; L-Carnitine [OTC]

Brand Names: Canada Carnitor®

Pharmacologic Category Dietary Supplement

Use
Oral: Primary systemic carnitine deficiency; acute and chronic treatment of patients with an inborn error of metabolism which results in secondary carnitine deficiency

I.V.: Acute and chronic treatment of patients with an inborn error of metabolism which results in secondary carnitine deficiency; prevention and treatment of carnitine deficiency in patients with end-stage renal disease (ESRD) who are undergoing hemodialysis.

Unlabeled Use Treatment of elevated ammonia levels, coma, and/or hepatic dysfunction due to valproic acid overdose/toxicity (Eyer, 2005; Mock, 2012; Perrott, 2010; Russell, 2007)

Local Anesthetic/Vasoconstrictor Precautions No information available to require special precautions

Effects on Dental Treatment Key adverse event(s) related to dental treatment: Taste perversion.

Effects on Bleeding No information available to require special precautions

Adverse Effects
Intravenous: Frequencies noted with hemodialysis patients.
>10%:
Cardiovascular: Hypertension (18% to 21%), chest pain (6% to 15%)
Central nervous system: Headache (3% to 37%), dizziness (10% to 18%), fever (5% to 12%)
Endocrine & metabolic: Hypercalcemia (6% to 15%)

◄ Gastrointestinal: Diarrhea (9% to 35%), vomiting (9% to 21%), abdominal pain (5% to 21%), nausea (5% to 12%)

Hematologic: Anemia (3% to 12%)

Neuromuscular & skeletal: Weakness (8% to 12%), paresthesia (3% to 12%)

Respiratory: Cough (9% to 18%), rhinitis (6% to 11%)

Miscellaneous: Infection (10% to 24%), accidental injury (≤12%)

1% to 10%:

Cardiovascular: Tachycardia (5% to 9%), palpitation (3% to 8%), peripheral edema (3% to 6%), atrial fibrillation (2% to 6%), ECG abnormality (2% to 6%), vascular disorder (2% to 6%)

Central nervous system: Depression (5% to 6%), vertigo (2% to 6%)

Dermatologic: Rash (3% to 5%)

Endocrine & metabolic: Parathyroid disorder (2% to 6%)

Gastrointestinal: Taste perversion (2% to 9%), weight loss (3% to 8%), anorexia (3% to 6%), gastrointestinal disorder (2% to 6%), melena (2% to 6%), weight gain (2% to 6%)

Hematologic: Hemorrhage (2% to 9%)

Ocular: Amblyopia (3% to 6%), eye disorder (3% to 6%)

Respiratory: Bronchitis (3% to 5%)

Miscellaneous: Allergic reaction (2% to 6%), drug dependence (≤6%)

Frequency not defined:

Central nervous system: Seizures

Gastrointestinal: Gastritis

Miscellaneous: Body odor

Oral: Frequency not defined:

Central nervous system: Seizures

Gastrointestinal: Abdominal cramps, diarrhea, nausea, vomiting

Miscellaneous: Body odor

General Dosage Range

I.V.:

Children: 50 mg/kg/day in divided doses (maximum: 300 mg/kg/day)

Adults: 50 mg/kg/day in divided doses (maximum: 300 mg/kg/day) **or** 20 mg/kg after each hemodialysis session

Oral:

Infants and Children: Initial: 50 mg/kg/day in divided doses; Maintenance: 50-100 mg/kg/day in divided doses (maximum: 3000 mg daily)

Adults: 990 mg (tablet) 2-3 times daily **or** 1000-3000 g daily (oral solution) in divided doses

Mechanism of Action Carnitine is a naturally occurring metabolic compound which functions as a carrier molecule for long-chain fatty acids within the mitochondria, facilitating energy production. Carnitine deficiency is associated with accumulation of excess acyl CoA esters and disruption of intermediary metabolism. Carnitine supplementation increases carnitine plasma concentrations. The effects on specific metabolic alterations have not been evaluated. ESRD patients on maintenance hemodialysis may have low plasma carnitine levels because of reduced intake of meat and dairy products, reduced renal synthesis, and dialytic losses. Certain clinical conditions (malaise, muscle weakness, cardiomyopathy and arrhythmias) in hemodialysis patients may be related to carnitine deficiency.

In patients with valproic acid toxicity, administration of exogenous carnitine shifts the metabolism of valproic acid towards β-oxidation and away from ω-oxidation and potentially hepatotoxic metabolite production.

Pharmacodynamics/Kinetics

Half-life Elimination 17.4 hours

Time to Peak Oral: 3.3 hours

Pregnancy Risk Factor B

Pregnancy Considerations Teratogenic effects were not observed in animal studies. There are no adequate and well-controlled studies in pregnant women. However, carnitine is a naturally occurring substance in mammalian metabolism.

Levocetirizine (LEE vo se TI ra zeen)

Brand Names: U.S. Xyzal®

Pharmacologic Category Histamine H_1 Antagonist; Histamine H_1 Antagonist, Second Generation; Piperazine Derivative

Use Relief of symptoms of perennial and seasonal allergic rhinitis; treatment of skin manifestations (uncomplicated) of chronic idiopathic urticaria

Local Anesthetic/Vasoconstrictor Precautions No information available to require special precautions

Effects on Dental Treatment Key adverse event(s) related to dental treatment: Xerostomia and changes in salivation (normal salivary flow resumes upon discontinuation).

Effects on Bleeding No information available to require special precautions

Adverse Effects

>10%: Gastrointestinal: Diarrhea (children 4% to 13%)

1% to 10%:

Central nervous system: Somnolence (2% to 6%), fever (children 4%), fatigue (1% to 4%)

Gastrointestinal: Constipation (children 7%), vomiting (children 4%), xerostomia (2% to 3%)

Neuromuscular & skeletal: Weakness (2%)

Otic: Otitis media (children 3%)

Respiratory: Nasopharyngitis (4% to 6%), cough (children 3%), epistaxis (children 2%), pharyngitis (1% to 2%)

The following potentially-severe adverse reactions have been reported with cetirizine and, therefore, may also occur with levocetirizine: Cholestasis, glomerulonephritis, hallucination, hypotension (severe), orofacial dyskinesia

General Dosage Range Dosage adjustment recommended in patients with renal impairment

Oral:

Children 6 months to 5 years: 1.25 mg once daily

Children 6-11 years: 2.5 mg once daily

Children ≥12 years and Adults: 2.5-5 mg once daily

Mechanism of Action Levocetirizine is an antihistamine which selectively competes with histamine for H_1-receptor sites on effector cells in the gastrointestinal tract, blood vessels, and respiratory tract. Levocetirizine, the active enantiomer of cetirizine, has twice the binding affinity at the H_1-receptor compared to cetirizine.

Pharmacodynamics/Kinetics

Onset of Action 1 hour

Duration of Action 24 hours

Half-life Elimination Children: ~6 hours; Adults: ~8-9 hours; Renal impairment: 11-34 hours; End-stage renal disease: 46 hours

Time to Peak Children: 1.2 hours; Adults: Oral solution: 0.5 hours, Tablet: 0.9 hours

Pregnancy Risk Factor B
Pregnancy Considerations Adverse events have not been observed in animal reproduction studies; therefore, the manufacturer classifies levocetirizine as pregnancy category B. The use of antihistamines for the treatment of rhinitis during pregnancy is generally considered to be safe at recommended doses. Information related to the use of levocitirizine during pregnancy is limited; therefore, other agents are preferred. Levocetirizine is the active enantiomer of cetirizine; refer to the Cetirizine monograph for additional information.

Levodopa, Carbidopa, and Entacapone
(lee voe DOE pa, kar bi DOE pa, & en TA ka pone)

Related Information
Carbidopa *on page 249*
Entacapone *on page 480*
Brand Names: U.S. Stalevo®
Brand Names: Canada Stalevo®
Pharmacologic Category Anti-Parkinson's Agent, COMT Inhibitor; Anti-Parkinson's Agent, Decarboxylase Inhibitor; Anti-Parkinson's Agent, Dopamine Precursor
Use Treatment of idiopathic Parkinson's disease
Local Anesthetic/Vasoconstrictor Precautions No information available to require special precautions
Effects on Dental Treatment No significant effects or complications reported
Effects on Bleeding No information available to require special precautions
Adverse Effects See individual agents.
General Dosage Range Oral: *Adults:* 1 tablet (50-200 mg levodopa/12.5-50 mg carbidopa/200 mg entacapone) at each dosing interval (maximum: 1600 mg/day entacapone or 300 mg/day carbidopa)
Mechanism of Action
Levodopa: The metabolic precursor of dopamine, a chemical depleted in Parkinson's disease. Levodopa is able to circulate in the plasma and cross the blood-brain-barrier (BBB), where it is converted by striatal enzymes to dopamine.
Carbidopa: Inhibits the peripheral plasma breakdown of levodopa by inhibiting its decarboxylation; increases available levodopa at the BBB
Entacapone: A reversible and selective inhibitor of catechol-O-methyltransferase (COMT). Alters the pharmacokinetics of levodopa, resulting in more sustained levodopa serum levels and increased concentrations available for absorption across the BBB.
Pregnancy Risk Factor C
Pregnancy Considerations Teratogenic effects were observed with levodopa, carbidopa, and entacapone in animal studies. There are case reports of levodopa crossing the placenta in humans. There are no adequate and well-controlled studies in pregnant women. Use during pregnancy only if potential benefit exceeds risks.

Levofloxacin (Systemic) (lee voe FLOKS a sin)

Related Information
Clinical Risk Related to Drugs Prolonging QT Interval *on page 1510*
Gastrointestinal Disorders *on page 1512*
Related Sample Prescriptions
Bacterial Infections and Periodontal Diseases *on page 1609*
Brand Names: U.S. Levaquin®

Brand Names: Canada APO-Levofloxacin; AVA-Levofloxacin; CO Levofloxacin; Levaquin®; Mylan-Levofloxacin; Novo-Levofloxacin; PMS-Levofloxacin; Sandoz-Levofloxacin
Generic Availability (U.S.) Yes
Pharmacologic Category Antibiotic, Quinolone; Respiratory Fluoroquinolone
Use Treatment of community-acquired pneumonia, including multidrug resistant strains of *S. pneumoniae* (MDRSP); nosocomial pneumonia; chronic bronchitis (acute bacterial exacerbation); acute bacterial rhinosinusitis (ABRS); prostatitis (chronic bacterial), urinary tract infection (uncomplicated or complicated); acute pyelonephritis; skin or skin structure infections (uncomplicated or complicated); reduce incidence or disease progression of inhalational anthrax (postexposure); prophylaxis and treatment of plague (pneumonic and septicemic) due to *Y. pestis*
Unlabeled Use Diverticulitis, enterocolitis (*Shigella* spp), epididymitis (nongonococcal), urethritis (nongonococcal), complicated intra-abdominal infections (in combination with metronidazole), Legionnaires' disease, peritonitis, PID (alternative therapy); traveler's diarrhea; oral phase treatment of prosthetic joint infection
Note: As of April 2007, the CDC no longer recommends the use of fluoroquinolones for the treatment of gonococcal disease due to increased prevalence of fluoroquinolone-resistant *Neisseria gonorrhoeae*.
Local Anesthetic/Vasoconstrictor Precautions
Levofloxacin is one of the drugs confirmed to prolong the QT interval and is accepted as having a risk of causing torsade de pointes. The risk of drug-induced torsade de pointes is extremely low when a single QT interval prolonging drug is prescribed. In terms of epinephrine, it is not known what effect vasoconstrictors in the local anesthetic regimen will have in patients with a known history of congenital prolonged QT interval or in patients taking any medication that prolongs the QT interval. Until more information is obtained, it is suggested that the clinician consult with the physician prior to the use of a vasoconstrictor in suspected patients, and that the vasoconstrictor (epinephrine, mepivacaine and levonordefrin [Carbocaine® 2% with Neo-Cobefrin®]) be used with caution.
Effects on Dental Treatment No significant effects or complications reported
Effects on Bleeding No information available to require special precautions
Adverse Effects 1% to 10%:
Cardiovascular: Chest pain (1%), edema (1%)
Central nervous system: Headache (6%), insomnia (4%), dizziness (3%)
Dermatologic: Rash (2%), pruritus (1%)
Gastrointestinal: Nausea (7%), diarrhea (5%), constipation (3%), abdominal pain (2%), dyspepsia (2%), vomiting (2%)
Genitourinary: Vaginitis (1%)
Local: Injection site reaction (1%)
Respiratory: Dyspnea (1%)
Miscellaneous: Moniliasis (1%)
Dosage Note: Sequential therapy (intravenous to oral) may be instituted based on prescriber's discretion.
Usual dosage range: Adults: Oral, I.V.: 250-500 mg every 24 hours; severe or complicated infections: 750 mg every 24 hours

Indication-specific dosing:

Infants ≥6 months and Children ≤4 years:

Community-acquired pneumonia (CAP) (IDSA/ PIDS, 2011): Note: May consider addition of van-comycin or clindamycin to empiric therapy if community-acquired MRSA suspected; alternative to ceftriaxone or cefotaxime in patients not fully immunized for *H. influenzae* type b and *S. pneumoniae*, or significant local resistance to penicillin in invasive pneumococcal strains.

S. pneumoniae (MICs to penicillin ≤2.0 mcg/mL), mild infection or step-down therapy (alternative to amoxicillin): Oral: 8-10 mg/kg/dose every 12 hours (maximum: 750 mg daily)

S. pneumoniae (MICs to penicillin ≥4.0 mcg/mL):
Moderate-to-severe infection (alternative to cef-triaxone): I.V.: 8-10 mg/kg/dose every 12 hours (maximum: 750 mg daily)

Mild infection, step-down therapy (preferred): Oral: 8-10 mg/kg/dose every 12 hours (maximum: 750 mg daily)

H. influenzae, moderate-to-severe infection (alternative to ampicillin, ceftriaxone, or cefotaxime): I.V.: 8-10 mg/kg/dose every 12 hours (maximum: 750 mg daily)

Atypical pathogens, moderate-to-severe infection (alternative to azithromycin) or empiric treatment (alternative to azithromycin +/- beta-lactam; should be limited to macrolide allergic/intolerant patients): Oral, I.V.: 8-10 mg/kg/dose every 12 hours (maximum: 750 mg daily)

Infants ≥6 months, Children, and Adults: Oral, I.V.:

Anthrax (inhalational, postexposure):

≤50 kg: 8 mg/kg every 12 hours for 60 days (do not exceed 250 mg/dose), beginning as soon as possible after exposure

>50 kg and Adults: 500 mg every 24 hours for 60 days, beginning as soon as possible after exposure

Plague (prophylaxis and treatment):

≤50 kg: 8 mg/kg every 12 hours for 10-14 days (do not exceed 250 mg/dose), beginning as soon as possible after exposure

>50 kg and Adults: 500 mg every 24 hours for 10-14 days, beginning as soon as possible after exposure. **Note:** Dose of 750 mg once daily may be considered if clinically warranted.

Children:

Acute bacterial rhinosinusitis (unlabeled use): Oral, I.V.: 10-20 mg/kg/day divided every 12-24 hours for 10-14 days (maximum: 500 mg daily). **Note:** Recommended in patients with a type I penicillin allergy, after failure of initial therapy or in patients at risk for antibiotic resistance (eg, daycare attendance, age <2 years, recent hospitalization, antibiotic use within the past month) (Chow, 2012).

Children 5-16 years:

Community-acquired pneumonia (CAP) (IDSA/ PIDS, 2011): Note: May consider addition of van-comycin or clindamycin to empiric therapy if community-acquired MRSA suspected; alternative to ceftriaxone or cefotaxime in patients not fully immunized for *H. influenzae* type b and *S. pneumoniae*, or significant local resistance to penicillin in invasive pneumococcal strains.

S. pneumoniae (MICs to penicillin ≤2.0 mcg/mL), mild infection or step-down therapy (alternative to amoxicillin): Oral: 8-10 mg/kg/dose once daily (maximum: 750 mg daily)

S. pneumoniae (MICs to penicillin ≥4.0 mcg/mL):
Moderate-to-severe infection (alternative to cef-triaxone): I.V.: 8-10 mg/kg/dose once daily (maximum: 750 mg daily)

Mild infection, step-down therapy (preferred): Oral: 8-10 mg/kg/dose once daily (maximum: 750 mg daily)

H. influenzae, moderate-to-severe infection (alternative to ampicillin, ceftriaxone, or cefotaxime): I.V.: 8-10 mg/kg/dose once daily (maximum: 750 mg daily)

Atypical pathogens:

Moderate-to-severe infection (alternative to azithromycin): I.V.: 8-10 mg/kg/dose once daily (maximum: 750 mg daily)

Mild infection, step-down therapy (alternative to azithromycin in adolescents with skeletal maturity): Oral: 500 mg once daily

Adults: Oral, I.V.:

Acute bacterial rhinosinusitis:

Manufacturer's recommendations: 750 mg every 24 hours for 5 days or 500 mg every 24 hours for 10-14 days

Alternate recommendations: 500 mg every 24 hours for 5-7 days (Chow, 2012)

***Chlamydia trachomatis* sexually-transmitted infections (unlabeled use) (CDC, 2010):** Oral: 500 mg every 24 hours for 7 days

Chronic bronchitis (acute bacterial exacerbation): Oral: 500 mg every 24 hours for 7 days; Canadian labeling (not in U.S. labeling) also includes a dosage regimen of 750 mg every 24 hours for 5 days

Diverticulitis, peritonitis (unlabeled use) (Solomkin, [IDSA] 2010): 750 mg every 24 hours for 7-10 days; use adjunctive metronidazole therapy

Epididymitis, nongonococcal (unlabeled use) (CDC, 2010): Oral: 500 mg once daily for 10 days

Gonococcal infection (unlabeled use) (CDC, 2010): As of April 2007, the CDC no longer recommends the use of fluoroquinolones for the treatment of uncomplicated or more serious gonococcal disease, unless no other options exist and susceptibility can be confirmed via culture.

Intra-abdominal infection, complicated, community-acquired (in combination with metronidazole) (unlabeled use) (Solomkin, [IDSA] 2010): I.V.: 750 mg once daily for 4-7 days (provided source controlled). **Note:** Avoid using in settings where *E. coli* susceptibility to fluoroquinolones is <90%.

Pelvic inflammatory disease (unlabeled use) (CDC, 2010): Oral: 500 mg once daily for 14 days with or without concomitant metronidazole; **Note:** The CDC recommends use as an alternative therapy only if standard parenteral cephalosporin therapy is not feasible and community prevalence of quinolone-resistant gonococcal organisms is low. Culture sensitivity must be confirmed.

Pneumonia:

Community-acquired (CAP): 500 mg every 24 hours for 7-14 days or 750 mg every 24 hours for 5 days (efficacy of 5-day regimen for MDRSP not established)

Healthcare-associated (HAP): 750 mg every 24 hours for 7-14 days

Prostatitis (chronic bacterial): Oral: 500 mg every 24 hours for 28 days

Skin and skin structure infections:

Uncomplicated: 500 mg every 24 hours for 7-10 days

Complicated: 750 mg every 24 hours for 7-14 days

Traveler's diarrhea (unlabeled use): Oral: 500 mg for one dose (Sanders, 2007)

Tuberculosis, drug-resistant tuberculosis, or intolerance to first-line agents (unlabeled use): Oral: 500-1000 mg every 24 hours (CDC, 2003)

Urethritis, nongonococcal (unlabeled use) (CDC, 2010): Oral: 500 mg every 24 hours for 7 days

Urinary tract infections:

Uncomplicated: 250 mg once daily for 3 days

Complicated, including pyelonephritis: 250 mg once daily for 10 days **or** 750 mg once daily for 5 days

Dosage adjustment in renal impairment: I.V., Oral:

Normal renal function dosing of 750 mg daily:

Cl_{cr} 20-49 mL/minute: Administer 750 mg every 48 hours

Cl_{cr} 10-19 mL/minute: Administer 750 mg initial dose, followed by 500 mg every 48 hours

Hemodialysis/chronic ambulatory peritoneal dialysis (CAPD): Administer 750 mg initial dose, followed by 500 mg every 48 hours; supplemental doses are not required following either hemodialysis or CAPD.

Normal renal function dosing of 500 mg daily:

Cl_{cr} 20-49 mL/minute: Administer 500 mg initial dose, followed by 250 mg every 24 hours

Cl_{cr} 10-19 mL/minute: Administer 500 mg initial dose, followed by 250 mg every 48 hours

Hemodialysis/chronic ambulatory peritoneal dialysis (CAPD): Administer 500 mg initial dose, followed by 250 mg every 48 hours; supplemental doses are not required following either hemodialysis or CAPD.

Normal renal function dosing of 250 mg daily:

Cl_{cr} 20-49 mL/minute: No dosage adjustment required

Cl_{cr} 10-19 mL/minute: Administer 250 mg every 48 hours (except in uncomplicated UTI, where no dosage adjustment is required)

Hemodialysis/chronic ambulatory peritoneal dialysis (CAPD): No information available

Continuous renal replacement therapy (CRRT) (Heintz, 2009; Trotman, 2005): Drug clearance is highly dependent on the method of renal replacement, filter type, and flow rate. Appropriate dosing requires close monitoring of pharmacologic response, signs of adverse reactions due to drug accumulation, as well as drug concentrations in relation to target trough (if appropriate). The following are general recommendations only (based on dialysate flow/ultrafiltration rates of 1-2 L/hour and minimal residual renal function) and should not supersede clinical judgment:

CVVH: Loading dose of 500-750 mg followed by 250 mg every 24 hours

CVVHD: Loading dose of 500-750 mg followed by 250-500 mg every 24 hours

CVVHDF: Loading dose of 500-750 mg followed by 250-750 mg every 24 hours

Dosage adjustment in hepatic impairment: I.V., Oral: No dosage adjustment provided in manufacturer's labeling (has not been studied). However, dosage adjustment unlikely due to limited hepatic metabolism.

Mechanism of Action As the S(-) enantiomer of the fluoroquinolone, ofloxacin, levofloxacin, inhibits DNA-gyrase in susceptible organisms thereby inhibits relaxation of supercoiled DNA and promotes breakage of DNA strands. DNA gyrase (topoisomerase II), is an essential bacterial enzyme that maintains the super-helical structure of DNA and is required for DNA replication and transcription, DNA repair, recombination, and transposition.

Contraindications Hypersensitivity to levofloxacin, any component of the formulation, or other quinolones

Canadian labeling: Additional contraindications (not in U.S. labeling): History of tendonitis or tendon rupture associated with use of any quinolone antimicrobial agent

Warnings/Precautions [U.S. Boxed Warning]: There have been reports of tendon inflammation and/or rupture with quinolone antibiotics; risk may be increased with concurrent corticosteroids, organ transplant recipients, and in patients >60 years of age. Rupture of the Achilles tendon sometimes requiring surgical repair has been reported most frequently; but other tendon sites (eg, rotator cuff, biceps) have also been reported. Strenuous physical activity, rheumatoid arthritis, and renal impairment may be an independent risk factor for tendonitis. Discontinue at first sign of tendon inflammation or pain. May occur even after discontinuation of therapy. Use with caution in patients with rheumatoid arthritis; may increase risk of tendon rupture. Safety of use in pediatric patients for >14 days of therapy has not been studied; increased incidence of musculoskeletal disorders (eg, arthralgia, tendon rupture) has been observed in children. CNS effects may occur (toxic psychoses, tremor, restlessness, anxiety, lightheadedness, paranoia, depression, nightmares, confusion, and very rarely hallucinations increased intracranial pressure (including pseudotumor cerebri, seizures, or toxic psychosis). Potential for seizures, although very rare, may be increased with concomitant NSAID therapy. Use with caution in individuals at risk of seizures, with known or suspected CNS disorders or renal dysfunction. Avoid excessive sunlight and take precautions to limit exposure (eg, loose fitting clothing, sunscreen); may cause moderate-to-severe phototoxicity reactions. Discontinue use if photosensitivity occurs.

Rare cases of torsade de pointes have been reported in patients receiving levofloxacin. Use caution in patients with known prolongation of QT interval, bradycardia, hypokalemia, hypomagnesemia, or in those receiving concurrent therapy with Class Ia or Class III antiarrhythmics.

Severe hypersensitivity reactions, including anaphylaxis, have occurred with quinolone therapy. Reactions may present as typical allergic symptoms after a single dose, or may manifest as severe idiosyncratic dermatologic, vascular, pulmonary, renal, hepatic, and/or hematologic events, usually after multiple doses. Prompt discontinuation of drug should occur if skin rash or other symptoms arise. Prolonged use may result in fungal or bacterial superinfection, including *C. difficile*-associated diarrhea (CDAD) and pseudomembranous colitis; CDAD has been observed >2 months postantibiotic treatment. Peripheral neuropathies have been linked to levofloxacin use; discontinue if numbness, tingling, or weakness develops. **[U.S. Boxed Warning]: Quinolones may exacerbate myasthenia gravis; avoid use (rare, potentially life-threatening weakness of respiratory muscles may occur).** Unrelated to hypersensitivity, severe hepatotoxicity (including acute hepatitis and fatalities) has been reported. Elderly patients may be at greater risk. Discontinue therapy immediately if signs and symptoms of hepatitis occur. Hemolytic reactions may (rarely) occur with quinolone use in patients with latent or actual G6PD deficiency.

Fluoroquinolones have been associated with the development of serious, and sometimes fatal, hypoglycemia, most often in elderly diabetics, but also in patients without diabetes. This occurred most frequently with gatifloxacin (no longer available systemically) but may occur at a lower frequency with other quinolones.

Drug Interactions

Metabolism/Transport Effects None known.

Avoid Concomitant Use

Avoid concomitant use of Levofloxacin (Systemic) with any of the following: BCG; Highest Risk QTc-Prolonging Agents; Ivabradine; Mifepristone; Strontium Ranelate

Increased Effect/Toxicity

Levofloxacin (Systemic) may increase the levels/effects of: Corticosteroids (Systemic); Highest Risk QTc-Prolonging Agents; Moderate Risk QTc-Prolonging Agents; Porfimer; Sulfonylureas; Varenicline; Vitamin K Antagonists

The levels/effects of Levofloxacin (Systemic) may be increased by: Insulin; Ivabradine; Mifepristone; Nonsteroidal Anti-Inflammatory Agents; Probenecid; QTc-Prolonging Agents (Indeterminate Risk and Risk Modifying)

Decreased Effect

Levofloxacin (Systemic) may decrease the levels/effects of: BCG; Didanosine; Mycophenolate; Sodium Picosulfate; Sulfonylureas; Typhoid Vaccine

The levels/effects of Levofloxacin (Systemic) may be decreased by: Antacids; Calcium Salts; Didanosine; Iron Salts; Lanthanum; Magnesium Salts; Multivitamins/Minerals (with ADEK, Folate, Iron); Quinapril; Sevelamer; Strontium Ranelate; Sucralfate; Zinc Salts

Dietary Considerations Tablets may be taken without regard to meals. Oral solution should be administered on an empty stomach (1 hour before or 2 hours after a meal). Take 2 hours before or 2 hours after multiple vitamins, antacids, or other products containing magnesium, aluminum, iron, or zinc.

Pharmacodynamics/Kinetics

Half-life Elimination ~6-8 hours

Time to Peak 1-2 hours

Pregnancy Risk Factor C

Pregnancy Considerations Adverse events have been observed in some animal studies; therefore, the manufacturer classifies levofloxacin as pregnancy category C. Levofloxacin crosses the placenta. Quinolone exposure during human pregnancy has been reported with other agents (see Ciprofloxacin [Systemic], Ofloxacin [Systemic], and Norfloxacin monographs). To date, no specific teratogenic effect or increased pregnancy risk has been identified; however, because of concerns of cartilage damage in immature animals exposed to quinolones and the limited levofloxacin specific data, levofloxacin should only be used during pregnancy if a safer option is not available.

Lactation Enters breast milk/not recommended

Breast-Feeding Considerations Based on data from a case report, small amounts of levofloxacin are excreted in breast milk. Breast-feeding is not recommended by the manufacturer. Levofloxacin is the L-isomer of ofloxacin. Ofloxacin has also been shown to have minimal concentrations in human milk. Nondose-related effects could include modification of bowel flora.

Dosage Forms

Infusion, premixed in D₅W [preservative free]: 250 mg (50 mL); 500 mg (100 mL); 750 mg (150 mL)

Levaquin®: 250 mg (50 mL); 500 mg (100 mL); 750 mg (150 mL)

Injection, solution [preservative free]: 25 mg/mL (20 mL, 30 mL)

Solution, oral: 25 mg/mL (100 mL, 200 mL, 480 mL)

Levaquin®: 25 mg/mL (480 mL)

Tablet, oral: 250 mg, 500 mg, 750 mg

Levaquin®: 250 mg, 500 mg, 750 mg

Dental Comment Levofloxacin is known to prolong the QT interval. The QT interval is measured as the time and distance between the Q point of the QRS complex and the end of the T wave in the ECG tracing. After adjustment for heart rate, the QT interval is defined as prolonged if it is more than 450 msec in men and 460 msec in women. A long QT syndrome was first described in the 1950s and 60s as a congenital syndrome involving QT interval prolongation and syncope and sudden death. Some of the congenital long QT syndromes were characterized by a peculiar electrocardiographic appearance of the QRS complex involving a premature atria beat followed by a pause, then a subsequent sinus beat showing marked QT prolongation and deformity. This type of cardiac arrhythmia was originally termed "torsade de pointes" (translated from the French as "twisting of the points"). Levofloxacin is considered as having a risk of causing torsade de pointes. Since it is not known what effect vasoconstrictors in the local anesthetic regimen will have in patients with a known history of congenital prolonged QT interval or in patients taking any medication that prolongs the QT interval, a medical consult is suggested.

LEVOleucovorin (lee voe loo koe VOR in)

Brand Names: U.S. Fusilev®

Pharmacologic Category Antidote; Chemotherapy Modulating Agent; Rescue Agent (Chemotherapy)

Use Treatment of advanced, metastatic colorectal cancer (palliative) in combination with fluorouracil; rescue agent after high-dose methotrexate therapy in osteosarcoma; antidote for impaired methotrexate elimination and for inadvertent overdosage of folic acid antagonists

Local Anesthetic/Vasoconstrictor Precautions No information available to require special precautions

Effects on Dental Treatment Key adverse event(s) related to dental treatment: Stomatitis and taste perversion.

Effects on Bleeding No information available to require special precautions

Adverse Effects Note: Adverse reactions reported with levoleucovorin either as a part of combination chemotherapy or following chemotherapy.

>10%:

Central nervous system: Fatigue (≤29%)

Dermatologic: Dermatitis (6% to 29%), alopecia (≤26%)

Gastrointestinal: Stomatitis (38% to 72%; grades 3/4: 6% to 12%), diarrhea (6% to 70%; grades 3/4: ≤19%), nausea (19% to 62%), vomiting (38% to 40%), anorexia/appetite decreased (≤24%), abdominal pain (≤14%)

Neuromuscular & skeletal: Weakness/malaise (≤29%)

1% to 10%:

Central nervous system: Confusion (6%)

Gastrointestinal: Dyspepsia (6%), taste perversion (6%), typhlitis (6%)

Neuromuscular & skeletal: Neuropathy (6%)

Renal: Renal function abnormal (6%)

Respiratory: Dyspnea (6%)

General Dosage Range I.V.: *Children and Adults:* Dosing varies greatly depending on indication

Mechanism of Action Levoleucovorin counteracts the toxic (and therapeutic) effects of folic acid antagonists (eg, methotrexate) which act by inhibiting dihydrofolate reductase. Levoleucovorin is the levo isomeric and pharmacologic active form of leucovorin (levoleucovorin does not require reduction by dihydrofolate reductase). A reduced derivative of folic acid, leucovorin supplies the necessary cofactor blocked by methotrexate.

Leucovorin enhances the activity (and toxicity) of fluorouracil by stabilizing the binding of 5-fluoro-2'-deoxyuridine-5'-monophosphate (FdUMP; a fluorouracil metabolite) to thymidylate synthetase resulting in inhibition of this enzyme.

Pharmacodynamics/Kinetics
Half-life Elimination 15 mg: 5-7 hours; 300 mg: elimination half life: 16-30 hours
Time to Peak Serum: I.V.: 0.9 hours
Pregnancy Risk Factor C
Pregnancy Considerations Animal reproduction studies have not been conducted. Levoleucovorin is the levo isomeric form of racemic leucovorin, a biologically active form of folic acid. Adequate amounts of folic acid are recommended during pregnancy. Refer to Folic Acid monograph.

Levonorgestrel (LEE voe nor jes trel)

Brand Names: U.S. Mirena®; My Way™; Next Choice®; Next Choice™ One Dose; Plan B® One Step; Skyla™
Brand Names: Canada Mirena®; Next Choice®; Nor-Levo®; Plan B®
Pharmacologic Category Contraceptive; Progestin
Use
Intrauterine device (IUD): Prevention of pregnancy; treatment of heavy menstrual bleeding in women who also choose to use an IUD for contraception
Oral: Emergency contraception following unprotected intercourse or possible contraceptive failure
Note: Oral products are approved for OTC use by women ≥17 years of age and available by prescription only for women <17 years of age.
Local Anesthetic/Vasoconstrictor Precautions No information available to require special precautions
Effects on Dental Treatment No significant effects or complications reported
Effects on Bleeding No information available to require special precautions
Adverse Effects Frequency not always defined.
Intrauterine device:
>10%:
Central nervous system: Headache (12%)
Dermatologic: Acne (15%)
Endocrine & metabolic: Ovarian cysts (13%), enlarged follicles (12%), amenorrhea (<1% to 12%, increases with duration of treatment)
Gastrointestinal: Abdominal pain (12%)
Genitourinary: Uterine/vaginal bleeding alterations (52%), intermenstrual bleeding/spotting (23%), vulvovaginitis (20%)
Miscellaneous: Ectopic pregnancy (≤50%)
1% to 10%:
Cardiovascular: Edema
Central nervous system: Depression (4%), migraine (2%), nervousness
Dermatologic: Alopecia (1%), eczema, hirsutism, pruritus, rash, urticaria

Endocrine & metabolic: Dysmenorrhea (9%), menorrhagia (6%), breast pain/tenderness (3% to 9%), libido decreased
Gastrointestinal: Nausea (6%), abdominal distension, weight gain
Genitourinary: Pelvic pain (6%), leukorrhea (5%), vaginal discharge (4%), pelvic infection (1%), cervicitis, dyspareunia, vaginitis
Hematologic: Anemia
Neuromuscular & skeletal: Back pain
Miscellaneous: IUD expulsion (3%)
Oral tablets:
>10%:
Central nervous system: Fatigue (13% to 17%), headache (10% to 17%), dizziness (10% to 11%)
Endocrine & metabolic: Heavier menstrual bleeding (14% to 31%), lighter menstrual bleeding (12%), breast tenderness (8% to 11%)
Gastrointestinal: Nausea (14% to 23%), abdominal pain (13% to 18%)
1% to 10%:
Endocrine & metabolic: Menses delayed (5%)
Gastrointestinal: Vomiting (6%), diarrhea (5%)
General Dosage Range
Intrauterine: *Adults:* Insert into uterine cavity, releases ~10-20 mcg daily over 5 years (Mirena®) **or** ~6 mcg daily over 3 years (Skyla™)
Oral: *Adults:* 0.75 mg every 12 hours for 2 doses **or** 1.5 mg as a single dose
Mechanism of Action Pregnancy may be prevented through several mechanisms: Thickening of cervical mucus, which inhibits sperm passage through the uterus and sperm survival; inhibition of ovulation, from a negative feedback mechanism on the hypothalamus, leading to reduced secretion of follicle stimulating hormone (FSH) and luteinizing hormone (LH); and inhibition of implantation. Levonorgestrel is not effective once the implantation process has begun.
Pharmacodynamics/Kinetics
Duration of Action Intrauterine device: Mirena®: Up to 5 years; Skyla™: Up to 3 years
Half-life Elimination Oral: ~24 hours
Time to Peak Oral: ~2 hours
Pregnancy Considerations Use during pregnancy is contraindicated. When pregnancies have continued following levonorgestrel exposure, congenital anomalies have been infrequent. Significant adverse effects on infant growth and development have not been observed (limited data). In doses larger than those used for oral contraception, progestins have been reported to increase the risk of masculinization of female genitalia.

Intrauterine device: Pregnancy should be ruled out prior to insertion. Women who become pregnant with an IUD in place risk septic abortion (septic shock and death may occur). Removal of the device is recommended, however, removal or manipulation of IUD may result in pregnancy loss. In addition, miscarriage, premature labor, and premature delivery may occur if pregnancy is continued with IUD in place. Following pregnancy, insertion of the device should not take place until 6 weeks postpartum or until involution of the uterus is complete. Consider waiting until 12 weeks postpartum if involution is substantially delayed. The device may be inserted immediately following a first trimester abortion. Following removal of the device, ~80% of women who wished to conceive became pregnant within 12 months.

◀ Oral tablet: A rapid return of fertility is expected following use for emergency contraception; routine contraceptive measures should be initiated or continued following use to ensure ongoing prevention of pregnancy. Barrier contraception is recommended immediately following emergency contraception. Short-term contraception (eg, oral hormonal contraceptive pills, patches, rings) may be started with barrier contraception or after the next menstrual period. Long term contraception (eg, IUD, depot medroxyprogesterone, progestin implant) should be started after the next menstrual period.

Prescribing and Access Restrictions Oral tablets for OTC use are limited to pharmacies or healthcare clinics with a valid license to distribute prescription products. Pharmacies are required to keep the product behind the counter.

Levorphanol (lee VOR fa nole)

Pharmacologic Category Analgesic, Opioid

Use Relief of moderate-to-severe pain; preoperative sedation/analgesia; management of chronic pain (eg, cancer) requiring opioid therapy

Local Anesthetic/Vasoconstrictor Precautions No information available to require special precautions

Effects on Dental Treatment Key adverse event(s) related to dental treatment: Xerostomia (normal salivary flow resumes upon discontinuation).

Effects on Bleeding No information available to require special precautions

Adverse Effects Frequency not defined.

Cardiovascular: Palpitation, hypotension, bradycardia, peripheral vasodilation, cardiac arrest, shock, tachycardia

Central nervous system: CNS depression, fatigue, drowsiness, dizziness, nervousness, headache, restlessness, anorexia, malaise, confusion, coma, convulsion, insomnia, amnesia, mental depression, hallucinations, paradoxical CNS stimulation, intracranial pressure (increased)

Dermatologic: Pruritus, urticaria, rash

Endocrine & metabolic: Antidiuretic hormone release

Gastrointestinal: Nausea, vomiting, dyspepsia, stomach cramps, xerostomia, constipation, abdominal pain, dry mouth, biliary tract spasm, paralytic ileus

Genitourinary: Decreased urination, urinary tract spasm, urinary retention

Neuromuscular & skeletal: Weakness

Ocular: Miosis, diplopia

Respiratory: Respiratory depression, apnea, hypoventilation, cyanosis

Miscellaneous: Histamine release, physical and psychological dependence

General Dosage Range Dosage adjustment recommended in patients with hepatic impairment

Oral: *Adults:* 2-4 mg every 6-8 hours as needed

Mechanism of Action Levorphanol tartrate is a synthetic opioid agonist that is classified as a morphinan derivative. Opioids interact with stereospecific opioid receptors in various parts of the central nervous system and other tissues. Analgesic potency parallels the affinity for these binding sites. These drugs do not alter the threshold or responsiveness to pain, but the perception of pain.

Pharmacodynamics/Kinetics

Onset of Action Oral: 10-60 minutes

Duration of Action 4-8 hours

Half-life Elimination 11-16 hours

Pregnancy Risk Factor C

Pregnancy Considerations Adverse events have been observed in animal reproduction studies. Neonates born to mothers receiving opioids during pregnancy should be monitored for neonatal withdrawal syndrome and respiratory depression.

Controlled Substance C-II

Levothyroxine (lee voe thye ROKS een)

Related Information

Endocrine Disorders and Pregnancy *on page 1517*

Brand Names: U.S. Levothroid®; Levoxyl®; Synthroid®; Tirosint®; Unithroid®

Brand Names: Canada Eltroxin®; Euthyrox; Levothyroxine Sodium; Levothyroxine Sodium for Injection; Synthroid®

Generic Availability (U.S.) Yes: Excludes capsule

Pharmacologic Category Thyroid Product

Use Replacement or supplemental therapy in hypothyroidism; pituitary TSH suppression

Unlabeled Use Management of hemodynamically unstable potential organ donors increasing the quantity of organs available for transplantation

Local Anesthetic/Vasoconstrictor Precautions No precautions with vasoconstrictor are necessary if patient is well controlled with levothyroxine

Effects on Dental Treatment No significant effects or complications reported

Effects on Bleeding No information available to require special precautions

Adverse Effects Frequency not defined.

Cardiovascular: Angina, arrhythmia, cardiac arrest, flushing, heart failure, hypertension, MI, palpitation, pulse increased, tachycardia

Central nervous system: Anxiety, emotional lability, fatigue, fever, headache, hyperactivity, insomnia, irritability, nervousness, pseudotumor cerebri (children), seizure (rare)

Dermatologic: Alopecia

Endocrine & metabolic: Fertility impaired, menstrual irregularities

Gastrointestinal: Abdominal cramps, appetite increased, diarrhea, vomiting, weight loss

Hepatic: Liver function tests increased

Neuromuscular & skeletal: Bone mineral density decreased, muscle weakness, tremor, slipped capital femoral epiphysis (children)

Respiratory: Dyspnea

Miscellaneous: Diaphoresis, heat intolerance, hypersensitivity (to inactive ingredients, symptoms include urticaria, pruritus, rash, flushing, angioedema, GI symptoms, fever, arthralgia, serum sickness, wheezing)

Levoxyl®: Choking, dysphagia, gagging

Dosage Doses should be adjusted based on clinical response and laboratory parameters.

Oral:

Infants and Children: Hypothyroidism: Daily dosage based on body weight and age as listed below:

1-3 months: 10-15 mcg/kg/day; if the infant is at risk for development of cardiac failure, use a lower starting dose of 25 mcg/day; if the initial serum T_4 is very low (<5 mcg/dL) begin treatment at a higher dosage of 50 mcg/day

3-6 months: 8-10 mcg/kg/day **or** 25-50 mcg/day

6-12 months: 6-8 mcg/kg/day **or** 50-75 mcg/day

1-5 years: 5-6 mcg/kg/day **or** 75-100 mcg/day

6-12 years: 4-5 mcg/kg/day **or** 100-125 mcg/day

>12 years: 2-3 mcg/kg/day **or** ≥150 mcg/day

Growth and puberty complete: 1.7 mcg/kg/day; refer to Adult dosing.
Dosing modifications:
Hyperactivity in older children may be minimized by starting at $1/4$ of the recommended dose and increasing each week by that amount until the full dose is achieved (4 weeks).
Children with severe or chronic hypothyroidism should be started at 25 mcg/day; adjust dose by 25 mcg every 2-4 weeks.

Adults (including children in whom growth and puberty are complete, healthy adults <50 years of age, and older adults who have been recently treated for hyperthyroidism or who have been hypothyroid for only a few months):
Hypothyroidism: ~1.7 mcg/kg/day; usual doses are ≤200 mcg/day (range: 100-125 mcg/day [70 kg adult]); doses ≥300 mcg/day are rare (consider poor compliance, malabsorption, and/or drug interactions). Titrate dose every 6 weeks.
Patients >50 years or patients with cardiac disease: Refer to Elderly dosing.
Severe hypothyroidism: Initial: 12.5-25 mcg/day; adjust dose by 25 mcg/day every 2-4 weeks as appropriate
Myxedema: Oral agents are not recommended for myxedema: Refer to I.V. dosing.
Subclinical hypothyroidism (if treated): 1 mcg/kg/day
TSH suppression:
Well-differentiated thyroid cancer: Highly individualized; Doses >2 mcg/kg/day may be needed to suppress TSH to <0.1 mIU/L in intermediate- to high-risk tumors. Low-risk tumors may be maintained at or slightly below the lower limit of normal (0.1-0.5 mIU/L) (Cooper, 2009).
Benign nodules and nontoxic multinodular goiter: Routine use of T_4 for TSH suppression is not recommended in patients with benign thyroid nodules. In patients deemed appropriate candidates, treatment should never be fully suppressive (TSH <0.1 mIU/L) (Cooper, 2009; Gharib, 2010). Avoid use if TSH is already suppressed.
Elderly: Hypothyroidism (elderly patients may require <1 mcg/kg/day):
>50 years without cardiac disease **or** <50 years with cardiac disease: Initial: 25-50 mcg/day; adjust dose by 12.5-25 mcg increments at 6- to 8-week intervals as needed
>50 years with cardiac disease: Initial: 12.5-25 mcg/day; adjust dose by 12.5-25 mcg increments at 4- to 6-week intervals (many clinicians prefer to adjust at 6- to 8-week intervals)
Note: Patients with combined hypothyroidism and cardiac disease should be monitored carefully for changes in stability.
I.M., I.V.: Children, Adults, Elderly: Hypothyroidism: 50% of the oral dose; alternatively, some clinicians administer up to 80% of the oral dose. **Note:** Bioavailability of the oral formulation is highly variable, but absorption has been measured to be ~80%, when the oral tablet formulation was administered in the recommended fasting state (Dickerson, 2010; Fish, 1987).
I.V.:
Adults: Myxedema coma or stupor: 200-500 mcg, then 100-300 mcg the next day if necessary; smaller doses should be considered in patients with cardiovascular disease
Elderly: Myxedema coma: Refer to adult dosing; lower doses may be needed

Dosage adjustment in renal impairment: No dosage adjustment provided in manufacturer's labeling.
Dosage adjustment in hepatic impairment: No dosage adjustment provided in manufacturer's labeling.
Mechanism of Action Levothyroxine (T_4) is a synthetic form of thyroxine, an endogenous hormone secreted by the thyroid gland. T_4 is converted to its active metabolite, L-triiodothyronine (T_3). Thyroid hormones (T_4 and T_3) then bind to thyroid receptor proteins in the cell nucleus and exert metabolic effects through control of DNA transcription and protein synthesis; involved in normal metabolism, growth, and development; promotes gluconeogenesis, increases utilization and mobilization of glycogen stores, and stimulates protein synthesis, increases basal metabolic rate
Contraindications Hypersensitivity to levothyroxine sodium or any component of the formulation; acute MI; thyrotoxicosis of any etiology; uncorrected adrenal insufficiency
Capsule: Additional contraindication: Inability to swallow capsules
Warnings/Precautions [U.S. Boxed Warning]: Thyroid supplements are ineffective and potentially toxic when used for the treatment of obesity or for weight reduction, especially in euthyroid patients. High doses may produce serious or even life-threatening toxic effects particularly when used with some anorectic drugs (eg, sympathomimetic amines). Routine use of T_4 for TSH suppression is not recommended in patients with benign thyroid nodules. In patients deemed appropriate candidates, treatment should never be fully suppressive (TSH <0.1 mIU/L). Use with caution and reduce dosage in patients with angina pectoris or other cardiovascular disease; decrease initial dose. Use cautiously in the elderly since they may be more likely to have compromised cardiovascular functions. Patients with adrenal insufficiency, myxedema, diabetes mellitus and insipidus may have symptoms exaggerated or aggravated. Chronic hypothyroidism predisposes patients to coronary artery disease. Long-term therapy can decrease bone mineral density. Levoxyl® may rapidly swell and disintegrate causing choking or gagging (should be administered with a full glass of water); use caution in patients with dysphagia or other swallowing disorders.
Drug Interactions
Metabolism/Transport Effects None known.
Avoid Concomitant Use
Avoid concomitant use of Levothyroxine with any of the following: Sodium Iodide I131
Increased Effect/Toxicity
Levothyroxine may increase the levels/effects of: Vitamin K Antagonists
Decreased Effect
Levothyroxine may decrease the levels/effects of: Sodium Iodide I131; Theophylline Derivatives

The levels/effects of Levothyroxine may be decreased by: Aluminum Hydroxide; Bile Acid Sequestrants; Calcium Polystyrene Sulfonate; Calcium Salts; CarBAMazepine; Estrogen Derivatives; Fosphenytoin; Iron Salts; Lanthanum; Multivitamins/Minerals (with ADEK, Folate, Iron); Orlistat; Phenytoin; Raloxifene; Rifampin; Sevelamer; Sodium Polystyrene Sulfonate; Sucralfate
Ethanol/Nutrition/Herb Interactions Food: Taking levothyroxine with enteral nutrition may cause reduced bioavailability and may lower serum thyroxine levels leading to signs or symptoms of hypothyroidism. Soybean flour (infant formula), cottonseed meal, walnuts, and dietary fiber may decrease absorption of

levothyroxine from the GI tract. Management: Take in the morning on an empty stomach at least 30 minutes before food. Consider an increase in dose if taken with enteral tube feed.

Dietary Considerations Should be taken on an empty stomach, at least 30 minutes before food.

Pharmacodynamics/Kinetics

Onset of Action Therapeutic: Oral: 3-5 days; I.V. 6-8 hours; Peak effect: I.V.: 24 hours

Half-life Elimination Euthyroid: 6-7 days; Hypothyroid: 9-10 days; Hyperthyroid: 3-4 days

Time to Peak Serum: 2-4 hours

Pregnancy Risk Factor A

Pregnancy Considerations Endogenous thyroid hormones minimally cross the placenta; the fetal thyroid becomes active around the end of the first trimester. Levothyroxine has not been shown to increase the risk of congenital abnormalities.

Uncontrolled maternal hypothyroidism may result in adverse neonatal outcomes (eg, premature birth, low birth weight, and respiratory distress) and adverse maternal outcomes (eg, spontaneous abortion, preeclampsia, stillbirth, and premature delivery). To prevent adverse events, normal maternal thyroid function should be maintained prior to conception and throughout pregnancy. Levothyroxine is considered the treatment of choice for the control of hypothyroidism during pregnancy. Due to alterations of endogenous maternal thyroid hormones, the levothyroxine dose may need to be increased during pregnancy and the dose usually needs to be decreased after delivery.

Lactation Enters breast milk/use caution

Breast-Feeding Considerations Endogenous thyroid hormones are minimally found in breast milk. The amount of endogenous thyroxine found in breast milk does not influence infant plasma thyroid values. Levothyroxine was not found to cause adverse events to the infant or mother during breast-feeding. Adequate thyroid hormone concentrations are required to maintain normal lactation. Appropriate levothyroxine doses should be continued during breast-feeding.

Dosage Forms

Capsule, soft gelatin, oral:

Tirosint®: 13 mcg, 25 mcg, 50 mcg, 75 mcg, 88 mcg, 100 mcg, 112 mcg, 125 mcg, 137 mcg, 150 mcg

Injection, powder for reconstitution: 100 mcg, 500 mcg

Tablet, oral: 25 mcg, 50 mcg, 75 mcg, 88 mcg, 100 mcg, 112 mcg, 125 mcg, 137 mcg, 150 mcg, 175 mcg, 200 mcg, 300 mcg

Levothroid®: 25 mcg, 50 mcg, 75 mcg, 88 mcg, 100 mcg, 112 mcg, 125 mcg, 137 mcg, 150 mcg, 175 mcg, 200 mcg, 300 mcg

Levoxyl®: 25 mcg, 50 mcg, 75 mcg, 88 mcg, 100 mcg, 112 mcg, 125 mcg, 137 mcg, 150 mcg, 175 mcg, 200 mcg

Synthroid®: 25 mcg, 50 mcg, 75 mcg, 88 mcg, 100 mcg, 112 mcg, 125 mcg, 137 mcg, 150 mcg, 175 mcg, 200 mcg, 300 mcg

Unithroid®: 25 mcg, 50 mcg, 75 mcg, 88 mcg, 100 mcg, 112 mcg, 125 mcg, 150 mcg, 175 mcg, 200 mcg, 300 mcg

Lidocaine (Systemic) (LYE doe kane)

Related Information

Oral Pain *on page 1558*

Recurrent Aphthous Stomatitis *on page 1618*

Brand Names: U.S. Xylocaine®; Xylocaine® Dental; Xylocaine® MPF

Brand Names: Canada Xylocard®

Generic Availability (U.S.) Yes

Pharmacologic Category Antiarrhythmic Agent, Class Ib; Local Anesthetic

Dental Use Amide-type injectable local anesthetic

Use Local and regional anesthesia by infiltration, nerve block, epidural, or spinal techniques; acute treatment of ventricular arrhythmias from myocardial infarction or cardiac manipulation (eg, cardiac surgery)

Note: The routine prophylactic use of lidocaine to prevent arrhythmia associated with fibrinolytic administration or to suppress isolated ventricular premature beats, couplets, runs of accelerated idioventricular rhythm, and nonsustained VT is not recommended (Antman, 2004).

Unlabeled Use

ACLS guidelines: Hemodynamically stable monomorphic ventricular tachycardia (VT) (preserved ventricular function); polymorphic VT (preserved ventricular function); drug-induced monomorphic VT; when amiodarone is not available, pulseless VT or ventricular fibrillation (VF) (unresponsive to defibrillation, CPR, and vasopressor administration)

PALS guidelines: When amiodarone is not available, pulseless VT or VF (unresponsive to defibrillation, CPR, and epinephrine administration); consider in patients with cocaine overdose to prevent arrhythmias secondary to MI

I.V. infusion for chronic pain syndrome

Local Anesthetic/Vasoconstrictor Precautions No information available to require special precautions

Effects on Dental Treatment Key adverse event(s) related to dental treatment: Metallic taste.

Effects on Bleeding No information available to require special precautions

Adverse Effects Effects vary with route of administration. Many effects are dose related.

Frequency not defined.

Cardiovascular: Arrhythmia, bradycardia, arterial spasms, cardiovascular collapse, defibrillator threshold increased, edema, flushing, heart block, hypotension, sinus node supression, vascular insufficiency (periarticular injections)

Central nervous system: Agitation, anxiety, apprehension, coma, confusion, disorientation, dizziness, drowsiness, euphoria, hallucinations, headache, hyperesthesia, hypoesthesia, lethargy, lightheadedness, nervousness, psychosis, seizure, slurred speech, somnolence, unconsciousness

Gastrointestinal: Metallic taste, nausea, vomiting

Local: Thrombophlebitis

Neuromuscular & skeletal: Paresthesia, transient radicular pain (subarachnoid administration; up to 1.9%), tremor, twitching, weakness

Otic: Tinnitus

Respiratory: Bronchospasm, dyspnea, respiratory depression or arrest

Miscellaneous: Allergic reactions, anaphylactic reaction, anaphylactoid reaction, sensitivity to temperature extremes

Following spinal anesthesia: Positional headache (3%), shivering (2%), double vision (<1%), cauda equina syndrome, hypotension, nausea, peripheral nerve symptoms, respiratory inadequacy

Dosage

Antiarrhythmic:

Children:

I.V., intraosseous (I.O.): **Note:** For use in VF or pulseless VT if amiodarone is not available; give after defibrillation attempts, CPR, and epinephrine:

Loading dose: 1 mg/kg (maximum: 100 mg); follow with continuous infusion; may administer second bolus of 0.5-1 mg/kg if delay between bolus and start of infusion is >15 minutes (PALS, 2000; PALS, 2010)

Continuous infusion: 20-50 mcg/kg/minute (PALS, 2010). Per the manufacturer, do not exceed 20 mcg/kg/minute in patients with shock, hepatic disease, cardiac arrest, or CHF.

Endotracheal: 2-3 mg/kg; flush with 5 mL of NS and follow with 5 assisted manual ventilations (PALS, 2010)

Adults (ACLS, 2010):

VF or pulseless VT (after defibrillation attempts, CPR, and vasopressor administration) if amiodarone is not available: I.V., intraosseous (I.O.): Initial: 1-1.5 mg/kg. If refractory VF or pulseless VT, repeat with 0.5-0.75 mg/kg bolus every 5-10 minutes (maximum cumulative dose: 3 mg/kg). Follow with continuous infusion (1-4 mg/minute) after return of perfusion. Reappearance of arrhythmia during constant infusion: 0.5 mg/kg bolus and reassessment of infusion (Zipes, 2000).

Endotracheal (loading dose only): 2-3.75 mg/kg (2-2.5 times the recommended I.V. dose); dilute in 5-10 mL NS or sterile water. **Note:** Absorption is greater with sterile water and results in less impairment of PaO_2.

Hemodynamically stable monomorphic VT: I.V.: 1-1.5 mg/kg; repeat with 0.5-0.75 mg/kg every 5-10 minutes as necessary (maximum cumulative dose: 3 mg/kg). Follow with continuous infusion of 1-4 mg/minute (or 14-57 mcg/kg/minute).

Note: Reduce maintenance infusion in patients with CHF, shock, or hepatic disease; initiate infusion at 10 mcg/kg/minute (maximum dose: 1.5 mg/minute or 20 mcg/kg/minute).

Anesthetic, local injectable: Children and Adults: Varies with procedure, degree of anesthesia needed, vascularity of tissue, duration of anesthesia required, and physical condition of patient; maximum: 4.5 mg/kg/dose not to exceed 300 mg; do not repeat within 2 hours.

Dosage adjustment in renal impairment: No dosage adjustment provided in manufacturer's labeling. However, accumulation of metabolites may be increased in renal dysfunction. Not dialyzable (0% to 5%) by hemo- or peritoneal dialysis; supplemental dose is not necessary.

Dosage adjustment in hepatic impairment: Use with caution; reduce maintenance infusion. Initial: 0.75 mg/minute or 10 mcg/kg/minute; maximum dose: 1.5 mg/minute or 20 mcg/kg/minute. Monitor lidocaine concentrations closely and adjust infusion rate as necessary; consider alternative therapy.

Mechanism of Action Class Ib antiarrhythmic; suppresses automaticity of conduction tissue, by increasing electrical stimulation threshold of ventricle, His-Purkinje system, and spontaneous depolarization of the ventricles during diastole by a direct action on the tissues; blocks both the initiation and conduction of nerve impulses by decreasing the neuronal membrane's permeability to sodium ions, which results in inhibition of depolarization with resultant blockade of conduction

Contraindications Hypersensitivity to lidocaine or any component of the formulation; hypersensitivity to another local anesthetic of the amide type; Adam-Stokes syndrome; Wolff-Parkinson-White syndrome; severe degrees of SA, AV, or intraventricular heart block (except in patients with a functioning artificial pacemaker); premixed injection may contain corn-derived dextrose and its use is contraindicated in patients with allergy to corn or corn-related products

Warnings/Precautions Use caution in patients with severe hepatic dysfunction or pseudocholinesterase deficiency; may have increased risk of lidocaine toxicity.

Intravenous: Constant ECG monitoring is necessary during I.V. administration. Use cautiously in hepatic impairment, HF, marked hypoxia, severe respiratory depression, hypovolemia, history of malignant hyperthermia, or shock. Increased ventricular rate may be seen when administered to a patient with atrial fibrillation. Correct electrolyte disturbances, especially hypokalemia or hypomagnesemia, prior to use and throughout therapy. Use is contraindicated in patients with Wolff-Parkinson-White syndrome and severe degrees of SA, AV, or intraventricular heart block (except in patients with a functioning artificial pacemaker). Correct any underlying causes of ventricular arrhythmias. Monitor closely for signs and symptoms of CNS toxicity. The elderly may be prone to increased CNS and cardiovascular side effects. Reduce dose in hepatic dysfunction and CHF.

Injectable anesthetic: Follow appropriate administration techniques so as not to administer any intravascularly. Continuous intra-articular infusion of local anesthetics after arthroscopic or other surgical procedures is **not** an approved use; chondrolysis (primarily in the shoulder joint) has occurred following infusion, with some cases requiring arthroplasty or shoulder replacement. Solutions containing antimicrobial preservatives should not be used for epidural or spinal anesthesia. Some solutions contain a bisulfite; avoid in patients who are allergic to bisulfite. Resuscitative equipment, medicine and oxygen should be available in case of emergency. Use products containing epinephrine cautiously in patients with significant vascular disease, compromised blood flow, or during or following general anesthesia (increased risk of arrhythmias). Adjust the dose for the elderly, pediatric, acutely ill, and debilitated patients.

Drug Interactions

Metabolism/Transport Effects Substrate of CYP1A2 (major), CYP2A6 (minor), CYP2B6 (minor), CYP2C9 (minor), CYP3A4 (major); **Note:** Assignment of Major/Minor substrate status based on clinically relevant drug interaction potential; **Inhibits** CYP1A2 (weak)

Avoid Concomitant Use

Avoid concomitant use of Lidocaine (Systemic) with any of the following: Conivaptan; Saquinavir

Increased Effect/Toxicity

Lidocaine (Systemic) may increase the levels/effects of: Prilocaine

The levels/effects of Lidocaine (Systemic) may be increased by: Abiraterone Acetate; Amiodarone; Beta-Blockers; Conivaptan; CYP1A2 Inhibitors (Moderate); CYP1A2 Inhibitors (Strong); CYP3A4 Inhibitors

(Moderate); CYP3A4 Inhibitors (Strong); Darunavir; Dasatinib; Deferasirox; Disopyramide; Hyaluronidase; Ivacaftor; Mifepristone; Saquinavir; Telaprevir

Decreased Effect

The levels/effects of Lidocaine (Systemic) may be decreased by: CYP1A2 Inducers (Strong); CYP3A4 Inducers (Strong); Cyproterone; Deferasirox; Etravirine; Herbs (CYP3A4 Inducers); Tocilizumab

Ethanol/Nutrition/Herb Interactions Herb/Nutraceutical: St John's wort may decrease lidocaine levels; avoid concurrent use.

Dietary Considerations Premixed injection may contain corn-derived dextrose and its use is contraindicated in patients with allergy to corn-related products.

Pharmacodynamics/Kinetics

Onset of Action Single bolus dose: 45-90 seconds

Duration of Action 10-20 minutes

Half-life Elimination Biphasic: Prolonged with congestive heart failure, liver disease, shock, severe renal disease; Initial: 7-30 minutes; Terminal: Infants, premature: 3.2 hours, Adults: 1.5-2 hours

Pregnancy Risk Factor B

Pregnancy Considerations Animal studies with lidocaine have not shown teratogenic effects. Lidocaine and the MEGX metabolite cross the placenta. Use is not contraindicated during labor and delivery. Topical lidocaine is used locally to provide analgesia prior to episiotomy and during repair of obstetric lacerations. Administration by the perineal route may result in greater absorption than administration by the epidural route. Adverse events have been reported in the infant following maternal administration, however, when used in appropriate doses, the risk to the fetus is low. Cumulative exposure from all routes of administration should be considered.

Lactation Enters breast milk/use caution (AAP rates "compatible"; AAP 2001 update pending)

Breast-Feeding Considerations Small amounts of lidocaine and the MEGX metabolite are found in breast milk. The actual amount may depend on route and duration of administration. When administered topically at recommended doses, the amount of lidocaine available to the nursing infant would not be expected to cause adverse events. Cumulative exposure from all routes of administration should be considered.

Dosage Forms

Infusion, premixed in D_5W: 0.4% [4 mg/mL] (250 mL, 500 mL); 0.8% [8 mg/mL] (250 mL)

Injection, solution: 1% [10 mg/mL] (2 mL, 10 mL, 20 mL, 30 mL, 50 mL); 2% [20 mg/mL] (2 mL, 5 mL, 20 mL, 50 mL)

Xylocaine®: 0.5% [5 mg/mL] (50 mL); 1% [10 mg/mL] (10 mL, 20 mL, 50 mL); 2% [20 mg/mL] (10 mL, 20 mL, 50 mL)

Xylocaine® Dental: 2% [20 mg/mL] (1.8 mL)

Injection, solution [preservative free]: 0.5% [5 mg/mL] (50 mL); 1% [10 mg/mL] (2 mL, 5 mL, 30 mL); 1.5% [15 mg/mL] (20 mL); 2% [20 mg/mL] (2 mL, 5 mL, 10 mL); 4% [40 mg/mL] (5 mL)

Xylocaine®: 2% [20 mg/mL] (5 mL)

Xylocaine® MPF: 0.5% [5 mg/mL] (50 mL); 1% [10 mg/mL] (2 mL, 5 mL, 10 mL, 30 mL); 1.5% [15 mg/mL] (10 mL, 20 mL); 2% [20 mg/mL] (2 mL, 5 mL, 10 mL); 4% [40 mg/mL] (5 mL)

Injection, solution, premixed in $D_{7.5}W$ [preservative free]: 5% [50 mg/mL] (2 mL)

References

Moore PA and Hersh EV, "Local Anesthetics: Pharmacology and Toxicity," *Dent Clin North Am*, 2010, 54(4):587-99.

Lidocaine (Topical) (LYE doe kane)

Related Information

Management of Patients Undergoing Cancer Therapy *on page 1596*

Viral Infections *on page 1575*

Brand Names: U.S. AneCream® [OTC]; Anestafoam™ [OTC] [DSC]; Band-Aid® Hurt Free™ Antiseptic Wash [OTC]; Burn Jel Plus [OTC]; Burn Jel® [OTC]; L-M-X® 4 [OTC]; L-M-X® 5 [OTC]; LidaMantle® [DSC]; Lidoderm®; LidoPatch™ [OTC]; LTA® 360; Premjact®; RectiCare™ [OTC]; Regenecare®; Regenecare® HA [OTC]; Solarcaine® cool aloe Burn Relief [OTC]; Topicaine® [OTC]; Unburn® [OTC]; Xylocaine®

Brand Names: Canada Betacaine®; Lidodan™; Lidoderm®; Maxilene®; Xylocaine®

Generic Availability (U.S.) Yes: Hydrochloride cream, jelly, ointment, solution

Pharmacologic Category Analgesic, Topical; Local Anesthetic

Dental Use Topical local anesthetic

Patch: Production of mild topical anesthesia of accessible mucous membranes of the mouth prior to superficial dental procedures

Oral topical solution (viscous): Reduce gagging during dental impressions and x-rays

Use

Rectal: Temporary relief of pain and itching due to anorectal disorders

Topical: Local anesthetic for oral mucous membrane; use in laser/cosmetic surgeries; minor burns, cuts, and abrasions of the skin

Oral topical solution (viscous): Topical anesthesia of irritated oral mucous membranes and pharyngeal tissue

Patch (Lidoderm®): Relief of allodynia (painful hypersensitivity) and chronic pain in postherpetic neuralgia

Patch (LidoPatch™): Temporary relief of localized pain

Local Anesthetic/Vasoconstrictor Precautions No information available to require special precautions

Effects on Dental Treatment Key adverse event(s) related to dental treatment: Metallic taste.

Effects on Bleeding No information available to require special precautions

Adverse Effects Frequency not defined. **Note:** Adverse effects vary with formulation and extent of systemic absorption; children may be at increased risk.

Cardiovascular: Cyanosis, tachycardia

Central nervous system: Anxiety, confusion, dizziness, lethargy, lightheadedness, somnolence

Dermatologic: Angioedema, bruising (topical patch), contact dermatitis, depigmentation (topical patch), edema of the skin, itching, petechia (topical patch), pruritus, rash, urticaria

Hematologic: Methemoglobinemia

Local: Irritation (topical patch)

Neuromuscular & skeletal: Pain exacerbation (topical patch), paresthesia, weakness

Respiratory: Hypoxia

Dental Usual Dosage Anesthesia, topical:

Postherpetic neuralgia: Adults: Patch: Apply patch to most painful area. Up to 3 patches may be applied in a single application. Patch may remain in place for up to 12 hours in any 24-hour period.

Dosage Anesthesia, topical:

Cream:

LidaMantle®: Skin irritation: Children and Adults: Apply a thin film to affected area 2-3 times/day as needed

L-M-X® 4: Skin irritation: Children ≥2 years and Adults: Apply up to 3-4 times daily to intact skin

L-M-X® 5: Relief of anorectal pain and itching: Children ≥12 years and Adults: Apply to affected area up to 6 times/day

Gel, ointment: Adults: Apply to affected area ≤4 times/day as needed (maximum dose: 4.5 mg/kg, not to exceed 300 mg)

Topical solution: Adults: Apply 1-5 mL (40-200 mg) to affected area

Jelly:

Children: Dose varies with age and weight (maximum dose: 4.5 mg/kg)

Adults (maximum dose: 30 mL [600 mg] in any 12-hour period):

Anesthesia of male urethra: 5-30 mL (100-600 mg)

Anesthesia of female urethra: 3-5 mL (60-100 mg)

Oral topical solution (viscous):

Infants and Children <3 years: 1.25 mL applied to area with a cotton-tipped applicator no more frequently than every 3 hours (maximum: 4 doses per 12-hour period)

Children ≥3 years: Should not exceed 4.5 mg/kg/dose (or 300 mg/dose); swished in the mouth and spit out no more frequently than every 3 hours (maximum: 4 doses per 12-hour period)

Adults:

Anesthesia of the mouth: 15 mL swished in the mouth and spit out no more frequently than every 3 hours (maximum: 8 doses per 24-hour period)

Anesthesia of the pharynx: 15 mL gargled no more frequently than every 3 hours (maximum: 8 doses per 24-hour period); may be swallowed

Patch: Adults:

Lidoderm®: Postherpetic neuralgia: Apply patch to most painful area. Up to 3 patches may be applied in a single application. Patch(es) may remain in place for up to 12 hours in any 24-hour period.

LidoPatch™: Pain (localized): Apply patch to painful area. Patch may remain in place for up to 12 hours in any 24-hour period. No more than 1 patch should be used in a 24-hour period.

Mechanism of Action Blocks both the initiation and conduction of nerve impulses by decreasing the neuronal membrane's permeability to sodium ions, which results in inhibition of depolarization with resultant blockade of conduction

Contraindications Hypersensitivity to lidocaine or any component of the formulation; hypersensitivity to another local anesthetic of the amide type

Warnings/Precautions Potentially life-threatening side effects (eg, irregular heart beat, seizures, coma, respiratory depression, death) have occurred when used prior to cosmetic procedures. Excessive dosing (application to large areas, application to denuded skin, or wearing of device for longer than recommended) may lead to increased absorption and systemic toxicity. Application to broken or inflamed skin may lead to increased systemic absorption; use caution. Use caution in patients with severe hepatic disease due to diminished ability to metabolize systemically-absorbed lidocaine.

When topical anesthetics are used prior to cosmetic or medical procedures, the lowest amount of anesthetic necessary for pain relief should be applied. High systemic levels and toxic effects (eg, methemoglobinemia, irregular heart beats, respiratory depression, seizures, death) have been reported in patients who (without supervision of a trained professional) have applied topical anesthetics in large amounts (or to large areas of the skin), left these products on for prolonged periods of time, or have used wraps/dressings to cover the skin following application.

Topical cream, liquid, gel, and ointment: Do not leave on large body areas for >2 hours. Not for ophthalmic use. Some products are not recommended for use on mucous membranes; consult specific product labeling.

Topical patch: To avoid accidental ingestion by children, store and dispose of products out of the reach of children.

Drug Interactions

Metabolism/Transport Effects Substrate of CYP1A2 (major), CYP2A6 (minor), CYP2B6 (minor), CYP2C9 (minor), CYP3A4 (major); **Note:** Assignment of Major/Minor substrate status based on clinically relevant drug interaction potential; **Inhibits** CYP1A2 (weak)

Avoid Concomitant Use

Avoid concomitant use of Lidocaine (Topical) with any of the following: Conivaptan

Increased Effect/Toxicity

Lidocaine (Topical) may increase the levels/effects of: Antiarrhythmic Agents (Class III); Prilocaine

The levels/effects of Lidocaine (Topical) may be increased by: Abiraterone Acetate; Antiarrhythmic Agents (Class III); Beta-Blockers; Conivaptan; CYP1A2 Inhibitors (Moderate); CYP1A2 Inhibitors (Strong); CYP3A4 Inhibitors (Moderate); CYP3A4 Inhibitors (Strong); Darunavir; Dasatinib; Deferasirox; Disopyramide; Ivacaftor; Mifepristone

Decreased Effect

The levels/effects of Lidocaine (Topical) may be decreased by: CYP1A2 Inducers (Strong); CYP3A4 Inducers (Strong); Cyproterone; Deferasirox; Herbs (CYP3A4 Inducers); Tocilizumab

Pharmacodynamics/Kinetics

Onset of Action Transdermal: ~4 hours

Time to Peak Transdermal (5%): 11 hours (following application of 3 patches)

Pregnancy Risk Factor B

Pregnancy Considerations Animal studies with systemic lidocaine have not shown teratogenic effects. Lidocaine and the MEGX metabolite cross the placenta. Topical lidocaine is used locally to provide analgesia prior to episiotomy and during repair of obstetric lacerations. Cumulative exposure from all routes of administration should be considered.

Lactation Enters breast milk/use caution (AAP rates "compatible"; AAP 2001 update pending)

Breast-Feeding Considerations When administered topically at recommended doses, the amount of lidocaine available to the nursing infant would not be expected to cause adverse events. Cumulative exposure from all routes of administration should be considered.

Dosage Forms

Aerosol, spray, topical:
Solarcaine® cool aloe Burn Relief [OTC]: 0.5% (127 g)

Cream, rectal:
L-M-X® 5 [OTC]: 5% (15 g, 30 g)

Cream, topical: 0.5% (0.9 g)
AneCream® [OTC]: 4% (5 g, 15 g, 30 g)
L-M-X® 4 [OTC]: 4% (5 g, 15 g, 30 g)
RectiCare™ [OTC]: 5% (30 g)

Gel, topical:
Burn Jel Plus [OTC]: 2.5% (118 mL)
Burn Jel® [OTC]: 2% (59 mL, 118 mL); 2% (3.5 g)
Regenecare®: 2% (14 g, 85 g)
Regenecare® HA [OTC]: 2% (85 g)
Solarcaine® cool aloe Burn Relief [OTC]: 0.5% (113 g, 226 g)
Topicaine® [OTC]: 4% (10 g, 30 g, 113 g); 5% (10 g, 30 g, 113 g)
Unburn® [OTC]: 2.5% (59 mL)

Jelly, topical: 2% (5 mL, 30 mL)

Jelly, topical [preservative free]: 2% (5 mL, 10 mL, 20 mL)

Ointment, topical: 5% (30 g, 35.4 g, 50 g)

Patch, topical:
Lidoderm®: 5% (30s)
LidoPatch™ [OTC]: 3.99% (3s)

Solution, topical: 4% [40 mg/mL] (50 mL)
Band-Aid® Hurt Free™ Antiseptic Wash [OTC]: 2% [20 mg/mL] (177 mL)
LTA® 360: 4% [40 mg/mL] (4 mL)
Premjact®: 9.6% (13 mL)
Xylocaine®: 4% [40 mg/mL] (50 mL)

Solution, topical [preservative free]: 4% [40 mg/mL] (4 mL)

Solution, viscous, oral topical: 2% [20 mg/mL] (20 mL, 100 mL, 500 mL)

Lidocaine and Epinephrine
(LYE doe kane & ep i NEF rin)

Related Information
EPINEPHrine (Systemic, Oral Inhalation) on page 482
Lidocaine (Systemic) on page 816
Oral Pain on page 1558

Brand Names: U.S. Lignospan® Forte; Lignospan® Standard; Xylocaine® MPF With Epinephrine; Xylocaine® With Epinephrine

Brand Names: Canada Xylocaine® With Epinephrine

Generic Availability (U.S.) Yes

Pharmacologic Category Local Anesthetic

Dental Use Amide-type anesthetic used for local infiltration anesthesia injection near nerve trunks to produce nerve block

Use Local infiltration anesthesia; AVS for nerve block

Local Anesthetic/Vasoconstrictor Precautions No information available to require special precautions

Effects on Dental Treatment It is common to misinterpret psychogenic responses to local anesthetic injection as an allergic reaction. Intraoral injections are perceived by many patients as a stressful procedure in dentistry. Common symptoms to this stress are diaphoresis, palpitations, hyperventilation. Patients may exhibit hypersensitivity to bisulfites contained in local anesthetic solution to prevent oxidation of epinephrine. In general, patients reacting to bisulfites have a history of asthma and their airways are hyper-reactive to asthmatic syndrome.

Degree of adverse effects in the CNS and cardiovascular system is directly related to the blood levels of lidocaine: Bradycardia, hypersensitivity reactions (rare; may be manifest as dermatologic reactions and edema at injection site), asthmatic syndromes

High blood levels: Anxiety, restlessness, disorientation, confusion, dizziness, tremors, seizures, CNS depression (resulting in somnolence, unconsciousness and possible respiratory arrest), nausea, and vomiting.

Effects on Bleeding No information available to require special precautions

Adverse Effects Degree of adverse effects in the central nervous system and cardiovascular system are directly related to the blood levels of lidocaine. The effects below are more likely to occur after systemic administration rather than infiltration.

Cardiovascular: Myocardial effects include a decrease in contraction force as well as a decrease in electrical excitability and myocardial conduction rate resulting in bradycardia and reduction in cardiac output.

Central nervous system: High blood levels result in anxiety, restlessness, disorientation, confusion, dizziness, tremor, and seizure. This is followed by depression of CNS resulting in somnolence, unconsciousness and possible respiratory arrest. In some cases, symptoms of CNS stimulation may be absent and the primary CNS effects are somnolence and unconsciousness.

Gastrointestinal: Nausea and vomiting may occur

Hypersensitivity reactions: Extremely rare, but may be manifest as dermatologic reactions and edema at injection site. Asthmatic syndromes have occurred. Patients may exhibit hypersensitivity to bisulfites contained in local anesthetic solution to prevent oxidation of epinephrine. In general, patients reacting to bisulfites have a history of asthma and their airways are hyper-reactive to asthmatic syndrome.

Psychogenic reactions: It is common to misinterpret psychogenic responses to local anesthetic injection as an allergic reaction. Intraoral injections are perceived by many patients as a stressful procedure in dentistry. Common symptoms to this stress are diaphoresis, palpitation, hyperventilation, generalized pallor and a fainting feeling

Dental Usual Dosage Dosage varies with the anesthetic procedure, degree of anesthesia needed, vascularity of tissue, duration of anesthesia required, and physical condition of patient.

Dental anesthesia, infiltration, or conduction block:
Children <12 years: 20-30 mg (1-1.5 mL) of lidocaine hydrochloride as a 2% solution with epinephrine 1:100,000; maximum: 4.5 mg of lidocaine hydrochloride/kg of body weight or 100-150 mg as a single dose

Children ≥12 years and Adults: Do not exceed 7 mg/kg body weight or 300 mg of lidocaine hydrochloride and 3 mcg (0.003 mg) of epinephrine/kg of body weight or 0.2 mg epinephrine per dental appointment. The effective anesthetic dose varies with procedure, intensity of anesthesia needed, duration of anesthesia required, and physical condition of the patient. Always use the lowest effective dose along with careful aspiration.

The following numbers of dental carpules (1.7 mL or 1.8 mL) provide the indicated amounts of lidocaine hydrochloride 2% and epinephrine 1:100,000 (see table):

# of Cartridges (1.7 mL or 1.8 mL)	Lidocaine HCl (2%) (mg)		Epinephrine 1:100,000 (mg)	
	(1.7 mL cartridge)	(1.8 mL cartridge)	(1.7 mL cartridge)	(1.8 mL cartridge)
1	34	36	0.017	0.018
2	68	72	0.034	0.036
3	102	108	0.051	0.054
4	136	144	0.068	0.072
5	170	180	0.085	0.090
6	204	216	0.102	0.108
7	238	252	0.119	0.126
8	272	288	0.136	0.144
9	306	324	0.153	0.162
10	340	360	0.170	0.180

For most routine dental procedures, lidocaine hydrochloride 2% with epinephrine 1:100,000 is preferred. When a more pronounced hemostasis is required, a 1:50,000 epinephrine concentration should be used. The following numbers of dental cartridges (1.7 mL or 1.8 mL) provide the indicated amounts of lidocaine hydrochloride 2% and epinephrine 1:50,000.

# of Cartridges (1.7 mL or 1.8 mL)	Lidocaine HCl (2%) (mg)		Epinephrine 1:50,000 (mg)	
	(1.7 mL cartridge)	(1.8 mL cartridge)	(1.7 mL cartridge)	(1.8 mL cartridge)
1	34	36	0.034	0.036
2	68	72	0.068	0.072
3	102	108	0.102	0.108
4	136	144	0.136	0.144
5	170	180	0.170	0.180
6	204	216	0.204	0.216

Dosage Dosage varies with the anesthetic procedure, degree of anesthesia needed, vascularity of tissue, duration of anesthesia required, and physical condition of patient.

Dental anesthesia, infiltration, or conduction block:
Children <12 years: 20-30 mg (1-1.5 mL) of lidocaine hydrochloride as a 2% solution with epinephrine 1:100,000; maximum: 4.5 mg of lidocaine hydrochloride/kg of body weight or 100-150 mg as a single dose
Children ≥12 years and Adults: Do not exceed 7 mg/kg body weight up to a maximum range of 300 mg (usual dental practice) to 500 mg (approved product labeling) of lidocaine hydrochloride and 3 mcg (0.003 mg) of epinephrine/kg of body weight or 0.2 mg epinephrine per dental appointment. The effective anesthetic dose varies with procedure, intensity of anesthesia needed, duration of anesthesia required, and physical condition of the patient. Always use the lowest effective dose along with careful aspiration.
Note: For most routine dental procedures, lidocaine hydrochloride 2% with epinephrine 1:100,000 is preferred. When a more pronounced hemostasis is required, a 1:50,000 epinephrine concentration should be used.

Dosage adjustment in renal impairment: No dosage adjustment provided in manufacturer's labeling. However, accumulation of metabolites may be increased in renal dysfunction.

Dosage adjustment in hepatic impairment: No dosage adjustment provided in manufacturer's labeling; use with caution.

Mechanism of Action Lidocaine blocks both the initiation and conduction of nerve impulses via decreased permeability of sodium ions; epinephrine increases the duration of action of lidocaine by causing vasoconstriction (via alpha effects) which slows the vascular absorption of lidocaine

Contraindications Hypersensitivity to lidocaine, epinephrine, or any component of the formulation; hypersensitivity to other local anesthetics of the amide type; myasthenia gravis; shock; cardiac conduction disease; angle-closure glaucoma

Warnings/Precautions Aspirate the syringe (injection solution for infiltration formulation) after tissue penetration and before injection to minimize chance of direct vascular injection. Use caution in endocrine, hepatic, or thyroid disease. Use with caution in the elderly, debilitated, acutely ill and pediatric patients. Avoid use in presence of flammable anesthetics. Avoid in patients with uncontrolled hyperthyroidism. Use minimal amounts in patients with significant cardiovascular problems (because of epinephrine component). Careful and constant monitoring of the patient's state of consciousness should be done following each local anesthetic injection; at such times, restlessness, anxiety, tinnitus, dizziness, blurred vision, tremors, depression, or drowsiness may be early warning signs of CNS toxicity. Treatment is primarily symptomatic and supportive. Continuous intra-articular infusion of local anesthetics after arthroscopic or other surgical procedures is **not** an approved use; chondrolysis (primarily in the shoulder joint) has occurred following infusion, with some cases requiring arthroplasty or shoulder replacement. Local anesthetics have been associated with rare occurrences of sudden respiratory arrest, seizures, and cardiac arrest. May contain sodium metabisulfite; use caution in patients with a sulfite allergy. Dental practitioners and/or clinicians using local anesthetic agents should be well trained in diagnosis and management of emergencies that may arise from the use of these agents. Resuscitative equipment, oxygen, and other resuscitative drugs should be available for immediate use.

Drug Interactions

Metabolism/Transport Effects Refer to individual components.

Avoid Concomitant Use

Avoid concomitant use of Lidocaine and Epinephrine with any of the following: Ergot Derivatives; Iobenguane I 123; Lurasidone

Increased Effect/Toxicity

Lidocaine and Epinephrine may increase the levels/ effects of: Bromocriptine; Lurasidone; Sympathomimetics

The levels/effects of Lidocaine and Epinephrine may be increased by: Antacids; AtoMOXetine; Beta-Blockers; Cannabinoids; Carbonic Anhydrase Inhibitors; COMT Inhibitors; Ergot Derivatives; Hyaluronidase; Inhalational Anesthetics; MAO Inhibitors; Serotonin/ Norepinephrine Reuptake Inhibitors; Tricyclic Antidepressants

◀

Decreased Effect

Lidocaine and Epinephrine may decrease the levels/ effects of: Benzylpenicilloyl Polylysine; Iobenguane I 123

The levels/effects of Lidocaine and Epinephrine may be decreased by: Alpha1-Blockers; Promethazine; Spironolactone

Pharmacodynamics/Kinetics

Onset of Action Peak effect: ~5 minutes

Duration of Action Dose and anesthetic procedure dependent: ~2 hours

Pregnancy Risk Factor B

Pregnancy Considerations See individual agents.

Lactation Lidocaine enters breast milk/use caution

Breast-Feeding Considerations Refer to Lidocaine (Systemic, Oral Inhalation) and Epinephrine (Systemic) monographs.

Dosage Forms

Injection, solution:

Generics:

0.5% / 1:200,000: Lidocaine hydrochloride 0.5% [5 mg/mL] and epinephrine 1:200,000 (50 mL)

1% / 1:100,000: Lidocaine hydrochloride 1% [10 mg/mL] and epinephrine 1:100,000 (20 mL, 30 mL, 50 mL)

2% / 1:100,000: Lidocaine hydrochloride 2% [20 mg/mL] and epinephrine 1:100,000 (30 mL, 50 mL)

Brands:

Xylocaine® with Epinephrine:

0.5% / 1:200,000: Lidocaine hydrochloride 0.5% [5 mg/mL] and epinephrine 1:200,000 (50 mL)

1% / 1:100,000: Lidocaine hydrochloride 1% [10 mg/mL] and epinephrine 1:100,000 (10 mL, 20 mL, 50 mL)

2% / 1:100,000: Lidocaine hydrochloride 2% [20 mg/mL] and epinephrine 1:100,000 (10 mL, 20 mL, 50 mL)

Injection, solution [preservative free]:

Generics:

1.5% / 1:200,000: Lidocaine hydrochloride 1.5% [15 mg/mL] and epinephrine 1:200,000 (5 mL, 30 mL)

2% / 1:200,000: Lidocaine hydrochloride 2% [20 mg/mL] and epinephrine 1:200,000 (20 mL)

Brands:

Xylocaine®-MPF with Epinephrine:

1% / 1:200,000: Lidocaine hydrochloride 1% [10 mg/mL] and epinephrine 1:200,000 (5 mL, 10 mL, 30 mL)

1.5% / 1:200,000: Lidocaine hydrochloride 1.5% [15 mg/mL] and epinephrine 1:200,000 (5 mL, 10 mL, 30 mL)

2% / 1:200,000: Lidocaine hydrochloride 2% [20 mg/mL] and epinephrine 1:200,000 (5 mL, 10 mL, 20 mL)

Injection, solution [for dental use]:

Generics:

2% / 1:50,000: Lidocaine hydrochloride 2% [20 mg/mL] and epinephrine 1:50,000 (1.7 mL, 1.8 mL)

2% / 1:100,000: Lidocaine hydrochloride 2% [20 mg/mL] and epinephrine 1:100,000 (1.7 mL, 1.8 mL)

Brands:

Lignospan® Forte: 2% / 1:50,000: Lidocaine hydrochloride 2% [20 mg/mL] and epinephrine 1:50,000 (1.7 mL)

Lignospan® Standard: 2% / 1:100,000: Lidocaine hydrochloride 2% [20 mg/mL] and epinephrine 1:100,000 (1.7 mL)

Dental Comment Oral paresthesia: The occurrence of oral paresthesia associated with 4% solutions of prilocaine or articaine, although rare, continue to be slightly more frequent than other local anesthetics. From 1999-2008, there were 182 cases of nonsurgical paresthesia (Gaffen, 2009). Of the cases, 172 involved mandibular block injection only. Another eight cases involved mandibular block combined with at least one other type of anesthetic injection. A single case involved infiltration around tooth number 35 and the final case involved infiltration and intraligamentary injection in the maxillary anterior region.

A 2010 report, reviewed adverse events submitted voluntarily over a 10-year period involving the dental local anesthetics articaine, bupivacaine, lidocaine, mepivacaine, and prilocaine in the United States. Lidocaine reported incidence: One case per 181,076,673 cartridges sold. The reported incidence of paresthesia was one case for 13,800,970 cartridges of all local anesthetics sold in the U.S. (Garisto, 2010).

References

Dower JS Jr, "A Review of Paresthesia in Association With Administration of Local Anesthesia," *Dent Today*, 2003, 22(2):64-9.

Finder RL and Moore PA, "Adverse Drug Reactions to Local Anesthesia," *Dent Clin North Am*, 2002, 46(4):747-57, x.

Gaffen AS and Haas DA, "Retrospective Review of Voluntary Reports of Nonsurgical Paresthesia in Dentistry," *J Can Dent Assoc*, 2009, 75(8):579.

Garisto GA, Gaffen AS, Lawrence HP, et al, "Occurrence of Paresthesia After Dental Local Anesthetic Administration in the United States," *J Am Dent Assoc*, 2010, 141(7):836-44.

Haas DA, "An Update on Local Anesthetics in Dentistry," *J Can Dent Assoc*, 2002, 68(9):546-51.

Jastak JT and Yagiela JA, "Vasoconstrictors and Local Anesthesia: A Review and Rationale for Use," *J Am Dent Assoc*, 1983, 107(4):623-30.

Nusstein J, Reader A, and Beck FM, "Anesthetic Efficacy of Different Volumes of Lidocaine With Epinephrine for Inferior Alveolar Nerve Blocks," *Gen Dent*, 2002, 50(4):372-5.

Wynn RL, "Epinephrine Interactions With Beta-Blockers," *Gen Dent*, 1994, 42(1):16, 18.

Lidocaine and Hydrocortisone

(LYE doe kane & hye droe KOR ti sone)

Related Information

Hydrocortisone (Topical) *on page 699*

Lidocaine (Topical) *on page 818*

Brand Names: U.S. AnaMantle HC® Cream; AnaMantle HC® Forte; AnaMantle HC® Gel; LidaMantle HC®; LidaMantle HC® Relief Pad™; LidoCort™; Peranex™ HC; Peranex™ HC Medi-Pad; RectaGel™ HC

Pharmacologic Category Anesthetic/Corticosteroid

Use Topical anti-inflammatory and anesthetic for skin disorders; rectal for the treatment of hemorrhoids, anal fissures, pruritus ani, or similar conditions

Local Anesthetic/Vasoconstrictor Precautions No information available to require special precautions

Effects on Dental Treatment No significant effects or complications reported

Effects on Bleeding No information available to require special precautions

General Dosage Range

Rectal: *Adults:* 1 applicatorful twice daily

Topical: *Adults:* Apply 2-3 times/day

Pregnancy Risk Factor C

Pregnancy Considerations See individual agents.

Lidocaine and Prilocaine
(LYE doe kane & PRIL oh kane)

Related Information
Lidocaine (Topical) *on page 818*
Prilocaine *on page 1139*
Brand Names: U.S. EMLA®; Oraqix®
Brand Names: Canada EMLA®
Generic Availability (U.S.) Yes: Cream
Pharmacologic Category Local Anesthetic
Dental Use
Periodontal gel (Oraqix®): Use in adults who require localized anesthesia in periodontal pockets during scaling and/or root planning.
Topical: Amide-type topical anesthetic for use on normal intact skin to provide local analgesia for minor procedures such as I.V. cannulation or venipuncture
Use
Topical anesthetic for use on normal intact skin to provide local analgesia for minor procedures such as I.V. cannulation or venipuncture; has also been used for painful procedures such as lumbar puncture and skin graft harvesting; for superficial minor surgery of genital mucous membranes and as an adjunct for local infiltration anesthesia in genital mucous membranes.
Periodontal gel: Topical anesthetic for use in periodontal pockets during scaling or root planning procedures
Local Anesthetic/Vasoconstrictor Precautions No information available to require special precautions
Effects on Dental Treatment Key adverse event(s) related to dental treatment: Application site reactions in the oral cavity in 52/391 patients (13%) included pain, soreness, irritation, numbness, ulcerations, vesicles, edema, abscess and/or redness in the treated area. The 13% represented adverse effects occurring in more than one patient. Each patient was counted only once per adverse event. Taste perversion also reported (2%) including complaints of bad or bitter taste for up to 4 hours after administration.
Effects on Bleeding No information available to require special precautions
Adverse Effects
Cream/patch: Frequency not defined.
Cardiovascular: Angioedema, hypotension
Central nervous system: Shock
Dermatologic: Burning, erythema, hyperpigmentation, itching, rash, urticaria
Genitourinary: Blistering of foreskin (rare)
Local: Burning, edema, stinging
Respiratory: Bronchospasm
Miscellaneous: Alteration in temperature sensation, hypersensitivity reactions

Periodontal gel:
>10%: Local: Application site reaction (1%, includes abscess, edema, irritation, numbness, pain, ulceration, vesicles)
1% to 10%:
Central nervous system: Fatigue (1%)
Gastrointestinal: Bitter taste (2%), nausea (1%)
Respiratory: Infection (1%)
Miscellaneous: Flu-like syndrome (1%), allergic reactions
Dental Usual Dosage Oraqix®: Gel: Apply on gingival margin around selected teeth using the blunt-tipped applicator included in package. Wait 30 seconds, then fill the periodontal pockets using the blunt-tipped applicator until gel becomes visible at the gingival margin. Wait another 30 seconds before starting treatment.

Maximum recommended dose: One treatment session: 5 cartridges (8.5 g)
Dosage Although the incidence of systemic adverse effects is very low, caution should be exercised, particularly when applying over large areas and leaving on for >2 hours
Children (intact skin):
Cream: Should **not** be used in neonates with a gestation age <37 weeks nor in infants <12 months of age who are receiving treatment with methemoglobin-inducing agents
Dosing is based on child's age and weight:
Age 0-3 months or <5 kg: Apply a maximum of 1 g over no more than 10 cm^2 of skin; leave on for no longer than 1 hour
Age 3 months to 12 months and >5 kg: Apply no more than a maximum 2 g total over no more than 20 cm^2 of skin; leave on for no longer than 4 hours
Age 1-6 years and >10 kg: Apply no more than a maximum of 10 g total over no more than 100 cm^2 of skin; leave on for no longer than 4 hours.
Age 7-12 years and >20 kg: Apply no more than a maximum 20 g total over no more than 200 cm^2 of skin; leave on for no longer than 4 hours.
Note: If a patient >3 months of age does not meet the minimum weight requirement, the maximum total dose should be restricted to the corresponding maximum based on patient weight.
Transdermal patch: Canadian labeling (not available in U.S.): **Note:** Should not be used in neonates with a gestation age <37 weeks nor in infants <12 months of age who are receiving treatment with methemoglobin-inducing agents
Dosing is based on child's age and weight: Apply patch(es) to skin area(s) <10 cm^2:
Age 0-3 months or <5 kg: Apply 1 patch and leave on for ~1 hour (do not exceed 1-hour application time); do not apply more than 1 patch at same time; safety of repeated dosing not established
Age 3 months to 12 months and >5 kg: Apply 1-2 patches for ~1 hour (maximum application time: 4 hours); do not apply more than 2 patches at the same time
Age 1-6 years and >10 kg: Apply 1 or more patches for minimum of 1 hour (maximum application time: 5 hours); maximum dose: 10 patches
Age 7-12 years and >20 kg: Apply 1 or more patches for a minimum of 1 hour (maximum application time: 5 hours); maximum dose: 20 patches
Note: If a patient >3 months of age does not meet the minimum weight requirement, the maximum total dose should be restricted to that which corresponds to the patient's weight.

Adults (intact skin): **Note:** Cream: Apply a thick layer to intact skin and cover with an occlusive dressing. Transdermal patch (CAN; not available in U.S.): Apply patch or patches to intact skin.
Minor dermal procedures (eg, I.V. cannulation or venipuncture):
Cream: Apply 2.5 g of cream ($1/2$ of the 5 g tube) over 20-25 cm^2 of skin surface area) for at least 1 hour
Transdermal patch: (Canadian labeling; not available in U.S.): Apply 1 or more patches to skin surface area <10 cm^2 for at least 1 hour (maximum application time: 5 hours)
Major dermal procedures (eg, more painful dermatological procedures involving a larger skin area such as split thickness skin graft harvesting): Apply 2 g of cream per 10 cm^2 of skin and allow to remain in contact with the skin for at least 2 hours.

◄ Adult male genital skin (eg, pretreatment prior to local anesthetic infiltration): Apply a thick layer of cream (1 g/10 cm²) to the skin surface for 15 minutes. Local anesthetic infiltration should be performed immediately after removal of cream

Note: Dermal analgesia can be expected to increase for up to 3 hours under occlusive dressing and persist for 1-2 hours after removal of the cream

Adult female genital mucous membranes: Minor procedures (eg, removal of condylomata acuminata, pretreatment for local anesthetic infiltration): Apply 5-10 g (thick layer) of cream for 5-10 minutes

Periodontal gel (Oraqix®): Adults: Apply on gingival margin around selected teeth using the blunt-tipped applicator included in package. Wait 30 seconds, then fill the periodontal pockets using the blunt-tipped applicator until gel becomes visible at the gingival margin. Wait another 30 seconds before starting treatment. May reapply; maximum recommended dose: One treatment session: 5 cartridges (8.5 g)

Mechanism of Action Local anesthetic action occurs by stabilization of neuronal membranes and inhibiting the ionic fluxes required for the initiation and conduction of impulses

Contraindications Hypersensitivity to amide-type anesthetic agents; hypersensitivity to any component of the formulation selected; application on mucous membranes or broken or inflamed skin; infants <1 month of age if gestational age is <37 weeks; infants <12 months of age receiving therapy with methemoglobin-inducing agents; children with congenital or idiopathic methemoglobinemia, or in children who are receiving medications associated with drug-induced methemoglobinemia (eg, acetaminophen [overdosage], benzocaine, chloroquine, dapsone, nitrofurantoin, nitroglycerin, nitroprusside, phenazopyridine, phenelzine, phenobarbital, phenytoin, quinine, sulfonamides)

Warnings/Precautions Use with caution in patients with severe hepatic impairment. Use with caution in the debilitated or acutely ill patients and the elderly. Use with caution in patients receiving class I and III antiarrhythmic drugs, since systemic absorption occurs and synergistic toxicity is possible. Although the incidence of systemic adverse reactions with EMLA® is very low, caution should be exercised, particularly when applying over large areas and leaving on for longer than 2 hours. Avoid use on open wounds or near the eyes.

When topical anesthetics are used prior to cosmetic or medical procedures, the lowest amount of anesthetic necessary for pain relief should be applied. High systemic levels and toxic effects (eg, methemoglobinemia, irregular heart beats, respiratory depression, seizures, death) have been reported in patients who (without supervision of a trained professional) have applied topical anesthetics in large amounts (or to large areas of the skin), left these products on for prolonged periods of time, or have used wraps/dressings to cover the skin following application.

Drug Interactions

Metabolism/Transport Effects Refer to individual components.

Avoid Concomitant Use

Avoid concomitant use of Lidocaine and Prilocaine with any of the following: Conivaptan

Increased Effect/Toxicity

Lidocaine and Prilocaine may increase the levels/effects of: Antiarrhythmic Agents (Class III); Prilocaine

The levels/effects of Lidocaine and Prilocaine may be increased by: Abiraterone Acetate; Antiarrhythmic Agents (Class III); Beta-Blockers; Conivaptan; CYP1A2 Inhibitors (Moderate); CYP1A2 Inhibitors (Strong); CYP3A4 Inhibitors (Moderate); CYP3A4 Inhibitors (Strong); Darunavir; Dasatinib; Deferasirox; Disopyramide; Hyaluronidase; Ivacaftor; Methemoglobinemia Associated Agents; Mifepristone

Decreased Effect

The levels/effects of Lidocaine and Prilocaine may be decreased by: CYP1A2 Inducers (Strong); CYP3A4 Inducers (Strong); Cyproterone; Deferasirox; Herbs (CYP3A4 Inducers); Tocilizumab

Pharmacodynamics/Kinetics

Onset of Action EMLA®: 1 hour; Peak effect: 2-3 hours

Duration of Action EMLA®: 1-2 hours after removal; Oraqix®: ~20 minutes

Pregnancy Risk Factor B

Pregnancy Considerations Refer to Lidocaine (Topical) monograph.

Lactation Lidocaine enters breast milk/use caution

Breast-Feeding Considerations See individual agents.

Dosage Forms

Cream, topical: Lidocaine 2.5% and prilocaine 2.5% (5 g, 30 g)

EMLA®: Lidocaine 2.5% and prilocaine 2.5% (5 g, 30 g)

Gel, periodontal:

Oraqix®: Lidocaine 2.5% and prilocaine 2.5% (1.7 g)

Dosage Forms: Canada

Patch, transdermal:

EMLA® Patch: Lidocaine 2.5% and prilocaine 2.5% per patch (2s, 20s)

References

Broadman LM, Soliman IE, Hannallah RS, et al, "Analgesic Efficacy of Eutectic Mixture of Local Anesthetics (EMLA®) vs Intradermal Infiltration Prior to Venous Cannulation in Children," Am J Anaesth, 1987, 34:S56.

Friskopp J and Huledal G, "Plasma Levels of Lidocaine and Prilocaine After Application of Oraqix, a New Intrapocket Anesthetic, in Patients With Advanced Periodontitis," J Clin Periodontol, 2001, 28(5):425-9.

Friskopp J, Nilsson M, and Isacsson G, "The Anesthetic Onset and Duration of a New Lidocaine/Prilocaine Gel Intra-Pocket Anesthetic (Oraqix) for Periodontal Scaling/Root Planing," J Clin Periodontol, 2001, 28(5):453-8.

Lidocaine and Tetracaine

(LYE doe kane & TET ra kane)

Related Information

Lidocaine (Topical) on page 818

Tetracaine (Topical) on page 1307

Brand Names: U.S. Synera®

Generic Availability (U.S.) No

Pharmacologic Category Analgesic, Topical; Local Anesthetic

Use Topical anesthetic for use on normal intact skin for minor procedures (eg, I.V. cannulation or venipuncture) and superficial dermatologic procedures

Local Anesthetic/Vasoconstrictor Precautions No information available to require special precautions

Effects on Dental Treatment No significant effects or complications reported

Effects on Bleeding No information available to require special precautions

Adverse Effects

>10%: Dermatologic: Erythema (71%), edema (12%), blanching (12%)

1% to 10%: Dermatologic: Application site reactions (contact dermatitis, rash, skin discoloration)

Dosage Transdermal patch: Children ≥3 years and Adults:

Venipuncture or intravenous cannulation: Prior to procedure, apply to intact skin for 20-30 minutes; **Note:** Adults can use another patch at a new location to facilitate venous access after a failed attempt; remove previous patch.

Superficial dermatological procedures: Prior to procedure, apply to intact skin for 30 minutes

Dosage adjustment in hepatic impairment: Use caution in patients with severe hepatic dysfunction.

Mechanism of Action Local anesthetic action occurs by stabilization of neuronal membranes and inhibiting the sodium ion fluxes required for the initiation and conduction of impulses. A heating mechanism within the patch enhances drug delivery.

Contraindications Hypersensitivity to lidocaine, tetracaine, amide or ester-type anesthetic agents, para-aminobenzoid acid (PABA), or any other component of the formulation

Warnings/Precautions Hypersensitivity or anaphylactic reactions may occur. Use with caution in patients receiving class I antiarrhythmic drugs, since systemic absorption occurs and synergistic toxicity is possible. Use with caution in patients who may be sensitive to systemic effects (eg, acutely ill, debilitated, elderly). If being used with other products containing local anesthetic, consider potential for additive effects. Avoid contact with eye; loss of protective reflexes may predispose to corneal irritation and/or abrasion. Application to broken or inflamed skin or mucous membranes may lead to increased systemic absorption. Use caution in patients with severe hepatic disease or pseudocholinesterase deficiency. Not for use at home. Methemoglobinemia has been reported with local anesthetics including tetracaine. Use caution in patients with lung diseases (asthma, bronchitis, emphysema, in smokers), inflamed/damaged mucosa, heart disease, children <12 months of age, concurrent use with methemoglobin-inducing medications, and hemoglobin or enzyme abnormalities.

When topical anesthetics are used prior to cosmetic or medical procedures, the lowest amount of anesthetic necessary for pain relief should be applied. High systemic levels and toxic effects (eg, methemoglobinemia, irregular heart beats, respiratory depression, seizures, death) have been reported in patients who (without supervision of a trained professional) have applied topical anesthetics in large amounts (or to large areas of the skin), left these products on for prolonged periods of time, or have used wraps/dressings to cover the skin following application.

Use caution when applying simultaneous or sequential application of multiple patches to adults; this practice is not recommended with children. May contain conducting metal (eg, aluminum); remove patch prior to MRI.

Drug Interactions

Metabolism/Transport Effects Refer to individual components.

Avoid Concomitant Use

Avoid concomitant use of Lidocaine and Tetracaine with any of the following: Conivaptan

Increased Effect/Toxicity

Lidocaine and Tetracaine may increase the levels/effects of: Antiarrhythmic Agents (Class III); Prilocaine

The levels/effects of Lidocaine and Tetracaine may be increased by: Abiraterone Acetate; Antiarrhythmic Agents (Class III); Beta-Blockers; Conivaptan; CYP1A2 Inhibitors (Moderate); CYP1A2 Inhibitors (Strong); CYP3A4 Inhibitors (Moderate); CYP3A4 Inhibitors (Strong); Darunavir; Dasatinib; Deferasirox; Disopyramide; Ivacaftor; Mifepristone

Decreased Effect

The levels/effects of Lidocaine and Tetracaine may be decreased by: CYP1A2 Inducers (Strong); CYP3A4 Inducers (Strong); Cyproterone; Deferasirox; Herbs (CYP3A4 Inducers); Tocilizumab

Pharmacodynamics/Kinetics

Onset of Action Within 20-30 minutes

Pregnancy Risk Factor B

Pregnancy Considerations See individual agents.

Lactation Lidocaine enters breast milk/use caution

Breast-Feeding Considerations Refer to Lidocaine (Topical) monograph.

Dosage Forms

Patch, transdermal:

Synera®: Lidocaine 70 mg and tetracaine 70 mg (10s)

Linaclotide (lin AK loe tide)

Brand Names: U.S. Linzess™

Pharmacologic Category Gastrointestinal Agent, Miscellaneous

Use Treatment of chronic idiopathic constipation (CIC); treatment of irritable bowel syndrome with constipation (IBS-C) in adults

Local Anesthetic/Vasoconstrictor Precautions No information available to require special precautions

Effects on Dental Treatment

Key adverse event(s) related to dental treatment: Upper respiratory tract infection and sinusitis

Effects on Bleeding No information available to require special precautions

Adverse Effects Adverse reactions reported with use in IBS-C and CIC.

>10%: Gastrointestinal: Diarrhea (16% to 20%; severe diarrhea: 2%)

1% to 10%:

Central nervous system: Headache (4%), fatigue (<2%)

Gastrointestinal: Abdominal pain (7%), flatulence (4% to 6%), abdominal distension (2% to 3%), viral gastroenteritis (≤3%), dyspepsia (<2%), fecal incontinence (<2%), gastroesophageal reflux disease (<2%), vomiting (<2%)

Respiratory: Upper respiratory tract infection (5%), sinusitis (3%)

General Dosage Range

Oral: *Adults:* 145 mcg or 290 mcg once daily

Mechanism of Action Linaclotide and its active metabolite bind and agonize guanylate cyclase-C on the luminal surface of intestinal epithelium. Intracellular and extracellular cyclic guanosine monophosphate (cGMP) concentrations are subsequently increased resulting in chloride and bicarbonate secretion into the intestinal lumen. Intestinal fluid increases and transit time is decreased.. Extracellular cGMP may decrease visceral pain by reducing pain-sensing nerve activity.

Pregnancy Risk Factor C

Pregnancy Considerations Adverse events were observed in some animal reproduction studies. Linaclotide and its metabolite are not measurable in plasma when used at recommended doses.

Linagliptin (lin a GLIP tin)

Brand Names: U.S. Tradjenta™
Brand Names: Canada Trajenta™
Pharmacologic Category Antidiabetic Agent, Dipeptidyl Peptidase IV (DPP-IV) Inhibitor
Use Management of type 2 diabetes mellitus (noninsulin dependent, NIDDM) as an adjunct to diet and exercise as monotherapy or in combination with other antidiabetic agents
Local Anesthetic/Vasoconstrictor Precautions No information available to require special precautions
Effects on Dental Treatment Linagliptin-dependent patients with diabetes should be appointed for dental treatment in the morning in order to minimize chance of stress-induced hypoglycemia.
Effects on Bleeding No information available to require special precautions
Adverse Effects
>10%: Endocrine & metabolic: Hypoglycemia (combined with metformin and/or sulfonylurea [15% to 23%]; monotherapy [<1% to 7%]; metformin [<1%], pioglitazone [<1%])
1% to 10%:
Central nervous system: Headache (6%)
Endocrine & metabolic: Hyperuricemia (3%), lipids increased (3%), triglycerides increased (2% to 3%), weight gain (2%)
Gastrointestinal: Constipation (2%)
Genitourinary: Urinary tract infection (3%)
Neuromuscular & skeletal: Arthralgia (6%), back pain (6%)
Respiratory: Nasopharyngitis (6% to 7%), cough (2%)
General Dosage Range Oral: *Adults:* 5 mg once daily
Concomitant use with insulin and/or insulin secretagogues (eg, sulfonylureas): Reduced dose of insulin and/or insulin secretagogues may be needed.
Mechanism of Action Linagliptin inhibits dipeptidyl peptidase IV (DPP-IV) enzyme resulting in prolonged active incretin levels. Incretin hormones (eg, glucagon-like peptide-1 [GLP-1] and glucose-dependent insulinotropic polypeptide [GIP]) regulate glucose homeostasis by increasing insulin synthesis and release from pancreatic beta cells and decreasing glucagon secretion from pancreatic alpha cells. Decreased glucagon secretion results in decreased hepatic glucose production. Under normal physiologic circumstances, incretin hormones are released by the intestine throughout the day and levels are increased in response to a meal; incretin hormones are rapidly inactivated by the DPP-IV enzyme.
Pharmacodynamics/Kinetics
Half-life Elimination Effective (therapeutic): ~12 hours; Terminal (DPP-IV saturable binding): >100 hours
Time to Peak 1.5 hours
Pregnancy Risk Factor B
Pregnancy Considerations Adverse events were not observed in animal reproduction studies, except with doses that were also maternally toxic. Maternal hyperglycemia can be associated with adverse effects in the fetus, including macrosomia, neonatal hyperglycemia, and hyperbilirubinemia; the risk of congenital malformations is increased when the Hb A_{1c} is above the normal range. Diabetes can also be associated with adverse effects in the mother. Poorly-treated diabetes may cause end-organ damage that may in turn negatively affect obstetric outcomes. Physiologic glucose levels should be maintained prior to and during pregnancy to decrease the risk of adverse events in the mother and the fetus. Until additional safety and efficacy data are obtained, the use of oral agents is generally not recommended as routine management of GDM or type 2 diabetes mellitus during pregnancy. Insulin is the drug of choice for the control of diabetes mellitus during pregnancy.

Linagliptin and Metformin
(lin a GLIP tin & met FOR min)

Brand Names: U.S. Jentadueto™
Pharmacologic Category Antidiabetic Agent, Biguanide; Antidiabetic Agent, Dipeptidyl Peptidase IV (DPP-IV) Inhibitor
Use Management of type 2 diabetes mellitus (noninsulin dependent, NIDDM) as an adjunct to diet and exercise in patients not adequately controlled on metformin or linagliptin monotherapy
Local Anesthetic/Vasoconstrictor Precautions No information available to require special precautions
Effects on Dental Treatment
Linagliptin-dependent patients with diabetes should be appointed for dental treatment in the morning in order to minimize chance of stress-induced hypoglycemia.
Metformin-dependent patients with diabetes (noninsulin dependent, Type 2) should be appointed for dental treatment in the morning in order to minimize chance of stress-induced hypoglycemia.
Effects on Bleeding No information available to require special precautions
Adverse Effects Reactions/percentages reported with combination product; also see individual agents.
1% to 10%:
Gastrointestinal: Diarrhea (6%)
Respiratory: Nasopharyngitis (6%)
Frequency not defined:
Dermatologic: Pruritus
Gastrointestinal: Appetite decreased, nausea, pancreatitis, vomiting
Respiratory: Cough
Miscellaneous: Hypersensitivity reactions
General Dosage Range Oral: *Adults:* Linagliptin 2.5 mg and metformin 500-1000 mg twice daily (maximum: 5 mg/day [linagliptin], 2000 mg/day [metformin])
Mechanism of Action
Linagliptin inhibits dipeptidyl peptidase IV (DPP-IV) enzymes resulting in prolonged active incretin levels. Incretin hormones [eg, glucagon-like peptide-1 (GLP-1) and glucose-dependent insulinotropic polypeptide (GIP)] regulate glucose homeostasis by increasing insulin synthesis and release from pancreatic beta cells and decreasing glucagon secretion from pancreatic alpha cells. Decreased glucagon secretion results in decreased hepatic glucose production. Under normal physiologic circumstances, incretin hormones are released by the intestine throughout the day and levels are increased in response to a meal; incretin hormones are rapidly inactivated by DPP-IV enzymes.

Metformin decreases hepatic glucose production, decreasing intestinal absorption of glucose, and improves insulin sensitivity (increases peripheral glucose uptake and utilization).
Pregnancy Risk Factor B
Pregnancy Considerations Adverse events were not observed in animal reproduction studies using this combination. Refer to individual agents.

Lincomycin (lin koe MYE sin)

Brand Names: U.S. Lincocin®
Brand Names: Canada Lincocin®
Pharmacologic Category Antibiotic, Lincosamide
Use Treatment of serious susceptible bacterial infections, mainly those caused by streptococci, pneumococci, and staphylococci in patients who are penicillin allergic or in whom use of a penicillin is inappropriate
Local Anesthetic/Vasoconstrictor Precautions No information available to require special precautions
Effects on Dental Treatment Key adverse event(s) related to dental treatment: Glossitis and stomatitis.
Effects on Bleeding No information available to require special precautions
Adverse Effects Frequency not defined.
Cardiovascular: Cardiopulmonary arrest and hypotension (related to rapid I.V. infusion; rare)
Central nervous system: Vertigo
Dermatologic: Dermatitis (includes exfoliative and vesiculobullous; rare), erythema multiforme (rare; some resembling SJS), rash, urticaria
Gastrointestinal: Colitis, diarrhea, glossitis, nausea, pruritus ani, stomatitis, vomiting
Genitourinary: Vaginitis
Hematologic: Agranulocytosis, aplastic anemia (rare), leukopenia, neutropenia, pancytopenia (rare), thrombocytopenic purpura
Hepatic: Jaundice, liver function tests abnormal (ie, ALT increased, AST increased)
Local: Injection site reactions (rare)
Otic: Tinnitus
Renal: Azotemia (rare), proteinuria (rare), oliguria (rare)
Miscellaneous: Hypersensitivity reactions (anaphylaxis, angioneurotic edema, serum sickness)
General Dosage Range Dosage adjustment recommended in patients with renal impairment
I.M.:
Children >1 month: 10 mg/kg every 12-24 hours
Adults: 600 mg every 12-24 hours
I.V.:
Children >1 month: 10-20 mg/kg/day divided every 8-12 hours
Adults: 600 mg to 1 g every 8-12 hours (maximum: 8 g daily)
Subconjunctival injection: Adults: 75 mg
Mechanism of Action Lincosamide antibiotic which was isolated from a strain of Streptomyces lincolnensis; lincomycin, like clindamycin, inhibits bacterial protein synthesis by specifically binding on the 50S subunit and affecting the process of peptide chain initiation. Since only one molecule of antibiotic can bind to a single ribosome, the concomitant use of erythromycin and lincomycin is not recommended.
Pharmacodynamics/Kinetics
Half-life Elimination Serum: ~5 hours; prolonged with renal or hepatic impairment
Time to Peak Serum: I.M.: 1 hour
Pregnancy Risk Factor C
Pregnancy Considerations Because teratogenicity studies have not been completed in animals, lincomycin is classified as pregnancy category C. Lincomycin crosses the placenta, but has not caused adverse fetal effects when given during all three trimesters of pregnancy or at term.

Lindane (LIN dane)

Brand Names: Canada Hexit™; PMS-Lindane
Pharmacologic Category Antiparasitic Agent, Topical; Pediculocide; Scabicidal Agent
Use Treatment of Sarcoptes scabiei (scabies), Pediculus capitis (head lice), and Phthirus pubis (crab lice); FDA recommends reserving lindane as a second-line agent or with inadequate response to other therapies
Local Anesthetic/Vasoconstrictor Precautions No information available to require special precautions
Effects on Dental Treatment No significant effects or complications reported
Effects on Bleeding No information available to require special precautions
Adverse Effects Frequency not defined (includes post-marketing and/or case reports).
Cardiovascular: Cardiac arrhythmia
Central nervous system: Ataxia, dizziness, headache, restlessness, seizure, pain
Dermatologic: Alopecia, contact dermatitis, skin and adipose tissue may act as repositories, eczematous eruptions, pruritus, urticaria
Gastrointestinal: Nausea, vomiting
Hematologic: Aplastic anemia
Hepatic: Hepatitis
Local: Burning and stinging
Neuromuscular & skeletal: Paresthesia
Renal: Hematuria
Respiratory: Pulmonary edema
General Dosage Range Topical:
Lotion: Children and Adults: Apply a thin layer; bathe and remove drug after 8-12 hours
Shampoo: Children and Adults: Apply to dry hair (maximum: 60 mL)
Mechanism of Action Directly absorbed by parasites and ova through the exoskeleton; stimulates the nervous system resulting in seizures and death of parasitic arthropods
Pharmacodynamics/Kinetics
Half-life Elimination Children: 17-22 hours
Time to Peak Serum: Children: 6 hours
Pregnancy Risk Factor C
Pregnancy Considerations There are no well-controlled studies in pregnant women.

Linezolid (li NE zoh lid)

Brand Names: U.S. Zyvox®
Brand Names: Canada Zyvoxam®
Pharmacologic Category Antibiotic, Oxazolidinone
Use Treatment of vancomycin-resistant Enterococcus faecium (VRE) infections, nosocomial pneumonia caused by Staphylococcus aureus (including MRSA) or Streptococcus pneumoniae (including multidrug-resistant strains [MDRSP]), complicated and uncomplicated skin and skin structure infections (including diabetic foot infections without concomitant osteomyelitis), and community-acquired pneumonia caused by susceptible gram-positive organisms
Unlabeled Use Treatment of prosthetic joint infection
Local Anesthetic/Vasoconstrictor Precautions
Linezolid has mild monoamine oxidase inhibitor properties. The clinician is reminded that vasoconstrictors have the potential to interact with MAO-Is to result in elevation of blood pressure. Caution is suggested.

Effects on Dental Treatment Key adverse event(s) related to dental treatment: Oral moniliasis, taste alteration, and tongue discoloration.

Effects on Bleeding No information available to require special precautions

Adverse Effects Percentages as reported in adults; frequency similar in pediatric patients

>10%:

Central nervous system: Headache (<1% to 11%)
Gastrointestinal: Diarrhea (3% to 11%)

1% to 10%:

Central nervous system: Insomnia (3%), dizziness (≤2%), fever (2%)

Dermatologic: Rash (2%)

Gastrointestinal: Nausea (3% to 10%), lipase increased (3% to 4%), vomiting (1% to 4%), constipation (2%), taste alteration (1% to 2%), amylase increased (<1% to 2%), tongue discoloration (≤1%), oral moniliasis (≤1%), pancreatitis

Genitourinary: Vaginal moniliasis (1% to 2%)

Hematologic: Thrombocytopenia (<1% to 10%), hemoglobin decreased (1% to 7%), leukopenia (<1% to 2%), neutropenia (≤1%)

Hepatic: ALT increased (2% to 10%), AST increased (2% to 5%), alkaline phosphatase increased (<1% to 4%), bilirubin increased (≤1%)

Renal: BUN increased (≤2%)

Miscellaneous: Fungal infection (≤1% to 2%), lactate dehydrogenase increased (<1% to 2%)

General Dosage Range

I.V.:

Children ≤11 years: 10 mg/kg (maximum dose: 600 mg) every 8 hours

Children ≥12 years and Adults: 600 mg every 12 hours

Oral:

Children <5 years: 10 mg/kg every 8 hours (maximum: 600 mg/dose)

Children 5-11 years: 10 mg/kg every 8-12 hours (maximum: 600 mg/dose)

Children ≥12 years and Adults: 400-600 mg every 12 hours

Mechanism of Action Inhibits bacterial protein synthesis by binding to bacterial 23S ribosomal RNA of the 50S subunit. This prevents the formation of a functional 70S initiation complex that is essential for the bacterial translation process. Linezolid is bacteriostatic against enterococci and staphylococci and bactericidal against most strains of streptococci.

Pharmacodynamics/Kinetics

Half-life Elimination Children ≥1 week (full-term) to 11 years: 1.5-3 hours; Adults: 4-5 hours

Time to Peak Adults: Oral: 1-2 hours

Pregnancy Risk Factor C

Pregnancy Considerations Adverse effects were observed in some animal reproduction studies at doses that were also maternally toxic. Information related to linezolid use during pregnancy is limited.

Liothyronine (lye oh THYE roe neen)

Related Information

Endocrine Disorders and Pregnancy on page 1517

Brand Names: U.S. Cytomel®; Triostat®

Brand Names: Canada Cytomel®

Pharmacologic Category Thyroid Product

Use

Oral: Replacement or supplemental therapy in hypothyroidism; management of nontoxic goiter; a diagnostic aid

I.V.: Treatment of myxedema coma/precoma

Unlabeled Use Management of hemodynamically unstable potential organ donors increasing the quantity of organs available for transplantation

Local Anesthetic/Vasoconstrictor Precautions No precautions with vasoconstrictor are necessary if patient is well controlled with liothyronine

Effects on Dental Treatment No significant effects or complications reported

Effects on Bleeding No information available to require special precautions

Adverse Effects 1% to 10%: Cardiovascular: Arrhythmia (6%), tachycardia (3%), cardiopulmonary arrest (2%), hypotension (2%), MI (2%)

General Dosage Range

I.V.: Adults: 10-50 mcg/dose

Oral:

Infants: Initial: 5 mcg/day; Usual maintenance dose: 20 mcg/day

Children 1-3 years: Initial: 5 mcg/day; Usual maintenance dose: 50 mcg/day

Children >3 years: Initial: 5 mcg/day; Maintenance: Up to 100 mcg/day

Adults: Initial 5-25 mcg/day; Maintenance range 5-100 mcg/day

Elderly: Initial: 5 mcg/day

Mechanism of Action Exact mechanism of action is unknown; however, it is believed the thyroid hormone exerts its many metabolic effects through control of DNA transcription and protein synthesis; involved in normal metabolism, growth, and development; promotes gluconeogenesis, increases utilization and mobilization of glycogen stores, and stimulates protein synthesis, increases basal metabolic rate

Pharmacodynamics/Kinetics

Onset of Action ~3 hours

Half-life Elimination 2.5 days

Pregnancy Risk Factor A

Pregnancy Considerations Endogenous thyroid hormones minimally cross the placenta; the fetal thyroid becomes active around the end of the first trimester. Liothyronine has not been found to increase the risk of teratogenic or adverse effects following maternal use during pregnancy.

Uncontrolled maternal hypothyroidism may result in adverse neonatal and maternal outcomes. To prevent adverse events, normal maternal thyroid function should be maintained prior to conception and throughout pregnancy. Levothyroxine is considered the treatment of choice for the control of hypothyroidism during pregnancy.

Liotrix (LYE oh triks)

Related Information

Endocrine Disorders and Pregnancy on page 1517

Brand Names: U.S. Thyrolar®

Brand Names: Canada Thyrolar®

Pharmacologic Category Thyroid Product

Use

Replacement or supplemental therapy in hypothyroidism (uniform mixture of T_4:T_3 in 4:1 ratio by weight)

Thyroid-stimulating hormone (TSH) suppressant therapy used in the management of thyroid cancer (levothyroxine is generally recommended for this indication); prevention or treatment of euthyroid goiters (eg, thyroid nodules, subacute or chronic lymphocytic thyroiditis [Hashimoto's], multinodular goiters)

Diagnostic agent in suppression tests to diagnose suspected mild hyperthyroidism or to demonstrate thyroid gland autonomy

Local Anesthetic/Vasoconstrictor Precautions No precautions with vasoconstrictor are necessary if patient is well controlled with liotrix

Effects on Dental Treatment No significant effects or complications reported

Effects on Bleeding No information available to require special precautions

Adverse Effects Frequency not defined.
Cardiovascular: Blood pressure increased, cardiac arrhythmia, chest pain, palpitation, tachycardia
Central nervous system: Anxiety, ataxia, fever, headache, insomnia, nervousness
Dermatologic: Alopecia, hyperhydrosis, pruritus, urticaria
Endocrine & metabolic: Changes in menstrual cycle, increased appetite, weight loss
Gastrointestinal: Abdominal cramps, constipation, diarrhea, nausea, vomiting
Neuromuscular & skeletal: Hand tremor, myalgia, tremor
Respiratory: Dyspnea
Miscellaneous: Allergic skin reactions (rare), diaphoresis

General Dosage Range Oral:
Children 0-6 months: Levothyroxine 12.5-25 mcg/Liothyronine 3.1-6.25 mcg once daily
Children 6-12 months: Levothyroxine 25-37.5 mcg/Liothyronine 6.25-9.35 mcg once daily
Children 1-5 years: Levothyroxine 37.5-50 mcg/Liothyronine 9.35-12.5 mcg once daily
Children 6-12 years: Levothyroxine 50-75 mcg/Liothyronine 12.5-18.75 mcg once daily
Children >12 years: Levothyroxine 75 mcg/Liothyronine 18.75 mcg once daily
Adults: Initial: Levothyroxine 25 mcg/Liothyronine 6.25 mcg once daily; Usual maintenance: Levothyroxine 50-100 mcg/Liothyronine 12.5-25 mcg once daily
Elderly: Initial: Levothyroxine 12.5-25 mcg/Liothyronine 3.1-6.25 mcg once daily

Mechanism of Action The primary active compound is T_3 (triiodothyronine), which may be converted from T_4 (thyroxine) and then circulates throughout the body to influence growth and maturation of various tissues. Liotrix is uniform mixture of synthetic T_4 and T_3 in 4:1 ratio; exact mechanism of action is unknown; however, it is believed the thyroid hormone exerts its many metabolic effects through control of DNA transcription and protein synthesis; involved in normal metabolism, growth, and development; promotes gluconeogenesis, increases utilization and mobilization of glycogen stores and stimulates protein synthesis, increases basal metabolic rate

Pharmacodynamics/Kinetics
Onset of Action Liothyronine (T_3): ~3 hours
Half-life Elimination
T_4: Euthyroid: 6-7 days; Hyperthyroid: 3-4 days; Hypothyroid: 9-10 days
T_3: 2.5 days
Time to Peak Serum: T_4: 2-4 hours; T_3: 2-3 days
Pregnancy Risk Factor A

Pregnancy Considerations Endogenous thyroid hormones minimally cross the placenta; the fetal thyroid becomes active around the end of the first trimester. Liotrix has not been found to increase the risk of adverse effects following maternal use during pregnancy.

Uncontrolled maternal hypothyroidism may result in adverse neonatal and maternal outcomes. To prevent adverse events, normal maternal thyroid function should be maintained prior to conception and throughout pregnancy. Levothyroxine is considered the treatment of choice for the control of hypothyroidism during pregnancy.

Liraglutide (lir a GLOO tide)

Brand Names: U.S. Victoza®
Brand Names: Canada Victoza®
Pharmacologic Category Antidiabetic Agent, Glucagon-Like Peptide-1 (GLP-1) Receptor Agonist
Use Treatment of type 2 diabetes mellitus (noninsulin dependent, NIDDM) to improve glycemic control
Local Anesthetic/Vasoconstrictor Precautions No information available to require special precautions
Effects on Dental Treatment Schedule type 1 and type 2 diabetic patients for dental treatment in the morning in order to minimize chance of stress-induced hypoglycemia.
Effects on Bleeding No information available to require special precautions
Adverse Effects Incidence reported in monotherapy trials unless otherwise specified.
>10%: Gastrointestinal: Nausea (28%), diarrhea (17%), vomiting (11%)
1% to 10%:
Central nervous system: Headache (9%)
Gastrointestinal: Constipation (10%)
Hepatic: Hyperbilirubinemia (monotherapy and combination trials: 4%)
Local: Injection site reactions (monotherapy and combination trials: 2% [includes rash, erythema])
Miscellaneous: Antiliraglutide antibodies (low titers [concentrations not requiring dilution of serum]; monotherapy and combination trials: 9%), cross-reacting antiliraglutide antibodies to native GLP-1 (monotherapy: 7%; combination trials: 5%)
General Dosage Range SubQ: *Adults:* Initial: 0.6 mg once daily; maintenance: 1.2-1.8 mg/day
Mechanism of Action Liraglutide is a long acting analog of human glucagon-like peptide-1 (GLP-1) (an incretin hormone) which increases glucose-dependent insulin secretion, decreases inappropriate glucagon secretion, increases B-cell growth/replication, slows gastric emptying, and decreases food intake. Liraglutide administration results in decreases in hemoglobin A_{1c} by approximately 1%.
Pharmacodynamics/Kinetics
Half-life Elimination ~13 hours
Time to Peak Plasma: 8-12 hours
Pregnancy Risk Factor C
Pregnancy Considerations Teratogenic in animal reproduction studies. There are no adequate or well-controlled studies in pregnant women; use only if potential benefit outweighs possible risk to the fetus.

Lisdexamfetamine (lis dex am FET a meen)

Brand Names: U.S. Vyvanse®

◄ **Brand Names: Canada** Vyvanse®

Pharmacologic Category Central Nervous System Stimulant

Use Treatment of attention-deficit/hyperactivity disorder (ADHD)

Local Anesthetic/Vasoconstrictor Precautions Use vasoconstrictor with caution in patients taking lisdexamfetamine. Amphetamines enhance the sympathomimetic response of epinephrine or mepivacaine and levonordefrin (Carbocaine® 2% with Neo-Cobefrin®) leading to potential hypertension and cardiotoxicity.

Effects on Dental Treatment Key adverse event(s) related to dental treatment: Xerostomia (normal salivary flow resumes upon discontinuation).

Lisdexamfetamine is a prodrug that is converted to the active component dextroamphetamine (a noncatecholamine, sympathomimetic amine); dextroamphetamine is known to increase blood pressure. Monitor blood pressure prior to using local anesthetic with vasoconstrictors.

Effects on Bleeding No information available to require special precautions

Adverse Effects

>10%:

Central nervous system: Insomnia (13% to 27%)

Gastrointestinal: Appetite decreased (children and adolescents 34% to 39%; adults 27%), xerostomia (adults 26%; children and adolescents 4% to 5%), abdominal pain (children 12%)

1% to 10%:

Cardiovascular: Blood pressure increased (adults 3%), heart rate increased (adults 2%)

Central nervous system: Irritability (children 10%), anxiety (adults 6%), dizziness (children 5%), jitteriness (adults 4%), affect lability (children 3%), agitation (adults 3%), restlessness (adults 3%), fever (children 2%), somnolence (children 2%), tic (children 2%)

Dermatologic: Hyperhidrosis (adults 3%), rash (children 3%)

Gastrointestinal: Vomiting (children 9%), weight loss (children and adolescents 9%; adults 3%), diarrhea (adults 7%), nausea (6% to 7%), anorexia (adults 5%)

Genitourinary: Erectile dysfunction (adults 3%), libido decreased (adults <2%)

Neuromuscular & skeletal: Tremor (adults 2%)

Respiratory: Dyspnea (adults 2%)

Additional adverse reaction associated with amphetamines; frequency not defined:

Cardiovascular: Hypertension, MI, sudden death, tachycardia

Central nervous system: Exacerbation of motor and phonic tics, overstimulation, stroke, Tourette's syndrome

Dermatologic: Stevens-Johnson syndrome, toxic epidermal necrolysis

Gastrointestinal: Abnormal taste, constipation

General Dosage Range Oral: *Children ≥6 years, Adolescents, and Adults:* Initial: 30 mg once daily; Maintenance: Up to 70 mg once daily

Mechanism of Action Lisdexamfetamine dimesylate is a prodrug that is converted to the active component dextroamphetamine (a noncatecholamine, sympathomimetic amine). Amphetamines are noncatecholamine, sympathomimetic amines that cause release of catecholamines (primarily dopamine and norepinephrine) from their storage sites in the presynaptic nerve terminals. A less significant mechanism may include their

ability to block the reuptake of catecholamines by competitive inhibition.

Pharmacodynamics/Kinetics

Half-life Elimination Lisdexamfetamine: <1 hour; Dextroamphetamine: 10-13 hours

Time to Peak T_{max}: Lisdexamfetamine: ~1 hour; dextroamphetamine: ~3.5 hours

Pregnancy Risk Factor C

Pregnancy Considerations Adverse effects have not been observed in animal reproduction studies. Lisdexamfetamine is converted to dextroamphetamine. The majority of human data is based on illicit amphetamine/methamphetamine exposure and not from therapeutic maternal use (Golub, 2005). Use of amphetamines during pregnancy may lead to an increased risk of premature birth and low birth weight; newborns may experience symptoms of withdrawal. Behavioral problems may also occur later in childhood (LaGasse, 2012).

Controlled Substance C-II

Lisinopril (lyse IN oh pril)

Related Information

Cardiovascular Diseases *on page 1492*

Brand Names: U.S. Prinivil®; Zestril®

Brand Names: Canada Apo-Lisinopril®; CO Lisinopril; Dom-Lisinopril; JAMP-Lisinopril; Mint-Lisinopril; Mylan-Lisinopril; PMS-Lisinopril; Prinivil®; PRO-Lisinopril; RAN™-Lisinopril; ratio-Lisinopril; ratio-Lisinopril P; ratio-Lisinopril Z; Riva-Lisinopril; Sandoz-Lisinopril; Teva-Lisinopril (Type P); Teva-Lisinopril (Type Z); Zestril®

Generic Availability (U.S.) Yes

Pharmacologic Category Angiotensin-Converting Enzyme (ACE) Inhibitor

Use Treatment of hypertension, either alone or in combination with other antihypertensive agents; adjunctive therapy in treatment of heart failure (afterload reduction); treatment of acute myocardial infarction within 24 hours in hemodynamically-stable patients to improve survival; treatment of left ventricular dysfunction after myocardial infarction

Local Anesthetic/Vasoconstrictor Precautions No information available to require special precautions

Effects on Dental Treatment Key adverse event(s) related to dental treatment: Orthostatic effects.

Effects on Bleeding No information available to require special precautions

Adverse Effects Note: Frequency ranges include data from hypertension and heart failure trials. Higher rates of adverse reactions have generally been noted in patients with heart failure. However, the frequency of adverse effects associated with placebo is also increased in this population.

1% to 10%:

Cardiovascular: Orthostatic effects (1%), hypotension (1% to 4%)

Central nervous system: Headache (4% to 6%), dizziness (5% to 12%), fatigue (3%)

Dermatologic: Rash (1% to 2%)

Endocrine & metabolic: Hyperkalemia (2% to 5%)

Gastrointestinal: Diarrhea (3% to 4%), nausea (2%), vomiting (1%), abdominal pain (2%)

Genitourinary: Impotence (1%)

Hematologic: Decreased hemoglobin (small)

Neuromuscular & skeletal: Chest pain (3%), weakness (1%)

Renal: BUN increased (2%); deterioration in renal function (in patients with bilateral renal artery stenosis or hypovolemia); serum creatinine increased (often transient)

Respiratory: Cough (4% to 9%); upper respiratory infection (1% to 2%)

Dosage Oral:

Heart failure: Adults: Initial: 2.5-5 mg once daily; then increase by no more than 10 mg increments at intervals no less than 2 weeks to a maximum daily dose of 40 mg. Usual maintenance: 5-40 mg/day as a single dose. Target dose: 20-40 mg once daily (ACC/AHA 2009 Heart Failure Guidelines)

Note: If patient has hyponatremia (serum sodium <130 mEq/L) or renal impairment (Cl_{cr} <30 mL/minute or creatinine >3 mg/dL), then initial dose should be 2.5 mg/day

Hypertension:

Children ≥6 years: Initial: 0.07 mg/kg once daily (up to 5 mg); increase dose at 1- to 2-week intervals; doses >0.61 mg/kg or >40 mg have not been evaluated.

Adults: Usual dosage range (JNC 7): 10-40 mg/day

Not maintained on diuretic: Initial: 10 mg/day

Maintained on diuretic: Initial: 5 mg/day

Note: Antihypertensive effect may diminish toward the end of the dosing interval especially with doses of 10 mg/day. An increased dose may aid in extending the duration of antihypertensive effect. Doses up to 80 mg/day have been used, but do not appear to give greater effect.

Patients taking diuretics should have them discontinued 2-3 days prior to initiating lisinopril if possible. Restart diuretic after blood pressure is stable if needed. If diuretic cannot be discontinued prior to therapy, begin with 5 mg with close supervision until stable blood pressure. In patients with hyponatremia (<130 mEq/L), start dose at 2.5 mg/day

Elderly: Consider lower initial doses (eg, 2.5-5 mg/day) and titrate to response (Aronow, 2011)

Acute myocardial infarction (within 24 hours in hemodynamically stable patients): Adults: 5 mg immediately, then 5 mg at 24 hours, 10 mg at 48 hours, and 10 mg every day thereafter for 6 weeks. Patients should continue to receive standard treatments such as thrombolytics, aspirin, and beta-blockers.

Dosage adjustment in renal impairment:

Heart failure: Adults: Cl_{cr} <30 mL/minute or creatinine >3 mg/dL: Initial: 2.5 mg/day

Hypertension:

Adults: Initial doses should be modified and upward titration should be cautious, based on response (maximum: 40 mg/day)

Cl_{cr} >30 mL/minute: Initial: 10 mg/day

Cl_{cr} 10-30 mL/minute: Initial: 5 mg/day

Hemodialysis: Initial: 2.5 mg/day; dialyzable (50%)

Children: Use in not recommended in pediatric patients with GFR <30 mL/minute/1.73 m^2

Dosage adjustment in hepatic impairment: No dosage adjustment provided in manufacturer's labeling.

Mechanism of Action Competitive inhibitor of angiotensin-converting enzyme (ACE); prevents conversion of angiotensin I to angiotensin II, a potent vasoconstrictor; results in lower levels of angiotensin II which causes an increase in plasma renin activity and a reduction in aldosterone secretion; a CNS mechanism may also be involved in hypotensive effect as angiotensin II increases adrenergic outflow from CNS; vasoactive kallikreins may be decreased in conversion to active hormones by ACE inhibitors, thus reducing blood pressure

Contraindications Hypersensitivity to lisinopril or any component of the formulation; angioedema related to previous treatment with an ACE inhibitor; patients with idiopathic or hereditary angioedema; concomitant use with aliskiren in patients with diabetes mellitus

Warnings/Precautions Anaphylactic reactions may occur rarely with ACE inhibitors. At any time during treatment (especially following first dose), angioedema may occur rarely with ACE inhibitors; it may involve the head and neck (potentially compromising airway) or the intestine (presenting with abdominal pain). African-Americans may be at an increased risk. Prolonged frequent monitoring may be required especially if tongue, glottis, or larynx are involved as they are associated with airway obstruction. Patients with a history of airway surgery may have a higher risk of airway obstruction. Aggressive early and appropriate management is critical. Use in patients with idiopathic or hereditary angioedema or previous angioedema associated with ACE inhibitor therapy is contraindicated. Severe anaphylactoid reactions may be seen during hemodialysis (eg, CVVHD) with high-flux dialysis membranes (eg, AN69), and rarely, during low density lipoprotein apheresis with dextran sulfate cellulose. Rare cases of anaphylactoid reactions have been reported in patients undergoing sensitization treatment with hymenoptera (bee, wasp) venom while receiving ACE inhibitors.

Symptomatic hypotension with or without syncope can occur with ACE inhibitors (usually with the first several doses); effects are most often observed in volume depleted patients; correct volume depletion prior to initiation; close monitoring of patient is required especially with initial dosing and dosing increases; blood pressure must be lowered at a rate appropriate for the patient's clinical condition. Initiation of therapy in patients with ischemic heart disease or cerebrovascular disease warrants close observation due to the potential consequences posed by falling blood pressure (eg, MI, stroke). Use with caution in hypertrophic cardiomyopathy with outflow tract obstruction, severe aortic stenosis, or before, during, or immediately after major surgery. **[U.S. Boxed Warning]: Drugs that act on the renin-angiotensin system can cause injury and death to the developing fetus. Discontinue as soon as possible once pregnancy is detected.**

Hyperkalemia may occur with ACE inhibitors; risk factors include renal dysfunction, diabetes mellitus, concomitant use of potassium-sparing diuretics, potassium supplements, and/or potassium-containing salts. Use cautiously, if at all, with these agents and monitor potassium closely. Cough may occur with ACE inhibitors. Other causes of cough should be considered (eg, pulmonary congestion in patients with heart failure) and excluded prior to discontinuation.

May be associated with deterioration of renal function and/or increases in serum creatinine, particularly in patients with low renal blood flow (eg, renal artery stenosis, heart failure) whose glomerular filtration rate (GFR) is dependent on efferent arteriolar vasoconstriction by angiotensin II; deterioration may result in oliguria, acute renal failure, and progressive azotemia. Small increases in serum creatinine may occur following initiation; consider discontinuation only in patients with progressive and/or significant deterioration in renal function. Use with caution in patients with unstented unilateral/bilateral renal artery stenosis. When unstented bilateral renal artery stenosis is present, use is generally avoided due to the elevated risk of deterioration in renal function unless possible benefits outweigh risks.

Concomitant use of an angiotensin receptor blocker (ARB) or renin inhibitor (eg, aliskiren) is associated with an increased risk of hypotension, hyperkalemia, and renal dysfunction; concomitant use with aliskiren should be avoided in patients with GFR <60 mL/minute and is contraindicated in patients with diabetes mellitus (regardless of GFR).

Rare toxicities associated with ACE inhibitors include cholestatic jaundice (which may progress to fulminant hepatic necrosis), agranulocytosis, neutropenia, or leukopenia with myeloid hypoplasia. Patients with collagen vascular diseases (especially with concomitant renal impairment) or renal impairment alone may be at increased risk for hematologic toxicity; periodically monitor CBC with differential in these patients. Safety and efficacy have not been established in children <6 years of age or children with a Cl_{cr} ≤30 mL/minute.

Drug Interactions
Metabolism/Transport Effects None known.

Avoid Concomitant Use There are no known interactions where it is recommended to avoid concomitant use.

Increased Effect/Toxicity
Lisinopril may increase the levels/effects of: Allopurinol; Amifostine; Antihypertensives; AzaTHIOprine; CycloSPORINE (Systemic); Ferric Gluconate; Gold Sodium Thiomalate; Hypotensive Agents; Iron Dextran Complex; Lithium; Nonsteroidal Anti-Inflammatory Agents; RiTUXimab; Sodium Phosphates

The levels/effects of Lisinopril may be increased by: Alfuzosin; Amifostine; Aliskiren; Angiotensin II Receptor Blockers; Canagliflozin; Diazoxide; DPP-IV Inhibitors; Eplerenone; Everolimus; Herbs (Hypotensive Properties); Loop Diuretics; MAO Inhibitors; Pentoxifylline; Phosphodiesterase 5 Inhibitors; Potassium Salts; Potassium-Sparing Diuretics; Prostacyclin Analogues; Sirolimus; Temsirolimus; Thiazide Diuretics; TiZANidine; Tolvaptan; Trimethoprim

Decreased Effect
The levels/effects of Lisinopril may be decreased by: Antacids; Aprotinin; Herbs (Hypertensive Properties); Icatibant; Lanthanum; Methylphenidate; Nonsteroidal Anti-Inflammatory Agents; Salicylates; Yohimbine

Ethanol/Nutrition/Herb Interactions
Food: Potassium supplements and/or potassium-containing salts may cause or worsen hyperkalemia. Management: Consult prescriber before consuming a potassium-rich diet, potassium supplements, or salt substitutes.

Herb/Nutraceutical: Some herbal medications may worsen hypertension (eg, licorice); others may increase the antihypertensive effect of lisinopril (eg, shepherd's purse). Management: Avoid bayberry, blue cohosh, cayenne, ephedra, ginger, ginseng (American), kola, licorice, and yohimbe. Avoid black cohosh, California poppy, coleus, golden seal, hawthorn, mistletoe, periwinkle, quinine, and shepherd's purse.

Dietary Considerations
Use potassium-containing salt substitutes cautiously in patients with diabetes, patients with renal dysfunction, or those maintained on potassium supplements or potassium-sparing diuretics.

Pharmacodynamics/Kinetics
Onset of Action 1 hour; Peak effect: Hypotensive: Oral: ~6 hours

Duration of Action 24 hours

Half-life Elimination 11-12 hours

Time to Peak ~7 hours

Pregnancy Risk Factor D

Pregnancy Considerations [U.S. Boxed Warning]: Drugs that act on the renin-angiotensin system can cause injury and death to the developing fetus. Discontinue as soon as possible once pregnancy is detected. Lisinopril crosses the placenta; teratogenic effects may occur following maternal use during pregnancy. Drugs that act on the renin-angiotensin system are associated with oligohydramnios. Oligohydramnios, due to decreased fetal renal function, may lead to fetal lung hypoplasia and skeletal malformations. Their use in pregnancy is also associated with anuria, hypotension, renal failure, skull hypoplasia, and death in the fetus/neonate. Chronic maternal hypertension itself is also associated with adverse events in the fetus/infant. ACE inhibitors are not recommended during pregnancy to treat maternal hypertension or heart failure. Use of an ACE inhibitor should also be avoided in any woman of reproductive age. Women who are planning a pregnancy should be considered for other medication options if an ACE inhibitor is currently prescribed or the ACE inhibitor should be discontinued as soon as possible once pregnancy is detected. The exposed fetus should be monitored for fetal growth, amniotic fluid volume, and organ formation. Infants exposed to an ACE inhibitor *in utero* should be monitored for hyperkalemia, hypotension, and oliguria.

Lactation Excretion in breast milk unknown/not recommended

Breast-Feeding Considerations It is not known if lisinopril is excreted in breast milk. Breast-feeding is not recommended by the manufacturer.

Dosage Forms
Tablet, oral: 2.5 mg, 5 mg, 10 mg, 20 mg, 30 mg, 40 mg
Prinivil®: 5 mg, 10 mg, 20 mg
Zestril®: 2.5 mg, 5 mg, 10 mg, 20 mg, 30 mg, 40 mg

Lisinopril and Hydrochlorothiazide
(lyse IN oh pril & hye droe klor oh THYE a zide)

Related Information
Hydrochlorothiazide *on page 687*
Lisinopril *on page 830*

Brand Names: U.S. Prinzide®; Zestoretic®

Brand Names: Canada Apo-Lisinopril®/Hctz; Mylan-Lisinopril/Hctz; Novo-Lisinopril/Hctz; Prinzide®; Sandoz-Lisinopril/Hctz; Teva-Lisinopril/Hctz (Type P); Teva-Lisinopril/Hctz (Type Z); Zestoretic®

Pharmacologic Category Angiotensin-Converting Enzyme (ACE) Inhibitor; Diuretic, Thiazide

Use Treatment of hypertension

Local Anesthetic/Vasoconstrictor Precautions No information available to require special precautions

Effects on Dental Treatment No significant effects or complications reported

Effects on Bleeding No information available to require special precautions

Adverse Effects See individual agents.

General Dosage Range Oral: *Adults:* Lisinopril 10-80 mg and hydrochlorothiazide 12.5-50 mg once daily

Pregnancy Risk Factor D

Pregnancy Considerations [U.S. Boxed Warning]: Drugs that act on the renin-angiotensin system can cause injury and death to the developing fetus. Discontinue as soon as possible once pregnancy is detected. See individual agents.

Lithium (LITH ee um)

Brand Names: U.S. Lithobid®

Brand Names: Canada Apo-Lithium® Carbonate; Apo-Lithium® Carbonate SR; Carbolith™; Duralith®; Euro-Lithium; Lithane™; Lithmax; PHL-Lithium Carbonate; PMS-Lithium Carbonate; PMS-Lithium Citrate

Generic Availability (U.S.) Yes

Pharmacologic Category Antimanic Agent

Use Management of bipolar disorders; treatment of mania in individuals with bipolar disorder (maintenance treatment prevents or diminishes intensity of subsequent episodes)

Unlabeled Use Potential augmenting agent for antidepressants; aggression, post-traumatic stress disorder, conduct disorder in children

Local Anesthetic/Vasoconstrictor Precautions No information available to require special precautions

Effects on Dental Treatment Key adverse event(s) related to dental treatment: Xerostomia and changes in salivation (normal salivary flow resumes upon discontinuation), salivary gland swelling, and metallic taste. Avoid NSAIDs if analgesics are required since lithium toxicity has been reported with concomitant administration; acetaminophen products (ie, singly or with opioids) are recommended.

Effects on Bleeding No information available to require special precautions

Adverse Effects Frequency not defined.

Cardiovascular: Cardiac arrhythmia, hypotension, sinus node dysfunction, flattened or inverted T waves (reversible), edema, bradycardia, syncope

Central nervous system: Blackout spells, coma, confusion, dizziness, dystonia, fatigue, headache, lethargy, pseudotumor cerebri, psychomotor retardation, restlessness, sedation, seizure, slowed intellectual functioning, slurred speech, stupor, tics, vertigo

Dermatologic: Dry or thinning of hair, folliculitis, alopecia, exacerbation of psoriasis, rash

Endocrine & metabolic: Euthyroid goiter and/or hypothyroidism, hyperthyroidism, hyperglycemia, diabetes insipidus

Gastrointestinal: Polydipsia, anorexia, nausea, vomiting, diarrhea, xerostomia, metallic taste, weight gain, salivary gland swelling, excessive salivation

Genitourinary: Incontinence, polyuria, glycosuria, oliguria, albuminuria

Hematologic: Leukocytosis

Neuromuscular & skeletal: Tremor, muscle hyperirritability, ataxia, choreoathetoid movements, hyperactive deep tendon reflexes, myasthenia gravis (rare)

Ocular: Nystagmus, blurred vision, transient scotoma

Miscellaneous: Coldness and painful discoloration of fingers and toes

Postmarketing and/or case reports: Drug-induced Brugada syndrome

Dosage Oral: **Note:** Monitor serum concentrations and clinical response (efficacy and toxicity) to determine proper dose. Each 5 mL of lithium citrate oral solution contains 8 mEq of lithium ion, equivalent to the amount of lithium in 300 mg of lithium carbonate immediate release capsules/tablets.

Children 6-12 years:

Bipolar disorder (unlabeled use): 15-60 mg/kg/day in 3-4 divided doses; dose not to exceed usual adult dosage

Conduct disorder (unlabeled use): 15-30 mg/kg/day in 3-4 divided doses; dose not to exceed usual adult dosage

Adults: Bipolar disorder: 900-2400 mg/day in 3-4 divided doses or 900-1800 mg/day (extended release) in 2 divided doses

Elderly: Bipolar disorder: Initial dose: 300 mg once or twice daily; increase weekly in increments of 300 mg/day, monitoring levels; rarely need >900-1200 mg/day

Dosage adjustment in renal impairment:

Cl_{cr} 10-50 mL/minute: Administer 50% to 75% of normal dose

Cl_{cr} <10 mL/minute: Administer 25% to 50% of normal dose

Hemodialysis: Dialyzable (50% to 100%); 4-7 times more efficient than peritoneal dialysis

Dosage adjustment in hepatic impairment: No dosage adjustment provided in manufacturer's labeling.

Mechanism of Action Alters cation transport across cell membrane in nerve and muscle cells and influences reuptake of serotonin and/or norepinephrine; second messenger systems involving the phosphatidylinositol cycle are inhibited; postsynaptic D2 receptor supersensitivity is inhibited

Contraindications Hypersensitivity to lithium or any component of the formulation; avoid use in patients with severe cardiovascular or renal disease, or with severe debilitation, dehydration, or sodium depletion

Warnings/Precautions [U.S. Boxed Warning]: Lithium toxicity is closely related to serum levels and can occur at therapeutic doses; serum lithium determinations are required to monitor therapy. Use with caution in patients with thyroid disease, mild-moderate renal impairment, or mild-moderate cardiovascular disease. Use caution in patients receiving medications which alter sodium excretion (eg, diuretics, ACE inhibitors, NSAIDs), or in patients with significant fluid loss (protracted sweating, diarrhea, or prolonged fever); temporary reduction or cessation of therapy may be warranted. Some elderly patients may be extremely sensitive to the effects of lithium, see Dosage. Chronic therapy results in diminished renal concentrating ability (nephrogenic DI); this is usually reversible when lithium is discontinued. Changes in renal function should be monitored, and re-evaluation of treatment may be necessary. Use caution in patients at risk of suicide (suicidal thoughts or behavior).

Use with caution in patients receiving neuroleptic medications - a syndrome resembling NMS has been associated with concurrent therapy. Lithium may impair the patient's alertness, affecting the ability to operate machinery or driving a vehicle. Neuromuscular-blocking agents should be administered with caution; the response may be prolonged.

Higher serum concentrations may be required and tolerated during an acute manic phase; however, the tolerance decreases when symptoms subside. Normal fluid and salt intake must be maintained during therapy.

Drug Interactions

Metabolism/Transport Effects None known.

Avoid Concomitant Use There are no known interactions where it is recommended to avoid concomitant use.

Increased Effect/Toxicity

Lithium may increase the levels/effects of: Antipsychotics; Highest Risk QTc-Prolonging Agents; Metoclopramide; Moderate Risk QTc-Prolonging Agents; Neuromuscular-Blocking Agents; Selective Serotonin Reuptake Inhibitors; Serotonin Modulators; Tricyclic Antidepressants

The levels/effects of Lithium may be increased by: ACE Inhibitors; Angiotensin II Receptor Blockers; Antipsychotics; Calcium Channel Blockers (Nondihydropyridine); CarBAMazepine; Desmopressin; Eplerenone; Fosphenytoin; Loop Diuretics; MAO Inhibitors; Methyldopa; Mifepristone; Nonsteroidal Anti-Inflammatory Agents; Phenytoin; Potassium Iodide; Thiazide Diuretics; Topiramate

Decreased Effect

Lithium may decrease the levels/effects of: Amphetamines; Antipsychotics; Desmopressin

The levels/effects of Lithium may be decreased by: Calcitonin; Calcium Polystyrene Sulfonate; Carbonic Anhydrase Inhibitors; Loop Diuretics; Sodium Bicarbonate; Sodium Chloride; Sodium Polystyrene Sulfonate; Theophylline Derivatives

Ethanol/Nutrition/Herb Interactions Food: Limit caffeine.

Dietary Considerations May be taken with meals to avoid GI upset; maintain adequate fluid intake.

Pharmacodynamics/Kinetics

Half-life Elimination 18-24 hours; can increase to more than 36 hours in elderly or with renal impairment

Time to Peak Serum: Nonsustained release: ~0.5-2 hours; extended release: 4-12 hours; syrup: 15-60 minutes

Pregnancy Risk Factor D

Pregnancy Considerations Adverse events have been observed in animal reproduction studies. Lithium crosses the placenta in concentrations similar to those in the maternal plasma (Newport, 2005). Cardiac malformations in the infant, including Ebstein's anomaly, are associated with use of lithium during the first trimester of pregnancy. Other adverse events including polyhydramnios, fetal/neonatal cardiac arrhythmias, hypoglycemia, diabetes insipidus, changes in thyroid function, premature delivery, floppy infant syndrome, or neonatal lithium toxicity are associated with lithium exposure when used later in pregnancy (ACOG, 2008). The incidence of adverse events may be associated with higher maternal doses (Newport, 2005).

Due to pregnancy-induced physiologic changes, women who are pregnant may require dose adjustments of lithium to achieve euthymia and avoid toxicity (ACOG, 2008; Grandjean, 2009; Yonkers, 2011).

For planned pregnancies, use of lithium during the first trimester should be avoided if possible (Grandjean, 2009). If lithium is needed during pregnancy, the minimum effective dose should be used, maternal serum concentrations should be monitored, and consideration should be given to start therapy after the period of organogenesis; lithium should be suspended 24-48 hours prior to delivery or at the onset of labor when delivery is spontaneous, then restarted when the patient is medically stable after delivery (ACOG, 2008; Grandjean, 2009; Newport, 2005). Fetal echocardiography should be considered if first trimester exposure occurs (ACOG, 2008).

Lactation Enters breast milk/not recommended

Breast-Feeding Considerations Lithium is excreted into breast milk and serum concentrations of nursing infants may be 10% to 50% of the maternal serum concentration (Grandjean, 2009). Hypotonia, hypothermia, cyanosis, electrocardiogram changes, and lethargy have been reported in nursing infants (ACOG, 2008). It is generally recommended that breast-feeding be avoided during maternal use of lithium; however, treatment may be continued in appropriately selected patients (Grandjean, 2009; Sharma, 2009; Viguera, 2007). The hydration status of the nursing infant and maternal serum concentrations of lithium should be monitored (ACOG, 2008). In addition, monitor the infant for lethargy, growth, and feeding problems; obtain infant serum concentrations only if clinical concerns arise (Bogen, 2012; Yonkers, 2011). Long-term effects on development and behavior have not been studied (ACOG, 2008; Grandjean, 2009).

Dosage Forms

Capsule, oral: 150 mg, 300 mg, 600 mg
Solution, oral: 8 mEq/5 mL (5 mL, 500 mL)
Tablet, oral: 300 mg, 600 mg
Tablet, extended release, oral: 300 mg, 450 mg
Lithobid®: 300 mg

L-Lysine (el LYE seen)

Related Information

Viral Infections *on page 1575*

Brand Names: U.S. Lysinyl [OTC]

Generic Availability (U.S.) Yes

Pharmacologic Category Nutritional Supplement

Dental Use Prevention of recurrent herpes simplex infection

Use Improves utilization of vegetable proteins; prevention of recurrent herpes simplex infection

Local Anesthetic/Vasoconstrictor Precautions No information available to require special precautions

Effects on Dental Treatment No significant effects or complications reported

Effects on Bleeding No information available to require special precautions

Dental Usual Dosage Recurrent herpes simplex infection: Adults: Oral: 500-3000 mg/day; begin treatment during early stage of recurrence.

Dosage Oral: Adults:
Supplement: 334-1500 mg/day
Prevention of recurrent herpes simplex infection: 500-3000 mg/day; begin treatment during early stage of recurrence

Pregnancy Considerations L-lysine crosses the placenta in humans (Ronzoni, 1999; Schneider, 1979). Lysine is an essential amino acid. The RDA for lysine is increased in pregnant women (IOM, 2005).

Breast-Feeding Considerations Lysine is an essential amino acid and is found in breast milk. The RDA for lysine is increased in breast-feeding women (IOM, 2005).

Dosage Forms

Capsule, oral: 500 mg
Lysinyl [OTC]: 500 mg
Powder, oral: (100 g)
Lysinyl [OTC]: (150 g)
Tablet, oral: 500 mg, 1000 mg

References

Griffith RS, Walsh DE, Myrmel KH, et al, "Success of L-Lysine Therapy in Frequently Recurrent Herpes Simplex Infection. Treatment and Prophylaxis," *Dermatologica*, 1987, 175(4):183-90.
"L-lysine," *Altern Med Rev*, 2007, 12(2):169-72.

Lodoxamide (loe DOKS a mide)

Brand Names: U.S. Alomide®
Brand Names: Canada Alomide®
Pharmacologic Category Mast Cell Stabilizer
Use Treatment of vernal keratoconjunctivitis, vernal conjunctivitis, and vernal keratitis
Local Anesthetic/Vasoconstrictor Precautions No information available to require special precautions
Effects on Dental Treatment No significant effects or complications reported
Effects on Bleeding No information available to require special precautions
Adverse Effects
>10%: Local: Transient burning, stinging, discomfort
1% to 10%:
Central nervous system: Headache
Ocular: Blurred vision, crystalline deposits, dry eye, edema, foreign body sensation, hyperemia, itching, tearing
General Dosage Range Ophthalmic: *Children >2 years and Adults:* Instill 1-2 drops in eye(s) 4 times/day
Mechanism of Action Mast cell stabilizer that inhibits the *in vivo* type I immediate hypersensitivity reaction to increase cutaneous vascular permeability associated with IgE and antigen-mediated reactions
Pregnancy Risk Factor B
Pregnancy Considerations No adverse events were observed in animal reproduction studies following oral administration. The amount of lodoxamide available systemically following ophthalmic administration is below the level of detection.

Lomitapide (loe MI ta pide)

Related Information
Cardiovascular Diseases *on page 1492*
Brand Names: U.S. Juxtapid™
Pharmacologic Category Antilipemic Agent, Microsomal Triglyceride Transfer Protein (MTP) Inhibitor
Use Adjunct to dietary therapy and other lipid-lowering treatments, including LDL apheresis where available, to reduce low-density lipoprotein cholesterol (LDL-C), total cholesterol, apolipoprotein B, and non-high-density lipoprotein cholesterol (non-HDL-C) in patients with homozygous familial hypercholesterolemia (HoFH)
Local Anesthetic/Vasoconstrictor Precautions No information available to require special precautions
Effects on Dental Treatment Key adverse event(s) related to dental treatment: Nasal congestion, nasopharyngitis, and pharyngolaryngeal pain
Effects on Bleeding No information available to require special precautions
Adverse Effects
>10%:
Cardiovascular: Chest pain (24%)
Central nervous system: Fatigue (17%)
Gastrointestinal: Diarrhea (79%; severe: 14%), nausea (65%), dyspepsia (38%), vomiting (34%; severe: 10%), abdominal pain (34%; severe: 7%), weight loss (24%), abdominal discomfort (21%; severe: 7%), abdominal distension (21%; severe: 7%), constipation (21%), flatulence (21%), gastroenteritis (14%)
Hepatic: Hepatic steatosis (increase in hepatic fat >5%: 78%; >20% fat increase: 13%), ALT increased (17%; severe: 10%), ALT and/or AST ≥3 times upper limit of normal (34%)
Neuromuscular & skeletal: Back pain (14%)

Respiratory: Nasopharyngitis (17%), pharyngolaryngeal pain (14%)
Miscellaneous: Influenza (21%)
1% to 10%:
Cardiovascular: Angina pectoris (10%), palpitation (10%)
Central nervous system: Dizziness (10%), fever (10%), headache (10%)
Gastrointestinal: Defecation urgency (10%), gastroesophageal reflux disease (10%), rectal tenesmus (10%)
Hepatic: Hepatotoxicity (severe: 10%)
Respiratory: Nasal congestion (10%)
General Dosage Range Dosage adjustment recommended in patients on concomitant therapy, with renal or hepatic impairment, or who develop toxicities.
Oral: *Adults:* 5-60 mg once daily
Mechanism of Action Lomitapide directly binds to and inhibits microsomal triglyceride transfer protein (MTP) which is located in the lumen of the endoplasmic reticulum. MTP inhibition prevents the assembly of apo-B containing lipoproteins in enterocytes and hepatocytes resulting in reduced production of chylomicrons and VLDL and subsequently reduces plasma LDL-C concentrations.
Pharmacodynamics/Kinetics
Half-life Elimination 39.7 hours
Time to Peak ~6 hours
Pregnancy Risk Factor X
Pregnancy Considerations Teratogenic effects have been observed in animal reproduction studies using doses lower than equivalent human doses. Use is contraindicated in pregnant women. Discontinue immediately if pregnancy occurs during treatment. Women of reproductive potential should have a negative pregnancy test prior to therapy and effective contraception must be used during treatment. Dose adjustment may be required for women using oral contraceptives.
Prescribing and Access Restrictions As a requirement of the REMS program, access to this medication is restricted. Prescribers must enroll in the Juxtapid™ REMS program and complete the Prescriber Training Module and complete, sign, and submit the Prescriber Enrollment Form to the Juxtapid™ REMS program. Pharmacies must educate all pharmacy staff involved in the dispensing of Juxtapid™ on the REMS program requirements, put processes in place to verify (prior to dispensing Juxtapid™) that the prescriber is certified and the Prescription Authorization Form is received with each new prescription. Pharmacies must also agree to be audited to ensure that all processes and procedures in place are being followed in accordance with the program and be able to provide prescription data to the REMS program.

Lomustine (loe MUS teen)

Brand Names: U.S. CeeNU®
Brand Names: Canada CeeNU®
Pharmacologic Category Antineoplastic Agent; Antineoplastic Agent, Alkylating Agent; Antineoplastic Agent, Alkylating Agent (Nitrosourea)
Use Treatment of primary and metastatic brain tumors (after surgery and/or radiation therapy); treatment of relapsed or refractory Hodgkin's disease (as part of a combination chemotherapy regimen)
Unlabeled Use Treatment of gastric cancer, metastatic melanoma

◀ Local Anesthetic/Vasoconstrictor Precautions No information available to require special precautions

Effects on Dental Treatment No significant effects or complications reported

Effects on Bleeding Delayed and cumulative myelo-suppression is the major adverse effect and includes thrombocytopenia and anemia. Medical consult recommended.

Adverse Effects
>10%:
Gastrointestinal: Nausea and vomiting, (onset: 3-6 hours after oral administration; duration: <24 hours)
Hematologic: Myelosuppression (dose-limiting, delayed, cumulative); leukopenia (65%; nadir: 5-6 weeks; recovery 6-8 weeks); thrombocytopenia (nadir: 4 weeks; recovery 5-6 weeks)
Frequency not defined: Acute leukemia, alkaline phosphatase increased, alopecia, anemia, ataxia, azotemia (progressive), bilirubin increased, blindness, bone marrow dysplasia, disorientation, dysarthria, hepatotoxicity, kidney size decreased, lethargy, optic atrophy, pulmonary fibrosis, pulmonary infiltrates, renal damage, renal failure, stomatitis, transaminases increased, visual disturbances

General Dosage Range Dosage adjustment recommended in patients with renal impairment or who develop toxicities
Oral: *Children and Adults:* 100-130 mg/m^2 as a single dose once every 6 weeks

Mechanism of Action Inhibits DNA and RNA synthesis via carbamylation of DNA polymerase, alkylation of DNA, and alteration of RNA, proteins, and enzymes

Pharmacodynamics/Kinetics
Duration of Action Marrow recovery: ~5-8 weeks
Half-life Elimination Parent drug: 16-24 hours; Active metabolite: 16-48 hours
Time to Peak Serum: Active metabolite: ~3 hours
Pregnancy Risk Factor D
Pregnancy Considerations Teratogenic effects and embryotoxicity have been observed in animal studies. There are no adequate and well-controlled studies in pregnant women. May cause fetal harm when administered to a pregnant woman. Women of childbearing potential should be advised to avoid pregnancy and should be advised of the potential harm to the fetus.

Loperamide (loe PER a mide)

Brand Names: U.S. Anti-Diarrheal [OTC]; Diamode [OTC]; Imodium® A-D EZ Chews [OTC]; Imodium® A-D for children [OTC]; Imodium® A-D [OTC]
Brand Names: Canada Apo-Loperamide®; Diarr-Eze; Dom-Loperamide; Imodium®; Loperacap; Novo-Loperamide; PMS-Loperamine; Rhoxal-loperamide; Rho®-Loperamine; Riva-Loperamide; Sandoz-Loperamide
Pharmacologic Category Antidiarrheal
Use Control and symptomatic relief of chronic diarrhea associated with inflammatory bowel disease and of acute nonspecific diarrhea; to reduce volume of ileostomy discharge
OTC labeling: Control of symptoms of diarrhea, including Traveler's diarrhea
Unlabeled Use Cancer treatment-induced diarrhea (eg, irinotecan induced); chronic diarrhea caused by bowel resection

Local Anesthetic/Vasoconstrictor Precautions No information available to require special precautions

Effects on Dental Treatment No significant effects or complications reported

Effects on Bleeding No information available to require special precautions

Adverse Effects 1% to 10%:
Central nervous system: Dizziness (1%)
Gastrointestinal: Constipation (2% to 5%), abdominal cramping (≤3%), nausea (≤3%)
Postmarketing and/or case reports: Abdominal distention, abdominal pain, allergic reactions, anaphylactic shock, anaphylactoid reactions, angioedema, bullous eruption (rare), drowsiness, dyspepsia, erythema multiforme (rare), fatigue, flatulence, hypersensitivity, paralytic ileus, megacolon, pruritus, rash, Stevens-Johnson syndrome (rare), toxic epidermal necrolysis (rare), toxic megacolon, urinary retention, urticaria, vomiting, xerostomia

General Dosage Range Oral:
Children 2-5 years (13-20 kg): Initial: 1 mg 3 times/day for first 24 hours; Maintenance: 0.1 mg/kg after each loose stool
Children 6-8 years (20-30 kg): Initial: 2 mg twice daily for first 24 hours; Maintenance: 0.1 mg/kg after each loose stool or 2 mg after first loose stool, followed by 1 mg after each subsequent stool (maximum: 4 mg/day)
Children 8-12 years (>30 kg): Initial: 2 mg 3 times/day for first 24 hours; Maintenance: 0.1 mg/kg after each loose stool
Children 9-11 years: 2 mg after first loose stool, followed by 1 mg after each subsequent stool (maximum: 6 mg/day)
Children ≥12 years: Initial: 4 mg after first loose stool, followed by 2 mg after each subsequent stool (maximum: 8 mg/day)
Adults: Initial: 4 mg followed by 2 mg after each loose stool (maximum: 8-16 mg/day) or 4-8 mg/day in divided doses

Mechanism of Action Acts directly on circular and longitudinal intestinal muscles, through the opioid receptor, to inhibit peristalsis and prolong transit time; reduces fecal volume, increases viscosity, and diminishes fluid and electrolyte loss; demonstrates antisecretory activity. Loperamide increases tone on the anal sphincter

Pharmacodynamics/Kinetics
Half-life Elimination 9-14 hours
Time to Peak Liquid: 2.5 hours; Capsule: 5 hours
Pregnancy Risk Factor C
Pregnancy Considerations Teratogenic effects were not observed in animal reproduction studies. Information related to loperamide use in pregnancy is limited and data is conflicting (Einarson, 2000; Källén, 2008). For acute diarrhea in pregnant women, some clinicians recommend oral rehydration and dietary changes; loperamide in small amounts may be used only if symptoms are disabling (Wald, 2003).

Loperamide and Simethicone
(loe PER a mide & sye METH i kone)

Related Information
Loperamide *on page 836*
Simethicone *on page 1236*
Brand Names: U.S. Imodium® Multi-Symptom Relief [OTC]
Brand Names: Canada Imodium® Advanced Multi-Symptom
Pharmacologic Category Antidiarrheal; Antiflatulent
Use Control of symptoms of diarrhea and gas (bloating, pressure, and cramps)

Local Anesthetic/Vasoconstrictor Precautions No information available to require special precautions

Effects on Dental Treatment No significant effects or complications reported

Effects on Bleeding No information available to require special precautions

Adverse Effects See individual agents.

General Dosage Range Oral:
Children 6-8 years (48-59 lbs): 1 caplet/tablet after first loose stool, followed by 1/2 caplet/tablet with each subsequent loose stool (maximum: 2 caplets or tablets/24 hours)
Children 9-11 years (60-95 lbs): 1 caplet/tablet after first loose stool, followed by 1/2 caplet/tablet with each subsequent loose stool (maximum: 3 caplets or tablets/24 hours)
Children ≥12 years and Adults: 1 caplet/tablet after each loose stool (maximum: 4 caplets or tablets/24 hours)

Mechanism of Action
Loperamide acts by slowing intestinal motility and by affecting water and electrolyte movement through the bowel.

Simethicone acts in the stomach and intestines by altering the surface tension of gas bubbles enabling them to coalesce thereby freeing and eliminating the gas more easily by belching or passing flatus.

Pregnancy Considerations See individual agents.

Lopinavir and Ritonavir
(loe PIN a veer & rit ON uh veer)

Related Information
HIV Infection and AIDS *on page 1520*
Ritonavir *on page 1204*
Brand Names: U.S. Kaletra®
Brand Names: Canada Kaletra®
Pharmacologic Category Antiretroviral Agent, Protease Inhibitor
Use Treatment of HIV infection in combination with other antiretroviral agents

Local Anesthetic/Vasoconstrictor Precautions No information available to require special precautions

Effects on Dental Treatment Key adverse event(s) related to dental treatment: Dysphagia.

Effects on Bleeding Increased bleeding has been reported in HIV-infected patients with hemophilia (types A and B). Pediatric patients (4%) reported thrombocytopenia and less than 2% of adults reported anemia.

Adverse Effects Data presented for short- and long-term combination antiretroviral therapy in both protease inhibitor experienced and naïve patients.

>10%:
Dermatologic: Rash (children 12%; adults ≤5%)
Endocrine & metabolic: Hypercholesterolemia (3% to 39%), triglycerides increased (3% to 36%)
Gastrointestinal: Diarrhea (7% to 28%; greater with once-daily dosing), abnormal taste/taste perversion (children 22%; adults <2%), vomiting (children 21%; adults 2% to 6%), nausea (5% to 16%), abdominal pain (1% to 11%)
Hepatic: GGT increased (10% to 29%), ALT increased (grade 3/4: 1% to 11%)
>2% to 10%:
Cardiovascular: Vasodilation (≤3%)
Central nervous system: Headache (2% to 6%), insomnia (≤3%)

Endocrine & metabolic: Hyperglycemia (≤5%), hyperuricemia (≤5%), sodium decreased or increased (children 3%)
Gastrointestinal: Amylase increased (3% to 8%), dyspepsia (≤6%), lipase increased (3% to 5%), flatulence (1% to 4%), weight loss (≤3%)
Hematologic: Platelets decreased (grade 3/4: 4% children), neutropenia (grade 3/4: 1% to 5%)
Hepatic: AST increased (grade 3/4: 2% to 10%), bilirubin increased (children 3%; adults 1%)
Neuromuscular & skeletal: Weakness (≤9%)

General Dosage Range Dosage adjustment recommended in patients on concomitant therapy
Oral:
Children 14 days to 6 months: Lopinavir 16 mg/kg or 300 mg/m² twice daily
Children 6 months to 18 years and <15 kg: 12 mg lopinavir/kg twice daily (maximum dose: Lopinavir 400 mg/ritonavir 100 mg)
Children 6 months to 18 years and 15-40 kg: 10 mg lopinavir/kg twice daily (maximum dose: Lopinavir 400 mg/ritonavir 100 mg)
Children 6 months to 18 years and >40 kg: Lopinavir 400 mg/ritonavir 100 mg twice daily
Adults: Lopinavir 400 mg/ritonavir 100 mg twice daily **or** lopinavir 800 mg/ritonavir 200 mg once daily

Mechanism of Action A coformulation of lopinavir and ritonavir. The lopinavir component binds to the site of HIV-1 protease activity and inhibits the cleavage of viral Gag-Pol polyprotein precursors into individual functional proteins required for infectious HIV. This results in the formation of immature, noninfectious viral particles. The ritonavir component inhibits the CYP3A metabolism of lopinavir, allowing increased plasma levels of lopinavir.

Pharmacodynamics/Kinetics
Half-life Elimination Lopinavir: 5-6 hours
Time to Peak Lopinavir: ~4 hours
Pregnancy Risk Factor C

Pregnancy Considerations Adverse events were not seen in animal reproduction studies, except at doses which were also maternally toxic. Lopinavir/ritonavir crosses the placenta; however, based on information collected by the Antiretroviral Pregnancy Registry, an increased risk of teratogenic effects has not been observed in humans. The DHHS Perinatal HIV Guidelines consider lopinavir/ritonavir to be the preferred protease inhibitor for use in antiretroviral-naive pregnant women. Due to a decrease in bioavailability, a dose increase is suggested during the second and third trimesters of pregnancy, especially in PI-experienced women. Monitor virologic response (and lopinavir serum concentrations if available) if the standard dose is used. Once-daily dosing is not recommended during pregnancy. A small increased risk of preterm birth has been associated with maternal use of protease inhibitor-based combination antiretroviral (ARV) therapy during pregnancy; however, the benefits of use generally outweigh this risk and protease inhibitors (PIs) should not be withheld if otherwise recommended. Hyperglycemia, new onset of diabetes mellitus, or diabetic ketoacidosis have been reported with PIs; it is not clear if pregnancy increases this risk.

Regardless of CD4 count or HIV RNA copy number, all HIV-infected pregnant women should receive a combination antepartum ARV drug regimen; this includes women who require therapy for their own health, as well as women who do not yet require therapy for their own health. ARV therapy should be started as soon as possible if required for the woman's health. Although earlier initiation may be more effective in reducing the perinatal transmission of HIV, also consider maternal conditions (eg, nausea and vomiting) and the potential risks of first trimester fetal exposure for specific agents. Plasma HIV RNA levels should be assessed at ~34-36 weeks gestation in order to help determine mode of delivery. If ARV therapy must be interrupted for <24 hours during the peripartum period, stop then restart all medications simultaneously in order to decrease the chance of developing resistance. Long-term follow-up is recommended for all infants exposed to ARV medications.

Healthcare providers are encouraged to enroll pregnant women exposed to antiretroviral medications in the Antiretroviral Pregnancy Registry (1-800-258-4263 or www.APRegistry.com). Healthcare providers caring for HIV-infected women and their infants may contact the National Perinatal HIV Hotline (888-448-8765) for clinical consultation (DHHS [perinatal], 2012).

Loratadine (lor AT a deen)

Brand Names: U.S. Alavert® Allergy 24 Hour [OTC]; Alavert® Children's Allergy [OTC]; Claritin® 24 Hour Allergy [OTC]; Claritin® Children's Allergy [OTC]; Claritin® Liqui-Gels® 24 Hour Allergy [OTC]; Claritin® Redi-Tabs® 24 Hour Allergy [OTC]; Loradamed [OTC]

Brand Names: Canada Apo-Loratadine®; Claritin®; Claritin® Kids

Pharmacologic Category Histamine H$_1$ Antagonist; Histamine H$_1$ Antagonist, Second Generation; Piperidine Derivative

Use Relief of nasal and non-nasal symptoms of seasonal allergic rhinitis; treatment of chronic idiopathic urticaria

Local Anesthetic/Vasoconstrictor Precautions No information available to require special precautions

Effects on Dental Treatment Key adverse event(s) related to dental treatment: Xerostomia (normal salivary flow resumes upon discontinuation) and stomatitis in children (2-5 years).

Effects on Bleeding No information available to require special precautions

Adverse Effects

Central nervous system: Headache (12% adults), somnolence (8% adults), nervousness (4% ages 6-12 years), fatigue (4% adults; 3% ages 6-12 years, 2% to 3% ages 2-5 years), malaise (2% ages 6-12 years)

Dermatologic: Rash (2% to 3% ages 2-5 years)

Gastrointestinal: Xerostomia (3% adults), stomatitis (2% to 3% ages 2-5 years), abdominal pain (2% ages 2-5 years)

Neuromuscular & skeletal: Hyperkinesia (3% ages 6-12 years)

Ocular: Conjunctivitis (2% ages 6-12 years)

Respiratory: Wheezing (4% ages 6-12 years), epistaxis (2% to 3% ages 2-5 years), pharyngitis (2% to 3% ages 2-5 years), dysphonia (2% ages 6-12 years), upper respiratory infection (2% ages 6-12 years)

Miscellaneous: Flu-like syndrome (2% to 3% ages 2-5 years), viral infection (2% to 3% ages 2-5 years)

General Dosage Range Dosage adjustment recommended in patients with hepatic or renal impairment

Oral:

Children 2-5 years: 5 mg once daily

Children ≥6 years and Adults: 10 mg once daily

Mechanism of Action Long-acting tricyclic antihistamine with selective peripheral histamine H$_1$-receptor antagonistic properties

Pharmacodynamics/Kinetics

Onset of Action 1-3 hours; Peak effect: 8-12 hours

Duration of Action >24 hours

Half-life Elimination 12-15 hours

Pregnancy Considerations Maternal use of loratadine has not been associated with an increased risk of major malformations. The use of antihistamines for the treatment of rhinitis during pregnancy is generally considered to be safe at recommended doses. Although safety data is limited, loratadine may be the preferred second generation antihistamine for the treatment of rhinitis or urticaria during pregnancy.

Loratadine and Pseudoephedrine
(lor AT a deen & soo doe e FED rin)

Related Information

Bacterial Infections on page 1562

Loratadine on page 838

Pseudoephedrine on page 1159

Brand Names: U.S. Alavert™ Allergy and Sinus [OTC]; Claritin-D® 12 Hour Allergy & Congestion [OTC]; Claritin-D® 24 Hour Allergy & Congestion [OTC]; Loratadine-D 12 Hour [OTC]

Brand Names: Canada Chlor-Tripolon ND®; Claritin® Extra; Claritin® Liberator

Generic Availability (U.S.) Yes

Pharmacologic Category Alpha/Beta Agonist; Decongestant; Histamine H$_1$ Antagonist; Histamine H$_1$ Antagonist, Second Generation; Piperidine Derivative

Use Temporary relief of symptoms of seasonal allergic rhinitis, other upper respiratory allergies, or the common cold

Local Anesthetic/Vasoconstrictor Precautions Use with caution since pseudoephedrine is a sympathomimetic amine which could interact with epinephrine to cause a pressor response

Effects on Dental Treatment Key adverse event(s) related to dental treatment: Pseudoephedrine: Xerostomia (normal salivary flow resumes upon discontinuation).

Effects on Bleeding No information available to require special precautions

Adverse Effects See individual agents.

Dosage Children ≥12 years and Adults: Oral:

Claritin-D® 12-Hour: 1 tablet every 12 hours

Alavert™ Allergy and Sinus, Claritin-D® 24-Hour: 1 tablet daily

Dosage adjustment in renal impairment: Cl$_{cr}$ ≤30 mL/minute:

Claritin-D® 12-Hour: 1 tablet daily

Claritin-D® 24-Hour: 1 tablet every other day

Dosage adjustment in hepatic impairment: Should be avoided

Contraindications Hypersensitivity to loratadine, pseudoephedrine, or any component of the formulation; use with or within 14 days of MAO inhibitors

Warnings/Precautions Use with caution in hypertension, diabetes mellitus, ischemic heart disease, increased intraocular pressure, hyperthyroidism, and prostatic hyperplasia. Use with caution in the elderly; may be more sensitive to adverse effects. Patients with swallowing difficulties (eg, upper GI narrowing or abnormal esophageal peristalsis) should not use Claritin-D® 24-Hour. Use caution with hepatic or renal impairment; dose adjustment may be required. Safety and efficacy have not been established in children <12 years of age. When used for self medication (OTC), notify healthcare provider if symptoms do not improve within 7 days or are accompanied by fever. Discontinue and contact healthcare provider if nervousness, dizziness or sleeplessness occur.

Drug Interactions

Metabolism/Transport Effects Refer to individual components.

Avoid Concomitant Use

Avoid concomitant use of Loratadine and Pseudoephedrine with any of the following: Aclidinium; Azelastine (Nasal); Ergot Derivatives; Iobenguane I 123; Ipratropium (Oral Inhalation); MAO Inhibitors; Paraldehyde; Tiotropium

Increased Effect/Toxicity

Loratadine and Pseudoephedrine may increase the levels/effects of: Alcohol (Ethyl); Anticholinergics; ARIPiprazole; Azelastine (Nasal); Bromocriptine; Buprenorphine; CNS Depressants; Metyrosine; Mirtazapine; Paraldehyde; Pramipexole; ROPINIRole; Rotigotine; Selective Serotonin Reuptake Inhibitors; Sympathomimetics; Tiotropium; Zolpidem

The levels/effects of Loratadine and Pseudoephedrine may be increased by: Aclidinium; Amiodarone; Antacids; AtoMOXetine; Cannabinoids; Carbonic Anhydrase Inhibitors; Droperidol; Ergot Derivatives; HydrOXYzine; Ipratropium (Oral Inhalation); Magnesium Sulfate; MAO Inhibitors; Perampanel; P-glycoprotein/ABCB1 Inhibitors; Pramlintide; Serotonin/Norepinephrine Reuptake Inhibitors; Sodium Oxybate

Decreased Effect

Loratadine and Pseudoephedrine may decrease the levels/effects of: Acetylcholinesterase Inhibitors (Central); Benzylpenicilloyl Polylysine; Betahistine; FentaNYL; Hyaluronidase; Iobenguane I 123

The levels/effects of Loratadine and Pseudoephedrine may be decreased by: Acetylcholinesterase Inhibitors (Central); Alpha1-Blockers; Amphetamines; Peginterferon Alfa-2b; P-glycoprotein/ABCB1 Inducers; Spironolactone

Ethanol/Nutrition/Herb Interactions Ethanol: May increase CNS depression; monitor for increased effects with coadministration. Caution patients about effects.

Dosage Forms

Tablet, extended release: Loratadine 10 mg and pseudoephedrine 240 mg

Alavert™ Allergy and Sinus [OTC]: Loratadine 5 mg and pseudoephedrine 120 mg

Claritin-D® 12 Hour Allergy & Congestion [OTC]: Loratadine 5 mg and pseudoephedrine 120 mg

Claritin-D® 24 Hour Allergy & Congestion [OTC]: Loratadine 10 mg and pseudoephedrine 240 mg

Loratadine-D 12 Hour [OTC]: Loratadine 5 mg and pseudoephedrine sulfate 120 mg

---

LORazepam (lor A ze pam)

Related Information

Management of the Patient With Anxiety or Depression *on page 1594*

Temporomandibular Dysfunction (TMD), Chronic Pain, and Fibromyalgia *on page 1590*

Related Sample Prescriptions

Sedation (Prior to Dental Treatment) *on page 1621*

Brand Names: U.S. Ativan®; Lorazepam Intensol™

Brand Names: Canada Apo-Lorazepam®; Ativan®; Dom-Lorazepam; Lorazepam Injection, USP; Novo-Lorazem; Nu-Loraz; PHL-Lorazepam; PMS-Lorazepam; PRO-Lorazepam

Generic Availability (U.S.) Yes

Pharmacologic Category Benzodiazepine

Dental Use Short-term relief of anxiety prior to dental appointment

Use

Oral: Management of anxiety disorders or short-term (≤4 months) relief of the symptoms of anxiety, anxiety associated with depressive symptoms, or insomnia due to anxiety or transient stress

I.V.: Status epilepticus, amnesia, sedation

Unlabeled Use Ethanol detoxification; psychogenic catatonia; partial complex seizures; agitation (I.V.); antiemetic for chemotherapy; rapid tranquilization of the agitated patient

Local Anesthetic/Vasoconstrictor Precautions No information available to require special precautions

Effects on Dental Treatment Key adverse event(s) related to dental treatment: Xerostomia (normal salivary flow resumes upon discontinuation).

Effects on Bleeding No information available to require special precautions

Adverse Effects

>10%:

Central nervous system: Sedation

Respiratory: Respiratory depression

1% to 10%:

Cardiovascular: Hypotension

Central nervous system: Akathisia, amnesia, ataxia, confusion, depression, disorientation, dizziness, headache

Dermatologic: Dermatitis, rash

Gastrointestinal: Changes in appetite, nausea, weight gain/loss

Neuromuscular & skeletal: Weakness

Ocular: Visual disturbances

Respiratory: Apnea, hyperventilation, nasal congestion

Dental Usual Dosage

Anxiety and sedation: Adults: Oral: 1-10 mg/day in 2-3 divided doses; usual dose: 2-6 mg/day in divided doses

Preoperative: Adults:

I.M.: 0.05 mg/kg administered 2 hours before surgery (maximum: 4 mg/dose)

I.V.: 0.044 mg/kg 15-20 minutes before surgery (usual maximum: 2 mg/dose)

Preprocedural anxiety: Adults: Oral: 1-2 mg 1 hour before procedure

Dosage

Antiemetic (unlabeled use):

Children 2-15 years: I.V.: 0.05 mg/kg (up to 2 mg/dose) prior to chemotherapy

Adults: Oral, I.V. (**Note:** May be administered sublingually; not a labeled route): 0.5-2 mg every 4-6 hours as needed

Anxiety, sedation, and procedural amnesia (unlabeled use in children except for oral use in children >12 years):

Infants and Children:

Oral, I.M.: Usual: 0.05 mg/kg/dose (range: 0.02-0.09 mg/kg) every 4-8 hours

I.V.: Usual: 0.05 mg/kg/dose (range: 0.02-0.09 mg/kg) every 4-8 hours; may use smaller doses (eg, 0.01-0.03 mg/kg) and repeat every 20 minutes, as needed to titrate to effect

Adults:

Oral: 1-10 mg/day in 2-3 divided doses; usual dose: 2-6 mg/day in divided doses or 1-2 mg 1 hour before procedure

I.M.: 0.05 mg/kg administered 2 hours before surgery (maximum: 4 mg/dose)

I.V.: 0.044 mg/kg 15-20 minutes before surgery (usual dose 2 mg; maximum: 4 mg/dose)

Elderly: Oral: Initial: 1-2 mg/day in divided doses; Beers Criteria: Avoid maintenance doses >3 mg/day

Insomnia: Adults: Oral: 2-4 mg at bedtime

Status epilepticus: I.V.:

Infants and Children (unlabeled use): 0.05-0.1 mg/kg (maximum: 4 mg/dose) slow I.V. (maximum rate: 2 mg/minute); may repeat every 10-15 minutes as needed (Hegenbarth, 2008; Sabo-Graham, 1998)

Adults: 4 mg/dose slow I.V. (maximum rate: 2 mg/minute); may repeat in 10-15 minutes; usual maximum dose: 8 mg. May be given I.M, but I.V. preferred.

Rapid tranquilization of agitated patient (unlabeled use): Adults: Oral, I.M.: 1-2 mg administered every 30-60 minutes; may be administered with an antipsychotic (eg, haloperidol) (Battaglia, 2005; De Fruyt, 2004)

Average total dose for tranquilization: 4-8 mg

Agitation in the ICU patient (unlabeled use): Adults: I.V.: Loading dose: 0.02-0.04 mg/kg (maximum single dose: 2 mg); Maintenance: 0.02-0.06 mg/kg every 2-6 hours as needed or 0.01-0.1 mg/kg/hour; maximum dose: ≤10 mg/hour (Barr, 2013)

Alcohol withdrawal syndrome (unlabeled use): Oral: 2 mg every 6 hours for 4 doses, then 1 mg every 6 hours for 8 additional doses (Mayo-Smith, 1997)

Alcohol withdrawal delirium (unlabeled use) (Mayo-Smith, 2004):

I.V.: 1-4 mg every 5-15 minutes until calm, then every hour as needed to maintain light somnolence

I.M.: 1-4 mg every 30-60 minutes until calm, then every hour as needed to maintain light somnolence

Dosage adjustment for lorazepam with concomitant medications: *Probenecid or valproic acid:* Reduce lorazepam dose by 50%

Dosage adjustment in renal impairment: I.V.: Risk of propylene glycol toxicity. Monitor closely if using for prolonged periods of time or at high doses.

Dosage adjustment in hepatic impairment: No dose reduction necessary.

Mechanism of Action Binds to stereospecific benzodiazepine receptors on the postsynaptic GABA neuron at several sites within the central nervous system, including the limbic system, reticular formation. Enhancement of the inhibitory effect of GABA on neuronal excitability results by increased neuronal membrane permeability to chloride ions. This shift in chloride ions results in hyperpolarization (a less excitable state) and stabilization.

Contraindications Hypersensitivity to lorazepam or any component of the formulation (cross-sensitivity with other benzodiazepines may exist); acute narrow-angle glaucoma; sleep apnea (parenteral); intra-arterial injection of parenteral formulation; severe respiratory insufficiency (except during mechanical ventilation)

Warnings/Precautions Use with caution in elderly or debilitated patients, patients with hepatic disease (including alcoholics) or renal impairment. In older adults, benzodiazepines increase the risk of impaired cognition, delirium, falls, fractures, and motor vehicle accidents. Due to increased sensitivity in this age group, avoid use for treatment of insomnia, agitation, or delirium. (Beers Criteria). Use with caution in patients with respiratory disease (COPD or sleep apnea) or limited pulmonary reserve, or impaired gag reflex. Initial doses in elderly or debilitated patients should be at the lower end of the dosing range. May worsen hepatic encephalopathy.

Causes CNS depression (dose-related) resulting in sedation, dizziness, confusion, or ataxia which may impair physical and mental capabilities. Patients must be cautioned about performing tasks which require mental alertness (eg, operating machinery or driving). Use with caution in patients receiving other CNS depressants or psychoactive agents. Effects with other sedative drugs or ethanol may be potentiated. Benzodiazepines have been associated with falls and traumatic injury and should be used with extreme caution in patients who are at risk of these events.

Lorazepam may cause anterograde amnesia. Paradoxical reactions, including hyperactive or aggressive behavior have been reported with benzodiazepines, particularly in adolescent/pediatric or psychiatric patients. Does not have analgesic, antidepressant, or antipsychotic properties.

Use caution in patients with depression, particularly if suicidal risk may be present. Pre-existing depression may worsen or emerge during therapy. Not recommended for use in primary depressive or psychotic disorders. Use with caution in patients with a history of drug dependence, alcoholism, or significant personality disorders. Benzodiazepines have been associated with dependence and acute withdrawal symptoms on discontinuation or reduction in dose. Acute withdrawal, including seizures, may be precipitated after administration of flumazenil to patients receiving long-term benzodiazepine therapy.

As a hypnotic agent, should be used only after evaluation of potential causes of sleep disturbance. Failure of sleep disturbance to resolve after 7-10 days may indicate psychiatric or medical illness. A worsening of insomnia or the emergence of new abnormalities of thought or behavior may represent unrecognized psychiatric or medical illness and requires immediate and careful evaluation.

Parenteral formulation of lorazepam contains polyethylene glycol which has resulted in toxicity during high-dose and/or longer-term infusions. Parenteral formulation also contains propylene glycol (PG); may be associated with dose-related toxicity and can occur ≥48 hours after initiation of lorazepam. Limited data suggest increased risk of PG accumulation at doses of ≥6 mg/hour for 48 hours or more (Nelson, 2008). Monitor for signs of toxicity which may include acute renal failure, lactic acidosis, and/or osmol gap. May consider using enteral delivery of lorazepam tablets to decrease the risk of PG toxicity (Lugo, 1999). Parenteral formulation also contains benzyl alcohol; avoid in neonates.

Drug Interactions

Metabolism/Transport Effects None known.

Avoid Concomitant Use

Avoid concomitant use of LORazepam with any of the following: Azelastine (Nasal); OLANZapine; Paraldehyde; Sodium Oxybate

Increased Effect/Toxicity

LORazepam may increase the levels/effects of: Alcohol (Ethyl); Azelastine (Nasal); Buprenorphine; CloZAPine; CNS Depressants; Fosphenytoin; Methotrimeprazine; Metyrosine; Mirtazapine; Paraldehyde; Phenytoin; Pramipexole; ROPINIRole; Rotigotine; Selective Serotonin Reuptake Inhibitors; Sodium Oxybate; Zolpidem

The levels/effects of LORazepam may be increased by: Divalproex; Droperidol; HydrOXYzine; Loxapine; Magnesium Sulfate; Methotrimeprazine; OLANZapine; Perampanel; Probenecid; Valproic Acid

Decreased Effect

The levels/effects of LORazepam may be decreased by: Theophylline Derivatives; Yohimbine

Ethanol/Nutrition/Herb Interactions

Ethanol: May increase CNS depression; monitor for increased effects with coadministration. Caution patients about effects.

Herb/Nutraceutical: Avoid valerian, St John's wort, kava kava, gotu kola (may increase CNS depression).

Pharmacodynamics/Kinetics

Onset of Action Hypnosis: I.M.: 20-30 minutes; Sedation: I.V.: 5-20 minutes; Anticonvulsant: I.V.: 5 minutes, oral: 30-60 minutes

Duration of Action 6-8 hours

Half-life Elimination Neonates: 40.2 hours; Older children: 10.5 hours; Adults: 12.9 hours; Elderly: 15.9 hours; End-stage renal disease: 32-70 hours

Time to Peak Oral: 2 hours

Pregnancy Risk Factor D

Pregnancy Considerations Teratogenic effects have been observed in some animal studies. Lorazepam and its metabolite cross the human placenta. Teratogenic effects in humans have been observed with some benzodiazepines (including lorazepam); however, additional studies are needed. The incidence of premature birth and low birth weights may be increased following maternal use of benzodiazepines; hypoglycemia and respiratory problems in the neonate may occur following exposure late in pregnancy. Neonatal withdrawal symptoms may occur within days to weeks after birth and "floppy infant syndrome" (which also includes withdrawal symptoms) have been reported with some benzodiazepines (including lorazepam). Elimination of lorazepam in the newborn infant is slow; following in utero exposure, term infants may excrete lorazepam for up to 8 days.

Lactation Enters breast milk/not recommended (AAP rates "of concern"; AAP 2001 update pending)

Breast-Feeding Considerations Drowsiness, lethargy, or weight loss in nursing infants have been observed in case reports following maternal use of some benzodiazepines.

Controlled Substance C-IV

Dosage Forms

Injection, solution: 2 mg/mL (1 mL, 10 mL); 4 mg/mL (1 mL, 10 mL)

Ativan®: 2 mg/mL (1 mL, 10 mL); 4 mg/mL (1 mL, 10 mL)

Solution, oral: 2 mg/mL (30 mL)

Lorazepam Intensol™: 2 mg/mL (30 mL)

Tablet, oral: 0.5 mg, 1 mg, 2 mg

Ativan®: 0.5 mg, 1 mg, 2 mg

Lorcaserin (lor KA ser in)

Generic Availability (U.S.) No

Pharmacologic Category Anorexiant; Serotonin 5-HT$_{2C}$ Receptor Agonist

Use Chronic weight management, as an adjunct to a reduced-calorie diet and increased physical activity, in patients with either an initial body mass index (BMI) of ≥30 kg/m^2 or an initial BMI of ≥27 kg/m^2 and at least one weight-related comorbid condition (eg, hypertension, dyslipidemia, type 2 diabetes)

Local Anesthetic/Vasoconstrictor Precautions No information available to require special precautions

Effects on Dental Treatment No significant effects or complications reported

Effects on Bleeding No information available to require special precautions

Adverse Effects

>10%:

Central nervous system: Headache (15% to 17%)

Endocrine & metabolic: Hypoglycemia (diabetic patients 29%; severe: 2%)

Hematologic: Lymphocytes decreased (12%)

Neuromuscular & skeletal: Back pain (6% to 12%)

Respiratory: Upper respiratory tract infection (14%), nasopharyngitis (11% to 13%)

1% to 10%:

Cardiovascular: Peripheral edema (5%), hypertension (5%), valvulopathy (at 1 year: 2.4%; placebo: 2.0%)

Central nervous system: Dizziness (7% to 9%), fatigue (7%), anxiety (4%), insomnia (4%), depression (2% to 3%; placebo: 2%), cognitive impairment (2%), psychiatric disorders (2%)

Dermatologic: Rash (2%)

Endocrine & metabolic: Diabetes mellitus exacerbation (3%), prolactin increased (<2 x ULN: 7%; 2 x ULN: 2%; 5 x ULN: <1%)

Gastrointestinal: Nausea (8% to 9%), diarrhea (7%), constipation (6%), xerostomia (5%), vomiting (4%), gastroenteritis (3%), toothache (3%), appetite decreased (2%)

Genitourinary: Urinary tract infection (7% to 9%)

Hematologic: Hemoglobin decreased (10%), neutrophils decreased (6%)

Neuromuscular & skeletal: Muscle spasms (5%), musculoskeletal pain (2%)

Ocular: Eye disorders (5%; diabetic patients 6%)

Respiratory: Cough (4% to 8%), oropharyngeal pain (4%), sinus congestion (3%)

Miscellaneous: Seasonal allergy (3%), stress (3%)

Dosage Weight management: Adults: Oral: 10 mg twice daily (maximum: 10 mg twice daily); evaluate response by week 12; if patient has not lost ≥5% of baseline body weight, discontinue therapy

Dosage adjustment in renal impairment: Note: Renal function was estimated in studies using ideal body weight (IBW) with the Cockcroft-Gault formula.

Mild impairment (Cl$_{cr}$ >50 mL/minute): No dosage adjustment necessary.

Moderate impairment (Cl$_{cr}$ 30-50 mL/minute): Use with caution; serum concentrations and half-life of major metabolites are increased.

Severe impairment (Cl$_{cr}$ <30 mL/minute): Use is not recommended.

ESRD: Use is not recommended; hemodialysis does not remove lorcaserin or M1 metabolite

Dosage adjustment in hepatic impairment:

Mild-to-moderate impairment (Child-Pugh score 5-9): No dosage adjustment necessary.

Severe impairment: Use with caution (has not been studied); undergoes extensive hepatic metabolism.

Mechanism of Action Lorcaserin is believed to activate serotonin 5-HT$_{2C}$ receptors, which stimulate pro-opiomelanocortin (POMC) neurons in the arcuate nucleus of the hypothalamus, leading to increased alpha-melanocortin stimulating hormone release at melanocortin-4 receptors and resulting in satiety and decreased food intake. At recommended doses, lorcaserin has greater affinity for 5-HT$_{2C}$ receptors compared to other 5-HT receptor subtypes (including 5-HT2A and

▶

5-HT$_{2B}$), the 5-HT receptor transporter, and 5-HT reuptake sites (Hurren, 2011).

Contraindications Pregnancy

Warnings/Precautions Use may cause confusion, somnolence, fatigue, and cognitive impairment (difficulty with concentration/attention/memory); patients must be cautioned about performing tasks which require mental alertness (eg, operating machinery or driving). Agents affecting the CNS have been associated with depression and suicidal ideation; monitor patients closely during use; discontinue for suicidal thoughts or behaviors. Priapism may occur with use; men with erections >4 hours should immediately discontinue lorcaserin and seek emergency medical attention to avoid irreversible damage to erectile tissue. Use with caution in men with conditions that increase the risk for priapism (eg, sickle cell anemia, multiple myeloma, leukemia) or men with anatomical penis deformities (eg, angulation, cavernosal fibrosis, Peyronie's disease). Rare WBC and RBC count decreases (including leukopenia, lymphopenia, neutropenia, anemia, decreases in hematocrit and hemoglobin) have been observed; consider monitoring CBC periodically during use. Increased prolactin levels may occur; obtain prolactin levels if signs or symptoms of hyperprolactinemia occur (eg, galactorrhea, gynecomastia).

Primary pulmonary hypertension (PPH) is a rare and frequently fatal pulmonary disease, which has been reported in patients receiving other centrally acting, serotonergic weight loss agents. Available data from clinical trials are inadequate to determine if lorcaserin increases the risk for pulmonary hypertension (due to the low incidence of PPH occurring in the general population); however, a theoretical risk cannot be excluded. Cardiac valvular disease has been associated with the use of agents exhibiting potent 5-HT$_{2B}$ agonist activity (eg, cabergoline, fenfluramine [not currently on the U.S. market], dexfenfluramine [not currently on the U.S. market]). Cardiac valvular disease is believed to result from activation of 5-HT$_{2B}$ receptors in interstitial cardiac cells. Lorcaserin has greater affinity for 5-HT$_{2C}$ receptors compared to 5-HT$_{2B}$ receptors (at therapeutic doses). However, a slight increase in incidence of regurgitant cardiac valve disease (mitral and/or aortic) has been observed with lorcaserin compared to placebo in some clinical trials (pooled RR: 1.16; 95% CI: 0.81-1.67). The incidence observed in both groups was low, making it difficult to ascertain the risk of valvular disease with lorcaserin therapy based on available data. Evaluate patients if signs/symptoms of valvular heart disease (eg, dyspnea, dependent edema, heart failure, new onset cardiac murmur) arise during therapy; consider discontinuing therapy if present. Use has not been studied in patients with hemodynamically-significant valvular heart disease. Do not use lorcaserin in combination with potent serotonergic and dopaminergic agents that are potent 5-HT$_{2B}$ receptor agonists (eg, cabergoline) due to the risk for cardiac valvulopathy.

Serotonin syndrome (SS)/neuroleptic malignant syndrome (NMS)-like reactions have occurred with serotonergic agents such as lorcaserin, particularly when used in combination with other serotonergic agents (eg, triptans, SNRIs, SSRIs, TCAs, bupropion, St John's wort, tryptophan), agents that impair metabolism of serotonin (eg, MOA inhibitors, dextromethorphan, tramadol, lithium), or antidopaminergic agents (eg, antipsychotics). Concurrent use with these agents should be avoided. If concomitant use cannot be avoided, coadminister with extreme caution, and closely monitor patients,

particularly during treatment initiation. Discontinue treatment (and any concomitant serotonergic and/or antidopaminergic agents) immediately if signs/symptoms of SS or NMS-like reactions arise.

Use with caution in patients with bradycardia or heart block (second or third degree); bradycardia has been observed rarely with use. Use with caution in patients with heart failure (has not been studied). Effect of lorcaserin on cardiovascular morbidity and mortality has not been established. Use with caution in patients with type 2 diabetes mellitus; weight loss from therapy may result in decreased requirements of antidiabetic agents and an increased risk of hypoglycemia; monitor blood glucose. Use with caution in patients with severe hepatic impairment (not studied); lorcaserin undergoes extensive hepatic metabolism. Use is not recommended in patients with severe renal impairment or end stage renal disease. Use with caution in patients with moderate renal impairment. Serum concentrations and principal metabolite (M1 and M5) half-lives are increased in renal impairment.

In short-term studies, euphoria, hallucinations, and dissociation have been observed with lorcaserin at supratherapeutic doses. Data suggest lorcaserin may produce psychic dependence. Physical dependence or a withdrawal syndrome has not been observed. Pharmacotherapy for weight loss should be used in conjunction with a comprehensive weight management program including diet and exercise. Discontinue if significant weight loss has not occurred (ie, <5% within the first 12 weeks of treatment). Concomitant use of lorcaserin with other agents intended for weight loss (eg, phentermine, orlistat, OTC, or herbal preparations) has not been evaluated; safety and efficacy of coadministration with other weight loss agents are unknown.

Drug Interactions

Metabolism/Transport Effects Inhibits CYP2D6 (moderate)

Avoid Concomitant Use

Avoid concomitant use of Lorcaserin with any of the following: Ergot Derivatives; Thioridazine

Increased Effect/Toxicity

Lorcaserin may increase the levels/effects of: CYP2D6 Substrates; Ergot Derivatives; Fesoterodine; Metoclopramide; Metoprolol; Nebivolol; Phosphodiesterase 5 Inhibitors; Serotonin Modulators; Thioridazine

The levels/effects of Lorcaserin may be increased by: Antipsychotics; BuPROPion; Propafenone

Decreased Effect

Lorcaserin may decrease the levels/effects of: Codeine; Tamoxifen

Pharmacodynamics/Kinetics

Half-life Elimination ~11 hours

Time to Peak 1.5-2 hours

Pregnancy Risk Factor X

Pregnancy Considerations Adverse fetal effects were observed in some animal reproduction studies. Due to the fact that weight loss during pregnancy offers no clinical benefit, lorcaserin is contraindicated in pregnancy. Obese and overweight women should be encouraged to participate in weight reduction programs prior to attempting pregnancy; weight gain during pregnancy should be determined by their prepregnancy BMI and current guidelines (ADA, 2009; IOM, 2009).

Lactation Excretion in breast milk unknown/ not recommended

Breast-Feeding Considerations Lorcaserin may alter maternal serum prolactin concentrations. It is not known if lorcaserin is excreted into breast milk. According to the manufacturer, the decision to continue or discontinue breast-feeding during therapy should take into account the risk of exposure to the infant and the benefits of treatment to the mother. Weight-loss therapy is generally not recommended for lactating women. Weight-loss programs which include physical activity and nutrition components should be discussed at the 6-week postpartum visit (ADA, 2009; IOM, 2009).

Product Availability Belviq®: FDA approved June 2012; anticipated availability is first quarter of 2013. Consult prescribing information for additional information. The DEA is currently evaluating Belviq® as a controlled substance, and the scheduling category is being determined.

Losartan (loe SAR tan)

Related Information
Cardiovascular Diseases *on page 1492*

Brand Names: U.S. Cozaar®

Brand Names: Canada Apo-Losartan; CO Losartan; Cozaar®; Mylan-Losartan; PMS-Losartan; Teva-Losartan

Generic Availability (U.S.) Yes

Pharmacologic Category Angiotensin II Receptor Blocker

Use Treatment of hypertension (HTN); treatment of diabetic nephropathy in patients with type 2 diabetes mellitus (noninsulin dependent, NIDDM) and a history of hypertension; stroke risk reduction in patients with HTN and left ventricular hypertrophy (LVH)

Unlabeled Use To slow the rate of progression of aortic-root dilation in pediatric patients with Marfan's syndrome; syndrome; heart failure patients intolerant of ACE inhibitors (only for Stages A [treatment of hypertension] or B [to reduce future cardiovascular events] heart failure per ACCF/AHA 2009 guidelines)

Local Anesthetic/Vasoconstrictor Precautions No information available to require special precautions

Effects on Dental Treatment Key adverse event(s) related to dental treatment: Orthostatic hypotension.

Effects on Bleeding No information available to require special precautions

Adverse Effects Note: The incidence of some adverse reactions varied based on the underlying disease state. Notations are made, where applicable, for data derived from trials conducted in diabetic nephropathy and hypertensive patients, respectively.

>10%:
Cardiovascular: Chest pain (12% diabetic nephropathy)
Central nervous system: Fatigue (14% diabetic nephropathy)
Endocrine: Hypoglycemia (14% diabetic nephropathy)
Gastrointestinal: Diarrhea (2% hypertension to 15% diabetic nephropathy)
Genitourinary: Urinary tract infection (13% diabetic nephropathy)
Hematologic: Anemia (14% diabetic nephropathy)
Neuromuscular & skeletal: Weakness (14% diabetic nephropathy), back pain (2% hypertension to 12% diabetic nephropathy)

Respiratory: Cough (≤3% to 11%; similar to placebo; incidence higher in patients with previous cough related to ACE inhibitor therapy)
1% to 10%:
Cardiovascular: Hypotension (7% diabetic nephropathy), orthostatic hypotension (4% hypertension to 4% diabetic nephropathy), first-dose hypotension (dose related: <1% with 50 mg, 2% with 100 mg)
Central nervous system: Dizziness (4%), hypoesthesia (5% diabetic nephropathy), fever (4% diabetic nephropathy), insomnia (1%)
Dermatology: Cellulitis (7% diabetic nephropathy)
Endocrine: Hyperkalemia (<1% hypertension to 7% diabetic nephropathy)
Gastrointestinal: Gastritis (5% diabetic nephropathy), weight gain (4% diabetic nephropathy), dyspepsia (1% to 4%), abdominal pain (2%), nausea (2%)
Neuromuscular & skeletal: Muscular weakness (7% diabetic nephropathy), knee pain (5% diabetic nephropathy), leg pain (1% to 5%), muscle cramps (1%), myalgia (1%)
Respiratory: Bronchitis (10% diabetic nephropathy), upper respiratory infection (8%), nasal congestion (2%), sinusitis (1% hypertension to 6% diabetic nephropathy)
Miscellaneous: Infection (5% diabetic nephropathy), flu-like syndrome (10% diabetic nephropathy)

Dosage Oral:
Hypertension:
Children 6-16 years:
U.S. labeling: 0.7 mg/kg once daily (maximum: 50 mg daily); doses >1.4 mg/kg (maximum: 100 mg) have not been studied
Canadian labeling:
≥20 kg to <50 kg: 25 mg once daily (maximum: 50 mg once daily)
≥50 kg: 50 mg once daily (maximum: 100 mg once daily)
Adults: Usual starting dose: 50 mg once daily; can be administered once or twice daily with total daily doses ranging from 25-100 mg
Patients receiving diuretics or with intravascular volume depletion: Usual initial dose: 25 mg once daily
Nephropathy in patients with type 2 diabetes and hypertension: Adults: Initial: 50 mg once daily; can be increased to 100 mg once daily based on blood pressure response
Stroke reduction (HTN with LVH): Adults: 50 mg once daily (maximum daily dose: 100 mg); may be used in combination with a thiazide diuretic
Aortic-root dilation with Marfan's syndrome (unlabeled use): Children 14 months to 16 years: Initial: 0.6 mg/kg/day; can be increased to a maximum of 1.4 mg/kg/day (not to exceed adult maximum of 100 mg daily) (Brooke, 2008)
Heart failure (unlabeled use): Adults: Initial: 12.5-25 mg once daily; target dose: 150 mg once daily (HFSA, 2010; Konstam, 2009) **or** an initial dose of 25-50 mg once daily; maximum dose: 50-100 mg once daily (ACCF/AHA, 2009); **Note:** The ACCF/AHA heart failure guidelines recommend losartan only in stages A and B heart failure.

Dosing adjustment in renal impairment:
Children: Use is not recommended if GFR <30 mL/minute/1.73 m^2
Adults: No dosage adjustment necessary.

Dosing adjustment in hepatic impairment:
Children 6-16 years:
U.S. labeling: No specific dosing recommendations are provided in the approved labeling, however it may be advisable to initiate therapy at a reduced dosage.
Canadian labeling: Use is not recommended.
Adults: Reduce the initial dose to 25 mg/day

Mechanism of Action As a selective and competitive, nonpeptide angiotensin II receptor antagonist, losartan blocks the vasoconstrictor and aldosterone-secreting effects of angiotensin II; losartan interacts reversibly at the AT1 and AT2 receptors of many tissues and has slow dissociation kinetics; its affinity for the AT1 receptor is 1000 times greater than the AT2 receptor. Angiotensin II receptor antagonists may induce a more complete inhibition of the renin-angiotensin system than ACE inhibitors, they do not affect the response to bradykinin, and are less likely to be associated with nonrenin-angiotensin effects (eg, cough and angioedema). Losartan increases urinary flow rate and in addition to being natriuretic and kaliuretic, increases excretion of chloride, magnesium, uric acid, calcium, and phosphate.

Contraindications Hypersensitivity to losartan or any component of the formulation; concomitant use with aliskiren in patients with diabetes mellitus

Warnings/Precautions [U.S. Boxed Warning]: Drugs that act on the renin-angiotensin system can cause injury and death to the developing fetus. Discontinue as soon as possible once pregnancy is detected. Avoid use or use a much smaller dose in patients who are volume-depleted; correct depletion first. Use with caution in patients with significant aortic/mitral stenosis. May cause hyperkalemia; avoid potassium supplementation unless specifically required by healthcare provider. May be associated with deterioration of renal function and/or increases in serum creatinine, particularly in patients with low renal blood flow (eg, renal artery stenosis, heart failure) whose glomerular filtration rate (GFR) is dependent on efferent arteriolar vasoconstriction by angiotensin II. Use caution in patients with unstented unilateral/bilateral renal artery stenosis. When unstented bilateral renal artery stenosis is present, use is generally avoided due to the elevated risk of deterioration in renal function unless possible benefits outweigh risks. Use with caution with pre-existing renal insufficiency. AUCs of losartan (not the active metabolite) are about 50% greater in patients with Cl_{cr} <30 mL/minute and are doubled in hemodialysis patients. Concomitant use of an angiotensin-converting enzyme (ACE) inhibitor or renin inhibitor (eg, aliskiren) is associated with an increased risk of hypotension, hyperkalemia, and renal dysfunction; concomitant use with aliskiren should be avoided in patients with GFR <60 mL/minute and is contraindicated in patients with diabetes mellitus (regardless of GFR).

At any time during treatment (especially following first dose), angioedema may occur rarely; may involve the head and neck (potentially compromising airway) or the intestine (presenting with abdominal pain). Patients with idiopathic or hereditary angioedema or previous angioedema associated with ACE-inhibitor therapy may be at an increased risk. Prolonged frequent monitoring may be required, especially if tongue, glottis, or larynx are involved, as they are associated with airway obstruction. Patients with a history of airway surgery may have a higher risk of airway obstruction. Aggressive early management is critical; intramuscular (I.M.) administration of epinephrine may be necessary.

When used to reduce the risk of stroke in patients with HTN and LVH, may not be effective in African-American population. Use caution with hepatic dysfunction, dose adjustment may be needed.

Drug Interactions
Metabolism/Transport Effects Substrate of CYP2C9 (major), CYP3A4 (major); **Note:** Assignment of Major/Minor substrate status based on clinically relevant drug interaction potential; **Inhibits** CYP1A2 (weak), CYP2C19 (weak), CYP2C8 (moderate), CYP2C9 (moderate), CYP3A4 (weak)

Avoid Concomitant Use
Avoid concomitant use of Losartan with any of the following: Pimozide

Increased Effect/Toxicity
Losartan may increase the levels/effects of: ACE Inhibitors; Amifostine; Antihypertensives; ARIPiprazole; Carvedilol; CycloSPORINE (Systemic); CYP2C8 Substrates; CYP2C9 Substrates; Hypoglycemic Agents; Hypotensive Agents; Lithium; Lomitapide; Nonsteroidal Anti-Inflammatory Agents; Pimozide; Potassium-Sparing Diuretics; RiTUXimab; Sodium Phosphates

The levels/effects of Losartan may be increased by: Alfuzosin; Aliskiren; Antifungal Agents (Azole Derivatives, Systemic); Canagliflozin; CYP2C9 Inhibitors (Moderate); CYP2C9 Inhibitors (Strong); Diazoxide; Eplerenone; Fluconazole; Herbs (Hypoglycemic Properties); Herbs (Hypotensive Properties); MAO Inhibitors; Mifepristone; Milk Thistle; Pentoxifylline; Phosphodiesterase 5 Inhibitors; Potassium Salts; Prostacyclin Analogues; Salicylates; Selective Serotonin Reuptake Inhibitors; Tolvaptan; Trimethoprim

Decreased Effect
The levels/effects of Losartan may be decreased by: CYP2C9 Inducers (Strong); CYP3A4 Inducers (Strong); Deferasirox; Herbs (CYP3A4 Inducers); Herbs (Hypertensive Properties); Loop Diuretics; Methylphenidate; Nonsteroidal Anti-Inflammatory Agents; Peginterferon Alfa-2b; Rifamycin Derivatives; Tocilizumab; Yohimbine

Ethanol/Nutrition/Herb Interactions Herb/Nutraceutical: St John's wort may decrease levels of losartan. Some herbal medications may worsen hypertension (eg, licorice); others may increase the antihypertensive effect of losartan (eg, shepherd's purse). Some herbal medications may increase the hypoglycemic effects of losartan (eg, alfalfa). Management: Avoid St John's wort. Avoid bayberry, blue cohosh, ginseng (American), kola, licorice, and yohimbe. Avoid black cohosh, California poppy, coleus, golden seal, hawthorn, mistletoe, periwinkle, quinine, and shepherd's purse. Avoid alfalfa, aloe, bilberry, bitter melon, burdock, celery, damiana, fenugreek, garcinia, garlic, ginger, ginseng (American), gymnema, marshmallow, and stinging nettle.

Dietary Considerations May be taken without regard to meals. Some products may contain potassium.

Pharmacodynamics/Kinetics
Onset of Action 6 hours
Half-life Elimination Losartan: 1.5-2 hours; E-3174: 6-9 hours
Time to Peak Serum: Losartan: 1 hour; E-3174: 3-4 hours
Pregnancy Risk Factor C (1st trimester); D (2nd and 3rd trimesters)
Pregnancy Considerations [U.S. Boxed Warning]: Drugs that act on the renin-angiotensin system can cause injury and death to the developing fetus. Discontinue as soon as possible once pregnancy

is detected. The use of drugs which act on the renin-angiotensin system are associated with oligohydramnios. Oligohydramnios, due to decreased fetal renal function, may lead to fetal lung hypoplasia and skeletal malformations. Use is also associated with anuria, hypotension, renal failure, skull hypoplasia, and death in the fetus/neonate. The exposed fetus should be monitored for fetal growth, amniotic fluid volume, and organ formation. Infants exposed *in utero* should be monitored for hyperkalemia, hypotension, and oliguria.

Lactation Excretion in breast milk unknown/not recommended

Breast-Feeding Considerations It is not known if losartan is found in breast milk; the manufacturer recommends discontinuing the drug or discontinuing nursing based on the importance of the drug to the mother.

Dosage Forms
Tablet, oral: 25 mg, 50 mg, 100 mg
Cozaar®: 25 mg, 50 mg, 100 mg

Losartan and Hydrochlorothiazide
(loe SAR tan & hye droe klor oh THYE a zide)

Related Information
Hydrochlorothiazide *on page 687*
Losartan *on page 843*
Brand Names: U.S. Hyzaar®
Brand Names: Canada Apo-Losartan/HCTZ; Hyzaar®; Hyzaar® DS; Mint-Losartan/HCTZ; Mint-Losartan/HCTZ DS; Mylan-Losartan/HCTZ; PMS-Losartan/HCTZ; Sandoz-Losartan HCT; Sandoz-Losartan HCT DS; Teva-Losartan/HCTZ
Generic Availability (U.S.) Yes
Pharmacologic Category Angiotensin II Receptor Blocker; Diuretic, Thiazide
Use Treatment of hypertension; stroke risk reduction in patients with HTN and left ventricular hypertrophy (LVH)
Local Anesthetic/Vasoconstrictor Precautions No information available to require special precautions
Effects on Dental Treatment No significant effects or complications reported
Effects on Bleeding No information available to require special precautions
Adverse Effects Based on clinical trials of the combination product in patients with essential hypertension. Also see individual agents.
1% to 10%:
Cardiovascular: Edema (1%), palpitation (1%)
Central nervous system: Dizziness (6%)
Dermatologic: Skin rash (1%)
Gastrointestinal: Abdominal pain (1%)
Neuromuscular & skeletal: Back pain (2%)
Respiratory: Upper respiratory infection (6%), cough (3%), sinusitis (1%)
Dosage Oral: Adults: Dose is individualized (combination substituted for individual components); dose may be titrated after 2-4 weeks of therapy
Hypertension/stroke reduction in hypertension (with LVH): Usual recommended starting dose of losartan: 50 mg once daily when used as monotherapy in patients who are not volume depleted

Dosage adjustment in renal impairment: $Cl_{cr} \leq 30$ mL/minute: Use of combination formulation not recommended
Dosage adjustment in hepatic impairment: Use is not recommended

Contraindications Hypersensitivity to losartan, hydrochlorothiazide, or any component of the formulation; sulfonamide-derived drugs; concomitant use with aliskiren in patients with diabetes mellitus; anuria
Warnings/Precautions See individual agents.
Drug Interactions
Metabolism/Transport Effects Refer to individual components.
Avoid Concomitant Use
Avoid concomitant use of Losartan and Hydrochlorothiazide with any of the following: Dofetilide; Pimozide
Increased Effect/Toxicity
Losartan and Hydrochlorothiazide may increase the levels/effects of: ACE Inhibitors; Allopurinol; Amifostine; Antihypertensives; ARIPiprazole; Benazepril; Calcium Salts; CarBAMazepine; Carvedilol; CycloSPORINE (Systemic); CYP2C8 Substrates; CYP2C9 Substrates; Dofetilide; Hypoglycemic Agents; Hypotensive Agents; Lithium; Lomitapide; Multivitamins/Minerals (with ADEK, Folate, Iron); Nonsteroidal Anti-Inflammatory Agents; OXcarbazepine; Pimozide; Porfimer; Potassium-Sparing Diuretics; RiTUXimab; Sodium Phosphates; Topiramate; Toremifene; Valsartan; Vitamin D Analogs

The levels/effects of Losartan and Hydrochlorothiazide may be increased by: Alcohol (Ethyl); Alfuzosin; Aliskiren; Analgesics (Opioid); Antifungal Agents (Azole Derivatives, Systemic); Barbiturates; Beta2-Agonists; Canagliflozin; Corticosteroids (Orally Inhaled); Corticosteroids (Systemic); CYP2C9 Inhibitors (Moderate); CYP2C9 Inhibitors (Strong); Eplerenone; Fluconazole; Herbs (Hypoglycemic Properties); Herbs (Hypotensive Properties); Licorice; MAO Inhibitors; Mifepristone; Milk Thistle; Pentoxifylline; Phosphodiesterase 5 Inhibitors; Potassium Salts; Prostacyclin Analogues; Salicylates; Selective Serotonin Reuptake Inhibitors; Tolvaptan; Trimethoprim; Valsartan
Decreased Effect
Losartan and Hydrochlorothiazide may decrease the levels/effects of: Antidiabetic Agents

The levels/effects of Losartan and Hydrochlorothiazide may be decreased by: Benazepril; Bile Acid Sequestrants; CYP2C9 Inducers (Strong); CYP3A4 Inducers (Strong); Deferasirox; Herbs (CYP3A4 Inducers); Herbs (Hypertensive Properties); Loop Diuretics; Methylphenidate; Nonsteroidal Anti-Inflammatory Agents; Peginterferon Alfa-2b; Rifamycin Derivatives; Tocilizumab; Yohimbine
Dietary Considerations Some products may contain potassium.
Pregnancy Risk Factor C/D (2nd and 3rd trimesters)
Pregnancy Considerations [U.S. Boxed Warning]: Drugs that act on the renin-angiotensin system can cause injury and death to the developing fetus. Discontinue as soon as possible once pregnancy is detected. Also see individual agents.
Lactation Enters breast milk/contraindicated
Dosage Forms
Tablet: 50/12.5: Losartan 50 mg and hydrochlorothiazide 12.5 mg; 100/12.5: Losartan 100 mg and hydrochlorothiazide 12.5 mg; 100/25: Losartan 100 mg and hydrochlorothiazide 25 mg
Hyzaar®: 50/12.5: Losartan 50 mg and hydrochlorothiazide 12.5 mg; 100/12.5: Losartan 100 mg and hydrochlorothiazide 12.5 mg; 100/25: Losartan 100 mg and hydrochlorothiazide 25 mg

Loteprednol (loe te PRED nol)

Brand Names: U.S. Alrex®; Lotemax®
Brand Names: Canada Alrex®; Lotemax®
Pharmacologic Category Corticosteroid, Ophthalmic
Use

Alrex®: Temporary relief of signs and symptoms of seasonal allergic conjunctivitis

Lotemax®: Treatment of postoperative inflammation and pain following ocular surgery; treatment of inflammatory conditions (eg, steroid-responsive inflammatory conditions of the palpebral and bulbar conjunctiva, cornea, and anterior segment of the globe such as allergic conjunctivitis, acne rosacea, superficial punctate keratitis, herpes zoster keratitis, iritis, cyclitis, selected infective conjunctivitis, when the inherent hazard of steroid use is accepted to obtain an advisable diminution in edema and inflammation)

Local Anesthetic/Vasoconstrictor Precautions No information available to require special precautions
Effects on Dental Treatment No significant effects or complications reported
Effects on Bleeding No information available to require special precautions
Adverse Effects
>10%:

Central nervous system: Headache (2% to <15%)
Ocular: Anterior chamber inflammation (5% to 25%), abnormal vision/blurring (5% to 15%), burning on instillation (5% to 15%), chemosis (5% to 15%), discharge (5% to 15%), dry eyes (5% to 15%), epiphora (5% to 15%), foreign body sensation (2% to 15%), itching (5% to 15%), photophobia (5% to 15%)
Respiratory: Pharyngitis (<15%), rhinitis (<15%)
1% to 5%: Ocular: Conjunctival hyperemia, conjunctivitis/irritation, corneal abnormalities, corneal edema, eyelid erythema, increased intraocular pressure, pain, papillae, uveitis
<1%: Cataract formation, changes in visual acuity and/or field defects, global perforation in disease which thins cornea or sclera, optic nerve damage, secondary ocular infection

General Dosage Range Ophthalmic: *Adults:* Ointment: Apply ~1/2 inch ribbon into affected eye(s) 4 times daily; Gel: Instill 1-2 drops into affected eye(s) 4 times daily; Suspension: Instill 1-2 drops into affected eye(s) 4 times daily
Mechanism of Action Corticosteroids inhibit the inflammatory response including edema, capillary dilation, leukocyte migration, and scar formation. Loteprednol is highly lipid soluble and penetrates cells readily to induce the production of lipocortins. These proteins modulate the activity of prostaglandins and leukotrienes.
Pharmacodynamics/Kinetics

Onset of Action Seasonal allergic conjunctivitis: Reduction of symptoms seen within 2 hours of instillation

Pregnancy Risk Factor C
Pregnancy Considerations Loteprednol was shown to be teratogenic in animal reproduction studies when administered orally. The amount of loteprednol absorbed systemically following ophthalmic administration is not known but expected to be <1 ng/mL.

Loteprednol and Tobramycin
(loe te PRED nol & toe bra MYE sin)

Related Information
Loteprednol *on page 846*
Brand Names: U.S. Zylet®
Pharmacologic Category Antibiotic/Corticosteroid, Ophthalmic
Use Treatment of steroid-responsive ocular inflammatory conditions where either a superficial bacterial ocular infection or the risk of a superficial bacterial ocular infection exists
Local Anesthetic/Vasoconstrictor Precautions No information available to require special precautions
Effects on Dental Treatment No significant effects or complications reported
Effects on Bleeding No information available to require special precautions
Adverse Effects Also see individual agents.
>10%:

Central nervous system: Headache (14%)
Ocular: Superficial punctate keratitis (15%)
4% to 10%:
Local: Burning & stinging (9%)
Ocular: Intraocular pressure increased (10%)
<4%:
Local: Discharge, itching
Ocular: Corneal deposits, eye disorders unspecified, eyelid disorder, lacrimation disorder, ocular discomfort, photophobia, secondary infection

General Dosage Range Ophthalmic: *Children and Adults:* Instill 1-2 drops into the affected eye(s) every 4-6 hours
Mechanism of Action See individual agents.
Pregnancy Risk Factor C
Pregnancy Considerations There are no adequate or well-controlled studies in pregnant women. Use only if the potential benefit to the mother justifies the potential risk to the fetus.

Lovastatin (LOE va sta tin)

Related Information
Cardiovascular Diseases *on page 1492*
Brand Names: U.S. Altoprev®; Mevacor®
Brand Names: Canada Apo-Lovastatin®; CO Lovastatin; Dom-Lovastatin; Gen-Lovastatin; Mevacor®; Mylan-Lovastatin; Novo-Lovastatin; Nu-Lovastatin; PHL-Lovastatin; PMS-Lovastatin; PRO-Lovastatin; RAN™-Lovastatin; ratio-Lovastatin; Riva-Lovastatin; Sandoz-Lovastatin
Generic Availability (U.S.) Yes: Excludes extended release tablet
Pharmacologic Category Antilipemic Agent, HMG-CoA Reductase Inhibitor
Use

Adjunct to dietary therapy to decrease elevated serum total and LDL-cholesterol concentrations in primary hypercholesterolemia

Primary prevention of coronary artery disease (patients without symptomatic disease with average to moderately elevated total and LDL-cholesterol and below average HDL-cholesterol); slow progression of coronary atherosclerosis in patients with coronary heart disease and reduce the risk of myocardial infarction, unstable angina, and coronary revascularization procedures.

Adjunct to dietary therapy in adolescent patients (10-17 years of age, females >1 year postmenarche) with heterozygous familial hypercholesterolemia having LDL >189 mg/dL, **or** LDL >160 mg/dL with positive family history of premature cardiovascular disease (CVD), **or** LDL >160 mg/dL with the presence of at least two other CVD risk factors

Local Anesthetic/Vasoconstrictor Precautions No information available to require special precautions

Effects on Dental Treatment No significant effects or complications reported

Effects on Bleeding No information available to require special precautions

Adverse Effects Percentages as reported with immediate release tablets; similar adverse reactions seen with extended release tablets.

>10%: Neuromuscular & skeletal: CPK increased (>2x normal) (11%)

1% to 10%:

Central nervous system: Headache (2% to 3%), dizziness (≤1%)

Dermatologic: Rash (≤1%)

Gastrointestinal: Flatulence (4% to 5%), constipation (2% to 4%), abdominal pain (2% to 3%), diarrhea (2% to 3%), nausea (2% to 3%), dyspepsia (1% to 2%)

Neuromuscular & skeletal: Myalgia (2% to 3%), weakness (1% to 2%), muscle cramps (≤1%)

Ocular: Blurred vision (≤1%)

Additional class-related events or case reports (not necessarily reported with lovastatin therapy): Alkaline phosphatase increased, alteration in taste, anaphylaxis, angioedema, anorexia, anxiety, arthritis, cataracts, chills, cholestatic jaundice, cirrhosis, depression, dryness of skin/mucous membranes, dyspnea, eosinophilia, erectile dysfunction, erythema multiforme, ESR increased, facial paresis, fatty liver, fever, flushing, fulminant hepatic necrosis, GGT increased, gynecomastia, hemolytic anemia, hepatic failure (fatal and nonfatal), hepatitis, hepatoma, hyperbilirubinemia, hypersensitivity reaction, immune-mediated necrotizing myopathy (IMNM), impaired extraocular muscle movement, impotence, interstitial lung disease, leukopenia, libido decreased, malaise, myopathy, nail changes, nodules, ophthalmoplegia, pancreatitis, peripheral nerve palsy, peripheral neuropathy, photosensitivity, polymyalgia rheumatica, positive ANA, psychic disturbance, purpura, renal failure (secondary to rhabdomyolysis), rhabdomyolysis, skin discoloration, Stevens-Johnson syndrome, systemic lupus erythematosus-like syndrome, thrombocytopenia, thyroid dysfunction, toxic epidermal necrolysis, transaminases increased, tremor, urticaria, vasculitis, vertigo

Dosage Oral:

Adolescents 10-17 years: Immediate release tablet:

LDL reduction <20%: Initial: 10 mg daily with evening meal

LDL reduction ≥20%: Initial: 20 mg daily with evening meal

Usual range: 10-40 mg once daily with evening meal, then adjust dose at 4-week intervals; maximum dose per manufacturer: 40 mg daily

Adults:

Immediate release: Initial: 20 mg once daily with evening meal, then adjust at 4-week intervals; maximum dose: 80 mg daily

Extended release: Initial: 20, 40, or 60 mg once daily at bedtime, then adjust at 4-week intervals; maximum dose: 60 mg daily

Note: Doses should be individualized according to the baseline LDL-cholesterol levels, the recommended goal of therapy, and patient response. For patients requiring smaller reductions in cholesterol, the use of the extended release tablet is not recommended; consider use of immediate release formulation.

Elderly: Immediate release: Refer to adult dosing; Extended release: Initial: 20 mg once daily at bedtime

Dosage adjustment for lovastatin with concomitant medications:

Amiodarone: Maximum recommended lovastatin dose (extended release and immediate release): 40 mg daily

Danazol, diltiazem, dronedarone, or verapamil: Initial lovastatin (immediate release) dose: 10 mg daily; Maximum recommended lovastatin (extended release and immediate release) dose: 20 mg daily

Lomitapide: Consider lovastatin dose reduction (per lomitapide manufacturer).

Dosage adjustment in renal impairment: Cl_{cr} <30 mL/minute: Use with caution and carefully consider doses >20 mg/day.

Dosage adjustment in hepatic impairment: No dosage adjustment provided in manufacturer's labeling (has not been studied).

Mechanism of Action Lovastatin acts by competitively inhibiting 3-hydroxyl-3-methylglutaryl-coenzyme A (HMG-CoA) reductase, the enzyme that catalyzes the rate-limiting step in cholesterol biosynthesis

Contraindications Hypersensitivity to lovastatin or any component of the formulation; active liver disease; unexplained persistent elevations of serum transaminases; concomitant use of strong CYP3A4 inhibitors (eg, clarithromycin, erythromycin, itraconazole, ketoconazole, nefazodone, posaconazole, voriconazole, protease inhibitors [including boceprevir and telaprevir], telithromycin); pregnancy; breast-feeding

Canadian labeling: Additional contraindications (not in U.S. labeling): Concomitant use of cyclosporine

Warnings/Precautions Secondary causes of hyperlipidemia should be ruled out prior to therapy. Liver enzyme tests should be obtained at baseline and as clinically indicated; routine periodic monitoring of liver enzymes is not necessary. Use with caution in patients who consume large amounts of ethanol or have a history of liver disease; use is contraindicated with active liver disease and with unexplained transaminase elevations. Rhabdomyolysis with or without acute renal failure has occurred. Risk of rhabdomyolysis is dose-related and increased with concurrent use of lipid-lowering agents which may also cause rhabdomyolysis (fibric acid derivatives or niacin at doses ≥1 g/day) or during concurrent use with potent CYP3A4 inhibitors. Use is contraindicated in patients taking strong CYP3A4 inhibitors. Concomitant use of lovastatin with some drugs may require cautious use, may not be recommended, may require dosage adjustments, or may be contraindicated. Increases in Hb A_{1c} and fasting blood glucose have been reported with HMG-CoA reductase inhibitors; however, the benefits of statin therapy far outweigh the risk of dysglycemia. Monitor closely if used with other drugs associated with myopathy (eg, colchicine). Patients should be instructed to report unexplained muscle pain or weakness; lovastatin should be discontinued if myopathy is suspected/confirmed. Immune-mediated necrotizing myopathy (IMNM), an autoimmune-mediated myopathy, has been reported (rarely) with HMG-CoA reductase inhibitor therapy. IMNM presents as proximal muscle weakness with elevated CPK levels, which persists despite discontinuation of HMG-CoA reductase inhibitor therapy; additionally, muscle biopsy may show necrotizing myopathy with limited inflammation; immunosuppressive therapy (eg, corticosteroids, azathioprine) may be used for treatment. The manufacturer recommends temporary discontinuation for elective major surgery, acute medical or surgical conditions, or in any patient experiencing an acute or serious condition predisposing to renal failure (eg, sepsis, hypotension, trauma, uncontrolled seizures). However, based upon current evidence, HMG-CoA reductase inhibitor therapy should be continued in the perioperative period unless risk outweighs cardioprotective benefit. Use with caution in patients with advanced age; these patients are predisposed to myopathy.

Drug Interactions

Metabolism/Transport Effects Substrate of CYP3A4 (major), P-glycoprotein; **Note:** Assignment of Major/Minor substrate status based on clinically relevant drug interaction potential; **Inhibits** CYP2C9 (weak), CYP3A4 (weak)

Avoid Concomitant Use

Avoid concomitant use of Lovastatin with any of the following: Boceprevir; CycloSPORINE (Systemic); CYP3A4 Inhibitors (Strong); Erythromycin (Systemic); Fusidic Acid; Gemfibrozil; Lomitapide; Mifepristone; Pimozide; Protease Inhibitors; Red Yeast Rice; Telaprevir

Increased Effect/Toxicity

Lovastatin may increase the levels/effects of: ARIPiprazole; DAPTOmycin; Diltiazem; Pazopanib; Pimozide; Trabectedin; Vitamin K Antagonists

The levels/effects of Lovastatin may be increased by: Amiodarone; Bezafibrate; Boceprevir; Colchicine; CycloSPORINE (Systemic); CYP3A4 Inhibitors (Moderate); CYP3A4 Inhibitors (Strong); Cyproterone; Danazol; Dasatinib; Diltiazem; Dronedarone; Erythromycin (Systemic); Fenofibrate; Fenofibric Acid; Fluconazole; Fusidic Acid; Gemfibrozil; Grapefruit Juice; Ivacaftor; Lomitapide; Macrolide Antibiotics; Mifepristone; Niacin; Niacinamide; P-glycoprotein/ABCB1 Inhibitors; Protease Inhibitors; QuiNINE; Ranolazine; Red Yeast Rice; Sildenafil; Telaprevir; Ticagrelor; Verapamil

Decreased Effect

Lovastatin may decrease the levels/effects of: Lanthanum

The levels/effects of Lovastatin may be decreased by: Antacids; Bosentan; CYP3A4 Inducers (Strong); Deferasirox; Efavirenz; Etravirine; Fosphenytoin; P-glycoprotein/ABCB1 Inducers; Phenytoin; Rifamycin Derivatives; St Johns Wort; Tocilizumab

Ethanol/Nutrition/Herb Interactions

Ethanol: Excessive ethanol consumption may have harmful hepatic effects. Management: Avoid excessive ethanol consumption.

Food: Food decreases the bioavailability of lovastatin extended release tablets and increases the bioavailability of lovastatin immediate release tablets. Lovastatin serum concentrations may be increased if taken with grapefruit juice. Management: Avoid concurrent intake of large quantities (>1 quart/day) of grapefruit juice. Red yeast rice contains an estimated 2.4 mg lovastatin per 600 mg rice.

Herb/Nutraceutical: St John's wort may decrease lovastatin levels.

Dietary Considerations Before initiation of therapy, patients should be placed on a standard cholesterol-lowering diet for 6 weeks and the diet should be continued during drug therapy. Avoid intake of large quantities of grapefruit juice (≥1 quart/day); may increase toxicity. Red yeast rice contains an estimated 2.4 mg lovastatin per 600 mg rice. Immediate release tablet should be taken with the evening meal.

Pharmacodynamics/Kinetics

Onset of Action LDL-cholesterol reductions: 3 days

Half-life Elimination 1.1-1.7 hours

Time to Peak Serum: Immediate release: 2-4 hours; extended release: 12-14 hours

Pregnancy Risk Factor X

Pregnancy Considerations Adverse events were observed in animal reproduction studies. There are reports of congenital anomalies following maternal use of HMG-CoA reductase inhibitors in pregnancy; however, maternal disease, differences in specific agents used, and the low rates of exposure limit the interpretation of the available data (Godfrey, 2012; Lecarpentier, 2012). Cholesterol biosynthesis may be important in fetal development; serum cholesterol and triglycerides increase normally during pregnancy. The discontinuation of lipid lowering medications temporarily during pregnancy is not expected to have significant impact on the long term outcomes of primary hypercholesterolemia treatment.

Use of lovastatin is contraindicated in pregnancy. HMG-CoA reductase inhibitors should be discontinued prior to pregnancy (ADA, 2013). If treatment of dyslipidemias is needed in pregnant women or in women of reproductive age, other agents are preferred (Berglund, 2012; NCEP, 2002). The manufacturer recommends administration to women of childbearing potential only when conception is highly unlikely and patients have been informed of potential hazards.

Lactation Excretion in breast milk unknown/contraindicated

Breast-Feeding Considerations It is not known if lovastatin is excreted into breast milk. Due to the potential for serious adverse reactions in a nursing infant, use while breast-feeding is contraindicated by the manufacturer.

Dosage Forms

Tablet, oral: 10 mg, 20 mg, 40 mg
Mevacor®: 20 mg, 40 mg

Tablet, extended release, oral:
Altoprev®: 20 mg, 40 mg, 60 mg

Loxapine (LOKS a peen)

Brand Names: U.S. Loxitane®

Brand Names: Canada Apo-Loxapine®; Dom-Loxapine; Loxapac; Nu-Loxapine; PHL-Loxapine; Xylac™

Pharmacologic Category Antipsychotic Agent, Typical

Use Management of psychotic disorders

Unlabeled Use Psychosis/agitation related to Alzheimer's dementia

Local Anesthetic/Vasoconstrictor Precautions Most pharmacology textbooks state that in presence of phenothiazines, systemic doses of epinephrine paradoxically decrease the blood pressure. This is the so called "epinephrine reversal" phenomenon. This has never been observed when epinephrine is given by infiltration as part of the anesthesia procedure. Loxapine is one of the drugs confirmed to prolong the QT interval and is accepted as having a risk of causing torsade de pointes. The risk of drug-induced torsade de pointes is extremely low when a single QT interval prolonging drug is prescribed. In terms of epinephrine, it is not known what effect vasoconstrictors in the local anesthetic regimen will have in patients with a known history of congenital prolonged QT interval or in patients taking any medication that prolongs the QT interval. Until more information is obtained, it is suggested that the clinician consult with the physician prior to the use of a vasoconstrictor in suspected patients, and that the vasoconstrictor (epinephrine, mepivacaine and levonordefrin [Carbocaine® 2% with Neo-Cobefrin®]) be used with caution.

Effects on Dental Treatment Key adverse event(s) related to dental treatment:

Xerostomia and changes in salivation (normal salivary flow resumes upon discontinuation).

Significant hypotension may occur, especially when the drug is administered parenterally; orthostatic hypotension is due to alpha-receptor blockade, the elderly are at greater risk for orthostatic hypotension.

Tardive dyskinesia: Prevalence rate may be 40% in elderly; development of the syndrome and the irreversible nature are proportional to duration and total cumulative dose over time. Extrapyramidal reactions are more common in elderly with up to 50% developing these reactions after 60 years of age. Drug-induced Parkinson's syndrome occurs often; akathisia is the most common extrapyramidal reaction in elderly.

Increased confusion, memory loss, psychotic behavior, and agitation frequently occur as a consequence of anticholinergic effects. Antipsychotic associated sedation in nonpsychotic patients is extremely unpleasant due to feelings of depersonalization, derealization, and dysphoria.

Effects on Bleeding No information available to require special precautions

Adverse Effects Frequency not defined.

Cardiovascular: ECG changes, edema, facial flushing, hyper-/hypotension, orthostatic hypotension, tachycardia, syncope

Central nervous system: Agitation, altered central temperature regulation, confusion, dizziness, drowsiness, extrapyramidal reactions (akathisia, akinesia, dystonia, pseudoparkinsonism, tardive dyskinesia), faintness, headache, hyperpyrexia, insomnia, lightheadedness, neuroleptic malignant syndrome (NMS), sedation, seizure, slurred speech, tension

Dermatologic: Alopecia, dermatitis, photosensitivity, pruritus, rash, seborrhea

Endocrine & metabolic: Amenorrhea, galactorrhea, gynecomastia, hyperprolactinemia, impotence, menstrual irregularity, polydipsia

Gastrointestinal: Adynamic ileus, constipation, nausea, vomiting, weight gain/loss, xerostomia

Genitourinary: Priapism (rare), urinary retention

Hematologic: Agranulocytosis, leukopenia, thrombocytopenia

Hepatic: ALT increased, AST increased, hepatitis, jaundice

Neuromuscular & skeletal: Gait instability, muscle twitching, numbness, paresthesia, weakness

Ocular: Blurred vision, ptosis

Respiratory: Dyspnea, nasal congestion

General Dosage Range Oral: *Adults:* Initial: 10 mg twice a day (up to 50 mg/day); Usual maintenance: 20-100 mg/day in 2-4 divided doses (maximum: 250 mg/day)

Mechanism of Action Loxapine is a dibenzoxazepine antipsychotic which blocks postsynaptic mesolimbic D_1 and D_2 receptors in the brain, and also possesses serotonin 5-HT_2 blocking activity

Pharmacodynamics/Kinetics

Onset of Action Oral, I.M.: Within 30 minutes; Peak effect: 1.5-3 hours

Duration of Action ~12 hours

Half-life Elimination Biphasic: Initial: 5 hours; Terminal: 19 hours

Pregnancy Considerations Antipsychotic use during the third trimester of pregnancy has a risk for abnormal muscle movements (extrapyramidal symptoms [EPS]) and withdrawal symptoms in newborns following delivery. Symptoms in the newborn may include agitation, feeding disorder, hypertonia, hypotonia, respiratory distress, somnolence, and tremor; these effects may be self-limiting or require hospitalization.

Product Availability

Adasuve™ oral inhalation: FDA approved December 2012; anticipated availability is early third quarter of 2013.

Adasuve™ is approved for the acute treatment of agitation associated with schizophrenia or bipolar I disorder.

Dental Comment Loxapine is known to prolong the QT interval. The QT interval is measured as the time and distance between the Q point of the QRS complex and the end of the T wave in the ECG tracing. After adjustment for heart rate, the QT interval is defined as prolonged if it is more than 450 msec in men and 460 msec in women. A long QT syndrome was first described in the 1950s and 60s as a congenital syndrome involving QT interval prolongation and syncope and sudden death. Some of the congenital long QT syndromes were characterized by a peculiar electrocardiographic appearance of the QRS complex involving a premature atria beat followed by a pause, then a subsequent sinus beat showing marked QT prolongation and deformity. This type of cardiac arrhythmia was originally termed "torsade de pointes" (translated from the French as "twisting of the points"). Loxapine is considered as having a risk of causing torsade de pointes. Since it is not known what effect vasoconstrictors in the local anesthetic regimen will have in patients with a known history of congenital prolonged QT interval or in patients taking any medication that prolongs the QT interval, a medical consult is suggested.

Lubiprostone (loo bi PROS tone)

Brand Names: U.S. Amitiza®

Pharmacologic Category Chloride Channel Activator; Gastrointestinal Agent, Miscellaneous

Use Treatment of chronic idiopathic constipation; treatment of irritable bowel syndrome with constipation in adult women

Local Anesthetic/Vasoconstrictor Precautions No information available to require special precautions

Effects on Dental Treatment Key adverse event(s) related to dental treatment: Xerostomia (normal salivary flow resumes upon discontinuation).

Effects on Bleeding No information available to require special precautions

Adverse Effects

>10%:

Central nervous system: Headache (3% to 11%)

Gastrointestinal: Nausea (7% to 29%; severe: 4%; dose related), diarrhea (7% to 12%; severe 2%)

1% to 10%:
Cardiovascular: Edema (3%), chest discomfort/pain (2%)
Central nervous system: Dizziness (3%), fatigue (2%)
Gastrointestinal: Abdominal pain (1% to 8%), abdominal distention (3% to 6%), flatulence (3% to 6%), vomiting (3%), loose stools (3%), dyspepsia (2%), xerostomia (1%)
Respiratory: Dyspnea (2% to 3%)

General Dosage Range Dosage adjustment recommended in hepatic impairment and in patients who develop toxicities

Oral:
Adults (females): 8 mcg twice daily **or** 24 mcg twice daily
Adults (males): 24 mcg twice daily

Mechanism of Action Bicyclic fatty acid that acts locally at the apical portion of the intestine as a chloride channel activator, increasing intestinal fluid secretion and intestinal motility. Does not alter serum sodium or potassium concentrations.

Pharmacodynamics/Kinetics
Half-life Elimination M3: 0.9-1.4 hours
Time to Peak Plasma: M3: ~1 hour

Pregnancy Risk Factor C
Pregnancy Considerations Animal reproduction studies suggest that lubiprostone may cause fetal loss; teratogenic effects were not observed.

Lurasidone (loo RAS i done)

Brand Names: U.S. Latuda®
Brand Names: Canada Latuda™
Pharmacologic Category Antipsychotic Agent, Atypical
Use Treatment of schizophrenia
Local Anesthetic/Vasoconstrictor Precautions No information available to require special precautions
Effects on Dental Treatment Key adverse event(s) related to dental treatment: Salivary hypersecretion has been reported (normal salivary flow resumes upon discontinuation)
Effects on Bleeding No information available to require special precautions
Adverse Effects
10%:
Central nervous system: Somnolence (dose-related: 8% to 27%), akathisia (dose-related: 6% to 22%)
Endocrine & metabolic: Fasting glucose increased (10% to 14%)
Neuromuscular & skeletal: Extrapyramidal symptoms (24% to 26%), parkinsonism (6% to 17%)
1% to 10%:
Cardiovascular: Tachycardia
Central nervous system: Insomnia (10%), agitation (5%), anxiety (5%), dizziness (4%), dystonia (≤7%), restlessness (1% to 3%)
Dermatologic: Pruritus, rash
Endocrine & metabolic: Prolactin increased (≥5 x ULN: females: 8%; males: 2%)
Gastrointestinal: Nausea (10%), vomiting (8%), weight gain (≥7% increase in baseline body weight: 6%), dyspepsia (6%), salivary hypersecretion (2%), abdominal pain, appetite decreased, diarrhea
Neuromuscular & skeletal: Back pain (3%), CPK increased
Ocular: Blurred vision
Renal: Creatinine increased (3%)

General Dosage Range Dosage adjustment recommended in patients with hepatic or renal impairment or on concomitant therapy.
Oral: Adults: Initial: 40 mg once daily (maximum: 160 mg daily)
Mechanism of Action Lurasidone is a benzoisothiazol-derivative atypical antipsychotic with mixed serotonin-dopamine antagonist activity. It exhibits high affinity for D_2, $5-HT_{2A}$, and $5-HT_7$ receptors; moderate affinity for $alpha_{2C}$-adrenergic receptors; and is a partial agonist for $5-HT_{1A}$ receptors. Lurasidone has no significant affinity for muscarinic M_1 and histamine H_1 receptors. The addition of serotonin antagonism to dopamine antagonism (classic neuroleptic mechanism) is thought to improve negative symptoms of psychoses and reduce the incidence of extrapyramidal side effects as compared to typical antipsychotics.
Pharmacodynamics/Kinetics
Half-life Elimination 18 hours; Main active metabolite, ID-14283 (exo-hydroxy metabolite), exhibits a half-life of 7.5-10 hours
Time to Peak 1-3 hours; steady state concentrations achieved within 7 days
Pregnancy Risk Factor B
Pregnancy Considerations No teratogenic or adverse developmental effects were observed in animal reproduction studies. Antipsychotic use during the third trimester of pregnancy has a risk for abnormal muscle movements (extrapyramidal symptoms [EPS]) and withdrawal symptoms in newborns following delivery. Symptoms in the newborn may include agitation, feeding disorder, hypertonia, hypotonia, respiratory distress, somnolence, and tremor; these effects may be self-limiting or require hospitalization. Healthcare providers are encouraged to enroll women 18-45 years of age exposed to lurasidone during pregnancy in the Atypical Antipsychotics Pregnancy Registry (866-961-2388 or http://www.womensmentalhealth.org/pregnancyregistry).

Lutropin Alfa (LOO troe pin AL fa)

Brand Names: U.S. Luveris® [DSC]
Pharmacologic Category Gonadotropin; Ovulation Stimulator
Use Stimulation of follicular development in infertile hypogonadotropic hypogonadal (HH) women with profound luteinizing hormone (LH) deficiency (<1.2 units/L); to be used in combination with follitropin alfa
Local Anesthetic/Vasoconstrictor Precautions No information available to require special precautions
Effects on Dental Treatment No significant effects or complications reported
Effects on Bleeding No information available to require special precautions
Adverse Effects
1% to 10%:
Central nervous system: Headache (10%), fatigue (3%)
Endocrine & metabolic: Ovarian hyperstimulation (6%), breast pain (5% to 6 %), dysmenorrhea (2% to 3%), ovarian disorder (2%)
Gastrointestinal: Nausea (7%), constipation (2% to 3%), diarrhea (2% to 3%)

Adverse events reported with gonadotropin or menotropin therapy: Adnexal torsion, arterial thromboembolism, congenital abnormalities, ectopic pregnancy, hemoperitoneum, ovarian enlargement (mild-to-moderate), ovarian neoplasms (infrequent), postpartum fever, premature labor, pulmonary complications, spontaneous abortion, vascular complications

General Dosage Range SubQ: *Adults (females):* 75 units daily

Mechanism of Action Lutropin alfa is a recombinant luteinizing hormone prepared using Chinese hamster cell ovaries. Administration leads to increased follicular estradiol secretion needed for follicle stimulating hormone induced follicular development.

Pharmacodynamics/Kinetics
Half-life Elimination Terminal: ~18 hours
Time to Peak 4-16 hours
Pregnancy Risk Factor X
Pregnancy Considerations Adverse events have been observed in animal reproduction studies. Ectopic pregnancy, congenital abnormalities, and multiple births have been reported.

Mafenide (MA fe nide)

Brand Names: U.S. Sulfamylon®
Pharmacologic Category Antibiotic, Topical
Use
Cream: Adjunctive antibacterial agent in the treatment of second- and third-degree burns
Solution: Adjunctive antibacterial agent for use under moist dressings over meshed autografts on excised burn wounds
Local Anesthetic/Vasoconstrictor Precautions No information available to require special precautions
Effects on Dental Treatment No significant effects or complications reported
Effects on Bleeding No information available to require special precautions
Adverse Effects Frequency not defined.
Cardiovascular: Edema, facial edema
Dermatologic: Erythema, maceration, pruritus, rash, urticaria
Endocrine & metabolic: Hyperchloremia, metabolic acidosis
Gastrointestinal: Diarrhea (following accidental ingestion)
Hematologic: Bleeding, bone marrow suppression, DIC, eosinophilia, hemolytic anemia, porphyria
Local: Blisters, burning sensation, excoriation, pain
Respiratory: Dyspnea, hyperventilation, pCO_2 decreased, tachypnea
Miscellaneous: Hypersensitivity
General Dosage Range Topical: *Children and Adults:* Apply to a thickness of approximately $1/16$" once or twice daily
Mechanism of Action As a sulfonamide, mafenide interferes with bacterial folic acid synthesis through competitive inhibition of para-aminobenzoic acid. Spectrum of activity encompasses both gram positive and negative organisms, including *Pseudomonas* and some anaerobes.
Pharmacodynamics/Kinetics
Time to Peak Serum: Cream 11%: 2-4 hours; Burn tissue: Cream 11%: 2 hours, Solution 5%: 4 hours
Pregnancy Risk Factor C
Pregnancy Considerations Teratogenic effects were not observed in animal studies using an oral preparation. Safety and efficacy have not been established in

pregnant women. The manufacturer does not recommended use in women of childbearing potential unless the burn area covers >20% of the total body surface or when benefits of treatment outweigh possible risks to the fetus.

Magaldrate and Simethicone (MAG al drate & sye METH i kone)

Related Information
Simethicone *on page 1236*
Pharmacologic Category Antacid; Antiflatulent
Use Relief of hyperacidity associated with peptic ulcer, gastritis, peptic esophagitis, and hiatal hernia which are accompanied by symptoms of gas
Local Anesthetic/Vasoconstrictor Precautions No information available to require special precautions
Effects on Dental Treatment Key adverse event(s) related to dental treatment: Chalky taste.
Effects on Bleeding No information available to require special precautions
Adverse Effects Frequency not defined.
Based on **magaldrate** component:
Central nervous system: Encephalopathy
Gastrointestinal: Constipation, chalky taste, stomach cramps, fecal impaction, diarrhea, nausea, vomiting, discoloration of feces (white speckles), rebound hyperacidity
Endocrine & metabolic: Hypophosphatemia, hypermagnesemia, milk-alkali syndrome
Neuromuscular & metabolic: Osteomalacia
Miscellaneous: Aluminum intoxication
Based on **simethicone** component: No data reported
General Dosage Range Oral: *Adults:* 5-10 mL (540-1080 mg magaldrate) between meals and at bedtime

Magnesium Carbonate, Calcium Carbonate, and Folic Acid (mag NEE zhum KAR bun ate, KAL see um KAR bun ate, & FOE lik AS id)

Related Information
Calcium Carbonate *on page 233*
Folic Acid *on page 626*
Brand Names: U.S. MagneBind® 400 Rx
Pharmacologic Category Calcium Salt; Electrolyte Supplement, Oral; Magnesium Salt; Vitamin; Vitamin, Water Soluble
Use Prevention or treatment of nutritional deficiencies
Local Anesthetic/Vasoconstrictor Precautions No information available to require special precautions
Effects on Dental Treatment No significant effects or complications reported
Effects on Bleeding No information available to require special precautions
General Dosage Range Oral: *Adults:* 1-3 tablets 3 times/day
Pregnancy Considerations See individual agents.

Magnesium Chloride (mag NEE zhum KLOR ide)

Brand Names: U.S. Chloromag®; Mag 64® [OTC]; Mag Delay™ [OTC]; Slow-Mag® [OTC]
Pharmacologic Category Electrolyte Supplement, Oral; Electrolyte Supplement, Parenteral; Magnesium Salt

Use Correction or prevention of hypomagnesemia; dietary supplement

Local Anesthetic/Vasoconstrictor Precautions No information available to require special precautions

Effects on Dental Treatment Key adverse event(s) related to dental treatment: Magnesium products may prevent GI absorption of tetracyclines by forming a large ionized chelated molecule with the tetracyclines in the stomach. Tetracyclines should be given at least 1 hour before magnesium.

Effects on Bleeding No information available to require special precautions

Adverse Effects Frequency not defined: Gastrointestinal: Diarrhea (excessive oral doses)

General Dosage Range

I.V.:
Children <50 kg: 0.3-0.5 mEq/kg/day
Children >50 kg: 10-30 mEq/day
Adults: 8-24 mEq/day added to TPN
Oral: RDA (elemental magnesium):
Children: 80-240 mg/day
Adults: 360-410 mg/day

Mechanism of Action Magnesium is important as a cofactor in many enzymatic reactions in the body involving protein synthesis and carbohydrate metabolism (at least 300 enzymatic reactions require magnesium). Actions on lipoprotein lipase have been found to be important in reducing serum cholesterol and on sodium/potassium ATPase in promoting polarization (eg, neuromuscular functioning).

Pregnancy Risk Factor C

Pregnancy Considerations Animal reproduction studies have not been conducted. Magnesium crosses the placenta; serum levels in the fetus correlate with those in the mother (Idama, 1998; Osada, 2002).

Magnesium Citrate (mag NEE zhum SIT rate)

Brand Names: U.S. Citroma® [OTC]
Brand Names: Canada Citro-Mag®
Pharmacologic Category Laxative, Saline; Magnesium Salt
Use Relieves occasional constipation
Unlabeled Use Evacuation of bowel prior to certain surgical and diagnostic procedures or overdose situations

Local Anesthetic/Vasoconstrictor Precautions No information available to require special precautions

Effects on Dental Treatment Key adverse event(s) related to dental treatment: Magnesium products may prevent GI absorption of tetracyclines by forming a large ionized chelated molecule with the tetracyclines in the stomach. Tetracyclines should be given at least 1 hour before magnesium.

Effects on Bleeding No information available to require special precautions

Adverse Effects Frequency not defined: Gastrointestinal: Abdominal pain, diarrhea, gas formation, nausea, vomiting

General Dosage Range Oral solution:
Children 2-6 years: 60-90 mL given once or in divided doses (maximum: 90 mL/24 hours)
Children 6-12 years: 90-210 mL given once or in divided doses
Children >12 years, Adolescents, and Adults: 195-300 mL given once or in divided doses

Mechanism of Action Promotes bowel evacuation by causing osmotic retention of fluid which distends the colon with increased peristaltic activity

Pharmacodynamics/Kinetics
Onset of Action Laxative effect: Oral solution: 0.5-6 hours

Pregnancy Considerations Magnesium crosses the placenta; serum concentrations in the fetus are similar to those in the mother (Osada, 2002; Idama, 1998). The American Gastroenterological Association considers the use of magnesium citrate as a laxative to be low risk in pregnancy, but long term use should be avoided (not the preferred treatment of chronic constipation) (Mahadevan, 2006).

Magnesium Gluconate
(mag NEE zhum GLOO koe nate)

Brand Names: U.S. Magonate® [OTC]; Magtrate® [OTC]; Mag®-G [OTC]
Pharmacologic Category Electrolyte Supplement, Oral; Magnesium Salt
Use Dietary supplement

Local Anesthetic/Vasoconstrictor Precautions No information available to require special precautions

Effects on Dental Treatment Key adverse event(s) related to dental treatment: Magnesium products may prevent GI absorption of tetracyclines by forming a large ionized chelated molecule with the tetracyclines in the stomach. Tetracyclines should be given at least 1 hour before magnesium.

Effects on Bleeding No information available to require special precautions

Adverse Effects Frequency not defined: Gastrointestinal: Diarrhea (excessive oral doses)

General Dosage Range Oral: RDA (elemental magnesium):
Children 1-13 years: 80-240 mg/day
Children ≥14 years and Adults: 310-420 mg/day

Mechanism of Action Magnesium is important as a cofactor in many enzymatic reactions in the body involving protein synthesis and carbohydrate metabolism (at least 300 enzymatic reactions require magnesium). Actions on lipoprotein lipase have been found to be important in reducing serum cholesterol and on sodium/potassium ATPase in promoting polarization (eg, neuromuscular functioning).

Pregnancy Considerations Magnesium crosses the placenta; serum concentrations in the fetus are similar to those in the mother (Idama, 1998; Osada, 2002).

Magnesium Hydroxide
(mag NEE zhum hye DROKS ide)

Brand Names: U.S. Fleet® Pedia-Lax™ Chewable Tablet [OTC]; Little Phillips'® Milk of Magnesia [OTC]; Milk of Magnesia [OTC]; Milk of Magnesium [OTC]; Phillips'® Milk of Magnesia [OTC]
Pharmacologic Category Antacid; Laxative; Magnesium Salt
Use Short-term treatment of occasional constipation and symptoms of hyperacidity, laxative

Local Anesthetic/Vasoconstrictor Precautions No information available to require special precautions

Effects on Dental Treatment Key adverse event(s) related to dental treatment: Magnesium products may prevent GI absorption of tetracyclines by forming a large ionized chelated molecule with the tetracyclines in the stomach. Tetracyclines should be given at least 1 hour before magnesium.

Effects on Bleeding No information available to require special precautions

General Dosage Range Oral:
Children 2-5 years: OTC laxative: Magnesium hydroxide 400 mg/5 mL: 5-15 mL/day
Children 6-11 years: OTC laxative: Magnesium hydroxide 400 mg/5 mL: 15-30 mL/day
Children ≥12 years and Adults: OTC laxative: Magnesium hydroxide 400 mg/5 mL: 30-60 mL/day

Mechanism of Action Promotes bowel evacuation by causing osmotic retention of fluid which distends the colon with increased peristaltic activity; reacts with hydrochloric acid in stomach to form magnesium chloride

Pharmacodynamics/Kinetics
Onset of Action Laxative: 30 minutes to 6 hours
Pregnancy Considerations Magnesium crosses the placenta; serum concentrations in the fetus are similar to those in the mother (Idama, 1998; Osada, 2002). The American Gastroenterological Association considers the use of magnesium containing antacids to be low risk in pregnancy (Mahadevan, 2006).

Magnesium Hydroxide and Mineral Oil
(mag NEE zhum hye DROKS ide & MIN er al oyl)

Related Information
Magnesium Hydroxide *on page 852*
Brand Names: U.S. Phillips'® M-O [OTC]
Pharmacologic Category Laxative
Use Short-term treatment of occasional constipation
Local Anesthetic/Vasoconstrictor Precautions No information available to require special precautions
Effects on Dental Treatment Key adverse event(s) related to dental treatment: Magnesium products may prevent GI absorption of tetracyclines by forming a large ionized chelated molecule with the tetracyclines in the stomach. Tetracyclines should be given at least 1 hour before magnesium.
Effects on Bleeding No information available to require special precautions
General Dosage Range Oral:
Children 6-11 years: 20-30 mL at bedtime
Children ≥12 years and Adults: 45-60 mL at bedtime
Pharmacodynamics/Kinetics
Onset of Action Laxative: 30 minutes to 6 hours hours
Pregnancy Considerations See individual agents.

Magnesium L-aspartate Hydrochloride
(mag NEE zhum el as PAR tate hye droe KLOR ide)

Brand Names: U.S. Maginex™ DS [OTC]; Maginex™ [OTC]
Pharmacologic Category Electrolyte Supplement, Oral; Magnesium Salt
Use Dietary supplement
Local Anesthetic/Vasoconstrictor Precautions No information available to require special precautions
Effects on Dental Treatment Key adverse event(s) related to dental treatment: Magnesium ions prevent GI absorption of tetracycline by forming a large, ionized, chelated molecule with the magnesium ion and tetracyclines in the stomach. Magnesium supplement should not be taken within 2-4 hours of oral tetracycline or other members of the tetracycline family.
Effects on Bleeding No information available to require special precautions
Adverse Effects Frequency not defined: Gastrointestinal: Abdominal cramps, diarrhea (excessive oral doses), gas formation

General Dosage Range Oral:
RDA (in terms of elemental magnesium):
Children 1-13 years: 80-240 mg daily
Children ≥14 years and Adults: 310-420 mg daily
Dietary supplement: OTC labeling (dosage in terms of magnesium-L-aspartate hydrochloride salt): *Adults:* One packet or 2 tablets (1230 mg) up to 3 times daily

Mechanism of Action Magnesium is important as a cofactor in many enzymatic reactions in the body involving protein synthesis and carbohydrate metabolism (at least 300 enzymatic reactions require magnesium). Actions on lipoprotein lipase have been found to be important in reducing serum cholesterol and on sodium/potassium ATPase in promoting polarization (eg, neuromuscular functioning).

Pregnancy Considerations Magnesium crosses the placenta; serum concentrations in the fetus are similar to those in the mother (Osada, 2002; Idama, 1998).

Magnesium Oxide (mag NEE zhum OKS ide)

Brand Names: U.S. Mag-Ox® 400 [OTC]; MAGnesium-Oxide™ [OTC]; Phillips'® Laxative Dietary Supplement Cramp-Free [OTC]; Uro-Mag® [OTC]
Pharmacologic Category Electrolyte Supplement, Oral; Magnesium Salt
Use Dietary supplement; relief of acid indigestion and upset stomach; short-term treatment of occasional constipation
Local Anesthetic/Vasoconstrictor Precautions No information available to require special precautions
Effects on Dental Treatment Key adverse event(s) related to dental treatment: Magnesium products may prevent GI absorption of tetracyclines by forming a large ionized chelated molecule with the tetracyclines in the stomach. Tetracyclines should be given at least 1 hour before magnesium.
Effects on Bleeding No information available to require special precautions
Adverse Effects Frequency not defined: Gastrointestinal: Diarrhea (excessive oral doses)
General Dosage Range Oral:
RDA (in terms of elemental magnesium):
Children 1-13 years: 80-240 mg daily
Children ≥14 years, Adolescents, and Adults: 310-420 mg daily
OTC labeling (dosing in terms of magnesium oxide salt): *Children ≥12 years, Adolescents, and Adults:* Dosage varies greatly depending on product.

Mechanism of Action Magnesium is important as a cofactor in many enzymatic reactions in the body involving protein synthesis and carbohydrate metabolism (at least 300 enzymatic reactions require magnesium). Actions on lipoprotein lipase have been found to be important in reducing serum cholesterol and on sodium/potassium ATPase in promoting polarization (eg, neuromuscular functioning).

Pregnancy Considerations Magnesium crosses the placenta; serum concentrations in the fetus are similar to those in the mother (Osada, 2002; Idama, 1998)

Magnesium Salicylate
(mag NEE zhum sa LIS i late)

Related Information
Temporomandibular Dysfunction (TMD), Chronic Pain, and Fibromyalgia *on page 1590*
Brand Names: U.S. Doan's® Extra Strength [OTC]; Keygesic [OTC]; Momentum® [OTC]

◀ **Generic Availability (U.S.)** Yes

Pharmacologic Category Salicylate

Use Mild-to-moderate pain, fever, various inflammatory conditions; relief of pain and inflammation of rheumatoid arthritis and osteoarthritis

Local Anesthetic/Vasoconstrictor Precautions No information available to require special precautions

Effects on Dental Treatment The dentist should be aware of the potential of abnormal coagulation. Caution should also be exercised in the use of NSAIDs in patients already on anticoagulant therapy with drugs such as warfarin (Coumadin®). See Effects on Bleeding.

Effects on Bleeding No information available to require special precautions

Adverse Effects Refer to Aspirin monograph.

Dosage Oral:

Children ≥12 years and Adults: Relief of mild-to-moderate pain:

Doan's® Extra Strength, Momentum®: Two caplets every 6 hours as needed (maximum: 8 caplets/24 hours)

Keygesic: One tablet every 4 hours as needed (maximum: 4 tablets/24 hours)

Contraindications Hypersensitivity to magnesium salicylate, salicylates, other NSAIDs, or any component of the formulation; advanced chronic renal dysfunction; concomitant use with uricosuric agents

In patients ≥65 years of age: Also contraindicated with a history of chronic salicylate use, carditis, chronic liver dysfunction

Warnings/Precautions [U.S. Boxed Warnings]: Use caution with hepatic dysfunction, hypoprothrombinemia, vitamin K deficiency, and prior to surgery. Surgical patients should avoid salicylates if possible, for 1-2 weeks prior to surgery, to reduce the risk of excessive bleeding. Use with caution with bleeding disorders, renal dysfunction, dehydration, gastritis, or peptic ulcer disease. Heavy ethanol use (>3 drinks/day) can increase bleeding risks. Avoid use in renal or hepatic failure. Discontinue use if tinnitus or impaired hearing occurs. Patients with sensitivity to tartrazine dyes, nasal polyps, and asthma may have an increased risk of salicylate sensitivity. Children and teenagers who have or are recovering from chickenpox or flu-like symptoms should not use this product. Changes in behavior (along with nausea and vomiting) may be an early sign of Reye's syndrome; patients should be instructed to contact their healthcare provider if these occur. The lowest effective dose should be used in patients ≥65 years of age. Safety and efficacy have not been established in children <12 years.

Drug Interactions

Metabolism/Transport Effects None known.

Avoid Concomitant Use There are no known interactions where it is recommended to avoid concomitant use.

Increased Effect/Toxicity

Magnesium Salicylate may increase the levels/effects of: Calcium Channel Blockers; Neuromuscular-Blocking Agents

The levels/effects of Magnesium Salicylate may be increased by: Alfacalcidol; Calcitriol; Calcium Channel Blockers

Decreased Effect

Magnesium Salicylate may decrease the levels/effects of: Bisphosphonate Derivatives; Deferiprone; Eltrombopag; Mycophenolate; Phosphate Supplements; Quinolone Antibiotics; Tetracycline Derivatives; Trientine

The levels/effects of Magnesium Salicylate may be decreased by: Trientine

Ethanol/Nutrition/Herb Interactions Refer to Aspirin monograph.

Pharmacodynamics/Kinetics

Half-life Elimination 2 hours; increased with repeated dosing

Time to Peak 1.5 hours

Pregnancy Considerations Refer to Aspirin monograph for additional information.

Breast-Feeding Considerations Salicylates are excreted into human milk. Refer to Aspirin monograph for additional information.

Dosage Forms

Caplet, oral:

Doan's® Extra Strength [OTC]: 580 mg

Momentum® [OTC]: 580 mg

Tablet, oral:

Keygesic [OTC]: 650 mg

Magnesium Sulfate (mag NEE zhum SUL fate)

Pharmacologic Category Anticonvulsant, Miscellaneous; Electrolyte Supplement, Parenteral; Magnesium Salt

Use Treatment and prevention of hypomagnesemia; prevention and treatment of seizures in severe preeclampsia or eclampsia, pediatric acute nephritis; torsade de pointes; treatment of cardiac arrhythmias (VT/VF) caused by hypomagnesemia; soaking aid

Unlabeled Use Asthma exacerbation (life-threatening)

Local Anesthetic/Vasoconstrictor Precautions No information available to require special precautions

Effects on Dental Treatment Key adverse event(s) related to dental treatment: Magnesium products may prevent GI absorption of tetracyclines by forming a large ionized chelated molecule with the tetracyclines in the stomach. Tetracyclines should be given at least 1 hour before magnesium.

Effects on Bleeding No information available to require special precautions

Adverse Effects Adverse effects on neuromuscular function may occur at lower concentrations in patients with neuromuscular disease (eg, myasthenia gravis). Frequency not defined:

Cardiovascular: Flushing (I.V.; dose related), hypotension (I.V.; rate related), vasodilation (I.V.; rate related)

Gastrointestinal: Diarrhea

General Dosage Range

I.V.: *Children and Adults:* Dosage varies greatly depending on indication

Oral: RDA (elemental magnesium):

Children 1-13 years: 80-240 mg/day

Children ≥14 years and Adults: 310-420 mg/day

I.M.: *Adults:* Hypomagnesemia: 1-4 g/day in divided doses

Topical: *Adults:* Soaking aid: Dissolve 2 cupfuls of powder per gallon of warm water

Mechanism of Action When taken orally, magnesium promotes bowel evacuation by causing osmotic retention of fluid which distends the colon with increased peristaltic activity; parenterally, magnesium decreases acetylcholine in motor nerve terminals and acts on myocardium by slowing rate of S-A node impulse formation and prolonging conduction time. Magnesium is necessary for the movement of calcium, sodium, and potassium in and out of cells, as well as stabilizing excitable membranes.

Intravenous magnesium may improve pulmonary function in patients with asthma; causes relaxation of bronchial smooth muscle independent of serum magnesium concentration.

Pharmacodynamics/Kinetics
Onset of Action Anticonvulsant: I.M.: 1 hour; Anticonvulsant: I.V.: Immediate
Duration of Action Anticonvulsant activity: I.M.: 3-4 hours; I.V.: 30 minutes
Pregnancy Risk Factor A/C (manufacturer dependent)
Pregnancy Considerations Animal reproduction studies have not been conducted; however, studies in pregnant women have not shown an increased risk of fetal abnormalities. Magnesium crosses the placenta; serum concentrations in the fetus are similar to those in the mother (Idama, 1998; Osada, 2002). Magnesium sulfate is used for the prevention and treatment of seizures in pregnant women with severe pre-eclampsia or eclampsia (ACOG, 2002). Magnesium sulfate may also be used prior to early preterm delivery to reduce the risk of cerebral palsy (ACOG, 2010; Reeves, 2011).

Maltodextrin (mal toe DEK strin)

Brand Names: U.S. Carrington® Oral Wound Rinse [OTC]; Multidex® [OTC]
Generic Availability (U.S.) No
Pharmacologic Category Anti-inflammatory, Locally Applied
Dental Use Oral: Management and relief of pain due to oral lesions (including mucositis/stomatitis), oral ulcers, or irritation; treatment of aphthous ulcers
Use Topical: Treatment of infected or noninfected wounds
Local Anesthetic/Vasoconstrictor Precautions No information available to require special precautions
Effects on Dental Treatment No significant effects or complications reported (see Dental Comment)
Effects on Bleeding No information available to require special precautions
Dental Usual Dosage Management of pain due to oral lesions: Adults: Oral: Carrington® Oral Wound Rinse: 15 mL, swish or gargle for ~1 minute, 4 times/day or more if needed
Dosage Adults:
Oral: Management of pain due to oral lesions: Carrington® Oral Wound Rinse: 15 mL, swish or gargle for ~1 minute, 4 times/day or more if needed
Topical: Wound dressing: Multidex®: After debridement and irrigation of wound, apply and cover with a nonadherent, nonocclusive dressing. Apply 1/4" thick dressing over entire shallow wound. Completely fill in deep wounds with dressing. May be applied to moist or dry, infected or noninfected wounds. Change dressing once or twice daily.
Mechanism of Action Forms a protective barrier over wound providing an environment which promotes tissue growth.
Contraindications Third-degree burns
Warnings/Precautions Oral: Avoid eating or drinking for 1 hour; products are not harmful if accidentally swallowed; notify healthcare provider if improvement is not seen within 7 days

Dietary Considerations Some products may contain phenylalanine.
Dosage Forms
Gel, topical [preservative free]:
Multidex® [OTC]: 7.1 mL (7.1 mL); 14.2 mL (14.2 mL); 85.2 mL (85.2 mL)
Powder, topical [preservative free]:
Multidex® [OTC]: 6 g (6 g); 12 g (12 g); 25 g (25 g); 45 g (45 g)
Powder for suspension, oral:
Carrington® Oral Wound Rinse [OTC]: 23 g
Solution, topical [preservative free]:
Multidex® [OTC]: 45 mL (45 mL)
Dental Comment Carrington® Oral Wound Rinse: Fill bottle with water to first arrow; shake vigorously until suspended; continue to fill to second arrow; shake well

---

Maprotiline (ma PROE ti leen)

Related Information
Vasoconstrictor Interactions With Antidepressants *on page 1650*
Brand Names: Canada Novo-Maprotiline; Teva-Maprotiline
Pharmacologic Category Antidepressant, Tetracyclic
Use Treatment of major depressive disorder (MDD) or of anxiety associated with depression
Unlabeled Use Chronic pain; panic attacks
Local Anesthetic/Vasoconstrictor Precautions Although maprotiline is not a tricyclic antidepressant, it does block norepinephrine reuptake within CNS synapses as part of its mechanisms. It has been suggested that vasoconstrictor be administered with caution and to monitor vital signs in dental patients taking antidepressants that affect norepinephrine in this way, including maprotiline. Epinephrine and levonordefrin have been shown to have an increased pressor response in combination with TCAs. Maprotiline is one of the drugs confirmed to prolong the QT interval and is accepted as having a risk of causing torsade de pointes. The risk of drug-induced torsade de pointes is extremely low when a single QT interval prolonging drug is prescribed. In epinephrine, it is not known what effect vasoconstrictors in the local anesthetic regimen will have in patients with a known history of congenital prolonged QT interval or in patients taking any medication that prolongs the QT interval. Until more information is obtained, it is suggested that the clinician consult with the physician prior to the use of a vasoconstrictor in suspected patients, and that the vasoconstrictor (epinephrine, mepivacaine and levonordefrin [Carbocaine® 2% with Neo-Cobefrin®]) be used with caution.
Effects on Dental Treatment Key adverse event(s) related to dental treatment: Xerostomia and changes in salivation (normal salivary flow resumes upon discontinuation).
Effects on Bleeding No information available to require special precautions
Adverse Effects
>10%:
Central nervous system: Drowsiness (16%)
Gastrointestinal: Xerostomia (22%)
1% to 10%:
Central nervous system: Dizziness (8%), nervousness (6%), fatigue (4%), headache (4%), anxiety (3%), agitation (2%), insomnia (2%)

Gastrointestinal: Constipation (6%), nausea (2%)
Neuromuscular & skeletal: Weakness (4%), tremor (3%)
Ocular: Blurred vision (4%)

General Dosage Range Oral:
Adults: Initial: 75-150 mg once daily; Maintenance: 75-225 mg/day as a single dose or in divided doses
Elderly: Initial: 25 mg/day; Maintenance: 50-75 mg/day

Mechanism of Action Traditionally believed to increase the synaptic concentration of norepinephrine in the central nervous system by inhibition of its reuptake by the presynaptic neuronal membrane. However, additional receptor effects have been found including desensitization of adenyl cyclase, down regulation of beta-adrenergic receptors, and down regulation of serotonin receptors.

Pharmacodynamics/Kinetics
Half-life Elimination Serum: 27-58 hours (mean: 51 hours)
Time to Peak Serum: Within 12 hours
Pregnancy Risk Factor B
Pregnancy Considerations Adverse effects were not seen in animal reproduction studies.

Dental Comment Maprotiline is known to prolong the QT interval. The QT interval is measured as the time and distance between the Q point of the QRS complex and the end of the T wave in the ECG tracing. After adjustment for heart rate, the QT interval is defined as prolonged if it is more than 450 msec in men and 460 msec in women. A long QT syndrome was first described in the 1950s and 60s as a congenital syndrome involving QT interval prolongation and syncope and sudden death. Some of the congenital long QT syndromes were characterized by a peculiar electrocardiographic appearance of the QRS complex involving a premature atria beat followed by a pause, then a subsequent sinus beat showing marked QT prolongation and deformity. This type of cardiac arrhythmia was originally termed "torsade de pointes" (translated from the French as "twisting of the points"). Maprotiline is considered as having a risk of causing torsade de pointes. Since it is not known what effect vasoconstrictors in the local anesthetic regimen will have in patients with a known history of congenital prolonged QT interval or in patients taking any medication that prolongs the QT interval, a medical consult is suggested.

Maraviroc (mah RAV er rock)

Related Information
HIV Infection and AIDS *on page 1520*
Brand Names: U.S. Selzentry®
Brand Names: Canada Celsentri™
Pharmacologic Category Antiretroviral Agent, CCR5 Antagonist
Use Treatment of CCR5-tropic HIV-1 infection, in combination with other antiretroviral agents
Local Anesthetic/Vasoconstrictor Precautions No information available to require special precautions
Effects on Dental Treatment Key adverse event(s) related to dental treatment: Stomatitis has been observed.
Effects on Bleeding No information available to require special precautions relative to hemostasis.

Adverse Effects
>10%:
Central nervous system: Fever (13%)
Dermatologic: Rash (11%)
Respiratory: Upper respiratory tract infection (23%), cough (14%)
2% to 10%:
Cardiovascular: Vascular hypertensive disorder (3%)
Central nervous system: Dizziness (9%; including postural dizziness), insomnia (8%), anxiety (4%), consciousness disturbances (4%), depression (4%), pain (4%)
Dermatologic: Folliculitis (4%), pruritus (4%), skin neoplasms (benign; 3%), erythema (2%)
Endocrine & metabolic: Lipodystrophy (3%)
Gastrointestinal: Appetite disorders (8%), constipation (6%)
Genitourinary: Urinary tract/bladder symptoms (3% to 5%), genital warts (2%)
Hematologic: Neutropenia (grades 3/4: 4%)
Hepatic: Transaminases increased (grades 3/4: 3% to 5%), bilirubin increased (grades 3/4: 6%)
Neuromuscular & skeletal: Joint disorders (7%), paresthesia (5%), peripheral neuropathy (4%), sensory abnormality (4%), muscle pain (3%)
Ocular: Conjunctivitis (2%), infection/inflammation (2%)
Otic: Otitis media (2%)
Respiratory: Bronchitis (7%), sinusitis (7%), respiratory tract/sinus disorder (3% to 6%), breathing abnormality (4%)
Miscellaneous: Herpes infection (8%), sweat gland disturbances (5%), influenza (2%)

General Dosage Range Dosage adjustment recommended in patients with renal impairment or on concomitant therapy
Oral: *Children ≥16 years and Adults:* 300 mg twice daily
Mechanism of Action Maraviroc, a CCR5 antagonist, selectively and reversibly binds to the chemokine (C-C motif receptor 5 [CCR5]) coreceptors located on human CD4 cells. CCR5 antagonism prevents interaction between the human CCR5 coreceptor and the gp120 subunit of the viral envelope glycoprotein, thereby inhibiting gp120 conformational change required for CCR5-tropic HIV-1 fusion with the CD4 cell and subsequent cell entry.

Pharmacodynamics/Kinetics
Half-life Elimination 14-18 hours
Time to Peak Plasma: 0.5-4 hours
Pregnancy Risk Factor B
Pregnancy Considerations Adverse fetal effects were not observed in animal reproduction studies. It is not known if maraviroc crosses the placenta. The DHHS Perinatal HIV Guidelines note there are insufficient data to recommend use in pregnancy.

Regardless of CD4 count or HIV RNA copy number, all HIV-infected pregnant women should receive a combination antepartum antiretroviral (ARV) drug regimen; this includes women who require therapy for their own health, as well as women who do not yet require therapy for their own health. ARV therapy should be started as soon as possible if required for the woman's health. Although earlier initiation may be more effective in reducing the perinatal transmission of HIV, also consider maternal conditions (eg, nausea and vomiting) and the potential risks of first trimester fetal exposure for specific agents. Plasma HIV RNA levels should be assessed at ~34-36 weeks gestation in order to help determine mode of delivery. If ARV therapy must be interrupted for <24 hours during the peripartum period, stop then restart all medications simultaneously in order to decrease the chance of developing resistance. Long-term follow-up is recommended for all infants exposed to ARV medications.

Healthcare providers are encouraged to enroll pregnant women exposed to antiretroviral medications in the Antiretroviral Pregnancy Registry (1-800-258-4263 or www.APRegistry.com). Healthcare providers caring for HIV-infected women and their infants may contact the National Perinatal HIV Hotline (888-448-8765) for clinical consultation (DHHS [perinatal], 2012).

m-Cresyl Acetate (em-KREE sil AS e tate)

Brand Names: U.S. Cresylate™
Pharmacologic Category Otic Agent, Anti-infective
Use Treatment of external otitis infections caused by susceptible bacteria or fungus
Local Anesthetic/Vasoconstrictor Precautions No information available to require special precautions
Effects on Dental Treatment No significant effects or complications reported
Effects on Bleeding No information available to require special precautions
Adverse Effects Frequency not defined: Otic: Irritation
General Dosage Range Dose reduction may be necessary in children.
Otic: *Children and Adults:* Instill 3-5 drops into the affected ear(s) 3 times daily
Mechanism of Action Creates an acidic environment which inhibits the growth of the bacteria or fungi

Measles, Mumps, and Rubella Virus Vaccine (MEE zels, mumpz & roo BEL a VYE rus vak SEEN)

Brand Names: U.S. M-M-R® II
Brand Names: Canada M-M-R® II; Priorix™
Pharmacologic Category Vaccine, Live (Viral)
Use Measles, mumps, and rubella prophylaxis
The Advisory Committee on Immunization Practices (ACIP) recommends routine vaccination for the following:
• All children (first dose given at 12-15 months of age)
• Adults born 1957 or later (without evidence of immunity or documentation of vaccination).
• Adults at higher risk for exposure to and transmission of measles mumps and rubella should receive special consideration for vaccination, unless an acceptable evidence of immunity exists. This includes international travelers, persons attending colleges and other post-high school education, persons working in healthcare facilities.
Local Anesthetic/Vasoconstrictor Precautions No information available to require special precautions
Effects on Dental Treatment No significant effects or complications reported
Effects on Bleeding No information available to require special precautions
Adverse Effects All serious adverse reactions must be reported to the U.S. Department of Health and Human Services (DHHS) Vaccine Adverse Event Reporting System (VAERS) 1-800-822-7967 or online at https://vaers.hhs.gov/esub/index. In Canada, adverse reactions may be reported to local provincial/territorial health agencies or to the Vaccine Safety Section at Public Health Agency of Canada (1-866-844-0018).

Frequency not defined:
Cardiovascular: Syncope, vasculitis
Central nervous system: Ataxia, dizziness, febrile seizure, fever, encephalitis, encephalopathy, Guillain-Barré syndrome, headache, irritability, malaise, measles inclusion body encephalitis, polyneuritis, polyneuropathy, seizure, subacute sclerosing panencephalitis,
Dermatologic: Angioneurotic edema, erythema multiforme, measles-like rash, pruritus, purpura, rash, Stevens-Johnson syndrome, urticaria
Endocrine & metabolic: Diabetes mellitus, parotitis
Gastrointestinal: Diarrhea, nausea, pancreatitis, sore throat, vomiting
Genitourinary: Epididymitis, orchitis
Hematologic: Leukocytosis, thrombocytopenia
Local: Injection site reactions which include burning, induration, redness, stinging, swelling, tenderness, wheal and flare, vesiculation
Neuromuscular & skeletal: Arthralgia/arthritis (variable; highest rates in women, 12% to 26% versus children, up to 3%), myalgia, paresthesia
Ocular: Conjunctivitis, ocular palsies, optic neuritis, papillitis, retinitis, retrobulbar neuritis
Otic: Nerve deafness, otitis media
Renal: Conjunctivitis, retinitis, optic neuritis, papillitis, retrobulbar neuritis
Respiratory: Bronchospasm, cough, pneumonia, pneumonitis, rhinitis
Miscellaneous: Anaphylactoid reactions, anaphylaxis, atypical measles, panniculitis, regional lymphadenopathy
General Dosage Range SubQ:
Children ≥12 months: 0.5 mL
Adults: Born ≥1957 without evidence of immunity: 0.5 mL for 1 or 2 doses
Mechanism of Action As a live, attenuated vaccine, MMR vaccine offers active immunity to disease caused by the measles, mumps, and rubella viruses.
Pregnancy Risk Factor C
Pregnancy Considerations Animal reproduction studies have not been conducted. It is not known whether this vaccine can cause fetal harm or affect reproduction capacity. Based on information collected following inadvertent administration during pregnancy, adverse events have not been observed following use of rubella or mumps vaccines. However, theoretical risks cannot be ruled out; do not administer to pregnant females. The Advisory Committee on Immunization Practices (ACIP) recommends that pregnancy should be avoided for 1 month following vaccination. Adverse events have been reported following natural infection in unvaccinated pregnant women. Measles infection during pregnancy may increase the risk of premature labor, spontaneous abortion and low birth weights. Rubella infection during the first trimester may lead to congenital rubella syndrome (includes auditory, ophthalmic, cardiac and neurologic defects), growth retardation, bone defects, hepatosplenomegaly, thrombocytopenia and/or purpuric skin lesions; fetal rubella infection can occur during any trimester of pregnancy. Maternal mumps infection during the first trimester may increase the risk of fetal death. Women of childbearing age without documentation of rubella vaccination or serologic evidence of immunity should be vaccinated (for women of childbearing potential, birth prior to 1957 is not acceptable evidence of immunity to rubella). Women who are pregnant should be vaccinated upon completion or termination of pregnancy, prior to discharge (CDC, 1998; CDC, 2001).

Measles, Mumps, Rubella, and Varicella Virus Vaccine
(MEE zels, mumpz, roo BEL a, & var i SEL a VYE rus vak SEEN)

Brand Names: U.S. ProQuad®
Brand Names: Canada Priorix-Tetra™
Pharmacologic Category Vaccine, Live (Viral)
Use To provide simultaneous active immunization against measles, mumps, rubella, and varicella

The Advisory Committee on Immunization Practices (ACIP) recommends routine vaccination against measles, mumps, rubella, and varicella in healthy children 12 months to 12 years of age. For children receiving their first dose at 12-47 months of age, either the MMRV combination vaccine or separate MMR and varicella vaccines can be used. (The ACIP prefers administration of separate MMR and varicella vaccines as the first dose in this age group unless the parent or caregiver expresses preference for the MMRV combination.) For children receiving the first dose at ≥48 months or their second dose at any age, use of MMRV is preferred.

Canadian labeling (not in U.S. labeling): MMRV combination vaccine is approved for use in healthy children 9 months to 6 years; may consider use in healthy children ≤12 years of age based upon prior experience with the separate component (live-attenuated MMR or live-attenuated varicella [OKA-strain]) vaccines.

Local Anesthetic/Vasoconstrictor Precautions No information available to require special precautions
Effects on Dental Treatment No significant effects or complications reported
Effects on Bleeding No information available to require special precautions
Adverse Effects All serious adverse reactions must be reported to the U.S. Department of Health and Human Services (DHHS) Vaccine Adverse Event Reporting System (VAERS) 1-800-822-7967 or online at https://vaers.hhs.gov/esub/index. In Canada, adverse reactions may be reported to local provincial/territorial health agencies or to the Vaccine Safety Section at Public Health Agency of Canada (1-866-844-0018). Percentages reported following one dose of ProQuad® at 12-23 months of age.

Also refer to Measles, Mumps, and Rubella Virus Vaccine (M-M-R® II) monograph for additional adverse reactions reported with this agents.
>10%:
Central nervous system: Fever ≥38.9°C (≥102°F) (22%)
Local: Injection site reaction: Pain/tenderness/soreness (22%), erythema (14%)
1% to 10%:
Central nervous system: Irritability (7%)
Dermatologic: Measles-like rash (3%), varicella-like rash (2%), rash (2%), viral exanthema (1%)
Gastrointestinal: Diarrhea (1%)
Local: Injection site reaction: Swelling (8%), bruising (2%)
Respiratory: Upper respiratory tract infection (1%)
General Dosage Range SubQ: *Children 12 months to 12 years:* 1 dose (0.5 mL)
Mechanism of Action A live, attenuated virus; offers active immunity to disease caused by the measles, mumps, rubella, and varicella-zoster virus.
Pregnancy Risk Factor C

Pregnancy Considerations Animal reproduction studies have not been conducted. Do not administer to pregnant females and pregnancy should be avoided for 3 months (per manufacturer labeling) following vaccination. The ACIP recommends that pregnancy should be avoided for 1 month following vaccination with any of the individual components of this vaccine. Refer to individual monographs. A pregnancy registry has been established for pregnant women exposed to varicella virus vaccine (800-986-8999). Refer to the Measles, Mumps, and Rubella Virus Vaccine monograph for additional information.

Mebendazole (me BEN da zole)

Brand Names: Canada Vermox®
Pharmacologic Category Anthelmintic
Use Treatment of *Ancylostoma duodenale* or *Necator amiericanus* (hookworms), *Ascaris lumbricoides* (roundworms), *Enterobius vermicularis* (pinworms), *Strongyloides stercoralis* (roundworm), *Taenia solium* (tapeworms), *Trichuris trichiura* (whipworms),
Unlabeled Use Treatment of *Ancylostoma caninum* (eosinophilic enterocolitis), *Capillaria philippinensis* (capillariasis), *Giardia duodenalis* (giardiasis), *Mansonella perstans* (filariasis), visceral larva migrans (toxocariasis)
Local Anesthetic/Vasoconstrictor Precautions No information available to require special precautions
Effects on Dental Treatment No significant effects or complications reported
Effects on Bleeding No information available to require special precautions
Adverse Effects Frequency not defined.
Central nervous system: Dizziness, drowsiness, headache, seizure
Dermatologic: Alopecia, angioedema, exanthema, itching, rash, Stevens-Johnson syndrome, toxic epidermal necrolysis, urticaria
Gastrointestinal: Abdominal pain, diarrhea, vomiting
Hematologic: Agranulocytosis, eosinophilia, hemoglobin decreased, leukopenia, neutropenia
Hepatic: Alkaline phosphatase increased, ALT increased, AST increased, GGT increased, hepatitis
Renal: BUN increased, cylindruria, glomerulonephritis, hematuria
Miscellaneous: Hypersensitivity reactions (anaphylactic, anaphylactoid)
General Dosage Range Oral: *Children ≥2 years and Adults:* 100 mg as a single dose **or** twice daily
Mechanism of Action Inhibits the formation of helminth microtubules; selectively and irreversibly blocks glucose uptake and other nutrients in susceptible adult intestine-dwelling helminths
Pharmacodynamics/Kinetics
Half-life Elimination 3-6 hours
Time to Peak Serum: 2-4 hours
Pregnancy Risk Factor C
Pregnancy Considerations Adverse events have been observed in animal reproduction studies; adverse pregnancy outcomes have not been observed following use in pregnancy (Diav-Citrin, 2003; Gyorkos, 2006). Treatment of pinworm in pregnancy may be considered; however, the CDC suggests postponing therapy until the third trimester when possible (CDC, 2010).

Mecasermin (mek a SER min)

Brand Names: U.S. Increlex®

Pharmacologic Category Growth Hormone

Use Treatment of growth failure in children with severe primary insulin-like growth factor-1 deficiency (IGF-1 deficiency; primary IGFD), or with growth hormone (GH) gene deletions who have developed neutralizing antibodies to GH

information available to require special precautions

No significant effects or complications reported

No information available to require special precautions

Adverse Effects ≥5%:

Cardiovascular: Cardiac murmur

Central nervous system: Dizziness, headache, seizure

Endocrine & metabolic: Hypoglycemia (42%), hyperglycemia, iron-deficiency anemia, ovarian cysts, thymus hypertrophy, thyromegaly

Gastrointestinal: Vomiting

Hepatic: Liver enzymes increased

Local: Injection site reactions: Bruising, erythema, hair growth, lipohypertrophy

Neuromuscular & skeletal: Arthralgia, bone pain, extremity pain, muscular atrophy

Ocular: Papilledema

Otic: Ear pain, hypoacusis, middle ear fluid, otitis media, serous otitis media, tympanometry abnormal

Renal: Hematuria

Respiratory: Tonsillar hypertrophy (15%), snoring

Miscellaneous: Lymphadenopathy

General Dosage Range SubQ: *Children ≥2 years:* Initial: 0.04-0.08 mg/kg twice daily; Maintenance: 0.04-0.12 mg/kg twice daily

Mechanism of Action Mecasermin is an insulin-like growth factor (IGF-1) produced using recombinant DNA technology to replace endogenous IGF-1. Endogenous IGF-1 circulates predominately bound to insulin-like growth factor-binding protein-3 (IGFBP-3) and a growth hormone-dependent acid-labile subunit (ALS). Acting at receptors in the liver and other tissues, endogenous growth hormone (GH) stimulates the synthesis and secretion of IGF-1. In patients with primary severe IGF-1 deficiency, growth hormone receptors in the liver are unresponsive to GH, leading to reduced endogenous IGF-I concentrations and decreased growth (skeletal, cell, and organ). Endogenous IGF-1 also suppresses liver glucose production, stimulates peripheral glucose utilization and has an inhibitory effect on insulin secretion.

Pharmacodynamics/Kinetics

Half-life Elimination Severe primary IGFD: Mecasermin: 5.8 hours; Mecasermin rinfabate: >12 hours

Pregnancy Risk Factor C

Pregnancy Considerations Teratogenic effects were not observed in animal studies

---

Meclizine (MEK li zeen)

Brand Names: U.S. Antivert®; Bonine® [OTC] [DSC]; Dramamine® Less Drowsy Formula [OTC]; Medi-Meclizine [OTC]; Trav-L-Tabs® [OTC]; VertiCalm™ [OTC]

Pharmacologic Category Antiemetic; Histamine H_1 Antagonist; Histamine H_1 Antagonist, First Generation; Piperazine Derivative

Use Prevention and treatment of symptoms of motion sickness; management of vertigo with diseases affecting the vestibular system

information available to require special precautions

Key adverse event(s) related to dental treatment: Slight to moderate drowsiness, thickening of bronchial secretions, significant xerostomia (normal salivary flow resumes upon discontinuation).

No information available to require special precautions

Adverse Effects Frequency not defined.

Central nervous system: Drowsiness, fatigue, headache

Gastrointestinal: Vomiting, xerostomia

Ocular: Blurred vision

Miscellaneous: Anaphylactoid reaction

General Dosage Range Oral: *Children ≥12 years and Adults:* 25-50 mg 1 hour before travel, may repeat every 24 hours if needed **or** 25-100 mg/day in divided doses

Mechanism of Action Has central anticholinergic action by blocking chemoreceptor trigger zone; decreases excitability of the middle ear labyrinth and blocks conduction in the middle ear vestibular-cerebellar pathways

Pharmacodynamics/Kinetics

Onset of Action ~1 hour (Wang, 2012)

Duration of Action ~24 hours (Wang, 2012)

Half-life Elimination 5 hours (Wang, 2011a; Wang, 2011)

Time to Peak Plasma: 3 hours (Wang, 2011a; Wang, 2011)

Pregnancy Risk Factor B

Pregnancy Considerations Adverse events have been observed in animal reproduction studies; however, an increased risk of fetal abnormalities has not been observed following maternal use of meclizine during pregnancy.

Meclofenamate (me kloe fen AM ate)

Related Information

Rheumatoid Arthritis, Osteoarthritis, and Osteoporosis *on page 1526*

Temporomandibular Dysfunction (TMD), Chronic Pain, and Fibromyalgia *on page 1590*

Brand Names: Canada Meclomen®

Generic Availability (U.S.) Yes

Pharmacologic Category Nonsteroidal Anti-inflammatory Drug (NSAID), Oral

Use Treatment of inflammatory disorders, arthritis, mild-to-moderate pain, dysmenorrhea

information available to require special precautions

The dentist should be aware of the potential of abnormal coagulation. Caution should also be exercised in the use of NSAIDs in patients already on anticoagulant therapy with drugs such as warfarin (Coumadin®). Recovery of platelet function usually occurs 1-2 days after discontinuation of NSAIDs. See Effects on Bleeding.

Nonselective NSAIDs such as meclofenamate inhibit platelet aggregation and prolong bleeding time in some patients. Unlike aspirin, the NSAID effect on platelet function is quantitatively less, of shorter duration, and reversible.

Adverse Effects

>10%:

Central nervous system: Dizziness

Dermatologic: Rash

Gastrointestinal: Abdominal cramps, heartburn, indigestion, nausea

1% to 10%:

Central nervous system: Headache, nervousness

Dermatologic: Itching
Endocrine & metabolic: Fluid retention
Gastrointestinal: Vomiting
Otic: Tinnitus

Dosage Children >14 years and Adults: Oral:

Mild-to-moderate pain: 50 mg every 4-6 hours; increases to 100 mg may be required; maximum dose: 400 mg

Rheumatoid arthritis and osteoarthritis: 50 mg every 4-6 hours; increase, over weeks, to 200-400 mg/day in 3-4 divided doses; do not exceed 400 mg/day; maximal benefit for any dose may not be seen for 2-3 weeks

Dosage adjustment in renal impairment: No dosage adjustment provided in manufacturer's labeling; use with caution.

Dosage adjustment in hepatic impairment: No dosage adjustment provided in manufacturer's labeling; use with caution.

Mechanism of Action Reversibly inhibits cyclooxygenase-1 and 2 (COX-1 and 2) enzymes, which results in decreased formation of prostaglandin precursors; has antipyretic, analgesic, and anti-inflammatory properties.

Other proposed mechanisms not fully elucidated (and possibly contributing to the anti-inflammatory effect to varying degrees) include inhibiting chemotaxis, altering lymphocyte activity, inhibiting neutrophil aggregation/activation, and decreasing proinflammatory cytokine levels.

Contraindications Hypersensitivity to meclofenamate, aspirin, other NSAIDs, or any component of the formulation; perioperative pain in the setting of coronary artery bypass graft (CABG) surgery

Warnings/Precautions NSAIDs are associated with an increased risk of adverse cardiovascular thrombotic events, including MI and stroke. Risk may be increased with duration of use or pre-existing cardiovascular risk factors or disease. Carefully evaluate individual cardiovascular risk profiles prior to prescribing. May cause new-onset hypertension or worsening of existing hypertension. Use caution with fluid retention. Avoid use in heart failure. Concurrent administration of ibuprofen, and potentially other nonselective NSAIDs, may interfere with aspirin's cardioprotective effect. Risk of MI and stroke may be increased with use following CABG surgery.

Platelet adhesion and aggregation may be decreased; may prolong bleeding time; patients with coagulation disorders or who are receiving anticoagulants should be monitored closely. Anemia may occur; patients on long-term NSAID therapy should be monitored for anemia. Rarely, NSAID use may cause severe blood dyscrasias (eg, agranulocytosis, aplastic anemia, thrombocytopenia).

NSAID use may compromise existing renal function; dose-dependent decreases in prostaglandin synthesis may result from NSAID use, reducing renal blood flow which may cause renal decompensation. NSAID use may increase the risk for hyperkalemia. Patients with impaired renal function, dehydration, heart failure, liver dysfunction, those taking diuretics, and ACE inhibitors, and the elderly are at greater risk of renal toxicity and hyperkalemia. Rehydrate patient before starting therapy; monitor renal function closely. Not recommended for use in patients with advanced renal disease. Long-term NSAID use may result in renal papillary necrosis.

NSAIDs may increase risk of gastrointestinal irritation, inflammation, ulceration, bleeding, and perforation. These events may occur at any time during therapy and without warning. Use caution with a history of GI disease (bleeding or ulcers), concurrent therapy with aspirin, anticoagulants and/or corticosteroids, smoking, use of alcohol, the elderly or debilitated patients. When used concomitantly with ≤325 mg of aspirin, a substantial increase in the risk of gastrointestinal complications (eg, ulcer) occurs; concomitant gastroprotective therapy (eg, proton pump inhibitors) is recommended (Bhatt, 2008).

Use the lowest effective dose for the shortest duration of time, consistent with individual patient goals, to reduce risk of cardiovascular or GI adverse events. Alternate therapies should be considered for patients at high risk.

NSAIDs may cause serious skin adverse events including exfoliative dermatitis, Stevens-Johnson syndrome (SJS) and toxic epidermal necrolysis (TEN); discontinue use at first sign of skin rash or hypersensitivity. Anaphylactoid reactions may occur, even without prior exposure; patients with "aspirin triad" (bronchial asthma, aspirin intolerance, rhinitis) may be at increased risk. Do not use in patients who experience bronchospasm, asthma, rhinitis, or urticaria with NSAID or aspirin therapy. Use caution in other forms of asthma.

Use with caution in patients with decreased hepatic function. Closely monitor patients with any abnormal LFT. Severe hepatic reactions (eg, fulminant hepatitis, liver failure) have occurred with NSAID use, rarely; discontinue if signs or symptoms of liver disease develop, or if systemic manifestations occur.

NSAIDS may cause drowsiness, dizziness, blurred vision and other neurologic effects which may impair physical or mental abilities; patients must be cautioned about performing tasks which require mental alertness (eg, operating machinery or driving). Discontinue use with blurred or diminished vision and perform ophthalmologic exam. Monitor vision with long-term therapy.

In the elderly, avoid chronic use (unless alternative agents ineffective and patient is able to receive concomitant gastroprotective agent); nonselective oral NSAID use is associated with an increased risk of GI bleeding and peptic ulcer disease in older adults in high risk category (eg, >75 years or age or receiving concomitant oral/parenteral corticosteroids, anticoagulants, or antiplatelet agents) (Beers Criteria).

Withhold for at least 4-6 half-lives prior to surgical or dental procedures.

Drug Interactions

Metabolism/Transport Effects None known.

Avoid Concomitant Use

Avoid concomitant use of Meclofenamate with any of the following: Floctafenine; Ketorolac (Nasal); Ketorolac (Systemic); NSAID (COX-2 Inhibitor); Omacetaxine

Increased Effect/Toxicity

Meclofenamate may increase the levels/effects of: Agents with Antiplatelet Properties; Aliskiren; Aminoglycosides; Anticoagulants; Bisphosphonate Derivatives; Collagenase (Systemic); CycloSPORINE (Systemic); Dabigatran Etexilate; Deferasirox; Desmopressin; Digoxin; Drotrecogin Alfa (Activated); Eplerenone; Haloperidol; Ibritumomab; Lithium; Methotrexate; Nonsteroidal Anti-Inflammatory Agents; NSAID (COX-2 Inhibitor); Omacetaxine; PEMEtrexed; Porfimer; Potassium-Sparing Diuretics; PRALAtrexate; Quinolone Antibiotics; Rivaroxaban; Salicylates; Thrombolytic Agents; Tositumomab and Iodine I 131 Tositumomab; Vancomycin; Vitamin K Antagonists

The levels/effects of Meclofenamate may be increased by: ACE Inhibitors; Angiotensin II Receptor Blockers; Antidepressants (Tricyclic, Tertiary Amine); Corticosteroids (Systemic); CycloSPORINE (Systemic); Dasatinib; Floctafenine; Glucosamine; Herbs (Anticoagulant/Antiplatelet Properties); Ketorolac (Nasal); Ketorolac (Systemic); Multivitamins/Minerals (with ADEK, Folate, Iron); Nonsteroidal Anti-Inflammatory Agents; Omega-3 Fatty Acids; Pentosan Polysulfate Sodium; Pentoxifylline; Probenecid; Prostacyclin Analogues; Selective Serotonin Reuptake Inhibitors; Serotonin/Norepinephrine Reuptake Inhibitors; Sodium Phosphates; Tipranavir; Treprostinil; Vitamin E

Decreased Effect

Meclofenamate may decrease the levels/effects of: ACE Inhibitors; Agents with Antiplatelet Properties; Aliskiren; Angiotensin II Receptor Blockers; Beta-Blockers; Eplerenone; HydrALAZINE; Loop Diuretics; Potassium-Sparing Diuretics; Salicylates; Selective Serotonin Reuptake Inhibitors; Thiazide Diuretics

The levels/effects of Meclofenamate may be decreased by: Bile Acid Sequestrants; Nonsteroidal Anti-Inflammatory Agents; Salicylates

Ethanol/Nutrition/Herb Interactions

Ethanol: Avoid ethanol (may enhance gastric mucosal irritation).

Herb/Nutraceutical: Avoid alfalfa, anise, bilberry, bladderwrack, bromelain, cat's claw, celery, chamomile, coleus, cordyceps, dong quai, evening primrose, fenugreek, feverfew, garlic, ginger, ginkgo biloba, ginseng (American, Panax, Siberian), grapeseed, green tea, guggul, horse chestnut seed, horseradish, licorice, prickly ash, red clover, reishi, SAMe (S-adenosylmethionine), sweet clover, turmeric, white willow (all have additional antiplatelet activity).

Dietary Considerations May be taken with food, milk, or antacids.

Pharmacodynamics/Kinetics

Duration of Action 2-4 hours

Half-life Elimination Meclofenamate sodium: 0.8-2.1 hours; metabolite I 15.3 hours

Time to Peak Serum: Meclofenamate sodium 0.5-1.5 hours; metabolite I 0.5-4 hours

Pregnancy Considerations NSAID exposure during the first trimester is not strongly associated with congenital malformations; however, cardiovascular anomalies and cleft palate have been observed following NSAID exposure in some studies. The use of an NSAID close to conception may be associated with an increased risk of miscarriage. Nonteratogenic effects have been observed following NSAID administration during the third trimester including myocardial degenerative changes, prenatal constriction of the ductus arteriosus, fetal tricuspid regurgitation, failure of the ductus arteriosus to close postnatally; renal dysfunction or failure, oligohydramnios; gastrointestinal bleeding or perforation, increased risk of necrotizing enterocolitis; intracranial bleeding (including intraventricular hemorrhage), platelet dysfunction with resultant bleeding; pulmonary hypertension. Because they may cause premature closure of the ductus arteriosus, use of NSAIDs late in pregnancy should be avoided (use after 31 or 32 weeks gestation is not recommended by some clinicians). The manufacture does not recommend the use of meclofenamate in the first or third trimesters of pregnancy. The chronic use of NSAIDs in women of reproductive age may be associated with infertility that is reversible upon discontinuation of the medication.

Lactation Enters breast milk/not recommended

Breast-Feeding Considerations Meclofenamate is excreted into breast milk in trace amounts. Breast-feeding is not recommended by the manufacturer.

Dosage Forms

Capsule, oral: 50 mg, 100 mg

Medium Chain Triglycerides
(mee DEE um chane trye GLIS er ides)

Brand Names: U.S. MCT Oil® [OTC]

Brand Names: Canada MCT Oil®

Pharmacologic Category Nutritional Supplement

Use Dietary supplement for those who cannot digest long chain fats; malabsorption associated with disorders such as pancreatic insufficiency, bile salt deficiency, short bowel syndrome, and bacterial overgrowth of the small bowel; induce ketosis as a prevention for seizures

Local Anesthetic/Vasoconstrictor Precautions No information available to require special precautions

Effects on Dental Treatment No significant effects or complications reported

Effects on Bleeding No information available to require special precautions

Adverse Effects Frequency not defined.

Endocrine & metabolic: HDL serum levels decreased and triglycerides serum levels increased (>6 months daily use)

Gastrointestinal: Abdominal pain, bloating, cramping, diarrhea, nausea

General Dosage Range Oral:

Infants: Initial: 0.5 mL every other feeding, then advance to every feeding, then increase in increments of 0.25-0.5 mL/feeding at intervals of 2-3 days as tolerated

Children: 45 mL/day in divided doses **or** ~39 mL with each meal **or** 50% to 70% (800-1120 kcal) of total calories (1600 kcal)

Adults: 45 mL/day in divided doses **or** 15 mL 3-4 times/day

Mechanism of Action MCTs are saturated fatty acids in chains of 6-12 carbon atoms. They are water soluble and can pass directly through intestinal cell membranes and blood stream. Once taken up by the liver, they are used for metabolic energy before being stored.

MedroxyPROGESTERone
(me DROKS ee proe JES te rone)

Related Information

Endocrine Disorders and Pregnancy *on page 1517*

Brand Names: U.S. Depo-Provera®; Depo-Provera® Contraceptive; depo-subQ provera 104®; Provera®

Brand Names: Canada Alti-MPA; Apo-Medroxy®; Depo-Prevera®; Depo-Provera®; Dom-Medroxyprogesterone; Gen-Medroxy; Medroxy; Medroxyprogesterone Acetate Injectable Suspension USP; Novo-Medrone; PMS-Medroxyprogesterone; Provera-Pak; Provera®; Teva-Medroxyprogesterone

Pharmacologic Category Contraceptive; Progestin

Use Secondary amenorrhea or abnormal uterine bleeding due to hormonal imbalance; reduction of endometrial hyperplasia in nonhysterectomized postmenopausal women receiving conjugated estrogens; prevention of pregnancy; management of endometriosis-associated pain; adjunctive therapy and palliative treatment of recurrent and metastatic endometrial carcinoma

Unlabeled Use Treatment of low-grade endometrial stromal sarcoma; treatment of paraphilia/hypersexuality

◀ **Local Anesthetic/Vasoconstrictor Precautions** No information available to require special precautions

Effects on Dental Treatment Progestins may predispose the patient to gingival bleeding.

Effects on Bleeding No information available to require special precautions

Adverse Effects Adverse effects as reported with any dosage form; percent ranges presented are noted with the MPA I.M. contraceptive injection:

>5%:

Central nervous system: Dizziness, headache, nervousness

Endocrine & metabolic: Libido decreased, menstrual irregularities (includes bleeding, amenorrhea, or both)

Gastrointestinal: Abdominal pain/discomfort, weight gain (>10 lbs at 24 months: 38%)

1% to 5%:

Cardiovascular: Edema

Central nervous system: Depression, fatigue, insomnia

Dermatologic: Acne, alopecia, rash

Endocrine & metabolic: Breast pain, hot flashes

Gastrointestinal: Bloating, nausea

Genitourinary: Dysmenorrhea, leukorrhea, vaginitis

Local: Injection site reaction (SubQ administration): Atrophy, induration, pain

Neuromuscular & skeletal: Arthralgia, backache, leg cramp, weakness

General Dosage Range Dosage adjustment recommended in patients with hepatic impairment.

I.M.:

Adolescents and Adults: Contraception: 150 mg every 3 months

Adults: Endometrial cancer: 400-1000 mg/week

Oral: *Adolescents and Adults:* 5-10 mg once daily

SubQ: *Adolescents and Adults:* 104 mg every 3 months (every 12-14 weeks)

Mechanism of Action Inhibits secretion of pituitary gonadotropins, which prevents follicular maturation and ovulation; causes endometrial thinning

Pharmacodynamics/Kinetics

Half-life Elimination Oral: 12-17 hours; I.M. (Depo-Provera® Contraceptive): ~50 days; SubQ: ~40 days

Time to Peak Oral: 2-4 hours; I.M. (Depo-Provera® Contraceptive): ~3 weeks; SubQ: ~1 week

Pregnancy Risk Factor X

Pregnancy Considerations In general, there is not an increased risk of birth defects following inadvertent use of the injectable medroxyprogesterone contraceptives early in pregnancy. There is an increased risk of minor birth defects in children whose mothers take progesterones during the first 4 months of pregnancy. Hypospadias has been reported in male babies and mild masculinization of the external genitalia has been reported in female babies exposed during the first trimester. High doses are used to impair fertility. Ectopic pregnancies have been reported with use of the MPA contraceptive injection. Median time to conception/return to ovulation following discontinuation of MPA contraceptive injection is 10 months following the last injection.

Mefenamic Acid (me fe NAM ik AS id)

Related Information

Rheumatoid Arthritis, Osteoarthritis, and Osteoporosis *on page 1526*

Temporomandibular Dysfunction (TMD), Chronic Pain, and Fibromyalgia *on page 1590*

Brand Names: U.S. Ponstel®

Brand Names: Canada Apo-Mefenamic®; Dom-Mefenamic Acid; Mefenamic-250; Nu-Mefenamic; PMS-Mefenamic Acid; Ponstan®

Generic Availability (U.S.) Yes

Pharmacologic Category Nonsteroidal Anti-inflammatory Drug (NSAID), Oral

Use Short-term relief of mild-to-moderate pain including primary dysmenorrhea

Local Anesthetic/Vasoconstrictor Precautions No information available to require special precautions

Effects on Dental Treatment The dentist should be aware of the potential of abnormal coagulation. Caution should also be exercised in the use of NSAIDs in patients already on anticoagulant therapy with drugs such as warfarin (Coumadin®). Recovery of platelet function usually occurs 1-2 days after discontinuation of NSAIDs. See Effects on Bleeding.

Effects on Bleeding Nonselective NSAIDs such as mefenamic acid inhibit platelet aggregation and prolong bleeding time in some patients. Unlike aspirin, the NSAID effect on platelet function is quantitatively less, of shorter duration, and reversible.

Adverse Effects 1% to 10%:

Central nervous system: Headache, nervousness, dizziness (3% to 9%)

Dermatologic: Itching, rash

Endocrine & metabolic: Fluid retention

Gastrointestinal: Abdominal cramps, heartburn, indigestion, nausea (1% to 10%), vomiting (1% to 10%), diarrhea (1% to 10%), constipation (1% to 10%), abdominal distress/cramping/pain (1% to 10%), dyspepsia (1% to 10%), flatulence (1% to 10%), gastric or duodenal ulcer with bleeding or perforation (1% to 10%), gastritis (1% to 10%)

Hematologic: Bleeding (1% to 10%)

Hepatic: LFTs increased (1% to 10%)

Otic: Tinnitus (1% to 10%)

Dosage Children >14 years and Adults: Oral: 500 mg to start then 250 mg every 6 hours as needed; maximum therapy: 1 week

Dosage adjustment in renal impairment: Use is not recommended.

Dosage adjustment in hepatic impairment: No dosage adjustment provided in manufacturer's labeling (has not been studied). However, adjustment may be necessary due to extensive hepatic metabolism.

Mechanism of Action Reversibly inhibits cyclooxygenase-1 and 2 (COX-1 and 2) enzymes, which results in decreased formation of prostaglandin precursors; has antipyretic, analgesic, and anti-inflammatory properties.

Other proposed mechanisms not fully elucidated (and possibly contributing to the anti-inflammatory effect to varying degrees) include inhibiting chemotaxis, altering lymphocyte activity, inhibiting neutrophil aggregation/activation, and decreasing proinflammatory cytokine levels.

Contraindications Hypersensitivity to mefenamic acid, aspirin, other NSAIDs, or any component of the formulation; perioperative pain in the setting of coronary artery bypass graft (CABG) surgery; active ulceration or chronic inflammation of the GI tract; renal disease

Warnings/Precautions [U.S. Boxed Warning]: NSAIDs are associated with an increased risk of adverse cardiovascular thrombotic events, including MI and stroke. Risk may be increased with duration of use or pre-existing cardiovascular risk factors or disease. Carefully evaluate individual cardiovascular risk profiles prior to prescribing. May cause new-onset hypertension or worsening of existing hypertension. Use caution with fluid retention. Avoid use in heart failure. Concurrent administration of ibuprofen, and potentially other nonselective NSAIDs, may interfere with aspirin's cardioprotective effect. **[U.S. Boxed Warning]: Use is contraindicated for treatment of perioperative pain in the setting of coronary artery bypass graft (CABG) surgery.** Risk of MI and stroke may be increased with use following CABG surgery.

Platelet adhesion and aggregation may be decreased; may prolong bleeding time; patients with coagulation disorders or who are receiving anticoagulants should be monitored closely. Anemia may occur; patients on long-term NSAID therapy should be monitored for anemia. Rarely, NSAID use may cause severe blood dyscrasias (eg, agranulocytosis, aplastic anemia, thrombocytopenia).

NSAID use may compromise existing renal function; dose-dependent decreases in prostaglandin synthesis may result from NSAID use, reducing renal blood flow which may cause renal decompensation. NSAID use may increase the risk for hyperkalemia. Patients with impaired renal function, dehydration, heart failure, liver dysfunction, those taking diuretics, and ACE inhibitors, and the elderly are at greater risk of renal toxicity and hyperkalemia. Rehydrate patient before starting therapy; monitor renal function closely. Contraindicated in patients with advanced renal disease. Long-term NSAID use may result in renal papillary necrosis.

[U.S. Boxed Warning]: NSAIDs may increase risk of gastrointestinal irritation, inflammation, ulceration, bleeding, and perforation. These events may occur at any time during therapy and without warning. Use caution with a history of GI disease (bleeding or ulcers), concurrent therapy with aspirin, anticoagulants and/or corticosteroids, smoking, use of alcohol, the elderly or debilitated patients. When used concomitantly with ≤325 mg of aspirin, a substantial increase in the risk of gastrointestinal complications (eg, ulcer) occurs; concomitant gastroprotective therapy (eg, proton pump inhibitors) is recommended (Bhatt, 2008).

Use the lowest effective dose for the shortest duration of time, consistent with individual patient goals, to reduce risk of cardiovascular or GI adverse events. Alternate therapies should be considered for patients at high risk.

NSAIDs may cause serious skin adverse events including exfoliative dermatitis, Stevens-Johnson syndrome (SJS) and toxic epidermal necrolysis (TEN); discontinue use at first sign of skin rash or hypersensitivity. Anaphylactoid reactions may occur, even without prior exposure; patients with "aspirin triad" (bronchial asthma, aspirin intolerance, rhinitis) may be at increased risk. Do not use in patients who experience bronchospasm, asthma, rhinitis, or urticaria with NSAID or aspirin therapy. Use caution in other forms of asthma.

Use with caution in patients with decreased hepatic function. Closely monitor patients with any abnormal LFT. Severe hepatic reactions (eg, fulminant hepatitis, liver failure) have occurred with NSAID use, rarely; discontinue if signs or symptoms of liver disease develop, or if systemic manifestations occur.

NSAIDS may cause drowsiness, dizziness, blurred vision and other neurologic effects which may impair physical or mental abilities; patients must be cautioned about performing tasks which require mental alertness (eg, operating machinery or driving). Discontinue use with blurred or diminished vision and perform ophthalmologic exam. Monitor vision with long-term therapy.

In the elderly, avoid chronic use (unless alternative agents ineffective and patient can receive concomitant gastroprotective agent); nonselective oral NSAID use is associated with an increased risk of GI bleeding and peptic ulcer disease in older adults in high risk category (eg, >75 years or age or receiving concomitant oral/parenteral corticosteroids, anticoagulants, or antiplatelet agents) (Beers Criteria).

Withhold for at least 4-6 half-lives prior to surgical or dental procedures.

Drug Interactions

Metabolism/Transport Effects Substrate of CYP2C9 (minor); **Note:** Assignment of Major/Minor substrate status based on clinically relevant drug interaction potential; **Inhibits** CYP2C9 (weak)

Avoid Concomitant Use

Avoid concomitant use of Mefenamic Acid with any of the following: Floctafenine; Ketorolac (Nasal); Ketorolac (Systemic); NSAID (COX-2 Inhibitor); Omacetaxine

Increased Effect/Toxicity

Mefenamic Acid may increase the levels/effects of: Agents with Antiplatelet Properties; Aliskiren; Aminoglycosides; Anticoagulants; Bisphosphonate Derivatives; Collagenase (Systemic); CycloSPORINE (Systemic); Dabigatran Etexilate; Deferasirox; Desmopressin; Digoxin; Drotrecogin Alfa (Activated); Eplerenone; Haloperidol; Ibritumomab; Lithium; Methotrexate; Nonsteroidal Anti-Inflammatory Agents; NSAID (COX-2 Inhibitor); Omacetaxine; PEMEtrexed; Porfimer; Potassium-Sparing Diuretics; PRALAtrexate; Quinolone Antibiotics; Rivaroxaban; Salicylates; Thrombolytic Agents; Tositumomab and Iodine I 131 Tositumomab; Vancomycin; Vitamin K Antagonists

The levels/effects of Mefenamic Acid may be increased by: ACE Inhibitors; Angiotensin II Receptor Blockers; Antidepressants (Tricyclic, Tertiary Amine); Corticosteroids (Systemic); CycloSPORINE (Systemic); Dasatinib; Floctafenine; Glucosamine; Herbs (Anticoagulant/Antiplatelet Properties); Ketorolac (Nasal); Ketorolac (Systemic); Multivitamins/Minerals (with ADEK, Folate, Iron); Nonsteroidal Anti-Inflammatory Agents; Omega-3 Fatty Acids; Pentosan Polysulfate Sodium; Pentoxifylline; Probenecid; Prostacyclin Analogues; Selective Serotonin Reuptake Inhibitors; Serotonin/Norepinephrine Reuptake Inhibitors; Sodium Phosphates; Tipranavir; Treprostinil; Vitamin E

Decreased Effect

Mefenamic Acid may decrease the levels/effects of: ACE Inhibitors; Agents with Antiplatelet Properties; Aliskiren; Angiotensin II Receptor Blockers; Beta-Blockers; Eplerenone; HydrALAZINE; Loop Diuretics; Potassium-Sparing Diuretics; Salicylates; Selective Serotonin Reuptake Inhibitors; Thiazide Diuretics

The levels/effects of Mefenamic Acid may be decreased by: Bile Acid Sequestrants; Nonsteroidal Anti-Inflammatory Agents; Salicylates

Ethanol/Nutrition/Herb Interactions

Ethanol: Avoid ethanol (may enhance gastric mucosal irritation).

Herb/Nutraceutical: Avoid alfalfa, anise, bilberry, bladderwrack, bromelain, cat's claw, celery, chamomile, coleus, cordyceps, dong quai, evening primrose, fenugreek, feverfew, garlic, ginger, ginkgo biloba, ginseng (American, Panax, Siberian), grapeseed, green tea, guggul, horse chestnut seed, horseradish, licorice, prickly ash, red clover, reishi, SAMe (S-adenosylmethionine), sweet clover, turmeric, white willow (all have additional antiplatelet activity).

Dietary Considerations May be taken with food, milk, or antacids.

Pharmacodynamics/Kinetics

Onset of Action Peak effect: 2-4 hours

Duration of Action ≤6 hours

Half-life Elimination ~2 hours

Time to Peak 2-4 hours

Pregnancy Risk Factor C

Pregnancy Considerations Adverse events were not observed in the initial animal reproduction studies; therefore, the manufacturer classifies mefenamic acid as pregnancy category C. NSAID exposure during the first trimester is not strongly associated with congenital malformations; however, cardiovascular anomalies and cleft palate have been observed following NSAID exposure in some studies. The use of an NSAID close to conception may be associated with an increased risk of miscarriage. Nonteratogenic effects have been observed following NSAID administration during the third trimester including myocardial degenerative changes, prenatal constriction of the ductus arteriosus, fetal tricuspid regurgitation, failure of the ductus arteriosus to close postnatally; renal dysfunction or failure, oligohydramnios; gastrointestinal bleeding or perforation, increased risk of necrotizing enterocolitis; intracranial bleeding (including intraventricular hemorrhage), platelet dysfunction with resultant bleeding; pulmonary hypertension. Because they may cause premature closure of the ductus arteriosus, use of NSAIDs late in pregnancy should be avoided (use after 31 or 32 weeks gestation is not recommended by some clinicians). The chronic use of NSAIDs in women of reproductive age may be associated with infertility that is reversible upon discontinuation of the medication.

Lactation Enters breast milk (trace amounts)/not recommended (AAP rates "compatible"; AAP 2001 update pending)

Breast-Feeding Considerations Trace amounts of mefenamic acid may be present in breast milk. Breast-feeding is not recommended by the manufacturer.

Dosage Forms

Capsule, oral: 250 mg

Ponstel®: 250 mg

Mefloquine (ME floe kwin)

Brand Names: Canada Apo-Mefloquine®; Lariam®

Pharmacologic Category Antimalarial Agent

Use Treatment of mild-to-moderate acute malarial infections (including treatment of chloroquine-resistant malaria) and prevention of malaria caused by *Plasmodium falciparum* or *P. vivax*

Note: Due to geographical resistance and cross-resistance, consult current CDC guidelines.

Unlabeled Use Treatment of uncomplicated, chloroquine-resistant *P. vivax* malaria

Local Anesthetic/Vasoconstrictor Precautions No information available to require special precautions

Effects on Dental Treatment No significant effects or complications reported

Effects on Bleeding No information available to require special precautions

Adverse Effects 1% to 10%:

Central nervous system: Chills, dizziness, fatigue, fever, headache

Dermatologic: Rash

Gastrointestinal: Vomiting (3%), abdominal pain, appetite decreased, diarrhea, nausea

Neuromuscular & skeletal: Myalgia

Otic: Tinnitus

General Dosage Range Oral:

Children ≥6 months: Prophylaxis: 5 mg/kg/once weekly (maximum: 250 mg/dose); Treatment: 20-25 mg/kg/day in 2 divided doses (maximum: 1250 mg)

Adults: Prophylaxis: 250 mg once weekly; Treatment: 1250 mg (5 tablets) as a single dose

Mechanism of Action Mefloquine is a quinoline-methanol compound structurally similar to quinine; mefloquine's effectiveness in the treatment and prophylaxis of malaria is due to the destruction of the asexual blood forms of the malarial pathogens that affect humans, *Plasmodium falciparum, P. vivax*

Pharmacodynamics/Kinetics

Half-life Elimination ~3 weeks (range: 2-4 weeks)

Time to Peak Plasma: ~17 hours (range: 6-24 hours)

Pregnancy Risk Factor B

Pregnancy Considerations Mefloquine crosses the placenta and is teratogenic in animals. Malaria infection in pregnant women may be more severe than in nonpregnant women. Clinical experience with mefloquine has not shown teratogenic or embryotoxic effects in humans; use with caution during pregnancy if travel to endemic areas cannot be postponed. Nonpregnant women of childbearing potential are advised to use contraception and avoid pregnancy during malaria prophylaxis and for 3 months thereafter. In case of an unplanned pregnancy, treatment with mefloquine is not considered a reason for pregnancy termination. CDC treatment guidelines are available for the use of mefloquine in the treatment of malaria during pregnancy (CDC, 2011).

Megestrol (me JES trole)

Brand Names: U.S. Megace®; Megace® ES

Brand Names: Canada Apo-Megestrol®; Megace®; Megace® OS; Nu-Megestrol

Pharmacologic Category Antineoplastic Agent, Hormone; Appetite Stimulant; Progestin

Use Palliative treatment of breast and endometrial carcinoma; treatment of anorexia, cachexia, or unexplained significant weight loss in patients with AIDS

Local Anesthetic/Vasoconstrictor Precautions No information available to require special precautions

Effects on Dental Treatment No significant effects or complications reported

Effects on Bleeding Thromboembolic events have been reported.

Adverse Effects Frequency not always defined.

Cardiovascular: Hypertension (≤8%), cardiomyopathy (1% to 3%), chest pain (1% to 3%), edema (1% to 3%), palpitation (1% to 3%), peripheral edema (1% to 3%), heart failure

Central nervous system: Headache (≤10%), insomnia (≤6%), fever (1% to 6%), pain (≤6%, similar to placebo), abnormal thinking (1% to 3%), confusion (1% to 3%), depression (1% to 3%), hypoesthesia (1% to 3%), seizure (1% to 3%), mood changes, malaise, lethargy

Dermatologic: Rash (2% to 12%), alopecia (1% to 3%), pruritus (1% to 3%), vesiculobullous rash (1% to 3%)

Endocrine & metabolic: Hyperglycemia (≤6%), gynecomastia (1% to 3%), adrenal insufficiency, amenorrhea, breakthrough bleeding, cervical erosion and secretions (changes), breast tenderness increased, Cushing's syndrome, diabetes, glucose intolerance, HPA axis suppression, hot flashes, hypercalcemia, menstrual flow changes, spotting, vaginal bleeding pattern changes

Gastrointestinal: Diarrhea (6% to 15%, similar to placebo), flatulence (≤10%), vomiting (≤6%), nausea (≤5%), dyspepsia (≤4%), abdominal pain (1% to 3%), constipation (1% to 3%), salivation increased (1% to 3%), xerostomia (1% to 3%), weight gain (not attributed to edema or fluid retention)

Genitourinary: Impotence (4% to 14%), decreased libido (≤5%), urinary incontinence (1% to 3%), urinary tract infection (1% to 3%), urinary frequency (≤2%)

Hematologic: Anemia (≤5%), leukopenia (1% to 3%)

Hepatic: Hepatomegaly (1% to 3%), LDH increased (1% to 3%), cholestatic jaundice, hepatotoxicity

Neuromuscular & skeletal: Weakness (2% to 6%), neuropathy (1% to 3%), paresthesia (1% to 3%), carpal tunnel syndrome

Ocular: Amblyopia (1% to 3%)

Renal: Albuminuria (1% to 3%)

Respiratory: Dyspnea (1% to 3%), cough (1% to 3%), pharyngitis (1% to 3%), pneumonia (≤2%), hyperpnea

Miscellaneous: Diaphoresis (1% to 3%), herpes infection (1% to 3%), infection (1% to 3%), moniliasis (1% to 3%), tumor flare

General Dosage Range Oral:

Adults (females): Tablet: 40-320 mg/day in divided doses

Adults (males/females): Suspension: 400-800 mg/day [Megace®] **or** 625 mg/day [Megace® ES]

Mechanism of Action A synthetic progestin with antiestrogenic properties which disrupt the estrogen receptor cycle. Megestrol interferes with the normal estrogen cycle and results in a lower LH titer. May also have a direct effect on the endometrium. Megestrol is an antineoplastic progestin thought to act through an antileutenizing effect mediated via the pituitary. May stimulate appetite by antagonizing the metabolic effects of catabolic cytokines.

Pharmacodynamics/Kinetics

Half-life Elimination 13-105 hours

Time to Peak Serum: 1-3 hours

Pregnancy Risk Factor D (tablet) / X (suspension)

Pregnancy Considerations Adverse effects were demonstrated in animal studies. Use during pregnancy is contraindicated (suspension).

Meloxicam (mel OKS i kam)

Related Information
Rheumatoid Arthritis, Osteoarthritis, and Osteoporosis *on page 1526*

Brand Names: U.S. Mobic®

Brand Names: Canada Apo-Meloxicam®; Auro-Meloxicam; Ava-Meloxicam; CO Meloxicam; Dom-Meloxicam; Mobicox®; Mobic®; Mylan-Meloxicam; Novo-Meloxicam; PHL-Meloxicam; PMS-Meloxicam; ratio-Meloxicam; Teva-Meloxicam

Generic Availability (U.S.) Yes:

Pharmacologic Category Nonsteroidal Anti-inflammatory Drug (NSAID), Oral

Use Relief of signs and symptoms of osteoarthritis, rheumatoid arthritis, and juvenile idiopathic arthritis (JIA)

Local Anesthetic/Vasoconstrictor Precautions No information available to require special precautions

Effects on Dental Treatment Key adverse event(s) related to dental treatment: Taste perversion, ulcerative stomatitis, and xerostomia (normal salivary flow resumes upon discontinuation). The dentist should be aware of the potential of abnormal coagulation. Caution should also be exercised in the use of NSAIDs in patients already on anticoagulant therapy with drugs such as warfarin (Coumadin®). See Effects on Bleeding.

Effects on Bleeding Nonselective NSAIDs such as meloxicam inhibit platelet aggregation and prolong bleeding time in some patients. Unlike aspirin, the NSAID effect on platelet function is quantitatively less, of shorter duration, and reversible.

Adverse Effects Percentages reported in adult patients; abdominal pain, diarrhea, fever, headache, pyrexia, and vomiting were reported more commonly in pediatric patients

2% to 10%:

Cardiovascular: Edema (≤5%)

Central nervous system: Headache (2% to 8%), pain (1% to 5%), dizziness (≤4%), insomnia (≤4%)

Dermatologic: Pruritus (≤3%), rash (≤3%)

Gastrointestinal: Dyspepsia (4% to 10%), diarrhea (2% to 8%), nausea (2% to 7%), abdominal pain (2% to 5%), constipation (≤3%), flatulence (≤3%), vomiting (≤3%)

Genitourinary: Urinary tract infection (≤7%), micturition (≤2%)

Hematologic: Anemia (≤4%)

Neuromuscular & skeletal: Arthralgia (≤5%), back pain (≤3%)

Respiratory: Upper respiratory infection (≤8%), cough (≤2%), pharyngitis (≤3%)

Miscellaneous: Flu-like syndrome (2% to 6%), falls (≤3%)

Dosage Oral:

Children ≥2 years: Juvenile idiopathic arthritis (JIA): 0.125 mg/kg/day; maximum dose: 7.5 mg/day

Adults: Osteoarthritis, rheumatoid arthritis: Initial: 7.5 mg once daily; some patients may receive additional benefit from increasing dose to 15 mg once daily; maximum dose: 15 mg/day

Elderly: Increased concentrations may occur in elderly patients (particularly in females); however, no specific dosage adjustment is recommended

Dosage adjustment in renal impairment:
Mild-to-moderate impairment: No specific dosage recommendations

Significant impairment (Cl$_{cr}$ ≤20 mL/minute): Patients with severe renal impairment have not been adequately studied; use not recommended.
Hemodialysis: Maximum dose: 7.5 mg/day

Dosage adjustment in hepatic impairment:
Mild-to-moderate hepatic impairment (Child-Pugh class A or B): No dosage adjustment is necessary
Severe hepatic impairment: Patients with severe hepatic impairment have not been adequately studied

Mechanism of Action Reversibly inhibits cyclooxygenase-1 and 2 (COX-1 and 2) enzymes, which results in decreased formation of prostaglandin precursors; has antipyretic, analgesic, and anti-inflammatory properties

Other proposed mechanisms not fully elucidated (and possibly contributing to the anti-inflammatory effect to varying degrees), include inhibiting chemotaxis, altering lymphocyte activity, inhibiting neutrophil aggregation/activation, and decreasing proinflammatory cytokine levels.

Contraindications Hypersensitivity (eg, asthma, urticaria, allergic-type reactions) to meloxicam, aspirin, other NSAIDs, or any component of the formulation; perioperative pain in the setting of coronary artery bypass graft (CABG) surgery

Warnings/Precautions [U.S. Boxed Warning]: NSAIDs are associated with an increased risk of adverse cardiovascular thrombotic events, including MI and stroke. Risk may be increased with duration of use or pre-existing cardiovascular risk factors or disease. Carefully evaluate individual cardiovascular risk profiles prior to prescribing. May cause new-onset hypertension or worsening of existing hypertension. Use caution with fluid retention. Avoid use in heart failure. Concurrent administration of ibuprofen, and potentially other nonselective NSAIDs, may interfere with aspirin's cardioprotective effect. **[U.S. Boxed Warning]: Use is contraindicated for treatment of perioperative pain in the setting of coronary artery bypass graft (CABG) surgery.** Risk of MI and stroke may be increased with use within the first 10-14 days following CABG surgery.

Platelet adhesion and aggregation may be decreased; may prolong bleeding time; patients with coagulation disorders or who are receiving anticoagulants should be monitored closely. Anemia may occur; patients on long-term NSAID therapy should be monitored for anemia. Rarely, NSAID use may cause severe blood dyscrasias (eg, agranulocytosis, aplastic anemia, thrombocytopenia).

NSAID use may compromise existing renal function; dose-dependent decreases in prostaglandin synthesis may result from NSAID use, reducing renal blood flow which may cause renal decompensation. NSAID use may increase the risk for hyperkalemia. Patients with impaired renal function, dehydration, heart failure, liver dysfunction, those taking diuretics, and ACE inhibitors, and the elderly are at greater risk of renal toxicity and hyperkalemia. Rehydrate patient before starting therapy; monitor renal function closely. Not recommended for use in patients with advanced renal disease. Long-term NSAID use may result in renal papillary necrosis.

[U.S. Boxed Warning]: NSAIDs may increase risk of gastrointestinal irritation, inflammation, ulceration, bleeding, and perforation. These events may occur at any time during therapy and without warning. Use caution with a history of GI disease (bleeding or ulcers), concurrent therapy with aspirin, anticoagulants and/or corticosteroids, smoking, use of alcohol, the elderly or debilitated patients. When used concomitantly with ≤325 mg of aspirin, a substantial increase in the risk of gastrointestinal complications (eg, ulcer) occurs; concomitant gastroprotective therapy (eg, proton pump inhibitors) is recommended (Bhatt, 2008).

Use the lowest effective dose for the shortest duration of time, consistent with individual patient goals, to reduce risk of cardiovascular or GI adverse events. Alternate therapies should be considered for patients at high risk.

NSAIDs may cause serious skin adverse events including exfoliative dermatitis, Stevens-Johnson syndrome (SJS) and toxic epidermal necrolysis (TEN); discontinue use at first sign of skin rash or hypersensitivity. Anaphylactoid reactions may occur, even without prior exposure; patients with "aspirin triad" (bronchial asthma, aspirin intolerance, rhinitis) may be at increased risk. Do not use in patients who experience bronchospasm, asthma, rhinitis, or urticaria with NSAID or aspirin therapy. Use caution in other forms of asthma.

Use with caution in patients with decreased hepatic function. Closely monitor patients with any abnormal LFT. Severe hepatic reactions (eg, fulminant hepatitis, liver failure) have occurred with NSAID use, rarely; discontinue if signs or symptoms of liver disease develop, or if systemic manifestations occur.

NSAIDS may cause drowsiness, dizziness, blurred vision and other neurologic effects which may impair physical or mental abilities; patients must be cautioned about performing tasks which require mental alertness (eg, operating machinery or driving). Discontinue use with blurred or diminished vision and perform ophthalmologic exam. Monitor vision with long-term therapy.

In the elderly, avoid chronic use (unless alternative agents ineffective and patient can receive concomitant gastroprotective agent); nonselective oral NSAID use is associated with an increased risk of GI bleeding and peptic ulcer disease in older adults in high risk category (eg, >75 years or age or receiving concomitant oral/parenteral corticosteroids, anticoagulants, or antiplatelet agents) (Beers Criteria).

Oral suspension formulation may contain sorbitol. Concomitant use with sodium polystyrene sulfonate (Kayexalate®) may cause intestinal necrosis (including fatal cases); combined use should be avoided. Withhold for at least 4-6 half-lives prior to surgical or dental procedures.

Drug Interactions
Metabolism/Transport Effects Substrate of CYP3A4 (minor); **Note:** Assignment of Major/Minor substrate status based on clinically relevant drug interaction potential; **Inhibits** CYP2C9 (weak)

Avoid Concomitant Use
Avoid concomitant use of Meloxicam with any of the following: Calcium Polystyrene Sulfonate; Floctafenine; Ketorolac (Nasal); Ketorolac (Systemic); NSAID (COX-2 Inhibitor); Omacetaxine; Sodium Polystyrene Sulfonate

Increased Effect/Toxicity
Meloxicam may increase the levels/effects of: Agents with Antiplatelet Properties; Aliskiren; Aminoglycosides; Anticoagulants; Bisphosphonate Derivatives; Calcium Polystyrene Sulfonate; Collagenase (Systemic); CycloSPORINE (Systemic); Dabigatran Etexilate; Deferasirox; Desmopressin; Digoxin; Drotrecogin Alfa (Activated); Eplerenone; Haloperidol; Ibritumomab; Lithium; Methotrexate; Nonsteroidal Anti-Inflammatory Agents; NSAID (COX-2 Inhibitor);

Omacetaxine; PEMEtrexed; Porfimer; Potassium-Sparing Diuretics; PRALAtrexate; Quinolone Antibiotics; Rivaroxaban; Salicylates; Sodium Polystyrene Sulfonate; Thrombolytic Agents; Tositumomab and Iodine I 131 Tositumomab; Vancomycin; Vitamin K Antagonists

The levels/effects of Meloxicam may be increased by: ACE Inhibitors; Angiotensin II Receptor Blockers; Antidepressants (Tricyclic, Tertiary Amine); Corticosteroids (Systemic); CycloSPORINE (Systemic); Dasatinib; Floctafenine; Glucosamine; Herbs (Anticoagulant/Antiplatelet Properties); Ketorolac (Nasal); Ketorolac (Systemic); Multivitamins/Minerals (with ADEK, Folate, Iron); Nonsteroidal Anti-Inflammatory Agents; Omega-3 Fatty Acids; Pentosan Polysulfate Sodium; Pentoxifylline; Probenecid; Prostacyclin Analogues; Selective Serotonin Reuptake Inhibitors; Serotonin/Norepinephrine Reuptake Inhibitors; Sodium Phosphates; Tipranavir; Treprostinil; Vitamin E; Voriconazole

Decreased Effect

Meloxicam may decrease the levels/effects of: ACE Inhibitors; Agents with Antiplatelet Properties; Aliskiren; Angiotensin II Receptor Blockers; Beta-Blockers; Eplerenone; HydrALAZINE; Loop Diuretics; Potassium-Sparing Diuretics; Salicylates; Selective Serotonin Reuptake Inhibitors; Thiazide Diuretics

The levels/effects of Meloxicam may be decreased by: Bile Acid Sequestrants; Nonsteroidal Anti-Inflammatory Agents; Salicylates

Ethanol/Nutrition/Herb Interactions

Ethanol: Avoid ethanol (may enhance gastric mucosal irritation).

Herb/Nutraceutical: Avoid alfalfa, anise, bilberry, bladderwrack, bromelain, cat's claw, celery, chamomile, coleus, cordyceps, dong quai, evening primrose, fenugreek, feverfew, garlic, ginger, ginkgo biloba, ginseng (American, Panax, Siberian), grapeseed, green tea, guggul, horse chestnut seed, horseradish, licorice, prickly ash, red clover, reishi, SAMe (S-adenosylmethionine), sweet clover, turmeric, white willow (all have additional antiplatelet activity).

Dietary Considerations Should be taken with food or milk to minimize gastrointestinal irritation.

Pharmacodynamics/Kinetics

Half-life Elimination Adults: 15-20 hours

Time to Peak Initial: 4-5 hours; Secondary: 12-14 hours

Pregnancy Risk Factor C/D ≥30 weeks gestation

Pregnancy Considerations Adverse events were not observed in the initial animal reproduction studies; therefore, the manufacturer classifies meloxicam as pregnancy category C (category D: ≥30 weeks gestation). Meloxicam crosses the placenta. NSAID exposure during the first trimester is not strongly associated with congenital malformations; however, cardiovascular anomalies and cleft palate have been observed following NSAID exposure in some studies. The use of an NSAID close to conception may be associated with an increased risk of miscarriage. Nonteratogenic effects have been observed following NSAID administration during the third trimester including myocardial degenerative changes, prenatal constriction of the ductus arteriosus, fetal tricuspid regurgitation, failure of the ductus arteriosus to close postnatally; renal dysfunction or failure, oligohydramnios; gastrointestinal bleeding or perforation, increased risk of necrotizing enterocolitis; intracranial bleeding (including intraventricular hemorrhage), platelet dysfunction with resultant bleeding;

pulmonary hypertension. Because they may cause premature closure of the ductus arteriosus, use of NSAIDs late in pregnancy should be avoided (use after 31 or 32 weeks gestation is not recommended by some clinicians). Product labeling for Mobic® specifically notes that use at ≥30 weeks gestation should be avoided and therefore classifies meloxicam as pregnancy category D at this time. The chronic use of NSAIDs in women of reproductive age may be associated with infertility that is reversible upon discontinuation of the medication.

Lactation Excretion in breast milk unknown/not recommended

Breast-Feeding Considerations It is not known whether meloxicam is excreted in human milk. Breast-feeding is not recommended by the manufacturer.

Dosage Forms

Suspension, oral: 7.5 mg/5 mL (100 mL)
  Mobic®: 7.5 mg/5 mL (100 mL)
Tablet, oral: 7.5 mg, 15 mg
  Mobic®: 7.5 mg, 15 mg

Melphalan (MEL fa lan)

Brand Names: U.S. Alkeran®
Brand Names: Canada Alkeran®
Pharmacologic Category Antineoplastic Agent, Alkylating Agent

Use Palliative treatment of multiple myeloma and nonresectable epithelial ovarian carcinoma

Unlabeled Use Treatment of Hodgkin lymphoma, light chain amyloidosis; conditioning regimen for autologous hematopoietic stem cell transplantation in adults with hematologic disorders (eg, multiple myeloma) and autologous marrow or stem cell transplantation in pediatric neuroblastoma and Ewing's sarcoma

Local Anesthetic/Vasoconstrictor Precautions No information available to require special precautions

Effects on Dental Treatment Key adverse event(s) related to dental treatment: Stomatitis.

Effects on Bleeding Severe myelosuppression including anemia and thrombocytopenia occurs which may result in bleeding. Medical consult recommended.

Adverse Effects

>10%:
  Gastrointestinal: Nausea/vomiting, diarrhea, oral ulceration
  Hematologic: Myelosuppression, leukopenia (nadir: 14-21 days; recovery: 28-35 days), thrombocytopenia (nadir: 14-21 days; recovery: 28-35 days), anemia
  Miscellaneous: Secondary malignancy (<2% to 20%; cumulative dose and duration dependent, includes acute myeloid leukemia, myeloproliferative syndrome, carcinoma)

1% to 10%: Miscellaneous: Hypersensitivity (I.V.: 2%; includes bronchospasm, dyspnea, edema, hypotension, pruritus, rash, tachycardia, urticaria)

General Dosage Range Dosage adjustment recommended in patients with renal impairment or who develop toxicities

I.V.: *Adults:* 16 mg/m² administered at 2-week intervals for 4 doses, then repeat at 4-week intervals

Oral: *Adults:* Dosage varies greatly depending on indication

Mechanism of Action Alkylating agent which is a derivative of mechlorethamine that inhibits DNA and RNA synthesis via formation of carbonium ions; crosslinks strands of DNA; acts on both resting and rapidly dividing tumor cells.

◀ **Pharmacodynamics/Kinetics**
Half-life Elimination Terminal: I.V.: 75 minutes; Oral: 1-2 hours
Time to Peak Serum: Oral: ~1-2 hours
Pregnancy Risk Factor D
Pregnancy Considerations Animal studies have demonstrated embryotoxicity and teratogenicity. Therapy may suppress ovarian function leading to amenorrhea. There are no adequate and well-controlled studies in pregnant women. May cause fetal harm if administered during pregnancy. Women of childbearing potential should be advised to avoid pregnancy while on melphalan therapy.

Memantine (me MAN teen)

Brand Names: U.S. Namenda®
Brand Names: Canada Apo-Memantine; CO Memantine; Ebixa®; PMS-Memantine; ratio-Memantine; Riva-Memantine; Sandoz-Memantine
Pharmacologic Category N-Methyl-D-Aspartate Receptor Antagonist
Use Treatment of moderate-to-severe dementia of the Alzheimer's type
Unlabeled Use Treatment of mild-to-moderate vascular dementia
Local Anesthetic/Vasoconstrictor Precautions No information available to require special precautions
Effects on Dental Treatment No significant effects or complications reported
Effects on Bleeding No information available to require special precautions
Adverse Effects 1% to 10%:
Cardiovascular: Hypertension (4%), cardiac failure, cerebrovascular accident, syncope, transient ischemic attack
Central nervous system: Dizziness (7%), confusion (6%), headache (6%), hallucinations (3%), pain (3%), somnolence (3%), fatigue (2%), aggressive reaction, ataxia, vertigo
Dermatologic: Rash
Gastrointestinal: Constipation (5%), vomiting (3%), weight loss
Genitourinary: Micturition
Hematologic: Anemia
Hepatic: Alkaline phosphatase increased
Neuromuscular & skeletal: Back pain (3%), hypokinesia
Ocular: Cataract, conjunctivitis
Respiratory: Cough (4%), dyspnea (2%), pneumonia
General Dosage Range Dosage adjustment recommended in patients with renal impairment
Oral: *Adults:* Initial: 5 mg once daily; Target: 20 mg daily in 2 divided doses
Mechanism of Action Glutamate, the primary excitatory amino acid in the CNS, may contribute to the pathogenesis of Alzheimer's disease (AD) by overstimulating various glutamate receptors leading to excitotoxicity and neuronal cell death. Memantine is an uncompetitive antagonist of the N-methyl-D-aspartate (NMDA) type of glutamate receptors, located ubiquitously throughout the brain. Under normal physiologic conditions, the (unstimulated) NMDA receptor ion channel is blocked by magnesium ions, which are displaced after agonist-induced depolarization. Pathologic or excessive receptor activation, as postulated to occur during AD, prevents magnesium from reentering and blocking the channel pore resulting in a chronically open state and excessive calcium influx. Memantine binds to the intra-pore magnesium site, but with longer dwell time, and thus functions as an effective receptor blocker only under conditions of excessive stimulation; memantine does not affect normal neurotransmission.
Pharmacodynamics/Kinetics
Half-life Elimination Terminal: ~60-80 hours; severe renal impairment (Cl$_{cr}$ 5-29 mL/minute): 117-156 hours
Time to Peak Serum: 3-7 hours
Pregnancy Risk Factor B
Pregnancy Considerations Teratogenic effects were not observed in animal studies. There are no studies in pregnant women.
Product Availability
Namenda XR™: FDA approved in June 2010; anticipated availability is May 2013. Consult prescribing information for additional information.
Namenda XR™ is an extended release capsule (once-daily administration) approved for the treatment of moderate-to-severe dementia associated with Alzheimer's disease

Meningococcal (Groups A / C / Y and W-135) Diphtheria Conjugate Vaccine
(me NIN joe kok al groops aye, see, why & dubl yoo won thur tee fyve dif THEER ee a KON joo gate vak SEEN)

Brand Names: U.S. Menactra®; Menveo®
Brand Names: Canada Menactra®; Menveo®
Pharmacologic Category Vaccine, Inactivated (Bacterial)
Use Provide active immunization of children and adults against invasive meningococcal disease caused by *N. meningitidis* serogroups A, C, Y, and W-135.

The Advisory Committee on Immunization Practices (ACIP) (CDC, 2013):
ACIP recommends routine vaccination of the following:
- Children and adolescents 11-18 years of age
- Persons ≥2 months of age who are at increased risk of meningococcal disease
- Persons (in all recommended age groups) at increased risk who are part of outbreaks caused by vaccine preventable serogroups
Those at increased risk of meningococcal disease include the following:
- Persons ≥2 months of age with medical conditions such as anatomical or functional asplenia or persistent compliment component deficiencies (eg, C$_5$-C$_9$, properdin, factor H, or factor D)
- Persons ≥9 months of age that travel to or reside in countries where meningococcal disease is hyperendemic or epidemic, especially if contact with the local population will be prolonged
- Unvaccinated or incompletely vaccinated first year college students living in residence halls
- Military recruits
- Microbiologists with occupational exposure

The Canadian National Advisory Committee on Immunization (NACI): NACI recommends a routine vaccination at ~12 years of age but no booster unless at a continued high risk of exposure. Either quadrivalent vaccine may be used; NACI does not have a preference. NACI recommends use of Menveo® (unlabeled use) for high risk persons 2 months to 2 years of age if vaccination with a quadrivalent vaccine is needed; may also be considered for use in persons ≥56 years of age (NACI, 39[1], 2013). Additional recommendations may be found at www.phac-aspc.gc.ca/publicat/ccdr-rmtc/13vol39/acs-dcc-1/index-eng.php

Local Anesthetic/Vasoconstrictor Precautions No information available to require special precautions

Effects on Dental Treatment No significant effects or complications reported

Effects on Bleeding No information available to require special precautions

Adverse Effects All serious adverse reactions must be reported to the U.S. Department of Health and Human Services (DHHS) Vaccine Adverse Event Reporting System (VAERS) 1-800-822-7967 or online at https://vaers.hhs.gov/esub/index. In Canada, adverse reactions may be reported to local provincial/territorial health agencies or to the Vaccine Safety Section at Public Health Agency of Canada (1-866-844-0018).

Actual percentages may vary by product and age group:
>10%:
   Central nervous system: Crying (abnormal), drowsiness, fatigue, fever, headache, irritability, malaise, sleepiness
   Gastrointestinal: Anorexia, diarrhea, nausea, vomiting
   Local: Injection site: Erythema, induration, pain, redness, swelling, tenderness
   Neuromuscular & skeletal: Arthralgia, myalgia
1% to 10%:
   Central nervous system: Chills
   Dermatologic: Rash
   Gastrointestinal: Eating changes
General Dosage Range I.M.:
   Children 9-23 months (Menactra®):0.5 mL/dose given as a 2-dose series, 3 months apart
   Children ≥2 years and Adults ≤55 years: 0.5 mL as a single dose
Mechanism of Action Induces immunity against meningococcal disease via the formation of bactericidal antibodies directed toward the polysaccharide capsular components of *Neisseria meningitidis* serogroups A, C, Y and W-135.
Pregnancy Risk Factor B/C (manufacturer dependent)
Pregnancy Considerations Animal reproduction studies have not been conducted with Menactra®. An isolated teratogenic effect was observed in an animal developmental toxicity study; not necessarily vaccine related. Carcinogenic or mutagenic studies have not been performed. Patients should contact the Sanofi Pasteur Inc vaccine registry at 1-800-822-2463 if they are pregnant or become aware they were pregnant at the time of Menactra® vaccination.

Adverse events were not observed in animal reproduction studies conducted with Menveo®. Patients should contact the Novartis Vaccines and Diagnostics Inc. pregnancy registry at 1-877-311-8972 if they are pregnant or become aware they were pregnant at the time of Menveo® vaccination.

Limited information is available following inadvertent use of meningococcal diphtheria conjugate vaccine during pregnancy. Inactivated bacterial vaccines have not been shown to cause increased risks to the fetus (CDC, 60[2], 2011). Pregnancy should not preclude vaccination if indicated (CDC, 2013).

Meningococcal Polysaccharide (Groups C and Y) and *Haemophilus* b Tetanus Toxoid Conjugate Vaccine
(me NIN joe kok al pol i SAK a ride groops see & why & he MOF i lus bee TET a nus TOKS oyd KON joo gate vak SEEN)

Pharmacologic Category Vaccine, Inactivated (Bacterial)

Use To provide active immunity to prevent invasive disease caused by meningococcal serogroups C and Y and *Haemophilus influenzae* type b

The Advisory Committee on Immunization Practices (ACIP) recommends vaccination only for infants 2-18 months of age who are at increased risk for meningococcal disease, including:
- Infants with persistent complement pathway deficiencies
- Infants with anatomic or functional asplenia, including sickle cell disease
- Infants in communities with serogroups C and Y meningococcal disease outbreaks
The ACIP does not recommend routine vaccination for infants not at increased risk for meningococcal disease. In addition, infants traveling to certain areas (eg, meningitis belt of sub-Saharan Africa) will require a meningococcal vaccine with serogroups A and W_{135}; vaccination with Hib-MenCY-TT will not be adequate (CDC, 2013).

Local Anesthetic/Vasoconstrictor Precautions No information available to require special precautions

Effects on Dental Treatment No significant effects or complications reported

Effects on Bleeding No information available to require special precautions

Adverse Effects All serious adverse reactions must be reported to the U.S. Department of Health and Human Services (DHHS) Vaccine Adverse Event Reporting System (VAERS) 1-800-822-7967 or online at https://vaers.hhs.gov/esub/index. In Canada, adverse reactions may be reported to local provincial/territorial health agencies or to the Vaccine Safety Section at Public Health Agency of Canada (1-866-844-0018).

>10%:
   Central nervous system: Irritability (62% to 71%), drowsiness (49% to 63%), fever ≥100.4°F/38°C (11% to 26%)
   Gastrointestinal: Appetite decreased (30% to 34%)
   Local: Injection site reactions: Pain (41% to 46%), redness (21% to 36%), swelling (15% to 25%)
General Dosage Range I.M.: *Infants ≥6 weeks and Children ≤18 months:* 0.5 mL/dose given as a four-dose series at 2, 4, 6, and 12-15 months of age
Mechanism of Action Provides active immunity against meningococcal disease via the formation of bactericidal antibodies directed toward the polysaccharide capsular components of *Neisseria meningitidis* serogroups C and Y; stimulates production of anticapsular antibodies and to *Haemophilus influenzae* type b
Pharmacodynamics/Kinetics
   Onset of Action Antibody response to the components of the vaccine occurs in ≥95% of children following the third dose and ≥98% following the fourth dose.
Pregnancy Risk Factor C
Pregnancy Considerations Animal reproduction studies have not been conducted.

◀ **Product Availability** MenHibrix®: FDA approved June 2012; availability expected April 2013. Consult prescribing information for additional information.

Meningococcal Polysaccharide Vaccine (Groups A, C, Y, and W-135)

(me NIN joe kok al pol i SAK a ride vak SEEN groops aye, see, why & dubl yoo won thur tee fyve)

Brand Names: U.S. Menomune®-A/C/Y/W-135

Brand Names: Canada Menomune®-A/C/Y/W-135

Pharmacologic Category Vaccine, Inactivated (Bacterial)

Use Provide active immunity to meningococcal serogroups contained in the vaccine

The Advisory Committee on Immunization Practices (ACIP) recommends routine vaccination for persons at increased risk for meningococcal disease. Meningococcal quadrivalent conjugate vaccine (MenACWY) is preferred; meningococcal polysaccharide vaccine (MPSV4) is preferred in meningococcal vaccine-naive adults ≥56 years of age requiring only a single vaccination (CDC, 2013).

Those at increased risk of meningococcal disease include the following:
- Persons ≥2 months of age with medical conditions such as anatomical or functional asplenia or persistent compliment component deficiencies (eg, C_5-C_9, properdin, factor H, or factor D)
- Persons ≥9 months of age that travel to or reside in countries where meningococcal disease is hyperendemic or epidemic, especially if contact with the local population will be prolonged
- Unvaccinated or incompletely vaccinated first year college students living in residence halls
- Military recruits
- Microbiologists with occupational exposure
- Persons (in all recommended age groups) at risk who are part of outbreaks caused by vaccine preventable serogroups

Local Anesthetic/Vasoconstrictor Precautions No information available to require special precautions

Effects on Dental Treatment No significant effects or complications reported

Effects on Bleeding No information available to require special precautions

Adverse Effects All serious adverse reactions must be reported to the U.S. Department of Health and Human Services (DHHS) Vaccine Adverse Event Reporting System (VAERS) 1-800-822-7967 or online at https://vaers.hhs.gov/esub/index. In Canada, adverse reactions may be reported to local provincial/territorial health agencies or to the Vaccine Safety Section at Public Health Agency of Canada (1-866-844-0018).

>10%:
Central nervous system: Headache (29% to 42%), fatigue (25% to 32%), malaise (17% to 22%), irritability (12%), drowsiness (11%)
Gastrointestinal: Diarrhea (10% to 14%)
Local: Injection site: Pain (26% to 48%), redness (6% to 16%), induration (4% to 11%)
Neuromuscular & skeletal: Arthralgia (5% to 16%)
1% to 10%:
Central nervous system: Chills (4% to 6%), fever (≤5%)

Dermatologic: Rash (≤3%)
Gastrointestinal: Anorexia (8% to 10%), vomiting (1% to 3%)
Local: Injection site: Swelling (3% to 8%)

General Dosage Range SubQ: *Children ≥2 years and Adults:* 0.5 mL as a single dose

Mechanism of Action Induces the formation of bactericidal antibodies to meningococcal antigens; the presence of these antibodies is strongly correlated with immunity to meningococcal disease caused by *Neisseria meningitidis* groups A, C, Y and W-135.

Pharmacodynamics/Kinetics

Onset of Action Antibody levels: 7-10 days

Duration of Action Antibodies against group A and C polysaccharides decline markedly (to prevaccination levels) over the first 3 years following a single dose of vaccine, especially in children <4 years of age

Pregnancy Risk Factor C

Pregnancy Considerations Animal reproduction studies have not been conducted. Inactivated bacterial vaccines have not been shown to cause increased risks to the fetus (CDC, 2011). Pregnancy should not preclude vaccination if indicated (CDC, 2013).

Menotropins (men oh TROE pins)

Brand Names: U.S. Menopur®; Repronex®

Brand Names: Canada Menopur®; Repronex®

Pharmacologic Category Gonadotropin; Ovulation Stimulator

Use Female:
In conjunction with hCG to induce ovulation and pregnancy in infertile females experiencing oligoanovulation or anovulation when the cause of anovulation is functional and not caused by primary ovarian failure (Repronex®)
Stimulation of multiple follicle development in ovulatory patients as part of an assisted reproductive technology (ART) (Menopur®, Repronex®)

Unlabeled Use Male: Stimulation of spermatogenesis in primary or secondary hypogonadotropic hypogonadism

Local Anesthetic/Vasoconstrictor Precautions No information available to require special precautions

Effects on Dental Treatment No significant effects or complications reported

Effects on Bleeding Has been associated with thrombotic events; however, no information available to require special precautions in dental procedures.

Adverse Effects Adverse effects may vary according to specific product, route, and/or dosage.
>10%:
Central nervous system: Headache (up to 34%)
Gastrointestinal: Abdominal pain (up to 18%), nausea (up to 12%)
Genitourinary: OHSS (up to 13%, dose related)
Local: Injection site reaction (4% to 12%)
1% to 10%:
Cardiovascular: Flushing
Central nervous system: Dizziness, malaise, migraine
Endocrine & metabolic: Breast tenderness, hot flashes, menstrual irregularities
Gastrointestinal: Abdominal cramping, abdominal fullness, constipation, diarrhea, enlarged abdomen, vomiting
Genitourinary: Ectopic pregnancy, ovarian disease, vaginal hemorrhage

Local: Injection site edema/pain
Neuromuscular & skeletal: Back pain
Respiratory: Cough increased, respiratory disorder
Miscellaneous: Infection, flu-like syndrome

Frequency not defined:
Cardiovascular: Stroke, tachycardia, thrombosis (venous or arterial)
Dermatologic: Angioedema, rash, urticaria
Genitourinary: Adnexal torsion, hemoperitoneum, ovarian enlargement
Neuromuscular & skeletal: Limb necrosis
Respiratory: Acute respiratory distress syndrome, atelectasis, dyspnea, embolism, laryngeal edema, pulmonary infarction, tachypnea
Miscellaneous: Allergic reaction, anaphylaxis

General Dosage Range
I.M.: *Adults:* Repronex®: Initial: 150 units **or** 225 units daily (maximum: 450 units/day; 12 days of therapy)
SubQ: *Adults:* Menopur®: Initial: 225 units daily (maximum: 450 units/day; 20 days of therapy); Repronex®: Initial: 150 units **or** 225 units daily (maximum: 450 units/day; 12 days of therapy)

Mechanism of Action Actions occur as a result of both follicle stimulating hormone (FSH) effects and luteinizing hormone (LH) effects; menotropins stimulate the development and maturation of the ovarian follicle (FSH), cause ovulation (LH), and stimulate the development of the corpus luteum (LH); in males it stimulates spermatogenesis (LH)

Pregnancy Risk Factor X
Pregnancy Considerations Ectopic pregnancy and congenital abnormalities have been reported. The incidence of congenital abnormality is similar during natural conception.

Menthol and Zinc Oxide (Topical)
(MEN thole & zink OKS ide)

Brand Names: U.S. Calmoseptine® [OTC]; Remedy® Calazime® [OTC]; Risamine™ [OTC]
Pharmacologic Category Protectant, Topical; Topical Skin Product
Use Provides a barrier to protect intact and/or injured skin from moisture, wound or fistula drainage, urine, or feces; diaper rash
Local Anesthetic/Vasoconstrictor Precautions No information available to require special precautions
Effects on Dental Treatment No significant effects or complications reported
Effects on Bleeding No information available to require special precautions
Adverse Effects Frequency not defined.
Dermatologic: Pruritus, rash, stinging (temporarily on application)
Miscellaneous: Hypersensitivity reactions
General Dosage Range Topical: *Children and Adults:* Apply thin layer 2-4 times/day or after each incontinent episode/diaper change

Mepenzolate (me PEN zoe late)

Brand Names: U.S. Cantil®
Brand Names: Canada Cantil®
Pharmacologic Category Anticholinergic Agent; Antispasmodic Agent, Gastrointestinal
Use Adjunctive treatment of peptic ulcer disease; has not been shown to be effective in contributing to the healing of peptic ulcer, preventing complications, or decreasing the rate of recurrence

Local Anesthetic/Vasoconstrictor Precautions No information available to require special precautions
Effects on Dental Treatment Key adverse event(s) related to dental treatment: Xerostomia (normal salivary flow resumes upon discontinuation), dry throat, dysphagia, and loss of taste.
Effects on Bleeding No information available to require special precautions
Adverse Effects Frequency not defined.
Cardiovascular: Palpitation, tachycardia
Central nervous system: Confusion, dizziness, drowsiness, headache, insomnia, nervousness
Dermatologic: Urticaria
Gastrointestinal: Bloating, constipation, delayed gastric emptying, loss of taste, nausea, vomiting, xerostomia
Genitourinary: Impotence, urinary hesitation, urinary retention
Neuromuscular & skeletal: Weakness
Ophthalmic: Blurred vision, cycloplegia, ocular tension increased, pupil dilation
Miscellaneous: Anaphylaxis, diaphoresis decreased, lactation suppressed
General Dosage Range Oral: *Adults:* 25-50 mg 4 times/day
Mechanism of Action Mepenzolate is a postganglionic parasympathetic inhibitor. It decreases gastric acid and pepsin secretion and suppresses spontaneous contractions of the colon.
Pregnancy Risk Factor B
Pregnancy Considerations Adverse events were not observed in animal reproduction studies.

Meperidine (me PER i deen)

Related Information
Management of the Patient With Anxiety or Depression *on page 1594*
Brand Names: U.S. Demerol®
Brand Names: Canada Demerol®
Generic Availability (U.S.) Yes
Pharmacologic Category Analgesic, Opioid
Dental Use Adjunct in preoperative intravenous conscious sedation in patients undergoing dental surgery; alternate oral opioid in patients allergic to codeine to treat moderate to moderate-severe pain
Use Management of moderate-to-severe pain; adjunct to anesthesia and preoperative sedation
Unlabeled Use Reduce postoperative shivering; reduce rigors from amphotericin B (conventional)
Local Anesthetic/Vasoconstrictor Precautions No information available to require special precautions
Effects on Dental Treatment Key adverse event(s) related to dental treatment: Xerostomia (normal salivary flow resumes upon discontinuation). See Dental Comment.
Effects on Bleeding No information available to require special precautions
Adverse Effects Frequency not defined.
Cardiovascular: Bradycardia, cardiac arrest, circulatory depression, hypotension, palpitation, shock, syncope, tachycardia
Central nervous system: Agitation, confusion, delirium, disorientation, dizziness, drowsiness, dysphoria, euphoria, fatigue, flushing, hallucinations, headache, intracranial pressure increased, lightheadedness, malaise, mental depression, nervousness, paradoxical CNS stimulation, restlessness, sedation, seizure (associated with metabolite accumulation), serotonin syndrome

Dermatologic: Pruritus, rash, urticaria

Gastrointestinal: Abdominal cramps, anorexia, biliary spasm, constipation, nausea, paralytic ileus, sphincter of Oddi spasm, vomiting, xerostomia

Genitourinary: Ureteral spasms, urinary retention

Local: Injection site reaction (including pain, wheal, and flare)

Neuromuscular & skeletal: Muscle twitching, myoclonus, tremor, weakness

Ocular: Visual disturbances

Respiratory: Dyspnea, respiratory arrest, respiratory depression

Miscellaneous: Anaphylaxis, diaphoresis, histamine release, hypersensitivity reactions, physical and psychological dependence

Dental Usual Dosage Pain (analgesic): Adults: Oral: Initial: Opiate-naive: 50 mg every 3-4 hours as needed; usual dosage range: 50-150 mg every 2-4 hours as needed (manufacturers recommendation; oral route is not recommended for acute pain)

Dosage Note: The American Pain Society (2008) and ISMP (2007) do not recommend meperidine's use as an analgesic. If use in acute pain (in patients without renal or CNS disease) cannot be avoided, treatment should be limited to ≤48 hours and doses should not exceed 600 mg/24 hours. Oral route is not recommended for treatment of acute or chronic pain. If I.V. route is required, consider a reduced dose. Patients with prior opioid exposure may require higher initial doses.

Children: Pain: Oral, I.M., SubQ: 1.1-1.8 mg/kg/dose every 3-4 hours as needed (maximum: 50-150 mg/dose)

Preoperatively: I.M., SubQ: 1.1-2.2 mg/kg given 30-90 minutes before the beginning of anesthesia (maximum: 50-150 mg/dose)

Adults:

Pain: Oral, I.M., SubQ: 50-150 mg every 3-4 hours as needed

Preoperatively: I.M., SubQ: 50-150 mg given 30-90 minutes before the beginning of anesthesia

Obstetrical analgesia: I.M., SubQ: 50-100 mg when pain becomes regular; may repeat at every 1-3 hours

Postoperative shivering (unlabeled use): I.V.: 25-50 mg once (Crowley, 2008; Kranke, 2002; Mercandante, 1994; Wang, 1999)

Elderly: Avoid use (American Pain Society, 2008; ISMP, 2007)

Dosing adjustment in renal impairment: Avoid use in renal impairment (American Pain Society, 2008; ISMP, 2007)

Dosing adjustment in hepatic impairment: Use with caution in severe hepatic impairment; consider a lower initial dose when initiating therapy. An increased opioid effect may be seen in patients with cirrhosis; dose reduction is more important for the oral than I.V. route.

Mechanism of Action Binds to opioid receptors in the CNS, causing inhibition of ascending pain pathways, altering the perception of and response to pain; produces generalized CNS depression

Contraindications Hypersensitivity to meperidine or any component of the formulation; use with or within 14 days of MAO inhibitors; severe respiratory insufficiency

Warnings/Precautions Oral meperidine is not recommended for acute/chronic pain management. Meperidine should not be used for acute/cancer pain because of the risk of neurotoxicity. Normeperidine (an active metabolite and CNS stimulant) may accumulate

and precipitate anxiety, tremors, or seizures; risk increases with CNS or renal dysfunction, prolonged use (>48 hours), and cumulative dose (>600 mg/24 hours). The Institute for Safe Medication Practice recommends avoiding the use of meperidine for pain control, especially in the elderly and renally-impaired (ISMP, 2007). In the elderly; meperidine is not an effective oral analgesic at commonly used doses; may cause neurotoxicity; other agents are preferred in the elderly (Beers Criteria).

May cause CNS depression, which may impair physical or mental abilities; patients must be cautioned about performing tasks which require mental alertness (eg, operating machinery or driving). Effects (eg, sedation, respiratory depression, hypotension) may be potentiated when used with other sedative/hypnotic drugs, general anesthetics, phenothiazines, or ethanol; consider reduced dose of meperidine if using concomitantly. Use only with extreme caution (if at all) in patients with head injury or increased intracranial pressure (ICP). Use caution with pulmonary, hepatic, or renal disorders, supraventricular tachycardias (including atrial flutter), acute abdominal conditions, delirium tremens, hypothyroidism, myxedema, toxic psychosis, kyphoscoliosis, morbid obesity, Addison's disease, seizure disorders, pheochromocytoma, BPH, or urethral stricture. Use with caution in patients with biliary tract dysfunction; acute pancreatitis may cause constriction of sphincter of Oddi. May cause hypotension (including orthostatic hypotension); use with caution in patients with depleted blood volume or drugs which may exaggerate hypotensive effects (including phenothiazines or general anesthetics).

An opioid-containing analgesic regimen should be tailored to each patient's needs and based upon the type of pain being treated (acute versus chronic), the route of administration, degree of tolerance for opioids (naive versus chronic user), age, weight, and medical condition. The optimal analgesic dose varies widely among patients. Some preparations contain sulfites which may cause allergic reaction. Tolerance or drug dependence may result from extended use. Healthcare provider should be alert to problems of abuse, misuse, and diversion. Concurrent use of agonist/antagonist analgesics may precipitate withdrawal symptoms and/or reduced analgesic efficacy in patients following prolonged therapy with mu opioid agonists. Abrupt discontinuation following prolonged use may also lead to withdrawal symptoms. Avoid use in the elderly.

Drug Interactions

Metabolism/Transport Effects None known.

Avoid Concomitant Use

Avoid concomitant use of Meperidine with any of the following: Azelastine (Nasal); MAO Inhibitors; Paraldehyde

Increased Effect/Toxicity

Meperidine may increase the levels/effects of: Alcohol (Ethyl); Alvimopan; Azelastine (Nasal); CNS Depressants; Desmopressin; Metoclopramide; Metyrosine; Paraldehyde; Pramipexole; ROPINIRole; Rotigotine; Selective Serotonin Reuptake Inhibitors; Serotonin Modulators; Thiazide Diuretics; Zolpidem

The levels/effects of Meperidine may be increased by: Amphetamines; Antipsychotic Agents (Phenothiazines); Antipsychotics; Barbiturates; HydrOXYzine; Magnesium Sulfate; MAO Inhibitors; Perampanel; Protease Inhibitors; Sodium Oxybate; Succinylcholine

Decreased Effect
Meperidine may decrease the levels/effects of: Pegvisomant

The levels/effects of Meperidine may be decreased by: Ammonium Chloride; Fosphenytoin; Mixed Agonist / Antagonist Opioids; Phenytoin; Protease Inhibitors

Ethanol/Nutrition/Herb Interactions
Ethanol: May increase CNS depression; monitor for increased effects with coadministration. Caution patients about effects.

Herb/Nutraceutical: Avoid valerian, St John's wort, kava kava, gotu kola (may increase CNS depression).

Pharmacodynamics/Kinetics
Onset of Action Onset of action: Analgesic: Oral, SubQ: 10-15 minutes; I.V.: ~5 minutes. Peak effect: SubQ.: ~1 hour; Oral: 2 hours

Duration of Action Oral, SubQ.: 2-4 hours

Half-life Elimination
Parent drug: Terminal phase: Adults: 2.5-4 hours, Liver disease: 7-11 hours

Normeperidine (active metabolite): 15-30 hours; can accumulate with high doses (>600 mg/day) or renal impairment

Pregnancy Risk Factor C

Pregnancy Considerations Animal reproduction studies have not been conducted. Meperidine is known to cross the placenta, which may result in respiratory or CNS depression in the newborn.

Lactation Enters breast milk/not recommended (AAP rates "compatible"; AAP 2001 update pending)

Breast-Feeding Considerations Meperidine is excreted in breast milk and may cause CNS and/or respiratory depression in the nursing infant.

Controlled Substance C-II

Dosage Forms
Injection, solution: 10 mg/mL (30 mL); 25 mg/mL (1 mL)

Demerol®: 25 mg/mL (1 mL); 25 mg/0.5 mL (0.5 mL); 50 mg/mL (1 mL, 1.5 mL, 2 mL, 30 mL); 75 mg/mL (1 mL); 100 mg/mL (1 mL, 20 mL)

Solution, oral: 50 mg/5 mL (500 mL)

Tablet, oral: 50 mg, 100 mg

Demerol®: 50 mg, 100 mg

Dental Comment Meperidine is not to be used as the opioid drug of first choice. It is recommended only to be used in codeine-allergic patients when an opioid analgesic is indicated. Meperidine is not an anti-inflammatory agent. Meperidine, as with other opioid analgesics, is recommended only for limited acute dosing (ie, 3 days or less); common adverse effects in the dental patient are nausea, sedation, and constipation. Meperidine has a significant addiction liability, especially when given long-term.

Mepivacaine (me PIV a kane)

Brand Names: U.S. Carbocaine®; Polocaine®; Polocaine® MPF

Brand Names: Canada Carbocaine®; Polocaine®

Generic Availability (U.S.) No

Pharmacologic Category Local Anesthetic

Use Local or regional analgesia; anesthesia by local infiltration, peripheral and central neural techniques (epidural and caudal); **not** for use in spinal anesthesia

Local Anesthetic/Vasoconstrictor Precautions No information available to require special precautions

Effects on Dental Treatment Key adverse event(s) related to dental treatment: Degree of adverse effects in the CNS and cardiovascular system is directly related to blood levels of mepivacaine (frequency not defined; more likely to occur after systemic administration rather than infiltration): Bradycardia, cardiovascular collapse, hypotension, myocardial depression, ventricular arrhythmias, nausea, vomiting, respiratory arrest, anaphylactoid reactions, blurred vision, heart block, transient stinging or burning at injection site

High blood levels: Anxiety, restlessness, disorientation, confusion, dizziness, and seizures, followed by CNS depression resulting in somnolence, unconsciousness, and possible respiratory arrest.

In some cases, symptoms of CNS stimulation may be absent and the primary CNS effects are somnolence and unconsciousness.

Effects on Bleeding No information available to require special precautions

Adverse Effects Degree of adverse effects in the CNS and cardiovascular system is directly related to the blood levels of mepivacaine, route of administration, and physical status of the patient. The effects below are more likely to occur after systemic administration rather than infiltration.

Cardiovascular: Bradycardia, cardiac arrest, cardiac output decreased, heart block, hyper-/hypotension, myocardial depression, syncope, tachycardia, ventricular arrhythmias

Central nervous system: Anxiety, chills, convulsions, depression, dizziness, excitation, restlessness, tremors

Dermatologic: Angioneurotic edema, diaphoresis, erythema, pruritus, urticaria

Gastrointestinal: Fecal incontinence, nausea, vomiting

Genitourinary: Incontinence, urinary retention

Neuromuscular & skeletal: Chondrolysis (continuous intra-articular administration), paralysis

Ocular: Blurred vision, pupil constriction

Otic: Tinnitus

Respiratory: Apnea, hypoventilation, sneezing

Miscellaneous: Allergic reaction, anaphylactoid reaction

Dosage
Injectable local anesthetic: Dose varies with procedure, degree of anesthesia needed, vascularity of tissue, duration of anesthesia required, and physical condition of patient. The smallest dose and concentration required to produce the desired effect should be used.

Children: Maximum single or total dose given for one procedure: 5-6 mg/kg; only concentrations <2% should be used in children <3 years or <14 kg (30 lbs)

Adults: Maximum single or total dose given for one procedure: 400 mg; 500 mg if epinephrine has been added (Barash, 2009)

Cervical, brachial, intercostal, pudendal nerve block: 5-40 mL of a 1% solution (maximum: 400 mg) **or** 5-20 mL of a 2% solution (maximum: 400 mg). For pudendal block, inject one-half the total dose each side.

Transvaginal block (paracervical plus pudendal): Up to 30 mL (total for both sides) of a 1% solution (maximum: 300 mg). Inject one-half the total dose each side.

Paracervical block: Up to 20 mL (total for both sides) of a 1% solution (maximum: 200 mg). Inject one-half the total dose to each side. This is the maximum recommended dose per 90-minute procedure; inject slowly with 5 minutes between sides.

Caudal and epidural block (preservative free solutions only): 15-30 mL of a 1% solution (maximum: 300 mg) **or** 10-25 mL of a 1.5% solution (maximum: 375 mg) **or** 10-20 mL of a 2% solution (maximum: 400 mg)

Infiltration: Up to 40 mL of a 1% solution (maximum: 400 mg); up to 50 mL if epinephrine has been added (maximum: 500 mg) (Barash, 2009); an equivalent amount of a 0.5% solution (prepared by diluting the 1% solution with NS) may be used for large areas

Peripheral nerve block to provide a surgical level of anesthesia (Miller, 2010):

Major nerve block (blockade of two or more distinct nerves, a nerve plexus, or very large nerves at more proximal sites: 30-50 mL of a 1% or 1.5% solution (maximum: 500 mg)

Minor nerve block (blockade of a single nerve [eg, ulnar or radial]): 5-20 mL of a 1% solution (maximum: 200 mg)

Therapeutic block: 1-5 mL of 1% solution (maximum: 50 mg) **or** 1-5 mL of 2% solution (maximum: 100 mg)

Elderly: Decreased doses suggested by manufacturer's labeling; however, no dosing adjustments provided. Refer to adult dosing.

Dosage adjustment in renal impairment: No dosage adjustment provided in manufacturer's labeling; use with caution.

Dosage adjustment in hepatic impairment: No dosage adjustment provided in manufacturer's labeling; use with caution.

Mechanism of Action Mepivacaine is an amide local anesthetic similar to lidocaine; like all local anesthetics, mepivacaine acts by preventing the generation and conduction of nerve impulses

Contraindications Hypersensitivity to mepivacaine, other amide-type local anesthetics, or any component of the formulation

Warnings/Precautions Careful and constant monitoring of the patient's state of consciousness should be done following each local anesthetic injection; at such times, restlessness, anxiety, tinnitus, dizziness, blurred vision, tremors, depression, or drowsiness may be early warning signs of CNS toxicity; treatment is primarily symptomatic and supportive. Continuous intra-articular infusion of local anesthetics after arthroscopic or other surgical procedures is **not** an approved use; chondrolysis (primarily in the shoulder joint) has occurred following infusion, with some cases requiring arthroplasty or shoulder replacement. Use with caution in patients with cardiac disease, hepatic or renal disease, or hyperthyroidism. Local anesthetics have been associated with rare occurrences of sudden respiratory arrest; convulsions due to systemic toxicity leading to cardiac arrest have been reported presumably due to intravascular injection. A test dose is recommended prior to epidural administration and all reinforcing doses with continuous catheter technique. Do not use solutions containing preservatives for caudal or epidural block. Use caution in debilitated, elderly, or acutely-ill patients; dose reduction may be required. Resuscitative equipment, oxygen, and other resuscitative drugs should be available for immediate use.

Drug Interactions

Metabolism/Transport Effects None known.

Avoid Concomitant Use There are no known interactions where it is recommended to avoid concomitant use.

Increased Effect/Toxicity

The levels/effects of Mepivacaine may be increased by: Beta-Blockers; Hyaluronidase

Decreased Effect There are no known significant interactions involving a decrease in effect.

Pharmacodynamics/Kinetics

Onset of Action Route and dose dependent: Range: 3-20 minute

Duration of Action Route and dose dependent: 2-2.5 hours

Half-life Elimination Neonates: 8.7-9 hours; Adults: 1.9-3 hours

Pregnancy Risk Factor C

Pregnancy Considerations Animal reproduction studies have not been conducted. Mepivacaine has been used in obstetrical analgesia.

Lactation Excretion in breast milk unknown/use caution

Dosage Forms

Injection, solution: 3% [30 mg/mL] (1.8 mL)

Carbocaine®: 1% [10 mg/mL] (50 mL); 2% [20 mg/mL] (50 mL); 3% [30 mg/mL] (1.7 mL)

Polocaine®: 1% [10 mg/mL] (50 mL); 2% [20 mg/mL] (50 mL)

Injection, solution [preservative free]:

Carbocaine®: 1% [10 mg/mL] (30 mL); 1.5% [15 mg/mL] (30 mL); 2% [20 mg/mL] (20 mL)

Polocaine® MPF: 1% [10 mg/mL] (30 mL); 1.5% [15 mg/mL] (30 mL); 2% [20 mg/mL] (20 mL)

References

Moore PA and Hersh EV, "Local Anesthetics: Pharmacology and Toxicity," *Dent Clin North Am*, 2010, 54(4):587-99.

Mepivacaine (Dental Anesthetic)
(me PIV a kane, DEN tl)

Related Information

Mepivacaine *on page 873*

Oral Pain *on page 1558*

Brand Names: U.S. Carbocaine®; Polocaine® Dental; Scandonest® 3% Plain

Brand Names: Canada Polocaine®

Generic Availability (U.S.) Yes

Pharmacologic Category Local Anesthetic

Dental Use Amide-type anesthetic used for local infiltration anesthesia; injection near nerve trunks to produce nerve block

Use Amide-type anesthetic used for local infiltration anesthesia; injection near nerve trunks to produce nerve block

Local Anesthetic/Vasoconstrictor Precautions No information available to require special precautions

Effects on Dental Treatment It is common to misinterpret psychogenic responses to local anesthetic injection as an allergic reaction. Intraoral injections are perceived by many patients as a stressful procedure in dentistry. Common symptoms to this stress are diaphoresis, palpitations, hyperventilation, generalized pallor, and a fainting feeling.

Degree of adverse effects in the CNS and cardiovascular system is directly related to the blood levels of mepivacaine.

Frequency not defined: Bradycardia and reduction in cardiac output, nausea, vomiting, tremors, asthmatic syndromes, hypersensitivity reactions (may manifest as dermatologic reactions and edema at injection site) High blood levels: Anxiety, restlessness, disorientation, confusion, dizziness, tremors and seizures, followed by CNS depression resulting in somnolence, unconsciousness and possible respiratory arrest. In some cases, symptoms of CNS stimulation may be absent and the primary CNS effects are somnolence and unconsciousness.

Effects on Bleeding No information available to require special precautions

Adverse Effects Degree of adverse effects in the CNS and cardiovascular system are directly related to the blood levels of local anesthetic.

Cardiovascular: Myocardial effects include a decrease in contraction force as well as a decrease in electrical excitability and myocardial conduction rate resulting in bradycardia and reduction in cardiac output

Central nervous system: High blood levels result in anxiety, restlessness, disorientation, confusion, dizziness, and seizure. This is followed by depression of CNS resulting in somnolence, unconsciousness and possible respiratory arrest. In some cases, symptoms of CNS stimulation may be absent and the primary CNS effects are somnolence and unconsciousness.

Gastrointestinal: Nausea and vomiting may occur

Hypersensitivity reactions: May manifest as dermatologic reactions and edema at injection site. Asthmatic syndromes have occurred.

Neuromuscular & skeletal: Tremors

Psychogenic reactions: It is common to misinterpret psychogenic responses to local anesthetic injection as an allergic reaction. Intraoral injection is perceived by many patients as a stressful procedure in dentistry. Common symptoms to this stress are diaphoresis, palpitation, hyperventilation, generalized pallor and a fainting feeling.

Dental Usual Dosage

Children <10 years: Up to 5-6 mg/kg of body weight; maximum pediatric dosage must be carefully calculated on the basis of patient's weight but must not exceed 270 mg (9 mL) of the 3% solution

Children >10 years and Adults:
Dental anesthesia, single site in upper or lower jaw: 54 mg (1.8 mL) as a 3% solution
Infiltration and nerve block of entire oral cavity: 270 mg (9 mL) as a 3% solution; up to a maximum of 6.6 mg/kg of body weight but not to exceed 300 mg per appointment. Manufacturer's maximum recommended dose is not more than 400 mg to normal healthy adults. The effective anesthetic dose varies with procedure, intensity of anesthesia needed, duration of anesthesia required, and physical condition of the patient. Always use the lowest effective dose along with careful aspiration.

The following number of dental carpules (1.8 mL) provide the indicated amounts of mepivacaine dental anesthetic 3%. See table.

# of Cartridges (1.8 mL)	mg Mepivacaine (3%)
1	54
2	108
3	162
4	216
5	270
6	324
7	378
8	432

Note: Adult and children doses of mepivacaine dental anesthetic cited from USP Dispensing Information (USP DI), 17th ed, The United States Pharmacopeial Convention, Inc, Rockville, MD, 1997, 138-9.

Dosage

Children <10 years: Up to 5-6 mg/kg of body weight; maximum pediatric dosage must be carefully calculated on the basis of patient's weight but must not exceed 270 mg (9 mL) of the 3% solution

Children >10 years and Adults:
Dental anesthesia, single site in upper or lower jaw: 54 mg (1.8 mL) as a 3% solution
Infiltration and nerve block of entire oral cavity: 270 mg (9 mL) as a 3% solution; up to a maximum of 6.6 mg/kg of body weight but not to exceed 300 mg per appointment. Manufacturer's maximum recommended dose is not more than 400 mg to normal healthy adults. The effective anesthetic dose varies with procedure, intensity of anesthesia needed, duration of anesthesia required, and physical condition of the patient. Always use the lowest effective dose along with careful aspiration.

Note: Adult and children doses of mepivacaine dental anesthetic cited from USP Dispensing Information (USP DI), 17th ed, The United States Pharmacopeial Convention, Inc, Rockville, MD, 1997, 138-9.

Dosage adjustment in renal impairment: No dosage adjustment provided in manufacturer's labeling; use with caution.

Dosage adjustment in hepatic impairment: No dosage adjustment provided in manufacturer's labeling; use with caution.

Mechanism of Action Local anesthetics bind selectively to the intracellular surface of sodium channels to block influx of sodium into the axon. As a result, depolarization necessary for action potential propagation and subsequent nerve function is prevented. The block at the sodium channel is reversible. When drug diffuses away from the axon, sodium channel function is restored and nerve propagation returns.

Contraindications Hypersensitivity to local anesthetics of the amide type or any component of the formulation

Warnings/Precautions Aspirate the syringe after tissue penetration and before injection to minimize chance of direct vascular injection

Pharmacodynamics/Kinetics

Onset of Action Upper jaw: 30-120 seconds; Lower jaw: 1-4 minutes

Duration of Action Upper jaw: 20 minutes; Lower jaw: 40 minutes

Half-life Elimination Serum: 1.9 hours

Pregnancy Risk Factor C

Pregnancy Considerations Animal reproduction studies have not been conducted.

Lactation Excretion in breast milk unknown/use caution

Breast-Feeding Considerations Usual infiltration doses of mepivacaine dental anesthetic given to nursing mothers has not been shown to affect the health of the nursing infant.

Dosage Forms

Injection, solution: 3% (1.8 mL)

Carbocaine®, Polocaine® Dental, Scandonest® 3%

Plain: 3% (1.7 mL)

Dental Comment Oral paresthesia: The occurrence of oral paresthesia associated with 4% solutions of prilocaine or articaine, although rare, continue to be slightly more frequent than other local anesthetics. From 1999-2008, there were 182 cases of nonsurgical paresthesia (Gaffen, 2009). Of the cases, 172 involved mandibular block injection only. Another eight cases involved mandibular block combined with at least one other type of anesthetic injection. A single case involved infiltration around tooth number 35 and the final case involved infiltration and intraligamentary injection in the maxillary anterior region.

A 2010 report, reviewed adverse events submitted voluntarily over a 10-year period involving the dental local anesthetics articaine, bupivacaine, lidocaine, mepivacaine, and prilocaine in the United States. Mepivacaine reported incidence: One case per 623,112,900 cartridges sold. The reported incidence of paresthesia was one case for 13,800,970 cartridges of all local anesthetics sold in the U.S. (Garisto, 2010).

References

Dower JS Jr, "A Review of Paresthesia in Association With Administration of Local Anesthesia," Dent Today, 2003, 22(2):64-9.

Finder RL and Moore PA, "Adverse Drug Reactions to Local Anesthesia," Dent Clin North Am, 2002, 46(4):747-57, x.

Gaffen AS and Haas DA, "Retrospective Review of Voluntary Reports of Nonsurgical Paresthesia in Dentistry," J Can Dent Assoc, 2009, 75(8):579.

Garisto GA, Gaffen AS, Lawrence HP, et al, "Occurrence of Paresthesia After Dental Local Anesthetic Administration in the United States," J Am Dent Assoc, 2010, 141(7):836-44.

Haas DA, "An Update on Local Anesthetics in Dentistry," J Can Dent Assoc, 2002, 68(9):546-51.

Mepivacaine and Levonordefrin

(me PIV a kane & lee voe nor DEF rin)

Related Information

Mepivacaine on page 873

Oral Pain on page 1558

Brand Names: U.S. Carbocaine® 2% with Neo-Cobefrin®; Scandonest® 2% L

Brand Names: Canada Carbocaine® 2% with Neo-Cobefrin®; Scandonest 2%® with Levonordefrin

Generic Availability (U.S.) No

Pharmacologic Category Local Anesthetic

Dental Use Amide-type anesthetic used for local infiltration anesthesia; injection near nerve trunks to produce nerve block

Use Amide-type anesthetic used for local infiltration anesthesia; injection near nerve trunks to produce nerve block

Local Anesthetic/Vasoconstrictor Precautions No information available to require special precautions

Effects on Dental Treatment It is common to misinterpret psychogenic responses to local anesthetic injection as an allergic reaction. Intraoral injections are perceived by many patients as a stressful procedure in dentistry. Common symptoms to this stress are diaphoresis, palpitations, hyperventilation, generalized pallor and a fainting feeling. Patients may exhibit hypersensitivity to bisulfites contained in local anesthetic solution to prevent oxidation of levonordefrin. In general, patients reacting to bisulfites have a history of asthma and their airways are hyper-reactive to asthmatic syndrome.

Degree of adverse effects in the CNS and cardiovascular system is directly related to the blood levels of mepivacaine (frequency not defined; more likely to occur after systemic administration rather than infiltration): Bradycardia and reduction in cardiac output, nausea, vomiting, tremors, hypersensitivity reactions (extremely rare; may be manifest as dermatologic reactions and edema at injection site), asthmatic syndromes

High blood levels: Anxiety, restlessness, disorientation, confusion, dizziness, and seizures, followed by CNS depression resulting in somnolence, unconsciousness and possible respiratory arrest.

In some cases, symptoms of CNS stimulation may be absent and the primary CNS effects are somnolence and unconsciousness.

Effects on Bleeding No information available to require special precautions

Adverse Effects Degree of adverse effects in the CNS and cardiovascular system are directly related to the blood levels of mepivacaine. The effects below are more likely to occur after systemic administration rather than infiltration.

Central nervous system: Disorientation, dizziness, drowsiness, excitation, nervousness, respiratory arrest, seizure, unconsciousness.

Neuromuscular & skeletal: Tremors

Ocular: Blurred vision

Miscellaneous: Allergic reactions, anaphylactoid reactions (rare)

Dental Usual Dosage Note: Dosage varies with the anesthetic procedure, degree of anesthesia needed, vascularity of tissue, duration of anesthesia required, and physical condition of patient. Always use the lowest effective dose along with careful aspiration.

Children: Calculate the weight-specific maximum mepivacaine dose; regardless of the patient's weight, the maximum pediatric **mepivacaine** dose is 6.6 mg/kg or 180 mg (whichever is less) during any single dental sitting

Weight-Specific Maximum Mepivacaine Dose (mg) = [Weight (**lbs**)/150] x 400

Adults: Injection: Usual dose: Mepivacaine 34 mg (1.7 mL) per site or mepivacaine 180 mg (9 mL) for entire oral cavity; maximum cumulative **mepivacaine** dose: 6.6 mg/kg or 400 mg (whichever is less) during any single dental sitting

The following numbers of dental carpules (1.7 mL) provide the indicated amounts of mepivacaine hydrochloride 2% and levonordefrin 1:20,000. See table.

# of Cartridges (1.7 mL)	Mepivacaine (mg) (2%)	Vasoconstrictor (mg) (Levonordefrin 1:20,000)
1	34	0.085
2	68	0.170
3	102	0.255
4	136	0.340
5	170	0.425
6	204	0.510
7	238	0.595
8	272	0.680
9	306	0.765
10	340	0.850

Dosage Note: Dosage varies with the anesthetic procedure, degree of anesthesia needed, vascularity of tissue, duration of anesthesia required, and physical condition of patient. Always use the lowest effective dose along with careful aspiration.

Children: Calculate the weight-specific maximum **mepivacaine** dose; regardless of the patient's weight, the maximum pediatric **mepivacaine** dose is 6.6 mg/kg or 180 mg (whichever is less) during any single dental sitting

Adults: Injection: Usual dose: Mepivacaine 34 mg (1.7 mL) per site or mepivacaine 180 mg (9 mL) for entire oral cavity; maximum cumulative **mepivacaine** dose: 6.6 mg/kg or 400 mg (whichever is less) during any single dental sitting

Dosage adjustment in renal impairment: No dosage adjustment provided in manufacturer's labeling; use with caution.

Dosage adjustment in hepatic impairment: No dosage adjustment provided in manufacturer's labeling; use with caution.

Mechanism of Action Local anesthetics bind selectively to the intracellular surface of sodium channels to block influx of sodium into the axon. As a result, depolarization necessary for action potential propagation and subsequent nerve function is prevented. The block at the sodium channel is reversible. When drug diffuses away from the axon, sodium channel function is restored and nerve propagation returns.

Levonordefrin prolongs the duration of the anesthetic actions of mepivacaine by causing vasoconstriction (alpha-adrenergic receptor agonist) of the vasculature surrounding the nerve axons. This prevents the diffusion of mepivacaine away from the nerves resulting in a longer retention in the axon.

Contraindications Hypersensitivity to local anesthetics of the amide-type or any component of the formulation

Warnings/Precautions Local anesthetics have been associated with rare occurrences of sudden respiratory arrest. Careful and constant monitoring of the patient's state of consciousness should be done following each local anesthetic injection; at such times, restlessness, anxiety, tinnitus, dizziness, blurred vision, tremors, depression, or drowsiness may be early warning signs of CNS toxicity. Treatment is primarily symptomatic and supportive. Convulsions due to systemic toxicity leading to cardiac arrest have also been reported, presumably following unintentional intravascular injection. Methemoglobinemia has been reported with local anesthetics including mepivacaine; clinically significant methemoglobinemia requires immediate treatment with oxygen and/or methylene blue.

Use with caution in patients with arteriosclerotic heart disease, cerebral vascular insufficiency, heart block, hypertension, and ischemic heart disease; minimal amounts of vasoconstrictor should be used in this patient population. Use with caution in patients with diabetes, hepatic or renal impairment, and hyperthyroidism. Use with caution in pediatric or elderly patients or in patients who are acutely ill or debilitated; reduce dose consistent with age and physical status. Use caution in patients with asthma; products may contains potassium metabisulfite which may cause severe hypersensitivity reactions (anaphylaxis) in some individuals. Use with caution and reduce dosage when administering to patients receiving other CNS depressants; effects with other sedative drugs may be potentiated.

Intravascular injections should be avoided; aspiration should be performed prior to administration; the needle must be repositioned until no return of blood can be elicited by aspiration; however, absence of blood in the syringe does not guarantee that intravascular injection has been avoided. To avoid serious adverse effects and high plasma levels, the lowest dosage resulting in effective anesthesia should be administered. Repeated doses may cause significant increases in blood levels with each repeated dose due to the possibility of accumulation of the drug or its metabolites. Tolerance to elevated blood levels varies with patient status. Dental practitioners using local anesthetic agents should be well trained in diagnosis and management of emergencies that may arise from the use of these agents. Resuscitative equipment, oxygen, and other resuscitative drugs should be available for immediate use.

Drug Interactions

Metabolism/Transport Effects None known.

Avoid Concomitant Use

Avoid concomitant use of Mepivacaine and Levonordefrin with any of the following: Ergot Derivatives; Iobenguane I 123

Increased Effect/Toxicity

Mepivacaine and Levonordefrin may increase the levels/effects of: Bromocriptine; Sympathomimetics

The levels/effects of Mepivacaine and Levonordefrin may be increased by: Antacids; AtoMOXetine; Beta-Blockers; Cannabinoids; Carbonic Anhydrase Inhibitors; Ergot Derivatives; Hyaluronidase; MAO Inhibitors; Serotonin/Norepinephrine Reuptake Inhibitors; Tricyclic Antidepressants

Decreased Effect

Mepivacaine and Levonordefrin may decrease the levels/effects of: Benzylpenicilloyl Polylysine; Iobenguane I 123

The levels/effects of Mepivacaine and Levonordefrin may be decreased by: Alpha1-Blockers; Spironolactone

Pharmacodynamics/Kinetics

Onset of Action Upper jaw: 30-120 seconds; Lower jaw: 1-4 minutes

Duration of Action

Upper jaw: 1-2.5 hours; Lower jaw: 2.5-5.5 hours

Infiltration: 50 minutes

Inferior alveolar block: 75 minutes

Pregnancy Risk Factor C

Pregnancy Considerations Animal reproduction studies have not been conducted with this combination.

Lactation Excretion unknown/use caution

◄ **Breast-Feeding Considerations** Usual infiltration doses of mepivacaine with levonordefrin given to nursing mothers has not been shown to affect the health of the nursing infant.

Dosage Forms

Injection, solution [for dental use]:
Carbocaine® 2% with Neo-Cobefrin®: Mepivacaine 2% and levonordefrin 1:20,000 (1.7 mL)
Scandonest® 2% L: Mepivacaine 2% and levonordefrin 1:20,000 (1.7 mL)

Dental Comment Oral paresthesia: The occurrence of oral paresthesia associated with 4% solutions of prilocaine or articaine, although rare, continue to be slightly more frequent than other local anesthetics. From 1999-2008, there were 182 cases of nonsurgical paresthesia (Gaffen, 2009). Of the cases, 172 involved mandibular block injection only. Another eight cases involved mandibular block combined with at least one other type of anesthetic injection. A single case involved infiltration around tooth number 35 and the final case involved infiltration and intraligamental injection in the maxillary anterior region.

A 2010 report, reviewed adverse events submitted voluntarily over a 10-year period involving the dental local anesthetics articaine, bupivacaine, lidocaine, mepivacaine, and prilocaine in the United States. Mepivacaine reported incidence: One case per 623,112,900 cartridges sold. The reported incidence of paresthesia was one case for 13,800,970 cartridges of all local anesthetics sold in the U.S. (Garisto, 2010).

References

Garisto GA, Gaffen AS, Lawrence HP, et al, "Occurrence of Paresthesia After Dental Local Anesthetic Administration in the United States," *J Am Dent Assoc*, 2010, 141(7):836-44.

Jastak JT and Yagiela JA, "Vasoconstrictors and Local Anesthesia: A Review and Rationale for Use," *J Am Dent Assoc*, 1983, 107 (4):623-30.

Wynn RL, "Epinephrine Interactions With Beta-Blockers," *Gen Dent*, 1994, 42(1):16, 18.

Meprobamate (me proe BA mate)

Brand Names: Canada Novo-Mepro

Generic Availability (U.S.) Yes

Pharmacologic Category Antianxiety Agent, Miscellaneous

Dental Use Treatment of muscle spasm associated with acute temporomandibular joint (TMJ) pain; management of dental anxiety disorders

Use Management of anxiety disorders

Unlabeled Use Demonstrated value for muscle contraction, headache, external sphincter spasticity, muscle rigidity, opisthotonos-associated with tetanus; treatment of muscle spasm associated with acute temporomandibular joint (TMJ) pain

Local Anesthetic/Vasoconstrictor Precautions No information available to require special precautions

Effects on Dental Treatment No significant effects or complications reported

Effects on Bleeding No information available to require special precautions

Adverse Effects Frequency not defined.

Cardiovascular: Arrhythmia EEG abnormalities, hypotensive crisis, peripheral edema, palpitation, syncope, tachycardia

Central nervous system: Ataxia, chills, dizziness, drowsiness, euphoria, fever, headache, overstimulation, paradoxical excitement, slurred speech, vertigo

Dermatologic: Angioneurotic edema, bruising, dermatitis, erythema multiforme, petechiae, purpura, rash, Stevens-Johnson syndrome

Gastrointestinal: Diarrhea, nausea, proctitis, stomatitis, vomiting

Hematologic: Agranulocytosis, aplastic anemia, eosinophilia, leukopenia, porphyria exacerbation, thrombocytopenic purpura

Neuromuscular & skeletal: Paresthesia, weakness

Ocular: Impairment of accommodation

Renal: Anuria, oliguria

Respiratory: Bronchospasm

Miscellaneous: Anaphylaxis, hypersensitivity

Dental Usual Dosage Muscle spasm (TMJ) pain or anxiety: Adults: Oral: 400 mg 3-4 times/day, up to 2400 mg/day

Dosage Oral:

Anxiety:
Children 6-12 years: 200-600 mg/day in 2-3 divided doses
Adults: 1200-1600 mg/day in 3-4 divided doses, up to 2400 mg/day

Muscle spasm (TMJ) pain (unlabeled use): Adults: 1200-1600 mg/day in 3-4 divided doses, up to 2400 mg/day

Dosing interval in renal impairment: No dosage adjustment provided in manufacturer's labeling; however, the following adjustments have been recommended (Aronoff, 2007): Adults:
Cl$_{cr}$ 10-50 mL/minute: Administer every 9-12 hours.
Cl$_{cr}$ <10 mL/minute: Administer every 12-18 hours.
Hemodialysis: No dosage adjustment necessary.
Peritoneal dialysis: Administer every 12-18 hours.
Continuous renal replacement therapy (CRRT): Administer every 9-12 hours.

Dosing adjustment in hepatic impairment: No dosage adjustment provided in manufacturer's labeling; use with caution.

Mechanism of Action Affects the thalamus and limbic system; also appears to inhibit multineuronal spinal reflexes

Contraindications Hypersensitivity to meprobamate, related compounds (including carisoprodol), or any component of the formulation; acute intermittent porphyria

Warnings/Precautions Physical and psychological dependence and abuse may occur; abrupt cessation may precipitate withdrawal. Use with caution in patients with depression or suicidal tendencies, or in patients with a history of drug abuse. May cause CNS depression, which may impair physical or mental abilities. Patients must be cautioned about performing tasks which require mental alertness (eg, operating machinery or driving). Effects with other sedative drugs or ethanol may be potentiated. Allergic reaction may occur in patients with history of dermatological condition (usually by fourth dose). Use with caution in patients with renal or hepatic impairment, or with a history of seizures. Avoid use in older adults; use associated with excessive sedation and high rate of physical dependence (Beers Criteria).

Drug Interactions

Metabolism/Transport Effects None known.

Avoid Concomitant Use

Avoid concomitant use of Meprobamate with any of the following: Azelastine (Nasal); Paraldehyde

Increased Effect/Toxicity

Meprobamate may increase the levels/effects of: Alcohol (Ethyl); Azelastine (Nasal); Buprenorphine; CNS Depressants; Methotrimeprazine; Metyrosine; Mirtazapine; Paraldehyde; Pramipexole; ROPINIRole; Rotigotine; Selective Serotonin Reuptake Inhibitors; Zolpidem

The levels/effects of Meprobamate may be increased by: Droperidol; HydrOXYzine; Magnesium Sulfate; Methotrimeprazine; Perampanel; Sodium Oxybate

Decreased Effect

The levels/effects of Meprobamate may be decreased by: Yohimbine

Ethanol/Nutrition/Herb Interactions

Ethanol: May increase CNS depression; monitor for increased effects with coadministration. Caution patients about effects.

Herb/Nutraceutical: Avoid valerian, St John's wort, kava kava, gotu kola (may increase CNS depression).

Pharmacodynamics/Kinetics

Onset of Action Sedation: ~1 hour

Half-life Elimination 10 hours

Pregnancy Considerations Meprobamate crosses the placenta and is found in cord blood in concentrations similar to those in the maternal plasma. Maternal use may be associated with congenital malformations; avoid use during pregnancy.

Lactation Enters breast milk

Breast-Feeding Considerations Breast milk concentrations are higher than maternal plasma concentrations.

Controlled Substance C-IV

Dosage Forms

Tablet, oral: 200 mg, 400 mg

Mercaptopurine (mer kap toe PURE een)

Brand Names: U.S. Purinethol® [DSC]

Brand Names: Canada Purinethol®

Pharmacologic Category Antineoplastic Agent, Antimetabolite; Antineoplastic Agent, Antimetabolite (Purine Analog); Immunosuppressant Agent

Use Maintenance treatment component of acute lymphoblastic leukemia (ALL)

Unlabeled Use Steroid-sparing agent for corticosteroid-dependent Crohn's disease (CD) and ulcerative colitis (UC); maintenance of remission in CD; fistulizing Crohn's disease; maintenance treatment in acute promyelocytic leukemia (APL); treatment component for non Hodgkin lymphoma (NHL), treatment of autoimmune hepatitis

Local Anesthetic/Vasoconstrictor Precautions No information available to require special precautions

Effects on Dental Treatment Key adverse event(s) related to dental treatment: Stomatitis and mucositis.

Effects on Bleeding Significant bleeding has been associated with drug-induced thrombocytopenia and altered hemostasis. Medical consult recommended.

Adverse Effects Frequency not defined.

Central nervous system: Drug fever

Dermatologic: Alopecia, hyperpigmentation, rash

Endocrine & metabolic: Hyperuricemia

Gastrointestinal: Anorexia, diarrhea, intestinal ulcers, mucositis/oral lesions (rare), nausea (minimal), pancreatitis, sprue-like symptoms, stomach pain, vomiting (minimal)

Genitourinary: Oligospermia

Hematologic: Myelosuppression (onset 7-10 days; nadir 14 days; recovery: 21 days); anemia, bleeding, granulocytopenia, leukopenia, marrow hypoplasia, thrombocytopenia

Hepatic: Hepatotoxicity, ascites, biliary stasis, hepatic damage/injury, hepatic encephalopathy, hepatic necrosis, hepatomegaly, intrahepatic cholestasis, jaundice, parenchymal cell necrosis, toxic hepatitis

Renal: Hyperuricosuria, renal toxicity

Miscellaneous: Hepatosplenic T cell lymphoma, immunosuppression, infection, secondary malignancy

General Dosage Range Dosage adjustment recommended in patients with hepatic or renal impairment or on concomitant therapy

Oral: *Children and Adults:* Maintenance: 1.5-2.5 mg/kg/day

Mechanism of Action Purine antagonist which inhibits DNA and RNA synthesis; acts as false metabolite and is incorporated into DNA and RNA, eventually inhibiting their synthesis; specific for the S phase of the cell cycle

Pharmacodynamics/Kinetics

Half-life Elimination Age dependent: Children: 21 minutes; Adults: 47 minutes

Time to Peak Serum: ~2 hours

Pregnancy Risk Factor D

Pregnancy Considerations May cause fetal harm if administered during pregnancy. Case reports of fetal loss have been noted with mercaptopurine administration during the first trimester; adverse effects have also been noted with second and third trimester use. Women of child bearing potential should avoid becoming pregnant during treatment.

Meropenem (mer oh PEN em)

Brand Names: U.S. Merrem® I.V.

Brand Names: Canada Merrem®

Pharmacologic Category Antibiotic, Carbapenem

Use

Treatment of intra-abdominal infections (complicated appendicitis and peritonitis); treatment of bacterial meningitis in pediatric patients ≥3 months of age caused by *S. pneumoniae*, *H. influenzae*, and *N. meningitidis*; treatment of complicated skin and skin structure infections caused by susceptible organisms

Canadian labeling: Additional indications (not in U.S. labeling): Treatment of lower respiratory tract infections (community-acquired and nosocomial pneumonias), complicated urinary tract infections, gynecologic infections (excluding chlamydia), and septicemia; treatment of bacterial meningitis in adults caused by *S. pneumoniae*, *H. influenzae*, and *N. meningitidis* (use in adult meningitis based on pediatric data)

Unlabeled Use *Burkholderia pseudomallei* (melioidosis), febrile neutropenia, liver abscess, otitis externa; treatment of prosthetic joint infection

Local Anesthetic/Vasoconstrictor Precautions No information available to require special precautions

Effects on Dental Treatment Key adverse event(s) related to dental treatment: Oral moniliasis (pediatric patients) and glossitis.

Effects on Bleeding No information available to require special precautions

Adverse Effects 1% to 10%:

Central nervous system: Headache (2% to 8%), pain (≤5%)

Dermatologic: Rash (2% to 3%, includes diaper-area moniliasis in infants), pruritus (1%)

Endocrine & metabolic: Hypoglycemia

Gastrointestinal: Diarrhea (4% to 7%), nausea/vomiting (1% to 8%), constipation (1% to 7%), oral moniliasis (up to 2% in pediatric patients), glossitis (1%)

Hematologic: Anemia (≤6%)

Local: Inflammation at the injection site (2%), phlebitis/thrombophlebitis (1%), injection site reaction (1%)

Respiratory: Apnea (1%), pharyngitis, pneumonia

Miscellaneous: Sepsis (2%), shock (1%)

General Dosage Range Dosage adjustment recommended in patients with renal impairment

I.V.:
Children ≥3 months and <50 kg: 10-40 mg/kg every 8 hours (maximum: 2 **g** every 8 hours)
Children ≥50 kg and Adults: 500 mg to 2 **g** every 8 hours

Mechanism of Action Inhibits bacterial cell wall synthesis by binding to several of the penicillin-binding proteins, which in turn inhibit the final transpeptidation step of peptidoglycan synthesis in bacterial cell walls, thus inhibiting cell wall biosynthesis; bacteria eventually lyse due to ongoing activity of cell wall autolytic enzymes (autolysins and murein hydrolases) while cell wall assembly is arrested

Pharmacodynamics/Kinetics

Half-life Elimination
Normal renal function: 1-1.5 hours
Cl$_{cr}$ 30-80 mL/minute: 1.9-3.3 hours
Cl$_{cr}$ 2-30 mL/minute: 3.82-5.7 hours

Time to Peak Tissue: 1 hour following infusion

Pregnancy Risk Factor B

Pregnancy Considerations Adverse events were not observed in animal reproduction studies. Incomplete transplacental transfer of meropenem was found using an *ex vivo* human perfusion model.

Mesalamine (me SAL a meen)

Brand Names: U.S. Apriso™; Asacol® HD; Asacol® [DSC]; Canasa®; Delzicol™; Lialda®; Pentasa®; Rowasa®; sfRowasa™

Brand Names: Canada 5-ASA; Asacol®; Asacol® 800; Mesasal®; Mezavant®; Novo-5 ASA; Novo-5 ASA-ECT; Pentasa®; Salofalk®; Salofalk® 5-ASA

Pharmacologic Category 5-Aminosalicylic Acid Derivative

Use
Oral:
Asacol®, Delzicol™, Lialda®, Mezavant®, Pentasa®: Treatment and maintenance of remission of mildly- to moderately-active ulcerative colitis
Apriso™: Maintenance of remission of ulcerative colitis
Asacol® HD: Treatment of moderately-active ulcerative colitis
Rectal: Treatment of active mild-to-moderate distal ulcerative colitis, proctosigmoiditis, or proctitis

Local Anesthetic/Vasoconstrictor Precautions No information available to require special precautions

Effects on Dental Treatment Key adverse event(s) related to dental treatment: Pharyngitis.

Effects on Bleeding No information available to require special precautions

Adverse Effects Adverse effects vary depending upon dosage form. Incidence usually on lower end with enema and suppository dosage forms.
>10%:
Central nervous system: Headache (2% to 35%), pain (≤14%)
Gastrointestinal: Abdominal pain (1% to 18%), eructation (16%), nausea (3% to 13%)

Respiratory: Pharyngitis (11%)
1% to 10%:
Cardiovascular: Chest pain (3%), peripheral edema (3%), vasodilation (≥2%)
Central nervous system: Dizziness (2% to 8%), fever (1% to 6%), chills (3%), malaise (2% to 3%), fatigue (<3%), vertigo (<3%), anxiety (≥2%), migraine (≥2%), nervousness (≥2%), paresthesia (≥2%), insomnia (2%)
Dermatologic: Skin rash (1% to 6%), pruritus (1% to 3%), alopecia (<3%), acne vulgaris (1% to 2%)
Endocrine & metabolic: Increased serum triglycerides (<3%)
Gastrointestinal: Diarrhea (2% to 8%), dyspepsia (1% to 6%), flatulence (1% to 6%), constipation (5%), vomiting (1% to 5%), exacerbation of ulcerative colitis (1% to 3%), rectal hemorrhage (<3%), abdominal distention (≥2%), gastroenteritis (≥2%), gastrointestinal hemorrhage (≥2%), abnormal stools (≥2%), tenesmus (≥2%), rectal pain (1% to 2%), hemorrhoids (1%)
Genitourinary: Polyuria (≥2%)
Hematologic & oncologic: Hematocrit/hemoglobin decreased (<3%)
Hepatic: Cholestatic hepatitis (<3%), increased serum transaminases (<3%), increased serum ALT (1%)
Infection: Infection (≥2%)
Local: Pain on insertion of enema tip (1%)
Musculoskeletal: Back pain (1% to 7%), hypertonia (5%), arthralgia (≤5%), myalgia (3%), weakness (≥2%), arthritis (2%), leg/joint pain (2%)
Ophthalmic: Visual disturbance (≥2%), conjunctivitis (2%)
Otic: Tinnitus (<3%), ear pain (≥2%)
Renal: Decreased creatinine clearance (<3%), hematuria (<3%)
Respiratory: Nasopharyngitis (1% to 4%), dyspnea (<3%), bronchitis (≥2%), sinusitis (≥2%), cough (≤2%)
Miscellaneous: Flu-like symptoms (1% to 5%), diaphoresis (3%), intolerance syndrome (3%)

General Dosage Range
Oral: *Adults:*
Capsule: Apriso™: 1.5 g once daily; Delzicol™: 800 mg 3 times daily or 1.6 g daily in 4 divided doses; Pentasa®: 1 g 4 times daily
Tablet: Asacol®: 800 mg 3 times daily or 1.6 g daily in divided doses; Asacol® HD: 1.6 g 3 times daily; Lialda®, Mezavant®: 2.4-4.8 g once daily
Rectal: *Adults:* Retention enema: 60 mL (4 g) at bedtime, retained overnight (~8 hours); Suppository: Insert 1000 mg at bedtime

Mechanism of Action Mesalamine (5-aminosalicylic acid) is the active component of sulfasalazine; the specific mechanism of action of mesalamine is unknown; however, it is thought that it modulates local chemical mediators of the inflammatory response, especially leukotrienes, and is also postulated to be a free radical scavenger or an inhibitor of tumor necrosis factor (TNF); action appears topical rather than systemic

Pharmacodynamics/Kinetics

Half-life Elimination 5-ASA: 0.5-10 hours; N-acetyl-5-ASA: 2-15 hours

Time to Peak
Capsule: Apriso™: ~4 hours; Delzicol™: 4-16 hours; Pentasa®: 3 hours
Rectal: 4-7 hours
Tablet: Asacol®: 4-12 hours; Asacol® HD: 10-16 hours; Lialda®: 9-12 hours; Mezavant®: 8 hours

Pregnancy Risk Factor B/C (product specific)

Pregnancy Considerations Animal reproduction studies with mesalamine have not demonstrated teratogenicity or fertility impairment. Dibutyl phthalate (DBP) is an inactive ingredient in the enteric coating of Asacol® and Asacol® HD; adverse effects in male rats were noted at doses greater than the recommended human dose. Mesalamine is known to cross the placenta. An increased rate of congenital malformations has not been observed in human studies. Preterm birth, still birth and decreased birth weight have been observed; however, these events may also be due to maternal disease.

Metaproterenol (met a proe TER e nol)

Related Information
Respiratory Diseases *on page 1514*

Brand Names: Canada Apo-Orciprenaline®; ratio-Orciprenaline®; Tanta-Orciprenaline®

Pharmacologic Category Beta$_2$ Agonist

Use Bronchodilator in reversible airway obstruction due to asthma or COPD

Local Anesthetic/Vasoconstrictor Precautions No information available to require special precautions

Effects on Dental Treatment Key adverse event(s) related to dental treatment: Bad taste and xerostomia (normal salivary flow resumes upon discontinuation).

Effects on Bleeding No information available to require special precautions

Adverse Effects
>10%:
Cardiovascular: Tachycardia (6% to 17%)
Central nervous system: Nervousness (5% to 20%), headache (1% to 7%)
Neuromuscular & skeletal: Tremor (2% to 17%)
1% to 10%:
Cardiovascular: Palpitation (4%)
Central nervous system: Dizziness (2%), insomnia (2%), fatigue (1%)
Gastrointestinal: Nausea (1% to 4%), diarrhea (1%)
Respiratory: Asthma exacerbation (2%)

General Dosage Range Oral:
Children <6 years: 1.3-2.6 mg/kg/day divided every 6-8 hours
Children 6-9 years (or <27 kg): 10 mg/dose 3-4 times/day
Children >9 years (or ≥27 kg) and Adults: 20 mg 3-4 times/day

Mechanism of Action Stimulates beta$_2$-receptors which increases the conversion of adenosine triphosphate (ATP) to 3'-5'-cyclic adenosine monophosphate (cAMP), resulting in bronchial smooth muscle relaxation

Pharmacodynamics/Kinetics
Onset of Action Bronchodilation: Oral: ~30 minutes; Peak effect: Oral: ~1 hour
Duration of Action ~2-6 hours

Pregnancy Risk Factor C

Pregnancy Considerations Teratogenic and embryotoxic effects have been observed in some animal studies. There are no adequate and well-controlled studies in pregnant women.

Metaxalone (me TAKS a lone)

Brand Names: U.S. Skelaxin®
Brand Names: Canada Skelaxin®
Generic Availability (U.S.) Yes
Pharmacologic Category Skeletal Muscle Relaxant

Use Relief of discomfort associated with acute, painful musculoskeletal conditions

Local Anesthetic/Vasoconstrictor Precautions No information available to require special precautions

Effects on Dental Treatment No significant effects or complications reported

Effects on Bleeding No information available to require special precautions

Adverse Effects Frequency not defined.
Central nervous system: Dizziness, drowsiness, headache, irritability, nervousness
Dermatologic: Rash (with or without pruritus)
Gastrointestinal: Gastrointestinal upset, nausea, vomiting
Hematologic: Hemolytic anemia, leukopenia
Hepatic: Jaundice
Miscellaneous: Hypersensitivity (including rare anaphylactoid reactions)

Dosage Oral: Children >12 years and Adults: Muscle discomfort: 800 mg 3-4 times/day
Dosage adjustment in renal impairment: Use caution in patients with mild-to-moderate renal impairment; contraindicated with significant impairment. No specific recommendation are provided in approved labeling.
Dosage adjustment in hepatic impairment: Use caution in patients with mild-to-moderate hepatic impairment; contraindicated with significant impairment. No specific recommendation are provided in approved labeling.

Mechanism of Action Precise mechanism has not been established; however, efficacy appears to result from disruption of the spasm-pain-spasm cycle, probably by a general CNS depressant effect. Does not have a direct effect on skeletal muscle.

Contraindications Hypersensitivity to metaxalone or any component of the formulation; significantly impaired hepatic or renal function, history of drug-induced hemolytic anemias or other anemias

Warnings/Precautions May cause CNS depression. CNS depressant effects may be augmented when used in conjunction with other depressants (eg, barbiturates, ethanol), when taken with food, or in the elderly. May impair mental and/or physical ability to perform hazardous tasks such as operating machinery or driving a motor vehicle. Use with caution in patients with impaired renal or hepatic function (contraindicated if significant impairment); routine monitoring of transaminases is recommended. An increase in bioavailability and half-life have been observed in female patients. Muscle relaxants are poorly tolerated by the elderly due to potent anticholinergic effects, sedation, and risk of fracture. Efficacy is questionable at dosages tolerated by elderly patients; avoid use (Beers Criteria). Safety and efficacy have not been established in children ≤12 years of age.

Drug Interactions
Metabolism/Transport Effects Substrate of CYP1A2 (minor), CYP2C19 (minor), CYP2C8 (minor), CYP2C9 (minor), CYP2D6 (minor), CYP2E1 (minor), CYP3A4 (minor); **Note:** Assignment of Major/Minor substrate status based on clinically relevant drug interaction potential

Avoid Concomitant Use
Avoid concomitant use of Metaxalone with any of the following: Azelastine (Nasal); Paraldehyde

Increased Effect/Toxicity

Metaxalone may increase the levels/effects of: Alcohol (Ethyl); Azelastine (Nasal); Buprenorphine; CNS Depressants; Methotrimeprazine; Metyrosine; Mirtazapine; Paraldehyde; Pramipexole; ROPINIRole; Rotigotine; Selective Serotonin Reuptake Inhibitors; Zolpidem

The levels/effects of Metaxalone may be increased by: Droperidol; HydrOXYzine; Magnesium Sulfate; Methotrimeprazine; Perampanel; Sodium Oxybate

Decreased Effect

The levels/effects of Metaxalone may be decreased by: Peginterferon Alfa-2b

Ethanol/Nutrition/Herb Interactions

Ethanol: May increase CNS depression; monitor for increased effects with coadministration. Caution patients about effects.

Food: Bioavailability may be increased (may increase CNS depression).

Herb/Nutraceutical: Avoid valerian, St John's wort, kava kava, gotu kola (may increase CNS depression).

Dietary Considerations Administration with food may increase serum concentrations.

Pharmacodynamics/Kinetics

Onset of Action ~1 hour

Duration of Action ~4-6 hours

Half-life Elimination 4-14 hours

Time to Peak T_{max}: ~3 hours

Pregnancy Considerations Teratogenic effects were not observed in animal studies. There are no adequate and well-controlled studies in pregnant women. Use during pregnancy (especially first trimester) only if benefits outweigh risks.

Lactation Excretion in breast milk unknown/not recommended

Dosage Forms

Tablet, oral: 800 mg

Skelaxin®: 800 mg

MetFORMIN (met FOR min)

Related Information

Endocrine Disorders and Pregnancy *on page 1517*

Brand Names: U.S. Fortamet®; Glucophage®; Glucophage® XR; Glumetza®; Riomet®

Brand Names: Canada Apo-Metformin®; Ava-Metformin; CO Metformin; Dom-Metformin; Glucophage®; Glumetza®; Glycon; JAMP-Metformin; JAMP-Metformin Blackberry; Med-Metformin; Mylan-Metformin; Novo-Metformin; Nu-Metformin; PHL-Metformin; PMS-Metformin; PRO-Metformin; Q-Metformin; RAN™-Metformin; ratio-Metformin; Riva-Metformin; Sandoz-Metformin FC

Generic Availability (U.S.) Yes: Excludes solution

Pharmacologic Category Antidiabetic Agent, Biguanide

Use Management of type 2 diabetes mellitus (noninsulin dependent, NIDDM) when hyperglycemia cannot be managed with diet and exercise alone.

Unlabeled Use Gestational diabetes mellitus (GDM); polycystic ovary syndrome (PCOS); prevention of type 2 diabetes mellitus

Local Anesthetic/Vasoconstrictor Precautions No information available to require special precautions

Effects on Dental Treatment Key adverse event(s) related to dental treatment: Taste disorder.

Metformin-dependent patients with diabetes (noninsulin dependent, Type 2) should be appointed for dental treatment in morning in order to minimize chance of stress-induced hypoglycemia.

Effects on Bleeding No information available to require special precautions

Adverse Effects

>10%:

Gastrointestinal: Diarrhea (IR tablet: 12% to 53%; ER tablet: 10% to 17%), nausea/vomiting (IR tablet: 7% to 26%; ER tablet: 7% to 9%), flatulence (12%)

Neuromuscular & skeletal: Weakness (9%)

1% to 10%:

Cardiovascular: Chest discomfort, flushing, palpitation

Central nervous system: Headache (6%), chills, dizziness, lightheadedness

Dermatologic: Rash

Endocrine & metabolic: Hypoglycemia

Gastrointestinal: Indigestion (7%), abdominal discomfort (6%), abdominal distention, abnormal stools, constipation, dyspepsia/ heartburn, taste disorder

Neuromuscular & skeletal: Myalgia

Respiratory: Dyspnea, upper respiratory tract infection

Miscellaneous: Decreased vitamin B_{12} levels (7%), increased diaphoresis, flu-like syndrome, nail disorder

Dosage

Type 2 diabetes management: **Note:** Allow 1-2 weeks between dose titrations: Generally, clinically significant responses are not seen at doses <1500 mg daily; however, a lower recommended starting dose and gradual increased dosage is recommended to minimize gastrointestinal symptoms.

Immediate release tablet or solution: Oral:

Children 10-16 years: Initial: 500 mg twice daily; increases in daily dosage should be made in increments of 500 mg at weekly intervals, given in divided doses, up to a maximum of 2000 mg daily

Children ≥17 years and Adults: Initial: 500 mg twice daily **or** 850 mg once daily; titrate in increments of 500 mg weekly or 850 mg every other week; may also titrate from 500 mg twice a day to 850 mg twice a day after 2 weeks

If a dose >2000 mg daily is required, it may be better tolerated in 3 divided doses. Maximum recommended dose 2550 mg daily.

Extended release tablet: Oral: **Note:** If glycemic control is not achieved at maximum dose, may divide dose and administer twice daily.

Children ≥17 years and Adults:

Fortamet®: Initial: 500-1000 mg once daily; dosage may be increased by 500 mg weekly; maximum dose: 2500 mg once daily

Glucophage® XR: Initial: 500 mg once daily; dosage may be increased by 500 mg weekly; maximum dose: 2000 mg once daily

Adults: Glumetza®: Initial: 1000 mg once daily; dosage may be increased by 500 mg weekly; maximum dose: 2000 mg once daily

Elderly: The initial and maintenance dosing should be conservative, due to the potential for decreased renal function. Generally, elderly patients should not be titrated to the maximum dose of metformin. Do not use in patients ≥80 years of age unless normal renal function has been established.

Transfer from other antidiabetic agents: No transition period is generally necessary except when transferring from chlorpropamide. When transferring from chlorpropamide, care should be exercised during the first 2 weeks because of the prolonged retention of chlorpropamide in the body, leading to overlapping drug effects and possible hypoglycemia.

Concomitant metformin and oral sulfonylurea therapy: If patients have not responded to 4 weeks of the maximum dose of metformin monotherapy, consider a gradual addition of an oral sulfonylurea, even if prior primary or secondary failure to a sulfonylurea has occurred. Continue metformin at the maximum dose. If adequate response has not occurred following 3 months of metformin and sulfonylurea combination therapy, consider switching to insulin with or without metformin.

Failed sulfonylurea therapy: Patients with prior failure on glyburide may be treated by gradual addition of metformin. Initiate with glyburide 20 mg and metformin 500 mg daily. Metformin dosage may be increased by 500 mg/day at weekly intervals, up to a maximum metformin dose (dosage of glyburide maintained at 20 mg daily).

Concomitant metformin and insulin therapy: Initial: 500 mg metformin once daily, continue current insulin dose; increase by 500 mg metformin weekly until adequate glycemic control is achieved

Maximum daily dose: Immediate release and solution: 2550 mg metformin; Extended release: 2000-2500 mg (varies by product)

Decrease insulin dose 10% to 25% when FPG <120 mg/dL; monitor and make further adjustments as needed

Type 2 diabetes prevention (unlabeled use): **Immediate release tablet or solution:** Oral: Adults: Initial: 850 mg once daily; Target: 850 mg twice daily (Knowler, 2002)

Dosing adjustment/comments in renal impairment: The plasma and blood half-life of metformin is prolonged and the renal clearance is decreased in proportion to the decrease in creatinine clearance. Per the manufacturer, metformin is contraindicated in the presence of renal dysfunction defined as a serum creatinine ≥1.5 mg/dL in males, or ≥1.4 mg/dL in females and in patients with abnormal clearance. The Canadian labeling recommends that metformin be avoided in patients with Cl_{cr} <60 mL/minute.

Dosing adjustment in hepatic impairment: Avoid metformin; liver disease is a risk factor for the development of lactic acidosis during metformin therapy.

Mechanism of Action Decreases hepatic glucose production, decreasing intestinal absorption of glucose and improves insulin sensitivity (increases peripheral glucose uptake and utilization)

Contraindications Hypersensitivity to metformin or any component of the formulation; renal disease or renal dysfunction (serum creatinine ≥1.5 mg/dL in males or ≥1.4 mg/dL in females) or abnormal creatinine clearance from any cause, including shock, acute myocardial infarction, or septicemia; acute or chronic metabolic acidosis with or without coma (including diabetic ketoacidosis)

Note: Temporarily discontinue in patients undergoing radiologic studies in which intravascular iodinated contrast media are utilized.

Warnings/Precautions [U.S. Boxed Warning]: Lactic acidosis is a rare, but potentially severe consequence of therapy with metformin. Lactic acidosis should be suspected in any patient with diabetes receiving metformin with evidence of acidosis but without evidence of ketoacidosis. Discontinue metformin in clinical situations predisposing to hypoxemia, including conditions such as cardiovascular collapse, respiratory failure, acute myocardial infarction, acute congestive heart failure, and septicemia. Use caution in patients with congestive heart failure requiring pharmacologic management, particularly in patients with unstable or acute CHF; risk of lactic acidosis may be increased secondary to hypoperfusion.

Metformin is substantially excreted by the kidney. The risk of accumulation and lactic acidosis increases with the degree of impairment of renal function. Patients with renal function below the limit of normal for their age should not receive metformin. In elderly patients, renal function should be monitored regularly; should not be initiated in patients ≥80 years of age unless normal renal function is confirmed. Use of concomitant medications that may affect renal function (ie, affect tubular secretion) may also affect metformin disposition. Metformin should be withheld in patients with dehydration and/or prerenal azotemia. Therapy should be suspended for any surgical procedures (resume only after normal oral intake resumed and normal renal function is verified). Therapy should be temporarily discontinued prior to or at the time of intravascular administration of iodinated contrast media (potential for acute alteration in renal function). Metformin should be withheld for 48 hours after the radiologic study and restarted only after renal function has been confirmed as normal. It may be necessary to discontinue metformin and administer insulin if the patient is exposed to stress (fever, trauma, infection, surgery).

Avoid use in patients with impaired liver function. Patient must be instructed to avoid excessive acute or chronic ethanol use; ethanol may potentiate metformin's effect on lactate metabolism. Administration of oral antidiabetic drugs has been reported to be associated with increased cardiovascular mortality; metformin does not appear to share this risk. Insoluble tablet shell of Glumetza® 1000 mg extended release tablet may remain intact and be visible in the stool. Other extended released tablets (Fortamet®, Glucophage® XR, Glumetza® 500 mg) may appear in the stool as a soft mass resembling the tablet.

Drug Interactions

Metabolism/Transport Effects None known.

Avoid Concomitant Use There are no known interactions where it is recommended to avoid concomitant use.

Increased Effect/Toxicity

MetFORMIN may increase the levels/effects of: Dalfampridine; Dofetilide

The levels/effects of MetFORMIN may be increased by: Carbonic Anhydrase Inhibitors; Cephalexin; Cimetidine; Dalfampridine; Glycopyrrolate; Iodinated Contrast Agents; LamoTRIgine; Pegvisomant; Trimethoprim

Decreased Effect

MetFORMIN may decrease the levels/effects of: Trospium

The levels/effects of MetFORMIN may be decreased by: Corticosteroids (Orally Inhaled); Corticosteroids (Systemic); Luteinizing Hormone-Releasing Hormone Analogs; Somatropin; Thiazide Diuretics

◄ **Ethanol/Nutrition/Herb Interactions**
Ethanol: Avoid or limit ethanol (incidence of lactic acidosis may be increased; may cause hypoglycemia).
Food: Food decreases the extent and slightly delays the absorption. May decrease absorption of vitamin B_{12} and/or folic acid.
Herb/Nutraceutical: Caution with chromium, garlic, gymnema (may cause hypoglycemia).

Dietary Considerations Drug may cause GI upset; take with food (to decrease GI upset). Take at the same time(s) each day. Dietary modification based on ADA recommendations is a part of therapy. Monitor for signs and symptoms of vitamin B_{12} and/or folic acid deficiency; supplementation may be required.

Pharmacodynamics/Kinetics
Onset of Action Within days; maximum effects up to 2 weeks
Half-life Elimination Plasma: 4-9 hours
Time to Peak Immediate release: 2-3 hours; Extended release: 7 hours (range: 4-8 hours)

Pregnancy Risk Factor B
Pregnancy Considerations Adverse events have not been observed in animal studies; therefore, metformin is classified as pregnancy category B. Metformin has been found to cross the placenta in concentrations which may be comparable to those found in the maternal plasma. Pharmacokinetic studies suggest that clearance of metformin may be increased during pregnancy and dosing may need adjusted in some women when used during the third trimester.

Fetal, neonatal, and maternal outcomes have been evaluated following maternal use of metformin for the treatment of GDM and type 2 diabetes. Available information suggests that metformin use during pregnancy may be safe as long as good glycemic control is maintained; however, many studies used metformin during the second or third trimester only. Maternal hyperglycemia can be associated with adverse effects in the fetus, including macrosomia, neonatal hyperglycemia, and hyperbilirubinemia; the risk of congenital malformations is increased when the Hb A_{1c} is above the normal range. Diabetes can also be associated with adverse effects in the mother. Poorly-treated diabetes may cause end-organ damage that may negatively affect obstetric outcomes. Physiologic glucose levels should be maintained prior to and during pregnancy to decrease the risk of adverse events in the mother and the fetus. Until additional safety and efficacy data are obtained, the use of oral agents is generally not recommended as routine management of GDM or type 2 diabetes mellitus during pregnancy. Insulin is the drug of choice for the control of diabetes mellitus during pregnancy.

Metformin has also been evaluated for the treatment of PCOS, a syndrome which may exhibit oligomenorrhea and, in some women, hyperinsulinemia. It is not recommended as first-line therapy; when used to treat infertility related to PCOS, current guidelines restrict the use of metformin to women with glucose intolerance. Because ovulation rates will likely improve in women with PCOS who are taking metformin, appropriate contraceptive measures should be discussed in women who are not attempting to conceive.

Lactation Enters breast milk/not recommended
Breast-Feeding Considerations Low amounts of metformin (generally ≤1% of the weight-adjusted maternal dose) are excreted into breast milk. Breast-feeding is not recommended by the manufacturer. Because breast milk concentrations of metformin stay relatively constant, avoiding nursing around peak plasma concentrations in the mother would not be helpful in reducing metformin exposure to the infant. Growth and development were not affected in infants born to mothers with PCOS and who took metformin while breast-feeding.

Dosage Forms
Solution, oral:
Riomet®: 100 mg/mL (118 mL, 473 mL)
Tablet, oral: 500 mg, 850 mg, 1000 mg
Glucophage®: 500 mg, 850 mg, 1000 mg
Tablet, extended release, oral: 500 mg, 750 mg, 1000 mg
Fortamet®: 500 mg, 1000 mg
Glucophage® XR: 500 mg, 750 mg
Glumetza®: 500 mg, 1000 mg

Methadone (METH a done)

Related Information
Clinical Risk Related to Drugs Prolonging QT Interval *on page 1510*
Brand Names: U.S. Dolophine®; Methadone Diskets®; Methadone Intensol™; Methadose®
Brand Names: Canada Metadol-D™; Metadol™
Pharmacologic Category Analgesic, Opioid
Use Management of moderate-to-severe pain when a continuous, around-the-clock opioid analgesic is needed for an extended period of time; detoxification and maintenance treatment of opioid addiction through a certified program
Local Anesthetic/Vasoconstrictor Precautions
Methadone is one of the drugs confirmed to prolong the QT interval and is accepted as having a risk of causing torsade de pointes. The risk of drug-induced torsade de pointes is extremely low when a single QT interval prolonging drug is prescribed. In terms of epinephrine, it is not known what effect vasoconstrictors in the local anesthetic regimen will have in patients with a known history of congenital prolonged QT interval or in patients taking any medication that prolongs the QT interval. Until more information is obtained, it is suggested that the clinician consult with the physician prior to the use of a vasoconstrictor in suspected patients, and that the vasoconstrictor (epinephrine, levonordefrin [Neo-Cobefrin®]) be used with caution.
Effects on Dental Treatment Key adverse event(s) related to dental treatment: Significant xerostomia (normal salivary flow resumes upon discontinuation) and glossitis.
Effects on Bleeding No information available to require special precautions
Adverse Effects Frequency not defined. During prolonged administration, adverse effects may decrease over several weeks; however, constipation and sweating may persist.
Cardiovascular: Arrhythmia, bigeminal rhythms, bradycardia, cardiac arrest, cardiomyopathy, ECG changes, edema, extrasystoles, faintness, flushing, heart failure, hypotension, palpitation, peripheral vasodilation, phlebitis, orthostatic hypotension, QT interval prolonged, shock, syncope, tachycardia, torsade de pointes, T-wave inversion, ventricular fibrillation, ventricular tachycardia
Central nervous system: Agitation, confusion, disorientation, dizziness, drowsiness, dysphoria, euphoria, hallucination, headache, insomnia, lightheadedness, sedation, seizure
Dermatologic: Hemorrhagic urticaria, pruritus, rash, urticaria

Endocrine & metabolic: Antidiuretic effect, amenorrhea, hypokalemia, hypomagnesemia, libido decreased

Gastrointestinal: Abdominal pain, anorexia, biliary tract spasm, constipation, glossitis, nausea, stomach cramps, vomiting, weight gain, xerostomia

Genitourinary: Impotence, urinary retention or hesitancy

Hematologic: Thrombocytopenia (reversible, reported in patients with chronic hepatitis)

Neuromuscular & skeletal: Weakness

Local: I.M./SubQ injection: Erythema, pain, swelling; I.V. injection: Hemorrhagic urticaria (rare), pruritus, urticaria, rash

Ocular: Miosis, visual disturbances

Respiratory: Pulmonary edema, respiratory depression, respiratory arrest

Miscellaneous: Death, diaphoresis, physical and psychological dependence

General Dosage Range Dosage adjustment recommended in patients with renal impairment or who develop toxicities

I.M.:
Adults: Initial: 2.5 mg every 8-12 hours
Elderly: 2.5 mg every 8-12 hours

I.V., SubQ: *Adults:* Initial: 2.5 mg every 8-12 hours

Oral:
Adults: Detoxification: Initial: Up to 40 mg/day; Maintenance: 80-120 mg/day; Pain: 2.5-10 mg every 4-12 hours as needed
Elderly: 2.5 mg every 8-12 hours

Mechanism of Action Binds to opiate receptors in the CNS, causing inhibition of ascending pain pathways, altering the perception of and response to pain; produces generalized CNS depression. Methadone has also been shown to have weak N-methyl-D-aspartate (NMDA) receptor antagonism (Callahan, 2004).

Pharmacodynamics/Kinetics

Onset of Action Oral: Analgesic: 0.5-1 hour; Parenteral: 10-20 minutes; Peak effect: Parenteral: 1-2 hours; Oral: Continuous dosing: 3-5 days

Duration of Action Analgesia: Oral: 4-8 hours (single-dose studies), increases to 22-48 hours with repeated doses; slow release from the liver and other tissues may prolong duration of action

Half-life Elimination Terminal: 8-59 hours; may be prolonged with alkaline pH, decreased during pregnancy

Time to Peak 1-7.5 hours

Pregnancy Risk Factor C

Pregnancy Considerations Teratogenic effects have been observed in some, but not all, animal studies. Data collected by the Teratogen Information System are complicated by maternal use of illicit drugs, nutrition, infection, and psychosocial circumstances. However, pregnant women in methadone treatment programs are reported to have improved fetal outcomes compared to pregnant women using illicit drugs. Methadone can be detected in the amniotic fluid, cord plasma, and newborn urine. Fetal growth, birth weight, length, and/or head circumference may be decreased in infants born to narcotic-addicted mothers treated with methadone during pregnancy. Growth deficits do not appear to persist; however, decreased performance on psychometric and behavioral tests has been found to continue into childhood. Abnormal fetal nonstress tests have also been reported. Withdrawal symptoms in the neonate may be observed up to 2-4 weeks after delivery. The manufacturer states that methadone should be used during pregnancy only if clearly needed. Because methadone clearance in pregnant women is increased and half-life is decreased during the 2nd and 3rd trimesters of pregnancy, withdrawal symptoms may be observed in the mother; dosage of methadone may need increased or dosing interval decreased during pregnancy.

Controlled Substance C-II

Prescribing and Access Restrictions When used for treatment of opioid addiction: May only be dispensed in accordance to guidelines established by the Substance Abuse and Mental Health Services Administration's (SAMHSA) Center for Substance Abuse Treatment (CSAT). Regulations regarding methadone use may vary by state and/or country. Obtain advice from appropriate regulatory agencies and/or consult with pain management/palliative care specialists.

Note: Regulatory Exceptions to the General Requirement to Provide Opioid Agonist Treatment (per manufacturer's labeling):
1. During inpatient care, when the patient was admitted for any condition other than concurrent opioid addiction, to facilitate the treatment of the primary admitting diagnosis.
2. During an emergency period of no longer than 3 days while definitive care for the addiction is being sought in an appropriately licensed facility.

Dental Comment This drug is known to prolong the QT interval. The QT interval is measured as the time and distance between the Q point of the QRS complex and the end of the T wave in the ECG tracing. After adjustment for heart rate, the QT interval is defined as prolonged if it is more than 450 msec in men and 460 msec in women. A long QT syndrome was first described in the 1950s and 60s as a congenital syndrome involving QT interval prolongation and syncope and sudden death. Some of the congenital long QT syndromes were characterized by a peculiar electrocardiographic appearance of the QRS complex involving a premature atria beat followed by a pause, then a subsequent sinus beat showing marked QT prolongation and deformity. This type of cardiac arrhythmia was originally termed "torsade de pointes" (translated from the French as "twisting of the points").

Prolongation of the QT interval is thought to result from delayed ventricular repolarization. The repolarization process within the myocardial cell is due to the efflux of intracellular potassium. The channels associated with this current can be blocked by many drugs and predispose the electrical propagation cycle to torsade de pointes.

Methamphetamine (meth am FET a meen)

Related Information
Management of the Chemically Dependent Patient *on page 1550*

Brand Names: U.S. Desoxyn®

Brand Names: Canada Desoxyn®

Pharmacologic Category Anorexiant; Central Nervous System Stimulant; Sympathomimetic

Use Treatment of attention-deficit/hyperactivity disorder (ADHD); short-term (few weeks) adjunct to caloric restriction in exogenous obesity

Pharmacotherapy for weight loss is recommended only for obese patients with a body mass index ≥ 30 kg/m^2, or ≥ 27 kg/m^2 in the presence of other risk factors such as hypertension, diabetes, and/or dyslipidemia or a high waist circumference; therapy should be used in conjunction with a comprehensive weight management program.

Unlabeled Use Narcolepsy

Local Anesthetic/Vasoconstrictor Precautions Use vasoconstrictor with caution in patients taking methamphetamine. Amphetamines enhance the sympathomimetic response of epinephrine and norepinephrine leading to potential hypertension and cardiotoxicity.

Effects on Dental Treatment Key adverse event(s) related to dental treatment: Xerostomia (normal salivary flow resumes upon discontinuation) and unpleasant taste. Up to 10% of patients taking methamphetamine may present with hypertension. Monitor blood pressure prior to using local anesthetic with vasoconstrictors.

Effects on Bleeding No information available to require special precautions

Adverse Effects Frequency not defined.

Cardiovascular: Hypertension, palpitation, tachycardia

Central nervous system: Dizziness, dysphoria, euphoria, exacerbation of motor and phonic tics and Tourette's syndrome, headache, insomnia, overstimulation, psychosis, restlessness

Dermatologic: Rash, urticaria

Endocrine & metabolic: Change in libido

Gastrointestinal: Anorexia, constipation, diarrhea, unpleasant taste, weight loss, xerostomia

Genitourinary: Impotence

Neuromuscular & skeletal: Tremor

Miscellaneous: Suppression of growth in children, tolerance and withdrawal with prolonged use

General Dosage Range Oral:

Children ≥6 years: ADHD: Initial: 5 mg 1-2 times daily; Usual maintenance: 20-25 mg daily

Children ≥12 years and Adults: Exogenous obesity: 5 mg before each meal

Mechanism of Action A sympathomimetic amine related to ephedrine and amphetamine with CNS stimulant activity; causes release of catecholamines (primarily dopamine and other catecholamines) from their storage sites in the presynaptic nerve terminals. Inhibits reuptake and metabolism of catecholamines through inhibition of monoamine transporters and oxidase.

Pharmacodynamics/Kinetics

Half-life Elimination 4-5 hours

Pregnancy Risk Factor C

Pregnancy Considerations Adverse effects have been observed in animal reproduction studies. Methamphetamine and amphetamine were detected in newborn tissues following intermittent maternal use of Desoxyn® during pregnancy (Garriott, 1973). The majority of human data is based on illicit amphetamine/methamphetamine exposure and not from therapeutic maternal use (Golub, 2005). Use of amphetamines during pregnancy may lead to an increased risk of premature birth and low birth weight; newborns may experience symptoms of withdrawal. Behavioral problems may also occur later in childhood (LaGasse, 2012).

Controlled Substance C-II

Methazolamide (meth a ZOE la mide)

Brand Names: U.S. Neptazane™

Brand Names: Canada Apo-Methazolamide®

Pharmacologic Category Carbonic Anhydrase Inhibitor; Diuretic, Carbonic Anhydrase Inhibitor; Ophthalmic Agent, Antiglaucoma

Use Treatment of chronic open-angle or secondary glaucoma; short-term therapy of acute angle-closure glaucoma prior to surgery

Local Anesthetic/Vasoconstrictor Precautions No information available to require special precautions

Effects on Dental Treatment Key adverse event(s) related to dental treatment: Xerostomia (normal salivary flow resumes upon discontinuation) and metallic taste.

Effects on Bleeding No information available to require special precautions

Adverse Effects Frequency not defined.

Central nervous system: Confusion, drowsiness, fatigue, fever, malaise, seizure

Dermatologic: Erythema multiforme, photosensitivity, rash, Stevens-Johnson syndrome, toxic epidermal necrolysis, urticaria

Endocrine & metabolic: Electrolyte imbalance, metabolic acidosis

Gastrointestinal: Appetite decreased, diarrhea, melena, nausea, taste alteration, vomiting

Genitourinary: Crystalluria, glycosuria, hematuria, polyuria, renal calculi

Hematologic: Agranulocytosis, aplastic anemia, bone marrow depression, hemolytic anemia, leukopenia, pancytopenia, thrombocytopenic purpura

Hepatic: Fulminant hepatic necrosis, hepatic insufficiency

Neuromuscular & skeletal: Flaccid paralysis, paresthesia

Ocular: Myopia

Otic: Hearing disturbance, tinnitus

Miscellaneous: Anaphylaxis, hypersensitivity

General Dosage Range Oral: *Adults:* 50-100 mg 2-3 times/day

Mechanism of Action Noncompetitive inhibition of the enzyme carbonic anhydrase; thought that carbonic anhydrase is located at the luminal border of cells of the proximal tubule. When the enzyme is inhibited, there is an increase in urine volume and a change to an alkaline pH with a subsequent decrease in the excretion of titratable acid and ammonia.

Pharmacodynamics/Kinetics

Onset of Action Slow in comparison with acetazolamide (2-4 hours); Peak effect: 6-8 hours

Duration of Action 10-18 hours

Half-life Elimination ~14 hours

Pregnancy Risk Factor C

Pregnancy Considerations Teratogenic in animal studies; however, there are no adequate and well-controlled studies in pregnant women.

Methenamine (meth EN a meen)

Brand Names: U.S. Hiprex®

Brand Names: Canada Dehydral®; Hiprex®; Mandelamine®; Urasal®

Pharmacologic Category Antibiotic, Miscellaneous

Use Prophylaxis or suppression of recurrent urinary tract infections; urinary tract discomfort secondary to hypermotility

Local Anesthetic/Vasoconstrictor Precautions No information available to require special precautions

Effects on Dental Treatment No significant effects or complications reported

Effects on Bleeding No information available to require special precautions

Adverse Effects <4%:

Dermatologic: Pruritus, rash

Gastrointestinal: Dyspepsia, nausea, vomiting

Hepatic: ALT increased (reversible; rare), AST increased (reversible; rare)

Note: Large doses (higher than recommended) have resulted in bladder irritation, frequent/painful micturition, albuminuria, and hematuria.

General Dosage Range Oral:
Hippurate:
Children ≥6 years: 0.5-1 g twice daily
Adults: 1 g twice daily
Mandelate:
Children >2-6 years: 50-75 mg/kg/day in 3-4 divided doses **or** 0.25 g/30 lb 4 times/day
Children 6-12 years: 50-75 mg/kg/day in 3-4 divided doses **or** 0.5 g 4 times/day
Children >12 years and Adults: 1 g 4 times/day
Mechanism of Action Methenamine is hydrolyzed to formaldehyde and ammonia in acidic urine; formaldehyde has nonspecific bactericidal action. Other components, hippuric acid or mandelic acid, aid in maintaining urine acidity and may aid in suppressing bacteria.
Pharmacodynamics/Kinetics
Half-life Elimination 3-6 hours
Pregnancy Risk Factor C (methenamine mandelate)
Pregnancy Considerations Methenamine hippurate did not cause adverse fetal effects in animals; animal reproduction studies have not been conducted with methenamine mandelate. Methenamine crosses the placenta and distributes to amniotic fluid. Adverse fetal effects were not observed in two human trials. Methenamine use has been shown to interfere with urine estriol concentrations if measured via acid hydrolysis. Use of enzyme hydrolysis prevents this lab interference.

Methenamine, Phenyl Salicylate, Methylene Blue, Benzoic Acid, and Hyoscyamine

(meth EN a meen, fen nil sa LIS i late, METH i leen bloo, ben ZOE ik AS id & hye oh SYE a meen)

Related Information
Hyoscyamine *on page 707*
Methenamine *on page 886*
Brand Names: U.S. Hyophen™; Prosed®/DS
Pharmacologic Category Antibiotic, Miscellaneous
Use Urinary tract discomfort secondary to hypermotility resulting from infection or diagnostic procedures
Local Anesthetic/Vasoconstrictor Precautions No information available to require special precautions
Effects on Dental Treatment Key adverse event(s) related to dental treatment: Xerostomia (normal salivary flow resumes upon discontinuation).
Effects on Bleeding No information available to require special precautions
Adverse Effects Frequency not defined.
Cardiovascular: Flushing, tachycardia
Central nervous system: Dizziness
Gastrointestinal: Discoloration of stool (blue), nausea, vomiting, xerostomia
Genitourinary: Discoloration of urine (blue), micturition difficulty, urinary retention (acute)
Ocular: Blurred vision
Respiratory: Dyspnea
General Dosage Range Oral: *Adults:* 1 tablet 4 times/day
Pregnancy Risk Factor C
Pregnancy Considerations Reproduction studies have not been conducted with this combination. Methenamine and hyoscyamine cross the placenta. Refer to individual monographs.

Methenamine, Sodium Biphosphate, Phenyl Salicylate, Methylene Blue, and Hyoscyamine

(meth EN a meen, SOW dee um bye FOS fate, fen nil sa LIS i late, METH i leen bloo, & hye oh SYE a meen)

Related Information
Hyoscyamine *on page 707*
Methenamine *on page 886*
Brand Names: U.S. Phosphasal™; Urelle®; Uribel™; Uta®
Pharmacologic Category Antibiotic, Miscellaneous
Use Treatment of symptoms of irritative voiding; relief of local symptoms associated with urinary tract infections; relief of urinary tract symptoms caused by diagnostic procedures
Local Anesthetic/Vasoconstrictor Precautions No information available to require special precautions
Effects on Dental Treatment Key adverse event(s) related to dental treatment: Xerostomia (normal salivary flow resumes upon discontinuation).
Effects on Bleeding No information available to require special precautions
Adverse Effects Frequency not defined.
Cardiovascular: Tachycardia, flushing
Central nervous system: Dizziness
Gastrointestinal: Xerostomia, nausea, vomiting
Genitourinary: Urinary retention (acute), micturition difficulty, discoloration of urine (blue)
Ocular: Blurred vision
Respiratory: Dyspnea
General Dosage Range Oral: *Adults:* 1 tablet 4 times/day
Pregnancy Risk Factor C
Pregnancy Considerations Reproduction studies have not been conducted with this combination. Methenamine and hyoscyamine cross the placenta. Refer to individual monographs.

Methimazole (meth IM a zole)

Related Information
Endocrine Disorders and Pregnancy *on page 1517*
Brand Names: U.S. Tapazole®
Brand Names: Canada Dom-Methimazole; PHL-Methimazole; Tapazole®
Pharmacologic Category Antithyroid Agent; Thioamide
Use Treatment of hyperthyroidism (including preparation for radioactive iodine therapy or thyroidectomy)
Unlabeled Use Treatment of Graves' disease
Local Anesthetic/Vasoconstrictor Precautions No information available to require special precautions
Effects on Dental Treatment Key adverse event(s) related to dental treatment: Abnormal taste and salivary gland swelling.
Effects on Bleeding No information available to require special precautions
Adverse Effects Frequency not defined.
Cardiovascular: ANCA-positive vasculitis, edema, leukocytoclastic vasculitis, periarteritis
Central nervous system: Drowsiness, fever, headache, neuritis, vertigo
Dermatologic: Alopecia, exfoliative dermatitis, pruritus, skin pigmentation, skin rash, urticaria
Endocrine & metabolic: Goiter, hypoglycemic coma

Gastrointestinal: Constipation, epigastric distress, loss of taste perception, nausea, salivary gland swelling, vomiting, weight gain

Hematologic: Agranulocytosis, aplastic anemia, granulocytopenia, hypoprothrombinemia, leukopenia, thrombocytopenia

Hepatic: Hepatic necrosis, hepatitis, jaundice

Neuromuscular & skeletal: Arthralgia, myalgia, paresthesia

Renal: Nephritis

Miscellaneous: Insulin autoimmune syndrome, lymphadenopathy, SLE-like syndrome

General Dosage Range Oral:

Children: Initial: 0.4 mg/kg/day in 3 divided doses; Maintenance: 0.2 mg/kg/day in 3 divided doses

Adults: Initial: 15-60 mg/day in 3 divided doses; Maintenance: 5-15 mg/day in 1-3 divided doses

Mechanism of Action Inhibits the synthesis of thyroid hormones by blocking the oxidation of iodine in the thyroid gland. As a result, methimazole inhibits the ability of iodine to combine with tyrosine to form thyroxine and triiodothyronine (T_3); does not inactivate circulating T_4 and T_3

Pharmacodynamics/Kinetics

Onset of Action Antithyroid: Oral: 12-18 hours (Clark, 2006)

Duration of Action 36-72 hours (Clark, 2006)

Half-life Elimination 4-6 hours

Time to Peak Serum concentration: 1-2 hours

Pregnancy Risk Factor D

Pregnancy Considerations Methimazole has been found to readily cross the placenta. Congenital anomalies, including esophageal atresia, choanal atresia, aplasia cutis, and iridic and retinal coloboma, have been observed in neonates born to mothers taking methimazole during pregnancy. Nonteratogenic adverse events, including fetal and neonatal hypothyroidism, have been observed following maternal methimazole use. The transfer of thyroid-stimulating immunoglobulins can stimulate the fetal thyroid *in utero* and transiently after delivery and may increase the risk of fetal or neonatal hyperthyroidism.

Uncontrolled maternal hyperthyroidism may result in adverse neonatal outcomes (eg, prematurity, low birth weight, infants born small for gestational age) and adverse maternal outcomes (eg, pre-eclampsia, congestive heart failure). To prevent adverse fetal and maternal events, normal maternal thyroid function should be maintained prior to conception and throughout pregnancy. Antithyroid treatment is recommended for the control of hyperthyroidism during pregnancy. Due to an increased risk of congenital anomalies with methimazole, propylthiouracil is considered first-line therapy, especially during the first trimester of pregnancy. The use of methimazole is an option during the second and third trimesters of pregnancy. If drug therapy is changed, maternal thyroid function should be monitored after 2 weeks and then every 2-4 weeks.

The severity of hyperthyroidism may fluctuate throughout pregnancy and may result in decreased dose requirements or discontinuation of methimazole 2-3 weeks prior to delivery.

Methocarbamol (meth oh KAR ba mole)

Related Information

Temporomandibular Dysfunction (TMD), Chronic Pain, and Fibromyalgia *on page 1590*

Brand Names: U.S. Robaxin®; Robaxin®-750

Brand Names: Canada Robaxin®

Generic Availability (U.S.) Yes: Tablet

Pharmacologic Category Skeletal Muscle Relaxant

Dental Use Treatment of muscle spasm associated with acute temporomandibular joint pain (TMJ)

Use Adjunctive treatment of muscle spasm associated with acute painful musculoskeletal conditions (eg, tetanus)

Local Anesthetic/Vasoconstrictor Precautions No information available to require special precautions

Effects on Dental Treatment Key adverse event(s) related to dental treatment: Metallic taste.

Effects on Bleeding No information available to require special precautions

Adverse Effects Frequency not defined.

Cardiovascular: Bradycardia, flushing, hypotension, syncope

Central nervous system: Amnesia, confusion, coordination impaired (mild), dizziness, drowsiness, fever, headache, insomnia, lightheadedness, sedation, seizures, vertigo

Dermatologic: Angioneurotic edema, pruritus, rash, urticaria

Gastrointestinal: Dyspepsia, metallic taste, nausea, vomiting

Hematologic: Leukopenia

Hepatic: Jaundice

Local: Pain at injection site, thrombophlebitis

Ocular: Blurred vision, conjunctivitis, diplopia, nystagmus

Respiratory: Nasal congestion

Miscellaneous: Hypersensitivity reactions including anaphylaxis

Dental Usual Dosage Muscle spasm associated with acute TMJ pain: Children ≥16 years and Adults: Oral: 1.5 g 4 times/day for 2-3 days (up to 8 g/day may be given in severe conditions), then decrease to 4-4.5 g/day in 3-6 divided doses

Dosage

Tetanus: I.V.:

Children: Recommended **only** for use in tetanus: 15 mg/kg/dose or 500 mg/m²/dose, may repeat every 6 hours if needed; maximum dose: 1.8 g/m²/day for 3 days only

Adults: Initial dose: 1-2 g by direct I.V. injection, which may be followed by an additional 1-2 g by infusion (maximum initial dose: 3 g total); followed by 1-2 g every 6 hours until oral administration by mouth or via NG tube is possible; total oral daily doses of up to 24 g may be needed; injection should not be used for more than 3 consecutive days

Muscle spasm:

Oral: Children ≥16 years and Adults: 1.5 g 4 times/day for 2-3 days (up to 8 g/day may be given in severe conditions), then decrease to 4-4.5 g/day in 3-6 divided doses

I.M., I.V.: Adults: Initial: 1 g; may repeat every 8 hours if oral administration not possible; maximum dose: 3 g/day for no more than 3 consecutive days. If condition persists, may repeat course of therapy after a drug-free interval of 48 hours.

Dosage adjustment in renal impairment: No dosage adjustment provided in manufacturer's labeling. However, administration of the parenteral formulation is contraindicated in patients with renal dysfunction due to the presence of polyethylene glycol.

Dosage adjustment in hepatic impairment: No dosage adjustment provided in manufacturer's labeling. However, elimination may be reduced in patients with cirrhosis.

Mechanism of Action Causes skeletal muscle relaxation by general CNS depression

Contraindications Hypersensitivity to methocarbamol or any component of the formulation; renal impairment (injection formulation)

Warnings/Precautions May cause CNS depression, which may impair physical or mental abilities; patients must be cautioned about performing tasks which require mental alertness (eg, operating machinery or driving). Effects may be potentiated when used with other sedative drugs or ethanol. Plasma protein binding and clearance are decreased and the half-life is increased in patients with hepatic impairment. Muscle relaxants are poorly tolerated by the elderly due to potent anticholinergic effects, sedation, and risk of fracture. Efficacy is questionable at dosages tolerated by elderly patients; avoid use (Beers Criteria).

Injection: Contraindicated in renal impairment. Contains polyethylene glycol. Rate of injection should not exceed 3 mL/minute; solution is hypertonic; avoid extravasation. Use with caution in patients with a history of seizures. Use caution with hepatic impairment. Vial stopper contains latex. Recommended only for the treatment of tetanus in pediatric patients.

Drug Interactions

Metabolism/Transport Effects None known.

Avoid Concomitant Use

Avoid concomitant use of Methocarbamol with any of the following: Azelastine (Nasal); Paraldehyde

Increased Effect/Toxicity

Methocarbamol may increase the levels/effects of: Alcohol (Ethyl); Azelastine (Nasal); Buprenorphine; CNS Depressants; Methotrimeprazine; Metyrosine; Mirtazapine; Paraldehyde; Pramipexole; ROPINIRole; Rotigotine; Selective Serotonin Reuptake Inhibitors; Zolpidem

The levels/effects of Methocarbamol may be increased by: Droperidol; HydrOXYzine; Magnesium Sulfate; Methotrimeprazine; Perampanel; Sodium Oxybate

Decreased Effect

Methocarbamol may decrease the levels/effects of: Pyridostigmine

Ethanol/Nutrition/Herb Interactions

Ethanol: May increase CNS depression; monitor for increased effects with coadministration. Caution patients about effects.

Herb/Nutraceutical: Avoid valerian, St John's wort, kava kava, gotu kola (may increase CNS depression).

Pharmacodynamics/Kinetics

Onset of Action Muscle relaxation: Oral: ~30 minutes

Half-life Elimination 1-2 hours

Time to Peak Serum: Oral: 1-2 hours

Pregnancy Risk Factor C

Pregnancy Considerations Animal reproduction studies have not been conducted. The manufacturer notes that fetal and congenital abnormalities have been rarely reported following *in utero* exposure. Use during pregnancy only if clearly needed.

Lactation Excretion in breast milk unknown/use caution

Dosage Forms

Injection, solution:
Robaxin®: 100 mg/mL (10 mL)
Tablet, oral: 500 mg, 750 mg
Robaxin®: 500 mg
Robaxin®-750: 750 mg

Methohexital (meth oh HEKS i tal)

Brand Names: U.S. Brevital® Sodium

Brand Names: Canada Brevital®

Generic Availability (U.S.) No

Pharmacologic Category Barbiturate; General Anesthetic

Dental Use Induction and maintenance of general anesthesia for short procedures

Use Induction of anesthesia; procedural sedation

Unlabeled Use Wada test

Local Anesthetic/Vasoconstrictor Precautions No information available to require special precautions

Effects on Dental Treatment No significant effects or complications reported

Effects on Bleeding No information available to require special precautions

Adverse Effects Frequency not defined.

Cardiovascular: Cardiorespiratory arrest, circulatory depression, hypotension, peripheral vascular collapse, tachycardia

Central nervous system: Anxiety, emergence delirium, headache, restlessness, seizure

Dermatologic: Erythema, pruritus, urticaria

Gastrointestinal: Abdominal pain, nausea, salivation, vomiting

Hepatic: Transaminases increased

Local: Injection site pain, nerve injury adjacent to injection site, thrombophlebitis

Neuromuscular & skeletal: Involuntary muscle movement, radial nerve palsy, rigidity, tremor, twitching

Respiratory: Apnea, bronchospasm, cough, dyspnea, hiccups, laryngospasm, respiratory depression, rhinitis

Miscellaneous: Anaphylaxis (rare)

Dental Usual Dosage Induction and maintenance of general anesthesia for short procedures: Doses must be titrated to effect: Adults: I.V.: Induction: 50-120 mg to start; 20-40 mg every 4-7 minutes

Dosage Doses must be titrated to effect.

Infants <1 month: Safety and efficacy not established.

Infants ≥1 month and Children:

Anesthesia induction:

I.M.: 6.6-10 mg/kg of a 5% solution

Rectal: Usual: 25 mg/kg of a 1% solution

I.V. (unlabeled dose): 1-2 mg/kg/dose of a 1% solution

Procedural sedation (unlabeled dose):

I.V.: Initial: 0.5 mg/kg; may repeat 0.5 mg/kg to a maximum total dose of 2 mg/kg

Rectal: 25 mg/kg of a 10% (100 mg/mL) solution given 5-15 minutes prior to procedure; maximum dose 500 mg

Adults: I.V.:

Induction: 1-1.5 mg/kg

Procedural sedation (unlabeled dose): 0.75-1 mg/kg; can redose 0.5 mg/kg every 2-5 minutes as needed (Bahn, 2005)

Wada test (unlabeled use): 3-4 mg over 3 seconds; following signs of recovery, administer a second dose of 2 mg over 2 seconds (Buchtel, 2002)

Elderly: I.V.: Refer to adult dosing. Reduce dose or administer at the low end of the dosage range.

▶

◀ **Dosage adjustment in renal impairment:** No dosage adjustment provided in manufacturer's labeling; use with caution.

Dosage adjustment in hepatic impairment: No dosage adjustment provided in manufacturer's labeling. However, adjustment may be necessary due to hepatic metabolism. Use with caution.

Mechanism of Action Ultra short-acting I.V. barbiturate anesthetic

Contraindications Hypersensitivity to barbiturates, methohexital, or any component of the formulation; porphyria (latent or manifest); patients in whom general anesthesia is contraindicated

Warnings/Precautions Use with caution in patients with liver impairment, renal impairment, cardiovascular disease (including heart failure), severe anemia, extreme obesity, or seizure disorder, the elderly and children. May cause hypotension; use with caution in hemodynamically unstable patients (hypotension or shock) or severe hypertension. May cause respiratory depression; use with caution in patients with pulmonary disease. Use with caution in patients with asthma and chronic obstructive pulmonary disease. Use with extreme caution in patients with ongoing status asthmaticus; hiccups, coughing, laryngospasm, and muscle twitching have occurred impairing ventilation.

Postmarketing studies have indicated that the use of hypnotic/sedative agents for sleep has been associated with hypersensitivity reactions including anaphylaxis as well as angioedema. Effects with other sedative drugs or ethanol may be potentiated. Repeated dosing or continuous infusions may cause cumulative effects. Ensure patient has intravenous access; extravasation or intra-arterial injection causes necrosis. **[U.S. Boxed Warning]: Should only be administered in hospitals or ambulatory care settings with continuous monitoring of respiratory function; resuscitative drugs, age- and size-appropriate and intubation equipment and trained personnel experienced in handling their use should be readily available. For deeply sedated patients, a healthcare provider other than the individual performing the procedure should be present to continuously monitor the patient.**

Drug Interactions

Metabolism/Transport Effects None known.

Avoid Concomitant Use

Avoid concomitant use of Methohexital with any of the following: Azelastine (Nasal); Paraldehyde

Increased Effect/Toxicity

Methohexital may increase the levels/effects of: Alcohol (Ethyl); Azelastine (Nasal); Buprenorphine; CNS Depressants; Fosphenytoin; Meperidine; Methadone; Metyrosine; Mirtazapine; Paraldehyde; Pramipexole; QuiNIDine; ROPINIRole; Rotigotine; Selective Serotonin Reuptake Inhibitors; Thiazide Diuretics; Zolpidem

The levels/effects of Methohexital may be increased by: Chloramphenicol; Divalproex; Droperidol; Felbamate; Fosphenytoin; HydrOXYzine; Magnesium Sulfate; Perampanel; Phenytoin; Primidone; Sodium Oxybate; Valproic Acid

Decreased Effect

Methohexital may decrease the levels/effects of: Acetaminophen; Beta-Blockers; Calcium Channel Blockers; Chloramphenicol; Contraceptives (Estrogens); Contraceptives (Progestins); Corticosteroids (Systemic); CycloSPORINE (Systemic); Disopyramide; Divalproex; Doxycycline; Etoposide; Etoposide Phosphate; Felbamate; Fosphenytoin; LamoTRIgine; Methadone; Phenytoin; Propafenone; QuiNIDine;

Teniposide; Theophylline Derivatives; Tricyclic Antidepressants; Valproic Acid; Vitamin K Antagonists

The levels/effects of Methohexital may be decreased by: Multivitamins/Minerals (with ADEK, Folate, Iron); Pyridoxine; Rifamycin Derivatives

Pharmacodynamics/Kinetics

Onset of Action I.V.: Immediate; I.M. (pediatrics): 2-10 minutes; Rectal (pediatrics): 5-15 minutes

Duration of Action Single dose: I.V.: 10-20 minutes; Rectal: 45 minutes

Pregnancy Risk Factor B

Pregnancy Considerations Animal studies have not shown fetal or maternal harm. There are no adequate and well-controlled studies in pregnant women. Methohexital crosses the placenta. Use only if potential benefit outweighs risk to fetus.

Lactation Enters breast milk/use caution

Breast-Feeding Considerations Methohexital is minimally excreted in breast milk and levels decline rapidly after administration. Interruption of breast-feeding is unnecessary.

Controlled Substance C-IV

Dosage Forms

Injection, powder for reconstitution:
Brevital® Sodium: 500 mg, 2.5 g

References
Dionne RA, Yagiela JA, Moore PA, et al, "Comparing Efficacy and Safety of Four Intravenous Sedation Regimens in Dental Outpatients," *Am Dent Assoc*, 2001, 132(6):740-51.

Methotrexate (meth oh TREKS ate)

Related Information
Rheumatoid Arthritis, Osteoarthritis, and Osteoporosis *on page 1526*

Brand Names: U.S. Rheumatrex®; Trexall™

Brand Names: Canada Apo-Methotrexate®; ratio-Methotrexate

Generic Availability (U.S.) Yes

Pharmacologic Category Antineoplastic Agent, Antimetabolite (Antifolate); Antirheumatic, Disease Modifying; Immunosuppressant Agent

Use
Oncology-related uses: Acute lymphoblastic leukemia (ALL) maintenance treatment, ALL meningeal leukemia (prophylaxis and treatment); treatment of trophoblastic neoplasms (gestational choriocarcinoma, chorioadenoma destruens and hydatidiform mole), breast cancer, head and neck cancer (epidermoid), cutaneous T-Cell lymphoma (advanced mycosis fungoides), lung cancer (squamous cell and small cell), advanced non-Hodgkin's lymphomas (NHL), osteosarcoma

Nononcology uses: Treatment of psoriasis (severe, recalcitrant, disabling) and severe rheumatoid arthritis (RA), including polyarticular-course juvenile idiopathic arthritis (JIA)

Unlabeled Use Treatment and maintenance of remission in Crohn's disease; management of ectopic pregnancy; dermatomyositis/polymyositis; treatment of bladder cancer, central nervous system tumors (including nonleukemic meningeal cancers), acute promyelocytic leukemia (maintenance treatment), soft tissue sarcoma (desmoid tumors); acute graft-versus-host disease (GVHD) prophylaxis; medical management of abortion; systemic lupus erythematosus; Takayasu arteritis

Local Anesthetic/Vasoconstrictor Precautions No information available to require special precautions

Effects on Dental Treatment Key adverse event(s) related to dental treatment: Ulcerative stomatitis, gingivitis, glossitis, and mucositis (dose dependent; appears 3-7 days post-therapy and resolves within 2 weeks). Dental professionals should note before prescribing NSAIDS that concurrent administration with methotrexate may cause severe bone marrow suppression, aplastic anemia, and GI toxicity (see Warnings/Precautions). Although the risk is lower at the methotrexate dosages used for rheumatoid conditions/psoriasis, the addition of an NSAID or salicylate may still lead to unexpected toxicities; caution is warranted.

Effects on Bleeding Suppression of hematopoiesis may cause myelosuppression including thrombocytopenia. Medical consult recommended.

Adverse Effects Note: Adverse reactions vary by route and dosage. Hematologic and/or gastrointestinal toxicities may be common at dosages used in chemotherapy; these reactions are much less frequent when used at typical dosages for rheumatic diseases.

>10%:
Central nervous system (with intrathecal administration or very high-dose therapy):
Arachnoiditis: Acute reaction manifested as severe headache, nuchal rigidity, vomiting, and fever; may be alleviated by reducing the dose
Subacute toxicity: 10% of patients treated with 12-15 mg of intrathecal methotrexate may develop this in the second or third week of therapy; consists of motor paralysis of extremities, cranial nerve palsy, seizure, or coma. This has also been seen in pediatric cases receiving very high-dose I.V. methotrexate.
Demyelinating encephalopathy: Seen months or years after receiving methotrexate; usually in association with cranial irradiation or other systemic chemotherapy
Dermatologic: Reddening of skin
Endocrine & metabolic: Hyperuricemia, oligospermia
Gastrointestinal: Ulcerative stomatitis, glossitis, gingivitis, nausea, vomiting, diarrhea, intestinal perforation, mucositis (dose dependent; appears in 3-7 days after therapy, resolving within 2 weeks)
Hematologic: Leukopenia, myelosuppression (nadir: 7-10 days), thrombocytopenia
Renal: Renal failure, azotemia, nephropathy
Respiratory: Pharyngitis
Miscellaneous: Immunosuppression
1% to 10%:
Cardiovascular: Vasculitis
Central nervous system: Dizziness, malaise, fever, chills
Dermatologic: Alopecia, rash, photosensitivity, depigmentation or hyperpigmentation of skin, pruritus, dermatitis
Endocrine & metabolic: Diabetes
Genitourinary: Cystitis
Hematologic: Hemorrhage
Hepatic: Cirrhosis (chronic therapy), liver function tests increased (chronic therapy), portal fibrosis (chronic therapy)
Neuromuscular & skeletal: Arthralgia
Ocular: Blurred vision
Renal: Renal dysfunction: Manifested by an abrupt rise in serum creatinine and BUN and a fall in urine output; more common with high-dose methotrexate, and may be due to precipitation of the drug.

Respiratory: Pneumonitis: Associated with fever, cough, and interstitial pulmonary infiltrates; treatment is to withhold methotrexate during the acute reaction; interstitial pneumonitis has been reported to occur with an incidence of 1% in patients with RA (dose 7.5-15 mg/week)
Miscellaneous: Infection

Dosage Details concerning dosing in combination regimens should also be consulted.
Note: Doses between 100-500 mg/m^2 **may require** leucovorin calcium rescue. Doses >500 mg/m^2 **require** leucovorin calcium rescue: Oral, I.M., I.V.: Leucovorin calcium 10-15 mg/m^2 every 6 hours for 8 or 10 doses, starting 24 hours after the start of methotrexate infusion. Continue until the methotrexate level is ≤0.1 micromolar (10^{-7} M). Some clinicians continue leucovorin calcium until the methotrexate level is <0.05 micromolar (5×10^{-8} M) or 0.01 micromolar (10^{-8} M).
If the 48-hour methotrexate level is >1 micromolar (10^{-6} M) or the 72-hour methotrexate level is >0.2 micromolar (2×10^{-7} M): I.V., I.M, Oral: Leucovorin calcium 100 mg/m^2 every 6 hours until the methotrexate level is ≤0.1 micromolar (10^{-7} M). Some clinicians continue leucovorin calcium until the methotrexate level is <0.05 micromolar (5×10^{-8} M) or 0.01 micromolar (10^{-8} M).

Children:
Dermatomyositis (unlabeled use): Oral: 15-20 mg/m^2/week as a single dose once weekly **or** 0.3-1 mg/kg/dose once weekly
GVHD (acute) prophylaxis (unlabeled use): I.V.: Refer to adult dosing.
Juvenile idiopathic arthritis (JIA): Oral, I.M.: 10 mg/m^2 once weekly, then 5-15 mg/m^2/week as a single dose **or** as 3 divided doses given 12 hours apart
Antineoplastic dosage range:
Oral, I.M.: 7.5-30 mg/m^2/week **or** every 2 weeks
I.V.: 10-18,000 mg/m^2 bolus dosing **or** continuous infusion over 6-42 hours
Pediatric solid tumors (high-dose): I.V.:
<12 years: 12-25 g/m^2
≥12 years: 8 g/m^2
Acute lymphocytic leukemia (intermediate-dose): I.V.: Loading: 100 mg/m^2 bolus dose, followed by 900 mg/m^2/day infusion over 23-41 hours.
Meningeal leukemia: I.T.: 6-12 mg/dose based on age.
Note: Optimal intrathecal chemotherapy dosing should be based on age rather than on body surface area (BSA); CSF volume correlates with age and not to BSA (Bleyer, 1983; Kerr, 2001):
<1 year: 6 mg/dose
1 year: 8 mg/dose
2 years: 10 mg/dose
≥3 years: 12 mg/dose

Adults:
Antineoplastic dosage range: I.V.: Range is wide from 30-40 mg/m^2/week to 100-12,000 mg/m^2 with leucovorin calcium rescue
Breast cancer: I.V.: 30-60 mg/m^2 days 1 and 8 every 3-4 weeks
Head and neck cancer: Oral, I.M., I.V.: 25-50 mg/m^2 once weekly
Lymphoma, non-Hodgkin's: I.V.:
30 mg/m^2 days 3 and 10 every 3 weeks **or**
120 mg/m^2 day 8 and 15 every 3-4 weeks **or**
200 mg/m^2 day 8 and 15 every 3 weeks **or**
400 mg/m^2 every 4 weeks for 3 cycles **or**
1 g/m^2 every 3 weeks **or**
1.5 g/m^2 every 4 weeks

Meningeal leukemia: I.T.: Usual dose: 12 mg/dose. **Note:** Optimal intrathecal chemotherapy dosing should be based on age rather than on body surface area (BSA); CSF volume correlates with age and not to BSA (Bleyer, 1983; Kerr, 2001).

Mycosis fungoides (cutaneous T-cell lymphoma): Oral, I.M.: Initial (early stages):
5-50 mg once weekly **or**
15-37.5 mg twice weekly

Osteosarcoma: I.V.: 8-12 g/m^2 weekly for 2-4 weeks

Psoriasis: **Note:** Some experts recommend concomitant folic acid 1-5 mg/day (except the day of methotrexate) to reduce hematologic, gastrointestinal, and hepatic adverse events related to methotrexate.
Oral: 2.5-5 mg/dose every 12 hours for 3 doses given weekly **or**
Oral, I.M., SubQ: 10-25 mg/dose given once weekly; titrate to lowest effective dose
Note: An initial test dose of 2.5-5 mg is recommended in patients with risk factors for hematologic toxicity or renal impairment (Kalb, 2009).

Rheumatoid arthritis: **Note:** Some experts recommend concomitant folic acid at a dose of at least 5 mg/week (except the day of methotrexate) to reduce hematologic, gastrointestinal, and hepatic adverse events related to methotrexate.
Oral (manufacturer labeling): 7.5 mg once weekly or 2.5 mg every 12 hours for 3 doses/week (dosage exceeding 20 mg/week may cause a higher incidence and severity of adverse events); *alternatively,* 10-15 mg once weekly, increased by 5 mg every 2-4 weeks to a maximum of 20-30 mg once weekly has been recommended by some experts (Visser, 2009)
I.M., SubQ (unlabeled route): 15 mg once weekly (dosage varies, similar to oral) (Braun, 2008)

Trophoblastic neoplasms:
Oral, I.M.: 15-30 mg/day for 5 days; repeat in 7 days for 3-5 courses
I.V.: 11 mg/m^2 days 1 through 5 every 3 weeks

Unlabeled uses:
Bladder cancer (unlabeled use): I.V.:
30 mg/m^2 day 1 and 8 every 3 weeks **or**
30 mg/m^2 day 1, 15, and 22 every 4 weeks
Crohn's disease, mild/moderate, corticosteroid-dependent or refractory (unlabeled use):
Remission induction or reduction of steroid use: I.M., SubQ: 25 mg once weekly (Lichtenstein, 2009)
Remission maintenance: I.M.: 15 mg once weekly (Feagan, 2000; Lichtenstein, 2009)
Dermatomyositis/polymyositis (unlabeled uses):
Oral: Initial: 7.5-15 mg/week, often adjunctively with high-dose corticosteroid therapy; may increase in weekly 2.5 mg increments to target dose of 10-25 mg/week (**Note:** Administration of folate 5-7 mg/week has been used to reduce side effects). (Briemberg, 2003; Newman, 1995; Wiendl, 2008)
I.V., I.M.: Doses of 20-60 mg/week have been employed if failure with oral therapy (doses >50 mg/week may require leucovorin calcium rescue) (Briemberg, 2003)
Ectopic pregnancy (unlabeled use): I.M.:
Single-dose regimen: Methotrexate 50 mg/m^2 on day 1; Measure serum hCG levels on days 4 and 7; if needed, repeat dose on day 7 (Barnhart, 2009)
Two-dose regimen: Methotrexate 50 mg/m^2 on day 1; Measure serum hCG levels on day 4 and administer a second dose of methotrexate 50 mg/m^2; Measure serum hCG levels on day 7 and if needed, administer a third dose of 50 mg/m^2 (Barnhart, 2009)

Multidose regimen: Methotrexate 1 mg/kg on day 1; leucovorin calcium 0.1 mg/kg I.M. on day 2; measure serum hCG on day 2; methotrexate 1 mg/kg on day 3; leucovorin calcium 0.1 mg/kg on day 4; measure serum hCG on day 4; continue up to a total of 4 courses based on hCG concentrations (Barnhart, 2009)

GVHD (acute) prophylaxis: I.V.: 15 mg/m^2/dose on day 1 and 10 mg/m^2/dose on days 3 and 6 after allogeneic transplant (in combination with cyclosporine and prednisone) (Chao, 1993; Chao, 2000; Ross, 1999) **or** 15 mg/m^2/dose on day 1 and 10 mg/m^2/dose on days 3, 6, and 11 after allogeneic transplant (in combination with cyclosporine) (Chao, 2000)

Nonleukemic meningeal cancer (unlabeled uses): I.T.: 10-12 mg/dose twice weekly for 4 weeks, then weekly for 4 weeks, then monthly (NCCN CNS cancer guidelines v.2.2009) **or** 12 mg/dose twice weekly for 4 weeks, then weekly for 4 doses, then monthly for 4 doses (Glantz, 1998) **or** 10 mg twice weekly for 4 weeks, then weekly for 1 month, then every 2 weeks for 2 months (Glantz, 1999)

Takayasu arteritis, refractory or relapsing disease (unlabeled use): Oral: Initial dose: 0.3 mg/kg/week (maximum: 15 mg/week), titrated by 2.5 mg increments every 1-2 weeks until reaching a maximum tolerated weekly dose of 25 mg (use in combination with a corticosteroid; Hoffman, 1994)

Elderly:
Meningeal leukemia: I.T.: Consider a dose reduction (CSF volume and turnover may decrease with age)
Rheumatoid arthritis/psoriasis: Oral: Initial: 5-7.5 mg/week, not to exceed 20 mg/week

Dosage adjustment for toxicity:
Nonhematologic toxicity: Diarrhea, stomatitis, or vomiting which may lead to dehydration: Discontinue until recovery
Hematologic toxicity:
Psoriasis, rheumatoid arthritis: Significant blood count decrease: Discontinue immediately.
Oncologic uses: Profound granulocytopenia and fever: Evaluate immediately; consider broad-spectrum parenteral antimicrobial coverage

Dosage adjustment in renal impairment: No dosage adjustment provided in the manufacturer's labeling. The following adjustments have been recommended:
Aronoff, 2007:
Children:
Cl$_{cr}$ 10-50 mL/minute/1.73 m^2: Administer 50% of dose
Cl$_{cr}$ <10 mL/minute/1.73 m^2: Administer 30% of dose
Hemodialysis: Administer 30% of dose
Continuous ambulatory peritoneal dialysis (CAPD): Administer 30% of dose
Continuous renal replacement therapy (CRRT): Administer 50% of dose
Adults:
Cl$_{cr}$ 10-50 mL/minute: Administer 50% of dose
Cl$_{cr}$ <10 mL/minute: Avoid use
Hemodialysis: Administer 50% of dose
Continuous renal replacement therapy (CRRT): Administer 50% of dose

Kintzel, 1995:
Cl$_{cr}$ 46-60 mL/minute: Administer 65% of normal dose
Cl$_{cr}$ 31-45 mL/minute: Administer 50% of normal dose
Cl$_{cr}$ <30 mL/minute: Avoid use

Dosage adjustment in hepatic impairment: No dosage adjustment provided in the manufacturer's labeling; use with caution. The following adjustments have been recommended (Floyd, 2006):

Bilirubin 3.1-5 mg/dL **or** transaminases >3 times ULN: Administer 75% of dose

Bilirubin >5 mg/dL: Avoid use

Mechanism of Action Methotrexate is a folate antimetabolite that inhibits DNA synthesis, repair, and cellular replication. Methotrexate irreversibly binds to dihydrofolate reductase, inhibiting the formation of reduced folates, and thymidylate synthetase, resulting in inhibition of purine and thymidylic acid synthesis. Methotrexate is cell cycle specific for the S phase of the cycle.

The MOA in the treatment of rheumatoid arthritis is unknown, but may affect immune function. In psoriasis, methotrexate is thought to target rapidly proliferating epithelial cells in the skin.

In Crohn's disease, it may have immune modulator and anti-inflammatory activity.

Contraindications Hypersensitivity to methotrexate or any component of the formulation; breast-feeding

Additional contraindications for patients with psoriasis or rheumatoid arthritis: Pregnancy, alcoholism, alcoholic liver disease or other chronic liver disease, immunodeficiency syndrome (overt or laboratory evidence); pre-existing blood dyscrasias (eg, bone marrow hypoplasia, leukopenia, thrombocytopenia, significant anemia)

Warnings/Precautions Hazardous agent - use appropriate precautions for handling and disposal (NIOSH, 2012).

[U.S. Boxed Warning]: Methotrexate has been associated with acute (elevated transaminases) and potentially fatal chronic (fibrosis, cirrhosis) hepatotoxicity. Risk is related to cumulative dose (≥1.5 g) and prolonged exposure. Monitor closely (with liver function tests, including serum albumin) for liver toxicities. Liver enzyme elevations may be noted, but may not be predictive of hepatic disease in long term treatment for psoriasis (but generally is predictive in rheumatoid arthritis [RA] treatment). With long-term use, liver biopsy may show histologic changes, fibrosis, or cirrhosis; periodic liver biopsy is recommended with long-term use for psoriasis patients with risk factors for hepatotoxicity and for persistent abnormal liver function tests in psoriasis patients without risk factors for hepatotoxicity and in RA patients; discontinue methotrexate with moderate-to-severe change in liver biopsy. Risk factors for hepatotoxicity include history of above moderate ethanol consumption, persistent abnormal liver chemistries, history of chronic liver disease (including hepatitis B or C), family history of inheritable liver disease, diabetes, obesity, hyperlipidemia, lack of folate supplementation during methotrexate therapy, cumulative methotrexate dose exceeding 1.5 g, continuous daily dosing of methotrexate and history of significant exposure to hepatotoxic drugs. Use caution with preexisting liver impairment; may require dosage reduction. Use caution when used with other hepatotoxic agents (azathioprine, retinoids, sulfasalazine). **[U.S. Boxed Warning]: Methotrexate elimination is reduced in patients with ascites and pleural effusions;** resulting in prolonged half-life and toxicity; may require dose reduction or discontinuation. Monitor closely for toxicity.

[U.S. Boxed Warning]: May cause renal damage leading to acute renal failure, especially with high-dose methotrexate; monitor renal function and methotrexate levels closely, maintain adequate hydration and urinary alkalinization. Use caution in osteosarcoma patients treated with high-dose methotrexate in combination with nephrotoxic chemotherapy (eg, cisplatin). **[U.S. Boxed Warning]: Methotrexate elimination is reduced in patients with renal impairment;** may require dose reduction or discontinuation; monitor closely for toxicity. **[U.S. Boxed Warning]: Tumor lysis syndrome may occur in patients with high tumor burden;** use appropriate prevention and treatment.

[U.S. Boxed Warning]: May cause potentially life-threatening pneumonitis (may occur at any time during therapy and at any dosage); monitor closely for pulmonary symptoms, particularly dry, nonproductive cough. Other potential symptoms include fever, dyspnea, hypoxemia, or pulmonary infiltrate. **[U.S. Boxed Warning]: Methotrexate elimination is reduced in patients with pleural effusions;** may require dose reduction or discontinuation. Monitor closely for toxicity.

[U.S. Boxed Warning]: Bone marrow suppression may occur, resulting in anemia, aplastic anemia, pancytopenia, leukopenia, neutropenia, and/or thrombocytopenia. Use caution in patients with pre-existing bone marrow suppression. Discontinue treatment (immediately) in RA or psoriasis if a significant decrease in hematologic components is noted. **[U.S. Boxed Warning]: Use of low dose methotrexate has been associated with the development of malignant lymphomas;** may regress upon treatment discontinuation; treat lymphoma appropriately if regression is not induced by cessation of methotrexate.

[U.S. Boxed Warning]: Diarrhea and ulcerative stomatitis may require treatment interruption; death from hemorrhagic enteritis or intestinal perforation has been reported. Use with caution in patients with peptic ulcer disease, ulcerative colitis.

May cause neurotoxicity including seizures (usually in pediatric ALL patients receiving intermediate-dose (1 g/m² methotrexate), leukoencephalopathy (usually with concurrent cranial irradiation) and stroke-like encephalopathy (usually with high-dose regimens). Chemical arachnoiditis (headache, back pain, nuchal rigidity, fever), myelopathy and chronic leukoencephalopathy may result from intrathecal administration.

[U.S. Boxed Warning]: Any dose level or route of administration may cause severe and potentially fatal dermatologic reactions, including toxic epidermal necrolysis, Stevens-Johnson syndrome, exfoliative dermatitis, skin necrosis, and erythema multiforme. Radiation dermatitis and sunburn may be precipitated by methotrexate administration. Psoriatic lesions may be worsened by concomitant exposure to ultraviolet radiation.

[U.S. Boxed Warning]: Concomitant administration with NSAIDs may cause severe bone marrow suppression, aplastic anemia, and GI toxicity. Do not administer NSAIDs prior to or during high dose methotrexate therapy; may increase and prolong serum methotrexate levels. Doses used for psoriasis may still lead to unexpected toxicities; use caution when administering NSAIDs or salicylates with lower doses of methotrexate for RA. Methotrexate may increase the levels and effects of mercaptopurine; may require dosage adjustments. Vitamins containing folate may ▶

decrease response to systemic methotrexate; folate deficiency may increase methotrexate toxicity. Concomitant use of proton pump inhibitors with methotrexate (primarily high-dose methotrexate) may elevate and prolong serum methotrexate and metabolite (hydroxymethotrexate) levels; may lead to toxicities; use with caution. Immunization may be ineffective during methotrexate treatment. Immunization with live vaccines is not recommended; cases of disseminated vaccinia infections due to live vaccines have been reported. **[U.S. Boxed Warning]: Concomitant methotrexate administration with radiotherapy may increase the risk of soft tissue necrosis and osteonecrosis.**

[U.S. Boxed Warnings]: Should be administered under the supervision of a physician experienced in the use of antimetabolite therapy; serious and fatal toxicities have occurred at all dose levels. Immune suppression may lead to potentially fatal opportunistic infections. Use methotrexate with extreme caution in patients with an active infection (contraindicated in patients with immunodeficiency syndrome). **[U.S. Boxed Warnings]: For rheumatoid arthritis and psoriasis, immunosuppressive therapy should only be used when disease is active and less toxic, traditional therapy is ineffective. Methotrexate formulations and/or diluents containing preservatives should not be used for intrathecal or high-dose methotrexate therapy. May cause fetal death or congenital abnormalities; do not use for psoriasis or RA treatment in pregnant women.** May cause impairment of fertility, oligospermia, and menstrual dysfunction. Toxicity from methotrexate or any immunosuppressive is increased in the elderly. Methotrexate injection may contain benzyl alcohol and should not be used in neonates. Errors have occurred (some resulting in death) when methotrexate was administered as "daily" dose instead of an intended "weekly" dose.

When used for intrathecal administration, should not be prepared during the preparation of any other agents; after preparation, store intrathecal medications in an isolated location or container clearly marked with a label identifying as "intrathecal" use only; delivery of intrathecal medications to the patient should only be with other medications intended for administration into the central nervous system (Jacobson, 2009).

Drug Interactions

Metabolism/Transport Effects Substrate of P-glycoprotein, SLCO1B1

Avoid Concomitant Use

Avoid concomitant use of Methotrexate with any of the following: Acitretin; BCG; CloZAPine; Natalizumab; Pimecrolimus; Tacrolimus (Topical); Tofacitinib

Increased Effect/Toxicity

Methotrexate may increase the levels/effects of: CloZAPine; CycloSPORINE (Systemic); Leflunomide; Loop Diuretics; Natalizumab; Theophylline Derivatives; Tofacitinib; Vaccines (Live); Vitamin K Antagonists

The levels/effects of Methotrexate may be increased by: Acitretin; Ciprofloxacin (Systemic); CycloSPORINE (Systemic); Denosumab; Eltrombopag; Loop Diuretics; Mipomersen; Nonsteroidal Anti-Inflammatory Agents; Penicillins; P-glycoprotein/ABCB1 Inhibitors; Pimecrolimus; Probenecid; Proton Pump Inhibitors; Roflumilast; Salicylates; SulfaSALAzine; Sulfonamide Derivatives; Tacrolimus (Topical); Trastuzumab; Trimethoprim

Decreased Effect

Methotrexate may decrease the levels/effects of: BCG; Cardiac Glycosides; Coccidioidin Skin Test; Loop Diuretics; Sapropterin; Sipuleucel-T; Vaccines (Inactivated); Vitamin K Antagonists

The levels/effects of Methotrexate may be decreased by: Bile Acid Sequestrants; Echinacea; P-glycoprotein/ABCB1 Inducers

Ethanol/Nutrition/Herb Interactions

Ethanol: Ethanol may be associated with increased liver injury. Management: Avoid ethanol.

Food: Methotrexate peak serum levels may be decreased if taken with food. Milk-rich foods may decrease methotrexate absorption. Folate may decrease drug response.

Herb/Nutraceutical: Echinacea has immunostimulant properties. Management: Avoid echinacea.

Dietary Considerations Some products may contain sodium.

Pharmacodynamics/Kinetics

Onset of Action Antirheumatic: 3-6 weeks; additional improvement may continue longer than 12 weeks

Half-life Elimination Low dose: 3-10 hours; High dose: 8-15 hours

Time to Peak Serum: Oral: 1-2 hours; I.M.: 30-60 minutes

Pregnancy Risk Factor X (psoriasis, rheumatoid arthritis)

Pregnancy Considerations [U.S. Boxed Warning]: Methotrexate may cause fetal death and/or congenital abnormalities. Studies in animals and pregnant women have shown evidence of fetal abnormalities; therefore, the manufacturer classifies methotrexate as pregnancy category X (for psoriasis or RA). A pattern of congenital malformations associated with maternal methotrexate use is referred to as the aminopterin/methotrexate syndrome. Features of the syndrome include CNS, skeletal, and cardiac abnormalities. Low birth weight and developmental delay have also been reported. The use of methotrexate may impair fertility and cause menstrual irregularities or oligospermia during treatment and following therapy. Methotrexate is approved for the treatment of trophoblastic neoplasms (gestational choriocarcinoma, chorioadenoma destruens, and hydatidiform mole) and has been used for the medical management of ectopic pregnancy and the medical management of abortion. **[U.S. Boxed Warning]: Use is contraindicated for the treatment of psoriasis or RA in pregnant women.** Pregnancy should be excluded prior to therapy in women of childbearing potential. Use for the treatment of neoplastic diseases only when the potential benefit to the mother outweighs the possible risk to the fetus. Pregnancy should be avoided for ≥3 months following treatment in male patients and ≥1 ovulatory cycle in female patients. A registry is available for pregnant women exposed to autoimmune medications including methotrexate. For additional information contact the Organization of Teratology Information Specialists, OTIS Autoimmune Diseases Study, at 877-311-8972.

Lactation Enters breast milk/contraindicated

Breast-Feeding Considerations Low amounts of methotrexate are excreted into breast milk. Due to the potential for serious adverse reactions in a breast-feeding infant, use is contraindicated in nursing mothers.

Dosage Forms

Injection, powder for reconstitution: 1 g

Injection, solution: 25 mg/mL (2 mL, 10 mL)

Injection, solution [preservative free]: 25 mg/mL (2 mL, 4 mL, 8 mL, 10 mL, 20 mL, 40 mL)
Tablet, oral: 2.5 mg
Rheumatrex®: 2.5 mg
Trexall™: 5 mg, 7.5 mg, 10 mg, 15 mg

Methotrimeprazine (meth oh trye MEP ra zeen)

Brand Names: Canada Apo-Methoprazine®; Novo-Meprazine; Nozinan®; PMS-Methotrimeprazine
Pharmacologic Category Analgesic, Nonopioid; Antimanic Agent; Antipsychotic Agent, Typical
Use Treatment of schizophrenia; psychosis; manic-depressive syndromes; anxiety or tension disorders; management of pain, including pain caused by neuralgia or cancer; adjunct to general anesthesia; management of nausea and vomiting; sedation
Local Anesthetic/Vasoconstrictor Precautions No information available to require special precautions (see Dental Comment)
Effects on Dental Treatment Key adverse event(s) related to dental treatment: Anticholinergic side effects can cause a reduction of saliva production or secretion, contributing to discomfort and dental disease (ie, caries, oral candidiasis, and periodontal disease). Phenothiazines can cause extrapyramidal reactions which may appear as muscle twitching or increased motor activity of the face, neck, or head.
Effects on Bleeding No information available to require special precautions
Adverse Effects Note: Frequencies not defined; some reactions listed are based on reports for other agents in this same pharmacologic class, and may not be specifically reported for methotrimeprazine.
Cardiovascular: Orthostatic hypotension, QT_c prolongation (rare), tachycardia, venous thromboembolism
Central nervous system: Dizziness, drowsiness; extrapyramidal symptoms (akathisia, dystonias, pseudoparkinsonism, tardive dyskinesia); headache, impairment of temperature regulation, neuroleptic malignant syndrome (NMS), seizure
Dermatologic: Photosensitivity (rare), rash
Endocrine & metabolic: Gynecomastia, hyperglycemia or glucose intolerance, libido changes, menstrual irregularity
Gastrointestinal: Constipation, ileus, nausea, necrotizing enterocolitis, vomiting, weight gain, xerostomia
Genitourinary: Ejaculatory disturbances or dysfunction, incontinence, polyuria, priapism, urinary retention
Hematologic: Agranulocytosis (rare), eosinophilia, hemolytic anemia, leukopenia, pancytopenia, thrombocytopenic purpura
Hepatic: Cholestatic jaundice, hepatotoxicity
Respiratory: Pulmonary embolus
Miscellaneous: Diaphoresis
General Dosage Range
I.M.:
Children: 0.063-0.125 mg/kg/day in 1-3 divided doses
Adults: 10-25 mg every 8 hours **or** 75-100 mg as a single dose
I.V.:
Children: 0.063 mg/kg in 250 mL D_5W infused at a rate of 20-40 drops/minute
Adults: 10-25 mg in 500 mL D_5W infused at a rate of 20-40 drops/minute
Oral:
Children: 0.25 mg/kg/day in 2-3 divided doses (maximum: 40 mg/day [children <12 years])

Adults: 6-75 mg/day in 2-3 divided doses (maximum: doses up to 1000 mg/day have been used) **or** 10-25 mg at bedtime
Mechanism of Action Aliphatic phenothiazine that antagonizes D1 and D2 dopamine receptor subtypes; also binds alpha-1, alpha-2, serotonin (5-HT$_1$ and 5-HT$_2$), and muscarinic (M$_1$ and M$_2$) receptors
Pharmacodynamics/Kinetics
Onset of Action Injection: 1 hour
Duration of Action 2-4 hours
Half-life Elimination 15-30 hours
Time to Peak Serum: I.M.: 0.5-1.5 hours; Oral: 1-3 hours
Pregnancy Considerations Antipsychotic use during the third trimester of pregnancy has a risk for abnormal muscle movements (extrapyramidal symptoms [EPS]) and withdrawal symptoms in newborns following delivery. Symptoms in the newborn may include agitation, feeding disorder, hypertonia, hypotonia, respiratory distress, somnolence, and tremor; these effects may be self-limiting or require hospitalization.
Product Availability Not available in U.S.
Dental Comment This drug is known to prolong the QT interval. The QT interval is measured as the time and distance between the Q point of the QRS complex and the end of the T wave in the ECG tracing. After adjustment for heart rate, the QT interval is defined as prolonged if it is more than 450 msec in men and 460 msec in women. A long QT syndrome was first described in the 1950s and 60s as a congenital syndrome involving QT interval prolongation and syncope and sudden death. Some of the congenital long QT syndromes were characterized by a peculiar electrocardiographic appearance of the QRS complex involving a premature atria beat followed by a pause, then a subsequent sinus beat showing marked QT prolongation and deformity. This type of cardiac arrhythmia was originally termed "torsade de pointes" (translated from the French as "twisting of the points").

Prolongation of the QT interval is thought to result from delayed ventricular repolarization. The repolarization process within the myocardial cell is due to the efflux of intracellular potassium. The channels associated with this current can be blocked by many drugs and predispose the electrical propagation cycle to torsade de pointes.

Methotrimeprazine is one of the drugs confirmed to prolong the QT interval and is accepted as having a risk of causing torsade de pointes. The risk of drug-induced torsade de pointes is extremely low when a single QT interval prolonging drug is prescribed. In terms of epinephrine, it is not known what effect vasoconstrictors in the local anesthetic regimen will have in patients with a known history of congenital prolonged QT interval or in patients taking any medication that prolongs the QT interval. Until more information is obtained, it is suggested that the clinician consult with the physician prior to the use of a vasoconstrictor in suspected patients, and that the vasoconstrictor (epinephrine, levonordefrin [Neo-Cobefrin®]) be used with caution.

Methscopolamine (meth skoe POL a meen)

Brand Names: U.S. Pamine®; Pamine® Forte
Brand Names: Canada Pamine®
Pharmacologic Category Anticholinergic Agent
Use Adjunctive therapy in the treatment of peptic ulcer

Local Anesthetic/Vasoconstrictor Precautions No information available to require special precautions
Effects on Dental Treatment Key adverse event(s) related to dental treatment: Xerostomia and changes in salivation (normal salivary flow resumes upon discontinuation), and dry throat and nose. Anticholinergic side effects can cause a reduction of saliva production or secretion, contributing to discomfort and dental disease (ie, caries, oral candidiasis and periodontal disease).
Effects on Bleeding No information available to require special precautions
Adverse Effects Frequency not defined.
Cardiovascular: Palpitation, tachycardia
Central nervous system: Headache, insomnia, flushing, nervousness, drowsiness, dizziness, confusion, fever, CNS stimulation may be produced with large doses
Dermatologic: Dry skin, urticaria
Endocrine & metabolic: Lactation suppressed
Gastrointestinal: Constipation, xerostomia, dry throat, dysphagia, nausea, vomiting, loss of taste
Genitourinary: Impotence, urinary hesitancy, urinary retention
Neuromuscular & skeletal: Weakness
Ocular: Blurred vision, cycloplegia, ocular tension increased, pupil dilation
Respiratory: Dry nose
Miscellaneous: Allergic reaction, diaphoresis decreased, hypersensitivity reactions, anaphylaxis
General Dosage Range Oral: *Adults:* 2.5-5 mg twice daily
Mechanism of Action Methscopolamine is a peripheral anticholinergic agent with limited ability to cross the blood-brain barrier and provides a peripheral blockade of muscarinic receptors. This agent reduces the volume and the total acid content of gastric secretions, inhibits salivation, and reduces gastrointestinal motility.
Pharmacodynamics/Kinetics
Onset of Action 1 hour
Duration of Action 4-6 hours
Pregnancy Risk Factor C
Pregnancy Considerations Animal reproduction studies have not been conducted. Methscopolamine is a derivative of scopolamine. Scopolamine is reported to cross the placenta; fetal toxicity noted in case reports.

Methsuximide (meth SUKS i mide)

Brand Names: U.S. Celontin®
Brand Names: Canada Celontin®
Pharmacologic Category Anticonvulsant, Succinimide
Use Control of absence (petit mal) seizures that are refractory to other drugs
Unlabeled Use Partial complex (psychomotor) seizures
Local Anesthetic/Vasoconstrictor Precautions No information available to require special precautions
Effects on Dental Treatment No significant effects or complications reported
Effects on Bleeding No information available to require special precautions
Adverse Effects Frequency not defined.
Cardiovascular: Hyperemia
Central nervous system: Aggressiveness, ataxia, confusion, depression, dizziness, drowsiness, hallucinations (auditory), headache, hypochondriacal behavior, insomnia, irritability, mental instability, mental slowness, nervousness, psychosis, suicidal behavior
Dermatologic: Pruritus, rash, Stevens-Johnson syndrome, urticaria

Gastrointestinal: Abdominal pain, anorexia, constipation, diarrhea, epigastric pain, nausea, vomiting, weight loss
Genitourinary: Hematuria (microscopic), proteinuria
Hematologic: Eosinophilia, leukopenia, monocytosis, pancytopenia
Ocular: Blurred vision, periorbital edema, photophobia
Miscellaneous: Hiccups, systemic lupus erythematosus
General Dosage Range Oral: *Adults:* Initial: 300 mg/day for 1 week; Maintenance: Up to 1.2 g/day in 2-4 divided doses
Mechanism of Action Increases the seizure threshold and suppresses paroxysmal spike-and-wave pattern in absence seizures; depresses nerve transmission in the motor cortex
Pharmacodynamics/Kinetics
Half-life Elimination 2-4 hours
Time to Peak Serum: 1-3 hours
Pregnancy Considerations Patients exposed to methsuximide during pregnancy are encouraged to enroll themselves into the NAAED Pregnancy Registry by calling 1-888-233-2334. Additional information is available at www.aedpregnancyregistry.org.

Methyclothiazide (meth i kloe THYE a zide)

Related Information
Cardiovascular Diseases *on page 1492*
Pharmacologic Category Diuretic, Thiazide
Use Management of hypertension; adjunctive therapy of edema
Local Anesthetic/Vasoconstrictor Precautions No information available to require special precautions
Effects on Dental Treatment Key adverse event(s) related to dental treatment: Orthostatic hypotension.
Effects on Bleeding No information available to require special precautions
Adverse Effects Frequency not defined.
Cardiovascular: Necrotizing angiitis, orthostatic hypotension
Central nervous system: Dizziness, fever, headache, vertigo
Dermatologic: Photosensitivity, purpura, rash, Stevens-Johnson syndrome, urticaria
Endocrine & metabolic: Electrolyte imbalance, hypercalcemia, hyperglycemia, hyperuricemia, hypokalemia
Gastrointestinal: Anorexia, constipation, diarrhea, epigastric distress, gastric irritation, nausea, pancreatitis, sialadenitis, vomiting
Genitourinary: Glycosuria
Hematologic: Agranulocytosis, aplastic anemia, hemolytic anemia, leukopenia, thrombocytopenia
Hepatic: Jaundice
Neuromuscular & skeletal: Cramping, muscle spasm, paresthesias, restlessness, weakness
Ocular: Blurred vision (transient), xanthopsia
Respiratory: Pneumonitis, pulmonary edema, respiratory distress
Miscellaneous: Anaphylactic reactions
General Dosage Range Oral: *Adults:* 2.5-10 mg once daily
Mechanism of Action Inhibits sodium reabsorption in the distal tubules causing increased excretion of sodium and water, as well as potassium and hydrogen ions
Pharmacodynamics/Kinetics
Onset of Action Diuresis: 2 hours; Peak effect: 6 hours
Duration of Action ~1 day
Pregnancy Risk Factor B

Pregnancy Considerations Adverse events were not observed in animal reproduction studies. Thiazide diuretics cross the placenta and are found in cord blood. Maternal use may cause fetal or neonatal jaundice, thrombocytopenia, or other adverse events observed in adults. Use of thiazide diuretics during normal pregnancies is not appropriate; use may be considered when edema is due to pathologic causes (as in the nonpregnant patient); monitor.

Methyl Aminolevulinate
(METH il a mee noe LEV ue lin ate)

Brand Names: U.S. Metvixia®
Brand Names: Canada Metvix®
Pharmacologic Category Photosensitizing Agent, Topical; Topical Skin Product
Use Treatment of thin and moderately thick, nonhyperkeratotic, nonpigmented actinic keratoses of the face and scalp; to be used in conjunction with red light illumination
Local Anesthetic/Vasoconstrictor Precautions No information available to require special precautions
Effects on Dental Treatment No significant effects or complications reported
Effects on Bleeding No information available to require special precautions
Adverse Effects Pain and burning begin during illumination and generally resolve completely within a few minutes or hours, but may last up to a few days. Erythema and other signs generally resolve within a few days up to 3 weeks.
>10%: Dermatologic: Skin burning/pain/discomfort (86%; severe: 20%), erythema (63%; severe 6%), scabbing/crusting/blister/erosions (29%), itching (22%), skin or eyelid edema (18%), skin exfoliation (14%)
1% to 10%:
Dermatologic: Skin warm (4%), hyperpigmentation (2%), skin hemorrhage (2%), skin tightness (2%)
Local: Application site discharge (2%)
General Dosage Range Topical: *Adults:* Apply up to 1 g once; repeat in 1 week
Mechanism of Action Methyl aminolevulinate (prodrug) is metabolically converted to photoactive porphyrins (PAPs), which accumulate in the skin lesions resulting in photosensitization. When exposed to light of appropriate wavelength and energy, the accumulated PAPs produce a photodynamic reaction, releasing oxygen singlets which result in local cytotoxicity.
Pregnancy Risk Factor C
Pregnancy Considerations Teratogenic effects have been demonstrated in animal reproduction studies using intravenous doses >900-fold higher than a human topical dose of 2 g. There are no adequate and well-controlled studies in pregnant women. Use during pregnancy only if clearly needed.

Methylcellulose (meth il SEL yoo lose)

Brand Names: U.S. Citrucel® [OTC]; Soluble Fiber Therapy [OTC]
Pharmacologic Category Fiber Supplement; Laxative; Laxative, Bulk-Producing
Use Adjunct in treatment of constipation
Local Anesthetic/Vasoconstrictor Precautions No information available to require special precautions
Effects on Dental Treatment No significant effects or complications reported

Effects on Bleeding No information available to require special precautions
General Dosage Range Oral:
Caplet:
Children 6-11 years: 1 caplet up to 6 times/day (maximum: 6 caplets/day)
Children ≥12 years and Adults: 2 caplets up to 6 times/day (maximum: 12 caplets/day)
Powder:
Children 6-11 years: 1 g (2-2.5 level teaspoons) up to 3 times/day
Children ≥12 years and Adults: 2 g (1 rounded or heaping tablespoon) up to 3 times/day
Pregnancy Considerations When administered with adequate fluids, use is considered safe for the treatment of occasional constipation during pregnancy (Wald, 2003).

Methyldopa (meth il DOE pa)

Related Information
Cardiovascular Diseases *on page 1492*
Brand Names: Canada Apo-Methyldopa®; Nu-Medopa
Pharmacologic Category Alpha$_2$-Adrenergic Agonist
Use Management of moderate-to-severe hypertension
Local Anesthetic/Vasoconstrictor Precautions No information available to require special precautions
Effects on Dental Treatment Key adverse event(s) related to dental treatment: Xerostomia (normal salivary flow resumes upon discontinuation). Anticholinergic side effects can cause a reduction of saliva production or secretion, contributing to discomfort and dental disease (ie, caries, oral candidiasis, and periodontal disease).
Effects on Bleeding No information available to require special precautions
Adverse Effects Frequency not defined.
Cardiovascular: Angina pectoris aggravation, bradycardia, carotid sinus hypersensitivity prolonged, heart failure, myocarditis, orthostatic hypotension, paradoxical pressor response (I.V. use), pericarditis, peripheral edema, symptoms of cerebrovascular insufficiency, vasculitis
Central nervous system: Bell's palsy, dizziness, drug fever, headache, lightheadedness, mental acuity decreased, mental depression, nightmares, parkinsonism, sedation
Dermatologic: Rash, toxic epidermal necrolysis
Endocrine & metabolic: Amenorrhea, breast enlargement, gynecomastia, hyperprolactinemia, lactation, libido decreased
Gastrointestinal: Abdominal distension, colitis, constipation, diarrhea, flatulence, nausea, pancreatitis, sialadenitis, sore or "black" tongue, vomiting, weight gain, xerostomia
Genitourinary: Impotence
Hematologic: Bone marrow suppression, eosinophilia, granulocytopenia, hemolytic anemia; positive tests for ANA, LE cells, rheumatoid factor, Coombs test (positive); leukopenia, thrombocytopenia
Hepatic: Abnormal LFTs, liver disorders (hepatitis), jaundice
Neuromuscular & skeletal: Arthralgia, choreoathetosis, myalgia, paresthesias, weakness
Renal: BUN increased
Respiratory: Nasal congestion
Miscellaneous: SLE-like syndrome
General Dosage Range Dosage adjustment recommended in patients with renal impairment

I.V.:
Children: 5-10 mg/kg/dose every 6-8 hours (maximum: 65 mg/kg/day; 3 g/day)
Adults: 250-500 mg every 6-8 hours (maximum: 1 g every 6 hours)

Oral:
Children: Initial: 10 mg/kg/day in 2-4 divided doses; Maintenance: Up to 65 mg/kg/day (maximum: 3 g/day)
Adults: Initial: 250 mg 2-3 times/day; Maintenance: 250-1000 mg/day in 2 divided doses (maximum: 3 g/day)

Mechanism of Action Stimulation of central alpha-adrenergic receptors by a false neurotransmitter (alpha-methylnorepinephrine) that results in a decreased sympathetic outflow to the heart, kidneys, and peripheral vasculature

Pharmacodynamics/Kinetics
Onset of Action Peak effect: Hypotensive: Oral, I.V.: 4-6 hours
Duration of Action Oral: Single-dose: 12-24, Multiple-dose: 24-48 hours; I.V.: 10-16 hours
Half-life Elimination 1.5-2 hours; End-stage renal disease: Prolonged (Myhre, 1982)
Time to Peak Plasma: Oral: 2-4 hours (Myhre, 1982)
Pregnancy Risk Factor B/C (injectable)
Pregnancy Considerations Adverse events have not been observed in animal reproduction studies. Methyldopa crosses the placenta and appears in cord blood. Methyldopa is considered an appropriate agent for the treatment of hypertension in pregnancy (ACOG, 2012).

Methyldopa and Hydrochlorothiazide
(meth il DOE pa & hye droe klor oh THYE a zide)

Related Information
Hydrochlorothiazide *on page 687*
Methyldopa *on page 897*
Brand Names: Canada Apo-Methazide®
Pharmacologic Category Alpha$_2$-Adrenergic Agonist; Diuretic, Thiazide
Use Management of moderate-to-severe hypertension
Local Anesthetic/Vasoconstrictor Precautions No information available to require special precautions
Effects on Dental Treatment Key adverse event(s) related to dental treatment: Anticholinergic side effects can cause a reduction of saliva production or secretion, contributing to discomfort and dental disease (ie, caries, oral candidiasis, and periodontal disease).
Effects on Bleeding No information available to require special precautions
Adverse Effects See individual agents.
General Dosage Range Oral: *Adults:* Methyldopa 250 mg and hydrochlorothiazide 15-25 mg twice daily **or** methyldopa 250 mg and hydrochlorothiazide 15 mg 3 times daily **or** methyldopa 500 mg and hydrochlorothiazide 30-50 mg once daily. Maximum daily dose, based on the hydrochlorothiazide content: Oral: 50 mg/day
Mechanism of Action
Methyldopa stimulates central alpha-adrenergic receptors by a false transmitter that results in a decreased sympathetic outflow to the heart, kidneys, and peripheral vasculature.
Hydrochlorothiazide inhibits sodium reabsorption in the distal tubules causing increased excretion of sodium and water as well as potassium and hydrogen ions.
Pregnancy Risk Factor C
Pregnancy Considerations See individual agents.

Methylergonovine (meth il er goe NOE veen)

Brand Names: U.S. Methergine® [DSC]
Brand Names: Canada Methergine®
Pharmacologic Category Ergot Derivative
Use Management of uterine atony, hemorrhage and subinvolution of the uterus following delivery of the placenta; control of uterine hemorrhage following delivery of the anterior shoulder in the second stage of labor
Local Anesthetic/Vasoconstrictor Precautions Use vasoconstrictor with caution in patients taking methylergonovine; this ergot alkaloid derivative causes constriction of peripheral blood vessels
Effects on Dental Treatment No significant effects or complications reported
Effects on Bleeding Thrombosis has been reported; however, there are no special precautions associated with bleeding related to dental procedures.
Adverse Effects Frequency not defined.
Cardiovascular: Acute MI, angina pectoris, arterial spasm, atrioventricular block, bradycardia, cerebrovascular accident, chest pain, hyper-/hypotension, palpitation, tachycardia, vasospasm, ventricular fibrillation
Central nervous system: Dizziness, hallucinations, headache, seizure
Dermatologic: Rash
Endocrine & metabolic: Water intoxication
Gastrointestinal: Abdominal pain, diarrhea, foul taste, nausea, vomiting
Local: Thrombophlebitis
Neuromuscular & skeletal: Leg cramps, paresthesia
Otic: Tinnitus
Renal: Hematuria
Respiratory: Dyspnea, nasal congestion
Miscellaneous: Anaphylaxis, diaphoresis
General Dosage Range
I.M., I.V.: *Adults:* 0.2 mg after delivery; may repeat every 2-4 hours
Oral: *Adults:* 0.2 mg 3-4 times daily in the puerperium
Mechanism of Action Increases the tone, rate and amplitude of contractions on the smooth muscles of the uterus, producing sustained contractions which shortens the third stage of labor and reduces blood loss.
Pharmacodynamics/Kinetics
Onset of Action Oxytocic: Oral: 5-10 minutes; I.M.: 2-5 minutes; I.V.: Immediately
Duration of Action Oral: ~3 hours; I.M.: ~3 hours; I.V.: 45 minutes
Half-life Elimination ~3 hours (range: 1.5-12.7 hours)
Time to Peak Serum: Oral: 0.3-2 hours; I.M.: 0.2-0.6 hours
Pregnancy Risk Factor C
Pregnancy Considerations Animal reproduction studies have not been conducted. Methylergonovine is intended for use after delivery of the infant; use is contraindicated during pregnancy.

Methylfolate (meth il FO late)

Brand Names: U.S. Deplin®
Generic Availability (U.S.) Yes
Pharmacologic Category Dietary Supplement
Use Medicinal food for the nutritional requirements of patients with suboptimal L-methylfolate and have major depressive disorder or who have or are at risk for hyperhomocysteinemia and have schizophrenia
Local Anesthetic/Vasoconstrictor Precautions No information available to require special precautions

Effects on Dental Treatment No significant effects or complications reported

Effects on Bleeding No information available to require special precautions

Dosage Oral: Adults: 7.5-15 mg daily

Mechanism of Action Methylfolate, or L-methylfolate, is the active form of folate in the body, which can be transported into peripheral tissues and across the blood-brain barrier. Folate is necessary for formation of numerous coenzymes in many metabolic systems, particularly for purine, pyrimidine, and nucleoprotein synthesis, and maintenance in erythropoiesis; stimulates WBC and platelet production in folate deficiency anemia.

Contraindications Hypersensitivity to any component of the formulation

Warnings/Precautions Folate administration is not appropriate for monotherapy with pernicious or other megaloblastic anemias when anemia is present with vitamin B_{12} deficiency. Doses >0.1 mg/day may obscure pernicious anemia with continuing irreversible nerve damage progression. Product is a medicinal food for use only under the supervision of a healthcare provider.

Drug Interactions

Metabolism/Transport Effects None known.

Avoid Concomitant Use

Avoid concomitant use of Methylfolate with any of the following: Raltitrexed

Increased Effect/Toxicity There are no known significant interactions involving an increase in effect.

Decreased Effect

Methylfolate may decrease the levels/effects of: CarBAMazepine; Divalproex; Fosphenytoin; PHENobarbital; Phenytoin; Primidone; Pyrimethamine; Raltitrexed; Valproic Acid

The levels/effects of Methylfolate may be decreased by: Cholestyramine Resin; Colestipol; SulfaSALAzine

Pregnancy Considerations Animal and human reproduction studies have not been located. Methylfolate is the active form of folic acid, which is required during pregnancy; folic acid deficiency may result in fetal harm.

Dosage Forms

Caplet, oral: L-methylfolate 15 mg
Deplin®: L-methylfolate 15 mg
Tablet, oral: L-methylfolate 7.5 mg, L-methylfolate 15 mg
Deplin®: L-methylfolate 7.5 mg

Methylfolate, Methylcobalamin, and Acetylcysteine
(meth il FO late meth il koe BAL a min & a se teel SIS teen)

Related Information

Acetylcysteine *on page 43*
Methylfolate *on page 898*
Brand Names: U.S. Cerefolin® NAC
Pharmacologic Category Dietary Supplement
Use Medicinal food for use in patients with neurovascular oxidative stress and/or hyperhomocysteinemia
Local Anesthetic/Vasoconstrictor Precautions No information available to require special precautions
Effects on Dental Treatment No significant effects or complications reported
Effects on Bleeding No information available to require special precautions
General Dosage Range Oral: *Children ≥12 years and Adults:* 1 caplet daily

---

Methylnaltrexone (meth il nal TREKS one)

Brand Names: U.S. Relistor®
Brand Names: Canada Relistor®
Pharmacologic Category Gastrointestinal Agent, Miscellaneous; Opioid Antagonist, Peripherally-Acting
Use Treatment of opioid-induced constipation in patients with advanced illness receiving palliative care with inadequate response to conventional laxative regimens
Local Anesthetic/Vasoconstrictor Precautions No information available to require special precautions
Effects on Dental Treatment No significant effects or complications reported
Effects on Bleeding No information available to require special precautions
Adverse Effects
>10%: Gastrointestinal: Abdominal pain (29%), flatulence (13%), nausea (12%)
1% to 10%:
Central nervous system: Dizziness (7%)
Dermatologic: Hyperhidrosis (7%)
Gastrointestinal: Diarrhea (6%)
General Dosage Range Dosage adjustment recommended in patients with renal impairment
SubQ:
Adults <38 kg and >114 kg: 0.15 mg/kg (round dose up to nearest 0.1 mL of volume) every other day as needed (maximum: 1 dose/24 hours)
Adults 38 to <62 kg: 8 mg every other day as needed (maximum: 1 dose/24 hours)
Adults 62-114 kg: 12 mg every other day as needed (maximum: 1 dose/24 hours)
Mechanism of Action An opioid receptor antagonist which blocks opioid binding at the mu receptor, methylnaltrexone is a quaternary derivative of naltrexone with restricted ability to cross the blood-brain barrier. It therefore functions as a peripheral acting opioid antagonist, including actions on the gastrointestinal tract to inhibit opioid-induced decreased gastrointestinal motility and delay in gastrointestinal transit time, thereby decreasing opioid-induced constipation. Does not affect opioid analgesic effects or induce opioid withdrawal symptoms.
Pharmacodynamics/Kinetics
Onset of Action Usually within 30-60 minutes (in responding patients)
Half-life Elimination Terminal: ~8 hours
Time to Peak SubQ: 30 minutes
Pregnancy Risk Factor B
Pregnancy Considerations Adverse effects were not observed in animal studies. There are no adequate and well-controlled studies in pregnant women.

Methylphenidate (meth il FEN i date)

Brand Names: U.S. Concerta®; Daytrana®; Metadate CD®; Metadate® ER; Methylin®; Quillivant™ XR; Ritalin LA®; Ritalin-SR®; Ritalin®
Brand Names: Canada Apo-Methylphenidate®; Apo-Methylphenidate® SR; Biphentin®; Concerta®; PHL-Methylphenidate; PMS-Methylphenidate; ratio-Methylphenidate; Ritalin®; Ritalin® SR; Sandoz-Methylphenidate SR; Teva-Methylphenidate ER-C
Generic Availability (U.S.) Yes: Extended release capsule, extended/sustained release tablet, immediate release tablet, immediate release oral solution
Pharmacologic Category Central Nervous System Stimulant

899

◀ **Use** U.S. labeling: Treatment of attention-deficit/hyperactivity disorder (ADHD); symptomatic management of narcolepsy (except Concerta®, Daytrana®, Metadate CD®, Ritalin LA®, and Quillivant™ XR)

Canadian labeling: Treatment of attention-deficit/hyperactivity disorder (ADHD); symptomatic management of narcolepsy (except Biphentin®, Concerta®)

Local Anesthetic/Vasoconstrictor Precautions No information available to require special precautions

Effects on Dental Treatment Key adverse event(s) related to dental treatment: Up to 10% of patients taking amphetamine-like drugs may present with hypertension. Monitor blood pressure prior to using local anesthetic with vasoconstrictors.

Effects on Bleeding No information available to require special precautions

Adverse Effects

All dosage forms: Frequency not always defined:

Cardiovascular: Angina, cardiac arrhythmia, cerebral arteritis, cerebral hemorrhage, cerebral occlusion, cerebrovascular accidents, hyper-/hypotension, MI, murmur, palpitation, pulse increased/decreased, Raynaud's phenomenon, tachycardia, vasculitis

Central nervous system: Motion sickness (children 2%), tic (children 2%), aggression, agitation, anger, anxiety, confusional state, depression, dizziness, drowsiness, emotional lability, fatigue, fever, headache, hypervigilance, insomnia, irritability, lethargy, nervousness, neuroleptic malignant syndrome (NMS) (rare), restlessness, stroke, tension, Tourette's syndrome (rare), toxic psychosis, tremor, vertigo

Dermatologic: Excoriation (children 4%), alopecia, erythema multiforme, exfoliative dermatitis, hyperhidrosis, rash, urticaria

Endocrine & metabolic: Dysmenorrhea, growth retardation, libido decreased

Gastrointestinal: Abdominal pain, anorexia, appetite decreased, bruxism, constipation, diarrhea, dyspepsia, nausea, vomiting, weight loss, xerostomia

Genitourinary: Erectile dysfunction

Hematologic: Anemia, leukopenia, pancytopenia, thrombocytopenia, thrombocytopenic purpura

Hepatic: Bilirubin increased, hepatic coma, liver function tests abnormal, transaminases increased

Neuromuscular & skeletal: Arthralgia, dyskinesia, muscle tightness, paresthesia

Ocular: Eye pain (children 2%), blurred vision, dry eyes, mydriasis, visual accommodation disturbance

Renal: Necrotizing vasculitis

Respiratory: Cough increased, dyspnea, pharyngitis, pharyngolaryngeal pain, rhinitis, sinusitis, upper respiratory tract infection

Miscellaneous: Accidental injury, hypersensitivity reactions

Transdermal system: Frequency of adverse events as reported in trials of 7-week duration. Incidence of some events higher with extended use.

>10%:

Central nervous system: Headache (≤15%; long-term use in children: 28%), insomnia (6% to 13%; long-term use in children: 30%), irritability (7% to 11%)

Gastrointestinal: Appetite decreased (26%), nausea (10% to 12%)

Miscellaneous: Viral infection (long-term use in children: 28%)

1% to 10%:

Cardiovascular: Tachycardia (≤1%)

Central nervous system: Tic (7%), dizziness (adolescents 6%), emotional instability (6%)

Gastrointestinal: Vomiting (3% to 10%), weight loss (6% to 9%), abdominal pain (5% to 7%), anorexia (5%; long-term use in children: 46%)

Local: Application site reaction

Respiratory: Nasal congestion (6%) nasopharyngitis (5%)

Dosage

ADHD:

Oral, immediate release (IR) products (tablets, chewable tablets, and solution): Children ≥6 years, Adolescents, and Adults: Initial: 5 mg twice daily, before breakfast and lunch; increase by 5-10 mg daily at weekly intervals; maximum dose: 60 mg daily (in 2-3 divided doses).

Oral, extended release (ER), sustained release (SR) products (capsules, tablets, and oral suspension):

Children ≥6 years and Adolescents <18 years: *Concerta®:*

Patients not currently taking methylphenidate: Initial: 18 mg once daily in the morning

Patients currently taking immediate release (IR) methylphenidate: Initial: **Note:** Dosing based on current regimen and clinical judgment; suggested dosing listed below:

- Patients taking IR methylphenidate 5 mg 2-3 times daily **or** (Canadian labeling; not in U.S. labeling) methylphenidate SR 20 mg daily: 18 mg once every morning

- Patients taking IR methylphenidate 10 mg 2-3 times daily **or** (Canadian labeling; not in U.S. labeling) methylphenidate SR 40 mg daily: 36 mg once every morning

- Patients taking IR methylphenidate 15 mg 2-3 times daily **or** (Canadian labeling; not in U.S. labeling) methylphenidate SR 60 mg daily: 54 mg once every morning

- Patients taking IR methylphenidate 20 mg 2-3 times daily: 72 mg once every morning

Dose adjustment: May increase dose in increments of 18 mg at weekly intervals. A dosage strength of 27 mg is available for situations in which a dosage between 18-36 mg is desired.

Maximum dose:

U.S. labeling: 54 mg daily in children 6-12 years **or** 2 mg/kg/day (up to 72 mg daily) in adolescents <18 years

Canadian labeling: 54 mg daily in children and adolescents 6-18 years

Children ≥6 years, Adolescents, and Adults:

Biphentin® (Canadian availability; not available in the U.S.): Patients not currently taking methylphenidate: Initial: 10-20 mg once daily; may be adjusted in 10 mg increments at weekly intervals. Maximum: 60 mg daily (children ≥6 years, adolescents) or 80 mg daily (adults). **Note:** In some children >60 kg, a maximum dose of 1 mg/kg/daily (not to exceed 80 mg daily) may be necessary; however, close monitoring for adverse events is required. Reduce dose or discontinue if adverse events arise.

Conversion from immediate release methylphenidate formulations to Biphentin®: Use equivalent total daily dose administered once daily.

Metadate® ER, Ritalin-SR®: May be given in place of immediate release products (duration of action ~8 hours), once the immediate release formulation daily dose is titrated and the titrated 8-hour dosage corresponds to sustained or extended release tablet size; maximum: 60 mg daily

Metadate CD®, Quillivant™ XR: Initial: 20 mg once daily; may be adjusted in 10-20 mg increments at weekly intervals; maximum: 60 mg daily

Ritalin LA®: Initial: 20 mg once daily (10 mg once daily may be considered for some patients); may be adjusted in 10 mg increments at weekly intervals; maximum: 60 mg daily

Conversion from immediate release or sustained release methylphenidate formulation to Ritalin LA®: Use equivalent total daily dose administered once daily.

Adolescent ≥18 years and Adults (<65 years): *Concerta®:*

Patients not currently taking methylphenidate: Initial:

U.S. labeling: 18-36 mg once every morning

Canadian labeling: 18 mg once every morning

Patients currently taking immediate release (IR) methylphenidate: Initial: **Note:** Dosing based on current regimen and clinical judgment; suggested dosing listed below:

- Patients taking IR methylphenidate 5 mg 2-3 times daily **or** (Canadian labeling; not in U.S. labeling) methylphenidate SR 20 mg daily: 18 mg once every morning
- Patients taking IR methylphenidate 10 mg 2-3 times daily **or** (Canadian labeling; not in U.S. labeling) methylphenidate SR 40 mg daily: 36 mg once every morning
- Patients taking IR methylphenidate 15 mg 2-3 times daily **or** (Canadian labeling; not in U.S. labeling) methylphenidate SR 60 mg daily: 54 mg once every morning
- Patients taking IR methylphenidate 20 mg 2-3 times daily: 72 mg once every morning

Dose adjustment: May increase dose in increments of 18 mg at weekly intervals. A dosage strength of 27 mg is available for situations in which a dosage between 18-36 mg is desired. Maximum dose: 72 mg daily.

Transdermal: (Daytrana®): Children ≥6 years and Adolescents <18 years: Initial: 10 mg patch once daily; remove up to 9 hours after application. Titrate based on response and tolerability; may increase to next transdermal dose no more frequently than every week. **Note:** Application should occur 2 hours prior to desired effect. Drug absorption may continue for a period of time after patch removal. The prescribing information recommends patients converting from another formulation of methylphenidate should be initiated at 10 mg regardless of their previous dose and titrated as needed due to the differences in bioavailability of the transdermal formulation. However, some clinicians have supported higher starting patch doses for patients converting from oral methylphenidate doses of >20 mg daily; for example, the 15 mg (18.75 cm^2) patch has been investigated to have the same effect as 22.5 mg daily of the immediate release preparation, 27 mg/day of the osmotic release preparation, or 20 mg daily of the encapsulated bead preparation (Arnold, 2007).

Narcolepsy: Oral: Children ≥6 years, Adolescents, Adults:

Immediate release tablets and solution (Methylin®, Ritalin®): Initial: 5 mg twice daily before breakfast and lunch; increase by 5-10 mg daily at weekly intervals; maximum dose: 60 mg daily (in 2-3 divided doses).

Extended and sustained release tablets (Metadate ER®, Ritalin-SR®): May be given in place of immediate release products (duration of action ~8 hours), once the immediate release formulation daily dose is titrated and the titrated 8-hour dosage corresponds to sustained or extended release tablet size; maximum: 60 mg daily.

Depression (unlabeled use): Oral: Adults: Initial: 2.5 mg every morning before 9 AM; dosage may be increased by 2.5-5 mg every 2-3 days as tolerated to a maximum of 20 mg daily; may be divided (ie, 7 AM and 12 noon), but should not be given after 12 noon; do not use sustained release product

Dosage adjustment in renal impairment:

Oral: No dosage adjustment provided in manufacturer's labeling (has not been studied); undergoes extensive metabolism to a renally eliminated metabolite with little or no pharmacologic activity.

Transdermal: No dosage adjustment provided in manufacturer's labeling (has not been studied).

Dosage adjustment in hepatic impairment:

Oral: No dosage adjustment provided in manufacturer's labeling (has not been studied).

Transdermal: No dosage adjustment provided in manufacturer's labeling (has not been studied).

Mechanism of Action Mild CNS stimulant; blocks the reuptake of norepinephrine and dopamine into presynaptic neurons; appears to stimulate the cerebral cortex and subcortical structures similar to amphetamines

Contraindications

U.S. labeling: Hypersensitivity to methylphenidate or any component of the formulation; marked anxiety, tension, and agitation; glaucoma; use during or within 14 days following MAO inhibitor therapy; family history or diagnosis of Tourette's syndrome or tics

Additional contraindications: Metadate CD® and Metadate® ER: Severe hypertension, heart failure, arrhythmia, hyperthyroidism, recent MI or angina; concomitant use of halogenated anesthetics

Canadian labeling: Hypersensitivity to methylphenidate or any component of the formulation; marked anxiety, tension, and agitation; glaucoma; use during or within 14 days following MAO inhibitor therapy; family history or diagnosis of Tourette's syndrome or tics; thyrotoxicosis, advanced arteriosclerosis, symptomatic cardiovascular disease, or moderate-to-severe hypertension

Additional contraindications: Ritalin® and Ritalin® SR: Pheochromocytoma

Warnings/Precautions CNS stimulant use has been associated with serious cardiovascular events (eg, sudden death in children and adolescents; sudden death, stroke, and MI in adults) in patients with pre-existing structural cardiac abnormalities or other serious heart problems. These products should be avoided in patients with known serious structural cardiac abnormalities, cardiomyopathy, serious heart rhythm abnormalities, or other serious cardiac problems that could further increase their risk of sudden death. Patients should be carefully evaluated for cardiac disease prior to initiation of therapy. Use of stimulants can cause an increase in blood pressure (average 2-4 mm Hg) and increases in heart rate (average 3-6 bpm), although some patients may have larger than average increases. Use caution with hypertension, hyperthyroidism, or other cardiovascular conditions that might be exacerbated by increases in blood pressure or heart rate. Some products are contraindicated in patients with heart failure, arrhythmias, severe hypertension, hyperthyroidism, angina, or recent MI.

Has demonstrated value as part of a comprehensive treatment program for ADHD. Use with caution in patients with bipolar disorder (may induce mixed/manic episode). May exacerbate symptoms of behavior and thought disorder in psychotic patients; new-onset psychosis or mania may occur with stimulant use; observe for symptoms of aggression and/or hostility. Use caution with seizure disorders (may reduce seizure threshold). Use caution in patients with history of ethanol or drug abuse. May exacerbate symptoms of behavior and thought disorder in psychotic patients. **[U.S. Boxed Warning]: Potential for drug dependency exists - avoid abrupt discontinuation in patients who have received for prolonged periods.** Visual disturbances have been reported (rare). Not labeled for use in children <6 years of age. Use of stimulants has been associated with suppression of growth in children; monitor growth rate during treatment.

Concerta® should not be used in patients with esophageal motility disorders or pre-existing severe gastrointestinal narrowing (small bowel disease, short gut syndrome, history of peritonitis, cystic fibrosis, chronic intestinal pseudo-obstruction, Meckel's diverticulum). Concomitant use of Metadate CD® and Metadate® ER with halogenated anesthetics is contraindicated; may cause sudden elevations in blood pressure; if surgery is planned, do not administer Metadate CD® or Metadate® ER on the day of surgery. Transdermal system may cause allergic contact sensitization, characterized by intense local reactions (edema, papules) that may spread beyond the patch site; sensitization may subsequently manifest systemically with other routes of methylphenidate administration; monitor closely. Avoid exposure of application site to any direct external heat sources (eg, hair dryers, heating pads, electric blankets); may increase the rate and extent of absorption and risk of overdose. Efficacy of transdermal methylphenidate therapy for >7 weeks has not been established. Potentially significant interactions may exist, requiring dose or frequency adjustment, additional monitoring, and/or selection of alternative therapy. Consult drug interactions database for more detailed information. Biphentin® (Canadian availability; not available in U.S.) controlled release capsules are not interchangeable with other controlled release formulations. Some dosage forms may contain lactose or sucrose; use with caution in patients intolerant to either component (some manufacturer labels recommend avoiding use in such patients).

Drug Interactions

Metabolism/Transport Effects Inhibits CYP2D6 (weak)

Avoid Concomitant Use

Avoid concomitant use of Methylphenidate with any of the following: Inhalational Anesthetics; Iobenguane I 123; MAO Inhibitors

Increased Effect/Toxicity

Methylphenidate may increase the levels/effects of: Anti-Parkinson's Agents (Dopamine Agonist); Antipsychotics; CloNIDine; Fosphenytoin; Inhalational Anesthetics; PHENobarbital; Phenytoin; Primidone; Sympathomimetics; Tricyclic Antidepressants; Vitamin K Antagonists

The levels/effects of Methylphenidate may be increased by: Antacids; Antipsychotics; AtoMOXetine; Cannabinoids; H2-Antagonists; MAO Inhibitors; Proton Pump Inhibitors

Decreased Effect

Methylphenidate may decrease the levels/effects of: Antihypertensives; Iobenguane I 123; Ioflupane I 123

Ethanol/Nutrition/Herb Interactions

Food: Food may increase oral absorption of immediate release tablet/solution and chewable tablet. Management: Administer 30-45 minutes before meals.

Herb/Nutraceutical: Ephedra may cause hypertension or arrhythmias and yohimbe has CNS stimulatory activity. Management: Avoid ephedra and yohimbe.

Dietary Considerations Administer immediate release (IR) tablet (Ritalin®), IR solution (Methylin®), chewable tablet (Methylin®), and sustained released tablet (Ritalin-SR®) 30-45 minutes before meals. Some products may contain phenylalanine.

Pharmacodynamics/Kinetics

Onset of Action Peak effect:

Immediate release tablet: Cerebral stimulation: ~2 hours

Controlled release capsule: Biphentin® (Canadian availability; not available in U.S.): Initial: within 1 hour

Extended release capsule: Metadate CD®, Ritalin LA®: Biphasic; initial peak similar to immediate release product, followed by second rising portion (corresponding to extended release portion)

Extended release tablet: Concerta®: Initial: 1-2 hours

Sustained release tablet: Ritalin-SR®: 4-7 hours

Transdermal: ~2 hours; may be expedited by the application of external heat

Duration of Action Immediate release tablet: 3-6 hours; Sustained release tablet: Ritalin-SR®: 8 hours; Extended release tablet: Metadate® ER: 8 hours, Concerta®: 12 hours; Controlled release capsule: Biphentin® (Canadian availability; not available in U.S.): ~10-12 hours

Half-life Elimination d-methylphenidate: 3-6 hours; l-methylphenidate: 1-3 hours

Time to Peak Biphentin® (Canadian availability; not available in U.S.): ~2-3 hours; Concerta®: C_{max}: 6-8 hours; Daytrana®: 7.5-10.5 hours; Quillivant™ XR: ~4 hours

Pregnancy Risk Factor C

Pregnancy Considerations Animal studies have shown teratogenic effects to the fetus. There are no adequate and well-controlled studies in pregnant women. Do not use in women of childbearing age unless the potential benefit outweighs the possible risk.

Lactation Enters breast milk/use caution

Breast-Feeding Considerations Methylphenidate excretion into breast milk has been noted in case reports. In both cases, the authors calculated the relative infant dose to be ≤0.2% of the weight adjusted maternal dose. Adverse events were not noted in either infant, however, both were older (6 months of age and 11 months of age) and exposure was limited.

Controlled Substance C-II

Dosage Forms

Capsule, extended release, oral: 10 mg, 20 mg, 30 mg, 40 mg, 50 mg, 60 mg

Metadate CD®: 10 mg, 20 mg, 30 mg, 40 mg, 50 mg, 60 mg

Ritalin LA®: 10 mg, 20 mg, 30 mg, 40 mg

Patch, transdermal:

Daytrana®: 10 mg/9 hours (30s); 15 mg/9 hours (30s); 20 mg/9 hours (30s); 30 mg/9 hours (30s)

Powder for suspension, extended release, oral:

Quillivant™ XR: 25 mg/5 mL (60 mL, 120 mL, 150 mL, 180 mL)

Solution, oral: 5 mg/5 mL (500 mL); 10 mg/mL (500 mL)
Methylin®: 5 mg/5 mL (500 mL); 10 mg/5 mL (500 mL)
Tablet, oral: 5 mg, 10 mg, 20 mg
Ritalin®: 5 mg, 10 mg, 20 mg
Tablet, chewable, oral:
Methylin®: 2.5 mg, 5 mg, 10 mg
Tablet, extended release, oral: 10 mg, 18 mg, 20 mg, 27 mg, 36 mg, 54 mg
Concerta®: 18 mg, 27 mg, 36 mg, 54 mg
Metadate® ER: 20 mg
Tablet, sustained release, oral: 20 mg
Ritalin-SR®: 20 mg
Dosage Forms: Canada
Capsule, controlled release, oral:
Biphentin®: 10 mg, 15 mg, 20 mg, 30 mg, 40 mg, 50 mg, 60 mg, 80 mg

---

MethylPREDNISolone (meth il pred NIS oh lone)

Related Information
Respiratory Diseases *on page 1514*
Related Sample Prescriptions
Erosive Lichen Planus, Other Biopsy-Proven Desquamative Oral Diseases, and Major Aphthae *on page 1618*
Brand Names: U.S. A-Methapred®; Depo-Medrol®; Medrol®; Medrol® Dosepak™; Solu-MEDROL®
Brand Names: Canada Depo-Medrol®; Medrol®; Methylprednisolone Acetate; Solu-Medrol®
Generic Availability (U.S.) Yes: Excludes preservative free injection
Pharmacologic Category Corticosteroid, Systemic
Dental Use Treatment of a variety of oral diseases of allergic, inflammatory, or autoimmune origin
Use Primarily as an anti-inflammatory or immunosuppressant agent in the treatment of a variety of diseases including those of hematologic, allergic, inflammatory, neoplastic, and autoimmune origin. Prevention and treatment of graft-versus-host disease following allogeneic bone marrow transplantation.
Unlabeled Use Acute spinal cord injury
Local Anesthetic/Vasoconstrictor Precautions No information available to require special precautions
Effects on Dental Treatment Key adverse event(s) related to dental treatment: Ulcerative esophagitis.
Effects on Bleeding No information available to require special precautions
Adverse Effects Frequency not defined.
Cardiovascular: Arrhythmias, bradycardia, cardiac arrest, cardiomegaly, circulatory collapse, congestive heart failure, edema, fat embolism, hypertension, hypertrophic cardiomyopathy in premature infants, myocardial rupture (post MI), syncope, tachycardia, thromboembolism, vasculitis
Central nervous system: Delirium, depression, emotional instability, euphoria, hallucinations, headache, intracranial pressure increased, insomnia, malaise, mood swings, nervousness, neuritis, personality changes, psychic disorders, pseudotumor cerebri (usually following discontinuation), seizure, vertigo
Dermatologic: Acne, allergic dermatitis, alopecia, dry scaly skin, ecchymoses, edema, erythema, hirsutism, hyper-/hypopigmentation, hypertrichosis, impaired wound healing, petechiae, rash, skin atrophy, sterile abscess, skin test reaction impaired, striae, urticaria

Endocrine & metabolic: Adrenal suppression, amenorrhea, carbohydrate intolerance increased, Cushing's syndrome, diabetes mellitus, fluid retention, glucose intolerance, growth suppression (children), hyperglycemia, hyperlipidemia, hypokalemia, hypokalemic alkalosis, menstrual irregularities, negative nitrogen balance, pituitary-adrenal axis suppression, protein catabolism, sodium and water retention
Gastrointestinal: Abdominal distention, appetite increased, bowel/bladder dysfunction (after intrathecal administration), gastrointestinal hemorrhage, gastrointestinal perforation, nausea, pancreatitis, peptic ulcer, perforation of the small and large intestine, ulcerative esophagitis, vomiting, weight gain
Hematologic: Leukocytosis (transient)
Hepatic: Hepatomegaly, transaminases increased
Local: Postinjection flare (intra-articular use), thrombophlebitis
Neuromuscular & skeletal: Arthralgia, arthropathy, aseptic necrosis (femoral and humoral heads), fractures, muscle mass loss, muscle weakness, myopathy (particularly in conjunction with neuromuscular disease or neuromuscular-blocking agents), neuropathy, osteoporosis, parasthesia, tendon rupture, vertebral compression fractures, weakness
Ocular: Cataracts, exophthalmoses, glaucoma, intraocular pressure increased
Renal: Glycosuria
Respiratory: Pulmonary edema
Miscellaneous: Abnormal fat disposition, anaphylactoid reaction, anaphylaxis, angioedema, avascular necrosis, diaphoresis, hiccups, hypersensitivity reactions, infections, secondary malignancy
Dental Usual Dosage Anti-inflammatory or immunosuppressive: Adults: Oral: 2-60 mg/day in 1-4 divided doses to start, followed by gradual reduction in dosage to the lowest possible level consistent with maintaining an adequate clinical response.
Dosage Dosing should be based on the lesser of ideal body weight or actual body weight
Children: **Only sodium succinate may be given I.V.;** methylprednisolone sodium succinate is highly soluble and has a rapid effect by I.M. and I.V. routes. Methylprednisolone acetate has a low solubility and has a sustained I.M. effect.
Acute spinal cord injury (unlabeled use): I.V. (sodium succinate): 30 mg/kg over 15 minutes, followed in 45 minutes by a continuous infusion of 5.4 mg/kg/hour for 23 hours. **Note:** Due to insufficient evidence of clinical efficacy (ie, preserving or improving spinal cord function), the routine use of methylprednisolone in the treatment of acute spinal cord injury is no longer recommended. If used in this setting, methylprednisolone should not be initiated >8 hours after the injury; not effective in penetrating trauma (eg, gunshot) (Consortium for Spinal Cord Medicine, 2008).
Anti-inflammatory or immunosuppressive: Oral, I.M., I.V. (sodium succinate): 0.5-1.7 mg/kg/day **or** 5-25 mg/m^2/day in divided doses every 6-12 hours; "Pulse" therapy: 15-30 mg/kg/dose over ≥30 minutes given once daily for 3 days
Asthma exacerbations, including status asthmaticus (emergency medical care or hospital doses) (NIH Asthma Guidelines, NAEPP, 2007): Children ≤12 years: Oral, I.V.: 1-2 mg/kg/day in 2 divided doses (maximum: 60 mg/day) until peak expiratory flow is 70% of predicted or personal best
Lupus nephritis: I.V. (sodium succinate): 30 mg/kg over ≥30 minutes every other day for 6 doses

◀ Adults: **Only sodium succinate may be given I.V.;** methylprednisolone sodium succinate is highly soluble and has a rapid effect by I.M. and I.V. routes. Methylprednisolone acetate has a low solubility and has a sustained I.M. effect.

Acute spinal cord injury (unlabeled use): I.V. (sodium succinate): 30 mg/kg over 15 minutes, followed in 45 minutes by a continuous infusion of 5.4 mg/kg/hour for 23 hours. **Note:** Due to insufficient evidence of clinical efficacy (ie, preserving or improving spinal cord function), the routine use of methylprednisolone in the treatment of acute spinal cord injury is no longer recommended. If used in this setting, methylprednisolone should not be initiated >8 hours after the injury; not effective in penetrating trauma (eg, gunshot) (Consortium for Spinal Cord Medicine, 2008).

Allergic conditions: Oral: Tapered-dosage schedule (eg, dose-pack containing 21 x 4 mg tablets):

Day 1: 24 mg on day 1 administered as 8 mg (2 tablets) before breakfast, 4 mg (1 tablet) after lunch, 4 mg (1 tablet) after supper, and 8 mg (2 tablets) at bedtime **OR** 24 mg (6 tablets) as a single dose or divided into 2 or 3 doses upon initiation (regardless of time of day)

Day 2: 20 mg on day 2 administered as 4 mg (1 tablet) before breakfast, 4 mg (1 tablet) after lunch, 4 mg (1 tablet) after supper, and 8 mg (2 tablets) at bedtime

Day 3: 16 mg on day 3 administered as 4 mg (1 tablet) before breakfast, 4 mg (1 tablet) after lunch, 4 mg (1 tablet) after supper, and 4 mg (1 tablet) at bedtime

Day 4: 12 mg on day 4 administered as 4 mg (1 tablet) before breakfast, 4 mg (1 tablet) after lunch, and 4 mg (1 tablet) at bedtime

Day 5: 8 mg on day 5 administered as 4 mg (1 tablet) before breakfast and 4 mg (1 tablet) at bedtime

Day 6: 4 mg on day 6 administered as 4 mg (1 tablet) before breakfast

Anti-inflammatory or immunosuppressive:

Oral: 2-60 mg/day in 1-4 divided doses to start, followed by gradual reduction in dosage to the lowest possible level consistent with maintaining an adequate clinical response.

I.M. (sodium succinate): 10-80 mg/day once daily

I.M. (acetate): 10-80 mg every 1-2 weeks

I.V. (sodium succinate): 10-40 mg over a period of several minutes and repeated I.V. or I.M. at intervals depending on clinical response; when high dosages are needed, give 30 mg/kg over a period ≥30 minutes and may be repeated every 4-6 hours for 48 hours.

Arthritis: Intra-articular (acetate): Administer every 1-5 weeks.

Large joints (eg, knee, ankle): 20-80 mg

Medium joints (eg, elbow, wrist): 10-40 mg

Small joints: 4-10 mg

Asthma exacerbations, including status asthmaticus (emergency medical care or hospital doses): Oral, I.V.: 40-80 mg/day in 1-2 divided doses until peak expiratory flow is 70% of predicted or personal best (NIH Asthma Guidelines, NAEPP, 2007)

Asthma, severe persistent, long-term control: Oral: 7.5-60 mg/day (or on alternate days) (NIH Asthma Guidelines, NAEPP, 2007)

Dermatitis, acute severe: I.M. (acetate): 80-120 mg as a single dose

Dermatitis, chronic: I.M. (acetate): 40-120 mg every 5-10 days

Dermatologic conditions (eg, keloids, lichen planus): Intralesional (acetate): 20-60 mg

Dermatomyositis/polymyositis: I.V. (sodium succinate): 1 g/day for 3-5 days for severe muscle weakness, followed by conversion to oral prednisone (Drake, 1996)

Lupus nephritis: High-dose "pulse" therapy: I.V. (sodium succinate): 0.5-1 g/day for 3 days (Ponticelli, 2010)

Pneumocystis pneumonia in AIDS patients: I.V.: 30 mg twice daily for 5 days, then 30 mg once daily for 5 days, then 15 mg once daily for 11 days

Dosage adjustment in renal impairment: No dosage adjustment provided in manufacturer's labeling; use with caution.

Hemodialysis effects: Slightly dialyzable (5% to 20%) Administer dose post-hemodialysis.

Dosage adjustment in hepatic impairment: No dosage adjustment provided in manufacturer's labeling.

Mechanism of Action In a tissue-specific manner, corticosteroids regulate gene expression subsequent to binding specific intracellular receptors and translocation into the nucleus. Corticosteroids exert a wide array of physiologic effects including modulation of carbohydrate, protein, and lipid metabolism and maintenance of fluid and electrolyte homeostasis. Moreover cardiovascular, immunologic, musculoskeletal, endocrine, and neurologic physiology are influenced by corticosteroids. Decreases inflammation by suppression of migration of polymorphonuclear leukocytes and reversal of increased capillary permeability.

Contraindications Hypersensitivity to methylprednisolone or any component of the formulation; systemic fungal infection (except intra-articular injection in localized joint conditions); administration of live virus vaccines. methylprednisolone formulations containing benzyl alcohol preservative are contraindicated in premature infants; I.M. administration in idiopathic thrombocytopenia purpura; intrathecal administration

Warnings/Precautions Use with caution in patients with thyroid disease, hepatic impairment, renal impairment, cardiovascular disease, diabetes, glaucoma, cataracts, myasthenia gravis, patients at risk for osteoporosis, patients at risk for seizures, or GI diseases (diverticulitis, peptic ulcer, ulcerative colitis) due to perforation risk. Not recommended for the treatment of optic neuritis; may increase frequency of new episodes. Use caution following acute MI (corticosteroids have been associated with myocardial rupture). Cardiomegaly and congestive heart failure have been reported following concurrent use of amphotericin B and hydrocortisone for the management of fungal infections.

Because of the risk of adverse effects, systemic corticosteroids should be used cautiously in the elderly in the smallest possible effective dose for the shortest duration. May affect growth velocity; growth should be routinely monitored in pediatric patients. Withdraw therapy with gradual tapering of dose.

May cause hypercorticism or suppression of hypothalamic-pituitary-adrenal (HPA) axis, particularly in younger children or in patients receiving high doses for prolonged periods. HPA axis suppression may lead to adrenal crisis. Withdrawal and discontinuation of a corticosteroid should be done slowly and carefully. Particular care is required when patients are transferred from systemic corticosteroids to inhaled products due to possible adrenal insufficiency or withdrawal from steroids, including an increase in allergic symptoms. Patients receiving >20 mg per day of prednisone (or equivalent) may be most susceptible. Fatalities have occurred due to adrenal insufficiency in asthmatic patients during and after transfer from systemic corticosteroids to aerosol steroids; aerosol steroids do not provide the systemic steroid needed to treat patients having trauma, surgery, or infections.

Acute myopathy has been reported with high dose corticosteroids, usually in patients with neuromuscular transmission disorders; may involve ocular and/or respiratory muscles; monitor creatine kinase; recovery may be delayed. Corticosteroid use may cause psychiatric disturbances, including depression, euphoria, insomnia, mood swings, and personality changes. Pre-existing psychiatric conditions may be exacerbated by corticosteroid use. Prolonged use of corticosteroids may also increase the incidence of secondary infection, cause activation of latent infections, mask acute infection (including fungal infections), prolong or exacerbate viral or parasitic infections, or limit response to vaccines. Exposure to chickenpox or measles should be avoided; corticosteroids should not be used to treat ocular herpes simplex. Corticosteroids should not be used for cerebral malaria or viral hepatitis. Close observation is required in patients with latent tuberculosis and/or TB reactivity; restrict use in active TB (only in conjunction with antituberculosis treatment). Amebiasis should be ruled out in any patient with recent travel to tropic climates or unexplained diarrhea prior to initiation of corticosteroids. Prolonged treatment with corticosteroids has been associated with the development of Kaposi's sarcoma (case reports); discontinuation may result in clinical improvement.

High-dose corticosteroids should not be used to manage acute head injury. Rare cases of anaphylactoid reactions have been observed in patients receiving corticosteroids. Avoid injection or leakage into the dermis; dermal and/or subdermal skin depression may occur at the site of injection. Avoid deltoid muscle injection; subcutaneous atrophy may occur. Some dosage forms contain benzyl alcohol which has been associated with "gasping syndrome" in neonates.

Drug Interactions

Metabolism/Transport Effects Substrate of CYP3A4 (minor); **Note:** Assignment of Major/Minor substrate status based on clinically relevant drug interaction potential; **Inhibits** CYP2C8 (weak), CYP3A4 (weak)

Avoid Concomitant Use

Avoid concomitant use of MethylPREDNISolone with any of the following: Aldesleukin; BCG; Mifepristone; Natalizumab; Pimecrolimus; Pimozide; Tacrolimus (Topical); Tofacitinib

Increased Effect/Toxicity

MethylPREDNISolone may increase the levels/effects of: Acetylcholinesterase Inhibitors; Amphotericin B; ARIPiprazole; CycloSPORINE (Systemic); Deferasirox; Leflunomide; Lomitapide; Loop Diuretics; Natalizumab; NSAID (COX-2 Inhibitor); NSAID (Nonselective); Pimozide; Thiazide Diuretics; Tofacitinib; Vaccines (Live); Warfarin

The levels/effects of MethylPREDNISolone may be increased by: Antifungal Agents (Azole Derivatives, Systemic); Aprepitant; Calcium Channel Blockers (Nondihydropyridine); CycloSPORINE (Systemic); CYP3A4 Inhibitors (Strong); Denosumab; Estrogen Derivatives; Fluconazole; Fosaprepitant; Indacaterol; Macrolide Antibiotics; Mifepristone; Neuromuscular-Blocking Agents (Nondepolarizing); Pimecrolimus;

Quinolone Antibiotics; Roflumilast; Salicylates; Tacrolimus (Topical); Telaprevir; Trastuzumab

Decreased Effect

MethylPREDNISolone may decrease the levels/effects of: Aldesleukin; Antidiabetic Agents; BCG; Calcitriol; Coccidioidin Skin Test; Corticorelin; CycloSPORINE (Systemic); Hyaluronidase; Isoniazid; Salicylates; Sipuleucel-T; Telaprevir; Vaccines (Inactivated)

The levels/effects of MethylPREDNISolone may be decreased by: Aminoglutethimide; Antacids; Barbiturates; Bile Acid Sequestrants; CarBAMazepine; Echinacea; Fosphenytoin; Mifepristone; Mitotane; Phenytoin; Primidone; Rifamycin Derivatives

Ethanol/Nutrition/Herb Interactions

Ethanol: Ethanol may increase gastric mucosal irritation. Management: Avoid ethanol.

Food: Methylprednisolone interferes with calcium absorption. May cause GI upset. Management: Administer with food. Limit caffeine.

Herb/Nutraceutical: St John's wort may decrease methylprednisolone levels. Cat's claw and echinacea have immunostimulant properties. Management: Avoid St John's wort, cat's claw, and echinacea.

Dietary Considerations Take with meals to decrease GI upset.; need diet rich in pyridoxine, vitamin C, vitamin D, folate, calcium, phosphorus, and protein.

Pharmacodynamics/Kinetics

Onset of Action Peak effect (route dependent): Oral: 1-2 hours; I.M.: 4-8 days; Intra-articular: 1 week; methylprednisolone sodium succinate is highly soluble and has a rapid effect by I.M. and I.V. routes

Duration of Action Route dependent: Oral: 30-36 hours; I.M.: 1-4 weeks; Intra-articular: 1-5 weeks; methylprednisolone acetate has a low solubility and has a sustained I.M. effect

Half-life Elimination 3-3.5 hours; reduced in obese

Pregnancy Considerations Adverse events have been observed with corticosteroids in animal reproduction studies. Methylprednisolone crosses the placenta. Some studies have shown an association between first trimester systemic corticosteroid use and oral clefts; adverse events in the fetus/neonate have been noted in case reports following large doses of systemic corticosteroids during pregnancy. Pregnant women exposed to methylprednisolone for antirejection therapy following a transplant may contact the National Transplantation Pregnancy Registry (NTPR) at 215-955-4820. Women exposed to methylprednisolone during pregnancy for the treatment of an autoimmune disease may contact the OTIS Autoimmune Diseases Study at 877-311-8972.

Lactation Enters breast milk/use caution

Breast-Feeding Considerations Low levels of methylprednisolone are excreted in breast milk

Dosage Forms

Injection, powder for reconstitution: 40 mg, 125 mg, 500 mg, 1 g
A-Methapred®: 40 mg, 125 mg
Solu-MEDROL®: 500 mg, 1 g, 2 g

Injection, powder for reconstitution [preservative free]:
Solu-MEDROL®: 40 mg, 125 mg, 500 mg, 1 g

Injection, suspension: 40 mg/mL (1 mL, 5 mL, 10 mL); 80 mg/mL (1 mL, 5 mL)
Depo-Medrol®: 20 mg/mL (5 mL); 40 mg/mL (1 mL, 5 mL, 10 mL); 80 mg/mL (5 mL)

Injection, suspension [preservative free]:
Depo-Medrol®: 80 mg/mL (1 mL)
Tablet, oral: 4 mg, 8 mg, 16 mg, 32 mg
Medrol®: 2 mg, 4 mg, 8 mg, 16 mg, 32 mg
Medrol® Dosepak™: 4 mg

MethylTESTOSTERone (meth il tes TOS te rone)

Brand Names: U.S. Android®; Methitest™; Testred®
Pharmacologic Category Androgen
Use
Male: Hypogonadism; delayed puberty; impotence and climacteric symptoms
Female: Palliative treatment of metastatic breast cancer
Unlabeled Use Hypogonadism (male); delayed puberty (male)
Local Anesthetic/Vasoconstrictor Precautions No information available to require special precautions
Effects on Dental Treatment No significant effects or complications reported
Effects on Bleeding No information available to require special precautions
Adverse Effects Frequency not defined.
Male: Gynecomastia, impotence, oligospermia (at high doses), priapism, prostatic carcinoma, prostatic hyperplasia, testicular atrophy, virilism
Female: Atrophy, breast soreness, hirsutism, menstrual problems (amenorrhea), virilism
Cardiovascular: Edema
Central nervous system: Anxiety, depression, headache
Dermatologic: Acne, "male pattern" baldness
Endocrine & metabolic: Hypercalcemia, hypercholesterolemia, libido (changes in)
Gastrointestinal: Nausea, vomiting
Hematologic: Polycythemia, suppression of clotting factors
Hepatic: Cholestatic hepatitis, hepatic dysfunction, hepatic necrosis, hepatocellular neoplasm (rare), jaundice, liver function tests (abnormal), peliosis hepatitis
Neuromuscular & skeletal: Paresthesia
Miscellaneous: Anaphylactoid reactions (rare)
General Dosage Range
Oral:
Adults (females): 50-200 mg/day
Adults (males): 10-50 mg/day
Mechanism of Action Stimulates receptors in organs and tissues to promote growth and development of male sex organs and maintains secondary sex characteristics in androgen-deficient males
Pregnancy Risk Factor X
Pregnancy Considerations Use is contraindicated in women who are or may become pregnant. May cause androgenic effects to the female fetus; clitoral hypertrophy, labial fusion, urogenital sinus defect, vaginal atresia, and ambiguous genitalia have been reported.
Controlled Substance C-III

Metipranolol (met i PRAN oh lol)

Brand Names: U.S. OptiPranolol®
Brand Names: Canada OptiPranolol®
Pharmacologic Category Beta-Blocker, Nonselective; Ophthalmic Agent, Antiglaucoma
Use Treatment of chronic open-angle glaucoma or ocular hypertension
Local Anesthetic/Vasoconstrictor Precautions No information available to require special precautions

Effects on Dental Treatment Metipranolol is a nonselective beta-blocker and may enhance the pressor response to epinephrine, resulting in hypertension and bradycardia. Many nonsteroidal anti-inflammatory drugs, such as ibuprofen and indomethacin, can reduce the hypotensive effect of beta-blockers after 3 or more weeks of therapy with the NSAID. Short-term NSAID use (ie, 3 days) requires no special precautions in patients taking beta-blockers.
Effects on Bleeding No information available to require special precautions
Adverse Effects Frequency not defined.
Cardiovascular: Angina, atrial fibrillation, bradycardia, hypertension, MI, palpitation
Central nervous system: Anxiety, depression, dizziness, headache, nervousness, somnolence
Dermatologic: Rash
Gastrointestinal: Nausea
Neuromuscular & skeletal: Arthritis, myalgia, weakness
Ocular: Abnormal vision, blepharitis, blurred vision, browache, conjunctivitis, discomfort, edema, eyelid dermatitis, photophobia, tearing, uveitis
Respiratory: Bronchitis, cough, dyspnea, epistaxis, rhinitis
Miscellaneous: Allergic reaction
General Dosage Range Ophthalmic: *Adults:* Instill 1 drop into affected eye(s) twice daily
Mechanism of Action Beta-adrenoceptor-blocking agent; lacks intrinsic sympathomimetic activity and membrane-stabilizing effects and possesses only slight local anesthetic activity; mechanism of action of metipranolol in reducing intraocular pressure appears to be via reduced production of aqueous humor. This effect may be related to a reduction in blood flow to the iris root-ciliary body. It remains unclear if the reduction in intraocular pressure observed with beta-blockers is actually secondary to beta-adrenoceptor blockade.
Pharmacodynamics/Kinetics
Onset of Action ≤30 minutes; Peak effect: Maximum: ~2 hours
Duration of Action Intraocular pressure reduction: Up to 24 hours
Half-life Elimination ~3 hours
Pregnancy Risk Factor C
Pregnancy Considerations Adverse events were observed in some animal reproduction studies.

Metoclopramide (met oh KLOE pra mide)

Brand Names: U.S. Metozolv™ ODT; Reglan®
Brand Names: Canada Apo-Metoclop®; Metoclopramide Hydrochloride Injection; Metoclopramide Omega; Nu-Metoclopramide; PMS-Metoclopramide
Pharmacologic Category Antiemetic; Gastrointestinal Agent, Prokinetic
Use
Oral: Symptomatic treatment of diabetic gastroparesis; gastroesophageal reflux
I.V., I.M.: Symptomatic treatment of diabetic gastroparesis; postpyloric placement of enteral feeding tubes; prevention and/or treatment of nausea and vomiting associated with chemotherapy, or postsurgery; to stimulate gastric emptying and intestinal transit of barium during radiological examination of the stomach/small intestine
Unlabeled Use Management of gastroparesis (regardless of etiology)
Local Anesthetic/Vasoconstrictor Precautions No information available to require special precautions

Effects on Dental Treatment Metoclopramide has relatively few adverse effects when used in low doses; however, extrapyramidal effects including akathisia (motor restlessness), acute dystonia (spasmodic contractures), pseudoparkinsonism, and tardive dyskinesia can occur. These effects are more likely in the elderly, patients taking other dopamine antagonists (including antipsychotic agents and some antiemetic agents), and patients with Parkinson's disease. Metoclopramide will increase gastric emptying which will aid in the absorption of orally administered anxiolytic or sedative agents used for minimal or moderate sedation as well as promote the emptying of the stomach following procedures during which blood may be swallowed causing GI upset.

Effects on Bleeding No information available to require special precautions

Adverse Effects Frequency not always defined.
   Cardiovascular: AV block, bradycardia, HF, fluid retention, flushing (following high I.V. doses), hyper-/hypotension, supraventricular tachycardia
   Central nervous system: Drowsiness (~10% to 70%; dose related), acute dystonic reactions (<1% to 25%; dose and age related), fatigue (2% to 10%), lassitude (~10%), restlessness (~10%), headache (4% to 5%), dizziness (1% to 4%), somnolence (2% to 3%), akathisia, confusion, depression, hallucinations (rare), insomnia, neuroleptic malignant syndrome (rare), Parkinsonian-like symptoms, suicidal ideation, seizure, tardive dyskinesia
   Dermatologic: Angioneurotic edema (rare), rash, urticaria
   Endocrine & metabolic: Amenorrhea, galactorrhea, gynecomastia, hyperprolactinemia, impotence
   Gastrointestinal: Nausea (4% to 6%), vomiting (1% to 2%), diarrhea
   Hematologic: Agranulocytosis, leukopenia, neutropenia, porphyria
   Hepatic: Hepatotoxicity (rare)
   Ocular: Visual disturbance
   Respiratory: Bronchospasm, laryngeal edema (rare), laryngospasm (rare)
   Miscellaneous: Allergic reactions, methemoglobinemia, sulfhemoglobinemia

General Dosage Range Dosage adjustment recommended in patients with renal impairment
   I.M.: *Adults:* 10-20 mg as a single dose **or** 10 mg before each meal and at bedtime
   I.V.:
      Children <6 years: 0.1 mg/kg as a single dose
      Children 6-14 years: 2.5-5 mg as a single dose
      Children >14 years: 10 mg as a single dose
      Adults: 10 mg before each meal and at bedtime **or** 1-2 mg/kg every 2-3 hours (maximum: 5 doses daily) **or** 10 mg as a single dose
   Oral: *Adults:* 10-15 mg up to 4 times daily

Mechanism of Action Blocks dopamine receptors and (when given in higher doses) also blocks serotonin receptors in chemoreceptor trigger zone of the CNS; enhances the response to acetylcholine of tissue in upper GI tract causing enhanced motility and accelerated gastric emptying without stimulating gastric, biliary, or pancreatic secretions; increases lower esophageal sphincter tone

Pharmacodynamics/Kinetics
   Onset of Action Oral: 30-60 minutes; I.V.: 1-3 minutes; I.M.: 10-15 minutes
   Duration of Action Therapeutic: 1-2 hours, regardless of route

Half-life Elimination Normal renal function: Children: ~4 hours; Adults: 5-6 hours (may be dose dependent)
Time to Peak Serum: Oral: 1-2 hours
Pregnancy Risk Factor B
Pregnancy Considerations Teratogenic effects were not observed in animal studies; however, there are no adequate and well-controlled studies in pregnant women. Crosses the placenta; available evidence suggests safe use during pregnancy.

Metolazone (me TOLE a zone)

Related Information
   Cardiovascular Diseases *on page 1492*
Brand Names: U.S. Zaroxolyn®
Brand Names: Canada Zaroxolyn®
Pharmacologic Category Diuretic, Thiazide-Related
Use Management of mild-to-moderate hypertension; treatment of edema in heart failure and nephrotic syndrome, impaired renal function

Local Anesthetic/Vasoconstrictor Precautions No information available to require special precautions

Effects on Dental Treatment Key adverse event(s) related to dental treatment: Xerostomia (normal salivary flow resumes upon discontinuation) and orthostatic hypotension.

Effects on Bleeding No information available to require special precautions

Adverse Effects Frequency not defined.
   Cardiovascular: Chest pain/discomfort, necrotizing angiitis, orthostatic hypotension, palpitation, syncope, venous thrombosis, vertigo, volume depletion
   Central nervous system: Chills, depression, dizziness, drowsiness, fatigue, headache, lightheadedness, restlessness
   Dermatologic: Petechiae, photosensitivity, pruritus, purpura, rash, skin necrosis, Stevens-Johnson syndrome, toxic epidermal necrolysis, urticaria
   Endocrine & metabolic: Gout attacks, hypercalcemia, hyperglycemia, hyperuricemia, hypochloremia, hypochloremic alkalosis, hypokalemia, hypomagnesemia, hyponatremia, hypophosphatemia
   Gastrointestinal: Abdominal bloating, abdominal pain, anorexia, constipation, diarrhea, epigastric distress, nausea, pancreatitis, vomiting, xerostomia
   Genitourinary: Impotence
   Hematologic: Agranulocytosis, aplastic/hypoplastic anemia, hemoconcentration, leukopenia, thrombocytopenia
   Hepatic: Cholestatic jaundice, hepatitis
   Neuromuscular & skeletal: Joint pain, muscle cramps/spasm, neuropathy, paresthesia, weakness
   Ocular: Blurred vision (transient)
   Renal: BUN increased, glucosuria

General Dosage Range Oral: *Adults:* 2.5-20 mg every 24 hours

Mechanism of Action Inhibits sodium reabsorption in the distal tubules causing increased excretion of sodium and water, as well as, potassium and hydrogen ions

Pharmacodynamics/Kinetics
   Onset of Action Diuresis: ~60 minutes
   Duration of Action ≥24 hours
   Half-life Elimination 20 hours
   Pregnancy Risk Factor B

◄ **Pregnancy Considerations** Teratogenic effects were not observed in animal studies. Metolazone crosses the placenta and appears in cord blood. Hypoglycemia, hypokalemia, hyponatremia, jaundice, and thrombocytopenia are reported as complications to the fetus or newborn following maternal use of thiazide diuretics.

Metoprolol (me toe PROE lole)

Related Information
Cardiovascular Diseases *on page 1492*
Brand Names: U.S. Lopressor®; Toprol-XL®
Brand Names: Canada Apo-Metoprolol (Type L®); Apo-Metoprolol SR®; Apo-Metoprolol®; Ava-Metoprolol; Ava-Metoprolol (Type L); Betaloc®; Dom-Metoprolol-B; Dom-Metoprolol-L; JAMP-Metoprolol-L; Lopresor SR®; Lopresor®; Metoprolol Tartrate Injection, USP; Metoprolol-25; Metoprolol-L; Mylan-Metoprolol (Type L); Nu-Metop; PMS-Metoprolol-B; PMS-Metoprolol-L; Riva-Metoprolol-L; Sandoz-Metoprolol (Type L); Sandoz-Metoprolol SR; Teva-Metoprolol
Generic Availability (U.S.) Yes
Pharmacologic Category Antianginal Agent; Beta-Blocker, Beta-1 Selective
Use Treatment of angina pectoris, hypertension, or hemodynamically-stable acute myocardial infarction
Extended release: Treatment of angina pectoris or hypertension; to reduce mortality/hospitalization in patients with heart failure (stable NYHA Class II or III) already receiving ACE inhibitors, diuretics, and/or digoxin
Unlabeled Use Treatment of ventricular arrhythmias, atrial ectopy; migraine prophylaxis, essential tremor; prevention of reinfarction and sudden death after myocardial infarction; prevention and treatment of atrial fibrillation and atrial flutter; multifocal atrial tachycardia; symptomatic treatment of hypertrophic obstructive cardiomyopathy; management of thyrotoxicosis
Local Anesthetic/Vasoconstrictor Precautions No information available to require special precautions
Effects on Dental Treatment Metoprolol is a cardioselective beta-blocker. Local anesthetic with vasoconstrictor can be safely used in patients medicated with metoprolol. Nonselective beta-blockers (ie, propranolol, nadolol) enhance the pressor response to epinephrine, resulting in hypertension and bradycardia; this has not been reported for metoprolol. Many nonsteroidal anti-inflammatory drugs, such as ibuprofen and indomethacin, can reduce the hypotensive effect of beta-blockers after 3 or more weeks of therapy with the NSAID. Short-term NSAID use (ie, 3 days) requires no special precautions in patients taking beta-blockers.
Effects on Bleeding No information available to require special precautions
Adverse Effects Frequency may not be defined.
Cardiovascular: Hypotension (1% to 27%), bradycardia (2% to 16%), first-degree heart block (P-R interval ≥0.26 sec; 5%), arterial insufficiency (usually Raynaud type; 1%), chest pain (1%), CHF (1%), edema (peripheral; 1%), palpitation (1%), syncope (1%)
Central nervous system: Dizziness (2% to 10%), fatigue (1% to 10%), depression (5%), confusion, hallucinations, headache, insomnia, memory loss (short-term), nightmares, sleep disturbances, somnolence, vertigo
Dermatology: Pruritus (5%), rash (5%), photosensitivity, psoriasis exacerbated
Endocrine & metabolic: Libido decreased, Peyronie's disease (<1%), diabetes exacerbated

Gastrointestinal: Diarrhea (5%), constipation (1%), flatulence (1%), gastrointestinal pain (1%), heartburn (1%), nausea (1%), xerostomia (1%), vomiting
Hematologic: Claudication
Neuromuscular & skeletal: Musculoskeletal pain
Ocular: Blurred vision, visual disturbances
Otic: Tinnitus
Respiratory: Dyspnea (1% to 3%), bronchospasm (1%), wheezing (1%), rhinitis, shortness of breath
Miscellaneous: Cold extremities (1%)

Other events reported with beta-blockers: Catatonia, emotional lability, fever, hypersensitivity reactions, laryngospasm, nonthrombocytopenic purpura, respiratory distress, thrombocytopenic purpura
Dosage
Children: Hypertension: Oral:
1-17 years: Immediate release tablet: (National High Blood Pressure Education Program Working Group on High Blood Pressure in Children and Adolescents, 2004): Initial: 1-2 mg/kg/day; maximum 6 mg/kg/day (≤200 mg/day); administer in 2 divided doses
≥6 years: Extended release tablet: Initial: 1 mg/kg once daily (maximum initial dose: 50 mg/day). Adjust dose based on patient response (maximum: 2 mg/kg/day or 200 mg/day)
Adults:
Angina: Oral:
Immediate release: Initial: 50 mg twice daily; usual dosage range: 50-200 mg twice daily; maximum: 400 mg/day; increase dose at weekly intervals to desired effect
Extended release: Initial: 100 mg/day (maximum: 400 mg/day)
Atrial fibrillation/flutter (ventricular rate control), supraventricular tachycardia (SVT) (acute treatment; unlabeled use; Antman, 2004; Fuster, 2006; Neumar, 2010): I.V.: 2.5-5 mg every 2-5 minutes (maximum total dose: 15 mg over a 10-15 minute period). **Note:** Initiate cautiously in patients with concomitant heart failure; avoid in patients with decompensated heart failure.
Maintenance: Oral (immediate release): 25-100 mg twice daily
Heart failure: Oral (extended release): Initial: 25 mg once daily (reduce to 12.5 mg once daily in NYHA class higher than class II); may double dosage every 2 weeks as tolerated (target dose: 200 mg/day)
Hypertension: Oral:
Immediate release: Initial: 50 mg twice daily; effective dosage range: 100-450 mg/day in 2-3 divided doses; increase dose at weekly intervals to desired effect; maximum: 450 mg/day; usual dosage range (JNC 7): 50-100 mg/day
Extended release: Initial: 25-100 mg once daily; increase doses at weekly (or longer) intervals to desired effect; maximum: 400 mg/day; usual dosage range (JNC 7): 50-100 mg/day
Hypertension/ventricular rate control: I.V. (in patients having nonfunctioning GI tract): Initial: 1.25-5 mg every 6-12 hours; titrate initial dose to response. Initially, low doses may be appropriate to establish response; however, although not routine, up to 15 mg administered as frequently as every 3 hours has been employed in patients with refractory tachycardia.

Myocardial infarction:

Acute: I.V.: 5 mg every 2 minutes for 3 doses in early treatment of myocardial infarction; thereafter, give 50 mg orally every 6 hours beginning 15 minutes after last I.V. dose and continue for 48 hours; then administer a maintenance dose of 100 mg twice daily. **Note:** Do not initiate this regimen in those with signs of heart failure, a low output state, increased risk of cardiogenic shock, or other contraindications (eg, second- or third-degree heart block). If initial I.V. dosing is not tolerated, may give 25-50 mg orally (depending on degree of intolerance) every 6 hours beginning 15 minutes after the last I.V. dose or as soon as clinical condition permits.

Secondary prevention (unlabeled use; Olsson, 1992): Oral: Immediate release: 25-100 mg twice daily; optimize dose based on heart rate and blood pressure; continue indefinitely.

Thyrotoxicosis (unlabeled use): Oral: Immediate release: 25-50 mg every 6 hours; may also consider administering extended release formulation (Bahn, 2011)

Elderly: Hypertension: Initiate at the lower end of the dosage range and titrate to response

Note: Switching dosage forms:

When switching from immediate release metoprolol to extended release, the same total daily dose of metoprolol should be used.

When switching between oral and intravenous dosage forms, equivalent beta-blocking effect is achieved when doses in a 2.5:1 (Oral:I.V.) ratio is used. For example, if the patient is receiving an oral dose of 25 mg twice daily (50 mg/day), this would translate to 5 mg I.V. every 6 hours; consider reducing initial I.V. dose to evaluate patient response.

Dosage adjustment in renal impairment: No dosage adjustment necessary.

Dosage adjustment in hepatic impairment: No dosage adjustment provided in manufacturer's labeling. However, reduced dose may be necessary due to extensive hepatic metabolism.

Mechanism of Action Selective inhibitor of beta$_1$-adrenergic receptors; competitively blocks beta$_1$-receptors, with little or no effect on beta$_2$-receptors at doses <100 mg; does not exhibit any membrane stabilizing or intrinsic sympathomimetic activity

Contraindications

Hypersensitivity to metoprolol, any component of the formulation, or other beta-blockers

Note: Additional contraindications are formulation and/or indication specific.

Immediate release tablets/injectable formulation:

Hypertension and angina: Sinus bradycardia; second- and third-degree heart block; cardiogenic shock; overt heart failure; sick sinus syndrome (except in patients with a functioning artificial pacemaker); severe peripheral arterial disease; pheochromocytoma (without alpha blockade)

Myocardial infarction: Severe sinus bradycardia (heart rate <45 beats/minute); significant first-degree heart block (P-R interval ≥0.24 seconds); second- and third-degree heart block; systolic blood pressure <100 mm Hg; moderate-to-severe cardiac failure

Extended release tablet: Severe bradycardia, second- and third degree heart block; cardiogenic shock; decompensated heart failure; sick sinus syndrome (except in patients with a functioning artificial pacemaker)

Warnings/Precautions [U.S. Boxed Warning]: Beta-blocker therapy should not be withdrawn abruptly (particularly in patients with CAD), but gradually tapered over 1-2 weeks to avoid acute tachycardia, hypertension, and/or ischemia. Consider pre-existing conditions such as sick sinus syndrome before initiating. Metoprolol commonly produces mild first-degree heart block (P-R interval >0.2-0.24 sec). May also produce severe first- (P-R interval ≥0.26 sec), second-, or third-degree heart block. Patients with acute MI (especially right ventricular MI) have a high risk of developing heart block of varying degrees. If severe heart block occurs, metoprolol should be discontinued and measures to increase heart rate should be employed. Symptomatic hypotension may occur with use. May precipitate or aggravate symptoms of arterial insufficiency in patients with PVD and Raynaud's disease; use with caution and monitor for progression of arterial obstruction. Potentially significant interactions may exist, requiring dose or frequency adjustment, additional monitoring, and/or selection of alternative therapy. Consult drug interactions database for more detailed information.

In general, beta-blockers should be avoided in patients with bronchospastic disease. Metoprolol, with B$_1$ selectivity, should be used cautiously in bronchospastic disease with close monitoring. Use cautiously in patients with diabetes because it can mask prominent hypoglycemic symptoms. May mask signs of hyperthyroidism (eg, tachycardia); if hyperthyroidism is suspected, carefully manage and monitor; abrupt withdrawal may exacerbate symptoms of hyperthyroidism or precipitate thyroid storm. Alterations in thyroid function tests may be observed. Use caution with hepatic dysfunction. Use with caution in patients with myasthenia gravis or psychiatric disease (may cause CNS depression). Although perioperative beta-blocker therapy is recommended prior to elective surgery in selected patients, use of high-dose extended release metoprolol in patients naïve to beta-blocker therapy undergoing noncardiac surgery has been associated with bradycardia, hypotension, stroke, and death. Chronic beta-blocker therapy should not be routinely withdrawn prior to major surgery. Use of beta-blockers may unmask cardiac failure in patients without a history of dysfunction. Adequate alpha-blockade is required prior to use of any beta-blocker for patients with untreated pheochromocytoma. May induce or exacerbate psoriasis. Use caution with history of severe anaphylaxis to allergens; patients taking beta-blockers may become more sensitive to repeated allergen challenges. Treatment of anaphylaxis (eg, epinephrine) in patients taking beta-blockers may be ineffective or promote undesirable effects. Bradycardia may be observed more frequently in elderly patients (>65 years of age); dosage reductions may be necessary.

Extended release: Use with caution in patients with compensated heart failure; monitor for a worsening of heart failure.

◀ **Drug Interactions**

Metabolism/Transport Effects Substrate of CYP2C19 (minor), CYP2D6 (major); **Note:** Assignment of Major/Minor substrate status based on clinically relevant drug interaction potential; **Inhibits** CYP2D6 (weak)

Avoid Concomitant Use

Avoid concomitant use of Metoprolol with any of the following: Floctafenine; Methacholine

Increased Effect/Toxicity

Metoprolol may increase the levels/effects of: Alpha-/Beta-Agonists (Direct-Acting); Alpha1-Blockers; Alpha2-Agonists; Amifostine; Antihypertensives; Antipsychotic Agents (Phenothiazines); ARIPiprazole; Bupivacaine; Cardiac Glycosides; Cholinergic Agonists; Ergot Derivatives; Fingolimod; Hypotensive Agents; Insulin; Lidocaine (Systemic); Lidocaine (Topical); Mepivacaine; Methacholine; Midodrine; RiTUXimab; Sulfonylureas

The levels/effects of Metoprolol may be increased by: Acetylcholinesterase Inhibitors; Alpha2-Agonists; Aminoquinolines (Antimalarial); Amiodarone; Anilidopiperidine Opioids; Antipsychotic Agents (Phenothiazines); Calcium Channel Blockers (Dihydropyridine); Calcium Channel Blockers (Nondihydropyridine); CYP2D6 Inhibitors; Darunavir; Diazoxide; Dipyridamole; Disopyramide; Dronedarone; Floctafenine; Herbs (Hypotensive Properties); MAO Inhibitors; Mirabegron; Pentoxifylline; Phosphodiesterase 5 Inhibitors; Propafenone; Prostacyclin Analogues; QuiNIDine; Reserpine; Selective Serotonin Reuptake Inhibitors

Decreased Effect

Metoprolol may decrease the levels/effects of: Beta2-Agonists; Theophylline Derivatives

The levels/effects of Metoprolol may be decreased by: Barbiturates; Herbs (Hypertensive Properties); Methylphenidate; Mirabegron; Nonsteroidal Anti-Inflammatory Agents; Peginterferon Alfa-2b; Rifamycin Derivatives; Yohimbine

Ethanol/Nutrition/Herb Interactions

Food: Food increases absorption. Metoprolol serum levels may be increased if taken with food. Management: Take immediate release tartrate tablets with food; succinate can be taken with or without food.

Herb/Nutraceutical: Some herbal medications may worsen hypertension (eg, licorice); others may increase the antihypertensive effect of metoprolol (eg, shepherd's purse). Management: Avoid bayberry, blue cohosh, cayenne, ephedra, ginger, ginseng (American), gotu kola, licorice, and yohimbe. Avoid black cohosh, California poppy, coleus, golden seal, hawthorn, mistletoe, periwinkle, quinine, and shepherd's purse.

Dietary Considerations Immediate release tablets should be taken with food. Extended release tablets may be taken without regard to meals.

Pharmacodynamics/Kinetics

Onset of Action Peak effect: Oral: 1-2 hours (Regårdh, 1980); I.V.: 20 minutes (when infused over 10 minutes)

Duration of Action Oral: Immediate release: Variable (dose-related; 50% reduction in maximum heart rate after single doses of 20, 50, and 100 mg occurred at 3.3, 5, and 6.4 hours, respectively), Extended release: ~24 hours; I.V.: 5-8 hours

Half-life Elimination 3-4 hours (7-9 hours in poor CYP2D6 metabolizers)

Pregnancy Risk Factor C

Pregnancy Considerations Adverse events were observed in animal studies; therefore, the manufacturer classifies metoprolol as pregnancy category C. Metoprolol crosses the placenta and can be detected in cord blood, amniotic fluid, and the serum of newborn infants. In a cohort study, an increased risk of cardiovascular defects was observed following maternal use of beta-blockers during pregnancy. Intrauterine growth restriction (IUGR), small placentas, as well as fetal/neonatal bradycardia, hypoglycemia, and/or respiratory depression have been observed following *in utero* exposure to beta-blockers as a class. Adequate facilities for monitoring infants at birth should be available. Untreated chronic maternal hypertension and pre-eclampsia are also associated with adverse events in the fetus, infant, and mother. The clearance of metoprolol is increased and serum concentrations and AUC of metoprolol are decreased during pregnancy. Metoprolol has been evaluated for the treatment of hypertension in pregnancy, but other agents may be more appropriate for use.

Lactation Enters breast milk/use caution (AAP rates "compatible"; AAP 2001 update pending)

Breast-Feeding Considerations Small amounts of metoprolol can be detected in breast milk. The manufacturer recommends that caution be exercised when administering metoprolol to nursing women.

Dosage Forms

Injection, solution: 1 mg/mL (5 mL)

  Lopressor®: 1 mg/mL (5 mL)

Injection, solution [preservative free]: 1 mg/mL (5 mL)

Tablet, oral: 25 mg, 50 mg, 100 mg

  Lopressor®: 50 mg, 100 mg

Tablet, extended release, oral: 25 mg, 50 mg, 100 mg, 200 mg

  Toprol-XL®: 25 mg, 50 mg, 100 mg, 200 mg

References

Foster CA and Aston SJ, "Propranolol-Epinephrine Interaction: A Potential Disaster," *Plast Reconstr Surg*, 1983, 72(1):74-8.

Wong DG, Spence JD, Lamki L, et al, "Effect of Nonsteroidal Anti-inflammatory Drugs on Control of Hypertension of Beta-Blockers and Diuretics," *Lancet*, 1986, 1(8488):997-1001.

Wynn RL, "Dental Nonsteroidal Anti-inflammatory Drugs and Prostaglandin-Based Drug Interactions, Part Two," *Gen Dent*, 1992, 40 (2):104, 106, 108.

Wynn RL, "Epinephrine Interactions With Beta-Blockers," *Gen Dent*, 1994, 42(1):16, 18.

Metoprolol and Hydrochlorothiazide

(me toe PROE lole & hye droe klor oh THYE a zide)

Related Information

Hydrochlorothiazide *on page 687*

Metoprolol *on page 908*

Brand Names: U.S. Dutoprol™; Lopressor HCT®

Pharmacologic Category Beta-Blocker, Beta-1 Selective; Diuretic, Thiazide

Use Treatment of hypertension (not recommended for initial treatment)

Local Anesthetic/Vasoconstrictor Precautions No information available to require special precautions

Effects on Dental Treatment

Metoprolol: Metoprolol is a cardioselective beta-blocker. Local anesthetic with vasoconstrictor can be safely used in patients medicated with metoprolol. Nonselective beta-blockers (ie, propranolol, nadolol) enhance the pressor response to epinephrine, resulting in hypertension and bradycardia; this has not been reported for metoprolol. Many nonsteroidal anti-inflammatory drugs, such as ibuprofen and indomethacin, can reduce the hypotensive effect of beta-blockers after 3 or more weeks of therapy with the NSAID. Short-term NSAID use (ie, 3 days) requires no special precautions in patients taking beta-blockers.

Hydrochlorothiazide: Key adverse event(s) related to dental treatment: Orthostatic hypotension and hypotension.

Effects on Bleeding No information available to require special precautions

Adverse Effects Reactions noted here have been reported with the combination product; see individual drug monographs for additional adverse reactions that may be expected from each agent.

1% to 10%:

Cardiovascular: Bradycardia (6%), edema (1%)

Central nervous system: Drowsiness (10%), headache (10%), vertigo (10%), dizziness (3% to 10%), fatigue (3% to 10%), abnormal dreams (1%)

Dermatologic: Purpura (1%)

Endocrine & metabolic: Hypokalemia (<10%), gout (1%)

Gastrointestinal: Anorexia (1%), constipation (1%), diarrhea (1%), nausea (1%), vomiting (1%), xerostomia (1%)

Genitourinary: Impotence (1%)

Neuromuscular & skeletal: Back pain (≤2%), myalgia (1%)

Ocular: Blurred vision (1%)

Otic: Earache (1%), tinnitus (1%)

Respiratory: Nasopharyngitis (≤3%), dyspnea (1%)

Miscellaneous: Flu-like syndrome (10%), diaphoresis (1%), exercise tolerance decreased (1%)

General Dosage Range Oral: *Adults:*

Metoprolol **tartrate** (immediate release) 50-200 mg and hydrochlorothiazide 12.5-50 mg administered daily as single or 2 divided doses (maximum: 200 mg/day [metoprolol tartrate] and 50 mg/day [hydrochlorothiazide])

Metoprolol **succinate** (extended release) 25-200 mg and hydrochlorothiazide 12.5-25 mg once daily (maximum: 200 mg [metoprolol succinate] and 25 mg/day [hydrochlorothiazide])

Mechanism of Action See individual agents.

Pregnancy Risk Factor C/D (expert analysis)

Pregnancy Considerations See individual agents.

MetroNIDAZOLE (Systemic)

(met roe NYE da zole)

Related Information

Bacterial Infections *on page 1562*

Gastrointestinal Disorders *on page 1512*

Periodontal Diseases *on page 1570*

Ulcerative, Erosive, and Painful Oral Mucosal Disorders *on page 1578*

Related Sample Prescriptions

Bacterial Infections and Periodontal Diseases *on page 1609*

Brand Names: U.S. Flagyl®; Flagyl® 375; Flagyl® ER

Brand Names: Canada Apo-Metronidazole®; Flagyl®; Florazole® ER

Generic Availability (U.S.) Yes: Excludes capsule, extended release tablet

Pharmacologic Category Amebicide; Antibiotic, Miscellaneous; Antiprotozoal, Nitroimidazole

Dental Use Treatment of oral soft tissue infections due to anaerobic bacteria including all anaerobic cocci, anaerobic gram-negative bacilli (*Bacteroides*), and gram-positive spore-forming bacilli (*Clostridium*). Useful as single agent or in combination with amoxicillin, amoxicillin/clavulanic acid, or ciprofloxacin in the

treatment of periodontitis associated with presence of *Actinobacillus actinomycetemcomitans* (AA). In aggressive periodontitis, greatest benefit is seen after 3 months of therapy. No benefit was seen after 6 months of therapy (Varela, 2011).

Use Treatment of susceptible anaerobic bacterial and protozoal infections in the following conditions: Amebiasis, symptomatic and asymptomatic trichomoniasis; skin and skin structure infections, bone and joint infections, CNS infections, endocarditis, gynecologic infections, intra-abdominal infections (as part of combination regimen), respiratory tract infections (lower), systemic anaerobic infections; treatment of antibiotic-associated pseudomembranous colitis (AAPC); as part of a multidrug regimen for *H. pylori* eradication to reduce the risk of duodenal ulcer recurrence; surgical prophylaxis (colorectal); useful as single agent or in combination with amoxicillin, amoxicillin/clavulanic acid, or ciprofloxacin in the treatment of periodontitis associated with the presence of *Actinobacillus actinomycetemcomitans* (AA).

Unlabeled Use Crohn's disease

Local Anesthetic/Vasoconstrictor Precautions No information available to require special precautions

Effects on Dental Treatment Key adverse event(s) related to dental treatment: Unusual/metallic taste, glossitis, stomatitis, xerostomia (normal salivary flow resumes upon discontinuation), and furry tongue.

Effects on Bleeding No information available to require special precautions

Adverse Effects Frequency not always defined.

Cardiovascular: Flattening of the T-wave, flushing, syncope

Central nervous system: Aseptic meningitis, ataxia, confusion, coordination impaired, depression, dizziness, encephalopathy, fever, headache, insomnia, irritability, seizure, vertigo

Dermatologic: Erythematous rash, pruritus, Stevens-Johnson syndrome, toxic epidermal necrolysis, urticaria

Endocrine & metabolic: Disulfiram-like reaction, dysmenorrhea

Gastrointestinal: Nausea (~12%), anorexia, abdominal cramping, constipation, diarrhea, epigastric distress, furry tongue, glossitis, pancreatitis (rare), proctitis, stomatitis, unusual/metallic taste, vomiting, xerostomia

Genitourinary: Cystitis, darkened urine (rare), dyspareunia, dysuria, incontinence, libido decreased, pelvic pressure, polyuria, vaginal dryness, vaginitis

Hematologic: Neutropenia (reversible), thrombocytopenia (reversible, rare)

Local: Thrombophlebitis

Neuromuscular & skeletal: Dysarthria, peripheral neuropathy, weakness

Ocular: Optic neuropathy

Respiratory: Nasal congestion, pharyngitis, rhinitis, sinusitis, pharyngitis

Miscellaneous: Flu-like syndrome, joint pains resembling serum sickness, moniliasis

Dental Usual Dosage

Anaerobic infections/abscess: Adults: Oral, I.V.: 500 mg every 6-8 hours, not to exceed 4 g/day

Periodontitis treatment (monotherapy or combination) associated with the presence of *Actinobacillus actinomycetemcomitans* (AA): Adults: Oral: 250-500 mg every 8 hours for 8-10 days used in addition to scaling and root planing (Varela, 2011)

Dosage

Infants and Children:

Amebiasis: Oral: 35-50 mg/kg/day in divided doses every 8 hours for 10 days

Trichomoniasis: Oral: 15-30 mg/kg/day in divided doses every 8 hours for 7 days

Anaerobic infections:

Oral: 15-35 mg/kg/day in divided doses every 8 hours

I.V.: 30 mg/kg/day in divided doses every 6 hours

Clostridium difficile (antibiotic-associated colitis): Oral: 30 mg/kg/day divided every 6 hours for 7-10 days; maximum dose: 2 g/day

Adults:

Anaerobic infections (diverticulitis, intra-abdominal, peritonitis, cholangitis, or abscess): Oral, I.V.: 500 mg every 6-8 hours, not to exceed 4 g/day; **Note:** Initial: 1 g I.V. loading dose may be administered

Amebiasis: Oral: 500-750 mg every 8 hours for 5-10 days

Antibiotic-associated pseudomembranous colitis: IDSA Guidelines (Cohen, 2010):

Mild-to-moderate infection: Oral: 500 mg 3 times/day for 10-14 days

Severe complicated infection: I.V.: 500 mg 3 times/day with oral vancomycin (recommended agent) for 10-14 days

Note: Due to the emergence of a new strain of *C. difficile*, some clinicians recommend converting to oral vancomycin therapy if the patient does not show a clear clinical response after 2 days of metronidazole therapy.

Giardiasis: 500 mg twice daily for 5-7 days

Helicobacter pylori eradication: Oral: 250-500 mg with meals and at bedtime for 14 days; requires combination therapy with at least one other antibiotic and an acid-suppressing agent (proton pump inhibitor or H_2 blocker)

Intra-abdominal infection, complicated, community-acquired, mild-to-moderate (in combination with cephalosporin or fluoroquinolone): I.V.: 500 mg every 8-12 hours **or** 1.5 g every 24 hours for for 4-7 days (provided source controlled)

Bacterial vaginosis or vaginitis due to *Gardnerella*, *Mobiluncus*: Oral: 500 mg twice daily (regular release) or 750 mg once daily (extended release tablet) for 7 days

Pelvic inflammatory disease (unlabeled use): Oral: 500 mg twice daily for 14 days (in combination with a cephalosporin and doxycycline) (CDC, 2010)

Periodontitis treatment (monotherapy or combination) associated with presence of *Actinobacillus actinomycetemcomitans* (AA): Oral: 250-500 mg every 8 hours for 8-10 days used in addition to scaling and root planing (Varela, 2011)

Trichomoniasis: Oral: 250 mg every 8 hours for 7 days **or** 375 mg twice daily for 7 days **or** 2 g as a single dose **or** 1 g twice daily for 2 doses (on same day)

Urethritis (unlabeled use): Oral: 2 g as a single dose with azithromycin (CDC, 2010)

Surgical prophylaxis (colorectal): I.V. 15 mg/kg 1 hour prior to surgery; followed by 7.5 mg/kg 6 and 12 hours after initial dose

Elderly: Use lower end of dosing recommendations for adults, do not administer as a single dose

Dosage adjustment in renal impairment: Cl_{cr} <10 mL/minute (not on dialysis): Recommendations vary: To reduce possible accumulation in patients receiving multiple doses, consider reduction to 50% of dose or administer normal dose every 12 hours; **Note:** Dosage reduction is unnecessary in short courses of therapy. Some references do not recommend reduction at any level of renal impairment (Lamp, 1999).

Intermittent hemodialysis (IHD) (administer after hemodialysis on dialysis days): Dialyzable (50% to 100%): 500 mg every 8-12 hours. **Note:** Dosing regimen highly dependent on clinical indication (trichomoniasis vs *C. difficile* colitis) (Heintz, 2009). **Note:** Dosing dependent on the assumption of thrice weekly, complete IHD sessions.

Peritoneal dialysis (PD): Dose as for Cl_{cr} <10 mL/minute

Continuous renal replacement therapy (CRRT) (Heintz, 2009; Trotman, 2005): Drug clearance is highly dependent on the method of renal replacement, filter type, and flow rate. Appropriate dosing requires close monitoring of pharmacologic response, signs of adverse reactions due to drug accumulation, as well as drug concentrations in relation to target trough (if appropriate). The following are general recommendations only (based on dialysate flow/ultrafiltration rates of 1-2 L/hour and minimal residual renal function) and should not supersede clinical judgment:

CVVH/CVVHD/CVVHDF: 500 mg every 6-12 hours (or per clinical indication; dosage reduction generally not necessary)

Dosage adjustment in hepatic disease: No specific dosage adjustment provided in the manufacturer's labeling; however, reduce dosage in severe liver disease. Use with caution.

Mechanism of Action After diffusing into the organism, interacts with DNA to cause a loss of helical DNA structure and strand breakage resulting in inhibition of protein synthesis and cell death in susceptible organisms

Contraindications Hypersensitivity to metronidazole, nitroimidazole derivatives, or any component of the formulation; pregnancy (first trimester)

Warnings/Precautions Use with caution in patients with severe liver impairment due to potential accumulation, blood dyscrasias; history of seizures, CHF or other sodium-retaining states; reduce dosage in patients with severe liver impairment, CNS disease, and consider dosage reduction in longer-term therapy with severe renal failure (Cl_{cr} <10 mL/minute); if *H. pylori* is not eradicated in patients being treated with metronidazole in a regimen, it should be assumed that metronidazole-resistance has occurred and it should not again be used; aseptic meningitis, encephalopathy, seizures, and neuropathies have been reported especially with increased doses and chronic treatment; monitor and consider discontinuation of therapy if symptoms occur.

[U.S. Boxed Warning]: Possibly carcinogenic based on animal data. Prolonged use may result in fungal or bacterial superinfection, including *C. difficile*-associated diarrhea (CDAD) and pseudomembranous colitis; CDAD has been observed >2 months postantibiotic treatment. The Infectious Disease Society of America (IDSA) recommends the use of oral metronidazole for initial treatment of mild-to-moderate *C. difficile* infection and the use of oral vancomycin for initial treatment of severe *C. difficile* infection with or without I.V. metronidazole depending on the presence of complications. May treat recurrent mild-to-moderate infection once with oral metronidazole; avoid use beyond first reoccurrence due to potential cumulative neurotoxicity (Cohen, 2010). Candidiasis infection (known or unknown) maybe more prominent during metronidazole treatment, antifungal treatment required. Disulfiram-like reactions to ethanol have been reported with oral metronidazole; avoid alcoholic beverages during therapy

Drug Interactions

Metabolism/Transport Effects Inhibits CYP2C9 (weak), CYP3A4 (moderate)

Avoid Concomitant Use

Avoid concomitant use of MetroNIDAZOLE (Systemic) with any of the following: BCG; Bosutinib; Disulfiram; Ivabradine; Lomitapide; Pimozide; Tolvaptan

Increased Effect/Toxicity

MetroNIDAZOLE (Systemic) may increase the levels/ effects of: Alcohol (Ethyl); ARIPiprazole; Avanafil; Bosutinib; Budesonide (Systemic, Oral Inhalation); Busulfan; Calcineurin Inhibitors; Colchicine; CYP3A4 Substrates; Eplerenone; Everolimus; FentaNYL; Fluorouracil (Systemic); Fosphenytoin; Halofantrine; Ivabradine; Ivacaftor; Lomitapide; Lurasidone; Phenytoin; Pimecrolimus; Pimozide; Propafenone; Ranolazine; Salmeterol; Saxagliptin; Tipranavir; Tolvaptan; Vilazodone; Vitamin K Antagonists; Zuclopenthixol

The levels/effects of MetroNIDAZOLE (Systemic) may be increased by: Disulfiram; Mebendazole

Decreased Effect

MetroNIDAZOLE (Systemic) may decrease the levels/ effects of: BCG; Ifosfamide; Mycophenolate; Sodium Picosulfate; Typhoid Vaccine

The levels/effects of MetroNIDAZOLE (Systemic) may be decreased by: Fosphenytoin; PHENobarbital; Phenytoin

Ethanol/Nutrition/Herb Interactions

Ethanol: The manufacturer recommends to avoid all ethanol or any ethanol-containing drugs (may cause disulfiram-like reaction characterized by flushing, headache, nausea, vomiting, sweating, or tachycardia).

Food: Peak antibiotic serum concentration lowered and delayed, but total drug absorbed not affected.

Dietary Considerations Take on an empty stomach. Drug may cause GI upset; if GI upset occurs, take with food. Extended release tablets should be taken on an empty stomach (1 hour before or 2 hours after meals). Some products may contain sodium. The manufacturer recommends that ethanol be avoided during treatment and for 3 days after therapy is complete.

Pharmacodynamics/Kinetics

Half-life Elimination Neonates: 25-75 hours; Others: 6-8 hours, prolonged with hepatic impairment; End-stage renal disease: 21 hours

Time to Peak Serum: Oral: Immediate release: 1-2 hours

Pregnancy Risk Factor B

Pregnancy Considerations Teratogenic effects have not been observed in animal reproduction studies. Metronidazole crosses the placenta and rapidly distributes into the fetal circulation. Although there have been a few reports of facial anomalies after *in utero* exposure, most studies have not found an increased risk of congenital abnormalities following maternal use of metronidazole during the first trimester of pregnancy. In studies that included women taking metronidazole during all trimesters of pregnancy, an increased risk of adverse fetal and neonatal outcomes has not been observed. Because metronidazole has been carcinogenic in some animal species, concern has been raised whether metronidazole should be used during pregnancy; however, a strong carcinogenic potential in humans has not been observed, including one study of prenatal exposure.

Metronidazole pharmacokinetics are similar between pregnant and nonpregnant patients. Bacterial vaginosis has been associated with adverse pregnancy outcomes (including preterm labor); metronidazole is recommended for the treatment of symptomatic bacterial vaginosis in pregnant patients. Vaginal trichomoniasis has been also associated with adverse pregnancy outcomes (including preterm labor). Treatment may relieve symptoms and prevent further sexual transmission; however, metronidazole has not resulted in reduced perinatal morbidity and should not be used solely to prevent preterm delivery. Some clinicians consider deferring therapy in asymptomatic women until >37 weeks gestation. Use of oral metronidazole is contraindicated during the first trimester (per the FDA approved labeling). Consult current CDC guidelines for appropriate use in pregnant women.

Lactation Enters breast milk/not recommended (AAP rates "of concern"; AAP 2001 update pending)

Breast-Feeding Considerations Metronidazole and its active metabolite are measurable in the breast milk and infant plasma. Milk concentrations are similar to those in the maternal plasma and are highly variable. Peak concentrations of metronidazole in breast milk occur ~2-4 hours after the oral dose. In studies, the calculated relative infant doses have ranged from 0.13% to 36% of the weight-adjusted maternal dose. Use of metronidazole in a lactating patient is not recommended by the manufacturer. If metronidazole is given, breast-feeding should be withheld for 12-24 hours after the dose (CDC, 2010).

Dosage Forms

Capsule, oral:
Flagyl® 375: 375 mg

Infusion, premixed iso-osmotic sodium chloride solution: 500 mg (100 mL)

Tablet, oral: 250 mg, 500 mg
Flagyl®: 250 mg, 500 mg

Tablet, extended release, oral:
Flagyl® ER: 750 mg

References

Eisenberg L, Suchow R, Coles RS, et al, "The Effects of Metronidazole Administration on Clinical and Microbiologic Parameters of Periodontal Disease," *Clin Prev Dent,* 1991, 13(1):28-34.

Herrera D, Sanz M, Jepsen S, et al, "A Systematic Review on the Effect of Systemic Antimicrobials as an Adjunct to Scaling and Root Planing in Periodontitis Patients," *J Clin Periodontol,* 2002, 29(Suppl 3):136-59.

Loesche WJ, Giordano JR, Hujoel P, et al, "Metronidazole in Periodontitis: Reduced Need for Surgery," *J Clin Periodontol,* 1992, 19 (2):103-12.

Loesche WJ, Schmidt E, Smith BA, et al, "Effects of Metronidazole on Periodontal Treatment Needs," *J Periodontol,* 1991, 62(4):247-57.

Varela VM, Heller D, Silva-Senem MX, et al, "Systemic Antimicrobials Adjunctive to a Repeated Mechanical and Antiseptic Therapy for Aggressive Periodontitis: A 6-Month Randomized Controlled Trial," *J Periodontol,* 2011, 82(8):1121-30.

Metronidazole and Nystatin
(met roe NYE da zole & nye STAT in)

Related Information

Nystatin (Topical) *on page 995*

Brand Names: Canada Flagystatin®

Pharmacologic Category Antifungal Agent, Vaginal; Antiprotozoal, Nitroimidazole

Use Treatment of mixed vaginal infection due to *T. vaginalis* and *C. albicans*

Local Anesthetic/Vasoconstrictor Precautions No information available to require special precautions

Effects on Dental Treatment Key adverse event(s) related to dental treatment: Taste disturbances (bitter) and coated tongue.

Effects on Bleeding No information available to require special precautions

Adverse Effects See individual agents.

General Dosage Range Intravaginal: *Adults:* Insert 1 applicatorful or tablet daily

Mechanism of Action See individual agents.

◀ **Pregnancy Considerations** Refer to individual agents.
Product Availability Not available in U.S.

Metyrosine (me TYE roe seen)

Brand Names: U.S. Demser®
Pharmacologic Category Tyrosine Hydroxylase Inhibitor
Use Short-term management of pheochromocytoma before surgery, long-term management when surgery is contraindicated or when chronic malignant pheochromocytoma exists
Local Anesthetic/Vasoconstrictor Precautions No information available to require special precautions
Effects on Dental Treatment Key adverse event(s) related to dental treatment: Xerostomia (normal salivary flow resumes upon discontinuation).
Effects on Bleeding No information available to require special precautions
Adverse Effects Frequency not always defined.
Cardiovascular: Peripheral edema
Central nervous system: Extrapyramidal symptoms (~10%), anxiety, confusion, depression, disorientation, headache, hallucination, parkinsonism, sedation
Dermatologic: Urticaria
Endocrine & metabolic: Galactorrhea, edema of the breasts
Gastrointestinal: Diarrhea (~10%), abdominal pain, nausea, salivation decreased, vomiting, xerostomia
Genitourinary: Crystalluria, dysuria, ejaculatory disturbances, impotence
Hematologic: Anemia, eosinophilia, thrombocytopenia, thrombocytosis
Hepatic: AST increased
Renal: Hematuria
Respiratory: Nasal congestion, pharyngeal edema
Miscellaneous: Hypersensitivity reactions, hyperstimulation after withdrawal
General Dosage Range Oral: *Children ≥12 years and Adults:* Initial: 250 mg 4 times/day; Usual maintenance: 2-3 g/day in 4 divided doses (maximum: 4 g/day)
Mechanism of Action Blocks the rate-limiting step in the biosynthetic pathway of catecholamines. It is a tyrosine hydroxylase inhibitor, blocking the conversion of tyrosine to dihydroxyphenylalanine. This inhibition results in decreased levels of endogenous catecholamines. Catecholamine biosynthesis is reduced by 35% to 80% in patients treated with metyrosine at recommended doses.
Pharmacodynamics/Kinetics
Half-life Elimination ~3-4 hours
Pregnancy Risk Factor C
Pregnancy Considerations Animal reproduction studies have not been conducted.

Mexiletine (meks IL e teen)

Brand Names: Canada Novo-Mexiletine
Pharmacologic Category Antiarrhythmic Agent, Class Ib
Use Management of serious ventricular arrhythmias; suppression of PVCs
Local Anesthetic/Vasoconstrictor Precautions No information available to require special precautions
Effects on Dental Treatment Key adverse event(s) related to dental treatment: Xerostomia (normal salivary flow resumes upon discontinuation).

Effects on Bleeding No information available to require special precautions
Adverse Effects
>10%:
Central nervous system: Lightheadedness (11% to 25%), dizziness (20% to 25%), nervousness (5% to 10%), incoordination (10%)
Gastrointestinal: GI distress (41%), nausea/vomiting (40%)
Neuromuscular & skeletal: Trembling, unsteady gait, tremor (13%), ataxia (10% to 20%)
1% to 10%:
Cardiovascular: Chest pain (3% to 8%), premature ventricular contractions (1% to 2%), palpitation (4% to 8%), angina (2%), proarrhythmia (10% to 15% in patients with malignant arrhythmia)
Central nervous system: Confusion, headache, insomnia (5% to 7%), depression (2%)
Dermatologic: Rash (4%)
Gastrointestinal: Constipation or diarrhea (4% to 5%), xerostomia (3%), abdominal pain (1%)
Neuromuscular & skeletal: Weakness (5%), numbness of fingers or toes (2% to 4%), paresthesia (2%), arthralgia (1%)
Ocular: Blurred vision (5% to 7%), nystagmus (6%)
Otic: Tinnitus (2% to 3%)
Respiratory: Dyspnea (3%)
General Dosage Range Dosage adjustment recommended in patients with hepatic impairment
Oral: *Adults:* Initial: 200 mg every 8 hours; Maintenance: 200-300 mg every 8 hours (maximum: 1.2 g/day)
Mechanism of Action Class IB antiarrhythmic, structurally related to lidocaine, which inhibits inward sodium current, decreases rate of rise of phase 0, increases effective refractory period/action potential duration ratio
Pharmacodynamics/Kinetics
Half-life Elimination Adults: 10-14 hours (average: 14.4 hours elderly, 12 hours younger adults); prolonged with hepatic impairment or heart failure
Time to Peak Serum: 2-3 hours
Pregnancy Risk Factor C
Pregnancy Considerations Adverse events were observed in some animal reproduction studies. A few case reports have demonstrated safe use of mexiletine in pregnant women.

Micafungin (mi ka FUN gin)

Related Information
Fungal Infections *on page 1573*
Brand Names: U.S. Mycamine®
Brand Names: Canada Mycamine®
Pharmacologic Category Antifungal Agent, Parenteral; Echinocandin
Use Treatment of esophageal candidiasis; *Candida* prophylaxis in patients undergoing hematopoietic stem cell transplant (HSCT); treatment of candidemia, acute disseminated candidiasis, and other *Candida* infections (peritonitis and abscesses)
Unlabeled Use Treatment of infections due to *Aspergillus* spp; prophylaxis of HIV-related esophageal candidiasis
Local Anesthetic/Vasoconstrictor Precautions No information available to require special precautions
Effects on Dental Treatment No significant effects or complications reported
Effects on Bleeding May cause thrombocytopenia in ≤15% of patients.

Adverse Effects
>10%:
Central nervous system: Fever (7% to 20%), headache (2% to 16%), dizziness (13%)
Endocrine & metabolic: Hypokalemia (14% to 18%), hypomagnesemia (6% to 13%)
Gastrointestinal: Diarrhea (8% to 23%), nausea (7% to 22%), vomiting (7% to 22%), mucosal inflammation (14%), constipation (11%)
Hematologic: Thrombocytopenia (4% to 15%), neutropenia (14%)
Local: Phlebitis (with peripheral administration; 5% to 19%)
1% to 10%:
Cardiovascular: Hypotension (6% to 10%), tachycardia (3% to 8%), hypertension (3% to 5%), peripheral edema (7%), edema (5%), bradycardia (3% to 5%), atrial fibrillation (3% to 5%)
Central nervous system: Insomnia (4% to 10%), anxiety (6%), fatigue (6%)
Dermatologic: Rash (2% to 9%), pruritus (6%)
Endocrine & metabolic: Hypocalcemia (7%), hypoglycemia (6% to 7%), hyperglycemia (6%), hypernatremia (4% to 6%), hyperkalemia (4% to 5%), fluid overload (5%)
Gastrointestinal: Abdominal pain (2% to 10%), anorexia (6%), dyspepsia (6%)
Hematologic: Anemia (3% to 10%), febrile neutropenia (6%)
Hepatic: AST increased (6%), ALT increased (5%), serum alkaline phosphatase increased (6% to 8%)
Neuromuscular & skeletal: Rigors (9%), back pain (5%)
Respiratory: Cough (8%), dyspnea (6%), epistaxis (6%)
Miscellaneous: Bacteremia (5% to 9%), sepsis (5% to 6%)
General Dosage Range I.V.: *Adults:* Prophylaxis: 50 mg daily; Treatment: 100-150 mg daily
Mechanism of Action Concentration-dependent inhibition of 1,3-beta-D-glucan synthase resulting in reduced formation of 1,3-beta-D-glucan, an essential polysaccharide comprising 30% to 60% of *Candida* cell walls (absent in mammalian cells); decreased glucan content leads to osmotic instability and cellular lysis
Pharmacodynamics/Kinetics
Half-life Elimination 11-21 hours
Pregnancy Risk Factor C
Pregnancy Considerations Visceral teratogenic and abortifacient effects were noted in animal studies. There are no adequate and well-controlled studies in pregnant women. Use only if benefit outweighs risk.

Miconazole (Oral) (mi KON a zole)

Related Information
Fungal Infections *on page 1573*
Brand Names: U.S. Oravig®
Pharmacologic Category Antifungal Agent, Oral Nonabsorbed
Use Treatment of oropharyngeal candidiasis
Local Anesthetic/Vasoconstrictor Precautions No information available to require special precautions
Effects on Dental Treatment Key adverse event(s) related to dental treatment: Application site reaction (including burning, discomfort, edema, glossodynia, pain, pruritus, toothache, ulceration), abnormal taste, oral discomfort, xerostomia and changes in salivation (normal salivary flow resumes upon discontinuation)

Effects on Bleeding No information available to require special precautions
Adverse Effects
>10%: Local: Application site reaction (10% to 12%; including burning, discomfort, edema, glossodynia, pain, pruritus, toothache, ulceration)
1% to 10%:
Central nervous system: Headache (5% to 8%), fatigue (3%), pain (1%)
Dermatologic: Pruritus (2%)
Gastrointestinal: Diarrhea (6% to 9%), nausea (1% to 7%), vomiting (1% to 4%), abnormal taste (3% to 4%), oral discomfort (3%), xerostomia (3%), abdominal pain (1% to 3%), ageusia (2%), gastroenteritis (1%)
Hematologic: Anemia (3%), lymphopenia (2%), neutropenia (1%)
Hepatic: GGT increased (1%)
Respiratory: Cough (3%), upper respiratory infection (2%), pharyngeal pain (1%)
General Dosage Range Buccal: *Children ≥16 years and Adults:* 50 mg (1 tablet) once daily
Mechanism of Action Inhibits biosynthesis of ergosterol, damaging the fungal cell wall membrane, which increases permeability causing leaking of nutrients
Pharmacodynamics/Kinetics
Duration of Action Buccal adhesion: 15 hours
Pregnancy Risk Factor C
Pregnancy Considerations Embryofetotoxicity has been observed in animal reproduction studies. There are no adequate and well-controlled studies in pregnant women. Use only if benefit outweighs risk.

Miconazole (Topical) (mi KON a zole)

Related Information
Fungal Infections *on page 1573*
Brand Names: U.S. 3M™ Cavilon™ Antifungal [OTC]; Aloe Vesta® Antifungal [OTC]; Baza® Antifungal [OTC]; Carrington® Antifungal [OTC]; Critic-Aid® Clear AF [OTC]; DermaFungal [OTC]; Dermagran® AF [OTC]; DiabetAid® Antifungal Foot Bath [OTC]; Fungoid® [OTC]; Lotrimin AF® [OTC]; Micaderm® [OTC]; Micatin® [OTC]; Micro-Guard® [OTC]; Miranel AF™ [OTC]; Mitrazol® [OTC]; Monistat® 1 Day or Night [OTC]; Monistat® 1 [OTC]; Monistat® 3 [OTC]; Monistat® 7 [OTC]; Neosporin® AF [OTC]; Podactin Cream [OTC]; Secura® Antifungal Extra Thick [OTC]; Secura® Antifungal Greaseless [OTC]; Ting® Spray Powder [OTC]; Zeasorb®-AF [OTC]
Brand Names: Canada Dermazole; Micatin®; Micozole; Monistat®; Monistat® 3
Pharmacologic Category Antifungal Agent, Topical; Antifungal Agent, Vaginal
Use Treatment of vulvovaginal candidiasis and a variety of skin and mucous membrane fungal infections
Local Anesthetic/Vasoconstrictor Precautions No information available to require special precautions
Effects on Dental Treatment No significant effects or complications reported
Effects on Bleeding No information available to require special precautions
Adverse Effects Frequency not defined.
Topical: Allergic contact dermatitis, burning, maceration
Vaginal: Abdominal cramps, burning, irritation, itching

General Dosage Range

Intravaginal: *Children ≥12 years and Adults:* Insert 1 applicatorful or suppository (100 mg or 200 mg) once daily at bedtime **or** insert 1 suppository (1200 mg) as a single dose.

Topical: *Children and Adults:* Apply twice daily **or** dissolve 1 effervescent tablet in ~1 gallon of water and soak feet for 15-30 minutes

Mechanism of Action Inhibits biosynthesis of ergosterol, damaging the fungal cell wall membrane, which increases permeability causing leaking of nutrients

Pregnancy Considerations Following vaginal administration, small amounts are absorbed systemically. Adverse fetal events have not been observed and vaginal products may be considered for the treatment of vulvovaginal candidiasis in pregnant women (CDC, 2010; Czeizel, 2004; Stevens, 2002). This product may weaken latex condoms and diaphragms (CDC, 2010).

Miconazole and Zinc Oxide

(mi KON a zole & zink OKS ide)

Related Information

Miconazole (Topical) *on page 915*
Zinc Oxide *on page 1421*

Brand Names: U.S. Vusion®

Pharmacologic Category Antifungal Agent, Topical

Use Adjunctive treatment of diaper dermatitis complicated by *Candida albicans* infection

Local Anesthetic/Vasoconstrictor Precautions No information available to require special precautions

Effects on Dental Treatment No significant effects or complications reported

Effects on Bleeding No information available to require special precautions

General Dosage Range Topical: *Children ≥4 weeks:* Apply to affected area with each diaper change (maximum therapy: 7 days)

Mechanism of Action

Miconazole inhibits the biosynthesis of ergosterol, damaging the fungal cell wall membrane.

Zinc oxide is a mild astringent with weak antiseptic properties.

Pregnancy Risk Factor C

Pregnancy Considerations Reproduction studies have not been conducted with this combination. See individual agents.

Midazolam (MID aye zoe lam)

Brand Names: Canada Apo-Midazolam®; Midazolam Injection

Generic Availability (U.S.) Yes

Pharmacologic Category Benzodiazepine

Dental Use Sedation component in I.V. conscious sedation in oral surgery patients; syrup formulation is used for children to help alleviate anxiety before a dental procedure

Use Preoperative sedation; moderate sedation prior to diagnostic or radiographic procedures; ICU sedation (continuous infusion); induction and maintenance of general anesthesia

Unlabeled Use Anxiety, status epilepticus, conscious sedation (intranasal route)

Local Anesthetic/Vasoconstrictor Precautions No information available to require special precautions

Effects on Dental Treatment No significant effects or complications reported

Effects on Bleeding No information available to require special precautions

Adverse Effects As reported in adults unless otherwise noted:

>10%: Respiratory: Decreased tidal volume and/or respiratory rate decrease, apnea (3% children)

1% to 10%:

Cardiovascular: Hypotension (3% children)

Central nervous system: Drowsiness (1%), oversedation, headache (1%), seizure-like activity (1% children)

Gastrointestinal: Nausea (3%), vomiting (3%)

Local: Pain and local reactions at injection site (4% I.M., 5% I.V.; severity less than diazepam)

Neuromuscular & skeletal: Myoclonic jerks (preterm infants)

Ocular: Nystagmus (1% children)

Respiratory: Cough (1%)

Miscellaneous: Physical and psychological dependence with prolonged use, hiccups (4%, 1% children), paradoxical reaction (2% children)

Dental Usual Dosage Adults:

Preoperative sedation:

I.M.: 0.07-0.08 mg/kg 30-60 minutes prior to surgery/procedure; usual dose: 5 mg; **Note:** Reduce dose in patients with COPD, high-risk patients, patients ≥60 years of age, and patients receiving other opioids or CNS depressants

I.V.: 0.02-0.04 mg/kg; repeat every 5 minutes as needed to desired effect or up to 0.1-0.2 mg/kg

Intranasal (not an approved route): 0.2 mg/kg (up to 0.4 mg/kg in some studies); administer 30-45 minutes prior to surgery/procedure

Conscious sedation: I.V.: Initial: 0.5-2 mg slow I.V. over at least 2 minutes; slowly titrate to effect by repeating doses every 2-3 minutes if needed; usual total dose: 2.5-5 mg; use decreased doses in elderly.

Healthy Adults <60 years: Initial: Some patients respond to doses as low as 1 mg; no more than 2.5 mg should be administered over a period of 2 minutes. Additional doses of midazolam may be administered after a 2-minute waiting period and evaluation of sedation after each dose increment. A total dose >5 mg is generally not needed. If opioids or other CNS depressants are administered concomitantly, the midazolam dose should be reduced by 30%.

Dosage

Children: The dose of midazolam needs to be individualized based on the patient's age, underlying diseases, and concurrent medications. Decrease dose (by ~30%) if opioids or other CNS depressants are administered concomitantly. Children <6 years may require higher doses and closer monitoring than older children; calculate dose based on ideal body weight.

Conscious sedation for procedures or preoperative sedation:

Oral, rectal: Children: 0.5-0.75 mg/kg as a single dose preprocedure (maximum: 20 mg); administer 20-30 minutes prior to procedure. Children <6 years or less cooperative patients may require as much as 1 mg/kg as a single dose; 0.25 mg/kg may suffice for children 6-16 years of age (Bozkurt, 2007).

Intranasal (unlabeled route): Children: 0.2-0.5 mg/kg (maximum total dose: 10 mg or 5 mg per nare); may be administered 10-20 minutes prior to procedure (Bozkurt, 2007; Chiaretti, 2011). **Note:** Use 5 mg/mL injectable concentrated solution to deliver dose. Due to the low pH of the solution, burning upon administration is likely to occur.

I.M.: Children: 0.1-0.15 mg/kg 30-60 minutes before surgery or procedure; range: 0.05-0.15 mg/kg; doses up to 0.5 mg/kg have been used in more anxious patients; maximum total dose: 10 mg

I.V.:

Infants <6 months: Limited information is available in nonintubated infants; dosing recommendations not clear; infants <6 months are at higher risk for airway obstruction and hypoventilation; titrate dose in small increments to desired effect

Infants 6 months to Children 5 years: Initial: 0.05-0.1 mg/kg; total dose of 0.6 mg/kg may be required; maximum total dose: 6 mg

Children 6-12 years: Initial: 0.025-0.05 mg/kg; total doses of 0.4 mg/kg may be required; maximum total dose: 10 mg

Children 12-16 years: Dose as adults; maximum total dose: 10 mg

Conscious sedation during mechanical ventilation: Children: Loading dose: 0.05-0.2 mg/kg, followed by initial continuous infusion: 0.06-0.12 mg/kg/hour (1-2 **mcg**/kg/minute); range in clinical trials: 0.024-0.564 mg/kg/hour (0.4-9.4 **mcg**/kg/minute) (Hartman, 2009)

Status epilepticus refractory to standard therapy (unlabeled use): **Note:** Intubation required; adjust dose based on hemodynamics, seizure activity, and EEG. Infants >2 months and Children: Loading dose: 0.15 mg/kg followed by a continuous infusion of 0.06 mg/kg/**hour** (1 **mcg**/kg/minute); titrate dose upward every 5 minutes until clinical seizure activity is controlled; mean infusion rate required in 24 children was 0.14 mg/kg/**hour** (2.3 **mcg**/kg/minute) with a range of 0.06-1.1 mg/kg/**hour** (1-18.3 **mcg**/kg/minute) (Rivera, 1993).

A more aggressive approach has been demonstrated to provide control of status epilepticus within 30 minutes of initiation: Loading dose: 0.5 mg/kg followed by 0.12 mg/kg/**hour** (2 **mcg**/kg/minute). If seizures persist or recur, administer 0.5 mg/kg bolus with an increase in the infusion rate to 0.24 mg/kg/**hour** (4 **mcg**/kg/minute); if seizures continue to persist/recur, administer 0.1 mg/kg bolus and increase infusion to 0.48 mg/kg/**hour** (8 **mcg**/kg/minute); continue to repeat this last incremental increase until seizure control or a maximum dose of 1.44 mg/kg/**hour** (24 **mcg**/kg/minute) is reached; do not allow >5 minutes to elapse between each dose increment while seizures persist (dose range within clinical trial: 0.12-1.92 mg/kg/**hour** or 2-32 **mcg**/kg/minute) (Morrison, 2006).

Status epilepticus, prehospital treatment (unlabeled use; Silbergleit, 2012): **Note:** Administered by paramedics when convulsions last >5 minutes **or** if convulsions are occurring after having intermittent seizures without regaining consciousness for >5 minutes. I.M.: Children and Adolescents:

13-40 kg: 5 mg once

>40 kg: Refer to adult dosing

Adults: The dose of midazolam needs to be individualized based on the patient's age, underlying diseases, and concurrent medications. Consider reducing dose by 20% to 50% in elderly, chronically ill, or debilitated patients and those receiving opioids or other CNS depressants.

Preoperative/preprocedural sedation: Healthy adults <60 years:

I.M.: 0.07-0.08 mg/kg 30-60 minutes prior to surgery/procedure; usual dose: 5 mg

I.V.: 0.02-0.04 mg/kg; repeat every 5 minutes as needed to desired effect or up to 0.1-0.2 mg/kg

Intranasal (unlabeled route): 0.1 mg/kg; administer 10-20 minutes prior to surgery/procedure (Uygur-Bayramiçli, 2002). **Note:** Use 5 mg/mL injectable solution to deliver dose. Due to the low pH of the solution, burning upon administration is likely to occur.

Conscious sedation: I.V.:

Manufacturer's labeling:

Healthy adults <60 years:

Initial: Some patients respond to doses as low as 1 mg; no more than 2.5 mg should be administered over a period of 2 minutes. Additional doses of midazolam may be administered after a 2-minute waiting period and evaluation of sedation after each dose increment. A total dose >5 mg is generally not needed.

Maintenance: 25% of dose used to reach sedative effect

Adults ≥60 years, debilitated, or chronically ill: Refer to elderly dosing.

Alternate recommendations: American Society for Gastrointestinal Endoscopy: Initial: 0.5-2 mg slow I.V. over at least 2 minutes; slowly titrate to effect by repeating doses every 2-3 minutes if needed; usual total dose: 2.5-5 mg (Waring, 2003)

Anesthesia: I.V.:

Induction: Adults <55 years:

Unpremedicated patients: 0.3-0.35 mg/kg over 20-30 seconds; after 2 minutes, may repeat if necessary at 25% of initial dose every 2 minutes, up to a total dose of 0.6 mg/kg in resistant cases

Premedicated patients: Usual dosage range: 0.05-0.2 mg/kg (Barash, 2009; Miller, 2010). Use of 0.2 mg/kg administered over 5-10 seconds has been shown to safely produce anesthesia within 30 seconds (Samuelson, 1981) and is recommended for ASA physical status P1 and P2 patients. When used with other anesthetic drugs (ie, co-induction), the dose is <0.1 mg/kg (Miller, 2010).

ASA physical status >P3 or debilitation: Reduce dose by at least 20% (Miller, 2010)

Maintenance: 0.05 mg/kg as needed (Miller, 2010), or continuous infusion 0.015-0.06 mg/kg/**hour** (0.25-1 **mcg**/kg/minute) (Barash, 2009; Miller, 2010)

Sedation in mechanically-ventilated patients: I.V.: Initial dose: 0.01-0.05 mg/kg (~0.5-4 mg); may repeat at 5- to 15-minute intervals until adequate sedation achieved; maintenance infusion: 0.02-0.1 mg/kg/**hour** (0.3-1.7 **mcg**/kg/minute). Titrate to reach desired level of sedation. Titration to maintain a light rather than a deep level of sedation is recommended unless clinically contraindicated (Barr, 2013). May consider a trial of daily awakening; if agitated after discontinuation of drip, then restart at 50% of the previous dose (Kress, 2000).

Status epilepticus refractory to standard therapy (unlabeled use): **Note:** Intubation required; adjust dose based on hemodynamics, seizure activity, and EEG. I.V.: 0.15-0.3 mg/kg (usual dose: 5-15 mg); may repeat every 10-15 minutes as needed **or** 0.2 mg/kg bolus followed by a continuous infusion of 0.05-0.6 mg/kg/**hour** (0.83-10 **mcg**/kg/minute) (Lowenstein, 2005; Meierkord, 2010)

Status epilepticus, prehospital treatment (unlabeled use): **Note:** Administered by paramedics when convulsions last >5 minutes **or** if convulsions are occurring after having intermittent seizures without regaining consciousness for >5 minutes. I.M.: 10 mg once (Silbergleit, 2012)

Elderly:

Anesthesia: I.V.: Induction: Adults >55 years:
Unpremedicated patients: Initial dose: 0.3 mg/kg
Premedicated patients: Reduce dose by at least 20% (Miller, 2010).

Conscious sedation: I.V.: Initial: 0.5 mg slow I.V.; give no more than 1.5 mg in a 2-minute period; if additional titration is needed, give no more than 1 mg over 2 minutes, waiting another 2 or more minutes to evaluate sedative effect; a total dose of >3.5 mg is rarely necessary

Preoperative/preprocedural sedation: Adults >60 years (without concomitant opioid administration): I.M.: 2-3 mg (or 0.02-0.05 mg/kg) 30-60 minutes prior to surgery/procedure; some may only require 1 mg (or 0.01 mg/kg) if anticipated intensity and duration of sedation is less critical.

Dosage adjustment in renal impairment: There are no dosage adjustments provided in manufacturer's labeling; however, patients with renal failure receiving a continuous infusion cannot adequately eliminate the active hydroxylated metabolites (eg, 1-hydroxymidazolam) contributing to prolonged sedation sometimes for days after discontinuation (Spina, 2007).

Intermittent hemodialysis: Supplemental dose is not necessary.

Continuous venovenous hemofiltration (CVVH): Unconjugated 1-hydroxymidazolam not effectively removed; 1-hydroxymidazolamglucuronide effectively removed; sieving coefficient = 0.45 (Swart, 2005).

Peritoneal dialysis: Significant drug removal is unlikely based on physiochemical characteristics.

Dosage adjustment in hepatic impairment:

Severe hepatic impairment (eg, cirrhosis): **Note:** Use with caution in patients with any degree of hepatic impairment; patients with hepatic encephalopathy likely to be more sensitive to midazolam.

Single dose (eg, induction): No dosage adjustment recommended; patients with hepatic impairment may be more sensitive compared to patients without hepatic impairment; anticipate longer duration of action (MacGilchrist, 1986; Trouvin, 1988).

Multiple dosing or continuous infusion: Expect longer duration of action and accumulation; based on patient response, dosage reduction likely to be necessary (Trouvin, 1988).

Mechanism of Action Binds to stereospecific benzodiazepine receptors on the postsynaptic GABA neuron at several sites within the central nervous system, including the limbic system, reticular formation. Enhancement of the inhibitory effect of GABA on neuronal excitability results by increased neuronal membrane permeability to chloride ions. This shift in chloride ions results in hyperpolarization (a less excitable state) and stabilization.

Contraindications Hypersensitivity to midazolam or any component of the formulation; intrathecal or epidural injection of parenteral forms containing preservatives (ie, benzyl alcohol); acute narrow-angle glaucoma; concurrent use of potent inhibitors of CYP3A4 (amprenavir, atazanavir, or ritonavir)

Per respective protease inhibitor manufacturer's labeling: Concurrent use of oral midazolam with amprenavir, atazanavir, darunavir, indinavir, lopinavir-ritonavir, nelfinavir, ritonavir, saquinavir, tipranavir and concurrent use of oral or injectable midazolam with fosamprenavir

Warnings/Precautions [U.S. Boxed Warning]: May cause severe respiratory depression, respiratory arrest, or apnea. Use with extreme caution, particularly in noncritical care settings. Appropriate resuscitative equipment and qualified personnel must be available for administration and monitoring. Initial dosing must be cautiously titrated and individualized, particularly in elderly or debilitated patients, patients with hepatic impairment (including alcoholics), or in renal impairment, particularly if other CNS depressants (including opiates) are used concurrently. **[U.S. Boxed Warning]: Initial doses in elderly or debilitated patients should be conservative; as little as 1 mg, but not to exceed 2.5 mg.** Use with caution in patients with respiratory disease or impaired gag reflex. Use during upper airway procedures may increase risk of hypoventilation. Prolonged responses have been noted following extended administration by continuous infusion (possibly due to metabolite accumulation) or in the presence of drugs which inhibit midazolam metabolism.

Causes CNS depression (dose-related) resulting in sedation, dizziness, confusion, or ataxia which may impair physical and mental capabilities. Patients must be cautioned about performing tasks which require mental alertness (eg, operating machinery or driving). A minimum of 1 day should elapse after midazolam administration before attempting these tasks. Use with caution in patients receiving other CNS depressants or psychoactive agents. Effects with other sedative drugs or ethanol may be potentiated. Benzodiazepines have been associated with falls and traumatic injury and should be used with extreme caution in patients who are at risk of these events (especially the elderly).

Use with caution in patients receiving CYP3A4 inhibitors; may result in more intense and prolonged sedation; consider reducing midazolam dose and anticipate potential for prolongation and intensity of effect. The concurrent use of all protease inhibitors is contraindicated with oral midazolam per their respective manufacturer's labeling. The concurrent use of fosamprenavir is contraindicated with both oral and parenteral forms of midazolam.

May cause hypotension - hemodynamic events are more common in pediatric patients or patients with hemodynamic instability. Hypotension and/or respiratory depression may occur more frequently in patients who have received opioid analgesics. Use with caution in obese patients, chronic renal failure, and HF. Does not protect against increases in heart rate or blood pressure during intubation. Should not be used in shock, coma, or acute alcohol intoxication. **[U.S. Boxed Warning]: Do not administer by rapid I.V. injection in neonates; severe hypotension and seizures have been reported; risk may be increased with concomitant fentanyl use.**

Avoid intra-arterial administration or extravasation of parenteral formulation. Some parenteral dosage forms may contain benzyl alcohol which has been associated with "gasping syndrome" in neonates. Some formulations may contain cherry flavoring.

Midazolam causes anterograde amnesia. Paradoxical reactions, including hyperactive or aggressive behavior have been reported with benzodiazepines, particularly in adolescent/pediatric or psychiatric patients; may consider treatment with flumazenil (Massanari, 1997). Does not have analgesic, antidepressant, or antipsychotic properties.

Benzodiazepines have been associated with dependence and acute withdrawal symptoms on discontinuation or reduction in dose. Acute withdrawal, including seizures, may be precipitated after administration of flumazenil to patients receiving long-term benzodiazepine therapy.

Drug Interactions

Metabolism/Transport Effects Substrate of CYP2B6 (minor), CYP3A4 (major); **Note:** Assignment of Major/Minor substrate status based on clinically relevant drug interaction potential; **Inhibits** CYP2C8 (weak), CYP2C9 (weak), CYP3A4 (weak)

Avoid Concomitant Use

Avoid concomitant use of Midazolam with any of the following: Azelastine (Nasal); Boceprevir; Cobicistat; Conivaptan; Efavirenz; Itraconazole; Ketoconazole (Systemic); OLANZapine; Paraldehyde; Pimozide; Protease Inhibitors; Sodium Oxybate; Telaprevir

Increased Effect/Toxicity

Midazolam may increase the levels/effects of: Alcohol (Ethyl); ARIPiprazole; Azelastine (Nasal); Buprenorphine; CloZAPine; CNS Depressants; Fosphenytoin; Lomitapide; Methotrimeprazine; Metyrosine; Mirtazapine; Paraldehyde; Phenytoin; Pimozide; Pramipexole; Propofol; ROPINIRole; Rotigotine; Selective Serotonin Reuptake Inhibitors; Sodium Oxybate; Zolpidem

The levels/effects of Midazolam may be increased by: Antifungal Agents (Azole Derivatives, Systemic); Aprepitant; AtorvaSTATin; Boceprevir; Calcium Channel Blockers (Nondihydropyridine); Cimetidine; Cobicistat; Conivaptan; Contraceptives (Estrogens); Contraceptives (Progestins); CYP3A4 Inhibitors (Moderate); CYP3A4 Inhibitors (Strong); Dasatinib; Droperidol; Efavirenz; Fosaprepitant; Grapefruit Juice; HydrOXYzine; Isoniazid; Itraconazole; Ivacaftor; Ketoconazole (Systemic); Macrolide Antibiotics; Magnesium Sulfate; Methotrimeprazine; Mifepristone; OLANZapine; Perampanel; Propofol; Protease Inhibitors; Proton Pump Inhibitors; Selective Serotonin Reuptake Inhibitors; Telaprevir

Decreased Effect

The levels/effects of Midazolam may be decreased by: CarBAMazepine; CYP3A4 Inducers (Strong); Deferasirox; Ginkgo Biloba; Rifamycin Derivatives; St Johns Wort; Theophylline Derivatives; Tocilizumab; Yohimbine

Ethanol/Nutrition/Herb Interactions

Ethanol: Ethanol may increase CNS depression. Management: Avoid ethanol.

Food: Grapefruit juice may increase serum concentrations of midazolam. Management: Avoid concurrent use of grapefruit juice with oral midazolam.

Herb/Nutraceutical: St John's wort may decrease midazolam levels and increase CNS depression; valerian, kava kava, and gotu kola may increase CNS depression. Management: Avoid concurrent use with St John's wort, valerian, kava kava, and gotu kola.

Dietary Considerations Avoid grapefruit juice with oral syrup.

Pharmacodynamics/Kinetics

Onset of Action I.M.: Sedation: ~15 minutes; I.V.: 3-5 minutes; Oral: 10-20 minutes; Intranasal: Children: 4-8 minutes (Lee-Kim, 2004); Peak effect: I.M.: 0.5-1 hour

Duration of Action I.M.: Up to 6 hours; Mean: 2 hours; Intranasal: Children: 18-41 minutes (Lee-Kim, 2004); I.V.: Single dose: <2 hours (dose-dependent) (Fragen, 1997); Cirrhosis: Up to 6 hours (MacGilcrhist, 1986)

Half-life Elimination 2-6 hours; prolonged in cirrhosis, congestive heart failure, obesity, renal failure, and elderly. **Note:** In patients with renal failure, reduced elimination of active hydroxylated metabolites leads to drug accumulation and prolonged sedation.

Pregnancy Risk Factor D

Pregnancy Considerations Adverse events were not observed in animal teratology studies. Midazolam has been found to cross the human placenta and can be detected in the serum of the umbilical vein and artery, as well as the amniotic fluid. Teratogenic effects have been observed with some benzodiazepines; however, additional studies are needed. The incidence of premature birth and low birth weights may be increased following maternal use of benzodiazepines; hypoglycemia and respiratory problems in the neonate may occur following exposure late in pregnancy. Neonatal withdrawal symptoms may occur within days to weeks after birth and "floppy infant syndrome" (which also includes withdrawal symptoms) have been reported with some benzodiazepines.

Lactation Enters breast milk/use caution (AAP rates "of concern"; AAP 2001 update pending)

Breast-Feeding Considerations Midazolam and hydroxymidazolam can be detected in breast milk. Based on information from two women, 2-3 months postpartum, the half-life of midazolam in breast milk is ~1 hour. Milk concentrations were below the limit of detection (<5 nmol/L) 4 hours after a single maternal dose of midazolam 15 mg. Drowsiness, lethargy, or weight loss in nursing infants have been observed in case reports following maternal use of some benzodiazepines.

Controlled Substance C-IV

Dosage Forms

Injection, solution: 1 mg/mL (2 mL, 5 mL, 10 mL); 5 mg/mL (1 mL, 2 mL, 5 mL, 10 mL)

Injection, solution [preservative free]: 1 mg/mL (2 mL, 5 mL); 5 mg/mL (1 mL, 2 mL)

Syrup, oral: 2 mg/mL (2.5 mL, 118 mL)

Dental Comment Compared to oral sedation, intranasal (IN) sedation resulted in greater irritability during the first 10-15 minutes after administration, but a faster onset and shorter duration of sedation with improved behavior following onset of sedation. (Johnson, 2010; Lee-Kim, 2004). Monitor oxygen saturation with midazolam. If desaturation occurs, reposition airway (head tilt, chin lift).

References

Dionne RA, Yagiela JA, Moore PA, et al, "Comparing Efficacy and Safety of Four Intravenous Sedation Regimens in Dental Outpatients," *Am Dent Assoc*, 2001, 132(6):740-51.
Johnson E, Briskie D, Majewski R, et al, "The Physiologic and Behavioral Effects of Oral and Intranasal Midazolam in Pediatric Dental Patients," *Pediatr Dent*, 2010, 32(3):229-38.
Lee-Kim SJ, Fadavi S, Punwani I, et al, "Nasal Versus Oral Midazolam Sedation for Pediatric Dental Patients," *J Dent Child (Chic)*, 2004, 71 (2):126-30.

Midodrine (MI doe dreen)

Brand Names: Canada Amatine®; Apo-Midodrine®

Pharmacologic Category Alpha$_1$ Agonist

Use *Orphan drug:* Treatment of symptomatic orthostatic hypotension

Unlabeled Use Management of urinary incontinence; vasovagal syncope; prevention of dialysis-induced hypotension

Local Anesthetic/Vasoconstrictor Precautions No information available to require special precautions

Effects on Dental Treatment Key adverse event(s) related to dental treatment: Xerostomia (normal salivary flow resumes upon discontinuation).

Effects on Bleeding No information available to require special precautions

Adverse Effects
>10%:
Cardiovascular: Supine hypertension (7% to 13%)
Dermatologic: Piloerection (13%), pruritus (12%)
Genitourinary: Urinary urgency, retention, or polyuria, dysuria (up to 13%)
Neuromuscular & skeletal: Paresthesia (18%)
1% to 10%:
Central nervous system: Chills (5%), pain (5%)
Dermatologic: Rash (2%)
Gastrointestinal: Abdominal pain

General Dosage Range Dosage adjustment recommended in patients with renal impairment
Oral: *Adults:* 10 mg 3 times/day (maximum: 40 mg/day)

Mechanism of Action Midodrine forms an active metabolite, desglymidodrine, which is an alpha$_1$-agonist. This agent increases arteriolar and venous tone resulting in a rise in standing, sitting, and supine systolic and diastolic blood pressure in patients with orthostatic hypotension.

Pharmacodynamics/Kinetics
Onset of Action ~1 hour
Duration of Action 2-3 hours
Half-life Elimination Desglymidodrine: ~3-4 hours; Midodrine: 25 minutes
Time to Peak Desglymidodrine: 1-2 hours; Midodrine: 30 minutes

Pregnancy Risk Factor C
Pregnancy Considerations Increased rate of embryo resorption and decreased fetal weight were observed in animal studies. Use during pregnancy should be avoided unless the potential benefit outweighs the risk to the fetus.

Mifepristone (mi FE pris tone)

Related Information
Clinical Risk Related to Drugs Prolonging QT Interval *on page 1510*
Brand Names: U.S. Korlym™; Mifeprex®
Pharmacologic Category Abortifacient; Antineoplastic Agent, Hormone Antagonist; Antiprogestin; Cortisol Receptor Blocker
Use
Korlym™: To control hyperglycemia occurring secondary to hypercortisolism in patients with endogenous Cushing's syndrome who have type 2 diabetes mellitus or glucose intolerance and who failed surgery or who are not surgical candidates
Mifeprex®: Medical termination of intrauterine pregnancy, through day 49 of pregnancy. Patients may need treatment with misoprostol and possibly surgery to complete therapy.
Unlabeled Use Treatment of unresectable meningioma; has been studied in the treatment of breast cancer and ovarian cancer; termination of pregnancy ≤63 days of pregnancy

Local Anesthetic/Vasoconstrictor Precautions
Mifepristone is one of the drugs confirmed to prolong the QT interval and is accepted as having a risk of causing torsade de pointes. The risk of drug-induced torsade de pointes is extremely low when a single QT interval prolonging drug is prescribed. In terms of epinephrine, it is not known what effect vasoconstrictors in the local anesthetic regimen will have in patients with a known history of congenital prolonged QT interval or in patients taking any medication that prolongs the QT interval. Until more information is obtained, it is suggested that the clinician consult with the physician prior to the use of a vasoconstrictor in suspected patients, and that the vasoconstrictor (epinephrine, mepivacaine and levonordefrin [Carbocaine® 2% with Neo-Cobefrin®]) be used with caution.
Effects on Dental Treatment No significant effects or complications reported
Effects on Bleeding No information available to require special precautions
Adverse Effects
Adverse events associated with treatment of hyperglycemia in patients with Cushing's syndrome:
>10%:
Cardiovascular: Peripheral edema (26%), hypertension (24%)
Central nervous system: Fatigue (48%), headache (44%), dizziness (22%), pain (14%)
Endocrine & metabolic: Hypokalemia (34% to 44%), endometrial hypertrophy (38%), thyroid function tests abnormal (18%)
Gastrointestinal: Nausea (48%), vomiting (26%), appetite decreased (20%), xerostomia (18%), diarrhea (12%)
Genitourinary: Vaginal bleeding (14%)
Neuromuscular & skeletal: Arthralgia (30%), back pain (16%), myalgia (14%), extremity pain (12%)
Respiratory: Dyspnea (16%), sinusitis (14%), nasopharyngitis (12%)
5% to 10%:
Cardiovascular: Edema, pitting edema
Central nervous system: Anxiety (10%), somnolence (10%), insomnia, malaise
Endocrine & metabolic: Hypoglycemia, triglycerides increased
Gastrointestinal: Anorexia (10%), constipation (10%), abdominal pain, GI reflux
Genitourinary: Vaginal hemorrhage, metrorrhagia
Neuromuscular & skeletal: Flank pain, malaise, musculoskeletal chest pain, weakness
Miscellaneous: Thirst
<5% or frequency not defined: Adrenal insufficiency (4%), pruritus (4%), rash (4%), HDL cholesterol decreased

Adverse events associated with treatment for termination of pregnancy: Note: Vaginal bleeding and uterine cramping are expected to occur when this medication is used to terminate a pregnancy; ~90% of women using this medication for this purpose also report adverse reactions on day 3 after the procedure. Bleeding or spotting occurs in most women for a period of 9-16 days. Up to 8% of women will experience some degree of bleeding or spotting for 30 days or more. In some cases, bleeding may be prolonged and heavy, potentially leading to hypovolemic shock.
Central nervous system: Headache (2% to 31%), dizziness (1% to 12%)

Gastrointestinal: Abdominal pain (cramping) (96%), nausea (43% to 61%), vomiting (18% to 26%), diarrhea (12% to 20%)

Genitourinary: Uterine cramping (83%)

1% to 10%:

Cardiovascular: Syncope (1%)

Central nervous system: Fatigue (10%), fever (4%), insomnia (3%), anxiety (2%), fainting (2%)

Gastrointestinal: Dyspepsia (3%)

Genitourinary: Uterine hemorrhage (5%), vaginitis (3%), pelvic pain (2%), endometriosis/salpingitis/pelvic inflammatory disease (1%)

Hematologic: Decreased hemoglobin >2 g/dL (6%), anemia (2%), leukorrhea (2%)

Neuromuscular & skeletal: Back pain (9%), rigors (3%), leg pain (2%), weakness (2%)

Respiratory: Sinusitis (2%)

Miscellaneous: Viral infection (4%)

General Dosage Range Dosage adjustment recommended in patients with hepatic or renal impairment or on concomitant therapy when treating hyperglycemia in patients with Cushing's syndrome.

Oral: *Adults:* Hyperglycemia in patients with Cushing's syndrome: 300-1200 mg once daily (maximum: 1200 mg once daily, not to exceed 20 mg/kg/day); Termination of pregnancy: Day 1: 600 mg (three 200 mg tablets) as a single dose

Mechanism of Action Mifepristone is a synthetic steroid. At low doses, it competitively binds to the intracellular progesterone receptor, blocking the effects of progesterone. When used for the termination of pregnancy, this leads to contraction-inducing activity in the myometrium. In the absence of progesterone, mifepristone acts as a partial progesterone agonist. At high doses used for the treatment of hyperglycemia in patients with Cushing's syndrome, mifepristone blocks the effect of cortisol at the glucocorticoid receptor (antagonizes the effects of cortisol on glucose metabolism) while at the same time increasing circulating cortisol concentrations.

Pharmacodynamics/Kinetics

Half-life Elimination Single dose: Terminal: 18 hours following a slower phase where 50% eliminated between 12-72 hours; Multiple doses (600 mg/day): 85 hours

Time to Peak Oral: 90 minutes; Range: Single dose: 1-2 hours, Multiple doses: 1-4 hours

Pregnancy Risk Factor X

Pregnancy Considerations Use of mifepristone in a pregnant woman will result in fetal loss. In addition, skull deformities were observed in rabbit reproduction studies and were most likely due to uterine contractions.

Korlym™: **[U.S. Boxed Warning]: Use of mifepristone will result in termination of pregnancy.** When used to control hyperglycemia in women with Cushing's syndrome, **pregnancy must be excluded prior to initiation of therapy. Nonhormonal contraception must be used during treatment and for 1 month after discontinuation of therapy unless the patient has had surgical sterilization. Pregnancy must be excluded if treatment is interrupted for ≥14 days.**

Mifeprex®: This medication is used to terminate pregnancy; there are no approved treatment indications for its use during pregnancy. In addition, skull defects, cranial nerve palsies, delayed growth and psychomotor development, facial malformations and limb defects have been reported following prostaglandin exposure (including misoprostol). If treatment fails, there is a risk of fetal malformation. In sexually active women, pregnancy can occur prior to the first menstrual period

following treatment. Appropriate contraception can be started as soon as termination of pregnancy is confirmed or before sexual intercourse is resumed.

Prescribing and Access Restrictions

Korlym™ is only available through a restricted access program. For prescriber registration and patient enrollment forms, please refer to https://www.korlymspark.com/login.aspx?ReturnUrl=%2fdefault.aspx or call 1-855-4Korlym (1-855-456-7596).

Mifeprex®: As a requirement of the REMS program, a medication guide must be given to the patient prior to receiving the medication. In addition, the manufacturer recommends distributing a patient agreement form which must be signed by the patient and prescriber confirming the patient's agreement to terminate her pregnancy. A signed copy of the patient agreement should be kept in the patient's medical record.

Mifeprex® is only available direct from Danco Laboratories' distributor. To obtain the product, please refer to, http://www.earlyoptionpill.com, or call 1-877-432-7596.

Investigators wishing to obtain the agent for use in oncology patients must apply for a patient-specific IND from the FDA.

Dental Comment Mifepristone is known to prolong the QT interval. The QT interval is measured as the time and distance between the Q point of the QRS complex and the end of the T wave in the ECG tracing. After adjustment for heart rate, the QT interval is defined as prolonged if it is more than 450 msec in men and 460 msec in women. A long QT syndrome was first described in the 1950s and 60s as a congenital syndrome involving QT interval prolongation and syncope and sudden death. Some of the congenital long QT syndromes were characterized by a peculiar electrocardiographic appearance of the QRS complex involving a premature atria beat followed by a pause, then a subsequent sinus beat showing marked QT prolongation and deformity. This type of cardiac arrhythmia was originally termed "torsade de pointes" (translated from the French as "twisting of the points"). Mifepristone is considered as having a risk of causing torsade de pointes. Since it is not known what effect vasoconstrictors in the local anesthetic regimen will have in patients with a known history of congenital prolonged QT interval or in patients taking any medication that prolongs the QT interval, a medical consult is suggested.

Miglitol (MIG li tol)

Related Information

Endocrine Disorders and Pregnancy *on page 1517*

Brand Names: U.S. Glyset®

Pharmacologic Category Antidiabetic Agent, Alpha-Glucosidase Inhibitor

Use Type 2 diabetes mellitus (noninsulin-dependent, NIDDM):

Monotherapy as an adjunct to diet to improve glycemic control in patients with type 2 diabetes mellitus (non-insulin-dependent, NIDDM) whose hyperglycemia cannot be managed with diet alone

Combination therapy with a sulfonylurea when diet plus either miglitol or a sulfonylurea alone do not result in adequate glycemic control. The effect of miglitol to enhance glycemic control is additive to that of sulfonylureas when used in combination

Local Anesthetic/Vasoconstrictor Precautions No information available to require special precautions

◄ Effects on Dental Treatment No significant effects or complications reported

Effects on Bleeding No information available to require special precautions

Adverse Effects

>10%: Gastrointestinal: Flatulence (42%), diarrhea (29%), abdominal pain (12%)

1% to 10%: Dermatologic: Rash (4%)

General Dosage Range Oral: *Adults:* Initial: 25 mg 3 times daily; Maintenance: 25-100 mg 3 times daily (maximum: 300 mg daily)

Mechanism of Action In contrast to sulfonylureas, miglitol does not enhance insulin secretion; the antihyperglycemic action of miglitol results from a reversible inhibition of membrane-bound intestinal alpha-glucosidases which hydrolyze oligosaccharides and disaccharides to glucose and other monosaccharides in the brush border of the small intestine. In patients with diabetes, this enzyme inhibition results in delayed glucose absorption and lowering of postprandial hyperglycemia.

Pharmacodynamics/Kinetics

Half-life Elimination ~2 hours

Time to Peak 2-3 hours

Pregnancy Risk Factor B

Pregnancy Considerations Adverse events have not been reported in animal reproduction studies; therefore, miglitol is classified as pregnancy category B. Information specific to the use of miglitol during pregnancy has not been located. Maternal hyperglycemia can be associated with adverse effects in the fetus, including macrosomia, neonatal hyperglycemia, and hyperbilirubinemia; the risk of congenital malformations is increased when the Hb A$_{1c}$ is above the normal range. Diabetes can also be associated with adverse effects in the mother. Poorly-treated diabetes may cause end-organ damage that may in turn negatively affect obstetric outcomes. Physiologic glucose levels should be maintained prior to and during pregnancy to decrease the risk of adverse events in the mother and the fetus. Until additional safety and efficacy data are obtained, the use of oral agents is generally not recommended as routine management of GDM or type 2 diabetes mellitus during pregnancy. Insulin is the drug of choice for the control of diabetes mellitus during pregnancy.

Miglustat (MIG loo stat)

Brand Names: U.S. Zavesca®

Brand Names: Canada Zavesca®

Pharmacologic Category Enzyme Inhibitor

Use Treatment of mild-to-moderate type 1 Gaucher disease when enzyme replacement therapy is not a therapeutic option

Canadian labeling: Additional use (not in U.S. labeling): Treatment to delay the progression of neurological manifestations in Niemann-Pick Type C disease

Local Anesthetic/Vasoconstrictor Precautions No information available to require special precautions

Effects on Dental Treatment No significant effects or complications reported

Effects on Bleeding No information available to require special precautions

Adverse Effects Percentages reported from open-label, uncontrolled monotherapy trials.

>10%:

Central nervous system: Headache (21% to 22%), dizziness (up to 11%)

Gastrointestinal: Diarrhea (89% to 100%), weight loss (39% to 67%), abdominal pain (18% to 67%), flatulence (29% to 50%), nausea (8% to 22%), vomiting (4% to 11%)

Neuromuscular & skeletal: Tremor (11% to 30%), weakness (17%), leg cramps (4% to 11%)

Ocular: Visual disturbances (up to 17%)

1% to 10%:

Central nervous system: Memory impairment (8%), migraine (up to 6%)

Endocrine & metabolic: Menstrual disorder (up to 6%)

Gastrointestinal: Abdominal distension (8%), constipation (8%), xerostomia (8%), bloating (up to 6%), anorexia (up to 7%), dyspepsia (up to 7%), epigastric pain (up to 6%)

Hematologic: Thrombocytopenia (6% to 7%)

Neuromuscular & skeletal: Back pain (8%), gait instability (8%), paresthesia (up to 7%)

General Dosage Range Dosage adjustment recommended in patients with renal impairment

Oral: *Adults:* 100 mg 1-3 times/day

Mechanism of Action Miglustat competitively and reversibly inhibits the enzyme needed to produce glycosphingolipids and decreases the rate of glycosphingolipid glucosylceramide formation. Glucosylceramide accumulates in type 1 Gaucher disease, causing complications specific to this disease.

Pharmacodynamics/Kinetics

Half-life Elimination 6-7 hours

Time to Peak Plasma: 2-2.5 hours

Pregnancy Risk Factor X

Pregnancy Considerations Decreased fetus weight, fetal loss, and difficult or delayed births were observed in animal studies. Women with reproduction potential should use effective contraception during therapy. In addition, adverse effects on spermatogenesis and reduced fertility were observed in male animal studies. The manufacturer recommends that male patients use reliable contraception during therapy and for 3 months following treatment.

Milnacipran (mil NAY ci pran)

Related Information

Vasoconstrictor Interactions With Antidepressants *on page 1650*

Brand Names: U.S. Savella®

Generic Availability (U.S.) No

Pharmacologic Category Antidepressant, Serotonin/Norepinephrine Reuptake Inhibitor

Use Management of fibromyalgia

Local Anesthetic/Vasoconstrictor Precautions Although milnacipran is not a tricyclic antidepressant, it blocks norepinephrine reuptake within the CNS synapses as part of the mechanism of action. It has been suggested that vasoconstrictors be administered with caution and vial signs monitored in dental patients taking antidepressants that affect norepinephrine in this way.

Effects on Dental Treatment Key adverse event(s) related to dental treatment: Xerostomia and changes in salivation (normal salivary flow resumes upon discontinuation) and taste perversion.

Effects on Bleeding Serotonin/norepinephrine reuptake inhibitors (SNRIs) may impair platelet aggregation resulting in increased risk of bleeding events, particularly if used concomitantly with aspirin or NSAIDs.

Adverse Effects

>10%:

Central nervous system: Headache (18%), insomnia (12%)

Endocrine & metabolic: Hot flashes (12%)

Gastrointestinal: Nausea (37%), constipation (16%)

1% to 10%:

Cardiovascular: Palpitation (7%), heart rate increased (6%), hypertension (5%), blood pressure increased (3%), flushing (3%), tachycardia (2%), peripheral edema (≥1%)

Central nervous system: Dizziness (10%), migraine (5%), chills (2%), tremor (2%), depression (≥1%), fatigue (≥1%), fever (≥1%), irritability (≥1%), somnolence (≥1%)

Dermatologic: Hyperhidrosis (9%), rash (3%)

Endocrine & metabolic: Hypercholesterolemia (≥1%)

Gastrointestinal: Vomiting (7%), xerostomia (5%), abdominal pain (3%), appetite decreased (2%), abdominal distension (≥1%), abnormal taste (≥1%), diarrhea (≥1%), dyspepsia (≥1%), flatulence (≥1%), gastroesophageal reflux disease (≥1%), weight changes (≥1%)

Genitourinary: Dysuria (≥2%), ejaculation disorder/failure (≥2%), erectile dysfunction (≥2%), libido decreased (≥2%), prostatitis (≥2%), scrotal pain (≥2%), testicular pain (≥2%), testicular swelling (≥2%), urethral pain (≥2%), urinary hesitation (≥2%), urinary retention (≥2%), urine flow decreased (≥2%), cystitis (≥1%), urinary tract infection (≥1%)

Neuromuscular & skeletal: Falling (≥1%)

Ocular: Blurred vision (2%)

Respiratory: Dyspnea (2%)

Miscellaneous: Night sweats (≥1%)

Dosage Oral: Adults: 50 mg twice daily (maximum dose: 200 mg/day)

Titration schedule: 12.5 mg once on day 1, then 12.5 mg twice daily on days 2-3, 25 mg twice daily on days 4-7, then 50 mg twice daily thereafter. Dose may be increased to 100 mg twice daily, based on individual response. Doses >200 mg/day have not been studied.

Discontinuation of therapy: Gradually taper dose. If intolerable symptoms occur following a dose reduction, consider resuming the previously prescribed dose and/or decrease dose at a more gradual rate.

Dosing adjustment in renal impairment:

Mild renal impairment: No dose adjustment is recommended

Moderate renal impairment: Use with caution

Severe renal impairment (Cl$_{cr}$ ≤29 mL/minute): Reduce maintenance dose to 25 mg twice daily; dose may be increased to 50 mg twice daily, based on individual tolerance

End-stage renal disease (ESRD): Use not recommended

Dosing adjustment in hepatic impairment:

Mild-to-moderate hepatic impairment: No dose adjustment is recommended

Severe hepatic impairment: Use with caution

Mechanism of Action Potent inhibitor of norepinephrine and serotonin reuptake (3:1). Milnacipran has no significant activity for serotonergic, alpha- and beta-adrenergic, muscarinic, histaminergic, dopaminergic, opiate, benzodiazepine, and GABA receptors. It does not possess MAO-inhibitory activity.

Contraindications Concomitant use or within 2 weeks of MAO inhibitors; uncontrolled narrow-angle glaucoma

Warnings/Precautions [U.S. Boxed Warning]: Milnacipran is a serotonin/norepinephrine reuptake inhibitor (SNRI) similar to SNRIs used to treat depression and other psychiatric disorders. Antidepressants increase the risk of suicidal thinking and behavior in children, adolescents, and young adults (18-24 years of age) with major depressive disorder (MDD) and other psychiatric disorders; consider risk prior to prescribing. Short-term studies did not show an increased risk in patients >24 years of age and showed a decreased risk in patients ≥65 years. Closely monitor for clinical worsening, suicidality, or unusual changes in behavior; the patient's family or caregiver should be instructed to closely observe the patient and communicate condition with healthcare provider. A medication guide should be dispensed with each prescription. **Milnacipran is not FDA approved for the treatment of major depressive disorder or for use in children.**

Suicide risks should be monitored in patients treated with SNRIs regardless of the indication. The possibility of a suicide attempt is inherent in major depression and may persist until remission occurs. Monitor for worsening of depression or suicidality, especially during initiation of therapy (generally first 1-2 months) or with dose increases or decreases. Use caution in high-risk patients. Worsening depression and severe abrupt suicidality that are not part of the presenting symptoms may require discontinuation or modification of drug therapy. The patient's family or caregiver should be alerted to monitor patients for the emergence of suicidality and associated behaviors (such as agitation, irritability, hostility, impulsivity, and hypomania) and call healthcare provider.

Patients with major depressive disorder were excluded from clinical trials evaluating milnacipran for fibromyalgia; however, mania has been reported in patients with mood disorders taking similar medications. May worsen psychosis in some patients or precipitate a shift to mania or hypomania in patients with bipolar disorder. Patients presenting with depressive symptoms should be screened for bipolar disorder. Monotherapy in patients with bipolar disorder should be avoided. **Milnacipran is not FDA approved for the treatment of bipolar depression.**

Serotonin syndrome and neuroleptic malignant syndrome (NMS)-like reactions have occurred with serotonin/norepinephrine reuptake inhibitors (SNRIs) and selective serotonin reuptake inhibitors (SSRIs) when used alone, and particularly when used in combination with serotonergic agents (eg, triptans) or antidopaminergic agents (eg, antipsychotics). Concurrent use with MAO inhibitors is contraindicated. May cause sustained increase in blood pressure or heart rate. Control preexisting hypertension and cardiovascular disease prior to initiation of milnacipran. Use caution in patients with renal impairment; dose reduction required in severe renal impairment. Use caution in patients with hepatic impairment. Avoid ethanol use. Use cautiously in patients with a history of seizures. May impair platelet aggregation, resulting in bleeding. May cause increased urinary resistance. Use caution in patients with a history of dysuria, especially males with prostatic hypertrophy, prostatitis, or other lower urinary tract disorders. Use caution in patients with controlled narrow-angle glaucoma; use is contraindicated with uncontrolled narrow-angle glaucoma.

Abrupt discontinuation or dosage reduction after extended therapy may lead to agitation, dysphoria, anxiety, and other symptoms. When discontinuing therapy, dosage should be tapered gradually. If intolerable symptoms occur following a decrease in dosage or upon discontinuation of therapy, then resuming the previous dose with a more gradual taper should be considered.

Drug Interactions

Metabolism/Transport Effects None known.

Avoid Concomitant Use

Avoid concomitant use of Milnacipran with any of the following: Iobenguane I 123; Linezolid; MAO Inhibitors; Methylene Blue

Increased Effect/Toxicity

Milnacipran may increase the levels/effects of: Alpha-/Beta-Agonists; Aspirin; Digoxin; Methylene Blue; Metoclopramide; NSAID (Nonselective); Serotonin Modulators; Vitamin K Antagonists

The levels/effects of Milnacipran may be increased by: Alcohol (Ethyl); Antipsychotics; ClomiPRAMINE; Linezolid; MAO Inhibitors

Decreased Effect

Milnacipran may decrease the levels/effects of: Alpha2-Agonists; Iobenguane I 123; Ioflupane I 123

Ethanol/Nutrition/Herb Interactions

Ethanol: Ethanol may increase CNS depression. Management: Avoid ethanol.

Herb/Nutraceutical: Some herbal medications may increase risk of serotonin syndrome and/or excessive sedation. Management: Avoid valerian, St John's wort, SAMe, kava kava, and tryptophan.

Dietary Considerations May be taken with or without food; food may improve tolerability.

Pharmacodynamics/Kinetics

Half-life Elimination 6-8 hours

Time to Peak Plasma: Oral: 2-4 hours

Pregnancy Risk Factor C

Pregnancy Considerations Adverse events were observed in some animal reproduction studies. Nonteratogenic effects in the newborn following SSRI/SNRI exposure late in the third trimester include respiratory distress, cyanosis, apnea, seizures, temperature instability, feeding difficulty, vomiting, hypoglycemia, hyper- or hypotonia, hyper-reflexia, jitteriness, irritability, constant crying, and tremor. Symptoms may be due to the toxicity of the SNRIs/SSRIs or a discontinuation syndrome and may be consistent with serotonin syndrome associated with SSRI treatment. The long-term effects of *in utero* SNRI/SSRI exposure on infant development and behavior are not known.

Women inadvertently exposed to milnacipran during pregnancy may be enrolled in the Savella Pregnancy Registry (877-643-3010 or http://www.savellapregnancyregistry.com).

Lactation Enters breast milk/use caution

Breast-Feeding Considerations Milnacipran is excreted into breast milk. The manufacturer recommends that caution be exercised when administering milnacipran to nursing women.

Dosage Forms

Combination package, oral:

Savella®: Tablet: 12.5 mg (5s), Tablet: 25 mg (8s), and Tablet: 50 mg (42s)

Tablet, oral:

Savella®: 12.5 mg, 25 mg, 50 mg, 100 mg

References

Gendreau RM, Thorn MD, Gendreau JF, et al, "Efficacy of Milnacipran in Patients With Fibromyalgia," *J Rheumatol*, 2005, 32(10):1975-85.
Vitton O, Gendreau M, Gendreau J, et al, "A Double-Blind Placebo-Controlled Trial of Milnacipran in the Treatment of Fibromyalgia," *Hum Psychopharmacol*, 2004, 19(Suppl 1):27-35.

Milrinone (MIL ri none)

Brand Names: Canada Milrinone Lactate Injection; Primacor®

Pharmacologic Category Phosphodiesterase-3 Enzyme Inhibitor

Use Short-term I.V. therapy of acutely-decompensated heart failure

Unlabeled Use Inotropic therapy for patients unresponsive to other acute heart failure therapies (eg, dobutamine); outpatient inotropic therapy for heart transplant candidates; palliation of symptoms in end-stage heart failure patients who cannot otherwise be discharged from the hospital and are not transplant candidates

Local Anesthetic/Vasoconstrictor Precautions No information available to require special precautions

Effects on Dental Treatment No significant effects or complications reported

Effects on Bleeding No information available to require special precautions

Adverse Effects

>10%: Cardiovascular: Ventricular arrhythmia (ectopy 9%, NSVT 3%, sustained ventricular tachycardia 1%, ventricular fibrillation <1%)

1% to 10%:

Cardiovascular: Supraventricular arrhythmia (4%), hypotension (3%), angina/chest pain (1%)

Central nervous system: Headache (3%)

General Dosage Range Dosage adjustment recommended in patients with renal impairment

I.V.: *Adults:* Loading dose (optional): 50 mcg/kg; Maintenance: 0.375-0.75 mcg/kg/minute

Mechanism of Action A selective phosphodiesterase inhibitor in cardiac and vascular tissue, resulting in vasodilation and inotropic effects with little chronotropic activity.

Pharmacodynamics/Kinetics

Onset of Action I.V.: 5-15 minutes

Half-life Elimination Normal renal function: ~2.5 hours; CVVH: 20.1 hours (Taniguchi, 2000)

Pregnancy Risk Factor C

Pregnancy Considerations Teratogenic effects have not been observed in animal reproduction studies; however, increased resorption was reported in some studies.

Minocycline (mi noe SYE kleen)

Related Sample Prescriptions

Bacterial Infections and Periodontal Diseases *on page 1609*

Brand Names: U.S. Dynacin®; Minocin®; Minocin® PAC; Solodyn®

Brand Names: Canada Apo-Minocycline®; Arestin Microspheres; Dom-Minocycline; Minocin®; Mylan-Minocycline; Novo-Minocycline; PHL-Minocycline; PMS-Minocycline; ratio-Minocycline; Riva-Minocycline; Sandoz-Minocycline

Generic Availability (U.S.) Yes: Excludes injection, pellet-filled capsule

Pharmacologic Category Antibiotic, Tetracycline Derivative

Use Treatment of susceptible bacterial infections of both gram-negative and gram-positive organisms; treatment of anthrax (inhalational, cutaneous, and gastrointestinal); moderate-to-severe acne; meningococcal (asymptomatic) carrier state; Rickettsial diseases (including Rocky Mountain spotted fever, Q fever); nongonococcal urethritis, gonorrhea; acute intestinal amebiasis; respiratory tract infection; skin/soft tissue infections; chlamydial infections

Extended release (Solodyn®): Only indicated for treatment of inflammatory lesions of non-nodular moderate-to-severe acne

Unlabeled Use Rheumatoid arthritis (patients with low disease activity of short duration); nocardiosis; alternative treatment for community-acquired MRSA infection; chronic oral antimicrobial suppression of prosthetic joint infection

Local Anesthetic/Vasoconstrictor Precautions No information available to require special precautions

Effects on Dental Treatment Key adverse event(s) related to dental treatment: Discoloration of teeth (children). Opportunistic "superinfection" with *Candida albicans*; tetracyclines are not recommended for use during pregnancy or in children ≤8 years of age since they have been reported to cause enamel hypoplasia and permanent teeth discoloration. The use of tetracycline's should only be used in these patients if other agents are contraindicated or alternative antimicrobials will not eradicate the organism. Long-term use associated with oral candidiasis.

Effects on Bleeding No information available to require special precautions

Adverse Effects Frequency not defined.

Cardiovascular: Myocarditis, pericarditis, vasculitis

Central nervous system: Bulging fontanels, dizziness, fatigue, fever, headache, hypoesthesia, malaise, mood changes, paresthesia, pseudotumor cerebri, sedation, seizure, somnolence, vertigo

Dermatologic: Alopecia, angioedema, drug rash with eosinophilia and systemic symptoms (DRESS), erythema multiforme, erythema nodosum, erythematous rash, exfoliative dermatitis, hyperpigmentation of nails, maculopapular rash, photosensitivity, pigmentation of the skin and mucous membranes, pruritus, Stevens-Johnson syndrome, toxic epidermal necrolysis, urticaria

Endocrine & metabolic: Thyroid cancer, thyroid discoloration, thyroid dysfunction

Gastrointestinal: Anorexia, diarrhea, dyspepsia, dysphagia, enamel hypoplasia, enterocolitis, esophageal ulcerations, esophagitis, glossitis, inflammatory lesions (oral/anogenital), moniliasis, nausea, oral cavity discoloration, pancreatitis, pseudomembranous colitis, stomatitis, tooth discoloration, vomiting, xerostomia

Genitourinary: Balanitis, vulvovaginitis

Hematologic: Agranulocytosis, eosinophilia, hemolytic anemia, leukopenia, neutropenia, pancytopenia, thrombocytopenia

Hepatic: Autoimmune hepatitis, hepatic cholestasis, hepatic failure, hepatitis, hyperbilirubinemia, jaundice, liver enzyme increases

Local: Injection site reaction (I.V. administration)

Neuromuscular & skeletal: Arthralgia, arthritis, bone discoloration, joint stiffness, joint swelling, myalgia

Otic: Hearing loss, tinnitus

Renal: Acute renal failure, BUN increased, interstitial nephritis

Respiratory: Asthma, bronchospasm, cough, dyspnea, pneumonitis, pulmonary infiltrate (with eosinophilia)

Miscellaneous: Anaphylaxis, hypersensitivity, lupus erythematosus, lupus-like syndrome, serum sickness

Dosage

Usual dosage range:

I.V.:

Children >8 years: Initial: 4 mg/kg, followed by 2 mg/kg/dose every 12 hours (maximum: 400 mg daily)

Adults: Initial: 200 mg, followed by 100 mg every 12 hours (maximum: 400 mg daily)

Oral:

Capsule or immediate release tablet:

Children >8 years: Oral: Initial: 4 mg/kg, followed by 2 mg/kg/dose every 12 hours (maximum: 400 mg daily)

Adults: Oral: Initial: 200 mg, followed by 100 mg every 12 hours; more frequent dosing intervals may be used (100-200 mg initially, followed by 50 mg 4 times daily)

Extended release tablet (Solodyn®): Children ≥12 years and Adults (≥45 kg): Oral: 45-135 mg once daily (weight based)

Indication-specific dosing:

Children ≥12 years and Adults:

Acne, inflammatory, non-nodular, moderate-to-severe (Solodyn®): Oral:

45-49 kg: 45 mg once daily

50-59 kg: 55 mg once daily

60-71 kg: 65 mg once daily

72-84 kg: 80 mg once daily

85-96 kg: 90 mg once daily

97-110 kg: 105 mg once daily

111-125 kg: 115 mg once daily

126-136 kg: 135 mg once daily

Note: Therapy should be continued for 12 weeks. Higher doses do not confer greater efficacy and may be associated with more acute vestibular side effects. Safety of use beyond 12 weeks has not been established.

Cellulitis (purulent) infection due to community-acquired MRSA (unlabeled use): Oral: Children >8 years: Initial: 4 mg/kg (maximum: 200 mg); Maintenance: 2 mg/kg/dose (maximum: 100 mg) every 12 hours for 5-10 days (Liu, 2011)

Adults:

Acne: Oral: Capsule or immediate-release tablet: 50-100 mg twice daily

Cellulitis (purulent) due to community-acquired MRSA (unlabeled use): Oral: Initial: 200 mg; Maintenance: 100 mg twice daily for 5-10 days (Liu, 2011)

Chlamydial or *Ureaplasma urealyticum* infection, uncomplicated: Oral, I.V.: Urethral, endocervical, or rectal: 100 mg every 12 hours for at least 7 days

Gonococcal infection, uncomplicated (males): Oral, I.V.:

Without urethritis or anorectal infection: Initial: 200 mg, followed by 100 mg every 12 hours for at least 4 days (cultures 2-3 days post-therapy)

Urethritis: 100 mg every 12 hours for 5 days

Meningococcal carrier state (manufacturer's labeling): Oral: 100 mg every 12 hours for 5 days. **Note:** CDC recommendations do not mention use of minocycline for eradicating nasopharyngeal carriage of meningococcal

***Mycobacterium marinum*:** Oral: 100 mg every 12 hours for 6-8 weeks

Nocardiosis, cutaneous (non-CNS) (unlabeled use): Oral: 100-200 mg every 12 hours

Prosthetic joint infection:

Staphylococci (oxacillin-sensitive or –resistant) oral phase treatment (after completion of pathogen-specific I.V. therapy) following 1-stage exchange:
Total ankle, elbow, hip, or shoulder arthroplasty: 100 mg twice daily for 3 months; **Note:** Must be used in combination with rifampin (Osmon, 2013)
Total knee arthroplasty: 100 mg twice daily for 6 months; **Note:** Must be used in combination with rifampin (Osmon, 2013)

Chronic oral antimicrobial suppression (unlabeled use): Oral:
Propionibacterium spp (alternative to penicillin or amoxicillin): 100 mg twice daily (Osmon, 2013)
Staphylococci (oxacillin-resistant): 100 mg twice daily (Osmon, 2013)

Rheumatoid arthritis (unlabeled use): Oral: 100 mg twice daily (O'Dell, 2001)

Syphilis: Oral, I.V.: Initial: 200 mg, followed by 100 mg every 12 hours for 10-15 days

Elderly: Refer to adult dosing.

Dosage adjustment in renal impairment: Use with caution; monitor BUN and creatinine clearance. Consider decreasing dose or increasing dosing interval (extended release).
Cl_{cr} <80 mL/minute: Do not exceed 200 mg daily

Dosage adjustment in hepatic impairment: No dosage adjustment provided in manufacturer's labeling; however, hepatotoxicity has been reported. Use with caution in patients with hepatic impairment.

Mechanism of Action Inhibits bacterial protein synthesis by binding with the 30S and possibly the 50S ribosomal subunit(s) of susceptible bacteria; cell wall synthesis is not affected

Rheumatoid arthritis: The mechanism of action of minocycline in rheumatoid arthritis is not completely understood. It is thought to have antimicrobial, anti-inflammatory, immunomodulatory, and chondroprotective effects. More specifically, it is thought to be a potent inhibitor of metalloproteinases, which are active in rheumatoid arthritis joint destruction.

Contraindications Hypersensitivity to minocycline, other tetracyclines, or any component of the formulation

Warnings/Precautions May be associated with increases in BUN secondary to antianabolic effects; use caution in patients with renal impairment (Cl_{cr} <80 mL/minute). Hepatotoxicity has been reported; use caution in patients with hepatic insufficiency. Autoimmune syndromes (eg, lupus-like, hepatitis, and vasculitis) have been reported; discontinue if symptoms occur. CNS effects (lightheadedness, vertigo) may occur; patients must be cautioned about performing tasks which require mental alertness (eg, operating machinery or driving). Pseudotumor cerebri has been (rarely) reported with tetracycline use; usually resolves with discontinuation. May cause photosensitivity; discontinue if skin erythema occurs. Prolonged use may result in fungal or bacterial superinfection, including *C. difficile*-associated diarrhea (CDAD) and pseudomembranous colitis; CDAD has been observed >2 months postantibiotic treatment. May cause tissue hyperpigmentation, enamel hypoplasia, or permanent tooth discoloration; use of tetracyclines should be avoided during tooth development (children <8 years of age) unless other drugs are not likely to be effective or are contraindicated. Do not use during pregnancy. In addition to affecting tooth development, tetracycline use has been associated with retardation of skeletal development and reduced bone growth. Rash, along with eosinophilia,

fever, and organ failure (Drug Rash with Eosinophilia and Systemic Symptoms [DRESS] syndrome) has been reported; discontinue treatment immediately if DRESS syndrome is suspected.

Drug Interactions

Metabolism/Transport Effects None known.

Avoid Concomitant Use
Avoid concomitant use of Minocycline with any of the following: BCG; Retinoic Acid Derivatives; Strontium Ranelate

Increased Effect/Toxicity
Minocycline may increase the levels/effects of: Mipomersen; Neuromuscular-Blocking Agents; Porfimer; Retinoic Acid Derivatives; Vitamin K Antagonists

Decreased Effect
Minocycline may decrease the levels/effects of: Atazanavir; BCG; Penicillins; Sodium Picosulfate; Typhoid Vaccine

The levels/effects of Minocycline may be decreased by: Antacids; Bile Acid Sequestrants; Bismuth; Bismuth Subsalicylate; Calcium Salts; Iron Salts; Lanthanum; Magnesium Salts; Multivitamins/Minerals (with ADEK, Folate, Iron); Quinapril; Strontium Ranelate; Sucralfate; Zinc Salts

Ethanol/Nutrition/Herb Interactions
Food: Minocycline serum concentrations are not significantly altered if taken with food or dairy products.
Herb/Nutraceutical: Avoid dong quai, St John's wort (may also cause photosensitization).

Dietary Considerations May be taken with or without food.

Pharmacodynamics/Kinetics

Half-life Elimination I.V.: 15-23 hours; Oral: 16 hours (range: 11-22 hours)

Time to Peak Capsule, pellet filled: 1-4 hours; Extended release tablet: 3.5-4 hours

Pregnancy Risk Factor D

Pregnancy Considerations Tetracyclines cross the placenta and accumulate in developing teeth and long tubular bones. Rare spontaneous reports of congenital anomalies, including limb reduction, have been reported following maternal minocycline use. Due to limited information, a causal association cannot be established. Tetracyclines may discolor fetal teeth following maternal use during pregnancy; the specific teeth involved and the portion of the tooth affected depends on the timing and duration of exposure relative to tooth calcification. As a class, tetracyclines are generally considered second-line antibiotics in pregnant women and their use should be avoided (Mylonas, 2011). Minocycline should not be used for the treatment of acne in pregnant women, or in males or females attempting to conceive a child.

Lactation Enters breast milk/not recommended

Breast-Feeding Considerations Minocycline is excreted in breast milk (Brogden, 1975). According to the manufacturer, the decision to continue or discontinue breast-feeding during therapy should take into account the risk of exposure to the infant and the benefits of treatment to the mother. Oral absorption is not affected by dairy products; therefore, oral absorption of minocycline by the breast-feeding infant would not be expected to be diminished by the calcium in the maternal milk. Nondose-related effects could include modification of bowel flora. There have been case reports of black discoloration of breast milk in women taking minocycline (Basler, 1985; Hunt, 1996).

Product Availability Ximino™ extended-release capsules: FDA approved July 2012; anticipated availability currently unknown. Consult prescribing information for additional information.

Dosage Forms

Capsule, oral: 50 mg, 75 mg, 100 mg

Capsule, pellet filled, oral:

Minocin®: 50 mg, 100 mg

Minocin® PAC: 50 mg, 100 mg

Injection, powder for reconstitution:

Minocin®: 100 mg

Tablet, oral: 50 mg, 75 mg, 100 mg

Dynacin®: 50 mg, 75 mg, 100 mg

Tablet, extended release, oral: 45 mg, 90 mg, 135 mg

Solodyn®: 55 mg, 65 mg, 80 mg, 105 mg, 115 mg

Minocycline Hydrochloride (Periodontal)

(mi noe SYE kleen hye droe KLOR ide pair ee oh DON tol)

Related Information

Minocycline *on page 924*

Periodontal Diseases *on page 1570*

Brand Names: U.S. Arestin®

Generic Availability (U.S.) No

Pharmacologic Category Antibiotic, Tetracycline Derivative

Dental Use Adjunct to scaling and root planing procedures for reduction of pocket depth in patients with adult periodontitis. May be used as part of a periodontal maintenance program which includes good oral hygiene, scaling, and root planing.

Use Adjunct to scaling and root planing procedures for reduction of pocket depth in patients with adult periodontitis. May be used as part of a periodontal maintenance program which includes good oral hygiene, scaling, and root planing.

Local Anesthetic/Vasoconstrictor Precautions No information available to require special precautions

Effects on Dental Treatment Key adverse event(s) related to dental treatment: Patients should avoid the following postadministration: Eating hard, crunchy, or sticky foods for 1 week; brushing for a 12-hour period; touching treated areas; use of interproximal cleaning devices for 10 days.

Effects on Bleeding No information available to require special precautions

Adverse Effects

>10%: Gastrointestinal: Tooth disorder (12%)

1% to 10%:

Central nervous system: Headache (9%), pain (4%)

Gastrointestinal: Dental caries (10%), dental pain (10%), gingivitis (9%), mouth ulceration (5%), dyspepsia (4%), mucous membrane disorder (3%)

Respiratory: Pharyngitis (4%)

Miscellaneous: Infection (8%), flu-like syndrome (5%)

Dental Usual Dosage Arestin® is a variable-dose product; dependent upon the size, shape, and number of pockets being treated.

Administration of Arestin® does not require local anesthesia. Professional subgingival administration is accomplished by inserting the unit-dose cartridge to the base of the periodontal pocket and then pressing the thumb ring in the handle mechanism to expel the powder while gradually withdrawing the tip from the base of the pocket. The handle mechanism should be sterilized between patients. Arestin® does not have to

be removed (it is bioresorbable) nor is an adhesive dressing required.

Dosage Variable-dose product; dependent upon the size, shape, and number of pockets being treated

Mechanism of Action Minocycline, a member of the tetracycline class of antibiotics, has a broad spectrum of activity. It is bacteriostatic and exerts its antimicrobial activity by inhibiting protein synthesis.

Contraindications Known hypersensitivity to minocycline, tetracyclines, or any component of the formulation; children <8 years of age

Warnings/Precautions Hypersensitivity reactions (eg, anaphylaxis, angioneurotic edema, urticaria, rash, swelling of the face, and pruritus) have been reported. Lupus-like, hepatitis, and vasculitis autoimmune syndromes have been reported with oral minocycline use; no further treatment should be given if symptoms occur. May cause photosensitivity; discontinue if skin erythema occurs. Use skin protection and avoid prolonged exposure to sunlight; do not use tanning equipment. Prolonged use may result in fungal or bacterial superinfection, including *C. difficile*-associated diarrhea (CDAD) and pseudomembranous colitis; CDAD has been observed >2 months postantibiotic treatment. May cause tissue hyperpigmentation, enamel hypoplasia, or permanent tooth discoloration; use of tetracyclines should be avoided during tooth development (children <8 years of age) unless other drugs are not likely to be effective or are contraindicated. Do not use during pregnancy. In addition to affecting tooth development, tetracycline use has been associated with retardation of skeletal development and reduced bone growth.

Use in an acutely abscessed periodontal pocket has not been studied and is not recommended. The effects of treatment for >6 months have not been studied. Should be used with caution in patients having a history of predisposition to oral candidiasis. Safety and effectiveness have not been established for the treatment of periodontitis in patients with coexistent oral candidiasis. Not clinically tested in immunocompromised patients (such as those immunocompromised by diabetes, chemotherapy, radiation therapy, or infection with HIV). Not clinically tested for use in the regeneration of alveolar bone, either in preparation for or in conjunction with the placement of endosseous (dental) implants or in the treatment of failing implants.

Pregnancy Risk Factor D

Pregnancy Considerations Refer to Warnings/Precautions.

Lactation Enters breast milk/not recommended

Dosage Forms

Powder, sustained release microspheres, subgingival:

Arestin®: 1 mg (12s)

Minoxidil (Systemic) (mi NOKS i dil)

Related Information

Cardiovascular Diseases *on page 1492*

Brand Names: Canada Loniten®

Pharmacologic Category Vasodilator, Direct-Acting

Use Management of severe hypertension (usually in combination with a diuretic and beta-blocker)

Local Anesthetic/Vasoconstrictor Precautions No information available to require special precautions

Effects on Dental Treatment No significant effects or complications reported

Effects on Bleeding No information available to require special precautions

Adverse Effects Frequency not always reported.

Cardiovascular: ECG changes (T-wave changes 60%), peripheral edema (7%), pericardial effusion with tamponade (3%), pericardial effusion without tamponade (3%), angina pectoris, heart failure, pericarditis, rebound hypertension (in children after a gradual withdrawal), sodium and water retention, tachycardia

Dermatologic: Hypertrichosis (common; 80%), bullous eruption (rare), rash, Stevens-Johnson syndrome (rare)

Endocrine & metabolic: Breast tenderness (rare; <1%)

Gastrointestinal: Nausea, vomiting, weight gain

Hematologic: Leukopenia (rare), thrombocytopenia (rare), transient decreased erythrocyte count (hemodilution), transient decreased hematocrit/hemoglobin (hemodilution)

Hepatic: Increased alkaline phosphatase

Renal: Transient increase in serum BUN and creatinine

Respiratory: Pulmonary edema

General Dosage Range Oral:

Children <12 years: Initial: 0.1-0.2 mg/kg once daily (maximum: 5 mg/day); Usual dosage range: 0.25-1 mg/kg/day in 1-2 divided doses (maximum: 50 mg/day)

Children ≥12 years and Adults: Initial: 5 mg once daily; Usual dosage range: 2.5-80 mg/day in 1-2 divided doses (maximum: 100 mg/day)

Elderly: Initial: 2.5 mg once daily

Mechanism of Action Produces vasodilation by directly relaxing arteriolar smooth muscle, with little effect on veins; effects may be mediated by cyclic AMP; stimulation of hair growth is secondary to vasodilation, increased cutaneous blood flow and stimulation of resting hair follicles

Pharmacodynamics/Kinetics

Onset of Action Hypotensive: ~30 minutes; Peak effect: 2-8 hours

Duration of Action 2-5 days

Half-life Elimination Adults: 3.5-4.2 hours

Pregnancy Risk Factor C

Pregnancy Considerations Adverse events were observed in some animal studies.

Mipomersen (mi poe MER sen)

Brand Names: U.S. Kynamro™

Pharmacologic Category Antihyperlipidemic Agent, Apolipoprotein B Antisense Oligonucleotide

Use Adjunct to dietary therapy and other lipid-lowering treatments to reduce low-density lipoprotein cholesterol (LDL-C), total cholesterol, apolipoprotein B, and non-high-density lipoprotein cholesterol (non-HDL-C) in patients with homozygous familial hypercholesterolemia (HoFH)

Local Anesthetic/Vasoconstrictor Precautions No information available to require special precautions

Effects on Dental Treatment No significant effects or complications reported

Effects on Bleeding No information available to require special precautions

Adverse Effects

>10%:

Central nervous system: Fatigue (15%), headache (12%)

Gastrointestinal: Nausea (14%)

Hepatic: ALT increased (≥3 x ULN to <5 x ULN: 12%; ≥5 x ULN to <10 x ULN: 3%; ≥10 x ULN: 1%)

Local: Injection site reactions: Erythema (59%), pain (56%), hematoma (32%), pruritus (29%), swelling (18%), discoloration (17%)

Miscellaneous: Antibody formation (38% to 72%), flu-like syndrome (13% to 66%)

1% to 10%:

Cardiovascular: Hypertension (7%), peripheral edema (5%), angina pectoris (4%), palpitations (3%)

Central nervous system: Fever (8%), chills (6%), insomnia (3%)

Gastrointestinal: Vomiting (4%), abdominal pain (3%)

Hepatic: Hepatic steatosis (7%), AST increased (≥3 x ULN to <5 x ULN: 7%; ≥5 x ULN to <10 x ULN: 3%)

Neuromuscular & skeletal: Limb pain (7%), musculoskeletal pain (4%)

Renal: Proteinuria (9%)

Miscellaneous: Neoplasms (4%, benign and malignant)

General Dosage Range SubQ *Adults:* 200 mg once weekly

Mechanism of Action Mipomersen is an oligonucleotide inhibitor of apo B-100 synthesis. ApoB is the main component of LDL-C and very low density lipoprotein (VLDL), which is the precursor to LDL-C. Mipomersen binds to the messenger ribonucleic acid (mRNA) of apoB in a sequence-specific manner which results in degradation (RNase H-mediated) or disruption of the mRNA thereby reducing formation of apoB.

Pharmacodynamics/Kinetics

Half-life Elimination 1-2 months

Time to Peak 3-4 hours

Pregnancy Risk Factor B

Pregnancy Considerations Adverse events have not been observed in animal reproduction studies. There are no adequate and well-controlled studies in pregnant women. Use during pregnancy only if clearly needed.

Prescribing and Access Restrictions As a requirement of the REMS program, access to this medication is restricted. Prescribers must enroll in the Kynamro™ REMS program and complete the prescriber training and complete, sign, and submit the Prescriber Enrollment Form to the Kynamro™ REMS program. The prescriber must then complete the Prescriber Training before activation within the Kynamro™ REMS program. Pharmacies must educate all pharmacy staff involved in the dispensing of Kynamro™ on the REMS program requirements, put processes in place to verify (prior to dispensing Kynamro™) that the prescriber is certified and the Prescription Authorization Form is received with each new prescription. Pharmacies must also agree to be audited to ensure that all processes and procedures in place are being followed in accordance with the program and be able to provide prescription data to the REMS program.

Mirabegron (mir a BEG ron)

Brand Names: U.S. Myrbetriq™

Pharmacologic Category Beta$_3$ Agonist

Use Treatment of overactive bladder (OAB) with symptoms of urinary frequency, urgency, or urge incontinence

Local Anesthetic/Vasoconstrictor Precautions No information available to require special precautions

Effects on Dental Treatment Key adverse event(s) related to dental treatment: Xerostomia (normal salivary flow resumes upon discontinuation)

Effects on Bleeding No information available to require special precautions

Adverse Effects
>10%: Cardiovascular: Hypertension (9% to 11%)

1% to 10%:

Cardiovascular: Tachycardia (2%)

Central nervous system: Headache (4%), dizziness (3%)

Gastrointestinal: Constipation (2% to 3%), xerostomia (3%), diarrhea (2%)

Genitourinary: Urinary tract infection (3% to 6%), cystitis (2%)

Neuromuscular & skeletal: Back pain (3%), arthralgia (2%)

Respiratory: Nasopharyngitis (4%), sinusitis (3%)

Miscellaneous: Flu-like syndrome (3%)

General Dosage Range Dosage adjustment recommended in patients with renal and hepatic impairment

Oral: *Adults:* Initial: 25 mg once daily; Maintenance: 25-50 mg once daily

Mechanism of Action Mirabegron, a beta-3 adrenergic receptor agonist, activates beta-3 adrenergic receptors in the bladder resulting in relaxation of the detrusor smooth muscle during the urine storage phase, thus increasing bladder capacity. At usual doses, mirabegron is believed to display selectivity for the beta-3 adrenergic receptor subtype compared to its affinity for the beta-1 and -2 adrenoceptor subtypes. Data have shown that beta-adrenoceptors, predominately the beta-3 subtype, mediate detrusor smooth muscle tone and promote the storage function of the human bladder.

Pharmacodynamics/Kinetics
Onset of Action Efficacy is seen within 8 weeks; steady state achieved within 7 days

Half-life Elimination ~50 hours

Time to Peak ~3.5 hours

Pregnancy Risk Factor C

Pregnancy Considerations Adverse effects were observed in some animal reproduction studies.

Mirtazapine (mir TAZ a peen)

Related Information
Vasoconstrictor Interactions With Antidepressants *on page 1650*

Brand Names: U.S. Remeron SolTab®; Remeron®

Brand Names: Canada Apo-Mirtazapine®; Auro-Mirtazapine; Ava-Mirtazapine; CO Mirtazapine; Dom-Mirtazapine; GD-Mirtazapine; Jamp-Mirtazapine; Mylan-Mirtazapine; Novo-Mirtazapine; PMS-Mirtazapine; PRO-Mirtazapine; ratio-Mirtazapine; Remeron®; Remeron® RD; Riva-Mirtazapine; Sandoz-Mirtazapine; Sandoz-Mirtazapine FC; ZYM-Mirtazapine

Pharmacologic Category Antidepressant, Alpha-2 Antagonist

Use Treatment of depression

Unlabeled Use Alzheimer's dementia-related depression; post-traumatic stress disorder (PTSD)

Local Anesthetic/Vasoconstrictor Precautions Although mirtazapine is not a tricyclic antidepressant, it results in increased norepinephrine release as part of its mechanisms. It has been suggested that vasoconstrictor be administered with caution and to monitor vital signs in dental patients taking antidepressants that affect norepinephrine in this way, including mirtazapine.

Effects on Dental Treatment Key adverse event(s) related to dental treatment: Significant xerostomia (normal salivary flow resumes upon discontinuation).

Effects on Bleeding No information available to require special precautions

Adverse Effects
>10%:

Central nervous system: Somnolence (54%)

Endocrine & metabolic: Cholesterol increased

Gastrointestinal: Xerostomia (25%), appetite increased (17%), constipation (13%), weight gain (12%; weight gain of >7% reported in 8% of adults, ≤49% of pediatric patients)

1% to 10%:

Cardiovascular: Peripheral edema (2%), edema (1%), hypertension, vasodilatation

Central nervous system: Dizziness (7%), abnormal dreams (4%), abnormal thoughts (3%), confusion (2%), agitation, amnesia, anxiety, apathy, depression, hyper/hypokinesia, hypoesthesia, malaise, vertigo

Dermatologic: Pruritus, rash

Endocrine & metabolic: Triglycerides increased

Gastrointestinal: Abdominal pain, anorexia, vomiting

Genitourinary: Urinary frequency (2%), urinary tract infection

Hepatic: SGPT increased (≥3 times ULN: 2%)

Neuromuscular & skeletal: Weakness (8%), back pain (2%), myalgia (2%), tremor (2%), arthralgia, myasthenia, paresthesia, twitching

Respiratory: Dyspnea (1%), cough increased, sinusitis

Miscellaneous: Flu-like syndrome (5%), thirst

General Dosage Range Oral: *Adults:* Initial: 15 mg nightly; Maintenance: 15-45 mg nightly

Mechanism of Action Mirtazapine is a tetracyclic antidepressant that works by its central presynaptic alpha$_2$-adrenergic antagonist effects, which results in increased release of norepinephrine and serotonin. It is also a potent antagonist of 5-HT$_2$ and 5-HT$_3$ serotonin receptors and H1 histamine receptors and a moderate peripheral alpha$_1$-adrenergic and muscarinic antagonist; it does not inhibit the reuptake of norepinephrine or serotonin.

Pharmacodynamics/Kinetics
Half-life Elimination 20-40 hours; increased with renal or hepatic impairment

Time to Peak Serum: ~2 hours

Pregnancy Risk Factor C

Pregnancy Considerations Adverse events were observed in some animal reproduction studies. A significant increase in major teratogenic effects has not been observed in humans following exposure to mirtazapine during pregnancy; however, some nonteratogenic adverse events (similar to those observed with SSRI agents) have been reported (Djulus, 2006; Einarson, 2009; Lennestål, 2007). Mirtazapine was found to cross the placenta following a maternal overdose (Hatzidaki, 2008).

The ACOG recommends that therapy with antidepressants during pregnancy be individualized; treatment of depression during pregnancy should incorporate the clinical expertise of the mental health clinician, obstetrician, primary healthcare provider, and pediatrician. According to the American Psychiatric Association (APA), the risks of medication treatment should be weighed against other treatment options and untreated depression. Consideration should be given to using agents with safety data in pregnancy. For women who discontinue antidepressant medications during pregnancy and who may be at high risk for postpartum depression, the medications can be restarted following delivery. Treatment algorithms have been developed by the ACOG and the APA for the management of depression in women prior to conception and during pregnancy (ACOG, 2008; APA, 2010; Yonkers, 2009).

Misoprostol (mye soe PROST ole)

Brand Names: U.S. Cytotec®
Brand Names: Canada Novo-Misoprostol; PMS-Misoprostol
Pharmacologic Category Prostaglandin
Use
Prevention of NSAID-induced gastric ulcers
Medical termination of pregnancy of ≤49 days in conjunction with mifepristone (refer to Mifepristone monograph for details)
Unlabeled Use Cervical ripening and labor induction (except in women with prior cesarean delivery or major uterine surgery); prevention of postpartum hemorrhage; treatment of postpartum hemorrhage; treatment of incomplete or missed abortion in women <12 weeks gestation
Local Anesthetic/Vasoconstrictor Precautions No information available to require special precautions
Effects on Dental Treatment No significant effects or complications reported
Effects on Bleeding No information available to require special precautions
Adverse Effects
>10%: Gastrointestinal: Diarrhea, abdominal pain
1% to 10%:
Central nervous system: Headache
Gastrointestinal: Constipation, dyspepsia, flatulence, nausea, vomiting
General Dosage Range Oral: *Adults:* 100-200 mcg 4 times daily
Mechanism of Action Misoprostol is a synthetic prostaglandin E_1 analog that replaces the protective prostaglandins consumed with prostaglandin-inhibiting therapies (eg, NSAIDs); has been shown to induce uterine contractions
Pharmacodynamics/Kinetics
Half-life Elimination Misoprostol acid: 20-40 minutes
Time to Peak Serum: Misoprostol acid: Fasting: 6-22 minutes
Pregnancy Risk Factor X
Pregnancy Considerations Teratogenic effects were not observed in animal reproduction studies. Congenital anomalies following first trimester exposure have been reported, including skull defects, cranial nerve palsies, falcial malformations, and limb defects. Misoprostol may produce uterine contractions; fetal death, uterine perforation, and abortion may occur. **[U.S. Boxed Warning]: Use of misoprostol during pregnancy may cause abortion, birth defects, or premature birth. It is not to be used to reduce NSAID-induced ulcers in a woman of childbearing potential unless she is capable of complying with effective contraceptive measures and is at high risk of developing gastric ulcers and/or their complications.** If needed, the patient must have a negative pregnancy test within 2 weeks of starting therapy, she must use effective contraception during treatment, and therapy should begin on the second or third day of next normal menstrual period. Written and verbal warnings concerning the hazards of misoprostol should be provided.

Misoprostol is FDA approved for the medical termination of pregnancy of ≤49 days in conjunction with mifepristone.

Because misoprostol may induce or augment uterine contractions, it has been used off-label as a cervical-ripening agent for induction of labor in women who have not had a prior cesarean delivery or major uterine surgery. Hyperstimulation of the uterus, uterine rupture, or adverse events in the fetus or mother may occur with this use.

MitoMYcin (Systemic) (mye toe MYE sin)

Brand Names: Canada Mitomycin For Injection; Mitomycin For Injection USP; Mutamycin®
Pharmacologic Category Antineoplastic Agent, Antibiotic
Use Treatment of adenocarcinoma of stomach or pancreas
Unlabeled Use Treatment of anal carcinoma (nonmetastatic), bladder cancer, cervical cancer (recurrent or metastatic), esophageal cancer, gastric cancer, non small cell lung cancer (NSCLC)
Local Anesthetic/Vasoconstrictor Precautions No information available to require special precautions
Effects on Dental Treatment Key adverse event(s) related to dental treatment: Stomatitis.
Effects on Bleeding Bone marrow toxicity (pancytopenia) including thrombocytopenia, leukopenia, and anemia has been reported in 64% of patients. Medical consult recommended.
Adverse Effects
>10%:
Central nervous system: Fever (14%)
Gastrointestinal: Nausea, vomiting and anorexia (14%)
Hematologic: Myelosuppression (64%; onset: 4 weeks; recovery: 8-10 weeks)
Miscellaneous: Thrombotic thrombocytopenic purpura (TTP)/hemolytic uremic syndrome (HUS) (≤15%)
1% to 10%:
Dermatologic: Alopecia, mucous membrane toxicity (4%)
Gastrointestinal: Stomatitis (4%)
Renal: Serum creatinine increased (2%)
General Dosage Range Dosage adjustment recommended in patients with renal impairment or who develop toxicities.
I.V.: *Adults:* 20 mg/m^2 every 6-8 weeks
Mechanism of Action Acts like an alkylating agent and produces DNA cross-linking (primarily with guanine and cytosine pairs); cell-cycle nonspecific; inhibits DNA and RNA synthesis; degrades preformed DNA, causes nuclear lysis and formation of giant cells. While not phase-specific *per se*, mitomycin has its maximum effect against cells in late G and early S phases.
Pharmacodynamics/Kinetics
Half-life Elimination 17-78 minutes; Terminal: 50 minutes
Pregnancy Considerations Teratogenic effects have been observed in animal reproduction studies.

Mitotane (MYE toe tane)

Brand Names: U.S. Lysodren®
Brand Names: Canada Lysodren®
Pharmacologic Category Antineoplastic Agent, Miscellaneous
Use Treatment of inoperable adrenocortical carcinoma
Unlabeled Use Treatment of Cushing's syndrome
Local Anesthetic/Vasoconstrictor Precautions No information available to require special precautions

Effects on Dental Treatment No significant effects or complications reported

Effects on Bleeding No information available to require special precautions

Adverse Effects The majority of adverse events are dose-dependent.

>10%:

Central nervous system: CNS depression (32%), lethargy/somnolence (25%), dizziness/vertigo (15%)

Dermatologic: Skin rash (15%)

Gastrointestinal: Anorexia (24%), nausea (39%), vomiting (37%), diarrhea (13%)

Neuromuscular & skeletal: Weakness (12%)

1% to 10%:

Central nervous system: Headache (5%), confusion (3%)

Neuromuscular & skeletal: Muscle tremor (3%)

General Dosage Range Dosage adjustment recommended in patients who develop toxicities

Oral: *Adults:* Initial: 2-6 g/day in divided doses; Maintenance: 9-10 g/day in 3-4 divided doses (maximum: 18 g/day)

Mechanism of Action Adrenolytic agent which causes adrenal cortical atrophy; affects mitochondria in adrenal cortical cells and decreases production of cortisol; also alters the peripheral metabolism of steroids

Pharmacodynamics/Kinetics

Half-life Elimination 18-159 days

Time to Peak Serum: 3-5 hours

Pregnancy Risk Factor C

Pregnancy Considerations Animal reproduction studies have not been conducted. There are no adequate and well-controlled studies in pregnant women. Use during pregnancy only if clearly needed.

MitoXANtrone (mye toe ZAN trone)

Brand Names: Canada Mitoxantrone Injection®

Pharmacologic Category Antineoplastic Agent, Anthracenedione

Use Initial treatment of acute nonlymphocytic leukemias (ANLL [includes myelogenous, promyelocytic, monocytic and erythroid leukemias]); treatment of advanced hormone-refractory prostate cancer; secondary progressive or relapsing-remitting multiple sclerosis (MS)

Canadian labeling: Additional uses (not in U.S. labeling): Treatment of metastatic breast cancer, relapsed leukemia (adults), lymphoma, and hepatocellular carcinoma

Unlabeled Use Treatment of Hodgkin lymphoma (refractory), non-Hodgkin lymphomas (NHL), acute lymphocytic leukemia (ALL), relapsed acute myeloid leukemia (AML), breast cancer (metastatic), pediatric acute myelogenous leukemia (AML), pediatric acute promyelocytic leukemia (APL); part of a conditioning regimen for autologous hematopoietic stem cell transplantation (HSCT)

Local Anesthetic/Vasoconstrictor Precautions No information available to require special precautions

Effects on Dental Treatment Key adverse event(s) related to dental treatment: Mucositis and stomatitis.

Effects on Bleeding Myelosuppression is an extension of the pharmacologic effects; therefore, thrombocytopenia (grades 3/4: 3% to 4%) is expected. Anemia may also occur. Medical consult recommended.

Adverse Effects Includes events reported with any indication; incidence varies based on treatment, dose, and/or concomitant medications

>10%:

Cardiovascular: Edema (10% to 30%), arrhythmia (3% to 18%), cardiac function changes (≤18%), ECG changes (≤11%)

Central nervous system: Fever (6% to 78%), pain (8% to 41%), fatigue (≤39%), headache (6% to 13%)

Dermatologic: Alopecia (20% to 61%), nail bed changes (≤11%), petechiae/bruising (6% to 11%)

Endocrine & metabolic: Menstrual disorder (26% to 61%), amenorrhea (28% to 53%), hyperglycemia (10% to 31%)

Gastrointestinal: Nausea (26% to 76%), vomiting (6% to 72%), diarrhea (14% to 47%), mucositis (10% to 29%; onset: ≤1 week), stomatitis (8% to 29%; onset: ≤1 week), anorexia (22% to 25%), weight gain/loss (13% to 17%), constipation (10% to 16%), GI bleeding (2% to 16%), abdominal pain (9% to 15%), dyspepsia (5% to 14%)

Genitourinary: Urinary tract infection (7% to 32%), abnormal urine (5% to 11%)

Hematologic: Neutropenia (79% to 100%; onset: ≤3 weeks; grade 4: 23% to 54%), leukopenia (9% to 100%), lymphopenia (72% to 95%), anemia/hemoglobin decreased (5% to 75%) thrombocytopenia (33% to 39%; grades 3/4: 3% to 4%), neutropenic fever (≤11%)

Hepatic: Alkaline phosphatase increased (≤37%), transaminases increased (5% to 20%), GGT increased (3% to 15%)

Neuromuscular & skeletal: Weakness (≤24%)

Renal: BUN increased (≤22%), creatinine increased (≤13%), hematuria (≤11%)

Respiratory: Upper respiratory tract infection (7% to 53%), pharyngitis (≤19%), dyspnea (6% to 18%), cough (5% to 13%)

Miscellaneous: Infection (4% to 60%), sepsis (ANLL 31% to 34%), fungal infection (9% to 15%)

1% to 10%:

Cardiovascular: CHF (≤5%), ischemia (≤5%), LVEF decreased (≤5%), hypertension (≤4%)

Central nervous system: Chills (≤5%), anxiety (5%), depression (5%), seizure (2% to 4%)

Dermatologic: Cutaneous mycosis (≤10%), skin infection (≤5%)

Endocrine & metabolic: Hypocalcemia (10%), hypokalemia (7% to 10%), hyponatremia (9%), menorrhagia (7%)

Gastrointestinal: Aphthosis (≤10%)

Genitourinary: Impotence (≤7%), sterility (≤5%)

Hematologic: Granulocytopenia (6%), hemorrhage (5% to 6%), secondary acute leukemias (≤3%; includes AML, APL)

Hepatic: Jaundice (3% to 7%)

Neuromuscular & skeletal: Back pain (6% to 8%), myalgia (≤5%), arthralgia (≤5%)

Ocular: Conjunctivitis (≤5%), blurred vision (≤3%)

Renal: Renal failure (≤8%), proteinuria (≤6%)

Respiratory: Rhinitis (10%), pneumonia (≤9%), sinusitis (≤6%)

Miscellaneous: Systemic infection (≤10%), diaphoresis (≤9%)

General Dosage Range I.V.: *Adults:* 12 mg/m²/day once daily for 2-3 days **or** 12-14 mg/m² every 3 weeks **or** 12 mg/m² every 3 months (multiple sclerosis; maximum lifetime cumulative dose: 140 mg/m²)

Mechanism of Action Related to the anthracyclines, mitoxantrone intercalates into DNA resulting in cross-links and strand breaks; binds to nucleic acids and inhibits DNA and RNA synthesis by template disordering and steric obstruction; replication is decreased by

◀ binding to DNA topoisomerase II and seems to inhibit the incorporation of uridine into RNA and thymidine into DNA; active throughout entire cell cycle (cell-cycle non-specific)

Pharmacodynamics/Kinetics

Half-life Elimination Terminal: 23-215 hours (median: ~75 hours); may be prolonged with hepatic impairment

Pregnancy Risk Factor D

Pregnancy Considerations Adverse effects were noted in animal reproduction studies. May cause fetal harm if administered to a pregnant woman. Pregnancy should be avoided while on treatment. Women with multiple sclerosis who are of reproductive potential should have a pregnancy test prior to each dose.

Modafinil (moe DAF i nil)

Brand Names: U.S. Provigil®

Brand Names: Canada Alertec®

Generic Availability (U.S.) Yes

Pharmacologic Category Central Nervous System Stimulant

Use Improve wakefulness in patients with excessive daytime sleepiness associated with narcolepsy and shift work sleep disorder (SWSD); adjunctive therapy for obstructive sleep apnea/hypopnea syndrome (OSAHS)

Unlabeled Use Attention-deficit/hyperactivity disorder (ADHD); treatment of fatigue in MS and other disorders

Local Anesthetic/Vasoconstrictor Precautions Use vasoconstrictor with caution. Patients may experience heart palpitations and increased heart rate when taking modafinil.

Effects on Dental Treatment Key adverse event(s) related to dental treatment: Xerostomia (normal salivary flow resumes upon discontinuation), oral ulceration, gingivitis, and taste perversion.

Effects on Bleeding No information available to require special precautions

Adverse Effects

>10%:

Central nervous system: Headache (adults 34%; children 20%; dose related)

Gastrointestinal: Appetite decreased (children 16%), abdominal pain (children 12%), nausea (11%)

1% to 10%:

Cardiovascular: Chest pain (3%), hypertension (3%), palpitation (2%), tachycardia (2%), vasodilation (2%), edema (1%)

Central nervous system: Nervousness (7%), dizziness (5%), anxiety (5%; dose related), insomnia (5%), depression (2%), somnolence (2%), chills (1%), agitation (1%), confusion (1%), emotional lability (1%), vertigo (1%)

Dermatologic: Rash (1%; includes some severe cases requiring hospitalization)

Gastrointestinal: Diarrhea (6%), dyspepsia (5%), weight loss (children 5%), xerostomia (4%), anorexia (4%), constipation (2%), flatulence (1%), mouth ulceration (1%), taste perversion (1%)

Genitourinary: Abnormal urine (1%), hematuria (1%), pyuria (1%)

Hematologic: Eosinophilia (1%)

Hepatic: LFTs abnormal (2%)

Neuromuscular & skeletal: Back pain (6%), paresthesia (2%), dyskinesia (1%), hyperkinesia (1%), hypertonia (1%), neck rigidity (1%), tremor (1%)

Ocular: Amblyopia (1%), eye pain (1%), vision abnormal (1%)

Respiratory: Rhinitis (7%), pharyngitis (4%), lung disorder (2%), asthma (1%), epistaxis (1%)

Miscellaneous: Flu-like syndrome (4%), thirst (1%), diaphoresis (1%), herpes simplex infection (1%)

Dosage

U.S. labeling:

Narcolepsy, obstructive sleep apnea/hypopnea syndrome (OSAHS): Adults: Oral: Initial: 200 mg as a single daily dose in the morning

Shift work sleep disorder (SWSD): Adults: Oral: Initial: 200 mg as a single dose taken ~1 hour prior to start of work shift

Note: Doses up to 400 mg daily, given as a single dose, have been well tolerated, but there is no consistent evidence that this dose confers additional benefit.

Canadian labeling:

Narcolepsy: Adults: Oral: Initial: 200 mg daily in 2 divided doses (first dose in the morning and second dose at noon [or no later than early afternoon]); may titrate dose upward in 100 mg increments as needed and tolerated (maximum single dose: < 300 mg; maximum daily dose: 400 mg). Single doses ≥300 mg and daily doses >400 mg are associated with increased side effects and are not recommended.

Obstructive sleep apnea: Adults: Oral: 200 mg once daily in the morning.

Shift work sleep disorder: Adults: Oral: 200 mg as a single dose taken ~1 hour prior to start of work shift

Unlabeled use: ADHD: 100-400 mg daily (Taylor, 2000)

Elderly: Elimination of modafinil and its metabolites may be reduced as a consequence of aging and as a result, consider initiating at lower doses in this patient population.

Dosing adjustment in renal impairment: Severe impairment: No dosage adjustment provided in manufacturer's labeling (insufficient data).

Dosing adjustment in hepatic impairment: Severe hepatic impairment: Dose should be reduced to one-half of that recommended for patients with normal liver function.

Mechanism of Action The exact mechanism of action is unclear, it does not appear to alter the release of dopamine or norepinephrine, it may exert its stimulant effects by decreasing GABA-mediated neurotransmission, although this theory has not yet been fully evaluated; several studies also suggest that an intact central alpha-adrenergic system is required for modafinil's activity; the drug increases high-frequency alpha waves while decreasing both delta and theta wave activity, and these effects are consistent with generalized increases in mental alertness

Contraindications Hypersensitivity to modafinil, armodafinil, or any component of the formulation

Canadian labeling: Additional contraindications (not in U.S. labeling): Patients in agitated states or with severe anxiety

Warnings/Precautions For use following complete evaluation of sleepiness and in conjunction with other standard treatments (eg, CPAP). The degree of sleepiness should be reassessed frequently; some patients may not return to a normal level of wakefulness. Use is not recommended with a history of angina, cardiac ischemia, recent history of myocardial infarction, left ventricular hypertrophy, or patients with mitral valve prolapse who have developed mitral valve prolapse syndrome with previous CNS stimulant use.

Serious and life-threatening rashes (including Stevens-Johnson syndrome and toxic epidermal necrolysis) have been reported with modafinil. Most cases have occurred within the first 5 weeks of therapy; however, rare cases have occurred after long-term use. No risk factors have been identified to predict occurrence or severity. Patients should be advised to discontinue at first sign of rash. The serious nature of these dermatologic adverse effects, as well reports of psychiatric events, resulted in the FDA's Pediatric Advisory Committee unanimously recommending that a specific warning against the use of modafinil in children be added to the manufacturer's labeling. Modafinil is not FDA-approved for use in pediatrics for any indication.

In addition, rare cases of multiorgan hypersensitivity reactions in association with modafinil use, and lone cases of angioedema and anaphylactoid reactions with armodafinil, have been reported. Signs and symptoms are diverse, reflecting the involvement of specific organs. Patients typically present with fever and rash associated with organ-system dysfunction. Patients should be advised to report any signs and symptoms related to these effects; discontinuation of therapy is recommended.

Caution should be exercised when modafinil is given to patients with a history of psychosis; may impair the ability to engage in potentially hazardous activities. Stimulants may unmask tics in individuals with coexisting Tourette's syndrome. Use caution with renal or hepatic impairment (dosage adjustment in severe hepatic dysfunction is recommended).

Drug Interactions
Metabolism/Transport Effects Substrate of CYP3A4 (major); **Note:** Assignment of Major/Minor substrate status based on clinically relevant drug interaction potential; **Inhibits** CYP1A2 (weak), CYP2A6 (weak), CYP2C19 (strong), CYP2C9 (weak), CYP2E1 (weak), CYP3A4 (weak); **Induces** CYP1A2 (weak/moderate), CYP2B6 (weak/moderate), CYP3A4 (weak/moderate)

Avoid Concomitant Use
Avoid concomitant use of Modafinil with any of the following: Axitinib; Bosutinib; Clopidogrel; Conivaptan; Iobenguane I 123; Pimozide

Increased Effect/Toxicity
Modafinil may increase the levels/effects of: ARIPiprazole; Citalopram; CYP2C19 Substrates; Lomitapide; Pimozide; Sympathomimetics

The levels/effects of Modafinil may be increased by: AtoMOXetine; Cannabinoids; Conivaptan; CYP3A4 Inhibitors (Moderate); CYP3A4 Inhibitors (Strong); Dasatinib; Ivacaftor; Linezolid; Mifepristone

Decreased Effect
Modafinil may decrease the levels/effects of: ARIPiprazole; Axitinib; Bosutinib; Clopidogrel; Contraceptives (Estrogens); CycloSPORINE (Systemic); Iobenguane I 123; Saxagliptin

The levels/effects of Modafinil may be decreased by: CYP3A4 Inducers (Strong); Deferasirox; Herbs (CYP3A4 Inducers); Tocilizumab

Ethanol/Nutrition/Herb Interactions
Ethanol: Avoid or limit ethanol.
Food: Delays absorption, but does not affect bioavailability.

Pharmacodynamics/Kinetics
Half-life Elimination Effective half-life: 15 hours
Time to Peak Serum: 2-4 hours
Pregnancy Risk Factor C

Pregnancy Considerations Embryotoxic effects have been observed in some, but not all animal studies. There are no adequate and well-controlled studies in pregnant women; use only when the potential risk of drug therapy is outweighed by the drug's benefits.

Healthcare providers are encouraged to register pregnant patients exposed to modafinil by calling 1-866-404-4106.

Efficacy of steroidal contraceptives (including depot and implantable contraceptives) may be decreased; alternate means of contraception should be considered during therapy and for 1 month after modafinil is discontinued.

Lactation Excretion in breast milk unknown/use caution
Controlled Substance C-IV
Dosage Forms
Tablet, oral: 100 mg, 200 mg
Provigil®: 100 mg, 200 mg
Dosage Forms: Canada
Tablet, oral: 100 mg
Alertec®: 100 mg

Moexipril (mo EKS i pril)

Related Information
Cardiovascular Diseases on page 1492
Brand Names: U.S. Univasc®
Pharmacologic Category Angiotensin-Converting Enzyme (ACE) Inhibitor
Use Treatment of hypertension, alone or in combination with thiazide diuretics
Local Anesthetic/Vasoconstrictor Precautions No information available to require special precautions
Effects on Dental Treatment No significant effects or complications reported
Effects on Bleeding No information available to require special precautions
Adverse Effects 1% to 10%:
Cardiovascular: Hypotension, peripheral edema
Central nervous system: Headache, dizziness, fatigue
Dermatologic: Flushing, rash
Endocrine & metabolic: Hyperkalemia, hyponatremia
Gastrointestinal: Diarrhea, nausea, heartburn
Genitourinary: Polyuria
Neuromuscular & skeletal: Myalgia
Renal: Reversible increases in creatinine or BUN
Respiratory: Cough, pharyngitis, upper respiratory infection, sinusitis
General Dosage Range Dosage adjustment recommended in patients with renal impairment
Oral: Adults: Initial: 3.75-7.5 mg once daily; Maintenance: 7.5-30 mg/day in 1 or 2 divided doses
Mechanism of Action Competitive inhibitor of angiotensin-converting enzyme (ACE); prevents conversion of angiotensin I to angiotensin II, a potent vasoconstrictor; results in lower levels of angiotensin II which causes an increase in plasma renin activity and a reduction in aldosterone secretion
Pharmacodynamics/Kinetics
Onset of Action Peak effect: 1-2 hours
Duration of Action >24 hours
Half-life Elimination Moexipril: 1 hour; Moexiprilat: 2-9 hours
Time to Peak 1.5 hours
Pregnancy Risk Factor D
Pregnancy Considerations [U.S. Boxed Warning]: Drugs that act on the renin-angiotensin system can cause injury and death to the developing fetus. ▶

◄ **Discontinue as soon as possible once pregnancy is detected.** Teratogenic effects may occur following maternal use during pregnancy. Drugs that act on the renin-angiotensin system are associated with oligohydramnios. Oligohydramnios, due to decreased fetal renal function, may lead to fetal lung hypoplasia and skeletal malformations. Their use in pregnancy is also associated with anuria, hypotension, renal failure, skull hypoplasia, and death in the fetus/neonate. Chronic maternal hypertension itself is also associated with adverse events in the fetus/infant. ACE inhibitors are not recommended during pregnancy to treat maternal hypertension or heart failure. Use of an ACE inhibitor should also be avoided in any woman of reproductive age. Women who are planning a pregnancy should be considered for other medication options if an ACE inhibitor is currently prescribed or the ACE inhibitor should be discontinued as soon as possible once pregnancy is detected. The exposed fetus should be monitored for fetal growth, amniotic fluid volume, and organ formation. Infants exposed to an ACE inhibitor *in utero* should be monitored for hyperkalemia, hypotension, and oliguria.

Moexipril and Hydrochlorothiazide
(mo EKS i pril & hye droe klor oh THYE a zide)

Related Information
Hydrochlorothiazide *on page 687*
Moexipril *on page 933*
Brand Names: U.S. Uniretic®
Brand Names: Canada Uniretic®
Pharmacologic Category Angiotensin-Converting Enzyme (ACE) Inhibitor; Diuretic, Thiazide
Use Treatment of hypertension; not indicated for initial treatment of hypertension
Local Anesthetic/Vasoconstrictor Precautions No information available to require special precautions
Effects on Dental Treatment No significant effects or complications reported
Effects on Bleeding No information available to require special precautions
Adverse Effects See individual agents.
General Dosage Range Oral: *Adults:* 7.5-30 mg of moexipril/day and ≤50 mg hydrochlorothiazide/day in a single or divided dose
Mechanism of Action See individual agents.
Pregnancy Risk Factor D
Pregnancy Considerations [U.S. Boxed Warning]: Drugs that act on the renin-angiotensin system can cause injury and death to the developing fetus. Discontinue as soon as possible once pregnancy is detected. Also see individual agents.

Mometasone (Oral Inhalation)
(moe MET a sone)

Related Information
Respiratory Diseases *on page 1514*
Brand Names: U.S. Asmanex® Twisthaler®
Brand Names: Canada Asmanex® Twisthaler®
Generic Availability (U.S.) No
Pharmacologic Category Corticosteroid, Inhalant (Oral)
Use Maintenance treatment of asthma as prophylactic therapy
Local Anesthetic/Vasoconstrictor Precautions No information available to require special precautions

Effects on Dental Treatment No significant effects or complications reported
Effects on Bleeding No information available to require special precautions
Adverse Effects
>10%:
  Central nervous system: Headache (17% to 22%), fatigue (1% to 13%), depression (11%)
  Neuromuscular & skeletal: Musculoskeletal pain (4% to 22%), arthralgia (13%)
  Respiratory: Sinusitis (5% to 22%), rhinitis (4% to 20%), upper respiratory infection (8% to 15%), pharyngitis (8% to 13%)
  Miscellaneous: Oral candidiasis (4% to 22%)
1% to 10%:
  Central nervous system: Fever (children 7%), pain (1% to <3%)
  Dermatologic: Bruising (children 2%)
  Gastrointestinal: Abdominal pain (2% to 6%), dyspepsia (3% to 5%), nausea (1% to 3%), vomiting (1% to ≤3%), anorexia (1% to <3%), dry throat (1% to <3%), gastroenteritis (1% to <3%)
  Genitourinary: Dysmenorrhea (4% to 9%), urinary tract infection (children 2%)
  Neuromuscular & skeletal: Back pain (3% to 6%), myalgia (2% to 3%)
  Ocular: Ocular pressure increased (3%), cataracts (1%)
  Otic: Earache (1% to <3%)
  Respiratory: Sinus congestion (9%), dysphonia (1% to <3%), epistaxis (1% to <3%), nasal irritation (1% to <3%)
  Miscellaneous: Flu-like syndrome (1% to <3%), infection (1% to <3%)
Dosage Oral inhalation: **Note:** Dosage forms available in the U.S. (110 mcg and 220 mcg Twisthaler®) deliver 100 and 200 mcg mometasone furoate per actuation respectively.
U.S. labeling:
  Children 4-11 years: 110 mcg once daily in the evening (maximum: 110 mcg/day)
  Children ≥12 years and Adults: Previous therapy:
    Bronchodilators or inhaled corticosteroids: Initial: 1 inhalation (220 mcg) daily (maximum: 2 inhalations or 440 mcg/day); may be given in the evening or in divided doses twice daily
    Oral corticosteroids: Initial: 440 mcg twice daily (maximum: 880 mcg/day); prednisone should be reduced no faster than 2.5 mg/day on a weekly basis, beginning after at least 1 week of mometasone furoate use
Canadian labeling: Children ≥12 years and Adults:
  Usual dose: 400 mcg once daily in the morning; maintenance: 200-400 mcg once daily in the morning. **Note:** Some patients (eg, previously receiving high-dose inhaled corticosteroids) may respond more favorably to 400 mcg daily administered in 2 divided doses.
  Severe asthma and requiring oral corticosteroids: Initial: 400 mcg twice daily; taper off oral corticosteroid gradually by decreasing daily prednisone dose by 1 mg/day (or equivalent of other corticosteroid) on a weekly basis, beginning after at least 1 week of mometasone furoate use; upon successful taper off of oral steroids, titrate mometasone to lowest effective dose.

NIH Asthma Guidelines (NIH, 2007): Children ≥12 years and Adults:

"Low" dose: 200 mcg/day

"Medium" dose: 400 mcg/day

"High" dose: >400 mcg/day

Note: Maximum effects may not be evident for 1-2 weeks or longer; dose should be titrated to effect, using the lowest possible dose

Mechanism of Action May depress the formation, release, and activity of endogenous chemical mediators of inflammation (kinins, histamine, liposomal enzymes, prostaglandins). Leukocytes and macrophages may have to be present for the initiation of responses mediated by the above substances. Inhibits the margination and subsequent cell migration to the area of injury, and also reverses the dilatation and increased vessel permeability in the area resulting in decreased access of cells to the sites of injury.

Contraindications Hypersensitivity to mometasone or any component of the formulation; hypersensitivity to milk proteins; primary treatment of status asthmaticus or acute bronchospasm

Canadian labeling: Additional contraindications (not in U.S. labeling): Untreated systemic fungal, bacterial, viral, or parasitic infections; active or quiet tuberculosis infection of the respiratory tract; ocular herpes simplex

Warnings/Precautions May cause hypercorticism or suppression of hypothalamic-pituitary-adrenal (HPA) axis, particularly in younger children or in patients receiving high doses for prolonged periods. HPA axis suppression may lead to adrenal crisis. Withdrawal and discontinuation of a corticosteroid should be done slowly and carefully. Particular care is required when patients are transferred from systemic corticosteroids to inhaled products due to possible adrenal insufficiency or withdrawal from steroids, including an increase in allergic symptoms. Patients receiving >20 mg per day of prednisone (or equivalent) may be most susceptible. Fatalities have occurred due to adrenal insufficiency in asthmatic patients during and after transfer from systemic corticosteroids to aerosol steroids; aerosol steroids do not provide the systemic steroid needed to treat patients having trauma, surgery, or infections. When transferring to oral inhaler, previously-suppressed allergic conditions (rhinitis, conjunctivitis, eczema) may be unmasked.

Bronchospasm may occur with wheezing after inhalation; if this occurs, stop steroid and treat with a fast-acting bronchodilator. Supplemental steroids (oral or parenteral) may be needed during stress or severe asthma attacks. Not to be used in status asthmaticus or for the relief of acute bronchospasm. Corticosteroid use may cause psychiatric disturbances, including depression, euphoria, insomnia, mood swings, and personality changes. Pre-existing psychiatric conditions may be exacerbated by corticosteroid use. Prolonged use of corticosteroids may also increase the incidence of secondary infection, mask acute infection (including fungal infections), prolong or exacerbate viral infections, or limit response to vaccines. Exposure to chickenpox should be avoided; corticosteroids should not be used to treat ocular herpes simplex. Corticosteroids should not be used for cerebral malaria or viral hepatitis. Close observation is required in patients with latent tuberculosis and/or TB reactivity; restrict use in active TB (only in conjunction with antituberculosis treatment). Canadian labeling contraindicates use in patients with untreated systemic fungal, bacterial, viral, or parasitic infections, active or quiet tuberculosis infection of the respiratory tract and ocular herpes simplex.

Prolonged treatment with corticosteroids has been associated with the development of Kaposi's sarcoma (case reports); if noted, discontinuation of therapy should be considered. Local oropharyngeal *Candida* infections have been reported; if occurs treat appropriately while continuing mometasone therapy. Patients should be instructed to rinse mouth after each use.

Reactions including, anaphylaxis, angioedema, pruritus, and rash have been reported; if these symptoms occur discontinue use. Use with caution in patients with thyroid disease, hepatic impairment, renal impairment, cardiovascular disease, diabetes, glaucoma, cataracts, myasthenia gravis, patients with or who are at risk for osteoporosis, patients at risk for seizures, or GI diseases (diverticulitis, peptic ulcer, ulcerative colitis) due to perforation risk. Use caution following acute MI (corticosteroids have been associated with myocardial rupture). Because of the risk of adverse effects, systemic corticosteroids should be used cautiously in the elderly in the smallest possible effective dose for the shortest duration.

Orally-inhaled corticosteroids may cause a reduction in growth velocity in pediatric patients (~1 centimeter per year [range: 0.3-1.8 cm per year] and related to dose and duration of exposure). To minimize the systemic effects of orally-inhaled corticosteroids, each patient should be titrated to the lowest effective dose. Growth should be routinely monitored in pediatric patients. Prior to use, the dose and duration of treatment should be based on the risk versus benefit for each individual patient. In general, use the smallest effective dose for the shortest duration of time to minimize adverse events. A gradual tapering of dose may be required prior to discontinuing therapy. There have been reports of systemic corticosteroid withdrawal symptoms (eg, joint/muscle pain, lassitude, depression) when withdrawing inhalation therapy. May contain lactose; very rare anaphylactic reactions have been reported in patients with severe milk protein allergy.

Drug Interactions

Metabolism/Transport Effects Substrate of CYP3A4 (minor); **Note:** Assignment of Major/Minor substrate status based on clinically relevant drug interaction potential

Avoid Concomitant Use

Avoid concomitant use of Mometasone (Oral Inhalation) with any of the following: Aldesleukin

Increased Effect/Toxicity

Mometasone (Oral Inhalation) may increase the levels/ effects of: Amphotericin B; Deferasirox; Loop Diuretics; Thiazide Diuretics

The levels/effects of Mometasone (Oral Inhalation) may be increased by: CYP3A4 Inhibitors (Strong); Telaprevir

Decreased Effect

Mometasone (Oral Inhalation) may decrease the levels/effects of: Aldesleukin; Antidiabetic Agents; Corticorelin; Hyaluronidase; Telaprevir

Dietary Considerations Asmanex® Twisthaler® contains lactose.

Pharmacodynamics/Kinetics

Half-life Elimination 5 hours

Pregnancy Risk Factor C

◄ **Pregnancy Considerations** Adverse events were observed in animal studies following topical and SubQ administration. Hypoadrenalism may occur in infants born to women receiving corticosteroids during pregnancy. Monitor these infants closely after birth. A decrease in fetal growth has not been observed with inhaled corticosteroid use during pregnancy. Inhaled corticosteroids are recommended for the treatment of asthma (most information available using budesonide) during pregnancy.

Lactation Excretion in breast milk unknown/use caution

Breast-Feeding Considerations Systemic corticosteroids are excreted in human milk; however, information for mometasone is not available. The use of inhaled corticosteroids is not considered a contraindication to breast-feeding.

Dosage Forms
Powder, for oral inhalation:
Asmanex® Twisthaler®: 110 mcg (7 doses, 30 doses); 220 mcg (14 doses, 30 doses, 60 doses, 120 doses)

Dosage Forms: Canada
Powder, for oral inhalation:
Asmanex® Twisthaler®: 200 mcg (30 doses, 60 doses); 400 mcg (30 doses, 60 doses)

Mometasone (Nasal) (moe MET a sone)

Brand Names: U.S. Nasonex®
Brand Names: Canada Apo-Mometasone®; Nasonex®
Pharmacologic Category Corticosteroid, Nasal
Use Treatment of nasal symptoms of seasonal and perennial allergic rhinitis; prevention of nasal symptoms associated with seasonal allergic rhinitis; treatment of nasal polyps in adults

Canadian labeling: Additional use (not in U.S. labeling): Treatment of mild-to-moderate uncomplicated rhinosinusitis or as adjunctive treatment (with antimicrobials) in acute rhinosinusitis

Unlabeled Use Adjunct to antibiotics in empiric treatment of acute bacterial rhinosinusitis (ABRS) (Chow, 2012)

Local Anesthetic/Vasoconstrictor Precautions No information available to require special precautions

Effects on Dental Treatment No significant effects or complications reported

Effects on Bleeding Shown to cause localized epistaxis (nosebleed) with prolonged use. The localized epistaxis is reversible following discontinuation of the drug. Impacts relating to the systemic circulation do not warrant special precautions.

Adverse Effects
>10%:
Central nervous system: Headache (17% to 26%)
Respiratory: Pharyngitis (8% to 13%), cough (nasal inhalation 7% to 13%), epistaxis (1% to 11%)
Miscellaneous: Viral infection (nasal inhalation 8% to 14%)
1% to 10%:
Gastrointestinal: Diarrhea, dyspepsia, vomiting
Genitourinary: Dysmenorrhea
Neuromuscular & skeletal: Musculoskeletal pain, myalgia
Ocular: Conjunctivitis
Otic: Otitis media
Respiratory: Asthma, nasal irritation, rhinitis, sinusitis, upper respiratory infection, wheezing
Miscellaneous: Flu-like syndrome

General Dosage Range Intranasal:
Children 2-11 years: 1 spray (50 mcg) in each nostril once daily
Children ≥12 years and Adults: 2 sprays (100 mcg) in each nostril once or twice daily

Mechanism of Action May depress the formation, release, and activity of endogenous chemical mediators of inflammation (kinins, histamine, liposomal enzymes, prostaglandins). Leukocytes and macrophages may have to be present for the initiation of responses mediated by the above substances. Inhibits the margination and subsequent cell migration to the area of injury, and also reverses the dilatation and increased vessel permeability in the area resulting in decreased access of cells to the sites of injury.

Pregnancy Risk Factor C

Pregnancy Considerations Adverse events were observed in animal studies following topical and SubQ administration. Hypoadrenalism may occur in infants born to women receiving corticosteroids during pregnancy. Monitor these infants closely after birth. A decrease in fetal growth has not been observed with inhaled corticosteroid use during pregnancy. Inhaled corticosteroids are recommended for the treatment of allergic rhinitis during pregnancy.

Mometasone and Formoterol
(moe MET a sone & for MOH te rol)

Related Information
Formoterol on page 629
Mometasone (Oral Inhalation) on page 934
Brand Names: U.S. Dulera®
Brand Names: Canada Zenhale™
Pharmacologic Category Beta₂ Agonist, Long-Acting; Beta₂-Adrenergic Agonist, Long-Acting; Corticosteroid, Inhalant (Oral)
Use Maintenance treatment of asthma where combination therapy is indicated
Local Anesthetic/Vasoconstrictor Precautions No information available to require special precautions
Effects on Dental Treatment Key adverse event(s) related to dental treatment: Formoterol: Xerostomia (normal salivary flow resumes upon discontinuation). Localized infections with Candida albicans or Aspergillus niger have occurred frequently in the mouth and pharynx with repetitive use of oral inhaler of corticosteroids. These infections may require treatment with appropriate antifungal therapy or discontinuance of treatment with corticosteroid inhaler.
Effects on Bleeding No information available to require special precautions
Adverse Effects Also see individual agents.
1% to 10%:
Central nervous system: Headache (≤5%)
Respiratory: Nasopharyngitis (5%), dysphonia (4% to 5%), sinusitis (2% to 3%)
General Dosage Range Inhalation: Children ≥12 years and Adults: 2 inhalations twice daily (maximum: 4 inhalations/day)
Mechanism of Action Formoterol relaxes bronchial smooth muscle by selective action on beta₂ receptors with little effect on heart rate. Formoterol has a long-acting effect. Mometasone is a corticosteroid which controls the rate of protein synthesis, depresses the migration of polymorphonuclear leukocytes/fibroblasts, and reverses capillary permeability and lysosomal stabilization at the cellular level to prevent or control inflammation.

Pregnancy Risk Factor C
Pregnancy Considerations See individual agents.

Monobenzone (mon oh BEN zone)

Pharmacologic Category Topical Skin Product
Use Final depigmentation in extensive vitiligo
Local Anesthetic/Vasoconstrictor Precautions No information available to require special precautions
Effects on Dental Treatment No significant effects or complications reported
Effects on Bleeding No information available to require special precautions
Adverse Effects Frequency not defined.
  Local: Burning sensation, depigmentation of skin distant to application site, dermatitis, irritation
General Dosage Range Topical: *Children ≥12 years and Adults:* Initial: Apply 2-3 times/day; once depigmentation obtained apply as needed (usually 2 times/week)
Mechanism of Action Increases excretion of melanin from melanocytes; causes melanocyte destruction and permanent depigmentation
Pharmacodynamics/Kinetics
  Onset of Action 1-4 months
Pregnancy Risk Factor C
Pregnancy Considerations Animal reproduction studies have not been conducted.

Montelukast (mon te LOO kast)

Related Information
  Respiratory Diseases *on page 1514*
Brand Names: U.S. Singulair®
Brand Names: Canada Apo-Montelukast; Dom-Montelukast; Dom-Montelukast FC; Jamp-Montelukast; Montelukast Sodium Tablets; Mylan-Montelukast; PMS-Montelukast; PMS-Montelukast FC; Sandoz-Montelukast; Sandoz-Montelukast Granules; Singulair®; Teva-Montelukast
Generic Availability (U.S.) Yes
Pharmacologic Category Leukotriene-Receptor Antagonist
Use Prophylaxis and chronic treatment of asthma; relief of symptoms of seasonal allergic rhinitis and perennial allergic rhinitis; prevention of exercise-induced bronchoconstriction
Local Anesthetic/Vasoconstrictor Precautions No information available to require special precautions
Effects on Dental Treatment Key adverse event(s) related to dental treatment: Dental pain.
Effects on Bleeding Postmarket safety evaluation has identified increased bleeding tendency and thrombocytopenia.
Adverse Effects
  Children ≥15 years and Adults:
    >10%: Central nervous system: Headache (18%)
    1% to 10%:
      Central nervous system: Dizziness (2%), fatigue (2%), fever (2%)
      Dermatologic: Rash (2%)
      Gastrointestinal: Dyspepsia (2%), dental pain (2%), gastroenteritis (2%)
      Hepatic: AST increased (2%), ALT increased (≥1%)
      Neuromuscular & skeletal: Weakness (2%)
      Respiratory: Nasal congestion (2%), cough (≥1%), epistaxis (≥1%), sinusitis (≥1%), upper respiratory infection (≥1%)

Children 2 to ≤14 years: ≥2%:
  Central nervous system: Fever, headache
  Dermatologic: Dermatitis, eczema, rash, urticaria
  Gastrointestinal: Abdominal pain, diarrhea, dyspepsia, gastroenteritis, nausea
  Ocular: Conjunctivitis
  Otic: Ear pain, otitis, otitis media
  Respiratory: Laryngitis, pharyngitis, pneumonia, rhinorrhea, sinusitis, upper respiratory infection
  Miscellaneous: Influenza, varicella, viral infection
Children 6-23 months: ≥2%: Respiratory: Cough, otitis media, pharyngitis, rhinitis, tonsillitis, upper respiratory infection, wheezing
Dosage Note: Patients with **both** asthma and allergic rhinitis should take only one dose in the evening.
Asthma: Oral:
  Children ≥1 to <2 years: 4 mg (oral granules) once daily (in the evening)
  Children ≥2 to <6 years: 4 mg (chewable tablet or oral granules) once daily (in the evening)
  Children ≥6 years and Adolescents <15 years: 5 mg (chewable tablet) once daily (in the evening)
  Adolescents ≥15 years and Adults: 10 mg once daily (in the evening)
Bronchoconstriction, exercise-induced (prevention): Note: Additional doses should not be administered within 24 hours. Daily administration to prevent exercise-induced bronchoconstriction has not been evaluated. Patients receiving montelukast for another indication should not take an additional dose to prevent exercise-induced bronchoconstriction. Oral:
  Children ≥6 years and Adolescents <15 years: 5 mg (chewable tablet) at least 2 hours prior to exercise
  Adolescents ≥15 years and Adults: 10 mg once daily at least 2 hours prior to exercise
Perennial allergic rhinitis: Oral:
  Children 6 months to <2 years: 4 mg (oral granules) once daily
  Children ≥2 to <6 years: 4 mg (chewable tablet or oral granules) once daily
  Children ≥6 years and Adolescents <15 years: 5 mg (chewable tablet) once daily
  Adolescents ≥15 years and Adults: 10 mg once daily
Seasonal allergic rhinitis: Oral:
  Children ≥2 to <6 years: 4 mg (chewable tablet or oral granules) once daily
  Children ≥6 years and Adolescents <15 years: 5 mg (chewable tablet) once daily
  Adolescents ≥15 years and Adults: 10 mg once daily
Dosage adjustment in renal impairment: No dosage adjustment necessary.
Dosage adjustment in hepatic impairment:
  Mild-to-moderate impairment: No dosage adjustment necessary.
  Severe impairment: No dosage adjustment provided in manufacturer's labeling; has not been studied.
Mechanism of Action Selective leukotriene receptor antagonist that inhibits the cysteinyl leukotriene receptor. Cysteinyl leukotrienes and leukotriene receptor occupation have been correlated with the pathophysiology of asthma, including airway edema, smooth muscle contraction, and altered cellular activity associated with the inflammatory process, which contribute to the signs and symptoms of asthma. Cysteinyl leukotrienes are also released from the nasal mucosa following allergen exposure leading to symptoms associated with allergic rhinitis.
Contraindications Hypersensitivity to montelukast or any component of the formulation

Warnings/Precautions Montelukast is not FDA approved for use in the reversal of bronchospasm in acute asthma attacks, including status asthmaticus; some studies, however, support its use as adjunctive therapy (Cylly, 2003; Ferreira, 2001; Harmancik 2006). Appropriate rescue medication should be available. Montelukast treatment should continue during acute asthma exacerbation. When inhaled or systemic corticosteroid reduction is considered in patients initiating or receiving montelukast, appropriate clinical monitoring and a gradual dose reduction of the steroid are recommended.

Postmarketing reports of behavioral changes (eg, agitation, aggression, anxiety, attention deficit, depression, hallucinations, hostility, insomnia, irritability, restlessness, sleep disturbance, suicide ideation/behavior) have been noted in pediatric, adolescent, and adult patients. In a retrospective analysis performed by Merck, serious behavior-related events were rare (Philip, 2009a); assess patients for behavioral changes. Patients should be instructed to notify the prescriber if behavioral changes occur.

Potentially significant drug-drug interactions may exist, requiring dose or frequency adjustment, additional monitoring, and/or selection of alternative therapy. In rare cases, patients on therapy with montelukast may present with systemic eosinophilia, sometimes presenting with clinical features of vasculitis consistent with Churg-Strauss syndrome, a condition which is often treated with systemic corticosteroid therapy. Healthcare providers should be alert to eosinophilia, vasculitic rash, worsening pulmonary symptoms, cardiac complications, and/or neuropathy presenting in their patients. A causal association between montelukast and these underlying conditions has not been established. Montelukast will not interrupt bronchoconstrictor response to aspirin or other NSAIDs; aspirin sensitive asthmatics should continue to avoid these agents. The chewable tablet contains phenylalanine.

Drug Interactions

Metabolism/Transport Effects Substrate of CYP2C9 (major), CYP3A4 (major); **Note:** Assignment of Major/Minor substrate status based on clinically relevant drug interaction potential; **Inhibits** CYP2C8 (weak), CYP2C9 (weak)

Avoid Concomitant Use There are no known interactions where it is recommended to avoid concomitant use.

Increased Effect/Toxicity
The levels/effects of Montelukast may be increased by: CYP2C9 Inhibitors (Moderate); CYP2C9 Inhibitors (Strong); Mifepristone

Decreased Effect
The levels/effects of Montelukast may be decreased by: CYP2C9 Inducers (Strong); CYP3A4 Inducers (Strong); Deferasirox; Herbs (CYP3A4 Inducers); Peginterferon Alfa-2b; Tocilizumab

Ethanol/Nutrition/Herb Interactions Herb/Nutraceutical: St John's wort may decrease montelukast levels.

Dietary Considerations Some products may contain phenylalanine.

Pharmacodynamics/Kinetics

Duration of Action >24 hours

Half-life Elimination 2.7-5.5 hours; Mild-to-moderate hepatic impairment: 7.4 hours

Time to Peak Tablet: 10 mg: 3-4 hours; Chewable tablet: 2-2.5 hours; granules: 1-3 hours (fasting) and 3.5 to ~9 hours (with high-fat meal)

Pregnancy Risk Factor B

Pregnancy Considerations Montelukast was not teratogenic in animal studies, however, there are no adequate and well-controlled studies in pregnant women. Based on limited data, structural defects have been reported in neonates exposed to montelukast *in utero*; however, a specific pattern and relationship to montelukast has not been established. Healthcare providers should report any prenatal exposures to the montelukast pregnancy registry at (800) 986-8999.

Lactation Excretion in breast milk unknown/use caution

Dosage Forms
Granules, oral: 4 mg/packet (30s)
Singulair®: 4 mg/packet (30s)
Tablet, oral: 10 mg
Singulair®: 10 mg
Tablet, chewable, oral: 4 mg, 5 mg
Singulair®: 4 mg, 5 mg

Morphine (Systemic) (MOR feen)

Related Information
Oxymorphone *on page 1037*

Brand Names: U.S. Astramorph/PF™; AVINza®; Duramorph; Infumorph 200; Infumorph 500; Kadian®; MS Contin®

Brand Names: Canada Doloral; Kadian®; M-Eslon®; M.O.S.-SR®; M.O.S.-Sulfate®; M.O.S.® 10; M.O.S.® 20; M.O.S.® 30; Morphine Extra Forte Injection; Morphine Forte Injection; Morphine HP®; Morphine LP® Epidural; Morphine SR; Morphine-EPD; MS Contin SRT; MS Contin®; MS-IR®; Novo-Morphine SR; PMS-Morphine Sulfate SR; ratio-Morphine; ratio-Morphine SR; Sandoz-Morphine SR; Statex®; Teva-Morphine SR

Generic Availability (U.S.) Yes: Excludes Avinza® extended release capsule

Pharmacologic Category Analgesic, Opioid

Use Relief of moderate-to-severe acute and chronic pain; relief of pain of myocardial infarction; relief of dyspnea of acute left ventricular failure and pulmonary edema; preanesthetic medication

Infumorph: Used in continuous microinfusion devices for intrathecal or epidural administration in treatment of intractable chronic pain

Extended release products: Moderate-to-severe pain when continuous, around-the-clock opioid analgesia is needed for an extended period of time

Note: Opioid tolerance: Use of morphine sulfate extended release tablets/capsules ≥90 mg, and/or the oral solution 100 mg/5 mL (20 mg/mL) should be reserved for opioid-tolerant patients (ie, already taking at least 60 mg daily of oral morphine equivalent for at least 1 week).

Local Anesthetic/Vasoconstrictor Precautions No information available to require special precautions

Effects on Dental Treatment Key adverse event(s) related to dental treatment: Xerostomia (normal salivary flow resumes upon discontinuation) and dysphagia. Anticholinergic side effects can cause a reduction of saliva production or secretion, contributing to discomfort and dental disease (ie, caries, oral candidiasis, and periodontal disease).

Effects on Bleeding No information available to require special precautions

Adverse Effects Note: Individual patient differences are unpredictable, and percentage may differ in acute pain (surgical) treatment. Reactions may be dose-, formulation, and/or route dependent.

Frequency not defined:

Cardiovascular: Circulatory depression, flushing, shock

Central nervous system: Dysphonia, physical and psychological dependence, sedation

Endocrine & metabolic: Antidiuretic hormone release, hypogonadism

Neuromuscular & skeletal: Bone mineral density decreased

>10%:

Cardiovascular: Bradycardia, hypotension

Central nervous system: Drowsiness (9% to 48%; tolerance usually develops to drowsiness with regular dosing for 1-2 weeks), dizziness (6% to 20%), fever (<3% to >10%), confusion, headache (following epidural or intrathecal use)

Dermatologic: Pruritus (may be dose related)

Gastrointestinal: Xerostomia (78%), constipation (9% to 40%; tolerance develops very slowly if at all), nausea (7% to 28%; tolerance usually develops to nausea and vomiting with chronic use), vomiting

Genitourinary: Urinary retention (16%; may be prolonged, up to 20 hours, following epidural or intrathecal use)

Hematologic: Anemia (following intrathecal use)

Local: Pain at injection site

Neuromuscular & skeletal: Weakness

Respiratory: Oxygen saturation decreased

Miscellaneous: Histamine release

1% to 10%:

Cardiovascular: Atrial fibrillation (<3%), chest pain (<3%), edema, hypertension, palpitation, peripheral edema, syncope, tachycardia, vasodilation

Central nervous system: Amnesia, agitation, anxiety, apathy, apprehension, ataxia, chills, coma, delirium, depression, dream abnormalities, euphoria, false sense of well being, hallucination, hypoesthesia, insomnia, lethargy, malaise, nervousness, restlessness, seizure, slurred speech, somnolence, vertigo

Dermatologic: Dry skin, rash, urticaria

Endocrine & metabolic: Gynecomastia (<3%), hypokalemia, hyponatremia, libido decreased

Gastrointestinal: Abdominal distension, abdominal pain, anorexia, biliary colic, diarrhea, dyspepsia, dysphagia, flatulence, gastroenteritis, GERD, GI irritation, paralytic ileus, rectal disorder, taste perversion, weight loss

Genitourinary: Bladder spasm, dysuria, ejaculation abnormal, impotence, urination decreased

Hematologic: Leukopenia (<3%), thrombocytopenia (<3%), hematocrit decreased

Hepatic: Liver function tests increased

Neuromuscular & skeletal: Arthralgia, back pain, bone pain, foot drop, gait abnormalities, paresthesia, rigors, skeletal muscle rigidity, tremor

Ocular: Amblyopia, conjunctivitis, eye pain, vision problems/disturbance

Renal: Oliguria

Respiratory: Asthma, atelectasis, dyspnea, hiccups, hypercapnia, hypoxia, pulmonary edema (noncardiogenic), respiratory depression, rhinitis

Miscellaneous: Diaphoresis, flu-like syndrome, infection, thirst, voice alteration, withdrawal syndrome

Dosage These are guidelines and do not represent the doses that may be required in all patients. Doses and dosage intervals should be titrated to pain relief/prevention.

Children >6 months and <50 kg: *Acute pain (moderate-to-severe):*

Oral (immediate release formulations): 0.15-0.3 mg/kg every 3-4 hours as needed. **Note:** The American Pain Society recommends an initial dose of 0.3 mg/kg for children with severe pain (American Pain Society [APS], 2008)

I.M., SubQ: 0.1-0.2 mg/kg; **Note:** Repeated SubQ administration causes local tissue irritation, pain, and induration. The use of I.M. injections is no longer recommended especially for repeated administration due to painful administration, variable absorption and lag time to peak effect.

I.V.: 0.05-0.3 mg/kg every 3-4 hours as needed, not to exceed 10 mg per dose

Continuous infusion: Initial: 10-30 **mcg/kg/hour**; titrate as needed to control pain

Patient-controlled analgesia (PCA) (APS, 2008): **Note:** Opioid-naive: Consider lower end of dosing range:

Usual concentration: 1 mg/mL

Demand dose: Usual: 0.02 mg/kg/dose; range: 0.01-0.03 mg/kg/dose

Lockout interval: 8-10 minutes

Usual basal rate: 0-0.03 mg/kg/hour

Adults:

Acute pain (moderate-to-severe):

Oral (immediate release formulations): Opioid-naive: Initial: **Note:** Usual dosage range: 10-30 mg every 4 hours as needed. Patients with prior opioid exposure may require higher initial doses.

Solution: 10-20 mg every 4 hours as needed

Tablet: 15-30 mg every 4 hours as needed

I.M., SubQ: **Note:** Repeated SubQ administration causes local tissue irritation, pain, and induration. The use of I.M. injections is no longer recommended especially for repeated administration due to painful administration, variable absorption and lag time to peak effect; other routes are more reliable and less painful (APS, 2008).

Initial: Opioid-naive: 5-10 mg every 4 hours as needed; usual dosage range: 5-15 mg every 4 hours as needed. Patients with prior opioid exposure may require higher initial doses.

I.V.: Initial: Opioid-naive: 2.5-5 mg every 3-4 hours; patients with prior opioid exposure may require higher initial doses. **Note:** Administration of 2-3 mg every 5 minutes until pain relief or if associated sedation, oxygen saturation <95%, or serious adverse event occurs may be appropriate in treating acute moderate-to-severe pain in settings such as the immediate postoperative period or the emergency department (Aubrun, 2012; Lvovschi, 2008); dose reduction in the immediate postoperative period (postanesthesia care unit) in the elderly is usually not necessary (Aubrun, 2002). A maximum cumulative dose (eg, 10 mg) prompting reevaluation of continued morphine use and/or dose should be included as part of any medication order intended for short-term use (eg, PACU orders). Refer to institution-specific protocols as appropriate.

Acute myocardial infarction, analgesia (unlabeled use): Initial management: 4-8 mg (lower doses in the elderly); subsequently may give 2-8 mg every 5-15 minutes as needed (O'Gara, 2012)

Critically-ill patients, analgesia (unlabeled dose): 2-4 mg every 1-2 hours **or** 4-8 mg every 3-4 hours as needed (Barr, 2013)

I.V., SubQ continuous infusion: 0.8-10 mg/hour; usual range: Up to 80 mg/hour. **Note:** May administer a loading dose (amount administered should depend on severity of pain) prior to initiating the infusion. A continuous (basal) infusion is not recommended in an opioid-naive patient (ISMP, 2009)

Continuous infusion for critically-ill patients: Usual dosage range: 2-30 mg/hour (Barr, 2013)

Patient-controlled analgesia (PCA) (APS, 2008): **Note:** In opioid-naive patients, consider lower end of dosing range:

Usual concentration: 1 mg/mL

Demand dose: Usual: 1 mg; range: 0.5-2.5 mg

Lockout interval: 5-10 minutes

Epidural: Pain management: **Note: Must be preservative-free.** Administer with extreme caution and in reduced dosage to geriatric or debilitated patients. Vigilant monitoring is particularly important in these patients.

Single-dose: **Lumbar region:** Astramorph/PF™, Duramorph: 30-100 mcg/kg (optimal range: 2.5-3.75 mg; may depend upon patient comorbidities; Bujedo, 2012; Sultan, 2011)

Continuous infusion (may be combined with bupivacaine): 0.2-0.4 mg/hour (Bujedo, 2012)

Continuous microinfusion (Infumorph):

Opioid-naive: Initial: 3.5-7.5 mg over 24 hours

Opioid-tolerant: Initial: 4.5-10 mg over 24 hours, titrate to effect; usual maximum is ~30 mg per 24 hours

Intrathecal (I.T.): **Note: Must be preservative-free.** Administer with extreme caution and in reduced dosage to geriatric or debilitated patients. I.T. dose is usually 1/10 (one-tenth) that of epidural dosage.

Opioid-naive: Single dose: Lumbar region: Astramorph/PF™, Duramorph: 0.1-0.3 mg (may provide adequate relief for up to 24 hours; APS, 2008); repeat doses are **not** recommended. If pain recurs within 24 hours of administration, use of an alternate route of administration is recommended. **Note:** Although product labeling recommends doses up to 1 mg, an analgesic ceiling exists with doses >0.3 mg and the risk of respiratory depression is higher with doses >0.3 mg (Rathmell, 2005).

Continuous microinfusion (Infumorph): Lumbar region: After initial in-hospital evaluation of response to single-dose injections (Astramorph/PF™, Duramorph) the initial dose of Infumorph is 0.2-1 mg over 24 hours

Opioid-tolerant: Continuous microinfusion (Infumorph): Lumbar region: Dosage range: 1-10 mg over 24 hours, titrate to effect; usual maximum is ~20 mg over 24 hours

Rectal: 10-20 mg every 3-4 hours

Chronic pain: **Note:** Patients taking opioids chronically may become tolerant and require doses higher than the usual dosage range to maintain the desired effect. Tolerance can be managed by appropriate dose titration. There is no optimal or maximal dose for morphine in chronic pain. The appropriate dose is one that relieves pain throughout its dosing interval without causing unmanageable side effects. Consider total daily dose, potency, prior opioid use, degree of opioid experience and tolerance, conversion from previous opioid (including opioid formulation), patient's general condition, concurrent medications, and type and severity of pain during prescribing process.

Oral (extended release formulations): A patient's morphine requirement should be established using immediate release formulations. Conversion to long-acting products may be considered when chronic, continuous treatment is required. Higher dosages should be reserved for use only in opioid-tolerant patients.

Capsules, extended release (Avinza®): Daily dose administered once daily (for best results, administer at same time each day)

Opioid-naive: Initial: 30 mg once daily; adjust in increments ≤30 mg daily every 4 days

Conversion from other oral morphine formulations to Avinza®: Total daily morphine dose given as once daily. The first dose of Avinza® may be taken with the last dose of the immediate release morphine. Maximum: 1600 mg daily due to fumaric acid content.

Capsules, extended release (Kadian®): **Note:** Not intended for use as an initial opioid in the management of pain; use immediate release formulations before initiation. Total daily oral morphine dose may be either administered once daily or in 2 divided doses daily (every 12 hours). The first dose of Kadian® may be taken with the last dose of the immediate release morphine.

Tablets, extended release (MS Contin®): Daily dose divided and administered every 8 or every 12 hours

Conversion from parenteral morphine or other opioids to extended release formulations: Substantial interpatient variability exists in relative potency. Therefore, it is safer to underestimate a patient's daily oral morphine requirement and provide breakthrough pain relief with immediate release morphine than to overestimate requirements. Consider the parenteral to oral morphine ratio or other oral or parenteral opioids to oral morphine conversions.

Elderly or debilitated patients: Use with caution; may require dose reduction.

Dosing adjustment in renal impairment:

Cl$_{cr}$ 10-50 mL/minute: Children and Adults: Administer at 75% of normal dose.

Cl$_{cr}$ <10 mL/minute: Children and Adults: Administer at 50% of normal dose.

Intermittent HD:

Children: Administer 50% of normal dose.

Adults: No dosage adjustment necessary.

Peritoneal dialysis: Children: Administer 50% of normal dose.

CRRT: Children and Adults: Administer 75% of normal dose, titrate.

Dosing adjustment/comments in hepatic disease: No dosage adjustment provided in manufacturer's labeling. Pharmacokinetics unchanged in mild liver disease; substantial extrahepatic metabolism may occur. In cirrhosis, increases in half-life and AUC suggest dosage adjustment required.

Mechanism of Action Binds to opioid receptors in the CNS, causing inhibition of ascending pain pathways, altering the perception of and response to pain; produces generalized CNS depression

Contraindications Note: Some contraindications are product specific. For details, please see detailed product prescribing information.

Hypersensitivity to morphine sulfate or any component of the formulation; severe respiratory depression, acute or severe asthma (in an unmonitored setting or without resuscitative equipment); known or suspected paralytic ileus

Additional contraindication information (based on formulation):

Epidural/intrathecal:

Astramorph/PF™, Duramorph: Upper airway obstruction

Astramorph/PF™, Duramorph, Infumorph: Usual contraindications related to neuraxial analgesia apply (eg, presence of infection at infusion site, concomitant anticoagulant therapy, uncontrolled bleeding diathesis)

Extended release: GI obstruction

Immediate release tablets/solution: Hypercarbia

Injectable formulation: Heart failure due to chronic lung disease, cardiac arrhythmias; increased intracranial pressure, head injuries, brain tumors; acute alcoholism, deliriums tremens; seizure disorders; use during labor when a premature birth is anticipated

Suppository: Severe CNS depression; cardiac arrhythmias, heart failure due to chronic lung disease; increased intracranial or cerebrospinal pressure, head injuries, brain tumor; acute alcoholism, delirium tremens; seizure disorder; use after biliary tract surgery, suspected surgical abdomen, surgical anastomosis; concurrent use or within 2 weeks of MAO inhibitors

Warnings/Precautions An opioid-containing analgesic regimen should be tailored to each patient's needs and based upon the type of pain being treated (acute versus chronic), the route of administration, degree of tolerance for opioids (naive versus chronic user), age, weight, and medical condition. The optimal analgesic dose varies widely among patients. Doses should be titrated to pain relief/prevention. When used as an epidural injection, monitor for delayed sedation. **[U.S. Boxed Warning]: Healthcare provider should be alert to problems of abuse, misuse, and diversion. [U.S. Boxed Warning]: Extended release formulations, concentrated oral solution (100 mg/5 mL): Fatal overdose of morphine can result from accidental ingestion, especially in children.**

[U.S. Boxed Warning]: Fatal respiratory depression may occur. Greatest risk during initiation and dose increases. Use with caution in patients (particularly elderly, debilitated) with impaired respiratory function (especially hypoxia or hypercapnia), COPD, other obstructive pulmonary disease, decreased respiratory reserve, kyphoscoliosis or other skeletal disorder which may alter respiratory function. Infants <3 months of age are more susceptible to respiratory depression, use with caution and generally in reduced doses in this age group.

Use caution in morbid obesity, adrenal insufficiency, CNS depression, coma, prostatic hyperplasia, thyroid dysfunction, urinary stricture, renal impairment, or severe hepatic dysfunction and in patients with hypersensitivity reactions to other phenanthrene derivative opioid agonists (codeine, hydrocodone, hydromorphone, levorphanol, oxycodone, oxymorphone). Use with caution in patients with biliary tract dysfunction including acute pancreatitis as may cause constriction of sphincter of Oddi. May obscure diagnosis or clinical course of patients with acute abdominal conditions. Some preparations contain sulfites which may cause allergic reactions.

May cause CNS depression, which may impair physical or mental abilities; patients must be cautioned about performing tasks which require mental alertness (eg, operating machinery or driving). Effects may be potentiated when used with other sedative drugs. **[U.S. Boxed Warning]: Do not administer Avinza® with alcoholic beverages or ethanol-containing prescription or nonprescription products, which may disrupt extended-release characteristic of product.**

May cause hypotension; use with caution in patients with hypovolemia, cardiovascular disease (including acute MI), circulatory shock, or drugs which may exaggerate hypotensive effects (including phenothiazines or general anesthetics). May cause orthostatic hypotension and syncope in ambulatory patients. Use with extreme caution in patients with head injury, intracranial lesions, or elevated intracranial pressure; exaggerated elevation of ICP may occur if respiratory drive is depressed and CO_2 retention occurs. Use with caution in patients with seizure disorders, may exacerbate pre-existing seizures. Tolerance or drug dependence may result from extended use. Concurrent use of agonist/antagonist analgesics may precipitate withdrawal symptoms and/or reduced analgesic efficacy in patients following prolonged therapy with mu opioid agonists. Abrupt discontinuation following prolonged use may also lead to withdrawal symptoms. Gradually wean dose over a short period of time. Elderly may be particularly susceptible to adverse effects. Use epidural/intrathecal formulations with extreme caution in the elderly.

[U.S. Boxed Warning]: Extended release dosage forms should not be crushed, dissolved, or chewed. Extended release products are not intended for "as needed (PRN)" use. Avinza® capsules contain fumaric acid; dangerous quantities of fumaric acid may be ingested when >1600 mg/day is used; serious renal toxicity may occur above the maximum dose. **Extended release products are not interchangeable;** when determining a generic equivalent or switching from one extended release product to another, review pharmacokinetic properties.

Highly concentrated oral solutions: **[U.S. Boxed Warning]: Check doses carefully when using highly concentrated oral solutions. The 100 mg/5 mL (20 mg/mL) concentration is indicated for use in opioid-tolerant patients only.**

Injections: Products are designed for administration by specific routes (ie, I.V., intrathecal, epidural). Use caution when prescribing, dispensing, or administering to use formulations only by intended route(s).

Astramorph/PF™, Duramorph, Infumorph: **[U.S. Boxed Warning]: Due to the risk of severe and/or sustained cardiopulmonary depressant effects, must be administered in a fully equipped room for resuscitation and staffed environment.** Naloxone injection should be immediately available. Patient should remain in this environment for at least 24 hours following the initial dose. **[U.S. Boxed Warning]: Accidental dermal exposure to Astramorph/PF™, Duramorph, Infumorph should be rinsed with water. Contaminated clothing should be removed.** For patients receiving Infumorph via microinfusion device, patient may be observed, as appropriate, for the first several days after catheter implantation. Thoracic epidural administration has been shown to dramatically increase the risk of early and late respiratory depression.

[U.S. Boxed Warning]: Improper or erroneous substitution of Infumorph for regular Duramorph is likely to result in serious overdosage, leading to seizures, respiratory depression and possibly a fatal outcome. Infumorph should only be used in microinfusion devices; not for I.V., I.M., or SubQ administration or for single-dose administration. Monitor closely, especially in the first 24 hours. Inflammatory masses (eg, granulomas), some resulting in severe neurologic impairment have occurred when receiving Infumorph via indwelling intrathecal catheter; monitor carefully for new neurologic signs/symptoms. **[U.S. Boxed Warning]:** Intrathecal dosage is usually 1/10 (one-tenth) that of epidural dosage.

Drug Interactions

Metabolism/Transport Effects Substrate of CYP2D6 (minor); **Note:** Assignment of Major/Minor substrate status based on clinically relevant drug interaction potential

Avoid Concomitant Use

Avoid concomitant use of Morphine (Systemic) with any of the following: Azelastine (Nasal); Paraldehyde

Increased Effect/Toxicity

Morphine (Systemic) may increase the levels/effects of: Alcohol (Ethyl); Alvimopan; Azelastine (Nasal); CNS Depressants; Desmopressin; Metyrosine; Mirtazapine; Paraldehyde; Pramipexole; ROPINIRole; Rotigotine; Selective Serotonin Reuptake Inhibitors; Thiazide Diuretics; Zolpidem

The levels/effects of Morphine (Systemic) may be increased by: Amphetamines; Antipsychotic Agents (Phenothiazines); Droperidol; HydrOXYzine; Magnesium Sulfate; Perampanel; Sodium Oxybate; Succinylcholine

Decreased Effect

Morphine (Systemic) may decrease the levels/effects of: Pegvisomant

The levels/effects of Morphine (Systemic) may be decreased by: Ammonium Chloride; Mixed Agonist / Antagonist Opioids; Peginterferon Alfa-2b; Rifamycin Derivatives

Ethanol/Nutrition/Herb Interactions

Ethanol: Alcoholic beverages or ethanol-containing products may disrupt extended release formulation resulting in rapid release of entire morphine dose. Ethanol may also increase CNS depression. Management: Avoid alcohol. **Do not administer Avinza® with alcoholic beverages or ethanol-containing prescription or nonprescription products.**

Food: Administration of oral morphine solution with food may increase bioavailability (ie, a report of 34% increase in morphine AUC when morphine oral solution followed a high-fat meal). The bioavailability of Avinza®, MS Contin®, or Kadian® does not appear to be affected by food. Management: Take consistently with or without meals.

Herb/Nutraceutical: Gotu kola, valerian, and kava kava may increase CNS depression. Management: Avoid gotu kola, valerian, and kava kava.

Dietary Considerations Morphine may cause GI upset; take with food if GI upset occurs. Be consistent when taking morphine with or without meals.

Pharmacodynamics/Kinetics

Onset of Action Patient dependent; dosing must be individualized: Oral (immediate release): ~30 minutes; I.V.: 5-10 minutes

Duration of Action Patient dependent; dosing must be individualized: Pain relief:

Immediate release formulations: 4 hours

Extended release capsule and tablet: 8-24 hours (formulation dependent)

Half-life Elimination Adults: Immediate release forms: 2-4 hours; Avinza® ~24 hours; Kadian®:11-13 hours

Time to Peak Avinza®: 30 minutes (maintained for 24 hours); Kadian®: ~10 hours

Pregnancy Risk Factor C

Pregnancy Considerations Teratogenic effects were not observed in animal studies; however reduced growth and behavioral abnormalities in offspring have been observed. Morphine crosses the human placenta. The frequency of congenital malformations has not been reported to be greater than expected in children from mothers treated with morphine during pregnancy. However, following *in utero* exposure, infants may exhibit withdrawal, decreased brain volume (reversible), small size, decreased ventilatory response to CO_2, and increased risk of sudden infant death syndrome. In patients with chronic, noncancer pain, minimal (if any) opioids should be used during pregnancy. Neonates born to mothers receiving chronic opioids during pregnancy should be monitored for neonatal withdrawal syndrome.

Lactation Enters breast milk/use caution (AAP rates "compatible"; AAP 2001 update pending)

Breast-Feeding Considerations Morphine concentrates in breast milk, with a milk to plasma AUC ratio of 2.5:1. Detectable serum levels of morphine can be found in infants following morphine administration to nursing mothers. Treatment of the mother with single doses of morphine is not expected to cause detrimental effects in nursing infants. Breast-feeding following chronic use or in neonates with hepatic or renal dysfunction may lead to higher levels of morphine in the infant and a risk of adverse effects.

Controlled Substance C-II

Dosage Forms

Capsule, extended release, oral: 10 mg, 20 mg, 30 mg, 50 mg, 60 mg, 80 mg, 100 mg, 200 mg

AVINza®: 30 mg, 45 mg, 60 mg, 75 mg, 90 mg, 120 mg

Kadian®: 10 mg, 20 mg, 30 mg, 40 mg, 50 mg, 60 mg, 70 mg, 80 mg, 100 mg, 130 mg, 150 mg, 200 mg

Injection, solution: 1 mg/mL (10 mL, 30 mL, 50 mL); 2 mg/mL (1 mL); 4 mg/mL (1 mL); 5 mg/mL (1 mL, 30 mL, 50 mL); 8 mg/mL (1 mL); 10 mg/mL (1 mL, 10 mL); 10 mg/0.7 mL (0.7 mL); 15 mg/mL (1 mL, 20 mL); 25 mg/mL (4 mL, 10 mL, 20 mL); 50 mg/mL (20 mL, 40 mL, 50 mL)

Injection, solution [preservative free]: 0.5 mg/mL (10 mL, 30 mL); 1 mg/mL (10 mL, 30 mL); 5 mg/mL (30 mL); 25 mg/mL (4 mL, 10 mL, 20 mL)

Astramorph/PF™: 0.5 mg/mL (2 mL, 10 mL); 1 mg/mL (2 mL, 10 mL)

Duramorph: 0.5 mg/mL (10 mL); 1 mg/mL (10 mL)

Infumorph 200: 10 mg/mL (20 mL)

Infumorph 500: 25 mg/mL (20 mL)

Solution, oral: 10 mg/5 mL (5 mL, 100 mL, 500 mL); 20 mg/5 mL (100 mL, 500 mL); 100 mg/5 mL (15 mL, 30 mL, 120 mL, 240 mL)

Suppository, rectal: 5 mg (12s); 10 mg (12s); 20 mg (12s); 30 mg (12s)

Tablet, oral: 15 mg, 30 mg

Tablet, extended release, oral: 15 mg, 30 mg, 60 mg, 100 mg, 200 mg

MS Contin®: 15 mg, 30 mg, 60 mg, 100 mg, 200 mg

Dosage Forms: Canada
Solution, oral:
Doloral: 1 mg/mL; 5 mg/mL [not available in U.S.]

Morrhuate Sodium (MOR yoo ate SOW dee um)

Pharmacologic Category Sclerosing Agent
Use Treatment of small, uncomplicated varicose veins of the lower extremities
Local Anesthetic/Vasoconstrictor Precautions No information available to require special precautions
Effects on Dental Treatment No significant effects or complications reported
Effects on Bleeding Shown to induce thrombosis and phlebosclerosis by directly damaging the endothelium and erythrocytes, activating platelets, and aggregating granulocytes at the venous wall endothelium.
Adverse Effects Frequency not defined.
Cardiovascular: Thrombosis, vascular collapse
Central nervous system: Dizziness, drowsiness, headache
Dermatologic: Urticaria
Gastrointestinal: Nausea, vomiting
Local: Burning or cramping at the site of injection, severe extravasation effects
Neuromuscular & skeletal: Weakness
Respiratory: Asthma, pulmonary embolism, respiratory depression
Miscellaneous: Anaphylaxis, hypersensitivity reactions
General Dosage Range I.V.: *Adults:* 50-250 mg
Mechanism of Action Morrhuate sodium causes inflammation of the vein's intima resulting in the formation of a thrombus. Occlusion secondary to the fibrous tissue and the thrombus results in the obliteration of the vein.
Pregnancy Risk Factor C
Pregnancy Considerations Animal reproduction studies have not been conducted.

Mouthwash (Antiseptic) (MOUTH wosh)

Related Information
Bacterial Infections *on page 1562*
Dentin Hypersensitivity, Acid Erosion, High Caries Index, Management of Alveolar Osteitis, and Xerostomia *on page 1582*
Periodontal Diseases *on page 1570*
Ulcerative, Erosive, and Painful Oral Mucosal Disorders *on page 1578*
Related Sample Prescriptions
Antimicrobial Oral Rinses *on page 1613*
Pharmacologic Category Antimicrobial Mouth Rinse; Antiplaque Agent; Mouthwash
Dental Use Aid in prevention and reduction of plaque and gingivitis; halitosis
Use Aid in prevention and reduction of plaque and gingivitis; halitosis
Local Anesthetic/Vasoconstrictor Precautions No information available to require special precautions
Effects on Dental Treatment No significant effects or complications reported (see Dental Comment)
Effects on Bleeding No information available to require special precautions
Adverse Effects No data reported

Dental Usual Dosage Plaque/gingivitis prevention: Adults: Oral: Rinse full strength for 30 seconds with 20 mL morning and night
Dosage Rinse full strength for 30 seconds with 20 mL morning and night
Contraindications Hypersensitivity to any component of the formulation
Dosage Forms
Rinse: 250 mL, 500 mL, 1000 mL
Dental Comment Active ingredients:
Listerine® Antiseptic: Thymol 0.064%, eucalyptus 0.092%, methyl salicylate 0.060%, menthol 0.042%, alcohol 26.9%, water, benzoic acid, poloxamer 407, sodium benzoate, caramel
Fresh Burst Listerine® Antiseptic: Thymol 0.064%, eucalyptus 0.092%, methyl salicylate 0.060%, menthol 0.042%, alcohol 26.9%, water, benzoic acid, poloxamer 407, sodium benzoate, flavoring, sodium, saccharin, sodium citrate, citric acid, D&C yellow #10, FD&C green #3
Cool Mint Listerine® Antiseptic: Thymol 0.064%, eucalyptus 0.092%, methyl salicylate 0.060%, menthol 0.042%, alcohol 26.9%, water, benzoic acid, poloxamer 407, sodium benzoate, flavoring, sodium, saccharin, sodium citrate, citric acid, FD&C green #3
The following information is endorsed on the label of the Listerine® products by the Council on Scientific Affairs, American Dental Association: "Listerine® Antiseptic has been shown to help prevent and reduce supragingival plaque accumulation and gingivitis when used in a conscientiously applied program of oral hygiene and regular professional care. Its effect on periodontitis has not been determined."

Moxifloxacin (Systemic) (moxs i FLOKS a sin)

Related Information
Bacterial Infections *on page 1562*
Clinical Risk Related to Drugs Prolonging QT Interval *on page 1510*
Brand Names: U.S. Avelox®; Avelox® ABC Pack; Avelox® I.V.
Brand Names: Canada Avelox®; Avelox® I.V.
Generic Availability (U.S.) No
Pharmacologic Category Antibiotic, Quinolone; Respiratory Fluoroquinolone
Use Treatment of mild-to-moderate community-acquired pneumonia, including multidrug-resistant *Streptococcus pneumoniae* (MDRSP); acute bacterial exacerbation of chronic bronchitis; acute bacterial rhinosinusitis (ABRS); complicated and uncomplicated skin and skin structure infections; complicated intra-abdominal infections
Unlabeled Use Treatment of *Legionella* pneumonia; treatment of mild-to-moderate community-acquired pneumonia (CAP), including multidrug-resistant *Streptococcus pneumoniae* (MDRSP) in adolescents with skeletal maturity; tuberculosis (second-line therapy)
Local Anesthetic/Vasoconstrictor Precautions Moxifloxacin is one of the drugs confirmed to prolong the QT interval and is accepted as having a risk of causing torsade de pointes. The risk of drug-induced torsade de pointes is extremely low when a single QT interval prolonging drug is prescribed. In terms of epinephrine, it is not known what effect vasoconstrictors in the local anesthetic regimen will have in patients with a known history of congenital prolonged QT interval or in patients taking any medication that prolongs the QT interval. Until more information is obtained, it is suggested that the clinician consult with the physician prior ▶

to the use of a vasoconstrictor in suspected patients, and that the vasoconstrictor (epinephrine, mepivacaine and levonordefrin [Carbocaine® 2% with Neo-Cobefrin®]) be used with caution.

Effects on Dental Treatment Key adverse event(s) related to dental treatment: Dry mouth, glossitis, stomatitis, and taste perversion.

Effects on Bleeding Anemia, prolonged prothrombin activation, prolonged activated partial thromboplastin time, increased platelet count, decreased hemoglobin, decreased hematocrit have been reported in a subset of all patients receiving systemic moxifloxacin at therapeutic concentrations. As a consequence, prothrombin time should be closely monitored during moxifloxacin therapy, especially if administered concomitantly with warfarin.

Adverse Effects

2% to 10%:

Central nervous system: Headache (≤4%), dizziness (3%), insomnia (2%)

Endocrine & metabolic: Chloride increased (≥2%), glucose decreased (≥2%), ionized calcium increased (≥2%)

Gastrointestinal: Nausea (7%), diarrhea (6%), amylase decreased (≥2%), constipation (2%), vomiting (2%), abdominal pain (1% to 2%)

Hematologic: Decreased serum levels of the following (≥2%): Basophils, eosinophils, hemoglobin, PT, RBC, neutrophils; increased serum levels of the following (≥2%): MCH, neutrophils, PT, WBC

Hepatic: Bilirubin decreased/increased (≥2%)

Renal: Albumin increased (≥2%)

Respiratory: PO_2 decreased (≥2%)

0.1% to <2%:

Cardiovascular: Angina, atrial fibrillation, bradycardia, cardiac arrest, edema, heart failure, hypertension, hypotension, palpitation, peripheral edema, QT_c prolongation, syncope, tachycardia

Central nervous system: Fever (1%), agitation, anxiety, chills, confusion, depression, disorientation, fatigue, hallucinations, hypoesthesia, lethargy, malaise, nervousness, pain, restlessness, somnolence, vertigo

Dermatologic: Allergic dermatitis, erythema, hyperhidrosis, pruritus, rash, urticaria

Endocrine & metabolic: Hypokalemia (1%), dehydration, hyperglycemia, hyperlipidemia, triglycerides increased, uric acid increased

Gastrointestinal: Dyspepsia (1%), abdominal discomfort, abdominal distension, amylase increased, anorexia, appetite decreased, flatulence, gastritis, gastroenteritis, gastroesophageal reflux disease, lactic dehydrogenase increased, lipase increased, taste perversion, xerostomia

Genitourinary: Dysuria, vaginitis, vulvovaginal candidiasis, vulvovaginal mycotic infection, vulvovaginal pruritus

Hematologic: Anemia (1%), eosinophilia, hematocrit decreased, leukocytosis, leukopenia, aPTT increased, thrombocythemia, thrombocytopenia

Hepatic: ALT increased (1%), AST increased, alkaline phosphatase increased, GGTP increased, liver function test abnormal

Local: Injection site extravasation, phlebitis

Neuromuscular & skeletal: Arthralgia, back pain, chest pain (noncardiac), facial pain, limb pain, muscle spasms, musculoskeletal pain, myalgia, paresthesia, tremor, weakness

Ocular: Blurred vision

Otic: Tinnitus

Renal: BUN increased, creatinine increased, renal failure

Respiratory: Asthma, bronchospasm, dyspnea, wheezing

Miscellaneous: Allergic reaction, candidiasis, fungal infection, night sweats, oral candidiasis

Dosage

Adolescents (unlabeled use): **Community-acquired pneumonia (CAP) due to atypical pathogens (M. pneumoniae, C. trachomatis, or C. pneumoniae), mild infection or step-down therapy in adolescents with skeletal maturity, (alternative to azithromycin) (IDSA/PIDS, 2011):** Oral: 400 mg once daily

Adults: Oral, I.V.: Usual dosage range: 400 mg every 24 hours

Indication-specific dosing:

Acute bacterial rhinosinusitis: 400 mg every 24 hours for 10 days or 5-7 days (Chow, 2012). **Note:** Recommended in patients with beta-lactam allergy; may also be used if initial therapy fails, in areas with high endemic rates of penicillin nonsusceptible *S. pneumoniae*, those with severe infections, age >65 years, recent hospitalization, antibiotic use within the past month, or who are immunocompromised.

Chronic bronchitis, acute bacterial exacerbation: 400 mg every 24 hours for 5 days

Community-acquired pneumonia (CAP) (including MDRSP): 400 mg every 24 hours for 7-14 days

Intra-abdominal infections, complicated: 400 mg every 24 hours for 5-14 days (initiate with I.V.); **Note:** 2010 IDSA guidelines recommend a treatment duration of 4-7 days (provided source controlled) for community-acquired, mild-to-moderate IAI

***M. genitalium* infections** (including confirmed cases or clinically significant persistent cervicitis, pelvic inflammatory disease or urethritis in patients who previously received azithromycin or doxycycline; unlabeled use): Oral, I.V.: 400 mg every 24 hours for 7-10 days (Manhart, 2011)

Skin and skin structure infections:

Complicated: 400 mg every 24 hours for 7-21 days

Uncomplicated: 400 mg every 24 hours for 7 days

Tuberculosis, drug-resistant tuberculosis, or intolerance to first-line agents (unlabeled use): Oral: 400 mg every 24 hours (*MMWR*, 2003)

Elderly: No dosage adjustments are required based on age

Dosage adjustment in renal impairment: No dosage adjustment required in renal impairment.

Poorly dialyzed; no supplemental dose or dosage adjustment necessary, including patients on intermittent hemodialysis, peritoneal dialysis, or continuous renal replacement therapy (eg, CVVHD).

Dosage adjustment in hepatic impairment: No dosage adjustment is required in mild, moderate, or severe hepatic insufficiency (Child-Pugh class A, B, or C); however, use with caution in this patient population secondary to the risk of QT prolongation.

Mechanism of Action Moxifloxacin is a DNA gyrase inhibitor, and also inhibits topoisomerase IV. DNA gyrase (topoisomerase II) is an essential bacterial enzyme that maintains the superhelical structure of DNA. DNA gyrase is required for DNA replication and transcription, DNA repair, recombination, and transposition; inhibition is bactericidal.

Contraindications Hypersensitivity to moxifloxacin, other quinolone antibiotics, or any component of the formulation

Warnings/Precautions [U.S. Boxed Warning]: There have been reports of tendon inflammation and/or rupture with quinolone antibiotics; risk may be increased with concurrent corticosteroids, organ transplant recipients, and in patients >60 years of age. Rupture of the Achilles tendon sometimes requiring surgical repair has been reported most frequently; but other tendon sites (eg, rotator cuff, biceps) have also been reported. Strenuous physical activity, rheumatoid arthritis, and renal impairment may be an independent risk factor for tendonitis. Discontinue at first sign of tendon inflammation or pain. Tendon rupture may occur even after discontinuation of therapy. Use with caution in patients with rheumatoid arthritis or renal impairment; may increase risk of tendon rupture.

Use with caution in patients with significant bradycardia or acute myocardial ischemia. Moxifloxacin causes a concentration-dependent QT prolongation. Do not exceed recommended dose or infusion rate. Avoid use with uncorrected hypokalemia, with other drugs that prolong the QT interval or induce bradycardia, or with class Ia or III antiarrhythmic agents. CNS effects may occur (tremor, restlessness, confusion, and very rarely hallucinations, increased intracranial pressure [including pseudotumor cerebri] or seizures). Use with caution in patients with known or suspected CNS disorder. Potential for seizures, although very rare, may be increased with concomitant NSAID therapy. Use with caution in individuals at risk of seizures. Use with caution in patients with mild, moderate, or severe hepatic impairment or liver cirrhosis; may increase the risk of QT prolongation. Fulminant hepatitis potentially leading to liver failure (including fatalities) has been reported with use. Use with caution in diabetes; glucose regulation may be altered.

Fluoroquinolones have been associated with the development of serious, and sometimes fatal, hypoglycemia, most often in elderly diabetics, but also in patients without diabetes. This occurred most frequently with gatifloxacin (no longer available systemically) but may occur at a lower frequency with other quinolones.

Severe hypersensitivity reactions, including anaphylaxis, have occurred with quinolone therapy. Reactions may present as typical allergic symptoms after a single dose, or may manifest as severe idiosyncratic dermatologic, vascular, pulmonary, renal, hepatic, and/or hematologic events, usually after multiple doses. Prompt discontinuation of drug should occur if skin rash or other symptoms arise. Avoid excessive sunlight and take precautions to limit exposure (eg, loose fitting clothing, sunscreen); may cause moderate-to-severe phototoxicity reactions. Discontinue use if photosensitivity occurs. Prolonged use may result in fungal or bacterial superinfection, including *C. difficile*-associated diarrhea (CDAD) and pseudomembranous colitis; CDAD has been observed >2 months postantibiotic treatment. **[U.S. Boxed Warning]: Quinolones may exacerbate myasthenia gravis; avoid use (rare, potentially life-threatening weakness of respiratory muscles may occur).** Peripheral neuropathy may rarely occur. Hemolytic reactions may (rarely) occur with quinolone use in patients with latent or actual G6PD deficiency. Adverse effects (eg, tendon rupture, QT changes) may be increased in the elderly. Some quinolones may exacerbate myasthenia gravis, use with caution (rare, potentially life-threatening weakness of respiratory muscles may occur). Safety and efficacy of systemically administered moxifloxacin (oral, intravenous) in patients <18 years of age have not been established.

Drug Interactions

Metabolism/Transport Effects None known.

Avoid Concomitant Use

Avoid concomitant use of Moxifloxacin (Systemic) with any of the following: BCG; Highest Risk QTc-Prolonging Agents; Ivabradine; Mifepristone; Strontium Ranelate

Increased Effect/Toxicity

Moxifloxacin (Systemic) may increase the levels/effects of: Corticosteroids (Systemic); Highest Risk QTc-Prolonging Agents; Moderate Risk QTc-Prolonging Agents; Porfimer; Sulfonylureas; Varenicline; Vitamin K Antagonists

The levels/effects of Moxifloxacin (Systemic) may be increased by: Insulin; Ivabradine; Mifepristone; Nonsteroidal Anti-Inflammatory Agents; Probenecid; QTc-Prolonging Agents (Indeterminate Risk and Risk Modifying)

Decreased Effect

Moxifloxacin (Systemic) may decrease the levels/effects of: BCG; Didanosine; Mycophenolate; Sodium Picosulfate; Sulfonylureas; Typhoid Vaccine

The levels/effects of Moxifloxacin (Systemic) may be decreased by: Antacids; Didanosine; Iron Salts; Lanthanum; Magnesium Salts; Multivitamins/Minerals (with ADEK, Folate, Iron); Quinapril; Sevelamer; Strontium Ranelate; Sucralfate; Zinc Salts

Ethanol/Nutrition/Herb Interactions Food: Absorption is not affected by administration with a high-fat meal or yogurt.

Dietary Considerations May be taken without regard to meals. Take 4 hours before or 8 hours after multiple vitamins, antacids, or other products containing magnesium, aluminum, iron, or zinc.
Avelox® I.V. infusion (premixed in sodium chloride 0.8%) contains sodium 34.2 mEq (~787 mg)/250 mL.

Pharmacodynamics/Kinetics

Half-life Elimination Single dose: Oral: 12-16 hours; I.V.: 8-15 hours

Pregnancy Risk Factor C

Pregnancy Considerations Adverse events have been observed in some animal studies; therefore, the manufacturer classifies moxifloxacin as pregnancy category C. Quinolone exposure during human pregnancy has been reported with other agents (see Ciprofloxacin [Systemic], Ofloxacin [Systemic], and Norfloxacin monographs). To date, no specific teratogenic effect or increased pregnancy risk has been identified; however, because of concerns of cartilage damage in immature animals exposed to quinolones and the limited moxifloxacin specific data, moxifloxacin should only be used during pregnancy if a safer option is not available.

Lactation Excretion in breast milk unknown/not recommended

Breast-Feeding Considerations It is not known if moxifloxacin is excreted into breast milk. Breast-feeding is not recommended by the manufacturer. Although there is no information on the use of moxifloxacin during breast-feeding, other quinolones are considered compatible. Nondose-related effects could include modification of bowel flora.

Dosage Forms

Infusion, premixed in sodium chloride 0.8% [preservative free]:
Avelox® I.V.: 400 mg (250 mL)

Tablet, oral:
Avelox®: 400 mg
Avelox® ABC Pack: 400 mg

◀ Dental Comment Moxifloxacin is known to prolong the QT interval. The QT interval is measured as the time and distance between the Q point of the QRS complex and the end of the T wave in the ECG tracing. After adjustment for heart rate, the QT interval is defined as prolonged if it is more than 450 msec in men and 460 msec in women. A long QT syndrome was first described in the 1950s and 60s as a congenital syndrome involving QT interval prolongation and syncope and sudden death. Some of the congenital long QT syndromes were characterized by a peculiar electrocardiographic appearance of the QRS complex involving a premature atria beat followed by a pause, then a subsequent sinus beat showing marked QT prolongation and deformity. This type of cardiac arrhythmia was originally termed "torsade de pointes" (translated from the French as "twisting of the points"). Moxifloxacin is considered as having a risk of causing torsade de pointes. Since it is not known what effect vasoconstrictors in the local anesthetic regimen will have in patients with a known history of congenital prolonged QT interval or in patients taking any medication that prolongs the QT interval, a medical consult is suggested.

Mucosal Coating Agent
(myoo KOH sul KOH ting AY gent)

Brand Names: U.S. Episil®; Gelclair® [DSC]; Mucotrol™; MuGard™

Pharmacologic Category Gastrointestinal Agent, Miscellaneous

Dental Use Management of oral mucosal pain caused by oral mucositis/stomatitis (resulting from chemotherapy or radiation therapy), irritation due to oral surgery, traumatic ulcers caused by braces/ill-fitting dentures or disease, diffuse aphthous ulcers (canker sores)

Use Management of oral mucosal pain caused by oral mucositis/stomatitis (resulting from chemotherapy or radiation therapy), irritation due to oral surgery, traumatic ulcers caused by braces/ill-fitting dentures or disease, diffuse aphthous ulcers (canker sores)

Local Anesthetic/Vasoconstrictor Precautions No information available to require special precautions

Effects on Dental Treatment No significant effects or complications reported

Effects on Bleeding No information available to require special precautions

Dental Usual Dosage Oral: Adults: Mucosal protection:
Episil®: Apply 1-3 pumps to the oral cavity 2-3 times daily, or as needed.
Gelclair®: Rinse, gargle, and spit 15 mL (1 single-use packet) mixed water 3 times daily, or as needed.
Mucotrol™: Slowly dissolve 1 wafer by swishing around in the mouth, 3 times daily, or as needed.
MuGard™: Rinse with 5 mL 4-6 times daily; may use up to 10 mL if needed to fully coat inside of month.

Dosage Oral: Adults: Mucosal protection:
Episil®: Apply 1-3 pumps to the oral cavity 2-3 times daily, or as needed.
Gelclair®: Rinse, gargle, and spit 15 mL (1 single-use packet) mixed in water 3 times daily, or as needed.
Mucotrol™: Slowly dissolve 1 wafer by swishing around in the mouth, 3 times daily, or as needed.
MuGard™: Rinse with 5 mL 4-6 times daily; may use up to 10 mL if needed to fully coat inside of month.

Mechanism of Action Adheres to the mucosal surface of mouth forming a protective film or coating over the irritated areas and lesions.

Contraindications Hypersensitivity to any component of the formulation

Additional product-specific contraindications: Episil®: Hypersensitivity to peanuts, soya, or peppermint oil

Warnings/Precautions May decrease absorption of sublingually administered medications. Episil® contains alcohol (may cause irritation when applied), propylene glycol (may cause skin irritation), and peppermint oil (may cause allergic reaction). For Gelclair®, Mucotrol™, and MuGard™, patients should avoid eating or drinking for at least 1 hour following use. Consult a physician if no improvement is seen after 7 days of use.

Drug Interactions

Metabolism/Transport Effects None known.

Avoid Concomitant Use There are no known interactions where it is recommended to avoid concomitant use.

Increased Effect/Toxicity There are no known significant interactions involving an increase in effect.

Decreased Effect There are no known significant interactions involving a decrease in effect.

Product Availability Gelclair®: U.S. availability expected in the first quarter of 2013

Dosage Forms
Gel-forming wafer, oral:
Mucotrol™: (21s, 45s)
Liquid, oral:
Episil®: (10 mL)
MuGard™: (5 mL, 240 mL)

Mupirocin (myoo PEER oh sin)

Brand Names: U.S. Bactroban Cream®; Bactroban Nasal®; Bactroban®; Centany®; Centany® AT

Brand Names: Canada Bactroban®

Pharmacologic Category Antibiotic, Topical

Use
Intranasal: Eradication of nasal colonization with MRSA in adult patients and healthcare workers
Topical: Treatment of impetigo or secondary infected traumatic skin lesions due to *S. aureus* and *S. pyogenes*

Unlabeled Use Intranasal: Surgical prophylaxis to prevent wound infections

Local Anesthetic/Vasoconstrictor Precautions No information available to require special precautions

Effects on Dental Treatment Key adverse event(s) related to dental treatment: Xerostomia (normal salivary flow resumes upon discontinuation) and taste perversion.

Effects on Bleeding No information available to require special precautions

Adverse Effects Frequency not defined.
Central nervous system: Dizziness, headache
Dermatologic: Cellulitis, dermatitis, dry skin, erythema, hives, pruritus, rash
Gastrointestinal: Abdominal pain, diarrhea, nausea, taste perversion, ulcerative stomatitis, xerostomia
Local: Burning, edema, pain, stinging, tenderness
Ocular: Blepharitis
Otic: Ear pain
Respiratory: Cough, pharyngitis, rhinitis, upper respiratory tract congestion
Miscellaneous: Secondary wound infection

General Dosage Range
Intranasal: *Children ≥12 years and Adults:* Approximately one-half of the ointment from the single-use tube should be applied into one nostril and the other half into the other nostril twice daily
Topical: *Children ≥2 months and Adults:* Apply to affected area 3 times/day

Mechanism of Action Binds to bacterial isoleucyl transfer-RNA synthetase resulting in the inhibition of protein synthesis

Pregnancy Risk Factor B

Pregnancy Considerations Teratogenic effects were not observed in animal studies. There are no adequate and well-controlled studies in pregnant women; use during pregnancy only if clearly needed.

Mycophenolate (mye koe FEN oh late)

Brand Names: U.S. CellCept®; Myfortic®

Brand Names: Canada Apo-Mycophenolate; Cell-Cept®; CO Mycophenolate; JAMP-Mycophenolate; Myfortic®; Mylan-Mycophenolate; Novo-Mycophenolate; Sandoz-Mycophenolate; Sandoz-Mycophenolate Mofetil

Pharmacologic Category Immunosuppressant Agent

Use Prophylaxis of organ rejection concomitantly with cyclosporine and corticosteroids in patients receiving allogeneic renal (CellCept®, Myfortic®), cardiac (Cell-Cept®), or hepatic (CellCept®) transplants

Unlabeled Use Treatment of rejection in liver transplant patients unable to tolerate tacrolimus or cyclosporine due to toxicity; treatment of recurrent or persistent rejection in heart transplant patients; treatment of moderate-severe psoriasis; treatment of lupus nephritis; treatment of myasthenia gravis; prevention of graft-versus-host disease (GVHD); treatment of refractory acute GVHD and chronic GVHD; treatment of refractory autoimmune hepatitis

Local Anesthetic/Vasoconstrictor Precautions No information available to require special precautions

Effects on Dental Treatment Key adverse event(s) related to dental treatment: Mouth ulceration, gum hyperplasia, gingivitis, dry mouth, dysphagia, oral moniliasis, and stomatitis.

Effects on Bleeding May be associated with hematologic effects, potentially including significant reduction in platelet counts with altered hemostasis. In patients who are under active treatment, medical consult is suggested.

Adverse Effects Data for incidence >20% as reported in adults following oral dosing of CellCept® alone in renal, cardiac, and hepatic allograft rejection studies. Profile in 3% to <20% range reflects use in combination with cyclosporine and corticosteroids. In general, lower doses used in renal rejection patients had less adverse effects than higher doses. Rates of adverse effects were similar for each indication, except for those unique to the specific organ involved. The type of adverse effects observed in pediatric patients was similar to those seen in adults, with the exception of abdominal pain, anemia, diarrhea, fever, hypertension, infection, pharyngitis, respiratory tract infection, sepsis, and vomiting; lymphoproliferative disorder was the only type of malignancy observed. Percentages of adverse reactions were similar in studies comparing CellCept® to Myfortic® in patients following renal transplant.

>20%:
Cardiovascular: Hypertension (28% to 78%), hypotension (33%), peripheral edema (27% to 64%), edema (27% to 28%), chest pain (26%), tachycardia (20% to 22%)
Central nervous system: Pain (31% to 76%), headache (16% to 54%), insomnia (41% to 52%), fever (21% to 52%), dizziness (29%), anxiety (28%)
Dermatologic: Rash (22%)

Endocrine & metabolic: Hyperglycemia (44% to 47%), hypercholesterolemia (41%), hypomagnesemia (39%), hypokalemia (32% to 37%), hypocalcemia (30%), hyperkalemia (22%)
Gastrointestinal: Abdominal pain (25% to 63%), nausea (20% to 55%), diarrhea (31% to 51%), constipation (19% to 41%), vomiting (33% to 34%), anorexia (25%), dyspepsia (22%)
Genitourinary: Urinary tract infection (37%)
Hematologic: Leukopenia (23% to 46%), anemia (26% to 43%; hypochromic 25%), leukocytosis (22% to 41%), thrombocytopenia (24% to 38%)
Hepatic: Liver function tests abnormal (25%), ascites (24%)
Neuromuscular & skeletal: Back pain (35% to 47%), weakness (35% to 43%), tremor (24% to 34%), paresthesia (21%)
Renal: Creatinine increased (39%), BUN increased (35%), kidney function abnormal (22% to 26%)
Respiratory: Dyspnea (31% to 37%), respiratory tract infection (22% to 37%), pleural effusion (34%), cough (31%), lung disorder (22% to 30%), sinusitis (26%)
Miscellaneous: Infection (18% to 27%), sepsis (27%), lactate dehydrogenase increased (23%), Candida (17% to 22%), herpes simplex (10% to 21%)
3% to <20%:
Cardiovascular: Angina, arrhythmia, arterial thrombosis, atrial fibrillation, atrial flutter, bradycardia, cardiac arrest, cardiac failure, CHF, extrasystole, facial edema, hyper-/hypovolemia, orthostatic hypotension, pallor, palpitation, pericardial effusion, peripheral vascular disorder, supraventricular extrasystoles, supraventricular tachycardia, syncope, thrombosis, vasodilation, vasospasm, venous pressure increased, ventricular extrasystole, ventricular tachycardia
Central nervous system: Agitation, chills with fever, confusion, delirium, depression, emotional lability, hallucinations, hypoesthesia, malaise, nervousness, psychosis, seizure, somnolence, thinking abnormal, vertigo
Dermatologic: Acne, alopecia, bruising, cellulitis, fungal dermatitis, hirsutism, petechia, pruritus, skin carcinoma, skin hypertrophy, skin ulcer, vesiculobullous rash
Endocrine & metabolic: Acidosis, alkalosis, Cushing's syndrome, dehydration, diabetes mellitus, gout, hypercalcemia, hyper-hypophosphatemia, hyperlipemia, hyperuricemia, hypochloremia, hypoglycemia, hyponatremia, hypoproteinemia, hypothyroidism, parathyroid disorder
Gastrointestinal: Abdomen enlarged, dysphagia, esophagitis, flatulence, gastritis, gastroenteritis, gastrointestinal hemorrhage, gastrointestinal moniliasis, gingivitis, gum hyperplasia, ileus, melena, mouth ulceration, oral moniliasis, stomach disorder, stomach ulcer, stomatitis, xerostomia, weight gain/loss
Genitourinary: Impotence, nocturia, pelvic pain, prostatic disorder, scrotal edema, urinary frequency, urinary incontinence, urinary retention, urinary tract disorder
Hematologic: Coagulation disorder, hemorrhage, neutropenia, pancytopenia, polycythemia, prothrombin time increased, thromboplastin time increased
Hepatic: Alkaline phosphatase increased, bilirubinemia, cholangitis, cholestatic jaundice, GGT increased, hepatitis, jaundice, liver damage, transaminases increased
Local: Abscess

Neuromuscular & skeletal: Arthralgia, hypertonia, joint disorder, leg cramps, myalgia, myasthenia, neck pain, neuropathy, osteoporosis

Ocular: Amblyopia, cataract, conjunctivitis, eye hemorrhage, lacrimation disorder, vision abnormal

Otic: Deafness, ear disorder, ear pain, tinnitus

Renal: Albuminuria, creatinine increased, dysuria, hematuria, hydronephrosis, oliguria, pyelonephritis, renal failure, renal tubular necrosis

Respiratory: Apnea, asthma, atelectasis, bronchitis, epistaxis, hemoptysis, hiccup, hyperventilation, hypoxia, respiratory acidosis, pharyngitis, pneumonia, pneumothorax, pulmonary edema, pulmonary hypertension, respiratory moniliasis, rhinitis, sputum increased, voice alteration

Miscellaneous: *Candida* (mucocutaneous 16% to 18%), CMV viremia/syndrome (12% to 14%), CMV tissue invasive disease (6% to 12%), herpes zoster cutaneous disease (4% to 10%), cyst, diaphoresis, flu-like syndrome, healing abnormal, hernia, ileus infection, neoplasm, peritonitis, thirst

General Dosage Range Dosage adjustment recommended in patient with renal impairment and who develop toxicities

I.V.: *Adults:* 1-1.5 g twice daily

Oral:

Cellcept®:

Children (suspension): 600 mg/m^2/dose twice daily (maximum: 1 g twice daily)

Children with BSA 1.25-1.5 m^2: 750 mg capsule twice daily

Children with BSA >1.5 m^2: 1 g capsule or tablet twice daily

Adults: 1-1.5 g twice daily

Myfortic®:

Children with BSA 1.19-1.58 m^2: 540 mg twice daily (maximum: 1080 mg daily)

Children with BSA >1.58 m^2 and Adults: 720 mg twice daily (maximum: 1440 mg daily)

Mechanism of Action MPA exhibits a cytostatic effect on T and B lymphocytes. It is an inhibitor of inosine monophosphate dehydrogenase (IMPDH) which inhibits *de novo* guanosine nucleotide synthesis. T and B lymphocytes are dependent on this pathway for proliferation.

Pharmacodynamics/Kinetics

Onset of Action Peak effect: Correlation of toxicity or efficacy is still being developed, however, one study indicated that 12-hour AUCs >40 mcg/mL/hour were correlated with efficacy and decreased episodes of rejection

Half-life Elimination

CellCept®: MPA: Oral: 18 hours; I.V.: 17 hours

Myfortic®: MPA: Oral: 8-16 hours; MPAG: 13-17 hours

Time to Peak Plasma: Oral: MPA:

CellCept®: 1-1.5 hours

Myfortic®: 1.5-2.75 hours

Pregnancy Risk Factor D

Pregnancy Considerations [U.S. Boxed Warning]: Mycophenolate is associated with an increased risk of congenital malformations and first trimester pregnancy loss when used by pregnant women. Females of reproductive potential must be counseled about pregnancy prevention and planning. Alternative agents should be considered for women planning a pregnancy. Adverse events have been reported in animal studies at doses less than the equivalent recommended human dose. In humans, the following congenital malformations have been reported: external ear abnormalities, cleft lip and palate, anomalies of the distal limbs, heart, esophagus and kidney. Spontaneous abortions have also been noted. Females of reproductive potential (girls who have entered puberty, women with a uterus who have not passed through clinically confirmed menopause) should have a negative pregnancy test with a sensitivity of ≥25 mIU/mL immediately before therapy and the test should be repeated 8-10 days later. Pregnancy tests should be repeated during routine follow-up visits. Acceptable forms of contraception should be used during treatment and for 6 weeks after therapy is discontinued. The effectiveness of hormonal contraceptive agents may be affected by mycophenolate.

Healthcare providers should report female exposures to mycophenolate during pregnancy or within 6 weeks of discontinuing therapy to the Mycophenolate Pregnancy Registry (800-617-8191). The National Transplantation Pregnancy Registry (NTPR, Temple University) is a registry for pregnant women taking immunosuppressants following any solid organ transplant. The NTPR encourages reporting of all immunosuppressant exposures during pregnancy in transplant recipients at 877-955-6877.

Nabumetone (na BYOO me tone)

Related Information

Rheumatoid Arthritis, Osteoarthritis, and Osteoporosis *on page 1526*

Temporomandibular Dysfunction (TMD), Chronic Pain, and Fibromyalgia *on page 1590*

Brand Names: Canada Apo-Nabumetone®; Gen-Nabumetone; Mylan-Nabumetone; Novo-Nabumetone; Relafen®; Rhoxal-nabumetone; Sandoz-Nabumetone

Generic Availability (U.S.) Yes

Pharmacologic Category Nonsteroidal Anti-inflammatory Drug (NSAID), Oral

Use Management of osteoarthritis and rheumatoid arthritis

Unlabeled Use Moderate pain

Local Anesthetic/Vasoconstrictor Precautions No information available to require special precautions

Effects on Dental Treatment Key adverse event(s) related to dental treatment: Xerostomia (normal salivary flow resumes upon discontinuation) and stomatitis. The dentist should be aware of the potential of abnormal coagulation. Caution should also be exercised in the use of NSAIDs in patients already on anticoagulant therapy with drugs such as warfarin (Coumadin®). See Effects on Bleeding.

Effects on Bleeding Nonselective NSAIDs, such as nabumetone, inhibit platelet aggregation and prolong bleeding time in some patients. Unlike aspirin, the NSAID effect on platelet function is quantitatively less, of shorter duration, and reversible. Normal platelet function should occur in ~5 elimination half-lives or in <10 hours after discontinuation of nabumetone. Concomitant use of other NSAIDs should be avoided.

Adverse Effects

>10%: Gastrointestinal: Diarrhea (14%), dyspepsia (13%), abdominal pain (12%)

1% to 10%:

Cardiovascular: Edema (3% to 9%)

Central nervous system: Dizziness (3% to 9%), headache (3% to 9%), fatigue (1% to 3%), insomnia (1% to 3%), nervousness (1% to 3%), somnolence (1% to 3%)

Dermatologic: Pruritus (3% to 9%), rash (3% to 9%)

Gastrointestinal: Constipation (3% to 9%), flatulence (3% to 9%), guaiac positive (3% to 9%), nausea (3% to 9%), gastritis (1% to 3%), stomatitis (1% to 3%), vomiting (1% to 3%), xerostomia (1% to 3%)

Otic: Tinnitus

Miscellaneous: Diaphoresis (1% to 3%)

Dosage Adults: Oral: 1000 mg/day; an additional 500-1000 mg may be needed in some patients to obtain more symptomatic relief; may be administered once or twice daily (maximum dose: 2000 mg/day)

Note: Patients <50 kg are less likely to require doses >1000 mg/day.

Dosage adjustment in renal impairment: In general, NSAIDs are not recommended for use in patients with advanced renal disease, but the manufacturer of nabumetone does provide some guidelines for adjustment in renal dysfunction:

Moderate impairment (Cl_{cr} 30-49 mL/minute): Initial dose: 750 mg/day; maximum dose: 1500 mg/day

Severe impairment (Cl_{cr} <30 mL/minute): Initial dose: 500 mg/day; maximum dose: 1000 mg/day

Dosage adjustment in hepatic impairment: No dosage adjustment provided in manufacturer's labeling (has not been studied). Prodrug activation and metabolism are hepatic function dependent and may be reduced in severe hepatic impairment.

Mechanism of Action Reversibly inhibits cyclooxygenase-1 and 2 (COX-1 and 2) enzymes, which results in decreased formation of prostaglandin precursors; has antipyretic, analgesic, and anti-inflammatory properties

Other proposed mechanisms not fully elucidated (and possibly contributing to the anti-inflammatory effect to varying degrees), include inhibiting chemotaxis, altering lymphocyte activity, inhibiting neutrophil aggregation/activation, and decreasing proinflammatory cytokine levels.

Contraindications Hypersensitivity to nabumetone, aspirin, other NSAIDs, or any component of the formulation; perioperative pain in the setting of coronary artery bypass graft (CABG) surgery

Warnings/Precautions [U.S. Boxed Warning]: NSAIDs are associated with an increased risk of adverse cardiovascular thrombotic events, including MI and stroke. Risk may be increased with duration of use or pre-existing cardiovascular risk factors or disease. Carefully evaluate individual cardiovascular risk profiles prior to prescribing. May cause new-onset hypertension or worsening of existing hypertension. Use caution with fluid retention. Avoid use in heart failure. Concurrent administration of ibuprofen, and potentially other nonselective NSAIDs, may interfere with aspirin's cardioprotective effect. **[U.S. Boxed Warning]: Use is contraindicated for treatment of perioperative pain in the setting of coronary artery bypass graft (CABG) surgery.** Risk of MI and stroke may be increased with use following CABG surgery.

Platelet adhesion and aggregation may be decreased; may prolong bleeding time; patients with coagulation disorders or who are receiving anticoagulants should be monitored closely. Anemia may occur; patients on long-term NSAID therapy should be monitored for anemia. Rarely, NSAID use may cause severe blood dyscrasias (eg, agranulocytosis, aplastic anemia, thrombocytopenia).

NSAID use may compromise existing renal function; dose-dependent decreases in prostaglandin synthesis may result from NSAID use, reducing renal blood flow which may cause renal decompensation. NSAID use may increase the risk for hyperkalemia. Patients with impaired renal function, dehydration, heart failure, liver dysfunction, those taking diuretics, and ACE inhibitors, and the elderly are at greater risk of renal toxicity and hyperkalemia. Rehydrate patient before starting therapy; monitor renal function closely. Not recommended for use in patients with advanced renal disease. Long-term NSAID use may result in renal papillary necrosis.

[U.S. Boxed Warning]: NSAIDs may increase risk of gastrointestinal irritation, inflammation, ulceration, bleeding, and perforation. These events may occur at any time during therapy and without warning. Use caution with a history of GI disease (bleeding or ulcers), concurrent therapy with aspirin, anticoagulants and/or corticosteroids, smoking, use of alcohol, the elderly or debilitated patients. When used concomitantly with ≤325 mg of aspirin, a substantial increase in the risk of gastrointestinal complications (eg, ulcer) occurs; concomitant gastroprotective therapy (eg, proton pump inhibitors) is recommended (Bhatt, 2008).

Use the lowest effective dose for the shortest duration of time, consistent with individual patient goals, to reduce risk of cardiovascular or GI adverse events. Alternate therapies should be considered for patients at high risk.

NSAIDs may cause serious skin adverse events including exfoliative dermatitis, Stevens-Johnson syndrome (SJS) and toxic epidermal necrolysis (TEN); discontinue use at first sign of skin rash or hypersensitivity. Anaphylactoid reactions may occur, even without prior exposure; patients with "aspirin triad" (bronchial asthma, aspirin intolerance, rhinitis) may be at increased risk. Do not use in patients who experience bronchospasm, asthma, rhinitis, or urticaria with NSAID or aspirin therapy. Use caution in other forms of asthma.

Use with caution in patients with decreased hepatic function. Closely monitor patients with any abnormal LFT. Severe hepatic reactions (eg, fulminant hepatitis, liver failure) have occurred with NSAID use, rarely; discontinue if signs or symptoms of liver disease develop, or if systemic manifestations occur.

NSAIDS may cause drowsiness, dizziness, blurred vision and other neurologic effects which may impair physical or mental abilities; patients must be cautioned about performing tasks which require mental alertness (eg, operating machinery or driving). Discontinue use with blurred or diminished vision and perform ophthalmologic exam. Monitor vision with long-term therapy.

In the elderly, avoid chronic use (unless alternative agents ineffective and patient can receive concomitant gastroprotective agent); nonselective oral NSAID use is associated with an increased risk of GI bleeding and peptic ulcer disease in older adults in high risk category (eg, >75 years or age or receiving concomitant oral/parenteral corticosteroids, anticoagulants, or antiplatelet agents) (Beers Criteria).

Withhold for at least 4-6 half-lives prior to surgical or dental procedures. May cause photosensitivity reactions.

Drug Interactions

Metabolism/Transport Effects None known.

Avoid Concomitant Use

Avoid concomitant use of Nabumetone with any of the following: Floctafenine; Ketorolac (Nasal); Ketorolac (Systemic); NSAID (COX-2 Inhibitor); Omacetaxine

Increased Effect/Toxicity

Nabumetone may increase the levels/effects of: Agents with Antiplatelet Properties; Aliskiren; Aminoglycosides; Anticoagulants; Bisphosphonate Derivatives; Collagenase (Systemic); CycloSPORINE (Systemic); Dabigatran Etexilate; Deferasirox; Desmopressin; Digoxin; Drotrecogin Alfa (Activated); Eplerenone; Haloperidol; Ibritumomab; Lithium; Methotrexate; Nonsteroidal Anti-Inflammatory Agents; NSAID (COX-2 Inhibitor); Omacetaxine; PEMEtrexed; Porfimer; Potassium-Sparing Diuretics; PRALAtrexate; Quinolone Antibiotics; Rivaroxaban; Salicylates; Thrombolytic Agents; Tositumomab and Iodine I 131 Tositumomab; Vancomycin; Vitamin K Antagonists

The levels/effects of Nabumetone may be increased by: ACE Inhibitors; Angiotensin II Receptor Blockers; Antidepressants (Tricyclic, Tertiary Amine); Corticosteroids (Systemic); CycloSPORINE (Systemic); Dasatinib; Floctafenine; Glucosamine; Herbs (Anticoagulant/Antiplatelet Properties); Ketorolac (Nasal); Ketorolac (Systemic); Multivitamins/Minerals (with ADEK, Folate, Iron); Nonsteroidal Anti-Inflammatory Agents; Omega-3 Fatty Acids; Pentosan Polysulfate Sodium; Pentoxifylline; Probenecid; Prostacyclin Analogues; Selective Serotonin Reuptake Inhibitors; Serotonin/Norepinephrine Reuptake Inhibitors; Sodium Phosphates; Tipranavir; Treprostinil; Vitamin E

Decreased Effect

Nabumetone may decrease the levels/effects of: ACE Inhibitors; Agents with Antiplatelet Properties; Aliskiren; Angiotensin II Receptor Blockers; Beta-Blockers; Eplerenone; HydrALAZINE; Loop Diuretics; Potassium-Sparing Diuretics; Salicylates; Selective Serotonin Reuptake Inhibitors; Thiazide Diuretics

The levels/effects of Nabumetone may be decreased by: Bile Acid Sequestrants; Nonsteroidal Anti-Inflammatory Agents; Salicylates

Ethanol/Nutrition/Herb Interactions

Ethanol: Avoid ethanol (may enhance gastric mucosal irritation).

Food: Nabumetone peak serum concentrations may be increased if taken with food or dairy products.

Herb/Nutraceutical: Avoid alfalfa, anise, bilberry, bladderwrack, bromelain, cat's claw, celery, chamomile, coleus, cordyceps, dong quai, evening primrose, fenugreek, feverfew, garlic, ginger, ginkgo biloba, ginseng (American, Panax, Siberian), grapeseed, green tea, guggul, horse chestnut seed, horseradish, licorice, prickly ash, red clover, reishi, SAMe (S-adenosylmethionine), sweet clover, turmeric, white willow (all have additional antiplatelet activity).

Pharmacodynamics/Kinetics

Onset of Action Several days

Half-life Elimination 6MNA: ~24 hours

Time to Peak Serum: 6MNA: Oral: 2.5-4 hours; Synovial fluid: 4-12 hours

Pregnancy Risk Factor C

Pregnancy Considerations Adverse events were not observed in the initial animal reproduction studies; therefore, the manufacturer classifies nabumetone as pregnancy category C. NSAID exposure during the first trimester is not strongly associated with congenital malformations; however, cardiovascular anomalies and cleft palate have been observed following NSAID exposure in some studies. The use of an NSAID close to conception may be associated with an increased risk of miscarriage. Nonteratogenic effects have been observed following NSAID administration during the third trimester including myocardial degenerative changes, prenatal constriction of the ductus arteriosus, fetal tricuspid regurgitation, failure of the ductus arteriosus to close postnatally; renal dysfunction or failure, oligohydramnios; gastrointestinal bleeding or perforation, increased risk of necrotizing enterocolitis; intracranial bleeding (including intraventricular hemorrhage), platelet dysfunction with resultant bleeding; pulmonary hypertension. Because they may cause premature closure of the ductus arteriosus, use of NSAIDs late in pregnancy should be avoided (use after 31 or 32 weeks gestation is not recommended by some clinicians). The chronic use of NSAIDs in women of reproductive age may be associated with infertility that is reversible upon discontinuation of the medication. A registry is available for pregnant women exposed to autoimmune medications including nabumetone. For additional information contact the Organization of Teratology Information Specialists, OTIS Autoimmune Diseases Study, at 877-311-8972.

Lactation Excretion in breast milk unknown/not recommended

Breast-Feeding Considerations It is not known if nabumetone or 6MNA are excreted into breast milk. Breast-feeding is not recommended by the manufacturer.

Dosage Forms

Tablet, oral: 500 mg, 750 mg

Nadolol (NAY doe lol)

Related Information

Cardiovascular Diseases *on page 1492*

Brand Names: U.S. Corgard®

Brand Names: Canada Alti-Nadolol; Apo-Nadol®; Corgard®; Novo-Nadolol; Teva-Nadolol

Pharmacologic Category Antianginal Agent; Beta-Blocker, Nonselective

Use Treatment of hypertension and angina pectoris; prophylaxis of migraine headaches

Unlabeled Use Primary and secondary prophylaxis of variceal hemorrhage; management of thyrotoxicosis

Local Anesthetic/Vasoconstrictor Precautions Use with caution; epinephrine has interacted with nonselective beta-blockers to result in initial hypertensive episode followed by bradycardia

Effects on Dental Treatment Nadolol is a nonselective beta-blocker and may enhance the pressor response to epinephrine, resulting in hypertension and bradycardia. Many nonsteroidal anti-inflammatory drugs, such as ibuprofen and indomethacin, can reduce the hypotensive effect of beta-blockers after 3 or more weeks of therapy with the NSAID. Short-term NSAID use (ie, 3 days) requires no special precautions in patients taking beta-blockers.

Effects on Bleeding No information available to require special precautions

Adverse Effects

>10%:

Central nervous system: Drowsiness, insomnia
Endocrine & metabolic: Decreased sexual ability

1% to 10%:

Cardiovascular: Bradycardia, palpitation, edema, CHF, reduced peripheral circulation
Central nervous system: Mental depression
Gastrointestinal: Diarrhea or constipation, nausea, vomiting, stomach discomfort
Respiratory: Bronchospasm
Miscellaneous: Cold extremities

General Dosage Range Dosage adjustment recommended in patients with renal impairment
Oral:
  Adults: Initial: 40 mg once daily; Maintenance: 40-320 mg once daily
  Elderly: Initial: 20 mg once daily; Maintenance: 20-240 mg once daily
Mechanism of Action Competitively blocks response to beta$_1$- and beta$_2$-adrenergic stimulation; does not exhibit any membrane stabilizing or intrinsic sympathomimetic activity. Nonselective beta-adrenergic blockers (propranolol, nadolol) reduce portal pressure by producing splanchnic vasoconstriction (beta$_2$ effect) thereby reducing portal blood flow.
Pharmacodynamics/Kinetics
  Duration of Action 17-24 hours
  Half-life Elimination Adults: 10-24 hours, prolonged with renal impairment; End-stage renal disease: 45 hours
  Time to Peak Serum: 2-4 hours
Pregnancy Risk Factor C
Pregnancy Considerations Adverse events were observed in some animal reproduction studies; therefore, the manufacturer classifies nadolol as pregnancy category C. Nadolol crosses the placenta and is measurable in infant serum after birth. In a cohort study, an increased risk of cardiovascular defects was observed following maternal use of beta-blockers during pregnancy. Intrauterine growth restriction (IUGR), small placentas, as well as fetal/neonatal bradycardia, hypoglycemia, and/or respiratory depression have been observed following *in utero* exposure to beta-blockers as a class. Adequate facilities for monitoring infants at birth should be available. Untreated chronic maternal hypertension and pre-eclampsia are also associated with adverse events in the fetus, infant, and mother. Nadolol is indicated for the treatment of hypertension, but due to its long half-life and potential effects to the fetus, other agents may be more appropriate for use during pregnancy.

Nadolol and Bendroflumethiazide
(NAY doe lol & ben droe floo meth EYE a zide)

Related Information
Nadolol *on page 950*
Brand Names: U.S. Corzide®
Pharmacologic Category Beta-Blocker, Nonselective; Diuretic, Thiazide
Use Treatment of hypertension; combination product should not be used for initial therapy
Local Anesthetic/Vasoconstrictor Precautions Use with caution; epinephrine has interacted with nonselective beta-blockers to result in initial hypertensive episode followed by bradycardia
Effects on Dental Treatment Nadolol is a nonselective beta-blocker and may enhance the pressor response to epinephrine, resulting in hypertension and bradycardia. Many nonsteroidal anti-inflammatory drugs, such as ibuprofen and indomethacin, can reduce the hypotensive effect of beta-blockers after 3 or more weeks of therapy with the NSAID. Short-term NSAID use (ie, 3 days) requires no special precautions in patients taking beta-blockers.
Effects on Bleeding No information available to require special precautions
Adverse Effects See individual agents.
General Dosage Range Dosage adjustment recommended in patients with renal impairment

Oral: *Adults:* Initial: Nadolol 40 mg and bendroflumethiazide 5 mg once daily; Maintenance: Nadolol 40-80 mg and bendroflumethiazide 5 mg once daily
Mechanism of Action See individual agents.
Pregnancy Risk Factor C
Pregnancy Considerations See individual agents.

Nadroparin (nad roe PA rin)

Related Information
Cardiovascular Diseases *on page 1492*
Brand Names: Canada Fraxiparine™; Fraxiparine™ Forte
Pharmacologic Category Low Molecular Weight Heparin
Use Prophylaxis of thromboembolic disorders (particularly deep venous thrombosis and pulmonary embolism) in general and orthopedic surgery; treatment of deep venous thrombosis; prevention of clotting during hemodialysis; treatment of unstable angina and non-Q-wave myocardial infarction
Local Anesthetic/Vasoconstrictor Precautions No information available to require special precautions
Effects on Dental Treatment Key adverse event(s) related to dental treatment: Bleeding is the major adverse effect of nadroparin. See Effects on Bleeding.
Effects on Bleeding As with all anticoagulants, bleeding is the major adverse effect of nadroparin. Hemorrhage may occur at virtually any site; risk is dependent on multiple variables including the intensity of anticoagulation and patient susceptibility. At the recommended doses, LMWHS do not significantly influence platelet aggregation or affect global clotting time (ie, PT or aPTT). Medical consult is suggested.
Adverse Effects Frequency not defined. **Note:** As with all anticoagulants, bleeding is the major adverse effect of nadroparin. Hemorrhage may occur at virtually any site. Risk is dependent on multiple variables.
  Cardiovascular: Arterial/venous thrombosis, thromboembolism
  Dermatologic: Angioedema (very rare), cutaneous necrosis (rare), rash
  Endocrine & metabolic: Hypoaldosteronism (causing hyperkalemia and/or hyponatremia)
  Genitourinary: Priapism (very rare)
  Hematological: Bleeding, eosinophilia (very rare), thrombocytopenia, thrombocytosis
  Hepatic: ALT increased, AST increased
  Local: Calcinosis, injection site hematoma, pain at injection site
  Neuromuscular & skeletal: Osteopenic effects
  Miscellaneous: Allergic reactions, anaphylactoid reactions (very rare)
  Postmarketing and/or case reports: Erythema, pruritus, urticaria
Dosage Adults: **Note:** Dose expressed as anti-Xa international units
  Prevention of clotting during hemodialysis: Single dose of 65 units/kg into arterial line at start of each dialysis session; may give additional dose if session lasts longer than 4 hours; adjust dose during subsequent dialysis sessions to plasma anti-Xa levels of 0.5-1 anti-Xa units/mL
  Patients at risk of hemorrhage: Administer 32.5 units/kg; may give additional smaller dose if session lasts longer than 4 hours; adjust dose during subsequent dialysis sessions to plasma anti-Xa levels of 0.2-0.4 anti-Xa units/mL.

Thromboprophylaxis therapy: SubQ:

General surgery: Initial: 2850 units administered 2-4 hours preoperatively; Maintenance: SubQ: 2850 units once daily. Continue therapy for at least 7 days and until ambulant or no longer at DVT risk.

Hip replacement surgery: 38 units/kg (maximum dose: 3800 units) administered 12 hours preoperatively and repeated at 12 hours postoperatively then followed by 38 units/kg once daily (maximum dose: 3800 units) up to and including postoperative day 3; postoperative day 4 begin 57 units/kg once daily (maximum dose: 5700 units). Continue therapy for at least 10 days and until ambulant or no longer at DVT risk.

Treatment of DVT: SubQ: 171 units/kg once daily (maximum dose: 17,100 units/day); expected plasma anti-Xa levels are 1.2-1.8 anti-Xa units/mL 3-4 hours postinjection. **Note:** Patients at an increased risk of bleeding should receive a dose of 86 units/kg every 12 hours with expected plasma anti-Xa levels of 0.5-1.1 anti-Xa units/mL 3-4 hours postinjection.

Treatment of unstable angina and non-Q-wave myocardial infarction (in conjunction with aspirin): Initial: I.V.: 86 units/kg bolus. Maintenance: SubQ: 86 units/kg every 12 hours (usual treatment duration: 6 days); plasma anti-Xa levels should be <1.2 anti-Xa units/mL 3-4 hours postinjection

Conversion to oral anticoagulation therapy: Continue nadroparin until therapeutic INR has been achieved with vitamin K antagonist (usually at least 5 days).

Dosage adjustment in renal impairment:

Cl_{cr} ≥50 mL/minute: No dosage adjustment necessary.

Cl_{cr} ≥30-50 mL/minute: Reduce dose by 25% to 33%

Cl_{cr} <30 mL/minute:

Prophylaxis: Reduce dose by 25% to 33%

Treatment: Use is contraindicated

Dosage adjustment in hepatic impairment: No dosage adjustment provided in manufacturer's labeling (has not been studied).

Mechanism of Action Nadroparin has high anti-Xa activity, but low anti-IIa activity. The greater ratio of anti-Xa activity has the potential to provide equivalent antithrombic efficacy with reduced hemorrhagic complications.

Contraindications Hypersensitivity to nadroparin, any component of the formulation, or to other low molecular weight heparins and/or heparin; acute infective endocarditis; active bleeding or increased risk of hemorrhage (hemostasis disorder); history of confirmed or suspected immunologically mediated heparin-induced thrombocytopenia (HIT) (delayed-onset severe thrombocytopenia) or positive *in vitro* test for antiplatelet antibodies in the presence of nadroparin; major blood clotting disorders; hemorrhagic tendency or other conditions involving increase risk of bleeding; organic lesions likely to bleed (active peptic ulceration); hemorrhagic cerebrovascular event (unless systemic emboli present); severe uncontrolled hypertension; diabetic or hemorrhagic retinopathy; injuries to or operations on the CNS, eyes, or ears; severe renal insufficiency (creatinine clearance <30 mL/minute when used for treatment); concomitant use of spinal/epidural anesthesia with repeated high-dose nadroparin

Note: Use of nadroparin in patients with current HIT or HIT with thrombosis is **not** recommended and considered contraindicated due to high cross-reactivity to heparin-platelet factor-4 antibody (Guyatt [ACCP], 2012; Warkentin, 1999).

Warnings/Precautions Spinal or epidural hematomas, including subsequent paralysis, may occur with recent or anticipated neuraxial anesthesia (epidural or spinal) or spinal puncture in patients anticoagulated with low molecular weight heparins (LMWHs) or heparinoids. Consider risk versus benefit prior to spinal procedures; risk is increased by concomitant agents which may alter hemostasis, the use of indwelling epidural catheters for analgesia, a history of spinal deformity or spinal surgery, as well as traumatic or repeated epidural or spinal punctures. Avoid lumbar puncture or spinal or epidural anesthesia for 12 hours following the last nadroparin prophylactic dose or 24 hours following the last nadroparin treatment dose. Nadroparin therapy should not be resumed for at least 2 hours after anesthesia procedures. Longer intervals should be considered for patients with renal impairment. Observe patient closely for bleeding if nadroparin is administered.

Not to be used interchangeably (unit for unit) with heparin or any other low molecular weight heparins (LMWHs). Cases of thrombocytopenia including thrombocytopenia with thrombosis have occurred. Use with caution in patients with history of thrombocytopenia (drug-induced or congenital) or platelet defects; monitor platelet count closely. Use is contraindicated in patients with a history of confirmed or suspected heparin-induced thrombocytopenia or positive *in vitro* test for antiplatelet antibodies in the presence of nadroparin. Discontinue therapy and consider alternative treatment if platelets are <100,000/mm³ and/or thrombosis develops. Prosthetic valve thrombosis has been reported in patients receiving thromboprophylaxis therapy with LMWHs. Pregnant women may be at increased risk.

Monitor patient closely for signs or symptoms of bleeding. Certain patients are at increased risk of bleeding. Risk factors include bacterial endocarditis; congenital or acquired bleeding disorders; active ulcerative or angiodysplastic GI diseases; severe uncontrolled hypertension; hemorrhagic stroke; recent brain, spinal, or ophthalmology surgery; concomitant treatment with platelet inhibitors; recent GI bleeding; thrombocytopenia or platelet defects; severe liver disease; hypertensive or diabetic retinopathy; or in patients undergoing invasive procedures (particularly knee surgery). Use with caution in patients with hepatic or renal disease, or with a history of peptic ulcer disease; use is contraindicated in patients with active ulceration or in severe renal insufficiency (when used for treatment of thromboembolic disorders, unstable angina, or NSTEMI).

Can cause hyperkalemia possibly by affecting aldosterone production; monitor for hyperkalemia. Cutaneous necrosis preceded by purpura or infiltrated or painful erythematous blotches has been reported rarely; discontinue treatment immediately if suspected. Packaging may contain natural latex rubber. Do **not** administer intramuscularly.

Drug Interactions

Metabolism/Transport Effects None known.

Avoid Concomitant Use

Avoid concomitant use of Nadroparin with any of the following: Apixaban; Dabigatran Etexilate; Omacetaxine; Rivaroxaban

Increased Effect/Toxicity

Nadroparin may increase the levels/effects of: Anticoagulants; Collagenase (Systemic); Deferasirox; Drotrecogin Alfa (Activated); Ibritumomab; Omacetaxine; Palifermin; Rivaroxaban; Tositumomab and Iodine I 131 Tositumomab

The levels/effects of Nadroparin may be increased by: 5-ASA Derivatives; Agents with Antiplatelet Properties; Apixaban; Dabigatran Etexilate; Dasatinib; Herbs (Anticoagulant/Antiplatelet Properties); Nonsteroidal Anti-Inflammatory Agents; Omega-3 Fatty Acids; Pentosan Polysulfate Sodium; Pentoxifylline; Prostacyclin Analogues; Salicylates; Thrombolytic Agents; Tipranavir; Vitamin E

Decreased Effect There are no known significant interactions involving a decrease in effect.

Ethanol/Nutrition/Herb Interactions Herb/Nutraceutical: Avoid cat's claw, dong quai, evening primrose, garlic, ginseng (all have anticoagulant or antiplatelet activity).

Pharmacodynamics/Kinetics

Duration of Action Anti-Xa activity: 18 hours

Half-life Elimination 3.5 hours (prolonged in renal impairment)

Time to Peak Serum: 3-6 hours

Pregnancy Considerations Adverse events were not observed in animal reproduction studies. Low molecular weight heparin (LMWH) does not cross the placenta; increased risks of fetal bleeding or teratogenic effects have not been reported. LMWH is recommended over unfractionated heparin for the treatment of acute venous thromboembolism (VTE) in pregnant women. LMWH is also recommended over unfractionated heparin for VTE prophylaxis in pregnant women with certain risk factors. LMWH should be discontinued prior to induction of labor or a planned cesarean delivery. When choosing therapy, fetal outcomes (ie, pregnancy loss, malformations), maternal outcomes (ie, VTE, hemorrhage), burden of therapy, and maternal preference should be considered (Guyatt, 2012).

Lactation Excretion in breast milk unknown/use caution

Breast-Feeding Considerations Small amounts of LMWH have been detected in breast milk; however, because it has a low oral bioavailability, it is unlikely to cause adverse events in a nursing infant. Use of LMWH may be continued in breast-feeding women (Guyatt, 2012).

Product Availability Not available in U.S.

Dosage Forms: Canada

Injection, solution:
Fraxiparine™: 9500 anti-Xa units/mL (0.2 mL, 0.3 mL, 0.4 mL, 0.6 mL, 0.8 mL, 1 mL)
Fraxiparine™ Forte: 19,000 anti-Xa units/mL (0.6 mL, 0.8 mL, 1 mL)

Nafarelin (naf a REL in)

Brand Names: U.S. Synarel®
Brand Names: Canada Synarel®
Pharmacologic Category Gonadotropin Releasing Hormone Agonist
Use Treatment of endometriosis, including pain and reduction of lesions; treatment of central precocious puberty (CPP; gonadotropin-dependent precocious puberty) in children of both sexes
Local Anesthetic/Vasoconstrictor Precautions No information available to require special precautions
Effects on Dental Treatment No significant effects or complications reported
Effects on Bleeding No information available to require special precautions
Adverse Effects Note: Adverse events may be more frequent in the first 6 weeks of treatment due to stimulation of the pituitary-gonadal axis. Sensitivity reactions included chest pain, pruritus, shortness of breath, rash.

CPP: 1% to 10%:
Central nervous system: Emotional lability (6%)
Dermatologic: Acne (10%), seborrhea (3%)
Endocrine & metabolic: Breast enlargement (8%; transient), vaginal bleeding (8%), hot flashes (3%; transient), vaginal discharge (3%)
Respiratory: Rhinitis (5%)
Miscellaneous: Pubic hair increased (5%; transient), body odor (4%), sensitivity reactions (3%)

Endometriosis:
>10%:
Central nervous system: Headache, emotional lability
Dermatologic: Acne
Endocrine & metabolic: Hot flashes (90%), hyperphosphatemia, hypertriglyceridemia, hypocalcemia, libido decreased
Genitourinary: Vaginal dryness
Hematologic: Leukopenia
1% to 10%:
Cardiovascular: Edema
Central nervous system: Depression, insomnia
Dermatologic: Hirsutism, seborrhea
Endocrine & metabolic: Breast size reduced, cholesterol increased, hyperlipidemia, libido increased
Gastrointestinal: Weight gain/loss
Neuromuscular & skeletal: Bone mineral density decreased, myalgia
Respiratory: Nasal irritation

General Dosage Range Nasal:
Children: 2 sprays (400 mcg) into each nostril twice daily; may increase to 3 sprays (600 mcg) into alternating nostrils 3 times/day
Adults: 1 spray (200 mcg) in 1-2 nostrils twice daily

Mechanism of Action Potent synthetic decapeptide analogue of gonadotropin-releasing hormone (GnRH; LHRH) which is approximately 200 times more potent than GnRH in terms of pituitary release of luteinizing hormone (LH) and follicle-stimulating hormone (FSH). Effects on the pituitary gland and sex hormones are dependent upon its length of administration. After acute administration, an initial stimulation of the release of LH and FSH from the pituitary is observed; an increase in androgens and estrogens subsequently follows. Continued administration of nafarelin, however, suppresses gonadotrope responsiveness to endogenous GnRH resulting in reduced secretion of LH and FSH and, secondarily, decreased ovarian and testicular steroid production.

Pharmacodynamics/Kinetics
Half-life Elimination ~3 hours; Metabolites: ~86 hours
Time to Peak Serum: 10-45 minutes
Pregnancy Risk Factor X
Pregnancy Considerations Major fetal abnormalities have been reported in some animal studies; a dose-related increase in fetal mortality and decrease in fetal weight was also observed. Ovulation is inhibited and menstruation is stopped when used appropriately for the treatment of endometriosis, however contraception is not assured. Nonhormonal contraception is recommended. Pregnancy should be excluded prior to initiating treatment. There is no evidence that pregnancy rates are enhanced or adversely affected by use.

Nafcillin (naf SIL in)

Pharmacologic Category Antibiotic, Penicillin
Use Treatment of infections such as osteomyelitis, septicemia, endocarditis, and CNS infections caused by susceptible strains of staphylococci species

Local Anesthetic/Vasoconstrictor Precautions No information available to require special precautions

Effects on Dental Treatment Key adverse event(s) related to dental treatment: Prolonged use of penicillins may lead to the development of oral candidiasis.

Effects on Bleeding Abnormal clinical bleeding episodes with concurrent platelet aggregation dysfunction have been observed during therapeutic use. This occurrence is enhanced during coexposure with epinephrine. As a result, the clinician should be mindful for adverse bleeding episodes in nafcillin-treated individuals, especially displaying "fight or flight" sympathetic responses (eg, high blood pressure, tachycardia). This reaction may be more likely with penicillins combined with a beta-lactamase inhibitor and/or with agents that have greater activity against specific enteric bacterial species.

Adverse Effects Frequency not defined.

Central nervous system: Neurotoxicity (high doses)

Gastrointestinal: *C. difficile*-associated diarrhea

Hematologic: Agranulocytosis, bone marrow depression, neutropenia

Local: Inflammation, pain, phlebitis, skin sloughing, swelling, and thrombophlebitis at the injection site; tissue necrosis with sloughing (SubQ extravasation)

Renal: Interstitial nephritis (rare), renal tubular damage (rare)

Miscellaneous: Anaphylaxis, hypersensitivity reactions (immediate and delayed; general incidence of 1% to 10% for penicillins), serum sickness

General Dosage Range I.M., I.V.: *Children and Adults:* Dosage varies greatly depending on indication

Mechanism of Action Interferes with bacterial cell wall synthesis during active multiplication, causing cell wall destruction and resultant bactericidal activity against susceptible bacteria; resistant to inactivation by staphylococcal penicillinase

Pharmacodynamics/Kinetics

Half-life Elimination

Neonates: <3 weeks: 2.2-5.5 hours; 4-9 weeks: 1.2-2.3 hours

Children 1 month to 14 years: 0.75-1.9 hours

Adults: Normal renal/hepatic function: 30-60 minutes

Time to Peak Serum: I.M.: 30-60 minutes

Pregnancy Risk Factor B

Pregnancy Considerations Adverse events have not been observed in animal reproduction studies. Information specific to nafcillin use in pregnancy is limited. Maternal use of penicillins has generally not resulted in an increased risk of birth defects.

Naftifine (NAF ti feen)

Brand Names: U.S. Naftin®

Pharmacologic Category Antifungal Agent, Topical

Use Topical treatment of tinea cruris (jock itch), tinea corporis (ringworm), and tinea pedis (athlete's foot)

Local Anesthetic/Vasoconstrictor Precautions No information available to require special precautions

Effects on Dental Treatment No significant effects or complications reported

Effects on Bleeding No information available to require special precautions

Adverse Effects 1% to 10%:

Dermatologic: Burning/stinging (5% to 6%), erythema (≤2%), pruritus (1% to 2%)

Local: Dryness (3%), irritation (2%)

General Dosage Range Topical: *Adults:* Cream: Apply once daily; Gel: Apply twice daily

Mechanism of Action Synthetic, broad-spectrum antifungal agent in the allylamine class; appears to have both fungistatic and fungicidal activity. Exhibits antifungal activity by selectively inhibiting the enzyme squalene epoxidase in a dose-dependent manner which results in a reduced synthesis of ergosterol, the primary sterol within the fungal membrane, and increased squalene in cells.

Pharmacodynamics/Kinetics

Half-life Elimination 2-3 days

Pregnancy Risk Factor B

Pregnancy Considerations Adverse events were not observed in animal reproduction studies following oral administration. Naftifine is absorbed systemically (4% to 6%) following topical administration.

Nalbuphine (NAL byoo feen)

Pharmacologic Category Analgesic, Opioid; Analgesic, Opioid Partial Agonist

Use Relief of moderate-to-severe pain; preoperative analgesia, postoperative and surgical anesthesia, and obstetrical analgesia during labor and delivery

Unlabeled Use Opioid-induced pruritus

Local Anesthetic/Vasoconstrictor Precautions No information available to require special precautions

Effects on Dental Treatment Key adverse event(s) related to dental treatment: Xerostomia and changes in salivation (normal salivary flow resumes upon discontinuation). Anticholinergic side effects can cause a reduction of saliva production or secretion, contributing to discomfort and dental disease (ie, caries, oral candidiasis, and periodontal disease).

Effects on Bleeding No information available to require special precautions

Adverse Effects

>10%: Central nervous system: Sedation (36%)

1% to 10%:

Central nervous system: Dizziness (5%), headache (3%)

Gastrointestinal: Nausea/vomiting (6%), xerostomia (4%)

Miscellaneous: Clamminess (9%)

General Dosage Range

I.M., SubQ: *Adults:* 10 mg/70 kg every 3-6 hours (maximum: 20 mg/dose; 160 mg/day)

I.V.: *Adults:* 10 mg/70 kg every 3-6 hours (maximum: 20 mg/dose; 160 mg/day) or 0.3-3 mg/kg over 10-15 minutes, then 0.25-0.5 mg/kg as required for anesthesia or 2.5-5 mg (1-2 doses)

Mechanism of Action Agonist of kappa opiate receptors and partial antagonist of mu opiate receptors in the CNS, causing inhibition of ascending pain pathways, altering the perception of and response to pain; produces generalized CNS depression

Pharmacodynamics/Kinetics

Onset of Action Peak effect: SubQ, I.M.: <15 minutes; I.V.: 2-3 minutes

Half-life Elimination 5 hours

Pregnancy Risk Factor C

Pregnancy Considerations Severe fetal bradycardia has been reported following use in labor/delivery. Fetal bradycardia may occur when administered earlier in pregnancy (not documented). Use only if clearly needed, with monitoring to detect and manage possible adverse fetal effects. Naloxone has been reported to reverse bradycardia. Newborn should be monitored for respiratory depression or bradycardia following nalbuphine use in labor.

Dental Comment **Sedation:** When administered following diazepam or midazolam, the depth of sedation is rarely increased; however, recovery is somewhat less complete than that observed when diazepam or midazolam is administered alone.

Naloxone (nal OKS one)

Brand Names: Canada Naloxone Hydrochloride Injection®; Naloxone Hydrochloride Injection® USP
Generic Availability (U.S.) Yes
Pharmacologic Category Antidote; Opioid Antagonist
Dental Use Reverse overdose effects of the two opioid agents, fentanyl and meperidine, used in the technique of I.V. conscious sedation
Use Complete or partial reversal of opioid drug effects, including respiratory depression; management of known or suspected opioid overdose; diagnosis of suspected opioid dependence or acute opioid overdose
Unlabeled Use Opioid-induced pruritus
Local Anesthetic/Vasoconstrictor Precautions No information available to require special precautions
Effects on Dental Treatment No significant effects or complications reported
Effects on Bleeding No information available to require special precautions
Adverse Effects Adverse reactions are related to reversing dependency and precipitating withdrawal. Withdrawal symptoms are the result of sympathetic excess. Adverse events occur secondarily to reversal (withdrawal) of narcotic analgesia and sedation.
Cardiovascular: Cardiac arrest, fever, flushing, hypertension, hypotension, tachycardia, ventricular fibrillation ventricular tachycardia
Central nervous system: Agitation, coma, crying (excessive [neonates]), encephalopathy, hallucination, irritability, nervousness, restlessness, seizure (neonates), tremulousness
Gastrointestinal: Abdominal cramps, diarrhea, nausea, vomiting
Local: Injection site reaction
Neuromuscular & skeletal: Ache, hyperreflexia (neonates), paresthesia, piloerection, tremor, weakness
Respiratory: Dyspnea, hypoxia, pulmonary edema, respiratory depression, rhinorrhea, sneezing
Miscellaneous: Diaphoresis, hot flashes, shivering, yawning
Dental Usual Dosage Opioid overdose: Adults: I.V.: 0.4-2 mg every 2-3 minutes as needed; may need to repeat doses every 20-60 minutes, if no response is observed after 10 mg, question the diagnosis. **Note:** Use 0.1-0.2 mg increments in patients who are opioid dependent and in postoperative patients to avoid large cardiovascular changes.
Dosage Note: Available routes of administration include I.V. (preferred), I.M., and SubQ; other available routes (unlabeled) include endotracheal, inhalation via nebulization (adults only), intranasal (adults only), and intraosseous (I.O.). Endotracheal administration is the least desirable and is supported by only anecdotal evidence (case report) (Neumar, 2010); nebulized naloxone has been shown to be an effective alternative to parenteral administration when needleless administration is desired (Weber, 2012):
Infants, Children, and Adolescents:
Opioid overdose (with standard PALS protocols):
I.V., intraosseous (I.O.) (unlabeled route), endotracheal (unlabeled route): **Note:** I.V. administration is preferred; I.O. and endotracheal routes are alternative routes recommended by the PALS guidelines (Kleinman, 2010)
<5 years or ≤20 kg (unlabeled dose): 0.1 mg/kg/dose (maximum dose: 2 mg); repeat every 2-3 minutes if needed (Hegenbarth, 2008; Kleinman, 2010)
≥5 years or >20 kg: 2 mg; if no response, repeat every 2-3 minutes. If no response is observed after 10 mg total, consider other causes of respiratory depression (Hegenbarth, 2008; Kleinman, 2010).
Continuous infusion (unlabeled dosing): I.V.: If continuous infusion is required, calculate dosage/hour based on effective intermittent dose used and duration of adequate response seen (Tenenbein, 1984) **or** use two-thirds ($2/3$) of the initial effective naloxone bolus on an hourly basis; titrate dose (typically 0.04-0.16 mg/kg/hour for 2-5 days in children); one-half ($1/2$) of the initial bolus dose should be readministered 15 minutes after initiation of the continuous infusion to prevent a drop in naloxone levels; increase infusion rate as needed to assure adequate ventilation and prevent withdrawal symptoms (Goldfrank, 1986). **Note:** The infusion should be discontinued by reducing the infusion in decrements of 25%; closely monitor the patient (eg, pulse oximetry) after each adjustment and after discontinuation of the infusion for recurrence of opioid-induced respiratory depression (Perry, 1996).
Reversal of respiratory depression with therapeutic opioid dosing: I.V.: 0.001-0.015 mg/kg/dose; dose may be repeated as needed (Hegenbarth, 2008; Kleinman, 2010)
Postoperative reversal: I.V.: 0.005-0.01 mg/kg (Fischer, 1974); may repeat every 2-3 minutes as needed based on response (adequate ventilation without significant pain)
Adults:
Opioid overdose (with standard ACLS protocols):
I.V., I.M., SubQ: Initial: 0.4-2 mg; may need to repeat doses every 2-3 minutes; after reversal, may need to readminister dose(s) at a later interval (ie, 20-60 minutes) depending on type/duration of opioid. If no response is observed after 10 mg total, consider other causes of respiratory depression. **Note:** May be given endotracheally (unlabeled route) as 2-2.5 times the initial I.V. dose (ie, 0.8-5 mg) (Neumar, 2010).
Continuous infusion (unlabeled dosing): I.V.: **Note:** For use with exposures to long-acting opioids (eg, methadone), sustained release product, and symptomatic body packers after initial naloxone response. Calculate dosage/hour based on effective intermittent dose used and duration of adequate response seen (Tenenbein, 1984) **or** use two-thirds ($2/3$) of the initial effective naloxone bolus on an hourly basis (typically 0.25-6.25 mg/hour); one-half ($1/2$) of the initial bolus dose should be readministered 15 minutes after initiation of the continuous infusion to prevent a drop in naloxone levels; adjust infusion rate as needed to assure adequate ventilation and prevent withdrawal symptoms (Goldfrank, 1986).
Inhalation via nebulization (unlabeled route): 2 mg; may repeat. Switch to I.V. or I.M. administration when possible (Weber, 2012).
Intranasal administration (unlabeled route): 2 mg (1 mg per nostril); may repeat in 5 minutes if respiratory depression persists. **Note:** Onset of action is slightly delayed compared to I.M. or I.V. routes (Kelly, 2005; Robertson, 2009; Vanden Hoek, 2010).

Reversal of respiratory depression with therapeutic opioid doses: I.V., I.M., SubQ.: Initial: 0.04-0.4 mg; may repeat until desired response achieved. If desired response is not observed after 0.8 mg total, consider other causes of respiratory depression. **Note:** May be given endotracheally (unlabeled route) as 2-2.5 times the initial I.V. dose (ie, 0.08-1 mg) (Neumar, 2010).

Continuous infusion (unlabeled dosing): I.V.: **Note:** For use with exposures to long-acting opioids (eg, methadone) or sustained release products. Calculate dosage/hour based on effective intermittent dose used and duration of adequate response seen (Tenenbein, 1984) **or** use two-thirds ($2/3$) of the initial effective naloxone bolus on an hourly basis (typically 0.2-0.6 mg/hour); one-half ($1/2$) of the initial bolus dose should be readministered 15 minutes after initiation of the continuous infusion to prevent a drop in naloxone levels; adjust infusion rate as needed to assure adequate ventilation and prevent withdrawal symptoms (Goldfrank, 1986).

Opioid-dependent patients being treated for cancer pain (NCCN guidelines, v.2.2011): I.V.: 0.04-0.08 mg (40-80 **mcg**) slow I.V. push; administer every 30-60 seconds until improvement in symptoms; if no response is observed after total naloxone dose 1 mg, consider other causes of respiratory depression. **Note:** May dilute 0.4 mg/mL (1 mL) ampul into 9 mL of normal saline for a total volume of 10 mL to achieve a 0.04 mg/mL (40 **mcg**/mL) concentration.

Postoperative reversal: I.V.: 0.1-0.2 mg every 2-3 minutes until desired response (adequate ventilation and alertness without significant pain). **Note:** Repeat doses may be needed within 1-2 hour intervals depending on type, dose, and timing of the last dose of opioid administered.

Opioid-induced pruritus (unlabeled use): I.V. infusion: 0.25 **mcg/kg/hour**; **Note:** Monitor pain control; verify that the naloxone is not reversing analgesia (Gan, 1997)

Dosage adjustment in renal impairment: No dosage adjustment provided in manufacturer's labeling.

Dosage adjustment in hepatic impairment: No dosage adjustment provided in manufacturer's labeling.

Mechanism of Action Pure opioid antagonist that competes and displaces narcotics at opioid receptor sites

Contraindications Hypersensitivity to naloxone or any component of the formulation

Warnings/Precautions Due to an association between naloxone and acute pulmonary edema, use with caution in patients with cardiovascular disease or in patients receiving medications with potential adverse cardiovascular effects (eg, hypotension, pulmonary edema, or arrhythmias). Administration of naloxone causes the release of catecholamines; may precipitate acute withdrawal or unmask pain in those who regularly take opioids. Excessive dosages should be avoided after use of opiates in surgery. Abrupt postoperative reversal may result in nausea, vomiting, sweating, tachycardia, hypertension, seizures, and other cardiovascular events (including pulmonary edema and arrhythmias). May precipitate withdrawal symptoms in patients addicted to opiates, including pain, hypertension, sweating, agitation, irritability; in neonates, symptoms may include shrill cry, failure to feed; carefully titrate dose to reverse hypoventilation; do not fully awaken patient or reverse analgesic effect (postoperative patient). Use caution in patients with history of seizures; avoid use in treatment of meperidine-induced seizures. Recurrence of respiratory depression is possible if the opioid involved is long-acting; observe patients until there is no reasonable risk of recurrent respiratory depression.

To prevent overdose deaths, there are initiatives to dispense naloxone for self- or buddy-administration to patients at risk of opioid overdose (eg, recipients of high-dose opioids, suspected or confirmed history of illicit opioid use) and individuals likely to be present in an overdose situation (eg, family members of illicit drug users) (Albert, 2011; Bennett, 2011). Needleless administration via nebulization and the intranasal route by first responders and bystanders has also been described (Doe-Simkins, 2009; Weber, 2012). Needleless administration provides an alternative route of administration in patients with venous scarring due to illicit drug use (eg, heroin). There is a low incidence of death following naloxone reversal of opioid toxicity in patients who refuse transport to a healthcare facility (Wampler, 2011).

Drug Interactions

Metabolism/Transport Effects None known.

Avoid Concomitant Use There are no known interactions where it is recommended to avoid concomitant use.

Increased Effect/Toxicity There are no known significant interactions involving an increase in effect.

Decreased Effect There are no known significant interactions involving a decrease in effect.

Pharmacodynamics/Kinetics

Onset of Action Endotracheal, I.M., SubQ: 2-5 minutes; Inhalation via nebulization: ~5 minutes (Mycyk, 2003); Intranasal: ~8-13 minutes (Kelley, 2005; Robertson, 2009); I.V.: ~2 minutes

Duration of Action Depending on route of administration, ~30-120 minutes; I.V. has a shorter duration of action than I.M. administration; since naloxone's action is shorter than that of most opioids, repeated doses are usually needed

Half-life Elimination Neonates: 3-4 hours; Adults: 0.5-1.5 hours

Pregnancy Risk Factor C

Pregnancy Considerations Adverse events were not observed in animal reproduction studies. Naloxone crosses the placenta. Consider the benefit to the mother and the risk to the fetus before administering to a pregnant woman who is known or suspected to be opioid dependent; may precipitate withdrawal in both the mother and fetus. In general, medications used as antidotes should take into consideration the health and prognosis of the mother (Bailey, 2003). Use caution in pregnant women with mild-to-moderate hypertension during labor; severe hypertension may occur.

Lactation Excretion in breast milk unknown/use caution

Breast-Feeding Considerations It is not known if naloxone is excreted into breast milk, however, systemic absorption following oral administration is low (Smith, 2012) and any exposure of naloxone to a nursing infant would therefore be limited. Since naloxone is used for opioid reversal, the opioid concentrations in the milk of a breast-feeding mother and potential transfer of the opioid to the infant should be considered.

Dosage Forms

Injection, solution: 0.4 mg/mL (1 mL, 10 mL)
Injection, solution [preservative free]: 0.4 mg/mL (1 mL)

Naltrexone (nal TREKS one)

Brand Names: U.S. ReVia®; Vivitrol®

Brand Names: Canada ReVia®

Pharmacologic Category Antidote; Opioid Antagonist

Use Treatment of ethanol dependence; prevention of relapse in opioid dependent patients, following opioid detoxification

Local Anesthetic/Vasoconstrictor Precautions No information available to require special precautions

Effects on Dental Treatment Key adverse event(s) related to dental treatment: Dry mouth.

Effects on Bleeding No information available to require special precautions

Adverse Effects Combined reporting of adverse events from oral and injectable formulations:

>10%:

Cardiovascular: Syncope (13%)

Central nervous system: Headache (3% to 25%), insomnia (3% to 14%), dizziness (4% to 13%), anxiety (2% to 12%), nervousness (4% to >10%)

Gastrointestinal: Nausea (10% to 33%), vomiting (3% to 14%), appetite decreased (14%), diarrhea (13%), abdominal pain (11%), abdominal cramping

Hepatic: ALT increased (13%)

Local: Injection site reaction (≤69%; includes bruising, induration, nodules, pain, pruritus, swelling, tenderness)

Neuromuscular & skeletal: Arthralgia (12%), CPK increased (11% to 39%)

Respiratory: Pharyngitis (7% to 11%)

1% to 10%:

Cardiovascular: Hypertension (5%)

Central nervous system: Suicidal thoughts (≤10%), depression (8%), somnolence (2% to 4%), fatigue (4%), chills, energy increased, feeling down, irritability

Dermatologic: Rash (6%)

Endocrine & metabolic: Polydipsia

Gastrointestinal: Dry mouth (5%), toothache (4%)

Genitourinary: Delayed ejaculation, impotency

Hepatic: AST increased (2% to 10%), GGT increased (7%)

Neuromuscular & skeletal: Muscle cramps (8%), back pain (6%)

Miscellaneous: Influenza (5%)

General Dosage Range

I.M.: *Adults:* 380 mg once every 4 weeks

Oral: *Adults:* 25-50 mg once daily

Mechanism of Action Naltrexone (a pure opioid antagonist) is a cyclopropyl derivative of oxymorphone similar in structure to naloxone and nalorphine (a morphine derivative); it acts as a competitive antagonist at opioid receptor sites, showing the highest affinity for mu receptors.

Pharmacodynamics/Kinetics

Duration of Action Oral: 50 mg: 24 hours; 100 mg: 48 hours; 150 mg: 72 hours; I.M.: 4 weeks

Half-life Elimination Oral: 4 hours; 6-beta-naltrexol: 13 hours; I.M.: naltrexone and 6-beta-naltrexol: 5-10 days

Time to Peak Serum: Oral: ~60 minutes; I.M.: Biphasic: ~2 hours (first peak), ~2-3 days (second peak)

Pregnancy Risk Factor C

Pregnancy Considerations Evidence of early fetal loss has been observed in animal studies with oral naltrexone. Reproduction studies have not been conduced using the sustained release I.M formulation. There are no adequate and well-controlled studies of naltrexone in pregnant women.

Naphazoline (Nasal) (naf AZ oh leen)

Brand Names: U.S. Privine® [OTC]

Pharmacologic Category Alpha$_1$ Agonist; Imidazoline Derivative

Use Temporary relief of nasal congestion associated with the common cold, upper respiratory allergies, or sinusitis

Local Anesthetic/Vasoconstrictor Precautions No information available to require special precautions

Effects on Dental Treatment No significant effects or complications reported

Effects on Bleeding No information available to require special precautions

Adverse Effects Frequency not defined.

Local: Transient stinging, nasal mucosa irritation, dryness, rebound congestion

Respiratory: Sneezing

General Dosage Range Intranasal: *Children ≥12 years and Adults:* Instill 1-2 drops or sprays every 6 hours if needed

Mechanism of Action Stimulates alpha-adrenergic receptors in the arterioles of the conjunctiva and the nasal mucosa to produce vasoconstriction

Pharmacodynamics/Kinetics

Onset of Action Decongestant: Topical: ~10 minutes

Duration of Action 2-6 hours

Naphazoline and Pheniramine

(naf AZ oh leen & fen NIR a meen)

Brand Names: U.S. Naphcon-A® [OTC]; Opcon-A® [OTC]; Visine-A® [OTC]

Brand Names: Canada Naphcon-A®; Visine® Advanced Allergy

Pharmacologic Category Alkylamine Derivative; Alpha$_1$ Agonist; Histamine H$_1$ Antagonist; Histamine H$_1$ Antagonist, First Generation; Imidazoline Derivative; Ophthalmic Agent, Vasoconstrictor

Use Treatment of ocular congestion, irritation, and itching

Local Anesthetic/Vasoconstrictor Precautions No information available to require special precautions

Effects on Dental Treatment No significant effects or complications reported

Effects on Bleeding No information available to require special precautions

Adverse Effects Frequency not defined: Ocular: Pupillary dilation, tingling

General Dosage Range Ophthalmic: *Children ≥6 years and Adults:* 1-2 drops into the affected eye(s) up to 4 times/day

Mechanism of Action

Pheniramine, a nonselective histamine antagonist, inhibits the effect of histamine on conjunctival epithelial cells by preventing its release from mast cells.

Naphazoline, an alpha$_1$-agonist, stimulates alpha-adrenergic receptors in the arterioles of the conjunctiva to produce vasoconstriction.

Naproxen (na PROKS en)

Related Information

Oral Pain on page 1558
Rheumatoid Arthritis, Osteoarthritis, and Osteoporosis on page 1526
Temporomandibular Dysfunction (TMD), Chronic Pain, and Fibromyalgia on page 1590

Related Sample Prescriptions

Mild/Moderate Oral Pain on page 1606
Moderate/Moderately Severe Oral Pain on page 1606

Brand Names: U.S. Aleve® [OTC]; All Day Relief [OTC]; Anaprox®; Anaprox® DS; EC-Naprosyn®; Mediproxen [OTC]; Midol® Extended Relief [OTC]; Naprelan®; Naprosyn®; Pamprin® Maximum Strength All Day Relief [OTC]

Brand Names: Canada Anaprox®; Anaprox® DS; Apo-Napro-Na DS®; Apo-Napro-Na®; Apo-Naproxen EC®; Apo-Naproxen SR®; Apo-Naproxen®; Mylan-Naproxen EC; Naprelan™; Naprosyn®; Naprosyn® E; Naprosyn® SR; Naproxen Sodium DS; Naproxen-NA; Naproxen-NA DF; PMS-Naproxen; PMS-Naproxen EC; PRO-Naproxen EC; Riva-Naproxen; Riva-Naproxen Sodium; Riva-Naproxen Sodium DS; Teva-Naproxen; Teva-Naproxen EC; Teva-Naproxen Sodium; Teva-Naproxen Sodium DS; Teva-Naproxen SR

Generic Availability (U.S.) Yes: Caplet, suspension, tablet

Pharmacologic Category Nonsteroidal Anti-inflammatory Drug (NSAID), Oral

Dental Use Management of pain and swelling

Use Management of ankylosing spondylitis, osteoarthritis, and rheumatoid disorders (including juvenile idiopathic arthritis [JIA]); acute gout; mild-to-moderate pain; tendonitis, bursitis; dysmenorrhea; fever

Unlabeled Use Migraine prophylaxis

Local Anesthetic/Vasoconstrictor Precautions No information available to require special precautions

Effects on Dental Treatment Key adverse event(s) related to dental treatment: Stomatitis.

Naproxen and naproxen sodium have the potential to interfere with the antiplatelet effect of low-dose aspirin. One study of naproxen and low-dose aspirin has suggested that naproxen may interfere with aspirin's antiplatelet activity when they are coadministered (Steinhubl, 2005). However, naproxen 500 mg administered 2 hours before or after aspirin 100 mg did not interfere with aspirin's antiplatelet effect. The FDA stated that there is no data looking at doses of naproxen <500 mg. Naproxen over-the-counter strength is 220 mg tablets.

The FDA has warned that ibuprofen can interfere with the antiplatelet effect of low-dose aspirin (81 mg/day), potentially rendering aspirin less effective when used for cardioprotection and stroke protection. In situations where these drugs could be used concomitantly, the FDA has proved the following information: Patients who use immediate release aspirin (not enteric-coated aspirin) and take single doses of ibuprofen 400 mg, should dose the ibuprofen at least 30 minutes or longer after aspirin ingestion or more than 8 hours before aspirin ingestion to avoid attenuation of aspirin's effect. Similar recommendations may hold for concomitant may hold for concomitant naproxen and aspirin use. See Effects on Bleeding.

Effects on Bleeding Nonselective NSAIDs, such as naproxen, inhibit platelet aggregation and prolong bleeding time in some patients. Unlike aspirin, the NSAID effect on platelet function is quantitatively less, of shorter duration, and reversible. Normal platelet function should occur in ~5 elimination half-lives or in <10 hours after discontinuation of naproxen. Concomitant use of other NSAIDs should be avoided.

Adverse Effects 1% to 10%:

Cardiovascular: Edema (3% to 9%), palpitations (<3%)
Central nervous system: Dizziness (3% to 9%), drowsiness (3% to 9%), headache (3% to 9%), lightheadedness (<3%), vertigo (<3%)
Dermatologic: Pruritus (3% to 9%), skin eruption (3% to 9%), ecchymosis (3% to 9%), purpura (<3%), rash
Endocrine & metabolic: Fluid retention (3% to 9%)
Gastrointestinal: Abdominal pain (3% to 9%), constipation (3% to 9%), nausea (3% to 9%), heartburn (3% to 9%), diarrhea (<3%), dyspepsia (<3%), stomatitis (<3%), flatulence, gross bleeding/perforation, indigestion, ulcers, vomiting
Genitourinary: Abnormal renal function
Hematologic: Hemolysis (3% to 9%), ecchymosis (3% to 9%), anemia, bleeding time increased
Hepatic: LFTs increased
Ocular: Visual disturbances (<3%)
Otic: Tinnitus (3% to 9%), hearing disturbances (<3%)
Respiratory: Dyspnea (3% to 9%)
Miscellaneous: Diaphoresis (<3%), thirst (<3%)

Dental Usual Dosage

Mild-to-moderate pain: Adults: Initial: 500 mg, then 250 mg every 6-8 hours; maximum: 1250 mg/day naproxen base

Pain/fever (OTC labeling): Children ≥12 years and Adults: 200 mg naproxen base every 8-12 hours; if needed, may take 400 mg naproxen base for the initial dose; maximum: 400 mg naproxen base in any 8- to 12-hour period or 600 mg naproxen base/24 hours

Dosage Note: Dosage expressed as naproxen base; 200 mg naproxen base is equivalent to 220 mg naproxen sodium.

Oral:

Children >2 years: Juvenile idiopathic arthritis: 10 mg/kg/day in 2 divided doses

Adults:

Gout, acute: Initial: 750 mg, followed by 250 mg every 8 hours until attack subsides. **Note:** EC-Naprosyn® is not recommended.

Migraine, acute (unlabeled use): Initial: 500-750 mg; an additional 250-500 mg may be given if needed (maximum: 1250 mg in 24 hours). **Note:** EC-Naprosyn® is not recommended.

Pain (mild-to-moderate), dysmenorrhea, acute tendonitis, bursitis: Initial: 500 mg, then 250 mg every 6-8 hours; maximum: 1250 mg/day naproxen base

Rheumatoid arthritis, osteoarthritis, and ankylosing spondylitis: 500-1000 mg/day in 2 divided doses; may increase to 1.5 g/day of naproxen base for limited time period

OTC labeling: Pain/fever: Children ≥12 years and Adults: 200 mg naproxen base every 8-12 hours; if needed, may take 400 mg naproxen base for the initial dose; maximum: 400 mg naproxen base in any 8- to 12-hour period or 600 mg naproxen base/24 hours

Dosing adjustment in renal impairment: Cl_{cr} <30 mL/minute: Use is not recommended

Mechanism of Action Reversibly inhibits cyclooxygenase-1 and 2 (COX-1 and 2) enzymes, which results in decreased formation of prostaglandin precursors; has antipyretic, analgesic, and anti-inflammatory properties

Other proposed mechanisms not fully elucidated (and possibly contributing to the anti-inflammatory effect to varying degrees), include inhibiting chemotaxis, altering lymphocyte activity, inhibiting neutrophil aggregation/activation, and decreasing proinflammatory cytokine levels.

Contraindications Hypersensitivity to naproxen, aspirin, other NSAIDs, or any component of the formulation; perioperative pain in the setting of coronary artery bypass graft (CABG) surgery

Warnings/Precautions [U.S. Boxed Warning]: NSAIDs are associated with an increased risk of adverse cardiovascular thrombotic events, including MI and stroke. Risk may be increased with duration of use or pre-existing cardiovascular risk factors or disease. Carefully evaluate individual cardiovascular risk profiles prior to prescribing. May cause new-onset hypertension or worsening of existing hypertension. Use caution with fluid retention. Avoid use in heart failure. Use the lowest effective dose for the shortest duration of time, consistent with individual patient goals, to reduce risk of cardiovascular or GI adverse events. Alternate therapies should be considered for patients at high risk. Concurrent administration of ibuprofen, and potentially other nonselective NSAIDs, may interfere with aspirin's cardioprotective effect. **[U.S. Boxed Warning]: Use is contraindicated for treatment of perioperative pain in the setting of coronary artery bypass graft (CABG) surgery.** Risk of MI and stroke may be increased with use following CABG surgery.

[U.S. Boxed Warning]: NSAIDs may increase risk of gastrointestinal irritation, inflammation, ulceration, bleeding, and perforation. These events may occur at any time during therapy and without warning. Use caution with a history of GI disease (bleeding or ulcers), concurrent therapy with aspirin, anticoagulants and/or corticosteroids, smoking, use of alcohol, the elderly or debilitated patients. When used concomitantly with ≤325 mg of aspirin, a substantial increase in the risk of gastrointestinal complications (eg, ulcer) occurs; concomitant gastroprotective therapy (eg, proton pump inhibitors) is recommended (Bhatt, 2008).

May increase the risk of aseptic meningitis, especially in patients with systemic lupus erythematosus (SLE) and mixed connective tissue disorders. Platelet adhesion and aggregation may be decreased; may prolong bleeding time; patients with coagulation disorders or who are receiving anticoagulants should be monitored closely. Anemia may occur; patients on long-term NSAID therapy should be monitored for anemia. Rarely, NSAID use may cause severe blood dyscrasias (eg, agranulocytosis, aplastic anemia, thrombocytopenia).

NSAID use may compromise existing renal function; dose-dependent decreases in prostaglandin synthesis may result from NSAID use, reducing renal blood flow which may cause renal decompensation. NSAID use may increase the risk for hyperkalemia. Patients with impaired renal function, dehydration, heart failure, liver dysfunction, those taking diuretics, and ACE inhibitors, and the elderly are at greater risk of renal toxicity and hyperkalemia. Rehydrate patient before starting therapy; monitor renal function closely. Not recommended for use in patients with advanced renal disease. Long-term NSAID use may result in renal papillary necrosis.

NSAIDs may cause serious skin adverse events including exfoliative dermatitis, Stevens-Johnson Syndrome (SJS) and toxic epidermal necrolysis (TEN); discontinue use at first sign of skin rash or hypersensitivity. Anaphylactoid reactions may occur, even without prior exposure; patients with "aspirin triad" (bronchial asthma, aspirin intolerance, rhinitis) may be at increased risk. Do not use in patients who experience bronchospasm, asthma, rhinitis, or urticaria with NSAID or aspirin therapy. Use caution in other forms of asthma.

Use with caution in patients with decreased hepatic function. Closely monitor patients with any abnormal LFT. Severe hepatic reactions (eg, fulminant hepatitis, liver failure) have occurred with NSAID use, rarely; discontinue if signs or symptoms of liver disease develop, or if systemic manifestations occur.

NSAIDS may cause drowsiness, dizziness, blurred vision and other neurologic effects which may impair physical or mental abilities; patients must be cautioned about performing tasks which require mental alertness (eg, operating machinery or driving). Discontinue use with blurred or diminished vision and perform ophthalmologic exam. Monitor vision with long-term therapy.

In the elderly, avoid chronic use (unless alternative agents ineffective and patient can receive concomitant gastroprotective agent); nonselective oral NSAID use is associated with an increased risk of GI bleeding and peptic ulcer disease in older adults in high risk category (eg, >75 years or age or receiving concomitant oral/parenteral corticosteroids, anticoagulants, or antiplatelet agents) (Beers Criteria).

Withhold for at least 4-6 half-lives prior to surgical or dental procedures. Safety and efficacy have not been established in children <2 years of age.

OTC labeling: Prior to self-medication, patients should contact healthcare provider if they have had recurring stomach pain or upset, ulcers, bleeding problems, asthma, high blood pressure, heart or kidney disease, other serious medical problems, are currently taking a diuretic, anticoagulant, other NSAIDs, or are ≥60 years of age. Recommended dosages and duration should not be exceeded, due to an increased risk of GI bleeding, MI, and stroke. Patients should stop use and consult a healthcare provider if symptoms get worse, newly appear, or continue; if an allergic reaction occurs; if feeling faint, vomit blood or have bloody/black stools; if having difficulty swallowing or heartburn, or if fever lasts for >3 days or pain >10 days. Consuming ≥3 alcoholic beverages/day or taking longer than recommended may increase the risk of GI bleeding. Not for self-medication (OTC use) in children <12 years of age.

Drug Interactions

Metabolism/Transport Effects Substrate of CYP1A2 (minor), CYP2C9 (minor); **Note:** Assignment of Major/Minor substrate status based on clinically relevant drug interaction potential

Avoid Concomitant Use

Avoid concomitant use of Naproxen with any of the following: Floctafenine; Ketorolac (Nasal); Ketorolac (Systemic); NSAID (COX-2 Inhibitor); Omacetaxine

Increased Effect/Toxicity

Naproxen may increase the levels/effects of: Agents with Antiplatelet Properties; Aliskiren; Aminoglycosides; Anticoagulants; Bisphosphonate Derivatives; Collagenase (Systemic); CycloSPORINE (Systemic); Dabigatran Etexilate; Deferasirox; Desmopressin; Digoxin; Drotrecogin Alfa (Activated); Eplerenone;

Haloperidol; Ibritumomab; Lithium; Methotrexate; Nonsteroidal Anti-Inflammatory Agents; NSAID (COX-2 Inhibitor); Omacetaxine; PEMEtrexed; Porfimer; Potassium-Sparing Diuretics; PRALAtrexate; Quinolone Antibiotics; Rivaroxaban; Salicylates; Thrombolytic Agents; Tositumomab and Iodine I 131 Tositumomab; Vancomycin; Vitamin K Antagonists

The levels/effects of Naproxen may be increased by: ACE Inhibitors; Angiotensin II Receptor Blockers; Antidepressants (Tricyclic, Tertiary Amine); Corticosteroids (Systemic); CycloSPORINE (Systemic); Dasatinib; Floctafenine; Glucosamine; Herbs (Anticoagulant/Antiplatelet Properties); Ketorolac (Nasal); Ketorolac (Systemic); Multivitamins/Minerals (with ADEK, Folate, Iron); Nonsteroidal Anti-Inflammatory Agents; Omega-3 Fatty Acids; Pentosan Polysulfate Sodium; Pentoxifylline; Probenecid; Prostacyclin Analogues; Selective Serotonin Reuptake Inhibitors; Serotonin/Norepinephrine Reuptake Inhibitors; Sodium Phosphates; Tipranavir; Treprostinil; Vitamin E

Decreased Effect

Naproxen may decrease the levels/effects of: ACE Inhibitors; Agents with Antiplatelet Properties; Aliskiren; Angiotensin II Receptor Blockers; Beta-Blockers; Eplerenone; HydrALAZINE; Loop Diuretics; Potassium-Sparing Diuretics; Salicylates; Selective Serotonin Reuptake Inhibitors; Thiazide Diuretics

The levels/effects of Naproxen may be decreased by: Bile Acid Sequestrants; Nonsteroidal Anti-Inflammatory Agents; Salicylates

Ethanol/Nutrition/Herb Interactions

Ethanol: Avoid ethanol (may enhance gastric mucosal irritation).

Food: Naproxen absorption rate/levels may be decreased if taken with food.

Herb/Nutraceutical: Avoid alfalfa, anise, bilberry, bladderwrack, bromelain, cat's claw, celery, chamomile, coleus, cordyceps, dong quai, evening primrose, fenugreek, feverfew, garlic, ginger, ginkgo biloba, ginseng (American, Panax, Siberian), grapeseed, green tea, guggul, horse chestnut seed, horseradish, licorice, prickly ash, red clover, reishi, SAMe (S-adenosylmethionine), sweet clover, turmeric, white willow (all have additional antiplatelet activity).

Dietary Considerations Drug may cause GI upset, bleeding, ulceration, perforation; take with food or milk to minimize GI upset.

Pharmacodynamics/Kinetics

Onset of Action Analgesic: 1 hour; Anti-inflammatory: ~2 weeks; Peak effect: Anti-inflammatory: 2-4 weeks

Duration of Action Analgesic: ≤7 hours; Anti-inflammatory: ≤12 hours

Half-life Elimination Normal renal function: 12-17 hours; End-stage renal disease: No change

Time to Peak Serum: 1-4 hours

Pregnancy Risk Factor C

Pregnancy Considerations Adverse events were not observed in the initial animal reproduction studies; therefore, the manufacturer classifies naproxen as pregnancy category C. Naproxen crosses the placenta and can be detected in fetal tissue and the serum of newborn infants following *in utero* exposure. NSAID exposure during the first trimester is not strongly associated with congenital malformations; however, cardiovascular anomalies and cleft palate have been observed following NSAID exposure in some studies. The use of a NSAID close to conception may be associated with an increased risk of miscarriage. Nonteratogenic effects have been observed following NSAID administration during the third trimester including: Myocardial degenerative changes, prenatal constriction of the ductus arteriosus, fetal tricuspid regurgitation, failure of the ductus arteriosus to close postnatally; renal dysfunction or failure, oligohydramnios; gastrointestinal bleeding or perforation, increased risk of necrotizing enterocolitis; intracranial bleeding (including intraventricular hemorrhage), platelet dysfunction with resultant bleeding; pulmonary hypertension. Because they may cause premature closure of the ductus arteriosus, use of NSAIDs late in pregnancy should be avoided (use after 31 or 32 weeks gestation is not recommended by some clinicians). The chronic use of NSAIDs in women of reproductive age may be associated with infertility that is reversible upon discontinuation of the medication. A registry is available for pregnant women exposed to autoimmune medications including naproxen. For additional information contact the Organization of Teratology Information Specialists, OTIS Autoimmune Diseases Study, at (877) 311-8972.

Lactation Enters breast milk/not recommended (AAP rates "compatible"; AAP 2001 update pending)

Breast-Feeding Considerations Small amounts of naproxen are excreted into breast milk. Naproxen has been detected in the urine of a breast-feeding infant. Breast-feeding is not recommended by the manufacturer. In a study which included 20 mother-infant pairs, there were two cases of drowsiness and one case of vomiting in the breast-fed infants. Maternal naproxen dose, duration, and relationship to breast-feeding were not provided.

Dosage Forms

Caplet, oral: 220 mg
Aleve® [OTC]: 220 mg
All Day Relief [OTC]: 220 mg
Midol® Extended Relief [OTC]: 220 mg
Pamprin® Maximum Strength All Day Relief [OTC]: 220 mg

Capsule, liquid gel, oral:
Aleve® [OTC]: 220 mg

Combination package, oral:
Naprelan®: Day 1-3: Tablet, controlled release: 750 mg (6s) [contains sodium 75 mg] and Day 4-10: Tablet, controlled release: 500 mg (14s) [contains sodium 50 mg]

Gelcap, oral:
Aleve® [OTC]: 220 mg

Suspension, oral: 125 mg/5 mL (500 mL)
Naprosyn®: 125 mg/5 mL (473 mL)

Tablet, oral: 220 mg, 250 mg, 275 mg, 375 mg, 500 mg, 550 mg
Aleve® [OTC]: 220 mg
Anaprox®: 275 mg
Anaprox® DS: 550 mg
Mediproxen [OTC]: 220 mg
Naprosyn®: 250 mg, 375 mg, 500 mg

Tablet, controlled release, oral:
Naprelan®: 375 mg, 500 mg, 750 mg

Tablet, delayed release, enteric coated, oral: 375 mg, 500 mg
EC-Naprosyn®: 375 mg, 500 mg

References

Brooks PM and Day RO, "Nonsteroidal Anti-inflammatory Drugs - Differences and Similarities," *N Engl J Med*, 1991, 324(24):1716-25.
Dionne R, "Additive Analgesia Without Opioid Side Effects," *Compend Contin Educ Dent*, 2000, 21(7):572-4, 576-7.

Dionne RA and Berthold CW, "Therapeutic Uses of Nonsteroidal Anti-inflammatory Drugs in Dentistry," *Crit Rev Oral Biol Med*, 2001, 12 (4):315-30.

Forbes JA, Keller CK, Smith JW, et al, "Analgesic Effect of Naproxen Sodium, Codeine, a Naproxen-Codeine Combination and Aspirin on the Postoperative Pain of Oral Surgery," *Pharmacotherapy*, 1986, 6 (5):211-8.

Nguyen AM, Graham DY, Gage T, et al, "Nonsteroidal Anti-inflammatory Drug Use in Dentistry: Gastrointestinal Implications," *Gen Dent*, 1999, 47(6):590-6.

Naproxen and Esomeprazole
(na PROKS en & es oh ME pray zol)

Related Information
Esomeprazole *on page 502*
Naproxen *on page 958*
Rheumatoid Arthritis, Osteoarthritis, and Osteoporosis *on page 1526*

Brand Names: U.S. Vimovo™
Brand Names: Canada Vimovo™
Pharmacologic Category Nonsteroidal Anti-inflammatory Drug (NSAID), Oral; Proton Pump Inhibitor; Substituted Benzimidazole
Use Reduction of the risk of NSAID-associated gastric ulcers in patients at risk of developing gastric ulcers who require an NSAID for the treatment of rheumatoid arthritis, osteoarthritis, and ankylosing spondylitis

Local Anesthetic/Vasoconstrictor Precautions No information available to require special precautions
Effects on Dental Treatment Key adverse event(s) related to dental treatment: Esomeprazole: Xerostomia (normal salivary flow resumes upon discontinuation)
Effects on Bleeding Nonselective NSAIDs, such as naproxen and esomeprazole, inhibit platelet aggregation and prolong bleeding time in some patients. Unlike aspirin, the NSAID effect on platelet function is quantitatively less, of shorter duration, and reversible. Normal platelet function should occur in ~5 elimination half-lives or in <10 hours after discontinuation of naproxen and esomeprazole. Concomitant use of other NSAIDs should be avoided.
Adverse Effects See individual agents.
General Dosage Range Oral: *Adults:* 1 tablet (naproxen 375-500 mg/esomeprazole 20 mg) twice daily; Maximum dose of esomeprazole: 40 mg daily
Mechanism of Action
Naproxen: Reversibly inhibits cyclooxygenase-1 and 2 (COX-1 and 2) enzymes, which result in decreased formation of prostaglandin precursors; has antipyretic, analgesic, and anti-inflammatory properties
Esomeprazole: Proton pump inhibitor which decreases acid secretion in gastric parietal cells
Pregnancy Risk Factor C/D ≥30 weeks gestation
Pregnancy Considerations Teratogenic effects were not observed with esomeprazole or naproxen in animal reproduction studies. Because they may cause premature closure of the ductus arteriosus, use of NSAIDs late in pregnancy should be avoided; use of this combination product is contraindicated the late stages of pregnancy. Refer to individual agents.

Naproxen and Pseudoephedrine
(na PROKS en & soo doe e FED rin)

Related Information
Naproxen *on page 958*
Pseudoephedrine *on page 1159*
Brand Names: U.S. Aleve®-D Sinus & Cold [OTC]; Aleve®-D Sinus & Headache [OTC]; Sudafed® 12 Hour Pressure + Pain [OTC]
Pharmacologic Category Decongestant/Analgesic

Use Temporary relief of cold, sinus, and flu symptoms (including nasal congestion, sinus congestion/pressure, headache, minor body aches and pains, and fever)
Local Anesthetic/Vasoconstrictor Precautions Use with caution since pseudoephedrine is a sympathomimetic amine which could interact with epinephrine to cause a pressor response.
Effects on Dental Treatment Key adverse event(s) related to dental treatment: Pseudoephedrine: Xerostomia (normal salivary flow resumes upon discontinuation).

The dentist should be aware of the potential of abnormal coagulation. See Effects on Bleeding.
Effects on Bleeding Nonselective NSAIDs, such as naproxen and pseudoephedrine, inhibit platelet aggregation and prolong bleeding time in some patients. Unlike aspirin, the NSAID effect on platelet function is quantitatively less, of shorter duration, and reversible. Normal platelet function should occur in ~5 elimination half-lives or in <10 hours after discontinuation of naproxen and pseudoephedrine. Concomitant use of other NSAIDs should be avoided.
Adverse Effects See individual agents.
General Dosage Range Oral: *Children ≥12 years and Adults:* 1 caplet (naproxen sodium 220 mg/pseudoephedrine 120 mg) every 12 hours (maximum: 2 caplets/day)
Mechanism of Action
Naproxen: Reversibly inhibits cyclooxygenase-1 and 2 (COX-1 and 2) enzymes, which result in decreased formation of prostaglandin precursors; has antipyretic, analgesic, and anti-inflammatory properties
Pseudoephedrine: Directly stimulates alpha-adrenergic receptors of respiratory mucosa causing vasoconstriction; directly stimulates beta-adrenergic receptors causing bronchial relaxation
Pregnancy Considerations See individual agents.

Naratriptan (NAR a trip tan)

Related Information
Temporomandibular Dysfunction (TMD), Chronic Pain, and Fibromyalgia *on page 1590*
Brand Names: U.S. Amerge®
Brand Names: Canada Amerge®; Sandoz-Naratriptan; Teva-Naratriptan
Pharmacologic Category Antimigraine Agent; Serotonin 5-HT$_{1B, 1D}$ Receptor Agonist
Use Treatment of acute migraine headache with or without aura
Unlabeled Use Short-term prevention of menstrually-associated migraines (MAMs)
Local Anesthetic/Vasoconstrictor Precautions No information available to require special precautions
Effects on Dental Treatment No significant effects or complications reported
Effects on Bleeding No information available to require special precautions
Adverse Effects 1% to 10%:
Central nervous system: Pain/pressure (2% to 4%), malaise/fatigue (2%), dizziness (1% to 2%), drowsiness (1% to 2%), vertigo (1%)
Gastrointestinal: Nausea (4% to 5%), hyposalivation (1%), vomiting (1%)
Neuromuscular & skeletal: Paresthesia (1% to 2%)
Ocular: Photophobia (1%)

◀ Miscellaneous: Ear/nose/throat infection (1%), pressure/tightness/heaviness sensations (1%), warm/cold temperature sensations (1%)

General Dosage Range Dosage adjustment recommended in patients with hepatic or renal impairment

Oral: *Adults:* 1-2.5 mg, may repeat after 4 hours (maximum: 5 mg/day)

Mechanism of Action Selective agonist for serotonin (5-HT$_{1B}$ and 5-HT$_{1D}$ receptors) in cranial arteries; causes vasoconstriction and reduces sterile inflammation associated with antidromic neuronal transmission correlating with relief of migraine

Pharmacodynamics/Kinetics

Onset of Action ~1-2 hours (Bomhof, 1999; Tfelt-Hansen, 2000)

Half-life Elimination 6 hours; increased in renal impairment (moderate impairment; mean: 11 hours; range: 7-20 hours); increased in hepatic impairment (moderate impairment: 8-16 hours)

Time to Peak 2-3 hours

Pregnancy Risk Factor C

Pregnancy Considerations There are no adequate and well-controlled studies using naratriptan in pregnant women. Use only if potential benefit to the mother outweighs the potential risk to the fetus. A pregnancy registry has been established to monitor outcomes of women exposed to naratriptan during pregnancy (800-336-2176). In animal studies, administration was associated with embryolethality, fetal abnormalities, and pup mortality and growth retardation. Tremors were observed in the offspring of female rats when exposed to naratriptan late in gestation.

Natalizumab (na ta LIZ u mab)

Brand Names: U.S. Tysabri®

Brand Names: Canada Tysabri®

Pharmacologic Category Gastrointestinal Agent, Miscellaneous; Monoclonal Antibody, Selective Adhesion-Molecule Inhibitor

Use Monotherapy for the treatment of relapsing forms of multiple sclerosis; treatment of moderately- to severely-active Crohn's disease

Canada labeling: Treatment of relapsing forms of multiple sclerosis

Local Anesthetic/Vasoconstrictor Precautions No information available to require special precautions

Effects on Dental Treatment No significant effects or complications reported

Effects on Bleeding No information available to require special precautions

Adverse Effects

>10%:

Central nervous system: Headache (32% to 38%), fatigue (10% to 27%), depression (≤19%)

Dermatologic: Rash (6% to 12%)

Gastrointestinal: Nausea (≤17%), gastroenteritis (≤11%), abdominal discomfort (≤11%)

Genitourinary: Urinary tract infection (3% to 21%)

Neuromuscular & skeletal: Arthralgia (8% to 19%), extremity pain (16%), back pain (≤12%)

Respiratory: Upper respiratory infection (≤22%), lower respiratory infection (≤17%)

Miscellaneous: Infusion-related reaction (11% to 24%), influenza (≤12%), flu-like syndrome (≤11%)

1% to 10%:

Cardiovascular: Peripheral edema (5% to 6%), chest discomfort (≤5%)

Central nervous system: Vertigo (≤6%), dysesthesia (3%), syncope (≤2%), somnolence (≤2%)

Dermatologic: Dermatitis (≤7%), pruritus (≤4%), urticaria (≤2%), dry skin (≤1%)

Endocrine & metabolic: Dysmenorrhea (2% to 6%), menstrual irregularities (≤5%), amenorrhea (≤2%), ovarian cyst (≤2%)

Gastrointestinal: Diarrhea (10%), dyspepsia (≤5%), abdominal pain (≤4%), constipation (≤4%), flatulence (≤3%), aphthous stomatitis (≤2%), weight changes (≤2%), cholelithiasis (≤1%), gingival infection (1%)

Genitourinary: Vaginitis/vaginal infections (4% to 10%), urinary frequency (≤9%), urinary incontinence (≤4%)

Hematologic: Hematoma (1%)

Hepatic: Transaminase increased (≤5%)

Local: Bleeding at injection site (≤3%)

Neuromuscular & skeletal: Muscle cramp (≤5%), tremor (1% to 3%), rigors (≤3%), joint swelling (≤2%)

Respiratory: Sinusitis (≤8%), cough (≤7%), tonsillitis (≤7%), pharyngolaryngeal pain (≤6%), epistaxis (2%)

Miscellaneous: Antibody formation (9% to 10%), tooth infection (≤9%), herpes infection (≤8%), viral infection (≤7%), hypersensitivity reactions (acute: 2% to 4%; serious acute: ≤1%; delayed: ≤5%), toothache (≤4%), serious infection (2% to 3%), night sweats (≤1%)

General Dosage Range I.V.: *Adults:* 300 mg every 4 weeks

Mechanism of Action Natalizumab is a monoclonal antibody against the alpha-4 subunit of integrin molecules. These molecules are important to adhesion and migration of cells from the vasculature into inflamed tissue. Natalizumab blocks integrin association with vascular receptors, limiting adhesion and transmigration of leukocytes. Efficacy in specific disorders may be related to reduction in specific inflammatory cell populations in target tissues. In multiple sclerosis, efficacy may be related to blockade of T-lymphocyte migration into the central nervous system; treatment results in a decreased frequency of relapse. In Crohn's disease, natalizumab decreases inflammation by binding to alpha-4 integrin, blocking adhesion and migration of leukocytes in the gut.

Pharmacodynamics/Kinetics

Half-life Elimination Crohn's disease: 3-17 days; Multiple sclerosis: 7-15 days

Pregnancy Risk Factor C

Pregnancy Considerations Adverse events have been observed in animal studies. There are no adequate and well-controlled studies in pregnant women. Use only if clearly needed. Pregnant women exposed to natalizumab should be enrolled in the Tysabri® Pregnancy Exposure Registry (800-456-2255).

Prescribing and Access Restrictions

U.S.: Tysabri® is deemed to have an approved REMS program. As a requirement of the REMS program, access to this medication is restricted. Patients must be enrolled in the Tysabri® Outreach Unified Commitment to Health (TOUCH™) Prescribing Program (800-456-2255) to receive natalizumab (MS-TOUCH™ for multiple sclerosis or CD-TOUCH™ for Crohn's disease). Healthcare providers must also register with the program in order to prescribe, dispense or administer natalizumab. Treatment must be reauthorized every 6 months. Natalizumab is available only through infusion centers registered with the TOUCH™ program; infusion center information is available at 1-800-456-2255.

Canada: Patients receiving natalizumab therapy for multiple sclerosis are to be enrolled in the Tysabri Care Program™ (888-827-2827). This program is associated with the prescribing, administration, and monitoring of Canadian patients receiving natalizumab. Clinicians are educated on the appropriate use of natalizumab and are expected to discuss the benefits/risks of therapy. Clinicians should evaluate patients every 6 months during treatment.

Natamycin (na ta MYE sin)

Brand Names: U.S. Natacyn®
Brand Names: Canada Natacyn®
Pharmacologic Category Antifungal Agent, Ophthalmic
Use Treatment of blepharitis, conjunctivitis, and keratitis caused by susceptible fungi (*Aspergillus*, *Candida*, *Cephalosporium*, *Fusarium*, and *Penicillium*)
Local Anesthetic/Vasoconstrictor Precautions No information available to require special precautions
Effects on Dental Treatment No significant effects or complications reported
Effects on Bleeding No information available to require special precautions
Adverse Effects Postmarketing and/or case reports: Allergic reaction, chest pain, corneal opacity, dyspnea, eye discomfort, edema, hyperemia, irritation and/or pain, foreign body sensation, parasthesia, tearing, vision changes
General Dosage Range Ophthalmic: *Adults:* Initial: Instill 1 drop in conjunctival sac every 1-2 hours for 3-4 days; Maintenance: 1 drop 4-8 times/day
Mechanism of Action Increases cell membrane permeability in susceptible fungi
Pregnancy Risk Factor C
Pregnancy Considerations Animal reproduction studies have not been conducted.

Nateglinide (na te GLYE nide)

Related Information
Endocrine Disorders and Pregnancy *on page 1517*
Brand Names: U.S. Starlix®
Brand Names: Canada Starlix®
Pharmacologic Category Antidiabetic Agent, Meglitinide Derivative
Use Management of type 2 diabetes mellitus (noninsulin dependent, NIDDM) as monotherapy when hyperglycemia cannot be managed by diet and exercise alone; in combination with metformin or a thiazolidinedione to lower blood glucose in patients whose hyperglycemia cannot be controlled by exercise, diet, or a single agent alone
Local Anesthetic/Vasoconstrictor Precautions No information available to require special precautions
Effects on Dental Treatment No significant effects or complications reported
Effects on Bleeding May increase overall bleeding times
Adverse Effects As reported with nateglinide monotherapy:
>10%: Respiratory: Upper respiratory infection (11%)
1% to 10%:
Central nervous system: Dizziness (4%)
Endocrine & metabolic: Hypoglycemia (2%), uric acid increased
Gastrointestinal: Diarrhea (3%), weight gain

Neuromuscular & skeletal: Back pain, (4%), arthropathy (3%)
Respiratory: Bronchitis (3%), cough (2%)
Miscellaneous: Flu-like syndrome (4%)
General Dosage Range Oral: *Adults:* 60-120 mg 3 times/day
Mechanism of Action A phenylalanine derivative, non-sulfonylurea hypoglycemic agent used in the management of type 2 diabetes mellitus (noninsulin dependent, NIDDM); stimulates insulin release from the pancreatic beta cells to reduce postprandial hyperglycemia; amount of insulin release is dependent upon existing glucose levels
Pharmacodynamics/Kinetics
Onset of Action Insulin secretion: ~20 minutes; Peak effect: 1 hour
Duration of Action 4 hours
Half-life Elimination 1.5 hours
Time to Peak ≤1 hour
Pregnancy Risk Factor C
Pregnancy Considerations Adverse events have been observed in animal reproduction studies; therefore, nateglinide is classified as pregnancy category C. Information describing the effects of nateglinide on pregnancy outcomes is limited. Maternal hyperglycemia can be associated with adverse effects in the fetus, including macrosomia, neonatal hyperglycemia, and hyperbilirubinemia; the risk of congenital malformations is increased when the Hb A_{1c} is above the normal range. Diabetes can also be associated with adverse effects in the mother. Poorly-treated diabetes may cause end-organ damage that may in turn negatively affect obstetric outcomes. Physiologic glucose levels should be maintained prior to and during pregnancy to decrease the risk of adverse events in the mother and the fetus. Until additional safety and efficacy data are obtained, the use of oral agents is generally not recommended as routine management of GDM or type 2 diabetes mellitus during pregnancy. Insulin is the drug of choice for the control of diabetes mellitus during pregnancy.

Nebivolol (ne BIV oh lole)

Related Information
Cardiovascular Diseases *on page 1492*
Brand Names: U.S. Bystolic®
Brand Names: Canada Bystolic®
Generic Availability (U.S.) No
Pharmacologic Category Beta-Blocker, Beta-1 Selective
Use Treatment of hypertension, alone or in combination with other agents
Unlabeled Use Heart failure
Local Anesthetic/Vasoconstrictor Precautions No information available to require special precautions
Effects on Dental Treatment Nebivolol is a cardioselective beta-blocker. Local anesthetic with vasoconstrictor can be safely used in patients medicated with nebivolol. Nonselective beta-blockers (ie, propranolol, nadolol) enhance the pressor response to epinephrine, resulting in hypertension and bradycardia; this has not been reported for nebivolol. Many nonsteroidal anti-inflammatory drugs, such as ibuprofen and indomethacin, can reduce the hypotensive effect of beta-blockers after 3 or more weeks of therapy with the NSAID. Short-term NSAID use (ie, 3 days) requires no special precautions in patients taking beta-blockers.
Effects on Bleeding No information available to require special precautions

◀ **Adverse Effects** 1% to 10%:

Cardiovascular: Peripheral edema (1%), bradycardia (≤1%), chest pain (≤1%)

Central nervous system: Headache (6% to 9%), fatigue (dose related; 2% to 5%), dizziness (2% to 4%), insomnia (1%)

Dermatologic: Rash (≤1%)

Endocrine & metabolic: HDL levels decreased, hypercholesterolemia, triglyceride levels increased, uric acid levels increased

Gastrointestinal: Diarrhea (dose related; 2% to 3%), nausea (1% to 3%), abdominal pain

Hematologic: Platelet count decreased

Neuromuscular & skeletal: Paresthesia, weakness

Renal: BUN increased

Respiratory: Dyspnea (≤1%)

Dosage

Adults: Oral:

U.S. labeling: Hypertension: Initial: 5 mg once daily; if initial response is inadequate, may be increased at 2-week intervals to a maximum dose of 40 mg once daily

Canadian labeling: Hypertension: Initial: 5 mg once daily; if initial response is inadequate, may be increased at 2-week intervals to a maximum dose of 20 mg once daily

Unlabeled use: Heart failure: Adults ≥70 years: Initial: 1.25 mg once daily; if tolerated, may increase by 2.5 mg at 1- to 2-week intervals to a maximum dose of 10 mg once daily (Flather, 2005). **Note:** Nebivolol has not been shown to reduce mortality in the general HF population.

Elderly: Refer to adult dosing.

Dosing adjustment in renal impairment: Severe impairment (Cl$_{cr}$ <30 mL/minute): Initial: 2.5 mg daily; if initial response is inadequate, may increase cautiously.

Dosage adjustment in hepatic impairment:

Moderate impairment (Child-Pugh class B): Initial: 2.5 mg daily; if initial response is inadequate, may increase cautiously

Severe impairment (Child-Pugh class C): Use is contraindicated.

Mechanism of Action Highly-selective inhibitor of beta$_1$-adrenergic receptors; at doses ≤10 mg nebivolol preferentially blocks beta$_1$-receptors. Nebivolol, unlike other beta-blockers, also produces an endothelium-derived nitric oxide-dependent vasodilation resulting in a reduction of systemic vascular resistance.

Contraindications Hypersensitivity to nebivolol or any component of the formulation; severe bradycardia; heart block greater than first-degree (except in patients with a functioning artificial pacemaker); cardiogenic shock; decompensated heart failure; sick sinus syndrome (unless a permanent pacemaker is in place); severe hepatic impairment (Child-Pugh class C)

Canadian labeling: Additional contraindications (not in U.S. labeling): Severe peripheral arterial circulatory disorders; sinoatrial block

Warnings/Precautions Use caution in patients with heart failure (HF); use gradual and careful titration; monitor for symptoms of congestive heart failure. Patients should be stabilized on HF regimen prior to initiation of beta-blocker; adjustment of other medications (ACE inhibitors and/or diuretics) may be required. **Note:** Nebivolol has not been shown to reduce morbidity or mortality in the general HF population. Use with caution in patients with myasthenia gravis, psychiatric disease (may cause CNS depression), bronchospastic

disease, undergoing anesthesia; and in those with impaired hepatic function. Bradycardia may be observed more frequently in elderly patients (>65 years of age); dosage reductions may be necessary. Nebivolol should not be withdrawn abruptly (particularly in patients with CAD), but gradually tapered over 1-2 weeks to avoid acute tachycardia, hypertension, and/or ischemia. Chronic beta-blocker therapy should not be routinely withdrawn prior to major surgery. Can precipitate or aggravate symptoms of arterial insufficiency in patients with PVD and Raynaud's disease. Use with caution and monitor for progression of arterial obstruction (Canadian labeling contraindicates use in severe peripheral vascular disease). Potentially significant interactions may exist, requiring dose or frequency adjustment, additional monitoring, and/or selection of alternative therapy.

Nebivolol, with beta$_1$-selectivity, may be used cautiously in bronchospastic disease with close monitoring. Use cautiously in patients with diabetes because it can mask prominent hypoglycemic symptoms. May mask signs of hyperthyroidism (eg, tachycardia); if hyperthyroidism is suspected, carefully manage and monitor; abrupt withdrawal may exacerbate symptoms of hyperthyroidism or precipitate thyroid storm. Dosage adjustment is required in patients with moderate hepatic or severe renal impairment. Adequate alpha-blockade is required prior to use of any beta-blocker for patients with untreated pheochromocytoma. May induce or exacerbate psoriasis. Use caution with history of severe anaphylaxis to allergens; patients taking beta-blockers may become more sensitive to repeated challenges. Treatment of anaphylaxis (eg, epinephrine) in patients taking beta-blockers may be ineffective or promote undesirable effects.

Drug Interactions

Metabolism/Transport Effects Substrate of CYP2D6 (minor); **Note:** Assignment of Major/Minor substrate status based on clinically relevant drug interaction potential

Avoid Concomitant Use

Avoid concomitant use of Nebivolol with any of the following: Floctafenine; Methacholine

Increased Effect/Toxicity

Nebivolol may increase the levels/effects of: Alpha-/Beta-Agonists (Direct-Acting); Alpha1-Blockers; Alpha2-Agonists; Amifostine; Antihypertensives; Antipsychotic Agents (Phenothiazines); Bupivacaine; Cardiac Glycosides; Cholinergic Agonists; Ergot Derivatives; Fingolimod; Hypotensive Agents; Insulin; Lidocaine (Systemic); Lidocaine (Topical); Mepivacaine; Methacholine; Midodrine; RiTUXimab; Sulfonylureas

The levels/effects of Nebivolol may be increased by: Acetylcholinesterase Inhibitors; Alpha2-Agonists; Aminoquinolines (Antimalarial); Amiodarone; Anilidopiperidine Opioids; Antipsychotic Agents (Phenothiazines); Calcium Channel Blockers (Dihydropyridine); Calcium Channel Blockers (Nondihydropyridine); CYP2D6 Inhibitors (Moderate); CYP2D6 Inhibitors (Strong); Diazoxide; Dipyridamole; Disopyramide; Dronedarone; Floctafenine; Herbs (Hypotensive Properties); MAO Inhibitors; Pentoxifylline; Phosphodiesterase 5 Inhibitors; Propafenone; Prostacyclin Analogues; QuiNIDine; Reserpine; Selective Serotonin Reuptake Inhibitors

Decreased Effect

Nebivolol may decrease the levels/effects of: Beta2-Agonists; Theophylline Derivatives

The levels/effects of Nebivolol may be decreased by: Barbiturates; Herbs (Hypertensive Properties); Methylphenidate; Nonsteroidal Anti-Inflammatory Agents; Peginterferon Alfa-2b; Rifamycin Derivatives; Yohimbine

Ethanol/Nutrition/Herb Interactions Herb/Nutraceutical: Avoid bayberry, blue cohosh, cayenne, ephedra, ginger, ginseng (American), kola, licorice (may worsen hypertension). Avoid black cohosh, California poppy, coleus, golden seal, hawthorn, mistletoe, periwinkle, quinine, shepherd's purse (may increase antihypertensive effect).

Dietary Considerations May be taken without regard to meals.

Pharmacodynamics/Kinetics

Half-life Elimination Terminal: 12 hours (extensive metabolizers) or 19 hours (poor metabolizers); up to 32 hours has been reported in poor metabolizers (Mangrella, 1998).

Time to Peak 1.5-4 hours

Pregnancy Risk Factor C

Pregnancy Considerations Adverse events have been observed in some animal reproduction studies; therefore, nebivolol is classified as pregnancy category C. In a cohort study, an increased risk of cardiovascular defects was observed following maternal use of beta-blockers during pregnancy. Intrauterine growth restriction (IUGR), small placentas, as well as fetal/neonatal bradycardia, hypoglycemia, and/or respiratory depression have been observed following *in utero* exposure to beta-blockers as a class. Adequate facilities for monitoring infants at birth should be available. Untreated chronic maternal hypertension and pre-eclampsia are also associated with adverse events in the fetus, infant, and mother. Information related to the use of nebivolol for the treatment of hypertension in pregnancy has not been located; other agents may be more appropriate for use.

Lactation Excretion in breast milk unknown/not recommended

Breast-Feeding Considerations It is not known if nebivolol is excreted into breast milk. Breast-feeding is not recommended by the manufacturer due to potential for beta-blockers to produce serious effects on nursing infants, especially bradycardia.

Dosage Forms
Tablet, oral:
Bystolic®: 2.5 mg, 5 mg, 10 mg, 20 mg

Nedocromil (ne doe KROE mil)

Brand Names: U.S. Alocril®
Brand Names: Canada Alocril®
Pharmacologic Category Mast Cell Stabilizer
Use Treatment of itching associated with allergic conjunctivitis
Local Anesthetic/Vasoconstrictor Precautions No information available to require special precautions
Effects on Dental Treatment Key adverse event(s) related to dental treatment: Unpleasant taste.
Effects on Bleeding No information available to require special precautions
Adverse Effects
>10%:
Central nervous system: Headache (40%)
Gastrointestinal: Unpleasant taste
Ocular: Burning, irritation, stinging
Respiratory: Nasal congestion

1% to 10%:
Ocular: Conjunctivitis, eye redness, photophobia
Respiratory: Asthma, rhinitis

General Dosage Range
Ophthalmic: *Children ≥3 years and Adults:* 1-2 drops in each eye twice daily

Mechanism of Action Inhibits the activation of and mediator release from a variety of inflammatory cell types associated with hypersensitivity reactions including eosinophils, neutrophils, macrophages, mast cells, monocytes, and platelets; it inhibits the release of histamine, leukotrienes, and slow-reacting substance of anaphylaxis.

Pregnancy Risk Factor B

Pregnancy Considerations There are no well-controlled studies in pregnant women. Animal studies show no evidence of teratogenicity or harm to fetus. Additionally, nedocromil has minimal systemic absorption.

Nefazodone (nef AY zoe done)

Related Information
Vasoconstrictor Interactions With Antidepressants *on page 1650*

Pharmacologic Category Antidepressant, Serotonin Reuptake Inhibitor/Antagonist

Use Treatment of depression

Unlabeled Use Post-traumatic stress disorder (PTSD)

Local Anesthetic/Vasoconstrictor Precautions Nefazodone inhibits reuptake of both serotonin and norepinephrine and also blocks some serotonin receptors. No precautions with vasoconstrictors appear to be necessary.

Effects on Dental Treatment Key adverse event(s) related to dental treatment: Significant xerostomia (normal salivary flow resumes upon discontinuation) and taste perversion.

Effects on Bleeding No information available to require special precautions

Adverse Effects
>10%:
Central nervous system: Headache, drowsiness, insomnia, agitation, dizziness
Gastrointestinal: Xerostomia, nausea, constipation
Neuromuscular & skeletal: Weakness

1% to 10%:
Cardiovascular: Bradycardia, hypotension, orthostatic hypotension, peripheral edema, vasodilation
Central nervous system: Chills, fever, incoordination, lightheadedness, confusion, memory impairment, abnormal dreams, decreased concentration, ataxia, psychomotor retardation, tremor
Dermatologic: Pruritus, rash
Endocrine & metabolic: Breast pain, impotence, libido decreased
Gastrointestinal: Gastroenteritis, vomiting, dyspepsia, diarrhea, increased appetite, thirst, taste perversion
Genitourinary: Urinary frequency, urinary retention
Hematologic: Hematocrit decreased
Neuromuscular & skeletal: Arthralgia, hypertonia, paresthesia, neck rigidity, tremor
Ocular: Blurred vision (9%), abnormal vision (7%), eye pain, visual field defect
Otic: Tinnitus
Respiratory: Bronchitis, cough, dyspnea, pharyngitis
Miscellaneous: Flu syndrome, infection

965

General Dosage Range Oral:

Adults: Initial: 200 mg/day in 2 divided doses; Maintenance: 300-600 mg/day in 2 divided doses

Elderly: Initial: 50 mg twice daily; Maintenance: 200-400 mg/day in 2 divided doses

Mechanism of Action Inhibits neuronal reuptake of serotonin and norepinephrine; also blocks 5-HT_2 and $alpha_1$ receptors; has no significant affinity for $alpha_2$, beta-adrenergic, 5-HT_{1A}, cholinergic, dopaminergic, or benzodiazepine receptors

Pharmacodynamics/Kinetics

Onset of Action Therapeutic: Up to 6 weeks

Half-life Elimination Parent drug: 2-4 hours; active metabolites persist longer

Time to Peak Serum: 1 hour, prolonged in presence of food

Pregnancy Risk Factor C

Pregnancy Considerations Adverse effects were observed in some animal reproduction studies. When nefazodone is taken during pregnancy, an increased risk of major malformations has not been observed in the limited number of pregnancies studied (Einarson, 2003; Einarson, 2009). The long-term effects of *in utero* exposure to nefazodone on infant development and behavior are not known.

The ACOG recommends that therapy with antidepressants during pregnancy be individualized; treatment of depression during pregnancy should incorporate the clinical expertise of the mental health clinician, obstetrician, primary healthcare provider, and pediatrician. According to the American Psychiatric Association (APA), the risks of medication treatment should be weighed against other treatment options and untreated depression. Consideration should be given to using agents with safety data in pregnancy. For women who discontinue antidepressant medications during pregnancy and who may be at high risk for postpartum depression, the medications can be restarted following delivery. Treatment algorithms have been developed by the ACOG and the APA for the management of depression in women prior to conception and during pregnancy (ACOG, 2008; APA, 2010; Yonkers, 2009).

Nelarabine (nel AY re been)

Brand Names: U.S. Arranon®

Brand Names: Canada Atriance™

Pharmacologic Category Antineoplastic Agent, Antimetabolite; Antineoplastic Agent, Antimetabolite (Purine Analog)

Use Treatment of relapsed or refractory T-cell acute lymphoblastic leukemia (ALL) and T-cell lymphoblastic lymphoma

Local Anesthetic/Vasoconstrictor Precautions No information available to require special precautions

Effects on Dental Treatment Key adverse event(s) related to dental treatment: Taste perversion and stomatitis.

Effects on Bleeding Chemotherapy may result in significant myelosuppression. Thrombocytopenia has been reported in 86% to 88% (grade 4: 22% to 32%). Nosebleeds have occurred in 8% of patients. In patients who are under active treatment with these agents, medical consult is suggested.

Adverse Effects Note: Pediatric adverse reactions fell within a range similar to adults except where noted.

>10%:

Cardiovascular: Peripheral edema (15%), edema (11%)

Central nervous system: Fatigue (50%), fever (23%), somnolence (7% to 23%; grades 2-4: 1% to 6%), dizziness (21%; grade 2: 8% adults), headache (15% to 17%; grades 2-4: 4% to 8%), hypoesthesia (6% to 17%; grades 2/3: children 5%, adults 12%), pain (11%)

Dermatologic: Petechiae (12%)

Endocrine & metabolic: Hypokalemia (11%)

Gastrointestinal: Nausea (41%), diarrhea (22%), vomiting (10% to 22%), constipation (21%)

Hematologic: Anemia (95% to 99%; grade 4: 10% to 14%), neutropenia (81% to 94%; grade 4: children 62%, adults 49%), thrombocytopenia (86% to 88%; grade 4: 22% to 32%), leukopenia (38%; grade 4: 7%), neutropenic fever (12%; grade 4: 1%)

Hepatic: Transaminases increased (12%; grade 3: 4%)

Neuromuscular & skeletal: Peripheral neuropathy (12% to 21%; grades 2/3: 11% to 14%), weakness (6% to 17%; grade 4: 1%), paresthesia (4% to 15%; grades 2/3: 3% to 4%), myalgia (13%)

Respiratory: Cough (25%), dyspnea (7% to 20%)

1% to 10%:

Cardiovascular: Hypotension (8%), sinus tachycardia (8%), chest pain (5%)

Central nervous system: Ataxia (2% to 9%; grades 2/3: children 1%, adults 8%), confusion (8%), insomnia (7%), depressed level of consciousness (6%; grades 2-4: 2%), depression (6%), seizure (grade 3: 1% adults; grade 4: 6% children), motor dysfunction (4%; grades 2/3: 2%), amnesia (3%; grade 2: 1%), balance disorder (2%; grade 2: 1%), sensory loss (1% to 2%), aphasia (grade 3: 1%), attention disturbance (1%), cerebral hemorrhage (grade 4: 1%), coma (grade 4: 1%), encephalopathy (grade 4: 1%), hemiparesis (grade 3: 1%), hydrocephalus (1%), intracranial hemorrhage (grade 4: 1%), lethargy (1%), leukoencephalopathy (grade 4: 1%), loss of consciousness (grade 3: 1%), mental impairment (1%), nerve paralysis (1%), neuropathic pain (1%), nerve palsy (1%), paralysis (1%), sciatica (1%), sensory disturbance (1%), speech disorder (1%)

Endocrine & Metabolic: Hypocalcemia (8%), dehydration (7%), hyper-/hypoglycemia (6%), hypomagnesemia (6%)

Gastrointestinal: Abdominal pain (9%), anorexia (9%), stomatitis (8%), abdominal distension (6%), taste perversion (3%)

Hepatic: Albumin decreased (10%), bilirubin increased (10%; grade 3: 7%, grade 4: 2%), AST increased (6%)

Neuromuscular & skeletal: Arthralgia (9%), back pain (8%), muscle weakness (8%), rigors (8%), limb pain (7%), abnormal gait (6%), noncardiac chest pain (5%), tremor (4% to 5%; grade 2: 2% to 3%), dysarthria (1%), hyporeflexia (1%), hypertonia (1%), incoordination (1%)

Ocular: Blurred vision (4%), nystagmus (1%)

Renal: Creatinine increased (6%)

Respiratory: Pleural effusion (10%), epistaxis (8%), pneumonia (8%), sinusitis (7%), wheezing (5%), sinus headache (3%)

Miscellaneous: Infection (5% to 9%)

General Dosage Range I.V.:

Children: 650 mg/m^2/dose on days 1 through 5; repeat every 21 days

Adults: 1500 mg/m^2/dose on days 1, 3, and 5; repeat every 21 days

Mechanism of Action Nelarabine, a prodrug of ara-G, is demethylated by adenosine deaminase to ara-G and then converted to ara-GTP. Ara-GTP is incorporated into the DNA of the leukemic blasts, leading to inhibition of DNA synthesis and inducing apoptosis. Ara-GTP appears to accumulate at higher levels in T-cells, which correlates to clinical response.

Pharmacodynamics/Kinetics

Half-life Elimination Children: Nelarabine: 13 minutes, Ara-G: 2 hours; Adults: Nelarabine: 18 minutes, Ara-G: 3 hours

Time to Peak Adults: 3-25 hours (of day 1)

Pregnancy Risk Factor D

Pregnancy Considerations Teratogenic effects were observed in animal reproduction studies. May cause fetal harm if administered during pregnancy. Women of childbearing potential should be advised to use effective contraception and avoid becoming pregnant during therapy.

Nelfinavir (nel FIN a veer)

Related Information

HIV Infection and AIDS *on page 1520*

Viral Infections *on page 1575*

Brand Names: U.S. Viracept®

Brand Names: Canada Viracept®

Generic Availability (U.S.) No

Pharmacologic Category Antiretroviral Agent, Protease Inhibitor

Use In combination with other antiretroviral therapy in the treatment of HIV infection

Local Anesthetic/Vasoconstrictor Precautions No information available to require special precautions

Effects on Dental Treatment Key adverse event(s) related to dental treatment: Mouth ulcers.

Effects on Bleeding Increased bleeding has been noted with protease inhibitors in patients with hemophilia A or B. No information available to require routine special precautions relative to hemostasis in other patients.

Adverse Effects Data presented on experience in adults, unless otherwise noted.

>10%: Gastrointestinal: Diarrhea (14% to 20%; children: 39% to 47%)

2% to 10%:

Dermatologic: Rash (1% to 3%)

Gastrointestinal: Nausea (3% to 7%), flatulence (1% to 5%)

Hematologic: Lymphocytes decreased (1% to 6%), neutrophils decreased (1% to 5%)

Dosage Oral:

Children 2-13 years: 45-55 mg/kg twice daily **or** 25-35 mg/kg 3 times/day (maximum: 2500 mg/day). If tablets are unable to be taken, use oral powder in small amount of water, milk (cow's or soy), formula, or dietary supplements; do not use acidic food/juice or store for >6 hours.

Adults: 750 mg 3 times/day or 1250 mg twice daily with meals in combination with other antiretroviral therapies. **Note:** The DHHS Perinatal HIV Guidelines do not recommend the 3 times/day dosing in pregnant women (DHHS [perinatal], 2012).

Dosage adjustment in renal impairment: No dosage adjustment provided in manufacturer's labeling (has not been studied). However, since <2% excreted in urine a dosage reduction would not be expected

Dosage adjustment in hepatic impairment: No dosage adjustment necessary in mild impairment (Child-Pugh class A); not recommended in patients with moderate-to-severe impairment (Child-Pugh class B or C)

Mechanism of Action Binds to the site of HIV-1 protease activity and inhibits cleavage of viral Gag-Pol polyprotein precursors into individual functional proteins required for infectious HIV. This results in the formation of immature, noninfectious viral particles.

Contraindications Hypersensitivity to nelfinavir or any component of the formulation; concurrent therapy with alfuzosin, amiodarone, cisapride, ergot derivatives, lovastatin, midazolam (oral), pimozide, quinidine, rifampin, sildenafil (when used for pulmonary artery hypertension [eg, Revatio®]), simvastatin, St John's wort, triazolam

Warnings/Precautions High potential for drug interactions; concomitant use of nelfinavir with some drugs may require cautious use, may not be recommended, may require dosage adjustments, or may be contraindicated.

Use caution with hepatic impairment; use not recommended with moderate-to-severe impairment. Warn patients that redistribution of body fat can occur. New-onset diabetes mellitus, exacerbation of diabetes, and hyperglycemia have been reported in HIV-infected patients receiving protease inhibitors. Use with caution in patients with hemophilia A or B; increased bleeding during protease inhibitor therapy has been reported. Patients may develop immune reconstitution syndrome resulting in the occurrence of an inflammatory response to an indolent or residual opportunistic infection during initial HIV treatment or activation of autoimmune disorders (eg, Graves' disease, polymyositis, Guillain-Barré syndrome) later in therapy; further evaluation and treatment may be required.

The oral powder contains phenylalanine.

Drug Interactions

Metabolism/Transport Effects Substrate of CYP2C19 (major), CYP2C9 (minor), CYP2D6 (minor), CYP3A4 (major), P-glycoprotein; **Note:** Assignment of Major/Minor substrate status based on clinically relevant drug interaction potential; **Inhibits** CYP1A2 (weak), CYP2B6 (weak), CYP2C19 (weak), CYP2C9 (weak), CYP2D6 (weak), CYP3A4 (strong), P-glycoprotein

Avoid Concomitant Use

Avoid concomitant use of Nelfinavir with any of the following: Ado-Trastuzumab Emtansine; Alfuzosin; Amiodarone; Apixaban; Avanafil; Axitinib; Bosutinib; Cabozantinib; Cisapride; Conivaptan; Crizotinib; Dronedarone; Eplerenone; Ergot Derivatives; Everolimus; Fluticasone (Oral Inhalation); Halofantrine; Ivabradine; Lapatinib; Lomitapide; Lovastatin; Lurasidone; Midazolam; Nilotinib; Nisoldipine; Pimozide; Pomalidomide; Proton Pump Inhibitors; QuiNIDine; Ranolazine; Red Yeast Rice; Regorafenib; Rifampin; Rivaroxaban; RomiDEPsin; Salmeterol; Silodosin; Simvastatin; St Johns Wort; Tamsulosin; Ticagrelor; Tolvaptan; Topotecan; Toremifene; Triazolam; VinCRIStine (Liposomal)

Increased Effect/Toxicity

Nelfinavir may increase the levels/effects of: Ado-Trastuzumab Emtansine; Alfuzosin; Almotriptan; Alosetron; ALPRAZolam; Amiodarone; Apixaban; ARIPiprazole; AtorvaSTATin; Avanafil; Axitinib; Azithromycin (Systemic); Bedaquiline; Bortezomib; Bosentan; Bosutinib; Brentuximab Vedotin; Brinzolamide; Budesonide (Nasal); Budesonide (Systemic, Oral Inhalation);

Cabozantinib; Calcium Channel Blockers (Dihydropyridine); Calcium Channel Blockers (Nondihydropyridine); CarBAMazepine; Cisapride; Clarithromycin; Colchicine; Conivaptan; Corticosteroids (Orally Inhaled); Crizotinib; CycloSPORINE (Systemic); CYP3A4 Substrates; Dabigatran Etexilate; Dienogest; Digoxin; Dronedarone; Dutasteride; Enfuvirtide; Enzalutamide; Eplerenone; Ergot Derivatives; Everolimus; FentaNYL; Fesoterodine; Fluticasone (Nasal); Fluticasone (Oral Inhalation); Fusidic Acid; GuanFACINE; Halofantrine; Iloperidone; Ivabradine; Ivacaftor; Ixabepilone; Lapatinib; Lomitapide; Lovastatin; Lumefantrine; Lurasidone; Maraviroc; Meperidine; MethylPREDNISolone; Midazolam; Mifepristone; Nefazodone; Nilotinib; Nisoldipine; Ospemifene; Paricalcitol; Pazopanib; P-glycoprotein/ABCB1 Substrates; Pimecrolimus; Pimozide; Pomalidomide; Ponatinib; Propafenone; Protease Inhibitors; Prucalopride; QuiNIDine; Ranolazine; Red Yeast Rice; Regorafenib; Rifabutin; Rivaroxaban; RomiDEPsin; Rosuvastatin; Ruxolitinib; Salmeterol; Saxagliptin; Sildenafil; Silodosin; Simvastatin; Sirolimus; SORAfenib; Tacrolimus (Systemic); Tacrolimus (Topical); Tadalafil; Tamsulosin; Temsirolimus; Tenofovir; Ticagrelor; Tofacitinib; Tolterodine; Tolvaptan; Topotecan; Toremifene; TraZODone; Triazolam; Tricyclic Antidepressants; Vardenafil; Vemurafenib; Vilazodone; VinCRIStine (Liposomal); Warfarin; Zuclopenthixol

The levels/effects of Nelfinavir may be increased by: Clarithromycin; CycloSPORINE (Systemic); Delavirdine; Enfuvirtide; Etravirine; Fusidic Acid; Lopinavir; P-glycoprotein/ABCB1 Inhibitors; Voriconazole

Decreased Effect

Nelfinavir may decrease the levels/effects of: Abacavir; Boceprevir; Clarithromycin; Contraceptives (Estrogens); Delavirdine; Divalproex; Etravirine; Ifosfamide; Lopinavir; Meperidine; Methadone; Phenytoin; Prasugrel; Pravastatin; Theophylline Derivatives; Ticagrelor; Valproic Acid; Warfarin; Zidovudine

The levels/effects of Nelfinavir may be decreased by: Antacids; Boceprevir; Bosentan; CarBAMazepine; CYP2C19 Inducers (Strong); CYP3A4 Inducers (Strong); Deferasirox; Fosphenytoin; Garlic; H2-Antagonists; Nevirapine; Peginterferon Alfa-2b; P-glycoprotein/ABCB1 Inducers; Proton Pump Inhibitors; Rifabutin; Rifampin; St Johns Wort; Tenofovir; Tocilizumab

Ethanol/Nutrition/Herb Interactions

Food: Nelfinavir taken with food increases plasma concentration time curve (AUC) by two- to threefold. Do not administer with acidic food or juice (orange juice, apple juice, or applesauce) since the combination may have a bitter taste.

Herb/Nutraceutical: St John's wort may decrease the levels/effects of protease inhibitors; concurrent use should probably be avoided.

Dietary Considerations Should be taken as scheduled with a meal. Some products may contain phenylalanine.

Pharmacodynamics/Kinetics

Half-life Elimination 3.5-5 hours

Time to Peak Serum: 2-4 hours

Pregnancy Risk Factor B

Pregnancy Considerations Adverse events were not observed in animal reproduction studies. Nelfinavir crosses the placenta. A modest increased risk of overall birth defects has been observed following first trimester exposure in humans according to data collected by the antiretroviral pregnancy registry. However, no pattern of defects has been detected. The DHHS Perinatal HIV Guidelines recommend nelfinavir to be used only in special circumstances during pregnancy for the prophylaxis of perinatal transmission in antiretroviral-naive women when alternative agents cannot be tolerated. A dose of 1250 mg twice daily has been shown to provide adequate plasma concentrations although lower and variable levels may occur late in pregnancy. A small increased risk of preterm birth has been associated with maternal use of protease inhibitor-based combination antiretroviral (ARV) therapy during pregnancy; however, the benefits of use generally outweigh this risk and protease inhibitors (PIs) should not be withheld if otherwise recommended. Hyperglycemia, new onset of diabetes mellitus, or diabetic ketoacidosis have been reported with PIs; it is not clear if pregnancy increases this risk.

Regardless of CD4 count or HIV RNA copy number, all HIV-infected pregnant women should receive a combination antepartum ARV drug regimen; this includes women who require therapy for their own health, as well as women who do not yet require therapy for their own health. ARV therapy should be started as soon as possible if required for the woman's health. Although earlier initiation may be more effective in reducing the perinatal transmission of HIV, also consider maternal conditions (eg, nausea and vomiting) and the potential risks of first trimester fetal exposure for specific agents. Plasma HIV RNA levels should be assessed at ~34-36 weeks gestation in order to help determine mode of delivery. If ARV therapy must be interrupted for <24 hours during the peripartum period, stop then restart all medications simultaneously in order to decrease the chance of developing resistance. Long-term follow-up is recommended for all infants exposed to ARV medications.

Healthcare providers are encouraged to enroll pregnant women exposed to antiretroviral medications in the Antiretroviral Pregnancy Registry (1-800-258-4263 or www.APRegistry.com). Healthcare providers caring for HIV-infected women and their infants may contact the National Perinatal HIV Hotline (888-448-8765) for clinical consultation (DHHS [perinatal], 2012).

Lactation Excretion in breast milk unknown/contraindicated

Breast-Feeding Considerations Maternal or infant antiretroviral therapy does not completely eliminate the risk of postnatal HIV transmission. In addition, multi-class-resistant virus has been detected in breast-feeding infants despite maternal therapy. Therefore, in the United States, where formula is accessible, affordable, safe, and sustainable, and the risk of infant mortality due to diarrhea and respiratory infections is low, complete avoidance of breast-feeding by HIV-infected women is recommended to decrease potential transmission of HIV (DHHS [perinatal], 2012).

Dosage Forms

Tablet, oral:

Viracept®: 250 mg, 625 mg

Neomycin (nee oh MYE sin)

Pharmacologic Category Ammonium Detoxicant; Antibiotic, Aminoglycoside; Antibiotic, Topical

Use Orally to prepare GI tract for surgery; treatment of diarrhea caused by *E. coli*; adjunct in the treatment of hepatic encephalopathy

Local Anesthetic/Vasoconstrictor Precautions No information available to require special precautions

Effects on Dental Treatment No significant effects or complications reported

Effects on Bleeding No information available to require special precautions

Adverse Effects

>10%: Gastrointestinal: Nausea, diarrhea, vomiting, irritation or soreness of the mouth or rectal area

General Dosage Range Oral:

Children: Encephalopathy: 50-100 mg/kg/day divided every 6-8 hours **or** 2.5-7 g/m^2/day divided every 4-6 hours (maximum: 12 g/day); Preoperative GI preparation: 75-90 mg/kg/day

Adults: Encephalopathy/hepatic insufficiency: 500 mg to 12 g/day in divided doses every 4-8 hours; Preoperative GI preparation: 1 g for 3-9 doses

Mechanism of Action Interferes with bacterial protein synthesis by binding to 30S ribosomal subunits

Pharmacodynamics/Kinetics

Half-life Elimination Age and renal function dependent: 3 hours

Time to Peak Serum: Oral: 1-4 hours

Pregnancy Risk Factor D

Pregnancy Considerations Aminoglycosides cross the placenta; however, neomycin has limited maternal absorption. Therefore the portion of an orally administered maternal dose available to cross the placenta is very low. Teratogenic effects have not been observed following maternal use of neomycin. Because of several reports of total irreversible bilateral congenital deafness in children whose mothers received another aminoglycoside (streptomycin) during pregnancy, the manufacturer classifies neomycin as pregnancy category D.

Neomycin and Polymyxin B
(nee oh MYE sin & pol i MIKS in bee)

Related Information

Neomycin *on page 968*

Polymyxin B *on page 1112*

Brand Names: U.S. Neosporin® G.U. Irrigant

Brand Names: Canada Neosporin® Irrigating Solution

Pharmacologic Category Antibiotic, Topical; Genitourinary Irrigant

Use Short-term as a continuous irrigant or rinse in the urinary bladder to prevent bacteriuria and gram-negative rod septicemia associated with the use of indwelling catheters

Local Anesthetic/Vasoconstrictor Precautions No information available to require special precautions

Effects on Dental Treatment No significant effects or complications reported

Effects on Bleeding No information available to require special precautions

Adverse Effects Frequency not defined.

Dermatologic: Contact dermatitis, erythema, rash, urticaria

Genitourinary: Bladder irritation

Local: Burning

Neuromuscular & skeletal: Neuromuscular blockade

Otic: Ototoxicity

Renal: Nephrotoxicity

General Dosage Range Irrigation (bladder): *Children and Adults:* Add 1 mL irrigant to 1 L isotonic saline solution (maximum: Usually no more than 1 L irrigant/day)

Mechanism of Action See individual agents.

Pregnancy Risk Factor D

Pregnancy Considerations Because of several reports of total irreversible bilateral congenital deafness in children whose mothers received streptomycin during pregnancy, the manufacturer classifies neomycin and polymyxin B as pregnancy risk factor D. See individual agents.

Neomycin, Polymyxin B, and Dexamethasone
(nee oh MYE sin, pol i MIKS in bee, & deks a METH a sone)

Related Information

Neomycin *on page 968*

Polymyxin B *on page 1112*

Brand Names: U.S. Maxitrol®

Brand Names: Canada Dioptrol®; Maxitrol®

Pharmacologic Category Antibiotic/Corticosteroid, Ophthalmic

Use Steroid-responsive inflammatory ocular conditions in which a corticosteroid is indicated and where bacterial infection or a risk of bacterial infection exists

Local Anesthetic/Vasoconstrictor Precautions No information available to require special precautions

Effects on Dental Treatment No significant effects or complications reported

Effects on Bleeding No information available to require special precautions

Adverse Effects See individual agents.

General Dosage Range Ophthalmic:

Ointment: *Adults:* Place ~1/2" ribbon in the conjunctival sac of the affected eye(s) 3-4 times/day or at bedtime as an adjunct with suspension

Suspension: *Children ≥2 years and Adults:* Instill 1-2 drops in the conjunctival sac of the affected eye(s) 4-6 times/day

Mechanism of Action See individual agents.

Pregnancy Risk Factor C

Pregnancy Considerations Animal reproduction studies have not been conducted with this combination. See individual agents.

Neomycin, Polymyxin B, and Gramicidin
(nee oh MYE sin, pol i MIKS in bee, & gram i SYE din)

Related Information

Neomycin *on page 968*

Polymyxin B *on page 1112*

Brand Names: U.S. Neosporin® Ophthalmic Solution

Brand Names: Canada Neosporin®; Optimyxin Plus®

Pharmacologic Category Antibiotic, Ophthalmic

Use Treatment of superficial ocular infection

Local Anesthetic/Vasoconstrictor Precautions No information available to require special precautions

Effects on Dental Treatment No significant effects or complications reported

Effects on Bleeding No information available to require special precautions

Adverse Effects Frequency not defined: Ocular: Transient irritation, burning, stinging, itching, inflammation, angioneurotic edema, urticaria, vesicular and maculopapular dermatitis

General Dosage Range Ophthalmic: *Children and Adults:* Instill 1-2 drops 4-6 times/day

◀ **Mechanism of Action** Interferes with bacterial protein synthesis by binding to 30S ribosomal subunits; binds to phospholipids, alters permeability, and damages the bacterial cytoplasmic membrane permitting leakage of intracellular constituents

Pregnancy Risk Factor C

Pregnancy Considerations Reproduction studies have not been conducted with this combination; therefore, Neomycin, Polymyxin B, and Gramicidin is classified as pregnancy category C. See individual monographs for Neomycin and Polymyxin B.

Neomycin, Polymyxin B, and Hydrocortisone
(nee oh MYE sin, pol i MIKS in bee, & hye droe KOR ti sone)

Related Information
Hydrocortisone (Topical) *on page 699*
Neomycin *on page 968*
Polymyxin B *on page 1112*
Brand Names: U.S. Cortisporin®; Cortomycin
Brand Names: Canada Cortimyxin®; Cortisporin® Otic
Pharmacologic Category Antibiotic, Ophthalmic; Antibiotic, Otic; Antibiotic, Topical; Antibiotic/Corticosteroid, Otic; Corticosteroid, Ophthalmic; Corticosteroid, Otic; Corticosteroid, Topical
Use Steroid-responsive inflammatory condition for which a corticosteroid is indicated and where bacterial infection or a risk of bacterial infection exists
Local Anesthetic/Vasoconstrictor Precautions No information available to require special precautions
Effects on Dental Treatment No significant effects or complications reported
Effects on Bleeding No information available to require special precautions
Adverse Effects Frequency not defined. For additional information, see individual agents.

Ophthalmic ointment:
Dermatologic: Delayed wound healing, rash
Ocular: Cataracts, corneal thinning, glaucoma, irritation, keratitis (bacterial), intraocular pressure increase, optic nerve damage, scleral thinning
Miscellaneous: Hypersensitivity (including anaphylaxis), secondary infection, sensitization to kanamycin, paromomycin, streptomycin, and gentamicin

Otic solution and suspension:
Dermatologic: Acneiform eruptions, allergic contact dermatitis, burning skin, dryness, folliculitis, hypertrichosis, hypopigmentation, irritation, maceration of skin, miliaria, ocular hypertension, perioral dermatitis, pruritus, skin atrophy, striae
Otic: Burning, ototoxicity, stinging
Renal: Nephrotoxicity
Miscellaneous: Hypersensitivity (including anaphylaxis), secondary infection, sensitization to karamycin, paromycin, streptomycin, and gentamicin

General Dosage Range
Ophthalmic: *Adults:* Instill 1-2 drops every 3-4 hours, or more frequently
Otic:
Children ≥2 years: Instill 3 drops into affected ear 3-4 times/day
Children ≥12 years and Adults: Instill 4 drops into affected ear 3-4 times/day
Topical: *Adults:* Apply a thin layer 1-4 times/day
Mechanism of Action See individual agents.
Pregnancy Risk Factor C

Pregnancy Considerations Animal reproduction studies have not been conducted with this combination. See individual agents.

Nepafenac (ne pa FEN ak)

Brand Names: U.S. Ilevro™; Nevanac®
Brand Names: Canada Nevanac®
Pharmacologic Category Nonsteroidal Anti-inflammatory Drug (NSAID), Ophthalmic
Use Treatment of pain and inflammation associated with cataract surgery
Local Anesthetic/Vasoconstrictor Precautions No information available to require special precautions
Effects on Dental Treatment The dentist should be aware of the potential of abnormal coagulation. Caution should also be exercised in the use of NSAIDs in patients already on anticoagulant therapy with drugs such as warfarin (Coumadin®). See Effects on Bleeding.
Effects on Bleeding Nonselective NSAIDs, such as nepafenac, inhibit platelet aggregation and prolong bleeding time in some patients. Unlike aspirin, the NSAID effect on platelet function is quantitatively less, of shorter duration, and reversible. Normal platelet function should occur in ~5 elimination half-lives or in <10 hours after discontinuation of nepafenac. Concomitant use of other NSAIDs should be avoided.
Adverse Effects 1% to 10%:
Cardiovascular: Hypertension (1% to 4%)
Central nervous system: Headache (1% to 4%)
Gastrointestinal: Nausea (1% to 4%), vomiting (1% to 4%)
Ocular: Capsular opacity (5% to 10%), foreign body sensation (5% to 10%), intraocular pressure increased (5% to 10%), sticky sensation (5% to 10%), visual acuity decreased (5% to 10%), conjunctival edema (1% to 5%), corneal edema (1% to 5%), dry eye (1% to 5%), lid margin crusting (1% to 5%), ocular discomfort (1% to 5%), ocular hyperemia (1% to 5%), ocular pain (1% to 5%), ocular pruritus (1% to 5%), photophobia (1% to 5%), tearing (1% to 5%), vitreous detachment (1% to 5%)
Respiratory: Sinusitis (1% to 4%)
General Dosage Range Ophthalmic: *Children ≥10 years, Adolescents, and Adults:*
Ilevro™: Instill 1 drop into affected eye(s) once daily
Nevanac®: Instill 1 drop into affected eye(s) 3 times/day
Mechanism of Action Nepafenac is a prodrug which once converted to amfenac inhibits prostaglandin synthesis by decreasing the activity of the enzyme, cyclooxygenase, which results in decreased formation of prostaglandin precursors.
Pregnancy Risk Factor C
Pregnancy Considerations Teratogenic events were not observed in animal reproduction studies. Exposure to nonsteroidal anti-inflammatory drugs late in pregnancy may lead to premature closure of the ductus arteriosus.
Product Availability Ilevro™ 0.3% ophthalmic suspension: FDA approved December 2012; availability anticipated in January 2013. Consult prescribing information for additional detail.

Nesiritide (ni SIR i tide)

Brand Names: U.S. Natrecor®
Pharmacologic Category Natriuretic Peptide, B-Type, Human

Use Treatment of acutely decompensated heart failure (HF) with dyspnea at rest or with minimal activity

Local Anesthetic/Vasoconstrictor Precautions No information available to require special precautions

Effects on Dental Treatment No significant effects or complications reported

Effects on Bleeding No information available to require special precautions

Adverse Effects Note: Frequencies cited below were recorded in VMAC trial, unless otherwise noted, at dosages similar to approved labeling. Higher frequencies have been observed in trials using higher dosages of nesiritide. The percentages marked with an asterisk (*) indicate frequency less than or equal to placebo or other standard therapy.

>10%:

Cardiovascular: Hypotension (total: 11% [27% in ASCEND-HF trial]; symptomatic: 4% [7% in ASCEND-HF trial] at recommended dose, up to 17% at higher doses)

Renal: Increased serum creatinine (28% with >0.5 mg/dL increase over baseline)

1% to 10%:

Cardiovascular: Ventricular tachycardia (3%)*, ventricular extrasystoles (3%)*, angina (2%)*, bradycardia (1%), tachycardia, atrial fibrillation, AV node conduction abnormalities

Central nervous system: Headache (8%)*, dizziness (3%), insomnia (2%)*, anxiety (3%), confusion, fever, paresthesia, somnolence, tremor

Dermatologic: Pruritus, rash

Gastrointestinal: Nausea (4%)*, abdominal pain (1%)*, vomiting (1%)*

Hematologic: Anemia

Local: Injection site reaction, catheter pain

Neuromuscular & skeletal: Back pain (4%), leg cramps

Ocular: Amblyopia

Respiratory: Apnea, cough increased, hemoptysis

Miscellaneous: Diaphoresis

General Dosage Range I.V.: *Adults:* Bolus: 2 mcg/kg; Infusion: Initial: 0.01 mcg/kg/minute (maximum: 0.03 mcg/kg/minute)

Mechanism of Action Binds to guanylate cyclase receptor on vascular smooth muscle and endothelial cells, increasing intracellular cyclic GMP, resulting in smooth muscle cell relaxation. Has been shown to produce dose-dependent reductions in pulmonary capillary wedge pressure (PCWP) and systemic arterial pressure.

Pharmacodynamics/Kinetics

Onset of Action PCWP reduction: 15 minutes (60% of 3-hour effect achieved within this time period); Peak effect: Within 1 hour

Duration of Action >60 minutes (up to several hours) for systolic blood pressure; hemodynamic effects persist longer than serum half-life would predict

Half-life Elimination Initial (distribution) ~2 minutes; Terminal: ~18 minutes

Pregnancy Risk Factor C

Pregnancy Considerations Adverse events were not observed in an animal reproduction study. Nesiritide is a recombinant B-type natriuretic peptide (rhBNP). BNP and NT-proBNP (which has been used as a marker of BNP), are endogenous peptides and NT-proBNP is measurable in the umbilical cord serum of normal pregnancies. Information related to the administration of nesiritide during pregnancy has not been located.

Nevirapine (ne VYE ra peen)

Related Information

HIV Infection and AIDS *on page 1520*

Brand Names: U.S. Viramune XR®; Viramune®

Brand Names: Canada Auro-Nevirapine; Mylan-Nevirapine; Teva-Nevirapine; Viramune XR®; Viramune®

Pharmacologic Category Antiretroviral Agent, Reverse Transcriptase Inhibitor (Non-nucleoside)

Use In combination therapy with other antiretroviral agents for the treatment of HIV-1

Local Anesthetic/Vasoconstrictor Precautions No information available to require special precautions

Effects on Dental Treatment Key adverse event(s) related to dental treatment: Ulcerative stomatitis and oral lesions.

Effects on Bleeding No information available to require special precautions relative to hemostasis.

Adverse Effects Note: Potentially life-threatening nevirapine-associated adverse effects may present with the following symptoms: Abrupt onset of flu-like symptoms, abdominal pain, jaundice, or fever with or without rash; may progress to hepatic failure with encephalopathy. Skin rash is present in ~50% of cases.

>10%:

Dermatologic: Rash (1% to 7%; grade 1/2: 13%; grade 3/4: 2%)

Endocrine & metabolic: Cholesterol increased (240-300 mg/dL: 18% to 19%; >300 mg/dL: 3% to 4%), LDL increased (160-190 mg/dL: 15%; >190 mg/dL: 5%)

Hematologic: Neutropenia (4% to 13%; grades 3/4: 1% to 2%)

Hepatic: ALT increased (2.6-5 x ULN: 10% to 13%; ≥5.1 x ULN: 6% to 7%), symptomatic hepatic events (including hepatitis and hepatic failure: 2% to 11%; risk higher in ARV-naive women with CD4 counts >250 cells/mm^3 and ARV-naive men with CD4 counts >400 cells/mm^3)

1% to 10%:

Central nervous system: Fatigue (≤5%), headache (1% to 4%), fever (1% to 2%)

Gastrointestinal: Nausea (<1% to 9%), amylase increased (1.6-5 x ULN: 7% to 8%; ≥5.1 x ULN: <1%), abdominal pain (≤2%), diarrhea (≤2%)

Hepatic: AST increased (≥5.1 x ULN: 4% to 5%)

Neuromuscular & skeletal: Arthralgia (2%)

General Dosage Range Dosage adjustment recommended in patients who are receiving hemodialysis.

Oral, immediate release:

Infants and Children <8 years: Initial: 150-200 mg/m^2/dose once daily (maximum: 200 mg daily); Maintenance: 150-200 mg/m^2/dose twice daily (maximum: 400 mg daily).

Children ≥8 years: Initial: 120-150 mg/m^2/dose once daily (maximum: 200 mg daily); Maintenance: 120-150 mg/m^2/dose twice daily (maximum: 400 mg daily)

Adolescents and Adults: Initial: 200 mg once daily; Maintenance: 200 mg twice daily

Oral, extended release:

Children 6 to <18 years: Maintenance:
0.58 m^2 to 0.83 m^2: 200 mg once daily
0.84 m^2 to 1.16 m^2: 300 mg once daily
≥1.17 m^2: 400 mg once daily (do not exceed 400 mg daily)

Adults: Maintenance: 400 mg once daily

◀ **Mechanism of Action** As a non-nucleoside reverse transcriptase inhibitor, nevirapine has activity against HIV-1 by binding to reverse transcriptase. It consequently blocks the RNA-dependent and DNA-dependent DNA polymerase activities including HIV-1 replication. It does not require intracellular phosphorylation for antiviral activity.

Pharmacodynamics/Kinetics

Half-life Elimination Decreases over 2- to 4-week time with chronic dosing due to autoinduction (ie, half-life = 45 hours initially and decreases to 25-30 hours)

Time to Peak Serum: Immediate release: 4 hours; Extended release:~24 hours

Pregnancy Risk Factor B

Pregnancy Considerations Teratogenic effects were not observed in animal reproduction studies. Nevirapine crosses the placenta. No increased risk of overall birth defects has been observed following first trimester exposure according to data collected by the antiretroviral pregnancy registry. Pharmacokinetics are not altered during pregnancy and dose adjustment is not needed. The DHHS Perinatal HIV Guidelines recommend nevirapine as the preferred NNRTI for use during pregnancy. Nevirapine may be initiated in pregnant women with a CD4$^+$ lymphocyte count <250/mm^3 or continued in women who are virologically suppressed and tolerating therapy once pregnancy is detected (regardless of CD4$^+$ lymphocyte count); however, **do not** initiate therapy in pregnant women with a CD4$^+$ lymphocyte count >250/mm^3 unless the benefit of therapy clearly outweighs the risk. Elevated transaminase concentrations at baseline may increase the risk of toxicity; the monitoring recommendation for transaminase levels is generally the same as in nonpregnant women. Hypersensitivity reactions (including hepatic toxicity and rash) are more common in women on NNRTI.

Regardless of CD4 count or HIV RNA copy number, all HIV-infected pregnant women should receive a combination antepartum antiretroviral (ARV) drug regimen; this includes women who require therapy for their own health, as well as women who do not yet require therapy for their own health. ARV therapy should be started as soon as possible if required for the woman's health. Although earlier initiation may be more effective in reducing the perinatal transmission of HIV), also consider maternal conditions (eg, nausea and vomiting) and the potential risks of first trimester fetal exposure for specific agents. Plasma HIV RNA levels should be assessed at ~34-36 weeks gestation in order to help determine mode of delivery. If ARV therapy must be interrupted for <24 hours during the peripartum period, stop then restart all medications simultaneously in order to decrease the chance of developing resistance. Long-term follow-up is recommended for all infants exposed to ARV medications.

Healthcare providers are encouraged to enroll pregnant women exposed to antiretroviral medications in the Antiretroviral Pregnancy Registry (1-800-258-4263 or www.APRegistry.com). Healthcare providers caring for HIV-infected women and their infants may contact the National Perinatal HIV Hotline (888-448-8765) for clinical consultation (DHHS [perinatal], 2012).

Niacin (NYE a sin)

Related Information
Cardiovascular Diseases *on page 1492*

Brand Names: U.S. Niacin-Time® [OTC]; Niacor®; Niaspan®; Slo-Niacin® [OTC]

Brand Names: Canada Niaspan®; Niaspan® FCT; Niodan

Generic Availability (U.S.) Yes

Pharmacologic Category Antilipemic Agent, Miscellaneous; Vitamin, Water Soluble

Use Treatment of dyslipidemias (Fredrickson types IIa and IIb or primary hypercholesterolemia) as mono- or adjunctive therapy; to lower the risk of recurrent MI in patients with a history of MI and hyperlipidemia; to slow progression or promote regression of coronary artery disease; treatment of hypertriglyceridemia in patients at risk of pancreatitis; dietary supplement

Unlabeled Use Treatment of pellagra

Local Anesthetic/Vasoconstrictor Precautions No information available to require special precautions

Effects on Dental Treatment No significant effects or complications reported

Effects on Bleeding Sustained-release niacin has been shown to prolong blood clotting times, as observed by significant clotting factor synthesis deficiency and coagulopathy defined by prothrombin times 1.5 times greater than control. Caution is advised in patients with bleeding disorders or those using other anticoagulant medications. Mild leukopenia and increased eosinophil levels have also been reported.

Adverse Effects Frequency not defined.

Cardiovascular: Arrhythmias, atrial fibrillation, edema, flushing, hypotension, orthostasis, palpitation, syncope (rare), tachycardia

Central nervous system: Chills, dizziness, headache, insomnia, migraine, nervousness, pain

Dermatologic: Acanthosis nigricans, burning skin, dry skin, hyperpigmentation, maculopapular rash, pruritus, rash, skin discoloration, urticaria

Endocrine & metabolic: Glucose tolerance decreased, gout, phosphorous levels decreased, hyperuricemia

Gastrointestinal: Abdominal pain, amylase increased, diarrhea, dyspepsia, eructation, flatulence, nausea, peptic ulcers, vomiting

Hematologic: Platelet counts decreased

Hepatic: Hepatic necrosis (rare), hepatitis, jaundice, transaminases increased (dose-related), prothrombin time increased, total bilirubin increased

Neuromuscular & skeletal: CPK increased, leg cramps, myalgia, myasthenia, myopathy (with concurrent HMG-CoA reductase inhibitor), paresthesia, rhabdomyolysis (with concurrent HMG-CoA reductase inhibitor; rare), weakness

Ocular: Blurred vision, cystoid macular edema, toxic amblyopia

Respiratory: Cough, dyspnea

Miscellaneous: Diaphoresis, hypersensitivity reactions (rare; includes anaphylaxis, angioedema, laryngismus, vesiculobullous rash), LDH increased

Dosage Oral: **Note:** Formulations of niacin (regular release versus extended release) are not interchangeable.

Children:

Pellagra (unlabeled use): 50-100 mg/dose 3 times/day (some experts prefer niacinamide for treatment due to more favorable side effect profile)

Adequate intake (National Academy of Sciences, 1998):

0-5 months: 2 mg/day

6-11 months: 3 mg/day

Recommended daily allowances (National Academy of Sciences, 1998):

1-3 years: 6 mg/day

4-8 years: 8 mg/day

9-13 years: 12 mg/day

14-18 years: Females: 14 mg/day; Males: 16 mg/day

≥19 years: Refer to adult dosing

Adults:

Recommended daily allowances (National Academy of Sciences, 1998):

≥19 years: Females: 14 mg/day; Males: 16 mg/day

Pregnancy (all ages): 18 mg/day

Lactation (all ages): 17 mg/day

Dietary supplement (OTC labeling): 50 mg twice daily or 100 mg once daily. **Note:** Many over-the-counter formulations exist.

Hyperlipidemia:

Regular release formulation (Niacor®): Initial: 250 mg once daily (with evening meal); increase frequency and/or dose every 4-7 days to desired response or first-level therapeutic dose (1.5-2 g/day in 2-3 divided doses); after 2 months, may increase at 2- to 4-week intervals to 3 g/day in 3 divided doses (maximum dose: 6 g/day [NCEP recommends 4.5 g/day] in 3 divided doses). Usual daily dose after titration (NCEP, 2002): 1.5-3 g/day. **Note:** Many over-the-counter formulations exist.

Sustained release (or controlled release) formulations: **Note:** Several over-the-counter formulations exist. Usual daily dose after titration (NCEP, 2002): 1-2 g/day

Extended release formulation (Niaspan®): Initial: 500 mg at bedtime for 4 weeks, then 1 g at bedtime for 4 weeks; adjust dose to response and tolerance; may increase dose every 4 weeks by 500 mg/day to a maximum of 2 g/day. Usual daily dose after titration (NCEP, 2002): 1-2 g once daily

If additional LDL-lowering is necessary with lovastatin or simvastatin: Recommended initial lovastatin or simvastatin dose: 20 mg/day (maximum lovastatin or simvastatin dose: 40 mg/day); **Note:** Lovastatin prescribing information recommends a maximum dose of 20 mg/day with concurrent use of niacin (>1 g/day).

Pellagra (unlabeled use): 50-100 mg 3-4 times/day; maximum: 500 mg/day (some experts prefer niacinamide for treatment due to more favorable side effect profile)

Dosage adjustment in renal impairment: No dosage adjustment provided in manufacturer's labeling (has not been studied); use with caution.

Dosage adjustment in hepatic impairment: No dosage adjustment provided in manufacturer's labeling (has not been studied). However, contraindicated in patients with significant or unexplained hepatic dysfunction, active liver disease or unexplained persistent transaminase elevations.

Dosage adjustment for hepatic toxicity: Transaminases rise ≥3 times ULN, either persistent or if symptoms of nausea, fever, and/or malaise occur: Discontinue therapy.

Mechanism of Action Component of two coenzymes which is necessary for tissue respiration, lipid metabolism, and glycogenolysis; inhibits the synthesis of very low density lipoproteins (VLDL) and low density lipoproteins (LDL); may also increase the rate of chylomicron triglyceride removal from plasma.

Contraindications Hypersensitivity to niacin, niacinamide, or any component of the formulation; active hepatic disease or significant or unexplained persistent elevations in hepatic transaminases; active peptic ulcer; arterial hemorrhage

Warnings/Precautions Use with caution in patients with unstable angina or MI, diabetes (may interfere with glucose control), renal disease, active gallbladder disease (can exacerbate), gout, or with anticoagulants (may slightly increase prothrombin time). Use with caution in patients with a past history of hepatic impairment and/or who consume substantial amounts of ethanol; contraindicated with active liver disease or unexplained persistent transaminase elevation. Rare cases of rhabdomyolysis have occurred during concomitant use with HMG-CoA reductase inhibitors. With concurrent use or if symptoms suggestive of myopathy occur, monitor creatine phosphokinase (CPK) and potassium; use with caution in patients with renal impairment, inadequately treated hypothyroidism, patients with diabetes or the elderly; risk for myopathy and rhabdomyolysis may be increased.

Immediate and extended or sustained release products are not interchangeable. Cases of severe hepatotoxicity have occurred when immediate release (crystalline) niacin products have been substituted with sustained-release (modified release, timed-release) niacin products at equivalent doses. Patients should be initiated with low doses (eg, 500 mg at bedtime) with titration to achieve desired response. Flushing and pruritus, common adverse effects of niacin, may be attenuated with a gradual increase in dose, and/or by taking aspirin (adults: 325 mg) or an NSAID 30-60 minutes before dosing. Compliance is enhanced with twice-daily dosing (extended-release product excluded). Prior to initiation, secondary causes for hypercholesterolemia (eg, poorly controlled diabetes mellitus, hypothyroidism) should be excluded; management with diet and other nonpharmacologic measures (eg, exercise or weight reduction) should be attempted prior to initiation. Use has not been evaluated in Fredrickson type I or III dyslipidemias.

Drug Interactions

Metabolism/Transport Effects None known.

Avoid Concomitant Use There are no known interactions where it is recommended to avoid concomitant use.

Increased Effect/Toxicity

Niacin may increase the levels/effects of: HMG-CoA Reductase Inhibitors

Decreased Effect

The levels/effects of Niacin may be decreased by: Bile Acid Sequestrants

Ethanol/Nutrition/Herb Interactions Ethanol: Avoid heavy use; avoid use around niacin dose.

Dietary Considerations Should be taken with meal; low-fat meal if treating hyperlipidemia. Avoid hot drinks around the time of niacin dose.

Pharmacodynamics/Kinetics

Half-life Elimination 25-45 minutes

Time to Peak Serum: Immediate release formulation: 30-60 minutes; extended release formulation: 4-5 hours

Pregnancy Risk Factor C

◄ **Pregnancy Considerations** Water soluble vitamins cross the placenta. When used as a dietary supplement, niacin requirements may be increased in pregnant women compared to nonpregnant women (IOM, 1998). Animal reproduction studies have not been conducted. It is not known if niacin at lipid-lowering doses is harmful to the developing fetus. If a woman becomes pregnant while receiving niacin for primary hypercholesterolemia, niacin should be discontinued. If a woman becomes pregnant while receiving niacin for hypertriglyceridemia, the benefits and risks of continuing niacin should be assessed on an individual basis.

Lactation Enters breast milk/consider risk:benefit

Breast-Feeding Considerations Niacin is excreted in human breast milk. When used as a dietary supplement, niacin requirements may be increased in nursing women compared to non-nursing women (IOM, 1998). Because lipid-lowering doses of niacin may cause serious adverse reactions in nursing infants, a decision should be made whether to discontinue nursing or discontinue the drug, taking into account the importance of the drug to the mother.

Dosage Forms

Caplet, timed release, oral: 500 mg

Capsule, oral: 50 mg, 250 mg

Capsule, extended release, oral: 250 mg, 500 mg

Capsule, timed release, oral: 250 mg, 400 mg, 500 mg

Tablet, oral: 50 mg, 100 mg, 250 mg, 500 mg
Niacor®: 500 mg

Tablet, controlled release, oral:
Slo-Niacin® [OTC]: 250 mg, 500 mg, 750 mg

Tablet, extended release, oral:
Niaspan®: 500 mg, 750 mg, 1000 mg

Tablet, timed release, oral: 250 mg, 500 mg, 750 mg, 1000 mg
Niacin-Time® [OTC]: 500 mg

Niacinamide (nye a SIN a mide)

Pharmacologic Category Vitamin, Water Soluble

Use Dietary supplement

Unlabeled Use Prophylaxis and treatment of pellagra

Local Anesthetic/Vasoconstrictor Precautions No information available to require special precautions

Effects on Dental Treatment No significant effects or complications reported

Effects on Bleeding No information available to require special precautions

General Dosage Range Oral:
Children: 10-50 mg every 6 hours
Adults: Initial: 100 mg every 6 hours; Maintenance: 50 mg every 8-12 hours

Mechanism of Action Used by the body as a source of niacin; is a component of two coenzymes which is necessary for tissue respiration, lipid metabolism, and glycogenolysis; does not have hypolipidemia or vaso-dilating effects.

Pharmacodynamics/Kinetics

Half-life Elimination 45 minutes

Time to Peak Serum: 20-70 minutes

Pregnancy Considerations Water-soluble vitamins cross the placenta (IOM, 1998).

Niacin and Lovastatin (NYE a sin & LOE va sta tin)

Related Information
Lovastatin *on page 846*
Niacin *on page 972*

Brand Names: U.S. Advicor®

Brand Names: Canada Advicor®

Generic Availability (U.S.) No

Pharmacologic Category Antilipemic Agent, HMG-CoA Reductase Inhibitor; Antilipemic Agent, Miscellaneous

Use For use when treatment with both extended-release niacin and lovastatin is appropriate in combination with a standard cholesterol-lowering diet:
Extended-release niacin: Adjunctive treatment of dyslipidemias (types IIa and IIb or primary hypercholesterolemia) to lower the risk of recurrent MI and/or slow progression of coronary artery disease, including combination therapy with other antidyslipidemic agents when additional triglyceride-lowering or HDL-increasing effects are desired; treatment of hypertriglyceridemia in patients at risk of pancreatitis
Lovastatin: Treatment of primary hypercholesterolemia (Frederickson types IIa and IIb); primary and secondary prevention of cardiovascular disease

Local Anesthetic/Vasoconstrictor Precautions No information available to require special precautions

Effects on Dental Treatment No significant effects or complications reported

Effects on Bleeding Sustained-release niacin has been shown to prolong blood clotting times, as observed by significant clotting factor synthesis deficiency and coagulopathy defined by prothrombin times 1.5 times greater than control. Caution is advised in patients with bleeding disorders or those using other anticoagulant medications. Mild leukopenia and increased eosinophil levels have also been reported. No additional warnings with lovastatin coadministration.

Adverse Effects See individual agents.

Dosage Dosage forms are a fixed combination of niacin and lovastatin.
Oral: Adults: Lowest dose: Niacin 500 mg/lovastatin 20 mg; may increase by not more than 500 mg (niacin) at 4-week intervals (maximum dose: Niacin 2000 mg/lovastatin 40 mg daily); should be taken at bedtime with a low-fat snack. **Note:** If therapy is interrupted for >7 days, reinstitution of therapy should begin with the lowest dose followed by retitration as needed.
Not for use as initial therapy of dyslipidemias. May be substituted for equivalent dose of Niaspan®; however, manufacturer does not recommend direct substitution with other niacin products.

Dosage adjustment for lovastatin component with concomitant medications:
Amiodarone: Maximum recommended lovastatin dose: 40 mg daily
Danazol, diltiazem, dronedarone, or verapamil: Initial lovastatin dose: 10 mg daily (dose unavailable with combination product; use separate components); Maximum recommended lovastatin dose: 20 mg daily

Dosage adjustment in renal impairment:
Mild-to-moderate impairment: No dosage adjustment required
Cl_{cr} <30 mL/minute: Use doses of lovastatin >20 mg daily with caution

Dosage adjustment in hepatic impairment: Do not use in active liver disease or unexplained persistent elevations of serum transaminases.

Mechanism of Action Lovastatin acts by competitively inhibiting 3-hydroxyl-3-methylglutaryl-coenzyme A (HMG-CoA) reductase, the enzyme that catalyzes the rate-limiting step in cholesterol biosynthesis. Niacin is a component of two coenzymes which is necessary for tissue respiration, lipid metabolism, and glycogenolysis; inhibits the synthesis of very low density lipoproteins.

Contraindications Hypersensitivity to lovastatin, niacin, or any component of the formulation; active liver disease; unexplained persistent elevations of serum transaminases; active peptic ulcer disease; arterial bleeding; pregnancy; breast-feeding; concomitant use of strong CYP3A4 inhibitors (eg, clarithromycin, erythromycin, itraconazole, ketoconazole, nefazodone, posaconazole, voriconazole, protease inhibitors including boceprevir and telaprevir, telithromycin).

Warnings/Precautions See individual agents.

Drug Interactions

Metabolism/Transport Effects Refer to individual components.

Avoid Concomitant Use
Avoid concomitant use of Niacin and Lovastatin with any of the following: Boceprevir; CycloSPORINE (Systemic); CYP3A4 Inhibitors (Strong); Erythromycin (Systemic); Fusidic Acid; Gemfibrozil; Lomitapide; Mifepristone; Pimozide; Protease Inhibitors; Red Yeast Rice; Telaprevir

Increased Effect/Toxicity
Niacin and Lovastatin may increase the levels/effects of: ARIPiprazole; DAPTOmycin; Diltiazem; HMG-CoA Reductase Inhibitors; Pazopanib; Pimozide; Trabectedin; Vitamin K Antagonists

The levels/effects of Niacin and Lovastatin may be increased by: Amiodarone; Bezafibrate; Boceprevir; Colchicine; CycloSPORINE (Systemic); CYP3A4 Inhibitors (Moderate); CYP3A4 Inhibitors (Strong); Cyproterone; Danazol; Dasatinib; Diltiazem; Dronedarone; Erythromycin (Systemic); Fenofibrate; Fenofibric Acid; Fluconazole; Fusidic Acid; Gemfibrozil; Grapefruit Juice; Ivacaftor; Lomitapide; Macrolide Antibiotics; Mifepristone; Niacin; Niacinamide; P-glycoprotein/ABCB1 Inhibitors; Protease Inhibitors; QuiNINE; Ranolazine; Red Yeast Rice; Sildenafil; Telaprevir; Ticagrelor; Verapamil

Decreased Effect
Niacin and Lovastatin may decrease the levels/effects of: Lanthanum

The levels/effects of Niacin and Lovastatin may be decreased by: Antacids; Bile Acid Sequestrants; Bosentan; CYP3A4 Inducers (Strong); Deferasirox; Efavirenz; Etravirine; Fosphenytoin; P-glycoprotein/ABCB1 Inducers; Phenytoin; Rifamycin Derivatives; St Johns Wort; Tocilizumab

Ethanol/Nutrition/Herb Interactions
Ethanol: Consumption of large amounts of ethanol may increase the risk of liver damage with HMG-CoA reductase inhibitors. Concurrent ingestion of ethanol may increase the risk of flushing associated with niacin.
Food: Lovastatin absorption may be decreased with food, however, the combination product is recommended to be taken with a low-fat snack at bedtime. Lovastatin serum concentrations may be increased if taken with grapefruit juice; avoid concurrent use. Concurrent ingestion of hot liquids may increase the risk of flushing associated with niacin.

Herb/Nutraceutical: St John's wort may decrease lovastatin levels. Red yeast rice contains an estimated 2.4 mg lovastatin per 600 mg rice.

Dietary Considerations Continue standard cholesterol-lowering diet during therapy. Should be taken with a low-fat snack.

Pregnancy Risk Factor X

Pregnancy Considerations Use during pregnancy is contraindicated. See individual agents.

Lactation Enters breast milk/contraindicated

Breast-Feeding Considerations Niacin is excreted in breast milk. The excretion of lovastatin is unknown. Use during breast-feeding is contraindicated. See individual agents.

Dosage Forms
Tablet, variable release, oral:
Advicor®: 500/20: Niacin 500 mg [extended release] and lovastatin 20 mg [immediate release]; 750/20: Niacin 750 mg [extended release] and lovastatin 20 mg [immediate release]; 1000/20: Niacin 1000 mg [extended release] and lovastatin 20 mg [immediate release]; 1000/40: Niacin 1000 mg [extended release] and lovastatin 40 mg [immediate release]

Niacin and Simvastatin
(NYE a sin & sim va STAT in)

Related Information
Niacin *on page 972*
Simvastatin *on page 1236*

Brand Names: U.S. Simcor®

Pharmacologic Category Antilipemic Agent, HMG-CoA Reductase Inhibitor; Antilipemic Agent, Miscellaneous

Use Reduce total cholesterol, LDL, Apo B, non-HDL, TG, and/or increase HDL in patients with primary hypercholesterolemia, mixed dyslipidemia, or hypertriglyceridemia in combination with standard cholesterol-lowering diet when simvastatin or niacin monotherapy is inadequate

Local Anesthetic/Vasoconstrictor Precautions No information available to require special precautions

Effects on Dental Treatment No significant effects or complications reported

Effects on Bleeding Sustained-release niacin has been shown to prolong blood clotting times, as observed by significant clotting factor synthesis deficiency and coagulopathy defined by prothrombin times 1.5 times greater than control. Caution is advised in patients with bleeding disorders or those using other anticoagulant medications. Mild leukopenia and increased eosinophil levels have also been reported. No additional warnings with simvastatin coadministration.

Adverse Effects Reactions/percentages reported with combination product; also see individual agents.
>10%: Cardiovascular: Flushing (≤59%)
1% to 10%:
Central nervous system: Headache (5%)
Dermatologic: Pruritus (3%)
Gastrointestinal: Diarrhea (3%), nausea (3%)
Neuromuscular & skeletal: Back pain (3%)

Frequency not defined: Alkaline phosphatase increased, amylase increased, bilirubin increased, creatinine kinase increased, fasting blood glucose increased, GGT increased, LDH increased, phosphorus decreased, platelets decreased, prothrombin time increased, thyroid function test abnormalities, transaminases increased, uric acid increased

General Dosage Range Oral: *Adults:* Niacin 500-2000 mg/simvastatin 20-40 mg once daily

Mechanism of Action

Niacin is a component of two coenzymes which is necessary for tissue respiration, lipid metabolism, and glycogenolysis; inhibits the synthesis of very low density lipoproteins.

Simvastatin is a derivative of lovastatin that acts by competitively inhibiting 3-hydroxy-3-methylglutaryl-coenzyme A (HMG-CoA) reductase, the enzyme that catalyzes the rate-limiting step in cholesterol biosynthesis.

Pregnancy Risk Factor X

Pregnancy Considerations Use is contraindicated in pregnant women. See individual agents.

NiCARdipine (nye KAR de peen)

Related Information

Calcium Channel Blockers and Gingival Hyperplasia *on page 1640*

Cardiovascular Diseases *on page 1492*

Brand Names: U.S. Cardene® I.V.; Cardene® SR

Pharmacologic Category Antianginal Agent; Calcium Channel Blocker; Calcium Channel Blocker, Dihydropyridine

Use Chronic stable angina (immediate-release product only); management of hypertension (immediate and sustained release products); parenteral only for short-term use when oral treatment is not feasible

Unlabeled Use Control of blood pressure in acute ischemic stroke and spontaneous intracranial hemorrhage, postoperative hypertension associated with carotid endarterectomy, perioperative hypertension, prevention of migraine headaches, subarachnoid hemorrhage associated cerebral vasospasm

Local Anesthetic/Vasoconstrictor Precautions No information available to require special precautions

Effects on Dental Treatment Key adverse event(s) related to dental treatment: Xerostomia (normal salivary flow resumes upon discontinuation). Other drugs of this class can cause gingival hyperplasia (ie, nifedipine). The first case of nicardipine-induced gingival hyperplasia has been reported in a child taking 40-50 mg daily for 20 months.

Effects on Bleeding No information available to require special precautions

Adverse Effects 1% to 10%:

Cardiovascular: Cardiovascular: Flushing (6% to 10%), peripheral edema (dose related; 6% to 8%), hypotension (I.V. 6%), increased angina (dose related; 6%), palpitation (3% to 4%), tachycardia (1% to 4%), vasodilation (1% to 5%), chest pain (I.V. 1%), ECG abnormal (I.V. 1%), extrasystoles (I.V. 1%), hemopericardium (I.V. 1%), hypertension (I.V. 1%), orthostasis (1%), supraventricular tachycardia (I.V. 1%), syncope (1%), ventricular extrasystoles (I.V. 1%), ventricular tachycardia (I.V. 1%)

Central nervous system: Headache (6% to 15%), dizziness (1% to 7%), hypoesthesia (1%), intracranial hemorrhage (1% plus), somnolence (1%)

Dermatologic: Rash (1%)

Endocrine & metabolic: Hypokalemia (I.V. 1%)

Gastrointestinal: Nausea (2% to 5%), vomiting (I.V. 5%), dyspepsia (oral 2%), abdominal pain (I.V. 1%), dry mouth (1%)

Genitourinary: Polyuria (1%)

Local: Injection site pain (I.V. 1%), injection site reaction (I.V. 1%)

Neuromuscular & skeletal: Weakness (1% to 6%), myalgia (1%), paresthesia (1%)

Renal: Hematuria (1%)

Respiratory: Dyspnea (1%)

Miscellaneous: Diaphoresis (1%)

General Dosage Range Dosage adjustment recommended in patients with hepatic or renal impairment

I.V.: *Adults:* Initial: 5 mg/hour; Maintenance: 3-15 mg/hour

Oral:

Immediate release: *Adults:* Initial: 20 mg 3 times/day; Maintenance: 20-40 mg 3 times/day

Sustained release: *Adults:* Initial: 30 mg twice daily; Maintenance: Up to 60 mg twice daily

Mechanism of Action Inhibits calcium ion from entering the "slow channels" or select voltage-sensitive areas of vascular smooth muscle and myocardium during depolarization, producing a relaxation of coronary vascular smooth muscle and coronary vasodilation; increases myocardial oxygen delivery in patients with vasospastic angina

Pharmacodynamics/Kinetics

Onset of Action Oral: 0.5-2 hours; I.V.: 10 minutes; Hypotension: ~20 minutes

Duration of Action I.V.: ≤8 hours; Oral: Immediate release capsules: ≤8 hours, Sustained release capsules: 8-12 hours

Half-life Elimination 2-4 hours

Time to Peak Serum: Oral: Immediate release: 30-120 minutes; Sustained release: 60-240 minutes

Pregnancy Risk Factor C

Pregnancy Considerations Adverse events were observed in some animal reproduction studies. Nicardipine has been used for the treatment of severe hypertension in pregnancy and pre-term labor. Nicardipine crosses the placenta; changes in fetal heart rate, neonatal hypotension and neonatal acidosis have been observed following maternal use (rare; based on limited data). Adverse effects reported in pregnant women are generally similar to those reported in non pregnant patients; however pulmonary edema has been observed.

Nicotine (nik oh TEEN)

Related Information

Management of the Chemically Dependent Patient *on page 1550*

Brand Names: U.S. Commit® [OTC]; NicoDerm® CQ® [OTC]; Nicorelief® [OTC]; Nicorette® [OTC]; Nicotrol® Inhaler; Nicotrol® NS; Thrive™ [OTC]

Brand Names: Canada Habitrol®; Nicoderm®; Nicorette®; Nicorette® Plus; Nicotrol®

Generic Availability (U.S.) Yes: Transdermal patch and gum

Pharmacologic Category Smoking Cessation Aid

Dental Use Treatment to aid smoking cessation for the relief of nicotine withdrawal symptoms (including nicotine craving)

Use Treatment to aid smoking cessation for the relief of nicotine withdrawal symptoms (including nicotine craving)

Unlabeled Use Management of ulcerative colitis (transdermal)

Local Anesthetic/Vasoconstrictor Precautions No information available to require special precautions

Effects on Dental Treatment Key adverse event(s) related to dental treatment: Chewing gum: Excessive salivation, mouth/throat soreness, jaw muscle ache, hiccups, tachycardia, headache (mild), vomiting, belching, nausea, xerostomia (normal salivary flow resumes upon discontinuation), dizziness, nervousness, GI distress, hoarseness, and muscle pain.

Effects on Bleeding No information available to require special precautions

Adverse Effects

Nasal spray/inhaler:

>10%:

Central nervous system: Headache (18% to 26%)

Gastrointestinal: Inhaler: Mouth/throat irritation (66%), dyspepsia (18%)

Respiratory: Inhaler: Cough (32%), rhinitis (23%)

1% to 10%:

Dermatologic: Acne (3%)

Endocrine & metabolic: Dysmenorrhea (3%)

Gastrointestinal: Flatulence (4%), gum problems (4%), diarrhea, hiccup, nausea, taste disturbance, tooth abrasions

Neuromuscular & skeletal: Back pain (6%), arthralgia (5%), jaw/neck pain

Respiratory: Nasal burning (nasal spray), sinusitis

Miscellaneous: Withdrawal symptoms

Adverse events previously reported in prescription labeling for chewing gum, lozenge and/or transdermal systems. Frequency not defined; may be product or dose specific:

Central nervous system: Concentration impaired, depression, dizziness, headache, insomnia, nervousness, pain

Gastrointestinal: Aphthous stomatitis, constipation, cough, diarrhea, dyspepsia, flatulence, gingival bleeding, glossitis, hiccups, jaw pain, nausea, salivation increased, stomatitis, taste perversion, tooth abrasions, ulcerative stomatitis, xerostomia

Dermatologic: Rash

Local: Application site reaction, local edema, local erythema

Neuromuscular & skeletal: Arthralgia, myalgia, paresthesia

Respiratory: Cough, sinusitis

Miscellaneous: Allergic reaction, diaphoresis

Dental Usual Dosage

Tobacco cessation (patients should be advised to completely stop smoking upon initiation of therapy): Adults:

Gum: Chew 1 piece of gum when urge to smoke, up to 24 pieces/day. Patients who smoke <25 cigarettes/day should start with 2-mg strength; patients smoking ≥25 cigarettes/day should start with the 4-mg strength. Use according to the following 12-week dosing schedule:

Weeks 1-6: Chew 1 piece of gum every 1-2 hours; to increase chances of quitting, chew at least 9 pieces/day during the first 6 weeks

Weeks 7-9: Chew 1 piece of gum every 2-4 hours

Weeks 10-12: Chew 1 piece of gum every 4-8 hours

Inhaler: Oral: Usually 6 to 16 cartridges per day; best effect was achieved by frequent continuous puffing (20 minutes); recommended duration of treatment is 3 months, after which patients may be weaned from the inhaler by gradual reduction of the daily dose over 6-12 weeks

Lozenge: Oral: Patients who smoke their first cigarette within 30 minutes of waking should use the 4 mg strength; otherwise the 2 mg strength is recommended. Use according to the following 12-week dosing schedule:

Weeks 1-6: One lozenge every 1-2 hours

Weeks 7-9: One lozenge every 2-4 hours

Weeks 10-12: One lozenge every 4-8 hours

Note: Use at least 9 lozenges/day during first 6 weeks to improve chances of quitting; do not use more than one lozenge at a time (maximum: 5 lozenges every 6 hours, 20 lozenges/day)

Spray: Nasal: 1-2 sprays/hour; do not exceed more than 5 doses (10 sprays) per hour [maximum: 40 doses/day (80 sprays); each dose (2 sprays) contains 1 mg of nicotine]

Transdermal patch: Topical: Apply new patch every 24 hours to nonhairy, clean, dry skin on the upper body or upper outer arm; each patch should be applied to a different site. **Note:** Adjustment may be required during initial treatment (move to higher dose if experiencing withdrawal symptoms; lower dose if side effects are experienced).

NicoDerm CQ®:

Patients smoking >10 cigarettes/day: Begin with step 1 (21 mg/day) for 6 weeks, **followed by** step 2 (14 mg/day) for 2 weeks; **finish with** step 3 (7 mg/day) for 2 weeks

Patients smoking ≤10 cigarettes/day: Begin with step 2 (14 mg/day) for 6 weeks, **followed by** step 3 (7 mg/day) for 2 weeks

Note: Patients who are receiving >600 mg/day of cimetidine: Decrease to the next lower patch size

Benefits of use of nicotine transdermal patches beyond 3 months have not been demonstrated

Dosage

Smoking deterrent: Patients should be advised to completely stop smoking upon initiation of therapy.

Oral:

Gum: Chew 1 piece of gum when urge to smoke, up to 24 pieces/day. Patients who smoke <25 cigarettes/day should start with 2-mg strength; patients smoking ≥25 cigarettes/day should start with the 4-mg strength. Use according to the following 12-week dosing schedule:

Weeks 1-6: Chew 1 piece of gum every 1-2 hours; to increase chances of quitting, chew at least 9 pieces/day during the first 6 weeks

Weeks 7-9: Chew 1 piece of gum every 2-4 hours

Weeks 10-12: Chew 1 piece of gum every 4-8 hours

Inhaler: Usually 6 to 16 cartridges per day; best effect was achieved by frequent continuous puffing (20 minutes); recommended duration of treatment is 3 months, after which patients may be weaned from the inhaler by gradual reduction of the daily dose over 6-12 weeks

Lozenge: Patients who smoke their first cigarette within 30 minutes of waking should use the 4 mg strength; otherwise the 2 mg strength is recommended. Use according to the following 12-week dosing schedule:

Weeks 1-6: One lozenge every 1-2 hours

Weeks 7-9: One lozenge every 2-4 hours

Weeks 10-12: One lozenge every 4-8 hours

Note: Use at least 9 lozenges/day during first 6 weeks to improve chances of quitting; do not use more than one lozenge at a time (maximum: 5 lozenges every 6 hours, 20 lozenges/day)

Topical:

Transdermal patch: Apply new patch every 24 hours to nonhairy, clean, dry skin on the upper body or upper outer arm; each patch should be applied to a different site. **Note:** Adjustment may be required during initial treatment (move to higher dose if experiencing withdrawal symptoms; lower dose if side effects are experienced).

NicoDerm CQ®:

Patients smoking >10 cigarettes/day: Begin with **step 1** (21 mg/day) for 6 weeks, followed by **step 2** (14 mg/day) for 2 weeks; finish with **step 3** (7 mg/day) for 2 weeks

Patients smoking ≤10 cigarettes/day: Begin with **step 2** (14 mg/day) for 6 weeks, followed by **step 3** (7 mg/day) for 2 weeks

Note: Patients receiving >600 mg/day of cimetidine: Decrease to the next lower patch size

Note: Benefits of use of nicotine transdermal patches beyond 3 months have not been demonstrated.

Nasal: Spray: 1-2 sprays/hour; do not exceed more than 5 doses (10 sprays) per hour [maximum: 40 doses/day (80 sprays); each dose (2 sprays) contains 1 mg of nicotine]

Mechanism of Action Nicotine is one of two naturally-occurring alkaloids which exhibit their primary effects via autonomic ganglia stimulation. The other alkaloid is lobeline which has many actions similar to those of nicotine but is less potent. Nicotine is a potent ganglionic and central nervous system stimulant, the actions of which are mediated via nicotine-specific receptors. Biphasic actions are observed depending upon the dose administered. The main effect of nicotine in small doses is stimulation of all autonomic ganglia; with larger doses, initial stimulation is followed by blockade of transmission. Biphasic effects are also evident in the adrenal medulla; discharge of catecholamines occurs with small doses, whereas prevention of catecholamines release is seen with higher doses as a response to splanchnic nerve stimulation. Stimulation of the central nervous system (CNS) is characterized by tremors and respiratory excitation. However, convulsions may occur with higher doses, along with respiratory failure secondary to both central paralysis and peripheral blockade to respiratory muscles.

Contraindications Hypersensitivity to nicotine or any component of the formulation; patients who are smoking during the postmyocardial infarction period; patients with life-threatening arrhythmias, or severe or worsening angina pectoris; active temporomandibular joint disease (gum); pregnancy; not for use in nonsmokers

Warnings/Precautions Hazardous agent - use appropriate precautions for handling and disposal (EPA, P-listed). Use caution in patients with hyperthyroidism, pheochromocytoma, or insulin-dependent diabetes. Use with caution in oropharyngeal inflammation and in patients with history of esophagitis, peptic ulcer, coronary artery disease, recent MI, serious cardiac arrhythmias, vasospastic disease, angina, hypertension, hyperthyroidism, pheochromocytoma, diabetes, severe renal dysfunction, and hepatic dysfunction. The oral inhaler and nasal spray should be used with caution in patients with bronchospastic disease (other forms of nicotine replacement may be preferred). Use of nasal product is not recommended with chronic nasal disorders (eg, allergy, rhinitis, nasal polyps, and sinusitis). Transdermal patch may contain conducting metal (eg, aluminum); remove patch prior to MRI. Cautious use of topical nicotine in patients with certain skin diseases. Hypersensitivity to the topical products can occur.

Dental problems may be worsened by chewing the gum. Urge patients to stop smoking completely when initiating therapy.

Drug Interactions

Metabolism/Transport Effects Substrate of CYP1A2 (minor), CYP2A6 (minor), CYP2B6 (minor), CYP2C19 (minor), CYP2C9 (minor), CYP2D6 (minor), CYP2E1 (minor), CYP3A4 (minor); **Note:** Assignment of Major/Minor substrate status based on clinically relevant drug interaction potential; **Inhibits** CYP2A6 (weak), CYP2E1 (weak)

Avoid Concomitant Use There are no known interactions where it is recommended to avoid concomitant use.

Increased Effect/Toxicity

Nicotine may increase the levels/effects of: Adenosine

The levels/effects of Nicotine may be increased by: Cimetidine

Decreased Effect

The levels/effects of Nicotine may be decreased by: Peginterferon Alfa-2b

Ethanol/Nutrition/Herb Interactions Food: Lozenge: Acidic foods/beverages decrease absorption of nicotine.

Dietary Considerations Some products may contain phenylalanine and/or sodium.

Pharmacodynamics/Kinetics

Onset of Action Intranasal: More closely approximate the time course of plasma nicotine levels observed after cigarette smoking than other dosage forms

Duration of Action Transdermal: 24 hours

Half-life Elimination 4 hours; Nasal spray: 1-2 hours

Time to Peak Serum: Transdermal: 8-9 hours; Nasal spray: 10-20 minutes

Pregnancy Risk Factor D (nasal)

Pregnancy Considerations Nicotine is teratogenic in animal studies. Nicotine exposure via cigarette smoke may cause increased ectopic pregnancy, low birth weight, increased risk of spontaneous abortion, increased perinatal mortality; increased aortic blood flow, increased heart rate, decreased uterine blood flow, and decreased breathing have been reported in the fetus. Smoking during pregnancy is associated with sudden infant death syndrome (SIDS), an increased risk of asthma, infantile colic, and childhood obesity. Women who are pregnant should be encouraged not to smoke. The use of nicotine replacement products to aid in smoking cessation has not been adequately studied in pregnant women (amount of nicotine exposure is varied). Nonpharmacologic treatments are recommended. If the benefits of nicotine replacement therapy outweigh the unknown risks, products with intermittent dosing are suggested to be tried first. If a patch is used, it is suggested to remove it overnight while sleeping to decrease fetal exposure.

Lactation Excretion in breast milk unknown/use caution

Breast-Feeding Considerations Nicotine from cigarette smoke is found in breast milk at 1.5-3 times the maternal plasma concentrations. The amount from nicotine replacement products is not known. Women who are breast-feeding are encouraged not to smoke.

Dosage Forms

Gum, chewing, oral: 2 mg (20s, 40s, 50s, 100s, 108s, 110s); 4 mg (20s, 40s, 48s, 50s, 100s, 108s, 110s)

Nicorelief® [OTC]: 2 mg (50s, 110s); 4 mg (50s, 110s)

Nicorette® [OTC]: 2 mg (40s, 48s, 50s, 100s, 108s, 110s, 168s, 170s, 192s, 200s, 216s); 4 mg (40s, 48s, 50s, 100s, 108s, 110s, 168s, 170s, 192s, 200s, 216s)

Thrive™ [OTC]: 2 mg (40s); 4 mg (40s)

Lozenge, oral:
Commit® [OTC]: 2 mg, 4 mg
Nicorelief® [OTC]: 2 mg, 4 mg
Nicorette® [OTC]: 4 mg
Oral inhalation system, for oral inhalation:
Nicotrol® Inhaler: 10 mg (10 mL)
Patch, transdermal: 7 mg/24 hours (7s, 14s, 30s); 14 mg/24 hours (7s, 14s, 30s); 21 mg/24 hours (7s, 14s, 30s)
NicoDerm® CQ® [OTC]: 7 mg/24 hours (14s); 14 mg/24 hours (14s); 21 mg/24 hours (7s, 14s)
Solution, intranasal:
Nicotrol® NS: 10 mg/mL (10 mL)

References

Davies GM, Willner P, James DL, et al, "Influence of Nicotine Gum on Acute Cravings for Cigarettes," *J Psychopharmacol*, 2004, 18 (1):83-7.
Li Wan Po A, "Transdermal Nicotine in Smoking Cessation. A Meta-Analysis," *Eur J Clin Pharmacol*, 1993, 45(6):519-28.
Transdermal Nicotine Study Group, "Transdermal Nicotine for Smoking Cessation. Six-Month Results From Two Multicenter Controlled Clinical Trials," *JAMA*, 1991, 266(22):3133-8.
Westman EC, Levin ED, and Rose JE, "The Nicotine Patch in Smoking Cessation," *Arch Intern Med*, 1993, 153(16):1917-23.

NIFEdipine (nye FED i peen)

Related Information

Calcium Channel Blockers and Gingival Hyperplasia *on page 1640*
Cardiovascular Diseases *on page 1492*
Brand Names: U.S. Adalat® CC; Afeditab® CR; Nifediac CC®; Nifedical XL®; Procardia XL®; Procardia®
Brand Names: Canada Adalat® XL®; Apo-Nifed PA®; Mylan-Nifedipine Extended Release; Nu-Nifed; Nu-Nifedipine-PA; PMS-Nifedipine
Generic Availability (U.S.) Yes
Pharmacologic Category Antianginal Agent; Calcium Channel Blocker; Calcium Channel Blocker, Dihydropyridine
Use Management of chronic stable or vasospastic angina; treatment of hypertension (sustained release products only)
Unlabeled Use Management of pulmonary hypertension, preterm labor, and Raynaud's phenomenon; prevention and treatment of high altitude pulmonary edema
Local Anesthetic/Vasoconstrictor Precautions No information available to require special precautions
Effects on Dental Treatment Nifedipine has been reported to cause 10% incidence of gingival hyperplasia; effects from 30-100 mg/day have appeared after 1-9 months. Discontinuation results in complete disappearance or marked regression of symptoms; symptoms will reappear upon remediation. Marked regression occurs after 1 week and complete disappearance of symptoms has occurred within 15 days. If a gingivectomy is performed and use of the drug is continued or resumed, hyperplasia usually will recur. The success of the gingivectomy usually requires that the medication be discontinued or that a switch to a noncalcium channel blocker be made. If for some reason nifedipine cannot be discontinued, hyperplasia has not recurred after gingivectomy when extensive plaque control was performed. If nifedipine is changed to another class of cardiovascular agent, the gingival hyperplasia will probably regress and resolve. Switching to another calcium channel blocker may result in continued hyperplasia.
Effects on Bleeding No information available to require special precautions

Adverse Effects

>10%:
Cardiovascular: Flushing (10% to 25%; extended release products 3% to 4%), peripheral edema (dose related 7% to 30%)
Central nervous system: Dizziness/lightheadedness/giddiness (10% to 27%), headache (10% to 23%)
Gastrointestinal: Nausea/heartburn (10% to 11%)
≥1% to 10%:
Cardiovascular: Palpitation (≤2% to 7%), transient hypotension (dose related 5%), CHF (2%)
Central nervous system: Nervousness/mood changes (≤2% to 7%), fatigue (6%), shakiness (≤2%), jitteriness (≤2%), sleep disturbances (≤2%), difficulties in balance (≤2%), fever (≤2%), chills (≤2%)
Dermatologic: Dermatitis (≤2%), pruritus (≤2%), urticaria (≤2%)
Endocrine & metabolic: Sexual difficulties (≤2%)
Gastrointestinal: Diarrhea (≤2%), constipation (≤2%), cramps (≤2%), flatulence (≤2%), gingival hyperplasia (≤10%)
Neuromuscular & skeletal: Muscle cramps/tremor (≤2% to 8%), weakness (<3%), inflammation (≤2%), joint stiffness (≤2%)
Ocular: Blurred vision (≤2%)
Respiratory: Cough/wheezing (6%), nasal congestion/sore throat (≤2% to 6%), chest congestion (≤2%), dyspnea (≤2%)
Miscellaneous: Diaphoresis (≤2%)

Dosage Oral:

Children 1-17 years:
High altitude pulmonary edema (unlabeled use; Pollard, 2001): **Note:** Treatment with nifedipine is only necessary if response to oxygen and/or descent is unsatisfactory; extended release preparation is preferred at equivalent dose with proper frequency adjustment:
Immediate release: 0.5 mg/kg/dose (maximum: 20 mg/dose) every 8 hours
Hypertension (unlabeled use): Extended release tablet: Initial: 0.25-0.5 mg/kg/day once daily or in 2 divided doses; maximum: 3 mg/kg/day up to 120 mg/day
Adults: **Note:** Dosage adjustments should occur at 7- to 14-day intervals, to allow for adequate assessment of new dose; when switching from immediate release to sustained release formulations, use same total daily dose.
Chronic stable or vasospastic angina:
Immediate release: Initial: 10 mg 3 times/day; usual dose: 10-20 mg 3 times/day; coronary artery spasm may require up to 20-30 mg 3-4 times/day; single doses >30 mg and total daily doses >120 mg are rarely needed; maximum: 180 mg/day; **Note:** Do not use for acute anginal episodes; may precipitate myocardial infarction
Extended release: Initial: 30 or 60 mg once daily; maximum: 120-180 mg/day
Hypertension: Extended release: Initial: 30 or 60 mg once daily; maximum: 90-120 mg/day
High altitude pulmonary edema (unlabeled use; Luks, 2010):
Prevention: Extended release: 30 mg every 12 hours starting the day before ascent and may be discontinued after staying at the same elevation for 5 days or if descent initiated
Treatment: Extended release: 30 mg every 12 hours
Pulmonary hypertension (unlabeled use; Galie, 2004): Extended release: Initial: 30 mg twice daily; may increase cautiously to 120-240 mg/day

◄ Raynaud's phenomenon (unlabeled use; Wigley, 2002): Extended release: Dosage range: 30-120 mg once daily

Elderly: Hypertension: Consider lower initial doses and titrate to response (Aronow, 2011)

Dosage adjustment in renal impairment: No dosage adjustment provided in manufacturer's labeling (has not been studied); use with caution.

Hemodialysis: Supplemental dose is not necessary

Peritoneal dialysis effects: Supplemental dose is not necessary

Dosage adjustment in hepatic impairment: No dosage adjustment provided in manufacturer's labeling (has not been studied); use with caution. Clearance of nifedipine is reduced in cirrhotic patients, which may lead to increased systemic exposure; monitor closely for adverse effects/toxicity and consider dose adjustments.

Mechanism of Action Inhibits calcium ion from entering the "slow channels" or select voltage-sensitive areas of vascular smooth muscle and myocardium during depolarization, producing a relaxation of coronary vascular smooth muscle and coronary vasodilation; increases myocardial oxygen delivery in patients with vasospastic angina; also reduces peripheral vascular resistance, producing a reduction in arterial blood pressure.

Contraindications Hypersensitivity to nifedipine or any component of the formulation; concomitant use with strong CYP3A4 inducers (eg, rifampin); cardiogenic shock; immediate release preparation for treatment of urgent or emergent hypertension (Chobanian, 2003); acute MI (Antman, 2004)

Warnings/Precautions Symptomatic hypotension with or without syncope can rarely occur; blood pressure must be lowered at a rate appropriate for the patient's clinical condition. **The use of immediate release nifedipine (sublingually or orally) in hypertensive emergencies and urgencies is neither safe nor effective.** Serious adverse events (eg, death, cerebrovascular ischemia, syncope, stroke, acute myocardial infarction, and fetal distress) have been reported. **Immediate release nifedipine should not be used for acute blood pressure reduction.**

Blood pressure lowering should be done at a rate appropriate for the patient's condition. Rapid drops in blood pressure can lead to arterial insufficiency. Increased angina and/or MI have occurred with initiation or dosage titration of dihydropyridine calcium channel blockers; use with caution in patients with obstructive coronary disease especially in the absence of concurrent beta-blockade. Use with caution before major surgery. Cardiopulmonary bypass, intraoperative blood loss or vasodilating anesthesia may result in severe hypotension and/or increased fluid requirements. Consider withdrawing nifedipine (>36 hours) before surgery if possible.

The most common side effect is peripheral edema; occurs within 2-3 weeks of starting therapy. Reflex tachycardia may occur with use. Use with caution in HF or severe aortic stenosis (especially with concomitant beta-adrenergic blocker), severe left ventricular dysfunction, renal impairment, hypertrophic cardiomyopathy (especially obstructive), concomitant therapy with beta-blockers or digoxin, and edema. Use caution in patients with severe hepatic impairment. Clearance of nifedipine is reduced in cirrhotic patients leading to increased systemic exposure; monitor closely for adverse effects/toxicity and consider dose adjustments.

Mild and transient elevations in liver function enzymes may be apparent within 8 weeks of therapy initiation. Abrupt withdrawal may cause rebound angina in patients with CAD. In the elderly, immediate release nifedipine should be avoided in due to potential to cause hypotension and risk of precipitating myocardial ischemia (Beers Criteria). Immediate release formulations should not be used to manage essential hypertension, adequate studies to evaluate outcomes have not been conducted. Avoid use of extended release tablets (Procardia XL®) in patients with known stricture/narrowing of the GI tract. Adalat® CC tablets contain lactose; do not use with galactose intolerance, Lapp lactase deficiency, or glucose-galactose malabsorption syndromes.

Use with caution in patients taking CYP3A4 inhibitors; may result in increased nifedipine concentrations; monitor for adverse effects/toxicity and consider dose adjustments. Use with strong CYP3A4 inducers (eg, rifampin, rifabutin, phenobarbital, phenytoin, carbamazepine, St John's wort) is contraindicated due to reduced bioavailability and efficacy.

Drug Interactions

Metabolism/Transport Effects Substrate of CYP2D6 (minor), CYP3A4 (major); **Note:** Assignment of Major/Minor substrate status based on clinically relevant drug interaction potential; **Inhibits** CYP1A2 (moderate), CYP2C9 (weak), CYP2D6 (weak), CYP3A4 (weak)

Avoid Concomitant Use

Avoid concomitant use of NIFEdipine with any of the following: Conivaptan; Grapefruit Juice; Pimozide; Pirfenidone

Increased Effect/Toxicity

NIFEdipine may increase the levels/effects of: Amifostine; Antihypertensives; ARIPiprazole; Atosiban; Beta-Blockers; Calcium Channel Blockers (Nondihydropyridine); CYP1A2 Substrates; Digoxin; Fosphenytoin; Hypotensive Agents; Lomitapide; Magnesium Salts; Neuromuscular-Blocking Agents (Nondepolarizing); Nitroprusside; Phenytoin; Pimozide; Pirfenidone; QuiNIDine; RiTUXimab; Tacrolimus (Systemic); VinCRIStine; VinCRIStine (Liposomal)

The levels/effects of NIFEdipine may be increased by: Alcohol (Ethyl); Alpha1-Blockers; Antifungal Agents (Azole Derivatives, Systemic); Calcium Channel Blockers (Nondihydropyridine); Cimetidine; Cisapride; Conivaptan; CycloSPORINE (Systemic); CYP3A4 Inhibitors (Moderate); CYP3A4 Inhibitors (Strong); Dasatinib; Diazoxide; Fluconazole; FLUoxetine; Grapefruit Juice; Herbs (Hypotensive Properties); Ivacaftor; Macrolide Antibiotics; Magnesium Salts; MAO Inhibitors; Mifepristone; Pentoxifylline; Phosphodiesterase 5 Inhibitors; Prostacyclin Analogues; Protease Inhibitors; QuiNIDine

Decreased Effect

NIFEdipine may decrease the levels/effects of: Clopidogrel; QuiNIDine

The levels/effects of NIFEdipine may be decreased by: Barbiturates; Calcium Salts; CarBAMazepine; CYP3A4 Inducers (Strong); Deferasirox; Herbs (CYP3A4 Inducers); Herbs (Hypertensive Properties); Melatonin; Methylphenidate; Nafcillin; Peginterferon Alfa-2b; Rifamycin Derivatives; Tocilizumab; Yohimbine

Ethanol/Nutrition/Herb Interactions

Ethanol: Ethanol may increase CNS depression and may increase the effects of nifedipine. Management: Avoid ethanol.

Food: Nifedipine serum levels may be decreased if taken with food. Food may decrease the rate but not the extent of absorption of Procardia XL®. Increased nifedipine concentrations resulting in therapeutic and vasodilator side effects, including severe hypotension and myocardial ischemia, may occur if nifedipine is taken by patients ingesting grapefruit. Management: Avoid grapefruit/grapefruit juice. Avoid caffeine.

Herb/Nutraceutical: St John's wort may decrease nifedipine levels. Some herbal medications (eg, licorice) may worsen hypertension; others may increase the antihypertensive effect of nifedipine (eg, shepherd's purse). Management: Avoid bayberry, blue cohosh, cayenne, ephedra, ginger, ginseng (American), kola, licorice, and yohimbe. Avoid black cohosh, California poppy, coleus, golden seal, hawthorn, mistletoe, periwinkle, quinine, and shepherd's purse.

Dietary Considerations Avoid grapefruit juice with all products.

Immediate release: Capsule is rapidly absorbed orally if it is administered without food, but may result in vasodilator side effects; if flushing is problematic, administration with low-fat meals may decrease. In general, can take with or without food.

Extended release: Adalat® CC, Afeditab® CR, Nifediac CC®: Take on an empty stomach (manufacturer recommendation). Other extended release products may not have this recommendation; consult product labeling.

Pharmacodynamics/Kinetics

Onset of Action Immediate release: ~20 minutes

Half-life Elimination Adults: Healthy: 2-5 hours; Cirrhosis: 7 hours; Elderly: 7 hours (extended release tablet)

Pregnancy Risk Factor C

Pregnancy Considerations Adverse events were observed in animal reproduction studies. Nifedipine crosses the placenta. Use in pregnancy only when clearly needed and when the benefits outweigh the potential hazard to the fetus. Hypotension, IUGR reported. IUGR probably related to maternal hypertension. Nifedipine has been evaluated for the treatment of preterm labor. Tocolytics may be used for the short-term (48 hour) prolongation of pregnancy to allow for the administration of antenatal steroids and should not be used prior to fetal viability or when the risks of use to the fetus or mother are greater than the risk of preterm birth (ACOG, 2012). Nifedipine is ineffective for maintenance tocolytic therapy (ACOG, 2012).

Lactation Enters breast milk/not recommended (AAP considers "compatible"; AAP 2001 update pending)

Dosage Forms

Capsule, softgel, oral: 10 mg, 20 mg

Procardia®: 10 mg

Tablet, extended release, oral: 30 mg, 60 mg, 90 mg

Adalat® CC: 30 mg, 60 mg, 90 mg

Afeditab® CR: 30 mg, 60 mg

Nifediac CC®: 90 mg

Nifedical XL®: 30 mg, 60 mg

Procardia XL®: 30 mg, 60 mg, 90 mg

References

Deen-Duggins L, Fry HR, Clay JR, et al, "Nifedipine-Associated Gingival Overgrowth: A Survey of the Literature and Report of Four Cases," *Quintessence Int*, 1996, 27(3):163-70.

Harel-Raviv M, Eckler M, Lalani K, et al, "Nifedipine-Induced Gingival Hyperplasia. A Comprehensive Review and Analysis," *Oral Surg Oral Med Oral Pathol Oral Radiol Endod*, 1995, 79(6):715-22.

Nery EB, Edson RG, Lee KK, et al, "Prevalence of Nifedipine-Induced Gingival Hyperplasia," *J Periodontol*, 1995, 66(7):572-8.

Nishikawa SJ, Tada H, Hamasaki A, et al, "Nifedipine-Induced Gingival Hyperplasia: A Clinical and In Vitro Study," *J Periodontol*, 1991, 62(1):30-5.

Silverstein LH, Koch JP, Lefkove MD, et al, "Nifedipine-Induced Gingival Enlargement Around Dental Implants: A Clinical Report," *J Oral Implantol*, 1995, 21(2):116-20.

Westbrook P, Bednarczyk EM, Carlson M, et al, "Regression of Nifedipine-Induced Gingival Hyperplasia Following Switch to a Same Class Calcium Channel Blocker, Isradipine," *J Periodontol*, 1997, 68 (7):645-50.

Wynn RL, "Calcium Channel Blockers and Gingival Hyperplasia-An Update," *Gen Dent*, 2009, 57(2):105-7.

Nilotinib (nye LOE ti nib)

Related Information

Clinical Risk Related to Drugs Prolonging QT Interval *on page 1510*

Brand Names: U.S. Tasigna®

Brand Names: Canada Tasigna®

Pharmacologic Category Antineoplastic Agent, Tyrosine Kinase Inhibitor

Use Treatment of newly-diagnosed Philadelphia chromosome-positive chronic myelogenous leukemia (Ph+ CML) in chronic phase; treatment of chronic and accelerated phase Ph+ CML refractory or intolerant to prior therapy (including imatinib)

Unlabeled Use Treatment of refractory gastrointestinal stromal tumor (GIST)

Local Anesthetic/Vasoconstrictor Precautions Nilotinib is one of the drugs confirmed to prolong the QT interval and is accepted as having a risk of causing torsade de pointes. The risk of drug-induced torsade de pointes is extremely low when a single QT interval prolonging drug is prescribed. In terms of epinephrine, it is not known what effect vasoconstrictors in the local anesthetic regimen will have in patients with a known history of congenital prolonged QT interval or in patients taking any medication that prolongs the QT interval. Until more information is obtained, it is suggested that the clinician consult with the physician prior to the use of a vasoconstrictor in suspected patients, and that the vasoconstrictor (epinephrine, mepivacaine and levonordefrin [Carbocaine® 2% with Neo-Cobefrin®]) be used with caution.

Effects on Dental Treatment Key adverse event(s) related to dental treatment: Mouth ulcerations, stomatitis

Effects on Bleeding Chemotherapy may result in significant myelosuppression. Thrombocytopenia (grades 3/4) occurs in 10% to 37% of patients (median duration 22 days). In patients who are under active treatment with these agents, medical consult is suggested.

Adverse Effects

>10%:

Cardiovascular: Peripheral edema (8% to 15%), hypertension (10% to 11%)

Central nervous system: Headache (20% to 35%), fatigue (21% to 32%), fever (11% to 28%), insomnia (7% to 12%)

Dermatologic: Rash (29% to 38%), pruritus (20% to 32%), alopecia (11% to 13%)

Endocrine & metabolic: Hypophosphatemia (grades 3/4: 5% to 17%), hyperglycemia (grades 3/4: 6% to 12%)

Gastrointestinal: Nausea (20% to 37%), vomiting (11% to 29%), diarrhea (14% to 28%), constipation (17% to 26%), lipase increased (1% to ≥10%; grades 3/4: 7% to 18%), abdominal pain (12% to 17%), anorexia (12% to 15%)

Hematologic: Neutropenia (grades 3/4: 12% to 42%; median duration: 15 days), thrombocytopenia (grades 3/4: 10% to 42%; median duration: 22 days), anemia (grades 3/4: 4% to 27%)

◀ Hepatic: Hyperbilirubinemia (≥10%; grades 3/4: 4% to 9%), ALT increased (≥10%; grades 3/4: 4%), AST increased (≥10%; grades 3/4: 1% to 3%)

Neuromuscular & skeletal: Arthralgia (16% to 26%), limb pain (11% to 20%), myalgia (14% to 19%), back pain (14% to 17%), weakness (11% to 16%), bone pain (14% to 15%), muscle spasm (11% to 15%), musculoskeletal pain (11% to 12%)

Respiratory: Cough (14% to 27%), nasopharyngitis (15% to 24%), dyspnea (9% to 15%), upper respiratory tract infection (≤15%), oropharyngeal pain (7% to 11%)

Miscellaneous: Night sweats (12% to 27%), flu-like syndrome (11%)

1% to 10%:

Cardiovascular: Arterial stenosis (5% to 6%), cerebrovascular accident (5% to 6%), peripheral arterial occlusive disease (5% to 6%), angina, arrhythmia (including AV block, atrial fibrillation, bradycardia, cardiac flutter, extrasystoles, and tachycardia), chest pain (including noncardiac), flushing, palpitation, QT interval prolonged

Central nervous system: Dizziness (10%), anxiety, depression, dysphonia, hypoesthesia, malaise, pain, vertigo

Dermatologic: Dry skin (>5% to <10%), acne, bruising, dermatitis (including allergic and acneiform), eczema, erythema, folliculitis, hyperhidrosis, skin papilloma, urticaria

Endocrine & metabolic: Hypokalemia (grades 3/4: ≤9%), hyponatremia (grades 3/4: ≤7%), hyperkalemia (grades 3/4: 2% to 6%), hypocalcemia (grades 3/4: ≤5%), albumin decreased (grades 3/4: ≤4%), diabetes mellitus, hypercalcemia, hypercholesterolemia, hyperlipidemia, hyperphosphatemia, hypomagnesemia

Gastrointestinal: Dyspepsia (4% to 10%), abdominal discomfort, abnormal taste, amylase increased, flatulence, pancreatitis, weight gain/loss

Genitourinary: Pollakuria

Hematologic: Lymphopenia, neutropenic fever, pancytopenia

Hepatic: Alkaline phosphatase increased (grades 3/4: ≤1%), GGT increased

Neuromuscular & skeletal: Paresthesia, peripheral neuropathy

Ocular: Eyelid edema (1%), conjunctivitis, dry eye, eye hemorrhage, periorbital edema, pruritus

Respiratory: Pleural effusion (≤1%), dyspnea (exertional), epistaxis

General Dosage Range Dosage adjustment recommended in patients with hepatic impairment, on concomitant therapy, or who develop toxicities

Oral: *Adults:* 300-400 mg twice daily

Mechanism of Action Selective tyrosine kinase inhibitor that targets BCR-ABL kinase, c-KIT and platelet derived growth factor receptor (PDGFR); does not have activity against the SRC family. Inhibits BCR-ABL mediated proliferation of leukemic cell lines by binding to the ATP-binding site of BCR-ABL and inhibiting tyrosine kinase activity. Nilotinib has activity in imatinib-resistant BCR-ABL kinase mutations.

Pharmacodynamics/Kinetics

Half-life Elimination ~15-17 hour

Time to Peak 3 hours

Pregnancy Risk Factor D

Pregnancy Considerations Animal reproduction studies have demonstrated embryo-fetal toxicity and maternal toxicity. Women of childbearing potential should be advised to use effective contraception during treatment.

Dental Comment Nilotinib is known to prolong the QT interval. The QT interval is measured as the time and distance between the Q point of the QRS complex and the end of the T wave in the ECG tracing. After adjustment for heart rate, the QT interval is defined as prolonged if it is more than 450 msec in men and 460 msec in women. A long QT syndrome was first described in the 1950s and 60s as a congenital syndrome involving QT interval prolongation and syncope and sudden death. Some of the congenital long QT syndromes were characterized by a peculiar electrocardiographic appearance of the QRS complex involving a premature atria beat followed by a pause, then a subsequent sinus beat showing marked QT prolongation and deformity. This type of cardiac arrhythmia was originally termed "torsade de pointes" (translated from the French as "twisting of the points"). Nilotinib is considered as having a risk of causing torsade de pointes. Since it is not known what effect vasoconstrictors in the local anesthetic regimen will have in patients with a known history of congenital prolonged QT interval or in patients taking any medication that prolongs the QT interval, a medical consult is suggested.

Nilutamide (ni LOO ta mide)

Brand Names: U.S. Nilandron®
Brand Names: Canada Anandron®
Pharmacologic Category Antiandrogen; Antineoplastic Agent, Antiandrogen
Use Treatment of metastatic prostate cancer (in combination with surgical castration)
Local Anesthetic/Vasoconstrictor Precautions No information available to require special precautions
Effects on Dental Treatment Key adverse event(s) related to dental treatment: Xerostomia (normal salivary flow resumes upon discontinuation).
Effects on Bleeding Although significant myelosuppression with associated altered hemostasis has been reported for many chemotherapeutic agents, myelosuppression is not common with nilutamide and no specific precautions appear to necessary.

Adverse Effects

>10%:

Central nervous system: Insomnia (16%), headache (14%)

Endocrine & metabolic: Hot flashes (28% to 67%)

Gastrointestinal: Nausea (10% to 24%), constipation (7% to 20%), anorexia (11%), abdominal pain (10%)

Genitourinary: Testicular atrophy (16%), libido decreased (11%)

Hepatic: AST increased (8% to 13%), ALT increased (8% to 9%)

Ocular: Impaired dark adaptation (13% to 57%)

Respiratory: Dyspnea (6% to 11%)

1% to 10%:

Cardiovascular: Hypertension (5% to 9%), chest pain (7%), heart failure (3%), angina (2%), edema (2%), syncope (2%)

Central nervous system: Dizziness (7% to 10%), depression (9%), hypoesthesia (5%), malaise (2%), nervousness (2%)

Dermatologic: Alopecia (6%), dry skin (5%), rash (5%), pruritus (2%)

Endocrine & metabolic: Alcohol intolerance (5%), hyperglycemia (4%)

Gastrointestinal: Vomiting (6%), diarrhea (2%), GI hemorrhage (2%), melena (2%), weight loss (2%), xerostomia (2%), dyspepsia

Genitourinary: Nocturia (7%)

Hematologic: Anemia (7%), haptoglobin increased (2%), leukopenia (2%)

Hepatic: Alkaline phosphatase increased (3%)

Neuromuscular & skeletal: Bone pain (6%), arthritis (2%), paresthesia (2%)

Ocular: Chromatopsia (9%), impaired light adaptation (8%), abnormal vision (6% to 7%), cataract (2%), photophobia (2%)

Renal: Hematuria (8%), BUN increased (2%), creatinine increased (2%)

Respiratory: Pneumonia (5%), cough (2%), interstitial pneumonitis (2%), rhinitis (2%)

Miscellaneous: Flu-like syndrome (7%), diaphoresis (6%)

General Dosage Range Oral: *Adults:* Initial: 300 mg once daily; Maintenance: 150 mg once daily

Mechanism of Action Nonsteroidal antiandrogen which blocks testosterone effects at the androgen receptor level, preventing androgen response.

Pharmacodynamics/Kinetics

Half-life Elimination Terminal: 38-59 hours; Metabolites: 59-126 hours

Pregnancy Risk Factor C

Pregnancy Considerations Animal reproduction studies have not been conducted. Not indicated for use in women.

NiMODipine (nye MOE di peen)

Related Information

Calcium Channel Blockers and Gingival Hyperplasia *on page 1640*

Brand Names: Canada Nimotop®

Pharmacologic Category Calcium Channel Blocker; Calcium Channel Blocker, Dihydropyridine

Use Vasospasm following subarachnoid hemorrhage from ruptured intracranial aneurysms

Local Anesthetic/Vasoconstrictor Precautions No information available to require special precautions

Effects on Dental Treatment Other drugs of this class can cause gingival hyperplasia (ie, nifedipine) but there have been no reports for nimodipine.

Effects on Bleeding No information available to require special precautions

Adverse Effects 1% to 10%:

Cardiovascular: Reductions in systemic blood pressure (1% to 8%)

Central nervous system: Headache (1% to 4%)

Dermatologic: Rash (1% to 2%)

Gastrointestinal: Diarrhea (2% to 4%), abdominal discomfort (2%)

General Dosage Range Dosage adjustment recommended in patients with hepatic impairment

Oral: *Adults:* 60 mg every 4 hours

Mechanism of Action Nimodipine shares the pharmacology of other calcium channel blockers; animal studies indicate that nimodipine has a greater effect on cerebral arterials than other arterials; this increased specificity may be due to the drug's increased lipophilicity and cerebral distribution as compared to nifedipine; inhibits calcium ion from entering the "slow channels" or select voltage sensitive areas of vascular smooth muscle and myocardium during depolarization

Pharmacodynamics/Kinetics

Half-life Elimination 1-2 hours; prolonged with renal impairment

Time to Peak Serum: ~1 hour

Pregnancy Risk Factor C

Pregnancy Considerations Use in pregnancy only when clearly needed and when the benefits outweigh the potential hazard to the fetus. Teratogenic and embryotoxic effects have been demonstrated in small animals. No well-controlled studies have been conducted in pregnant women.

Nisoldipine (nye SOL di peen)

Related Information

Calcium Channel Blockers and Gingival Hyperplasia *on page 1640*

Cardiovascular Diseases *on page 1492*

Brand Names: U.S. Sular®

Pharmacologic Category Calcium Channel Blocker; Calcium Channel Blocker, Dihydropyridine

Use Management of hypertension, alone or in combination with other antihypertensive agents

Local Anesthetic/Vasoconstrictor Precautions No information available to require special precautions

Effects on Dental Treatment Key adverse event(s) related to dental treatment: Xerostomia (normal salivary flow resumes upon discontinuation).

Unlike other calcium channel blockers, information is sparse as to whether nisoldipine causes gingival hyperplasia. Consultation with physician is suggested if hyperplasia is observed in patients taking nisoldipine.

Effects on Bleeding No information available to require special precautions

Adverse Effects

>10%:

Cardiovascular: Peripheral edema (dose related; 7% to 29%)

Central nervous system: Headache (22%)

1% to 10%:

Cardiovascular: Vasodilation (4%), palpitation (3%), angina exacerbation (2%), chest pain (2%)

Central nervous system: Dizziness (3% to 10%)

Dermatologic: Rash (2%)

Gastrointestinal: Nausea (2%)

Respiratory: Pharyngitis (5%), sinusitis (3%)

General Dosage Range Dosage adjustment recommended in patients with hepatic impairment

Oral:

Adults:

Sular® (Geomatrix® delivery system): Initial: 17 mg once daily; Maintenance: 17-34 mg once daily (maximum: 34 mg/day)

Nisoldipine extended-release (original formulation): Initial: 20 mg once daily; Maintenance: 10-40 mg once daily (maximum: 60 mg/day)

Elderly: Sular® (Geomatrix® delivery system): Initial: 8.5 mg once daily; Nisoldipine extended-release (original formulation): Initial: 10 mg once daily

Mechanism of Action As a dihydropyridine calcium channel blocker, structurally similar to nifedipine, nisoldipine impedes the movement of calcium ions into vascular smooth muscle and cardiac muscle. Dihydropyridines are potent vasodilators and are not as likely to suppress cardiac contractility and slow cardiac conduction as other calcium antagonists such as verapamil and diltiazem; nisoldipine is 5-10 times as potent a vasodilator as nifedipine.

Pharmacodynamics/Kinetics

Duration of Action >24 hours

Half-life Elimination 9-18 hours

Time to Peak 4-14 hours

Pregnancy Risk Factor C

Pregnancy Considerations Animal studies have demonstrated fetotoxic but not teratogenic effects. There are no adequate and well-controlled studies in pregnant women. Use during pregnancy only if potential benefit to the mother outweighs potential risk to the fetus.

Nitazoxanide (nye ta ZOX a nide)

Brand Names: U.S. Alinia®

Pharmacologic Category Antiprotozoal

Use Treatment of diarrhea caused by *Cryptosporidium parvum* or *Giardia lamblia*

Unlabeled Use Alternative treatment for *Clostridium difficile*-associated diarrhea (CDAD)

Local Anesthetic/Vasoconstrictor Precautions No information available to require special precautions

Effects on Dental Treatment No significant effects or complications reported

Effects on Bleeding No information available to require special precautions

Adverse Effects Rates of adverse effects were similar to those reported with placebo.

1% to 10%:

Central nervous system: Headache (1% to 3%)

Gastrointestinal: Abdominal pain (7% to 8%), diarrhea (2% to 4%), nausea (3%), vomiting (1%)

General Dosage Range Oral:

Children 1-3 years: 100 mg every 12 hours (oral suspension)

Children 4-11 years: 200 mg every 12 hours (oral suspension)

Children ≥12 years and Adults: 500 mg every 12 hours (oral suspension or tablets)

Mechanism of Action Nitazoxanide is rapidly metabolized to the active metabolite tizoxanide *in vivo*. Activity may be due to interference with the pyruvate:ferredoxin oxidoreductase (PFOR) enzyme-dependent electron transfer reaction which is essential to anaerobic metabolism. *In vitro*, nitazoxanide and tizoxanide inhibit the growth of sporozoites and oocysts of *Cryptosporidium parvum* and trophozoites of *Giardia lamblia*.

Pharmacodynamics/Kinetics

Time to Peak Plasma: Tizoxanide and tizoxanide glucuronide: 1-4 hours

Pregnancy Risk Factor B

Pregnancy Considerations Teratogenic effects were not observed in animal reproduction studies.

Nitisinone (ni TIS i known)

Brand Names: U.S. Orfadin®

Pharmacologic Category 4-Hydroxyphenylpyruvate Dioxygenase Inhibitor

Use Treatment of hereditary tyrosinemia type 1 (HT-1) as an adjunct to dietary restriction of tyrosine and phenylalanine

Local Anesthetic/Vasoconstrictor Precautions No information available to require special precautions

Effects on Dental Treatment No significant effects or complications reported

Effects on Bleeding Thrombocytopenia occurs in about 3% of patients and may be due to underlying liver disease.

Adverse Effects 1% to 10%:

Dermatologic: Alopecia (1%), dry skin (1%), exfoliative dermatitis (1%), maculopapular rash (1%), pruritus (1%)

Hematologic: Thrombocytopenia (3%), leukopenia (3%), epistaxis (1%), granulocytopenia (1%), porphyria (1%)

Hepatic: Hepatic neoplasm (8%), hepatic failure (7%)

Ocular: Conjunctivitis (2%), corneal opacity (2%), keratitis (2%), photophobia (2%), blepharitis (1%), cataracts (1%), eye pain (1%)

General Dosage Range Oral: *Infants, Children, and Adults:* 1-2 mg/kg/day in 2 divided doses

Mechanism of Action In patients with HT-1, tyrosine metabolism is interrupted due to a lack of the enzyme (fumarylacetoacetate hydrolase) needed in the last step of tyrosine degradation. Toxic metabolites of tyrosine accumulate and cause liver and kidney toxicity. Nitisinone competitively inhibits 4-hydroxyphenyl-pyruvate dioxygenase, an enzyme present early in the tyrosine degradation pathway, thereby preventing the build-up of the toxic metabolites.

Pharmacodynamics/Kinetics

Half-life Elimination Terminal: 54 hours (healthy volunteers)

Time to Peak 3 hours (healthy volunteers)

Pregnancy Risk Factor C

Pregnancy Considerations Adverse events were observed in some animal reproduction studies.

Prescribing and Access Restrictions Distributed by Rare Disease Therapeutics, Inc; for information regarding acquisition of product, call Accredo Health Group, Inc at 1-888-454-8860

Nitrazepam (nye TRA ze pam)

Brand Names: Canada Apo-Nitrazepam®; Mogadon; Nitrazadon®; Sandoz-Nitrazepam

Pharmacologic Category Benzodiazepine

Use Short-term management of insomnia; treatment of myoclonic seizures

Local Anesthetic/Vasoconstrictor Precautions No information available to require special precautions.

Effects on Dental Treatment Key adverse event(s) related to dental treatment: Excessive salivation has been reported. The mechanism of this effect is unknown, since many benzodiazepines cause xerostomia rather than salivation excess.

Effects on Bleeding No information available to require special precautions

Adverse Effects Frequency not defined.

Cardiovascular: Hypotension, palpitation

Central nervous system: Agitation, aggressiveness, amnesia, ataxia, confusion, delusions, depression, disorientation, dizziness, excitement, fatigue, hallucination, hangover, headache, hyperactivity, irritability, lethargy, lightheadedness, nervousness, nightmares, psychoses, rage, restlessness, sedation, staggering

Dermatologic: Cutaneous reactions

Endocrine & metabolic: Changes in libido

Gastrointestinal: Constipation, diarrhea, excessive salivation, heartburn, nausea, vomiting

Hematologic: Granulocytopenia, leukopenia

Hepatic: Hepatic function tests abnormal

Neuromuscular & skeletal: Delirium tremens, falling, muscle spasticity increased, muscle weakness

Ocular: Blurred vision

Respiratory: Aspiration, bronchial hypersecretion, dyspnea

Miscellaneous: Anaphylaxis/anaphylactoid reactions (angioedema, dyspnea, throat closing, nausea/vomiting)

General Dosage Range Oral:
Children ≤30 kg: 0.3-1 mg/kg/day in 3 divided doses
Adults: 5-10 mg once daily
Elderly: 2.5-5 mg once daily
Mechanism of Action Binds to stereospecific benzodiazepine receptors on the postsynaptic GABA neuron at several sites within the CNS, including the limbic system, reticular formation. Enhancement of the inhibitory effect of GABA on neuronal excitability results by increased neuronal membrane permeability to chloride ions. This shift in chloride ions results in hyperpolarization (a less excitable state) and stabilization.
Pharmacodynamics/Kinetics
Onset of Action 20-50 minutes
Half-life Elimination 30 hours, Elderly/ill patients: 40 hours
Time to Peak ~3 hours
Pregnancy Considerations Use during pregnancy is not recommended. Nitrazepam crosses the human placenta. Teratogenic effects have been observed with some benzodiazepines; however, additional studies are needed. The incidence of premature birth and low birth weights may be increased following maternal use of benzodiazepines; hypoglycemia and respiratory problems in the neonate may occur following exposure late in pregnancy. Neonatal withdrawal symptoms may occur within days to weeks after birth and "floppy infant syndrome" (which also includes withdrawal symptoms) have been reported with some benzodiazepines.
Product Availability Not available in U.S.
Controlled Substance CDSA IV

Nitric Oxide (NYE trik OKS ide)

Brand Names: U.S. INOmax®
Brand Names: Canada INOmax®
Pharmacologic Category Vasodilator, Pulmonary
Use Treatment of term and near-term (>34 weeks) neonates with hypoxic respiratory failure associated with pulmonary hypertension; used concurrently with ventilatory support and other agents
Unlabeled Use Treatment of adult respiratory distress syndrome (ARDS); acute vasodilator testing in pulmonary artery hypertension (PAH); right ventricular dysfunction after cardiac surgery
Local Anesthetic/Vasoconstrictor Precautions No information available to require special precautions
Effects on Dental Treatment No significant effects or complications reported
Effects on Bleeding No information available to require special precautions
Adverse Effects
>10%:
Cardiovascular: Hypotension (13%)
Miscellaneous: Withdrawal syndrome (12%)
1% to 10%:
Dermatologic: Cellulitis (5%)
Endocrine & metabolic: Hyperglycemia (8%)
Genitourinary: Hematuria (8%)
Respiratory: Atelectasis (9% - same as placebo), stridor (5%)
Miscellaneous: Sepsis (7%), infection (6%)
General Dosage Range Inhalation: *Neonates (up to 14 days old):* 20 ppm
Mechanism of Action In neonates with persistent pulmonary hypertension, nitric oxide improves oxygenation. Nitric oxide relaxes vascular smooth muscle by binding to the heme moiety of cytosolic guanylate cyclase, activating guanylate cyclase and increasing intracellular levels of cyclic guanosine 3',5'-monophosphate, which leads to vasodilation. When inhaled, pulmonary vasodilation occurs and an increase in the partial pressure of arterial oxygen results. Dilation of pulmonary vessels in well ventilated lung areas redistributes blood flow away from lung areas where ventilation/perfusion ratios are poor.
Pregnancy Risk Factor C
Pregnancy Considerations Reproduction studies have not been conducted.

Nitrofurantoin (nye troe fyoor AN toyn)

Brand Names: U.S. Furadantin®; Macrobid®; Macrodantin®
Brand Names: Canada Apo-Nitrofurantoin®; Macrobid®; Macrodantin®; Novo-Furantoin; Teva-Nitrofurantoin
Pharmacologic Category Antibiotic, Miscellaneous
Use Prevention and treatment of urinary tract infections caused by susceptible strains of *E. coli, S. aureus, Enterococcus, Klebsiella,* and *Enterobacter*
Local Anesthetic/Vasoconstrictor Precautions No information available to require special precautions
Effects on Dental Treatment No significant effects or complications reported
Effects on Bleeding No information available to require special precautions
Adverse Effects Frequency not defined.
Cardiovascular: Cyanosis, ECG changes (nonspecific ST/T wave changes, bundle branch block)
Central nervous system: Bulging fontanels (infants), chills, confusion, depression, dizziness, drowsiness, fever, headache, malaise, pseudotumor cerebri, psychotic reaction, vertigo
Dermatologic: Alopecia, angioedema, erythema multiforme, exfoliative dermatitis, pruritus, rash (eczematous, erythematous, maculopapular), Stevens-Johnson syndrome, urticaria
Endocrine & metabolic: Hyperphosphatemia
Gastrointestinal: Abdominal pain, anorexia, *C. difficile* colitis, constipation, diarrhea, dyspepsia, flatulence, nausea, pancreatitis, pseudomembranous colitis, sialadenitis, vomiting
Genitourinary: Urine discoloration (brown)
Hematologic: Agranulocytosis, aplastic anemia, eosinophilia, glucose-6-phosphate dehydrogenase deficiency anemia, granulocytopenia, hemoglobin decreased, hemolytic anemia, leukopenia, megaloblastic anemia, thrombocytopenia
Hepatic: Hepatitis, hepatic necrosis, transaminases increased, jaundice (cholestatic)
Neuromuscular & skeletal: Arthralgia, myalgia, numbness, paresthesia, peripheral neuropathy, weakness
Ocular: Amblyopia, nystagmus, optic neuritis
Respiratory: Cough, dyspnea, pneumonitis, pulmonary fibrosis (with long-term use), pulmonary infiltration
Miscellaneous: Acute pulmonary reaction (symptoms include chills, chest pain, cough, dyspnea, fever, and eosinophilia), anaphylaxis, hypersensitivity (including acute pulmonary hypersensitivity), lupus-like syndrome, superinfections (eg, *Pseudomonas* or *Candida*)
General Dosage Range Oral:
Children >1 month: Furadantin®, Macrodantin®: 5-7 mg/kg/day divided every 6 hours (maximum: 400 mg/day) **or** 1-2 mg/kg/day divided every 12-24 hours (maximum: 100 mg/day)
Children >12 years: Macrobid®: 100 mg twice daily

Adults: Furadantin®, Macrodantin®: 50-100 mg every 6 hours **or** once daily; Macrobid®: 100 mg twice daily

Mechanism of Action Inhibits several bacterial enzyme systems including acetyl coenzyme A interfering with metabolism and possibly cell wall synthesis

Pharmacodynamics/Kinetics

Half-life Elimination 20-60 minutes; prolonged with renal impairment

Pregnancy Risk Factor B (contraindicated at term)

Pregnancy Considerations Because adverse effects have not been observed in animals, nitrofurantoin is classified pregnancy category B. Nitrofurantoin crosses the placenta, but very little reaches the amniotic fluid. Most published experiences with nitrofurantoin use during pregnancy have failed to identify any increased obstetric or teratogenic risks. Isolated reports of a potential increased risk for cardiovascular defects and a case report of upper limb paralysis have not been replicated in other studies. Use of nitrofurantoin during pregnancy has been generally well tolerated with rare reports of maternal toxicity including severe pulmonary reactions or hematologic adverse effects. Nitrofurantoin is contraindicated in pregnant patients at term (38-42 weeks gestation), during labor and delivery, or when the onset of labor is imminent due to the possibility of hemolytic anemia in the neonate.

Nitroglycerin (nye troe GLI ser in)

Related Information
Cardiovascular Diseases *on page 1492*

Brand Names: U.S. Minitran™; Nitro-Bid®; Nitro-Dur®; Nitro-Time®; Nitrolingual®; NitroMist®; Nitrostat®; Rectiv®

Brand Names: Canada Minitran™; Mylan-Nitro Sublingual Spray; Nitro-Dur®; Nitroglycerin Injection, USP; Nitrol®; Nitrostat®; Rho®-Nitro Pump Spray; Transderm-Nitro®; Trinipatch®

Generic Availability (U.S.) Yes: Capsule, infusion, injection, patch, solution

Pharmacologic Category Antianginal Agent; Vasodilator

Use Treatment or prevention of angina pectoris

Intravenous (I.V.) administration: Treatment or prevention of angina pectoris; acute decompensated heart failure (especially when associated with acute myocardial infarction); perioperative hypertension (especially during cardiovascular surgery); induction of intraoperative hypotension

Intra-anal administration (Rectiv™ ointment): Treatment of moderate-to-severe pain associated with chronic anal fissure

Unlabeled Use Short-term management of pulmonary hypertension (I.V.); esophageal spastic disorders; uterine relaxation

Local Anesthetic/Vasoconstrictor Precautions No information available to require special precautions

Effects on Dental Treatment Key adverse event(s) related to dental treatment: Xerostomia (normal salivary flow resumes upon discontinuation).

Effects on Bleeding No information available to require special precautions

Adverse Effects Frequency not defined.

Cardiovascular: Flushing, hypotension, orthostatic hypotension, peripheral edema, syncope, tachycardia

Central nervous system: Headache (common), dizziness, lightheadedness

Gastrointestinal: Nausea, vomiting, xerostomia

Neuromuscular & skeletal: Paresthesia, weakness

Respiratory: Dyspnea, pharyngitis, rhinitis

Miscellaneous: Diaphoresis

Dosage Note: Hemodynamic and antianginal tolerance often develop within 24-48 hours of continuous nitrate administration. Nitrate-free interval (10-12 hours/day) is recommended to avoid tolerance development; gradually decrease dose in patients receiving NTG for prolonged period to avoid withdrawal reaction.

Adults:

Angina/coronary artery disease:

Oral: Initial: 2.5-6.5 mg 3-4 times/day; may titrate up to 26 mg 4 times/day

I.V.: 5 mcg/minute, increase by 5 mcg/minute every 3-5 minutes to 20 mcg/minute; if no response at 20 mcg/minute, may increase by 10-20 mcg/minute every 3-5 minutes (generally accepted maximum dose: 400 mcg/minute)

Sublingual: 0.3-0.6 mg every 5 minutes for maximum of 3 doses in 15 minutes; may also use prophylactically 5-10 minutes prior to activities which may provoke an attack

Topical ointment: 1/2" upon rising and 1/2" 6 hours later; if necessary, the dose may be doubled to 1" and subsequently doubled again to 2" if response is inadequate. Doses of 1/2" to 2" were used in clinical trials. Recommended maximum: 2 doses/day; include a nitrate free-interval ~10-12 hours/day.

Topical patch, transdermal: Initial: 0.2-0.4 mg/hour, titrate to 0.4-0.8 mg/hour; tolerance is minimized by using a patch-on period of 12-14 hours and patch-off period of 10-12 hours

Translingual: 1-2 sprays onto or under tongue every 3-5 minutes for maximum of 3 doses in 15 minutes, may also be used prophylactically 5-10 minutes prior to activities which may provoke an angina attack

Anal fissure, chronic (0.4% ointment): Intra-anal: 1 inch (equals 1.5 mg of nitroglycerin) every 12 hours for up to 3 weeks

Esophageal spastic disorders (unlabeled use): Sublingual: 0.3-0.6 mg (Swamy, 1977)

Uterine relaxation (unlabeled use): I.V. bolus: 100-200 mcg; may repeat dose every 2 minutes as necessary (Axemo, 1998; Chandraharan, 2005)

Elderly: In general, dose selection should be cautious, usually starting at the low end of the dosing range

Dosage adjustment in renal impairment: No dosage adjustment provided in manufacturer's labeling.

Dosage adjustment in hepatic impairment: No dosage adjustment provided in manufacturer's labeling.

Mechanism of Action Nitroglycerin forms free radical nitric oxide. In smooth muscle, nitric oxide activates guanylate cyclase which increases guanosine 3'5' monophosphate (cGMP) leading to dephosphorylation of myosin light chains and smooth muscle relaxation. Produces a vasodilator effect on the peripheral veins and arteries with more prominent effects on the veins. Primarily reduces cardiac oxygen demand by decreasing preload (left ventricular end-diastolic pressure); may modestly reduce afterload; dilates coronary arteries and improves collateral flow to ischemic regions. For use in rectal fissures, intra-anal administration results in decreased sphincter tone and intra-anal pressure.

Contraindications Hypersensitivity to organic nitrates or any component of the formulation (includes adhesives for transdermal product); concurrent use with phosphodiesterase-5 (PDE-5) inhibitors (sildenafil, tadalafil, or vardenafil); increased intracranial pressure; severe anemia

Additional contraindications for I.V. product: Constrictive pericarditis; pericardial tamponade; restrictive cardiomyopathy

Note: According to the 2010 American Heart Association guidelines for the treatment of acute coronary syndromes, nitrates are considered contraindicated in the following conditions: Hypotension (SBP <90 mm Hg or ≥30 mm Hg below baseline), extreme bradycardia (<50 bpm), tachycardia in the absence of heart failure (>100 bpm), and right ventricular infarction (O'Connor, 2010).

Warnings/Precautions Severe hypotension can occur. Use with caution in volume depletion, moderate hypotension, and extreme caution with inferior wall MI and suspected right ventricular involvement. Use considered contraindicated in patients with severe hypotension (SBP <90 mm Hg or ≥30 mm Hg below baseline), extreme bradycardia (<50 bpm), and right ventricular MI (O'Connor, 2010). Avoid use in patients with hypertrophic cardiomyopathy (HCM) with outflow tract obstruction; nitrates may reduce preload, exacerbating obstruction and cause hypotension or syncope and/or worsening of heart failure (Gersh, 2011).

Paradoxical bradycardia and increased angina pectoris can accompany hypotension. Orthostatic hypotension can also occur. Ethanol can accentuate this. Tolerance does develop to nitrates and appropriate dosing is needed to minimize this (drug-free interval). Avoid use of long-acting agents in acute MI or acute HF; cannot easily reverse effects. Nitrates may aggravate angina caused by hypertrophic cardiomyopathy. Nitroglycerin may precipitate or aggravate increased intracranial pressure and subsequently may worsen clinical outcomes in patients with neurologic injury (eg, intracranial hemorrhage, traumatic brain injury). Nitroglycerin transdermal patches may contain conducting metal (eg, aluminum); remove patch prior to MRI. Avoid concurrent use with PDE-5 inhibitors. When nitrate administration becomes medically necessary, may administer nitrates only if 24 hours have elapsed after use of sildenafil or vardenafil (48 hours after tadalafil use) (Trujillo, 2007).

Use caution when treating rectal anal fissures with nitroglycerin ointment formulation in patients with suspected or known significant cardiovascular disorders (eg, cardiomyopathies, heart failure, acute MI); intra-anal nitroglycerin administration may decrease systolic blood pressure and decrease arterial vascular resistance.

Drug Interactions

Metabolism/Transport Effects None known.

Avoid Concomitant Use

Avoid concomitant use of Nitroglycerin with any of the following: Ergot Derivatives; Phosphodiesterase 5 Inhibitors

Increased Effect/Toxicity

Nitroglycerin may increase the levels/effects of: Ergot Derivatives; Hypotensive Agents; Prilocaine; Rosiglitazone

The levels/effects of Nitroglycerin may be increased by: Alfuzosin; Phosphodiesterase 5 Inhibitors

Decreased Effect

Nitroglycerin may decrease the levels/effects of: Alteplase; Heparin

The levels/effects of Nitroglycerin may be decreased by: Ergot Derivatives

Ethanol/Nutrition/Herb Interactions

Ethanol: Avoid ethanol (may increase the hypotensive effects of nitroglycerin). Monitor.

Herb/Nutraceutical: Avoid bayberry, blue cohosh, cayenne, ephedra, ginger, ginseng (American), kola, licorice (may worsen hypertension). Avoid black cohosh, California poppy, coleus, golden seal, hawthorn, mistletoe, periwinkle, quinine, shepherd's purse (may cause hypotension).

Pharmacodynamics/Kinetics

Onset of Action Sublingual tablet: 1-3 minutes; Translingual spray: Similar to sublingual tablet; Extended release: ~60 minutes; Topical: 15-30 minutes; Transdermal: ~30 minutes; I.V.: Immediate

Peak effect: Sublingual tablet: 5 minutes; Translingual spray: 4-10 minutes; Extended release: 2.5-4 hours; Topical: ~60 minutes; Transdermal: 120 minutes; I.V.: Immediate

Duration of Action Sublingual tablet: At least 25 minutes; Translingual spray: Similar to sublingual tablet; Extended release: 4-8 hours (Gibbons, 2002); Topical: 7 hours; Transdermal: 10-12 hours; I.V.: 3-5 minutes

Half-life Elimination ~1-4 minutes

Pregnancy Risk Factor C

Pregnancy Considerations Increased fetal mortality has been observed in animal studies using isosorbide mononitrate and isosorbide dinitrate at doses much higher than those used in humans. Toxic effects were not observed in animal studies following topical administration of nitroglycerin. There are no adequate and well-controlled studies in pregnant women.

Lactation Excretion in breast milk unknown/use caution

Dosage Forms

Aerosol, spray, translingual: 400 mcg/spray (4.1 g, 8.5 g)
NitroMist®: 400 mcg/spray (8.5 g)

Capsule, extended release, oral: 2.5 mg, 6.5 mg, 9 mg
Nitro-Time®: 2.5 mg, 6.5 mg, 9 mg

Infusion, premixed in D₅W: 25 mg (250 mL); 50 mg (250 mL, 500 mL); 100 mg (250 mL)

Injection, solution: 5 mg/mL (5 mL, 10 mL)

Ointment, rectal:
Rectiv®: 0.4% (30 g)

Ointment, topical:
Nitro-Bid®: 2% (1 g, 30 g, 60 g)

Patch, transdermal: 0.1 mg/hr (30s); 0.2 mg/hr (30s); 0.4 mg/hr (30s); 0.6 mg/hr (30s)
Minitran™: 0.1 mg/hr (30s); 0.2 mg/hr (30s); 0.4 mg/hr (30s); 0.6 mg/hr (30s)
Nitro-Dur®: 0.1 mg/hr (30s); 0.2 mg/hr (30s); 0.3 mg/hr (30s); 0.4 mg/hr (30s); 0.6 mg/hr (30s); 0.8 mg/hr (30s)

Solution, translingual: 0.4 mg/spray (4.9 g, 12 g)
Nitrolingual®: 0.4 mg/spray (4.9 g, 12 g)

Tablet, sublingual:
Nitrostat®: 0.3 mg, 0.4 mg, 0.6 mg

Nitroprusside (nye troe PRUS ide)

Brand Names: U.S. Nitropress®
Brand Names: Canada Nipride®
Pharmacologic Category Vasodilator
Use Management of hypertensive crises; acute decompensated heart failure (HF); used for controlled hypotension to reduce bleeding during surgery
Unlabeled Use Management of hypertension during acute ischemic stroke
Local Anesthetic/Vasoconstrictor Precautions No information available to require special precautions

Effects on Dental Treatment No significant effects or complications reported

Effects on Bleeding No information available to require special precautions

Adverse Effects Frequency not defined.

Cardiovascular: Bradycardia, ECG changes, flushing, hypotension (excessive), palpitation, substernal distress, tachycardia

Central nervous system: Apprehension, dizziness, headache, intracranial pressure increased, restlessness

Dermatologic: Rash

Endocrine & metabolic: Metabolic acidosis (secondary to cyanide toxicity), hypothyroidism

Gastrointestinal: Abdominal pain, ileus, nausea, retching, vomiting

Hematologic: Methemoglobinemia, platelet aggregation decreased

Local: Injection site irritation

Neuromuscular & skeletal: Hyperreflexia (secondary to thiocyanate toxicity), muscle twitching

Ocular: Miosis (secondary to thiocyanate toxicity)

Otic: Tinnitus (secondary to thiocyanate toxicity)

Respiratory: Hyperoxemia (secondary to cyanide toxicity)

Miscellaneous: Cyanide toxicity, diaphoresis, thiocyanate toxicity

General Dosage Range I.V.: *Children and Adults:* Initial: 0.3 mcg/kg/minute; Usual dose: 3 mcg/kg/minute (maximum: 10 mcg/kg/minute)

Mechanism of Action Causes peripheral vasodilation by direct action on venous and arteriolar smooth muscle, thus reducing peripheral resistance; will increase cardiac output by decreasing afterload; reduces aortal and left ventricular impedance

Pharmacodynamics/Kinetics

Onset of Action Hypotensive effect: <2 minutes

Duration of Action Hypotensive effect: 1-10 minutes

Half-life Elimination Nitroprusside, circulatory: ~2 minutes; Thiocyanate, elimination: ~3 days (may be doubled or tripled in renal failure)

Pregnancy Risk Factor C

Pregnancy Considerations Animal studies have shown that nitroprusside may cross the placental barrier and result in fetal cyanide levels that are dose-related to maternal nitroprusside levels. However, information related to use in pregnancy is limited.

Nitrous Oxide (NYE trus OKS ide)

Related Information

Management of the Patient With Anxiety or Depression *on page 1594*

Generic Availability (U.S.) Yes

Pharmacologic Category Dental Gases; General Anesthetic

Dental Use Induction of sedation and analgesia in anxious dental patients

Use Sedation, analgesia, and amnesia; principal adjunct to inhalation and intravenous general anesthesia

Local Anesthetic/Vasoconstrictor Precautions No information available to require special precautions

Effects on Dental Treatment No significant effects or complications reported

Effects on Bleeding No information available to require special precautions

Adverse Effects An increased risk of renal and hepatic diseases and peripheral neuropathy similar to that of vitamin B_{12} deficiency have been reported in dental personnel who work in areas where nitrous oxide is frequently used without an enclosed gas scavenging system

Methionine synthase, a vitamin B_{12} dependent enzyme, is inactivated following prolonged administration of nitrous oxide, and the subsequent interference with DNA synthesis prevents production of both leukocytes and red blood cells by bone marrow. These effects do not occur within the time frame of clinical use.

Female dental personnel who were exposed to unscavenged nitrous oxide for more than 5 hours/week were significantly less fertile than women who were not exposed, or who were exposed to lower levels of scavenged or unscavenged nitrous oxide. Fertility was measured by the number of menstrual cycles, without use of contraception, required to become pregnant. Women who were exposed to nitrous oxide for more than 5 hours/week were only 41% as likely as unexposed women to conceive during each monthly cycle.

Frequency not defined:

Cardiovascular: Hypotension

Central nervous system: Headache, dizziness, confusion, CNS excitation

Gastrointestinal: Possibly nausea and vomiting

Respiratory: Apnea

Dental Usual Dosage Sedation and analgesia: Children and Adults: Concentrations of 25% to 50% nitrous oxide with oxygen

Dosage Children and Adults:

Surgical: For sedation and analgesia: Concentrations of 25% to 50% nitrous oxide with oxygen. For general anesthesia, concentrations of 40% to 70% via mask or endotracheal tube. Minimal alveolar concentration (MAC), which can be considered the ED_{50} of inhalational anesthetics, is 105%; therefore delivery in a hyperbaric chamber is necessary to use as a complete anesthetic. When administered at 70%, reduces the MAC of other anesthetics by half.

Dental: For sedation and analgesia: Concentrations of 25% to 50% nitrous oxide with oxygen

Mechanism of Action General CNS depressant action; may act similarly as inhalant general anesthetics by stabilizing axonal membranes to partially inhibit action potentials leading to sedation; may partially act on opiate receptor systems to cause mild analgesia; central sympathetic stimulating action supports blood pressure, systemic vascular resistance, and cardiac output; it does not depress carbon dioxide drive to breath. Nitrous oxide increases cerebral blood flow and intracranial pressure while decreasing hepatic and renal blood flow; has analgesic action similar to morphine.

Contraindications Hypersensitivity to nitrous oxide or any component of the formulation; nitrous oxide should not be administered without oxygen

Warnings/Precautions Nausea and vomiting occurs postoperatively in ~15% of patients. Prolonged use may produce bone marrow suppression and/or neurologic dysfunction. Oxygen should be briefly administered during emergence from prolonged anesthesia with nitrous oxide to prevent diffusion hypoxia. Patients with vitamin B_{12} deficiency (pernicious anemia) and those with other nutritional deficiencies (alcoholics) are at increased risk of developing neurologic disease and bone marrow suppression with exposure to nitrous oxide. May be associated with abuse and/or addiction.

Drug Interactions

Metabolism/Transport Effects None known.

Avoid Concomitant Use There are no known interactions where it is recommended to avoid concomitant use.

Increased Effect/Toxicity There are no known significant interactions involving an increase in effect.

Decreased Effect There are no known significant interactions involving a decrease in effect.

Pharmacodynamics/Kinetics

Onset of Action Inhalation: 2-5 minutes

Pregnancy Considerations Nitrous oxide crosses the placenta in concentrations ~80% of those in the maternal plasma. The half-life in the neonate is ~3 minutes and it is quickly eliminated from neonatal lungs with the onset of breathing (Rooks, 2011). Infertility, spontaneous abortion, and congenital abnormalities have been reported following prolonged occupational exposure (Becker, 2008; Brodsky, 1986; Rooks, 2011). Adverse events are related to dose and duration of exposure and risks may be decreased with proper administration procedures (Rooks, 2011). May be used when needed for dental treatments that cannot be postponed during pregnancy; use for labor analgesia is considered acceptable (Becker, 2008; Rooks, 2011). Avoid use in pregnant women during the first two trimesters of pregnancy, those with medical conditions that increase the risk of vitamin B_{12} deficiency, or infertile women undergoing *in vitro* fertilization (Brodsky, 1986; Rooks, 2011).

Dosage Forms

Supplied in blue cylinders

Nizatidine (ni ZA ti deen)

Related Information

Gastrointestinal Disorders *on page 1512*

Brand Names: U.S. Axid®

Brand Names: Canada Apo-Nizatidine®; Axid®; Gen-Nizatidine; Novo-Nizatidine; Nu-Nizatidine; PMS-Nizatidine

Pharmacologic Category Histamine H_2 Antagonist

Use Treatment and maintenance of duodenal ulcer; treatment of benign gastric ulcer; treatment of gastroesophageal reflux disease (GERD)

Unlabeled Use Part of a multidrug regimen for *H. pylori* eradication to reduce the risk of duodenal ulcer recurrence

Local Anesthetic/Vasoconstrictor Precautions No information available to require special precautions

Effects on Dental Treatment Key adverse event(s) related to dental treatment: Xerostomia (normal salivary flow resumes upon discontinuation).

Effects on Bleeding No information available to require special precautions

Adverse Effects

>10%: Central nervous system: Headache (16%)

1% to 10%:

Central nervous system: Anxiety, dizziness, fever (reported in children), insomnia, irritability (reported in children), somnolence, nervousness

Dermatologic: Pruritus, rash

Gastrointestinal: Abdominal pain, anorexia, constipation, diarrhea, dry mouth, flatulence, heartburn, nausea, vomiting

Respiratory: Reported in children: Cough, nasal congestion, nasopharyngitis

General Dosage Range Dosage adjustment recommended in patients with renal impairment

Oral:

Children ≥12 years: 150 mg twice daily

Adults: 300 mg/day in 1-2 divided doses **or** 75 mg twice daily (OTC dosing)

Mechanism of Action Competitive inhibition of histamine at H_2-receptors of the gastric parietal cells resulting in reduced gastric acid secretion, gastric volume and hydrogen ion concentration reduced. In healthy volunteers, nizatidine suppresses gastric acid secretion induced by pentagastrin infusion or food.

Pharmacodynamics/Kinetics

Half-life Elimination 1-2 hours; prolonged with renal impairment

Time to Peak Plasma: 0.5-3.0 hours

Pregnancy Risk Factor B

Pregnancy Considerations Adverse events have not been observed in animal reproduction studies; therefore, the nizatidine is classified as pregnancy category B. Nizatidine crosses the placenta. An increased risk of congenital malformations or adverse events in the newborn has generally not been observed following maternal use of nizatidine during pregnancy. Histamine H_2 antagonists have been evaluated for the treatment of gastroesophageal reflux disease (GERD), as well as gastric and duodenal ulcers during pregnancy. Although if needed, nizatidine is not the agent of choice. Histamine H_2 antagonists may be used for aspiration prophylaxis prior to cesarean delivery.

Nonoxynol 9 (non OKS i nole nine)

Brand Names: U.S. Conceptrol® [OTC]; Delfen® [OTC]; Encare® [OTC]; Gynol II® Extra Strength [OTC]; Gynol II® [OTC]; Today® [OTC]; VCF® [OTC]

Pharmacologic Category Contraceptive; Spermicide

Use Prevention of pregnancy

Local Anesthetic/Vasoconstrictor Precautions No information available to require special precautions

Effects on Dental Treatment No significant effects or complications reported

Effects on Bleeding No information available to require special precautions

Adverse Effects Frequency not defined: Genitourinary: Irritation, burning, or itching of mucous membranes (including vaginal/urethral)

General Dosage Range Intravaginal: *Adolescents and Adults:* Insert 1 applicatorful, film, suppository, or sponge 10 minutes to 3 hours prior to intercourse [product specific]

Mechanism of Action

Nonoxynol 9 is a surfactant which prevents pregnancy by damaging the cell membrane of sperm; some product formulations may also provide a physical barrier

Pregnancy Considerations Use of spermicides has not been associated with birth defects (FDA, 1986).

Norepinephrine (nor ep i NEF rin)

Brand Names: U.S. Levophed®

Brand Names: Canada Levophed®

Pharmacologic Category Alpha/Beta Agonist

Use Treatment of shock which persists after adequate fluid volume replacement; severe hypotension

Local Anesthetic/Vasoconstrictor Precautions No information available to require special precautions

Effects on Dental Treatment No significant effects or complications reported

Effects on Bleeding Norepinephrine has been shown to cause platelet hyper-reactivity and enhance platelet-mediated coagulation associated with thrombotic risk.

Adverse Effects Frequency not defined.
Cardiovascular: Arrhythmias, bradycardia, peripheral (digital) ischemia
Central nervous system: Anxiety, headache (transient)
Local: Skin necrosis (with extravasation)
Respiratory: Dyspnea, respiratory difficulty

General Dosage Range I.V.:
Children: Initial: 0.05-0.1 mcg/kg/minute; Maintenance: Titrate to desired effect (maximum: 2 mcg/kg/minute)
Adults: Initial: 8-12 mcg/minute; Maintenance: Titrate to desired effect (usual maintenance range: 2-4 mcg/minute)

Mechanism of Action Stimulates beta$_1$-adrenergic receptors and alpha-adrenergic receptors causing increased contractility and heart rate as well as vasoconstriction, thereby increasing systemic blood pressure and coronary blood flow; clinically, alpha effects (vasoconstriction) are greater than beta effects (inotropic and chronotropic effects)

Pharmacodynamics/Kinetics
Onset of Action I.V.: Very rapid-acting
Duration of Action Vasopressor: 1-2 minutes
Pregnancy Risk Factor C
Pregnancy Considerations Animal reproduction studies have not been conducted. Norepinephrine is an endogenous catecholamine and crosses the placenta (Minzter, 2010; Wang, 1999).

Norethindrone (nor ETH in drone)

Related Information
Endocrine Disorders and Pregnancy *on page 1517*
Brand Names: U.S. Aygestin®; Camila®; Errin®; Heather; Jolivette®; Nor-QD®; Nora-BE®; Ortho Micronor®
Brand Names: Canada Micronor®; Norlutate®
Pharmacologic Category Contraceptive; Progestin
Use Treatment of amenorrhea; abnormal uterine bleeding; endometriosis; prevention of pregnancy
Local Anesthetic/Vasoconstrictor Precautions No information available to require special precautions
Effects on Dental Treatment Until we know more about the mechanism of interaction, caution is required in prescribing antibiotics to female dental patients taking progestin-only hormonal contraceptives.
Effects on Bleeding Norethindrone has been shown to enhance the risk of thrombosis, as assessed by significant increases in prothrombin fragments 1+2, thrombin-antithrombin complex, and D-dimer. These increases were higher during the first 3 months of therapy and gradually declined following prolonged therapy (>3 months). Medical consult is suggested for patients who are under active norethindrone treatment.

Adverse Effects Frequency not defined.
Cardiovascular: Cerebral embolism, cerebral thrombosis, DVT, edema
Central nervous system: Depression, dizziness, headache, insomnia, migraine, mood swings
Dermatologic: Acne, chloasma, hirsutism, melasma, pruritus, rash, urticaria
Endocrine & metabolic: Amenorrhea, breakthrough bleeding, breast enlargement/tenderness, menstrual flow changes, spotting
Gastrointestinal: Nausea, weight gain/loss
Genitourinary: Cervical erosion changes, cervical secretion changes
Hepatic: Cholestatic jaundice, liver function test abnormalities

Ocular: Optic neuritis (with or without vision loss), retinal vascular thrombosis
Respiratory: Pulmonary embolism
Miscellaneous: Anaphylactic/anaphylactoid reactions

General Dosage Range Oral:
Norethindrone: *Children (postmenarche) and Adults:* 0.35 mg every day
Norethindrone acetate: *Adolescents and Adults:* 2.5-15 mg once daily for 5-14 days of menstrual cycle

Mechanism of Action Inhibits secretion of pituitary gonadotropin (LH) which prevents follicular maturation and ovulation

Pharmacodynamics/Kinetics
Half-life Elimination ~8 hours
Time to Peak 1-2 hours
Pregnancy Risk Factor X
Pregnancy Considerations First trimester exposure may cause genital abnormalities including hypospadias in male infants and mild virilization of external female genitalia. Significant adverse events related to growth and development have not been observed (limited studies). Use is contraindicated during pregnancy. May be started immediately postpartum if not breast-feeding.

Norethindrone and Mestranol
(nor eth IN drone & MES tra nole)

Related Information
Endocrine Disorders and Pregnancy *on page 1517*
Norethindrone *on page 990*
Brand Names: U.S. Necon® 1/50; Norinyl® 1+50
Brand Names: Canada Ortho-Novum® 1/50
Pharmacologic Category Contraceptive; Estrogen and Progestin Combination
Use Prevention of pregnancy
Unlabeled Use Treatment of hypermenorrhea (menorrhagia); pain associated with endometriosis; dysmenorrhea; dysfunctional uterine bleeding
Local Anesthetic/Vasoconstrictor Precautions No information available to require special precautions
Effects on Dental Treatment When prescribing antibiotics, patient must be advised to use additional methods of birth control if on hormonal contraceptives.
Effects on Bleeding Norethindrone has been shown to enhance the risk of thrombosis, as assessed by significant increases in prothrombin fragments 1+2, thrombin-antithrombin complex, and D-dimer. These increases were higher during the first 3 months of therapy and gradually declined following prolonged therapy (>3 months). Medical consult is suggested for patients who are under active norethindrone treatment.

Adverse Effects Frequency not defined.
Cardiovascular: Arterial thromboembolism, cerebral hemorrhage, cerebral thrombosis, edema, hypertension, mesenteric thrombosis, MI
Central nervous system: Depression, dizziness, headache, migraine, nervousness, premenstrual syndrome, stroke
Dermatologic: Acne, erythema multiforme, erythema nodosum, hirsutism, loss of scalp hair, melasma (may persist), rash (allergic)
Endocrine & metabolic: Amenorrhea, breakthrough bleeding, breast enlargement, breast secretion, breast tenderness, carbohydrate intolerance, lactation decreased (postpartum), glucose tolerance decreased, libido changes, menstrual flow changes, sex hormone-binding globulins (SHBG) increased, spotting, temporary infertility (following discontinuation), thyroid-binding globulin increased, triglycerides increased

Gastrointestinal: Abdominal cramps, appetite changes, bloating, cholestasis, colitis, gallbladder disease, jaundice, nausea, vomiting, weight gain/loss

Genitourinary: Cervical erosion changes, cervical secretion changes, cystitis-like syndrome, vaginal candidiasis, vaginitis

Hematologic: Antithrombin III decreased, folate levels decreased, hemolytic uremic syndrome, norepinephrine induced platelet aggregability increased, porphyria, prothrombin increased; factors VII, VIII, IX, and X increased

Hepatic: Benign liver tumors, Budd-Chiari syndrome, cholestatic jaundice, hepatic adenomas

Local: Thrombophlebitis

Ocular: Cataracts, change in corneal curvature (steepening), contact lens intolerance, optic neuritis, retinal thrombosis

Renal: Impaired renal function

Respiratory: Pulmonary thromboembolism

Miscellaneous: Hemorrhagic eruption

General Dosage Range Oral:

21-tablet package: *Children (menarche) and Adults:* 1 tablet daily for 21 days, followed by 7 days off

28-tablet package: *Children (menarche) and Adults:* 1 tablet daily

Mechanism of Action Combination oral contraceptives inhibit ovulation via a negative feedback mechanism on the hypothalamus, which alters the normal pattern of gonadotropin secretion of a follicle-stimulating hormone (FSH) and luteinizing hormone by the anterior pituitary. The follicular phase FSH and midcycle surge of gonadotropins are inhibited. In addition, combination hormonal contraceptives produce alterations in the genital tract, including changes in the cervical mucus, rendering it unfavorable for sperm penetration even if ovulation occurs. Changes in the endometrium may also occur, producing an unfavorable environment for nidation. Combination hormonal contraceptive drugs may alter the tubal transport of the ova through the fallopian tubes. Progestational agents may also alter sperm fertility.

Pregnancy Risk Factor X

Pregnancy Considerations Pregnancy should be ruled out prior to treatment and discontinued if pregnancy occurs. In general, the use of combination hormonal contraceptives when inadvertently taken early in pregnancy have not been associated with teratogenic effects. Hormonal contraceptives may be less effective in obese patients. An increase in oral contraceptive failure was noted in women with a BMI >27.3 kg/m^2. Similar findings were noted in patients weighing ≥90 kg (198 lb) using the contraceptive patch.

Due to increased risk of venous thromboembolism (VTE) postpartum, combination hormonal contraceptives should not be started in any woman <21 days following delivery. Women without risk factors for VTE and who are not breast-feeding may start combination hormonal contraceptives during 21-42 days postpartum. After 42 days postpartum, restrictions for use are not related to postpartum status and should be based on other medical conditions (CDC, 2011).

Norfloxacin (nor FLOKS a sin)

Brand Names: U.S. Noroxin®

Brand Names: Canada Apo-Norflox®; CO Norfloxacin; Norfloxacine®; Novo-Norfloxacin; PMS-Norfloxacin; Riva-Norfloxacin

Pharmacologic Category Antibiotic, Quinolone

Use Uncomplicated and complicated urinary tract infections caused by susceptible gram-negative and gram-positive bacteria; sexually-transmitted disease (eg, uncomplicated urethral and cervical gonorrhea) caused by *N. gonorrhoeae*; prostatitis due to *E. coli*

Note: As of April 2007, the CDC no longer recommends the use of fluoroquinolones for the treatment of gonococcal disease.

Unlabeled Use Shigella dysentery type 1

Local Anesthetic/Vasoconstrictor Precautions Norfloxacin is one of the drugs confirmed to prolong the QT interval and is accepted as having a risk of causing torsade de pointes. The risk of drug-induced torsade de pointes is extremely low when a single QT interval prolonging drug is prescribed. In terms of epinephrine, it is not known what effect vasoconstrictors in the local anesthetic regimen will have in patients with a known history of congenital prolonged QT interval or in patients taking any medication that prolongs the QT interval. Until more information is obtained, it is suggested that the clinician consult with the physician prior to the use of a vasoconstrictor in suspected patients, and that the vasoconstrictor (epinephrine, mepivacaine and levonordefrin [Carbocaine® 2% with Neo-Cobefrin®]) be used with caution.

Effects on Dental Treatment No significant effects or complications reported

Effects on Bleeding Norfloxacin has been shown to alter leukocyte populations (reduce neutrophils and increase eosinophils). In more than 1 in 1000 patients, norfloxacin has been shown to reduce clotting ability through reduction in blood platelet concentrations. May also reduce the erythrocyte concentration following extended treatment.

Adverse Effects

>1% to 10%:

Central nervous system: Dizziness (2% to 3%), headache (2% to 3%)

Gastrointestinal: Nausea (3% to 4%), abdominal cramping (2%)

Hematologic: Eosinophilia (1% to 2%)

Hepatic: Liver enzymes increased (1% to 2%)

≥0.3% to 1%:

Central nervous system: Fever, somnolence

Dermatologic: Hyperhidrosis, pruritus, rash

Gastrointestinal: Abdominal pain, anorectal pain, anorexia, constipation, diarrhea, dyspepsia, flatulence, loose stools, vomiting, xerostomia

Hematologic: Hematocrit/hemoglobin decreased (1%), leukopenia (1%), thrombocytopenia (1%)

Neuromuscular & skeletal: Back pain, paresthesia, weakness

Renal: Proteinuria (1%)

General Dosage Range Dosage adjustment recommended in patients with renal impairment

Oral: *Adults:* 400 mg every 12 hours **or** 800 mg as a single dose

Mechanism of Action Norfloxacin is a DNA gyrase inhibitor. DNA gyrase is an essential bacterial enzyme that maintains the superhelical structure of DNA. DNA gyrase is required for DNA replication and transcription, DNA repair, recombination, and transposition; bactericidal

Pharmacodynamics/Kinetics

Half-life Elimination 3-4 hours; Renal impairment (Cl_{cr} ≤30 mL/minute): 6.5 hours; Elderly: 4 hours

Time to Peak Serum: 1-2 hours

Pregnancy Risk Factor C

◄ **Pregnancy Considerations** Adverse events have been observed in some animal studies; therefore, the manufacturer classifies norfloxacin as pregnancy category C. Norfloxacin crosses the placenta, distributing to cord blood and amniotic fluid. An increased risk of teratogenic effects has not been observed in animals or humans following norfloxacin use during pregnancy; however, because of concerns of cartilage damage in immature animals, norfloxacin should only be used during pregnancy if a safer option is not available.

Dental Comment Norfloxacin is known to prolong the QT interval. The QT interval is measured as the time and distance between the Q point of the QRS complex and the end of the T wave in the ECG tracing. After adjustment for heart rate, the QT interval is defined as prolonged if it is more than 450 msec in men and 460 msec in women. A long QT syndrome was first described in the 1950s and 60s as a congenital syndrome involving QT interval prolongation and syncope and sudden death. Some of the congenital long QT syndromes were characterized by a peculiar electrocardiographic appearance of the QRS complex involving a premature atria beat followed by a pause, then a subsequent sinus beat showing marked QT prolongation and deformity. This type of cardiac arrhythmia was originally termed "torsade de pointes" (translated from the French as "twisting of the points"). Norfloxacin is considered as having a risk of causing torsade de pointes. Since it is not known what effect vasoconstrictors in the local anesthetic regimen will have in patients with a known history of congenital prolonged QT interval or in patients taking any medication that prolongs the QT interval, a medical consult is suggested.

Nortriptyline (nor TRIP ti leen)

Related Information
Vasoconstrictor Interactions With Antidepressants *on page 1650*

Brand Names: U.S. Pamelor™

Brand Names: Canada Apo-Nortriptyline®; Ava-Nortriptyline; Aventyl®; Dom-Nortriptyline; Norventyl; Nu-Nortriptyline; PMS-Nortriptyline; Teva-Nortriptyline

Generic Availability (U.S.) Yes

Pharmacologic Category Antidepressant, Tricyclic (Secondary Amine)

Dental Use Treatment of myofascial pain, neuralgia, burning mouth syndrome

Use Treatment of symptoms of depression

Unlabeled Use Chronic pain (including neuropathic pain), myofascial pain, burning mouth sydrome, anxiety disorders, attention-deficit/hyperactivity disorder (ADHD); enuresis; adjunctive therapy for smoking cessation

Local Anesthetic/Vasoconstrictor Precautions Nortriptyline is one of the drugs confirmed to prolong the QT interval and is accepted as having a risk of causing torsade de pointes. In terms of epinephrine, it is not known what effect vasoconstrictors in the local anesthetic regimen will have in patients with a known history of congenital prolonged QT interval or in patients taking any medication that prolongs the QT interval. Until more information is obtained, it is suggested that the clinician consult with the physician prior to the use of a vasoconstrictor in suspected patients, and that the vasoconstrictor (epinephrine, mepivacaine and levonordefrin [Carbocaine® 2% with Neo-Cobefrin®]) be used with caution. See Dental Comment.

Effects on Dental Treatment Key adverse event(s) related to dental treatment: Xerostomia (normal salivary flow resumes upon discontinuation), black tongue, and unpleasant taste. Long-term treatment with TCAs, such as nortriptyline, increases the risk of caries by reducing salivation and salivary buffer capacity.

Effects on Bleeding No information available to require special precautions

Adverse Effects Frequency not defined.

Cardiovascular: Arrhythmia, flushing, heart block, hypertension, MI, orthostatic hypotension, palpitation, tachycardia

Central nervous system: Agitation, anxiety, ataxia, confusion, delirium, delusions, disorientation, dizziness, drowsiness, EEG changes, exacerbation of psychosis, extrapyramidal symptoms, fatigue, hallucinations, headache, hypomania, incoordination, insomnia, nightmares, panic, restlessness, seizure

Dermatologic: Alopecia, itching, petechiae, photosensitivity, rash, urticaria

Endocrine & metabolic: Blood sugar increased/decreased, breast enlargement, galactorrhea, gynecomastia, libido increased/decreased, sexual dysfunction, SIADH

Gastrointestinal: Abdominal cramps, anorexia, black tongue, constipation, diarrhea, epigastric distress, nausea, paralytic ileus, stomatitis, taste disturbance, vomiting, weight gain/loss, xerostomia

Genitourinary: Delayed micturition, impotence, nocturia, polyuria, testicular edema, urinary retention

Hematologic: Agranulocytosis (rare), eosinophilia, purpura, thrombocytopenia

Hepatic: Cholestatic jaundice, transaminases increased

Neuromuscular & skeletal: Numbness, paresthesia, peripheral neuropathy, tingling, tremor, weakness

Ocular: Blurred vision, disturbances in accommodation, eye pain, mydriasis

Otic: Tinnitus

Miscellaneous: Allergic reactions (eg, general edema or of the face/tongue), diaphoresis (excessive), withdrawal symptoms

Dental Usual Dosage Myofascial pain, neuralgia, burning mouth syndrome (unlabeled use): Adults: Initial: 10-25 mg at bedtime; dosage may be increased by 25 mg/day weekly, if tolerated; usual maintenance dose: 75 mg as a single bedtime dose or 2 divided doses

Dosage Oral:

Nocturnal enuresis: Children (unlabeled use): 10-20 mg/day; titrate to a maximum of 40 mg/day

Depression: Children (unlabeled use): 1-3 mg/kg/day

Depression:

Adults: 25 mg 3-4 times/day up to 150 mg/day; doses may be given once daily

Elderly: Initial: 30-50 mg/day, given as a single daily dose or in divided doses. **Note:** Nortriptyline is one of the best tolerated TCAs in the elderly.

Myofascial pain, neuralgia, burning mouth syndrome (unlabeled uses): Adults: Initial: 10-25 mg at bedtime; dosage may be increased by 25 mg/day weekly, if tolerated; usual maintenance dose: 75 mg as a single bedtime dose or 2 divided doses

Chronic urticaria, angioedema, nocturnal pruritus (unlabeled use): Adults: Oral: 75 mg/day

Smoking cessation (unlabeled use; Fiore, 2008): Adults: Initial: 25 mg/day; titrate dose to 75-100 mg/day 10-28 days prior to selected "quit" date; continue therapy for ≥12 weeks after "quit" day

MAO inhibitor recommendations:
Switching to or from an MAO inhibitor intended to treat psychiatric disorders:
Allow 14 days to elapse between discontinuing an MAO inhibitor intended to treat psychiatric disorders and initiation of nortriptyline.

Allow 14 days to elapse between discontinuing nortriptyline and initiation of an MAO inhibitor intended to treat psychiatric disorders.

Use with other MAO inhibitors (linezolid or I.V. methylene blue):
Do not initiate nortriptyline in patients receiving linezolid or I.V. methylene blue; consider other interventions for psychiatric condition.

If urgent treatment with linezolid or I.V. methylene blue is required in a patient already receiving nortriptyline and potential benefits outweigh potential risks, discontinue nortriptyline promptly and administer linezolid or I.V. methylene blue. Monitor for serotonin syndrome for 2 weeks or until 24 hours after the last dose of linezolid or I.V. methylene blue, whichever comes first. May resume nortriptyline 24 hours after the last dose of linezolid or I.V. methylene blue.

Dosage adjustment in renal impairment: No dosage adjustment provided in manufacturer's labeling.

Dosage adjustment in hepatic impairment: Lower doses and slower titration dependent on individualization of dosage is recommended

Mechanism of Action Traditionally believed to increase the synaptic concentration of serotonin and/or norepinephrine in the central nervous system by inhibition of their reuptake by the presynaptic neuronal membrane. However, additional receptor effects have been found including desensitization of adenyl cyclase, down regulation of beta-adrenergic receptors, and down regulation of serotonin receptors.

Contraindications Hypersensitivity to nortriptyline and similar chemical class, or any component of the formulation; use in a patient during the acute recovery phase of MI; use of MAO inhibitors intended to treat psychiatric disorders (concurrently or within 14 days of discontinuing either nortriptyline or the MAO inhibitor); initiation of nortriptyline in a patient receiving linezolid or intravenous methylene blue

Warnings/Precautions [U.S. Boxed Warning]: Antidepressants increase the risk of suicidal thinking and behavior in children, adolescents, and young adults (18-24 years of age) with major depressive disorder (MDD) and other psychiatric disorders; consider risk prior to prescribing. Short-term studies did not show an increased risk in patients >24 years of age and showed a decreased risk in patients ≥65 years. Closely monitor for clinical worsening, suicidality, or unusual changes in behavior; the patient's family or caregiver should be instructed to closely observe the patient and communicate condition with healthcare provider. A medication guide should be dispensed with each prescription. **Nortriptyline is not FDA approved for use in children.**

The possibility of a suicide attempt is inherent in major depression and may persist until remission occurs. Monitor for worsening of depression or suicidality, especially during initiation of therapy (generally first 1-2 months) or with dose increases or decreases. Use caution in high-risk patients. Worsening depression and severe abrupt suicidality that are not part of the presenting symptoms may require discontinuation or modification of drug therapy. The patient's family or caregiver should be alerted to monitor patients for the emergence of suicidality and associated behaviors (such as agitation, irritability, hostility, impulsivity, and hypomania) and call healthcare provider.

May worsen psychosis in some patients or precipitate a shift to mania or hypomania in patients with bipolar disorder. Patients presenting with depressive symptoms should be screened for bipolar disorder. Monotherapy in patients with bipolar disorder should be avoided. **Nortriptyline is not FDA approved for the treatment of bipolar depression.**

Potentially life-threatening serotonin syndrome (SS) has occurred with serotonergic agents (eg, SSRIs, SNRIs), particularly when used in combination with other serotonergic agents (eg, triptans, TCAs, fentanyl, lithium, tramadol, buspirone, St John's wort, tryptophan) or agents that impair metabolism of serotonin (eg, MOA inhibitors intended to treat psychiatric disorders, other MAO inhibitors [ie, linezolid and intravenous methylene blue]). Discontinue treatment (and any concomitant serotonergic agent) immediately if signs/symptoms arise. TCAs may rarely cause bone marrow suppression; monitor for any signs of infection and obtain CBC if symptoms (eg, fever, sore throat) evident. The risk of sedation and orthostatic effects are low relative to other antidepressants. However, nortriptyline may result in impaired performance of tasks requiring alertness (eg, operating machinery or driving). The degree of anticholinergic blockade produced by this agent is moderate relative to other cyclic antidepressants, however, caution should still be used in patients with urinary retention, benign prostatic hyperplasia, narrow-angle glaucoma, xerostomia, visual problems, constipation, or history of bowel obstruction. May cause orthostatic hypotension (risk is low relative to other antidepressants) or conduction disturbances. Use with caution in patients with a history of cardiovascular disease (including previous MI, stroke, tachycardia, or conduction abnormalities). The risk conduction abnormalities with this agent is moderate relative to other antidepressants.

Consider discontinuing, when possible, prior to elective surgery. Therapy should not be abruptly discontinued in patients receiving high doses for prolonged periods. May alter glucose regulation - use caution in patients with diabetes. Use caution in patients with a previous seizure disorder or condition predisposing to seizures such as brain damage, alcoholism, or concurrent therapy with other drugs which lower the seizure threshold. May increase the risks associated with electroconvulsive therapy. Use with caution in hyperthyroid patients or those receiving thyroid supplementation. Use with caution in patients with hepatic or renal dysfunction.

Use caution in elderly patients; may cause or exacerbate syndrome of inappropriate antidiuretic hormone secretion or hyponatremia; monitor sodium closely with initiation or dosage adjustments in older adults. May be inappropriate in older adults depending on comorbidities (eg, dementia, delirium) due to its potent anticholinergic effects (Beers Criteria).

Drug Interactions
Metabolism/Transport Effects Substrate of CYP1A2 (minor), CYP2C19 (minor), CYP2D6 (major), CYP3A4 (minor); **Note:** Assignment of Major/Minor substrate status based on clinically relevant drug interaction potential; **Inhibits** CYP2D6 (weak), CYP2E1 (weak)

Avoid Concomitant Use
Avoid concomitant use of Nortriptyline with any of the following: Aclidinium; Iobenguane I 123; Ipratropium (Oral Inhalation); Linezolid; MAO Inhibitors; Methylene Blue; Tiotropium

Increased Effect/Toxicity
Nortriptyline may increase the levels/effects of: Alpha-/Beta-Agonists (Direct-Acting); Alpha1-Agonists; Amphetamines; Anticholinergics; Beta2-Agonists; Desmopressin; Highest Risk QTc-Prolonging Agents; Methylene Blue; Metoclopramide; Moderate Risk QTc-Prolonging Agents; QuiNIDine; Serotonin Modulators; Sodium Phosphates; Sulfonylureas; Tiotropium; TraMADol; Vitamin K Antagonists; Yohimbine

The levels/effects of Nortriptyline may be increased by: Abiraterone Acetate; Aclidinium; Altretamine; Antipsychotics; BuPROPion; Cimetidine; Cinacalcet; Cobicistat; CYP2D6 Inhibitors (Moderate); CYP2D6 Inhibitors (Strong); Dexmethylphenidate; Divalproex; DULoxetine; Ipratropium (Oral Inhalation); Linezolid; Lithium; MAO Inhibitors; Methylphenidate; Metoclopramide; Metyrosine; Mifepristone; Pramlintide; Protease Inhibitors; QuiNIDine; Selective Serotonin Reuptake Inhibitors; Terbinafine (Systemic); Valproic Acid

Decreased Effect
Nortriptyline may decrease the levels/effects of: Acetylcholinesterase Inhibitors (Central); Alpha2-Agonists; Iobenguane I 123

The levels/effects of Nortriptyline may be decreased by: Acetylcholinesterase Inhibitors (Central); Barbiturates; CarBAMazepine; Peginterferon Alfa-2b; St Johns Wort

Ethanol/Nutrition/Herb Interactions
Ethanol: May increase CNS depression; monitor for increased effects with coadministration. Caution patients about effects.

Herb/Nutraceutical: Avoid valerian, St John's wort, tryptophan, SAMe, kava kava (may increase risk of serotonin syndrome and/or excessive sedation).

Pharmacodynamics/Kinetics
Onset of Action Therapeutic: 1-3 weeks

Half-life Elimination 28-31 hours

Time to Peak Serum: 7-8.5 hours

Pregnancy Considerations Animal reproduction studies are inconclusive. Nortriptyline and its metabolites cross the human placenta and can be detected in cord blood. According to the manufacturer, the decision to use nortriptyline during pregnancy or in women of childbearing potential should take into account the potential benefits and possible risks. Treatment algorithms have been developed by the ACOG and the APA for the management of depression in women prior to conception and during pregnancy.

Lactation Enters breast milk/not recommended (AAP rates "of concern"; AAP 2001 update pending)

Breast-Feeding Considerations Nortriptyline is excreted into breast milk and the M/P ratio ranged from 0.87 to 3.71 in one study. Based on available information, nortriptyline has not been detected in the serum of nursing infants, however low levels of the active metabolite E-10-hydroxynortriptyline have been detected in the serum of newborns following breast-feeding.

Dosage Forms
Capsule, oral: 10 mg, 25 mg, 50 mg, 75 mg
 Pamelor™: 10 mg, 25 mg, 50 mg, 75 mg
Solution, oral: 10 mg/5 mL (473 mL)

Dental Comment Nortriptyline is known to prolong the QT interval. The QT interval is measured as the time and distance between the Q point of the QRS complex and the end of the T wave in the ECG tracing. After adjustment for heart rate, the QT interval is defined as prolonged if it is more than 450 msec in men and 460 msec in women. A long QT syndrome was first described in the 1950s and 60s as a congenital syndrome involving QT interval prolongation and syncope and sudden death. Some of the congenital long QT syndromes were characterized by a peculiar electrocardiographic appearance of the QRS complex involving a premature atria beat followed by a pause, then a subsequent sinus beat showing marked QT prolongation and deformity. This type of cardiac arrhythmia was originally termed "torsade de pointes" (translated from the French as "twisting of the points"). Nortriptyline is considered as having a risk of causing torsade de pointes. Since it is not known what effect vasoconstrictors in the local anesthetic regimen will have in patients with a known history of congenital prolonged QT interval or in patients taking any medication that prolongs the QT interval, a medical consult is suggested.

References
Buchanan J and Zakrzewska J, "Burning Mouth Syndrome," *Clin Evid (online)*, March 14, 2008. Available at http://www.ncbi.nlm.nih.gov/pmc/articles/PMC2907957/pdf/2008-1301.pdf.

Jastak JT and Yagiela JA, "Vasoconstrictors and Local Anesthesia: A Review and Rationale for Use," *J Am Dent Assoc*, 1983, 107 (4):623-30.

Minguez Serra MP, Salort Llorca C, Silvestre Donat FJ, "Pharmacological Treatment of Burning Mouth Syndrome: A Review and Update," *Med Oral Patol Oral Cir Bucal*, 2007, 12(4):E299-304.

Rundegren J, van Dijken J, Mörnstad H, et al, "Oral Conditions in Patients Receiving Long-Term Treatment With Cyclic Antidepressant Drugs," *Swed Dent J*, 1985, 9(2):55-64.

Yagiela JA, "Adverse Drug Interactions in Dental Practice: Interactions Associated With Vasoconstrictors. Part V of a Series," *J Am Dent Assoc*, 1999, 130(5):701-9.

Nylidrin (NYE li drin)

Brand Names: Canada Arlidin®

Pharmacologic Category Vasodilator, Peripheral

Use Considered "possibly effective" for increasing blood supply to treat peripheral disease (arteriosclerosis obliterans, diabetic vascular disease, nocturnal leg cramps, Raynaud's disease, frost bite, ischemic ulcer, thrombophlebitis) and circulatory disturbances of the inner ear (cochlear ischemia, macular or ampullar ischemia, etc)

Local Anesthetic/Vasoconstrictor Precautions No information available to require special precautions

Effects on Dental Treatment No significant effects or complications reported

Effects on Bleeding No information available to require special precautions

Adverse Effects
1% to 10%:
 Central nervous system: Nervousness
 Neuromuscular & skeletal: Trembling

General Dosage Range Oral: *Adults:* 3-12 mg 3-4 times/day

Mechanism of Action Nylidrin is a peripheral vasodilator; this results from direct relaxation of vascular smooth muscle and beta-agonist action. Nylidrin does not appear to affect cutaneous blood flow; it reportedly increases heart rate and cardiac output; cutaneous blood flow is not enhanced to any appreciable extent.

Pregnancy Considerations Animal reproduction studies have not been conducted. Nylidrin has been evaluated for use as a tocolytic (Kurki, 1991).

Nystatin (Oral) (nye STAT in)

Related Information
Fungal Infections *on page 1573*
Related Sample Prescriptions
Fungal Infections Requiring Topical Therapy *on page 1614*
Brand Names: Canada PMS-Nystatin
Generic Availability (U.S.) Yes
Pharmacologic Category Antifungal Agent, Oral Nonabsorbed
Dental Use Treatment of susceptible cutaneous, mucocutaneous, and oral cavity fungal infections normally caused by the *Candida* species
Use Treatment of susceptible cutaneous, mucocutaneous, and oral cavity fungal infections normally caused by the *Candida* species
Local Anesthetic/Vasoconstrictor Precautions No information available to require special precautions
Effects on Dental Treatment No significant effects or complications reported
Effects on Bleeding No information available to require special precautions
Adverse Effects 1% to 10%: Gastrointestinal: Diarrhea, nausea, stomach pain, vomiting
Dental Usual Dosage Oral candidiasis: Suspension (swish and swallow orally):
Premature infants: 100,000 units 4 times/day; paint suspension into recesses of the mouth
Infants: 200,000 units 4 times/day or 100,000 units to each side of mouth 4 times/day; paint suspension into recesses of the mouth
Children and Adults: 400,000-600,000 units 4 times/day; swish in the mouth and retain for as long as possible (several minutes) before swallowing
Dosage Oral:
Oral candidiasis:
Suspension:
Premature infants: 100,000 units 4 times/day; paint suspension into recesses of the mouth
Infants: 200,000 units 4 times/day or 100,000 units to each side of mouth 4 times/day; paint suspension into recesses of the mouth
Children and Adults: 400,000-600,000 units 4 times/day; swish in the mouth and retain for as long as possible (several minutes) before swallowing
Powder for compounding: Children and Adults: 1/8 teaspoon (500,000 units) to equal approximately 1/2 cup of water; give 4 times/day
Intestinal infections: Adults: 500,000-1,000,000 units every 8 hours

Dosage adjustment in renal impairment: No dosage adjustment provided in manufacturer's labeling.
Dosage adjustment in hepatic impairment: No dosage adjustment provided in manufacturer's labeling.
Mechanism of Action Binds to sterols in fungal cell membrane, changing the cell wall permeability allowing for leakage of cellular contents
Contraindications Hypersensitivity to nystatin or any component of the formulation
Drug Interactions
Metabolism/Transport Effects None known.
Avoid Concomitant Use There are no known interactions where it is recommended to avoid concomitant use.
Increased Effect/Toxicity There are no known significant interactions involving an increase in effect.

Decreased Effect
Nystatin (Oral) may decrease the levels/effects of:
Saccharomyces boulardii
Pharmacodynamics/Kinetics
Onset of Action Symptomatic relief from candidiasis: 24-72 hours
Pregnancy Risk Factor C
Pregnancy Considerations Animal reproduction studies have not been conducted. Adverse events in the fetus or newborn have not been reported following maternal use of vaginal nystatin during pregnancy. Absorption following oral use is poor.
Lactation Excretion in breast milk unknown/use caution
Breast-Feeding Considerations Excretion into breast milk is not known; however, absorption following oral use is poor.
Dosage Forms
Powder, for prescription compounding: 50 million units (10 g); 150 million units (30 g); 500 million units (100 g)
Suspension, oral: 100,000 units/mL (5 mL, 60 mL, 3 mL, 480 mL)
Tablet, oral: 500,000 units

Nystatin (Topical) (nye STAT in)

Related Information
Fungal Infections *on page 1573*
Related Sample Prescriptions
Fungal Infections Requiring Topical Therapy *on page 1614*
Brand Names: U.S. Nyamyc®; Nystop®; Pedi-Dri®; Pediaderm™ AF
Brand Names: Canada Candistatin®; Nyaderm
Generic Availability (U.S.) Yes
Pharmacologic Category Antifungal Agent, Topical; Antifungal Agent, Vaginal
Use Treatment of susceptible cutaneous and mucocutaneous fungal infections normally caused by the *Candida* species
Local Anesthetic/Vasoconstrictor Precautions No information available to require special precautions
Effects on Dental Treatment No significant effects or complications reported
Effects on Bleeding No information available to require special precautions
Adverse Effects Frequency not defined: Dermatologic: Contact dermatitis, Stevens-Johnson syndrome
Dental Usual Dosage Mucocutaneous infections: Children and Adults: Topical: Apply 2-3 times/day to affected areas; very moist topical lesions are treated best with powder
Dosage
Mucocutaneous infections: Children and Adults: Topical: Apply 2-3 times/day to affected areas; very moist topical lesions are treated best with powder
Vaginal infections: Adults: Vaginal tablets: Insert 1 tablet/day at bedtime for 2 weeks
Mechanism of Action Binds to sterols in fungal cell membrane, changing the cell wall permeability allowing for leakage of cellular contents
Contraindications Hypersensitivity to nystatin or any component of the formulation

Drug Interactions
Metabolism/Transport Effects None known.
Avoid Concomitant Use There are no known interactions where it is recommended to avoid concomitant use.
Increased Effect/Toxicity There are no known significant interactions involving an increase in effect.
Decreased Effect There are no known significant interactions involving a decrease in effect.
Pharmacodynamics/Kinetics
Onset of Action Symptomatic relief from candidiasis: 24-72 hours
Pregnancy Risk Factor A (vaginal)/C (topical)
Pregnancy Considerations Animal reproduction studies have not been conducted. Adverse events in the fetus or newborn have not been reported following maternal use of vaginal nystatin during pregnancy. Absorption following oral use is poor and nystatin is not absorbed following application to mucous membranes or intact skin.
Lactation Excretion in breast milk unknown/not recommended
Breast-Feeding Considerations Excretion into breast milk is not known; however, absorption following oral use is poor and nystatin is not absorbed following application to mucous membranes or intact skin.
Dosage Forms
Cream, topical: 100,000 units/g (15 g, 30 g)
Pediaderm™ AF: 100,000 units/g (30 g)
Ointment, topical: 100,000 units/g (15 g, 30 g)
Powder, topical: 100,000 units/g (15 g, 30 g, 60 g)
Nyamyc®: 100,000 units/g (15 g, 30 g, 60 g)
Nystop®: 100,000 units/g (15 g, 30 g, 60 g)
Pedi-Dri®: 100,000 units/g (56.7 g)

Nystatin and Triamcinolone (nye STAT in & trye am SIN oh lone)

Related Information
Fungal Infections on page 1573
Nystatin (Topical) on page 995
Triamcinolone (Topical) on page 1359
Related Sample Prescriptions
Angular Cheilitis on page 1614
Generic Availability (U.S.) Yes
Pharmacologic Category Antifungal Agent, Topical; Corticosteroid, Topical
Dental Use Treatment of angular cheilitis and cutaneous candidiasis
Use Treatment of cutaneous candidiasis
Local Anesthetic/Vasoconstrictor Precautions No information available to require special precautions
Effects on Dental Treatment No significant effects or complications reported
Effects on Bleeding No information available to require special precautions
Adverse Effects Frequency not defined.
Dermatologic: Acne, allergic dermatitis, dryness, folliculitis, hypertrichosis, hypopigmentation, maceration of the skin, miliaria, perioral dermatitis, skin atrophy, striae
Local: Burning, irritation, itching
Miscellaneous: Increased incidence of secondary infection
Dental Usual Dosage Angular cheilitis and cutaneous candidiasis: Children and Adults: Topical: Apply sparingly 2-4 times/day. Therapy should be discontinued when control is achieved; if no improvement is seen, reassessment of diagnosis may be necessary.

Dosage Children and Adults: Topical: Apply sparingly to affected area(s) twice daily. Therapy should be discontinued when control is achieved or if symptoms persist for >25 days of therapy.
Mechanism of Action Nystatin is an antifungal agent that binds to sterols in fungal cell membrane, changing the cell wall permeability allowing for leakage of cellular contents. Triamcinolone is a synthetic corticosteroid; it decreases inflammation by suppression of migration of polymorphonuclear leukocytes and reversal of increased capillary permeability. It suppresses the immune system reducing activity and volume of the lymphatic system. It suppresses adrenal function at high doses.
Contraindications Hypersensitivity to nystatin, triamcinolone, or any component of the formulation
Warnings/Precautions Avoid use of occlusive dressings; limit therapy to least amount necessary for effective therapy, pediatric patients may be more susceptible to HPA axis suppression due to larger BSA to weight ratio
Drug Interactions
Metabolism/Transport Effects None known.
Avoid Concomitant Use
Avoid concomitant use of Nystatin and Triamcinolone with any of the following: Aldesleukin
Increased Effect/Toxicity
Nystatin and Triamcinolone may increase the levels/effects of: Deferasirox

The levels/effects of Nystatin and Triamcinolone may be increased by: Telaprevir
Decreased Effect
Nystatin and Triamcinolone may decrease the levels/effects of: Aldesleukin; Corticorelin; Hyaluronidase; Telaprevir
Pregnancy Risk Factor C
Pregnancy Considerations See individual agents.
Lactation Excretion in breast milk unknown/use caution
Breast-Feeding Considerations See individual agents.
Dosage Forms
Cream: Nystatin 100,000 units and triamcinolone 0.1% (15 g, 30 g, 60 g)
Ointment: Nystatin 100,000 units and triamcinolone 0.1% (15 g, 30 g, 60 g)

Ocriplasmin (ok ri PLAZ min)

Brand Names: U.S. Jetrea®
Pharmacologic Category Ophthalmic Agent; Vitreolytic
Use Treatment of symptomatic vitreomacular adhesion (VMA)
Local Anesthetic/Vasoconstrictor Precautions No information available to require special precautions
Effects on Dental Treatment No significant effects or complications reported
Effects on Bleeding No information available to require special precautions
Adverse Effects
>10%: Ocular: Blurred vision (5% to 20%), conjunctival hemorrhage (5% to 20%), eye pain (5% to 20%), macular hole (5% to 20%), photopsia (5% to 20%), retinal edema (5% to 20%), visual acuity decreased (5% to 20%; ≥3-line decrease 6%), visual impairment (5% to 20%), vitreous floaters (5% to 20%)

1% to 10%: Ocular: Intraocular inflammation (7%), anterior chamber cell (2% to 5%), cataract (2% to 5%), conjunctival hyperemia (2% to 5%), dry eyes (2% to 5%), intraocular pressure increased (2% to 5%), iritis (2% to 5%), macular edema (2% to 5%), metamorphopsia (2% to 5%), ocular discomfort (2% to 5%), photophobia (2% to 5%), retinal degeneration (2% to 5%), vitreous detachment (2% to 5%), dyschromatopsia (2%), a-wave and b-wave amplitude decreased (1%)

General Dosage Range Intravitreal: *Adults:* 0.125 mg once

Mechanism of Action Ocriplasmin is a recombinant form of human plasmin that acts as a proteolytic within the vitreous body and vitreoretinal interface. Protein matrix components responsible for the vitreomacular adhesion (eg, laminin, fibronectin, and collagen) are lysed by ocriplasmin.

Pregnancy Risk Factor C

Pregnancy Considerations Animal reproduction studies have not been conducted. Systemic exposure following a single intravitreal injection is expected to be low.

Octreotide (ok TREE oh tide)

Brand Names: U.S. SandoSTATIN LAR®; SandoSTATIN®

Brand Names: Canada Octreotide Acetate Injection; Octreotide Acetate Omega; Sandostatin LAR®; Sandostatin®

Pharmacologic Category Antidiarrheal; Antidote; Somatostatin Analog

Use Control of symptoms (diarrhea and flushing) in patients with metastatic carcinoid tumors; treatment of watery diarrhea associated with vasoactive intestinal peptide-secreting tumors (VIPomas); treatment of acromegaly

Unlabeled Use Treatment of AIDS-associated diarrhea (including *Cryptosporidiosis*), chemotherapy-induced diarrhea, graft-versus-host disease (GVHD) associated diarrhea, postgastrectomy dumping syndrome; control of bleeding of esophageal varices; second-line treatment for thymic malignancies; Cushing's syndrome (ectopic); insulinomas; small bowel fistulas; islet cell tumors; Zollinger-Ellison syndrome; congenital hyperinsulinism; hypothalamic obesity; treatment of hypoglycemia secondary to sulfonylurea poisoning; treatment of malignant bowel obstruction

Local Anesthetic/Vasoconstrictor Precautions Octreotide is one of the drugs confirmed to prolong the QT interval and is accepted as having a risk of causing torsade de pointes. The risk of drug-induced torsade de pointes is extremely low when a single QT interval prolonging drug is prescribed. In terms of epinephrine, it is not known what effect vasoconstrictors in the local anesthetic regimen will have in patients with a known history of congenital prolonged QT interval or in patients taking any medication that prolongs the QT interval. Until more information is obtained, it is suggested that the clinician consult with the physician prior to the use of a vasoconstrictor in suspected patients, and that the vasoconstrictor (epinephrine, mepivacaine and levonordefrin [Carbocaine® 2% with Neo-Cobefrin®]) be used with caution.

Effects on Dental Treatment Key adverse event(s) related to dental treatment: Xerostomia (normal salivary flow resumes upon discontinuation), gingivitis, glossitis, stomatitis, taste perversion, and dysphagia.

Effects on Bleeding No information available to require special precautions

Adverse Effects Adverse reactions vary by route of administration and dosage form. Frequency of cardiac, endocrine, and gastrointestinal adverse reactions was generally higher in acromegalics.

>16%:
Cardiovascular: Sinus bradycardia (19% to 25%), chest pain (≤20%; non-depot formulations)
Central nervous system: Fatigue (1% to 32%), headache (6% to 30%), malaise (16% to 20%), fever (16% to 20%), dizziness (5% to 20%)
Dermatologic: Pruritus (≤18%)
Endocrine & metabolic: Hyperglycemia (2% to 27%)
Gastrointestinal: Abdominal pain (5% to 61%), loose stools (5% to 61%), nausea (5% to 61%), diarrhea (34% to 61%), flatulence (≤38%), cholelithiasis (13% to 38%; length of therapy dependent), biliary sludge (24%; length of therapy dependent), constipation (9% to 21%), vomiting (4% to 21%), biliary duct dilatation (12%)
Local: Injection site pain (2% to 50%; dose and formulation related)
Neuromuscular & skeletal: Back pain (1% to 27%), arthropathy (8% to 19%), myalgia (≤18%)
Respiratory: Upper respiratory infection (10% to 23%), dyspnea (≤20%; non-depot formulations)
Miscellaneous: Antibodies to octreotide (up to 25%; no efficacy change), flu symptoms (1% to 20%)

5% to 15%:
Cardiovascular: Hypertension (≤13%), conduction abnormalities (9% to 10%), arrhythmia (3% to 9%), palpitation, peripheral edema
Central nervous system: Pain (4% to 15%), anxiety, confusion, hypoesthesia, insomnia
Dermatologic: Rash (15%; depot formulation), alopecia (≤13%)
Endocrine & metabolic: Hypothyroidism (≤12%; non-depot formulations), goiter (≤8%; non-depot formulations)
Gastrointestinal: Dyspepsia (4% to 6%), feces discoloration (4% to 6%), steatorrhea (4% to 6%), tenesmus (4% to 6%), anorexia, cramping
Hematologic: Anemia (≤15%; non-depot formulations: <1%)
Neuromuscular & skeletal: Arthralgia, myalgia, paresthesia, rigors, weakness
Otic: Earache
Renal: Renal calculus
Respiratory: Cough, pharyngitis, rhinitis, sinusitis
Miscellaneous: Allergy, diaphoresis

1% to 4%:
Cardiovascular: Angina, cardiac failure, edema, flushing, hematoma, phlebitis
Central nervous system: Abnormal gait, amnesia, depression, dysphonia, hallucinations, nervousness, neuralgia, somnolence, vertigo
Dermatologic: Acne, bruising, cellulitis
Endocrine & metabolic: Hypoglycemia (2% to 4%), hypokalemia, hypoproteinemia, gout, cachexia, breast pain, impotence
Gastrointestinal: Colitis, diverticulitis, dysphagia, fat malabsorption, gastritis, gastroenteritis, gingivitis, glossitis, melena, stomatitis, taste perversion, xerostomia
Genitourinary: Incontinence, pollakiuria (non-depot formulations), urinary tract infection
Local: Injection site hematoma
Neuromuscular & skeletal: Hyperkinesia, hypertonia, joint pain, neuropathy, tremor

Ocular: Blurred vision, visual disturbance

Otic: Tinnitus

Renal: Albuminuria, renal abscess

Respiratory: Bronchitis, epistaxis

Miscellaneous: Bacterial infection, cold symptoms, moniliasis

General Dosage Range Dosage adjustment recommended in patients with hepatic or renal impairment

I.M.: *Adults:* Depot: 20 mg every 4 weeks (maximum: 40 mg every 2 weeks)

I.V., SubQ: *Adults:* 50-1500 mcg/day in 2-4 divided doses

Mechanism of Action Mimics natural somatostatin by inhibiting serotonin release, and the secretion of gastrin, VIP, insulin, glucagon, secretin, motilin, and pancreatic polypeptide. Decreases growth hormone and IGF-1 in acromegaly. Octreotide provides more potent inhibition of growth hormone, glucagon, and insulin as compared to endogenous somatostatin. Also suppresses LH response to GnRH, secretion of thyroid-stimulating hormone and decreases splanchnic blood flow.

Pharmacodynamics/Kinetics

Duration of Action SubQ: 6-12 hours

Half-life Elimination 1.7-1.9 hours; Increased in elderly patients; Cirrhosis: Up to 3.7 hours; Fatty liver disease: Up to 3.4 hours; Renal impairment: Up to 3.1 hours

Time to Peak Plasma: SubQ: 0.4 hours (0.7 hours acromegaly); I.M.: 1 hour

Pregnancy Risk Factor B

Pregnancy Considerations Teratogenic effects were not observed in animal studies. Octreotide crosses the human placenta; data concerning use in pregnancy is limited. Women of childbearing potential should use adequate contraception during treatment with octreotide; normalization of IGF-1 and GH may restore fertility in women with acromegaly. In case reports of acromegalic women who received normal doses of octreotide during pregnancy, no congenital malformations were reported.

Dental Comment Octreotide is known to prolong the QT interval. The QT interval is measured as the time and distance between the Q point of the QRS complex and the end of the T wave in the ECG tracing. After adjustment for heart rate, the QT interval is defined as prolonged if it is more than 450 msec in men and 460 msec in women. A long QT syndrome was first described in the 1950s and 60s as a congenital syndrome involving QT interval prolongation and syncope and sudden death. Some of the congenital long QT syndromes were characterized by a peculiar electrocardiographic appearance of the QRS complex involving a premature atria beat followed by a pause, then a subsequent sinus beat showing marked QT prolongation and deformity. This type of cardiac arrhythmia was originally termed "torsade de pointes" (translated from the French as "twisting of the points"). Octreotide is considered as having a risk of causing torsade de pointes. Since it is not known what effect vasoconstrictors in the local anesthetic regimen will have in patients with a known history of congenital prolonged QT interval or in patients taking any medication that prolongs the QT interval, a medical consult is suggested.

Ofatumumab (oh fa TOOM yoo mab)

Brand Names: U.S. Arzerra™

Brand Names: Canada Arzerra™

Pharmacologic Category Antineoplastic Agent, Monoclonal Antibody; Monoclonal Antibody

Use Treatment of refractory chronic lymphocytic leukemia (CLL)

Local Anesthetic/Vasoconstrictor Precautions No information available to require special precautions

Effects on Dental Treatment No significant effects or complications reported

Effects on Bleeding Thrombocytopenia is not frequently observed (<1%) although it can rarely be seen. Neutropenia may be prolonged >2 weeks. In patients who are under active treatment with this agent, medical consult is suggested.

Adverse Effects

>10%:

Central nervous system: Fever (20%), fatigue (15%)

Dermatologic: Rash (14%)

Gastrointestinal: Diarrhea (18%), nausea (11%)

Hematologic: Neutropenia (≥grade 3: 42%; grade 4: 18%; may be prolonged >2 weeks), anemia (16%; grades 3/4: 5%)

Respiratory: Pneumonia (23%), cough (19%), dyspnea (14%), bronchitis (11%), upper respiratory tract infection (11%)

Miscellaneous: Infection (70%; includes bacterial, fungal or viral; ≥grade 3: 29%), infusion reaction (first infusion [300 mg]: 44%; second infusion [2000 mg]: 29%)

1% to 10%:

Cardiovascular: Peripheral edema (9%), hypertension (5%), hypotension (5%), tachycardia (5%)

Central nervous system: Chills (8%), insomnia (7%), headache (6%)

Dermatologic: Urticaria (8%), hyperhidrosis (5%)

Neuromuscular & skeletal: Back pain (8%), muscle spasm (5%)

Respiratory: Nasopharyngitis (8%), sinusitis (5%)

Miscellaneous: Sepsis (8%), herpes zoster (6%)

General Dosage Range Dosage adjustment recommended in patients who develop toxicities

I.V.: *Adults:* 300 mg week 1, followed 1 week later by 2000 mg once weekly for 7 doses (doses 2-8), followed 4 weeks later by 2000 mg once every 4 weeks for 4 doses (doses 9-12; for a total of 12 doses)

Mechanism of Action Ofatumumab is a monoclonal antibody which binds specifically the extracellular (large and small) loops of the CD20 molecule (which is expressed on normal B lymphocytes and in B-cell CLL) resulting in potent complement-dependent cell lysis and antibody-dependent cell-mediated toxicity in cells that overexpress CD20.

Pharmacodynamics/Kinetics

Half-life Elimination Between dose 4 and dose 12: ~14 days (range: 2-62 days)

Pregnancy Risk Factor C

Pregnancy Considerations Teratogenicity was not observed in animal reproduction studies, although prolonged depletion of circulating B cells was observed in animal offspring. There are no adequate and well-controlled studies in pregnant women. Use in pregnancy only if the potential benefit to the mother outweighs the potential risk to the fetus.

Ofloxacin (Systemic) (oh FLOKS a sin)

Related Information

Clinical Risk Related to Drugs Prolonging QT Interval *on page 1510*

Brand Names: Canada Apo-Oflox®; Novo-Ofloxacin

Pharmacologic Category Antibiotic, Quinolone

Use Quinolone antibiotic for the treatment of acute exacerbations of chronic bronchitis, community-acquired pneumonia, skin and skin structure infections (uncomplicated), urethral and cervical gonorrhea (acute, uncomplicated), urethritis and cervicitis (nongonococcal), mixed infections of the urethra and cervix, pelvic inflammatory disease (acute), cystitis (uncomplicated), urinary tract infections (complicated), prostatitis

Note: As of April 2007, the CDC no longer recommends the use of fluoroquinolones for the treatment of gonococcal disease.

Unlabeled Use Epididymitis (nongonococcal), leprosy, Traveler's diarrhea

Local Anesthetic/Vasoconstrictor Precautions Ofloxacin (Systemic) is one of the drugs confirmed to prolong the QT interval and is accepted as having a risk of causing torsade de pointes. The risk of drug-induced torsade de pointes is extremely low when a single QT interval prolonging drug is prescribed. In terms of epinephrine, it is not known what effect vasoconstrictors in the local anesthetic regimen will have in patients with a known history of congenital prolonged QT interval or in patients taking any medication that prolongs the QT interval. Until more information is obtained, it is suggested that the clinician consult with the physician prior to the use of a vasoconstrictor in suspected patients, and that the vasoconstrictor (epinephrine, mepivacaine and levonordefrin [Carbocaine® 2% with Neo-Cobefrin®]) be used with caution.

Effects on Dental Treatment Key adverse event(s) related to dental treatment: Xerostomia (normal salivary flow resumes upon discontinuation) and abnormal taste.

Effects on Bleeding Quinolone antibiotic administration has not been shown to independently effect bleeding; however, ofloxacin has been shown to potentiate the hypoprothrombinemic effect of warfarin and other coumarin anticoagulants. The hypoprothrombinemic mechanism may involve inhibition of coumarin metabolism and/or depletion of certain clotting factors due to suppression of vitamin K-producing intestinal flora.

Adverse Effects 1% to 10%:

Cardiovascular: Chest pain (1% to 3%)

Central nervous system: Headache (1% to 9%), insomnia (3% to 7%), dizziness (1% to 5%), fatigue (1% to 3%), somnolence (1% to 3%), sleep disorders (1% to 3%), nervousness (1% to 3%), pyrexia (1% to 3%)

Dermatologic: Rash/pruritus (1% to 3%)

Gastrointestinal: Diarrhea (1% to 4%), vomiting (1% to 4%), GI distress (1% to 3%), abdominal cramps (1% to 3%), flatulence (1% to 3%), abnormal taste (1% to 3%), xerostomia (1% to 3%), appetite decreased (1% to 3%), nausea (3% to 10%), constipation (1% to 3%)

Genitourinary: Vaginitis (1% to 5%), external genital pruritus in women (1% to 3%)

Ocular: Visual disturbances (1% to 3%)

Respiratory: Pharyngitis (1% to 3%)

Miscellaneous: Trunk pain

General Dosage Range Dosage adjustment recommended in patients with hepatic or renal impairment

Oral: *Adults:* 200-400 mg every 12 hours

Mechanism of Action Ofloxacin is a DNA gyrase inhibitor. DNA gyrase is an essential bacterial enzyme that maintains the superhelical structure of DNA. DNA gyrase is required for DNA replication and transcription, DNA repair, recombination, and transposition; bactericidal

Pharmacodynamics/Kinetics

Half-life Elimination Biphasic: 4-5 hours and 20-25 hours (accounts for <5%); prolonged with renal impairment

Pregnancy Risk Factor C

Pregnancy Considerations Adverse events have been observed in some animal studies; therefore, the manufacturer classifies ofloxacin as pregnancy category C. Ofloxacin crosses the placenta and produces measurable concentrations in the amniotic fluid. An increased risk of teratogenic effects has not been observed in animals or humans following ofloxacin use during pregnancy; however, because of concerns of cartilage damage in immature animals, ofloxacin should only be used during pregnancy if a safer option is not available. Serum concentrations of ofloxacin may be lower during pregnancy than in nonpregnant patients.

Dental Comment Ofloxacin (Systemic) is known to prolong the QT interval. The QT interval is measured as the time and distance between the Q point of the QRS complex and the end of the T wave in the ECG tracing. After adjustment for heart rate, the QT interval is defined as prolonged if it is more than 450 msec in men and 460 msec in women. A long QT syndrome was first described in the 1950s and 60s as a congenital syndrome involving QT interval prolongation and syncope and sudden death. Some of the congenital long QT syndromes were characterized by a peculiar electrocardiographic appearance of the QRS complex involving a premature atria beat followed by a pause, then a subsequent sinus beat showing marked QT prolongation and deformity. This type of cardiac arrhythmia was originally termed "torsade de pointes" (translated from the French as "twisting of the points"). Ofloxacin (Systemic) is considered as having a risk of causing torsade de pointes. Since it is not known what effect vasoconstrictors in the local anesthetic regimen will have in patients with a known history of congenital prolonged QT interval or in patients taking any medication that prolongs the QT interval, a medical consult is suggested.

OLANZapine (oh LAN za peen)

Brand Names: U.S. ZyPREXA®; ZyPREXA® IntraMuscular; ZyPREXA® Relprevv™; ZyPREXA® Zydis®

Brand Names: Canada Apo-Olanzapine ODT®; Apo-Olanzapine®; Ava-Olanzapine; CO Olanzapine; CO Olanzapine ODT; Mylan-Olanzapine; Olanzapine ODT; PHL-Olanzapine; PHL-Olanzapine ODT; PMS-Olanzapine; PMS-Olanzapine ODT; Riva-Olanzapine; Riva-Olanzapine ODT; Sandoz-Olanzapine; Sandoz-Olanzapine ODT; Teva-Olanzapine; Teva-Olanzapine OD; Zyprexa®; Zyprexa® Intramuscular; Zyprexa® Zydis®

Generic Availability (U.S.) Yes: Excludes Injection (powder for suspension, extended release)

Pharmacologic Category Antimanic Agent; Antipsychotic Agent, Atypical

Use

Oral: Treatment of the manifestations of schizophrenia; treatment of acute or mixed mania episodes associated with bipolar I disorder (as monotherapy or in combination with lithium or valproate); maintenance treatment of bipolar disorder; in combination with fluoxetine for treatment-resistant or bipolar I depression

I.M., extended-release (Zyprexa® Relprevv™): Treatment of schizophrenia

I.M., short-acting (Zyprexa® IntraMuscular): Treatment of acute agitation associated with schizophrenia and bipolar I mania

◄ **Unlabeled Use** Treatment of psychosis/schizophrenia in children; chronic pain; prevention of chemotherapy-associated delayed nausea or vomiting; psychosis/agitation related to Alzheimer's dementia; acute treatment of delirium

Local Anesthetic/Vasoconstrictor Precautions No information available to require special precautions

Effects on Dental Treatment No significant effects or complications reported

Effects on Bleeding No information available to require special precautions

Adverse Effects

Oral: Unless otherwise noted, adverse events are reported for placebo-controlled trials in adult patients on monotherapy:

>10%:

Central nervous system: Somnolence (dose dependent; 20% to 39%; adolescents 39% to 48%), extrapyramidal symptoms (dose dependent; ≤32%), dizziness (11% to 18%), headache (adolescents 17%), fatigue (adolescents 3% to 14%), insomnia (12%)

Endocrine & metabolic: Prolactin increased (30%; adolescents 47%)

Gastrointestinal: Weight gain (5% to 6%, has been reported as high as 40%; adolescents 29% to 31%), appetite increased (3% to 6%; adolescents 17% to 29%), xerostomia (dose dependent; 3% to 22%), constipation (9% to 11%), dyspepsia (7% to 11%)

Hepatic: ALT increased ≥3 x ULN (adolescents 12%; adults 5%)

Neuromuscular & skeletal: Weakness (dose dependent; 8% to 20%)

Miscellaneous: Accidental injury (12%)

1% to 10%:

Cardiovascular: Chest pain, hypertension, orthostatic hypotension, peripheral edema, tachycardia

Central nervous system: Fever, personality changes, restlessness (adolescents)

Dermatologic: Bruising

Endocrine & metabolic: Breast-related events ([adolescents] discharge, enlargement, galactorrhea, gynecomastia, lactation disorder); menstrual-related events (amenorrhea, hypomenorrhea, menstruation delayed, oligomenorrhea); sexual function-related events (anorgasmia, ejaculation delayed, erectile dysfunction, changes in libido, abnormal orgasm, sexual dysfunction)

Gastrointestinal: Abdominal pain (adolescents), diarrhea (adolescents), flatulence, nausea (dose dependent), vomiting

Genitourinary: Incontinence, UTI

Hepatic: Hepatic enzymes increased

Neuromuscular & skeletal: Abnormal gait, akathisia, articulation impairment, back pain, falling, hypertonia, joint/extremity pain, muscle stiffness (adolescents), tremor (dose dependent)

Ocular: Amblyopia

Respiratory: Cough, epistaxis (adolescents), pharyngitis, respiratory tract infection (adolescents), rhinitis, sinusitis (adolescents)

Injection: Unless otherwise noted, adverse events are reported for placebo-controlled trials in adult patients on extended-release I.M. injection (Zyprexa® Relprevv™). Also refer to adverse reactions noted with oral therapy.

>10%: Central nervous system: Headache (13% to 18%), sedation (8% to 13%)

1% to 10%:

Cardiovascular: Hypertension, hypotension (short-acting), orthostatic hypotension (short-acting), QT prolongation

Central nervous system: Abnormal dreams, abnormal thinking, auditory hallucination, dizziness, dysarthria, extrapyramidal symptoms, fatigue, fever, pain, restlessness, somnolence

Dermatologic: Acne

Gastrointestinal: Abdominal pain, appetite increased, diarrhea, flatulence, nausea, vomiting, weight gain, xerostomia

Genitourinary: Vaginal discharge

Hepatic: Liver enzymes increased

Local: Injection site pain

Neuromuscular & skeletal: Arthralgia, back pain, muscle spasms, stiffness, tremor, weakness (short-acting)

Otic: Ear pain

Respiratory: Cough, nasal congestion, nasopharyngitis, pharyngolaryngeal pain, sneezing, upper respiratory tract infection

Miscellaneous: Toothache, tooth infection, viral infection

<1%, postmarketing, and/or case reports (limited to important or life-threatening): CPK increased, post-injection delirium/sedation syndrome, syncope (short-acting)

Dosage

Adolescents ≥13 years: Schizophrenia/bipolar disorder: Oral: Initial: 2.5-5 mg once daily; adjust by 2.5-5 mg/day to target dose of 10 mg/day; dosing range: 2.5-20 mg/day

Adults:

Agitation (acute, associated with bipolar I mania or schizophrenia): Short-acting I.M. injection: Initial dose: 10 mg (a lower dose of 5-7.5 mg may be considered when clinical factors warrant); additional doses (up to 10 mg) may be considered, however, 2-4 hours should be allowed between doses to evaluate response (maximum total daily dose: 30 mg, per manufacturer's recommendation)

Bipolar I acute mixed or manic episodes: Oral:

Monotherapy: Initial: 10-15 mg once daily; increase by 5 mg/day at intervals of not less than 24 hours. Maintenance: 5-20 mg/day; recommended maximum dose: 20 mg/day.

Combination therapy (with lithium or valproate): Initial: 10 mg once daily; dosing range: 5-20 mg/day; recommended maximum dose: 20 mg/day.

Depression:

Depression associated with bipolar disorder (in combination with fluoxetine): Oral: Initial: 5 mg in the evening; adjust as tolerated to usual range of 5-12.5 mg/day. See **"Note"**

Treatment-resistant depression (in combination with fluoxetine): Oral: Initial: 5 mg in the evening; adjust as tolerated to range of 5-20 mg/day. See **"Note"**

Note: When using individual components of fluoxetine with olanzapine rather than fixed dose combination product (Symbyax®), approximate dosage correspondence is as follows:

Olanzapine 2.5 mg + fluoxetine 20 mg = Symbyax® 3/25

Olanzapine 5 mg + fluoxetine 20 mg = Symbyax® 6/25

Olanzapine 12.5 mg + fluoxetine 20 mg = Symbyax® 12/25

Olanzapine 5 mg + fluoxetine 50 mg = Symbyax® 6/50

Olanzapine 12.5 mg + fluoxetine 50 mg = Symbyax® 12/50

Schizophrenia:

Oral: Initial: 5-10 mg once daily (increase to 10 mg once daily within 5-7 days); thereafter, adjust by 5 mg/day at 1-week intervals, up to a recommended maximum of 20 mg/day. Maintenance: 10-20 mg once daily. Doses of 30-50 mg/day have been used; however, doses >10 mg/day have not demonstrated better efficacy, and safety and efficacy of doses >20 mg/day have not been evaluated.

Extended-release I.M. injection: **Note:** Establish tolerance to oral olanzapine prior to changing to extended-release I.M. injection. Maximum dose: 300 mg/2 weeks or 405 mg/4 weeks

Patients established on oral olanzapine 10 mg/day: Initial dose: 210 mg every 2 weeks for 4 doses or 405 mg every 4 weeks for 2 doses; Maintenance dose: 150 mg every 2 weeks or 300 mg every 4 weeks

Patients established on oral olanzapine 15 mg/day: Initial dose: 300 mg every 2 weeks for 4 doses; Maintenance dose: 210 mg every 2 weeks or 405 mg every 4 weeks

Patients established on oral olanzapine 20 mg/day: Initial and maintenance dose: 300 mg every 2 weeks

Delirium (unlabeled use): Oral: 5 mg daily for up to 5 days (NICE, 2010)

Prevention of chemotherapy-associated delayed nausea or vomiting (unlabeled use; in combination with a corticosteroid and serotonin [5-HT$_3$] antagonist): Oral: 10 mg once daily for 3-5 days, beginning on day 1 of chemotherapy **or** 5 mg once daily for 2 days before chemotherapy, followed by 10 mg once daily (beginning on the day of chemotherapy) for 3-8 days

Elderly:

Short-acting I.M., Oral: Consider lower starting dose of 2.5-5 mg/day for elderly or debilitated patients; may increase as clinically indicated and tolerated with close monitoring of orthostatic blood pressure

Extended release I.M.: Consider lower starting dose of 150 mg every 4 weeks for elderly or debilitated patients; increase dose with caution as clinically indicated.

Delirium (unlabeled use): Patients >60 years: 2.5 mg daily for up to 5 days (NICE, 2010)

Psychosis/agitation related to Alzheimer's dementia (unlabeled use): Oral: Initial: 2.5-5 mg/day (Sultzer, 2008)

Dosage adjustment in renal impairment: No adjustment required. Not removed by dialysis.

Dosage adjustment in hepatic impairment: Dosage adjustment may be necessary; however, there are no specific recommendations. Monitor closely.

Mechanism of Action Olanzapine is a second generation thienobenzodiazepine antipsychotic which displays potent antagonism of serotonin 5-HT$_{2A}$ and 5-HT$_{2C}$, dopamine D$_{1-4}$, histamine H$_1$ and alpha$_1$-adrenergic receptors. Olanzapine shows moderate antagonism of 5-HT$_3$ and muscarinic M$_{1-5}$ receptors, and weak binding to GABA-A, BZD, and beta-adrenergic receptors. Although the precise mechanism of action in schizophrenia and bipolar disorder is not known, the efficacy of olanzapine is thought to be mediated through combined antagonism of dopamine and serotonin type 2 receptor sites.

Contraindications There are no contraindications listed in the manufacturer's labeling.

Canadian labeling: Hypersensitivity to olanzapine or any component of the formulation

Warnings/Precautions [U.S. Boxed Warning]: Elderly patients with dementia-related psychosis treated with antipsychotics are at an increased risk of death compared to placebo. Most deaths appeared to be either cardiovascular (eg, heart failure, sudden death) or infectious (eg, pneumonia) in nature. In addition, an increased incidence of cerebrovascular effects (eg, transient ischemic attack, stroke) has been reported in studies of placebo-controlled trials of olanzapine in elderly patients with dementia-related psychosis. Olanzapine is not approved for the treatment of dementia-related psychosis.

Moderate to highly sedating, use with caution in disorders where CNS depression is a feature; patients must be cautioned about performing tasks which require mental alertness (eg, operating machinery or driving). Use caution in patients with cardiac disease. Use with caution in Parkinson's disease, predisposition to seizures, or severe hepatic or renal disease. Life-threatening arrhythmias have occurred with therapeutic doses of some neuroleptics. May induce orthostatic hypotension; use caution with history of cardiovascular disease, hemodynamic instability, prior myocardial infarction, or ischemic heart disease. Increases in cholesterol and triglycerides have been noted. Use with caution in patients with pre-existing abnormal lipid profile. Esophageal dysmotility and aspiration have been associated with antipsychotic use; use with caution in patients at risk of aspiration pneumonia. May increase prolactin levels; clinical significance of hyperprolactinemia in patients with breast cancer or other prolactin-dependent tumors is unknown. Significant weight gain (>7% of baseline weight) may occur; monitor waist circumference and BMI. Impaired core body temperature regulation may occur; caution with strenuous exercise, heat exposure, dehydration, and concomitant medication possessing anticholinergic effects.

Leukopenia, neutropenia, and agranulocytosis (sometimes fatal) have been reported in clinical trials and postmarketing reports with antipsychotic use; presence of risk factors (eg, pre-existing low WBC or history of drug-induced leuko-/neutropenia) should prompt periodic blood count assessment. Discontinue therapy at first signs of blood dyscrasias or if absolute neutrophil count <1000/mm^3.

May cause anticholinergic effects; use with caution in patients with decreased gastrointestinal motility, urinary retention, BPH, xerostomia, or narrow-angle glaucoma. Relative to other neuroleptics, olanzapine has a moderate potency of cholinergic blockade. May cause extrapyramidal symptoms (EPS), although risk of these reactions is lower relative to other neuroleptics. Risk of dystonia (and probably other EPS) may be greater with increased doses, use of conventional antipsychotics, males, and younger patients. May be associated with neuroleptic malignant syndrome (NMS). May cause extreme and life-threatening hyperglycemia; use with caution in patients with diabetes or other disorders of glucose regulation; monitor. Olanzapine levels may be lower in patients who smoke; the manufacturer does not require dosage adjustments, although dosage adjustments may be considered. Use in adolescent patients ≥13 years of age may result in increased weight gain and sedation, as well as greater increases in LDL cholesterol, total cholesterol, triglycerides, prolactin, and liver transaminase levels when compared to adults. ▸

Adolescent patients should be maintained on the lowest dose necessary.

Use in elderly patients with dementia is associated with an increased risk of mortality and cerebrovascular accidents; avoid antipsychotic use for behavioral problems associated with dementia unless alternative nonpharmacologic therapies have failed and patient may harm self or others. In addition, use may cause or exacerbate syndrome of inappropriate antidiuretic hormone secretion or hyponatremia; monitor sodium closely with initiation or dosage adjustments in older adults. May also be inappropriate in older adults depending on comorbidities (eg, dementia, delirium) due to its potent anticholinergic effects (Beers Criteria).

The possibility of a suicide attempt is inherent in psychotic illness or bipolar disorder; use caution in high-risk patients during initiation of therapy. Prescriptions should be written for the smallest quantity consistent with good patient care.

There are two Zyprexa® formulations for intramuscular injection: Zyprexa® Relprevv™ is an extended-release formulation and Zyprexa® Intramuscular is short-acting:

Extended-release I.M. injection (Zyprexa® Relprevv™): Monitor for post injection delirium/sedation syndrome; patients should be continuously watched (≥3 hours) for symptoms of olanzapine overdose. Only available through a restricted drug distribution program.

Short-acting I.M. injection (Zyprexa® IntraMuscular): Patients should remain recumbent if drowsy/dizzy until hypotension, bradycardia, and/or hypoventilation have been ruled out. Concurrent use of I.M./I.V. benzodiazepines is not recommended (fatalities have been reported, though causality not determined).

Drug Interactions

Metabolism/Transport Effects Substrate of CYP1A2 (major), CYP2D6 (minor); **Note:** Assignment of Major/Minor substrate status based on clinically relevant drug interaction potential; **Inhibits** CYP1A2 (weak), CYP2C19 (weak), CYP2C9 (weak), CYP2D6 (weak), CYP3A4 (weak)

Avoid Concomitant Use

Avoid concomitant use of OLANZapine with any of the following: Aclidinium; Azelastine (Nasal); Benzodiazepines; Ipratropium (Oral Inhalation); Metoclopramide; Paraldehyde; Pimozide; Tiotropium

Increased Effect/Toxicity

OLANZapine may increase the levels/effects of: Alcohol (Ethyl); Anticholinergics; ARIPiprazole; Azelastine (Nasal); Benzodiazepines; Buprenorphine; CNS Depressants; Lomitapide; Methotrimeprazine; Methylphenidate; Paraldehyde; Pimozide; Serotonin Modulators; Tiotropium; Zolpidem

The levels/effects of OLANZapine may be increased by: Abiraterone Acetate; Acetylcholinesterase Inhibitors (Central); Aclidinium; CYP1A2 Inhibitors (Moderate); CYP1A2 Inhibitors (Strong); Deferasirox; Droperidol; FluvoxaMINE; HydrOXYzine; Ipratropium (Oral Inhalation); LamoTRIgine; Lithium formulations; Magnesium Sulfate; Methotrimeprazine; Methylphenidate; Metoclopramide; Metyrosine; Perampanel; Pramlintide; Sodium Oxybate; Tetrabenazine

Decreased Effect

OLANZapine may decrease the levels/effects of: Amphetamines; Anti-Parkinson's Agents (Dopamine Agonist); Quinagolide

The levels/effects of OLANZapine may be decreased by: CYP1A2 Inducers (Strong); Cyproterone; Lithium formulations; Peginterferon Alfa-2b

Ethanol/Nutrition/Herb Interactions

Ethanol: May increase CNS depression; monitor for increased effects with coadministration. Caution patients about effects.

Herb/Nutraceutical: Avoid dong quai, St John's wort (may also cause photosensitization). Avoid kava kava, gotu kola, valerian, St John's wort (may increase CNS depression).

Dietary Considerations Tablets may be taken without regard to meals. Some products may contain phenylalanine.

Pharmacodynamics/Kinetics

Half-life Elimination 21-54 hours; approximately 1.5 times greater in elderly; Extended-release injection: ~30 days

Time to Peak Maximum plasma concentrations after I.M. administration are 5 times higher than maximum plasma concentrations produced by an oral dose.
Extended-release injection: ~7 days
Short-acting injection: 15-45 minutes
Oral: ~6 hours

Pregnancy Risk Factor C

Pregnancy Considerations No evidence of teratogenicity reported in animal studies. However, fetal toxicity and prolonged gestation have been observed. Antipsychotic use during the third trimester of pregnancy has a risk for abnormal muscle movements (extrapyramidal symptoms [EPS]) and withdrawal symptoms in newborns following delivery. Symptoms in the newborn may include agitation, feeding disorder, hypertonia, hypotonia, respiratory distress, somnolence, and tremor; these effects may be self-limiting or require hospitalization. There are no adequate and well-controlled studies in pregnant women. Healthcare providers are encouraged to enroll women 18-45 years of age exposed to olanzapine during pregnancy in the Atypical Antipsychotics Pregnancy Registry (1-866-961-2388 or http://www.womensmentalhealth.org/pregnancyregistry).

Lactation Enters breast milk/not recommended

Breast-Feeding Considerations At steady-state concentrations, it is estimated that a breast-fed infant may be exposed to ~2% of the maternal dose.

Prescribing and Access Restrictions As a requirement of the REMS program, only prescribers, healthcare facilities, and pharmacies registered with the Zyprexa® Relprevv™ Patient Care Program are able to prescribe, distribute, or dispense Zyprexa® Relprevv™ for patients who are enrolled in and meet all conditions of the program. Zyprexa® Relprevv™ must be administered at a registered healthcare facility. Prescribers will need to be recertified every 3 years. Contact the Zyprexa® Relprevv™ Patient Care Program at 1-877-772-9390.

Dosage Forms

Injection, powder for reconstitution: 10 mg
ZyPREXA® IntraMuscular: 10 mg

Injection, powder for suspension, extended release:
ZyPREXA® Relprevv™: 210 mg, 300 mg, 405 mg

Tablet, oral: 2.5 mg, 5 mg, 7.5 mg, 10 mg, 15 mg, 20 mg
ZyPREXA®: 2.5 mg, 5 mg, 7.5 mg, 10 mg, 15 mg, 20 mg

Tablet, orally disintegrating, oral: 5 mg, 10 mg, 15 mg, 20 mg
ZyPREXA® Zydis®: 5 mg, 10 mg, 15 mg, 20 mg

Olanzapine and Fluoxetine
(oh LAN za peen & floo OKS e teen)

Related Information
FLUoxetine *on page 608*
OLANZapine *on page 999*
Vasoconstrictor Interactions With Antidepressants *on page 1650*

Brand Names: U.S. Symbyax®

Pharmacologic Category Antidepressant, Selective Serotonin Reuptake Inhibitor; Antipsychotic Agent, Atypical

Use Treatment of depressive episodes associated with bipolar I disorder; treatment-resistant depression (unresponsive to 2 trials of different antidepressants in the current episode)

Local Anesthetic/Vasoconstrictor Precautions Although caution should be used in patients taking tricyclic antidepressants, no interactions have been reported with vasoconstrictors and fluoxetine, a non-tricyclic antidepressant which acts to increase serotonin; no precautions appear to be needed. Fluoxetine is one of the drugs confirmed to prolong the QT interval and is accepted as having a risk of causing torsade de pointes. The risk of drug-induced torsade de pointes is extremely low when a single QT interval prolonging drug is prescribed. In terms of epinephrine, it is not known what effect vasoconstrictors in the local anesthetic regimen will have in patients with a known history of congenital prolonged QT interval or in patients taking any medication that prolongs the QT interval. Until more information is obtained, it is suggested that the clinician consult with the physician prior to the use of a vasoconstrictor in suspected patients, and that the vasoconstrictor (epinephrine, mepivacaine and levonordefrin [Carbocaine® 2% with Neo-Cobefrin®]) be used with caution.

Effects on Dental Treatment Key adverse event(s) related to dental treatment: Xerostomia or salivation increased (normal salivary flow resumes upon discontinuation), tooth disorder, and taste perversion. See Effects on Bleeding.

Effects on Bleeding May impair platelet aggregation resulting in increased risk of bleeding events, particularly if used concomitantly with aspirin, NSAIDs, warfarin, or other anticoagulants. Bleeding related to SSRI use has been reported to range from relatively minor bruising and epistaxis to life-threatening hemorrhage. Routine interruption of therapy for most dental procedures is not warranted. In medically complicated patients or extensive oral surgery, the decision to interrupt therapy must be based on the risk to benefit in an individual patient and a medical consult is suggested. If therapy is continued without interruption, the clinician should anticipate the potential for a prolonged bleeding time.

Adverse Effects As reported with combination product (also see individual agents):
>10%:
Central nervous system: Somnolence (14%), fatigue (12%)
Endocrine & metabolic: Hyperprolactinemia (28%), bicarbonate decreased (14%)
Gastrointestinal: Weight gain (25%), appetite increased (20%), xerostomia (15%)
Hepatic: Hyperbilirubinemia (15%)
1% to 10%:
Cardiovascular: Peripheral edema (9%), edema (3%), vasodilation (≥1%)

Central nervous system: Sedation (8%), attention disturbance (5%), hypersomnia (5%), restlessness (4%), lethargy (3%), pain in extremity (3%), fever (2%), nervousness (2%), pain (2%), thinking abnormal (2%), chills (≥1%), amnesia (≥1%)
Dermatologic: Photosensitivity (≥1%), ecchymosis (≥1%)
Endocrine & metabolic: Hypoalbuminemia (3%), uric acid levels increased (3%), hypophosphatemia (2%), breast pain (≥1%), menorrhagia (≥1%)
Gastrointestinal: Flatulence (3%), abdominal distension (2%), diarrhea (≥1%), taste perversion (≥1%), weight loss (≥1%)
Genitourinary: Erectile dysfunction (2%), urinary frequency (≥1%), urinary incontinence (≥1%)
Hematologic: Hemoglobin decreased (3%), lymphocytopenia (2%)
Hepatic: ALT increased (3%)
Neuromuscular & skeletal: Tremor (9%), arthralgia (4%), weakness (3%), stiffness (2%), neck rigidity (≥1%)
Ocular: Blurred vision (5%)
Renal: Glucosuria (4%)
Respiratory: Sinusitis (2%)

Frequency not defined: Alkaline phosphate increased, AST increased, cholesterol increased, GGT increased, hyperglycemia, hyponatremia, orthostatic hypotension, triglycerides increased

General Dosage Range Dosage adjustment recommended in patients with hepatic impairment
Oral:
Adults: Initial: Olanzapine 6 mg and fluoxetine 25 mg once daily; Maintenance: Olanzapine 6-12 mg and fluoxetine 25-50 mg once daily
Elderly >65 years: Initial: Olanzapine 3-6 mg and fluoxetine 25 mg once daily

Mechanism of Action Olanzapine is a second generation thienobenzodiazepine antipsychotic which displays potent antagonism of serotonin 5-HT$_{2A}$ and 5-HT$_{2C}$, dopamine D$_{1-4}$, histamine H$_1$ and alpha$_1$-adrenergic receptors. Olanzapine shows moderate antagonism of 5-HT$_3$ and muscarinic M$_{1-5}$ receptors, and weak binding to GABA-A, BZD, and beta-adrenergic receptors. Fluoxetine inhibits CNS neuron serotonin reuptake; minimal or no effect on reuptake of norepinephrine or dopamine; does not significantly bind to alpha-adrenergic, histamine, or cholinergic receptors. The enhanced antidepressant effect of the combination may be due to synergistic increases in serotonin, norepinephrine, and dopamine.

Pregnancy Risk Factor C

Pregnancy Considerations A decrease in fetal weight, testicular degeneration and atrophy, depletion of epididymal sperm, and infertility in males was reported in some animal reproduction studies using this combination. Use during pregnancy is not recommended. Refer to individual agents for additional information.

Dental Comment Fluoxetine is known to prolong the QT interval. The QT interval is measured as the time and distance between the Q point of the QRS complex and the end of the T wave in the ECG tracing. After adjustment for heart rate, the QT interval is defined as prolonged if it is more than 450 msec in men and 460 msec in women. A long QT syndrome was first described in the 1950s and 60s as a congenital syndrome involving QT interval prolongation and syncope and sudden death. Some of the congenital long QT syndromes were characterized by a peculiar ▶

electrocardiographic appearance of the QRS complex involving a premature atria beat followed by a pause, then a subsequent sinus beat showing marked QT prolongation and deformity. This type of cardiac arrhythmia was originally termed "torsade de pointes" (translated from the French as "twisting of the points"). Fluoxetine is considered as having a risk of causing torsade de pointes. Since it is not known what effect vasoconstrictors in the local anesthetic regimen will have in patients with a known history of congenital prolonged QT interval or in patients taking any medication that prolongs the QT interval, a medical consult is suggested.

Olmesartan (ole me SAR tan)

Related Information
Cardiovascular Diseases on page 1492
Brand Names: U.S. Benicar®
Brand Names: Canada Olmetec®
Pharmacologic Category Angiotensin II Receptor Blocker
Use Treatment of hypertension with or without concurrent use of other antihypertensive agents
Local Anesthetic/Vasoconstrictor Precautions No information available to require special precautions
Effects on Dental Treatment No significant effects or complications reported
Effects on Bleeding No information available to require special precautions
Adverse Effects 1% to 10%:
Central nervous system: Dizziness (3%), headache
Endocrine & metabolic: Hyperglycemia, hypertriglyceridemia
Gastrointestinal: Diarrhea
Neuromuscular & skeletal: Back pain, CPK increased
Renal: Hematuria
Respiratory: Bronchitis, pharyngitis, rhinitis, sinusitis
Miscellaneous: Flu-like syndrome
General Dosage Range Oral:
Children 6-16 years:
20 kg to <35 kg: Initial: 10 mg once daily (maximum: 20 mg once daily)
≥35 kg: Initial: 20 mg once daily (maximum: 40 mg once daily)
Adolescents >16 years and Adults: Initial: 20 mg once daily; Maintenance: 20-40 mg once daily
Elderly: Initial: 5-20 mg once daily
Mechanism of Action As a selective and competitive, nonpeptide angiotensin II receptor antagonist, olmesartan blocks the vasoconstrictor and aldosterone-secreting effects of angiotensin II; olmesartan interacts reversibly at the AT1 and AT2 receptors of many tissues and has slow dissociation kinetics; its affinity for the AT1 receptor is 12,500 times greater than the AT2 receptor. Angiotensin II receptor antagonists may induce a more complete inhibition of the renin-angiotensin system than ACE inhibitors, they do not affect the response to bradykinin, and are less likely to be associated with nonrenin-angiotensin effects (eg, cough and angioedema). Olmesartan increases urinary flow rate and, in addition to being natriuretic and kaliuretic, increases excretion of chloride, magnesium, uric acid, calcium, and phosphate.
Pharmacodynamics/Kinetics
Half-life Elimination Terminal: 13 hours
Time to Peak 1-2 hours
Pregnancy Risk Factor D

Pregnancy Considerations [U.S. Boxed Warning]: Drugs that act on the renin-angiotensin system can cause injury and death to the developing fetus. Discontinue as soon as possible once pregnancy is detected. The use of drugs which act on the renin-angiotensin system are associated with oligohydramnios. Oligohydramnios, due to decreased fetal renal function, may lead to fetal lung hypoplasia and skeletal malformations. Use is also associated with anuria, hypotension, renal failure, skull hypoplasia, and death in the fetus/neonate. The exposed fetus should be monitored for fetal growth, amniotic fluid volume, and organ formation. Infants exposed in utero should be monitored for hyperkalemia, hypotension, and oliguria.

Olmesartan, Amlodipine, and Hydrochlorothiazide
(ole me SAR tan, am LOE di peen, & hye droe klor oh THYE a zide)

Related Information
AmLODIPine on page 88
Hydrochlorothiazide on page 687
Olmesartan on page 1004
Brand Names: U.S. Tribenzor™
Pharmacologic Category Angiotensin II Receptor Blocker; Antianginal Agent; Calcium Channel Blocker; Calcium Channel Blocker, Dihydropyridine; Diuretic, Thiazide
Use Treatment of hypertension (not for initial therapy)
Local Anesthetic/Vasoconstrictor Precautions No information available to require special precautions
Effects on Dental Treatment Fewer reports of gingival hyperplasia with amlodipine than with other CCBs (usually resolves upon discontinuation); consultation with physician is suggested.
Effects on Bleeding No information available to require special precautions
Adverse Effects Reactions/percentages reported with combination product; also see individual agents.
1% to 10%:
Cardiovascular: Edema (8%), syncope (1%)
Central nervous system: Dizziness (6% to 9%), headache (6%), fatigue (4%)
Gastrointestinal: Diarrhea (3%), nausea (3%)
Neuromuscular & skeletal: Muscle spasms (3%), joint swelling (2%)
Renal: Urinary tract infection (2%)
Respiratory: Nasopharyngitis (4%), upper respiratory tract infection (3%)
General Dosage Range Oral: Adults: Amlodipine 5-10 mg and olmesartan 20-40 mg and hydrochlorothiazide 12.5-25 mg once daily (maximum: 10 mg/day [amlodipine]; 25 mg/day [hydrochlorothiazide]; 40 mg/day [olmesartan])
Mechanism of Action
Amlodipine inhibits calcium ion from entering the "slow channels" or select voltage-sensitive areas of vascular smooth muscle and myocardium during depolarization, producing a relaxation of coronary vascular smooth muscle and coronary vasodilation; increases myocardial oxygen delivery in patients with vasospastic angina. Amlodipine directly acts on vascular smooth muscle to produce peripheral arterial vasodilation reducing peripheral vascular resistance and blood pressure.

Olmesartan produces direct antagonism of the angiotensin II receptors, unlike the ACE inhibitors. It displaces angiotensin II from the AT1 receptor and produces its blood pressure-lowering effects by antagonizing AT1-induced vasoconstriction, aldosterone release, catecholamine release, arginine vasopressin release, water intake, and hypertrophic responses. This action results in more efficient blockade of the cardiovascular effects of angiotensin II and fewer side effects than the ACE inhibitors.

Hydrochlorothiazide inhibits sodium reabsorption in the distal tubules causing increased excretion of sodium and water as well as potassium and hydrogen ions.

Pregnancy Risk Factor D
Pregnancy Considerations [U.S. Boxed Warning]: Drugs that act on the renin-angiotensin system can cause injury and death to the developing fetus. Discontinue as soon as possible once pregnancy is detected. Also see individual agents.

Olmesartan and Hydrochlorothiazide
(ole me SAR tan & hye droe klor oh THYE a zide)

Related Information
Hydrochlorothiazide on page 687
Olmesartan on page 1004
Brand Names: U.S. Benicar HCT®
Brand Names: Canada Olmetec Plus®
Pharmacologic Category Angiotensin II Receptor Blocker; Diuretic, Thiazide
Use Treatment of hypertension (not recommended for initial treatment)
Local Anesthetic/Vasoconstrictor Precautions No information available to require special precautions
Effects on Dental Treatment No significant effects or complications reported
Effects on Bleeding No information available to require special precautions
Adverse Effects Frequencies reported with combination product. See individual monographs for additional adverse effects reported with each agent.
Cardiovascular: Chest pain, peripheral edema
Central nervous system: Dizziness (9%), vertigo
Dermatologic: Rash
Endocrine & metabolic: Hyperuricemia (4%), hyperglycemia, hyperlipidemia
Gastrointestinal: Nausea (3%), abdominal pain, dyspepsia, gastroenteritis, diarrhea
Genitourinary: Hematuria
Hepatic: Transaminases increased
Neuromuscular & skeletal: Back pain, arthritis, arthralgia, myalgia
Respiratory: Upper respiratory infection (7%), cough
Miscellaneous: CPK increased
<1%, postmarketing, and/or case reports: Acute renal failure, alopecia, angioedema, anaphylactic reactions, BUN increased, creatinine increased, diarrhea, facial edema, hyperkalemia, pruritus, rhabdomyolysis, urticaria, vomiting, weakness
General Dosage Range Oral: Adults: Olmesartan 20-40 mg and hydrochlorothiazide 12.5-25 mg once daily (maximum: 25 mg/day [hydrochlorothiazide]; 40 mg/day [olmesartan])
Mechanism of Action Olmesartan blocks the vasoconstrictor and aldosterone-secreting effects of angiotensin II. Hydrochlorothiazide inhibits sodium reabsorption in the distal tubules causing increased excretion of sodium and water as well as potassium and hydrogen ions.

Pregnancy Risk Factor D
Pregnancy Considerations [U.S. Boxed Warning]: Drugs that act on the renin-angiotensin system can cause injury and death to the developing fetus. Discontinue as soon as possible once pregnancy is detected. Also see individual agents.

Olopatadine (Nasal) (oh la PAT a deen)

Brand Names: U.S. Patanase®
Pharmacologic Category Histamine H_1 Antagonist; Histamine H_1 Antagonist, Second Generation; Piperidine Derivative
Use Treatment of the symptoms of seasonal allergic rhinitis
Local Anesthetic/Vasoconstrictor Precautions No information available to require special precautions
Effects on Dental Treatment Key adverse event(s) related to dental treatment: Taste perversion.
Effects on Bleeding No information available to require special precautions
Adverse Effects
>10%:
Gastrointestinal: Bitter taste (13%; children 1%)
Respiratory: Epistaxis (3% to 25%)
1% to 10%:
Central nervous system: Depression (2%), fatigue (1%), somnolence (1%)
Dermatologic: Rash (children 1%)
Gastrointestinal: Weight gain (1%), xerostomia (1%)
Genitourinary: Urinary tract infection (1%)
Neuromuscular & skeletal: CPK increased (1%)
Respiratory: Nasal ulceration (9% to 10%), upper respiratory tract infection (children 3%), pharyngolaryngeal pain (2%), postnasal drip (2%), cough (1%), throat irritation (1%)
Miscellaneous: Influenza (1%)
General Dosage Range Intranasal:
Children 6-11 years: 1 spray into each nostril twice daily
Children ≥12 years, Adolescents, and Adults: 2 sprays into each nostril twice daily
Mechanism of Action Selective histamine H_1-antagonist; inhibits release of histamine from mast cells.
Pharmacodynamics/Kinetics
Onset of Action 30 minutes in seasonal allergy patients
Half-life Elimination 8-12 hours
Time to Peak Serum: 15 minutes to 2 hours
Pregnancy Risk Factor C
Pregnancy Considerations Adverse effects were observed in animal reproduction studies when using doses greater than the equivalent maximum recommended human dose.

Olopatadine (Ophthalmic) (oh la PAT a deen)

Brand Names: U.S. Pataday™; Patanol®
Brand Names: Canada Pataday™; Patanol®
Pharmacologic Category Histamine H_1 Antagonist; Histamine H_1 Antagonist, Second Generation; Piperidine Derivative
Use Treatment of the signs and symptoms of allergic conjunctivitis
Local Anesthetic/Vasoconstrictor Precautions No information available to require special precautions
Effects on Dental Treatment No significant effects or complications reported

◀ **Effects on Bleeding** No information available to require special precautions

Adverse Effects

>5%:
Central nervous system: Cold syndrome (up to 10%), headache (up to 7%)
Respiratory: Pharyngitis (up to 10%)

≤5%:
Gastrointestinal: Nausea, taste perversion
Neuromuscular & skeletal: Back pain, weakness
Ocular: Blurred vision, burning, conjunctivitis, dry eyes, eye pain, eyelid edema, foreign body sensation, hyperemia, keratitis, ocular pruritus, stinging
Respiratory: Cough, rhinitis, sinusitis
Miscellaneous: Flu-like syndrome, hypersensitivity, infection

General Dosage Range Ophthalmic:
Children ≥3 years, Adolescents, and Adults: Patanol®: Instill 1 drop into each affected eye twice daily
Children ≥2 years, Adolescents, and Adults: Pataday™: Instill 1 drop into each affected eye once daily

Mechanism of Action Selective histamine H₁-antagonist; inhibits release of histamine from mast cells. Inhibits histamine induced effects on conjunctival epithelial cells.

Pharmacodynamics/Kinetics
Half-life Elimination ~3 hours

Pregnancy Risk Factor C

Pregnancy Considerations Adverse effects were observed in animal reproduction studies when using doses greater than the equivalent maximum recommended ocular human dose.

Olsalazine (ole SAL a zeen)

Brand Names: U.S. Dipentum®
Brand Names: Canada Dipentum®
Pharmacologic Category 5-Aminosalicylic Acid Derivative

Use Maintenance of remission of ulcerative colitis in patients intolerant to sulfasalazine

Local Anesthetic/Vasoconstrictor Precautions No information available to require special precautions

Effects on Dental Treatment No significant effects or complications reported

Effects on Bleeding No information available to require special precautions

Adverse Effects
>10%: Gastrointestinal: Diarrhea (11% to 17%; dose related)
1% to 10%:
Central nervous system: Depression (2%), dizziness/vertigo (1%)
Dermatologic: Rash (2%), pruritus (1%)
Gastrointestinal: Abdominal pain/cramps (10%), nausea (5%), bloating (2%), stomatitis (1%), vomiting (1%)
Neuromuscular & skeletal: Arthralgia (4%)
Respiratory: Upper respiratory infection (2%)

General Dosage Range Oral: *Adults:* 1 g/day in 2 divided doses

Mechanism of Action Mesalamine (5-aminosalicylic acid) is the active component of olsalazine; the specific mechanism of action of mesalamine is unknown; however, it is thought that it modulates local chemical mediators of the inflammatory response, especially leukotrienes, and is also postulated to be a free radical scavenger or an inhibitor of tumor necrosis factor (TNF); action appears topical rather than systemic.

Pharmacodynamics/Kinetics
Half-life Elimination 54 minutes
Time to Peak ~1 hour
Pregnancy Risk Factor C
Pregnancy Considerations Animal studies have demonstrated fetal developmental toxicities. There are no well-controlled studies in pregnant women. Use during pregnancy only if clearly necessary.

Omacetaxine (oh ma se TAX een)

Brand Names: U.S. Synribo™
Pharmacologic Category Antineoplastic Agent, Cephalotaxine; Antineoplastic Agent, Protein Synthesis Inhibitor

Use Treatment of chronic or accelerated phase chronic myelogenous leukemia (CML) in patients resistant and/or intolerant to ≥2 tyrosine kinase inhibitors

Local Anesthetic/Vasoconstrictor Precautions Use vasoconstrictor with caution; patients may experience tachycardia and palpitations when taking omacetaxine

Effects on Dental Treatment Key adverse event(s) related to dental treatment: Abnormal taste, aphthous stomatitis, gingival bleeding, gingival pain, gingivitis, mouth ulceration, mouth hemorrhage, mucosal inflammation, oral pain, stomatitis, and xerostomia (normal salivary flow resumes upon discontinuation) have been reported.

Effects on Bleeding Chemotherapy may result in significant myelosuppression, potentially including significant reduction in platelet counts. Thrombocytopenia has been reported (grades 3/4: 49% to 88%). Gingival and GI bleeding have been reported. In patients who are under active treatment with these agents, medical consult is suggested.

Adverse Effects
>10%:
Cardiovascular: Peripheral edema (13%)
Central nervous system: Fatigue (26% to 31%), fever (24% to 29%), headache (13% to 19%), chills (13%)
Dermatologic: Alopecia (15%)
Endocrine & metabolic: Uric acid increased (grades 3/4: 56% to 57%), hyperglycemia (grades 3/4: 10% to 15%; hyperosmolar nonketotic hyperglycemia: <1%)
Gastrointestinal: Diarrhea (35% to 42%), nausea (27% to 32%), constipation (15%), vomiting (12% to 15%), abdominal pain (13% to 14%), anorexia (13%)
Hematologic: Thrombocytopenia (grades 3/4: 49% to 88%), neutropenia (grades 3/4: 18% to 81%), anemia (grades 3/4: 36% to 80%), leukocytes decreased (grades 3/4: 61% to 72%), neutropenic fever (10% to 20%; grades 3/4: 10% to 16%), lymphopenia (17%; grades 3/4: 16%)
Local: Injection site reactions (22% to 34%)
Neuromuscular & skeletal: Weakness (23% to 24%), arthralgia (19%), limb pain (11% to 13%), back pain (11%)
Renal: Creatinine increased (grades 3/4: 9% to 16%)
Respiratory: Cough (≤16%), epistaxis (11% to 15%), dyspnea (11%)
Miscellaneous: Infection (46% to 56%; grades 3/4: 11% to 20%)
1% to 10%:
Cardiovascular: Acute coronary syndrome, angina pectoris, arrhythmia, bradycardia, cerebral hemorrhage, chest pain, edema, hyper-/hypotension, palpitations, tachycardia, ventricular extrasystoles

Central nervous system: Insomnia (10%), anxiety, agitation, confusion, depression, dizziness, dysphonia, hyperthermia, hypoesthesia, lethargy, malaise, mental status change, pain, seizures

Dermatologic: Bruising, burning sensation, dry skin, erythema, hyperhidrosis, hyperpigmentation, petechiae, pruritus, purpura, rash, skin exfoliation, skin lesions, skin ulceration

Endocrine & metabolic: Glucose decreased (grades 3/4: 6% to 8%), dehydration, diabetes mellitus, gout, hot flashes

Gastrointestinal: Abdominal distension, abnormal taste, anal fissure, aphthous stomatitis, appetite decreased, dyspepsia, dysphagia, gastritis, gastroesophageal reflux disease, GI bleeding, gingival bleeding, gingival pain, gingivitis, hemorrhoids, melena, mouth ulceration, mouth hemorrhage, mucosal inflammation, oral pain, stomatitis, xerostomia

Genitourinary: Dysuria

Hematologic: Bone marrow failure (10%; grades 3/4: 10%), hematoma

Hepatic: Bilirubin increased (grades 3/4: 6% to 9%), ALT increased (grades 3/4: 2% to 6%)

Neuromuscular & skeletal: Bone pain, muscle spasms, muscle weakness, musculoskeletal chest pain, musculoskeletal discomfort, musculoskeletal pain myalgia, paresthesia, sciatica, stiffness, tremor

Ocular: Blurred vision, cataract, conjunctival hemorrhage, conjunctivitis, diplopia, dry eyes, eye pain, eyelid edema, lacrimation increased

Otic: Ear hemorrhage, ear pain, tinnitus

Respiratory: Hemoptysis, nasal congestion, pharyngolaryngeal pain, rales, rhinorrhea, sinus congestion

Miscellaneous: Flu-like syndrome, hypersensitivity reactions, night sweats, transfusion reaction

General Dosage Range SubQ: *Adults:* Induction: 1.25 mg/m^2 twice daily for 14 days of a 28-day treatment cycle; Maintenance: 1.25 mg/m^2 twice daily for 7 consecutive days of a 28-day treatment cycle

Mechanism of Action Omacetaxine is a reversible protein synthesis inhibitor which binds to the A-site cleft of the ribosomal subunit to interfere with chain elongation and inhibit protein synthesis. It acts independently of BCR-ABL1 kinase-binding activity, and has demonstrated activity against tyrosine kinase inhibitor-resistant BCR-ABL mutations.

Pharmacodynamics/Kinetics

Onset of Action
Chronic phase CML: Mean time to major cytogenetic response: 3.5 months
Accelerated phase CML: Mean time to response: 2.3 months

Duration of Action
Chronic phase CML: Median duration of major cytogenetic response: 12.5 months
Accelerated phase CML: Median duration of complete hematologic response: 4.7 months

Half-life Elimination ~6 hours

Time to Peak SubQ: ~30 minutes

Pregnancy Risk Factor D

Pregnancy Considerations Adverse events were observed in animal reproduction studies at doses less than the equivalent human dose (based on BSA). Based on the mechanism of action, omacetaxine may cause fetal harm if administered during pregnancy. Women of reproductive potential should avoid pregnancy during therapy.

Omalizumab (oh mah lye ZOO mab)

Related Information
Respiratory Diseases *on page 1514*
Brand Names: U.S. Xolair®
Brand Names: Canada Xolair®
Pharmacologic Category Monoclonal Antibody, Anti-Asthmatic
Use Treatment of moderate-to-severe, persistent allergic asthma in patients with a positive skin test or *in vitro* reactivity to a perennial aeroallergen and not adequately controlled with inhaled corticosteroids
Local Anesthetic/Vasoconstrictor Precautions No information available to require special precautions
Effects on Dental Treatment No significant effects or complications reported
Effects on Bleeding No information available to require special precautions
Adverse Effects
>10%: Local: Injection site reaction (45%; placebo 43%; severe 12%). Most reactions occurred within 1 hour, lasted <8 days, and decreased in frequency with additional dosing.
1% to 10%:
Central nervous system: Pain (7%), fatigue (3%), dizziness (3%)
Dermatologic: Dermatitis (2%), pruritus (2%)
Neuromuscular & skeletal: Arthralgia (8%), leg pain (4%), arm pain (2%), fracture (2%)
Otic: Earache (2%)
General Dosage Range SubQ:
Pretreatment serum IgE ≥30-100 units/mL:
Children ≥12 years and Adults 30-90 kg: 150 mg every 4 weeks
Children ≥12 years and Adults >90-150 kg: 300 mg every 4 weeks
Pretreatment serum IgE >100-200 units/mL:
Children ≥12 years and Adults 30-90 kg: 300 mg every 4 weeks
Children ≥12 years and Adults >90-150 kg: 225 mg every 2 weeks
Pretreatment serum IgE >200-300 units/mL:
Children ≥12 years and Adults 30-60 kg: 300 mg every 4 weeks
Children ≥12 years and Adults >60-90 kg: 225 mg every 2 weeks
Children ≥12 years and Adults >90-150 kg: 300 mg every 2 weeks
Pretreatment serum IgE >300-400 units/mL:
Children ≥12 years and Adults 30-70 kg: 225 mg every 2 weeks
Children ≥12 years and Adults >70-90 kg: 300 mg every 2 weeks
Children ≥12 years and Adults >90 kg: Do not administer dose
Pretreatment serum IgE >400-500 units/mL:
Children ≥12 years and Adults 30-70 kg: 300 mg every 2 weeks
Children ≥12 years and Adults >70-90 kg: 375 mg every 2 weeks
Children ≥12 years and Adults >90 kg: Do not administer dose
Pretreatment serum IgE >500-600 units/mL:
Children ≥12 years and Adults 30-60 kg: 300 mg every 2 weeks
Children ≥12 years and Adults >60-70 kg: 375 mg every 2 weeks
Children ≥12 years and Adults >70 kg: Do not administer dose

Pretreatment serum IgE >600-700 units/mL:

Children ≥12 years and Adults 30-60 kg: 375 mg every 2 weeks

Children ≥12 years and Adults >60 kg: Do not administer dose

Mechanism of Action Omalizumab is an IgG monoclonal antibody (recombinant DNA derived) which inhibits IgE binding to the high-affinity IgE receptor on mast cells and basophils. By decreasing bound IgE, the activation and release of mediators in the allergic response (early and late phase) is limited. Serum free IgE levels and the number of high-affinity IgE receptors are decreased. Long-term treatment in patients with allergic asthma showed a decrease in asthma exacerbations and corticosteroid usage.

Pharmacodynamics/Kinetics

Half-life Elimination 26 days (asthma patients)

Time to Peak 7-8 days

Pregnancy Risk Factor B

Pregnancy Considerations Teratogenic effects were not observed in animal studies. There are no adequate and well-controlled studies in pregnant women. IgG molecules are known to cross the placenta; use during pregnancy only if clearly needed. A registry has been established to monitor outcomes of women exposed to omalizumab during pregnancy or within 8 weeks prior to pregnancy (866-496-5247).

Omega-3-Acid Ethyl Esters
(oh MEG a three AS id ETH il ES ters)

Related Information

Cardiovascular Diseases *on page 1492*

Brand Names: U.S. Lovaza®

Pharmacologic Category Antilipemic Agent, Omega-3 Fatty Acids

Use Lovaza®: Adjunct to diet therapy in the treatment of hypertriglyceridemia (≥500 mg/dL)

Note: The Endocrine Society recommends that omega-3 fatty acids such as Lovaza® may be considered for triglyceride levels >1000 mg/dL and may be used alone or in combination with HMG-CoA reductase inhibitors (Berglund, 2012). A number of OTC formulations containing omega-3 fatty acids are marketed as nutritional supplements; these do not have FDA-approved indications and may not contain the same amounts of the active ingredient.

Unlabeled Use Lovaza®: Treatment of IgA nephropathy

Local Anesthetic/Vasoconstrictor Precautions No information available to require special precautions

Effects on Dental Treatment No significant effects or complications reported

Effects on Bleeding Prolongation of bleeding time has been observed in some clinical studies; however, there is no scientific evidence to warrant discontinuance prior to dental surgery. The clinician should anticipate the potential for slower clotting times.

Adverse Effects Frequency not always defined.

Dermatologic: Pruritis, rash

Gastrointestinal: Eructation (4%), taste perversion (4%), dyspepsia (3%), constipation, vomiting

Hepatic: ALT increased, AST increased

Dosage Oral: Adults:

Hypertriglyceridemia: 4 g/day as a single daily dose or in 2 divided doses

Treatment of IgA nephropathy (unlabeled use): 4 g/day (Donadio, 2001)

Dosage adjustment in renal impairment: No dosage adjustment provided in manufacturer's labeling (has not been studied).

Dosage adjustment in hepatic impairment: No dosage adjustment provided in manufacturer's labeling (has not been studied).

Mechanism of Action Mechanism has not been completely defined. Possible mechanisms include inhibition of acyl CoA:1,2 diacylglycerol acyltransferase, increased hepatic beta-oxidation, a reduction in the hepatic synthesis of triglycerides, or an increase in plasma lipoprotein lipase activity.

Contraindications Hypersensitivity (eg, anaphylactic reaction) to omega-3-acid ethyl esters or any component of the formulation

Warnings/Precautions Use with caution in patients with known allergy or sensitivity to fish and/or shellfish. Should be used as an adjunct to diet therapy and exercise and only in those with very high triglyceride levels (≥500 mg/dL). The Endocrine Society guidelines for the treatment of hypertriglyceridemia recommends that omega-3 fatty acids such as Lovaza® may be considered for triglyceride levels >1000 mg/dL and may be used alone or in combination with HMG-CoA reductase inhibitors (Berglund, 2012). Treatment of primary metabolic disorders (eg, diabetes, thyroid disease) and/or evaluation of the patient's medication regimen for possible etiologic agents should be completed prior to a decision to initiate therapy. Secondary causes of hyperlipidemia should be ruled out prior to therapy. If triglyceride levels do not adequately respond after 2 months of treatment with omega-3-acid ethyl esters, discontinue treatment. ALT may be increased without ALT increasing. May increase LDL levels; periodically monitor LDL levels. Prolongation of bleeding time has been observed in some clinical studies; use with caution in patients with coagulopathy or in those receiving therapeutic anticoagulation; monitor INR. Omega-3-acid ethyl esters are not indicated for the treatment of atrial fibrillation (AF) or flutter; recurrent AF or flutter may occur in patients with symptomatic paroxysmal or persistent AF treated with omega-3-acid ethyl esters; more frequent occurrences were observed with omega-3-acid ethyl esters in the first 2 to 3 months of therapy compared to placebo in clinical trials. However, the clinical significance of these results is uncertain.

Drug Interactions

Metabolism/Transport Effects None known.

Avoid Concomitant Use There are no known interactions where it is recommended to avoid concomitant use.

Increased Effect/Toxicity

Omega-3-Acid Ethyl Esters may increase the levels/ effects of: Agents with Antiplatelet Properties; Anticoagulants

Decreased Effect There are no known significant interactions involving a decrease in effect.

Ethanol/Nutrition/Herb Interactions

Ethanol: Monitor ethanol use (alcohol use may increase triglycerides).

Dietary Considerations May be taken with or without food. Dietary modification is important in the control of severe hypertriglyceridemia. Maintain standard cholesterol-lowering diet during therapy.

Pregnancy Risk Factor C

Pregnancy Considerations In some animal studies, embryocidal and maternal effects have been observed at high doses. There are no adequate or well-controlled studies in pregnant women. Use during pregnancy only if potential benefit outweighs possible risk.

Lactation Excretion in breast milk unknown/use caution

Dosage Forms
Capsule, liquid gel, oral:
Lovaza®: 1 g

Omeprazole (oh MEP ra zole)

Related Information
Esomeprazole on page 502
Gastrointestinal Disorders on page 1512

Brand Names: U.S. First®-Omeprazole; PriLOSEC OTC® [OTC]; PriLOSEC®

Brand Names: Canada Apo-Omeprazole®; Ava-Omeprazole; Dom-Omeprazole DR; Losec®; Mylan-Omeprazole; PMS-Omeprazole; PMS-Omeprazole DR; Q-Omeprazole; RAN™-Omeprazole; ratio-Omeprazole; Sandoz-Omeprazole; Teva-Omeprazole

Generic Availability (U.S.) Yes: Excludes granules for suspension

Pharmacologic Category Proton Pump Inhibitor; Substituted Benzimidazole

Use Short-term (4-8 weeks) treatment of active duodenal ulcer disease or active benign gastric ulcer; treatment of heartburn and other symptoms associated with gastroesophageal reflux disease (GERD); short-term (4-8 weeks) treatment of endoscopically-diagnosed erosive esophagitis; maintenance healing of erosive esophagitis; long-term treatment of pathological hypersecretory conditions (eg, Zollinger-Ellison syndrome); as part of a multidrug regimen for H. pylori eradication to reduce the risk of duodenal ulcer recurrence

OTC labeling: Short-term treatment of frequent, uncomplicated heartburn occurring ≥2 days/week

Unlabeled Use Healing NSAID-induced ulcers; prevention of NSAID-induced ulcer; stress-ulcer prophylaxis in the critically-ill

Local Anesthetic/Vasoconstrictor Precautions No information available to require special precautions

Effects on Dental Treatment Key adverse event(s) related to dental treatment: Taste perversion, dry mouth, esophageal candidiasis, and mucosal atrophy (tongue).

Effects on Bleeding No information available to require special precautions

Adverse Effects 1% to 10%:
Central nervous system: Headache (7%), dizziness (2%)
Dermatologic: Rash (2%)
Gastrointestinal: Abdominal pain (5%), diarrhea (4%), nausea (4%), vomiting (3%), flatulence (3%), acid regurgitation (2%), constipation (2%)
Neuromuscular & skeletal: Back pain (1%), weakness (1%)
Respiratory: Upper respiratory infection (2%), cough (1%)

Dosage Oral:
Children 1-16 years: GERD or other acid-related disorders:
5 kg to <10 kg: 5 mg once daily
10 kg to <20 kg: 10 mg once daily
≥20 kg: 20 mg once daily
Adults:
Active duodenal ulcer: 20 mg once daily for 4-8 weeks
Gastric ulcers: 40 mg once daily for 4-8 weeks

Symptomatic GERD (without esophageal lesions): 20 mg once daily for up to 4 weeks
Erosive esophagitis: 20 mg once daily for 4-8 weeks; maintenance of healing: 20 mg once daily for up to 12 months total therapy (including treatment period of 4-8 weeks)
Helicobacter pylori eradication: Dose varies with regimen:
Manufacturer labeling: 40 mg once daily administered with clarithromycin 500 mg 3 times daily for 14 days or 20 mg twice daily administered with amoxicillin 1000 mg and clarithromycin 500 mg twice daily for 10 days. **Note:** Presence of ulcer at time of therapy initiation may necessitate an additional 14-18 days of omeprazole 20 mg daily (monotherapy) after completion of combination therapy.
American College of Gastroenterology guidelines (Chey, 2007):
Nonpenicillin allergy: 20 mg twice daily administered with amoxicillin 1000 mg and clarithromycin 500 mg twice daily for 10-14 days
Penicillin allergy: 20 mg twice daily administered with clarithromycin 500 mg and metronidazole 500 mg twice daily for 10-14 days or 20 mg once or twice daily administered with bismuth subsalicylate 525 mg and metronidazole 250 mg plus tetracycline 500 mg 4 times daily for 10-14 days
Pathological hypersecretory conditions: Initial: 60 mg once daily; doses up to 120 mg 3 times daily have been administered; administer daily doses >80 mg in divided doses
NSAID-induced ulcer treatment (unlabeled use): 20 mg once daily for 4-8 weeks; Maintenance: 20 mg once daily for up to 6 months (Hawkey, 1998)
NSAID-induced ulcer prophylaxis (unlabeled use): 20 mg once daily for up to 6 months (Cullen, 1998)
Stress-ulcer prophylaxis (ICU patients; unlabeled use): 40 mg once daily; periodically evaluate patient for continued need (Levy, 1997)
Frequent heartburn (OTC labeling): 20 mg once daily for 14 days; treatment may be repeated after 4 months if needed

Dosage adjustment in hepatic impairment: No dosage adjustment provided in manufacturer's labeling. However, based on increased bioavailability, a dosage reduction should be considered, especially for maintenance of healing of erosive esophagitis.

Mechanism of Action Proton pump inhibitor; suppresses gastric basal and stimulated acid secretion by inhibiting the parietal cell H+/K+ ATP pump

Contraindications Hypersensitivity to omeprazole, other substituted benzimidazole proton pump inhibitors, or any component of the formulation

Warnings/Precautions Use of proton pump inhibitors (PPIs) may increase the risk of gastrointestinal infections (eg, Salmonella, Campylobacter). Relief of symptoms does not preclude the presence of a gastric malignancy. Atrophic gastritis (by biopsy) has been noted with long-term omeprazole therapy. In long-term (2-year) studies in rats, omeprazole produced a dose-related increase in gastric carcinoid tumors. While available endoscopic evaluations and histologic examinations of biopsy specimens from human stomachs have not detected a risk from short-term exposure to omeprazole, further human data on the effect of sustained hypochlorhydria and hypergastrinemia are needed to rule out the possibility of an increased risk for the development of tumors in humans receiving long-term therapy. Use of PPIs may increase risk of Clostridium difficile-associated diarrhea (CDAD), especially in hospitalized patients; consider CDAD diagnosis in patients with persistent diarrhea that does not improve. Use the lowest dose and shortest duration of PPI therapy appropriate for the condition being treated.

PPIs may diminish the therapeutic effect of clopidogrel, thought to be due to reduced formation of the active metabolite of clopidogrel. The manufacturer of clopidogrel recommends either avoidance both omeprazole (even when scheduled 12 hours apart) and esomeprazole or use of a PPI with comparatively less effect on the active metabolite of clopidogrel (eg, pantoprazole). In contrast to these warnings, others have recommended the continued use of PPIs, regardless of the degree of inhibition, in patients with a history of GI bleeding or multiple risk factors for GI bleeding who are also receiving clopidogrel since no evidence has established clinically meaningful differences in outcome; however, a clinically-significant interaction cannot be excluded in those who are poor metabolizers of clopidogrel (Abraham, 2010; Levine, 2011). Additionally, concomitant use of omeprazole with some drugs may require cautious use, may not be recommended, or may require dosage adjustments.

Increased incidence of osteoporosis-related bone fractures of the hip, spine, or wrist may occur with PPI therapy. Patients on high-dose (multiple daily doses) or long-term (≥1 year) therapy should be monitored. Use the lowest effective dose for the shortest duration of time, use vitamin D and calcium supplementation, and follow appropriate guidelines to reduce risk of fractures in patients at risk.

Hypomagnesemia, reported rarely, usually with prolonged PPI use of >3 months (most cases >1 year of therapy); may be symptomatic or asymptomatic; severe cases may cause tetany, seizures, and cardiac arrhythmias. Consider obtaining serum magnesium concentrations prior to beginning long-term therapy, especially if taking concomitant digoxin, diuretics, or other drugs known to cause hypomagnesemia; and periodically thereafter. Hypomagnesemia may be corrected by magnesium supplementation, although discontinuation of omeprazole may be necessary; magnesium levels typically return to normal within 1 week of stopping. Serum chromogranin A levels may be increased if assessed while patient on omeprazole; may lead to diagnostic errors related to neuroendocrine tumors.

Decreased *H. pylori* eradication rates have been observed with short-term (≤7 days) combination therapy. The American College of Gastroenterology recommends 10-14 days of therapy (triple or quadruple) for eradication of *H. pylori* (Chey, 2007). Bioavailability may be increased in Asian populations and patients with hepatic dysfunction; consider dosage reductions, especially for maintenance healing of erosive esophagitis. Bioavailability may be increased in the elderly. When used for self-medication (OTC), do not use for >14 days.

Drug Interactions
Metabolism/Transport Effects Substrate of CYP2A6 (minor), CYP2C19 (major), CYP2C9 (minor), CYP2D6 (minor), CYP3A4 (minor); **Note:** Assignment of Major/Minor substrate status based on clinically relevant drug interaction potential; **Inhibits** CYP1A2 (weak), CYP2C19 (moderate), CYP2C9 (moderate), CYP2D6 (weak), CYP3A4 (weak); **Induces** CYP1A2 (weak/moderate)

Avoid Concomitant Use
Avoid concomitant use of Omeprazole with any of the following: Clopidogrel; Dasatinib; Delavirdine; Erlotinib;

Nelfinavir; Pimozide; Ponatinib; Posaconazole; Rifampin; Rilpivirine; Risedronate; St Johns Wort

Increased Effect/Toxicity
Omeprazole may increase the levels/effects of: Amphetamines; ARIPiprazole; Benzodiazepines (metabolized by oxidation); Carvedilol; Cilostazol; Citalopram; CloZAPine; CycloSPORINE (Systemic); CYP2C19 Substrates; CYP2C9 Substrates; Dexmethylphenidate; Escitalopram; Fosphenytoin; Lomitapide; Methotrexate; Methylphenidate; Phenytoin; Pimozide; Raltegravir; Risedronate; Saquinavir; Tacrolimus (Systemic); Vitamin K Antagonists; Voriconazole

The levels/effects of Omeprazole may be increased by: Fluconazole; Ketoconazole (Systemic); Voriconazole

Decreased Effect
Omeprazole may decrease the levels/effects of: Atazanavir; Bisphosphonate Derivatives; Bosutinib; Cefditoren; Clopidogrel; CloZAPine; Dabigatran Etexilate; Dasatinib; Delavirdine; Erlotinib; Gefitinib; Indinavir; Iron Salts; Itraconazole; Ketoconazole (Systemic); Mesalamine; Multivitamins/Minerals (with ADEK, Folate, Iron); Mycophenolate; Nelfinavir; Nilotinib; Ponatinib; Posaconazole; Rilpivirine; Risedronate; Vismodegib

The levels/effects of Omeprazole may be decreased by: CYP2C19 Inducers (Strong); Peginterferon Alfa-2b; Rifampin; St Johns Wort; Tipranavir

Ethanol/Nutrition/Herb Interactions
Ethanol: Avoid ethanol (may cause gastric mucosal irritation).
Food: Food delays absorption.
Herb/Nutraceutical: Avoid use of St John's wort (may decrease efficacy of omeprazole).

Dietary Considerations
Should be taken on an empty stomach; best if taken before breakfast.

Pharmacodynamics/Kinetics
Onset of Action Antisecretory: ~1 hour; Peak effect: Within 2 hours
Duration of Action Up to 72 hours; 50% of maximum effect at 24 hours; after stopping treatment, secretory activity gradually returns over 3-5 days
Half-life Elimination 0.5-1 hour; hepatic impairment: ~3 hours
Time to Peak Plasma: 0.5-3.5 hours

Pregnancy Risk Factor C
Pregnancy Considerations Adverse events were observed in some animal reproduction studies. Based on data collected by the Teratogen Information System (TERIS), it was concluded that therapeutic doses used during pregnancy would be unlikely to pose a substantial teratogenic risk (quantity/quality of data: fair). Because the possibility of harm still exists, the manufacturer recommends use during pregnancy only if the potential benefit to the mother outweighs the possible risk to the fetus.

Lactation Enters breast milk/not recommended
Breast-Feeding Considerations Following administration of omeprazole 20 mg, peak concentrations detected in the breast milk were <7% of the maternal serum concentration.

Dosage Forms
Capsule, delayed release, oral: 10 mg, 20 mg, 40 mg
PriLOSEC®: 10 mg, 20 mg, 40 mg
Granules for suspension, delayed release, oral:
PriLOSEC®: 2.5 mg/packet (30s); 10 mg/packet (30s)

Powder for suspension, oral:
First®-Omeprazole: 2 mg/mL (90 mL, 150 mL, 300 mL)
Tablet, delayed release, oral: 20 mg
PriLOSEC OTC® [OTC]: 20 mg

Omeprazole and Sodium Bicarbonate
(oh MEP ra zole & SOW dee um bye KAR bun ate)

Related Information
Gastrointestinal Disorders *on page 1512*
Omeprazole *on page 1009*
Sodium Bicarbonate *on page 1244*
Brand Names: U.S. Zegerid OTC™ [OTC]; Zegerid®
Pharmacologic Category Proton Pump Inhibitor; Substituted Benzimidazole
Use Short-term (4-8 weeks) treatment of active duodenal ulcer or active benign gastric ulcer; treatment of heartburn and other symptoms associated with gastroesophageal reflux disease (GERD); short-term (4-8 weeks) treatment of endoscopically-diagnosed erosive esophagitis; maintenance healing of erosive esophagitis; reduction of risk of upper gastrointestinal bleeding in critically-ill patients

OTC labeling: Short-term (2 weeks) treatment of frequent (2 days/week), uncomplicated heartburn
Local Anesthetic/Vasoconstrictor Precautions No information available to require special precautions
Effects on Dental Treatment Key adverse event(s) related to dental treatment: Oral candidiasis.
Effects on Bleeding No information available to require special precautions
Adverse Effects
Percentages of adverse events reported from a controlled clinical trial of 359 critically-ill patients receiving the oral powder for suspension
>10%:
Central nervous system: Pyrexia (20%)
Endocrine & metabolic: Hypokalemia (12%), hyperglycemia (11%)
Respiratory: Nosocomial pneumonia (11%)
1% to 10%:
Cardiovascular: Hypotension (10%), hypertension (8%), atrial fibrillation (6%), ventricular tachycardia (5%), bradycardia (4%), tachycardia (3%), supraventricular tachycardia (3%), edema (3%)
Central nervous system: Hyperpyrexia (5%), agitation (3%)
Dermatological: Rash (6%), decubitus ulcer (3%)
Endocrine & metabolic: Hypomagnesemia (10%), hypocalcemia (6%), hypophosphatemia (6%), fluid overload (5%), hypoglycemia (3%), hyponatremia (4%), hypernatremia (2%), hyperkalemia (2%)
Gastrointestinal: Constipation (5%), diarrhea (4%), hypomotility (2%)
Genitourinary: Urinary tract infection (2%)
Hematological: Thrombocytopenia (10%), anemia (8%), anemia increased (2%)
Hepatic: LFTs increased (2%)
Respiratory: ARDS (3%), respiratory failure (2%), pneumothorax (1%)
Miscellaneous: Sepsis (5%), oral candidiasis (4%), candidal infection (2%)
General Dosage Range Oral: *Adults:* 20-40 mg/day in 1-2 divided doses
Mechanism of Action Suppresses gastric basal and stimulated acid secretion by inhibiting the parietal cell H+/K+ ATP pump

Pharmacodynamics/Kinetics
Onset of Action Antisecretory: ~1 hour; Peak antisecretory effect: 2 hours; Full therapeutic effect: 1-4 days
Duration of Action 72 hours
Half-life Elimination ~1 hour (range: 0.4-3.2 hours); Hepatic dysfunction: ~3 hours
Time to Peak Serum: ~30 minutes
Pregnancy Risk Factor C
Pregnancy Considerations Adverse events were observed in some animal reproduction studies with omeprazole. Based on data collected by the Teratogen Information System (TERIS), it was concluded that therapeutic doses used during pregnancy would be unlikely to pose a substantial teratogenic risk (quantity/ quality of data: fair). Because the possibility of harm still exists, the manufacturer recommends use during pregnancy only if the potential benefit to the mother outweighs the possible risk to the fetus. Chronic use of sodium bicarbonate-containing products may lead to systemic alkalosis, edema, and weight gain; metabolic alkalosis and fluid overload may occur in mother and fetus.

Omeprazole, Clarithromycin, and Amoxicillin
(oh MEP ra zole, kla RITH roe mye sin, & a moks i SIL in)

Brand Names: U.S. Omeclamox-Pak®
Pharmacologic Category Antibiotic, Macrolide Combination; Antibiotic, Penicillin; Gastrointestinal Agent, Miscellaneous; Proton Pump Inhibitor; Substituted Benzimidazole
Use Eradication of *H. pylori* infection in patients with duodenal ulcer disease (active or a history of up to 1 year)
Local Anesthetic/Vasoconstrictor Precautions Clarithromycin is one of the drugs confirmed to prolong the QT interval and is accepted as having a risk of causing torsade de pointes. In terms of epinephrine, it is not known what effect vasoconstrictors in the local anesthetic regimen will have in patients with a known history of congenital prolonged QT interval or in patients taking any medication that prolongs the QT interval. Until more information is obtained, it is suggested that the clinician consult with the physician prior to the use of a vasoconstrictor in suspected patients, and that the vasoconstrictor (epinephrine, mepivacaine and levonordefrin [Carbocaine® 2% with Neo-Cobefrin®]) be used with caution. See Dental Comment.
Effects on Dental Treatment No significant effects or complications reported
Effects on Bleeding No information available to require special precautions
Adverse Effects Note: Frequencies noted refer to experience with combination therapy. Also see individual agents.
>10%: Gastrointestinal: Diarrhea (14%)
1% to 10%:
Central nervous system: Headache (7%)
Gastrointestinal: Abnormal taste (10%)
General Dosage Range Oral: *Adults:* Omeprazole 20 mg, clarithromycin 500 mg, and amoxicillin 1000 mg twice daily ▶

Mechanism of Action Triple therapy with amoxicillin, clarithromycin, and omeprazole has demonstrated *in vitro* activity against most susceptible strains of *H. pylori*. Omeprazole, a proton pump inhibitor, suppresses gastric acid secretion via inhibition of the parietal cell H+/K+ ATP pump; clarithromycin, an antibacterial agent, binds to the 50s ribosomal subunit of susceptible microorganisms resulting in inhibition of protein synthesis; amoxicillin, an antibacterial agent, inhibits bacterial cell wall synthesis.

Pregnancy Risk Factor C

Pregnancy Considerations Adverse events were observed in animal reproduction studies using clarithromycin or omeprazole. Refer to individual monographs for additional information.

Dental Comment Clarithromycin is known to prolong the QT interval. The QT interval is measured as the time and distance between the Q point of the QRS complex and the end of the T wave in the ECG tracing. After adjustment for heart rate, the QT interval is defined as prolonged if it is more than 450 msec in men and 460 msec in women. A long QT syndrome was first described in the 1950s and 60s as a congenital syndrome involving QT interval prolongation and syncope and sudden death. Some of the congenital long QT syndromes were characterized by a peculiar electrocardiographic appearance of the QRS complex involving a premature atria beat followed by a pause, then a subsequent sinus beat showing marked QT prolongation and deformity. This type of cardiac arrhythmia was originally termed "torsade de pointes" (translated from the French as "twisting of the points"). Clarithromycin is considered as having a risk of causing torsade de pointes. Since it is not known what effect vasoconstrictors in the local anesthetic regimen will have in patients with a known history of congenital prolonged QT interval or in patients taking any medication that prolongs the QT interval, a medical consult is suggested.

OnabotulinumtoxinA
(oh nuh BOT yoo lin num TOKS in aye)

Brand Names: U.S. Botox®; Botox® Cosmetic

Brand Names: Canada Botox®; Botox® Cosmetic

Generic Availability (U.S.) No

Pharmacologic Category Neuromuscular Blocker Agent, Toxin; Ophthalmic Agent, Toxin

Use Treatment of strabismus and blepharospasm associated with dystonia (including benign essential blepharospasm or VII nerve disorders) in patients ≥12 years of age; treatment of cervical dystonia (spasmodic torticollis) in patients ≥16 years of age; temporary improvement in the appearance of lines/wrinkles of the face (moderate-to-severe glabellar lines associated with corrugator and/or procerus muscle activity) in adult patients ≤65 years of age; treatment of severe primary axillary hyperhidrosis in adults not adequately controlled with topical treatments; treatment of focal spasticity (specifically upper limb spasticity) in adults; prophylaxis of chronic migraine headache (≥15 days/month with ≥4 hours/day headache duration) in adults; treatment of urinary incontinence due to detrusor overactivity associated with neurologic conditions in adults; treatment of overactive bladder (with symptoms of urge urinary incontinence, urgency, and frequency) in adults with an inadequate response or intolerance to anticholinergic medication.

Canadian labeling: Additional use (not in U.S. labeling): Dynamic equinus foot deformity in pediatric cerebral palsy patients; treatment of forehead, lateral canthus, and glabellar lines in adults >65 years of age

Unlabeled Use Treatment of oromandibular dystonia, spasmodic dysphonia (laryngeal dystonia) and other dystonias (ie, writer's cramp, focal task-specific dystonias); treatment of dynamic muscle contracture in pediatric cerebral palsy patients

Local Anesthetic/Vasoconstrictor Precautions No information available to require special precautions

Effects on Dental Treatment Key adverse event(s) related to dental treatment: Xerostomia (normal salivary flow resumes upon discontinuation), facial pain, and facial weakness. Effects occur in ~1 week and may last up to several months

Effects on Bleeding No information available to require special precautions

Adverse Effects Adverse effects usually occur in 1 week and may last up to several months

>10%:
Bladder dysfunction:
Genitourinary: Urinary tract infection (18% to 49%), urinary retention (17%)
Cervical dystonia:
Central nervous system: Pain (32%), headache (≤11%)
Gastrointestinal: Dysphagia (19%)
Neuromuscular & skeletal: Focal weakness (17%), neck pain (11%)
Respiratory: Upper respiratory infection (12%)
Other indications (blepharospasm, primary axillary hyperhidrosis, strabismus):
Ocular: Ptosis (blepharospasm 21%; strabismus 1% to 38%), vertical deviation (strabismus 17%)

1% to 10%:
Bladder dysfunction:
Gastrointestinal: Constipation (4%)
Genitourinary: Dysuria (4% to 9%), urinary retention (6%), bacteriuria (4%), hematuria (4%), residual urine volume increased (not requiring catheterization: 3%)
Neuromuscular & skeletal: Muscular weakness (4%), gait disturbance (3%), muscle spasm (2%)
Cervical dystonia:
Central nervous system: Dizziness, drowsiness, fever, malaise, speech disorder
Gastrointestinal: Nausea, xerostomia
Local: Injection site reaction: Soreness
Neuromuscular & skeletal: Back pain, hypertonia, numbness, stiffness, weakness
Ocular: Diplopia, ptosis
Respiratory: Cough, dyspnea, rhinitis
Miscellaneous: Flu-like syndrome
Cerebral palsy spasticity:
Central nervous system: Pain (1% to 2%), fever (1%), lethargy (1%)
Neuromuscular & skeletal: Falling, weakness
Chronic migraines:
Cardiovascular: Hypertension (2%)
Central nervous system: Headache (5%), worsening migraine (4%), facial paresis (2%)
Neuromuscular & skeletal: Neck pain (9%), stiffness (4%), weakness (4%), myalgia (3%), musculoskeletal pain (3%), muscle spasm (2%)
Ocular: Eyelid ptosis (4%)
Respiratory: Bronchitis (3%)
Miscellaneous: Injection site pain (3%)

Focal spasticity:
Central nervous system: Fatigue
Gastrointestinal: Nausea
Neuromuscular & skeletal: Pain in extremity, weakness
Respiratory: Bronchitis
Other indications (blepharospasm, primary axillary hyperhidrosis, reduction of glabellar lines, strabismus):
Cardiovascular: Hypertension
Central nervous system: Anxiety, dizziness, fever, headache, pain
Dermatologic: Pruritus, rash, skin tightness
Gastrointestinal: Dyspepsia, nausea
Local: Injection site reaction: Hemorrhage, pain, soreness
Neuromuscular & skeletal: Back pain, facial pain, neck pain, weakness
Ocular: Diplopia, irritation/tearing (includes dry eye, lagophthalmos, photophobia); keratitis, ptosis, superficial punctate keratitis
Respiratory: Pharyngitis
Miscellaneous: Flu-like syndrome, infection, nonaxillary sweating

Dosage Note: The lowest recommended dose should be used when initiating treatment (regardless of indication). In adults treated for more than one indication, the maximum cumulative dose should be ≤360 units/3 months. Canadian labeling recommends a maximum cumulative dose of 6 units/kg (adults up to 360 units; children up to 200 units) over 3 months in patients receiving additional treatment for noncosmetic indications.

Bladder dysfunction: Adults: Intradetrusor: **Note:** Prophylactic antimicrobial therapy (excluding aminoglycosides) should be administered 1-3 days prior to, on the day of, and for 1-3 days following onabotulinumtoxinA administration to decrease risk of UTI.
Detrusor overactivity associated with neurologic condition: 30 injections of 1 mL (recommended concentration: ~6.7 units/mL) for a total dose of 200 units/30 mL (maximum: 200 units); for the final injection, ~1 mL of sterile NS should be injected to ensure that the remaining medication in the needle is delivered to the bladder; may consider retreatment with diminishing effect but no sooner than 12 weeks from previous administration (median time until second treatment in studies: 42-48 weeks).
Overactive bladder: 20 injections of 0.5 mL (recommended concentration: 10 units/mL) for a total dose of 100 units/10 mL (maximum: 100 units); for the final injection, ~1 mL of sterile NS should be injected to ensure that the remaining medication in the needle is delivered to the bladder; may consider retreatment with diminishing effect but no sooner than 12 weeks from the previous administration (median time until second treatment in studies: ~24 weeks)

Blepharospasm:
Botox®: Children ≥12 years and Adults: I.M.: Initial dose: 1.25-2.5 units injected into the medial and lateral pretarsal orbicularis oculi of the upper lid and lateral pretarsal orbicularis oculi of lower lid
Dose may be increased up to twice the previous dose if the response from the initial dose lasted ≤2 months; maximum dose per site: 5 units. Tolerance may occur if treatments are given more often than every 3 months, but the effect is not usually permanent.
Cumulative dose:
U.S. labeling: ≤200 units in 30-day period
Canadian labeling (not in U.S. labeling): Botox®: ≤200 units in 2-month period

Cervical dystonia:
Children ≥16 years and Adults: I.M.: For dosing guidance, the mean dose is 236 units (25th to 75th percentile range 198-300 units) divided among the affected muscles in patients previously treated with botulinum toxin (maximum: ≤50 units/site). Initial dose in previously untreated patients should be lower. Sequential dosing should be based on the patient's head and neck position, localization of pain, muscle hypertrophy, patient response, and previous adverse reactions. The total dose injected into the sternocleidomastoid muscles should be ≤100 units to decrease the occurrence of dysphagia.
Canadian labeling (not in U.S. labeling): Botox®: Children ≥16 years and Adults: I.M.: Effective range of 200-360 units has been used in clinical practice; administer no more frequently than every 2 months
Chronic migraine: Adults: I.M.: Administer 5 units/0.1 mL per site. Recommended total dose is 155 units once every 12 weeks. Each 155 unit dose should be equally divided and administered bilaterally, into 31 total sites as described below (refer to prescribing information for specific diagrams of recommended injection sites):
Corrugator: 5 units to each side (2 sites)
Procerus: 5 units (1 site only)
Frontalis: 10 units to each side (divided into 2 sites/side)
Temporalis: 20 units to each side (divided into 4 sites/side)
Occipitalis: 15 units to each side (divided into 3 sites/side)
Cervical paraspinal: 10 units to each side (divided into 2 sites/side)
Trapezius: 15 units to each side (divided into 3 sites/side)
Strabismus: Children ≥12 years and Adults: I.M.: **Note:** Several minutes prior to injection, administration of local anesthetic and ocular decongestant drops are recommended.
Initial dose:
Vertical muscles and for horizontal strabismus <20 prism diopters: 1.25-2.5 units in any one muscle
Horizontal strabismus of 20-50 prism diopters: 2.5-5 units in any one muscle
Persistent VI nerve palsy ≥1 month: 1.25-2.5 units in the medial rectus muscle
Re-examine patients 7-14 days after each injection to assess the effect of that dose. Subsequent doses for patients experiencing incomplete paralysis of the target may be increased up to twice the previous administered dose. The maximum recommended dose as a single injection for any one muscle is 25 units. Do not administer subsequent injections until the effects of the previous dose are gone.
Primary axillary hyperhidrosis: Adults ≥18 years: Intradermal: 50 units/axilla. Injection area should be defined by standard staining techniques. Injections should be evenly distributed into multiple sites (10-15), administered in 0.1-0.2 mL aliquots, ~1-2 cm apart. May repeat when clinical effect diminishes.
Spasticity (cerebral palsy related [dynamic equinus foot deformity]): Canadian labeling [not approved in U.S. labeling]: Children ≥2 years: I.M.: 4 units/kg (total dose) divided into two injections into medial and lateral heads of the gastrocnemius of affected leg; if clinically indicated, may repeat every 2 months (maximum dose: 200 units); in diplegia, the recommended dose is 6 units/kg (total dose) divided between affected limbs

◄ **Spasticity (focal):** Adults ≥18 years: I.M.: Individualize dose based on patient size, extent, and location of muscle involvement, degree of spasticity, local muscle weakness, and response to prior treatment. In clinical trials, total doses up to 360 units (Botox®) were administered as separate injections typically divided among selected muscles; may repeat therapy at ≥3 months with appropriate dosage based upon the clinical condition of patient at time of retreatment.

Suggested guidelines for the treatment of upper limb spasticity. The lowest recommended starting dose should be used and ≤50 units/site should be administered. **Note:** Dose listed is total dose administered as individual or separate intramuscular injection(s):

Biceps brachii: 100-200 units (divided into 4 sites)
Flexor digitorum profundus: 30-50 units (1 site)
Flexor digitorum sublimes: 30-50 units (1 site)
Flexor carpi radialis: 12.5-50 units (1 site)
Flexor carpi ulnaris: 12.5-50 units (1 site)

Suggested guidelines for the treatment of stroke-related upper limb spasticity: Canadian labeling: **Note:** Dose listed is total dose administered as individual or separate intramuscular injection(s):

Biceps brachii: 100-200 units (up to 4 sites)
Flexor digitorum profundus: 15-50 units (1-2 sites)
Flexor digitorum sublimes: 15-50 units (1-2 sites)
Flexor carpi radialis: 15-60 units (1-2 sites)
Flexor carpi ulnaris: 10-50 units (1-2 sites)
Adductor pollicis: 20 units (1-2 sites)
Flexor pollicis longus: 20 units (1-2 sites)

Cosmetic uses:

Reduction of glabellar lines: Adults ≤65 years: I.M.: An effective dose is determined by gross observation of the patient's ability to activate the superficial muscles injected. The location, size and use of muscles may vary markedly among individuals. Inject 0.1 mL (4 units) dose into each of five sites, two in each corrugator muscle and one in the procerus muscle for a total dose 0.5 mL (20 units) administered no more frequently than every 3-4 months. **Note:** Treatment of adults >65 years is approved in the Canadian labeling.

Reduction of forehead lines (Canadian labeling; not in U.S. labeling): Adults: I.M.: Inject 2-6 units into each of four sites in the frontalis muscle every 1-2 cm along either side of forehead crease and 2-3 cm above eyebrows for total dose of 24 units.

Reduction of lateral canthus lines (Canadian labeling; not in U.S. labeling): Adults: I.M.: Inject 2-6 units into each of 1-3 injection sites, lateral to the lateral orbital rim.

Elderly: No specific adjustment recommended; initiate therapy at lowest recommended dose

Mechanism of Action OnabotulinumtoxinA (previously known as botulinum toxin type A) is a neurotoxin produced by *Clostridium botulinum*, spore-forming anaerobic bacillus, which appears to affect only the presynaptic membrane of the neuromuscular junction in humans, where it prevents calcium-dependent release of acetylcholine and produces a state of denervation. Muscle inactivation persists until new fibrils grow from the nerve and form junction plates on new areas of the muscle-cell walls. Intradetrusor injection affects efferent pathways of detrusor activity by inhibiting release of acetylcholine. Intradermal injection results in temporary sweat gland denervation, reducing local sweating.

Contraindications Hypersensitivity to botulinum toxin, or any component of the formulation; infection at the proposed injection site(s); intradetrusor injection in patients with a urinary tract infection; intradetrusor injection in patients with urinary retention and in patients with post-void residual (PVR) urine volume >200 mL who are not routinely performing clean intermittent self-catheterization

Warnings/Precautions [U.S. Boxed Warning]: Distant spread of botulinum toxin beyond the site of injection has been reported; dysphagia and breathing difficulties have occurred and may be life threatening; other symptoms reported include blurred vision, diplopia, dysarthria, dysphonia, generalized muscle weakness, ptosis, and urinary incontinence which may develop within hours or weeks following injection. The risk is likely greatest in children treated for the unapproved use of spasticity. Systemic effects have occurred following use in approved and unapproved uses, including low doses. Immediate medical attention required if respiratory, speech, or swallowing difficulties appear. Higher doses or more frequent administration may result in neutralizing antibody formation and loss of efficacy. Use caution in patients with bleeding disorders and/or receiving anticoagulation therapy. May impair ability to drive and/or operate machinery; if loss of strength, muscle weakness, or impaired vision occurs, patients should avoid driving or engaging in other hazardous activities.

Product contains albumin and may carry a remote risk of virus transmission. Use caution if there is excessive weakness or atrophy at the proposed injection site(s); use is contraindicated if infection is present at injection site. Serious events (including fatalities) have been observed with direct injection into the esophagus, stomach, salivary glands and oro-lingual-pharyngeal region. Use caution when administering in close proximity to the lungs; pneumothorax has been reported following administration near the thorax. Have appropriate support in case of anaphylactic reaction. Use with caution in patients with neuromuscular diseases (such as myasthenia gravis or Lambert-Eaton syndrome), neuropathic disorders (such as amyotrophic lateral sclerosis), patients taking aminoglycosides, neuromuscular-blocking agents, or other drugs that interfere with neuromuscular transmission and patients with pre-existing cardiovascular disease (rare reports of arrhythmia and MI). Long-term effects of chronic therapy are unknown. Botulinum products (abobotulinumtoxinA, onabotulinumtoxinA, rimabotulinumtoxinB) are not interchangeable; potency units are specific to each preparation and cannot be compared or converted to any other botulinum product.

Cervical dystonia: Dysphagia is common. It may be severe requiring alternative feeding methods and may persist anywhere from 2 weeks up to 5 months after administration. Risk factors include smaller neck muscle mass, bilateral injections into the sternocleidomastoid muscle, or injections into the levator scapulae. Use extreme caution in patients with pre-existing respiratory disease; may weaken accessory muscles that are necessary for these patients to maintain adequate ventilation. Risk of aspiration resulting from severe dysphagia is increased in patients with decreased respiratory function.

Bladder dysfunction (overactive bladder or detrusor overactivity associated with a neurologic condition): Rule out acute urinary tract infection (UTI) prior to treatment; appropriate prophylactic antimicrobial therapy is required prior to, during, and following treatment. Discontinue antiplatelet therapy at least 3 days prior to administration. An increased incidence of urinary retention and need for catheterization has been observed in patients receiving therapy for bladder dysfunction; due to the risk of urinary retention, treatment should only be used in patients able and willing to initiate post-treatment catheterization, if required. Therapy in patients with overactive bladder increases the incidence of urinary tract infections; clinical trials for overactive bladder excluded patients with >2 UTIs in the previous 6 months and those taking chronic antibiotics for prophylaxis of recurrent UTIs. Consider risks vs. benefits when contemplating use in these patients or patients experiencing recurrent UTIs during treatment. Patients with diabetes had an increased incidence of urinary retention and urinary tract infection. Patients experiencing difficulty in voiding should be instructed to consult their healthcare provider. Autonomic dysreflexia has been observed with therapy in patients with detrusor overactivity associated with a neurologic condition; acts as stimuli to trigger an exaggerated sympathetic and parasympathetic response. Clinical presentation often includes headache, a marked increase in blood pressure, and diaphoresis; prompt treatment may be required in patients presenting with severe symptoms (eg, hypertensive crisis).

Episodic migraines: Safety and efficacy have not been established in patients with 14 or fewer headaches per month.

Ocular disease: Blepharospasm: Reduced blinking from injection of the orbicularis muscle can lead to corneal exposure and ulceration. Strabismus: Retrobulbar hemorrhages may occur from needle penetration into orbit. Spatial disorientation, double vision, or past-pointing may occur if one or more extraocular muscles are paralyzed. Covering the affected eye may help. Careful testing of corneal sensation, avoidance of lower lid injections, and treatment of epithelial defects are necessary. Use with caution in angle closure glaucoma.

Primary axillary hyperhidrosis: Evaluate for secondary causes prior to treatment (eg, hyperthyroidism). Safety and efficacy for treatment of hyperhidrosis in other areas of the body have not been established.

Temporary reduction in glabellar lines: Do not use more frequently than every 3 months (Canadian labeling states not to use more frequently than every 2 months). Patients with marked facial asymmetry, ptosis, excessive dermatochalasis, deep dermal scarring, thick sebaceous skin, or the inability to substantially lessen glabellar lines by physically spreading them apart were excluded from clinical trials. Use with caution in patients with surgical alterations to the facial anatomy. Reduced blinking from injection of the orbicularis muscle can lead to corneal exposure and ulceration. Spatial disorientation, double vision, or past pointing may occur if one or more extraocular muscles are paralyzed.

Drug Interactions

Metabolism/Transport Effects None known.

Avoid Concomitant Use There are no known interactions where it is recommended to avoid concomitant use.

Increased Effect/Toxicity

OnabotulinumtoxinA may increase the levels/effects of: AbobotulinumtoxinA; RimabotulinumtoxinB

The levels/effects of OnabotulinumtoxinA may be increased by: Aminoglycosides; Anticholinergic Agents; Neuromuscular-Blocking Agents

Decreased Effect There are no known significant interactions involving a decrease in effect.

Pharmacodynamics/Kinetics

Onset of Action Blepharospasm: ~3-4 days; Cervical dystonia: ~2 weeks; Detrusor overactivity associated with neurologic condition: ~2 weeks; Reduction of glabellar lines (Botox® Cosmetic): 1-2 days, increasing in intensity during first week; Spasticity: Focal and cerebral palsy related: <2 weeks; Strabismus: ~1-2 days

Duration of Action Blepharospasm: ~3-4 months; Cervical dystonia: ≤3-4 months; Detrusor overactivity associated with neurologic condition: ~42-48 weeks; Reduction of glabellar lines (Botox® Cosmetic): ~3-4 months; Spasticity: ~3-3.5 months; Strabismus: ~2-6 weeks; Primary axillary hyperhidrosis: 201 days (mean)

Time to Peak Blepharospasm: 1-2 weeks; Cervical dystonia: ~6 weeks; Spasticity (focal): 4-6 weeks; Strabismus: Within first week

Pregnancy Risk Factor C

Pregnancy Considerations Decreased fetal body weight, delayed ossification, maternal toxicity, abortions, and fetal malformations were observed in animal studies. Human reproduction studies have not been conducted. Avoid use in pregnancy. Based on limited case reports, adverse fetal effects have not been observed with inadvertent administration during pregnancy. It is currently recommended to ensure adequate contraception in women of childbearing potential.

Lactation Excretion in breast milk unknown/use caution

Dosage Forms

Injection, powder for reconstitution [preservative free]:

Botox®: *Clostridium botulinum* type A neurotoxin complex 100 units, *Clostridium botulinum* type A neurotoxin complex 200 units

Botox® Cosmetic: *Clostridium botulinum* type A neurotoxin complex 100 units, *Clostridium botulinum* type A neurotoxin complex 50 units

Dosage Forms: Canada

Injection, powder for reconstitution [preservative free]:

Botox®: Botulinum toxin A 50 units, 100 units, 200 units

Botox Cosmetic®: Botulinum toxin A 50 unit, 100 units, 200 units

Dental Comment Cote and associates, published a paper describing all serious adverse reactions reported to the FDA (Cote, 2005). Included in the 217 serious effects reported, there were 28 deaths and 17 seizures. The deaths were attributed to heart attacks, cerebrovascular accident, pulmonary embolisms, pneumonia, or unknown causes. There were 1031 adverse effects reported after cosmetic use, 36 were of a serious nature. These included focal facial paralysis, muscle weakness, dysphagia, flu-like symptoms, and allergic reactions.

In contrast to the Cote study, the Naumann study reviewed the adverse reactions described and reported in randomized, controlled trials of onabotulinumtoxinA. They reviewed 36 studies involving 2309 subjects through the years 1966-2003. Of the 2309 subjects, 1425 received onabotulinumtoxinA treatment. No study reported severe adverse events. The only adverse event occurring significantly more often than with placebo was focal weakness.

References

Batra RS, Dover JS, and Arndt KA, "Adverse Event Reporting for Botulinum Toxin Type A," *J Am Acad Dermatol*, 2005, 53(6):1080-2.

Coté TR, Mohan AK, Polder JA, et al, "Botulinum Toxin Type A Injections: Adverse Events Reported to the U.S. Food and Drug Administration in Therapeutic and Cosmetic Cases," *J Am Acad Dermatol*, 2005, 53(3):407-15.

Naumann M and Jankovic J, "Safety of Botulinum Toxin Type A: A Systematic Review and Meta-Analysis," *Curr Med Res Opin*, 2004, 20(7):981-90.

Ondansetron (on DAN se tron)

Related Information

Clinical Risk Related to Drugs Prolonging QT Interval *on page 1510*

Brand Names: U.S. Zofran®; Zofran® ODT; Zuplenz®

Brand Names: Canada Apo-Ondansetron®; CO Ondansetron; Dom-Ondansetron; JAMP-Ondansetron; Mint-Ondansetron; Mylan-Ondansetron; Ondansetron Injection; Ondansetron Injection USP; Ondansetron-Odan; Ondansetron-Omega; PHL-Ondansetron; PMS-Ondansetron; RAN™-Ondansetron; ratio-Ondansetron; Sandoz-Ondansetron; Teva-Ondansetron; Zofran®; Zofran® ODT; ZYM-Ondansetron

Pharmacologic Category Antiemetic; Selective 5-HT$_3$ Receptor Antagonist

Use

I.V.: Prevention of nausea and vomiting associated with initial and repeat courses of emetogenic cancer chemotherapy (including high-dose cisplatin); prevention of postoperative nausea and/or vomiting (PONV); treatment of PONV if no prophylactic dose of ondansetron received

Oral: Prevention of nausea and vomiting associated with highly emetogenic cancer chemotherapy (including high-dose cisplatin); prevention of nausea and vomiting associated with initial and repeat courses of moderately emetogenic cancer chemotherapy; prevention of nausea and vomiting associated with radiotherapy (either total body irradiation, single high-dose fraction to the abdomen, or daily fractions to the abdomen); prevention of PONV

Unlabeled Use Hyperemesis gravidarum (severe or refractory); breakthrough treatment of nausea and vomiting associated with chemotherapy

Local Anesthetic/Vasoconstrictor Precautions Ondansetron is one of the drugs confirmed to prolong the QT interval and is accepted as having a risk of causing torsade de pointes. The risk of drug-induced torsade de pointes is extremely low when a single QT interval prolonging drug is prescribed. In terms of epinephrine, it is not known what effect vasoconstrictors in the local anesthetic regimen will have in patients with a known history of congenital prolonged QT interval or in patients taking any medication that prolongs the QT interval. Until more information is obtained, it is suggested that the clinician consult with the physician prior to the use of a vasoconstrictor in suspected patients, and that the vasoconstrictor (epinephrine, mepivacaine and levonordefrin [Carbocaine® 2% with Neo-Cobefrin®]) be used with caution.

Effects on Dental Treatment Ondansetron is an alternative to phenothiazines (ie, promethazine) for the treatment of moderate-to-severe postoperative nausea and vomiting. Ondansetron prolongs the QT interval in a dose-dependent manner. Avoid ondansetron in patients with congenital long QT syndrome.

Effects on Bleeding No information available to require special precautions

Adverse Effects Note: Percentages reported in adult patients.

>10%:

Central nervous system: Headache (9% to 27%), malaise/fatigue (9% to 13%)

Gastrointestinal: Constipation (6% to 11%)

1% to 10%:

Central nervous system: Drowsiness (8%), fever (2% to 8%), dizziness (7%), anxiety (6%), cold sensation (2%)

Dermatologic: Pruritus (2% to 5%), rash (1%)

Gastrointestinal: Diarrhea (2% to 7%)

Genitourinary: Gynecological disorder (7%), urinary retention (5%)

Hepatic: ALT increased (>2 times ULN: 1% to 5%), AST increased (>2 times ULN: 1% to 5%)

Local: Injection site reaction (4%; pain, redness, burning)

Neuromuscular & skeletal: Paresthesia (2%)

Respiratory: Hypoxia (9%)

General Dosage Range Dosage adjustment recommended in patients with hepatic impairment

I.M.: *Adults:* 4 mg as a single dose

I.V.:

Infants 1-6 months: 0.1 mg/kg as a single dose

Children 6 months to 12 years and ≤40 kg: 0.1 mg/kg as a single dose **or** 0.15 mg/kg/dose (maximum: 16 mg/dose) for 3 doses

Children 6 months to 12 years and >40 kg and Children >12 years to 18 years: 4 mg as a single dose **or** 0.15 mg/kg/dose (maximum: 16 mg/dose) for 3 doses

Adults: 0.15 mg/kg/dose (maximum: 16 mg/dose) for 3 doses **or** 4 mg as a single dose

Oral:

Children 4-11 years: 4 mg every 4 hours for 3 doses (day 1), then 4 mg every 8 hours for 1-2 days

Children ≥12 years and Adults: 16 mg or 24 mg as a single dose **or** 8 mg every 8-12 hours

Mechanism of Action Selective 5-HT$_3$-receptor antagonist, blocking serotonin, both peripherally on vagal nerve terminals and centrally in the chemoreceptor trigger zone

Pharmacodynamics/Kinetics

Onset of Action ~30 minutes

Half-life Elimination Children <15 years: 2-7 hours; Adults: 3-6 hours

Mild-to-moderate hepatic impairment (Child-Pugh classes A and B): Adults: 12 hours

Severe hepatic impairment (Child-Pugh class C): Adults: 20 hours

Time to Peak Oral: ~2 hours; Oral soluble film: ~1 hour

Pregnancy Risk Factor B

Pregnancy Considerations Teratogenic effects were not observed in animal reproduction studies. Ondansetron readily crosses the human placenta in the first trimester of pregnancy and can be detected in fetal tissue (Siu, 2006). The use of ondansetron for the treatment of nausea and vomiting of pregnancy (NVP) has been evaluated. Although a significant increase in birth defects has not been described in case reports and some studies (Ferreira, 2012; Pasternak, 2013), other studies have shown a possible association with ondansetron exposure and adverse fetal events (Anderka, 2012; Einarson, 2004). Additional studies are needed to determine safety to the fetus, particularly during the first trimester. Based on available data, use is generally reserved for severe NVP (hyperemesis gravidarum) or when conventional treatments are not effective (ACOG, 2004; Koren, 2012; Levicheck, 2002; Tan, 2011). Because a dose-dependent QT-interval prolongation occurs with use, the manufacturer recommends ECG monitoring in patients with electrolyte abnormalities (which can be associated with some cases of NVP; Koren, 2012).

Dental Comment Ondansetron is a safer alternative than phenothiazines (ie, promethazine) for the treatment of moderate-to-severe postoperative nausea and vomiting. The cost can be a limitation.

Ondansetron is known to prolong the QT interval. The QT interval is measured as the time and distance between the Q point of the QRS complex and the end of the T wave in the ECG tracing. After adjustment for heart rate, the QT interval is defined as prolonged if it is more than 450 msec in men and 460 msec in women. A long QT syndrome was first described in the 1950s and 60s as a congenital syndrome involving QT interval prolongation and syncope and sudden death. Some of the congenital long QT syndromes were characterized by a peculiar electrocardiographic appearance of the QRS complex involving a premature atria beat followed by a pause, then a subsequent sinus beat showing marked QT prolongation and deformity. This type of cardiac arrhythmia was originally termed "torsade de pointes" (translated from the French as "twisting of the points"). Ondansetron is considered as having a risk of causing torsade de pointes. Since it is not known what effect vasoconstrictors in the local anesthetic regimen will have in patients with a known history of congenital prolonged QT interval or in patients taking any medication that prolongs the QT interval, a medical consult is suggested.

Opium Tincture (OH pee um TING chur)

Pharmacologic Category Analgesic, Opioid; Antidiarrheal

Use Treatment of diarrhea in adults

Local Anesthetic/Vasoconstrictor Precautions No information available to require special precautions

Effects on Dental Treatment No significant effects or complications reported

Effects on Bleeding No information available to require special precautions

Adverse Effects Frequency not defined.

Cardiovascular: Palpitation, hypotension, bradycardia, peripheral vasodilation

Central nervous system: Drowsiness, dizziness, restlessness, headache, malaise, CNS depression, intracranial pressure increased, insomnia, mental depression

Gastrointestinal: Nausea, vomiting, constipation, anorexia, stomach cramps, biliary tract spasm

Genitourinary: Urination decreased, urinary tract spasm

Neuromuscular & skeletal: Weakness

Ocular: Miosis

Respiratory: Respiratory depression

Miscellaneous: Histamine release, physical and psychological dependence

General Dosage Range

Oral: Opium tincture 10% contains morphine 10 mg/mL. Use caution in ordering, dispensing, and/or administering. The following doses are expressed in **mg** (milligram) dosing units of morphine.

Adults: Usual: 6 **mg** of undiluted opium tincture (10 mg/mL) 4 times daily

Mechanism of Action Contains many narcotic alkaloids including morphine; its mechanism for gastric motility inhibition is primarily due to this morphine content; it results in a decrease in digestive secretions, an increase in GI muscle tone, and therefore a reduction in GI propulsion

Pharmacodynamics/Kinetics

Duration of Action 4-5 hours

Pregnancy Risk Factor C

Pregnancy Considerations Animal reproduction studies have not been conducted.

Controlled Substance C-II

Oprelvekin (oh PREL ve kin)

Brand Names: U.S. Neumega®

Pharmacologic Category Biological Response Modulator; Human Growth Factor

Use Prevention of severe thrombocytopenia; reduce the need for platelet transfusions following myelosuppressive chemotherapy for nonmyeloid malignancy

Local Anesthetic/Vasoconstrictor Precautions No information available to require special precautions

Effects on Dental Treatment Key adverse event(s) related to dental treatment: Oral moniliasis.

Effects on Bleeding No information available to require special precautions

Adverse Effects

>10%:

Cardiovascular: Tachycardia (children 84%; adults 20%), edema (59%), cardiomegaly (children 21%), vasodilation (19%), atrial arrhythmia (12% to 15%), palpitation (14%), syncope (13%)

Central nervous system: Neutropenic fever (48%), headache (41%), dizziness (38%), fever (36%), insomnia (33%)

Dermatologic: Rash (25%)

Endocrine & metabolic: Fluid retention

Gastrointestinal: Nausea/vomiting (77%), diarrhea (43%), mucositis (43%), oral moniliasis (14%), weight gain (due to fluid retention)

Hematologic: Anemia (dilutional; onset: 3-5 days; duration: ≤1 week)

Neuromuscular & skeletal: Weakness (severe 14%), periostitis (children 11%), arthralgia

Ocular: Conjunctival injection/redness/swelling (children 57%; adults 19%), papilledema (children 16%; adults 1%)

Respiratory: Dyspnea (48%), rhinitis (42%), cough (29%), pharyngitis (25%)

1% to 10%: Respiratory: Pleural effusion (10%)

General Dosage Range Dosage adjustment recommended in patients with renal impairment

SubQ: *Adults:* 50 mcg/kg once daily

Mechanism of Action Oprelvekin is a thrombopoietic growth factor which stimulates multiple stages of megakaryocytopoiesis and thrombopoiesis, resulting in proliferation of megakaryocyte progenitors and megakaryocyte maturation, thereby increasing platelet production.

Pharmacodynamics/Kinetics

Half-life Elimination Terminal: 5-9 hours

Time to Peak Serum: 1-6 hours

Pregnancy Risk Factor C

Pregnancy Considerations Animal studies have demonstrated adverse fetal effects. There are no adequate and well-controlled studies in pregnant women. Use during pregnancy only if the potential benefits outweigh the potential risk to the fetus.

Orlistat (OR li stat)

Brand Names: U.S. Alli® [OTC]; Xenical®
Brand Names: Canada Xenical®
Pharmacologic Category Lipase Inhibitor
Use Management of obesity, including weight loss and weight management, when used in conjunction with a reduced-calorie and low-fat diet; reduce the risk of weight regain after prior weight loss; indicated for obese patients with an initial body mass index (BMI) ≥30 kg/m² or ≥27 kg/m² in the presence of other risk factors (eg, diabetes, dyslipidemia, hypertension)
Local Anesthetic/Vasoconstrictor Precautions No information available to require special precautions
Effects on Dental Treatment No significant effects or complications reported
Effects on Bleeding No information available to require special precautions
Adverse Effects Note: The frequency of most adverse reactions (especially gastrointestinal effects) decreases over time.
>10%:
Central nervous system: Headache (≤31%)
Gastrointestinal: Oily spotting (4% to 27%), abdominal pain/discomfort (≤26%), flatus with discharge (2% to 24%), fecal urgency (3% to 22%), fatty/oily stool (6% to 20%), oily evacuation (2% to 12%), defecation increased (3% to 11%)
Neuromuscular & skeletal: Back pain (≤14%)
Respiratory: Upper respiratory infection (26% to 38%)
Miscellaneous: Influenza (≤40%)
1% to 10%:
Cardiovascular: Pedal edema (≤3%)
Central nervous system: Fatigue (3% to 7%), anxiety (3% to 5%), sleep disorder (≤4%)
Dermatologic: Dry skin (≤2%)
Endocrine & metabolic: Menstrual irregularities (≤10%)
Gastrointestinal: Nausea (4% to 8%), fecal incontinence (2% to 8%), infectious diarrhea (≤5%), rectal pain/discomfort (3% to 5%), tooth disorder (3% to 4%), gingival disorder (2% to 4%)
Genitourinary: Urinary tract infection (6% to 8%), vaginitis (3% to 4%)
Neuromuscular & skeletal: Myalgia (≤4%)
Otic: Otitis (3% to 4%)
Respiratory: Lower respiratory infection (≤8%)
General Dosage Range Oral:
Children ≥12 years and Adults: Xenical®: 120 mg 3 times/day
Adults: Alli™ (OTC labeling): 60 mg 3 times/day
Mechanism of Action A reversible inhibitor of gastric and pancreatic lipases, thus inhibiting absorption of dietary fats by 30% (at doses of 120 mg 3 times/day).
Pharmacodynamics/Kinetics
Onset of Action 24-48 hours
Duration of Action 48-72 hours
Half-life Elimination 1-2 hours
Time to Peak Serum: ~8 hours
Pregnancy Risk Factor X
Pregnancy Considerations Adverse events were not observed in animal reproduction studies. Although orlistat is minimally absorbed, weight-loss therapy is not recommended for pregnant women. Obese and overweight women should be encouraged to participate in weight reduction programs prior to attempting pregnancy; weight gain during pregnancy should be determined by their prepregnancy BMI and current guidelines (ADA, 2009; IOM, 2009). Use of orlistat is contraindicated in pregnant women.

Orphenadrine (or FEN a dreen)

Related Information
Temporomandibular Dysfunction (TMD), Chronic Pain, and Fibromyalgia *on page 1590*
Brand Names: U.S. Norflex™
Brand Names: Canada Norflex™; Orphenace®; Rhoxal-orphenrine
Generic Availability (U.S.) Yes
Pharmacologic Category Skeletal Muscle Relaxant
Use Treatment of muscle spasm associated with acute painful musculoskeletal conditions
Local Anesthetic/Vasoconstrictor Precautions No information available to require special precautions
Effects on Dental Treatment The peripheral anticholinergic effects of orphenadrine may decrease or inhibit salivary flow; normal salivation will return with cessation of drug therapy.
Effects on Bleeding No information available to require special precautions
Adverse Effects Frequency not defined.
Cardiovascular: Palpitation, tachycardia
Central nervous system: Agitation, dizziness, drowsiness, euphoria, hallucination, headache, mental confusion
Dermatologic: Pruritus, urticaria
Gastrointestinal: Constipation, gastric irritation, nausea, vomiting, xerostomia
Genitourinary: Urination hesitancy, urinary retention
Hematologic: Aplastic anemia (rare)
Neuromuscular & skeletal: Tremor, weakness
Ocular: Blurred vision, intraocular pressure increased, nystagmus, pupil dilation
Respiratory: Nasal congestion
Miscellaneous: Anaphylactic reaction (injection, rare), hypersensitivity
Dosage
Adults:
Oral: 100 mg twice daily
I.M., I.V.: 60 mg every 12 hours
Elderly: Use caution; generally not recommended for use in the elderly
Mechanism of Action Indirect skeletal muscle relaxant thought to work by central atropine-like effects; has some euphorigenic and analgesic properties
Contraindications Hypersensitivity to orphenadrine or any component of the formulation; glaucoma; GI obstruction, stenosing peptic ulcer; prostatic hypertrophy, bladder neck obstruction; cardiospasm; myasthenia gravis
Warnings/Precautions Use with caution in patients with HF, cardiac decompensation, coronary insufficiency, tachycardia or cardiac arrhythmias. May cause CNS depression, which may impair physical or mental abilities. Muscle relaxants are poorly tolerated by the elderly due to potent anticholinergic effects, sedation, and risk of fracture. Efficacy is questionable at dosages tolerated by elderly patients; avoid use (Beers Criteria). Potential for abuse; use with caution in patients with history of drug abuse. Solution for injection contains sodium bisulfite which may cause allergic reaction in some individuals. Has not been evaluated for continuous long-term use; monitor closely.
Drug Interactions
Metabolism/Transport Effects Substrate of CYP1A2 (minor), CYP2B6 (minor), CYP2D6 (minor), CYP3A4 (minor); **Note:** Assignment of Major/Minor substrate status based on clinically relevant drug interaction potential; **Inhibits** CYP1A2 (weak),

CYP2A6 (weak), CYP2B6 (weak), CYP2C19 (weak), CYP2C9 (weak), CYP2D6 (weak), CYP2E1 (weak), CYP3A4 (weak)

Avoid Concomitant Use

Avoid concomitant use of Orphenadrine with any of the following: Aclidinium; Azelastine (Nasal); Ipratropium (Oral Inhalation); Paraldehyde; Pimozide; Potassium Chloride; Tiotropium

Increased Effect/Toxicity

Orphenadrine may increase the levels/effects of: AbobotulinumtoxinA; Alcohol (Ethyl); Anticholinergics; ARIPiprazole; Azelastine (Nasal); Buprenorphine; Cannabinoids; CNS Depressants; Lomitapide; Methotrimeprazine; Metyrosine; Mirabegron; Mirtazapine; OnabotulinumtoxinA; Paraldehyde; Pimozide; Potassium Chloride; Pramipexole; RimabotulinumtoxinB; ROPINIRole; Rotigotine; Selective Serotonin Reuptake Inhibitors; Tiotropium; Topiramate; Zolpidem

The levels/effects of Orphenadrine may be increased by: Aclidinium; Droperidol; HydrOXYzine; Ipratropium (Oral Inhalation); Magnesium Sulfate; Methotrimeprazine; Perampanel; Pramlintide; Sodium Oxybate

Decreased Effect

Orphenadrine may decrease the levels/effects of: Acetylcholinesterase Inhibitors (Central); Secretin

The levels/effects of Orphenadrine may be decreased by: Acetylcholinesterase Inhibitors (Central); Peginterferon Alfa-2b

Ethanol/Nutrition/Herb Interactions

Ethanol: Avoid ethanol (may increase CNS depression). Herb/Nutraceutical: Avoid valerian, St John's wort, kava kava, gotu kola (may increase CNS depression).

Pharmacodynamics/Kinetics

Onset of Action Peak effect: Oral: Within 2-4 hours

Duration of Action 4-6 hours

Half-life Elimination 14-16 hours

Pregnancy Risk Factor C

Pregnancy Considerations Animal reproduction studies have not been conducted. There are no adequate and well-controlled studies in pregnant women. Use during pregnancy only if clearly needed.

Lactation Excretion in breast milk unknown/use caution

Dosage Forms

Injection, solution: 30 mg/mL (2 mL)

Norflex™: 30 mg/mL (2 mL)

Injection, solution [preservative free]: 30 mg/mL (2 mL)

Tablet, extended release, oral: 100 mg

Orphenadrine, Aspirin, and Caffeine
(or FEN a dreen, AS pir in, & KAF een)

Related Information

Aspirin *on page 135*

Caffeine *on page 229*

Orphenadrine *on page 1018*

Pharmacologic Category Skeletal Muscle Relaxant

Use Relief of discomfort associated with skeletal muscular conditions

Local Anesthetic/Vasoconstrictor Precautions No information available to require special precautions

Effects on Dental Treatment Key adverse event(s) related to dental treatment: The peripheral anticholinergic effects of orphenadrine may decrease or inhibit salivary flow; normal salivation will return with cessation of drug therapy.

Aspirin: As with all drugs which may affect hemostasis, bleeding is associated with aspirin. Other serious reactions are idiosyncratic, related to allergy or individual sensitivity (see Effects on Bleeding).

Effects on Bleeding Aspirin irreversibly inhibits platelet aggregation which can prolong bleeding. Upon discontinuation, normal platelet function returns only when new platelets are released (~7-10 days). However, in the case of dental surgery, there is no scientific evidence to support discontinuation of aspirin.

General Dosage Range Oral: *Adults:* 1-2 tablets 3-4 times/day

Pregnancy Considerations See individual agents.

Dental Comment There is no scientific evidence to warrant discontinuance of aspirin prior to dental surgery. Patients taking one aspirin tablet daily as an antithrombotic and who require dental surgery should be given special consideration in consultation with the physician before removal of the aspirin relative to prevention of postoperative bleeding.

Oseltamivir (oh sel TAM i vir)

Related Information

Systemic Viral Diseases *on page 1537*

Brand Names: U.S. Tamiflu®

Brand Names: Canada Tamiflu®

Pharmacologic Category Antiviral Agent; Neuraminidase Inhibitor

Use Treatment of uncomplicated acute illness due to influenza (A or B) infection in children ≥2 weeks and adults who have been symptomatic for no more than 2 days; prophylaxis against influenza (A or B) infection in children ≥1 year of age and adults

The Advisory Committee on Immunization Practices (ACIP) recommends that **treatment** be considered for the following:

• Persons with severe, complicated or progressive illness

• Hospitalized persons

• Persons at higher risk for influenza complications:
  - Children <2 years of age (highest risk in children <6 months of age)
  - Adults ≥65 years of age
  - Persons with chronic disorders of the pulmonary (including asthma) or cardiovascular systems (except hypertension)
  - Persons with chronic metabolic diseases (including diabetes mellitus), hepatic disease, renal dysfunction, hematologic disorders (including sickle cell disease), or immunosuppression (including immunosuppression caused by medications or HIV)
  - Persons with neurologic/neuromuscular conditions (including conditions such as spinal cord injuries, seizure disorders, cerebral palsy, stroke, mental retardation, moderate to severe developmental delay, or muscular dystrophy) which may compromise respiratory function, the handling of respiratory secretions, or that can increase the risk of aspiration
  - Pregnant or postpartum women (≤2 weeks after delivery)
  - Persons <19 years of age on long-term aspirin therapy
  - American Indians and Alaskan Natives
  - Persons who are morbidly obese (BMI ≥40)
  - Residents of nursing homes or other chronic care facilities

▶

• Use may also be considered for previously healthy, nonhigh-risk outpatients with confirmed or suspected influenza based on clinical judgment when treatment can be started within 48 hours of illness onset.

The ACIP recommends that **prophylaxis** be considered for the following:
• Postexposure prophylaxis may be considered for family or close contacts of suspected or confirmed cases, who are at higher risk of influenza complications, and who have not been vaccinated against the circulating strain at the time of the exposure.
• Postexposure prophylaxis may be considered for unvaccinated healthcare workers who had occupational exposure without protective equipment.
• Pre-exposure prophylaxis should only be used for persons at very high risk of influenza complications who cannot be otherwise protected at times of high risk for exposure.
• Prophylaxis should also be administered to all eligible residents of institutions that house patients at high risk when needed to control outbreaks.

The ACIP recommends that treatment and prophylaxis be given to children <1 year of age when indicated.

Local Anesthetic/Vasoconstrictor Precautions No information available to require special precautions

Effects on Dental Treatment No significant effects or complications reported

Effects on Bleeding No information available to require special precautions

Adverse Effects
>10%: Gastrointestinal: Vomiting (2% to 15%)
1% to 10%:
Gastrointestinal: Nausea (4% to 10%), abdominal pain (2% to 5%), diarrhea (1% to 3%)
Ocular: Conjunctivitis (1%)
Respiratory: Epistaxis (1%)

General Dosage Range Dosage adjustment recommended in patients with renal impairment
Oral:
Infants ≥2 weeks: 3 mg/kg/dose twice daily
Children 1-12 years and ≤15 kg: 30 mg once or twice daily
Children 1-12 years and >15 to ≤23 kg: 45 mg once or twice daily
Children 1-12 years and >23 to ≤40 kg: 60 mg once or twice daily
Children 1-12 years and >40 kg, Adolescents, and Adults: 75 mg once or twice daily

Mechanism of Action Oseltamivir, a prodrug, is hydrolyzed to the active form, oseltamivir carboxylate (OC). OC inhibits influenza virus neuraminidase, an enzyme known to cleave the budding viral progeny from its cellular envelope attachment point (neuraminic acid) just prior to release.

Pharmacodynamics/Kinetics
Half-life Elimination Oseltamivir: 1-3 hours; Oseltamivir carboxylate: 6-10 hours

Pregnancy Risk Factor C

Pregnancy Considerations In animal reproduction studies, a dose-dependent increase in the rates of minor skeleton abnormalities was found in exposed offspring. The rate of each abnormality remained within the background rate of occurrence in the species studied. Oseltamivir phosphate and its active metabolite oseltamivir carboxylate cross the placenta (*in vitro* data). An increased risk of adverse neonatal outcomes has generally not been observed following maternal use of oseltamivir during pregnancy. Untreated influenza infection is associated with an increased risk of adverse events to the fetus and an increased risk of complications or death to the mother. Oseltamivir and zanamivir are currently recommended for the treatment or prophylaxis of influenza in pregnant women and women up to 2 weeks postpartum. Oseltamivir and zanamivir are currently recommended as an adjunct to vaccination and should not be used as a substitute for vaccination in pregnant women (consult current CDC guidelines).

Ospemifene (os PEM i feen)

Pharmacologic Category Selective Estrogen Receptor Modulator (SERM)
Use Treatment of moderate-to-severe dyspareunia due to vulvar and vaginal atrophy (VVA) of menopause
Local Anesthetic/Vasoconstrictor Precautions No information available to require special precautions
Effects on Dental Treatment No significant effects or complications reported
Effects on Bleeding Ospemifene has been associated with thromboembolic adverse events. There is no information available to require special precautions for dental procedures.
Adverse Effects 1% to 10%:
Dermatologic: Hyperhidrosis (2%)
Endocrine & metabolic: Hot flashes (8%)
Genitourinary: Vaginal discharge (4%), genital discharge (1%)
Neuromuscular & skeletal: Muscle spasm (3%)
General Dosage Range Oral: *Adults (postmenopausal females):* 60 mg once daily
Mechanism of Action Ospemifene is a selective estrogen receptor modulator (SERM); it activates estrogen pathways in some tissues and blocks estrogen pathways in others, and specifically has agonistic effects on the endometrium. In women with VVA, ospemifene was shown to improve vaginal changes associated with the decrease in natural estrogen production associated with menopause (improves vaginal maturation index, decreases vaginal pH) and significantly decreased the most bothersome moderate-to-severe subjective findings reported by women (vaginal dryness and dyspareunia) after 12 weeks of therapy (Bachmann, 2010).
Pharmacodynamics/Kinetics
Onset of Action A significant decrease in vaginal dryness and dyspareunia were observed after 12 weeks of therapy (Bachmann, 2010).
Half-life Elimination ~26 hours
Time to Peak ~2 hours (range: 1-8 hours)
Pregnancy Risk Factor X
Pregnancy Considerations Adverse events were observed in animal reproduction studies. Use is contraindicated in women who are or may become pregnant. Ospemifene is currently approved only for the treatment of moderate-to-severe dyspareunia due to vulvar and vaginal atrophy (VVA) of menopause.
Product Availability Osphena™: FDA approved February 2013; anticipated availability is June 2013. Consult prescribing information for additional information.

Oxacillin (oks a SIL in)

Pharmacologic Category Antibiotic, Penicillin
Use Treatment of infections such as osteomyelitis, septicemia, endocarditis, and CNS infections caused by susceptible strains of *Staphylococcus*
Local Anesthetic/Vasoconstrictor Precautions No information available to require special precautions

Effects on Dental Treatment Key adverse event(s) related to dental treatment: Prolonged use of penicillins may lead to development of oral candidiasis.

Effects on Bleeding No information available to require special precautions

Adverse Effects Frequency not defined.

Central nervous system: Fever

Dermatologic: Rash

Gastrointestinal: Nausea, diarrhea, vomiting

Hematologic: Eosinophilia, leukopenia, neutropenia, thrombocytopenia, agranulocytosis

Hepatic: Hepatotoxicity, AST increased

Renal: Acute interstitial nephritis, hematuria

Miscellaneous: Serum sickness-like reactions

General Dosage Range I.M., I.V.:

Children: 100-200 mg/kg/day in divided doses every 6 hours (maximum: 12 g/day)

Adults: 250-2000 mg every 4-6 hours

Mechanism of Action Inhibits bacterial cell wall synthesis by binding to one or more of the penicillin-binding proteins (PBPs); which in turn inhibits the final transpeptidation step of peptidoglycan synthesis in bacterial cell walls, thus inhibiting cell wall biosynthesis. Bacteria eventually lyse due to ongoing activity of cell wall autolytic enzymes (autolysins and murein hydrolases) while cell wall assembly is arrested.

Pharmacodynamics/Kinetics

Half-life Elimination Children 1 week to 2 years: 0.9-1.8 hours; Adults: 23-60 minutes; prolonged with renal impairment and in neonates

Time to Peak Serum: I.M.: 30-60 minutes

Pregnancy Risk Factor B

Pregnancy Considerations Adverse events have not been observed in animal reproduction studies. Oxacillin is distributed into the amniotic fluid and is detected in cord blood. Maternal use of penicillins has generally not resulted in an increased risk of adverse fetal effects.

Oxaliplatin (ox AL i pla tin)

Brand Names: U.S. Eloxatin®

Brand Names: Canada Eloxatin®

Pharmacologic Category Antineoplastic Agent, Alkylating Agent; Antineoplastic Agent, Platinum Analog

Use Treatment of stage III colon cancer (adjuvant) after complete resection of primary tumor; treatment of advanced colorectal cancer

Unlabeled Use Treatment of esophageal cancer, gastric cancer, hepatobiliary cancer (advanced), non-Hodgkin's lymphoma (refractory), ovarian cancer (advanced, platinum-pretreated), pancreatic cancer (advanced), testicular cancer (refractory)

Local Anesthetic/Vasoconstrictor Precautions No information available to require special precautions

Effects on Dental Treatment Key adverse event(s) related to dental treatment: Stomatitis, dysphagia, mucositis, and taste perversion.

Effects on Bleeding Chemotherapy may result in significant myelosuppression, potentially including significant reduction in platelet counts (infrequent, <1%) and altered hemostasis. In patients who are under active treatment with these agents, medical consult is suggested.

Adverse Effects Percentages reported with monotherapy.

>10%:

Central nervous system: Fatigue (61%), fever (25%), pain (14%), headache (13%), insomnia (11%)

Gastrointestinal: Nausea (64%), diarrhea (46%), vomiting (37%), abdominal pain (31%), constipation (31%), anorexia (20%), stomatitis (14%)

Hematologic: Anemia (64%; grades 3/4: 1%), thrombocytopenia (30%; grades 3/4: 3%), leukopenia (13%)

Hepatic: AST increased (54%; grades 3/4: 4%), ALT increased (36%; grades 3/4: 1%), total bilirubin increased (13%; grades 3/4: 5%)

Neuromuscular & skeletal: Peripheral neuropathy (may be dose limiting; 76%; acute 65%; grades 3/4: 5%; persistent 43%; grades 3/4: 3%), back pain (11%)

Respiratory: Dyspnea (13%), cough (11%)

1% to 10%:

Cardiovascular: Edema (10%), chest pain (5%), peripheral edema (5%), flushing (3%), thromboembolism (2%)

Central nervous system: Dizziness (7%)

Dermatologic: Rash (5%), alopecia (3%), hand-foot syndrome (1%)

Endocrine & metabolic: Dehydration (5%), hypokalemia (3%)

Gastrointestinal: Dyspepsia (7%), taste perversion (5%), flatulence (3%), mucositis (2%), gastroesophageal reflux (1%), dysphagia (acute 1% to 2%)

Genitourinary: Dysuria (1%)

Hematologic: Neutropenia (7%)

Local: Injection site reaction (9%; redness/swelling/pain)

Neuromuscular & skeletal: Rigors (9%), arthralgia (7%)

Ocular: Abnormal lacrimation (1%)

Renal: Serum creatinine increased (5% to 10%)

Respiratory: URI (7%), rhinitis (6%), epistaxis (2%), pharyngitis (2%), pharyngolaryngeal dysesthesia (grades 3/4: 1% to 2%)

Miscellaneous: Allergic reactions (3%); hypersensitivity (includes urticaria, pruritus, facial flushing, shortness of breath, bronchospasm, diaphoresis, hypotension, syncope: grades 3/4: 2% to 3%); hiccup (2%)

General Dosage Range Dosage adjustment recommended in patients with renal impairment or who develop toxicities

I.V.: *Adults:* 85 mg/m^2 every 2 weeks

Mechanism of Action Oxaliplatin, a platinum derivative, is an alkylating agent. Following intracellular hydrolysis, the platinum compound binds to DNA forming cross-links which inhibit DNA replication and transcription, resulting in cell death. Cytotoxicity is cell-cycle nonspecific.

Pharmacodynamics/Kinetics

Half-life Elimination Terminal: 391 hours

Pregnancy Risk Factor D

Pregnancy Considerations Decreased fetal weight, decreased ossification, and increased fetal deaths were observed in animal reproduction studies at one-tenth the equivalent human dose. Women of childbearing potential should be advised to avoid pregnancy and use effective contraception during treatment.

Canadian labeling: Use in pregnant women is contraindicated in the Canadian labeling. Males should be advised not to father children during and for up to 6 months following therapy. May cause permanent infertility in males. Prior to initiating therapy, advise males desiring to father children, to seek counseling on sperm storage.

Oxandrolone (oks AN droe lone)

Brand Names: U.S. Oxandrin®

Pharmacologic Category Androgen

Use Adjunctive therapy to promote weight gain after weight loss following extensive surgery, chronic infections, or severe trauma, and in some patients who, without definite pathophysiologic reasons, fail to gain or to maintain normal weight; to offset protein catabolism with prolonged corticosteroid administration; relief of bone pain associated with osteoporosis

Local Anesthetic/Vasoconstrictor Precautions No information available to require special precautions

Effects on Dental Treatment No significant effects or complications reported

Effects on Bleeding No information available to require special precautions

Adverse Effects Frequency not defined.

Cardiovascular: Edema

Central nervous system: Depression, excitation, insomnia

Dermatologic: Acne (females and prepubertal males)

Also reported in females: Hirsutism, male-pattern baldness

Endocrine & metabolic: Electrolyte imbalances, glucose intolerance, gonadotropin secretion inhibited, gynecomastia, HDL decreased, LDL increased, libido changes

Also reported in females: Clitoral enlargement, menstrual irregularities

Genitourinary:

Prepubertal males: Increased or persistent erections, penile enlargement

Postpubertal males: Bladder irritation, epididymitis, impotence, oligospermia, priapism (chronic), testicular atrophy, testicular function

Hematologic: Prothrombin time increased, suppression of clotting factors

Hepatic: Alkaline phosphatase increased, ALT increased, AST increased, bilirubin increased, cholestatic jaundice, hepatic necrosis (rare), hepatocellular neoplasms, peliosis hepatis (with long-term therapy)

Neuromuscular & skeletal: CPK increased, premature closure of epiphyses (in children)

Renal: Creatinine excretion increased

Miscellaneous: Bromsulfophthalein retention, habituation, voice alteration (deepening, in females)

General Dosage Range Oral:

Children: ≤0.1 mg/kg/day

Adults: 2.5-20 mg daily in 2-4 divided doses

Elderly: 5 mg twice daily

Mechanism of Action Synthetic testosterone derivative with similar androgenic and anabolic actions

Pharmacodynamics/Kinetics

Half-life Elimination 10-13 hours

Pregnancy Risk Factor X

Pregnancy Considerations Use is contraindicated in women who are or may become pregnant; masculinization of the fetus has been reported.

Controlled Substance C-III

Oxaprozin (oks a PROE zin)

Related Information

Rheumatoid Arthritis, Osteoarthritis, and Osteoporosis *on page 1526*

Temporomandibular Dysfunction (TMD), Chronic Pain, and Fibromyalgia *on page 1590*

Brand Names: U.S. Daypro®

Brand Names: Canada Apo-Oxaprozin®; Daypro®

Generic Availability (U.S.) Yes

Pharmacologic Category Nonsteroidal Anti-inflammatory Drug (NSAID)

Use Management of signs and symptoms of osteoarthritis, rheumatoid arthritis, and juvenile idiopathic arthritis (JIA)

Local Anesthetic/Vasoconstrictor Precautions No information available to require special precautions

Effects on Dental Treatment The dentist should be aware of the potential of abnormal coagulation. Caution should also be exercised in the use of NSAIDs in patients already on anticoagulant therapy with drugs such as warfarin (Coumadin®). See Effects on Bleeding.

Effects on Bleeding Nonselective NSAIDs, such as oxaprozin, inhibit platelet aggregation and prolong bleeding time in some patients. Unlike aspirin, the NSAID effect on platelet function is quantitatively less, of shorter duration, and reversible. Normal platelet function should occur in ~5 elimination half-lives or in <10 hours after discontinuation of oxaprozin. Concomitant use of other NSAIDs should be avoided.

Adverse Effects

1% to 10%:

Cardiovascular: Edema

Central nervous system: Confusion, depression, dizziness, headache, sedation, sleep disturbance, somnolence

Dermatologic: Pruritus, rash

Gastrointestinal: Abdominal distress, abdominal pain, anorexia, constipation, diarrhea, dyspepsia, flatulence, gastrointestinal ulcer, gross bleeding with perforation, heartburn, nausea, vomiting

Hematologic: Anemia, bleeding time increased

Hepatic: Liver enzymes increased

Otic: Tinnitus

Renal: Dysuria, renal function abnormal, urinary frequency

Dosage Oral: **Note:** Individualize dosage to lowest effective dose for the shortest duration to minimize adverse effects.

Children 6-16 years: Juvenile idiopathic arthritis (JIA):

22-31 kg: 600 mg once daily

32-54 kg: 900 mg once daily

≥55 kg: 1200 mg once daily

Adults: Osteoarthritis, rheumatoid arthritis: 1200 mg once daily. **Note:** Patients with low body weight should start with 600 mg daily. A one-time loading dose of 1200-1800 mg (≤26 mg/kg) may be used when a quick onset of action is desired.

Maximum doses:

Patient <50 kg: Maximum: 1200 mg daily

Patient >50 kg with normal renal/hepatic function and low risk of peptic ulcer: Maximum: 1800 mg daily or 26 mg/kg/day (whichever is lower) in divided doses

Dosing adjustment in renal impairment: In general, NSAIDs are not recommended for use in patients with advanced renal disease but the manufacturer of oxaprozin does provide some guidelines for adjustment in renal dysfunction.

Severe renal impairment or on dialysis: 600 mg once daily; may increase cautiously to 1200 mg daily with close monitoring

Dosing adjustment in hepatic impairment: Use caution in patients with severe hepatic impairment.

Mechanism of Action Reversibly inhibits cyclooxygenase-1 and 2 (COX-1 and 2) enzymes, which results in decreased formation of prostaglandin precursors; has antipyretic, analgesic, and anti-inflammatory properties.

Other proposed mechanisms not fully elucidated (and possibly contributing to the anti-inflammatory effect to varying degrees) include inhibiting chemotaxis, altering lymphocyte activity, inhibiting neutrophil aggregation/activation, and decreasing proinflammatory cytokine levels.

Contraindications Hypersensitivity to oxaprozin, aspirin, other NSAIDs, or any component of the formulation; perioperative pain in the setting of coronary artery bypass graft (CABG) surgery

Warnings/Precautions [U.S. Boxed Warning]: NSAIDs are associated with an increased risk of adverse cardiovascular thrombotic events, including MI and stroke. Risk may be increased with duration of use or pre-existing cardiovascular risk factors or disease. Carefully evaluate individual cardiovascular risk profiles prior to prescribing. May cause new onset hypertension or worsening of existing hypertension. Use caution with fluid retention. Avoid use in heart failure. Concurrent administration of ibuprofen, and potentially other nonselective NSAIDs, may interfere with aspirin's cardioprotective effect. **[U.S. Boxed Warning]: Use is contraindicated for treatment of perioperative pain in the setting of coronary artery bypass graft (CABG) surgery.** Risk of MI and stroke may be increased with use following CABG surgery.

Platelet adhesion and aggregation may be decreased; may prolong bleeding time; patients with coagulation disorders or who are receiving anticoagulants should be monitored closely. Anemia may occur; patients on long-term NSAID therapy should be monitored for anemia. Rarely, NSAID use may cause severe blood dyscrasias (eg, agranulocytosis, aplastic anemia, thrombocytopenia).

NSAID use may compromise existing renal function; dose-dependent decreases in prostaglandin synthesis may result from NSAID use, reducing renal blood flow which may cause renal decompensation. NSAID use may increase the risk for hyperkalemia. Patients with impaired renal function, dehydration, heart failure, liver dysfunction, those taking diuretics, and ACE inhibitors, and the elderly are at greater risk of renal toxicity and hyperkalemia. In the elderly, may be inappropriate for long-term use due to potential for GI bleeding, hypertension, heart failure, and renal failure (Beers Criteria). Rehydrate patient before starting therapy; monitor renal function closely. Not recommended for use in patients with advanced renal disease. Long-term NSAID use may result in renal papillary necrosis.

[U.S. Boxed Warning]: NSAIDs may increase risk of gastrointestinal irritation, inflammation, ulceration, bleeding, and perforation. These events may occur at any time during therapy and without warning. Use caution with a history of GI disease (bleeding or ulcers);

concurrent therapy with aspirin, anticoagulants, and/or corticosteroids; smoking; use of alcohol; and the elderly or debilitated patients. When used concomitantly with ≤325 mg of aspirin, a substantial increase in the risk of gastrointestinal complications (eg, ulcer) occurs; concomitant gastroprotective therapy (eg, proton pump inhibitors) is recommended (Bhatt, 2008).

Use the lowest effective dose for the shortest duration of time, consistent with individual patient goals, to reduce risk of cardiovascular or GI adverse events. Alternate therapies should be considered for patients at high risk.

NSAIDs may cause serious skin adverse events including exfoliative dermatitis, Stevens-Johnson syndrome (SJS), and toxic epidermal necrolysis (TEN); discontinue use at first sign of skin rash or hypersensitivity. Anaphylactoid reactions may occur, even without prior exposure; patients with "aspirin triad" (bronchial asthma, aspirin intolerance, rhinitis) may be at increased risk. Do not use in patients who experience bronchospasm, asthma, rhinitis, or urticaria with NSAID or aspirin therapy. Use caution in other forms of asthma.

Use with caution in patients with decreased hepatic function. Closely monitor patients with any abnormal LFT. Severe hepatic reactions (eg, fulminant hepatitis, liver failure) have occurred with NSAID use, rarely; discontinue if signs or symptoms of liver disease develop, or if systemic manifestations occur.

NSAIDS may cause drowsiness, dizziness, blurred vision and other neurologic effects which may impair physical or mental abilities; patients must be cautioned about performing tasks which require mental alertness (eg, operating machinery or driving). Discontinue use with blurred or diminished vision and perform ophthalmologic exam. Monitor vision with long-term therapy.

In the elderly, avoid chronic use (unless alternative agents ineffective and patient can receive concomitant gastroprotective agent); nonselective oral NSAID use is associated with an increased risk of GI bleeding and peptic ulcer disease in older adults in high risk category (eg, >75 years or age or receiving concomitant oral/parenteral corticosteroids, anticoagulants, or antiplatelet agents) (Beers Criteria).

Withhold for at least 4-6 half-lives prior to surgical or dental procedures. May cause mild photosensitivity reactions.

Drug Interactions

Metabolism/Transport Effects None known.

Avoid Concomitant Use

Avoid concomitant use of Oxaprozin with any of the following: Floctafenine; Ketorolac (Nasal); Ketorolac (Systemic); NSAID (COX-2 Inhibitor); Omacetaxine

Increased Effect/Toxicity

Oxaprozin may increase the levels/effects of: Agents with Antiplatelet Properties; Aliskiren; Aminoglycosides; Anticoagulants; Bisphosphonate Derivatives; Collagenase (Systemic); CycloSPORINE (Systemic); Dabigatran Etexilate; Deferasirox; Desmopressin; Digoxin; Drotrecogin Alfa (Activated); Eplerenone; Haloperidol; Ibritumomab; Lithium; Methotrexate; Nonsteroidal Anti-Inflammatory Agents; NSAID (COX-2 Inhibitor); Omacetaxine; PEMEtrexed; Porfimer; Potassium-Sparing Diuretics; PRALAtrexate; Quinolone Antibiotics; Rivaroxaban; Salicylates; Thrombolytic Agents; Tositumomab and Iodine I 131 Tositumomab; Vancomycin; Vitamin K Antagonists

The levels/effects of Oxaprozin may be increased by: ACE Inhibitors; Angiotensin II Receptor Blockers; Antidepressants (Tricyclic, Tertiary Amine); Corticosteroids (Systemic); CycloSPORINE (Systemic); Dasatinib; Floctafenine; Glucosamine; Herbs (Anticoagulant/Antiplatelet Properties); Ketorolac (Nasal); Ketorolac (Systemic); Multivitamins/Minerals (with ADEK, Folate, Iron); Nonsteroidal Anti-Inflammatory Agents; Omega-3 Fatty Acids; Pentosan Polysulfate Sodium; Pentoxifylline; Probenecid; Prostacyclin Analogues; Selective Serotonin Reuptake Inhibitors; Serotonin/Norepinephrine Reuptake Inhibitors; Sodium Phosphates; Tipranavir; Treprostinil; Vitamin E

Decreased Effect

Oxaprozin may decrease the levels/effects of: ACE Inhibitors; Agents with Antiplatelet Properties; Aliskiren; Angiotensin II Receptor Blockers; Beta-Blockers; Eplerenone; HydrALAZINE; Loop Diuretics; Potassium-Sparing Diuretics; Salicylates; Selective Serotonin Reuptake Inhibitors; Thiazide Diuretics

The levels/effects of Oxaprozin may be decreased by: Bile Acid Sequestrants; Nonsteroidal Anti-Inflammatory Agents; Salicylates

Ethanol/Nutrition/Herb Interactions

Ethanol: Avoid ethanol (may enhance gastric mucosal irritation).

Herb/Nutraceutical: Avoid alfalfa, anise, bilberry, bladderwrack, bromelain, cat's claw, celery, chamomile, coleus, cordyceps, dong quai, evening primrose, fenugreek, feverfew, garlic, ginger, ginkgo biloba, ginseng (American, Panax, Siberian), grapeseed, green tea, guggul, horse chestnut seed, horseradish, licorice, prickly ash, red clover, reishi, SAMe (S-adenosylmethionine), sweet clover, turmeric, white willow (all have additional antiplatelet activity).

Pharmacodynamics/Kinetics

Half-life Elimination 41-55 hours

Time to Peak 2-3 hours

Pregnancy Risk Factor C

Pregnancy Considerations Adverse events were not observed in the initial animal reproduction studies; therefore, the manufacturer classifies oxaprozin as pregnancy category C. NSAID exposure during the first trimester is not strongly associated with congenital malformations; however, cardiovascular anomalies and cleft palate have been observed following NSAID exposure in some studies. The use of an NSAID close to conception may be associated with an increased risk of miscarriage. Nonteratogenic effects have been observed following NSAID administration during the third trimester including myocardial degenerative changes, prenatal constriction of the ductus arteriosus, fetal tricuspid regurgitation, failure of the ductus arteriosus to close postnatally; renal dysfunction or failure, oligohydramnios; gastrointestinal bleeding or perforation, increased risk of necrotizing enterocolitis; intracranial bleeding (including intraventricular hemorrhage), platelet dysfunction with resultant bleeding; pulmonary hypertension. Because they may cause premature closure of the ductus arteriosus, use of NSAIDs late in pregnancy should be avoided (use after 31 or 32 weeks gestation is not recommended by some clinicians). The chronic use of NSAIDs in women of reproductive age may be associated with infertility that is reversible upon discontinuation of the medication. A registry is available for pregnant women exposed to autoimmune medications including oxaprozin. For additional information, contact the Organization of Teratology Information Specialists, OTIS Autoimmune Diseases Study, at 877-311-8972.

Lactation Excretion in breast milk unknown/not recommended

Breast-Feeding Considerations The amount of oxaprozin found in breast milk is not known; however, distribution into breast milk would be expected. Breast-feeding is not recommended by the manufacturer.

Dosage Forms

Caplet, oral: 600 mg

Daypro®: 600 mg

Tablet, oral: 600 mg

Oxazepam (oks A ze pam)

Brand Names: Canada Apo-Oxazepam®; Bio-Oxazepam; Novoxapram®; Oxpam®; Oxpram®; PMS-Oxazepam; Riva-Oxazepam

Generic Availability (U.S.) Yes

Pharmacologic Category Benzodiazepine

Use Management of anxiety disorders, including anxiety associated with depression; management of ethanol withdrawal

Local Anesthetic/Vasoconstrictor Precautions No information available to require special precautions

Effects on Dental Treatment Key adverse event(s) related to dental treatment: Xerostomia (normal salivary flow resumes upon discontinuation).

Effects on Bleeding No information available to require special precautions

Adverse Effects Frequency not defined.

Cardiovascular: Syncope (rare), edema

Central nervous system: Drowsiness, ataxia, dizziness, vertigo, memory impairment, headache, paradoxical reactions (excitement, stimulation of effect), lethargy, amnesia, euphoria

Dermatologic: Rash

Endocrine & metabolic: Decreased libido, menstrual irregularities

Genitourinary: Incontinence

Hematologic: Leukopenia, blood dyscrasias

Hepatic: Jaundice

Neuromuscular & skeletal: Dysarthria, tremor, reflex slowing

Ocular: Blurred vision, diplopia

Miscellaneous: Drug dependence

Dosage Oral:

Children >12 years, Adolescents, and Adults:

Anxiety, mild-to-moderate: 10-15 mg 3-4 times daily

Anxiety, severe or associated with depression: 15-30 mg 3-4 times daily

Ethanol withdrawal: 15-30 mg 3-4 times daily

Elderly: Anxiety: Initial: 10 mg 3 times daily. If necessary, increase cautiously to 15 mg 3-4 times daily. Dose titration should be slow to evaluate sensitivity.

Dosage adjustment in renal impairment: No dosage adjustment provided in manufacturer's labeling

Hemodialysis: Not dialyzable (0% to 5%) (Greenblatt, 1981; Mokhlesi, 2003)

Dosage adjustment in hepatic impairment: No dosage adjustment provided in manufacturer's labeling; however, pharmacokinetic studies have shown that hepatic dysfunction is not expected to significantly decrease clearance (Furlan, 1999; Greenblatt, 1981).

Mechanism of Action Binds to stereospecific benzodiazepine receptors on the postsynaptic GABA neuron at several sites within the central nervous system, including the limbic system, reticular formation. Enhancement of the inhibitory effect of GABA on neuronal excitability results by increased neuronal membrane permeability to chloride ions. This shift in chloride ions results in hyperpolarization (a less excitable state) and stabilization.

Contraindications Hypersensitivity to oxazepam or any component of the formulation (cross-sensitivity with other benzodiazepines may exist)

Warnings/Precautions May cause hypotension (rare) - use with caution in patients with cardiovascular or cerebrovascular disease, or in patients who would not tolerate transient decreases in blood pressure.

Use with caution in elderly or debilitated patients, patients with hepatic disease (including alcoholics). In older adults, benzodiazepines increase the risk of impaired cognition, delirium, falls, fractures, and motor vehicle accidents. Due to increased sensitivity in this age group, avoid use for treatment of insomnia, agitation, or delirium. (Beers Criteria). However, relative to other benzodiazepines, oxazepam possesses a short half-life and lacks an active metabolite which may be preferable in the elderly if benzodiazepine use is required for anxiety (Flint, 2005). Kinetics were not altered in patients of advanced age compared to younger patients, except in patients >80 years of age where an increased half-life was observed due to an increased volume of distribution and a decrease in unbound clearance. Use with caution in patients with respiratory disease or impaired gag reflex.

May cause CNS depression which may impair physical and mental capabilities. Patients must be cautioned about performing tasks which require mental alertness (eg, operating machinery or driving). Use with caution in patients receiving other CNS depressants or psychoactive agents; effects with other sedative drugs or ethanol may be potentiated. Benzodiazepines have been associated with falls and traumatic injury and should be used with extreme caution in patients who are at risk of these events.

Use caution in patients with depression, particularly if suicidal risk may be present. Use with caution in patients with a history of drug abuse or acute alcoholism; potential for drug dependency exists. Tolerance, psychological and physical dependence may occur with prolonged use. Rebound or withdrawal symptoms may occur following abrupt discontinuation or large decreases in dose. Use caution when reducing dose or withdrawing therapy; decrease slowly and monitor for withdrawal symptoms. Flumazenil may cause withdrawal in patients receiving long-term benzodiazepine therapy.

Benzodiazepines have been associated with transient amnesia. Paradoxical reactions, including hyperactive or aggressive behavior have been reported with benzodiazepines, particularly in adolescent/pediatric or psychiatric patients. Does not have analgesic, antidepressant, or antipsychotic properties; not indicated for use in the treatment of psychosis.

Drug Interactions

Metabolism/Transport Effects None known.

Avoid Concomitant Use

Avoid concomitant use of Oxazepam with any of the following: Azelastine (Nasal); OLANZapine; Paraldehyde; Sodium Oxybate

Increased Effect/Toxicity

Oxazepam may increase the levels/effects of: Alcohol (Ethyl); Azelastine (Nasal); Buprenorphine; CloZAPine; CNS Depressants; Fosphenytoin; Methotrimeprazine; Metyrosine; Mirtazapine; Paraldehyde;

Phenytoin; Pramipexole; ROPINIRole; Rotigotine; Selective Serotonin Reuptake Inhibitors; Sodium Oxybate; Zolpidem

The levels/effects of Oxazepam may be increased by: Droperidol; HydrOXYzine; Magnesium Sulfate; Methotrimeprazine; OLANZapine; Perampanel

Decreased Effect

The levels/effects of Oxazepam may be decreased by: Theophylline Derivatives; Yohimbine

Ethanol/Nutrition/Herb Interactions

Ethanol: May increase CNS depression; monitor for increased effects with coadministration. Caution patients about effects.

Herb/Nutraceutical: Avoid valerian, St John's wort, kava kava, gotu kola (may increase CNS depression).

Pharmacodynamics/Kinetics

Half-life Elimination ~8 hours

Time to Peak Serum: ~3 hours

Pregnancy Considerations Oxazepam crosses the placenta. Teratogenic effects have been observed with some benzodiazepines; however, additional studies are needed. The incidence of premature birth and low birth weights may be increased following maternal use of benzodiazepines; hypoglycemia and respiratory problems in the neonate may occur following exposure late in pregnancy. Neonatal withdrawal symptoms may occur within days to weeks after birth and "floppy infant syndrome" (which also includes withdrawal symptoms) have been reported with some benzodiazepines.

Breast-Feeding Considerations Drowsiness, lethargy, or weight loss in nursing infants have been observed in case reports following maternal use of some benzodiazepines.

Controlled Substance C-IV

Dosage Forms

Capsule, oral: 10 mg, 15 mg, 30 mg

OXcarbazepine (ox car BAZ e peen)

Brand Names: U.S. Oxtellar XR™; Trileptal®

Brand Names: Canada Apo-Oxcarbazepine®; Trileptal®

Pharmacologic Category Anticonvulsant, Miscellaneous

Use

Oxtellar XR™: Adjunctive therapy in the treatment of partial seizures in patients with epilepsy

Trileptal®: Monotherapy or adjunctive therapy in the treatment of partial seizures in patients with epilepsy

Unlabeled Use Bipolar disorder; treatment of neuropathic pain

Local Anesthetic/Vasoconstrictor Precautions No information available to require special precautions

Effects on Dental Treatment No significant effects or complications reported

Effects on Bleeding No information available to require special precautions

Adverse Effects As reported in adults with doses of up to 2400 mg/day (includes patients on monotherapy, adjunctive therapy, and those not previously on AEDs); incidence in children was similar.

>10%:

Central nervous system: Dizziness (22% to 49%), somnolence (20% to 36%), headache (13% to 32%), ataxia (5% to 31%), fatigue (12% to 15%), vertigo (6% to 15%)

Gastrointestinal: Vomiting (7% to 36%), nausea (15% to 29%), abdominal pain (10% to 13%)

Neuromuscular & skeletal: Abnormal gait (5% to 17%), tremor (3% to 16%)

Ocular: Diplopia (14% to 40%), nystagmus (7% to 26%), abnormal vision (4% to 14%)

1% to 10%:

Cardiovascular: Hypotension (≤2%), leg edema (1% to 2%)

Central nervous system: Nervousness (2% to 5%), amnesia (4%), abnormal thinking (≤4%), insomnia (2% to 4%), fever (3%), speech disorder (1% to 3%), abnormal feelings (≤2%), EEG abnormalities (≤2%), agitation (1% to 2%), confusion (1% to 2%)

Dermatologic: Rash (4%), acne (1% to 2%)

Endocrine & metabolic: Hyponatremia (1% to 3%)

Gastrointestinal: Diarrhea (5% to 7%), dyspepsia (5% to 6%), constipation (2% to 6%), taste perversion (5%), xerostomia (3%), gastritis (1% to 2%), weight gain (1% to 2%)

Genitourinary: Micturition (2%)

Neuromuscular & skeletal: Weakness (3% to 6%), back pain (4%), falling down (4%), abnormal coordination (1% to 4%), dysmetria (1% to 3%), sprains/strains (≤2%), muscle weakness (1% to 2%)

Ocular: Abnormal accommodation (≤2%)

Respiratory: Upper respiratory tract infection (7%), rhinitis (2% to 5%), chest infection (4%), epistaxis (4%), sinusitis (4%)

General Dosage Range Dosage adjustment recommended in patients with renal impairment

Oral:

Children 2-3 years and <20 kg: Immediate release (Trileptal®): Initial: 8-20 mg/kg/day (maximum: 600 mg daily) in 2 divided doses; Maintenance: maximum of 60 mg/kg/day in 2 divided doses

Children 2-3 years and ≥20 kg: Immediate release (Trileptal®): Initial: 8-10 mg/kg/day (maximum: 600 mg daily) in 2 divided doses; Maintenance: maximum of 60 mg/kg/day in 2 divided doses

Children 4-16 years: Immediate release (Trileptal®): Initial: 8-10 mg/kg/day (maximum: 600 mg daily) in 2 divided doses; Maintenance: Dependent on patient weight and indication

Children 6-17 years and ≤29 kg: Extended release (Oxtellar XR™): Initial: 8-10 mg/kg once daily (maximum: 600 mg daily in the first week); Maintenance: up to 900 mg once daily

Children 6-17 years and ≥29.1-39 kg: Extended release (Oxtellar XR™): Initial: 8-10 mg/kg once daily (maximum: 600 mg daily in the first week); Maintenance: up to 1200 mg once daily

Children 6-17 years and >39 kg: Extended release (Oxtellar XR™): Initial: 8-10 mg/kg once daily (maximum: 600 mg daily in the first week); Maintenance: up to 1800 mg once daily

Children >16 years and Adults: Immediate release (Trileptal®): Initial: 600 mg daily in 2 divided doses; Maintenance: 1200-2400 mg daily in 2 divided doses (maximum: 2400 mg daily)

Children >17 years and Adults: Extended release (Oxtellar XR™): Initial: 600 mg once daily; Maintenance: 1200-2400 mg once daily (maximum: 2400 mg daily)

Mechanism of Action Pharmacological activity results from both oxcarbazepine and its monohydroxy metabolite (MHD). Precise mechanism of anticonvulsant effect has not been defined. Oxcarbazepine and MHD block voltage-sensitive sodium channels, stabilizing hyperexcited neuronal membranes, inhibiting repetitive firing, and decreasing the propagation of synaptic impulses. These actions are believed to prevent the spread of seizures. Oxcarbazepine and MHD also increase potassium conductance and modulate the activity of high-voltage activated calcium channels.

Pharmacodynamics/Kinetics

Half-life Elimination Immediate release: Parent drug: 2 hours; MHD: 9 hours; renal impairment (Cl$_{cr}$ 30 mL/minute): MHD: 19 hours; Extended release: Parent drug: 7-11 hours; MHD: 9-11 hours

Clearance of MHD is increased in younger children (~80% in children 2-4 years of age) and approaches that of adults by ~13 years of age

Time to Peak Serum (median): Immediate release: Tablets: 4.5 hours; Oral suspension: 6 hours

Pregnancy Risk Factor C

Pregnancy Considerations Adverse events have been observed in animal reproduction studies; therefore, the manufacturer classifies oxcarbazepine as pregnancy category C. Oxcarbazepine, the active metabolite MHD and the inactive metabolite DHD, crosses the placenta and can be detected in the newborn. An increased risk in the overall rate of major congenital malformations has not been observed following maternal use of oxcarbazepine. Available studies have not been large enough to determine if there is an increased risk of specific defects. In general, the risk of teratogenic effects is higher with AED polytherapy than monotherapy. Plasma concentrations of MHD gradually decrease due to physiologic changes which occur during pregnancy; patients should be monitored during pregnancy and postpartum. Oxcarbazepine may decrease plasma concentrations of hormonal contraceptives.

Patients exposed to oxcarbazepine during pregnancy are encouraged to enroll themselves into the AED Pregnancy Registry by calling 1-888-233-2334. Additional information is available at www.aedpregnancy-registry.org.

Oxiconazole (oks i KON a zole)

Brand Names: U.S. Oxistat®

Brand Names: Canada Oxistat®

Pharmacologic Category Antifungal Agent, Topical

Use

Cream: Treatment of tinea pedis (athlete's foot), tinea cruris (jock itch), tinea corporis (ringworm), and tinea (pityriasis) versicolor

Lotion: Treatment of tinea pedis (athlete's foot), tinea cruris (jock itch), tinea corporis (ringworm)

Local Anesthetic/Vasoconstrictor Precautions No information available to require special precautions

Effects on Dental Treatment No significant effects or complications reported

Effects on Bleeding No information available to require special precautions

Adverse Effects 1% to 10%:

Dermatologic: Pruritus (<2%)

Local: Burning (≤1%)

General Dosage Range Topical: *Children ≥12 years, Adolescents, and Adults:* Apply to affected areas 1-2 times daily

Mechanism of Action The cytoplasmic membrane integrity of fungi is destroyed by oxiconazole which exerts a fungicidal activity through inhibition of ergosterol synthesis. Effective for treatment of tinea pedis, tinea cruris, tinea corporis, and tinea versicolor. Active against *Trichophyton rubrum*, *Trichophyton mentagrophytes*, *Trichophyton violaceum*, *Microsporum canis*, *Microsporum audouinii*, *Microsporum gypseum*,

Epidermophyton floccosum, Candida albicans, and *Malassezia furfur.*

Pregnancy Risk Factor B

Pregnancy Considerations When administered orally, teratogenic effects were not observed in animal reproduction studies.

Oxybutynin (oks i BYOO ti nin)

Brand Names: U.S. Ditropan XL®; Gelnique 3%™; Gelnique®; Oxytrol®

Brand Names: Canada Apo-Oxybutynin®; Ditropan XL®; Dom-Oxybutynin; Gelnique®; Mylan-Oxybutynin; Novo-Oxybutynin; Nu-Oxybutyn; Oxybutyn; Oxybutynine; Oxytrol®; PHL-Oxybutynin; PMS-Oxybutynin; Riva-Oxybutynin; Uromax®

Pharmacologic Category Antispasmodic Agent, Urinary

Use Antispasmodic for neurogenic bladder (urgency, frequency, leakage, urge incontinence, dysuria); extended release formulation also indicated for treatment of symptoms associated with detrusor overactivity due to a neurological condition (eg, spina bifida)

Local Anesthetic/Vasoconstrictor Precautions No information available to require special precautions

Effects on Dental Treatment Key adverse event(s) related to dental treatment: Xerostomia and changes in salivation (normal salivary flow resumes upon discontinuation), and taste perversion.

Effects on Bleeding No information available to require special precautions

Adverse Effects

Oral:

>10%:
  Central nervous system: Dizziness (4% to 17%), somnolence (2% to 14%)
  Gastrointestinal: Xerostomia (29% to 71%; dose related), constipation (7% to 15%), nausea (2% to 12%)

1% to 10%:
  Cardiovascular: Arrhythmia (sinus; 1% to <5%), blood pressure change (increased/decreased; 1% to <5%), chest pain (1% to <5%), edema (1% to <5%), flushing (1% to <5%), palpitation (1% to <5%), peripheral edema (1% to <5%)
  Central nervous system: Headache (6% to 10%), nervousness (1% to 7%), pain (1% to 7%), insomnia (1% to 6%), confusion (1% to <5%), depression (1% to <5%), fatigue (1% to <5%)
  Dermatologic: Dry skin (1% to <5%), pruritus (1% to <5%)
  Endocrine & metabolic: Fluid retention (1% to <5%), hyperglycemia (1% to <5%)
  Gastrointestinal: Diarrhea (1% to 9%), dyspepsia (5% to 7%), abdominal pain (1% to <5%), abnormal taste (1% to <5%), dry throat (1% to <5%), dysphagia (1% to <5%), eructation (1% to <5%), flatulence (1% to <5%), gastrointestinal reflux disease (1% to <5%), vomiting (1% to <5%)
  Genitourinary: Urinary hesitation (9%), urinary tract infection (5% to 7%), urinary retention (6%), cystitis (1% to <5%), dysuria (1% to <5%), pollakiuria (1% to <5%)
  Neuromuscular & skeletal: Weakness (1% to 7%), arthralgia (1% to <5%), back pain (1% to <5%), extremity pain (1% to <5%), flank pain (1% to <5%)
  Ocular: Blurred vision (1% to 10%), dry eyes (3% to 6%), eye irritation (1% to <5%), keratoconjunctivitis sicca (1% to <5%)

Respiratory: Asthma (1% to <5%), bronchitis (1% to <5%), cough (1% to <5%), hoarseness (1% to <5%), nasal congestion (1% to <5%), nasal dryness (1% to <5%), nasopharyngitis (1% to <5%), pharyngolaryngeal pain (1% to <5%), sinus congestion (1% to <5%), upper respiratory tract infection (1% to <5%)
  Miscellaneous: Fungal infection (1% to <5%), thirst (1% to <5%)

Topical gel:

>10%:
  Gastrointestinal: Xerostomia (7% to 12%)
  Local: Application site reaction (4% to 14%; includes dermatitis, erythema, irritation, pain, papules, pruritus, rash)

1% to 10%:
  Central nervous system: Dizziness (2% to 3%), fatigue (2%), headache (2%)
  Dermatologic: Pruritus (1%)
  Gastrointestinal: Gastroenteritis (2%), constipation (1%)
  Genitourinary: Urinary tract infection (5% to 7%)
  Ocular: Conjunctivitis (4%), blurred vision (<2%), dry eyes (<2%)
  Respiratory: Nasopharyngitis (3% to 5%)

Transdermal:

>10%: Local: Application site reaction (17%), pruritus (14%)

1% to 10%:
  Gastrointestinal: Xerostomia (4% to 10%), constipation (3%), diarrhea (3%)
  Genitourinary: Dysuria (2%)
  Local: Erythema (6% to 8%), rash (3%), vesicles (3%)
  Ocular: Vision changes (3%)

General Dosage Range

Oral:

Extended release:
  Children ≥6 years: 5 mg once daily (maximum: 20 mg/day)
  Adults: Initial: 5-10 mg once daily; Maintenance: 5-30 mg once daily (maximum: 30 mg/day)

Immediate release:
  Children ≥5 years: 5 mg 2-3 times/day (maximum: 15 mg/day)
  Adults: 5 mg 2-4 times/day (maximum: 20 mg/day)
  Elderly: 2.5 mg 2-3 times/day

Topical gel: *Adults:* Gelnique 3%™: Apply 3 pumps (84 mg) once daily; Gelnique® 10%: Apply contents of 1 sachet (100 mg/g) once daily

Transdermal: *Adults:* Apply one 3.9 mg/day patch twice weekly

Mechanism of Action Direct antispasmodic effect on smooth muscle, also inhibits the action of acetylcholine on smooth muscle (exhibits 1/5 the anticholinergic activity of atropine, but is 4-10 times the antispasmodic activity); does not block effects at skeletal muscle or at autonomic ganglia; increases bladder capacity, decreases uninhibited contractions, and delays desire to void, therefore, decreases urgency and frequency

Pharmacodynamics/Kinetics

Onset of Action Onset of action: Oral: 30-60 minutes; Peak effect: 3-6 hours

Duration of Action 6-10 hours (up to 24 hours for extended release oral formulation)

Half-life Elimination I.V.: ~2 hours (parent drug), 7-8 hours (metabolites); Oral: Immediate release: ~2-3 hours; Extended release: ~13 hours; Transdermal: 30-64 hours

Time to Peak Serum: Oral: Immediate release: ~60 minutes; Extended release: 4-6 hours; Transdermal: 24-48 hours

Pregnancy Risk Factor B

Pregnancy Considerations Teratogenic effects were not observed in animal reproduction studies.

Product Availability Oxytrol® for Women: FDA approved January 2013; availability anticipated in the fall of 2013. Oxytrol® for Women is an over-the-counter (OTC) transdermal patch indicated for the treatment of overactive bladder.

Oxychlorosene (oks i KLOR oh seen)

Brand Names: U.S. Clorpactin® WCS-90 [OTC]

Pharmacologic Category Antibiotic, Topical

Use Treatment of localized infections

Local Anesthetic/Vasoconstrictor Precautions No information available to require special precautions

Effects on Dental Treatment No significant effects or complications reported

Effects on Bleeding No information available to require special precautions

General Dosage Range Topical: *Adults:* Apply by irrigation, instillation, spray, soaks, or wet compresses

OxyCODONE (oks i KOE done)

Related Information

Oral Pain *on page 1558*

Brand Names: U.S. Oxecta™; OxyCONTIN®; Roxicodone®

Brand Names: Canada Apo-Oxycodone CR; CO Oxycodone CR; Oxy.IR®; OxyContin®; OxyNEO™; PMS-Oxycodone; PMS-Oxycodone CR; Supeudol®

Generic Availability (U.S.) Yes: Excludes controlled release tablet

Pharmacologic Category Analgesic, Opioid

Dental Use Treatment of postoperative pain

Use Management of moderate-to-severe pain, normally used in combination with nonopioid analgesics

OxyContin® is indicated for around-the-clock management of moderate-to-severe pain when a continuous analgesic is needed for an extended period of time.

Local Anesthetic/Vasoconstrictor Precautions No information available to require special precautions

Effects on Dental Treatment Key adverse event(s) related to dental treatment: Xerostomia (normal salivary flow resumes upon discontinuation).

Effects on Bleeding No information available to require special precautions

Adverse Effects Note: Percentages as reported with OxyContin®

>10%:

Central nervous system: Somnolence (23%), dizziness (13%)

Dermatologic: Pruritus (13%)

Gastrointestinal: Constipation (23%), nausea (23%), vomiting (12%)

1% to 10%:

Cardiovascular: Orthostatic hypotension (1% to 5%)

Central nervous system: Headache (7%), abnormal dreams (1% to 5%), anxiety (1% to 5%), chills (1% to 5%), confusion (1% to 5%), dysphoria (1% to 5%), euphoria (1% to 5%), fever (1% to 5%), insomnia (1% to 5%), nervousness (1% to 5%), thought abnormalities (1% to 5%)

Dermatologic: Rash (1% to 5%)

Gastrointestinal: Xerostomia (6%), abdominal pain (1% to 5%), anorexia (1% to 5%), diarrhea (1% to 5%), dyspepsia (1% to 5%), gastritis (1% to 5%)

Neuromuscular & skeletal: Weakness (6%), twitching (1% to 5%)

Respiratory: Dyspnea (1% to 5%), hiccups (1% to 5%)

Miscellaneous: Diaphoresis (5%)

Dental Usual Dosage Postoperative pain: Adults: Oral: 5 mg every 6 hours as needed

Dosage Oral: **Note:** All doses should be titrated to appropriate effect:

Children (unlabeled use): Immediate release, initial dose: 0.1-0.2 mg/kg/dose (moderate pain) or 0.2 mg/kg/dose (severe pain) (APS 6th edition). For severe chronic pain, administer on a regularly scheduled basis, every 4-6 hours, at the lowest dose that will achieve adequate analgesia.

Adults:

Immediate release: Initial: 5-15 mg every 4-6 hours as needed; dosing range: 5-20 mg per dose (APS 6th edition). For severe chronic pain, administer on a regularly scheduled basis, every 4-6 hours, at the lowest dose that will achieve adequate analgesia.

Controlled release: **Note:** 60 mg and 80 mg strengths, a single dose >40 mg, or a total dose of >80 mg daily are for use only in opioid-tolerant patients.

Opioid naive: Initial: 10 mg every 12 hours

Concurrent CNS depressants: Reduce usual initial oxycodone dose by one-third ($1/3$) to one-half ($1/2$)

Conversion from transdermal fentanyl: For each 25 mcg/hour transdermal dose, substitute 10 mg controlled release oxycodone every 12 hours; should be initiated 18 hours after the removal of the transdermal fentanyl patch

Currently on opioids: Use standard conversion chart to convert daily opioid dose to oxycodone equivalent. Initiate controlled release oxycodone with one-half ($1/2$) the estimated oxycodone daily dose (mg/day) and provide rescue medication in the form of immediate release oxycodone. Divide the initial controlled release oxycodone daily dose in 2 (for twice-daily dosing, usually every 12 hours) and round down to nearest dosage form.

Dose adjustment: Doses may be adjusted by changing the total daily dose (not by changing the dosing interval). Doses may be adjusted every 1-2 days and may be increased by 25% to 50%. Dose should be gradually tapered when no longer required in order to prevent withdrawal.

Multiplication factors for converting the daily dose of current oral opioid to the daily dose of oral oxycodone:

Current opioid mg/day dose x factor = Oxycodone mg/day dose

Codeine mg/day oral dose **x** 0.15 = Oxycodone mg/day dose

Hydrocodone mg/day oral dose **x** 0.9 = Oxycodone mg/day dose

Hydromorphone mg/day oral dose **x** 4 = Oxycodone mg/day dose

Levorphanol mg/day oral dose **x** 7.5 = Oxycodone mg/day dose

Meperidine mg/day oral dose **x** 0.1 = Oxycodone mg/day dose

Methadone mg/day oral dose **x** 1.5 = Oxycodone mg/day dose

Morphine mg/day oral dose **x** 0.5 = Oxycodone mg/day dose

Note: Divide the oxycodone mg/day dose into the appropriate dosing interval for the specific form being used.

Dosage adjustment in renal impairment: Serum concentrations are increased ~50% in patients with Cl_{cr} <60 mL/minute; adjust dose based on clinical situation.

Dosage adjustment in hepatic impairment:

Immediate release: Reduced initial doses may be necessary (use a conservative approach to initial dosing); adjust dose based on clinical situation.

Controlled release: Decrease initial dose to one-third ($^1/_3$) to one-half ($^1/_2$) the usual starting dose; titrate carefully.

Mechanism of Action Binds to opiate receptors in the CNS, causing inhibition of ascending pain pathways, altering the perception of and response to pain; produces generalized CNS depression

Contraindications Hypersensitivity to oxycodone or any component of the formulation; significant respiratory depression; hypercarbia; acute or severe bronchial asthma; paralytic ileus (known or suspected); GI obstruction

Warnings/Precautions May cause CNS depression, which may impair physical or mental abilities; patients must be cautioned about performing tasks which require mental alertness (eg, operating machinery or driving). Effects may be potentiated when used with other sedative drugs or ethanol. Use with caution in patients with hypersensitivity reactions to other phenanthrene derivative opioid agonists (morphine, hydrocodone, hydromorphone, levorphanol, oxymorphone), respiratory diseases including asthma, emphysema, or COPD. Use with caution in pancreatitis or biliary tract disease, acute alcoholism (including delirium tremens), morbid obesity, adrenocortical insufficiency, history of seizure disorders, CNS depression/coma, kyphoscoliosis (or other skeletal disorder which may alter respiratory function), hypothyroidism (including myxedema), prostatic hyperplasia, urethral stricture, and toxic psychosis. May obscure diagnosis or clinical course of patients with acute abdominal conditions.

Use with caution in the elderly, debilitated, or cachectic patients, and hepatic or renal dysfunction. Hemodynamic effects (hypotension, orthostasis) may be exaggerated in patients with hypovolemia, concurrent vasodilating drugs, or in patients with head injury. Monitor for symptoms of hypotension following initiation or dose titration. Respiratory depressant effects and capacity to elevate CSF pressure may be exaggerated in presence of head injury, other intracranial lesion, or pre-existing intracranial pressure.

Concomitant use with CYP3A4 inhibitors may result in increased effects and potentially fatal respiratory depression. Concurrent use of agonist/antagonist analgesics may precipitate withdrawal symptoms and/or reduced analgesic efficacy in patients following prolonged therapy with mu opioid agonists. Abrupt discontinuation following prolonged use may also lead to withdrawal symptoms. Healthcare provider should be alert to problems of abuse, misuse, and diversion; abuse of products by crushing, chewing, snorting, or injecting may result in severe overdose, adverse effects, or death.

Controlled-release tablets: OxyContin® is not intended for use as an "as needed" analgesic or for the treatment of mild pain, acute pain, or postoperative pain requiring short-term analgesia (should be used postoperatively only if the patient has received it prior to surgery or if severe, persistent pain is anticipated). **[U.S. Boxed Warning]: May cause potentially life-threatening respiratory depression even with therapeutic use. Ensure proper dosing and titration; monitor for respiratory depression especially within the first 24-72 hours of initiation or dose escalation. Oxycodone controlled-release tablets should only be prescribed by healthcare professionals familiar with the use of potent opioids for chronic pain. Do NOT crush, break, chew or dissolve controlled-release tablets (may result in a potentially fatal overdose);** 60 mg and 80 mg strengths, a single dose >40 mg, or a total dose of >80 mg/day are for use only in opioid-tolerant patients. Tablets may be difficult to swallow and could become lodged in throat; patients with swallowing difficulties may be at increased risk. Cases of intestinal obstruction or diverticulitis exacerbation have also been reported, including cases requiring medical intervention to remove the tablet; patients with an underlying GI disease (eg, esophageal cancer, colon cancer) may be at increased risk. **[U.S. Boxed Warning]: Accidental exposure may result in fatal overdose of oxycodone, especially in children. [U.S. Boxed Warning]: Healthcare provider should be alert to problems of abuse, misuse, and diversion. Tolerance or drug dependence may result from extended use. Patients should be assessed for risk of abuse or addiction prior to therapy and all patients should be monitored for signs of misuse, abuse, and addiction. Risk of opioid abuse is increased in patients with a history or family history of alcohol or drug abuse or mental illness.**

Oral solutions: **[U.S. Boxed Warning]: Highly concentrated oral solution (20 mg/mL) should only be used in opioid tolerant patients (taking ≥30 mg/day of oxycodone or equivalent for ≥1 week). [U.S. Boxed Warning]: Orders for oxycodone oral solutions (20 mg/mL or 5 mg/5 mL) should be clearly written to include the intended dose (in mg vs mL) and the intended product concentration to be dispensed to avoid potential dosing errors. Products should be stored out of reach of children; seek immediate medical care in the event of accidental ingestion.**

Drug Interactions

Metabolism/Transport Effects Substrate of CYP2D6 (minor), CYP3A4 (major); **Note:** Assignment of Major/Minor substrate status based on clinically relevant drug interaction potential

Avoid Concomitant Use

Avoid concomitant use of OxyCODONE with any of the following: Azelastine (Nasal); Conivaptan; Paraldehyde

Increased Effect/Toxicity

OxyCODONE may increase the levels/effects of: Alcohol (Ethyl); Alvimopan; Azelastine (Nasal); CNS Depressants; Desmopressin; Metyrosine; Mirtazapine; Paraldehyde; Pramipexole; ROPINIRole; Rotigotine; Selective Serotonin Reuptake Inhibitors; Thiazide Diuretics; Zolpidem

The levels/effects of OxyCODONE may be increased by: Amphetamines; Antipsychotic Agents (Phenothiazines); Conivaptan; CYP3A4 Inhibitors (Moderate); CYP3A4 Inhibitors (Strong); Dasatinib; Droperidol; HydrOXYzine; Ivacaftor; Magnesium Sulfate; Mifepristone; Perampanel; Sodium Oxybate; Succinylcholine; Voriconazole

Decreased Effect

OxyCODONE may decrease the levels/effects of: Pegvisomant

The levels/effects of OxyCODONE may be decreased by: Ammonium Chloride; CYP3A4 Inducers (Strong); Deferasirox; Mixed Agonist / Antagonist Opioids; Rifampin; St Johns Wort; Tocilizumab

Ethanol/Nutrition/Herb Interactions

Ethanol: May increase CNS depression; monitor for increased effects with coadministration. Caution patients about effects.

Herb/Nutraceutical: Avoid valerian, St John's wort, kava kava, gotu kola (may increase CNS depression).

Dietary Considerations Instruct patient to avoid high-fat meals when taking some products (food has no effect on the reformulated OxyContin®).

Pharmacodynamics/Kinetics

Onset of Action Pain relief: Immediate release: 10-15 minutes; Peak effect: Immediate release: 0.5-1 hour

Duration of Action Immediate release: 3-6 hours; Controlled release: ≤12 hours

Half-life Elimination Immediate release: 2-4 hours; Controlled release: ~5 hours

Time to Peak Plasma: Immediate release: 1.2-1.9 hours; Controlled release: 4-5 hours

Pregnancy Risk Factor B

Pregnancy Considerations Adverse events were not observed in animal reproduction studies. Opioids cross the placenta; respiratory depression and withdrawal symptoms may occur in the neonate following use during pregnancy. Controlled release formulations should not be used immediately prior to or during labor.

Lactation Enters breast milk/not recommended

Breast-Feeding Considerations Sedation and/or respiratory depression may occur in the infant; symptoms of opioid withdrawal may occur following the cessation of breast-feeding.

Controlled Substance C-II

Prescribing and Access Restrictions As a requirement of the REMS program, healthcare providers who prescribe OxyContin® need to receive training on the proper use and potential risks of OxyContin®. For training, please refer to http://www.oxycontinrems.com. Prescribers will need retraining every 2 years or following any significant changes to the OxyContin® REMS program.

Dosage Forms

Capsule, oral: 5 mg

Solution, oral: 5 mg/5 mL (5 mL, 100 mL, 500 mL); 20 mg/mL (30 mL)

Tablet, oral: 5 mg, 10 mg, 15 mg, 20 mg, 30 mg
Oxecta™: 5 mg, 7.5 mg
Roxicodone®: 15 mg, 30 mg

Tablet, controlled release, oral:
OxyCONTIN®: 10 mg, 15 mg, 20 mg, 30 mg, 40 mg, 60 mg, 80 mg

Oxycodone and Acetaminophen
(oks i KOE done & a seet a MIN oh fen)

Related Information

Acetaminophen on page 27
Oral Pain on page 1558
OxyCODONE on page 1028

Related Sample Prescriptions

Severe Oral Pain on page 1606

Brand Names: U.S. Endocet®; Magnacet®; Percocet®; Primlev™; Roxicet™; Roxicet™ 5/500; Tylox® [DSC]

Brand Names: Canada Endocet®; Novo-Oxycodone Acet; Oxycocet®; Percocet®; Percocet®-Demi; PMS-Oxycodone-Acetaminophen

Generic Availability (U.S.) Yes: Excludes caplet and solution

Pharmacologic Category Analgesic Combination (Opioid)

Dental Use Treatment of postoperative pain

Use Management of moderate-to-severe pain

Local Anesthetic/Vasoconstrictor Precautions No information available to require special precautions

Effects on Dental Treatment Key adverse event(s) related to dental treatment: Nausea, sedation, constipation, and xerostomia (normal salivary flow resumes upon discontinuation). See Dental Comment.

Effects on Bleeding No information available to require special precautions

Adverse Effects Frequency not defined (also see individual agents): Allergic reaction, constipation, dizziness, dysphoria, euphoria, lightheadedness, nausea, pruritus, respiratory depression, sedation, skin rash, vomiting

Dental Usual Dosage

Note: Initial dose is based on the **oxycodone** content; however, the maximum daily dose is based on the **acetaminophen** content.

Management of pain: Doses should be given every 4-6 hours as needed and titrated to appropriate analgesic effects.

Mild-to-moderate pain:

Children: Initial dose, **based on oxycodone content:** 0.05-0.1 mg/kg/dose

Maximum acetaminophen dose: Children <45 kg: 90 mg/kg/day; children >45 kg: 4 g/day

Adults: Initial dose, **based on oxycodone content:** 2.5-5 mg

Severe pain:

Children: Initial dose, **based on oxycodone content:** 0.3 mg/kg/dose

Adults: Initial dose, **based on oxycodone content:** 10-30 mg. Do not exceed acetaminophen 4 g/day.

Elderly: Doses should be titrated to appropriate analgesic effects: Initial dose, **based on oxycodone content:** 2.5-5 mg every 6 hours. Do not exceed acetaminophen 4 g/day.

Dosage adjustment in hepatic impairment: Dose should be reduced in patients with severe liver disease.

Dosage Oral: Doses should be given every 4-6 hours as needed and titrated to appropriate analgesic effects.

Note: Initial dose is based on the **oxycodone** content; however, the maximum daily dose is based on the **acetaminophen** content.

Children: Maximum acetaminophen dose: Children <45 kg: 90 mg/kg/day; children >45 kg: 4 g/day

Mild-to-moderate pain: Initial dose, **based on oxycodone content:** 0.05-0.1 mg/kg/dose

Severe pain: Initial dose, **based on oxycodone content:** 0.3 mg/kg/dose

Adults:

Mild-to-moderate pain: Initial dose, **based on oxycodone content:** 2.5-5 mg

Severe pain: Initial dose, **based on oxycodone content:** 10-30 mg. Do not exceed acetaminophen 4 g/day.

Elderly: Doses should be titrated to appropriate analgesic effects: Initial dose, **based on oxycodone content:** 2.5-5 mg every 6 hours. Do not exceed acetaminophen 4 g/day.

Dosage adjustment in hepatic impairment: Dose should be reduced in patients with severe liver disease.

Mechanism of Action

Oxycodone, as with other narcotic (opiate) analgesics, blocks pain perception in the cerebral cortex by binding to specific receptor molecules (opiate receptors) within the neuronal membranes of synapses. This binding results in a decreased synaptic chemical transmission throughout the CNS thus inhibiting the flow of pain sensations into the higher centers. Mu and kappa are the two subtypes of the opiate receptor to which oxycodone binds to cause analgesia.

Acetaminophen inhibits the synthesis of prostaglandins in the CNS and peripherally blocks pain impulse generation; produces antipyresis from inhibition of hypothalamic heat-regulating center.

Contraindications

Hypersensitivity to oxycodone, acetaminophen, or any component of the formulation; severe respiratory depression (in absence of resuscitative equipment or ventilatory support); pregnancy (prolonged periods or high doses at term)

Warnings/Precautions

Use with caution in patients with hypersensitivity reactions to other phenanthrene-derivative opioid agonists (morphine, codeine, hydrocodone, hydromorphone, levorphanol, oxymorphone); respiratory diseases including asthma, emphysema, COPD; severe liver or renal insufficiency; hypothyroidism; Addison's disease; seizure disorder; toxic psychosis; morbid obesity; CNS depression/coma; biliary tract impairment; prostatic hyperplasia; or urethral stricture. May obscure diagnosis or clinical course of patients with acute abdominal conditions. Some preparations contain sulfites which may cause allergic reactions. May be habit-forming. Causes sedation; caution must be used in performing tasks which require alertness (eg, operating machinery or driving). Effects may be potentiated when used with other sedative drugs or ethanol. May cause hypotension. Concurrent use of agonist/antagonist analgesics may precipitate withdrawal symptoms and/or reduced analgesic efficacy in patients following prolonged therapy with mu opioid agonists. Abrupt discontinuation following prolonged use may also lead to withdrawal symptoms.

Use with caution in patients with head injury and increased intracranial pressure (respiratory depressant effects increased and may also elevate CSF pressure).

Enhanced analgesia has been seen in elderly and debilitated patients on therapeutic doses of narcotics. Duration of action may be increased in the elderly. The elderly may be particularly susceptible to the CNS depressant and constipating effects of narcotics.

[U.S. Boxed Warning]: Acetaminophen may cause severe hepatotoxicity, potentially requiring liver transplant or resulting in death; hepatotoxicity is usually associated with excessive acetaminophen intake (>4 g/day). Risk is increased with alcohol use, pre-existing liver disease, and intake of more than one source of acetaminophen-containing medications. Chronic daily dosing in adults has also resulted in liver damage in some patients. Hypersensitivity and anaphylactic reactions have been reported with acetaminophen use; discontinue immediately if symptoms of allergic or hypersensitivity reactions occur. Use with caution in patients with known G6PD deficiency.

Drug Interactions

Metabolism/Transport Effects Refer to individual components.

Avoid Concomitant Use

Avoid concomitant use of Oxycodone and Acetaminophen with any of the following: Azelastine (Nasal); Conivaptan; Paraldehyde; Pimozide

Increased Effect/Toxicity

Oxycodone and Acetaminophen may increase the levels/effects of: Alcohol (Ethyl); Alvimopan; ARIPiprazole; Azelastine (Nasal); Busulfan; CNS Depressants; Dasatinib; Desmopressin; Imatinib; Lomitapide; Metyrosine; Mipomersen; Mirtazapine; Paraldehyde; Pimozide; Pramipexole; Prilocaine; ROPINIRole; Rotigotine; Selective Serotonin Reuptake Inhibitors; SORAfenib; Thiazide Diuretics; Vitamin K Antagonists; Zolpidem

The levels/effects of Oxycodone and Acetaminophen may be increased by: Amphetamines; Antipsychotic Agents (Phenothiazines); Conivaptan; CYP3A4 Inhibitors (Moderate); CYP3A4 Inhibitors (Strong); Dasatinib; Droperidol; HydrOXYzine; Imatinib; Isoniazid; Ivacaftor; Magnesium Sulfate; Metyrapone; Mifepristone; Perampanel; Probenecid; Sodium Oxybate; SORAfenib; Succinylcholine; Voriconazole

Decreased Effect

Oxycodone and Acetaminophen may decrease the levels/effects of: Pegvisomant

The levels/effects of Oxycodone and Acetaminophen may be decreased by: Ammonium Chloride; Anticonvulsants (Hydantoin); Barbiturates; CarBAMazepine; Cholestyramine Resin; CYP3A4 Inducers (Strong); Deferasirox; Mixed Agonist / Antagonist Opioids; Peginterferon Alfa-2b; Rifampin; St Johns Wort; Tocilizumab

Ethanol/Nutrition/Herb Interactions Ethanol: Excessive intake of ethanol may increase the risk of acetaminophen-induced hepatotoxicity. Avoid ethanol or limit to <3 drinks/day. Ethanol may also increase CNS depression; monitor for increased effects with co-administration. Caution patients about effects.

Pregnancy Risk Factor C

Pregnancy Considerations Use of opioids during pregnancy may produce physical dependence in the neonate; respiratory depression may occur in the newborn if opioids are used prior to delivery (especially high doses).

Lactation Enters breast milk/use caution

Breast-Feeding Considerations

Oxycodone: Excreted in breast milk. If occasional doses are used during breast-feeding, monitor infant for sedation, GI effects, and changes in feeding pattern. Acetaminophen: May be taken while breast-feeding.

Controlled Substance C-II

Dosage Forms

Caplet, oral: Oxycodone 5 mg and acetaminophen 500 mg

Roxicet™ 5/500: Oxycodone 5 mg and acetaminophen 500 mg

Capsule, oral: Oxycodone 5 mg and acetaminophen 500 mg

Solution, oral: Oxycodone 5 mg and acetaminophen 325 mg per 5 mL

Roxicet™: Oxycodone 5 mg and acetaminophen 325 mg per 5 mL

Tablet, oral: 2.5/325: Oxycodone hydrochloride 2.5 mg and acetaminophen 325 mg; 5/325: Oxycodone hydrochloride 5 mg and acetaminophen 325 mg; 7.5/325: Oxycodone hydrochloride 7.5 mg and acetaminophen 325 mg; 7.5/500: Oxycodone hydrochloride 7.5 mg and acetaminophen 500 mg; 10/325: Oxycodone hydrochloride 10 mg and acetaminophen 325 mg; 10/650: Oxycodone hydrochloride 10 mg and acetaminophen 650 mg

Endocet® 5/325 [scored]: Oxycodone 5 mg and acetaminophen 325 mg

Endocet® 7.5/325: Oxycodone 7.5 mg and acetaminophen 325 mg

Endocet® 7.5/500: Oxycodone 7.5 mg and acetaminophen 500 mg

Endocet® 10/325: Oxycodone 10 mg and acetaminophen 325 mg

Endocet® 10/650: Oxycodone 10 mg and acetaminophen 650 mg

Magnacet® 5/400: Oxycodone 5 mg and acetaminophen 400 mg

Magnacet® 10/400: Oxycodone 10 mg and acetaminophen 400 mg

Percocet® 2.5/325: Oxycodone 2.5 mg and acetaminophen 325 mg

Percocet® 5/325 [scored]: Oxycodone 5 mg and acetaminophen 325 mg

Percocet® 7.5/325: Oxycodone 7.5 mg and acetaminophen 325 mg

Percocet® 7.5/500: Oxycodone 7.5 mg and acetaminophen 500 mg

Percocet® 10/325: Oxycodone 10 mg and acetaminophen 325 mg

Percocet® 10/650: Oxycodone 10 mg and acetaminophen 650 mg

Primlev™ 5/300: Oxycodone 5 mg and acetaminophen 300 mg

Primlev™ 7.5/300: Oxycodone 7.5 mg and acetaminophen 300 mg

Primlev™ 10/300: Oxycodone 10 mg and acetaminophen 300 mg

Roxicet™ [scored]: Oxycodone 5 mg and acetaminophen 325 mg

Dental Comment Oxycodone, as with other opioid analgesics, is recommended only for limited acute dosing (ie, 3 days or less). Oxycodone has an addictive liability, especially when given long-term. The acetaminophen component requires use with caution in patients with alcoholic liver disease.

Hepatotoxicity caused by acetaminophen is potentiated by chronic alcohol consumption. People who are taking acetaminophen, even at therapeutic doses, and consume alcohol are at risk of developing hepatotoxicity.

Acetaminophen may increase the levels and enhance the anticoagulant effects of vitamin K antagonists acenocoumarol and warfarin (Coumadin®). Studies have reported that acetaminophen has increased the INR in warfarin treated patients with daily acetaminophen doses as low as 2 g, particularly when taking acetaminophen for >1 week (Antlitz, 1968; Boeijinga, 1982; Gebauer, 2003; Hylek, 1998; Rubin, 1984). In addition, case reports of bleeding as a result of increased INR have been published (Bagheri, 1999; Bartle, 1991). There is no known mechanism of the interaction; furthermore, some studies have failed to demonstrate this interaction (Gadisseur, 2003; Kwan, 1995; van den Bemt, 2002). In terms of risk, the data suggest that acetaminophen and warfarin could interact in some clinically significant manner but that the benefits of concomitant use of acetaminophen for pain control in dental patients taking warfarin usually outweigh the risks. An appropriate monitoring plan should be in place to identify potential negative effects and dosage adjustments may be necessary in a minority of patients. The interaction may be more likely to occur with daily acetaminophen doses of >1.3 g for >1 week.

There are no reports of acetaminophen interacting with antiplatelet drugs such as aspirin, clopidogrel (Plavix®), or prasugrel (Effient™). Also, there are no reports of acetaminophen in combination with hydrocodone, codeine, or oxycodone interacting with warfarin (Coumadin®).

References

Antlitz AM, Mead JA Jr, and Tolentino MA, "Potentiation of Oral Anticoagulant Therapy by Acetaminophen," *Curr Ther Res Clin Exp*, 1968, 10(10):501-7.

Bagheri H, Bernhard NB, and Montastruc JL, "Potentiation of the Acenocoumarol Anticoagulant Effect by Acetaminophen," *Ann Pharmacother*, 1999, 33(4):506.

Bartle WR and Blakely JA, "Potentiation of Warfarin Anticoagulation by Acetaminophen," *JAMA*, 1991, 265(10):1260.

Boeijinga JJ, Boerstra EE, Ris P, et al, "Interaction Between Paracetamol and Coumarin Anticoagulants," *Lancet*, 1982, 1(8270):506.

Gadisseur AP, Van Der Meer FJ, and Rosendaal FR, "Sustained Intake of Paracetamol (Acetaminophen) During Oral Anticoagulant Therapy With Coumarins Does Not Cause Clinically Important INR Changes: A Randomized Double-Blind Clinical Trial," *J Thromb Haemost*, 2003, 1(4):714-7.

Gebauer MG, Nyfort-Hansen K, Henschke PJ, et al, "Warfarin and Acetaminophen Interaction," *Pharmacotherapy*, 2003, 23(1):109-12.

Hylek EM, Heiman H, Skates SJ, et al, "Acetaminophen and Other Risk Factors for Excessive Warfarin Anticoagulation," *JAMA*, 1998, 279(9):657-62.

Kwan D, Bartle WR, and Walker SE, "The Effects of Acute and Chronic Acetaminophen Dosing on the Pharmacodynamics and Pharmacokinetics of (R)- and (S)-Warfarin," *Clin Pharmacol Ther*, 1995, 57:212.

Rubin RN, Mentzer RL, and Budzynski AZ, "Potentiation of Anticoagulant Effect of Warfarin by Acetaminophen (Tylenol®)," *Clin Res*, 1984, 32:698a.

van den Bemt PM, Geven LM, Kuitert NA, et al, "The Potential Interaction Between Oral Anticoagulants and Acetaminophen in Everyday Practice," *Pharm World Sci*, 2002, 24(5):201-4.

Oxycodone and Aspirin
(oks i KOE done & AS pir in)

Related Information
Aspirin *on page 135*
Oral Pain *on page 1558*
OxyCODONE *on page 1028*

Brand Names: U.S. Endodan®; Percodan®

Brand Names: Canada Endodan®; Oxycodan®; Percodan®

Generic Availability (U.S.) Yes

Pharmacologic Category Analgesic Combination (Opioid)

Dental Use Treatment of postoperative pain

Use Management of moderate- to moderately-severe pain

Local Anesthetic/Vasoconstrictor Precautions No information available to require special precautions

Effects on Dental Treatment Key adverse event(s) related to dental treatment: Nausea, sedation, constipation, and xerostomia (normal salivary flow resumes upon discontinuation). May have anticoagulant effects which may affect bleeding time. The elderly are a high-risk population for adverse effects from NSAIDs. As many as 60% of elderly patients with GI complications from NSAIDs can develop peptic ulceration and/or hemorrhage asymptomatically. Concomitant disease and drug use contribute to the risk of GI adverse effects. Enhanced analgesia has been seen with therapeutic doses of opioids; duration of action may be increased. Elderly may also be particularly susceptible to the CNS depressant effects of opioids. See Effects on Bleeding and Dental Comment.

Effects on Bleeding Aspirin irreversibly inhibits platelet aggregation which can prolong bleeding. Upon discontinuation, normal platelet function returns only when new platelets are released (~7-10 days). However, in the case of dental surgery, there is no scientific evidence to support discontinuation of aspirin.

Adverse Effects Note: Also see individual agents
Frequency not defined.

Cardiovascular: Circulatory depression, hypotension, shock

Central nervous system: Dizziness, drowsiness, dysphoria, euphoria, lightheadedness, sedation

Dermatologic: Pruritus

Gastrointestinal: Constipation, nausea, vomiting

Respiratory: Apnea, respiratory arrest, respiratory depression

Dental Usual Dosage

Analgesic: Oral (based on oxycodone combined salts):
Children: Maximum oxycodone: 5 mg/dose; maximum aspirin dose should not exceed 4 g/day. Doses should be given every 6 hours as needed.

Mild-to-moderate pain: Initial dose, **based on oxycodone content:** 0.05-0.1 mg/kg/dose

Severe pain: Initial dose, **based on oxycodone content:** 0.3 mg/kg/dose

Adults: Percodan®: 1 tablet every 6 hours as needed for pain; maximum aspirin dose should not exceed 4 g/day.

Dosage Oral:

Children (dose based on total oxycodone content): Oxycodone 0.1-0.2 mg/kg/dose (maximum oxycodone: 5 mg/dose; maximum aspirin: 4 g/day). Doses should be given every 4-6 hours as needed (American Pain Society, 2008)

Adults: One tablet every 6 hours as needed for pain; maximum aspirin dose should not exceed 4 g/day

Dosing adjustment in renal impairment: Use with caution. Avoid use of aspirin in patients with Cl$_{cr}$ <10 mL/minute.

Dosing adjustment in hepatic impairment: Use with caution. Avoid use of aspirin-containing products in severe impairment.

Mechanism of Action

Oxycodone, as with other narcotic (opiate) analgesics, blocks pain perception in the cerebral cortex by binding to specific receptor molecules (opiate receptors) within the neuronal membranes of synapses. This binding results in a decreased synaptic chemical transmission throughout the CNS, thus inhibiting the flow of pain sensations into the higher centers. Mu and kappa are the two subtypes of the opiate receptor to which oxycodone binds to cause analgesia.

Aspirin inhibits prostaglandin synthesis by decreasing the activity of the enzyme, cyclooxygenase, which results in decreased formation of prostaglandin precursors, acts on the hypothalamic heat-regulating center to reduce fever, blocks thromboxane synthetase action which prevents formation of the platelet-aggregating substance thromboxane A$_2$

Contraindications Hypersensitivity to oxycodone, salicylates, other NSAIDs, or any component of the formulation; patients with the syndrome of asthma, rhinitis, and nasal polyps; inherited or acquired bleeding disorders (including factor VII and factor IX deficiency); do not use in children and teenagers in the presence of viral infections (chickenpox or flu symptoms), with or without fever, due to a potential association with Reye's syndrome; significant respiratory depression; hypercarbia; known or suspected paralytic ileus; acute or severe bronchial asthma

Warnings/Precautions Use with caution in patients with hypersensitivity reactions to other phenanthrene-derivative opioid agonists (morphine, hydrocodone, hydromorphone, levorphanol, oxycodone, oxymorphone), respiratory diseases including asthma, emphysema, or COPD. Use with caution in pancreatitis or biliary tract disease, acute alcoholism (including delirium tremens), adrenocortical insufficiency, CNS depression/coma, kyphoscoliosis (or other skeletal disorder which may alter respiratory function), hypothyroidism (including myxedema), seizure disorder, morbid obesity, prostatic hyperplasia, urethral stricture, and toxic psychosis. May obscure diagnosis or clinical course of patients with acute abdominal conditions.

Causes sedation; caution must be used in performing tasks which require alertness (eg, operating machinery or driving). Effects may be potentiated when used with other sedative drugs or ethanol. Use with caution in elderly or debilitated patients. Use with caution in patients with renal and/or hepatic impairment; avoid use of aspirin-containing products in patients with severe hepatic or renal dysfunction. Hemodynamic effects (hypotension, orthostasis) may be exaggerated in patients with dehydration, hypovolemia, concurrent vasodilating drugs, or in patients with head injury. Respiratory depressant effects and capacity to elevate CSF pressure may be exaggerated in presence of head injury, other intracranial lesion, or pre-existing elevation of intracranial pressure. Tolerance or drug dependence may result from extended use. Healthcare provider should be alert to problems of abuse, misuse, and diversion. Taper dose gradually to avoid withdrawal symptoms in physically-dependent patients.

Use with caution in patients with platelet and bleeding disorders, erosive gastritis, or peptic ulcer disease. Heavy ethanol use (>3 drinks/day) can increase bleeding risks. Discontinue use if tinnitus or impaired hearing occurs. Patients with sensitivity to tartrazine dyes, nasal polyps, and asthma may have an increased risk of salicylate sensitivity. Surgical patients should avoid ASA if possible, for 1-2 weeks prior to surgery, to reduce the risk of excessive bleeding.

Drug Interactions

Metabolism/Transport Effects Refer to individual components.

Avoid Concomitant Use

Avoid concomitant use of Oxycodone and Aspirin with any of the following: Azelastine (Nasal); Conivaptan; Floctafenine; Influenza Virus Vaccine (Live/Attenuated); Ketorolac (Nasal); Ketorolac (Systemic); Omacetaxine; Paraldehyde

Increased Effect/Toxicity

Oxycodone and Aspirin may increase the levels/effects of: Alcohol (Ethyl); Alendronate; Alvimopan; Anticoagulants; Azelastine (Nasal); Carbonic Anhydrase Inhibitors; CNS Depressants; Collagenase (Systemic); Corticosteroids (Systemic); Dabigatran Etexilate; Desmopressin; Divalproex; Drotrecogin Alfa (Activated); Heparin; Hypoglycemic Agents; Ibritumomab; Methotrexate; Metyrosine; Mirtazapine; NSAID (COX-2 Inhibitor); Omacetaxine; Paraldehyde; PRALAtrexate; Pramipexole; Rivaroxaban; ROPINIRole; Rotigotine; Salicylates; Selective Serotonin Reuptake Inhibitors; Thiazide Diuretics; Thrombolytic Agents; Ticagrelor; Tositumomab and Iodine I 131 Tositumomab; Valproic Acid; Varicella Virus-Containing Vaccines; Vitamin K Antagonists; Zolpidem

◀ The levels/effects of Oxycodone and Aspirin may be increased by: Agents with Antiplatelet Properties; Ammonium Chloride; Amphetamines; Antidepressants (Tricyclic, Tertiary Amine); Antipsychotic Agents (Phenothiazines); Calcium Channel Blockers (Nondihydropyridine); Conivaptan; CYP3A4 Inhibitors (Moderate); CYP3A4 Inhibitors (Strong); Dasatinib; Droperidol; Floctafenine; Ginkgo Biloba; Glucosamine; Herbs (Anticoagulant/Antiplatelet Properties); HydrOXYzine; Influenza Virus Vaccine (Live/Attenuated); Ivacaftor; Ketorolac (Nasal); Ketorolac (Systemic); Loop Diuretics; Magnesium Sulfate; Mifepristone; Multivitamins/Minerals (with ADEK, Folate, Iron); NSAID (Nonselective); Omega-3 Fatty Acids; Pentosan Polysulfate Sodium; Pentoxifylline; Perampanel; Potassium Acid Phosphate; Prostacyclin Analogues; Selective Serotonin Reuptake Inhibitors; Serotonin/Norepinephrine Reuptake Inhibitors; Sodium Oxybate; Succinylcholine; Tipranavir; Treprostinil; Vitamin E; Voriconazole

Decreased Effect
Oxycodone and Aspirin may decrease the levels/effects of: ACE Inhibitors; Hyaluronidase; Loop Diuretics; Multivitamins/Minerals (with ADEK, Folate, Iron); NSAID (Nonselective); Pegvisomant; Probenecid; Ticagrelor; Tiludronate

The levels/effects of Oxycodone and Aspirin may be decreased by: Ammonium Chloride; Corticosteroids (Systemic); CYP3A4 Inducers (Strong); Deferasirox; Floctafenine; Ketorolac (Nasal); Ketorolac (Systemic); Mixed Agonist / Antagonist Opioids; NSAID (Nonselective); Rifampin; St Johns Wort; Tocilizumab

Dietary Considerations Take without regard to meals.
Pregnancy Risk Factor B (oxycodone); D (aspirin)
Pregnancy Considerations See individual agents.
Lactation Enters breast milk/not recommended
Breast-Feeding Considerations See individual agents.
Controlled Substance C-II
Dosage Forms
  Tablet: Oxycodone hydrochloride 4.8355 mg and aspirin 325 mg
  Endodan®, Percodan®: Oxycodone hydrochloride 4.8355 mg and aspirin 325 mg
Dental Comment Oxycodone, as with other opioid analgesics, is recommended only for limited acute dosing (ie, 3 days or less). Oxycodone has an addictive liability, especially when given long-term. The oxycodone with aspirin could have anticoagulant effects and could possibly affect bleeding times.

There is no scientific evidence to warrant discontinuance of aspirin prior to dental surgery. Patients taking one aspirin tablet daily as an antithrombotic and who require dental surgery should be given special consideration in consultation with the physician before removal of the aspirin relative to prevention of postoperative bleeding.

Oxycodone and Ibuprofen
(oks i KOE done & eye byoo PROE fen)

Related Information
  Ibuprofen on page 711
  Oral Pain on page 1558
  OxyCODONE on page 1028
Related Sample Prescriptions
  Severe Oral Pain on page 1606
Generic Availability (U.S.) Yes

Pharmacologic Category Analgesic Combination (Opioid); Nonsteroidal Anti-inflammatory Drug (NSAID), Oral
Dental Use Short-term (≤3-5 days) management of acute, moderate-to-severe pain
Use Short-term (≤7 days) management of acute, moderate-to-severe pain
Local Anesthetic/Vasoconstrictor Precautions No information available to require special precautions
Effects on Dental Treatment Key adverse event(s) related to dental treatment: Nausea, sedation, dizziness. See Dental Comment.

The dentist should be aware of the potential of abnormal coagulation. Caution should also be exercised in the use of NSAIDs in patients already on anticoagulant therapy with drugs such as warfarin (Coumadin®). See Effects on Bleeding.

Effects on Bleeding Nonselective NSAIDs, such as oxycodone and ibuprofen, inhibit platelet aggregation and prolong bleeding time in some patients. Unlike aspirin, the NSAID effect on platelet function is quantitatively less, of shorter duration, and reversible. Normal platelet function should occur in ~5 elimination half-lives or in <10 hours after discontinuation of oxycodone and ibuprofen. Concomitant use of other NSAIDs should be avoided.

Adverse Effects
  >10%:
    Central nervous system: Dizziness (5% to 19%), somnolence (7% to 17%)
    Gastrointestinal: Nausea (9% to 25%)
  2% to 10%:
    Cardiovascular: Vasodilation (<1% to 3%)
    Central nervous system: Headache (10%), fever (3%)
    Gastrointestinal: Vomiting (5%), constipation (<1% to 5%), diarrhea (2%), dyspepsia (<1% to 2%), flatulence (1%)
    Neuromuscular & skeletal: Weakness (<1% to 3%)
    Miscellaneous: Diaphoresis (2%)

Dental Usual Dosage Pain: Adults: Oral: Take 1 tablet as needed (maximum: 4 tablets/24 hours); do not take for longer than 7 days
Dosage Oral: Adults: Pain: Take 1 tablet as needed (maximum: 4 tablets/24 hours); do not take for longer than 7 days
Mechanism of Action
  Oxycodone: Binds to opiate receptors in the CNS, causing inhibition of ascending pain pathways, altering the perception of and response to pain; produces generalized CNS depression
  Ibuprofen: Reversibly inhibits cyclooxygenase-1 and 2 (COX-1 and 2) enzymes, which result in decreased formation of prostaglandin precursors; has antipyretic, analgesic, and anti-inflammatory properties
Contraindications Hypersensitivity to oxycodone, ibuprofen, aspirin, other NSAIDs, or any component of the formulation; paralytic ileus (known or suspected); perioperative pain in the setting of coronary artery bypass graft (CABG) surgery; significant respiratory depression; hypercarbia, acute/severe bronchial asthma
Warnings/Precautions Causes sedation; caution must be used in performing tasks which require alertness (eg, operating machinery or driving). Effects may be potentiated when used with other sedative drugs or ethanol. Use with caution in patients with hypersensitivity reactions to other phenanthrene-derivative opioid agonists and in patients with respiratory diseases. Use with caution in pancreatitis or biliary tract disease, acute alcoholism, adrenocortical insufficiency, CNS

depression/coma, kyphoscoliosis (or other skeletal disorder which may alter respiratory function), hypothyroidism, seizure disorder, morbid obesity, prostatic hyperplasia, urethral stricture, and toxic psychosis. Use with caution in the elderly, debilitated, severe hepatic or renal dysfunction. Hemodynamic effects (hypotension, orthostasis) may be exaggerated in patients with hypovolemia, concurrent vasodilating drugs, or in patients with head injury. Respiratory depressant effects and capacity to elevate CSF pressure may be exaggerated in presence of head injury, other intracranial lesion, or pre-existing increased intracranial pressure. Opioids may suppress cough reflex; use with caution during postoperative period and in patients with pulmonary disease. Patients with acute abdominal condition should use this agent cautiously. Tolerance or drug dependence may result from extended use. Concurrent use of agonist/antagonist analgesics may precipitate withdrawal symptoms and/or reduced analgesic efficacy in patients following prolonged therapy with mu opioid agonists. Abrupt discontinuation following prolonged use may also lead to withdrawal symptoms.

[U.S. Boxed Warning]: NSAIDs are associated with an increased risk of adverse cardiovascular thrombotic events, including MI and stroke. New-onset or worsening of pre-existing hypertension may occur. Risk may be increased with duration of use or pre-existing cardiovascular risk factors or disease. Use caution with fluid retention. Avoid use in heart failure. Use of NSAIDs can compromise existing renal function. Rehydrate patient before starting therapy. Monitor renal function closely. Ibuprofen is not recommended for patients with advanced renal disease. **[U.S. Boxed Warning]: Use is contraindicated for treatment of perioperative pain in the setting of coronary artery bypass graft (CABG) surgery.** Risk of MI and stroke may be increased with use following CABG surgery.

[U.S. Boxed Warning]: NSAIDs may increase risk of gastrointestinal irritation, inflammation, ulceration, bleeding, and perforation. Use caution with a history of GI disease (bleeding or ulcers), concurrent therapy with aspirin, anticoagulants and/or corticosteroids, smoking, use of alcohol, the elderly or debilitated patients. When used concomitantly with ≤325 mg of aspirin, a substantial increase in the risk of gastrointestinal complications (eg, ulcer) occurs; concomitant gastroprotective therapy (eg, proton pump inhibitors) is recommended (Bhatt, 2008). May increase the risk of aseptic meningitis, especially in patients with systemic lupus erythematosus (SLE) and mixed connective tissue disorders. Platelet adhesion and aggregation may be decreased; may prolong bleeding time; patients with coagulation disorders or who are receiving anticoagulants should be monitored closely. Anemia may occur; patients on long-term NSAID therapy should be monitored for anemia. Rarely, NSAID use may cause severe blood dyscrasias (eg, agranulocytosis, aplastic anemia, thrombocytopenia).

NSAID use may compromise existing renal function; dose-dependent decreases in prostaglandin synthesis may result from NSAID use, reducing renal blood flow which may cause renal decompensation. NSAID use may increase the risk for hyperkalemia. Patients with impaired renal function, dehydration, heart failure, liver dysfunction, those taking diuretics, and ACE inhibitors, and the elderly are at greater risk of renal toxicity and hyperkalemia. Rehydrate patient before starting therapy; monitor renal function closely. Not recommended

for use in patients with advanced renal disease. Long-term NSAID use may result in renal papillary necrosis.

NSAIDS may cause drowsiness, dizziness, blurred vision and other neurologic effects which may impair physical or mental abilities; patients must be cautioned about performing tasks which require mental alertness (eg, operating machinery or driving). Discontinue use with blurred or diminished vision and perform ophthalmologic exam. Monitor vision with long-term therapy.

NSAIDs may cause serious skin adverse events including exfoliative dermatitis, Stevens-Johnson Syndrome (SJS) and toxic epidermal necrolysis (TEN); discontinue use at first sign of skin rash or hypersensitivity. Anaphylactoid reactions may occur, even without prior exposure; patients with "aspirin triad" (bronchial asthma, aspirin intolerance, rhinitis) may be at increased risk. Do not use in patients who experience bronchospasm, asthma, rhinitis, or urticaria with NSAID or aspirin therapy. Use caution in other forms of asthma.

Withhold for at least 4-6 half-lives prior to surgical or dental procedures.

The elderly are at increased risk for adverse effects (especially peptic ulceration, CNS effects, renal toxicity) from NSAIDs even at low doses.

Drug Interactions

Metabolism/Transport Effects Refer to individual components.

Avoid Concomitant Use

Avoid concomitant use of Oxycodone and Ibuprofen with any of the following: Azelastine (Nasal); Conivaptan; Floctafenine; Ketorolac (Nasal); Ketorolac (Systemic); NSAID (COX-2 Inhibitor); Omacetaxine; Paraldehyde

Increased Effect/Toxicity

Oxycodone and Ibuprofen may increase the levels/effects of: Agents with Antiplatelet Properties; Alcohol (Ethyl); Aliskiren; Alvimopan; Aminoglycosides; Anticoagulants; Azelastine (Nasal); Bisphosphonate Derivatives; CNS Depressants; Collagenase (Systemic); CycloSPORINE (Systemic); Dabigatran Etexilate; Deferasirox; Desmopressin; Digoxin; Drotrecogin Alfa (Activated); Eplerenone; Haloperidol; Ibritumomab; Lithium; Methotrexate; Metyrosine; Mirtazapine; Nonsteroidal Anti-Inflammatory Agents; NSAID (COX-2 Inhibitor); Omacetaxine; Paraldehyde; PEMEtrexed; Porfimer; Potassium-Sparing Diuretics; PRALAtrexate; Pramipexole; Quinolone Antibiotics; Rivaroxaban; ROPINIRole; Rotigotine; Salicylates; Selective Serotonin Reuptake Inhibitors; Thiazide Diuretics; Thrombolytic Agents; Tositumomab and Iodine I 131 Tositumomab; Vancomycin; Vitamin K Antagonists; Zolpidem

The levels/effects of Oxycodone and Ibuprofen may be increased by: ACE Inhibitors; Amphetamines; Angiotensin II Receptor Blockers; Antidepressants (Tricyclic, Tertiary Amine); Antipsychotic Agents (Phenothiazines); Conivaptan; Corticosteroids (Systemic); CycloSPORINE (Systemic); CYP3A4 Inhibitors (Moderate); CYP3A4 Inhibitors (Strong); Dasatinib; Droperidol; Floctafenine; Glucosamine; Herbs (Anticoagulant/Antiplatelet Properties); HydrOXYzine; Ivacaftor; Ketorolac (Nasal); Ketorolac (Systemic); Magnesium Sulfate; Mifepristone; Multivitamins/Minerals (with ADEK, Folate, Iron); Nonsteroidal Anti-Inflammatory Agents; Omega-3 Fatty Acids; Pentosan Polysulfate Sodium; Pentoxifylline; Perampanel; Probenecid; Prostacyclin Analogues; Selective Serotonin Reuptake Inhibitors;

Serotonin/Norepinephrine Reuptake Inhibitors; Sodium Oxybate; Sodium Phosphates; Succinylcholine; Tipranavir; Treprostinil; Vitamin E; Voriconazole

Decreased Effect

Oxycodone and Ibuprofen may decrease the levels/ effects of: ACE Inhibitors; Agents with Antiplatelet Properties; Aliskiren; Angiotensin II Receptor Blockers; Beta-Blockers; Eplerenone; HydrALAZINE; Imatinib; Loop Diuretics; Pegvisomant; Potassium-Sparing Diuretics; Salicylates; Selective Serotonin Reuptake Inhibitors

The levels/effects of Oxycodone and Ibuprofen may be decreased by: Ammonium Chloride; Bile Acid Sequestrants; CYP3A4 Inducers (Strong); Deferasirox; Mixed Agonist / Antagonist Opioids; Nonsteroidal Anti-Inflammatory Agents; Rifampin; Salicylates; St Johns Wort; Tocilizumab

Ethanol/Nutrition/Herb Interactions

Based on **oxycodone** component: Ethanol: May increase CNS depression; monitor for increased effects with coadministration. Caution patients about effects.

Based on **ibuprofen** component:

Ethanol: Avoid ethanol (may enhance gastric mucosal irritation).

Food: Food or milk are recommended to decrease gastric irritation.

Herb/Nutraceutical: Avoid alfalfa, anise, bilberry, bladderwrack, bromelain, cat's claw, celery, chamomile, coleus, cordyceps, dong quai, evening primrose, fenugreek, feverfew, garlic, ginger, ginkgo biloba, ginseng (American, Panax, Siberian), grapeseed, green tea, guggul, horse chestnut seed, horseradish, licorice, prickly ash, red clover, reishi, SAMe (S-adenosylmethionine), sweet clover, turmeric, white willow (all have additional antiplatelet activity).

Dietary Considerations Take without regard to meals.

Pharmacodynamics/Kinetics

Half-life Elimination Ibuprofen: 1.8-2.6 hours; Oxycodone: 3.1-3.7 hours

Time to Peak Serum: Ibuprofen: 1.6-3.1 hours; Oxycodone 1.3-2.1 hours

Pregnancy Risk Factor C/D ≥30 weeks gestation

Pregnancy Considerations Refer to individual agents.

Lactation Enters breast milk/not recommended

Breast-Feeding Considerations Refer to individual agents.

Controlled Substance C-II

Dosage Forms

Tablet: Oxycodone 5 mg and ibuprofen 400 mg

Dental Comment The combination of oxycodone and ibuprofen in this dose form is appropriate for the management of moderate-to-severe pain when the concomitant anti-inflammatory action of ibuprofen is desired. Oxycodone is recommended only for limited acute dosing (ie, ≤3 days). Oxycodone has an addictive liability, especially when given long term.

Oxygen (OKS i jen)

Generic Availability (U.S.) Yes

Pharmacologic Category Dental Gases

Dental Use Administered as a supplement with nitrous oxide to ensure adequate ventilation during sedation; a resuscitative agent for medical emergencies in dental office

Use Treatment of various clinical disorders, both respiratory and nonrespiratory; relief of arterial hypoxia and secondary complications; treatment of pulmonary hypertension, polycythemia secondary to hypoxemia, chronic disease states complicated by anemia, cancer, migraine headaches, coronary artery disease, seizure disorders, sickle-cell crisis, and sleep apnea

Local Anesthetic/Vasoconstrictor Precautions No information available to require special precautions

Effects on Dental Treatment No significant effects or complications reported

Effects on Bleeding No information available to require special precautions

Adverse Effects No data reported

Dental Usual Dosage Administered as a supplement with nitrous oxide to ensure adequate ventilation during sedation: Children and Adults: Average rate of 2 L/minute

Dosage Children and Adults: Average rate of 2 L/minute

Mechanism of Action Increased oxygen in tidal volume and oxygenation of tissues at molecular level

Contraindications No data reported

Warnings/Precautions Oxygen-induced hypoventilation is the greatest potential hazard of oxygen therapy. In patients with severe COPD, the respiratory drive results from hypoxic stimulation of the carotid chemoreceptors. If this hypoxic drive is diminished by excessive oxygen therapy, hypoventilation may occur and further carbon dioxide retention with possible cessation of ventilation.

Dosage Forms

Liquid system with large reservoir holding 75-100 lb of liquid oxygen; compressed gas system consisting of high-pressure tank; tank sizes are "H" (6900 L of oxygen), "E" (622 L of oxygen) and "D" (356 L of oxygen)

Oxymetazoline (Nasal) (oks i met AZ oh leen)

Related Information

Bacterial Infections *on page 1562*

Related Sample Prescriptions

Sinus Infection Treatment *on page 1611*

Brand Names: U.S. 12 Hour Nasal Relief [OTC]; 4-Way® 12 Hour [OTC]; Afrin® Extra Moisturizing [OTC]; Afrin® Original [OTC]; Afrin® Severe Congestion [OTC]; Afrin® Sinus [OTC]; Dristan® [OTC]; Duramist Plus [OTC]; Neo-Synephrine® Nighttime12-Hour [OTC]; Nostrilla® [OTC]; NRS® [OTC]; Vicks® Sinex® VapoSpray 12-Hour; Vicks® Sinex® VapoSpray 12-Hour Ultra-Fine Mist [OTC]; Vicks® Sinex® VapoSpray Moisturizing 12-Hour UltraFine Mist [OTC]

Brand Names: Canada Claritin® Allergic Decongestant; Dristan® Long Lasting Nasal; Drixoral® Nasal

Generic Availability (U.S.) Yes: Intranasal solution (spray)

Pharmacologic Category Adrenergic Agonist Agent; Decongestant; Imidazoline Derivative

Dental Use Symptomatic relief of nasal mucosal congestion

Use Adjunctive therapy for nasal congestion, associated with acute or chronic rhinitis, the common cold, sinusitis, hay fever, or other allergies

Local Anesthetic/Vasoconstrictor Precautions No information available to require special precautions

Effects on Dental Treatment No significant effects or complications reported

Effects on Bleeding No information available to require special precautions

Adverse Effects Frequency not defined.

Respiratory: Dryness of the nasal mucosa, nasal irritation (temporary), rebound congestion (chronic use), sneezing

Dental Usual Dosage Symptomatic relief of nasal mucosal congestion: Children ≥6 years and Adults: Intranasal: Instill 2-3 sprays into each nostril twice daily for ≤3 days

Dosage Intranasal: Children ≥6 years and Adults: Instill 2-3 sprays into each nostril twice daily for ≤3 days

Mechanism of Action Stimulates alpha-adrenergic receptors in the arterioles of the nasal mucosa to produce vasoconstriction

Contraindications Hypersensitivity to oxymetazoline or any component of the formulation

Warnings/Precautions Rebound congestion may occur with extended use. Use with caution in the presence of hypertension, diabetes, hyperthyroidism, heart disease, coronary artery disease, or benign prostatic hyperplasia.

Drug Interactions

Metabolism/Transport Effects None known.

Avoid Concomitant Use

Avoid concomitant use of Oxymetazoline (Nasal) with any of the following: Ergot Derivatives; Iobenguane I 123; MAO Inhibitors

Increased Effect/Toxicity

Oxymetazoline (Nasal) may increase the levels/effects of: Sympathomimetics

The levels/effects of Oxymetazoline (Nasal) may be increased by: AtoMOXetine; Cannabinoids; Ergot Derivatives; MAO Inhibitors; Tricyclic Antidepressants

Decreased Effect

Oxymetazoline (Nasal) may decrease the levels/ effects of: FentaNYL; Iobenguane I 123

The levels/effects of Oxymetazoline (Nasal) may be decreased by: Alpha1-Blockers

Pharmacodynamics/Kinetics

Onset of Action Within seconds

Duration of Action Up to 12 hours

Pregnancy Considerations Adverse fetal or neonatal effects have not been observed following normal maternal doses of oxymetazoline during the third trimester of pregnancy. Adverse events have been noted in case reports following large doses or extended use. Decongestants are not the preferred agents for the treatment of rhinitis during pregnancy. Short-term (<3 days) use of intranasal oxymetazoline may be beneficial to some patients although its safety during pregnancy has not been studied.

Dosage Forms

Solution, intranasal: 0.05% (15 mL, 30 mL)
12 Hour Nasal Relief [OTC]: 0.05% (15 mL, 30 mL)
4-Way® 12 Hour [OTC]: 0.05% (15 mL)
Afrin® Extra Moisturizing [OTC]: 0.05% (15 mL)
Afrin® Original [OTC]: 0.05% (15 mL, 30 mL)
Afrin® Severe Congestion [OTC]: 0.05% (15 mL)
Afrin® Sinus [OTC]: 0.05% (15 mL)
Dristan® [OTC]: 0.05% (15 mL)
Duramist Plus [OTC]: 0.05% (15 mL)
Neo-Synephrine® Nighttime12-Hour [OTC]: 0.05% (15 mL)
Nostrilla® [OTC]: 0.05% (15 mL)
NRS® [OTC]: 0.05% (15 mL, 30 mL)

Vicks® Sinex® VapoSpray 12-Hour: 0.05% (15 mL)
Vicks® Sinex® VapoSpray 12-Hour UltraFine Mist [OTC]: 0.05% (15 mL)
Vicks® Sinex® VapoSpray Moisturizing 12-Hour Ultra-Fine Mist [OTC]: 0.05% (15 mL)

Oxymetholone (oks i METH oh lone)

Brand Names: U.S. Anadrol®-50

Pharmacologic Category Anabolic Steroid

Use Treatment of anemias caused by deficient red cell production

Local Anesthetic/Vasoconstrictor Precautions No information available to require special precautions

Effects on Dental Treatment No significant effects or complications reported

Effects on Bleeding No information available to require special precautions

Adverse Effects Frequency not defined.

Cardiovascular: Coronary artery disease, peripheral edema

Central nervous system: Chills, excitation, insomnia

Dermatologic: Acne, hirsutism (women), hyperpigmentation, male-pattern baldness (postpubertal males, women)

Endocrine & metabolic: Amenorrhea, clitoromegaly, glucose tolerance decreased, gynecomastia, HDL-cholesterol decreased, hypercalcemia, hyperchloremia, hyperkalemia, hypernatremia, hyperphosphatemia, LDL-cholesterol increased, libido increased/ decreased, menstrual irregularities, virilism (women)

Gastrointestinal: Diarrhea, nausea, vomiting

Genitourinary: Bladder irritability, epididymitis, impotence, oligospermia, penile enlargement, penile erections increased (prepubertal males), priapism, prostate cancer, prostatic hyperplasia (elderly males), seminal volume decreased, testicular atrophy, testicular dysfunction

Hematologic: Bleeding, INR increased, iron-deficiency anemia, leukemia, prothrombin time increased, clotting factors (II, V, VII, X) suppressed

Hepatic: Alkaline phosphatase increased, bilirubin increased, cholestatic hepatitis, cholestatic jaundice, hepatic failure, hepatic necrosis, hepatocellular carcinoma, liver cell tumors, peliosis hepatis, transaminases increased

Neuromuscular & skeletal: Creatine phosphokinase increased, premature closure of epiphysis (children)

Renal: Creatinine increased

Respiratory: Hoarseness (women)

Miscellaneous: Voice deepening (women)

General Dosage Range Oral: Children and Adults: 1-5 mg/kg once daily

Mechanism of Action Enhances production of erythropoietin in patients with anemias which are due to bone marrow failure; stimulates erythropoiesis in anemias due to deficient red cell production

Pregnancy Risk Factor X

Pregnancy Considerations Oligospermia or amenorrhea may occur resulting in an impairment of fertility. Use is contraindicated in women who are or may become pregnant.

Controlled Substance C-III

Oxymorphone (oks i MOR fone)

Related Information

Oral Pain on page 1558

Brand Names: U.S. Opana®; Opana® ER

Pharmacologic Category Analgesic, Opioid

Use
Parenteral: Management of moderate-to-severe acute pain; analgesia during labor; preoperative medication; anesthesia support; relief of anxiety in patients with dyspnea associated with pulmonary edema secondary to acute left ventricular failure

Oral, regular release: Management of moderate-to-severe acute pain

Oral, extended release: Management of moderate-to-severe pain in patients requiring around-the-clock opioid treatment for an extended period of time

Local Anesthetic/Vasoconstrictor Precautions No information available to require special precautions

Effects on Dental Treatment Key adverse event(s) related to dental treatment: Xerostomia (normal salivary flow resumes upon discontinuation). Anticholinergic side effects can cause a reduction of saliva production or secretion, contributing to discomfort and dental disease (ie, caries, oral candidiasis, and periodontal disease).

Effects on Bleeding No information available to require special precautions

Adverse Effects Incidence usually on higher end with extended release (ER) tablet.
>10%:
Central nervous system: Somnolence (9% to 19%), dizziness (7% to 18%), fever (1% to 14%), headache (7% to 12%)
Dermatologic: Pruritus (8% to 15%)
Gastrointestinal: Nausea (19% to 33%), constipation (4% to 28%), vomiting (9% to 16%)
1% to 10%:
Cardiovascular: Hypotension (<10%), tachycardia (<10%), edema (<10%), flushing (<10%), hypertension (<10%)
Central nervous system: Anxiety (1% to <10%), sedation (1% to <10%), depression (<10%), disorientation (<10%), lethargy (<10%), nervousness (<10%), restlessness (<10%), fatigue (≤4%), insomnia (≤4%), confusion (3%)
Endocrine & metabolic: Dehydration (<10%)
Gastrointestinal: Abdominal distension (<10%), flatulence (1% to <10%), xerostomia (1% to <10%), dyspepsia (<10%), weight loss (<10%), diarrhea (≤4%), abdominal pain (≤3%), appetite decreased (≤3%)
Neuromuscular & skeletal: Weakness (<10%)
Ocular: Blurred vision (<10%)
Respiratory: Hypoxia (<10%), dyspnea (<10%)
Miscellaneous: Diaphoresis (1% to <10%)

General Dosage Range Dosage adjustment recommended in patients with hepatic or renal impairment
I.M., SubQ: *Adults:* Initial: 0.5 mg; Maintenance: 1-1.5 mg every 4-6 hours as needed
I.V.: *Adults:* Initial: 0.5 mg
Oral:
Extended release: *Adults (opioid-naive):* Initial: 5 mg every 12 hours; Maintenance: Titrate upward with 5-10 mg every 12 hours at 3-7 day intervals until desired response
Immediate release: *Adults (opioid-naive):* Initial: 5-10 mg every 4-6 hours; Maintenance: Titrate upward to desired response

Mechanism of Action Oxymorphone hydrochloride is a potent narcotic analgesic with uses similar to those of morphine. The drug is a semisynthetic derivative of morphine (phenanthrene derivative) and is closely related to hydromorphone chemically (Dilaudid®).

Pharmacodynamics/Kinetics
Onset of Action Parenteral: 5-10 minutes
Duration of Action Analgesic: Parenteral: 3-6 hours
Half-life Elimination Oral: Immediate release: 7-9 hours; Extended release: 9-11 hours
Pregnancy Risk Factor C
Pregnancy Considerations Teratogenic effects were not observed in animal studies; however, decreased fetal weight, decreased litter size, increased stillbirths, and increased neonatal death were noted. Chronic opioid use during pregnancy may lead to a withdrawal syndrome in the neonate. Symptoms include irritability, hyperactivity, loss of sleep pattern, abnormal crying, tremor, vomiting, diarrhea, weight loss, or failure to gain weight.
Controlled Substance C-II

Oxytocin (oks i TOE sin)

Brand Names: U.S. Pitocin®
Brand Names: Canada Oxytocin for injection
Pharmacologic Category Oxytocic Agent
Use Induction of labor in patients with a medical indication; stimulation or reinforcement of labor; adjunctive therapy in management of abortion; to produce uterine contractions during the third stage of labor; control of postpartum bleeding
Local Anesthetic/Vasoconstrictor Precautions No information available to require special precautions
Effects on Dental Treatment No significant effects or complications reported
Effects on Bleeding No information available to require special precautions
Adverse Effects Frequency not defined.
Fetus or neonate:
Cardiovascular: Arrhythmias (including premature ventricular contractions), bradycardia
Central nervous system: Brain or CNS damage (permanent), neonatal seizure
Hepatic: Neonatal jaundice
Ocular: Neonatal retinal hemorrhage
Miscellaneous: Fetal death, low Apgar score (5 minute)
Mother:
Cardiovascular: Arrhythmias (including premature ventricular contractions), hypertensive episodes
Gastrointestinal: Nausea, vomiting
Genitourinary: Pelvic hematoma, postpartum hemorrhage, uterine hypertonicity, tetanic contraction of the uterus, uterine rupture, uterine spasm
Hematologic: Afibrinogenemia (fatal)
Miscellaneous: Anaphylactic reaction, subarachnoid hemorrhage; severe water intoxication with convulsions, coma, and death is associated with a slow oxytocin infusion over 24 hours
General Dosage Range
I.M.: *Adults:* Total dose of 10 units after delivery of the placenta
I.V.: *Adults:* Dosage varies greatly depending on indication
Mechanism of Action Oxytocin stimulates uterine contraction by activating G-protein-coupled receptors that trigger increases in intracellular calcium levels in uterine myofibrils. Oxytocin also increases local prostaglandin production, further stimulating uterine contraction.
Pharmacodynamics/Kinetics
Onset of Action Uterine contractions: I.M.: 3-5 minutes; I.V.: ~1 minute
Duration of Action I.M.: 2-3 hour; I.V.: 1 hour
Half-life Elimination 1-6 minutes; decreased in late pregnancy and during lactation

Pregnancy Risk Factor C (manufacturer specific)
Pregnancy Considerations [U.S. Boxed Warning]:
**To be used for medical rather than elective induction
of labor.** Animal reproduction studies have not been
conducted. When used as indicated, teratogenic effects
would not be expected. Nonteratogenic adverse reactions are reported in the neonate as well as the mother.

PACLitaxel (pac li TAKS el)

Brand Names: Canada Apo-Paclitaxel®; Paclitaxel for
Injection; Paclitaxel Injection USP
Pharmacologic Category Antineoplastic Agent, Anti-
microtubular; Antineoplastic Agent, Natural Source
(Plant) Derivative; Antineoplastic Agent, Taxane Derivative
Use Treatment of breast, nonsmall cell lung, and ovarian
cancers; treatment of AIDS-related Kaposi's sarcoma
(KS)
Unlabeled Use Treatment of bladder, cervical, small cell
lung, and head and neck cancers; treatment of
(unknown primary) adenocarcinoma
Local Anesthetic/Vasoconstrictor Precautions No
information available to require special precautions
Effects on Dental Treatment Key adverse event(s)
related to dental treatment: Severe, potentially dose-
limiting mucositis and stomatitis.
Effects on Bleeding Chemotherapy may result in
significant myelosuppression, potentially including significant reduction in platelet counts (thrombocytopenia
grades 3/4: 1% to 7%) and altered hemostasis. Bleeding
in seen in ~14% of patients. In patients who are under
active treatment with these agents, medical consult is
suggested.
Adverse Effects Percentages reported with single-
agent therapy. **Note:** Myelosuppression is dose related,
schedule related, and infusion-rate dependent
(increased incidences with higher doses, more frequent
doses, and longer infusion times) and, in general, rapidly reversible upon discontinuation.
>10%:
Cardiovascular: Flushing (28%), ECG abnormal (14%
to 23%), edema (21%), hypotension (4% to 12%)
Dermatologic: Alopecia (87%), rash (12%)
Gastrointestinal: Nausea/vomiting (52%), diarrhea
(38%), mucositis (17% to 35%; grades 3/4: up to
3%), stomatitis (15%; most common at doses
>390 mg/m^2), abdominal pain (with intraperitoneal
paclitaxel)
Hematologic: Neutropenia (78% to 98%; grade 4: 14%
to 75%; onset 8-10 days, median nadir 11 days,
recovery 15-21 days), leukopenia (90%; grade 4:
17%), anemia (47% to 90%; grades 3/4: 2% to
16%), thrombocytopenia (4% to 20%; grades 3/4:
1% to 7%), bleeding (14%)
Hepatic: Alkaline phosphatase increased (22%), AST
increased (19%)
Local: Injection site reaction (erythema, tenderness,
skin discoloration, swelling: 13%)
Neuromuscular & skeletal: Peripheral neuropathy
(42% to 70%; grades 3/4: up to 7%), arthralgia/
myalgia (60%), weakness (17%)
Renal: Creatinine increased (observed in KS patients
only: 18% to 34%; severe: 5% to 7%)
Miscellaneous: Hypersensitivity reaction (31% to 45%;
grades 3/4: up to 2%), infection (15% to 30%)

1% to 10%:
Cardiovascular: Bradycardia (3%), tachycardia (2%),
hypertension (1%), rhythm abnormalities (1%), syn-
cope (1%), venous thrombosis (1%)
Dermatologic: Nail changes (2%)
Hematologic: Febrile neutropenia (2%)
Hepatic: Bilirubin increased (7%)
Respiratory: Dyspnea (2%)
General Dosage Range Dosage adjustment recommended in patients with hepatic impairment or who
develop toxicities
I.V.: *Adults:* Dosage varies greatly depending on indication
Mechanism of Action Paclitaxel promotes microtubule
assembly by enhancing the action of tubulin dimers,
stabilizing existing microtubules, and inhibiting their
disassembly, interfering with the late G$_2$ mitotic phase,
and inhibiting cell replication. In addition, the drug can
distort mitotic spindles, resulting in the breakage of
chromosomes. Paclitaxel may also suppress cell proliferation and modulate immune response.
Pharmacodynamics/Kinetics
Half-life Elimination
1- to 6-hour infusion: Mean (beta): 6.4 hours
3-hour infusion: Mean (terminal): 13.1-20.2 hours
24-hour infusion: Mean (terminal): 15.7-52.7 hours
Pregnancy Risk Factor D
Pregnancy Considerations Adverse events (embryotoxicity, fetal toxicity, and maternal toxicity) have been
observed in animal reproduction studies at doses less
than the recommended human dose. An *ex vivo* human
placenta perfusion model illustrated that paclitaxel
crossed the placenta at term. Placental transfer was
low and affected by the presence of albumin; higher
albumin concentrations resulted in lower paclitaxel placental transfer (Berveiller, 2012). Women of childbearing
potential should be advised to avoid becoming pregnant. A pregnancy registry is available for all cancers
diagnosed during pregnancy at Cooper Health
(877-635-4499).

PACLitaxel (Protein Bound)
(pac li TAKS el PROE teen bownd)

Brand Names: U.S. Abraxane®
Brand Names: Canada Abraxane® for Injectable Suspension
Pharmacologic Category Antineoplastic Agent, Antimicrotubular; Antineoplastic Agent, Natural Source
(Plant) Derivative; Antineoplastic Agent, Taxane Derivative
Use Treatment of refractory (metastatic) or relapsed
(within 6 months of adjuvant therapy) breast cancer;
first-line treatment of locally advanced or metastatic
nonsmall cell lung cancer (NSCLC) (in combination with
carboplatin) in patients ineligible for curative surgery or
radiation therapy
Unlabeled Use Treatment of recurrent or persistent
ovarian, fallopian tube, or primary peritoneal cancers;
metastatic pancreatic cancer
Local Anesthetic/Vasoconstrictor Precautions No
information available to require special precautions
Effects on Dental Treatment Key adverse event(s)
related to dental treatment: Mucositis.
Effects on Bleeding Chemotherapy may result in
significant myelosuppression, potentially including significant reduction in platelet counts (thrombocytopenia
grades 3/4: <1%) and altered hemostasis. In patients
who are under active treatment with these agents,
medical consult is suggested.

Adverse Effects Adverse reactions and incidences reported are associated with monotherapy unless otherwise stated.

>10%:

Cardiovascular: ECG abnormal (60%; 35% in patients with a normal baseline)

Central nervous system: Fatigue (25% combination therapy for NSCLC)

Dermatologic: Alopecia (56% [combination therapy for NSCLC] to 90%)

Gastrointestinal: Nausea (27% to 30%; grades 3/4: 3%), diarrhea (15% to 27%; grades 3/4: <1%), vomiting (12% to 18%; grades 3/4: 4%), appetite decreased (17% combination therapy for NSCLC), constipation (16% combination therapy for NSCLC)

Hematologic: Neutropenia (80%; grades 3/4: 34%; combination therapy for NSCLC: 85%; grades 3/4: 47%), anemia (33%; grades 3/4: 1%; combination therapy for NSCLC: 98%; grades 3/4: 28%), thrombocytopenia (2%; grades 3/4: <1%; combination therapy for NSCLC: 68%; grades 3/4: 18%), myelosuppression (dose-related)

Hepatic: AST increased (39%), alkaline phosphatase increased (36%), GGT increased (grades 3/4: 14%)

Neuromuscular & skeletal: Sensory neuropathy (71%; grades 3/4: 10%; dose dependent; cumulative), weakness (47%; severe 8%; combination therapy for NSCLC: 16%), myalgia/arthralgia (44%; combination therapy for NSCLC: 10% to 13%)

Ocular: Vision disturbance (13%; severe [keratitis, blurred vision]: 1%)

Renal: Creatinine increased (11%; severe 1%)

Respiratory: Dyspnea (12%)

Miscellaneous: Infection (24%; primarily included oral candidiasis, respiratory tract infection, and pneumonia)

1% to 10%:

Cardiovascular: Edema/fluid retention (10%), peripheral edema (10% combination therapy for NSCLC), hypotension (5%), cardiovascular events (grades 3/4: 3%; included chest pain, cardiac arrest, supraventricular tachycardia, thrombosis, pulmonary thromboembolism, pulmonary emboli, and hypertension)

Dermatologic: Rash (10% combination therapy NSCLC)

Gastrointestinal: Mucositis (7%; grades 3/4: <1%)

Hematologic: Bleeding (2%), neutropenic fever (2%)

Hepatic: Bilirubin increased (7%)

Neuromuscular & skeletal: Peripheral neuropathy (grade 3: 10%; combination therapy for NSCLC: 3%)

Respiratory: Cough (7%), epistaxis (7% combination therapy for NSCLC)

Miscellaneous: Hypersensitivity reaction (4%, includes anaphylactic reactions, chest pain, dyspnea, flushing, hypotension; severe: <1%)

General Dosage Range Dosage adjustment recommended in patients with hepatic impairment or who develop toxicities

I.V.: *Adults:* Dosage varies greatly depending on indication.

Mechanism of Action Albumin-bound paclitaxel nanoparticle formulation; paclitaxel promotes microtubule assembly by enhancing the action of tubulin dimers, stabilizing existing microtubules, and inhibiting their disassembly, interfering with the late G_2 mitotic phase, and inhibiting cell replication. May also distort mitotic spindles, resulting in the breakage of chromosomes. Paclitaxel may also suppress cell proliferation and modulate immune response.

Pharmacodynamics/Kinetics

Half-life Elimination Terminal: 27 hours

Pregnancy Risk Factor D

Pregnancy Considerations Adverse events were observed in animal reproduction studies. An *ex vivo* human placenta perfusion model illustrated that paclitaxel (non-protein bound preparation) crossed the placenta at term. Placental transfer was low and affected by the presence of albumin; higher albumin concentrations resulted in lower paclitaxel placental transfer (Berveiller, 2012). Women of childbearing potential should be advised to avoid becoming pregnant during therapy; may cause fetal harm if administered during pregnancy. Additionally, testicular atrophy/degeneration was observed in animal studies; males should be advised to not father a child during therapy. A pregnancy registry is available for all cancers diagnosed during pregnancy at Cooper Health (877-635-4499).

Palifermin (pal ee FER min)

Brand Names: U.S. Kepivance®

Brand Names: Canada Kepivance®

Generic Availability (U.S.) No

Pharmacologic Category Keratinocyte Growth Factor

Dental Use Decrease the incidence and duration of severe oral mucositis associated with hematologic malignancies in patients receiving myelotoxic therapy requiring hematopoietic stem cell support (when the preparative regimen is expected to result in mucositis ≥grade 3 in most patients)

Note: Use (safety and efficacy) is not established for nonhematologic malignancies; use is not recommended with conditioning regimens containing melphalan 200 mg/m²

Use Decrease the incidence and duration of severe oral mucositis associated with hematologic malignancies in patients receiving myelotoxic therapy requiring hematopoietic stem cell support (when the preparative regimen is expected to result in mucositis ≥grade 3 in most patients)

Note: Use (safety and efficacy) is not established for nonhematologic malignancies; use is not recommended with conditioning regimens containing melphalan 200 mg/m²

Local Anesthetic/Vasoconstrictor Precautions No information available to require special precautions

Effects on Dental Treatment Key adverse event(s) related to dental treatment: Taste alteration, mouth/tongue discoloration or thickness. See Dental Comment.

Effects on Bleeding No information available to require special precautions

Adverse Effects

>10%:

Cardiovascular: Edema (28%)

Central nervous system: Fever (39%); pain (16%); dysesthesia (oral hyperesthesia, hypoesthesia, and paresthesia 12%)

Dermatologic: Rash (62%; grade 3: 3%), pruritus (35%), erythema (32%)

Gastrointestinal: Serum amylase increased (62%, grades 3/4: 38%), serum lipase increased (28%, grades 3/4: 11%), mouth/tongue discoloration or thickness (17%), taste alteration (16%)

1% to 10%:

Neuromuscular & skeletal: Arthralgia (10%)

Miscellaneous: Antibody formation (2%)

Dental Usual Dosage Oral mucositis: Adults: I.V.: 60 mcg/kg/day for 3 consecutive days before and after myelotoxic therapy; total of 6 doses

Dosage I.V.: Adults: Oral mucositis associated with hematopoietic stem cell transplant (HSCT) conditioning regimens: 60 mcg/kg/day for 3 consecutive days before and 3 consecutive days after myelotoxic therapy; total of 6 doses (Spielberger, 2004)

Note: Administer first 3 doses prior to myelotoxic therapy, with the 3rd dose given 24-48 hours before beginning the myelotoxic conditioning regimen. Administer the last 3 doses after completion of the conditioning regimen, with the first of these doses after but on the same day as HSCT infusion and at least 4 days after the most recent dose of palifermin.

Dosage adjustment in renal impairment: No adjustment necessary

Dosage adjustment in hepatic impairment: No dosage adjustment provided in the manufacturer's labeling (has not been studied).

Mechanism of Action Palifermin is a recombinant keratinocyte growth factor (KGF) produced in *E. coli*. Endogenous KGF is produced by mesenchymal cells in response to epithelial tissue injury. KGF binds to the KGF receptor resulting in proliferation, differentiation and migration of epithelial cells in multiple tissues, including (but not limited to) the tongue, buccal mucosa, esophagus, and salivary gland.

Contraindications There are no contraindications listed within the manufacturer's U.S. product labeling.

Canadian labeling: Hypersensitivity to palifermin, *E. coli*-derived proteins, or any component of the formulation

Warnings/Precautions Hazardous agent - use appropriate precautions for handling and disposal (NIOSH, 2012). Edema, erythema, pruritus, rash, oral/perioral dysesthesia, taste alteration, tongue discoloration, and tongue thickening may occur (median onset of cutaneous toxicities following initial dose is 6 days; median duration is 5 days); instruct patients to report mucocutaneous effects. Safety and efficacy have not been established with nonhematologic malignancies; effect on the growth of keratinocyte growth factor (KGF) receptor expressing, nonhematopoietic human tumors is not known. Palifermin has been shown to enhance epithelial tumor cell lines *in vitro*. Do not administer within 24 hours before, during, or after myelotoxic chemotherapy. If administered during or within 24 hours of (before or after) chemotherapy, palifermin may increase the severity and duration of mucositis due to the increased sensitivity of rapidly-dividing epithelial cells.

Drug Interactions

Metabolism/Transport Effects None known.

Avoid Concomitant Use

Avoid concomitant use of Palifermin with any of the following: Heparin

Increased Effect/Toxicity

The levels/effects of Palifermin may be increased by: Heparin; Heparin (Low Molecular Weight)

Decreased Effect There are no known significant interactions involving a decrease in effect.

Pharmacodynamics/Kinetics

Onset of Action Epithelial cell proliferation (dose-dependent): 48 hours

Half-life Elimination 4.5 hours (range: 3.3-5.7 hours)

Pregnancy Risk Factor C

Pregnancy Considerations Palifermin has been shown to be embryotoxic in animal reproduction studies at doses also associated with maternal toxicity. Use in pregnancy only if the potential benefit outweighs the potential risk for the fetus.

Lactation Excretion in breast milk unknown/not recommended

Breast-Feeding Considerations According to the manufacturer labeling, the decision to discontinue palifermin or discontinue breast-feeding during treatment should take into account the benefits of treatment to the mother.

Dosage Forms

Injection, powder for reconstitution [preservative free]:

Kepivance®: 6.25 mg

Dental Comment Palifermin works at the cellular level by protecting the epithelial cells lining the mouth and throat from damage caused by chemotherapy and radiation and by stimulating the growth and development of new epithelial cells to build up the mucosal barrier.

Paliperidone (pal ee PER i done)

Related Information

Clinical Risk Related to Drugs Prolonging QT Interval *on page 1510*

Brand Names: U.S. Invega®; Invega® Sustenna®

Brand Names: Canada Invega®; Invega® Sustenna®

Pharmacologic Category Antipsychotic Agent, Atypical

Use

Oral: Treatment of schizophrenia; acute treatment of schizoaffective disorder (monotherapy or adjunctive therapy to mood stabilizers and/or antidepressants)

Injection: Treatment of schizophrenia

Unlabeled Use Psychosis/agitation related to Alzheimer's dementia

Local Anesthetic/Vasoconstrictor Precautions Paliperidone is one of the drugs confirmed to prolong the QT interval and is accepted as having a risk of causing torsade de pointes. The risk of drug-induced torsade de pointes is extremely low when a single QT interval prolonging drug is prescribed. In terms of epinephrine, it is not known what effect vasoconstrictors in the local anesthetic regimen will have in patients with a known history of congenital prolonged QT interval or in patients taking any medication that prolongs the QT interval. Until more information is obtained, it is suggested that the clinician consult with the physician prior to the use of a vasoconstrictor in suspected patients, and that the vasoconstrictor (epinephrine, mepivacaine and levonordefrin [Carbocaine® 2% with Neo-Cobefrin®]) be used with caution.

Effects on Dental Treatment Key adverse event(s) related to dental treatment: Significant xerostomia and changes in salivation (normal salivary flow resumes upon discontinuation).

Effects on Bleeding No information available to require special precautions

Adverse Effects Unless otherwise noted, frequency of adverse effects is reported for the oral/I.M. formulation in adults.

>10%:
  Cardiovascular: Tachycardia (1% to 14%)
  Central nervous system: EPS (≤26%; dose dependent), insomnia (10% to 15%), headache (6% to 15%), parkinsonism (3% to 14%; dose dependent), somnolence (adolescents 9% to 26%; adults 1% to 12%; dose dependent)
  Neuromuscular & skeletal: Tremor (2% to 12%)
3% to 10%:
  Cardiovascular: Orthostatic hypotension (1% to 4%; dose dependent), bundle branch block (≤3%)
  Central nervous system: Agitation (4% to 10%), akathisia (adolescents 4% to 17%; adults 1% to 10%; dose dependent), anxiety (adolescents ≤9%; adults 3% to 8%), dizziness (1% to 6%), dystonia (1% to 5%; dose dependent), dysarthria (1% to 4%; dose dependent), fatigue (adolescents ≤4%), sleep disorder (≤3%), lethargy (adolescents ≤3%)
  Endocrine & metabolic: Amenorrhea (adolescents ≤6%), galactorrhea (adolescents ≤4%), gynecomastia (adolescents ≤3%)
  Gastrointestinal: Weight gain (1% to 9%; dose dependent), nausea (2% to 8%), dyspepsia (5% to 6%), vomiting (adolescents ≤11%; adults 2% to 5%), constipation (1% to 5%), salivation increased (adolescents ≤6%; adults ≤4%; dose dependent), appetite increased (2% to 3%), toothache (1% to 3%), abdominal pain (≤3%), diarrhea (≤3%), xerostomia (≤3%); tongue swelling (adolescents ≤3%), tongue paralysis (adolescents ≤3%)
  Local: I.M. formulation: Injection site reaction (≤10%)
  Neuromuscular & skeletal: Hyperkinesia (2% to 10% dose dependent), dyskinesia (1% to 9%), weakness (≤4%), myalgia (≤4% dose dependent), back pain (1% to 3%), extremity pain (≤3%)
  Ocular: Blurred vision (adolescents ≤3%)
  Respiratory: Nasopharyngitis (≤5%; dose dependent), upper respiratory tract infection (1% to 4%), cough (≤3%; dose dependent), rhinitis (1% to 3%; dose dependent)

General Dosage Range Dosage adjustment recommended in patients with renal impairment
I.M.: *Adults:* Initial: 234 mg, then 156 mg 1 week later; Maintenance: 39-234 mg monthly
Oral: *Adolescents 12-17 years and Adults:* 3-12 mg once daily (maximum: 12 mg daily)

Mechanism of Action Paliperidone is considered a benzisoxazole atypical antipsychotic as it is the primary active metabolite of risperidone. As with other atypical antipsychotics, its therapeutic efficacy is believed to result from mixed central serotonergic and dopaminergic antagonism. The addition of serotonin antagonism to dopamine antagonism (classic neuroleptic mechanism) is thought to improve negative symptoms of psychoses and reduce the incidence of extrapyramidal side effects. Similar to risperidone, paliperidone demonstrates high affinity to α_1, D_2, H_1, and 5-HT$_{2C}$ receptors, and low affinity for muscarinic and 5-HT$_{1A}$ receptors. In contrast to risperidone, paliperidone displays nearly 10-fold lower affinity for α_2 and 5-HT$_{2A}$ receptors, and nearly three- to fivefold less affinity for 5-HT$_{1A}$ and 5-HT$_{1D}$, respectively.

Pharmacodynamics/Kinetics
Half-life Elimination
  Oral: 23 hours; 24-51 hours with renal impairment (Cl$_{cr}$ <80 mL/minute)
  I.M. (following a single-dose administration): Range: 25-49 days
  Time to Peak Oral: ~24 hours; I.M.: 13 days
Pregnancy Risk Factor C

Pregnancy Considerations Adverse events were not observed in animal reproduction studies. Antipsychotic use during the third trimester of pregnancy has a risk for extrapyramidal symptoms (EPS) and withdrawal symptoms in newborns following delivery. Symptoms in the newborn may include agitation, feeding disorder, hypertonia, hypotonia, respiratory distress, somnolence, and tremor. These effects may be self-limiting and allow recovery within hours or days with no specific treatment, or they may be severe requiring prolonged hospitalization. Paliperidone may cause hyperprolactinemia, which may decrease reproductive function in both males and females. Paliperidone is the active metabolite of risperidone; refer to Risperidone monograph for additional information.

The ACOG recommends that therapy during pregnancy be individualized; treatment with psychiatric medications during pregnancy should incorporate the clinical expertise of the mental health clinician, obstetrician, primary healthcare provider, and pediatrician. Safety data related to atypical antipsychotics during pregnancy is limited and routine use is not recommended. However, if a woman is inadvertently exposed to an atypical antipsychotic while pregnant, continuing therapy may be preferable to switching to a typical antipsychotic that the fetus has not yet been exposed to; consider risk:benefit (ACOG, 2008).

Healthcare providers are encouraged to enroll women 18-45 years of age exposed to paliperidone during pregnancy in the Atypical Antipsychotics Pregnancy Registry (1-866-961-2388 or http://www.womensmental-health.org/pregnancyregistry).

Dental Comment Paliperidone is known to prolong the QT interval. The QT interval is measured as the time and distance between the Q point of the QRS complex and the end of the T wave in the ECG tracing. After adjustment for heart rate, the QT interval is defined as prolonged if it is more than 450 msec in men and 460 msec in women. A long QT syndrome was first described in the 1950s and 60s as a congenital syndrome involving QT interval prolongation and syncope and sudden death. Some of the congenital long QT syndromes were characterized by a peculiar electrocardiographic appearance of the QRS complex involving a premature atria beat followed by a pause, then a subsequent sinus beat showing marked QT prolongation and deformity. This type of cardiac arrhythmia was originally termed "torsade de pointes" (translated from the French as "twisting of the points"). Paliperidone is considered as having a risk of causing torsade de pointes. Since it is not known what effect vasoconstrictors in the local anesthetic regimen will have in patients with a known history of congenital prolonged QT interval or in patients taking any medication that prolongs the QT interval, a medical consult is suggested.

Palivizumab (pah li VIZ u mab)

Brand Names: U.S. Synagis®
Brand Names: Canada Synagis®
Pharmacologic Category Monoclonal Antibody
Use Prevention of serious lower respiratory tract disease caused by respiratory syncytial virus (RSV) in infants and children at high risk of RSV disease

The American Academy of Pediatrics recommends RSV prophylaxis with palivizumab during RSV season for:
- Infants <3 months of age who were born between 32 and 34 6/7 weeks gestational age and have one of the following:
  - Day care attendance
  - One or more siblings <5 years of age living in the same household
- Infants <6 months of age who were born between 29 and 31 6/7 weeks gestational age
- Infants <12 months of age who were born <28 weeks gestational age
- Infants <12 months of age with congenital airway abnormality or neuromuscular disorder that decreases the ability to manage airway secretions
- Infants and children <24 months of age with chronic lung disease (CLD) necessitating medical therapy within 6 month prior to the beginning of RSV season
- Infants and children ≤24 months of age with congenital heart disease and one of the following:
  - Receiving medication to treat congestive heart failure
  - Moderate-to-severe pulmonary hypertension
  - Cyanotic heart disease

Local Anesthetic/Vasoconstrictor Precautions No information available to require special precautions

Effects on Dental Treatment No significant effects or complications reported

Effects on Bleeding No information available to require special precautions

Adverse Effects
>10%:
Central nervous system: Fever (27%)
Dermatologic: Rash (12%)
1% to 10%: Miscellaneous: Antibody formation (1% to 2%)

General Dosage Range I.M.: *Children <2 years:* 15 mg/kg monthly

Mechanism of Action Exhibits neutralizing and fusion-inhibitory activity against RSV; these activities inhibit RSV replication in laboratory and clinical studies

Pharmacodynamics/Kinetics
Half-life Elimination Children <24 months: 20 days

Pregnancy Risk Factor C

Pregnancy Considerations Not for adult use; reproduction studies have not been conducted

---

Palonosetron (pal oh NOE se tron)

Brand Names: U.S. Aloxi®
Pharmacologic Category Antiemetic; Selective 5-HT₃ Receptor Antagonist

Use Prevention of chemotherapy-associated nausea and vomiting; indicated for prevention of acute (highly-emetogenic therapy) as well as acute and delayed (moderately-emetogenic therapy) nausea and vomiting; prevention of postoperative nausea and vomiting (PONV)

Local Anesthetic/Vasoconstrictor Precautions No information available to require special precautions

Effects on Dental Treatment No significant effects or complications reported

Effects on Bleeding No information available to require special precautions

Adverse Effects Adverse events may vary according to indication.
1% to 10%:
Cardiovascular: QT prolongation (chemotherapy-associated <1%; PONV 1% to 5%), bradycardia (chemotherapy-associated 1%; PONV 4%), hypotension (≤1%), sinus bradycardia (≤1%), tachycardia (non-sustained) (≤1%)
Central nervous system: Headache (chemotherapy-associated 5% to 9%; PONV 3%), anxiety (1%), dizziness (≤1%)
Dermatologic: Pruritus (≤1%)
Endocrine & metabolic: Hyperkalemia (1%)
Gastrointestinal: Constipation (2% to 5%), diarrhea (≤1%), flatulence (≤1%)
Genitourinary: Urinary retention (≤1%)
Hepatic: ALT increased (≤1%; transient), AST increased (≤1%; transient)
Neuromuscular & skeletal: Weakness (1%)

General Dosage Range I.V.: *Adults:* 0.25 mg or 0.075 mg as a single dose

Mechanism of Action Selective 5-HT₃ receptor antagonist, blocking serotonin, both on vagal nerve terminals in the periphery and centrally in the chemoreceptor trigger zone

Pharmacodynamics/Kinetics
Half-life Elimination I.V.: Terminal: ~40 hours

Pregnancy Risk Factor B

Pregnancy Considerations Teratogenic effects were not observed in animal studies. There are no adequate and well-controlled studies in pregnant women; use during pregnancy only if clearly needed.

Pamidronate (pa mi DROE nate)

Brand Names: U.S. Aredia®
Brand Names: Canada Aredia®; Pamidronate Disodium Omega; Pamidronate Disodium®; PMS-Pamidronate
Pharmacologic Category Antidote; Bisphosphonate Derivative

Use Treatment of moderate or severe hypercalcemia associated with malignancy (in conjunction with adequate hydration) with or without bone metastases; treatment of osteolytic bone lesions associated with multiple myeloma or metastatic breast cancer; moderate-to-severe Paget's disease of bone

Unlabeled Use Treatment of osteogenesis imperfecta; treatment of symptomatic bone metastases of thyroid cancer; prevention of bone loss associated with androgen deprivation treatment in prostate cancer

Local Anesthetic/Vasoconstrictor Precautions No information available to require special precautions

Effects on Dental Treatment Osteonecrosis of the jaw (ONJ), generally associated with local infection and/or tooth extraction and often with delayed healing, has been reported in patients taking bisphosphonates. Symptoms included nonhealing extraction socket or an exposed jawbone. Most reported cases of bisphosphonate-associated osteonecrosis have been in cancer patients treated with intravenous bisphosphonates. However, some have occurred in patients with postmenopausal osteoporosis taking oral bisphosphonates. Dental surgery, particularly tooth extraction, may increase the risk for ONJ. Patients who develop ONJ while on bisphosphonate therapy should receive care by an oral surgeon. See Dental Comment.

Effects on Bleeding No information available to require special precautions

◀ **Adverse Effects Note:** Actual percentages may vary by indication; treatment for multiple myeloma is associated with higher percentage.

\>10%:

Central nervous system: Fever (18% to 39%; transient), fatigue (≤37%), headache (≤26%), insomnia (≤22%)

Endocrine & metabolic: Hypophosphatemia (≤18%), hypokalemia (4% to 18%), hypomagnesemia (4% to 12%), hypocalcemia (≤12%)

Gastrointestinal: Nausea (≤54%), vomiting (≤36%), anorexia (≤26%), abdominal pain (≤23%), dyspepsia (≤23%)

Genitourinary: Urinary tract infection (≤19%)

Hematologic: Anemia (≤43%), granulocytopenia (≤20%)

Local: Infusion site reaction (≤18%; includes induration, pain, redness and swelling)

Neuromuscular & skeletal: Myalgia (≤26%), weakness (≤22%), arthralgia (≤14%), osteonecrosis of the jaw (cancer patients: 1% to 11%)

Renal: Serum creatinine increased (≤19%)

Respiratory: Dyspnea (≤30%), cough (≤26%), upper respiratory tract infection (≤24%), sinusitis (≤16%), pleural effusion (≤11%)

1% to 10%:

Cardiovascular: Atrial fibrillation (≤6%), hypertension (≤6%), syncope (≤6%), tachycardia (≤6%), atrial flutter (≤1%), cardiac failure (≤1%), edema (≤1%)

Central nervous system: Somnolence (≤6%), psychosis (≤4%), seizure (≤2%)

Endocrine & metabolic: Hypothyroidism (≤6%)

Gastrointestinal: Constipation (≤6%), gastrointestinal hemorrhage (≤6%), diarrhea (≤1%), stomatitis (≤1%)

Hematologic: Leukopenia (≤4%), neutropenia (≤1%), thrombocytopenia (≤1%)

Neuromuscular & skeletal: Back pain, bone pain

Renal: Uremia (≤4%)

Respiratory: Rales (≤6%), rhinitis (≤6%)

Miscellaneous: Moniliasis (≤6%)

General Dosage Range Dosage adjustment recommended in patients with renal impairment

I.V.: *Adults:* 60-90 mg as a single dose, may repeat every 3-4 weeks **or** 30 mg daily for 3 consecutive days

Mechanism of Action Nitrogen-containing bisphosphonate; inhibits bone resorption and decreases mineralization by disrupting osteoclast activity (Gralow, 2009; Rogers, 2011)

Pharmacodynamics/Kinetics

Onset of Action

Hypercalcemia of malignancy (HCM): ≤24 hours for decrease in albumin-corrected serum calcium; maximum effect: ≤7 days

Paget's disease: ~1 month for ≥50% decrease in serum alkaline phosphatase

Duration of Action HCM: 7-14 days; Paget's disease: 1-372 days

Half-life Elimination 21-35 hours

Pregnancy Risk Factor D

Pregnancy Considerations Pamidronate has been shown to cross the placenta and cause adverse effects in animal reproduction studies. Bisphosphonates are expected to cross the human placenta. Bisphosphonates are incorporated into the bone matrix and gradually released over time. Theoretically, there may be a risk of fetal harm when pregnancy follows the completion of therapy. Based on limited case reports, serum calcium levels in the newborn may be transiently altered if pamidronate is administered during pregnancy; shortened gestational age and low birth weight have also

been noted, but significant fetal toxicity has not been observed. Women of childbearing potential should be advised to avoid becoming pregnant during therapy. Monitoring of calcium concentrations in the mother during pregnancy and in the neonate after birth are recommended if therapy is required (Stathopoulos, 2011).

Dental Comment The American Association of Oral and Maxillofacial Surgeons position paper on bisphosphonate-related osteonecrosis of the jaws, 2009 update, stated that I.V. bisphosphonate exposure in the setting of managing malignancy remains the major risk factor for the development of ONJ. After reviewing case series, case-controlled studies, and cohort studies, the estimates of the cumulative incidence of I.V. bisphosphonate-associated ONJ ranges from 0.8% to 12%.

Two reports have attempted to assess more accurately the percent of cancer patients developing ONJ after bisphosphonate treatment. Maerevoet et al, reported that among 194 patients treated with Zometa® every 3-4 weeks, nine developed ONJ. Before receiving Zometa®, six had received Aredia® 90 mg every 3-4 weeks. The median duration of treatment with Aredia® was 39 months and for Zometa® 18 months. The incidence of ONJ in these patients was calculated to be 4.6%. Durie et al, described the results of a survey by the International Myeloma Foundation in 2004 to assess the risk factors of ONJ. Out of 1203 respondents, 904 had myeloma and 299 had breast cancer. Of the myeloma patients, 62 developed ONJ and 54 had suspicious findings. Of the breast cancer patients, 13 had ONJ and 23 had suspicious findings. The total number of cases of either ONJ or suspicious findings was 152. ONJ developed in 10% of 211 patients receiving Zometa® compared to 4% of 413 receiving Aredia®. The mean time to onset of ONJ among patients taking Zometa® was 18 months; the mean time to onset after Aredia® was 6 years. It should be noted that an early report by authors from Novartis Pharmaceuticals Corporation stressed that Aredia® and Zometa® had been used in 2.5 million patients world wide and reports of ONJ during their extensive use had been rare (Tarassoff, 2003). In addition, these authors stated that review of the reported cases revealed multiple risk factors for avascular necrosis. McMahon et al, followed up with a report that, along with other factors, bisphosphonates are additional stressors of bone health that can tip the balance to osteonecrosis. They suggested that the prevention of ONJ should be stressed such as the elimination of chronic dental infections prior to chemotherapy and bisphosphonate use in cancer patients.

According to the 2011 report by the American Dental Association (ADA), the incidence of BP-associated ONJ remains low and the benefits of using oral bisphosphonates significantly outweighs the risk of developing BP-associated ONJ for treatment and prevention of osteoporosis and cancer treatment (Hellstein, 2011). The full 47 page report can be accessed at http://www.ada.org/sections/professionalResources/pdfs/topics_AR-ONJ_report.pdf.

The ADA review of 2011 stated the incidence of oral BP-associated ONJ was one case for every 1000 individuals exposed to oral bisphosphonates (0.1%) (Hellstein, 2011).

Pancrelipase (pan kre LYE pase)

Brand Names: U.S. Creon®; Pancreaze™; Pancrelipase™; Pertzye™; Ultresa™; Viokace™; Zenpep®
Brand Names: Canada Cotazym®; Creon®; Pancrease® MT; Ultrase®; Ultrase® MT; Viokase®
Pharmacologic Category Enzyme
Use Treatment of exocrine pancreatic insufficiency (EPI) due to conditions such as cystic fibrosis (Creon®, Pancreaze™, Pertzye™, Ultresa™, Zenpep®); chronic pancreatitis (Creon®, Viokace™); or pancreatectomy (Creon®, Viokace™)

Note: Viokace™ must be administered with a proton pump inhibitor (PPI) since it is not enteric coated.
Local Anesthetic/Vasoconstrictor Precautions No information available to require special precautions
Effects on Dental Treatment No significant effects or complications reported
Effects on Bleeding No information available to require special precautions
Adverse Effects The following adverse reactions were reported in a short-term safety studies; actual frequency varies with different products; adverse events, particularly gastrointestinal events, were often greater with placebo:
>10%:
 Central nervous system: Headache (3% to 15%)
 Gastrointestinal: Abdominal pain (3% to 18%)
 Neuromuscular & skeletal: Neck pain (14%)
 Otic: Ear pain (11%)
 Respiratory: Nasal congestion (14%), beta-hemolytic streptococcal infection (11%)
 Miscellaneous: Lymphadenopathy (11%)
1% to 10%:
 Cardiovascular: Peripheral edema (3%)
 Central nervous system: Dizziness (4% to 6%)
 Dermatologic: Rash (3%)
 Endocrine & metabolic: Hyperglycemia (4% to 8%), diabetes mellitus exacerbation (4%), hypoglycemia (4%)
 Gastrointestinal: Dyspepsia (10%), diarrhea (≤10%), flatulence (3% to 9%), anal itching (7%), biliary tract stones (7%), early satiety (6%), vomiting (6%), weight loss (3% to 6%), upper abdominal pain (≤5%), feces abnormal (≤4%)
 Hematologic: Anemia (3%)
 Hepatic: Ascites (3%), hydrocholecystis (3%)
 Renal: Renal cyst (3%)
 Respiratory: Cough (4% to 10%), epistaxis (7%), pharyngolaryngeal pain (7%), nasopharyngitis (4%)
 Miscellaneous: Viral infection (3%)
General Dosage Range Oral:
 Infants ≤1 year: Lipase 2000-4000 units per 120 mL of formula or per breast-feeding
 Children >1 and <4 years: Lipase 1000-2500 units/kg/meal; Maximum: Lipase ≤2500 units/kg/**meal or** lipase ≤10,000 units/kg/**day or** lipase <4000 units/g of fat daily
 Children ≥4 years, Adolescents, and Adults: Lipase 500-2500 units/kg/meal **or** lipase 72,000 units/meal (while consuming ≥100 g of fat per day); Maximum: Lipase ≤2500 units/kg/**meal or** lipase ≤10,000 units/kg/**day or** lipase <4000 units/g of fat daily

Mechanism of Action Pancrelipase is a natural product harvested from the porcine pancreatic glands. It contains a combination of lipase, amylase, and protease. Products are formulated to dissolve in the more basic pH of the duodenum so that they may act locally to break down fats, protein, and starch.
Pregnancy Risk Factor C
Pregnancy Considerations Reproduction studies have not been conducted. Nutrition should be optimized in pregnancy; in cystic fibrosis patients with malabsorption, pancreatic enzyme replacement is not considered to cause a risk to the pregnancy.

Panitumumab (pan i TOOM yoo mab)

Brand Names: U.S. Vectibix®
Brand Names: Canada Vectibix®
Pharmacologic Category Antineoplastic Agent, Monoclonal Antibody; Epidermal Growth Factor Receptor (EGFR) Inhibitor
Use Monotherapy in treatment of EGFR-expressing refractory metastatic colorectal cancer with disease progression on or following fluoropyrimidine-, oxaliplatin-, and irinotecan-based regimens
Panitumumab is not indicated for the treatment of patients with *KRAS* mutation-positive metastatic colorectal cancer or patients in which *KRAS* mutation status is unknown. Subset analyses (retrospective) in metastatic colorectal cancer trials have not shown a benefit with EGFR inhibitor treatment in patients whose tumors have codon 12 or 13 *KRAS* mutations.
Unlabeled Use Treatment of metastatic colorectal cancer (KRAS wild-type) in combination with other chemotherapy agents
Local Anesthetic/Vasoconstrictor Precautions No information available to require special precautions
Effects on Dental Treatment Key adverse event(s) related to dental treatment: Stomatitis and mucositis.
Effects on Bleeding Although significant myelosuppression with associated altered hemostasis has been reported for many chemotherapeutic agents, myelosuppression is not common with panitumumab and no specific precautions appear to necessary.
Adverse Effects
>10%:
 Cardiovascular: Peripheral edema (12%)
 Central nervous system: Fatigue (26%)
 Dermatologic: Skin toxicity (90%; grades 3/4: 14% to 16%), erythema (65%; grades 3/4: 5%), acneiform rash (57%; grades 3/4: 7%), pruritus (57%; grades 3/4: 2%), nail toxicity (29%; grades 3/4: 2%), exfoliation (25%; grades 3/4: 2%), paronychia (25%), rash (22%; grades 3/4: 1%), fissures (20%; grades 3/4: 1%), acne (13%; grades 3/4: 1%)
 Endocrine & metabolic: Hypomagnesemia (38%; grades 3/4: 4%)
 Gastrointestinal: Abdominal pain (25%), nausea (23%), diarrhea (21%; grades 3/4: 2%), constipation (21%), vomiting (19%)
 Ocular: Ocular toxicity (15%)
 Respiratory: Cough (14%)
1% to 10%:
 Dermatologic: Dry skin (10%)
 Gastrointestinal: Stomatitis (7%), mucositis (6%)
 Ocular: Eyelash growth (6%), conjunctivitis (4%), ocular hyperemia (3%), lacrimation increased (2%), eye/eye lid irritation (1%)
 Miscellaneous: Antibody formation (≤5%), infusion reactions (3%; grades 3/4: 1%)

◄ **General Dosage Range** Dosage adjustment recommended in patients who develop toxicities
I.V.: *Adults:* 6 mg/kg every 14 days

Mechanism of Action Recombinant human IgG2 monoclonal antibody which binds specifically to the epidermal growth factor receptor (EGFR, HER1, c-ErbB-1) and competitively inhibits the binding of epidermal growth factor (EGF) and other ligands. Binding to the EGFR blocks phosphorylation and activation of intracellular tyrosine kinases, resulting in inhibition of cell survival, growth, proliferation and transformation. EGFR signal transduction results in *KRAS* wild-type activation; cells with *KRAS* mutations appear to be unaffected by EGFR inhibition.

Pharmacodynamics/Kinetics
Half-life Elimination ~7.5 days (range: 4-11 days)
Pregnancy Risk Factor C

Pregnancy Considerations Animal reproduction studies have demonstrated adverse fetal effects. Based on animal studies, panitumumab may disrupt normal menstrual cycles. IgG is known to cross the placenta; therefore, it is possible the developing fetus may be exposed to panitumumab. Because panitumumab inhibits epidermal growth factor (EGF), a component of fetal development, adverse effects on pregnancy would be expected. Panitumumab should only be given to a pregnant woman if the potential benefit justifies the potential risk to the fetus. Women of childbearing potential should use effective contraception during and for 6 months after treatment. Women who become pregnant during panitumumab treatment are encouraged to enroll in Amgen's Pregnancy Surveillance Program (1-800-772-6436).

Pantoprazole (pan TOE pra zole)

Related Information
Gastrointestinal Disorders *on page 1512*
Brand Names: U.S. Protonix®; Protonix® I.V.
Brand Names: Canada Apo-Pantoprazole®; Ava-Pantoprazole; CO Pantoprazole; Mylan-Pantoprazole; Pantoloc®; Pantoprazole for Injection; Panto™ I.V.; PMS-Pantoprazole; Q-Pantoprazole; RAN™-Pantoprazole; ratio-Pantoprazole; Riva-Pantoprazole; Sandoz-Pantoprazole; Tecta®; Teva-Pantoprazole
Generic Availability (U.S.) Yes: Excludes granules for suspension
Pharmacologic Category Proton Pump Inhibitor; Substituted Benzimidazole
Use
Oral: Short-term (up to 8 weeks) treatment and maintenance of healing of erosive esophagitis associated with GERD; reduction in relapse rates of daytime and nighttime heartburn symptoms in GERD; hypersecretory disorders associated with Zollinger-Ellison syndrome or other GI hypersecretory disorders
I.V.: Short-term treatment (7-10 days) of patients with gastroesophageal reflux disease (GERD) and a history of erosive esophagitis; hypersecretory disorders associated with Zollinger-Ellison syndrome or other GI hypersecretory disorders

Canadian labeling: Additional use (not in U.S. labeling): Oral: Peptic ulcer disease (eg, duodenal or gastric ulcer); adjunct treatment with antibiotics for *Helicobacter pylori* eradication; prevention of GI lesions in patients receiving prolonged NSAID therapy

Unlabeled Use Peptic ulcer disease, active ulcer bleeding (parenteral formulation); adjunct treatment with antibiotics for *Helicobacter pylori* eradication; stress-ulcer prophylaxis in the critically-ill
Local Anesthetic/Vasoconstrictor Precautions No information available to require special precautions
Effects on Dental Treatment No significant effects or complications reported
Effects on Bleeding No information available to require special precautions
Adverse Effects
>10%: Central nervous system: Headache (adults 12%; children >4%)
1% to 10%:
Cardiovascular: Facial edema (≤4%), generalized edema (≤2%)
Central nervous system: Dizziness (≤4%), vertigo (≤4%), depression (≤2%), fever (adults ≤2%; children >4%)
Dermatologic: Rash (adults ≤2%; children >4%), urticaria (≤4%), photosensitivity (≤2%), pruritus (≤2%)
Endocrine & metabolic: Triglycerides increased (≤4%)
Gastrointestinal: Diarrhea (≤9%), abdominal pain (children >4%), vomiting (≥4%), constipation (≤4%), flatulence (children ≤4%), nausea (children ≤4%), xerostomia (≤2%)
Hematologic: Leukopenia (≤2%), thrombocytopenia (≤2%)
Hepatic: Liver function tests abnormal (≤4%), hepatitis (≤2%)
Local: Injection site reaction (thrombophlebitis ≤2%)
Neuromuscular & skeletal: Arthralgia (≤4%), myalgia (≤4%), CPK increased (≤4%)
Ocular: Blurred vision (≤2%)
Respiratory: Upper respiratory tract infection (children >4%)
Miscellaneous: Allergic reaction (≤4%)
Dosage
Oral:
Children ≥5 years: Erosive esophagitis associated with GERD:
≥15 to <40 kg: 20 mg once daily for up to 8 weeks
≥40 kg: 40 mg once daily for up to 8 weeks
Adults:
Erosive esophagitis associated with GERD:
Treatment: 40 mg once daily for up to 8 weeks; an additional 8 weeks may be used in patients who have not healed after an 8-week course. **Note:** Canadian labeling recommends initial treatment for up to 4 weeks and an additional 4 weeks in patients who have not healed after the initial 4-week course. Lower doses (20 mg once daily) have been used successfully in mild GERD treatment (Dettmer, 1998).
Maintenance of healing: 40 mg once daily (U.S. labeling) or 20-40 mg once daily (Canadian labeling); 20 mg once daily has been used successfully in maintenance of healing (Escourrou, 1999). **Note:** Has not been studied beyond 12 months.
Hypersecretory disorders (including Zollinger-Ellison): Initial: 40 mg twice daily; adjust dose based on patient needs; doses up to 240 mg daily have been administered
Helicobacter pylori eradication (unlabeled use in U.S.):
American College of Gastroenterology guidelines (Chey, 2007):
Nonpenicillin allergy: 40 mg twice daily administered with amoxicillin 1000 mg *and* clarithromycin 500 mg twice daily for 10-14 days

Penicillin allergy: 40 mg twice daily administered with clarithromycin 500 mg *and* metronidazole 500 mg twice daily for 10-14 days **or** 40 mg once or twice daily administered with bismuth subsalicylate 525 mg *and* metronidazole 250 mg *plus* tetracycline 500 mg 4 times daily for 10-14 days

Canadian labeling: 40 mg twice daily administered with clarithromycin 500 mg twice daily *and* either metronidazole 500 mg **or** amoxicillin 1000 mg twice daily for 7 days

Peptic ulcer disease (Canadian labeling): Treatment: 40 mg once daily for 2 weeks (duodenal ulcer) or 4 weeks (gastric ulcer); may extend therapy for an additional 2 or 4 weeks (based on indication) for inadequate healing

Prevention of GI lesions associated with NSAID use (Canadian labeling): 20 mg once daily

Symptomatic GERD (Canadian labeling): Treatment: 40 mg once daily for up to 4 weeks; failure to achieve adequate symptom relief after the initial 4 weeks of therapy warrants further evaluation

I.V.:

Erosive esophagitis associated with GERD: 40 mg once daily for 7-10 days

Hypersecretory disorders: 80 mg every 12 hours; adjust dose based on acid output measurements; 160-240 mg daily in divided doses has been used for a limited period (up to 7 days)

Prevention of rebleeding in peptic ulcer bleed (unlabeled use) (Barkun, 2010; Zargar, 2006): 80 mg, followed by 8 mg/hour infusion for 72 hours. **Note:** A daily infusion of 40 mg does not raise gastric pH sufficiently to enhance coagulation in active GI bleeds.

Elderly: Dosage adjustment not required

Dosage adjustment in renal impairment: No dosage adjustment necessary; pantoprazole is not removed by hemodialysis

Dosage adjustment in hepatic impairment:

U.S. labeling: No dosage adjustment necessary; doses >40 mg daily have not been evaluated in patients with hepatic impairment.

Canadian labeling:

Mild-moderate impairment: No dosage adjustment necessary.

Severe impairment: I.V., Oral: Manufacturer labeling suggests a maximum dose of 20 mg daily.

Mechanism of Action Suppresses gastric acid secretion by inhibiting the parietal cell H^+/K^+ ATP pump

Contraindications Hypersensitivity to pantoprazole, substituted benzimidazole proton pump inhibitors, or any component of the formulation

Warnings/Precautions Use of proton pump inhibitors (PPIs) may increase the risk of gastrointestinal infections (eg, *Salmonella, Campylobacter*). Relief of symptoms does not preclude the presence of a gastric malignancy. Long-term pantoprazole therapy (especially in patients who were *H. pylori* positive) has caused biopsy-proven atrophic gastritis. Benign and malignant neoplasia has been observed in long-term rodent studies; while not reported in humans, the relevance of these findings in regards to tumorigenicity in humans is not known. Use of PPIs may increase risk of *Clostridium difficile*-associated diarrhea (CDAD), especially in hospitalized patients; consider CDAD diagnosis in patients with persistent diarrhea that does not improve. Use the lowest dose and shortest duration of PPI therapy appropriate for the condition being treated. Prolonged treatment (typically >3 years) may lead to vitamin B_{12} malabsorption and subsequent deficiency. Intravenous

preparation contains edetate sodium (EDTA); use caution in patients who are at risk for zinc deficiency if other EDTA-containing solutions are coadministered. Decreased *H. pylori* eradication rates have been observed with short-term (≤7 days) combination therapy. The American College of Gastroenterology recommends 10-14 days of therapy (triple or quadruple) for eradication of *H. pylori* (Chey, 2007).

PPIs may diminish the therapeutic effect of clopidogrel, thought to be due to reduced formation of the active metabolite of clopidogrel. The manufacturer of clopidogrel recommends either avoidance of both omeprazole (even when scheduled 12 hours apart) and esomeprazole or use of a PPI with comparatively less effect on the active metabolite of clopidogrel. Of the PPIs, pantoprazole has the lowest degree of CYP2C19 inhibition *in vitro* (Li, 2004) and has been shown to have less effect on conversion of clopidogrel to its active metabolite compared to omeprazole (Angiolillo, 2011). In contrast to these warnings, others have recommended the continued use of PPIs, regardless of the degree of inhibition, in patients with a history of GI bleeding or multiple risk factors for GI bleeding who are also receiving clopidogrel since no evidence has established clinically meaningful differences in outcome; however, a clinically-significant interaction cannot be excluded in those who are poor metabolizers of clopidogrel (Abraham, 2010; Levine, 2011). Concomitant use of pantoprazole with some drugs may require cautious use, may not be recommended, or may require dosage adjustments.

Increased incidence of osteoporosis-related bone fractures of the hip, spine, or wrist may occur with PPI therapy. Patients on high-dose or long-term therapy (≥1 year) should be monitored. Use the lowest effective dose for the shortest duration of time, use vitamin D and calcium supplementation, and follow appropriate guidelines to reduce risk of fractures in patients at risk. Thrombophlebitis and hypersensitivity reactions including anaphylaxis, Stevens-Johnson syndrome, and toxic epidermal necrolysis have been reported with IV administration.

Hypomagnesemia, reported rarely, usually with prolonged PPI use of >3 months (most cases >1 year of therapy); may be symptomatic or asymptomatic; severe cases may cause tetany, seizures, and cardiac arrhythmias. Consider obtaining serum magnesium concentrations prior to beginning long-term therapy, especially if taking concomitant digoxin, diuretics, or other drugs known to cause hypomagnesemia; and periodically thereafter. Hypomagnesemia may be corrected by magnesium supplementation, although discontinuation of pantoprazole may be necessary; magnesium levels typically return to normal within 2 weeks of stopping.

Drug Interactions

Metabolism/Transport Effects Substrate of CYP2C19 (major), CYP2D6 (minor), CYP3A4 (minor); **Note:** Assignment of Major/Minor substrate status based on clinically relevant drug interaction potential; **Inhibits** BCRP, CYP2C19 (weak); **Induces** CYP1A2 (weak/moderate)

Avoid Concomitant Use

Avoid concomitant use of Pantoprazole with any of the following: Dasatinib; Delavirdine; Erlotinib; Nelfinavir; Ponatinib; Posaconazole; Rilpivirine; Risedronate

Increased Effect/Toxicity

Pantoprazole may increase the levels/effects of: Amphetamines; Dexmethylphenidate; Methotrexate; Methylphenidate; Raltegravir; Risedronate; Saquinavir; Topotecan; Voriconazole

The levels/effects of Pantoprazole may be increased by: Fluconazole; Ketoconazole (Systemic); Voriconazole

Decreased Effect

Pantoprazole may decrease the levels/effects of: Atazanavir; Bisphosphonate Derivatives; Bosutinib; Cefditoren; Clopidogrel; Dabigatran Etexilate; Dasatinib; Delavirdine; Erlotinib; Gefitinib; Indinavir; Iron Salts; Itraconazole; Ketoconazole (Systemic); Mesalamine; Multivitamins/Minerals (with ADEK, Folate, Iron); Mycophenolate; Nelfinavir; Nilotinib; Ponatinib; Posaconazole; Rilpivirine; Risedronate; Vismodegib

The levels/effects of Pantoprazole may be decreased by: CYP2C19 Inducers (Strong); Peginterferon Alfa-2b; Tipranavir

Ethanol/Nutrition/Herb Interactions

Ethanol: Avoid ethanol (may cause gastric mucosal irritation).

Herb/Nutraceutical: Prolonged treatment (typically >3 years) may lead to vitamin B_{12} malabsorption and subsequent deficiency.

Dietary Considerations

Oral: May be taken with or without food; best if taken before breakfast.

I.V.: Due to EDTA in preparation, zinc supplementation may be needed in patients prone to zinc deficiency.

Pharmacodynamics/Kinetics

Half-life Elimination 1 hour; increased to 3.5-10 hours with CYP2C19 deficiency

Time to Peak Oral: 2.5 hours

Pregnancy Risk Factor B

Pregnancy Considerations Teratogenic effects were not observed in animal reproduction studies. There are no adequate and well-controlled studies in pregnant women. Use in pregnancy only if clearly needed.

Lactation Enters breast milk/not recommended

Breast-Feeding Considerations Not recommended due to carcinogenicity in animal studies.

Dosage Forms

Granules for suspension, delayed release, enteric coated, oral:
Protonix®: 40 mg/packet (30s)

Injection, powder for reconstitution: 40 mg
Protonix® I.V.: 40 mg

Tablet, delayed release, oral: 20 mg, 40 mg
Protonix®: 20 mg, 40 mg

Dosage Forms: Canada

Tablet, enteric coated:
Tecta®: 40 mg

Papaverine (pa PAV er een)

Pharmacologic Category Vasodilator

Use Various vascular spasms associated with smooth muscle spasms as in myocardial infarction, angina, peripheral and pulmonary embolism, peripheral vascular disease; cerebral angiospastic states; visceral spasms (ureteral, biliary, and GI colic). **Note:** Labeled uses have fallen out of favor; safer and more effective alternatives are available.

Unlabeled Use Prevention of vasospasm during harvesting mammary arteries for coronary artery bypass graft surgery

Local Anesthetic/Vasoconstrictor Precautions No information available to require special precautions

Effects on Dental Treatment No significant effects or complications reported

Effects on Bleeding No information available to require special precautions

Adverse Effects Frequency not defined.

Cardiovascular: Arrhythmias (with rapid I.V. use), flushing, mild hypertension, tachycardia

Central nervous system: Headache, malaise, sedation, vertigo

Dermatologic: Rash

Gastrointestinal: Abdominal distress, anorexia, constipation, diarrhea, nausea

Hepatic: Cirrhosis, hepatic hypersensivity, hepatitis (rare)

Respiratory: Apnea (with rapid I.V. use)

Miscellaneous: Diaphoresis

General Dosage Range I.M., I.V.: Adults: 30-120 mg, may repeat dose every 3 hours

Mechanism of Action Smooth muscle spasmolytic producing a generalized smooth muscle relaxation including: vasodilatation, gastrointestinal sphincter relaxation, bronchiolar muscle relaxation, and potentially a depressed myocardium (with large doses); muscle relaxation may occur due to inhibition or cyclic nucleotide phosphodiesterase, increasing cyclic AMP; muscle relaxation is unrelated to nerve innervation; papaverine increases cerebral blood flow in normal subjects; oxygen uptake is unaltered

Pregnancy Risk Factor C

Pregnancy Considerations Teratogenic effects have not been observed in animal reproduction studies.

Papillomavirus (Types 6, 11, 16, 18) Vaccine (Human, Recombinant)
(pap ih LO ma VYE rus typs six e LEV en SIX teen AYE teen vak SEEN YU man ree KOM be nant)

Related Information

Systemic Viral Diseases on page 1537

Brand Names: U.S. Gardasil®

Brand Names: Canada Gardasil®

Pharmacologic Category Vaccine, Inactivated (Viral)

Use

U.S. labeling:

Females ≥9 years and ≤26 years of age: Prevention of cervical, vulvar, vaginal, and anal cancer caused by HPV types 16 and 18; genital warts caused by HPV types 6 and 11; cervical adenocarcinoma in situ, and vulvar, vaginal, cervical, or anal intraepithelial neoplasia caused by HPV types 6, 11, 16, and 18

Males ≥9 years and ≤26 years of age: Prevention of genital warts caused by human papillomavirus (HPV) types 6 and 11; anal cancer caused by HPV types 16 and 18, and anal intraepithelial neoplasia caused by HPV types 6, 11, 16, and 18

Canadian labeling:

Females ≥9 years and ≤26 years of age: Prevention of anal cancer caused by HPV types 16 and 18; anal intraepithelial neoplasia caused by HPV types 6, 11, 16, and 18

Females ≥9 years and ≤45 years of age: Prevention of cervical, vulvar, and vaginal cancer caused by HPV types 16 and 18; genital warts caused by HPV types 6 and 11; cervical adenocarcinoma in situ, vulvar, vaginal, or cervical intraepithelial neoplasia caused by HPV types 6, 11, 16, and 18

Males ≥9 years and ≤26 years of age: Prevention of anal cancer caused by HPV types 16 and 18; anal intraepithelial neoplasia caused by HPV types 6, 11, 16, and 18; genital warts caused by HPV types 6 and 11

The Advisory Committee on Immunization Practices (ACIP) recommends routine vaccination for females and males 11-12 years of age; catch-up vaccination is recommended for females 13-26 years of age and males 13-21 years of age. Males 22-26 years may also be vaccinated. The ACIP also recommends routine vaccination for men who have sex with men (MSM) through 26 years of age (CDC, 59[20], 2010; CDC, 60 [50], 2011). Vaccination is also recommended for immunocompromised persons or MSM through 26 years of age who were not previously vaccinated when they were younger. Although not specifically recommended for their profession, health care providers within the recommended age groups should also receive the HPV vaccine (CDC, 2013).

Local Anesthetic/Vasoconstrictor Precautions No information available to require special precautions

Effects on Dental Treatment No significant effects or complications reported

Effects on Bleeding No information available to require special precautions

Adverse Effects All serious adverse reactions must be reported to the U.S. Department of Health and Human Services (DHHS) Vaccine Adverse Event Reporting System (VAERS) 1-800-822-7967 or online at https://vaers.hhs.gov/esub/index. In Canada, adverse reactions may be reported to local provincial/territorial health agencies or to the Vaccine Safety Section at Public Health Agency of Canada (1-866-844-0018).

>10%:
Central nervous system: Headache (12% to 28%), fever (8% to 13%)
Local: Injection site: Pain (61% to 84%), erythema (17% to 25%), swelling (14% to 25%)

1% to 10%:
Central nervous system: Dizziness (1% to 4%), malaise (1%), insomnia (1%)
Gastrointestinal: Nausea (2% to 7%), diarrhea (3% to 4%), vomiting (1% to 2%), toothache (2%)
Local: Injection site: Bruising (3%), pruritus (3%), hematoma (1%)
Neuromuscular & skeletal: Arthralgia (1%), myalgia (≤1%)
Respiratory: Pharyngolaryngeal pain (3%), cough (2%), nasal congestion (1%)

General Dosage Range I.M.: *Children ≥9 years and Adults ≤26 years:* 0.5 mL initial dose, followed by 0.5 mL 2 and 6 months later

Mechanism of Action Contains inactive human papillomavirus (HPV) proteins HPV 6 L1, HPV 11 L1, HPV 16 L1, and HPV 18 L1 which produce neutralizing antibodies to prevent cervical cancer, cervical adenocarcinoma, cervical, vaginal and vulvar neoplasia, and genital warts caused by HPV.

Pharmacodynamics/Kinetics
Onset of Action Peak seroconversion was observed 1 month following the last dose of vaccine
Duration of Action Not well defined; at least 5 years

Pregnancy Risk Factor B

Pregnancy Considerations Teratogenic effects were not observed in animal studies. In clinical trials, women who were found to be pregnant before the completion of the 3-dose regimen were instructed to defer any remaining dose until pregnancy resolution. Pregnancies detected within 30 days of vaccination had a higher rate of congenital anomalies (pyloric stenosis, congenital megacolon, congenital hydronephrosis, hip dysplasia, club foot) than the placebo group. Pregnancies with

onset beyond 30 days of vaccination had a rate of congenital anomalies consistent with the general population. Overall, the type of teratogenic events were the same as those generally observed for this age group. Administration of the vaccine in pregnancy is not recommended; until additional information is available, the vaccine series (or completion of the series) should be delayed until pregnancy is completed. Pregnancy testing is not required prior to administration of the vaccine (CDC, 2013).

A registry has been established for women exposed to the HPV vaccine during pregnancy (1-800-986-8999).

Papillomavirus (Types 16, 18) Vaccine (Human, Recombinant)
(pap ih LO ma VYE rus typs SIX teen AYE teen vak SEEN YU man ree KOM be nant)

Related Information
Systemic Viral Diseases *on page 1537*
Brand Names: U.S. Cervarix®
Brand Names: Canada Cervarix®
Pharmacologic Category Vaccine, Inactivated (Viral)
Use Females 9 through 25 years of age: Prevention of cervical cancer, cervical adenocarcinoma *in situ*, and cervical intraepithelial neoplasia caused by human papillomavirus (HPV) types 16, 18

The Advisory Committee on Immunization Practices (ACIP) recommends routine vaccination for females 11-12 years of age; catch-up vaccination is recommended for females 13-25 years of age (CDC, 59[20], 2010). Vaccination is also recommended for immunocompromised females through 26 years of age who were not previously vaccinated when they were younger. Although not specifically recommended for their profession, female health care providers within the recommended age groups should also receive the HPV vaccine (CDC, 2013).

Local Anesthetic/Vasoconstrictor Precautions No information available to require special precautions

Effects on Dental Treatment No significant effects or complications reported

Effects on Bleeding No information available to require special precautions

Adverse Effects All serious adverse reactions must be reported to the U.S. Department of Health and Human Services (DHHS) Vaccine Adverse Event Reporting System (VAERS) 1-800-822-7967 or online at https://vaers.hhs.gov/esub/index. In Canada, adverse reactions may be reported to local provincial/territorial health agencies or to the Vaccine Safety Section at Public Health Agency of Canada (1-866-844-0018).

>10%:
Central nervous system: Fatigue (55%)
Local: Injection site reactions: Pain (92%), redness (48%), swelling (44%)
Neuromuscular & skeletal: Myalgia (49%), arthralgia (21%)

1% to 10%:
Dermatologic: Urticaria (7%)
Local: Injection site: Pruritus (1%)
Respiratory: Nasopharyngitis (4%), pharyngolaryngeal pain (3%), upper respiratory tract infection (2%), pharyngitis (1%)
Miscellaneous: Influenza (3%), chlamydia infection (2%), vaginal infection (1%)

◄ **Note:** The following occurred more often with the placebo (percentages reported with Cervarix®): Headache (5% to 53%); gastrointestinal symptoms (abdominal pain, diarrhea, nausea, vomiting) (28%); fever (13%); rash (10%); dizziness (2%); dysmenorrhea (2%); back pain (1%); injection site bruising (1%)

General Dosage Range I.M.: *Children ≥9 years and Adults ≤25 years (females):* 0.5 mL initial dose, followed by 0.5 mL 1 and 6 months later

Mechanism of Action Contains inactive human papillomavirus (HPV) proteins HPV 16 L1, and HPV 18 L1 which produce neutralizing antibodies to prevent cervical cancer, cervical adenocarcinoma, and cervical neoplasia cause by HPV.

Pharmacodynamics/Kinetics

Onset of Action Peak seroconversion was observed 1 month following the last dose of vaccine

Duration of Action Not well defined; >5 years

Pregnancy Risk Factor B

Pregnancy Considerations Adverse events were not observed in animal reproduction studies. Vaccination with papilloma virus vaccine is not recommended in pregnant women. In clinical trials, pregnancy testing was conducted prior to each vaccine administration and vaccination was discontinued if the woman was found to be pregnant; women were also instructed to avoid pregnancy for 2 months after receiving the vaccine. Pregnancies detected within 30 days prior or 45 days after vaccination had a higher rate of spontaneous abortions. A registry has been established for women exposed to Cervarix® during pregnancy (888-452-9622).

Administration of the vaccine in pregnancy is not recommended; until additional information is available, the vaccine series (or completion of the series) should be delayed until pregnancy is completed. Pregnancy testing is not required prior to administration of the vaccine (CDC, 2013).

Paregoric (par e GOR ik)

Pharmacologic Category Analgesic, Opioid

Use Treatment of diarrhea

Local Anesthetic/Vasoconstrictor Precautions No information available to require special precautions

Effects on Dental Treatment No significant effects or complications reported

Effects on Bleeding No information available to require special precautions

Adverse Effects Frequency not defined.
Cardiovascular: Hypotension, peripheral vasodilation
Central nervous system: CNS depression, dizziness, drowsiness, headache, increased intracranial pressure, insomnia, malaise, mental depression, restlessness
Gastrointestinal: Anorexia, biliary tract spasm, constipation, nausea, stomach cramps, vomiting
Genitourinary: Decreased urination, ureteral spasms, urinary tract spasm
Hepatic: Increased liver function tests
Neuromuscular & skeletal: Weakness
Ocular: Miosis
Respiratory: Respiratory depression
Miscellaneous: Physical and psychological dependence, histamine release

General Dosage Range Oral:
Children: 0.25-0.5 mL/kg 1-4 times daily
Adults: 5-10 mL 1-4 times daily

Mechanism of Action Increases smooth muscle tone in GI tract, decreases motility and peristalsis, diminishes digestive secretions

Pregnancy Risk Factor C

Pregnancy Considerations Refer to Morphine (Systemic) monograph.

Controlled Substance C-III

Paricalcitol (pah ri KAL si tole)

Brand Names: U.S. Zemplar®
Brand Names: Canada Zemplar®
Pharmacologic Category Vitamin D Analog
Use
I.V.: Prevention and treatment of secondary hyperparathyroidism associated with stage 5 chronic kidney disease (CKD)
Oral: Prevention and treatment of secondary hyperparathyroidism associated with stage 3 and 4 CKD and stage 5 CKD patients on hemodialysis or peritoneal dialysis

Local Anesthetic/Vasoconstrictor Precautions No information available to require special precautions

Effects on Dental Treatment Key adverse event(s) related to dental treatment: Xerostomia (normal salivary flow resumes upon discontinuation).

Effects on Bleeding No information available to require special precautions

Adverse Effects
>10%:
Gastrointestinal: Nausea (5% to 13%), diarrhea (7% to 12%)
Miscellaneous: Infection (bacterial, fungal, viral: 3% to 15%)
2% to 10%:
Cardiovascular: Edema (7%), hypertension (7%), hypervolemia (5%), hypotension (5%), palpitation (3%), chest pain (3%), peripheral edema (3%), syncope (3%)
Central nervous system: Pain (8%), dizziness (5% to 7%), chills (5%), insomnia (5%), lightheadedness (5%), vertigo (5%), fever (3% to 5%), headache (3% to 5%), anxiety (3%), depression (3%)
Dermatologic: Rash (6%), bruising (3%), skin ulcer (3%)
Endocrine & metabolic: Dehydration (3%), hypoglycemia (3%)
Gastrointestinal: Vomiting (5% to 8%), GI bleeding (5%), constipation (4% to 5%), abdominal pain (4%), dyspepsia (3%), xerostomia (3%)
Genitourinary: Urinary tract infection (3%)
Neuromuscular & skeletal: Arthritis (5%), weakness (3% to 5%), back pain (4%), leg cramps (3%)
Renal: Uremia (3%)
Respiratory: Pneumonia (5%), rhinitis (5%), oropharyngeal pain (4%), bronchitis (3%), cough (3%), sinusitis (3%)
Miscellaneous: Allergic reaction (6%), flu-like syndrome (5%), peritonitis (5%), sepsis (5%)

General Dosage Range Dosage adjustment recommended in patients with renal impairment
I.V.: *Children ≥5 years and Adults:* 0.04-0.24 mcg/kg (2.8-16.8 mcg) every other day during dialysis
Oral: *Adults:* 1-2 mcg/day **or** 2-4 mcg 3 times/week

Mechanism of Action Decreased renal conversion of vitamin D to its primary active metabolite (1,25-hydroxyvitamin D) in chronic renal failure leads to reduced activation of vitamin D receptor (VDR), which subsequently removes inhibitory suppression of parathyroid hormone (PTH) release; increased serum PTH (secondary hyperparathyroidism) reduces calcium excretion and enhances bone resorption. Paricalcitol is a synthetic vitamin D analog which binds to and activates the VDR in kidney, parathyroid gland, intestine and bone, thus reducing PTH levels and improving calcium and phosphate homeostasis.

Pharmacodynamics/Kinetics

Half-life Elimination

Healthy subjects: Oral: 4-6 hours; I.V.: 5-7 hours
Stage 3 and 4 CKD: Oral: 14-20 hours
Stage 5 CKD: Oral: 14-20 hours; I.V.: 14-15 hours

Time to Peak Plasma: 3 hours; Delayed by food

Pregnancy Risk Factor C

Pregnancy Considerations There are no adequate and well-controlled studies in pregnant women; use during pregnancy only if potential benefit to mother outweighs possible risk to fetus.

Paromomycin (par oh moe MYE sin)

Brand Names: Canada Humatin®
Pharmacologic Category Amebicide
Use Treatment of acute and chronic intestinal amebiasis; hepatic coma
Unlabeled Use Treatment of cryptosporidiosis
Local Anesthetic/Vasoconstrictor Precautions No information available to require special precautions
Effects on Dental Treatment No significant effects or complications reported
Effects on Bleeding No information available to require special precautions

Adverse Effects

1% to 10%: Gastrointestinal: Diarrhea, abdominal cramps, nausea, vomiting, heartburn

General Dosage Range Oral: *Children and Adults:* Dosage varies greatly depending on indication

Mechanism of Action Acts directly on ameba; has antibacterial activity against normal and pathogenic organisms in the GI tract; interferes with bacterial protein synthesis by binding to 30S ribosomal subunits

Pregnancy Considerations Paromomycin is poorly absorbed when given orally. Because it does not reach the maternal serum, it would not be expected to adversely affect the fetus. No adverse effects were observed in two infants whose mothers took paromomycin during pregnancy.

PARoxetine (pa ROKS e teen)

Related Information

Management of the Patient With Anxiety or Depression *on page 1594*
Vasoconstrictor Interactions With Antidepressants *on page 1650*

Brand Names: U.S. Paxil CR®; Paxil®; Pexeva®
Brand Names: Canada Apo-Paroxetine®; CO Paroxetine; Dom-Paroxetine; Mylan-Paroxetine; Novo-Paroxetine; Paxil CR®; Paxil®; PHL-Paroxetine; PMS-Paroxetine; ratio-Paroxetine; Riva-Paroxetine; Sandoz-Paroxetine; Teva-Paroxetine
Generic Availability (U.S.) Yes: Excludes suspension, tablet (mesylate)
Pharmacologic Category Antidepressant, Selective Serotonin Reuptake Inhibitor
Use Treatment of major depressive disorder (MDD); treatment of panic disorder with or without agoraphobia; obsessive-compulsive disorder (OCD); social anxiety

disorder (social phobia); generalized anxiety disorder (GAD); post-traumatic stress disorder (PTSD); premenstrual dysphoric disorder (PMDD)

Unlabeled Use May be useful in eating disorders, impulse control disorders; vasomotor symptoms of menopause; treatment of obsessive-compulsive disorder (OCD) in children; treatment of mild dementia-associated agitation in nonpsychotic patients; treatment of paraphilia/hypersexuality

Local Anesthetic/Vasoconstrictor Precautions Although caution should be used in patients taking tricyclic antidepressants, no interactions have been reported with vasoconstrictor and paroxetine, a nontricyclic antidepressant which acts to increase serotonin; no precautions appear to be needed

Effects on Dental Treatment Key adverse event(s) related to dental treatment: Xerostomia and changes in salivation (normal salivary flow resumes upon discontinuation), postural hypotension, and abnormal taste. Problems with SSRI-induced bruxism have been reported and may preclude their use; clinicians attempting to evaluate any patient with bruxism or involuntary muscle movement, who is simultaneously being treated with an SSRI drug, should be aware of the potential association. Prolonged use may decrease or inhibit salivary flow; normal salivation resumes upon discontinuation. See Effects on Bleeding.

Effects on Bleeding May impair platelet aggregation resulting in increased risk of bleeding events, particularly if used concomitantly with aspirin, NSAIDs, warfarin, or other anticoagulants. Bleeding related to SSRI use has been reported to range from relatively minor bruising and epistaxis to life-threatening hemorrhage. Routine interruption of therapy for most dental procedures is not warranted. In medically complicated patients or extensive oral surgery, the decision to interrupt therapy must be based on the risk to benefit in an individual patient and a medical consult is suggested. If therapy is continued without interruption, the clinician should anticipate the potential for a prolonged bleeding time.

Adverse Effects Frequency varies by dose and indication. Adverse reactions reported as a composite of all indications.

>10%:

Central nervous system: Somnolence (15% to 24%), insomnia (11% to 24%), headache (17% to 18%), dizziness (6% to 14%)

Endocrine & metabolic: Libido decreased (3% to 15%)

Gastrointestinal: Nausea (19% to 26%), xerostomia (9% to 18%), constipation (5% to 16%), diarrhea (9% to 12%)

Genitourinary: Ejaculatory disturbances (13% to 28%)

Neuromuscular & skeletal: Weakness (12% to 22%), tremor (4% to 11%)

Miscellaneous: Diaphoresis (5% to 14%)

1% to 10%:

Cardiovascular: Vasodilation (2% to 4%), chest pain (3%), palpitation (2% to 3%), hypertension (≥1%), tachycardia (≥1%)

Central nervous system: Nervousness (4% to 9%), anxiety (5%), agitation (3% to 5%), abnormal dreams (3% to 4%), concentration impaired (3% to 4%), yawning (2% to 4%), depersonalization (≤3%), amnesia (2%), chills (2%), emotional lability (≥1%), vertigo (≥1%), confusion (1%)

Dermatologic: Rash (2% to 3%), pruritus (≥1%)

Endocrine & metabolic: Orgasmic disturbance (2% to 9%), dysmenorrhea (5%)

Gastrointestinal: Appetite decreased (5% to 9%), dyspepsia (2% to 5%), flatulence (4%), abdominal pain (4%), appetite increased (2% to 4%), vomiting (2% to 3%), taste perversion (2%), weight gain (≥1%)

Genitourinary: Genital disorder (male 10%; female 2% to 9%), impotence (2% to 9%), urinary frequency (2% to 3%), urinary tract infection (2%)

Neuromuscular & skeletal: Paresthesia (4%), myalgia (2% to 4%), back pain (3%), myoclonus (2% to 3%), myopathy (2%), myasthenia (1%), arthralgia (≥1%)

Ocular: Blurred vision (4%), abnormal vision (2% to 4%)

Otic: Tinnitus (≥1%)

Respiratory: Respiratory disorder (≤7%), pharyngitis (4%), sinusitis (≤4%), rhinitis (3%)

Miscellaneous: Infection (5% to 6%)

Dosage Oral:

Children ≥8 years:

Obsessive-compulsive disorder (unlabeled use): Initial: 10 mg/day; titrate every 7-14 days in 10 mg/day increments as necessary to a maximum 60 mg/day; trials have typically continued for a 10- to 12-week treatment course (Geller, 2004; Rosenberg, 1999)

Social anxiety disorder (unlabeled use): Initial: 2.5-10 mg/day; titrate every ≥7 days in 5-10 mg/day increments to a maximum of 50 mg/day; trials have typically continued for a 16-week treatment course (Mancini, 1999; Wagner, 2004)

Adults:

Major depressive disorder:

Paxil®, Pexeva®: Initial: 20 mg once daily, preferably in the morning; increase if needed by 10 mg/day increments at intervals of at least 1 week; maximum dose: 50 mg/day

Paxil CR®: Initial: 25 mg once daily; increase if needed by 12.5 mg/day increments at intervals of at least 1 week; maximum dose: 62.5 mg/day

Generalized anxiety disorder (Paxil®, Pexeva®): Initial: 20 mg once daily, preferably in the morning (if dose is increased, adjust in increments of 10 mg/day at 1-week intervals); doses of 20-50 mg/day were used in clinical trials, however, no greater benefit was seen with doses >20 mg.

Obsessive-compulsive disorder (Paxil®, Pexeva®): Initial: 20 mg once daily, preferably in the morning; increase if needed by 10 mg/day increments at intervals of at least 1 week; recommended dose: 40 mg/day; range: 20-60 mg/day; maximum dose: 60 mg/day

Panic disorder:

Paxil®, Pexeva®: Initial: 10 mg once daily, preferably in the morning; increase if needed by 10 mg/day increments at intervals of at least 1 week; recommended dose: 40 mg/day; range: 10-60 mg/day; maximum dose: 60 mg/day

Paxil CR®: Initial: 12.5 mg once daily; increase if needed by 12.5 mg/day at intervals of at least 1 week; maximum dose: 75 mg/day

Premenstrual dysphoric disorder (Paxil CR®): Initial: 12.5 mg once daily in the morning; may be increased to 25 mg/day; dosing changes should occur at intervals of at least 1 week. May be given daily throughout the menstrual cycle or limited to the luteal phase.

Post-traumatic stress disorder (PTSD) (Paxil®): Initial: 20 mg once daily, preferably in the morning; increase if needed by 10 mg/day increments at intervals of at least 1 week; range: 20-50 mg. Limited data suggest doses of 40 mg/day were not more efficacious than 20 mg/day.

Social anxiety disorder:

Paxil®: Initial: 20 mg once daily, preferably in the morning; recommended dose: 20 mg/day; range: 20-60 mg/day; doses >20 mg may not have additional benefit

Paxil CR®: Initial: 12.5 mg once daily, preferably in the morning; may be increased by 12.5 mg/day at intervals of at least 1 week; maximum dose: 37.5 mg/day

Vasomotor symptoms of menopause (unlabeled use, Paxil CR®): 12.5-25 mg/day

Elderly:

Paxil®, Pexeva®: Initial: 10 mg/day; increase if needed by 10 mg/day increments at intervals of at least 1 week; maximum dose: 40 mg/day

Paxil CR®: Initial: 12.5 mg/day; increase if needed by 12.5 mg/day increments at intervals of at least 1 week; maximum dose: 50 mg/day

Note: Upon discontinuation of paroxetine therapy, gradually taper dose:

Paxil®, Pexeva®: 10 mg/day at weekly intervals; when 20 mg/day dose is reached, continue for 1 week before treatment is discontinued. Some patients may need to be titrated to 10 mg/day for 1 week before discontinuation.

Paxil CR®: Patients receiving 37.5 mg/day in clinical trials had their dose decreased by 12.5 mg/day to a dose of 25 mg/day and remained at a dose of 25 mg/day for 1 week before treatment was discontinued.

MAO inhibitor recommendations:

Switching to or from an MAO inhibitor intended to treat psychiatric disorders:

Allow 14 days to elapse between discontinuing an MAO inhibitor intended to treat psychiatric disorders and initiation of paroxetine.

Allow 14 days to elapse between discontinuing paroxetine and initiation of an MAO inhibitor intended to treat psychiatric disorders.

Use with other MAO inhibitors (linezolid or I.V. methylene blue):

Do not initiate paroxetine in patients receiving linezolid or I.V. methylene blue; consider other interventions for psychiatric condition.

If urgent treatment with linezolid or I.V. methylene blue is required in a patient already receiving paroxetine and potential benefits outweigh potential risks, discontinue paroxetine promptly and administer linezolid or I.V. methylene blue. Monitor for serotonin syndrome for 2 weeks or until 24 hours after the last dose of linezolid or I.V. methylene blue, whichever comes first. May resume paroxetine 24 hours after the last dose of linezolid or I.V. methylene blue.

Dosage adjustment in renal impairment: Adults:

Cl_{cr} 30-60 mL/minute: Plasma concentration is 2 times that seen in normal function. There are no dosage adjustments provided in manufacturer's labeling.

Severe impairment (Cl_{cr} <30 mL/minute): Mean plasma concentration is ~4 times that seen in normal function.

Paxil®, Pexeva®: Initial: 10 mg/day; increase if needed by 10 mg/day increments at intervals of at least 1 week; maximum dose: 40 mg/day

Paxil CR®: Initial: 12.5 mg/day; increase if needed by 12.5 mg/day increments at intervals of at least 1 week; maximum dose: 50 mg/day

Dosage adjustment in hepatic impairment: Adults: In hepatic dysfunction, plasma concentration is 2 times that seen in normal function.

Mild-to-moderate impairment: There are no dosage adjustments provided in manufacturer's labeling.

Severe impairment:

Paxil®, Pexeva®: Initial: 10 mg/day; increase if needed by 10 mg/day increments at intervals of at least 1 week; maximum dose: 40 mg/day

Paxil CR®: Initial: 12.5 mg/day; increase if needed by 12.5 mg/day increments at intervals of at least 1 week; maximum dose: 50 mg/day

Mechanism of Action Paroxetine is a selective serotonin reuptake inhibitor, chemically unrelated to tricyclic, tetracyclic, or other antidepressants; presumably, the inhibition of serotonin reuptake from brain synapse stimulated serotonin activity in the brain

Contraindications Hypersensitivity to paroxetine or any component of the formulation; use of MAO inhibitors intended to treat psychiatric disorders (concurrently or within 14 days of discontinuing either paroxetine or the MAO inhibitor); initiation of paroxetine in a patient receiving linezolid or intravenous methylene blue; concurrent use with thioridazine or pimozide

Warnings/Precautions Hazardous agent - use appropriate precautions for handling and disposal (NIOSH, 2012). **[U.S. Boxed Warning]: Antidepressants increase the risk of suicidal thinking and behavior in children, adolescents, and young adults (18-24 years of age) with major depressive disorder (MDD) and other psychiatric disorders;** consider risk prior to prescribing. Short-term studies did not show an increased risk in patients >24 years of age and showed a decreased risk in patients ≥65 years. Closely monitor patients for clinical worsening, suicidality, or unusual changes in behavior, particularly during the initial 1-2 months of therapy or during periods of dosage adjustments (increases or decreases); the patient's family or caregiver should be instructed to closely observe the patient and communicate with healthcare provider. A medication guide concerning the use of antidepressants should be dispensed with each prescription. **Paroxetine is not FDA approved for use in children.**

The possibility of a suicide attempt is inherent in major depression and may persist until remission occurs. Patients treated with antidepressants (for any indication) should be observed for clinical worsening and suicidality, especially during the initial few months of a course of drug therapy, or at times of dose changes, either increases or decreases. Use caution in high-risk patients. Worsening depression and severe abrupt suicidality that are not part of the presenting symptoms may require discontinuation or modification of drug therapy. The patient's family or caregiver should be alerted to monitor patients for the emergence of suicidality and associated behaviors (such as agitation, irritability, hostility, impulsivity, and hypomania) and call healthcare provider.

May worsen psychosis in some patients or precipitate a shift to mania or hypomania in patients with bipolar disorder. Patients presenting with depressive symptoms should be screened for bipolar disorder. Monotherapy in patients with bipolar disorder should be avoided. **Paroxetine is not FDA approved for the treatment of bipolar depression.**

Potentially life-threatening serotonin syndrome (SS) has occurred with serotonergic agents (eg, SSRIs, SNRIs), particularly when used in combination with other serotonergic agents (eg, triptans, TCAs, fentanyl, lithium, tramadol, buspirone, St John's wort, tryptophan) or agents that impair metabolism of serotonin (eg, MOA

inhibitors intended to treat psychiatric disorders, other MAO inhibitors [ie, linezolid and intravenous methylene blue]). Discontinue treatment (and any concomitant serotonergic agent) immediately if signs/symptoms arise.

Paroxetine may increase the risks associated with electroconvulsive therapy. Has a low potential to impair cognitive or motor performance - use caution when operating hazardous machinery or driving. Symptoms of agitation and/or restlessness may occur during initial few weeks of therapy. Low potential for sedation or anticholinergic effects relative to cyclic antidepressants.

Use caution in elderly patients; may cause or exacerbate syndrome of inappropriate antidiuretic hormone secretion or hyponatremia; monitor sodium closely with initiation or dosage adjustments in older adults. Medication associated with potent anticholinergic properties which may be inappropriate in older adults depending on comorbidities (eg, dementia, delirium) (Beers Criteria).

Use caution in patients with a previous seizure disorder or condition predisposing to seizures such as brain damage, alcoholism, or concurrent therapy with other drugs which lower the seizure threshold. Use with caution in patients with hepatic dysfunction. May cause SIADH; volume depletion and/or diuretics may increase risk. Potentially significant interactions may exist, requiring dose or frequency adjustment, additional monitoring, and/or selection of alternative therapy. Consult drug interactions database for more detailed information. Use with caution in patients with renal insufficiency or other concurrent illness (due to limited experience); dose reduction recommended with severe renal impairment. May cause or exacerbate sexual dysfunction. Use caution in patients with narrow-angle glaucoma. Avoid use in the first trimester of pregnancy.

Upon discontinuation of paroxetine therapy, gradually taper dose and monitor for discontinuation symptoms (eg, dizziness, dysphoric mood, irritability, agitation, confusion, paresthesias). If intolerable symptoms occur following a decrease in dosage or upon discontinuation of therapy, then resuming the previous dose with a more gradual taper should be considered.

Drug Interactions

Metabolism/Transport Effects Substrate of CYP2D6 (major); **Note:** Assignment of Major/Minor substrate status based on clinically relevant drug interaction potential; **Inhibits** CYP1A2 (weak), CYP2B6 (moderate), CYP2C19 (weak), CYP2C9 (weak), CYP2D6 (strong), CYP3A4 (weak)

Avoid Concomitant Use

Avoid concomitant use of PARoxetine with any of the following: Iobenguane I 123; Linezolid; MAO Inhibitors; Methylene Blue; Pimozide; Tamoxifen; Thioridazine; Tryptophan

Increased Effect/Toxicity

PARoxetine may increase the levels/effects of: Agents with Antiplatelet Properties; Anticoagulants; Antidepressants (Serotonin Reuptake Inhibitor/Antagonist); ARIPiprazole; Aspirin; AtoMOXetine; Beta-Blockers; BusPIRone; CarBAMazepine; CloZAPine; Collagenase (Systemic); CYP2B6 Substrates; CYP2D6 Substrates; Dabigatran Etexilate; Desmopressin; Dextromethorphan; Drotrecogin Alfa (Activated); DULoxetine; Fesoterodine; Galantamine; Highest Risk QTc-Prolonging Agents; Hypoglycemic Agents; Ibritumomab; Lomitapide; Methadone; Methylene Blue; Metoclopramide; Metoprolol; Mexiletine; Moderate

Risk QTc-Prolonging Agents; NSAID (COX-2 Inhibitor); NSAID (Nonselective); Pimozide; Propafenone; RisperiDONE; Rivaroxaban; Salicylates; Serotonin Modulators; Tetrabenazine; Thioridazine; Thrombolytic Agents; Tositumomab and Iodine I 131 Tositumomab; TraMADol; Tricyclic Antidepressants; Vitamin K Antagonists

The levels/effects of PARoxetine may be increased by: Abiraterone Acetate; Alcohol (Ethyl); Analgesics (Opioid); Antipsychotics; ARIPiprazole; Asenapine; BusPIRone; Cimetidine; CNS Depressants; Cobicistat; CYP2D6 Inhibitors (Moderate); CYP2D6 Inhibitors (Strong); Dasatinib; DULoxetine; Glucosamine; Herbs (Anticoagulant/Antiplatelet Properties); Linezolid; Lithium; MAO Inhibitors; Metoclopramide; Metyrosine; Mifepristone; Multivitamins/Minerals (with ADEK, Folate, Iron); Omega-3 Fatty Acids; Pentosan Polysulfate Sodium; Pentoxifylline; Pravastatin; Prostacyclin Analogues; Tipranavir; TraMADol; Tryptophan; Vitamin E

Decreased Effect

PARoxetine may decrease the levels/effects of: Aprepitant; Fosaprepitant; Iobenguane I 123; Ioflupane I 123; Tamoxifen

The levels/effects of PARoxetine may be decreased by: Aprepitant; CarBAMazepine; Cyproheptadine; Darunavir; Fosamprenavir; Fosaprepitant; NSAID (COX-2 Inhibitor); NSAID (Nonselective); Peginterferon Alfa-2b

Ethanol/Nutrition/Herb Interactions

Ethanol: May increase CNS depression; monitor for increased effects with coadministration. Caution patients about effects.

Food: Peak concentration is increased, but bioavailability is not significantly altered by food.

Herb/Nutraceutical: Avoid valerian, St John's wort, tryptophan, SAMe, kava kava.

Dietary Considerations May be taken without regard to meals.

Pharmacodynamics/Kinetics

Onset of Action Depression: The onset of action is within a week, however, individual response varies greatly and full response may not be seen until 8-12 weeks after initiation of treatment.

Half-life Elimination 21 hours (3-65 hours)

Time to Peak Immediate release: 5.2-8.1 hours; controlled release: 6-10 hours

Pregnancy Risk Factor D

Pregnancy Considerations Studies in pregnant women have demonstrated a risk to the fetus. Paroxetine crosses the placenta. An increased risk of teratogenic effects, including cardiovascular defects, may be associated with maternal use of paroxetine or other SSRIs; however, available information is conflicting. Nonteratogenic effects in the newborn following SSRI/SNRI exposure late in the third trimester include respiratory distress, cyanosis, apnea, seizures, temperature instability, feeding difficulty, vomiting, hypoglycemia, hypo- or hypertonia, hyper-reflexia, jitteriness, irritability, constant crying, and tremor. Symptoms may be due to the toxicity of the SSRIs/SNRIs or a discontinuation syndrome and may be consistent with serotonin syndrome associated with SSRI treatment. Persistent pulmonary hypertension of the newborn (PPHN) has also been reported with SSRI exposure. The long-term effects of *in utero* SSRI exposure on infant development and behavior are not known.

Due to pregnancy-induced physiologic changes, some pharmacokinetic parameters of paroxetine may be altered. The maternal CYP2D6 genotype also influences paroxetine plasma concentrations during pregnancy.

The manufacturer suggests discontinuing paroxetine or switching to another antidepressant unless the benefits of therapy justify continuing treatment during pregnancy; consider other treatment options for women who are planning to become pregnant. The ACOG recommends that therapy with SSRIs or SNRIs during pregnancy be individualized; treatment of depression during pregnancy should incorporate the clinical expertise of the mental health clinician, obstetrician, primary healthcare provider, and pediatrician. The ACOG also recommends that therapy with paroxetine be avoided during pregnancy if possible and that fetuses exposed in early pregnancy be assessed with a fetal echocardiography. According to the American Psychiatric Association (APA), the risks of medication treatment should be weighed against other treatment options and untreated depression. The use of paroxetine is not recommended as first line therapy during pregnancy. For women who discontinue antidepressant medications during pregnancy and who may be at high risk for postpartum depression, the medications can be restarted following delivery. Treatment algorithms have been developed by the ACOG and the APA for the management of depression in women prior to conception and during pregnancy.

Lactation Enters breast milk/use caution (AAP rates "of concern"; AAP 2001 update pending)

Breast-Feeding Considerations Paroxetine is excreted in breast milk and concentrations in the hindmilk are higher than in foremilk. Paroxetine has not been detected in the serum of nursing infants. Adverse reactions have been reported in nursing infants exposed to some SSRIs. The manufacturer recommends that caution be exercised when administering paroxetine to nursing women. Maternal use of an SSRI during pregnancy may cause delayed milk secretion. The American Academy of Breastfeeding Medicine suggests that paroxetine may be considered for the treatment of postpartum depression in appropriately selected women who are nursing. Mothers should be monitored for changes in symptoms and infants should be monitored for growth. The long-term effects on development and behavior have not been studied.

Dosage Forms

Suspension, oral:
Paxil®: 10 mg/5 mL (250 mL)

Tablet, oral: 10 mg, 20 mg, 30 mg, 40 mg
Paxil®: 10 mg, 20 mg, 30 mg, 40 mg
Pexeva®: 10 mg, 20 mg, 30 mg, 40 mg

Tablet, controlled release, enteric coated, oral: 12.5 mg, 25 mg, 37.5 mg
Paxil CR®: 12.5 mg, 25 mg, 37.5 mg

Tablet, extended release, enteric coated, oral: 12.5 mg, 25 mg, 37.5 mg

---

Pasireotide (pas i REE oh tide)

Related Information

Clinical Risk Related to Drugs Prolonging QT Interval *on page 1510*

Brand Names: U.S. Signifor®

Pharmacologic Category Somatostatin Analog

Use Treatment of Cushing's disease in patients for whom pituitary surgery is not an option or has not been curative

Local Anesthetic/Vasoconstrictor Precautions Pasireotide is one of the drugs confirmed to prolong the QT interval and is accepted as having a risk of causing torsade de pointes. In terms of epinephrine, it is not known what effect vasoconstrictors in the local anesthetic regimen will have in patients with a known history of congenital prolonged QT interval or in patients taking any medication that prolongs the QT interval. Until more information is obtained, it is suggested that the clinician consult with the physician prior to the use of a vasoconstrictor in suspected patients, and that the vasoconstrictor (epinephrine, mepivacaine and levonor-defrin [Carbocaine® 2% with Neo-Cobefrin®]) be used with caution. See Dental Comment.

Effects on Dental Treatment No significant effects or complications reported

Effects on Bleeding No information available to require special precautions

Adverse Effects

>10%:

Central nervous system: Headache (28%), fatigue (19%)

Dermatologic: Alopecia (12%)

Endocrine & metabolic: Hyperglycemia (40%), diabetes mellitus (18%), Hb A_{1c} increased (11%)

Gastrointestinal: Diarrhea (58%), nausea (52%), cholelithiasis (30%), abdominal pain (24%)

Hepatic: Prothrombin time increased (2% to 33%)

Local: Injection site reactions (17%; including pain, erythema, hematoma, hemorrhage, pruritus)

Neuromuscular & skeletal: Weakness (11%)

Respiratory: Nasopharyngitis (13%)

1% to 10%:

Cardiovascular: Hypertension (10%), peripheral edema (10%), hypotension (7%), bradycardia (6%), QT prolongation (6%; >480 msec 2%)

Central nervous system: Anxiety (9%), dizziness (9%), insomnia (9%), vertigo (6%)

Dermatologic: Pruritus (8%), dry skin (6%)

Endocrine & metabolic: Hypercholesterolemia (10%), hypoglycemia (9%), type 2 diabetes mellitus (9%), adrenal insufficiency (6%), hypokalemia (6%), hypothyroidism (4%)

Gastrointestinal: Appetite decreased (10%), constipation (7%), lipase increased (7%), vomiting (7%), abdominal distension (6%), amylase increased (2%)

Hematologic: Anemia (4%)

Hepatic: ALT increased (10%), GGT increased (10%), AST increased (6%), bilirubin increased (2%)

Neuromuscular & skeletal: Myalgia (9%), arthralgia (8%), back pain (6%), limb pain (6%)

Miscellaneous: Flu-like syndrome (9%)

General Dosage Range Dosage adjustment recommended in patients with hepatic impairment.

SubQ: *Adults:* Initial: 0.6 mg or 0.9 mg twice daily; titrate based on response and tolerability. Recommended dosage range: 0.3-0.9 mg twice daily.

Mechanism of Action Synthetic cyclohexapeptide analogue of somatostatin which is a peptide inhibitor of multiple endocrine, neuroendocrine, and exocrine mechanisms. Binds to somatostatin receptor (sst_{1-5}), with high affinity for the sst_1, sst_2, sst_3 subtypes, and highest affinity for the sst_5 subtype, resulting in inhibition of ACTH secretion which leads to decreased cortisol secretion.

Pharmacodynamics/Kinetics

Half-life Elimination ~12 hours

Time to Peak Plasma: 0.25-0.5 hours

Pregnancy Risk Factor C

Pregnancy Considerations Adverse events were observed in animal reproduction studies.

Dental Comment Pasireotide is known to prolong the QT interval. The QT interval is measured as the time and distance between the Q point of the QRS complex and the end of the T wave in the ECG tracing. After adjustment for heart rate, the QT interval is defined as prolonged if it is more than 450 msec in men and 460 msec in women. A long QT syndrome was first described in the 1950s and 60s as a congenital syndrome involving QT interval prolongation and syncope and sudden death. Some of the congenital long QT syndromes were characterized by a peculiar electrocardiographic appearance of the QRS complex involving a premature atria beat followed by a pause, then a subsequent sinus beat showing marked QT prolongation and deformity. This type of cardiac arrhythmia was originally termed "torsade de pointes" (translated from the French as "twisting of the points"). Pasireotide is considered as having a risk of causing torsade de pointes. Since it is not known what effect vasoconstrictors in the local anesthetic regimen will have in patients with a known history of congenital prolonged QT interval or in patients taking any medication that prolongs the QT interval, a medical consult is suggested.

Pazopanib (paz OH pa nib)

Related Information

Clinical Risk Related to Drugs Prolonging QT Interval *on page 1510*

Brand Names: U.S. Votrient™

Brand Names: Canada Votrient™

Pharmacologic Category Antineoplastic Agent, Tyrosine Kinase Inhibitor; Vascular Endothelial Growth Factor (VEGF) Inhibitor

Use Treatment of advanced renal cell cancer (RCC); treatment of advanced soft tissue sarcoma (STS) (in patients previously treated with chemotherapy)

Unlabeled Use Treatment of advanced, differentiated thyroid cancer

Local Anesthetic/Vasoconstrictor Precautions Hypertension can occur with the use of this drug, particularly early in the treatment course. Monitor for hypertension prior to using local anesthetic with vasoconstrictor; medical consult if necessary.

Pazopanib is one of the drugs confirmed to prolong the QT interval and is accepted as having a risk of causing torsade de pointes. The risk of drug-induced torsade de pointes is extremely low when a single QT interval prolonging drug is prescribed. In terms of epinephrine, it is not known what effect vasoconstrictors in the local anesthetic regimen will have in patients with a known history of congenital prolonged QT interval or in patients taking any medication that prolongs the QT interval. Until more information is obtained, it is suggested that the clinician consult with the physician prior to the use of a vasoconstrictor in suspected patients, and that the vasoconstrictor (epinephrine, mepivacaine and levonor-defrin [Carbocaine® 2% with Neo-Cobefrin®]) be used with caution.

Effects on Dental Treatment Key adverse event(s) related to dental treatment: Taste alteration.

◀ **Effects on Bleeding** Chemotherapy may result in significant myelosuppression, potentially including significant reduction in platelet counts (thrombocytopenia grades 3/4: <1%) and altered hemostasis. Hemorrhagic events have been reported. In patients who are under active treatment with these agents, medical consult is suggested.

Adverse Effects

>10%:

Cardiovascular: Hypertension (40% to 42%; grade 3: 4% to 7%), peripheral edema (14%)

Central nervous system: Fatigue (19% to 65%), headache (10% to 23%), dizziness (11%)

Dermatologic: Hair color change (38% to 39%), rash (8% to 18%), alopecia (8% to 12%), palmar-plantar erythrodysesthesia (6% to 11%), skin depigmentation (3% to 11%)

Endocrine & metabolic: Hyperglycemia (41% to 45%), hypophosphatemia (34%), hyponatremia (31%), thyroid-stimulating hormone (TSH) increased (27%), hypomagnesemia (26%), hypoglycemia (17%), hyperkalemia (16%)

Gastrointestinal: Diarrhea (52% to 59%; grade 3: 3% to 5%; grade 4: <1%), nausea (26% to 56%), weight loss (9% to 48%), anorexia (22% to 40%), vomiting (21% to 33%), taste alteration (8% to 28%), lipase increased (4% to 27%), abdominal pain (11% to 23%), mucositis (12%), stomatitis (11%)

Hematologic: Leukopenia (37% to 44%; grade 3: ≤1%), lymphocytopenia (31% to 43%; grade 3: 4% to 10%; grade 4: <1%), thrombocytopenia (32% to 36%; grade 3: ≤3%; grade 4: ≤1%), neutropenia (33% to 34%; grade 3: 1% to 4%; grade 4: <1%)

Hepatic: AST increased (51% to 53%; grade 3: 5% to 7%; grade 4: <3%), ALT increased (46% to 53%; grade 3: 8% to 10%; grade 4: 2%), bilirubin increased (29% to 36%; grade 3: ≤3%; grade 4: <1%), albumin decreased (34%), alkaline phosphatase increased (32%)

Neuromuscular & skeletal: Musculoskeletal pain (23%), myalgia (23%), weakness (14%)

Respiratory: Dyspnea (20%), cough (17%)

Miscellaneous: Tumor pain (29%)

1% to 10%:

Cardiovascular: Chest pain (5% to 10%), left ventricular dysfunction (≤8%), venous thrombosis (≤5%), MI/ischemia (2%), QT prolongation (1% to 2%), facial edema (1%), transient ischemic event (≤1%)

Central nervous system: Insomnia (9%), dysphonia (4% to 8%), chills (5%)

Dermatologic: Dry skin (6%), nail disorder (5%)

Endocrine & metabolic: Hypothyroidism (4% to 8%)

Gastrointestinal: Dyspepsia (5% to 7%), mouth hemorrhage (3%), rectal hemorrhage (1% to 2%)

Ocular: Blurred vision (5%)

Renal: Proteinuria (1% to 9%), hematuria (4%)

Respiratory: Epistaxis (2% to 8%), pneumothorax (≤3%), hemoptysis (2%), PE (fatal; 1%)

General Dosage Range Dosage adjustment recommended in patients with hepatic impairment, on concomitant therapy, or who develop toxicities

Oral: *Adults:* 800 mg once daily

Mechanism of Action Tyrosine kinase (multikinase) inhibitor; limits tumor growth via inhibition of angiogenesis angiogenesis by inhibiting cell surface vascular endothelial growth factor receptors (VEGFR-1, VEGFR-2, VEGFR-3), platelet-derived growth factor receptors (PDGFR-alpha and -beta), fibroblast growth factor receptor (FGFR-1 and -3), cytokine receptor (cKIT), interleukin-2 receptor inducible T-cell kinase, leukocyte-specific protein tyrosine kinase (Lck), and transmembrane glycoprotein receptor tyrosine kinase (c-Fms)

Pharmacodynamics/Kinetics

Half-life Elimination ~31 hours

Time to Peak Plasma: 2-4 hours

Pregnancy Risk Factor D

Pregnancy Considerations Adverse effects were observed in animal reproduction studies. Based on its mechanism of action, pazopanib would be expected to cause fetal harm if administered to a pregnant woman. Women of childbearing potential should avoid becoming pregnant during treatment.

Dental Comment Pazopanib is known to prolong the QT interval. The QT interval is measured as the time and distance between the Q point of the QRS complex and the end of the T wave in the ECG tracing. After adjustment for heart rate, the QT interval is defined as prolonged if it is more than 450 msec in men and 460 msec in women. A long QT syndrome was first described in the 1950s and 60s as a congenital syndrome involving QT interval prolongation and syncope and sudden death. Some of the congenital long QT syndromes were characterized by a peculiar electrocardiographic appearance of the QRS complex involving a premature atria beat followed by a pause, then a subsequent sinus beat showing marked QT prolongation and deformity. This type of cardiac arrhythmia was originally termed "torsade de pointes" (translated from the French as "twisting of the points"). Pazopanib is considered as having a risk of causing torsade de pointes. Since it is not known what effect vasoconstrictors in the local anesthetic regimen will have in patients with a known history of congenital prolonged QT interval or in patients taking any medication that prolongs the QT interval, a medical consult is suggested.

Pegademase Bovine (peg A de mase BOE vine)

Brand Names: U.S. Adagen®

Brand Names: Canada Adagen®

Pharmacologic Category Enzyme

Use Enzyme replacement therapy for adenosine deaminase (ADA) deficiency in patients with severe combined immunodeficiency disease (SCID) who are not candidates for or who have failed bone marrow transplant

Local Anesthetic/Vasoconstrictor Precautions No information available to require special precautions

Effects on Dental Treatment No significant effects or complications reported

Effects on Bleeding No information available to require special precautions

Adverse Effects Postmarketing and/or case reports: Autoimmune hemolytic anemia, erythema (injection site), hemolytic anemia, thrombocythemia, urticaria

General Dosage Range I.M.: *Children:* First dose: 10 units/kg; Second dose: 15 units/kg 7 days after first dose; Third dose: 20 units/kg 7 days after second dose; Maintenance: 20 units/kg/week (maximum: 30 units/kg/week)

Mechanism of Action Adenosine deaminase is an enzyme that catalyzes the deamination of both adenosine and deoxyadenosine. Hereditary lack of adenosine deaminase activity results in severe combined immunodeficiency disease, a fatal disorder of infancy characterized by profound defects of both cellular and humoral immunity. It is estimated that 25% of patients with the autosomal recessive form of severe combined immunodeficiency lack adenosine deaminase. Pegademase bovine is a (modified) enzyme replacement for adenosine deaminase deficiency.

Pharmacodynamics/Kinetics

Half-life Elimination Plasma ADA half-life (following administration): Range: 3 to >6 days

Time to Peak Plasma adenosine deaminase activity: 2-3 days

Pregnancy Risk Factor C

Pregnancy Considerations Animal studies have not been conducted. There are no adequate and well-controlled studies in pregnant women. The benefits versus risks should be considered carefully before initiating pegademase bovine therapy in pregnant women.

Pegaptanib (peg AP ta nib)

Brand Names: U.S. Macugen®

Brand Names: Canada Macugen®

Pharmacologic Category Ophthalmic Agent; Vascular Endothelial Growth Factor (VEGF) Inhibitor

Use Treatment of neovascular (wet) age-related macular degeneration (AMD)

Local Anesthetic/Vasoconstrictor Precautions No information available to require special precautions

Effects on Dental Treatment No significant effects or complications reported

Effects on Bleeding No information available to require special precautions

Adverse Effects

10% to 40%:

Cardiovascular: Hypertension

Ocular: Anterior chamber inflammation, blurred vision, cataract, conjunctival hemorrhage, corneal edema, eye discharge, eye irritation, eye pain, intraocular pressure increased, ocular discomfort, punctate keratitis, visual acuity decreased, visual disturbance, vitreous floaters, vitreous opacities

1% to 10%:

Cardiovascular: Carotid artery occlusion (1% to 5%), cerebrovascular accident (1% to 5%), chest pain (1% to 5%), transient ischemic attack (1% to 5%)

Central nervous system: Dizziness (6% to 10%), headache (6% to 10%), vertigo (1% to 5%)

Dermatologic: Contact dermatitis (1% to 5%)

Endocrine & metabolic: Diabetes mellitus (1% to 5%)

Gastrointestinal: Diarrhea (6% to 10%), nausea (6% to 10%), dyspepsia (1% to 5%), vomiting (1% to 5%)

Genitourinary: Urinary retention (1% to 5%)

Neuromuscular & skeletal: Arthritis (1% to 5%), bone spur (1% to 5%)

Ocular: Blepharitis (6% to 10%), conjunctivitis (6% to 10%), photopsia (6% to 10%), vitreous disorder (6% to 10%), allergic conjunctivitis (1% to 5%), conjunctival edema (1% to 5%), corneal abrasion (1% to 5%), corneal deposits (1% to 5%), corneal epithelium disorder (1% to 5%), endophthalmitis (1% to 5%), eye inflammation (1% to 5%), eye swelling (1% to 5%), eyelid irritation (1% to 5%), meibomianitis (1% to 5%), mydriasis (1% to 5%), periorbital hematoma (1% to 5%), retinal edema (1% to 5%), vitreous hemorrhage (1% to 5%)

Otic: Hearing loss (1% to 5%)

Renal: Urinary tract infection (6% to 10%)

Respiratory: Bronchitis (6% to 10%), pleural effusion (1% to 5%)

Miscellaneous: Contusion (1% to 5%)

General Dosage Range Intravitreous: *Adults:* 0.3 mg into affected eye every 6 weeks

Mechanism of Action Pegaptanib is an apatamer, an oligonucleotide covalently bound to polyethylene glycol, which can adopt a three-dimensional shape and bind to vascular endothelial growth factor (VEGF). Pegaptanib binds to extracellular VEGF, inhibiting VEGF from binding to its receptors and thereby suppressing neovascularization and slowing vision loss.

Pharmacodynamics/Kinetics

Half-life Elimination Plasma: 6-14 days

Pregnancy Risk Factor B

Pregnancy Considerations Teratogenic effects were not reported in animal studies. There are no adequate and well-controlled studies in pregnant women.

Pegaspargase (peg AS par jase)

Related Information

Asparaginase (*E. coli*) *on page 134*

Brand Names: U.S. Oncaspar®

Pharmacologic Category Antineoplastic Agent, Miscellaneous; Enzyme

Use Treatment of acute lymphocytic leukemia (ALL); treatment of ALL with previous hypersensitivity to native L-asparaginase

Local Anesthetic/Vasoconstrictor Precautions No information available to require special precautions

Effects on Dental Treatment No significant effects or complications reported

Effects on Bleeding Although significant myelosuppression with associated altered hemostasis has been reported for many chemotherapeutic agents, myelosuppression is not common with pegaspargase and no specific precautions appear to necessary.

Adverse Effects

>5%:

Cardiovascular: Edema

Central nervous system: Fever, malaise

Dermatologic: Rash

Gastrointestinal: Nausea, vomiting

Hematologic: Coagulopathy (7%; grades 3/4: 2%)

Hepatic: Transaminases increased (11%; grades 3/4: 3%)

Miscellaneous: Allergic reactions (including bronchospasm, chills, dyspnea, edema, erythema, hypotension, rash, swelling, urticaria; no prior asparaginase hypersensitivity: 1% to 10%; grades 3/4: 2%; prior asparaginase hypersensitivity: 32%; grades 3/4: 8%)

1% to 5%:

Cardiovascular: Hypotension, peripheral edema, tachycardia, thrombosis (4%)

Central nervous system: Chills, CNS thrombosis (2% to 4%; grades 3/4: 3%), CNS hemorrhage (2%), headache, seizure

Dermatologic: Lip edema, urticaria

Endocrine & metabolic: Hyperglycemia (3% to 5%; grades 3/4: ≤5%), hyperuricemia, hypoglycemia, hypoproteinemia

Gastrointestinal: Abdominal pain, anorexia, diarrhea, pancreatitis (1% to 2%; grades 3/4: 2%)

Hematologic: Anticoagulant effect decreased, disseminated intravascular coagulation (DIC), fibrinogen decreased, hemolytic anemia, leukopenia, pancytopenia, thrombocytopenia, thromboplastin increased, myelosuppression

Hepatic: Liver function tests abnormal (grades 3/4: 5%), hyperbilirubinemia (grades 3/4: 2%), jaundice

Local: Injection site hypersensitivity, pain or reaction

Neuromuscular & skeletal: Arthralgia, limb pain, myalgia, paresthesia

◀ Respiratory: Dyspnea

Miscellaneous: Anaphylactic reactions, night sweats

General Dosage Range I.M., I.V.: *Children and Adults:* 2500 units/m^2 every 14 days

Mechanism of Action Pegaspargase is a modified version of asparaginase. Leukemic cells, especially lymphoblasts, require exogenous asparagine; normal cells can synthesize asparagine. Asparaginase contains L-asparaginase amidohydrolase type EC-2 which inhibits protein synthesis by deaminating asparagine to aspartic acid and ammonia in the plasma and extracellular fluid and therefore deprives tumor cells of the amino acid for protein synthesis. Asparaginase is cycle-specific for the G$_1$ phase of the cell cycle.

Pharmacodynamics/Kinetics

Onset of Action

Asparagine depletion: I.M.: Within 4 days

Duration of Action Asparagine depletion: I.M.: ~21 days; I.V. (in asparaginase naive adults): 2-4 weeks

Half-life Elimination I.M.: ~5.5-6 days; unaffected by age, renal or hepatic function; half-life decreased to 1.8-3.2 days in patients with previous hypersensitivity to native L-asparaginase; I.V.: Adults (asparaginase naive): 7 days

Time to Peak I.M.: 3-4 days

Pregnancy Risk Factor C

Pregnancy Considerations Reproduction studies have not been conducted with pegaspargase.

Pegfilgrastim (peg fil GRA stim)

Brand Names: U.S. Neulasta®

Brand Names: Canada Neulasta®

Pharmacologic Category Colony Stimulating Factor

Use To decrease the incidence of infection, by stimulation of granulocyte production, in patients with non-myeloid malignancies receiving myelosuppressive therapy associated with a significant risk of febrile neutropenia

Local Anesthetic/Vasoconstrictor Precautions No information available to require special precautions

Effects on Dental Treatment No significant effects or complications reported

Effects on Bleeding No information available to require special precautions. Medical consultation may be necessary to confirm adequate platelet counts.

Adverse Effects

>10%:

Cardiovascular: Peripheral edema (12%)

Central nervous system: Headache (16%)

Gastrointestinal: Vomiting (13%)

Neuromuscular & skeletal: Bone pain (31% to 57%), myalgia (21%), arthralgia (16%), weakness (13%)

1% to 10%:

Gastrointestinal: Constipation (10%)

Miscellaneous: Antibody formation (1% to 6%)

General Dosage Range SubQ:

Children: 100 mcg/kg (maximum dose: 6 mg) once per chemotherapy cycle

Adolescents >45 kg and Adults: 6 mg once per chemotherapy cycle

Mechanism of Action Stimulates the production, maturation, and activation of neutrophils, pegfilgrastim activates neutrophils to increase both their migration and cytotoxicity. Pegfilgrastim has a prolonged duration of effect relative to filgrastim and a reduced renal clearance.

Pharmacodynamics/Kinetics

Half-life Elimination SubQ: Adults: 15-80 hours; Children (100 mcg/kg dose): ~20-30 hours (range: up to 68 hours)

Pregnancy Risk Factor C

Pregnancy Considerations Animal studies have demonstrated adverse effects and fetal loss. There are no adequate and well-controlled studies in pregnant women; use only if potential benefit to mother justifies the potential risk to the fetus.

Peginesatide (peg in ESS a tide)

Brand Names: U.S. Omontys®

Pharmacologic Category Colony Stimulating Factor; Erythropoiesis-Stimulating Agent (ESA); Growth Factor

Use Treatment of anemia due to chronic kidney disease (CKD) in patients receiving dialysis

Note: Peginesatide is **not** indicated for use under the following conditions:

- CKD patients not receiving dialysis
- Cancer patients with anemia that is not due to CKD
- As a substitute for RBC transfusion in patients requiring immediate correction of anemia

Note: Peginesatide has not demonstrated improved symptoms, physical functioning, or health-related quality of life.

Local Anesthetic/Vasoconstrictor Precautions No information available to require special precautions

Effects on Dental Treatment No significant effects or complications reported

Effects on Bleeding Although erythropoietin stimulating agents (ESAs) have been associated with thromboembolic events, there is no information available to require special precautions for dental procedures.

Adverse Effects

>10%:

Cardiovascular: Hypotension (14%), hypertension (13%), procedural hypotension (11%)

Central nervous system: Headache (15%), fever (12%)

Endocrine & metabolic: Hyperkalemia (11%)

Gastrointestinal: Diarrhea (18%), nausea (17%), vomiting (15%)

Neuromuscular & skeletal: Muscle spasms (15%), arthralgia (11%), back pain (11%), extremity pain (11%)

Respiratory: Dyspnea (18%), cough (16%), upper respiratory tract infection (11%)

Miscellaneous: Arteriovenous fistula site complication (16%)

1% to 10%: Miscellaneous: Peginesatide-specific binding antibodies (1%)

General Dosage Range I.V., SubQ: *Adults:* Initial: 0.04 mg/kg once monthly; maintenance: 2-20 mg/month

Mechanism of Action Peginesatide, a pegylated synthetic peptide, binds to the human erythropoietin receptor to induce erythropoiesis by stimulating the division and differentiation of committed erythroid progenitor cells; induces the release of reticulocytes from the bone marrow into the bloodstream, where they mature to erythrocytes. There is a dose response relationship with this effect. This results in an increase in reticulocyte counts followed by a rise in hemoglobin levels.

Pharmacodynamics/Kinetics

Half-life Elimination I.V.: Healthy subjects: 25 hours, Dialysis patients: 47.9 hours; SubQ: Healthy patients: 53 hours

Time to Peak SubQ: ~48 hours

Pregnancy Risk Factor C

Pregnancy Considerations Adverse events were observed in animal reproduction studies with maternal exposure similar to that observed with human doses.

Peginterferon Alfa-2a
(peg in ter FEER on AL fa too aye)

Related Information
Systemic Viral Diseases *on page 1537*
Brand Names: U.S. Pegasys®
Brand Names: Canada Pegasys®
Pharmacologic Category Interferon
Use Treatment of chronic hepatitis C (CHC), in combination with ribavirin (unless contraindicated or significant intolerance to ribavirin), in patients ≥5 years of age with compensated liver disease and not previously treated with alfa interferons, in patients with histological evidence of cirrhosis (Child-Pugh class A) and compensated liver disease; treatment of adults coinfected with CHC and clinically-stable HIV disease (CD4 count >100 cells/mm^3); treatment (monotherapy) of adults with HBeAg-positive and HBeAg-negative chronic hepatitis B with compensated liver disease and evidence of viral replication and liver inflammation
Local Anesthetic/Vasoconstrictor Precautions No information available to require special precautions
Effects on Dental Treatment Key adverse event(s) related to dental treatment: Xerostomia (normal salivary flow resumes upon discontinuation).
Effects on Bleeding Thrombocytopenia may occur in patients. Monitor for the potential for increased bleeding.
Adverse Effects Note: Percentages are reported for peginterferon alfa-2a in chronic hepatitis C (CHC) patients. Other percentages indicated as "with ribavirin" or "in HIV/CHC" are those which significantly exceed incidence reported for peginterferon monotherapy in CHC patients.
>10%:
Central nervous system: Headache (54%), fatigue (56%), fever (37%; 41% with ribavirin; 54% in hepatitis B), insomnia (19%; 30% with ribavirin), depression (18%), dizziness (16%), irritability/anxiety/nervousness (19%; 33% with ribavirin), pain (11%)
Dermatologic: Alopecia (23%; 28% with ribavirin), pruritus (12%; 19% with ribavirin), dermatitis (16% with ribavirin)
Endocrine & metabolic: Growth suppression (children) percentile decrease (≥15 percentiles), weight (43%), height (25%)
Gastrointestinal: Nausea/vomiting (24%), anorexia (17%; 24% with ribavirin), diarrhea (16%), weight loss (16% in HIV/CHC), abdominal pain (15%)
Hematologic: Neutropenia (21%; 27% with ribavirin; 40% in HIV/CHC), lymphopenia (14% with ribavirin), anemia (11% with ribavirin; 14% in HIV/CHC)
Hepatic: ALT increases 5-10 x ULN during treatment (25% to 27% in hepatitis B); ALT increases >10 x ULN during treatment (12% to 18% in hepatitis B); ALT increases 5-10 x ULN after treatment (13% to 16% in hepatitis B); ALT increases >10 x ULN after treatment (7% to 12% in hepatitis B)
Local: Injection site reaction (22%)
Neuromuscular & skeletal: Weakness (56%; 65% with ribavirin), myalgia (37%), rigors (35%; 25% to 27% in hepatitis B), arthralgia (28%)
Respiratory: Dyspnea (13% with ribavirin)
1% to 10%:
Central nervous system: Concentration impaired (8%), memory impaired (5%), mood alteration (3%; 9% in HIV/CHC)

Dermatologic: Dermatitis (8%), rash (5%), dry skin (4%; 10% with ribavirin), eczema (1%; 5% with ribavirin)
Endocrine & metabolic: Hypothyroidism (3% to 4%), hyperthyroidism (≤1%)
Gastrointestinal: Xerostomia (6%), dyspepsia (<1%; 6% with ribavirin), weight loss (4%; 10% with ribavirin)
Hematologic: Thrombocytopenia (5%; 8% in HIV/CHC), lymphopenia (3%), anemia (2%)
Hepatic: Hepatic decompensation (2% in CHC/HIV)
Neuromuscular & skeletal: Back pain (9%)
Ocular: Blurred vision (4%)
Respiratory: Cough (4%; 10% with ribavirin), dyspnea (4%), exertional dyspnea (4% with ribavirin)
Miscellaneous: Diaphoresis (6%), bacterial infection (3%; 5% in HIV/CHC)
General Dosage Range Dosage adjustment recommended in patients with hepatic or renal impairment or who develop toxicities
SubQ:
Children ≥5 years: 180 mcg/1.73 m^2 x BSA once weekly (maximum dose: 180 mcg)
Adults: 180 mcg once weekly
Mechanism of Action Alpha interferons are a family of proteins, produced by nucleated cells that have antiviral, antiproliferative, and immune-regulating activity. There are 16 known subtypes of alpha interferons. Interferons interact with cells through high affinity cell surface receptors. Following activation, multiple effects can be detected including induction of gene transcription. Interferons inhibit cellular growth, alter the state of cellular differentiation, interfere with oncogene expression, alter cell surface antigen expression, increase phagocytic activity of macrophages, and augment cytotoxicity of lymphocytes for target cells.
Pharmacodynamics/Kinetics
Half-life Elimination Terminal: 50-160 hours; increased with renal dysfunction
Time to Peak Serum: 72-96 hours
Pregnancy Risk Factor C / X in combination with ribavirin
Pregnancy Considerations Reproduction studies with pegylated interferon alfa have not been conducted. Animal studies with nonpegylated interferon alfa-2b have demonstrated abortifacient effects. Disruption of the normal menstrual cycle was also observed in animal studies; therefore, the manufacturer recommends that reliable contraception is used in women of childbearing potential. Alfa interferon is endogenous to normal amniotic fluid. *In vitro* administration studies have reported that when administered to the mother, it does not cross the placenta. Case reports of use in pregnant women are limited. The Perinatal HIV Guidelines Working Group does not recommend that peginterferon-alfa be used during pregnancy. Peginterferon monotherapy should only be used in pregnancy when the potential benefit to the mother justifies the possible risk to the fetus. **[U.S. Boxed Warning]: Combination therapy with ribavirin may cause birth defects; avoid pregnancy in females and female partners of male patients;** combination therapy with ribavirin is contraindicated in pregnancy (refer to Ribavirin monograph); a pregnancy registry has been established for women inadvertently exposed to ribavirin while pregnant (800-593-2214).

Peginterferon Alfa-2a and Ribavirin
(peg in ter FEER on AL fa too aye & rye ba VYE rin)

Related Information

Peginterferon Alfa-2a *on page 1059*
Ribavirin *on page 1190*
Systemic Viral Diseases *on page 1537*

Brand Names: Canada Pegasys® RBV

Pharmacologic Category Antiviral Agent; Interferon

Use Combination therapy for the treatment of chronic hepatitis C (HCV) in patients without cirrhosis and patients with compensated cirrhosis; includes patients coinfected with stable HIV disease

Local Anesthetic/Vasoconstrictor Precautions No information available to require special precautions

Effects on Dental Treatment Key adverse event(s) related to dental treatment: Xerostomia (normal salivary flow resumes upon discontinuation), glossitis, stomatitis, mouth ulcerations, taste disturbances, and cheilitis.

Effects on Bleeding Thrombocytopenia may occur in patients. Monitor for the potential for increased bleeding.

Adverse Effects Adverse reactions as reported with use of the combination product. Also see individual agents.

>10%:

Central nervous system: Fatigue (40% to 49%), headache (35% to 48%), fever (37% to 41%), insomnia (19% to 32%), rigors (16% to 30%), irritability (15% to 28%), depression (17% to 22%), dizziness (7% to 15%)

Dermatologic: Alopecia (10% to 25%), pruritus (4% to 25%), dermatitis (1% to 16%), dry skin (4% to 13%)

Gastrointestinal: Nausea (24% to 29%), anorexia (20% to 27%), diarrhea (14% to 16%), weight loss (2% to 16%)

Hematologic: Hemolytic anemia (≤14%), neutropenia (3% to 11%)

Local: Injection site reaction (10% to 28%)

Neuromuscular & skeletal: Myalgia (32% to 42%), weakness (15% to 26%), arthralgia (16% to 22%)

Respiratory: Cough (3% to 13%), dyspnea (3% to 13%)

1% to 10%:

Cardiovascular: Chest pain (≥1% to ≤5%), flushing (≥1% to ≤5%), hypertension (≥1% to ≤5%), palpitation (≥1% to ≤5%), peripheral edema (≥1% to ≤5%), syncope (≥1% to ≤5%), tachycardia (≥1% to ≤5%)

Central nervous system: Pain (6% to 10%), impaired concentration (2% to 10%), anxiety (8%), mood altered (≤8%), malaise (3% to 6%), emotional disorder (≤5%), aggression (≥1% to ≤5%), confusion (≥1% to ≤5%), hyper-/hypoesthesia (≥1% to ≤5%), lethargy (≥1% to ≤5%), migraine (≥1% to ≤5%), nightmares (≥1% to ≤5%), somnolence (≥1% to ≤5%), suicidal ideation (≥1% to ≤5%), vertigo (≥1% to ≤5%), impaired memory (1% to 5%), nervousness (≤3%), affect lability (HIV-HCV coinfection: ≥1% to ≤3%), apathy (HIV-HCV coinfection: ≥1% to ≤3%)

Dermatologic: Rash (5% to 9%), eczema (≥1% to ≤5%), photosensitivity (≥1% to ≤5%), psoriasis (≥1% to ≤5%), urticaria (≥1% to ≤5%)

Endocrine & metabolic: Libido decreased (2% to 5%), dehydration (≥1% to ≤5%), hot flashes (≥1% to ≤5%), hyperthyroidism (≥1% to ≤5%), impotence (≥1% to ≤5%), hypothyroidism (≤4%), lactic acidosis (HIV-HCV coinfection: ≥1% to ≤3%)

Gastrointestinal: Abdominal pain (7% to 10%), vomiting (7% to 8%), xerostomia (5% to 8%), appetite decreased (≤7%), dyspepsia (2% to 6%), constipation (≥1% to ≤5%), dysphagia (≥1% to ≤5%), flatulence (≥1% to ≤5%), glossitis (≥1% to ≤5%), mouth ulceration (≥1% to ≤5%), stomatitis (≥1% to ≤5%), taste disturbance (≥1% to ≤5%), cheilitis (HIV-HCV coinfection: ≥1% to ≤3%)

Genitourinary: Chromaturia (HIV-HCV coinfection: ≥1% to ≤3%)

Hematologic: Thrombocytopenia (≥1% to 8%), bleeding (gingival) (≥1% to ≤5%)

Neuromuscular & skeletal: Back pain (3% to 5%), arthritis (≥1% to ≤5%), bone pain (≥1% to ≤5%), muscle cramps (≥1% to ≤5%), muscle weakness (≥1% to ≤5%), musculoskeletal pain (≥1% to ≤5%), neck pain (≥1% to ≤5%), paresthesia (≥1% to ≤5%), tremor (≥1% to ≤5%)

Ocular: Eye inflammation (≥1% to ≤5%), eye pain (≥1% to ≤5%), vision blurred (≥1% to ≤5%), xerophthalmia (≥1% to ≤5%)

Otic: Earache (≥1% to ≤5%), tinnitus (≥1% to ≤5%)

Respiratory: Bronchitis (≥1% to ≤5%), epistaxis (≥1% to ≤5%), nasal congestion (≥1% to ≤5%), nasopharyngitis (≥1% to ≤5%), pharyngolaryngeal pain (≥1% to ≤5%), rhinitis (≥1% to ≤5%), sinus congestion (≥1% to ≤5%), throat sore (≥1% to ≤5%), upper respiratory infection (≥1% to ≤5%), pneumonia (HIV-HCV coinfection: ≥1% to ≤3%)

Miscellaneous: Diaphoresis (2% to 5%), flu-like syndrome (≥1% to ≤5%), herpes simplex (≥1% to ≤5%), lymphadenopathy (≥1% to ≤5%), night sweats (≥1% to ≤5%), oral candidiasis (≥1% to ≤5%), thirst (≥1% to ≤5%), acquired lipodystrophy (HIV-HCV coinfection: ≥1% to ≤3%)

Use of alfa interferons has been associated with rare cases of autoimmune diseases, including idiopathic thrombocytopenic purpura, thyroiditis, rheumatoid arthritis, systemic lupus erythematosus, vasculitis, and Vogt-Koyanagi-Harada syndrome

General Dosage Range Dosage adjustment recommended in patients with hepatic or renal impairment or who develop toxicities

SubQ: Peginterferon Alfa-2a: *Adults:* 180 mcg/week

Oral: Ribavirin:

Adults <75 kg: 800-1000 mg/day in 2 divided doses

Adults ≥75 kg: 800-1200 mg/day in 2 divided doses

Mechanism of Action

Peginterferon Alfa-2a: Alpha interferons are a family of proteins, produced by nucleated cells that have antiviral, antiproliferative, and immune-regulating activity. There are 16 known subtypes of alpha interferons. Interferons interact with cells through high affinity cell surface receptors. Following activation, multiple effects can be detected including induction of gene transcription. Inhibits cellular growth, alters the state of cellular differentiation, interferes with oncogene expression, alters cell surface antigen expression, increases phagocytic activity of macrophages, and augments cytotoxicity of lymphocytes for target cells.

Ribavirin: Inhibits replication of RNA and DNA viruses; inhibits influenza virus RNA polymerase activity and inhibits the initiation and elongation of RNA fragments resulting in inhibition of viral protein synthesis.

Pregnancy Considerations Use during pregnancy is contraindicated. Abortifacient and teratogenic effects have been reported in women receiving interferons. Women of childbearing potential should not be treated unless two reliable forms of contraception are used. In addition, male patients and their female partners must also use two reliable forms of contraception. Pregnancy must be avoided during treatment and for 6 months following therapy.

Product Availability Not available in U.S.

Peginterferon Alfa-2b
(peg in ter FEER on AL fa too bee)

Related Information
Systemic Viral Diseases *on page 1537*

Brand Names: U.S. PegIntron®; PegIntron™ Redipen®; Sylatron™

Brand Names: Canada PegIntron®

Pharmacologic Category Interferon

Use
PegIntron®: Treatment of chronic hepatitis C (CHC; in combination with ribavirin) in patients who have compensated liver disease; treatment of chronic hepatitis C (as monotherapy) in adult patients with compensated liver disease who have never received alfa interferons and are intolerant to ribavirin or have contraindications to ribavirin. **Note:** Combination therapy with ribavirin provides better response rates than peginterferon monotherapy

Sylatron™: Adjuvant treatment of melanoma (with microscopic or gross nodal involvement within 84 days of definitive surgical resection, including complete lymphadenectomy)

Local Anesthetic/Vasoconstrictor Precautions No information available to require special precautions

Effects on Dental Treatment Key adverse event(s) related to dental treatment: Xerostomia (normal salivary flow resumes upon discontinuation).

Effects on Bleeding Thrombocytopenia may occur in patients. Monitor for the potential for increased bleeding.

Adverse Effects Note: Percentages reported for adults receiving monotherapy unless noted:

>10%:
Central nervous system: Fatigue (52% to 94%), fever (22% to 75%), headache (56% to 70%), chills (≤63%), depression (29% to 59%; may be severe), dizziness (12% to 35%), anxiety/emotional liability/irritability (28%), insomnia (23%), olfactory nerve disorder (≤23%)

Dermatologic: Rash (6% to 36%), alopecia (22% to 34%), pruritus (12%), dry skin (11%)

Gastrointestinal: Anorexia (20% to 69%), nausea (26% to 64%), taste perversion (≤38%), diarrhea (18% to 37%), vomiting (7% to 26%), abdominal pain (8% to 15%), weight loss (11%)

Hematologic: Neutropenia (6% to 70%; grade 4: 1%), thrombocytopenia (7% to 20%; grades 3/4: <4%), anemia (6%; in combination with ribavirin: 12% to 47%)

Hepatic: ALT/AST increased (10% to 77%), alkaline phosphatase increased (≤23%)

Local: Injection site inflammation/reaction (23% to 62%)

Neuromuscular & skeletal: Myalgia (54% to 68%), weakness (52%), arthralgia (23% to 51%), musculoskeletal pain (28%), rigors (23%), paresthesia (21%)

Miscellaneous: Binding antibodies (melanoma patients 35%), viral infection (11%)

1% to 10%:
Cardiovascular: Chest pain (6%), flushing (6%), bundle branch block (4%), myocardial infarction (4%), supraventricular arrhythmia (4%), ventricular tachycardia (4%)

Central nervous system: Concentration impaired (10%), malaise (7%), nervousness (4%), agitation (2%), suicidal behavior (ideation/attempt/suicide ≤2%)

Endocrine & metabolic: Hypothyroidism (5%), menstrual disorder (4%), hyperthyroidism (3%)

Gastrointestinal: Dyspepsia (6%), xerostomia (6%), constipation (1%)

Hepatic: GGT increased (8%), hepatomegaly (6%)

Local: Injection site pain (2% to 3%)

Ocular: Conjunctivitis (4%), blurred vision (2%)

Renal: Proteinuria (≤7%)

Respiratory: Pharyngitis (10%), cough (5% to 8%), sinusitis (7%), dyspnea (4% to 6%), rhinitis (2%)

Miscellaneous: Diaphoresis (6%), neutralizing antibodies (≤2%)

General Dosage Range Dosage adjustment recommended in patients with renal impairment or who develop toxicities

SubQ: Melanoma:
Adults: Initial: 6 mcg/kg/week; Maintenance: 3 mcg/kg/week

SubQ: Chronic hepatitis C:
Children ≥3 years: 60 mcg/m^2/week (in combination with ribavirin)

Adults: Peginterferon monotherapy (based on average weekly dose of 1 mcg/kg):
Adults ≤45 kg: 40 mcg once weekly
Adults 46-56 kg: 50 mcg once weekly
Adults 57-72 kg: 64 mcg once weekly
Adults 73-88 kg: 80 mcg once weekly
Adults 89-106 kg: 96 mcg once weekly
Adults 107-136 kg: 120 mcg once weekly
Adults 137-160 kg: 150 mcg once weekly

Adults: Combination therapy with ribavirin (based on average weekly dose of 1.5 mcg/kg):
Adults <40 kg: 50 mcg once weekly (with ribavirin 800 mg/day)
Adults 40-50 kg: 64 mcg once weekly (with ribavirin 800 mg/day)
Adults 51-60 kg: 80 mcg once weekly (with ribavirin 800 mg/day)
Adults 61-65 kg: 96 mcg once weekly (with ribavirin 800 mg/day)
Adults 66-75 kg: 96 mcg once weekly (with ribavirin 1000 mg/day)
Adults 76-80 kg: 120 mcg once weekly (with ribavirin 1000 mg/day)
Adults 81-85 kg: 120 mcg once weekly (with ribavirin 1200 mg/day)
Adults 86-105 kg: 150 mcg once weekly (with ribavirin 1200 mg/day)
Adults >105 kg: 1.5 mcg/kg once weekly (with ribavirin 1400 mg/day)

Mechanism of Action Alpha interferons are a family of proteins, produced by nucleated cells, that have antiviral, antiproliferative, and immune-regulating activity. There are 16 known subtypes of alpha interferons. Interferons interact with cells through high affinity cell surface receptors. Following activation, multiple effects can be detected including induction of gene transcription. Inhibits cellular growth, alters the state of cellular differentiation, interferes with oncogene expression, ▶

alters cell surface antigen expression, increases phag-ocytic activity of macrophages, and augments cytotox-icity of lymphocytes for target cells.

Pharmacodynamics/Kinetics
Half-life Elimination CHC: ~40 hours (range: 22-60 hours); Melanoma: ~43-51 hours
Time to Peak CHC: 15-44 hours

Pregnancy Risk Factor C / X in combination with ribavirin

Pregnancy Considerations Reproduction studies with pegylated interferon alfa have not been conducted. Animal reproduction studies with nonpegylated inter-feron alfa-2b have demonstrated abortifacient effects. Disruption of the normal menstrual cycle was also observed in animal studies; therefore, the manufacturer recommends that reliable contraception is used in women of childbearing potential. Alfa interferon is endogenous to normal amniotic fluid. *In vitro* adminis-tration studies have reported that when administered to the mother, it does not cross the placenta. Case reports of use in pregnant women are limited. The Perinatal HIV Guidelines Working Group does not recommend that peginterferon alfa be used during pregnancy. Peginter-feron alfa-2b monotherapy should only be used in pregnancy when the potential benefit to the mother justifies the possible risk to the fetus. **[U.S. Boxed Warning]: Combination therapy with ribavirin may cause birth defects and/or fetal mortality; avoid pregnancy in females and female partners of male patients;** combination therapy with ribavirin is contra-indicated in pregnancy. Two forms of contraception should be used during combination therapy; patients should have monthly pregnancy tests. A pregnancy registry has been established for women inadvertently exposed to ribavirin while pregnant (800-593-2214).

Pegloticase (peg LOE ti kase)

Brand Names: U.S. Krystexxa™
Pharmacologic Category Enzyme; Enzyme, Urate-Oxidase (Recombinant)
Use Treatment of chronic gout refractory to conventional therapy
Local Anesthetic/Vasoconstrictor Precautions No information available to require special precautions
Effects on Dental Treatment No significant effects or complications reported
Effects on Bleeding No information available to require special precautions
Adverse Effects
>10%:
Dermatologic: Bruising (11%), urticaria (11%)
Gastrointestinal: Nausea (12%)
Miscellaneous: Antibody formation (antipegloticase antibodies: 92%; antiPEG antibodies: 42%), gout flare (74% within the first 3 months), infusion reac-tions (26%)
1% to 10%:
Cardiovascular: Chest pain (6% to 10%)
Dermatologic: Erythema (10%), pruritus (10%)
Gastrointestinal: Constipation (6%), vomiting (5%)
Respiratory: Dyspnea (7%), nasopharyngitis (7%)
Miscellaneous: Anaphylaxis (≤7%)
Frequency not defined: Anemia, diarrhea, headache, muscle spasms, nephrolithiasis
General Dosage Range I.V.: *Adults:* 8 mg every 2 weeks

Mechanism of Action Pegloticase is a pegylated recombinant form of urate-oxidase enzyme, also known as uricase (an enzyme normally absent in humans and high primates), which converts uric acid to allantoin (an inactive and water soluble metabolite of uric acid); it does not inhibit the formation of uric acid.

Pharmacodynamics/Kinetics
Onset of Action ~24 hours following the first dose, serum uric acid concentrations decreased
Duration of Action >300 hours (12.5 days)
Half-life Elimination Median: ~14 days
Pregnancy Risk Factor C
Pregnancy Considerations Adequate animal repro-duction studies have not been conducted. There are no adequate and well-controlled studies in pregnant women. Use during pregnancy only if the benefit to the mother outweigh the potential risk to the fetus.

PEMEtrexed (pem e TREKS ed)

Brand Names: U.S. Alimta®
Brand Names: Canada Alimta®
Pharmacologic Category Antineoplastic Agent, Anti-metabolite; Antineoplastic Agent, Antimetabolite (Anti-folate)
Use Treatment of unresectable malignant pleural meso-thelioma (in combination with cisplatin); treatment of locally advanced or metastatic **non**squamous nonsmall cell lung cancer (NSCLC; as initial treatment in combi-nation with cisplatin, as single-agent maintenance treat-ment after 4 cycles of initial platinum-based double therapy, and single-agent treatment after prior chemo-therapy)

Note: Not indicated for the treatment of **squamous** cell NSCLC

Unlabeled Use Treatment of bladder cancer (meta-static), cervical cancer (recurrent or metastatic), ovarian cancer (recurrent or persistent), thymic malignancies; treatment of malignant pleural mesothelioma (either as a single agent or in combination with carboplatin)
Local Anesthetic/Vasoconstrictor Precautions No information available to require special precautions
Effects on Dental Treatment Key adverse event(s) related to dental treatment: Dysphagia, esophagitis, odynophagia, and stomatitis.
Effects on Bleeding Chemotherapy may result in significant myelosuppression, potentially including sig-nificant reduction in platelet counts (thrombocytopenia grades 3/4: 2%) and altered hemostasis. In patients who are under active treatment with these agents, medical consult is suggested.
Adverse Effects
>10%:
Central nervous system: Fatigue (18% to 34%; dose-limiting)
Dermatologic: Rash/desquamation (10% to 14%)
Gastrointestinal: Nausea (12% to 31%), anorexia (19% to 22%), vomiting (6% to 16%), stomatitis (5% to 15%), diarrhea (5% to 13%)
Hematologic: Anemia (15% to 19%; grades 3/4: 3% to 5%), leukopenia (6% to 12%; grades 3/4: 2% to 4%), neutropenia (6% to 11%; grades 3/4: 3% to 5%; dose-limiting; nadir: 8-10 days; recovery: 4-8 days after nadir)
Respiratory: Pharyngitis (15%)
Central nervous system: Fatigue (25% to 34%; dose-limiting)
Dermatologic: Rash/desquamation (10% to 14%)

Gastrointestinal: Nausea (19% to 31%), anorexia (19% to 22%), vomiting (9% to 16%), stomatitis (7% to 15%), diarrhea (5% to 13%)

Hematologic: Anemia (15% to 19%; grades 3/4: 3% to 4%), leukopenia (6% to 12%; grades 3/4: 2% to 4%), neutropenia (6% to 11%; grades 3/4: 3% to 5%; dose-limiting; nadir: 8-10 days; recovery: 4-8 days after nadir)

Respiratory: Pharyngitis (15%)

1% to 10%:

Cardiovascular: Edema (1% to 5%)

Central nervous system: Fever (1% to 8%)

Dermatologic: Pruritus (1% to 7%), alopecia (1% to 6%), erythema multiforme (≤5%)

Gastrointestinal: Constipation (1% to 6%), weight loss (1%), abdominal pain (≤5%)

Hematologic: Thrombocytopenia (1% to 8%; grades 3/4: 2%; dose-limiting), febrile neutropenia (grades 3/4: 2%)

Hepatic: ALT increased (8% to 10%; grades 3/4: ≤2%), AST increased (7% to 8%; grades 3/4: ≤1%)

Neuromuscular & skeletal: Sensory neuropathy (≤9%), motor neuropathy (≤5%)

Ocular: Conjunctivitis (≤5%), lacrimation increased (≤5%)

Renal: Creatinine increased/creatinine clearance decreased (1% to 5%)

Miscellaneous: Allergic reaction/hypersensitivity (≤5%), infection (≤5%), sepsis (1%)

General Dosage Range Dosage adjustment recommended in patients with hepatic impairment, on concomitant therapy, or who develop toxicities

I.V.: *Adults:* 500 mg/m^2 on day 1 of each 21-day cycle

Mechanism of Action Antifolate; disrupts folate-dependent metabolic processes essential for cell replication. Inhibits thymidylate synthase (TS), dihydrofolate reductase (DHFR), glycinamide ribonucleotide formyltransferase (GARFT), and aminoimidazole carboxamide ribonucleotide formyltransferase (AICARFT), the enzymes involved in folate metabolism and DNA synthesis, resulting in inhibition of purine and thymidine nucleotide and protein synthesis.

Pharmacodynamics/Kinetics

Half-life Elimination Normal renal function: 3.5 hours; Cl$_{cr}$ 40-59 mL/minute: 5.3-5.8 hours

Pregnancy Risk Factor D

Pregnancy Considerations Adverse effects (embryotoxicity, fetotoxicity and teratogenicity) were observed in animal reproduction studies. Based on the mechanism of action, may cause fetal harm if administered to a pregnant woman. Women of childbearing potential should have a negative serum pregnancy test prior to treatment and should use effective contraceptive measures to avoid becoming pregnant during treatment. Irreversible infertility has been reported in males; prior to receiving treatment, males should be counseled on sperm storage. The Canadian labeling recommends that males receiving therapy use effective contraceptive measures and not father a child during, and for up to 6 months after therapy.

Penbutolol (pen BYOO toe lole)

Brand Names: U.S. Levatol®

Brand Names: Canada Levatol®

Pharmacologic Category Beta-Blocker With Intrinsic Sympathomimetic Activity

Use Treatment of mild-to-moderate arterial hypertension

Local Anesthetic/Vasoconstrictor Precautions No information available to require special precautions

Effects on Dental Treatment Key adverse event(s) related to dental treatment: Xerostomia (normal salivary flow resumes upon discontinuation). Penbutolol is a nonselective beta-blocker and may enhance the pressor response to epinephrine, resulting in hypertension and bradycardia. Many nonsteroidal anti-inflammatory drugs, such as ibuprofen and indomethacin, can reduce the hypotensive effect of beta-blockers after 3 or more weeks of therapy with the NSAID. Short-term NSAID use (ie, 3 days) requires no special precautions in patients taking beta-blockers.

Effects on Bleeding No information available to require special precautions

Adverse Effects 1% to 10%:

Cardiovascular: CHF, arrhythmia

Central nervous system: Mental depression, headache, dizziness, fatigue

Gastrointestinal: Nausea, diarrhea, dyspepsia

Neuromuscular & skeletal: Arthralgia

General Dosage Range Oral: *Adults:* Initial: 20 mg once daily; Maintenance: 10-40 mg once daily (maximum: 80 mg/day)

Mechanism of Action Blocks both beta$_1$- and beta$_2$-receptors and has mild intrinsic sympathomimetic activity; has negative inotropic and chronotropic effects and can significantly slow AV nodal conduction

Pharmacodynamics/Kinetics

Onset of Action Peak effect: 1.3-3 hours

Duration of Action >20 hours

Half-life Elimination Penbutolol: 5 hours; Conjugated metabolite: ~20 hours with normal renal function, 100 hours with end-stage renal disease

Time to Peak Plasma: 2-3 hours

Pregnancy Risk Factor C

Pregnancy Considerations Adverse events were observed in animal reproduction studies; therefore, the manufacturer classifies penbutolol as pregnancy category C. In a cohort study, an increased risk of cardiovascular defects was observed following maternal use of beta-blockers during pregnancy. Intrauterine growth restriction (IUGR), small placentas, as well as fetal/neonatal bradycardia, hypoglycemia, and/or respiratory depression have been observed following *in utero* exposure to beta-blockers as a class. Adequate facilities for monitoring infants at birth should be available. Untreated chronic maternal hypertension and pre-eclampsia are also associated with adverse events in the fetus, infant, and mother. Protein binding of penbutolol is decreased during the 2nd and 3rd trimesters of pregnancy. Limited information is available related to the use of penbutolol for the treatment of hypertension in pregnancy; other agents may be more appropriate for use.

Penciclovir (pen SYE kloe veer)

Related Information

Systemic Viral Diseases *on page 1537*
Viral Infections *on page 1575*

Related Sample Prescriptions

Herpes Simplex (Recurrent) *on page 1616*

Brand Names: U.S. Denavir®

Generic Availability (U.S.) No

Pharmacologic Category Antiviral Agent

Dental Use Topical treatment of recurrent herpes simplex labialis (cold sores)

Use Topical treatment of recurrent herpes simplex labialis (cold sores)

Local Anesthetic/Vasoconstrictor Precautions No information available to require special precautions

Effects on Dental Treatment No significant effects or complications reported

Effects on Bleeding No information available to require special precautions

Adverse Effects
>10%: Dermatologic: Mild erythema (50%)
1% to 10%:
Central nervous system: Headache (5%)
Local: Application site reaction (1%)

Dental Usual Dosage Treatment of herpes simplex labialis (cold sores): Children ≥12 years and Adults: Topical: Apply cream at the first sign or symptom of cold sore (eg, tingling, swelling); apply every 2 hours during waking hours for 4 days

Dosage Children ≥12 years and Adults: Topical: Apply cream at the first sign or symptom of cold sore (eg, tingling, swelling); apply every 2 hours during waking hours for 4 days

Mechanism of Action In cells infected with HSV-1 or HSV-2, viral thymidine kinase phosphorylates penciclovir to a monophosphate form which, in turn, is converted to penciclovir triphosphate by cellular kinases. Penciclovir triphosphate inhibits HSV polymerase competitively with deoxyguanosine triphosphate. Consequently, herpes viral DNA synthesis and, therefore, replication are selectively inhibited

Contraindications Hypersensitivity to the penciclovir or any component of the formulation

Warnings/Precautions Penciclovir should only be used on herpes labialis on the lips and face; because no data are available, application to mucous membranes is not recommended. Avoid application in or near eyes since it may cause irritation. The effect of penciclovir has not been established in immunocompromised patients.

Drug Interactions

Metabolism/Transport Effects None known.

Avoid Concomitant Use There are no known interactions where it is recommended to avoid concomitant use.

Increased Effect/Toxicity There are no known significant interactions involving an increase in effect.

Decreased Effect There are no known significant interactions involving a decrease in effect.

Pregnancy Risk Factor B

Pregnancy Considerations Adverse events have not been observed in animal reproduction studies following intravenous administration.

Lactation Excretion in breast milk unknown/not recommended

Breast-Feeding Considerations According to the manufacturer, the decision to continue or discontinue breast-feeding during therapy should take into account the risk of exposure to the infant and the benefits of treatment to the mother.

Dosage Forms
Cream, topical:
Denavir®: 1% (1.5 g, 5 g)

PenicillAMINE (pen i SIL a meen)

Brand Names: U.S. Cuprimine®; Depen®
Brand Names: Canada Cuprimine®
Pharmacologic Category Chelating Agent
Use Treatment of Wilson's disease, cystinuria; adjunctive treatment of severe, active rheumatoid arthritis

Canadian labeling: Additional use (not in U.S. labeling): Treatment of chronic lead poisoning

Local Anesthetic/Vasoconstrictor Precautions No information available to require special precautions

Effects on Dental Treatment Key adverse event(s) related to dental treatment: Oral ulcerations, glossitis, gingivostomatitis, and taste alteration.

Effects on Bleeding No information available to require special precautions

Adverse Effects Frequency not always defined and may vary by indication.
Cardiovascular: Vasculitis
Central nervous system: Anxiety, agitation, fever, Guillain-Barré syndrome, hyperpyrexia, psychiatric disturbances, worsening neurologic symptoms
Dermatologic: Alopecia, cheilosis, dermatomyositis, drug eruptions, exfoliative dermatitis, lichen planus, pemphigus, pruritus, rash (early and late: 5%), skin friability increased, toxic epidermal necrolysis, urticaria, wrinkling (excessive), yellow nail syndrome
Endocrine & metabolic: Hypoglycemia, thyroiditis
Gastrointestinal: Diarrhea (17%), taste alteration (12%), anorexia, epigastric pain, gingivostomatitis, glossitis, nausea, oral ulcerations, pancreatitis, peptic ulcer reactivation, vomiting
Hematologic: Thrombocytopenia (4%), leukopenia (2%), agranulocytosis, aplastic anemia, eosinophilia, hemolytic anemia, leukocytosis, monocytosis, red cell aplasia, sideroblastic anemia, thrombotic thrombocytopenia purpura, thrombocytosis
Hepatic: Alkaline phosphatase increased, hepatic failure, intrahepatic cholestasis, toxic hepatitis
Local: Thrombophlebitis, white papules at venipuncture and surgical sites
Neuromuscular & skeletal: Arthralgia, dystonia, myasthenia gravis, muscle weakness, neuropathies, polyarthralgia (migratory, often with objective synovitis), polymyositis
Ocular: Diplopia, extraocular muscle weakness, optic neuritis, ptosis, visual disturbances
Otic: Tinnitus
Renal: Proteinuria (6%), Goodpasture's syndrome, hematuria, nephrotic syndrome, renal failure, renal vasculitis
Respiratory: Asthma, interstitial pneumonitis, pulmonary fibrosis, obliterative bronchiolitis
Miscellaneous: Allergic alveolitis, anetoderma, elastosis perforans serpiginosa, lupus-like syndrome, lactic dehydrogenase increased, lymphadenopathy, mammary hyperplasia, positive ANA test

General Dosage Range Dosage adjustment recommended in patients with renal impairment
Oral:
Children: 30 mg/kg/day in 4 divided doses
Adults: Dosage varies greatly depending on indication
Mechanism of Action Chelates with lead, copper, mercury and other heavy metals to form stable, soluble complexes that are excreted in urine; depresses circulating IgM rheumatoid factor, depresses T-cell but not B-cell activity; combines with cystine to form a compound which is more soluble, thus cystine calculi are prevented
Pharmacodynamics/Kinetics
Onset of Action Rheumatoid arthritis: 2-3 months; Wilson's disease: 1-3 months
Half-life Elimination 1.7-7 hours (Roberts, 2008)
Time to Peak Serum: 1-3 hours
Pregnancy Risk Factor D

Pregnancy Considerations Birth defects, including congenital cutix laxa and associated defects, have been reported in infants following penicillamine exposure during pregnancy. Use for the treatment of rheumatoid arthritis during pregnancy is contraindicated. Use for the treatment of cystinuria only if the possible benefits to the mother outweigh the potential risks to the fetus. Continued treatment of Wilson's disease during pregnancy protects the mother against relapse. Discontinuation has detrimental maternal and fetal effects. Daily dosage should be limited to 750 mg. For planned cesarean section, reduce dose to 250 mg/day for the last 6 weeks of pregnancy, and continue at this dosage until wound healing is complete.

Penicillin G Benzathine
(pen i SIL in jee BENZ a theen)

Related Information
Sexually-Transmitted Diseases *on page 1536*
Brand Names: U.S. Bicillin® L-A
Brand Names: Canada Bicillin® L-A
Pharmacologic Category Antibiotic, Penicillin
Use Active against some gram-positive organisms, few gram-negative organisms such as *Neisseria gonorrhoeae*, and some anaerobes and spirochetes; used in the treatment of syphilis; used only for the treatment of mild to moderately-severe upper respiratory tract infections caused by organisms susceptible to low concentrations of penicillin G or for prophylaxis of infections caused by these organisms; primary and secondary prevention of rheumatic fever
Local Anesthetic/Vasoconstrictor Precautions No information available to require special precautions
Effects on Dental Treatment No significant effects or complications reported
Effects on Bleeding No information available to require special precautions
Adverse Effects Frequency not defined.
Cardiovascular: Cardiac arrest, cerebral vascular accident, cyanosis, gangrene, hypotension, pallor, palpitations, syncope, tachycardia, vasodilation, vasospasm, vasovagal reaction
Central nervous system: Anxiety, coma, confusion, dizziness, euphoria, fatigue, headache, nervousness, pain, seizure, somnolence
  In addition, a syndrome of CNS symptoms has been reported which includes: Severe agitation with confusion, hallucinations (auditory and visual), and fear of death (Hoigne's syndrome); other symptoms include cyanosis, dizziness, palpitations, psychosis, seizures, tachycardia, taste disturbance, tinnitus
Gastrointestinal: Bloody stool, intestinal necrosis, nausea, vomiting
Genitourinary: Impotence, priapism
Hepatic: AST increased
Local: Injection site reactions: Abscess, atrophy, bruising, cellulitis, edema, hemorrhage, inflammation, lump, necrosis, pain, skin ulcer
Neuromuscular & skeletal: Arthritis exacerbation, joint disorder, neurovascular damage, numbness, periostitis, rhabdomyolysis, transverse myelitis, tremor, weakness
Ocular: Blindness, blurred vision
Renal: BUN increased, creatinine increased, hematuria, myoglobinuria, neurogenic bladder, proteinuria, renal failure
Miscellaneous: Diaphoresis, hypersensitivity reactions, Jarisch-Herxheimer reaction, lymphadenopathy, mottling, warmth

General Dosage Range I.M.:
Children ≤27 kg: 600,000 units/dose
Children >27 kg: 1.2 million units/dose
Adults: 1.2-2.4 million units as a single dose
Mechanism of Action Interferes with bacterial cell wall synthesis during active multiplication, causing cell wall death and resultant bactericidal activity against susceptible bacteria
Pharmacodynamics/Kinetics
Duration of Action Dose dependent: 1-4 weeks; larger doses result in more sustained levels
Time to Peak Serum: 12-24 hours
Pregnancy Risk Factor B
Pregnancy Considerations Adverse events have not been observed in animal reproduction studies. Penicillin crosses the placenta and distributes into amniotic fluid. Maternal use of penicillins has generally not resulted in an increased risk of adverse fetal effects. Penicillin G is the drug of choice for treatment of syphilis during pregnancy.

Penicillin G Benzathine and Penicillin G Procaine
(pen i SIL in jee BENZ a theen & pen i SIL in jee PROE kane)

Related Information
Penicillin G Benzathine *on page 1065*
Penicillin G Procaine *on page 1066*
Brand Names: U.S. Bicillin® C-R; Bicillin® C-R 900/300
Pharmacologic Category Antibiotic, Penicillin
Use May be used in specific situations in the treatment of streptococcal infections; primary prevention of rheumatic fever
Local Anesthetic/Vasoconstrictor Precautions No information available to require special precautions
Effects on Dental Treatment No significant effects or complications reported
Effects on Bleeding No information available to require special precautions
Adverse Effects See individual agents.
General Dosage Range I.M.:
Children <14 kg: 600,000 units/dose
Children 14-27 kg: 900,000 units to 1.2 million units as a single dose
Children >27 kg and Adults: 2.4 million units/dose
Mechanism of Action Inhibits bacterial cell wall synthesis by binding to one or more of the penicillin-binding proteins (PBPs); which in turn inhibits the final transpeptidation step of peptidoglycan synthesis in bacterial cell walls, thus inhibiting cell wall biosynthesis. Bacteria eventually lyse due to ongoing activity of cell wall autolytic enzymes (autolysins and murein hydrolases) while cell wall assembly is arrested.
Pharmacodynamics/Kinetics
Time to Peak Serum: I.M.: Within 3 hours
Pregnancy Risk Factor B
Pregnancy Considerations See individual agents.

Penicillin G (Parenteral/Aqueous)
(pen i SIL in jee, pa REN ter al, AYE kwee us)

Related Information
Sexually-Transmitted Diseases *on page 1536*
Brand Names: U.S. Pfizerpen®
Brand Names: Canada Crystapen®
Pharmacologic Category Antibiotic, Penicillin

◄ **Use** Treatment of infections (including sepsis, pneumonia, pericarditis, endocarditis, meningitis, anthrax) caused by susceptible organisms; active against some gram-positive organisms, generally not *Staphylococcus aureus*; some gram-negative organisms such as *Neisseria gonorrhoeae*, and some anaerobes and spirochetes

Local Anesthetic/Vasoconstrictor Precautions No information available to require special precautions

Effects on Dental Treatment No significant effects or complications reported

Effects on Bleeding No information available to require special precautions

Adverse Effects Frequency not defined.

Central nervous system: Coma (high doses), hyperreflexia (high doses), seizures (high doses)

Dermatologic: Contact dermatitis, rash

Endocrine & metabolic: Electrolyte imbalance (high doses)

Gastrointestinal: Pseudomembranous colitis

Hematologic: Neutropenia, positive Coombs' hemolytic anemia (rare, high doses)

Local: Injection site reaction, phlebitis, thrombophlebitis

Neuromuscular & skeletal: Myoclonus (high doses)

Renal: Acute interstitial nephritis (high doses), renal tubular damage (high doses)

Miscellaneous: Anaphylaxis, hypersensitivity reactions (immediate and delayed), Jarisch-Herxheimer reaction, serum sickness

General Dosage Range Dosage adjustment recommended in patients with renal impairment

I.M., I.V.:

Infants ≥1 month and Children: 100,000-400,000 units/kg/day in divided doses every 4-6 hours (maximum: 24 million units/day)

Adults: 2-30 million units/day in divided doses every 4-6 hours

Mechanism of Action Interferes with bacterial cell wall synthesis during active multiplication, causing cell wall death and resultant bactericidal activity against susceptible bacteria

Pharmacodynamics/Kinetics

Half-life Elimination

Neonates: <6 days old: 3.2-3.4 hours; 7-13 days old: 1.2-2.2 hours; >14 days old: 0.9-1.9 hours

Children and Adults: Normal renal function: 30-50 minutes

End-stage renal disease: 3.3-5.1 hours

Time to Peak Serum: I.M.: ~30 minutes; I.V.: ~1 hour

Pregnancy Risk Factor B

Pregnancy Considerations Adverse events have not been observed in animal reproduction studies. Penicillin crosses the placenta and distributes into amniotic fluid. Maternal use of penicillins has generally not resulted in an increased risk of adverse fetal effects. Penicillin G is the drug of choice for treatment of syphilis during pregnancy and penicillin G (parenteral/aqueous) is the drug of choice for the prevention of early-onset Group B Streptococcal (GBS) disease in newborns (consult current guidelines).

Penicillin G Procaine (pen i SIL in jee PROE kane)

Brand Names: Canada Pfizerpen-AS®; Wycillin®

Pharmacologic Category Antibiotic, Penicillin

Use Treatment of moderately-severe infections due to *Treponema pallidum* and other penicillin G-sensitive microorganisms that are susceptible to low, but prolonged serum penicillin concentrations; anthrax due to

Bacillus anthracis (postexposure) to reduce the incidence or progression of disease following exposure to aerolized *Bacillus anthracis*

Local Anesthetic/Vasoconstrictor Precautions No information available to require special precautions

Effects on Dental Treatment No significant effects or complications reported

Effects on Bleeding No information available to require special precautions

Adverse Effects Frequency not defined.

Cardiovascular: Conduction disturbances, myocardial depression, vasodilation

Central nervous system: CNS stimulation, confusion, drowsiness, myoclonus, seizure

Hematologic: Hemolytic anemia, neutropenia, positive Coombs' reaction

Local: Pain at injection site, sterile abscess at injection site, thrombophlebitis

Renal: Interstitial nephritis

Miscellaneous: Hypersensitivity reactions, Jarisch-Herxheimer reaction, pseudoanaphylactic reactions, serum sickness

General Dosage Range Dosage adjustment recommended in patients with renal impairment

I.M.:

Children: 25,000-50,000 units/kg/day in divided doses 1-2 times/day (maximum: 4.8 million units/day)

Adults: 0.6-4.8 million units/day in divided doses every 12-24 hours

Mechanism of Action Inhibits bacterial cell wall synthesis by binding to one or more of the penicillin-binding proteins (PBPs); which in turn inhibits the final transpeptidation step of peptidoglycan synthesis in bacterial cell walls, thus inhibiting cell wall biosynthesis. Bacteria eventually lyse due to ongoing activity of cell wall autolytic enzymes (autolysins and murein hydrolases) while cell wall assembly is arrested.

Pharmacodynamics/Kinetics

Duration of Action Therapeutic: 15-24 hours

Time to Peak Serum: 1-4 hours

Pregnancy Risk Factor B

Pregnancy Considerations Adverse events have not been observed in animal reproduction studies. Penicillin crosses the placenta and distributes into amniotic fluid. Maternal use of penicillins has generally not resulted in an increased risk of adverse fetal effects.

Penicillin V Potassium
(pen i SIL in vee poe TASS ee um)

Related Information

Bacterial Infections *on page 1562*

Viral Infections *on page 1575*

Related Sample Prescriptions

Bacterial Infections and Periodontal Diseases *on page 1609*

Brand Names: Canada Apo-Pen VK®; Novo-Pen-VK; Nu-Pen-VK

Generic Availability (U.S.) Yes

Pharmacologic Category Antibiotic, Penicillin

Dental Use Antibiotic of first choice in treatment of common orofacial infections caused by aerobic gram-positive cocci and anaerobes. These orofacial infections include cellulitis, periapical abscess, periodontal abscess, acute suppurative pulpitis, oronasal fistula, pericoronitis, osteitis, osteomyelitis, postsurgical and post-traumatic infection. **Note: This agent is no longer recommended for dental procedure prophylaxis.**

Use Treatment of infections caused by susceptible organisms involving the respiratory tract, otitis media, sinusitis, skin, and urinary tract; prophylaxis in rheumatic fever

Unlabeled Use Chronic antimicrobial suppression of prosthetic joint infection

Local Anesthetic/Vasoconstrictor Precautions No information available to require special precautions

Effects on Dental Treatment Key adverse event(s) related to dental treatment: Oral candidiasis (prolonged use).

Effects on Bleeding No information available to require special precautions

Adverse Effects >10%: Gastrointestinal: Mild diarrhea, vomiting, nausea, oral candidiasis

Dental Usual Dosage Note: No longer recommended for dental procedure prophylaxis

Orofacial infections: Oral:

Children <12 years: 25-50 mg/kg/day in divided doses every 6-8 hours (maximum dose: 3000 mg daily)

Children ≥12 years and Adults: 125-500 mg every 6-8 hours

Dosage

Usual dosage range:

Children <12 years: Oral: 25-50 mg/kg/day in divided doses every 6-8 hours (maximum dose: 3000 mg daily)

Children ≥12 years and Adults: Oral: 125-500 mg every 6-8 hours

Indication-specific dosing:

Infants >3 months and Children: Oral:

Community-acquired pneumonia (CAP) due to group A *Streptococcus*, mild infection or step-down therapy (preferred) (IDSA/PIDS, 2011): 50-75 mg/kg/day in 3-4 divided doses

Children: Oral:

Pharyngitis (streptococcal) (IDSA guidelines):

Acute treatment: 250 mg 2-3 times daily for 10 days

Chronic carrier treatment, group A streptococci: 50 mg/kg/day in 4 divided doses (maximum: 2000 mg daily) for 10 days in combination with oral rifampin (Shulman, 2012)

Prophylaxis of pneumococcal infections:

Children <5 years: 125 mg twice daily

Children ≥5 years: 250 mg twice daily

Prophylaxis of recurrent rheumatic fever:

Children <5 years: 125 mg twice daily

Children ≥5 years: 250 mg twice daily

Adolescents: Oral:

Pharyngitis (streptococcal), acute treatment (IDSA guidelines): Refer to adult dosing.

Adults: Oral:

Actinomycosis:

Mild: 2000-4000 mg daily in 4 divided doses for 8 weeks

Surgical: 2000-4000 mg in 4 divided doses for 6-12 months (after I.V. penicillin G therapy of 4-6 weeks)

Erysipelas: 500 mg 4 times daily

Periodontal infections: 250-500 mg every 6 hours for 5-7 days

Note: Efficacy of antimicrobial therapy in periapical abscess is questionable; the American Academy of Periodontology recommends use of antibiotic therapy only when systemic symptoms (eg, fever, lymphadenopathy) are present or in immunocompromised patients.

Pharyngitis (streptococcal):

Manufacturer's labeling: 500 mg 3-4 times daily for 10 days

Acute treatment, group A streptococci (IDSA guidelines): 250 mg 4 times daily or 500 mg twice daily for 10 days (Shulman, 2012)

Chronic carrier treatment, group A streptococcal (IDSA guidelines): 500 mg 4 times daily (maximum: 2000 mg daily) for 10 days in combination with oral rifampin (Shulman, 2012)

Prophylaxis of pneumococcal or recurrent rheumatic fever infections: 250 mg twice daily

Prosthetic joint infection (unlabeled use): *Chronic oral antimicrobial suppression (Enterococcus spp [penicillin-susceptible], streptococci [beta-hemolytic], Propionibacterium spp):* 500 mg 2-4 times daily (Osmon, 2013)

Dosing interval in renal impairment: Cl_{cr} <10 mL/minute: Administer 250 mg every 6 hours

Mechanism of Action Inhibits bacterial cell wall synthesis by binding to one or more of the penicillin-binding proteins (PBPs); which in turn inhibits the final transpeptidation step of peptidoglycan synthesis in bacterial cell walls, thus inhibiting cell wall biosynthesis. Bacteria eventually lyse due to ongoing activity of cell wall autolytic enzymes (autolysins and murein hydrolases) while cell wall assembly is arrested.

Contraindications Hypersensitivity to penicillin or any component of the formulation

Warnings/Precautions Use with caution in patients with severe renal impairment (modify dosage) or history of seizures. Serious and occasionally severe or fatal hypersensitivity (anaphylactoid) reactions have been reported in patients on penicillin therapy, especially with a history of beta-lactam hypersensitivity, history of sensitivity to multiple allergens, or previous IgE-mediated reactions (eg, anaphylaxis, angioedema, urticaria). Use with caution in asthmatic patients. Extended duration of therapy or use associated with high serum concentrations may be associated with an increased risk for some adverse reactions. Prolonged use may result in fungal or bacterial superinfection, including *C. difficile*-associated diarrhea (CDAD) and pseudomembranous colitis; CDAD has been observed >2 months postantibiotic treatment.

Drug Interactions

Metabolism/Transport Effects None known.

Avoid Concomitant Use

Avoid concomitant use of Penicillin V Potassium with any of the following: BCG

Increased Effect/Toxicity

Penicillin V Potassium may increase the levels/effects of: Methotrexate; Vitamin K Antagonists

The levels/effects of Penicillin V Potassium may be increased by: Probenecid

Decreased Effect

Penicillin V Potassium may decrease the levels/effects of: BCG; Mycophenolate; Sodium Picosulfate; Typhoid Vaccine

The levels/effects of Penicillin V Potassium may be decreased by: Fusidic Acid; Tetracycline Derivatives

Ethanol/Nutrition/Herb Interactions Food: Decreases drug absorption rate; decreases drug serum concentration. Management: Take on an empty stomach 1 hour before or 2 hours after meals around-the-clock to promote less variation in peak and trough serum levels.

Dietary Considerations Take on an empty stomach 1 hour before or 2 hours after meals.

Pharmacodynamics/Kinetics
Half-life Elimination 30 minutes; prolonged with renal impairment
Time to Peak Serum: 0.5-1 hour
Pregnancy Considerations Penicillin crosses the placenta and distributes into amniotic fluid. Maternal use of penicillins has generally not resulted in an increased risk of adverse fetal effects. Due to pregnancy-induced physiologic changes, some pharmacokinetic parameters of penicillin V may be altered in the second and third trimester. Higher doses or increased dosing frequency may be required.
Lactation Enters breast milk
Breast-Feeding Considerations Penicillin V is excreted into breast milk (low concentrations) and may be detected in the urine of some breast-feeding infants. Loose stools and rash have been reported in nursing infants.
Dosage Forms
Powder for solution, oral: 125 mg/5 mL (100 mL, 200 mL); 250 mg/5 mL (100 mL, 200 mL)
Tablet, oral: 250 mg, 500 mg
References
Wynn RL and Bergman SA, "Antibiotics and Their Use in the Treatment of Orofacial Infections, Part I," *Gen Dent*, 1994, 42(5):398, 400, 402.
Wynn RL and Bergman SA, "Antibiotics and Their Use in the Treatment of Orofacial Infections, Part II," *Gen Dent*, 1994, 42(6):498-502.
Wynn RL, Bergman SA, Meiller TF, et al, "Antibiotics in Treating Oral-Facial Infections of Odontogenic Origin: An Update," *Gen Dent*, 2001, 49(3):238-40, 242, 244 passim.

Pentafluoropropane and Tetrafluoroethane
(pen ta flure oh PRO pane & tet ra flure oh ETH ane)

Brand Names: U.S. Gebauer's Instant Ice™ [OTC]; Gebauer's Pain Ease®; Gebauer's Spray and Stretch®
Pharmacologic Category Anesthetic, Topical
Use Management of myofascial pain, restricted motion, and muscle tension; temporary relief of muscle spasm and minor sports injuries (eg, bruises, contusions, cuts/abrasions, swelling, minor sprains, strains); control of pain associated with injections or minor surgical procedures
Local Anesthetic/Vasoconstrictor Precautions No information available to require special precautions
Effects on Dental Treatment No significant effects or complications reported
Effects on Bleeding No information available to require special precautions
Adverse Effects Frequency not defined.
Dermatologic: Skin irritation, skin pigmentation change, frostbite
General Dosage Range Topical: *Adults:* Spray over affected area at a rate of ~4 inches/second (10 cm/second); reapply as needed
Mechanism of Action
Vapocoolant (skin refrigerant) and counterirritant
Pharmacodynamics/Kinetics
Duration of Action Anesthetic effect: Seconds to 1 minute
Pregnancy Considerations Animal reproduction studies have not been conducted.

Pentamidine (pen TAM i deen)

Related Information
Clinical Risk Related to Drugs Prolonging QT Interval *on page 1510*
Brand Names: U.S. Nebupent®; Pentam® 300

Pharmacologic Category Antifungal Agent; Antiprotozoal
Use
I.M., I.V.: Treatment of pneumonia caused by *Pneumocystis jirovecii* pneumonia (PCP)
Inhalation: Prevention of PCP in high-risk, HIV-infected patients either with a history of PCP or with a CD4+ count ≤200/mm^3
Unlabeled Use Prevention of PCP in nonHIV-infected patients; treatment of African trypanosomiasis, cutaneous leishmaniasis, and amebic meningoencephalitis
Local Anesthetic/Vasoconstrictor Precautions
Pentamidine is one of the drugs confirmed to prolong the QT interval and is accepted as having a risk of causing torsade de pointes. The risk of drug-induced torsade de pointes is extremely low when a single QT interval prolonging drug is prescribed. In terms of epinephrine, it is not known what effect vasoconstrictors in the local anesthetic regimen will have in patients with a known history of congenital prolonged QT interval or in patients taking any medication that prolongs the QT interval. Until more information is obtained, it is suggested that the clinician consult with the physician prior to the use of a vasoconstrictor in suspected patients, and that the vasoconstrictor (epinephrine, mepivacaine and levonordefrin [Carbocaine® 2% with Neo-Cobefrin®]) be used with caution.
Effects on Dental Treatment No significant effects or complications reported
Effects on Bleeding Has been shown to induce anemia, leukopenia, and thrombocytopenia (3%). Hemolytic anemia has also been observed following parenteral pentamidine administration. Rare but potentially life-threatening blood clot formation has also been observed in less than 1% of treated patients.
Adverse Effects
Aerosol:
>10%:
Central nervous system: Fatigue (66%), fever (51%), dizziness/lightheadedness (45%)
Gastrointestinal: Appetite decreased (50%)
Respiratory: Cough (1% to 63%), dyspnea (48%), wheezing (32%)
Miscellaneous: Infection (15%)
1% to 10%:
Central nervous system: Headache
Gastrointestinal: Diarrhea, nausea, oral candida, taste alteration
Hematologic: Anemia
Respiratory: Bronchitis, chest pain, pharyngitis, sinusitis, upper respiratory tract infection
Miscellaneous: Herpes infection, influenza, night sweats

Injection:
>10%:
Local: Local reactions at I.M. injection site (11%; includes sterile abscess, necrosis, pain, induration)
Renal: Renal function impaired (29%), creatinine increased (24%)
1% to 10%:
Cardiovascular: Hypotension (5%)
Central nervous system: Confusion/hallucinations (2%)
Dermatologic: Rash (3%)
Endocrine & metabolic: Hypoglycemia (6%)
Gastrointestinal: Nausea/anorexia (6%), taste alteration (2%)
Hematologic: Leukopenia (10%), thrombocytopenia (3%), anemia (1%)

Hepatic: Liver function tests increased (9%)
Renal: Azotemia (9%), BUN increased (7%)

General Dosage Range Dosage adjustment recommended in patients with renal impairment

I.M.: *Children >4 months and Adults:* 4 mg/kg once daily for 14-21 days

I.V.:
Children >4 months and Adults: 4 mg/kg once daily for 14-21 days

Inhalation: *Children >16 years and Adults:* 300 mg/dose every 4 weeks

Mechanism of Action Interferes with microbial RNA/DNA, phospholipids and protein synthesis, through inhibition of oxidative phosphorylation and/or interference with incorporation of nucleotides and nucleic acids into RNA and DNA

Pharmacodynamics/Kinetics

Half-life Elimination I.V.: 5-8 hours; I.M.: 7-11 hours; may be prolonged with severe renal impairment

Pregnancy Risk Factor C

Pregnancy Considerations Animal reproduction studies were not conducted by the manufacturer; therefore, pentamidine is classified pregnancy category C. In postmarketing studies, pentamidine was embryocidal but not teratogenic when administered to animals. Pentamidine crosses the human placenta. Administration via the aerosolized route may minimize maternal serum concentrations. Concern regarding occupational exposure of pregnant healthcare workers has been discussed in the literature. Pregnant healthcare workers should avoid aerolized exposure if possible. If avoidance is not possible, they should wear a mask and gloves and ensure proper ventilation. Pentamidine may be used in pregnancy for prophylaxis or treatment of PCP if the patient is unable to take first line medications.

Dental Comment Pentamidine is known to prolong the QT interval. The QT interval is measured as the time and distance between the Q point of the QRS complex and the end of the T wave in the ECG tracing. After adjustment for heart rate, the QT interval is defined as prolonged if it is more than 450 msec in men and 460 msec in women. A long QT syndrome was first described in the 1950s and 60s as a congenital syndrome involving QT interval prolongation and syncope and sudden death. Some of the congenital long QT syndromes were characterized by a peculiar electrocardiographic appearance of the QRS complex involving a premature atria beat followed by a pause, then a subsequent sinus beat showing marked QT prolongation and deformity. This type of cardiac arrhythmia was originally termed "torsade de pointes" (translated from the French as "twisting of the points"). Pentamidine is considered as having a risk of causing torsade de pointes. Since it is not known what effect vasoconstrictors in the local anesthetic regimen will have in patients with a known history of congenital prolonged QT interval or in patients taking any medication that prolongs the QT interval, a medical consult is suggested.

Pentastarch (PEN ta starch)

Brand Names: Canada Pentaspan®
Pharmacologic Category Plasma Volume Expander, Colloid
Use Adjunctive treatment in the management of shock
Local Anesthetic/Vasoconstrictor Precautions No information available to require special precautions

Effects on Dental Treatment No significant effects or complications reported
Effects on Bleeding No information available to require special precautions
Adverse Effects Frequency not defined.
Cardiovascular: Angina, edema, tachycardia
Central nervous system: Anxiety, chills, dizziness, fatigue, fever, headache, insomnia, malaise, shakiness
Dermatologic: Acne
Endocrine & metabolic: Amylase increased
Gastrointestinal: Diarrhea, nausea, weight gain (temporary)
Hematologic: Coagulation disorder, hemorrhage
Hepatic: Bilirubin increased
Neuromuscular & skeletal: Paresthesia, weakness
Respiratory: Nasal congestion
Miscellaneous: Anaphylactic/anaphylactoid reaction, hypersensitivity (hypotension, urticaria, wheezing)

General Dosage Range I.V.: *Adults:* 500-2000 mL/day (maximum daily dose: 28 mL/kg or 2000 mL)

Mechanism of Action Produces plasma volume expansion by virtue of its highly colloidal starch structure

Pharmacodynamics/Kinetics

Onset of Action Volume expansion: Within 1 hour

Duration of Action 18-24 hours (improves hemodynamic status for 12-18 hours)

Half-life Elimination ~2 days

Pregnancy Considerations Adverse events were observed in animal reproduction studies.

Product Availability Not available in U.S.

Pentazocine (pen TAZ oh seen)

Brand Names: U.S. Talwin®
Brand Names: Canada Talwin®
Pharmacologic Category Analgesic, Opioid; Analgesic, Opioid Partial Agonist
Use Relief of moderate-to-severe pain; has also been used as a sedative prior to surgery and as a supplement to surgical anesthesia
Local Anesthetic/Vasoconstrictor Precautions No information available to require special precautions
Effects on Dental Treatment Key adverse event(s) related to dental treatment: Xerostomia (normal salivary flow resumes upon discontinuation).
Effects on Bleeding No information available to require special precautions
Adverse Effects Frequency not defined.
Cardiovascular: Circulatory depression, facial edema, flushing, hyper-/hypotension, shock, syncope, systemic vascular resistance increased, tachycardia
Central nervous system: Chills, CNS depression, confusion, disorientation, dizziness, drowsiness, euphoria, excitement, hallucinations, headache, insomnia, irritability, lightheadedness, malaise, nightmares, sedation
Dermatologic: Dermatitis, erythema multiforme, pruritus, rash, Stevens-Johnson syndrome, toxic epidermal necrolysis, urticaria
Gastrointestinal: Abdominal distress, anorexia, constipation, diarrhea, nausea, taste alteration, vomiting, xerostomia
Genitourinary: Urinary retention
Hematologic: Agranulocytosis (rare), eosinophilia, WBCs decreased
Local: Injection site reaction (tissue damage and irritation)
Neuromuscular & skeletal: Paresthesia, tremor, weakness
Ocular: Blurred vision, diplopia, miosis, nystagmus

Otic: Tinnitus

Respiratory: Dyspnea, respiratory depression (rare)

Miscellaneous: Anaphylaxis, diaphoresis, physical and psychological dependence

General Dosage Range Dosage adjustment recommended in patients with renal impairment

I.M.:

Children 1-16 years: 0.5 mg/kg preoperatively

Adults: 30-60 mg every 3-4 hours (maximum: 360 mg/day; 60 mg/dose) **or** 30 mg once

I.V.: *Adults:* 30 mg every 3-4 hours (maximum: 360 mg/day; 30 mg/dose) **or** 20 mg every 2-3 hours as needed (maximum total dose: 60 mg)

SubQ: *Adults:* 30 mg every 3-4 hours (maximum: 360 mg/day; 60 mg/dose)

Mechanism of Action Agonist of kappa opiate receptors and partial agonist of mu opiate receptors in the CNS, causing inhibition of ascending pain pathways, altering the perception of and response to pain; produces analgesia, respiratory depression and sedation similar to opioids

Pharmacodynamics/Kinetics

Onset of Action I.M., SubQ: 15-20 minutes; I.V.: 2-3 minutes

Duration of Action 2-3 hours

Half-life Elimination 2-3 hours; prolonged with hepatic impairment

Pregnancy Risk Factor C

Pregnancy Considerations Pentazocine was not found to be teratogenic in animal studies. Pentazocine has been shown to cross the human placenta. Use should be avoided during labor and delivery of premature infants. Abstinence syndromes in the newborn have been reported after long-term use of pentazocine during pregnancy. Other adverse effects in the newborn have been reported following abuse of pentazocine during pregnancy; these effects may be due to pentazocine, other drugs abused, the mother's lifestyle, or a combination of all factors.

Controlled Substance C-IV

Pentazocine and Acetaminophen

(pen TAZ oh seen & a seet a MIN oh fen)

Related Information

Acetaminophen *on page 27*

Pentazocine *on page 1069*

Generic Availability (U.S.) Yes

Pharmacologic Category Analgesic Combination (Opioid); Analgesic, Opioid Partial Agonist

Dental Use Relief of mild-to-moderate pain

Use Relief of mild-to-moderate pain

Local Anesthetic/Vasoconstrictor Precautions No information available to require special precautions

Effects on Dental Treatment No significant effects or complications reported (see Dental Comment)

Effects on Bleeding No information available to require special precautions

Adverse Effects Adverse reactions attributed to pentazocine 50 mg. Frequency not defined. See Acetaminophen monograph for acetaminophen-related reactions.

Cardiovascular: Circulatory depression, facial edema, flushing, hyper-/hypotension, syncope, tachycardia

Central nervous system: Chills, confusion, depression, disorientation, dizziness, drowsiness, euphoria, excitement, hallucinations, headache, insomnia, intracranial pressure increased, irritability, lightheadedness, nightmares, sedation, seizure

Dermatologic: Dermatitis, erythema multiforme, pruritus, rash, Stevens-Johnson syndrome, toxic epidermal necrolysis, urticaria

Gastrointestinal: Abdominal distress, anorexia, biliary spasm, constipation, diarrhea, nausea, vomiting, xerostomia

Genitourinary: Urinary retention

Hematologic: Agranulocytosis, eosinophilia, WBCs decreased

Neuromuscular & skeletal: Paresthesia, tremor, weakness

Ocular: Blurred vision, miosis

Otic: Tinnitus

Respiratory: Respiratory depression

Miscellaneous: Anaphylaxis, diaphoresis, physical and psychological dependence, withdrawal syndrome

Dental Usual Dosage Analgesic: Adults: Oral: 1 caplet every 4 hours (maximum: 6 caplets/day)

Dosage Note: Maximum daily intake of acetaminophen from all sources should not exceed 4 g.

Oral: Children ≥12 years and Adults: Analgesic: One caplet (pentazocine 25 mg/acetaminophen 650 mg) every 4 hours as needed (maximum: 6 caplets/day)

Dosage adjustment in renal impairment: Use with caution. Manufacturer labeling does not provide specific dosing recommendations; less frequent administration may be necessary.

Dosage adjustment in hepatic impairment: Use with caution. Manufacturer labeling does not provide specific dosing recommendations; less frequent administration may be necessary.

Mechanism of Action

Pentazocine: Agonist of kappa opiate receptors and partial agonist of mu opiate receptors in the CNS, causing inhibition of ascending pain pathways, altering the perception of and response to pain; produces analgesia, respiratory depression and sedation similar to opioids

Acetaminophen: Inhibits the synthesis of prostaglandins in the central nervous system and peripherally blocks pain impulse generation

Contraindications Hypersensitivity to pentazocine, acetaminophen, or any component of the formulation; hypersensitivity to sulfites (contains metabisulfite)

Warnings/Precautions Contains sodium metabisulfite; may cause allergic-type reactions including anaphylaxis; potential for elevating CSF pressure due to respiratory effects which may be exaggerated in presence of head injury, intracranial lesions, or pre-existing increase in intracranial lesions. May cause CNS depression, which may impair physical or mental abilities; patients must be cautioned about performing tasks which require mental alertness (eg, operating machinery or driving). Effects may be potentiated when used with other sedative drugs or ethanol. Confusion, disorientation, and visual hallucinations have occurred in some patients, but usually clears within a few hours; observe patients closely. **[U.S. Boxed Warning]: Acetaminophen may cause severe hepatotoxicity, potentially requiring liver transplant or resulting in death; hepatotoxicity is usually associated with excessive acetaminophen intake (>4 g/day).** Risk is increased with alcohol use, pre-existing liver disease, and intake of more than one source of acetaminophen-containing medications. Chronic daily dosing in adults has also resulted in liver damage in some patients. Hypersensitivity and anaphylactic reactions have been reported with acetaminophen use; discontinue immediately if symptoms of allergic or hypersensitivity reactions occur. May cause psychological and physical dependence. May obscure diagnosis or clinical course of patients with acute abdominal conditions. Use with caution in patients with respiratory depression, G6PD deficiency, biliary tract impairment, adrenal insufficiency, prostatic hyperplasia, urinary stricture, ethanol abuse, CNS depression, coma, myocardial infarction, porphyria, hypothyroidism, severely limited respiratory reserve, severe bronchial asthma, other obstructive respiratory conditions or cyanosis, impaired renal function, patients prone to seizures. Use with caution in elderly or debilitated patients. Abrupt discontinuation may result in withdrawal symptoms; taper dose to decrease risk of withdrawal symptoms. Pentazocine may precipitate opiate withdrawal symptoms in patients who have been receiving opiates regularly. Pentazocine clearance may be increased in tobacco smokers.

Drug Interactions

Metabolism/Transport Effects Refer to individual components.

Avoid Concomitant Use

Avoid concomitant use of Pentazocine and Acetaminophen with any of the following: Azelastine (Nasal); Paraldehyde; Pimozide

Increased Effect/Toxicity

Pentazocine and Acetaminophen may increase the levels/effects of: Alcohol (Ethyl); Alvimopan; ARIPiprazole; Azelastine (Nasal); Busulfan; CNS Depressants; Dasatinib; Desmopressin; Imatinib; Lomitapide; Metyrosine; Mipomersen; Mirtazapine; Paraldehyde; Pimozide; Pramipexole; Prilocaine; ROPINIRole; Rotigotine; Selective Serotonin Reuptake Inhibitors; SORAfenib; Thiazide Diuretics; Vitamin K Antagonists; Zolpidem

The levels/effects of Pentazocine and Acetaminophen may be increased by: Amphetamines; Antipsychotic Agents (Phenothiazines); Dasatinib; Droperidol; HydrOXYzine; Imatinib; Isoniazid; Magnesium Sulfate; Metyrapone; Perampanel; Probenecid; Sodium Oxybate; SORAfenib; Succinylcholine

Decreased Effect

Pentazocine and Acetaminophen may decrease the levels/effects of: Analgesics (Opioid); Pegvisomant

The levels/effects of Pentazocine and Acetaminophen may be decreased by: Ammonium Chloride; Anticonvulsants (Hydantoin); Barbiturates; CarBAMazepine; Cholestyramine Resin; Peginterferon Alfa-2b

Ethanol/Nutrition/Herb Interactions

Ethanol: Avoid ethanol (may increase CNS depression). Herb/Nutraceutical: Avoid valerian, St John's wort, kava kava, gotu kola (may increase CNS depression).

Pregnancy Risk Factor C

Pregnancy Considerations See individual agents.

Lactation Pentazocine and acetaminophen enter breast milk/use caution

Breast-Feeding Considerations See individual agents.

Controlled Substance C-IV

Dosage Forms

Tablet: Pentazocine 25 mg and acetaminophen 650 mg

Dental Comment Hepatotoxicity caused by acetaminophen is potentiated by chronic alcohol consumption. People who are taking acetaminophen, even at therapeutic doses, and consume alcohol are at risk of developing hepatotoxicity.

Acetaminophen may increase the levels and enhance the anticoagulant effects of vitamin K antagonists acenocoumarol and warfarin (Coumadin®). Studies have reported that acetaminophen has increased the INR in warfarin treated patients with daily acetaminophen doses as low as 2 g, particularly when taking acetaminophen for >1 week (Antlitz, 1968; Boeijinga, 1982; Gebauer, 2003; Hylek, 1998; Rubin, 1984). In addition, case reports of bleeding as a result of increased INR have been published (Bagheri, 1999; Bartle, 1991). There is no known mechanism of the interaction; furthermore, some studies have failed to demonstrate this interaction (Gadisseur, 2003; Kwan, 1995; van den Bemt, 2002). In terms of risk, the data suggest that acetaminophen and warfarin could interact in some clinically significant manner but that the benefits of concomitant use of acetaminophen for pain control in dental patients taking warfarin usually outweigh the risks. An appropriate monitoring plan should be in place to identify potential negative effects and dosage adjustments may be necessary in a minority of patients. The interaction may be more likely to occur with daily acetaminophen doses of >1.3 g for >1 week.

There are no reports of acetaminophen interacting with antiplatelet drugs such as aspirin, clopidogrel (Plavix®), or prasugrel (Effient™). Also, there are no reports of acetaminophen in combination with hydrocodone, codeine, or oxycodone interacting with warfarin (Coumadin®).

References

Antlitz AM, Mead JA Jr, and Tolentino MA, "Potentiation of Oral Anticoagulant Therapy by Acetaminophen," *Curr Ther Res Clin Exp*, 1968, 10(10):501-7.

Bagheri H, Bernhard NB, and Montastruc JL, "Potentiation of the Acenocoumarol Anticoagulant Effect by Acetaminophen," *Ann Pharmacother*, 1999, 33(4):506.

Bartle WR and Blakely JA, "Potentiation of Warfarin Anticoagulation by Acetaminophen," *JAMA*, 1991, 265(10):1260.

Boeijinga JJ, Boerstra EE, Ris P, et al, "Interaction Between Paracetamol and Coumarin Anticoagulants," *Lancet*, 1982, 1(8270):506.

Gadisseur AP, Van Der Meer FJ, and Rosendaal FR, "Sustained Intake of Paracetamol (Acetaminophen) During Oral Anticoagulant Therapy With Coumarins Does Not Cause Clinically Important INR Changes: A Randomized Double-Blind Clinical Trial," *J Thromb Haemost*, 2003, 1(4):714-7.

Gebauer MG, Nyfort-Hansen K, Henschke PJ, et al, "Warfarin and Acetaminophen Interaction," *Pharmacotherapy*, 2003, 23(1):109-12.

Hylek EM, Heiman H, Skates SJ, et al, "Acetaminophen and Other Risk Factors for Excessive Warfarin Anticoagulation," *JAMA*, 1998, 279(9):657-62.

Kwan D, Bartle WR, and Walker SE, "The Effects of Acute and Chronic Acetaminophen Dosing on the Pharmacodynamics and Pharmacokinetics of (R)- and (S)-Warfarin," *Clin Pharmacol Ther*, 1995, 57:212.

Rubin RN, Mentzer RL, and Budzynski AZ, "Potentiation of Anticoagulant Effect of Warfarin by Acetaminophen (Tylenol®)," *Clin Res*, 1984, 32:698a.

van den Bemt PM, Geven LM, Kuitert NA, et al, "The Potential Interaction Between Oral Anticoagulants and Acetaminophen in Everyday Practice," *Pharm World Sci*, 2002, 24(5):201-4.

PENTobarbital (pen toe BAR bi tal)

Brand Names: U.S. Nembutal®

Brand Names: Canada Nembutal® Sodium

Pharmacologic Category Anticonvulsant, Barbiturate; Barbiturate

Use Sedative/hypnotic; refractory status epilepticus

Unlabeled Use Barbiturate coma in patients with severe brain injury (eg, hemorrhagic stroke, traumatic brain injury) and increased intracranial pressure

Local Anesthetic/Vasoconstrictor Precautions No information available to require special precautions

Effects on Dental Treatment No significant effects or complications reported

Effects on Bleeding No information available to require special precautions

Adverse Effects Frequency not defined.

Cardiovascular: Bradycardia, hypotension, syncope

Central nervous system: Abnormal thinking, agitation, anxiety, ataxia, CNS excitation, confusion, depression, dizziness, drowsiness, fever, hallucinations, headache, hyperkinesia, insomnia, nervousness, nightmares, psychiatric disturbances, somnolence

Dermatologic: Angioedema, exfoliative dermatitis, rash

Gastrointestinal: Constipation, nausea, vomiting

Hematologic: Megaloblastic anemia

Hepatic: Hepatotoxicity

Local: Injection site reactions

Respiratory: Apnea (especially with rapid I.V. use), hypoventilation, laryngospasm, respiratory depression

Miscellaneous: Gangrene with inadvertent intra-arterial injection, hypersensitivity reactions

General Dosage Range
I.M.:
Children: 2-6 mg/kg (maximum: 100 mg/dose)
Adults: 150-200 mg
I.V.:
Children:
Hypnotic/sedative: 1-6 mg/kg
Refractory status epilepticus: Loading dose: 5-15 mg/kg; Maintenance infusion: 0.5-5 mg/kg/hour
Adults:
Hypnotic/sedative: 100 mg; may repeat (maximum total dose: 500 mg)
Refractory status epilepticus: Loading dose: 10-15 mg/kg; Maintenance infusion: 0.5-10 mg/kg/hour

Mechanism of Action Barbiturate with sedative, hypnotic, and anticonvulsant properties. Barbiturates depress the sensory cortex, decrease motor activity, alter cerebellar function, and produce drowsiness, sedation, and hypnosis. In high doses, barbiturates exhibit anticonvulsant activity; barbiturates produce dose-dependent respiratory depression; reduce brain metabolism and cerebral blood flow in order to decrease intracranial pressure

Pharmacodynamics/Kinetics
Onset of Action I.M.: 10-15 minutes (Krauss, 2006); I.V.: Almost immediate, within 3-5 minutes (Krauss, 2006)
Duration of Action I.V.: Variable
Half-life Elimination Terminal: Children: 26 ± 16 hours (Schaible, 1982); Adults: Healthy: 22 hours (average; Ehrnebo, 1974); (range: 15-50 hours; dose dependent)
Pregnancy Risk Factor D
Pregnancy Considerations Barbiturates can be detected in the placenta, fetal liver and fetal brain. Fetal and maternal blood concentrations may be similar following parenteral administration. An increased incidence of fetal abnormalities may occur following maternal use. When used during the third trimester of pregnancy, withdrawal symptoms may occur in the neonate including seizures and hyperirritability; symptoms may be delayed up to 14 days. Use during labor does not impair uterine activity; however, respiratory depression may occur in the newborn; resuscitation equipment should be available, especially for premature infants.
Controlled Substance C-II

Pentosan Polysulfate Sodium
(PEN toe san pol i SUL fate SOW dee um)

Brand Names: U.S. Elmiron®
Brand Names: Canada Elmiron®
Pharmacologic Category Analgesic, Urinary

Use Relief of bladder pain or discomfort due to interstitial cystitis
Local Anesthetic/Vasoconstrictor Precautions No information available to require special precautions
Effects on Dental Treatment No significant effects or complications reported
Effects on Bleeding Pentosan polysulfate sodium is a low-molecular weight heparin-like compound with anticoagulant and fibrinolytic effects. Medical consult is suggested.
Adverse Effects 1% to 10%:
Central nervous system: Headache (3%), dizziness (1%)
Dermatologic: Alopecia (4%), rash (3%)
Gastrointestinal: Rectal hemorrhage (6%), diarrhea (4%), nausea (4%), abdominal pain (2%), dyspepsia (2%)
Hepatic: Liver function test abnormalities (1%; dose related)
General Dosage Range Oral: *Children ≥16 years and Adults:* 100 mg 3 times/day
Mechanism of Action Although pentosan polysulfate sodium is a low-molecular weight heparinoid, it is not known whether these properties play a role in its mechanism of action in treating interstitial cystitis; the drug appears to adhere to the bladder wall mucosa where it may act as a buffer to protect the tissues from irritating substances in the urine.
Pharmacodynamics/Kinetics
Half-life Elimination 20-27 hours
Time to Peak Serum: 2 hours (range: 0.6-120 hours)
Pregnancy Risk Factor B
Pregnancy Considerations No adverse events were noted in animal reproduction studies; however, reversible limb bud abnormalities were noted during *in vitro* animal studies. There are no adequate and well-controlled studies in pregnant women. Use with caution and only if clearly needed during pregnancy. Based on limited data, pentosan polysulfate does not appear to cross the placenta.

Pentostatin (pen toe STAT in)

Brand Names: U.S. Nipent®
Brand Names: Canada Nipent®
Pharmacologic Category Antineoplastic Agent, Antibiotic; Antineoplastic Agent, Antimetabolite (Purine Analog)
Use Treatment of hairy cell leukemia
Unlabeled Use Treatment of cutaneous T-cell lymphoma, chronic lymphocytic leukemia (CLL), and acute and chronic graft-versus-host-disease (GVHD)
Local Anesthetic/Vasoconstrictor Precautions No information available to require special precautions
Effects on Dental Treatment Key adverse event(s) related to dental treatment: Stomatitis.
Effects on Bleeding Chemotherapy may result in significant myelosuppression, potentially including significant reduction in platelet counts (thrombocytopenia: 6% to 32%) and altered hemostasis. In patients who are under active treatment with these agents, medical consult is suggested.
Adverse Effects
>10%:
Central nervous system: Fever (42% to 46%), fatigue (29% to 42%), pain (8% to 20%), chills (11% to 19%), headache (13% to 17%), CNS toxicity (1% to 11%)
Dermatologic: Rash (26% to 43%), pruritus (10% to 21%), skin disorder (4% to 17%)

Gastrointestinal: Nausea/vomiting (22% to 63%), diarrhea (15% to 17%), anorexia (13% to 16%), abdominal pain (4% to 16%), stomatitis (5% to 12%)

Hematologic: Myelosuppression (nadir: 7 days; recovery: 10-14 days), leukopenia (22% to 60%), anemia (8% to 35%), thrombocytopenia (6% to 32%)

Hepatic: Transaminases increased (2% to 19%)

Neuromuscular & skeletal: Myalgia (11% to 19%), weakness (10% to 12%)

Respiratory: Cough (17% to 20%), upper respiratory infection (13% to 16%), rhinitis (10% to 11%), dyspnea (8% to 11%)

Miscellaneous: Infection (7% to 36%), allergic reaction (2% to 11%)

1% to 10%:

Cardiovascular: Chest pain (3% to 10%), facial edema (3% to 10%), hypotension (3% to 10%), peripheral edema (3% to 10%), angina (<3%), arrhythmia (<3%), AV block (<3%), bradycardia (<3%), cardiac arrest (<3%), deep thrombophlebitis (<3%), heart failure (<3%), hypertension (<3%), pericardial effusion (<3%), sinus arrest (<3%), syncope (<3%), tachycardia (<3%), vasculitis (<3%), ventricular extrasystoles (<3%)

Central nervous system: Anxiety (3% to 10%), confusion (3% to 10%), depression (3% to 10%), dizziness (3% to 10%), insomnia (3% to 10%), nervousness (3% to 10%), somnolence (3% to 10%), abnormal dreams/thinking (<3%), amnesia (<3%), ataxia (<3%), emotional lability (<3%), encephalitis (<3%), hallucination (<3%), hostility (<3%), meningism (<3%), neuritis (<3%), neurosis (<3%), seizure (<3%), vertigo (<3%)

Dermatologic: Cellulitis (6%), furunculosis (4%), dry skin (3% to 10%), urticaria (3% to 10%), acne (<3%), alopecia (<3%), eczema (<3%), petechial rash (<3%), photosensitivity (<3%), abscess (2%)

Endocrine & metabolic: Amenorrhea (<3%), hypercalcemia (<3%), hyponatremia (<3%), gout (<3%), libido decreased/loss (<3%)

Gastrointestinal: Dyspepsia (3% to 10%) flatulence (3% to 10%), gingivitis (3% to 10%), constipation (<3%), dysphagia (<3%), glossitis (<3%), ileus (<3%), taste perversion (<3%), oral moniliasis (2%)

Genitourinary: Urinary tract infection (3%), impotence (<3%)

Hematologic: Agranulocytosis (3% to 10%), hemorrhage (3% to 10%), acute leukemia (<3%), aplastic anemia (<3%), hemolytic anemia (<3%)

Local: Phlebitis (<3%)

Neuromuscular & skeletal: Arthralgia (3% to 10%), paresthesia (3% to 10%), arthritis (<3%), dysarthria (<3%), hyperkinesia (<3%), neuralgia (<3%), neuropathy (<3%), paralysis (<3%), twitching (<3%), osteomyelitis (1%)

Ocular: Conjunctivitis (4%), amblyopia (<3%), eyes nonreactive (<3%), lacrimation disorder (<3%), photophobia (<3%), retinopathy (<3%), vision abnormal (<3%), watery eyes (<3%), xerophthalmia (<3%)

Otic: Deafness (<3%), earache (<3%), labyrinthitis (<3%), tinnitus (<3%)

Renal: Creatinine increased (3% to 10%), nephropathy (<3%), renal failure (<3%), renal insufficiency (<3%), renal function abnormal (<3%), renal stone (<3%)

Respiratory: Pharyngitis (8% to 10%), sinusitis (6%), pneumonia (5%), asthma (3% to 10%), bronchitis (3%), bronchospasm (<3%), laryngeal edema (<3%), pulmonary embolus (<3%)

Miscellaneous: Diaphoresis (8% to 10%), herpes zoster (8%), viral infection (≤8%), bacterial infection (5%), herpes simplex (4%), sepsis (3%), flu-like syndrome (<3%)

General Dosage Range Dosage adjustment recommended in patients with renal impairment

I.V.: *Adults:* 4 mg/m^2 every 2 weeks

Mechanism of Action Pentostatin is a purine antimetabolite that inhibits adenosine deaminase, preventing the deamination of adenosine to inosine. Accumulation of deoxyadenosine (dAdo) and deoxyadenosine 5'-triphosphate (dATP) results in a reduction of purine metabolism and DNA synthesis and cell death.

Pharmacodynamics/Kinetics

Half-life Elimination

Distribution half-life: 11-85 minutes

Terminal: 3-7 hours

Renal impairment (Cl$_{cr}$ <50 mL/minute): 4-18 hours

Pregnancy Risk Factor D

Pregnancy Considerations Animal studies have demonstrated teratogenicity, maternal toxicity, and fetal loss. There are no adequate and well-controlled studies in pregnant women. Women of childbearing potential should be advised to avoid becoming pregnant.

Pentoxifylline (pen toks IF i lin)

Brand Names: U.S. TRENtal®

Brand Names: Canada Pentoxifylline SR; Trental®

Pharmacologic Category Blood Viscosity Reducer Agent

Use Treatment of intermittent claudication on the basis of chronic occlusive arterial disease of the limbs; may improve function and symptoms, but not intended to replace more definitive therapy

Note: The American College of Chest Physicians (ACCP) discourages the use of pentoxifylline for the treatment of intermittent claudication refractory to exercise therapy (and smoking cessation) (Guyatt, 2012).

Unlabeled Use Severe alcoholic hepatitis; venous leg ulcers (with compression therapy)

Local Anesthetic/Vasoconstrictor Precautions No information available to require special precautions

Effects on Dental Treatment No significant effects or complications reported

Effects on Bleeding Pentoxifylline is a methylxanthine derivative with potent hemorrheologic properties. Pentoxifylline has been shown to decrease platelet aggregation and adhesion, and enhances plasminogen activator while decreasing fibrinogen and alpha$_2$-antiplasmin.

Adverse Effects 1% to 10%: Gastrointestinal: Nausea (2%), vomiting (1%)

General Dosage Range Dosage adjustment recommended in patients with renal impairment

Oral: *Adults:* 400 mg 2-3 times/day

Mechanism of Action Reduces blood viscosity via increased leukocyte and erythrocyte deformability and decreased neutrophil adhesion/activation; improves peripheral tissue oxygenation presumably through enhanced blood flow.

Pharmacodynamics/Kinetics

Half-life Elimination Parent drug: 24-48 minutes; Metabolites: 60-96 minutes

Time to Peak Serum: 2-4 hours

Pregnancy Risk Factor C

Pregnancy Considerations Teratogenic effects were not observed in animal studies. There are no adequate and well-controlled studies in pregnant women.

Perampanel (per AM pa nel)

Pharmacologic Category AMPA Glutamate Receptor Antagonist; Anticonvulsant, Miscellaneous

Use Adjunctive therapy in the treatment of partial-onset seizures (with or without generalized seizures)

Local Anesthetic/Vasoconstrictor Precautions No information available to require special precautions

Effects on Dental Treatment Key adverse event(s) related to dental treatment: Cough, upper respiratory tract infection, and oropharyngeal pain

Effects on Bleeding No information available to require special precautions

Adverse Effects

>10%: Central nervous system: Dizziness (16% to 43%), somnolence (9% to 18%), headache (13%), fatigue (8% to 12%), irritability (4% to 12%)

1% to 10%:

Cardiovascular: Peripheral edema (2%)

Central nervous system: Ataxia (1% to 8%), vertigo (3% to 5%), balance impaired (≤5%), gait disturbance (4%), anxiety (2% to 4%), aggression (2% to 3%), hypersomnia (1% to 3%), anger (≤3%), hypoesthesia (≤3%), confusion (2%), coordination impaired (≤2%), euphoria (≤2%), memory impaired (≤2%), mood changes (1% to 2%)

Dermatologic: Bruising (≤2%), skin laceration (≤2%)

Endocrine & metabolic: Hyponatremia (≤2%)

Gastrointestinal: Weight gain (4% to 9%), nausea (6% to 8%), vomiting (4%), constipation (3%)

Neuromuscular & skeletal: Falling (5% to 10%), back pain (5%), dysarthria (1% to 4%), myalgia (3%), arthralgia (≤3%), limb pain (≤3%), limb injury (2%), musculoskeletal pain (2%), weakness (2%), paresthesia (≤2%)

Ocular: Blurred vision (3% to 4%), diplopia (3%)

Respiratory: Cough (4%), upper respiratory tract infection (4%), oropharyngeal pain (2%)

Miscellaneous: Head injury (3%)

General Dosage Range Dosage adjustment recommended in patients with hepatic impairment and on concomitant therapy.

Oral: *Children ≥12 years, Adolescents, and Adults*: Initial: 2 mg once daily at bedtime; maintenance dose: 8-12 mg once daily

Mechanism of Action The exact mechanism by which perampanel exerts antiseizure activity is not definitively known; it is a noncompetitive antagonist of the ionotropic alpha-amino-3-hydroxy-5-methyl-4-isoxazolepropionic acid (AMPA) glutamate receptor on postsynaptic neurons. Glutamate is a primary excitatory neurotransmitter in the central nervous center causing many neurological disorders from neuronal over excitation.

Pharmacodynamics/Kinetics

Half-life Elimination 105 hours

Time to Peak 0.5-2.5 hours

Pregnancy Risk Factor C

Pregnancy Considerations Adverse events were observed in animal reproduction studies at doses equivalent to the human dose (based on BSA). Contraceptives containing levonorgestrel may be less effective; additional nonhormonal forms of contraception are recommended during perampanel therapy.

Patients exposed to perampanel during pregnancy are encouraged to enroll in the North American Antiepileptic Drug (NAAED) Pregnancy Registry by calling 1-888-233-2334. Additional information is available at www.aedpregnancyregistry.org.

Product Availability Fycompa™: FDA approved October 2012; anticipated availability currently unknown. Consult prescribing information for additional information.

Periciazine (per ee CYE ah zeen)

Brand Names: Canada Neuleptil®

Pharmacologic Category Antipsychotic Agent, Typical, Phenothiazine, Piperidine

Use Adjunctive therapy in selected psychotic patients to control prevailing hostility, impulsivity, or aggression

Local Anesthetic/Vasoconstrictor Precautions
Most pharmacology textbooks state that in presence of phenothiazines, systemic doses of epinephrine paradoxically decrease the blood pressure. This is the so called "epinephrine reversal" phenomenon. This has never been observed when epinephrine is given by infiltration as part of the anesthesia procedure. See Dental Comment.

Effects on Dental Treatment Key adverse event(s) related to dental treatment:

Significant hypotension may occur, especially when the drug is administered parenterally. Orthostatic hypotension is due to alpha-receptor blockade; elderly are at greater risk.

Tardive dyskinesia: Prevalence rate may be 40% in elderly; development of the syndrome and the irreversible nature are proportional to duration and total cumulative dose over time. Extrapyramidal reactions are more common in elderly with up to 50% developing these reactions after 60 years of age. Drug-induced Parkinson's syndrome occurs often; akathisia is the most common extrapyramidal reaction in elderly.

Increased confusion, memory loss, psychotic behavior, and agitation frequently occur as a consequence of anticholinergic effects. Antipsychotic-associated sedation in nonpsychotic patients is extremely unpleasant due to feelings of depersonalization, derealization, and dysphoria.

Effects on Bleeding No information available to require special precautions

Adverse Effects Frequency not defined; listing includes adverse reactions reported with other agents from the phenothiazine class.

Cardiovascular: Arrhythmias, AV block, cardiac arrest, ECG changes, edema, hypotension, orthostatic hypotension, paroxysmal tachycardia, QT_c prolongation, syncope, tachycardia, ventricular fibrillation

Central nervous system: Aggressive behavior, agitation, anxiety, bizarre dreams, cerebral edema, depression, dizziness, drowsiness, EEG changes, excitement, extrapyramidal symptoms (tremor, akathisia, dystonia, dyskinesia, oculogyric, opisthotonos, hyper-reflexia, pseudo-Parkinsonism, rigidity, sialorrhea); fatigue, fever, headache, insomnia, NMS, paradoxical psychosis, restlessness, seizure, sleep disturbance, tardive dyskinesia, temperature regulation impaired

Dermatologic: Angioedema, dermatitis, eczema, epithelial keratopathy, erythema, exfoliative dermatitis, photosensitivity, pruritus, rash, seborrhea, skin pigmentation (prolonged therapy), urticaria

Endocrine & metabolic: Delayed ovulation, galactorrhea, gynecomastia, hyperglycemia, libido changes, menstrual irregularities, thirst

Gastrointestinal: Adynamic ileus, anorexia, appetite increased, constipation, diarrhea, fecal impaction, nausea, paralytic ileus, salivation, vomiting, weight changes, xerostomia

Genitourinary: Bladder paralysis, ejaculation disturbance, impotence, incontinence, polyuria, priapism, urinary retention

Hematologic: Agranulocytosis, anemia, eosinophilia, granulocytopenia, leukopenia, neutropenia, pancytopenia, thrombocytopenia

Hepatic: Cholestasis, cholestatic jaundice, jaundice

Ocular: Blurred vision, corneal deposits (prolonged therapy), glaucoma, lenticular deposits, pigmentary retinopathy (prolonged therapy)

Respiratory: Asthma, laryngeal edema, nasal congestion, pneumonia, pneumonitis

Miscellaneous: Diaphoresis increased, lupus-like syndrome

Dosage Oral:

Children ≥5 years: Psychosis: Initial: 2.5-10 mg in the morning, followed by 5-30 mg in the evening. In general, lower dosage should be used on initiation and gradually increased based on effect and tolerance.

Adults: Psychosis: Initial: 5-20 mg in the morning, followed by 10-40 mg in the evening. Maintenance: Decrease dose to lowest effective dose. **Note:** Reduced doses (2.5-15 mg in the morning and 5-30 mg in the evening) may be considered. In general, lower dosage should be used on initiation and gradually increased based on effect and tolerance.

Elderly: Initial: ~5 mg/day; may increase dose gradually based on effect and tolerance. Doses >30 mg/day are rarely needed. Also see adult dosing.

Mechanism of Action Blocks postsynaptic mesolimbic dopaminergic receptors in the brain; depresses the release of hypothalamic and hypophyseal hormones.

Contraindications Hypersensitivity to periciazine, phenothiazine derivatives, or any component of the formulation; altered states of consciousness or comatose states particularly when due to intoxication with CNS depressant medications; hepatic dysfunction; circulatory collapse; blood dyscrasias; patients receiving spinal or regional anesthesia

Warnings/Precautions Use caution in cardiovascular disease. May alter cardiac conduction (life-threatening arrhythmias have occurred with therapeutic doses of phenothiazines); QT prolongation has been reported rarely with periciazine. Use with caution in patients with electrolyte abnormalities (eg, hypokalemia, hypomagnesemia), hypothyroidism, familial long QT syndrome, concomitant medications which may augment QT prolongation, or any underlying cardiac abnormality which may also potentiate risk. May cause orthostatic hypotension; use with caution in patients at risk of this effect or those who would not tolerate transient hypotensive episodes (cerebrovascular disease, cardiovascular disease, or other medications which may predispose). Phenothiazines have been associated with worsening of pheochromocytoma; use caution.

Elderly patients with dementia-related psychosis treated with antipsychotics are at an increased risk of death compared to placebo. Most deaths appeared to be either cardiovascular (eg, heart failure, sudden death) or infectious (eg, pneumonia) in nature. An increased incidence of cerebrovascular adverse events (including fatalities) has been reported in elderly patients with dementia-related psychosis. Periciazine is not approved for use in elderly patients with dementia. Use with caution in Parkinson's disease (may be more sensitive

to adverse effects), hemodynamic instability, and predisposition to seizures. Esophageal dysmotility and aspiration have been associated with antipsychotic use; use with caution in patients at risk of pneumonia (eg, Alzheimer's disease). May cause extrapyramidal symptoms, including pseudoparkinsonism, acute dystonic reactions, akathisia, and tardive dyskinesia. Risk for developing tardive dyskinesia is increased in elderly patients. Consider therapy discontinuation with signs/symptoms of tardive dyskinesia. May be associated with neuroleptic malignant syndrome (NMS); monitor for mental status changes, fever, muscle rigidity, and/or autonomic instability (risk may be increased in patients with Parkinson's disease or Lewy body dementia). Discontinue treatment immediately with onset of NMS; recurrence has been reported in patients rechallenged with antipsychotic therapy.

Use associated with increased prolactin levels; clinical significance of hyperprolactinemia in patients with breast cancer or other prolactin-dependent tumors is unknown. Phenothiazines may cause anticholinergic effects (confusion, agitation, constipation, xerostomia, blurred vision, urinary retention); therefore, use with caution in patients with decreased gastrointestinal motility, paralytic ileus, urinary retention, BPH, xerostomia, glaucoma or other visual problems. Conditions which also may be exacerbated by cholinergic blockade include narrow-angle glaucoma (screening is recommended) and worsening of myasthenia gravis. May alter temperature regulation; use caution with strenuous exercise, heat exposure, dehydration, and concomitant medication possessing anticholinergic effects. May mask toxicity of other drugs or conditions (eg, intestinal obstruction, Reye's syndrome, brain tumor) due to antiemetic effects.

Check blood counts periodically and discontinue at first signs of blood dyscrasias; use is contraindicated in patients with blood dyscrasias. May be sedating; use with caution in disorders where CNS depression is a feature (risk may be lower than with other phenothiazines); caution patients about performing tasks which require mental alertness.

Prolonged therapy may cause pigmentary retinopathy, corneal deposits, and/or changes in skin pigmentation. Patients experiencing hypersensitivity to phenothiazines in general should not be rechallenged unless deemed clinically necessary.

Drug Interactions

Metabolism/Transport Effects None known.

Avoid Concomitant Use

Avoid concomitant use of Periciazine with any of the following: Aclidinium; Azelastine (Nasal); Ipratropium (Oral Inhalation); Metoclopramide; Paraldehyde; Tiotropium

Increased Effect/Toxicity

Periciazine may increase the levels/effects of: Alcohol (Ethyl); Analgesics (Opioid); Anticholinergics; Antidepressants (Serotonin Reuptake Inhibitor/Antagonist); Azelastine (Nasal); Beta-Blockers; CNS Depressants; Highest Risk QTc-Prolonging Agents; Methotrimeprazine; Methylphenidate; Moderate Risk QTc-Prolonging Agents; Paraldehyde; Porfimer; Serotonin Modulators; Tiotropium; Zolpidem

The levels/effects of Periciazine may be increased by: Acetylcholinesterase Inhibitors (Central); Aclidinium; Antidepressants (Serotonin Reuptake Inhibitor/Antagonist); Antimalarial Agents; Beta-Blockers; Droperidol; HydrOXYzine; Ipratropium (Oral Inhalation); Lithium formulations; Magnesium Sulfate; Methotrimeprazine; Methylphenidate; Metoclopramide; Metyrosine; Mifepristone; Perampanel; Pramlintide; Sodium Oxybate; Tetrabenazine

Decreased Effect

Periciazine may decrease the levels/effects of: Amphetamines; Anti-Parkinson's Agents (Dopamine Agonist); Quinagolide

The levels/effects of Periciazine may be decreased by: Antacids; Anti-Parkinson's Agents (Dopamine Agonist); Lithium formulations

Ethanol/Nutrition/Herb Interactions

Ethanol: Avoid ethanol (may increase CNS depression). Herb/Nutraceutical: Avoid kava kava, valerian, St John's wort, gotu kola (may increase CNS depression). Avoid dong quai, St John's wort (may also cause photosensitization). Cigarette smoking may decrease the serum concentrations of periciazine.

Pregnancy Considerations Teratogenic effects were observed in some animal studies. Safety and efficacy have not been established in pregnant women. Use of antipsychotic agents during the third trimester may increase the risk of extrapyramidal and/or withdrawal symptoms (eg, hypertonia, tremor, agitation, respiratory distress) in newborns. Reported adverse events have ranged from self-limiting to severe.

Product Availability Not available in U.S.

Dosage Forms: Canada

Capsule, oral:

Neuleptil®: 5 mg, 10 mg, 20 mg

Solution, oral [drops]:

Neuleptil®: 10 mg/mL

Dental Comment This drug is known to prolong the QT interval. The QT interval is measured as the time and distance between the Q point of the QRS complex and the end of the T wave in the ECG tracing. After adjustment for heart rate, the QT interval is defined as prolonged if it is more than 450 msec in men and 460 msec in women. A long QT syndrome was first described in the 1950s and 60s as a congenital syndrome involving QT interval prolongation and syncope and sudden death. Some of the congenital long QT syndromes were characterized by a peculiar electrocardiographic appearance of the QRS complex involving a premature atria beat followed by a pause, then a subsequent sinus beat showing marked QT prolongation and deformity. This type of cardiac arrhythmia was originally termed "torsade de pointes" (translated from the French as "twisting of the points").

Prolongation of the QT interval is thought to result from delayed ventricular repolarization. The repolarization process within the myocardial cell is due to the efflux of intracellular potassium. The channels associated with this current can be blocked by many drugs and predispose the electrical propagation cycle to torsade de pointes.

Periciazine is one of the drugs confirmed to prolong the QT interval and is accepted as having a risk of causing torsade de pointes. The risk of drug-induced torsade de pointes is extremely low when a single QT interval prolonging drug is prescribed. In terms of epinephrine, it is not known what effect vasoconstrictors in the local anesthetic regimen will have in patients with a known history of congenital prolonged QT interval or in patients taking any medication that prolongs the QT interval. Until more information is obtained, it is suggested that the clinician consult with the physician prior to the use of a vasoconstrictor in suspected patients, and that the vasoconstrictor (epinephrine, levonordefrin [Neo-Cobefrin®]) be used with caution.

Perindopril Erbumine

(per IN doe pril er BYOO meen)

Related Information

Cardiovascular Diseases *on page 1492*

Brand Names: U.S. Aceon®

Brand Names: Canada Apo-Perindopril®; Coversyl®

Pharmacologic Category Angiotensin-Converting Enzyme (ACE) Inhibitor

Use Treatment of hypertension; reduction of cardiovascular mortality or nonfatal myocardial infarction in patients with stable coronary artery disease

Canadian labeling: Additional use (unlabeled use in U.S.): Treatment of mild-moderate (NYHA I-III) heart failure

Unlabeled Use To delay the progression of nephropathy and reduce risks of cardiovascular events in hypertensive patients with type 1 or 2 diabetes mellitus

Local Anesthetic/Vasoconstrictor Precautions No information available to require special precautions

Effects on Dental Treatment No significant effects or complications reported

Effects on Bleeding No information available to require special precautions

Adverse Effects

>10%:

Central nervous system: Headache (24%)

Respiratory: Cough (incidence is higher in women, 3:1) (12%)

1% to 10%:

Cardiovascular: Edema (4%), chest pain (2%), ECG abnormal (2%), palpitation (1%)

Central nervous system: Dizziness (8%, less than placebo), sleep disorders (3%), depression (2%), fever (2%), nervousness (1%), somnolence (1%)

Dermatologic: Rash (2%)

Endocrine & metabolic: Hyperkalemia (1%, less than placebo), triglycerides increased (1%), menstrual disorder (1%)

Gastrointestinal: Diarrhea (4%), abdominal pain (3%), nausea (2%), vomiting (2%), dyspepsia (2%), flatulence (1%)

Genitourinary: Urinary tract infection (3%), sexual dysfunction (male 1%)

Hepatic: ALT increased (2%)

Neuromuscular & skeletal: Weakness (8%), back pain (6%), lower extremity pain (5%), upper extremity pain (3%), hypertonia (3%), paresthesia (2%), joint pain (1%), myalgia (1%), arthritis (1%), neck pain (1%)

Renal: Proteinuria (2%)

Respiratory: Upper respiratory tract infection (9%), sinusitis (5%), rhinitis (5%), pharyngitis (3%)

Otic: Tinnitus (2%), ear infection (1%)

Miscellaneous: Viral infection (3%), seasonal allergy (2%)

Note: Some reactions occurred at an incidence >1% but ≤ placebo.

Additional adverse effects that have been reported with **ACE inhibitors** include agranulocytosis (especially in patients with renal impairment or collagen vascular disease), neutropenia, anemia, bullous pemphigoid, cardiac arrest, eosinophilic pneumonitis, exfoliative dermatitis, falls, hepatic failure, hyponatremia, jaundice, pancreatitis (acute), pancytopenia, pemphigus, psoriasis, thrombocytopenia; decreases in creatinine clearance in some elderly hypertensive patients or those with chronic renal failure, and worsening of renal function in patients with bilateral renal artery stenosis or hypovolemic patients (diuretic therapy). In addition, a syndrome which may include fever, myalgia, arthralgia, interstitial nephritis, vasculitis, rash, eosinophilia and positive ANA, and elevated ESR has been reported with ACE inhibitors.

General Dosage Range Dosage adjustment recommended in patients with renal impairment

Oral: *Adults:* Initial: 2-4 mg once daily; Maintenance: 4-8 mg/day in 1-2 divided doses (maximum: 16 mg/day)

Mechanism of Action Perindopril is a prodrug for perindoprilat, which acts as a competitive inhibitor of angiotensin-converting enzyme (ACE); prevents conversion of angiotensin I to angiotensin II, a potent vasoconstrictor; results in lower levels of angiotensin II which, in turn, causes an increase in plasma renin activity and a reduction in aldosterone secretion

Pharmacodynamics/Kinetics

Onset of Action Peak effect: 1-2 hours

Half-life Elimination Parent drug: 1.5-3 hours; Metabolite: Effective: 3-10 hours, Terminal: 30-120 hours

Time to Peak Chronic therapy: Perindopril: 1 hour; Perindoprilat: 3-7 hours (maximum perindoprilat serum levels are 2-3 times higher and T_{max} is shorter following chronic therapy); CHF: Perindoprilat: 6 hours

Pregnancy Risk Factor D

Pregnancy Considerations [U.S. Boxed Warning]: Drugs that act on the renin-angiotensin system can cause injury and death to the developing fetus. Discontinue as soon as possible once pregnancy is detected. Perindopril crosses the placenta; teratogenic effects may occur following maternal use during pregnancy. Drugs that act on the renin-angiotensin system are associated with oligohydramnios. Oligohydramnios, due to decreased fetal renal function, may lead to fetal lung hypoplasia and skeletal malformations. Their use in pregnancy is also associated with anuria, hypotension, renal failure, skull hypoplasia, and death in the fetus/neonate. Chronic maternal hypertension itself is also associated with adverse events in the fetus/infant. ACE inhibitors are not recommended during pregnancy to treat maternal hypertension or heart failure. Use of an ACE inhibitor should also be avoided in any woman of reproductive age. Women who are planning a pregnancy should be considered for other medication options if an ACE inhibitor is currently prescribed or the ACE inhibitor should be discontinued as soon as possible once pregnancy is detected. The exposed fetus should be monitored for fetal growth, amniotic fluid volume, and organ formation. Infants exposed to an ACE inhibitor *in utero* should be monitored for hyperkalemia, hypotension, and oliguria.

Perindopril Erbumine and Indapamide
(per IN doe pril er BYOO meen & in DAP a mide)

Related Information

Indapamide *on page 733*

Perindopril Erbumine *on page 1076*

Brand Names: Canada Coversyl® Plus; Coversyl® Plus HD; Coversyl® Plus LD

Pharmacologic Category Angiotensin-Converting Enzyme (ACE) Inhibitor; Diuretic, Thiazide-Related

Use Treatment of hypertension

Note: Coversyl® Plus LD may be used as initial treatment; Coversyl® Plus and Coversyl® Plus HD are not indicated for initial treatment of hypertension.

Local Anesthetic/Vasoconstrictor Precautions No information available to require special precautions

Effects on Dental Treatment Key adverse event(s) related to dental treatment: Indapamide: Orthostatic hypotension, palpitations, flushing, rhinorrhea, and xerostomia and changes in salivation (normal salivary flow resumes upon discontinuation).

Effects on Bleeding No information available to require special precautions

Adverse Effects Note: Observed with perindopril/indapamide; also see individual agents.

1% to 10%:

Central nervous system: Dizziness (1% to 2%)

Endocrine & metabolic: Hypokalemia (2% to 7%), hyperkalemia (1%)

Gastrointestinal: Nausea (2%), vomiting (2%), dyspepsia (≤1%)

Renal: BUN increased (2% to 4%)

Respiratory: Cough (3% to 5%), upper respiratory infection (2%)

General Dosage Range Oral: *Adults:* Perindopril 2-8 mg/indapamide 0.625-2.5 mg once daily

Mechanism of Action See individual agents.

Pregnancy Considerations [Canadian Boxed Warning]: Drugs that act on the renin-angiotensin system can cause injury and death to the developing fetus. Discontinue as soon as possible once pregnancy is detected. Use is contraindicated during the second and third trimesters of pregnancy. Also see individual agents.

Product Availability Not available in U.S.

Permethrin (per METH rin)

Brand Names: U.S. A200® Lice [OTC]; Nix® Complete Lice Treatment System [OTC]; Nix® Creme Rinse Lice Treatment [OTC]; Nix® Creme Rinse [OTC]; Nix® Lice Control Spray [OTC]; Rid® [OTC]

Brand Names: Canada Kwellada-P™; Nix®

Pharmacologic Category Antiparasitic Agent, Topical; Pediculocide; Scabicidal Agent

Use Single-application treatment of infestation with *Pediculus humanus capitis* (head louse) and its nits or *Sarcoptes scabiei* (scabies); indicated for prophylactic use during epidemics of lice

Local Anesthetic/Vasoconstrictor Precautions No information available to require special precautions

Effects on Dental Treatment No significant effects or complications reported

Effects on Bleeding No information available to require special precautions

Adverse Effects 1% to 10%:

Dermatologic: Pruritus, erythema, rash of the scalp

Local: Burning, stinging, tingling, numbness or scalp discomfort, edema

General Dosage Range Topical:
Cream: *Children and Adults:* Apply from head to toe, leave on 8-14 hours before washing off with water; May reapply in 1 week if live mites appear
Liquid (lotion or cream rinse): *Children >2 months and Adults:* Apply a sufficient volume to saturate the hair and scalp, leave on for 10 minutes before rinsing off with water; May reapply in 1 week if lice or nits still present

Mechanism of Action Inhibits sodium ion influx through nerve cell membrane channels in parasites resulting in delayed repolarization and thus paralysis and death of the pest

Pregnancy Risk Factor B

Pregnancy Considerations Adverse effects have not been observed in oral animal reproduction studies. The amount of permethrin available systemically following topical application is ≤2%. The CDC considers the use of permethrin or pyrethrins with piperonyl butoxide the drugs of choice for the treatment of pubic lice during pregnancy (CDC, 2010).

Perphenazine (per FEN a zeen)

Brand Names: Canada Apo-Perphenazine®
Pharmacologic Category Antiemetic; Antipsychotic Agent, Typical, Phenothiazine
Use Treatment of schizophrenia; severe nausea and vomiting
Unlabeled Use Psychosis; psychosis/agitation related to Alzheimer's dementia (risks vs benefits)
Local Anesthetic/Vasoconstrictor Precautions Most pharmacology textbooks state that in presence of phenothiazines, systemic doses of epinephrine paradoxically decrease the blood pressure. This is the so called "epinephrine reversal" phenomenon. This has never been observed when epinephrine is given by infiltration as part of the anesthesia procedure.
Effects on Dental Treatment Key adverse event(s) related to dental treatment:
Significant hypotension may occur, especially when the drug is administered parenterally; orthostatic hypotension is due to alpha-receptor blockade, the elderly are at greater risk for orthostatic hypotension.
Tardive dyskinesia: Prevalence rate may be 40% in elderly; development of the syndrome and the irreversible nature are proportional to duration and total cumulative dose over time. Extrapyramidal reactions are more common in elderly with up to 50% developing these reactions after 60 years of age. Drug-induced Parkinson's syndrome occurs often; akathisia is the most common extrapyramidal reaction in elderly.
Effects on Bleeding No information available to require special precautions
Adverse Effects Frequency not defined.
Cardiovascular: Bradycardia, cardiac arrest, ECG changes, hyper-/hypotension, orthostatic hypotension, pallor, peripheral edema, sudden death, tachycardia
Central nervous system: Bizarre dreams, catatonic-like states, cerebral edema, dizziness, drowsiness, extrapyramidal symptoms (pseudoparkinsonism, akathisia, dystonias, tardive dyskinesia), faintness, headache, hyperactivity, hyperpyrexia, impairment of temperature regulation, insomnia, lethargy, neuroleptic malignant syndrome (NMS), nocturnal confusion, paradoxical excitement, paranoid reactions, restlessness, seizure
Dermatologic: Discoloration of skin (blue-gray), photosensitivity

Endocrine & metabolic: Amenorrhea, breast enlargement, hyper-/hypoglycemia, galactorrhea, lactation, libido changes, gynecomastia, menstrual irregularity, parotid swelling (rare), SIADH
Gastrointestinal: Adynamic ileus, anorexia, appetite increased, constipation, diarrhea, fecal impaction, obstipation, nausea, salivation, vomiting, weight gain, xerostomia
Genitourinary: Bladder paralysis, ejaculatory disturbances, incontinence, polyuria, urinary retention
Hematologic: Agranulocytosis, eosinophilia, hemolytic anemia, leukopenia, pancytopenia, thrombocytopenic purpura
Hepatic: Hepatotoxicity, jaundice
Neuromuscular & skeletal: Muscle weakness
Ocular: Blurred vision, cornea and lens changes, epithelial keratopathies, glaucoma, mydriasis, myosis, photophobia, pigmentary retinopathy
Renal: Glycosuria
Respiratory: Nasal congestion
Miscellaneous: Allergic reactions, diaphoresis, systemic lupus erythematosus-like syndrome
General Dosage Range Oral: *Adults:* 4-16 mg 2-4 times/day (maximum: 64 mg/day)
Mechanism of Action Perphenazine is a piperazine phenothiazine antpsychotic which blocks postsynaptic mesolimbic dopaminergic receptors in the brain; exhibits alpha-adrenergic blocking effect and depresses the release of hypothalamic and hypophyseal hormones
Pharmacodynamics/Kinetics
Half-life Elimination Perphenazine: 9-12 hours; 7-hydroxyperphenazine: 10-19 hours
Time to Peak Serum: Perphenazine: 1-3 hours; 7-hydroxyperphenazine: 2-4 hours
Pregnancy Considerations Jaundice or hyper-/hyporeflexia have been reported in newborn infants following maternal use of phenothiazines. Antipsychotic use during the third trimester of pregnancy has a risk for abnormal muscle movements (extrapyramidal symptoms [EPS]) and withdrawal symptoms in newborns following delivery. Symptoms in the newborn may include agitation, feeding disorder, hypertonia, hypotonia, respiratory distress, somnolence, and tremor; these effects may be self-limiting or require hospitalization.

Pertuzumab (per TU zoo mab)

Brand Names: U.S. Perjeta™
Pharmacologic Category Antineoplastic Agent, Anti-HER2; Antineoplastic Agent, Monoclonal Antibody
Use Treatment of HER2-positive metastatic breast cancer (in combination with trastuzumab and docetaxel) in patients who have not received prior anti-HER2 therapy or chemotherapy to treat metastatic disease
Local Anesthetic/Vasoconstrictor Precautions No information available to require special precautions
Effects on Dental Treatment Key adverse event(s) related to dental treatment: A significant number of patients have experienced mucosal inflammation (28%), stomatitis (19%), or abnormal taste (18%)
Effects on Bleeding Although significant myelosuppression with associated altered hemostasis has been reported for many chemotherapeutic agents, myelosuppression is not common with pertuzumab and no specific precautions appear necessary.

Adverse Effects Note: Reactions reported in combination therapy with trastuzumab and docetaxel unless otherwise noted.
>10%:
Central nervous system: Fatigue (38%), headache (21%), fever (19%; grades 3/4: 1%), dizziness (13%)
Dermatologic: Rash (34%; grades 3/4: <1%), pruritus (14%), dry skin (11%)
Gastrointestinal: Diarrhea (67%; grades 3/4: 8%), appetite decreased (29%), mucosal inflammation (28%), nausea (monotherapy 24%), stomatitis (19%), abnormal taste (18%), vomiting (monotherapy 15%), abdominal pain (monotherapy 12%)
Hematologic: Neutropenia (53%; grades 3/4: 49%), anemia (23%; grades 3/4: 3%), neutropenic fever (14%; grades 3/4: 13%)
Respiratory: Upper respiratory tract infection (17%; grades 3/4: <1%)
Miscellaneous: Infusion reactions (13%; grades 3/4: <1%), hypersitivity reactions (10% to 11%; grades 3/4: 2%)
1% to 10%:
Dermatologic: Paronychia (7%)
Gastrointestinal: Anorexia (monotherapy 5%)
General Dosage Range I.V.: *Adults:* Initial: 840 mg; Maintenance: 420 mg every 3 weeks
Mechanism of Action Pertuzumab is a recombinant humanized monoclonal antibody which targets the extracellular human epidermal growth factor receptor 2 protein (HER2) dimerization domain. Inhibits HER2 dimerization and blocks HER downstream signaling halting cell growth and initiating apoptosis. Pertuzumab binds to a different HER2 epitope than trastuzumab so that when pertuzumab is combined with trastuzumab, a more complete inhibition of HER2 signaling occurs (Baselga, 2012).
Pharmacodynamics/Kinetics
Half-life Elimination Terminal: 18 days
Pregnancy Risk Factor D
Pregnancy Considerations May cause fetal harm if administered during pregnancy. **[U.S. Boxed Warning]: Pertuzumab exposure during pregnancy may result in embryo-fetal mortality and birth defects. Oligohydramnios has been observed in animal reproduction studies. Advise patients of the risks and the need for effective contraception.** Verify pregnancy status prior to treatment initiation. Effective contraception should be used during therapy and for 6 months after treatment. Advise patients to immediately report to healthcare provider if pregnancy is suspected during treatment. Effects during pregnancy are likely to occur in all 3 trimesters. If administered during pregnancy, monitor for oligohydramnios (if oligohydramnios occurs, fetal testing is indicated). Report pregnancies exposed to pertuzumab to the Genentech Adverse Event Line (1-888-835-2555). Women exposed to pertuzumab during pregnancy are encouraged to enroll in MotHER (the Pregnancy Registry; 1-800-690-6720).

Phenazopyridine (fen az oh PEER i deen)

Brand Names: U.S. AZO Standard® Maximum Strength [OTC] [DSC]; AZO Standard® [OTC] [DSC]; AZO Urinary Pain Relief™ Maximum Strength [OTC]; AZO Urinary Pain Relief™ [OTC]; Azo-Gesic™ [OTC]; Baridium [OTC]; Phenazo [OTC]; Pyridium®; Urinary Pain Relief [OTC]
Pharmacologic Category Analgesic, Urinary

Use Symptomatic relief of urinary burning, itching, frequency, and urgency in association with urinary tract infection or following urologic procedures
Local Anesthetic/Vasoconstrictor Precautions No information available to require special precautions
Effects on Dental Treatment No significant effects or complications reported
Effects on Bleeding No information available to require special precautions
Adverse Effects 1% to 10%:
Central nervous system: Headache, dizziness
Gastrointestinal: Stomach cramps
General Dosage Range Dosage adjustment recommended in patients with renal impairment
Oral:
Children: 12 mg/kg/day in 3 divided doses
Adults: 100-200 mg 3 times/day
Mechanism of Action An azo dye which exerts local anesthetic or analgesic action on urinary tract mucosa through an unknown mechanism
Pregnancy Risk Factor B
Pregnancy Considerations Phenazopyridine crosses the placenta. Adverse events have not been observed in animal reproduction studies.

Phendimetrazine (fen dye ME tra zeen)

Brand Names: U.S. Bontril® PDM; Bontril® Slow-Release
Brand Names: Canada Bontril®; Plegine®; Statobex®
Pharmacologic Category Anorexiant; Sympathomimetic
Use Short-term (few weeks) adjunct in exogenous obesity

Pharmacotherapy for weight loss is recommended only for obese patients with a body mass index ≥30 kg/m^2, or ≥27 kg/m^2 in the presence of other risk factors such as hypertension, diabetes, and/or dyslipidemia or a high waist circumference; therapy should be used in conjunction with a comprehensive weight management program.
Local Anesthetic/Vasoconstrictor Precautions Use vasoconstrictor with caution in patients taking phendimetrazine. Phendimetrazine can enhance the sympathomimetic response to epinephrine leading to potential hypertension and cardiotoxicity.
Effects on Dental Treatment Key adverse event(s) related to dental treatment: Xerostomia (normal salivary flow resumes upon discontinuation).
Effects on Bleeding No information available to require special precautions
Adverse Effects Frequency not defined.
Cardiovascular: Flushing, hypertension, ischemic events, palpitation, tachycardia, valvular disease (regurgitant)
Central nervous system: Agitation, dizziness, headache, insomnia, overstimulation, psychosis, restlessness
Endocrine & metabolic: Changes in libido
Gastrointestinal: Constipation, diarrhea, nausea, stomach pain, xerostomia
Genitourinary: Dysuria, urinary frequency
Neuromuscular & skeletal: Tremor
Ocular: Blurred vision, mydriasis
Respiratory: Primary pulmonary hypertension
Miscellaneous: Diaphoresis, tachyphylaxis

General Dosage Range Oral:
Capsule: *Adolescents 17 years and Adults:* 105 mg once daily before breakfast
Tablet: *Adults:* 17.5-35 mg 2-3 times/day, 1 hour before meals (maximum: 70 mg 3 times/day)
Mechanism of Action Phendimetrazine is a sympathomimetic amine with pharmacologic properties similar to the amphetamines. The mechanism of action in reducing appetite appears to be secondary to CNS effects, including stimulation of the hypothalamus to release norepinephrine.
Pharmacodynamics/Kinetics
Half-life Elimination Bontril® PDM: ~2 hours; Bontril® Slow Release: ~10 hours
Pregnancy Risk Factor X
Pregnancy Considerations Animal reproduction studies have not been conducted. Use is contraindicated during pregnancy. The risks of using appetite-suppressing drugs in pregnant women are not known. Weight loss therapy is generally not recommended for pregnant women. Obese and overweight women should be encouraged to participate in weight reduction programs prior to attempting pregnancy; weight gain during pregnancy should be determined by their prepregnancy BMI and current guidelines.
Controlled Substance C-III

Phenelzine (FEN el zeen)

Related Information
Vasoconstrictor Interactions With Antidepressants *on page 1650*
Brand Names: U.S. Nardil®
Brand Names: Canada Nardil®
Pharmacologic Category Antidepressant, Monoamine Oxidase Inhibitor
Use Symptomatic treatment of atypical, nonendogenous, or neurotic depression
Local Anesthetic/Vasoconstrictor Precautions Attempts should be made to avoid use of vasoconstrictor due to possibility of hypertensive episodes with monoamine oxidase inhibitors
Effects on Dental Treatment Key adverse event(s) related to dental treatment: Orthostatic hypotension, xerostomia and changes in salivation (normal salivary flow resumes upon discontinuation). Avoid use as an analgesic due to toxic reactions with MAO inhibitors.
Effects on Bleeding No information available to require special precautions
Adverse Effects Frequency not defined.
Cardiovascular: Edema, orthostatic hypotension
Central nervous system: Anxiety (acute), ataxia, coma, delirium, dizziness, drowsiness, euphoria, fatigue, fever, headache, hyper-reflexia, hypersomnia, insomnia, mania, schizophrenia, seizure, twitching
Dermatologic: Pruritus, rash
Endocrine & metabolic: Decreased sexual ability (anorgasmia, ejaculatory disturbances, impotence), hypermetabolic syndrome, hypernatremia
Gastrointestinal: Constipation, weight gain, xerostomia
Genitourinary: Urinary retention
Hematologic: Leukopenia
Hepatic: Jaundice, necrotizing hepatocellular necrosis (rare), transaminases increased
Neuromuscular & skeletal: Myoclonia, paresthesia, tremor, weakness
Ocular: Blurred vision, glaucoma, nystagmus
Respiratory: Edema (glottis)

Miscellaneous: Diaphoresis, lupus-like syndrome, transient cardiac or respiratory depression (following ECT), withdrawal syndrome (nausea, vomiting, malaise)
General Dosage Range Oral: *Adults:* Initial: 45 mg/day in 3 divided doses; Maintenance: 15-90 mg/day in 1-3 divided doses
Mechanism of Action Thought to act by increasing endogenous concentrations of norepinephrine, dopamine, and serotonin through inhibition of the enzyme (monoamine oxidase) responsible for the breakdown of these neurotransmitters
Pharmacodynamics/Kinetics
Onset of Action Therapeutic: 2-4 weeks; geriatric patients receiving an average of 55 mg/day developed a mean platelet MAO activity inhibition of about 85%.
Duration of Action May continue to have a therapeutic effect and interactions 2 weeks after discontinuing therapy
Half-life Elimination 12 hours
Pregnancy Risk Factor C
Pregnancy Considerations Safe use during pregnancy has not been established; use only if benefits outweigh the risks.

PHENobarbital (fee noe BAR bi tal)

Brand Names: Canada PMS-Phenobarbital
Generic Availability (U.S.) Yes
Pharmacologic Category Anticonvulsant, Barbiturate; Barbiturate
Use Management of generalized tonic-clonic (grand mal), status epilepticus, and partial seizures; sedative/hypnotic
Note: Use to treat insomnia is not recommended (Schutte-Rodin, 2008)
Unlabeled Use Prevention and treatment of neonatal hyperbilirubinemia and lowering of bilirubin in chronic cholestasis; neonatal seizures
Local Anesthetic/Vasoconstrictor Precautions No information available to require special precautions
Effects on Dental Treatment No significant effects or complications reported
Effects on Bleeding No information available to require special precautions
Adverse Effects Frequency not defined.
Cardiovascular: Bradycardia, hypotension, syncope
Central nervous system: Agitation, anxiety, ataxia, CNS excitation or depression, confusion, dizziness drowsiness, hallucinations, "hangover" effect, headache, hyperkinesia, impaired judgment, insomnia, lethargy, nervousness, nightmares, somnolence
Dermatologic: Exfoliative dermatitis, rash, Stevens-Johnson syndrome
Gastrointestinal: Nausea, vomiting, constipation
Hematologic: Agranulocytosis, thrombocytopenia, megaloblastic anemia
Local: Pain at injection site, thrombophlebitis with I.V. use
Renal: Oliguria
Respiratory: Laryngospasm, respiratory depression, apnea (especially with rapid I.V. use), hypoventilation
Miscellaneous: Gangrene with inadvertent intra-arterial injection
Dosage
Children:
Sedation: Oral: 2 mg/kg 3 times/day
Preoperative sedation: Oral, I.M., I.V.: 1-3 mg/kg 1-1.5 hours before procedure

Adults:
Sedation: Oral, I.M.: 30-120 mg/day in 2-3 divided doses
Preoperative sedation: I.M.: 100-200 mg 1-1.5 hours before procedure

Anticonvulsant: Status epilepticus: **Loading dose:** I.V.:
Infants and Children: 15-20 mg/kg (maximum: 1000 mg/dose, maximum rate ≤30 mg/minute in children <60 kg); may repeat dose after 15 minutes as needed (maximum total dose: 40 mg/kg)
Adults: 10-20 mg/kg (maximum rate ≤60 mg/minute in patients ≥60 kg); may repeat dose in 20-minute intervals as needed (maximum total dose: 30 mg/kg)

Anticonvulsant maintenance dose: Oral, I.V.:
Infants: 5-8 mg/kg/day in 1-2 divided doses
Children:
1-5 years: 6-8 mg/kg/day in 1-2 divided doses
5-12 years: 4-6 mg/kg/day in 1-2 divided doses
Children >12 years and Adults: 1-3 mg/kg/day in divided doses or 50-100 mg 2-3 times/day

Sedative/hypnotic withdrawal (unlabeled use): Initial daily requirement is determined by substituting phenobarbital 30 mg for every 100 mg pentobarbital used during tolerance testing; then daily requirement is decreased by 10% of initial dose
Elderly or debilitated: Initiate at the lowest recommended dose.

Dosing adjustment in renal impairment: Cl$_{cr}$ <10 mL/minute: Administer every 12-16 hours
Hemodialysis: Moderately dialyzable (20% to 50%)
Dosing adjustment in hepatic impairment: Reduce dose in patients with hepatic impairment.

Mechanism of Action Long-acting barbiturate with sedative, hypnotic, and anticonvulsant properties. Barbiturates depress the sensory cortex, decrease motor activity, alter cerebellar function, and produce drowsiness, sedation, and hypnosis. In high doses, barbiturates exhibit anticonvulsant activity; barbiturates produce dose-dependent respiratory depression.

Contraindications Hypersensitivity to barbiturates or any component of the formulation; marked hepatic impairment; dyspnea or airway obstruction; porphyria (manifest and latent); intra-arterial administration, subcutaneous administration (not recommended); use in patients with a history of sedative/hypnotic addiction is not recommended; nephritic patients (large doses)

Warnings/Precautions Potential for drug dependency exists, abrupt cessation may precipitate withdrawal, including status epilepticus in epileptic patients. Do not administer to patients in acute pain. Use caution in debilitated, renal or hepatic dysfunction, and pediatric patients. May cause paradoxical responses, including agitation and hyperactivity, particularly in acute pain and pediatric patients. Avoid use in the eldely due to risk of overdose with low dosages, tolerance to sleep effects, and increased risk of physical dependence (Beers Criteria). Use with caution in patients with depression or suicidal tendencies, or in patients with a history of drug abuse. Tolerance, psychological and physical dependence may occur with prolonged use. May cause CNS depression, which may impair physical or mental abilities. Effects with other sedative drugs or ethanol may be potentiated. May cause respiratory depression or hypotension, particularly when administered intravenously. Use with caution in hemodynamically unstable patients (hypovolemic shock, CHF) or patients with respiratory disease. Due to its long half-life and risk of dependence, phenobarbital is not recommended as a sedative in the elderly. Use has been associated with cognitive deficits

in children. Use with caution in patients with hypoadrenalism. Intra-arterial administration may cause reactions ranging from transient pain to gangrene and is contraindicated. Subcutaneous administration may cause tissue irritation (eg, redness, tenderness, necrosis) and is not recommended.

Drug Interactions
Metabolism/Transport Effects Substrate of CYP2C19 (major), CYP2C9 (minor), CYP2E1 (minor); **Note:** Assignment of Major/Minor substrate status based on clinically relevant drug interaction potential; **Induces** CYP1A2 (strong), CYP2A6 (strong), CYP2B6 (strong), CYP2C8 (strong), CYP2C9 (strong), CYP3A4 (strong)

Avoid Concomitant Use
Avoid concomitant use of PHENobarbital with any of the following: Apixaban; Axitinib; Azelastine (Nasal); Bedaquiline; Boceprevir; Bortezomib; Bosutinib; Cabozantinib; Crizotinib; Darunavir; Dronedarone; Enzalutamide; Etravirine; Everolimus; Itraconazole; Ivacaftor; Lapatinib; Lurasidone; Mifepristone; Nilotinib; Paraldehyde; Pazopanib; Perampanel; Pirfenidone; Pomalidomide; Ponatinib; Praziquantel; Ranolazine; Regorafenib; Rilpivirine; Rivaroxaban; Roflumilast; RomiDEPsin; SORAfenib; Telaprevir; Ticagrelor; Tofacitinib; Tolvaptan; Toremifene; Vandetanib; VinCRIStine (Liposomal); Voriconazole

Increased Effect/Toxicity
PHENobarbital may increase the levels/effects of: Alcohol (Ethyl); Azelastine (Nasal); Buprenorphine; Clarithromycin; CNS Depressants; Fosphenytoin; Ifosfamide; Meperidine; Methadone; Metyrosine; Mirtazapine; Paraldehyde; Pramipexole; Prilocaine; QuiNIDine; ROPINIRole; Rotigotine; Selective Serotonin Reuptake Inhibitors; Thiazide Diuretics; Zolpidem

The levels/effects of PHENobarbital may be increased by: Carbonic Anhydrase Inhibitors; Chloramphenicol; Clarithromycin; Cosyntropin; CYP2C19 Inhibitors (Moderate); CYP2C19 Inhibitors (Strong); Dexmethylphenidate; Divalproex; Droperidol; Felbamate; Fosphenytoin; HydrOXYzine; Magnesium Sulfate; Methylphenidate; OXcarbazepine; Perampanel; Phenytoin; Primidone; QuiNINE; Rufinamide; Sodium Oxybate; Telaprevir; Valproic Acid

Decreased Effect
PHENobarbital may decrease the levels/effects of: Acetaminophen; Apixaban; ARIPiprazole; Axitinib; Bedaquiline; Bendamustine; Beta-Blockers; Boceprevir; Bortezomib; Bosutinib; Brentuximab Vedotin; Cabozantinib; Calcium Channel Blockers; Canagliflozin; Chloramphenicol; Clarithromycin; Cobicistat; Contraceptives (Estrogens); Contraceptives (Progestins); Corticosteroids (Systemic); Crizotinib; CycloSPORINE (Systemic); CYP1A2 Substrates; CYP2B6 Substrates; CYP2C8 Substrates; CYP2C9 Substrates; CYP3A4 Substrates; Darunavir; Dasatinib; Deferasirox; Diclofenac (Systemic); Disopyramide; Divalproex; Doxycycline; Dronedarone; Elvitegravir; Enzalutamide; Etoposide; Etoposide Phosphate; Etravirine; Everolimus; Exemestane; Felbamate; Fosphenytoin; Gefitinib; Griseofulvin; GuanFACINE; Imatinib; Irinotecan; Itraconazole; Ivacaftor; Ixabepilone; Lacosamide; LamoTRIgine; Lapatinib; Linagliptin; Lopinavir; Lurasidone; Maraviroc; Methadone; MetroNIDAZOLE (Systemic); Mifepristone; Nilotinib; OXcarbazepine; Pazopanib; Perampanel; Phenytoin; Pirfenidone; Pomalidomide; Ponatinib; Praziquantel; Propafenone; QuiNIDine; QuiNINE; Ranolazine; Regorafenib; Rilpivirine; Rivaroxaban; Roflumilast; RomiDEPsin; Rufinamide; Saxagliptin; SORAfenib; SUNItinib; Tadalafil; ▶

Telaprevir; Teniposide; Theophylline Derivatives; Ticagrelor; Tipranavir; Tofacitinib; Tolvaptan; Toremifene; Treprostinil; Tricyclic Antidepressants; Ulipristal; Valproic Acid; Vandetanib; Vemurafenib; VinCRIStine (Liposomal); Vitamin K Antagonists; Voriconazole; Zonisamide; Zuclopenthixol

The levels/effects of PHENobarbital may be decreased by: Amphetamines; Cholestyramine Resin; CYP2C19 Inducers (Strong); Folic Acid; Ketorolac (Nasal); Ketorolac (Systemic); Leucovorin Calcium-Levoleucovorin; Levomefolate; Mefloquine; Methylfolate; Multivitamins/Minerals (with ADEK, Folate, Iron); Pyridoxine; Rifamycin Derivatives; Telaprevir; Tipranavir

Ethanol/Nutrition/Herb Interactions
Ethanol: May increase CNS depression; monitor for increased effects with coadministration. Caution patients about effects.
Food: May cause decrease in vitamin D and calcium.
Herb/Nutraceutical: Avoid evening primrose (seizure threshold decreased). Avoid valerian, St John's wort, kava kava, gotu kola (may increase CNS depression).
Dietary Considerations Vitamin D: Loss in vitamin D due to malabsorption; increase intake of foods rich in vitamin D. Supplementation of vitamin D and/or calcium may be necessary. Injection may contain sodium.
Pharmacodynamics/Kinetics
Onset of Action Oral: Hypnosis: 20-60 minutes; I.V.: ~5 minutes; Peak effect: I.V.: ~30 minutes
Duration of Action Oral: 6-10 hours; I.V.: 4-10 hours
Half-life Elimination Neonates: 45-500 hours; Infants: 20-133 hours; Children: 37-73 hours; Adults: 53-140 hours
Time to Peak Serum: Oral: 1-6 hours
Pregnancy Risk Factor B/D (manufacturer dependent)
Pregnancy Considerations Barbiturates can be detected in the placenta, fetal liver, and fetal brain. Fetal and maternal blood concentrations may be similar following parenteral administration. An increased incidence of fetal abnormalities may occur following maternal use. The use of folic acid throughout pregnancy and vitamin K during the last month of pregnancy is recommended; epilepsy itself, number of medications, genetic factors, or a combination of these probably influence the teratogenicity of anticonvulsant therapy. When used during the third trimester of pregnancy, withdrawal symptoms may occur in the neonate, including seizures and hyperirritability; symptoms of withdrawal may be delayed in the neonate up to 14 days after birth. Use during labor does not impair uterine activity; however, respiratory depression may occur in the newborn; resuscitation equipment should be available, especially for premature infants.
Lactation Enters breast milk/use caution (AAP recommends use "with caution"; AAP 2001 update pending)
Breast-Feeding Considerations Phenobarbital is excreted into breast milk. Infantile spasms and other withdrawal symptoms have been reported following the abrupt discontinuation of breast-feeding.
Controlled Substance C-IV
Dosage Forms
Elixir, oral: 20 mg/5 mL (5 mL, 7.5 mL, 15 mL, 473 mL, 480 mL)
Injection, solution: 65 mg/mL (1 mL); 130 mg/mL (1 mL)
Tablet, oral: 15 mg, 16.2 mg, 30 mg, 32.4 mg, 60 mg, 100 mg

Phenol (FEE nol)

Brand Names: U.S. Castellani Paint Modified [OTC]; Cepastat® Extra Strength [OTC]; Cepastat® [OTC]; Cheracol® Spray [OTC]; Chloraseptic® Kids Sore Throat Spray [OTC]; Chloraseptic® Mouth Pain [OTC]; Chloraseptic® Sore Throat Gargle [OTC]; Chloraseptic® Sore Throat Spray [OTC]; Pain-A-Lay® [OTC]; Phenaseptic [OTC]; Phenol EZ® [OTC]; Ulcerease® [OTC]; Vicks® Formula 44® Sore Throat [OTC]
Brand Names: Canada P & S™ Liquid Phenol
Pharmacologic Category Anesthetic, Topical
Use Relief of sore throat pain, mouth, gum, and throat irritations; antiseptic; topical anesthetic
Local Anesthetic/Vasoconstrictor Precautions No information available to require special precautions
Effects on Dental Treatment No significant effects or complications reported
Effects on Bleeding No information available to require special precautions
General Dosage Range
Oral:
Children 2-12 years:
Chloraseptic®: 3 sprays onto throat or affected area; may repeat every 2 hours
Chloraseptic® for Kids: 5 sprays onto throat or affected area; may repeat every 2 hours
Children >3 years: Ulcerease®: Gargle or swish for 15 seconds, then expectorate; may repeat every 2 hours
Children 6-12 years:
Cēpastat® Extra Strength: Up to 1 lozenge every 2 hours as needed (maximum: 10 lozenges/24 hours)
Cēpastat®: Up to 1 lozenge every 2 hours as needed (maximum: 18 lozenges/24 hours)
Pain-A-Lay® Gargle: Using gauze pad, apply 10 mL to affected area, or gargle or swish for 15 seconds, then expectorate
Children ≥12 years and Adults:
Cēpastat® Extra Strength, Cēpastat®: Up to 2 lozenges every 2 hours as needed
Cheracol®, Pain-A-Lay® Spray: Spray directly in throat; rinse for 15 seconds then expectorate; may repeat every 2 hours
Chloraseptic®: 5 sprays onto throat or affected area; may repeat every 2 hours
Chloraseptic® Gargle, Cēpastat® Mouth Pain, Pain-A-Lay® Gargle, Ulcerease®: Gargle or swish for 15 seconds, then expectorate; may repeat every 2 hours
Topical: *Adults:* Apply small amount to affected area 1-3 times/day
Pregnancy Considerations Phenol is systemically absorbed following oral ingestion, inhalation, or application to the skin. Fetotoxic effects have been observed in animal reproduction studies (Bruce, 1987).

Phenoxybenzamine (fen oks ee BEN za meen)

Brand Names: U.S. Dibenzyline®
Pharmacologic Category Alpha$_1$ Blocker; Antidote
Use Symptomatic management of pheochromocytoma
Unlabeled Use Micturition problems associated with neurogenic bladder, functional outlet obstruction, and partial prostate obstruction; treatment of hypertensive crisis caused by sympathomimetic amines
Local Anesthetic/Vasoconstrictor Precautions No information available to require special precautions

Effects on Dental Treatment Key adverse event(s) related to dental treatment: Xerostomia (normal salivary flow resumes upon discontinuation).

Effects on Bleeding No information available to require special precautions

Adverse Effects Frequency not defined.

Cardiovascular: Orthostatic hypotension, tachycardia

Central nervous system: Drowsiness, fatigue

Gastrointestinal: GI irritation

Genitourinary: Inhibition of ejaculation

Ocular: Miosis

Respiratory: Nasal congestion

General Dosage Range Oral: *Adults:* Initial: 10 mg twice daily; Maintenance: 10-40 mg 1-3 times/day (maximum: 240 mg/day)

Mechanism of Action Produces long-lasting noncompetitive alpha-adrenergic blockade of postganglionic synapses in exocrine glands and smooth muscle; relaxes urethra and increases opening of the bladder

Pharmacodynamics/Kinetics

Duration of Action I.V.: ≥3 days

Half-life Elimination I.V.: 24 hours

Pregnancy Risk Factor C

Pregnancy Considerations Adequate animal reproduction studies have not been conducted. It is not known whether phenoxybenzamine can cause fetal harm when administered to a pregnant woman or can affect reproduction capacity.

Phentermine (FEN ter meen)

Brand Names: U.S. Adipex-P®; Suprenza™

Pharmacologic Category Anorexiant; Central Nervous System Stimulant; Sympathomimetic

Use Short-term (few weeks) adjunct therapy in obese patients with an initial body mass index (BMI) ≥30 kg/m² or ≥27 kg/m² in the presence of other risk factors (eg, diabetes, hyperlipidemia, controlled hypertension); therapy should be used in conjunction with a comprehensive weight management program.

Local Anesthetic/Vasoconstrictor Precautions Use vasoconstrictor with caution in patients taking phentermine. Amphetamines enhance the sympathomimetic response of epinephrine and norepinephrine leading to potential hypertension and cardiotoxicity.

Effects on Dental Treatment Key adverse event(s) related to dental treatment: Xerostomia (normal salivary flow resumes upon discontinuation) and unpleasant taste. Up to 10% of patients may present with hypertension. The use of local anesthetic without vasoconstrictor is recommended in these patients. See Dental Comment.

Effects on Bleeding No information available to require special precautions

Adverse Effects Frequency not defined.

Cardiovascular: Hypertension, ischemic events, palpitation, primary pulmonary hypertension and/or regurgitant cardiac valvular disease, tachycardia

Central nervous system: Dizziness, dysphoria, euphoria, headache, insomnia, overstimulation, psychosis, restlessness

Dermatologic: Urticaria

Endocrine & metabolic: Changes in libido

Gastrointestinal: Constipation, diarrhea, unpleasant taste, xerostomia

Genitourinary: Impotence

Neuromuscular & skeletal: Tremor

General Dosage Range Oral: *Children >16 years and Adults:* 15-37.5 mg/day

Mechanism of Action Phentermine is a sympathomimetic amine with pharmacologic properties similar to the amphetamines. The mechanism of action in reducing appetite appears to be secondary to CNS effects, including stimulation of the hypothalamus to release norepinephrine.

Pharmacodynamics/Kinetics

Time to Peak Orally disintegrating tablet: 3-4.4 hours

Pregnancy Risk Factor X

Pregnancy Considerations Animal reproduction studies have not been conducted. Use is contraindicated during pregnancy. The risks of using appetite suppressing drugs in pregnant women are not known and limited information is available about the use of phentermine in pregnancy. Weight loss therapy is generally not recommended for pregnant women. Obese and overweight women should be encouraged to participate in weight reduction programs prior to attempting pregnancy; weight gain during pregnancy should be determined by their prepregnancy BMI and current guidelines.

Controlled Substance C-IV

Dental Comment Many diet physicians have prescribed fenfluramine ("fen") and phentermine ("phen"). When taken together the combination is known as "fen-phen". The diet drug dexfenfluramine (Redux®) is chemically similar to fenfluramine (Pondimin®) and was also used in combination with phentermine called "Redux-phen". While each of the three drugs alone had approval from the FDA for sale in the treatment of obesity, neither combination had an official approval. The use of the combinations in the treatment of obesity was considered an "off-label" use. Reports in medical literature have been accumulating for some years about significant side effects associated with fenfluramine and dexfenfluramine. In 1997, the manufacturers, at the urging of the FDA, agreed to voluntarily withdraw the drugs from the market. The action was based on findings from physicians who evaluated patients taking fenfluramine and dexfenfluramine with echocardiograms. The findings indicated that approximately 30% of patients had abnormal echocardiograms, even though they had no symptoms. This was a much higher than expected percentage of abnormal test results. This conclusion was based on a sample of 291 patients examined by five different physicians. Under normal conditions, fewer than 1% of patients would be expected to show signs of heart valve disease. The findings suggested that fenfluramine and dexfenfluramine were the likely cause of heart valve problems of the type that promoted FDA's earlier warnings concerning "fen-phen". The earlier warning included the following: The mitral valve and other valves in the heart are damaged by a strange white coating and allow blood to flow back, causing heart muscle damage. In several cases, valve replacement surgery has been done. As a rule, the person must, thereafter for life, be on a blood thinner to prevent clots from the mechanical valve. This type of valve damage had only been seen before in persons who were exposed to large amounts of serotonin. The fenfluramine increases the availability of serotonin.

Phentermine and Topiramate
(FEN ter meen & toe PYRE a mate)

Brand Names: U.S. Qsymia™

Pharmacologic Category Anorexiant; Anticonvulsant, Miscellaneous; Sympathomimetic

◄ **Use** Chronic weight management, as an adjunct to a reduced-calorie diet and increased physical activity, in patients with either an initial body mass index (BMI) of ≥30 kg/m² **or** an initial BMI of ≥27 kg/m² and at least one weight-related comorbid condition (eg, hypertension, dyslipidemia, type 2 diabetes)

Local Anesthetic/Vasoconstrictor Precautions Use vasoconstrictor with caution in patients taking phentermine and topiramate. Phentermine is a sympathomimetic amine with pharmacologic properties similar to amphetamines. The phentermine component may enhance the sympathomimetic response of epinephrine and levonordefrin leading to potential hypertension and cardiotoxicity.

Effects on Dental Treatment Key adverse event(s) related to dental treatment: The following effects were reported more frequently than placebo during 1 year of treatment (n=1580): Paresthesia (experienced by ≤20% of patients), dysgeusia (metallic taste, experienced by ≤9% of patients), and dry mouth (experienced by ≤19% of patients). The paresthesia was characterized as tingling in hands, feet, or face.

Effects on Bleeding No information available to require special precautions

Adverse Effects As reported with combination product (also see individual agents):

>10%:

Central nervous system: Headache (10% to 11%), insomnia (6% to 11%)

Endocrine & metabolic: Serum bicarbonate decreased (6% to 13%; marked reductions [to <17 mEq/L] ≤1%)

Gastrointestinal: Xerostomia (7% to 19%), constipation (8% to 16%)

Neuromuscular & skeletal: Paresthesia (4% to 20%)

Respiratory: Upper respiratory tract infection (12% to 16%), nasopharyngitis (9% to 13%)

1% to 10%:

Cardiovascular: Palpitations (1% to 2%), chest discomfort (≤2%)

Central nervous system: Dizziness (3% to 9%), anxiety (3% to 8%), depression (3% to 8%), fatigue (4% to 6%), attention disturbance (2% to 4%), irritability (2% to 4%), hypoesthesia (1% to 4%)

Dermatologic: Alopecia (2% to 4%), rash (2% to 3%)

Endocrine & metabolic: Hypokalemia (≤3%), dysmenorrhea (≤2%)

Gastrointestinal: Abnormal taste (1% to 9%), nausea (4% to 7%), diarrhea (5% to 6%), dyspepsia (2% to 3%), gastroenteritis (1% to 3%), GERD (1% to 3%), appetite decreased (2%), oral paresthesia (≤2%)

Genitourinary: Urinary tract infection (3% to 5%)

Neuromuscular & skeletal: Back pain (5% to 7%), muscle spasm (3%), musculoskeletal pain (2% to 3%), neck pain (2%)

Ocular: Blurred vision (4% to 6%), dry eyes (1% to 3%), eye pain (2%)

Renal: Creatinine increased (2% to 8%), kidney stones (≤1%)

Respiratory: Sinusitis (7% to 8%), bronchitis (4% to 7%), cough (5%), pharyngolaryngeal pain (3%), sinus congestion (3%), nasal congestion (2%)

Miscellaneous: Influenza (4% to 8%), thirst (2%)

Dosage Weight management: Adults: Oral: Initial: Phentermine 3.75 mg/topiramate 23 mg once daily for 14 days. Increase dose to phentermine 7.5 mg/topiramate 46 mg once daily for 12 weeks then evaluate weight loss. If 3% of baseline body weight has not been lost, discontinue use or increase dose to phentermine 11.25 mg/topiramate 69 mg once daily for 14 days,

and then to phentermine 15 mg/topiramate 92 mg once daily. Evaluate weight loss after 12 weeks on phentermine 15 mg/topiramate 92 mg; if 5% of baseline body weight has not been lost at dose of phentermine 15 mg/topiramate 92 mg gradually discontinue therapy (eg, 1 dose every other day for at least 1 week).

Dosage adjustment in renal impairment: Note: Renal function should be estimated using the Cockcroft-Gault formula with actual body weight.

Mild impairment (Cl_cr ≥50 mL/minute): No dosage adjustment necessary.

Moderate-to-severe impairment (Cl_cr <50 mL/minute): Maximum dose: Phentermine 7.5 mg/topiramate 46 mg once daily

Dialysis: Use is not recommended (has not been studied).

Dosage adjustment in hepatic impairment:

Mild impairment (Child-Pugh class A): No dosage adjustment necessary.

Moderate impairment (Child-Pugh class B): Maximum dose: Phentermine 7.5 mg/topiramate 46 mg once daily

Severe impairment (Child-Pugh class C): Use is not recommended (has not been studied).

Mechanism of Action

Phentermine: A sympathomimetic amine with pharmacologic properties similar to amphetamines. The mechanism of action in reducing appetite appears to be secondary to CNS effects, including stimulation of the hypothalamus to release norepinephrine.

Topiramate: Effect on weight management may be due to its effects on appetite suppression and satiety enhancement and based on a combination of potential mechanisms: blocks neuronal voltage-dependent sodium channels, enhances GABA(A) activity, antagonizes AMPA/kainate glutamate receptors, and weakly inhibits carbonic anhydrase.

Contraindications Hypersensitivity or idiosyncrasy to phentermine or other sympathomimetic amines or any component of the formulation; hyperthyroidism; glaucoma; use during or within 14 days following MAO inhibitor therapy; pregnancy

Warnings/Precautions Antiepileptics, including topiramate, are associated with an increased risk of suicidal behavior/thoughts with use (regardless of indication); avoid use in patients with a history of suicide attempts or current suicidal ideation; patients should be monitored for signs/symptoms of depression, suicidal tendencies, and other unusual behavior changes during therapy. Use can increase resting heart rate; monitor closely when starting or increasing dosage and in patients with cardiac or cerebrovascular disease. Reduce dose or discontinue use with a sustained increase in resting heart rate. Use with caution in patients with hepatic or renal impairment; dose adjustment may be required. Avoid use in patients with severe hepatic impairment (Child-Pugh class C). May increase serum creatinine; peak increases from baseline were observed after 4-8 weeks of treatment. Monitor serum creatinine prior to and during treatment. For persistent elevations, dose reduction or discontinuation may be necessary. May decrease serum bicarbonate concentrations; risk may be increased in patients with a predisposing condition (eg, diarrhea, renal disease, severe respiratory disorders, ketogenic diet, status epilepticus, surgery) or concurrent treatment with other carbonic anhydrase inhibitors. Monitor serum electrolytes and bicarbonate prior to and during treatment. Reduce dose or discontinue use if persistent metabolic acidosis develops. Monitor for complications of chronic acidosis (eg, nephrolithiasis); kidney stones have been reported; the risk of this event may be reduced by increasing fluid intake. Use with caution in patients with type 2 diabetes mellitus; antidiabetic agent requirements (eg, insulin or oral hypoglycemic agents) may be decreased with weight loss, anorexigens, and concomitant dietary restrictions. Monitor blood glucose levels prior to and during treatment. Weight loss in conjunction with antihypertensive therapy may increase the risk of hypotension in hypertensive patients; monitor blood pressure and adjust antihypertensive treatment as necessary.

Cognitive dysfunction (including attention or memory difficulties) and psychiatric disturbances (mood disorders including anxiety, depression, or insomnia) may occur with use; incidence may be related to rapid titration and higher doses. Patients must be cautioned about performing tasks which require mental alertness (eg, operating machinery or driving). Risk may be increased in patients with a history of depression; dose reduction or discontinuation may be necessary. Topiramate has been associated with acute myopia and secondary angle-closure glaucoma in adults and children, typically within 1 month of initiation but may occur at any time; discontinue in patients with acute onset of decreased visual acuity or ocular pain. Topiramate may be associated (rarely) with severe oligohidrosis and hyperthermia; use caution and monitor closely during strenuous exercise, during exposure to high environmental temperature, or in patients receiving drugs with anticholinergic activity.

Use can cause hypokalemia; use caution with concurrent use of hydrochlorothiazide or furosemide as risk of hypokalemia may be increased; monitor potassium closely. Avoid use of other sedative drugs or ethanol; CNS effects may be potentiated. Phentermine is pharmacologically related to the amphetamines, which have a high abuse potential; prolonged use may lead to dependency. Prescriptions should be written for the smallest quantity consistent with good patient care to minimize the possibility of overdose. Avoid abrupt withdrawal of anticonvulsants (including topiramate); therapy should be withdrawn/tapered slowly to minimize the potential of increased seizure frequency. Tapering doses over at least 1 week (1 dose every other day) is recommended.

Drug Interactions
Metabolism/Transport Effects Refer to individual components.

Avoid Concomitant Use
Avoid concomitant use of Phentermine and Topiramate with any of the following: Axitinib; Carbonic Anhydrase Inhibitors; Iobenguane I 123; MAO Inhibitors; Paraldehyde

Increased Effect/Toxicity
Phentermine and Topiramate may increase the levels/effects of: Alpha-/Beta-Agonists; Amphetamines; Analgesics (Opioid); Anticonvulsants (Barbiturate); Anticonvulsants (Hydantoin); Carbonic Anhydrase Inhibitors; CNS Depressants; Flecainide; Fosphenytoin; Lithium; Memantine; MetFORMIN; Metyrosine; Paraldehyde; Phenytoin; Pramipexole; Primidone; QuiNIDine; ROPINIRole; Rotigotine; Sympathomimetics; Valproic Acid; Zolpidem

The levels/effects of Phentermine and Topiramate may be increased by: Alcohol (Ethyl); Alkalinizing Agents; Antacids; Anticholinergic Agents; AtoMOXetine; Cannabinoids; Carbonic Anhydrase Inhibitors; Divalproex;

Loop Diuretics; Magnesium Sulfate; MAO Inhibitors; Perampanel; Proton Pump Inhibitors; Salicylates; Sodium Oxybate; Thiazide Diuretics; Tricyclic Antidepressants

Decreased Effect
Phentermine and Topiramate may decrease the levels/effects of: Antihistamines; Axitinib; Contraceptives (Estrogens); Contraceptives (Progestins); Ethosuximide; Iobenguane I 123; Ioflupane I 123; Methenamine; PHENobarbital; Phenytoin; Primidone; Saxagliptin

The levels/effects of Phentermine and Topiramate may be decreased by: Ammonium Chloride; Antipsychotics; CarBAMazepine; Fosphenytoin; Gastrointestinal Acidifying Agents; Ketorolac (Nasal); Ketorolac (Systemic); Lithium; Mefloquine; Methenamine; Multivitamins/Minerals (with ADEK, Folate, Iron); Phenytoin

Dietary Considerations Take with or without food in the morning; avoid taking in the late evening. Most effective when combined with a low calorie diet, increased physical activity and behavior modification counseling.

Pregnancy Risk Factor X

Pregnancy Considerations Based on human data, topiramate may cause fetal harm if used during pregnancy. Use of this combination product is contraindicated in pregnant women. Females of reproductive potential should have a negative pregnancy test prior to and monthly during therapy. Effective contraception should be used during treatment. If irregular bleeding or spotting occurs while using hormonal contraceptives during pregnancy, patients should be instructed to continue the contraceptive (contraceptive failure is not expected) and notify their health care provider if symptoms become troubling.

The risks of using appetite suppressing drugs in pregnant women are not known. Weight loss therapy is generally not recommended for pregnant women (NHLBI, 1998). Obese women should participate in weight reduction programs prior to attempting pregnancy (ACOG, 2005). Refer to individual monographs for additional information.

Healthcare providers are encouraged to enroll women exposed to Qsymia™ during pregnancy in the Qsymia™ Pregnancy Surveillance Program (888-998-4887).

Lactation Excreted in breast milk/not recommended

Breast-Feeding Considerations Topiramate and amphetamines are excreted in breast milk. Due to the potential for adverse effects, the manufacturer recommends to discontinue therapy or discontinue nursing. Weight loss therapy is generally not recommended for lactating women (NHLBI, 1998). Refer to individual monographs for additional information.

Controlled Substance C-IV

Dosage Forms
Capsule, extended release, oral:
  Qsymia™: 3.75/23: Phentermine 3.75 mg [immediate release] and topiramate 23 mg [extended release]
  Qsymia™: 7.5/46: Phentermine 7.5 mg [immediate release] and topiramate 46 mg [extended release]
  Qsymia™: 11.25/69: Phentermine 11.25 mg [immediate release] and topiramate 69 mg [extended release]
  Qsymia™: 15/92: Phentermine 15 mg [immediate release] and topiramate 92 mg [extended release]

◀ **Dental Comment** According to product labeling, phentermine and topiramate can cause an increase in resting heart rate. A higher percentage of overweight and obese adults taking phentermine and topiramate experienced heart rate increases from baseline of more than 5, 10, 15, and 20 beats per minute compared to placebo-treated overweight and obese adults. The clinical significance of a heart rate elevation with treatment is presently unclear. Regular measurement of resting heart rate is recommended for all patients taking phentermine and topiramate. Product labeling states that patients should inform healthcare provider of palpitations or feelings of a racing heartbeat while at rest during treatment.

Phentolamine (fen TOLE a meen)

Related Information
Oral Pain on page 1558
Brand Names: U.S. OraVerse™
Brand Names: Canada Regitine®; Rogitine®
Generic Availability (U.S.) Yes: Excludes injection, solution
Pharmacologic Category Alpha$_1$ Blocker
Dental Use Reversal of soft tissue anesthesia and the associated functional deficits resulting from a local dental anesthetic containing a vasoconstrictor
Use Diagnosis of pheochromocytoma and treatment of hypertension associated with pheochromocytoma or other forms of hypertension caused by excess sympathomimetic amines; prevention and treatment of dermal necrosis after extravasation of drugs with alpha-adrenergic effects (ie, dopamine, epinephrine, norepinephrine, phenylephrine)

OraVerse™: Reversal of soft tissue anesthesia and the associated functional deficits resulting from a local dental anesthetic containing a vasoconstrictor
Unlabeled Use Treatment of pralidoxime-induced hypertension
Local Anesthetic/Vasoconstrictor Precautions Although the alpha-adrenergic blocking effects could antagonize epinephrine, there is no information available to require special precautions
Effects on Dental Treatment Key adverse event(s) related to dental treatment: The most common reaction that was greater than controls was injection site pain (~4% to 6%). A few incidences of paresthesia associated with OraVerse™ have been reported. These incidences were mild and transient, and resolved during the same time period. Orthostatic hypotension has also been reported.
Effects on Bleeding No information available to require special precautions
Adverse Effects Frequency not always defined.
Cardiovascular: Arrhythmia, flushing, hypertension (OraVerse™), hypotension, orthostatic hypotension, tachycardia (OraVerse™ ≤6%), bradycardia (OraVerse™ ≤4%)
Central nervous system: Dizziness, headache (OraVerse™ ≤6%)
Dermatologic: Pruritus (OraVerse™)
Gastrointestinal: Nausea, vomiting, diarrhea
Local: Injection site pain (OraVerse™ 4% to 6%)
Neuromuscular & skeletal: Paresthesia (OraVerse™), weakness
Respiratory: Nasal congestion

Dental Usual Dosage Reversal of soft tissue (lip, tongue) anesthesia (OraVerse™): Infiltration or block technique:submucosal oral injection:
Children: 15-30 kg: 0.2 mg maximum dose
Children >30 kg and <12 years: 0.4 mg maximum dose
Adults: **Note:** Dose is based upon the number of cartridges of local anesthetic administered. Infiltration or block injection:
0.2 mg if one-half cartridge of anesthesia was administered
0.4 mg if 1 cartridge of anesthesia was administered
0.8 mg if 2 cartridges of anesthesia were administered
Dosage
Treatment of alpha-adrenergic agonist drug extravasation: SubQ:
Children: Infiltrate area with a small amount (eg, 1 mL given in 0.2 mL aliquots) of a 0.5-1 mg/mL solution (made by diluting 5-10 mg in 10 mL of NS) within 12 hours of extravasation; in general, do not exceed 0.1-0.2 mg/kg or 5 mg total
Adults: Infiltrate area with small amount of solution made by diluting 5-10 mg in 10 mL 0.9% sodium chloride within 12 hours of extravasation; in general, do not exceed 0.1-0.2 mg/kg (5 mg total); typically doses of ≤5 mg are effective; a case using 50 mg for a large extravasation has been reported (Cooper, 1989).
If dose is effective, normal skin color should return to the blanched area within 1 hour
Diagnosis of pheochromocytoma: I.M., I.V.:
Children: 0.05-0.1 mg/kg/dose, maximum single dose: 5 mg
Adults: 5 mg
Surgery for pheochromocytoma: Hypertension: I.M., I.V.:
Children: 0.05-0.1 mg/kg/dose given 1-2 hours before procedure; repeat as needed every 2-4 hours until hypertension is controlled; maximum single dose: 5 mg
Adults: 5 mg given 1-2 hours before procedure and repeated as needed every 2-4 hours
Hypertensive crisis: Adults: 5-20 mg
Treatment of pralidoxime-induced hypertension (unlabeled use): I.V.:
Children: 1 mg
Adults and Elderly: 5 mg
Reversal of soft tissue (lip, tongue) anesthesia (OraVerse™): Infiltration or block technique: Submucosal oral injection:
Children: 15-30 kg: 0.2 mg maximum dose
Children >30 kg and <12 years: 0.4 mg maximum dose
Adults: **Note:** Dose is based upon the number of cartridges of local anesthetic administered. Infiltration or block injection:
0.2 mg if one-half cartridge of anesthesia was administered
0.4 mg if 1 cartridge of anesthesia was administered
0.8 mg if 2 cartridges of anesthesia were administered
Mechanism of Action Competitively blocks alpha-adrenergic receptors to produce brief antagonism of circulating epinephrine and norepinephrine to reduce hypertension caused by alpha effects of these catecholamines; also has a positive inotropic and chronotropic effect on the heart
OraVerse™: Causes vasodilation and increased blood flow in injection area via alpha-adrenergic blockade to accelerate reversal of soft tissue anesthetic

Contraindications Hypersensitivity to phentolamine or any component of the formulation; renal impairment; coronary or cerebral arteriosclerosis; concurrent use with phosphodiesterase-5 (PDE-5) inhibitors including sildenafil (>25 mg), tadalafil, or vardenafil

OraVerse™: There are no contraindications listed in the manufacturer's labeling.

Warnings/Precautions Myocardial infarction, cerebrovascular spasm, and cerebrovascular occlusion have occurred following administration; use with caution in patients with gastritis or peptic ulcer, tachycardia, or a history of cardiac arrhythmias. Discontinue if symptoms of angina occur or worsen. OraVerse™: Efficacy has not been established in children <6 years of age or <15 kg (33 pounds).

Drug Interactions

Metabolism/Transport Effects None known.

Avoid Concomitant Use

Avoid concomitant use of Phentolamine with any of the following: Alpha1-Blockers

Increased Effect/Toxicity

Phentolamine may increase the levels/effects of: Alpha1-Blockers; Amifostine; Antihypertensives; Calcium Channel Blockers; RiTUXimab

The levels/effects of Phentolamine may be increased by: Beta-Blockers; Diazoxide; Herbs (Hypotensive Properties); MAO Inhibitors; Pentoxifylline; Phosphodiesterase 5 Inhibitors; Prostacyclin Analogues

Decreased Effect

Phentolamine may decrease the levels/effects of: Alpha-/Beta-Agonists; Alpha1-Agonists

The levels/effects of Phentolamine may be decreased by: Herbs (Hypertensive Properties); Methylphenidate; Yohimbine

Pharmacodynamics/Kinetics

Onset of Action I.M.: 15-20 minutes; I.V.: Immediate Peak effect: OraVerse™: 10-20 minutes

Duration of Action I.M.: 30-45 minutes; I.V.: 15-30 minutes

Half-life Elimination 19 minutes

Pregnancy Risk Factor C

Pregnancy Considerations Adverse events were observed in some oral animal reproduction studies. Diagnosing and treating pheochromocytoma is critical for favorable maternal and fetal outcomes (Schenker, 1971; Schenker, 1982).

Lactation Excretion in breast milk unknown/use caution

Dosage Forms

Injection, powder for reconstitution: 5 mg

Injection, solution [preservative free]: OraVerse™: 0.4 mg/1.7 mL (1.7 mL)

Dental Comment OraVerse™ (solution for injection/dental cartridge) is administered as a submucosal injection and is not to be confused with phentolamine used as an intramuscular or intravenous injection for the treatment of hypertension associated with pheochromocytoma.

In adolescents >12 years and adults, OraVerse™ reduced the median time to recovery of normal sensation in the lower lip by 85 minutes compared to control. OraVerse™ reduced the median time to recovery of normal sensation in the upper lip by 83 minutes. Within 1 hour after administration, 41% of patients reported normal lower lip sensation as compared to 7% in the control group and 59% of patients given OraVerse™ reported normal upper lip sensation as compared to 12% in the control group.

In children 6-11 years of age, the median time to normal sensation was reduced by 75 minutes after OraVerse™ administration, a 56% acceleration of the time to normal sensation.

Phenylephrine (Systemic) (fen il EF rin)

Brand Names: U.S. Medi-First® Sinus Decongestant [OTC]; Medi-Phenyl [OTC]; PediaCare® Children's Decongestant [OTC]; Sudafed PE® Children's [OTC]; Sudafed PE® Congestion [OTC]; Sudafed PE™ Nasal Decongestant [OTC]; Sudogest™ PE [OTC]

Pharmacologic Category Alpha-Adrenergic Agonist

Use Treatment of hypotension, vascular failure in shock; as a vasoconstrictor in regional analgesia; supraventricular tachycardia (**Note:** Not for routine use in treatment of supraventricular tachycardias); as a decongestant [OTC]

Local Anesthetic/Vasoconstrictor Precautions Use with caution since phenylephrine is a sympathomimetic amine which could interact with epinephrine to cause a pressor response

Effects on Dental Treatment Key adverse event(s) related to dental treatment: Tachycardia, palpitations (use vasoconstrictor with caution), and xerostomia (normal salivary flow resumes upon discontinuation).

Effects on Bleeding No information available to require special precautions

Adverse Effects Frequency not defined.

Injection:

Cardiovascular: Arrhythmia (rare), decreased cardiac output, hypertension, pallor, precordial pain or discomfort, reflex bradycardia, severe peripheral and visceral vasoconstriction

Central nervous system: Anxiety, dizziness, excitability, giddiness, headache, insomnia, nervousness, restlessness

Endocrine & metabolic: Metabolic acidosis

Gastrointestinal: Gastric irritation, nausea

Local: I.V.: Extravasation which may lead to necrosis and sloughing of surrounding tissue, blanching of skin

Neuromuscular & skeletal: Paresthesia, pilomotor response, tremor, weakness

Renal: Decreased renal perfusion, reduced urine output

Respiratory: Respiratory distress

Miscellaneous: Hypersensitivity reactions (including rash, urticaria, leukopenia, agranulocytosis, thrombocytopenia)

Oral: Central nervous system: Anxiety, dizziness, excitability, giddiness, headache, insomnia, nervousness, restlessness

General Dosage Range

I.V.:

Children: Bolus: 5-20 mcg/kg/dose every 10-15 minutes as needed; Infusion: 0.1-0.5 mcg/kg/minute

Adults: Bolus: 100-500 mcg/dose every 10-15 minutes as needed (maximum: 500 mcg); Infusion: Initial: 100-180 mcg/minute

Oral:

Children 4 to <6 years: 2.5 mg every 4 hours as needed (maximum: 15 mg/24 hours)

Children 6 to <12 years: 5 mg every 4 hours as needed (maximum: 30 mg/24 hours)

Children ≥12 years and Adults: 10 mg every 4 hours as needed (maximum: 60 mg/24 hours)

◄ **Mechanism of Action** Potent, direct-acting alpha-adrenergic agonist with virtually no beta-adrenergic activity; produces systemic arterial vasoconstriction. Such increases in systemic vascular resistance result in dose dependent increases in systolic and diastolic blood pressure and reductions in heart rate and cardiac output especially in patients with heart failure.

Pharmacodynamics/Kinetics

Onset of Action

Blood pressure increase/vasoconstriction: I.M., SubQ: 10-15 minutes; I.V.: Immediate

Nasal decongestant: Oral: 15-30 minutes (Kollar, 2007)

Duration of Action

Blood pressure increase/vasoconstriction: I.M.: 1-2 hours; I.V.: ~15-20 minutes; SubQ: 50 minutes

Nasal decongestant: Oral: ≤4 hours (Kollar, 2007)

Half-life Elimination Alpha phase: ~5 minutes; Terminal phase: 2-3 hours (Hengstmann, 1982; Kanfer, 1993)

Time to Peak Oral: 0.75-2 hours (Kanfer, 1993)

Pregnancy Risk Factor C

Pregnancy Considerations Animal reproduction studies have not been conducted; therefore, the manufacturer classifies phenylephrine as pregnancy category C. Phenylephrine crosses the placenta at term. Maternal use of phenylephrine during the first trimester of pregnancy is not strongly associated with an increased risk of fetal malformations; maternal dose and duration of therapy were not reported in available publications. Phenylephrine is available over-the-counter (OTC) for the symptomatic relief of nasal congestion. Decongestants are not the preferred agents for the treatment of rhinitis during pregnancy. Oral phenylephrine should be avoided during the first trimester of pregnancy; short-term use (<3 days) of intranasal phenylephrine may be beneficial to some patients although its safety during pregnancy has not been studied. Phenylephrine injection is used at delivery for the prevention and/or treatment of maternal hypotension associated with spinal anesthesia in women undergoing cesarean section. Phenylephrine may be associated with a more favorable fetal acid base status than ephedrine; however, overall fetal outcomes appear to be similar. Nausea or vomiting may be less with phenylephrine than ephedrine but is also dependent upon blood pressure control. Phenylephrine may be preferred in the absence of maternal bradycardia.

Phenylephrine (Topical) (fen il EF rin)

Brand Names: U.S. Anu-Med [OTC]; Formulation R™ [OTC]; Medicone® Suppositories [OTC]; Preparation H® [OTC]; Rectacaine [OTC]; Tronolane® Suppository [OTC]

Pharmacologic Category Alpha-Adrenergic Agonist

Use For OTC use as treatment of hemorrhoids

Local Anesthetic/Vasoconstrictor Precautions No information available to require special precautions

Effects on Dental Treatment No significant effects or complications reported

Effects on Bleeding No information available to require special precautions

Adverse Effects Rare systemic effects may occur.

General Dosage Range Rectal: *Children >12 years and Adults:* Ointment: Apply up to 4 times/day; Suppository: Insert 1 up to 4 times/day

Mechanism of Action Potent, direct-acting alpha-adrenergic agonist with virtually no beta-adrenergic activity; produces local vasoconstriction.

Pregnancy Considerations When administered intravenously, phenylephrine crosses the placenta. Refer to the Phenylephrine (Systemic) monograph for details. There is limited information available supporting the use of topical agents for the treatment of hemorrhoids. Products containing phenylephrine should be used with caution in pregnant women, especially patients with hypertension or diabetes.

Phenylephrine and Zinc Sulfate
(fen il EF rin & zingk SUL fate)

Related Information

Zinc Sulfate *on page 1422*

Brand Names: Canada Zincfrin®

Pharmacologic Category Adrenergic Agonist Agent

Use Soothe, moisturize, and remove redness due to minor eye irritation

Local Anesthetic/Vasoconstrictor Precautions No information available to require special precautions

Effects on Dental Treatment No significant effects or complications reported

Effects on Bleeding No information available to require special precautions

General Dosage Range Ophthalmic: *Adults:* Instill 1-2 drops in eye(s) 2-4 times/day as needed

Product Availability Not available in U.S.

Phenytoin (FEN i toyn)

Related Information

Fosphenytoin *on page 636*

Brand Names: U.S. Dilantin-125®; Dilantin®; Phenytek®

Brand Names: Canada Dilantin®; Novo-Phenytoin; Taro-Phenytoin; Tremytoine Inj

Generic Availability (U.S.) Yes

Pharmacologic Category Anticonvulsant, Hydantoin

Use Management of generalized tonic-clonic (grand mal), complex partial seizures; prevention of seizures following neurosurgery

Unlabeled Use Prevention of early (within 1 week) post-traumatic seizures (PTS) following traumatic brain injury

Local Anesthetic/Vasoconstrictor Precautions No information available to require special precautions

Effects on Dental Treatment Gingival hyperplasia is a common problem observed during the first 6 months of phenytoin therapy appearing as gingivitis or gum inflammation. To minimize severity and growth rate of gingival tissue begin a program of professional cleaning and patient plaque control within 10 days of starting anticonvulsant therapy.

Effects on Bleeding No information available to require special precautions

Adverse Effects I.V. effects: Hypotension, bradycardia, cardiac arrhythmia, cardiovascular collapse (especially with rapid I.V. use), venous irritation and pain, thrombophlebitis

Effects not related to plasma phenytoin concentrations: Hypertrichosis, gingival hypertrophy, thickening of facial features, carbohydrate intolerance, folic acid deficiency, peripheral neuropathy, vitamin D deficiency, osteomalacia, systemic lupus erythematosus

Concentration-related effects: Nystagmus, blurred vision, diplopia, ataxia, slurred speech, dizziness, drowsiness, lethargy, coma, rash, fever, nausea, vomiting, gum tenderness, confusion, mood changes, folic acid depletion, osteomalacia, hyperglycemia

Related to elevated concentrations:
>20 mcg/mL: Far lateral nystagmus
>30 mcg/mL: 45° lateral gaze nystagmus and ataxia
>40 mcg/mL: Decreased mentation
>100 mcg/mL: Death

Cardiovascular: Bradycardia, cardiac arrhythmia, cardiovascular collapse, hypotension

Central nervous system: Dizziness, drowsiness, headache, insomnia, psychiatric changes, slurred speech

Dermatologic: Rash

Gastrointestinal: Constipation, gingival hyperplasia, enlargement of lips, nausea, taste disturbance, vomiting

Genitourinary: Peyronie's disease

Hematologic: Agranulocytosis, granulocytopenia, leukopenia, pancytopenia, thrombocytopenia

Hepatic: Hepatitis

Local: I.V. administration: Inflammation, irritation, necrosis, sloughing, tenderness, thrombophlebitis

Neuromuscular & skeletal: Paresthesia, peripheral neuropathy, tremor

Ocular: Blurred vision, diplopia, nystagmus

Rarely seen effects: Anaphylaxis, blood dyscrasias, coarsening of facial features, DRESS, dyskinesias, hepatitis, Hodgkin lymphoma, hypertrichosis, immunoglobulin abnormalities, lymphadenopathy, lymphoma, macrocytosis, megaloblastic anemia, periarteritis nodosa, pseudolymphoma, SLE-like syndrome, Stevens-Johnson syndrome, toxic epidermal necrolysis, venous irritation and pain

Dosage Note: Phenytoin base (eg, oral suspension, chewable tablets) contains ~8% more drug than phenytoin sodium (~92 mg base is equivalent to 100 mg phenytoin sodium). Dosage adjustments and closer serum monitoring may be necessary when switching dosage forms.

Status epilepticus: I.V.:
Infants and Children: Loading dose: 15-20 mg/kg, then begin maintenance therapy usually 12 hours after loading dose
Adolescents and Adults: Loading dose: Manufacturer recommends 10-15 mg/kg; however, 15-20 mg/kg at a maximum rate of 50 mg/minute is generally recommended (Kalvianines, 2007; Lowenstein, 2005); initial maintenance dose: I.V. or Oral: 100 mg every 6-8 hours

Anticonvulsant (nonemergent use): Oral:
Loading dose: Children, Adolescents, and Adults: 15-20 mg/kg; consider prior phenytoin serum concentrations and/or recent dosing history if available; administer oral loading dose in 3 divided doses given every 2-4 hours to decrease GI adverse effects and to ensure complete oral absorption

Maintenance dose:
Infants and Children: Initial maintenance dose: 5 mg/kg/day in 2-3 divided doses; usual maintenance dose range: 4-8 mg/kg/day; maximum daily dose: 300 mg. Some experts suggest higher maintenance doses may be necessary in infant and young children (range: 8-10 mg/kg/day in divided doses).

Adolescents and Adults: Initial maintenance dose: 300 mg daily in 3 divided doses; may also administer in 1-2 divided doses using extended release formulation; adjust dosage based on individual requirements; usual maintenance dose range: 300-600 mg daily

Dosage adjustment in obesity: Adults: Loading dose: Use adjusted body weight (ABW) correction based on a pharmacokinetic study of phenytoin loading doses in obese patients (Abernethy, 1985). The larger correction factor (ie, 1.33) is due to a doubling of V_d estimated in these obese patients.

ABW = [(Actual body weight – IBW) x 1.33] + IBW

Maintenance doses should be based on ideal body weight, conventional daily doses with adjustments based upon therapeutic drug monitoring and clinical effectiveness. (Abernethy, 1985; Erstad, 2002; Erstad, 2004)

Dosing adjustment in renal impairment: No dosage adjustment provided in manufacturer's labeling; <5% excreted as unchanged drug. Serum concentration may be difficult to interpret in renal failure. Monitoring of free (unbound) concentrations or adjustment to allow interpretation is recommended.

Dosage adjustment in hepatic impairment: No dosage adjustment provided in manufacturer's labeling; undergoes hepatic metabolism and clearance may be decreased. Monitor free phenytoin levels closely. Dosage adjustments may be necessary.

Mechanism of Action Stabilizes neuronal membranes and decreases seizure activity by increasing efflux or decreasing influx of sodium ions across cell membranes in the motor cortex during generation of nerve impulses; prolongs effective refractory period and suppresses ventricular pacemaker automaticity, shortens action potential in the heart

Contraindications Hypersensitivity to phenytoin, other hydantoins, or any component of the formulation; concurrent use of delavirdine (due to loss of virologic response and possible resistance to delavirdine or other non-nucleoside reverse transcriptase inhibitors [NNRTIs])

I.V.: Sinus bradycardia, sinoatrial block, second- and third-degree heart block, Adams-Stokes syndrome

Warnings/Precautions Antiepileptics are associated with an increased risk of suicidal behavior/thoughts with use (regardless of indication); patients should be monitored for signs/symptoms of depression, suicidal tendencies, and other unusual behavior changes during therapy and instructed to inform their healthcare provider immediately if symptoms occur.

[U.S. Boxed Warning]: Phenytoin must be administered slowly. Intravenous administration should not exceed 50 mg/minute in adult patients. In pediatric patients, intravenous administration rate should not exceed 1-3 mg/kg/minute or 50 mg/minute whichever is slower. Hypotension and severe cardiac arrhythmias (eg, heart block, ventricular tachycardia, ventricular fibrillation) may occur with rapid administration; adverse cardiac events have been reported at or below the recommended infusion rate. Cardiac monitoring is necessary during and after administration of intravenous phenytoin; reduction in rate of administration or discontinuation of infusion may be necessary. For non-emergency use, intravenous phenytoin should be administered more slowly; the use of oral phenytoin should be used whenever possible. I.V. form may cause soft tissue irritation and inflammation, and skin necrosis at I.V. site; avoid I.V. administration in small veins. The "purple glove syndrome" (ie, discoloration with edema and pain of distal limb) may occur following peripheral I.V. administration of phenytoin; may or may not be associated with drug extravasation; symptoms may resolve spontaneously; however, skin necrosis and limb ischemia may occur; interventions such as fasciotomies, skin grafts, and amputation (rare) may be required. May increase frequency of petit mal seizures; use with caution in patients with porphyria; discontinue if rash or lymphadenopathy occurs; a spectrum of hematologic effects have been reported with use (eg, agranulocytosis, neutropenia, leukopenia, thrombocytopenia, pancytopenia, and anemias); use with caution in patients with hepatic dysfunction, hypothyroidism, or underlying cardiac disease; I.V. use is contraindicated in patients with sinus bradycardia, sinoatrial block, or second- and third-degree heart block; use with caution in elderly or debilitated patients, or in any condition associated with low serum albumin levels, which will increase the free fraction of phenytoin in the serum and, therefore, the pharmacologic response. Sedation, confusional states, or cerebellar dysfunction (loss of motor coordination) may occur at higher total serum concentrations, or at lower total serum concentrations when the free fraction of phenytoin is increased. Effects with other sedative drugs or ethanol may be potentiated. Abrupt withdrawal may precipitate status epilepticus. Severe reactions, including toxic epidermal necrolysis and Stevens-Johnson syndromes, although rarely reported, have resulted in fatalities; drug should be discontinued if there are any signs of rash and evaluate for signs and symptoms of drug reaction with eosinophilia and systemic symptoms (DRESS). Patients of Asian descent with the variant *HLA-B*1502* may be at an increased risk of developing Stevens-Johnson syndrome and/or toxic epidermal necrolysis. Chronic use of phenytoin has been associated with decreased bone mineral density (osteopenia, osteoporosis, and osteomalacia) and bone fractures. Chronic use may result in decreased vitamin D concentrations due to hepatic enzyme induction and may lead to hypocalcemia and hypophosphatemia; monitor as appropriate and consider implementing vitamin D and calcium supplementation.

Drug Interactions

Metabolism/Transport Effects Substrate of CYP2C19 (major), CYP2C9 (major), CYP3A4 (minor); **Note:** Assignment of Major/Minor substrate status based on clinically relevant drug interaction potential; **Induces** CYP2B6 (strong), CYP2C19 (strong), CYP2C8 (strong), CYP2C9 (strong), CYP3A4 (strong)

Avoid Concomitant Use

Avoid concomitant use of Phenytoin with any of the following: Apixaban; Axitinib; Azelastine (Nasal); Bedaquiline; Boceprevir; Bortezomib; Bosutinib; Cabozantinib; Crizotinib; Darunavir; Delavirdine; Dronedarone; Enzalutamide; Etravirine; Everolimus; Ivacaftor; Lapatinib; Lurasidone; Mifepristone; Nilotinib; Paraldehyde; Pazopanib; Pomalidomide; Ponatinib; Praziquantel; Ranolazine; Regorafenib; Rilpivirine; Rivaroxaban; Roflumilast; RomiDEPsin; SORAfenib; Telaprevir; Ticagrelor; Tofacitinib; Tolvaptan; Toremifene; Vandetanib; VinCRIStine (Liposomal)

Increased Effect/Toxicity

Phenytoin may increase the levels/effects of: Azelastine (Nasal); Barbiturates; Buprenorphine; Clarithromycin; CNS Depressants; Fosamprenavir; Ifosfamide; Lithium; Methotrimeprazine; Metyrosine; Mirtazapine; Paraldehyde; Pramipexole; Prilocaine; ROPINIRole; Rotigotine; Selective Serotonin Reuptake Inhibitors; Vecuronium; Vitamin K Antagonists; Zolpidem

The levels/effects of Phenytoin may be increased by: Alcohol (Ethyl); Allopurinol; Amiodarone; Antifungal Agents (Azole Derivatives, Systemic); Benzodiazepines; Calcium Channel Blockers; Capecitabine; CarBAMazepine; Carbonic Anhydrase Inhibitors; CeFAZolin; Chloramphenicol; Cimetidine; Clarithromycin; Cosyntropin; CYP2C19 Inhibitors (Moderate); CYP2C19 Inhibitors (Strong); CYP2C9 Inhibitors (Moderate); CYP2C9 Inhibitors (Strong); Delavirdine; Dexmethylphenidate; Disulfiram; Droperidol; Efavirenz; Ethosuximide; Felbamate; Floxuridine; Fluconazole; Fluorouracil (Systemic); Fluorouracil (Topical); FLUoxetine; FluvoxaMINE; Halothane; HydrOXYzine; Isoniazid; Magnesium Sulfate; Methotrimeprazine; Methylphenidate; MetroNIDAZOLE (Systemic); Mifepristone; OXcarbazepine; Proton Pump Inhibitors; Rufinamide; Sertraline; Sodium Oxybate; Sulfonamide Derivatives; Tacrolimus (Systemic); Telaprevir; Ticlopidine; Topiramate; TraZODone; Trimethoprim; Vitamin K Antagonists

Decreased Effect

Phenytoin may decrease the levels/effects of: Acetaminophen; Amiodarone; Antifungal Agents (Azole Derivatives, Systemic); Apixaban; ARIPiprazole; Axitinib; Bedaquiline; Boceprevir; Bortezomib; Bosutinib; Brentuximab Vedotin; Busulfan; Cabozantinib; Canagliflozin; CarBAMazepine; Caspofungin; Chloramphenicol; Clarithromycin; CloZAPine; Cobicistat; Contraceptives (Estrogens); Contraceptives (Progestins); Crizotinib; CycloSPORINE (Systemic); CYP2B6 Substrates; CYP2C19 Substrates; CYP2C8 Substrates; CYP2C9 Substrates; CYP3A4 Substrates; Darunavir; Dasatinib; Deferasirox; Delavirdine; Diclofenac (Systemic); Disopyramide; Divalproex; Doxycycline; Dronedarone; Efavirenz; Elvitegravir; Ethosuximide; Etoposide; Etoposide Phosphate; Etravirine; Everolimus; Exemestane; Felbamate; Flunarizine; Gefitinib; GuanFACINE; HMG-CoA Reductase Inhibitors; Imatinib; Irinotecan; Ivacaftor; Ixabepilone; Lacosamide; LamoTRIgine; Lapatinib; Levodopa; Linagliptin; Loop Diuretics; Lopinavir; Lurasidone; Maraviroc; Mebendazole; Meperidine; Methadone; MethylPREDNISolone; MetroNIDAZOLE (Systemic); Metyrapone; Mexiletine; Mifepristone; Nilotinib; OXcarbazepine; Pazopanib; Perampanel; Pomalidomide; Ponatinib; Praziquantel; PrednisoLONE (Systemic); PredniSONE; Primidone; QUEtiapine; QuiNIDine; QuiNINE; Ranolazine; Regorafenib; Rilpivirine; Ritonavir; Rivaroxaban; Roflumilast; RomiDEPsin; Rufinamide; Saxagliptin; Sertraline; Sirolimus; SORAfenib; SUNItinib; Tacrolimus (Systemic); Tadalafil; Telaprevir; Temsirolimus; Teniposide; Theophylline Derivatives; Thyroid Products; Ticagrelor; Tipranavir; Tofacitinib; Tolvaptan; Topiramate; Toremifene; TraZODone; Treprostinil; Ulipristal; Valproic Acid; Vandetanib; Vecuronium; Vemurafenib; VinCRIStine; VinCRIStine (Liposomal); Zonisamide; Zuclopenthixol

The levels/effects of Phenytoin may be decreased by: Alcohol (Ethyl); Amphetamines; Antacids; Barbiturates; CarBAMazepine; Ciprofloxacin (Systemic); CISplatin; Colesevelam; CYP2C19 Inducers (Strong); CYP2C9 Inducers (Strong); Diazoxide; Divalproex; Enzalutamide; Folic Acid; Fosamprenavir; Ketorolac (Nasal); Ketorolac (Systemic); Leucovorin Calcium-Levoleucovorin; Levomefolate; Lopinavir; Mefloquine; Methylfolate; Multivitamins/Minerals (with ADEK, Folate, Iron); Nelfinavir; Peginterferon Alfa-2b; Pyridoxine; Rifamycin Derivatives; Ritonavir; Telaprevir; Theophylline Derivatives; Tipranavir; Valproic Acid; Vigabatrin; VinCRIStine

Ethanol/Nutrition/Herb Interactions

Ethanol:

Acute use: Ethanol inhibits metabolism of phenytoin and may also increase CNS depression. Management: Avoid or limit ethanol. Caution patients about effects.

Chronic use: Ethanol stimulates metabolism of phenytoin. Management: Avoid or limit ethanol.

Food: Phenytoin serum concentrations may be altered if taken with food. If taken with enteral nutrition, phenytoin serum concentrations may be decreased. Tube feedings decrease bioavailability. Phenytoin may decrease calcium, folic acid, and vitamin D levels. Supplementing folic acid may lower the seizure threshold. Management: Hold tube feedings 1-2 hours before and 1-2 hours after phenytoin administration. Do not supplement folic acid. Consider vitamin D supplementation. Take preferably on an empty stomach.

Herb/Nutraceutical: Evening primrose may decrease the seizure threshold; other herbal medications may increase CNS depression. Management: Avoid evening primrose, valerian, St John's wort, kava kava, and gotu kola.

Dietary Considerations

Folic acid: Phenytoin may decrease mucosal uptake of folic acid; to avoid folic acid deficiency and megaloblastic anemia, some clinicians recommend giving patients on anticonvulsants prophylactic doses of folic acid and cyanocobalamin. Folic acid 0.5 mg/day has been shown to reduce the incidence of phenytoin-induced gingival overgrowth in children (Arya, 2011). However, folate supplementation may increase seizures in some patients (dose dependent). Discuss with healthcare provider prior to using any supplements.

Calcium: Hypocalcemia has been reported in patients taking prolonged high-dose therapy with an anticonvulsant. Some clinicians have given an additional 4000 units/week of vitamin D (especially in those receiving poor nutrition and getting no sun exposure) to prevent hypocalcemia.

Vitamin D: Phenytoin interferes with vitamin D metabolism and osteomalacia may result; may need to supplement with vitamin D

Tube feedings: Tube feedings decrease phenytoin absorption. To avoid decreased serum levels with continuous NG feeds, hold feedings for 1-2 hours prior to and 1-2 hours after phenytoin administration, if possible. There is a variety of opinions on how to administer phenytoin with enteral feedings. Be **consistent** throughout therapy.

Injection may contain sodium.

Pharmacodynamics/Kinetics

Onset of Action I.V.: ~0.5-1 hour

Half-life Elimination Range: 7-42 hours; **Note:** Elimination is not first-order (ie, follows Michaelis-Menten pharmacokinetics); half-life increases with increasing phenytoin concentrations; best described using parameters such as V_{max} (metabolic capacity) and Km (constant equal to the concentration at which the rate of metabolism is $1/2$ of V_{max}).

Time to Peak Serum (formulation dependent): Oral: Extended-release capsule: 4-12 hours; Immediate release preparation: 2-3 hours

Pregnancy Risk Factor D

Pregnancy Considerations Phenytoin crosses the placenta. Congenital malformations (including a pattern of malformations termed the "fetal hydantoin syndrome" or "fetal anticonvulsant syndrome") have been reported in infants. Isolated cases of malignancies (including neuroblastoma) and coagulation defects in the neonate

following delivery have also been reported. Epilepsy itself, the number of medications, genetic factors, or a combination of these probably influence the teratogenicity of anticonvulsant therapy.

Total plasma concentrations of phenytoin are decreased by 56% in the mother during pregnancy; unbound plasma (free) concentrations are decreased by 31%. Because protein binding is decreased, monitoring of unbound plasma concentrations is recommended. Concentrations should be monitored through the 8th week postpartum. The use of folic acid throughout pregnancy and vitamin K during the last month of pregnancy is recommended.

Patients exposed to phenytoin during pregnancy are encouraged to enroll themselves into the AED Pregnancy Registry by calling 1-888-233-2334. Additional information is available at www.aedpregnancyregistry.org.

Lactation Enters breast milk/not recommended (AAP rates "compatible"; AAP 2001 update pending)

Breast-Feeding Considerations Phenytoin is excreted in breast milk; however, the amount to which the infant is exposed is considered small. The manufacturers of phenytoin do not recommend breast-feeding during therapy. Women should be counseled of the possible risks and benefits associated with breast-feeding while on phenytoin.

Dosage Forms

Capsule, extended release, oral: 100 mg, 200 mg, 300 mg

Dilantin®: 30 mg, 100 mg

Phenytek®: 200 mg, 300 mg

Injection, solution: 50 mg/mL (2 mL, 5 mL)

Suspension, oral: 100 mg/4 mL (4 mL); 125 mg/5 mL (237 mL, 240 mL)

Dilantin-125®: 125 mg/5 mL (240 mL)

Tablet, chewable, oral: 50 mg

Dilantin®: 50 mg

Physostigmine (fye zoe STIG meen)

Pharmacologic Category Acetylcholinesterase Inhibitor; Antidote

Use Reversal of central nervous system anticholinergic syndrome

Note: Physostigmine should only be used to reverse toxic, life-threatening delirium caused by pure anticholinergic agents (ie, atropine, diphenhydramine, dimenhydrinate, *Atropa belladonna* [deadly nightshade], or jimson weed [*Datura* spp]). Consultation with a clinical toxicologist or poison control center is recommended in patients who require physostigmine administration.

Local Anesthetic/Vasoconstrictor Precautions No information available to require special precautions

Effects on Dental Treatment Key adverse event(s) related to dental treatment: Salivation.

Effects on Bleeding No information available to require special precautions

Adverse Effects Frequency not defined.

Cardiovascular: Asystole, bradycardia, palpitation

Central nervous system: Hallucinations, nervousness, restlessness, seizure

Gastrointestinal: Defecation, diarrhea, nausea, salivation, stomach pain, vomiting

Genitourinary: Urinary frequency

Neuromuscular & skeletal: Twitching

Ocular: Lacrimation, miosis

Respiratory: Bronchospasm, dyspnea, pulmonary edema, respiratory distress, respiratory paralysis

Miscellaneous: Diaphoresis, hypersensitivity

General Dosage Range

I.M.:

Children: Initial: 0.02 mg/kg, may repeat every 5-10 minutes until response occurs (maximum total dose: 2 mg)

Adults: Initial: 0.5-2 mg, may repeat every 10-30 minutes until response occurs

I.V.:

Children: Initial: 0.02 mg/kg, may repeat every 5-10 minutes until response occurs (maximum total dose: 2 mg)

Adults: Initial: 0.5-2 mg, may repeat every 10-30 minutes until response occurs

Mechanism of Action Physostigmine is a carbamate which inhibits the enzyme acetylcholinesterase and prolongs the central and peripheral effects of acetylcholine

Pharmacodynamics/Kinetics

Onset of Action Approximately several minutes

Duration of Action 45-60 minutes

Pregnancy Considerations In general, medications used as antidotes should take into consideration the health and prognosis of the mother; antidotes should be administered to pregnant women if there is a clear indication for use and should not be withheld because of fears of teratogenicity (Bailey, 2003).

Phytonadione (fye toe na DYE one)

Brand Names: U.S. Mephyton®

Brand Names: Canada AquaMEPHYTON®; Konakion; Mephyton®

Pharmacologic Category Vitamin, Fat Soluble

Use Prevention and treatment of hypoprothrombinemia caused by vitamin K antagonist (VKA)-induced (eg, warfarin-induced) or other drug-induced vitamin K deficiency, altered activity, or altered metabolism; hypoprothrombinemia caused by malabsorption or inability to synthesize vitamin K; prophylaxis and treatment of hemorrhagic disease of the newborn

Unlabeled Use Treatment of hypoprothrombinemia caused by long-acting anticoagulant rodenticides (LAARs)

Local Anesthetic/Vasoconstrictor Precautions No information available to require special precautions

Effects on Dental Treatment Key adverse event(s) related to dental treatment: Abnormal taste.

Effects on Bleeding Phytonadione is a synthetic form of vitamin K and has been used as an antidote to reverse warfarin-induced bleeding complications or endogenous vitamin K deficiencies.

Adverse Effects Frequency not defined.

Cardiovascular: Cyanosis, flushing, hyper-/hypotension

Central nervous system: Dizziness

Dermatologic: Erythematous skin eruptions, pruritus, scleroderma-like lesions

Endocrine & metabolic: Hyperbilirubinemia (newborn; greater than recommended doses)

Gastrointestinal: Abnormal taste

Local: Injection site reactions

Respiratory: Dyspnea

Miscellaneous: Diaphoresis, hypersensitivity reactions, nonimmunologic anaphylaxis (formerly known as anaphylactoid reaction), sweating

General Dosage Range

I.M.:

Newborns: Prophylaxis: 0.5-1 mg within 1 hour of birth; Treatment: 1 mg/dose/day

Adults: Initial: 2.5-25 mg/dose (maximum: 50 mg)

I.V.: *Adults:* Initial: 2.5-25 mg/dose (maximum: 50 mg)

Oral: *Adults:* Initial: 2.5-25 mg/dose (maximum: 50 mg)

SubQ:

Newborns: 1 mg/dose/day

Adults: Initial: 2.5-25 mg/dose (maximum: 50 mg)

Mechanism of Action Promotes liver synthesis of clotting factors (II, VII, IX, X); however, the exact mechanism as to this stimulation is unknown. Menadiol is a water soluble form of vitamin K; phytonadione has a more rapid and prolonged effect than menadione; menadiol sodium diphosphate (K_4) is half as potent as menadione (K_3).

Pharmacodynamics/Kinetics

Onset of Action

Onset of action: Increased coagulation factors: Oral: 6-10 hours; I.V.: 1-2 hours

Peak effect: INR values return to normal: Oral: 24-48 hours; I.V.: 12-14 hours

Pregnancy Risk Factor C

Pregnancy Considerations Animal reproduction studies have not been conducted.

Pilocarpine (Systemic) (pye loe KAR peen)

Related Information

Dentin Hypersensitivity, Acid Erosion, High Caries Index, Management of Alveolar Osteitis, and Xerostomia *on page 1582*

Management of Patients Undergoing Cancer Therapy *on page 1596*

Brand Names: U.S. Salagen®

Brand Names: Canada Salagen®

Generic Availability (U.S.) Yes

Pharmacologic Category Cholinergic Agonist

Dental Use Treatment of xerostomia caused by radiation therapy in patients with head and neck cancer and from Sjögren's syndrome

Use Symptomatic treatment of xerostomia caused by salivary gland hypofunction resulting from radiotherapy for cancer of the head and neck or Sjögren's syndrome

Local Anesthetic/Vasoconstrictor Precautions No information available to require special precautions

Effects on Dental Treatment Key adverse event(s) related to dental treatment: Increased salivation (therapeutic effect). See Dental Comment.

Effects on Bleeding No information available to require special precautions

Adverse Effects

>10%:

Cardiovascular: Flushing (8% to 13%)

Central nervous system: Chills (3% to 15%), dizziness (5% to 12%), headache (11%)

Gastrointestinal: Nausea (6% to 15%)

Genitourinary: Urinary frequency (9% to 12%)

Neuromuscular & skeletal: Weakness (2% to 12%)

Respiratory: Rhinitis (5% to 14%)

Miscellaneous: Diaphoresis (29% to 68%)

1% to 10%:

Cardiovascular: Edema (<1% to 5%), facial edema, hypertension (3%), palpitation, tachycardia

Central nervous system: Pain (4%), fever, somnolence

Dermatologic: Pruritus, rash

Gastrointestinal: Diarrhea (4% to 7%), dyspepsia (7%), vomiting (3% to 4%), constipation, flatulence, glossitis, salivation increased, stomatitis, taste perversion

Genitourinary: Vaginitis, urinary incontinence

Neuromuscular & skeletal: Myalgias, tremor

Ocular: Lacrimation (6%), amblyopia (4%), abnormal vision, blurred vision, conjunctivitis

Otic: Tinnitus

Respiratory: Cough increased, dysphagia, epistaxis, sinusitis

Miscellaneous: Allergic reaction, voice alteration

Dental Usual Dosage Treatment of xerostomia: Adults: Oral: 1-2 tablets 3-4 times/day not to exceed 30 mg/day (minimum 90-day therapy required for optimum effects)

Dosage Oral: Adults: Xerostomia:

Following head and neck cancer: 5 mg 3 times/day, titration up to 10 mg 3 times/day may be considered for patients who have not responded adequately; do not exceed 2 tablets/dose

Sjögren's syndrome: 5 mg 4 times/day

Dosage adjustment in hepatic impairment:

Moderate impairment: 5 mg 2 times/day regardless of indication; adjust dose based on response and tolerability

Severe impairment (Child-Pugh score >10): Contraindicated

Contraindications Hypersensitivity to pilocarpine or any component of the formulation; uncontrolled asthma; angle-closure glaucoma, severe hepatic impairment

Warnings/Precautions Use caution with cardiovascular disease; patients may have difficulty compensating for transient changes in hemodynamics or rhythm induced by pilocarpine. Use caution with controlled asthma, chronic bronchitis, or COPD; may increase airway resistance, bronchial smooth muscle tone, and bronchial secretions. Use caution with cholelithiasis, biliary tract disease, and nephrolithiasis; adjust dose with moderate hepatic impairment.

Drug Interactions

Metabolism/Transport Effects Inhibits CYP2A6 (weak), CYP2E1 (weak), CYP3A4 (weak)

Avoid Concomitant Use

Avoid concomitant use of Pilocarpine (Systemic) with any of the following: Pimozide

Increased Effect/Toxicity

Pilocarpine (Systemic) may increase the levels/effects of: ARIPiprazole; Lomitapide; Pimozide

The levels/effects of Pilocarpine (Systemic) may be increased by: Acetylcholinesterase Inhibitors; Beta-Blockers

Decreased Effect There are no known significant interactions involving a decrease in effect.

Ethanol/Nutrition/Herb Interactions Food: Avoid administering with high-fat meal; fat decreases the rate of absorption, maximum concentration and increases the time it takes to reach maximum concentration.

Dietary Considerations Avoid taking with a high-fat meal.

Pharmacodynamics/Kinetics

Onset of Action 20 minutes

Duration of Action 3-5 hours

Half-life Elimination 0.76-1.35 hours; increased with hepatic impairment

Pregnancy Risk Factor C

Pregnancy Considerations Adverse events were observed in some animal studies.

Lactation Excretion in breast milk unknown/not recommended

Dosage Forms

Tablet, oral: 5 mg, 7.5 mg

Salagen®: 5 mg, 7.5 mg

Dental Comment Pilocarpine may have potential as a salivary stimulant in individuals suffering from xerostomia induced by antidepressants and other medications. At the present time however, the FDA has not approved pilocarpine for use in drug-induced xerostomia (clinical studies required). In an attempt to discern the efficacy of pilocarpine as a salivary stimulant in patients suffering from Sjögren's syndrome (SS), Rhodus and Schuh studied 9 patients with SS given daily doses of pilocarpine over a 6-week period. A dose of 5 mg daily produced a significant overall increase in both whole unstimulated salivary flow and parotid stimulated salivary flow. These results support the use of pilocarpine to increase salivary flow in patients with SS.

References

Davies AN and Singer J, "A Comparison of Artificial Saliva and Pilocarpine in Radiation-Induced Xerostomia," *J Laryngol Otol,* 1994, 108(8):663-5.

Fox PC, Atkinson JC, Macynski AA, et al, "Pilocarpine Treatment of Salivary Gland Hypofunction and Dry Mouth (Xerostomia)," *Arch Intern Med,* 1991, 151(6):1149-52.

Johnson JT, Ferretti GA, Nethery WJ, et al, "Oral Pilocarpine for Postirradiation Xerostomia in Patients With Head and Neck Cancer," *N Engl J Med,* 1993, 329(6):390-5.

Mosqueda-Taylor A, Luna-Ortiz K, Irigoyen-Camacho ME, et al, "Effect of Pilocarpine Hydrochloride on Salivary Production in Previously Irradiated Head and Neck Cancer Patients," *Med Oral,* 2004, 9 (3):204-11.

Nelson JD, Friedlaender M, Yeatts RP, et al, "Oral Pilocarpine for Symptomatic Relief of Keratoconjunctivitis Sicca in Patients with Sjögren's Syndrome. The MGI PHARMA Sjögren's Syndrome Study Group," *Adv Exp Med Biol,* 1998, 438:979-83.

Rhodus NL and Schuh MJ, "Effects of Pilocarpine on Salivary Flow in Patients With Sjögren's Syndrome," *Oral Surg Oral Med Oral Pathol,* 1991, 72(5):545-9.

Rieke JW, Hafermann MD, Johnson JT, et al, "Oral Pilocarpine for Radiation-Induced Xerostomia: Integrated Efficacy and Safety Results From Two Prospective Randomized Clinical Trials," *Int J Radiat Oncol Biol Phys,* 1995, 31(3):661-9.

Rousseau P, "Pilocarpine in Radiation-Induced Xerostomia," *Am J Hosp Palliat Care,* 1995, 12(2):38-9.

Schuller DE, Stevens P, Clausen KP, et al, "Treatment of Radiation Side Effects With Oral Pilocarpine," *J Surg Oncol,* 1989, 42(4):272-6.

Wiseman LR and Faulds D, "Oral Pilocarpine: A Review of Its Pharmacological Properties and Clinical Potential in Xerostomia," *Drugs,* 1995, 49(1):143-55.

Pimecrolimus (pim e KROE li mus)

Brand Names: U.S. Elidel®

Brand Names: Canada Elidel®

Generic Availability (U.S.) No

Pharmacologic Category Calcineurin Inhibitor; Immunosuppressant Agent; Topical Skin Product

Use Short-term and intermittent long-term treatment of mild-to-moderate atopic dermatitis in patients not responsive to conventional therapy or when conventional therapy is not appropriate

Unlabeled Use Second-line treatment of oral lichen planus; treatment of intertriginous and facial psoriasis

Local Anesthetic/Vasoconstrictor Precautions No information available to require special precautions

Effects on Dental Treatment No significant effects or complications reported

Effects on Bleeding No information available to require special precautions

Adverse Effects

>10%:

Central nervous system: Headache (7% to 25%), fever (1% to 13%)

Local: Burning at application site (2% to 26%; tends to resolve/improve as lesions resolve)

Respiratory: Nasopharyngitis (8% to 27%), cough (2% to 16%), upper respiratory tract infection (4% to 19%), bronchitis (≤11%)

Miscellaneous: Influenza (3% to 13%)
1% to 10%:
Dermatologic: Skin infection (2% to 6%), folliculitis (1% to 6%), impetigo (2% to 4%), skin papilloma (warts) (≤3%), acne (≤2%), herpes simplex dermatitis (≤2%), molluscum contagiosum (≤2%), urticaria (≤1%)
Endocrine & metabolic: Dysmenorrhea (1% to 2%)
Gastrointestinal: Diarrhea (1% to 8%), gastroenteritis (≤7%), abdominal pain (≤4%), constipation (≤4%)
Local: Irritation at application site (≤6%), pruritus at application site (1% to 6%), erythema at application site (≤2%)
Ocular: Eye infection (≤1%)
Otic: Ear infection (1% to 6%), otitis media (1% to 3%)
Respiratory: Pharyngitis (1% to 8%), asthma (1% to 4%), asthma aggravated (≤4%), nasal congestion (1% to 3%), sinusitis (1% to 3%), epistaxis (≤3%), dyspnea (≤2%), pneumonia (≤2%), rhinorrhea (≤2%), wheezing (≤1%)
Miscellaneous: Viral infection (≤7%), tonsillitis (≤6%), hypersensitivity (3% to 5%), herpes simplex infection (≤4%), bacterial infection (1% to 2%)

Dosage
Atopic dermatitis (mild-to-moderate): Children ≥2 years, Adolescents, and Adults: Topical: Apply thin layer to affected area twice daily; rub in gently and completely. **Note:** Limit application to involved areas. Continue as long as signs and symptoms persist; discontinue if resolution occurs; re-evaluate if symptoms persist >6 weeks.
Oral lichen planus (unlabeled use): Adults: Topical: Apply twice daily for 1 month (Passeron, 2007; Volz, 2008)
Psoriasis (unlabeled use): Adults: Topical: Apply twice daily (Gribetz, 2004; Menter, 2009)

Mechanism of Action Penetrates inflamed epidermis to inhibit T cell activation by blocking transcription of proinflammatory cytokine genes such as interleukin-2, interferon gamma (Th1-type), interleukin-4, and interleukin-10 (Th2-type). Pimecrolimus binds to the intracellular protein FKBP-12, inhibiting calcineurin, which blocks cytokine transcription and inhibits T-cell activation. Prevents release of inflammatory cytokines and mediators from mast cells *in vitro* after stimulation by antigen/IgE.

Contraindications Hypersensitivity to pimecrolimus or any component of the formulation

Warnings/Precautions [U.S. Boxed Warning]: Topical calcineurin inhibitors (including pimecrolimus) have been associated with rare cases of lymphoma and skin malignancy. Avoid use on malignant or premalignant skin conditions (eg, cutaneous T-cell lymphoma). Topical calcineurin agents are considered second-line therapies in the treatment of atopic dermatitis/eczema, and should be limited to use in patients who have failed treatment with other therapies. **[U.S. Boxed Warning]: They should be used for short-term and intermittent treatment using the minimum amount necessary for the control of symptoms should be used.** Application should be limited to involved areas. Diagnosis should be reconfirmed if sign/symptoms do not improve within 6 weeks of treatment. Safety of intermittent use for >1 year has not been established.

May cause local symptoms (eg, burning, soreness, stinging) during first few days of treatment; usually self-resolving. Should not be used in immunocompromised patients. Do not apply to areas of active bacterial or viral infection; local infections at the treatment site should be resolved prior to therapy. Patients with atopic dermatitis are predisposed to skin infections, and pimecrolimus therapy has been associated with risk of developing eczema herpeticum, varicella zoster, and herpes simplex. Papilloma/warts have been observed with use; discontinue pimecrolimus until resolution if worsening or do not respond to conventional treatment. Pimecrolimus may be associated with development of lymphadenopathy; possible infectious causes should be investigated. Discontinue use in patients with unknown cause of lymphadenopathy or acute infectious mononucleosis. Not recommended for use in patients with skin disease which may increase the potential for systemic absorption (eg, Netherton's syndrome). Avoid artificial or natural sunlight exposure, even when pimecrolimus is not on the skin. Safety not established in patients with generalized erythroderma. **[U.S. Boxed Warning]: The use of pimecrolimus in children <2 years of age is not recommended,** particularly since the effect on immune system development is unknown.

Drug Interactions
Metabolism/Transport Effects Substrate of CYP3A4 (minor); **Note:** Assignment of Major/Minor substrate status based on clinically relevant drug interaction potential

Avoid Concomitant Use
Avoid concomitant use of Pimecrolimus with any of the following: Immunosuppressants

Increased Effect/Toxicity
Pimecrolimus may increase the levels/effects of: Immunosuppressants

The levels/effects of Pimecrolimus may be increased by: CYP3A4 Inhibitors (Moderate); CYP3A4 Inhibitors (Strong)

Decreased Effect There are no known significant interactions involving a decrease in effect.

Ethanol/Nutrition/Herb Interactions Ethanol: Avoid ethanol (topical pimecrolimus may increase the potential for experiencing facial flushing following the consumption of alcoholic beverages).

Pregnancy Risk Factor C
Pregnancy Considerations Adverse events were not observed in animal reproduction studies following topical application. Experience with pimecrolimus use in pregnant women is limited.

Lactation Excretion in breast milk unknown/not recommended
Breast-Feeding Considerations It is not known if pimecrolimus is excreted in breast milk. Due to the potential for serious adverse reactions in the nursing infant, breast-feeding is not recommended.

Dosage Forms
Cream, topical:
Elidel® 1% (30 g, 60 g, 100 g)

Pimozide (PI moe zide)

Related Information
Clinical Risk Related to Drugs Prolonging QT Interval *on page 1510*
Brand Names: U.S. Orap®
Brand Names: Canada Apo-Pimozide®; Orap®; PMS-Pimozide
Pharmacologic Category Antipsychotic Agent, Typical
Use Suppression of severe motor and phonic tics in patients with Tourette's disorder who have failed to respond satisfactorily to standard treatment

Unlabeled Use Psychosis; reported use in individuals with delusions focused on physical symptoms (ie, preoccupation with parasitic infestation); Huntington's chorea

Local Anesthetic/Vasoconstrictor Precautions Pimozide is one of the drugs confirmed to prolong the QT interval and is accepted as having a risk of causing torsade de pointes. The risk of drug-induced torsade de pointes is extremely low when a single QT interval prolonging drug is prescribed. In terms of epinephrine, it is not known what effect vasoconstrictors in the local anesthetic regimen will have in patients with a known history of congenital prolonged QT interval or in patients taking any medication that prolongs the QT interval. Until more information is obtained, it is suggested that the clinician consult with the physician prior to the use of a vasoconstrictor in suspected patients, and that the vasoconstrictor (epinephrine, mepivacaine and levonordefrin [Carbocaine® 2% with Neo-Cobefrin®]) be used with caution.

Effects on Dental Treatment Key adverse event(s) related to dental treatment: Tourette's disorder: Xerostomia and increased salivation (normal salivary flow resumes upon discontinuation), taste disturbance, and dysphagia.

Effects on Bleeding No information available to require special precautions

Adverse Effects

Frequencies as reported in adults (limited data) and/ or children with Tourette's disorder:

>10%:

Central nervous system: Sedation (70%), akathisia (40%), akinesia (40%), drowsiness (35%), behavior changes (22% to 25%), somnolence (up to 25% in children)

Gastrointestinal: Xerostomia (25%), constipation (20%)

Genitourinary: Impotence (15%)

Neuromuscular & skeletal: Muscle tightness (15%), weakness (14%)

Ocular: Accommodation decreased (20%), visual disturbance (3% to 20%)

1% to 10%:

Cardiovascular: Abnormal ECG (3%)

Central nervous system: Depression (10%), insomnia (10%), speech disorder (10%), nervousness (5% to 6%), headache (3% to 5%), dreams abnormal (3%), hyperkinesias (3%)

Dermatologic: Rash (3%)

Gastrointestinal: Salivation increased (6%), appetite increased (5%), diarrhea (5%), taste disturbance (5%), thirst (5%), dysphagia (3%)

Neuromuscular & skeletal: Rigidity (10%), stooped posture (10%), handwriting change (5%), myalgia (3%), torticollis (3%), tremor (3%)

Ocular: Photophobia (5%)

Frequency not defined, postmarketing, and/or case reports (some reported for disorders other than Tourette's disorder): Anorexia, blurred vision, cataracts, chest pain, diaphoresis, dizziness, excitement; extrapyramidal symptoms (dystonia, pseudoparkinsonism, tardive dyskinesia); GI distress, gingival hyperplasia (case report), hemolytic anemia, hyper-/hypotension, hyponatremia, libido decreased, nausea, neuroleptic malignant syndrome, nocturia, orthostatic hypotension, palpitation, periorbital edema, polyuria, QT_c prolongation, seizure, skin irritation, syncope, tachycardia, ventricular arrhythmia, vomiting, weight gain/loss

General Dosage Range Dosage adjustment recommended in patients who develop toxicities or those with a CYP2D6 poor metabolizer status.

Oral:

Children 2-12 years: Initial: 0.05 mg/kg once daily (preferably bedtime); Maintenance: 2-4 mg once daily (maximum: 10 mg/day [0.2 mg/kg/day])

Children >12 years and Adults: Initial: 1-2 mg in divided doses (maximum: 10 mg/day [0.2 mg/kg/day])

Mechanism of Action Pimozide, a diphenylbutylperidine conventional antipsychotic, is a potent centrally-acting dopamine-receptor antagonist resulting in its characteristic neuroleptic effects

Pharmacodynamics/Kinetics

Half-life Elimination ~55 hours

Time to Peak Serum: 6-8 hours (range: 4-12 hours)

Pregnancy Risk Factor C

Pregnancy Considerations Adverse events were observed in some animal reproduction studies. Antipsychotic use during the third trimester of pregnancy has a risk for abnormal muscle movements (extrapyramidal symptoms [EPS]) and withdrawal symptoms in newborns following delivery. Symptoms in the newborn may include agitation, feeding disorder, hypertonia, hypotonia, respiratory distress, somnolence, and tremor; these effects may be self-limiting or require hospitalization. There are no adequate and well-controlled studies in pregnant women. Use only if potential benefit justifies risk to the fetus.

Dental Comment Pimozide is known to prolong the QT interval. The QT interval is measured as the time and distance between the Q point of the QRS complex and the end of the T wave in the ECG tracing. After adjustment for heart rate, the QT interval is defined as prolonged if it is more than 450 msec in men and 460 msec in women. A long QT syndrome was first described in the 1950s and 60s as a congenital syndrome involving QT interval prolongation and syncope and sudden death. Some of the congenital long QT syndromes were characterized by a peculiar electrocardiographic appearance of the QRS complex involving a premature atria beat followed by a pause, then a subsequent sinus beat showing marked QT prolongation and deformity. This type of cardiac arrhythmia was originally termed "torsade de pointes" (translated from the French as "twisting of the points"). Pimozide is considered as having a risk of causing torsade de pointes. Since it is not known what effect vasoconstrictors in the local anesthetic regimen will have in patients with a known history of congenital prolonged QT interval or in patients taking any medication that prolongs the QT interval, a medical consult is suggested.

Pindolol (PIN doe lole)

Related Information

Cardiovascular Diseases *on page 1492*

Brand Names: Canada Apo-Pindol®; Dom-Pindolol; Mylan-Pindolol; Novo-Pindol; Nu-Pindol; PMS-Pindolol; Sandoz-Pindolol; Teva-Pindolol; Visken®

Pharmacologic Category Beta-Blocker With Intrinsic Sympathomimetic Activity

Use Treatment of hypertension, alone or in combination with other agents

Unlabeled Use Potential augmenting agent for antidepressants; ventricular arrhythmias/tachycardia, antipsychotic-induced akathisia, situational anxiety; aggressive behavior associated with dementia

◀ **Local Anesthetic/Vasoconstrictor Precautions**
Use with caution; epinephrine has interacted with non-selective beta-blockers to result in initial hypertensive episode followed by bradycardia

Effects on Dental Treatment Pindolol is a nonselective beta-blocker and may enhance the pressor response to epinephrine, resulting in hypertension and bradycardia. Many nonsteroidal anti-inflammatory drugs, such as ibuprofen and indomethacin, can reduce the hypotensive effect of beta-blockers after 3 or more weeks of therapy with the NSAID. Short-term NSAID use (ie, 3 days) requires no special precautions in patients taking beta-blockers.

Effects on Bleeding No information available to require special precautions

Adverse Effects
1% to 10%:
Cardiovascular: Edema (6%), chest pain (3%), bradycardia (≤2%), heart block (≤2%), hypotension (≤2%), syncope (≤2%), tachycardia (≤2%), palpitation (≤1%)
Central nervous system: Insomnia (10%), dizziness (9%), fatigue (8%), nervousness (7%), nightmares/vivid dreams (5%), anxiety (≤2%), lethargy (≤2%)
Dermatologic: Hyperhidrosis (≤2%), pruritus (1%)
Gastrointestinal: Nausea (5%), diarrhea (≤2%), vomiting (≤2%), weight gain (≤2%)
Genitourinary: Impotence (≤2%)
Hematologic: Claudication (≤2%)
Hepatic: ALT increased (7%), AST increased (7%)
Neuromuscular & skeletal: Muscle pain (10%), arthralgia (7%), weakness (4%), paresthesia (3%), muscle cramps (3%)
Ocular: Burning eyes (≤2%), visual disturbances (≤2%), eye discomfort (≤2%)
Renal: Polyuria (≤2%)
Respiratory: Dyspnea (5%), wheezing (≤2%)
Miscellaneous: Cold extremities (≤2%)
Other adverse reactions (noted with other beta-adrenergic-blocking agents that should be considered potential adverse events with pindolol): Agranulocytosis, alopecia, catatonia, clouded sensorium, disorientation, emotional lability, fever, intensification of pre-existing AV block, ischemic colitis, laryngospasm, mental depression, mesenteric artery thrombosis, nonthrombocytopenic purpura, Peyronie's disease, rash (erythematous), respiratory distress, short-term memory loss, thrombocytopenic purpura

General Dosage Range Dosage adjustment recommended in patients with hepatic impairment
Oral:
Adults: Initial: 5 mg twice daily; Maintenance: 10-40 mg twice daily (maximum: 60 mg/day)
Elderly: Initial: 5 mg once daily

Mechanism of Action Blocks both beta$_1$- and beta$_2$-receptors and has mild intrinsic sympathomimetic activity; pindolol has negative inotropic and chronotropic effects and can significantly slow AV nodal conduction. Augmentive action of antidepressants thought to be mediated via a serotonin 1A autoreceptor antagonist.

Pharmacodynamics/Kinetics
Half-life Elimination 3-4 hours; prolonged with advanced age, and cirrhosis (range: 2.5-30 hours)
Time to Peak Serum: ~1 hour
Pregnancy Risk Factor B
Pregnancy Considerations Adverse effects were not observed in animal reproduction studies. Pindolol crosses placenta and is measurable in the cord blood and amniotic fluid. In a cohort study, an increased risk of cardiovascular defects was observed following maternal use of beta-blockers during pregnancy. Intrauterine

growth restriction (IUGR), small placentas, as well as fetal/neonatal bradycardia, hypoglycemia, and/or respiratory depression have been observed following in utero exposure to beta-blockers as a class. Adequate facilities for monitoring infants at birth should be available. Untreated chronic maternal hypertension and pre-eclampsia are also associated with adverse events in the fetus, infant, and mother. The clearance and volume of distribution of pindolol are increased during pregnancy. Pindolol has been evaluated for the treatment of hypertension in pregnancy but other agents may be more appropriate for use.

Pindolol and Hydrochlorothiazide (PIN doe lole & hye droe klor oh THYE a zide)

Related Information
Hydrochlorothiazide on page 687
Pindolol on page 1095
Brand Names: Canada Viskazide®
Pharmacologic Category Beta-Blocker With Intrinsic Sympathomimetic Activity; Diuretic, Thiazide
Use Treatment of hypertension; not for initial therapy
Local Anesthetic/Vasoconstrictor Precautions
Use with caution; epinephrine has interacted with non-selective beta-blockers to result in initial hypertensive episode followed by bradycardia
Effects on Dental Treatment Pindolol is a nonselective beta-blocker and may enhance the pressor response to epinephrine, resulting in hypertension and bradycardia. Many nonsteroidal anti-inflammatory drugs, such as ibuprofen and indomethacin, can reduce the hypotensive effect of beta-blockers after 3 or more weeks of therapy with the NSAID. Short-term NSAID use (ie, 3 days) requires no special precautions in patients taking beta-blockers.
Effects on Bleeding No information available to require special precautions
Adverse Effects See individual agents.
General Dosage Range Oral: Adults: Usual dose: Pindolol 10-20 mg and hydrochlorothiazide 25-100 mg once daily (maximum daily dose: Pindolol 20 mg/hydrochlorothiazide 100 mg)
Mechanism of Action
Pindolol: Blocks both beta$_1$- and beta$_2$-receptors and has mild intrinsic sympathomimetic activity; has negative inotropic and chronotropic effects and can significantly slow AV nodal conduction. Augmentive action of antidepressants thought to be mediated via a serotonin 1A autoreceptor antagonism.
Hydrochlorothiazide: Inhibits sodium reabsorption in the distal tubules causing increased excretion of sodium and water as well as potassium and hydrogen ions
Pregnancy Considerations See individual agents.
Product Availability Not available in U.S.

Pioglitazone (pye oh GLI ta zone)

Related Information
Endocrine Disorders and Pregnancy on page 1517
Brand Names: U.S. Actos®
Brand Names: Canada Accel-Pioglitazone; Actos®; Apo-Pioglitazone®; Auro-Pioglitazone; Ava-Pioglitazone; CO Pioglitazone; Dom-Pioglitazone; JAMP-Pioglitazone; Mint-Pioglitazone; Mylan-Pioglitazone; Novo-Pioglitazone; PHL-Pioglitazone; PMS-Pioglitazone; PRO-Pioglitazone; RAN™-Pioglitazone; ratio-Pioglitazone; Sandoz-Pioglitazone; Teva-Pioglitazone; ZYM-Pioglitazone

Generic Availability (U.S.) Yes

Pharmacologic Category Antidiabetic Agent, Thiazolidinedione

Use Type 2 diabetes mellitus (noninsulin dependent, NIDDM), monotherapy or combination therapy: Adjunct to diet and exercise, to improve glycemic control

Local Anesthetic/Vasoconstrictor Precautions No information available to require special precautions

Effects on Dental Treatment Key adverse event(s) related to dental treatment: Tooth disorder. Pioglitazone-dependent diabetics should be appointed for dental treatment in morning in order to minimize chance of stress-induced hypoglycemia.

Effects on Bleeding No information available to require special precautions

Adverse Effects Adverse reactions and incidences reported are associated with monotherapy unless otherwise stated.

>10%:
Cardiovascular: Edema (combination trials: ≤27%)
Endocrine and metabolic: Hypoglycemia (combination trials: ≤27%)
Respiratory: Upper respiratory tract infection (13%)
1% to 10%:
Cardiovascular: Heart failure (combination trials: ≤8%)
Central nervous system: Headache (9%)
Neuromuscular & skeletal: Fractures (females: ≤5%), myalgia (5%)
Respiratory: Sinusitis (6%), pharyngitis (5%)
Frequency not defined: HDL-cholesterol increased, hematocrit/hemoglobin decreased, serum triglycerides decreased, weight gain/loss

Dosage Type 2 diabetes: Adults: Oral:
Initial:
U.S. labeling: Monotherapy or combination therapy: 15-30 mg once daily
Patients with heart failure (NYHA Class I or II): Monotherapy or combination therapy: 15 mg once daily
Note: Not recommended in patients with symptomatic heart failure
Canadian labeling: Monotherapy or combination therapy (with a sulfonylurea or metformin): 15-30 mg once daily
Dosage titration: If response is inadequate based on HbA1c, the dosage may be increased in 15 mg increments with careful monitoring of adverse effects (eg, weight gain, edema, signs/symptoms of heart failure); maximum recommended dose: 45 mg once daily
Dosage adjustment for hypoglycemia with combination therapy:
With an insulin secretagogue (eg, sulfonylurea): Decrease the insulin secretagogue dose.
With insulin: Decrease insulin dose by 10% to 25%
Dosage adjustment with strong CYP2C8 inhibitors (eg, gemfibrozil): Maximum recommended dose: 15 mg once daily

Dosage adjustment in renal impairment: No dosage adjustment necessary.

Dosage adjustment in hepatic impairment: No dosage adjustment necessary (mean AUC values are unaffected in Child-Pugh grade B/C compared to healthy subjects); however, liver injury has been associated with use.

U.S. labeling:
Prior to initiation: Evaluate liver tests (ALT, AST, alkaline phosphatase, total bilirubin) and if abnormal, initiate with caution.

During therapy: If liver injury is suspected (eg, fatigue, jaundice, dark urine): Interrupt therapy, measure serum liver tests, and investigate possible etiologies:
If ALT >3 x ULN **and** without alternative etiologies: Do not reinitiate therapy.
If ALT >3 x ULN **and** total bilirubin >2 x ULN **and** without alternative etiologies: Do not reinitiate therapy (these patients are at increased risk for severe drug-induced hepatotoxicity).
If ALT elevated (but <3 x ULN) **or** total bilirubin elevated (but <2 x ULN) **and** with an alternative etiology: May reinitiate with caution.
Canadian labeling:
Severe hepatic impairment: Use is contraindicated.
Prior to initiation:
If ALT > 2.5 x ULN or clinical evidence of active liver disease: Do not initiate therapy.
If ALT 1-2.5 x ULN: Initiate therapy with caution and investigate etiology of liver enzyme elevation.
During therapy:
If ALT levels >3 x ULN: Recheck levels immediately and if ALT elevation >3 x ULN persists, discontinue therapy.
If ALT 1-2.5 x ULN: Continue therapy with caution and investigate etiology of liver enzyme elevation.

Mechanism of Action Thiazolidinedione antidiabetic agent that lowers blood glucose by improving target cell response to insulin, without increasing pancreatic insulin secretion. It has a mechanism of action that is dependent on the presence of insulin for activity. Pioglitazone is a potent and selective agonist for peroxisome proliferator-activated receptor-gamma (PPARgamma). Activation of nuclear PPARgamma receptors influences the production of a number of gene products involved in glucose and lipid metabolism. PPARgamma is abundant in the cells within the renal collecting tubules; fluid retention results from stimulation by thiazolidinediones which increases sodium reabsorption.

Contraindications Hypersensitivity to pioglitazone or any component of the formulation; NYHA Class III/IV heart failure (initiation of therapy)

Canadian labeling: Additional contraindications (not is U.S. labeling): Any stage of heart failure (eg, NYHA Class I, II, III, IV); serious hepatic impairment; active bladder cancer; history of bladder cancer; uninvestigated macroscopic hematuria; pregnancy

Warnings/Precautions [U.S. Boxed Warning]: Thiazolidinediones, including pioglitazone, may cause or exacerbate heart failure; closely monitor for signs and symptoms of heart failure (eg, rapid weight gain, dyspnea, edema), particularly after initiation or dose increases; if heart failure develops, treat accordingly and consider dose reduction or discontinuation of pioglitazone. Not recommended for use in any patient with symptomatic heart failure. Initiation of therapy is contraindicated in patients with NYHA class III or IV heart failure. If used in patients with NYHA class I or II (systolic heart failure), initiate at lowest dosage and monitor closely. In Canada, use in any stage of heart failure (NYHA I, II, III, IV) is contraindicated.. Dose reduction or discontinuation is recommended if heart failure suspected. Dose-related edema and weight gain observed with use; use with caution in patients with edema; monitor for signs/symptoms of heart failure.

Should not be used in diabetic ketoacidosis. Mechanism requires the presence of insulin; therefore use in type 1 diabetes is not recommended. Use with caution in premenopausal, anovulatory women - may result in a resumption of ovulation, increasing the risk of pregnancy. Use with caution in patients with anemia (may reduce hemoglobin and hematocrit). Increased incidence of bone fractures in females treated with pioglitazone; majority of fractures occurred in the lower limb and distal upper limb. Clinical trial data suggest an increased risk of bladder cancer in patients exposed to pioglitazone; risk may be increased with duration of use. Avoid use in patients with active bladder cancer and consider risks vs. benefits prior to initiating therapy in patients with a history of bladder cancer. In Canada, use is contraindicated in patients with active or a history of bladder cancer.

Hepatic failure, including fatalities, has been reported. Monitor for signs/symptoms of liver injury closely during therapy; discontinuation of therapy may be necessary. Due to this risk, serum liver function tests (ALT, AST, alkaline phosphatase, and total bilirubin) should be obtained prior to initiation in all patients. In patients with abnormal hepatic tests, therapy should be initiated with caution (Canadian labeling recommends avoiding use in patients with baseline ALT >3 x ULN). During therapy, if signs/symptoms of liver injury (eg, fatigue, anorexia, jaundice, dark urine, right upper abdominal discomfort) arise, interrupt pioglitazone therapy, obtain liver tests immediately, and evaluate alternative etiologies. Depending on the results of the liver tests and whether an alternative etiology is identified, discontinuation of therapy may be recommended. U.S. labeling states that routine periodic monitoring of serum liver tests during therapy is not necessary unless patient has liver disease or signs/symptoms of liver injury arise during use (Canadian labeling recommends periodic monitoring of liver enzymes in all patients per clinical judgment). Macular edema has been reported with thiazolidinedione use, including pioglitazone. Patients should be seen by an ophthalmologist if any visual symptoms arise during therapy and all diabetic patients should have regular eye exams.

Concomitant administration of pioglitazone with a strong CYP2C8 inhibitor increases pioglitazone exposure 3-fold; dosage adjustments are recommended if pioglitazone is coadministered with a strong CYP2C8 inhibitor (eg, gemfibrozil).Risk of hypoglycemia is increased when pioglitazone is combined with insulin or other diabetic medications; dosage adjustment of concomitant hypoglycemic agents may be necessary. Canadian labeling (not in U.S. labeling) states use with insulin **or** as part of triple therapy (pioglitazone in combination with a sulfonylurea and metformin) is not indicated. Use in pediatrics is not recommended; risks and adverse effects have not been evaluated in this population and there is a lack of long-term safety data.

Drug Interactions

Metabolism/Transport Effects Substrate of CYP2C8 (major), CYP3A4 (minor); **Note:** Assignment of Major/Minor substrate status based on clinically relevant drug interaction potential; **Inhibits** CYP2C19 (weak), CYP2C8 (moderate), CYP2C9 (weak); **Induces** CYP3A4 (weak/moderate)

Avoid Concomitant Use
Avoid concomitant use of Pioglitazone with any of the following: Axitinib

Increased Effect/Toxicity
Pioglitazone may increase the levels/effects of: CYP2C8 Substrates; Hypoglycemic Agents

The levels/effects of Pioglitazone may be increased by: CYP2C8 Inhibitors (Moderate); CYP2C8 Inhibitors (Strong); Deferasirox; Gemfibrozil; Herbs (Hypoglycemic Properties); Insulin; MAO Inhibitors; Mifepristone; Pegvisomant; Pregabalin; Salicylates; Selective Serotonin Reuptake Inhibitors; Trimethoprim

Decreased Effect
Pioglitazone may decrease the levels/effects of: ARIPiprazole; Axitinib; Saxagliptin

The levels/effects of Pioglitazone may be decreased by: Bile Acid Sequestrants; Corticosteroids (Orally Inhaled); Corticosteroids (Systemic); CYP2C8 Inducers (Strong); Loop Diuretics; Luteinizing Hormone-Releasing Hormone Analogs; Rifampin; Somatropin; Thiazide Diuretics

Ethanol/Nutrition/Herb Interactions
Ethanol: Caution with ethanol (may cause hypoglycemia).
Food: Peak concentrations are delayed when administered with food, but the extent of absorption is not affected. Pioglitazone may be taken without regard to meals.
Herb/Nutraceutical: Caution with alfalfa, aloe, bilberry, bitter melon, burdock, celery, damiana, fenugreek, garcinia, garlic, ginger, ginseng (American), gymnema, marshmallow, and stinging nettle (may cause hypoglycemia).

Dietary Considerations Dietary modification based on ADA recommendations is a part of therapy.

Pharmacodynamics/Kinetics
Onset of Action Delayed; Peak effect: Glucose control: Several weeks
Half-life Elimination Parent drug: 3-7 hours; Total: 16-24 hours
Time to Peak ~2 hours; delayed with food

Pregnancy Risk Factor C

Pregnancy Considerations Pioglitazone is classified as pregnancy category C due to adverse effects observed in animal studies. The use of pioglitazone in pregnant women is limited to very few case reports where pregnancy occurred during treatment for polycystic ovarian syndrome (PCOS); details concerning fetal outcomes are limited. Thiazolidinediones may cause ovulation in anovulatory premenopausal women, increasing the risk of pregnancy; adequate contraception in premenopausal women is recommended. Maternal hyperglycemia can be associated with adverse effects in the fetus, including macrosomia, neonatal hyperglycemia, and hyperbilirubinemia; the risk of congenital malformations is increased when the Hb A_{1c} above the normal range. Diabetes can also be associated with adverse effects in the mother. Poorly-treated diabetes may cause end-organ damage that may in turn negatively affect obstetric outcomes. Physiologic glucose levels should be maintained prior to and during pregnancy to decrease the risk of adverse events in the mother and the fetus. Until additional safety and efficacy data are obtained, the use of oral agents is generally not recommended as routine management of GDM or type 2 diabetes mellitus during pregnancy. Insulin is the drug of choice for the control of diabetes mellitus during pregnancy.

Lactation Excretion in breast milk unknown/not recommended

Breast-Feeding Considerations It is not known if pioglitazone is excreted in breast milk. Breast-feeding is not recommended by the manufacturer.

Dosage Forms
Tablet, oral: 15 mg, 30 mg, 45 mg
Actos®: 15 mg, 30 mg, 45 mg

Pioglitazone and Glimepiride
(pye oh GLI ta zone & GLYE me pye ride)

Related Information
Glimepiride *on page 658*
Pioglitazone *on page 1096*
Brand Names: U.S. Duetact™
Pharmacologic Category Antidiabetic Agent, Sulfonylurea; Antidiabetic Agent, Thiazolidinedione; Hypoglycemic Agent, Oral
Use Management of type 2 diabetes mellitus (noninsulin dependent, NIDDM) as an adjunct to diet and exercise in patients already treated with a thiazolidinedione and a sulfonylurea or who have inadequate control on either agent alone
Local Anesthetic/Vasoconstrictor Precautions No information available to require special precautions
Effects on Dental Treatment Pioglitazone-dependent patients with diabetes (noninsulin dependent, type 2) or glimepiride-dependent patients with diabetes (noninsulin dependent, type 2) should be appointed for dental treatment in morning in order to minimize chance of stress-induced hypoglycemia.
Effects on Bleeding No information available to require special precautions
Adverse Effects Also see individual agents.
>10%:
Cardiovascular: Peripheral edema (6% to 12%)
Endocrine & metabolic: Hypoglycemia (13% to 16%)
Gastrointestinal: Weight gain (9% to 13%)
Respiratory: Upper respiratory tract infection (12% to 15%)
1% to 10%:
Central nervous system: Headache (4% to 7%)
Gastrointestinal: Diarrhea (4% to 6%), nausea (4% to 5%)
Genitourinary: Urinary tract infection (6% to 7%)
Hematologic: Anemia (≤2%)
Neuromuscular & skeletal: Limb pain (4% to 5%)
General Dosage Range Dosage adjustment recommended in patients with renal impairment
Oral:
Adults:
Patients inadequately controlled on **glimepiride** alone: Initial dose: Pioglitazone 30 mg and glimepiride 2-4 mg once daily (maximum: 45 mg/day [pioglitazone]; 8 mg/day [glimepiride])
Patients inadequately controlled on **pioglitazone** alone: Initial dose: Pioglitazone 30 mg and glimepiride 2 mg once daily (maximum: 45 mg/day [pioglitazone]; 8 mg/day [glimepiride])
Elderly: Initial: Glimepiride 1 mg/day prior to initiating Duetact™
Mechanism of Action
Pioglitazone: A thiazolidinedione that lowers blood glucose by improving target cell response to insulin, without increasing pancreatic insulin secretion. It has a mechanism of action that is dependent on the presence of insulin for activity.

Glimepiride: A sulfonylurea that stimulates insulin release from the pancreatic beta cells; reduces glucose output from the liver; insulin sensitivity is increased at peripheral target sites.
Pregnancy Risk Factor C
Pregnancy Considerations Animal reproduction studies have not been conducted with this combination; therefore, pioglitazone/glimepiride is classified as pregnancy category C. See individual agents.

Pioglitazone and Metformin
(pye oh GLI ta zone & met FOR min)

Related Information
MetFORMIN *on page 882*
Pioglitazone *on page 1096*
Brand Names: U.S. Actoplus Met®; Actoplus Met® XR
Generic Availability (U.S.) Yes: Excludes variable release tablet
Pharmacologic Category Antidiabetic Agent, Biguanide; Antidiabetic Agent, Thiazolidinedione
Use Management of type 2 diabetes mellitus (noninsulin dependent, NIDDM) in patients already receiving a thiazolidinedione and metformin or who have inadequate control on either agent
Local Anesthetic/Vasoconstrictor Precautions No information available to require special precautions
Effects on Dental Treatment Pioglitazone-dependent patients with diabetes (noninsulin dependent, type 2) or metformin-dependent patients with diabetes (noninsulin dependent, type 2) should be appointed for dental treatment in morning in order to minimize chance of stress-induced hypoglycemia.
Effects on Bleeding No information available to require special precautions
Adverse Effects Also see individual agents. Percentages of adverse effects as reported with the combination product.
>10%:
Cardiovascular: Edema (lower limb, 3% to 11%)
Respiratory: Upper respiratory infection (12% to 16%)
1% to 10%:
Central nervous system: Headache (2% to 6%), dizziness (5%)
Endocrine & metabolic: Weight gain (3% to 7%)
Gastrointestinal: Diarrhea (5% to 6%), nausea (4% to 6%)
Genitourinary: Urinary tract infection (5% to 6%)
Hematologic: Anemia (≤2%)
Respiratory: Sinusitis (4% to 5%)
Dosage Type 2 diabetes mellitus:
Adults: Oral: Initial dose should be based on current dose of pioglitazone and/or metformin
Immediate release tablet:
Initial: Pioglitazone 15 mg plus metformin 500 mg twice daily **or** pioglitazone 15 mg plus metformin 850 mg tablets once or twice daily
Patients with heart failure (NYHA Class I or II): Initial: Pioglitazone 15 mg plus metformin 500 mg once daily **or** pioglitazone 15 mg plus metformin 850 mg once daily. **Note:** Not recommended in patients with symptomatic heart failure.
Dose titration: If necessary, may titrate gradually with careful monitoring of adverse effects (eg, weight gain, edema, signs/symptoms of heart failure). Maximum daily dose: Pioglitazone 45 mg/metformin 2550 mg. **Note:** Metformin daily doses >2000 mg may be better tolerated if given 3 times daily.

Variable release tablet: Initial: Pioglitazone 15-30 mg plus metformin 1000 mg once daily with evening meal. If necessary, titrate gradually with careful monitoring of adverse effects (eg, weight gain, edema, signs/symptoms of heart failure). Maximum daily dose: Pioglitazone 45 mg/metformin 2000 mg.

Elderly: *Immediate release or variable release tablet:* The initial and maintenance dosing should be conservative, due to the potential for decreased renal function (monitor). Generally, elderly patients should not be titrated to the maximum; do not use in patients ≥80 years of age unless normal renal function has been established.

Dosage adjustment for hypoglycemia with combination therapy:
With an insulin secretagogue (eg, sulfonylurea): Decrease the insulin secretagogue dose.
With insulin: Decrease insulin dose by 10% to 25%.

Dosage adjustment with strong CYP2C8 inhibitors (eg, gemfibrozil): Maximum recommended dose: Pioglitazone 15 mg plus metformin 850 mg daily

Dosage adjustment in renal impairment: *Immediate release or variable release tablet:* Contraindicated in patients with renal disease or renal dysfunction (serum creatinine ≥1.5 mg/dL in males or ≥1.4 mg/dL in females or abnormal clearance).

Dosage adjustment in hepatic impairment: *Immediate release or variable release:* Not recommended in hepatic impairment due to potential for lactic acidosis associated with metformin component.

Mechanism of Action

Pioglitazone is a thiazolidinedione antidiabetic agent that lowers blood glucose by improving target cell response to insulin, without increasing pancreatic insulin secretion. It has a mechanism of action that is dependent on the presence of insulin for activity.

Metformin decreases hepatic glucose production, decreasing intestinal absorption of glucose, and improves insulin sensitivity (increases peripheral glucose uptake and utilization).

Contraindications Hypersensitivity to pioglitazone, metformin, or any component of the formulation; NYHA Class III/IV heart failure (initiation of therapy); renal disease or renal dysfunction (serum creatinine ≥1.5 mg/dL in males or ≥1.4 mg/dL in females, or abnormal creatinine clearance which may also result from conditions such as cardiovascular collapse, acute myocardial infarction, and septicemia); acute or chronic metabolic acidosis with or without coma (including diabetic ketoacidosis); concurrent iodinated radiocontrast administration (manufacturer recommends temporary discontinuation of metformin)

Warnings/Precautions [U.S. Boxed Warning]: Lactic acidosis is a rare, but potentially severe consequence of therapy with metformin. Lactic acidosis should be suspected in any patient with diabetes receiving metformin with evidence of acidosis but without evidence of ketoacidosis. Discontinue metformin in clinical situations predisposing to hypoxemia, including conditions such as cardiovascular collapse, respiratory failure, acute myocardial infarction, acute congestive heart failure, and septicemia.

Metformin is substantially excreted by the kidney. The risk of accumulation and lactic acidosis increases with the degree of impairment of renal function. Patients with renal function below the limit of normal for their age should not receive metformin. In elderly patients, renal function should be monitored regularly; should not be used in any patient ≥80 years of age unless normal renal function is confirmed. Use of concomitant medications that may affect renal function (ie, affect tubular secretion) may also affect metformin disposition. Metformin should be withheld in patients with dehydration and/or prerenal azotemia. Metformin therapy should be temporarily discontinued prior to or at the time of intravascular administration of iodinated contrast media (potential for acute alteration in renal function). Metformin should be withheld for 48 hours after the radiologic study and restarted only after renal function has been confirmed as normal.

[U.S. Boxed Warning]: Thiazolidinediones, including pioglitazone, may cause or exacerbate heart failure; closely monitor for signs and symptoms of heart failure (eg, rapid weight gain, dyspnea, edema), particularly after initiation or dose increases; if heart failure develops, treat accordingly and consider dose reduction or discontinuation. Not recommended for use in any patient with symptomatic heart failure; initiation of therapy is contraindicated in patients with NYHA class III or IV heart failure. If used in patients with NYHA class I or II (systolic) heart failure, initiate at lowest dosage and monitor closely. In addition, metformin should be used with caution in patients with heart failure requiring pharmacologic management, particularly in unstable or acute heart failure due to risk of lactic acidosis secondary to hypoperfusion. Dose reduction or discontinuation is recommended if heart failure suspected. Dose-related edema and weight gain observed with pioglitazone use; use with caution in patients with edema; monitor for signs/symptoms of heart failure.

Avoid metformin use in patients with impaired liver function due to potential for lactic acidosis. Hepatic failure, including fatalities, has been reported with pioglitazone. Monitor for signs/symptoms of liver injury closely during therapy; discontinuation of therapy may be necessary. Due to the possible risk of drug-induced liver injury with pioglitazone use, serum liver tests (ALT, AST, alkaline phosphatase, and total bilirubin) should be obtained prior to initiation in all patients. In patients with abnormal hepatic tests, therapy should be initiated with caution. During therapy, if signs/symptoms of liver injury (eg, fatigue, anorexia, jaundice, dark urine, right upper abdominal discomfort) arise, interrupt therapy, obtain liver tests immediately, and evaluate alternative etiologies. Routine periodic monitoring of serum liver tests during therapy is not necessary unless patient has liver disease or signs/symptoms of liver injury arise during use. Idiosyncratic hepatotoxicity has been reported with another thiazolidinedione agent (troglitazone); avoid use in patients who previously experienced jaundice during troglitazone therapy. Instruct patients to avoid excessive acute or chronic ethanol use; ethanol may potentiate metformin's effect on lactate metabolism.

Mechanism of pioglitazone requires the presence of insulin; therefore, use in type 1 diabetes (insulin dependent, IDDM) or diabetic ketoacidosis is not recommended. It may be necessary to discontinue metformin and administer insulin if the patient is exposed to stress (fever, trauma, infection, surgery). Increased incidence of bone fractures in females treated with pioglitazone; majority of fractures occurred in the lower limb and distal upper limb. Consider risk of fracture prior to initiation and during use. Clinical trial data suggest an increased risk of bladder cancer in patients exposed to pioglitazone; risk may be increased with duration of use. Avoid use in patients with active bladder cancer and consider risks vs benefits prior to initiating therapy in patients with a history of bladder cancer.

Pioglitazone may decrease hemoglobin/hematocrit; effects may be related to increased plasma volume. Metformin may impair vitamin B_{12} absorption; monitor for anemia. Use pioglitazone with caution in premenopausal, anovulatory women; may result in a resumption of ovulation, increasing the risk of pregnancy. Macular edema has been reported with thiazolidinedione use, including pioglitazone. Patients should be seen by an ophthalmologist if any visual symptoms arise during therapy and all diabetic patients should have regular eye exams. The risk of hypoglycemia is increased when pioglitazone is combined with insulin or other diabetic medications; dosage adjustment of concomitant hypoglycemic agents may be necessary. Concomitant administration of pioglitazone with a strong CYP2C8 inhibitor increases pioglitazone exposure 3-fold; dosage adjustments are recommended if coadministered with a strong CYP2C8 inhibitor (eg, gemfibrozil).

Drug Interactions
Metabolism/Transport Effects Refer to individual components.

Avoid Concomitant Use
Avoid concomitant use of Pioglitazone and Metformin with any of the following: Axitinib

Increased Effect/Toxicity
Pioglitazone and Metformin may increase the levels/effects of: CYP2C8 Substrates; Dalfampridine; Dofetilide; Hypoglycemic Agents

The levels/effects of Pioglitazone and Metformin may be increased by: Carbonic Anhydrase Inhibitors; Cephalexin; Cimetidine; CYP2C8 Inhibitors (Moderate); CYP2C8 Inhibitors (Strong); Dalfampridine; Deferasirox; Gemfibrozil; Glycopyrrolate; Herbs (Hypoglycemic Properties); Insulin; Iodinated Contrast Agents; LamoTRIgine; MAO Inhibitors; Mifepristone; Pegvisomant; Pregabalin; Salicylates; Selective Serotonin Reuptake Inhibitors; Trimethoprim

Decreased Effect
Pioglitazone and Metformin may decrease the levels/effects of: ARIPiprazole; Axitinib; Saxagliptin; Trospium

The levels/effects of Pioglitazone and Metformin may be decreased by: Bile Acid Sequestrants; Corticosteroids (Orally Inhaled); Corticosteroids (Systemic); CYP2C8 Inducers (Strong); Loop Diuretics; Luteinizing Hormone-Releasing Hormone Analogs; Rifampin; Somatropin; Thiazide Diuretics

Ethanol/Nutrition/Herb Interactions See individual agents.

Dietary Considerations Immediate release tablets should be administered with meals. Variable release tablets should be administered with the evening meal. Avoid ethanol. Dietary modification based on ADA recommendations is a part of therapy. Monitor for signs and symptoms of vitamin B_{12} and/or folic acid deficiency; supplementation may be required.

Pregnancy Risk Factor C

Pregnancy Considerations Animal reproduction studies were not conducted with this combination; therefore, pioglitazone/metformin is classified as pregnancy category C. See individual agents.

Lactation
Metformin: Enters breast milk/not recommended
Pioglitazone: Excretion in breast milk unknown/not recommended

Breast-Feeding Considerations See individual agents.

Dosage Forms
Tablet, oral: 15/500: Pioglitazone 15 mg and metformin hydrochloride 500 mg; 15/850: Pioglitazone 15 mg and metformin hydrochloride 850 mg
Actoplus Met®: 15/500: Pioglitazone 15 mg and metformin 500 mg; 15/850: Pioglitazone 15 mg and metformin 850 mg

Tablet, variable release, oral:
Actoplus Met® XR: 15/1000: Pioglitazone 15 mg and metformin 1000 mg; 30/1000: Pioglitazone 30 mg and metformin 1000 mg

---

Piperacillin (pi PER a sil in)

Brand Names: Canada Piperacillin for Injection, USP
Pharmacologic Category Antibiotic, Penicillin
Use Treatment of susceptible infections such as septicemia, acute and chronic respiratory tract infections, skin and soft tissue infections, and urinary tract infections due to susceptible strains of *Pseudomonas*, *Proteus*, and *Escherichia coli* and *Enterobacter*; active against some streptococci and some anaerobic bacteria; febrile neutropenia (as part of combination regimen)

Local Anesthetic/Vasoconstrictor Precautions No information available to require special precautions

Effects on Dental Treatment Key adverse event(s) related to dental treatment: Prolonged use of penicillins may lead to development of oral candidiasis.

Effects on Bleeding May inhibit platelet aggregation (dose related). The clinical significance may be greater with those penicillins that are combined with a beta-lactamase inhibitor and/or with agents that have greater activity against specific enteric bacterial species.

Adverse Effects Frequency not defined.
Central nervous system: Confusion, convulsions, drowsiness, fever, Jarisch-Herxheimer reaction
Dermatologic: Rash, toxic epidermal necrolysis, urticaria
Endocrine & metabolic: Electrolyte imbalance, hypokalemia
Hematologic: Abnormal platelet aggregation and prolonged PT (high doses), agranulocytosis, Coombs' reaction (positive), hemolytic anemia, pancytopenia
Local: Thrombophlebitis
Neuromuscular & skeletal: Myoclonus
Renal: Acute interstitial nephritis, acute renal failure
Miscellaneous: Anaphylaxis, hypersensitivity reactions

General Dosage Range Dosage adjustment recommended in patients with renal impairment

I.M., I.V.:
Children: 200-300 mg/kg/day in divided doses every 4-6 hours
Adults: 2-4 g/dose every 4-6 hours (maximum: 24 g/day)

Mechanism of Action Inhibits bacterial cell wall synthesis by binding to one or more of the penicillin-binding proteins (PBPs); which in turn inhibits the final transpeptidation step of peptidoglycan synthesis in bacterial cell walls, thus inhibiting cell wall biosynthesis. Bacteria eventually lyse due to ongoing activity of cell wall autolytic enzymes (autolysins and murein hydrolases) while cell wall assembly is arrested.

Pharmacodynamics/Kinetics

Half-life Elimination Dose dependent; prolonged with moderately severe renal or hepatic impairment:

Neonates: 1-5 days old: 3.6 hours; >6 days old: 2.1-2.7 hours

Children: 1-6 months: 0.79 hour; 6 months to 12 years: 0.39-0.5 hour

Adults: 36-80 minutes

Time to Peak Serum: I.M.: 30-50 minutes

Pregnancy Considerations Adverse events have not been observed in animal reproduction studies. Maternal use of penicillins has generally not resulted in an increased risk of adverse fetal effects. Piperacillin crosses the placenta and distributes into the amniotic fluid. Due to pregnancy induced physiologic changes, some pharmacokinetic parameters of piperacillin may be altered. At term, the apparent volume of distribution of piperacillin is increased and peak concentrations are significantly lower. Total clearance is normal to increased at term. These changes continue into the early postpartum period.

Piperacillin and Tazobactam
(pi PER a sil in & ta zoe BAK tam)

Related Information

Piperacillin *on page 1101*

Brand Names: U.S. Zosyn®

Brand Names: Canada AJ-PIP/TAZ; Piperacillin and Tazobactam for Injection; Tazocin®

Pharmacologic Category Antibiotic, Penicillin

Use Treatment of moderate-to-severe infections caused by susceptible organisms, including infections of the lower respiratory tract (community-acquired pneumonia, nosocomial pneumonia); uncomplicated and complicated skin and skin structures (including diabetic foot infections); gynecologic (endometritis, pelvic inflammatory disease); and intra-abdominal infections (appendicitis with rupture/abscess, peritonitis). Tazobactam expands activity of piperacillin to include beta-lactamase producing strains of *S. aureus*, *H. influenzae*, *E. coli*, *Bacteroides* spp, and other gram-positive and gram-negative aerobic and anaerobic bacteria.

Unlabeled Use Treatment of moderate-to-severe infections caused by susceptible organisms, including urinary tract infections, bone and joint infections, septicemia, endocarditis, and cystic fibrosis exacerbations

Local Anesthetic/Vasoconstrictor Precautions No information available to require special precautions

Effects on Dental Treatment Key adverse event(s) related to dental treatment: Prolonged use of penicillins may lead to development of oral candidiasis.

Effects on Bleeding May inhibit platelet aggregation (dose related). The clinical significance may be greater with those penicillins that are combined with a beta-lactamase inhibitor and/or with agents that have greater activity against specific enteric bacterial species.

Adverse Effects

>10%: Gastrointestinal: Diarrhea (7% to 11%)

1% to 10%:

Cardiovascular: Hypertension (2%), chest pain (1%), edema (1%)

Central nervous system: Insomnia (7%), headache (8%), fever (2% to 5%), agitation (2%), pain (2%), anxiety (1% to 2%), dizziness (1% to 2%)

Dermatologic: Rash (4%), pruritus (3%)

Gastrointestinal: Constipation (1% to 8%), nausea (7%), vomiting (3% to 4%), dyspepsia (3%), stool changes (2%), abdominal pain (1% to 2%)

Hepatic: AST increased (1%)

Local: Local reaction (3%), phlebitis (1%)

Respiratory: Pharyngitis (2%), dyspnea (1%), rhinitis (1%)

Miscellaneous: Moniliasis (2%), sepsis (2%), infection (2%)

General Dosage Range Dosage adjustment recommended in patients with renal impairment

I.V.:

Children 2-8 months: 80 mg/kg every 8 hours

Children ≥9 months and ≤40 kg: 100 mg/kg every 8 hours

Children >40 kg: 4.5 g every 8 hours **or** 3.375 g every 6 hours

Adults: 3.375 g every 6 hours **or** 4.5 g every 6-8 hours (maximum: 18 g/day)

Mechanism of Action Piperacillin inhibits bacterial cell wall synthesis by binding to one or more of the penicillin-binding proteins (PBPs); which in turn inhibits the final transpeptidation step of peptidoglycan synthesis in bacterial cell walls, thus inhibiting cell wall biosynthesis. Bacteria eventually lyse due to ongoing activity of cell wall autolytic enzymes (autolysins and murein hydrolases) while cell wall assembly is arrested. Piperacillin exhibits time-dependent killing. Tazobactam inhibits many beta-lactamases, including staphylococcal penicillinase and Richmond-Sykes types 2, 3, 4, and 5, including extended spectrum enzymes; it has only limited activity against class 1 beta-lactamases other than class 1C types.

Pharmacodynamics/Kinetics

Half-life Elimination Piperacillin and tazobactam: 0.7-1.2 hours (unaffected by dose or duration of infusion)

Time to Peak Immediately following completion of 30-minute infusion

Pregnancy Risk Factor B

Pregnancy Considerations Adverse events have not been observed in animal reproduction studies. Piperacillin and tazobactam both cross the placenta and are found in the fetal serum, placenta, amniotic fluid, and fetal urine. When used during pregnancy, the clearance and volume of distribution of piperacillin/tazobactam are increased; half-life and AUC are decreased. Piperacillin/tazobactam is approved for the treatment of postpartum gynecologic infections, including endometritis or pelvic inflammatory disease, caused by susceptible organisms.

Pipotiazine (pip oh TYE a zeen)

Brand Names: Canada Piportil® L₄

Pharmacologic Category Antipsychotic Agent, Typical, Phenothiazine, Piperidine

Use Maintenance treatment of schizophrenia

Local Anesthetic/Vasoconstrictor Precautions No information available to require special precautions

Effects on Dental Treatment Key adverse event(s) related to dental treatment: Xerostomia and changes in salivation (normal salivary flow resumes upon discontinuation).

Effects on Bleeding No information available to require special precautions

Adverse Effects Frequency not defined.

Cardiovascular: Cardiac arrest, ECG changes, edema, hypotension, QT$_c$ prolongation, syncope, tachycardia, venous thromboembolism

Central nervous system: Agitation, anxiety, bizarre dreams, cerebral edema, depression, dizziness, drowsiness, EEG changes, excitement, extrapyramidal symptoms (akathisia, dyskinesia, dystonia, hyperreflexia, oculogyric crisis, opisthotonos, pseudoparkinsonism, rigidity, sialorrhea, tremor), fatigue, fever, headache, insomnia, paradoxical psychosis, restlessness, seizure, sleep disturbance, tardive dyskinesia

Dermatologic: Angioedema, eczema, epithelial keratopathy erythema, exfoliative dermatitis, dermatitis, photosensitivity, pruritus, rash, seborrhea, skin pigmentation (prolonged therapy), urticaria

Endocrine & metabolic: Galactorrhea, glucose intolerance, gynecomastia, hyperglycemia, libido (changes in), menstrual irregularities, thirst

Gastrointestinal: Adynamic ileus, anorexia, appetite increased, constipation, fecal impaction, nausea, salivation, vomiting, weight changes, xerostomia

Genitourinary: Bladder paralysis, impotence, incontinence, polyuria, priapism, urinary retention

Hematologic: Agranulocytosis, anemia, eosinophilia, leukopenia, pancytopenia, thrombocytopenia

Hepatic: Biliary stasis, cholestatic jaundice

Ocular: Blurred vision, corneal deposits (prolonged therapy), glaucoma, lenticular deposits, pigmentary retinopathy (prolonged therapy)

Respiratory: Nasal congestion, pneumonia, pneumonitis, pulmonary embolism

Miscellaneous: Diaphoresis increased, lupus-like syndrome

General Dosage Range I.M.:

Adults: Initial: 50-100 mg; Maintenance: 25-250 mg every 3-4 weeks

Elderly >50 years: Initial: <50 mg is recommended

Mechanism of Action Blocks postsynaptic mesolimbic dopaminergic receptors in the brain; depresses the release of hypothalamic and hypophyseal hormones. Relative to other piperidine phenothiazines, pipotiazine appears to be less sedating, with less potential to potentiate other CNS depressants, and may possess a lower propensity to cause hypotension. However, it has a relatively high propensity for cause extrapyramidal reactions. Pipotiazine palmitate is an ester of pipotiazine with a prolonged duration of action.

Pharmacodynamics/Kinetics

Onset of Action I.M.: 2-3 days

Duration of Action 3-6 weeks

Pregnancy Considerations Antipsychotic use during the third trimester of pregnancy has a risk for abnormal muscle movements (extrapyramidal symptoms [EPS]) and withdrawal symptoms in newborns following delivery. Symptoms in the newborn may include agitation, feeding disorder, hypertonia, hypotonia, respiratory distress, somnolence, and tremor; these effects may be self-limiting or require hospitalization.

Product Availability Not available in U.S.

Pirbuterol (peer BYOO ter ole)

Related Information

Respiratory Diseases *on page 1514*

Brand Names: U.S. Maxair® Autohaler®

Pharmacologic Category Beta$_2$ Agonist

Use Prevention and treatment of reversible bronchospasm including asthma

Local Anesthetic/Vasoconstrictor Precautions No information available to require special precautions

Effects on Dental Treatment Key adverse event(s) related to dental treatment: Xerostomia (normal salivary flow resumes upon discontinuation) and taste changes.

Effects on Bleeding No information available to require special precautions

Adverse Effects

>10%:

Central nervous system: Nervousness (7%)

Endocrine & metabolic: Serum glucose increased, serum potassium decreased

Neuromuscular & skeletal: Trembling (6%)

1% to 10%:

Cardiovascular: Palpitation (2%), tachycardia (1%)

Central nervous system: Headache (2%), dizziness (1%)

Gastrointestinal: Nausea (2%)

Respiratory: Cough (1%)

General Dosage Range Inhalation: *Children ≥12 years and Adults:* Prevention: 2 inhalations every 4-6 hours; Treatment: 2 inhalations at an interval of at least 1-3 minutes, followed by a third inhalation (maximum: 12 inhalations/day)

Mechanism of Action Pirbuterol is a beta$_2$-adrenergic agonist with a similar structure to albuterol, specifically a pyridine ring has been substituted for the benzene ring in albuterol. The increased beta$_2$ selectivity of pirbuterol results from the substitution of a tertiary butyl group on the nitrogen of the side chain, which additionally imparts resistance of pirbuterol to degradation by monoamine oxidase and provides a lengthened duration of action in comparison to the less selective previous beta-agonist agents.

Pharmacodynamics/Kinetics

Onset of Action Peak effect: Therapeutic: Oral: 2-3 hours with peak serum concentration of 6.2-9.8 mcg/L; Inhalation: 0.5-1 hour

Half-life Elimination 2-3 hours

Pregnancy Risk Factor C

Pregnancy Considerations Adverse events have been observed in some animal reproduction studies with oral administration. Beta-agonists may interfere with uterine contractility if administered during labor.

Pirfenidone

Brand Names: Canada Esbriet™

Pharmacologic Category Anti-inflammatory Agent; Antifibrotic Agent

Use Treatment of mild-to-moderate idiopathic pulmonary fibrosis

Local Anesthetic/Vasoconstrictor Precautions No information available to require special precautions

Effects on Dental Treatment No significant effects or complications reported

Effects on Bleeding No information available to require special precautions

Adverse Effects

>10%:

Central nervous system: Fatigue (22%)

Dermatologic: Rash (29%), photosensitivity reaction (12%)

Gastrointestinal: Nausea (33%), diarrhea (22%), dyspepsia (17%)

≥3% to 10%:

Central nervous system: Headache (10%), dizziness (9%), insomnia (4%), somnolence (3%)

Dermatologic: Macular rash (4%), pruritus (4%), sunburn (4%), erythema (3%)

Endocrine & metabolic: Hot flush (3%)

Gastrointestinal: Abdominal distension (9%), anorexia (9%), vomiting (9%), appetite decreased (8%), abdominal/stomach discomfort (3% to 8%), GERD (6%), weight loss (6%), abdominal pain (5% to 6%), flatulence (5%)

Hepatic: GGT increased (5%), ALT increased (4%), AST increased (3%)

Neuromuscular & skeletal: Weakness (6%)

Respiratory: Dyspnea (4%), upper respiratory tract infection (3%)

≥1% to <3%:

Central nervous system: Fever, lethargy, malaise

Cardiovascular: Angina pectoris, edema

Dermatologic: Dry skin, erythematous rash, hyperhidrosis, maculopapular rash, skin exfoliation, urticaria

Endocrine & metabolic: Dyslipidemia, gout, hyper-/hypoglycemia, hyper-/hyponatremia, hyperlipidemia, hypertriglyceridemia, hypokalemia, LDH increased, vitamin D deficiency

Gastrointestinal: Appetite increased, frequent bowel movements, gastritis, taste abnormal

Genitourinary: Urinary tract infection, vaginal infection

Hepatic: Liver function test abnormal

Neuromuscular & skeletal: Arthralgia, CPK increased, myalgia, chest pain (noncardiac), paresthesia, tremor

Respiratory: Cough, sinusitis, throat irritation

Miscellaneous: Influenza

Mechanism of Action Precise mechanisms of action have not been fully elucidated; however, pirfenidone may exert antifibrotic properties by decreasing fibroblast proliferation and the production of fibrosis-associated proteins and cytokines; may decrease the formation and accumulation of extracellular matrix (ie, collagen) in response to transforming growth factor-beta and platelet derived growth factor. Pirfenidone is also believed to exert anti-inflammatory properties by decreasing the accumulation of inflammatory cells resulting from a variety of stimuli.

Pharmacodynamics/Kinetics

Half-life Elimination ~2.4 hours

Time to Peak 30 minutes (fasting); prolonged to 3.5 hours by food (Rubino, 2009)

Pregnancy Considerations Animal reproductive studies have demonstrated placental transfer of pirfenidone and/or its metabolites to the fetus as well as prolonged gestation and decreased fetal viability. The manufacturer labeling recommends avoiding use of pirfenidone during pregnancy.

Product Availability Not Available in the U.S.

Piroxicam (peer OKS i kam)

Related Information

Rheumatoid Arthritis, Osteoarthritis, and Osteoporosis on page 1526

Temporomandibular Dysfunction (TMD), Chronic Pain, and Fibromyalgia on page 1590

Brand Names: U.S. Feldene®

Brand Names: Canada Apo-Piroxicam®; Dom-Piroxicam; Novo-Pirocam; Nu-Pirox; PMS-Piroxicam

Generic Availability (U.S.) Yes

Pharmacologic Category Nonsteroidal Anti-inflammatory Drug (NSAID), Oral

Use Symptomatic treatment of acute and chronic rheumatoid arthritis and osteoarthritis

Canadian labeling: Additional use (not in U.S. labeling): Symptomatic treatment of ankylosing spondylitis

Local Anesthetic/Vasoconstrictor Precautions No information available to require special precautions

Effects on Dental Treatment The dentist should be aware of the potential of abnormal coagulation. Caution should also be exercised in the use of NSAIDs in patients already on anticoagulant therapy with drugs such as warfarin (Coumadin®). See Effects on Bleeding.

Effects on Bleeding Nonselective NSAIDs, such as piroxicam, inhibit platelet aggregation and prolong bleeding time in some patients. Unlike aspirin, the NSAID effect on platelet function is quantitatively less, of shorter duration, and reversible. Normal platelet function should occur in ~5 elimination half-lives or in <10 hours after discontinuation of piroxicam. Concomitant use of other NSAIDs should be avoided.

Adverse Effects Reported with piroxicam or other NSAIDS:

1% to 10%:

Cardiovascular: Edema

Central nervous system: Dizziness, headache

Dermatologic: Pruritus, rash

Gastrointestinal: Abdominal pain, anorexia, bleeding, constipation, diarrhea, dyspepsia, flatulence, heartburn, nausea, perforation, ulcer, vomiting

Hematologic: Anemia, bleeding time increased

Hepatic: Liver enzymes increased

Otic: Tinnitus

Renal: Renal function abnormal

Dosage Osteoarthritis, rheumatoid arthritis: Adults: Oral: 10-20 mg daily in 1-2 divided doses (maximum dose: 20 mg daily)

Ankylosing spondylitis (Canadian labeling; not an approved use in U.S. labeling): Adults: Oral: 10-20 mg daily in 1-2 divided doses (maximum dose: 20 mg daily)

Elderly: Refer to adult dosing. Initiate therapy cautiously at low end of dosing range.

Dosing adjustment in renal impairment:

Mild-to-moderate impairment:

U.S. labeling: No dosage adjustment provided in manufacturer's labeling.

Canadian labeling: No specific dosage adjustment provided in manufacturer's labeling; however, a dosage reduction is recommended. Caution and close monitoring is advised for patients with Cl$_{cr}$ <60 mL/minute. Use is contraindicated in patients with deteriorating renal disease.

Severe impairment:

U.S. labeling: Use is not recommended (has not been studied); if therapy must be initiated, close monitoring is recommended.

Canadian labeling: Use is contraindicated in severe impairment (Cl$_{cr}$ <30 mL/minute) or in patients with deteriorating renal disease.

Dosing adjustment in hepatic impairment: No specific dosage adjustment provided in manufacturer's labeling; however, a dosage reduction is recommended. **Note:** Canadian labeling contraindicates use in severe impairment or in patients with active liver disease.

Mechanism of Action Reversibly inhibits cyclooxyge-nase-1 and 2 (COX-1 and 2) enzymes, which results in decreased formation of prostaglandin precursors; has antipyretic, analgesic, and anti-inflammatory properties

Other proposed mechanisms not fully elucidated (and possibly contributing to the anti-inflammatory effect to varying degrees), include inhibiting chemotaxis, altering lymphocyte activity, inhibiting neutrophil aggregation/activation, and decreasing proinflammatory cytokine levels.

Contraindications Hypersensitivity or asthma-type reactions to piroxicam, aspirin, other NSAIDs or any component of the formulation; perioperative pain in the setting of coronary artery bypass graft (CABG) surgery; active gastrointestinal bleeding

Canadian labeling: Additional contraindications (not in U.S. labeling): Recent or recurrent history of GI bleeding; active GI inflammatory disease; inflammatory bowel disease; cerebrovascular bleeding or other bleeding disorders; severe liver impairment or active liver disease; severe renal impairment (Cl_{cr} <30 mL/minute) or deteriorating renal disease; known hyperkalemia; children and adolescents <16 years of age; use in the third trimester of pregnancy; breast-feeding, severe uncontrolled heart failure

Warnings/Precautions [U.S. Boxed Warning]: NSAIDs are associated with an increased risk of adverse cardiovascular thrombotic events, including MI and stroke. Risk may be increased with duration of use or pre-existing cardiovascular risk factors or disease. Carefully evaluate individual cardiovascular risk profiles prior to prescribing. May cause new-onset hypertension or worsening of existing hypertension. Use caution with fluid retention or heart failure. Use is contraindicated in severe heart failure. Concurrent administration of ibuprofen, and potentially other nonselective NSAIDs, may interfere with aspirin's cardioprotective effect. **[U.S. Boxed Warning]: Use is contraindicated for treatment of perioperative pain in the setting of coronary artery bypass graft (CABG) surgery.** Risk of MI and stroke may be increased with use following CABG surgery.

Platelet adhesion and aggregation may be decreased; may prolong bleeding time; patients with coagulation disorders or who are receiving anticoagulants should be monitored closely. Anemia may occur; patients on long-term NSAID therapy should be monitored for anemia. Rarely, NSAID use may cause severe blood dyscrasias (eg, agranulocytosis, aplastic anemia, thrombocytopenia).

NSAID use may compromise existing renal function; dose-dependent decreases in prostaglandin synthesis may result from NSAID use, reducing renal blood flow which may cause renal decompensation. NSAID use may increase the risk for hyperkalemia. Patients with impaired renal function, dehydration, heart failure, liver dysfunction, those taking diuretics, and ACE inhibitors, and the elderly are at greater risk of renal toxicity and hyperkalemia. Rehydrate patient before starting therapy; monitor renal function closely. Use is contraindicated in severe renal failure (Canadian labeling also contraindicates use in patients with deteriorating renal disease or known hyperkalemia). Long-term NSAID use may result in renal papillary necrosis.

[U.S. Boxed Warning]: NSAIDs may increase risk of gastrointestinal irritation, inflammation, ulceration, bleeding, and perforation. These events may occur at any time during therapy and without warning. Use caution with a history of GI disease (bleeding or ulcers), concurrent therapy with aspirin, anticoagulants and/or corticosteroids, smoking, use of alcohol, the elderly or debilitated patients. When used concomitantly with ≤325 mg of aspirin, a substantial increase in the risk of gastrointestinal complications (eg, ulcer) occurs; concomitant gastroprotective therapy (eg, proton pump inhibitors) is recommended (Bhatt, 2008). Use is contraindicated with active peptic ulcers.

Use the lowest effective dose for the shortest duration of time, consistent with individual patient goals, to reduce risk of cardiovascular or GI adverse events. Alternate therapies should be considered for patients at high risk.

NSAIDs may cause serious skin adverse events including exfoliative dermatitis, Stevens-Johnson syndrome (SJS) and toxic epidermal necrolysis (TEN); discontinue use at first sign of skin rash or hypersensitivity. Anaphylactoid reactions may occur, even without prior exposure; patients with "aspirin triad" (bronchial asthma, aspirin intolerance, rhinitis) may be at increased risk. Do not use in patients who experience bronchospasm, asthma, rhinitis, or urticaria with NSAID or aspirin therapy. Use caution with other forms of asthma. A serum sickness-like reaction can rarely occur; watch for arthralgias, pruritus, fever, fatigue, and rash.

Use with caution in patients with decreased hepatic function (contraindicated in severe hepatic impairment). Closely monitor patients with any abnormal LFT. Severe hepatic reactions (eg, fulminant hepatitis, liver failure) have occurred with NSAID use, rarely; discontinue if signs or symptoms of liver disease develop, or if systemic manifestations occur. Use with caution in poor CYP2C9 metabolizers as hepatic metabolism may be reduced resulting in elevated serum concentrations.

NSAIDS may cause drowsiness, dizziness, blurred vision and other neurologic effects which may impair physical or mental abilities; patients must be cautioned about performing tasks which require mental alertness (eg, operating machinery or driving). Discontinue use with blurred or diminished vision and perform ophthalmologic exam. Monitor vision with long-term therapy.

In the elderly, avoid chronic use (unless alternative agents ineffective and patient can receive concomitant gastroprotective agent); nonselective oral NSAID use is associated with an increased risk of GI bleeding and peptic ulcer disease in older adults in high risk category (eg, >75 years or age or receiving concomitant oral/parenteral corticosteroids, anticoagulants, or antiplatelet agents) (Beers Criteria).

Withhold for at least 4-6 half-lives prior to surgical or dental procedures.

Drug Interactions

Metabolism/Transport Effects Substrate of CYP2C9 (major); **Note:** Assignment of Major/Minor substrate status based on clinically relevant drug interaction potential; **Inhibits** CYP2C9 (weak)

Avoid Concomitant Use

Avoid concomitant use of Piroxicam with any of the following: Floctafenine; Ketorolac (Nasal); Ketorolac (Systemic); NSAID (COX-2 Inhibitor); Omacetaxine

Increased Effect/Toxicity

Piroxicam may increase the levels/effects of: Agents with Antiplatelet Properties; Aliskiren; Aminoglycosides; Anticoagulants; Bisphosphonate Derivatives; Collagenase (Systemic); CycloSPORINE (Systemic); Dabigatran Etexilate; Deferasirox; Desmopressin;

Digoxin; Drotrecogin Alfa (Activated); Eplerenone; Haloperidol; Ibritumomab; Lithium; Methotrexate; Nonsteroidal Anti-Inflammatory Agents; NSAID (COX-2 Inhibitor); Omacetaxine; PEMEtrexed; Porfimer; Potassium-Sparing Diuretics; PRALAtrexate; Quinolone Antibiotics; Rivaroxaban; Salicylates; Thrombolytic Agents; Tositumomab and Iodine I 131 Tositumomab; Vancomycin; Vitamin K Antagonists

The levels/effects of Piroxicam may be increased by: ACE Inhibitors; Angiotensin II Receptor Blockers; Antidepressants (Tricyclic, Tertiary Amine); Corticosteroids (Systemic); CycloSPORINE (Systemic); CYP2C9 Inhibitors (Moderate); CYP2C9 Inhibitors (Strong); Dasatinib; Floctafenine; Glucosamine; Herbs (Anticoagulant/Antiplatelet Properties); Ketorolac (Nasal); Ketorolac (Systemic); Mifepristone; Multivitamins/Minerals (with ADEK, Folate, Iron); Nonsteroidal Anti-Inflammatory Agents; Omega-3 Fatty Acids; Pentosan Polysulfate Sodium; Pentoxifylline; Probenecid; Prostacyclin Analogues; Selective Serotonin Reuptake Inhibitors; Serotonin/Norepinephrine Reuptake Inhibitors; Sodium Phosphates; Tipranavir; Treprostinil; Vitamin E

Decreased Effect
Piroxicam may decrease the levels/effects of: ACE Inhibitors; Agents with Antiplatelet Properties; Aliskiren; Angiotensin II Receptor Blockers; Beta-Blockers; Eplerenone; HydrALAZINE; Loop Diuretics; Potassium-Sparing Diuretics; Salicylates; Selective Serotonin Reuptake Inhibitors; Thiazide Diuretics

The levels/effects of Piroxicam may be decreased by: Bile Acid Sequestrants; CYP2C9 Inducers (Strong); Nonsteroidal Anti-Inflammatory Agents; Peginterferon Alfa-2b; Salicylates

Ethanol/Nutrition/Herb Interactions
Ethanol: Avoid ethanol (may enhance gastric mucosal irritation).
Food: Onset of effect may be delayed if piroxicam is taken with food.
Herb/Nutraceutical: Avoid alfalfa, anise, bilberry, bladderwrack, bromelain, cat's claw, celery, chamomile, coleus, cordyceps, dong quai, evening primrose, fenugreek, feverfew, garlic, ginger, ginkgo biloba, ginseng (American, Panax, Siberian), grapeseed, green tea, guggul, horse chestnut seed, horseradish, licorice, prickly ash, red clover, reishi, SAMe (S-adenosylmethionine), sweet clover, turmeric, white willow (all have additional antiplatelet activity).

Dietary Considerations May be taken with food to decrease GI adverse effect.

Pharmacodynamics/Kinetics
Half-life Elimination 50 hours
Time to Peak 3-5 hours

Pregnancy Risk Factor C

Pregnancy Considerations Adverse events were not observed in the initial animal reproduction studies; therefore, the manufacturer classifies piroxicam as pregnancy category C. NSAID exposure during the first trimester is not strongly associated with congenital malformations; however, cardiovascular anomalies and cleft palate have been observed following NSAID exposure in some studies. The use of a NSAID close to conception may be associated with an increased risk of miscarriage. Nonteratogenic effects have been observed following NSAID administration during the third trimester including: Myocardial degenerative changes, prenatal constriction of the ductus arteriosus, fetal tricuspid regurgitation, failure of the ductus arteriosus to close postnatally; renal dysfunction or failure, oligohydramnios; gastrointestinal bleeding or perforation, increased risk of necrotizing enterocolitis; intracranial bleeding (including intraventricular hemorrhage), platelet dysfunction with resultant bleeding; pulmonary hypertension. Because they may cause premature closure of the ductus arteriosus, use of NSAIDs late in pregnancy should be avoided (use after 31 or 32 weeks gestation is not recommended by some clinicians). The chronic use of NSAIDs in women of reproductive age may be associated with infertility that is reversible upon discontinuation of the medication.

Lactation Enters breast milk/not recommended (AAP rates "compatible"; AAP 2001 update pending)

Breast-Feeding Considerations Piroxicam is excreted into breast milk. Breast-feeding is not recommended by the manufacturer.

Dosage Forms
Capsule, oral: 10 mg, 20 mg
  Feldene®: 10 mg, 20 mg

Pitavastatin (pi TA va sta tin)

Related Information
Cardiovascular Diseases *on page 1492*
Brand Names: U.S. Livalo®
Generic Availability (U.S.) No
Pharmacologic Category Antilipemic Agent, HMG-CoA Reductase Inhibitor
Use Adjunct to dietary therapy to reduce elevations in total cholesterol (TC), LDL-C, apolipoprotein B (Apo B), and triglycerides (TG), and to increase low HDL-C in patients with primary hyperlipidemia and mixed dyslipidemia
Local Anesthetic/Vasoconstrictor Precautions No information available to require special precautions
Effects on Dental Treatment No significant effects or complications reported
Effects on Bleeding No information available to require special precautions
Adverse Effects
2% to 10%:
  Gastrointestinal: Constipation (2% to 4%), diarrhea (2% to 3%)
  Neuromuscular & skeletal: Back pain (1% to 4%), myalgia (2% to 3%), pain in extremities (1% to 2%)
Additional class-related events or case reports (not necessarily reported with pitavastatin therapy): Cataracts, cirrhosis, dermatomyositis, eosinophilia, extraocular muscle movement impaired, fulminant hepatic necrosis, gynecomastia, hypersensitivity syndrome (symptoms may include anaphylaxis, angioedema, arthralgia, erythema multiforme, eosinophilia, hemolytic anemia, immune-mediated necrotizing myopathy (IMNM), interstitial lung disease, lupus syndrome, photosensitivity, polymyalgia rheumatica, positive ANA, purpura, Stevens-Johnson syndrome, toxic epidermal necrolysis, urticaria, vasculitis), ophthalmoplegia, peripheral nerve palsy, rhabdomyolysis, renal failure (secondary to rhabdomyolysis), thyroid dysfunction, tremor, vertigo
Dosage Oral: **Note:** Doses should be individualized according to the baseline LDL-cholesterol levels, the recommended goal of therapy, and patient response; adjustments should be made at intervals of 4 weeks.
Adults: Primary hyperlipidemia and mixed dyslipidemia: Initial: 2 mg once daily; may be increased to maximum 4 mg once daily

Dosage adjustment with concomitant medications:
  Erythromycin: Pitavastatin dose should not exceed 1 mg once daily
  Rifampin: Pitavastatin dose should not exceed 2 mg once daily

Dosing adjustment in renal impairment:
  Cl_{cr} 15-60 mL/minute/1.73 m^2 (not receiving hemodialysis): Initial: 1 mg once daily; maximum: 2 mg once daily
  ESRD: Initial: 1 mg once daily; maximum: 2 mg once daily

Dosing adjustment in hepatic impairment: Contraindicated in active liver disease or in patients with unexplained persistent elevations of serum transaminases

Mechanism of Action Inhibitor of 3-hydroxy-3-methylglutaryl coenzyme A (HMG-CoA) reductase, the rate-limiting enzyme in cholesterol synthesis (reduces the production of mevalonic acid from HMG-CoA); this then results in a compensatory increase in the expression of LDL receptors on hepatocyte membranes and a stimulation of LDL catabolism

Contraindications Hypersensitivity to pitavastatin or any component of the formulation; active liver disease including unexplained persistent elevations of hepatic transaminases; concurrent use with cyclosporine; pregnancy; breast-feeding

Warnings/Precautions Secondary causes of hyperlipidemia should be ruled out prior to therapy. Pitavastatin has not been studied when the primary lipid abnormality is chylomicron elevation (Fredrickson types I and V) or in familial dysbetalipoproteinemia (Fredrickson type III). May cause hepatic dysfunction; in all patients, liver function must be monitored prior to initiation of therapy; repeat LFTs if clinically indicated thereafter; routine periodic monitoring of liver enzymes is not necessary. Use with caution in patients who consume large amounts of ethanol or have a history of liver disease; use is contraindicated in patients with active liver disease or unexplained persistent elevations of serum transaminases. If serious hepatotoxicity with clinical symptoms and/or hyperbilirubinemia or jaundice occurs during treatment, interrupt therapy. If an alternate etiology is not identified, do not restart pitavastatin.

Myopathy and rhabdomyolysis with acute renal failure have occurred with use. Risk is dose related and is increased with concurrent use of lipid-lowering agents which may cause rhabdomyolysis (fibric acid derivatives or niacin at doses ≥1 g/day) or during concurrent use with erythromycin or protease inhibitors. Use caution in patients with renal impairment, inadequately treated hypothyroidism, and those taking other drugs associated with myopathy (eg, colchicine); these patients are predisposed to myopathy. Monitor closely if used with other drugs associated with myopathy. Weigh the risk versus benefit when combining any of these drugs with pitavastatin. Immune-mediated necrotizing myopathy (IMNM), an autoimmune-mediated myopathy, has been reported (rarely) with HMG-CoA reductase inhibitor therapy. IMNM presents as proximal muscle weakness with elevated CPK levels, which persists despite discontinuation of HMG-CoA reductase inhibitor therapy; additionally, muscle biopsy may show necrotizing myopathy with limited inflammation; immunosuppressive therapy (eg, corticosteroids, azathioprine) may be used for treatment. The manufacturer recommends temporary discontinuation for elective major surgery, acute medical or surgical conditions, or in any patient experiencing an acute or serious condition predisposing to renal failure (eg, sepsis, hypotension, trauma, uncontrolled seizures). However, based upon current evidence, HMG-CoA reductase inhibitor therapy should be continued in the perioperative period unless risk outweighs cardioprotective benefit. Patients should be instructed to report unexplained muscle pain, tenderness, weakness, or brown urine. Concurrent use with cyclosporine is contraindicated. Ensure patient is on the lowest effective pitavastatin dose. Use with caution in elderly patients, as these patients are predisposed to myopathy. Increases in Hb A_{1c} and fasting blood glucose have been reported with HMG-CoA reductase inhibitors; however, the benefits of statin therapy far outweigh the risk of dysglycemia.

Drug Interactions

Metabolism/Transport Effects Substrate of SLCO1B1, UGT1A3, UGT2B7

Avoid Concomitant Use
Avoid concomitant use of Pitavastatin with any of the following: CycloSPORINE (Systemic); Fusidic Acid; Gemfibrozil; Red Yeast Rice

Increased Effect/Toxicity
Pitavastatin may increase the levels/effects of: DAPTOmycin; Pazopanib; Trabectedin; Vitamin K Antagonists

The levels/effects of Pitavastatin may be increased by: Atazanavir; Bezafibrate; Boceprevir; Colchicine; CycloSPORINE (Systemic); Danazol; Eltrombopag; Fenofibrate; Fenofibric Acid; Fusidic Acid; Gemfibrozil; Macrolide Antibiotics; Niacin; Niacinamide; Red Yeast Rice; Rifamycin Derivatives; Sildenafil; Telaprevir

Decreased Effect
Pitavastatin may decrease the levels/effects of: Lanthanum

The levels/effects of Pitavastatin may be decreased by: Antacids; Bosentan; St Johns Wort

Ethanol/Nutrition/Herb Interactions
Ethanol: Avoid excessive ethanol consumption (due to potential hepatic effects).
Food: Red yeast rice contains an estimated 2.4 mg lovastatin per 600 mg rice.

Dietary Considerations May be taken with or without food; may take without regard to time of day. Red yeast rice contains an estimated 2.4 mg lovastatin per 600 mg rice.

Pharmacodynamics/Kinetics
Half-life Elimination ~12 hours
Time to Peak ~1 hour

Pregnancy Risk Factor X

Pregnancy Considerations Adverse events were observed in some animal reproduction studies. There are reports of congenital anomalies following maternal use of HMG-CoA reductase inhibitors in pregnancy; however, maternal disease, differences in specific agents used, and the low rates of exposure limit the interpretation of the available data (Godfrey, 2012; Lecarpentier, 2012). Cholesterol biosynthesis may be important in fetal development; serum cholesterol and triglycerides increase normally during pregnancy. The discontinuation of lipid lowering medications temporarily during pregnancy is not expected to have significant impact on the long term outcomes of primary hypercholesterolemia treatment.

◄ Use of pitavastatin is contraindicated in pregnancy. HMG-CoA reductase inhibitors should be discontinued prior to pregnancy (ADA, 2013). If treatment of dyslipidemias is needed in pregnant women or in women of reproductive age, other agents are preferred (Berglund, 2012; NCEP, 2002). The manufacturer recommends administration to women of childbearing potential only when conception is highly unlikely and patients have been informed of potential hazards.

Lactation Excretion in breast milk unknown/contraindicated

Breast-Feeding Considerations It is not known if pitavastatin is excreted into breast milk. Due to the potential for serious adverse reactions in a nursing infant, use while breast-feeding is contraindicated by the manufacturer.

Dosage Forms
Tablet, oral:
Livalo®: 1 mg, 2 mg, 4 mg

Plerixafor (pler IX a fore)

Brand Names: U.S. Mozobil™
Pharmacologic Category Hematopoietic Stem Cell Mobilizer
Use Mobilization of hematopoietic stem cells (HSC) for collection and subsequent autologous transplantation (in combination with filgrastim) in patients with non-Hodgkin's lymphoma (NHL) and multiple myeloma (MM)
Local Anesthetic/Vasoconstrictor Precautions No information available to require special precautions
Effects on Dental Treatment Key adverse event(s) related to dental treatment: Xerostomia (normal salivary flow resumes upon discontinuation).
Effects on Bleeding No information available to require special precautions
Adverse Effects Adverse reactions reported with filgrastim combination therapy.
>10%:
Central nervous system: Fatigue (27%), headache (22%), dizziness (11%)
Gastrointestinal: Diarrhea (37%), nausea (34%)
Local: Injection site reactions (34%, including erythema, hematoma, hemorrhage, induration, inflammation, irritation, pain, paresthesia, pruritus, rash, swelling, urticaria)
Neuromuscular & skeletal: Arthralgia (13%)
5% to 10%:
Central nervous system: Insomnia (7%)
Gastrointestinal: Vomiting (10%), flatulence (7%)
General Dosage Range Dosage adjustment recommended in patients with renal impairment
SubQ: *Adults:* 0.24 mg/kg/day (maximum dose: 40 mg/day)
Mechanism of Action Reversibly inhibits binding of stromal cell-derived factor-1-alpha (SDF-1α), expressed on bone marrow stromal cells, to the CXC chemokine receptor 4 (CXCR4), resulting in mobilization of hematopoietic stem and progenitor cells from bone marrow into peripheral blood. Plerixafor used in combination with filgrastim results in synergistic increase in CD34+ cell mobilization. Mobilized CD34+ cells are capable of engrafting with extended repopulating capacity.
Pharmacodynamics/Kinetics
Onset of Action Peak CD34+ mobilization: Plerixafor monotherapy: 6-9 hours after administration; Plerixafor + filgrastim: 10-14 hours
Duration of Action WBC counts return toward baseline at ~24 after administration

Half-life Elimination Terminal: 3-6 hours
Time to Peak Plasma: SubQ: 30-60 minutes
Pregnancy Risk Factor D
Pregnancy Considerations Adverse effects (including fetal mortality, decreased fetal weights, and teratogenicity) have been reported in animal studies. May cause fetal harm if administered to pregnant women. There are no adequate and well-controlled studies in pregnant women. Women of childbearing potential should use effective contraceptive measures to avoid becoming pregnant during treatment.

Pneumococcal Conjugate Vaccine (10-Valent) (noo moe KOK al KON ju gate vak SEEN, ten vay lent)

Brand Names: Canada Synflorix™
Pharmacologic Category Vaccine, Inactivated (Bacterial)
Use Immunization of infants and children against *Streptococcus pneumoniae* infection and invasive diseases caused by serotypes included in the vaccine
Local Anesthetic/Vasoconstrictor Precautions No information available to require special precautions
Effects on Dental Treatment No significant effects or complications reported
Effects on Bleeding No information available to require special precautions
Adverse Effects In Canada, adverse reactions may be reported to local provincial/territorial health agencies or to the Vaccine Safety Section at Public Health Agency of Canada (1-866-844-0018).
Frequency not always defined:
>10%:
Central nervous system: Irritability (51% to 66%), drowsiness (33% to 58%), fever (≥38°C rectally ages <2 years: 26% to 37%)
Gastrointestinal: Loss of appetite (17% to 31%)
Local: Injection site reactions: Pain (23% to 57%), redness (38% to 53%), swelling (28% to 37%)
1% to 10%:
Central nervous system: Fever (>39°C rectally age <2 years: 2% to 3%; ≥38°C rectally age 2-5 years)
Local: Injection site induration
General Dosage Range I.M.:
Infants 6 weeks to 6 months: 0.5 mL dose at 2, 4 and 6 months (minimum interval of 1 month between each of the first 3 doses), followed by booster dose of 0.5 mL administered at 12-15 months (minimum interval of 6 months between doses 3 and 4) **or** 0.5 mL dose at 2 and 4 months (minimum interval of 2 months between doses 1 and 2), followed by an additional 0.5 mL dose at 11-12 months (minimum interval of 6 months between doses 2 and 3)
Infants 7-11 months (previously unvaccinated): 0.5 mL for 2 doses administered at least 1 month apart, followed by a third dose administered after 1 year of age (minimum interval of 2 months between doses 2 and 3)
Children 12 months to <6 years (previously unvaccinated): 0.5 mL for a total of 2 doses administered at least 2 months apart
Mechanism of Action Promotes active immunization against invasive disease caused by *S. pneumoniae* capsular serotypes 1, 4, 5, 6B, 7F, 9V, 14, 18C, 19F, and 23F, all which are individually conjugated to a carrier protein (protein D, tetanus toxoid, or diphtheria toxoid); the aluminum salt, a mineral adjuvant, enhances the antibody response.

Pregnancy Considerations Animal reproduction studies have not been conducted. Inactivated vaccines have not been shown to cause increased risks to the fetus (CDC, 2011). This product is indicated for use in infants and toddlers.

Product Availability Not available in the U.S.

Pneumococcal Conjugate Vaccine (13-Valent)
(noo moe KOK al KON ju gate vak SEEN, thur TEEN vay lent)

Brand Names: U.S. Prevnar 13®
Brand Names: Canada Prevnar 13®
Pharmacologic Category Vaccine, Inactivated (Bacterial)
Use
Immunization of children 6 weeks through 17 years of age against *Streptococcus pneumoniae* infection caused by serotypes included in the vaccine

Immunization of children 6 weeks through 5 years of age against otitis media caused by *Streptococcus pneumoniae* serotypes 4, 6B, 9V, 14, 18C, 19F, and 23F

Immunization of adults ≥50 years against pneumococcal pneumonia and invasive disease caused by *Streptococcus pneumoniae* serotypes included in the vaccine

The Advisory Committee on Immunization Practices (ACIP) recommends routine vaccination for the following (CDC 59[RR-11], 2010):
All children age 2-59 months
Children 60-71 months with underlying medical conditions including:
Immunocompetent children with chronic heart disease (particularly cyanotic congenital heart disease and heart failure), chronic lung disease (including asthma if treated with high dose corticosteroids), diabetes, cerebrospinal fluid leaks, or cochlear implants
Children with functional or anatomic asplenia, including sickle cell disease or other hemoglobinopathies, congenital or acquired asplenia, or splenic dysfunction.
Children with immunocompromising conditions including congenital immunodeficiency (includes B or T cell deficiency, compliment deficiencies and phagocytic disorders; excludes chronic granulomatous disease),HIV infection, chronic renal failure, nephrotic syndrome, leukemia, lymphoma, Hodgkin disease, generalized malignancies, solid organ transplant, or other diseases requiring immunosuppressive drugs (including long term systemic corticosteroids and radiation therapy)
Children who received ≥1 dose of PCV7
Children 6-18 years of age at increased risk for invasive pneumococcal disease due to anatomic or functional asplenia (including sickle cell disease), HIV infection or other immunocompromising conditions, cochlear implant, or cerebrospinal fluid leaks (regardless of prior receipt of PCV7 or PPSV23). Routine use is not recommended for healthy children ≥5 years of age.

Adults ≥19 years of age: The ACIP also recommends routine vaccination for adults ≥19 years of age with the following underlying medical conditions (CDC, 2012):
Immunocompetent persons with cerebrospinal fluid leaks or cochlear implants

Persons with functional or anatomic asplenia, including sickle cell disease or other hemoglobinopathies, congenital or acquired asplenia
Persons with immunocompromising conditions including congenital or acquired immunodeficiency (includes B or T cell deficiency, compliment deficiencies and phagocytic disorders; excludes chronic granulomatous disease), HIV infection, chronic renal failure, nephrotic syndrome, leukemia, lymphoma, Hodgkin disease, generalized malignancies, solid organ transplant, multiple myeloma, or other diseases requiring immunosuppressive drugs (including long term systemic corticosteroids and radiation therapy)

Local Anesthetic/Vasoconstrictor Precautions No information available to require special precautions
Effects on Dental Treatment No significant effects or complications reported
Effects on Bleeding No information available to require special precautions
Adverse Effects All serious adverse reactions must be reported to the U.S. Department of Health and Human Services (DHHS) Vaccine Adverse Event Reporting System (VAERS) 1-800-822-7967 or online at https://vaers.hhs.gov/esub/index.

>10%:
Central nervous system: Chills, drowsiness, fatigue, fever, headache, insomnia, irritability
Dermatologic: Rash
Gastrointestinal: Appetite decreased
Local: Erythema, limitation of arm motion, pain, swelling, tenderness
Neuromuscular & skeletal: Arthralgia, myalgia
1% to 10%:
Dermatologic: Hives
Gastrointestinal: Diarrhea, vomiting
Adverse reactions observed with PCV7 which may also be seen with PCV-13: Anaphylactic reaction, angioneurotic edema, apnea, breath holding, edema, hypotonic hyporesponsive episode, injection site reaction (dermatitis, pruritus), lymphadenopathy (localized), shock
General Dosage Range I.M.:
Infants 2-6 months: 0.5 mL at approximately 2-month intervals for 3 consecutive doses, followed by a fourth dose of 0.5 mL at 12-15 months of age
Infants 7-11 months (previously unvaccinated): 0.5 mL for a total of 3 doses, 2 doses at least 4 weeks apart, followed by a third dose at 12-15 months (at least 2 months after second dose)
Children 12-23 months (previously unvaccinated) and Children 24-71 months (previously unvaccinated) with underlying conditions: 0.5 mL for a total of 2 doses, separated by at least 8 weeks
Healthy Children 24-59 months (previously unvaccinated) and Children 6-18 years at high risk for invasive pneumococcal disease: 0.5 mL as a single dose
Children 14 months-71 months (previously completing vaccination with PCV7): 0.5 mL supplemental dose
Children 6 through 17 years: 0.5 mL as a single dose
Adults ≥50 years: 0.5 mL as a single dose
Mechanism of Action Promotes active immunization against invasive disease caused by *S. pneumoniae* capsular serotypes 1, 3, 4, 5, 6A, 6B, 7F, 9V, 14, 18C, 19A, 19F, and 23F, all which are individually conjugated to CRM197 protein
Pregnancy Risk Factor B

Pregnancy Considerations Animal reproduction studies have not shown adverse fetal effects. Inactivated vaccines have not been shown to cause increased risks to the fetus (CDC, 2011).

Podofilox (poe DOF il oks)

Brand Names: U.S. Condylox®
Brand Names: Canada Condyline™; Wartec®
Pharmacologic Category Keratolytic Agent; Topical Skin Product
Use Treatment of external genital warts
Local Anesthetic/Vasoconstrictor Precautions No information available to require special precautions
Effects on Dental Treatment No significant effects or complications reported
Effects on Bleeding No information available to require special precautions
General Dosage Range Topical: *Adults:* Apply twice daily for 3 consecutive days, then withhold use for 4 consecutive days; May repeat cycle up to 4 times
Pregnancy Risk Factor C
Pregnancy Considerations Adverse events have not been observed in animal reproduction studies with topical administration.

Podophyllum Resin (po DOF fil um REZ in)

Brand Names: U.S. Podocon-25®
Brand Names: Canada Podofilm®
Pharmacologic Category Keratolytic Agent
Use Topical treatment of soft external genital (venereal) warts (condylomata acuminata); compound benzoin tincture generally is used as the medium for topical application
Local Anesthetic/Vasoconstrictor Precautions No information available to require special precautions
Effects on Dental Treatment No significant effects or complications reported
Effects on Bleeding No information available to require special precautions
Adverse Effects
Central nervous system: Coma, fever, polyneuritis
Gastrointestinal: Paralytic ileus
Hematologic: Leukopenia, thrombocytopenia
Neuromuscular & skeletal: Paresthesia
Miscellaneous: Death
General Dosage Range Topical: *Children and Adults:* Applied by physician only
Mechanism of Action Directly affects epithelial cell metabolism by arresting mitosis through binding to a protein subunit of spindle microtubules (tubulin)
Pregnancy Considerations Reports in pregnant women have shown evidence of fetal abnormalities, fetal death, and stillbirth; use is contraindicated in women who are or may become pregnant

Polidocanol (pol i DOE kuh nol)

Brand Names: U.S. Asclera™
Pharmacologic Category Sclerosing Agent
Use Treatment of small, uncomplicated varicose veins of the lower extremities
Local Anesthetic/Vasoconstrictor Precautions No information available to require special precautions
Effects on Dental Treatment No significant effects or complications reported

Effects on Bleeding No information available to require special precautions
Adverse Effects
>10%: Local: Hematoma (42%), irritation (41%), discoloration (38%), pain (24%), pruritus (19%), warmth (16%)
1% to 10%: Local: Neovascularization (8%), injection site thrombosis (6%)
General Dosage Range I.V.: *Adults:* 0.1-0.3 mL injection (0.5% or 1% solution) per session (maximum: 10 mL/session)
Mechanism of Action Acts by irritation of the vein intimal endothelium and causes thrombosis formation leading to occlusion of the injected vein
Pharmacodynamics/Kinetics
Half-life Elimination 1.5 hours
Pregnancy Risk Factor C
Pregnancy Considerations Teratogenic effects were reported in some animal reproduction studies. There are no adequate and well-controlled studies in pregnant women. Polidocanol should not be used in pregnant women.

Poliovirus Vaccine (Inactivated) (POE lee oh VYE rus vak SEEN, in ak ti VAY ted)

Brand Names: U.S. IPOL®
Brand Names: Canada Imovax® Polio
Pharmacologic Category Vaccine, Inactivated (Viral)
Use Active immunization against poliomyelitis caused by poliovirus types 1, 2 and 3. **Note:** Combination products containing polio vaccine are also available and may be preferred in certain age groups if recipients are likely to be susceptible to the agents contained within each vaccine.

The Advisory Committee on Immunization Practices (ACIP) recommends routine vaccination for the following:
• All children (first dose given at 2 months of age)

Routine immunization of adults in the United States is generally not recommended. Adults with previous wild poliovirus disease, who have never been immunized, or those who are incompletely immunized may receive inactivated poliovirus vaccine if they fall into one of the following categories:
• Travelers to regions or countries where poliomyelitis is endemic or epidemic
• Healthcare workers in close contact with patients who may be excreting poliovirus
• Laboratory workers handling specimens that may contain poliovirus
• Members of communities or specific population groups with diseases caused by wild poliovirus
• Incompletely vaccinated or unvaccinated adults in a household or with other close contact with children receiving oral poliovirus (may be at increased risk of vaccine associated paralytic poliomyelitis)
Local Anesthetic/Vasoconstrictor Precautions No information available to require special precautions
Effects on Dental Treatment No significant effects or complications reported
Effects on Bleeding No information available to require special precautions
Adverse Effects All serious adverse reactions must be reported to the U.S. Department of Health and Human Services (DHHS) Vaccine Adverse Event Reporting System (VAERS) 1-800-822-7967 or online at https://vaers.hhs.gov/esub/index. In Canada,

adverse reactions may be reported to local provincial/territorial health agencies or to the Vaccine Safety Section at Public Health Agency of Canada (1-866-844-0018).

Percentages noted with concomitant administration of DTP or DTaP vaccine and observed within 48 hours of injection.

>10%:
Central nervous system: Irritability (7% to 65%; most common in infants 2 months of age), tiredness (4% to 61%)
Gastrointestinal: Anorexia (1% to 17%)
Local: Injection Site: Tenderness (≤29%), swelling (≤11%)
1% to 10%:
Central nervous system: Fever >39°C (≤4%)
Gastrointestinal: Vomiting (1% to 3%)
Local: Injection site: Erythema (≤3%)
Miscellaneous: Persistent crying (≤1% reported within 72 hours)

General Dosage Range I.M., SubQ:
Children: Primary immunization: Administer three 0.5 mL doses at 2, 4, and 6-18 months of age; do not administer more frequently than 4 weeks apart (preferably given more than 8 weeks apart). Booster dose: 0.5 mL at 4-6 years of age; Minimum interval between booster and previous dose is 6 months.
Adults (previously unvaccinated): Two 0.5 mL doses administered at 1- to 2-month intervals followed by a third dose 6-12 months later.

Pregnancy Risk Factor C
Pregnancy Considerations Animal reproduction studies have not been conducted. Although adverse effects of IPV have not been documented in pregnant women or their fetuses, vaccination of pregnant women should be avoided on theoretical grounds. Pregnant women at increased risk for infection and requiring immediate protection against polio may be administered the vaccine.

Polycarbophil (pol i KAR boe fil)

Brand Names: U.S. Equalactin® [OTC]; Fiber-Lax [OTC]; Fiber-Tabs™ [OTC]; FiberCon® [OTC]; Fibertab [OTC]; Konsyl® Fiber [OTC]
Pharmacologic Category Antidiarrheal; Fiber Supplement; Laxative, Bulk-Producing
Use Treatment of constipation or diarrhea
Local Anesthetic/Vasoconstrictor Precautions No information available to require special precautions
Effects on Dental Treatment Oral medication should be given at least 1 hour prior to taking the bulk-producing laxative in order to prevent decreased absorption of medication.
Effects on Bleeding No information available to require special precautions
Adverse Effects Frequency not defined: Gastrointestinal: Abdominal fullness
General Dosage Range Oral:
Children 6-12 years: 625 mg calcium polycarbophil 1-4 times/day
Children ≥12 years and Adults: 1250 mg calcium polycarbophil 1-4 times/day
Mechanism of Action Restoring a more normal moisture level and providing bulk in the patient's intestinal tract

Pregnancy Considerations When administered with adequate fluids, use is considered safe for the treatment of occasional constipation during pregnancy (Wald, 2003).

Polyethylene Glycol 3350 (pol i ETH i leen GLY kol 3350)

Brand Names: U.S. Dulcolax Balance® [OTC]; MiraLAX® [OTC]
Pharmacologic Category Laxative, Osmotic
Use Treatment of occasional constipation in adults
Unlabeled Use Treatment of constipation in children; bowel preparation before colonoscopy
Local Anesthetic/Vasoconstrictor Precautions No information available to require special precautions
Effects on Dental Treatment No significant effects or complications reported
Effects on Bleeding No information available to require special precautions
Adverse Effects Frequency not defined.
Dermatologic: Urticaria
Gastrointestinal: Abdominal bloating, cramping, diarrhea, flatulence, nausea
General Dosage Range Oral: *Adults:* 17 g of powder (~1 heaping tablespoon) dissolved in 4-8 ounces of beverage once daily (maximum use: 1 week)
Mechanism of Action An osmotic agent, polyethylene glycol 3350 causes water retention in the stool; increases stool frequency.
Pharmacodynamics/Kinetics
Onset of Action Oral: 24-96 hours
Pregnancy Risk Factor C
Pregnancy Considerations Reproduction studies have not been conducted in animals or in humans.

Polyethylene Glycol-Electrolyte Solution (pol i ETH i leen GLY kol ee LEK troe lite soe LOO shun)

Brand Names: U.S. Colyte®; GaviLyte™-C; GaviLyte™-G; GaviLyte™-N; GoLYTELY®; MoviPrep®; NuLYTELY®; TriLyte®
Brand Names: Canada Colyte™; Klean-Prep®; PegLyte®
Pharmacologic Category Laxative, Osmotic
Use Bowel cleansing prior to GI examination
Unlabeled Use Whole bowel irrigation (WBI) in the following toxic ingestions: Packets of illicit drugs (body packers, body stuffers), potentially toxic sustained-release or enteric-coated agents, substantial amounts of iron (AACT, 2004)
Local Anesthetic/Vasoconstrictor Precautions No information available to require special precautions
Effects on Dental Treatment No significant effects or complications reported
Effects on Bleeding No information available to require special precautions
Adverse Effects
>10%:
Central nervous system: Malaise (18% to 27%)
Gastrointestinal: Abdominal distension (<60%), anal irritation (<52%), nausea (14% to 47%), abdominal pain (13% to 39%), vomiting (7% to 12%)
Neuromuscular & skeletal: Rigors (34%)
Miscellaneous: Thirst (<47%)

◀ 1% to 10%:
Central nervous system: Dizziness (7%), headache (2%)
Gastrointestinal: Dyspepsia (1% to 3%)

General Dosage Range

Nasogastric tube:
Children ≥6 months: 25 mL/kg/hour until rectal effluent is clear
Adults: 20-30 mL/minute (1.2-1.8 L/hour) until rectal effluent is clear

Oral:
Children ≥6 months: (GaviLyte™-N, NuLYTELY®, TriLyte®): 25 mL/kg/hour (some studies have used up to 40 mL/kg/hour) for 4-10 hours until rectal effluent is clear (maximum total dose: 4 L)
Adults: CoLyte®, GaviLyte™-C, GaviLyte™-G, GaviLyte™-N, GoLYTELY®, NuLYTELY®, TriLyte®: 240 mL (8 oz) every 10 minutes, until 4 L are consumed or the rectal effluent is clear; MoviPrep®: 240 mL (8 oz) every 15 minutes until 1 L consumed; repeat 1 time

Mechanism of Action Induces catharsis by strong electrolyte and osmotic effects

Pharmacodynamics/Kinetics
Onset of Action Oral: ~1-2 hours

Pregnancy Risk Factor C

Pregnancy Considerations Reproduction studies have not been conducted in animals or in humans.

Poly-L-Lactic Acid (POL i el LAK tik AS id)

Brand Names: U.S. Sculptra®; Sculptra® Aesthetic
Pharmacologic Category Cosmetic Agent, Implant
Use Restoration and/or correction of facial lipoatrophy in patients with HIV; correction of shallow to deep nasolabial fold contour deficiencies and other facial wrinkles in immunocompetent patients
Local Anesthetic/Vasoconstrictor Precautions No information available to require special precautions
Effects on Dental Treatment No significant effects or complications reported
Effects on Bleeding No information available to require special precautions
Adverse Effects
>10%:
Dermatologic: Bruising (1% to 65%)
Hematologic: Hematoma (up to 28%)
Local: Injection site: Edema (3% to 81%), tenderness (81%), redness (78%), pain (71%), papules (3% to 52%), bleeding (34%), pruritus (20%), nodules (3%)
Miscellaneous: Discomfort (up to 19%)
1% to 10%:
Central nervous system: Fever (<5%)
Local: erythema (up to 10%), injection site reactions (<5%)
Postmarketing/case reports: Allergic reaction, angioedema, brittle nails, colitis, ectropion, fatigue, hair breakage, hypersensitivity reaction, hypertrophy, joint aches, malaise, periorbital nodules, photosensitivity, rash, scar/skin discoloration, skin infection, skin roughness, skin sarcoidosis, telangiectasia, urticaria, visible nodules
Injection site reactions: Abscess, atrophy, discharge, fat atrophy, granuloma, induration

General Dosage Range Intradermal, SubQ:
Adults:
Sculptra® Aesthetic: 0.1-0.2 mL per individual injection to a maximum of 2.5 mL per nasolabial fold as a single treatment; may repeat treatment at ≥3-week intervals up to 4 times
Sculptra®: 0.05-0.2 mL per individual injection, ~20 injections may be needed per cheek, usually involves 3-6 treatments separated by ≥2 weeks
Mechanism of Action Poly-L-lactic acid is an immunologically inert synthetic polymer. It increases dermal thickness by causing a local reaction leading to an increase in collagen deposits. It is eventually degraded and undergoes resorption.
Pharmacodynamics/Kinetics
Onset of Action Weeks to months for full effect of treatment
Pregnancy Considerations Safety for use during pregnancy has not been established.

Polymyxin B (pol i MIKS in bee)

Pharmacologic Category Antibiotic, Irrigation; Antibiotic, Miscellaneous
Use Treatment of acute infections caused by susceptible strains of *Pseudomonas aeruginosa*; used occasionally for gut decontamination; parenteral use of polymyxin B has mainly been replaced by less toxic antibiotics, reserved for life-threatening infections caused by organisms resistant to the preferred drugs (eg, pseudomonal meningitis - intrathecal administration)
Local Anesthetic/Vasoconstrictor Precautions No information available to require special precautions
Effects on Dental Treatment No significant effects or complications reported
Effects on Bleeding No information available to require special precautions
Adverse Effects Frequency not defined.
Cardiovascular: Facial flushing
Central nervous system: Neurotoxicity (irritability, drowsiness, ataxia, perioral paresthesia, numbness of the extremities, and blurred vision); dizziness, drug fever, meningeal irritation with intrathecal administration
Dermatologic: Urticarial rash
Endocrine & metabolic: Hypocalcemia, hyponatremia, hypokalemia, hypochloremia
Local: Pain at injection site
Neuromuscular & skeletal: Neuromuscular blockade, weakness
Renal: Nephrotoxicity
Respiratory: Respiratory arrest
Miscellaneous: Anaphylactoid reaction
General Dosage Range Dosage adjustment recommended in patients with renal impairment
I.M.:
Children <2 years: Up to 40,000 units/kg/day divided every 6 hours
Children ≥2 years and Adults: 25,000-30,000 units/kg/day divided every 4-6 hours (maximum: 2,000,000 units/day)
I.V.:
Children <2 years: Up to 40,000 units/kg/day divided every 12 hours
Children ≥2 years and Adults: 15,000-25,000 units/kg/day divided every 12 hours (maximum: 2,000,000 units/day)

Intrathecal:
Children <2 years: 20,000 units/day for 3-4 days, then 25,000 units every other day
Children ≥2 years and Adults: 50,000 units/day for 3-4 days, then every other day
Irrigation: *Adults:*
Bladder: 20 mg (equal to 200,000 units) added to 1 L of normal saline as continuous irrigant or rinse
Topical: 500,000 units/L of normal saline (maximum: 2 million units/day)
Ophthalmic: *Children ≥2 years and Adults:* Initial: 1-3 drops/hour; Reduce to 1-2 drops 4-6 times/day based on response
Otic: *Children and Adults:* 1-2 drops 3-4 times/day
Mechanism of Action Binds to phospholipids, alters permeability, and damages the bacterial cytoplasmic membrane permitting leakage of intracellular constituents
Pharmacodynamics/Kinetics
Half-life Elimination 6 hours; 2-3 days with anuria
Time to Peak Serum: I.M.: ~2 hours
Pregnancy Risk Factor B
Pregnancy Considerations [U.S. Boxed Warning]: Safety in pregnant women has not been established. A teratogenic potential has not been identified for polymyxin B, but very limited data is available. Based on the relative toxicity compared to other antibiotics, systemic use in pregnancy cannot be recommended. Due to limited absorption through the maternal skin, limited fetal exposure would be expected after topical polymyxin use.

Polysaccharide-Iron Complex
(pol i SAK a ride-EYE ern KOM pleks)

Brand Names: U.S. Ferrex™ 150 Plus [OTC]; Ferrex™ 150 [OTC]; Nu-Iron® 150 [OTC]; Poly-Iron 150 [OTC]; ProFe [OTC]
Pharmacologic Category Iron Salt
Use Prevention and treatment of iron-deficiency anemias
Local Anesthetic/Vasoconstrictor Precautions No information available to require special precautions
Effects on Dental Treatment No significant effects or complications reported
Effects on Bleeding No information available to require special precautions
Adverse Effects
>10%: Gastrointestinal: Stomach cramping, constipation, nausea, vomiting, dark stools, GI irritation, epigastric pain, nausea
1% to 10%:
Gastrointestinal: Heartburn, diarrhea
Genitourinary: Discolored urine
Miscellaneous: Staining of teeth
General Dosage Range Oral:
Children ≥6 years: 50-100 mg once daily or in divided doses
Adults: 100-300 mg/day in 1-2 divided doses
Pregnancy Considerations It is recommended that pregnant women meet the dietary requirements of iron with diet and/or supplements in order to prevent adverse events associated with iron deficiency anemia in pregnancy. Treatment of iron deficiency anemia in pregnant women is the same as in nonpregnant women and in most cases, oral iron preparations may be used. Except in severe cases of maternal anemia, the fetus achieves normal iron stores regardless of maternal concentrations.

Polysaccharide-Iron Complex and Folic Acid
(pol i SAK a ride-EYE ern KOM pleks & FOE lik AS id)

Brand Names: U.S. NovaFerrum®
Pharmacologic Category Iron Salt
Use Prevention and treatment of iron-deficiency anemias
Local Anesthetic/Vasoconstrictor Precautions No information available to require special precautions
Effects on Dental Treatment No significant effects or complications reported
Effects on Bleeding No information available to require special precautions
Adverse Effects Frequency not defined.
Gastrointestinal: Abdominal pain, constipation, dark stools, diarrhea, nausea, vomiting
Miscellaneous: Hypersensitivity reaction
General Dosage Range Oral: *Children >12 years and Adults:* Iron deficiency: 5 mL daily
Pregnancy Considerations It is recommended that pregnant women meet the dietary requirements of iron with diet and/or supplements in order to prevent adverse events associated with iron-deficiency anemia in pregnancy. Treatment of iron-deficiency anemia in pregnant women is the same as in nonpregnant women, and in most cases, oral iron preparations may be used. Except in severe cases of maternal anemia, the fetus achieves normal iron stores regardless of maternal concentrations.

Polysaccharide-Iron Complex, Vitamin B12, and Folic Acid
(pol i SAK a ride-EYE ern KOM pleks, VYE ta min bee twelve & FOE lik AS id)

Brand Names: U.S. Ferrex™ 150 Forte; Ferrex™ 150 Forte Plus; Maxaron® Forte; Poly-Iron 150 Forte; Polysaccharide Iron 150 Forte
Pharmacologic Category Iron Salt
Use Prevention and treatment of iron-deficiency anemias and/or nutritional megaloblastic anemias
Local Anesthetic/Vasoconstrictor Precautions No information available to require special precautions
Effects on Dental Treatment No significant effects or complications reported
Effects on Bleeding No information available to require special precautions
Adverse Effects Frequency not defined.
Gastrointestinal: Abdominal pain, constipation, dark stools, diarrhea, epigastric pain, GI irritation, nausea, stomach cramping, vomiting
Genitourinary: Discolored urine
Miscellaneous: Hypersensitivity reaction
General Dosage Range Oral: *Adults:* 1-2 capsules daily
Pregnancy Considerations It is recommended that pregnant women meet the dietary requirements of iron with diet and/or supplements in order to prevent adverse events associated with iron-deficiency anemia in pregnancy. Treatment of iron-deficiency anemia in pregnant women is the same as in nonpregnant women, and in most cases, oral iron preparations may be used. Except in severe cases of maternal anemia, the fetus achieves normal iron stores regardless of maternal concentrations.

Polyvinylpyrrolidone and Sodium Hyaluronate

(pol e VI nil pi ROL i don & SOW dee um hye al yoor ON ate)

Brand Names: U.S. Ameseal™

Generic Availability (U.S.) No

Pharmacologic Category Protectant, Topical

Dental Use Treatment of mouth ulcers

Local Anesthetic/Vasoconstrictor Precautions No information available to require special precautions

Effects on Dental Treatment No significant effects or complications reported

Effects on Bleeding No information available to require special precautions

Dental Usual Dosage Spray: Direct the spray applicator towards the lesions and spray 3 times or as needed to cover the affected area. Repeat throughout the day as necessary.

Mechanism of Action Polyvinylpyrrolidone (PVP) sets up a barrier at application site to protect ulcer from irritants and irritation

Dosage Forms Excipient information presented when available (limited, particularly for generics); consult specific product labeling.

Solution, topical [spray]: 15 mL

Pomalidomide (poe ma LID oh mide)

Brand Names: U.S. Pomalyst®

Pharmacologic Category Angiogenesis Inhibitor; Antineoplastic Agent; Immunomodulator, Systemic

Use Treatment of multiple myeloma in patients who have received at least two prior therapies (including lenalidomide and bortezomib) and have continued disease progression on or within 60 days of completion of the last therapy

Local Anesthetic/Vasoconstrictor Precautions No information available to require special precautions

Effects on Dental Treatment No significant effects or complications reported

Effects on Bleeding Chemotherapy may result in significant myelosuppression, neutropenia (50% to 52%; grades 3/4: 43% to 47%), anemia (38%; grades 3/4: 22%), thrombocytopenia (25%; grades 3/4: 22%), leukopenia (11%; grades 3/4: 6%). In patients who are under active treatment with these agents, medical consult is suggested.

Adverse Effects

>10%:

Cardiovascular: Peripheral edema (23%)

Central nervous system: Fatigue (55%), dizziness (18% to 20%), fever (19%), neuropathy (18%), headache (13%), confusion (10% to 12%), anxiety (11%)

Dermatologic: Skin rash (22%), pruritus (15%)

Endocrine & metabolic: Hypercalcemia (21%), hyperglycemia (12%)

Gastrointestinal: Constipation (36%), nausea (36%), diarrhea (34%), decreased appetite (22%), vomiting (14%), weight loss (14%)

Hematologic & oncologic: Neutropenia (50% to 52%; grades 3/4: 43% to 47%), anemia (38%; grades 3/4: 22%), thrombocytopenia (25%; grades 3/4: 22%), leukopenia (11%; grades 3/4: 6%)

Musculoskeletal: Back pain (32%), musculoskeletal chest pain (22%), muscle spasm (19%), arthralgia (16%), ostealgia (12%), myasthenia (12%), musculoskeletal pain (11%)

Renal: Increased serum creatinine (15%), renal failure (15%)

Respiratory: Dyspnea (34%), upper respiratory tract infection (32%), pneumonia (23%), epistaxis (15%), cough (14%)

1% to 10%:

Cardiovascular: Thrombosis (venous thrombosis, pulmonary embolism, 3%), atrial fibrillation (2%)

Central nervous system: Peripheral neuropathy (10%), chills (9%), insomnia (7%), pain (6%)

Dermatologic: Xeroderma (9%), hyperhidrosis (6%)

Endocrine & metabolic: Hypokalemia (10%), hyponatremia (10%), hypocalcemia (6%), dehydration (5%)

Gastrointestinal: Weight gain (1%)

Genitourinary: Urinary tract infection (8%)

Hematologic & oncologic: Lymphocytopenia (4%; grades 3/4: 2%), febrile neutropenia (3% to 5%)

Infection: Sepsis (6%)

Musculoskeletal: Tremor (9%), limb pain (5%)

Miscellaneous: Night sweats (5%)

Frequency not defined: Acute myelocytic leukemia, hyperbilirubinemia, hyperkalemia, increased serum ALT, interstitial pulmonary disease, neutropenic sepsis, pelvic pain, *Pneumocystis jiroveci* pneumonia, respiratory syncytial virus infection, urinary retention, vertigo

General Dosage Range Dosage adjustment recommended in patients who develop toxicities.

Oral: *Adults:* 4 mg once daily on days 1-21 of 28-day cycles

Mechanism of Action Induces cell cycle arrest and apoptosis directly in multiple myeloma cells; enhances T cell- and natural killer (NK) cell-mediated cytotoxicity; inhibits production of proinflammatory cytokines tumor necrosis factor-α (TNF-α), IL-1, IL-6, and IL-12; inhibits angiogenesis (Zhu, 2013)

Pharmacodynamics/Kinetics

Half-life Elimination ~9.5 hours (healthy subjects); ~7.5 hours (multiple myeloma patients)

Time to Peak 2-3 hours

Pregnancy Risk Factor X

Pregnancy Considerations [U.S. Boxed Warning]: Pomalidomide is an analogue of thalidomide (a known human teratogen) and may cause severe birth defects or embryo-fetal death if taken during pregnancy. Pomalidomide cannot be used in women who are pregnant or may become pregnant during therapy. Obtain 2 negative pregnancy tests prior to initiation of treatment; 2 forms of contraception (or abstain from heterosexual intercourse) must be used at least 4 weeks prior to, during, and for ≥4 weeks after pomalidomide treatment (and during treatment interruptions) in females of reproductive potential. Distribution is restricted; physicians, pharmacists, and patients must be registered with the Pomalyst® REMS ™ Program. Studies in animals have shown evidence of fetal abnormalities and use is contraindicated in women who are or may become pregnant. Women of childbearing potential should be treated only if they are able to comply with the conditions of the Pomalyst® REMS ™ Program. Reliable contraception is required even with a history of infertility (unless due to hysterectomy or if ≥24 consecutive months postmenopausal (natural). Pregnancy tests should be performed 10-14 days and 24 hours prior to beginning therapy; weekly for the first 4 weeks and then every 4 weeks (every 2 weeks if menstrual cycle irregular) thereafter and during therapy interruptions. Pomalidomide must be immediately discontinued for a missed period, abnormal pregnancy test or abnormal menstrual bleeding; refer patient to a reproductive toxicity specialist if pregnancy occurs during treatment. Pomalidomide is present in the semen of males taking this medication. Males (including those vasectomized) should use a latex or synthetic condom during any sexual contact with women of childbearing age during treatment, during treatment interruptions, and for 28 days after discontinuation. Male patients should not donate sperm. Any suspected fetal exposure should be reported to the FDA via the MedWatch program (1-800-332-1088) and to Celgene Corporation (1-888-423-5436).

Prescribing and Access Restrictions As a requirement of the REMS program, access to this medication is restricted. Pomalidomide is approved for marketing in the U.S. only under a Food and Drug Administration (FDA) approved, restricted distribution program called Pomalyst REMS™ (celgeneriskmanagement.com or 1-888-423-5436). Physicians, pharmacies, and patients must be registered; a maximum 28-day supply may be dispensed; a new prescription is required each time it is filled; pregnancy testing is required for women of childbearing potential.

Ponatinib (poe NA ti nib)

Brand Names: U.S. Iclusig®

Pharmacologic Category Antineoplastic Agent, Tyrosine Kinase Inhibitor

Use Treatment of chronic myelogenous leukemia (CML) in chronic, accelerated, or blast phase that is resistant or intolerant to prior tyrosine kinase inhibitor therapy; treatment of Philadelphia chromosome-positive (Ph+) acute lymphoblastic leukemia (ALL) that is resistant or intolerant to prior tyrosine kinase inhibitor therapy

Local Anesthetic/Vasoconstrictor Precautions Ponatinib may cause hypertension; monitor blood pressure prior to vasoconstrictor use

Effects on Dental Treatment Key adverse event(s) related to dental treatment: Oral mucositis

Effects on Bleeding Chemotherapy may result in significant myelosuppression, potentially including significant reduction in platelet counts (thrombocytopenia grades 3/4: 36% to 57%) and altered hemostasis. In patients who are under active treatment with these agents, medical consult is suggested.

Adverse Effects

>10%:
Cardiovascular: Hypertension (53% to 71%), peripheral edema (13% to 22%; grades 3/4: ≤1%), heart failure (6% to 15%; including ejection fraction decreased, pulmonary edema, cardiogenic shock, cardiopulmonary failure), arterial ischemia (3% to 13%; grades 3/4: ≤7%; including cardiac, cerebro-, and peripheral-vascular events)
Central nervous system: Fatigue or weakness (31% to 39%), headache (25% to 39%), fever (23% to 32%), pain (6% to 16%), chills (7% to 13%), insomnia (7% to 12%), dizziness (3% to 11%)
Dermatologic: Rash (34% to 54%), dry skin (24% to 39%), cellulitis (≤11%)
Endocrine & metabolic: Glucose increased (58%), phosphorus decreased (57%), calcium decreased (52%), sodium decreased (29%), glucose decreased (24%), potassium decreased (16%), potassium increased (15%), bicarbonate decreased (11%)

Gastrointestinal: Abdominal pain (34% to 49%), constipation (24% to 47%), lipase increased (41%; grades 3/4: 15%), nausea (22% to 32%), appetite decreased (8% to 31%), diarrhea (13% to 26%), vomiting (13% to 24%), oral mucositis (9% to 23%), weight loss (5% to 13%), gastrointestinal hemorrhage (2% to 11%; grades 3/4: ≤6%)
Genitourinary: Urinary tract infection (≤12%)
Hematologic: Neutropenia (grades 3/4: 24% to 63%), leukopenia (grades 3/4: 14% to 63%), thrombocytopenia (grades 3/4: 36% to 57%), anemia (grades 3/4: 9% to 55%), lymphopenia (grades 3/4: 10% to 37%), neutropenic fever (1% to 25%), hemorrhage (24%; grades 3/4: 4% to 5%; including cerebral and gastrointestinal)
Hepatic: ALT increased (53%; grades 3/4: 8%), AST increased (41%; grades 3/4: 4%), alkaline phosphatase increased (37%), albumin decreased (28%), bilirubin increased (19%)
Neuromuscular & skeletal: Arthralgia (13% to 31%), myalgia (6% to 22%), limb pain (9% to 17%), back pain (11% to 16%), peripheral neuropathy (6% to 13%), muscle spasm (5% to 13%), bone pain (9% to 12%)
Respiratory: Dyspnea (6% to 21%), pleural effusion (3% to 19%; grades 3/4: ≤3%), cough (6% to 18%), pneumonia (3% to 13%), nasopharyngitis (3% to 12%), upper respiratory tract infection (≤11%)
Miscellaneous: Sepsis (1% to 22%)

1% to 10%:
Cardiovascular: Myocardial infarction or other cardiac ischemic event (5%), supraventricular tachyarrhythmia (5%), atrial fibrillation (4%), venous thromboembolism (3%; including deep vein thrombosis, pulmonary embolism, portal vein thrombosis, and retinal vein thrombosis), pericardial effusion (1% to 3%), cerebral hemorrhage (2%), peripheral ischemia (2%), stroke or TIA (2%), bradyarrhythmia (1%; symptomatic)
Endocrine & metabolic: Sodium increased (10%), hyperuricemia (7%), calcium increased (5%), triglycerides increased (3%)
Gastrointestinal: Pancreatitis (6%; grade 3: 5%), amylase increased (3%)
Renal: Creatinine increased (7%)

General Dosage Range Dosage adjustment recommended in patients on concomitant therapy or who develop toxicities.

Oral: *Adults:* 45 mg once daily

Mechanism of Action Ponatinib is a pan-BCR-ABL tyrosine kinase inhibitor with *in vitro* activity against cells expressing native or mutant BCR-ABL (including T315I); it also inhibits VEGFR, FGFR, PDGFR, FGFR, EPH, and SRC kinases, as well as KIT, RET, TIE2, and FLT3.

Pharmacodynamics/Kinetics

Half-life Elimination ~24 hours (range: 12-66 hours)

Time to Peak ≤6 hours

Pregnancy Risk Factor D

Pregnancy Considerations Adverse events were observed in animal reproduction studies when administered in doses lower than or equivalent to the normal human dose. Based on its mechanism of action, adverse effects on pregnancy would be expected. Women of childbearing potential should be advised to avoid pregnancy during therapy.

Prescribing and Access Restrictions Patient access and support is available through the ARIAD PASS program. Information regarding program enrollment may be found at http://www.ariadpass.com/healthcare-professional or by calling 1-855-447-PASS (7277).

Poractant Alfa (por AKT ant AL fa)

Brand Names: U.S. Curosurf®
Brand Names: Canada Curosurf®
Pharmacologic Category Lung Surfactant
Use Treatment of respiratory distress syndrome (RDS) in premature infants
Local Anesthetic/Vasoconstrictor Precautions No information available to require special precautions
Effects on Dental Treatment No significant effects or complications reported
Effects on Bleeding No information available to require special precautions
Adverse Effects Frequency not defined.
Cardiovascular: Bradycardia, hypotension
Respiratory: Endotracheal tube blockage, oxygen desaturation
General Dosage Range Intratracheal: *Premature infants:* Initial: 2.5 mL/kg of birth weight, up to 2 subsequent doses of 1.25 mL/kg birth weight can be administered at 12-hour intervals if needed; Maximum total dose: 5 mL/kg
Mechanism of Action Endogenous pulmonary surfactant reduces surface tension at the air-liquid interface of the alveoli during ventilation and stabilizes the alveoli against collapse at resting transpulmonary pressures. A deficiency of pulmonary surfactant in preterm infants results in respiratory distress syndrome characterized by poor lung expansion, inadequate gas exchange, and atelectasis. Poractant alpha compensates for the surfactant deficiency and restores surface activity to the infant's lungs. It reduces mortality and pneumothoraces associated with RDS.

Porfimer (POR fi mer)

Brand Names: U.S. Photofrin®
Brand Names: Canada Photofrin®
Pharmacologic Category Antineoplastic Agent, Miscellaneous
Use Palliation in patients with obstructing (partial or complete) esophageal cancer; treatment of microinvasive endobronchial nonsmall cell lung cancer (NSCLC); reduction of obstruction and palliation in patients with obstructing (partial or complete) NSCLC; ablation of high-grade dysplasia in Barrett's esophagus

Canadian labeling (additional use; not in U.S. labeling): Second-line treatment of recurrent, superficial papillary bladder cancer
Unlabeled Use Treatment of actinic keratoses and low-risk basal and squamous cell skin cancers
Local Anesthetic/Vasoconstrictor Precautions No information available to require special precautions
Effects on Dental Treatment Key adverse event(s) related to dental treatment: Dysphagia.
Effects on Bleeding No information available to require special precautions
Adverse Effects
>10%:
Cardiovascular: Chest pain (5% to 31%), edema (3% to 18%)
Central nervous system: Fever (8% to 31%), pain (1% to 22%), insomnia (5% to 14%)
Dermatologic: Photosensitivity reaction (19% to 69%)
Gastrointestinal: Esophageal stricture/stenosis (6% to 38%), nausea (24% to 37%), vomiting (17% to 31%), constipation (5% to 24%), dysphagia (10% to 24%), mucositis (≤20%), abdominal pain (5% to 20%)

Hematologic: Anemia (32% in esophageal cancer patients)
Neuromuscular & skeletal: Back pain (3% to 11%)
Respiratory: Pleural effusion (5% to 32%), dyspnea (7% to 30%), bronchial obstruction/mucus plug (21%), pneumonia (6% to 18%), hemoptysis (7% to 16%), cough (5% to 15%), bronchostenosis (11%), pharyngitis (11%)
5% to 10%:
Cardiovascular: Atrial fibrillation, cardiac failure (esophageal cancer), hyper-/hypotension, tachycardia
Central nervous system: Anxiety, confusion, dysphonia
Endocrine & metabolic: Dehydration
Gastrointestinal: Anorexia, diarrhea, dyspepsia, eructation, esophageal edema, esophageal pain, esophagitis, hematemesis, melena, odynophagia, weight loss
Genitourinary: Urinary tract infection
Neuromuscular & skeletal: Weakness
Respiratory: Bronchial ulceration, bronchitis, fatal massive hemoptysis, respiratory insufficiency, tracheoesophageal fistula
Miscellaneous: Hiccups, moniliasis, tumor hemorrhage, surgical complication
Common adverse reactions observed in papillary bladder cancer (Canadian labeling; not an approved use in the U.S.):
Cardiovascular: Peripheral edema
Central nervous system: Anxiety, insomnia, pain
Gastrointestinal: Constipation, nausea
Genitourinary: Bladder contracture (irreversible), dysuria, genital edema, micturition frequency, nocturia, suprapubic pain, urinary incontinence, urinary tract infection, urinary urgency
Renal: Hematuria
General Dosage Range I.V.: *Adults:* 2 mg/kg, followed by endoscopic exposure to the appropriate laser light
Mechanism of Action Porfimer's cytotoxic activity is dependent on light and oxygen. Following administration, the drug is selectively retained in neoplastic tissues. Exposure of the drug to laser light at wavelengths >630 nm results in the production of oxygen free-radicals. Release of thromboxane A_2, leading to vascular occlusion and ischemic necrosis, may also occur.
Pharmacodynamics/Kinetics
Half-life Elimination First dose: 17 days; Second dose: 30 days
Pregnancy Risk Factor C
Pregnancy Considerations Animal studies have shown maternal and fetal toxicity, but no major malformations. There are no adequate and well-controlled studies in pregnant women. Use during pregnancy only if the potential benefit outweighs the potential risk to the fetus. Effective contraception is recommended for women of childbearing potential.

Posaconazole (poe sa KON a zole)

Related Information
Fungal Infections *on page 1573*
Related Sample Prescriptions
Fungal Infections Requiring Systemic Therapy *on page 1614*
Brand Names: U.S. Noxafil®
Brand Names: Canada Posanol™
Generic Availability (U.S.) No
Pharmacologic Category Antifungal Agent, Oral

Dental Use Treatment of oropharyngeal candidiasis (including patients refractory to itraconazole and/or fluconazole)

Use

U.S. labeling: Prophylaxis of invasive *Aspergillus* and *Candida* infections in severely-immunocompromised patients (eg, hematopoietic stem cell transplant [HSCT] recipients with graft-versus-host disease [GVHD] or those with prolonged neutropenia secondary to chemotherapy for hematologic malignancies); treatment of oropharyngeal candidiasis (including patients refractory to itraconazole and/or fluconazole)

Canadian labeling: Prophylaxis of invasive *Aspergillus* and *Candida* infections in severely-immunocompromised patients (eg, hematopoietic stem cell transplant [HSCT] recipients with graft-versus-host disease [GVHD] or those with prolonged neutropenia); treatment of invasive aspergillosis in patients refractory to or intolerant of itraconazole or amphotericin B; treatment of oropharyngeal candidiasis

Unlabeled Use Salvage therapy of refractory or relapsed invasive fungal infections; mucormycosis; pulmonary infection (nonimmunosuppressed)

Local Anesthetic/Vasoconstrictor Precautions No information available to require special precautions

Effects on Dental Treatment Key adverse event(s) related to dental treatment: Xerostomia (normal salivary flow resumes upon discontinuation), abnormal taste, mucositis.

Effects on Bleeding No information available to require special precautions

Adverse Effects Note: Percentages reflect data from use in comparator trials with multiple concomitant conditions and medications; some adverse reactions may be due to underlying condition(s).

>10%:

Cardiovascular: Hypertension (18%), edema (9% to 15%), hypotension (14%), tachycardia (12%)

Central nervous system: Fever (6% to 45%), headache (8% to 28%), fatigue (3% to 17%), insomnia (1% to 17%), dizziness (11%), pain (1% to 11%)

Endocrine & metabolic: Hypokalemia (≤30%), hypomagnesemia (18%), dehydration (1% to 11%), hyperglycemia (11%)

Gastrointestinal: Diarrhea (10% to 42%), nausea (9% to 38%), vomiting (7% to 29%), abdominal pain (5% to 27%), constipation (21%), anorexia (2% to 19%), mucositis (17%), weight loss (1% to 14%), oral candidiasis (1% to 12%)

Hematologic: Thrombocytopenia (29%), anemia (2% to 25%), neutropenia (4% to 23%), neutropenic fever (20%)

Hepatic: ALT increased (6% to 17%)

Neuromuscular & skeletal: Rigors (≤20%), musculoskeletal pain (16%), weakness (2% to 13%), arthralgia (11%)

Respiratory: Cough (3% to 25%), dyspnea (1% to 20%), epistaxis (14%), pharyngitis (12%)

Miscellaneous: Bacteremia (18%), herpes simplex (3% to 15%), CMV infection (14%)

1% to 10%:

Central nervous system: Anxiety (9%)

Endocrine & metabolic: Hypocalcemia (9%)

Gastrointestinal: Dyspepsia (10%)

Genitourinary: Vaginal hemorrhage (10%)

Hepatic: Hyperbilirubinemia (7% to 10%), AST increased (3% to 4%), alkaline phosphatase increased (1% to 3%)

Neuromuscular & skeletal: Back pain (10%)

Respiratory: Pneumonia (3% to 10%), upper respiratory infection (7%)

Miscellaneous: Diaphoresis (2% to 10%)

Dental Usual Dosage Children ≥13 years and Adults: Oral:

Oropharyngeal candidiasis: Initial: 100 mg twice daily for 1 day; maintenance dose: 100 mg once daily for 13 days

Refractory oropharyngeal candidiasis: 400 mg twice daily

Dosage

Aspergillosis, invasive:

Prophylaxis: Children ≥13 years, Adolescents, and Adults: Oral: 200 mg 3 times daily; duration of therapy is based on recovery from neutropenia or immunosuppression; initiate posaconazole in patients with acute myelogenous leukemia (AML) or myelodysplastic syndromes (MDS) several days before the anticipated onset of neutropenia (eg, at the time of chemotherapy initiation) and discontinue once neutropenia is resolved (Cornely, 2007; NCCN, 2009).

Treatment (refractory to or intolerant of conventional therapy):

U.S. unlabeled use: Adults: Oral: 200 mg 4 times daily initially; after disease stabilization, may decrease frequency to 400 mg twice daily (Walsh, 2007). **Note:** Duration of therapy should be a minimum of 6-12 weeks or throughout period of immunosuppression and until lesions have resolved (Walsh, 2008).

Canadian labeling: Children ≥13 years, Adolescents, and Adults: Oral: 400 mg twice daily; in patients unable to tolerate food or nutritional supplement, administer 200 mg 4 times daily; duration of therapy is based on severity of underlying disease, recovery from immunosuppression, and clinical response.

Candidal infections: Children ≥13 years, Adolescents, and Adults: Oral:

U.S. labeling:

Prophylaxis: 200 mg 3 times daily; duration of therapy is based on recovery from neutropenia or immunosuppression

Treatment:

Oropharyngeal infection: Initial: 100 mg twice daily for 1 day; maintenance: 100 mg once daily for 13 days

Refractory oropharyngeal infection: 400 mg twice daily; duration of therapy is based on underlying disease and clinical response

Canadian labeling:

Prophylaxis: 200 mg 3 times daily; duration of therapy is based on recovery from neutropenia or immunosuppression

Treatment: Oropharyngeal infection: Initial: 100 mg twice daily for 1 day; maintenance: 100 mg once daily for 13 days

Mucormycosis (unlabeled use): Adults: Oral: 800 mg daily in 2 or 4 divided doses; duration of therapy is based on response and risk of relapse due to immunosuppression (Greenburg, 2006)

Cryptococcal infections: Adults: Oral:

Pulmonary, nonimmunosuppressed (unlabeled use): 400 mg twice daily. **Note:** Fluconazole is considered first-line treatment (Perfect, 2010).

Salvage treatment of relapsed infection (unlabeled use): 400 mg twice daily (or 200 mg 4 times daily) for 10-12 weeks. **Note:** Salvage treatment should only be started after an appropriate course of an induction regimen (Perfect, 2010).

Dosage adjustment in renal impairment:
Mild-to-moderate renal insufficiency (Cl$_{cr}$ 20-80 mL/minute/1.73 m^2): No adjustment necessary

Severe renal insufficiency (Cl$_{cr}$ <20 mL/minute/1.73 m^2): No adjustment necessary; however, monitor for breakthrough fungal infections due to variability in posaconazole exposure.

Dosage adjustment in hepatic impairment:
Mild-to-severe hepatic insufficiency (Child-Pugh class A, B, or C): No adjustment necessary

Clinical signs and symptoms of liver disease due to posaconazole: Consider discontinuing therapy

Mechanism of Action Interferes with fungal cytochrome P450 (latosterol-14α-demethylase) activity, decreasing ergosterol synthesis (principal sterol in fungal cell membrane) and inhibiting fungal cell membrane formation.

Contraindications Hypersensitivity to posaconazole, other azole antifungals, or any component of the formulation; coadministration of sirolimus, cisapride, ergot alkaloids, pimozide, quinidine, or a HMG-CoA reductase inhibitor metabolized by CYP3A4 (eg, atorvastatin, lovastatin, simvastatin)

Warnings/Precautions Hepatic dysfunction has occurred, ranging from reversible mild/moderate increases of ALT, AST, alkaline phosphatase, total bilirubin, and/or clinical hepatitis to severe reactions (cholestasis, hepatic failure including death). Consider discontinuation of therapy in patients who develop clinical evidence of liver disease that may be secondary to posaconazole. Use caution in patients with an increased risk of arrhythmia (long QT syndrome, concurrent QT$_c$-prolonging drugs, hypokalemia). Correct electrolyte abnormalities (eg, potassium, magnesium, and calcium) before initiating therapy. Concurrent use with cyclosporine or tacrolimus may significantly increase cyclosporine/tacrolimus concentrations and may result in rare serious adverse events (eg, nephrotoxicity, leukoencephalopathy, and death); dose reduction and close monitoring are recommended with initiation of posaconazole therapy. Concurrent use with midazolam may increase midazolam concentrations and potentiate midazolam-related adverse effects.

U.S. labeling contraindicates use in patients with hypersensitivity to other azole antifungal agents; Canadian labeling does not contraindicate use, but recommends using caution in hypersensitivity with other azole antifungal agents; cross-reaction may occur, but has not been established. Consider alternative therapy or closely monitor for breakthrough fungal infections in patients receiving drugs that decrease absorption or increase the metabolism of posaconazole or in any patient unable to eat or tolerate an oral liquid nutritional supplement. Use caution in severe renal impairment or GI disturbances; monitor for breakthrough fungal infections.

Drug Interactions
Metabolism/Transport Effects Inhibits CYP3A4 (strong)

Avoid Concomitant Use
Avoid concomitant use of Posaconazole with any of the following: Ado-Trastuzumab Emtansine; Alfuzosin; Apixaban; AtorvaSTATin; Avanafil; Axitinib; Bosutinib; Cabozantinib; Cisapride; Conivaptan; Crizotinib; Dihydroergotamine; Dofetilide; Dronedarone; Efavirenz; Eletriptan; Eplerenone; Ergoloid Mesylates; Ergonovine; Ergotamine; Everolimus; Fluticasone (Oral Inhalation); Halofantrine; Ivabradine; Lapatinib; Lomitapide; Lovastatin; Lurasidone; Methadone; Methylergonovine; Nilotinib; Nisoldipine; Pimozide; Pomalidomide; Proton Pump Inhibitors; QuiNIDine; Ranolazine; Red Yeast Rice; Regorafenib; Rivaroxaban; RomiDEPsin; Salmeterol; Silodosin; Simvastatin; Sirolimus; Tamsulosin; Ticagrelor; Tolvaptan; Toremifene; VinCRIStine (Liposomal)

Increased Effect/Toxicity
Posaconazole may increase the levels/effects of: Ado-Trastuzumab Emtansine; Alfentanil; Alfuzosin; Almotriptan; Alosetron; Antineoplastic Agents (Vinca Alkaloids); Apixaban; Aprepitant; ARIPiprazole; Atazanavir; AtorvaSTATin; Avanafil; Axitinib; Bedaquiline; Benzodiazepines (metabolized by oxidation); Boceprevir; Bortezomib; Bosentan; Bosutinib; Brentuximab Vedotin; Brinzolamide; Budesonide (Nasal); Budesonide (Systemic, Oral Inhalation); BusPIRone; Busulfan; Cabozantinib; Calcium Channel Blockers; CarBAMazepine; Cardiac Glycosides; Cilostazol; Cinacalcet; Cisapride; Colchicine; Conivaptan; Corticosteroids (Orally Inhaled); Corticosteroids (Systemic); Crizotinib; CycloSPORINE (Systemic); CYP3A4 Substrates; Dienogest; Dihydroergotamine; DOCEtaxel; Dofetilide; Dronedarone; Dutasteride; Eletriptan; Enzalutamide; Eplerenone; Ergoloid Mesylates; Ergonovine; Ergotamine; Erlotinib; Eszopiclone; Etravirine; Everolimus; FentaNYL; Fesoterodine; Fluticasone (Nasal); Fluticasone (Oral Inhalation); Fosamprenavir; Fosaprepitant; Fosphenytoin; Gefitinib; GlipiZIDE; GuanFACINE; Halofantrine; Iloperidone; Imatinib; Irinotecan; Ivabradine; Ivacaftor; Ixabepilone; Lapatinib; Lomitapide; Losartan; Lovastatin; Lumefantrine; Lurasidone; Macrolide Antibiotics; Maraviroc; Methadone; Methylergonovine; MethylPREDNISolone; Mifepristone; Nilotinib; Nisoldipine; Ospemifene; Paricalcitol; Pazopanib; Phenytoin; Pimecrolimus; Pimozide; Pomalidomide; Ponatinib; Propafenone; QuiNIDine; Ramelteon; Ranolazine; Red Yeast Rice; Regorafenib; Repaglinide; Rifamycin Derivatives; Ritonavir; Rivaroxaban; RomiDEPsin; Ruxolitinib; Salmeterol; Saxagliptin; Sildenafil; Silodosin; Simvastatin; Sirolimus; Solifenacin; SORAfenib; SUNItinib; Tacrolimus (Systemic); Tacrolimus (Topical); Tadalafil; Tamsulosin; Telaprevir; Temsirolimus; Ticagrelor; Tofacitinib; Tolterodine; Tolvaptan; Toremifene; Vardenafil; Vemurafenib; Vilazodone; VinCRIStine (Liposomal); Vitamin K Antagonists; Ziprasidone; Zolpidem; Zuclopenthixol

The levels/effects of Posaconazole may be increased by: Boceprevir; Etravirine; Grapefruit Juice; Macrolide Antibiotics; Telaprevir

Decreased Effect
Posaconazole may decrease the levels/effects of: Amphotericin B; Ifosfamide; Prasugrel; Saccharomyces boulardii; Ticagrelor

The levels/effects of Posaconazole may be decreased by: Didanosine; Efavirenz; Etravirine; Fosamprenavir; Fosphenytoin; H2-Antagonists; Metoclopramide; Phenytoin; Proton Pump Inhibitors; Rifamycin Derivatives; Sucralfate

Ethanol/Nutrition/Herb Interactions Food: Bioavailability increased ~3 times when posaconazole is administered with a nonfat meal or an oral liquid nutritional supplement; increased ~4 times when administered with a high-fat meal. Grapefruit juice may decrease the levels/effects of posaconazole. Management: Must be administered with or within 20 minutes of a full meal or an oral liquid nutritional supplement, or may be administered with an acidic carbonated beverage (eg, ginger ale). Consider alternative antifungal therapy in patients with inadequate oral intake or severe diarrhea/vomiting. Avoid concurrent use of grapefruit juice.

Dietary Considerations Give during or within 20 minutes following a full meal or liquid nutritional supplement; alternatively, posaconazole may be administered with an acidic carbonated beverage (eg, ginger ale). Consider alternative antifungal therapy in patients with inadequate oral intake or severe diarrhea/vomiting; if alternative therapy is not an option, closely monitoring for breakthrough fungal infections. Adequate posaconazole absorption from GI tract and subsequent plasma concentrations are dependent on food for efficacy. Lower average plasma concentrations have been associated with an increased risk of treatment failure.

Pharmacodynamics/Kinetics
Half-life Elimination 35 hours (range: 20-66 hours)
Time to Peak ~3-5 hours

Pregnancy Risk Factor C

Pregnancy Considerations Posaconazole has been shown to be teratogenic in animal studies. There are no adequate and well-controlled studies in pregnant women. Use only if the benefit to the mother justifies potential risk to the fetus.

Lactation Excretion in breast milk unknown/not recommended

Breast-Feeding Considerations Excretion in breast milk has not been investigated; use only if the benefit to the mother justifies potential risk to the fetus.

Dosage Forms
Suspension, oral:
  Noxafil®: 40 mg/mL (123 mL)

Dental Comment This drug is known to prolong the QT interval. The QT interval is measured as the time and distance between the Q point of the QRS complex and the end of the T wave in the ECG tracing. After adjustment for heart rate, the QT interval is defined as prolonged if it is more than 450 msec in men and 460 msec in women. A long QT syndrome was first described in the 1950s and 60s as a congenital syndrome involving QT interval prolongation and syncope and sudden death. Some of the congenital long QT syndromes were characterized by a peculiar electrocardiographic appearance of the QRS complex involving a premature atria beat followed by a pause, then a subsequent sinus beat showing marked QT prolongation and deformity. This type of cardiac arrhythmia was originally termed "torsade de pointes" (translated from the French as "twisting of the points").

Prolongation of the QT interval is thought to result from delayed ventricular repolarization. The repolarization process within the myocardial cell is due to the efflux of intracellular potassium. The channels associated with this current can be blocked by many drugs and predispose the electrical propagation cycle to torsade de pointes.

Posaconazole is one of the drugs confirmed to prolong the QT interval and is accepted as having a risk of causing torsade de pointes. The risk of drug-induced torsade de pointes is extremely low when a single QT interval prolonging drug is prescribed. In terms of epinephrine, it is not known what effect vasoconstrictors in the local anesthetic regimen will have in patients with a known history of congenital prolonged QT interval or in patients taking any medication that prolongs the QT interval. Until more information is obtained, it is suggested that the clinician consult with the physician prior to the use of a vasoconstrictor in suspected patients, and that the vasoconstrictor (epinephrine, levonordefrin [Neo-Cobefrin®]) be used with caution.

Potassium Acetate (poe TASS ee um AS e tate)

Pharmacologic Category Electrolyte Supplement, Parenteral

Use Potassium deficiency; to avoid chloride when high concentration of potassium is needed, source of bicarbonate

Local Anesthetic/Vasoconstrictor Precautions No information available to require special precautions

Effects on Dental Treatment No significant effects or complications reported

Effects on Bleeding No information available to require special precautions

Adverse Effects Frequency not defined.
Cardiovascular: Arrhythmias, EEG abnormalities, heart block, hypotension
Central nervous system: Confusion, listlessness
Neuromuscular & skeletal: Paralysis, paresthesia, weakness
Local: Local tissue necrosis with extravasation

General Dosage Range I.V.:
Children: 2-5 mEq/kg/day; Intermittent infusion: 0.5-1 mEq/kg/dose (maximum: 30 mEq/dose) to infuse at 0.3-0.5 mEq/kg/hour (maximum: 1 mEq/kg/hour)
Adults: 40-100 mEq/day; Intermittent infusion: 5-10 mEq/dose (maximum: 40 mEq/dose) to infuse over 2-3 hours (maximum: 40 mEq over 1 hour)

Mechanism of Action Potassium is the major cation of intracellular fluid and is essential for the conduction of nerve impulses in heart, brain, and skeletal muscle; contraction of cardiac, skeletal and smooth muscles; maintenance of normal renal function, acid-base balance, carbohydrate metabolism, and gastric secretion

Pregnancy Risk Factor C

Pregnancy Considerations Animal reproduction studies have not been conducted. Potassium requirements are the same in pregnant and nonpregnant women. Adverse events have not been observed following use of potassium supplements in healthy women with normal pregnancies. Use caution in pregnant women with other medical conditions (eg, pre-eclampsia; may be more likely to develop hyperkalemia) (IOM, 2004).

Potassium Acid Phosphate
(poe TASS ee um AS id FOS fate)

Brand Names: U.S. K-Phos® Original
Pharmacologic Category Urinary Acidifying Agent
Use Acidifies urine and lowers urinary calcium concentration; reduces odor and rash caused by ammoniacal urine; increases the antibacterial activity of methenamine

Local Anesthetic/Vasoconstrictor Precautions No information available to require special precautions

Effects on Dental Treatment No significant effects or complications reported

Effects on Bleeding No information available to require special precautions

Adverse Effects
>10%: Gastrointestinal: Diarrhea, nausea, stomach pain, flatulence, vomiting
1% to 10%:
  Cardiovascular: Bradycardia
  Endocrine & metabolic: Hyperkalemia
  Local: Local tissue necrosis with extravasation
  Neuromuscular & skeletal: Weakness
  Respiratory: Dyspnea

◄ **General Dosage Range Oral:** *Adults:* 1000 mg dissolved in 6-8 oz of water 4 times/day

Mechanism of Action The principal intracellular cation; involved in transmission of nerve impulses, muscle contractions, enzyme activity, and glucose utilization

Pregnancy Risk Factor C

Pregnancy Considerations Animal reproduction studies have not been conducted.

Potassium Bicarbonate
(poe TASS ee um bye KAR bun ate)

Brand Names: U.S. K-Effervescent

Pharmacologic Category Electrolyte Supplement, Oral

Use Potassium deficiency, hypokalemia

Local Anesthetic/Vasoconstrictor Precautions No information available to require special precautions

Effects on Dental Treatment No significant effects or complications reported

Effects on Bleeding No information available to require special precautions

General Dosage Range Oral:
Children: 1-4 mEq/kg/day
Adults: 25 mEq 2-4 times/day

Pregnancy Risk Factor C

Pregnancy Considerations Animal reproduction studies have not been conducted. Potassium requirements are the same in pregnant and nonpregnant women. Adverse events have not been observed following use of potassium supplements in healthy women with normal pregnancies. Use caution in pregnant women with other medical conditions (eg, pre-eclampsia; may be more likely to develop hyperkalemia) (IOM, 2004).

Potassium Bicarbonate and Potassium Chloride
(poe TASS ee um bye KAR bun ate & poe TASS ee um KLOR ide)

Related Information
Potassium Bicarbonate *on page 1120*
Potassium Chloride *on page 1120*

Pharmacologic Category Electrolyte Supplement, Oral

Use Treatment or prevention of hypokalemia

Local Anesthetic/Vasoconstrictor Precautions No information available to require special precautions

Effects on Dental Treatment No significant effects or complications reported

Effects on Bleeding No information available to require special precautions

Adverse Effects Frequency not defined: Gastrointestinal: Abdominal discomfort, diarrhea, nausea, vomiting

General Dosage Range
Oral:
Children: 1-4 mEq/kg/day in divided doses
Adults: Prevention: 16-24 mEq/day in 2-4 divided doses; Treatment: 40-100 mEq/day in 2-4 divided doses

Pregnancy Risk Factor C

Pregnancy Considerations Animal reproduction studies have not been conducted with this combination. Refer to individual agents.

Potassium Bicarbonate and Potassium Citrate
(poe TASS ee um bye KAR bun ate & poe TASS ee um SIT rate)

Related Information
Potassium Bicarbonate *on page 1120*
Potassium Citrate *on page 1121*

Brand Names: U.S. Effer-K®; Klor-Con®/EF

Pharmacologic Category Electrolyte Supplement, Oral

Use Treatment or prevention of hypokalemia, particularly when it is necessary to avoid chloride or the acid/base status requires bicarbonate

Local Anesthetic/Vasoconstrictor Precautions No information available to require special precautions

Effects on Dental Treatment No significant effects or complications reported

Effects on Bleeding No information available to require special precautions

Adverse Effects Frequency not defined.
Gastrointestinal: Abdominal pain, diarrhea, nausea, vomiting
Endocrine & metabolic: Hyperkalemia and associated manifestations (eg, cardiac arrhythmias, etc)

General Dosage Range
Oral: *Adults:* Prevention: 10-80 mEq/day in 1-4 divided doses; Treatment: 40-100 mEq/day in 2-4 divided doses

Mechanism of Action Potassium is needed for the conduction of nerve impulses in heart, brain, and skeletal muscle; contraction of cardiac, skeletal and smooth muscles; maintenance of normal renal function

Pregnancy Risk Factor C

Pregnancy Considerations Animal reproduction studies have not been conducted with this combination. See individual agents.

Potassium Chloride (poe TASS ee um KLOR ide)

Brand Names: U.S. K-Tab®; Kaon-CL® 10; Klor-Con®; Klor-Con® 10; Klor-Con® 8; Klor-Con® M10; Klor-Con® M15; Klor-Con® M20; Klor-Con®/25; microK®; microK® 10

Brand Names: Canada Apo-K®; K-10®; K-Dur®; Micro-K Extencaps®; Roychlor®; Slo-Pot; Slow-K®

Pharmacologic Category Electrolyte Supplement, Oral; Electrolyte Supplement, Parenteral

Use Treatment or prevention of hypokalemia

Local Anesthetic/Vasoconstrictor Precautions No information available to require special precautions

Effects on Dental Treatment No significant effects or complications reported

Effects on Bleeding No information available to require special precautions

Adverse Effects Frequency not defined.
Dermatologic: Rash
Endocrine & metabolic: Hyperkalemia
Gastrointestinal: Abdominal pain/discomfort, diarrhea, flatulence, GI bleeding (oral), GI obstruction (oral), GI perforation (oral), nausea, vomiting

General Dosage Range
I.V.:
Children: Initial: 0.5-1 mEq/kg/dose (maximum dose: 40 mEq); repeat as needed based on lab values
Adults: Intermittent infusion: ≤10 mEq/hour; repeat as needed based on lab values (maximum: 200 mEq/day)

Oral:
Children: 1-2 mEq/kg/day in 1-2 divided doses or as needed based on lab values
Adults: Initial: 6-10 mEq/dose (maximum: 40 mEq/dose); Maintenance: 40-100 mEq/day in divided doses or as needed based on lab values
Mechanism of Action Potassium is the major cation of intracellular fluid and is essential for the conduction of nerve impulses in heart, brain, and skeletal muscle; contraction of cardiac, skeletal and smooth muscles; maintenance of normal renal function, acid-base balance, carbohydrate metabolism, and gastric secretion
Pregnancy Risk Factor C
Pregnancy Considerations Reproduction studies have not been conducted. Potassium requirements are the same in pregnant and nonpregnant women. Adverse events have not been observed following use of potassium supplements in healthy women with normal pregnancies. Use caution in pregnant women with other medical conditions (eg, pre-eclampsia; may be more likely to develop hyperkalemia) (IOM, 2004). Potassium supplementation (that does not cause maternal hyperkalemia) would not be expected to cause adverse fetal events.

Potassium Citrate (poe TASS ee um SIT rate)

Brand Names: U.S. Urocit®-K
Brand Names: Canada Urocit®-K
Pharmacologic Category Alkalinizing Agent, Oral
Use Prevention of uric acid nephrolithiasis; prevention of calcium renal stones in patients with hypocitraturia; urinary alkalinizer when sodium citrate is contraindicated
Local Anesthetic/Vasoconstrictor Precautions No information available to require special precautions
Effects on Dental Treatment No significant effects or complications reported
Effects on Bleeding No information available to require special precautions
Adverse Effects Frequency not defined.
Endocrine & metabolic: Hyperkalemia
Gastrointestinal: Abdominal discomfort, diarrhea, nausea, vomiting
General Dosage Range Oral: *Adults:*
Immediate release: 10-20 mEq 3 times/day or 15 mEq 4 times/day (maximum: 100 mEq/day)
Extended release: 15-30 mEq 2 times/day or 10-20 mEq 3 times/day (maximum: 100 mEq/day)
Pregnancy Risk Factor C
Pregnancy Considerations Animal reproduction studies have not been conducted.

Potassium Citrate and Citric Acid
(poe TASS ee um SIT rate & SI trik AS id)

Related Information
Potassium Citrate *on page 1121*
Brand Names: U.S. Cytra-K
Pharmacologic Category Alkalinizing Agent, Oral
Use Treatment of metabolic acidosis; alkalinizing agent in conditions where long-term maintenance of an alkaline urine is desirable
Local Anesthetic/Vasoconstrictor Precautions No information available to require special precautions
Effects on Dental Treatment No significant effects or complications reported
Effects on Bleeding No information available to require special precautions

General Dosage Range Oral:
Children: 5-15 mL after meals and at bedtime
Adults: 15-30 mL **or** 1 packet dissolved in water after meals and at bedtime
Pregnancy Considerations Refer to potassium citrate monograph for information.

Potassium Gluconate
(poe TASS ee um GLOO coe nate)

Pharmacologic Category Electrolyte Supplement, Oral
Use Dietary supplement
Local Anesthetic/Vasoconstrictor Precautions No information available to require special precautions
Effects on Dental Treatment No significant effects or complications reported
Effects on Bleeding No information available to require special precautions
General Dosage Range Oral: *Adults:* One tablet daily
Mechanism of Action Potassium is the major cation of intracellular fluid and is essential for the conduction of nerve impulses in heart, brain, and skeletal muscle; contraction of cardiac, skeletal and smooth muscles; maintenance of normal renal function, acid-base balance, carbohydrate metabolism, and gastric secretion
Pregnancy Considerations Potassium requirements are the same in pregnant and non-pregnant women. Adverse events have not been observed following use of potassium supplements in healthy women with normal pregnancies. Use caution in pregnant women with other medical conditions (eg, pre-eclampsia; may be more likely to develop hyperkalemia) (IOM, 2004).

Potassium Iodide (poe TASS ee um EYE oh dide)

Related Information
Endocrine Disorders and Pregnancy *on page 1517*
Brand Names: U.S. iOSAT™ [OTC]; SSKI®; ThyroSafe® [OTC]; Thyroshield® [OTC]
Pharmacologic Category Antidote; Antithyroid Agent; Expectorant
Use Expectorant for the symptomatic treatment of chronic pulmonary diseases complicated by mucous; block thyroidal uptake of radioactive isotopes of iodine in a nuclear radiation emergency
Unlabeled Use Lymphocutaneous and cutaneous sporotrichosis; reduce thyroid vascularity prior to thyroidectomy; management of thyrotoxic crisis; block thyroidal uptake of radioactive isotopes of iodine after therapeutic or diagnostic exposure to radioactive iodine
Local Anesthetic/Vasoconstrictor Precautions No information available to require special precautions
Effects on Dental Treatment Key adverse event(s) related to dental treatment: Metallic taste.
Effects on Bleeding No information available to require special precautions
Adverse Effects Frequency not defined.
Cardiovascular: Cardiac arrhythmia
Central nervous system: Confusion, fatigue, fever, numbness, tingling sensation
Dermatologic: Skin rash, urticaria
Endocrine & metabolic: Goiter, hyperthyroidism (prolonged use), hypothyroidism (prolonged use), myxedema
Gastrointestinal: Diarrhea, enlargement of salivary glands, gastric distress, gastrointestinal hemorrhage, metallic taste, nausea, stomach pain, vomiting

◀ Hematologic & oncologic: Lymphedema, thyroid adenoma

Hypersensitivity: Hypersensitivity reaction (angioedema, cutaneous and mucosal hemorrhage, serum sickness-like symptoms)

Musculoskeletal: Weakness

Respiratory: Dyspnea, wheezing

Miscellaneous: Iodine poisoning (with prolonged treatment/high doses)

General Dosage Range Oral:

Infants <1 month: iOSAT™, ThyroSafe®, ThyroShield®: 16.25 mg once daily

Infants 1-12 months and Children 1-3 years: iOSAT™, ThyroSafe®, ThyroShield®: 32.5 mg once daily

Children 3-12 years and Children 12-18 years weighing <68 kg: iOSAT™, ThyroSafe®, ThyroShield®: 65 mg once daily

Children 12-18 years weighing ≥68 kg and Adults: iOSAT™, ThyroSafe®, ThyroShield®: 130 mg once daily

Adults: SSKI®: 300-600 mg 3-4 times daily

Mechanism of Action Reduces viscosity of mucus by increasing respiratory tract secretions; inhibits secretion of thyroid hormone, fosters colloid accumulation in thyroid follicles. Following radioactive iodine exposure, potassium iodide blocks the uptake of radioactive iodine by the thyroid, reducing the risk of thyroid cancer.

Pharmacodynamics/Kinetics

Onset of Action Hyperthyroidism: 24-48 hours; Peak effect: 10-15 days after continuous therapy

Duration of Action Radioactive iodine exposure: Each dose has a duration of ~24 hours

Pregnancy Risk Factor D

Pregnancy Considerations Iodide crosses the placenta (may cause hypothyroidism and goiter in fetus/newborn). Use as an expectorant during pregnancy is contraindicated by the AAP. Use for protection against thyroid cancer secondary to radioactive iodine exposure is considered acceptable based upon risk:benefit, keeping in mind the dose and duration. In general, medications used as antidotes should take into consideration the health and prognosis of the mother (Bailey, 2003). Pregnant women should take as instructed by public officials and contact their physician. Repeat dosing should be avoided if possible. Refer to Iodine monograph for additional information.

Potassium Iodide and Iodine
(poe TASS ee um EYE oh dide & EYE oh dine)

Related Information

Iodine *on page 755*

Potassium Iodide *on page 1121*

Pharmacologic Category Antithyroid Agent

Use Topical antiseptic

Unlabeled Use Reduce thyroid vascularity prior to thyroidectomy and management of thyrotoxic crisis; block thyroidal uptake of radioactive isotopes of iodine in a radiation emergency or after therapeutic/diagnostic use of radioactive iodine

Local Anesthetic/Vasoconstrictor Precautions No information available to require special precautions

Effects on Dental Treatment Key adverse event(s) related to dental treatment: Metallic taste.

Effects on Bleeding No information available to require special precautions

Adverse Effects Frequency not defined.

Cardiovascular: Irregular heart beat

Central nervous system: Confusion, tiredness, fever

Dermatologic: Skin rash

Endocrine & metabolic: Goiter, salivary gland swelling/tenderness, thyroid adenoma, swelling of neck/throat, myxedema, lymph node swelling, hyper-/hypothyroidism

Gastrointestinal: Diarrhea, gastrointestinal bleeding, metallic taste, nausea, stomach pain, stomach upset, vomiting

Neuromuscular & skeletal: Numbness, tingling, weakness, joint pain

Miscellaneous: Chronic iodine poisoning (with prolonged treatment/high doses); iodism, hypersensitivity reactions (angioedema, cutaneous and mucosal hemorrhage, serum sickness-like symptoms)

General Dosage Range Topical: *Adults:* Apply directly to area(s) requiring antiseptic

Mechanism of Action In hyperthyroidism, iodine temporarily inhibits thyroid hormone synthesis and secretion into the circulation; use also decreases thyroid gland size and vascularity. Serum T_4 and T_3 concentrations can be reduced for several weeks with use but effect will not be maintained.

Following radioactive iodine exposure, potassium iodide blocks uptake of radioiodine by the thyroid, reducing the risk of thyroid cancer.

Pharmacodynamics/Kinetics

Onset of Action Hyperthyroidism: 24-48 hours; Peak effect: 10-15 days after continuous therapy

Pregnancy Risk Factor D (potassium iodide)

Pregnancy Considerations Iodide crosses the placenta (may cause hypothyroidism and goiter in fetus/newborn). Use for protection against thyroid cancer secondary to radioactive iodine exposure is considered acceptable based upon risk:benefit, keeping in mind the dose and duration. Repeat dosing should be avoided if possible. Refer to Iodine for additional information.

Potassium P-Aminobenzoate
(poe TASS ee um pe a mee noe BEN zoe ate)

Brand Names: U.S. Potaba®

Pharmacologic Category Vitamin, Water Soluble

Use Presently, all indications are classified by the FDA as "possibly effective."

Treatment of scleroderma, dermatomyositis, morphea, linear scleroderma, pemphigus, Peyronie's disease

Local Anesthetic/Vasoconstrictor Precautions No information available to require special precautions

Effects on Dental Treatment No significant effects or complications reported

Effects on Bleeding No information available to require special precautions

Adverse Effects Frequency not defined.

Central nervous system: Fever

Dermatologic: Rash

Gastrointestinal: Anorexia, nausea

Miscellaneous: Hypersensitivity reaction

General Dosage Range Oral:

Children: 1 g/10 pounds of weight/day in divided doses

Adults: 12 g/day in 4-6 divided doses

Mechanism of Action P-aminobenzoate is a member of the vitamin B complex family. It may have an antifibrotic effect due to increased oxygen uptake at the tissue level.

Pregnancy Considerations Safety for use in pregnancy has not been established.

Potassium Phosphate (poe TASS ee um FOS fate)

Brand Names: U.S. Neutra-Phos®-K [OTC] [DSC]
Pharmacologic Category Electrolyte Supplement, Parenteral
Use Treatment and prevention of hypophosphatemia; **Note:** The concomitant amount of potassium must be calculated into the total electrolyte content. For each 1 mmol of phosphate, ~1.5 mEq of potassium will be administered. Therefore, if ordering 30 mmol of potassium phosphate, the patient will receive ~45 mEq of potassium.
Local Anesthetic/Vasoconstrictor Precautions No information available to require special precautions
Effects on Dental Treatment No significant effects or complications reported
Effects on Bleeding No information available to require special precautions
Adverse Effects Frequency not defined.
  Cardiovascular: Arrhythmia, bradycardia, chest pain, ECG changes, edema, heart block, hypotension
  Central nervous system: Listlessness, mental confusion, tetany (with large doses of phosphate)
  Endocrine & metabolic: Hyperkalemia
  Gastrointestinal: Diarrhea, nausea, stomach pain, vomiting
  Genitourinary: Urine output decreased
  Local: Phlebitis
  Neuromuscular & skeletal: Paralysis, paresthesia, weakness
  Renal: Acute renal failure
  Respiratory: Dyspnea
General Dosage Range
  I.V.:
    Children: 0.08-1 mmol phosphate/kg **or** Parenteral nutrition Infusion: 0.5-2 mmol/kg/24 hours
    Adults: 0.08-1 mmol phosphate/kg **or** Parenteral nutrition: Infusion: 20-40 mmol/24 hours
Pregnancy Risk Factor C
Pregnancy Considerations Reproduction studies have not been conducted. Phosphorus requirements are the same in pregnant and nonpregnant women (IOM, 1997). Although this product is not used for potassium supplementation, adverse events have not been observed following use of potassium supplements in healthy women with normal pregnancies. Use caution in pregnant women with other medical conditions (eg, pre-eclampsia; may be more likely to develop hyperkalemia) (IOM, 2004).

Potassium Phosphate and Sodium Phosphate
(poe TASS ee um FOS fate & SOW dee um FOS fate)

Related Information
  Potassium Phosphate *on page 1123*
  Sodium Phosphates *on page 1248*
Brand Names: U.S. K-Phos® MF; K-Phos® Neutral; K-Phos® No. 2; Phos-NaK; Phospha 250™ Neutral
Pharmacologic Category Electrolyte Supplement, Oral
Use Phosphorus supplement; to increase urinary phosphate and pyrophosphate; to acidify the urine to lower calcium concentrations; to increase the antibacterial activity of methenamine; reduce odor and rash caused by ammonia in urine
Local Anesthetic/Vasoconstrictor Precautions No information available to require special precautions

Effects on Dental Treatment No significant effects or complications reported
Effects on Bleeding No information available to require special precautions
Adverse Effects Frequency not defined.
  Cardiovascular: Bradycardia, arrhythmia, chest pain, edema, tachycardia
  Central nervous system: Mental confusion, tetany (with large doses of phosphate), headache, dizziness, seizure
  Endocrine & metabolic: Hyperkalemia, alkalosis
  Gastrointestinal: Diarrhea, nausea, stomach pain, flatulence, vomiting, throat pain, weight gain
  Genitourinary: Urine output decreased
  Local: Phlebitis
  Neuromuscular & skeletal: Weakness, arthralgia, bone pain, paralysis, paresthesia, pain/weakness of extremities, muscle cramps
  Renal: Acute renal failure
  Respiratory: Dyspnea
  Miscellaneous: Thirst
General Dosage Range Oral:
  Children ≥4 years and Adolescents: 250 mg elemental phosphorus 4 times daily
  Adults: 250-500 mg elemental phosphorus 4 times daily; may be increased to 250 mg elemental phosphorus every 2 hours (maximum daily dose: 2000 mg elemental phosphorus)
Pregnancy Risk Factor C
Pregnancy Considerations Animal reproduction studies have not been conducted.

Povidone-Iodine (Topical)
(POE vi done EYE oh dyne)

Related Information
  Management of Patients Undergoing Cancer Therapy *on page 1596*
Brand Names: U.S. Betadine® Swab Aids [OTC]; Betadine® [OTC]; Operand® Povidone-Iodine [OTC]; Povidine™ [OTC]; Summer's Eve® Medicated Douche [OTC]; Vagi-Gard® [OTC]
Brand Names: Canada Betadine®; Proviodine
Pharmacologic Category Antiseptic, Topical; Antiseptic, Vaginal; Topical Skin Product
Use External antiseptic with broad microbicidal spectrum for the prevention or treatment of topical infections associated with surgery, burns, minor cuts/scrapes; relief of minor vaginal irritation
Local Anesthetic/Vasoconstrictor Precautions No information available to require special precautions
Effects on Dental Treatment No significant effects or complications reported
Effects on Bleeding No information available to require special precautions
Adverse Effects Frequency not defined. Also refer to Iodine monograph.
  Local: Edema, irritation, pruritus, rash
General Dosage Range
  Intravaginal: *Adults:* Insert 0.3% solution vaginally once daily
  Topical: *Adults:* Apply to affected area as needed **or** apply to wet skin or hands, scrub for ~5 minutes, then rinse
Mechanism of Action Povidone-iodine is known to be a powerful broad spectrum germicidal agent effective against a wide range of bacteria, viruses, fungi, protozoa, and spores.

◄ **Pregnancy Considerations** Vaginal products should not be used during pregnancy. Absorbed systemically as iodine. Transient hypothyroidism in the newborn has been reported following topical or vaginal use prior to delivery. Refer to Iodine for additional information.

PRALAtrexate (pral a TREX ate)

Brand Names: U.S. Folotyn®

Pharmacologic Category Antineoplastic Agent, Antimetabolite (Antifolate)

Use Treatment of relapsed or refractory peripheral T-cell lymphoma (PTCL)

Unlabeled Use Treatment of relapsed or refractory cutaneous T-cell lymphomas (mycosis fungoides [MF] and Sézary syndrome [SS])

Local Anesthetic/Vasoconstrictor Precautions No information available to require special precautions

Effects on Dental Treatment Key adverse event(s) related to dental treatment: Mucositis and stomatitis

Effects on Bleeding No information available to require special precautions

Adverse Effects

>10%:

Cardiovascular: Edema (30%)

Central nervous system: Fatigue (36%), fever (32%)

Dermatologic: Rash (15%; grades 3/4: 0%), pruritus (14%; grade 3: 2%; grade 4: 0%)

Endocrine & metabolic: Hypokalemia (15%)

Gastrointestinal: Mucositis (70%; grade 3: 17%; grade 4: 4%), nausea (40%), constipation (33%), vomiting (25%), diarrhea (21%), anorexia (15%), abdominal pain (12%)

Hematologic: Thrombocytopenia (41%; grade 3: 14%; grade 4: 19%), anemia (34%; grade 3: 15%; grade 4: 2%), neutropenia (24%; grade 3: 13%; grade 4: 7%), leukopenia (11%; grade 3: 3%; grade 4: 4%)

Hepatic: Transaminases increased (13%; grade 3: 5%; grade 4: 0%)

Neuromuscular & skeletal: Limb pain (12%), back pain (11%)

Respiratory: Cough (28%), epistaxis (26%), dyspnea (19%), pharyngolaryngeal pain (14%)

Miscellaneous: Night sweats (11%), infection

1% to 10%:

Cardiovascular: Tachycardia (10%)

Endocrine & metabolic: Dehydration (serious >3%)

Hematologic: Neutropenic fever (serious >3%)

Neuromuscular & skeletal: Weakness (10%)

Respiratory: Upper respiratory infection (10%)

Miscellaneous: Sepsis (serious >3%)

General Dosage Range Dosage adjustment recommended in patients with renal impairment, hepatic impairment, or who develop toxicities.

I.V.: *Adults:* 30 mg/m² once weekly for 6 weeks of a 7-week treatment cycle

Mechanism of Action Antifolate analog; inhibits DNA, RNA, and protein synthesis by selectively entering cells expressing reduced folate carrier (RFC-1), is polyglutamylated by folylpolyglutamate synthetase (FPGS) and then competes for the DHFR-folate binding site to inhibit dihydrofolate reductase (DHFR)

Pharmacodynamics/Kinetics

Half-life Elimination 12-18 hours

Pregnancy Risk Factor D

Pregnancy Considerations Adverse effects were observed in animal reproduction studies. May cause fetal harm if administered to a pregnant woman.

Pramipexole (pra mi PEKS ole)

Brand Names: U.S. Mirapex®; Mirapex® ER®

Brand Names: Canada Apo-Pramipexole®; Ava-Pramipexole; CO Pramipexole; Mirapex®; PMS-Pramipexole; Sandoz-Pramipexole; Teva-Pramipexole

Pharmacologic Category Anti-Parkinson's Agent, Dopamine Agonist

Use

Immediate release: Treatment of the signs and symptoms of idiopathic Parkinson's disease; treatment of moderate-to-severe primary Restless Legs Syndrome (RLS)

Extended release: Treatment of the signs and symptoms of idiopathic Parkinson's disease

Unlabeled Use Treatment of depression in bipolar disorder; treatment of fibromyalgia

Local Anesthetic/Vasoconstrictor Precautions No information available to require special precautions

Effects on Dental Treatment Key adverse event(s) related to dental treatment: Xerostomia (normal salivary flow resumes upon discontinuation) and dysphagia.

Effects on Bleeding No information available to require special precautions

Adverse Effects

Parkinson's disease: Actual frequency may be dependent on dose and/or formulation:

>10%:

Cardiovascular: Orthostatic hypotension (dose related; ≤53%)

Central nervous system: Somnolence (dose related; 9% to 36%), extrapyramidal syndrome (28%), insomnia (4% to 27%), dizziness (2% to 26%), hallucinations (5% to 17%), abnormal dreams (11%), headache (4% to 7%)

Gastrointestinal: Nausea (dose related; 11% to 28%), constipation (dose related; 6% to 14%)

Neuromuscular & skeletal: Dyskinesia (17% to 47%), weakness (1% to 14%)

Miscellaneous: Accidental injury (17%)

1% to 10%:

Cardiovascular: Edema (2% to 8%), chest pain (3%)

Central nervous system: Confusion (4% to 10%), dystonia (2% to 8%), fatigue (6%), amnesia (dose related; 4% to 6%), sudden onset of sleep (3% to 6%), vertigo (2% to 4%), hypesthesia (3%), abnormal thinking (2% to 3%), akathisia (2% to 3%), malaise (2% to 3%), paranoia (2%), sleep disorder (1% to 3%), depression (≤2%), delusions (1%), fever (1%), myoclonus (1%)

Endocrine & metabolic: Libido decreased (1%)

Gastrointestinal: Xerostomia (4% to 7%), anorexia (1% to 5%), vomiting (4%), abdominal discomfort/pain (1% to 4%), dyspepsia (3%), appetite increased (2% to 3%), dysphagia (2%), weight loss (2%), salivary hypersecretion (≤2%), diarrhea (1% to 2%)

Genitourinary: Urinary frequency (6%), urinary tract infection (4%), impotence (2%), urinary incontinence (2%)

Neuromuscular & skeletal: Gait abnormalities (7%), hypertonia (7%), muscle spasm (3% to 5%), falls (4%), arthritis (3%), tremor (3%), back pain (2% to 3%), bursitis (2%), muscle twitching (2%), balance abnormalities (≤2%), CPK increased (1%), myasthenia (1%)

Ocular: Accommodation abnormalities (4%), vision abnormalities (3%), diplopia (1%)

Respiratory: Dyspnea (4%), cough (3%), rhinitis (3%), pneumonia (2%)

Restless legs syndrome: Actual frequency may be dependent on dose:

>10%:

Central nervous system: Headache (16%), insomnia (9% to 13%)

Gastrointestinal: Nausea (11% to 27%)

1% to 10%:

Central nervous system: Fatigue (3% to 9%), abnormal dreams (1% to 8%), somnolence (6%)

Gastrointestinal: Diarrhea (1% to 7%), constipation (4%), xerostomia (3%)

Neuromuscular & skeletal: Limb pain (3% to 7%)

Respiratory: Nasal congestion (≤6%)

Miscellaneous: Influenza (1% to 7%)

General Dosage Range Dosage adjustment recommended in patients with renal impairment

Oral: Immediate release: *Adults:* Initial: 0.125 mg 3 times daily **or** 0.125 mg once daily before bedtime; Maintenance: 0.5-1.5 mg 3 times daily **or** 0.125-0.5 mg once daily before bedtime

Oral: Extended release: *Adults:* 0.375-4.5 mg once daily

Mechanism of Action Pramipexole is a nonergot dopamine agonist with specificity for the D_2 subfamily dopamine receptor, and has also been shown to bind to D_3 and D_4 receptors. By binding to these receptors, it is thought that pramipexole can stimulate dopamine activity on the nerves of the striatum and substantia nigra.

Pharmacodynamics/Kinetics

Half-life Elimination 8.5 hours; Elderly: 12 hours

Time to Peak Serum: Immediate release: ~2 hours; Extended release: 6 hours

Pregnancy Risk Factor C

Pregnancy Considerations Early embryonic loss and postnatal growth inhibition were observed in animal studies. There are no adequate and well-controlled studies in pregnant women.

Pramlintide (PRAM lin tide)

Brand Names: U.S. SymlinPen®

Pharmacologic Category Amylinomimetic; Antidiabetic Agent

Use

Adjunctive treatment with mealtime insulin in type 1 diabetes mellitus (insulin dependent, IDDM) patients who have failed to achieve desired glucose control despite optimal insulin therapy

Adjunctive treatment with mealtime insulin in type 2 diabetes mellitus (noninsulin dependent, NIDDM) patients who have failed to achieve desired glucose control despite optimal insulin therapy, with or without concurrent sulfonylurea and/or metformin

Local Anesthetic/Vasoconstrictor Precautions No information available to require special precautions

Effects on Dental Treatment No significant effects or complications reported

Effects on Bleeding No information available to require special precautions

Adverse Effects

>10%:

Central nervous system: Headache (5% to 13%)

Gastrointestinal: Nausea (28% to 48%), vomiting (7% to 11%), anorexia (≤17%)

Endocrine & metabolic: Severe hypoglycemia (type 1 diabetes ≤17%)

Miscellaneous: Inflicted injury (8% to 14%)

1% to 10%:

Central nervous system: Fatigue (3% to 7%), dizziness (2% to 6%)

Endocrine & metabolic: Severe hypoglycemia (type 2 diabetes ≤8%)

Gastrointestinal: Abdominal pain (2% to 8%)

Respiratory: Pharyngitis (3% to 5%), cough (2% to 6%)

Neuromuscular & skeletal: Arthralgia (2% to 7%)

Miscellaneous: Allergic reaction (≤6%)

General Dosage Range SubQ: *Adults:*

Type 1 diabetes mellitus (insulin dependent, IDDM): Initial: 15 mcg immediately prior to meals; Target dose: 30-60 mcg prior to meals

Type 2 diabetes mellitus (noninsulin dependent, NIDDM): Initial: 60 mcg immediately prior to meals; after 3-7 days increase to 120 mcg prior to meals

Mechanism of Action Synthetic analog of human amylin cosecreted with insulin by pancreatic beta cells; reduces postprandial glucose increases via the following mechanisms: 1) prolongation of gastric emptying time, 2) reduction of postprandial glucagon secretion, and 3) reduction of caloric intake through centrally-mediated appetite suppression

Pharmacodynamics/Kinetics

Duration of Action 3 hours

Half-life Elimination ~48 minutes

Time to Peak 20 minutes

Pregnancy Risk Factor C

Pregnancy Considerations Adverse events have been observed in animal reproduction studies. Based on *in vitro* data, pramlintide has a low potential to cross the placenta. Maternal hyperglycemia can be associated with adverse effects in the fetus, including macrosomia, neonatal hyperglycemia, and hyperbilirubinemia; the risk of congenital malformations is increased when the Hb A_{1c} is above the normal range. Diabetes can also be associated with adverse effects in the mother. Poorly-treated diabetes may cause end-organ damage that may in turn negatively affect obstetric outcomes. Physiologic glucose levels should be maintained prior to and during pregnancy to decrease the risk of adverse events in the mother and the fetus. Until additional safety and efficacy data are obtained, the use of pramlintide is generally not recommended in the routine management of diabetes mellitus during pregnancy. Insulin is the drug of choice for the control of diabetes mellitus during pregnancy.

Pramoxine (pra MOKS een)

Brand Names: U.S. Caladryl® Clear™ [OTC]; Callergy Clear [OTC]; Curasore® [OTC]; Dermarest® Eczema Medicated Moisturizer [OTC]; Itch-X® [OTC]; Prax® [OTC]; Proctofoam® NS [OTC]; Sarna® Sensitive [OTC]; Soothing Care™ Itch Relief [OTC]; Summer's Eve® Anti-Itch Maximum Strength [OTC]; Tronolane® Cream [OTC]; Tucks® Hemorrhoidal [OTC]

Pharmacologic Category Local Anesthetic

Use Temporary relief of pain and itching associated with hemorrhoids, burns, minor cuts, scrapes, or minor skin irritations

Local Anesthetic/Vasoconstrictor Precautions No information available to require special precautions

Effects on Dental Treatment No significant effects or complications reported

Effects on Bleeding No information available to require special precautions

General Dosage Range Topical:
Children ≥2 years and Adults: Lotion, cream: Apply up to 3-4 times daily
Children ≥12 years and Adults: Hemorrhoidal foam, ointment, wipes: Apply up to 5 times daily
Mechanism of Action Pramoxine, like other anesthetics, decreases the neuronal membrane's permeability to sodium ions; both initiation and conduction of nerve impulses are blocked, thus depolarization of the neuron is inhibited
Pharmacodynamics/Kinetics
Onset of Action 3-5 minutes

Pramoxine and Hydrocortisone
(pra MOKS een & hye droe KOR ti sone)

Related Information
Hydrocortisone (Topical) *on page 699*
Pramoxine *on page 1125*
Brand Names: U.S. Analpram E™; Analpram HC®; Epifoam®; Pramosone E™; Pramosone®; ProCort®; ProctoFoam® HC; Zypram™
Brand Names: Canada Pramox® HC; Proctofoam™-HC
Pharmacologic Category Anesthetic/Corticosteroid
Use Relief of inflammatory and pruritic manifestations of corticosteroid-responsive dermatoses
Local Anesthetic/Vasoconstrictor Precautions No information available to require special precautions
Effects on Dental Treatment No significant effects or complications reported
Effects on Bleeding No information available to require special precautions
Adverse Effects See individual agents.
General Dosage Range Rectal, topical: *Adults:* Apply to affected areas 3-4 times/day
Mechanism of Action See individual agents.
Pregnancy Risk Factor C
Pregnancy Considerations Adverse events have been observed with corticosteroids in animal reproduction studies. Rectal use of pramoxine and hydrocortisone for the treatment of hemorrhoids in the third trimester of pregnancy was not shown to affect birth weight (Ebrahimi, 2011). Also refer to Hydrocortisone (Topical) monograph.

Prasugrel (PRA soo grel)

Related Information
Antiplatelet and Anticoagulation Considerations in Dentistry *on page 1503*
Cardiovascular Diseases *on page 1492*
Brand Names: U.S. Effient®
Brand Names: Canada Effient®
Generic Availability (U.S.) No
Pharmacologic Category Antiplatelet Agent; Antiplatelet Agent, Thienopyridine
Use Reduces rate of thrombotic cardiovascular events (including stent thrombosis) in patients who are to be managed with percutaneous coronary intervention (PCI) for unstable angina (UA), non-ST-segment elevation MI (NSTEMI), or ST-elevation MI (STEMI)
Unlabeled Use Initial treatment of UA/NSTEMI in patients undergoing PCI with allergy or major gastrointestinal intolerance to aspirin (**Note:** Dual antiplatelet therapy with another P2Y12 receptor inhibitor is not recommended in this situation [Jneid, 2012].)

Local Anesthetic/Vasoconstrictor Precautions No information available to require special precautions
Effects on Dental Treatment Key adverse event(s) related to dental treatment: May cause bleeding during invasive dental procedures and medical consultation is suggested prior to any consideration of discontinuation. If possible, manage bleeding without discontinuing therapy; premature discontinuation of treatment may increase the risk for cardiac adverse effects.
Aspirin in combination with clopidogrel (Plavix®), prasugrel (Effient®), or ticagrelor (Brilinta™) is the primary prevention strategy against stent thrombosis after placement of drug-eluting metal stents in coronary patients. Premature discontinuation of combination antiplatelet therapy (ie, dual antiplatelet therapy) strongly increases the risk of a catastrophic event of stent thrombosis leading to myocardial infarction and/or death, so says a science advisory issued in January 2007 from the American Heart Association in collaboration with the American Dental Association and other professional healthcare organizations. The advisory stresses a 12-month therapy of dual antiplatelet therapy after placement of a drug-eluting stent in order to prevent thrombosis at the stent site. Any elective surgery should be postponed for 1 year after stent implantation, and if surgery must be performed, consideration should be given to continuing the antiplatelet therapy during the perioperative period in high-risk patients with drug-eluting stents.
This advisory was issued from a science panel made up of representatives from the American Heart Association (AHA), the American College of Cardiology, the Society for Cardiovascular Angiography and Interventions, the American College of Surgeons, the American Dental Association (ADA), and the American College of Physicians (Grines, 2007).
Effects on Bleeding Prasugrel blocks platelet aggregation and may prolong bleeding time. Inhibition is irreversible; on discontinuation of prasugrel, normal platelet function returns only when new platelets are released from the bone marrow. Normal platelet function will occur within 5-9 days of discontinuation. There is no scientific evidence to warrant the discontinuance of prasugrel prior to dental surgery.

Dual antiplatelet therapy: Aspirin irreversibly inhibits platelet aggregation which can prolong bleeding. Upon discontinuation, normal platelet function returns only when new platelets are released (~7-10 days). However, in the case of dental surgery, there is no scientific evidence to support discontinuation of aspirin. The discontinuation of aspirin may place the patient at risk for a thrombotic event or other cardiovascular complication. In particular, aspirin should **not** be discontinued in patients with cardiac stents that have not completed their full course of dual antiplatelet therapy (eg, aspirin and clopidogrel [prasugrel or ticagrelor]); patient-specific situations need to be discussed with cardiologist. When feasible, postponement of dental surgery until the completion of dual antiplatelet therapy should be considered. Any modification of aspirin therapy should be discussed with the prescribing physician.
Adverse Effects As with all drugs which may affect hemostasis, bleeding is associated with prasugrel. Hemorrhage may occur at virtually any site. Risk is dependent on multiple variables, including patient susceptibility and concurrent use of multiple agents which alter hemostasis.

2% to 10%:
  Cardiovascular: Hypertension (8%), hypotension (4%), atrial fibrillation (3%), bradycardia (3%), noncardiac chest pain (3%), peripheral edema (3%)
  Central nervous system: Headache (6%), dizziness (4%), fatigue (4%), fever (3%), extremity pain (3%)
  Dermatologic: Rash (3%)
  Endocrine & metabolic: Hypercholesterolemia/hyperlipidemia (7%)
  Gastrointestinal: Nausea (5%), diarrhea (2%), gastrointestinal hemorrhage (2%)
  Hematologic: Leukopenia (3%), anemia (2%)
  Neuromuscular & skeletal: Back pain (5%)
  Respiratory: Epistaxis (6%), dyspnea (5%), cough (4%)

Dosage Oral:
  Adults: Acute coronary syndrome (ACS): Oral:
  Percutaneous coronary intervention (PCI) for ACS: Loading dose: 60 mg administered promptly (as soon as coronary anatomy is known or before if risk for bleeding is low and need for CABG considered unlikely) and no later than 1 hour after PCI; Maintenance dose: 10 mg once daily (in combination with aspirin 81-325 mg/day day; 81 mg/day recommended [Levine, 2011]). For patients with STEMI, a loading dose may also be administered if PCI is performed >24 hours after treatment with a fibrin-specific thrombolytic (ie, alteplase, reteplase, tenecteplase) (O'Gara, 2013).
  Duration of prasugrel (in combination with aspirin) after stent placement: **Premature interruption of therapy may result in stent thrombosis with subsequent fatal or nonfatal MI.** Those with ACS receiving either stent type (bare metal [BMS] or drug-eluting stent [DES]) or those receiving a DES for a non-ACS indication, prasugrel for at least 12 months is recommended. Those receiving a BMS for a non-ACS indication should be given at least 1 month and ideally up to 12 months; if patient is at increased risk of bleeding, give for a minimum of 2 weeks. A duration >12 months, regardless of indication, may be considered in patients with DES placement (Jneid, 2012; Levine, 2011).
  Maintenance dosing in low body weight (ie, <60 kg) individuals: Due to a higher incidence of bleeding in patients weighing <60 kg, a maintenance dose of 5 mg once daily may be considered. In aspirin-treated patients weighing <60 kg (mean: 56.4 ± 3.7 kg) with stable coronary artery disease, the use of prasugrel 5 mg once daily was shown to reduce platelet reactivity to a similar extent as prasugrel 10 mg administered once daily to patients >60 kg (mean: 84.7 ± 14.9 kg); clinical events were not evaluated (Erlinge, 2012). In patients with ACS (medically managed) treated with aspirin, a 5 mg daily maintenance dose (after a 30 mg loading dose) in patients <60 kg did not demonstrate a significant difference in the composite primary end point of death from cardiovascular causes, MI, or stroke compared to patients >60 kg treated with a 10 mg maintenance dose; bleeding risk was not increased (Roe, 2012).
  Elderly: Refer to adult dosing. Patients ≥75 years: Use not recommended; may be considered in high-risk situations (eg, patients with diabetes or history of MI)

Dosing adjustment in renal impairment: No dosage adjustment necessary

Dosing adjustment in hepatic impairment: No dosage adjustment necessary for mild-to-moderate hepatic impairment; use in severe hepatic impairment has not been evaluated

Mechanism of Action Prasugrel is a prodrug that is metabolized to both active (R-138727) and inactive metabolites. The active metabolite irreversibly blocks the $P2Y_{12}$ component of ADP receptors on the platelet, which prevents activation of the GPIIb/IIIa receptor complex, thereby reducing platelet activation and aggregation. Platelet aggregation returns to baseline within 5-9 days of discontinuation.

Contraindications Hypersensitivity (eg, anaphylaxis) to prasugrel or any component of the formulation; active pathological bleeding such as peptic ulcer or intracranial hemorrhage; history of transient ischemic attack (TIA) or stroke

Warnings/Precautions [U.S. Boxed Warning]: May cause significant or fatal bleeding. Use is contraindicated in patients with active pathological bleeding or history of TIA or stroke. Use with caution in patients who may be at risk of increased bleeding, including patients with active PUD, recent or recurrent GI bleeding, severe hepatic impairment, end-stage renal disease (ESRD), trauma, or surgery. Additional risk factors include body weight <60 kg, CABG or other surgical procedure, concomitant use of medications that increase risk of bleeding.

[U.S. Boxed Warning]: In patients ≥75 years of age, use is not recommended due to increased risk of fatal and intracranial bleeding and uncertain benefit; use may be considered in high-risk situations (eg, patients with diabetes or history of MI). Risk of bleeding is increased in older adults (Beers Criteria). **[U.S. Boxed Warning]: Do not initiate therapy in patients likely to undergo urgent CABG surgery; when possible, discontinue ≥7 days prior to any surgery; increased risk of bleeding.** The American College of Chest Physicians (ACCP) recommends discontinuing prasugrel 5 days before surgery (Guyatt, 2012). When urgent CABG is necessary, the ACCF/AHA CABG guidelines suggest that it may be reasonable to perform surgery within 7 days of discontinuing prasugrel (Hillis, 2011).

Because of structural similarities, cross-reactivity is possible among the thienopyridines (clopidogrel, prasugrel, and ticlopidine); use with caution or avoid in patients with previous thienopyridine hypersensitivity. Use of prasugrel is contraindicated in patients with hypersensitivity (eg, anaphylaxis) to prasugrel. If necessary, discontinue therapy for active bleeding, elective surgery, stroke, or TIA; reinitiate therapy as soon as possible unless patient suffers stroke or TIA where subsequent use is contraindicated. If possible, manage bleeding without discontinuing prasugrel. Use caution in concurrent treatment with oral anticoagulants (eg, warfarin), NSAIDs, or fibrinolytic agents; bleeding risk is increased. Use with caution in patients with severe hepatic impairment or end-stage renal disease (experience is limited and generally are at higher risk for bleeding). Cases of thrombotic thrombocytopenic purpura (TTP) (usually occurring within the first 2 weeks of therapy), resulting in some fatalities, have been reported with prasugrel; urgent plasmapheresis is required. In patients <60 kg, risk of bleeding increased; consider lower maintenance dose.

◄ **Drug Interactions**
Metabolism/Transport Effects Substrate of CYP2B6 (minor), CYP3A4 (minor); **Note:** Assignment of Major/Minor substrate status based on clinically relevant drug interaction potential; **Inhibits** CYP2B6 (weak)

Avoid Concomitant Use There are no known interactions where it is recommended to avoid concomitant use.

Increased Effect/Toxicity
Prasugrel may increase the levels/effects of: Agents with Antiplatelet Properties; Anticoagulants; Collagenase (Systemic); Dabigatran Etexilate; Drotrecogin Alfa (Activated); Ibritumomab; Rivaroxaban; Salicylates; Thrombolytic Agents; Tositumomab and Iodine I 131 Tositumomab

The levels/effects of Prasugrel may be increased by: Dasatinib; Glucosamine; Herbs (Anticoagulant/Antiplatelet Properties); Multivitamins/Minerals (with ADEK, Folate, Iron); Nonsteroidal Anti-Inflammatory Agents; Omega-3 Fatty Acids; Pentosan Polysulfate Sodium; Pentoxifylline; Prostacyclin Analogues; Tipranavir; Vitamin E

Decreased Effect
The levels/effects of Prasugrel may be decreased by: CYP3A4 Inhibitors (Strong); Nonsteroidal Anti-Inflammatory Agents; Ranitidine; Rifampin

Dietary Considerations May be taken without regard to meals.

Pharmacodynamics/Kinetics
Onset of Action Inhibition of platelet aggregation (IPA): Dose dependent: 60 mg loading dose: <30 minutes; median time to reach 20% IPA: 30 minutes (Brandt, 2007)

Peak effect: Time to maximal IPA: Dose-dependent: **Note:** Degree of IPA based on adenosine diphosphate (ADP) concentration used during light aggregometry: 60 mg loading dose: Occurs 4 hours post administration; mean IPA (ADP 5 μmol/L): 78.8%: mean IPA (ADP 20 micromole/L): 84.1%

Duration of Action Duration of effect: >3 days; platelet aggregation gradually returns to baseline values over 5-9 days after discontinuation; reflective of new platelet production

Half-life Elimination Half-life elimination: Active metabolite: ~7 hours (range 2-15 hours)

Time to Peak Active metabolite: ~30 minutes (peak plasma levels begin to decrease at ~24 hours); with high-fat/high-calorie meal: 1.5 hours

Pregnancy Risk Factor B

Pregnancy Considerations There are no adequate and well-controlled studies in pregnant women. Use during pregnancy only if the benefits justify the risk to the fetus.

Lactation Excretion in breast milk unknown/consider risk:benefit

Dosage Forms
Tablet, oral:
Effient®: 5 mg, 10 mg

Dental Comment There is no scientific evidence to warrant the discontinuance of prasugrel prior to dental surgery. Patients requiring dental surgery who are taking 1 tablet daily as an antithrombotic or taking 1 tablet daily in combination with aspirin should be given special consideration in consultation with their healthcare provider.

References
Brandt JT, Payne CD, Wiviott SD, et al, "A Comparison of Prasugrel and Clopidogrel Loading Doses on Platelet Function: Magnitude of Platelet Inhibition is Related to Active Metabolite Formation," *Am Heart J*, 2007, 153(1):66.e9-16.

Pravastatin (prav a STAT in)

Related Information
Cardiovascular Diseases *on page 1492*
Brand Names: U.S. Pravachol®
Brand Names: Canada Apo-Pravastatin®; CO Pravastatin; Dom-Pravastatin; JAMP-Pravastatin; Mint-Pravastatin; Mylan-Pravastatin; Novo-Pravastatin; Nu-Pravastatin; PHL-Pravastatin; PMS-Pravastatin; Pravachol®; RAN™-Pravastatin; ratio-Pravastatin; Riva-Pravastatin; Sandoz-Pravastatin; Teva-Pravastatin; ZYM-Pravastatin
Generic Availability (U.S.) Yes
Pharmacologic Category Antilipemic Agent, HMG-CoA Reductase Inhibitor
Use Use with dietary therapy for the following:
Primary prevention of coronary events: In hypercholesterolemic patients without established coronary heart disease to reduce cardiovascular morbidity (myocardial infarction, coronary revascularization procedures) and mortality.

Secondary prevention of cardiovascular events in patients with established coronary heart disease: To slow the progression of coronary atherosclerosis; to reduce cardiovascular morbidity (myocardial infarction, coronary vascular procedures) and to reduce mortality; to reduce the risk of stroke and transient ischemic attacks

Hyperlipidemias: Reduce elevations in total cholesterol, LDL-C, apolipoprotein B, and triglycerides (elevations of 1 or more components are present in Fredrickson type IIa, IIb, III, and IV hyperlipidemias)

Heterozygous familial hypercholesterolemia (HeFH): In pediatric patients, 8-18 years of age, with HeFH having LDL-C ≥190 mg/dL **or** LDL ≥160 mg/dL with positive family history of premature cardiovascular disease (CVD) or 2 or more CVD risk factors in the pediatric patient

Local Anesthetic/Vasoconstrictor Precautions No information available to require special precautions

Effects on Dental Treatment No significant effects or complications reported

Effects on Bleeding No information available to require special precautions

Adverse Effects As reported in short-term trials; safety and tolerability with long-term use were similar to placebo

1% to 10%:
Cardiovascular: Chest pain (4%)
Central nervous system: Headache (2% to 6%), fatigue (4%), dizziness (1% to 3%)
Dermatologic: Rash (4%)
Gastrointestinal: Nausea/vomiting (7%), diarrhea (6%), heartburn (3%)
Hepatic: Transaminases increased (>3x normal on two occasions: 1%)
Neuromuscular & skeletal: Myalgia (2%)
Respiratory: Cough (3%)
Miscellaneous: Influenza (2%)
Additional class-related events or case reports (not necessarily reported with pravastatin therapy): Angioedema, blood glucose increased, cataracts, depression, diabetes mellitus (new onset), dyspnea, eosinophilia, erectile dysfunction, facial paresis, glycosylated

hemoglobin (Hb A$_{1c}$) increased, hypersensitivity reaction, immune-mediated necrotizing myopathy (IMNM), impaired extraocular muscle movement, impotence, interstitial lung disease, leukopenia, malaise, memory loss, ophthalmoplegia, paresthesia, peripheral neuropathy, photosensitivity, psychic disturbance, skin discoloration, thrombocytopenia, thyroid dysfunction, toxic epidermal necrolysis, transaminases increased, vomiting

Dosage Oral: **Note:** Doses should be individualized according to the baseline LDL-cholesterol levels, the recommended goal of therapy, and patient response; adjustments should be made at intervals of 4 weeks or more; doses may need adjusted based on concomitant medications

Children: HeFH:

8-13 years: 20 mg/day

14-18 years: 40 mg/day

Dosage adjustment for pravastatin with concomitant medications (clarithromycin, cyclosporine): Refer to adult dosing.

Adults: Hyperlipidemias, primary prevention of coronary events, secondary prevention of cardiovascular events: Initial: 40 mg once daily; titrate dosage to response; usual range: 10-80 mg; (maximum dose: 80 mg once daily)

Dosage adjustment for pravastatin with concomitant medications:

Clarithromycin: Limit daily pravastatin dose to 40 mg/day

Cyclosporine: Initial: 10 mg pravastatin daily, titrate with caution (maximum dose: 20 mg/day)

Elderly: No specific dosage recommendations. Clearance is reduced in the elderly, resulting in an increase in AUC between 25% to 50%. However, substantial accumulation is not expected.

Dosing adjustment in renal impairment: Significant impairment: Initial dose: 10 mg/day

Dosing adjustment in hepatic impairment: Contraindicated in active liver disease or in patients with unexplained persistent elevations of serum transaminases

Mechanism of Action Pravastatin is a competitive inhibitor of 3-hydroxy-3-methylglutaryl coenzyme A (HMG-CoA) reductase, which is the rate-limiting enzyme involved in *de novo* cholesterol synthesis.

Contraindications Hypersensitivity to pravastatin or any component of the formulation; active liver disease; unexplained persistent elevations of serum transaminases; pregnancy; breast-feeding

Warnings/Precautions Secondary causes of hyperlipidemia should be ruled out prior to therapy. Liver function must be monitored by periodic laboratory assessment. Rhabdomyolysis with acute renal failure has occurred. Risk may be increased with concurrent use of other drugs which may cause rhabdomyolysis (including colchicine, gemfibrozil, fibric acid derivatives, or niacin at doses ≥1 g/day). Discontinue in any patient in which CPK levels are markedly elevated (>10 times ULN) or if myopathy is suspected/diagnosed. Immune-mediated necrotizing myopathy (IMNM), an autoimmune-mediated myopathy, has been reported (rarely) with HMG-CoA reductase inhibitor therapy. IMNM presents as proximal muscle weakness with elevated CPK levels, which persists despite discontinuation of HMG-CoA reductase inhibitor therapy; additionally, muscle biopsy may show necrotizing myopathy with limited inflammation; immunosuppressive therapy (eg, corticosteroids, azathioprine) may be used for treatment. The manufacturer recommends temporary discontinuation for elective major surgery, acute medical or surgical conditions, or in any patient experiencing an acute or serious condition predisposing to renal failure (eg, sepsis, hypotension, trauma, uncontrolled seizures). However, based upon current evidence, HMG-CoA reductase inhibitor therapy should be continued in the perioperative period unless risk outweighs cardioprotective benefit. Use with caution in patients with advanced age, these patients are predisposed to myopathy. Use caution in patients with previous liver disease or heavy ethanol use. If serious hepatotoxicity with clinical symptoms and/or hyperbilirubinemia or jaundice occurs during treatment, interrupt therapy. If an alternate etiology is not identified, do not restart pravastatin. Liver enzyme tests should be obtained at baseline and as clinically indicated; routine periodic monitoring of liver enzymes is not necessary. Increases in Hb A$_{1c}$ and fasting blood glucose have been reported with HMG-CoA reductase inhibitors; however, the benefits of statin therapy far outweigh the risk of dysglycemia. Treatment in patients <8 years of age is not recommended.

Drug Interactions

Metabolism/Transport Effects Substrate of CYP3A4 (minor), P-glycoprotein, SLCO1B1; **Note:** Assignment of Major/Minor substrate status based on clinically relevant drug interaction potential; **Inhibits** CYP2C9 (weak), CYP2D6 (weak), CYP3A4 (weak)

Avoid Concomitant Use

Avoid concomitant use of Pravastatin with any of the following: Fusidic Acid; Gemfibrozil; Pimozide; Red Yeast Rice

Increased Effect/Toxicity

Pravastatin may increase the levels/effects of: ARIPiprazole; CycloSPORINE (Systemic); DAPTOmycin; Lomitapide; PARoxetine; Pazopanib; Pimozide; Trabectedin; Vitamin K Antagonists

The levels/effects of Pravastatin may be increased by: Bezafibrate; Boceprevir; Colchicine; CycloSPORINE (Systemic); Darunavir; Eltrombopag; Fenofibrate; Fenofibric Acid; Fusidic Acid; Gemfibrozil; Itraconazole; Niacin; Niacinamide; P-glycoprotein/ABCB1 Inhibitors; Red Yeast Rice; Telaprevir

Decreased Effect

Pravastatin may decrease the levels/effects of: Lanthanum

The levels/effects of Pravastatin may be decreased by: Antacids; Bile Acid Sequestrants; Efavirenz; Fosphenytoin; Nelfinavir; P-glycoprotein/ABCB1 Inducers; Phenytoin; Rifamycin Derivatives; Saquinavir

Ethanol/Nutrition/Herb Interactions

Ethanol: Consumption of large amounts of ethanol may increase the risk of liver damage with HMG-CoA reductase inhibitors.

Food: Red yeast rice contains an estimated 2.4 mg lovastatin per 600 mg rice.

Herb/Nutraceutical: St John's wort may decrease pravastatin levels.

Dietary Considerations May be taken without regard to meals. Before initiation of therapy, patients should be placed on a standard cholesterol-lowering diet for 6 weeks and the diet should be continued during drug therapy. Red yeast rice contains an estimated 2.4 mg lovastatin per 600 mg rice.

Pharmacodynamics/Kinetics

Onset of Action Several days; Peak effect: 4 weeks

Half-life Elimination 77 hours (including all metabolites); pravastatin: ~2-3 hours (Pan, 1990); 3α-hydroxy-iso-pravastatin: ~1.5 hours (Gustavson, 2005)

Time to Peak Serum: 1-1.5 hours

Pregnancy Risk Factor X
Pregnancy Considerations Adverse events were observed in some animal reproduction studies. There are reports of congenital anomalies following maternal use of HMG-CoA reductase Inhibitors in pregnancy; however, maternal disease, differences in specific agents used, and the low rates of exposure limit the interpretation of the available data (Godfrey, 2012; Lecarpentier, 2012). Cholesterol biosynthesis may be important in fetal development; serum cholesterol and triglycerides increase normally during pregnancy. The discontinuation of lipid lowering medications temporarily during pregnancy is not expected to have significant impact on the long term outcomes of primary hypercholesterolemia treatment.

Use of pravastatin is contraindicated in pregnancy. HMG-CoA reductase Inhibitors should be discontinued prior to pregnancy (ADA, 2013). If treatment of dyslipidemias is needed in pregnant women or in women of reproductive age, other agents are preferred (Berglund, 2012; NCEP, 2002). The manufacturer recommends administration to women of childbearing potential only when conception is highly unlikely and patients have been informed of potential hazards.
Lactation Enters breast milk/contraindicated
Breast-Feeding Considerations A small amount of pravastatin is excreted into breast milk. Data is available from eight lactating females administered pravastatin 20 mg twice daily for 2.5 days. After the fifth dose, maximum maternal serum concentrations were ~40 ng/mL (pravastatin) and ~26 ng/mL (metabolite) and maximum milk concentrations were ~3.9 ng/mL (pravastatin) and ~2.1 ng/mL (metabolite). Maximum milk concentrations were detected ~3 hours after the dose (Pan, 1988). Due to the potential for serious adverse reactions in a nursing infant, use while breast-feeding is contraindicated by the manufacturer.
Dosage Forms
Tablet, oral: 10 mg, 20 mg, 40 mg, 80 mg
Pravachol®: 20 mg, 40 mg, 80 mg

Praziquantel (pray zi KWON tel)

Brand Names: U.S. Biltricide®
Brand Names: Canada Biltricide®
Pharmacologic Category Anthelmintic
Use Treatment of all stages of schistosomiasis caused by all *Schistosoma* species; treatment of infection (clonorchiasis and opisthorchiasis) due to liver flukes
Unlabeled Use Cysticercosis and many intestinal tapeworms
Local Anesthetic/Vasoconstrictor Precautions No information available to require special precautions
Effects on Dental Treatment No significant effects or complications reported
Effects on Bleeding No information available to require special precautions
Adverse Effects Frequency not defined.
Central nervous system: Dizziness, fever, headache, malaise
Dermatologic: Urticaria (rare)
Gastrointestinal: Abdominal discomfort, nausea
General Dosage Range Oral: *Children ≥4 years and Adults:* 20 mg/kg/dose 2-3 times/day for 1 day at 4- to 6-hour intervals **or** 25 mg/kg 3 times/day for 1 day

Mechanism of Action Increases the cell permeability to calcium in schistosomes, causing strong contractions and paralysis of worm musculature leading to detachment of suckers from the blood vessel walls and to dislodgment
Pharmacodynamics/Kinetics
Half-life Elimination Parent drug: 0.8-1.5 hours; Metabolites: 4.5 hours
Time to Peak Serum: 1-3 hours
Pregnancy Risk Factor B
Pregnancy Considerations Adverse effects have not been observed in animal reproduction studies. There are no adequate and well-controlled studies in pregnant women. Use in pregnant women only if clearly needed.

Prazosin (PRAZ oh sin)

Related Information
Cardiovascular Diseases *on page 1492*
Brand Names: U.S. Minipress®
Brand Names: Canada Apo-Prazo®; Minipress®; Novo-Prazin; Nu-Prazo; Teva-Prazosin
Pharmacologic Category Alpha₁ Blocker
Use Treatment of hypertension
Unlabeled Use Post-traumatic stress disorder (PTSD) related nightmares and sleep disruption; benign prostatic hyperplasia; Raynaud's syndrome
Local Anesthetic/Vasoconstrictor Precautions No information available to require special precautions
Effects on Dental Treatment Key adverse event(s) related to dental treatment: Significant xerostomia (normal salivary flow resumes upon discontinuation). Significant orthostatic hypotension is a possibility; monitor patient when getting out of dental chair.
Effects on Bleeding No information available to require special precautions
Adverse Effects
>4%:
Cardiovascular: Palpitation (5%)
Central nervous system: Dizziness (10%), headache (8%), drowsiness (8%)
Endocrine & metabolic: Decreased energy (7%)
Gastrointestinal: Nausea (5%)
Neuromuscular & skeletal: Weakness (7%)
1% to 4%:
Cardiovascular: Edema, orthostatic hypotension, syncope
Central nervous system: Depression, nervousness, vertigo
Dermatologic: Rash
Gastrointestinal: Constipation, diarrhea, vomiting, xerostomia
Genitourinary: Urinary frequency
Ocular: Blurred vision, reddened sclera
Respiratory: Dyspnea, epistaxis, nasal congestion
General Dosage Range Oral: *Adults:* Initial: 1 mg/dose 2-3 times/day; Maintenance: 2-20 mg/day in divided doses 2-3 times/day (maximum: 20 mg/day) (JNC 7)
Mechanism of Action Competitively inhibits postsynaptic alpha-adrenergic receptors which results in vasodilation of veins and arterioles and a decrease in total peripheral resistance and blood pressure
Pharmacodynamics/Kinetics
Onset of Action Anithypertensive: ~2 hours; Peak effect: Antihypertensive: 2-4 hours

Duration of Action 10-24 hours

Half-life Elimination 2-3 hours; prolonged with congestive heart failure

Time to Peak Plasma: ~3 hours

Pregnancy Risk Factor C

Pregnancy Considerations Teratogenic effects were not observed in animal studies. Limited use in pregnant women has not demonstrated any fetal abnormalities or adverse effects (Dommisse, 1983).

Prednicarbate (pred ni KAR bate)

Brand Names: U.S. Dermatop®

Brand Names: Canada Dermatop®

Pharmacologic Category Corticosteroid, Topical

Use Relief of the inflammatory and pruritic manifestations of corticosteroid-responsive dermatoses (medium potency topical corticosteroid)

Local Anesthetic/Vasoconstrictor Precautions No information available to require special precautions

Effects on Dental Treatment No significant effects or complications reported

Effects on Bleeding No information available to require special precautions

Adverse Effects 1% to 10%: Dermatologic: Skin atrophy (children 8%; adults 1%), mild telangiectasia (children 5%), shininess (children 3%), thinness (children 3%)

General Dosage Range Topical:

Children ≥1 year and Adults: Cream: Apply a thin film to affected area twice daily

Children ≥10 year and Adults: Ointment: Apply a thin film to affected area twice daily

Mechanism of Action Topical corticosteroids have anti-inflammatory, antipruritic, vasoconstrictive, and antiproliferative actions

Pregnancy Risk Factor C

Pregnancy Considerations There are no adequate and well-controlled studies using prednicarbate during pregnancy. However, intrauterine growth retardation has been reported with other topical steroids. Avoid use in large amounts for long periods of time during pregnancy.

PrednisoLONE (Systemic) (pred NISS oh lone)

Related Information

PredniSONE *on page 1133*

Respiratory Diseases *on page 1514*

Brand Names: U.S. Flo-Pred™; Millipred™; Millipred™ DP; Orapred ODT®; Orapred®; Pediapred®; Veripred™ 20

Brand Names: Canada Hydeltra T.B.A.®; Novo-Prednisolone; Pediapred®

Generic Availability (U.S.) Yes: Excludes orally disintegrating tablet, oral suspension, tablet

Pharmacologic Category Corticosteroid, Systemic

Dental Use Treatment of a variety of oral diseases of allergic, inflammatory, or autoimmune origin

Use Treatment of endocrine disorders, rheumatic disorders, collagen diseases, allergic states, respiratory diseases, hematologic disorders, neoplastic diseases, edematous states, and gastrointestinal diseases; resolution of acute exacerbations of multiple sclerosis; management of fulminating or disseminated tuberculosis and trichinosis; acute or chronic solid organ rejection

Unlabeled Use Severe alcoholic hepatitis; Bell's palsy; acute exacerbations of chronic obstructive pulmonary disease (COPD)

Local Anesthetic/Vasoconstrictor Precautions No information available to require special precautions

Effects on Dental Treatment Key adverse event(s) related to dental treatment: Ulcerative esophagitis.

Effects on Bleeding No information available to require special precautions

Adverse Effects Frequency not defined.

Cardiovascular: Cardiomyopathy, CHF, edema, facial edema, hypertension

Central nervous system: Headache, insomnia, malaise, nervousness, pseudotumor cerebri, psychic disorders, seizure, vertigo

Dermatologic: Bruising, facial erythema, hirsutism, petechiae, skin test reaction suppression, thin fragile skin, urticaria

Endocrine & metabolic: Carbohydrate tolerance decreased, Cushing's syndrome, diabetes mellitus, growth suppression, hyperglycemia, hypernatremia, hypokalemia, hypokalemic alkalosis, menstrual irregularities, negative nitrogen balance, pituitary adrenal axis suppression

Gastrointestinal: Abdominal distention, increased appetite, indigestion, nausea, pancreatitis, peptic ulcer, ulcerative esophagitis, weight gain

Hepatic: LFTs increased (usually reversible)

Neuromuscular & skeletal: Arthralgia, aseptic necrosis (humeral/femoral heads), fractures, muscle mass decreased, muscle weakness, osteoporosis, steroid myopathy, tendon rupture, weakness

Ocular: Cataracts, exophthalmus, eyelid edema, glaucoma, intraocular pressure increased, irritation

Respiratory: Epistaxis

Miscellaneous: Diaphoresis increased, impaired wound healing

Dental Usual Dosage Anti-inflammatory or immunosuppressive dose: Oral:

Children: 0.1-2 mg/kg/day in divided doses 1-4 times/day

Adults: Usual range: 5-60 mg/day

Dosage Dose depends upon condition being treated and response of patient; dosage for infants and children should be based on severity of the disease and response of the patient rather than on strict adherence to dosage indicated by age, weight, or body surface area. Oral dosage expressed in terms of prednisolone base. Consider alternate day therapy for long-term therapy. Discontinuation of long-term therapy requires gradual withdrawal by tapering the dose. Patients undergoing unusual stress while receiving corticosteroids should receive increased doses prior to, during, and after the stressful situation.

Children: Oral:

Acute asthma: 1-2 mg/kg/day in divided doses 1-2 times daily for 3-5 days

Anti-inflammatory or immunosuppressive dose: 0.1-2 mg/kg/day in divided doses 1-4 times daily

Nephrotic syndrome:

Initial (first 3 episodes): 2 mg/kg/day or 60 mg/m^2/day (maximum: 80 mg daily) in divided doses 3-4 times daily until urine is protein free for 3 consecutive days (maximum: 28 days); followed by 1-1.5 mg/kg/dose or 40 mg/m^2/dose given every other day for 4 weeks

Maintenance (long-term maintenance dose for frequent relapses): 0.5-1 mg/kg/dose given every other day for 3-6 months

Adults: Oral:
Usual range: 5-60 mg daily
Multiple sclerosis: 200 mg/day for 1 week followed by 80 mg every other day for 1 month
Rheumatoid arthritis: Initial: 5-7.5 mg daily; adjust dose as necessary
Acute exacerbations of chronic obstructive pulmonary disease (COPD) (unlabeled use): 30-40 mg daily for 10-14 days (GOLD guidelines, 2013)
Bell's palsy (unlabeled use): 60 mg daily for 5 days, followed by 10 mg daily for 5 days (Berg, 2012)
Severe alcoholic hepatitis (Maddrey Discriminant Function [MDF] score ≥32) (unlabeled use): 40 mg daily for 28 days, followed by a 2-week taper (O'Shea, 2010)
Elderly: Use lowest effective dose
Dosing adjustment in hyperthyroidism: Prednisolone dose may need to be increased to achieve adequate therapeutic effects

Hemodialysis: Slightly dialyzable (5% to 20%); administer dose posthemodialysis
Peritoneal dialysis: Supplemental dose is not necessary
Mechanism of Action Decreases inflammation by suppression of migration of polymorphonuclear leukocytes and reversal of increased capillary permeability; suppresses the immune system by reducing activity and volume of the lymphatic system
Contraindications Hypersensitivity to prednisolone or any component of the formulation; acute superficial herpes simplex keratitis; live or attenuated virus vaccines (with immunosuppressive doses of corticosteroids); systemic fungal infections; varicella
Warnings/Precautions May cause hypercorticism or suppression of hypothalamic-pituitary-adrenal (HPA) axis, particularly in younger children or in patients receiving high doses for prolonged periods. HPA axis suppression may lead to adrenal crisis. Withdrawal and discontinuation of a corticosteroid should be done slowly and carefully. Particular care is required when patients are transferred from systemic corticosteroids to inhaled products due to possible adrenal insufficiency or withdrawal from steroids, including an increase in allergic symptoms. Patients receiving >20 mg per day of prednisone (or equivalent) may be most susceptible. Fatalities have occurred due to adrenal insufficiency in asthmatic patients during and after transfer from systemic corticosteroids to aerosol steroids; aerosol steroids do **not** provide the systemic steroid needed to treat patients having trauma, surgery, or infections.

Acute myopathy has been reported with high dose corticosteroids, usually in patients with neuromuscular transmission disorders; may involve ocular and/or respiratory muscles; monitor creatine kinase; recovery may be delayed. Corticosteroid use may cause psychiatric disturbances, including depression, euphoria, insomnia, mood swings, and personality changes. Pre-existing psychiatric conditions may be exacerbated by corticosteroid use. Prolonged use of corticosteroids may also increase the incidence of secondary infection, mask acute infection (including fungal infections), prolong or exacerbate viral infections, or limit response to vaccines. Exposure to chickenpox should be avoided; corticosteroids should not be used to treat ocular herpes simplex. Corticosteroids should not be used for cerebral malaria or viral hepatitis. Close observation is required in patients with latent tuberculosis and/or TB reactivity; restrict use in active TB (only in conjunction with antituberculosis treatment). Prolonged use of corticosteroids may result in glaucoma; cataract formation may

occur. Prolonged treatment with corticosteroids has been associated with the development of Kaposi's sarcoma (case reports); if noted, discontinuation of therapy should be considered.

Use with caution in patients with thyroid disease, hepatic impairment, renal impairment, cardiovascular disease, diabetes, glaucoma, cataracts, myasthenia gravis, patients at risk for osteoporosis, patients at risk for seizures, or GI diseases (diverticulitis, peptic ulcer, ulcerative colitis) due to perforation risk. Use caution following acute MI (corticosteroids have been associated with myocardial rupture). Because of the risk of adverse effects, systemic corticosteroids should be used cautiously in the elderly in the smallest possible effective dose for the shortest duration. Withdraw therapy with gradual tapering of dose. May affect growth velocity; growth should be routinely monitored in pediatric patients.

Drug Interactions
Metabolism/Transport Effects Substrate of CYP3A4 (minor); **Note:** Assignment of Major/Minor substrate status based on clinically relevant drug interaction potential; **Inhibits** CYP3A4 (weak)
Avoid Concomitant Use
Avoid concomitant use of PrednisoLONE (Systemic) with any of the following: Aldesleukin; BCG; Mifepristone; Natalizumab; Pimecrolimus; Pimozide; Tacrolimus (Topical); Tofacitinib
Increased Effect/Toxicity
PrednisoLONE (Systemic) may increase the levels/ effects of: Acetylcholinesterase Inhibitors; Amphotericin B; ARIPiprazole; CycloSPORINE (Systemic); Deferasirox; Leflunomide; Lomitapide; Loop Diuretics; Natalizumab; NSAID (COX-2 Inhibitor); NSAID (Nonselective); Pimozide; Thiazide Diuretics; Tofacitinib; Vaccines (Live); Warfarin

The levels/effects of PrednisoLONE (Systemic) may be increased by: Antifungal Agents (Azole Derivatives, Systemic); Aprepitant; Calcium Channel Blockers (Nondihydropyridine); CycloSPORINE (Systemic); Denosumab; Estrogen Derivatives; Fluconazole; Fosaprepitant; Indacaterol; Macrolide Antibiotics; Mifepristone; Neuromuscular-Blocking Agents (Nondepolarizing); Pimecrolimus; Quinolone Antibiotics; Ritonavir; Roflumilast; Salicylates; Tacrolimus (Topical); Telaprevir; Trastuzumab
Decreased Effect
PrednisoLONE (Systemic) may decrease the levels/ effects of: Aldesleukin; Antidiabetic Agents; BCG; Calcitriol; Coccidioidin Skin Test; Corticorelin; CycloSPORINE (Systemic); Hyaluronidase; Isoniazid; Salicylates; Sipuleucel-T; Telaprevir; Vaccines (Inactivated)

The levels/effects of PrednisoLONE (Systemic) may be decreased by: Aminoglutethimide; Antacids; Barbiturates; Bile Acid Sequestrants; Echinacea; Fosphenytoin; Mifepristone; Mitotane; Phenytoin; Primidone; Rifamycin Derivatives
Ethanol/Nutrition/Herb Interactions
Ethanol: Avoid ethanol (may increase gastric mucosal irritation).
Food: Prednisolone interferes with calcium absorption. Limit caffeine.
Herb/Nutraceutical: St John's wort may decrease prednisolone levels. Avoid cat's claw, echinacea (have immunostimulant properties).

Dietary Considerations Should be taken after meals or with food or milk to decrease GI effects; increase dietary intake of pyridoxine, vitamin C, vitamin D, folate, calcium, and phosphorus.

Pharmacodynamics/Kinetics

Duration of Action 18-36 hours

Half-life Elimination 3.6 hours; End-stage renal disease: 3-5 hours

Pregnancy Risk Factor C/D (Flo-Pred™)

Pregnancy Considerations Adverse events have been observed with corticosteroids in animal reproduction studies. Prednisolone crosses the placenta; prior to reaching the fetus, prednisolone is converted by placental enzymes to prednisone. As a result, the amount of prednisolone reaching the fetus is ~8-10 times lower than the maternal serum concentration (healthy women at term; similar results observed with preterm pregnancies complicated by HELLP syndrome). Human studies have shown an association between first trimester corticosteroid use and oral clefts. Additional adverse events in the fetus/neonate, including low birth weight, have been noted in case reports following large doses of systemic corticosteroids during pregnancy. Women exposed to prednisolone during pregnancy for the treatment of an autoimmune disease may contact the OTIS Autoimmune Diseases Study at 877-311-8972.

Lactation Enters breast milk/use caution (AAP rates "compatible"; AAP 2001 update pending)

Breast-Feeding Considerations Prednisolone is excreted into breast milk with peak concentrations occurring ~1 hour after the maternal dose. The milk/plasma ratio was found to be 0.2 with doses ≥30 mg/day and 0.1 with doses <30 mg/day. Following a maternal dose of prednisolone 80 mg/day, a breast-feeding infant would ingest <0.1% of the dose.

Dosage Forms

Solution, oral: 5 mg/5 mL (120 mL); 15 mg/5 mL (237 mL, 240 mL, 473 mL, 480 mL); 25 mg/5 mL (237 mL)
Millipred™: 10 mg/5 mL (237 mL)
Orapred®: 15 mg/5 mL (20 mL, 237 mL)
Pediapred®: 5 mg/5 mL (120 mL)
Veripred™ 20: 20 mg/5 mL (237 mL)

Suspension, oral:
Flo-Pred™: 15 mg/5 mL (52 mL)

Tablet, oral:
Millipred™: 5 mg
Millipred™ DP: 5 mg

Tablet, orally disintegrating, oral:
Orapred ODT®: 10 mg, 15 mg, 30 mg

Prednisolone and Gentamicin
(pred NIS oh lone & jen ta MYE sin)

Brand Names: U.S. Pred-G®

Pharmacologic Category Antibiotic/Corticosteroid, Ophthalmic

Use Treatment of steroid responsive inflammatory conditions where either a superficial bacterial ocular infection or the risk of bacterial ocular infection exists

Local Anesthetic/Vasoconstrictor Precautions No information available to require special precautions

Effects on Dental Treatment No significant effects or complications reported

Effects on Bleeding No information available to require special precautions

Adverse Effects Frequency not defined.
Dermatologic: Delayed wound healing
Local: Discomfort, irritation

Ocular: Glaucoma, intraocular pressure increased, optic nerve damage (infrequent), posterior subcapsular cataract formation, superficial punctate keratitis
Miscellaneous: Secondary infection

General Dosage Range Ophthalmic: *Adults:*
Ointment: Apply 1/2" ribbon into the conjunctival sac of the affected eye(s) 1-3 times/day
Suspension: Initial: Instill 1 drop into the conjunctival sac of the affected eye(s) every hour for 1-2 days; Maintenance: 1 drop 2-4 times/day

Pregnancy Risk Factor C

Pregnancy Considerations See individual agents.

PredniSONE (PRED ni sone)

Related Information
PrednisoLONE (Systemic) *on page 1131*
Respiratory Diseases *on page 1514*
Rheumatoid Arthritis, Osteoarthritis, and Osteoporosis *on page 1526*
Ulcerative, Erosive, and Painful Oral Mucosal Disorders *on page 1578*

Related Sample Prescriptions
Erosive Lichen Planus, Other Biopsy-Proven Desquamative Oral Diseases, and Major Aphthae *on page 1618*

Brand Names: U.S. PredniSONE Intensol™; Rayos®

Brand Names: Canada Apo-Prednisone®; Novo-Prednisone; Winpred™

Generic Availability (U.S.) Yes

Pharmacologic Category Corticosteroid, Systemic

Dental Use Treatment of a variety of oral diseases of allergic, inflammatory, or autoimmune origin

Use Treatment of a variety of diseases, including:
Allergic conditions: Atopic dermatitis, drug hypersensitivity reactions, allergic rhinitis, serum sickness, adjunctive treatment of anaphylaxis
Dermatologic diseases: Bullous dermatitis herpetiformis, contact dermatitis, exfoliative erythroderma, mycosis fungoides, pemphigus, severe erythema multiforme (Stevens-Johnson syndrome), severe seborrheic dermatitis (immediate release only)
Endocrine conditions: Congenital adrenal hyperplasia, hypercalcemia of malignancy, nonsuppurative thyroiditis, adrenocortical insufficiency
Gastrointestinal diseases: Crohn's disease, ulcerative colitis
Hematologic diseases: Acquired (autoimmune) hemolytic anemia, Diamond-Blackfan anemia, idiopathic thrombocytopenic purpura, pure red cell aplasia, secondary thrombocytopenia
Infectious diseases: Trichinosis with neurologic or myocardial involvement, tuberculosis meningitis with subarachnoid block or impending block
Neoplastic conditions: Acute leukemia, aggressive lymphomas
Nervous system conditions (delayed release only): Acute exacerbations of multiple sclerosis, cerebral edema associated with primary or metastatic brain tumor, craniotomy or head injury
Ophthalmic conditions:
Immediate release only: Allergic conjunctivitis, keratitis, allergic corneal marginal ulcers, herpes zoster ophthalmicus, iritis and iridocyclitis, chorioretinitis, anterior segment inflammation, diffuse posterior uveitis and choroiditis, optic neuritis
Delayed release only: Uveitis, and ocular inflammatory conditions

Organ transplantation-related conditions (delayed release only): Solid organ rejection

Pulmonary diseases: Aspiration pneumonitis, asthma, pulmonary tuberculosis, symptomatic sarcoidosis

Immediate release only: Loeffler's syndrome not manageable by other means, berylliosis

Delayed release only: Acute exacerbations of chronic obstructive pulmonary disease (COPD), allergic bronchopulmonary aspergillosis, hypersensitivity pneumonitis, idiopathic bronchiolitis obliterans with organizing pneumonia, idiopathic eosinophilic pneumonias, idiopathic pulmonary fibrosis, *Pneumocystis jiroveci* (formerly *carinii*) pneumonia (PCP)

Renal conditions: Nephrotic syndrome (idiopathic or related to lupus erythematosus), without uremia

Rheumatologic conditions, short-term therapy: Psoriatic arthritis, rheumatoid and juvenile arthritis, ankylosing spondylitis, acute gouty arthritis, systemic lupus erythematosus, dermatomyositis/polymyositis

Immediate release only: Bursitis, tenosynovitis, posttraumatic osteoarthritis, synovitis of osteoarthritis, epicondolyitis acute rheumatic carditis

Delayed release only: Polymyalgia rheumatica, relapsing polychondritis, Sjogren's syndrome, vasculitis

Rheumatologic conditions, maintenance therapy: Rheumatoid and juvenile arthritis, systemic lupus erythematosus, dermatomyositis/polymyositis

Immediate release only: Acute rheumatic carditis

Delayed release only: Ankylosing spondylitis, polymyalgia rheumatic, psoriatic arthritis, relapsing polychondritis, Sjogren's syndrome, vasculitis

Unlabeled Use Autoimmune hepatitis; adjunctive therapy for pain management in immunocompetent patients with herpes zoster; Takayasu arteritis; giant cell arteritis; Grave's ophthalmopathy prophylaxis; subacute thyroiditis; thyrotoxicosis (type II amiodarone-induced); acute exacerbation of chronic obstructive pulmonary disease (COPD) (immediate release products)

Local Anesthetic/Vasoconstrictor Precautions No information available to require special precautions

Effects on Dental Treatment No significant effects or complications reported

Effects on Bleeding No information available to require special precautions

Adverse Effects Frequency not defined.

Cardiovascular: Congestive heart failure (in susceptible patients), hypertension

Central nervous system: Emotional instability, headache, intracranial pressure increased (with papilledema), psychic derangements (including euphoria, insomnia, mood swings, personality changes, severe depression), seizure, vertigo

Dermatologic: Bruising, facial erythema, petechiae, thin fragile skin, urticaria, wound healing impaired

Endocrine & metabolic: Adrenocortical and pituitary unresponsiveness (in times of stress), carbohydrate intolerance, Cushing's syndrome, diabetes mellitus, fluid retention, growth suppression (in children), hypokalemic alkalosis, hypothyroidism enhanced, menstrual irregularities, negative nitrogen balance due to protein catabolism, potassium loss, sodium retention

Gastrointestinal: Abdominal distension, pancreatitis, peptic ulcer (with possible perforation and hemorrhage), ulcerative esophagitis

Hepatic: ALT increased, AST increased, alkaline phosphatase increased

Neuromuscular & skeletal: Aseptic necrosis of femoral and humeral heads, muscle mass loss, muscle weakness, osteoporosis, pathologic fracture of long bones, steroid myopathy, tendon rupture (particularly Achilles tendon), vertebral compression fractures

Ocular: Exophthalmos, glaucoma, intraocular pressure increased, posterior subcapsular cataracts

Miscellaneous: Allergic reactions, anaphylactic reactions, diaphoresis, hypersensitivity reactions, infections, Kaposi's sarcoma

Dental Usual Dosage

Anti-inflammatory or immunosuppressive dose: Children: Oral: 0.05-2 mg/kg/day divided 1-4 times/day

Immunosuppression/chemotherapy adjunct: Adults: Oral: Range: 5-60 mg/day in divided doses 1-4 times/day

Dosage Oral:

General dosing range: Children and Adults: Initial: 5-60 mg daily: **Note:** Dose depends upon condition being treated and response of patient; dosage for infants and children should be based on severity of the disease and response of the patient rather than on strict adherence to dosage indicated by age, weight, or body surface area. Consider alternate day therapy for long-term therapy. Discontinuation of long-term therapy requires gradual withdrawal by tapering the dose. Prednisone taper (other regimens also available):

Day 1: 30 mg divided as 10 mg before breakfast, 5 mg at lunch, 5 mg at dinner, 10 mg at bedtime

Day 2: 5 mg at breakfast, 5 mg at lunch, 5 mg at dinner, 10 mg at bedtime

Day 3: 5 mg 4 times daily (with meals and at bedtime)

Day 4: 5 mg 3 times daily (breakfast, lunch, bedtime)

Day 5: 5 mg 2 times daily (breakfast, bedtime)

Day 6: 5 mg before breakfast

Indication-specific dosing:

Children:

Acute asthma (NIH guidelines, 2007):

0-11 years 1-2 mg/kg/day for 3-10 days (maximum: 60 mg daily)

≥12 years: Refer to Adults dosing

Autoimmune hepatitis (unlabeled use; Czaja, 2002): Initial treatment: 2 mg/kg/day for 2 weeks (maximum: 60 mg daily), followed by a taper over 6-8 weeks to a dose of 0.1-0.2 mg/kg/day or 5 mg daily

Nephrotic syndrome (Pediatric Nephrology Panel recommendations [Hogg, 2000]): Initial: 2 mg/kg/day or 60 mg/m^2/day given every day in 1-3 divided doses (maximum: 80 mg daily) until urine is protein free or for 4-6 weeks; followed by maintenance dose: 2 mg/kg/dose or 40 mg/m^2/dose given every other day in the morning; gradually taper and discontinue after 4-6 weeks. **Note:** No definitive treatment guidelines exist. Dosing is dependent on institution protocols and individual response.

PCP pneumonia (AIDS*info* guidelines, 2008): 1 mg/kg twice daily for 5 days, *followed by* 0.5-1 mg/kg twice daily for 5 days, *followed by* 0.5 mg/kg once daily for 11-21 days

Adolescents and Adults:

PCP pneumonia (AIDS*info* guidelines, 2008): Note: Begin within 72 hours of PCP therapy: 40 mg twice daily for 5 days, *followed by* 40 mg once daily for 5 days, *followed by* 20 mg once daily for 11 days or until antimicrobial regimen is completed

Adults:

Acute asthma (NIH guidelines, 2007): 40-60 mg daily for 3-10 days; administer as single or 2 divided doses

Acute exacerbations of chronic obstructive pulmonary disease (COPD) (unlabeled use for immediate release products; unlabeled dose): 30-40 mg once daily (based on prednisolone equivalency) for 10-14 days (GOLD guidelines, 2013).

Anaphylaxis, adjunctive treatment (Lieberman, 2005): 0.5 mg/kg

Antineoplastic: Usual range: 10 mg daily to 100 mg/m²/day (depending on indication). **Note:** Details concerning dosing in combination regimens should also be consulted.

Autoimmune hepatitis (unlabeled use; Czaja, 2002): Initial treatment: 60 mg daily for 1 week, *followed by* 40 mg daily for 1 week, *then* 30 mg daily for 2 weeks, *then* 20 mg daily. Half this dose should be given when used in combination with azathioprine

Crohn's disease, moderate/severe (unlabeled use): 40-60 mg daily until resolution of symptoms and resumption of weight gain (usual duration: 7-28 days) (Lichtenstein, 2009)

Dermatomyositis/polymyositis: Oral: 1 mg/kg daily (range: 0.5-1.5 mg/kg/day), often in conjunction with steroid-sparing therapies; depending on response/tolerance, consider slow tapering after 2-8 weeks depending on response; taper regimens vary widely, but often involve 5-10 mg decrements per week and may require 6-12 months to reach a low once-daily or every-other-day dose to prevent disease flare (Briemberg, 2003; Hengstman, 2009; Iorizzo, 2008; Wiendl, 2008)

Giant cell arteritis (unlabeled use): Oral: Initial: 40-60 mg daily; typically requires 1-2 years of treatment, but may begin to taper after 2-3 months; alternative dosing of 30-40 mg daily has demonstrated similar efficacy (Hiratzka, 2010)

Graves' ophthalmopathy prophylaxis (unlabeled use): 0.4-0.5 mg/kg/day, starting 1-3 days after radioactive iodine treatment, and continued for 1 month, then gradually taper over 2 months (Bahn, 2011)

Herpes zoster (unlabeled use; Dworkin, 2007): 60 mg daily for 7 days, *followed by* 30 mg daily for 7 days, *then* 15 mg daily for 7 days

Idiopathic thrombocytopenia purpura (American Society of Hematology, 1997): 1-2 mg/kg/day

Lupus nephritis, induction (Hahn, 2012): Oral:
Class III-IV lupus nephritis: 0.5-1 mg/kg/day (after glucocorticoid pulse) tapered after a few weeks to lowest effective dose, in combination with an immunosuppressive agent

Class V lupus nephritis: 0.5 mg/kg/day for 6 months in combination mycophenolate mofetil; if not improved after 6 months, use 0.5-1 mg/kg/day (after a glucocorticoid pulse) for an additional 6 months in combination with cyclophosphamide

Rheumatoid arthritis (American College of Rheumatology, 2002): ≤10 mg daily

Subacute thyroiditis (unlabeled use): 40 mg daily for 1-2 weeks; gradually taper over 2-4 weeks or longer depending on clinical response. **Note:** NSAIDs should be considered first-line therapy in such patients (Bahn, 2011).

Takayasu arteritis (unlabeled use): Oral: Initial: 40-60 mg daily; taper to lowest effective dose when ESR and CRP levels are normal; usual duration: 1-2 years (Hiratzka, 2010)

Thyrotoxicosis (type II amiodarone-induced; unlabeled use): 40 mg daily for 14-28 days; gradually taper over 2-3 months depending on clinical response (Bahn, 2011)

Tuberculosis, severe, paradoxical reactions (unlabeled dose, AIDS*info* guidelines, 2008): 1 mg/kg/day, gradually reduce after 1-2 weeks

Elderly: Use the lowest effective dose

Dosing adjustment in hepatic impairment: Prednisone is inactive and must be metabolized by the liver to prednisolone. This conversion may be impaired in patients with liver disease, however, prednisolone levels are observed to be higher in patients with severe liver failure than in normal patients. Therefore, compensation for the inadequate conversion of prednisone to prednisolone occurs.

Dosing adjustment in hyperthyroidism: Prednisone dose may need to be increased to achieve adequate therapeutic effects

Hemodialysis: Supplemental dose is not necessary

Peritoneal dialysis: Supplemental dose is not necessary

Mechanism of Action Decreases inflammation by suppression of migration of polymorphonuclear leukocytes and reversal of increased capillary permeability; suppresses the immune system by reducing activity and volume of the lymphatic system; suppresses adrenal function at high doses. Antitumor effects may be related to inhibition of glucose transport, phosphorylation, or induction of cell death in immature lymphocytes. Antiemetic effects are thought to occur due to blockade of cerebral innervation of the emetic center via inhibition of prostaglandin synthesis.

Contraindications Hypersensitivity to any component of the formulation; systemic fungal infections; administration of live or live attenuated vaccines with immunosuppressive doses of prednisone

Warnings/Precautions May cause hypercorticism or suppression of hypothalamic-pituitary-adrenal (HPA) axis, particularly in younger children or in patients receiving high doses for prolonged periods. HPA axis suppression may lead to adrenal crisis. Withdrawal and discontinuation of a corticosteroid should be done slowly and carefully. Particular care is required when patients are transferred from systemic corticosteroids to inhaled products due to possible adrenal insufficiency or withdrawal from steroids, including an increase in allergic symptoms. Patients receiving >20 mg per day of prednisone (or equivalent) may be most susceptible. Fatalities have occurred due to adrenal insufficiency in asthmatic patients during and after transfer from systemic corticosteroids to aerosol steroids; aerosol steroids do **not** provide the systemic steroid needed to treat patients having trauma, surgery, or infections.

Acute myopathy has been reported with high dose corticosteroids, usually in patients with neuromuscular transmission disorders; may involve ocular and/or respiratory muscles; monitor creatine kinase; recovery may be delayed. Prolonged use of corticosteroids may increase the incidence of secondary infection, mask acute infection (including fungal infections), prolong or exacerbate viral infections, or limit response to vaccines. Exposure to chickenpox should be avoided. Corticosteroids should not be used to treat ocular herpes simplex or cerebral malaria. Close observation is required in patients with latent tuberculosis and/or TB reactivity; restrict use in active TB (only in conjunction with antituberculosis treatment). Prolonged treatment with corticosteroids has been associated with the development of Kaposi's sarcoma (case reports); if noted, discontinuation of therapy should be considered. Prolonged use may cause posterior subcapsular cataracts, glaucoma (with possible nerve damage) and may increase the risk for ocular infections. Corticosteroid use may cause psychiatric disturbances, including depression, euphoria, insomnia, mood swings, and personality changes. Pre-existing psychiatric conditions may be exacerbated by corticosteroid use.

Use with caution in patients with HF, diabetes, GI diseases (diverticulitis, peptic ulcer, ulcerative colitis; due to risk of perforation), hepatic impairment, myasthenia gravis, MI, patients with or who are at risk for osteoporosis, seizure disorders or thyroid disease. May affect growth velocity; growth should be routinely monitored in pediatric patients.

Prior to use, the dose and duration of treatment should be based on the risk versus benefit for each individual patient. In general, use the smallest effective dose for the shortest duration of time to minimize adverse events. A gradual tapering of dose may be required prior to discontinuing therapy.

Drug Interactions

Metabolism/Transport Effects Substrate of CYP3A4 (minor); **Note:** Assignment of Major/Minor substrate status based on clinically relevant drug interaction potential; **Induces** CYP2C19 (weak/moderate), CYP3A4 (weak/moderate)

Avoid Concomitant Use

Avoid concomitant use of PredniSONE with any of the following: Aldesleukin; Axitinib; BCG; Mifepristone; Natalizumab; Pimecrolimus; Tacrolimus (Topical); Tofacitinib

Increased Effect/Toxicity

PredniSONE may increase the levels/effects of: Acetylcholinesterase Inhibitors; Amphotericin B; Cyclo-SPORINE (Systemic); Deferasirox; Leflunomide; Loop Diuretics; Natalizumab; NSAID (COX-2 Inhibitor); NSAID (Nonselective); Thiazide Diuretics; Tofacitinib; Vaccines (Live); Warfarin

The levels/effects of PredniSONE may be increased by: Antifungal Agents (Azole Derivatives, Systemic); Aprepitant; Calcium Channel Blockers (Nondihydropyridine); CycloSPORINE (Systemic); Denosumab; Estrogen Derivatives; Fluconazole; Fosaprepitant; Indacaterol; Macrolide Antibiotics; Mifepristone; Neuromuscular-Blocking Agents (Nondepolarizing); Pimecrolimus; Quinolone Antibiotics; Ritonavir; Roflumilast; Salicylates; Tacrolimus (Topical); Telaprevir; Trastuzumab

Decreased Effect

PredniSONE may decrease the levels/effects of: Aldesleukin; Antidiabetic Agents; ARIPiprazole; Axitinib; BCG; Calcitriol; Coccidioidin Skin Test; Corticorelin; CycloSPORINE (Systemic); Hyaluronidase; Isoniazid; Salicylates; Sipuleucel-T; Telaprevir; Vaccines (Inactivated)

The levels/effects of PredniSONE may be decreased by: Aminoglutethimide; Antacids; Barbiturates; Bile Acid Sequestrants; Echinacea; Fosphenytoin; Mifepristone; Mitotane; Phenytoin; Primidone; Rifamycin Derivatives; Somatropin; Tesamorelin

Ethanol/Nutrition/Herb Interactions

Ethanol: Avoid ethanol (may increase gastric mucosal irritation)

Food: Prednisone interferes with calcium absorption. Limit caffeine.

Herb/Nutraceutical: St John's wort may decrease prednisone levels. Avoid cat's claw, echinacea (have immunostimulant properties).

Dietary Considerations Should be taken after meals or with food or milk; may require increased dietary intake of pyridoxine, vitamin C, vitamin D, folate, calcium, and phosphorus; may require decreased dietary intake of sodium

Pharmacodynamics/Kinetics

Half-life Elimination Normal renal function: ~3.5 hours

Time to Peak Oral: Immediate release tablet: 2 hours; Delayed release tablet (Rayos®): 6-6.5 hours

Pregnancy Considerations Adverse events have been observed with corticosteroids in animal reproduction studies. Prednisone and prednisolone cross the human placenta. In the mother, prednisone is converted to the active metabolite prednisolone by the liver. Prior to reaching the fetus, prednisolone is converted by placental enzymes back to prednisone. As a result, the level of prednisone remaining in the maternal serum and reaching the fetus are similar; however, the amount of prednisolone reaching the fetus is ~8-10 times lower than the maternal serum concentration (healthy women at term). Some studies have shown an association between first trimester prednisone use and oral clefts; adverse events in the fetus/neonate have been noted in case reports following large doses of systemic corticosteroids during pregnancy. Pregnant women exposed to prednisone for antirejection therapy following a transplant may contact the National Transplantation Pregnancy Registry (NTPR) at 215-955-4820. Women exposed to prednisone during pregnancy for the treatment of an autoimmune disease (eg, rheumatoid arthritis) may contact the OTIS Autoimmune Diseases Study at 877-311-8972.

Lactation Enters breast milk/AAP rates "compatible" (AAP 2001 update pending)

Breast-Feeding Considerations Prednisone and its metabolite prednisolone are found in low concentrations in breast milk. Peak milk concentrations of both were found ~2 hours after the maternal dose in one case report. In a study which included 6 mother/infant pairs, adverse events were not observed in nursing infants (maternal prednisone dose not provided).

Dosage Forms

Solution, oral: 1 mg/mL (5 mL, 120 mL, 500 mL)
PredniSONE Intensol™: 5 mg/mL (30 mL)

Tablet, oral: 1 mg, 2.5 mg, 5 mg, 10 mg, 20 mg, 50 mg

Tablet, delayed release, oral:
Rayos®: 1 mg, 2 mg, 5 mg

Pregabalin (pre GAB a lin)

Brand Names: U.S. Lyrica®

Brand Names: Canada GD-Pregabalin; Lyrica®; PMS-Pregabalin; RAN™-Pregabalin; Riva-Pregabalin; Teva-Pregabalin

Generic Availability (U.S.) No

Pharmacologic Category Analgesic, Miscellaneous; Anticonvulsant, Miscellaneous

Use Management of neuropathic pain associated with diabetic peripheral neuropathy or with spinal cord injury; management of postherpetic neuralgia; adjunctive therapy for partial-onset seizure disorder; management of fibromyalgia

Local Anesthetic/Vasoconstrictor Precautions No information available to require special precautions

Effects on Dental Treatment Key adverse event(s) related to dental treatment: Xerostomia and changes in salivation (normal salivary flow resumes upon discontinuation).

Effects on Bleeding May be associated with thrombocytopenia (3%). No information available to require routine special precautions

Adverse Effects Note: Frequency of adverse effects may be influenced by dose or concurrent therapy. In add-on trials in epilepsy, frequency of CNS and visual adverse effects were higher than those reported in pain management trials. Range noted below is inclusive of all trials.

>10%:

Cardiovascular: Peripheral edema (≤16%)

Central nervous system: Dizziness (8% to 45%), somnolence (4% to 36%), ataxia (1% to 20%), headache (5% to 14%), fatigue (5% to 11%)

Gastrointestinal: Weight gain (≤16%), xerostomia (1% to 15%)

Neuromuscular & skeletal: Tremor (≤11%)

Ocular: Blurred vision (1% to 12%), diplopia (≤12%)

Miscellaneous: Infection (3% to 14%), accidental injury (2% to 11%)

1% to 10%:

Cardiovascular: Edema (≤8%), chest pain (1% to 4%), hypertension (2%), hypotension (2%)

Central nervous system: Neuropathy (2% to 9%), thinking abnormal (≤9%), confusion (≤7%), euphoria (≤7%), speech disorder (≤7%), attention disturbance (4% to 6%), amnesia (≤6%), incoordination (≤6%), pain (2% to 5%), insomnia (4%), memory impaired (1% to 4%), vertigo (1% to 4%), hypoesthesia (2% to 3%), feeling abnormal (1% to 3%), anxiety (2%), lethargy (1% to 2%), drunk feeling (1% to 2%), disorientation (≤2%), depersonalization (≥1%), fever (≥1%), hypertonia (≥1%), sedation (≥1%), stupor (≥1%), nervousness (≤1%)

Dermatologic: Decubitus ulcer (3%), facial edema (≤3%), bruising (≥1%), pruritus (≥1%)

Endocrine & metabolic: Fluid retention (2% to 3%), hypoglycemia (1% to 3%), libido decreased (≥1%)

Gastrointestinal: Constipation (≤10%), appetite increased (2% to 7%), nausea (5%), flatulence (≤3%), vomiting (1% to 3%), abdominal distension (2%), abdominal pain (≥1%), gastroenteritis (≥1%)

Genitourinary: Incontinence (≤3%), anorgasmia (≥1%), impotence (≥1%), urinary frequency (≥1%)

Hematologic: Thrombocytopenia (≥1%)

Neuromuscular & skeletal: Balance disorder (2% to 9%), abnormal gait (≤8%), weakness (2% to 7%), arthralgia (3% to 6%), twitching (≤5%), muscle spasm (2% to 4%), myoclonus (≤4%), CPK increased (3%), neck pain (3%), pain in extremity (3%), joint swelling (2%), paresthesia (2%), leg cramps (≥1%), myalgia (≥1%), myasthenia (1%)

Ocular: Visual abnormalities (≤5%), eye disorder (≤2%), conjunctivitis (≥1%), nystagmus (≥1%)

Otic: Otitis media (≥1%), tinnitus (≥1%)

Respiratory: Nasopharyngitis (8%), sinusitis (4% to 7%), pharyngolaryngeal pain (1% to 3%), bronchitis (≤3%), dyspnea (≤3%)

Miscellaneous: Flu-like syndrome (1% to 2%), allergic reaction (≥1%)

Dosage Oral: Adults: **Note:** When discontinuing, taper off gradually over at least 1 week.

Fibromyalgia:

U.S. labeling: Initial: 150 mg daily in divided doses (75 mg twice daily); may be increased to 300 mg daily (150 mg twice daily) within 1 week based on tolerability and effect; may be further increased to 450 mg daily (225 mg twice daily). Maximum dose: 450 mg daily (dosages up to 600 mg daily were evaluated with no significant additional benefit and an increase in adverse effects)

Canadian labeling: Initial: 150 mg daily in divided doses (75 mg twice daily); may be increased to 300 mg daily (150 mg twice daily) after 1 week based on tolerability and effect; may be further increased to 450 mg daily (225 mg twice daily). The manufacturer labeling suggests that patients with severe ongoing symptoms may receive up to a maximum of 600 mg daily (300 mg twice daily). However, dosages up to 600 mg daily have been evaluated with no significant additional benefit and an increase in adverse effects.

Neuropathic pain, diabetes-associated:

U.S. labeling: Initial: 150 mg daily in divided doses (50 mg 3 times daily); may be increased within 1 week based on tolerability and effect; maximum dose: 300 mg daily in 3 divided doses (dosages up to 600 mg daily were evaluated with no significant additional benefit and an increase in adverse effects)

Canadian labeling: Initial: 150 mg daily in divided doses (50 mg 3 times daily or 75 mg twice daily); may be increased after 1 week based on tolerability and effect to 300 mg daily (150 mg twice daily). The manufacturer labeling suggests that patients with severe ongoing symptoms may receive up to a maximum of 600 mg daily (300 mg twice daily). However, dosages up to 600 mg daily have been evaluated with no significant additional benefit and an increase in adverse effects.

Neuropathic pain, spinal cord injury associated: Initial: 150 mg daily in divided doses (75 mg twice daily); may be increased to 300 mg daily (150 mg twice daily) within 1 week based on tolerability and effect; further titration to 600 mg daily (300 mg twice daily) after 2-3 weeks may be considered in patients who do not experience sufficient relief of pain provided they are able to tolerate pregabalin. Maximum dose: 600 mg daily

Partial-onset seizures (adjunctive therapy): Initial: 150 mg daily in divided doses (75 mg twice daily or 50 mg 3 times daily); may be increased based on tolerability and effect (optimal titration schedule has not been defined). Maximum dose: 600 mg daily

Postherpetic neuralgia: Initial: 150 mg daily in divided doses (75 mg twice daily or 50 mg 3 times daily); may be increased to 300 mg daily within 1 week based on tolerability and effect; further titration (to 600 mg daily) after 2-4 weeks may be considered in patients who do not experience sufficient relief of pain provided they are able to tolerate pregabalin. Maximum dose: 600 mg daily

Dosage adjustment in renal impairment: Renal function may be estimated using the Cockcroft-Gault formula. Then determine recommended dosage regimen based on the indication-specific total daily dose for normal renal function (Cl_{cr} ≥60 mL/minute). For example, if the indication-specific daily dose is 450 mg daily for normal renal function, the daily dose should be reduced to 225 mg daily (in 2-3 divided doses) for a creatinine clearance of 30-60 mL/minute (see table on next page).

Pregabalin Renal Impairment Dosing

Cl$_{cr}$ (mL/minute)	Total Pregabalin Daily Dose (mg/day)				Dosing Frequency
≥60 (normal renal function)	150	300	450	600	2-3 divided doses
30-60	75	150	225	300	2-3 divided doses
15-30	25-50	75	100-150	150	1-2 divided doses
<15	25	25-50	50-75	75	Single daily dose

Posthemodialysis supplementary dosage (as a single additional dose):
25 mg/day schedule: Single supplementary dose of 25 mg **or** 50 mg
25-50 mg/day schedule: Single supplementary dose of 50 mg **or** 75 mg
50-75 mg/day schedule: Single supplementary dose of 75 mg **or** 100 mg
75 mg/day schedule: Single supplementary dose of 100 mg **or** 150 mg

Dosage adjustment in hepatic impairment: No dosage adjustment provided in manufacturer's labeling; however, undergoes negligible metabolism and dosage adjustments would not likely be necessary.

Mechanism of Action Binds to alpha$_2$-delta subunit of voltage-gated calcium channels within the CNS, inhibiting excitatory neurotransmitter release. Although structurally related to GABA, it does not bind to GABA or benzodiazepine receptors. Exerts antinociceptive and anticonvulsant activity. Decreases symptoms of painful peripheral neuropathies and, as adjunctive therapy in partial seizures, decreases the frequency of seizures. Pregabalin may also affect descending noradrenergic and serotonergic pain transmission pathways from the brainstem to the spinal cord.

Contraindications Hypersensitivity to pregabalin or any component of the formulation

Warnings/Precautions Antiepileptics are associated with an increased risk of suicidal behavior/thoughts with use (regardless of indication); patients should be monitored for signs/symptoms of depression, suicidal tendencies, and other unusual behavior changes during therapy and instructed to inform their healthcare provider immediately if symptoms occur.

Angioedema has been reported; may be life threatening; use with caution in patients with a history of angioedema episodes. Concurrent use with other drugs known to cause angioedema (eg, ACE inhibitors) may increase risk. Hypersensitivity reactions, including skin redness, blistering, hives, rash, dyspnea, and wheezing have been reported; discontinue treatment of hypersensitivity occurs. Dizziness and somnolence are commonly reported; effects generally occur shortly after initiation and occur more frequently at higher doses. Patients must be cautioned about performing tasks which require mental alertness (eg, operating machinery or driving). Visual disturbances (blurred vision, decreased acuity and visual field changes) have been associated with pregabalin therapy; patients should be instructed to notify their physician if these effects are noted.

Pregabalin has been associated with increases in CPK and rare cases of rhabdomyolysis. Patients should be instructed to notify their prescriber if unexplained muscle pain, tenderness, or weakness, particularly if fever and/or malaise are associated with these symptoms. Use may cause peripheral edema or weight gain; use with caution in patients with heart failure (NYHA Class III or IV) due to limited data in this patient population. In addition, effect on weight gain/edema may be additive with the thiazolidinedione class of antidiabetic agents; use caution when coadministering these agents, particularly in patients with prior cardiovascular disease. May decrease platelet count or prolong PR interval.

Has been noted to be tumorigenic (increased incidence of hemangiosarcoma) in animal studies; significance of these findings in humans is unknown. Pregabalin has been associated with discontinuation symptoms following abrupt cessation, and increases in seizure frequency (when used as an antiepileptic) may occur. Should not be discontinued abruptly; dosage tapering over at least 1 week is recommended. Use caution in renal impairment; dosage adjustment required.

Drug Interactions

Metabolism/Transport Effects None known.

Avoid Concomitant Use

Avoid concomitant use of Pregabalin with any of the following: Azelastine (Nasal); Paraldehyde

Increased Effect/Toxicity

Pregabalin may increase the levels/effects of: Alcohol (Ethyl); Antidiabetic Agents (Thiazolidinedione); Azelastine (Nasal); Buprenorphine; CNS Depressants; Methotrimeprazine; Metyrosine; Mirtazapine; Paraldehyde; Pramipexole; ROPINIRole; Rotigotine; Selective Serotonin Reuptake Inhibitors; Zolpidem

The levels/effects of Pregabalin may be increased by: Droperidol; HydrOXYzine; Magnesium Sulfate; Methotrimeprazine; Perampanel; Sodium Oxybate

Decreased Effect

The levels/effects of Pregabalin may be decreased by: Ketorolac (Nasal); Ketorolac (Systemic); Mefloquine

Ethanol/Nutrition/Herb Interactions

Ethanol: May increase CNS depression; monitor for increased effects with coadministration. Caution patients about effects.

Herb/Nutraceutical: Avoid valerian, St John's wort, kava kava, gotu kola (may increase CNS depression).

Dietary Considerations May be taken with or without food.

Pharmacodynamics/Kinetics

Onset of Action Pain management: Effects may be noted as early as the first week of therapy

Half-life Elimination 6.3 hours

Time to Peak 1.5 hours (3 hours with food)

Pregnancy Risk Factor C

Pregnancy Considerations Increased incidence of fetal abnormalities, particularly skeletal malformations, were observed in animal studies. Male-mediated teratogenicity has been observed in animal reproduction studies; implications in humans are not defined. Impaired male and female fertility has been noted in animal studies.

Patients exposed to pregabalin during pregnancy are encouraged to enroll themselves into the North American Antiepileptic Drug (NAAED) Pregnancy Registry by calling 1-888-233-2334. Additional information is available at www.aedpregnancyregistry.org.

Lactation Excretion in breast milk unknown/not recommended

Controlled Substance C-V

Dosage Forms

Capsule, oral:
Lyrica®: 25 mg, 50 mg, 75 mg, 100 mg, 150 mg, 200 mg, 225 mg, 300 mg

Solution, oral:
Lyrica®: 20 mg/mL (473 mL)

References

Hill CM, Balkenohl M, Thomas DW, et al, "Pregabalin in Patients With Postoperative Dental Pain," *Eur J Pain*, 2001, 5(2):119-24.

Prilocaine (PRIL oh kane)

Related Information

Oral Pain *on page 1558*

Brand Names: U.S. Citanest® Plain Dental

Brand Names: Canada Citanest® Plain

Generic Availability (U.S.) No

Pharmacologic Category Local Anesthetic

Dental Use Amide-type anesthetic used for local infiltration anesthesia; injection near nerve trunks to produce nerve block

Use Amide-type anesthetic used for local infiltration anesthesia; injection near nerve trunks to produce nerve block

Local Anesthetic/Vasoconstrictor Precautions No information available to require special precautions

Effects on Dental Treatment It is common to misinterpret psychogenic responses to local anesthetic injection as an allergic reaction. Intraoral injections are perceived by many patients as a stressful procedure in dentistry. Common symptoms to this stress are diaphoresis, palpitations, hyperventilation, generalized pallor and a fainting feeling.

Degree of adverse effects in the CNS and cardiovascular system is directly related to blood levels of prilocaine (frequency not defined; more likely to occur after systemic administration rather than infiltration): Bradycardia and reduction in cardiac output, hypersensitivity reactions (may be manifest as dermatologic reactions and edema at injection site), asthmatic syndromes

High blood levels: Anxiety, restlessness, disorientation, confusion, dizziness, tremors, and seizures, followed by CNS depression, resulting in somnolence, unconsciousness and possible respiratory arrest; nausea and vomiting

In some cases, symptoms of CNS stimulation may be absent and the primary CNS effects are somnolence and unconsciousness.

Effects on Bleeding No information available to require special precautions

Adverse Effects Degree of adverse effects in the central nervous system and cardiovascular system are directly related to the blood levels of local anesthetic. The effects below are more likely to occur after systemic administration rather than infiltration.

Cardiovascular: Myocardial effects include a decrease in contraction force as well as a decrease in electrical excitability and myocardial conduction rate resulting in bradycardia and reduction in cardiac output.

Central nervous system: High blood levels result in anxiety, restlessness, disorientation, confusion, dizziness, tremor, and seizure. This is followed by depression of CNS resulting in somnolence, unconsciousness and possible respiratory arrest. Nausea and vomiting may also occur. In some cases, symptoms of CNS stimulation may be absent and the primary CNS effects are somnolence and unconsciousness.

Hypersensitivity reactions: May be manifest as dermatologic reactions and edema at injection site. Asthmatic syndromes have occurred.

Psychogenic reactions: It is common to misinterpret psychogenic responses to local anesthetic injection as an allergic reaction. Intraoral injections are perceived by many patients as a stressful procedure in dentistry. Common symptoms to this stress are diaphoresis, palpitation, hyperventilation, generalized pallor and a fainting feeling

Dental Usual Dosage

Children <10 years: Doses >40 mg (1 mL) as a 4% solution per procedure rarely needed

Children >10 years and Adults: Dental anesthesia, infiltration, or conduction block: Initial: 40-80 mg (1-2 mL) as a 4% solution; up to a maximum of 400 mg (10 mL) as a 4% solution within a 2-hour period. Manufacturer's maximum recommended dose is not more than 600 mg to normal healthy adults. The effective anesthetic dose varies with procedure, intensity of anesthesia needed, duration of anesthesia required and physical condition of the patient. Always use the lowest effective dose along with careful aspiration.

The following numbers of dental carpules (1.8 mL) provide the indicated amounts of prilocaine hydrochloride 4%. See table.

Prilocaine

# of Cartridges (1.8 mL)	mg Prilocaine (4%)
1	72
2	144
3	216
4	288
5	360
6	432
7	504
8	576

Note: Adult and children doses of prilocaine hydrochloride cited from *USP Dispensing Information (USP DI)*, 17th ed, The United States Pharmacopeial Convention, Inc, Rockville, MD, 1997, 139.

Dosage

Children <10 years: Doses >40 mg (1 mL) as a 4% solution per procedure rarely needed

Children >10 years and Adults: Dental anesthesia, infiltration, or conduction block: Initial: 40-80 mg (1-2 mL) as a 4% solution; up to a maximum of 400 mg (10 mL) as a 4% solution within a 2-hour period. Manufacturer's maximum recommended dose is not more than 600 mg to normal healthy adults. The effective anesthetic dose varies with procedure, intensity of anesthesia needed, duration of anesthesia required and physical condition of the patient. Always use the lowest effective dose along with careful aspiration.

Note: Adult and children doses of prilocaine hydrochloride cited from *USP Dispensing Information (USP DI)*, 17th ed, The United States Pharmacopeial Convention, Inc, Rockville, MD, 1997, 139.

Mechanism of Action Local anesthetics bind selectively to the intracellular surface of sodium channels to block influx of sodium into the axon. As a result, depolarization necessary for action potential propagation and subsequent nerve function is prevented. The block at the sodium channel is reversible. When drug diffuses away from the axon, sodium channel function is restored and nerve propagation returns.

Contraindications Hypersensitivity to local anesthetics of the amide type or any component of the formulation

Warnings/Precautions Methemoglobinemia has been reported. Careful and constant monitoring of the patient's state of consciousness should be done following each local anesthetic injection; at such times, restlessness, anxiety, tinnitus, dizziness, blurred vision, tremors, depression, or drowsiness may be early warning signs of CNS toxicity. Treatment is primarily symptomatic and supportive. Intravascular injections should be avoided. Local anesthetics have been associated with rare occurrences of sudden respiratory arrest, seizures, and cardiac arrest. Use with caution in patients with cardiovascular disease or hepatic impairment. Use with caution in acutely ill, debilitated, pediatric or elderly patients. Aspirate the syringe after tissue penetration and before injection to minimize chance of direct vascular injection. Resuscitative equipment, oxygen, and other resuscitative drugs should be available for immediate use.

Drug Interactions

Metabolism/Transport Effects None known.

Avoid Concomitant Use There are no known interactions where it is recommended to avoid concomitant use.

Increased Effect/Toxicity

The levels/effects of Prilocaine may be increased by: Hyaluronidase; Methemoglobinemia Associated Agents

Decreased Effect There are no known significant interactions involving a decrease in effect.

Pharmacodynamics/Kinetics

Onset of Action Infiltration: ~2 minutes; Inferior alveolar nerve block: ~3 minutes

Duration of Action Infiltration: Complete anesthesia for procedures lasting 20 minutes; Inferior alveolar nerve block: ~2.5 hours

Half-life Elimination 10-150 minutes; prolonged with hepatic or renal impairment

Pregnancy Risk Factor B

Pregnancy Considerations Adverse events have not been observed in animal reproduction studies.

Breast-Feeding Considerations Usual infiltration doses of prilocaine given to nursing mothers has not been shown to affect the health of the nursing infant.

Dosage Forms

Injection, solution:

Citanest® Plain Dental: 4% [40 mg/mL] (1.8 mL)

References

Haas DA, "An Update on Local Anesthetics in Dentistry," *J Can Dent Assoc*, 2002, 68(9):546-51.

Jastak JT and Yagiela JA, "Vasoconstrictors and Local Anesthesia: A Review and Rationale for Use," *J Am Dent Assoc*, 1983, 107 (4):623-30.

Moore PA and Hersh EV, "Local Anesthetics: Pharmacology and Toxicity," *Dent Clin North Am*, 2010, 54(4):587-99.

Wahl MJ, Schmitt MM, Overton DA, et al, "Injection Pain of Bupivacaine With Epinephrine vs. Prilocaine Plain," *J Am Dent Assoc*, 2002, 133(12):1652-6.

Prilocaine and Epinephrine

(PRIL oh kane & ep i NEF rin)

Related Information

EPINEPHrine (Systemic, Oral Inhalation) *on page 482*

Oral Pain *on page 1558*

Prilocaine *on page 1139*

Brand Names: U.S. Citanest® Forte Dental

Brand Names: Canada Citanest® Forte

Generic Availability (U.S.) No

Pharmacologic Category Local Anesthetic

Dental Use Amide-type anesthetic used for local infiltration anesthesia; injection near nerve trunks to produce nerve block

Use Amide-type anesthetic used for local infiltration anesthesia; injection near nerve trunks to produce nerve block

Local Anesthetic/Vasoconstrictor Precautions No information available to require special precautions

Effects on Dental Treatment It is common to misinterpret psychogenic responses to local anesthetic injection as an allergic reaction. Intraoral injections are perceived by many patients as a stressful procedure in dentistry. Common symptoms to this stress are diaphoresis, palpitations, hyperventilation, generalized pallor and a fainting feeling. Patients may exhibit hypersensitivity to bisulfites contained in local anesthetic solution to prevent oxidation of epinephrine. In general, patients reacting to bisulfites have a history of asthma and their airways are hyper-reactive to asthmatic syndrome.

Degree of adverse effects in the CNS and cardiovascular system is directly related to blood levels of prilocaine (frequency not defined; more likely to occur after systemic administration rather than infiltration): Bradycardia and reduction in cardiac output, hypersensitivity reactions (extremely rare; may be manifest as dermatologic reactions and edema at injection site), asthmatic syndromes

High blood levels: Anxiety, restlessness, disorientation, confusion, dizziness, tremors, and seizures, followed by CNS depression, resulting in somnolence, unconsciousness and possible respiratory arrest; nausea and vomiting

In some cases, symptoms of CNS stimulation may be absent and the primary CNS effects are somnolence and unconsciousness.

Effects on Bleeding No information available to require special precautions

Adverse Effects Degree of adverse effects in the CNS and cardiovascular system are directly related to the blood levels of prilocaine. The effects below are more likely to occur after systemic administration rather than infiltration.

Cardiovascular: Bradycardia, cardiovascular collapse, edema, hypotension

Central nervous system: Apprehension, confusion, dizziness, drowsiness, euphoria, lightheadedness, nervousness, seizures, unconsciousness

Dermatologic: Urticaria

Gastrointestinal: Vomiting

Ocular: Blurred vision, double vision

Otic: Tinnitus

Neuromuscular & skeletal: Tremors, twitching

Respiratory: Respiratory arrest, respiratory depression

Miscellaneous: Allergic reactions (rare), anaphylactoid reactions, sensation of warm/cold

Dental Usual Dosage

Children <10 years: Doses >40 mg (1 mL) of prilocaine hydrochloride as a 4% solution with epinephrine 1:200,000 are rarely needed

Children >10 years and Adults: Dental anesthesia, infiltration, or conduction block: Initial: 40-80 mg (1-2 mL) of prilocaine hydrochloride as a 4% solution with epinephrine 1:200,000; up to a maximum of 400 mg (10 mL) of prilocaine hydrochloride within a 2-hour period. The effective dental dose varies with procedure, intensity of anesthesia needed, duration of anesthesia required, and physical condition of the patient. Always use the lowest effective dose along with careful aspiration.

The following numbers of dental carpules (1.7 mL) provide the indicated amounts of prilocaine hydrochloride 4% and epinephrine 1:200,000. See table.

Prilocaine With Epinephrine

# of Cartridges (1.7 mL/ cartridge)	mg Prilocaine (4%)	mg Vasoconstrictor (Epinephrine 1:200,000)
1	68	0.0085
2	136	0.017
3	204	0.0255
4	272	0.034
5	340	0.0425
6	408	0.051
7	476	0.0595
8	544	0.068

Dosage

Children <10 years: Doses >40 mg (1 mL) of prilocaine hydrochloride as a 4% solution with epinephrine 1:200,000 are rarely needed for procedures involving a single tooth, in a maxillary infiltration for 2-3 teeth, or for an entire quadrant with a mandibular block.

Children >10 years and Adults: Dental anesthesia, infiltration, or conduction block:

Initial: 40-80 mg (1-2 mL) of prilocaine hydrochloride as a 4% solution with epinephrine 1:200,000

Maximum dose (weight-based) within a 2-hour period: Prilocaine hydrochloride:

<70 kg: 8 mg/kg

≥70 kg: 600 mg (15 mL) or 8 cartridges

Note: The effective anesthetic dose varies with procedure, intensity of anesthesia needed, duration of anesthesia required, and physical condition of the patient. Always use the lowest effective dose along with careful aspiration prior to administration.

Mechanism of Action Local anesthetics bind selectively to the intracellular surface of sodium channels to block influx of sodium into the axon. As a result, depolarization necessary for action potential propagation and subsequent nerve function is prevented. The block at the sodium channel is reversible. When drug diffuses away from the axon, sodium channel function is restored and nerve propagation returns.

Epinephrine prolongs the duration of the anesthetic actions of prilocaine by causing vasoconstriction (alpha-adrenergic receptor agonist) of the vasculature surrounding the nerve axons. This prevents the diffusion of prilocaine away from the nerves resulting in a longer retention in the axon.

Contraindications Hypersensitivity to local anesthetics of the amide-type or any component of the formulation; congenital or idiopathic methemoglobinemia

Warnings/Precautions Should be avoided in patients with uncontrolled hyperthyroidism. Should be used in minimal amounts in patients with significant cardiovascular problems (because of epinephrine component). Aspirate the syringe after tissue penetration and before injection to minimize chance of direct vascular injection

Drug Interactions

Metabolism/Transport Effects Refer to individual components.

Avoid Concomitant Use

Avoid concomitant use of Prilocaine and Epinephrine with any of the following: Ergot Derivatives; Iobenguane I 123; Lurasidone

Increased Effect/Toxicity

Prilocaine and Epinephrine may increase the levels/ effects of: Bromocriptine; Lurasidone; Sympathomimetics

The levels/effects of Prilocaine and Epinephrine may be increased by: Antacids; AtoMOXetine; Beta-Blockers; Cannabinoids; Carbonic Anhydrase Inhibitors; COMT Inhibitors; Ergot Derivatives; Hyaluronidase; Inhalational Anesthetics; MAO Inhibitors; Serotonin/ Norepinephrine Reuptake Inhibitors; Tricyclic Antidepressants

Decreased Effect

Prilocaine and Epinephrine may decrease the levels/ effects of: Benzylpenicilloyl Polylysine; Iobenguane I 123

The levels/effects of Prilocaine and Epinephrine may be decreased by: Alpha1-Blockers; Promethazine; Spironolactone

Pharmacodynamics/Kinetics

Onset of Action Infiltration: <2 minutes; Inferior alveolar nerve block: <3 minutes

Duration of Action Infiltration: ~2.25 hours; Inferior alveolar nerve block: ~3 hours

Pregnancy Risk Factor B

Pregnancy Considerations Adverse events were not observed in animal reproduction studies.

Lactation Excretion in breast milk unknown/use caution

Breast-Feeding Considerations Usual infiltration doses of prilocaine with epinephrine given to nursing mothers has not been shown to affect the health of the nursing infant.

Dosage Forms

Injection, solution [for dental use]:

Citanest® Forte Dental: Prilocaine 4% and epinephrine 1:200,000 (1.7 mL)

Dental Comment Oral paresthesia: The occurrence of oral paresthesia associated with 4% solutions of prilocaine or articaine, although rare, continue to be slightly more frequent than other local anesthetics. From 1999-2008, there were 182 cases of nonsurgical paresthesia (Gaffen, 2009). Of the cases, 172 involved mandibular block injection only. Another eight cases involved mandibular block combined with at least one other type of anesthetic injection. A single case involved infiltration around tooth number 35 and the final case involved infiltration and intraligamentary injection in the maxillary anterior region.

A 2010 report, reviewed adverse events submitted voluntarily over a 10-year period involving the dental local anesthetics articaine, bupivacaine, lidocaine, mepivacaine, and prilocaine in the United States. Prilocaine reported incidence: One case per 2,070,678 cartridges sold. The reported incidence of paresthesia was one case for 13,800,970 cartridges of all local anesthetics sold in the U.S. (Garisto, 2010).

References

Dower JS Jr, "A Review of Paresthesia in Association With Administration of Local Anesthesia," Dent Today, 2003, 22(2):64-9.

Finder RL and Moore PA, "Adverse Drug Reactions to Local Anesthesia," Dent Clin North Am, 2002, 46(4):747-57, x.

Gaffen AS and Haas DA, "Retrospective Review of Voluntary Reports of Nonsurgical Paresthesia in Dentistry," J Can Dent Assoc, 2009, 75(8):579.

Garisto GA, Gaffen AS, Lawrence HP, et al, "Occurrence of Paresthesia After Dental Local Anesthetic Administration in the United States," J Am Dent Assoc, 2010, 141(7):836-44.

Haas DA, "An Update on Local Anesthetics in Dentistry," J Can Dent Assoc, 2002, 68(9):546-51.

Jastak JT and Yagiela JA, "Vasoconstrictors and Local Anesthesia: A Review and Rationale for Use," J Am Dent Assoc, 1983, 107 (4):623-30.

Primaquine (PRIM a kween)

Pharmacologic Category Aminoquinoline (Antimalarial)
Use Prevention of relapse of *P. vivax* malaria
Unlabeled Use Prevention of relapse of *P. ovale* malaria; prevention of malaria; treatment of uncomplicated *P. vivax* and *P. ovale* malaria; treatment of *Pneumocystis jirovecii* pneumonia (PCP); prevention of malaria
Local Anesthetic/Vasoconstrictor Precautions No information available to require special precautions
Effects on Dental Treatment No significant effects or complications reported
Effects on Bleeding No information available to require special precautions.
Adverse Effects Frequency not defined.
Cardiovascular: Arrhythmias (rare)
Central nervous system: Headache
Dermatologic: Pruritus
Gastrointestinal: Abdominal cramps, dyspepsia, nausea, vomiting
Hematologic: Agranulocytosis, anemia, hemolytic anemia (in patients with G6PD deficiency), leukopenia, leukocytosis, methemoglobinemia (in NADH-methemoglobin reductase-deficient individuals)
Ocular: Interference with visual accommodation
General Dosage Range Oral:
Children: 0.5 mg/kg once daily for 14 days (maximum dose: 30 mg/day)
Adults: 30 mg once daily for 14 days; Alternative regimen (recommended for mild G6PD deficiency): 45 mg once weekly for 8 weeks
Mechanism of Action Eliminates the primary tissue exoerythrocytic forms of *P. ovale* and *P. vivax*; disrupts mitochondria and binds to DNA
Pharmacodynamics/Kinetics
Half-life Elimination 3.7-9.6 hours
Time to Peak Serum: 1-2 hours
Pregnancy Considerations Animal reproduction studies have not been conducted. Primaquine use is not recommended in pregnant women per CDC Guidelines. Consult current CDC guidelines for the treatment of malaria during pregnancy.

Primidone (PRI mi done)

Brand Names: U.S. Mysoline®
Brand Names: Canada Apo-Primidone®
Pharmacologic Category Anticonvulsant, Miscellaneous; Barbiturate
Use Management of grand mal, psychomotor, and focal seizures
Unlabeled Use Benign familial tremor (essential tremor)
Local Anesthetic/Vasoconstrictor Precautions No information available to require special precautions
Effects on Dental Treatment No significant effects or complications reported
Effects on Bleeding Primidone has been associated with clotting factor defects in children, including elevated prothrombin time, elevated partial thromboplastin time, and diminished factors V, VII, or X. These defects are reversible; clotting factors return to normal after discontinuation of primidone.
Adverse Effects Frequency not defined.
Central nervous system: Ataxia, drowsiness, emotional disturbances, fatigue, hyperirritability, suicidal ideation, vertigo

Dermatologic: Morbilliform skin eruptions
Gastrointestinal: Anorexia, nausea, vomiting
Genitourinary: Impotence
Hematologic: Agranulocytosis, granulocytopenia, megaloblastic anemia (idiosyncratic), red cell aplasia/hypoplasia
Ocular: Diplopia, nystagmus
General Dosage Range Dosage adjustment recommended in patients with renal impairment
Oral:
Children <8 years: Initial: 50 mg once daily at bedtime; Maintenance: 375-750 mg/day (10-25 mg/kg/day) in 3-4 divided doses
Children ≥8 years and Adults: Initial: 100-125 mg/day at bedtime; Maintenance: 750-1500 mg/day in 3-4 divided doses (maximum: 2 g/day)
Mechanism of Action Decreases neuron excitability, raises seizure threshold similar to phenobarbital; primidone has two active metabolites, phenobarbital and phenylethylmalonamide (PEMA); PEMA may enhance the activity of phenobarbital
Pharmacodynamics/Kinetics
Half-life Elimination Age dependent: Primidone: Mean: 5-15 hours (variable); PEMA: 16 hours (variable)
Time to Peak Serum:~3 hours (variable)
Pregnancy Considerations Primidone and its metabolites (PEMA, phenobarbital, and p-hydroxyphenobarbital) cross the placenta; neonatal serum concentrations at birth are similar to those in the mother. Withdrawal symptoms may occur in the neonate and may be delayed due to the long half-life of primidone and its metabolites. Use may be associated with birth defects and adverse events; the use of folic acid throughout pregnancy and vitamin K during the last month of pregnancy is recommended. Epilepsy itself, number of medications, genetic factors, or a combination of these probably influence the teratogenicity of anticonvulsant therapy.

Patients exposed to primidone during pregnancy are encouraged to enroll themselves into the NAAED Pregnancy Registry by calling 1-888-233-2334. Additional information is available at www.aedpregnancyregistry.org.

Probenecid (proe BEN e sid)

Brand Names: Canada Benuryl™
Pharmacologic Category Uricosuric Agent
Use Treatment of hyperuricemia associated with gout or gouty arthritis; prolongation and elevation of beta-lactam plasma levels (eg, uncomplicated gonococcal infection)
Unlabeled Use Prolongation and elevation of beta-lactam plasma levels (eg, neurosyphilis, pelvic inflammatory disease)
Local Anesthetic/Vasoconstrictor Precautions No information available to require special precautions
Effects on Dental Treatment Key adverse event(s) related to dental treatment: Sore gums.
Effects on Bleeding No information available to require special precautions
Adverse Effects Frequency not defined.
Cardiovascular: Flushing
Central nervous system: Dizziness, fever, headache
Dermatologic: Alopecia, dermatitis, pruritus, rash
Gastrointestinal: Anorexia, dyspepsia, gastroesophageal reflux, nausea, sore gums, vomiting
Genitourinary: Hematuria, polyuria

Hematologic: Anemia, aplastic anemia, hemolytic anemia (in G6PD deficiency), leukopenia

Hepatic: Hepatic necrosis

Neuromuscular & skeletal: Costovertebral pain, gouty arthritis (acute)

Renal: Nephrotic syndrome, renal colic

Miscellaneous: Anaphylaxis, hypersensitivity

General Dosage Range Avoid use if Cl$_{cr}$ <30 mL/minute.

Oral:

Children 2-14 years: Prolong penicillin serum levels: Initial: 25 mg/kg then 40 mg/kg/day given 4 times/day (maximum: 500 mg/dose)

Children >50 kg and Adults:

Gonorrhea, PID: 1 g as a single dose

Gout: Initial: 250 mg twice daily (maximum: 2 g/day)

Neurosyphilis: 500 mg 4 times/day for 10-14 days

Prolong PCN levels: 500 mg 4 times/day

Mechanism of Action Competitively inhibits the reabsorption of uric acid at the proximal convoluted tubule, thereby promoting its excretion and reducing serum uric acid levels; increases plasma levels of weak organic acids (penicillins, cephalosporins, or other beta-lactam antibiotics) by competitively inhibiting their renal tubular secretion

Pharmacodynamics/Kinetics

Onset of Action Effect on penicillin levels: 2 hours

Half-life Elimination Dose dependent: Normal renal function: 6-12 hours

Time to Peak Serum: 2-4 hours

Pregnancy Considerations Probenecid crosses the placenta; adverse fetal events have not been reported.

Procainamide (pro KANE a mide)

Related Information

Clinical Risk Related to Drugs Prolonging QT Interval on page 1510

Brand Names: Canada Apo-Procainamide®; Procainamide Hydrochloride Injection, USP; Procan SR®

Pharmacologic Category Antiarrhythmic Agent, Class Ia

Use

Intravenous: Treatment of life-threatening ventricular arrhythmias

Oral (Canadian labeling; not available in U.S.): Treatment of supraventricular arrhythmias. **Note:** In the treatment of atrial fibrillation, use only when preferred treatment is ineffective or cannot be used. Use in paroxysmal atrial tachycardia when reflex stimulation or other measures are ineffective.

Unlabeled Use

Paroxysmal supraventricular tachycardia (PSVT); prevent recurrence of ventricular tachycardia; symptomatic premature ventricular contractions

ACLS guidelines: I.V.: Treatment of the following arrhythmias in patients with preserved left ventricular function: Stable monomorphic VT; pre-excited atrial fibrillation; stable wide complex regular tachycardia (likely VT)

PALS guidelines: I.V.: Tachycardia with pulses and poor perfusion (probable SVT [unresponsive to vagal maneuvers and adenosine or synchronized cardioversion]; probable VT [unresponsive to synchronized cardioversion or adenosine])

Local Anesthetic/Vasoconstrictor Precautions

Procainamide is one of the drugs confirmed to prolong the QT interval and is accepted as having a risk of causing torsade de pointes. The risk of drug-induced torsade de pointes is extremely low when a single QT interval prolonging drug is prescribed. In terms of epinephrine, it is not known what effect vasoconstrictors in the local anesthetic regimen will have in patients with a known history of congenital prolonged QT interval or in patients taking any medication that prolongs the QT interval. Until more information is obtained, it is suggested that the clinician consult with the physician prior to the use of a vasoconstrictor in suspected patients, and that the vasoconstrictor (epinephrine, mepivacaine and levonordefrin [Carbocaine® 2% with Neo-Cobefrin®]) be used with caution.

Effects on Dental Treatment Key adverse event(s) related to dental treatment: Taste disorder.

Effects on Bleeding Patients may develop procainamide-induced syndrome, which causes prolonged thrombin and Reptilase® clotting times of plasma. Clinical manifestations of procainamide-induced syndrome subside following procainamide cessation.

Adverse Effects >1%:

Cardiovascular: Hypotension (I.V. up to 5%)

Dermatologic: Rash

Gastrointestinal: Diarrhea (oral: 3% to 4%), nausea (oral: 3% to 4%), taste disorder (oral: 3% to 4%), vomiting (oral: 3% to 4%)

Miscellaneous: Positive ANA (≤50%), SLE-like syndrome (≤30%, increased incidence with long-term therapy or slow acetylators; syndrome may include abdominal pain, arthralgia, arthritis, chills, fever, hepatomegaly, myalgia, pericarditis, pleural effusion, pulmonary infiltrates, rash)

General Dosage Range Dosage adjustment recommended in patients with hepatic or renal impairment

I.M.:

Children: 20-30 mg/kg/day divided every 4-6 hours (maximum: 4 g/day)

Adults: 50 mg/kg/day divided every 3-6 hours or 0.5-1 g every 4-8 hours

I.V.:

Children: Loading dose: 3-6 mg/kg/dose over 5 minutes (maximum: 100 mg/dose), may repeat every 5-10 minutes to maximum of 15 mg/kg/load; Infusion: 20-80 mcg/kg/minute (maximum: 2 g/day)

Adults: Loading dose: 15-18 mg/kg administered as slow infusion over 25-30 minutes or 100 mg/dose at a rate not to exceed 50 mg/minute repeated every 5 minutes as needed (maximum total dose: 1 g); Infusion: 1-4 mg/minute

Mechanism of Action Decreases myocardial excitability and conduction velocity and may depress myocardial contractility, by increasing the electrical stimulation threshold of ventricle, His-Purkinje system and through direct cardiac effects

Pharmacodynamics/Kinetics

Onset of Action I.M. 10-30 minutes

Half-life Elimination

Procainamide (hepatic acetylator, phenotype, cardiac and renal function dependent): Children: 1.7 hours; Adults: 2.5-4.7 hours; Anephric: 11 hours

NAPA (renal function dependent): Children: 6 hours; Adults: 6-8 hours; Anephric: 42 hours

Time to Peak Serum: I.M.: 15-60 minutes

Pregnancy Risk Factor C

Pregnancy Considerations Animal reproduction studies have not been conducted. Procainamide crosses the placenta; procainamide and its active metabolite (N-acetyl procainamide) can be detected in the cord blood and neonatal serum.

Dental Comment Procainamide is known to prolong the QT interval. The QT interval is measured as the time and distance between the Q point of the QRS complex and the end of the T wave in the ECG tracing. After adjustment for heart rate, the QT interval is defined as prolonged if it is more than 450 msec in men and 460 msec in women. A long QT syndrome was first described in the 1950s and 60s as a congenital syndrome involving QT interval prolongation and syncope and sudden death. Some of the congenital long QT syndromes were characterized by a peculiar electrocardiographic appearance of the QRS complex involving a premature atria beat followed by a pause, then a subsequent sinus beat showing marked QT prolongation and deformity. This type of cardiac arrhythmia was originally termed "torsade de pointes" (translated from the French as "twisting of the points"). Procainamide is considered as having a risk of causing torsade de pointes. Since it is not known what effect vasoconstrictors in the local anesthetic regimen will have in patients with a known history of congenital prolonged QT interval or in patients taking any medication that prolongs the QT interval, a medical consult is suggested.

Procarbazine (proe KAR ba zeen)

Brand Names: U.S. Matulane®
Brand Names: Canada Matulane®; Natulan®
Pharmacologic Category Antineoplastic Agent, Alkylating Agent
Use Treatment of Hodgkin's disease
Unlabeled Use Treatment of non-Hodgkin's lymphoma, brain tumors
Local Anesthetic/Vasoconstrictor Precautions No information available to require special precautions
Effects on Dental Treatment Key adverse event(s) related to dental treatment: Xerostomia (normal salivary flow resumes upon discontinuation), stomatitis, and dysphagia.
Effects on Bleeding Chemotherapy may result in significant myelosuppression, potentially including significant reduction in platelet counts and altered hemostasis. In patients who are under active treatment with these agents, medical consult is suggested.
Adverse Effects Most frequencies not defined.
Cardiovascular: Edema, flushing, hypotension, syncope, tachycardia
Central nervous system: Apprehension, ataxia, chills, coma, confusion, depression, dizziness, drowsiness, fatigue, fever, hallucination, headache, insomnia, lethargy, nervousness, nightmares, pain, seizure, slurred speech
Dermatologic: Alopecia, dermatitis, hyperpigmentation, petechiae, pruritus, purpura, rash, urticaria
Endocrine & metabolic: Gynecomastia (in prepubertal and early pubertal males)
Hematologic: Eosinophilia; hemolysis (in patients with G6PD deficiency); hemolytic anemia; myelosuppression (leukopenia, anemia, thrombocytopenia); pancytopenia
Gastrointestinal: Abdominal pain, anorexia, constipation, diarrhea, dysphagia, hematemesis, melena; nausea and vomiting ([60% to 90%], increasing the dose in a stepwise fashion over several days may minimize); stomatitis, xerostomia
Genitourinary: Azoospermia (reported with combination chemotherapy), hematuria, nocturia, polyuria, reproductive dysfunction (>10%)
Hepatic: Hepatic dysfunction, jaundice

Neuromuscular & skeletal: Arthralgia, falling, foot drop, myalgia, neuropathy, paresthesia, reflex diminished, tremor, unsteadiness, weakness
Ocular: Diplopia, inability to focus, nystagmus, papilledema, photophobia, retinal hemorrhage
Otic: Hearing loss
Respiratory: Cough, epistaxis, hemoptysis, hoarseness, pleural effusion, pneumonitis, pulmonary toxicity (<1%)
Miscellaneous: Allergic reaction, diaphoresis, herpes, infection, secondary malignancies (2% to 15%; reported with combination therapy)
General Dosage Range Dosage adjustment recommended in patients with hepatic impairment
Oral:
Children: 100 mg/m^2/day for 14 days and repeated every 4 weeks
Adults: Initial: 2-4 mg/kg/day in single or divided doses for 7 days, then increase dose to 4-6 mg/kg/day; Maintenance: 1-2 mg/kg/day
Mechanism of Action Mechanism of action is not clear, methylating of nucleic acids; inhibits DNA, RNA, and protein synthesis; may damage DNA directly and suppresses mitosis; metabolic activation required by host
Pharmacodynamics/Kinetics
Half-life Elimination 1 hour
Time to Peak 1 hour
Pregnancy Risk Factor D
Pregnancy Considerations Animal studies have demonstrated teratogenic effects. There are no adequate and well-controlled studies in pregnant women. There are, however, case reports of fetal malformations in the offspring of pregnant women exposed to procarbazine as part of a combination chemotherapy regimen. Women of childbearing potential should avoid becoming pregnant during treatment.

Prochlorperazine (proe klor PER a zeen)

Related Information
Management of the Patient With Anxiety or Depression on page 1594
Brand Names: U.S. Compro®
Brand Names: Canada Apo-Prochlorperazine®; Nu-Prochlor; PMS-Prochlorperazine; Sandoz-Prochlorperazine
Generic Availability (U.S.) Yes
Pharmacologic Category Antiemetic; Antipsychotic Agent, Typical, Phenothiazine
Use Management of nausea and vomiting; psychotic disorders, including schizophrenia and anxiety; nonpsychotic anxiety
Unlabeled Use Behavioral syndromes in dementia; psychosis/agitation related to Alzheimer's dementia
Local Anesthetic/Vasoconstrictor Precautions May lower seizure threshold; use caution when administering prochlorperazine in combination with other agents that reduce seizure threshold (ie, local anesthetics). Due to prochlorperazine induced alpha-adrenergic blockade, administration of local anesthetics containing vasoconstrictors (epinephrine or levonordefrin), causes unopposed stimulation of beta-adrenergic receptors in heart and peripheral blood vessels that may result in tachycardia, peripheral vasodilation, or hypotension. Effects on blood pressure are greater in combination with epinephrine than levonordefrin.

Effects on Dental Treatment Key adverse event(s) related to dental treatment: Xerostomia and changes in salivation (normal salivary flow resumes upon discontinuation).

Significant hypotension may occur, especially when the drug is administered parenterally or following administration of local anesthetics containing vasoconstrictors (ie, epinephrine or levonordefrin); orthostatic hypotension is due to alpha-receptor blockade, the elderly are at greater risk for orthostatic hypotension.

Significant sedation can occur and may be increased in the elderly and in patients taking other CNS depressants (ie, opioid analgesics or benzodiazepines).

Extrapyramidal effects including akathisia (motor restlessness), acute dystonia (spasmodic contractures), pseudoparkinsonism, and tardive dyskinesia can occur with 1 dose. These effects are more likely in the elderly, patients taking other dopamine antagonists (including antipsychotic agents and some antiemetic agents), and patients with Parkinson's disease.

Due to increased risk of adverse effects and drug interactions especially with opioid analgesics, reserve use for patients with moderate-to-severe postoperative nausea and vomiting, who cannot afford ondansetron, and for whom promethazine did not provide adequate control.

Effects on Bleeding No information available to require special precautions

Adverse Effects Reported with prochlorperazine or other phenothiazines. Frequency not defined.

Cardiovascular: Cardiac arrest, cerebral edema, hypotension, peripheral edema, Q-wave distortions, sudden death, T-wave distortions

Central nervous system: Agitation, altered cerebrospinal fluid proteins, catatonia, coma, cough reflex suppressed, dizziness, drowsiness, fever (mild [I.M.]), headache, hyperpyrexia, impairment of temperature regulation, insomnia, neuroleptic malignant syndrome (NMS), oculogyric crisis, opisthotonos, restlessness, seizure, somnolence, tremulousness

Dermatologic: Angioedema, contact dermatitis, epithelial keratopathy, erythema, eczema, exfoliative dermatitis, itching, photosensitivity, skin pigmentation, urticaria

Endocrine & metabolic: Amenorrhea, galactorrhea, gynecomastia, glucosuria, hyper-/hypoglycemia, lactation, libido (changes in), menstrual irregularity

Gastrointestinal: Appetite increased, atonic colon, constipation, ileus, nausea, obstipation, vomiting, weight gain, xerostomia

Genitourinary: Ejaculating dysfunction, ejaculatory disturbances, impotence, priapism, urinary retention

Hematologic: Agranulocytosis, aplastic anemia, eosinophilia, hemolytic anemia, leukopenia, pancytopenia, thrombocytopenic purpura

Hepatic: Biliary stasis, cholestatic jaundice, hepatotoxicity

Neuromuscular & skeletal: Dystonias (torticollis, carpopedal spasm, trismus, protrusion of tongue); extrapyramidal symptoms (pseudoparkinsonism, akathisia, dystonias, tardive dyskinesia, hyperreflexia); SLE-like syndrome, tremor

Ocular: Blurred vision, lenticular/corneal deposits, miosis, mydriasis, pigmentary retinopathy

Respiratory: Asthma, laryngeal edema, nasal congestion

Miscellaneous: Allergic reactions, asphyxia, diaphoresis

Dosage Note: Injection solution mesylate formulation has Canadian availability (not available in U.S.).

Antiemetic: Children (therapy >1 day usually not required): **Note:** Use is contraindicated in children <9 kg or <2 years:

Oral, rectal:
9-13 kg: 2.5 mg 1-2 times/day as needed (maximum: 7.5 mg/day)
>13-18 kg: 2.5 mg 2-3 times/day as needed (maximum: 10 mg/day)
>18-39 kg: 2.5 mg 3 times/day or 5 mg 2 times/day as needed (maximum: 15 mg/day)

I.M. (as edisylate): 0.13 mg/kg/dose; convert to oral therapy as soon as possible

I.M. (as mesylate): 0.14 mg/kg/dose; convert to oral therapy at equivalent or greater dose (if necessary) as soon as possible

Antiemetic: Adults:
Oral (tablet): 5-10 mg 3-4 times/day; usual maximum: 40 mg/day; larger doses may rarely be required

I.M. (as edisylate): 5-10 mg every 3-4 hours; usual maximum: 40 mg/day

I.M. (as mesylate): 5-10 mg 2-3 times/day; usual maximum: 40 mg/day

I.V. (as edisylate): 2.5-10 mg; maximum: 10 mg/dose or 40 mg/day; may repeat dose every 3-4 hours as needed

Rectal:
U.S. labeling: 25 mg twice daily
Canadian labeling: 5-10 mg 3-4 times/day

Surgical nausea/vomiting: Adults: **Note:** Should not exceed 40 mg/day

I.M. (as edisylate): 5-10 mg 1-2 hours before anesthesia induction or to control symptoms during or after surgery; may repeat once if necessary

I.M. (as mesylate): 5-10 mg 1-2 hours before anesthesia induction; may repeat once if needed during surgery; postoperatively: 5-10 mg every 3-4 hours as needed up to maximum of 40 mg daily

I.V. (as edisylate): 5-10 mg 15-30 minutes before anesthesia induction or to control symptoms during or after surgery; may repeat once if necessary

I.V. (as mesylate): 20 mg/L of I.V. solution during surgery or postoperatively; usual maximum: 30 mg daily

Rectal (unlabeled use; Golembiewski, 2005): 25 mg

Antipsychotic:
Children 2-12 years (contraindicated in children <9 kg or <2 years):

Oral, rectal: 2.5 mg 2-3 times/day; do not give more than 10 mg the first day; increase dosage as needed to maximum daily dose of 20 mg for 2-5 years and 25 mg for 6-12 years

I.M. (as edisylate): 0.13 mg/kg/dose; convert to oral therapy as soon as possible

I.M. (as mesylate): 0.14 mg/kg/dose; convert to oral therapy at equivalent or greater dose (if necessary) as soon as possible

Adults:
Oral: 5-10 mg 3-4 times/day; titrate dose slowly every 2-3 days; doses up to 150 mg/day may be required in some patients for treatment of severe disturbances

I.M. (as edisylate): Initial: 10-20 mg; if necessary repeat initial dose every 2-4 hours to gain control; more than 3-4 doses are rarely needed. If parenteral administration is still required; give 10-20 mg every 4-6 hours; convert to oral therapy as soon as possible

◀ I.M. (as mesylate): Initial: 10-20 mg; if necessary repeat initial dose every 2-4 hours to gain control; more than 3-4 doses are rarely needed; convert to oral therapy as soon as possible

Nonpsychotic anxiety: Oral (tablet): Adults: Usual dose: 5 mg 3-4 times/day; do not exceed 20 mg/day or administer >12 weeks

Elderly: Initiate at lower end of dosage range; titrate slowly and cautiously. Refer to adult dosing.

Dosage adjustment in renal impairment:
U.S. labeling: No dosage adjustment provided in manufacturer's labeling.
Canadian labeling: Use is contraindicated.

Dosage adjustment in hepatic impairment:
U.S. labeling: No dosage adjustment provided in manufacturer's labeling; systemic exposure may be increased as drug undergoes hepatic metabolism.
Canadian labeling: Use is contraindicated.

Mechanism of Action Prochlorperazine is a piperazine phenothiazine antipsychotic which blocks postsynaptic mesolimbic dopaminergic D_1 and D_2 receptors in the brain, including the chemoreceptor trigger zone; exhibits a strong alpha-adrenergic and anticholinergic blocking effect and depresses the release of hypothalamic and hypophyseal hormones; believed to depress the reticular activating system, thus affecting basal metabolism, body temperature, wakefulness, vasomotor tone and emesis

Contraindications Hypersensitivity to prochlorperazine or any component of the formulation (cross-reactivity between phenothiazines may occur); coma or presence of large amounts of CNS depressants (eg, alcohol, narcotics, barbiturates); pediatric surgery; children <2 years of age or <9 kg

Canadian labeling: Additional contraindications (not in U.S. labeling): Presence of circulatory collapse; severe cardiovascular disorders; altered state of consciousness; concomitant use of high dose hypnotics; severe depression; presence of blood dyscrasias, hepatic or renal impairment, or pheochromocytoma; suspected or established subcortical brain damage with or without hypothalamic damage

Warnings/Precautions [U.S. Boxed Warning]: Elderly patients with dementia-related psychosis treated with antipsychotics are at an increased risk of death compared to placebo. Most deaths appeared to be either cardiovascular (eg, heart failure, sudden death) or infectious (eg, pneumonia) in nature. Prochlorperazine is not approved for the treatment of dementia-related psychosis. May cause extrapyramidal symptoms (EPS), including pseudoparkinsonism, acute dystonic reactions, akathisia, and tardive dyskinesia. Risk of dystonia (and possibly other EPS) may be greater with increased doses, use of conventional antipsychotics, males, and younger patients. Risk of tardive dyskinesia and potential for irreversibility often associated with total cumulative dose and therapy duration and may also be increased in elderly patients (particularly elderly women); antipsychotics may also mask signs/symptoms of tardive dyskinesia. Consider therapy discontinuation with signs/symptoms of tardive dyskinesia. Antipsychotic use has been associated with esophageal dysmotility and aspiration; use with caution in patients at risk of pneumonia (ie, Alzheimer's disease).

May be sedating and impair physical or mental abilities; use with caution in disorders where CNS depression is a feature. Effects with other sedative drugs or ethanol may be potentiated. Use with caution in Parkinson's disease; hemodynamic instability; predisposition to seizures;

subcortical brain damage; and in severe cardiac, hepatic, or renal disease. Canadian labeling contraindicates use in patients with severe cardiac disease, hepatic or renal impairment, subcortical brain damage, and circulatory collapse. May alter temperature regulation, obscure intestinal obstruction or brain tumor or mask toxicity of other drugs. May alter cardiac conduction. Hypotension may occur following administration, particularly when parenteral form is used or in high dosages. May cause orthostatic hypotension; use with caution in patients at risk of this effect or in those who would not tolerate transient hypotensive episodes (cerebrovascular disease, cardiovascular disease, hypovolemia, or concurrent medication use which may predispose to hypotension/bradycardia).

Leukopenia, neutropenia, and agranulocytosis (sometimes fatal) have been reported in clinical trials and postmarketing reports with antipsychotic use; presence of risk factors (eg, pre-existing low WBC or history of drug-induced leuko-/neutropenia) should prompt periodic blood count assessment. Discontinue therapy at first signs of blood dyscrasias or if absolute neutrophil count <1000/mm^3.

Due to its potent anticholinergic effects, may be inappropriate in older adults depending on comorbidities (eg, dementia, delirium) (Beers Criteria). Use with caution in patients with decreased gastrointestinal motility, urinary retention, BPH, xerostomia, or visual problems. Conditions which also may be exacerbated by cholinergic blockade include narrow-angle glaucoma and worsening of myasthenia gravis. Use caution with exposure to heat. May cause pigmentary retinopathy, and lenticular and corneal deposits, particularly with prolonged therapy. Use associated with increased prolactin levels; clinical significance of hyperprolactinemia in patients with breast cancer or other prolactin-dependent tumors is unknown. Avoid use in patients with signs/symptoms suggestive of Reye's syndrome. Children with acute illness or dehydration are more susceptible to neuromuscular reactions; use cautiously. May be associated with neuroleptic malignant syndrome (NMS). Some dosage forms may contain benzyl alcohol which has been associated with "gasping syndrome" in neonates. Some dosage forms may contain sodium sulfite.

Drug Interactions

Metabolism/Transport Effects None known.

Avoid Concomitant Use
Avoid concomitant use of Prochlorperazine with any of the following: Aclidinium; Azelastine (Nasal); Dofetilide; Ipratropium (Oral Inhalation); Metoclopramide; Paraldehyde; Tiotropium

Increased Effect/Toxicity
Prochlorperazine may increase the levels/effects of: Alcohol (Ethyl); Analgesics (Opioid); Anticholinergics; Antidepressants (Serotonin Reuptake Inhibitor/Antagonist); Azelastine (Nasal); Beta-Blockers; CNS Depressants; Dofetilide; Methotrimeprazine; Methylphenidate; Paraldehyde; Porfimer; Serotonin Modulators; Tiotropium; Zolpidem

The levels/effects of Prochlorperazine may be increased by: Acetylcholinesterase Inhibitors (Central); Aclidinium; Antidepressants (Serotonin Reuptake Inhibitor/Antagonist); Antimalarial Agents; Beta-Blockers; Deferoxamine; Droperidol; HydrOXYzine; Ipratropium (Oral Inhalation); Lithium formulations; Magnesium Sulfate; Methotrimeprazine; Methylphenidate; Metoclopramide; Metyrosine; Perampanel; Pramlintide; Sodium Oxybate; Tetrabenazine

Decreased Effect

Prochlorperazine may decrease the levels/effects of: Amphetamines; Anti-Parkinson's Agents (Dopamine Agonist); Quinagolide

The levels/effects of Prochlorperazine may be decreased by: Antacids; Anti-Parkinson's Agents (Dopamine Agonist); Lithium formulations

Ethanol/Nutrition/Herb Interactions

Ethanol: May increase CNS depression; monitor for increased effects with coadministration. Caution patients about effects.

Herb/Nutraceutical: Avoid dong quai, St John's wort (may also cause photosensitization). Avoid kava kava, gotu kola, valerian, St John's wort (may increase CNS depression).

Dietary Considerations Increase dietary intake of riboflavin; should be administered with food or water. Rectal suppositories may contain coconut and palm oil.

Pharmacodynamics/Kinetics

Onset of Action Oral: 30-40 minutes; I.M.: 10-20 minutes; Rectal: ~60 minutes

Peak antiemetic effect: I.V.: 30-60 minutes

Duration of Action Rectal: 3-12 hours; I.M., Oral: 3-4 hours

Half-life Elimination Oral: 6-10 hours (single dose), 14-22 hours (repeated dosing) (Isah, 1991); I.V.: 6-10 hours (Isah, 1991; Taylor, 1987)

Pregnancy Considerations Jaundice or hyper-/hyporeflexia have been reported in newborn infants following maternal use of phenothiazines. Antipsychotic use during the third trimester of pregnancy has a risk for abnormal muscle movements (extrapyramidal symptoms [EPS]) and withdrawal symptoms in newborns following delivery. Symptoms in the newborn may include agitation, feeding disorder, hypertonia, hypotonia, respiratory distress, somnolence, and tremor; these effects may be self-limiting or require hospitalization.

Lactation Excretion in breast milk unknown/use caution

Breast-Feeding Considerations Other phenothiazines are excreted in human milk; excretion of prochlorperazine is not known.

Dosage Forms

Injection, solution: 5 mg/mL (2 mL, 10 mL)

Suppository, rectal: 25 mg (12s)

Compro®: 25 mg (12s)

Tablet, oral: 5 mg, 10 mg

Dosage Forms: Canada

Injection, solution 5 mg/mL (2 mL)

Suppository, rectal: 10 mg (10s)

Procyclidine (proe SYE kli deen)

Brand Names: Canada PHL-Procyclidine; PMS-Procyclidine

Pharmacologic Category Anti-Parkinson's Agent, Anticholinergic; Anticholinergic Agent

Use Relieves symptoms of parkinsonian syndrome and drug-induced extrapyramidal symptoms

Effects on Dental Treatment Key adverse event(s) related to dental treatment: Xerostomia (normal salivary flow resumes upon discontinuation) and dry throat and nose. Prolonged use of antidyskinetics may decrease or inhibit salivary flow, contributing to discomfort and dental disease (ie, caries, oral candidiasis, and periodontal disease).

Effects on Bleeding No information available to require special precautions

Adverse Effects Frequency not defined.

Cardiovascular: Tachycardia

Central nervous system: Acute toxic psychosis, agitation, concentration impaired, confusion, disorientation, giddiness, hallucinations, lightheadedness, memory impaired, restlessness, slurred speech

Dermatologic: Rash

Gastrointestinal: Constipation, epigastric distress, nausea, parotitis (secondary to xerostomia), vomiting, xerostomia

Genitourinary: Dysuria

Neuromuscular & skeletal: Weakness

Ocular: Blurred vision, mydriasis

Miscellaneous: Allergic reaction

General Dosage Range Oral:

Adults: Initial: 2.5 mg 3 times/day; Maintenance: Up to 30 mg/day in 3-4 divided doses

Elderly: Initial: 2.5 mg 1-2 times/day

Mechanism of Action Thought to act by blocking excess acetylcholine at cerebral synapses; many of its effects are due to its pharmacologic similarities with atropine; it exerts an antispasmodic effect on smooth muscle, is a potent mydriatic; inhibits salivation

Pharmacodynamics/Kinetics

Onset of Action 30-40 minutes

Duration of Action 4-6 hours

Half-life Elimination ~12.5 hours

Time to Peak ~1 hour

Pregnancy Considerations Safe use during pregnancy has not been established. Potential benefits of therapy should be weighed against potential risks to fetus.

Product Availability Not available in U.S.

Progesterone (proe JES ter one)

Brand Names: U.S. Crinone®; Endometrin®; First™-Progesterone VGS 100; First™-Progesterone VGS 200; First™-Progesterone VGS 25; First™-Progesterone VGS 400; First™-Progesterone VGS 50; Prometrium®

Brand Names: Canada Crinone®; Prometrium®

Pharmacologic Category Progestin

Use

Oral: Prevention of endometrial hyperplasia in nonhysterectomized, postmenopausal women who are receiving conjugated estrogen tablets; secondary amenorrhea

I.M.: Amenorrhea; abnormal uterine bleeding due to hormonal imbalance

Intravaginal gel: Part of assisted reproductive technology (ART) for infertile women with progesterone deficiency; secondary amenorrhea

Vaginal tablet: Part of ART for infertile women with progesterone deficiency

Unlabeled Use Reduce the risk of recurrent spontaneous preterm birth in appropriately selected women

Effects on Dental Treatment Key adverse event(s) related to dental treatment: Progestins may predispose the patient to gingival bleeding.

Effects on Bleeding No information available to require special precautions

Adverse Effects

Injection (I.M.):

Cardiovascular: Cerebral edema, cerebral thrombosis, edema

Central nervous system: Depression, fever, insomnia, somnolence

Dermatologic: Acne, allergic rash (rare), alopecia, hirsutism, pruritus, rash, urticaria

Endocrine & metabolic: Amenorrhea, breakthrough bleeding, breast tenderness, galactorrhea, menstrual flow changes, spotting

Gastrointestinal: Nausea, weight gain/loss

Genitourinary: Cervical erosion changes, cervical secretion changes

Hepatic: Cholestatic jaundice

Local: Injection site: Irritation, pain, redness

Ocular: Optic neuritis, retinal thrombosis

Respiratory: Pulmonary embolism

Miscellaneous: Anaphylactoid reactions

Oral capsule (percentages reported when used in combination with or cycled with conjugated estrogens):

>10%:

Central nervous system: Headache (16% to 31%), dizziness (15% to 24%), depression (19%)

Endocrine & metabolic: Breast tenderness (27%), breast pain (6% to 16%)

Gastrointestinal: Abdominal pain (10% to 20%), abdominal bloating (8% to 12%)

Genitourinary: Urinary problems (11%)

Neuromuscular & skeletal: Joint pain (20%), musculoskeletal pain (12%)

Miscellaneous: Viral infection (12%)

5% to 10%:

Cardiovascular: Chest pain (7%)

Central nervous system: Fatigue (8%), irritability (8%), worry (8%)

Gastrointestinal: Nausea/vomiting (8%), diarrhea (7% to 8%)

Genitourinary: Vaginal discharge (10%)

Respiratory: Cough (8%)

<5%: Breast biopsy, breast cancer, cholecystectomy, constipation

Vaginal gel (percentages reported with ART); also refer to oral capsule reactions listing for additional effects noted with progesterone:

>10%:

Central nervous system: Somnolence (27%), headache (13% to 17%), nervousness (16%), depression (11%)

Endocrine & metabolic: Breast enlargement (40%), breast pain (13%), libido decreased (11%)

Gastrointestinal: Constipation (27%), nausea (7% to 22%), cramps (15%), abdominal pain (12%)

Genitourinary: Perineal pain (17%), nocturia (13%)

5% to 10%:

Central nervous system: Pain (8%), dizziness (5%)

Gastrointestinal: Diarrhea (8%), bloating (7%), vomiting (5%)

Genitourinary: Vaginal discharge (7%), dyspareunia (6%), genital moniliasis (5%), genital pruritus (5%)

Neuromuscular & skeletal: Arthralgia (8%)

Vaginal tablet (percentages reported with ART); also refer to oral capsule reactions listing for additional effects noted with progesterone:

>10%:

Gastrointestinal: Abdominal pain (12%)

Miscellaneous: Post-oocyte retrieval pain (25% to 28%)

1% to 10%:

Central nervous system: Headache (3% to 4%), fatigue (2% to 3%)

Endocrine & metabolic: Ovarian hyperstimulation syndrome (7%)

Gastrointestinal: Nausea (7% to 8%), abdominal distension (4%), constipation (2% to 3%), vomiting (2% to 3%)

Genitourinary: Uterine spasm (3% to 4%), vaginal bleeding (3%), urinary tract infection (1% to 2%)

General Dosage Range

I.M.: *Adults (females):* 5-10 mg/day for 6 doses

Intravaginal: *Adults (females):*

ART: 90 mg (8% gel) once or twice daily or 100 mg (vaginal tablet) 2-3 times/day

Secondary amenorrhea: 45 mg (4% gel) every other day, may increase to 90 mg (8% gel) every other day if needed (maximum: 6 doses)

Oral: *Adults (females):*

Amenorrhea: 400 mg once daily in the evening for 10 days

Endometrial hyperplasia prevention: 200 mg once daily in the evening for 12 days sequentially per 28-day cycle

Mechanism of Action Natural steroid hormone that induces secretory changes in the endometrium, promotes mammary gland development, relaxes uterine smooth muscle, blocks follicular maturation and ovulation, and maintains pregnancy. When used as part of an ART program in the luteal phase, progesterone supports embryo implantation.

Pharmacodynamics/Kinetics

Half-life Elimination Vaginal gel: 5-20 minutes

Time to Peak Oral: Within 3 hours; I.M.: ~8 hours; Vaginal tablet: ~17-24 hours

Pregnancy Risk Factor B (Prometrium®; none established for vaginal gel, vaginal tablet, or injection

Pregnancy Considerations Adverse events were not observed following oral administration in animal reproduction studies. There is an increased risk of minor birth defects in children whose mothers take progesterones during the first 4 months of pregnancy. Hypospadias has been reported in male and mild masculinization of the external genitalia has been reported in female babies exposed during the first trimester. Cleft lip, cleft palate, congenital heart disease, patent ductus arteriosus, ventricular septal defect, intrauterine death, and spontaneous abortion have been noted in case reports following use of oral progesterone during pregnancy. High doses of progesterone would be expected to impair fertility. Use of vaginal progesterone may be considered to decrease the risk of recurrent spontaneous preterm birth in women with a singleton pregnancy and prior spontaneous preterm singleton birth; use is not recommended as an intervention for women with multiple gestations (ACOG, 2012). The vaginal gel and tablet are indicated for use in ART. The oral capsules are contraindicated for use during pregnancy.

Promethazine (proe METH a zeen)

Brand Names: U.S. Phenadoz®; Phenergan; Promethegan™

Brand Names: Canada Bioniche Promethazine; Histantil; Phenergan; PMS-Promethazine

Pharmacologic Category Antiemetic; Histamine H_1 Antagonist; Histamine H_1 Antagonist, First Generation; Phenothiazine Derivative

Use Symptomatic treatment of various allergic conditions; antiemetic; motion sickness; sedative; adjunct to postoperative analgesia and anesthesia

Unlabeled Use Treatment of nausea and vomiting of pregnancy (NVP)

Local Anesthetic/Vasoconstrictor Precautions
Promethazine may lower seizure threshold; use caution administering promethazine in combination with other agents that reduce seizure threshold (ie, local anesthetics). Due to promethazine induced alpha-adrenergic blockade, administration of local anesthetics containing the vasoconstrictors epinephrine or levonordefrin, causes unopposed stimulation of beta-adrenergic receptors in heart and peripheral blood vessels that may result in tachycardia and peripheral vasodilation causing hypotension. Effects on blood pressure are greater in combination with epinephrine than levonordefrin.

Effects on Dental Treatment Key adverse event(s) related to dental treatment: Xerostomia (normal salivary flow resumes upon discontinuation).

Significant hypotension may occur, especially when the drug is administered parenterally or following administration of local anesthetics containing vasoconstrictors (ie, epinephrine or levonordefrin); orthostatic hypotension is due to alpha-receptor blockade, the elderly are at greater risk for orthostatic hypotension.

Significant sedation can occur and may be increased in the elderly and in patients taking or administered other CNS depressants (ie, opioid analgesics or benzodiazepines).

Extrapyramidal effects including akathisia (motor restlessness), acute dystonia (spasmodic contractures), pseudoparkinsonism, and tardive dyskinesia can occur with a single dose. These effects are more likely in the elderly, patients taking other dopamine antagonists (including antipsychotic agents and some antiemetic agents), and patients with Parkinson's disease.

Promethazine is a less expensive alternative for moderate-to-severe postoperative nausea than ondansetron but with a greater chance of adverse effects and drug interactions especially with opioid analgesics.

Effects on Bleeding No information available to require special precautions

Adverse Effects Frequency not defined.
Cardiovascular: Bradycardia, hyper-/hypotension, non-specific QT changes, orthostatic hypotension, tachycardia,
Central nervous system: Agitation akathisia, catatonic states, confusion, delirium, disorientation, dizziness, drowsiness, dystonias, euphoria, excitation, extrapyramidal symptoms, faintness, fatigue, hallucinations, hysteria, insomnia, lassitude, pseudoparkinsonism, tardive dyskinesia, nervousness, neuroleptic malignant syndrome, nightmares, sedation, seizure, somnolence
Dermatologic: Angioneurotic edema, dermatitis, photosensitivity, skin pigmentation (slate gray), urticaria
Endocrine & metabolic: Amenorrhea, breast engorgement, gynecomastia, hyperglycemia, lactation
Gastrointestinal: Constipation, nausea, vomiting, xerostomia
Genitourinary: Ejaculatory disorder, impotence, urinary retention
Hematologic: Agranulocytosis, leukopenia, thrombocytopenia, thrombocytopenic purpura
Hepatic: Jaundice
Local: Abscess, distal vessel spasm, gangrene, injection site reactions (burning, edema, erythema, pain), palsies, paralysis, phlebitis, sensory loss, thrombophlebitis, tissue necrosis, venous thrombosis
Neuromuscular & skeletal: Incoordination, tremor
Ocular: Blurred vision, corneal and lenticular changes, diplopia, epithelial keratopathy, pigmentary retinopathy

Otic: Tinnitus
Respiratory: Apnea, asthma, nasal congestion, respiratory depression

General Dosage Range
I.M., I.V.:
Children ≥2 years: 0.25-1 mg/kg 4-6 times/day as needed (maximum: 25 mg/dose; sedation: 50 mg/dose)
Adults: 12.5-75 mg/dose as a single dose **or** 12.5-50 mg every 4-6 hours as needed

Oral, rectal:
Children ≥2 years:
Allergic reactions: 0.1 mg/kg every 6 hours (maximum: 12.5 mg) during the day and 0.5 mg/kg (maximum: 25 mg/dose) at bedtime as needed
Antiemetic: 0.25-1 mg/kg 4-6 times/day as needed (maximum: 25 mg/dose)
Motion sickness: 0.5 mg/kg 30 minutes to 1 hour before departure, then every 12 hours as needed (maximum: 25 mg twice daily)
Sedation: 12.5-25 mg as single dose (maximum: 25 mg/dose)
Adults: 6.25-25 mg every 4-8 hours as needed **or** 12.5-50 mg as a single dose **or** 25 mg 30-60 minutes before departure, then every 12 hours as needed

Mechanism of Action Phenothiazine derivative; blocks postsynaptic mesolimbic dopaminergic receptors in the brain; exhibits a strong alpha-adrenergic blocking effect and depresses the release of hypothalamic and hypophyseal hormones; competes with histamine for the H_1-receptor; muscarinic-blocking effect may be responsible for antiemetic activity; reduces stimuli to the brainstem reticular system

Pharmacodynamics/Kinetics
Onset of Action Oral, I.M.: ~20 minutes; I.V.: ~5 minutes
Duration of Action Usually 4-6 hours (up to 12 hours)
Half-life Elimination I.M.: ~10 hours; I.V.: 9-16 hours; Suppositories, syrup: 16-19 hours (range: 4-34 hours) (Strenkoski-Nox, 2000)
Time to Peak Maximum serum concentration: Suppositories: 6.7-8.6 hours; Syrup: 4.4 hours (Strenkoski-Nox, 2000)

Pregnancy Risk Factor C
Pregnancy Considerations Teratogenic effects were not observed in animal reproduction studies. Promethazine crosses the placenta. Maternal promethazine use has generally not resulted in an increased risk of birth defects. Platelet aggregation may be inhibited in newborns following maternal use of promethazine within 2 weeks of delivery. Promethazine is used for the treatment of nausea and vomiting of pregnancy (refer to current guidelines). Promethazine is also indicated for use during labor for obstetric sedation and may be used alone or as an adjunct to narcotic analgesics.

Dental Comment Sedation: When used alone as a sedative agent the degree of sedation is often mild. As a sedative agent, promethazine is effective in managing pediatric patients that require mild anxiety control. It is ineffective when used alone in children with extreme apprehension or for the disruptive, unmanageable child. A more profound sedation will occur if promethazine is administered in combination with an opioid or benzodiazepine. If promethazine is combined with an opioid, the dose of the opioid should be decreased by 25% to 50%.

Promethazine and Codeine
(proe METH a zeen & KOE deen)

Related Information
Codeine *on page 344*
Promethazine *on page 1148*
Pharmacologic Category Analgesic, Opioid; Antitussive; Histamine H$_1$ Antagonist; Histamine H$_1$ Antagonist, First Generation; Phenothiazine Derivative
Use Temporary relief of coughs and upper respiratory symptoms associated with allergy or the common cold
Local Anesthetic/Vasoconstrictor Precautions No information available to require special precautions
Effects on Dental Treatment Although promethazine is a phenothiazine derivative, extrapyramidal reactions or tardive dyskinesias are not seen with the use of this drug.
Effects on Bleeding No information available to require special precautions
Adverse Effects See individual agents.
General Dosage Range Oral:
Children 6-11 years: 2.5-5 mL every 4-6 hours (maximum: 30 mL/day)
Children ≥12 years and Adults: 5 mL every 4-6 hours (maximum: 30 mL/day)
Pregnancy Risk Factor C
Pregnancy Considerations Reproduction studies have not been conducted with this combination. See individual agents.
Controlled Substance C-V

Promethazine and Dextromethorphan
(proe METH a zeen & deks troe meth OR fan)

Related Information
Dextromethorphan *on page 406*
Promethazine *on page 1148*
Pharmacologic Category Antitussive; Histamine H$_1$ Antagonist; Histamine H$_1$ Antagonist, First Generation; Phenothiazine Derivative
Use Temporary relief of coughs and upper respiratory symptoms associated with allergy or the common cold
Local Anesthetic/Vasoconstrictor Precautions No information available to require special precautions
Effects on Dental Treatment Although promethazine is a phenothiazine derivative, extrapyramidal reactions or tardive dyskinesias are not seen with the use of this drug.
Effects on Bleeding No information available to require special precautions
General Dosage Range Oral:
Children 2-6 years: 1.25-2.5 mL every 4-6 hours (maximum: 10 mL/day)
Children 6-12 years: 2.5-5 mL every 4-6 hours (maximum: 20 mL/day)
Adults: 5 mL every 4-6 hours (maximum: 30 mL/day)
Pregnancy Risk Factor C
Pregnancy Considerations Reproduction studies have not been conducted with this combination. Refer to individual monographs.

Promethazine and Phenylephrine
(proe METH a zeen & fen il EF rin)

Related Information
Phenylephrine (Systemic) *on page 1087*
Promethazine *on page 1148*
Brand Names: U.S. Promethazine VC

Pharmacologic Category Alpha-Adrenergic Agonist; Decongestant; Histamine H$_1$ Antagonist; Histamine H$_1$ Antagonist, First Generation; Phenothiazine Derivative
Use Temporary relief of upper respiratory symptoms associated with allergy or the common cold
Local Anesthetic/Vasoconstrictor Precautions
Phenylephrine: Use with caution since phenylephrine is a sympathomimetic amine which could interact with epinephrine to cause a pressor response
Promethazine: No information available to require special precautions
Effects on Dental Treatment Key adverse event(s) related to dental treatment: Phenylephrine: Tachycardia, palpitations, xerostomia (normal salivary flow resumes upon discontinuation); use vasoconstrictor with caution. Although promethazine is a phenothiazine derivative, extrapyramidal reactions or tardive dyskinesias are not seen with the use of this drug.
Effects on Bleeding No information available to require special precautions
Adverse Effects See individual agents.
General Dosage Range Oral:
Children 2-6 years: 1.25-2.5 mL every 4-6 hours (maximum: 7.5 mL/day)
Children 6-12 years: 2.5-5 mL every 4-6 hours (maximum: 30 mL/day)
Children >12 years and Adults: 5 mL every 4-6 hours (maximum: 30 mL/day)
Pregnancy Risk Factor C
Pregnancy Considerations Reproduction studies have not been conducted with this combination. Refer to individual monographs.

Promethazine, Phenylephrine, and Codeine
(proe METH a zeen, fen il EF rin, & KOE deen)

Related Information
Codeine *on page 344*
Phenylephrine (Systemic) *on page 1087*
Promethazine *on page 1148*
Pharmacologic Category Alpha-Adrenergic Agonist; Analgesic, Opioid; Antitussive; Decongestant; Histamine H$_1$ Antagonist; Histamine H$_1$ Antagonist, First Generation; Phenothiazine Derivative
Use Temporary relief of coughs and upper respiratory symptoms including nasal congestion associated with allergy or the common cold
Local Anesthetic/Vasoconstrictor Precautions
Phenylephrine: Use with caution since phenylephrine is a sympathomimetic amine which could interact with epinephrine to cause a pressor response
Promethazine: No information available to require special precautions
Effects on Dental Treatment Key adverse event(s) related to dental treatment: Phenylephrine: Tachycardia, palpitations, xerostomia (normal salivary flow resumes upon discontinuation); use vasoconstrictor with caution. Although promethazine is a phenothiazine derivative, extrapyramidal reactions or tardive dyskinesias are not seen with the use of this drug.
Effects on Bleeding No information available to require special precautions
Adverse Effects See individual agents.
General Dosage Range Oral:
Children 6-11 years: 2.5-5 mL every 4-6 hours (maximum: 30 mL/day)
Children ≥12 years and Adults: 5 mL every 4-6 hours (maximum: 30 mL/day)

Pregnancy Risk Factor C
Pregnancy Considerations Reproduction studies have not been conducted with this combination. See individual agents.
Controlled Substance C-V

Propafenone (pro PAF en one)

Related Information
Clinical Risk Related to Drugs Prolonging QT Interval *on page 1510*
Brand Names: U.S. Rythmol®; Rythmol® SR
Brand Names: Canada Apo-Propafenone®; Mylan-Propafenone; PMS-Propafenone; Rythmol® Gen-Propafenone
Pharmacologic Category Antiarrhythmic Agent, Class Ic
Use Treatment of life-threatening ventricular arrhythmias; treatment of paroxysmal atrial fibrillation/flutter (PAF) or paroxysmal supraventricular tachycardia (PSVT) in patients with disabling symptoms and without structural heart disease
Extended release capsule: Prolong the time to recurrence of symptomatic atrial fibrillation in patients without structural heart disease
Unlabeled Use Cardioversion of recent-onset atrial fibrillation (single dose); supraventricular tachycardia in patients with Wolff-Parkinson-White syndrome
Local Anesthetic/Vasoconstrictor Precautions In some patients, propafenone has been reported to induce new or worsened arrhythmias (proarrhythmic effect). It is suggested that vasoconstrictors be used with caution since epinephrine has the potential to stimulate the heart rate when given in the anesthetic regimen. The manufacturer notes that propafenone may increase the QT interval; however, due to QRS prolongation; changes in the QT interval are difficult to interpret. Cases of torsade de pointes have been reported. The risk of drug-induced torsade de pointes is extremely low when a single QT interval prolonging drug is prescribed. In terms of epinephrine, it is not known what effect vasoconstrictors in the local anesthetic regimen will have in patients with a known history of congenital prolonged QT interval or in patients taking any medication that prolongs the QT interval. Until more information is obtained, it is suggested that the clinician consult with the physician prior to the use of a vasoconstrictor in suspected patients, and that the vasoconstrictor (epinephrine, mepivacaine and levonordefrin [Carbocaine® 2% with Neo-Cobefrin®]) be used with caution.
Effects on Dental Treatment Key adverse event(s) related to dental treatment: Unusual taste and significant xerostomia (normal salivary flow resumes upon discontinuation).
Effects on Bleeding No information available to require special precautions
Adverse Effects 1% to 10%:
Cardiovascular: New or worsened arrhythmia (proarrhythmic effect) (2% to 10%), angina (2% to 5%), CHF (1% to 4%), ventricular tachycardia (1% to 3%), palpitation (1% to 3%), AV block (first-degree) (1% to 3%), syncope (1% to 2%), increased QRS interval (1% to 2%), chest pain (1% to 2%), PVCs (1% to 2%), bradycardia (1% to 2%), edema (0% to 1%), bundle branch block (0% to 1%), atrial fibrillation (1%), hypotension (0% to 1%), intraventricular conduction delay (0% to 1%)

Central nervous system: Dizziness (4% to 15%), fatigue (2% to 6%), headache (2% to 5%), ataxia (0% to 2%), insomnia (0% to 2%), anxiety (1% to 2%), drowsiness (1%)
Dermatologic: Rash (1% to 3%)
Gastrointestinal: Nausea/vomiting (2% to 11%), unusual taste (3% to 23%), constipation (2% to 7%), dyspepsia (1% to 3%), diarrhea (1% to 3%), xerostomia (1% to 2%), anorexia (1% to 2%), abdominal pain (1% to 2%), flatulence (0% to 1%)
Neuromuscular & skeletal: Tremor (0% to 1%), arthralgia (0% to 1%), weakness (1% to 2%)
Ocular: Blurred vision (1% to 6%)
Respiratory: Dyspnea (2% to 5%)
Miscellaneous: Diaphoresis (1%)
General Dosage Range Dosage adjustment recommended in patients with hepatic impairment
Oral:
Extended release: *Adults:* Initial: 225 mg every 12 hours; Maintenance: 225-425 mg every 12 hours
Immediate release: *Adults:* Initial: 150 mg every 8 hours; Maintenance: 150-300 mg every 8 hours
Mechanism of Action Propafenone is a class 1c antiarrhythmic agent which possesses local anesthetic properties, blocks the fast inward sodium current, and slows the rate of increase of the action potential. Prolongs conduction and refractoriness in all areas of the myocardium, with a slightly more pronounced effect on intraventricular conduction; it prolongs effective refractory period, reduces spontaneous automaticity and exhibits some beta-blockade activity.
Pharmacodynamics/Kinetics
Half-life Elimination Extensive metabolizers: 2-10 hours; Poor metabolizers: 10-32 hours
Time to Peak Serum: IR: 3.5 hours; ER: 3-8 hours
Pregnancy Risk Factor C
Pregnancy Considerations There are no adequate and well-controlled studies in pregnant women; use only if potential benefit to the mother justifies potential risk to the fetus.
Dental Comment Propafenone may prolong the QT interval. The QT interval is measured as the time and distance between the Q point of the QRS complex and the end of the T wave in the ECG tracing. After adjustment for heart rate, the QT interval is defined as prolonged if it is more than 450 msec in men and 460 msec in women. A long QT syndrome was first described in the 1950s and 60s as a congenital syndrome involving QT interval prolongation and syncope and sudden death. Some of the congenital long QT syndromes were characterized by a peculiar electrocardiographic appearance of the QRS complex involving a premature atria beat followed by a pause, then a subsequent sinus beat showing marked QT prolongation and deformity. This type of cardiac arrhythmia was originally termed "torsade de pointes" (translated from the French as "twisting of the points"). Propafenone is considered as having a risk of causing torsade de pointes. Since it is not known what effect vasoconstrictors in the local anesthetic regimen will have in patients with a known history of congenital prolonged QT interval or in patients taking any medication that prolongs the QT interval, a medical consult is suggested.

Propantheline (proe PAN the leen)

Generic Availability (U.S.) Yes
Pharmacologic Category Anticholinergic Agent
Dental Use Induce dry field (xerostomia) in oral cavity

Use Adjunctive treatment of peptic ulcer

Unlabeled Use Decreased salivation and drooling

Local Anesthetic/Vasoconstrictor Precautions No information available to require special precautions

Effects on Dental Treatment Key adverse event(s) related to dental treatment: Significant xerostomia (therapeutic effect; normal salivary flow resumes upon discontinuation), dry throat, nasal dryness, and dysphagia.

Effects on Bleeding No information available to require special precautions

Adverse Effects Frequency not defined.

Cardiovascular: Palpitation, tachycardia

Central nervous system: Confusion, dizziness, drowsiness, headache, insomnia, nervousness

Endocrine & metabolic: Suppression of lactation

Gastrointestinal: Bloated feeling, constipation, loss of taste, nausea, vomiting, xerostomia

Genitourinary: Impotence, urinary hesitancy, urinary retention

Neuromuscular & skeletal: Weakness

Ocular: Blurred vision, cycloplegia, mydriasis, ocular tension increased

Miscellaneous: Allergic reactions, anaphylaxis, diaphoresis decreased

Dental Usual Dosage Antisecretory: Oral:

Children: 1-2 mg/kg/day in 3-4 divided doses

Adults: 15 mg 3 times/day before meals or food and 30 mg at bedtime

Elderly: 7.5 mg 3 times/day before meals and at bedtime

Dosage Oral:

Antisecretory (unlabeled use):

Children: 1-2 mg/kg/day in 3-4 divided doses

Adults: 15 mg 3 times/day before meals or food and 30 mg at bedtime

Elderly: 7.5 mg 3 times/day before meals and at bedtime

Antispasmodic:

Children: 2-3 mg/kg/day in divided doses every 4-6 hours and at bedtime

Adults: 15 mg 3 times/day before meals or food and 30 mg at bedtime

Mechanism of Action Competitively blocks the action of acetylcholine at postganglionic parasympathetic receptor sites

Contraindications Severe ulcerative colitis, toxic megacolon, obstructive disease of the GI or urinary tract; glaucoma; myasthenia gravis; unstable cardiovascular adjustment in acute hemorrhage; intestinal atony of elderly or debilitated patients

Warnings/Precautions May cause drowsiness and/or blurred vision, which may impair physical or mental abilities; patients must be cautioned about performing tasks which require mental alertness (eg, operating machinery or driving). Use with caution in patients with hyperthyroidism, hiatal hernia with reflux esophagitis, autonomic neuropathy, hepatic, cardiac, or renal disease, hypertension, GI infections, or other endocrine diseases. Avoid use in the elderly due to potent anticholinergic adverse effects and uncertain effectiveness (Beers Criteria). Heat prostration may occur in the presence of increased environmental temperature; use caution in hot weather and/or exercise. Diarrhea may be a sign of incomplete intestinal obstruction, treatment should be discontinued if this occurs.

Drug Interactions

Metabolism/Transport Effects None known.

Avoid Concomitant Use

Avoid concomitant use of Propantheline with any of the following: Aclidinium; Ipratropium (Oral Inhalation); Potassium Chloride; Tiotropium

Increased Effect/Toxicity

Propantheline may increase the levels/effects of: AbobotulinumtoxinA; Anticholinergics; Cannabinoids; Mirabegron; OnabotulinumtoxinA; Potassium Chloride; RimabotulinumtoxinB; Tiotropium; Topiramate

The levels/effects of Propantheline may be increased by: Aclidinium; Ipratropium (Oral Inhalation); MAO Inhibitors; Pramlintide

Decreased Effect

Propantheline may decrease the levels/effects of: Acetylcholinesterase Inhibitors (Central); Secretin

The levels/effects of Propantheline may be decreased by: Acetylcholinesterase Inhibitors (Central)

Dietary Considerations Should be taken 30 minutes before meals so that the drug's peak effect occurs at the proper time. The tablet (15 mg) contains lactose 23.2 mg.

Pharmacodynamics/Kinetics

Onset of Action 30-45 minutes

Duration of Action 4-6 hours

Half-life Elimination Serum: Average: 1.6 hours

Pregnancy Risk Factor C

Pregnancy Considerations Animal reproduction studies have not been conducted.

Lactation Excretion in breast milk unknown/use caution

Dosage Forms

Tablet, oral: 15 mg

Proparacaine (proe PAR a kane)

Brand Names: U.S. Alcaine®

Brand Names: Canada Alcaine®; Diocaine®

Pharmacologic Category Local Anesthetic, Ophthalmic

Use Anesthesia for tonometry, gonioscopy; suture removal from cornea; removal of corneal foreign body; cataract extraction, glaucoma surgery; short operative procedure involving the cornea and conjunctiva

Local Anesthetic/Vasoconstrictor Precautions No information available to require special precautions

Effects on Dental Treatment No significant effects or complications reported

Effects on Bleeding No information available to require special precautions

Adverse Effects 1% to 10%: Local: Burning, stinging, redness

General Dosage Range Ophthalmic: *Children and Adults:* Instill 1-2 drops of 0.5% solution in eye once or instill 1 drop of 0.5% solution in eye every 5-10 minutes for 5-7 doses

Mechanism of Action Prevents initiation and transmission of impulse at the nerve cell membrane by decreasing ion permeability through stabilizing

Pharmacodynamics/Kinetics

Onset of Action ~20 seconds

Duration of Action 15-20 minutes

Pregnancy Risk Factor C

Pregnancy Considerations Animal reproduction studies have not been conducted.

Proparacaine and Fluorescein
(proe PAR a kane & FLURE e seen)

Related Information
Proparacaine *on page 1152*
Brand Names: U.S. Flucaine
Pharmacologic Category Diagnostic Agent; Local Anesthetic
Use Anesthesia for tonometry, gonioscopy; suture removal from cornea; removal of corneal foreign body; cataract extraction, glaucoma surgery
Local Anesthetic/Vasoconstrictor Precautions No information available to require special precautions
Effects on Dental Treatment No significant effects or complications reported
Effects on Bleeding No information available to require special precautions
Adverse Effects 1% to 10%: Local: Burning, stinging of eye
General Dosage Range Ophthalmic: *Children and Adults:* Instill 1 drop in each eye every 5-10 minutes for 5-7 doses **or** instill 1-2 drops in each eye once
Mechanism of Action Prevents initiation and transmission of impulse at the nerve cell membrane by decreasing ion permeability through stabilizing
Pharmacodynamics/Kinetics
Onset of Action ~20 seconds
Duration of Action 15-20 minutes

Propofol (PROE po fole)

Brand Names: U.S. Diprivan®
Brand Names: Canada Diprivan®
Pharmacologic Category General Anesthetic
Use Induction of anesthesia in patients ≥3 years of age; maintenance of anesthesia in patients >2 months of age; in adults, for monitored anesthesia care sedation during procedures; sedation in intubated, mechanically-ventilated ICU patients
Unlabeled Use Postoperative antiemetic; refractory delirium tremens (case reports)
Local Anesthetic/Vasoconstrictor Precautions No information available to require special precautions
Effects on Dental Treatment No significant effects or complications reported
Effects on Bleeding No information available to require special precautions
Adverse Effects
>10%:
Cardiovascular: Hypotension (children 17%; adults 3% to 26%)
Central nervous system: Movement (children 17%; adults 3% to 10%)
Local: Injection site burning, stinging, or pain (children 10%; adults 18%)
Respiratory: Apnea lasting 30-60 seconds (children 10%; adults 24%), apnea lasting >60 seconds (children 5%; adults 12%)
1% to 10%:
Cardiovascular: Hypertension (children 8%), arrhythmia (1% to 3%), bradycardia (1% to 3%), cardiac output decreased (1% to 3%; concurrent opioid use increases incidence), tachycardia (1% to 3%)

Dermatologic: Pruritus (1% to 3%), rash (children 5%; adults 1% to 3%)
Endocrine & metabolic: Hypertriglyceridemia (3% to 10%)
Respiratory: Respiratory acidosis during weaning (3% to 10%)
General Dosage Range I.V.: *Children and Adults:* Dosage varies greatly depending on indication
Mechanism of Action Propofol is a short-acting, lipophilic intravenous general anesthetic. The drug is unrelated to any of the currently used barbiturate, opioid, benzodiazepine, arylcyclohexylamine, or imidazole intravenous anesthetic agents. Propofol causes global CNS depression, presumably through agonism of GABA$_A$ receptors and perhaps reduced glutamatergic activity through NMDA receptor blockade.
Pharmacodynamics/Kinetics
Onset of Action Anesthetic: Bolus infusion (dose dependent): 9-51 seconds (average: 30 seconds)
Duration of Action Dose and rate dependent: 3-10 minutes
Half-life Elimination Biphasic: Initial: 40 minutes; Terminal: 4-7 hours (after 10-day infusion, may be up to 1-3 days)
Pregnancy Risk Factor B
Pregnancy Considerations Propofol should only be used in pregnancy if clearly needed. Propofol is not recommended for obstetrics, including cesarean section deliveries. Propofol crosses the placenta and may be associated with neonatal CNS and respiratory depression.

Propranolol (proe PRAN oh lole)

Related Information
Cardiovascular Diseases *on page 1492*
Endocrine Disorders and Pregnancy *on page 1517*
Brand Names: U.S. Inderal® LA; InnoPran XL®
Brand Names: Canada Apo-Propranolol®; Dom-Propranolol; Inderal®; Inderal® LA; Novo-Pranol; Nu-Propranolol; PMS-Propranolol; Propranolol Hydrochloride Injection, USP; Teva-Propranolol
Generic Availability (U.S.) Yes
Pharmacologic Category Antianginal Agent; Antiarrhythmic Agent, Class II; Beta-Adrenergic Blocker, Nonselective
Use Management of hypertension; angina pectoris; pheochromocytoma; essential tremor; supraventricular arrhythmias (such as atrial fibrillation and flutter, AV nodal reentrant tachycardias), ventricular tachycardias (catecholamine-induced arrhythmias, digoxin toxicity); prevention of myocardial infarction; migraine headache prophylaxis; symptomatic treatment of hypertrophic subaortic stenosis (hypertrophic obstructive cardiomyopathy)
Unlabeled Use Tremor due to Parkinson's disease; aggressive behavior (not recommended for dementia-associated aggression), anxiety, schizophrenia; antipsychotic-induced akathisia; primary and secondary prophylaxis of variceal hemorrhage; acute panic; thyrotoxicosis; tetralogy of Fallot (TOF) hypercyanotic spells
Local Anesthetic/Vasoconstrictor Precautions Use with caution; epinephrine has interacted with nonselective beta-blockers to result in initial hypertensive episode followed by bradycardia

Effects on Dental Treatment Propranolol is a non-selective beta-blocker and may enhance the pressor response to epinephrine, resulting in hypertension and bradycardia. Many nonsteroidal anti-inflammatory drugs, such as ibuprofen and indomethacin, can reduce the hypotensive effect of beta-blockers after 3 or more weeks of therapy with the NSAID. Short-term NSAID use (ie, 3 days) requires no special precautions in patients taking beta-blockers.

Effects on Bleeding No information available to require special precautions

Adverse Effects Frequency not defined.

Cardiovascular: Angina, arterial insufficiency, AV conduction disturbance increased, bradycardia, cardiogenic shock, CHF, hypotension, impaired myocardial contractility, mesenteric arterial thrombosis (rare), Raynaud's syndrome, syncope

Central nervous system: Amnesia, catatonia, cognitive dysfunction, confusion, depression, dizziness, emotional lability, fatigue, hallucinations, hypersomnolence, insomnia, lethargy, lightheadedness, psychosis, vertigo, vivid dreams

Dermatologic: Alopecia, contact dermatitis, cutaneous ulcers, eczematous eruptions, erythema multiforme, exfoliative dermatitis, hyperkeratosis, nail changes, oculomucocutaneous reactions, pruritus, psoriasiform eruptions, rash, Stevens-Johnson syndrome, toxic epidermal necrolysis, ulcers, ulcerative lichenoid, urticaria

Endocrine & metabolic: Hyper-/hypoglycemia, hyperkalemia, hyperlipidemia

Gastrointestinal: Anorexia, cramping, constipation, diarrhea, ischemic colitis, nausea, stomach discomfort, vomiting

Genitourinary: Impotence, interstitial nephritis (rare), oliguria (rare), Peyronie's disease, proteinuria (rare)

Hematologic: Agranulocytosis, nonthrombocytopenic purpura, thrombocytopenia, thrombocytopenic purpura

Hepatic: Alkaline phosphatase increased, transaminases increased

Neuromuscular & skeletal: Arthropathy, carpal tunnel syndrome (rare), myotonus, paresthesia, polyarthritis, weakness

Ocular: Hyperemia of the conjunctiva, mydriasis, visual acuity decreased, visual disturbances, xerophthalmia

Renal: BUN increased

Respiratory: Bronchospasm, dyspnea, laryngospasm, pharyngitis, pulmonary edema, respiratory distress, wheezing

Miscellaneous: Anaphylactic/anaphylactoid allergic reaction, cold extremities, lupus-like syndrome (rare)

Dosage

Akathisia (unlabeled use): Oral: Adults: 30-120 mg/day in 2-3 divided doses

Essential tremor: Oral: Adults: 40 mg twice daily initially; maintenance doses: Usually 120-320 mg/day

Hypertension:

Oral:

Children (unlabeled use): Initial: 0.5-1 mg/kg/day in divided doses every 6-12 hours; increase gradually every 5-7 days; maximum: 16 mg/kg/24 hours

Adults: Initial: 40 mg twice daily; increase dosage every 3-7 days; usual dose: 120-240 mg divided in 2-3 doses/day; maximum daily dose: 640 mg; usual dosage range (JNC 7): 40-160 mg/day in 2 divided doses

Extended release formulations:

Inderal® LA: Initial: 80 mg once daily; usual maintenance: 120-160 mg once daily; maximum daily dose: 640 mg; usual dosage range (JNC 7): 60-180 mg/day once daily

InnoPran XL®: Initial: 80 mg once daily at bedtime; if initial response is inadequate, may be increased at 2-3 week intervals to a maximum dose of 120 mg

Elderly: Consider lower initial doses and titrate to response (Aronow, 2011)

Hypertrophic subaortic stenosis: Oral: Adults: 20-40 mg 3-4 times/day

Inderal® LA: 80-160 mg once daily

Migraine headache prophylaxis: Oral:

Children (unlabeled use): Initial: 2-4 mg/kg/day or ≤35 kg: 10-20 mg 3 times/day
>35 kg: 20-40 mg 3 times/day

Adults: Initial: 80 mg/day divided every 6-8 hours; increase by 20-40 mg/dose every 3-4 weeks to a maximum of 160-240 mg/day given in divided doses every 6-8 hours; if satisfactory response not achieved within 6 weeks of starting therapy, drug should be withdrawn gradually over several weeks

Inderal® LA: Initial: 80 mg once daily; effective dose range: 160-240 mg once daily

Post-MI mortality reduction: Oral: Adults: Initial: 40 mg 3 times/day; usual dosage range: 180-240 mg/day in 3-4 divided doses

Pheochromocytoma: Oral: Adults: 30-60 mg/day in divided doses

Stable angina: Oral: Adults: 80-320 mg/day in doses divided 2-4 times/day

Inderal® LA: Initial: 80 mg once daily; maximum dose: 320 mg once daily

Tachyarrhythmias:

Oral:

Children (unlabeled use): Initial: 0.5-1 mg/kg/day in divided doses every 6-8 hours; titrate dosage upward every 3-7 days; usual dose: 2-6 mg/kg/day; higher doses may be needed; do not exceed 16 mg/kg/day or 60 mg/day

Adults: 10-30 mg/dose every 6-8 hours

Elderly: Initial: 10 mg twice daily; increase dosage every 3-7 days; usual dosage range: 10-320 mg given in 2 divided doses

I.V.:

Children (unlabeled use): 0.01-0.1 mg/kg/dose slow IVP over 10 minutes; maximum dose: 1 mg for infants; 3 mg for children

Adults: 1-3 mg/dose slow IVP; repeat every 2-5 minutes up to a total of 5 mg; titrate initial dose to desired response

or

0.5-1 mg over 1 minute; may repeat, if necessary, up to a total maximum dose of 0.1 mg/kg (ACLS guidelines, 2010)

Note: Once response achieved or maximum dose administered, additional doses should not be given for at least 4 hours.

Elderly: Use caution; initiate at lower end of the dosing range.

Hypercyanotic spells (TOF) (unlabeled use): Children:

Oral: Palliation: Initial: 1 mg/kg/day every 6 hours; if ineffective, may increase dose after 1 week by 1 mg/kg/day to a maximum of 5 mg/kg/day; if patient becomes refractory, may increase slowly to a maximum of 10-15 mg/kg/day. Allow 24 hours between dosing changes.

I.V.: 0.01-0.2 mg/kg/dose infused over 10 minutes; maximum dose: 5 mg

Thyroid storm (unlabeled use):

Children: 0.5 mg/kg/dose every 4-8 hours; titrate to effective dose (Eyal, 2008)

Adults:

Oral: 60-80 mg every 4 hours; may consider the use of an intravenous shorter-acting beta-blocker (ie, esmolol) (Bahn, 2011)

I.V.: 0.5-1 mg administered over 10 minutes every 3 hours (Gardner, 2011)

Thyrotoxicosis (unlabeled use): Oral:

Children: 10-40 mg every 6 hours; titrate to effective dose (Eyal, 2008)

Adolescents and Adults: Oral: 10-40 mg/dose every 6-8 hours; may also consider administering extended or sustained release formulations (Bahn, 2011)

Variceal hemorrhage prophylaxis (unlabeled use; Garcia-Tsao, 2007): Oral: Adults:

Primary prophylaxis: Initial: 20 mg twice daily; adjust to maximal tolerated dose. **Note:** Risk factors for hemorrhage include Child-Pugh class B/C or variceal red wale markings on endoscopy.

Secondary prophylaxis: Initial: 20 mg twice daily; adjust to maximal tolerated dose

Dosing adjustment in renal impairment:
Not dialyzable (0% to 5%); supplemental dose is not necessary.
Peritoneal dialysis effects: Supplemental dose is not necessary.

Dosing adjustment in hepatic disease: Marked slowing of heart rate may occur in chronic liver disease with conventional doses; low initial dose and regular heart rate monitoring

Mechanism of Action Nonselective beta-adrenergic blocker (class II antiarrhythmic); competitively blocks response to beta$_1$- and beta$_2$-adrenergic stimulation which results in decreases in heart rate, myocardial contractility, blood pressure, and myocardial oxygen demand. Nonselective beta-adrenergic blockers (propranolol, nadolol) reduce portal pressure by producing splanchnic vasoconstriction (beta$_2$ effect) thereby reducing portal blood flow.

Contraindications Hypersensitivity to propranolol, beta-blockers, or any component of the formulation; uncompensated congestive heart failure (unless the failure is due to tachyarrhythmias being treated with propranolol), cardiogenic shock, severe sinus bradycardia or heart block greater than first-degree (except in patients with a functioning artificial pacemaker), severe hyperactive airway disease (asthma or COPD)

Warnings/Precautions Consider pre-existing conditions such as sick sinus syndrome before initiating. Administer cautiously in compensated heart failure and monitor for a worsening of the condition (efficacy of propranolol in HF has not been demonstrated). **[U.S. Boxed Warning]: Beta-blocker therapy should not be withdrawn abruptly (particularly in patients with CAD), but gradually tapered to avoid acute tachycardia, hypertension, and/or ischemia.** Chronic beta-blocker therapy should not be routinely withdrawn prior to major surgery. May precipitate or aggravate symptoms of arterial insufficiency in patients with PVD and Raynaud's disease; use with caution and monitor for progression of arterial obstruction. Bradycardia may be observed more frequently in elderly patients (>65 years of age); dosage reductions may be necessary. Use caution with concurrent use of digoxin, verapamil, or diltiazem; bradycardia or heart block can occur. Avoid concurrent I.V. use of both agents. Use with caution in patients receiving inhaled anesthetic agents known to depress myocardial contractility.

Use cautiously in patients with diabetes because it can mask prominent hypoglycemic symptoms. May mask signs of hyperthyroidism (eg, tachycardia); if hyperthyroidism is suspected, carefully manage and monitor; abrupt withdrawal may exacerbate symptoms of hyperthyroidism or precipitate thyroid storm. May alter thyroid-function tests. Use with caution in myasthenia gravis or psychiatric disease (may cause CNS depression). Use cautiously in renal and hepatic dysfunction; dosage adjustment required in hepatic impairment. In general, patients with bronchospastic disease should not receive beta-blockers; if used at all, should be used cautiously with close monitoring. Adequate alpha-blockade is required prior to use of any beta-blocker for patients with untreated pheochromocytoma. May induce or exacerbate psoriasis. Use caution with history of severe anaphylaxis to allergens; patients taking beta-blockers may become more sensitive to repeated challenges. Treatment of anaphylaxis (eg, epinephrine) in patients taking beta-blockers may be ineffective or promote undesirable effects.

Drug Interactions

Metabolism/Transport Effects Substrate of CYP1A2 (major), CYP2C19 (minor), CYP2D6 (major), CYP3A4 (minor); **Note:** Assignment of Major/Minor substrate status based on clinically relevant drug interaction potential; **Inhibits** CYP1A2 (weak), CYP2D6 (weak), P-glycoprotein

Avoid Concomitant Use

Avoid concomitant use of Propranolol with any of the following: Beta2-Agonists; Bosutinib; Floctafenine; Methacholine; Pomalidomide; Topotecan; VinCRIStine (Liposomal)

Increased Effect/Toxicity

Propranolol may increase the levels/effects of: Alpha-/Beta-Agonists (Direct-Acting); Alpha1-Blockers; Alpha2-Agonists; Amifostine; Antihypertensives; Antipsychotic Agents (Phenothiazines); ARIPiprazole; Bosutinib; Bupivacaine; Cardiac Glycosides; Cholinergic Agonists; Colchicine; Dabigatran Etexilate; Ergot Derivatives; Everolimus; Fingolimod; Hypotensive Agents; Insulin; Lidocaine (Systemic); Lidocaine (Topical); Mepivacaine; Methacholine; Midodrine; P-glycoprotein/ABCB1 Substrates; Pomalidomide; Prucalopride; RiTUXimab; Rivaroxaban; Rizatriptan; Sulfonylureas; Topotecan; VinCRIStine (Liposomal); ZOLMitriptan

The levels/effects of Propranolol may be increased by: Abiraterone Acetate; Acetylcholinesterase Inhibitors; Alcohol (Ethyl); Alpha2-Agonists; Aminoquinolines (Antimalarial); Amiodarone; Anilidopiperidine Opioids; Antipsychotic Agents (Phenothiazines); Calcium Channel Blockers (Dihydropyridine); Calcium Channel Blockers (Nondihydropyridine); CYP1A2 Inhibitors (Moderate); CYP1A2 Inhibitors (Strong); CYP2D6 Inhibitors (Moderate); CYP2D6 Inhibitors (Strong); Darunavir; Deferasirox; Diazoxide; Dipyridamole; Disopyramide; Dronedarone; Floctafenine; FluvoxaMINE; Herbs (Hypotensive Properties); Lacidipine; MAO Inhibitors; Pentoxifylline; Phosphodiesterase 5 Inhibitors; Propafenone; Prostacyclin Analogues; QuiNIDine; Reserpine; Selective Serotonin Reuptake Inhibitors; Zileuton

Decreased Effect

Propranolol may decrease the levels/effects of: Beta2-Agonists; Lacidipine; Theophylline Derivatives

The levels/effects of Propranolol may be decreased by: Alcohol (Ethyl); Barbiturates; Bile Acid Sequestrants; CYP1A2 Inducers (Strong); Cyproterone; Herbs (Hypertensive Properties); Methylphenidate; Nonsteroidal Anti-Inflammatory Agents; Peginterferon Alfa-2b; Rifamycin Derivatives; Yohimbine

Ethanol/Nutrition/Herb Interactions

Cigarette: Smoking may decrease plasma levels of propranolol by increasing metabolism. Management: Avoid smoking.

Ethanol: Ethanol may increase or decrease plasma levels of propranolol. Reports are variable and have shown both enhanced as well as inhibited hepatic metabolism (of propranolol). Management: Caution advised with consumption of ethanol and monitor for heart rate and/or blood pressure changes.

Food: Propranolol serum levels may be increased if taken with food. Protein-rich foods may increase bioavailability; a change in diet from high carbohydrate/low protein to low carbohydrate/high protein may result in increased oral clearance. Management: Tablets (immediate release) should be taken on an empty stomach. Capsules (extended release) may be taken with or without food, but be consistent with regard to food.

Herb/Nutraceutical: Dong quai has estrogenic activity. Some herbal medications may worsen hypertension (eg, licorice); others may enhance the antihypertensive effect of propranolol (eg, shepherd's purse). Management: Avoid dong quai if using for hypertension. Avoid bayberry, blue cohosh, cayenne, ephedra, ginger, ginseng (American), gotu kola, licorice, and yohimbe. Avoid black cohosh, california poppy, coleus, garlic, golden seal, hawthorn, mistletoe, periwinkle, quinine, and shepherd's purse.

Dietary Considerations Tablets (immediate release) should be taken on an empty stomach; capsules (extended release) may be taken with or without food, but should always be taken consistently (with food or on an empty stomach)

Pharmacodynamics/Kinetics

Onset of Action Beta-blockade: Oral: 1-2 hours

Duration of Action Immediate release: 6-12 hours; Extended-release formulations: ~24-27 hours

Half-life Elimination Neonates and Infants: Possible increased half-life; Children: 3.9-6.4 hours; Adults: Immediate release formulation: 3-6 hours; Extended-release formulations: 8-10 hours

Time to Peak Immediate release: 1-4 hours; Extended-release formulations: ~6-14 hours

Pregnancy Risk Factor C

Pregnancy Considerations Adverse events have been observed in some animal reproduction studies; therefore, the manufacturer classifies propranolol as pregnancy category C. Propranolol crosses the placenta and is measurable in the newborn serum following maternal use during pregnancy. In a cohort study, an increased risk of cardiovascular defects was observed following maternal use of beta-blockers during pregnancy. Intrauterine growth restriction (IUGR), small placentas, as well as fetal/neonatal bradycardia, hypoglycemia, and/or respiratory depression have been observed following *in utero* exposure to beta-blockers as a class. Adequate facilities for monitoring infants at birth should be available. Untreated chronic maternal hypertension and pre-eclampsia are also associated with adverse events in the fetus, infant, and mother. The peak maternal serum concentrations of propranolol and the active metabolite 4-hydroxypropranolol do not change during pregnancy; peak serum concentrations

of naphthoxylactic acid are lower in the third trimester when compared to postpartum. Propranolol is recommended for use in the management of thyrotoxicosis in pregnancy. Propranolol has been evaluated for the treatment of hypertension in pregnancy, but other agents may be more appropriate for use. Propranolol has also been used in the management of hypertrophic obstructive cardiomyopathy in pregnancy and has been studied for use as an adjunctive agent in the management of dysfunctional labor (dystocia).

Lactation Enters breast milk/use caution (AAP rates "compatible"; AAP 2001 update pending)

Breast-Feeding Considerations Propranolol is excreted into breast milk with peak concentrations occurring ~2-3 hours after an oral dose. The inactive metabolites of propranolol have also been detected in breast milk. The manufacturer recommends that caution be exercised when administering propranolol to nursing women. Due to immature hepatic metabolism in newborns, breast-feeding infants should be monitored for adverse events.

Dosage Forms

Capsule, extended release, oral: 60 mg, 80 mg, 120 mg, 160 mg
InnoPran XL®: 80 mg, 120 mg

Capsule, sustained release, oral:
Inderal® LA: 60 mg, 80 mg, 120 mg, 160 mg

Injection, solution: 1 mg/mL (1 mL)

Injection, solution [preservative free]: 1 mg/mL (1 mL)

Solution, oral: 4 mg/mL (500 mL); 8 mg/mL (500 mL)

Tablet, oral: 10 mg, 20 mg, 40 mg, 60 mg, 80 mg

References

Foster CA and Aston SJ, "Propranolol-Epinephrine Interaction: A Potential Disaster," *Plast Reconstr Surg*, 1983, 72(1):74-8.

Wong DG, Spence JD, Lamki L, et al, "Effect of Nonsteroidal Anti-inflammatory Drugs on Control of Hypertension of Beta-Blockers and Diuretics," *Lancet*, 1986, 1(8488):997-1001.

Wynn RL, "Dental Nonsteroidal Anti-inflammatory Drugs and Prostaglandin-Based Drug Interactions, Part Two," *Gen Dent*, 1992, 40 (2):104, 106, 108.

Wynn RL, "Epinephrine Interactions With Beta-Blockers," *Gen Dent*, 1994, 42(1):16, 18.

Propranolol and Hydrochlorothiazide
(proe PRAN oh lole & hye droe klor oh THYE a zide)

Related Information
Hydrochlorothiazide *on page 687*
Propranolol *on page 1153*

Pharmacologic Category Beta-Blocker, Nonselective; Diuretic, Thiazide

Use Management of hypertension

Local Anesthetic/Vasoconstrictor Precautions Use with caution; epinephrine has interacted with nonselective beta-blockers to result in initial hypertensive episode followed by bradycardia

Effects on Dental Treatment Noncardioselective beta-blockers (ie, propranolol, nadolol) enhance the pressor response to epinephrine, resulting in hypertension and bradycardia. Many nonsteroidal anti-inflammatory drugs, such as ibuprofen and indomethacin, can reduce the hypotensive effect of beta-blockers after 3 or more weeks of therapy with the NSAID. Short-term NSAID use (ie, 3 days) requires no special precautions in patients taking beta-blockers.

Effects on Bleeding No information available to require special precautions

Adverse Effects See individual agents.

General Dosage Range Oral: *Adults:* Propranolol 80-160 mg/day and hydrochlorothiazide 12.5-50 mg/day in 2 divided doses

Pregnancy Risk Factor C

Pregnancy Considerations Reproduction studies have not been conducted for this combination. See individual agents.

Propylhexedrine (proe pil HEKS e dreen)

Brand Names: U.S. Benzedrex® [OTC]
Pharmacologic Category Adrenergic Agonist Agent
Use Topical nasal decongestant
Local Anesthetic/Vasoconstrictor Precautions No information available to require special precautions
Effects on Dental Treatment No significant effects or complications reported
Effects on Bleeding No information available to require special precautions
Adverse Effects Frequency not defined.
Local: Nasal: Burning, stinging
Respiratory: Sneezing, nasal discharge increased
General Dosage Range Oral: *Children ≥6 years and Adults:* 2 inhalations in each nostril, not more frequently than every 2 hours

Propylthiouracil (proe pil thye oh YOOR a sil)

Related Information
Endocrine Disorders and Pregnancy *on page 1517*
Brand Names: Canada Propyl-Thyracil®
Pharmacologic Category Antithyroid Agent; Thioamide
Use Adjunctive therapy in patients intolerant of methimazole to ameliorate hyperthyroidism symptoms in preparation for surgical treatment or radioactive iodine therapy; treatment of hyperthyroidism in patients intolerant of methimazole and not candidates for surgical/radiotherapy
Unlabeled Use Management of Graves' disease, thyrotoxic crisis, or thyroid storm
Local Anesthetic/Vasoconstrictor Precautions No information available to require special precautions
Effects on Dental Treatment Key adverse event(s) related to dental treatment: Loss of taste perception.
Effects on Bleeding Propylthiouracil administration may cause a bishydroxycoumarin-like hypocoagulable condition that is clinically observed by hemorrhagic diathesis. The syndrome is usually responsive to vitamin K therapy. It is suggested that all patients receiving propylthiouracil have their prothrombin times evaluated.
Adverse Effects Frequency not defined.
Cardiovascular: Periarteritis, vasculitis (ANCA-positive, cutaneous, leukocytoclastic)
Central nervous system: Drowsiness, drug fever, fever, headache, neuritis, vertigo
Dermatologic: Alopecia, erythema nodosum, exfoliative dermatitis, pruritus, skin pigmentation, skin rash, skin ulcers, urticaria
Endocrine & metabolic: Goiter, weight gain
Gastrointestinal: Constipation, loss of taste, nausea, sialoadenopathy, splenomegaly, stomach pain, taste perversion, vomiting
Hematologic: Agranulocytosis, aplastic anemia, bleeding, granulocytopenia, hypoprothrombinemia, leukopenia, thrombocytopenia
Hepatic: Acute liver failure, cholestatic jaundice, hepatitis
Neuromuscular & skeletal: Arthralgia, myalgia, paresthesia

Renal: Acute renal failure, glomerulonephritis, nephritis
Respiratory: Alveolar hemorrhage, interstitial pneumonitis
Miscellaneous: Lymphadenopathy, SLE-like syndrome
General Dosage Range Oral:
Children 6-10 years: 50-150 mg/day
Children >10 years: 150-300 mg/day
Adults: Initial: 300-900 mg/day in 3 divided doses; Maintenance: 100-150 mg/day
Mechanism of Action Inhibits the synthesis of thyroid hormones by blocking the oxidation of iodine in the thyroid gland; blocks synthesis of thyroxine and triiodothyronine
Pharmacodynamics/Kinetics
Duration of Action 12-24 hours
Half-life Elimination ~1 hour
Time to Peak 1-2 hours
Pregnancy Risk Factor D
Pregnancy Considerations Propylthiouracil has been found to readily cross the placenta. Teratogenic effects have not been observed; however, nonteratogenic adverse effects, including fetal and neonatal hypothyroidism, goiter, and hyperthyroidism, have been reported following maternal propylthiouracil use. The transfer of thyroid-stimulating immunoglobulins can stimulate the fetal thyroid *in utero* and transiently after delivery and may increase the risk of fetal or neonatal hyperthyroidism.

Uncontrolled maternal hyperthyroidism may result in adverse neonatal outcomes (eg, prematurity, low birth weight) and adverse maternal outcomes (eg, preeclampsia, congestive heart failure, stillbirth, and abortion). To prevent adverse fetal and maternal events, normal maternal thyroid function should be maintained prior to conception and throughout pregnancy. Antithyroid treatment is recommended for the control of hyperthyroidism during pregnancy. Propylthiouracil is considered first-line therapy, especially during the first trimester. Due to an increased risk of liver toxicity, use of methimazole may be preferred during the second and third trimesters. If drug therapy is changed, maternal thyroid function should be monitored after 2 weeks and then every 2-4 weeks. Propylthiouracil, along with other medications, is used for the treatment of thyroid storm in pregnant women; alternative therapy is recommended if oral administration is not possible.

The pharmacokinetics of propylthiouracil are not significantly changed during pregnancy; however, the severity of hyperthyroidism may fluctuate throughout pregnancy. Doses of propylthiouracil may be decreased as pregnancy progresses and discontinued weeks to months prior to delivery.

Protamine (PROE ta meen)

Pharmacologic Category Antidote
Use Treatment of heparin overdosage; neutralize heparin during surgery or dialysis procedures
Unlabeled Use Treatment of low molecular weight heparin (LMWH) overdose
Local Anesthetic/Vasoconstrictor Precautions No information available to require special precautions
Effects on Dental Treatment No significant effects or complications reported

◄ **Effects on Bleeding** Administration reverses the effect of heparin anticoagulants to permit general surgical treatment (eg, abdominal or orthopedic surgery). Risk of bleeding is dependent on multiple variables, including the intensity of anticoagulation and patient susceptibility. The need to address the effects of anticoagulation for dental surgery is based on a complex risk to benefit assessment; medical consult is suggested.

Adverse Effects Frequency not defined.

Cardiovascular: Sudden fall in blood pressure, bradycardia, flushing, hypotension

Central nervous system: Lassitude

Gastrointestinal: Nausea, vomiting

Hematologic: Hemorrhage

Respiratory: Dyspnea, pulmonary hypertension

Miscellaneous: Hypersensitivity reactions

General Dosage Range I.V.: *Children and Adults:* 1 mg of protamine neutralizes ~100 units of heparin (maximum dose: 50 mg)

Mechanism of Action Combines with strongly acidic heparin to form a stable complex (salt) neutralizing the anticoagulant activity of both drugs

Pharmacodynamics/Kinetics

Onset of Action I.V.: Heparin neutralization: ~5 minutes

Half-life Elimination ~7 minutes

Pregnancy Risk Factor C

Pregnancy Considerations Animal reproduction studies have not been conducted. In general, medications used as antidotes should take into consideration the health and prognosis of the mother (Bailey, 2004). Protamine sulfate may be used during delivery to reduce the risk of bleeding following maternal use of heparin or low molecular weight heparin (LMWH) (Bates, 2012).

Protein C Concentrate (Human)
(PROE teen cee KON suhn trate HYU man)

Brand Names: U.S. Ceprotin

Pharmacologic Category Anticoagulant; Blood Product Derivative; Enzyme; Protein C

Use Replacement therapy for severe congenital protein C deficiency for the prevention and/or treatment of venous thromboembolism and purpura fulminans

Local Anesthetic/Vasoconstrictor Precautions No information available to require special precautions

Effects on Dental Treatment No significant effects or complications reported

Effects on Bleeding As with all drugs which may affect hemostasis, bleeding may be associated with protein C administration. Risk is dependent on multiple variables. Medical consult is suggested.

Adverse Effects As with all drugs which may affect hemostasis, bleeding may be associated with protein C administration. Hemorrhage may occur at virtually any site. Risk is dependent on multiple variables, including the concurrent use of multiple agents that alter hemostasis and patient susceptibility. Frequency not defined.

Central nervous system: Lightheadedness

Hematologic: Bleeding

Miscellaneous: Hypersensitivity reactions (itching and rash)

Postmarketing and/or case reports: Fever, hemothorax, hypotension, hyperhidrosis, restlessness

General Dosage Range I.V.: *Children and Adults:* Initial: 100-120 units, followed by 60-80 units every 6 hours for 3 doses; maintenance: 45-60 units every 6 hours (short-term) or every 12 hours (short-to-long term)

Mechanism of Action Converted to activated protein C (APC). APC is a serine protease which inactivates factors Va and VIIIa, limiting thrombotic formation. *In vitro* data also suggest inhibition of plasminogen activator inhibitor-1 (PAF-1) resulting in profibrinolytic activity, inhibition of macrophage production of tumor necrosis factor, blocking of leukocyte adhesion, and limitation of thrombin-induced inflammatory responses.

Pharmacodynamics/Kinetics

Half-life Elimination Median: 9.8 hours; range 4.9-14.7 hours

Time to Peak Plasma: T_{max}: 0.5 hours

Pregnancy Risk Factor C

Pregnancy Considerations Reproductive studies have not been performed. It is unknown if administration during pregnancy will result in fetal harm.

Protriptyline (proe TRIP ti leen)

Related Information
Vasoconstrictor Interactions With Antidepressants *on page 1650*

Brand Names: U.S. Vivactil®

Pharmacologic Category Antidepressant, Tricyclic (Secondary Amine)

Use Treatment of depression

Local Anesthetic/Vasoconstrictor Precautions Use with caution; epinephrine and levonordefrin have been shown to have an increased pressor response in combination with TCAs. Protriptyline is one of the drugs confirmed to prolong the QT interval and is accepted as having a risk of causing torsade de pointes. The risk of drug-induced torsade de pointes is extremely low when a single QT interval prolonging drug is prescribed. In terms of epinephrine, it is not known what effect vasoconstrictors in the local anesthetic regimen will have in patients with a known history of congenital prolonged QT interval or in patients taking any medication that prolongs the QT interval. Until more information is obtained, it is suggested that the clinician consult with the physician prior to the use of a vasoconstrictor in suspected patients, and that the vasoconstrictor (epinephrine, mepivacaine and levonordefrin [Carbocaine® 2% with Neo-Cobefrin®]) be used with caution.

Effects on Dental Treatment Key adverse event(s) related to dental treatment: Xerostomia and changes in salivation (normal salivary flow resumes upon discontinuation), unpleasant taste, and trouble with gums. Long-term treatment with TCAs, such as protriptyline, increases the risk of caries by reducing salivation and salivary buffer capacity.

Effects on Bleeding No information available to require special precautions

Adverse Effects Frequency not defined.

Cardiovascular: Arrhythmias, heart block, hyper-/hypotension, MI, palpitation, stroke, tachycardia

Central nervous system: Agitation, anxiety, ataxia, confusion, delirium, delusions, dizziness, drowsiness, EPS, exacerbation of psychosis, fatigue, hallucinations, headache, hypomania, incoordination, insomnia, nightmares, panic, restlessness, seizure

Dermatologic: Alopecia, itching, petechiae, photosensitivity, rash, urticaria

Endocrine & metabolic: Breast enlargement, galactorrhea, gynecomastia, increased or decreased libido, syndrome of inappropriate ADH secretion (SIADH)

Gastrointestinal: Anorexia, constipation, decreased lower esophageal sphincter tone may cause GE reflux, diarrhea, heartburn, increased appetite, nausea, trouble with gums, unpleasant taste, vomiting, weight gain/loss, xerostomia

Genitourinary: Difficult urination, impotence, testicular edema

Hematologic: Agranulocytosis, eosinophilia, leukopenia, purpura, thrombocytopenia

Hepatic: Cholestatic jaundice, increased liver enzymes

Neuromuscular & skeletal: Fine muscle tremor, numbness, tingling, tremor, weakness

Ocular: Blurred vision, eye pain, increased intraocular pressure

Otic: Tinnitus

Miscellaneous: Allergic reactions, excessive diaphoresis

General Dosage Range Oral:
Adolescents: 15-20 mg/day
Adults: 15-60 mg/day in 3-4 divided doses
Elderly: Initial: 5-10 mg/day; Maintenance: 15-20 mg/day

Mechanism of Action Increases the synaptic concentration of serotonin and/or norepinephrine in the central nervous system by inhibition of their reuptake by the presynaptic neuronal membrane

Pharmacodynamics/Kinetics
Half-life Elimination 54-92 hours (average: 74 hours)
Time to Peak Serum: 24-30 hours

Pregnancy Considerations Adverse events have not been observed in animal reproduction studies.

Dental Comment Protriptyline is known to prolong the QT interval. The QT interval is measured as the time and distance between the Q point of the QRS complex and the end of the T wave in the ECG tracing. After adjustment for heart rate, the QT interval is defined as prolonged if it is more than 450 msec in men and 460 msec in women. A long QT syndrome was first described in the 1950s and 60s as a congenital syndrome involving QT interval prolongation and syncope and sudden death. Some of the congenital long QT syndromes were characterized by a peculiar electrocardiographic appearance of the QRS complex involving a premature atria beat followed by a pause, then a subsequent sinus beat showing marked QT prolongation and deformity. This type of cardiac arrhythmia was originally termed "torsade de pointes" (translated from the French as "twisting of the points"). Protriptyline is considered as having a risk of causing torsade de pointes. Since it is not known what effect vasoconstrictors in the local anesthetic regimen will have in patients with a known history of congenital prolonged QT interval or in patients taking any medication that prolongs the QT interval, a medical consult is suggested.

Prucalopride (proo KAL oh pride)

Brand Names: Canada Resotran™
Pharmacologic Category Serotonin 5-HT$_4$ Receptor Agonist
Use Treatment of chronic idiopathic constipation in adult females with inadequate response to laxatives
Unlabeled Use Opioid-induced constipation in chronic pain (noncancer) patients
Local Anesthetic/Vasoconstrictor Precautions No information available to require special precautions
Effects on Dental Treatment No significant effects or complications reported

Effects on Bleeding No information available to require special precautions
Adverse Effects
>10%:
Central nervous system: Headache (22%)
Gastrointestinal: Nausea (17%), abdominal pain (12%), diarrhea (12%)
1% to 10%:
Cardiovascular: Palpitation (1%; similar to placebo)
Central nervous system: Dizziness (4%), fatigue (3%), fever (1%), malaise (1%)
Genitourinary: Pollakiuria (1%)
Gastrointestinal: Upper abdominal pain (5%), flatulence (5%), vomiting (5%), dyspepsia (3%), bowel sounds abnormal (2%), anorexia (1%), gastroenteritis (1%)
Neuromuscular & skeletal: Muscle spasms (2%)

General Dosage Range Dosage adjustment recommended in patients with renal impairment.
Oral:
Adults (females ≥18 years): 2 mg once daily
Elderly (females >65 years): Initial: 1 mg once daily; maintenance: 1-2 mg once daily

Mechanism of Action Prucalopride is a selective, high affinity 5-HT$_4$ receptor agonist whose action at the receptor site promotes cholinergic and nonadrenergic, noncholinergic neurotransmission by enteric neurons leading to stimulation of the peristaltic reflex, intestinal secretions, and gastrointestinal motility.

Pharmacodynamics/Kinetics
Half-life Elimination ~24 hours; terminal half-life increases to 34, 43, and 47 hours in mild, moderate, and severe renal impairment, respectively
Time to Peak 2-3 hours

Pregnancy Considerations Reproductive animal studies did not demonstrate adverse effects. Spontaneous abortion has been observed in pregnant women during clinical trials, although a causal association with prucalopride has not been established. Use during pregnancy is not recommended. Women of childbearing potential should employ effective contraception during therapy. An additional method of contraception is recommended for patients experiencing severe diarrhea and receiving oral contraceptives due to the potential for decreased efficacy of the oral contraceptive; cases of unintended pregnancies have been reported with prucalopride.

Product Availability Not available in U.S.

Pseudoephedrine (soo doe e FED rin)

Related Information
Bacterial Infections *on page 1562*
Related Sample Prescriptions
Sinus Infection Treatment *on page 1611*
Brand Names: U.S. Children's Nasal Decongestant [OTC]; Nexafed® [OTC]; Oranyl [OTC]; Silfedrine Children's [OTC]; Sudafed® 12 Hour [OTC]; Sudafed® 24 Hour [OTC]; Sudafed® Children's [OTC]; Sudafed® Maximum Strength Nasal Decongestant [OTC]; SudoTab® [OTC]; SudoGest 12 Hour [OTC]; SudoGest Children's [OTC] [DSC]; SudoGest [OTC]
Brand Names: Canada Balminil Decongestant; Benylin® D for Infants; Contac® Cold 12 Hour Relief Non Drowsy; Drixoral® ND; Eltor®; PMS-Pseudoephedrine; Pseudofrin; Robidrine®; Sudafed® Decongestant
Generic Availability (U.S.) Yes: Excludes extended release products

Pharmacologic Category Alpha/Beta Agonist; Decongestant

Dental Use Temporary symptomatic relief of nasal congestion due to common cold, upper respiratory allergies, and sinusitis; also promotes nasal or sinus drainage

Use Temporary symptomatic relief of nasal congestion due to common cold, upper respiratory allergies, and sinusitis; also promotes nasal or sinus drainage

Local Anesthetic/Vasoconstrictor Precautions Use with caution since pseudoephedrine is a sympathomimetic amine which could interact with epinephrine to cause a pressor response

Effects on Dental Treatment Key adverse event(s) related to dental treatment: Xerostomia (normal salivary flow resumes upon discontinuation).

Effects on Bleeding No information available to require special precautions

Adverse Effects Frequency not defined.

Cardiovascular: Arrhythmia, cardiovascular collapse with hypotension, hypertension, palpitation, tachycardia

Central nervous system: Chills, confusion, coordination impaired, dizziness, drowsiness, excitability, fatigue, hallucination, headache, insomnia, nervousness, neuritis, restlessness, seizure, transient stimulation, vertigo

Dermatologic: Photosensitivity, rash, urticaria

Gastrointestinal: Anorexia, constipation, diarrhea, dry throat, ischemic colitis, nausea, vomiting, xerostomia

Genitourinary: Difficult urination, dysuria, polyuria, urinary retention

Hematologic: Agranulocytosis, hemolytic anemia, thrombocytopenia

Neuromuscular & skeletal: Tremor, weakness

Ocular: Blurred vision, diplopia

Otic: Tinnitus

Respiratory: Chest/throat tightness, dry nose, dyspnea, nasal congestion, thickening of bronchial secretions, wheezing

Miscellaneous: Anaphylaxis, diaphoresis

Dosage Oral: General dosing guidelines:

Children:

4-5 years: 15 mg every 4-6 hours: maximum: 60 mg/24 hours

6-12 years: 30 mg every 4-6 hours; maximum: 120 mg/24 hours

Children >12 years and Adults: Immediate release: 60 mg every 4-6 hours; Extended release: 120 mg every 12 hours **or** 240 mg every 24 hours; maximum: 240 mg/24 hours

Dosing adjustment in renal impairment: Consider reducing dose

Mechanism of Action Directly stimulates alpha-adrenergic receptors of respiratory mucosa causing vasoconstriction; directly stimulates beta-adrenergic receptors causing bronchial relaxation, increased heart rate and contractility

Contraindications Hypersensitivity to pseudoephedrine or any component of the formulation; with or within 14 days of MAO inhibitor therapy

Warnings/Precautions Use with caution in the elderly; may be more sensitive to adverse effects; administer with caution to patients with hypertension, hyperthyroidism, diabetes mellitus, cardiovascular disease, ischemic heart disease, increased intraocular pressure, prostatic hyperplasia, seizure disorders, or renal impairment. When used for self-medication (OTC), notify healthcare provider if symptoms do not improve within 7 days or are accompanied by fever. Discontinue and contact healthcare provider if nervousness, dizziness, or

sleeplessness occur. Some products may contain sodium. Not for OTC use in children <4 years of age.

Drug Interactions

Metabolism/Transport Effects None known.

Avoid Concomitant Use

Avoid concomitant use of Pseudoephedrine with any of the following: Ergot Derivatives; Iobenguane I 123; MAO Inhibitors

Increased Effect/Toxicity

Pseudoephedrine may increase the levels/effects of: Bromocriptine; Sympathomimetics

The levels/effects of Pseudoephedrine may be increased by: Antacids; AtoMOXetine; Cannabinoids; Carbonic Anhydrase Inhibitors; Ergot Derivatives; MAO Inhibitors; Serotonin/Norepinephrine Reuptake Inhibitors

Decreased Effect

Pseudoephedrine may decrease the levels/effects of: Benzylpenicilloyl Polylysine; FentaNYL; Iobenguane I 123

The levels/effects of Pseudoephedrine may be decreased by: Alpha1-Blockers; Spironolactone

Ethanol/Nutrition/Herb Interactions

Food: Onset of effect may be delayed if pseudoephedrine is taken with food.

Herb/Nutraceutical: Avoid ephedra, yohimbe (may cause hypertension).

Dietary Considerations Some products may contain sodium. May be taken with or without food.

Pharmacodynamics/Kinetics

Onset of Action Decongestant: Oral: 30 minutes (Chua, 1989); Peak effect: Decongestant: Oral: ~1-2 hours (Chua, 1989)

Duration of Action Immediate release tablet: 3-8 hours (Chua, 1989)

Half-life Elimination Varies by urine pH and flow rate; alkaline urine decreases renal elimination of pseudoephedrine (Kanfer, 1993)

Children: ~3 hours (urine pH ~6.5) (Simons, 1996)

Adults: 9-16 hours (pH 8); 3-6 hours (pH 5) (Chua, 1989)

Time to Peak

Children (immediate release) ~2 hours (Simons, 1996)

Adults (immediate release): 1-3 hours (dose dependent) (Kanfer, 1993)

Pregnancy Considerations Use of pseudoephedrine during the first trimester may be associated with a possible risk of gastroschisis, small intestinal atresia, and hemifacial microsomia due to pseudoephedrine's vasoconstrictive effects; additional studies are needed to define the magnitude of risk. Single doses of pseudoephedrine were not found to adversely affect the fetus during the third trimester of pregnancy (limited data); however, fetal tachycardia was noted in a case report following maternal use of an extended release product for multiple days. Decongestants are not the preferred agents for the treatment of rhinitis during pregnancy. Oral pseudoephedrine should be avoided during the first trimester.

Lactation Enters breast milk (AAP rates "compatible"; AAP 2001 update pending)

Breast-Feeding Considerations Pseudoephedrine is excreted into breast milk in concentrations that are ~4% of the weight adjusted maternal dose. The time to maximum milk concentration is ~1-2 hours after the maternal dose. Irritability has been reported in nursing infants (limited data; dose, duration, relationship to breast-feeding not provided). Milk production may be decreased in some women.

Dosage Forms

Caplet, extended release, oral:
Sudafed® 12 Hour [OTC]: 120 mg

Liquid, oral: 30 mg/5 mL (473 mL)
Children's Nasal Decongestant [OTC]: 30 mg/5 mL (118 mL)
Silfedrine Children's [OTC]: 15 mg/5 mL (118 mL, 237 mL)
Sudafed® Children's [OTC]: 15 mg/5 mL (118 mL)

Syrup, oral: 30 mg/5 mL (118 mL)

Tablet, oral: 30 mg
Nexafed® [OTC]: 30 mg
Oranyl [OTC]: 30 mg
Sudafed® Maximum Strength Nasal Decongestant [OTC]: 30 mg
Sudo-Tab® [OTC]: 30 mg
SudoGest [OTC]: 30 mg, 60 mg

Tablet, extended release, oral:
Sudafed® 24 Hour [OTC]: 240 mg
SudoGest 12 Hour [OTC]: 120 mg

Pseudoephedrine and Codeine
(soo doe e FED rin & KOE deen)

Related Information
Codeine on page 344
Pseudoephedrine on page 1159

Brand Names: U.S. Codar® D; EndaCof-DC; Notuss®-DC

Pharmacologic Category Antitussive/Decongestant

Use Temporary symptomatic relief of congestion and cough due to upper respiratory infections including common cold, bronchitis, sinusitis, and influenza

Local Anesthetic/Vasoconstrictor Precautions Use with caution since pseudoephedrine is a sympathomimetic amine which could interact with epinephrine or mepivacaine and levonordefrin (Carbocaine® 2% with Neo-Cobefrin®) to cause a pressor response.

Effects on Dental Treatment Key adverse event(s) related to dental treatment: Xerostomia (normal salivary flow resumes upon discontinuation).

Effects on Bleeding No information available to require special precautions

Adverse Effects Frequency not defined.
Cardiovascular: Arrhythmia, heart rate decreased/increased, hypertension, pallor, palpitation, tightness of chest
Central nervous system: Confusion, coordination impaired, dizziness, drowsiness, euphoria, excitation, fatigue, headache, hysteria, insomnia, irritability, lightheadedness, nervousness, neuritis, restlessness, sedation, seizure, vertigo
Dermatologic: Photosensitivity, pruritus, rash, urticaria
Endocrine & metabolic: Early menses
Gastrointestinal: Abdominal pain, anorexia, constipation, diarrhea, epigastric distress, nausea, vomiting
Genitourinary: Dysuria, polyuria, urinary retention
Neuromuscular & skeletal: Paresthesia, tremor, weakness
Ocular: Blurred vision, diplopia
Otic: Acute labyrinthitis, tinnitus
Respiratory: Dyspnea, nasal congestion, thickening of bronchial secretions, wheezing
Miscellaneous: Diaphoresis

General Dosage Range Oral:
Children 6-11 years: 2.5-5 mL every 4-6 hours as needed (maximum: 20 mL/24 hours)
Children ≥12 years and Adults: 5-10 mL every 4-6 hours as needed (maximum: 40 mL/24 hours)

Mechanism of Action
Pseudoephedrine directly stimulates alpha-adrenergic receptors of respiratory mucosa causing vasoconstriction; directly stimulates beta-adrenergic receptors causing bronchial relaxation
Codeine is an antitussive that controls cough by depressing the medullary cough center

Pregnancy Risk Factor C

Pregnancy Considerations Refer to Codeine monograph.

Controlled Substance Liquid: C-V

Pseudoephedrine and Dextromethorphan
(soo doe e FED rin & deks troe meth OR fan)

Related Information
Dextromethorphan on page 406
Pseudoephedrine on page 1159

Brand Names: U.S. Pedia Relief Cough and Cold [OTC]; Sudafed® Children's Cold & Cough [OTC]

Brand Names: Canada Balminil DM D; Benylin® DM-D; Koffex DM-D; Novahistex® DM Decongestant; Novahistine® DM Decongestant; Robitussin® Childrens Cough & Cold

Pharmacologic Category Antitussive/Decongestant

Use Temporary symptomatic relief of nasal congestion and cough due to common cold, hay fever, upper respiratory allergies

Local Anesthetic/Vasoconstrictor Precautions Use with caution since pseudoephedrine is a sympathomimetic amine which could interact with epinephrine to cause a pressor response

Effects on Dental Treatment Key adverse event(s) related to dental treatment: Pseudoephedrine: Xerostomia (normal salivary flow resumes upon discontinuation).

Effects on Bleeding No information available to require special precautions

Adverse Effects See individual agents.

General Dosage Range Oral:
Children 2-6 years: 15 mg (based on pseudoephedrine) every 4-6 hours (maximum: 60 mg/day)
Children 6-12 years: 30 mg (based on pseudoephedrine) every 4-6 hours (maximum: 120 mg/day)
Children ≥12 years and Adults: 60 mg (based on pseudoephedrine) every 4-6 hours (maximum: 240 mg/day)

Pseudoephedrine and Ibuprofen
(soo doe e FED rin & eye byoo PROE fen)

Related Information
Ibuprofen on page 711
Pseudoephedrine on page 1159

Brand Names: U.S. Advil® Cold & Sinus [OTC]; Proprinal® Cold and Sinus [OTC]

Brand Names: Canada Advil® Cold & Sinus; Advil® Cold & Sinus Daytime; Children's Advil® Cold; Sudafed® Sinus Advance

Pharmacologic Category Decongestant/Analgesic

Use For temporary relief of cold, sinus, and flu symptoms (including nasal congestion, sinus pressure, headache, minor body aches and pains, and fever)

Local Anesthetic/Vasoconstrictor Precautions Use with caution since pseudoephedrine is a sympathomimetic amine which could interact with epinephrine to cause a pressor response

Effects on Dental Treatment Key adverse event(s) related to dental treatment: Pseudoephedrine: Xerostomia (normal salivary flow resumes upon discontinuation).

The dentist should be aware of the potential of abnormal coagulation. Caution should also be exercised in the use of NSAIDs in patients already on anticoagulant therapy with drugs such as warfarin (Coumadin®). See Effects on Bleeding.

Effects on Bleeding Nonselective NSAIDs, such as pseudoephedrine and ibuprofen, inhibit platelet aggregation and prolong bleeding time in some patients. Unlike aspirin, the NSAID effect on platelet function is quantitatively less, of shorter duration, and reversible. Normal platelet function should occur in ~5 elimination half-lives or in <10 hours after discontinuation of pseudoephedrine and ibuprofen. Concomitant use of other NSAIDs should be avoided.

Adverse Effects See individual agents.

General Dosage Range Oral: *Children ≥12 years and Adults:* 1-2 doses (ibuprofen 200 mg and pseudoephedrine 30 mg per dose) every 4-6 hours as needed (maximum: 6 doses/day)

Pregnancy Considerations Refer to individual agents.

Pyrantel Pamoate (pi RAN tel PAM oh ate)

Brand Names: U.S. Pin-X® [OTC]; Reese's Pinworm Medicine [OTC]
Brand Names: Canada Combantrin™
Pharmacologic Category Anthelmintic
Use Treatment of pinworms caused by *Enterobius vermicularis* (alternative agent; not preferred therapy)
Unlabeled Use Treatment of hookworms caused by *Ancylostoma caninum, Ancylostoma duodenale,* and *Necator americanus); Moniliformis;* roundworms caused by *Ascaris lumbricoides; Trichostrongylus*
Local Anesthetic/Vasoconstrictor Precautions No information available to require special precautions
Effects on Dental Treatment No significant effects or complications reported
Effects on Bleeding No information available to require special precautions
Adverse Effects Frequency not defined.
Central nervous system: Dizziness, headache
Gastrointestinal: Abdominal cramps, diarrhea, nausea, vomiting
General Dosage Range Oral: *Children ≥2 years and Adults:* 11 mg/kg as a single dose (maximum: 1 g/dose)
Mechanism of Action Causes the release of acetylcholine and inhibits cholinesterase; acts as a depolarizing neuromuscular blocker, paralyzing the helminths
Pharmacodynamics/Kinetics
Time to Peak Serum: 1-3 hours
Pregnancy Considerations Pyrantel pamoate has minimal systemic absorption. Systemic absorption would be required in order for pyrantel pamoate to cross the placenta and reach the fetus.

Pyrazinamide (peer a ZIN a mide)

Brand Names: Canada Tebrazid™
Pharmacologic Category Antitubercular Agent

Use Adjunctive treatment of tuberculosis in combination with other antituberculosis agents
Local Anesthetic/Vasoconstrictor Precautions No information available to require special precautions
Effects on Dental Treatment No significant effects or complications reported
Effects on Bleeding No information available to require special precautions
Adverse Effects 1% to 10%:
Central nervous system: Malaise
Gastrointestinal: Anorexia, nausea, vomiting
Neuromuscular & skeletal: Arthralgia, myalgia
General Dosage Range Dosage adjustment recommended in patients with renal impairment
Oral:
Children: 15-30 mg/kg once daily (maximum: 2 g/day) **or** 50 mg/kg/dose twice weekly (maximum: 2 g/dose)
Adults 40-55 kg: 1000 mg once daily **or** 2000 mg twice weekly **or** 1500 mg 3 times/week
Adults 56-75 kg: 1500 mg once daily **or** 3000 mg twice weekly **or** 2500 mg 3 times/week
Adults 76-90 kg: 2000 mg once daily (maximum dose regardless of weight) **or** 4000 mg twice weekly (maximum dose regardless of weight) **or** 3000 mg 3 times/week (maximum dose regardless of weight)
Mechanism of Action Converted to pyrazinoic acid in susceptible strains of *Mycobacterium* which lowers the pH of the environment; exact mechanism of action has not been elucidated
Pharmacodynamics/Kinetics
Half-life Elimination 9-10 hours
Time to Peak Serum: Within 2 hours
Pregnancy Risk Factor C
Pregnancy Considerations Teratogenic effects have not been observed in animal reproduction studies. Due to the risk of tuberculosis to the fetus, treatment is recommended when the probability of maternal disease is moderate to high. Although not recommended as the initial treatment regimen, the use of pyrazinamide during pregnancy is recommended by The World Health Organization (Blumberg, 2003).

Pyrethrins and Piperonyl Butoxide
(pye RE thrins & pi PER oh nil byo TOKS ide)

Brand Names: U.S. A-200® Lice Treatment Kit [OTC]; A-200® Maximum Strength [OTC]; Licide® [OTC]; Pronto® Complete Lice Removal System [OTC]; Pronto® Plus Lice Killing Mousse Plus Vitamin E [OTC]; Pronto® Plus Lice Killing Mousse Shampoo Plus Natural Extracts and Oils [OTC]; Pronto® Plus Warm Oil Treatment and Conditioner [OTC]; RID® Maximum Strength [OTC]
Brand Names: Canada Pronto® Lice Control; R & C™ II; R & C™ Shampoo/Conditioner; RID® Mousse
Pharmacologic Category Antiparasitic Agent, Topical; Pediculocide; Shampoo, Pediculocide
Use Treatment of *Pediculus humanus* infestations (head lice, body lice, pubic lice, and their eggs)
Local Anesthetic/Vasoconstrictor Precautions No information available to require special precautions
Effects on Dental Treatment No significant effects or complications reported
Effects on Bleeding No information available to require special precautions
Adverse Effects Frequency not defined.
Dermatologic: Pruritus
Local: Burning, stinging, irritation with repeat use

General Dosage Range Topical: *Children and Adults:* Apply to infested area, keep on for 10 minutes, wash, and rinse; may repeat once in a 24-hour period and then again in 7-10 days

Mechanism of Action Pyrethrins are derived from flowers that belong to the chrysanthemum family. The mechanism of action on the neuronal membranes of lice is similar to that of DDT. Piperonyl butoxide is usually added to pyrethrin to enhance the product's activity by decreasing the metabolism of pyrethrins in arthropods.

Pharmacodynamics/Kinetics

Onset of Action ~30 minutes

Pregnancy Risk Factor C

Pregnancy Considerations Pregnant women may be treated with pyrethrins and piperonyl butoxide (CDC, 2010).

Pyridostigmine (peer id oh STIG meen)

Brand Names: U.S. Mestinon®; Mestinon® Timespan®; Regonol®

Brand Names: Canada Mestinon®; Mestinon®-SR

Pharmacologic Category Acetylcholinesterase Inhibitor

Use Symptomatic treatment of myasthenia gravis; antagonism of nondepolarizing neuromuscular blockers

Military use: Pretreatment for Soman nerve gas exposure

Local Anesthetic/Vasoconstrictor Precautions No information available to require special precautions

Effects on Dental Treatment Key adverse event(s) related to dental treatment: Dysphagia.

Effects on Bleeding No information available to require special precautions

Adverse Effects Frequency not defined.

Cardiovascular: Arrhythmias (especially bradycardia), AV block, cardiac arrest, decreased carbon monoxide, flushing, hypotension, nodal rhythm, nonspecific ECG changes, syncope, tachycardia

Central nervous system: Convulsions, dizziness, drowsiness, dysphonia, headache, loss of consciousness

Dermatologic: Skin rash, thrombophlebitis (I.V.), urticaria

Gastrointestinal: Abdominal pain, diarrhea, dysphagia, flatulence, hyperperistalsis, nausea, salivation, stomach cramps, vomiting

Genitourinary: Urinary urgency

Neuromuscular & skeletal: Arthralgia, dysarthria, fasciculations, muscle cramps, myalgia, spasms, weakness

Ocular: Amblyopia, lacrimation, small pupils

Respiratory: Bronchial secretions increased, bronchiolar constriction, bronchospasm, dyspnea, laryngospasm, respiratory arrest, respiratory depression, respiratory muscle paralysis

Miscellaneous: Allergic reactions, anaphylaxis, diaphoresis increased

General Dosage Range

I.M.:
Children: 0.05-0.15 mg/kg/dose
Adults: ~1/30th of oral dose

I.V.:
Children: 0.05-0.25 mg/kg/dose
Adults: IVP: ~1/30th of oral dose **or** 0.1-0.25 mg/kg/dose (usual: 10-20 mg); Infusion: 2 mg/hour with gradual titration in increments of 0.5-1 mg/hour (maximum: 4 mg/hour)

Oral:
Immediate release:
Children: 7 mg/kg/day divided into 5-6 doses

Adults: 60-1500 mg/day in 5-6 divided doses (usual: 600 mg/day)
Sustained release: *Adults:* 180-540 mg once or twice daily (doses separated by at least 6 hours)

Mechanism of Action Inhibits destruction of acetylcholine by acetylcholinesterase which facilitates transmission of impulses across myoneural junction

Pharmacodynamics/Kinetics

Onset of Action Oral, I.M.: 15-30 minutes; I.V. injection: 2-5 minutes

Duration of Action Oral: Up to 6-8 hours (due to slow absorption); I.V.: 2-3 hours

Half-life Elimination 1-2 hours; Renal failure: ≤6 hours

Pregnancy Risk Factor B

Pregnancy Considerations Safety has not been established for use during pregnancy. The potential benefit to the mother should outweigh the potential risk to the fetus. When pyridostigmine is needed in myasthenic mothers, giving dose parenterally 1 hour before completion of the second stage of labor may facilitate delivery and protect the neonate during the immediate postnatal state.

Pyridoxine (peer i DOKS een)

Brand Names: U.S. Aminoxin® [OTC]; Pyri-500 [OTC]

Pharmacologic Category Vitamin, Water Soluble

Use Prevention and treatment of vitamin B_6 deficiency

Unlabeled Use Treatment and prophylaxis of neurological toxicities (ie, seizures, coma) associated with isoniazid and Gyromitrin-containing mushroom (false morel) overdose/toxicity; nausea and vomiting of pregnancy; prevention of peripheral neuropathy associated with isoniazid therapy for *Mycobacterium tuberculosis*

Local Anesthetic/Vasoconstrictor Precautions No information available to require special precautions

Effects on Dental Treatment No significant effects or complications reported

Effects on Bleeding No information available to require special precautions

Adverse Effects Frequency not defined.

Central nervous system: Headache, seizure (following very large I.V. doses), somnolence

Endocrine & metabolic: Acidosis, folic acid decreased

Gastrointestinal: Nausea

Hepatic: AST increased

Neuromuscular & skeletal: Neuropathy, paresthesia

Miscellaneous: Allergic reactions

General Dosage Range

I.M., I.V.: *Adults:* 10-20 mg/day

Oral:
Infants 1-6 months: Adequate intake: 0.1 mg/day
Infants 7-12 months: Adequate intake: 0.3 mg/day
Children 1-3 years: RDA: 0.5 mg
Children 4-8 years: RDA: 0.6 mg
Children 9-13 years: RDA: 1 mg
Children 14-18 years: RDA: 1.2 mg (females); 1.3 mg (males)
Adults 19-50 years: RDA: 1.3 mg
Adults ≥51 years: RDA: 1.5 mg (females); 1.7 mg (males)
Pregnancy: RDA: 1.9 mg
Lactation: RDA: 2 mg

Mechanism of Action Precursor to pyridoxal, which functions in the metabolism of proteins, carbohydrates, and fats; pyridoxal also aids in the release of liver and muscle-stored glycogen and in the synthesis of GABA (within the central nervous system) and heme

◄ **Pharmacodynamics/Kinetics**
Half-life Elimination Biologic: 15-20 days
Pregnancy Risk Factor A
Pregnancy Considerations Water soluble vitamins cross the placenta. Maternal pyridoxine plasma concentrations may decrease as pregnancy progresses and requirements may be increased in pregnant women (IOM, 1998). Pyridoxine is used to treat nausea and vomiting of pregnancy (Neibyl, 2010). In addition to being a dietary supplement, pyridoxine is also used as an antidote. In general, medications used as antidotes should take into consideration the health and prognosis of the mother (Bailey, 2003).

Pyrimethamine (peer i METH a meen)

Brand Names: U.S. Daraprim®
Brand Names: Canada Daraprim®
Pharmacologic Category Antimalarial Agent
Use Prophylaxis of malaria due to susceptible strains of plasmodia; used in conjunction with a sulfonamide for the treatment of uncomplicated malaria due to susceptible strains of plasmodia (alternative agent; not preferred therapy); synergistic combination with sulfonamide in treatment of toxoplasmosis
Local Anesthetic/Vasoconstrictor Precautions No information available to require special precautions
Effects on Dental Treatment Key adverse event(s) related to dental treatment: Xerostomia (normal salivary flow resumes upon discontinuation). Atrophic glossitis has been reported.
Effects on Bleeding No information available to require special precautions
Adverse Effects Frequency not defined.
Cardiovascular: Arrhythmias (large doses)
Dermatologic: Erythema multiforme, rash, Stevens-Johnson syndrome, toxic epidermal necrolysis
Gastrointestinal: Anorexia, atrophic glossitis, vomiting
Hematologic: Leukopenia, megaloblastic anemia, pancytopenia, pulmonary eosinophilia, thrombocytopenia
Genitourinary: Hematuria
Miscellaneous: Anaphylaxis
General Dosage Range Oral:
Children <4 years: Malaria prophylaxis: 6.25 mg once weekly (maximum: 25 mg/dose)
Children 4-10 years: Malaria prophylaxis: 12.5 mg once weekly (maximum: 25 mg/dose); Malaria treatment: 25 mg daily
Children >10 years: Malaria prophylaxis: 25 mg once weekly; Malaria treatment: 25 mg daily
Children: Toxoplasmosis treatment: Loading dose: 1 mg/kg/day divided into 2 equal doses for 2-4 days; Maintenance: 0.5 mg/kg/day divided into 2 doses (maximum: 25 mg/day)
Adults: Malaria prophylaxis: 25 mg once weekly; Malaria treatment: 25-50 mg daily; Toxoplasmosis treatment: Initial: 50-75 mg/day; Maintenance: 12.5-37.5 mg/day
Mechanism of Action Inhibits parasitic dihydrofolate reductase, resulting in inhibition of vital tetrahydrofolic acid synthesis
Pharmacodynamics/Kinetics
Onset of Action ~1 hour
Half-life Elimination 80-95 hours
Time to Peak Serum: 1.5-8 hours
Pregnancy Risk Factor C

Pregnancy Considerations Teratogenic effects have been observed in animal reproduction studies. If administered during pregnancy (ie, for toxoplasmosis), supplementation of folate is strongly recommended. Pregnancy should be avoided during therapy.

Pyrithione Zinc (peer i THYE one zingk)

Brand Names: U.S. BetaMed™ [OTC]; DermaZinc™ [OTC]; DHS™ Zinc [OTC]; Head & Shoulders® Citrus Breeze 2-in-1 [OTC]; Head & Shoulders® Citrus Breeze [OTC]; Head & Shoulders® Classic Clean 2-in-1 [OTC]; Head & Shoulders® Classic Clean [OTC]; Head & Shoulders® Dry Scalp 2-in-1 [OTC]; Head & Shoulders® Dry Scalp Care 2-in-1 [OTC]; Head & Shoulders® Dry Scalp Care [OTC]; Head & Shoulders® Dry Scalp [OTC]; Head & Shoulders® Extra Volume [OTC]; Head & Shoulders® intensive solutions 2 in 1 [OTC]; Head & Shoulders® intensive solutions for dry/damaged hair [OTC]; Head & Shoulders® intensive solutions for fine/oily hair [OTC]; Head & Shoulders® intensive solutions for normal hair [OTC]; Head & Shoulders® Ocean Lift 2-in-1 [OTC]; Head & Shoulders® Ocean Lift [OTC]; Head & Shoulders® Refresh 2-in-1 [OTC]; Head & Shoulders® Refresh [OTC]; Head & Shoulders® Restoring Shine 2 in 1 [OTC]; Head & Shoulders® Restoring Shine [OTC]; Head & Shoulders® Sensitive Care 2 in 1 [OTC]; Head & Shoulders® Sensitive Care [OTC]; Head & Shoulders® Smooth & Silky 2-in-1 [OTC]; Head & Shoulders® Smooth & Silky [OTC]; Selsun blue® Itchy Dry Scalp [OTC]; Skin Care™ [OTC]; T/Gel® Daily Control 2 in 1 Dandruff Shampoo Plus Conditioner [OTC]; T/Gel® Daily Control Dandruff Shampoo [OTC]; Zincon® [OTC]; ZNP® [OTC]
Pharmacologic Category Topical Skin Product
Use Relieves the itching, irritation, and scalp flaking associated with dandruff and/or seborrheal dermatitis
Local Anesthetic/Vasoconstrictor Precautions No information available to require special precautions
Effects on Dental Treatment No significant effects or complications reported
Effects on Bleeding No information available to require special precautions
General Dosage Range Topical: Adults: Apply at least twice weekly

Quazepam (KWAZ e pam)

Brand Names: U.S. Doral®
Brand Names: Canada Doral®
Pharmacologic Category Benzodiazepine
Use Treatment of insomnia
Local Anesthetic/Vasoconstrictor Precautions No information available to require special precautions
Effects on Dental Treatment Key adverse event(s) related to dental treatment: Xerostomia (normal salivary flow resumes upon discontinuation) and abnormal taste perception.
Effects on Bleeding No information available to require special precautions
Adverse Effects
>10%: Central nervous system: Daytime drowsiness (12%)
<10%:
Central nervous system: Headache (5%), dizziness (2%), fatigue (2%)
Gastrointestinal: Xerostomia (2%), dyspepsia (1%)

Frequency not defined. **Note:** Asterisked (*) reactions are those reported with benzodiazepines.

Cardiovascular: Palpitation

Central nervous system: Abnormal thinking, agitation, amnesia, anxiety, apathy, ataxia, confusion, depression, dystonia*, euphoria, hallucinations*, hyper-/hypokinesia, incoordination, irritability*, malaise, nervousness, nightmare, paranoid reaction, sleep disturbances*, slurred speech*, speech disorder, stimulation*

Dermatologic: Pruritus, rash

Endocrine & metabolic: Libido decreased, menstrual irregularities*

Gastrointestinal: Abdominal pain, abnormal taste perception, anorexia, constipation, diarrhea, nausea

Genitourinary: Impotence, incontinence, urinary retention*

Hepatic: Jaundice*

Neuromuscular & skeletal: Dysarthria*, muscle spasticity*, tremor, weakness

Ocular: Abnormal vision, cataract

Miscellaneous: Drug dependence, withdrawal*

General Dosage Range Oral:
Adults: 7.5-15 mg at bedtime
Elderly: Initial: 7.5 mg at bedtime

Mechanism of Action Binds to stereospecific benzodiazepine receptors on the postsynaptic GABA neuron at several sites within the central nervous system, including the limbic system, reticular formation. Enhancement of the inhibitory effect of GABA on neuronal excitability results by increased neuronal membrane permeability to chloride ions. This shift in chloride ions results in hyperpolarization (a less excitable state) and stabilization.

Pharmacodynamics/Kinetics

Half-life Elimination Serum: Quazepam, 2-oxoquasepam: 39 hours; N-desalkyl-2-oxoquazepam: 73 hours

Time to Peak ~2 hours

Pregnancy Risk Factor X

Pregnancy Considerations Although information specific to the use of quazepam has not been located, all benzodiazepines are assumed to cross the placenta. Teratogenic effects have been observed with some benzodiazepines; however, additional studies are needed. The incidence of premature birth and low birth weights may be increased following maternal use of benzodiazepines; hypoglycemia and respiratory problems in the neonate may occur following exposure late in pregnancy. Neonatal withdrawal symptoms may occur within days to weeks after birth and "floppy infant syndrome" (which also includes withdrawal symptoms) have been reported with some benzodiazepines. Use during pregnancy is contraindicated.

Controlled Substance C-IV

QUEtiapine (kwe TYE a peen)

Related Information
Clinical Risk Related to Drugs Prolonging QT Interval *on page 1510*

Brand Names: U.S. SEROquel XR®; SEROquel®

Brand Names: Canada Apo-Quetiapine®; Auro-Quetiapine; Ava-Quetiapine; CO Quetiapine; Dom-Quetiapine; JAMP-Quetiapine; Mylan-Quetiapine; PHL-Quetiapine; PMS-Quetiapine; PRO-Quetiapine; ratio-Quetiapine; Riva-Quetiapine; Sandoz-Quetiapine; Seroquel XR®; Seroquel®; Teva-Quetiapine; Teva-Quetiapine XR

Generic Availability (U.S.) Yes: Excludes extended release tablet

Pharmacologic Category Antipsychotic Agent, Atypical

Use Treatment of schizophrenia; treatment of acute manic or mixed episodes associated with bipolar I disorder (as monotherapy or in combination with lithium or divalproex); maintenance treatment of bipolar I disorder (in combination with lithium or divalproex); treatment of acute depressive episodes associated with bipolar disorder; adjunctive treatment of major depressive disorder

Unlabeled Use Autism; delirium in the critically-ill patient; psychosis/agitation related to Alzheimer's dementia

Local Anesthetic/Vasoconstrictor Precautions Quetiapine is one of the drugs confirmed to prolong the QT interval and is accepted as having a risk of causing torsade de pointes. The risk of drug-induced torsade de pointes is extremely low when a single QT interval prolonging drug is prescribed. In terms of epinephrine, it is not known what effect vasoconstrictors in the local anesthetic regimen will have in patients with a known history of congenital prolonged QT interval or in patients taking any medication that prolongs the QT interval. Until more information is obtained, it is suggested that the clinician consult with the physician prior to the use of a vasoconstrictor in suspected patients, and that the vasoconstrictor (epinephrine, mepivacaine and levonordefrin [Carbocaine® 2% with Neo-Cobefrin®]) be used with caution.

Effects on Dental Treatment Key adverse event(s) related to dental treatment: Xerostomia (normal salivary flow resumes upon discontinuation).

Effects on Bleeding No information available to require special precautions

Adverse Effects Actual frequency may be dependent upon dose and/or indication. Unless otherwise noted, frequency of adverse effects is reported for adult patients; spectrum and incidence of adverse effects similar in children (with significant exceptions noted).

>10%:

Cardiovascular: Diastolic blood pressure increased (children and adolescents, 41%), systolic blood pressure increased (children and adolescents, 15%)

Central nervous system: Somnolence (18% to 57%), headache (7% to 21%), agitation (5% to 20%), dizziness (1% to 18%), fatigue (3% to 14%), extrapyramidal symptoms (1% to 13%)

Endocrine & metabolic: Triglycerides increased (≥200 mg/dL, 8% to 22%), HDL cholesterol decreased (≤40 mg/dL, 6% to 19%), total cholesterol increased (≥240 mg/dL, 7% to 18%), LDL cholesterol increased (≥160 mg/dL, 4% to 17%), hyperglycemia (≥200 mg/dL post glucose challenge or fasting glucose ≥126 mg/dL, 2% to 12%)

Gastrointestinal: Xerostomia (9% to 44%), weight gain (dose related; 3% to 23%), appetite increased (2% to 12%), constipation (6% to 11%)

1% to 10%:

Cardiovascular: Orthostatic hypotension (2% to 7%; children and adolescents <1%), tachycardia (1% to 6%), syncope (<5%), palpitation (4%), peripheral edema (4%), hypotension (3%), hypertension (1% to 2%)

Central nervous system: Insomnia (9%), akathisia (≤8%), pain (1% to 7%), dystonia (≤6%), lethargy (1% to 5%), tardive dyskinesia (<5%), anxiety (2% to 4%), irritability (1% to 4%), parkinsonism (≤4%), abnormal dreams (2% to 3%), depression (1% to 3%), hypersomnia (1% to 3%), abnormal thinking (2%), ataxia (2%), attention disturbance (2%), coordination impaired (2%), disorientation (2%), hypoesthesia (2%), mental impairment (2%), migraine (2%), sluggishness (2%), vertigo (2%), confusion (1% to 2%), restlessness (1% to 2%), fever (1% to 2%), chills (1%)

Dermatologic: Rash (4%), hyperhidrosis (2%)

Endocrine & metabolic: Hyperprolactinemia (4%), libido decreased (≤2%), hypothyroidism (≤2%), female lactation (1%)

Gastrointestinal: Nausea (7% to 8%), abdominal pain (dose related; 4% to 7%), dyspepsia (dose related; 2% to 7%), vomiting (1% to 6%), drooling (<5%), gastroenteritis (2% to 4%), toothache (2% to 3%), appetite decreased (2%), dysphagia (2%), flatulence (2%), GERD (2%), anorexia (≥1%), abnormal taste (1%), abdominal distension (≤1%)

Genitourinary: Pollakiuria (2%), urinary tract infection (2%), impotence (1%)

Hematologic: Neutropenia (≤2%), leukopenia (≥1%), hemorrhage (1%)

Hepatic: Transaminases increased (1% to 6%), GGT increased (1%)

Neuromuscular & skeletal: Weakness (2% to 10%), tremor (2% to 8%), back pain (3% to 5%), dysarthria (1% to 5%), hypertonia (4%), twitching (4%), dyskinesia (≤4%), arthralgia (1% to 4%), paresthesia (3%), muscle spasm (1% to 3%), limb pain (2%), myalgia (2%), neck pain (2%), neck rigidity (1%)

Ocular: Blurred vision (1% to 4%), amblyopia (2% to 3%)

Otic: Ear pain (1% to 2%)

Respiratory: Pharyngitis (4% to 6%), nasal congestion (5%), rhinitis (3% to 4%), upper respiratory tract infection (2% to 3%), sinus congestion (2%), sinus headache (2%), sinusitis (2%), cough (3%), dyspnea (≥1%), dry throat (1%)

Miscellaneous: Diaphoresis (2%), restless legs syndrome (2%), flu-like syndrome (1% to 2%), lymphadenopathy (1%)

Dosage Oral:

Children ≥10 years: **Note:** Total daily doses may also be divided into 3 doses per day.

Bipolar disorder:

Mania: Immediate release tablet: Initial: 25 mg twice daily on day 1; increase to 50 mg twice daily on day 2, further increasing by 100 mg/day each day until a target dose of 400 mg/day is reached on day 5. May increase up to 600 mg/day at increments ≤100 mg/day; however, no additional benefit seen with 600 mg/day. Usual dosage range: 400-600 mg/day.

Maintenance therapy: Immediate release tablet: Continue therapy at lowest dose needed to maintain remission; periodically assess maintenance treatment needs.

Autism (unlabeled use): 100-350 mg/day (1.6-5.2 mg/kg/day) (Martin, 1999)

Adolescents ≥13 years: **Note:** Total daily doses may also be divided into 3 doses per day: Schizophrenia: Immediate release tablet: Initial: 25 mg twice daily on day 1; increase to 50 mg twice daily on day 2, further increasing by 100 mg/day each day until a target dose of 400 mg/day is reached on day 5. May increase up to

800 mg/day at increments ≤100 mg/day; however, no additional benefit seen with 800 mg/day. Usual dosage range: 400-800 mg/day; periodically assess maintenance treatment needs.

Adults:

Bipolar disorder:

Depression:

Immediate release tablet: Initial: 50 mg once daily the first day; increase to 100 mg once daily on day 2, further increasing by 100 mg/day each day until a target dose of 300 mg once daily is reached by day 4. Further increases up to 600 mg once daily by day 8 have been evaluated in clinical trials, but no additional antidepressant efficacy was noted.

Extended release tablet: Initial: 50 mg/day the first day; increase to 100 mg on day 2, further increasing by 100 mg/day each day until a target dose of 300 mg/day is reached by day 4.

Mania:

Immediate release tablet: Initial: 50 mg twice daily on day 1, increase dose in increments of 100 mg/day to 200 mg twice daily on day 4; may increase to a target dose of 800 mg/day by day 6 at increments ≤200 mg/day. Usual dosage range: 400-800 mg/day.

Extended release tablet: Initial: 300 mg on day 1; increase to 600 mg on day 2 and adjust dose to 400-800 mg once daily on day 3, depending on response and tolerance.

Maintenance therapy: Immediate release tablet: 200-400 mg twice daily with lithium or divalproex; **Note:** Average time of stabilization was 15 weeks in clinical trials.

Major depressive disorder (adjunct to antidepressants): Extended release tablet: Initial: 50 mg once daily; may be increased to 150 mg on day 3. Usual dosage range: 150-300 mg/day

Schizophrenia/psychoses:

Immediate release tablet: Initial: 25 mg twice daily; followed by increases in the total daily dose on the second and third day in increments of 25-50 mg divided 2-3 times/day, if tolerated, to a target dose of 300-400 mg/day in 2-3 divided doses by day 4. Make further adjustments as needed at intervals of at least 2 days in adjustments of 25-50 mg divided twice daily. Usual maintenance range: 300-800 mg/day.

Extended release tablet: Initial: 300 mg once daily; increase in increments of up to 300 mg/day (in intervals of ≥1 day). Usual maintenance range: 400-800 mg/day.

Note: Dose reductions should be attempted periodically to establish lowest effective dose in patients with psychosis. Patients being restarted after 1 week of no drug need to be titrated as above.

ICU delirium: Initial: 50 mg twice daily; may increase as necessary on a daily basis in increments of 50 mg twice daily to a maximum dose of 400 mg/day (Devlin, 2010)

Elderly: 40% lower mean oral clearance of quetiapine in adults >65 years of age; higher plasma levels expected and, therefore, dosage adjustment may be needed; elderly patients usually require 50-200 mg/day of immediate release tablets or 50 mg/day of extended release tablets with a slower titration schedule. Increase immediate release dose by 25-50 mg/day or extended release dose by 50 mg/day to effective dose, based on clinical response and tolerability. If initiated with immediate release tablets, patient may transition to extended release formulation (at equivalent total daily dose) when effective dose has been reached. See **"Note"** in adult dosing.

Psychosis/agitation related to Alzheimer's dementia (unlabeled use): Initial: 12.5-50 mg/day; if necessary, gradually increase as tolerated not to exceed 200-300 mg/day (Rabins, 2007)

Dosing comments in renal insufficiency: 25% lower mean oral clearance of quetiapine than normal subjects; however, plasma concentrations similar to normal subjects receiving the same dose; no dosage adjustment required

Dosing comments in hepatic insufficiency: 30% lower mean oral clearance of quetiapine than normal subjects; higher plasma levels expected in hepatically impaired subjects; dosage adjustment may be needed

Immediate release tablet: Initial: 25 mg/day, increase dose by 25-50 mg/day to effective dose, based on clinical response and tolerability to patient. If initiated with immediate-release formulation, patient may transition to extended-release formulation (at equivalent total daily dose) when effective dose has been reached.

Extended release tablet: Initial: 50 mg/day; increase dose by 50 mg/day to effective dose, based on clinical response and tolerability to patient.

Mechanism of Action Quetiapine is a dibenzothiazepine atypical antipsychotic. It has been proposed that this drug's antipsychotic activity is mediated through a combination of dopamine type 2 (D_2) and serotonin type 2 (5-HT_2) antagonism. It is an antagonist at multiple neurotransmitter receptors in the brain: Serotonin 5-HT_{1A} and 5-HT_2, dopamine D_1 and D_2, histamine H_1, and adrenergic alpha$_1$- and alpha$_2$-receptors; but appears to have no appreciable affinity at cholinergic muscarinic and benzodiazepine receptors. Norquetiapine, an active metabolite, differs from its parent molecule by exhibiting high affinity for muscarinic M1 receptors.

Antagonism at receptors other than dopamine and 5-HT_2 with similar receptor affinities may explain some of the other effects of quetiapine. The drug's antagonism of histamine H_1-receptors may explain the somnolence observed. The drug's antagonism of adrenergic alpha$_1$-receptors may explain the orthostatic hypotension observed.

Contraindications There are no contraindications listed in manufacturer's labeling.

Canadian labeling: Hypersensitivity to quetiapine or any component of the formulation

Warnings/Precautions [U.S. Boxed Warning]: Antidepressants increase the risk of suicidal thinking and behavior in children, adolescents, and young adults (18-24 years of age) with major depressive disorder (MDD) and other psychiatric disorders; consider risk prior to prescribing. Short-term studies did not show an increased risk in patients >24 years of age and showed a decreased risk in patients ≥65 years. Closely monitor all patients for clinical worsening, suicidality, or unusual changes in behavior; particularly during the initial 1-2 months of therapy or during periods of dosage adjustments (increased or decreases); the patient's family or caregiver should be instructed to closely observe the patient and communicate condition with healthcare provider. A medication guide concerning the use of antidepressants should be dispensed with each prescription.

[U.S. Boxed Warning]: Elderly patients with dementia-related psychosis treated with antipsychotics are at an increased risk of death compared to placebo. Most deaths appeared to be either cardiovascular (eg, heart failure, sudden death) or infectious (eg, pneumonia) in nature. Quetiapine is not approved for the treatment of dementia-related psychosis.

Leukopenia, neutropenia, and agranulocytosis (sometimes fatal) have been reported in clinical trials and postmarketing reports with antipsychotic use; presence of risk factors (eg, pre-existing low WBC or history of drug-induced leuko-/neutropenia) should prompt periodic blood count assessment. Discontinue therapy at first signs of blood dyscrasias or if absolute neutrophil count <1000/mm^3.

May be sedating, use with caution in disorders where CNS depression is a feature. Use with caution in Parkinson's disease. May induce orthostatic hypotension associated with dizziness, tachycardia, and, in some cases, syncope, especially during the initial dose titration period. Should be used with particular caution in patients with known cardiovascular disease (history of MI or ischemic heart disease, heart failure, or conduction abnormalities), cerebrovascular disease, or conditions that predispose to hypotension. Use has been associated with QT prolongation; postmarketing reports have occurred in patients with concomitant illness, quetiapine overdose, or who were receiving concomitant therapy known to affect QT interval or cause electrolyte imbalance. Esophageal dysmotility and aspiration have been associated with antipsychotic use; use with caution in patients at risk of aspiration pneumonia (eg, Alzheimer's disease). May cause dose-related decreases in thyroid levels, including cases requiring thyroid replacement therapy. Development of cataracts has been observed in animal studies; lens changes have been observed in humans during long-term treatment. Lens examination on initiation of therapy and every 6 months thereafter is recommended.

Due to anticholinergic effects, use with caution in patients with decreased gastrointestinal motility, urinary retention, BPH, xerostomia, visual problems, and narrow-angle glaucoma. Relative to other antipsychotics, quetiapine has a moderate potency of cholinergic blockade. May cause extrapyramidal symptoms (EPS), pseudoparkinsonism, and/or tardive dyskinesia. Risk of dystonia (and probably other EPS) may be greater with increased doses, use of conventional antipsychotics, males, and younger patients. Impaired core body temperature regulation may occur; caution with strenuous exercise, heat exposure, dehydration, and concomitant medication possessing anticholinergic effects. Neuroleptic malignant syndrome (NMS) is a potentially fatal symptom complex that has been reported in association with administration of antipsychotic drugs. Clinical manifestations of NMS are hyperpyrexia, muscle rigidity, altered mental status, and evidence of autonomic instability (irregular pulse or blood pressure, tachycardia, diaphoresis, and cardiac dysrhythmia). Management of NMS should include immediate discontinuation of antipsychotic drugs and other drugs not essential to concurrent therapy, intensive symptomatic treatment and medication monitoring, and treatment of any concomitant medical problems for which specific treatment are available.

Use caution in patients with a history of seizures. May cause decreases in total free thyroxine, elevations of liver enzymes, cholesterol levels, and/or triglyceride increases. Rare cases of priapism have been reported. May increase prolactin levels; clinical significance of hyperprolactinemia in patients with breast cancer or other prolactin-dependent tumors is unknown.

Use in elderly patients with dementia is associated with an increased risk of mortality and cerebrovascular accidents; avoid antipsychotic use for behavioral problems associated with dementia unless alternative nonpharmacologic therapies have failed and patient may harm self or others. In addition, use may cause or exacerbate syndrome of inappropriate antidiuretic hormone secretion or hyponatremia; monitor sodium closely with initiation or dosage adjustments in older adults (Beers Criteria).

May cause hyperglycemia; in some cases may be extreme and associated with ketoacidosis, hyperosmolar coma, or death. Use with caution in patients with diabetes or other disorders of glucose regulation; monitor for worsening of glucose control. Significant weight gain has been observed with antipsychotic therapy; incidence varies with product. Monitor waist circumference and BMI. Patients using immediate release tablets may be switched to extended release tablets at the same total daily dose taken once daily. Dosage adjustments may be necessary based on response and tolerability. May cause withdrawal symptoms (rare) with abrupt cessation; gradually taper dose during discontinuation.

Drug Interactions

Metabolism/Transport Effects Substrate of CYP2D6 (minor), CYP3A4 (major); **Note:** Assignment of Major/Minor substrate status based on clinically relevant drug interaction potential

Avoid Concomitant Use

Avoid concomitant use of QUEtiapine with any of the following: Aclidinium; Azelastine (Nasal); Conivaptan; Highest Risk QTc-Prolonging Agents; Ipratropium (Oral Inhalation); Ivabradine; Metoclopramide; Mifepristone; Moderate Risk QTc-Prolonging Agents; Paraldehyde; Tiotropium

Increased Effect/Toxicity

QUEtiapine may increase the levels/effects of: Alcohol (Ethyl); Anticholinergics; Azelastine (Nasal); Buprenorphine; CNS Depressants; Highest Risk QTc-Prolonging Agents; Methotrimeprazine; Methylphenidate; Paraldehyde; Serotonin Modulators; Tiotropium; Zolpidem

The levels/effects of QUEtiapine may be increased by: Acetylcholinesterase Inhibitors (Central); Aclidinium; Conivaptan; CYP3A4 Inhibitors (Moderate); CYP3A4 Inhibitors (Strong); Dasatinib; HydrOXYzine; Ipratropium (Oral Inhalation); Ivabradine; Ivacaftor; Lithium formulations; Magnesium Sulfate; Methotrimeprazine; Methylphenidate; Metoclopramide; Metyrosine; Mifepristone; Moderate Risk QTc-Prolonging Agents; Perampanel; Pramlintide; QTc-Prolonging Agents (Indeterminate Risk and Risk Modifying); Sodium Oxybate; Tetrabenazine

Decreased Effect

QUEtiapine may decrease the levels/effects of: Amphetamines; Anti-Parkinson's Agents (Dopamine Agonist); Quinagolide

The levels/effects of QUEtiapine may be decreased by: CYP3A4 Inducers (Strong); Deferasirox; Fosphenytoin; Lithium formulations; Peginterferon Alfa-2b; Phenytoin; Tocilizumab

Ethanol/Nutrition/Herb Interactions

Ethanol: May increase CNS depression; monitor for increased effects with coadministration. Caution patients about effects.

Food: In healthy volunteers, administration of quetiapine (immediate release) with food resulted in an increase in the peak serum concentration and AUC by 25% and 15%, respectively, compared to the fasting state. Administration of the extended release formulation with a high-fat meal (~800-1000 calories) resulted in an increase in peak serum concentration by 44% to 52% and AUC by 20% to 22% for the 50 mg and 300 mg tablets; administration with a light meal (≤300 calories) had no significant effect on the C_{max} or AUC.

Herb/Nutraceutical: St John's wort may decrease quetiapine levels. Avoid valerian, St John's wort, kava kava, gotu kola (may increase CNS depression).

Dietary Considerations Immediate-release tablet may be taken without regard to meals. Extended release tablet should be taken without food or with a light meal (≤300 calories).

Pharmacodynamics/Kinetics

Half-life Elimination

Mean: Terminal: Quetiapine: ~6 hours; Extended release: ~7 hours

Metabolite: N-desalkyl quetiapine: 9-12 hours

Time to Peak Plasma: Immediate release: 1.5 hours; Extended release: 6 hours

Pregnancy Risk Factor C

Pregnancy Considerations Quetiapine was embryo and fetal toxic, but not teratogenic in animal reproduction studies. Congenital malformations have not been observed in humans (based on limited data). The long term effects of *in utero* exposure on infant development and behavior are not known. Antipsychotic use during the third trimester of pregnancy has a risk for abnormal muscle movements (extrapyramidal symptoms [EPS]) and withdrawal symptoms in newborns following delivery. Symptoms in the newborn may include agitation, feeding disorder, hypertonia, hypotonia, respiratory distress, somnolence, and tremor; these effects may be self-limiting or require hospitalization. Treatment algorithms have been developed by the ACOG and the APA for the management of depression in women prior to conception and during pregnancy (Yonkers, 2009). Healthcare providers are encouraged to enroll women 18-45 years of age exposed to quetiapine during pregnancy in the Atypical Antipsychotics Pregnancy Registry (1-866-961-2388 or http://www.womensmentalhealth.org/pregnancyregistry).

Lactation Enters breast milk/not recommended

Breast-Feeding Considerations Based on information from 8 mother/infant pairs, concentrations of quetiapine in breast milk have been reported as 0-170 µg/L. The estimated exposure to the breast-feeding infant would be up to 1 mg/kg/day (relative infant dose up to 0.43% based on a weight adjusted maternal dose of 400 mg/day).

Dosage Forms

Tablet, oral: 25 mg, 50 mg, 100 mg, 200 mg, 300 mg, 400 mg

SEROquel®: 25 mg, 50 mg, 100 mg, 200 mg, 300 mg, 400 mg

Tablet, extended release, oral:

SEROquel XR®: 50 mg, 150 mg, 200 mg, 300 mg, 400 mg

Dental Comment Quetiapine is known to prolong the QT interval. The QT interval is measured as the time and distance between the Q point of the QRS complex and the end of the T wave in the ECG tracing. After adjustment for heart rate, the QT interval is defined as prolonged if it is more than 450 msec in men and 460 msec in women. A long QT syndrome was first described in the 1950s and 60s as a congenital syndrome involving QT interval prolongation and syncope and sudden death. Some of the congenital long QT syndromes were characterized by a peculiar electrocardiographic appearance of the QRS complex involving a premature atria beat followed by a pause, then a subsequent sinus beat showing marked QT prolongation and deformity. This type of cardiac arrhythmia was originally termed "torsade de pointes" (translated from the French as "twisting of the points"). Quetiapine is considered as having a risk of causing torsade de pointes. Since it is not known what effect vasoconstrictors in the local anesthetic regimen will have in patients with a known history of congenital prolonged QT interval or in patients taking any medication that prolongs the QT interval, a medical consult is suggested.

Quinagolide (kwin AG o lide)

Brand Names: Canada Norprolac®
Pharmacologic Category Hyperprolactinemia Agent, Dopamine (D_2) Agonist
Use Treatment of hyperprolactinemia due to prolactin-secreting pituitary tumors (microadenoma or macroadenoma) or idiopathic in nature
Local Anesthetic/Vasoconstrictor Precautions No information available to require special precautions
Effects on Dental Treatment No significant effects or complications reported
Effects on Bleeding No information available to require special precautions
Adverse Effects
>10%:
  Central nervous system: Dizziness, fatigue, headache
  Gastrointestinal: Nausea, vomiting
1% to 10%:
  Cardiovascular: Edema (2%), flushing (1%), hypotension (1%), palpitation (1%), syncope (1%)
  Central nervous system: Sedation (3%), insomnia (2%), concentration decreased (1%), malaise (1%), mood lability (1%)
  Gastrointestinal: Abdominal pain/discomfort (3%), constipation (3%), anorexia (2%), dyspepsia (2%), diarrhea (1%), weight gain (1%)
  Endocrine & metabolic: Breast pain (1%)
  Neuromuscular & skeletal: Weakness (3%), extremity pain (1%)
  Respiratory: Nasal congestion (2%)
General Dosage Range Oral: *Adults:* Initial: 0.025 mg/day for 3 days followed by 0.05 mg/day for 3 days; Maintenance (begin day 7): Usual range 0.075-0.15 mg/day (maximum: 0.9 mg/day)
Mechanism of Action Selective dopamine D_2 receptor agonist that exerts a direct inhibitory effect on cells (lactotrophs) in the anterior pituitary gland which synthesize and secrete prolactin; not an ergot alkaloid
Pharmacodynamics/Kinetics
  Onset of Action 2 hours; maximum effect: 4-6 hours
  Duration of Action >24 hours
  Half-life Elimination 11.5 hours; steady state: 17 hours
  Time to Peak 30-60 minutes

Pregnancy Considerations Animal studies revealed no embryotoxic or teratogenic effects. Fertility may be restored with treatment. Discontinue use with confirmed pregnancy unless medically necessary to continue. No increase in the incidence of abortion has been seen with a discontinuation of the drug during pregnancy. The reinstitution of therapy may be necessary in patients who display symptoms of tumor enlargement (headaches, visual field changes).
Product Availability Not available in U.S.

Quinapril (KWIN a pril)

Related Information
  Cardiovascular Diseases *on page 1492*
Brand Names: U.S. Accupril®
Brand Names: Canada Accupril®
Generic Availability (U.S.) Yes
Pharmacologic Category Angiotensin-Converting Enzyme (ACE) Inhibitor
Use Treatment of hypertension; treatment of heart failure
Unlabeled Use Treatment of left ventricular dysfunction after myocardial infarction; pediatric hypertension; to delay the progression of nephropathy and reduce risks of cardiovascular events in hypertensive patients with type 1 or 2 diabetes mellitus
Local Anesthetic/Vasoconstrictor Precautions No information available to require special precautions
Effects on Dental Treatment No significant effects or complications reported
Effects on Bleeding No information available to require special precautions
Adverse Effects Note: Frequency ranges include data from hypertension and heart failure trials. Higher rates of adverse reactions have generally been noted in patients with CHF. However, the frequency of adverse effects associated with placebo is also increased in this population.

1% to 10%:
  Cardiovascular: Hypotension (3%), chest pain (2%), first-dose hypotension (up to 3%)
  Central nervous system: Dizziness (4% to 8%), headache (2% to 6%), fatigue (3%)
  Dermatologic: Rash (1%)
  Endocrine & metabolic: Hyperkalemia (2%)
  Gastrointestinal: Vomiting/nausea (1% to 2%), diarrhea (2%)
  Neuromuscular & skeletal: Myalgias (2% to 5%), back pain (1%)
  Renal: BUN/serum creatinine increased (2%, transient elevations may occur with a higher frequency), worsening of renal function (in patients with bilateral renal artery stenosis or hypovolemia)
  Respiratory: Upper respiratory symptoms, cough (2% to 4%; up to 13% in some studies), dyspnea (2%)
Dosage Oral:
  Children (unlabeled use): Hypertension: Initial 5-10 mg once daily; maximum: 80 mg/day
  Adults:
    Heart failure: Initial: 5 mg once or twice daily, titrated at weekly intervals to 20-40 mg daily in 2 divided doses; target dose (heart failure): 20 mg twice daily (ACC/AHA 2009 Heart Failure Guidelines)

Hypertension: Initial: 10-20 mg once daily, adjust according to blood pressure response at peak and trough blood levels; initial dose may be reduced to 5 mg in patients receiving diuretic therapy if the diuretic is continued; usual dose range (JNC 7): 10-40 mg once daily

Elderly: Initial: 2.5-5 mg/day; increase dosage at increments of 2.5-5 mg at 1- to 2-week intervals.

Dosing adjustment in renal impairment: Lower initial doses should be used; after initial dose (if tolerated), administer initial dose twice daily; may be increased at weekly intervals to optimal response:

Heart failure: Initial:

Cl_{cr} >30 mL/minute: Administer 5 mg/day

Cl_{cr} 10-30 mL/minute: Administer 2.5 mg/day

Hypertension: Initial:

Cl_{cr} >60 mL/minute: Administer 10 mg/day

Cl_{cr} 30-60 mL/minute: Administer 5 mg/day

Cl_{cr} 10-30 mL/minute: Administer 2.5 mg/day

Dosing comments in hepatic impairment: In patients with alcoholic cirrhosis, hydrolysis of quinapril to quinaprilat is impaired; however, the subsequent elimination of quinaprilat is unaltered.

Mechanism of Action Competitive inhibitor of angiotensin-converting enzyme (ACE); prevents conversion of angiotensin I to angiotensin II, a potent vasoconstrictor; results in lower levels of angiotensin II which causes an increase in plasma renin activity and a reduction in aldosterone secretion; a CNS mechanism may also be involved in hypotensive effect as angiotensin II increases adrenergic outflow from CNS; vasoactive kallikreins may be decreased in conversion to active hormones by ACE inhibitors, thus reducing blood pressure

Contraindications

U.S. labeling: Hypersensitivity to quinapril or any component of the formulation; angioedema related to previous treatment with an ACE inhibitor; concomitant use with aliskiren in patients with diabetes mellitus

Canadian labeling: Hypersensitivity to quinapril or any component of the formulation; angioedema related to previous treatment with an ACE inhibitor; concomitant use with aliskiren in patients with diabetes mellitus (type 1 or 2) or with moderate-to-severe renal impairment (GFR <60 mL/minute/1.73 m^2); women who are pregnant, intend to become pregnant, or of childbearing potential and not using adequate contraception; breast-feeding

Warnings/Precautions Anaphylactic reactions may occur rarely with ACE inhibitors. At any time during treatment (especially following first dose) angioedema may occur rarely with ACE inhibitors; it may involve the head and neck (potentially compromising airway) or the intestine (presenting with abdominal pain). African-Americans and patients with idiopathic or hereditary angioedema may be at an increased risk. Prolonged frequent monitoring may be required especially if tongue, glottis, or larynx are involved as they are associated with airway obstruction. Patients with a history of airway surgery may have a higher risk of airway obstruction. Aggressive early and appropriate management is critical. Use in patients with previous angioedema associated with ACE inhibitor therapy is contraindicated. Severe anaphylactoid reactions may be seen during hemodialysis (eg, CVVHD) with high-flux dialysis membranes (eg, AN69), and rarely, during low density lipoprotein apheresis with dextran sulfate cellulose. Rare cases of anaphylactoid reactions have been reported in patients undergoing sensitization treatment with hymenoptera (bee, wasp) venom while receiving ACE inhibitors.

Symptomatic hypotension with or without syncope can occur with ACE inhibitors (usually with the first several doses); effects are most often observed in volume-depleted patients; close monitoring of patient is required especially with initial dosing and dosing increases; blood pressure must be lowered at a rate appropriate for the patient's clinical condition. Initiation of therapy in patients with ischemic heart disease or cerebrovascular disease warrants close observation due to the potential consequences posed by falling blood pressure (eg, MI, stroke). Use with caution in hypertrophic cardiomyopathy with outflow tract obstruction, severe aortic stenosis, or before, during, or immediately after major surgery. **[U.S. Boxed Warning]: Drugs that act on the renin-angiotensin system can cause injury and death to the developing fetus. Discontinue as soon as possible once pregnancy is detected.**

Hyperkalemia may occur with ACE inhibitors; risk factors include renal dysfunction, diabetes mellitus, concomitant use of potassium-sparing diuretics, potassium supplements, and/or potassium-containing salts. Use cautiously, if at all, with these agents and monitor potassium closely. Cough may occur with ACE inhibitors. Other causes of cough should be considered (eg, pulmonary congestion in patients with heart failure) and excluded prior to discontinuation.

May be associated with deterioration of renal function and/or increases in serum creatinine, particularly in patients with low renal blood flow (eg, renal artery stenosis, heart failure) whose glomerular filtration rate (GFR) is dependent on efferent arteriolar vasoconstriction by angiotensin II; deterioration may result in oliguria, acute renal failure, and progressive azotemia. Small increases in serum creatinine may occur following initiation; consider discontinuation only in patients with progressive and/or significant deterioration in renal function. Use with caution in patients with unstented unilateral/bilateral renal artery stenosis. When unstented bilateral renal artery stenosis is present, use is generally avoided due to the elevated risk of deterioration in renal function unless possible benefits outweigh risks. Concomitant use of an angiotensin receptor blocker (ARB) or renin inhibitor (eg, aliskiren) is associated with an increased risk of hypotension, hyperkalemia, and renal dysfunction; concomitant use with aliskiren should be avoided in patients with GFR <60 mL/minute and is contraindicated in patients with diabetes mellitus (regardless of GFR).

Rare toxicities associated with ACE inhibitors include cholestatic jaundice (which may progress to fulminant hepatic necrosis), agranulocytosis, neutropenia, or leukopenia with myeloid hypoplasia. Patients with collagen vascular diseases (especially with concomitant renal impairment) or renal impairment alone may be at increased risk for hematologic toxicity; periodically monitor CBC with differential in these patients.

Drug Interactions

Metabolism/Transport Effects None known.

Avoid Concomitant Use There are no known interactions where it is recommended to avoid concomitant use.

Increased Effect/Toxicity

Quinapril may increase the levels/effects of: Allopurinol; Amifostine; Antihypertensives; AzaTHIOprine; CycloSPORINE (Systemic); Ferric Gluconate; Gold Sodium Thiomalate; Hypotensive Agents; Iron Dextran

Complex; Lithium; Nonsteroidal Anti-Inflammatory Agents; RiTUXimab; Sodium Phosphates

The levels/effects of Quinapril may be increased by: Alfuzosin; Aliskiren; Angiotensin II Receptor Blockers; Canagliflozin; Diazoxide; DPP-IV Inhibitors; Eplerenone; Everolimus; Herbs (Hypotensive Properties); Loop Diuretics; MAO Inhibitors; Pentoxifylline; Phosphodiesterase 5 Inhibitors; Potassium Salts; Potassium-Sparing Diuretics; Prostacyclin Analogues; Sirolimus; Temsirolimus; Thiazide Diuretics; TiZANidine; Tolvaptan; Trimethoprim

Decreased Effect

Quinapril may decrease the levels/effects of: Quinolone Antibiotics; Tetracycline Derivatives

The levels/effects of Quinapril may be decreased by: Antacids; Aprotinin; Herbs (Hypertensive Properties); Icatibant; Lanthanum; Methylphenidate; Nonsteroidal Anti-Inflammatory Agents; Salicylates; Yohimbine

Ethanol/Nutrition/Herb Interactions

Food: Potassium supplements and/or potassium-containing salts may cause or worsen hyperkalemia. Management: Consult prescriber before consuming a potassium-rich diet, potassium supplements, or salt substitutes.

Herb/Nutraceutical: Some herbal medications may worsen hypertension (eg, licorice); others may increase the antihypertensive effects of quinapril (eg, shepherd's purse). Management: Avoid bayberry, blue cohosh, cayenne, ephedra, ginger, ginseng (American), kola, licorice, and yohimbe. Avoid black cohosh, California poppy, coleus, golden seal, hawthorn, mistletoe, periwinkle, quinine, and shepherd's purse.

Pharmacodynamics/Kinetics

Onset of Action 1 hour

Duration of Action 24 hours

Half-life Elimination Quinapril: 0.8 hours; Quinaprilat: 3 hours; increases as Cl_{cr} decreases

Time to Peak Serum: Quinapril: 1 hour; Quinaprilat: ~2 hours

Pregnancy Risk Factor D

Pregnancy Considerations [U.S. Boxed Warning]: Drugs that act on the renin-angiotensin system can cause injury and death to the developing fetus. Discontinue as soon as possible once pregnancy is detected. Quinapril crosses the placenta; teratogenic effects may occur following maternal use during pregnancy. Drugs that act on the renin-angiotensin system are associated with oligohydramnios. Oligohydramnios, due to decreased fetal renal function, may lead to fetal lung hypoplasia and skeletal malformations. Their use in pregnancy is also associated with anuria, hypotension, renal failure, skull hypoplasia, and death in the fetus/neonate. Chronic maternal hypertension itself is also associated with adverse events in the fetus/infant. ACE inhibitors are not recommended during pregnancy to treat maternal hypertension or heart failure. Use of an ACE inhibitor should also be avoided in any woman of reproductive age. Women who are planning a pregnancy should be considered for other medication options if an ACE inhibitor is currently prescribed or the ACE inhibitor should be discontinued as soon as possible once pregnancy is detected. The exposed fetus should be monitored for fetal growth, amniotic fluid volume, and organ formation. Infants exposed to an ACE inhibitor *in utero* should be monitored for hyperkalemia, hypotension, and oliguria.

Lactation Enters breast milk/use caution

Breast-Feeding Considerations Quinapril is excreted in breast milk. The manufacturer recommends that caution be exercised when administering quinapril to nursing women.

Dosage Forms

Tablet, oral: 5 mg, 10 mg, 20 mg, 40 mg

Accupril®: 5 mg, 10 mg, 20 mg, 40 mg

Quinapril and Hydrochlorothiazide
(KWIN a pril & hye droe klor oh THYE a zide)

Related Information

Hydrochlorothiazide *on page 687*

Quinapril *on page 1169*

Brand Names: U.S. Accuretic®

Brand Names: Canada Accuretic®

Pharmacologic Category Angiotensin-Converting Enzyme (ACE) Inhibitor; Diuretic, Thiazide

Use Treatment of hypertension (not for initial therapy)

Local Anesthetic/Vasoconstrictor Precautions No information available to require special precautions

Effects on Dental Treatment No significant effects or complications reported

Effects on Bleeding No information available to require special precautions

Adverse Effects 1% to 10%:

Central nervous system: Dizziness (5%), somnolence (1%)

Neuromuscular & skeletal: Weakness (1%)

Renal: Serum creatinine increased (3%), blood urea nitrogen increased (4%)

Respiratory: Cough (3%), bronchitis (1%)

General Dosage Range Oral: *Adults:* Initial: 10-20 mg quinapril and 12.5 mg hydrochlorothiazide once daily; Maintenance: 5-40 mg quinapril and 6.25-25 mg hydrochlorothiazide once daily

Pregnancy Risk Factor D

Pregnancy Considerations [U.S. Boxed Warning]: Drugs that act on the renin-angiotensin system can cause injury and death to the developing fetus. Discontinue as soon as possible once pregnancy is detected. Also see individual agents.

QuiNIDine (KWIN i deen)

Related Information

Clinical Risk Related to Drugs Prolonging QT Interval *on page 1510*

Brand Names: Canada Apo-Quinidine®; BioQuin® Durules™; Novo-Quinidin; Quinate®

Pharmacologic Category Antiarrhythmic Agent, Class Ia; Antimalarial Agent

Use

Quinidine gluconate and sulfate salts: Conversion and prevention of relapse into atrial fibrillation and/or flutter; suppression of ventricular arrhythmias. **Note:** Due to proarrhythmic effects, use should be reserved for life-threatening arrhythmias. Moreover, the use of quinidine has largely been replaced by more effective/safer antiarrhythmic agents and/or nonpharmacologic therapies (eg, radiofrequency ablation).

Quinidine gluconate (I.V. formulation): Conversion of atrial fibrillation/flutter and ventricular tachycardia. **Note:** The use of I.V. quinidine gluconate for these indications has been replaced by more effective/safer antiarrhythmic agents (eg, amiodarone and procainamide).

Quinidine gluconate (I.V. formulation) and quinidine sulfate: Treatment of malaria (*Plasmodium falciparum*)

◀ **Unlabeled Use** Paroxysmal supraventricular tachycardia, paroxysmal AV junctional rhythm, and symptomatic atrial or ventricular premature contractions; short QT syndrome; Brugada syndrome

Local Anesthetic/Vasoconstrictor Precautions Quinidine is one of the drugs confirmed to prolong the QT interval and is accepted as having a risk of causing torsade de pointes. The risk of drug-induced torsade de pointes is extremely low when a single QT interval prolonging drug is prescribed. In terms of epinephrine, it is not known what effect vasoconstrictors in the local anesthetic regimen will have in patients with a known history of congenital prolonged QT interval or in patients taking any medication that prolongs the QT interval. Until more information is obtained, it is suggested that the clinician consult with the physician prior to the use of a vasoconstrictor in suspected patients, and that the vasoconstrictor (epinephrine, mepivacaine and levonordefrin [Carbocaine® 2% with Neo-Cobefrin®]) be used with caution.

Effects on Dental Treatment When taken over a long period of time, the anticholinergic side effects from quinidine can cause a reduction of saliva production or secretion contributing to discomfort and dental disease (ie, caries, oral candidiasis, and periodontal disease).

Effects on Bleeding Quinidine has been shown to induce thrombocytopenia through the generation of both drug-dependent and drug-independent antibodies. In general, quinidine-induced thrombocytopenia is reversible following 9 days of discontinuation.

Adverse Effects

Frequency not defined: Hypotension, syncope

>10%:
Cardiovascular: QT_c prolongation (modest prolongation is common, however, excessive prolongation is rare and indicates toxicity)
Central nervous system: Lightheadedness (15%)
Gastrointestinal: Diarrhea (35%), upper GI distress, bitter taste, diarrhea, anorexia, nausea, vomiting, stomach cramping (22%)

1% to 10%:
Cardiovascular: Angina (6%), palpitation (7%), new or worsened arrhythmia (proarrhythmic effect)
Central nervous system: Syncope (1% to 8%), headache (7%), fatigue (7%), sleep disturbance (3%), tremor (2%), nervousness (2%), incoordination (1%)
Dermatologic: Rash (5%)
Neuromuscular & skeletal: Weakness (5%)
Ocular: Blurred vision
Otic: Tinnitus
Respiratory: Wheezing

Note: Cinchonism, a syndrome which may include tinnitus, high-frequency hearing loss, deafness, vertigo, blurred vision, diplopia, photophobia, headache, confusion, and delirium has been associated with quinidine use. Usually associated with chronic toxicity, this syndrome has also been described after brief exposure to a moderate dose in sensitive patients. Vomiting and diarrhea may also occur as isolated reactions to therapeutic quinidine levels.

General Dosage Range Dosages expressed in terms of the salt. Dosage adjustment recommended in patients with renal impairment.
I.V.: Quinidine gluconate: *Children and Adults:* 10 mg/kg bolus followed by 0.02 mg/kg/minute **or** 24 mg/kg bolus followed by 12 mg/kg every 8 hours
Oral:
Immediate release: Quinidine sulfate: *Adults:* Initial: 200-400 mg/dose every 6 hours

Extended release:
Quinidine gluconate: *Adults:* Initial: 324 mg every 8-12 hours
Quinidine sulfate: *Adults:* Initial: 300 mg every 8-12 hours

Mechanism of Action Class Ia antiarrhythmic agent; depresses phase O of the action potential; decreases myocardial excitability and conduction velocity, and myocardial contractility by decreasing sodium influx during depolarization and potassium efflux in repolarization; also reduces calcium transport across cell membrane

Pharmacodynamics/Kinetics
Half-life Elimination Plasma: Children: 3-4 hours; Adults: 6-8 hours; prolonged with elderly, cirrhosis, and congestive heart failure
Time to Peak Serum: Sulfate: 2 hours; Gluconate: 3-6 hours

Pregnancy Risk Factor C

Pregnancy Considerations Animal reproduction studies have not been conducted. Quinidine crosses the placenta and can be detected in the amniotic fluid, cord blood, and neonatal serum. Quinidine is indicated for use in the treatment of severe malaria infection in pregnant women (CDC, 2011; Smereck, 2011) and has also been used to treat arrhythmias in pregnancy when other agents are ineffective (European Society of Cardiology, 2003).

Dental Comment Quinidine is known to prolong the QT interval. The QT interval is measured as the time and distance between the Q point of the QRS complex and the end of the T wave in the ECG tracing. After adjustment for heart rate, the QT interval is defined as prolonged if it is more than 450 msec in men and 460 msec in women. A long QT syndrome was first described in the 1950s and 60s as a congenital syndrome involving QT interval prolongation and syncope and sudden death. Some of the congenital long QT syndromes were characterized by a peculiar electrocardiographic appearance of the QRS complex involving a premature atria beat followed by a pause, then a subsequent sinus beat showing marked QT prolongation and deformity. This type of cardiac arrhythmia was originally termed "torsade de pointes" (translated from the French as "twisting of the points"). Quinidine is considered as having a risk of causing torsade de pointes. Since it is not known what effect vasoconstrictors in the local anesthetic regimen will have in patients with a known history of congenital prolonged QT interval or in patients taking any medication that prolongs the QT interval, a medical consult is suggested.

QuiNINE (KWYE nine)

Related Information
Clinical Risk Related to Drugs Prolonging QT Interval *on page 1510*
Brand Names: U.S. Qualaquin®
Brand Names: Canada Apo-Quinine®; Novo-Quinine; Quinine-Odan
Pharmacologic Category Antimalarial Agent
Use In conjunction with other antimalarial agents, treatment of uncomplicated chloroquine-resistant *P. falciparum* malaria
Unlabeled Use Treatment of *Babesia microti* infection in conjunction with clindamycin; treatment of uncomplicated chloroquine-resistant *P. vivax* malaria (in conjunction with other antimalarial agents)

Local Anesthetic/Vasoconstrictor Precautions Quinine is one of the drugs confirmed to prolong the QT interval and is accepted as having a risk of causing torsade de pointes. The risk of drug-induced torsade de pointes is extremely low when a single QT interval prolonging drug is prescribed. In terms of epinephrine, it is not known what effect vasoconstrictors in the local anesthetic regimen will have in patients with a known history of congenital prolonged QT interval or in patients taking any medication that prolongs the QT interval. Until more information is obtained, it is suggested that the clinician consult with the physician prior to the use of a vasoconstrictor in suspected patients, and that the vasoconstrictor (epinephrine, mepivacaine and levonordefrin [Carbocaine® 2% with Neo-Cobefrin®]) be used with caution.

Effects on Dental Treatment No significant effects or complications reported

Effects on Bleeding Quinine has been shown to induce platelet-reactive monoclonal antibodies responsible for immune thrombocytopenia, leading to prolonged bleeding times. This drug-dependent antibody generation leads to the destruction of endogenous platelets. Quinine-induced thrombocytopenia can be treated through the discontinuation of the drug. Severe cases require a platelet transfusion.

Adverse Effects

Frequency not defined.

Cardiovascular: Atrial fibrillation, atrioventricular block, bradycardia, cardiac arrest, chest pain, hypotension, irregular rhythm, nodal escape beats, orthostatic hypotension, palpitation, QT prolongation, syncope, tachycardia, torsade de pointes, unifocal premature ventricular contractions, U waves, vasodilation, ventricular fibrillation, ventricular tachycardia

Central nervous system: Aphasia, ataxia, chills, coma, confusion, disorientation, dizziness, dystonic reaction, fever, flushing, headache, mental status altered, restlessness, seizure, suicide, vertigo

Dermatologic: Acral necrosis, allergic contact dermatitis, bullous dermatitis, bruising, cutaneous rash (urticaria, papular, scarlatinal), cutaneous vasculitis, exfoliative dermatitis, erythema multiforme, petechiae, photosensitivity, pruritus, Stevens-Johnson syndrome, toxic epidermal necrolysis

Endocrine & metabolic: Hypoglycemia

Gastrointestinal: Abdominal pain, anorexia, diarrhea, esophagitis, gastric irritation, nausea, vomiting

Hematologic: Agranulocytosis, aplastic anemia, coagulopathy, disseminated intravascular coagulation, hemolytic anemia, hemolytic uremic syndrome, hemorrhage, hypoprothrombinemia, idiopathic thrombocytopenic purpura, leukopenia, neutropenia, pancytopenia, thrombocytopenia, thrombotic thrombocytopenic purpura

Hepatic: Granulomatous hepatitis, hepatitis, jaundice, liver function test abnormalities

Neuromuscular & skeletal: Myalgia, tremor, weakness

Ocular: Blindness, blurred vision (with or without scotomata), color vision disturbance, diminished visual fields, diplopia, night blindness, optic neuritis, photophobia, pupillary dilation, vision loss (sudden)

Otic: Deafness, hearing impaired, tinnitus

Renal: Acute interstitial nephritis, hemoglobinuria, renal failure, renal impairment

Respiratory: Asthma, dyspnea, pulmonary edema

Miscellaneous: Black water fever, diaphoresis, hypersensitivity reaction, lupus anticoagulant, lupus-like syndrome

General Dosage Range Dosage adjustment recommended in patients with renal impairment

Oral:

Children: 30 mg/kg/day divided every 8 hours

Adults: 648 mg every 8 hours

Mechanism of Action Depresses oxygen uptake and carbohydrate metabolism; intercalates into DNA, disrupting the parasite's replication and transcription; cardiovascular effects similar to quinidine

Pharmacodynamics/Kinetics

Half-life Elimination

Children: ~3 hours in healthy subjects; ~12 hours with malaria

Healthy adults: 10-13 hours

Healthy elderly subjects: 18 hours

Time to Peak

Children: Serum: 2 hours in healthy subjects; 4 hours with malaria

Adults: Serum: 2-4 hours in healthy subjects; 1-11 hours with malaria

Pregnancy Risk Factor C

Pregnancy Considerations Teratogenic effects have been reported in some animal studies. Quinine crosses the human placenta. Cord plasma to maternal plasma quinine ratios have been reported as 0.18-0.46 and should not be considered therapeutic to the infant. Teratogenic effects, optic nerve hypoplasia, and deafness have been reported in the infant following maternal use of very high doses; however, therapeutic doses used for malaria are generally considered safe. Quinine may also cause significant hypoglycemia when used during pregnancy. Malaria infection in pregnant women may be more severe than in nonpregnant women. Because *P. falciparum* malaria can cause maternal death and fetal loss, pregnant women traveling to malaria-endemic areas must use personal protection against mosquito bites. Quinine may be used for the treatment of malaria in pregnant women; consult current CDC guidelines. Pregnant women should be advised not to travel to areas of *P. falciparum* resistance to chloroquine.

Dental Comment Quinine is known to prolong the QT interval. The QT interval is measured as the time and distance between the Q point of the QRS complex and the end of the T wave in the ECG tracing. After adjustment for heart rate, the QT interval is defined as prolonged if it is more than 450 msec in men and 460 msec in women. A long QT syndrome was first described in the 1950s and 60s as a congenital syndrome involving QT interval prolongation and syncope and sudden death. Some of the congenital long QT syndromes were characterized by a peculiar electrocardiographic appearance of the QRS complex involving a premature atria beat followed by a pause, then a subsequent sinus beat showing marked QT prolongation and deformity. This type of cardiac arrhythmia was originally termed "torsade de pointes" (translated from the French as "twisting of the points"). Quinine is considered as having a risk of causing torsade de pointes. Since it is not known what effect vasoconstrictors in the local anesthetic regimen will have in patients with a known history of congenital prolonged QT interval or in patients taking any medication that prolongs the QT interval, a medical consult is suggested.

Quinupristin and Dalfopristin
(kwi NYOO pris tin & dal FOE pris tin)

Brand Names: U.S. Synercid®
Brand Names: Canada Synercid®

Pharmacologic Category Antibiotic, Streptogramin

Use Treatment of complicated skin and skin structure infections caused by methicillin-susceptible *Staphylococcus aureus* or *Streptococcus pyogenes*

Unlabeled Use Treatment of persistent MRSA bacteremia associated with vancomycin failure

Local Anesthetic/Vasoconstrictor Precautions No information available to require special precautions

Effects on Dental Treatment No significant effects or complications reported

Effects on Bleeding No information available to require special precautions

Adverse Effects

>10%:

Hepatic: Hyperbilirubinemia (3% to 35%)

Local: Local pain (40% to 44%), inflammation at infusion site (38% to 42%), local edema (17% to 18%), infusion site reaction (12% to 13%)

Neuromuscular & skeletal: Arthralgia (up to 47%), myalgia (up to 47%)

1% to 10%:

Central nervous system: Pain (2% to 3%), headache (2%)

Dermatologic: Rash (3%), pruritus (2%)

Endocrine & metabolic: Hyperglycemia (1%)

Gastrointestinal: Nausea (3% to 5%), vomiting (3% to 4%), diarrhea (3%)

Hematologic: Anemia (3%)

Hepatic: GGT increased (2%), LDH increased (3%)

Local: Thrombophlebitis (2%)

Neuromuscular & skeletal: CPK increased (2%)

General Dosage Range I.V.: *Children ≥12 years and Adults:* 7.5 mg/kg every 12 hours

Mechanism of Action Quinupristin/dalfopristin inhibits bacterial protein synthesis by binding to different sites on the 50S bacterial ribosomal subunit thereby inhibiting protein synthesis

Pharmacodynamics/Kinetics

Half-life Elimination Quinupristin: 0.85 hour; Dalfopristin: 0.7 hour (mean elimination half-lives, including metabolites: 3 and 1 hours, respectively)

Pregnancy Risk Factor B

Pregnancy Considerations Because adverse effects were not observed in animal reproduction studies, quinupristin/dalfopristin is classified pregnancy category B. There are no adequate and well-controlled studies of quinupristin/dalfopristin in pregnant women.

RABEprazole (ra BEP ra zole)

Related Information

Gastrointestinal Disorders *on page 1512*

Brand Names: U.S. AcipHex®

Brand Names: Canada Apo-Rabeprazole®; Pariet®; Pat-Rabeprazole; PMS-Rabeprazole EC; PRO-Rabeprazole; Rabeprazole EC; RAN™-Rabeprazole; Riva-Rabeprazole EC; Sandoz-Rabeprazole; Teva-Rabeprazole EC

Generic Availability (U.S.) No

Pharmacologic Category Proton Pump Inhibitor; Substituted Benzimidazole

Use Short-term (4-8 weeks) treatment and maintenance of erosive or ulcerative gastroesophageal reflux disease (GERD); symptomatic GERD; short-term (up to 4 weeks) treatment of duodenal ulcers; long-term treatment of pathological hypersecretory conditions, including Zollinger-Ellison syndrome; *H. pylori* eradication (in combination therapy)

Canadian labeling: Additional uses (not in U.S. labeling): Treatment of nonerosive reflux disease (NERD); treatment of gastric ulcers

Unlabeled Use Maintenance of healing and prevention of relapse for duodenal ulcer; treatment and prevention of NSAID-induced ulcer

Local Anesthetic/Vasoconstrictor Precautions No information available to require special precautions

Effects on Dental Treatment No significant effects or complications reported

Effects on Bleeding No information available to require special precautions

Adverse Effects Frequency not always defined.

1% to 10%:

Cardiovascular: Peripheral edema

Central nervous system: Headache (2% to 10%), pain (3%), dizziness

Gastrointestinal: Diarrhea (2% to 5%), nausea (2% to 5%), abdominal pain (4%), vomiting (4%), flatulence (3%), constipation (2%), xerostomia

Hepatic: Hepatic encephalopathy, hepatic enzymes increased, hepatitis

Neuromuscular & skeletal: Arthralgia, myalgia

Respiratory: Pharyngitis (3%)

Miscellaneous: Infection (2%)

Dosage Oral:

Children ≥12 years: *U.S. labeling:* Short-term treatment of GERD: 20 mg once daily for ≤8 weeks

Adults >18 years and Elderly:

Erosive/ulcerative GERD: Treatment: 20 mg once daily for 4-8 weeks; if inadequate response, may repeat up to an additional 8 weeks; maintenance: 20 mg once daily

Canadian labeling: 20 mg once daily for 4 weeks; if inadequate response, may repeat for an additional 4 weeks (lack of symptom control after 4 weeks warrants further evaluation); maintenance: 10 mg once daily (maximum: 20 mg once daily)

Symptomatic GERD: Treatment: 20 mg once daily for 4 weeks; if inadequate response, may repeat for an additional 4 weeks

Canadian labeling: 10 mg once daily (maximum: 20 mg once daily) for 4 weeks; lack of symptom control after 4 weeks warrants further evaluation

Duodenal ulcer: 20 mg daily before breakfast for 4 weeks; additional therapy may be required for some patients

Gastric ulcers (*Canadian labeling*): 20 mg once daily up to 6 weeks; additional therapy may be required for some patients

Helicobacter pylori eradication:

Manufacturer labeling: 20 mg twice daily administered with amoxicillin 1000 mg *and* clarithromycin 500 mg twice daily for 7 days

American College of Gastroenterology guidelines (Chey, 2007):

Nonpenicillin allergy: 20 mg twice daily administered with amoxicillin 1000 mg *and* clarithromycin 500 mg twice daily for 10-14 days

Penicillin allergy: 20 mg twice daily administered with clarithromycin 500 mg *and* metronidazole 500 mg twice daily for 10-14 days **or** 20 mg once or twice daily administered with bismuth subsalicylate 525 mg *and* metronidazole 250 mg *plus* tetracycline 500 mg 4 times/day for 10-14 days

Hypersecretory conditions: 60 mg once daily; dose may need to be adjusted as necessary. Doses as high as 100 mg once daily and 60 mg twice daily have been used, and continued as long as necessary (up to 1 year in some patients).

NERD (*Canadian labeling*): Treatment: 10 mg (maximum: 20 mg once daily) for 4 weeks; lack of symptom control after 4 weeks warrants further evaluation

Dosage adjustment in renal impairment: No dosage adjustment necessary

Dosage adjustment in hepatic impairment:
Mild-to-moderate: No dosage adjustment necessary.
Severe: No dosage adjustment provided in manufacturer's labeling (has not been studied). Use with caution.

Mechanism of Action Potent proton pump inhibitor; suppresses gastric acid secretion by inhibiting the parietal cell H+/K+ ATP pump

Contraindications Hypersensitivity to rabeprazole, other substituted benzimidazoles proton pump inhibitors, or any component of the formulation

Warnings/Precautions Use of proton pump inhibitors (PPIs) may increase the risk of gastrointestinal infections (eg, *Salmonella, Campylobacter*). Use caution in severe hepatic impairment. Relief of symptoms with rabeprazole does not preclude the presence of a gastric malignancy. Use of PPIs may increase risk of *Clostridium difficile*-associated diarrhea (CDAD), especially in hospitalized patients; consider CDAD diagnosis in patients with persistent diarrhea that does not improve. Use the lowest dose and shortest duration of PPI therapy appropriate for the condition being treated. Decreased *H. pylori* eradication rates have been observed with short-term (≤7 days) combination therapy. The American College of Gastroenterology recommends 10-14 days of therapy (triple or quadruple) for eradication of *H. pylori* (Chey, 2007).

PPIs may diminish the therapeutic effect of clopidogrel, thought to be due to reduced formation of the active metabolite of clopidogrel. The manufacturer of clopidogrel recommends either avoidance of both omeprazole (even when scheduled 12 hours apart) and esomeprazole or use of a PPI with comparatively less effect on the active metabolite of clopidogrel. Avoidance of rabeprazole appears prudent due to potent *in vitro* CYP2C19 inhibition (Li, 2004) and lack of sufficient comparative *in vivo* studies with other PPIs. In contrast to these warnings, others have recommended the continued use of PPIs, regardless of the degree of inhibition, in patients with a history of GI bleeding or multiple risk factors for GI bleeding who are also receiving clopidogrel since no evidence has established clinically meaningful differences in outcome; however, a clinically-significant interaction cannot be excluded in those who are poor metabolizers of clopidogrel (Abraham, 2010; Levine, 2011). Concomitant use of rabeprazole with some drugs may require cautious use, may not be recommended, or may require dosage adjustments.

Increased incidence of osteoporosis-related bone fractures of the hip, spine, or wrist may occur with PPI therapy. Patients on high-dose (multiple daily doses) or long-term therapy (≥1 year) should be monitored. Use the lowest effective dose for the shortest duration of time, use vitamin D and calcium supplementation, and follow appropriate guidelines to reduce risk of fractures in patients at risk.

Hypomagnesemia, reported rarely, usually with prolonged PPI use of >3 months (most cases >1 year of therapy); may be symptomatic or asymptomatic; severe cases may cause tetany, seizures, and cardiac arrhythmias. Consider obtaining serum magnesium concentrations prior to beginning long-term therapy, especially if taking concomitant digoxin, diuretics, or other drugs known to cause hypomagnesemia; and periodically thereafter. Hypomagnesemia may be corrected by magnesium supplementation, although discontinuation of rabeprazole may be necessary; magnesium levels typically return to normal within 1 week of stopping.

Drug Interactions

Metabolism/Transport Effects Substrate of CYP2C19 (major), CYP3A4 (major); **Note:** Assignment of Major/Minor substrate status based on clinically relevant drug interaction potential; **Inhibits** CYP2C19 (weak), CYP2C8 (moderate), CYP2D6 (weak), CYP3A4 (weak)

Avoid Concomitant Use
Avoid concomitant use of RABEprazole with any of the following: Dasatinib; Delavirdine; Erlotinib; Nelfinavir; Pimozide; Ponatinib; Posaconazole; Rilpivirine; Risedronate

Increased Effect/Toxicity
RABEprazole may increase the levels/effects of: Amphetamines; ARIPiprazole; CYP2C8 Substrates; Dexmethylphenidate; Lomitapide; Methotrexate; Methylphenidate; Pimozide; Raltegravir; Risedronate; Saquinavir; Tacrolimus (Systemic); Voriconazole

The levels/effects of RABEprazole may be increased by: Fluconazole; Ketoconazole (Systemic); Voriconazole

Decreased Effect
RABEprazole may decrease the levels/effects of: Atazanavir; Bisphosphonate Derivatives; Bosutinib; Cefditoren; Clopidogrel; Dabigatran Etexilate; Dasatinib; Delavirdine; Erlotinib; Gefitinib; Indinavir; Iron Salts; Itraconazole; Ketoconazole (Systemic); Mesalamine; Multivitamins/Minerals (with ADEK, Folate, Iron); Mycophenolate; Nelfinavir; Nilotinib; Ponatinib; Posaconazole; Rilpivirine; Risedronate; Vismodegib

The levels/effects of RABEprazole may be decreased by: CYP2C19 Inducers (Strong); CYP3A4 Inducers (Strong); Deferasirox; Herbs (CYP3A4 Inducers); Tipranavir; Tocilizumab

Ethanol/Nutrition/Herb Interactions
Ethanol: Avoid ethanol (may cause gastric mucosal irritation).
Food: High-fat meals may delay absorption, but C_{max} and AUC are not altered.
Herb/Nutraceutical: St John's wort may increase the metabolism and thus decrease the levels/effects of rabeprazole.

Dietary Considerations May be taken without regard to meals; best if taken before breakfast.

Pharmacodynamics/Kinetics
Onset of Action Within 1 hour
Duration of Action 24 hours
Half-life Elimination Dose dependent: 1-2 hours
Time to Peak Plasma: 2-5 hours

Pregnancy Risk Factor B

Pregnancy Considerations Not shown to be teratogenic in animal studies, however, adequate and well-controlled studies have not been done in humans; use during pregnancy only if clearly needed

Lactation Excretion in breast milk unknown/not recommended

Product Availability Aciphex Sprinkle (delayed-release capsule): FDA approved March 2013; anticipated availability currently unknown. Consult prescribing information for additional information.

Dosage Forms
Tablet, delayed release, enteric coated, oral:
AcipHex®: 20 mg

◄ **Dosage Forms: Canada**
Tablet, delayed release, enteric coated:
Pariet®: 10 mg, 20 mg

Rabies Immune Globulin (Human)
(RAY beez i MYUN GLOB yoo lin, HYU man)

Brand Names: U.S. HyperRAB® S/D; Imogam® Rabies-HT

Brand Names: Canada HyperRAB® S/D; Imogam® Rabies Pasteurized

Pharmacologic Category Blood Product Derivative; Immune Globulin

Use Part of postexposure prophylaxis of persons with rabies exposure. Provides passive immunity until active immunity with rabies vaccine is established. Not for use in persons with a history of pre-exposure vaccination, history of postexposure prophylaxis, or previous vaccination with rabies vaccine and documentation of antibody response.

Local Anesthetic/Vasoconstrictor Precautions No information available to require special precautions

Effects on Dental Treatment No significant effects or complications reported

Effects on Bleeding No information available to require special precautions

Adverse Effects Frequency not defined.
Central nervous system: Fever (mild), headache, malaise
Dermatologic: Angioneurotic edema, rash
Local: Injection site: Pain, stiffness, soreness, tenderness
Renal: Nephrotic syndrome
Miscellaneous: Anaphylaxis

General Dosage Range Local wound infiltration/ I.M.: *Children and Adults:* 20 units/kg in a single dose

Mechanism of Action Rabies immune globulin is a solution of globulins dried from the plasma or serum of selected adult human donors who have been immunized with rabies vaccine and have developed high titers of rabies antibody. It generally contains 10% to 18% of protein of which not less than 80% is monomeric immunoglobulin G.

Pregnancy Risk Factor C

Pregnancy Considerations Reproduction studies have not been conducted. Pregnancy is not a contraindication to postexposure prophylaxis.

Rabies Vaccine (RAY beez vak SEEN)

Brand Names: U.S. Imovax® Rabies; RabAvert®
Brand Names: Canada Imovax® Rabies; RabAvert®
Pharmacologic Category Vaccine, Inactivated (Viral)
Use Pre-exposure and postexposure vaccination against rabies

The Advisory Committee on Immunization Practices (ACIP) recommends a primary course of prophylactic immunization (pre-exposure vaccination) for the following:

• Persons with continuous risk of infection, including rabies research laboratory and biologics production workers
• Persons with frequent risk of infection in areas where rabies is enzootic, including rabies diagnostic laboratory workers, cavers, veterinarians and their staff, and animal control and wildlife workers; persons who frequently handle bats

• Persons with infrequent risk of infection, including veterinarians and animal control staff with terrestrial animals in areas where rabies infection is rare, veterinary students, and travelers visiting areas where rabies is enzootic and immediate access to medical care and biologicals is limited

The ACIP recommends the use of postexposure vaccination for a particular person be assessed by the severity and likelihood versus the actual risk of acquiring rabies. Consideration should include the type of exposure, epidemiology of rabies in the area, species of the animal, circumstances of the incident, and the availability of the exposing animal for observation or rabies testing. Postexposure vaccination is used in both previously vaccinated and previously unvaccinated individuals.

Local Anesthetic/Vasoconstrictor Precautions No information available to require special precautions

Effects on Dental Treatment No significant effects or complications reported

Effects on Bleeding No information available to require special precautions

Adverse Effects All serious adverse reactions must be reported to the U.S. Department of Health and Human Services (DHHS) Vaccine Adverse Event Reporting System (VAERS) 1-800-822-7967 or online at https://vaers.hhs.gov/esub/index. In Canada, adverse reactions may be reported to local provincial/ territorial health agencies or to the Vaccine Safety Section at Public Health Agency of Canada (1-866-844-0018).

>10%:
Central nervous system: Dizziness, headache, malaise
Gastrointestinal: Abdominal pain, nausea
Local: Erythema, itching, pain, swelling
Neuromuscular & skeletal: Myalgia
Miscellaneous: Lymphadenopathy
Uncommon, frequency not defined, postmarketing, and/ or case reports:
Cardiovascular: Circulatory reactions, edema, palpitation
Central nervous system: Chills, fatigue, fever >38°C (100°F), Guillain-Barré syndrome, encephalitis, meningitis, multiple sclerosis, myelitis, neuroparalysis, seizures, vertigo
Dermatologic: Pruritus, urticaria, urticaria pigmentosa
Endocrine & metabolic: Hot flashes
Gastrointestinal: Diarrhea, vomiting
Local: Hematoma, limb swelling (extensive)
Neuromuscular & skeletal: Arthralgia, limb pain, monoarthritis, neuropathy, paralysis (transient), paresthesias (transient), weakness
Ocular: Retrobulbar neuritis, visual disturbances
Respiratory: Bronchospasm, dyspnea, wheezing
Miscellaneous: Allergic reactions, anaphylaxis, hypersensitivity reactions, serum sickness, swollen lymph nodes

General Dosage Range I.M.: *Children and Adults:* 1 mL

Mechanism of Action Rabies vaccine is an inactivated virus vaccine which promotes immunity by inducing an active immune response. The production of specific antibodies requires about 7-10 days to develop. Rabies immune globulin or antirabies serum, equine (ARS) is given in conjunction with rabies vaccine to provide immune protection until an antibody response can occur.

Pharmacodynamics/Kinetics
Onset of Action I.M.: Rabies antibody: ~7-10 days; Peak effect: ~30-60 days
Duration of Action ≥1 year
Pregnancy Risk Factor C
Pregnancy Considerations Animal reproduction studies have not been conducted. Pregnancy is not a contraindication to postexposure prophylaxis. Pre-exposure prophylaxis during pregnancy may also be considered if risk of rabies is great.

Raloxifene (ral OKS i feen)

Related Information
Endocrine Disorders and Pregnancy *on page 1517*
Rheumatoid Arthritis, Osteoarthritis, and Osteoporosis *on page 1526*
Brand Names: U.S. Evista®
Brand Names: Canada Apo-Raloxifene®; Evista®; Novo-Raloxifene; Teva-Raloxifene
Generic Availability (U.S.) No
Pharmacologic Category Selective Estrogen Receptor Modulator (SERM)
Use Prevention and treatment of osteoporosis in postmenopausal women; risk reduction for invasive breast cancer in postmenopausal women with osteoporosis and in postmenopausal women with high risk for invasive breast cancer
Local Anesthetic/Vasoconstrictor Precautions No information available to require special precautions
Effects on Dental Treatment No significant effects or complications reported
Effects on Bleeding Has been associated with thromboembolic adverse events. No information available to require routine special precautions for dental procedures.
Adverse Effects Note: Raloxifene has been associated with increased risk of thromboembolism (DVT, PE) and superficial thrombophlebitis; risk is similar to reported risk of HRT
>10%:
Cardiovascular: Peripheral edema (3% to 14%)
Endocrine & metabolic: Hot flashes (8% to 29%)
Neuromuscular & skeletal: Arthralgia (11% to 16%), leg cramps/muscle spasm (6% to 12%)
Miscellaneous: Flu syndrome (14% to 15%), infection (11%)
1% to 10%:
Cardiovascular: Chest pain (3%), venous thromboembolism (1% to 2%)
Central nervous system: Insomnia (6%)
Dermatologic: Rash (6%)
Endocrine & metabolic: Breast pain (4%)
Gastrointestinal: Weight gain (9%), abdominal pain (7%), vomiting (5%), flatulence (2% to 3%), cholelithiasis (≤3%), gastroenteritis (≤3%)
Genitourinary: Vaginal bleeding (6%), leukorrhea (3%), urinary tract disorder (3%), uterine disorder (3%), vaginal hemorrhage (3%), endometrial disorder (≤3%)
Neuromuscular & skeletal: Myalgia (8%), tendon disorder (4%)
Respiratory: Bronchitis (10%), sinusitis (10%), pharyngitis (8%), pneumonia (3%), laryngitis (≤2%)
Miscellaneous: Diaphoresis (3%)
Dosage Adults: Females: Oral:
Osteoporosis: 60 mg once daily
Invasive breast cancer risk reduction: 60 mg once daily for 5 years per ASCO guidelines (Visvanathan, 2009)

Dosage adjustment in renal impairment: Moderate-to-severe impairment: Use caution; safety and efficacy have not been established.
Dosage adjustment in hepatic impairment: Mild impairment (Child-Pugh class A): Plasma concentrations were higher and correlated with total bilirubin. Safety and efficacy in hepatic insufficiency have not been established.
Mechanism of Action A selective estrogen receptor modulator (SERM), meaning that it affects some of the same receptors that estrogen does, but not all, and in some instances, it antagonizes or blocks estrogen; it acts like estrogen to prevent bone loss and has the potential to block some estrogen effects in the breast and uterine tissues. Raloxifene decreases bone resorption, increasing bone mineral density and decreasing fracture incidence.
Contraindications History of or current venous thromboembolic disorders (including DVT, PE, and retinal vein thrombosis); pregnancy or women who could become pregnant; breast-feeding
Warnings/Precautions Hazardous agent - use appropriate precautions for handling and disposal (NIOSH, 2012). **[U.S. Boxed Warning]: May increase the risk for DVT or PE; use contraindicated in patients with history of or current venous thromboembolic disorders.** Use with caution in patients at high risk for venous thromboembolism; the risk for DVT and PE are higher in the first 4 months of treatment. Discontinue at least 72 hours prior to and during prolonged immobilization (postoperative recovery or prolonged bedrest). **[U.S. Boxed Warning]: The risk of death due to stroke may be increased in women with coronary heart disease or in women at risk for coronary events;** use with caution in patients with cardiovascular disease. Not be used for the prevention of cardiovascular disease. Use caution with moderate-to-severe renal dysfunction, hepatic impairment, unexplained uterine bleeding, and in women with a history of elevated triglycerides in response to treatment with oral estrogens (or estrogen/progestin). Safety with concomitant estrogen therapy has not been established. Safety and efficacy in premenopausal women or men have not been established. Not indicated for treatment of invasive breast cancer, to reduce the risk of recurrence of invasive breast cancer or to reduce the risk of noninvasive breast cancer. The efficacy (for breast cancer risk reduction) in women with inherited BRCA1 and BRCA1 mutations has not been established.
Drug Interactions
Metabolism/Transport Effects None known.
Avoid Concomitant Use
Avoid concomitant use of Raloxifene with any of the following: Ospemifene
Increased Effect/Toxicity
Raloxifene may increase the levels/effects of: Ospemifene
Decreased Effect
Raloxifene may decrease the levels/effects of: Levothyroxine; Ospemifene

The levels/effects of Raloxifene may be decreased by: Bile Acid Sequestrants
Ethanol/Nutrition/Herb Interactions Ethanol: Avoid ethanol (may increase risk of osteoporosis).
Dietary Considerations May be taken without regard to meals. Osteoporosis prevention or treatment: Ensure adequate calcium and vitamin D intake; postmenopausal women should consume ~1500 mg/day of elemental calcium and 400-800 units/day of vitamin D.

Pharmacodynamics/Kinetics
Onset of Action 8 weeks
Half-life Elimination 28-33 hours
Pregnancy Risk Factor X
Pregnancy Considerations Animal studies have demonstrated teratogenicity and fetal loss. There are no adequate and well-controlled studies in pregnant women. Raloxifene should not be used by women who are or may become pregnant.
Lactation Excretion in breast milk unknown/contraindicated
Dosage Forms
Tablet, oral:
Evista®: 60 mg

Raltegravir (ral TEG ra vir)

Related Information
HIV Infection and AIDS *on page 1520*
Brand Names: U.S. Isentress®
Brand Names: Canada Isentress®
Pharmacologic Category Antiretroviral Agent, Integrase Inhibitor
Use Treatment of HIV-1 infection in combination with other antiretroviral agents
Local Anesthetic/Vasoconstrictor Precautions No information available to require special precautions
Effects on Dental Treatment No significant effects or complications reported
Effects on Bleeding No information available to require special precautions related to hemostasis.
Adverse Effects 2% to 10%:
Central nervous system: Insomnia (4%), headache (2%)
Endocrine & metabolic: Glucose increased (126-250 mg/dL: 3% to 10%; 251-500 mg/dL: 2% to 3%)
Gastrointestinal: Lipase increased (1.6-3 x ULN: 5%; 3.1-5 x ULN: 2%), nausea (3%), amylase increased (1.6-2 x ULN: 2%; 2.1-5 x ULN: 4%)
Hematologic: Absolute neutrophil count decreased (grade 2: 3% to 4%; grade 3: 2% to 3%), platelets decreased (grade 2: 2% to 3%)
Hepatic: AST increased (2.6-5 x ULN: 4% to 9%, 5.1-10 x ULN: 2% to 4%), hyperbilirubinemia (1.6-2.5 x ULN: 4% to 6%; 2.6-5 x ULN: 1% to 3%), ALT increased (2.6-5 x ULN: 6% to 9%; 5.1-10 x ULN: 4% to 6%), alkaline phosphatase increased (2.6-5 x ULN: 1% to 2%)
Note: Incidence of liver function abnormalities higher with hepatitis B and/or C coinfection.
Neuromuscular & skeletal: Creatine kinase increased (6.0-9.9 x ULN: 2%; 10-19.9 x ULN: 4%; ≥20 x ULN: 3%)
General Dosage Range Dosage adjustment recommended in patients on concomitant therapy
Oral:
Children 2 to <6 years: Chewable tablet: Weight-based dosing: 75-300 mg twice daily
Children 6 to <12 years: Chewable tablet: Weight-based dosing: 75-300 mg twice daily; if ≥25 kg, refer to weight-based dosing or adult dosing
Adolescents ≥12 years and Adults: Film-coated tablet: 400 mg twice daily
Mechanism of Action Incorporation of viral DNA into the host cell's genome is required to produce a self-replicating provirus and propagation of infectious virion particles. The viral cDNA strand produced by reverse transcriptase is subsequently processed and inserted into the human genome by the enzyme HIV-1 integrase (encoded by the pol gene of HIV). Raltegravir inhibits the catalytic activity of integrase, thus preventing integration of the proviral gene into human DNA.
Pharmacodynamics/Kinetics
Half-life Elimination ~9 hours
Time to Peak Film-coated tablet: ~3 hours
Pregnancy Risk Factor C
Pregnancy Considerations Adverse events were observed in some animal reproduction studies. Raltegravir crosses the placenta and can be detected in neonatal serum after delivery. Standard doses appear to be appropriate in pregnant women. The DHHS Perinatal HIV Guidelines note that raltegravir may be used under special circumstances in pregnant women (eg, when preferred or alternative agents cannot be used).

Regardless of CD4 count or HIV RNA copy number, all HIV-infected pregnant women should receive a combination antepartum antiretroviral (ARV) drug regimen; this includes women who require therapy for their own health, as well as women who do not yet require therapy for their own health. ARV therapy should be started as soon as possible if required for the woman's health. Although earlier initiation may be more effective in reducing the perinatal transmission of HIV, also consider maternal conditions (eg nausea and vomiting) and the potential risks of first trimester fetal exposure for specific agents. Plasma HIV RNA levels should be assessed at ~34-36 weeks gestation in order to help determine mode of delivery. If ARV therapy must be interrupted for <24 hours during the peripartum period, stop then restart all medications simultaneously in order to decrease the chance of developing resistance. Long-term follow-up is recommended for all infants exposed to ARV medications.

Healthcare providers are encouraged to enroll pregnant women exposed to antiretroviral medications in the Antiretroviral Pregnancy Registry (1-800-258-4263 or www.APRegistry.com). Healthcare providers caring for HIV-infected women and their infants may contact the National Perinatal HIV Hotline (888-448-8765) for clinical consultation (DHHS [perinatal], 2012).

Ramelteon (ra MEL tee on)

Brand Names: U.S. Rozerem®
Generic Availability (U.S.) No
Pharmacologic Category Hypnotic, Miscellaneous
Use Treatment of insomnia characterized by difficulty with sleep onset
Local Anesthetic/Vasoconstrictor Precautions No information available to require special precautions
Effects on Dental Treatment Key adverse event(s) related to dental treatment: Taste perversion.
Effects on Bleeding No information available to require special precautions
Adverse Effects 1% to 10%:
Central nervous system: Dizziness (4% to 5%), somnolence (3% to 5%), fatigue (3% to 4%), insomnia worsened (3%), depression (2%)
Endocrine & metabolic: Serum cortisol decreased (1%)
Gastrointestinal: Nausea (3%), taste perversion (2%)
Neuromuscular & skeletal: Myalgia (2%), arthralgia (2%)
Respiratory: Upper respiratory infection (3%)
Miscellaneous: Influenza (1%)
Dosage Oral: Adults: One 8 mg tablet within 30 minutes of bedtime
Dosage adjustment in renal impairment: No dosage adjustment required

Dosage adjustment in hepatic impairment: No adjustment required for mild-to-moderate impairment; use caution. Not recommended with severe impairment.

Mechanism of Action Potent, selective agonist of melatonin receptors MT_1 and MT_2 (with little affinity for MT_3) within the suprachiasmic nucleus of the hypothalamus, an area responsible for determination of circadian rhythms and synchronization of the sleep-wake cycle. Agonism of MT_1 is thought to preferentially induce sleepiness, while MT_2 receptor activation preferentially influences regulation of circadian rhythms. Ramelteon is eightfold more selective for MT_1 than MT_2 and exhibits nearly sixfold higher affinity for MT_1 than melatonin, presumably allowing for enhanced effects on sleep induction.

Contraindications History of angioedema with previous ramelteon therapy (do not rechallenge); concurrent use with fluvoxamine

Warnings/Precautions Symptomatic treatment of insomnia should be initiated only after careful evaluation of potential causes of sleep disturbance. Failure of sleep disturbance to resolve after a reasonable period of treatment may indicate psychiatric and/or medical illness. Because of the rapid onset of action, administer immediately prior to bedtime or after the patient has gone to bed and is having difficulty falling asleep. Hypnotics/sedatives have been associated with abnormal thinking and behavior changes including decreased inhibition, aggression, bizarre behavior, agitation, hallucinations, and depersonalization. These changes may occur unpredictably and may indicate previously unrecognized psychiatric disorders; evaluate appropriately. Postmarketing studies have indicated that the use of hypnotic/sedative agents (including ramelteon) for sleep has been associated with hypersensitivity reactions including anaphylaxis as well as angioedema. Do not rechallenge patients who have developed angioedema with ramelteon therapy. An increased risk for hazardous sleep-related activities such as sleep-driving; cooking and eating food, and making phone calls while asleep have also been noted. Use caution with pre-existing depression or other psychiatric conditions. Caution when using with other CNS depressants; avoid engaging in hazardous activities or activities requiring mental alertness. Not recommended for use in patients with severe sleep apnea or COPD. Use caution with moderate hepatic impairment; not recommended in patients with severe impairment. May cause disturbances of hormonal regulation. Use caution when administered concomitantly with strong CYP1A2 inhibitors.

Drug Interactions

Metabolism/Transport Effects Substrate of CYP1A2 (major), CYP2C19 (minor), CYP3A4 (minor); **Note:** Assignment of Major/Minor substrate status based on clinically relevant drug interaction potential

Avoid Concomitant Use

Avoid concomitant use of Ramelteon with any of the following: Azelastine (Nasal); FluvoxaMINE; Paraldehyde; Sodium Oxybate

Increased Effect/Toxicity

Ramelteon may increase the levels/effects of: Alcohol (Ethyl); Azelastine (Nasal); Buprenorphine; CNS Depressants; Methotrimeprazine; Metyrosine; Mirtazapine; Paraldehyde; Pramipexole; ROPINIRole; Rotigotine; Selective Serotonin Reuptake Inhibitors; Sodium Oxybate; Zolpidem

The levels/effects of Ramelteon may be increased by: Abiraterone Acetate; Antifungal Agents (Azole Derivatives, Systemic); CYP1A2 Inhibitors (Moderate); CYP1A2 Inhibitors (Strong); Deferasirox; Droperidol; Fluconazole; FluvoxaMINE; HydrOXYzine; Magnesium Sulfate; Methotrimeprazine; Perampanel

Decreased Effect

The levels/effects of Ramelteon may be decreased by: Rifamycin Derivatives

Ethanol/Nutrition/Herb Interactions

Ethanol: May increase CNS depression. Management: Avoid or limit ethanol.

Food: Taking with high-fat meal delays T_{max} and increases AUC (~31%). Management: Do not take with a high-fat meal.

Herb/Nutraceutical: Some herbal medications may increase CNS depression. Management: Avoid valerian, St John's wort, kava kava, and gotu kola.

Dietary Considerations Do not take with high-fat meal.

Pharmacodynamics/Kinetics

Onset of Action 30 minutes

Half-life Elimination Ramelteon: 1-2.6 hours; M-II: 2-5 hours

Time to Peak Median: 0.5-1.5 hours

Pregnancy Risk Factor C

Pregnancy Considerations Animal studies have demonstrated teratogenic effects. May cause disturbances of reproductive hormonal regulation (eg, disruption of menses or decreased libido). There are no adequate and well-controlled studies in pregnant women.

Lactation Excretion in breast milk unknown/use caution

Dosage Forms

Tablet, oral:
Rozerem®: 8 mg

Ramipril (RA mi pril)

Related Information

Cardiovascular Diseases *on page 1492*

Brand Names: U.S. Altace®

Brand Names: Canada Altace®; Apo-Ramipril®; Ava-Ramipril; CO Ramipril; Dom-Ramipril; JAMP-Ramipril; Mylan-Ramipril; PHL-Ramipril; PMS-Ramipril; RAN™-Ramipril; ratio-Ramipril; Sandoz-Ramipril; Teva-Ramipril

Generic Availability (U.S.) Yes

Pharmacologic Category Angiotensin-Converting Enzyme (ACE) Inhibitor

Use Treatment of hypertension, alone or in combination with thiazide diuretics; treatment of left ventricular dysfunction after MI; to reduce risk of MI, stroke, and death in patients at increased risk for these events

Unlabeled Use Treatment of heart failure; to delay the progression of nephropathy and reduce risks of cardiovascular events in hypertensive patients with type 1 or 2 diabetes mellitus

Local Anesthetic/Vasoconstrictor Precautions No information available to require special precautions

Effects on Dental Treatment No significant effects or complications reported

Effects on Bleeding No information available to require special precautions

Adverse Effects Note: Frequency ranges include data from hypertension and heart failure trials. Higher rates of adverse reactions have generally been noted in patients with CHF. However, the frequency of adverse effects associated with placebo is also increased in this population.

◀ >10%: Respiratory: Cough increased (7% to 12%)

1% to 10%:

Cardiovascular: Hypotension (11%), angina (up to 3%), orthostatic hypotension (2%), syncope (up to 2%)

Central nervous system: Headache (1% to 5%), dizziness (2% to 4%), fatigue (2%), vertigo (up to 2%)

Endocrine & metabolic: Hyperkalemia (1% to 10%)

Gastrointestinal: Nausea/vomiting (1% to 2%)

Neuromuscular & skeletal: Chest pain (noncardiac) (1%)

Renal: Renal dysfunction (1%), serum creatinine increased (1% to 2%), BUN increased (<1% to 3%); transient increases of creatinine and/or BUN may occur more frequently

Respiratory: Cough (estimated 1% to 10%)

Worsening of renal function may occur in patients with bilateral renal artery stenosis or in hypovolemia. In addition, a syndrome which may include fever, myalgia, arthralgia, interstitial nephritis, vasculitis, rash, eosinophilia and positive ANA, and elevated ESR has been reported with ACE inhibitors. Risk of pancreatitis and agranulocytosis may be increased in patients with collagen vascular disease or renal impairment.

Dosage Oral:

Adults:

Heart failure (unlabeled use): Initial: 1.25-2.5 mg once daily; target dose: 10 mg once daily (ACC/AHA 2009 Heart Failure Guidelines)

Hypertension: 2.5-5 mg once daily, maximum: 20 mg/day

LV dysfunction postmyocardial infarction: Initial: 2.5 mg twice daily titrated upward, if possible, to 5 mg twice daily

Reduction in risk of MI, stroke, and death from cardiovascular causes: Initial: 2.5 mg once daily for 1 week, then 5 mg once daily for the next 3 weeks, then increase as tolerated to 10 mg once daily (may be given as divided dose)

Elderly: Adjust for renal function for elderly since glomerular filtration rates are decreased; may see exaggerated hypotensive effects if renal clearance is not considered. In the management of hypertension, consider lower initial doses and titrate to response (Aronow, 2011).

Note: The dose of any concomitant diuretic should be reduced. If the diuretic cannot be discontinued, initiate therapy with 1.25 mg. After the initial dose, the patient should be monitored carefully until blood pressure has stabilized.

Dosing adjustment in renal impairment:

Cl_{cr} <40 mL/minute: Administer 25% of normal dose.

Renal failure and heart failure: Administer 1.25 mg once daily, increasing to 1.25 mg twice daily up to 2.5 mg twice daily as tolerated.

Renal failure and hypertension: Administer 1.25 mg once daily, titrated upward as possible; maximum daily dose 5 mg

Mechanism of Action Ramipril is an ACE inhibitor which prevents the formation of angiotensin II from angiotensin I and exhibits pharmacologic effects that are similar to captopril. Ramipril must undergo enzymatic saponification by esterases in the liver to its biologically active metabolite, ramiprilat. The pharmacodynamic effects of ramipril result from the high-affinity, competitive, reversible binding of ramiprilat to angiotensin-converting enzyme, thus preventing the formation of the potent vasoconstrictor angiotensin II.

This isomerized enzyme-inhibitor complex has a slow rate of dissociation, which results in high potency and a long duration of action; a CNS mechanism may also be involved in the hypotensive effect as angiotensin II increases adrenergic outflow from CNS; vasoactive kallikreins may be decreased in conversion to active hormones by ACE inhibitors, thus reducing blood pressure

Contraindications Hypersensitivity to ramipril or any component of the formulation; prior hypersensitivity (including angioedema) to ACE inhibitors; concomitant use with aliskiren in patients with diabetes mellitus

Warnings/Precautions Anaphylactic reactions may occur rarely with ACE inhibitors. At any time during treatment (especially following first dose) angioedema may occur rarely with ACE inhibitors; it may involve the head and neck (potentially compromising airway) or the intestine (presenting with abdominal pain). African-Americans and patients with idiopathic or hereditary angioedema may be at an increased risk. Prolonged frequent monitoring may be required especially if tongue, glottis, or larynx are involved as they are associated with airway obstruction. Patients with a history of airway surgery may have a higher risk of airway obstruction. Aggressive early and appropriate management is critical. Use in patients with previous angioedema associated with ACE inhibitor therapy is contraindicated. Severe anaphylactoid reactions may be seen during hemodialysis (eg, CVVHD) with high-flux dialysis membranes (eg, AN69), and rarely, during low density lipoprotein apheresis with dextran sulfate cellulose. Rare cases of anaphylactoid reactions have been reported in patients undergoing sensitization treatment with hymenoptera (bee, wasp) venom while receiving ACE inhibitors.

Symptomatic hypotension with or without syncope can occur with ACE inhibitors (usually with the first several doses); effects are most often observed in volume-depleted patients; close monitoring of patient is required especially with initial dosing and dosing increases; blood pressure must be lowered at a rate appropriate for the patient's clinical condition. Initiation of therapy in patients with ischemic heart disease or cerebrovascular disease warrants close observation due to the potential consequences posed by falling blood pressure (eg, MI, stroke). Use with caution in hypertrophic cardiomyopathy with outflow tract obstruction, severe aortic stenosis, or before, during, or immediately after major surgery. **[U.S. Boxed Warning]: Drugs that act on the renin-angiotensin system can cause injury and death to the developing fetus. Discontinue as soon as possible once pregnancy is detected.**

Hyperkalemia may occur with ACE inhibitors; risk factors include renal dysfunction, diabetes mellitus, concomitant use of potassium-sparing diuretics, potassium supplements, and/or potassium containing salts. Use cautiously, if at all, with these agents and monitor potassium closely. Cough may occur with ACE inhibitors. Other causes of cough should be considered (eg, pulmonary congestion in patients with heart failure) and excluded prior to discontinuation.

May be associated with deterioration of renal function and/or increases in serum creatinine, particularly in patients with low renal blood flow (eg, renal artery stenosis, heart failure) whose glomerular filtration rate (GFR) is dependent on efferent arteriolar vasoconstriction by angiotensin II; deterioration may result in oliguria, acute renal failure, and progressive azotemia. Small increases in serum creatinine may occur following initiation; consider discontinuation only in patients with progressive and/or significant deterioration in renal function. Use with caution in patients with unstented unilateral/bilateral renal artery stenosis. When unstented bilateral renal artery stenosis is present, use is generally avoided due to the elevated risk of deterioration in renal function unless possible benefits outweigh risks. Concomitant use of an angiotensin receptor blocker (ARB) or renin inhibitor (eg, aliskiren) is associated with an increased risk of hypotension, hyperkalemia, and renal dysfunction; concurrent use with telmisartan is not recommended; concomitant use with aliskiren should be avoided in patients with GFR <60 mL/minute and is contraindicated in patients with diabetes mellitus (regardless of GFR).

Rare toxicities associated with ACE inhibitors include cholestatic jaundice (which may progress to fulminant hepatic necrosis), agranulocytosis, neutropenia, or leukopenia with myeloid hypoplasia. Patients with collagen vascular diseases (especially with concomitant renal impairment) or renal impairment alone may be at increased risk for hematologic toxicity; periodically monitor CBC with differential in these patients.

Drug Interactions
Metabolism/Transport Effects None known.
Avoid Concomitant Use There are no known interactions where it is recommended to avoid concomitant use.

Increased Effect/Toxicity
Ramipril may increase the levels/effects of: Allopurinol; Amifostine; Antihypertensives; AzaTHIOprine; CycloSPORINE (Systemic); Ferric Gluconate; Gold Sodium Thiomalate; Hypotensive Agents; Iron Dextran Complex; Lithium; Nonsteroidal Anti-Inflammatory Agents; RiTUXimab; Sodium Phosphates

The levels/effects of Ramipril may be increased by: Alfuzosin; Aliskiren; Angiotensin II Receptor Blockers; Canagliflozin; Diazoxide; DPP-IV Inhibitors; Eplerenone; Everolimus; Herbs (Hypotensive Properties); Loop Diuretics; MAO Inhibitors; Pentoxifylline; Phosphodiesterase 5 Inhibitors; Potassium Salts; Potassium-Sparing Diuretics; Prostacyclin Analogues; Sirolimus; Telmisartan; Temsirolimus; Thiazide Diuretics; TiZANidine; Tolvaptan; Trimethoprim

Decreased Effect
The levels/effects of Ramipril may be decreased by: Aprotinin; Herbs (Hypertensive Properties); Icatibant; Lanthanum; Methylphenidate; Nonsteroidal Anti-Inflammatory Agents; Salicylates; Yohimbine

Ethanol/Nutrition/Herb Interactions Herb/Nutraceutical: Avoid bayberry, blue cohosh, cayenne, ephedra, ginger, ginseng (American), kola, licorice (may worsen hypertension). Avoid black cohosh, California poppy, coleus, golden seal, hawthorn, mistletoe, periwinkle, quinine, shepherd's purse (may have increased antihypertensive effect).

Pharmacodynamics/Kinetics
Onset of Action 1-2 hours
Duration of Action 24 hours
Half-life Elimination Ramiprilat: Effective: 13-17 hours; Terminal: >50 hours
Time to Peak Serum: Ramipril: ~1 hour; Ramiprilat: 2-4 hours
Pregnancy Risk Factor D
Pregnancy Considerations [U.S. Boxed Warning]: **Drugs that act on the renin-angiotensin system can cause injury and death to the developing fetus. Discontinue as soon as possible once pregnancy is detected.** Ramipril crosses the placenta; teratogenic effects may occur following maternal use during pregnancy. Drugs that act on the renin-angiotensin system are associated with oligohydramnios. Oligohydramnios, due to decreased fetal renal function, may lead to fetal lung hypoplasia and skeletal malformations. Their use in pregnancy is also associated with anuria, hypotension, renal failure, skull hypoplasia, and death in the fetus/neonate. Chronic maternal hypertension itself is also associated with adverse events in the fetus/infant. ACE inhibitors are not recommended during pregnancy to treat maternal hypertension or heart failure. Use of an ACE inhibitor should also be avoided in any woman of reproductive age. Women who are planning a pregnancy should be considered for other medication options if an ACE inhibitor is currently prescribed or the ACE inhibitor should be discontinued as soon as possible once pregnancy is detected. The exposed fetus should be monitored for fetal growth, amniotic fluid volume, and organ formation. Infants exposed to an ACE inhibitor in utero should be monitored for hyperkalemia, hypotension, and oliguria.

Lactation Excretion in breast milk unknown/not recommended

Breast-Feeding Considerations Ramipril and its metabolites were not detected in breast milk following a single oral dose of 10 mg. It is not known if multiple doses will produce detectable levels. Breast-feeding is not recommended by the manufacturer.

Dosage Forms
Capsule, oral: 1.25 mg, 2.5 mg, 5 mg, 10 mg
Altace®: 1.25 mg, 2.5 mg, 5 mg, 10 mg

Ramipril and Felodipine
(RA mi pril & fe LOE di peen)

Related Information
Felodipine *on page 571*
Ramipril *on page 1179*
Brand Names: Canada Altace® Plus Felodipine
Pharmacologic Category Angiotensin-Converting Enzyme (ACE) Inhibitor; Calcium Channel Blocker; Calcium Channel Blocker, Dihydropyridine
Use Treatment of hypertension when combination therapy is appropriate (not for initial therapy)
Local Anesthetic/Vasoconstrictor Precautions No information available to require special precautions
Effects on Dental Treatment No significant effects or complications reported
Effects on Bleeding No information available to require special precautions
Adverse Effects Incidence observed with combination product. Also see individual agents.
1% to 10%:
Cardiovascular: Vasodilation (3%), peripheral edema (2%), palpitation (1%)
Central nervous system: Headache (8%), dizziness (3%), vertigo (2%)
Gastrointestinal: Nausea (2%), abdominal pain (1%), diarrhea (1%)
Neuromuscular & skeletal: Back pain (2%), weakness (2%)
Respiratory: Cough (6%), bronchitis (3%), upper respiratory infection (1%)
Miscellaneous: Infection (2%), flu-like syndrome (2%) ▶

◀ **General Dosage Range** Dosage adjustment recommended in patients with hepatic or renal impairment

Oral:

Adults: Ramipril 2.5-10 mg and felodipine ER 2.5-10 mg once daily

Elderly: Initial: Felodipine ER: 2.5 mg daily (maximum: 10 mg/day)

Mechanism of Action

Ramipril is an ACE inhibitor which first undergoes enzymatic saponification by esterases in the liver, to its active metabolite ramiprilat. The pharmacodynamic effects of ramipril result from the high-affinity, competitive, reversible binding of ramiprilat to angiotensin-converting enzyme thus preventing the formation of the potent vasoconstrictor angiotensin II from angiotensin I. This isomerized enzyme-inhibitor complex has a slow rate of dissociation, which results in high potency and a long duration of action; a CNS mechanism may also be involved in the hypotensive effect as angiotensin II increases adrenergic outflow from CNS; vasoactive kallikreins may be decreased in conversion to active hormones by ACE inhibitors, thus reducing blood pressure

Felodipine inhibits calcium ions from entering the "slow channels" or select voltage-sensitive areas of vascular smooth muscle and myocardium during depolarization, producing a relaxation of coronary vascular smooth muscle and coronary vasodilation, increases myocardial oxygen delivery in patients with vasospastic angina.

Pregnancy Considerations Use is contraindicated in pregnancy. See individual agents.

Product Availability Not available in U.S.

Ranibizumab (ra nib i ZUE mab)

Brand Names: U.S. Lucentis®

Brand Names: Canada Lucentis®

Pharmacologic Category Angiogenesis Inhibitor; Monoclonal Antibody; Ophthalmic Agent; Vascular Endothelial Growth Factor (VEGF) Inhibitor

Use Treatment of neovascular (wet) age-related macular degeneration (AMD); treatment of macular edema following retinal vein occlusion (RVO); diabetic macular edema (DME)

Local Anesthetic/Vasoconstrictor Precautions No information available to require special precautions

Effects on Dental Treatment No significant effects or complications reported

Effects on Bleeding No information available to require special precautions in dental procedures.

Adverse Effects Note: Rates of ocular adverse reactions reported for control group when percentages overlapped with treatment group.

As reported with AMD, RVO, and DME studies:

>10%:

Cardiovascular: Arterial thromboembolic events (AMD trials during first year: 2%; control: 1%; DME trials at 3 years: 11%; control rate not given)

Ocular: Conjunctival hemorrhage (48% to 74%; control: 32% to 60%), eye pain (17% to 35%; control 12% to 30%), vitreous floaters (7% to 27%), intraocular pressure increased (7% to 24%), blurred vision/visual disturbance (5% to 18%), intraocular inflammation (1% to 18%; control 3% to 8%), foreign body sensation (7% to 16%; control: 5% to 14%)

Note: Cataract, blepharitis, dry eye, eye irritation, lacrimation increased, maculopathy, ocular hyperemia, pruritus, and vitreous detachment occurred in

>10% of patients, but also occurred either in similar percentages to the control or more often in the control in some studies.

1% to 10%:

Cardiovascular: Stroke (AMD trials during 2 years: 3%; control: 1%; DME trials at 3 years: 2%; control rate not given)

Ocular: Retinal degeneration (1% to 8%), injection site hemorrhage (≤5%)

Note: Conjunctival hyperemia, ocular discomfort, posterior capsule opacification, and retinal disorder occurred in 1% to 10% of patients, but also occurred in similar percentages to the control or more often in the control in some of the studies.

Miscellaneous: Ranibizumab antibodies (1% to 8%), influenza (3% to 7%; control: 2% to 5%)

General Dosage Range Intravitreal: *Adults:* 0.3 mg or 0.5 mg once every 1-3 months

Mechanism of Action Ranibizumab is a recombinant humanized monoclonal antibody fragment which binds to and inhibits human vascular endothelial growth factor A (VEGF-A). Ranibizumab inhibits VEGF from binding to its receptors and thereby suppressing neovascularization and slowing vision loss.

Pharmacodynamics/Kinetics

Half-life Elimination Vitreous: ~9 days

Pregnancy Risk Factor C

Pregnancy Considerations Adverse fetal effects have been observed in some animal reproduction studies. Based on its mechanism of action, adverse effects on pregnancy would be expected. Canadian labeling recommends that women of childbearing potential use effective contraception during therapy and to wait 3 months after therapy before trying to conceive.

Ranitidine (ra NI ti deen)

Related Information

Gastrointestinal Disorders *on page 1512*

Brand Names: U.S. Zantac 150® [OTC]; Zantac 75® [OTC]; Zantac®; Zantac® EFFERdose®

Brand Names: Canada Acid Reducer; Apo-Ranitidine®; CO Ranitidine; Dom-Ranitidine; Myl-Ranitidine; Mylan-Ranitidine; Nu-Ranit; PHL-Ranitidine; PMS-Ranitidine; Ranitidine Injection, USP; RAN™-Ranitidine; ratio-Ranitidine; Riva-Ranitidine; Sandoz-Ranitidine; ScheinPharm Ranitidine; Teva-Ranitidine; Zantac 75®; Zantac Maximum Strength Non-Prescription; Zantac®

Generic Availability (U.S.) Yes: Excludes effervescent tablet, premixed infusion

Pharmacologic Category Histamine H_2 Antagonist

Use

Zantac®: Short-term and maintenance therapy of duodenal ulcer, gastric ulcer, gastroesophageal reflux disease (GERD), active benign ulcer, erosive esophagitis, and pathological hypersecretory conditions; as part of a multidrug regimen for *H. pylori* eradication to reduce the risk of duodenal ulcer recurrence

Zantac 75® [OTC]: Relief of heartburn, acid indigestion, and sour stomach

Unlabeled Use Recurrent postoperative ulcer, upper GI bleeding, prevention of acid-aspiration pneumonitis during surgery, and prevention of stress-induced ulcers

Local Anesthetic/Vasoconstrictor Precautions No information available to require special precautions

Effects on Dental Treatment No significant effects or complications reported

Effects on Bleeding No information available to require special precautions

Adverse Effects Frequency not defined.

Cardiovascular: Asystole, atrioventricular block, bradycardia (with rapid I.V. administration), premature ventricular beats, tachycardia, vasculitis

Central nervous system: Agitation, dizziness, depression, hallucinations, headache, insomnia, malaise, mental confusion, somnolence, vertigo

Dermatologic: Alopecia, erythema multiforme, rash

Endocrine & metabolic: Prolactin levels increased

Gastrointestinal: Abdominal discomfort/pain, constipation, diarrhea, nausea, necrotizing enterocolitis (VLBW neonates; Guillet, 2006), pancreatitis, vomiting

Hematologic: Acquired immune hemolytic anemia, acute porphyritic attack, agranulocytosis, aplastic anemia, granulocytopenia, leukopenia, pancytopenia, thrombocytopenia

Hepatic: Cholestatic hepatitis, hepatic failure, hepatitis, jaundice

Local: Transient pain, burning or itching at the injection site

Neuromuscular & skeletal: Arthralgia, involuntary motor disturbance, myalgia

Ocular: Blurred vision

Renal: Acute interstitial nephritis, serum creatinine increased

Respiratory: Pneumonia (causal relationship not established)

Miscellaneous: Anaphylaxis, angioneurotic edema, hypersensitivity reactions (eg, bronchospasm, fever, eosinophilia)

Dosage

Children 1 month to 16 years:

Duodenal and gastric ulcer:

Oral:

Treatment: 4-8 mg/kg/day divided twice daily; maximum: 300 mg/day

Maintenance: 2-4 mg/kg/day once daily; maximum: 150 mg/day

I.V.: 2-4 mg/kg/day divided every 6-8 hours; maximum: 200 mg/day

GERD and erosive esophagitis:

Oral: 5-10 mg/kg/day divided twice daily; maximum: GERD: 300 mg/day, erosive esophagitis: 600 mg/day

I.V. (unlabeled): 2-4 mg/kg/day divided every 6-8 hours; maximum: 200 mg/day **or as an alternative**

Continuous infusion: Initial: 1 mg/kg/dose for one dose followed by infusion of 0.08-0.17 mg/kg/hour or 2-4 mg/kg/day

Children ≥12 years: Prevention of heartburn: Oral: Zantac 75® [OTC]: 75 mg 30-60 minutes before eating food or drinking beverages which cause heartburn; maximum: 150 mg/24 hours; do not use for more than 14 days

Adults:

Duodenal ulcer: Oral: Treatment: 150 mg twice daily, or 300 mg once daily after the evening meal or at bedtime; maintenance: 150 mg once daily at bedtime

Helicobacter pylori eradication: 150 mg twice daily; requires combination therapy

Pathological hypersecretory conditions:

Oral: 150 mg twice daily; adjust dose or frequency as clinically indicated; doses of up to 6 g/day have been used

I.V.: Continuous infusion for Zollinger-Ellison: Initial: 1 mg/kg/hour; measure gastric acid output at 4 hours, if >10 mEq or if patient is symptomatic, increase dose in increments of 0.5 mg/kg/hour; doses of up to 2.5 mg/kg/hour (or 220 mg/hour) have been used

Gastric ulcer, benign: Oral: 150 mg twice daily; maintenance: 150 mg once daily at bedtime

GERD: Oral: 150 mg twice daily

Erosive esophagitis: Oral: Treatment: 150 mg 4 times/day; maintenance: 150 mg twice daily

Prevention of heartburn: Oral: Zantac 75® [OTC]: 75 mg 30-60 minutes before eating food or drinking beverages which cause heartburn; maximum: 150 mg in 24 hours; do not use for more than 14 days

Stress ulcer prophylaxis, ICU patients (unlabeled use; ASHP, 1999): **Note:** Intended for patients with associated risk factors (eg, coagulopathy, mechanical ventilation for >48 hours, severe sepsis); discontinue use once risk factors have resolved. The Surviving Sepsis Campaign guidelines suggest the use of proton pump inhibitors rather than H_2 antagonist therapy (Dellinger, 2013).

Oral, nasogastric (NG) tube: 150 mg twice daily; may administer a 300 mg loading dose prior to maintenance dosing (Pemberton, 1993)

I.V.: Intermittent bolus: 50 mg every 6-8 hours (Cook, 1998; Geus 1993)

Patients not able to take oral medication:

I.M.: 50 mg every 6-8 hours

I.V.: Intermittent bolus or infusion: 50 mg every 6-8 hours

Continuous I.V. infusion: 6.25 mg/hour

Elderly: Ulcer healing rates and incidence of adverse effects are similar in the elderly, when compared to younger patients; dosing adjustments not necessary based on age alone

Dosing adjustment in renal impairment: Adults: Cl_{cr} <50 mL/minute:

Oral: 150 mg every 24 hours; adjust dose cautiously if needed

I.V.: 50 mg every 18-24 hours; adjust dose cautiously if needed

Hemodialysis: Adjust dosing schedule so that dose coincides with the end of hemodialysis

Stress ulcer prophylaxis (ASHP, 1999): Cl_{cr} <50 mL/minute:

Oral, nasogastric (NG) tube: 150 mg 1-2 times daily

I.V.: Intermittent bolus: 50 mg every 12-24 hours

Dosing adjustment/comments in hepatic disease: Patients with hepatic impairment may have minor changes in ranitidine half-life, distribution, clearance, and bioavailability; dosing adjustments not necessary, monitor

Mechanism of Action Competitive inhibition of histamine at H_2-receptors of the gastric parietal cells, which inhibits gastric acid secretion, gastric volume, and hydrogen ion concentration are reduced. Does not affect pepsin secretion, pentagastrin-stimulated intrinsic factor secretion, or serum gastrin.

Contraindications Hypersensitivity to ranitidine or any component of the formulation

Warnings/Precautions Ranitidine has been associated with confusional states (rare). Use with caution in patients with hepatic impairment; use with caution in renal impairment, dosage modification required. Avoid use in patients with history of acute porphyria (may precipitate attacks); long-term therapy may be associated with vitamin B_{12} deficiency. Symptoms of GI distress may be associated with a variety of conditions; symptomatic response to H_2 antagonists does not rule out the potential for significant pathology (eg, malignancy). EFFERdose® formulation contains phenylalanine.

◀ **Drug Interactions**
Metabolism/Transport Effects Substrate of CYP1A2 (minor), CYP2C19 (minor), CYP2D6 (minor), P-glycoprotein; **Note:** Assignment of Major/Minor substrate status based on clinically relevant drug interaction potential; **Inhibits** CYP1A2 (weak), CYP2D6 (weak)

Avoid Concomitant Use
Avoid concomitant use of Ranitidine with any of the following: Dasatinib; Delavirdine; Ponatinib; Risedronate

Increased Effect/Toxicity
Ranitidine may increase the levels/effects of: ARIPiprazole; Dexmethylphenidate; Methylphenidate; Procainamide; Risedronate; Saquinavir; Sulfonylureas; Varenicline; Warfarin

The levels/effects of Ranitidine may be increased by: P-glycoprotein/ABCB1 Inhibitors

Decreased Effect
Ranitidine may decrease the levels/effects of: Atazanavir; Bosutinib; Cefditoren; Cefpodoxime; Cefuroxime; Dasatinib; Delavirdine; Erlotinib; Fosamprenavir; Gefitinib; Indinavir; Iron Salts; Itraconazole; Ketoconazole (Systemic); Mesalamine; Multivitamins/Minerals (with ADEK, Folate, Iron); Nelfinavir; Nilotinib; Ponatinib; Posaconazole; Prasugrel; Rilpivirine; Vismodegib

The levels/effects of Ranitidine may be decreased by: Peginterferon Alfa-2b; P-glycoprotein/ABCB1 Inducers

Ethanol/Nutrition/Herb Interactions
Ethanol: Avoid ethanol (may cause gastric mucosal irritation).
Food: Does not interfere with absorption of ranitidine.

Dietary Considerations Some products may contain phenylalanine and/or sodium. Oral dosage forms may be taken with or without food.

Pharmacodynamics/Kinetics
Half-life Elimination
Oral: Normal renal function: 2.5-3 hours; Cl_{cr} 25-35 mL/minute: 4.8 hours
I.V.: Normal renal function: 2-2.5 hours
Time to Peak Serum: Oral: 2-3 hours; I.M.: ≤15 minutes

Pregnancy Risk Factor B
Pregnancy Considerations Adverse events were not observed in animal studies; therefore, ranitidine is classified as pregnancy category B. Ranitidine crosses the placenta. An increased risk of congenital malformations or adverse events in the newborn has generally not been observed following maternal use of ranitidine during pregnancy. Histamine H_2 antagonists have been evaluated for the treatment of gastroesophageal reflux disease (GERD) as well as gastric and duodenal ulcers during pregnancy. If needed, ranitidine is the agent of choice. Histamine H_2 antagonists may be used for aspiration prophylaxis prior to cesarean delivery.

Lactation Enters breast milk/use caution
Breast-Feeding Considerations Ranitidine is excreted into breast milk. The manufacturer recommends that caution be exercised when administering ranitidine to nursing women. Peak milk concentrations of ranitidine occur ~5.5 hours after the dose (case report).

Dosage Forms
Capsule, oral: 150 mg, 300 mg
Infusion, premixed in 1/2 NS [preservative free]:
Zantac®: 50 mg (50 mL)
Injection, solution: 25 mg/mL (2 mL, 6 mL, 40 mL)
Zantac®: 25 mg/mL (2 mL, 6 mL, 40 mL)

Syrup, oral: 15 mg/mL (1 mL, 5 mL, 10 mL, 120 mL, 473 mL, 474 mL, 480 mL)
Zantac®: 15 mg/mL (480 mL)
Tablet, oral: 75 mg, 150 mg, 300 mg
Zantac 150® [OTC]: 150 mg
Zantac 75® [OTC]: 75 mg
Zantac®: 150 mg, 300 mg
Tablet for solution, oral:
Zantac® EFFERdose®: 25 mg

Ranolazine (ra NOE la zeen)

Related Information
Clinical Risk Related to Drugs Prolonging QT Interval *on page 1510*
Brand Names: U.S. Ranexa®
Pharmacologic Category Antianginal Agent; Cardiovascular Agent, Miscellaneous
Use Treatment of chronic angina
Local Anesthetic/Vasoconstrictor Precautions Ranolazine is one of the drugs confirmed to prolong the QT interval and is accepted as having a risk of causing torsade de pointes. The risk of drug-induced torsade de pointes is extremely low when a single QT interval prolonging drug is prescribed. In terms of epinephrine, it is not known what effect vasoconstrictors in the local anesthetic regimen will have in patients with a known history of congenital prolonged QT interval or in patients taking any medication that prolongs the QT interval. Until more information is obtained, it is suggested that the clinician consult with the physician prior to the use of a vasoconstrictor in suspected patients, and that the vasoconstrictor (epinephrine, mepivacaine and levonordefrin [Carbocaine® 2% with Neo-Cobefrin®]) be used with caution.
Effects on Dental Treatment Key adverse event(s) related to dental treatment: Xerostomia (normal salivary flow resumes upon discontinuation).
Effects on Bleeding No information available to require special precautions
Adverse Effects >0.5% to 10%:
Cardiovascular: Bradycardia (≤4%), hypotension (≤4%), orthostatic hypotension (≤4%), palpitation (≤4%), peripheral edema (≤4%), QT_c prolongation (>500 msec: ≤1%)
Central nervous system: Headache (≤6%), dizziness (1% to 6%), confusion (≤4%), vasovagal attacks (≤4%), vertigo (≤4%)
Dermatologic: Hyperhidrosis (≤4%)
Gastrointestinal: Constipation (≤9%), abdominal pain (≤4%), anorexia (≤4%), dyspepsia (≤4%), nausea (≤4%; dose related), vomiting (≤4%), xerostomia (≤4%)
Neuromuscular: Weakness (≤4%)
Ocular: Blurred vision (≤4%)
Otic: Tinnitus (≤4%)
Renal: Hematuria (≤4%)
Respiratory: Dyspnea (≤4%)
General Dosage Range Dosage adjustment recommended in patients on concomitant therapy
Oral: *Adults:* Initial: 500 mg twice daily; Maintenance: 500-1000 mg twice daily (maximum: 2000 mg/day)
Mechanism of Action Ranolazine exerts antianginal and anti-ischemic effects without changing hemodynamic parameters (heart rate or blood pressure). At therapeutic levels, ranolazine inhibits the late phase of the inward sodium channel (late I_{Na}) in ischemic cardiac myocytes during cardiac repolarization reducing intracellular sodium concentrations and thereby reducing calcium influx via Na^+-Ca^{2+} exchange. Decreased

intracellular calcium reduces ventricular tension and myocardial oxygen consumption. It is thought that ranolazine produces myocardial relaxation and reduces anginal symptoms through this mechanism although this is uncertain. At higher concentrations, ranolazine inhibits the rapid delayed rectifier potassium current (I_{Kr}) thus prolonging the ventricular action potential duration and subsequent prolongation of the QT interval.

Pharmacodynamics/Kinetics

Half-life Elimination Ranolazine: Terminal: 7 hours; Metabolites (activity undefined): 6-22 hours

Time to Peak 2-5 hours

Pregnancy Risk Factor C

Pregnancy Considerations Adverse effects were observed in animal studies. There are no adequate and well-controlled studies in pregnant women.

Dental Comment Ranolazine is known to prolong the QT interval. The QT interval is measured as the time and distance between the Q point of the QRS complex and the end of the T wave in the ECG tracing. After adjustment for heart rate, the QT interval is defined as prolonged if it is more than 450 msec in men and 460 msec in women. A long QT syndrome was first described in the 1950s and 60s as a congenital syndrome involving QT interval prolongation and syncope and sudden death. Some of the congenital long QT syndromes were characterized by a peculiar electrocardiographic appearance of the QRS complex involving a premature atria beat followed by a pause, then a subsequent sinus beat showing marked QT prolongation and deformity. This type of cardiac arrhythmia was originally termed "torsade de pointes" (translated from the French as "twisting of the points"). Ranolazine is considered as having a risk of causing torsade de pointes. Since it is not known what effect vasoconstrictors in the local anesthetic regimen will have in patients with a known history of congenital prolonged QT interval or in patients taking any medication that prolongs the QT interval, a medical consult is suggested.

Rasagiline (ra SA ji leen)

Brand Names: U.S. Azilect®

Brand Names: Canada Azilect®

Pharmacologic Category Anti-Parkinson's Agent, MAO Type B Inhibitor

Use Treatment of idiopathic Parkinson's disease (initial monotherapy or as adjunct to levodopa)

Local Anesthetic/Vasoconstrictor Precautions Rasagiline in approved doses of 0.5-1 mg daily should not inhibit type-A MAO; however, the possibility exists of nonselective MAO inhibition at higher doses and/or in certain sensitive individuals. Therefore, attempts should be made to avoid use of vasoconstrictors due to possibility of hypertensive episodes.

Effects on Dental Treatment Key adverse event(s) related to dental treatment: Xerostomia and changes in salivation (normal salivary flow resumes upon discontinuation). Anticholinergic side effects can cause a reduction of saliva production or secretion, contributing to discomfort and dental disease (ie, caries, oral candidiasis, and periodontal disease). May cause orthostatic hypotension particularly during the first 2 months of therapy.

Effects on Bleeding No information available to require special precautions

Adverse Effects Unless otherwise noted, the following adverse reactions are as reported for monotherapy. Spectrum of adverse events was generally similar with adjunctive (levodopa) therapy, though the incidence tended to be higher.

>10%:

Cardiovascular: Orthostatic hypotension (6% to 13% adjunct therapy, dose dependent)

Central nervous system: Dyskinesia (18% adjunct therapy), headache (14%)

Gastrointestinal: Nausea (10% to 12% adjunct therapy)

1% to 10%:

Cardiovascular: Angina, bundle branch block, chest pain, syncope

Central nervous system: Depression (5%), hallucinations (4% to 5% adjunct therapy), fever (3%), malaise (2%), vertigo (2%), anxiety, dizziness

Dermatologic: Bruising (2%), alopecia, skin carcinoma, vesiculobullous rash

Endocrine & metabolic: Impotence, libido decreased

Gastrointestinal: Constipation (4% to 9% adjunct therapy), weight loss (2% to 9% adjunct therapy; dose dependent), dyspepsia (7%), xerostomia (2% to 6% adjunct therapy; dose dependent), gastroenteritis (3%), anorexia, diarrhea, gastrointestinal hemorrhage, vomiting

Genitourinary: Hematuria, urinary incontinence

Hematologic: Leukopenia

Hepatic: Liver function tests increased

Neuromuscular & skeletal: Arthralgia (7%), neck pain (2%), arthritis (2%), paresthesia (2%), abnormal gait, hyperkinesias, hypertonia, neuropathy, tremor, weakness

Ocular: Conjunctivitis (3%)

Renal: Albuminuria

Respiratory: Rhinitis (3%), asthma, cough increased

Miscellaneous: Fall (5%), flu-like syndrome (5%), allergic reaction

General Dosage Range Dosage adjustment recommended in patients with hepatic impairment or on concomitant therapy

Oral: *Adults:* 0.5-1 mg once daily

Mechanism of Action Potent, irreversible and selective inhibitor of brain monoamine oxidase (MAO) type B, which plays a major role in the catabolism of dopamine. Inhibition of dopamine depletion in the striatal region of the brain reduces the symptomatic motor deficits of Parkinson's disease. There is also experimental evidence of rasagiline conferring neuroprotective effects (antioxidant, antiapoptotic), which may delay onset of symptoms and progression of neuronal deterioration.

Pharmacodynamics/Kinetics

Onset of Action Therapeutic: Within 1 hour

Duration of Action ~1 week (irreversible inhibition); may require ~14-40 days for complete restoration of (brain) MAO-B activity

Half-life Elimination ~1.3-3 hours (no correlation with biologic effect due to irreversible inhibition)

Time to Peak ~1 hour

Pregnancy Risk Factor C

Pregnancy Considerations Animal studies have documented decreased offspring survival and birth weight. An increased incidence of teratogenic effects, embryo-fetal deaths, and cardiovascular abnormalities were also noted with rasagiline in combination with levodopa/carbidopa. There are no adequate and well-controlled studies in pregnant women.

Rasburicase (ras BYOOR i kayse)

Brand Names: U.S. Elitek®
Brand Names: Canada Fasturtec®
Pharmacologic Category Enzyme; Enzyme, Urate-Oxidase (Recombinant)
Use Initial management of uric acid levels in patients with leukemia, lymphoma, and solid tumor malignancies receiving chemotherapy expected to result in tumor lysis and elevation of plasma uric acid
Local Anesthetic/Vasoconstrictor Precautions No information available to require special precautions
Effects on Dental Treatment Key adverse event(s) related to dental treatment: Mucositis.
Effects on Bleeding No information available to require special precautions
Adverse Effects
>10%:
 Cardiovascular: Peripheral edema (≤50%), fluid overload (≤12%)
 Central nervous system: Fever (46%; serious: 5%), headache (26%), anxiety (≤24%)
 Dermatologic: Rash (13%; serious: 1%)
 Endocrine & metabolic: Hypophosphatemia (≤17%)
 Gastrointestinal: Vomiting (50%), nausea (27%), abdominal pain (20%), constipation (20%), diarrhea (20%), mucositis (15%; serious: 2%)
 Hepatic: Hyperbilirubinemia (≤16%), ALT increased (≤11%)
 Respiratory: Pharyngolaryngeal pain (≤14%)
 Miscellaneous: Antibody formation (healthy volunteers: 61% to 64%; patients with malignancies: 11%), sepsis (≤12%; serious: 3% to 5%)
1% to 10%:
 Cardiovascular: Ischemic coronary disorder, supraventricular arrhythmia
 Endocrine & metabolic: Hyperphosphatemia (≤10%)
 Gastrointestinal: Abdominal/gastrointestinal infection
 Hematologic: Neutropenic fever (serious: 4%), neutropenia (serious: 2%)
 Respiratory: Respiratory distress (serious: 3%), pulmonary hemorrhage, respiratory failure
 Miscellaneous: Hypersensitivity (≤4%)
General Dosage Range I.V.: *Children and Adults:* 0.2 mg/kg once daily
Mechanism of Action Rasburicase is a recombinant urate-oxidase enzyme, which converts uric acid to allantoin (an inactive and soluble metabolite of uric acid); it does not inhibit the formation of uric acid.
Pharmacodynamics/Kinetics
 Onset of Action Uric acid levels decrease within 4 hours of initial administration
 Half-life Elimination ~16-23 hours
Pregnancy Risk Factor C
Pregnancy Considerations Adverse effects were observed in animal reproduction studies. There are no adequate and well-controlled studies in pregnant women. Use during pregnancy only if the benefit to the mother outweighs the potential risk to the fetus.

Regorafenib (re goe RAF e nib)

Brand Names: U.S. Stivarga®
Brand Names: Canada Stivarga®
Pharmacologic Category Antineoplastic Agent, Tyrosine Kinase Inhibitor; Vascular Endothelial Growth Factor (VEGF) Inhibitor

Use
U.S. labeling: Treatment of metastatic colorectal cancer in patients previously treated with fluoropyrimidine-, oxaliplatin-, and irinotecan-based chemotherapy, anti-VEGF therapy, or anti-EGFR therapy (if *KRAS* wild type); treatment of locally-advanced, unresectable, or metastatic gastrointestinal stromal tumor (GIST) in patients previously treated with imatinib and sunitinib

Canadian labeling: Treatment of metastatic colorectal cancer in patients previously treated with fluoropyrimidine-, oxaliplatin-, and irinotecan-based chemotherapy, anti-VEGF therapy, or anti-EGFR therapy (if *KRAS* wild type)
Local Anesthetic/Vasoconstrictor Precautions Use vasoconstrictor with caution; patients may experience significant hypertension when taking regorafenib
Effects on Dental Treatment Key adverse event(s) related to dental treatment: Mucositis, xerostomia (normal salivary flow resumes upon discontinuation), and taste disturbance
Effects on Bleeding Chemotherapy may result in significant myelosuppression, potentially including significant reduction in platelet counts and altered hemostasis. Thrombocytopenia has been reported (41%; grade 3: 2%; grade 4: <1%). Bleeding has been reported in 21% in patients. In patients who are under active treatment with these agents, medical consult is suggested.
Adverse Effects
>10%:
 Cardiovascular: Hypertension (30% to 59%; grade ≥3: 8% to 28%)
 Central nervous system: Fatigue (52% to 64%), dysphonia (30% to 39%), pain (29%), fever (21% to 28%), headache (10% to 16%)
 Dermatologic: Palmar-plantar erythrodysesthesia (45% to 67%; grade ≥3: 17% to 22%), rash (26% to 30%; grade ≥3: 6% to 7%), alopecia (8% to 24%)
 Endocrine & metabolic: Hypocalcemia (17% to 59%), hypophosphatemia (55% to 57%), hyponatremia (30%), hypokalemia (21% to 26%), hypothyroidism (4% to 18%)
 Gastrointestinal: Appetite decreased (31% to 47%), lipase increased (14% to 46%), diarrhea (43% to 47%), mucositis (33% to 40%), weight loss (14% to 32%), amylase increased (26%), nausea (20%), vomiting (17%)
 Hematologic: Anemia (79%; grade 3: 5%; grade 4: 1%), lymphopenia (30% to 54%; grade 3: 8% to 9%), thrombocytopenia (13% to 41%; grade 3: 1% to 2%; grade 4: <1%), INR increased (24%), hemorrhage (11% to 21%; grade ≥3: 2% to 4%), neutropenia (3% to 16%; grade 3: 1% to 2%)
 Hepatic: AST increased (58% to 65%; grade 3: 3% to 5%; grade 4: 1%), ALT increased (39% to 45%; grade 3: 4% to 5%; grade 4: 1%), hyperbilirubinemia (33% to 45%)
 Neuromuscular & skeletal: Stiffness (14%)
 Renal: Proteinuria (33% to 60%; grade 3: 3%)
 Miscellaneous: Infection (31% to 32%; grade ≥3: 5% to 9%)
1% to 10%:
 Cardiovascular: Myocardial ischemia and infarction (1%)
 Gastrointestinal: Taste disturbance (8%), xerostomia (5%), gastroesophageal reflux (1%)
 Neuromuscular & skeletal: Tremor (2%)
 Respiratory: Dyspnea (2%)

General Dosage Range Dosage adjustment recommended in patients who develop toxicities

Oral: *Adults:* 160 mg once daily

Mechanism of Action Regorafenib is a multikinase inhibitor; it targets kinases involved with tumor angiogenesis, oncogenesis, and maintenance of the tumor microenvironment which results in inhibition of tumor growth. Specifically, it inhibits VEGF receptors 1-3, KIT, PDGFR-alpha, PDGFR-beta, RET, FGFR1 and 2, TIE2, DDR2, TrkA, Eph2A, RAF-1. BRAF, BRAF^V600E, SAPK2, PTK5, and Abl.

Pharmacodynamics/Kinetics

Half-life Elimination Regorafenib: 28 hours (range: 14-58 hours); M-2 metabolite: 25 hours (range: 14-32 hours); M-5 metabolite: 51 hours (range: 32-70 hours)

Time to Peak 4 hours

Pregnancy Risk Factor D

Pregnancy Considerations In animal reproduction studies, teratogenic effects were observed with doses less than the equivalent human dose. Patients (male and female) should use effective contraception during therapy and for at least 2 months following treatment.

Prescribing and Access Restrictions Regorafenib is available only through the REACH support program. Information regarding program enrollment may be found at http://www.stivarga-us.com/access_stivarga.html or by calling 1-866-639-2827.

Remifentanil (rem i FEN ta nil)

Brand Names: U.S. Ultiva®
Brand Names: Canada Ultiva®
Pharmacologic Category Analgesic, Opioid; Anilidopiperidine Opioid
Use Analgesic for use during the induction and maintenance of general anesthesia; for continued analgesia into the immediate postoperative period; analgesic component of monitored anesthesia
Unlabeled Use Management of pain in mechanically-ventilated patients
Local Anesthetic/Vasoconstrictor Precautions No information available to require special precautions
Effects on Dental Treatment No significant effects or complications reported
Effects on Bleeding No information available to require special precautions
Adverse Effects Frequency of adverse events may vary based on surgical procedures and rate of infusion.
>10%:
Cardiovascular: Hypotension (2% to 19%), bradycardia (1% to 7%; dose dependent)
Central nervous system: Headache (<2% to 18%)
Dermatologic: Pruritus (<2% to 18%)
Gastrointestinal: Nausea (<36% to 44%), vomiting (<16% to 22%)
Neuromuscular & skeletal: Muscle rigidity (<1% to 11%; includes chest wall rigidity)
1% to 10%:
Cardiovascular: Hypertension (1% to 2%; dose dependent), tachycardia (≤1%; dose dependent), flushing (1%)
Central nervous system: Fever (<5%), dizziness (<5%), postoperative pain (<2%), chills (1%), agitation (≤1%)
Local: Pain at injection site (1%)
Respiratory: Respiratory depression (<7%), apnea (<3%), hypoxia (≤1%)
Miscellaneous: Diaphoresis (6%), shivering (<5%), warm sensation (1%)

General Dosage Range I.V.:
Infants Birth to 2 months: Infusion: 0.4-1 mcg/kg/minute; Supplemental bolus dose: ≤1 mcg/kg
Children 1-12 years: Infusion: 0.05-1.3 mcg/kg/minute; Bolus: 1 mcg/kg every 2-5 minutes
Adults: Infusion: 0.025-4 mcg/kg/minute; Bolus: 0.5-1 mcg/kg every 2-5 minutes
Elderly: Doses should be decreased by 50% and titrated
Mechanism of Action Binds with stereospecific mu-opioid receptors at many sites within the CNS, increases pain threshold, alters pain reception, inhibits ascending pain pathways
Pharmacodynamics/Kinetics
Onset of Action I.V.: 1-3 minutes
Half-life Elimination Dose dependent: Terminal: 10-20 minutes; effective: 3-10 minutes
Pregnancy Risk Factor C
Pregnancy Considerations Adverse events were not observed in animal reproduction studies. Remifentanil has been shown to cross the placenta; fetal and maternal concentrations may be similar. Maternal apnea, as well as neonatal respiratory depression and sedation, may occur (Montgomery, 2006).
Controlled Substance C-II

Repaglinide (re PAG li nide)

Related Information
Endocrine Disorders and Pregnancy *on page 1517*
Brand Names: U.S. Prandin®
Brand Names: Canada CO-Repaglinide; Gluco-Norm®; PMS-Repaglinide; Sandoz-Repaglinide
Pharmacologic Category Antidiabetic Agent, Meglitinide Derivative
Use Management of type 2 diabetes mellitus (noninsulin dependent, NIDDM) as an adjunct to diet and exercise; may be used in combination with metformin or thiazolidinediones
Local Anesthetic/Vasoconstrictor Precautions No information available to require special precautions
Effects on Dental Treatment Key adverse event(s) related to dental treatment: Tooth disorder.
Effects on Bleeding No information available to require special precautions
Adverse Effects
>10%:
Central nervous system: Headache (9% to 11%)
Endocrine & metabolic: Hypoglycemia (16% to 31%)
Respiratory: Upper respiratory tract infection (10% to 16%)
1% to 10%:
Cardiovascular: Ischemia (4%), chest pain (2% to 3%)
Gastrointestinal: Diarrhea (4% to 5%), constipation (2% to 3%)
Genitourinary: Urinary tract infection (2% to 3%)
Neuromuscular & skeletal: Back pain (5% to 6%), arthralgia (3% to 6%)
Respiratory: Sinusitis (3% to 6%), bronchitis (2% to 6%)
Miscellaneous: Allergy (1% to 2%)
General Dosage Range Dosage adjustment recommended in patients with renal impairment
Oral: *Adults:* Initial: 0.5-2 mg before each meal; Maintenance: 0.5-4 mg before each meal (maximum: 16 mg/day)
Mechanism of Action Nonsulfonylurea hypoglycemic agent which blocks ATP-dependent potassium channels, depolarizing the membrane and facilitating calcium entry through calcium channels. Increased intracellular

calcium stimulates insulin release from the pancreatic beta cells. Repaglinide-induced insulin release is glucose-dependent.

Pharmacodynamics/Kinetics

Onset of Action Single dose: Increased insulin levels: ~15-60 minutes

Duration of Action 4-6 hours

Half-life Elimination ~1 hour

Time to Peak Plasma: ~1 hour

Pregnancy Risk Factor C

Pregnancy Considerations Adverse events have been observed in some animal studies; therefore, repaglinide is classified as pregnancy category C. Information describing the effects of repaglinide on pregnancy outcomes is limited. Maternal hyperglycemia can be associated with adverse effects in the fetus, including macrosomia, neonatal hyperglycemia, and hyperbilirubinemia; the risk of congenital malformations is increased when the Hb A_{1c} is above the normal range. Diabetes can also be associated with adverse effects in the mother. Poorly-treated diabetes may cause end-organ damage that may in turn negatively affect obstetric outcomes. Physiologic glucose levels should be maintained prior to and during pregnancy to decrease the risk of adverse events in the mother and the fetus. Until additional safety and efficacy data are obtained, the use of oral agents is generally not recommended as routine management of GDM or type 2 diabetes mellitus during pregnancy. Insulin is the drug of choice for the control of diabetes mellitus during pregnancy.

Repaglinide and Metformin
(re PAG li nide & met FOR min)

Related Information

MetFORMIN *on page 882*

Repaglinide *on page 1187*

Brand Names: U.S. PrandiMet®

Pharmacologic Category Antidiabetic Agent, Biguanide; Antidiabetic Agent, Meglitinide Derivative; Hypoglycemic Agent, Oral

Use Management of type 2 diabetes mellitus (noninsulin dependent, NIDDM), as an adjunct to diet and exercise, in patients currently receiving or not adequately controlled on metformin and/or a meglitinide

Local Anesthetic/Vasoconstrictor Precautions No information available to require special precautions

Effects on Dental Treatment Key adverse event(s) related to dental treatment: Patients with diabetes (noninsulin dependent, type 2) taking repaglinide and metformin combination should schedule dental treatment in morning in order to minimize stress-induced hypoglycemia

Effects on Bleeding No information available to require special precautions

Adverse Effects Note: The following information reflects the frequency of adverse effects experienced by patients who received the repaglinide/metformin fixed-dose combination product. Also see individual agents.

>10%:

Central nervous system: Headache (22%)

Endocrine & metabolic: Hypoglycemia (33%)

Gastrointestinal: Diarrhea (19%), nausea (15%)

Respiratory: Upper respiratory tract infection (11%)

General Dosage Range Oral: *Adults:* Repaglinide 1-2 mg and metformin 500 mg 2-3 times daily with meals (maximum single dose: 4 mg/dose [repaglinide], 1000 mg/dose [metformin]; maximum daily dose: 10 mg/day [repaglinide], 2500 mg/day [metformin])

Mechanism of Action Combination therapy; repaglinide and metformin act to improve glycemic control via two different mechanisms of action:

Repaglinide is a nonsulfonylurea hypoglycemic agent which stimulates insulin release by blocking ATP-dependent potassium channels, depolarizing the membrane and facilitating calcium entry through calcium channels; increased intracellular calcium stimulates insulin release from the pancreatic beta cells.

Metformin prevents hyperglycemia by decreasing hepatic glucose production, decreasing intestinal absorption of glucose, and improving insulin sensitivity via increased peripheral glucose uptake and utilization.

Pregnancy Risk Factor C

Pregnancy Considerations Reproduction studies have not been conducted with this combination; therefore, repaglinide/metformin is classified as pregnancy category C. See individual agents.

Reserpine (re SER peen)

Pharmacologic Category Central Monoamine-Depleting Agent; Rauwolfia Alkaloid

Use Management of mild-to-moderate hypertension; treatment of agitated psychotic states (schizophrenia)

Unlabeled Use Management of tardive dyskinesia

Local Anesthetic/Vasoconstrictor Precautions No information available to require special precautions

Effects on Dental Treatment Key adverse event(s) related to dental treatment: Xerostomia and changes in salivation (normal salivary flow resumes upon discontinuation).

Effects on Bleeding No information available to require special precautions

Adverse Effects Frequency not defined.

Cardiovascular: Arrhythmia, bradycardia, chest pain, hypotension, peripheral edema, PVC, syncope

Central nervous system: Dizziness, drowsiness, dull sensorium, fatigue, headache, mental depression, nightmares, nervousness, parkinsonism, paradoxical anxiety

Dermatologic: Flushing of skin, pruritus, purpura, rash

Endocrine & metabolic: Gynecomastia, weight gain

Gastrointestinal: Anorexia, diarrhea, dry mouth, gastric acid secretion increased, nausea, salivation increased, vomiting

Genitourinary: Impotence, libido decreased

Hematologic: Thrombocytopenia purpura

Neuromuscular & skeletal: Muscle ache

Ocular: Blurred vision, optic atrophy

Respiratory: Dyspnea, epistaxis, nasal congstion

General Dosage Range Oral:

Adults: Initial: 0.5 mg once daily; Maintenance: 0.05-0.5 mg once daily

Elderly: Initial: 0.05 mg once daily

Mechanism of Action Reduces blood pressure via depletion of sympathetic biogenic amines (norepinephrine and dopamine); this also commonly results in sedative effects

Pharmacodynamics/Kinetics

Onset of Action Antihypertensive: 3-6 days

Duration of Action 2-6 weeks

Half-life Elimination 50-100 hours

Pregnancy Risk Factor C

Pregnancy Considerations Reserpine crosses the placenta. Teratogenic events have been observed in animal reproduction studies with parenteral administration. Nonteratogenic effects in the newborn following reserpine exposure include anorexia, cyanosis, nasal congestion, and increased respiratory tract secretions.

Retapamulin (re te PAM ue lin)

Brand Names: U.S. Altabax™
Pharmacologic Category Antibiotic, Pleuromutilin; Antibiotic, Topical
Use Treatment of impetigo caused by susceptible strains of *S. pyogenes* or methicillin-susceptible *S. aureus*
Local Anesthetic/Vasoconstrictor Precautions No information available to require special precautions
Effects on Dental Treatment No significant effects or complications reported
Effects on Bleeding No information available to require special precautions
Adverse Effects 1% to 10%:
  Central nervous system: Headache (1% to 2%)
  Dermatologic: Eczema (infants, children, and adolescents 1%)
  Gastrointestinal: Diarrhea (1% to 2%), nausea (1%)
  Local: Application site irritation (adults 2%), application site pruritus (infants, children, and adolescents 2%)
  Respiratory: Nasopharyngitis (1% to 2%)
General Dosage Range Topical: *Children ≥9 months and Adults:* Apply to affected area twice daily. Total treatment area should not exceed 2% of total body surface area.
Mechanism of Action Primarily bacteriostatic. Inhibits normal bacterial protein biosynthesis by binding at a unique site (protein L3) on the ribosomal 50S subunit; prevents formation of active 50S ribosomal subunits by inhibiting peptidyl transfer and blocking P-site interactions at this site
Pregnancy Risk Factor B
Pregnancy Considerations Teratogenic effects were not observed in animal studies.

Reteplase (RE ta plase)

Related Information
  Cardiovascular Diseases *on page 1492*
Brand Names: U.S. Retavase® Half-Kit; Retavase® Kit
Brand Names: Canada Retavase®
Pharmacologic Category Thrombolytic Agent
Use Management of ST-elevation myocardial infarction (STEMI) for the improvement of ventricular function, the reduction of the incidence of CHF, and the reduction of mortality following STEMI
  Recommended criteria for treatment of STEMI (ACCF/ AHA; O'Gara, 2013): Ischemic symptoms within 12 hours of treatment or evidence of ongoing ischemia 12-24 hours after symptom onset with a large area of myocardium at risk or hemodynamic instability.
  STEMI ECG definition: New ST-segment elevation at the J point in at least 2 contiguous leads of ≥2 mm (0.2 mV) in men or ≥1.5 mm (0.15 mV) in women in leads V$_2$-V$_3$ and/or of ≥1 mm (0.1 mV) in other contiguous precordial leads or limb leads on ECG. New or presumably new left bundle branch block (LBBB) may interfere with ST-elevation analysis and should not be considered diagnostic in isolation.
  At non-PCI-capable hospitals, the ACCF/AHA recommends thrombolytic therapy administration when the anticipated first medical contact (FMC)-to-device time at a PCI-capable hospital is >120 minutes due to unavoidable delays.
Local Anesthetic/Vasoconstrictor Precautions No information available to require special precautions
Effects on Dental Treatment Key adverse event(s) related to dental treatment: Bleeding is the most frequent adverse effect of reteplase. See Effects on Bleeding.
Effects on Bleeding Bleeding is the most frequent adverse effect associated with reteplase. It is unlikely that ambulatory patients presenting for dental treatment will be taking intravenous anticoagulant therapy.
Adverse Effects Bleeding is the most frequent adverse effect associated with reteplase. Heparin and aspirin have been administered concurrently with reteplase in clinical trials. The incidence of adverse events is a reflection of these combined therapies, and is comparable to comparison thrombolytics.

>10%: Local: Injection site bleeding (5% to 49%)
1% to 10%:
  Gastrointestinal: Bleeding (2% to 9%)
  Genitourinary: Bleeding (1% to 10%)
  Hematologic: Anemia (1% to 3%)
Other adverse effects noted are frequently associated with MI (and therefore may or may not be attributable to Retavase®) and include arrhythmia, AV block, cardiac arrest, cardiogenic shock, embolism, heart failure, hypotension, myocardial rupture, mitral regurgitation, pericardial effusion, pericarditis, pulmonary edema, recurrent ischemia, reinfarction, tamponade, thrombosis
General Dosage Range I.V.: *Adults:* 10 units; repeat after 30 minutes
Mechanism of Action Reteplase is a nonglycosylated form of tPA produced by recombinant DNA technology using *E. coli*; it initiates local fibrinolysis by binding to fibrin in a thrombus (clot) and converts entrapped plasminogen to plasmin
Pharmacodynamics/Kinetics
  Onset of Action Thrombolysis: 30-90 minutes
  Half-life Elimination 13-16 minutes
Pregnancy Risk Factor C
Pregnancy Considerations Adverse events have been observed in some animal reproduction studies. The risk of bleeding may be increased in pregnant women.

Rh$_O$(D) Immune Globulin
(ar aych oh (dee) i MYUN GLOB yoo lin)

Brand Names: U.S. HyperRHO™ S/D Full Dose; HyperRHO™ S/D Mini-Dose; MICRhoGAM® UF Plus; RhoGAM® UF Plus; Rhophylac®; WinRho® SDF
Brand Names: Canada WinRho® SDF
Pharmacologic Category Blood Product Derivative; Immune Globulin
Use
  Suppression of Rh isoimmunization: Use in the following situations when an Rh$_O$(D)-negative individual is exposed to Rh$_O$(D)-positive blood: During delivery of an Rh$_O$(D)-positive infant; abortion; amniocentesis; chorionic villus sampling; ruptured tubal pregnancy; abdominal trauma; hydatidiform mole; transplacental hemorrhage. Used when the mother is Rh$_O$(D)-negative, the father of the child is either Rh$_O$(D)-positive or Rh$_O$(D)-unknown, or the baby is either Rh$_O$(D)-positive or Rh$_O$(D)-unknown.

◀ Transfusion: Suppression of Rh isoimmunization in Rh₀(D)-negative individuals transfused with Rh₀(D) antigen-positive RBCs or blood components containing Rh₀(D) antigen-positive RBCs

Treatment of idiopathic thrombocytopenic purpura (ITP): Used intravenously in the following nonsplenectomized Rh₀(D)-positive individuals: Children with acute or chronic ITP, adults with chronic ITP, and children and adults with ITP secondary to HIV infection

Local Anesthetic/Vasoconstrictor Precautions No information available to require special precautions

Effects on Dental Treatment No significant effects or complications reported

Effects on Bleeding No information available to require special precautions

Adverse Effects Frequency not defined.

Cardiovascular: Hyper-/hypotension, pallor, tachycardia, vasodilation

Central nervous system: Chills, dizziness, fever, headache, malaise, somnolence

Dermatologic: Pruritus, rash

Gastrointestinal: Abdominal pain, diarrhea, nausea, vomiting

Hematologic: Haptoglobin decreased, hemoglobin decreased (patients with ITP), intravascular hemolysis (patients with ITP)

Hepatic: Bilirubin increased, LDH increased

Local: Injection site reaction: Discomfort, induration, mild pain, redness, swelling

Neuromuscular & skeletal: Arthralgia, back pain, hyperkinesia, myalgia, weakness

Renal: Acute renal insufficiency

Miscellaneous: Anaphylaxis, diaphoresis, infusion-related reactions, positive anti-C antibody test (transient), shivering

General Dosage Range I.M., I.V.: *Children and Adults:* Dosage varies greatly depending on indication

Mechanism of Action

Rh suppression: Prevents isoimmunization by suppressing the immune response and antibody formation by Rh₀(D) negative individuals to Rh₀(D) positive red blood cells.

ITP: Not completely characterized; Rh₀(D) immune globulin is thought to form anti-D-coated red blood cell complexes which bind to macrophage Fc receptors within the spleen; blocking or saturating the spleens ability to clear antibody-coated cells, including platelets. In this manner, platelets are spared from destruction.

Pharmacodynamics/Kinetics

Onset of Action Onset of platelet increase: ITP: Platelets should rise within 1-2 days; Peak effect: In 7-14 days

Duration of Action Suppression of Rh isoimmunization: ~12 weeks; Treatment of ITP: 30 days (variable)

Half-life Elimination ~24-30 days

Time to Peak Plasma: I.M.: 5-10 days; I.V. (WinRho® SDF): ≤2 hours

Pregnancy Risk Factor C

Pregnancy Considerations Animal studies have not been conducted. Available evidence suggests that Rh₀(D) immune globulin administration during pregnancy does not harm the fetus or affect future pregnancies.

Ribavirin (rye ba VYE rin)

Related Information

Systemic Viral Diseases *on page 1537*

Brand Names: U.S. Copegus®; Rebetol®; Ribasphere®; Ribasphere® RibaPak®; Virazole®

Brand Names: Canada Virazole®

Pharmacologic Category Antiviral Agent

Use

Inhalation: Treatment of hospitalized infants and young children with respiratory syncytial virus (RSV) infections; specially indicated for treatment of severe lower respiratory tract RSV infections in patients with an underlying compromising condition (prematurity, cardiopulmonary disease, or immunosuppression)

Oral capsule: In combination with interferon alfa 2b (pegylated or nonpegylated) injection for the treatment of chronic hepatitis C in interferon alfa-naive or experienced-patients with compensated liver disease. Patients likely to fail retreatment after a prior failed course include previous nonresponders, those who received previous pegylated interferon treatment, patients who have significant bridging fibrosis or cirrhosis, or those with genotype 1 infection.

Oral solution: In combination with interferon alfa-2b (pegylated or nonpegylated) injection for the treatment of chronic hepatitis C in interferon alfa-naive or experienced patients ≥3 years of age with compensated liver disease. Patients likely to fail retreatment after a prior failed course include previous nonresponders, those who received previous pegylated interferon treatment, patients who have significant bridging fibrosis or cirrhosis, or those with genotype 1 infection.

Oral tablet: In combination with peginterferon alfa-2a (Pegasys®) injection for the treatment of chronic hepatitis C in patients with compensated liver disease who were previously untreated with alpha interferons, and in adult chronic hepatitis C patients coinfected with HIV.

Unlabeled Use

Inhalation: Treatment for RSV in adult hematopoietic stem cell or heart/lung transplant recipients

Used in other viral infections including influenza A and B and adenovirus

Local Anesthetic/Vasoconstrictor Precautions No information available to require special precautions

Effects on Dental Treatment Key adverse event(s) related to dental treatment: Xerostomia (normal salivary flow resumes upon discontinuation) and taste perversion.

Effects on Bleeding No information available to require special precautions

Adverse Effects

Inhalation:

1% to 10%:

Central nervous system: Fatigue, headache, insomnia

Gastrointestinal: Nausea, anorexia

Hematologic: Anemia

Oral (all adverse reactions are documented while receiving combination therapy with alfa interferons; percentages as reported in adults unless noted, most common pediatric adverse reactions were similar to adults); asterisked (*) percentages are those similar to interferon therapy alone:

>10%:

Central nervous system: Fatigue (60% to 70% [30% in pediatric patients])*, headache (43% to 66%)*, fever (32% to 55%)*, insomnia (26% to 41% [9% in pediatric patients]), depression (20% to 36%)*, irritability (23% to 33%), dizziness (14% to 26%), impaired concentration (10% to 21%)*, emotional lability (7% to 12%)*

Dermatologic: Alopecia (27% to 36% [17% in pediatric patients]), pruritus (13% to 29% [11% in pediatric patients]), rash (5% to 28%), dry skin (10% to 24%), dermatitis (≤16%)

Endocrine and metabolic: Growth suppression (pediatric) percentile decrease (≥15 percentiles: weight 43%; height 25%), hyperuricemia (33% to 38%)

Gastrointestinal: Nausea (25% to 47% [18% in pediatric patients]), anorexia (21% to 32%), weight decrease (10% to 29%), vomiting (9% to 25%)*, diarrhea (10% to 22%), dyspepsia (6% to 16%), abdominal pain (8% to 13%), xerostomia (≤12%), RUQ pain (≤12%)

Hematologic: Leukopenia (6% to 45%), neutropenia (8% to 42%; grade 4: 2% to 11%; 40% with HIV coinfection), hemoglobin decreased (11% to 35%), anemia (11% to 17%), thrombocytopenia (<1% to 15%), lymphopenia (12% to 14%), hemolytic anemia (10% to 13%)

Hepatic: Bilirubin increase (10% to 32%)

Neuromuscular & skeletal: Myalgia (40% to 64% [17% in pediatric patients])*, rigors (25% to 48%), arthralgia (22% to 34%)*, musculoskeletal pain (19% to 28% [35% in pediatric patients])

Respiratory: Upper respiratory tract infection (60% in pediatric patients), dyspnea (13% to 26%), cough (7% to 23%), pharyngitis (≤13%), sinusitis (≤12%)*

Miscellaneous: Flu-like syndrome (13% to 18% [up to 91% in pediatric patients])*, viral infection (≤12%), diaphoresis (≤11%)

1% to 10%:

Cardiovascular: Chest pain (5% to 9%)*, flushing (≤4%)

Central nervous system: Pain (≤10%), mood alteration (≤6%; 9% with HIV coinfection), agitation (5% to 8%), nervousness (6%)*, memory impairment (≤6%), malaise (≤6%), suicidal ideation (adolescents: 2%; adults: 1%)

Dermatologic: Eczema (4% to 5%)

Endocrine & metabolic: Menstrual disorder (≤7%), hypothyroidism (≤5%)

Gastrointestinal: Taste perversion (4% to 9%), constipation (5%)

Hepatic: Hepatomegaly (4%), transaminases increased (1% to 3%), hepatic decompensation (2% with HIV coinfection)

Neuromuscular & skeletal: Weakness (9% to 10%), back pain (5%)

Ocular: Blurred vision (≤6%), conjunctivitis (≤5%)

Respiratory: Rhinitis (≤8%), exertional dyspnea (≤7%)

Miscellaneous: Fungal infection (≤6%), bacterial infection (3% to 5%)

Note: Incidence of headache, fever, suicidal ideation, and vomiting are higher in children.

General Dosage Range Dosage adjustment recommended in patients with renal impairment and in patients who develop toxicities.

Inhalation: *Children:* 20 mg/mL (6 **g** in 300 mL) solution; continuous: 12-18 hours daily

Oral capsules:
Children 47-59 kg: 800 mg daily
Children 60-73 kg: 1000 mg daily
Children >73 kg: 1200 mg daily
Adults: 800-1400 mg daily

Oral solution:
Children <47 kg: 15 mg/kg/day in 2 divided doses
Adults: 800-1400 mg daily

Oral tablet (Copegus®):
Children 23-33 kg: 400 mg daily
Children 34-46 kg: 600 mg daily
Children 47-59 kg: 800 mg daily
Children 60-74 kg: 1000 mg daily
Children ≥75 kg: 1200 mg daily
Adults: 800-1200 mg daily

Oral tablet (Ribasphere®): *Adults:* 800-1200 mg daily

Mechanism of Action Inhibits replication of RNA and DNA viruses; inhibits influenza virus RNA polymerase activity and inhibits the initiation and elongation of RNA fragments resulting in inhibition of viral protein synthesis

Pharmacodynamics/Kinetics

Half-life Elimination Plasma:
Children: Inhalation: 6.5-11 hours
Adults: Oral:
Capsule, single dose (Rebetol®, Ribasphere®): 24 hours in healthy adults, 44 hours with chronic hepatitis C infection (increases to ~298 hours at steady state)
Tablet, single dose (Copegus®): ~120-170 hours

Time to Peak Serum: Inhalation: At end of inhalation period; Oral capsule: Multiple doses: 3 hours; Tablet: 2 hours

Pregnancy Risk Factor X

Pregnancy Considerations [U.S. Boxed Warning]: Significant teratogenic effects have been observed in all animal studies at ~0.01 times the maximum recommended daily human dose. Use is contraindicated in pregnancy. Negative pregnancy test is required before initiation and monthly thereafter. Avoid pregnancy in female patients and female partners of male patients during therapy by using two effective forms of contraception; continue contraceptive measures for at least 6 months after completion of therapy. If patient or female partner becomes pregnant during treatment, she should be counseled about potential risks of exposure. If pregnancy occurs during use or within 6 months after treatment, report to the ribavirin pregnancy registry (800-593-2214).

Riboflavin (RYE boe flay vin)

Brand Names: U.S. Ribo-100 [OTC]
Generic Availability (U.S.) Yes
Pharmacologic Category Vitamin, Water Soluble
Use Dietary supplement
Unlabeled Use Migraine prophylaxis
Local Anesthetic/Vasoconstrictor Precautions No information available to require special precautions
Effects on Dental Treatment No significant effects or complications reported
Effects on Bleeding No information available to require special precautions
Adverse Effects Frequency not defined: Genitourinary: Discoloration of urine (yellow-orange)
Dosage Oral:
Dietary supplement: Adults: 100 mg once or twice daily
Adequate intake:
1-6 months: 0.3 mg/day
7-12 months: 0.4 mg/day

Recommended daily intake:
1-3 years: 0.5 mg
4-8 years: 0.6 mg
9-13 years: 0.9 mg
14-18 years: Females: 1 mg; Males: 1.3 mg
≥19 years: Females: 1.1 mg; Males: 1.3 mg
Pregnancy: 1.4 mg
Lactation 1.6 mg

Mechanism of Action Component of flavoprotein enzymes that work together, which are necessary for normal tissue respiration; also needed for activation of pyridoxine and conversion of tryptophan to niacin

Warnings/Precautions Riboflavin deficiency often occurs in the presence of other B vitamin deficiencies.

Drug Interactions
Metabolism/Transport Effects None known.
Avoid Concomitant Use There are no known interactions where it is recommended to avoid concomitant use.
Increased Effect/Toxicity There are no known significant interactions involving an increase in effect.
Decreased Effect There are no known significant interactions involving a decrease in effect.

Dietary Considerations Dietary sources of riboflavin include liver, kidney, dairy products, green vegetables, eggs, whole grain cereals, yeast, and mushroom.

Pregnancy Considerations Water-soluble vitamins cross the placenta. Riboflavin requirements may be increased in pregnant women compared to nonpregnant women (IOM, 1998).

Breast-Feeding Considerations Riboflavin is found in breast milk. Concentrations may be influenced by supplements or maternal deficiency. Riboflavin requirements may be increased in nursing women compared to non-nursing women (IOM, 1998).

Dosage Forms
Tablet, oral: 25 mg, 50 mg, 100 mg
Ribo-100 [OTC]: 100 mg

Rifabutin (rif a BYOO tin)

Related Information
Systemic Viral Diseases on page 1537
Brand Names: U.S. Mycobutin®
Brand Names: Canada Mycobutin®
Pharmacologic Category Antibiotic, Miscellaneous; Antitubercular Agent
Use Prevention of disseminated Mycobacterium avium complex (MAC) in patients with advanced HIV infection
Unlabeled Use Utilized in multidrug regimens for treatment of MAC; alternative to rifampin as prophylaxis for latent tuberculosis infection (LTBI) or part of multidrug regimen for treatment active tuberculosis infection
Local Anesthetic/Vasoconstrictor Precautions No information available to require special precautions
Effects on Dental Treatment Key adverse event(s) related to dental treatment: Saliva (reddish orange).
Effects on Bleeding No information available to require special precautions
Adverse Effects
>10%:
Dermatologic: Rash (11%)
Genitourinary: Discoloration of urine (30%)
Hematologic: Neutropenia (25%), leukopenia (17%)
1% to 10%:
Central nervous system: Headache (3%), fever (2%)
Gastrointestinal: Nausea (3% to 6%), abdominal pain (4%), dyspepsia (3%), eructation (3%), taste perversion (3%), vomiting (3%), flatulence (2%)

Hematologic: Thrombocytopenia (5%)
Hepatic: ALT increased (7% to 9%; incidence less than placebo), AST increased (7% to 9%; incidence less than placebo)
Neuromuscular & skeletal: Myalgia (2%)

General Dosage Range Dosage adjustment recommended in patients with renal impairment or on concomitant therapy
Oral:
Children <6 years: 5 mg/kg once daily
Children ≥6 years and Adults: 300 mg once daily

Mechanism of Action Inhibits DNA-dependent RNA polymerase at the beta subunit which prevents chain initiation

Pharmacodynamics/Kinetics
Half-life Elimination Terminal: 45 hours (range: 16-69 hours)
Time to Peak Serum: 2-4 hours
Pregnancy Risk Factor B
Pregnancy Considerations Adverse events were seen in some animal reproduction studies.

Rifampin (rif AM pin)

Related Information
Rifapentine on page 1193
Brand Names: U.S. Rifadin®
Brand Names: Canada Rifadin®; Rofact™
Pharmacologic Category Antibiotic, Miscellaneous; Antitubercular Agent
Use Management of active tuberculosis in combination with other agents; elimination of meningococci from the nasopharynx in asymptomatic carriers
Unlabeled Use Prophylaxis of Haemophilus influenzae type b infection; Legionella pneumonia; used in combination with other anti-infectives in the treatment of staphylococcal infections; treatment of M. leprae infections; used in combination with penicillin for the treatment of chronic carriers of pharyngeal group A streptococci
Local Anesthetic/Vasoconstrictor Precautions No information available to require special precautions
Effects on Dental Treatment No significant effects or complications reported
Effects on Bleeding Rifampin doses >600 mg may be associated with more adverse events including hemolytic anemia and thrombocytopenia.
Adverse Effects
1% to 10%:
Dermatologic: Rash (1% to 5%)
Gastrointestinal (1% to 2%): Anorexia, cramps, diarrhea, epigastric distress, flatulence, heartburn, nausea, pseudomembranous colitis, pancreatitis, vomiting
Hepatic: LFTs increased (up to 14%)
Frequency not defined:
Cardiovascular: Edema, flushing
Central nervous system: Ataxia, behavioral changes, concentration impaired, confusion, dizziness, drowsiness, fatigue, fever, headache, numbness, psychosis
Dermatologic: Pemphigoid reaction, pruritus, urticaria
Endocrine & metabolic: Adrenal insufficiency, menstrual disorders
Hematologic: Agranulocytosis (rare), DIC, eosinophilia, hemoglobin decreased, hemolysis, hemolytic anemia, leukopenia, thrombocytopenia (especially with high-dose therapy)
Hepatic: Hepatitis (rare), jaundice

Neuromuscular & skeletal: Myalgia, osteomalacia, weakness

Ocular: Exudative conjunctivitis, visual changes

Renal: Acute renal failure, BUN increased, hemoglobinuria, hematuria, interstitial nephritis, uric acid increased

Miscellaneous: Flu-like syndrome

General Dosage Range I.V., Oral:

Children <12 years: 10-20 mg/kg/day in 1-2 divided doses **or** 10-20 mg/kg twice weekly (maximum: 600 mg/day)

Children ≥12 years and Adults: 10 mg/kg/day **or** 10 mg/kg 2-3 times/week **or** 600 mg every 12-24 hours

Mechanism of Action Inhibits bacterial RNA synthesis by binding to the beta subunit of DNA-dependent RNA polymerase, blocking RNA transcription

Pharmacodynamics/Kinetics

Duration of Action ≤24 hours

Half-life Elimination 3-4 hours, prolonged with hepatic impairment; End-stage renal disease: 1.8-11 hours

Time to Peak Serum: Oral: 2-4 hours

Pregnancy Risk Factor C

Pregnancy Considerations Teratogenic effects have been reported in animal studies. Rifampin crosses the human placenta. Due to the risk of tuberculosis to the fetus, treatment is recommended when the probability of maternal disease is moderate to high. Postnatal hemorrhages have been reported in the infant and mother with isoniazid administration during the last few weeks of pregnancy.

Rifampin and Isoniazid
(rif AM pin & eye soe NYE a zid)

Related Information

Isoniazid *on page 766*

Rifampin *on page 1192*

Brand Names: U.S. IsonaRif™; Rifamate®

Brand Names: Canada Rifamate®

Pharmacologic Category Antibiotic, Miscellaneous

Use Management of active tuberculosis; see individual agents for additional information

Local Anesthetic/Vasoconstrictor Precautions No information available to require special precautions

Effects on Dental Treatment No significant effects or complications reported

Effects on Bleeding Rifampin doses >600 mg may be associated with more adverse events including hemolytic anemia and thrombocytopenia.

General Dosage Range Oral: *Adults:* 2 capsules (rifampin 300 mg/isoniazid 150 mg/capsule) once daily

Pregnancy Risk Factor C

Pregnancy Considerations Refer to Rifampin monograph.

Rifampin, Isoniazid, and Pyrazinamide
(rif AM pin, eye soe NYE a zid, & peer a ZIN a mide)

Related Information

Isoniazid *on page 766*

Pyrazinamide *on page 1162*

Rifampin *on page 1192*

Brand Names: U.S. Rifater®

Brand Names: Canada Rifater®

Pharmacologic Category Antibiotic, Miscellaneous

Use Initial phase, short-course treatment of pulmonary tuberculosis; see individual agents for additional information

Local Anesthetic/Vasoconstrictor Precautions No information available to require special precautions

Effects on Dental Treatment No significant effects or complications reported

Effects on Bleeding Rifampin doses >600 mg may be associated with more adverse events including hemolytic anemia and thrombocytopenia.

Adverse Effects See individual agents.

Note: During clinical trial evaluation, the frequency of cardiorespiratory events (eg, chest pain, hemoptysis, palpitation, chest tightness, and pneumothorax) was higher with the combination product (7%) than that reported with individual agents (2%); frequency of central and peripheral nervous system events (eg, sweating, headache, insomnia, paresthesia, and anxiety) were also higher with the combination product (4%) than that reported with individual agents (3%).

General Dosage Range Oral:

Children ≥15 years and Adults ≤44 kg: 4 tablets (rifampin 120 mg/isoniazid 50 mg/pyrazinamide 300 mg per tablet) once daily

Children ≥15 years and Adults 45-54 kg: 5 tablets (rifampin 120 mg/isoniazid 50 mg/pyrazinamide 300 mg per tablet) once daily

Children ≥15 years and Adults ≥55 kg: 6 tablets (rifampin 120 mg/isoniazid 50 mg/pyrazinamide 300 mg per tablet) once daily

Mechanism of Action

Rifampin inhibits bacterial mRNA synthesis by binding to the beta subunit of DNA-dependent RNA polymerase, blocking transcription

Isoniazid inhibits mycolic acid synthesis resulting in disruption of the bacterial cell wall

Pyrazinamide is converted to pyrazinoic acid in susceptible strains of *Mycobacterium* which lowers the pH of the environment; exact mechanism of action has not been elucidated

Pregnancy Risk Factor C

Pregnancy Considerations Animal reproduction studies have not been conducted with this combination. See individual agents.

Rifapentine (rif a PEN teen)

Related Information

Rifampin *on page 1192*

Brand Names: U.S. Priftin®

Brand Names: Canada Priftin®

Pharmacologic Category Antitubercular Agent

Use Treatment of pulmonary tuberculosis; rifapentine must always be used in conjunction with at least one other antituberculosis drug to which the isolate is susceptible; it may also be necessary to add additional agents (eg, streptomycin, ethambutol) until susceptibility is known.

Unlabeled Use Treatment of latent tuberculosis infection (LTBI) in combination with isoniazid

Local Anesthetic/Vasoconstrictor Precautions No information available to require special precautions

Effects on Dental Treatment No significant effects or complications reported

Effects on Bleeding No information available to require special precautions

◀ **Adverse Effects** Frequency may vary based on treatment phase; adverse reaction data is based on rifapentine combination therapy.

>10%:

Endocrine & metabolic: Hyperuricemia (≤32%; most likely due to pyrazinamide from initiation phase)

Genitourinary: Hematuria (10% to 18%), pyuria (11% to 22%), urinary tract infection (7% to 13%)

Hematologic: Neutropenia (6% to 13%), lymphopenia (3% to 13%)

1% to 10%:

Cardiovascular: Chest pain (3% to 6%), edema (1%)

Central nervous system: Fatigue (≤1%), fever (≤1%)

Dermatologic: Acne (≤3%), maculopapular rash (2%), pruritus (1%)

Endocrine & metabolic: Hypoglycemia (5% to 10%), hyperglycemia (1% to 4%)

Gastrointestinal: Anorexia (3%), nausea (1% to 3%), abdominal pain (1% to 2%), constipation (1% to 2%), diarrhea (1% to 2%), hemorrhoids (1%), hyperphosphatemia (1%)

Genitourinary: Urinary casts (4% to 8%), cystitis (1%)

Hematologic: Thrombocytosis (≤6%), leukopenia (4% to 6%), leukocytosis (2% to 3%), neutrophilia (1% to 3%), thrombocytopenia (1% to 3%), polycythemia (≤2%), lymphadenopathy (≤1%)

Hepatic: ALT increased (2% to 7%), AST increased (2% to 6%)

Neuromuscular & skeletal: Back pain (4% to 7%), pain (3% to 6%), arthrosis (1%), gout (1%), tremor (1%)

Ocular: Conjunctivitis (2% to 3%)

Respiratory: Hemoptysis (8%), cough (6% to 8%), bronchitis (3%), pharyngitis (1% to 2%), epistaxis (1%) pleuritis (1%)

Miscellaneous: Influenza (3% to 8%), injury (1% to 5%), infection (1% to 3%), diaphoresis (2%), herpes zoster (1%)

General Dosage Range Oral: *Adults:* 600 mg once or twice weekly

Mechanism of Action Inhibits DNA-dependent RNA polymerase in susceptible strains of *Mycobacterium tuberculosis* (MTB) (but not in mammalian cells). Rifapentine is bactericidal against both intracellular and extracellular MTB organisms.

Pharmacodynamics/Kinetics

Half-life Elimination Rifapentine: 12-15 hours; 25-desacetyl rifapentine: 11-16 hours

Time to Peak Serum: 5-6 hours

Pregnancy Risk Factor C

Pregnancy Considerations Teratogenic effects have been observed in animal reproduction studies. Postnatal hemorrhages have been reported in the infant and mother with rifampin (another rifamycin) administration during the last few weeks of pregnancy. Due to the risk of tuberculosis to the fetus, treatment is recommended when the probability of maternal disease is moderate to high. The CDC does not currently recommend rifapentine as part of the treatment regimen due to insufficient data in pregnant women (CDC, 2003).

Rifaximin (rif AX i min)

Brand Names: U.S. Xifaxan®

Pharmacologic Category Antibiotic, Miscellaneous

Use Treatment of travelers' diarrhea caused by noninvasive strains of *E. coli*; reduction in the risk of overt hepatic encephalopathy (HE) recurrence

Unlabeled Use Treatment of hepatic encephalopathy; alternative treatment for *Clostridium difficile*-associated diarrhea (CDAD)

Local Anesthetic/Vasoconstrictor Precautions No information available to require special precautions

Effects on Dental Treatment No significant effects or complications reported

Effects on Bleeding No information available to require special precautions

Adverse Effects Note: Frequency of adverse events generally higher following treatment for hepatic encephalopathy (HE). Percentages are presented for HE unless otherwise stated.

>10%:

Cardiovascular: Peripheral edema (15%)

Central nervous system: Dizziness (13%), fatigue (12%)

Hepatic: Ascites (11%)

Gastrointestinal: Nausea (14%)

2% to 10%:

Cardiovascular: Chest pain (>2% to 5%), edema (>2% to 5%), hypotension (>2% to 5%)

Central nervous system: Headache (travelers' diarrhea 10%), depression (7%), fever (6%), amnesia (>2% to 5%), attention disturbance (>2% to 5%), confusion (>2% to 5%), hypoesthesia (>2% to 5%), pain (>2% to 5%), tremor (>2% to 5%), vertigo (>2% to 5%)

Dermatological: Pruritus (9%), rash (5%), cellulitis (>2% to 5%)

Endocrine and metabolism: Hyper-/hypoglycemia (>2% to 5%), hyperkalemia (>2% to 5%), hyponatremia (>2% to 5%)

Gastrointestinal: Abdominal pain (>2% to 9%), abdominal tenderness (>2% to 5%), anorexia (>2% to 5%), dehydration (>2% to 5%), esophageal varices (>2% to 5%), weight gain (>2% to 5%), xerostomia (>2% to 5%)

Hematologic: Anemia (8%)

Neuromuscular & skeletal: Muscle spasms (9%), arthralgia (6%), myalgia (>2% to 5%)

Respiratory: Nasopharyngitis (7%), dyspnea (6%), epistaxis(>2% to 5%), pneumonia (>2% to 5%), rhinitis (>2% to 5%), upper respiratory tract infection (>2% to 5%)

Miscellaneous: Influenza-like illness (>2% to 5%)

General Dosage Range Oral:

Children ≥12 years: 200 mg 3 times/day

Adults: 200 mg 3 times/day **or** 550 mg 2 times/day

Mechanism of Action Rifaximin inhibits bacterial RNA synthesis by binding to bacterial DNA-dependent RNA polymerase.

Pharmacodynamics/Kinetics

Half-life Elimination ~2-5 hours

Time to Peak Hepatic encephalopathy prevention: ~1 hour

Pregnancy Risk Factor C

Pregnancy Considerations Adverse events have been observed in animal reproduction studies; therefore, the manufacturer classifies rifaximin as pregnancy category C. Due to the limited oral absorption of rifaximin in patients with normal hepatic function, exposure to the fetus is expected to be extremely low.

Rilonacept (ri LON a sept)

Brand Names: U.S. Arcalyst®

Pharmacologic Category Interleukin-1 Inhibitor

Use Treatment of cryopyrin-associated periodic syndromes (CAPS) including familial cold autoinflammatory syndrome (FCAS) and Muckle-Wells syndrome (MWS)

Local Anesthetic/Vasoconstrictor Precautions No information available to require special precautions

Effects on Dental Treatment No significant effects or complications reported

Effects on Bleeding No information available to require special precautions

Adverse Effects
>10%:
Local: Injection site reactions (48%; majority mild-moderate; typically lasting 1-2 days; characterized by erythema, bruising, dermatitis, inflammation, pain, pruritus, swelling, urticaria, vesicles, warmth, and hemorrhage)
Respiratory: Upper respiratory tract infection (26%)
Miscellaneous: Infection (48% during winter months; 18% during summer months; antibody formation to rilonacept (35%)
1% to 10%:
Central nervous system: Hypoesthesia (9%)
Respiratory: Cough (9%), sinusitis (9%)

General Dosage Range SubQ:
Children ≥12 years: Loading dose 4.4 mg/kg (maximum dose: 320 mg); Maintenance dose: 2.2 mg/kg once weekly (maximum dose: 160 mg)
Adults: Loading dose: 320 mg; Maintenance dose: 160 mg once weekly

Mechanism of Action Cryopyrin-associated periodic syndromes (CAPS) refers to rare genetic syndromes caused by mutations in the nucleotide-binding domain, leucine rich family (NLR), pyrin domain containing 3 (NLRP-3) gene or the cold-induced autoinflammatory syndrome-1 (CIAS1) gene. Cryopyrin, a protein encoded by this gene, regulates interleukin-1 beta (IL-1β) activation. Deficiency of cryopyrin results in excessive inflammation. Rilonacept reduces inflammation by binding to IL-1β (some binding of IL-1α and IL-1 receptor antagonist) and preventing interaction with cell surface receptors.

Pharmacodynamics/Kinetics
Onset of Action Steady state reached by 6 weeks
Pregnancy Risk Factor C
Pregnancy Considerations Animal studies have demonstrated teratogenic effects and fetal loss. There are no adequate and well-controlled studies in pregnant women. Use during pregnancy only if potential benefit to the mother outweighs potential risk to the fetus.

Rilpivirine (ril pi VIR een)

Related Information
Clinical Risk Related to Drugs Prolonging QT Interval *on page 1510*
HIV Infection and AIDS *on page 1520*
Brand Names: U.S. Edurant®
Brand Names: Canada Edurant®
Pharmacologic Category Antiretroviral Agent, Reverse Transcriptase Inhibitor (Non-nucleoside)
Use Treatment of HIV-1 infections in treatment-naive patients with HIV-1 RNA ≤100,000 copies/mL in combination with at least 2 other antiretroviral agents

Local Anesthetic/Vasoconstrictor Precautions Rilpivirine is one of the drugs confirmed to prolong the QT interval and is accepted as having a risk of causing torsade de pointes. The risk of drug-induced torsade de pointes is extremely low when a single QT interval prolonging drug is prescribed. In terms of epinephrine,

it is not known what effect vasoconstrictors in the local anesthetic regimen will have in patients with a known history of congenital prolonged QT interval or in patients taking any medication that prolongs the QT interval. Until more information is obtained, it is suggested that the clinician consult with the physician prior to the use of a vasoconstrictor in suspected patients, and that the vasoconstrictor (epinephrine, mepivacaine and levonordefrin [Carbocaine® 2% with Neo-Cobefrin®]) be used with caution.

Effects on Dental Treatment No significant effects or complications reported

Effects on Bleeding No information available to require special precautions

Adverse Effects
>10%:
Endocrine & metabolic: Cholesterol increased (7% to 17%; grade 3: <1%), LDL increased (5% to 14%; grade 3: 1%)
Hepatic: ALT increased (5% to 18%; grade 3/4: 1%), AST increased (4% to 16%; grade 3/4: 1% to 2%)
2% to 10%:
Central nervous system: Depressive disorders (depression, depressed mood, dysphoria, mood changes, negative thoughts, suicide attempts, suicidal ideation) (4% to 9%; grades 3/4: 1%), headache (3%), insomnia (3%), abnormal dreams (2%), fatigue (2%)
Dermatologic: Rash (3%)
Endocrine & metabolic: Triglycerides increased (2%; grade 3/4: ≤1%)
Gastrointestinal: Abdominal pain (2%)
Hepatic: Total bilirubin increased (3% to 5%; grade 3/4: ≤1%)
Renal: Creatinine increased (1% to 6%; grade 3/4: ≤1%)

General Dosage Range Oral: *Adults:* 25 mg once daily

Mechanism of Action As a non-nucleoside reverse transcriptase inhibitor, rilpivirine has activity against HIV-1 by binding to reverse transcriptase. It consequently blocks the RNA-dependent and DNA-dependent DNA polymerase activities, including HIV-1 replication. It does not require intracellular phosphorylation for antiviral activity.

Pharmacodynamics/Kinetics
Half-life Elimination ~50 hours
Time to Peak Plasma: 4-5 hours
Pregnancy Risk Factor B
Pregnancy Considerations No evidence of fetal toxicity has been noted in animal reproduction studies. Available data in pregnant women are insufficient and the DHHS Perinatal HIV Guidelines do not recommend use unless other alternatives are not available. Hypersensitivity reactions (including hepatic toxicity and rash) are more common in women on NNRTI therapy; it is not known if pregnancy increases this risk.

Regardless of CD4 count or HIV RNA copy number, all HIV-infected pregnant women should receive a combination antepartum antiretroviral (ARV) drug regimen; this includes women who require therapy for their own health, as well as women who do not yet require therapy for their own health. ARV therapy should be started as soon as possible if required for the woman's health. Although earlier initiation may be more effective in reducing the perinatal transmission of HIV), also consider maternal conditions (eg, nausea and vomiting) and the potential risks of first trimester fetal exposure for specific agents. Plasma HIV RNA levels should be assessed at ~34-36 weeks gestation in order to help determine mode of delivery. If ARV therapy must be interrupted for <24 hours during the peripartum period, stop then restart all medications simultaneously in order to decrease the chance of developing resistance. Long-term follow-up is recommended for all infants exposed to ARV medications.

Healthcare providers are encouraged to enroll pregnant women exposed to antiretroviral medications in the Antiretroviral Pregnancy Registry (1-800-258-4263 or www.APRegistry.com). Healthcare providers caring for HIV-infected women and their infants may contact the National Perinatal HIV Hotline (888-448-8765) for clinical consultation (DHHS [perinatal], 2012).

Dental Comment Rilpivirine is known to prolong the QT interval. The QT interval is measured as the time and distance between the Q point of the QRS complex and the end of the T wave in the ECG tracing. After adjustment for heart rate, the QT interval is defined as prolonged if it is more than 450 msec in men and 460 msec in women. A long QT syndrome was first described in the 1950s and 60s as a congenital syndrome involving QT interval prolongation and syncope and sudden death. Some of the congenital long QT syndromes were characterized by a peculiar electrocardiographic appearance of the QRS complex involving a premature atria beat followed by a pause, then a subsequent sinus beat showing marked QT prolongation and deformity. This type of cardiac arrhythmia was originally termed "torsade de pointes" (translated from the French as "twisting of the points"). Rilpivirine is considered as having a risk of causing torsade de pointes. Since it is not known what effect vasoconstrictors in the local anesthetic regimen will have in patients with a known history of congenital prolonged QT interval or in patients taking any medication that prolongs the QT interval, a medical consult is suggested.

Riluzole (RIL yoo zole)

Brand Names: U.S. Rilutek®
Brand Names: Canada Apo-Riluzole®; Mylan-Riluzole; Rilutek®
Pharmacologic Category Glutamate Inhibitor
Use Treatment of amyotrophic lateral sclerosis (ALS); riluzole can extend survival or time to tracheostomy
Local Anesthetic/Vasoconstrictor Precautions No information available to require special precautions
Effects on Dental Treatment Key adverse event(s) related to dental treatment: Oral moniliasis and stomatitis.
Effects on Bleeding No information available to require special precautions
Adverse Effects
>10%:
Gastrointestinal: Nausea (16%)
Neuromuscular & skeletal: Weakness (19%)
1% to 10%:
Cardiovascular: Hypertension (5%), peripheral edema (3%), tachycardia (3%)
Central nervous system: Dizziness (4%), somnolence (2%), vertigo (2%), malaise (1%)
Dermatologic: Pruritus (4%), eczema (2%), exfoliative dermatitis (1%)
Gastrointestinal: Abdominal pain (5%), vomiting (4%), flatulence (3%), oral moniliasis (1%), stomatitis (1%), tooth caries (1%)
Genitourinary: Urinary tract infection (3%), dysuria (1%)

Hepatic: Liver function tests increased (8% >3 x ULN; 2% >5 x ULN)
Neuromuscular & skeletal: Arthralgia (4%), paresthesia (circumoral; 2%), tremor (1%)
Respiratory: Lung function decreased (10%), cough increased (3%)
General Dosage Range Oral: *Adults:* 50 mg every 12 hours
Mechanism of Action Mechanism of action is not known. Pharmacologic properties include inhibitory effect on glutamate release, inactivation of voltage-dependent sodium channels; and ability to interfere with intracellular events that follow transmitter binding at excitatory amino acid receptors
Pharmacodynamics/Kinetics
Half-life Elimination 12 hours
Pregnancy Risk Factor C
Pregnancy Considerations Impaired fertility, decreased implantation, increased intrauterine death, and adverse effects on offspring growth and viability were observed in animal studies. There are no adequate or well-controlled studies in pregnant women.

RimabotulinumtoxinB
(rime uh BOT yoo lin num TOKS in bee)

Brand Names: U.S. Myobloc®
Pharmacologic Category Neuromuscular Blocker Agent, Toxin
Use Treatment of cervical dystonia (spasmodic torticollis)
Unlabeled Use Treatment of cervical dystonia in patients who have developed resistance to onabotulinumtoxinA or abobotulinumtoxinA
Local Anesthetic/Vasoconstrictor Precautions No information available to require special precautions
Effects on Dental Treatment Key adverse event(s) related to dental treatment: Xerostomia (normal salivary flow resumes upon discontinuation), stomatitis, and abnormal taste.
Effects on Bleeding No information available to require special precautions
Adverse Effects
>10%:
Central nervous system: Headache (10% to 16%), pain (≤13%)
Gastrointestinal: Dysphagia (10% to 25%; severe dysphagia: 3%), xerostomia (3% to 34%; severe xerostomia: 6%)
Local: Injection site pain (12% to 16%)
Neuromuscular & skeletal: Neck pain (≤17%)
Miscellaneous: Infection (≤19%), antibody formation (~10% to 18%, at 12 and 18 months, respectively)
1% to 10%:
Cardiovascular: Chest pain, edema, peripheral edema, vasolidation
Central nervous system: Dizziness (3% to 6%), anxiety, chills, confusion, fever, hyperesthesia, malaise, migraine, somnolence, tremor, vertigo
Dermatologic: Pruritus, bruising
Endocrine & metabolic: Hypercholesterolemia
Gastrointestinal: Nausea (≤10%), dyspepsia (≤10%,) glossitis, stomatitis, taste perversion, vomiting
Genitourinary: Cystitis, urinary tract infection, vaginal moniliasis
Hematologic: Serum neutralizing activity
Neuromuscular & skeletal: Torticollis (≤8%), arthralgia (≤7%), back pain (≤7%), myasthenia (≤6%), weakness (≤6%), arthritis, hernia
Ocular: Amblyopia, vision abnormal
Otic: Otitis media, tinnitus

Respiratory: Cough (3% to 7%; placebo 3%), dyspnea, pneumonia

Miscellaneous: Flu-like syndrome (6% to 9%), abscess, allergic reaction, cyst, neoplasm, viral infection

General Dosage Range I.M.: *Adults:* Initial: 2500-5000 units divided among the affected muscles

Mechanism of Action RimabotulinumtoxinB (previously known as botulinum toxin type B) is a neurotoxin produced by *Clostridium botulinum*, spore-forming anaerobic bacillus. It cleaves synaptic Vesicle Association Membrane Protein (VAMP; synaptobrevin) which is a component of the protein complex responsible for docking and fusion of the synaptic vesicle to the presynaptic membrane. By blocking neurotransmitter release, rimabotulinumtoxinB paralyzes the muscle.

Pharmacodynamics/Kinetics

Duration of Action 12-16 weeks

Pregnancy Risk Factor C (manufacturer)

Pregnancy Considerations Reproduction studies have not been conducted. Based on limited case reports using onabotulinumtoxinA, adverse fetal effects have not been observed with inadvertent administration during pregnancy. It is currently recommended to ensure adequate contraception in women of childbearing years.

Rimantadine (ri MAN ta deen)

Related Information

Systemic Viral Diseases *on page 1537*

Brand Names: U.S. Flumadine®

Brand Names: Canada Flumadine®

Pharmacologic Category Antiviral Agent; Antiviral Agent, Adamantane

Use Prophylaxis (adults and children >1 year of age) and treatment (adults) of influenza A viral infection (per manufacturer labeling; also refer to current ACIP guidelines for recommendations during current flu season)

Note: In certain circumstances, the ACIP recommends use of rimantadine in combination with oseltamivir for the treatment or prophylaxis of influenza A infection when resistance to oseltamivir is suspected.

Local Anesthetic/Vasoconstrictor Precautions No information available to require special precautions

Effects on Dental Treatment Key adverse event(s) related to dental treatment: Xerostomia (normal salivary flow resumes upon discontinuation).

Effects on Bleeding No information available to require special precautions

Adverse Effects 1% to 10%:

Central nervous system: Insomnia (2% to 3%), concentration impaired (≤2%), dizziness (1% to 2%), nervousness (1% to 2%), fatigue (1%), headache (1%)

Gastrointestinal: Nausea (3%), anorexia (2%), vomiting (2%), xerostomia (2%), abdominal pain (1%)

Neuromuscular & skeletal: Weakness (1%)

General Dosage Range Dosage adjustment recommended in patients with hepatic or renal impairment

Oral:

Children 1-9 years: 5 mg/kg/day in 1-2 divided doses (maximum: 150 mg/day)

Children ≥10 years and <40 kg: 5 mg/kg/day in 2 divided doses

Children ≥10 years and Adults: 100 mg twice daily

Elderly: 100 mg daily

Mechanism of Action Exerts its inhibitory effect on three antigenic subtypes of influenza A virus (H1N1, H2N2, H3N2) early in the viral replicative cycle, possibly inhibiting the uncoating process; it has no activity against influenza B virus and is two- to eightfold more active than amantadine

Pharmacodynamics/Kinetics

Onset of Action Antiviral activity: No data exist establishing a correlation between plasma concentration and antiviral effect

Half-life Elimination 25.4 hours; prolonged with elderly, severe liver and severe renal impairment

Time to Peak 6 hours

Pregnancy Risk Factor C

Pregnancy Considerations Animal data suggest embryotoxicity, maternal toxicity, and offspring mortality at doses 7-11 times the recommended human dose. There are no adequate and well-controlled studies in pregnant women.

Influenza infection may be more severe in pregnant women. Untreated influenza infection is associated with an increased risk of adverse events to the fetus and an increased risk of complications or death to the mother. Oseltamivir and zanamivir are currently recommended for the treatment or prophylaxis influenza in pregnant women and women up to 2 weeks postpartum. Appropriate antiviral agents are currently recommended as an adjunct to vaccination and should not be used as a substitute for vaccination in pregnant women (consult current CDC guidelines).

Healthcare providers are encouraged to refer women exposed to influenza vaccine, or who have taken an antiviral medication during pregnancy to the Vaccines and Medications in Pregnancy Surveillance System (VAMPSS) by contacting The Organization of Teratology Information Specialists (OTIS) at (877) 311-8972.

Rimexolone (ri MEKS oh lone)

Brand Names: U.S. Vexol®

Brand Names: Canada Vexol®

Pharmacologic Category Corticosteroid, Ophthalmic

Use Treatment of inflammation after ocular surgery and the treatment of anterior uveitis

Local Anesthetic/Vasoconstrictor Precautions No information available to require special precautions

Effects on Dental Treatment No significant effects or complications reported

Effects on Bleeding No information available to require special precautions

Adverse Effects

1% to 5%: Ocular: Blurred vision, discharge, discomfort, pain, increased intraocular pressure, foreign body sensation, hyperemia, pruritus

<2%:

Cardiovascular: Hypotension

Central nervous system: Headache

Gastrointestinal: Taste perversion

Respiratory: Pharyngitis, rhinitis

Frequency not defined: Cataracts, damage to the optic nerve, defects in visual activity, perforation of globe, secondary ocular infection

General Dosage Range Ophthalmic: *Adults:* Instill 1-2 drops 4 times/day **or** instill 1-2 drops every 1-2 hours during waking hours

Mechanism of Action Decreases inflammation by suppression of migration of polymorphonuclear leukocytes and reversal of increased capillary permeability

◄ **Pregnancy Risk Factor** C
Pregnancy Considerations Rimexolone was shown to be teratogenic in animal reproduction studies when administered subcutaneously. The amount of rimexolone absorbed systemically following ophthalmic administration is not known.

Risedronate (ris ED roe nate)

Related Information
Osteonecrosis of the Jaw *on page 1529*
Rheumatoid Arthritis, Osteoarthritis, and Osteoporosis *on page 1526*
Brand Names: U.S. Actonel®; Atelvia™
Brand Names: Canada Actonel®; Actonel® DR; Apo-Risedronate®; Dom-Risedronate; Novo-Risedronate; PMS-Risedronate; ratio-Risedronate; Riva-Risedronate; Sandoz-Risedronate; Teva-Risedronate
Generic Availability (U.S.) No
Pharmacologic Category Bisphosphonate Derivative
Use
Actonel®: Treatment of Paget's disease of the bone; treatment and prevention of glucocorticoid-induced osteoporosis; treatment and prevention of osteoporosis in postmenopausal women; treatment of osteoporosis in men
Atelvia™: Treatment of osteoporosis in postmenopausal women
Local Anesthetic/Vasoconstrictor Precautions No information available to require special precautions
Effects on Dental Treatment Osteonecrosis of the jaw (ONJ), generally associated with local infection and/or tooth extraction and often with delayed healing, has been reported in patients taking bisphosphonates. Symptoms included nonhealing extraction socket or an exposed jawbone. Most reported cases of bisphosphonate-associated osteonecrosis have been in cancer patients treated with intravenous bisphosphonates. However, some have occurred in patients with postmenopausal osteoporosis taking oral bisphosphonates. Dental surgery, particularly tooth extraction, may increase the risk for ONJ. Patients who develop ONJ while on bisphosphonate therapy should receive care by an oral surgeon. See Dental Comment.
Effects on Bleeding No information available to require special precautions
Adverse Effects Frequency may vary with product, dose, and indication.
>10%:
Cardiovascular: Hypertension (11%)
Central nervous system: Headache (3% to 18%)
Dermatologic: Rash (8% to 12%)
Endocrine & metabolic: Serum PTH levels increased (transient; <30%)
Gastrointestinal: Diarrhea (5% to 20%), nausea (4% to 13%), constipation (3% to 13%), abdominal pain (2% to 12%), dyspepsia (4% to 11%)
Genitourinary: Urinary tract infection (11%)
Neuromuscular & skeletal: Arthralgia (7% to 33%), back pain (6% to 28%)
Miscellaneous: Infection (≤31%)
1% to 10%:
Cardiovascular: Peripheral edema (8%), chest pain (5% to 7%), arrhythmia (2%)
Central nervous system: Depression (7%), dizziness (3% to 7%)
Endocrine & metabolic: Hypocalcemia (≤5%), hypophosphatemia (<3%)

Gastrointestinal: Vomiting (2% to 5%), gastritis (3%), duodenitis (≤1%), glossitis (≤1%)
Genitourinary: Prostatic hyperplasia (5%; benign), nephrolithiasis (3%)
Neuromuscular & skeletal: Joint disorder (7%), myalgia (2% to 7%), neck pain (5%), muscle spasm (1% to 2%)
Ocular: Cataract (7%)
Respiratory: Bronchitis (3% to 10%), pharyngitis (6%), rhinitis (6%), dyspnea (4%)
Miscellaneous: Flu-like syndrome (10%), acute phase reaction (≤8%; includes fever, influenza-like illness)
Dosage Oral: Adults: **Note:** Patients should receive supplemental calcium and vitamin D if dietary intake is inadequate.
Immediate release tablet:
Paget's disease of bone: 30 mg once daily for 2 months
Retreatment may be considered (following post-treatment observation of at least 2 months) if relapse occurs, or if treatment fails to normalize serum alkaline phosphatase. For retreatment, the dose and duration of therapy are the same as for initial treatment. No data are available on more than one course of retreatment.
Osteoporosis (postmenopausal) prevention and treatment: 5 mg once daily **or** 35 mg once weekly **or** 150 mg once a month
Osteoporosis (males) treatment: 35 mg once weekly
Osteoporosis (glucocorticoid-induced) prevention and treatment: 5 mg once daily
Delayed release tablet: Osteoporosis (postmenopausal) treatment: 35 mg once weekly

Dosage adjustment in renal impairment:
Cl$_{cr}$ ≥30 mL/minute: No adjustment required
Cl$_{cr}$ <30 mL/minute: **Not** recommended for use
Dosage adjustment in hepatic impairment: No studies performed in hepatic impairment; no dosage adjustment necessary due to lack of hepatic metabolism
Mechanism of Action A bisphosphonate which inhibits bone resorption via actions on osteoclasts or on osteoclast precursors; decreases the rate of bone resorption, leading to an indirect increase in bone mineral density. In Paget's disease, characterized by disordered resorption and formation of bone, inhibition of resorption leads to an indirect decrease in bone formation; but the newly-formed bone has a more normal architecture.
Contraindications Hypersensitivity to risedronate, bisphosphonates, or any component of the formulation; hypocalcemia; inability to stand or sit upright for at least 30 minutes; abnormalities of the esophagus which delay esophageal emptying, such as stricture or achalasia
Warnings/Precautions Bisphosphonates may cause upper gastrointestinal disorders such as dysphagia, esophagitis, esophageal ulcer, and gastric ulcer; risk increases in patients unable to comply with dosing instructions. Use with caution in patients with dysphagia, esophageal disease, gastritis, duodenitis, or ulcers (may worsen underlying condition). Discontinue if new or worsening symptoms occur. Use caution in patients with renal impairment (not recommended in patients with a Cl$_{cr}$ <30 mL/minute). Hypocalcemia must be corrected before therapy initiation with risedronate. Ensure adequate calcium and vitamin D intake, especially for patients with Paget's disease in whom the pretreatment rate of bone turnover may be greatly elevated.

Bisphosphonate therapy has been associated with osteonecrosis, primarily of the jaw. Risk factors for osteonecrosis of the jaw (ONJ) include invasive dental procedures (eg, tooth extraction, dental implants, boney surgery); a diagnosis of cancer, with concomitant chemotherapy or corticosteroids; poor oral hygiene, ill-fitting dentures; and comorbid disorders (anemia, coagulopathy, infection, pre-existing dental disease). Most reported cases occurred after I.V. bisphosphonate therapy; however, cases have been reported following oral therapy. A dental exam and preventative dentistry should be performed prior to placing patients with risk factors on chronic bisphosphonate therapy. The manufacturer's labeling states that discontinuing bisphosphonates in patients requiring invasive dental procedures may reduce the risk of ONJ. However, other experts suggest that there is no evidence that discontinuing therapy reduces the risk of developing ONJ (Assael, 2009). The benefit/risk must be assessed by the treating physician and/or dentist/surgeon prior to any invasive dental procedure. Patients developing ONJ while on bisphosphonates should receive care by an oral surgeon.

Atypical femur fractures have been reported in patients receiving bisphosphonates for treatment/prevention of osteoporosis. The fractures include subtrochanteric femur (bone just below the hip joint) and diaphyseal femur (long segment of the thigh bone). Some patients experience prodromal pain weeks or months before the fracture occurs. It is unclear if bisphosphonate therapy is the cause for these fractures, although the majority have been reported in patients taking bisphosphonates. Patients receiving long-term (>3-5 years) therapy may be at an increased risk. Discontinue bisphosphonate therapy in patients who develop a femoral shaft fracture.

Infrequently, severe (and occasionally debilitating) bone, joint, and/or muscle pain have been reported during bisphosphonate treatment. The onset of pain ranged from a single day to several months. Consider discontinuing therapy in patients who experience severe symptoms; symptoms usually resolve upon discontinuation. Some patients experienced recurrence when rechallenged with same drug or another bisphosphonate; avoid use in patients with a history of these symptoms in association with bisphosphonate therapy.

When using for glucocorticoid-induced osteoporosis, evaluate sex steroid hormonal status prior to treatment initiation; consider appropriate hormone replacement if necessary. Not approved for use in pediatric patients with osteogenesis imperfecta due to lack of efficacy in reducing the risk of fracture.

Drug Interactions

Metabolism/Transport Effects None known.

Avoid Concomitant Use

Avoid concomitant use of Risedronate with any of the following: H2-Antagonists; Proton Pump Inhibitors

Increased Effect/Toxicity

Risedronate may increase the levels/effects of: Deferasirox; Phosphate Supplements; SUNItinib

The levels/effects of Risedronate may be increased by: Aminoglycosides; H2-Antagonists; Nonsteroidal Anti-Inflammatory Agents; Proton Pump Inhibitors

Decreased Effect

The levels/effects of Risedronate may be decreased by: Antacids; Calcium Salts; Iron Salts; Magnesium Salts; Multivitamins/Minerals (with ADEK, Folate, Iron); Proton Pump Inhibitors

Ethanol/Nutrition/Herb Interactions

Ethanol: Avoid ethanol (may increase risk of osteoporosis).

Food: Food reduces absorption (similar to other bisphosphonates); mean oral bioavailability is decreased when given with food.

Dietary Considerations Ensure adequate calcium and vitamin D intake. Take immediate release tablet with at least 6 oz of **plain water** (not mineral water) ≥30 minutes before the first food or drink of the day other than water. Take delayed release tablet with at least 4 ounces of **plain water** immediately **after** breakfast.

Pharmacodynamics/Kinetics

Onset of Action May require weeks

Half-life Elimination Initial: 1.5 hours; Terminal: 480-561 hours

Time to Peak Serum: 1-3 hours

Pregnancy Risk Factor C

Pregnancy Considerations Teratogenic and nonteratogenic embryo/fetal effects have been reported in animal studies. There are no adequate and well-controlled studies in pregnant women. Bisphosphonates are incorporated into the bone matrix and gradually released over time. Theoretically, there may be a risk of fetal harm when pregnancy follows the completion of therapy. Based on limited case reports with pamidronate, serum calcium levels in the newborn may be altered if administered during pregnancy.

Lactation Excretion in breast milk unknown/not recommended

Breast-Feeding Considerations The manufacturer recommends discontinuing nursing or discontinuing risedronate.

Dosage Forms

Tablet, oral:

Actonel®: 5 mg, 30 mg, 35 mg, 150 mg

Tablet, delayed release, oral:

Atelvia™: 35 mg

Dental Comment A review of 2408 published cases of bisphosphonate-associated osteonecrosis of the jaw bone (BP-associated ONJ) was done by Filleul, 2010. BP therapy was associated with 89% of the cases to treat malignancies and 11% of the cases to treat nonmalignant conditions. Information on the specific bisphosphonate used was available for 1694 of the patients. Intravenous therapy (primarily zoledronic acid) was received by 88% of the patients and 12% received oral treatment (primarily alendronate). Of all the cases of BP-associated ONJ, 67% were preceded by tooth extraction and for 26% of patients, there was no predisposing factor identified.

A 2010 retrospective case review reported the prevalence of BP-associated ONJ in patients using alendronate-type drugs was one out of 952 patients or ~0.1% (Lo, 2010). Of the 8572 respondents, nine cases of ONJ were identified; five had developed ONJ spontaneously and four developed ONJ after tooth extraction. When extrapolated to patient-years of bisphosphonate exposure, this prevalence rate of 0.1% equates to a frequency of 28 cases per 100,000 person-years of oral bisphosphonate treatment. An Australian group (Mavrokokki, 2007), identified the frequency of BP-associated ONJ in osteoporotic patients, mainly taking weekly oral alendronate, was 1 in 8470 to 1 in 2260 (0.01% to 0.04%) patients. If extractions were carried out, the calculated frequency was 1 in 1130 to 1 in 296 (0.09% to 0.34%) patients. The median time to onset of ONJ in alendronate patients was 24 months.

According to the 2011 report by the American Dental Association (ADA), the incidence of BP-associated ONJ remains low and the benefits of using oral bisphosphonates significantly outweighs the risk of developing BP-associated ONJ for treatment and prevention of osteoporosis and cancer treatment (Hellstein, 2011). The full 47 page report can be accessed at http://www.ada.org/sections/professionalResources/pdfs/topics_AR-ONJ_report.pdf.

The ADA review of 2011 stated the incidence of oral BP-associated ONJ was one case for every 1000 individuals exposed to oral bisphosphonates (0.1%) (Hellstein, 2011).

References

Durie BG, Katz M, and Crowley J, "Osteonecrosis of the Jaw and Bisphosphonates," *N Engl J Med*, 2005, 353(1):99-102.

Filleul O, Crompot E, and Saussez S, "Bisphosphonate-Induced Osteonecrosis of the Jaw: A Review of 2,400 Patient Cases," *J Cancer Res Clin Oncol*, 2010, 136(8):1117-24.

Hellstein JW, Adler RA, Edwards B, et al, "Managing the Care of Patients Receiving Antiresorptive Therapy for Prevention and Treatment of Osteoporosis: Executive Summary of Recommendations From the American Dental Association Council on Scientific Affairs," *J Am Dent Assoc*, 2011, 142(11):1243-51.

Hellstein JW, Adler RA, Edwards B, et al, "Managing the Care of Patients Receiving Antiresorptive Therapy for Prevention and Treatment of Osteoporosis: Recommendations From the American Dental Association Council on Scientific Affairs," 2011, Available at http://www.ada.org/sections/professionalResources/pdfs/topics_ARONJ_report.pdf. Accessed February 2013.

Lo JC, O'Ryan FS, Gordon NP, et al, "Prevalence of Osteonecrosis of the Jaw in Patients With Oral Bisphosphonate Exposure," *J Oral Maxillofac Surg*, 2010, 68(2):243-53.

Marx RE, Sawatari Y, Fortin M, et al, "Bisphosphonate-Induced Exposed Bone (Osteonecrosis/Osteopetrosis) of the Jaws: Risk Factors, Recognition, Prevention, and Treatment," *J Oral Maxillofac Surg*, 2005, 63(11):1567-75.

Mavrokokki T, Cheng A, Stein B, et al, "Nature and Frequency of Bisphosphonate-Associated Osteonecrosis of the Jaws in Australia," *J Oral Maxillofac Surg*, 2007, 65(3):415-23.

Ruggiero SL, Dodson TB, Assael LA, et al, "American Association of Oral and Maxillofacial Surgeons Position Paper on Bisphosphonate-Related Osteonecrosis of the Jaws-2009 Update," *J Oral Maxillofac Surg*, 2009, 67(5 Suppl):2-12.

Ruggiero S, Gralow J, Marx RE, et al, "Practical Guidelines for the Prevention, Diagnosis, and Treatment of Osteonecrosis of the Jaw in Patients With Cancer," *J Clin Oncol*, 2006, 2(1):7-14.

RisperiDONE (ris PER i done)

Related Information

Clinical Risk Related to Drugs Prolonging QT Interval *on page 1510*

Brand Names: U.S. RisperDAL®; RisperDAL® Consta®; RisperDAL® M-Tab®

Brand Names: Canada Apo-Risperidone®; Ava-Risperidone; CO Risperidone; Dom-Risperidone; JAMP-Risperidone; Mint-Risperidon; Mylan-Risperidone; Novo-Risperidone; PHL-Risperidone; PMS-Risperidone; PMS-Risperidone ODT; PRO-Risperidone; RAN™-Risperidone; ratio-Risperidone; Risperdal®; Risperdal® Consta®; Risperdal® M-Tab®; Riva-Risperidone; Sandoz-Risperidone; Teva-Risperidone

Generic Availability (U.S.) Yes: Excludes injection

Pharmacologic Category Antimanic Agent; Antipsychotic Agent, Atypical

Use

Oral: Treatment of schizophrenia; treatment of acute mania or mixed episodes associated with bipolar I disorder (as monotherapy in children or adults, or in combination with lithium or valproate in adults); treatment of irritability/aggression associated with autistic disorder

Injection: Treatment of schizophrenia; maintenance treatment of bipolar I disorder in adults as monotherapy or in combination with lithium or valproate

Unlabeled Use Treatment of Tourette's syndrome; psychosis/agitation related to Alzheimer's dementia; post-traumatic stress disorder (PTSD)

Local Anesthetic/Vasoconstrictor Precautions RisperiDONE is one of the drugs confirmed to prolong the QT interval and is accepted as having a risk of causing torsade de pointes. The risk of drug-induced torsade de pointes is extremely low when a single QT interval prolonging drug is prescribed. In terms of epinephrine, it is not known what effect vasoconstrictors in the local anesthetic regimen will have in patients with a known history of congenital prolonged QT interval or in patients taking any medication that prolongs the QT interval. Until more information is obtained, it is suggested that the clinician consult with the physician prior to the use of a vasoconstrictor in suspected patients, and that the vasoconstrictor (epinephrine, mepivacaine, and levonordefrin [Carbocaine® 2% with Neo-Cobefrin®]) be used with caution.

Effects on Dental Treatment Key adverse event(s) related to dental treatment: Significant xerostomia (normal salivary flow resumes upon discontinuation) and toothache.

Effects on Bleeding No information available to require special precautions

Adverse Effects

>10%:

Central nervous system: Sedation (children 12% to 63%; adults 5% to 11%), parkinsonism (children: 28% to 62%; adults 8% to 25%), somnolence (adults 5% to 41%; children 4% to 11%), insomnia (≤32%), fatigue (children 18% to 31%; adults 1% to 9%), headache (12% to 21%), anxiety (≤8% or 16%), dizziness (3% to 16%), fever (children 16%; adults 1% to 2%), akathisia (5% to 11%)

Gastrointestinal: Appetite increased (children 4% to 44%; adults 4%), weight gain (≥7% kg increase from baseline: children 8% to 33%; adults 4% to 21%), vomiting (children 10% to 20%; adults <4%), constipation (5% to 17%), nausea (5% to 16%), abdominal pain (children 6% to 16%; adults <4%), drooling (children 12%; adults <4%)

Genitourinary: Urinary incontinence (children 5% to 22%; adults <4%), enuresis (children 16%; adults <1%)

Neuromuscular & skeletal: Tremor (adults ≤24%; children ≤11%)

Respiratory: Nasopharyngitis (children 19%; adults ≤4%), cough (children ≤17%; adults ≤4%), rhinorrhea (children 12%; adults <4%)

1% to 10%:

Cardiovascular: Atrioventricular block first degree (<4%), bradycardia (<4%), bundle branch block (<4%), chest pain (<4%), ECG changes (<4%), facial edema (<4%), hypotension (<4%), orthostatic hypotension (<4%), palpitation (<4%), QT prolongation (<4%), tachycardia (adults <4%; children <1%), hypertension (≤3%), peripheral edema (≤3%), syncope (1% to 2%)

Central nervous system: Gait disturbance (4%), pain (1% to 4%), attention span decreased (≤4%), agitation (<4%), akinesia (<4%), coordination impaired (<4%), depression (<4%), malaise (<4%), nervousness (<4%), postural dizziness (<4%), seizure (<4%), sleep disturbances (<4%), sluggishness (<4%), vertigo (<4%), lethargy (2%), hypoesthesia (≤2%)

Dermatologic: Rash (<4% to 8%), eczema (<4%), pruritus (<4%), dry skin (≤3%), acne (<1% to 2%)

Endocrine & metabolic: Menorrhea (≤4%), breast discomfort (<4%), ejaculation disorder/delayed (<4%), erectile dysfunction (<4%), galactorrhea (<4%), gynecomastia (<4%), hyperglycemia (<4%), hyperprolactinemia (<4%), libido decreased (<4%), menstrual irregularities (<4%), sexual dysfunction (<4%)

Gastrointestinal: Dyspepsia (3% to 10%), xerostomia (≤7% to 10%), salivation increased (1% to 10%), diarrhea (<4% to 8%), appetite decreased (≤6%), anorexia (<1% to <4%), weight loss (≤4%), gastritis (<4%), gastroenteritis (<4%), toothache (≤3%)

Genitourinary: Cystitis (<4%), glucosuria (<4%), urinary tract infection (<4%)

Hematologic: Anemia (<4%), neutropenia (<4%)

Hepatic: ALT increased (<4%), AST increased (<4%), GGT increased (<4%)

Local: Abscess (<4%); injection site induration, pain, reaction, swelling (<4%)

Neuromuscular & skeletal: Dystonia (2% to 6%), limb pain (2% to 6%), dyskinesia (adults ≤6%; children <1%), arthralgia (2% to 4%), back pain (≤4%), buttock pain (<4%), dysarthria (<4%), hypokinesia (<4%), musculoskeletal chest pain (<4%), myalgia (<4%), neck pain (<4%), paresthesia (<4%), posture abnormal (<4%), tardive dyskinesia (<4%), weakness (<4%), creatine phosphokinase increased (≤2%)

Ocular: Blurred vision (2% to 7%), conjunctivitis (<4%), visual acuity reduced (<4%)

Otic: Earache (≤4%), otitis media (<4%)

Respiratory: Nasal congestion (≤6% to 10%), pharyngolaryngeal pain (3% to 10%), rhinitis (<4% to 9%), respiratory infection (≤6% to 8%), bronchitis (<4%), dyspnea (<4%), pharyngitis (<4%), pneumonia (<4%), sinusitis (<4%), epistaxis (≤2%)

Miscellaneous: Thirst (children ≤7%; adults <1%), flu-like syndrome (<4%), hypersensitivity (<4%), infection (<4%), viral infection (<4%)

Dosage Note: When reinitiating treatment after discontinuation, the initial titration schedule should be followed.

Oral:

Children ≥5 years and Adolescents: Autism:

<15 kg: Use with caution; specific dosing recommendations not available

15 to <20 kg: Initial: 0.25 mg daily; may increase dose to 0.5 mg daily after ≥4 days, maintain dose for ≥14 days. In patients not achieving sufficient clinical response, may increase dose by 0.25 mg daily in ≥2-week intervals. Doses ranging from 0.5-3 mg daily have been evaluated; however, therapeutic effect reached plateau at 1 mg daily in clinical trials. Following clinical response, consider gradually lowering dose. May be administered once daily or in divided doses twice daily.

≥20 kg: Initial: 0.5 mg daily; may increase dose to 1 mg daily after ≥4 days, maintain dose for ≥14 days. In patients not achieving sufficient clinical response, may increase dose by 0.5 mg daily in ≥2-week intervals. Doses ranging from 0.5-3 mg daily have been evaluated; however, therapeutic effect reached plateau at 2.5 mg daily (3 mg daily in children >45 kg) in clinical trials. Following clinical response, consider gradually lowering dose. May be administered once daily or in divided doses twice daily.

Children and Adolescents:

Schizophrenia: Adolescents 13-17 years: Initial: 0.5 mg once daily; dose may be adjusted in increments of 0.5-1 mg daily at intervals ≥24 hours to a dose of 3 mg daily. Doses ranging from 1-6 mg daily have been evaluated, however, doses >3 mg daily

do not confer additional benefit and are associated with increased adverse events.

Bipolar mania: Children and Adolescents 10-17 years: Initial: 0.5 mg once daily; dose may be adjusted in increments of 0.5-1 mg daily at intervals ≥24 hours to a dose of 1-2.5 mg daily. Doses ranging from 0.5-6 mg daily have been evaluated; however doses >2.5 mg daily do not confer additional benefit and are associated with increased adverse events.

Maintenance: No dosing recommendation available for treatment >3 weeks duration

Adolescents and Adults: Tourette's syndrome (unlabeled use): Initial: 0.25 mg once daily for 2 days, then 0.25 mg twice daily for 3 days, then 0.5 mg twice daily for 2 days; titrate slowly thereafter in increments/decrements ≤0.5 mg twice daily and at intervals ≥3 days; maximum dose: 6 mg daily (Dion, 2002)

Adults:

Schizophrenia:

Initial: 2 mg daily in 1-2 divided doses; may be increased by 1-2 mg daily at intervals ≥24 hours to a recommended dosage range of 4-8 mg daily; may be given as a single daily dose once maintenance dose is achieved; daily dosages >6 mg do not appear to confer any additional benefit, and the incidence of extrapyramidal symptoms is higher than with lower doses. Further dose adjustments should be made in increments/decrements of 1-2 mg daily on a weekly basis. Dose range studied in clinical trials: 4-16 mg daily.

Maintenance: Recommended dosage range: 2-8 mg daily

Bipolar mania:

Initial: 2-3 mg once daily; if needed, adjust dose by 1 mg daily in intervals ≥24 hours; dosing range: 1-6 mg daily

Maintenance: No dosing recommendation available for treatment >3 weeks duration.

Post-traumatic stress disorder (PTSD) (unlabeled use): 0.5-8 mg daily (Bandelow, 2008; Benedek, 2009)

Elderly:

Initial: 0.5 mg twice daily; titration should progress slowly in increments of no more than 0.5 mg twice daily; increases to dosages >1.5 mg twice daily should occur at intervals of ≥1 week.

Note: Additional monitoring of renal function and orthostatic blood pressure may be warranted. If once-a-day dosing in the elderly or debilitated patient is considered, a twice daily regimen should be used to titrate to the target dose, and this dose should be maintained for 2-3 days prior to attempts to switch to a once-daily regimen.

Psychosis/agitation related to Alzheimer's dementia (unlabeled use): Initial: 0.25-1 mg daily; if necessary, gradually increase as tolerated not to exceed 1.5-2 mg daily; doses >1 mg daily are associated with higher rates of extrapyramidal symptoms (Rabins, 2007)

I.M.: **Note:** Oral risperidone (or other antipsychotic) should be administered with the initial injection of Risperdal® Consta® and continued for 3 weeks (then discontinued) to maintain adequate therapeutic plasma concentrations prior to main release phase of risperidone from injection site. When switching from depot administration to a short-acting formulation, administer short-acting agent in place of the next regularly-scheduled depot injection.

Adults: Schizophrenia, bipolar I maintenance (Risperdal® Consta®): Initial: 25 mg every 2 weeks; if unresponsive, some may benefit from larger doses (37.5-50 mg); maximum dose: 50 mg every 2 weeks. Dosage adjustments should not be made more frequently than every 4 weeks. A lower initial dose of 12.5 mg may be appropriate in some patients (eg, demonstrated poor tolerability to other psychotropic medications).

Elderly (Risperdal® Consta®): 25 mg every 2 weeks; a lower initial dose of 12.5 mg may be appropriate in some patients

Dosing adjustment in renal impairment: Adults:

Oral: Cl_{cr} <30 mL/minute: Starting dose of 0.5 mg twice daily; titration should progress slowly in increments of no more than 0.5 mg twice daily; increases to dosages >1.5 mg twice daily should occur at intervals of ≥1 week. Clearance of the active moiety is decreased by 60% in patients with moderate-to-severe renal disease (Cl_{cr} <60 mL/minute) compared to healthy subjects.

I.M.: Initiate with **oral** dosing (0.5 mg twice daily for 1 week then 2 mg daily for 1 week); if tolerated, begin 25 mg **I.M.** every 2 weeks; continue oral dosing for 3 weeks after the first I.M. injection. An initial I.M. dose of 12.5 mg may also be considered.

Dosing adjustment in hepatic impairment: Adults:

Oral: Child-Pugh class C: Starting dose of 0.5 mg twice daily; titration should progress slowly in increments of no more than 0.5 mg twice daily; increases to dosages >1.5 mg twice daily should occur at intervals of ≥1 week. The mean free fraction of risperidone in plasma was increased by 35% in patients with hepatic impairment compared to healthy subjects.

I.M.: Initiate with **oral** dosing (0.5 mg twice daily for 1 week then 2 mg daily for 1 week); if tolerated, begin 25 mg **I.M.** every 2 weeks; continue oral dosing for 3 weeks after the first I.M. injection. An initial I.M. dose of 12.5 mg may also be considered.

Mechanism of Action Risperidone is a benzisoxazole atypical antipsychotic with mixed serotonin-dopamine antagonist activity that binds to $5-HT_2$-receptors in the CNS and in the periphery with a very high affinity; binds to dopamine-D_2 receptors with less affinity. The binding affinity to the dopamine-D_2 receptor is 20 times lower than the $5-HT_2$ affinity. The addition of serotonin antagonism to dopamine antagonism (classic neuroleptic mechanism) is thought to improve negative symptoms of psychoses and reduce the incidence of extrapyramidal side effects. Alpha$_1$, alpha$_2$ adrenergic, and histaminergic receptors are also antagonized with high affinity. Risperidone has low to moderate affinity for $5-HT_{1C}$, $5-HT_{1D}$, and $5-HT_{1A}$ receptors, weak affinity for D_1 and no affinity for muscarinics or beta$_1$ and beta$_2$ receptors

Contraindications Hypersensitivity to risperidone or any component of the formulation

Warnings/Precautions Hazardous agent - use appropriate precautions for handling and disposal (NIOSH, 2012). **[U.S. Boxed Warning]: Elderly patients with dementia-related psychosis treated with antipsychotics are at an increased risk of death compared to placebo.** Most deaths appeared to be either cardiovascular (eg, heart failure, sudden death) or infectious (eg, pneumonia) in nature. In addition, an increased incidence of cerebrovascular effects (eg, transient ischemic attack, cerebrovascular accidents) has been reported in studies of placebo-controlled trials of risperidone in elderly patients with dementia-related

psychosis. Risperidone is not approved for the treatment of dementia-related psychosis.

Leukopenia, neutropenia, and agranulocytosis (sometimes fatal) have been reported in clinical trials and postmarketing reports with antipsychotic use; presence of risk factors (eg, pre-existing low WBC or history of drug-induced leuko-/neutropenia) should prompt periodic blood count assessment. Discontinue therapy at first signs of blood dyscrasias or if absolute neutrophil count <1000/mm^3.

Low to moderately sedating, use with caution in disorders where CNS depression is a feature. Use with caution in Parkinson's disease. Caution in patients with predisposition to seizures. Use with caution in renal or hepatic dysfunction; dose reduction recommended. Esophageal dysmotility and aspiration have been associated with antipsychotic use; use with caution in patients at risk of aspiration pneumonia (ie, Alzheimer's disease). Risperidone is associated with greater increases in prolactin levels as compared to other antipsychotic agents; clinical significance of hyperprolactinemia in patients with breast cancer or other prolactin-dependent tumors is unknown. May alter temperature regulation. May mask toxicity of other drugs or conditions (eg, intestinal obstruction, Reyes syndrome, brain tumor) due to antiemetic effects. Neutropenia has been reported with antipsychotic use, including fatal cases of agranulocytosis. Pre-existing myelosuppression (disease or drug-induced) increases risk and these patients should have frequent CBC monitoring; decreased blood counts in absence of other causative factors should prompt discontinuation of therapy.

Use with caution in patients with cardiovascular diseases (eg, heart failure, history of myocardial infarction or ischemia, cerebrovascular disease, conduction abnormalities). May cause orthostatic hypotension; use with caution in patients at risk of this effect (eg, concurrent medication use which may predispose to hypotension/bradycardia or presence of hypovolemia) or in those who would not tolerate transient hypotensive episodes. May alter cardiac conduction (low risk relative to other neuroleptics); life-threatening arrhythmias have occurred with therapeutic doses of neuroleptics.

May cause anticholinergic effects (confusion, agitation, constipation, xerostomia, blurred vision, urinary retention); therefore, they should be used with caution in patients with decreased gastrointestinal motility, urinary retention, BPH, xerostomia, or visual problems (including narrow-angle glaucoma). Relative to other neuroleptics, risperidone has a low potency of cholinergic blockade.

May cause extrapyramidal symptoms (EPS), including pseudoparkinsonism, acute dystonic reactions, akathisia, and tardive dyskinesia (risk of these reactions is low relative to other neuroleptics, and is dose dependent). Risk of dystonia (and probably other EPS) may be greater with increased doses, use of conventional antipsychotics, males, and younger patients. Risk of neuroleptic malignant syndrome (NMS) may be increased in patients with Parkinson's disease or Lewy body dementia; monitor for symptoms of confusion, obtundation, postural instability and extrapyramidal symptoms. May cause hyperglycemia; in some cases may be extreme and associated with ketoacidosis, hyperosmolar coma, or death. Use with caution in patients with diabetes or other disorders of glucose regulation; monitor for worsening of glucose control. Dyslipidemia has been reported with atypical antipsychotics; risk profile may differ between agents. Discrepant results have been reported in clinical trials, regarding lipid changes associated with risperidone (American Diabetes Association, 2004). Significant weight gain has been observed with antipsychotic therapy; incidence varies with product. Monitor waist circumference and BMI. Rare cases of priapism have been reported.

Use in elderly patients with dementia is associated with an increased risk of mortality and cerebrovascular accidents; avoid antipsychotic use for behavioral problems associated with dementia unless alternative nonpharmacologic therapies have failed and patient may harm self or others. In addition, use may cause or exacerbate syndrome of inappropriate antidiuretic hormone secretion or hyponatremia; monitor sodium closely with initiation or dosage adjustments in older adults (Beers Criteria).

The possibility of a suicide attempt is inherent in psychotic illness or bipolar disorder; use caution in high-risk patients during initiation of therapy. Prescriptions should be written for the smallest quantity consistent with good patient care. Long-term effects on growth or sexual maturation have not been evaluated. Vehicle used in injectable (polylactide-co-glycolide microspheres) has rarely been associated with retinal artery occlusion in patients with abnormal arteriovenous anastomosis.

Drug Interactions

Metabolism/Transport Effects Substrate of CYP2D6 (major), CYP3A4 (minor), P-glycoprotein; **Note:** Assignment of Major/Minor substrate status based on clinically relevant drug interaction potential; **Inhibits** CYP2D6 (weak), CYP3A4 (weak)

Avoid Concomitant Use

Avoid concomitant use of RisperiDONE with any of the following: Aclidinium; Azelastine (Nasal); Highest Risk QTc-Prolonging Agents; Ipratropium (Oral Inhalation); Ivabradine; Metoclopramide; Mifepristone; Paraldehyde; Tiotropium

Increased Effect/Toxicity

RisperiDONE may increase the levels/effects of: Alcohol (Ethyl); Anticholinergics; ARIPiprazole; Azelastine (Nasal); Buprenorphine; CNS Depressants; Highest Risk QTc-Prolonging Agents; Lomitapide; Methotrimeprazine; Methylphenidate; Moderate Risk QTc-Prolonging Agents; Paliperidone; Paraldehyde; Serotonin Modulators; Tiotropium; Zolpidem

The levels/effects of RisperiDONE may be increased by: Abiraterone Acetate; Acetylcholinesterase Inhibitors (Central); Aclidinium; CYP2D6 Inhibitors (Moderate); CYP2D6 Inhibitors (Strong); Darunavir; Divalproex; HydrOXYzine; Ipratropium (Oral Inhalation); Ivabradine; Lithium formulations; Loop Diuretics; Magnesium Sulfate; Methotrimeprazine; Methylphenidate; Metoclopramide; Metyrosine; Mifepristone; Perampanel; P-glycoprotein/ABCB1 Inhibitors; Pramlintide; QTc-Prolonging Agents (Indeterminate Risk and Risk Modifying); Selective Serotonin Reuptake Inhibitors; Sodium Oxybate; Tetrabenazine; Valproic Acid; Verapamil

Decreased Effect

RisperiDONE may decrease the levels/effects of: Amphetamines; Anti-Parkinson's Agents (Dopamine Agonist); Quinagolide

The levels/effects of RisperiDONE may be decreased by: CarBAMazepine; Lithium formulations; Peginterferon Alfa-2b; P-glycoprotein/ABCB1 Inducers

Ethanol/Nutrition/Herb Interactions

Ethanol: Ethanol may increase CNS depression. Management: Limit or avoid ethanol.

Food: Oral solution is not compatible with beverages containing tannin or pectinate (cola or tea). Management: Administer oral solution with water, coffee, orange juice, or low-fat milk.

Herb/Nutraceutical: Some herbal medications may increase CNS depression. Management: Avoid kava kava, gotu kola, valerian, and St John's wort.

Dietary Considerations May be taken without regard to meals. Some products may contain phenylalanine.

Pharmacodynamics/Kinetics

Half-life Elimination Active moiety (risperidone and its active metabolite 9-hydroxyrisperidone)

Oral: 20 hours (mean)

Extensive metabolizers: Risperidone: 3 hours; 9-hydroxyrisperidone: 21 hours

Poor metabolizers: Risperidone: 20 hours; 9-hydroxyrisperidone: 30 hours

Injection: 3-6 days; related to microsphere erosion and subsequent absorption of risperidone

Time to Peak Plasma: Oral: Risperidone: Within 1 hour; 9-hydroxyrisperidone: Extensive metabolizers: 3 hours; Poor metabolizers: 17 hours

Pregnancy Risk Factor C

Pregnancy Considerations An increased risk of teratogenic effects was not observed in animal reproduction studies; however, an increase in pup mortality was observed following peri-postnatal exposure. In human studies, risperidone and its metabolite cross the placenta (Newport, 2007). An increased risk of teratogenic effects has not been observed following maternal use of risperidone (limited data) (Coppola, 2007). Agenesis of the corpus callosum has been noted in one case report of an infant exposed *in utero*. Antipsychotic use during the third trimester of pregnancy has a risk for extrapyramidal symptoms (EPS) and withdrawal symptoms in newborns following delivery. Symptoms in the newborn may include agitation, feeding disorder, hypertonia, hypotonia, respiratory distress, somnolence, and tremor. These effects may be self-limiting and allow recovery within hours or days with no specific treatment, or they may be severe requiring prolonged hospitalization. When using Risperdal® Consta®, patients should notify healthcare provider if they become or intend to become pregnant during therapy or within 12 weeks of last injection. Risperidone may cause hyperprolactinemia, which may decrease reproductive function in both males and females.

The ACOG recommends that therapy during pregnancy be individualized; treatment with psychiatric medications during pregnancy should incorporate the clinical expertise of the mental health clinician, obstetrician, primary healthcare provider, and pediatrician. Safety data related to atypical antipsychotics during pregnancy is limited and routine use is not recommended. However, if a woman is inadvertently exposed to an atypical antipsychotic while pregnant, continuing therapy may be preferable to switching to a typical antipsychotic that the fetus has not yet been exposed to; consider risk:benefit (ACOG, 2008).

Healthcare providers are encouraged to enroll women 18-45 years of age exposed to risperidone during pregnancy in the Atypical Antipsychotics Pregnancy Registry (1-866-961-2388 or http://www.womensmentalhealth.org/pregnancyregistry).

Lactation Enters breast milk/not recommended

Breast-Feeding Considerations Risperidone and its metabolite are excreted in breast milk; it is recommended that women not breast-feed during therapy or for 12 weeks after the last injection if using Risperdal® Consta®.

Dosage Forms

Injection, microspheres for reconstitution, extended release:

RisperDAL® Consta®: 12.5 mg, 25 mg, 37.5 mg, 50 mg

Solution, oral: 1 mg/mL (30 mL)

RisperDAL®: 1 mg/mL (30 mL)

Tablet, oral: 0.25 mg, 0.5 mg, 1 mg, 2 mg, 3 mg, 4 mg

RisperDAL®: 0.25 mg, 0.5 mg, 1 mg, 2 mg, 3 mg, 4 mg

Tablet, orally disintegrating, oral: 0.25 mg, 0.5 mg, 1 mg, 2 mg, 3 mg, 4 mg

RisperDAL® M-Tab®: 0.5 mg, 1 mg, 2 mg, 3 mg, 4 mg

Dental Comment RisperiDONE is known to prolong the QT interval. The QT interval is measured as the time and distance between the Q point of the QRS complex and the end of the T wave in the ECG tracing. After adjustment for heart rate, the QT interval is defined as prolonged if it is more than 450 msec in men and 460 msec in women. A long QT syndrome was first described in the 1950s and 60s as a congenital syndrome involving QT interval prolongation and syncope and sudden death. Some of the congenital long QT syndromes were characterized by a peculiar electrocardiographic appearance of the QRS complex involving a premature atria beat followed by a pause, then a subsequent sinus beat showing marked QT prolongation and deformity. This type of cardiac arrhythmia was originally termed "torsade de pointes" (translated from the French as "twisting of the points"). RisperiDONE is considered as having a risk of causing torsade de pointes. Since it is not known what effect vasoconstrictors in the local anesthetic regimen will have in patients with a known history of congenital prolonged QT interval or in patients taking any medication that prolongs the QT interval, a medical consult is suggested.

Ritonavir (ri TOE na veer)

Related Information

HIV Infection and AIDS *on page 1520*

Brand Names: U.S. Norvir®

Brand Names: Canada Norvir®; Norvir® SEC

Pharmacologic Category Antiretroviral Agent, Protease Inhibitor

Use Treatment of HIV infection; should always be used as part of a multidrug regimen

Unlabeled Use Used as a pharmacokinetic "booster" for other protease inhibitors

Local Anesthetic/Vasoconstrictor Precautions No information available to require special precautions

Effects on Dental Treatment Key adverse event(s) related to dental treatment: Xerostomia (normal salivary flow resumes upon discontinuation) and taste perversion.

Effects on Bleeding Increased bleeding has been noted with protease inhibitors in patients with hemophilia A or B. No information available to require routine special precautions relative to hemostasis in other patients.

Adverse Effects Percentages as reported for combined experiences in both treatment-naive and experienced adults:

>10%:

Endocrine & metabolic: Hypercholesterolemia (>240 mg/dL: 37% to 45%), triglycerides increased (>800 mg/dL: 17% to 34%; >1500 mg/dL: 1% to 13%)

Gastrointestinal: Nausea (26% to 30%), diarrhea (15% to 23%), vomiting (14% to 17%), taste perversion (7% to 11%)

Hepatic: GGT increased (5% to 20%)

Neuromuscular & skeletal: Weakness (10% to 15%), creatine phosphokinase increased (9% to 12%)

2% to 10%:

Cardiovascular: Vasodilation (2%), syncope (1% to 2%)

Central nervous system: Headache (6% to 7%), fever (1% to 5%), dizziness (3% to 4%), insomnia (2% to 3%), somnolence (2% to 3%), depression (2%), anxiety (up to 2%), malaise (1% to 2%)

Dermatologic: Rash (up to 4%)

Endocrine & metabolic: Uric acid increased (up to 4%)

Gastrointestinal: Abdominal pain (6% to 8%), anorexia (2% to 8%), dyspepsia (up to 6%), local throat irritation (2% to 3%), flatulence (1% to 2%)

Hepatic: Transaminases increased (6% to 10%)

Neuromuscular & skeletal: Paresthesia (3% to 7%), arthralgia (up to 2%), myalgia (2%)

Respiratory: Pharyngitis (≤1% to 3%)

Miscellaneous: Diaphoresis (2% to 3%)

General Dosage Range Dosage adjustment recommended in patients on concurrent therapy

Oral:

Infants >1 month and Children: Initial: 250 mg/m^2 twice daily; Maintenance: 350-400 mg/m^2 twice daily (maximum dose: 1200 mg daily)

Adolescents and Adults: 300-600 mg twice daily (maximum: 1200 mg daily)

Mechanism of Action Binds to the site of HIV-1 protease activity and inhibits cleavage of viral Gag-Pol polyprotein precursors into individual functional proteins required for infectious HIV. This results in the formation of immature, noninfectious viral particles.

Pharmacodynamics/Kinetics

Half-life Elimination 3-5 hours

Time to Peak Oral solution: 2 hours (fasted); 4 hours (nonfasted)

Pregnancy Risk Factor B

Pregnancy Considerations Adverse events were observed in animal reproduction studies only with doses which were also maternally toxic. Ritonavir crosses the placenta in minimal amounts; no increased risk of overall birth defects has been observed following first trimester exposure according to data collected by the antiretroviral pregnancy registry. Early studies have shown lower plasma levels during pregnancy compared to postpartum. The DHHS Perinatal HIV Guidelines consider ritonavir to be a preferred protease inhibitor (PI) for use during pregnancy when used as a booster for other PIs. The oral solution contains alcohol and therefore may not be the best formulation for use in pregnancy. A small increased risk of preterm birth has been associated with maternal use of protease inhibitor-based combination antiretroviral (ARV) therapy during pregnancy; however, the benefits of use generally outweigh this risk and PIs should not be withheld if otherwise recommended. Hyperglycemia, new onset of diabetes mellitus, or diabetic ketoacidosis have been reported with protease inhibitors; it is not clear if pregnancy increases this risk.

Regardless of CD4 count or HIV RNA copy number, all HIV-infected pregnant women should receive a combination antepartum ARV drug regimen; this includes women who require therapy for their own health, as well as women who do not yet require therapy for their own health. ARV therapy should be started as soon as possible if required for the woman's health. Although earlier initiation may be more effective in reducing the perinatal transmission of HIV, also consider maternal conditions (eg, nausea and vomiting) and the potential risks of first trimester fetal exposure for specific agents. Plasma HIV RNA levels should be assessed at ~34-36 weeks gestation in order to help determine mode of delivery. If ARV therapy must be interrupted for <24 hours during the peripartum period, stop then restart all medications simultaneously in order to decrease the chance of developing resistance. Long-term follow-up is recommended for all infants exposed to ARV medications.

Healthcare providers are encouraged to enroll pregnant women exposed to antiretroviral medications in the Antiretroviral Pregnancy Registry (1-800-258-4263 or www.APRegistry.com). Healthcare providers caring for HIV-infected women and their infants may contact the National Perinatal HIV Hotline (888-448-8765) for clinical consultation (DHHS [perinatal], 2012).

RiTUXimab (ri TUK si mab)

Brand Names: U.S. Rituxan®
Brand Names: Canada Rituxan®
Pharmacologic Category Antineoplastic Agent, Monoclonal Antibody; Antirheumatic Miscellaneous; Immunosuppressant Agent; Monoclonal Antibody
Use
Treatment of CD20-positive non-Hodgkin lymphomas (NHL):
Relapsed or refractory, low-grade or follicular B-cell NHL (as a single agent)
Follicular B-cell NHL, previously untreated (in combination with first-line chemotherapy, and as single-agent maintenance therapy if response to first-line rituximab with chemotherapy)
Nonprogressing, low-grade B-cell NHL (as a single agent after first-line CVP treatment)
Diffuse large B-cell NHL, previously untreated (in combination with CHOP chemotherapy [or other anthracycline-based regimen])
Treatment of CD20-positive chronic lymphocytic leukemia (CLL) (in combination with fludarabine and cyclophosphamide)
Treatment of moderately- to severely-active rheumatoid arthritis (in combination with methotrexate) in adult patients with inadequate response to one or more TNF antagonists
Treatment of granulomatosis with polyangiitis (GPA; Wegener's granulomatosis) (in combination with glucocorticoids)
Treatment of microscopic polyangiitis (MPA) (in combination with glucocorticoids)
Unlabeled Use Treatment of Burkitt's lymphoma, central nervous system lymphoma, Hodgkin's lymphoma (lymphocyte predominant); mucosal associated lymphoid tissue (MALT) lymphoma (gastric and nongastric), splenic marginal zone lymphoma; Waldenström's macroglobulinemia (WM); post-transplant lymphoproliferative disorder (PTLD); autoimmune hemolytic anemia

(AIHA) in children; chronic immune thrombocytopenic purpura (ITP); refractory pemphigus vulgaris; treatment of steroid-refractory chronic graft-versus-host disease (GVHD); refractory lupus nephritis; relapsed/refractory thrombotic thrombocytopenic purpura-hemolytic uremic syndrome (TTP-HUS), resistant idiopathic membranous nephropathy (IMN), refractory nephrotic syndrome (children)
Local Anesthetic/Vasoconstrictor Precautions No information available to require special precautions
Effects on Dental Treatment No significant effects or complications reported
Effects on Bleeding Chemotherapy may result in significant myelosuppression, potentially including significant reduction in platelet counts (thrombocytopenia grades 3/4: 2% to 11%) and altered hemostasis. In patients who are under active treatment with these agents, medical consult is suggested.
Adverse Effects Note: Patients treated with rituximab for rheumatoid arthritis (RA) may experience fewer adverse reactions.
>10%:
Cardiovascular: Peripheral edema (8% to 16%), hypertension (6% to 12%)
Central nervous system: Fever (5% to 53%), fatigue (13% to 39%), chills (3% to 33%), headache (17% to 19%), insomnia (≤14%), pain (12%)
Dermatologic: Rash (10% to 17%; grades 3/4: 1%), pruritus (5% to 17%), angioedema (11%; grades 3/4: 1%)
Gastrointestinal: Nausea (8% to 23%), diarrhea (10% to 17%), abdominal pain (2% to 14%), weight gain (11%)
Hematologic: Cytopenias (grades 3/4: ≤48%; may be prolonged), lymphopenia (48%; grades 3/4: 40%; median duration 14 days), anemia (8% to 35%; grades 3/4: 3%), leukopenia (NHL: 14%; grades 3/4: 4%; CLL: grades 3/4: 23%; GPA/MPA: 10%), neutropenia (NHL: 14%; grades 3/4: 4% to 6%; median duration 13 days; CLL: grades 3/4: 30% to 49%), neutropenic fever (CLL: grades 3/4: 9% to 15%), thrombocytopenia (12%; grades 3/4: 2% to 11%)
Hepatic: ALT increased (≤13%)
Neuromuscular & skeletal: Neuropathy (≤30%), weakness (2% to 26%), muscle spasm (≤17%), arthralgia (6% to 13%)
Respiratory: Cough (13%), rhinitis (3% to 12%), epistaxis (≤11%)
Miscellaneous: Infusion-related reactions (lymphoma: first dose 77%; decreases with subsequent infusions; may include angioedema, bronchospasm, chills, dizziness, fever, headache, hyper-/hypotension, myalgia, nausea, pruritus, rash, rigors, urticaria, and vomiting; reactions reported are lower [first infusion: 32%] in RA; CLL: 59%; grades 3/4: 7% to 9%; GPA/MPA: 12%); infection (19% to 62%; grades 3/4: 4%; bacterial: 19%; viral 10%; fungal: 1%; human anti-chimeric antibody (HACA) positive (1% to 23%), night sweats (15%)
1% to 10%:
Cardiovascular: Hypotension (10%; grades 3/4: 2%), flushing (5%)
Central nervous system: Dizziness (10%), anxiety (2% to 5%), migraine (RA: 2%)
Dermatologic: Urticaria (2% to 8%)
Endocrine & metabolic: Hyperglycemia (9%)
Gastrointestinal: Vomiting (10%), dyspepsia (RA: 3%)
Neuromuscular & skeletal: Back pain (10%), myalgia (10%), paresthesia (2%)

Respiratory: Dyspnea (≤10%), throat irritation (2% to 9%), bronchospasm (8%), dyspnea (7%), upper respiratory tract infection (RA: 7%), sinusitis (6%)

Miscellaneous: LDH increased (7%)

General Dosage Range I.V.: *Adults:* Dosage varies greatly depending on indication

Mechanism of Action Rituximab is a monoclonal antibody directed against the CD20 antigen on B-lymphocytes. CD20 regulates cell cycle initiation; and, possibly, functions as a calcium channel. Rituximab binds to the antigen on the cell surface, activating complement-dependent B-cell cytotoxicity; and to human Fc receptors, mediating cell killing through an antibody-dependent cellular toxicity. B-cells are believed to play a role in the development and progression of rheumatoid arthritis. Signs and symptoms of RA are reduced by targeting B-cells and the progression of structural damage is delayed.

Pharmacodynamics/Kinetics

Duration of Action Detectable in serum 3-6 months after completion of treatment; B-cell recovery begins ~6 months following completion of treatment; median B-cell levels return to normal by 12 months following completion of treatment

Half-life Elimination

CLL: Median terminal half-life: 32 days (range: 14-62 days)

NHL: Median terminal half-life: 22 days (range: 6-52 days)

RA: Mean terminal half-life: 18 days (range: 5-78 days)

GPA/MPA: 23 days (range: 9-49 days)

Pregnancy Risk Factor C

Pregnancy Considerations Animal reproduction studies have demonstrated adverse effects including decreased (reversible) B-cells and immunosuppression. IgG molecules are known to cross the placenta (rituximab is an engineered IgG molecule) and rituximab has been detected in the serum of infants exposed in utero. B-Cell lymphocytopenia lasting <6 months may occur in exposed infants. Retrospective case reports of inadvertent pregnancy during rituximab treatment (often combined with concomitant teratogenic therapies) describe premature births, and infant hematologic abnormalities and infections; no specific pattern of birth defects has been observed (limited data). Effective contraception should be used during and for 12 months following treatment. Healthcare providers are encouraged to enroll women with rheumatoid arthritis exposed to rituximab during pregnancy in the OTIS AutoImmune Diseases Study by contacting the Organization of Teratology Information Specialists (877-311-8972).

Rivaroxaban (riv a ROX a ban)

Related Information

Antiplatelet and Anticoagulation Considerations in Dentistry *on page 1503*

Brand Names: U.S. Xarelto®

Brand Names: Canada Xarelto®

Pharmacologic Category Factor Xa Inhibitor

Use Postoperative thromboprophylaxis in patients who have undergone hip or knee replacement surgery; prevention of stroke and systemic embolism in patients with nonvalvular atrial fibrillation; treatment of deep vein thrombosis (DVT) and pulmonary embolism (PE); to reduce the risk of recurrent DVT and/or PE

Canadian labeling: Postoperative thromboprophylaxis in patients who have undergone hip or knee replacement surgery; prevention of stroke and systemic embolism in patients with nonvalvular atrial fibrillation; treatment of DVT without symptomatic PE

Local Anesthetic/Vasoconstrictor Precautions No information available to require special precautions

Effects on Dental Treatment Key adverse event(s) related to dental treatment: Surgical site bleeding may occur. See Effects on Bleeding.

Effects on Bleeding Rivaroxaban inhibits platelet activation and fibrin clot formation via direct, selective, and reversible inhibition of factor Xa. As with all anticoagulants, bleeding is the major adverse effect of rivaroxaban. Hemorrhage may occur at virtually any site; risk is dependent on multiple variables including the intensity of anticoagulation and patient susceptibility. Medical consult is suggested.

Adverse Effects 1% to 10%:

Cardiovascular: Peripheral edema (≤6%)

Central nervous system: Dizziness (≤6%), headache (3% to 5%), pyrexia (1% to 3%), fatigue (≤3%), syncope (≤2%)

Dermatologic: Bruising (3%), pruritus (≤2%), rash (2%), blister (1%)

Gastrointestinal: Diarrhea (≤5%), constipation (≤3%), abdominal pain (≤2%), nausea (1% to 3%), dyspepsia (≤2%), vomiting (≤2%), oropharyngeal pain (≤1%), toothache (≤1%)

Genitourinary: Hematuria (≤4%), urinary tract infection (≤1%)

Hematologic: Bleeding (atrial fibrillation: 21% [major: 6%]; DVT prophylaxis: 5% to 6% [major: <1%]; DVT treatment: 6% to 10% [major: 1%]), thrombocytopenia (<100,000/mm^3 or <50% baseline: 3%), hematoma (≤3%), anemia (1% to 3%)

Local: Wound secretion (≤3%)

Neuromuscular & skeletal: Extremity pain (≤5%), back pain (≤4%), osteoarthritis (≤2%), muscle spasm (1%)

Respiratory: Epistaxis (4% to 10%), hemoptysis (≤1%), sinusitis (≤1%)

General Dosage Range Oral: *Adults:* 10-20 mg/day

Mechanism of Action Inhibits platelet activation and fibrin clot formation via direct, selective and reversible inhibition of factor Xa (FXa) in both the intrinsic and extrinsic coagulation pathways. FXa, as part of the prothrombinase complex consisting also of factor Va, calcium ions, factor II and phospholipid, catalyzes the conversion of prothrombin to thrombin. Thrombin both activates platelets and catalyzes the conversion of fibrinogen to fibrin.

Pharmacodynamics/Kinetics

Half-life Elimination Terminal: 5-9 hours; Elderly: 11-13 hours

Time to Peak Plasma: 2-4 hours

Pregnancy Risk Factor C

Pregnancy Considerations Adverse events were observed in animal reproduction studies. Data are insufficient to evaluate the safety of oral factor Xa inhibitors during pregnancy; use during pregnancy should be avoided (Guyatt, 2012). Use may increase the risk of pregnancy related hemorrhage. Clinicians should note that the anticoagulant effect cannot be easily monitored or readily reversed. Prompt clinical evaluation is warranted with any unexplained decrease in hemoglobin, hematocrit or blood pressure, or fetal distress. Pregnancy planning should be discussed if use is needed in women of reproductive potential. Use during pregnancy is contraindicated in the Canadian labeling.

Dental Comment At this time there are no coagulation parameters for rivaroxaban to predict the extent of bleeding. Increased bleeding may occur during invasive dental procedures in patients taking a 10 mg daily dose of rivaroxaban. Currently, postsurgical treatment with rivaroxaban is ~12 days for knee replacement patients and ~35 days for hip replacement patients. Medical consult is suggested prior to dental invasive procedures. There are no reports of interactions between the anticoagulant and amoxicillin, cephalexin, cefazolin, ampicillin, or clindamycin; therefore, any of these preprocedural antibiotics can safely be used in patients taking rivaroxaban.

Rivastigmine (ri va STIG meen)

Brand Names: U.S. Exelon®
Brand Names: Canada Apo-Rivastigmine®; Exelon®; Mylan-Rivastigmine; Novo-Rivastigmine; PMS-Rivastigmine; ratio-Rivastigmine; Sandoz-Rivastigmine
Pharmacologic Category Acetylcholinesterase Inhibitor (Central)
Use Treatment of mild-to-moderate dementia associated with Alzheimer's disease or Parkinson's disease
Unlabeled Use Severe dementia associated with Alzheimer's disease; Lewy body dementia
Local Anesthetic/Vasoconstrictor Precautions No information available to require special precautions
Effects on Dental Treatment No significant effects or complications reported
Effects on Bleeding No information available to require special precautions
Adverse Effects Note: Many concentration-related effects are reported at a lower frequency by transdermal route.
>10%:
  Central nervous system: Dizziness (1% to 21%), headache (3% to 17%)
  Gastrointestinal: Nausea (5% to 47%), vomiting (5% to 31%), diarrhea (<1% to 19%), anorexia (3% to 17%), abdominal pain (1% to 13%)
1% to 10%:
  Cardiovascular: Syncope (3%), hypertension (3%)
  Central nervous system: Fatigue (1% to 9%), insomnia (1% to 9%), confusion (8%), falling (6% to 8%), depression (4% to 6%), agitation (5%), anxiety (2% to 5%), malaise (5%), somnolence (4% to 5%), hallucinations (4%), aggressiveness (2% to 3%), parkinsonism symptoms worsening (2% to 3%), psychomotor hyperactivity (3%), vertigo (≤2%), paranoia (>1%)
  Dermatologic: Application site reactions (including erythema <1% to 6%)
  Gastrointestinal: Dyspepsia (9%), appetite decreased (3% to 9%), weight loss (3% to 8%), constipation (5%), flatulence (4%), dehydration (2%), eructation (2%)
  Genitourinary: Urinary tract infection (1% to 7%), urinary incontinence (2% to 3%)
  Neuromuscular & skeletal: Weakness (2% to 6%), tremor (1%; up to 10% in Parkinson's patients), back pain (>1%)
  Respiratory: Rhinitis (4%)
  Miscellaneous: Accidental trauma (10%), diaphoresis (4%), flu-like syndrome (3%)
General Dosage Range
  Oral: *Adults:* Initial: 1.5 mg twice daily; Maintenance: 1.5-6 mg twice daily (maximum: 12 mg daily)

Transdermal patch: *Adults:* Initial: 4.6 mg/24 hours; Maintenance: (9.5-13.3) mg/24 hours (maximum dose: 13.3 mg/24 hours)
Mechanism of Action A deficiency of cortical acetylcholine is thought to account for some of the symptoms of Alzheimer's disease and the dementia of Parkinson's disease; rivastigmine increases acetylcholine in the central nervous system through reversible inhibition of its hydrolysis by cholinesterase
Pharmacodynamics/Kinetics
  Duration of Action Anticholinesterase activity (CSF): ~10 hours (6 mg oral dose)
  Half-life Elimination Oral: 1.5 hours; Transdermal patch: 3 hours (after removal)
  Time to Peak Oral: 1 hour; Transdermal patch: 8-16 hours following first dose
Pregnancy Risk Factor B
Pregnancy Considerations Adverse events were observed in some animal reproduction studies. Use in women of reproductive age is not recommended.

Rizatriptan (rye za TRIP tan)

Related Information
  Temporomandibular Dysfunction (TMD), Chronic Pain, and Fibromyalgia *on page 1590*
Brand Names: U.S. Maxalt-MLT®; Maxalt®
Brand Names: Canada Apo-Rizatriptan®; CO Rizatriptan; CO Rizatriptan ODT; JAMP-Rizatriptan; Mar-Rizatriptan; Maxalt RPD™; Maxalt™; Mylan-Rizatriptan ODT; Sandoz-Rizatriptan ODT
Generic Availability (U.S.) Yes
Pharmacologic Category Antimigraine Agent; Serotonin 5-HT$_{1B, 1D}$ Receptor Agonist
Use Acute treatment of migraine with or without aura
Local Anesthetic/Vasoconstrictor Precautions No information available to require special precautions
Effects on Dental Treatment Key adverse event(s) related to dental treatment: Xerostomia (normal salivary flow resumes upon discontinuation).
Effects on Bleeding No information available to require special precautions
Adverse Effects 1% to 10%:
  Cardiovascular: Chest pain (<2% to 3%), flushing (>1%), palpitation (>1%)
  Central nervous system: Dizziness (4% to 9%), somnolence (4% to 8%), fatigue (adults 4% to 7%; children >1%), pain (3%), headache (≤2%), euphoria (>1%), hypoesthesia (>1%)
  Dermatologic: Skin flushing
  Gastrointestinal: Nausea (4% to 6%), xerostomia (3%), abdominal discomfort (children >1%), diarrhea (>1%), vomiting (>1%)
  Neuromuscular & skeletal: Weakness (4% to 7%), paresthesia (3% to 4%); neck, throat, and jaw pain/tightness/pressure (≤2%), tremor (>1%)
  Respiratory: Dyspnea (>1%)
  Miscellaneous: Feeling of heaviness (<1% to 2%)
Dosage Note: In patients with risk factors for coronary artery disease, following adequate evaluation to establish the absence of coronary artery disease, the initial dose should be administered in a setting where response may be evaluated (physician's office or similarly staffed setting). ECG monitoring may be considered.
  Children 6-17 years: Oral: **Note:** Safety and efficacy of multiple rizatriptan doses in a 24-hour period have not been established for pediatric patients.
    <40 kg: 5 mg as a single dose

≥40 kg: 10 mg as a single dose

Dose adjustment with concomitant propranolol therapy:
<40 kg: Use not recommended
≥40 kg: 5 mg as a single dose (maximum: 5 mg/24 hours)

Adults: Oral: 5-10 mg, repeat after 2 hours if significant relief is not attained; maximum: 30 mg/24 hours

Dose adjustment with concomitant propranolol therapy: 5 mg/dose (maximum: 15 mg/24 hours)

Dosage adjustment in renal impairment: No dosage adjustment provided in manufacturer's labeling; however, the AUC was 44% greater in patients on hemodialysis.

Dosage adjustment in hepatic impairment: No dosage adjustment provided in manufacturer's labeling; however, plasma concentrations are increased by 30% in patients with moderate hepatic dysfunction.

Mechanism of Action Selective agonist for serotonin ($5-HT_{1B}$ and $5-HT_{1D}$ receptors) in cranial arteries; causes vasoconstriction and reduces sterile inflammation associated with antidromic neuronal transmission correlating with relief of migraine

Contraindications Hypersensitivity to rizatriptan or any component of the formulation; documented ischemic heart disease or other significant cardiovascular disease; coronary artery vasospasm (including Prinzmetal's angina); history of stroke or transient ischemic attack; peripheral vascular disease; ischemic bowel disease; uncontrolled hypertension; basilar or hemiplegic migraine; during or within 2 weeks of MAO inhibitors; during or within 24 hours of treatment with another $5-HT_1$ agonist, or an ergot-containing or ergot-type medication (eg, methysergide, dihydroergotamine)

Warnings/Precautions Only indicated for treatment of acute migraine; not for the prevention of migraines or the treatment of cluster headache. If a patient does not respond to the first dose, the diagnosis of migraine should be reconsidered. Coronary artery vasospasm, transient ischemia, myocardial infarction, ventricular tachycardia/fibrillation, cardiac arrest, and death have been reported with $5-HT_1$ agonist administration. Patients who experience sensations of chest pain/pressure/tightness or symptoms suggestive of angina following dosing should be evaluated for coronary artery disease or Prinzmetal's angina before receiving additional doses; if dosing is resumed and similar symptoms recur, monitor with ECG. Should not be given to patients who have risk factors for CAD (eg, hypertension, hypercholesterolemia, smoker, obesity, diabetes, strong family history of CAD, menopause, male >40 years of age) without adequate cardiac evaluation. Patients with suspected CAD should have cardiovascular evaluation to rule out CAD before considering use; if cardiovascular evaluation is "satisfactory," first dose should be given in the healthcare provider's office (consider ECG monitoring). Periodic evaluation of cardiovascular status should be done in all patients. Significant elevation in blood pressure, including hypertensive crisis, has also been reported on rare occasions in patients with and without a history of hypertension. Cerebral/subarachnoid hemorrhage, stroke, peripheral vascular ischemia, gastrointestinal ischemia/infarction, splenic infarction and Raynaud's syndrome have been reported with $5-HT_1$ agonist administration. Use is contraindicated in patients with a history of stroke or transient ischemic attack. Rarely, partial vision loss and blindness (transient and permanent) have been reported with $5-HT_1$ agonists.

Use with caution in elderly or patients with hepatic or renal impairment (including dialysis patients). Symptoms of agitation, confusion, hallucinations, hyperreflexia, myoclonus, shivering, and tachycardia may occur with concomitant proserotonergic drugs (eg, SSRIs/SNRIs or triptans) or agents which reduce rizatriptan's metabolism. Concurrent use of serotonin precursors (eg, tryptophan) is not recommended. If concomitant administration with SSRIs is warranted, monitor closely, especially at initiation and with dose increases. Overuse of medications for acute migraine, including $5-HT_1$ agonists, may lead to headache exacerbation. Maxalt-MLT® tablets contain phenylalanine.

Drug Interactions

Metabolism/Transport Effects None known.

Avoid Concomitant Use

Avoid concomitant use of Rizatriptan with any of the following: Ergot Derivatives; MAO Inhibitors

Increased Effect/Toxicity

Rizatriptan may increase the levels/effects of: Ergot Derivatives; Metoclopramide; Serotonin Modulators

The levels/effects of Rizatriptan may be increased by: Antipsychotics; Ergot Derivatives; MAO Inhibitors; Propranolol

Decreased Effect There are no known significant interactions involving a decrease in effect.

Ethanol/Nutrition/Herb Interactions Food: Food delays absorption.

Dietary Considerations Some products may contain phenylalanine.

Pharmacodynamics/Kinetics

Onset of Action Most patients have response to treatment within 2 hours

Half-life Elimination 2-3 hours

Time to Peak Maxalt®: 1-1.5 hours (delayed up to 0.7 hour with Maxalt-MLT®)

Pregnancy Risk Factor C

Pregnancy Considerations A pregnancy registry has been established to monitor outcomes of women exposed to rizatriptan during pregnancy (800-986-8999). Preliminary data from the pregnancy registry does not show an increased risk of congenital malformations (Fiore, 2005). In some animal studies, administration was associated with decreased weight gain, developmental toxicity and increased mortality in the offspring. Teratogenic effects were not observed.

Lactation Excretion in breast milk unknown/use caution

Dosage Forms

Tablet, oral: 5 mg, 10 mg
Maxalt®: 5 mg, 10 mg
Tablet, orally disintegrating, oral: 5 mg, 10 mg
Maxalt-MLT®: 5 mg, 10 mg

Roflumilast (roe FLUE mi last)

Brand Names: U.S. Daliresp®
Brand Names: Canada Daxas™
Pharmacologic Category Phosphodiesterase-4 Enzyme Inhibitor
Use Adjunct to bronchodilator therapy in the maintenance treatment of severe chronic obstructive pulmonary disease (COPD) associated with chronic bronchitis
Local Anesthetic/Vasoconstrictor Precautions No information available to require special precautions
Effects on Dental Treatment No significant effects or complications reported
Effects on Bleeding No information available to require special precautions

Adverse Effects

2% to 10%:

Central nervous system: Headache (4%), dizziness (2%), insomnia (2%)

Gastrointestinal: Diarrhea (10%), weight loss (8%; 7%: >10% loss), nausea (5%), appetite decreased (2%)

Neuromuscular & skeletal: Back pain (3%)

Miscellaneous: Influenza (3%)

General Dosage Range Oral: *Adults:* 500 mcg once daily

Mechanism of Action Roflumilast and its active N-oxide metabolite selectively inhibit phosphodiesterase-4 (PDE4) leading to an accumulation of cyclic AMP (cAMP) within inflammatory and structural cells important in the pathogenesis of COPD. Anti-inflammatory effects include suppression of cytokine release and inhibition of lung infiltration by neutrophils and other leukocytes. Pulmonary remodeling and mucociliary malfunction are also attenuated.

Pharmacodynamics/Kinetics

Half-life Elimination 17 hours; N-oxide metabolite: 30 hours

Time to Peak ~1 hour (delayed by food); N-oxide metabolite: ~8 hours

Pregnancy Risk Factor C

Pregnancy Considerations Animal studies have demonstrated reproductive toxicity (incomplete ossification, post-implantive losses) at doses greater than the human recommended dose. There are no adequate and well controlled studies in pregnant women. Avoid use during pregnancy.

RomiDEPsin (roe mi DEP sin)

Related Information

Clinical Risk Related to Drugs Prolonging QT Interval *on page 1510*

Brand Names: U.S. Istodax®

Pharmacologic Category Antineoplastic Agent, Histone Deacetylase Inhibitor

Use Treatment of refractory cutaneous T-cell lymphoma (CTCL) and refractory peripheral T-cell lymphoma (PTCL)

Local Anesthetic/Vasoconstrictor Precautions Romidepsin is one of the drugs confirmed to prolong the QT interval and is accepted as having a risk of causing torsade de pointes. The risk of drug-induced torsade de pointes is extremely low when a single QT interval prolonging drug is prescribed. In terms of epinephrine, it is not known what effect vasoconstrictors in the local anesthetic regimen will have in patients with a known history of congenital prolonged QT interval or in patients taking any medication that prolongs the QT interval. Until more information is obtained, it is suggested that the clinician consult with the physician prior to the use of a vasoconstrictor in suspected patients, and that the vasoconstrictor (epinephrine, mepivacaine and levonordefrin [Carbocaine® 2% with Neo-Cobefrin®]) be used with caution.

Effects on Dental Treatment Key adverse event(s) related to dental treatment: Taste alteration.

Effects on Bleeding Chemotherapy may result in significant myelosuppression, potentially including significant reduction in platelet counts (thrombocytopenia grades 3/4: ≤36%) and altered hemostasis. In patients who are under active treatment with these agents, medical consult is suggested.

Adverse Effects

>10%:

Cardiovascular: ST-T wave changes (2% to 63%), hypotension (7% to 23%)

Central nervous system: Fatigue (53% to 77%), fever (20% to 47%), headache (15% to 34%), chills (11% to 17%)

Dermatologic: Pruritus (7% to 31%), dermatitis/exfoliative dermatitis (4% to 27%)

Endocrine & metabolic: Hypocalcemia (4% to 52%), hyperglycemia (2% to 51%), hypoalbuminemia (3% to 48%), hyperuricemia (≤33%), hypomagnesemia (22% to 28%), hypermagnesemia (≤27%), hypophosphatemia (≤27%), hypokalemia (6% to 20%), hyponatremia (≤20%)

Gastrointestinal: Nausea (56% to 86%; grades 3/4: 2% to 6%), anorexia (23% to 54%), vomiting (34% to 52%; grades 3/4: ≤10%), taste alteration (15% to 40%), constipation (12% to 40%), diarrhea (20% to 36%), weight loss (10% to 15%), abdominal pain (13% to 14%)

Hematologic: Anemia (19% to 72%; grades 3/4: 3% to 28%), thrombocytopenia (17% to 72%; grades 3/4: ≤36%), neutropenia (11% to 66%; grades 3/4: 4% to 47%), lymphopenia (4% to 57%; grades 3/4: ≤37%), leukopenia (4% to 55%; grades 3/4: ≤45%)

Hepatic: AST increased (3% to 28%), ALT increased (3% to 22%)

Neuromuscular & skeletal: Weakness (53% to 77%)

Respiratory: Cough (18% to 21%), dyspnea (13% to 21%)

Miscellaneous: Infection (46% to 54%; grades 3/4: 11% to 33%)

1% to 10%:

Cardiovascular: Peripheral edema (6% to 10%), tachycardia (≤10%), chest pain, DVT, edema, QT prolongation, supraventricular arrhythmia, syncope, ventricular arrhythmia

Dermatologic: Cellulitis

Endocrine & metabolic: Dehydration

Gastrointestinal: Stomatitis (6% to 10%)

Hematologic: Neutropenic fever

Hepatic: Hyperbilirubinemia

Respiratory: Hypoxia, pneumonia, pneumonitis, pulmonary embolism

Miscellaneous: Central line infection, hypersensitivity, sepsis, tumor lysis syndrome (1% to 2%)

General Dosage Range Dosage adjustment recommended in patients who develop toxicities

I.V.: *Adults:* 14 mg/m^2 days 1, 8, and 15 of a 28-day treatment cycle

Mechanism of Action Histone deacetylase inhibitor; catalyzes acetyl group removal from protein lysine residues (including histone and transcription factors). Inhibition of histone deacetylase results in accumulation of acetyl groups, leading to alterations in chromatin structure and transcription factor activation causing termination of cell growth (induces arrest in cell cycle at G_1 and G_2/M phases) leading to cell death.

Pharmacodynamics/Kinetics

Half-life Elimination ~3 hours

Pregnancy Risk Factor D

Pregnancy Considerations Adverse events were observed in animal reproduction studies. Based on the mechanism of action, romidepsin may cause fetal harm if administered during pregnancy.

◀ **Dental Comment** Romidepsin is known to prolong the QT interval. The QT interval is measured as the time and distance between the Q point of the QRS complex and the end of the T wave in the ECG tracing. After adjustment for heart rate, the QT interval is defined as prolonged if it is more than 450 msec in men and 460 msec in women. A long QT syndrome was first described in the 1950s and 60s as a congenital syndrome involving QT interval prolongation and syncope and sudden death. Some of the congenital long QT syndromes were characterized by a peculiar electrocardiographic appearance of the QRS complex involving a premature atria beat followed by a pause, then a subsequent sinus beat showing marked QT prolongation and deformity. This type of cardiac arrhythmia was originally termed "torsade de pointes" (translated from the French as "twisting of the points"). Romidepsin is considered as having a risk of causing torsade de pointes. Since it is not known what effect vasoconstrictors in the local anesthetic regimen will have in patients with a known history of congenital prolonged QT interval or in patients taking any medication that prolongs the QT interval, a medical consult is suggested.

RomiPLOStim (roe mi PLOE stim)

Brand Names: U.S. Nplate®
Brand Names: Canada Nplate®
Pharmacologic Category Colony Stimulating Factor; Thrombopoietic Agent
Use Treatment of thrombocytopenia in patients with chronic immune (idiopathic) thrombocytopenia purpura (ITP) who have had insufficient response to corticosteroids, immune globulin, or splenectomy

Note: Should be used only when the degree of thrombocytopenia and clinical condition increase the risk for bleeding; should not be used in attempt to normalize platelet counts; **not** indicated for the treatment of thrombocytopenia due to myelodysplastic syndrome or any cause of thrombocytopenia other than chronic ITP.

Local Anesthetic/Vasoconstrictor Precautions No information available to require special precautions
Effects on Dental Treatment No significant effects or complications reported
Effects on Bleeding Romiplostim is used for treatment of thrombocytopenia; dosing is established to increase platelet counts and reduce the risk of bleeding. Bleeding is not expected with therapy; however, upon discontinuation of therapy, rebound thrombocytopenia may occur and risk of bleeding is increased; monitor closely.
Adverse Effects
>10%:
  Central nervous system: Headache (35%), dizziness (17%), insomnia (16%)
  Gastrointestinal: Abdominal pain (11%)
  Hematologic: Circulating myeloblasts increased (MDS patients: 17%)
  Neuromuscular & skeletal: Arthralgia (26%), myalgia (14%), limb pain (13%)
1% to 10%:
  Gastrointestinal: Dyspepsia (7%)
  Hematologic: Rebound thrombocytopenia (7%), AML (MDS patients: 4% to 6%), bone marrow reticulin formation/deposition (4%)
  Neuromuscular & skeletal: Shoulder pain (8%), paresthesia (6%)
  Miscellaneous: Antibody formation (romiplostim 6%; TPO 4%)

General Dosage Range SubQ: *Adults:* Initial: 1 mcg/kg once weekly; adjust dose by 1 mcg/kg/week increments to achieve platelet count ≥50,000/mm³ and reduce the risk of bleeding; Maximum: 10 mcg/kg/week
Mechanism of Action Thrombopoietin (TPO) peptide mimetic which increases platelet counts in ITP by binding to and activating the human TPO receptor.
Pharmacodynamics/Kinetics
  Onset of Action Platelet count increase: SubQ: 4-9 days; Peak platelet count increase: Days 12-16
  Duration of Action Platelet counts return to baseline by day 28
  Half-life Elimination Median: 3.5 days (range: 1-34 days)
  Time to Peak SubQ: Median: 14 hours (range: 7-50 hours)
Pregnancy Risk Factor C
Pregnancy Considerations Adverse effects were observed in animal reproduction studies. Use during pregnancy only if the potential benefit to the mother outweighs the potential risk to the fetus. The Nplate® pregnancy registry has been established to monitor outcomes of women exposed to romiplostim during pregnancy (1-800-772-6436).

ROPINIRole (roe PIN i role)

Brand Names: U.S. Requip®; Requip® XL™
Brand Names: Canada CO Ropinirole; JAMP-Ropinirole; PMS-Ropinirole; RAN™-Ropinirole; Requip®
Pharmacologic Category Anti-Parkinson's Agent, Dopamine Agonist
Use Treatment of idiopathic Parkinson's disease; in patients with early Parkinson's disease who were not receiving concomitant levodopa therapy as well as in patients with advanced disease on concomitant levodopa; treatment of moderate-to-severe primary Restless Legs Syndrome (RLS)
Local Anesthetic/Vasoconstrictor Precautions No information available to require special precautions
Effects on Dental Treatment Key adverse event(s) related to dental treatment: Xerostomia and increased salivation (normal salivary flow resumes upon discontinuation) and dysphagia.
Effects on Bleeding No information available to require special precautions
Adverse Effects
  Data inclusive of trials in early Parkinson's disease (without levodopa) and Restless Legs Syndrome:
  >10%:
    Cardiovascular: Syncope (1% to 12%)
    Central nervous system: Somnolence (11% to 40%), dizziness (6% to 40%), fatigue (8% to 11%)
    Gastrointestinal: Nausea (immediate release: 40% to 60%; extended release: 19%), vomiting (11% to 12%)
    Miscellaneous: Viral infection (11%)
  1% to 10%:
    Cardiovascular: Dependent/leg edema (2% to 7%), orthostasis (1% to 6%), hypertension (5%), chest pain (4%), flushing (3%), palpitation (3%), peripheral ischemia (2% to 3%), atrial fibrillation (2%), extrasystoles (2%), hypotension (2%), tachycardia (2%)
    Central nervous system: Pain (3% to 8%), headache (extended release: 6%), confusion (5%), hallucinations (up to 5%; dose related), hypoesthesia (4%), amnesia (3%), malaise (3%), yawning (3%), concentration impaired (2%), vertigo (2%)
    Dermatologic: Hyperhidrosis (3%)

Gastrointestinal: Dyspepsia (4% to 10%), abdominal pain (3% to 7%), constipation (≥5%), xerostomia (3% to 5%), diarrhea (5%), anorexia (4%), flatulence (3%)

Genitourinary: Urinary tract infection (5%), impotence (3%)

Hepatic: Alkaline phosphatase increased (3%)

Neuromuscular & skeletal: Weakness (6%), arthralgia (4%), muscle cramps (3%), paresthesia (3%), hyperkinesia (2%)

Ocular: Abnormal vision (6%), xerophthalmia (2%)

Respiratory: Pharyngitis (6% to 9%), rhinitis (4%), sinusitis (4%), bronchitis (3%), dyspnea (3%), influenza (3%), cough (3%), nasal congestion (2%)

Miscellaneous: Diaphoresis increased (3% to 6%)

Advanced Parkinson's disease (with levodopa):
>10%:

Central nervous system: Dizziness (immediate release: 26%; extended-release: 8%), somnolence (immediate release: 20%, extended release: 7%), headache (17%)

Gastrointestinal: Nausea (immediate release: 30%; extended-release: 11%)

Neuromuscular & skeletal: Dyskinesias (immediate release: 34%; extended-release: 13%; dose related)

1% to 10%:

Cardiovascular: Hypotension (2% to 5%; including orthostatic), peripheral edema (4%), syncope (3%), hypertension (3%; dose related)

Central nervous system: Hallucinations (7% to 10%; dose related), confusion (9%), anxiety (2% to 6%), amnesia (5%), nervousness (5%), pain (5%), vertigo (4%), abnormal dreaming (3%), paresis (3%), aggravated parkinsonism, insomnia

Gastrointestinal: Abdominal pain (6% to 9%), vomiting (7%), constipation (4% to 6%), diarrhea (3% to 5%), xerostomia (2% to 5%), dysphagia (2%), flatulence (2%), salivation increased (2%), weight loss (2%)

Genitourinary: Urinary tract infection (6%), pyuria (2%), urinary incontinence (2%)

Hematologic: Anemia (2%)

Neuromuscular & skeletal: Falls (2% to 10%; dose related), arthralgia (7%), tremor (6%), hypokinesia (5%), paresthesia (5%), arthritis (3%), back pain (3%)

Ocular: Diplopia (2%)

Respiratory: Upper respiratory tract infection (9%), dyspnea (3%)

Miscellaneous: Injury, diaphoresis increased (7%), viral infection, increased drug level (7%)

Other adverse effects (all phase 2/3 trials for Parkinson's disease and Restless Leg Syndrome): ≥1%: Asthma, BUN increased, depression, gastroenteritis, gastrointestinal reflux, irritability, migraine, muscle spasm, myalgia, neck pain, neuralgia, osteoarthritis, pharyngolaryngeal pain, rash, rigors, sleep disorder, tendonitis

General Dosage Range Oral: *Adults:*

Parkinson's:

Immediate release: Initial: 0.25 mg 3 times/day; Maintenance: 0.75-24 mg/day in 3 divided doses

Extended release: Initial: 2 mg once daily; Maintenance: 2-24 mg once daily (maximum: 24 mg/day)

Restless legs: Immediate release: Initial: 0.25 mg prior to bedtime; Maintenance: 0.25-4 mg prior to bedtime

Mechanism of Action Ropinirole has a high relative *in vitro* specificity and full intrinsic activity at the D_2 and D_3 dopamine receptor subtypes, binding with higher affinity to D_3 than to D_2 or D_4 receptor subtypes; relevance of D_3 receptor binding in Parkinson's disease is unknown. Ropinirole has moderate *in vitro* affinity for opioid receptors. Ropinirole and its metabolites have negligible *in vitro* affinity for dopamine D_1, 5-HT$_1$, 5-HT$_2$, benzodiazepine, GABA, muscarinic, alpha$_1$-, alpha$_2$-, and beta-adrenoreceptors. Although precise mechanism of action of ropinirole is unknown, it is believed to be due to stimulation of postsynaptic dopamine D_2-type receptors within the caudate putamen in the brain. Ropinirole caused decreases in systolic and diastolic blood pressure at doses >0.25 mg. The mechanism of ropinirole-induced postural hypotension is believed to be due to D_2-mediated blunting of the noradrenergic response to standing and subsequent decrease in peripheral vascular resistance.

Pharmacodynamics/Kinetics

Half-life Elimination ~6 hours

Time to Peak Immediate release: ~1-2 hours; Extended release: 6-10 hours; T_{max} increased by 2.5-3 hours when drug taken with food

Pregnancy Risk Factor C

Pregnancy Considerations Teratogenic effects have been observed in animal studies. There are no adequate and well-controlled studies in pregnant women; use only if potential benefit outweighs the risk to the fetus.

Ropivacaine (roe PIV a kane)

Related Information

Oral Pain *on page 1558*

Brand Names: U.S. Naropin®

Brand Names: Canada Naropin®

Pharmacologic Category Local Anesthetic

Use Local anesthetic for use in surgery, postoperative pain management, and obstetrical procedures when local or regional anesthesia is needed

Local Anesthetic/Vasoconstrictor Precautions No information available to require special precautions (see Dental Comment)

Effects on Dental Treatment No significant effects or complications reported

Effects on Bleeding No information available to require special precautions

Adverse Effects

>10%:

Cardiovascular: Hypotension (dose-related and age-related: 32% to 69%), bradycardia (6% to 20%)

Gastrointestinal: Nausea (11% to 29%), vomiting (7% to 14%)

Neuromuscular & skeletal: Back pain (7% to 16%)

1% to 10%:

Cardiovascular: Hypertension, tachycardia, chest pain (1% to 5%)

Central nervous system: Fever (3% to 9%), headache (5% to 8%), dizziness (3%), chills (2% to 3%), anxiety (1%), lightheadedness

Dermatologic: Pruritus (1% to 5%)

Endocrine & metabolic: Hypokalemia

Genitourinary: Urinary retention (1% to 5%), urinary tract infection (1% to 5%)

Hematologic: Anemia (6%)

Neuromuscular & skeletal: Paresthesia (2% to 6%), hypoesthesia, rigors, circumoral paresthesia

Renal: Oliguria

Respiratory: Dyspnea

Miscellaneous: Shivering

General Dosage Range

Epidural:

Lumbar: Adults: 10-30 mL of 0.2% to 1% solution **or** 15-20 mL of 0.75% solution; Infusion: 6-14 mL/hour of 0.2% solution, with incremental injections of 10-15 mL/hour of 0.2% solution

Thoracic: Adults: 5-15 mL of 0.5% or 0.75% solution; Infusion: 6-14 mL/hour of 0.2% solution

Field Block: *Adults:* 1-40 mL (5-200 mg) of 0.5% solution

Infiltration: *Adults:* 1-100 mL of 0.2% solution **or** 1-40 mL of 0.5% solution

Nerve Block: *Adults:* Major: 35-50 mL (175-250 mg) of 0.5 % solution **or** 10-40 mL (75-300 mg) of 0.75% solution; Minor: 1-100 mL of 0.2% solution **or** 1-40 mL of 0.5% solution

Mechanism of Action Blocks both the initiation and conduction of nerve impulses by decreasing the neuronal membrane's permeability to sodium ions, which results in inhibition of depolarization with resultant blockade of conduction

Pharmacodynamics/Kinetics

Onset of Action Anesthesia (route dependent): 3-15 minutes

Duration of Action Dose and route dependent: 3-15 hours

Half-life Elimination Epidural: 5-7 hours; I.V.: Terminal: 111 ± 62 minutes (Lee, 1989)

Pregnancy Risk Factor B

Pregnancy Considerations Teratogenic events were not observed in animal studies. When used for epidural block during labor and delivery, systemically absorbed ropivacaine may cross the placenta, resulting in varying degrees of fetal or neonatal effects (eg, CNS or cardiovascular depression). Fetal or neonatal adverse events include fetal bradycardia (12%), neonatal jaundice (8%), low Apgar scores (3%), fetal distress (2%), neonatal respiratory disorder (3%). Maternal hypotension may also result from systemic absorption. In cases of hypotension, position pregnant woman in left lateral decubitus position to prevent aortocaval compression by the gravid uterus. Epidural anesthesia may prolong the second stage of labor.

Dental Comment Not available with vasoconstrictor (epinephrine) and not available in dental (1.8 mL) carpules

---

Rosiglitazone (roh si GLI ta zone)

Related Information

Endocrine Disorders and Pregnancy *on page 1517*

Brand Names: U.S. Avandia®

Brand Names: Canada Avandia®

Generic Availability (U.S.) No

Pharmacologic Category Antidiabetic Agent, Thiazolidinedione

Use Type 2 diabetes mellitus (noninsulin dependent, NIDDM):

Monotherapy: Improve glycemic control as an adjunct to diet and exercise

Note: Canadian labeling approves use as monotherapy only when metformin is contraindicated or not tolerated.

Combination therapy: **Note:** Use when diet, exercise, and a single agent do not result in adequate glycemic control.

U.S. labeling: In combination with a sulfonylurea, metformin, or sulfonylurea plus metformin

Canadian labeling: In combination with metformin; in combination with a sulfonylurea only when metformin use is contraindicated or not tolerated

Local Anesthetic/Vasoconstrictor Precautions No information available to require special precautions

Effects on Dental Treatment Rosiglitazone-dependent patients with diabetes should be appointed for dental treatment in morning in order to minimize chance of stress-induced hypoglycemia.

Effects on Bleeding Rosiglitazone has been demonstrated to induce severe thrombocytopenia (rare). Analysis of the patient's serum shows rosiglitazone-induced antibody, responsible for thrombocytopenia, confirming an immune-mediated platelet depletion.

Adverse Effects Note: The rate of certain adverse reactions (eg, anemia, edema, hypoglycemia) may be higher with some combination therapies.

>10%: Endocrine & metabolic: HDL-cholesterol increased, LDL-cholesterol increased, total cholesterol increased, weight gain

1% to 10%:

Cardiovascular: Edema (5%), hypertension (4%); heart failure/CHF (up to 2% to 3% in patients receiving insulin; incidence likely higher in patients with pre-existing HF; myocardial ischemia (3%; incidence likely higher in patients with preexisting CAD)

Central nervous system: Headache (6%)

Endocrine & metabolic: Hypoglycemia (1% to 3%; combination therapy with insulin: 12% to 14%)

Gastrointestinal: Diarrhea (3%)

Hematologic: Anemia (2%)

Neuromuscular & skeletal: Fractures (up to 9%; incidence greater in females; usually upper arm, hand, or foot), arthralgia (5%), back pain (4% to 5%)

Respiratory: Upper respiratory tract infection (4% to 10%), nasopharyngitis (6%)

Miscellaneous: Injury (8%)

Dosage Oral:

Adults: **Note:** All patients should be initiated at the lowest recommended dose.

Monotherapy: Initial: 4 mg daily as a single daily dose or in divided doses twice daily. If response is inadequate after 8-12 weeks of treatment, the dosage may be increased to 8 mg daily as a single daily dose or in divided doses twice daily. In clinical trials, the 4 mg twice-daily regimen resulted in the greatest reduction in fasting plasma glucose and Hb A_{1c}.

Combination therapy: When adding rosiglitazone to existing therapy, continue current dose(s) of previous agents:

U.S. labeling: With sulfonylureas or metformin (or sulfonylurea plus metformin): Initial: 4 mg daily as a single daily dose or in divided doses twice daily. If response is inadequate after 8-12 weeks of treatment, the dosage may be increased to 8 mg daily as a single daily dose or in divided doses twice daily. Reduce dose of sulfonylurea if hypoglycemia occurs. It is unlikely that the dose of metformin will need to be reduced due to hypoglycemia.

Canadian labeling:

With metformin: Initial: 4 mg daily as a single daily dose or in divided doses twice daily. If response is inadequate after 8-12 weeks of treatment, the dosage may be increased to 8 mg daily as a single daily dose or in divided doses twice daily.

With a sulfonylurea: 4 mg daily as a single daily dose or in divided doses twice daily. Dose should not exceed 4 mg daily when using in combination with a sulfonylurea. Reduce dose of sulfonylurea if hypoglycemia occurs.

Elderly: No dosage adjustment is recommended

Dosage adjustment in renal impairment: No dosage adjustment is required

Dosage comment in hepatic impairment: Clearance is significantly lower in hepatic impairment. Therapy should not be initiated if the patient exhibits active liver disease or increased transaminases (ALT >2.5 times the upper limit of normal) at baseline.

Mechanism of Action Thiazolidinedione antidiabetic agent that lowers blood glucose by improving target cell response to insulin, without increasing pancreatic insulin secretion. It has a mechanism of action that is dependent on the presence of insulin for activity. Rosiglitazone is an agonist for peroxisome proliferator-activated receptor-gamma (PPARgamma). Activation of nuclear PPARgamma receptors influences the production of a number of gene products involved in glucose and lipid metabolism. PPARgamma is abundant in the cells within the renal collecting tubules; fluid retention results from stimulation by thiazolidinediones which increases sodium reabsorption.

Contraindications NYHA Class III/IV heart failure (initiation of therapy)

Canadian labeling: Hypersensitivity to rosiglitazone or any component of the formulation; any stage of heart failure (eg, NYHA Class I, II, III, IV); serious hepatic impairment; pregnancy

Warnings/Precautions [U.S. Boxed Warning]: Thiazolidinediones, including rosiglitazone, may cause or exacerbate congestive heart failure; closely monitor for signs/symptoms of congestive heart failure (eg, rapid weight gain, dyspnea, edema), particularly after initiation or dose increases. Not recommended for use in any patient with symptomatic heart failure. In the U.S., initiation of therapy is contraindicated in patients with NYHA class III or IV heart failure; in Canada use is contraindicated in patients with any stage of heart failure (NYHA Class I, II, III, IV). Use with caution in patients with edema; may increase plasma volume and/or cause fluid retention, leading to heart failure. Dose-related weight gain observed with use; mechanism unknown but likely associated with fluid retention and fat accumulation. Use may also be associated with an increased risk of angina and MI. Use caution in patients at risk for cardiovascular events and monitor closely. Discontinue if any deterioration in cardiac status occurs.

[U.S. Boxed Warning]: Due to cardiovascular risks, rosiglitazone-containing medications are only available through the Avandia-Rosiglitazone Medicines Access Program™. Patients and prescribers must be registered with and meet conditions of the program. Call 1-800-282-6342 or visit www.avandia.com for more information.

Should not be used in diabetic ketoacidosis. Mechanism requires the presence of insulin; therefore, use in type 1 diabetes (insulin dependent, IDDM) is not recommended. Combination therapy with other hypoglycemic agents may increase risk for hypoglycemic events; dose reduction with the concomitant agent may be warranted. Concomitant use with nitrates is not recommended due to increased risk of myocardial ischemia. Avoid use with insulin due to an increased risk of edema, congestive

heart failure, and myocardial ischemic events. Do not initiate in patients with stable ischemic heart disease due to an increased risk of cardiovascular complications (Fihn, 2012).

Use with caution in patients with elevated transaminases (AST or ALT); do not initiate in patients with active liver disease or ALT >2.5 times ULN at baseline; evaluate patients with ALT ≤2.5 times ULN at baseline or during therapy for cause of enzyme elevation; during therapy, if ALT >3 times ULN, reevaluate levels promptly and discontinue if elevation persists or if jaundice occurs at any time during use. Idiosyncratic hepatotoxicity has been reported with another thiazolidinedione agent (troglitazone); avoid use in patients who previously experienced jaundice during troglitazone therapy. Monitoring should include periodic determinations of liver function. Increased incidence of bone fractures in females treated with rosiglitazone observed during analysis of long-term trial; majority of fractures occurred in the upper arm, hand, and foot (differing from the hip or spine fractures usually associated with postmenopausal osteoporosis). May decrease hemoglobin/hematocrit and/or WBC count (slight); effects may be related to increased plasma volume and/or dose related; use with caution in patients with anemia.

Rosiglitazone has been associated with new onset and/or worsening of macular edema in patients with diabetes. Rosiglitazone should be used with caution in patients with a pre-existing macular edema or diabetic retinopathy. Discontinuation of rosiglitazone should be considered in any patient who reports visual deterioration. In addition, ophthalmological consultation should be initiated in these patients. Use with caution in premenopausal, anovulatory women; may result in resumption of ovulation, increasing the risk of pregnancy. Safety and efficacy in pediatric patients have not been established.

Additional Canadian warnings (not included in U.S. labeling): If glycemic control is inadequate, rosiglitazone may be added to metformin or a sulfonylurea (if metformin use is contraindicated or not tolerated); use of triple therapy (rosiglitazone in combination with both metformin and a sulfonylurea) is not indicated due to increased risks of heart failure and fluid retention.

Drug Interactions

Metabolism/Transport Effects Substrate of CYP2C8 (major), CYP2C9 (minor); **Note:** Assignment of Major/Minor substrate status based on clinically relevant drug interaction potential; **Inhibits** CYP2C19 (weak), CYP2C8 (moderate), CYP2C9 (weak)

Avoid Concomitant Use There are no known interactions where it is recommended to avoid concomitant use.

Increased Effect/Toxicity

Rosiglitazone may increase the levels/effects of: CYP2C8 Substrates; Hypoglycemic Agents

The levels/effects of Rosiglitazone may be increased by: CYP2C8 Inhibitors (Moderate); CYP2C8 Inhibitors (Strong); Deferasirox; Gemfibrozil; Herbs (Hypoglycemic Properties); Insulin; MAO Inhibitors; Mifepristone; Pegvisomant; Pregabalin; Salicylates; Selective Serotonin Reuptake Inhibitors; Trimethoprim; Vasodilators (Organic Nitrates)

Decreased Effect

The levels/effects of Rosiglitazone may be decreased by: Bile Acid Sequestrants; Corticosteroids (Orally Inhaled); Corticosteroids (Systemic); CYP2C8 Inducers (Strong); Loop Diuretics; Luteinizing

◄ Hormone-Releasing Hormone Analogs; Rifampin; Somatropin; Thiazide Diuretics

Ethanol/Nutrition/Herb Interactions

Ethanol: Avoid ethanol (may cause hypoglycemia).

Food: Peak concentrations are lower by 28% and delayed when administered with food, but these effects are not believed to be clinically significant.

Herb/Nutraceutical: Avoid alfalfa, aloe, bilberry, bitter melon, burdock, celery, damiana, fenugreek, garcinia, garlic, ginger, ginseng (American), gymnema, marshmallow, stinging nettle (may cause hypoglycemia).

Dietary Considerations Management of type 2 diabetes mellitus (noninsulin dependent, NIDDM) should include diet control. May be taken without regard to meals.

Pharmacodynamics/Kinetics

Onset of Action Delayed; Maximum effect: Up to 12 weeks

Half-life Elimination 3-4 hours

Time to Peak 1 hour; delayed with food

Pregnancy Risk Factor C

Pregnancy Considerations Rosiglitazone is classified as pregnancy category C due to adverse effects observed in initial animal studies. Rosiglitazone has been found to cross the placenta during the first trimester of pregnancy. Inadvertent use early in pregnancy has not shown adverse fetal effects although in the majority of cases, the medication was stopped as soon as pregnancy was detected. Thiazolidinediones may cause ovulation in anovulatory premenopausal women, increasing the risk of pregnancy; adequate contraception in premenopausal women is recommended. Maternal hyperglycemia can be associated with adverse effects in the fetus, including macrosomia, neonatal hyperglycemia, and hyperbilirubinemia; the risk of congenital malformations is increased when the Hb A_{1c} is above the normal range. Diabetes can also be associated with adverse effects in the mother. Poorly-treated diabetes may cause end-organ damage that may in turn negatively affect obstetric outcomes. Physiologic glucose levels should be maintained prior to and during pregnancy to decrease the risk of adverse events in the mother and the fetus. Until additional safety and efficacy data are obtained, the use of oral agents is generally not recommended as routine management of GDM or type 2 diabetes mellitus during pregnancy. Insulin is the drug of choice for the control of diabetes mellitus during pregnancy.

Lactation Excretion in breast milk unknown/not recommended

Breast-Feeding Considerations It is not known if rosiglitazone is excreted in breast milk. Breast-feeding is not recommended by the manufacturer.

Prescribing and Access Restrictions As a requirement of the REMS program, the prescribing and dispensing of any rosiglitazone-containing medication in the U.S. requires physician and patient enrollment in the Avandia-Rosiglitazone Medicines Access Program™. Complete program details are available at www.avandia.com or by calling the program Coordinating Center at 800-282-6342.

Health Canada requires written informed consent for new and current patients receiving rosiglitazone.

Dosage Forms

Tablet, oral:

Avandia®: 2 mg, 4 mg, 8 mg

Rosiglitazone and Glimepiride
(roh si GLI ta zone & GLYE me pye ride)

Related Information

Glimepiride *on page 658*

Rosiglitazone *on page 1212*

Brand Names: U.S. Avandaryl®

Brand Names: Canada Avandaryl®

Pharmacologic Category Antidiabetic Agent, Sulfonylurea; Antidiabetic Agent, Thiazolidinedione

Use Management of type 2 diabetes mellitus (noninsulin dependent, NIDDM) as an adjunct to diet and exercise

Local Anesthetic/Vasoconstrictor Precautions No information available to require special precautions

Effects on Dental Treatment Dependent patients with diabetes (noninsulin dependent, type 2) should be appointed for dental treatment in the morning in order to minimize chance of stress-induced hypoglycemia.

Effects on Bleeding Rosiglitazone has been demonstrated to induce severe thrombocytopenia (rare). Analysis of the patient's serum shows rosiglitazone-induced antibody, responsible for thrombocytopenia, confirming an immune-mediated platelet depletion.

Adverse Effects Percentages below refer to combination Avandaryl®. Also see individual agents.

1% to 10%:

Cardiovascular: Edema (3%), hypertension (2% to 3%)

Central nervous system: Headache (3% to 6%)

Endocrine & metabolic: Hypoglycemia (4% to 6%)

Respiratory: Nasopharyngitis (4% to 5%)

General Dosage Range Dosage adjustment recommended in patients with hepatic or renal impairment

Oral:

Adults: Initial: Rosiglitazone 4 mg and glimepiride 1-2 mg once daily; Maintenance: Rosiglitazone 4-8 mg and glimepiride 1-4 mg once daily

Elderly: Initial: Rosiglitazone 4 mg and glimepiride 1 mg once daily

Mechanism of Action

Rosiglitazone is a thiazolidinedione antidiabetic agent that lowers blood glucose by improving target cell response to insulin, without increasing pancreatic insulin secretion. It has a mechanism of action that is dependent on the presence of insulin for activity.

Glimepiride stimulates insulin release from the pancreatic beta cells; reduces glucose output from the liver; insulin sensitivity is increased at peripheral target sites.

Pregnancy Risk Factor C

Pregnancy Considerations Animal reproduction studies have not been conducted with this combination; therefore, rosiglitazone/glimepiride is classified as pregnancy category C. See individual agents.

Prescribing and Access Restrictions

As a requirement of the REMS program, the prescribing and dispensing of any rosiglitazone-containing medication in the U.S. requires physician and patient enrollment in the Avandia-Rosiglitazone Medicines Access Program™. Complete program details are available at www.avandia.com or by calling the program Coordinating Center at 800-282-6342.

Health Canada requires written informed consent for new and current patients receiving rosiglitazone.

Rosiglitazone and Metformin
(roh si GLI ta zone & met FOR min)

Related Information
MetFORMIN *on page 882*
Rosiglitazone *on page 1212*
Brand Names: U.S. Avandamet®
Brand Names: Canada Avandamet®
Pharmacologic Category Antidiabetic Agent, Biguanide; Antidiabetic Agent, Thiazolidinedione
Use Management of type 2 diabetes mellitus (noninsulin dependent, NIDDM) as an adjunct to diet and exercise in patients where dual rosiglitazone and metformin therapy is appropriate
Local Anesthetic/Vasoconstrictor Precautions No information available to require special precautions
Effects on Dental Treatment Dependent diabetics (noninsulin dependent, type 2) should be appointed for dental treatment in the morning in order to minimize chance of stress-induced hypoglycemia.
Effects on Bleeding Rosiglitazone has been demonstrated to induce severe thrombocytopenia (rare). Analysis of the patient's serum shows rosiglitazone-induced antibody, responsible for thrombocytopenia, confirming an immune-mediated platelet depletion.
Adverse Effects Also see individual agents. Percentages of adverse effects as reported with the combination product.
>10%:
Central nervous system: Headache (7% to 11%)
Gastrointestinal: Nausea/vomiting (16%), diarrhea (13% to 14%)
Respiratory: Upper respiratory tract infection (9% to 16%)
1% to 10%:
Cardiovascular: Edema (6%)
Central nervous system: Dizziness (8%), fatigue (6%)
Endocrine & metabolic: Hypoglycemia (3%)
Gastrointestinal: Dyspepsia (10%), abdominal pain (5%), loose stools (5%), constipation (5%)
Hematologic: Anemia (4% to 7%)
Neuromuscular & skeletal: Arthralgia (5%), back pain (5%)
Respiratory: Sinusitis (6%), nasopharyngitis (6%)
Miscellaneous: Injury (8%), viral infection (5%), flu-like syndrome (1%)
General Dosage Range Oral: *Adults:* Initial: Rosiglitazone 2 mg and metformin 500 mg once or twice daily; may increase by 2 mg/500 mg per day after 4 weeks (maximum: rosiglitazone 8 mg/day; metformin 2000 mg/day)
Mechanism of Action Rosiglitazone is a thiazolidinedione antidiabetic agent that lowers blood glucose by improving target cell response to insulin, without increasing pancreatic insulin secretion. It has a mechanism of action that is dependent on the presence of insulin for activity. Metformin decreases hepatic glucose production, decreases intestinal absorption of glucose, and improves insulin sensitivity (increases peripheral glucose uptake and utilization).
Pregnancy Risk Factor C
Pregnancy Considerations Animal reproduction studies were not conducted with this combination; therefore, rosiglitazone/metformin is classified as pregnancy category C. Refer to individual agents.

Prescribing and Access Restrictions
As a requirement of the REMS program, the prescribing and dispensing of any rosiglitazone-containing medication in the U.S. requires physician and patient enrollment in the Avandia-Rosiglitazone Medicines Access Program™. Complete program details are available at www.avandia.com or by calling the program Coordinating Center at 800-282-6342.

Health Canada requires written informed consent for new and current patients receiving rosiglitazone.

Rosuvastatin (roe soo va STAT in)

Related Information
Cardiovascular Diseases *on page 1492*
Brand Names: U.S. Crestor®
Brand Names: Canada Apo-Rosuvastatin; CO Rosuvastatin; Crestor®; Jamp-Rosuvastatin; Mylan-Rosuvastatin; PMS-Rosuvastatin; RAN™-Rosuvastatin; Sandoz-Rosuvastatin; Teva-Rosuvastatin
Pharmacologic Category Antilipemic Agent, HMG-CoA Reductase Inhibitor
Use
Treatment of dyslipidemias:
Used with dietary therapy for hyperlipidemias to reduce elevations in total cholesterol (TC), LDL-C, apolipoprotein B, nonHDL-C, and triglycerides (TG) in patients with primary hypercholesterolemia (elevations of 1 or more components are present in Fredrickson type IIa, IIb, and IV hyperlipidemias); increase HDL-C; treatment of primary dysbetalipoproteinemia (Fredrickson type III hyperlipidemia); treatment of homozygous familial hypercholesterolemia (FH); to slow progression of atherosclerosis as an adjunct to diet to lower TC and LDL-C
Heterozygous familial hypercholesterolemia (HeFH): In adolescent patients (10-17 years of age, females >1 year postmenarche) with HeFH having LDL-C >190 mg/dL or LDL >160 mg/dL with positive family history of premature cardiovascular disease (CVD), or ≥2 other CVD risk factors.
Primary prevention of cardiovascular disease: To reduce the risk of stroke, myocardial infarction, or arterial revascularization procedures in patients without clinically evident coronary heart disease or lipid abnormalities but with all of the following: 1) an increased risk of cardiovascular disease based on age ≥50 years old in men and ≥60 years old in women, 2) hsCRP ≥2 mg/L, and 3) the presence of at least one additional cardiovascular disease risk factor such as hypertension, low HDL-C, smoking, or a family history of premature coronary heart disease.
Secondary prevention of cardiovascular disease: To slow progression of atherosclerosis
Local Anesthetic/Vasoconstrictor Precautions No information available to require special precautions
Effects on Dental Treatment No significant effects or complications reported
Effects on Bleeding No information available to require special precautions
Adverse Effects
>10%: Neuromuscular & skeletal: Myalgia (3% to 13%)
2% to 10%:
Central nervous system: Headache (6%), dizziness (4%)
Gastrointestinal: Nausea (3%), abdominal pain (2%), constipation (2%)
Hepatic: ALT increased (2%; >3 times ULN)

◀ Neuromuscular & skeletal: Arthralgia (4% to 10%), CPK increased (3%; >10 x ULN: Children 3%), weakness (3%)

Adverse reactions reported with other HMG-CoA reductase inhibitors (not necessarily reported with rosuvastatin therapy) include a hypersensitivity syndrome (symptoms may include anaphylaxis, angioedema, arthralgia, erythema multiforme, eosinophilia, hemolytic anemia, immune-mediated necrotizing myopathy (IMNM), interstitial lung disease, lupus syndrome, photosensitivity, polymyalgia rheumatica, positive ANA, purpura, Stevens-Johnson syndrome, toxic epidermal necrolysis, urticaria, vasculitis)

General Dosage Range Dosage adjustment recommended in patients with renal impairment, on concomitant therapy, or who develop toxicities

Oral:

Children 10-17 years (females >1 year postmenarche): Initial: 5-20 mg once daily (maximum: 20 mg daily)

Adults: Initial: 5-20 mg once daily; Maintenance: 5-40 mg once daily (maximum: 40 mg daily)

Mechanism of Action Inhibitor of 3-hydroxy-3-methylglutaryl coenzyme A (HMG-CoA) reductase, the rate-limiting enzyme in cholesterol synthesis (reduces the production of mevalonic acid from HMG-CoA); this then results in a compensatory increase in the expression of LDL receptors on hepatocyte membranes and a stimulation of LDL catabolism

Pharmacodynamics/Kinetics

Onset of Action Within 1 week; maximal at 4 weeks

Half-life Elimination 19 hours

Time to Peak Plasma: 3-5 hours

Pregnancy Risk Factor X

Pregnancy Considerations Adverse events were observed in some animal reproduction studies. There are reports of congenital anomalies following maternal use of HMG-CoA reductase inhibitors in pregnancy; however, maternal disease, differences in specific agents used, and the low rates of exposure limit the interpretation of the available data (Godfrey, 2012; Lecarpentier, 2012). Cholesterol biosynthesis may be important in fetal development; serum cholesterol and triglycerides increase normally during pregnancy. The discontinuation of lipid lowering medications temporarily during pregnancy is not expected to have significant impact on the long term outcomes of primary hypercholesterolemia treatment.

Use of rosuvastatin is contraindicated in pregnancy. HMG-CoA reductase inhibitors should be discontinued prior to pregnancy (ADA, 2013). If treatment of dyslipidemias is needed in pregnant women or in women of reproductive age, other agents are preferred (Berglund, 2012; NCEP, 2002). The manufacturer recommends administration to women of childbearing potential only when conception is highly unlikely and patients have been informed of potential hazards.

Rotavirus Vaccine (ROE ta vye rus vak SEEN)

Brand Names: U.S. Rotarix®; RotaTeq®
Brand Names: Canada Rotarix®; RotaTeq®
Pharmacologic Category Vaccine, Live (Viral)
Use Prevention of rotavirus gastroenteritis in infants and children

The Advisory Committee on Immunization Practices (ACIP) recommends routine vaccination of all infants (CDC, 2009).

Local Anesthetic/Vasoconstrictor Precautions No information available to require special precautions

Effects on Dental Treatment No significant effects or complications reported

Effects on Bleeding No information available to require special precautions

Adverse Effects All serious adverse reactions must be reported to the U.S. Department of Health and Human Services (DHHS) Vaccine Adverse Event Reporting System (VAERS) 1-800-822-7967 or online at https://vaers.hhs.gov/esub/index.

Note: Ranges reported; actual percentage may vary between products.

>10%:

Central nervous system: Fever ≥38.1°C (17% to 43%; equal to or less than placebo), fussiness/irritability (3% to 52%)

Gastrointestinal: Diarrhea (4% to 24%), vomiting (3% to 15%)

Otic: Otitis media (15%)

1% to 10%:

Gastrointestinal: Flatulence (2%)

Respiratory: Nasopharyngitis (7%), bronchospasm (1%)

General Dosage Range Oral:

Infants 6-24 weeks: Rotarix®: A total of two 1 mL doses administered at 2 and 4 months of age

Infants 6-32 weeks: RotaTeq®: A total of three 2 mL doses given at 2, 4, and 6 months of age

Mechanism of Action A live vaccine; replicates in the small intestine and promotes active immunity to rotavirus gastroenteritis. Rotarix® is specifically indicated for prevention of rotavirus gastroenteritis caused by serotypes G1, G3, G4, and G9 and RotaTeq® is specifically indicated for prevention of rotavirus gastroenteritis caused by serotypes G1, G2, G3, and G4. However, vaccines may provide immunity to other serotypes.

Pharmacodynamics/Kinetics

Onset of Action Seroconversion:

Rotarix®: Antirotavirus IgA antibodies were noted 1-2 months following completion of the 2-dose series in 77% to 87% of infants.

RotaTeq®: A threefold increase in antirotavirus IgA was noted following completion of the 3-dose regimen in 93% to 100% of infants.

Duration of Action Following administration of rotavirus vaccine, efficacy of protecting against any grade of rotavirus gastroenteritis through two seasons was 70% to 79%.

Pregnancy Risk Factor C

Pregnancy Considerations Reproduction studies have not been conducted. Not indicated for use in women of reproductive age. Infants living in households with pregnant women may be vaccinated (CDC, 2009).

Rotigotine (roe TIG oh teen)

Brand Names: U.S. Neupro®
Pharmacologic Category Anti-Parkinson's Agent, Dopamine Agonist
Use Treatment of the signs and symptoms of idiopathic Parkinson's disease (early-stage to advanced-stage disease); treatment of moderate-to-severe primary restless legs syndrome (RLS)

Local Anesthetic/Vasoconstrictor Precautions No information available to require special precautions

Effects on Dental Treatment Key adverse event(s) related to dental treatment: Xerostomia and changes in salivation (normal salivary flow resumes upon discontinuation). Dopamine agonists may cause orthostatic hypotension and syncope. Parkinson's disease patients should be carefully assisted from the chair and observed for signs of orthostatic hypotension.

Effects on Bleeding No information available to require special precautions

Adverse Effects

>10%:

Cardiovascular: Peripheral edema (dose related; 2% to 14%)

Central nervous system: Somnolence (dose related; 5% to 32%), dizziness (5% to 23%), headache (8% to 18%), fatigue (6% to 18%), orthostatic hypotension (1% to 18%), sleep disorder (disturbance in initiating/maintaining sleep; dose related; 2% to 14%), hallucinations (dose related; 7% to 14%), insomnia (5% to 11%)

Dermatologic: Application site reactions (dose related; 27% to 46%), hyperhidrosis (dose related; 1% to 11%)

Gastrointestinal: Nausea (dose related; 15% to 48%), vomiting (dose related; 2% to 20%)

Neuromuscular & skeletal: Dyskinesia (dose related; 14% to 17%), arthralgia (8% to 11%)

1% to 10%:

Cardiovascular: Hypertension (dose related; 1% to 5%), T-wave abnormalities on ECG (≤3%), syncope

Central nervous system: Abnormal dreams (dose related; 1% to 7%), nightmare (dose related; 3% to 5%), depression (≤5%), vertigo (1% to 4%), early morning awakening (dose related; ≤3%), balance disorder (2% to 3%), lethargy (1% to 2%), postural dizziness (1% to 2%), sleep attacks (dose related; ≤2%)

Dermatologic: Pruritus (3% to 7%), erythema (dose related; ≤6%), pruritic rash (dose related; ≤3%)

Endocrine & metabolic: Hot flash (≤3%), serum ferritin decreased (dose related; 1% to 2%); serum glucose decreased

Gastrointestinal: Constipation (2% to 9%), weight gain (2% to 9%), diarrhea (5% to 7%), anorexia (≤8%), xerostomia (dose related; 3% to 7%), appetite decreased (≤3%), dyspepsia (dose related; ≤3%), weight loss (dose related; ≤3%)

Genitourinary: Erectile dysfunction (dose related; ≤3%), urinary WBC positive (≤3%)

Hematologic: Contusion (dose related; ≤4%), hemoglobin decreased, hematocrit decreased

Neuromuscular & skeletal: Paresthesia (dose related 5% to 6%), tremor (3% to 4%), weakness (3% to 4%), muscle spasms (dose related; 1% to 4%), musculoskeletal pain (2%)

Ocular: Vision changes

Otic: Tinnitus (≤3%)

Renal: BUN increased

Respiratory: Nasopharyngitis (7% to 10%), upper respiratory tract infection (≤5%), cough (3%), nasal congestion (3%), sinus congestion (2% to 3%), sinusitis (dose related; ≤3%), pharyngolaryngeal pain (≤2%)

Miscellaneous: Hiccups (dose related; 2% to 3%)

General Dosage Range

Transdermal: *Adults:* 1-4 mg/24 hours; Maintenance (usual): 1-8 mg/24 hours (maximum: varies by indication)

Mechanism of Action Rotigotine is a nonergot dopamine agonist with specificity for D_3-, D_2-, and D_1-dopamine receptors. Although the precise mechanism of action of rotigotine is unknown, it is believed to be due to stimulation of postsynaptic dopamine D_2-type auto receptors within the substantia nigra in the brain, leading to improved dopaminergic transmission in the motor areas of the basal ganglia, notably the caudate nucleus/putamen regions.

Pharmacodynamics/Kinetics

Half-life Elimination After removal of patch: ~5-7 hours

Time to Peak 15-18 hours; can occur 4-27 hours post application

Pregnancy Risk Factor C

Pregnancy Considerations Adverse events were observed in animal reproduction studies.

Rufinamide (roo FIN a mide)

Brand Names: U.S. Banzel®

Brand Names: Canada Banzel™

Pharmacologic Category Anticonvulsant, Triazole Derivative

Use Adjunctive therapy in the treatment of generalized seizures of Lennox-Gastaut syndrome

Local Anesthetic/Vasoconstrictor Precautions No information available to require special precautions

Effects on Dental Treatment No significant effects or complications reported

Effects on Bleeding No information available to require special precautions

Adverse Effects

>10%:

Cardiovascular: QT shortening (46% to 65%; dose related)

Central nervous system: Headache (16% to 27%), somnolence (11% to 24%), dizziness (3% to 19%), fatigue (9% to 16%)

Gastrointestinal: Vomiting (5% to 17%), nausea (7% to 12%)

1% to 10%:

Central nervous system: Ataxia (4% to 5%), seizure (children 5%), status epilepticus (≤4%), aggression (children 3%), anxiety (adults 3%), attention disturbance (children 3%), hyperactivity (children 3%), vertigo (adults 3%)

Dermatologic: Rash (children 4%), pruritus (children 3%)

Gastrointestinal: Appetite decreased (≥1% to 5%), abdominal pain (3%), constipation (adults 3%), dyspepsia (adults 3%), appetite increased (≥1%)

Hematologic: Leukopenia (≤4%), anemia (≥1%)

Neuromuscular & skeletal: Tremor (adults 6%), back pain (adults 3%), gait disturbance (1% to 3%)

Ocular: Diplopia (4% to 9%), blurred vision (adults 6%), nystagmus (adults 6%)

Otic: Otitis media (children 3%)

Renal: Pollakiuria (≥1%)

Respiratory: Nasopharyngitis (children 5%), bronchitis (children 3%), sinusitis (children 3%)

Miscellaneous: Influenza (children 5%)

General Dosage Range Oral:

Children ≥4 years: Initial: 10 mg/kg/day in 2 equally divided doses (maximum: 45 mg/kg/day or 3200 mg/day)

Adults: Initial: 400-800 mg/day in 2 equally divided doses (maximum: 3200 mg/day)

◄ **Mechanism of Action** A triazole-derivative antiepileptic whose exact mechanism is unknown. *In vitro*, it prolongs the inactive state of the sodium channels, thereby limiting repetitive firing of sodium-dependent action potentials mediating anticonvulsant effects.

Pharmacodynamics/Kinetics

Half-life Elimination ~6-10 hours

Time to Peak 4-6 hours

Pregnancy Risk Factor C

Pregnancy Considerations Adverse effects were seen in animal studies. There are no adequate and well-controlled studies in pregnant women; use during pregnancy only if clearly needed. Hormonal contraceptives may be less effective with concurrent rufinamide use; additional forms of nonhormonal contraceptives should be used.

Patients exposed to rufinamide during pregnancy are encouraged to enroll themselves into the AED Pregnancy Registry by calling 1-888-233-2334. Additional information is available at www.aedpregnancyregistry.org.

Ruxolitinib (rux oh LI ti nib)

Brand Names: U.S. Jakafi™

Brand Names: Canada Jakavi™

Pharmacologic Category Antineoplastic Agent, Janus Associated Kinase Inhibitor; Antineoplastic Agent, Tyrosine Kinase Inhibitor; Janus Associated Kinase Inhibitor

Use Treatment of intermediate or high-risk myelofibrosis, including primary myelofibrosis, post-polycythemia vera (post-PV) myelofibrosis and post-essential thrombocythemia (post-ET) myelofibrosis

Local Anesthetic/Vasoconstrictor Precautions No information available to require special precautions

Effects on Dental Treatment No significant effects or complications reported

Effects on Bleeding Chemotherapy may result in significant myelosuppression, potentially including significant reduction in platelet counts and altered hemostasis. In patients who are under active treatment with these agents, medical consult is suggested.

Adverse Effects

>10%:

Cardiovascular: Peripheral edema (22%)

Central nervous system: Dizziness (15% to 18%), headache (10% to 15%), insomnia (12%)

Dermatologic: Bruising (19% to 23%)

Endocrine & metabolic: Cholesterol increased (17%; grade 2: <1%)

Gastrointestinal: Diarrhea (23%), constipation (13%), nausea (13%), vomiting (12%)

Hematologic: Anemia (96%; grade 3: 34%; grade 4: 11%), thrombocytopenia (70%; grade 3: 9%; grade 4: 4%), neutropenia (19%; grade 3: 5%; grade 4: 2%)

Hepatic: ALT increased (25%; grades 2/3: 2%), AST increased (17%; grade 2: <1%)

Respiratory: Dyspnea (16%), nasopharyngitis (16%)

1% to 10%:

Gastrointestinal: Flatulence (5%)

Genitourinary: Urinary tract infection (9%)

Miscellaneous: Herpes zoster infection (2%)

General Dosage Range Dosage adjustment recommended in patients with hepatic impairment, renal impairment, on concomitant strong CYP3A4 inhibitor therapy, or who develop toxicities.

Oral: *Adults:* 15-20 mg twice daily; maximum dose: 25 mg twice daily

Mechanism of Action Kinase inhibitor which selectively inhibits Janus Associated Kinases (JAKs), JAK1 and JAK2. JAK1 and JAK2 mediate signaling of cytokine and growth factors responsible for hematopoiesis and immune function; JAK mediated signaling involves recruitment of STATs (signal transducers and activators of transcription) to cytokine receptors which leads to modulation of gene expression. In myelofibrosis, JAK1/2 activity is dysregulated; ruxolitinib modulates the affected JAK1/2 activity.

Pharmacodynamics/Kinetics

Half-life Elimination Ruxolitinib: 2.8-3 hours (hepatic impairment: 5 hours); Ruxolitinib + metabolites: ~6 hours

Pregnancy Risk Factor C

Pregnancy Considerations Increased resorptions (late) and reduced fetal weights were observed in animal reproduction studies. Use during human pregnancy only if the potential treatment benefits outweigh risks.

Prescribing and Access Restrictions Available through specialty/network pharmacies. Further information may be obtained from the manufacturer, Incyte, at 1-855-452-5234 or at www.Jakafi.com.

Saccharomyces boulardii
(sak roe MYE sees boo LAR dee)

Brand Names: U.S. Florastor® Kids [OTC]; Florastor® [OTC]

Pharmacologic Category Dietary Supplement; Probiotic

Use Promote maintenance of normal microflora in the gastrointestinal tract; used in management of bloating, gas, and diarrhea, particularly to decrease the incidence of diarrhea associated with antibiotic use

Local Anesthetic/Vasoconstrictor Precautions No information available to require special precautions

Effects on Dental Treatment No significant effects or complications reported

Effects on Bleeding No information available to require special precautions

Adverse Effects Frequency not defined.

Gastrointestinal: Constipation, flatulence

Miscellaneous: Thirst

General Dosage Range Oral: *Children and Adults:* 250 mg twice daily

Mechanism of Action S. boulardii, a nonpathogenic live yeast probiotic, acts as temporary flora to help reestablish the normal gastrointestinal microflora. May also modulate the immune system by inducing cytokines and suppress pathogenic bacteria growth.

Pharmacodynamics/Kinetics

Onset of Action Yeast cell release from capsules/powder: 30 minutes

Duration of Action Yeast cells cleared in 5-7 days

Sacrosidase (sak ROE si dase)

Brand Names: U.S. Sucraid®

Brand Names: Canada Sucraid®

Pharmacologic Category Enzyme, Gastrointestinal

Use Oral replacement therapy in sucrase deficiency, as seen in congenital sucrase-isomaltase deficiency (CSID)

Local Anesthetic/Vasoconstrictor Precautions No information available to require special precautions

Effects on Dental Treatment No significant effects or complications reported

Effects on Bleeding No information available to require special precautions

Adverse Effects

1% to 10%:

Central nervous system: Headache, insomnia, nervousness

Endocrine & metabolic: Dehydration

Gastrointestinal: Abdominal pain, constipation, diarrhea, nausea, vomiting

General Dosage Range Oral:

Infants ≥5 months and Children ≤15 kg: 8500 units (1 mL) per meal or snack

Children >15 kg, Adolescents, and Adults: 17,000 units (2 mL) per meal or snack

Mechanism of Action Sacrosidase is a naturally-occurring gastrointestinal enzyme derived from baker's yeast (*Saccharomyces cerevisiae*) which breaks down the disaccharide sucrose to its monosaccharide components. Hydrolysis is necessary to allow absorption of these nutrients.

Pregnancy Risk Factor C

Pregnancy Considerations Animal reproduction studies have not been conducted. Should be administered to a pregnant woman only when indicated.

Prescribing and Access Restrictions Sucraid® is not available in retail pharmacies or via mail-order pharmacies. To obtain the product, please refer to http://www.sucraid.net/how-to-order-sucraid or call 1-866-740-2743.

Salicylic Acid (sal i SIL ik AS id)

Brand Names: U.S. Aliclen™; Beta Sal® [OTC]; Clean & Clear® Advantage® Acne Cleanser [OTC]; Clean & Clear® Advantage® Acne Spot Treatment [OTC]; Clean & Clear® Advantage® Invisible Acne Patch [OTC]; Clean & Clear® Advantage® Oil-Free Acne [OTC]; Clean & Clear® Blackhead Clearing Daily Cleansing [OTC]; Clean & Clear® Blackhead Clearing Scrub [OTC]; Clean & Clear® Deep Cleaning [OTC]; Clean & Clear® Dual Action Moisturizer [OTC]; Clean & Clear® Invisible Blemish Treatment [OTC]; Compound W® One Step Invisible Strip [OTC]; Compound W® One Step Wart Remover for Feet [OTC]; Compound W® One-Step Wart Remover for Kids [OTC]; Compound W® One-Step Wart Remover [OTC]; Compound W® [OTC]; Curad® Mediplast® [OTC]; Denorex® Extra Strength Protection 2-in-1 [OTC]; Denorex® Extra Strength Protection [OTC]; Dermarest® Psoriasis Medicated Moisturizer [OTC]; Dermarest® Psoriasis Medicated Scalp Treatment [OTC]; Dermarest® Psoriasis Medicated Shampoo/Conditioner [OTC]; Dermarest® Psoriasis Medicated Skin Treatment [OTC]; Dermarest® Psoriasis Overnight Treatment [OTC]; DHS™ Sal [OTC]; Dr. Scholl's® Callus Removers [OTC]; Dr. Scholl's® Clear Away® One Step Wart Remover [OTC]; Dr. Scholl's® Clear Away® Plantar Wart Remover For Feet [OTC]; Dr. Scholl's® Clear Away® Wart Remover Fast-Acting [OTC]; Dr. Scholl's® Clear Away® Wart Remover Invisible Strips [OTC]; Dr. Scholl's® Clear Away® Wart Remover [OTC]; Dr. Scholl's® Corn Removers [OTC]; Dr. Scholl's® Corn/Callus Remover [OTC]; Dr. Scholl's® Extra Thick Corn Removers [OTC]; Dr. Scholl's® Extra-Thick Callus Removers [OTC]; Dr. Scholl's® For Her Corn Removers [OTC]; Dr. Scholl's® OneStep Callus Removers [OTC]; Dr. Scholl's® OneStep Corn Removers [OTC]; Dr. Scholl's® Small Corn Removers [OTC]; Dr. Scholl's® Ultra-Thin Corn Removers [OTC]; DuoFilm® [OTC]; Freezone® [OTC]; Fung-O® [OTC]; Gets-It® [OTC];

Gordofilm [OTC]; Hydrisalic® [OTC]; Ionil Plus® [OTC]; Ionil® [OTC]; Keralyt®; Keralyt® [OTC]; Lupi-Care® Dandruff [OTC]; LupiCare® Psoriasis [OTC]; MG217® Sal-Acid [OTC]; Mosco® Callus & Corn Remover [OTC]; Mosco® One Step Corn Remover [OTC]; Neutrogena® Acne Stress Control [OTC]; Neutrogena® Advanced Solutions™ [OTC]; Neutrogena® Blackhead Eliminating™ 2-in-1 Foaming Pads [OTC]; Neutrogena® Blackhead Eliminating™ Daily Scrub [OTC]; Neutrogena® Blackhead Eliminating™ [OTC]; Neutrogena® Body Clear® [OTC]; Neutrogena® Clear Pore™ Oil-Controlling Astringent [OTC]; Neutrogena® Maximum Strength T/Sal® [OTC]; Neutrogena® Oil-Free Acne Stress Control [OTC]; Neutrogena® Oil-Free Acne Wash 60 Second Mask Scrub [OTC]; Neutrogena® Oil-Free Acne Wash Cream Cleanser [OTC]; Neutrogena® Oil-Free Acne Wash Foam Cleanser [OTC]; Neutrogena® Oil-Free Acne Wash [OTC]; Neutrogena® Oil-Free Acne [OTC]; Neutrogena® Oil-Free Anti-Acne [OTC]; Neutrogena® Rapid Clear® Acne Defense [OTC]; Neutrogena® Rapid Clear® Acne Eliminating [OTC]; Neutrogena® Rapid Clear® [OTC]; OXY® Body Wash [OTC]; OXY® Chill Factor® [OTC]; OXY® Daily Cleansing [OTC]; OXY® Daily [OTC]; OXY® Face Wash [OTC]; OXY® Maximum Daily Cleansing [OTC]; OXY® Maximum [OTC]; OXY® Post-Shave [OTC]; OXY® Spot Treatment [OTC]; OXY® [OTC]; P&S® [OTC]; Palmer's® Skin Success Acne Cleanser [OTC]; Sal-Plant® [OTC]; Salactic® [OTC]; Salex®; Salvax; Scalpicin® Anti-Itch [OTC]; Selsun blue® Deep Cleaning Micro-Bead Scrub [OTC]; Selsun blue® Naturals Island Breeze [OTC]; Selsun blue® Naturals Itchy Dry Scalp [OTC]; Stridex® Essential Care® [OTC]; Stridex® Facewipes To Go® [OTC]; Stridex® Maximum Strength [OTC]; Stridex® Sensitive Skin [OTC]; Thera-Sal [OTC] [DSC]; Tinamed® Corn and Callus Remover [OTC]; Tinamed® Wart Remover [OTC]; Trans-Ver-Sal® [OTC]; Virasal®; Wart-Off® Maximum Strength [OTC]; Zapzyt® Acne Wash [OTC]; Zapzyt® Pore Treatment [OTC]

Brand Names: Canada Duofilm®; Duoforte® 27; Occlusal™-HP; Sebcur®; Soluver®; Soluver® Plus; Trans-Plantar®; Trans-Ver-Sal®

Pharmacologic Category Acne Products; Keratolytic Agent; Topical Skin Product, Acne

Use Topically for its keratolytic effect in controlling seborrheic dermatitis or psoriasis of body and scalp, dandruff, and other scaling dermatoses; also used to remove warts, corns, and calluses; acne

Local Anesthetic/Vasoconstrictor Precautions No information available to require special precautions

Effects on Dental Treatment No significant effects or complications reported

Effects on Bleeding No information available to require special precautions

Adverse Effects Frequency not defined.

Central nervous system: Dizziness, headache, mental confusion

Local: Burning and irritation at site of exposure on normal tissue, peeling, scaling

Otic: Tinnitus

Respiratory: Hyperventilation

General Dosage Range Topical: *Children and Adults:* Dosage varies greatly depending on product

Mechanism of Action Produces desquamation of hyperkeratotic epithelium via dissolution of the intercellular cement which causes the cornified tissue to swell, soften, macerate, and desquamate. Salicylic acid is keratolytic at concentrations of 3% to 6%; it becomes destructive to tissue at concentrations >6%.

◀ Concentrations of 6% to 60% are used to remove corns and warts and in the treatment of psoriasis and other hyperkeratotic disorders.

Pharmacodynamics/Kinetics

Time to Peak Serum: Within 5 hours of application with occlusion

Pregnancy Risk Factor C

Pregnancy Considerations Adverse events have been observed in animal reproduction studies when administered orally. Salicylates cross the placenta (Ostensen, 1998). Systemic absorption of topically applied salicylic acid varies depending on duration and vehicle (9% to 25%) (Akhavan, 2003).

Saliva Substitute (sa LYE va SUB stee tute)

Related Information

Dentin Hypersensitivity, Acid Erosion, High Caries Index, Management of Alveolar Osteitis, and Xerostomia *on page 1582*

Management of Patients Undergoing Cancer Therapy *on page 1596*

Brand Names: U.S. Aquoral™; Biotene® Moisturizing Mouth Spray [OTC]; Biotene® Oral Balance® [OTC]; Caphosol®; Entertainer's Secret® [OTC]; Moi-Stir® [OTC]; Mouth Kote® [OTC]; NeutraSal®; Numoisyn™; Oasis®; SalivaSure™ [OTC]

Generic Availability (U.S.) No

Pharmacologic Category Gastrointestinal Agent, Miscellaneous

Dental Use Relief of dry mouth and throat in xerostomia

Use Relief of dry mouth and throat in xerostomia or hyposalivation; adjunct to standard oral care in relief of symptoms associated with chemotherapy or radiation therapy-induced mucositis

Local Anesthetic/Vasoconstrictor Precautions No information available to require special precautions

Effects on Dental Treatment No significant effects or complications reported

Effects on Bleeding No information available to require special precautions

Adverse Effects Frequency not defined.

Central nervous system: Altered speech

Gastrointestinal: Abnormal taste, digestive problems (minor), dysphagia

Dosage

Mucositis (due to high-dose chemotherapy or radiation therapy): Adults: Oral:

Caphosol®, NeutraSal®: Swish and spit 4-10 doses daily (use for the duration of chemo- or radiation therapy)

Xerostomia: Adults: Oral: Use as needed, or product-specific dosing:

Aquoral™: 2 sprays 3-4 times daily

Biotene® Oral Balance® gel: Apply one-half inch length onto tongue and spread evenly; repeat as often as needed

Caphosol®, NeutraSal®: Swish and spit 2-10 doses daily

Entertainer's Secret®: Spray as often as needed

Mouth Kote® spray: Spray 3-5 times, swish for 8-10 seconds, then spit or swallow; use as often as needed

Numoisyn™ liquid: Use 2 mL as needed

Numoisyn™ lozenges: Dissolve 1 lozenge slowly; maximum 16 lozenges daily

Oasis® mouthwash: Rinse mouth with ~30 mL twice daily or as needed; do not swallow

Oasis® spray: 1-2 sprays as needed; maximum 60 sprays daily

SalivaSure™: Dissolve 1 lozenge slowly as needed; for severe symptoms, 1 lozenge per hour is recommended

Mechanism of Action Protein or electrolyte mixtures which restore/replace saliva, lubricate, moisten, clean, and/or provide a coating on oral mucosa

Contraindications

Numoisyn™ liquid: Hypersensitivity to saliva substitute or any component of the formulation.

Numoisyn™ lozenges: Fructose intolerance

Drug Interactions

Metabolism/Transport Effects None known.

Avoid Concomitant Use There are no known interactions where it is recommended to avoid concomitant use.

Increased Effect/Toxicity There are no known significant interactions involving an increase in effect.

Decreased Effect There are no known significant interactions involving a decrease in effect.

Dietary Considerations

Caphosol®: Contains sodium 75 mg/30 mL dose

Moi-Stir®: Contains sodium: 6.47 mEq/120 mL, potassium: 1.93 mEq/120 mL, magnesium: 0.128 mEq/120 mL

Dosage Forms

Liquid, oral:

Biotene® Oral Balance® [OTC]: Water, starch, sunflower oil, propylene glycol, xylitol, glycerine, purified milk extract

Numoisyn™: Water, sorbitol, linseed extract, *Chondrus crispus*, methylparaben, sodium benzoate, potassium sorbate, dipotassium phosphate, propylparaben

Lozenge, oral:

Numoisyn™: Sorbitol 0.3 g/lozenge, polyethylene glycol, malic acid, sodium citrate, calcium phosphate dibasic, hydrogenated cottonseed oil, citric acid, magnesium stearate, silicon dioxide

SalivaSure™ [OTC]: Xylitol, citric acid, apple acid, sodium citrate dihydrate, sodium carboxymethylcellulose, dibasic calcium phosphate, silica colloidal, magnesium stearate, stearic acid

Powder, for reconstitution, oral:

NeutraSal®: Sodium, phosphates, calcium, chloride, bicarbonate, silicon dioxide

Solution, oral:

Caphosol®: Dibasic sodium phosphate 0.032%, monobasic sodium phosphate 0.009%, calcium chloride 0.052%, sodium chloride 0.569%, purified water

Entertainer's Secret® [OTC]: Sodium carboxymethylcellulose, aloe vera gel, glycerin (60 mL)

Solution, oral [mouthwash/gargle]:

Oasis®: Water, glycerin, sorbitol, poloxamer 338, PEG-60, hydrogenated castor oil, copovidone, sodium benzoate, carboxymethylcellulose

Solution, oral [spray]:

Aquoral™: Oxidized glycerol triesters and silicon dioxide

Biotene® Moisturizing Mouth Spray [OTC]: Water, polyglycitol, propylene glycol, sunflower oil, xylitol, milk protein extract, potassium sorbate, acesulfame K, potassium thiocyanate, lysozyme, lactoferrin, lactoperoxidase

Moi-Stir® [OTC]: Water, sorbitol, sodium carboxymethylcellulose, methylparaben, propylparaben, potassium chloride, dibasic sodium phosphate, calcium chloride, magnesium chloride, sodium chloride

Mouth Kote® [OTC]: Water, xylitol, sorbitol, yerba santa, citric acid, ascorbic acid, sodium saccharin, sodium benzoate

Oasis®: Glycerin, cetylpyridinium, copovidone

Salmeterol (sal ME te role)

Related Information
Respiratory Diseases *on page 1514*

Brand Names: U.S. Serevent® Diskus®

Brand Names: Canada Serevent® Diskhaler® Disk; Serevent® Diskus®

Pharmacologic Category Beta$_2$ Agonist; Beta$_2$-Adrenergic Agonist, Long-Acting

Use Maintenance treatment of asthma and prevention of bronchospasm (as concomitant therapy) in patients with reversible obstructive airway disease, including patients with symptoms of nocturnal asthma; prevention of exercise-induced bronchospasm (monotherapy may be indicated in patients without persistent asthma); maintenance treatment of bronchospasm associated with COPD

Local Anesthetic/Vasoconstrictor Precautions No information available to require special precautions

Effects on Dental Treatment Key adverse event(s) related to dental treatment: Xerostomia (normal salivary flow resumes upon discontinuation), dental pain, and oropharyngeal candidiasis.

Effects on Bleeding No information available to require special precautions

Adverse Effects

>10%:
Central nervous system: Headache (13% to 17%)
Neuromuscular & skeletal: Pain (1% to 12%)

1% to 10%:
Cardiovascular: Hypertension (4%), edema (1% to 3%), pallor
Central nervous system: Dizziness (4%), sleep disturbance (1% to 3%), fever (1% to 3%), anxiety (1% to 3%), migraine (1% to 3%)
Dermatologic: Rash (1% to 4%), contact dermatitis (1% to 3%), eczema (1% to 3%), urticaria (3%), photodermatitis (1% to 2%)
Endocrine & metabolic: Hyperglycemia (1% to 3%)
Gastrointestinal: Throat irritation (7%), nausea (1% to 3%), dyspepsia (1% to 3%), dental pain (1% to 3%), gastrointestinal infection (1% to 3%), oropharyngeal candidiasis (1% to 3%), xerostomia (1% to 3%)
Hepatic: Liver enzymes increased
Neuromuscular & skeletal: Muscular cramps/spasm (3%), articular rheumatism (1% to 3%), arthralgia (1% to 3%), joint pain (1% to 3%), muscular stiffness (1% to 3%), paresthesia (1% to 3%), rigidity (1% to 3%)
Ocular: Keratitis/conjunctivitis (1% to 3%)
Respiratory: Nasal congestion (4% to 9%), tracheitis/bronchitis (7%), pharyngitis (≤6%), cough (5%), influenza (5%), viral respiratory tract infection (5%), sinusitis (4% to 5%), rhinitis (4% to 5%), asthma (3% to 4%)

General Dosage Range Inhalation: *Children ≥4 years and Adults:* 1 inhalation (50 mcg) twice daily

Mechanism of Action Relaxes bronchial smooth muscle by selective action on beta$_2$-receptors with little effect on heart rate; salmeterol acts locally in the lung.

Pharmacodynamics/Kinetics
Onset of Action Asthma: 30-48 minutes, COPD: 2 hours; Peak effect: Asthma: 3 hours, COPD: 2-5 hours
Duration of Action 12 hours

Half-life Elimination 5.5 hours
Time to Peak Serum: ~20 minutes
Pregnancy Risk Factor C
Pregnancy Considerations Animal studies have demonstrated (dose-dependent) teratogenicity. There are no adequate and well-controlled studies in pregnant women. Beta-agonists may interfere with uterine contractility if administered during labor. Use only if clearly needed.

Salsalate (SAL sa late)

Related Information
Temporomandibular Dysfunction (TMD), Chronic Pain, and Fibromyalgia *on page 1590*

Brand Names: Canada Amigesic®; Salflex®

Generic Availability (U.S.) Yes

Pharmacologic Category Salicylate

Use Treatment of rheumatoid arthritis, osteoarthritis, and related rheumatic disorders

Local Anesthetic/Vasoconstrictor Precautions No information available to require special precautions

Effects on Dental Treatment The dentist should be aware of the potential of abnormal coagulation. Caution should also be exercised in the use of NSAIDs in patients already on anticoagulant therapy with drugs such as warfarin (Coumadin®). See Effects on Bleeding.

Effects on Bleeding Nonacetylated salicylate formulations are known to reversibly decrease platelet aggregation via mechanisms different than observed with aspirin. Caution should also be exercised in the use of NSAIDs in patients already on anticoagulant therapy with drugs such as warfarin (Coumadin®). Unlike most salicylates/NSAIDs, salsalate does not interfere with platelet aggregation and presumably carries less risk of bleeding and/or effect on concurrent warfarin therapy.

With respect to surgery, dental practitioners should note that recommendations differ between general surgery (eg, appendectomy, hip replacement) and dental surgery. NSAIDs should be avoided (if possible) in general surgery patients for 3-5 half-lives of the drug (usually 1-3 days) prior to surgery to reduce the risk of excessive bleeding. However, there is no scientific evidence to warrant discontinuance of NSAIDs prior to dental surgery. In medically complicated patients or extensive oral surgery, the decision to interrupt therapy must be based on the risk to benefit in an individual patient and a medical consult is suggested. Routine interruption of NSAID therapy for most dental procedures is not warranted. If therapy is continued without interruption, the clinician should anticipate the potential for slower clotting times.

Adverse Effects Frequency not defined.
Cardiovascular: Hypotension
Central nervous system: Vertigo
Dermatologic: Angioedema, rash, Stevens-Johnson syndrome, toxic epidermal necrolysis, urticaria
Gastrointestinal: Abdominal pain, diarrhea, GI bleeding, GI perforation, GI ulceration, nausea
Hematologic: Anemia
Hepatic: Hepatitis, liver function abnormal
Otic: Hearing impairment, tinnitus
Renal: Creatinine clearance decreased, nephritis
Respiratory: Bronchospasm
Miscellaneous: Anaphylactic shock

◀ **Dosage** Oral:
Adults: 3 g/day in 2-3 divided dose
Elderly: May require lower dosage

Mechanism of Action Weakly inhibits cyclooxygenase enzymes, which results in decreased formation of prostaglandin precursors; has antipyretic, analgesic, and anti-inflammatory properties

Other proposed mechanisms not fully elucidated (and possibly contributing to the anti-inflammatory effect to varying degrees) include inhibiting chemotaxis, altering lymphocyte activity, inhibiting neutrophil aggregation/activation, and decreasing proinflammatory cytokine levels.

Contraindications Hypersensitivity to salsalate or any component of the formulation; asthma, urticaria, or allergic reaction to aspirin or NSAIDs; perioperative pain in the setting of coronary artery bypass graft (CABG) surgery

Warnings/Precautions [U.S. Boxed Warning]: NSAIDs are associated with an increased risk of adverse cardiovascular thrombotic events, including fatal MI and stroke. Risk may be increased with duration of use or pre-existing cardiovascular risk factors or disease. Carefully evaluate individual cardiovascular risk profiles prior to prescribing. May cause new-onset hypertension or worsening of existing hypertension. Response to ACE inhibitors, thiazides, or loop diuretics may be impaired with concurrent use of NSAIDs. Use caution with fluid retention. Avoid use in heart failure. Concurrent administration of salsalate, and potentially other nonselective NSAIDs, may interfere with aspirin's cardioprotective effect. **[U.S. Boxed Warning]: Use is contraindicated for treatment of perioperative pain in the setting of coronary artery bypass graft (CABG) surgery.** Risk of MI and stroke may be increased with use following CABG surgery. Use the lowest effective dose for the shortest duration of time, consistent with individual patient goals, to reduce risk of cardiovascular or GI adverse events. Alternate therapies should be considered for patients at high risk.

NSAID use may compromise existing renal function; dose-dependent decreases in prostaglandin synthesis may result from NSAID use, reducing renal blood flow which may cause renal decompensation. Patients with impaired renal function, dehydration, heart failure, liver dysfunction, those taking diuretics, and ACE inhibitors, and the elderly are at greater risk of renal toxicity. Rehydrate patient before starting therapy; monitor renal function closely. Not recommended for use in patients with advanced renal disease. Long-term NSAID use may result in renal papillary necrosis.

[U.S. Boxed Warning]: NSAIDs may increase risk of gastrointestinal irritation, inflammation, ulceration, bleeding, and perforation. These events may occur at any time during therapy and without warning. Use caution with a history of GI disease (bleeding or ulcers), concurrent therapy with aspirin, anticoagulants and/or corticosteroids, smoking, use of ethanol, the elderly or debilitated patients. When used concomitantly with ≤325 mg of aspirin, a substantial increase in the risk of gastrointestinal complications (eg, ulcer) occurs; concomitant gastroprotective therapy (eg, proton pump inhibitors) is recommended (Bhatt, 2008).

Use with caution in patients with platelet and bleeding disorders.

NSAIDs may cause serious skin adverse events including exfoliative dermatitis, Stevens-Johnson Syndrome (SJS) and toxic epidermal necrolysis (TEN); discontinue use at first sign of skin rash or hypersensitivity. Patients with sensitivity to tartrazine dyes, nasal polyps, and asthma may have an increased risk of salicylate sensitivity. Anaphylactoid reactions may occur, even without prior exposure; patients with "aspirin triad" (bronchial asthma, aspirin intolerance, rhinitis) may be at increased risk. Do not use in patients who experience bronchospasm, asthma, rhinitis, or urticaria with NSAID or aspirin therapy. Use caution in other forms of asthma.

Use with caution in patients with decreased hepatic function. Closely monitor patients with any abnormal LFT. Severe hepatic reactions (eg, fulminant hepatitis, liver failure) have occurred with NSAID use, rarely; discontinue if signs or symptoms of liver disease develop, or if systemic manifestations occur.

Children and teenagers who have or are recovering from chickenpox or flu-like symptoms should not use this product. Changes in behavior (along with nausea and vomiting) may be an early sign of Reye's syndrome; patients should be instructed to contact their healthcare provider if these occur.

Drug Interactions

Metabolism/Transport Effects None known.

Avoid Concomitant Use

Avoid concomitant use of Salsalate with any of the following: Influenza Virus Vaccine (Live/Attenuated)

Increased Effect/Toxicity

Salsalate may increase the levels/effects of: Anticoagulants; Carbonic Anhydrase Inhibitors; Corticosteroids (Systemic); Divalproex; Drotrecogin Alfa (Activated); Hypoglycemic Agents; Methotrexate; PRALAtrexate; Salicylates; Thrombolytic Agents; Valproic Acid; Varicella Virus-Containing Vaccines

The levels/effects of Salsalate may be increased by: Agents with Antiplatelet Properties; Ammonium Chloride; Calcium Channel Blockers (Nondihydropyridine); Ginkgo Biloba; Herbs (Anticoagulant/Antiplatelet Properties); Influenza Virus Vaccine (Live/Attenuated); Loop Diuretics; NSAID (Nonselective); Potassium Acid Phosphate; Treprostinil

Decreased Effect

Salsalate may decrease the levels/effects of: ACE Inhibitors; Hyaluronidase; Loop Diuretics; NSAID (Nonselective); Probenecid

The levels/effects of Salsalate may be decreased by: Corticosteroids (Systemic); NSAID (Nonselective)

Ethanol/Nutrition/Herb Interactions

Ethanol: Avoid ethanol (may enhance gastric mucosal irritation).

Food: Salsalate peak serum levels may be delayed if taken with food.

Herb/Nutraceutical: Avoid cat's claw, dong quai, evening primrose, feverfew, garlic, ginger, ginkgo, red clover, horse chestnut, green tea, ginseng (all have additional antiplatelet activity).

Dietary Considerations May be taken with food to decrease GI distress.

Pharmacodynamics/Kinetics

Onset of Action Therapeutic: 3-4 days of continuous dosing

Half-life Elimination 7-8 hours

Pregnancy Risk Factor C

Pregnancy Considerations Adverse events have not been observed in animal reproduction studies. Due to the known effects of salicylates (closure of ductus arteriosus), use during late pregnancy should be avoided.

Lactation Enters breast milk/use caution

Breast-Feeding Considerations Salsalate is metabolized to salicylic acid which is excreted in breast milk in concentrations equivalent to maternal blood concentrations. An infant may ingest up to 80% per kg body weight as the mother is taking.

Dosage Forms
Tablet, oral: 500 mg, 750 mg

Sapropterin (sap roe TER in)

Brand Names: U.S. Kuvan™
Pharmacologic Category Enzyme Cofactor
Use Adjunct to dietary management in the treatment of tetrahydrobiopterin (BH4) responsive phenylketonuria (PKU)

Local Anesthetic/Vasoconstrictor Precautions No information available to require special precautions

Effects on Dental Treatment No significant effects or complications reported

Effects on Bleeding No information available to require special precautions

Adverse Effects
>10%:
Central nervous system: Headache (15%)
Respiratory: Rhinorrhea (11%)
1% to 10%:
Gastrointestinal: Diarrhea (8%), vomiting (8%), nausea
Dermatologic: Bruising (5%)
Hematologic: Neutropenia (4%)
Respiratory: Pharyngolaryngeal pain (10%), cough (7%), nasal congestion (4%)

General Dosage Range Oral: *Children ≥4 years and Adults:* 10 mg/kg once daily; Maintenance range: 5-20 mg/kg/day

Mechanism of Action Sapropterin is a synthetic form of the cofactor BH4 (tetrahydrobiopterin) for the enzyme phenylalanine hydroxylase (PAH). PAH hydroxylates phenylalanine to form tyrosine. BH4 activates residual PAH enzyme, improving normal phenylalanine metabolism and decreasing phenylalanine levels in sapropterin responders.

Pharmacodynamics/Kinetics
Onset of Action Within 24 hours; maximum effect: 1-2 months
Duration of Action 24 hours
Half-life Elimination ~7 hours (range: 4-17 hours)

Pregnancy Risk Factor C

Pregnancy Considerations Statistically significant teratogenic effects were not observed in animal studies; however, there are no adequate and well-controlled studies in pregnant women. High levels of maternal phenylalanine are associated with congenital heart disease, developmental delay, facial dysmorphism, learning difficulties, and microcephaly. Phenylalanine concentrations should be normalized prior to conception and dietary control with proper supplementation are recommended during pregnancy. Some clinicians recommend that dietary control be achieved for at least 4 weeks prior to conception; however, studies suggest that as long as control is achieved by 10 weeks of pregnancy, teratogenic effects of untreated maternal phenylketonuria can be decreased. The effects of sapropterin on pregnancy have not been determined.

Pregnant women exposed to sapropterin are encouraged to enroll in the Kuvan™ pregnancy registry.

Saquinavir (sa KWIN a veer)

Related Information
Clinical Risk Related to Drugs Prolonging QT Interval *on page 1510*
HIV Infection and AIDS *on page 1520*
Brand Names: U.S. Invirase®
Brand Names: Canada Invirase®
Pharmacologic Category Antiretroviral Agent, Protease Inhibitor
Use Treatment of HIV infection; used in combination with ritonavir and other antiretroviral agents

Local Anesthetic/Vasoconstrictor Precautions Saquinavir is one of the drugs confirmed to prolong the QT interval and is accepted as having a risk of causing torsade de pointes. The risk of drug-induced torsade de pointes is extremely low when a single QT interval prolonging drug is prescribed. In terms of epinephrine, it is not known what effect vasoconstrictors in the local anesthetic regimen will have in patients with a known history of congenital prolonged QT interval or in patients taking any medication that prolongs the QT interval. Until more information is obtained, it is suggested that the clinician consult with the physician prior to the use of a vasoconstrictor in suspected patients, and that the vasoconstrictor (epinephrine, mepivacaine and levonordefrin [Carbocaine® 2% with Neo-Cobefrin®]) be used with caution.

Effects on Dental Treatment Key adverse event(s) related to dental treatment: Buccal mucosa ulceration and taste alteration.

Effects on Bleeding Increased bleeding has been noted with protease inhibitors in patients with hemophilia A or B. No information available to require routine special precautions relative to hemostasis in other patients.

Adverse Effects
Incidence data shown for saquinavir soft gel capsule formulation (no longer available) in combination with ritonavir.
10%: Gastrointestinal: Nausea (11%)
1% to 10%:
Cardiovascular: Chest pain
Central nervous system: Fatigue (6%), fever (3%), anxiety, depression, headache, insomnia, pain
Dermatologic: Pruritus (3%), rash (3%), dry lips/skin (2%), eczema (2%), verruca
Endocrine & metabolic: Lipodystrophy (5%), hyperglycemia (3%), hypoglycemia, hyperkalemia, libido disorder, serum amylase increased
Gastrointestinal: Diarrhea (8%), vomiting (7%), abdominal pain (6%), constipation (2%), abdominal discomfort, appetite decreased, buccal mucosa ulceration, dyspepsia, flatulence, taste alteration
Hepatic: AST increased, ALT increased, bilirubin increased
Neuromuscular & skeletal: Back pain (2%), CPK increased, paresthesia, weakness
Renal: Creatinine kinase increased
Respiratory: Pneumonia (5%), bronchitis (3%), sinusitis (3%)
Miscellaneous: Influenza (3%)

◄ **Incidence not currently defined (limited to significant reactions; reported for hard or soft gel capsule with/without ritonavir)**

Cardiovascular: Cyanosis, heart valve disorder (including murmur), hyper-/hypotension, peripheral vasoconstriction, prolonged QT interval, prolonged PR interval, syncope, thrombophlebitis

Central nervous system: Agitation, amnesia, ataxia, confusion, hallucination, hyper-/hyporeflexia, myelopolyradiculoneuritis, neuropathies, poliomyelitis, progressive multifocal encephalopathy, psychosis, seizures, somnolence, speech disorder, suicide attempt

Dermatologic: Alopecia, bullous eruption, dermatitis, erythema, maculopapular rash, photosensitivity, Stevens-Johnson syndrome, skin ulceration, urticaria

Endocrine & metabolic: Dehydration, diabetes, electrolyte changes, TSH increased

Gastrointestinal: Ascites, colic, dysphagia, esophagitis, bloody stools, gastritis, intestinal obstruction, hemorrhage (rectal), pancreatitis, stomatitis

Genitourinary: impotence, prostate enlarged, hematuria, UTI

Hematologic; Acute myeloblastic leukemia, anemia (including hemolytic), leukopenia, neutropenia, pancytopenia, splenomegaly, thrombocytopenia

Hepatic: Alkaline phosphatase increased, GGT increased, hepatitis, hepatomegaly, hepatosplenomegaly, jaundice, liver disease exacerbation

Neuromuscular & skeletal: Arthritis, LDH increased

Ocular: Blepharitis, visual disturbance

Otic: Otitis, hearing decreased, tinnitus

Renal: Nephrolithiasis, renal calculus

Respiratory: Dyspnea, hemoptysis, pharyngitis, upper respiratory tract infection

Miscellaneous: Immune reconstitution syndrome, infections (bacterial, fungal, viral)

General Dosage Range Dosage adjustment recommended in patients on concomitant therapy

Oral: *Children >16 years and Adults:* 1000 mg twice daily

Mechanism of Action Binds to the site of HIV-1 protease activity and inhibits cleavage of viral Gag-Pol polyprotein precursors into individual functional proteins required for infectious HIV. This results in the formation of immature, noninfectious viral particles.

Pregnancy Risk Factor B

Pregnancy Considerations Adverse events were not observed in animal reproduction studies. Saquinavir crosses the human placenta in minimal amounts. Based on limited data, saquinavir administered twice daily with ritonavir 100 mg twice daily provide adequate levels in pregnant women. The DHHS Perinatal HIV Guidelines consider saquinavir and ritonavir to be an alternative combination for use during pregnancy; use without ritonavir is **not** recommended. A small increased risk of preterm birth has been associated with maternal use of protease inhibitor-based combination antiretroviral (ARV) therapy during pregnancy; however, the benefits of use generally outweigh this risk and protease inhibitors (PIs) should not be withheld if otherwise recommended. Hyperglycemia, new onset of diabetes mellitus, or diabetic ketoacidosis have been reported with PIs; it is not clear if pregnancy increases this risk.

Regardless of CD4 count or HIV RNA copy number, all HIV-infected pregnant women should receive a combination antepartum ARV drug regimen; this includes women who require therapy for their own health, as well as women who do not yet require therapy for their own health. ARV therapy should be started as soon as

possible if required for the woman's health. Although earlier initiation may be more effective in reducing the perinatal transmission of HIV, also consider maternal conditions (eg, nausea and vomiting) and the potential risks of first trimester fetal exposure for specific agents. Plasma HIV RNA levels should be assessed at ~34-36 weeks gestation in order to help determine mode of delivery. If ARV therapy must be interrupted for <24 hours during the peripartum period, stop then restart all medications simultaneously in order to decrease the chance of developing resistance. Long-term follow-up is recommended for all infants exposed to ARV medications.

Healthcare providers are encouraged to enroll pregnant women exposed to antiretroviral medications in the Antiretroviral Pregnancy Registry (1-800-258-4263 or www.APRegistry.com). Healthcare providers caring for HIV-infected women and their infants may contact the National Perinatal HIV Hotline (888-448-8765) for clinical consultation (DHHS [perinatal], 2012).

Dental Comment Saquinavir is known to prolong the QT interval. The QT interval is measured as the time and distance between the Q point of the QRS complex and the end of the T wave in the ECG tracing. After adjustment for heart rate, the QT interval is defined as prolonged if it is more than 450 msec in men and 460 msec in women. A long QT syndrome was first described in the 1950s and 60s as a congenital syndrome involving QT interval prolongation and syncope and sudden death. Some of the congenital long QT syndromes were characterized by a peculiar electrocardiographic appearance of the QRS complex involving a premature atria beat followed by a pause, then a subsequent sinus beat showing marked QT prolongation and deformity. This type of cardiac arrhythmia was originally termed "torsade de pointes" (translated from the French as "twisting of the points"). Saquinavir is considered as having a risk of causing torsade de pointes. Since it is not known what effect vasoconstrictors in the local anesthetic regimen will have in patients with a known history of congenital prolonged QT interval or in patients taking any medication that prolongs the QT interval, a medical consult is suggested.

Sargramostim (sar GRAM oh stim)

Brand Names: U.S. Leukine®
Brand Names: Canada Leukine®
Pharmacologic Category Colony Stimulating Factor
Use

Acute myelogenous leukemia (AML) following induction chemotherapy in older adults (≥55 years of age) to shorten time to neutrophil recovery and to reduce the incidence of severe and life-threatening infections and infections resulting in death

Bone marrow transplant (allogeneic or autologous) failure or engraftment delay

Myeloid reconstitution after allogeneic bone marrow transplantation

Myeloid reconstitution after autologous bone marrow transplantation: Non-Hodgkin's lymphoma (NHL), acute lymphoblastic leukemia (ALL), Hodgkin's lymphoma

Peripheral stem cell transplantation: Mobilization and myeloid reconstitution following autologous peripheral stem cell transplantation

Local Anesthetic/Vasoconstrictor Precautions No information available to require special precautions

Effects on Dental Treatment Key adverse event(s) related to dental treatment: Dysphagia.

Effects on Bleeding No information available to require special precautions. Medical consultation may be considered to confirm adequate platelet counts.

Adverse Effects

>10%:

Cardiovascular: Hypertension (34%), pericardial effusion (4% to 25%), edema (13% to 25%), chest pain (15%), peripheral edema (11%), tachycardia (11%)

Central nervous system: Fever (81%), malaise (57%), headache (26%), chills (25%), anxiety (11%), insomnia (11%)

Dermatologic: Rash (44%), pruritus (23%)

Endocrine & metabolic: Hyperglycemia (25%), hypercholesterolemia (17%), hypomagnesemia (15%)

Gastrointestinal: Diarrhea (≤89%), nausea (58% to 70%), vomiting (46% to 70%), abdominal pain (38%), weight loss (37%), anorexia (13%), hematemesis (13%), dysphagia (11%), gastrointestinal hemorrhage (11%)

Genitourinary: Urinary tract disorder (14%)

Hepatic: Hyperbilirubinemia (30%)

Neuromuscular & skeletal: Weakness (66%), bone pain (21%), arthralgia (11% to 21%) myalgia (18%)

Ocular: Eye hemorrhage (11%)

Renal: BUN increased (23%), serum creatinine increased (15%)

Respiratory: Pharyngitis (23%), epistaxis (17%), dyspnea (15%)

1% to 10%: Respiratory: Pleural effusion (1%)

General Dosage Range

I.V.: *Children and Adults:* Infusion: 250 mcg/m²/day (maximum: 500 mcg/m²/day)

SubQ: *Children and Adults:* 250 mcg/m² once daily

Mechanism of Action Stimulates proliferation, differentiation and functional activity of neutrophils, eosinophils, monocytes, and macrophages, as indicated.

Pharmacodynamics/Kinetics

Onset of Action Increase in WBC: 7-14 days

Duration of Action WBCs return to baseline within 1 week of discontinuing drug

Half-life Elimination I.V.: 60 minutes; SubQ: 2.7 hours

Time to Peak Serum: SubQ: 1-3 hours

Pregnancy Risk Factor C

Pregnancy Considerations Clinical effects to the fetus: Animal reproduction studies have not been conducted. It is not known whether sargramostim can cause fetal harm when administered to a pregnant woman or can affect reproductive capability. Sargramostim should be given to a pregnant woman only if clearly needed.

Saxagliptin (sax a GLIP tin)

Related Information

Endocrine Disorders and Pregnancy *on page 1517*

Brand Names: U.S. Onglyza™

Brand Names: Canada Onglyza™

Generic Availability (U.S.) No

Pharmacologic Category Antidiabetic Agent, Dipeptidyl Peptidase IV (DPP-IV) Inhibitor

Use Treatment of type 2 diabetes mellitus (noninsulin dependent, NIDDM) as an adjunct to diet and exercise as monotherapy or in combination therapy with other antidiabetic agents to improve glycemic control

Local Anesthetic/Vasoconstrictor Precautions No information available to require special precautions

Effects on Dental Treatment Key adverse event(s) related to dental treatment: Saxagliptin dependent patients with diabetes should be appointed for dental treatment in the morning in order to minimize chance of stress-induced hypoglycemia.

Effects on Bleeding No information available to require special precautions

Adverse Effects Note: Frequencies and adverse reactions reported with monotherapy unless otherwise noted.

1% to 10%:

Cardiovascular: Peripheral edema (≤4%; incidence increased in conjunction with thiazolidinediones: ≤8%)

Central nervous system: Headache (7%)

Endocrine & metabolic: Hypoglycemia (≤6%; incidence increased in conjunction with insulin secretagogues: ≤15%)

Gastrointestinal: Abdominal pain (2%), gastroenteritis (2%), vomiting (2%)

Genitourinary: Urinary tract infection (7%)

Hematologic: Lymphopenia (≤2%; dose related)

Respiratory: Sinusitis (3%)

Miscellaneous: Hypersensitivity reactions (2%; including urticaria and facial edema)

Dosage Oral: Adults: Type 2 diabetes: 2.5-5 mg once daily

Concomitant use with strong CYP3A4/5 inhibitors: 2.5 mg once daily

Concomitant use with insulin or insulin secretagogues: Reduced dose of insulin or insulin secretagogues (eg, sulfonylureas) may be needed

Dosage adjustment in renal impairment:

Note: Renal function may be estimated using the Cockcroft-Gault formula or the MDRD formula for dosage adjustment purposes.

Cl_{cr} >50 mL/minute: No dosage adjustment necessary

Cl_{cr} ≤50 mL/minute: 2.5 mg once daily

ESRD requiring hemodialysis:

U.S. labeling: 2.5 mg once daily; administer post-dialysis

Canadian labeling: Use is not recommended.

Peritoneal dialysis: Not studied

Dosage adjustment in hepatic impairment:

U.S. labeling: Mild-to-severe impairment: No dosage adjustment necessary.

Canadian labeling:

Mild impairment: No dosage adjustment provided in manufacturer's labeling.

Moderate-to-severe impairment: Use is not recommended.

Mechanism of Action Saxagliptin inhibits dipeptidyl peptidase IV (DPP-IV) enzyme resulting in prolonged active incretin levels. Incretin hormones (eg, glucagon-like peptide-1 [GLP-1] and glucose-dependent insulinotropic polypeptide [GIP]) regulate glucose homeostasis by increasing insulin synthesis and release from pancreatic beta cells and decreasing glucagon secretion from pancreatic alpha cells. Decreased glucagon secretion results in decreased hepatic glucose production. Under normal physiologic circumstances, incretin hormones are released by the intestine throughout the day and levels are increased in response to a meal; incretin hormones are rapidly inactivated by the DPP-IV enzyme.

Contraindications Hypersensitivity to saxagliptin or any component of the formulation

◄ Canadian labeling: Additional contraindications (not in U.S. labeling): Diabetic ketoacidosis, diabetic coma/precoma, type 1 diabetes mellitus

Warnings/Precautions Use with caution in patients with moderate-to-severe renal dysfunction, end-stage renal disease (ESRD) requiring hemodialysis, and in patients taking strong CYP3A4/5 inhibitors (eg, atazanavir, clarithromycin, indinavir, itraconazole, nefazodone, nelfinavir, ritonavir, saquinavir, telithromycin [also see Drug Interactions]); dosing adjustment required. Clinical trials included only a limited number of patients with heart failure (HF). No specific recommendations regarding this population are provided in the U.S. manufacturer labeling (Canadian labeling recommends against use in this population). Use caution when used in conjunction with insulin or insulin secretagogues (eg, sulfonylureas); risk of hypoglycemia is increased. Monitor blood glucose closely; dosage adjustments of insulin or the insulin secretagogue may be necessary. Rare hypersensitivity reactions, including anaphylaxis, angioedema, and/or exfoliative dermatologic reactions have been reported; discontinue if signs/symptoms of severe hypersensitivity reactions occur. Cases of acute pancreatitis have been reported; discontinue immediately if suspected. Contains lactose; Canadian labeling recommends avoiding use in patients with galactose intolerance, Lapp lactase deficiency, or glucose-galactose malabsorption syndromes.

Drug Interactions

Metabolism/Transport Effects Substrate of CYP3A4 (major), P-glycoprotein; **Note:** Assignment of Major/Minor substrate status based on clinically relevant drug interaction potential

Avoid Concomitant Use There are no known interactions where it is recommended to avoid concomitant use.

Increased Effect/Toxicity

Saxagliptin may increase the levels/effects of: ACE Inhibitors; Hypoglycemic Agents

The levels/effects of Saxagliptin may be increased by: CYP3A4 Inhibitors (Moderate); CYP3A4 Inhibitors (Strong); Dasatinib; Herbs (Hypoglycemic Properties); Ivacaftor; MAO Inhibitors; Mifepristone; Pegvisomant; P-glycoprotein/ABCB1 Inhibitors; Salicylates; Selective Serotonin Reuptake Inhibitors

Decreased Effect

The levels/effects of Saxagliptin may be decreased by: Corticosteroids (Orally Inhaled); Corticosteroids (Systemic); CYP3A4 Inducers; Loop Diuretics; Luteinizing Hormone-Releasing Hormone Analogs; P-glycoprotein/ABCB1 Inducers; Somatropin; Thiazide Diuretics

Dietary Considerations May be taken without regard to meals. Individualized medical nutrition therapy (MNT) is an integral part of therapy (ADA, 2013).

Pharmacodynamics/Kinetics

Duration of Action 24 hours

Half-life Elimination Saxagliptin: 2.5 hours; 5-hydroxy saxagliptin: 3.1 hours

Time to Peak Plasma: Saxagliptin: 2 hours; 5-hydroxy saxagliptin: 4 hours

Pregnancy Risk Factor B

Pregnancy Considerations Teratogenic effects were not observed in animal studies. However, there are no adequate and well-controlled studies in pregnant women.

Lactation Excretion in breast milk unknown/use caution

Breast-Feeding Considerations It is not known if saxagliptin is excreted in breast milk. The manufacturer recommends that caution be exercised when administering saxagliptin to nursing women.

Dosage Forms

Tablet, oral:

Onglyza™: 2.5 mg, 5 mg

Saxagliptin and Metformin (sax a GLIP tin & met FOR min)

Related Information

MetFORMIN *on page 882*

Saxagliptin *on page 1225*

Brand Names: U.S. Kombiglyze™ XR

Pharmacologic Category Antidiabetic Agent, Biguanide; Antidiabetic Agent, Dipeptidyl Peptidase IV (DPP-IV) Inhibitor

Use Management of type 2 diabetes mellitus (noninsulin dependent, NIDDM) as an adjunct to diet and exercise when treatment with both saxagliptin and metformin is appropriate

Local Anesthetic/Vasoconstrictor Precautions No information available to require special precautions

Effects on Dental Treatment Key adverse event(s) related to dental treatment: Saxagliptin- and metformin-dependent patients with diabetes should be appointed for dental treatment in the morning in order to minimize chance of stress-induced hypoglycemia.

Effects on Bleeding No information available to require special precautions

Adverse Effects See individual agents.

General Dosage Range Dosage adjustment recommended in patients on concomitant therapy

Oral: *Adults:* Saxagliptin 2.5-5 mg and metformin 500-2000 mg once daily (maximum: 5 mg/day [saxagliptin], 2000 mg/day [metformin])

Mechanism of Action

Saxagliptin inhibits dipeptidyl peptidase IV (DPP-IV) enzyme resulting in prolonged active incretin levels. Incretin hormones (eg, glucagon-like peptide-1 [GLP-1] and glucose-dependent insulinotropic polypeptide [GIP]) regulate glucose homeostasis by increasing insulin synthesis and release from pancreatic beta cells and decreasing glucagon secretion from pancreatic alpha cells. Decreased glucagon secretion results in decreased hepatic glucose production. Under normal physiologic circumstances, incretin hormones are released by the intestine throughout the day and levels are increased in response to a meal; incretin hormones are rapidly inactivated by the DPP-IV enzyme.

Metformin decreases hepatic glucose production, decreasing intestinal absorption of glucose and improves insulin sensitivity (increases peripheral glucose uptake and utilization).

Pregnancy Risk Factor B

Pregnancy Considerations Reproduction studies have not been conducted with this combination. Adverse events were not observed in animal studies of the individual agents; therefore, saxagliptin/metformin is classified as pregnancy category B. See individual agents.

Scopolamine (Systemic) (skoe POL a meen)

Brand Names: U.S. Transderm Scōp®

Brand Names: Canada Buscopan®; Scopolamine Hydrobromide Injection; Transderm-V®

Pharmacologic Category Anticholinergic Agent

Use

Scopolamine base: Transdermal: Prevention of nausea/vomiting associated with motion sickness and recovery from anesthesia and surgery

Scopolamine hydrobromide: Injection: Preoperative medication to produce amnesia, sedation, tranquilization, antiemetic effects, and decrease salivary and respiratory secretions

Scopolamine butylbromide [not available in the U.S.]: Oral/injection: Treatment of smooth muscle spasm of the genitourinary or gastrointestinal tract; injection may also be used prior to radiological/diagnostic procedures to prevent spasm

Unlabeled Use Scopolamine base: Transdermal: Breakthrough treatment of nausea and vomiting associated with chemotherapy

Local Anesthetic/Vasoconstrictor Precautions No information available to require special precautions

Effects on Dental Treatment Key adverse event(s) related to dental treatment: Significant xerostomia (normal salivary flow resumes upon discontinuation), dry throat (transdermal), and dysphagia.

Effects on Bleeding No information available to require special precautions

Adverse Effects Frequency not defined.

Cardiovascular: Bradycardia, flushing, orthostatic hypotension, tachycardia

Central nervous system: Acute toxic psychosis (rare), agitation (rare), ataxia, confusion, delusion (rare), disorientation, dizziness, drowsiness, fatigue, hallucination (rare), headache, irritability, loss of memory, paranoid behavior (rare), restlessness, sedation

Dermatologic: Drug eruptions, dry skin, dyshidrosis, erythema, pruritus, rash, urticaria

Endocrine & metabolic: Thirst

Gastrointestinal: Constipation, diarrhea, dry throat, dysphagia, nausea, vomiting, xerostomia

Genitourinary: Dysuria, urinary retention

Neuromuscular & skeletal: Tremor, weakness

Ocular: Accommodation impaired, blurred vision, conjunctival infection, cycloplegia, dryness, glaucoma (narrow-angle), increased intraocular pain, itching, photophobia, pupil dilation, retinal pigmentation

Respiratory: Dry nose, dyspnea

Miscellaneous: Anaphylaxis (rare), anaphylactic shock (rare), angioedema, diaphoresis decreased, heat intolerance, hypersensitivity reactions

General Dosage Range

I.M., I.V., SubQ:

Children 6 months to 3 years: 0.1-0.15 mg

Children 3-6 years: 0.2-0.3 mg

Adults: 0.3-0.65 mg (single dose) **or** 0.6 mg 3-4 times/day

Transdermal: *Adults:* Apply 1 patch every 3 days as needed

Mechanism of Action Blocks the action of acetylcholine at parasympathetic sites in smooth muscle, secretory glands and the CNS; increases cardiac output, dries secretions, antagonizes histamine and serotonin

Pharmacodynamics/Kinetics

Onset of Action Oral, I.M.: 0.5-1 hour; I.V.: 10 minutes; Transdermal: 6-8 hours

Duration of Action I.M., I.V., SubQ: 4 hours

Half-life Elimination Butylbromide: ~5-11 hours; Hydrobromide: ~1-4 hours; Scopolamine base: 9.5 hours

Time to Peak Hydrobromide: I.M.: ~20 minutes, SubQ: ~15 minutes; Butylbromide: Oral: ~2 hours; Scopolamine base: Transdermal: 24 hours

Pregnancy Risk Factor C

Pregnancy Considerations Teratogenic effects were not observed in animal studies; embryotoxic events were observed in some studies. Scopolamine crosses the placenta; may cause respiratory depression and/or neonatal hemorrhage when used during pregnancy. Transdermal scopolamine has been used as an adjunct to epidural anesthesia for cesarean delivery without adverse CNS effects on the newborn. Parenteral administration does not increase the duration of labor or affect uterine contractions. Except when used prior to cesarean section, use during pregnancy only if the benefit to the mother outweighs the potential risk to the fetus.

Secobarbital (see koe BAR bi tal)

Brand Names: U.S. Seconal®

Pharmacologic Category Barbiturate

Use Preanesthetic agent; short-term treatment of insomnia

Local Anesthetic/Vasoconstrictor Precautions No information available to require special precautions

Effects on Dental Treatment No significant effects or complications reported

Effects on Bleeding No information available to require special precautions

Adverse Effects 1% to 10%: Central nervous system: Somnolence (1% to 3%)

General Dosage Range Oral: *Adults:* 100 mg at bedtime **or** 200-300 mg 1-2 hours before procedure

Mechanism of Action Depresses CNS activity by binding to barbiturate site at GABA-receptor complex enhancing GABA activity, depressing reticular activity system; higher doses may be gabamimetic

Pharmacodynamics/Kinetics

Onset of Action Onset of hypnosis: Oral: 10-15 minutes

Duration of Action Oral: 3-4 hours

Half-life Elimination 15-40 hours, mean: 28 hours

Pregnancy Risk Factor D

Pregnancy Considerations Barbiturates can be detected in the placenta, fetal liver, and fetal brain. Fetal and maternal blood concentrations may be similar following parenteral administration. An increased incidence of fetal abnormalities may occur following maternal use. When used during the third trimester of pregnancy, withdrawal symptoms may occur in the neonate including seizures and hyperirritability; symptoms may be delayed up to 14 days. Use during labor does not impair uterine activity; however, respiratory depression may occur in the newborn; resuscitation equipment should be available, especially for premature infants.

Controlled Substance C-II

Secretin (SEE kr tin)

Brand Names: U.S. ChiRhoStim®

Pharmacologic Category Diagnostic Agent

Use Secretin-stimulation testing to aid in diagnosis of pancreatic exocrine dysfunction; diagnosis of gastrinoma (Zollinger-Ellison syndrome); facilitation of endoscopic retrograde cholangiopancreatography (ERCP) visualization

Local Anesthetic/Vasoconstrictor Precautions No information available to require special precautions

Effects on Dental Treatment No significant effects or complications reported

Effects on Bleeding No information available to require special precautions

Adverse Effects 1% to 10%:

Cardiovascular: Flushing (1%)

Gastrointestinal: Nausea (1% to 2%), abdominal discomfort (≤1%), abdominal pain (≤1%), vomiting (≤1%)

Miscellaneous: Bleeding (sphincterectomy, 1%)

General Dosage Range I.V.: *Adults:* Test dose: 0.1 mL (0.2-0.4 mcg); Diagnostic dose: 0.2-0.4 mcg/kg

Mechanism of Action Human and porcine secretin are both synthetically derived products and are equally potent on an osmolar basis. Secretin is a hormone which is normally secreted by duodenal mucosa and upper jejunal mucosa. It increases the volume and bicarbonate content of pancreatic juice; stimulates the flow of hepatic bile with a high bicarbonate concentration; stimulates gastrin release in patients with Zollinger-Ellison syndrome.

Pharmacodynamics/Kinetics

Onset of Action Peak output of pancreatic secretions: ~30 minutes

Duration of Action Human: 1.5-2 hours; Porcine: 1-1.5 hours

Half-life Elimination Human: 45 minutes; Porcine: 27 minutes

Pregnancy Risk Factor C

Pregnancy Considerations Reproduction studies have not been conducted.

Selegiline (se LE ji leen)

Brand Names: U.S. Eldepryl®; Emsam®; Zelapar®

Brand Names: Canada Apo-Selegiline®; Gen-Selegiline; Mylan-Selegiline; Novo-Selegiline; Nu-Selegiline

Pharmacologic Category Anti-Parkinson's Agent, MAO Type B Inhibitor; Antidepressant, Monoamine Oxidase Inhibitor

Use Adjunct in the management of parkinsonian patients in which levodopa/carbidopa therapy is deteriorating (oral products); treatment of major depressive disorder (transdermal product)

Unlabeled Use Early Parkinson's disease; attention-deficit/hyperactivity disorder (ADHD)

Local Anesthetic/Vasoconstrictor Precautions Selegiline in doses of 10 mg a day or less does not inhibit type-A MAO. Therefore, there are no precautions with the use of vasoconstrictors.

Effects on Dental Treatment Key adverse event(s) related to dental treatment: Xerostomia and changes in salivation (normal salivary flow resumes upon discontinuation). Anticholinergic side effects can cause a reduction of saliva production or secretion, contributing to discomfort and dental disease (ie, caries, oral candidiasis, and periodontal disease).

Orally disintegrating tablet: Dysphagia, stomatitis, and taste perversion.

Effects on Bleeding No information available to require special precautions

Adverse Effects Unless otherwise noted, the percentage of adverse events is reported for the transdermal patch (**Note:** ODT = orally disintegrating tablet, Oral = capsule/tablet)

>10%:

Central nervous system: Headache (18%; ODT 7%; oral 4%), insomnia (12%; ODT 7%), dizziness (oral 14%; ODT 11%)

Gastrointestinal: Nausea (oral 20%; ODT 11%)

Local: Application site reaction (24%)

1% to 10%:

Cardiovascular: Hypotension (including postural 3% to 10%), palpitation (oral 2%), chest pain (≥1%; ODT 2%), hypertension (≥1%; ODT 3%), peripheral edema (≥1%)

Central nervous system: Pain (ODT 8%; oral 2%), hallucinations (oral 6%; ODT 4%), confusion (oral 6%; ODT 4%), vivid dreams (oral 4%), ataxia (ODT 3%), somnolence (ODT 3%), lethargy (oral 2%), agitation (≥1%), amnesia (≥1%), paresthesia (≥1%), thinking abnormal (≥1%), depression (<1%; ODT 2%)

Dermatologic: Rash (4%), bruising (≥1%; ODT 2%), pruritus (≥1%), acne (≥1%)

Endocrine & metabolic: Weight loss (5%; oral 2%), hypokalemia (ODT 2%), sexual side effects (≤1%)

Gastrointestinal: Diarrhea (9%; ODT 2%; oral 2%), xerostomia (8%; oral 6%; ODT 4%), stomatitis (ODT 5%), abdominal pain (oral 8%), dyspepsia (4%; ODT 5%), dysphagia (ODT 2%), dental caries (ODT 2%), constipation (≥1%; ODT 4%), flatulence (≥1%; ODT 2%), anorexia (≥1%), gastroenteritis (≥1%), taste perversion (≥1%; ODT 2%), vomiting (≥1%; ODT 3%)

Genitourinary: Urinary retention (oral 2%), dysmenorrhea (≥1%), metrorrhagia (≥1%), UTI (≥1%), urinary frequency (≥1%)

Neuromuscular & skeletal: Dyskinesia (ODT 6%), back pain (ODT 5%; oral 2%), ataxia (<1%; ODT 3%), leg cramps (ODT 3%; oral 2%), myalgia (≥1%; ODT 3%), neck pain (≥1%), tremor (<1%; ODT 3%)

Otic: Tinnitus (≥1%)

Respiratory: Rhinitis (ODT 7%), pharyngitis (3%; ODT 4%), sinusitis (3%), cough (≥1%), bronchitis (≥1%), dyspnea (<1%; ODT 3%)

Miscellaneous: Diaphoresis (≥1%)

General Dosage Range

Oral:

Capsule/Tablet: *Adults:* 5 mg twice daily

Disintegrating tablet: *Adults:* Initial: 1.25 mg daily; Maintenance: 1.25-2.5 mg daily (maximum: 2.5 mg daily)

Transdermal:

Adults: Initial: 6 mg once daily; Maintenance: 6-12 mg once daily (maximum: 12 mg/day)

Elderly: 6 mg once daily

Mechanism of Action Potent, irreversible inhibitor of monoamine oxidase (MAO). Plasma concentrations achieved via administration of oral dosage forms in recommended doses confer selective inhibition of MAO type B, which plays a major role in the metabolism of dopamine; selegiline may also increase dopaminergic activity by interfering with dopamine reuptake at the synapse. When administered transdermally in recommended doses, selegiline achieves higher blood levels and effectively inhibits both MAO-A and MAO-B, which blocks catabolism of other centrally-active biogenic amine neurotransmitters.

Pharmacodynamics/Kinetics

Onset of Action Therapeutic: Oral: Within 1 hour

Duration of Action Oral: 24-72 hours

Half-life Elimination 18-25 hours

Pregnancy Risk Factor C

Pregnancy Considerations Teratogenic and adverse behavioral events were noted in animal studies. There are no adequate and well-controlled studies in pregnant women.

Selenium (se LEE nee um)

Related Information

Trace Elements *on page 1345*

Brand Names: U.S. SE Aspartate [OTC]; Se-100 [OTC]; Selenicaps; Selenimin

Pharmacologic Category Trace Element, Parenteral

Use Trace metal supplement

Local Anesthetic/Vasoconstrictor Precautions No information available to require special precautions

Effects on Dental Treatment No significant effects or complications reported

Effects on Bleeding No information available to require special precautions

Adverse Effects Frequency not defined: Local: Irritation

General Dosage Range

I.V.:

Children: 3 mcg/kg/day added to TPN

Adults: Metabolically stable: 20-40 mcg/day added to TPN; Deficiency from prolonged TPN support: 100 mcg/day

Oral:

Children: Adequate intake: 1-6 months: 15 mcg/day, 7-12 months: 20 mcg/day; Recommended daily allowance: 1-3 years: 20 mcg/day, 4-8 years: 30 mcg/day, 9-13 years 40 mcg/day, ≥14 years

Adults: Recommended daily allowance: 55 mcg/day; Pregnancy: 60 mcg/day; Lactation: 70 mcg/day

Mechanism of Action Part of glutathione peroxidase which protects cell components from oxidative damage due to peroxidases produced in cellular metabolism

Pregnancy Risk Factor C

Pregnancy Considerations Adverse events were seen with high doses in animal studies. Selenium is found in the placenta and cord blood. Teratogenic effects have not been observed with nontoxic doses in humans (IOM, 2000).

Senna (SEN na)

Brand Names: U.S. Black Draught® [OTC]; Evac-U-Gen® [OTC]; ex-lax® Maximum Strength [OTC]; ex-lax® [OTC]; Fleet® Pedia-Lax™ Quick Dissolve [OTC]; Fletcher's® [OTC]; Geri-kot [OTC]; Little Tummys® Laxative [OTC]; Perdiem® Overnight Relief [OTC]; Senexon® [OTC]; Senna-Lax [OTC]; SennaGen [OTC]; Senokot® [OTC]

Pharmacologic Category Laxative, Stimulant

Use Short-term treatment of constipation; evacuate the colon for bowel or rectal examinations

Local Anesthetic/Vasoconstrictor Precautions No information available to require special precautions

Effects on Dental Treatment No significant effects or complications reported

Effects on Bleeding No information available to require special precautions

Adverse Effects Frequency not defined: Gastrointestinal: Abdominal cramps, diarrhea, nausea, vomiting

General Dosage Range Oral:

Children 2-6 years: Initial: 3.75 mg once daily; Maintenance: 3.75-15 mg/day in 1-2 divided doses (maximum: 15 mg/day) **or** 5-10 mL (33.3 mg/mL) up to twice daily

Children 6-12 years: Initial: 8.6 mg once daily; Maintenance: 8.6-50 mg/day in 1-2 divided doses (maximum: 50 mg/day) **or** 10-30 mL (33.3 mg/mL) up to twice daily

Children ≥12 years and Adults: Initial: 15 mg once daily; Maintenance: 15-100 mg/day in 1-2 divided doses (maximum: 100 mg/day) **or** 130 mg as a single dose

Pregnancy Considerations An increased risk of congenital abnormalities was not observed following maternal use of senna during pregnancy (Acs, 2009). Short-term use of senna is generally considered safe during pregnancy (Mahadevan, 2006).

Sertaconazole (ser ta KOE na zole)

Brand Names: U.S. Ertaczo®

Pharmacologic Category Antifungal Agent, Topical

Use Topical treatment of tinea pedis (athlete's foot)

Local Anesthetic/Vasoconstrictor Precautions No information available to require special precautions

Effects on Dental Treatment No significant effects or complications reported

Effects on Bleeding No information available to require special precautions

Adverse Effects 1% to 10%: Dermatologic: Burning, contact dermatitis, dry skin, tenderness

General Dosage Range Topical: *Children ≥12 years and Adults:* Apply twice daily

Mechanism of Action Alters fungal cell wall membrane permeability; inhibits the CYP450-dependent synthesis of ergosterol

Pregnancy Risk Factor C

Pregnancy Considerations Adverse events were not observed in animal reproduction studies following oral administration. No studies have been conducted using the topical formulation on pregnant women.

Sertraline (SER tra leen)

Related Information

Management of the Patient With Anxiety or Depression *on page 1594*

Vasoconstrictor Interactions With Antidepressants *on page 1650*

Brand Names: U.S. Zoloft®

Brand Names: Canada Apo-Sertraline®; CO Sertraline; Dom-Sertraline; GD-Sertraline; Mylan-Sertraline; Nu-Sertraline; PHL-Sertraline; PMS-Sertraline; ratio-Sertraline; Riva-Sertraline; Sandoz-Sertraline; Teva-Sertraline; Zoloft®

Generic Availability (U.S.) Yes

Pharmacologic Category Antidepressant, Selective Serotonin Reuptake Inhibitor

Use Treatment of major depression; obsessive-compulsive disorder (OCD); panic disorder; post-traumatic stress disorder (PTSD); premenstrual dysphoric disorder (PMDD); social anxiety disorder

Unlabeled Use Eating disorders; generalized anxiety disorder (GAD); impulse control disorders; treatment of mild dementia-associated agitation in nonpsychotic patients; treatment of paraphilia/hypersexuality

Local Anesthetic/Vasoconstrictor Precautions Although caution should be used in patients taking tricyclic antidepressants, no interactions have been reported with vasoconstrictor and sertraline, a nontricyclic antidepressant which acts to increase serotonin; no precautions appear to be needed

Effects on Dental Treatment Key adverse event(s) related to dental treatment: Xerostomia (normal salivary flow resumes upon discontinuation) (see Effects on Bleeding and Dental Comment).

Effects on Bleeding May impair platelet aggregation resulting in increased risk of bleeding events, particularly if used concomitantly with aspirin, NSAIDs, warfarin, or other anticoagulants. Bleeding related to SSRI use has been reported to range from relatively minor bruising and epistaxis to life-threatening hemorrhage. Routine interruption of therapy for most dental procedures is not warranted. In medically complicated patients or extensive oral surgery, the decision to interrupt therapy must be based on the risk to benefit in an individual patient and a medical consult is suggested. If therapy is continued without interruption, the clinician should anticipate the potential for a prolonged bleeding time.

Adverse Effects

>10%:
Central nervous system: Dizziness, fatigue, headache, insomnia, somnolence
Endocrine & metabolic: Libido decreased
Gastrointestinal: Anorexia, diarrhea, nausea, xerostomia
Genitourinary: Ejaculatory disturbances
Neuromuscular & skeletal: Tremors
Miscellaneous: Diaphoresis
1% to 10%:
Cardiovascular: Chest pain, palpitation
Central nervous system: Agitation, anxiety, hypoesthesia, malaise, nervousness, pain
Dermatologic: Rash
Endocrine & metabolic: Impotence
Gastrointestinal: Appetite increased, constipation, dyspepsia, flatulence, vomiting, weight gain
Neuromuscular & skeletal: Back pain, hypertonia, myalgia, paresthesia, weakness
Ocular: Visual difficulty, abnormal vision
Otic: Tinnitus
Respiratory: Rhinitis
Miscellaneous: Yawning

Pediatric patients: Additional adverse reactions reported in pediatric patients (frequency >2%): Aggressiveness, epistaxis, hyperkinesia, purpura, sinusitis, urinary incontinence

Dosage Oral:

Children and Adolescents: Obsessive-compulsive disorder:
6-12 years: Initial: 25 mg once daily
13-17 years: Initial: 50 mg once daily
Note: May increase daily dose, at intervals of not less than 1 week, to a maximum of 200 mg/day. If somnolence is noted, give at bedtime.
Adults:
Depression/obsessive-compulsive disorder: Oral: Initial: 50 mg/day (see **"Note"** above)
Panic disorder, post-traumatic stress disorder, social anxiety disorder: Initial: 25 mg once daily; increase to 50 mg once daily after 1 week; maximum dose: 200 mg/day
Premenstrual dysphoric disorder: 50 mg/day either daily throughout menstrual cycle **or** limited to the luteal phase of menstrual cycle, depending on physician assessment. Patients not responding to 50 mg/day may benefit from dose increases (50 mg increments per menstrual cycle) up to 150 mg/day when dosing throughout menstrual cycle **or** up to 100 mg day when dosing during luteal phase only. If a 100 mg/day dose has been established with luteal phase dosing, a 50 mg/day titration step for 3 days should be utilized at the beginning of each luteal phase dosing period.

Elderly: Depression/obsessive-compulsive disorder: Start treatment with 25 mg/day in the morning and increase by 25 mg/day increments every 2-3 days if tolerated to 50-100 mg/day; additional increases may be necessary; maximum dose: 200 mg/day. **Note:** Patients with Alzheimer's dementia-related depression may require a lower starting dosage of 12.5 mg/day, with titration intervals of 1-2 weeks, up to 150-200 mg/day maximum.

MAO inhibitor recommendations:
Switching to or from an MAO inhibitor intended to treat psychiatric disorders:
Allow 14 days to elapse between discontinuing an MAO inhibitor intended to treat psychiatric disorders and initiation of sertraline.
Allow 14 days to elapse between discontinuing sertraline and initiation of an MAO inhibitor intended to treat psychiatric disorders.
Use with other MAO inhibitors (linezolid or I.V. methylene blue):
Do not initiate sertraline in patients receiving linezolid or I.V. methylene blue; consider other interventions for psychiatric condition.
If urgent treatment with linezolid or I.V. methylene blue is required in a patient already receiving sertraline and potential benefits outweigh potential risks, discontinue sertraline promptly and administer linezolid or I.V. methylene blue. Monitor for serotonin syndrome for 2 weeks or until 24 hours after the last dose of linezolid or I.V. methylene blue, whichever comes first. May resume sertraline 24 hours after the last dose of linezolid or I.V. methylene blue.

Dosage adjustment/comment in renal impairment: Multiple-dose pharmacokinetics are unaffected by renal impairment.
Hemodialysis: Not removed by hemodialysis
Dosage adjustment/comment in hepatic impairment: Sertraline is extensively metabolized by the liver; caution should be used in patients with hepatic impairment; a lower dose or less frequent dosing should be used.

Mechanism of Action Antidepressant with selective inhibitory effects on presynaptic serotonin (5-HT) reuptake and only very weak effects on norepinephrine and dopamine neuronal uptake. *In vitro* studies demonstrate no significant affinity for adrenergic, cholinergic, GABA, dopaminergic, histaminergic, serotonergic, or benzodiazepine receptors.

Contraindications Hypersensitivity to sertraline or any component of the formulation; use of MAO inhibitors intended to treat psychiatric disorders (concurrently or within 14 days of discontinuing either sertraline or the MAO inhibitor); initiation of sertraline in a patient receiving linezolid or intravenous methylene blue; concurrent use of pimozide; concurrent use of sertraline oral concentrate with disulfiram

Warnings/Precautions [U.S. Boxed Warning]: Antidepressants increase the risk of suicidal thinking and behavior in children, adolescents, and young adults (18-24 years of age) with major depressive disorder (MDD) and other psychiatric disorders; consider risk prior to prescribing. Short-term studies did not show an increased risk in patients >24 years of age and showed a decreased risk in patients ≥65 years. Closely monitor patients for clinical worsening, suicidality, or unusual changes in behavior, particularly during the initial 1-2 months of therapy or during periods of dosage adjustments (increases or decreases); the patient's family or caregiver should be instructed to closely observe the patient and communicate condition with healthcare provider. A medication guide concerning the use of antidepressants should be dispensed with each prescription. **Sertraline is not FDA approved for use in children with major depressive disorder (MDD). However, it is approved for the treatment of obsessive-compulsive disorder (OCD) in children ≥6 years of age.**

The possibility of a suicide attempt is inherent in major depression and may persist until remission occurs. Use caution in high-risk patients. Worsening depression and severe abrupt suicidality that are not part of the presenting symptoms may require discontinuation or modification of drug therapy. The patient's family or caregiver should be alerted to monitor patients for the emergence of suicidality and associated behaviors (such as agitation, irritability, hostility, impulsivity, and hypomania) and call healthcare provider.

May worsen psychosis in some patients or precipitate a shift to mania or hypomania in patients with bipolar disorder. Patients presenting with depressive symptoms should be screened for bipolar disorder. Monotherapy in patients with bipolar disorder should be avoided. **Sertraline is not FDA approved for the treatment of bipolar depression.**

Potentially life-threatening serotonin syndrome (SS) has occurred with serotonergic agents (eg, SSRIs, SNRIs), particularly when used in combination with other serotonergic agents (eg, triptans, TCAs, fentanyl, lithium, tramadol, buspirone, St John's wort, tryptophan) or agents that impair metabolism of serotonin (eg, MOA inhibitors intended to treat psychiatric disorders, other MAO inhibitors [ie, linezolid and intravenous methylene blue]). Discontinue treatment (and any concomitant serotonergic agent) immediately if signs/symptoms arise. Has a very low potential to impair cognitive or motor performance. However, caution patients regarding activities requiring alertness until response to sertraline is known. Does not appear to potentiate the effects of alcohol, however, ethanol use is not advised.

Use caution in patients with a previous seizure disorder or condition predisposing to seizures such as brain damage, alcoholism, or concurrent therapy with other drugs which lower the seizure threshold. May increase the risks associated with electroconvulsive therapy. May cause mydriasis which can exacerbate narrow angle glaucoma. Use with caution in patients with hepatic or renal dysfunction and in elderly patients. May cause hyponatremia/SIADH (elderly at increased risk); volume depletion (diuretics may increase risk). Use with caution in patients with renal insufficiency or other concurrent illness (due to limited experience). Use caution in elderly patients; may cause or exacerbate syndrome of inappropriate antidiuretic hormone secretion or hyponatremia; monitor sodium closely with initiation or dosage adjustments in older adults (Beers Criteria). Sertraline acts as a mild uricosuric; use with caution in patients at risk of uric acid nephropathy. Use with caution in patients where weight loss is undesirable. May cause or exacerbate sexual dysfunction. Potentially significant interactions may exist, requiring dose or frequency adjustment, additional monitoring, and/or selection of alternative therapy.

Use oral concentrate formulation with caution in patients with latex sensitivity; dropper dispenser contains dry natural rubber. Monitor growth in pediatric patients. Discontinuation symptoms (eg, dysphoric mood, irritability, agitation, confusion, anxiety, insomnia, hypomania) may occur upon abrupt discontinuation. Taper dose when discontinuing therapy.

Drug Interactions

Metabolism/Transport Effects Substrate of CYP2B6 (minor), CYP2C19 (minor), CYP2C9 (minor), CYP2D6 (major), CYP3A4 (minor); **Note:** Assignment of Major/Minor substrate status based on clinically relevant drug interaction potential; **Inhibits** CYP1A2 (weak), CYP2B6 (moderate), CYP2C19 (moderate), CYP2C8 (weak), CYP2C9 (weak), CYP2D6 (moderate), CYP3A4 (moderate)

Avoid Concomitant Use

Avoid concomitant use of Sertraline with any of the following: Bosutinib; Clopidogrel; Disulfiram; Iobenguane I 123; Ivabradine; Linezolid; Lomitapide; MAO Inhibitors; Methylene Blue; Pimozide; Thioridazine; Tolvaptan; Tryptophan

Increased Effect/Toxicity

Sertraline may increase the levels/effects of: Agents with Antiplatelet Properties; Anticoagulants; Antidepressants (Serotonin Reuptake Inhibitor/Antagonist); Aspirin; Avanafil; Beta-Blockers; Bosutinib; Budesonide (Systemic, Oral Inhalation); BusPIRone; CarBAMazepine; CloZAPine; Colchicine; Collagenase (Systemic); CYP2B6 Substrates; CYP2C19 Substrates; CYP2D6 Substrates; CYP3A4 Substrates; Dabigatran Etexilate; Desmopressin; Dextromethorphan; Drotrecogin Alfa (Activated); Eplerenone; Everolimus; Fesoterodine; Fosphenytoin; Galantamine; Halofantrine; Highest Risk QTc-Prolonging Agents; Hypoglycemic Agents; Ibritumomab; Ivabradine; Ivacaftor; Lomitapide; Methadone; Methylene Blue; Metoclopramide; Metoprolol; Moderate Risk QTc-Prolonging Agents; NSAID (COX-2 Inhibitor); NSAID (Nonselective); Phenytoin; Pimecrolimus; Pimozide; Ranolazine; RisperiDONE; Rivaroxaban; Salicylates; Salmeterol; Saxagliptin; Serotonin Modulators; Thioridazine; Thrombolytic Agents; Tolvaptan; Tositumomab and Iodine I 131 Tositumomab; TraMADol; Tricyclic Antidepressants; Vitamin K Antagonists

The levels/effects of Sertraline may be increased by: Abiraterone Acetate; Alcohol (Ethyl); Analgesics (Opioid); Antipsychotics; BusPIRone; Cimetidine; CNS Depressants; Cobicistat; CYP2D6 Inhibitors (Moderate); CYP2D6 Inhibitors (Strong); Dasatinib; Disulfiram; Glucosamine; Grapefruit Juice; Herbs (Anticoagulant/Antiplatelet Properties); Linezolid; Lithium; Macrolide Antibiotics; MAO Inhibitors; Metoclopramide; Metyrosine; Mifepristone; Multivitamins/Minerals (with ADEK, Folate, Iron); Omega-3 Fatty Acids; Pentosan Polysulfate Sodium; Pentoxifylline; Prostacyclin Analogues; Tipranavir; TraMADol; Tryptophan; Vitamin E

Decreased Effect

Sertraline may decrease the levels/effects of: Clopidogrel; Ifosfamide; Iobenguane I 123; Ioflupane I 123; Tamoxifen

The levels/effects of Sertraline may be decreased by: CarBAMazepine; Cyproheptadine; Darunavir; Efavirenz; Fosphenytoin; NSAID (COX-2 Inhibitor); NSAID (Nonselective); Peginterferon Alfa-2b; Phenytoin

Ethanol/Nutrition/Herb Interactions

Ethanol: May increase CNS depression; monitor for increased effects with coadministration. Caution patients about effects.

Food: Sertraline average peak serum levels may be increased if taken with food.

◀ Herb/Nutraceutical: Avoid valerian, St John's wort, tryptophan, kava kava, gotu kola (may increase CNS depression and/or risk of serotonin syndrome).

Pharmacodynamics/Kinetics

Onset of Action Depression: The onset of action is within a week, however, individual response varies greatly and full response may not be seen until 8-12 weeks after initiation of treatment.

Half-life Elimination Sertraline: 26 hours; N-desmethylsertraline: 66 hours (range: 62-104 hours)

Time to Peak Plasma: Sertraline: 4.5-8.4 hours

Pregnancy Risk Factor C

Pregnancy Considerations Adverse events have been observed in animal reproduction studies. Sertraline crosses the human placenta. An increased risk of teratogenic effects, including cardiovascular defects, may be associated with maternal use of sertraline or other SSRIs; however, available information is conflicting. Nonteratogenic effects in the newborn following SSRI/SNRI exposure late in the third trimester include respiratory distress, cyanosis, apnea, seizures, temperature instability, feeding difficulty, vomiting, hypoglycemia, hypo- or hypertonia, hyper-reflexia, jitteriness, irritability, constant crying, and tremor. Symptoms may be due to the toxicity of the SSRIs/SNRIs or a discontinuation syndrome and may be consistent with serotonin syndrome associated with SSRI treatment. Persistent pulmonary hypertension of the newborn (PPHN) has also been reported with SSRI exposure. The long-term effects of *in utero* SSRI exposure on infant development and behavior are not known.

Due to pregnancy-induced physiologic changes, women who are pregnant may require adjusted doses of sertraline to achieve euthymia. The ACOG recommends that therapy with SSRIs or SNRIs during pregnancy be individualized; treatment of depression during pregnancy should incorporate the clinical expertise of the mental health clinician, obstetrician, primary healthcare provider, and pediatrician. According to the American Psychiatric Association (APA), the risks of medication treatment should be weighed against other treatment options and untreated depression. For women who discontinue antidepressant medications during pregnancy and who may be at high risk for postpartum depression, the medications can be restarted following delivery. Treatment algorithms have been developed by the ACOG and the APA for the management of depression in women prior to conception and during pregnancy.

Lactation Enters breast milk/use caution (AAP rates "of concern"; AAP 2001 update pending)

Breast-Feeding Considerations Sertraline and desmethylsertraline are excreted in breast milk. Adverse events have been reported in nursing infants exposed to some SSRIs. The American Academy of Breastfeeding Medicine suggests that sertraline may be considered for the treatment of postpartum depression in appropriately selected women who are nursing. Infants exposed to sertraline while breast-feeding generally receive a low relative dose and serum concentrations are not detectable in most infants. Sertraline concentrations in the hindmilk are higher than in foremilk. If the benefits of the mother receiving the sertraline and breast-feeding outweigh the risks, the mother may consider pumping and discarding breast milk with the feeding 7-9 hours after the daily dose to decrease sertraline exposure to the infant. The long-term effects on development and behavior have not been studied. The manufacturer recommends that caution be exercised when administering sertraline to nursing women. Maternal use of an SSRI during pregnancy may cause delayed milk secretion.

Dosage Forms

Solution, oral: 20 mg/mL (60 mL)
Zoloft®: 20 mg/mL (60 mL)

Tablet, oral: 25 mg, 50 mg, 100 mg
Zoloft®: 25 mg, 50 mg, 100 mg

Dental Comment Problems with SSRI-induced bruxism have been reported and may preclude their use; clinicians attempting to evaluate any patient with bruxism or involuntary muscle movement, who is simultaneously being treated with an SSRI drug, should be aware of the potential association.

Sevelamer (se VEL a mer)

Brand Names: U.S. Renagel®; Renvela®

Brand Names: Canada Renagel®

Pharmacologic Category Phosphate Binder

Use Reduction or control of serum phosphorous in patients with chronic kidney disease on hemodialysis

Local Anesthetic/Vasoconstrictor Precautions No information available to require special precautions

Effects on Dental Treatment No significant effects or complications reported

Effects on Bleeding No information available to require special precautions

Adverse Effects

>10%: Gastrointestinal: Vomiting (22%), nausea (20%), diarrhea (19%), dyspepsia (16%)

1% to 10%:
Endocrine & metabolic: Hypercalcemia (5% to 7%)
Gastrointestinal: Abdominal pain (9%), flatulence (8%), constipation (8%)
Miscellaneous: Peritonitis (peritoneal dialysis: 8%)

General Dosage Range Oral: *Adults:* Initial: 800-1600 mg 3 times/day; Maintenance: Up to 2400-14,000 mg/day in 3 divided doses

Mechanism of Action Sevelamer (a polymeric compound) binds phosphate within the intestinal lumen, limiting absorption and decreasing serum phosphate concentrations without altering calcium, aluminum, or bicarbonate concentrations.

Pharmacodynamics/Kinetics

Onset of Action Reduction in serum phosphorus has been demonstrated after 1-2 weeks (Burke, 1997; Chertow, 1997).

Pregnancy Risk Factor C

Pregnancy Considerations Animal studies have shown reduced or irregular ossification of fetal bones. Because sevelamer may cause a reduction in the absorption of some vitamins, it should be used with caution in pregnant women.

Sildenafil (sil DEN a fil)

Brand Names: U.S. Revatio®; Viagra®

Brand Names: Canada Apo-Sildenafil®; CO Sildenafil; GD-Sildenafil; PMS-Sildenafil; ratio-Sildenafil R; Revatio®; Teva-Sildenafil; Viagra®

Generic Availability (U.S.) Yes: Tablet

Pharmacologic Category Phosphodiesterase-5 Enzyme Inhibitor

Use

Revatio®: Treatment of pulmonary arterial hypertension (PAH) (WHO Group I) to improve exercise ability and delay clinical worsening. Efficacy established based upon short-term studies (12-16 weeks).

Viagra®: Treatment of erectile dysfunction (ED)

Unlabeled Use Pulmonary hypertension (WHO Group II, III, and IV); persistent pulmonary hypertension after recent left ventricular assist device placement

Local Anesthetic/Vasoconstrictor Precautions No information available to require special precautions

Effects on Dental Treatment No significant effects or complications reported

Effects on Bleeding No information available to require special precautions

Adverse Effects Based upon normal doses for either indication or route. (Adverse effects such as flushing, diarrhea, myalgia, and visual disturbances may be increased with adult doses >100 mg/24 hours.)

>10%:

Central nervous system: Headache (16% to 46%)

Gastrointestinal: Dyspepsia (7% to 17%; dose related)

2% to 10%:

Cardiovascular: Flushing (10%)

Central nervous system: Insomnia (≤7%), pyrexia (6%), dizziness (2%)

Dermatologic: Erythema (6%), rash (2%)

Gastrointestinal: Diarrhea (3% to 9%), gastritis (≤3%)

Genitourinary: Urinary tract infection (3%)

Hepatic: LFTs increased

Neuromuscular & skeletal: Myalgia (≤7%), paresthesia (≤3%)

Ocular: Abnormal vision (color changes, blurred vision, or increased sensitivity to light 3% to 11%; dose related)

Respiratory: Epistaxis (9% to 13%), dyspnea exacerbated (≤7%), nasal congestion (4%), rhinitis (4%), sinusitis (3%)

Dosage

I.V.: Adults: Pulmonary arterial hypertension (PAH) (Revatio®): 10 mg 3 times/day

Oral:

Adults:

Erectile dysfunction (Viagra®): Usual dose: 50 mg once daily 1 hour (range: 30 minutes to 4 hours) before sexual activity; dosing range: 25-100 mg once daily

PAH (Revatio®): 20 mg 3 times/day, taken 4-6 hours apart; maximum recommended dose: 20 mg 3 times/day

Elderly >65 years: Use with caution.

Revatio®: Refer to adult dosing.

Viagra®: Starting dose of 25 mg should be considered.

Dosage considerations for patients stable on alpha-blockers: Viagra®: Initial 25 mg

Dosage adjustment for concomitant use of potent CYP34A inhibitors:

Revatio®:

Erythromycin: No dosage adjustment

Itraconazole, ketoconazole: Not recommended

Protease inhibitors: Contraindicated

Viagra®:

Erythromycin, itraconazole, ketoconazole: Starting dose of 25 mg should be considered

Protease inhibitors: Maximum sildenafil dose: 25 mg every 48 hours

Dosage adjustment in renal impairment:

Revatio®: Dose adjustment not necessary

Viagra®: Cl_{cr} <30 mL/minute: Starting dose of 25 mg should be considered

Dosage adjustment in hepatic impairment:

Revatio®: Child-Pugh class A or B: Dose adjustment not necessary; not studied in severe impairment (Child-Pugh class C)

Viagra®: Child-Pugh class A or B: Starting dose of 25 mg should be considered; not studied in severe impairment (Child-Pugh class C)

Mechanism of Action

Erectile dysfunction: Does not directly cause penile erections, but affects the response to sexual stimulation. The physiologic mechanism of erection of the penis involves release of nitric oxide (NO) in the corpus cavernosum during sexual stimulation. NO then activates the enzyme guanylate cyclase, which results in increased levels of cyclic guanosine monophosphate (cGMP), producing smooth muscle relaxation and inflow of blood to the corpus cavernosum. Sildenafil enhances the effect of NO by inhibiting phosphodiesterase type 5 (PDE-5), which is responsible for degradation of cGMP in the corpus cavernosum; when sexual stimulation causes local release of NO, inhibition of PDE-5 by sildenafil causes increased levels of cGMP in the corpus cavernosum, resulting in smooth muscle relaxation and inflow of blood to the corpus cavernosum; at recommended doses, it has no effect in the absence of sexual stimulation.

Pulmonary arterial hypertension (PAH): Inhibits phosphodiesterase type 5 (PDE-5) in smooth muscle of pulmonary vasculature where PDE-5 is responsible for the degradation of cyclic guanosine monophosphate (cGMP). Increased cGMP concentration results in pulmonary vasculature relaxation; vasodilation in the pulmonary bed and the systemic circulation (to a lesser degree) may occur.

Contraindications Hypersensitivity to sildenafil or any component of the formulation; concurrent use (regularly/intermittently) of organic nitrates in any form (eg, nitroglycerin, isosorbide dinitrate); concurrent use with a protease inhibitor regimen when sildenafil used for pulmonary artery hypertension (eg, Revatio®)

Warnings/Precautions Decreases in blood pressure may occur due to vasodilator effects; use with caution in patients with left ventricular outflow obstruction (aortic stenosis or hypertrophic obstructive cardiomyopathy), those on antihypertensive therapy, with resting hypotension (BP <90/50 mm Hg), fluid depletion, or autonomic dysfunction; may be more sensitive to hypotensive actions. Patients should be hemodynamically stable prior to initiating therapy at the lowest possible dose. Avoid or limit concurrent substantial alcohol consumption as this may increase the risk of symptomatic hypotension. Use with caution in patients with uncontrolled hypertension (>170/110 mm Hg); life-threatening arrhythmias, stroke or MI within the last 6 months; cardiac failure or coronary artery disease causing unstable angina; safety and efficacy have not been studied in these patients. There is a degree of cardiac risk associated with sexual activity; therefore, physicians should consider the cardiovascular status of their patients prior to initiating any treatment for erectile dysfunction. If pulmonary edema occurs when treating pulmonary arterial hypertension (PAH), consider the possibility of pulmonary veno-occlusive disease (PVOD); continued use is not recommended in patient with PVOD.

Sildenafil should be used with caution in patients with anatomical deformation of the penis (angulation, cavernosal fibrosis, or Peyronie's disease) and in patients who have conditions which may predispose them to priapism (sickle cell anemia, multiple myeloma, leukemia). All patients should be instructed to seek medical attention if erection persists >4 hours.

Vision loss may occur rarely and be a sign of nonarteritic anterior ischemic optic neuropathy (NAION). Risk may be increased with history of vision loss. Other risk factors for NAION include low cup-to-disc ratio ("crowded disc"), coronary artery disease, diabetes, hypertension, hyperlipidemia, smoking, and age >50 years. May cause dose-related impairment of color discrimination. Use caution in patients with retinitis pigmentosa; a minority have genetic disorders of retinal phosphodiesterases (no safety information available). Sudden decrease or loss of hearing has been reported rarely; hearing changes may be accompanied by tinnitus and dizziness. A direct relationship between therapy and vision or hearing loss has not been determined.

The potential underlying causes of erectile dysfunction should be evaluated prior to treatment. The safety and efficacy of sildenafil with other treatments for erectile dysfunction have not been established; use is not recommended. Efficacy with concurrent bosentan therapy has not been evaluated; use with caution. Use with caution in patients taking strong CYP3A4 inhibitors or alpha-blockers. Concomitant use with all forms of nitrates is contraindicated. If nitrate administration is medically necessary, it is not known when nitrates can be safely administered following the use of sildenafil (per manufacturer); the ACC/AHA 2007 guidelines supports administration of nitrates only if 24 hours have elapsed.

Avoid abrupt discontinuation, especially if used as monotherapy in PAH as exacerbation may occur. Use caution in patients with bleeding disorders or with active peptic ulcer disease; safety and efficacy have not been established. Efficacy has not be established for treatment of pulmonary hypertension associated with sickle cell disease. Use with caution in the elderly, or patients with renal or hepatic dysfunction; dose adjustment may be needed. Use of Revatio®, especially chronic use, is not recommended in children. Increased mortality seen in long-term (mean: 3 years) study at high dose (20-80 mg [depending upon weight] 3 times/day).

Drug Interactions

Metabolism/Transport Effects Substrate of CYP1A2 (minor), CYP2C19 (minor), CYP2C9 (minor), CYP2D6 (minor), CYP2E1 (minor), CYP3A4 (major); **Note:** Assignment of Major/Minor substrate status based on clinically relevant drug interaction potential; **Inhibits** CYP2C9 (weak), CYP3A4 (weak)

Avoid Concomitant Use

Avoid concomitant use of Sildenafil with any of the following: Alprostadil; Amyl Nitrite; Boceprevir; Cobicistat; Phosphodiesterase 5 Inhibitors; Pimozide; Telaprevir; Vasodilators (Organic Nitrates)

Increased Effect/Toxicity

Sildenafil may increase the levels/effects of: Alpha1-Blockers; Alprostadil; Amyl Nitrite; Antihypertensives; ARIPiprazole; Bosentan; HMG-CoA Reductase Inhibitors; Lomitapide; Phosphodiesterase 5 Inhibitors; Pimozide; Vasodilators (Organic Nitrates)

The levels/effects of Sildenafil may be increased by: Alcohol (Ethyl); Boceprevir; Cobicistat; CYP3A4 Inhibitors (Moderate); CYP3A4 Inhibitors (Strong); Dasatinib; Erythromycin (Systemic); Fluconazole; Itraconazole; Ivacaftor; Ketoconazole (Systemic); Lorcaserin; Mifepristone; Posaconazole; Protease Inhibitors; Sapropterin; Telaprevir; Voriconazole

Decreased Effect

The levels/effects of Sildenafil may be decreased by: Bosentan; CYP3A4 Inducers (Strong); Deferasirox; Etravirine; Herbs (CYP3A4 Inducers); Peginterferon Alfa-2b; Tocilizumab

Ethanol/Nutrition/Herb Interactions Ethanol: Substantial consumption of ethanol may increase the risk of hypotension and orthostasis. Lower ethanol consumption has not been associated with significant changes in blood pressure or increase in orthostatic symptoms. Management: Avoid or limit ethanol consumption.

Food: Avoid grapefruit juice.

Herb/Nutraceutical: St John's wort may decrease sildenafil levels. Management: Avoid St John's wort.

Dietary Considerations Avoid grapefruit juice.

Pharmacodynamics/Kinetics

Onset of Action ~60 minutes

Duration of Action 2-4 hours

Half-life Elimination ~4 hours; the elderly and those with severe renal impairment have reduced clearance of sildenafil and its active N-desmethyl metabolite

Time to Peak 30-120 minutes; delayed by 60 minutes with a high-fat meal

Pregnancy Risk Factor B

Pregnancy Considerations Teratogenic effects were not observed in animal studies. There are no adequate and well-controlled studies in pregnant women. Less than 0.001% appears in the semen.

Lactation Excretion in breast milk unknown/use caution

Breast-Feeding Considerations It is not known if sildenafil is excreted in breast milk. The manufacturer recommends that caution be exercised when administering sildenafil to nursing women.

Dosage Forms

Injection, solution:
Revatio®: 0.8 mg/mL (12.5 mL)
Tablet, oral: 20 mg
Revatio®: 20 mg
Viagra®: 25 mg, 50 mg, 100 mg

Silodosin (SI lo doe sin)

Brand Names: U.S. Rapaflo®
Brand Names: Canada Rapaflo®
Pharmacologic Category Alpha₁ Blocker
Use Treatment of signs and symptoms of benign prostatic hyperplasia (BPH)

Local Anesthetic/Vasoconstrictor Precautions No information available to require special precautions

Effects on Dental Treatment Key adverse event(s) related to dental treatment: Postural hypotension, particularly with initial dosing; dizziness; nasal congestion or rhinitis

Effects on Bleeding No information available to require special precautions

Adverse Effects

>10%: Miscellaneous: Retrograde ejaculation (28%)
1% to 10%:
Cardiovascular: Orthostatic hypotension (3%; increased in elderly ≥65 years up to 5%)
Central nervous system: Dizziness (3%), headache (2%), insomnia (1% to 2%)
Gastrointestinal: Diarrhea (3%), abdominal pain (1% to 2%)

Genitourinary: PSA increased (1% to 2%)

Neuromuscular & skeletal: Weakness (1% to 2%)

Respiratory: Nasal congestion (2%), nasopharyngitis (2%), rhinorrhea (1% to 2%), sinusitis (1% to 2%)

General Dosage Range Dosage adjustment recommended in patients with renal impairment

Oral: *Adults:* Males: 8 mg once daily

Mechanism of Action Silodosin is a selective antagonist of alpha$_{1A}$-adrenoreceptors in the prostate and bladder. Smooth muscle tone in the prostate is mediated by alpha$_{1A}$-adrenoreceptors; blocking them leads to relaxation of smooth muscle in the bladder neck and prostate causing an improvement of urine flow and decreased symptoms of BPH. Approximately 75% of the alpha1-receptors in the prostate are of the alpha$_{1A}$ subtype.

Pharmacodynamics/Kinetics

Half-life Elimination Healthy volunteers: Silodosin: ~13 hours (mean); KMD-3213G: ~24 hours

Time to Peak Silodosin: ~3 hours; KMD-3213G: ~5.5 hours (Lepor, 2010)

Pregnancy Risk Factor B

Pregnancy Considerations Teratogenic effects were not observed in animal studies; however, silodosin is not approved for use in women.

Silver Nitrate (SIL ver NYE trate)

Generic Availability (U.S.) Yes

Pharmacologic Category Antibiotic, Topical; Cauterizing Agent, Topical; Topical Skin Product, Antibacterial

Use Astringent, cauterization of wounds, germicidal, removal of granulation tissue, corns and warts

Local Anesthetic/Vasoconstrictor Precautions No information available to require special precautions

Effects on Dental Treatment No significant effects or complications reported

Effects on Bleeding No information available to require special precautions

Adverse Effects Frequency not defined.

Dermatologic: Burning and skin irritation, staining of the skin

Hematologic: Methemoglobinemia

Dosage Children and Adults:

Sticks: Apply to mucous membranes and other moist skin surfaces only on area to be treated

Topical solution: Usual: Apply a cotton applicator dipped in solution on the affected area 2-3 times/week for 2-3 weeks

Mechanism of Action Free silver ions precipitate bacterial proteins by combining with chloride in tissue forming silver chloride; coagulates cellular protein to form an eschar; silver ions or salts or colloidal silver preparations can inhibit the growth of both gram-positive and gram-negative bacteria. This germicidal action is attributed to the precipitation of bacterial proteins by liberated silver ions. Silver nitrate coagulates cellular protein to form an eschar, and this mode of action is the postulated mechanism for control of benign hematuria, rhinitis, and recurrent pneumothorax.

Contraindications Hypersensitivity to silver nitrate or any component of the formulation; not for use on broken skin, cuts, or wounds

Warnings/Precautions Do not use applicator sticks on the eyes. Prolonged use may result in skin discoloration. Silver nitrate is a caustic agent and inappropriate use may cause chemical burns. Skin contact time with applicator sticks should be extremely short when used in neonates or on thin delicate skin contact.

Drug Interactions

Metabolism/Transport Effects None known.

Avoid Concomitant Use

Avoid concomitant use of Silver Nitrate with any of the following: BCG

Increased Effect/Toxicity There are no known significant interactions involving an increase in effect.

Decreased Effect

Silver Nitrate may decrease the levels/effects of: BCG; Sodium Picosulfate

Dosage Forms

Applicator sticks, topical: Silver nitrate 75% and potassium 25%

Solution, topical: 0.5% (960 mL); 10% (30 mL); 25% (30 mL); 50% (30 mL)

Silver Sulfadiazine (SIL ver sul fa DYE a zeen)

Brand Names: U.S. Silvadene®; SSD™; Thermazene®

Brand Names: Canada Flamazine®

Pharmacologic Category Antibiotic, Topical

Use Prevention and treatment of infection in second and third degree burns

Local Anesthetic/Vasoconstrictor Precautions No information available to require special precautions

Effects on Dental Treatment No significant effects or complications reported

Effects on Bleeding No information available to require special precautions

Adverse Effects Frequency not defined.

Dermatologic: Discoloration of skin, erythema multiforme, itching, photosensitivity, rash

Hematologic: Agranulocytosis, aplastic anemia, hemolytic anemia, leukopenia

Hepatic: Hepatitis

Renal: Interstitial nephritis

Miscellaneous: Allergic reactions may be related to sulfa component

General Dosage Range Topical: *Children and Adults:* Apply to a thickness of 1/16" once or twice daily

Mechanism of Action Acts upon the bacterial cell wall and cell membrane. Bactericidal for many gram-negative and gram-positive bacteria and is effective against yeast. Active against *Pseudomonas aeruginosa, Pseudomonas maltophilia, Enterobacter* species, *Klebsiella* species, *Serratia* species, *Escherichia coli, Proteus mirabilis, Morganella morganii, Providencia rettgeri, Proteus vulgaris, Providencia* species, *Citrobacter* species, *Acinetobacter calcoaceticus, Staphylococcus aureus, Staphylococcus epidermidis, Enterococcus* species, *Candida albicans, Corynebacterium diphtheriae,* and *Clostridium perfringens*

Pharmacodynamics/Kinetics

Half-life Elimination 10 hours; prolonged with renal impairment

Time to Peak Serum: 3-11 days of continuous therapy

Pregnancy Risk Factor B

Pregnancy Considerations Adverse events were not observed in animal reproduction studies. Because of the theoretical increased risk for hyperbilirubinemia and kernicterus, sulfadiazine is contraindicated for use near term, on premature infants, or on newborn infants during the first 2 months of life (refer to Sulfadiazine monograph).

Simethicone (sye METH i kone)

Brand Names: U.S. Equalizer Gas Relief [OTC]; Gas Free Extra Strength [OTC]; Gas Relief Ultra Strength [OTC]; Gas-X® Children's Tongue Twisters™ [OTC]; Gas-X® Extra Strength [OTC]; Gas-X® Maximum Strength [OTC]; Gas-X® Thin Strips™ [OTC]; Gas-X® [OTC]; Gax-X® Infant [OTC]; Infantaire Gas [OTC]; Infants Gas Relief Drops [OTC] [DSC]; Little Tummys® Gas Relief [OTC]; Mi-Acid Gas Relief [OTC]; Mylanta® Gas Maximum Strength [OTC]; Mylicon® Infants' [OTC]; Mytab Gas Maximum [OTC]; Mytab Gas [OTC]; Phazyme® Ultra Strength [OTC]

Brand Names: Canada Ovol®; Phazyme™

Pharmacologic Category Antiflatulent

Use Postoperative gas pain or for use in endoscopic examination; relief of bloating, pressure, and discomfort of gas

Local Anesthetic/Vasoconstrictor Precautions No information available to require special precautions

Effects on Dental Treatment No significant effects or complications reported

Effects on Bleeding No information available to require special precautions

Adverse Effects No data reported

General Dosage Range Oral:

Infants and Children <2 years or <11 kg: 20 mg 4 times/day, as needed

Children >2 years or >11 kg: 40 mg 4 times/day, as needed

Children >12 years and Adults: 40-360 mg after meals and at bedtime, as needed

Mechanism of Action Decreases the surface tension of gas bubbles thereby disperses and prevents gas pockets in the GI system

Pregnancy Considerations Simethicone is not absorbed systemically following oral administration. Systemic absorption would be required in order for simethicone to cross the placenta and reach the fetus.

Simvastatin (sim va STAT in)

Related Information
Cardiovascular Diseases *on page 1492*

Brand Names: U.S. Zocor®

Brand Names: Canada Apo-Simvastatin®; Ava-Simvastatin; CO Simvastatin; Dom-Simvastatin; JAMP-Simvastatin; Mint-Simvastatin; Mylan-Simvastatin; Nu-Simvastatin; PHL-Simvastatin; PMS-Simvastatin; Q-Simvastatin; RAN™-Simvastatin; ratio-Simvastatin; Riva-Simvastatin; Sandoz-Simvastatin; Simvastatin-Odan; Taro-Simvastatin; Teva-Simvastatin; Zocor®; ZYM-Simvastatin

Generic Availability (U.S.) Yes

Pharmacologic Category Antilipemic Agent, HMG-CoA Reductase Inhibitor

Use Used with dietary therapy for the following:

Secondary prevention of cardiovascular events in hypercholesterolemic patients with established coronary heart disease (CHD) or at high risk for CHD: To reduce cardiovascular morbidity (myocardial infarction, coronary/noncoronary revascularization procedures) and mortality; to reduce the risk of stroke

Hyperlipidemias: To reduce elevations in total cholesterol (total-C), LDL-C, apolipoprotein B, triglycerides, and VLDL-C, and to increase HDL-C in patients with primary hypercholesterolemia (elevations of 1 or more components are present in Fredrickson type IIa, IIb, III,

and IV hyperlipidemias); treatment of homozygous familial hypercholesterolemia

Heterozygous familial hypercholesterolemia (HeFH): In adolescent patients (10-17 years of age, females >1 year postmenarche) with HeFH having LDL-C ≥190 mg/dL or LDL-C ≥160 mg/dL with positive family history of premature cardiovascular disease (CVD), or 2 or more CVD risk factors in the adolescent patient

Local Anesthetic/Vasoconstrictor Precautions No information available to require special precautions

Effects on Dental Treatment No significant effects or complications reported

Effects on Bleeding No information available to require special precautions

Adverse Effects

1% to 10%:

Cardiovascular: Atrial fibrillation (6%; placebo 5%), edema (3%; placebo 2%)

Central nervous system: Headache (3% to 7%), vertigo (5%)

Dermatologic: Eczema (5%)

Gastrointestinal: Abdominal pain (7%), constipation (2% to 7%), gastritis (5%), nausea (5%)

Hepatic: Transaminases increased (>3 x ULN; 1%)

Neuromuscular & skeletal: CPK increased (>3 x normal; 5%), myalgia (4%)

Respiratory: Upper respiratory infections (9%), bronchitis (7%)

Additional class-related events or case reports (not necessarily reported with simvastatin therapy): Alteration in taste, anorexia, anxiety, bilirubin increased, cataracts, cholestatic jaundice, cirrhosis, decreased libido, depression, erectile dysfunction/impotence, facial paresis, fatty liver, fulminant hepatic necrosis, gynecomastia, hepatoma, hyperbilirubinemia, immune-mediated necrotizing myopathy (IMNM), impaired extraocular muscle movement, increased CPK (>10 x normal), interstitial lung disease, ophthalmoplegia, peripheral nerve palsy, psychic disturbance, renal failure (secondary to rhabdomyolysis), thyroid dysfunction, tremor, vertigo

Dosage Oral: **Note:** Doses should be individualized according to the baseline LDL-cholesterol levels, the recommended goal of therapy, and the patient's response; adjustments should be made at intervals of 4 weeks or more; doses may need adjusted based on concomitant medications

Children 10-17 years (females >1 year postmenarche): HeFH: 10 mg once daily in the evening; range: 10-40 mg/day (maximum: 40 mg/day)

Dosage adjustment for simvastatin with concomitant amiodarone, amlodipine, diltiazem, dronedarone, lomitapide, ranolazine, or verapamil: Refer to drug-specific dosing in adult dosing section

Adults:

Note: Dosing limitation: Simvastatin 80 mg is limited to patients that have been taking this dose for >12 consecutive months without evidence of myopathy and are not currently taking or beginning to take a simvastatin dose-limiting or contraindicated interacting medication. If patient is unable to achieve low-density lipoprotein cholesterol (LDL-C) goal using the 40 mg dose of simvastatin, increasing to 80 mg dose is not recommended. Instead, switch patient to an alternative LDL-C-lowering treatment providing greater LDL-C reduction.

Homozygous familial hypercholesterolemia: 40 mg once daily in the evening

Prevention of cardiovascular events, hyperlipidemias: 10-20 mg once daily in the evening; range: 5-40 mg/day

Patients requiring only moderate reduction of LDL-C may be started at 5-10 mg once daily in the evening; adjust to achieve recommended LDL-C goal

Patients requiring reduction of >40% of LDL-C may be started at 40 mg once daily in the evening; adjust to achieve recommended LDL-C goal

Patients with CHD or at high risk for cardiovascular events (patients with diabetes, PVD, history of stroke or other cerebrovascular disease): Dosing should be started at 40 mg once daily in the evening; start simultaneously with diet therapy.

Dosage adjustment with concomitant medications:
Note: Patients currently tolerating and requiring a dose of simvastatin 80 mg who require initiation of an interacting drug with a dose cap for simvastatin should be switched to an alternative statin with less potential for drug-drug interaction.

Amiodarone, amlodipine, or ranolazine: Simvastatin dose should **not** exceed 20 mg/day

Diltiazem, dronedarone, or verapamil: Simvastatin dose should **not** exceed 10 mg/day

Lomitapide: Simvastatin dose should not exceed 20 mg/day (or 40 mg daily for those who previously tolerated simvastatin 80 mg daily for ≥1 year without evidence of muscle toxicity)

Dosage adjustment in Chinese patients on niacin doses ≥1 g/day: Use caution with simvastatin doses exceeding 20 mg/day; because of an increased risk of myopathy, do not administer simvastatin 80 mg concurrently.

Dosing adjustment in renal impairment:
Manufacturer's recommendations:

Mild-to-moderate renal impairment: No dosage adjustment necessary; simvastatin does not undergo significant renal excretion

Severe renal impairment: Cl_{cr} <30 mL/minute: Initial: 5 mg/day with close monitoring

Alternative recommendation: No dosage adjustment necessary for any degree of renal impairment (Aronoff, 2007)

Mechanism of Action Simvastatin is a methylated derivative of lovastatin that acts by competitively inhibiting 3-hydroxy-3-methylglutaryl-coenzyme A (HMG-CoA) reductase, the enzyme that catalyzes the rate-limiting step in cholesterol biosynthesis

Contraindications Hypersensitivity to simvastatin or any component of the formulation; active liver disease; unexplained persistent elevations of serum transaminases (eg, clarithromycin, erythromycin, itraconazole, ketoconazole, nefazodone, posaconazole, voriconazole, protease inhibitors [including boceprevir and telaprevir], telithromycin), cyclosporine, danazol, and gemfibrozil; pregnancy; breast-feeding

Warnings/Precautions Secondary causes of hyperlipidemia should be ruled out prior to therapy. Liver enzyme tests should be obtained at baseline and as clinically indicated; routine periodic monitoring of liver enzymes is not necessary. Use with caution in patients who consume large amounts of ethanol or have a history of liver disease; use is contraindicated with active liver disease and with unexplained transaminase elevations. Rhabdomyolysis with acute renal failure has occurred. Risk of rhabdomyolysis is dose-related and increased with high doses (80 mg), concurrent use of lipid-lowering agents which may also cause rhabdomyolysis (other fibrates or niacin doses ≥1 g/day), or

moderate-to-strong CYP3A4 inhibitors (eg, amiodarone, grapefruit juice in large quantities, or verapamil), age ≥65 years, female gender, uncontrolled hypothyroidism, and renal dysfunction. In Chinese patients, do not use high-dose simvastatin (80 mg) if concurrently taking niacin ≥1 g/day; may increase risk of myopathy. Immune-mediated necrotizing myopathy (IMNM), an autoimmune-mediated myopathy, has been reported (rarely) with HMG-CoA reductase inhibitor therapy. IMNM presents as proximal muscle weakness with elevated CPK levels, which persists despite discontinuation of HMG-CoA reductase inhibitor therapy; additionally, muscle biopsy may show necrotizing myopathy with limited inflammation; immunosuppressive therapy (eg, corticosteroids, azathioprine) may be used for treatment. Concomitant use of simvastatin with some drugs may require cautious use, may not be recommended, may require dosage adjustments, or may be contraindicated. If concurrent use of a contraindicated interacting medication is unavoidable, treatment with simvastatin should be suspended during use or consider the use of an alternative HMG-CoA reductase inhibitor void of CYP3A4 metabolism. Monitor closely if used with other drugs associated with myopathy (eg, colchicine). Increases in Hb A_{1c} and fasting blood glucose have been reported with HMG-CoA reductase inhibitors; however, the benefits of statin therapy far outweigh the risk of dysglycemia. The manufacturer recommends temporary discontinuation for elective major surgery, acute medical or surgical conditions, or in any patient experiencing an acute or serious condition predisposing to renal failure (eg, sepsis, hypotension, trauma, uncontrolled seizures). However, based upon current evidence, HMG-CoA reductase inhibitor therapy should be continued in the perioperative period unless risk outweighs cardioprotective benefit. Use with caution in patients with severe renal impairment; initial dosage adjustment is necessary; monitor closely.

Drug Interactions

Metabolism/Transport Effects Substrate of CYP3A4 (major), SLCO1B1; **Note:** Assignment of Major/Minor substrate status based on clinically relevant drug interaction potential; **Inhibits** CYP2C8 (weak), CYP2C9 (weak), CYP2D6 (weak)

Avoid Concomitant Use
Avoid concomitant use of Simvastatin with any of the following: Boceprevir; CycloSPORINE (Systemic); CYP3A4 Inhibitors (Strong); Erythromycin (Systemic); Fusidic Acid; Gemfibrozil; Mifepristone; Protease Inhibitors; Red Yeast Rice; Telaprevir

Increased Effect/Toxicity
Simvastatin may increase the levels/effects of: ARIPiprazole; DAPTOmycin; Diltiazem; Pazopanib; Trabectedin; Vitamin K Antagonists

The levels/effects of Simvastatin may be increased by: Amiodarone; AmLODIPine; Bezafibrate; Boceprevir; Colchicine; CycloSPORINE (Systemic); CYP3A4 Inhibitors (Moderate); CYP3A4 Inhibitors (Strong); Cyproterone; Danazol; Dasatinib; Diltiazem; Dronedarone; Eltrombopag; Erythromycin (Systemic); Fenofibrate; Fenofibric Acid; Fluconazole; Fusidic Acid; Gemfibrozil; Grapefruit Juice; Green Tea; Imatinib; Ivacaftor; Lomitapide; Macrolide Antibiotics; Mifepristone; Niacin; Niacinamide; Protease Inhibitors; QuiNINE; Ranolazine; Red Yeast Rice; Sildenafil; Telaprevir; Ticagrelor; Verapamil

Decreased Effect
Simvastatin may decrease the levels/effects of: Lanthanum

The levels/effects of Simvastatin may be decreased by: Antacids; Bosentan; CYP3A4 Inducers (Strong); Deferasirox; Efavirenz; Etravirine; Fosphenytoin; Phenytoin; Rifamycin Derivatives; St Johns Wort; Tocilizumab

Ethanol/Nutrition/Herb Interactions
Ethanol: Excessive ethanol consumption has the potential to cause hepatic effects. Management: Avoid or limit ethanol consumption.
Food: Simvastatin serum concentration may be increased when taken with grapefruit juice. Red yeast rice contains an estimated 2.4 mg lovastatin per 600 mg rice. Management: Avoid concurrent intake of large quantities of grapefruit juice (>1 quart/day).
Herb/Nutraceutical: St John's wort may decrease simvastatin levels. Management: Avoid St John's wort.

Dietary Considerations May be taken without regard to meals. Red yeast rice contains an estimated 2.4 mg lovastatin per 600 mg rice.

Pharmacodynamics/Kinetics
Onset of Action >3 days; Peak effect: 2 weeks
Half-life Elimination Unknown
Time to Peak 1.3-2.4 hours
Pregnancy Risk Factor X
Pregnancy Considerations Adverse events were not observed in animal reproduction studies. There are reports of congenital anomalies following maternal use of HMG-CoA reductase inhibitors in pregnancy; however, maternal disease, differences in specific agents used, and the low rates of exposure limit the interpretation of the available data (Godfrey, 2012; Lecarpentier, 2012). Cholesterol biosynthesis may be important in fetal development; serum cholesterol and triglycerides increase normally during pregnancy. The discontinuation of lipid lowering medications temporarily during pregnancy is not expected to have significant impact on the long term outcomes of primary hypercholesterolemia treatment.

Use of simvastatin is contraindicated in pregnancy. HMG-CoA reductase inhibitors should be discontinued prior to pregnancy (ADA, 2013). If treatment of dyslipidemias is needed in pregnant women or in women of reproductive age, other agents are preferred (Berglund, 2012; NCEP, 2002). The manufacturer recommends administration to women of childbearing potential only when conception is highly unlikely and patients have been informed of potential hazards.

Lactation Excretion in breast milk unknown/contraindicated

Breast-Feeding Considerations It is not known if simvastatin is excreted into breast milk. Due to the potential for serious adverse reactions in a nursing infant, breast-feeding is contraindicated by the manufacturer.

Dosage Forms
Tablet, oral: 5 mg, 10 mg, 20 mg, 40 mg, 80 mg
Zocor®: 5 mg, 10 mg, 20 mg, 40 mg, 80 mg

Sincalide (SIN ka lide)

Brand Names: U.S. Kinevac®
Pharmacologic Category Diagnostic Agent
Use Postevacuation cholecystography; gallbladder bile sampling; stimulate pancreatic secretion for analysis; accelerate the transit of barium through the small bowel
Local Anesthetic/Vasoconstrictor Precautions No information available to require special precautions
Effects on Dental Treatment No significant effects or complications reported

Effects on Bleeding No information available to require special precautions
Adverse Effects
>10%: Gastrointestinal: Abdominal pain (20%), cramps, nausea (20%)
1% to 10%: Central nervous system: Dizziness (2%)
General Dosage Range
I.M.: Adults: 0.1 mcg/kg
I.V.: Adults: 0.02-0.04 mcg/kg as a single dose; may repeat 0.04 mcg/kg once or 0.12 mcg/kg as a single dose
Mechanism of Action Stimulates contraction of the gallbladder; inhibits gastric emptying by causing pyloric contraction, and increases intestinal motility; stimulates pancreatic secretion; causes smooth muscle contraction
Pharmacodynamics/Kinetics
Onset of Action Contraction of the gallbladder: ~5-15 minutes
Duration of Action ~1 hour
Pregnancy Risk Factor B
Pregnancy Considerations Fetal harm was not observed in animal studies. There are no adequate and well-controlled studies in pregnant women. Because of its effect on smooth muscle, use during pregnancy should be avoided (may cause spontaneous abortion or premature labor). Use during pregnancy only if clearly needed. Should not be administered near term; may induce labor.

Sinecatechins (sin e KAT e kins)

Brand Names: U.S. Veregen®
Pharmacologic Category Immunomodulator, Topical; Topical Skin Product
Use Treatment of external genital and perianal warts secondary to condylomata acuminata
Local Anesthetic/Vasoconstrictor Precautions No information available to require special precautions
Effects on Dental Treatment No significant effects or complications reported
Effects on Bleeding No information available to require special precautions
Adverse Effects
>10%:
Dermatologic: Erythema (70%), pruritus (69%), edema (45%), vesicular rash (20%)
Local: Burning (67%), pain/discomfort (56%), erosion/ulceration (49%), induration (35%)
1% to 10%:
Dermatologic: Desquamation (5%), rash (1%), scar formation (1%)
Local: Discharge (3%), lymphadenitis (3%), bleeding (2%), reaction (2%), irritation (1%)
Miscellaneous: Phimosis (uncircumcised males; 3%), hypersensitivity (2%)
General Dosage Range Topical: Adults: Apply a thin layer (~0.5 cm strand) 3 times/day
Mechanism of Action The mechanism by which sinecatechins ointment aids in the clearance of genital and perianal warts is unknown. Antioxidant properties have been demonstrated in vitro; however, the significance of this finding is not known.
Pregnancy Risk Factor C
Pregnancy Considerations Teratogenic effects were not observed in animal studies. There are no adequate and well-controlled studies in pregnant women; use only if possible benefit outweighs potential risk to the fetus. Sinecatechins ointment may weaken condoms and diaphragms.

Sipuleucel-T (si pu LOO sel tee)

Brand Names: U.S. Provenge®
Pharmacologic Category Cellular Immunotherapy, Autologous
Use Treatment of metastatic hormone-refractory prostate cancer in patients who are asymptomatic or minimally symptomatic
Local Anesthetic/Vasoconstrictor Precautions No information available to require special precautions
Effects on Dental Treatment No significant effects or complications reported
Effects on Bleeding No information available to require special precautions
Adverse Effects Note: Initial infusion-related events usually present within the first 24 hours after administration.
>10%:
Central nervous system: Chills (53%), fatigue (41%), fever (31%), headache (18%), dizziness (12%), pain (12%)
Gastrointestinal: Nausea (22%), vomiting (13%)
Hematologic: Anemia (13%)
Neuromuscular & skeletal: Back pain (30%), myalgia (12%), weakness (11%)
Miscellaneous: Acute infusion reaction (71%; grade 3: 4%), citrate toxicity (15%)
1% to 10%:
Cardiovascular: Hypertension (8%)
Central nervous system: Stroke (hemorrhagic or ischemic: 4%)
Dermatologic: Rash (5%)
Neuromuscular & skeletal: Muscle spasm (8%), neck pain (6%), tremor (5%)
Renal: Hematuria (8%)
Respiratory: Dyspnea (9%), cough (6%), upper respiratory tract infection (6%)
Miscellaneous: Flu-like syndrome (10%), diaphoresis (5%)
General Dosage Range I.V.: *Adults (males):* ≥50 million autologous CD54+ cells activated with PAP-GM-CSF; dose administered at ~2 week intervals for a total of 3 doses
Mechanism of Action Autologous cellular immunotherapy which stimulates an immune response against an antigen (PAP) expressed in most prostate cancer tissues. Peripheral blood is collected (~3 days prior to infusion) from the patient via leukapheresis, from which peripheral blood mononuclear cells (PBMCs) are isolated. Antigen presenting cell (APC) precursors, consisting of CD54-positive cells that include dendritic cells, are isolated from the PBMCs. The APCs are then activated (*in vitro*) with a recombinant human fusion protein, PAP-GM-CSF (also termed PA2024), composed of an antigen specific for prostate cancer, prostatic acid phosphatase (PAP) linked to granulocyte-macrophage colony-stimulating factor (GM-CSF) and cultured for ~40 hours. The final product, sipuleucel-T, is reinfused into the patient, inducing T-cell immunity to tumors that express PAP.
Pregnancy Considerations Animal reproduction studies have not been conducted. Not indicated for use in women.
Prescribing and Access Restrictions Patients may receive Sipuleucel-T at a participating site. Physicians must go through an inservice and register to prescribe the treatment; patients must also complete an enrollment form. Information on registration and enrollment is available at 1-877-336-3736.

Sirolimus (sir OH li mus)

Brand Names: U.S. Rapamune®
Brand Names: Canada Rapamune®
Generic Availability (U.S.) No
Pharmacologic Category Immunosuppressant Agent; mTOR Kinase Inhibitor
Use Prophylaxis of organ rejection in patients receiving renal transplants
Unlabeled Use Prophylaxis of organ rejection in heart transplant recipients; prevention acute graft-versus-host disease (GVHD) in allogeneic stem cell transplantation; treatment of refractory acute or chronic GVHD; treatment of soft tissue sarcoma (chordoma, angiomyolipoma, or lymphangioleiomyomatosis)
Local Anesthetic/Vasoconstrictor Precautions No information available to require special precautions
Effects on Dental Treatment Key adverse event(s) related to dental treatment: Mouth ulceration, oral moniliasis, stomatitis, gingival hyperplasia, gingivitis, and dysphagia.
Effects on Bleeding Thrombocytopenia (15% to 30%) has been associated with use; severe thrombocytopenia (rare) may be associated with delayed coagulation. Consultation to ensure adequate platelet counts may be considered in patients with signs/symptoms or a history of thrombocytopenia.
Adverse Effects Incidence of many adverse effects is dose related.
>20%:
Cardiovascular: Peripheral edema (54% to 58%), hypertension (45% to 49%), edema (18% to 20%)
Central nervous system: Headache (34%), pain (20% to 33%), insomnia (13% to 22%)
Dermatologic: Acne (22%)
Endocrine & metabolic: Hypertriglyceridemia (45% to 57%), hypercholesterolemia (43% to 46%)
Gastrointestinal: Constipation (36% to 38%), abdominal pain (29% to 36%), diarrhea (25% to 36%), nausea (25% to 31%)
Genitourinary: Urinary tract infection (26% to 33%)
Hematologic: Anemia (23% to 33%), thrombocytopenia (14% to 30%)
Neuromuscular & skeletal: Arthralgia (25% to 31%)
Renal: Serum creatinine increased (39% to 40%)
3% to 20%:
Cardiovascular: Atrial fibrillation, CHF, DVT, facial edema, hypervolemia, hypotension, orthostatic hypotension, palpitation, peripheral vascular disorder, syncope, tachycardia, thrombosis, vasodilation
Central nervous system: Anxiety, chills, confusion, depression, dizziness, emotional lability, hypoesthesia, malaise, neuropathy, somnolence
Dermatologic: Rash (10% to 20%), skin carcinoma (up to 3%; includes basal cell carcinoma, squamous cell carcinoma, melanoma), cellulitis, dermal ulcer, dermatitis (fungal), ecchymosis, hirsutism, pruritus, skin hypertrophy, wound healing abnormal
Endocrine & metabolic: Acidosis, Cushing's syndrome, dehydration, diabetes mellitus, glycosuria, hypercalcemia, hyperglycemia, hyperphosphatemia, hypocalcemia, hypoglycemia, hypokalemia, hypomagnesemia, hyponatremia
Gastrointestinal: Abdomen enlarged, anorexia, dysphagia, eructation, esophagitis, flatulence, gastritis, gastroenteritis, gingival hyperplasia, gingivitis, ileus, mouth ulceration, oral moniliasis, stomatitis, weight loss

Genitourinary: Impotence, pelvic pain, scrotal edema, testis disorder

Hematologic: Hemolytic-uremic syndrome, hemorrhage, leukopenia, leukocytosis, polycythemia, TTP

Hepatic: Abnormal liver function tests, alkaline phosphatase increased, LDH increased

Local: Thrombophlebitis

Neuromuscular & skeletal: Arthrosis, bone necrosis, CPK increased, hyper-/hypotonia, leg cramps, myalgia, osteoporosis, paresthesia, tetany

Ocular: Abnormal vision, cataract, conjunctivitis

Otic: Ear pain, otitis media, tinnitus

Renal: Albuminuria, bladder pain, BUN increased, dysuria, hematuria, hydronephrosis, kidney pain, nephropathy (toxic), nocturia, oliguria, pyelonephritis, pyuria, tubular necrosis, urinary frequency, urinary incontinence, urinary retention

Respiratory: Asthma, atelectasis, bronchitis, cough, epistaxis, hypoxia, lung edema, pleural effusion, pneumonia, pulmonary embolism, rhinitis, sinusitis

Miscellaneous: Lymphoproliferative disease/lymphoma (1% to 3%), abscess, diaphoresis, flu-like syndrome, hernia, herpesvirus infection, infection (including opportunistic), lymphadenopathy, lymphocele, peritonitis, sepsis

Dosage Oral:

Low-to-moderate immunologic risk renal transplant patients: Children ≥13 years and Adults: Dosing by body weight:

<40 kg: Loading dose: 3 mg/m^2 on day 1, followed by maintenance dosing of 1 mg/m^2 once daily

≥40 kg: Loading dose: 6 mg on day 1; maintenance: 2 mg once daily

High immunologic risk renal transplant patients: Adults: Loading dose: Up to 15 mg on day 1; maintenance: 5 mg/day; obtain trough concentration between days 5-7 and adjust accordingly. Continue concurrent cyclosporine/sirolimus therapy for 1 year following transplantation. Further adjustment of the regimen must be based on clinical status.

Dosage adjustment: Sirolimus dosages should be adjusted to maintain trough concentrations within desired range based on risk and concomitant therapy. Maximum daily dose: 40 mg. Dosage should be adjusted at intervals of 7-14 days to account for the long half-life of sirolimus. In general, dose proportionality may be assumed. New sirolimus dose **equals** current dose **multiplied by** (target concentration **divided by** current concentration). **Note:** If large dose increase is required, consider loading dose calculated as:

Loading dose **equals** (new maintenance dose **minus** current maintenance dose) **multiplied by** 3

Maximum dose in 1 day: 40 mg; if required dose is >40 mg (due to loading dose), divide loading dose over 2 days. Whole blood concentrations should not be used as the sole basis for dosage adjustment (monitor clinical signs/symptoms, tissue biopsy, and laboratory parameters).

Maintenance therapy after withdrawal of cyclosporine: Cyclosporine withdrawal is not recommended in high immunological risk patients. Following 2-4 months of combined therapy, withdrawal of cyclosporine may be considered in low-to-moderate immunologic risk patients. Cyclosporine should be discontinued over 4-8 weeks, and a necessary increase in the dosage of sirolimus (up to fourfold) should be anticipated due to removal of metabolic inhibition by cyclosporine and to maintain adequate immunosuppressive effects.

Dose-adjusted trough target concentrations are typically 16-24 ng/mL for the first year post-transplant and 12-20 ng/mL thereafter (measured by chromatographic methodology).

GVHD prophylaxis (unlabeled use): 12 mg loading dose on day -3, followed by 4 mg daily (target trough level: 3-12 ng/mL); taper off after 6-9 months (Armand, 2008; Cutler, 2007)

Treatment of refractory acute GVHD (unlabeled use): 4-5 mg/m^2 for 14 days (no loading dose) (Benito, 2001)

Treatment of chronic GVHD (unlabeled use): 6 mg loading dose, followed by 2 mg daily (target trough level: 7-12 ng/mL) for 6-9 months (Couriel, 2005)

Dosage adjustment in renal impairment: No dosage adjustment (in loading or maintenance dose) is necessary in renal impairment. However, adjustment of regimen (including discontinuation of therapy) should be considered when used concurrently with cyclosporine and elevated or increasing serum creatinine is noted.

Dosage adjustment in hepatic impairment:

Loading dose: No adjustment required

Maintenance dose:

Mild-to-moderate hepatic impairment: reduce maintenance dose by ~33%

Severe hepatic impairment: reduce maintenance dose by ~50%

Mechanism of Action Sirolimus inhibits T-lymphocyte activation and proliferation in response to antigenic and cytokine stimulation and inhibits antibody production. Its mechanism differs from other immunosuppressants. Sirolimus binds to FKBP-12, an intracellular protein, to form an immunosuppressive complex which inhibits the regulatory kinase, mTOR (mammalian target of rapamycin). This inhibition suppresses cytokine mediated T-cell proliferation, halting progression from the G1 to the S phase of the cell cycle. It inhibits acute rejection of allografts and prolongs graft survival.

Contraindications Hypersensitivity to sirolimus or any component of the formulation

Warnings/Precautions Hazardous agent - use appropriate precautions for handling and disposal (NIOSH, 2012). **[U.S. Boxed Warning]: Immunosuppressive agents, including sirolimus, increase the risk of infection and may be associated with the development of lymphoma.** Immune suppression may also increase the risk of opportunistic infections (including activation of latent viral infections including BK virus-associated nephropathy), fatal infections, and sepsis. Prophylactic treatment for *Pneumocystis jirovecii* pneumonia (PCP) should be administered for 1 year post-transplant; prophylaxis for cytomegalovirus (CMV) should be taken for 3 months post-transplant in patients at risk for CMV. Progressive multifocal leukoencephalopathy (PML), an opportunistic CNS infection caused by reactivation of the JC virus, has been reported in patients receiving immunosuppressive therapy, including sirolimus. Clinical findings of PML include apathy, ataxia, cognitive deficiency, confusion, and hemiparesis; promptly evaluate any patient presenting with neurological changes; consider decreasing the degree of immunosuppression with consideration to the risk of organ rejection in transplant patients.

[U.S. Boxed Warning]: Sirolimus is not recommended for use in liver or lung transplantation. Bronchial anastomotic dehiscence cases have been reported in lung transplant patients when sirolimus was used as part of an immunosuppressive

regimen; **most of these reactions were fatal. Studies indicate an association with an increase risk of hepatic artery thrombosis (HAT), graft failure, and increased mortality (with evidence of infection) in liver transplant patients when sirolimus is used in combination with cyclosporine and/or tacrolimus.** Most cases of HAT occurred within 30 days of transplant.

In renal transplant patients, *de novo* use without cyclosporine has been associated with higher rates of acute rejection. Sirolimus should be used in combination with cyclosporine (and corticosteroids) initially. Cyclosporine may be withdrawn in low-to-moderate immunologic risk patients after 2-4 months, in conjunction with an increase in sirolimus dosage. In high immunologic risk patients, use in combination with cyclosporine and corticosteroids is recommended for the first year. Safety and efficacy of combination therapy with cyclosporine in high immunologic risk patients has not been studied beyond 12 months of treatment; adjustment of immunosuppressive therapy beyond 12 months should be considered based on clinical judgement. Monitor renal function closely when combined with cyclosporine; consider dosage adjustment or discontinue in patients with increasing serum creatinine.

May increase serum creatinine and decrease GFR. Use caution when used concurrently with medications which may alter renal function. May delay recovery of renal function in patients with delayed allograft function. Increased urinary protein excretion has been observed when converting renal transplant patients from calcineurin inhibitors to sirolimus during maintenance therapy. A higher level of proteinuria prior to sirolimus conversion correlates with a higher degree of proteinuria after conversion. In some patients, proteinuria may reach nephrotic levels; nephrotic syndrome (new onset) has been reported. Increased risk of BK viral-associated nephropathy which may impair renal function and cause graft loss; consider decreasing immunosuppressive burden if evidence of deteriorating renal function.

Use caution with hepatic impairment; a reduction in the maintenance dose is recommended. Has been associated with an increased risk of fluid accumulation and lymphocele; peripheral edema, lymphedema, ascites, and pleural and pericardial effusions (including significant effusions and tamponade) were reported; use with caution in patients in whom fluid accumulation may be poorly tolerated, such as in cardiovascular disease (heart failure or hypertension) and pulmonary disease. Cases of interstitial lung disease (eg, pneumonitis, bronchiolitis obliterans organizing pneumonia [BOOP], pulmonary fibrosis) have been observed; risk may be increased with higher trough levels. Avoid concurrent use of strong CYP3A4 and/or P-glycoprotein (P-gp) inhibitors (eg, clarithromycin, erythromycin, telithromycin, itraconazole, ketoconazole, voriconazole) and strong inducers of CYP3A4 and/or P-gp (eg, rifampin, rifabutin). Concurrent use with a calcineurin inhibitor (cyclosporine, tacrolimus) may increase the risk of calcineurin inhibitor-induced hemolytic uremic syndrome/thrombotic thrombocytopenic purpura/thrombotic microangiopathy (HUS/TTP/TMA).

Hypersensitivity reactions, including anaphylactic/anaphylactoid reactions, angioedema, exfoliative dermatitis, and hypersensitivity vasculitis have been reported. Concurrent use with other drugs known to cause angioedema (eg, ACE inhibitors) may increase risk. Immunosuppressant therapy is associated with an increased risk of skin cancer; limit sun and ultraviolet light exposure; use appropriate sun protection. May increase serum lipids (cholesterol and triglycerides); use with caution in patients with hyperlipidemia. May be associated with wound dehiscence and impaired healing; use caution in the perioperative period. Patients with a body mass index (BMI) >30 kg/m^2 are at increased risk for abnormal wound healing.

Sirolimus tablets and oral solution are not bioequivalent, due to differences in absorption. Clinical equivalence was seen using 2 mg tablet and 2 mg solution. It is not known if higher doses are also clinically equivalent. Monitor sirolimus levels if changes in dosage forms are made. **[U.S. Boxed Warning]: Should only be used by physicians experienced in immunosuppressive therapy and management of transplant patients. Adequate laboratory and supportive medical resources must be readily available.** Sirolimus concentrations are dependent on the assay method (eg, chromatographic and immunoassay) used; assay methods are not interchangeable. Variations in methods to determine sirolimus whole blood concentrations, as well as interlaboratory variations, may result in improper dosage adjustments, which may lead to subtherapeutic or toxic levels. Determine the assay method used to assure consistency (or accommodations if changes occur), and for monitoring purposes, be aware of alterations to assay method or reference range. The manufacturer recommends high performance liquid chromatography (HPLC) as the reference standard to determine sirolimus trough concentrations.

Drug Interactions

Metabolism/Transport Effects Substrate of CYP3A4 (major), P-glycoprotein; **Note:** Assignment of Major/Minor substrate status based on clinically relevant drug interaction potential; **Inhibits** CYP3A4 (weak)

Avoid Concomitant Use

Avoid concomitant use of Sirolimus with any of the following: BCG; CloZAPine; Conivaptan; Crizotinib; Enzalutamide; Mifepristone; Natalizumab; Pimecrolimus; Pimozide; Posaconazole; Tacrolimus (Topical); Tofacitinib; Vaccines (Live); Voriconazole

Increased Effect/Toxicity

Sirolimus may increase the levels/effects of: ACE Inhibitors; ARIPiprazole; CloZAPine; CycloSPORINE (Systemic); Leflunomide; Lomitapide; Natalizumab; Pimozide; Tacrolimus (Systemic); Tacrolimus (Topical); Tofacitinib; Vaccines (Live)

The levels/effects of Sirolimus may be increased by: Boceprevir; Conivaptan; Crizotinib; CycloSPORINE (Systemic); CYP3A4 Inhibitors (Moderate); CYP3A4 Inhibitors (Strong); Dasatinib; Denosumab; Fluconazole; Itraconazole; Ivacaftor; Ketoconazole (Systemic); Macrolide Antibiotics; Mifepristone; P-glycoprotein/ABCB1 Inhibitors; Pimecrolimus; Posaconazole; Protease Inhibitors; Roflumilast; Tacrolimus (Systemic); Tacrolimus (Topical); Telaprevir; Trastuzumab; Voriconazole

Decreased Effect

Sirolimus may decrease the levels/effects of: BCG; Coccidioidin Skin Test; Sipuleucel-T; Tacrolimus (Systemic); Vaccines (Inactivated); Vaccines (Live)

The levels/effects of Sirolimus may be decreased by: CYP3A4 Inducers (Strong); Deferasirox; Echinacea; Efavirenz; Enzalutamide; Fosphenytoin; Herbs (CYP3A4 Inducers); P-glycoprotein/ABCB1 Inducers; Phenytoin; Rifampin; Tocilizumab

◀ **Ethanol/Nutrition/Herb Interactions**
Food: Grapefruit juice may decrease clearance of siro-limus. Ingestion with high-fat meals decreases peak concentrations but increases AUC by 23% to 35%. Management: Avoid grapefruit juice. Take consistently (either with or without food) to minimize variability.

Herb/Nutraceutical: St John's wort may decrease siroli-mus levels. Some herbal medications have immunos-timulant properties (eg, echinacea). Herbs with hypoglycemic properties may increase the risk of sirolimus-induced hypoglycemia (eg, alfalfa). Manage-ment: Avoid St John's wort, cat's claw, and echinacea. Avoid alfalfa, aloe, bilberry, bitter melon, burdock, celery, damiana, fenugreek, garcinia, garlic, ginger, ginseng (American), gymnema, marshmallow, and stinging nettle.

Dietary Considerations Take consistently (with or without food) to minimize variability of absorption.

Pharmacodynamics/Kinetics
Half-life Elimination Half-life elimination: Mean: 62 hours (range; 46-78 hours); extended in hepatic impairment (Child-Pugh class A or B) to 113 hours

Time to Peak Oral solution: 1-3 hours; Tablet: 1-6 hours

Pregnancy Risk Factor C

Pregnancy Considerations Animal studies have demonstrated embryotoxicity and fetotoxicity, as evi-denced by increased mortality, reduced fetal weights and delayed ossification. There are no adequate and well-controlled studies in pregnant women. Effective contraception must be initiated before therapy with sirolimus and continued for 12 weeks after discontinua-tion.

The National Transplantation Pregnancy Registry (NTPR, Temple University) is a registry for pregnant women taking immunosuppressants following any solid organ transplant. The NTPR encourages reporting of all immunosuppressant exposures during pregnancy in transplant recipients at 877-955-6877.

Lactation Excretion in breast milk unknown/not recom-mended

Breast-Feeding Considerations Due to the potential for adverse reactions in the breast-fed infant, including possible immunosuppression, breast-feeding is not rec-ommended.

Dosage Forms
Solution, oral:
Rapamune®: 1 mg/mL (60 mL)
Tablet, oral:
Rapamune®: 0.5 mg, 1 mg, 2 mg

SitaGLIPtin (sit a GLIP tin)

Related Information
Endocrine Disorders and Pregnancy on page 1517
Brand Names: U.S. Januvia®
Brand Names: Canada Januvia®
Generic Availability (U.S.) No
Pharmacologic Category Antidiabetic Agent, Dipep-tidyl Peptidase IV (DPP-IV) Inhibitor
Use Management of type 2 diabetes mellitus (noninsulin dependent, NIDDM) as an adjunct to diet and exercise as monotherapy or in combination therapy with other antidiabetic agents
Local Anesthetic/Vasoconstrictor Precautions No information available to require special precautions

Effects on Dental Treatment Sitagliptin-dependent patients with diabetes should be appointed for dental treatment in morning in order to minimize chance of stress-induced hypoglycemia.

Effects on Bleeding No information available to require special precautions

Adverse Effects As reported with monotherapy: 1% to 10%:
Cardiovascular: Peripheral edema (2%)
Endocrine & metabolic: Hypoglycemia (1%)
Gastrointestinal: Diarrhea (4%), constipation (3%), nau-sea (2%)
Neuromuscular & skeletal: Osteoarthritis (1%)
Respiratory: Nasopharyngitis (5%), pharyngitis (1%), upper respiratory tract infection (viral; 1%)

Dosage Oral: Adults: Type 2 diabetes: 100 mg once daily
Concomitant use with insulin and/or insulin secreta-gogues (eg, sulfonylureas): Reduced dose of insulin and/or insulin secretagogues may be needed.

Dosage adjustment in renal impairment: Note: Renal function may be estimated using the Cockcroft-Gault formula for dosage adjustment purposes.
Cl_{cr} ≥50 mL/minute: No dosage adjustment necessary.
Cl_{cr} ≥30 to <50 mL/minute (approximate S_{cr} of >1.7 to ≤3.0 mg/dL [males] or >1.5 to ≤2.5 mg/dL [females]): 50 mg once daily
Cl_{cr} <30 mL/minute (approximate S_{cr} of >3.0 mg/dL [males] or >2.5 mg/dL [females]): 25 mg once daily
ESRD requiring hemodialysis or peritoneal dialysis: 25 mg once daily; administered without regard to timing of hemodialysis

Dosage adjustment in hepatic impairment:
Mild-to-moderate impairment (Child-Pugh score 7-9): No dosage adjustment required
Severe impairment (Child-Pugh score >9): Not studied

Mechanism of Action Sitagliptin inhibits dipeptidyl peptidase IV (DPP-IV) enzyme resulting in prolonged active incretin levels. Incretin hormones (eg, glucagon-like peptide-1 [GLP-1] and glucose-dependent insulino-tropic polypeptide [GIP]) regulate glucose homeostasis by increasing insulin synthesis and release from pan-creatic beta cells and decreasing glucagon secretion from pancreatic alpha cells. Decreased glucagon secre-tion results in decreased hepatic glucose production. Under normal physiologic circumstances, incretin hor-mones are released by the intestine throughout the day and levels are increased in response to a meal; incretin hormones are rapidly inactivated by the DPP-IV enzyme.

Contraindications Serious hypersensitivity (eg, ana-phylaxis, angioedema) to sitagliptan or any component of the formulation

Warnings/Precautions Avoid use in type 1 diabetes mellitus (insulin dependent, IDDM) and diabetic ketoa-cidosis (DKA) due to lack of efficacy in these popula-tions. Use caution when used in conjunction with insulin or insulin secretagogues; risk of hypoglycemia is increased. Monitor blood glucose closely; dosage adjustments of insulin or insulin secretagogues may be necessary. Use with caution in patients with moder-ate-to-severe renal dysfunction and end-stage renal disease (ESRD) requiring hemodialysis or peritoneal dialysis; dosing adjustment required. Safety and efficacy have not been established in severe hepatic dysfunc-tion.

Rare hypersensitivity reactions, including anaphylaxis, angioedema, and/or severe dermatologic reactions (such as Stevens-Johnson syndrome), have been reported in postmarketing surveillance; discontinue if signs/symptoms of hypersensitivity reactions occur. Use with caution if patient has experienced angioedema with other DPP-IV inhibitor use. Cases of acute pancreatitis (including hemorrhagic and necrotizing with some fatalities) have been reported with use; monitor for signs/symptoms of pancreatitis. Discontinue use immediately if pancreatitis is suspected and initiate appropriate management. Use with caution in patients with a history of pancreatitis (not known if this population is at greater risk).

Clinical trials included only a limited number of patients with heart failure (HF). No specific recommendations regarding this population are provided in the approved U.S. labeling (Canadian labeling recommends against use in this population). Diabetes self-management education (DSME) is essential to maximize the effectiveness of therapy.

Drug Interactions
Metabolism/Transport Effects Substrate of P-glycoprotein
Avoid Concomitant Use There are no known interactions where it is recommended to avoid concomitant use.
Increased Effect/Toxicity
SitaGLIPtin may increase the levels/effects of: ACE Inhibitors; Digoxin; Hypoglycemic Agents

The levels/effects of SitaGLIPtin may be increased by: Herbs (Hypoglycemic Properties); MAO Inhibitors; Pegvisomant; P-glycoprotein/ABCB1 Inhibitors; Salicylates; Selective Serotonin Reuptake Inhibitors
Decreased Effect
The levels/effects of SitaGLIPtin may be decreased by: Corticosteroids (Orally Inhaled); Corticosteroids (Systemic); Loop Diuretics; Luteinizing Hormone-Releasing Hormone Analogs; P-glycoprotein/ABCB1 Inducers; Somatropin; Thiazide Diuretics
Dietary Considerations May be taken with or without food. Individualized medical nutrition therapy (MNT) based on ADA recommendations is an integral part of therapy.
Pharmacodynamics/Kinetics
Half-life Elimination 12 hours
Time to Peak 1-4 hours
Pregnancy Risk Factor B
Pregnancy Considerations Adverse events have not been observed in animal reproduction studies; therefore, sitagliptan is classified as pregnancy category B. There are no adequate and well controlled studies in pregnant women. Maternal hyperglycemia can be associated with adverse effects in the fetus, including macrosomia, neonatal hyperglycemia, and hyperbilirubinemia; the risk of congenital malformations is increased when the Hb A_{1c} is above the normal range. Diabetes can also be associated with adverse effects in the mother. Poorly-treated diabetes may cause end-organ damage that may in turn negatively affect obstetric outcomes. Physiologic glucose levels should be maintained prior to and during pregnancy to decrease the risk of adverse events in the mother and the fetus. Until additional safety and efficacy data are obtained, the use of oral agents is generally not recommended as routine management of GDM or type 2 diabetes mellitus during pregnancy. Insulin is the drug of choice for the control of diabetes mellitus during pregnancy. Health professionals are encouraged to report any prenatal exposure to

sitagliptin by contacting Merck's pregnancy registry (1-800-986-8999).
Lactation Excretion in breast milk unknown/use caution
Breast-Feeding Considerations It is not known if sitagliptin is excreted in breast milk. The manufacturer recommends that caution be used if administered to breast-feeding women.
Dosage Forms
Tablet, oral:
Januvia®: 25 mg, 50 mg, 100 mg

Sitagliptin and Metformin
(sit a GLIP tin & met FOR min)

Related Information
MetFORMIN *on page 882*
SitaGLIPtin *on page 1242*
Brand Names: U.S. Janumet®; Janumet® XR
Brand Names: Canada Janumet®
Pharmacologic Category Antidiabetic Agent, Biguanide; Antidiabetic Agent, Dipeptidyl Peptidase IV (DPP-IV) Inhibitor; Hypoglycemic Agent, Oral
Use Management of type 2 diabetes mellitus (noninsulin dependent, NIDDM) as an adjunct to diet and exercise in patients not adequately controlled on metformin or sitagliptin monotherapy
Local Anesthetic/Vasoconstrictor Precautions No information available to require special precautions
Effects on Dental Treatment Sitagliptin- and metformin-dependent patients with diabetes (noninsulin dependent, Type 2) should be appointed for dental treatment in morning in order to minimize chance of stress-induced hypoglycemia.
Effects on Bleeding No information available to require special precautions
Adverse Effects See individual agents.
General Dosage Range Oral: *Adults:*
Immediate release: Sitagliptin 50 mg and metformin 500-1000 mg twice daily (maximum: 100 mg/day [sitagliptin], 2000 mg/day [metformin])
Extended release: Sitagliptin 100 mg and metformin 1000-2000 mg once daily (maximum: 100 mg/day [sitagliptin], 2000 mg/day [metformin])
Mechanism of Action Sitagliptin inhibits dipeptidyl peptidase IV (DPP-IV) enzymes resulting in prolonged active incretin levels. Incretin hormones [eg, glucagon-like peptide-1 (GLP-1) and glucose-dependent insulinotropic polypeptide (GIP)] regulate glucose homeostasis by increasing insulin synthesis and release from pancreatic beta cells and decreasing glucagon secretion from pancreatic alpha cells. Decreased glucagon secretion results in decreased hepatic glucose production. Under normal physiologic circumstances, incretin hormones are released by the intestine throughout the day and levels are increased in response to a meal; incretin hormones are rapidly inactivated by DPP-IV enzymes.

Metformin decreases hepatic glucose production, decreasing intestinal absorption of glucose, and improves insulin sensitivity (increases peripheral glucose uptake and utilization).
Pregnancy Risk Factor B
Pregnancy Considerations Reproduction studies have not been conducted with this combination. Adverse events were not observed in animal studies of the individual agents; therefore, sitagliptin/metformin is classified as pregnancy category B. See individual agents. Health professionals are encouraged to report any prenatal exposure to Janumet® by contacting Merck's pregnancy registry (1-800-986-8999).

Sitagliptin and Simvastatin
(sit a GLIP tin & sim va STAT in)

Brand Names: U.S. Juvisync™

Pharmacologic Category Antidiabetic Agent, Dipeptidyl Peptidase IV (DPP-IV) Inhibitor; Antilipemic Agent, HMG-CoA Reductase Inhibitor

Use For use when treatment with both sitagliptin and simvastatin is appropriate:

Sitagliptin: Management of type 2 diabetes mellitus (noninsulin dependent, NIDDM) as an adjunct to diet and exercise as monotherapy or in combination therapy with other antidiabetic agents

Simvastatin: Used with dietary therapy for the following: Secondary prevention of cardiovascular events in hypercholesterolemic patients with established coronary heart disease (CHD) or at high risk for CHD: To reduce cardiovascular morbidity (myocardial infarction, coronary/noncoronary revascularization procedures) and mortality; to reduce the risk of stroke

Hyperlipidemias: To reduce elevations in total cholesterol (total-C), LDL-C, apolipoprotein B, triglycerides, and VLDL-C, and to increase HDL-C in patients with primary hypercholesterolemia (elevations of 1 or more components are present in Fredrickson type IIa, IIb, III, and IV hyperlipidemias); treatment of homozygous familial hypercholesterolemia

Local Anesthetic/Vasoconstrictor Precautions No information available to require special precautions

Effects on Dental Treatment Sitagliptin-dependent patients with diabetes should be appointed for dental treatment in morning in order to minimize chance of stress-induced hypoglycemia.

Effects on Bleeding No information available to require special precautions

Adverse Effects See individual agents.

General Dosage Range Dosage adjustment recommended in patients on concomitant therapy or with renal impairment.

Oral: *Adults:* Initial: Sitagliptin 100 mg and simvastatin 40 mg once daily

Mechanism of Action

Simvastatin: A methylated derivative of lovastatin that acts by competitively inhibiting 3-hydroxy-3-methylglutaryl-coenzyme A (HMG-CoA) reductase, the enzyme that catalyzes the rate-limiting step in cholesterol biosynthesis

Sitagliptin: Inhibits dipeptidyl peptidase IV (DPP-IV) enzyme resulting in prolonged active incretin levels. Incretin hormones (eg, glucagon-like peptide-1 [GLP-1] and glucose-dependent insulinotropic polypeptide [GIP]) regulate glucose homeostasis by increasing insulin synthesis and release from pancreatic beta cells and decreasing glucagon secretion from pancreatic alpha cells. Decreased glucagon secretion results in decreased hepatic glucose production. Under normal physiologic circumstances, incretin hormones are released by the intestine throughout the day and levels are increased in response to a meal; incretin hormones are rapidly inactivated by the DPP-IV enzyme.

Pregnancy Risk Factor X

Pregnancy Considerations Use is contraindicated in pregnant women. See individual agents.

Sodium Bicarbonate
(SOW dee um bye KAR bun ate)

Brand Names: U.S. Brioschi® [OTC]; Neut®

Pharmacologic Category Alkalinizing Agent; Antacid; Electrolyte Supplement, Oral; Electrolyte Supplement, Parenteral

Use Management of metabolic acidosis; gastric hyperacidity; as an alkalinization agent for the urine; treatment of hyperkalemia; management of overdose of certain drugs, including tricyclic antidepressants and aspirin

Unlabeled Use Prevention of contrast-induced nephropathy (CIN)

Local Anesthetic/Vasoconstrictor Precautions No information available to require special precautions

Effects on Dental Treatment No significant effects or complications reported

Effects on Bleeding No information available to require special precautions

Adverse Effects Frequency not defined.
Cardiovascular: Cerebral hemorrhage, CHF (aggravated), edema
Central nervous system: Tetany
Gastrointestinal: Belching, flatulence (with oral), gastric distension
Endocrine & metabolic: Hypernatremia, hyperosmolality, hypocalcemia, hypokalemia, increased affinity of hemoglobin for oxygen-reduced pH in myocardial tissue necrosis when extravasated, intracranial acidosis, metabolic alkalosis, milk-alkali syndrome (especially with renal dysfunction)
Respiratory: Pulmonary edema

General Dosage Range
I.V.: *Children and Adults:* Dosage varies greatly depending on indication
Oral:
Children: 1-10 mEq/kg/day as a single dose **or** divided every 4-6 hours
Adults <60 years: 0.5-200 mEq/kg/day in 4-5 divided doses **or** 325 mg to 2 g 1-4 times/day (maximum: 16 g [200 mEq] day)
Adults ≥60 years: 0.5-100 mEq/kg/day in 4-6 divided doses **or** 325 mg to 2 g 1-4 times/day (maximum: 8 g [100 mEq] day)

Mechanism of Action Dissociates to provide bicarbonate ion which neutralizes hydrogen ion concentration and raises blood and urinary pH

Pharmacodynamics/Kinetics
Onset of Action Oral: Rapid; I.V.: 15 minutes
Duration of Action Oral: 8-10 minutes; I.V.: 1-2 hours
Pregnancy Risk Factor C

Pregnancy Considerations Animal reproduction studies have not been conducted. The use of sodium bicarbonate in pregnant women for the management of cardiac arrest and metabolic acidosis is the same as in nonpregnant women (Campbell, 2009; Vanden Hoek, 2010). Antacids containing sodium bicarbonate should not be used during pregnancy due to their potential to cause metabolic alkalosis and fluid overload (Mahadevan, 2007).

Sodium Chloride (SOW dee um KLOR ide)

Brand Names: U.S. 4-Way® Saline Moisturizing Mist [OTC]; Altachlore [OTC]; Altamist [OTC]; Ayr® Allergy & Sinus [OTC]; Ayr® Baby Saline [OTC]; Ayr® Saline Nasal Gel [OTC]; Ayr® Saline No-Drip [OTC]; Ayr® Saline [OTC]; Deep Sea [OTC]; Entsol® [OTC]; HuMist® [OTC]; HyperSal®; Little Noses® Saline [OTC]; Little Noses® Sterile Saline Nasal Mist [OTC]; Little Noses® Stuffy Nose Kit [OTC]; Muro 128® [OTC]; Na-Zone® [OTC]; NebuSal™; Ocean® for Kids [OTC]; Ocean® [OTC]; Pretz® [OTC]; Rhinaris® [OTC]; Safe

Wash™ [OTC]; Saline Mist [OTC]; Saljet® [OTC]; Sea Soft Nasal Mist [OTC]; Simply Saline® Baby [OTC]; Simply Saline® [OTC]; Sochlor™ [OTC]; Syrex; Wound Wash Saline™ [OTC]

Pharmacologic Category Electrolyte Supplement, Parenteral; Genitourinary Irrigant; Irrigant; Lubricant, Ocular; Sodium Salt

Use

Parenteral: Restores sodium ion in patients with restricted oral intake (especially hyponatremia states or low salt syndrome).

Concentrated sodium chloride: Additive for parenteral fluid therapy

Hypertonic sodium chloride: For severe hyponatremia and hypochloremia

Hypotonic sodium chloride: Hydrating solution

Normal saline: Restores water/sodium losses

Ophthalmic: Reduces corneal edema

Inhalation: Restores moisture to pulmonary system; loosens and thins congestion caused by colds or allergies; diluent for bronchodilator solutions that require dilution before inhalation

Intranasal: Restores moisture to nasal membranes

Irrigation: Wound cleansing, irrigation, and flushing

Unlabeled Use Parenteral: Hypertonic saline: Refractory elevated intracranial pressure (ICP) due to various etiologies (eg, subarachnoid hemorrhage, neoplasm); transtentorial herniation syndrome; traumatic brain injury with elevated ICP. **Note:** May be used in patients in whom mannitol may not be recommended (eg, renal failure).

Local Anesthetic/Vasoconstrictor Precautions No information available to require special precautions

Effects on Dental Treatment No significant effects or complications reported

Effects on Bleeding No information available to require special precautions

Adverse Effects Frequency not defined.

Cardiovascular: Congestive heart failure, transient hypotension (especially with adult administration of 23.4% NaCl)

Central nervous system: Central pontine myelinolysis (due to rapid correction of hyponatremia)

Endocrine & metabolic: Dilution of serum electrolytes, extravasation, hypernatremia, hypervolemia, hypokalemia, overhydration

Gastrointestinal: Nausea, vomiting (oral use)

Local: Thrombosis, phlebitis, extravasation

Respiratory: Bronchospasm (inhalation with hypertonic solutions), pulmonary edema

General Dosage Range

I.V.: *Children and Adults:* Dosage varies greatly depending on indication

Inhalation: *Children ≥2 years and Adults:* 1-3 sprays (1-3 mL)

Intranasal: *Children ≥2 years and Adults:* 2-3 sprays in each nostril as needed

Irrigation: *Children ≥2 years and Adults:* 1-3 L/day **or** spray affected area

Ophthalmic: *Adults:* Ointment: Apply once or more daily; Solution: Instill 1-2 drops into affected eye(s) every 3-4 hours

Mechanism of Action Principal extracellular cation; functions in fluid and electrolyte balance, osmotic pressure control, and water distribution

Pregnancy Risk Factor C

Pregnancy Considerations Animal reproduction studies have not been conducted. Sodium requirements do not change during pregnancy (IOM, 2004). Nasal saline rinses may be used for the treatment of pregnancy rhinitis (Wallace, 2008)

Sodium Chondroitin Sulfate and Sodium Hyaluronate
(SOW de um kon DROY tin SUL fate & SOW de um hye al yoor ON ate)

Brand Names: U.S. DisCoVisc®; Viscoat®

Pharmacologic Category Ophthalmic Agent, Viscoelastic

Use Ophthalmic surgical aid in the anterior segment during cataract extraction and intraocular lens implantation

Local Anesthetic/Vasoconstrictor Precautions No information available to require special precautions

Effects on Dental Treatment No significant effects or complications reported

Effects on Bleeding No information available to require special precautions

Adverse Effects Frequency not defined: Ocular: Intraocular pressure increased

General Dosage Range Ophthalmic: *Adults:* Carefully introduce into anterior chamber during surgery

Mechanism of Action Ophthalmic viscosurgical device which modulates the interactions between adjacent tissues by space creation, tissue stabilization, balancing pressure, and providing protection of the corneal endothelial cells during surgery.

Sodium Citrate and Citric Acid
(SOW dee um SIT rate & SI trik AS id)

Brand Names: U.S. Cytra-2; Oracit®; Shohl's Solution (Modified)

Brand Names: Canada PMS-Dicitrate

Pharmacologic Category Alkalinizing Agent, Oral

Use Treatment of metabolic acidosis; alkalinizing agent in conditions where long-term maintenance of an alkaline urine is desirable

Local Anesthetic/Vasoconstrictor Precautions No information available to require special precautions

Effects on Dental Treatment No significant effects or complications reported

Effects on Bleeding No information available to require special precautions

Adverse Effects Frequency not defined. Generally well tolerated with normal renal function.

Central nervous system: Tetany

Endocrine & metabolic: Metabolic alkalosis

Gastrointestinal: Diarrhea, nausea, vomiting

General Dosage Range Oral:

Infants and Children: 2-3 mEq/kg/day in 3-4 divided doses **or** 5-15 mL after meals and at bedtime

Adults: 10-30 mL after meals and at bedtime

Pregnancy Risk Factor Not established

Pregnancy Considerations Use caution with toxemia of pregnancy.

Sodium Hypochlorite Solution
(SOW dee um hye poe KLOR ite soe LOO shun)

Brand Names: U.S. Atrapro™ Dermal; Dakin's Solution; Di-Dak-Sol

Pharmacologic Category Disinfectant, Antibacterial (Topical)

◄ **Use**
Atrapro™ Dermal (0.004%): Management (via debridement) of wounds such as stage I-IV pressure ulcers; partial and full thickness wounds; diabetic foot ulcers; post surgical and donor sites; first- and second-degree burns
Dakin's Solution (0.125%, 0.25%, 0.5%); Di-Dak-Sol (0.0125%): Prevention/treatment of skin and tissue infections, cuts, abrasions, skin ulcers; pre- and post-surgery
Local Anesthetic/Vasoconstrictor Precautions No information available to require special precautions
Effects on Dental Treatment No significant effects or complications reported
Effects on Bleeding No information available to require special precautions
Adverse Effects Frequency not defined.
Dermatologic: Irritating to skin
Hematologic: Dissolves blood clots, delays clotting
General Dosage Range
Topical: *Children and Adults:*
Atrapro™ Dermal spray: Apply to affected area 3 times daily.
Dakin's solution, Di-Dak-Sol: Via irrigation: Lightly-to-moderately exudative wounds: Apply once daily; Highly exudative or contaminated wounds: Apply twice daily

---

Sodium Iodide I131 (SOW dee um EYE oh dide)

Related Information
Endocrine Disorders and Pregnancy *on page 1517*
Brand Names: U.S. Hicon™; Iodotope®
Pharmacologic Category Antithyroid Agent; Radiopharmaceutical
Use For diagnostic use with the radioactive iodide (RAI) uptake test to evaluate thyroid function; treatment of hyperthyroidism and select cases of thyroid cancer
Unlabeled Use Graves' disease; toxic multinodular goiter; toxic thyroid adenoma
Local Anesthetic/Vasoconstrictor Precautions No information available to require special precautions
Effects on Dental Treatment Key adverse event(s) related to dental treatment: Salivary gland pain and swelling; decreased salivation and taste, mucositis (see Dental Comment)
Effects on Bleeding No information available to require special precautions
Adverse Effects Frequency not defined, dose dependent.
Cardiovascular: Chest pain, tachycardia
Dermatologic: Alopecia, itching, rash, urticaria
Endocrine & metabolic: Acute thyroid crisis, infertility (transient; may be permanent in males with repeated or high dose), thyroiditis
Gastrointestinal: Nausea (high dose used in treatment of thyroid cancer), sialoadenitis (high dose used in treatment of thyroid cancer), sore throat, swallowing pain, taste (metallic), taste (unpleasant), vomiting
Hematologic: Anemia, blood dyscrasia, leukopenia, myelosuppression (high dose used in treatment of thyroid cancer), thrombocytopenia
Neuromuscular & skeletal: Neck tenderness/swelling
Respiratory: Bronchospasm, cough
Miscellaneous: Allergic reactions, anaphylaxis, chromosomal abnormalities, hypersensitivity reactions, immunosuppression, radiation sickness
General Dosage Range Oral: *Adults:* Dosage varies greatly depending on product

Pregnancy Risk Factor X
Pregnancy Considerations Iodine-131 crosses the placenta and may cause severe and irreversible hypothyroidism in neonates. Pregnancy should be ruled out prior to therapy. Effective contraception is recommended for 12 months following treatment for cancer, 6-12 months following treatment for hyperthyroidism.
Dental Comment Loss of saliva and sialolithiasis may develop. If this persists may lead to excessive dental caries. Immediately after treatment there may be pain and tenderness of the salivary gland, mucositis, and neck pain and swelling. All of these effects are dose-related and are typically temporary. Although very rare, other malignancies may develop including in the salivary glands. Hydration of patient and efforts to increase salivary flow may be advised after treatment.

Sodium Nitrite and Sodium Thiosulfate
(SOW dee um NYE trite & SOW dee um thye oh SUL fate)

Brand Names: U.S. Nithiodote™
Pharmacologic Category Antidote
Use Acute, life-threatening cyanide poisoning
Local Anesthetic/Vasoconstrictor Precautions No information available to require special precautions
Effects on Dental Treatment No significant effects or complications reported
Effects on Bleeding No information available to require special precautions
Adverse Effects Frequency not defined.
Sodium nitrite:
Cardiovascular: Arrhythmias, cyanosis, flushing, hypotension, palpitations, syncope, tachycardia
Central nervous system: Anxiety, coma, confusion, dizziness, fatigue, headache, lightheadedness, seizure
Dermatologic: Urticaria
Endocrine & metabolic: Acidosis
Gastrointestinal: Abdominal pain, nausea, vomiting
Hematologic: Methemoglobinemia
Local: Injection site tingling
Neuromuscular & skeletal: Numbness, paresthesia, weakness
Ocular: Blurred vision
Respiratory: Dyspnea, tachypnea
Miscellaneous: Diaphoresis
Sodium thiosulfate:
Cardiovascular: Hypotension
Central nervous system: Disorientation, headache
Gastrointestinal: Nausea, salty taste, vomiting
Hematologic: Bleeding time prolonged
Miscellaneous: Warmth
General Dosage Range
I.V.:
Children:
Sodium nitrite: 6 mg/kg (maximum: 300 mg); may repeat at one-half the original dose if needed
Sodium thiosulfate: 7 g/m^2 (maximum: 12.5 g); may repeat at one-half the original dose if needed
Adults:
Sodium nitrite: 300 mg; may repeat at one-half the original dose if needed
Sodium thiosulfate: 12.5 g; may repeat at one-half the original dose if needed
Mechanism of Action
Sodium nitrite: Promotes the formation of methemoglobin which competes with cytochrome oxidase for the cyanide ion. Cyanide combines with methemoglobin to form cyanomethemoglobin, thereby freeing the

cytochrome oxidase and allowing aerobic metabolism to continue.

Sodium thiosulfate: Serves as a sulfur donor in rhodanese-catalyzed formation of thiocyanate (much less toxic than cyanide).

Pharmacodynamics/Kinetics

Onset of Action Sodium nitrite: Peak effect: Methemoglobinemia: 30-60 minutes

Duration of Action Sodium nitrite: Methemoglobinemia: ~55 minutes

Half-life Elimination Thiosulfate: ~3 hours; Thiocyanate: ~3 days; Renal impairment: ≤9 days

Pregnancy Risk Factor C

Pregnancy Considerations Teratogenic effects have been observed following maternal exposure to high concentrations of sodium nitrite in drinking water. Teratogenic effects were not observed in animal reproduction studies of sodium nitrite or sodium thiosulfate. Embryotoxic and nonteratogenic effects were observed in animal reproduction studies of sodium nitrite. Methemoglobin reductase is lower in the fetus compared to adults and may result in adverse effects due to nitrite-induced prenatal hypoxia. There are no adequate and well-controlled studies of Nithiodote™ in pregnant women. In general, medications used as antidotes should take into consideration the health and prognosis of the mother (Bailey, 2003).

Sodium Oxybate (SOW dee um ox i BATE)

Brand Names: U.S. Xyrem®
Brand Names: Canada Xyrem®
Pharmacologic Category Central Nervous System Depressant
Use Treatment of cataplexy and excessive daytime sleepiness in patients with narcolepsy

Local Anesthetic/Vasoconstrictor Precautions No information available to require special precautions

Effects on Dental Treatment Key adverse event(s) related to dental treatment: Tooth ache (see Dental Comment).

Effects on Bleeding No information available to require special precautions

Adverse Effects
>10%:
Central nervous system: Dizziness (9% to 15%)
Gastrointestinal: Nausea (8% to 20% dose related), vomiting (2% to 11%; dose related)

1% to 10%:
Cardiovascular: Peripheral edema (≤3%)
Central nervous system: Somnolence (1% to 8%), attention disturbance (≤4%; dose related), drunk feeling (≤3%; dose related), irritability (≤3%; dose related), pain (≤3%), sleep paralysis (≤3%), sleepwalking (≤3%; dose related), disorientation (1% to 3%; dose related), anxiety (1% to 2%)
Dermatologic: Hyperhidrosis (1% to 3%)
Gastrointestinal: Diarrhea (3% to 4%), abdominal pain (1% to 3%)
Genitourinary: Enuresis (3% to 7%; dose related)
Neuromuscular & skeletal: Tremor (≤5%), pain in extremity (1% to 3%), paresthesia (1% to 3%; dose related)

General Dosage Range Dosage adjustment recommended in patients with hepatic impairment
Oral: *Adults:* Initial: 4.5 g daily in 2 equal doses given at bedtime and 2.5-4 hours later; Maintenance: 4.5-9 g daily (maximum: 9 g daily)

Mechanism of Action Sodium oxybate is derived from gamma aminobutyric acid (GABA) and acts as an inhibitory chemical transmitter in the brain. May function through specific receptors for gamma hydroxybutyrate (GHB) and GABA (B).

Pharmacodynamics/Kinetics
Half-life Elimination 30-60 minutes
Time to Peak 30-75 minutes
Pregnancy Risk Factor C
Pregnancy Considerations Adverse effects have been reported with maternal use throughout pregnancy. The injection formulation, when used as an anesthetic during labor and delivery, was shown to cross the placenta in concentrations ≤25% of maternal levels; a slight decrease in Apgar scores due to sleepiness in the neonate was observed. Sodium oxybate was not detected in infant blood 30 minutes after delivery.

Controlled Substance C-I (illicit use); C-III (medical use)

Prescribing and Access Restrictions Sodium oxybate is deemed to have an approved REMS program. As a requirement of the REMS program, access to this medication is restricted. Sodium oxybate oral solution will be available only to prescribers and patients enrolled in the Xyrem® Patient Success Program® and dispensed to the patient through the designated centralized pharmacy (1-866-997-3688). Prior to dispensing the first prescription, prescribers will be sent educational materials to be reviewed with the patient and enrollment forms for the postmarketing surveillance program. Patients must be seen at least every 3 months; prescriptions can be written for a maximum of 3 months (the first prescription may only be written for a 1-month supply).

Dental Comment Sodium oxybate is a known substance of abuse. When used illegally, it has been referred to as a "date-rape drug". The dentist should be aware of patients showing signs of CNS depression, as with all other drugs in this class.

Sodium Phenylbutyrate
(SOW dee um fen il BYOO ti rate)

Brand Names: U.S. Buphenyl®
Pharmacologic Category Urea Cycle Disorder (UCD) Treatment Agent
Use Adjunctive therapy in the chronic management of patients with urea cycle disorder involving deficiencies of carbamoylphosphate synthetase, ornithine transcarbamylase, or argininosuccinic acid synthetase

Local Anesthetic/Vasoconstrictor Precautions No information available to require special precautions

Effects on Dental Treatment Key adverse event(s) related to dental treatment: Abnormal taste.

Effects on Bleeding No information available to require special precautions

Adverse Effects
>10%: Endocrine & metabolic: Amenorrhea/menstrual dysfunction (23%), acidosis (14%), hypoalbuminemia (11%)

1% to 10%:
Cardiovascular: Syncope (≤2%)
Central nervous system: Depression (≤2%), headache (≤2%)
Dermatologic: Rash (≤2%)
Endocrine & metabolic: Alkalosis (7%), hyperchloremia (7%), hypophosphatemia (6%), total protein decreased (3%), hyperuricemia (2%), hyperphosphatemia (2%), hypernatremia (1%), hypokalemia (1%), hyperbilirubinemia (1%)

◀

Gastrointestinal: Anorexia (4%), abnormal taste (3%), abdominal pain (≤2%), gastritis (≤2%), nausea (≤2%), vomiting (≤2%)

Hematologic: Anemia (9%), leukocytosis (4%), leukopenia (4%), thrombocytopenia (3%), thrombocytosis (1%)

Hepatic: Alkaline phosphatase increased (6%), transaminases increased (4%)

Renal: Renal tubular acidosis (≤2%)

Miscellaneous: Offensive body odor (3%)

General Dosage Range Oral:

Children <20 kg: Powder: 450-600 mg/kg/day administered in equally divided amounts with each meal or feeding, 3-6 times daily (maximum: 20 g/day)

Children ≥20 kg and Adults: 9.9-13 g/m²/day, administered in equally divided amounts with each meal, 3-6 times daily (maximum: 20 g/day)

Mechanism of Action Sodium phenylbutyrate is a prodrug which is rapidly converted to phenylacetate, followed by conjugation with glutamine to form phenylacetylglutamine; phenylacetylglutamine serves as a substitute for urea as it is clears nitrogenous waste from the body when excreted in the urine.

Pharmacodynamics/Kinetics

Half-life Elimination Phenylbutyrate: 0.8 hours; Phenylacetate: 1.2 hours

Time to Peak Plasma: Phenylbutyrate: ~1.4 hour; Phenylacetate: ~4 hours

Pregnancy Risk Factor C

Pregnancy Considerations Animal reproduction studies have not been conducted.

Sodium Phosphates (SOW dee um FOS fates)

Brand Names: U.S. Fleet® Enema Extra® [OTC]; Fleet® Enema [OTC]; Fleet® Pedia-Lax™ Enema [OTC]; LaCrosse Complete [OTC]; OsmoPrep®; Visicol®

Brand Names: Canada Fleet Enema®

Pharmacologic Category Cathartic; Electrolyte Supplement, Parenteral; Laxative, Bowel Evacuant

Use

Oral solution, rectal: Short-term treatment of constipation

Oral tablets (OsmoPrep®, Visicol®): Bowel cleansing prior to colonoscopy

I.V.: Source of phosphate in large volume I.V. fluids and parenteral nutrition; treatment and prevention of hypophosphatemia

Local Anesthetic/Vasoconstrictor Precautions No information available to require special precautions

Effects on Dental Treatment No significant effects or complications reported

Effects on Bleeding No information available to require special precautions

Adverse Effects Frequency not always defined.

Central nervous system: Dizziness, headache

Gastrointestinal: Bloating (31% to 47%), nausea (26% to 35%), abdominal pain (23% to 30%), vomiting (4% to 7%), mucosal bleeding, superficial mucosal ulcerations

Endocrine & metabolic: Hyperphosphatemia (≤96%), hypocalcemia (on colonoscopy day; 47%), hypophosphatemia (2-3 days postcolonoscopy; 34%), hypokalemia (on colonoscopy day; 28%), hypernatremia

General Dosage Range

I.V.:

Children: 0.08-1 mmol phosphate/kg **or** Parenteral nutrition: Infusion: 0.5-2 mmol/kg/24 hours

Adults: 0.08-1 mmol phosphate/kg **or** Parenteral nutrition: Infusion: 20-40 mmol/24 hours

Oral:

Solution:

Children 5-9 years: 7.5 mL as a single dose (maximum single daily dose: 7.5 mL)

Children 10-11 years: 15 mL as a single dose (maximum single daily dose: 15 mL)

Children ≥12 years and Adults: 15 mL as a single dose (maximum single daily dose: 45 mL)

Tablet: *Adults:*

Visicol®: 40 tablets in divided doses as directed beginning evening before colonoscopy

OsmoPrep®: 32 tablets in divided doses as directed beginning evening before colonoscopy

Rectal:

Children 2-4 years: One-half contents of one 2.25 oz pediatric enema

Children 5-11 years: Contents of one 2.25 oz pediatric enema

Children ≥12 years and Adults: Contents of one 4.5-ounce enema as a single dose

Mechanism of Action As a laxative, exerts osmotic effect in the small intestine by drawing water into the lumen of the gut, producing distention and promoting peristalsis and evacuation of the bowel; phosphorous participates in bone deposition, calcium metabolism, utilization of B complex vitamins, and as a buffer in acid-base equilibrium

Pharmacodynamics/Kinetics

Onset of Action Cathartic: 3-6 hours; Rectal: 2-5 minutes

Pregnancy Risk Factor C

Pregnancy Considerations Reproduction studies have not been conducted with these products. Use with caution in pregnant women.

Sodium Picosulfate, Magnesium Oxide, and Citric Acid

(SOW dee um pye ko SUL fate mag NEE zhum OKS ide & SI trik AS id)

Brand Names: U.S. Prepopik™

Brand Names: Canada Oral Purgative; Pico-Salax®; Picodan; Picoflo; Purg-Odan™

Pharmacologic Category Laxative, Osmotic; Laxative, Stimulant

Use Bowel cleansing prior to colonoscopy

Canadian labeling: Additional uses (not in U.S. labeling): Bowel cleansing prior to x-ray examination, endoscopy, or surgery

Local Anesthetic/Vasoconstrictor Precautions No information available to require special precautions

Effects on Dental Treatment No significant effects or complications reported

Effects on Bleeding No information available to require special precautions

Adverse Effects

>10%:

Endocrine & metabolic: Hypermagnesemia (9% to 12%)

Renal: GFR decreased (≤48 hours after colonoscopy: 10% to 29%)

1% to 10%:
Central nervous system: Headache (2% to 3%)
Endocrine & metabolic: Hypokalemia (5% to 7%), hypochloremia (1% to 4%), hyponatremia (1% to 4%)
Gastrointestinal: Nausea (3%), vomiting (1%)
Renal: Serum creatinine increased (<1% to 5%)

General Dosage Range Oral: *Adults:* Two 150 mL (5 oz) doses

Mechanism of Action

Sodium picosulfate, a prodrug, is hydrolyzed by colonic bacteria to an active metabolite which stimulates colonic peristalsis.

Magnesium oxide and citric acid react to create magnesium citrate which induces catharsis by the osmotic effects of the unabsorbed ions in the GI tract.

Pharmacodynamics/Kinetics

Half-life Elimination Sodium picosulfate: ~7.5 hours

Time to Peak Sodium picosulfate: ~7 hours; Magnesium: 10 hours

Pregnancy Risk Factor B

Pregnancy Considerations Adverse events were not observed in animal reproduction studies using doses similar to a human dose.

Sodium Tetradecyl (SOW dee um tetra DEK il)

Brand Names: U.S. Sotradecol®
Brand Names: Canada Trombovar®
Pharmacologic Category Sclerosing Agent
Use Treatment of small, uncomplicated varicose veins of the lower extremities
Local Anesthetic/Vasoconstrictor Precautions No information available to require special precautions
Effects on Dental Treatment No significant effects or complications reported
Effects on Bleeding No information available to require special precautions
Adverse Effects Frequency not defined.
Central nervous system: Headache
Dermatologic: Discoloration at site of injection, sloughing and tissue necrosis following extravasation
Gastrointestinal: Nausea, vomiting
Local: Pain, itching, or ulceration at injection site
Miscellaneous: Allergic reaction (including hives, asthma, hay fever); anaphylactic shock

General Dosage Range I.V.: *Adults:* 0.5-2 mL in each vein (maximum: 10 mL per treatment session)

Mechanism of Action Acts by irritation of the vein intimal endothelium and causes thrombosis formation leading to occlusion of the injected vein

Pregnancy Risk Factor C

Pregnancy Considerations Reproduction studies have not been conducted.

Sodium Thiosulfate (SOW dee um thye oh SUL fate)

Pharmacologic Category Antidote
Use Treatment of cyanide poisoning
Unlabeled Use Management of mechlorethamine extravasation
Local Anesthetic/Vasoconstrictor Precautions No information available to require special precautions
Effects on Dental Treatment No significant effects or complications reported
Effects on Bleeding No information available to require special precautions

Adverse Effects Frequency not defined
Cardiovascular: Hypotension
Central nervous system: Disorientation, headache
Gastrointestinal: Nausea, salty taste, vomiting
Hematologic: Bleeding time prolonged
Miscellaneous: Warmth

General Dosage Range I.V.:
Children: 7 g/m^2 (maximum: 12.5 g); may repeat at one-half the original dose if needed
Adults: 12.5 g; may repeat at one-half the original dose if needed

Mechanism of Action

Cyanide toxicity: Serves as a sulfur donor in rhodanese-catalyzed formation of thiocyanate (much less toxic than cyanide)

Mechlorethamine extravasation: Neutralizes the reactive species of mechlorethamine; reduces the formation of hydroxyl radicals

Pharmacodynamics/Kinetics

Half-life Elimination Thiosulfate: ~3 hours; Thiocyanate: ~3 days; Renal impairment: ≤9 days

Pregnancy Risk Factor C

Pregnancy Considerations Teratogenic effects were not observed in animal reproduction studies of sodium thiosulfate. In general, medications used as antidotes should take into consideration the health and prognosis of the mother (Bailey, 2003).

Solifenacin (sol i FEN a sin)

Brand Names: U.S. VESIcare®
Pharmacologic Category Anticholinergic Agent
Use Treatment of overactive bladder with symptoms of urinary frequency, urgency, or urge incontinence
Local Anesthetic/Vasoconstrictor Precautions No information available to require special precautions
Effects on Dental Treatment Key adverse event(s) related to dental treatment: Xerostomia (normal salivary flow resumes upon discontinuation). Prolonged xerostomia may contribute to discomfort and dental disease (eg, caries, periodontal disease, and oral candidiasis).
Effects on Bleeding No information available to require special precautions

Adverse Effects
>10%: Gastrointestinal: Xerostomia (11% to 28%; dose-related), constipation (5% to 13%; dose-related)
1% to 10%:
Cardiovascular: Edema (≤1%), hypertension (≤1%)
Central nervous system: Headache (3% to 6%), fatigue (1% to 2%), depression (≤1%)
Gastrointestinal: Dyspepsia (1% to 4%), nausea (2% to 3%), upper abdominal pain (1% to 2%)
Genitourinary: Urinary tract infection (3% to 5%), urinary retention (≤1%)
Ocular: Blurred vision (4% to 5%), dry eyes (≤2%)
Respiratory: Cough (≤1%)
Miscellaneous: Influenza (≤2%)

General Dosage Range Dosage adjustment recommended in patients with hepatic or renal impairment and on concomitant therapy
Oral: *Adults:* 5-10 mg/day

Mechanism of Action Inhibits muscarinic receptors resulting in decreased urinary bladder contraction, increased residual urine volume, and decreased detrusor muscle pressure.

Pharmacodynamics/Kinetics

Half-life Elimination 45-68 hours following chronic dosing; prolonged in severe renal (Cl_{cr} <30 mL/minute) or moderate hepatic (Child-Pugh class B) impairment

Time to Peak Plasma: 3-8 hours

Pregnancy Risk Factor C

Pregnancy Considerations Decreased fetal weight, increased incidence of cleft palate, and delayed physical development were observed in some animal studies. There are no adequate or well-controlled studies in pregnant women. Use during pregnancy only if the benefit to the mother outweighs the potential risk to the fetus.

Somatropin (soe ma TROE pin)

Brand Names: U.S. Genotropin Miniquick®; Genotropin®; Humatrope®; Norditropin FlexPro®; Norditropin® NordiFlex®; Nutropin AQ Pen®; Nutropin AQ®; Nutropin AQ® NuSpin™; Nutropin®; Omnitrope®; Saizen®; Serostim®; Tev-Tropin®; Zorbtive®

Brand Names: Canada Humatrope®; Norditropin Simplexx; Nutropin AQ Pen®; Nutropin AQ® NuSpin™; Nutropin®; Nutropin® AQ; Omnitrope®; Saizen®; Serostim®

Pharmacologic Category Growth Hormone

Use

Children:

Treatment of growth failure due to inadequate endogenous growth hormone secretion (Genotropin®, Humatrope®, Norditropin®, Nutropin®, Nutropin AQ®, Omnitrope®, Saizen®, Tev-Tropin®)

Treatment of short stature associated with Turner syndrome (Genotropin®, Humatrope®, Norditropin®, Nutropin®, Nutropin AQ®, Omnitrope®)

Treatment of Prader-Willi syndrome (Genotropin®, Omnitrope®)

Treatment of growth failure associated with chronic renal insufficiency (CRI) up until the time of renal transplantation (Nutropin®, Nutropin AQ®)

Treatment of growth failure in children born small for gestational age who fail to manifest catch-up growth by 2 years of age (Genotropin®, Omnitrope®) or by 2-4 years of age (Humatrope®, Norditropin®)

Treatment of idiopathic short stature (nongrowth hormone-deficient short stature) defined by height standard deviation score (SDS) ≤-2.25 and growth rate not likely to attain normal adult height (Genotropin®, Humatrope®, Nutropin®, Nutropin AQ®, Omnitrope®)

Treatment of short stature or growth failure associated with short stature homeobox gene (SHOX) deficiency (Humatrope®)

Treatment of short stature associated with Noonan syndrome (Norditropin®)

Adults:

HIV patients with wasting or cachexia with concomitant antiviral therapy (Serostim®)

Replacement of endogenous growth hormone in patients with adult growth hormone deficiency who meet both of the following criteria (Genotropin®, Humatrope®, Norditropin®, Nutropin®, Nutropin AQ®, Omnitrope®, Saizen®):

Biochemical diagnosis of adult growth hormone deficiency by means of a subnormal response to a standard growth hormone stimulation test (peak growth hormone ≤5 mcg/L). Confirmatory testing may not be required in patients with congenital/genetic growth hormone deficiency or multiple pituitary hormone deficiencies due to organic diseases.

and

Adult-onset: Patients who have adult growth hormone deficiency whether alone or with multiple hormone deficiencies (hypopituitarism) as a result of pituitary disease, hypothalamic disease, surgery, radiation therapy, or trauma

or

Childhood-onset: Patients who were growth hormone deficient during childhood, confirmed as an adult before replacement therapy is initiated

Treatment of short-bowel syndrome (Zorbtive®)

Unlabeled Use Pediatric HIV patients with wasting/cachexia (Serostim®); HIV-associated adipose redistribution syndrome (HARS) (Serostim®)

Local Anesthetic/Vasoconstrictor Precautions No information available to require special precautions

Effects on Dental Treatment No significant effects or complications reported

Effects on Bleeding No information available to require special precautions

Adverse Effects

Growth hormone deficiency: Adverse reactions reported with growth hormone deficiency vary greatly by age. Generally, percentages are less in pediatric patients than adults, and many of the reactions reported in adults are dose related. Percentages reported also vary by product. Below is a listing by age group; events reported more commonly overall are noted with an asterisk (*).

Children: Antibodies development, arthralgia, benign intracranial hypertension, edema, eosinophilia, glycosuria, Hb A_{1c} increased, headache, hematoma, hematuria, hyperglycemia (mild), hypertriglyceridemia, hypoglycemia, hypothyroidism, injection site reaction, intracranial tumor, leg pain, lipoatrophy, leukemia, meningioma, muscle pain, papilledema, pseudotumor cerebri, psoriasis exacerbation, rash, scoliosis progression, seizure, slipped capital femoral epiphysis, weakness

Adults: Acne, ALT increased, AST increased, arthralgia*, back pain, bronchitis, carpal tunnel syndrome, chest pain, cough, depression, diabetes mellitus (type 2), diaphoresis, dizziness, edema*, fatigue, flu-like syndrome*, gastritis, glucose intolerance, glucosuria, headache*, hyperglycemia (mild), hypertension, hypoesthesia, hypothyroidism, infection, insomnia, insulin resistance, joint disorder, leg edema, muscle pain, myalgia*, nausea, pain in extremities, paresthesia*, peripheral edema*, pharyngitis, retinopathy, rhinitis, skeletal pain*, stiffness in extremities, surgical procedure, upper respiratory tract infection, weakness

Additional/postmarketing reactions observed with growth hormone deficiency: Gynecomastia, increased growth of pre-existing nevi, pancreatitis

HARS: Serostim®: Limited to >10%: Edema (peripheral) (19% to 45%), arthralgia (28% to 37%), pain (extremity) (5% to 19%), hypoesthesia (9% to 15%), headache (4% to 14%), blood glucose increased (4% to 14%), paresthesia (11% to 13%), myalgia (3% to 13%)

Idiopathic short stature: Percentages reported using Humatrope® versus placebo: Myalgia (24%), scoliosis (19%), otitis media (16%), arthralgia (11%), arthrosis (11%), hyperlipidemia (8%), gynecomastia (5%), hip pain (3%), hypertension (3%). Additional adverse reactions listed as reported using other products from ISS NCGS Cohort (frequencies <1%): Aggressiveness, benign intracranial hypertension, diabetes, edema, hair loss, headache, injection site reaction

Prader-Willi syndrome: Genotropin® (frequency not defined): Aggressiveness, arthralgia, edema, hair loss, headache, benign intracranial hypertension, myalgia; fatalities associated with use in this population have been reported

Turner syndrome: Percentages reported using Humatrope® compared to untreated patients. Additional adverse reactions reported from other products, frequency not specified: Surgical procedures (45%), otitis media (43%), ear disorders (18%), joint pain, respiratory illness, urinary tract infection

HIV patients with wasting or cachexia: Serostim® (limited to ≥5%): Musculoskeletal disorders (arthralgia, arthrosis, myalgia: 78%), peripheral edema (26%), headache (13%), nausea (9%), paresthesia (8%), edema (6%), gynecomastia (6%), hypoesthesia (5%)

Short-bowel syndrome: Zorbtive® (limited to >10%): Peripheral edema (69% to 81%), facial edema (44% to 50%), arthralgia (31% to 44%), nausea (13% to 31%), injection site pain (up to 31%), flatulence (25%), injection site reaction (19% to 25%), abdominal pain (13% to 25%), vomiting (19%), pain (6% to 19%), chest pain (up to 19%), dehydration (up to 19%), infection (up to 19%), rhinitis (up to 19%), hearing symptoms (13%), dizziness (6% to 13%), rash (6% to 13%), diaphoresis (up to 13%), generalized edema (up to 13%), malaise (up to 13%), moniliasis (up to 13%), myalgia (up to 13%)

SHOX deficiency: Humatrope®: Arthralgia (11%), gynecomastia (8%), excessive cutaneous nevi (7%), scoliosis (4%)

Small for gestational age: Genotropin®, Humatrope® (frequency not defined): Mild, transient hyperglycemia; benign intracranial hypertension (rare); central precocious puberty; jaw prominence (rare); aggravation of pre-existing scoliosis (rare); injection site reactions; progression of pigmented nevi; carpal tunnel syndrome (rare) diabetes mellitus (rare); otitis media; headache; slipped capital femoral epiphysis

General Dosage Range I.M., SubQ: *Children and Adults:* Dosage varies greatly depending on indication

Mechanism of Action Somatropin is a purified polypeptide hormones of recombinant DNA origin; somatropin contains the identical sequence of amino acids found in human growth hormone; human growth hormone assists growth of linear bone, skeletal muscle, and organs by stimulating chondrocyte proliferation and differentiation, lipolysis, protein synthesis, and hepatic glucose output; stimulates erythropoietin which increases red blood cell mass; exerts both insulin-like and diabetogenic effects; enhances the transmucosal transport of water, electrolytes, and nutrients across the gut

Pharmacodynamics/Kinetics

Duration of Action Maintains supraphysiologic levels for 18-20 hours

Half-life Elimination Preparation and route of administration dependent; SubQ: ~2-4 hours

Pregnancy Risk Factor B/C (depending upon manufacturer)

Pregnancy Considerations Teratogenic effects were not observed in animal studies. Reproduction studies have not been conducted with all agents. During normal pregnancy, maternal production of endogenous growth hormone decreases as placental growth hormone production increases. Data with somatropin use during pregnancy is limited.

SORAfenib (sor AF e nib)

Brand Names: U.S. NexAVAR®
Brand Names: Canada Nexavar®
Pharmacologic Category Antineoplastic Agent, Tyrosine Kinase Inhibitor; Vascular Endothelial Growth Factor (VEGF) Inhibitor
Use Treatment of advanced renal cell cancer (RCC); treatment of unresectable hepatocellular cancer (HCC)
Unlabeled Use Treatment of advanced thyroid cancer, recurrent or metastatic angiosarcoma, resistant gastrointestinal stromal tumor (GIST)
Local Anesthetic/Vasoconstrictor Precautions Sorafenib may cause hypertension; monitor blood pressure prior to vasoconstrictor use
Effects on Dental Treatment Key adverse event(s) related to dental treatment: Mouth pain, mucositis, stomatitis, xerostomia (normal salivary flow resumes upon discontinuation), and dysphagia.
Effects on Bleeding Chemotherapy may result in significant myelosuppression, potentially including significant reduction in platelet counts (thrombocytopenia grades 3/4: 1% to 4%) and altered hemostasis. In patients who are under active treatment with these agents, medical consult is suggested.

Adverse Effects
>10%:
Cardiovascular: Hypertension (9% to 17%; grade 3: 3% to 4%; grade 4: <1%; onset: ~3 weeks)
Central nervous system: Fatigue (37% to 46%), sensory neuropathy (≤13%), pain (11%)
Dermatologic: Rash/desquamation (19% to 40%; grade 3: ≤1%), hand-foot syndrome (21% to 30%; grade 3: 6% to 8%), alopecia (14% to 27%), pruritus (14% to 19%), dry skin (10% to 11%), erythema
Endocrine & metabolic: Hypoalbuminemia (≤59%), hypophosphatemia (35% to 45%; grade 3: 11% to 13%; grade 4: <1%), hypocalcemia (12% to 27%)
Gastrointestinal: Diarrhea (43% to 55%; grade 3: 2% to 10%; grade 4: <1%), lipase increased (40% to 41% [usually transient]), amylase increased (30% to 34% [usually transient]), abdominal pain (11% to 31%), weight loss (10% to 30%), anorexia (16% to 29%), nausea (23% to 24%), vomiting (15% to 16%), constipation (14% to 15%)
Hematologic: Lymphopenia (23% to 47%; grades 3/4: ≤13%), thrombocytopenia (12% to 46%; grades 3/4: 1% to 4%), INR increased (≤42%), neutropenia (≤18%; grades 3/4: ≤5%), hemorrhage (15% to 18%; grade 3: 2% to 3%; grade 4: ≤2%), leukopenia
Hepatic: Liver dysfunction (≤11%; grade 3: 2%; grade 4: 1%)
Neuromuscular & skeletal: Muscle pain, weakness
Respiratory: Dyspnea (≤14%), cough (≤13%)

1% to 10%:

Cardiovascular: Cardiac ischemia/infarction (≤3%), heart failure (2%; congestive), flushing

Central nervous system: Headache (≤10%), depression, fever

Dermatologic: Acne, exfoliative dermatitis

Gastrointestinal: Appetite decreased, dyspepsia, dysphagia, esophageal varices bleeding (2%), glossodynia, mucositis, stomatitis, xerostomia

Genitourinary: Erectile dysfunction

Hematologic: Anemia

Hepatic: Transaminases increased (transient)

Neuromuscular & skeletal: Joint pain (≤10%), arthralgia, myalgia

Renal: Renal failure

Respiratory: Hoarseness

Miscellaneous: Flu-like syndrome

General Dosage Range Dosage adjustments recommended in patients with hepatic or renal impairment, or who develop toxicities

Oral: *Adults:* 400 mg twice daily

Mechanism of Action Multikinase inhibitor; inhibits tumor growth and angiogenesis by inhibiting intracellular Raf kinases (CRAF, BRAF, and mutant BRAF), and cell surface kinase receptors (VEGFR-1, VEGFR-2, VEGFR-3, PDGFR-beta, cKIT, FLT-3, and RET)

Pharmacodynamics/Kinetics

Half-life Elimination 25-48 hours

Time to Peak ~3 hours

Pregnancy Risk Factor D

Pregnancy Considerations Animal reproduction studies have demonstrated teratogenicity and fetal loss. Based on its mechanism of action and because sorafenib inhibits angiogenesis, a critical component of fetal development, adverse effects on pregnancy would be expected. Women of childbearing potential should be advised to avoid pregnancy. Men and women of reproductive potential should use effective birth control during treatment and for at least 2 weeks after treatment is discontinued.

Sorbitol (SOR bi tole)

Pharmacologic Category Genitourinary Irrigant; Laxative, Osmotic

Use Genitourinary irrigant in transurethral prostatic resection or other transurethral resection or other transurethral surgical procedures; diuretic; humectant; sweetening agent; hyperosmotic laxative; facilitate the passage of sodium polystyrene sulfonate through the intestinal tract

Local Anesthetic/Vasoconstrictor Precautions No information available to require special precautions

Effects on Dental Treatment Key adverse event(s) related to dental treatment: Xerostomia (normal salivary flow resumes upon discontinuation).

Effects on Bleeding No information available to require special precautions

Adverse Effects Frequency not defined.

Cardiovascular: Edema

Endocrine & metabolic: Fluid and electrolyte losses, hyperglycemia, lactic acidosis

Gastrointestinal: Abdominal discomfort, diarrhea, dry mouth, nausea, vomiting, xerostomia

General Dosage Range

Oral:

Children 2-11 years: 2 mL/kg (70% solution) as a single dose

Children ≥12 years and Adults: 30-150 mL (70% solution) as a single dose

Rectal:

Children 2-11 years: 30-60 mL (25% to 30% solution) as a single dose

Children ≥12 years and Adults: 120 mL (25% to 30% solution) as a single dose

Topical: *Adults:* 3% to 3.3% as a transurethral irrigation

Mechanism of Action A polyalcoholic sugar with osmotic cathartic actions

Pharmacodynamics/Kinetics

Onset of Action 0.25-1 hour

Pregnancy Risk Factor C

Pregnancy Considerations Animal reproduction studies have not been conducted.

Sotalol (SOE ta lole)

Related Information

Clinical Risk Related to Drugs Prolonging QT Interval *on page 1510*

Brand Names: U.S. Betapace AF®; Betapace®; Sorine®

Brand Names: Canada Apo-Sotalol®; CO Sotalol; Dom-Sotalol; Med-Sotalol; Mylan-Sotalol; Novo-Sotalol; Nu-Sotalol; PHL-Sotalol; PMS-Sotalol; PRO-Sotalol; ratio-Sotalol; Rhoxal-sotalol; Riva-Sotalol; Rylosol; Sandoz-Sotalol; ZYM-Sotalol

Pharmacologic Category Antiarrhythmic Agent, Class II; Antiarrhythmic Agent, Class III; Beta-Adrenergic Blocker, Nonselective

Use Treatment of documented ventricular arrhythmias (ie, sustained ventricular tachycardia), that in the judgment of the physician are life-threatening; maintenance of normal sinus rhythm in patients with symptomatic atrial fibrillation and atrial flutter who are currently in sinus rhythm. Manufacturer states substitutions should not be made for Betapace AF® since Betapace AF® is distributed with a patient package insert specific for atrial fibrillation/flutter.

Injection: Substitution for oral sotalol in those who are unable to take sotalol orally

Unlabeled Use Fetal tachycardia; alternative antiarrhythmic for the treatment of atrial fibrillation in patients with hypertrophic cardiomyopathy (HCM)

Local Anesthetic/Vasoconstrictor Precautions Use with caution; epinephrine has interacted with nonselective beta-blockers to result in initial hypertensive episode followed by bradycardia. Sotalol is one of the drugs confirmed to prolong the QT interval and is accepted as having a risk of causing torsade de pointes. The risk of drug-induced torsade de pointes is extremely low when a single QT interval prolonging drug is prescribed. In terms of epinephrine, it is not known what effect vasoconstrictors in the local anesthetic regimen will have in patients with a known history of congenital prolonged QT interval or in patients taking any medication that prolongs the QT interval. Until more information is obtained, it is suggested that the clinician consult with the physician prior to the use of a vasoconstrictor in suspected patients, and that the vasoconstrictor (epinephrine, mepivacaine and levonordefrin [Carbocaine® 2% with Neo-Cobefrin®]) be used with caution.

Effects on Dental Treatment Sotalol is a nonselective beta-blocker and may enhance the pressor response to epinephrine, resulting in hypertension and bradycardia. Many nonsteroidal anti-inflammatory drugs, such as ibuprofen and indomethacin, can reduce the hypotensive effect of beta-blockers after 3 or more weeks of therapy with the NSAID. Short-term NSAID use (ie, 3 days) requires no special precautions in patients taking beta-blockers.

Adverse Effects Note: No clinical experience with I.V. sotalol; however, since exposure is similar between I.V. and oral sotalol, adverse reactions are expected to be similar.

>10%:
Cardiovascular: Bradycardia (13% to 16%), chest pain (3% to 16%), palpitation (14%)
Central nervous system: Fatigue (20%), dizziness (20%), lightheadedness (12%)
Neuromuscular & skeletal: Weakness (13%)
Respiratory: Dyspnea (21%)

1% to 10%:
Cardiovascular: Edema (8%), abnormal ECG (7%), hypotension (6%), proarrhythmia (5%), syncope (5%), CHF (5%), torsade de pointes (dose related; 1% to 4%), peripheral vascular disorders (3%), ventricular tachycardia worsened (1%), QT_c interval prolongation (dose related)
Central nervous system: Headache (8%), sleep problems (8%), mental confusion (6%), anxiety (4%), depression (4%)
Dermatologic: Itching/rash (5%)
Endocrine & metabolic: Sexual ability decreased (3%)
Gastrointestinal: Nausea/vomiting (10%), diarrhea (7%), stomach discomfort (3% to 6%), flatulence (2%)
Genitourinary: Impotence (2%)
Hematologic: Bleeding (2%)
Neuromuscular & skeletal: Extremity pain (7%), paresthesia (4%), back pain (3%)
Ocular: Visual problems (5%)
Respiratory: Upper respiratory problems (5% to 8%), asthma (2%)

General Dosage Range Dosage adjustment recommended in patients with renal impairment or who develop toxicities
I.V.: *Adults:* Initial: 75 mg twice daily; Maintenance: 75-150 mg twice daily (maximum: 300 mg/day)
Oral:
Children ≤2 years: Dosage should be adjusted (decreased) by plotting of the child's age on a logarithmic scale; **Note:** Refer to manufacturer's package labeling
Children >2 years: Initial: 90 mg/m^2/day in 3 divided doses; Maintenance: 90-180 mg/m^2/day in 3 divided doses (maximum: 180 mg/m^2/day)
Adults: Initial: 80 mg twice daily; Maintenance: 240-320 mg/day in 2-3 divided doses (maximum: 320 mg/day)

Mechanism of Action
Beta-blocker which contains both beta-adrenoreceptor-blocking (Vaughan Williams Class II) and cardiac action potential prolongation (Vaughan Williams Class III) properties
Class II effects: Increased sinus cycle length, slowed heart rate, decreased AV nodal conduction, and increased AV nodal refractoriness Sotalol has both beta$_1$- and beta$_2$-receptor blocking activity. The beta-blocking effect of sotalol is a noncardioselective (half maximal at about 80 mg/day and maximal at doses of 320-640 mg/day). Significant beta-blockade occurs at oral doses as low as 25 mg/day.

Class III effects: Prolongation of the atrial and ventricular monophasic action potentials, and effective refractory prolongation of atrial muscle, ventricular muscle, and atrioventricular accessory pathways in both the antegrade and retrograde directions. Sotalol is a racemic mixture of *d*- and *l*-sotalol; both isomers have similar Class III antiarrhythmic effects while the *l*-isomer is responsible for virtually all of the beta-blocking activity. The Class III effects are seen only at oral doses ≥160 mg/day

Pharmacodynamics/Kinetics
Onset of Action Oral: Rapid, 1-2 hours; when administered I.V. for ongoing VT over 5 minutes, onset of action is ~5-10 minutes (Ho, 1994)
Duration of Action 8-16 hours
Half-life Elimination 12 hours; Children: 9.5 hours; terminal half-life decreases with age <2 years (time to steady state may be ≥1 week in neonates); increases with renal dysfunction
Time to Peak Serum: Oral: 2.5-4 hours
Pregnancy Risk Factor B
Pregnancy Considerations Adverse events were not observed in the initial animal reproduction studies; therefore, the manufacturer classifies sotalol as pregnancy category B. Sotalol crosses the placenta and is found in amniotic fluid. In a cohort study, an increased risk of cardiovascular defects was observed following maternal use of beta-blockers during pregnancy. Intrauterine growth restriction (IUGR), small placentas, as well as fetal/neonatal bradycardia, hypoglycemia, and/or respiratory depression have been observed following *in utero* exposure to beta-blockers as a class. Adequate facilities for monitoring infants at birth should be available. Untreated chronic maternal hypertension and preeclampsia are also associated with adverse events in the fetus, infant, and mother; however, sotalol is currently not recommended for the initial treatment of hypertension in pregnancy. Because sotalol crosses the placenta in concentrations similar to the maternal serum, it has been used for the treatment of fetal atrial flutter or fetal supraventricular tachycardia without hydrops. The clearance of sotalol is increased during the third trimester of pregnancy, but other pharmacokinetic parameters do not significantly differ from nonpregnant values.

Dental Comment Sotalol is known to prolong the QT interval. The QT interval is measured as the time and distance between the Q point of the QRS complex and the end of the T wave in the ECG tracing. After adjustment for heart rate, the QT interval is defined as prolonged if it is more than 450 msec in men and 460 msec in women. A long QT syndrome was first described in the 1950s and 60s as a congenital syndrome involving QT interval prolongation and syncope and sudden death. Some of the congenital long QT syndromes were characterized by a peculiar electrocardiographic appearance of the QRS complex involving a premature atria beat followed by a pause, then a subsequent sinus beat showing marked QT prolongation and deformity. This type of cardiac arrhythmia was originally termed "torsade de pointes" (translated from the French as "twisting of the points"). Sotalol is considered as having a risk of causing torsade de pointes. Since it is not known what effect vasoconstrictors in the local anesthetic regimen will have in patients with a known history of congenital prolonged QT interval or in patients taking any medication that prolongs the QT interval, a medical consult is suggested.

Spiramycin (speer a MYE sin)

Brand Names: Canada Rovamycine®

Pharmacologic Category Antibiotic, Macrolide

Use Treatment of infections of the respiratory tract, buccal cavity, skin and soft tissues due to susceptible organisms. *N. gonorrhoeae*: as an alternate choice of treatment for gonorrhea in patients allergic to the penicillins. Before treatment of gonorrhea, the possibility of concomitant infection due to *T. pallidum* should be excluded.

Unlabeled Use Treatment of *Toxoplasma gondii* to prevent transmission from mother to fetus

Local Anesthetic/Vasoconstrictor Precautions No information available to require special precautions

Effects on Dental Treatment No significant effects or complications reported

Effects on Bleeding No information available to require special precautions

Adverse Effects Frequency not defined.

Dermatologic: Angioedema (rare), pruritus, rash, urticaria

Gastrointestinal: Diarrhea, nausea, pseudomembranous colitis (rare), vomiting

Hepatic: Transaminases increased

Neuromuscular & skeletal: Paresthesia (rare)

Miscellaneous: Anaphylactic shock (rare)

General Dosage Range Oral:

Children: 150,000 units/kg/day in 2-3 divided doses

Adults: 6,000,000-15,000,000 units/day in 2 divided doses **or** 12,000,000-13,500,000 units as a single dose

Mechanism of Action Inhibits growth of susceptible organisms; mechanism not established.

Pregnancy Risk Factor Not assigned (other macrolides rated B); C per expert analysis

Pregnancy Considerations Crosses placenta. Specific safety information is not available. However, spiramycin has been used to treat *Toxoplasma gondii* to prevent transmission from mother to fetus.

Product Availability Not available in U.S.

Spironolactone (speer on oh LAK tone)

Related Information

Cardiovascular Diseases *on page 1492*

Brand Names: U.S. Aldactone®

Brand Names: Canada Aldactone®; Novo-Spiroton; Teva-Spironolactone

Generic Availability (U.S.) Yes

Pharmacologic Category Diuretic, Potassium-Sparing; Selective Aldosterone Blocker

Use Management of edema associated with excessive aldosterone excretion; hypertension; primary hyperaldosteronism; hypokalemia; cirrhosis of liver accompanied by edema or ascites; nephrotic syndrome; severe heart failure (NYHA class III-IV) to increase survival and reduce hospitalization when added to standard therapy

Unlabeled Use Female acne (adjunctive therapy); hirsutism; hypertension (pediatric); diuretic (pediatric)

Local Anesthetic/Vasoconstrictor Precautions No information available to require special precautions

Effects on Dental Treatment No significant effects or complications reported

Effects on Bleeding No information available to require special precautions

Adverse Effects Frequency not defined.

Cardiovascular: Vasculitis

Central nervous system: Ataxia, confusion, drowsiness, fever, headache, lethargy

Dermatologic: Drug rash with eosinophilia and systemic symptoms (DRESS), maculopapular or erythematous cutaneous eruptions, Stevens-Johnson syndrome, toxic epidermal necrolysis, urticaria

Endocrine & metabolic: Amenorrhea, gynecomastia, hyperkalemia, impotence, irregular menses, postmenopausal bleeding

Gastrointestinal: Cramps, diarrhea, gastritis, gastric bleeding, nausea, ulceration, vomiting

Hematologic: Agranulocytosis

Hepatic: Cholestatic/hepatocellular toxicity

Renal: BUN increased, renal dysfunction, renal failure

Miscellaneous: Anaphylactic reaction, breast cancer

Dosage Oral:

Children:

Diuretic, hypertension (unlabeled use): Children 1-17 years: Initial: 1 mg/kg/day divided every 12-24 hours (maximum dose: 3.3 mg/kg/day, up to 100 mg/day)

Diagnosis of primary aldosteronism (unlabeled use): 125-375 mg/m²/day in divided doses

Adults:

Edema: 25-200 mg/day in 1-2 divided doses

Hypokalemia: 25-100 mg daily

Hypertension (JNC 7): 25-50 mg/day in 1-2 divided doses

Diagnosis of primary aldosteronism: Long test: 400 mg daily for 3-4 weeks; short test: 400 mg daily for 4 days; maintenance until surgical correction: 100-400 mg/day in 1-2 divided doses

Heart failure, severe (NYHA class III-IV; with ACE inhibitor and a loop diuretic ± digoxin): 12.5-25 mg/day; maximum daily dose: 50 mg. If 25 mg once daily not tolerated, reduce to 25 mg every other day was the lowest maintenance dose possible.

Note: If potassium >5 mEq/L or serum creatinine >4 mg/dL, discontinue or interrupt therapy.

Acne in women (unlabeled use): 25-200 mg once daily

Hirsutism in women (unlabeled use): 50-200 mg/day in 1-2 divided doses (Koulouri, 2008; Martin, 2008)

Elderly: Indication specific: Initial: 12.5-50 mg/day in 1-2 divided doses, increasing by 25-50 mg every 5 days as needed; adjust for renal impairment

Dosing interval in renal impairment: Heart failure:

Cl_{cr} 31-50 mL/minute: Decrease initial dose to 12.5 mg once daily

Cl_{cr} <30 mL/minute: Not recommended

Mechanism of Action Competes with aldosterone for receptor sites in the distal renal tubules, increasing sodium chloride and water excretion while conserving potassium and hydrogen ions; may block the effect of aldosterone on arteriolar smooth muscle as well

Contraindications Anuria; acute renal insufficiency; significant impairment of renal excretory function; hyperkalemia

Warnings/Precautions Monitor serum potassium closely in patients being treated for heart failure. Avoid potassium supplements, potassium-containing salt substitutes, a diet rich in potassium, or other drugs that can cause hyperkalemia. Excess amounts can lead to profound diuresis with fluid and electrolyte loss; close medical supervision and dose evaluation are required. Watch for and correct electrolyte disturbances; adjust dose to avoid dehydration. In cirrhosis, avoid electrolyte and acid/base imbalances that might lead to hepatic encephalopathy. Gynecomastia is related to dose and duration of therapy. Discontinue use prior to adrenal vein catheterization. When evaluating a heart failure patient for spironolactone treatment, creatinine should be ≤2.5 mg/dL in men or ≤2 mg/dL in women and potassium <5 mEq/L. Discontinue or interrupt therapy if serum potassium >5 mEq/L or serum creatinine >4 mg/dL. **[U.S. Boxed Warning]: Shown to be a tumorigen in chronic toxicity animal studies. Avoid unnecessary use.**

In the elderly, avoid use of doses >25 mg/day in patients with heart failure or in patients with reduced renal function (Cl$_{cr}$ <30 mL/minute); risk of hyperkalemia is increased for heart failure patients receiving >25 mg/day, particularly if taking concomitant medications such as NSAIDS, ACE inhibitor, angiotensin receptor blocker, or potassium supplements (Beers Criteria).

Drug Interactions

Metabolism/Transport Effects None known.

Avoid Concomitant Use
Avoid concomitant use of Spironolactone with any of the following: CycloSPORINE (Systemic); Tacrolimus (Systemic)

Increased Effect/Toxicity
Spironolactone may increase the levels/effects of: ACE Inhibitors; Amifostine; Ammonium Chloride; Antihypertensives; Cardiac Glycosides; CycloSPORINE (Systemic); Digoxin; Hypotensive Agents; Neuromuscular-Blocking Agents (Nondepolarizing); RiTUXimab; Sodium Phosphates; Tacrolimus (Systemic)

The levels/effects of Spironolactone may be increased by: Alfuzosin; Angiotensin II Receptor Blockers; Canagliflozin; Diazoxide; Drospirenone; Eplerenone; Herbs (Hypotensive Properties); MAO Inhibitors; Nitrofurantoin; Nonsteroidal Anti-Inflammatory Agents; Pentoxifylline; Phosphodiesterase 5 Inhibitors; Potassium Salts; Prostacyclin Analogues; Tolvaptan; Trimethoprim

Decreased Effect
Spironolactone may decrease the levels/effects of: Abiraterone Acetate; Alpha-/Beta-Agonists; Cardiac Glycosides; Mitotane; QuiNIDine

The levels/effects of Spironolactone may be decreased by: Herbs (Hypertensive Properties); Methylphenidate; Nonsteroidal Anti-Inflammatory Agents; Yohimbine

Ethanol/Nutrition/Herb Interactions
Ethanol: Increases risk of orthostasis.
Food: Food increases absorption.
Herb/Nutraceutical: Avoid natural licorice (due to mineralocorticoid activity)

Dietary Considerations Should be taken with food to decrease gastrointestinal irritation and to increase absorption. Excessive potassium intake (eg, salt substitutes, low-salt foods, bananas, nuts) should be avoided.

Pharmacodynamics/Kinetics

Duration of Action 2-3 days

Half-life Elimination Spironolactone: 78-84 minutes; Canrenone: 10-23 hours; 7-alpha-spirolactone: 7-20 hours

Time to Peak Serum: 3-4 hours (primarily as the active metabolite)

Pregnancy Risk Factor C

Pregnancy Considerations Teratogenic effects were not observed in animal studies; however, doses used were less than or equal to equivalent doses in humans. The antiandrogen effects of spironolactone have been shown to cause feminization of the male fetus in animal studies. Two case reports did not demonstrate this effect in humans however, the authors caution that adequate data is lacking. Use of diuretics during normal pregnancies is not appropriate; use may be considered when edema is due to pathologic causes (as in the nonpregnant patient); monitor.

Lactation Enters breast milk/not recommended (AAP rates "compatible"; AAP 2001 update pending)

Breast-Feeding Considerations The active metabolite of spironolactone has been found in breast milk. Effects to humans are not known; however, this metabolite was found to be carcinogenic in rats. The manufacturer recommends discontinuing spironolactone or using an alternative method of feeding.

Dosage Forms
Tablet, oral: 25 mg, 50 mg, 100 mg
Aldactone®: 25 mg, 50 mg, 100 mg

Stavudine (STAV yoo deen)

Related Information
HIV Infection and AIDS *on page 1520*

Brand Names: U.S. Zerit®

Brand Names: Canada Zerit®

Pharmacologic Category Antiretroviral Agent, Reverse Transcriptase Inhibitor (Nucleoside)

Use Treatment of HIV infection in combination with other antiretroviral agents

Local Anesthetic/Vasoconstrictor Precautions No information available to require special precautions

Effects on Dental Treatment No significant effects or complications reported

Effects on Bleeding No information available to require special precautions relative to hemostasis.

Adverse Effects Adverse reactions reported below represent experience with combination therapy with other nucleoside analogues and protease inhibitors.

>10%:
Central nervous system: Headache (25% to 46%)
Dermatologic: Rash (18% to 30%)
Gastrointestinal: Nausea (43% to 53%; less than comparator group), vomiting (18% to 30%; less than comparator group), diarrhea (34% to 45%)
Hepatic: Hyperbilirubinemia (65% to 68%; grade 3/4: 7% to 16%), AST increased (42% to 53%; grade 3/4: 5% to 7%), ALT increased (40% to 50%; grade 3/4: 6% to 8%), GGT increased (15% to 28%; grade 3/4: 2% to 5%)
Neuromuscular & skeletal: Peripheral neuropathy (8% to 21%)
Miscellaneous: Amylase increased (21% to 31%; grade 3/4: 4% to 8%), lipase increased (~27%; grade 3/4: 5% to 6%)

General Dosage Range Dosage adjustment recommended in patients with renal impairment.
Oral:
Newborns (Birth to 13 days): 0.5 mg/kg every 12 hours
Children ≥14 days and <30 kg: 1 mg/kg every 12 hours
Children and Adults 30-59 kg: 30 mg every 12 hours
Children and Adults ≥60 kg: 40 mg every 12 hours

Mechanism of Action Stavudine is a thymidine analog which interferes with HIV viral DNA dependent DNA polymerase resulting in inhibition of viral replication; nucleoside reverse transcriptase inhibitor

Pharmacodynamics/Kinetics

Half-life Elimination HIV-infected Children: 0.96 hours, HIV-infected Adults: 1.6 hours

Time to Peak Serum: 1 hour

Pregnancy Risk Factor C

Pregnancy Considerations Adverse events were observed in some animal reproduction studies. Stavudine crosses the placenta. No increased risk of overall birth defects has been observed following first trimester exposure according to data collected by the antiretroviral pregnancy registry. Pharmacokinetics of stavudine are not significantly altered during pregnancy; dose adjustments are not needed. Cases of lactic acidosis/hepatic steatosis syndrome related to mitochondrial toxicity have been reported in pregnant women with prolonged use of nucleoside analogues. It is not known if pregnancy itself potentiates this known side effect; however, women may be at increased risk of lactic acidosis and liver damage. In addition, these adverse events are similar to other rare but life-threatening syndromes which occur during pregnancy (eg, HELLP syndrome). Combination treatment with didanosine may also contribute to the risk of lactic acidosis, and should be considered only if benefit outweighs risk. Hepatic enzymes and electrolytes should be monitored in women receiving nucleoside analogues and clinicians should watch for early signs of the syndrome. In addition, mitochondrial dysfunction may develop in infants following *in utero* exposure. The DHHS Perinatal HIV Guidelines recommend stavudine to be used only in special circumstances during pregnancy; do not use with didanosine or zidovudine.

Regardless of CD4 count or HIV RNA copy number, all HIV-infected pregnant women should receive a combination antepartum antiretroviral (ARV) drug regimen; this includes women who require therapy for their own health, as well as women who do not yet require therapy for their own health. ARV therapy should be started as soon as possible if required for the woman's health. Although earlier initiation may be more effective in reducing the perinatal transmission of HIV), also consider maternal conditions (eg, nausea and vomiting) and the potential risks of first trimester fetal exposure for specific agents. Plasma HIV RNA levels should be assessed at ~34-36 weeks gestation in order to help determine mode of delivery. If ARV therapy must be interrupted for <24 hours during the peripartum period, stop then restart all medications simultaneously in order to decrease the chance of developing resistance. Long-term follow-up is recommended for all infants exposed to ARV medications.

Healthcare providers are encouraged to enroll pregnant women exposed to antiretroviral medications in the Antiretroviral Pregnancy Registry (1-800-258-4263 or www.APRegistry.com). Healthcare providers caring for HIV-infected women and their infants may contact the National Perinatal HIV Hotline (888-448-8765) for clinical consultation (DHHS [perinatal], 2012).

Streptomycin (strep toe MYE sin)

Brand Names: Canada Streptomycin for Injection
Pharmacologic Category Antibiotic, Aminoglycoside; Antitubercular Agent
Use Part of combination therapy of active tuberculosis; used in combination with other agents for treatment of bacteremia caused by susceptible gram-negative bacilli, brucellosis, chancroid granuloma inguinale, *H. influenzae* (respiratory, endocardial, meningeal infections), *K. pneumoniae*, plague, streptococcal or enterococcal endocarditis, tularemia, urinary tract infections (caused by *A. aerogenes, E. coli, E. faecalis, K. pneumoniae, Proteus* spp)

Unlabeled Use Buruli ulcer (*Mycobacterium ulcerans*), Ménière's disease, *Mycobacterium kansasii* infection; *Mycobacterium avium* complex (MAC)

Local Anesthetic/Vasoconstrictor Precautions No information available to require special precautions

Effects on Dental Treatment No significant effects or complications reported

Effects on Bleeding No information available to require special precautions

Adverse Effects Frequency not defined.
Cardiovascular: Hypotension
Central nervous system: Drug fever, headache, neurotoxicity, paresthesia of face
Dermatologic: Angioedema, exfoliative dermatitis, skin rash, urticaria
Gastrointestinal: Nausea, vomiting
Hematologic: Eosinophilia, hemolytic anemia, leukopenia, pancytopenia, thrombocytopenia
Neuromuscular & skeletal: Arthralgia, tremor, weakness
Ocular: Amblyopia
Otic: Ototoxicity (auditory), ototoxicity (vestibular)
Renal: Azotemia, nephrotoxicity
Respiratory: Difficulty in breathing
Miscellaneous: Anaphylaxis

General Dosage Range Dosage adjustment recommended in patients with renal impairment
I.M.:
Children: Tuberculosis: 20-40 mg/kg given daily (maximum: 1 g daily) **or** 25-30 mg/kg 2-3 times weekly (maximum: 1.5 g daily)
Adults: Tuberculosis: 15 mg/kg/day **or** 25-30 mg/kg 2-3 times weekly; Other indications: 1-2 g daily in 2 divided doses

Mechanism of Action Inhibits bacterial protein synthesis by binding directly to the 30S ribosomal subunits causing faulty peptide sequence to form in the protein chain

Pharmacodynamics/Kinetics
Half-life Elimination Adults: ~5 hours
Time to Peak I.M.: Within 1 hour
Pregnancy Risk Factor D

Pregnancy Considerations Streptomycin crosses the placenta. Many case reports of hearing impairment in children exposed *in utero* have been published. Impairment has ranged from mild hearing loss to bilateral deafness. Because of several reports of total irreversible bilateral congenital deafness in children whose mothers received streptomycin during pregnancy, the manufacturer classifies streptomycin as pregnancy risk factor D.

Streptozocin (strep toe ZOE sin)

Brand Names: U.S. Zanosar®
Brand Names: Canada Zanosar®
Pharmacologic Category Antineoplastic Agent, Alkylating Agent
Use Treatment of metastatic islet cell carcinoma of the pancreas (symptomatic or progressive disease)
Unlabeled Use Treatment of metastatic adrenal carcinoma

Local Anesthetic/Vasoconstrictor Precautions No information available to require special precautions

Effects on Dental Treatment No significant effects or complications reported

Effects on Bleeding Chemotherapy may result in significant myelosuppression, potentially including significant reduction in platelet counts and altered hemostasis. In patients who are under active treatment with these agents, medical consult is suggested.

Adverse Effects Frequency not defined.

Endocrine & metabolic: Glucose intolerance, hyper-/hypoglycemia, hypoalbuminemia, hypophosphatemia

Gastrointestinal: Diarrhea, nausea, vomiting

Hepatic: LDH increased, transaminases increased

Local: Injection site reactions (burning, edema, erythema, inflammation, irritation, tenderness)

Renal: Anuria, azotemia, BUN increased, creatinine increased, glycosuria, nephrotoxicity, proteinuria, renal dysfunction, renal tubular acidosis

General Dosage Range Dosage adjustment recommended in patients with renal impairment or who develop toxicities.

I.V.: *Adults:* 500 mg/m^2 for 5 consecutive days every 6 weeks **or** 1000-1500 mg/m^2 once weekly (maximum dose: 1500 mg/m^2)

Mechanism of Action Inhibits DNA synthesis by alkylation and cross-linking the strands of DNA, and by possible protein modification; cell cycle nonspecific

Pharmacodynamics/Kinetics

Onset of Action 1500 mg/m^2 once weekly: Onset of response: 17 days; median time to maximum response: 35 days

Half-life Elimination <1 hour

Pregnancy Risk Factor D

Pregnancy Considerations Teratogenic events have been observed in animal reproduction studies.

Succinylcholine (suks in il KOE leen)

Brand Names: U.S. Anectine®; Quelicin®

Brand Names: Canada Quelicin®

Pharmacologic Category Neuromuscular Blocker Agent, Depolarizing

Use To facilitate both rapid sequence and routine endotracheal intubation and to relax skeletal muscles during surgery

Note: Does not relieve pain or produce sedation

Unlabeled Use To reduce the intensity of muscle contractions of electroconvulsive therapy (ECT)

Local Anesthetic/Vasoconstrictor Precautions No information available to require special precautions

Effects on Dental Treatment No significant effects or complications reported

Effects on Bleeding No information available to require special precautions

Adverse Effects Frequency not defined.

Cardiovascular: Arrhythmias, bradycardia (higher with second dose, more frequent in children), cardiac arrest, hyper-/hypotension, tachycardia

Dermatologic: Rash

Endocrine & metabolic: Hyperkalemia

Gastrointestinal: Salivation (excessive)

Neuromuscular & skeletal: Jaw rigidity, muscle fasciculation, postoperative muscle pain, rhabdomyolysis (with possible myoglobinuric acute renal failure)

Ocular: Intraocular pressure increased

Renal: Acute renal failure (secondary to rhabdomyolysis)

Respiratory: Apnea, respiratory depression (prolonged)

Miscellaneous: Anaphylaxis, malignant hyperthermia

Causes of prolonged neuromuscular blockade: Excessive drug administration; cumulative drug effect, decreased metabolism/excretion (hepatic and/or renal impairment); accumulation of active metabolites; electrolyte imbalance (hypokalemia, hypocalcemia, hypermagnesemia, hypernatremia); hypothermia; drug interactions; increased sensitivity to muscle relaxants

(eg, neuromuscular disorders such as myasthenia gravis or polymyositis)

General Dosage Range Dosage adjustment recommended in patients with renal or hepatic impairment

I.M.: *Children and Adults:* Up to 3-4 mg/kg (maximum: 150 mg total dose)

I.V.:

Smaller Children: Intermittent: Initial: 2 mg/kg/dose; Maintenance: 0.3-0.6 mg/kg/dose every 5-10 minutes as needed

Older Children and Adolescents: Intermittent: Initial: 1 mg/kg/dose; Maintenance: 0.3-0.6 mg/kg every 5-10 minutes as needed

Adults: Intubation: 0.6 mg/kg (range: 0.3-1.1 mg/kg); Rapid sequence intubation: 1-1.5 mg/kg

Mechanism of Action Acts similar to acetylcholine, produces depolarization of the motor endplate at the myoneural junction which causes sustained flaccid skeletal muscle paralysis produced by state of accommodation that develops in adjacent excitable muscle membranes

Pharmacodynamics/Kinetics

Onset of Action I.M.: 2-3 minutes; I.V.: Complete muscular relaxation: 30-60 seconds

Duration of Action I.M.: 10-30 minutes; I.V.: 4-6 minutes with single administration

Pregnancy Risk Factor C

Pregnancy Considerations Reproduction studies have not been conducted. Small amounts cross the placenta. Sensitivity to succinylcholine may be increased due to a ~24% decrease in plasma cholinesterase activity during pregnancy and several days postpartum.

Sucralfate (soo KRAL fate)

Related Information

Management of Patients Undergoing Cancer Therapy *on page 1596*

Brand Names: U.S. Carafate®

Brand Names: Canada Apo-Sucralfate; Dom-Sucralfate; Novo-Sucralate; Nu-Sucralate; PMS-Sucralate; Sucralfate-1; Sulcrate®; Sulcrate® Suspension Plus; Teva-Sucralfate

Generic Availability (U.S.) Yes

Pharmacologic Category Gastrointestinal Agent, Miscellaneous

Use Short-term (≤8 weeks) management of duodenal ulcers; maintenance therapy for duodenal ulcers

Unlabeled Use Gastric ulcers; suspension may be used topically for treatment of stomatitis due to cancer chemotherapy and other causes of esophageal and gastric erosions; GERD, esophagitis; treatment of NSAID mucosal damage; prevention of stress ulcers; postsclerotherapy for esophageal variceal bleeding

Local Anesthetic/Vasoconstrictor Precautions No information available to require special precautions

Effects on Dental Treatment No significant effects or complications reported

Effects on Bleeding No information available to require special precautions

Adverse Effects 1% to 10%: Gastrointestinal: Constipation (2%)

Dosage Oral:

Children (unlabeled use): Doses of 40-80 mg/kg/day divided every 6 hours have been used

Stomatitis (unlabeled use): 5-10 mL (1 g/10 mL suspension), swish and spit or swish and swallow 4 times/day

Adults:
  Stress ulcer (unlabeled use):
    Prophylaxis: 1 g 4 times/day
    Treatment: 1 g every 4 hours
  Duodenal ulcer:
    Treatment: 1 g 4 times/day on an empty stomach and at bedtime for 4-8 weeks, or alternatively 2 g twice daily; treatment is recommended for 4-8 weeks in adults
    Maintenance: Prophylaxis: 1 g twice daily
  Stomatitis (unlabeled use): 10 mL (1 g/10 mL suspension), swish and spit or swish and swallow 4 times/day

Dosage comment in renal impairment: Aluminum salt is minimally absorbed (<5%), however, may accumulate in renal failure

Mechanism of Action Forms a complex by binding with positively charged proteins in exudates, forming a viscous paste-like, adhesive substance. This selectively forms a protective coating that acts locally to protect the gastric lining against peptic acid, pepsin, and bile salts.

Contraindications Hypersensitivity to sucralfate or any component of the formulation

Warnings/Precautions Because sucralfate acts locally at the ulcer site, successful therapy with sucralfate should not be expected to alter the posthealing frequency of recurrence or the severity of duodenal ulceration. Use with caution in patients with chronic renal failure; sucralfate is an aluminum complex, small amounts of aluminum are absorbed following oral administration. Excretion of aluminum may be decreased in patients with chronic renal failure. Because of the potential for sucralfate to alter the absorption of some drugs, separate administration (take other medication 2 hours before sucralfate) should be considered when alterations in bioavailability are believed to be critical.

Drug Interactions
Metabolism/Transport Effects None known.

Avoid Concomitant Use
Avoid concomitant use of Sucralfate with any of the following: Multivitamins/Minerals (with ADEK, Folate, Iron); Vitamin D Analogs

Increased Effect/Toxicity
The levels/effects of Sucralfate may be increased by: Multivitamins/Minerals (with ADEK, Folate, Iron); Vitamin D Analogs

Decreased Effect
Sucralfate may decrease the levels/effects of: Antifungal Agents (Azole Derivatives, Systemic); Digoxin; Eltrombopag; Furosemide; Levothyroxine; Phosphate Supplements; QuiNIDine; Quinolone Antibiotics; Tetracycline Derivatives; Vitamin K Antagonists

Ethanol/Nutrition/Herb Interactions Food: Sucralfate may interfere with absorption of vitamin A, vitamin D, vitamin E, and vitamin K.

Dietary Considerations Take with water on an empty stomach.

Pharmacodynamics/Kinetics
Onset of Action Paste formation and ulcer adhesion: 1-2 hours
Duration of Action Up to 6 hours

Pregnancy Risk Factor B
Pregnancy Considerations Teratogenic effects were not observed in animal studies. Sucralfate is only minimally absorbed following oral administration.

Lactation Excretion in breast milk unknown/use caution

Dosage Forms
Suspension, oral: 1 g/10 mL (10 mL)
  Carafate®: 1 g/10 mL (420 mL)
Tablet, oral: 1 g
  Carafate®: 1 g

SUFentanil (soo FEN ta nil)

Brand Names: U.S. Sufenta®
Brand Names: Canada Sufentanil Citrate Injection, USP; Sufenta®
Pharmacologic Category Analgesic, Opioid; Anilidopiperidine Opioid; General Anesthetic
Use Analgesic supplement in maintenance of general anesthesia; epidural analgesic in conjunction with a local anesthetic
Local Anesthetic/Vasoconstrictor Precautions No information available to require special precautions
Effects on Dental Treatment Key adverse event(s) related to dental treatment: Orthostatic hypotension.
Effects on Bleeding No information available to require special precautions

Adverse Effects
>10%: Dermatologic: Pruritus (epidural: 25%)
1% to 10%:
  Cardiovascular: Bradycardia (dose related; 3% to 9%), hyper-/hypotension (3% to 9%; more common with I.V. administration)
  Central nervous system: Somnolence (3% to 9%), CNS depression, confusion
  Gastrointestinal: Nausea (3% to 9%), vomiting (3% to 9%)
  Neuromuscular & skeletal: Chest wall rigidity (dose related; 3% to 9%)
  Ocular: Blurred vision

General Dosage Range
I.V.:
  Children 2-12 years: 10-25 mcg/kg with 100% O_2; Maintenance: Up to 1-2 mcg/kg total dose
  Adults: 1-2 mcg/kg with N_2O/O_2; Maintenance: 5-20 mcg/kg as needed
  Epidural: *Adults:* 10-15 mcg (maximum: 3 doses)

Mechanism of Action Binds to opioid receptors throughout the CNS. Once receptor binding occurs, effects are exerted by opening K+ channels and inhibiting Ca++ channels. These mechanisms increase pain threshold, alter pain perception, inhibit ascending pain pathways; short-acting narcotic; dose-related inhibition of catecholamine release (up to 30 mcg/kg) controls sympathetic response to surgical stress.

Pharmacodynamics/Kinetics
Onset of Action Analgesia: I.V.: 1-3 minutes; Epidural: 10 minutes
Duration of Action Dose dependent; Epidural:10-15 mcg with bupivacaine: 1.7 hours
Half-life Elimination Neonates: 5-10 hours; Infants & Children: 55-139 minutes; Adults: 164 minutes

Pregnancy Risk Factor C
Pregnancy Considerations Animal studies suggest embryocidal effects when given I.V. for a period of 10 days to >30 days. No evidence of teratogenic effects observed in animals. Administration of epidural sufenanil with bupivacaine with or without epinephrine is indicated in labor and delivery. Intravenous use or larger epidural doses are not recommended in pregnant women.

Controlled Substance C-II

Sulconazole (sul KON a zole)

Brand Names: U.S. Exelderm®
Brand Names: Canada Exelderm®
Pharmacologic Category Antifungal Agent, Topical
Use Treatment of superficial fungal infections of the skin, including tinea cruris (jock itch), tinea corporis (ringworm), tinea versicolor, and tinea pedis (athlete's foot, cream only)
Local Anesthetic/Vasoconstrictor Precautions No information available to require special precautions
Effects on Dental Treatment No significant effects or complications reported
Effects on Bleeding No information available to require special precautions
Adverse Effects 1% to 10%:
Dermatologic: Itching
Local: Burning, stinging, redness
General Dosage Range Topical: *Adults:* Apply a small amount to affected area once or twice daily
Mechanism of Action Substituted imidazole derivative which inhibits metabolic reactions necessary for the synthesis of ergosterol, an essential membrane component. The end result is usually fungistatic; however, sulconazole may act as a fungicide in *Candida albicans* and *Candida parapsilosis* during certain growth phases.
Pregnancy Risk Factor C
Pregnancy Considerations Adverse events have been observed in animal reproduction studies with large doses administered orally. Systemic absorption is limited following topical administration.

Sulfabenzamide, Sulfacetamide, and Sulfathiazole

(sul fa BENZ a mide, sul fa SEE ta mide, & sul fa THYE a zole)

Brand Names: U.S. V.V.S.®
Pharmacologic Category Antibiotic, Vaginal
Use Treatment of *Haemophilus vaginalis* vaginitis
Local Anesthetic/Vasoconstrictor Precautions No information available to require special precautions
Effects on Dental Treatment No significant effects or complications reported
Effects on Bleeding No information available to require special precautions
Adverse Effects Frequency not defined.
Dermatologic: Pruritus, urticaria, Stevens-Johnson syndrome
Local: Local irritation
Miscellaneous: Allergic reactions
General Dosage Range Intravaginal: *Adults:* Insert 1/4 to 1 applicatorful twice daily
Mechanism of Action Interferes with microbial folic acid synthesis and growth via inhibition of para-aminobenzoic acid metabolism

Sulfacetamide (Ophthalmic)

(sul fa SEE ta mide)

Brand Names: U.S. Bleph®-10; Sulfamide
Brand Names: Canada AK Sulf Liq; Bleph 10 DPS; Diosulf™; PMS-Sulfacetamide; Sodium Sulamyd
Pharmacologic Category Antibiotic, Ophthalmic
Use Treatment and prophylaxis of conjunctivitis and other superficial ocular infections due to susceptible organisms; adjunctive treatment with systemic sulfonamides for therapy of trachoma

Local Anesthetic/Vasoconstrictor Precautions No information available to require special precautions
Effects on Dental Treatment No significant effects or complications reported
Effects on Bleeding No information available to require special precautions
Adverse Effects Frequency not defined.
Cardiovascular: Edema
Ocular (following ophthalmic application): Burning, conjunctivitis, conjunctival hyperemia, corneal ulcers, irritation, stinging
Miscellaneous: Allergic reactions, systemic lupus erythematosus
General Dosage Range Ophthalmic: *Children >2 months and Adults:* Solution: Instill 1-2 drops up to every 2-3 hours and at bedtime; Ointment: Instill 1/2" (1.25 cm) ribbon every 3-4 hours and at bedtime
Mechanism of Action Interferes with bacterial growth by inhibiting bacterial folic acid synthesis through competitive antagonism of PABA
Pregnancy Risk Factor C
Pregnancy Considerations Animal reproduction studies have not been conducted. Use of systemic sulfonamides during pregnancy may cause kernicterus in the newborn. Use during pregnancy only if clearly needed.

Sulfacetamide and Prednisolone

(sul fa SEE ta mide & pred NIS oh lone)

Related Information
Sulfacetamide (Ophthalmic) *on page 1259*
Brand Names: U.S. Blephamide®
Brand Names: Canada AK Cide Oph; Blephamide®; Dioptimyd®
Pharmacologic Category Antibiotic/Corticosteroid, Ophthalmic
Use Steroid-responsive inflammatory ocular conditions in which a corticosteroid is indicated and where infection is present or there is a risk of infection
Local Anesthetic/Vasoconstrictor Precautions No information available to require special precautions
Effects on Dental Treatment No significant effects or complications reported
Effects on Bleeding No information available to require special precautions
Adverse Effects Frequency not defined. Also see individual agents.
Dermatologic: Stevens-Johnson syndrome, toxic epidermal necrolysis, wound healing delayed
Hematologic: Agranulocytosis, aplastic anemia
Hepatic: Hepatic necrosis (fulminant)
Local: Irritation
Ocular: Accommodation loss, anterior uveitis (acute), intraocular pressure elevation, glaucoma, globe perforation, mydriasis, optic nerve damage (infrequent), posterior subcapsular cataract formation, ptosis
Miscellaneous: Allergic reactions, hypercorticoidism (systemic; rare), secondary infections (bacterial, fungal)
General Dosage Range Ophthalmic: *Children ≥6 years and Adults:*
Ointment: Apply ~1/2" ribbon 3-4 times/day and 1-2 times at night
Solution, suspension: Instill 2 drops every 4 hours

◄ **Mechanism of Action** Interferes with bacterial growth by inhibiting bacterial folic acid synthesis through competitive antagonism of PABA; decreases inflammation by suppression of migration of polymorphonuclear leukocytes and reversal of increased capillary permeability; suppresses the immune system by reducing activity and volume of the lymphatic system

Pregnancy Risk Factor C

Pregnancy Considerations Animal reproduction studies have not been conducted with sulfacetamide. See individual agents.

SulfADIAZINE (sul fa DYE a zeen)

Pharmacologic Category Antibiotic, Sulfonamide Derivative

Use Treatment of the following conditions (per product labeling): Chancroid, trachoma, inclusion conjunctivitis, nocardiosis, urinary tract infections, toxoplasmosis encephalitis, malaria, meningococcal meningitis, acute otitis media, rheumatic fever (prophylaxis), meningitis (adjunctive)

Refer to current guidelines for appropriate use.

Local Anesthetic/Vasoconstrictor Precautions No information available to require special precautions

Effects on Dental Treatment No significant effects or complications reported

Effects on Bleeding No information available to require special precautions

Adverse Effects Frequency not defined.

Cardiovascular: Allergic myocarditis, periarteritis nodosa

Central nervous system: Ataxia, chills, convulsions, depression, fever, hallucinations, headache, insomnia, vertigo

Dermatologic: Epidermal necrolysis, erythema multiforme, exfoliative dermatitis, photosensitivity, pruritus, purpura, rash, skin eruptions, Stevens-Johnson syndrome, urticaria

Endocrine & metabolic: Hypoglycemia, thyroid function disturbance

Gastrointestinal: Abdominal pain, anorexia, diarrhea, nausea, pancreatitis, stomatitis, vomiting

Genitourinary: Crystalluria, stone formation, toxic nephrosis with oliguria and anuria

Hematologic: Agranulocytopenia, aplastic anemia, hemolytic anemia, hypoprothrombinemia, leukopenia, methemoglobinemia, thrombocytopenia

Hepatic: Hepatitis

Neuromuscular & skeletal: Arthralgia, peripheral neuritis

Ocular: Conjunctival/scleral injection, periorbital edema

Otic: Tinnitus

Renal: Diuresis

Miscellaneous: Anaphylactoid reactions, lupus erythematosus, serum sickness-like reactions

General Dosage Range Oral:

Children >2 months: Initial: 75 mg/kg; Maintenance: 150 mg/kg/day (maximum: 6 g/24 hours)

Children <30 kg and Adults <30 kg: 0.5 g/day (rheumatic fever prophylaxis)

Children ≥30 kg and Adults ≥30 kg: 1 g/day (rheumatic fever prophylaxis)

Adults: 2-4 g/day in divided doses

Mechanism of Action Interferes with bacterial growth by inhibiting bacterial folic acid synthesis through competitive antagonism of PABA

Pharmacodynamics/Kinetics

Half-life Elimination 10 hours

Time to Peak Within 3-6 hours

Pregnancy Risk Factor C

Pregnancy Considerations Adverse events have been observed in animal reproduction studies; therefore, the manufacturer classifies sulfadiazine as pregnancy category C. Sulfadiazine crosses the placenta. Available studies and case reports have failed to show an increased risk for congenital malformations after use. Sulfadiazine is indicated for use in children <2 months of age for the treatment of congenital toxoplasmosis and may be used in pregnancy for the maternal treatment of *Toxoplasmic gondii* encephalitis and as an alternative agent for the secondary prevention of rheumatic fever. Because of the theoretical increased risk for hyperbilirubinemia and kernicterus, sulfadiazine is contraindicated by the manufacturer for use near term. Neonatal healthcare providers should be informed if maternal sulfonamide therapy is used near the time of delivery.

Sulfadoxine and Pyrimethamine
(sul fa DOKS een & peer i METH a meen)

Related Information

Pyrimethamine on page 1164

Brand Names: U.S. Fansidar® [DSC]

Pharmacologic Category Antimalarial Agent

Use Treatment of *Plasmodium falciparum* malaria in patients in whom chloroquine resistance is suspected; malaria prophylaxis for travelers to areas where chloroquine-resistant malaria is endemic

Local Anesthetic/Vasoconstrictor Precautions No information available to require special precautions

Effects on Dental Treatment Key adverse event(s) related to dental treatment: Atrophic glossitis.

Effects on Bleeding No information available to require special precautions

Adverse Effects Frequency not defined.

Cardiovascular: Myocarditis (allergic), pericarditis (allergic), periorbital edema

Central nervous system: Ataxia, hallucinations, headache, polyneuritis, seizure

Dermatologic: Photosensitivity, Stevens-Johnson syndrome, erythema multiforme, toxic epidermal necrolysis, rash

Endocrine & metabolic: Thyroid function dysfunction

Gastrointestinal: Anorexia, atrophic glossitis, gastritis, pancreatitis, vomiting

Genitourinary: Crystalluria

Hematologic: Megaloblastic anemia, leukopenia, thrombocytopenia, pancytopenia

Hepatic: Hepatic necrosis, hepatitis

Neuromuscular & skeletal: Tremors

Renal: BUN increased, interstitial nephritis, renal failure, serum creatinine increased

Respiratory: Respiratory failure, alveolitis (resembling eosinophilic or allergic)

Miscellaneous: Anaphylactoid reaction, drug fever, hypersensitivity, Lupus-like syndrome, periarteritis nodosum

General Dosage Range Oral:

Children 2-11 months: 1/4 tablet as a single dose

Children 1-3 years: 1/2 tablet as a single dose

Children 4-8 years: 1 tablet as a single dose

Children 9-14 years: 2 tablets as a single dose

Children >14 years and Adults: 3 tablets as a single dose

Mechanism of Action Sulfadoxine interferes with bacterial folic acid synthesis and growth via competitive inhibition of para-aminiobenzoic acid; pyrimethamine inhibits microbial dihydrofolate reductase, resulting in inhibition of tetrahydrofolic acid synthesis

Pharmacodynamics/Kinetics

Half-life Elimination Pyrimethamine: 80-95 hours; Sulfadoxine: 5-8 days

Time to Peak Serum: 2-8 hours

Pregnancy Risk Factor C

Pregnancy Considerations Adverse events have been observed in animal reproduction studies. Pyrimethamine and sulfadoxine both cross the placenta. Prophylactic use near term is contraindicated by the manufacturer.

Sulfamethoxazole and Trimethoprim
(sul fa meth OKS a zole & trye METH oh prim)

Related Information
Trimethoprim *on page 1365*

Brand Names: U.S. Bactrim™; Bactrim™ DS; Septra® DS

Brand Names: Canada Apo-Sulfatrim®; Apo-Sulfatrim® DS; Apo-Sulfatrim® Pediatric; Novo-Trimel; Novo-Trimel D.S.; Nu-Cotrimox; Septra® Injection

Generic Availability (U.S.) Yes

Pharmacologic Category Antibiotic, Miscellaneous; Antibiotic, Sulfonamide Derivative

Use
Oral treatment of urinary tract infections due to *E. coli*, *Klebsiella* and *Enterobacter* sp, *M. morganii*, *P. mirabilis* and *P. vulgaris*; acute otitis media in children; acute exacerbations of chronic bronchitis in adults due to susceptible strains of *H. influenzae* or *S. pneumoniae*; treatment and prophylaxis of *Pneumocystis jirovecii* pneumonia (PCP); traveler's diarrhea due to enterotoxigenic *E. coli*; treatment of enteritis caused by *Shigella flexneri* or *Shigella sonnei*

I.V. treatment of severe or complicated infections when oral therapy is not feasible, for documented PCP, empiric treatment of PCP in immune compromised patients; treatment of documented or suspected shigellosis, typhoid fever, or other infections caused by susceptible bacteria

Unlabeled Use Cholera and *Salmonella*-type infections and nocardiosis; chronic prostatitis; as prophylaxis in neutropenic patients with *P. jirovecii* infections, in leukemia patients, and in patients following renal transplantation, to decrease incidence of PCP; treatment of *Cyclospora* infection, typhoid fever, *Nocardia asteroides* infection; prophylaxis against urinary tract infection; alternative treatment for MRSA infections; oral phase treatment of prosthetic joint infection; chronic antimicrobial suppression of prosthetic joint infection

Local Anesthetic/Vasoconstrictor Precautions No information available to require special precautions

Effects on Dental Treatment Key adverse event(s) related to dental treatment: Stomatitis.

Effects on Bleeding No information available to require special precautions

Adverse Effects The most common adverse reactions include gastrointestinal upset (nausea, vomiting, anorexia) and dermatologic reactions (rash or urticaria). Rare, life-threatening reactions have been associated with co-trimoxazole, including severe dermatologic reactions, blood dyscrasias, and hepatotoxic reactions. Most other reactions listed are rare, however, frequency cannot be accurately estimated.

Cardiovascular: Allergic myocarditis

Central nervous system: Apathy, aseptic meningitis, ataxia, chills, depression, fatigue, fever, hallucinations, headache, insomnia, kernicterus (in neonates), nervousness, peripheral neuritis, seizure, vertigo

Dermatologic: Photosensitivity, pruritus, rash, skin eruptions, urticaria; rare reactions include erythema multiforme, exfoliative dermatitis, Henoch-Schönlein purpura (IgA vasculitis), Stevens-Johnson syndrome, and toxic epidermal necrolysis

Endocrine & metabolic: Hyperkalemia (generally at high dosages), hypoglycemia (rare), hyponatremia

Gastrointestinal: Abdominal pain, anorexia, diarrhea, glottitis, nausea, pancreatitis, pseudomembranous colitis, stomatitis, vomiting

Hematologic: Agranulocytosis, aplastic anemia, eosinophilia, hemolysis (with G6PD deficiency), hemolytic anemia, hypoprothrombinemia, leukopenia, megaloblastic anemia, methemoglobinemia, neutropenia, thrombocytopenia

Hepatic: Hepatotoxicity (including hepatitis, cholestasis, and hepatic necrosis), hyperbilirubinemia, transaminases increased

Neuromuscular & skeletal: Arthralgia, myalgia, rhabdomyolysis, weakness

Otic: Tinnitus

Renal: BUN increased, crystalluria, diuresis (rare), interstitial nephritis, nephrotoxicity (in association with cyclosporine), renal failure, serum creatinine increased, toxic nephrosis (with anuria and oliguria)

Respiratory: Cough, dyspnea, pulmonary infiltrates

Miscellaneous: Allergic reaction, anaphylaxis, angioedema, periarteritis nodosa (rare), serum sickness, systemic lupus erythematosus (rare)

Dosage Dosage recommendations are based on the trimethoprim component. Double-strength tablets are equivalent to sulfamethoxazole 800 mg and trimethoprim 160 mg.

Usual dosage ranges:

Children >2 months: Manufacturer's labeling:

Mild-to-moderate infections: Oral: 8 mg TMP/kg/day in divided doses every 12 hours

Serious infection:

Oral: 15-20 mg TMP/kg/day in divided doses every 6 hours

I.V.: 8-12 mg TMP/kg/day in divided doses every 6-12 hours

Adults:

Oral: 1-2 double-strength tablets (sulfamethoxazole 800 mg; trimethoprim 160 mg) every 12-24 hours

I.V.: 8-20 mg TMP/kg/day divided every 6-12 hours

Indication-specific dosing:

Children >2 months:

Acute otitis media: Oral: 8 mg TMP/kg/day in divided doses every 12 hours for 10 days. **Note:** Recommended by the American Academy of Pediatrics as an alternative agent in penicillin-allergic patients at a dose of 6-10 mg TMP/kg/day (AOM guidelines, 2004).

Cyclosporiasis (unlabeled use): Oral, I.V.: 5 mg TMP/kg twice daily for 7-10 days (*Red Book*, 2009)

Pneumocystis jirovecii:

Treatment: Oral, I.V.: 15-20 mg TMP/kg/day in divided doses every 6-8 hours for 21 days

Prophylaxis: Oral, 150 mg TMP/m^2/day in divided doses every 12 hours and administered for 3 days/week on consecutive or alternate days; an alternative dosing regimen allows for same dose to be administered in 2 divided doses daily (maximum: trimethoprim 320 mg and sulfamethoxazole 1600 mg daily) (CDC, 2009)

Shigellosis: Note: Due to reported widespread resistance, empiric therapy with sulfamethoxazole and trimethoprim is not recommended (CDC-NARMS, 2010; WHO, 2005).

Oral:

Manufacturer's recommendation: 8 mg TMP/kg/day in divided doses every 12 hours for 5 days

Alternate recommendations (unlabeled dose): 10 mg TMP/kg/day in divided doses every 12 hours for 5 days (Ashkenazi, 1993)

I.V.: 8-10 mg TMP/kg/day in divided doses every 6, 8, or 12 hours for up to 5 days

Skin/soft tissue infection due to community-acquired MRSA (unlabeled use): Oral: 4-6 mg TMP/kg/dose every 12 hours for 5-10 days (Liu, 2011); **Note:** If beta-hemolytic *Streptococcus* spp are also suspected, a beta-lactam antibiotic should be added to the regimen (Liu, 2011)

Toxoplasmosis primary prophylaxis in HIV-exposed/infected patients (unlabeled use; CDC, 2009): Oral: 150 mg TMP/m^2/day in 2 divided doses (preferred) or 150 mg TMP/m^2/day in a single dose 3 times/week on consecutive days; or 150 mg TMP/m^2/day in 2 divided doses 3 times/week on alternate days

Urinary tract infection:

Treatment:

Oral: 8 mg TMP/kg/day in divided doses every 12 hours

I.V.: 8-10 mg TMP/kg/day in divided doses every 6, 8, or 12 hours for up to 14 days with serious infections

Prophylaxis: Oral: 2 mg TMP/kg/dose daily or 5 mg TMP/kg/dose twice weekly

Adults:

Chronic bronchitis (acute): Oral: One double-strength tablet every 12 hours for 10-14 days

Cyclosporiasis (unlabeled use): Oral, I.V.: 160 mg TMP twice daily for 7-10 days. **Note:** AIDS patients: Oral: One double-strength tablet 2-4 times/day for 10 days, then 1 double-strength tablet 3 times/week for 10 weeks (Pape, 1994; Verdier, 2000)

Granuloma inguinale (donovanosis) (unlabeled use): Oral: One double-strength tablet every 12 hours for at least 3 weeks and until lesions have healed (CDC, 2010)

Isosporiasis (*Isospora belli* infection) in HIV-positive patients (unlabeled use; CDC, 2009):

Treatment: Oral, I.V.: 160 mg TMP 4 times/day for 10 days or 160 mg TMP 2 times/day for 7-10 days. May increase dose and/or duration up to 3-4 weeks if symptoms worsen or persist

Secondary prophylaxis (in patients with CD4+ count <200 /microL): Oral: 160 mg TMP 3 times/week (preferred) or alternatively, 160 mg TMP daily or 320 mg TMP 3 times/week

Meningitis (bacterial): I.V.: 10-20 mg TMP/kg/day in divided doses every 6-12 hours

Nocardia (unlabeled use): Oral, I.V.:

Cutaneous infections: 5-10 mg TMP/kg/day in 2-4 divided doses

Severe infections (pulmonary/cerebral): 15 mg TMP/kg/day in 2-4 divided doses for 3-4 weeks, then 10 mg TMP/kg/day in 2-4 divided doses. Treatment duration is controversial; an average of 7 months has been reported.

Note: Therapy for severe infection may be initiated I.V. and converted to oral therapy (frequently converted to approximate dosages of oral solid dosage forms: 2 DS tablets every 8-12 hours). Although not widely available, sulfonamide levels should be considered in patients with questionable absorption, at risk for dose-related toxicity, or those with poor therapeutic response.

Osteomyelitis due to MRSA (unlabeled use): Oral, I.V.: 3.5-4 mg TMP/kg/dose every 8-12 hours for a minimum of 8 weeks with rifampin 600 mg once daily (Liu, 2011)

Pneumocystis jirovecii pneumonia (PCP): Oral: Manufacturer's labeling:

Prophylaxis: 160 mg TMP daily

Treatment: 15-20 mg TMP/kg/day divided every 6 hours for 14-21 days

Pneumocystis jirovecii pneumonia (PCP) prophylaxis and treatment in HIV-positive patients (CDC, 2009): **Note:** Sulfamethoxazole and trimethoprim is the preferred regimen for this indication.

Prophylaxis: Oral: 80-160 mg TMP daily **or** alternatively, 160 mg TMP 3 times/week

Treatment:

Mild-to-moderate: Oral: 15-20 mg TMP/kg/day in 3 divided doses for 21 days **or** alternatively, 320 mg TMP 3 times/day for 21 days

Moderate-to-severe: Oral, I.V.: 15-20 mg TMP/kg/day in 3-4 divided doses for 21 days

Prosthetic joint infection (unlabeled use): Oral phase treatment (after completion of pathogen-specific I.V. therapy) following debridement and prosthesis retention or 1-stage exchange:

Total ankle, elbow, hip, or shoulder arthroplasty: 160 mg TMP 2 times daily for 3 months. **Note:** Must be used in combination with rifampin (Cordero-Ampuero, 2007; Osmon, 2013).

Total knee arthroplasty: Adults: 160 mg TMP 2 times daily for 6 months. **Note:** Must be used in combination with rifampin (Cordero-Ampuero, 2007; Osmon, 2013).

Sepsis: I.V.: 20 mg TMP/kg/day divided every 6 hours

Septic arthritis due to MRSA (unlabeled use): Oral, I.V.: 3.5-4 mg TMP/kg/dose every 8-12 hours for 3-4 weeks (some experts combine with rifampin) (Liu, 2011)

Shigellosis: Note: Due to reported widespread resistance, empiric therapy with sulfamethoxazole and trimethoprim is not recommended (CDC-NARMS, 2010; WHO, 2005).

Oral: One double-strength tablet every 12 hours for 5 days

I.V.: 8-10 mg TMP/kg/day in divided doses every 6, 8, or 12 hours for up to 5 days

Skin/soft tissue infection due to community-acquired MRSA (unlabeled use): Oral: 1-2 double-strength tablets every 12 hours for 5-10 days (Liu, 2011); **Note:** If beta-hemolytic *Streptococcus* spp are also suspected, a beta-lactam antibiotic should be added to the regimen (Liu, 2011)

Stenotrophomonas maltophilia **(ventilator-associated pneumonia):** I.V.: Most clinicians have utilized 12-15 mg TMP/kg/day for the treatment of VAP caused by *Stenotrophomonas maltophilia*. Higher doses (up to 20 mg TMP/kg/day) have been mentioned for treatment of severe infection in patients with normal renal function (Looney, 2009; Vartivarian, 1989; Wood, 2010)

Toxoplasma gondii **encephalitis (unlabeled use; CDC, 2009):** Oral:
Primary prophylaxis: Oral: 160 mg TMP daily (preferred) **or** 160 mg TMP 3 times/week **or** 80 mg TMP daily
Treatment (alternative to sulfadiazine, pyrimethamine and leucovorin calcium): Oral, I.V.: 5 mg/kg TMP twice daily

Travelers' diarrhea: Oral: One double-strength tablet every 12 hours for 5 days

Urinary tract infection:
Oral: One double-strength tablet every 12 hours
Duration of therapy: Uncomplicated: 3-5 days; Complicated: 7-10 days
Pyelonephritis: 14 days
Prostatitis: Acute: 2 weeks; Chronic: 2-3 months
I.V.: 8-10 mg TMP/kg/day in divided doses every 6, 8, or 12 hours for up to 14 days with severe infections

Dosing adjustment in renal impairment: Oral, I.V.:
Manufacturer's recommendation: Children and Adults:
Cl_{cr} >30 mL/minute: No dosage adjustment required
Cl_{cr} 15-30 mL/minute: Administer 50% of recommended dose
Cl_{cr} <15 mL/minute: Use is not recommended
Alternate recommendations:
Cl_{cr} 15-30 mL/minute:
Treatment: Administer full daily dose (divided every 12 hours) for 24-48 hours, then decrease daily dose by 50% and administer every 24 hours **(Note:** For serious infections including *Pneumocystis jirovecii* pneumonia (PCP), full daily dose is given in divided doses every 6-8 hours for 2 days, followed by reduction to 50% daily dose divided every 12 hours) (Nahata, 1995).
PCP prophylaxis: One-half single-strength tablet (40 mg trimethoprim) daily **or** 1 single-strength tablet (80 mg trimethoprim) daily or 3 times weekly (Masur, 2002).
Cl_{cr} <15 mL/minute:
Treatment: Administer full daily dose every 48 hours (Nahata, 1995)
PCP prophylaxis: One-half single-strength tablet (40 mg trimethoprim) daily **or** 1 single-strength tablet (80 mg trimethoprim) 3 times weekly (Masur, 2002). While the guidelines do acknowledge the alternative of giving 1 single-strength tablet daily, this may be inadvisable in the uremic/ESRD patient.
GFR <10 mL/minute/1.73 m^2: Children: Use is not recommended, but if required, administer 5-10 mg trimethoprim/kg every 24 hours (Aronoff, 2007).
Intermittent Hemodialysis (IHD) (administer after hemodialysis on dialysis days):
Children: Use is not recommended, but if required, administer 5-10 mg trimethoprim/kg every 24 hours (Aronoff, 2007).
Adults: 2.5-10 mg/kg trimethoprim every 24 hours or 5-20 mg/kg trimethoprim 3 times weekly after IHD. **Note:** Dosing is highly dependent upon indication for use (eg, treatment of cystitis versus treatment of PCP pneumonia (Heinz, 2009).

PCP prophylaxis: One single-strength tablet (80 mg trimethoprim) after each dialysis session (Masur, 2002)
Note: Dosing dependent on the assumption of 3 times/week, complete IHD sessions.
Peritoneal dialysis (PD):
Use Cl_{cr} <15 mL/minute dosing recommendations. Not significantly removed by PD; supplemental dosing is not required (Aronoff, 2007):
GFR <10 mL/minute/1.73 m^2: Children: Use is not recommended, but if required 5-10 mg TMP/kg every 24 hours.
Exit-site and tunnel infections: Oral: One single-strength tablet daily (Li, 2010)
Intraperitoneal: Loading dose: TMP-SMX 320/1600 mg/L; Maintenance: TMP-SMX 80/400 mg/L (Aronoff, 2007; Warady, 2000)
Peritonitis: Oral: One double-strength tablet twice daily (Li, 2010)
Continuous renal replacement therapy (CRRT) (Heintz, 2009; Trotman, 2005): Drug clearance is highly dependent on the method of renal replacement, filter type, and flow rate. Appropriate dosing requires close monitoring of pharmacologic response, signs of adverse reactions due to drug accumulation, as well as drug concentrations in relation to target trough (if appropriate). The following are general recommendations only (based on dialysate flow/ultrafiltration rates of 1-2 L/hour and minimal residual renal function) and should not supersede clinical judgment:
CVVH/CVVHD/CVVHDF: 2.5-7.5 mg/kg of TMP every 12 hours. **Note:** Dosing regimen dependent on clinical indication. Critically-ill patients with *P. jirovecii* pneumonia receiving CVVHDF may require up to 10 mg/kg every 12 hours (Heintz, 2009).

Mechanism of Action Sulfamethoxazole interferes with bacterial folic acid synthesis and growth via inhibition of dihydrofolic acid formation from para-aminobenzoic acid; trimethoprim inhibits dihydrofolic acid reduction to tetrahydrofolate resulting in sequential inhibition of enzymes of the folic acid pathway

Contraindications Hypersensitivity to any sulfa drug, trimethoprim, or any component of the formulation; megaloblastic anemia due to folate deficiency; infants <2 months of age; marked hepatic damage or severe renal disease (if patient not monitored); pregnancy (at term); breast-feeding

Warnings/Precautions Use with caution in patients with G6PD deficiency, impaired renal or hepatic function or potential folate deficiency (malnourished, chronic anticonvulsant therapy, or elderly); maintain adequate hydration to prevent crystalluria; adjust dosage in patients with renal impairment. Injection vehicle contains benzyl alcohol and sodium metabisulfite.

Chemical similarities are present among sulfonamides, sulfonylureas, carbonic anhydrase inhibitors, thiazides, and loop diuretics (except ethacrynic acid). Use in patients with sulfonamide allergy is specifically contraindicated in product labeling, however, a risk of cross-reaction exists in patients with allergy to any of these compounds; avoid use when previous reaction has been severe.

Fatalities associated with severe reactions including Stevens-Johnson syndrome, toxic epidermal necrolysis, hepatic necrosis, agranulocytosis, aplastic anemia, and other blood dyscrasias; discontinue use at first sign of rash or serious adverse reactions. Elderly patients appear at greater risk for more severe adverse reactions. May cause hypoglycemia, particularly in malnourished, or patients with renal or hepatic impairment. Use with caution in patients with porphyria or thyroid dysfunction. Potentially significant interactions may exist, requiring dose or frequency adjustment, additional monitoring, and/or selection of alternative therapy. Slow acetylators may be more prone to adverse reactions. Caution in patients with allergies or asthma. May cause hyperkalemia (associated with high doses of trimethoprim). Incidence of adverse effects appears to be increased in patients with AIDS. Prolonged use may result in fungal or bacterial superinfection, including *C. difficile*-associated diarrhea (CDAD) and pseudomembranous colitis; CDAD has been observed >2 months postantibiotic treatment. Avoid concomitant use with leucovorin when treating *Pneumocystis jirovecii* pneumonia (PCP) in HIV patients; may increase risk of treatment failure and death.

Drug Interactions
Metabolism/Transport Effects Refer to individual components.

Avoid Concomitant Use
Avoid concomitant use of Sulfamethoxazole and Trimethoprim with any of the following: BCG; Dofetilide; Leucovorin Calcium-Levoleucovorin; Methenamine; Potassium P-Aminobenzoate; Procaine

Increased Effect/Toxicity
Sulfamethoxazole and Trimethoprim may increase the levels/effects of: ACE Inhibitors; Amantadine; Angiotensin II Receptor Blockers; Antidiabetic Agents (Thiazolidinedione); AzaTHIOprine; Carvedilol; CycloSPORINE (Systemic); CYP2C8 Substrates; CYP2C9 Substrates; Dapsone (Systemic); Dapsone (Topical); Dofetilide; Eplerenone; Fosphenytoin; Highest Risk QTc-Prolonging Agents; LamiVUDine; Memantine; Mercaptopurine; MetFORMIN; Methotrexate; Moderate Risk QTc-Prolonging Agents; Phenytoin; Porfimer; PRALAtrexate; Prilocaine; Procainamide; Repaglinide; Spironolactone; Sulfonylureas; Varenicline; Vitamin K Antagonists

The levels/effects of Sulfamethoxazole and Trimethoprim may be increased by: Amantadine; CYP2C9 Inhibitors (Moderate); CYP2C9 Inhibitors (Strong); Dapsone (Systemic); Memantine; Methenamine; Mifepristone

Decreased Effect
Sulfamethoxazole and Trimethoprim may decrease the levels/effects of: BCG; CycloSPORINE (Systemic); Sodium Picosulfate; Typhoid Vaccine

The levels/effects of Sulfamethoxazole and Trimethoprim may be decreased by: CYP2C9 Inducers (Strong); CYP3A4 Inducers (Strong); Deferasirox; Herbs (CYP3A4 Inducers); Leucovorin Calcium-Levoleucovorin; Peginterferon Alfa-2b; Potassium P-Aminobenzoate; Procaine; Tocilizumab

Ethanol/Nutrition/Herb Interactions Herb/Nutraceutical: Avoid dong quai; St John's wort (may diminish effects and also cause photosensitization).

Dietary Considerations Should be taken with 8 oz of water. May be taken without regard to meals.

Pharmacodynamics/Kinetics
Half-life Elimination SMX: 9 hours, TMP: 6-17 hours; both are prolonged in renal failure

Time to Peak Serum: Within 1-4 hours

Pregnancy Risk Factor C

Pregnancy Considerations Adverse events have been observed in animal reproduction studies; therefore, the manufacturer classifies TMP-SMX as pregnancy category C. TMP-SMX crosses the placenta and distributes to amniotic fluid. Due to trimethoprim's

potential effect on folic acid metabolism, TMP-SMX should only be used during pregnancy if the benefit justifies the potential risk. The use of dihydrofolate reductase inhibitors, including trimethoprim, during pregnancy may increase the risk of congenital anomalies including cardiovascular defects, oral clefts, urinary tract anomalies, and neural tube defects. Folic acid supplementation may decrease this risk. A few case reports have described additional congenital anomalies after TMP-SMX exposure, but none of these have proven causality. Most studies and case reports have failed to show an increased risk for congenital malformations after use of TMP-SMX. Per the manufacturer, TMP-SMX is contraindicated in late pregnancy because sulfonamides pass the placenta and may cause kernicterus in the newborn, but this has not been observed specifically with SMX. Neonatal healthcare providers should be informed if maternal sulfonamide therapy is used near the time of delivery. TMP-SMX may be used in pregnancy for prophylaxis or treatment of *Pneumocystis jirovecii* pneumonia (PCP), the prophylaxis of *Toxoplasmic gondii* encephalitis (TE), and may prevent fetal loss in patients with Q fever (*Coxiella burnetii*). The pharmacokinetics of TMP-SMX are similar to nonpregnant values in early pregnancy.

Lactation Enters breast milk/contraindicated (AAP rates "compatible"; AAP 2001 update pending)

Breast-Feeding Considerations Small amounts of TMP and SMX are transferred to breast milk. Per the manufacturer, TMP-SMX is contraindicated in nursing mothers since sulfonamides cross into the milk and may cause kernicterus in the newborn. Because TMP-SMX has therapeutic indications for infants ≥2 months of age, kernicterus after exposure via breast-feeding would not be expected in healthy infants of this age group; however, sulfonamides should not be used while nursing an infant with G6PD deficiency or hyperbilirubinemia. Nondose related effects could include modification of bowel flora.

Dosage Forms The 5:1 ratio (SMX:TMP) remains constant in all dosage forms.
Injection, solution: Sulfamethoxazole 80 mg and trimethoprim 16 mg per mL (5 mL, 10 mL, 30 mL)
Suspension, oral: Sulfamethoxazole 200 mg and trimethoprim 40 mg per 5 mL
Tablet: Sulfamethoxazole 400 mg and trimethoprim 80 mg
  Bactrim™: Sulfamethoxazole 400 mg and trimethoprim 80 mg
Tablet, double-strength: Sulfamethoxazole 800 mg and trimethoprim 160 mg
  Bactrim™ DS, Septra® DS: Sulfamethoxazole 800 mg and trimethoprim 160 mg

---

Sulfanilamide (sul fa NIL a mide)

Brand Names: U.S. AVC™
Pharmacologic Category Antifungal Agent, Vaginal
Use Treatment of vulvovaginitis caused by *Candida albicans*
Local Anesthetic/Vasoconstrictor Precautions No information available to require special precautions
Effects on Dental Treatment No significant effects or complications reported
Effects on Bleeding No information available to require special precautions
General Dosage Range Intravaginal: *Adults:* 1 applicatorful once or twice daily

Mechanism of Action Interferes with microbial folic acid synthesis and growth via inhibition of para-aminiobenzoic acid metabolism; exerts a bacteriostatic action

Pregnancy Risk Factor C

Pregnancy Considerations Adverse events have been observed in animal reproduction studies with sulfonamides, including sulfanilamide. Sulfonamides cross the placenta and distribute to amniotic fluid. The fetal concentration is 50% to 90% of that measured in the maternal blood. Because of the theoretical increased risk for hyperbilirubinemia and kernicterus, neonatal healthcare providers should be informed if maternal sulfonamide therapy is used near the time of delivery.

SulfaSALAzine (sul fa SAL a zeen)

Brand Names: U.S. Azulfidine EN-tabs®; Azulfidine®; Sulfazine; Sulfazine EC

Brand Names: Canada Apo-Sulfasalazine®; PMS-Sulfasalazine; Salazopyrin En-Tabs®; Salazopyrin®

Pharmacologic Category 5-Aminosalicylic Acid Derivative

Use

U.S. labeling: Treatment of mild-to-moderate ulcerative colitis or as adjunctive therapy in severe ulcerative colitis; enteric coated tablets are also used for rheumatoid arthritis (including juvenile idiopathic arthritis [JIA]) in patients who inadequately respond to analgesics and NSAIDs

Canadian labeling: Adjunctive therapy in severe ulcerative colitis, distal ulcerative colitis or proctitis, and Crohn's disease; enteric coated tablets are also used for rheumatoid arthritis unsuccessfully treated with first-line therapy

Unlabeled Use Ankylosing spondylitis, Crohn's disease, psoriasis, psoriatic arthritis

Local Anesthetic/Vasoconstrictor Precautions No information available to require special precautions

Effects on Dental Treatment No significant effects or complications reported

Effects on Bleeding Sulfasalazine has been shown to induce a rare but potentially serious autoimmune thrombocytopenia, as detected by a significant decrease in platelet counts. Sulfasalazine-induced thrombocytopenia can be resolved by discontinuation of the drug.

Adverse Effects

>10%:

Central nervous system: Headache

Dermatologic: Rash

Gastrointestinal: Anorexia, dyspepsia, gastric distress, nausea, vomiting

Genitourinary: Oligospermia (reversible)

1% to 10%:

Cardiovascular: Cyanosis

Central nervous system: Dizziness, fever

Dermatologic: Pruritus, urticaria

Gastrointestinal: Abdominal pain, stomatitis

Hematologic: Heinz body anemia, hemolytic anemia, leukopenia, thrombocytopenia

Hepatic: Liver function tests abnormal

General Dosage Range Oral:

Delayed release:

Children ≥6 years: Initial: 1/4 to 1/3 of expected maintenance dose; Maintenance: 30-50 mg/kg/day in 2 divided doses (maximum: 2 g daily)

Adults: Initial: 0.5-1 g daily; Maintenance: 2 g/day in 2 divided doses (maximum: 3 g daily)

Immediate release:

Children ≥6 years: Initial: 40-60 mg/kg/day in 3-6 divided doses; Maintenance: 30 mg/kg/day in 4 divided doses

Adults: Initial: 3-4 g daily in evenly divided doses at ≤8-hour intervals; Maintenance: 2 g daily in divided doses at ≤8-hour intervals

Mechanism of Action 5-aminosalicylic acid (5-ASA) is the active component of sulfasalazine; the specific mechanism of action of 5-ASA is unknown; however, it is thought that it modulates local chemical mediators of the inflammatory response, especially leukotrienes, and is also postulated to be a free radical scavenger or an inhibitor of tumor necrosis factor (TNF); action appears topical rather than systemic

Pharmacodynamics/Kinetics

Half-life Elimination Sulfasalazine: 5.7-10 hours (prolonged in elderly); Sulfapyridine: 14.8 hours (slow acetylators) and 10.4 hours (fast acetylators)

Time to Peak Sulfasalazine: 3-12 hours (mean: 6 hours); Metabolites: ~10 hours

Pregnancy Risk Factor B

Pregnancy Considerations Adverse events have not been observed in animal reproduction studies. Sulfasalazine and sulfapyridine cross the placenta; a potential for kernicterus in the newborn exists. Agranulocytosis was noted in an infant following maternal use of sulfasalazine during pregnancy. Based on available data, an increase in fetal malformations has not been observed following maternal use of sulfasalazine for the treatment of inflammatory bowel disease or ulcerative colitis.

Sulfonated Phenolics in Aqueous Solution
(SUL fo NATE ed fe NOL iks in AYE kwee us so LU shun)

Related Information

Ulcerative, Erosive, and Painful Oral Mucosal Disorders *on page 1578*

Brand Names: U.S. Debacterol®

Generic Availability (U.S.) No

Pharmacologic Category Aphthous Ulcer Treatment Agent

Dental Use Therapeutic cauterization in the treatment of oral mucosal lesions (aphthous stomatitis, gingivitis, moderate-to-severe periodontitis)

Use Treatment of ulcerating oral lesions such as recurrent aphthous stomatitis (canker sores)

Local Anesthetic/Vasoconstrictor Precautions No information available to require special precautions

Effects on Dental Treatment No significant effects or complications reported

Effects on Bleeding No information available to require special precautions

Dental Usual Dosage Apply applicator tip to the lesion as directed (see Dental Comment)

Dosage Topical: Children ≥12 years and Adults: Oral ulcers: Apply 1 coated applicator swab to ulcer for 5-10 seconds. **Note:** Not recommended to apply more than 1 treatment to each ulcer; however, if ulcer pain returns shortly after rinsing with water, 1 repeat application may be used.

Mechanism of Action Semiviscous, chemical cautery agent which provides controlled, focal debridement and sterilization of necrotic tissues; relieving pain, sealing damaged tissue, and providing local antiseptic action

Contraindications There are no contraindications listed in the manufacturer's labeling.

◀ **Warnings/Precautions** Do not use if allergic to sulfur in any form. For topical use only. Debacterol® is not intended for the treatment of cold sores and fever blisters. Prolonged use of Debacterol® on normal tissue should be avoided. If ingested, do not induce vomiting; immediately dilute liquids (no more than 8 ounces in adults and 4 ounces in children) and get medical help or contact a Poison Control Center. Avoid contact with eyes. If eye exposure occurs, immediately remove contact lenses, irrigate eyes for at least 15 minutes with lukewarm water, and contact a physician. If excess irritation occurs, rinse with a sodium bicarbonate (baking soda) solution (1/2 teaspoonful mixed in 120 mL [4 oz] water); if irritation persists, contact healthcare provider.

Drug Interactions

Metabolism/Transport Effects None known.

Avoid Concomitant Use There are no known interactions where it is recommended to avoid concomitant use.

Increased Effect/Toxicity There are no known significant interactions involving an increase in effect.

Decreased Effect There are no known significant interactions involving a decrease in effect.

Dosage Forms

Solution, topical [for oral mucosa]:
Debacterol®: Sulfonated phenolics 50% and sulfuric acid 30% (1.5 mL) [for professional use only]

Swab, topical [for oral mucosa]:
Debacterol®: Sulfonated phenolics 50% and sulfuric acid 30% (12s) (0.2 mL) [for professional use only]

Dental Comment Prior to application/treatment, the ulcerated mucosal area should be thoroughly dried using the drying swab. After drying lesion, hold applicator "swab" with the colored ring end up. Bend the colored ring tip gently to the side until it snaps to release liquid inside. Liquid flows down into the white tip applicator. Apply the Debacterol® coated applicator tip to the dried ulcer area for at least 5 seconds, but no more than 10 seconds. Use rolling motion to completely cover the entire ulcer bed and ulcer rim. A "stinging" sensation is experienced immediately upon application. Debacterol® will not harm normal mucosa when used as directed. Thoroughly rinse out the mouth with water and spit out the rinse water. If the ulcer pain returns shortly after rinsing with water, it is an indication that some part of the ulcer was not covered. Repeat application one more time following directions above. One application per ulcer is usually sufficient. If excess irritation occurs during use, a rinse with sodium bicarbonate (baking soda) solution will neutralize the reaction (use 1/2 teaspoon in 120 mL water). It is not recommended that more than one Debacterol® treatment session be performed on an individual ulcer.

References

Rhodus NL and Bereuter J, "An Evaluation of a Chemical Cautery Agent and an Anti-inflammatory Ointment for the Treatment of Recurrent Aphthous Stomatitis: A Pilot Study," *Quintessence Int*, 1998, 29(12):769-73.

Sulfur and Salicylic Acid
(SUL fyoor & sal i SIL ik AS id)

Brand Names: U.S. ala seb [OTC]; Pernox® Lemon [OTC]; Pernox® Regular [OTC]; Sebex [OTC]; Sebulex® [OTC]

Pharmacologic Category Antiseborrheic Agent, Topical

Use Therapeutic shampoo for dandruff and seborrheic dermatitis; acne skin cleanser

Local Anesthetic/Vasoconstrictor Precautions No information available to require special precautions

Effects on Dental Treatment No significant effects or complications reported

Effects on Bleeding No information available to require special precautions

Adverse Effects Local: Topical preparations containing 2% to 5% sulfur generally are well tolerated, local irritation may occur, concentration >15% is very irritating to the skin, higher concentration (eg, 10% or higher) may cause systemic toxicity (eg, headache, vomiting, muscle cramps, dizziness, collapse)

Mechanism of Action Salicylic acid works synergistically with sulfur in its keratolytic action to break down keratin and promote skin peeling

Pregnancy Considerations Refer to salicylic acid monograph.

Sulindac (SUL in dak)

Related Information

Rheumatoid Arthritis, Osteoarthritis, and Osteoporosis *on page 1526*

Temporomandibular Dysfunction (TMD), Chronic Pain, and Fibromyalgia *on page 1590*

Brand Names: U.S. Clinoril®

Brand Names: Canada Apo-Sulin®; Novo-Sundac; Nu-Sulindac; Nu-Sundac; Teva-Sulindac

Generic Availability (U.S.) Yes

Pharmacologic Category Nonsteroidal Anti-inflammatory Drug (NSAID), Oral

Use Management of inflammatory diseases including osteoarthritis, rheumatoid arthritis, acute gouty arthritis, ankylosing spondylitis, acute painful shoulder (bursitis/tendonitis)

Unlabeled Use Management of preterm labor

Local Anesthetic/Vasoconstrictor Precautions No information available to require special precautions

Effects on Dental Treatment The dentist should be aware of the potential of abnormal coagulation. Caution should also be exercised in the use of NSAIDs in patients already on anticoagulant therapy with drugs such as warfarin (Coumadin®). See Effects on Bleeding.

Effects on Bleeding Nonselective NSAIDs, such as sulindac, inhibit platelet aggregation and prolong bleeding time in some patients. Unlike aspirin, the NSAID effect on platelet function is quantitatively less, of shorter duration, and reversible. Normal platelet function should occur in ~5 elimination half-lives or in <10 hours after discontinuation of sulindac. Concomitant use of other NSAIDs should be avoided.

Adverse Effects 1% to 10%:

Cardiovascular: Edema (1% to 3%)

Central nervous system: Dizziness (3% to 9%), headache (3% to 9%), nervousness (1% to 3%)

Dermatologic: Rash (3% to 9%), pruritus (1% to 3%)

Gastrointestinal: GI pain (10%), constipation (3% to 9%), diarrhea (3% to 9%), dyspepsia (3% to 9%), nausea (3% to 9%), abdominal cramps (1% to 3%), anorexia (1% to 3%), flatulence (1% to 3%), vomiting (1% to 3%)

Otic: Tinnitus (1% to 3%)

Dosage Oral:

Children: Dose not established

Adults: **Note:** Maximum daily dose: 400 mg

Osteoarthritis, rheumatoid arthritis, ankylosing spondylitis: 150 mg twice daily

Acute painful shoulder (bursitis/tendonitis): 200 mg twice daily; usual treatment: 7-14 days

Acute gouty arthritis: 200 mg twice daily; usual treatment: 7 days

Dosing adjustment in renal impairment: Not recommended with advanced renal impairment; if required, decrease dose and monitor closely

Dosing adjustment in hepatic impairment: Dose reduction is necessary; discontinue if abnormal liver function tests occur

Mechanism of Action Reversibly inhibits cyclooxygenase-1 and 2 (COX-1 and 2) enzymes, which results in decreased formation of prostaglandin precursors; has antipyretic, analgesic, and anti-inflammatory properties

Other proposed mechanisms not fully elucidated (and possibly contributing to the anti-inflammatory effect to varying degrees), include inhibiting chemotaxis, altering lymphocyte activity, inhibiting neutrophil aggregation/activation, and decreasing proinflammatory cytokine levels.

Contraindications Hypersensitivity or allergic-type reactions to sulindac, aspirin, other NSAIDs, or any component of the formulation; perioperative pain in the setting of coronary artery bypass graft (CABG) surgery

Warnings/Precautions [U.S. Boxed Warning]: NSAIDs are associated with an increased risk of adverse cardiovascular thrombotic events, including MI and stroke. Use caution with fluid retention. Avoid use in heart failure. Concurrent administration of ibuprofen, and potentially other nonselective NSAIDs, may interfere with aspirin's cardioprotective effect. May cause new-onset hypertension or worsening of existing hypertension. NSAID use may compromise existing renal function; dose-dependent decreases in prostaglandin synthesis may result from NSAID use, reducing renal blood flow which may cause renal decompensation. NSAID use may increase the risk for hyperkalemia. Patients with impaired renal function, dehydration, heart failure, liver dysfunction, those taking diuretics, and ACE inhibitors, and the elderly are at greater risk of renal toxicity and hyperkalemia. Rehydrate patient before starting therapy; monitor renal function closely. Not recommended for use in patients with advanced renal disease. Long-term NSAID use may result in renal papillary necrosis. Use caution in patients with renal lithiasis; sulindac metabolites have been reported as components of renal stones. Maintain adequate hydration in patients with a history of renal stones. Use with caution in patients with decreased hepatic function. May require dosage adjustment in hepatic dysfunction; sulfide and sulfone metabolites may accumulate. The elderly are at increased risk for adverse effects. **[U.S. Boxed Warning]: Use is contraindicated for treatment of perioperative pain in the setting of coronary artery bypass graft (CABG) surgery.** Risk of MI and stroke may be increased with use following CABG surgery.

[U.S. Boxed Warning]: NSAIDs may increase risk of gastrointestinal irritation, inflammation, ulceration, bleeding, and perforation. Use the lowest effective dose for the shortest duration of time, consistent with individual patient goals, to reduce risk of cardiovascular or GI adverse events. When used concomitantly with ≤325 mg of aspirin, a substantial increase in the risk of gastrointestinal complications (eg, ulcer) occurs; concomitant gastroprotective therapy (eg, proton pump inhibitors) is recommended (Bhatt, 2008). Pancreatitis has been reported; discontinue with suspected pancreatitis.

Avoid chronic use in the elderly (unless alternative agents ineffective and patient can receive concomitant gastroprotective agent); nonselective oral NSAID use is associated with an increased risk of GI bleeding and peptic ulcer disease in older adults in high risk category (eg, >75 years or age or receiving concomitant oral/parenteral corticosteroids, anticoagulants, or antiplatelet agents) (Beers Criteria).

NSAIDS may cause drowsiness, dizziness, blurred vision and other neurologic effects which may impair physical or mental abilities; patients must be cautioned about performing tasks which require mental alertness (eg, operating machinery or driving). Discontinue use with blurred or diminished vision and perform ophthalmologic exam. Monitor vision with long-term therapy.

Platelet adhesion and aggregation may be decreased, may prolong bleeding time; patients with coagulation disorders or who are receiving anticoagulants should be monitored closely. Anemia may occur; patients on long-term NSAID therapy should be monitored for anemia. Rarely, NSAID use may cause severe blood dyscrasias (eg, agranulocytosis, aplastic anemia, thrombocytopenia). NSAIDs may cause serious skin adverse events including exfoliative dermatitis, Stevens-Johnson syndrome (SJS) and toxic epidermal necrolysis (TEN); discontinue use at first sign of skin rash or hypersensitivity. Anaphylactoid reactions may occur. Do not use in patients who experience bronchospasm, asthma, rhinitis, or urticaria with NSAID or aspirin therapy. Use caution in other forms of asthma. May increase the risk of aseptic meningitis, especially in patients with systemic lupus erythematosus (SLE) and mixed connective tissue disorders.

Withhold for at least 4-6 half-lives prior to surgical or dental procedures.

Drug Interactions

Metabolism/Transport Effects None known.

Avoid Concomitant Use

Avoid concomitant use of Sulindac with any of the following: Floctafenine; Ketorolac (Nasal); Ketorolac (Systemic); NSAID (COX-2 Inhibitor); Omacetaxine

Increased Effect/Toxicity

Sulindac may increase the levels/effects of: Agents with Antiplatelet Properties; Aliskiren; Aminoglycosides; Anticoagulants; Bisphosphonate Derivatives; Collagenase (Systemic); CycloSPORINE (Systemic); Dabigatran Etexilate; Deferasirox; Desmopressin; Digoxin; Drotrecogin Alfa (Activated); Eplerenone; Haloperidol; Ibritumomab; Methotrexate; Nonsteroidal Anti-Inflammatory Agents; NSAID (COX-2 Inhibitor); Omacetaxine; PEMEtrexed; Porfimer; Potassium-Sparing Diuretics; PRALAtrexate; Quinolone Antibiotics; Rivaroxaban; Salicylates; Thrombolytic Agents; Tositumomab and Iodine I 131 Tositumomab; Vancomycin; Vitamin K Antagonists

The levels/effects of Sulindac may be increased by: ACE Inhibitors; Angiotensin II Receptor Blockers; Antidepressants (Tricyclic, Tertiary Amine); Corticosteroids (Systemic); CycloSPORINE (Systemic); Dasatinib; Dimethyl Sulfoxide; Floctafenine; Glucosamine; Herbs (Anticoagulant/Antiplatelet Properties); Ketorolac (Nasal); Ketorolac (Systemic); Multivitamins/Minerals (with ADEK, Folate, Iron); Nonsteroidal Anti-Inflammatory Agents; Omega-3 Fatty Acids; Pentosan Polysulfate Sodium; Pentoxifylline; Probenecid; Prostacyclin Analogues; Selective Serotonin Reuptake Inhibitors; Serotonin/Norepinephrine Reuptake Inhibitors; Sodium Phosphates; Tipranavir; Treprostinil; Vitamin E

Decreased Effect

Sulindac may decrease the levels/effects of: ACE Inhibitors; Agents with Antiplatelet Properties; Aliskiren; Angiotensin II Receptor Blockers; Beta-Blockers; Eplerenone; HydrALAZINE; Loop Diuretics; Potassium-Sparing Diuretics; Salicylates; Selective Serotonin Reuptake Inhibitors; Thiazide Diuretics

The levels/effects of Sulindac may be decreased by: Bile Acid Sequestrants; Nonsteroidal Anti-Inflammatory Agents; Salicylates

Ethanol/Nutrition/Herb Interactions

Ethanol: Avoid ethanol (may enhance gastric mucosal irritation).

Herb/Nutraceutical: Avoid alfalfa, anise, bilberry, bladderwrack, bromelain, cat's claw, celery, chamomile, coleus, cordyceps, dong quai, evening primrose, fenugreek, feverfew, garlic, ginger, ginkgo biloba, ginseng (American, Panax, Siberian), grapeseed, green tea, guggul, horse chestnut seed, horseradish, licorice, prickly ash, red clover, reishi, SAMe (S-adenosylmethionine), sweet clover, turmeric, white willow (all have additional antiplatelet activity).

Dietary Considerations Drug may cause GI upset, bleeding, ulceration, perforation; take with food or milk to minimize GI upset.

Pharmacodynamics/Kinetics

Half-life Elimination Sulindac: ~8 hours; Sulfide metabolite: ~16 hours

Time to Peak Sulindac: 3-4 hours; Sulfide and sulfone metabolites: 5-6 hours

Pregnancy Risk Factor C

Pregnancy Considerations Adverse events were not observed in the initial animal reproduction studies; therefore, the manufacturer classifies sulindac as pregnancy category C. Sulindac and the sulfide metabolite have been found to cross the placenta. NSAID exposure during the first trimester is not strongly associated with congenital malformations; however, cardiovascular anomalies and cleft palate have been observed following NSAID exposure in some studies. The use of an NSAID in the first trimester may be associated with an increased risk of miscarriage. Nonteratogenic effects have been observed following NSAID administration during the third trimester including myocardial degenerative changes, prenatal constriction of the ductus arteriosus, failure of the ductus arteriosus to close postnatally, and fetal tricuspid regurgitation; renal dysfunction or failure, oligohydramnios; gastrointestinal bleeding or perforation, increased risk of necrotizing enterocolitis; intracranial bleeding, platelet dysfunction with resultant bleeding; or pulmonary hypertension. Because they may cause premature closure of the ductus arteriosus, use of NSAIDs late in pregnancy should be avoided (use after 31-32 weeks gestation is not recommended by some clinicians). Sulindac has been used in the management of preterm labor. The chronic use of NSAIDs in women of reproductive age may be associated with infertility that is reversible upon discontinuation of the medication. A registry is available for pregnant women exposed to autoimmune medications including sulindac. For additional information contact the Organization of Teratology Information Specialists, OTIS Autoimmune Diseases Study, at (877) 311-8972.

Lactation Excretion in breast milk unknown/not recommended

Breast-Feeding Considerations It is not known if sulindac is excreted into breast milk. Breast-feeding is not recommended by the manufacturer.

Dosage Forms

Tablet, oral: 150 mg, 200 mg

Clinoril®: 200 mg

SUMAtriptan (soo ma TRIP tan)

Related Information

Temporomandibular Dysfunction (TMD), Chronic Pain, and Fibromyalgia *on page 1590*

Brand Names: U.S. Alsuma™; Imitrex®; Sumavel® DosePro®

Brand Names: Canada Apo-Sumatriptan®; Ava-Sumatriptan; CO Sumatriptan; Dom-Sumatriptan; Imitrex®; Imitrex® DF; Imitrex® Injection; Imitrex® Nasal Spray; Mylan-Sumatriptan; PHL-Sumatriptan; PMS-Sumatriptan; Riva-Sumatriptan; Sandoz-Sumatriptan; Sumatriptan Injection; Sumatriptan Sun Injection; Sumatryx; Taro-Sumatriptan; Teva-Sumatriptan; Teva-Sumatriptan DF

Generic Availability (U.S.) Yes

Pharmacologic Category Antimigraine Agent; Serotonin 5-HT$_{1B, 1D}$ Receptor Agonist

Use

Intranasal, Oral, SubQ: Acute treatment of migraine with or without aura

SubQ: Acute treatment of cluster headache episodes

Local Anesthetic/Vasoconstrictor Precautions No information available to require special precautions

Effects on Dental Treatment Key adverse event(s) related to dental treatment: Bad taste, dysphagia, hyposalivation (tablet), mouth/tongue discomfort (injection).

Effects on Bleeding No information available to require special precautions

Adverse Effects

Injection:

>10%:

Central nervous system: Dizziness (12%), warm/hot sensation (11%)

Local: Injection site reaction (≤86%; includes bleeding, bruising, edema, and erythema)

Neuromuscular & skeletal: Paresthesia (5% to 14%)

1% to 10%:

Cardiovascular: Chest discomfort/tightness/pressure (2% to 5%)

Central nervous system: Burning sensation (7%), feeling of heaviness (7%), flushing (7%), pressure sensation (7%), feeling of tightness (5%), drowsiness (3%), feeling strange (2%), headache (2%), tight feeling in head (2%), anxiety (1%), cold sensation (1%), malaise/fatigue (1%)

Gastrointestinal: Nausea/vomiting (4%), abdominal discomfort (1%), dysphagia (1%)

Neuromuscular & skeletal: Neck pain/stiffness (5%), numbness (5%), weakness (5%), jaw discomfort (2%), myalgia (2%), muscle cramps (1%)

Ocular: Vision alterations (1%)

Respiratory: Throat discomfort (3%), nasal disorder/discomfort (2%), bronchospasm (1%)

Miscellaneous: Diaphoresis (2%)

Nasal spray:

>10%: Gastrointestinal: Bad taste (13% to 24%), nausea (11% to 13%), vomiting (11% to 13%)

1% to 10%:

Central nervous system: Dizziness (1% to 2%)

Respiratory: Nasal disorder/discomfort (2% to 4%), throat discomfort (1% to 2%)

Tablet:

1% to 10%:

Cardiovascular: Chest pain/tightness/heaviness/pressure (1% to 2%), palpitation (1%), syncope (1%)

Central nervous system: Burning (1%), dizziness (>1%), drowsiness (>1%), malaise/fatigue (2% to 3%), headache (>1%), nonspecified pain (1% to 2%, placebo 1%), vertigo (<1% to 2%), migraine (>1%), sleepiness (>1%)

Gastrointestinal: Diarrhea (1%), nausea (>1%), vomiting (>1%), hyposalivation (>1%)

Hematologic: Hemolytic anemia (1%)

Neuromuscular & skeletal: Neck, throat, and jaw pain/tightness/pressure (2% to 3%), paresthesia (3% to 5%), myalgia (1%), numbness (1%)

Otic: Ear hemorrhage (1%), hearing loss (1%), sensitivity to noise (1%), tinnitus (1%)

Renal: Hematuria (1%)

Respiratory: Allergic rhinitis (1%), dyspnea (1%), nasal inflammation (1%), nose/throat hemorrhage (1%), sinusitis (1%), upper respiratory inflammation (1%)

Miscellaneous: Hypersensitivity reactions (1%), nonspecified pressure/tightness/heaviness (1% to 3%, placebo 2%); warm/cold sensation (2% to 3%, placebo 2%)

Dosage

Adults:

Oral: A single dose of 25 mg, 50 mg, or 100 mg (taken with fluids). If a satisfactory response has not been obtained at 2 hours, a second dose may be administered. Results from clinical trials show that initial doses of 50 mg and 100 mg are more effective than doses of 25 mg, and that 100 mg doses do not provide a greater effect than 50 mg and may have increased incidence of side effects. Although doses of up to 300 mg/day have been studied, the total daily dose should not exceed 200 mg. The safety of treating an average of >4 headaches in a 30-day period have not been established.

Intranasal: A single dose of 5 mg, 10 mg, or 20 mg administered in one nostril. A 10 mg dose may be achieved by administering a single 5 mg dose in each nostril. If headache returns, the dose may be repeated once after 2 hours, not to exceed a total daily dose of 40 mg. In clinical trials, a greater number of patients responded to initial doses of 20 mg versus 5 or 10 mg. The safety of treating an average of >4 headaches in a 30-day period has not been established.

SubQ: Initial: Up to 6 mg; may repeat if needed ≥1 hour after initial dose (maximum: Two 6 mg injections per 24-hour period). However, controlled clinical trials have failed to document a benefit with administration of a second 6 mg dose in nonresponders.

Elderly: Use is not recommended (due to increased potential for adverse effects).

Dosage adjustment in renal impairment: No dosage adjustments are recommended.

Dosage adjustment in hepatic impairment:

Mild-to-moderate hepatic impairment:

Oral: Bioavailability of oral sumatriptan is increased with liver disease. If treatment is needed, do not exceed single doses of 50 mg.

Nasal spray: Has not been studied in patients with hepatic impairment, however, because the spray does not undergo first-pass metabolism, levels would not be expected to be altered.

Subcutaneous: Has been studied and pharmacokinetics were not altered in patients with hepatic impairment compared to healthy patients.

Severe hepatic impairment: Oral, nasal, and subcutaneous (limited to Imitrex® injection, per prescribing information) formulations are contraindicated with severe hepatic impairment.

Mechanism of Action Selective agonist for serotonin (5-HT$_{1B}$ and 5-HT$_{1D}$ receptors) in cranial arteries; causes vasoconstriction and reduces neurogenic inflammation associated with antidromic neuronal transmission correlating with relief of migraine

Contraindications Hypersensitivity to sumatriptan or any component of the formulation; patients with ischemic heart disease or signs or symptoms of ischemic heart disease (including Prinzmetal's angina, angina pectoris, myocardial infarction, silent myocardial ischemia); cerebrovascular syndromes (including strokes, transient ischemic attacks); peripheral vascular disease (including ischemic bowel disease); uncontrolled hypertension; use within 24 hours of ergotamine derivatives; use within 24 hours of another 5-HT$_1$ agonist; concurrent administration or within 2 weeks of discontinuing an MAO type A inhibitors (oral and nasal sumatriptan only; see Warnings/Precautions); management of hemiplegic or basilar migraine; severe hepatic impairment (oral and nasal sumatriptan, and injectable Imitrex® only); not for I.V. administration

Warnings/Precautions Sumatriptan is only indicated for the acute treatment of migraine or cluster headache (product dependent); not indicated for migraine prophylaxis, or for the treatment of hemiplegic or basilar migraine. Acute migraine agents (eg, triptans, opioids, ergotamine, or a combination of the agents) used for 10 or more days per month may lead to worsening of headaches (medication overuse headache); withdrawal treatment may be necessary in the setting of overuse. May cause CNS depression, such as dizziness, weakness, or drowsiness, which may impair physical or mental abilities; patients must be cautioned about performing tasks which require mental alertness (eg, operating machinery or driving). If a patient does not respond to the first dose, the diagnosis of migraine or cluster headache should be reconsidered; rule out underlying neurologic disease in patients with atypical headache and in patients with no prior history of migraine or cluster headache. Cardiac events (coronary artery vasospasm, transient ischemia, myocardial infarction, ventricular tachycardia/fibrillation, cardiac arrest and death), cerebral/subarachnoid hemorrhage, and stroke have been reported with 5-HT$_1$ agonist administration. Patients who experience sensations of chest pain/pressure/tightness or symptoms suggestive of angina following dosing should be evaluated for coronary artery disease or Prinzmetal's angina before receiving additional doses; if dosing is resumed and similar symptoms recur, monitor with ECG. Do not give to patients with risk factors for CAD until a cardiovascular evaluation has been performed; if evaluation is satisfactory, the healthcare provider should administer the first dose (consider ECG monitoring) and cardiovascular status should be periodically evaluated.

Significant elevation in blood pressure, including hypertensive crisis, has also been reported on rare occasions in patients with and without a history of hypertension; use is contraindicated in patients with uncontrolled hypertension. Vasospasm-related reactions have been reported other than coronary artery vasospasm. Peripheral vascular ischemia and colonic ischemia with abdominal pain and bloody diarrhea have occurred. Transient and permanent blindness and significant partial vision loss have been very rarely reported. Use with caution in patients with a history of seizure disorder or in

◄

patients with a lowered seizure threshold. Use the oral formulation with caution (and with dosage limitations) in patients with hepatic impairment where treatment is necessary and advisable. Presystemic clearance of orally administered sumatriptan is reduced in hepatic impairment, leading to increased plasma concentrations; dosage reduction of the oral product is recommended. Non-oral routes of administration (nasal, subcutaneous formulations) do not undergo similar hepatic first-pass metabolism and are not expected to result in significantly altered pharmacokinetics in patients with hepatic impairment. Use of the oral, nasal, or Imitrex® injectable is contraindicated in severe hepatic impairment.

Symptoms of agitation, confusion, hallucinations, hyperreflexia, myoclonus, shivering, and tachycardia (serotonin syndrome) may occur with concomitant proserotonergic drugs (ie, SSRIs/SNRIs or triptans) or agents which reduce sumatriptan's metabolism. Concurrent use of serotonin precursors (eg, tryptophan) is not recommended. If concomitant administration with SSRIs is warranted, monitor closely, especially at initiation and with dose increases. Concurrent use with an MAO inhibitor may result in increased sumatriptan concentrations and increased risk for dose-related adverse effects (eg, serotonin syndrome); use with oral or nasal sumatriptan is contraindicated. Although generally not recommended, if concomitant use of MAO inhibitors with injectable sumatriptan is deemed necessary, careful monitoring and appropriate dosage adjustments are required. I.V. administration is contraindicated due to the potential to cause coronary vasospasm. Not recommended for use in elderly patients; older adults are at a higher risk for coronary artery disease and may be more likely to have reduced hepatic function.

Drug Interactions

Metabolism/Transport Effects None known.

Avoid Concomitant Use

Avoid concomitant use of SUMAtriptan with any of the following: Ergot Derivatives; MAO Inhibitors

Increased Effect/Toxicity

SUMAtriptan may increase the levels/effects of: Ergot Derivatives; Metoclopramide; Serotonin Modulators

The levels/effects of SUMAtriptan may be increased by: Antipsychotics; Ergot Derivatives; MAO Inhibitors

Decreased Effect There are no known significant interactions involving a decrease in effect.

Pharmacodynamics/Kinetics

Onset of Action Oral: ~30 minutes; Nasal: ~15-30 minutes; SubQ: ~10 minutes

Half-life Elimination ~2-2.5 hours

Time to Peak Oral: 2-2.5 hours; SubQ: 12 minutes (range: 4-20 minutes)

Pregnancy Risk Factor C

Pregnancy Considerations There are no adequate and well-controlled studies using sumatriptan in pregnant women. Use only if potential benefit to the mother outweighs the potential risk to the fetus. A pregnancy registry has been established to monitor outcomes of women exposed to sumatriptan during pregnancy (800-336-2176). Preliminary data from the registry do not suggest a greater risk of birth defects than the general population and so far a specific pattern of malformations has not been identified. However, sample sizes are small and studies are ongoing. In some (but not all) animal studies, administration was associated with embryolethality, fetal malformations and pup mortality.

Lactation Enters breast milk/use caution (AAP rates "compatible"; AAP 2001 update pending)

Breast-Feeding Considerations The amount of sumatriptan an infant would be exposed to following breast-feeding is considered to be small (although the mean milk-to-plasma ratio is ~4.9, weight adjusted doses estimates suggest breast-fed infants receive 3.5% of a maternal dose). Expressing and discarding the milk for 8-12 hours after a single dose is suggested to reduce the amount present even further. The half-life of sumatriptan in breast milk is 2.22 hours.

Product Availability Zecuity™ (transdermal system): FDA approved January 2013; availability anticipated in fourth quarter of 2013. Refer to prescribing information for additional information.

Dosage Forms

Injection, solution: 4 mg/0.5 mL (0.5 mL); 6 mg/0.5 mL (0.5 mL)

Alsuma™: 6 mg/0.5 mL (0.5 mL)

Imitrex®: 4 mg/0.5 mL (0.5 mL); 6 mg/0.5 mL (0.5 mL)

Sumavel® DosePro®: 6 mg/0.5 mL (0.5 mL)

Injection, solution [preservative free]: 6 mg/0.5 mL (0.5 mL)

Solution, intranasal: 5 mg/0.1 mL (6s); 20 mg/0.1 mL (6s)

Imitrex®: 5 mg/0.1 mL (6s); 20 mg/0.1 mL (6s)

Tablet, oral: 25 mg, 50 mg, 100 mg

Imitrex®: 25 mg, 50 mg, 100 mg

Sumatriptan and Naproxen
(soo ma TRIP tan & na PROKS en)

Related Information

Naproxen *on page 958*

SUMAtriptan *on page 1268*

Brand Names: U.S. Treximet®

Pharmacologic Category Antimigraine Agent; Nonsteroidal Anti-inflammatory Drug (NSAID), Oral; Serotonin 5-HT$_{1B, 1D}$ Receptor Agonist

Use Acute treatment of migraine with or without aura

Local Anesthetic/Vasoconstrictor Precautions No information available to require special precautions

Effects on Dental Treatment The dentist should be aware of the potential of abnormal coagulation. Caution should also be exercised in the use of NSAIDs in patients already on anticoagulant therapy with drugs such as warfarin (Coumadin®). See Effects on Bleeding.

Effects on Bleeding Nonselective NSAIDs, such as sumatriptan and naproxen, inhibit platelet aggregation and prolong bleeding time in some patients. Unlike aspirin, the NSAID effect on platelet function is quantitatively less, of shorter duration, and reversible. Normal platelet function should occur in ~5 elimination half-lives or in <10 hours after discontinuation of sumatriptan and naproxen. Concomitant use of other NSAIDs should be avoided.

Adverse Effects >1% to 10%:

Cardiovascular: Chest pain/discomfort (3%), palpitation (>1%)

Central nervous system: Dizziness (4%), somnolence (3%), fatigue (≥1%)

Gastrointestinal: Nausea (3%), dyspepsia (2%), xerostomia (2%), abdominal pain (≥1%)

Neuromuscular & skeletal: Neck, throat, and jaw pain/tightness/pressure (3%), paresthesia (2%), weakness (≥1%), muscle tightness (>1%)

Miscellaneous: Feeling hot (>1%)

General Dosage Range Oral: *Adults:* 1 tablet (sumatriptan 85 mg and naproxen 500 mg); may repeat in 2 hours if needed (maximum: 2 tablets/24 hours)

Mechanism of Action

Sumatriptan: Selective agonist for serotonin (5-HT$_{1B}$ and 5-HT$_{1D}$ receptors) in cranial arteries; causes vasoconstriction and reduces sterile inflammation associated with antidromic neuronal transmission correlating with relief of migraine

Naproxen: Reversibly inhibits cyclooxygenase-1 and 2 (COX-1 and 2) enzymes, which result in decreased formation of prostaglandin precursors; has antipyretic, analgesic, and anti-inflammatory properties

Pregnancy Risk Factor C

Pregnancy Considerations Adverse events were observed in animal studies. There are no well-controlled studies in pregnant women. Women exposed to this combination during pregnant are encouraged to contact the Treximet® Pregnancy Registry (800-336-2176). Also refer to individual agents.

SUNItinib (su NIT e nib)

Related Information

Clinical Risk Related to Drugs Prolonging QT Interval *on page 1510*

Brand Names: U.S. Sutent®

Brand Names: Canada Sutent®

Pharmacologic Category Antineoplastic Agent, Tyrosine Kinase Inhibitor; Vascular Endothelial Growth Factor (VEGF) Inhibitor

Use Treatment of gastrointestinal stromal tumor (GIST) intolerant to or with disease progression on imatinib; treatment of advanced renal cell cancer (RCC); treatment of advanced, metastatic or unresectable pancreatic neuroendocrine tumors (PNET)

Unlabeled Use Treatment of advanced thyroid cancer; treatment of non-GIST soft tissue sarcomas

Local Anesthetic/Vasoconstrictor Precautions Hypertension can occur with the use of this drug, particularly early in the treatment course. Monitor for hypertension prior to using local anesthetic with vasoconstrictor; medical consult if necessary.

Sunitinib is one of the drugs confirmed to prolong the QT interval and is accepted as having a risk of causing torsade de pointes. The risk of drug-induced torsade de pointes is extremely low when a single QT interval prolonging drug is prescribed. In terms of epinephrine, it is not known what effect vasoconstrictors in the local anesthetic regimen will have in patients with a known history of congenital prolonged QT interval or in patients taking any medication that prolongs the QT interval. Until more information is obtained, it is suggested that the clinician consult with the physician prior to the use of a vasoconstrictor in suspected patients, and that the vasoconstrictor (epinephrine, mepivacaine and levonordefrin [Carbocaine® 2% with Neo-Cobefrin®]) be used with caution.

Effects on Dental Treatment Key adverse event(s) related to dental treatment: Xerostomia (normal salivary flow resumes upon discontinuation), mucositis/stomatitis, taste perversion, and oral pain.

Effects on Bleeding Chemotherapy may result in significant myelosuppression, potentially including significant reduction in platelet counts (thrombocytopenia grades 3/4: 5% to 9%) and altered hemostasis. Bleeding has been reported in 18% to 37% of patients. In patients who are under active treatment with these agents, medical consult is suggested.

Adverse Effects

>10%:

Cardiovascular: Hypertension (15% to 34%; grade 3: 4% to 13%), peripheral edema (24%), LVEF decreased (11% to 16%; grades 3/4: 1% to 3%), heart failure (≤15%), chest pain (13%)

Central nervous system: Fatigue (33% to 62%), headache (≤23%), fever (≤22%), insomnia (15% to 18%), chills (14%), depression (11%), dizziness (11%)

Dermatologic: Skin discoloration (25% to 30%), rash (14% to 29%), hand-foot syndrome (14% to 29%; grades 3/4: 4% to 8%), hair color changes (7% to 29%), dry skin (≤23%), alopecia (5% to 14%), erythema (12%), pruritus (12%)

Endocrine & metabolic: Hyperglycemia (23% to 71%), hyperuricemia (≤46%), hypocalcemia (34% to 42%), hypoalbuminemia (28% to 41%), hypophosphatemia (≤36%), hyponatremia (≤29%), hypoglycemia (17% to 22%), hypokalemia (12% to 21%), hypomagnesemia (≤19%), hyperkalemia (≤18%), hypothyroidism (4% to 16%; grades 3/4: ≤2%), hypercalcemia (13%), hypernatremia (10% to 13%)

Gastrointestinal: Diarrhea (40% to 66%), nausea (45% to 58%), lipase increased (17% to 56%), anorexia (33% to 48%), mucositis/stomatitis (29% to 48%), taste perversion (21% to 47%), abdominal pain (39%), vomiting (34% to 39%), amylase increased (17% to 35%), dyspepsia (15% to 34%), constipation (20% to 23%), weight loss (16%), flatulence (14%), oral pain (6% to 14%), xerostomia (13%), GERD/reflux (12%), glossodynia (11%)

Hematologic: Anemia (26% to 79%; grades 3/4: ≤8%), leukopenia (78%; grades 3/4: 8%), neutropenia (53% to 77%; grades 3/4: 10% to 17%), lymphopenia (38% to 68%; grades 3/4: ≤18%), thrombocytopenia (38% to 68%; grades 3/4: 5% to 9%), hemorrhage/bleeding (18% to 37%)

Hepatic: AST increased (39% to 72%; grades 3/4: 2% to 5%), alkaline phosphatase increased (24% to 63%; grades 3/4: 2% to 10%), ALT increased (39% to 61%; grades 3/4: 2% to 4%), hyperbilirubinemia (10% to 37%; grades 3/4 ≤1%)

Neuromuscular & skeletal: Creatine kinase increased (49%), limb pain (14% to 40%), weakness (22% to 34%), arthralgia (15% to 30%), back pain (≤28%), myalgia (14%)

Renal: Creatinine increased (12% to 70%)

Respiratory: Cough (27%), dyspnea (26%), epistaxis (21%), nasopharyngitis (14%), upper respiratory tract infection (11%)

1% to 10%:

Cardiovascular: Venous thrombotic events (1% to 3%), DVT (2% to 3%)

Gastrointestinal: Hemorrhoids (10%), pancreatitis (1%)

Respiratory: Pulmonary embolism (2%)

Miscellaneous: Flu-like syndrome (5%)

General Dosage Range Dosage adjustment recommended in patients with renal impairment, on concomitant therapy, or who develop toxicities

Oral: *Adults:* 50 mg once daily for 4 weeks of a 6-week treatment cycle **or** 37.5 mg once daily, continuous daily dosing

Mechanism of Action Exhibits antitumor and antiangiogenic properties by inhibiting multiple receptor tyrosine kinases, including platelet-derived growth factors (PDGFRα and PDGFRβ), vascular endothelial growth factors (VEGFR1, VEGFR2, and VEGFR3), FMS-like tyrosine kinase-3 (FLT3), colony-stimulating factor type 1 (CSF-1R), and glial cell-line-derived neurotrophic factor receptor (RET).

Pharmacodynamics/Kinetics
Half-life Elimination Terminal: Sunitinib: 40-60 hours; SU12662: 80-110 hours

Time to Peak 6-12 hours

Pregnancy Risk Factor D

Pregnancy Considerations Animal reproduction studies have demonstrated teratogenicity, embryotoxicity, and fetal loss. Because sunitinib inhibits angiogenesis, a critical component of fetal development, adverse effects on pregnancy would be expected. Women of childbearing potential should be advised to avoid pregnancy if receiving sunitinib.

Dental Comment Sunitinib is known to prolong the QT interval. The QT interval is measured as the time and distance between the Q point of the QRS complex and the end of the T wave in the ECG tracing. After adjustment for heart rate, the QT interval is defined as prolonged if it is more than 450 msec in men and 460 msec in women. A long QT syndrome was first described in the 1950s and 60s as a congenital syndrome involving QT interval prolongation and syncope and sudden death. Some of the congenital long QT syndromes were characterized by a peculiar electrocardiographic appearance of the QRS complex involving a premature atria beat followed by a pause, then a subsequent sinus beat showing marked QT prolongation and deformity. This type of cardiac arrhythmia was originally termed "torsade de pointes" (translated from the French as "twisting of the points"). Sunitinib is considered as having a risk of causing torsade de pointes. Since it is not known what effect vasoconstrictors in the local anesthetic regimen will have in patients with a known history of congenital prolonged QT interval or in patients taking any medication that prolongs the QT interval, a medical consult is suggested.

Tacrolimus (Systemic) (ta KROE li mus)

Brand Names: U.S. Hecoria™; Prograf®

Brand Names: Canada Advagraf®; Prograf®

Generic Availability (U.S.) Yes: Capsule

Pharmacologic Category Calcineurin Inhibitor; Immunosuppressant Agent

Use

U.S. labeling: Prevention of organ rejection in heart (Prograf® only), and kidney or liver (Hecoria™, Prograf®) transplant recipients

Canadian labeling:

Prograf®: Prevention of organ rejection in heart, kidney, or liver transplant recipients; treatment of refractory rejection in kidney or liver transplant recipients; treatment of active rheumatoid arthritis in adult patients nonresponsive to disease-modifying antirheumatic drug (DMARD) therapy or when DMARD therapy is inappropriate

Advagraf®: Prevention of organ rejection in kidney transplant recipients

Unlabeled Use Prevention of organ rejection in lung, small bowel transplant recipients; prevention and treatment of graft-versus-host disease (GVHD) in allogenic hematopoietic stem cell transplantation

Local Anesthetic/Vasoconstrictor Precautions No information available to require special precautions

Effects on Dental Treatment Key adverse event(s) related to dental treatment: Stomatitis, oral moniliasis, dysphagia, and esophagitis (including ulcerative).

Effects on Bleeding Thrombocytopenia (14% to 24%) has been associated with use; severe thrombocytopenia (rare) may be associated with delayed coagulation.

Consultation to ensure adequate platelet counts may be considered in patients with signs/symptoms or a history of thrombocytopenia.

Adverse Effects As reported for kidney, liver, and heart transplantation:

≥15%:

Cardiovascular: Hypertension (13% to 62%), edema (peripheral 11% to 36%), chest pain (19%), edema (18%), pericardial effusion (heart transplant 15%)

Central nervous system: Headache (24% to 64%), insomnia (30% to 64%), pain (24% to 63%), fever (19% to 48%), postprocedural pain (kidney transplant 29%), dizziness (19%)

Dermatologic: Pruritus (15% to 36%), rash (10% to 24%)

Endocrine & metabolic: New-onset diabetes after transplant (75% kidney transplant), hypophosphatemia (28% to 49%), hypomagnesemia (16% to 48%), hyperglycemia (21% to 47%), hyperkalemia (13% to 45%), hyperlipemia (10% to 31%), hypokalemia (13% to 29%), diabetes mellitus (24% to 26%), post-transplant diabetes mellitus (heart transplant 13% to 22%; kidney transplant 20%; liver transplant 11% to 18%)

Gastrointestinal: Diarrhea (25% to 72%), abdominal pain (29% to 59%), nausea (32% to 46%), constipation (23% to 36%), anorexia (7% to 34%), vomiting (14% to 29%), dyspepsia (18% to 28%)

Genitourinary: Urinary tract infection (16% to 34%)

Hematologic: Anemia (5% to 50%), leukopenia (13% to 48%), leukocytosis (8% to 32%), thrombocytopenia (14% to 24%)

Hepatic: Liver function tests abnormal (6% to 36%), ascites (7% to 27%)

Local: Incision site complication (kidney transplant 28%)

Neuromuscular & skeletal: Tremor (15% to 56%; heart transplant 15%), weakness (11% to 52%), paresthesia (17% to 40%), back pain (17% to 30%), arthralgia (25%)

Renal: Abnormal kidney function (36% to 56%), creatinine increased (23% to 45%), BUN increased (12% to 30%), oliguria (18% to 19%)

Respiratory: Atelectasis (5% to 28%), pleural effusion (30% to 36%), dyspnea (5% to 29%), cough increased (18%), bronchitis (17%)

Miscellaneous: Infection (24% to 45%), CMV infection (heart transplant 32%), graft dysfunction (kidney transplant 24%)

<15%:

Cardiovascular: Abnormal ECG (QRS or ST segment abnormal), arrhythmia, atrial fibrillation, atrial flutter, bradycardia, cardiopulmonary failure, deep thrombophlebitis, heart failure, heart rate decreased, hemorrhage, hemorrhagic stroke, hypervolemia, hypotension, orthostatic hypotension, peripheral vascular disorder, phlebitis, syncope, tachycardia, thrombosis, vasodilation

Central nervous system: Abnormal dreams, abnormal thinking, agitation, amnesia, anxiety, chills, confusion, depression, emotional lability, encephalopathy, flaccid paralysis, hallucinations, mood elevated, nervousness, psychosis, quadriparesis, seizure, somnolence, vertigo

Dermatologic: Acne, alopecia, bruising, cellulitis, exfoliative dermatitis, fungal dermatitis, hirsutism, photosensitivity reaction, skin discoloration, skin disorder, skin neoplasm, skin ulcer, wound healing impaired

Endocrine & metabolic: Acidosis, alkalosis, bicarbonate decreased, Cushing's syndrome, dehydration, gout, hypercholesterolemia, hyper-/hypocalcemia, hyponatremia, hyperphosphatemia, hyperuricemia, hypoproteinemia, serum iron decreased

Gastrointestinal: Appetite increased, cramps, duodenitis, dysphagia, enlarged abdomen, esophagitis (including ulcerative), flatulence, gastritis, gastroesophagitis, GI perforation/hemorrhage, ileus, oral moniliasis, pancreatic pseudocyst, rectal disorder, stomatitis, weight gain

Genitourinary: Bladder spasm, cystitis, dysuria, nocturia, urge incontinence, urinary frequency, urinary incontinence, urinary retention, vaginitis

Hematologic: Coagulation disorder, decreased prothrombin, hypochromic anemia, polycythemia

Hepatic: Alkaline phosphatase increased, bilirubinemia, cholangitis, cholestatic jaundice, GGT increased, hepatitis (including granulomatous), jaundice, LDH increased, liver damage

Local: Phlebitis

Neuromuscular & skeletal: Hypertonia, incoordination, joint disorder, leg cramps, monoparesis, myalgia, myasthenia, myoclonus, nerve compression, neuropathy, osteoporosis, quadriparesis

Ocular: Abnormal vision, amblyopia

Otic: Ear pain, otitis media, tinnitus

Renal: Acute renal failure, albuminuria, BK nephropathy, hematuria, hydronephrosis, renal tubular necrosis, toxic nephropathy

Respiratory: Asthma, emphysema, lung disorder, lung function decreased, pharyngitis, pneumonia, pneumothorax, pulmonary edema, respiratory disorder, rhinitis, sinusitis, voice alteration

Miscellaneous: Abscess, abnormal healing, allergic reaction, crying, diaphoresis, flu-like syndrome, generalized spasm, hernia, herpes simplex, hiccups, peritonitis, sepsis, writing impaired

Dosage

Oral:

Prevention of organ rejection in transplant recipients: The initial dose of tacrolimus should begin no sooner than 6 hours after liver and heart transplant and within 24 hours of kidney transplant (but may be delayed until renal function has recovered). Adjunctive therapy with corticosteroids is recommended early post-transplant. I.V. route should only be used in patients not able to take oral medications and continued only until oral medication can be tolerated; anaphylaxis has been reported with I.V. administration. If switching from I.V. to oral, the oral dose should be started 8-12 hours after stopping the infusion.

Children: Patients without pre-existing renal or hepatic dysfunction have required (and tolerated) higher doses than adults to achieve similar blood concentrations. It is recommended that therapy be initiated at the **high end** of the recommended adult I.V. and oral dosing ranges; dosage adjustments may be required.

Liver transplant: Initial dose: 0.15-0.20 mg/kg/day in 2 divided doses, given every 12 hours

Adults:

Heart transplant: Initial dose: 0.075 mg/kg/day in 2 divided doses, given every 12 hours. Use in combination with azathioprine or mycophenolate mofetil is recommended.

Kidney transplant:

U.S. labeling: Initial dose: 0.2 mg/kg/day in combination with azathioprine **or** 0.1 mg/kg/day in combination with mycophenolate mofetil. Administer in 2 divided doses, given every 12 hours; African-American patients may require larger doses to maintain trough concentration.

Canadian labeling:

Prograf®: Initial: 0.2-0.3 mg/kg/day in 2 divided doses, given every 12 hours in combination with corticosteroids and other immunosuppressive agents.

Advagraf®: Initial: 0.15-0.2 mg/kg/day. Administer once daily in combination with corticosteroids and mycophenolate mofetil (MMF) in *de novo* kidney transplant recipients. Antibody induction therapy should also be used.

Conversion from Prograf® to Advagraf®: Initiate Advagraf® therapy using previously established total daily dose of Prograf®. Administer once daily.

Liver transplant: Initial dose: 0.1-0.15 mg/kg/day in 2 divided doses, given every 12 hours

Prevention of graft-versus-host disease (unlabeled use): Children and Adults: Convert from I.V. to oral dose (1:4 ratio): Multiply total daily I.V. dose times 4 and administer in 2 divided oral doses per day, every 12 hours (Uberti, 1999; Yanik, 2000).

Rheumatoid arthritis: Canadian labeling (not in U.S. labeling): Adults: 3 mg once daily; carefully monitor serum creatinine during therapy

Treatment of graft-versus-host disease (unlabeled use): Adults: 0.06 mg/kg twice daily (Furlong, 2000; Przepiorka, 1999)

I.V.:

Prevention of organ rejection in transplant recipients: The initial dose of tacrolimus should begin no sooner than 6 hours after liver and heart transplant and within 24 hours of kidney transplant (but may be delayed until renal function has recovered). Adjunctive therapy with corticosteroids is recommended early post-transplant. I.V. route should only be used in patients not able to take oral medications and continued only until oral medication can be tolerated; anaphylaxis has been reported with I.V. administration. If switching from I.V. to oral, the oral dose should be started 8-12 hours after stopping the infusion.

Children: It is recommended that therapy be initiated at the **high end** of the dosing range.

Liver transplant: Initial dose: 0.03-0.05 mg/kg/day as a continuous infusion

Adults: It is recommended that therapy be initiated at the **lower end** of the dosing range.

Heart transplant: Initial dose: 0.01 mg/kg/day as a continuous infusion. Use in combination with azathioprine or mycophenolate mofetil is recommended.

Kidney transplant: Initial dose: 0.03-0.05 mg/kg/day as a continuous infusion. Use in combination with azathioprine or mycophenolate mofetil is recommended.

Liver transplant: Initial dose: 0.03-0.05 mg/kg/day as a continuous infusion.

Prevention of graft-versus-host disease (unlabeled use): Children and Adults: Initial: 0.03 mg/kg/day (based on lean body weight) as continuous infusion. Treatment should begin at least 24 hours prior to stem cell infusion and continued only until oral medication can be tolerated (Przepiorka, 1999; Yanik, 2000).

Treatment of graft-versus-host disease (unlabeled use): Adults: Initial: 0.03 mg/kg/day (based on lean body weight) as continuous infusion (Furlong, 2000; Przepiorka, 1999)

Dosing adjustment in renal impairment: Systemic therapy: Evidence suggests that lower doses should be used; patients should receive doses at the lowest value of the recommended I.V. and oral dosing ranges; further reductions in dose below these ranges may be required.

Kidney transplant: Tacrolimus therapy in patients with postoperative oliguria should begin no sooner than 6 hours and within 24 hours post-transplant, but may be delayed until renal function has recovered.

Hemodialysis: Not removed by hemodialysis; supplemental dose is not necessary.

Peritoneal dialysis: Significant drug removal is unlikely based on physiochemical characteristics.

Dosing adjustment in hepatic impairment: Systemic therapy: Use of tacrolimus in liver transplant recipients experiencing post-transplant hepatic impairment may be associated with increased risk of developing renal insufficiency related to high whole blood levels of tacrolimus. The presence of moderate-to-severe hepatic dysfunction (serum bilirubin >2 mg/dL; Child-Pugh score ≥10) appears to affect the metabolism of tacrolimus. The half-life of the drug was prolonged and the clearance reduced after I.V. administration. The bioavailability of tacrolimus was also increased after oral administration. The higher plasma concentrations as determined by ELISA, in patients with severe hepatic dysfunction are probably due to the accumulation of metabolites of lower activity. These patients should be monitored closely and dosage adjustments should be considered. Some evidence indicates that lower doses could be used in these patients.

Mechanism of Action Suppresses cellular immunity (inhibits T-lymphocyte activation), by binding to an intracellular protein, FKBP-12 and complexes with calcineurin dependent proteins to inhibit calcineurin phosphatase activity

Contraindications Hypersensitivity to tacrolimus or any component of the formulation

Warnings/Precautions Hazardous agent: Use appropriate precautions for handling and disposal (NIOSH, 2012). **[U.S. Boxed Warning]: Risk of developing infections (including bacterial, viral [including CMV], fungal, and protozoal infections [including opportunistic infections]) is increased.** Latent viral infections may be activated, including BK virus (associated with polyoma virus-associated nephropathy [PVAN]) and JC virus (associated with progressive multifocal leukoencephalopathy [PML]); may result in serious adverse effects. The risk of CMV disease is increased for patients who are CMV-seronegative prior to transplant and receive a graft from a CMV-seropositive donor. Consider reduction in immunosuppression if PVAN, PML, CMV viremia and/or CMV disease occurs. **[U.S. Boxed Warning]: Immunosuppressive therapy may result in the development of lymphoma and other malignancies (predominantly skin malignancies).** The risk for new-onset diabetes and insulin-dependent post-transplant diabetes mellitus (PTDM) is increased with tacrolimus use after transplantation, including in patients without pretransplant history of diabetes mellitus; insulin dependence may be reversible; increased risk in African-American and Hispanic kidney transplant patients. Nephrotoxicity has has been reported, especially with higher doses; to avoid excess nephrotoxicity do not administer simultaneously with other nephrotoxic drugs (eg, sirolimus, cyclosporine). Neurotoxicity may occur especially when used in high doses; tremor headache, coma and delirium have been reported and are associated with serum concentrations.

Seizures may also occur. Posterior reversible encephalopathy syndrome (PRES) may also occur; symptoms (altered mental status, headache, hypertension, seizures, and visual disturbances) are reversible with dose reduction or discontinuation of therapy; stabilize blood pressure and reduce dose with suspected or confirmed PRES diagnosis.

Pure red cell aplasia (PRCA) has been reported in patients receiving tacrolimus. Use with caution in patients with risk factors for PRCA including parvovirus B19 infection, underlying disease, or use of concomitant medications associated with PRCA (eg, mycophenolate). Discontinuation of therapy should be considered with diagnosis of PRCA. Monitoring of serum concentrations (trough for oral therapy) is essential to prevent organ rejection and reduce drug-related toxicity. Use caution in renal or hepatic dysfunction, dosing adjustments may be required. Delay initiation of therapy in kidney transplant patients if postoperative oliguria occurs; begin therapy no sooner than 6 hours and within 24 hours post-transplant, but may be delayed until renal function has recovered. Use may be associated with the development of hypertension (common); hyperkalemia has been reported; avoid use of potassium-sparing diuretics. Myocardial hypertrophy has been reported (rare). Potentially significant drug-drug/drug-food interactions may exist, requiring dose or frequency adjustment, additional monitoring, and/or selection of alternative therapy. In liver transplantation, the tacrolimus dose and target range should be reduced to minimize the risk of nephrotoxicity when used in combination with everolimus.

Each mL of injection contains polyoxyl 60 hydrogenated castor oil (HCO-60) (200 mg) and dehydrated alcohol USP 80% v/v. Anaphylaxis has been reported with the injection, use should be reserved for those patients not able to take oral medications. Patients should not be immunized with live vaccines during or shortly after treatment and should avoid close contact with recently vaccinated (live vaccine) individuals. Oral formulations contain lactose; the Canadian labeling does not recommend use of these products in patients who may be lactose intolerant (eg, Lapp lactase deficiency, glucose-galactose malabsorption, galactose intolerance). **[U.S. Boxed Warning]: Should be administered under the supervision of a physician experienced in immunosuppressive therapy and organ transplantation in a facility appropriate for monitoring and managing therapy.**

Drug Interactions

Metabolism/Transport Effects Substrate of CYP3A4 (major), P-glycoprotein; **Note:** Assignment of Major/Minor substrate status based on clinically relevant drug interaction potential; **Inhibits** CYP3A4 (weak), P-glycoprotein

Avoid Concomitant Use

Avoid concomitant use of Tacrolimus (Systemic) with any of the following: BCG; Bosutinib; CloZAPine; Conivaptan; Crizotinib; CycloSPORINE (Systemic); Enzalutamide; Eplerenone; Grapefruit Juice; Mifepristone; Natalizumab; Pimecrolimus; Pimozide; Pomalidomide; Potassium-Sparing Diuretics; Silodosin; Tacrolimus (Topical); Temsirolimus; Tofacitinib; Topotecan; Vaccines (Live); VinCRIStine (Liposomal)

Increased Effect/Toxicity

Tacrolimus (Systemic) may increase the levels/effects of: ARIPiprazole; Bosutinib; CloZAPine; Colchicine; CycloSPORINE (Systemic); Dabigatran Etexilate; Everolimus; Fenofibrate; Fenofibric Acid;

Fosphenytoin; Highest Risk QTc-Prolonging Agents; Leflunomide; Lomitapide; Moderate Risk QTc-Prolonging Agents; Natalizumab; P-glycoprotein/ABCB1 Substrates; Phenytoin; Pimozide; Pomalidomide; Prucalopride; Rivaroxaban; Silodosin; Sirolimus; Temsirolimus; Tofacitinib; Topotecan; Vaccines (Live); VinCRIStine (Liposomal)

The levels/effects of Tacrolimus (Systemic) may be increased by: Antidepressants (Serotonin Reuptake Inhibitor/Antagonist); Boceprevir; Calcium Channel Blockers (Dihydropyridine); Calcium Channel Blockers (Nondihydropyridine); Chloramphenicol; Clotrimazole (Oral); Conivaptan; Crizotinib; CycloSPORINE (Systemic); CYP3A4 Inhibitors (Moderate); CYP3A4 Inhibitors (Strong); Danazol; Dasatinib; Denosumab; Eplerenone; Ertapenem; Fluconazole; Grapefruit Juice; Itraconazole; Ivacaftor; Ketoconazole (Systemic); Macrolide Antibiotics; MetroNIDAZOLE (Systemic); Mifepristone; P-glycoprotein/ABCB1 Inhibitors; Pimecrolimus; Posaconazole; Potassium-Sparing Diuretics; Protease Inhibitors; Proton Pump Inhibitors; Ranolazine; Roflumilast; Sirolimus; Tacrolimus (Topical); Telaprevir; Temsirolimus; Trastuzumab; Voriconazole

Decreased Effect
Tacrolimus (Systemic) may decrease the levels/effects of: BCG; Coccidioidin Skin Test; Sipuleucel-T; Vaccines (Inactivated); Vaccines (Live)

The levels/effects of Tacrolimus (Systemic) may be decreased by: Caspofungin; Cinacalcet; CYP3A4 Inducers (Strong); Deferasirox; Echinacea; Efavirenz; Enzalutamide; Fosphenytoin; P-glycoprotein/ABCB1 Inducers; Phenytoin; Rifamycin Derivatives; Sirolimus; St Johns Wort; Temsirolimus; Tocilizumab

Ethanol/Nutrition/Herb Interactions
Food: Food decreases rate and extent of absorption. High-fat meals have most pronounced effect (37% decrease in AUC, 77% decrease in C_{max}). Grapefruit juice, a CYP3A4 inhibitor, may increase serum level and/or toxicity of tacrolimus. Management: Administer with or without food, but be consistent. Avoid concurrent use of grapefruit juice.

Herb/Nutraceutical: St John's wort may reduce tacrolimus serum concentrations. Management: Avoid St John's wort.

Dietary Considerations
Capsule: Administer with or without food; be consistent with timing and composition of meals, food decreases bioavailability. Avoid grapefruit juice.

Pharmacodynamics/Kinetics
Half-life Elimination Variable, 23-46 hours in healthy volunteers; 2.1-36 hours in transplant patients

Time to Peak 0.5-6 hours

Pregnancy Risk Factor C

Pregnancy Considerations
Adverse events were observed in animal reproduction studies. Tacrolimus crosses the human placenta and is measurable in the cord blood, amniotic fluid, and newborn serum. Tacrolimus concentrations in the placenta may be higher than the maternal serum. No consistent pattern of congenital anomalies has been observed. Transient neonatal hyperkalemia and renal dysfunction have been reported.

The National Transplantation Pregnancy Registry (NTPR, Temple University) is a registry for pregnant women taking immunosuppressants following any solid organ transplant. The NTPR encourages reporting of all immunosuppressant exposures during pregnancy in transplant recipients at 877-955-6877.

Lactation Enters breast milk/not recommended

Breast-Feeding Considerations
Concentrations of tacrolimus in breast milk are lower than that of the maternal serum. The low bioavailability of tacrolimus following oral absorption may also decrease the amount of exposure to a nursing infant.

Dosage Forms
Capsule, oral: 0.5 mg, 1 mg, 5 mg
  Hecoria™: 0.5 mg, 1 mg, 5 mg
  Prograf®: 0.5 mg, 1 mg, 5 mg
Injection, solution:
  Prograf®: 5 mg/mL (1 mL)
Dosage Forms: Canada
Capsule, oral:
  Advagraf®: 0.5 mg, 1 mg, 3 mg, 5 mg

Tacrolimus (Topical) (ta KROE li mus)

Brand Names: U.S. Protopic®
Brand Names: Canada Protopic®
Generic Availability (U.S.) No
Pharmacologic Category Calcineurin Inhibitor; Immunosuppressant Agent; Topical Skin Product
Dental Use Treatment of severe ulcerative or vesicobullous lesions (usually in consult with patient's physician)
Use Moderate-to-severe atopic dermatitis in immunocompetent patients not responsive to conventional therapy or when conventional therapy is not appropriate

Canadian labeling: Additional use (not in U.S. labeling): Maintenance therapy to prevent flares and extend flare-free intervals in patients with moderate-to-severe atopic dermatitis who are responsive to initial therapy and experiencing ≥5 flares per year

Local Anesthetic/Vasoconstrictor Precautions No information available to require special precautions
Effects on Dental Treatment No significant effects or complications reported
Effects on Bleeding No information available to require special precautions
Adverse Effects As reported in children and adults, unless otherwise noted:
>10%:
  Central nervous system: Headache (5% to 20%), fever (1% to 21%)
  Dermatologic: Skin burning (43% to 58%; tends to improve as lesions resolve), pruritus (41% to 46%), erythema (12% to 28%)
  Respiratory: Increased cough (children 18%)
  Miscellaneous: Flu-like syndrome (23% to 31%), allergic reaction (4% to 12%)
1% to 10%:
  Cardiovascular: Peripheral edema (adults 3% to 4%)
  Central nervous system: Hyperesthesia (adults 3% to 7%), pain (1% to 2%)
  Dermatologic: Skin tingling (2% to 8%), acne (adults 4% to 7%), localized flushing (following ethanol consumption; adults 3% to 7%), folliculitis (2% to 6%), urticaria (1% to 6%), rash (2% to 5%), pustular rash (2% to 4%), vesiculobullous rash (children 4%), contact dermatitis (3% to 4%), cyst (adults 1% to 3%), eczema herpeticum (1% to 2%), fungal dermatitis ▶

(adults 1% to 2%), sunburn (adults 1% to 2%), alopecia (adults 1% to 2%), dry skin (children 1%)

Endocrine & metabolic: Dysmenorrhea (adult females 4%)

Gastrointestinal: Diarrhea (3% to 5%), dyspepsia (adults 1% to 4%), abdominal pain (children 3%), vomiting (adults 1%), gastroenteritis (adults 2%), nausea (children 1%)

Neuromuscular & skeletal: Paresthesia (adults 3%), myalgia (adults 2% to 3%), weakness (adults 2% to 3%), arthralgia (adults 1% to 3%), back pain (adults 2%)

Ocular: Conjunctivitis (2% adults)

Otic: Otitis media (12% children)

Respiratory: Rhinitis (6% children), sinusitis (2% to 4% adults), bronchitis (2% adults), pneumonia (1% adults)

Miscellaneous: Varicella/herpes zoster (1% to 5%), lymphadenopathy (3% children)

Dosage Topical: Atopic dermatitis (moderate-to-severe): Treatment:

Children ≥2-15 years: Apply thin layer of 0.03% ointment to affected area twice daily; rub in gently and completely. Discontinue use when symptoms have cleared. If no improvement within 6 weeks, patients should be re-examined to confirm diagnosis.

Children >15 years and Adults: Apply thin layer of 0.03% or 0.1% ointment to affected area twice daily; rub in gently and completely. Discontinue use when symptoms have cleared. If no improvement within 6 weeks, patients should be re-examined to confirm diagnosis.

Maintenance therapy (Canadian labeling; not in U.S. labeling):

Children ≥2-15 years: Apply one application (thin layer of 0.03% ointment) to areas usually affected twice a week, allowing 2-3 days between applications (eg, one application on Monday and Thursday). Reevaluate after 12 months. Safety of maintenance therapy >12 months has not been established.

Children >15 years and Adults: Apply one application (thin layer of 0.03% or 0.1% ointment) to areas usually affected twice a week, allowing 2-3 days between applications (eg, one application on Monday and Thursday). Re-evaluate after 12 months. Safety of maintenance therapy >12 months has not been established.

Note: Patients experiencing flares should resume twice daily treatment.

Mechanism of Action Suppresses cellular immunity (inhibits T-lymphocyte activation), by binding to an intracellular protein, FKBP-12 and complexes with calcineurin dependent proteins to inhibit calcineurin phosphatase activity

Contraindications Hypersensitivity to tacrolimus or any component of the formulation

Warnings/Precautions Hazardous agent - use appropriate precautions for handling and disposal (NIOSH, 2012). **[U.S. Boxed Warning]: Topical calcineurin inhibitors have been associated with rare cases of malignancy (including skin and lymphoma); therefore, it should be limited to short-term and intermittent treatment using the minimum amount necessary for the control of symptoms and only on involved areas. Use in children <2 years of age is not recommended, children ages 2-15 should only use the 0.03% ointment.** Avoid use on malignant or premalignant skin conditions (eg cutaneous T-cell lymphoma). Should not be used in immunocompromised patients. Do not apply to areas of active bacterial or viral infection; infections at the treatment site should be cleared prior to therapy. Topical calcineurin agents are considered second-line therapies in the treatment of atopic dermatitis/eczema, and should be limited to use in patients who have failed treatment with other therapies. Patients with atopic dermatitis are predisposed to skin infections, and tacrolimus therapy has been associated with risk of developing eczema herpeticum, varicella zoster, and herpes simplex. If atopic dermatitis is not improved in <6 weeks, re-evaluate to confirm diagnosis. May be associated with development of lymphadenopathy; possible infectious causes should be investigated. Discontinue use in patients with unknown cause of lymphadenopathy or acute infectious mononucleosis. Acute renal failure has been observed (rarely) with topical use. Not recommended for use in patients with skin disease which may increase systemic absorption (eg, Netherton's syndrome). Minimize sunlight exposure during treatment. Safety not established in patients with generalized erythroderma. Safety of intermittent use for >1 year has not been established, particularly since the effect on immune system development is unknown. Should not be used in immunocompromised patients; safety and efficacy have not been evaluated.

Drug Interactions

Metabolism/Transport Effects Substrate of CYP3A4 (minor), P-glycoprotein; **Note:** Assignment of Major/Minor substrate status based on clinically relevant drug interaction potential

Avoid Concomitant Use

Avoid concomitant use of Tacrolimus (Topical) with any of the following: CycloSPORINE (Systemic); Immunosuppressants; Sirolimus; Temsirolimus

Increased Effect/Toxicity

Tacrolimus (Topical) may increase the levels/effects of: Alcohol (Ethyl); CycloSPORINE (Systemic); Immunosuppressants; Sirolimus; Temsirolimus

The levels/effects of Tacrolimus (Topical) may be increased by: Antidepressants (Serotonin Reuptake Inhibitor/Antagonist); Antifungal Agents (Azole Derivatives, Systemic); Calcium Channel Blockers (Nondihydropyridine); CycloSPORINE (Systemic); Danazol; Fluconazole; Grapefruit Juice; Macrolide Antibiotics; Protease Inhibitors; Sirolimus; Temsirolimus

Decreased Effect There are no known significant interactions involving a decrease in effect.

Ethanol/Nutrition/Herb Interactions Ethanol: Localized flushing (redness, warm sensation) may occur at application site of topical tacrolimus following ethanol consumption.

Pregnancy Risk Factor C

Pregnancy Considerations Adverse events were observed in animal reproduction studies. Tacrolimus crosses the human placenta and is measurable in the cord blood, amniotic fluid, and newborn serum following systemic use. Refer to the Tacrolimus (Systemic) monograph for additional information.

Lactation Enters breast milk/not recommended

Breast-Feeding Considerations Tacrolimus is excreted into breast milk following systemic administration. Refer to the Tacrolimus (Systemic) monograph for additional information.

Dosage Forms

Ointment, topical:

Protopic®: 0.03% (30 g, 60 g, 100 g); 0.1% (30 g, 60 g, 100 g)

Tadalafil (tah DA la fil)

Brand Names: U.S. Adcirca®; Cialis®
Brand Names: Canada Adcirca®; Cialis®
Generic Availability (U.S.) No
Pharmacologic Category Phosphodiesterase-5 Enzyme Inhibitor

Use
Adcirca®: Treatment of pulmonary arterial hypertension (PAH) (WHO Group I) to improve exercise ability
Cialis®: Treatment of erectile dysfunction (ED); treatment of signs and symptoms of benign prostatic hyperplasia (BPH)

Local Anesthetic/Vasoconstrictor Precautions No information available to require special precautions

Effects on Dental Treatment No significant effects or complications reported

Effects on Bleeding No information available to require special precautions

Adverse Effects Based upon usual doses for either indication. For erectile dysfunction, similar adverse events are reported with once-daily versus intermittent dosing, but are generally lower than with doses used intermittently.

>10%:
Cardiovascular: Flushing (1% to 13%; dose related)
Central nervous system: Headache (3% to 42%; dose related)
Gastrointestinal: Dyspepsia (1% to 13%), nausea (10% to 11%)
Neuromuscular & skeletal: Myalgia (1% to 14%; dose related), back pain (2% to 12%), extremity pain (1% to 11%)
Respiratory: Respiratory tract infection (3% to 13%), nasopharyngitis (2% to 13%)

2% to 10%:
Cardiovascular: Hypertension (1% to 3%)
Gastrointestinal: Gastroenteritis (viral; 3% to 5%), GERD (1% to 3%), abdominal pain (1% to 2%), diarrhea (1% to 2%)
Genitourinary: Urinary tract infection (≤2%)
Respiratory: Nasal congestion (≤9%), cough (2% to 4%), bronchitis (≤2%)
Miscellaneous: Flu-like syndrome (2% to 5%)

Dosage Oral: Adults:
Benign prostatic hyperplasia (with or without concomitant erectile dysfunction) (Cialis®): 5 mg once daily
Dosing adjustment with concomitant medications: CYP3A4 inhibitors (strong): 2.5 mg once daily; maximum: 2.5 mg once daily

Erectile dysfunction (Cialis®):
As-needed dosing: 10 mg (U.S. labeling) or 20 mg (Canadian labeling) at least 30 minutes prior to anticipated sexual activity (dosing range: 5-20 mg); to be given as one single dose and not given more than once daily. **Note:** Erectile function may be improved for up to 36 hours following a single dose; adjust dose.
Once-daily dosing: 2.5 mg once daily (U.S. labeling) or 5 mg once daily (Canadian labeling) to be given at approximately the same time daily without regard to timing of sexual activity. Dose may be adjusted based on tolerability (dosage range: 2.5-5 mg/day).
Dosing adjustment with concomitant medications:
U.S. labeling: Alpha₁-blockers: If stabilized on either alpha-blockers or tadalafil therapy, initiate new therapy with the other agent at the lowest possible dose.

Canadian labeling: Nonselective alpha-blockers (eg, doxazosin): *As-needed dosing:* 10 mg at least 30 minutes prior to anticipated sexual activity
CYP3A4 inhibitors (strong):
As-needed dosing:
U.S. labeling: Maximum: 10 mg, not to be given more frequently than every 72 hours
Canadian labeling: 10 mg, not to be given more frequently than every 48 hours (maximum 3 doses/week); may increase to 20 mg if lower dose is tolerated but ineffective. Discontinue use if 10 mg dose is not tolerated.
Once-daily dosing:
U.S. labeling: 2.5 mg once daily; maximum: 2.5 mg once daily
Canadian labeling: 2.5-5 mg once daily

Pulmonary arterial hypertension (Adcirca®): 40 mg once daily

Dosing adjustment with concomitant medications:
Coadministration with protease inhibitor regimen:
Concurrent use with atazanavir/ritonavir, darunavir/ritonavir, fosamprenavir, ritonavir, saquinavir/ritonavir, tipranavir/ritonavir:
Coadministration of tadalafil in patients currently receiving one of these protease inhibitor regimens for at least 1 week: Initiate tadalafil at 20 mg once daily; increase to 40 mg once daily based on individual tolerability.
Coadministration of one of these protease inhibitor regimens in patients currently receiving tadalafil: Discontinue tadalafil at least 24 hours prior to the initiation of the protease inhibitor regimen. After at least 1 week of the protease inhibitor regimen, resume tadalafil at 20 mg once daily; increase to 40 mg once daily based on individual tolerability.
Concurrent use with indinavir or nelfinavir:
Patient receiving indinavir/nelfinavir when initiating tadalafil: Initiate tadalafil at 20 mg once daily; increase to 40 mg once daily based on individual tolerability
Patient receiving tadalafil when initiating indinavir/nelfinavir: Adjust tadalafil to 20 mg once daily; increase to 40 mg once daily based on individual tolerability

Elderly: No dose adjustment for patients >65 years of age in the absence of renal or hepatic impairment

Dosage adjustment in renal impairment:
Benign prostatic hyperplasia (with or without concomitant erectile dysfunction) (Cialis®):
Cl_{cr} ≥51 mL/minute: No dosage adjustment necessary
Cl_{cr} 30-50 mL/minute: Initial: 2.5 mg once daily; maximum: 5 mg once daily
Cl_{cr} <30 mL/minute: Use not recommended
ESRD requiring hemodialysis: Use not recommended
Erectile dysfunction (Cialis®):
As-needed use:
U.S. labeling:
Cl_{cr} ≥51 mL/minute: No dosage adjustment necessary
Cl_{cr} 30-50 mL/minute: Initial: 5 mg once daily; maximum: 10 mg (not to be given more frequently than every 48 hours)
Cl_{cr} <30 mL/minute: Maximum: 5 mg (not to be given more frequently than every 72 hours)
ESRD requiring hemodialysis: Maximum: 5 mg (not to be given more frequently than every 72 hours)

Canadian labeling:

Cl_{cr} >80 mL/minute: No dosage adjustment necessary

Cl_{cr} ≥31-80 mL/minute: 10 mg, not to be given more frequently than every 48 hours (maximum 3 doses/week); may increase to 20 mg if lower dose is tolerated but ineffective. Discontinue use if 10 mg dose is not tolerated.

Cl_{cr} <30 mL/minute: Use with extreme caution; has not been adequately studied

ESRD requiring hemodialysis: Use with extreme caution; has not been adequately studied

Once-daily use:

Cl_{cr} ≥31 mL/minute: No dosage adjustment necessary

Cl_{cr} <30 mL/minute: Use not recommended

ESRD requiring hemodialysis: Use not recommended

Pulmonary arterial hypertension (Adcirca®):

Cl_{cr} >80 mL/minute: No dosage adjustment necessary

Cl_{cr} 31-80 mL/minute: Initial: 20 mg once daily; increase to 40 mg once daily based on individual tolerability

Cl_{cr} <30 mL/minute: Avoid use due to increased tadalafil exposure, limited clinical experience, and lack of ability to influence clearance by dialysis.

Dosage adjustment in hepatic impairment:

Benign prostatic hyperplasia (with or without concomitant erectile dysfunction) (Cialis®):

Mild-to-moderate impairment (Child-Pugh class A or B): Use with caution

Severe impairment (Child-Pugh class C): Use is not recommended

Erectile dysfunction (Cialis®):

As-needed use:

U.S. labeling:

Mild-to-moderate impairment (Child-Pugh class A or B): Use with caution; dose should not exceed 10 mg once daily

Severe impairment (Child-Pugh class C): Use is not recommended

Canadian labeling:

Mild-to-moderate impairment (Child-Pugh class A or B): 10 mg, not to be given more frequently than every 48 hours (maximum 3 doses/week); may increase to 20 mg if lower dose is tolerated but ineffective. Discontinue use if 10 mg dose is not tolerated.

Severe impairment (Child-Pugh class C): Use with extreme caution; has not been adequately studied

Once-daily use:

U.S. labeling:

Mild-to-moderate impairment (Child-Pugh class A or B): Use with caution

Severe impairment (Child-Pugh class C): Use is not recommended

Canadian labeling:

Mild-to-moderate impairment (Child-Pugh class A or B): No dosage adjustment necessary

Severe impairment (Child-Pugh class C): Use with extreme caution; has not been adequately studied

Pulmonary arterial hypertension (Adcirca®):

Mild-to-moderate impairment (Child-Pugh class A or B): Use with caution; consider initial dose of 20 mg once daily

Severe impairment (Child-Pugh class C): Avoid use; has not been studied in patients with severe hepatic cirrhosis.

Mechanism of Action

BPH: Exact mechanism unknown; effects likely due to PDE-5 mediated reduction in smooth muscle and endothelial cell proliferation, decreased nerve activity, and increased smooth muscle relaxation and tissue perfusion of the prostate and bladder

Erectile dysfunction: Does not directly cause penile erections, but affects the response to sexual stimulation. The physiologic mechanism of erection of the penis involves release of nitric oxide (NO) in the corpus cavernosum during sexual stimulation. NO then activates the enzyme guanylate cyclase, which results in increased levels of cyclic guanosine monophosphate (cGMP), producing smooth muscle relaxation and inflow of blood to the corpus cavernosum. Tadalafil enhances the effect of NO by inhibiting phosphodiesterase type 5 (PDE-5), which is responsible for degradation of cGMP in the corpus cavernosum; when sexual stimulation causes local release of NO, inhibition of PDE-5 by tadalafil causes increased levels of cGMP in the corpus cavernosum, resulting in smooth muscle relaxation and inflow of blood to the corpus cavernosum. At recommended doses, it has no effect in the absence of sexual stimulation.

PAH: Inhibits phosphodiesterase type 5 (PDE-5) in smooth muscle of pulmonary vasculature where PDE-5 is responsible for the degradation of cyclic guanosine monophosphate (cGMP). Increased cGMP concentration results in pulmonary vasculature relaxation; vasodilation in the pulmonary bed and the systemic circulation (to a lesser degree) may occur.

Contraindications Known serious hypersensitivity to tadalafil or any component of the formulation; concurrent use (regularly/intermittently) of organic nitrates in any form (eg, nitroglycerin, isosorbide dinitrate)

Warnings/Precautions There is a degree of cardiac risk associated with sexual activity; therefore, physicians should consider the cardiovascular status of their patients prior to initiation. Use is not recommended in patients with hypotension (<90/50 mm Hg), uncontrolled hypertension (>170/100 mm Hg), NYHA class II-IV heart failure within the last 6 months, uncontrolled arrhythmias, stroke within the last 6 months, MI within the last 3 months, unstable angina or angina during sexual intercourse; safety and efficacy have not been evaluated in these patients. Safety and efficacy in PAH have not been evaluated in patients with clinically significant aortic and/or mitral valve disease, life-threatening arrhythmias, hypotension (<90/50 mm Hg), uncontrolled hypertension, significant left ventricular dysfunction, pericardial constriction, restrictive or congestive cardiomyopathy, symptomatic coronary artery disease. Use caution in patients with left ventricular outflow obstruction (eg, aortic stenosis, hypertrophic obstructive cardiomyopathy); may be more sensitive to vasodilator effects.

Patients experiencing anginal chest pain after tadalafil administration should seek immediate medical attention. Concomitant use (regularly/intermittently) with all forms of nitrates is contraindicated. When used for BPH, erectile dysfunction, or PAH and nitrate administration is medically necessary following use, at least 48 hours should elapse after the tadalafil dose and nitrate administration. When used for PAH, per the manufacturer, nitrate may be administered within 48 hours of tadalafil. For both situations, administration of nitrates should only be done under close medical supervision with hemodynamic monitoring.

Concurrent use with alpha-adrenergic antagonist therapy may cause symptomatic hypotension; patients should be hemodynamically stable prior to initiating tadalafil therapy at the lowest possible dose. Avoid or limit concurrent substantial alcohol consumption as this may increase the risk of symptomatic hypotension. When used for BPH or erectile dysfunction, use caution in patients receiving strong CYP3A4 inhibitors. When used for PAH, avoid use in patients taking strong CYP3A4 inducers/inhibitors. Use in patients receiving or about to receive ritonavir requires dosage adjustment or interruption of therapy, respectively. Canadian labeling does not recommend use of tadalafil in patients with PAH who are also receiving protease inhibitors.

Pulmonary vasodilators may exacerbate the cardiovascular status in patients with pulmonary veno-occlusive disease (PVOD); use is not recommended. In patients with unrecognized PVOD, signs of pulmonary edema should prompt investigation into this diagnosis. Use with caution in patients with mild-to-moderate hepatic impairment; dosage adjustment/limitation is needed. Use is not recommended in patients with severe hepatic impairment or cirrhosis. Use with caution in patients with renal impairment; dosage adjustment/limitation is needed. Safety and efficacy with other tadalafil brands or other PDE-5 inhibitors (ie, sildenafil and vardenafil) have not been established. Patients should be informed not to take with other tadalafil brands or other PDE-5 inhibitors. Use caution in patients with bleeding disorders or peptic ulcer disease due to effect on platelets (bleeding).

When used to treat BPH or erectile dysfunction, potential underlying causes of BPH or erectile dysfunction should be evaluated prior to treatment. Use with caution in patients with anatomical deformation of the penis (angulation, cavernosal fibrosis, or Peyronie's disease), or who have conditions which may predispose them to priapism (sickle cell anemia, multiple myeloma, leukemia). Instruct patients to seek immediate medical attention if erection persists >4 hours. Safety and efficacy with other tadalafil brands or other PDE-5 inhibitors (ie, sildenafil and vardenafil) have not been established. Patients should be informed not to take with other tadalafil brands or other PDE-5 inhibitors. The safety and efficacy of tadalafil with other treatments for erectile dysfunction have not been studied and are, therefore, not recommended as combination therapy.

Rare cases of nonarteritic anterior ischemic optic neuropathy (NAION) have been reported; risk may be increased with history of vision loss or NAION in one eye. Other risk factors for NAION include heart disease, diabetes, hypertension, smoking, age >50 years, or history of certain eye problems. Sudden decrease or loss of hearing has been reported rarely; hearing changes may be accompanied by tinnitus and dizziness. A direct relationship between therapy and vision or hearing loss has not been determined. Instruct patients to seek medical assistance for sudden loss of vision in one or both eyes, sudden decrease in hearing, or sudden loss of hearing.

Patients with genetic retinal disorders (eg, retinitis pigmentosa) were not evaluated in clinical trials; use is not recommended. Use with caution in the elderly.

Drug Interactions

Metabolism/Transport Effects Substrate of CYP3A4 (major); **Note:** Assignment of Major/Minor substrate status based on clinically relevant drug interaction potential

Avoid Concomitant Use
Avoid concomitant use of Tadalafil with any of the following: Alprostadil; Amyl Nitrite; Phosphodiesterase 5 Inhibitors; Vasodilators (Organic Nitrates)

Increased Effect/Toxicity
Tadalafil may increase the levels/effects of: Alpha1-Blockers; Alprostadil; Amyl Nitrite; Antihypertensives; Bosentan; Phosphodiesterase 5 Inhibitors; Vasodilators (Organic Nitrates)

The levels/effects of Tadalafil may be increased by: Alcohol (Ethyl); Boceprevir; Cobicistat; CYP3A4 Inhibitors (Moderate); CYP3A4 Inhibitors (Strong); Dasatinib; Fluconazole; Itraconazole; Ivacaftor; Ketoconazole (Systemic); Lorcaserin; Mifepristone; Posaconazole; Ritonavir; Sapropterin; Telaprevir; Voriconazole

Decreased Effect
The levels/effects of Tadalafil may be decreased by: Bosentan; CYP3A4 Inducers (Strong); Etravirine

Ethanol/Nutrition/Herb Interactions Ethanol: Substantial consumption of ethanol may increase the risk of hypotension and orthostasis. Lower ethanol consumption has not been associated with significant changes in blood pressure or increase in orthostatic symptoms. Management: Avoid or limit ethanol consumption.

Food: Rate and extent of absorption are not affected by food. Grapefruit juice may increase serum levels/toxicity of tadalafil. Management: Use of grapefruit juice should be limited or avoided.

Herb/Nutraceutical: St John's wort may decrease the levels/effectiveness of tadalafil. Management: Avoid or use caution with concomitant use.

Dietary Considerations May be taken with or without food.

Pharmacodynamics/Kinetics
Onset of Action Within 1 hour
Peak effect: Pulmonary artery vasodilation: 75-90 minutes (Ghofrani, 2004)

Duration of Action Erectile dysfunction: Up to 36 hours

Half-life Elimination 15-17.5 hours; Pulmonary hypertension (not receiving bosentan): 35 hours

Time to Peak Plasma: ~2-4 hours (range: 30 minutes to 8 hours)

Pregnancy Risk Factor B

Pregnancy Considerations Teratogenic events were not reported in animal reproduction studies. Postnatal development and pup survival was decreased at some doses. There are no adequate and well-controlled studies in pregnant women. Less than 0.0005% is found in the semen of healthy males.

Lactation Excretion in breast milk unknown/use caution

Breast-Feeding Considerations It is not known if tadalafil is excreted in breast milk. The manufacturer recommends that caution be exercised when administering tadalafil to nursing women.

Dosage Forms
Tablet, oral:
Adcirca®: 20 mg
Cialis®: 2.5 mg, 5 mg, 10 mg, 20 mg

Tafluprost (TA floo prost)

Brand Names: U.S. Zioptan™
Pharmacologic Category Ophthalmic Agent, Antiglaucoma; Prostaglandin, Ophthalmic

Use Reduction of intraocular pressure (IOP) in patients with open-angle glaucoma or ocular hypertension

Local Anesthetic/Vasoconstrictor Precautions No information available to require special precautions

Effects on Dental Treatment No significant effects or complications reported

Effects on Bleeding No information available to require special precautions

Adverse Effects
>10%: Ocular: Conjunctival hyperemia (4% to 20%)
1% to 10%:
Central nervous system: Headache (6%)
Genitourinary: Urinary tract infection (2%)
Ocular: Stinging/irritation (7%), conjunctivitis (5%), cataract (3%), dry eye (3%), ocular pain (3%), eyelash darkening (2%), eyelash growth (2%), vision blurred (2%)
Respiratory: Common cold (4%), cough (3%)

General Dosage Range Ophthalmic: *Adults:* One drop in the affected eye(s) once daily

Mechanism of Action Tafluprost acid is a fluorinated prostaglandin F_2-alpha analog believed to reduce intraocular pressure by increasing outflow of aqueous humor via the uveoscleral pathway; exact mechanism by which it reduces IOP is unknown.

Pharmacodynamics/Kinetics
Onset of Action Reduction of intraocular pressure (IOP): 2-4 hours; Peak effect: Maximum reduction of IOP: ~12 hours
Time to Peak Plasma: ~10 minutes
Pregnancy Risk Factor C
Pregnancy Considerations Teratogenic effects were observed in animal reproduction studies following I.V. administration. Effective contraception during treatment is recommended for women of childbearing potential.

Taliglucerase Alfa (tal i GLOO ser ase AL fa)

Brand Names: U.S. Elelyso™
Pharmacologic Category Enzyme
Use Long-term enzyme replacement therapy for patients with type 1 Gaucher's disease

Local Anesthetic/Vasoconstrictor Precautions No information available to require special precautions

Effects on Dental Treatment No significant effects or complications reported

Effects on Bleeding No information available to require special precautions

Adverse Effects
≥10%:
Central nervous system: Headache (11% to 19%)
Genitourinary: Urinary tract infection/pyelonephritis (9% to 11%)
Neuromuscular & skeletal: Arthralgia (11% to 13%), back pain (3% to 11%), limb pain (≤11%)
Respiratory: Upper respiratory tract infection/nasopharyngitis (18% to 22%), pharyngitis (4% to 19%)
Miscellaneous: IgG antibody formation (14% to 53%), infusion reactions (44% to 46%, including headache [16%], chest discomfort/pain [6%], asthenia [7%], back pain/arthralgia [7%], urticaria [7%], flushing [6%], erythema [5%], fatigue [5%], blood pressure increased [5%]), flu-like syndrome (4% to 13%)
>2% to <10%:
Cardiovascular: Chest discomfort, flushing, peripheral edema
Central nervous system: Dizziness, fatigue, insomnia, pain
Dermatologic: Erythema, pruritus, rash, skin irritation

Gastrointestinal: Abdominal pain, diarrhea, nausea, throat irritation
Hepatic: ALT increased
Local: Infusion site pain
Neuromuscular & skeletal: Bone pain, muscle spasm, musculoskeletal discomfort/pain, paresthesia, weakness
Respiratory: Dyspnea, pharyngolaryngeal pain

General Dosage Range I.V.: *Adults:* Initial: 60 units/kg every 2 weeks; range: 11-73 units/kg every 2 weeks

Mechanism of Action Taliglucerase alfa is an analogue of glucocerebrosidase; it is produced by recombinant DNA technology using plant (carrot) cell culture. Glucocerebrosidase is an enzyme deficient in Gaucher's disease. It is needed to catalyze the hydrolysis of glucocerebroside to glucose and ceramide, thereby reducing liver and spleen size and improving anemia and thrombocytopenia.

Pharmacodynamics/Kinetics
Half-life Elimination 19-29 minutes (dose-dependent; increased with higher doses)
Pregnancy Risk Factor B
Pregnancy Considerations Adverse events were not observed in animal reproduction studies.
Prescribing and Access Restrictions Product access is restricted to the Gaucher Personal Support (GPS) program. Healthcare providers and patients may obtain additional information by contacting the GPS program at 855-353-5976.

Tamoxifen (ta MOKS i fen)

Brand Names: U.S. Soltamox™
Brand Names: Canada Apo-Tamox®; Mylan-Tamoxifen; Nolvadex®-D; PMS-Tamoxifen; Teva-Tamoxifen
Generic Availability (U.S.) Yes
Pharmacologic Category Antineoplastic Agent, Estrogen Receptor Antagonist; Selective Estrogen Receptor Modulator (SERM)
Use Treatment of metastatic (female and male) breast cancer; adjuvant treatment of breast cancer after primary treatment with surgery and radiation; reduce risk of invasive breast cancer in women with ductal carcinoma *in situ* (DCIS) after surgery and radiation; reduce the incidence of breast cancer in women at high risk
Unlabeled Use Treatment of mastalgia, gynecomastia, ovarian cancer, endometrial cancer, uterine sarcoma, and desmoid tumors; risk reduction in women with Paget's disease of the breast (with DCIS or without associated cancer); induction of ovulation; treatment of precocious puberty in females, secondary to McCune-Albright syndrome

Local Anesthetic/Vasoconstrictor Precautions No information available to require special precautions

Effects on Dental Treatment No significant effects or complications reported

Effects on Bleeding Although significant myelosuppression with associated altered hemostasis has been reported for many chemotherapeutic agents, myelosuppression is not common with tamoxifen and no specific precautions appear to necessary.

Adverse Effects
>10%:
Cardiovascular: Vasodilation (41%), flushing (33%), hypertension (11%), peripheral edema (11%)
Central nervous system: Mood changes (12% to 18%), pain (3% to 16%), depression (2% to 12%)
Dermatologic: Skin changes (6% to 19%), rash (13%)

Endocrine & metabolic: Hot flashes (3% to 80%), fluid retention (32%), altered menses (13% to 25%), amenorrhea (16%)

Gastrointestinal: Nausea (5% to 26%), weight loss (23%), vomiting (12%)

Genitourinary: Vaginal discharge (13% to 55%), vaginal bleeding (2% to 23%)

Neuromuscular & skeletal: Weakness (18%), arthritis (14%), arthralgia (11%)

Respiratory: Pharyngitis (14%)

Miscellaneous: Lymphedema (11%)

1% to 10%:

Cardiovascular: Chest pain (5%), venous thrombotic events (5%), edema (4%), cardiovascular ischemia (3%), angina (2%), deep venous thrombus (≤2%), MI (1%)

Central nervous system: Insomnia (9%), dizziness (8%), headache (8%), anxiety (6%), fatigue (4%)

Dermatologic: Alopecia (≤5%)

Endocrine & metabolic: Oligomenorrhea (9%), breast pain (6%), menstrual disorder (6%), breast neoplasm (5%), hypercholesterolemia (4%)

Gastrointestinal: Abdominal pain (9%), weight gain (9%), constipation (4% to 8%), diarrhea (7%), dyspepsia (6%), throat irritation (oral solution 5%), abdominal cramps (1%), anorexia (1%)

Genitourinary: Urinary tract infection (10%), leukorrhea (9%), vaginal hemorrhage (6%), vaginitis (5%), vulvovaginitis (5%), ovarian cyst (3%)

Hematologic: Thrombocytopenia (≤10%), anemia (5%)

Hepatic: AST increased (5%), serum bilirubin increased (2%)

Neuromuscular & skeletal: Back pain (10%), bone pain (6% to 10%), osteoporosis (7%), fracture (7%), arthrosis (5%), joint disorder (5%), myalgia (5%), paresthesia (5%), musculoskeletal pain (3%)

Ocular: Cataract (7%)

Renal: Serum creatinine increased (≤2%)

Respiratory: Cough (4% to 9%), dyspnea (8%), bronchitis (5%), sinusitis (5%)

Miscellaneous: Infection/sepsis (≤9%), diaphoresis (6%), flu-like syndrome (6%), cyst (5%), neoplasm (5%), allergic reaction (3%)

Dosage Oral: **Note:** For the treatment of breast cancer, patients receiving both tamoxifen and chemotherapy, should receive treatment sequentially, with tamoxifen following completion of chemotherapy.

Children: Females: Precocious puberty and McCune-Albright syndrome (unlabeled use): A dose of 20 mg/day has been reported in patients 2-10 years of age; safety and efficacy have not been established for treatment of longer than 1 year duration (Eugster, 2003)

Adults:

Breast cancer treatment:

Adjuvant therapy (females): 20 mg once daily for 5 years

Metastatic (males and females): 20-40 mg/day (doses >20 mg should be given in 2 divided doses). **Note:** Although the FDA-approved labeling recommends dosing up to 40 mg/day, clinical benefit has not been demonstrated with doses above 20 mg/day (Bratherton, 1984).

Premenopausal women: Duration of treatment is 5 years (NCCN Breast Cancer guidelines v.1.2011)

Postmenopausal women: Duration of tamoxifen treatment is 2-3 years followed by an aromatase inhibitor (AI) to complete 5 years; if contraindications or intolerant to AI, may take tamoxifen for the full 5 years **or** extended therapy: 4.5-6 years of tamoxifen followed by 5 years of an AI (NCCN Breast Cancer guidelines v.1.2011)

DCIS (females), to reduce the risk for invasive breast cancer: 20 mg once daily for 5 years

Breast cancer risk reduction (pre- and postmenopausal high-risk females): 20 mg once daily for 5 years

Induction of ovulation (unlabeled use): 20 mg once daily (range: 20-80 mg once daily) for 5 days (Steiner, 2005)

Paget's disease of the breast (risk reduction; with DCIS or without associated cancer): 20 mg once daily for 5 years (NCCN Breast Cancer Guidelines, v.1.2011)

Dosage adjustment for DVT, pulmonary embolism, cerebrovascular accident, or prolonged immobilization: Discontinue tamoxifen (NCCN Breast Cancer Risk Reduction Guidelines, v.2.2010)

Mechanism of Action Competitively binds to estrogen receptors on tumors and other tissue targets, producing a nuclear complex that decreases DNA synthesis and inhibits estrogen effects; nonsteroidal agent with potent antiestrogenic properties which compete with estrogen for binding sites in breast and other tissues; cells accumulate in the G_0 and G_1 phases; therefore, tamoxifen is cytostatic rather than cytocidal.

Contraindications Hypersensitivity to tamoxifen or any component of the formulation; concurrent warfarin therapy or history of deep vein thrombosis or pulmonary embolism (when tamoxifen is used for breast cancer risk reduction in women at high risk for breast cancer and in women with DCIS)

Warnings/Precautions Hazardous agent - use appropriate precautions for handling and disposal (NIOSH, 2012). **[U.S. Boxed Warning]: Serious and life-threatening events (including stroke, pulmonary emboli, and uterine malignancy) have occurred at an incidence greater than placebo during use for breast cancer risk reduction in women at high-risk for breast cancer and in women with DCIS;** these events are rare, but require consideration in risk:benefit evaluation. An increased incidence of thromboembolic events, including DVT and pulmonary embolism, has been associated with use for breast cancer; risk is increased with concomitant chemotherapy; use with caution in individuals with a history of thromboembolic events. Thrombocytopenia and/or leukopenia may occur; neutropenia and pancytopenia have been reported rarely. Although the relationship to tamoxifen therapy is uncertain, rare hemorrhagic episodes have occurred in patients with significant thrombocytopenia. Use with caution in patients with hyperlipidemias; infrequent postmarketing cases of hyperlipidemias have been reported. Decreased visual acuity, retinal vein thrombosis, retinopathy, corneal changes, color perception changes, and increased incidence of cataracts (and the need for cataract surgery), have been reported. Hypercalcemia has occurred in patients with bone metastasis, usually within a few weeks of therapy initiation; institute appropriate hypercalcemia management; discontinue if severe. Local disease flare and increased bone and tumor pain may occur in patients with metastatic breast cancer; may be associated with (good) tumor response.

Tamoxifen is associated with a high potential for drug interactions, including CYP- and Pgp-mediated interactions. Decreased efficacy and an increased risk of breast cancer recurrence has been reported with concurrent moderate or strong CYP2D6 inhibitors (Aubert, 2009; Dezentje, 2009). Concomitant use with select SSRIs may result in decreased tamoxifen efficacy.

Strong CYP2D6 inhibitors (eg, fluoxetine, paroxetine) and moderate CYP2D6 inhibitors (eg, sertraline) are reported to interfere with transformation to the active metabolite endoxifen. Weak CYP2D6 inhibitors (eg, venlafaxine, citalopram) have minimal effect on the conversion to endoxifen (Jin, 2005; NCCN Breast Cancer Risk Reduction Guidelines v.2.2010); escitalopram is also a weak CYP2D6 inhibitor. Lower plasma concentrations of endoxifen (active metabolite) have been observed in patients associated with reduced CYP2D6 activity (Jin, 2005) and may be associated with reduced efficacy. In a retrospective analysis of breast cancer patients taking tamoxifen and SSRIs, concomitant use of paroxetine and tamoxifen was associated with an increased risk of death due to breast cancer (Kelly, 2010).

Tamoxifen use may be associated with changes in bone mineral density (BMD) and the effects may be dependent upon menstrual status. In postmenopausal women, tamoxifen use is associated with a protective effect on bone mineral density (BMD), preventing loss of BMD which lasts over the 5-year treatment period. In premenopausal women, a decline (from baseline) in BMD mineral density has been observed in women who continued to menstruate; may be associated with an increased risk of fractures. Liver abnormalities such as cholestasis, fatty liver, hepatitis, and hepatic necrosis have occurred. Hepatocellular carcinomas have been reported in some studies; relationship to treatment is unclear. Tamoxifen is associated with an increased incidence of uterine or endometrial cancers. Endometrial hyperplasia, polyps, endometriosis, uterine fibroids, and ovarian cysts have occurred. Monitor and promptly evaluate any report of abnormal vaginal bleeding. Amenorrhea and menstrual irregularities have been reported with tamoxifen use.

Drug Interactions

Metabolism/Transport Effects Substrate of CYP2A6 (minor), CYP2B6 (minor), CYP2C9 (major), CYP2D6 (major), CYP2E1 (minor), CYP3A4 (major); **Note:** Assignment of Major/Minor substrate status based on clinically relevant drug interaction potential; **Inhibits** CYP2B6 (weak), CYP2C8 (moderate), CYP2C9 (weak), CYP3A4 (weak), P-glycoprotein

Avoid Concomitant Use

Avoid concomitant use of Tamoxifen with any of the following: Bosutinib; Conivaptan; CYP2D6 Inhibitors (Strong); Ospemifene; Pimozide; Pomalidomide; Silodosin; Topotecan; VinCRIStine (Liposomal); Vitamin K Antagonists

Increased Effect/Toxicity

Tamoxifen may increase the levels/effects of: ARIPiprazole; Bosutinib; Colchicine; CYP2C8 Substrates; Dabigatran Etexilate; Everolimus; Highest Risk QTc-Prolonging Agents; Lomitapide; Mipomersen; Moderate Risk QTc-Prolonging Agents; P-glycoprotein/ABCB1 Substrates; Pimozide; Pomalidomide; Prucalopride; Rivaroxaban; Silodosin; Topotecan; VinCRIStine (Liposomal); Vitamin K Antagonists

The levels/effects of Tamoxifen may be increased by: Abiraterone Acetate; Conivaptan; CYP2C9 Inhibitors (Moderate); CYP2C9 Inhibitors (Strong); CYP3A4 Inhibitors (Moderate); CYP3A4 Inhibitors (Strong); Darunavir; Dasatinib; Ivacaftor; Mifepristone

Decreased Effect

Tamoxifen may decrease the levels/effects of: Anastrozole; Letrozole; Ospemifene

The levels/effects of Tamoxifen may be decreased by: Aminoglutethimide; Bexarotene (Systemic); CYP2C9 Inducers (Strong); CYP2D6 Inhibitors (Moderate); CYP2D6 Inhibitors (Strong); CYP3A4 Inducers (Strong); Deferasirox; Herbs (CYP2D6 Inducers); Peginterferon Alfa-2b; Rifamycin Derivatives; Tocilizumab

Ethanol/Nutrition/Herb Interactions

Food: Grapefruit juice may decrease the metabolism of tamoxifen. Management: Avoid grapefruit juice.

Herb/Nutraceutical: Black cohosh and dong quai have estrogenic properties. St John's wort may decrease levels/effects of tamoxifen. Management: Avoid black cohosh and dong quai in estrogen-dependent tumors. Avoid St John's wort.

Dietary Considerations Tablets and oral solution may be taken with or without food. Avoid grapefruit and grapefruit juice.

Pharmacodynamics/Kinetics

Half-life Elimination Tamoxifen: ~5-7 days; N-desmethyl tamoxifen: ~14 days

Time to Peak Serum: ~5 hours

Pregnancy Risk Factor D

Pregnancy Considerations Animal studies have demonstrated fetal adverse effects and fetal loss. There have been reports of vaginal bleeding, birth defects and fetal loss in pregnant women. Tamoxifen use during pregnancy may have a potential long term risk to the fetus of a DES-like syndrome. For sexually-active women of childbearing age, initiate during menstruation (negative β-hCG immediately prior to initiation in women with irregular cycles). Tamoxifen may induce ovulation. Barrier or nonhormonal contraceptives are recommended. Pregnancy should be avoided during treatment and for 2 months after treatment has been discontinued.

Lactation Excretion in breast milk unknown/not recommended

Breast-Feeding Considerations It is not known if tamoxifen is excreted in breast milk, however, it has been shown to inhibit lactation. Due to the potential for adverse reactions, women taking tamoxifen should not breast-feed.

Dosage Forms

Solution, oral:

Soltamox™: 10 mg/5 mL (150 mL)

Tablet, oral: 10 mg, 20 mg

Tamsulosin (tam SOO loe sin)

Brand Names: U.S. Flomax®

Brand Names: Canada Ava-Tamsulosin CR; Flomax® CR; JAMP-Tamsulosin; Mylan-Tamsulosin; RAN™-Tamsulosin; ratio-Tamsulosin; Sandoz-Tamsulosin; Sandoz-Tamsulosin CR; Teva-Tamsulosin

Generic Availability (U.S.) Yes

Pharmacologic Category Alpha$_1$ Blocker

Use Treatment of signs and symptoms of benign prostatic hyperplasia (BPH)

Unlabeled Use Symptomatic treatment of bladder outlet obstruction or dysfunction; facilitation of expulsion of ureteral stones

Local Anesthetic/Vasoconstrictor Precautions No information available to require special precautions

Effects on Dental Treatment Key adverse event(s) related to dental treatment: Orthostatic hypotension and tooth disorder.

Effects on Bleeding No information available to require special precautions

Adverse Effects

>10%:

Cardiovascular: Orthostatic hypotension (6% to 19%),

Central nervous system: Headache (19% to 21%), dizziness (15% to 17%)

Genitourinary: Abnormal ejaculation (8% to 18%)

Respiratory: Rhinitis (13% to 18%)

Miscellaneous: Infection (9% to 11%)

1% to 10%:

Cardiovascular: Chest pain (4%)

Central nervous system: Somnolence (3% to 4%), insomnia (1% to 2%), vertigo (≤1%)

Endocrine & metabolic: Libido decreased (1% to 2%)

Gastrointestinal: Diarrhea (4% to 6%), nausea (3% to 4%), gum pain, toothache

Neuromuscular & skeletal: Weakness (8% to 9%), back pain (7% to 8%)

Ocular: Blurred vision (≤2%)

Respiratory: Pharyngitis (5% to 6%), cough (3% to 5%), sinusitis (2% to 4%)

Dosage Oral: Adults:

Benign prostatic hyperplasia (BPH): 0.4 mg once daily ~30 minutes after the same meal each day; dose may be increased after 2-4 weeks to 0.8 mg once daily in patients who fail to respond. If therapy is interrupted for several days, restart with 0.4 mg once daily.

Bladder outlet obstruction symptoms (unlabeled use): 0.4 mg once daily (Rossi, 2001)

Ureteral stones, expulsion (unlabeled use): 0.4 mg once daily, discontinue after successful expulsion (average time to expulsion was 1-2 weeks) (Agrawal, 2009; Ahmed, 2010). **Note:** Patients with stones >10 mm were excluded from studies.

Dosage adjustment in renal impairment:

Cl_{cr} ≥10 mL/minute: No adjustment needed

Cl_{cr} <10 mL/minute: Not studied

Dosage adjustment in hepatic impairment:

Mild-to-moderate impairment: No adjustment needed

Severe impairment: Not studied

Mechanism of Action Tamsulosin is an antagonist of alpha$_{1A}$-adrenoreceptors in the prostate. Smooth muscle tone in the prostate is mediated by alpha$_{1A}$-adrenoreceptors; blocking them leads to relaxation of smooth muscle in the bladder neck and prostate causing an improvement of urine flow and decreased symptoms of BPH. Approximately 75% of the alpha$_1$-receptors in the prostate are of the alpha$_{1A}$ subtype.

Contraindications Hypersensitivity to tamsulosin or any component of the formulation

Warnings/Precautions Not intended for use as an antihypertensive drug. May cause significant orthostatic hypotension and syncope, especially with first dose; anticipate a similar effect if therapy is interrupted for a few days, if dosage is rapidly increased, or if another antihypertensive drug (particularly vasodilators) or a PDE-5 inhibitor (eg, sildenafil, tadalafil, vardenafil) is introduced. "First-dose" orthostatic hypotension may occur 4-8 hours after dosing; may be dose related. Patients should be cautioned about performing hazardous tasks when starting new therapy or adjusting dosage upward. Discontinue if symptoms of angina occur or worsen. Rule out prostatic carcinoma before beginning therapy with tamsulosin. Intraoperative floppy iris syndrome has been observed in cataract surgery patients who were on or were previously treated with alpha$_1$-blockers; causality has not been established and there appears to be no benefit in discontinuing alpha-blocker therapy prior to surgery; instruct patients to inform ophthalmologist of tamsulosin use when considering eye surgery. Priapism has been associated with use (rarely). Rarely, patients with a sulfa allergy have also developed an allergic reaction to tamsulosin; avoid use when previous reaction has been severe.

Drug Interactions

Metabolism/Transport Effects Substrate of CYP2D6 (minor), CYP3A4 (major); **Note:** Assignment of Major/Minor substrate status based on clinically relevant drug interaction potential

Avoid Concomitant Use

Avoid concomitant use of Tamsulosin with any of the following: Alpha1-Blockers; CYP3A4 Inhibitors (Strong)

Increased Effect/Toxicity

Tamsulosin may increase the levels/effects of: Alpha1-Blockers; Calcium Channel Blockers

The levels/effects of Tamsulosin may be increased by: Beta-Blockers; CYP3A4 Inhibitors (Moderate); CYP3A4 Inhibitors (Strong); Dasatinib; Ivacaftor; MAO Inhibitors; Mifepristone; Phosphodiesterase 5 Inhibitors

Decreased Effect

Tamsulosin may decrease the levels/effects of: Alpha-/Beta-Agonists; Alpha1-Agonists

The levels/effects of Tamsulosin may be decreased by: CYP3A4 Inducers (Strong); Deferasirox; Herbs (CYP3A4 Inducers); Peginterferon Alfa-2b; Tocilizumab

Ethanol/Nutrition/Herb Interactions

Food: Fasting increases bioavailability by 30% and peak concentration 40% to 70%. Management: Administer 30 minutes after the same meal each day.

Herb/Nutraceutical: St John's wort may decrease the levels/effects of tamsulosin. Some herbal medications have hypotensive properties or may increase the hypotensive effect of tamsulosin. Limited information is available regarding combination with saw palmetto. Management: Avoid St John's wort, black cohosh, California poppy, coleus, golden seal, hawthorn, mistletoe, periwinkle, quinine, and shepherd's purse. Avoid saw palmetto.

Dietary Considerations Take once daily, 30 minutes after the same meal each day.

Pharmacodynamics/Kinetics

Half-life Elimination Healthy volunteers: 9-13 hours; Target population: 14-15 hours

Time to Peak Fasting: 4-5 hours; With food: 6-7 hours Steady-state: By the fifth day of once daily dosing

Pregnancy Risk Factor B

Pregnancy Considerations Teratogenic effects were not observed in animal studies.

Dosage Forms

Capsule, oral: 0.4 mg

Flomax®: 0.4 mg

Tapentadol (ta PEN ta dol)

Related Information

Endocrine Disorders and Pregnancy *on page 1517*
Oral Pain *on page 1558*

Brand Names: U.S. Nucynta®; Nucynta® ER

Brand Names: Canada Nucynta® IR; Nucynta™ CR

Generic Availability (U.S.) No

Pharmacologic Category Analgesic, Opioid

Dental Use Management of moderate-to-severe acute pain

◄ **Use**

Immediate release formulation: Relief of moderate-to-severe acute pain

Long acting formulation: Relief of moderate-to-severe chronic pain or neuropathic pain associated with diabetic peripheral neuropathy (DPN) when continuous, around-the-clock analgesia is necessary for an extended period of time

Local Anesthetic/Vasoconstrictor Precautions
Although part of the mechanism of tapentadol inhibits the reuptake of norepinephrine, there is no information available to require any special precautions.

Effects on Dental Treatment Key adverse effect(s) related to dental treatment: Xerostomia (normal salivary flow resumes upon discontinuation)

Effects on Bleeding No information available to require special precautions

Adverse Effects

Immediate release:

>10%:

Central nervous system: Dizziness (24%), somnolence (15%)

Gastrointestinal: Nausea (30%), vomiting (18%)

1% to 10%:

Central nervous system: Fatigue (3%), insomnia (2%), anxiety (1%), confusion (1%), dreams abnormal (1%), lethargy (1%)

Dermatologic: Pruritus (3% to 5%), hyperhidrosis (3%), rash (1%)

Endocrine & metabolic: Hot flushes (1%)

Gastrointestinal: Constipation (8%), xerostomia (4%), appetite decreased (2%), dyspepsia (2%)

Genitourinary: Urinary tract infection (1%)

Neuromuscular & skeletal: Arthralgia (1%), tremor (1%)

Respiratory: Nasopharyngitis (1%), upper respiratory tract infection (1%)

Extended release:

>10%:

Central nervous system: Dizziness (17% to 18%), headache (10% to 15%), somnolence (12% to 14%)

Gastrointestinal: Nausea (21% to 27%), constipation (13% to 17%), vomiting (8% to 12%)

1% to 10%:

Cardiovascular: Hypotension (1%)

Central nervous system: Fatigue (9%), anxiety (2% to 5%), insomnia (4%), irritability (2%), lethargy (2%), abnormal dreams (1% to 2%), vertigo (1% to 2%), attention disturbances (1%), chills (1%), depression/depressed mood (1%), hypoesthesia (1%), nervousness (1%), sedation (1%), withdrawal syndrome (1%)

Dermatologic: Pruritus (1% to 8%), hyperhidrosis (3% to 5%), rash (1%)

Endocrine & metabolic: Hot flushes (2% to 3%)

Gastrointestinal: Diarrhea (7%), xerostomia (7%), appetite decreased (2% to 6%), dyspepsia (1% to 3%), abdominal discomfort (1%)

Genitourinary: Erectile dysfunction (1%)

Neuromuscular & skeletal: Tremor (1% to 3%), weakness (2%)

Ocular: Vision blurred (1%)

Respiratory: Dyspnea (1%)

Dental Usual Dosage Adults: 50-100 mg every 4-6 hours as need for acute pain

Dosage Adults: **Note:** Dose and dosage intervals should be individualized according to pain severity with respect to patient's previous experience with similar opioid analgesics. To reduce the risk of withdrawal symptoms, it is recommended to taper the dose when discontinuing therapy.

Acute moderate-severe pain: Oral: *Immediate release:* Day 1: 50-100 mg every 4-6 hours as needed; may administer a second dose ≥1 hour after the initial dose (maximum dose on first day: 700 mg daily); Day 2 and subsequent dosing: 50-100 mg every 4-6 hours as needed (maximum: 600 mg daily)

Chronic moderate-severe pain (U.S. and Canadian labeling), neuropathic pain associated with diabetic peripheral neuropathy (U.S. labeling): Oral: *Extended release:*

Opioid naive: Initial: 50 mg twice daily (recommended interval: every 12 hours)

Opioid experienced: No adequate data on converting patients from other opioids to tapentadol extended release. In general, begin with a dose that is 50% of the estimated daily tapentadol requirement and use immediate release rescue medications to supplement dose. Per the Canadian product labeling, comparable pain relief was observed between tapentadol CR and oxycodone CR at a dose ratio of 5:1 in clinical studies.

Conversion from Nucynta® immediate release to extended release: Convert using same total daily dose but divide into 2 equal doses and administer twice daily (recommended interval: ~12 hours) (maximum dose: 500 mg daily).

Dose titration: Titrate in increments of 50 mg no more frequently than twice daily every 3 days to effective dose (therapeutic range: 100-250 mg twice daily) (maximum dose: 500 mg daily)

Elderly: Initial: Consider initiating at lower range of dosing. Refer to adult dosing.

Dosage adjustment in renal impairment:

Mild-moderate renal impairment: No dosage adjustment necessary.

Severe renal impairment: Not recommended (not studied); use is contraindicated in the Canadian labeling

Dosage adjustment in hepatic impairment:

Mild hepatic impairment: No dosage adjustment necessary.

Moderate hepatic impairment:

Immediate release: Initial: 50 mg every 8 hours or longer (maximum: 3 doses/24 hours). Further treatment for maintenance of analgesia may be achieved by either shortening or lengthening the dosing interval.

Extended release: Initial: 50 mg every 24 hours or longer; maximum: 100 mg once daily

Severe hepatic impairment: Not recommended (not studied); use is contraindicated in the Canadian labeling.

Mechanism of Action Binds to μ-opiate receptors in the CNS causing inhibition of ascending pain pathways, altering the perception of and response to pain; also inhibits the reuptake of norepinephrine, which also modifies the ascending pain pathway

Contraindications Hypersensitivity to tapentadol or any component of the formulation; significant respiratory depression; acute or severe asthma or hypercapnia in unmonitored settings or in absence of resuscitative equipment or ventilatory support; known or suspected paralytic ileus; use with or within 14 days of MAO inhibitors

Canadian labeling: Additional contraindications (not in U.S. labeling): Hypersensitivity to opioids; acute respiratory depression, cor pulmonale; gastrointestinal obstruction or any disease/condition that affects bowel transit (eg, ileus of any type, strictures); severe renal impairment (Cl_{cr} <30 mL/minute); severe hepatic impairment (Child-Pugh class C); mild, intermittent, or short-duration pain that can be managed with alternative pain medication; management of perioperative pain (controlled release tablets); acute alcoholism, delirium tremens, and seizure disorders; severe CNS depression, increased cerebrospinal or intracranial pressure or head injury; pregnancy; breast-feeding; use during labor/delivery

Warnings/Precautions Use with caution in patients with respiratory disease or respiratory compromise (eg, asthma, chronic obstructive pulmonary disease [COPD], cor pulmonale, sleep apnea, severe obesity, kyphoscoliosis, hypoxia, hypercapnia); critical respiratory depression may occur, even at therapeutic dosages. Use with caution in debilitated or cachectic patients; there is a greater potential for critical respiratory depression, even at therapeutic dosages. Use with extreme caution in patients with head injury, intracranial lesions, or elevated intracranial pressure (ICP); exaggerated elevation of ICP may occur. Use caution in patients with a history of seizures or conditions predisposing patients to seizures; patients with a history of seizures were excluded in clinical trials of tapentadol. Tramadol, an analgesic with similar pharmacologic properties to tapentadol, has been associated with seizures, particularly in patients with predisposing factors.

Serotonin syndrome (SS) may occur when used in combination with serotonergic agents. Signs of SS may include agitation, tachycardia, hyperthermia, nausea, and vomiting. Avoid use with serotonergic agents such as TCAs, triptans, venlafaxine, trazodone, lithium, sibutramine, meperidine, dextromethorphan, St John's wort, SNRIs, and SSRIs. Use is contraindicated with or within 14 days of MAO inhibitor therapy. Opioids may obscure diagnosis or clinical course of patients with acute abdominal conditions. May cause CNS depression, which may impair physical or mental abilities; patients must be cautioned about performing tasks which require mental alertness (eg, operating machinery or driving). Effects may be potentiated when used with other sedative drugs or ethanol.

Use with caution in patients with adrenal insufficiency (including Addison's disease), patients with biliary tract dysfunction or acute pancreatitis (opioids may cause spasm of the sphincter of Oddi), patients with CNS depression or coma, patients with hypothyroidism, prostatic hyperplasia and/or urinary stricture. Use opioids with caution in the elderly; consider decreasing initial dose. May have a greater potential for critical respiratory depression. Serum concentrations are increased in hepatic impairment; use with caution in patients with moderate hepatic impairment (dosage adjustment required). Not recommended for use in severe hepatic impairment (not studied). Use with caution in patients with mild-to-moderate renal impairment; no dosage

adjustments recommended. Not recommended for use in severe renal impairment (not studied).

During dosage adjustments, immediate release tramadol may be used as rescue medication (maximum dose: 400 mg/day); fentanyl should not be used as rescue medication (Canadian labeling recommendations; not in U.S. labeling).

Prolonged use increases risk of abuse, addiction, and withdrawal symptoms. An opioid-containing regimen should be tailored to each patient's needs with respect to degree of tolerance for opioids (naïve versus chronic user), age, weight, and medical condition. Abrupt discontinuation may lead to withdrawal symptoms. Symptoms may be decreased by tapering prior to discontinuation. Mixed agonist/antagonist opioids may diminish the analgesic effect of tapentadol or precipitate withdrawal symptoms.

Extended release tablets:
[U.S. Boxed Warning]: Respiratory depression, possibly fatal, may occur. Proper dosing, titration, and monitoring are essential. Extended release tablets must be swallowed whole and should NOT be split, crushed, broken, chewed, or dissolved in order to avoid rapid release and potential for fatal dose. Risk for respiratory depression is greatest during the initiation of therapy or with dose increases. Use is contraindicated in patients with significant respiratory depression or conditions that may increase that risk. Extended release tablets may cause severe hypotension; use with caution in patients with risk factors (eg. hypovolemia, concomitant use of other hypotensive agents). Avoid use in patients with circulatory shock.

[U.S. Boxed Warning]: Accidental exposure, especially in children, may lead to fatal overdose. Not intended for use as an as-needed analgesic; **not** intended for the management of acute or postoperative pain; approved for the treatment of chronic pain only (not an as-needed basis).

[U.S. Boxed Warning]: Use of alcohol may increase tapentadol systemic exposure which may lead to possible fatal overdose. Avoid alcohol or alcohol containing medications during therapy.

[U.S. Boxed Warning]: Healthcare provider should be alert to problems of abuse, misuse, and diversion. Potential for abuse may be increased in patients with a history of or family history of substance abuse or mental illness. Use with caution in patients with a history of drug abuse or acute alcoholism. Tolerance, psychological and physical dependence may occur with prolonged use.

Drug Interactions

Metabolism/Transport Effects Substrate of CYP2C9 (minor), CYP2D6 (minor); **Note:** Assignment of Major/Minor substrate status based on clinically relevant drug interaction potential

Avoid Concomitant Use
Avoid concomitant use of Tapentadol with any of the following: Alcohol (Ethyl); Azelastine (Nasal); MAO Inhibitors; Paraldehyde

Increased Effect/Toxicity
Tapentadol may increase the levels/effects of: Alvimopan; Azelastine (Nasal); CNS Depressants; Desmopressin; MAO Inhibitors; Metoclopramide; Metyrosine; Paraldehyde; Pramipexole; ROPINIRole; Rotigotine; Selective Serotonin Reuptake Inhibitors; Serotonin Modulators; Thiazide Diuretics; Zolpidem

◀ *The levels/effects of Tapentadol may be increased by:*
Alcohol (Ethyl); Amphetamines; Antipsychotic Agents (Phenothiazines); Antipsychotics; HydrOXYzine; Magnesium Sulfate; Perampanel; Sodium Oxybate; Succinylcholine

Decreased Effect

Tapentadol may decrease the levels/effects of: Pegvisomant

The levels/effects of Tapentadol may be decreased by:
Ammonium Chloride; Antiemetics (5HT3 Antagonists); Mixed Agonist / Antagonist Opioids; Peginterferon Alfa-2b

Ethanol/Nutrition/Herb Interactions

Ethanol: May increase CNS depression; monitor for increased effects with coadministration. Caution patients about effects. Bioavailability of extended release tablets may be increased by alcohol; combined use should be avoided.

Food: When administered after a high fat/calorie meal, the AUC and C_{max} increased by 25% and 16%, respectively; may administer without regard to meals.

Herb/Nutraceutical: Avoid St John's wort (may increase CNS depression and risk of serotonin syndrome).

Dietary Considerations May be taken without regard to meals.

Pharmacodynamics/Kinetics

Half-life Elimination Immediate release: ~4 hours; Long acting formulations: ~5-6 hours

Time to Peak Plasma: Immediate release: 1.25 hours; Long acting formulations: 3-6 hours

Pregnancy Risk Factor C

Pregnancy Considerations Adverse events were observed in animal reproduction studies. Not recommended for use during labor and delivery. Use of opioids during pregnancy may produce physical dependence in the neonate. Symptoms of opioid withdrawal may include excessive crying, diarrhea, fever, hyper-reflexia, irritability, respiratory rate increased, sneezing, tremors, vomiting, or yawning; respiratory depression may occur in the newborn if opioids are used prior to delivery. Use in pregnant women is contraindicated in the Canadian labeling.

Lactation Excretion in breast milk unknown/not recommended

Breast-Feeding Considerations Limited information available on the excretion of tapentadol in human milk; however, data suggests it may be excreted in human milk. The possibility of sedation or respiratory depression in the nursing infant should be considered. Use while breast-feeding is contraindicated in the Canadian labeling.

Product Availability Nucynta® Oral Solution: FDA approved October 2012; anticipated availability currently unknown. Refer to prescribing information for additional information.

Controlled Substance C-II

Dosage Forms

Tablet, oral:
Nucynta®: 50 mg, 75 mg, 100 mg
Tablet, extended release, oral:
Nucynta® ER: 50 mg, 100 mg, 150 mg, 200 mg, 250 mg

Dosage Forms: Canada

Tablet, controlled release, oral:
Nucynta™ CR: 50 mg, 100 mg, 150 mg, 200 mg, 250 mg

Dental Comment Tapentadol is classified as an opioid analgesic having a unique ability to bind to μ-opiate receptors and to also inhibit the reuptake of norepinephrine. It shares many properties of the traditional opioid drugs including addiction liability. A report by Kleinert et al, showed that single doses of tapentadol ≥75 mg effectively reduced moderate-to-severe postoperative dental pain in a dose related fashion and were well tolerated compared to 60 mg morphine. The study showed that tapentadol was a highly effective, centrally acting analgesic with a favorable side effect profile with rapid onset of action.

References

Kleinert R, Lange C, Steup A, et al, "Single Dose Analgesic Efficacy of Tapentadol in Postsurgical Dental Pain: The Results of a Randomized, Double-Blind, Placebo-Controlled Study," *Anesth Analg,* 2008, 107(6):2048-55.

Tazarotene (taz AR oh teen)

Brand Names: U.S. Avage®; Tazorac®
Brand Names: Canada Tazorac®
Pharmacologic Category Acne Products; Keratolytic Agent; Topical Skin Product, Acne
Use Topical treatment of facial acne vulgaris; topical treatment of stable plaque psoriasis; mitigation (palliation) of facial skin wrinkling, facial mottled hyper-/hypopigmentation, and benign facial lentigines
Local Anesthetic/Vasoconstrictor Precautions No information available to require special precautions
Effects on Dental Treatment No significant effects or complications reported
Effects on Bleeding No information available to require special precautions
Adverse Effects Percentage of incidence varies with formulation and/or strength:

>10%: Dermatologic: Burning/stinging, desquamation, dry skin, erythema, irritation, pruritus, skin pain, worsening of psoriasis
1% to 10%:
Cardiovascular: Peripheral edema
Dermatologic: Cheilitis, contact dermatitis, discoloration, eczema, fissuring, inflammation, localized bleeding, rash
Endocrine & metabolic: Hypertriglyceridemia
Frequency not defined: Dermatologic: Photosensitization

General Dosage Range Topical: *Children ≥12 years and Adults:* Apply a pea-sized amount or thin film **or** 2 mg/cm^2 once daily
Mechanism of Action Synthetic, acetylenic retinoid which modulates differentiation and proliferation of epithelial tissue and exerts some degree of anti-inflammatory and immunological activity
Pharmacodynamics/Kinetics
Duration of Action Therapeutic: Psoriasis: Effects have been observed for up to 3 months after a 3-month course of topical treatment
Half-life Elimination 18 hours
Pregnancy Risk Factor X
Pregnancy Considerations May cause fetal harm if administered to a pregnant woman. A negative pregnancy test should be obtained within 2 weeks prior to treatment; treatment should begin during a normal menstrual period.

Teduglutide (te due GLOO tide)

Brand Names: U.S. Gattex®

Pharmacologic Category Glucagon-Like Peptide-2 (GLP-2) Analog

Use Treatment of short bowel syndrome (SBS) in patients requiring parenteral nutrition support

Local Anesthetic/Vasoconstrictor Precautions No information available to require special precautions

Effects on Dental Treatment No significant effects or complications reported

Effects on Bleeding No information available to require special precautions

Adverse Effects

>10%:

Central nervous system: Headache (16%)

Endocrine & metabolic: Fluid overload (12%)

Gastrointestinal: Stoma complications (42%), abdominal pain (30% to 38%), nausea (18% to 25%), abdominal distension (14% to 20%), vomiting (12%)

Local: Injection site reaction (12% to 22%)

Respiratory: Upper respiratory tract infection (12% to 26%)

1% to 10%:

Central nervous system: Sleep disturbances (5%)

Dermatologic: Cutaneous hemorrhage (5%)

Gastrointestinal: Flatulence (9%), appetite disorders (7%), intestinal obstruction/stenosis (4%), colorectal polyps (2%)

Respiratory: Cough (5%)

Miscellaneous: Hypersensitivity reactions (8%)

General Dosage Range Dosage adjustment recommended in patients with renal impairment.

SubQ: *Adults:* 0.05 mg/kg once daily

Mechanism of Action Teduglutide is an analog of glucagon-like peptide-2 (GLP-2), which is secreted in the distal intestine. Endogenous GLP-2 increases intestinal and portal blood flow while inhibiting gastric acid secretion and reducing gastric motility, thereby reducing intestinal losses and improving intestinal absorption. Teduglutide binds and activates GLP-2 receptors, resulting in release of mediators including insulin-like growth factor (IGF)-1, nitric oxide and keratinocyte growth factor (KGF).

Pharmacodynamics/Kinetics

Half-life Elimination 1.3 hours

Time to Peak Plasma: 3-5 hours

Pregnancy Risk Factor B

Pregnancy Considerations Adverse events were not observed in animal reproduction studies.

Tegaserod (teg a SER od)

Brand Names: U.S. Zelnorm®

Brand Names: Canada Zelnorm® [DSC]

Pharmacologic Category Serotonin 5-HT$_4$ Receptor Agonist

Use Emergency treatment of irritable bowel syndrome with constipation (IBS-C) and chronic idiopathic constipation (CIC) in women (<55 years of age) in which no alternative therapy exists

Local Anesthetic/Vasoconstrictor Precautions No information available to require special precautions

Effects on Dental Treatment No significant effects or complications reported

Effects on Bleeding No information available to require special precautions

Adverse Effects

>10%:

Central nervous system: Headache (15%)

Gastrointestinal: Abdominal pain (12%)

1% to 10%:

Central nervous system: Dizziness (4%), migraine (2%)

Gastrointestinal: Diarrhea (9%; severe <1%), nausea (8%), flatulence (6%)

Neuromuscular & skeletal: Back pain (5%), arthropathy (2%), leg pain (1%)

General Dosage Range Oral: *Adults (females <55 years of age):* 6 mg twice daily

Mechanism of Action Tegaserod is a partial neuronal 5-HT$_4$ receptor agonist. Its action at the receptor site leads to stimulation of the peristaltic reflex and intestinal secretion, and moderation of visceral sensitivity.

Pharmacodynamics/Kinetics

Half-life Elimination I.V.: 11 ± 5 hours

Time to Peak 1 hour

Pregnancy Risk Factor B

Pregnancy Considerations Safety and efficacy have not been established in pregnant women. Use during pregnancy only if clearly needed.

Prescribing and Access Restrictions Available in U.S. under an emergency investigational new drug (IND) process. Emergency situations are defined as immediately life-threatening or requiring hospitalization. Physicians with patients who may qualify can contact the FDA's Division of Drug Information via email (druginfo@fda.hhs.gov). The FDA may either deny the request or authorize shipment of Zelnorm® by Novartis. Additional information can be found at http://www.fda.gov/Drugs/DrugSafety/PostmarketDrugSafetyInformationforPatientsandProviders/ucm103223.htm.

Telaprevir (tel A pre vir)

Related Information

Systemic Viral Diseases *on page 1537*

Brand Names: U.S. Incivek™

Brand Names: Canada Incivek™

Generic Availability (U.S.) No

Pharmacologic Category Antiviral Agent; Protease Inhibitor

Use Treatment of genotype 1 chronic hepatitis C (in combination with peginterferon alfa and ribavirin) in adult patients with compensated liver disease (including cirrhosis) who are treatment naive or who have received previous interferon-based treatment, including null or partial responders, and treatment relapsers.

Local Anesthetic/Vasoconstrictor Precautions No information available to require special precautions

Effects on Dental Treatment Key adverse event(s) related to dental treatment: Abnormal taste

Effects on Bleeding No information available to require special precautions

Adverse Effects

>10%:

Central nervous system: Fatigue (56%)

Dermatologic: Rash (56%), pruritus (47%)

Endocrine and Metabolic: Hyperuricemia (<12.1 mg/dL: 66%; ≥12.1 mg/dL: 7%)

Gastrointestinal: Nausea (39%), diarrhea (26%), vomiting (13%), hemorrhoids (12%), anorectal discomfort (11%)

Hematologic: Anemia (36%), lymphopenia (15%)

Hepatic: Hyperbilirubinemia (<2.6 x ULN: 37%; ≥2.6 x ULN: 4%)

1% to 10%:

Gastrointestinal: Abnormal taste (10%), anal pruritus (6%)

Hematologic: Thrombocytopenia (3%)

Dosage Oral: Adults: 750 mg 3 times/day (in combination with peginterferon alfa and ribavirin)

Treatment-naive or prior relapse patients: **Note:** Relapse includes patients with an undetectable HCV-RNA upon completion of treatment (non-telaprevir based regimen) but with detectable HCV-RNA during the follow up period.

Weeks 1-12: Triple therapy: Telaprevir 750 mg 3 times/day in combination with peginterferon alfa and ribavirin

Weeks 13-23 (based on HCV-RNA results at weeks 4 and 12):

HCV-RNA **undetectable** (level less than ~10-15 units/mL) at both weeks 4 and 12 (eRVR): Dual therapy: Peginterferon alfa and ribavirin only (through week 24)

HCV-RNA **detectable** (level greater than ~10-15 units/mL but ≤1000 units/mL) at week 4 and/or week 12: Dual therapy: Peginterferon alfa and ribavirin only (through week 48 discussed below)

HCV-RNA **detectable** (level >1000 units/mL) at week 4 or week 12 (treatment futility): Discontinue telaprevir, peginterferon alfa and ribavirin at week 12

Weeks ≥24 (based on HCV-RNA results at week 24):

HCV-RNA **detectable** (level greater than ~10-15 units/mL but ≤1000 units/mL) at week 4 and/or week 12: Peginterferon alfa with concomitant ribavirin only (through week 48)

HCV-RNA **detectable** (level greater than ~10-15 units/mL) at week 24 (treatment futility): Discontinue peginterferon alfa and concomitant ribavirin

Treatment naïve patients with cirrhosis, compensated:

Weeks 1-12: Triple therapy: Telaprevir 750 mg 3 times/day in combination with peginterferon alfa and ribavirin

Weeks 13-24 (based on HCV-RNA results at weeks 4 and 12):

HCV-RNA **undetectable** at both weeks 4 and 12 (eRVR): Dual therapy: Peginterferon alfa and ribavirin only (through week 48 discussed below)

HCV-RNA **detectable** (level greater than ~10-15 units/mL but ≤1000 units/mL) at week 4 and/or week 12: Dual therapy: Peginterferon alfa and ribavirin only (through week 48 discussed below)

HCV-RNA **detectable** (level >1000 units/mL) at week 4 or week 12 (treatment futility): Discontinue telaprevir, peginterferon alfa and ribavirin at week 12

Weeks ≥ 24 (based on HCV-RNA results at week 24):

HCV-RNA **undetectable** at week 24: Peginterferon alfa with concomitant ribavirin only (through week 48)

HCV-RNA **detectable** (level greater than ~10-15 units/mL) at week 24 (treatment futility): Discontinue peginterferon alfa and ribavirin

Previously-treated patients (partial response or null responders): **Note:** Previously treated does not include prior treatment with telaprevir. Partial response includes patients with a >2-log$_{10}$ HCV-RNA decrease by week 12 but a nonsustained virologic response thereafter. Null response includes patients with a <2-log$_{10}$ HCV-RNA decrease at week 12.

Weeks 1-12: Triple therapy: Telaprevir 750 mg 3 times/day with peginterferon alfa and ribavirin

Weeks 13-48 (based on HCV-RNA results at weeks 4 and 12):

HCV-RNA **undetectable** (level less than ~10-15 units/mL) or detectable (level ≤1000 units/mL) at both weeks 4 and 12: Dual therapy: Peginterferon alfa and ribavirin only (through week 48)

HCV-RNA **detectable** (level >1000 units/mL) at week 4 or week 12: Discontinue telaprevir, peginterferon alfa, and ribavirin at week 12

HCV-RNA **detectable** (level greater than ~10-15 units/mL) at week 24: Discontinue peginterferon alfa and concomitant ribavirin

Dosage adjustment in renal impairment:

Telaprevir: No dosage adjustment necessary. Not studied in patients with Cl$_{cr}$ ≤50 mL/minute or in hemodialysis.

Peginterferon Alfa and Ribavirin: Refer to individual monographs.

Dosage adjustment in hepatic impairment: Telaprevir:

Mild impairment (Child-Pugh class A): No dosage adjustment necessary.

Moderate or severe impairment (Child-Pugh class B or C): Not studied

Peginterferon Alfa and Ribavirin: Refer to individual monographs.

Mechanism of Action Binds reversibly to nonstructural protein 3 (NS 3) serine protease and inhibits replication of the hepatitis C virus. Considered a direct-acting antiviral treatment for HCV, also called a specifically targeted antiviral therapy for HCV (STAT-C).

Contraindications Combination treatment with ribavirin: Pregnancy; male partners of pregnant women

Coadministration with CYP 3A4 highly dependent substrates (alfuzosin, cisapride, ergot derivatives, lovastatin, midazolam [oral], pimozide, sildenafil/tadalafil [when used for treatment of pulmonary arterial hypertension], simvastatin, triazolam), or strong CYP 3A4 inducers (rifampin, St John's wort)

Canadian labeling: Additional contraindications (not in U.S. labeling): Hypersensitivity to telaprevir or any component of the formulation; coadministration with amiodarone, atorvastatin, eletriptan, flecainide, propafenone, quinidine, terfenadine, vardenafil

Also refer to Peginterferon Alfa and Ribavirin monographs for individual product contraindications.

Warnings/Precautions [U.S. Boxed Warning] Serious skin reactions (some fatal) including Stevens-Johnson syndrome (SJS), drug reaction with eosinophilia and systemic symptoms (DRESS), and toxic epidermal necrolysis (TEN), have been reported with telaprevir combination therapy. Fatal cases have been reported in patients with progressive rash and systemic symptoms who received ongoing therapy after diagnoses of serious skin reactions. Discontinue telaprevir, peginterferon alfa, and ribavirin immediately for serious skin reactions (including rash with systemic symptoms or a progressive severe rash). Rash has been typically observed within first 4 weeks of therapy initiation but may occur at any time. Severe rashes (other than DRESS, SJS) are generalized, bullous, vesicular or ulcerative; may also have an eczematous appearance. Discontinue telaprevir (may continue peginterferon alfa and ribavirin) for severe rash or for mild-to-moderate rash that progresses; if no improvement in rash within 1 week of stopping telaprevir, interruption or discontinuation of peginterferon alfa and/or ribavirin should be considered (or sooner if clinically indicated). May use oral antihistamines/topical corticosteroids for rash treatment; do not use systemic corticosteroids. Do not restart telaprevir if discontinued due to any skin reaction.

Anemia has been reported with peginterferon alfa and ribavirin; addition of telaprevir is associated with further hemoglobin decreases. Low hemoglobin levels were measured during the first 4 weeks of treatment, and the lowest at the end of telaprevir treatment (week 12). Dose modifications of ribavirin were needed more often in patients also taking telaprevir. Assess complete blood count (CBC) pretreatment, at weeks 2, 4, 8, and 12, and when clinically indicated. May require ribavirin dose reduction, interruption or discontinuation of treatment; if ribavirin dose reductions are inadequate, may consider discontinuing telaprevir. Do not reduce telaprevir dose. If ribavirin is discontinued, telaprevir must also be discontinued. Do not restart telaprevir if ribavirin therapy is reinitiated.

Avoid pregnancy in female patients and female partners of male patients, during therapy, and for at least 6 months after treatment; two forms of nonhormonal contraception should be used. Hormonal contraceptives may not be effective in patients taking telaprevir or for two weeks after discontinuing therapy. Safety and efficacy have not been established in patients who have uncompensated cirrhosis, received organ transplants, or been coinfected with hepatitis B or HIV, or who have failed to respond to other NS3/4A inhibitors. Monotherapy is not effective for chronic hepatitis C infection. Not recommended in moderate or severe hepatic impairment (Child-Pugh class B or C) or decompensated hepatic disease. Potentially significant drug interactions may exist, requiring dose or frequency adjustments, additional monitoring, and/or selection of alternative therapy. Consult drug interactions database for more detailed information.

Drug Interactions

Metabolism/Transport Effects Substrate of CYP3A4 (major), P-glycoprotein; **Note:** Assignment of Major/Minor substrate status based on clinically relevant drug interaction potential; **Inhibits** CYP3A4 (strong), P-glycoprotein, SLCO1B1

Avoid Concomitant Use

Avoid concomitant use of Telaprevir with any of the following: Ado-Trastuzumab Emtansine; Alfuzosin; Apixaban; AtorvaSTATin; Avanafil; Axitinib; Bosutinib; Cabozantinib; CarBAMazepine; Cisapride; Conivaptan; Crizotinib; Darunavir; Dihydroergotamine; Dronedarone; Eplerenone; Ergoloid Mesylates; Ergonovine; Ergotamine; Everolimus; Fluticasone (Oral Inhalation); Fosamprenavir; Fosphenytoin; Halofantrine; Ivabradine; Lapatinib; Lomitapide; Lopinavir; Lovastatin; Lurasidone; Methylergonovine; Midazolam; Nilotinib; Nisoldipine; PHENobarbital; Phenytoin; Pimozide; Pomalidomide; Ranolazine; Red Yeast Rice; Regorafenib; Rifabutin; Rifampin; Rivaroxaban; RomiDEPsin; Salmeterol; Sildenafil; Silodosin; Simvastatin; St Johns Wort; Tamsulosin; Ticagrelor; Tolvaptan; Topotecan; Toremifene; Triazolam; VinCRIStine (Liposomal)

Increased Effect/Toxicity

Telaprevir may increase the levels/effects of: Ado-Trastuzumab Emtansine; Alfuzosin; Almotriptan; Alosetron; ALPRAZolam; Amiodarone; Apixaban; ARIPiprazole; Atazanavir; AtorvaSTATin; Avanafil; Axitinib; Bedaquiline; Bepridil [Off Market]; Bortezomib; Bosentan; Bosutinib; Brentuximab Vedotin; Brinzolamide; Budesonide (Nasal); Budesonide (Systemic, Oral Inhalation); Cabozantinib; CarBAMazepine; Cisapride; Clarithromycin; Colchicine; Conivaptan; Corticosteroids; Corticosteroids (Orally Inhaled); Corticosteroids (Systemic); Crizotinib; CycloSPORINE (Systemic); CYP3A4 Substrates; Dabigatran Etexilate; Dienogest; Digoxin; Dihydroergotamine; Dronedarone;

Dutasteride; Enzalutamide; Eplerenone; Ergoloid Mesylates; Ergonovine; Ergotamine; Erythromycin (Systemic); Everolimus; FentaNYL; Fesoterodine; Flecainide; Fluticasone (Nasal); Fluticasone (Oral Inhalation); Fluvastatin; Fosphenytoin; GuanFACINE; Halofantrine; Iloperidone; Itraconazole; Ivabradine; Ivacaftor; Ixabepilone; Ketoconazole (Systemic); Lapatinib; Lidocaine (Systemic); Lomitapide; Lovastatin; Lumefantrine; Lurasidone; Maraviroc; Methylergonovine; MethylPREDNISolone; Midazolam; Mifepristone; Nilotinib; Nisoldipine; Ospemifene; Paricalcitol; Pazopanib; P-glycoprotein/ABCB1 Substrates; PHENobarbital; Phenytoin; Pimecrolimus; Pimozide; Pitavastatin; Pomalidomide; Ponatinib; Posaconazole; Pravastatin; Propafenone; Prucalopride; QuiNIDine; Ranolazine; Red Yeast Rice; Regorafenib; Repaglinide; Rifabutin; Rivaroxaban; RomiDEPsin; Rosuvastatin; Ruxolitinib; Salmeterol; Saxagliptin; Sildenafil; Silodosin; Simvastatin; Sirolimus; SORAfenib; Tacrolimus (Systemic); Tadalafil; Tamsulosin; Telithromycin; Tenofovir; Ticagrelor; Tofacitinib; Tolterodine; Tolvaptan; Topotecan; Toremifene; TraZODone; Triazolam; Vardenafil; Vemurafenib; Vilazodone; VinCRIStine (Liposomal); Voriconazole; Warfarin; Zuclopenthixol

The levels/effects of Telaprevir may be increased by: Clarithromycin; CYP3A4 Inhibitors (Moderate); CYP3A4 Inhibitors (Strong); Dasatinib; Erythromycin (Systemic); Itraconazole; Ketoconazole (Systemic); P-glycoprotein/ABCB1 Inhibitors; Posaconazole; Ritonavir; Telithromycin; Voriconazole

Decreased Effect

Telaprevir may decrease the levels/effects of: Contraceptives (Estrogens); Contraceptives (Progestins); Darunavir; Efavirenz; Escitalopram; Fosamprenavir; Fosphenytoin; Ifosfamide; Methadone; PHENobarbital; Phenytoin; Prasugrel; Ticagrelor; Voriconazole; Warfarin; Zolpidem

The levels/effects of Telaprevir may be decreased by: Atazanavir; Bosentan; CarBAMazepine; Corticosteroids; Corticosteroids (Systemic); CYP3A4 Inducers (Strong); Darunavir; Deferasirox; Efavirenz; Etravirine; Fosamprenavir; Fosphenytoin; Lopinavir; P-glycoprotein/ABCB1 Inducers; PHENobarbital; Phenytoin; Rifabutin; Rifampin; Ritonavir; St Johns Wort; Tocilizumab

Dietary Considerations Take with a meal (not low fat).

Pharmacodynamics/Kinetics

Half-life Elimination Plasma: Adults: ~4-5 hours (single dose); steady state: ~9-11 hours

Time to Peak 4-5 hours

Pregnancy Risk Factor B / X (in combination with ribavirin)

Pregnancy Considerations Adverse events were not observed in telaprevir animal developmental studies; however, telaprevir must not be used as monotherapy (must be used in combination with peginterferon alfa and ribavirin). Significant ribavirin teratogenic effects have been observed in all animal studies at ~0.01 times the maximum recommended daily human dose. Use of ribavirin is contraindicated in pregnancy. In addition, animal studies with interferons have demonstrated abortifacient effects. Negative pregnancy test is required before initiation and monthly thereafter. Hormonal contraceptive measures may not be effective in patients taking telaprevir or for 2 weeks after discontinuing therapy. Avoid pregnancy in female patients and female partners of male patients during therapy by using two effective nonhormonal forms of contraception; continue contraceptive measures for at least 6 months after completion of therapy. If patient or female partner becomes pregnant during treatment, she should be counseled about potential risks of exposure. If pregnancy occurs during use or within 6 months after treatment, report to the ribavirin pregnancy registry (800-593-2214).

Lactation Excretion in breast milk unknown/not recommended

Breast-Feeding Considerations It is not known if telaprevir or ribavirin are excreted into breast milk. The manufacturer recommends that breast-feeding be discontinued prior to the initiation of treatment.

Dosage Forms
Tablet, oral:
Incivek™: 375 mg

Telavancin (tel a VAN sin)

Related Information
Clinical Risk Related to Drugs Prolonging QT Interval *on page 1510*

Brand Names: U.S. Vibativ™

Pharmacologic Category Glycopeptide

Use Treatment of complicated skin and skin structure infections caused by susceptible gram-positive organisms including methicillin-susceptible or -resistant *Staphylococcus aureus*, vancomycin-susceptible *Enterococcus faecalis*, and *Streptococcus pyogenes*, *Streptococcus agalactiae*, or *Streptococcus anginosus* group

Local Anesthetic/Vasoconstrictor Precautions
Telavancin is one of the drugs confirmed to prolong the QT interval and is accepted as having a risk of causing torsade de pointes. The risk of drug-induced torsade de pointes is extremely low when a single QT interval prolonging drug is prescribed. In terms of epinephrine, it is not known what effect vasoconstrictors in the local anesthetic regimen will have in patients with a known history of congenital prolonged QT interval or in patients taking any medication that prolongs the QT interval. Until more information is obtained, it is suggested that the clinician consult with the physician prior to the use of a vasoconstrictor in suspected patients, and that the vasoconstrictor (epinephrine, mepivacaine and levonordefrin [Carbocaine® 2% with Neo-Cobefrin®]) be used with caution.

Effects on Dental Treatment Key adverse event(s) related to dental treatment: Metallic or abnormal taste

Effects on Bleeding Although there are no reports of enhanced bleeding, telavancin may interfere with tests used to monitor coagulation (eg, prothrombin time, INR, activated partial thromboplastin time, activated clotting time, and coagulation-based factor Xa tests). Thrombocytopenia occurs in 7% of patients.

Adverse Effects
>10%:
Central nervous system: Insomnia (13%), psychiatric disorder (12%), headache (11%)
Gastrointestinal: Metallic/soapy taste (33%), nausea (27%), vomiting (14%)
Genitourinary: Foamy urine (13%)
1% to 10%:
Central nervous system: Dizziness (6%)
Dermatologic: Pruritus (3% to 6%), rash (4%)
Endocrine & metabolic: Hypokalemia (7%)
Gastrointestinal: Diarrhea (7%), appetite decreased (3%), abdominal pain (2%)
Hematologic: Thrombocytopenia (7%)
Local: Infusion site pain (4%), infusion site erythema (3%)

Neuromuscular & skeletal: Paresthesia (5%), rigors (4%)
Renal: Serum creatinine increased (8%), microalbuminuria (7%)
Respiratory: Dyspnea (8%)

General Dosage Range Dosage adjustment recommended in patients with renal impairment
I.V.: *Adults:* 10 mg/kg every 24 hours

Mechanism of Action Exerts concentration-dependent bactericidal activity; inhibits bacterial cell wall synthesis by blocking polymerization and cross-linking of peptidoglycan by binding to D-Ala-D-Ala portion of cell wall. Unlike vancomycin, additional mechanism involves disruption of membrane potential and changes cell permeability due to presence of lipophilic side chain moiety.

Pharmacodynamics/Kinetics
Half-life Elimination 6.6-9.6 hours

Pregnancy Risk Factor C

Pregnancy Considerations [U.S. Boxed Warning]: Based on animal data, adverse developmental outcomes have been observed. Prior to use, women of childbearing potential should have a serum pregnancy test. Use of telavancin is not recommended during pregnancy unless the potential benefit to the mother outweighs the possible risk to the fetus. Telavancin crosses the placenta. In women of childbearing potential, effective contraception should be used during therapy. Healthcare providers are encouraged to enroll women exposed to telavancin during pregnancy in the Vibativ Pregnancy Registry (888-658-4228).

Product Availability Vibativ™: Temporarily not commercially available; anticipated date of availability is unknown.

Dental Comment Telavancin is known to prolong the QT interval. The QT interval is measured as the time and distance between the Q point of the QRS complex and the end of the T wave in the ECG tracing. After adjustment for heart rate, the QT interval is defined as prolonged if it is more than 450 msec in men and 460 msec in women. A long QT syndrome was first described in the 1950s and 60s as a congenital syndrome involving QT interval prolongation and syncope and sudden death. Some of the congenital long QT syndromes were characterized by a peculiar electrocardiographic appearance of the QRS complex involving a premature atria beat followed by a pause, then a subsequent sinus beat showing marked QT prolongation and deformity. This type of cardiac arrhythmia was originally termed "torsade de pointes" (translated from the French as "twisting of the points"). Telavancin is considered as having a risk of causing torsade de pointes. Since it is not known what effect vasoconstrictors in the local anesthetic regimen will have in patients with a known history of congenital prolonged QT interval or in patients taking any medication that prolongs the QT interval, a medical consult is suggested.

Telbivudine (tel BI vyoo deen)

Related Information
HIV Infection and AIDS *on page 1520*
Systemic Viral Diseases *on page 1537*

Brand Names: U.S. Tyzeka®
Brand Names: Canada Sebivo®

Pharmacologic Category Antiretroviral Agent, Reverse Transcriptase Inhibitor (Nucleoside)

Use Treatment of chronic hepatitis B with evidence of viral replication and either persistent transaminase elevations or histologically-active disease

Local Anesthetic/Vasoconstrictor Precautions No information available to require special precautions

Effects on Dental Treatment No significant effects or complications reported

Effects on Bleeding No information available to require special precautions regarding hemostasis.

Adverse Effects

>10%:

Central nervous system: Fatigue (13%)

Neuromuscular & skeletal: CPK increased (79%; grades 3/4: 13%)

1% to 10%:

Central nervous system: Headache (10%), dizziness (4%), fever (4%), insomnia (3%)

Dermatologic: Rash (4%), pruritus (2%)

Endocrine & metabolic: Lipase increased (grades 3/4: 2%)

Gastrointestinal: Abdominal pain (3% to 6%), diarrhea (6%), nausea (5%), abdominal distension (3%), dyspepsia (3%)

Hematologic: Neutropenia (grades 3/4: 2%)

Hepatic: ALT increased (grades 3/4: 5% to 7%), AST increased (grades 3/4: 6%)

Neuromuscular & skeletal: Arthralgia (4%), back pain (4%), myalgia (3%)

Respiratory: Cough (6%), pharyngolaryngeal pain (5%)

General Dosage Range Dosage adjustment recommended in patients with renal impairment

Oral: *Children ≥16 years and Adults:* 600 mg once daily

Mechanism of Action Telbivudine, a synthetic thymidine nucleoside analogue (L-enantiomer of thymidine), is intracellularly phosphorylated to the active triphosphate form, which competes with the natural substrate, thymidine 5'-triphosphate, to inhibit hepatitis B viral DNA polymerase; enzyme inhibition blocks reverse transcriptase activity thereby reducing viral DNA replication.

Pharmacodynamics/Kinetics

Half-life Elimination Terminal: 40-49 hours

Time to Peak 1-4 hours

Pregnancy Risk Factor B

Pregnancy Considerations Teratogenic effects have not been observed in animal studies. There are no adequate and well-controlled studies in pregnant women. Health professionals are encouraged to contact the antiretroviral pregnancy registry to monitor outcomes of pregnant women exposed to antiretroviral medications (1-800-258-4263).

Product Availability Tyzeka® oral solution: FDA approved April 2009; anticipated availability is currently undetermined

---

Telithromycin (tel ith roe MYE sin)

Related Information

Clinical Risk Related to Drugs Prolonging QT Interval *on page 1510*

Brand Names: U.S. Ketek®

Brand Names: Canada Ketek®

Generic Availability (U.S.) No

Pharmacologic Category Antibiotic, Ketolide

Use Treatment of community-acquired pneumonia (mild-to-moderate) caused by susceptible strains of *Streptococcus pneumoniae* (including multidrug-resistant isolates), *Haemophilus influenzae*, *Chlamydophila pneumoniae*, *Moraxella catarrhalis*, and *Mycoplasma pneumoniae*

Local Anesthetic/Vasoconstrictor Precautions Telithromycin is one of the drugs confirmed to prolong the QT interval and is accepted as having a risk of causing torsade de pointes. The risk of drug-induced torsade de pointes is extremely low when a single QT interval prolonging drug is prescribed. In terms of epinephrine, it is not known what effect vasoconstrictors in the local anesthetic regimen will have in patients with a known history of congenital prolonged QT interval or in patients taking any medication that prolongs the QT interval. Until more information is obtained, it is suggested that the clinician consult with the physician prior to the use of a vasoconstrictor in suspected patients, and that the vasoconstrictor (epinephrine, mepivacaine and levonordefrin [Carbocaine® 2% with Neo-Cobefrin®]) be used with caution.

Effects on Dental Treatment Key adverse event(s) related to dental treatment: Xerostomia (normal salivary flow resumes upon discontinuation), glossitis, stomatitis, and tooth discoloration.

Effects on Bleeding No information available to require special precautions

Adverse Effects

>10%: Gastrointestinal: Diarrhea (10% to 11%)

2% to 10%:

Central nervous system: Headache (2% to 6%), dizziness (3% to 4%)

Gastrointestinal: Nausea (7% to 8%), vomiting (2% to 3%), loose stools (2%), dysgeusia (2%)

≥0.2% to <2%:

Central nervous system: Fatigue, insomnia, somnolence, vertigo

Dermatologic: Rash

Gastrointestinal: Abdominal distension, abdominal pain, anorexia, constipation, dyspepsia, flatulence, gastritis, gastroenteritis, GI upset, glossitis, stomatitis, watery stools, xerostomia

Genitourinary: Vaginal candidiasis

Hematologic: Platelets increased

Hepatic: Transaminases increased

Ocular: Blurred vision, accommodation delayed, diplopia

Miscellaneous: Candidiasis, diaphoresis increased

Dosage Oral:

Children ≥13 years and Adults: Tonsillitis/pharyngitis (unlabeled use; Canadian indication): 800 mg once daily for 5 days

Adults: Community-acquired pneumonia: 800 mg once daily for 7-10 days

Dosage adjustment in renal impairment:

U.S. product labeling: Cl_{cr} <30 mL/minute, including dialysis: 600 mg once daily; when renal impairment is accompanied by hepatic impairment, reduce dosage to 400 mg once daily

Canadian product labeling: Cl_{cr} <30 mL/minute: Reduce dose to 400 mg once daily

Hemodialysis: Administer following dialysis

Dosage adjustment in hepatic impairment: No adjustment recommended, unless concurrent severe renal impairment is present

Mechanism of Action Inhibits bacterial protein synthesis by binding to two sites on the 50S ribosomal subunit. Telithromycin has also been demonstrated to alter secretion of IL-1alpha and TNF-alpha; the clinical significance of this immunomodulatory effect has not been evaluated.

Contraindications Hypersensitivity to telithromycin, macrolide antibiotics, or any component of the formulation; myasthenia gravis; history of hepatitis and/or jaundice associated with telithromycin or other macrolide antibiotic use; concurrent use of colchicine (if patient has concomitant renal or hepatic impairment), cisapride, pimozide, lovastatin, or simvastatin

Warnings/Precautions Acute hepatic failure and severe liver injury, including hepatitis and hepatic necrosis (leading to some fatalities) have been reported, in some cases after only a few doses; if signs/symptoms of hepatitis or liver damage occur, discontinue therapy and initiate liver function tests. **[U.S. Boxed Warning]: Life-threatening (including fatal) respiratory failure has occurred in patients with myasthenia gravis;** use in these patients is contraindicated. May prolong QT$_c$ interval, leading to a risk of ventricular arrhythmias; closely-related antibiotics have been associated with malignant ventricular arrhythmias and torsade de pointes. Avoid in patients with prolongation of QT$_c$ interval due to congenital causes, history of long QT syndrome, uncorrected electrolyte disturbances (hypokalemia or hypomagnesemia), significant bradycardia (<50 bpm), or concurrent therapy with QT$_c$-prolonging drugs (eg, class Ia and class III antiarrhythmics). Avoid use in patients with a prior history of confirmed cardiogenic syncope or ventricular arrhythmias while receiving macrolide antibiotics or other QT$_c$-prolonging drugs. May cause severe visual disturbances (eg, changes in accommodation ability, diplopia, blurred vision). May cause loss of consciousness (possibly vagal-related); caution patients that these events may interfere with ability to operate machinery or drive, and to use caution until effects are known. Use caution in renal impairment; severe impairment (Cl$_{cr}$ <30 mL/minute) requires dosage adjustment. Pseudomembranous colitis has been reported. Safety and efficacy not established in pediatric patients <13 years of age per Canadian approved labeling and <18 years of age per U.S. approved labeling.

Drug Interactions

Metabolism/Transport Effects Substrate of CYP1A2 (minor), CYP3A4 (major); **Note:** Assignment of Major/Minor substrate status based on clinically relevant drug interaction potential; **Inhibits** CYP2D6 (weak), CYP3A4 (strong)

Avoid Concomitant Use

Avoid concomitant use of Telithromycin with any of the following: Ado-Trastuzumab Emtansine; Alfuzosin; Apixaban; Avanafil; Axitinib; BCG; Bosutinib; Cabozantinib; Cisapride; Conivaptan; Crizotinib; Disopyramide; Dronedarone; Eplerenone; Everolimus; Fluticasone (Oral Inhalation); Halofantrine; Highest Risk QTc-Prolonging Agents; Ivabradine; Lapatinib; Lomitapide; Lovastatin; Lurasidone; Mifepristone; Moderate Risk QTc-Prolonging Agents; Nilotinib; Nisoldipine; Pimozide; Pomalidomide; QuiNINE; Ranolazine; Red Yeast Rice; Regorafenib; Rivaroxaban; RomiDEPsin; Salmeterol; Silodosin; Simvastatin; Tamsulosin; Terfenadine; Ticagrelor; Tolvaptan; Toremifene; VinCRIStine (Liposomal)

Increased Effect/Toxicity

Telithromycin may increase the levels/effects of: Ado-Trastuzumab Emtansine; Alfentanil; Alfuzosin; Almotriptan; Alosetron; Antifungal Agents (Azole Derivatives, Systemic); Antineoplastic Agents (Vinca Alkaloids); Apixaban; ARIPiprazole; Avanafil; Axitinib; Bedaquiline; Benzodiazepines (metabolized by oxidation); Bortezomib; Bosutinib; Brentuximab Vedotin; Brinzolamide; Budesonide (Nasal); Budesonide (Systemic, Oral Inhalation); BusPIRone; Cabozantinib; Calcium Channel Blockers; CarBAMazepine; Cardiac Glycosides; Cilostazol; Cisapride; CloZAPine; Cobicistat; Colchicine; Conivaptan; Corticosteroids (Orally Inhaled); Corticosteroids (Systemic); Crizotinib; CycloSPORINE (Systemic); CYP3A4 Substrates; Dienogest; Disopyramide; Dronedarone; Dutasteride; Eletriptan; Enzalutamide; Eplerenone; Ergot Derivatives; Everolimus; FentaNYL; Fesoterodine; Fluticasone (Nasal); Fluticasone (Oral Inhalation); GuanFACINE; Halofantrine; Highest Risk QTc-Prolonging Agents; HMG-CoA Reductase Inhibitors; Iloperidone; Ivabradine; Ivacaftor; Ixabepilone; Lapatinib; Lomitapide; Lovastatin; Lumefantrine; Lurasidone; Maraviroc; MethylPREDNISolone; Mifepristone; Nilotinib; Nisoldipine; Ospemifene; Paricalcitol; Pazopanib; Pimecrolimus; Pimozide; Pomalidomide; Ponatinib; Propafenone; QuiNIDine; QuiNINE; Ranolazine; Red Yeast Rice; Regorafenib; Repaglinide; Rifamycin Derivatives; Rivaroxaban; RomiDEPsin; Ruxolitinib; Salmeterol; Saxagliptin; Selective Serotonin Reuptake Inhibitors; Sildenafil; Silodosin; Simvastatin; Sirolimus; SORAfenib; Tacrolimus (Systemic); Tacrolimus (Topical); Tadalafil; Tamsulosin; Telaprevir; Temsirolimus; Terfenadine; Ticagrelor; Tofacitinib; Tolterodine; Tolvaptan; Toremifene; Vardenafil; Vemurafenib; Verapamil; Vilazodone; VinCRIStine (Liposomal); Vitamin K Antagonists; Zopiclone; Zuclopenthixol

The levels/effects of Telithromycin may be increased by: Antifungal Agents (Azole Derivatives, Systemic); Cobicistat; CYP3A4 Inhibitors (Moderate); CYP3A4 Inhibitors (Strong); Dasatinib; Ivabradine; Mifepristone; Moderate Risk QTc-Prolonging Agents; QTc-Prolonging Agents (Indeterminate Risk and Risk Modifying); Telaprevir

Decreased Effect

Telithromycin may decrease the levels/effects of: BCG; Clopidogrel; Ifosfamide; Prasugrel; Sodium Picosulfate; Ticagrelor; Typhoid Vaccine

The levels/effects of Telithromycin may be decreased by: CYP3A4 Inducers (Strong); Deferasirox; Etravirine; Herbs (CYP3A4 Inducers); Tocilizumab

Ethanol/Nutrition/Herb Interactions Herb/Nutraceutical: St John's wort: May decrease the levels/effects of telithromycin.

Dietary Considerations May be taken with or without food.

Pharmacodynamics/Kinetics

Half-life Elimination 10 hours

Time to Peak Plasma: 1 hour

Pregnancy Risk Factor C

Pregnancy Considerations Because adverse effects were observed in some animal studies, telithromycin is classified pregnancy category C. There are no adequate and well-controlled studies of telithromycin in pregnant women.

Lactation Excretion in breast milk unknown/use caution

Breast-Feeding Considerations It is not known if telithromycin is excreted in breast milk. The manufacturer recommends caution if using telithromycin in a breast-feeding woman.

Dosage Forms

Tablet, oral:

Ketek®: 300 mg, 400 mg

Dosage Forms: Canada

Tablet:

Ketek®: 400 mg

Dental Comment Telithromycin is known to prolong the QT interval. The QT interval is measured as the time and distance between the Q point of the QRS complex and the end of the T wave in the ECG tracing. After adjustment for heart rate, the QT interval is defined as prolonged if it is more than 450 msec in men and 460 msec in women. A long QT syndrome was first described in the 1950s and 60s as a congenital syndrome involving QT interval prolongation and syncope and sudden death. Some of the congenital long QT syndromes were characterized by a peculiar electrocardiographic appearance of the QRS complex involving a premature atria beat followed by a pause, then a subsequent sinus beat showing marked QT prolongation and deformity. This type of cardiac arrhythmia was originally termed "torsade de pointes" (translated from the French as "twisting of the points"). Telithromycin is considered as having a risk of causing torsade de pointes. Since it is not known what effect vasoconstrictors in the local anesthetic regimen will have in patients with a known history of congenital prolonged QT interval or in patients taking any medication that prolongs the QT interval, a medical consult is suggested.

Telmisartan (tel mi SAR tan)

Related Information

Cardiovascular Diseases *on page 1492*

Brand Names: U.S. Micardis®

Brand Names: Canada Micardis®; Mylan-Telmisartan; PMS-Telmisartan; Sandoz-Telmisartan; Teva-Telmisartan

Generic Availability (U.S.) No

Pharmacologic Category Angiotensin II Receptor Blocker

Use Treatment of hypertension (may be used alone or in combination with other antihypertensive agents); cardiovascular risk reduction in patients ≥55 years of age unable to take ACE inhibitors and who are at high risk of major cardiovascular events (eg, MI, stroke, death)

Local Anesthetic/Vasoconstrictor Precautions No information available to require special precautions

Effects on Dental Treatment No significant effects or complications reported

Effects on Bleeding No information available to require special precautions

Adverse Effects May be associated with worsening of renal function in patients dependent on renin-angiotensin-aldosterone system.

1% to 10%:

Cardiovascular: Intermittent claudication (7%; placebo 6%), chest pain (≥1%), hypertension (≥1%), peripheral edema (≥1%)

Central nervous system: Dizziness (≥1%), fatigue (≥1%), headache (≥1%), pain (≥1%)

Dermatologic: Skin ulcer (3%; placebo 2%)

Gastrointestinal: Diarrhea (3%), abdominal pain (≥1%), dyspepsia (≥1%), nausea (≥1%)

Genitourinary: Urinary tract infection (≥1%)

Neuromuscular & skeletal: Back pain (3%), myalgia (≥1%)

Respiratory: Upper respiratory infection (7%), sinusitis (3%), cough (≥1%), pharyngitis (1%)

Dosage Oral:

Adults:

Hypertension: Initial: 40 mg once daily; usual maintenance dose range: 20-80 mg/day. Patients with volume depletion should be initiated on the lower dosage with close supervision.

Cardiovascular risk reduction: Initial: 80 mg once daily. **Note:** It is unknown whether doses <80 mg/day are associated with a reduction in risk of cardiovascular morbidity or mortality.

Elderly:

Hypertension: Initial: 20 mg/day; usual maintenance dose range: 20-80 mg/day

Cardiovascular risk reduction: Initial 80 mg once daily

Dosage adjustment in renal impairment: No adjustment required; hemodialysis patients are more susceptible to orthostatic hypotension

Dosage adjustment in hepatic impairment: Initiate therapy with low dose; titrate slowly and monitor closely.

Canadian labeling: Recommended initial dose: 40 mg/day

Mechanism of Action Angiotensin II acts as a vasoconstrictor. In addition to causing direct vasoconstriction, angiotensin II also stimulates the release of aldosterone. Once aldosterone is released, sodium as well as water are reabsorbed. The end result is an elevation in blood pressure. Telmisartan is a nonpeptide AT1 angiotensin II receptor antagonist. This binding prevents angiotensin II from binding to the receptor thereby blocking the vasoconstriction and the aldosterone secreting effects of angiotensin II.

Contraindications Hypersensitivity to telmisartan or any component of the formulation; concomitant use with aliskiren in patients with diabetes mellitus

Canadian labeling: Additional contraindications: Second and third trimesters of pregnancy; breast-feeding; fructose intolerance

Warnings/Precautions [U.S. Boxed Warning]: Drugs that act on the renin-angiotensin system can cause injury and death to the developing fetus. Discontinue as soon as possible once pregnancy is detected. May cause hyperkalemia; avoid potassium supplementation unless specifically required by healthcare provider. Avoid use or use a smaller dose in patients who are volume depleted; correct depletion first. May be associated with deterioration of renal function and/or increases in serum creatinine, particularly in patients with low renal blood flow (eg, renal artery stenosis, heart failure) whose glomerular filtration rate (GFR) is dependent on efferent arteriolar vasoconstriction by angiotensin II. Use with caution in unstented unilateral/bilateral renal artery stenosis. When unstented bilateral renal artery stenosis is present, use is generally avoided due to the elevated risk of deterioration in renal function unless possible benefits outweigh risks. Use with caution with pre-existing renal insufficiency; significant aortic/mitral stenosis. Concomitant use of an angiotensin-converting enzyme (ACE) inhibitor or renin inhibitor (eg, aliskiren) is associated with an increased risk of hypotension, hyperkalemia, and renal dysfunction; concurrent use with ramipril is

◀ not recommended; concomitant use with aliskiren should be avoided in patients with GFR <60 mL/minute and is contraindicated in patients with diabetes mellitus (regardless of GFR). Use with caution in patients who have biliary obstructive disorders or hepatic dysfunction. Product contains sorbitol. The Canadian labeling (not in U.S. labeling) contraindicates use in fructose intolerant patients.

Drug Interactions

Metabolism/Transport Effects Inhibits CYP2C19 (weak)

Avoid Concomitant Use There are no known interactions where it is recommended to avoid concomitant use.

Increased Effect/Toxicity

Telmisartan may increase the levels/effects of: ACE Inhibitors; Amifostine; Antihypertensives; Cardiac Glycosides; CycloSPORINE (Systemic); Hypotensive Agents; Lithium; Nonsteroidal Anti-Inflammatory Agents; Potassium-Sparing Diuretics; Ramipril; RiTUXimab; Sodium Phosphates

The levels/effects of Telmisartan may be increased by: Alfuzosin; Aliskiren; Canagliflozin; Diazoxide; Eplerenone; Herbs (Hypotensive Properties); MAO Inhibitors; Pentoxifylline; Phosphodiesterase 5 Inhibitors; Potassium Salts; Prostacyclin Analogues; Tolvaptan; Trimethoprim

Decreased Effect

The levels/effects of Telmisartan may be decreased by: Herbs (Hypertensive Properties); Methylphenidate; Nonsteroidal Anti-Inflammatory Agents; Yohimbine

Ethanol/Nutrition/Herb Interactions Herb/Nutraceutical: Some herbal medications may have hypertensive or hypotensive properties; others may increase or decrease the antihypertensive effect of telmisartan. Management: Avoid bayberry, blue cohosh, cayenne, ephedra, ginger, ginseng (American), kola, licorice, and yohimbe. Avoid black cohosh, California poppy, coleus, golden seal, hawthorn, mistletoe, periwinkle, quinine, and shepherd's purse.

Dietary Considerations May be taken without regard to meals. Product contains sorbitol.

Pharmacodynamics/Kinetics

Onset of Action 1-2 hours; Peak effect: 0.5-1 hours

Duration of Action Up to 24 hours

Half-life Elimination Terminal: 24 hours

Time to Peak Plasma: 0.5-1 hours

Pregnancy Risk Factor D

Pregnancy Considerations [U.S. Boxed Warning]: Drugs that act on the renin-angiotensin system can cause injury and death to the developing fetus. Discontinue as soon as possible once pregnancy is detected. The use of drugs which act on the renin-angiotensin system are associated with oligohydramnios. Oligohydramnios, due to decreased fetal renal function, may lead to fetal lung hypoplasia and skeletal malformations. Use is also associated with anuria, hypotension, renal failure, skull hypoplasia, and death in the fetus/neonate. The exposed fetus should be monitored for fetal growth, amniotic fluid volume, and organ formation. Infants exposed *in utero* should be monitored for hyperkalemia, hypotension, and oliguria.

Lactation Excretion in breast milk unknown/not recommended

Dosage Forms

Tablet, oral:

Micardis®: 20 mg, 40 mg, 80 mg

Telmisartan and Amlodipine
(tel mi SAR tan & am LOE di peen)

Related Information

AmLODIPine *on page 88*

Telmisartan *on page 1293*

Brand Names: U.S. Twynsta®

Brand Names: Canada Twynsta®

Pharmacologic Category Angiotensin II Receptor Blocker; Antianginal Agent; Calcium Channel Blocker; Calcium Channel Blocker, Dihydropyridine

Use Treatment of hypertension, including initial treatment in patients who will require multiple antihypertensives for adequate control

Local Anesthetic/Vasoconstrictor Precautions No information available to require special precautions

Effects on Dental Treatment Key adverse event(s) related to dental treatment: Fewer reports of gingival hyperplasia reported with amlodipine use than with other calcium channel blockers (usually resolves upon discontinuation); consult with healthcare provider. Orthostatic hypotension has been reported; monitor patient for dizziness while rising from dental chair.

Effects on Bleeding No information available to require special precautions

Adverse Effects Reactions/percentages reported with combination product; also see individual agents.

>10%: Cardiovascular: Peripheral edema (dose related: 1% to 11%)

1% to 10%:

Cardiovascular: Orthostatic hypotension (6%), edema (<2%), hypotension (<2%), syncope (<2%)

Central nervous system: Dizziness (3%)

Neuromuscular & skeletal: Back pain (2%)

General Dosage Range Oral: *Adults:* Amlodipine 5-10 mg and telmisartan 40-80 mg once daily (maximum: 10 mg/day [amlodipine]; 80 mg/day [telmisartan])

Mechanism of Action

Telmisartan is a nonpeptide AT1 (angiotensin II type 1) receptor antagonist. Angiotensin II acts as a vasoconstrictor. In addition to causing direct vasoconstriction, angiotensin II also stimulates the release of aldosterone. Once aldosterone is released, sodium and water are reabsorbed. The end result is an elevation in blood pressure. Telmisartan binding to AT1 prevents angiotensin II from binding to the receptor thereby blocking the vasoconstriction and the aldosterone secreting effects of angiotensin II.

Amlodipine inhibits calcium ion from entering the "slow channels" or select voltage-sensitive areas of vascular smooth muscle and myocardium during depolarization, producing a relaxation of coronary vascular smooth muscle and coronary vasodilation; increases myocardial oxygen delivery in patients with vasospastic angina. Amlodipine directly acts on vascular smooth muscle to produce peripheral arterial vasodilation reducing peripheral vascular resistance and blood pressure.

Pregnancy Risk Factor D

Pregnancy Considerations [U.S. Boxed Warning]: Drugs that act on the renin-angiotensin system can cause injury and death to the developing fetus. Discontinue as soon as possible once pregnancy is detected. Also see individual agents.

Telmisartan and Hydrochlorothiazide
(tel mi SAR tan & hye droe klor oh THYE a zide)

Related Information

Hydrochlorothiazide *on page 687*

Telmisartan *on page 1293*

Brand Names: U.S. Micardis® HCT

Brand Names: Canada Micardis® Plus; Mylan-Telmisartan HCTZ; Telmisartan HCTZ; Teva-Telmisartan HCTZ

Pharmacologic Category Angiotensin II Receptor Blocker; Diuretic, Thiazide

Use Treatment of hypertension; combination product should not be used for initial therapy

Local Anesthetic/Vasoconstrictor Precautions No information available to require special precautions

Effects on Dental Treatment No significant effects or complications reported

Effects on Bleeding No information available to require special precautions

Adverse Effects The following reactions have been reported with the combination product; see individual agents for additional adverse reactions that may be expected from each agent.

2% to 10%:

Central nervous system: Dizziness (5%), fatigue (3%)

Gastrointestinal: Diarrhea (3%), nausea (2%)

Renal: BUN increased (3%)

Respiratory: Upper respiratory tract infection (8%), sinusitis (4%)

Miscellaneous: Flu-like syndrome (2%)

<2%: Abdominal pain, back pain, bilirubin increased, bronchitis, dyspepsia, hematocrit decreased, hemoglobin decreased, hypokalemia, liver enzymes increased, orthostatic hypotension, pharyngitis, rash, serum creatinine increased, tachycardia, vomiting; rhabdomyolysis has been reported (rarely) with angiotensin-receptor antagonists

General Dosage Range Oral: *Adults:* Initial: Telmisartan 80 mg and hydrochlorothiazide 12.5-25 mg once daily; Maintenance: Telmisartan 80-160 mg and hydrochlorothiazide 12.5-25 mg once daily

Mechanism of Action

Telmisartan: Telmisartan is an angiotensin receptor antagonist. Angiotensin II acts as a vasoconstrictor. In addition to causing direct vasoconstriction, angiotensin II also stimulates the release of aldosterone. Once aldosterone is released, sodium as well as water are reabsorbed. The end result is an elevation in blood pressure. Telmisartan binds to the AT1 angiotensin II receptor. This binding prevents angiotensin II from binding to the receptor thereby blocking the vasoconstriction and the aldosterone secreting effects of angiotensin II.

Hydrochlorothiazide: Inhibits sodium reabsorption in the distal tubules causing increased excretion of sodium and water as well as potassium and hydrogen ions

Pregnancy Risk Factor D

Pregnancy Considerations [U.S. Boxed Warning]: Drugs that act on the renin-angiotensin system can cause injury and death to the developing fetus. Discontinue as soon as possible once pregnancy is detected. Also see individual agents.

Temazepam (te MAZ e pam)

Brand Names: U.S. Restoril™

Brand Names: Canada Apo-Temazepam®; CO Temazepam; Dom-Temazepam; Gen-Temazepam; Novo-Temazepam; Nu-Temazepam; PHL-Temazepam; PMS-Temazepam; ratio-Temazepam; Restoril™

Generic Availability (U.S.) Yes

Pharmacologic Category Benzodiazepine

Use Short-term treatment of insomnia

Unlabeled Use Treatment of anxiety

Local Anesthetic/Vasoconstrictor Precautions No information available to require special precautions

Effects on Dental Treatment Key adverse event(s) related to dental treatment: Significant xerostomia (normal salivary flow resumes upon discontinuation).

Effects on Bleeding No information available to require special precautions

Adverse Effects

1% to 10%:

Central nervous system: Anxiety, confusion, dizziness, drowsiness, euphoria, fatigue, hangover, headache, lethargy, vertigo

Dermatologic: Rash

Endocrine & metabolic: Libido decreased

Gastrointestinal: Diarrhea

Neuromuscular & skeletal: Dysarthria, weakness

Ocular: Blurred vision

Miscellaneous: Diaphoresis

Dosage Oral:

Adults: Usual dose: 15-30 mg at bedtime; some patients may respond to 7.5 mg in transient insomnia

Elderly or debilitated patients: Initial: 7.5 mg at bedtime

Mechanism of Action Binds to stereospecific benzodiazepine receptors on the postsynaptic GABA neuron at several sites within the central nervous system, including the limbic system, reticular formation. Enhancement of the inhibitory effect of GABA on neuronal excitability results by increased neuronal membrane permeability to chloride ions. This shift in chloride ions results in hyperpolarization (a less excitable state) and stabilization.

Contraindications Hypersensitivity to temazepam or any component of the formulation (cross-sensitivity with other benzodiazepines may exist); narrow-angle glaucoma (not in product labeling, however, benzodiazepines are contraindicated); pregnancy

Warnings/Precautions As a hypnotic, should be used only after evaluation of potential causes of sleep disturbance. Failure of sleep disturbance to resolve after 7-10 days may indicate psychiatric or medical illness. A worsening of insomnia or the emergence of new abnormalities of thought or behavior may represent unrecognized psychiatric or medical illness and requires immediate and careful evaluation.

Use with caution in debilitated patients, patients with hepatic disease (including alcoholics), or renal impairment. In older adults, benzodiazepines increase the risk of impaired cognition, delirium, falls, fractures, and motor vehicle accidents. Due to increased sensitivity in this age group, avoid use for treatment of insomnia, agitation, or delirium. (Beers Criteria). Use with caution in patients with respiratory disease, or impaired gag reflex. Avoid use inpatients with sleep apnea.

Causes CNS depression (dose-related) resulting in sedation, dizziness, confusion, or ataxia which may impair physical and mental capabilities. Patients must be cautioned about performing tasks which require mental alertness (eg, operating machinery or driving). Use with caution in patients receiving other CNS depressants or psychoactive agents. Postmarketing studies have indicated that the use of hypnotic/sedative agents for sleep has been associated with hypersensitivity reactions including anaphylaxis as well as angioedema. An increased risk for hazardous sleep-related activities such as sleep-driving; cooking and eating food, and making phone calls while asleep have also been noted. Effects with other sedative drugs or ethanol may be potentiated. Benzodiazepines have been associated with falls and traumatic injury and should be used with extreme caution in patients who are at risk of these events.

Use caution in patients with suicidal risk. Use with caution in patients with a history of drug dependence. Benzodiazepines have been associated with dependence and acute withdrawal symptoms on discontinuation or reduction in dose (may occur after as little as 10 days). Acute withdrawal, including seizures, may be precipitated after administration of flumazenil to patients receiving long-term benzodiazepine therapy.

Benzodiazepines have been associated with anterograde amnesia. Paradoxical reactions, including hyperactive or aggressive behavior, have been reported with benzodiazepines, particularly in adolescent/pediatric or psychiatric patients. Does not have analgesic, antidepressant, or antipsychotic properties.

Drug Interactions

Metabolism/Transport Effects Substrate of CYP2B6 (minor), CYP2C19 (minor), CYP2C9 (minor), CYP3A4 (minor); **Note:** Assignment of Major/Minor substrate status based on clinically relevant drug interaction potential

Avoid Concomitant Use

Avoid concomitant use of Temazepam with any of the following: Azelastine (Nasal); OLANZapine; Paraldehyde; Sodium Oxybate

Increased Effect/Toxicity

Temazepam may increase the levels/effects of: Alcohol (Ethyl); Azelastine (Nasal); Buprenorphine; CloZAPine; CNS Depressants; Fosphenytoin; Methotrimeprazine; Metyrosine; Mirtazapine; Paraldehyde; Phenytoin; Pramipexole; ROPINIRole; Rotigotine; Selective Serotonin Reuptake Inhibitors; Sodium Oxybate; Zolpidem

The levels/effects of Temazepam may be increased by: Droperidol; HydrOXYzine; Magnesium Sulfate; Methotrimeprazine; OLANZapine; Perampanel

Decreased Effect

The levels/effects of Temazepam may be decreased by: Theophylline Derivatives; Yohimbine

Ethanol/Nutrition/Herb Interactions

Ethanol: May increase CNS depression; monitor for increased effects with coadministration. Caution patients about effects.

Food: Serum levels may be increased by grapefruit juice.

Herb/Nutraceutical: St John's wort may decrease temazepam levels. Avoid valerian, St John's wort, kava kava, gotu kola (may increase CNS depression).

Pharmacodynamics/Kinetics

Half-life Elimination 9.5-12.4 hours

Time to Peak Serum: 2-3 hours

Pregnancy Risk Factor X

Pregnancy Considerations Adverse events were observed in animal reproduction studies. Although information specific to the use of temazepam has not been located, all benzodiazepines are assumed to cross the placenta. Teratogenic effects have been observed with some benzodiazepines; however, additional studies are needed. The incidence of premature birth and low birth weights may be increased following maternal use of benzodiazepines; hypoglycemia and respiratory problems in the neonate may occur following exposure late in pregnancy. Neonatal withdrawal symptoms may occur within days to weeks after birth and "floppy infant syndrome" (which also includes withdrawal symptoms) have been reported with some benzodiazepines. Use during pregnancy is contraindicated.

Lactation Enters breast milk/use caution (AAP rates "of concern"; AAP 2001 update pending)

Breast-Feeding Considerations Information is available from a study conducted in 10 nursing women, <2 weeks postpartum. All women were given temazepam 10-20 mg at bedtime for ≥2 nights. Samples were obtained 10-21 hours after a dose. Temazepam was not found in the milk of nine mothers (maternal serum concentrations 8-59 mcg/L). Temazepam was detected in the milk of one patient whose serum concentration was 234 mcg/mL at ~14 hours after the dose; milk concentrations were 28 mcg/L (pre-feed) and 26 mcg/L (post-feed). Oxazepam concentrations were 9 mcg/mL in the maternal serum and below the limit of detection in breast milk. Adverse events were not noted in any nursing infants. Drowsiness, lethargy, or weight loss in nursing infants have been observed in case reports following maternal use of some benzodiazepines.

Controlled Substance C-IV

Dosage Forms

Capsule, oral: 7.5 mg, 15 mg, 22.5 mg, 30 mg
Restoril™: 7.5 mg, 15 mg, 22.5 mg, 30 mg

Temozolomide (te moe ZOE loe mide)

Brand Names: U.S. Temodar®

Brand Names: Canada Ahi-Temozolomide Capsules; Temodal®

Pharmacologic Category Antineoplastic Agent, Alkylating Agent (Triazene)

Use Treatment of newly-diagnosed glioblastoma multiforme (initially in combination with radiotherapy, then as maintenance treatment); treatment of refractory anaplastic astrocytoma

Canadian labeling (not an approved indication in the U.S.): Treatment of recurrent or progressive glioblastoma multiforme

Unlabeled Use Treatment of recurrent glioblastoma multiforme, low-grade astrocytoma, low-grade oligodendroglioma, anaplastic oligodendroglioma, metastatic CNS lesions, refractory primary CNS lymphoma, advanced or metastatic melanoma, cutaneous T-cell lymphomas (mycosis fungoides [MF] and Sézary syndrome [SS]), advanced neuroendocrine tumors (carcinoid or islet cell), Ewing's sarcoma (recurrent or progressive), soft tissue sarcomas (extremity/retroperitoneal/intra-abdominal or hemangiopericytoma/solitary fibrous tumor), treatment of pediatric neuroblastoma

Local Anesthetic/Vasoconstrictor Precautions No information available to require special precautions

Effects on Dental Treatment Key adverse event(s) related to dental treatment: Stomatitis, dysphagia, and taste perversion.

Effects on Bleeding Chemotherapy may result in significant myelosuppression, potentially including significant reduction in platelet counts and altered hemostasis. In patients who are under active treatment with these agents, medical consult is suggested.

Adverse Effects Note: With CNS malignancies, it may be difficult to distinguish between CNS adverse events caused by temozolomide versus the effects of progressive disease.

>10%:

Cardiovascular: Peripheral edema (11%)

Central nervous system: Fatigue (34% to 61%), headache (23% to 41%), seizure (6% to 23%), hemiparesis (18%), fever (13%), dizziness (5% to 12%), coordination abnormality (11%)

Dermatologic: Alopecia (55%), rash (8% to 13%)

Gastrointestinal: Nausea (49% to 53%; grades 3/4: 1% to 10%), vomiting (29% to 42%; grades 3/4: 2% to 6%), constipation (22% to 33%), anorexia (9% to 27%), diarrhea (10% to 16%)

Hematologic: Lymphopenia (grades 3/4: 55%), thrombocytopenia (grades 3/4: adults: 4% to 19%; children: 25%), neutropenia (grades 3/4: adults: 8% to 14%; children: 20%), leukopenia (grades 3/4: 11%)

Neuromuscular & skeletal: Weakness (7% to 13%)

Miscellaneous: Viral infection (11%)

1% to 10%:

Central nervous system: Amnesia (10%), insomnia (4% to 10%), somnolence (9%), ataxia (8%), paresis (8%), anxiety (7%), memory impairment (7%), depression (6%), confusion (5%)

Dermatologic: Pruritus (5% to 8%), dry skin (5%), radiation injury (2% maintenance phase after radiotherapy), erythema (1%)

Endocrine & metabolic: Hypercorticism (8%), breast pain (females 6%)

Gastrointestinal: Stomatitis (9%), abdominal pain (5% to 9%), dysphagia (7%), taste perversion (5%), weight gain (5%)

Genitourinary: Incontinence (8%), urinary tract infection (8%), urinary frequency (6%)

Hematologic: Anemia (grades 3/4: 4%)

Neuromuscular & skeletal: Paresthesia (9%), back pain (8%), abnormal gait (6%), arthralgia (6%), myalgia (5%)

Ocular: Blurred vision (5% to 8%), diplopia (5%), vision abnormality (visual deficit/vision changes 5%)

Respiratory: Pharyngitis (8%), upper respiratory tract infection (8%), cough (5% to 8%), sinusitis (6%), dyspnea (5%)

Miscellaneous: Allergic reaction (≤3%)

General Dosage Range Dosage adjustment recommended in patients who develop toxicities.

I.V., Oral: *Adults:* Dosage varies greatly depending on indication

Mechanism of Action Temozolomide is a prodrug which is rapidly and nonenzymatically converted to the active alkylating metabolite MTIC [(methyl-triazene-1-yl)-imidazole-4-carboxamide]; this conversion is spontaneous, nonenzymatic, and occurs under physiologic conditions in all tissues to which it distributes. The cytotoxic effects of MTIC are manifested through alkylation (methylation) of DNA at the O^6, N^7 guanine positions which lead to DNA double strand breaks and apoptosis. Non-cell cycle specific.

Pharmacodynamics/Kinetics

Half-life Elimination Mean: Parent drug: 1.8 hours

Time to Peak Oral: Empty stomach: 1 hour; with food (high-fat meal): 2.25 hours

Pregnancy Risk Factor D

Pregnancy Considerations May cause fetal harm when administered to pregnant women. Animal studies, at doses less than used in humans, resulted in numerous birth defects. Testicular toxicity was demonstrated in animal studies using smaller doses than recommended for cancer treatment. There are no adequate and well-controlled studies in pregnant women. Male and female patients should avoid pregnancy while receiving drug.

Temsirolimus (tem sir OH li mus)

Brand Names: U.S. Torisel®

Brand Names: Canada Torisel®

Pharmacologic Category Antineoplastic Agent, mTOR Kinase Inhibitor

Use Treatment of advanced renal cell cancer (RCC)

Local Anesthetic/Vasoconstrictor Precautions No information available to require special precautions

Effects on Dental Treatment Key adverse event(s) related to dental treatment: Effects on oral cavity including mucositis, stomatitis, and taste disturbances.

Effects on Bleeding Thrombocytopenia has been associated with use; severe thrombocytopenia (grades 3/4: 1%) may be associated with delayed coagulation. Consultation to ensure adequate platelet counts may be considered in patients with signs/symptoms or a history of thrombocytopenia.

Adverse Effects

>10%:

Cardiovascular: Edema (35%), peripheral edema (27%), chest pain (16%)

Central nervous system: Pain (28%), fever (24%), headache (15%), insomnia (12%)

Dermatologic: Rash (47%), pruritus (19%), nail disorder/thinning (14%), dry skin (11%)

Endocrine & metabolic: Hyperglycemia (26% to 89%; grades 3/4: 16%), hypercholesterolemia (24% to 87%; grades 3/4: 2%), hypertriglyceridemia (83%; grades 3/4: 44%), hypophosphatemia (49%; grades 3/4: 18%), hyperlipidemia (27%), hypokalemia (21%; grades 3/4: 5%)

Gastrointestinal: Mucositis (41%), nausea (37%), anorexia (32%), diarrhea (27%), abdominal pain (21%), constipation (20%), stomatitis (20%), taste disturbance (20%), vomiting (19%), weight loss (19%)

Genitourinary: Urinary tract infection (15%)

Hematologic: Anemia (45% to 94%; grades 3/4: 20%), lymphopenia (53%; grades 3/4: 16%), thrombocytopenia (14% to 40%; grades 3/4: 1%; dose-limiting toxicity), leukopenia (6% to 32%; grades 3/4: 1%), neutropenia (7% to 19%; grades 3/4: 3% to 5%)

Hepatic: Alkaline phosphatase increased (68%; grades 3/4: 3%), AST increased (8% to 38%; grades 3/4: 1% to 2%)

Neuromuscular & skeletal: Weakness (51%), back pain (20%), arthralgia (18%)

Renal: Creatinine increased (14% to 57%; grades 3/4: 3%)

Respiratory: Dyspnea (28%), cough (26%), epistaxis (12%), pharyngitis (12%)

Miscellaneous: Infection (20% to 27%; includes abscess, bronchitis, cellulitis, herpes simplex, herpes zoster)

1% to 10%:

Cardiovascular: Hypertension, thrombophlebitis, venous thromboembolism (includes DVT and PE)

Central nervous system: Chills, depression
Dermatologic: Acne, wound healing impaired
Gastrointestinal: Bowel perforation
Hepatic: Hyperbilirubinemia
Neuromuscular & skeletal: Myalgia
Ocular: Conjunctivitis
Respiratory: Interstitial lung disease (ILD), pneumonia, rhinitis, upper respiratory tract infection
Miscellaneous: Allergic/hypersensitivity/infusion reaction (includes anaphylaxis, apnea, chest pain, dyspnea, flushing, hypotension, loss of consciousness)

General Dosage Range Dosage adjustment recommended in patients with hepatic impairment, on concomitant therapy, or who develop toxicities
I.V.: *Adults:* 25 mg once weekly

Mechanism of Action Temsirolimus and its active metabolite, sirolimus, are targeted inhibitors of mTOR (mammalian target of rapamycin) kinase activity. Temsirolimus (and sirolimus) bind to FKBP-12, an intracellular protein, to form a complex which inhibits mTOR signaling, halting the cell cycle at the G1 phase in tumor cells. In renal cell carcinoma, mTOR inhibition also exhibits anti-angiogenesis activity by reducing levels of HIF-1 and HIF-2 alpha (hypoxia inducible factors) and vascular endothelial growth factor (VEGF).

Pharmacodynamics/Kinetics
Half-life Elimination Temsirolimus: ~17 hours; Sirolimus: ~55 hours
Time to Peak Temsirolimus: At end of infusion; Sirolimus: 0.5-2 hours after temsirolimus infusion

Pregnancy Risk Factor D
Pregnancy Considerations Embryotoxicity and fetotoxicity (as evidenced by increased mortality, reduced fetal weights, and delayed ossification) occurred in animal reproduction studies at oral doses lower than the usual human dose. Women of childbearing potential should be advised to avoid pregnancy. Men and women should use effective birth control during temsirolimus treatment, and continue for 3 months after temsirolimus discontinuation.

Tenecteplase (ten EK te plase)

Related Information
Cardiovascular Diseases *on page 1492*
Brand Names: U.S. TNKase®
Brand Names: Canada TNKase®
Pharmacologic Category Thrombolytic Agent
Use Management of ST-elevation myocardial infarction (STEMI) for the lysis of thrombi in the coronary vasculature to restore perfusion and reduce mortality.
Recommended criteria for treatment of STEMI (ACCF/AHA; O'Gara, 2013): Ischemic symptoms within 12 hours of treatment or evidence of ongoing ischemia 12-24 hours after symptom onset with a large area of myocardium at risk or hemodynamic instability.
STEMI ECG definition: New ST-segment elevation at the J point in at least 2 contiguous leads of ≥2 mm (0.2 mV) in men or ≥1.5 mm (0.15 mV) in women in leads V_2-V_3 and/or of ≥1 mm (0.1 mV) in other contiguous precordial leads or limb leads on ECG. New or presumably new left bundle branch block (LBBB) may interfere with ST-elevation analysis and should not be considered diagnostic in isolation.
At non-PCI-capable hospitals, the ACCF/AHA recommends thrombolytic therapy administration when the anticipated first medical contact (FMC)-to-device time at a PCI-capable hospital is >120 minutes due to unavoidable delays.

Local Anesthetic/Vasoconstrictor Precautions No information available to require special precautions
Effects on Dental Treatment Key adverse event(s) related to dental treatment: Bleeding is the most frequent adverse effect of tenecteplase. See Effects on Bleeding.
Effects on Bleeding Bleeding is the most frequent adverse effect associated with tenecteplase. It is unlikely that ambulatory patients presenting for dental treatment will be taking intravenous anticoagulant therapy.
Adverse Effects As with all drugs which may affect hemostasis, bleeding is the major adverse effect associated with tenecteplase. Hemorrhage may occur at virtually any site. Risk is dependent on multiple variables, including the dosage administered, concurrent use of multiple agents which alter hemostasis, and patient predisposition. Rapid lysis of coronary artery thrombi by thrombolytic agents may be associated with reperfusion-related arterial and/or ventricular arrhythmia. The incidence of stroke and bleeding increase in patients >65 years.

>10%:
Hematologic: Bleeding (22% minor: ASSENT-2 trial)
Local: Hematoma (12% minor)
1% to 10%:
Central nervous system: Stroke (2%)
Gastrointestinal: Epistaxis (2% minor), GI hemorrhage (1% major, 2% minor)
Genitourinary: GU bleeding (4% minor)
Hematologic: Bleeding (5% major: ASSENT-2 trial)
Local: Bleeding at catheter puncture site (4% minor), hematoma (2% minor)
Respiratory: Pharyngeal bleeding (3% minor)
Additional cardiovascular events associated with use in MI: Arrhythmia, AV block, cardiac arrest, cardiac tamponade, cardiogenic shock, embolism, electromechanical dissociation, fever, heart failure, hypotension, mitral regurgitation, myocardial reinfarction, myocardial rupture, nausea, pericardial effusion, pericarditis, pulmonary edema, recurrent myocardial ischemia, thrombosis, vomiting

General Dosage Range I.V.:
Adults <60 kg: 30 mg as a single dose
Adults ≥60 to <70 kg: 35 mg as a single dose
Adults ≥70 to <80 kg: 40 mg as a single dose
Adults ≥80 to <90 kg: 45 mg as a single dose
Adults ≥90 kg: 50 mg as a single dose

Mechanism of Action Promotes initiation of fibrinolysis by binding to fibrin and converting plasminogen to plasmin. Tenecteplase is essentially alteplase with the exception of 3 point mutations and is more fibrin specific, more resistant to plasminogen activator inhibitor -1 (PAI-1), with a longer duration of action compared to alteplase. Produced by recombinant DNA technology using a mammalian cell line (Chinese hamster ovary cells).

Pharmacodynamics/Kinetics
Half-life Elimination Biphasic: Initial: 20-24 minutes; Terminal: 90-130 minutes

Pregnancy Risk Factor C
Pregnancy Considerations Adverse events have been observed in some animal reproduction studies. The risk of bleeding may be increased in pregnant women. Administer to pregnant women only if the potential benefits justify the risk to the fetus.

Teniposide (ten i POE side)

Brand Names: U.S. Vumon®
Brand Names: Canada Vumon®
Pharmacologic Category Antineoplastic Agent, Podophyllotoxin Derivative
Use Treatment of refractory childhood acute lymphoblastic leukemia (ALL) in combination with other chemotherapy
Unlabeled Use Treatment of refractory acute lymphoblastic leukemia (ALL) in adults
Local Anesthetic/Vasoconstrictor Precautions No information available to require special precautions
Effects on Dental Treatment Key adverse event(s) related to dental treatment: Mucositis.
Effects on Bleeding Chemotherapy may result in significant myelosuppression, including significant thrombocytopenia (85%), and altered hemostasis. In patients who are under active treatment with these agents, medical consult is suggested.
Adverse Effects
>10%:
   Gastrointestinal: Mucositis (76%), diarrhea (33%), nausea/vomiting (29%; mild to moderate)
   Hematologic: Neutropenia (95%), leukopenia (89%), anemia (88%), thrombocytopenia (85%), myelosuppression (75%)
   Miscellaneous: Infection (12%)
1% to 10%:
   Cardiovascular: Hypotension (2%; associated with rapid [<30 minutes] infusions)
   Central nervous system: Fever (3%)
   Dermatologic: Alopecia (9%; usually reversible), rash (3%)
   Hematologic: Bleeding (5%)
   Miscellaneous: Hypersensitivity reactions (5%; includes bronchospasm, chills, dyspnea, fever, flushing, hyper-/hypotension, tachycardia, or urticaria)
General Dosage Range I.V.: *Children:* 165 mg/m^2 twice weekly for 8-9 doses **or** 250 mg/m^2 weekly for 4-8 weeks
Mechanism of Action Teniposide does not inhibit microtubular assembly; it has been shown to delay transit of cells through the S phase and arrest cells in late S or early G$_2$ phase, preventing cells from entering mitosis. Teniposide is a topoisomerase II inhibitor, and appears to cause DNA strand breaks by inhibition of strand-passing and DNA ligase action.
Pharmacodynamics/Kinetics
Half-life Elimination Children: 5 hours
Pregnancy Risk Factor D
Pregnancy Considerations Adverse effects were observed in animal reproduction studies. May cause fetal harm if administered during pregnancy. Women of childbearing potential should avoid becoming pregnant during teniposide treatment.

Tenofovir (te NOE fo veer)

Related Information
HIV Infection and AIDS *on page 1520*
Systemic Viral Diseases *on page 1537*
Brand Names: U.S. Viread®
Brand Names: Canada Viread®
Pharmacologic Category Antiretroviral Agent, Reverse Transcriptase Inhibitor (Nucleotide)

Use
U.S. labeling: Management of HIV infections in combination with at least two other antiretroviral agents in patients ≥2 years of age; treatment of chronic hepatitis B virus (HBV) in patients with compensated or decompensated liver disease in patients ≥12 years of age

Canadian labeling: Management of HIV infections in combination with at least two other antiretroviral agents in patients ≥12 years of age; treatment of chronic hepatitis B virus (HBV) in patients with compensated or decompensated liver disease in patients ≥18 years of age
Local Anesthetic/Vasoconstrictor Precautions No information available to require special precautions
Effects on Dental Treatment No significant effects or complications reported
Effects on Bleeding No information available to require special precautions regarding hemostasis.
Adverse Effects Frequencies listed are treatment-emergent adverse effects noted at higher frequency than in the placebo group or comparator group. Only adverse events from treatment-naive studies which varied significantly were noted (eg, rash event). Patients treated for chronic hepatitis B had similar reactions and frequencies.

>10%:
   Central nervous system: Insomnia (3% to 4%; decompensated liver disease 18%), pain (7% to 13%), dizziness (3%; treatment naive 8%; decompensated liver disease 13%), depression (4% to 8%; treatment naive 9% to 11%), fever (2% to 4%; treatment naive 8%; decompensated liver disease 11%)
   Dermatologic: Rash event (includes maculopapular, pustular, or vesiculobullous rash, pruritus or urticaria 5% to 7%; treatment naive 18%)
   Endocrine & metabolic: Triglycerides increased (grades 3/4: 11%; treatment naive 4%)
   Gastrointestinal: Abdominal pain (4% to 7%; decompensated liver disease 22%), nausea (8% to 11%; decompensated liver disease 20%), diarrhea (11% to 16%), vomiting (4% to 7%; decompensated liver disease 13%)
   Neuromuscular & skeletal: Creatine kinase increased (9% to 12%), weakness (7% to 11%)
1% to 10%:
   Cardiovascular: Chest pain (3%)
   Central nervous system: Fatigue (9%), headache (5% to 8%), anxiety (6%)
   Endocrine & metabolic: Hyperglycemia (grades 3/4: 3%)
   Gastrointestinal: Serum amylase increased (grades 3/4: 4% to 7%; treatment naive 8% to 9%), anorexia (3% to 4%), dyspepsia (3% to 4%), flatulence (3% to 4%), weight loss (2% to 4%)
   Genitourinary: Hematuria (grades 3/4: 3% to 7%)
   Hematologic: Neutropenia (1% to 3%)
   Hepatic: Transaminases increased (2% to 5%), alkaline phosphatase increased (1%)
   Neuromuscular & skeletal: Back pain (3% to 4%; treatment naive 9%), peripheral neuropathy (3% to 5%), myalgia (3% to 4%)
   Renal: Serum creatinine increased (decompensated liver disease 9%), renal failure (decompensated liver disease 7%), glycosuria (grades 3/4: 3%)
   Respiratory: Upper respiratory tract infection (8%), sinusitis (8%), nasopharyngitis (5%), pneumonia (2% to 3%; treatment naive 5%)
   Miscellaneous: Diaphoresis (3%)

General Dosage Range Dosage adjustment recommended in patients with renal impairment

Oral:

Children 2 to <12 years: 8 mg/kg once daily (maximum: 300 mg once daily)

Children ≥12 years (and ≥35 kg), Adolescents, and Adults: 300 mg once daily

Mechanism of Action Tenofovir disoproxil fumarate (TDF) is an analog of adenosine 5'-monophosphate; it interferes with the HIV viral RNA dependent DNA polymerase resulting in inhibition of viral replication. TDF is first converted intracellularly by hydrolysis to tenofovir and subsequently phosphorylated to the active tenofovir diphosphate; nucleotide reverse transcriptase inhibitor. Tenofovir inhibits replication of HBV by inhibiting HBV polymerase.

Pharmacodynamics/Kinetics

Half-life Elimination ~17 hours

Time to Peak Serum: Fasting: 36-84 minutes; With food: 96-144 minutes

Pregnancy Risk Factor B

Pregnancy Considerations Adverse events were not observed in rat and rabbit reproduction studies. Decreased fetal growth and reduced fetal bone porosity were observed in monkeys. Clinical studies in children have shown bone demineralization with chronic use. Tenofovir crosses the human placenta. No increased risk of overall birth defects has been observed following first trimester exposure according to data collected by the antiretroviral pregnancy registry. Limited data indicate decreased maternal bioavailability during the third trimester. Cases of lactic acidosis/hepatic steatosis syndrome related to mitochondrial toxicity have been reported in pregnant women with prolonged use of nucleoside analogues. It is not known if pregnancy itself potentiates this known side effect; however, women may be at increased risk of lactic acidosis and liver damage. In addition, these adverse events are similar to other rare but life-threatening syndromes which occur during pregnancy (eg, HELLP syndrome). Hepatic enzymes and electrolytes should be monitored in women receiving nucleoside analogues and clinicians should watch for early signs of the syndrome. In addition, mitochondrial dysfunction may develop in infants following *in utero* exposure. Renal function should also be monitored. The DHHS Perinatal HIV Guidelines consider tenofovir to be an alternative NRTI in dual nucleoside combination regimens. The DHHS Perinatal HIV Guidelines consider emtricitabine plus tenofovir, or lamivudine plus tenofovir as recommended dual NRTI/NtRTI backbones for HIV/HBV coinfected pregnant women. Hepatitis B flare may occur if tenofovir is discontinued postpartum.

Regardless of CD4 count or HIV RNA copy number, all HIV-infected pregnant women should receive a combination antepartum antiretroviral (ARV) drug regimen; this includes women who require therapy for their own health, as well as women who do not yet require therapy for their own health. ARV therapy should be started as soon as possible if required for the woman's health. Although earlier initiation may be more effective in reducing the perinatal transmission of HIV), also consider maternal conditions (eg, nausea and vomiting) and the potential risks of first trimester fetal exposure for specific agents. Plasma HIV RNA levels should be assessed at ~34-36 weeks gestation in order to help determine mode of delivery. If ARV therapy must be interrupted for <24 hours during the peripartum period, stop then restart all medications simultaneously in order to decrease the chance of developing resistance. Long-term follow-up is recommended for all infants exposed to ARV medications.

Healthcare providers are encouraged to enroll pregnant women exposed to antiretroviral medications in the Antiretroviral Pregnancy Registry (1-800-258-4263 or www.APRegistry.com). Healthcare providers caring for HIV-infected women and their infants may contact the National Perinatal HIV Hotline (888-448-8765) for clinical consultation (DHHS [perinatal], 2012).

Terazosin (ter AY zoe sin)

Related Information

Cardiovascular Diseases *on page 1492*

Brand Names: Canada Apo-Terazosin®; Dom-Terazosin; Hytrin®; Nu-Terazosin; PHL-Terazosin; PMS-Terazosin; ratio-Terazosin; Teva-Terazosin

Generic Availability (U.S.) Yes

Pharmacologic Category Alpha$_1$ Blocker

Use Management of mild-to-moderate hypertension; alone or in combination with other agents such as diuretics or beta-blockers; benign prostate hyperplasia (BPH)

Unlabeled Use Pediatric hypertension

Local Anesthetic/Vasoconstrictor Precautions No information available to require special precautions

Effects on Dental Treatment Key adverse event(s) related to dental treatment: Xerostomia (normal salivary flow resumes upon discontinuation) and orthostatic hypotension.

Effects on Bleeding No information available to require special precautions

Adverse Effects

>10%:

Central nervous system: Dizziness (9% to 19%)

Neuromuscular & skeletal: Muscle weakness (7% to 11%)

1% to 10%:

Cardiovascular: Peripheral edema (1% to 6%), orthostatic hypotension (1% to 4%), palpitation (≤4%), tachycardia (≤2%), syncope (≤1%

Central nervous system: Somnolence (4% to 5%), vertigo (1%)

Gastrointestinal: Nausea (2% to 4%), weight gain (≤1%)

Genitourinary: Impotence (≤2%), libido decreased (≤1%)

Neuromuscular & skeletal: Extremity pain (≤4%), paresthesia (≤3%), back pain (≤2%)

Ocular: Blurred vision (≤2%)

Respiratory: Nasal congestion (2% to 6%), dyspnea (2% to 3%), sinusitis (≤3%)

Dosage Oral: **Note:** If drug is discontinued for greater than several days, consider beginning with initial dose and retitrate as needed.

Hypertension:

Children (unlabeled use): Initial: 1 mg once daily; gradually increase dose as necessary, up to maximum of 20 mg/day

Adults: Initial: 1 mg at bedtime; slowly increase dose to achieve desired blood pressure, up to 20 mg/day; usual dose range (JNC 7): 1-20 mg once daily. **Note:** Dosage may be given on a twice daily regimen if response is diminished at 24 hours and hypotension is observed at 2-4 hours following a dose.

Elderly: Consider lower initial doses (eg, immediate release: 0.5 mg once daily) and titrate to response (Aronow, 2011)

Benign prostatic hyperplasia: Adults: Initial: 1 mg at bedtime; thereafter, titrate upwards, if needed, over several weeks, balancing therapeutic benefit with terazosin-induced postural hypotension; most patients require 10 mg day; if no response after 4-6 weeks of 10 mg/day, may increase to 20 mg/day

Dosage adjustment with concurrent medication:
Concurrent use with a diuretic or other antihypertensive agent (especially verapamil): Dosage reduction may be needed when adding
Concurrent use with PDE-5 inhibitors: Initiate PDE-5 inhibitor therapy at the lowest dose due to additive orthostatic and blood pressure lowering effects

Dosage adjustment in renal impairment: No dosage adjustment necessary.
Hemodialysis: No supplemental dose necessary.
Dosage adjustment in hepatic impairment: No dosage adjustment provided in manufacturer's labeling.
Mechanism of Action Alpha$_1$-specific blocking agent with minimal alpha$_2$ effects; this allows peripheral postsynaptic blockade, with the resultant decrease in arterial tone, while preserving the negative feedback loop which is mediated by the peripheral presynaptic alpha$_2$-receptors; terazosin relaxes the smooth muscle of the bladder neck, thus reducing bladder outlet obstruction
Contraindications Hypersensitivity to terazosin or any component of the formulation
Warnings/Precautions Can cause significant orthostatic hypotension and syncope, especially with first dose; anticipate a similar effect if therapy is interrupted for a few days, if dosage is rapidly increased, or if another antihypertensive drug (particularly vasodilators) or a PDE-5 inhibitor is introduced. Discontinue if symptoms of angina occur or worsen. Patients should be cautioned about performing hazardous tasks when starting new therapy or adjusting dosage upward. Prostate cancer should be ruled out before starting for BPH. Intraoperative floppy iris syndrome has been observed in cataract surgery patients who were on or were previously treated with alpha$_1$-blockers. Causality has not been established and there appears to be no benefit in discontinuing alpha-blocker therapy prior to surgery. Priapism has been associated with use (rarely). In the elderly, avoid use as an antihypertensive due to high risk of orthostatic hypotension; alternative agents preferred due to a more favorable risk/benefit profile (Beers Criteria).
Drug Interactions
Metabolism/Transport Effects None known.
Avoid Concomitant Use
Avoid concomitant use of Terazosin with any of the following: Alpha1-Blockers
Increased Effect/Toxicity
Terazosin may increase the levels/effects of: Alpha1-Blockers; Amifostine; Antihypertensives; Calcium Channel Blockers; Hypotensive Agents; RiTUXimab

The levels/effects of Terazosin may be increased by: Beta-Blockers; Diazoxide; Herbs (Hypotensive Properties); MAO Inhibitors; Pentoxifylline; Phosphodiesterase 5 Inhibitors; Prostacyclin Analogues
Decreased Effect
Terazosin may decrease the levels/effects of: Alpha-/Beta-Agonists; Alpha1-Agonists

The levels/effects of Terazosin may be decreased by: Herbs (Hypertensive Properties); Methylphenidate; Yohimbine

Ethanol/Nutrition/Herb Interactions Herb/Nutraceutical: Avoid dong quai if using for hypertension (has estrogenic activity). Avoid ephedra, yohimbe, ginseng (may worsen hypertension). Avoid saw palmetto. Avoid garlic (may have increased antihypertensive effect).
Dietary Considerations May be taken without regard to meals at the same time each day.
Pharmacodynamics/Kinetics
Onset of Action 1-2 hours
Half-life Elimination ~12 hours
Time to Peak Serum: ~1 hour
Pregnancy Risk Factor C
Pregnancy Considerations Teratogenic effects have not been observed in animal studies. Decreased fetal weight and increased risk of fetal mortality were noted in some animal reproduction studies. There are no adequate and well-controlled studies in pregnant women. Use only if benefit outweighs risk.
Lactation Excretion in breast milk unknown/use caution
Breast-Feeding Considerations It is not known if terazosin is excreted in breast milk. The manufacturer recommends that caution be exercised when administering terazosin to nursing women.
Dosage Forms
Capsule, oral: 1 mg, 2 mg, 5 mg, 10 mg

Terbinafine (Systemic) (TER bin a feen)

Brand Names: U.S. LamISIL®; Terbinex™
Brand Names: Canada Apo-Terbinafine®; Auro-Terbinafine; CO Terbinafine; Dom-Terbinafine; GD-Terbinafine; JAMP-Terbinafine; Lamisil®; Mylan-Terbinafine; Nu-Terbinafine; PHL-Terbinafine; PMS-Terbinafine; Q-Terbinafine; Riva-Terbinafine; Sandoz-Terbinafine; Teva-Terbinafine
Pharmacologic Category Antifungal Agent, Oral
Use Treatment of onychomycosis of the toenail or fingernail due to susceptible dermatophytes; treatment of tinea capitis

Canadian labeling: Additional use (not in U.S. labeling): Severe tineal skin infections unresponsive to topical therapy
Local Anesthetic/Vasoconstrictor Precautions No information available to require special precautions
Effects on Dental Treatment Key adverse event(s) related to dental treatment: Taste disturbance.
Effects on Bleeding No information available to require special precautions
Adverse Effects Adverse events listed for tablets unless otherwise specified. Granules were studied in patients 4-12 years of age.
>10%: Central nervous system: Headache (13%; granules 7%)
1% to 10%:
Central nervous system: Fever (granules 7%)
Dermatologic: Rash (6%; granules 2%), pruritus (3%; granules 1%), urticaria (1%)
Gastrointestinal: Diarrhea (6%; granules 3%), vomiting (<1%; granules 5%), dyspepsia (4%), taste disturbance (3%), abdominal pain (2%; granules 2% to 4%), nausea (granules 2%), toothache (granules 1%)
Hepatic: Liver enzyme abnormalities (3%)
Respiratory: Nasopharyngitis (granules 10%), cough (granules 6%), upper respiratory tract infection (granules 5%), nasal congestion (granules 2%), pharyngeal pain (granules 2%), rhinorrhea (granules 2%)
Miscellaneous: Influenza (granules 2%)

General Dosage Range

Oral granules: *Children ≥4 years:*
<25 kg: 125 mg once daily for 6 weeks
25-35 kg: 187.5 mg once daily for 6 weeks
>35 kg: 250 mg once daily for 6 weeks
Oral tablet: *Adults:* 250 mg once daily for 6-12 weeks

Mechanism of Action Synthetic allylamine derivative which inhibits squalene epoxidase, a key enzyme in sterol biosynthesis in fungi. This results in a deficiency in ergosterol within the fungal cell wall and results in fungal cell death.

Pharmacodynamics/Kinetics

Half-life Elimination Terminal half-life: 200-400 hours; very slow release of drug from skin and adipose tissues occurs; effective half-life: ~36 hours; Children: 27-31 hours

Time to Peak Plasma: Within 2 hours

Pregnancy Risk Factor B

Pregnancy Considerations Adverse events were not observed in animal reproduction studies. Avoid use in pregnancy since treatment of onychomycosis is postponable.

Terbutaline (ter BYOO ta leen)

Brand Names: Canada Bricanyl® Turbuhaler®
Pharmacologic Category Beta$_2$ Agonist
Use Bronchodilator in reversible airway obstruction and bronchial asthma
Unlabeled Use Injection: Tocolytic agent (short-term [≤72 hours]) prevention or management of preterm labor
Local Anesthetic/Vasoconstrictor Precautions No information available to require special precautions
Effects on Dental Treatment Key adverse event(s) related to dental treatment: Xerostomia (normal salivary flow resumes upon discontinuation) and bad taste in mouth.
Effects on Bleeding No information available to require special precautions

Adverse Effects
>10%:
Central nervous system: Nervousness, restlessness
Endocrine & metabolic: Serum glucose increased, serum potassium decreased
Neuromuscular & skeletal: Trembling
1% to 10%:
Cardiovascular: Tachycardia, hypertension
Central nervous system: Dizziness, drowsiness, headache, insomnia
Gastrointestinal: Xerostomia, nausea, vomiting, bad taste in mouth
Neuromuscular & skeletal: Muscle cramps, weakness
Miscellaneous: Diaphoresis

General Dosage Range Dosage adjustment recommended in patients with renal impairment
Oral:
Children 12-15 years: 2.5 mg every 6 hours 3 times/day (maximum: 7.5 mg/day)
Children >15 years and Adults: 2.5-5 mg every 6 hours 3 times/day (maximum: 15 mg/day)
SubQ:
Children <12 years: 0.005-0.01 mg/kg/dose to a maximum of 0.4 mg/dose; may repeat in 15-20 minutes
Children ≥12 years and Adults: 0.25 mg/dose; may repeat in 15-30 minutes (maximum: 0.5 mg/4-hour period)

Mechanism of Action Relaxes bronchial and uterine smooth muscle by action on beta$_2$-receptors with less effect on heart rate

Pharmacodynamics/Kinetics

Onset of Action Oral: 30-45 minutes; SubQ: 6-15 minutes; Inhalation: 5 minutes (maximum effect: 15-60 minutes)

Duration of Action Inhalation: 4-7 hours

Half-life Elimination 11-16 hours

Pregnancy Risk Factor C

Pregnancy Considerations Adverse events have been observed in animal reproduction studies. Terbutaline crosses the placenta; umbilical cord concentrations are ~11% to 48% of maternal blood levels. **[U.S. Boxed Warning]:** Terbutaline is not FDA approved for and should not be used for prolonged tocolysis (>48-72 hours). Use for maintenance tocolysis should not be done in the outpatient setting. Adverse events observed in pregnant women include arrhythmias, increased heart rate, hyperglycemia (transient), hypokalemia, myocardial ischemia, and pulmonary edema. Heart rate may be increased in the fetus and hypoglycemia may occur in the neonate. Terbutaline has been used in the management of preterm labor. Tocolytics may be used for the short-term (48 hour) prolongation of pregnancy to allow for the administration of antenatal steroids and should not be used prior to fetal viability or when the risks of use to the fetus or mother are greater than the risk of preterm birth (ACOG, 2012).

Terconazole (ter KONE a zole)

Brand Names: U.S. Terazol® 3; Terazol® 7
Brand Names: Canada Terazol®
Pharmacologic Category Antifungal Agent, Vaginal
Use Local treatment of vulvovaginal candidiasis
Local Anesthetic/Vasoconstrictor Precautions No information available to require special precautions
Effects on Dental Treatment No significant effects or complications reported
Effects on Bleeding No information available to require special precautions

Adverse Effects
>10%: Central nervous system: Headache
1% to 10%:
Central nervous system: Chills, fever, pain
Gastrointestinal: Abdominal pain
Genitourinary: Dysmenorrhea; vulvar/vaginal burning, irritation, or itching

General Dosage Range Intravaginal: *Adults:* Insert 1 applicatorful or suppository at bedtime

Mechanism of Action Triazole ketal antifungal agent; involves inhibition of fungal cytochrome P450. Specifically, terconazole inhibits cytochrome P450-dependent 14-alpha-demethylase which results in accumulation of membrane disturbing 14-alpha-demethylsterols and ergosterol depletion.

Pregnancy Risk Factor C

Pregnancy Considerations Following vaginal administration, terconazole is absorbed systemically; use should be avoided during the first trimester of pregnancy. Although the manufacturer recommends that use should be avoided during the first trimester of pregnancy due to systemic absorption, vaginal products may be considered for the treatment of vulvovaginal candidiasis in pregnant women (CDC, 2010). This product may weaken latex condoms and diaphragms (CDC, 2010).

Teriflunomide (ter i FLOO noh mide)

Brand Names: U.S. Aubagio®

Pharmacologic Category Pyrimidine Synthesis Inhibitor

Use Treatment of relapsing forms of multiple sclerosis (MS)

Local Anesthetic/Vasoconstrictor Precautions Use vasoconstrictor with caution; patients may experience significant hypertension and palpitations when taking teriflunomide

Effects on Dental Treatment Key adverse event(s) related to dental treatment: Abnormal taste, aphthous stomatitis, and toothache have been reported.

Effects on Bleeding Thrombocytopenia has been reported.

Adverse Effects

>10%:
Central nervous system: Headache (19% to 22%)
Dermatologic: Alopecia (10% to 13%)
Endocrine & metabolic: Hypophosphatemia (5% to 18%)
Gastrointestinal: Diarrhea (15% to 18%), nausea (9% to 14%)
Hematologic: Neutropenia (2% to 15%)
Hepatic: ALT increased (12% to 14%)
Miscellaneous: Influenza (12%)

1% to 10%:
Cardiovascular: Hypertension (4%), palpitation (2% to 3%)
Central nervous system: Anxiety (3% to 4%)
Dermatologic: Pruritus (3% to 4%), acne (3%), burning sensation (2% to 3%)
Endocrine & metabolic: Hyperkalemia (1%)
Gastrointestinal: Abdominal pain (5% to 6%), toothache (4%), viral gastroenteritis (2% to 4%), weight loss (2% to 3%), abdominal distension (1% to 2%)
Genitourinary: Cystitis (2% to 4%)
Hematologic: Thrombocytopenia (10%), lymphocytopenia (7% to 10%), leukopenia (1% to 2%)
Hepatic: GGT increased (3% to 5%), AST increased (2% to 3%)
Neuromuscular & skeletal: Paresthesia (9% to 10%), musculoskeletal pain (4% to 5%), myalgia (3% to 4%), sciatica (3%), carpal tunnel syndrome (1% to 3%), peripheral neuropathy (1% to 2%)
Ocular: Blurred vision (3%), conjunctivitis (3%)
Renal: Renal failure (transient, 1%)
Respiratory: Upper respiratory tract infection (9%), bronchitis (8%), sinusitis (6%)
Miscellaneous: Herpes simplex (4%), seasonal allergy (2% to 3%)

General Dosage Range Oral: *Adults:* 7 mg or 14 mg once daily

Mechanism of Action Teriflunomide is an immunomodulatory agent that inhibits pyrimidine synthesis, resulting in antiproliferative and anti-inflammatory effects. It may reduce the number of activated lymphocytes in the CNS.

Pharmacodynamics/Kinetics

Half-life Elimination Median: 18-19 days; enterohepatic recycling appears to contribute to the long half-life of this agent, since activated charcoal and cholestyramine substantially reduce plasma half-life

Time to Peak Plasma: 1-4 hours

Pregnancy Risk Factor X

Pregnancy Considerations Adverse events have been observed in animal reproduction studies conducted using doses lower than the expected human exposure. **[U.S. Boxed Warning]: Based on animal data, teriflunomide may cause major birth defects if used in pregnant women. Teriflunomide is contraindicated in pregnant women or women of childbearing potential who are not using reliable contraception. Pregnancy must be avoided during therapy or prior to completing the accelerated elimination treatment protocol.** Pregnancy must be excluded prior to initiating treatment. Women of childbearing potential should not receive therapy until pregnancy has been excluded, they have been counseled concerning fetal risk, and reliable contraceptive measures have been confirmed. Following treatment, pregnancy should be avoided until undetectable serum concentrations (<0.02 mg/L) are verified. This may be accomplished by the use of an enhanced drug elimination procedure using cholestyramine or activated charcoal powder. If pregnancy occurs during treatment, discontinue therapy and initiate the accelerated elimination procedure. Pregnant women exposed to teriflunomide should be registered with the pregnancy registry (800-745-4447, option 2). Teriflunomide is also found in semen. Males and their female partners should use reliable contraception during therapy. Males taking teriflunomide who wish to father a child should consider discontinuing therapy and using the accelerated elimination procedure to decrease the potential risk of fetal exposure. (**Note:** Without use of the accelerated elimination procedure, teriflunomide may remain in the serum for up to 2 years)

Teriparatide (ter i PAR a tide)

Related Information
Rheumatoid Arthritis, Osteoarthritis, and Osteoporosis *on page 1526*

Brand Names: U.S. Forteo®

Brand Names: Canada Forteo®

Pharmacologic Category Parathyroid Hormone Analog

Use Treatment of osteoporosis in postmenopausal women at high risk of fracture; treatment of primary or hypogonadal osteoporosis in men at high risk of fracture; treatment of glucocorticoid-induced osteoporosis in men and women at high risk for fracture

Local Anesthetic/Vasoconstrictor Precautions No information available to require special precautions

Effects on Dental Treatment Key adverse event(s) related to dental treatment: May have beneficial effects for treatment of osteoporosis in patients with osteonecrosis of the jaw due to bisphosphonates; however, teriparatide may have cost constraints.

Effects on Bleeding No information available to require special precautions

Adverse Effects

>10%: Endocrine & metabolic: Hypercalcemia (transient increases noted 4-6 hours postdose [women 11%; men 6%])

1% to 10%:
Cardiovascular: Orthostatic hypotension (5%; transient), chest pain (3%), syncope (3%)
Central nervous system: Dizziness (8%), insomnia (4% to 5%), anxiety (≤4%), depression (4%), vertigo (4%)
Dermatologic: Rash (5%)
Endocrine & metabolic: Hyperuricemia (3%)
Gastrointestinal: Nausea (9% to 14%), gastritis (≤7%), dyspepsia (5%), vomiting (3%)
Neuromuscular & skeletal: Arthralgia (10%), weakness (9%), leg cramps (3%)
Respiratory: Rhinitis (10%), pharyngitis (6%), dyspnea (4% to 6%), pneumonia (4% to 6%)

Miscellaneous: Antibodies to teriparatide (3% of women in long-term treatment; hypersensitivity reactions or decreased efficacy were not associated in preclinical trials), herpes zoster (≤3%)

General Dosage Range
SubQ: *Adults:* 20 mcg once daily

Mechanism of Action Teriparatide is a recombinant formulation of endogenous parathyroid hormone (PTH), containing a 34-amino-acid sequence which is identical to the N-terminal portion of this hormone. The pharmacologic activity of teriparatide, which is similar to the physiologic activity of PTH, includes stimulating osteoblast function, increasing gastrointestinal calcium absorption, and increasing renal tubular reabsorption of calcium. Treatment with teriparatide results in increased bone mineral density, bone mass, and strength. In postmenopausal women, teriparatide has been shown to decrease osteoporosis-related fractures.

Pharmacodynamics/Kinetics
Half-life Elimination I.V.: 5 minutes; SubQ: ~1 hour
Time to Peak Serum: ~30 minutes
Pregnancy Risk Factor C
Pregnancy Considerations Adverse events were observed in animal studies; the effect on human fetal development has not been studied. Teriparatide is not indicated for use in pregnant or premenopausal women.

Tesamorelin (tes a moe REL in)

Brand Names: U.S. Egrifta®
Pharmacologic Category Growth Hormone Releasing Factor
Use Reduction of excess abdominal fat in HIV-infected patients with lipodystrophy
Local Anesthetic/Vasoconstrictor Precautions No information available to require special precautions
Effects on Dental Treatment No significant effects or complications reported
Effects on Bleeding No information available to require special precautions
Adverse Effects Note: The incidence of adverse reactions generally decreases with treatment continued beyond 26 weeks.
10%:
Local: Injection site reactions (6% to 25%; includes erythema [1% to 9%], pruritus [2% to 8%], pain [4%], irritation [3%], hemorrhage [2%], swelling [2%], urticaria [2%], rash [1%])
Neuromuscular & skeletal: Arthralgia (13%)
1% to 10%:
Cardiovascular: Peripheral edema (2% to 6%), hypertension (1% to 2%), chest pain (1%), palpitation (1%)
Central nervous system: Hypoesthesia (2% to 4%), depression (2%), pain (2%), insomnia (1%)
Dermatologic: Rash (4%), pruritus (1% to 2%), urticaria (1%)
Endocrine & metabolic: Hb A_{1c} increased (5%), hot flush (1%), hyperglycemia
Gastrointestinal: Nausea (4%), vomiting (2% to 3%), dyspepsia (2%), abdominal pain (1%)
Neuromuscular & skeletal: Pain in extremity (3% to 6%), myalgia (1% to 6%), paresthesia (2% to 5%), carpal tunnel syndrome (2%), creatine phosphokinase increased (2%), muscle stiffness (2%), musculoskeletal pain (2%), joint stiffness (2%), peripheral neuropathy (2%), joint swelling (1%), muscle spasm (1%), muscle strain (1%)
Miscellaneous: Hypersensitivity reactions (1% to 4%), night sweats (1%)

General Dosage Range SubQ: *Adults:* 2 mg once daily

Mechanism of Action Tesamorelin binds to pituitary growth hormone-releasing factor (GRF) receptors and stimulates the secretion of endogenous growth hormone which has anabolic and lipolytic properties. Growth hormone exerts its effects by interacting with receptors on target cells such as osteoblasts, myocytes, hepatocytes, and adipocytes to promote the reduction of total fat mass. These effects are primarily mediated by IGF-1 produced in the liver and in peripheral tissues.

Pharmacodynamics/Kinetics
Half-life Elimination Healthy adults: 26 minutes; HIV-infected patients: 38 minutes
Time to Peak 9 minutes
Pregnancy Risk Factor X
Pregnancy Considerations Adverse effects were noted in animal reproduction studies. During pregnancy, there is an increased deposition of visceral adipose tissue due to metabolic and hormonal changes. Tesamorelin decreases the deposition of visceral fat and could potentially cause harm to the unborn fetus. Therefore, use during pregnancy is contraindicated; if pregnancy occurs during treatment, discontinue tesamorelin.
Prescribing and Access Restrictions In order to prescribe Egrifta™, healthcare providers must call the Axis Center at 1-877-714-2947. Egrifta™ is only available through specialty pharmacy distribution.

Testosterone (tes TOS ter one)

Brand Names: U.S. Androderm®; AndroGel®; Axiron®; Delatestryl®; Depo®-Testosterone; First®-Testosterone; First®-Testosterone MC; Fortesta™; Striant®; Testim®; Testopel®
Brand Names: Canada Andriol®; Androderm®; AndroGel®; Andropository; Delatestryl®; Depotest® 100; Everone® 200; PMS-Testosterone; Testim®
Pharmacologic Category Androgen
Use
Injection: Androgen replacement therapy in the treatment of delayed male puberty; male hypogonadism (primary or hypogonadotropic); inoperable metastatic female breast cancer (enanthate only)
Pellet: Androgen replacement therapy in the treatment of delayed male puberty; male hypogonadism (primary or hypogonadotropic)
Buccal system, topical gel, topical solution, transdermal system: Male hypogonadism (primary or hypogonadotropic)
Capsule (not available in U.S.): Conditions associated with a deficiency or absence of endogenous testosterone
Local Anesthetic/Vasoconstrictor Precautions No information available to require special precautions
Effects on Dental Treatment Key adverse event(s) related to dental treatment: Buccal administration: Bitter taste, gum edema, gum or mouth irritation, gum tenderness, and taste perversion.
Effects on Bleeding No information available to require special precautions
Adverse Effects Frequency not always defined.
Cardiovascular: Deep venous thrombosis, edema, hypertension, vasodilation
Central nervous system: Abnormal dreams, aggressive behavior, anger, amnesia, anxiety, blood pressure increased/decreased, chills, depression, dizziness, emotional lability, excitation, fatigue, headache,

hostility, insomnia, malaise, memory loss, mood swings, nervousness, seizure, sleep apnea, sleeplessness

Dermatologic: Acne, alopecia, contact dermatitis, dry skin, erythema, folliculitis, hair discoloration, hirsutism (increase in pubic hair growth), pruritus, rash, seborrhea

Endocrine & metabolic: Breast pain/soreness, gonadotropin secretion decreased, growth acceleration, gynecomastia, hot flashes, hypercalcemia, hyperchloremia, hypercholesterolemia, hyper-/hypoglycemia, hyper-/hypokalemia, hyperlipidemia, hypernatremia, inorganic phosphate retention, libido changes, menstrual problems (including amenorrhea), virilism, water retention

Gastrointestinal: Appetite increased, diarrhea, gastroesophageal reflux, GI bleeding, GI irritation, nausea, taste disorder, vomiting, weight gain

Following buccal administration (most common): Bitter taste, gum edema, gum or mouth irritation, gum pain, gum tenderness, taste perversion

Genitourinary: Bladder irritability, impotence, oligospermia, penile erections (spontaneous), priapism, prostatic carcinoma, prostatic hyperplasia, prostatitis, PSA increased, testicular atrophy, urination impaired

Hepatic: Bilirubin increased, cholestatic hepatitis, cholestatic jaundice, hepatic dysfunction, hepatic necrosis, hepatocellular neoplasms, liver function test changes, peliosis hepatis

Hematologic: Anemia, bleeding, hematocrit/hemoglobin increased, leukopenia, polycythemia, suppression of clotting factors

Local: Application site reaction (gel, solution), injection site inflammation/pain

Transdermal system: Pruritus at application site (17% to 37%), burn-like blisters under system (12%), erythema at application site (≤7%), vesicles at application site (6%), allergic contact dermatitis to system (4%), burning at application site (3%), induration at application site (3%), exfoliation at application site (<3%)

Neuromuscular & skeletal: Back pain, hemarthrosis, hyperkinesias, paresthesia, weakness

Ocular: Lacrimation increased

Renal: Creatinine increased, hematuria, polyuria

Respiratory: Dyspnea, nasopharyngitis

Miscellaneous: Anaphylactoid reactions, diaphoresis, hypersensitivity reactions, smell disorder

General Dosage Range

Buccal: *Adults (males):* 30 mg every 12 hours

I.M.: *Adolescents and Adults (males):* 50-400 mg every 2-4 weeks

SubQ: *Adolescents and Adults (males):* 150-450 mg every 3-6 months

Transdermal: *Adults (males):* Androderm®: Apply 2-7.5 mg daily; AndroGel® 1%: Apply 50-100 mg daily; AndroGel® 1.62%: Apply 20.25-81 mg daily; Axiron®: Apply 30-120 mg daily; Fortesta™: Apply 10-70 mg daily; Testim®: 5-10 g (50-100 mg testosterone) applied once daily

Mechanism of Action Principal endogenous androgen responsible for promoting the growth and development of the male sex organs and maintaining secondary sex characteristics in androgen-deficient males

Pharmacodynamics/Kinetics

Duration of Action Route and ester dependent; I.M.: Cypionate and enanthate esters have longest duration, ≤2-4 weeks; gel: 24-48 hours

Half-life Elimination Variable: 10-100 minutes

Pregnancy Risk Factor X

Pregnancy Considerations Testosterone may cause adverse effects, including masculinization of the female fetus, if used during pregnancy. Females who are or may become pregnant should also avoid skin-to-skin contact to areas where testosterone has been applied topically on another person.

Controlled Substance C-III

Tetanus Immune Globulin (Human)
(TET a nus i MYUN GLOB yoo lin HYU man)

Brand Names: U.S. HyperTET™ S/D

Brand Names: Canada HyperTET™ S/D

Pharmacologic Category Immune Globulin

Use Prophylaxis against tetanus following injury in patients where immunization status is not known or uncertain

The Advisory Committee on Immunization Practices (ACIP) recommends passive immunization with TIG for the following:

• Persons with a wound that is not clean or minor and in whom contraindications to a tetanus-toxoid containing vaccine exist and they have not completed a primary series of tetanus toxoid immunization.

• Persons who are wounded in bombings or similar mass casualty events who have penetrating injuries or nonintact skin exposure and who cannot confirm receipt of a tetanus booster within the previous 5 years. In case of shortage, use should be reserved for persons ≥60 years of age.

Local Anesthetic/Vasoconstrictor Precautions No information available to require special precautions

Effects on Dental Treatment No significant effects or complications reported

Effects on Bleeding No information available to require special precautions

Adverse Effects Frequency not defined.

Central nervous system: Temperature increased

Dermatologic: Angioneurotic edema (rare)

Local: Injection site: Pain, soreness, tenderness

Renal: Nephritic syndrome (rare)

Miscellaneous: Anaphylactic shock (rare)

General Dosage Range I.M.:

Children <7 years: Prophylaxis: 4 units/kg

Children ≥7 years: Prophylaxis: 250 units

Children: Treatment: 500-6000 units

Adults: Prophylaxis: 250 units; Treatment: 500-6000 units

Mechanism of Action Passive immunity toward tetanus

Pregnancy Risk Factor C

Pregnancy Considerations Animal reproduction studies have not been conducted. Tetanus immune globulin and a tetanus toxoid containing vaccine are recommended by the ACIP as part of the standard wound management to prevent tetanus in pregnant women.

Tetanus Toxoid (Adsorbed)
(TET a nus TOKS oyd, ad SORBED)

Pharmacologic Category Vaccine, Inactivated (Bacterial)

Use Active immunization against tetanus when combination antigen preparations are not indicated; tetanus prophylaxis in wound management. **Note:** Tetanus and diphtheria toxoids for adult use (Td) is the preferred immunizing agent for most adults and for children after their seventh birthday. Young children should receive trivalent DTaP (diphtheria/tetanus/acellular pertussis) as part of their childhood immunization program, unless pertussis is contraindicated, then DT is warranted.

Local Anesthetic/Vasoconstrictor Precautions No information available to require special precautions

Effects on Dental Treatment No significant effects or complications reported

Effects on Bleeding No information available to require special precautions

Adverse Effects All serious adverse reactions must be reported to the U.S. Department of Health and Human Services (DHHS) Vaccine Adverse Event Reporting System (VAERS) 1-800-822-7967 or online at https://vaers.hhs.gov/esub/index.

Frequency not defined.

Cardiovascular: Hypotension

Central nervous system: Brachial neuritis, fever, malaise, pain

Gastrointestinal: Nausea

Local: Edema, induration (with or without tenderness), rash, redness, urticaria, warmth

Neuromuscular: Arthralgia, Guillain-Barré syndrome

Miscellaneous: Anaphylactic reaction, Arthus-type hypersensitivity reaction

General Dosage Range I.M.: *Children ≥7 years and Adults:* Initial: 0.5 mL; repeat at 4-8 weeks after first dose and 6-12 months after second dose

Mechanism of Action Tetanus toxoid preparations contain the toxin produced by virulent tetanus bacilli (detoxified growth products of *Clostridium tetani*). The toxin has been modified by treatment with formaldehyde so that it has lost toxicity but still retains ability to act as antigen and produce active immunity; the aluminum salt, a mineral adjuvant, delays the rate of absorption and prolongs and enhances its properties; duration ~10 years.

Pharmacodynamics/Kinetics

Duration of Action Primary immunization: ~10 years

Pregnancy Risk Factor C

Pregnancy Considerations Animal studies have not been conducted. Inactivated bacterial vaccines have not been shown to cause increased risks to the fetus (CDC, 2011). The ACIP recommends vaccination in previously unvaccinated women or in women with an incomplete vaccination series, whose child may be born in unhygienic conditions. Tetanus immune globulin and a tetanus toxoid-containing vaccine are recommended by the ACIP as part of the standard wound management to prevent tetanus in pregnant women. Vaccination using Td is preferred.

Tetrabenazine (tet ra BEN a zeen)

Related Information

Clinical Risk Related to Drugs Prolonging QT Interval *on page 1510*

Brand Names: U.S. Xenazine®

Brand Names: Canada Nitoman™

Pharmacologic Category Central Monoamine-Depleting Agent

Use Treatment of chorea associated with Huntington's disease

Canadian labeling: Treatment of hyperkinetic movement disorders, including Huntington's chorea, hemiballismus, senile chorea, Tourette syndrome, and tardive dyskinesia

Local Anesthetic/Vasoconstrictor Precautions Tetrabenazine is one of the drugs confirmed to prolong the QT interval and is accepted as having a risk of causing torsade de pointes. The risk of drug-induced torsade de pointes is extremely low when a single QT interval prolonging drug is prescribed. In terms of epinephrine, it is not known what effect vasoconstrictors in the local anesthetic regimen will have in patients with a known history of congenital prolonged QT interval or in patients taking any medication that prolongs the QT interval. Until more information is obtained, it is suggested that the clinician consult with the physician prior to the use of a vasoconstrictor in suspected patients, and that the vasoconstrictor (epinephrine, mepivacaine and levonordefrin [Carbocaine® 2% with Neo-Cobefrin®]) be used with caution.

Effects on Dental Treatment

Key adverse event(s) related to dental treatment: Orthostatic hypotension has been reported; monitor patient during erect posture from dental chair and dysphagia.

Effects on Bleeding No information available to require special precautions

Adverse Effects Note: Many adverse effects are dose-related and may resolve at lower dosages. Adverse effects reported for adults with chorea associated with Huntington's disease.

>10%:

Central nervous system: Extrapyramidal symptoms (15% to 33%), sedation (31%), somnolence (31%), fatigue (22%), insomnia (22%), akathisia (19%), depression (19%), anxiety (15%)

Gastrointestinal: Nausea (13%)

Neuromuscular & skeletal: Falls (15%)

Respiratory: Upper respiratory tract infection (11%)

1% to 10%:

Central nervous system: Parkinsonism (3% to 10%), irritability (9%), dizziness (4%), headache (4%), obsessive reaction (4%)

Dermatologic: Bruising (6%)

Gastrointestinal: Dysphagia (4% to 10%), vomiting (6%), appetite decreased (4%), diarrhea (2%)

Genitourinary: Dysuria (4%)

Neuromuscular & skeletal: Balance difficulty (9%), bradykinesia (9%), dysarthria (4%), gait disturbance (4%)

Respiratory: Bronchitis (4%), dyspnea (4%)

General Dosage Range Dosage adjustment recommended in patients on concomitant therapy or who develop toxicities

Oral: *Adults:* 12.5 mg once daily; Maintenance: 25-100 mg/day in 2-3 divided doses

Mechanism of Action Within basal ganglia, interferes with and depletes monoamine neurotransmitters (including dopamine, serotonin, and norepinephrine) in presynaptic vesicles (likely through actions on vesicle monoamine transporter). Tetrabenazine inhibits presynaptic dopamine release and also blocks CNS dopamine receptors. The effects resemble reserpine but with less peripheral activity and a shorter duration of action. Treatment results in symptomatic improvement of hyperkinetic movement disorders, including Huntington's chorea, hemiballismus, senile chorea, tic and Gille's de la Tourette syndrome, and tardive dyskinesia.

Pharmacodynamics/Kinetics

Duration of Action 16-24 hours (at steady-state); chorea may recur within 12-18 hours after discontinuation

Half-life Elimination Alpha-HTBZ: 4-8 hours; Beta-HTBZ: 2-4 hours (increased with hepatic impairment)

Time to Peak Within 1-1.5 hours

Pregnancy Risk Factor C

Pregnancy Considerations Adverse events were observed in some animal studies. There are no adequate and well-controlled studies in pregnant women. Avoid use in pregnant women unless the potential benefit justifies the potential risk to the fetus.

Prescribing and Access Restrictions Xenazine® is available only through specialty pharmacies. For more information regarding the procurement of Xenazine®, healthcare providers, patients, and caregivers may contact the Xenazine® Information Center (XIC) at 1-888-882-6013 or at:

Healthcare providers: http://www.xenazineusa.com/ HCP/PrescribingXenazine/Default.aspx

Patients and caregivers: http://www.xenazineusa.com/ AboutXenazine/Getting-Your-Prescription.aspx

Dental Comment Tetrabenazine is known to prolong the QT interval. The QT interval is measured as the time and distance between the Q point of the QRS complex and the end of the T wave in the ECG tracing. After adjustment for heart rate, the QT interval is defined as prolonged if it is more than 450 msec in men and 460 msec in women. A long QT syndrome was first described in the 1950s and 60s as a congenital syndrome involving QT interval prolongation and syncope and sudden death. Some of the congenital long QT syndromes were characterized by a peculiar electro-cardiographic appearance of the QRS complex involving a premature atria beat followed by a pause, then a subsequent sinus beat showing marked QT prolongation and deformity. This type of cardiac arrhythmia was originally termed "torsade de pointes" (translated from the French as "twisting of the points"). Tetrabenazine is considered as having a risk of causing torsade de pointes. Since it is not known what effect vasoconstrictors in the local anesthetic regimen will have in patients with a known history of congenital prolonged QT interval or in patients taking any medication that prolongs the QT interval, a medical consult is suggested.

Tetracaine (Systemic) (TET ra kane)

Brand Names: Canada Pontocaine®
Generic Availability (U.S.) Yes
Pharmacologic Category Local Anesthetic
Dental Use Ester-type local anesthetic
Use Spinal anesthesia
Local Anesthetic/Vasoconstrictor Precautions No information available to require special precautions
Effects on Dental Treatment No significant effects or complications reported
Effects on Bleeding No information available to require special precautions
Adverse Effects Frequency not defined. **Note:** Adverse effects listed are those characteristics of local anesthetics. Systemic adverse effects are generally associated with excessive doses or rapid absorption.

Cardiovascular: Cardiac arrest, hypotension
Central nervous system: Chills, convulsions, dizziness, drowsiness, nervousness, unconsciousness
Dermatologic: Urticaria
Gastrointestinal: Nausea, vomiting
Hematologic: Methemoglobinemia
Neuromuscular & skeletal: Tremors
Ocular: Blurred vision, pupil constriction
Otic: Tinnitus
Respiratory: Respiratory arrest
Miscellaneous: Allergic reaction, anaphylaxis

Dosage Injection: Adults: Spinal anesthesia: **Note:** Dosage varies with the anesthetic procedure, the degree of anesthesia required, and the individual patient response; it is administered by subarachnoid injection for spinal anesthesia.

Perineal anesthesia: 5 mg
Perineal and lower extremities: 10 mg
Anesthesia extending up to costal margin: 15 mg; doses up to 20 mg may be given, but are reserved for exceptional cases
Low spinal anesthesia (saddle block): 2-5 mg

Mechanism of Action Ester local anesthetic blocks both the initiation and conduction of nerve impulses by decreasing the neuronal membrane's permeability to sodium ions, which results in inhibition of depolarization with resultant blockade of conduction

Contraindications Hypersensitivity to tetracaine, ester-type anesthetics, aminobenzoic acid, or any component of the formulation; injection should not be used when spinal anesthesia is contraindicated

Warnings/Precautions Use with caution in patients with cardiac disease (especially rhythm disturbances, heart block, or shock), hyperthyroidism, and abnormal or decreased levels of plasma esterases. Use of the lowest effective dose is recommended. Acutely ill, elderly, debilitated, obstetric patients, or patients with increased intra-abdominal pressure may require decreased doses. Dental practitioners and/or clinicians using local anesthetic agents should be well-trained in diagnosis and management of emergencies that may arise from the use of these agents. Resuscitative equipment, oxygen, and other resuscitative drugs should be available for immediate use.

Drug Interactions

Metabolism/Transport Effects None known.

Avoid Concomitant Use There are no known interactions where it is recommended to avoid concomitant use.

Increased Effect/Toxicity
The levels/effects of Tetracaine (Systemic) may be increased by: Hyaluronidase

Decreased Effect There are no known significant interactions involving a decrease in effect.

Pregnancy Risk Factor C

Pregnancy Considerations Animal reproduction studies have not been conducted.

Lactation Excretion in breast milk unknown/use caution

Breast-Feeding Considerations It is not known if tetracaine (systemic) is excreted in breast milk. The manufacturer recommends that caution be exercised when administering tetracaine (systemic) to nursing women.

Dosage Forms
Injection, solution [preservative free]: 1% [10 mg/mL] (2 mL)

Tetracaine (Topical) (TET ra kane)

Related Information
Oral Pain *on page 1558*
Ulcerative, Erosive, and Painful Oral Mucosal Disorders *on page 1578*
Brand Names: U.S. Pontocaine® [DSC]
Brand Names: Canada Ametop™; Pontocaine®
Generic Availability (U.S.) No
Pharmacologic Category Local Anesthetic
Dental Use Ester-type local anesthetic; applied to throat for various diagnostic procedures and on cold sores and fever blisters for pain

Use Applied to nose and throat for diagnostic procedures

Local Anesthetic/Vasoconstrictor Precautions No information available to require special precautions

Effects on Dental Treatment No significant effects or complications reported

Effects on Bleeding No information available to require special precautions

Adverse Effects Frequency not defined. **Note:** Adverse effects listed are those characteristics of local anesthetics. Systemic adverse effects are generally associated with excessive doses or rapid absorption.

Cardiovascular: Cardiac arrest, hypotension

Central nervous system: Chills, convulsions, dizziness, drowsiness, nervousness, unconsciousness

Dermatologic: Urticaria

Gastrointestinal: Nausea, vomiting

Hematologic: Methemoglobinemia

Neuromuscular & skeletal: Tremors

Ocular: Blurred vision, pupil constriction

Otic: Tinnitus

Respiratory: Respiratory arrest

Miscellaneous: Allergic reaction, anaphylaxis

Dental Usual Dosage Topical mucous membranes (rhinolaryngology): Adults: Used as a 0.25% or 0.5% solution by direct application or nebulization; total dose should not exceed 20 mg

Dosage Adults: Topical mucous membranes (rhinolaryngology): Used as a 0.25% or 0.5% solution by direct application or nebulization; total dose should not exceed 20 mg

Mechanism of Action Ester local anesthetic blocks both the initiation and conduction of nerve impulses by decreasing the neuronal membrane's permeability to sodium ions, which results in inhibition of depolarization with resultant blockade of conduction

Contraindications Hypersensitivity to tetracaine, ester-type anesthetics, aminobenzoic acid, or any component of the formulation

Warnings/Precautions For topical use only. Use with caution in patients with cardiac disease, hyperthyroidism, and abnormal or decreased levels of plasma esterases. Use of the lowest effective dose is recommended. Use caution in acutely ill, elderly, debilitated, or obstetric patients. Dental practitioners and/or clinicians using local anesthetic agents should be well trained in diagnosis and management of emergencies that may arise from the use of these agents. Resuscitative equipment, oxygen, and other resuscitative drugs should be available for immediate use.

Drug Interactions

Metabolism/Transport Effects None known.

Avoid Concomitant Use There are no known interactions where it is recommended to avoid concomitant use.

Increased Effect/Toxicity There are no known significant interactions involving an increase in effect.

Decreased Effect There are no known significant interactions involving a decrease in effect.

Pharmacodynamics/Kinetics

Onset of Action Anesthetic: Rhinolaryngology: 5-10 minutes

Duration of Action Rhinolaryngology: ~30 minutes

Pregnancy Risk Factor C

Pregnancy Considerations Animal reproduction studies have not been conducted.

Lactation Excretion in breast milk unknown/use caution

Dosage Forms

Solution, topical:

Pontocaine® 2% [20 mg/mL] (30 mL, 118 mL)

Tetracycline (tet ra SYE kleen)

Related Information

Bacterial Infections *on page 1562*

Gastrointestinal Disorders *on page 1512*

Periodontal Diseases *on page 1570*

Ulcerative, Erosive, and Painful Oral Mucosal Disorders *on page 1578*

Brand Names: Canada Apo-Tetra®; Nu-Tetra

Generic Availability (U.S.) Yes: Capsule

Pharmacologic Category Antibiotic, Tetracycline Derivative

Dental Use Treatment of periodontitis associated with presence of *Actinobacillus actinomycetemcomitans* (AA); as adjunctive therapy in recurrent aphthous ulcers

Use Treatment of susceptible bacterial infections of both gram-positive and gram-negative organisms; also infections due to *Mycoplasma*, *Chlamydia*, and *Rickettsia*; indicated for acne, exacerbations of chronic bronchitis, and treatment of gonorrhea and syphilis in patients who are allergic to penicillin; as part of a multidrug regimen for *H. pylori* eradication to reduce the risk of duodenal ulcer recurrence

Unlabeled Use Treatment of periodontitis associated with presence of *Actinobacillus actinomycetemcomitans* (AA)

Local Anesthetic/Vasoconstrictor Precautions No information available to require special precautions

Effects on Dental Treatment Key adverse event(s) related to dental treatment: Esophagitis, superinfections, and candidal superinfection. Opportunistic "superinfection" with *Candida albicans*; tetracyclines are not recommended for use during pregnancy or in children ≤8 years of age since they have been reported to cause enamel hypoplasia and permanent teeth discoloration. The use of tetracyclines should only be used in these patients if other agents are contraindicated or alternative antimicrobials will not eradicate the organism. Long-term use associated with oral candidiasis.

Effects on Bleeding No information available to require special precautions

Adverse Effects Frequency not defined.

Cardiovascular: Pericarditis

Central nervous system: Bulging fontanels in infants, increased intracranial pressure, paresthesia, pseudotumor cerebri

Dermatologic: Exfoliative dermatitis, photosensitivity, pigmentation of nails, pruritus

Gastrointestinal: Abdominal cramps, anorexia, antibiotic-associated pseudomembranous colitis, diarrhea, discoloration of teeth and enamel hypoplasia (young children), esophagitis, nausea, pancreatitis, staphylococcal enterocolitis, vomiting

Hematologic: Thrombophlebitis

Hepatic: Hepatotoxicity

Renal: Acute renal failure, azotemia, renal damage

Miscellaneous: Anaphylaxis, candidal superinfection, hypersensitivity reactions, superinfection

Dental Usual Dosage Periodontitis: Adults: Oral: 250 mg every 6 hours until improvement (usually 10 days)

Dosage

Usual dosage range:

Children >8 years: Oral: 25-50 mg/kg/day in divided doses every 6 hours

Adults: Oral: 250-500 mg/dose every 6 hours

Indication-specific dosing:
Children ≥8 years: Oral:
Malaria, severe, treatment (unlabeled use): 25 mg/kg/day in divided doses every 6 hours (maximum dose: 250 mg every 6 hours) for 7 days with quinidine gluconate. **Note:** Quinidine gluconate duration is region specific; consult CDC for current recommendations (CDC, 2009).
Malaria, uncomplicated, treatment (unlabeled use): 25 mg/kg/day in divided doses every 6 hours (maximum dose: 250 mg every 6 hours) for 7 days with quinine sulfate. **Note:** Quinine sulfate duration is region specific; consult CDC for current recommendations (CDC, 2009).
Adults: Oral:
Acne: 250-500 twice daily
Chronic bronchitis, acute exacerbation: 500 mg 4 times/day
Erlichiosis: 500 mg 4 times/day for 7-14 days
Malaria, severe, treatment (unlabeled use): Oral: 250 mg 4 times/day for 7 days with quinidine gluconate. **Note:** Quinidine gluconate duration is region specific; consult CDC for current recommendations (CDC, 2009).
Malaria, uncomplicated, treatment (unlabeled use): Oral: 250 mg 4 times/day for 7 days with quinine sulfate. **Note:** Quinine sulfate duration is region specific; consult CDC for current recommendations (CDC, 2009).
Peptic ulcer disease: Eradication of *Helicobacter pylori*: 500 mg 2-4 times/day depending on regimen; requires combination therapy with at least one other antibiotic and an acid-suppressing agent (proton pump inhibitor or H₂ blocker)
Periodontitis (unlabeled use): 250 mg every 6 hours until improvement (usually 10 days)
Vibrio cholerae: 500 mg 4 times/day for 3 days

Dosing interval in renal impairment:
Cl_{cr} 50-80 mL/minute: Administer every 8-12 hours
Cl_{cr} 10-50 mL/minute: Administer every 12-24 hours
Cl_{cr} <10 mL/minute: Administer every 24 hours
Dialysis: Slightly dialyzable (5% to 20%) via hemo- and peritoneal dialysis or via continuous arteriovenous or venovenous hemofiltration; no supplemental dosage necessary
Dosing adjustment in hepatic impairment: Use caution; no dosing adjustment required
Mechanism of Action Inhibits bacterial protein synthesis by binding with the 30S and possibly the 50S ribosomal subunit(s) of susceptible bacteria; may also cause alterations in the cytoplasmic membrane
Contraindications Hypersensitivity to tetracycline or any component of the formulation
Warnings/Precautions Hazardous agent - use appropriate precautions for handling and disposal (NIOSH, 2012). Use with caution in patients with renal or hepatic impairment (eg, elderly); dosage modification required in patients with renal impairment since it may increase BUN as an antianabolic agent. Hepatotoxicity has been reported rarely; risk may be increased in patients with pre-existing hepatic or renal impairment. Pseudotumor cerebri has been reported with tetracycline use (usually resolves with discontinuation); outdated drug can cause nephropathy; use protective measure to avoid photosensitivity. Prolonged use may result in fungal or bacterial superinfection, including *C. difficile*-associated diarrhea (CDAD) and pseudomembranous colitis; CDAD has been observed >2 months postantibiotic treatment. May cause tissue hyperpigmentation, enamel hypoplasia, or permanent tooth discoloration; use of

tetracyclines should be avoided during tooth development (children <8 years of age) unless other drugs are not likely to be effective or are contraindicated. Do not use during pregnancy. In addition to affecting tooth development, tetracycline use has been associated with retardation of skeletal development and reduced bone growth.
Drug Interactions
Metabolism/Transport Effects Substrate of CYP3A4 (major); **Note:** Assignment of Major/Minor substrate status based on clinically relevant drug interaction potential; **Inhibits** CYP3A4 (moderate)
Avoid Concomitant Use
Avoid concomitant use of Tetracycline with any of the following: BCG; Bosutinib; Ivabradine; Lomitapide; Pimozide; Retinoic Acid Derivatives; Strontium Ranelate; Tolvaptan
Increased Effect/Toxicity
Tetracycline may increase the levels/effects of: ARIPiprazole; Avanafil; Bosutinib; Budesonide (Systemic, Oral Inhalation); Colchicine; CYP3A4 Substrates; Eplerenone; Everolimus; FentaNYL; Halofantrine; Ivabradine; Ivacaftor; Lomitapide; Lurasidone; Mipomersen; Neuromuscular-Blocking Agents; Pimecrolimus; Pimozide; Porfimer; Propafenone; Ranolazine; Retinoic Acid Derivatives; Salmeterol; Saxagliptin; Tolvaptan; Vilazodone; Vitamin K Antagonists; Zuclopenthixol
Decreased Effect
Tetracycline may decrease the levels/effects of: Atovaquone; BCG; Ifosfamide; Penicillins; Sodium Picosulfate; Typhoid Vaccine

The levels/effects of Tetracycline may be decreased by: Antacids; Bile Acid Sequestrants; Bismuth; Bismuth Subsalicylate; Calcium Salts; CYP3A4 Inducers (Strong); Deferasirox; Herbs (CYP3A4 Inducers); Iron Salts; Lanthanum; Magnesium Salts; Multivitamins/Minerals (with ADEK, Folate, Iron); Quinapril; Strontium Ranelate; Sucralfate; Tocilizumab; Zinc Salts
Ethanol/Nutrition/Herb Interactions
Food: Serum concentrations may be decreased if taken with dairy products. Take on an empty stomach 1 hour before or 2 hours after meals to increase total absorption. Administer around-the-clock to promote less variation in peak and trough serum levels.
Herb/Nutraceutical: Dong quai and St John's wort may also cause photosensitization. Management: Avoid dong quai and St John's wort.
Dietary Considerations Take on an empty stomach (ie, 1 hour prior to, or 2 hours after meals). Take at least 1-2 hours prior to, or 4 hours after antacid.
Pharmacodynamics/Kinetics
Half-life Elimination Normal renal function: 8-11 hours; End-stage renal disease: 57-108 hours
Time to Peak Serum: Oral: 2-4 hours
Pregnancy Risk Factor D
Pregnancy Considerations Tetracyclines cross the placenta and accumulate in developing teeth and long tubular bones. Tetracyclines may discolor fetal teeth following maternal use during pregnancy; the specific teeth involved and the portion of the tooth affected depends on the timing and duration of exposure relative to tooth calcification. The pharmacokinetics of tetracycline are not altered in pregnant patients with normal renal function. Hepatic toxicity during pregnancy, potentially associated with tetracycline use, has been widely reported in the literature. As a class, tetracyclines are generally considered second-line antibiotics in pregnant

women and their use should be avoided (Mylonas, 2011; Whalley, 1966; Whalley, 1970).

Lactation Enters breast milk/not recommended (AAP rates "compatible"; AAP 2001 update pending)

Breast-Feeding Considerations Tetracycline is excreted into breast milk (Matsuda, 1984). According to the manufacturer, the decision to continue or discontinue breast-feeding during therapy should take into account the risk of exposure to the infant and the benefits of treatment to the mother. Tetracycline binds to calcium. The calcium in the maternal milk will decrease the amount of tetracycline absorbed by the breast-feeding infant (Mitrano, 2009). Nondose-related effects could include modification of bowel flora.

Dosage Forms

Capsule, oral: 250 mg, 500 mg

References

Gordon JM and Walker CB, "Current Status of Systemic Antibiotic Usage in Destructive Periodontal Disease," *J Periodontol*, 1993, 64 (8 Suppl): 760-71.

Rams TE and Slots J, "Antibiotics in Periodontal Therapy: An Update," *Compendium*, 1992, 13(12):1130, 1132, 1134.

Seymour RA and Heasman PA, "Pharmacological Control of Periodontal Disease. II. Antimicrobial Agents," *J Dent*, 1995, 23(1):5-14

Seymour RA and Heasman PA, "Tetracyclines in the Management of Periodontal Diseases. A Review," *J Clin Periodontol*, 1995, 22 (1):22-35.

Tetrahydrocannabinol and Cannabidiol

(TET ra hye droe can NAB e nol & can nab e DYE ol)

Brand Names: Canada Sativex®

Pharmacologic Category Analgesic, Miscellaneous

Use Adjunctive treatment of neuropathic pain or spasticity in multiple sclerosis; adjunctive treatment of moderate-to-severe pain in advanced cancer

Local Anesthetic/Vasoconstrictor Precautions No information available to require special precautions

Effects on Dental Treatment Key adverse event(s) related to dental treatment: Xerostomia and changes in salivation (normal salivary flow resumes upon discontinuation), abnormal taste, oral pain, orthostatic hypotension; administered as buccal spray, associated with irritation to the buccal (oral) mucosa.

Effects on Bleeding No information available to require special precautions

Adverse Effects

>10%:

Central nervous system: Dizziness (12% to 25%), somnolence (8% to 15%), fatigue (13%)

Gastrointestinal: Nausea (10% to 12%)

1% to 10%:

Cardiovascular: Hypotension (5%), palpitation (1%), syncope (1%), tachycardia (1%)

Central nervous system: Confusion (7%), vertigo (5% to 7%), disorientation (4%), attention disturbance (3% to 4%), depression (3%), headache (3%), impaired balance (3%), insomnia (3%), panic attack (3%), euphoria (2% to 3%), hallucination (≤3%), dissociation (2%), feeling abnormal (2%), lethargy (2%), amnesia (1%), malaise (1%), memory impairment (1%), paranoia (1%), suicidal ideation (1%)

Gastrointestinal: Vomiting (4% to 8%), diarrhea (6% to 7%), xerostomia (6%), glossodynia (3%), oral candidiasis (3%), taste abnormal (3%), anorexia (2%), constipation (2%), mouth ulceration (2%), oral mucosal disorder (2%), tooth discoloration (2%), abdominal pain (1%), appetite increased (1%), stomatitis (1%)

Genitourinary: Urinary retention (5%)

Hepatic: Hepatic function tests abnormal (5%)

Neuromuscular & skeletal: Weakness (5% to 6%), dysarthria (2%), fall (2%)

Ocular: Vision blurred (2%)

Renal: Hematuria (3%)

Respiratory: Throat irritation (1%)

Miscellaneous: Drunken feeling (3%)

General Dosage Range Dosage adjustment recommended in patients who develop toxicities

Buccal: *Adults:* Initial: 1 spray twice daily; Maintenance: Usual: 4-8 sprays daily (usual maximum: 12 sprays daily)

Mechanism of Action Stimulates cannabinoid receptors CB1 and CB2 in the CNS and dorsal root ganglia as well as other sites in the body. Cannabinoid receptors in the pain pathways of the brain and spinal cord mediate cannabinoid-induced analgesia. Peripheral CB2 receptors modulate immune function through cytokine release.

Pharmacodynamics/Kinetics

Half-life Elimination Biphasic: Initial: 1-2 hours; Terminal: 24-36 hours (or longer) secondary to redistribution from fatty tissue

Time to Peak 2-4 hours

Pregnancy Considerations Cannabinoids have been associated with reproductive toxicity. Animal studies indicate possible effects on fetal development and spermatogenesis. Use in pregnancy is contraindicated. Women of childbearing potential and males who are capable of causing pregnancy should use a reliable form of contraception for the duration of treatment and for 3 months following discontinuation.

Product Availability Not available in U.S.

Controlled Substance CDSA-II

Tetrahydrozoline (Nasal) (tet ra hye DROZ a leen)

Brand Names: U.S. Tyzine®; Tyzine® Pediatric

Pharmacologic Category Adrenergic Agonist Agent; Decongestant; Imidazoline Derivative

Use Symptomatic relief of nasal congestion

Local Anesthetic/Vasoconstrictor Precautions No information available to require special precautions

Effects on Dental Treatment No significant effects or complications reported

Effects on Bleeding No information available to require special precautions

Adverse Effects

>10%:

Local: Transient stinging

Respiratory: Sneezing

1% to 10%:

Cardiovascular: Hypertension, palpitation, tachycardia

Central nervous system: Headache

Neuromuscular & skeletal: Tremor

Ocular: Blurred vision

General Dosage Range Intranasal:

Children 2-6 years: Instill 2-3 drops (0.05%) into each nostril every 4-6 hours as needed (maximum: Every 3 hours)

Children >6 years and Adults: Instill 2-4 drops (0.1%) **or** 3-4 sprays (0.1%) into each nostril every 3-4 hours as needed (maximum: Every 3 hours)

Mechanism of Action Stimulates alpha-adrenergic receptors in the arterioles of the nasal mucosa to produce vasoconstriction

Pharmacodynamics/Kinetics

Onset of Action Decongestant: 4-8 hours

Pregnancy Risk Factor C

Pregnancy Considerations Animal reproduction studies have not been conducted.

Tetrastarch (TET ra starch)

Brand Names: U.S. Voluven®
Brand Names: Canada Volulyte®; Voluven®
Pharmacologic Category Plasma Volume Expander, Colloid
Use Blood volume expander used in treatment and prevention of hypovolemia
Local Anesthetic/Vasoconstrictor Precautions No information available to require special precautions
Effects on Dental Treatment No significant effects or complications reported
Effects on Bleeding Tetrastarch has caused prolongation of activated partial thromboplastin time (aPTT); coagulation factors prolonged. Monitor patient for increased bleeding; medical consult is suggested. It is unlikely that ambulatory patients presenting for dental treatment will be receiving intravenous blood volume expander.
Adverse Effects 1% to 10%
Dermatologic: Pruritus (dose dependent; may be delayed), rash
Gastrointestinal: Amylase levels increased
Hematologic: Anemia, aPTT increased, coagulation factors prolonged, hemorrhage from wound site, PT prolonged
General Dosage Range I.V. infusion:
Children <2 years: Average dose: 7-25 mL/kg
Children >12 years and Adults: Maximum dose: 50 mL/kg/day (or up to 3500 mL per day in a 70 kg patient)
Mechanism of Action Produces plasma volume expansion by virtue of its highly colloidal starch structure
Pharmacodynamics/Kinetics
Duration of Action ≥6 hours
Half-life Elimination 12 hours
Pregnancy Risk Factor C
Pregnancy Considerations Adverse events have been observed in animal reproduction studies.

Thalidomide (tha LI doe mide)

Related Information
HIV Infection and AIDS *on page 1520*
Ulcerative, Erosive, and Painful Oral Mucosal Disorders *on page 1578*
Brand Names: U.S. Thalomid®
Brand Names: Canada Thalomid®
Generic Availability (U.S.) No
Pharmacologic Category Angiogenesis Inhibitor; Antineoplastic Agent; Immunomodulator, Systemic
Use Treatment of newly-diagnosed multiple myeloma; treatment and maintenance of cutaneous manifestations of erythema nodosum leprosum (ENL)
Unlabeled Use Treatment of refractory Crohn's disease; treatment of chronic graft-versus-host disease (GVHD) in hematopoietic stem cell transplantation; AIDS-related aphthous stomatitis; Waldenström's macroglobulinemia; maintenance therapy of multiple myeloma (following autologous stem cell transplant); systemic light chain amyloidosis
Local Anesthetic/Vasoconstrictor Precautions No information available to require special precautions
Effects on Dental Treatment Key adverse event(s) related to dental treatment: Oral moniliasis (HIV-seropositive patients), toothache, xerostomia (normal salivary flow resumes upon discontinuation), and aphthous stomatitis.

Effects on Bleeding No information available to require special precautions
Adverse Effects
>10%:
Cardiovascular: Edema (57%), thrombosis/embolism (23%; grade 3: 13%, grade 4: 9%), hypotension (16%)
Central nervous system: Fatigue (79%; grade 3: 14%, grade 4: 3%), somnolence (36% to 38%), dizziness (4% to 20%), sensory neuropathy (54%), confusion (28%), anxiety/agitation (9% to 26%), fever (19% to 23%), motor neuropathy (22%), headache (13% to 19%)
Dermatologic: Rash/desquamation (21% to 30%; grade 3: 4%), dry skin (21%), maculopapular rash (4% to 19%), acne (3% to 11%)
Endocrine & metabolic: Hypocalcemia (72%)
Gastrointestinal: Constipation (3% to 55%), nausea (4% to 28%), anorexia (3% to 28%), weight loss (23%), weight gain (22%), diarrhea (4% to 19%), oral moniliasis (4% to 11%)
Hematologic: Leukopenia (17% to 35%), neutropenia (31%), anemia (6% to 13%), lymphadenopathy (6% to 13%)
Hepatic: AST increased (3% to 25%), bilirubin increased (14%)
Neuromuscular & skeletal: Muscle weakness (40%), tremor (4% to 26%), weakness (6% to 22%), myalgia (17%), paresthesia (6% to 16%), arthralgia (13%)
Renal: Hematuria (11%)
Respiratory: Dyspnea (42%)
Miscellaneous: Diaphoresis (13%)
1% to 10%:
Cardiovascular: Peripheral edema (3% to 8%), facial edema (4%)
Central nervous system: Insomnia (9%), nervousness (3% to 9%), malaise (8%), vertigo (8%), pain (3% to 8%)
Dermatologic: Dermatitis (fungal 4% to 9%), pruritus (3% to 8%), nail disorder (3% to 4%)
Endocrine & metabolic: Hyperlipemia (6% to 9%)
Gastrointestinal: Xerostomia (8% to 9%), flatulence (8%), tooth pain (4%)
Genitourinary: Impotence (3% to 8%)
Hepatic: LFTs abnormal (9%)
Neuromuscular & skeletal: Neuropathy (8%), back pain (4% to 6%), neck pain (4%), neck rigidity (4%)
Renal: Albuminuria (3% to 8%)
Respiratory: Pharyngitis (4% to 8%), rhinitis (4%), sinusitis (3% to 8%)
Miscellaneous: Infection (6% to 8%)
Dosage
Children ≥3 years: Oral: Chronic graft-versus-host disease (refractory), treatment (unlabeled second-line use; limited data): 3 mg/kg 4 times daily (dose adjusted to goal thalidomide concentration of ≥5 mcg/mL 2 hours postdose) (Vogelsang, 1992) **or** Initial: 3-6 mg/kg/day in 2-4 divided doses; target dose 12 mg/kg/day; Maximum daily dose: 800 mg (Rovelli, 1998)
Children ≥12 years and Adults: Oral: Cutaneous erythema nodosum leprosum (ENL): Initial: 100-300 mg once daily at bedtime
Adjustments to initial dose:
Patients weighing <50 kg: Initiate at lower end of the dosing range
Severe cutaneous reaction or patients previously requiring high dose may be initiated at 400 mg daily; doses may be divided

Duration and tapering/maintenance:

Maintenance: Dosing should continue until active reaction subsides (usually at least 2 weeks), then tapered in 50 mg decrements every 2-4 weeks

Patients who flare during tapering or with a history of requiring prolonged maintenance should be maintained on the minimum dosage necessary to control the reaction. Efforts to taper should be repeated every 3-6 months, in decrements of 50 mg every 2-4 weeks.

Adults: Oral:

Multiple myeloma: **Note:** Details concerning dosing for multiple myeloma with combination regimens should also be consulted.

200 mg once daily at bedtime (in combination with dexamethasone 40 mg daily on days 1-4, 9-12, and 17-20 of a 28-day treatment cycle)

In combination with bortezomib and dexamethasone (unlabeled combination): Induction therapy: 100 mg once daily for the first 14 days, then 200 mg once daily for 3 (21-day) cycles (Cavo, 2010) **or** 100 mg once daily for up to 8 (21-day) cycles (Kaufman, 2010)

In combination with melphalan and prednisone (unlabeled combination in U.S.): 200-400 mg once daily (Facon, 2007) **or** 100 mg once daily (Palumbo, 2008)

Canadian labeling: Adults ≥65 years: 200 mg once daily; maximum: 12 six-week cycles (in combination with melphalan and prednisone)

Multiple myeloma, maintenance (following autologous stem cell transplant; unlabeled use): 200 mg once daily starting 3-6 months after transplant; continue until disease progression or unacceptable toxicity (Brinker, 2006) or 100 mg once daily starting 42-60 days following transplant; increase to 200 mg once daily after 2 weeks if tolerated; continue for up to 12 months (in combination with prednisolone) (Spencer, 2009)

AIDS-related aphthous stomatitis (unlabeled use): 200 mg once daily at bedtime for up to 8 weeks, if no response, then 200 mg twice daily for 4 weeks (Jacobson, 1997)

Chronic graft-versus-host disease (refractory), treatment (unlabeled second-line use; optimum dose not determined): Initial: 100 mg once daily at bedtime, with dose escalation up to 400 mg daily in 3-4 divided doses (Wolff, 2010) **or** Initial: 50-100 mg 3 times daily; maximum dose: 600-1200 mg daily (Kulkarni, 2003) **or** 200 mg 4 times daily (dose adjusted to goal thalidomide concentration of ≥5 mcg/mL 2 hours postdose) (Vogelsang, 1992) **or** 100-300 mg 4 times daily (Parker, 1995)

Crohn's disease, refractory (unlabeled use): 50-100 mg once daily at bedtime (Vasiliauskas, 1999) **or** 200-300 mg once daily at bedtime (Ehrenpreis, 1999)

Systemic light chain amyloidosis (unlabeled use): 200 mg once daily (starting dose 50-100 mg once daily; titrate at 4-week intervals) in combination with cyclophosphamide and dexamethasone (Wechalekar, 2007)

Waldenström's macroglobulinemia (unlabeled use): 200 mg once daily for up to 52 weeks (in combination with rituximab) (Treon, 2008)

Dosing adjustment for toxicity:

ANC ≤750/mm³: Withhold treatment if clinically appropriate

Multiple myeloma:

U.S. labeling: Constipation, oversedation, peripheral neuropathy: Temporarily withhold or continue with a reduced dose

Canadian labeling:

ANC <1500/mm³: Withhold melphalan and prednisone for 1 week; resume melphalan and prednisone after 1 week if ANC >1500/mm³ **or** if ANC 1000-1500/mm³ reduce melphalan dose by 50% **or** if ANC <1000/mm³ adjust chemotherapy dose based on clinical status of patient.

Constipation, oversedation: Temporarily withhold thalidomide treatment or continue with a reduced dose

Peripheral neuropathy, Grade 1 (paresthesia, weakness and/or loss of reflexes) without loss of function): Evaluate patient and consider dose reduction with worsening of symptoms; symptom improvement may not follow dose reduction, however.

Peripheral neuropathy, Grade 2 (interferes with function but not with daily activities), Grade 3 (interferes with daily activities), or Grade 4 (disabling neuropathy): Discontinue thalidomide treatment

Thromboembolic events: Withhold therapy and initiate standard anticoagulant treatment; may resume thalidomide therapy at original dose following stabilization of patient and resolution of thromboembolic event; maintain anticoagulant treatment for duration of thalidomide therapy

Unlabeled recommendation (Richardson, 2012): Peripheral neuropathy:

Grade 1: Reduce dose by 50%

Grade 2: Temporarily interrupt therapy; once resolved to ≤ grade 1, resume therapy with a 50% dosage reduction (if clinically appropriate)

Grade 3 or higher: Discontinue therapy

Dosing adjustment in renal impairment: No adjustment is required for patients with renal impairment and on dialysis (per manufacturer). In a study of 6 patients with end-stage renal disease on dialysis, although clearance was increased by dialysis, a supplemental dose was not needed (Eriksson, 2003).

Multiple myeloma: An evaluation of 29 newly-diagnosed myeloma patients with renal failure (serum creatinine ≥2 mg/dL) treated with thalidomide and dexamethasone (some also received cyclophosphamide) found that toxicities and efficacy were similar to patients with normal renal function (Seol, 2010). A study evaluating induction therapy with thalidomide and dexamethasone in 31 newly-diagnosed myeloma patients with renal failure (Cl$_{cr}$ <50 mL/minute), including 16 patients with severe renal impairment (Cl$_{cr}$ <30 mL/minute) and 7 patients on chronic hemodialysis found that toxicities were similar to patients without renal impairment and that thalidomide and dexamethasone could be administered safely (Tosi, 2009).

Dosing adjustment in hepatic impairment: No dosage adjustment provided in manufacturer's labeling (has not been studied). However, thalidomide does not appear to undergo significant hepatic metabolism.

Mechanism of Action Immunomodulatory and antiangiogenic characteristics; immunologic effects may vary based on conditions; may suppress excessive tumor necrosis factor-alpha production in patients with ENL, yet may increase plasma tumor necrosis factor-alpha levels in HIV-positive patients. In multiple myeloma, thalidomide is associated with an increase in natural killer cells and increased levels of interleukin-2 and interferon gamma. Other proposed mechanisms of action include suppression of angiogenesis, prevention of free-radical-mediated DNA damage, increased cell mediated cytotoxic effects, and altered expression of cellular adhesion molecules.

Contraindications Hypersensitivity to thalidomide or any component of the formulation; pregnancy

Canadian labeling: Additional contraindications (not in U.S. labeling): Hypersensitivity to lenalidomide; breast-feeding

Warnings/Precautions Hazardous agent - use appropriate precautions for handling and disposal (NIOSH, 2012).

[U.S. Boxed Warning]: Associated with an increased risk for venous thromboembolism, including deep vein thrombosis (DVT) and pulmonary embolism (PE) in multiple myeloma patients; the risk is increased when used in combination with dexamethasone. Monitor for signs and symptoms of thromboembolism (shortness of breath, chest pain, or arm or leg swelling) and instruct patients to seek prompt medical attention with development of these symptoms. Patients at risk may benefit from prophylactic anticoagulation. The NCCN multiple myeloma guidelines (v.1.2013) recommend anticoagulant prophylaxis with thalidomide-based therapy. Anticoagulant prophylaxis should be individualized and selected based on the venous thromboembolism risk of the combination treatment regimen, using the safest and easiest to administer (Palumbo, 2008). The Canadian labeling recommends anticoagulant prophylaxis for at least the first 5 months of thalidomide-based therapy. Patients with a high tumor burden may be at risk for tumor lysis syndrome; monitor closely; institute appropriate management for hyperuricemia.

May cause neutropenia; avoid initiating therapy if ANC <750/mm³; monitor blood counts. Persistent neutropenia may require treatment interruption. Anemia and thrombocytopenia have also been observed. May cause bradycardia; use with caution in patients with cardiovascular disease. May require dose reduction or discontinuation. Use caution when administering with concomitant medications which may decrease heart rate. Stevens-Johnson syndrome (SJS) and toxic epidermal necrolysis (TEN) have been reported (may be fatal); withhold therapy and evaluate with skin rashes; permanently discontinue if rash is exfoliative, purpuric, bullous or if SJS or TEN is suspected. Hypersensitivity, including erythematous macular rash, possibly associated with fever, tachycardia and hypotension has been reported. May require treatment interruption for severe reactions; discontinue if recurs with rechallenge.

Associated with the development of peripheral neuropathy, which may be irreversible; generally occurs following chronic use (over months), but may occur with short-term use; onset may be delayed. Use caution with other medications which may also cause peripheral neuropathy. Monitor for signs/symptoms of neuropathy monthly for the first 3 months of therapy and regularly thereafter. Electrophysiological testing may be considered at baseline and every 6 months to detect asymptomatic neuropathy. Consider immediate discontinuation (if clinically appropriate) in patients who develop neuropathy. Reinitiate therapy only if neuropathy returns to baseline; may require dosage reduction or permanent discontinuation. Seizures have been reported in postmarketing data; use caution in patients with a history of seizures, concurrent therapy with drugs which alter seizure threshold, or conditions which predispose to seizures. May cause dizziness, drowsiness, and/or

somnolence; caution patients about performing tasks which require mental alertness (eg, operating machinery or driving). Avoid concomitant medications which may exacerbate these symptoms; dose reductions may be necessary for excessive drowsiness or somnolence. May cause orthostatic hypotension; use with caution in patients who would not tolerate transient hypotensive episodes. When arising from a recumbent position, advise patients to sit upright for a few minutes prior to standing. Constipation may commonly occur. May require treatment interruption or dosage reduction. Certain adverse reactions (constipation, fatigue, weakness, nausea, hypokalemia, hyperglycemia, DVT, pulmonary embolism, atrial fibrillation) are more likely in elderly patients. In studies conducted prior to the use of highly active antiretroviral therapy, use was associated with increased viral loads in HIV infected patients. Monitor viral load after the 1st and 3rd months of therapy and every 3 months thereafter.

Potentially significant interactions may exist, requiring dose or frequency adjustment, additional monitoring, and/or selection of alternative therapy. Consult drug interactions database for more detailed information. Patients should not donate blood during thalidomide treatment and for 1 month after therapy discontinuation

[U.S. Boxed Warning]: Thalidomide may cause severe birth defects or embryo-fetal death if taken during pregnancy. Thalidomide cannot be used in women who are pregnant or may become pregnant during therapy as even a single dose may cause birth defects. In order to decrease the risk of fetal exposure, thalidomide is available only through a special restricted distribution program (Thalomid REMS™). Use is contraindicated in women who are or may become pregnant. Pregnancy must be excluded prior to therapy initiation with 2 negative pregnancy tests. Women of reproductive potential must avoid pregnancy 4 weeks prior to therapy, during therapy, during therapy interruptions, and for ≥4 weeks after therapy is discontinued; two reliable methods of birth control, or abstinence from heterosexual intercourse, must be used. Males taking thalidomide (even those vasectomized) must use a latex or synthetic condom during any sexual contact with women of childbearing potential and for up to 28 days following discontinuation of therapy. Males taking thalidomide must not donate sperm. Some forms of contraception may not be appropriate in certain patients. An intrauterine device (IUD) or implantable contraceptive may increase the risk of infection or bleeding; estrogen containing products may increase the risk of thromboembolism.

[U.S. Boxed Warning]: Thalidomide should only be prescribed to patients who can understand and comply with the conditions of the Thalomid REMS™ program. Prescribers, patients, and pharmacies must be certified with the program to prescribe or dispense thalidomide.

Drug Interactions

Metabolism/Transport Effects None known.

Avoid Concomitant Use

Avoid concomitant use of Thalidomide with any of the following: Abatacept; Anakinra; Azelastine (Nasal); BCG; Canakinumab; Certolizumab Pegol; CloZAPine; Natalizumab; Paraldehyde; Pimecrolimus; Rilonacept; Tacrolimus (Topical); Tocilizumab; Tofacitinib; Vaccines (Live)

Increased Effect/Toxicity

Thalidomide may increase the levels/effects of: Abatacept; Alcohol (Ethyl); Anakinra; Azelastine (Nasal); Buprenorphine; Canakinumab; Certolizumab Pegol; CloZAPine; CNS Depressants; Leflunomide; Methotrimeprazine; Metyrosine; Mirtazapine; Natalizumab; Pamidronate; Paraldehyde; Pramipexole; Rilonacept; ROPINIRole; Rotigotine; Selective Serotonin Reuptake Inhibitors; Tofacitinib; Vaccines (Live); Zoledronic Acid; Zolpidem

The levels/effects of Thalidomide may be increased by: Denosumab; Dexamethasone (Systemic); Droperidol; HydrOXYzine; Magnesium Sulfate; Methotrimeprazine; Perampanel; Pimecrolimus; Roflumilast; Sodium Oxybate; Tacrolimus (Topical); Tocilizumab; Trastuzumab

Decreased Effect

Thalidomide may decrease the levels/effects of: BCG; Coccidioidin Skin Test; Sipuleucel-T; Vaccines (Inactivated); Vaccines (Live)

The levels/effects of Thalidomide may be decreased by: Echinacea

Ethanol/Nutrition/Herb Interactions

Ethanol: May increase CNS depression; monitor for increased effects with coadministration. Caution patients about effects.

Herb/Nutraceutical: Avoid cat's claw and echinacea (have immunostimulant properties; consider therapy modifications).

Dietary Considerations Should be taken at least 1 hour after the evening meal.

Pharmacodynamics/Kinetics

Half-life Elimination 5.5-7.3 hours

Time to Peak Plasma: 2-5 hours

Pregnancy Risk Factor X

Pregnancy Considerations [U.S. Boxed Warning]: Thalidomide may cause severe birth defects or embryo-fetal death if taken during pregnancy. Thalidomide cannot be used in women who are pregnant or may become pregnant during therapy as even a single dose may cause birth defects. In order to decrease the risk of fetal exposure, thalidomide is available only through a special restricted distribution program (Thalomid REMS™). Reproduction studies in animals and data from pregnant women have shown evidence of fetal abnormalities; use is contraindicated in women who are or may become pregnant. Anomalies observed in humans include amelia, phocomelia, bone defects, ear and eye abnormalities, facial palsy, congenital heart defects, urinary and genital tract malformations; mortality in ~40% of infants at or shortly after birth has also been reported.

Women of reproductive potential must avoid pregnancy 4 weeks prior to therapy, during therapy, during therapy interruptions, and for ≥4 weeks after therapy is discontinued. Two forms of effective contraception or total abstinence from heterosexual intercourse must be used by females who are not infertile or who have not had a hysterectomy. A negative pregnancy test (sensitivity of at least 50 mIU/mL) 10-14 days prior to therapy, within 24 hours prior to beginning therapy, weekly during the first 4 weeks, and every 4 weeks (every 2 weeks for women with irregular menstrual cycles) thereafter is required for women of childbearing potential. Thalidomide must be immediately discontinued for a missed period, abnormal pregnancy test or abnormal menstrual bleeding; refer patient to a reproductive toxicity specialist if pregnancy occurs during treatment.

Females of reproductive potential must also avoid contact with thalidomide capsules.

Thalidomide is also present in the semen of males. Males (even those vasectomized) must use a latex or synthetic condom during any sexual contact with women of childbearing potential and for up to 28 days following discontinuation of therapy. Males taking thalidomide must not donate sperm.

The parent or legal guardian for patients between 12-18 years of age must agree to ensure compliance with the required guidelines.

If pregnancy occurs during treatment, thalidomide must be immediately discontinued and the patient referred to a reproductive toxicity specialist. Any suspected fetal exposure to thalidomide must be reported to the FDA via the MedWatch program (1-800-FDA-1088) and to Celgene Corporation (1-888-423-5436). In Canada, thalidomide is available only through a restricted-distribution program called RevAid® (1-888-738-2431).

Lactation Excretion in breast milk unknown/not recommended

Breast-Feeding Considerations It is not known if thalidomide is excreted in breast milk. Due to the potential for serious adverse reactions in the infant, a decision should be made to discontinue nursing or discontinue treatment with thalidomide, taking into account the importance of treatment to the mother. Use in breast-feeding women is contraindicated in the Canadian labeling.

Prescribing and Access Restrictions U.S.: As a requirement of the REMS program, access to this medication is restricted. Thalidomide is approved for marketing only under a special distribution program, the Thalomid REMS™ (www.celgeneriskmanagment.com or 1-888-423-5436), which has been approved by the FDA. Prescribers, patients, and pharmacies must be certified with the program to prescribe or dispense thalidomide. No more than a 4-week supply should be dispensed. Blister packs should be dispensed intact (do not repackage capsules). Prescriptions must be filled within 7 days (for females of reproductive potential) or within 30 days (for all other patients) after authorization number obtained. Subsequent prescriptions may be filled only if fewer than 7 days of therapy remain on the previous prescription. A new prescription is required for further dispensing (a telephone prescription may not be accepted.) Pregnancy testing is required for females of childbearing potential.

Canada: Access to thalidomide is restricted through a controlled distribution program called RevAid®. Only physicians and pharmacists enrolled in this program are authorized to prescribe or dispense thalidomide. Patients must be enrolled in the program by their physicians. Further information is available at www.RevAid.ca or by calling 1-888-738-2431.

Dosage Forms

Capsule, oral:

Thalomid®: 50 mg, 100 mg, 150 mg, 200 mg

References

Hamuryudan V, Mat C, Saip S, et al, "Thalidomide in the Treatment of the Mucocutaneous Lesions of the Behçet Syndrome. A Randomized, Double-Blind, Placebo-Controlled Trial," *Ann Intern Med*, 1998, 128(6):443-50.

Jacobson JM, Greenspan JS, Spritzler J, et al, "Thalidomide for the Treatment of Oral Aphthous Ulcers in Patients With Human Immunodeficiency Virus Infection. National Institute of Allergy and Infectious Diseases AIDS Clinical Trials Group," *N Engl J Med*, 1997, 336 (21):1487-93.

Schuler U and Ehninger G, "Thalidomide: Rationale for Renewed Use in Immunological Disorders," *Drug Saf*, 1995, 12(6):364-9.

Theophylline (thee OFF i lin)

Related Information

Aminophylline *on page 79*

Respiratory Diseases *on page 1514*

Brand Names: U.S. Elixophyllin® Elixir; Theo-24®

Brand Names: Canada Apo-Theo LA®; Novo-Theophyl SR; PMS-Theophylline; Pulmophylline; ratio-Theo-Bronc; Teva-Theophylline SR; Theo ER; Theolair; Uniphyl

Pharmacologic Category Phosphodiesterase Enzyme Inhibitor, Nonselective

Use Treatment of symptoms and reversible airway obstruction due to chronic asthma, or other chronic lung diseases

Note: The Global Initiative for Asthma Guidelines (2009) and the National Heart, Lung and Blood Institute Guidelines (2007) do not recommend oral theophylline as a long-term control medication for asthma in children ≤5 years of age; use has been shown to be effective as an add-on (but not preferred) agent in older children and adults with severe asthma treated with inhaled or oral glucocorticoids. The guidelines do not recommend theophylline for the treatment of exacerbations of asthma.

The Global Initiative for Chronic Obstructive Lung Disease Guidelines (2013) suggest that while higher doses of slow release formulations of theophylline have been proven to be effective for use in COPD, it is not a preferred agent due to its potential for toxicity.

Local Anesthetic/Vasoconstrictor Precautions No information available to require special precautions

Effects on Dental Treatment Prescribe erythromycin products with caution to patients taking theophylline products. Erythromycin will delay the normal metabolic inactivation of theophyllines leading to increased blood levels; this has resulted in nausea, vomiting, and CNS restlessness. Azithromycin does not cause these effects in combination with theophylline products.

Effects on Bleeding No information available to require special precautions

Adverse Effects Frequency not defined. Adverse events observed at therapeutic serum levels:

Cardiovascular: Flutter, tachycardia

Central nervous system: Headache, hyperactivity (children), insomnia, restlessness, seizures, status epilepticus (nonconvulsive)

Endocrine & metabolic: Hypercalcemia (with concomitant hyperthyroid disease)

Gastrointestinal: Nausea, reflux or ulcer aggravation, vomiting

Genitourinary: Difficulty urinating (elderly males with prostatism)

Neuromuscular & skeletal: Tremor

Renal: Diuresis (transient)

General Dosage Range

I.V.:

Infants 6-52 weeks: mg/kg/hour = (0.008) (age in weeks) + 0.21

Children 1-9 years: 0.8 mg/kg/hour

Children 9-12 years and Adolescents 12-16 years (cigarette or marijuana smokers): 0.7 mg/kg/hour

Adolescents 12-16 years (nonsmokers): 0.5 mg/kg/hour; maximum: 900 mg/day unless serum levels indicate need for larger dose

Adults 16-60 years (otherwise healthy, nonsmokers): 0.4 mg/kg/hour; maximum: 900 mg/day unless serum levels indicate need for larger dose

Adults >60 years: 0.3 mg/kg/hour; maximum: 400 mg/day unless serum levels indicate need for larger dose

Oral solution:

Full-term Infants and Infants <26 weeks: Total daily dose (mg) = [(0.2 x age in weeks) +5] x (weight in kg); divide dose into 3 equal amounts and administer at 8-hour intervals

Full-term Infants and Infants ≥26 weeks and <52 weeks: Total daily dose (mg) = [(0.2 x age in weeks) +5] x (weight in kg); divide dose into 4 equal amounts and administer at 6-hour intervals

Children ≥1 year and <45 kg: Initial: 10-14 mg/kg/day in divided doses (maximum dose: 300 mg/day); titrate to maintenance dose: 20 mg/kg/day in divided doses every 4-6 hours (maximum dose: 600 mg/day)

Children >45 kg and Adults: Initial: 300 mg/day in divided doses; titrate to maintenance dose: 600 mg/day in divided doses every 6-8 hours

Oral extended release formulations:

Children ≥1 year and <45 kg: Initial: 10-14 mg/kg once daily (maximum dose: 300 mg/day); titrate to maintenance dose: 20 mg/kg once daily (maximum dose: 600 mg/day)

Children >45 kg and Adults: 300-600 mg once daily

Mechanism of Action Causes bronchodilatation, diuresis, CNS and cardiac stimulation, and gastric acid secretion by blocking phosphodiesterase which increases tissue concentrations of cyclic adenine monophosphate (cAMP) which in turn promotes catecholamine stimulation of lipolysis, glycogenolysis, and gluconeogenesis and induces release of epinephrine from adrenal medulla cells

Pharmacodynamics/Kinetics

Onset of Action I.V.: <30 minutes

Half-life Elimination Highly variable and age, liver and cardiac function, lung disease, and smoking history dependent

Premature infants, postnatal age 3-15 days: 30 hours (range: 17-43 hours)

Premature infants, postnatal age 25-57 days: 20 hours (range: 9.4-30.6 hours)

Children 6-17 years: 3.7 hours (range: 1.5-5.9 hours)

Adults 16-60 years with asthma, nonsmoking, otherwise healthy: 8.7 hours (range: 6.1-12.8 hours)

Time to Peak Serum: Oral: Liquid: 1 hour

Pregnancy Risk Factor C

Pregnancy Considerations Teratogenic effects were observed in animal reproduction studies. Theophylline crosses the placenta; adverse effects may be seen in the newborn. Use is generally safe when used at the recommended doses (serum concentrations 5-12 mcg/mL) however maternal adverse events may be increased and efficacy may be decreased in pregnant women. Theophylline metabolism may change during pregnancy; the half-life is similar to that observed in otherwise healthy, nonsmoking adults with asthma during the first and second trimesters (~8.7 hours), but may increase to 13 hours (range: 8-18 hours) during the third trimester. The volume of distribution is also increased during the third trimester. Monitor serum levels. The recommendations for the use of theophylline in pregnant women with asthma are similar to those used in non-pregnant adults (National Heart, Lung, and Blood Institute Guidelines, 2004).

Thiamine (THYE a min)

Brand Names: Canada Betaxin®

Pharmacologic Category Vitamin, Water Soluble

Use Treatment of thiamine deficiency including beriberi, Wernicke's encephalopathy, Korsakoff's syndrome, neuritis associated with pregnancy, or in alcoholic patients; dietary supplement

Local Anesthetic/Vasoconstrictor Precautions No information available to require special precautions

Effects on Dental Treatment Key adverse event(s) related to dental treatment: Tightness of the throat.

Effects on Bleeding No information available to require special precautions

Adverse Effects Adverse reactions reported with injection. Frequency not defined.

Cardiovascular: Cyanosis

Central nervous system: Restlessness

Dermatologic: Angioneurotic edema, pruritus, urticaria

Gastrointestinal: Hemorrhage into GI tract, nausea, tightness of the throat

Local: Induration and/or tenderness at the injection site (following I.M. administration)

Neuromuscular & skeletal: Weakness

Respiratory: Pulmonary edema

Miscellaneous: Anaphylactic/hypersensitivity reactions (following I.V. administration), diaphoresis, warmth

General Dosage Range

I.M., I.V.:

Children: 10-25 mg/dose daily (thiamine deficiency)

Adults: 5-30 mg/dose 3 times/day (thiamine deficiency) **or** 50-250 mg/day (Wernicke's encephalopathy)

Oral:

Infants: 0.2-0.3 mg/day (adequate intake)

Children: 0.5-1.4 mg/day (recommended daily intake) **or** 5-50 mg/day (thiamine deficiency)

Adults: 1.1-1.4 mg/day (recommended daily intake) **or** 5-30 mg/day in 1-3 divided doses (thiamine deficiency)

Mechanism of Action An essential coenzyme in carbohydrate metabolism by combining with adenosine triphosphate to form thiamine pyrophosphate

Pregnancy Risk Factor A

Pregnancy Considerations Water soluble vitamins cross the placenta. Thiamine requirements may be increased during pregnancy (IOM, 1998). Severe nausea and vomiting (hyperemesis gravidarum) may lead to thiamine deficiency manifested as Wernicke's encephalopathy (Chiossi, 2006).

Thioguanine (thye oh GWAH neen)

Brand Names: U.S. Tabloid®

Brand Names: Canada Lanvis®

Pharmacologic Category Antineoplastic Agent, Antimetabolite (Purine Analog)

Use Treatment of acute myelogenous (nonlymphocytic) leukemia (AML)

Unlabeled Use Treatment of pediatric acute lymphoblastic leukemia (ALL)

Local Anesthetic/Vasoconstrictor Precautions No information available to require special precautions

Effects on Dental Treatment Key adverse event(s) related to dental treatment: Stomatitis.

Effects on Bleeding Chemotherapy may result in significant myelosuppression, potentially including significant reduction in platelet counts and altered hemostasis. In patients who are under active treatment with these agents, medical consult is suggested.

Adverse Effects Frequency not defined.

Endocrine & metabolic: Fluid retention, hyperuricemia (common)

Gastrointestinal: Anorexia, intestinal necrosis, intestinal perforation, nausea, splenomegaly, stomatitis, vomiting, weight gain

Hematologic: Anemia (may be delayed), bleeding, granulocytopenia, leukopenia (common; may be delayed), marrow hypoplasia, pancytopenia, thrombocytopenia (common; may be delayed)

Hepatic: Ascites, esophageal varices, hepatic necrosis (centrilobular), hepatic sinusoidal obstruction syndrome (SOS; veno-occlusive disease), hepatitis, hepatomegaly [tender], hepatoportal sclerosis, hepatotoxicity, hyperbilirubinemia, jaundice, LFTs increased, nodular regenerative hyperplasia, peliosis hepatitis, periportal fibrosis, portal hypertension

Miscellaneous: Infection

Mechanism of Action Purine analog that is incorporated into DNA and RNA resulting in the blockage of synthesis and metabolism of purine nucleotides

Pharmacodynamics/Kinetics

Half-life Elimination Terminal: 5-9 hours

Time to Peak Serum: Within 8 hours; predominantly metabolite(s)

Pregnancy Risk Factor D

Pregnancy Considerations Animal studies have demonstrated adverse effects. There are no adequate and well-controlled studies in pregnant women. May cause fetal harm if administered during pregnancy. Women of childbearing potential should avoid becoming pregnant during treatment.

Thiopental (thye oh PEN tal)

Brand Names: U.S. Pentothal® [DSC]

Pharmacologic Category Anticonvulsant, Barbiturate; Barbiturate; General Anesthetic

Use Induction of anesthesia; control of convulsive states; treatment of elevated intracranial pressure

Local Anesthetic/Vasoconstrictor Precautions No information available to require special precautions

Effects on Dental Treatment No significant effects or complications reported

Effects on Bleeding No information available to require special precautions

Adverse Effects Frequency not defined.

Cardiovascular: Bradycardia, hypotension, syncope

Central nervous system: Drowsiness, lethargy, CNS excitation or depression, impaired judgment, "hangover" effect, confusion, somnolence, agitation, hyperkinesia, ataxia, nervousness, headache, insomnia, nightmares, hallucinations, anxiety, dizziness, shivering

Dermatologic: Rash, exfoliative dermatitis, Stevens-Johnson syndrome

Gastrointestinal: Nausea, vomiting, constipation

Hematologic: Agranulocytosis, thrombocytopenia, megaloblastic anemia, immune hemolytic anemia (rare)

Local: Pain at injection site, thrombophlebitis with I.V. use

Renal: Oliguria

Respiratory: Laryngospasm, respiratory depression, apnea (especially with rapid I.V. use), hypoventilation, apnea, sneezing, cough, bronchospasm

Miscellaneous: Gangrene with inadvertent intra-arterial injection, anaphylaxis, anaphylactic reactions

General Dosage Range Dosage adjustment recommended in patients with renal impairment

I.V.:

Infants <1 year: Anesthesia induction: 5-8 mg/kg

Children 1-12 years: Anesthesia induction: 5-6 mg/kg; Maintenance: 1 mg/kg as needed **or** 1.5-5 mg/kg/dose, repeat as needed

Children >12 years: Maintenance: 1 mg/kg as needed **or** 1.5-5 mg/kg/dose, repeat as needed

Adults: Anesthesia induction: 3-5 mg/kg; Maintenance: 25-100 mg as needed **or** 1.5-5 mg/kg/dose, repeat as needed **or** 75-250 mg/dose, repeat as needed

Mechanism of Action Short-acting barbiturate with sedative, hypnotic, and anticonvulsant properties. Barbiturates depress the sensory cortex, decrease motor activity, alter cerebellar function, and produce drowsiness, sedation, and hypnosis. In high doses, barbiturates exhibit anticonvulsant activity; barbiturates produce dose-dependent respiratory depression.

Pharmacodynamics/Kinetics

Onset of Action Anesthetic: I.V.: 30-60 seconds

Duration of Action 5-30 minutes

Half-life Elimination 3-11.5 hours; decreased in children

Pregnancy Risk Factor C

Product Availability Pentothal® (thiopental injection): Hospira Pharmaceuticals, the sole manufacturer, has discontinued all Pentothal® products. Product is currently unavailable in the U.S. and in Canada.

Controlled Substance C-III

Thioridazine (thye oh RID a zeen)

Related Information

Clinical Risk Related to Drugs Prolonging QT Interval *on page 1510*

Pharmacologic Category Antipsychotic Agent, Typical, Phenothiazine

Use Management of schizophrenic patients who fail to respond adequately to treatment with other antipsychotic drugs, either because of insufficient effectiveness or the inability to achieve an effective dose due to intolerable adverse effects from those medications

Unlabeled Use Behavior problems (children); severe psychoses (children); schizophrenia/psychoses (children); depressive disorders/dementia (children and adults); behavioral symptoms associated with dementia (elderly); psychosis/agitation related to Alzheimer's dementia

Local Anesthetic/Vasoconstrictor Precautions Most pharmacology textbooks state that in presence of phenothiazines, systemic doses of epinephrine paradoxically decrease the blood pressure. This is the so called "epinephrine reversal" phenomenon. This has never been observed when epinephrine is given by infiltration as part of the anesthesia procedure. Thioridazine is one of the drugs confirmed to prolong the QT interval and is accepted as having a risk of causing torsade de pointes. The risk of drug-induced torsade de pointes is extremely low when a single QT interval prolonging drug is prescribed. In terms of epinephrine, it is not known what effect vasoconstrictors in the local anesthetic regimen will have in patients with a known history of congenital prolonged QT interval or in patients taking any medication that prolongs the QT interval. Until more information is obtained, it is suggested that the clinician consult with the physician prior to the use of a vasoconstrictor in suspected patients, and that the vasoconstrictor (epinephrine, mepivacaine and levonordefrin [Carbocaine® 2% with Neo-Cobefrin®]) be used with caution.

Effects on Dental Treatment Key adverse event(s) related to dental treatment: Xerostomia and changes in salivation (normal salivary flow resumes upon discontinuation). Significant hypotension may occur, especially when the drug is administered parenterally; orthostatic hypotension is due to alpha-receptor blockade, the elderly are at greater risk for orthostatic hypotension.

Tardive dyskinesia; Prevalence rate may be 40% in elderly; development of the syndrome and the irreversible nature are proportional to duration and total cumulative dose over time. Extrapyramidal reactions are more common in elderly with up to 50% developing these reactions after 60 years of age. Drug-induced Parkinson's syndrome occurs often; akathisia is the most common extrapyramidal reaction in elderly.

Effects on Bleeding No information available to require special precautions

Adverse Effects Frequency not defined.

Cardiovascular: Hypotension, orthostatic hypotension, peripheral edema, ECG changes

Central nervous system: EPS (pseudoparkinsonism, akathisia, dystonias, tardive dyskinesia), dizziness, drowsiness, neuroleptic malignant syndrome (NMS), impairment of temperature regulation, lowering of seizure threshold, seizure

Dermatologic: Increased sensitivity to sun, rash, discoloration of skin (blue-gray)

Endocrine & metabolic: Changes in menstrual cycle, libido (changes in), breast pain, galactorrhea, amenorrhea

Gastrointestinal: Constipation, weight gain, nausea, vomiting, stomach pain, xerostomia, nausea, vomiting, diarrhea

Genitourinary: Difficulty in urination, ejaculatory disturbances, urinary retention, priapism

Hematologic: Agranulocytosis, leukopenia

Hepatic: Cholestatic jaundice, hepatotoxicity

Neuromuscular & skeletal: Tremor

Ocular: Pigmentary retinopathy, blurred vision, cornea and lens changes

Respiratory: Nasal congestion

General Dosage Range Oral:

Children >2-12 years: 0.5-3 mg/kg/day in 2-3 divided doses **or** 10-25 mg 2-3 times/day (maximum: 3 mg/kg/day)

Children >12 years and Adults: Initial: 50-100 mg 3 times/day; Maintenance: 150-800 mg/day in 2-4 divided doses (maximum: 800 mg/day) **or** Initial: 25 mg 3 times/day; Maintenance: 20-200 mg/day

Elderly: Initial: 10-25 mg 1-2 times/day; Maintenance: 10-400 mg/day in 1-2 divided doses (maximum: 400 mg/day)

Mechanism of Action Thioridazine is a piperidine phenothiazine which blocks postsynaptic mesolimbic dopaminergic receptors in the brain; exhibits a strong alpha-adrenergic blocking effect and depresses the release of hypothalamic and hypophyseal hormones

Pharmacodynamics/Kinetics

Duration of Action 4-5 days

Half-life Elimination 21-25 hours

Time to Peak Serum: ~1 hour

Pregnancy Risk Factor C

Pregnancy Considerations Jaundice or hyper-/hyporeflexia have been reported in newborn infants following maternal use of phenothiazines. Antipsychotic use during the third trimester of pregnancy has a risk for abnormal muscle movements (extrapyramidal symptoms [EPS]) and withdrawal symptoms in new-borns following delivery. Symptoms in the newborn may include agitation, feeding disorder, hypertonia, hypotonia, respiratory distress, somnolence, and tremor; these effects may be self-limiting or require hospitalization.

Dental Comment Thioridazine is known to prolong the QT interval. The QT interval is measured as the time and distance between the Q point of the QRS complex and the end of the T wave in the ECG tracing. After adjustment for heart rate, the QT interval is defined as prolonged if it is more than 450 msec in men and 460 msec in women. A long QT syndrome was first described in the 1950s and 60s as a congenital syndrome involving QT interval prolongation and syncope and sudden death. Some of the congenital long QT syndromes were characterized by a peculiar electrocardiographic appearance of the QRS complex involving a premature atria beat followed by a pause, then a subsequent sinus beat showing marked QT prolongation and deformity. This type of cardiac arrhythmia was originally termed "torsade de pointes" (translated from the French as "twisting of the points"). Thioridazine is considered as having a risk of causing torsade de pointes. Since it is not known what effect vasoconstrictors in the local anesthetic regimen will have in patients with a known history of congenital prolonged QT interval or in patients taking any medication that prolongs the QT interval, a medical consult is suggested.

Thiotepa (thye oh TEP a)

Pharmacologic Category Antineoplastic Agent, Alkylating Agent

Use Treatment of superficial papillary bladder cancer; palliative treatment of adenocarcinoma of breast or ovary; controlling intracavitary effusions caused by metastatic tumors

Unlabeled Use Intrathecal treatment of leptomeningeal metastases

Local Anesthetic/Vasoconstrictor Precautions No information available to require special precautions

Effects on Dental Treatment No significant effects or complications reported

Effects on Bleeding Chemotherapy may result in significant myelosuppression, potentially including significant reduction in platelet counts and altered hemostasis. In patients who are under active treatment with these agents, medical consult is suggested.

Adverse Effects Frequency not defined.

Central nervous system: Chills, dizziness, fatigue, fever, headache

Dermatologic: Alopecia, contact dermatitis, depigmentation (with topical treatment), dermatitis, rash, urticaria

Endocrine & metabolic: Amenorrhea, spermatogenesis inhibition

Gastrointestinal: Abdominal pain, anorexia, nausea, vomiting

Genitourinary: Dysuria, urinary retention

Hematologic: Anemia, bleeding, leukopenia, thrombocytopenia

Local: Injection site pain

Neuromuscular & skeletal: Weakness

Ocular: Blurred vision, conjunctivitis

Renal: Hematuria

Respiratory: Asthma, epistaxis, laryngeal edema, wheezing

Miscellaneous: Allergic reaction, anaphylactic shock, infection

General Dosage Range Dosage adjustment recommended in patients who develop toxicities

I.V.: *Adults:* 0.3-0.4 mg/kg every 1-4 weeks

Intracavitary: *Adults:* 0.6-0.8 mg/kg

Intravesical: *Adults:* 60 mg retained for 2 hours once weekly for 4 weeks

Mechanism of Action Alkylating agent that reacts with DNA phosphate groups to produce cross-linking of DNA strands leading to inhibition of DNA, RNA, and protein synthesis; mechanism of action has not been explored as thoroughly as the other alkylating agents, it is presumed that the aziridine rings open and react as nitrogen mustard; reactivity is enhanced at a lower pH

Pharmacodynamics/Kinetics

Half-life Elimination Terminal: Dose-dependent clearance: ~2 hours

Pregnancy Risk Factor D

Pregnancy Considerations Animal reproduction studies have demonstrated teratogenicity and fetal loss. There are no adequate and well-controlled studies in pregnant women. May cause harm if administered during pregnancy. Effective contraception is recommended for men and women of childbearing potential.

Thiothixene (thye oh THIKS een)

Brand Names: Canada Navane®

Pharmacologic Category Antipsychotic Agent, Typical

Use Management of schizophrenia

Unlabeled Use Psychotic disorders (children); rapid tranquilization of the agitated patient (children); non-psychotic patient, dementia behavior (elderly); psychosis/agitation related to Alzheimer's dementia

Local Anesthetic/Vasoconstrictor Precautions Most pharmacology textbooks state that in presence of phenothiazines, systemic doses of epinephrine paradoxically decrease the blood pressure. This is the so called "epinephrine reversal" phenomenon. This has never been observed when epinephrine is given by infiltration as part of the anesthesia procedure. Thiothixene is one of the drugs confirmed to prolong the QT interval and is accepted as having a risk of causing torsade de pointes. The risk of drug-induced torsade de pointes is extremely low when a single QT interval prolonging drug is prescribed. In terms of epinephrine, it is not known what effect vasoconstrictors in the local anesthetic regimen will have in patients with a known history of congenital prolonged QT interval or in patients taking any medication that prolongs the QT interval. Until more information is obtained, it is suggested that the clinician consult with the physician prior to the use of a vasoconstrictor in suspected patients, and that the vasoconstrictor (epinephrine, mepivacaine and levonordefrin [Carbocaine® 2% with Neo-Cobefrin®]) be used with caution.

Effects on Dental Treatment Key adverse event(s) related to dental treatment: Xerostomia and changes in salivation (normal salivary flow resumes upon discontinuation), significant hypotension may occur, especially when the drug is administered parenterally; orthostatic hypotension is due to alpha-receptor blockade, the elderly are at greater risk for orthostatic hypotension.

Tardive dyskinesia: Prevalence rate may be 40% in elderly; development of the syndrome and the irreversible nature are proportional to duration and total cumulative dose over time. Extrapyramidal reactions are more common in elderly with up to 50% developing these reactions after 60 years of age. Drug-induced

Parkinson's syndrome occurs often; akathisia is the most common extrapyramidal reaction in elderly.

Effects on Bleeding No information available to require special precautions

Adverse Effects Frequency not defined.

Cardiovascular: Hypotension, nonspecific ECG changes, syncope, tachycardia

Central nervous system: Agitation, dizziness, drowsiness, extrapyramidal symptoms (akathisia, dystonias, lightheadedness, pseudoparkinsonism, tardive dyskinesia), insomnia restlessness

Dermatologic: Discoloration of skin (blue-gray), photosensitivity, pruritus, rash, urticaria

Endocrine & metabolic: Amenorrhea, breast pain, libido (changes in), changes in menstrual cycle, galactorrhea, gynecomastia, hyper-/hypoglycemia, hyperprolactinemia, lactation

Gastrointestinal: Constipation, nausea, salivation increased, stomach pain, vomiting, weight gain, xerostomia

Genitourinary: Difficulty in urination, ejaculatory disturbances, impotence

Hematologic: Leukocytes, leukopenia

Neuromuscular & skeletal: Tremors

Ocular: Blurred vision, pigmentary retinopathy

Respiratory: Nasal congestion

Miscellaneous: Diaphoresis

General Dosage Range Oral: *Adults:* Initial: 6-10 mg/day in 2-3 divided doses; Maintenance: 20-60 mg/day in 2-3 divided doses (maximum: 60 mg/day)

Mechanism of Action Thiothixene is a thioxanthene antipsychotic which elicits antipsychotic activity by postsynaptic blockade of CNS dopamine receptors resulting in inhibition of dopamine-mediated effects; also has alpha-adrenergic blocking activity

Pharmacodynamics/Kinetics

Half-life Elimination >24 hours with chronic use

Pregnancy Considerations Antipsychotic use during the third trimester of pregnancy has a risk for abnormal muscle movements (extrapyramidal symptoms [EPS]) and withdrawal symptoms in newborns following delivery. Symptoms in the newborn may include agitation, feeding disorder, hypertonia, hypotonia, respiratory distress, somnolence, and tremor; these effects may be self-limiting or require hospitalization.

Dental Comment Thiothixene is known to prolong the QT interval. The QT interval is measured as the time and distance between the Q point of the QRS complex and the end of the T wave in the ECG tracing. After adjustment for heart rate, the QT interval is defined as prolonged if it is more than 450 msec in men and 460 msec in women. A long QT syndrome was first described in the 1950s and 60s as a congenital syndrome involving QT interval prolongation and syncope and sudden death. Some of the congenital long QT syndromes were characterized by a peculiar electrocardiographic appearance of the QRS complex involving a premature atria beat followed by a pause, then a subsequent sinus beat showing marked QT prolongation and deformity. This type of cardiac arrhythmia was originally termed "torsade de pointes" (translated from the French as "twisting of the points"). Thiothixene is considered as having a risk of causing torsade de pointes. Since it is not known what effect vasoconstrictors in the local anesthetic regimen will have in patients with a known history of congenital prolonged QT interval or in patients taking any medication that prolongs the QT interval, a medical consult is suggested.

Thrombin (Topical) (THROM bin, TOP i kal)

Related Information
Antiplatelet and Anticoagulation Considerations in Dentistry *on page 1503*

Brand Names: U.S. Evithrom®; Recothrom®; Thrombi-Gel®; Thrombi-Pad®; Thrombin-JMI®; Thrombin-JMI® Epistaxis Kit; Thrombin-JMI® Pump Spray Kit; Thrombin-JMI® Syringe Spray Kit

Generic Availability (U.S.) No

Pharmacologic Category Blood Product Derivative; Hemostatic Agent

Dental Use Hemostasis whenever minor bleeding from capillaries and small venules is accessible

Use Hemostasis whenever minor bleeding from capillaries and small venules is accessible

Thrombi-Gel®; Thrombi-Pad®: Temporary control as trauma dressing for moderate-to-severe bleeding wounds; control of surface bleeding from vascular access sites and percutaneous catheter/tubes

Local Anesthetic/Vasoconstrictor Precautions No information available to require special precautions

Effects on Dental Treatment No significant effects or complications reported

Effects on Bleeding General dental procedures and simple restorative procedures are not associated with bleeding; therefore, there is no contraindication to general dental treatment for most patients with bleeding disorders. However, after dental extractions and other dental surgeries including deep scaling, block anesthesia, and large fillings, in patients with hemophilia, drugs such as topical thrombin may be useful in controlling bleeding. A carefully coordinated strategy between the dental and medical team may be required to ensure adequate procedures for hemostasis.

Adverse Effects Frequency not defined.

Dermatologic: Pruritus

Gastrointestinal: Nausea, vomiting

Hematologic: Bleeding, aPTT increased, INR increased, lymphocyte count decreased, neutrophil count increased, PT prolonged

Local: Incision site complication

Miscellaneous: Antibody development, hypersensitivity reactions

Dental Usual Dosage Topical: Hemostasis: **Note:** For topical use only; do not administer intravenously or intra-arterially:

Evithrom®: Children and Adults: Dose depends on area to be treated; up to 10 mL was used with absorbable gelatin sponge in clinical studies

Recothrom®: Adults: Dose depends on area to be treated

Thrombi-Gel® 10, 40, 100: Adults: Wet product with up to 3 mL, 10 mL, or 20 mL, respectively, of 0.9% sodium chloride or SWFI; apply directly over source of the bleeding with manual pressure

Thrombi-Pad®: Adults: Apply pad directly over source of bleeding; may apply dry or wetted with up to 10 mL of 0.9% sodium chloride. If desired, product may be left in place for up to 24 hours; do not leave in the body.

Thrombin-JMI®: Adults:

Solution: Use 1000-2000 units/mL of solution where bleeding is profuse; use 100 units/mL for bleeding from skin or mucosal surfaces

Powder: May apply powder directly to the site of bleeding or on oozing surfaces

◀ **Dosage** Topical: Hemostasis: **Note:** For topical use only; do not administer intravenously or intra-arterially:

Evithrom®: Children, Adolescents, and Adults: Dose depends on area to be treated; up to 10 mL was used with absorbable gelatin sponge in clinical studies

Recothrom®: Infants ≥1 month, Children, Adolescents, and Adults: Dose depends on area to be treated

Thrombi-Gel® 10, 40, 100: Adults: Wet product with up to 3 mL, 10 mL, or 20 mL, respectively, of 0.9% sodium chloride or SWFI; apply directly over source of the bleeding with manual pressure

Thrombi-Pad®: Adults: Apply pad directly over source of bleeding; may apply dry or wetted with up to 10 mL of 0.9% sodium chloride. If desired, product may be left in place for up to 24 hours; do not leave in the body.

Thrombin-JMI®: Adults:

Solution: Use 1000-2000 units/mL of solution where bleeding is profuse; use 100 units/mL for bleeding from skin or mucosal surfaces

Powder: May apply powder directly to the site of bleeding or on oozing surfaces

Mechanism of Action Activates platelets and catalyzes the conversion of fibrinogen to fibrin to promote hemostasis.

Contraindications Hypersensitivity to thrombin or any component of the formulation; not for direct injection into the circulatory system (for topical use only); additionally,

Evithrom® is also contraindicated in patients with known anaphylactic or severe systemic reactions to blood products; also contraindicated for the treatment of severe or brisk arterial bleeding

Recothrom® is also contraindicated in patients with hypersensitivity to hamster proteins; also contraindicated for the treatment of massive or brisk arterial bleeding

Thrombi-Gel®: Should not be used in closure of skin incisions, due to possible interference with healing of skin edges.

Thrombin-JMI® and Thrombi-Pad® are also contraindicated in patients with hypersensitivity to material of bovine origin.

Warnings/Precautions For topical use only. Do not inject intravenously or intra-arterially. Intravascular clotting, possibly leading to death, may occur following injection. Powder and solution formulations may be used in combination with absorbable gelatin sponges

[U.S. Boxed Warning]: Bovine-source topical thrombin may be associated with abnormal hemostasis, ranging from asymptomatic laboratory alterations to severe bleeding and/or thrombosis. Abnormalities appear to be immunologically mediated; repeated applications increase risk. Consult expert in coagulation disorders if laboratory evidence and/or signs and symptoms of bleeding are noted. Re-exposure of patients who develop antibodies to bovine thrombin preparations should be avoided. Evithrom® is a product of human plasma; may potentially contain infectious agents which could transmit disease. Screening of donors, as well as testing and/or inactivation or removal of certain viruses, reduces the risk. Infections thought to be transmitted by this product should be reported to the manufacturer. Recothrom® should be used with caution in patients with known hypersensitivity to snake proteins (manufacturing process uses an enzyme isolated from a snake protein); the potential for allergic reaction theoretically exists. Do not use Thrombi-Gel® or Thrombi-Pad® in the presence of infection; use caution in areas of contamination. Thrombi-Pad® is nonabsorbable; do not leave in the body.

Drug Interactions

Metabolism/Transport Effects None known.

Avoid Concomitant Use There are no known interactions where it is recommended to avoid concomitant use.

Increased Effect/Toxicity There are no known significant interactions involving an increase in effect.

Decreased Effect There are no known significant interactions involving a decrease in effect.

Pregnancy Risk Factor C

Pregnancy Considerations Adequate reproduction studies have not been conducted. Reproduction studies conducted with the solvent/detergent used in processing the human-derived product showed adverse events in animals. Only residual levels of the solvent/detergent would be expected to remain in the finished product.

Dosage Forms

Pad, topical [preservative free]:
Thrombi-Pad® 3x3: ≥200 units

Powder for reconstitution, topical:
Thrombin-JMI®: 5000 units, 20,000 units
Thrombin-JMI® Epistaxis kit: 5000 units
Thrombin-JMI® Pump Spray Kit: 20,000 units
Thrombin-JMI® Syringe Spray Kit: 5000 units; 20,000 units

Powder for reconstitution, topical [preservative free]:
Recothrom®: 5000 units; 20,000 units

Solution, topical:
Evithrom®: 800-1200 units/mL (2 mL, 5 mL, 20 mL)

Sponge, topical [preservative free]:
Thrombi-Gel® 10: ≥1000 units (10s)
Thrombi-Gel® 40: ≥1000 units (5s)
Thrombi-Gel® 100: ≥2000 units (5s)

Thyroid, Desiccated (THYE roid DES i kay tid)

Related Information

Endocrine Disorders and Pregnancy on page 1517

Brand Names: U.S. Armour® Thyroid; Nature-Throid™; Westhroid™

Pharmacologic Category Thyroid Product

Use Replacement or supplemental therapy in hypothyroidism; pituitary TSH suppressants (thyroid nodules, thyroiditis, multinodular goiter, thyroid cancer)

Local Anesthetic/Vasoconstrictor Precautions No precautions with vasoconstrictor are necessary if patient is well controlled with thyroid preparations

Effects on Dental Treatment No significant effects or complications reported

Effects on Bleeding No information available to require special precautions

General Dosage Range Oral:
Children 0-6 months: 15-30 mg/day **or** 4.8-6 mg/kg/day
Children 6-12 months: 30-45 mg/day **or** 3.6-4.8 mg/kg/day
Children 1-5 years: 45-60 mg/day **or** 3-3.6 mg/kg/day
Children 6-12 years: 60-90 mg/day **or** 2.4-3 mg/kg/day
Children >12 years: >90 mg/day **or** 1.2-1.8 mg/kg/day
Adults: Initial: 15-30 mg/day; Maintenance: 60-120 mg/day

Mechanism of Action The primary active compound is T_3 (triiodothyronine), which may be converted from T_4 (thyroxine) and then circulates throughout the body to influence growth and maturation of various tissues; exact mechanism of action is unknown; however, it is believed the thyroid hormone exerts its many metabolic effects through control of DNA transcription and protein synthesis; involved in normal metabolism, growth, and development; promotes gluconeogenesis, increases utilization and mobilization of glycogen stores and stimulates protein synthesis, increases basal metabolic rate

Pharmacodynamics/Kinetics
Onset of Action Liothyronine (T_3): ~3 hours
Half-life Elimination Serum:
T_4: Euthyroid: 6-7 days; Hyperthyroid: 3-4 days; Hypothyroid: 9-10 days
T_3: 2.5 days
Time to Peak Serum: T_4: 2-4 hours; T_3: 2-3 days
Pregnancy Risk Factor A
Pregnancy Considerations
Endogenous thyroid hormones minimally cross the placenta; the fetal thyroid becomes active around the end of the first trimester. Liothyronine has not been found to increase the risk of teratogenic or adverse effects following maternal use during pregnancy.

Uncontrolled maternal hypothyroidism may result in adverse neonatal and maternal outcomes. To prevent adverse events, normal maternal thyroid function should be maintained prior to conception and throughout pregnancy. Levothyroxine is considered the treatment of choice for the control of hypothyroidism during pregnancy.

Thyrotropin Alpha (thye roe TROH pin AL fa)

Brand Names: U.S. Thyrogen®
Brand Names: Canada Thyrogen®
Pharmacologic Category Diagnostic Agent
Use An adjunctive diagnostic tool for serum thyroglobulin (Tg) testing (with or without radioiodine imaging) in patients with well-differentiated thyroid cancer; adjunctive treatment for radioiodine ablation of thyroid tissue remnants after total or near-total thyroidectomy in patients with well-differentiated thyroid cancer without evidence of metastatic disease

Potential clinical uses include: Patients with an undetectable Tg on thyroid hormone suppressive therapy to exclude the diagnosis of residual or recurrent thyroid cancer, patients requiring serum Tg testing and radioiodine imaging who are unwilling to undergo thyroid hormone withdrawal testing and whose treating physician believes that use of a less sensitive test is justified, patients who are either unable to mount an adequate endogenous TSH response to thyroid hormone withdrawal or in whom withdrawal is medically contraindicated, and patients without evidence of metastatic disease to ablate thyroid remnants (in combination with radioiodine [I^{131}]) following near-total thyroidectomy.

Local Anesthetic/Vasoconstrictor Precautions No information available to require special precautions
Effects on Dental Treatment No significant effects or complications reported
Effects on Bleeding No information available to require special precautions
Adverse Effects
>10%: Gastrointestinal: Nausea (3% to 12%)
1% to 10%:
Central nervous system: Headache (1% to 7%), dizziness (≤3%), fatigue (1% to 3%), insomnia (≤2%)
Endocrine & metabolic: Hypercholesterolemia (≤3%), cholesterol abnormal (≤1%)
Gastrointestinal: Vomiting (1% to 3%), diarrhea (≤1%)
Neuromuscular & skeletal: Paresthesia (≤2%), weakness (≤2%)
Respiratory: Nasopharyngitis (≤1%)

Adverse reactions which may be related to local edema or hemorrhage at metastatic sites: Acute visual loss, enlargement of locally-recurring papillary carcinoma (accompanied by dyspnea, stridor, or dysphonia), hemiplegia, hemiparesis, laryngeal edema with respiratory distress, pain
General Dosage Range I.M.: *Children >16 years and Adults:* 0.9 mg, followed 24 hours later by a second 0.9 mg dose
Mechanism of Action Thyrotropin alfa, derived from a recombinant DNA source, has the identical amino acid sequence as endogenous human thyroid stimulating hormone (TSH). As a diagnostic tool in conjunction with serum thyroglobulin (Tg) testing, thyrotropin alfa stimulates the secretion of Tg from any remaining thyroid tissues (remnants). Under conditions of successful thyroidectomy and complete ablation, very little serum Tg should be detected under TSH stimulatory conditions; conversely, elevated Tg levels suggest the presence of remnant thyroid tissues. Since the source of TSH is exogenous, stimulation of Tg synthesis can be achieved in euthyroid patients, avoiding the need for thyroid hormone withdrawal.

As an adjunctive agent for radioiodine ablation treatment of thyroid cancer tissue remnants, thyrotropin alfa binds to TSH receptors on these tissues, stimulating the uptake and organification of iodine, including radiolabeled iodine (I^{131}). Cancerous tissue is destroyed via gamma emission from the radioiodine concentrated in these tissues.

Pharmacodynamics/Kinetics
Half-life Elimination 25 ± 10 hours
Time to Peak Median: 10 hours (range: 3-24 hours)
Pregnancy Risk Factor C
Pregnancy Considerations
Animal reproduction studies have not been conducted. Effects on the fetus or pregnant woman are unknown.

TiaGABine (tye AG a been)

Brand Names: U.S. Gabitril®
Pharmacologic Category Anticonvulsant, Miscellaneous
Use Adjunctive therapy in adults and children ≥12 years of age in the treatment of partial seizures
Local Anesthetic/Vasoconstrictor Precautions No information available to require special precautions
Effects on Dental Treatment Key adverse event(s) related to dental treatment: Stomatitis, gingivitis, and mouth ulceration.
Effects on Bleeding No information available to require special precautions
Adverse Effects
>10%:
Central nervous system: Concentration decreased, dizziness, nervousness, somnolence
Gastrointestinal: Nausea
Neuromuscular & skeletal: Weakness, tremor
1% to 10%:
Cardiovascular: Chest pain, edema, hypertension, palpitation, peripheral edema, syncope, tachycardia, vasodilation
Central nervous system: Agitation, ataxia, chills, confusion, difficulty with memory, confusion, depersonalization, depression, euphoria, hallucination, hostility, insomnia, malaise, migraine, paranoid reaction, personality disorder, speech disorder
Dermatologic: Alopecia, bruising, dry skin, pruritus, rash

Gastrointestinal: Abdominal pain, diarrhea, gingivitis, increased appetite, mouth ulceration, stomatitis, vomiting, weight gain/loss

Neuromuscular & skeletal: Abnormal gait, arthralgia, dysarthria, hyper-/hypokinesia, hyper-/hypotonia, myasthenia, myalgia, myoclonus, neck pain, paresthesia, reflexes decreased, stupor, twitching, vertigo

Ocular: Abnormal vision, amblyopia, nystagmus

Otic: Ear pain, hearing impairment, otitis media, tinnitus

Respiratory: Bronchitis, cough, dyspnea, epistaxis, pneumonia

Miscellaneous: Allergic reaction, cyst, diaphoresis, flu-like syndrome, lymphadenopathy

General Dosage Range Dosage adjustment recommended in patients on concomitant therapy

Oral:

Children 12-18 years: Initial: 4 mg once daily; Maintenance: 8-32 mg/day in 2-4 divided doses

Adults: Initial: 4 mg once daily; Maintenance: 8-56 mg/day in 2-4 divided doses

Mechanism of Action The exact mechanism by which tiagabine exerts antiseizure activity is not definitively known; however, *in vitro* experiments demonstrate that it enhances the activity of gamma aminobutyric acid (GABA), the major neuroinhibitory transmitter in the nervous system; it is thought that binding to the GABA uptake carrier inhibits the uptake of GABA into presynaptic neurons, allowing an increased amount of GABA to be available to postsynaptic neurons; based on *in vitro* studies, tiagabine does not inhibit the uptake of dopamine, norepinephrine, serotonin, glutamate, or choline

Pharmacodynamics/Kinetics

Half-life Elimination 2-5 hours when administered with enzyme inducers; 7-9 hours when administered without enzyme inducers

Time to Peak Plasma: 45 minutes

Pregnancy Risk Factor C

Pregnancy Considerations Patients exposed to tiagabine during pregnancy are encouraged to enroll themselves into the AED Pregnancy Registry by calling 1-888-233-2334. Additional information is available at www.aedpregnancyregistry.org.

Ticagrelor (tye KA grel or)

Related Information

Antiplatelet and Anticoagulation Considerations in Dentistry *on page 1503*

Cardiovascular Diseases *on page 1492*

Brand Names: U.S. Brilinta™

Brand Names: Canada Brilinta™

Pharmacologic Category Antiplatelet Agent; Antiplatelet Agent, Cyclopentyltriazolopyrimidine

Use Used in conjunction with aspirin for secondary prevention of thrombotic events in patients with unstable angina (UA), non-ST-elevation myocardial infarction (NSTEMI), or ST-elevation myocardial infarction (STEMI) managed medically or with percutaneous coronary intervention (PCI) and/or coronary artery bypass graft (CABG)

Unlabeled Use In patients with allergy or major gastrointestinal intolerance to aspirin, initial treatment of UA/NSTEMI; **Note:** Dual antiplatelet therapy with another P2Y$_{12}$ receptor inhibitor is not recommended in this situation (Jneid, 2012).

Local Anesthetic/Vasoconstrictor Precautions No information available to require special precautions

Effects on Dental Treatment No significant effects or complications reported (see Dental Comment)

Aspirin in combination with clopidogrel (Plavix®), prasugrel (Effient®), or ticagrelor (Brilinta™) is the primary prevention strategy against stent thrombosis after placement of drug-eluting metal stents in coronary patients. Premature discontinuation of combination antiplatelet therapy (ie, dual antiplatelet therapy) strongly increases the risk of a catastrophic event of stent thrombosis leading to myocardial infarction and/or death, so says a science advisory issued in January 2007 from the American Heart Association in collaboration with the American Dental Association and other professional healthcare organizations. The advisory stresses a 12-month therapy of dual antiplatelet therapy after placement of a drug-eluting stent in order to prevent thrombosis at the stent site. Any elective surgery should be postponed for 1 year after stent implantation, and if surgery must be performed, consideration should be given to continuing the antiplatelet therapy during the perioperative period in high-risk patients with drug-eluting stents.

This advisory was issued from a science panel made up of representatives from the American Heart Association (AHA), the American College of Cardiology, the Society for Cardiovascular Angiography and Interventions, the American College of Surgeons, the American Dental Association (ADA), and the American College of Physicians (Grines, 2007).

Effects on Bleeding Ticagrelor is an antiplatelet agent similar in actions to clopidogrel. Major bleeding has been reported with a frequency of 12% of individuals (as composite of major fatal or life-threatening and other major bleeding events). Minor bleeding has occurred in ~5% of patients; also reported have been anemia, hematoma, and postprocedural hemorrhage (2%).

Dual antiplatelet therapy: Aspirin irreversibly inhibits platelet aggregation which can prolong bleeding. Upon discontinuation, normal platelet function returns only when new platelets are released (~7-10 days). However, in the case of dental surgery, there is no scientific evidence to support discontinuation of aspirin. The discontinuation of aspirin may place the patient at risk for a thrombotic event or other cardiovascular complication. In particular, aspirin should **not** be discontinued in patients with cardiac stents that have not completed their full course of dual antiplatelet therapy (eg, aspirin and clopidogrel [prasugrel or ticagrelor]); patient-specific situations need to be discussed with cardiologist. When feasible, postponement of dental surgery until the completion of dual antiplatelet therapy should be considered. Any modification of aspirin therapy should be discussed with the prescribing physician.

Adverse Effects Note: As with all drugs which may affect hemostasis, bleeding is associated with ticagrelor. Hemorrhage may occur at virtually any site. Risk is dependent on multiple variables, including the concurrent use of multiple agents which alter hemostasis and patient susceptibility.

Frequencies as reported in PLATO trial versus clopidogrel:

>10%: Respiratory: Dyspnea (≤14%)

1% to 10%:

Cardiovascular: Ventricular pauses (6%; 2% after 1 month of therapy), atrial fibrillation (4%), hypertension (4%), angina (3%), hypotension (3%), bradycardia (1% to 3%), cardiac failure (2%), peripheral edema (2%), ventricular tachycardia (2%), palpitation (1%), syncope (1%), ventricular extrasystoles (1%), ventricular fibrillation (1%)

Central nervous system: Headache (7%), dizziness (5%), fatigue (3%), fever (3%), anxiety (2%), insomnia (2%), vertigo (2%), depression (1%)

Dermatologic: Bruising (2% to 4%), rash (2%), pruritus (1%), subcutaneous or dermal bleeding

Endocrine & metabolic: Hypokalemia (2%), diabetes mellitus (1%), dyslipidemia (1%), hypercholesterolemia (1%)

Gastrointestinal: Diarrhea (4%), nausea (4%), vomiting (3%), abdominal pain (2%), constipation (2%), dyspepsia (2%), GI hemorrhage

Genitourinary: Urinary tract infection (2%), urinary tract bleeding

Hematologic: Major bleeding (12%; composite of major fatal/life threatening and other major bleeding events), minor bleeding (~5%), anemia (2%), hematoma (2%), postprocedural hemorrhage (2%)

Local: Puncture site hematoma (2%)

Neuromuscular & skeletal: Back pain (4%), noncardiac chest pain (4%), extremity pain (2%), arthralgia (2%), musculoskeletal pain (2%), weakness (2%), myalgia (1%)

Renal: Creatinine increased (7%; mechanism undetermined), hematuria (2%), renal failure (1%)

Respiratory: Epistaxis (6%), cough (5%), nasopharyngitis (2%), bronchitis (1%), pneumonia (1%)

General Dosage Range Oral: *Adults:* Loading dose: 180 mg; Maintenance: 90 mg twice daily

Mechanism of Action
Reversibly and noncompetitively binds the adenosine diphosphate (ADP) P2Y$_{12}$ receptor on the platelet surface which prevents ADP-mediated activation of the GPIIb/IIIa receptor complex thereby reducing platelet aggregation. Due to the reversible antagonism of the P2Y$_{12}$ receptor, recovery of platelet function is likely to depend on serum concentrations of ticagrelor and its active metabolite.

Pharmacodynamics/Kinetics
Onset of Action Inhibition of platelet aggregation (IPA): 180 mg loading dose: ~41% within 30 minutes (similar to clopidogrel 600 mg at 8 hours); Peak effect: Time to maximal IPA: 180 mg loading dose: IPA ~88% at 2 hours post administration

Duration of Action IPA: 180 mg loading dose: 87% to 89% maintained from 2-8 hours; 24 hours after the last maintenance dose, IPA is 58% (similar to maintenance clopidogrel)

Time after discontinuation when IPA is 30%: ~56 hours; IPA 10%: ~110 hours (Gurbel, 2009). Mean IPA observed with ticagrelor at 3 days post-discontinuation was comparable to that observed with clopidogrel at 5 days post discontinuation.

Half-life Elimination Parent drug: ~7 hours; active metabolite: ~9 hours

Time to Peak Parent drug: ~1.5 hours; active metabolite (AR-C124910XX): ~2.5 hours

Pregnancy Risk Factor C

Pregnancy Considerations Fetal mortality and/or abnormalities were observed in animal studies at doses greater than maximum recommended human doses. There are no adequate and well-controlled studies in pregnant women. Use only if potential benefits outweigh potential risk to fetus. The Canadian labeling recommends women of childbearing potential use appropriate contraceptive measures.

Dental Comment Premature discontinuation of ticagrelor therapy may increase the risk of cardiac events (eg, stent thrombosis with subsequent fatal or nonfatal myocardial infarction). Duration of therapy, in general, is determined by the type of stent placed (bare metal or drug eluting) and whether an acute coronary syndrome event was ongoing at the time of placement. Patient-specific situations need to be discussed with healthcare provider.

Patients taking ticagrelor may have shortness of breath.

If patient is taking aspirin along with ticagrelor, aspirin dose should not exceed 100 mg/day. Patient should also avoid taking any other medicine containing aspirin. The manufacturer implemented REMS components to alert physicians to the risk of using higher doses of aspirin while taking ticagrelor.

Ticarcillin and Clavulanate Potassium
(tye kar SIL in & klav yoo LAN ate poe TASS ee um)

Brand Names: U.S. Timentin®
Brand Names: Canada Timentin®
Pharmacologic Category Antibiotic, Penicillin
Use Treatment of lower respiratory tract, urinary tract, skin and skin structures, bone and joint, gynecologic (endometritis) and intra-abdominal (peritonitis) infections, and septicemia caused by susceptible organisms. Clavulanate expands activity of ticarcillin to include beta-lactamase producing strains of *S. aureus, H. influenzae, Bacteroides* species, and some other gram-negative bacilli

Local Anesthetic/Vasoconstrictor Precautions No information available to require special precautions

Effects on Dental Treatment Key adverse event(s) related to dental treatment: Prolonged use of penicillins may lead to development of oral candidiasis.

Effects on Bleeding May inhibit platelet aggregation (dose related). No information available to require special precautions

Adverse Effects Frequency not defined.
Central nervous system: Confusion, drowsiness, fever, headache, Jarisch-Herxheimer reaction, seizure

Dermatologic: Erythema multiforme, pruritus, rash, Stevens-Johnson syndrome, toxic epidermal necrolysis, urticaria

Endocrine & metabolic: Electrolyte imbalance

Gastrointestinal: *Clostridium difficile* colitis, diarrhea, nausea, vomiting

Hematologic: Bleeding, eosinophilia, hemolytic anemia, leukopenia, neutropenia, positive Coombs' reaction, prothrombin time prolonged, thrombocytopenia

Hepatic: Hepatotoxicity, jaundice

Local: Injection site reaction (pain, burning, induration); thrombophlebitis

Neuromuscular & skeletal: Myoclonus

Renal: BUN increased, interstitial nephritis (acute), serum creatinine increased

Miscellaneous: Anaphylaxis, hypersensitivity reactions

General Dosage Range Dosage adjustment recommended in patients with hepatic or renal impairment
I.V.:
Children and Adults <60 kg: 200-300 mg of ticarcillin component/kg/day in divided doses every 4-6 hours
Children ≥60 kg and Adults: 3.1 g (ticarcillin 3 g plus clavulanic acid 0.1 g) every 4-6 hours (maximum: 24 g of ticarcillin component/day)

Mechanism of Action Inhibits bacterial cell wall synthesis by binding to one or more of the penicillin-binding proteins (PBPs); which in turn inhibits the final transpeptidation step of peptidoglycan synthesis in bacterial cell walls, thus inhibiting cell wall biosynthesis. Bacteria eventually lyse due to ongoing activity of cell wall autolytic enzymes (autolysins and murein hydrolases) while cell wall assembly is arrested.

◀ **Pharmacodynamics/Kinetics**
Half-life Elimination Ticarcillin: 1.1 hours; Clavulanic acid: 1.1 hours

Pregnancy Risk Factor B

Pregnancy Considerations Adverse events were not observed in animal reproduction studies. Ticarcillin and clavulanate cross the placenta. Maternal use of penicillins has generally not resulted in an increased risk of adverse fetal effects. Ticarcillin/clavulanate is approved for the treatment of postpartum gynecologic infections, including endometritis, caused by susceptible organisms.

Ticlopidine (tye KLOE pi deen)

Related Information
Antiplatelet and Anticoagulation Considerations in Dentistry on page 1503

Brand Names: Canada Apo-Ticlopidine®; Dom-Ticlopidine; Gen-Ticlopidine; Mylan-Ticlopidine; Novo-Ticlopidine; Nu-Ticlopidine; PMS-Ticlopidine; Sandoz-Ticlopidine; Teva-Ticlopidine

Pharmacologic Category Antiplatelet Agent; Antiplatelet Agent, Thienopyridine

Use Platelet aggregation inhibitor that reduces the risk of thrombotic stroke in patients who have had a stroke or stroke precursors (**Note:** Due to its association with life-threatening hematologic disorders, ticlopidine should be reserved for patients who are intolerant to aspirin, or who have failed aspirin therapy); adjunctive therapy (with aspirin) following successful coronary stent implantation to reduce the incidence of subacute stent thrombosis.

Unlabeled Use Protection of aortocoronary bypass grafts, diabetic microangiopathy, ischemic heart disease, prevention of postoperative DVT, reduction of graft loss following renal transplant

Local Anesthetic/Vasoconstrictor Precautions No information available to require special precautions

Effects on Dental Treatment No significant effects or complications reported; if a patient is to undergo elective surgery and an antiplatelet effect is not desired, ticlopidine should be discontinued at least 7 days prior to surgery.

Effects on Bleeding Ticlopidine blocks platelet aggregation and may prolong bleeding time. Inhibition is irreversible; on discontinuation, normal platelet function returns only when new platelets are released from the bone marrow. Dental practitioners should note that recommendations differ between general surgery (eg, appendectomy, hip replacement) and dental surgery. Prior to elective general surgery, it may be temporarily discontinued (usually for 5-10 days) to restore platelet function. However, routine interruption of therapy for noninvasive dental procedures is NOT warranted and there is no scientific evidence to warrant the discontinuance of ticlopidine prior to dental surgery. In particular, ticlopidine should NOT be discontinued in patients with cardiac stents that have not completed their full course of dual antiplatelet therapy (aspirin, clopidogrel/ticlopidine); patient specific situations need to be discussed with cardiologist. When feasible, postponement of dental surgery until the completion of dual antiplatelet therapy should be considered.

Adverse Effects As with all drugs which may affect hemostasis, bleeding is associated with ticlopidine. Hemorrhage may occur at virtually any site. Risk is dependent on multiple variables, including the use of multiple agents which alter hemostasis and patient susceptibility.

>10%:
Endocrine & metabolic: Total cholesterol increased (increases of ~8% to 10% within 1 month of therapy), triglycerides increased
Gastrointestinal: Diarrhea (13%)

1% to 10%:
Central nervous system: Dizziness (1%)
Dermatologic: Rash (5%), purpura (2%), pruritus (1%)
Gastrointestinal: Nausea (7%), dyspepsia (7%), gastrointestinal pain (4%), vomiting (2%), flatulence (2%), anorexia (1%)
Hematologic: Neutropenia (2%)
Hepatic: Alkaline phosphatase increased (>2 x upper limit of normal; 8%), abnormal liver function test (1%)

General Dosage Range Oral: *Adults:* 250 mg twice daily

Mechanism of Action Ticlopidine requires *in vivo* biotransformation to an unidentified active metabolite. This active metabolite irreversibly blocks the P2Y12 component of ADP receptors, which prevents activation of the GPIIb/IIIa receptor complex, thereby reducing platelet aggregation. Platelets blocked by ticlopidine are affected for the remainder of their lifespan.

Pharmacodynamics/Kinetics
Onset of Action ~6 hours; Peak effect: 3-5 days; serum levels do not correlate with clinical antiplatelet activity

Half-life Elimination 13 hours

Time to Peak ~2 hours

Pregnancy Risk Factor B

Pregnancy Considerations Teratogenic effects have not been observed in animal reproduction studies; a case report has demonstrated the safe use of ticlopidine in pregnant women (Ueno, 2001).

Tigecycline (tye ge SYE kleen)

Brand Names: U.S. Tygacil®
Brand Names: Canada Tygacil®
Pharmacologic Category Antibiotic, Glycylcycline

Use Treatment of complicated skin and skin structure infections caused by susceptible organisms, including methicillin-resistant *Staphylococcus aureus* and vancomycin-sensitive *Enterococcus faecalis*; complicated intra-abdominal infections (cIAI); community-acquired pneumonia

Local Anesthetic/Vasoconstrictor Precautions No information available to require special precautions

Effects on Dental Treatment Key adverse events(s) related to dental treatment: Tigecycline is structurally similar to tetracycline. Therefore, tigecycline is not recommended for use in pregnancy or in children ≤8 years of age. Permanent discoloration of the teeth may occur if used during tooth development.

Effects on Bleeding No information available to require special precautions

Adverse Effects Note: Frequencies relative to placebo are not available; some frequencies are lower than those experienced with comparator drugs.

>10%: Gastrointestinal: Nausea (26%; severe: 1%), vomiting (18%; severe: 1%), diarrhea (12%)

2% to 10%:

Central nervous system: Headache (6%), dizziness (3%)

Dermatologic: Rash (3%)

Endocrine & metabolic: Hypoproteinemia (5%)

Gastrointestinal: Abdominal pain (6%), dyspepsia (2%)

Hematologic: Anemia (4%)

Hepatic: ALT increased (5%), AST increased (4%), alkaline phosphatase increased (4%), amylase increased (3%), bilirubin increased (2%)

Local: Phlebitis (3%)

Neuromuscular & skeletal: Weakness (3%)

Renal: BUN increased (3%)

Miscellaneous: Infection (8%), abnormal healing (4%), abscess (3%)

General Dosage Range Dosage adjustment recommended in patients with hepatic impairment

I.V.: *Adults:* Initial: 100 mg as a single dose; Maintenance: 50 mg every 12 hours

Mechanism of Action A glycylcycline antibiotic that binds to the 30S ribosomal subunit of susceptible bacteria, thereby, inhibiting protein synthesis. Generally considered bacteriostatic; however, bactericidal activity has been demonstrated against isolates of *S. pneumoniae* and *L. pneumophila*. Tigecycline is a derivative of minocycline (9-t-butylglycylamido minocycline), and while not classified as a tetracycline, it may share some class-associated adverse effects. Tigecycline has demonstrated activity against a variety of gram-positive and -negative bacterial pathogens including methicillin-resistant staphylococci.

Pharmacodynamics/Kinetics

Half-life Elimination Single dose: 27 hours; following multiple doses: 42 hours

Pregnancy Risk Factor D

Pregnancy Considerations Because adverse effects were observed in animals and because of the potential for permanent tooth discoloration, tigecycline is classified pregnancy category D. Tigecycline frequently causes nausea and vomiting and, therefore, may not be ideal for use in a patient with pregnancy-related nausea.

Tiludronate (tye LOO droe nate)

Related Information

Osteonecrosis of the Jaw *on page 1529*

Brand Names: U.S. Skelid®

Pharmacologic Category Bisphosphonate Derivative

Use Treatment of Paget's disease of the bone (osteitis deformans) in patients who have a level of serum alkaline phosphatase (SAP) at least twice the upper limit of normal, or who are symptomatic, or who are at risk for future complications of their disease

Local Anesthetic/Vasoconstrictor Precautions No information available to require special precautions

Effects on Dental Treatment Osteonecrosis of the jaw (ONJ), generally associated with local infection and/or tooth extraction and often with delayed healing, has been reported in patients taking bisphosphonates. Symptoms included nonhealing extraction socket or an exposed jawbone. Most reported cases of bisphosphonate-associated osteonecrosis have been in cancer patients treated with intravenous bisphosphonates. However, some have occurred in patients with postmenopausal osteoporosis taking oral bisphosphonates. Dental surgery, particularly tooth extraction, may increase the risk for ONJ. Patients who develop ONJ

while on bisphosphonate therapy should receive care by an oral surgeon. See Dental Comment.

Effects on Bleeding No information available to require special precautions

Adverse Effects 1% to 10%:

Cardiovascular: Chest pain (3%), edema (3%), peripheral edema (3%), flushing, hypertension, syncope

Central nervous system: Anxiety, fatigue, insomnia, nervousness, somnolence, vertigo

Dermatologic: Rash (3%), skin disorder (3%), pruritus

Endocrine & metabolic: Hyperparathyroidism (3%)

Gastrointestinal: Nausea (9%), diarrhea (9%), dyspepsia (5%), vomiting (4%), flatulence (3%), abdominal pain, anorexia, constipation, gastritis, xerostomia

Genitourinary: Urinary tract infection

Neuromuscular & skeletal: Paresthesia (4%), arthrosis (3%), fractures, muscle spasm, weakness

Ocular: Cataract (3%), conjunctivitis (3%), glaucoma (3%)

Respiratory: Rhinitis (5%), sinusitis (5%), pharyngitis (3%), bronchitis

Miscellaneous: Accidental injury (4%), infection (3%), diaphoresis

General Dosage Range Oral: *Adults:* 400 mg once daily

Mechanism of Action Inhibition of normal and abnormal bone resorption. Inhibits osteoclasts through at least two mechanisms: disruption of the cytoskeletal ring structure, possibly by inhibition of protein-tyrosine-phosphatase, thus leading to the detachment of osteoclasts from the bone surface area and the inhibition of the osteoclast proton pump.

Pharmacodynamics/Kinetics

Onset of Action Delayed, may require several weeks

Half-life Elimination Healthy volunteers: Single dose: 50 hours; Cl_{cr} 11-18 mL/minute: 205 hours; Pagetic patients: Repeated dosing: 150 hours

Time to Peak Plasma: Within 2 hours

Pregnancy Risk Factor C

Pregnancy Considerations Teratogenic and nonteratogenic embryo/fetal effects have been reported in animal studies. There are no adequate and well-controlled studies in pregnant women. Bisphosphonates are incorporated into the bone matrix and gradually released over time. Theoretically, there may be a risk of fetal harm when pregnancy follows the completion of therapy. Based on limited case reports with pamidronate, serum calcium levels in the newborn may be altered if bisphosphonates are administered during pregnancy.

Dental Comment A review of 2408 published cases of bisphosphonate-associated osteonecrosis of the jaw bone (BP-associated ONJ) was done by Filleul, 2010. BP therapy was associated with 89% of the cases to treat malignancies and 11% of the cases to treat nonmalignant conditions. Information on the specific bisphosphonate used was available for 1694 of the patients. Intravenous therapy (primarily zoledronic acid) was received by 88% of the patients and 12% received oral treatment (primarily alendronate). Of all the cases of BP-associated ONJ, 67% were preceded by tooth extraction and for 26% of patients, there was no predisposing factor identified.

A 2010 retrospective case review reported the prevalence of BP-associated ONJ in patients using alendronate-type drugs was one out of 952 patients or ~0.1% (Lo, 2010). Of the 8572 respondents, nine cases of ONJ were identified; five had developed ONJ spontaneously and four developed ONJ after tooth extraction. When extrapolated to patient-years of bisphosphonate exposure, this prevalence rate of 0.1% equates to a frequency of 28 cases per 100,000 person-years of oral bisphosphonate treatment. An Australian group (Mavrokokki, 2007), identified the frequency of BP-associated ONJ in osteoporotic patients, mainly taking weekly oral alendronate, was 1 in 8470 to 1 in 2260 (0.01% to 0.04%) patients. If extractions were carried out, the calculated frequency was 1 in 1130 to 1 in 296 (0.09% to 0.34%) patients. The median time to onset of ONJ in alendronate patients was 24 months.

According to the 2011 report by the American Dental Association (ADA), the incidence of BP-associated ONJ remains low and the benefits of using oral bisphosphonates significantly outweighs the risk of developing BP-associated ONJ for treatment and prevention of osteoporosis and cancer treatment (Hellstein, 2011). The full 47 page report can be accessed at http://www.ada.org/sections/professionalResources/pdfs/topics_AR-ONJ_report.pdf.

The ADA review of 2011 stated the incidence of oral BP-associated ONJ was one case for every 1000 individuals exposed to oral bisphosphonates (0.1%) (Hellstein, 2011).

Timolol (Systemic) (TIM oh lol)

Related Information
Cardiovascular Diseases *on page 1492*

Brand Names: Canada Apo-Timol®; Nu-Timolol; Teva-Timolol

Pharmacologic Category Beta-Blocker, Nonselective

Use Treatment of hypertension and angina; to reduce mortality following myocardial infarction; prophylaxis of migraine

Local Anesthetic/Vasoconstrictor Precautions
Epinephrine has interacted with nonselective beta-blockers, such as propranolol, to result in initial hypertensive episode followed by bradycardia. Timolol is also a nonselective beta-blocker. The significance of a potential systemic interaction is well known and cautionary use of epinephrine is advised.

Effects on Dental Treatment Key adverse event(s) related to dental treatment: Xerostomia (normal salivary flow resumes upon discontinuation).

Timolol is a nonselective beta-blocker and may enhance the pressor response to epinephrine, resulting in hypertension and bradycardia. Many nonsteroidal anti-inflammatory drugs, such as ibuprofen and indomethacin, can reduce the hypotensive effect of beta-blockers after 3 or more weeks of therapy with the NSAID. Short-term NSAID use (ie, 3 days) requires no special precautions in patients taking beta-blockers.

Effects on Bleeding No information available to require special precautions

Adverse Effects 1% to 10%:
Cardiovascular: Bradycardia
Central nervous system: Fatigue, dizziness
Respiratory: Dyspnea

Frequency not defined:
Cardiovascular: Angina pectoris, arrhythmia, cardiac failure, cardiac arrest, cerebral vascular accident, cerebral ischemia, edema, hypotension, heart block, palpitation, Raynaud's phenomenon
Central nervous system: Anxiety, confusion, depression, disorientation, hallucinations, insomnia, memory loss, nervousness, nightmares, somnolence

Dermatologic: Alopecia, angioedema, pseudopemphigoid, psoriasiform rash, psoriasis exacerbation, rash, urticaria
Endocrine & metabolic: Hypoglycemia masked, libido decreased
Gastrointestinal: Anorexia, diarrhea, dyspepsia, nausea, xerostomia
Genitourinary: Impotence, retoperitoneal fibrosis
Hematologic: Claudication
Neuromuscular & skeletal: Myasthenia gravis exacerbation, paresthesia
Ocular: Blepharitis, conjunctivitis, corneal sensitivity decreased, cystoid macular edema, diplopia, dry eyes, foreign body sensation, keratitis, ocular discharge, ocular pain, ptosis, refractive changes, tearing, visual disturbances
Otic: Tinnitus
Respiratory: Bronchospasm, cough, nasal congestion, pulmonary edema, respiratory failure
Miscellaneous: Allergic reactions, cold hands/feet, Peyronie's disease, systemic lupus erythematosus

General Dosage Range Oral: *Adults:* Initial: 10 mg twice daily; Maintenance: 20-60 mg/day in 2 divided doses (maximum: 60 mg/day)

Mechanism of Action Blocks both $beta_1$- and $beta_2$-adrenergic receptors; reduces blood pressure by blocking adrenergic receptors and decreasing sympathetic outflow, produces a negative chronotropic and inotropic activity through an unknown mechanism

Pharmacodynamics/Kinetics
Onset of Action Hypotensive: 15-45 minutes; Peak effect: 0.5-2.5 hours

Duration of Action ~4 hours

Half-life Elimination 2-2.7 hours; prolonged with renal impairment

Time to Peak Plasma: 1-2 hours

Pregnancy Risk Factor C

Pregnancy Considerations Adverse events were not observed in the initial animal reproduction studies; therefore, the manufacturer classifies timolol as pregnancy category C. Timolol crosses the placenta and decreased fetal heart rate has been observed following maternal use of oral and ophthalmic timolol during pregnancy. In a cohort study, an increased risk of cardiovascular defects was observed following maternal use of beta-blockers during pregnancy. Intrauterine growth restriction (IUGR), small placentas, as well as fetal/neonatal bradycardia, hypoglycemia, and/or respiratory depression have been observed following *in utero* exposure to beta-blockers as a class. Adequate facilities for monitoring infants at birth should be available. Untreated chronic maternal hypertension and pre-eclampsia are also associated with adverse events in the fetus, infant, and mother; however, timolol is currently not recommended for the initial treatment of hypertension in pregnancy. If timolol is required for the treatment of glaucoma during pregnancy, the minimum effective dose should be used in combination with punctual occlusion to decrease exposure to the fetus.

Timolol (Ophthalmic) (TIM oh lol)

Brand Names: U.S. Betimol®; Istalol®; Timolol GFS; Timoptic-XE®; Timoptic®; Timoptic® in OcuDose®

Brand Names: Canada Apo-Timop®; Dom-Timolol; Mylan-Timolol; Novo-Timol; PMS-Timolol; Sandoz-Timolol; Tim-AK; Timolol Maleate-EX; Timoptic-XE®; Timoptic®

Pharmacologic Category Beta-Blocker, Nonselective; Ophthalmic Agent, Antiglaucoma

Use Treatment of elevated intraocular pressure such as glaucoma or ocular hypertension

Local Anesthetic/Vasoconstrictor Precautions Epinephrine has interacted with nonselective beta-blockers, such as propranolol, to result in initial hypertensive episode followed by bradycardia. Timolol is also a nonselective beta-blocker. The significance of a potential systemic interaction with epinephrine is unknown. However, it is suggested that cautionary procedures be used, particularly if vasoconstrictor is used immediately following a dose of timolol taken by the patient.

Effects on Dental Treatment Key adverse event(s) related to dental treatment: Xerostomia (normal salivary flow resumes upon discontinuation).

Timolol is a nonselective beta-blocker and may enhance the pressor response to epinephrine, resulting in hypertension and bradycardia.

Effects on Bleeding No information available to require special precautions

Adverse Effects

>10%: Ocular: Burning, stinging

Frequency not defined:

Cardiovascular: Angina pectoris, arrhythmia, bradycardia, cardiac arrest, cardiac failure, cerebral ischemia, cerebral vascular accident, edema, heart block, hypertension, hypotension, palpitation, Raynaud's phenomenon

Central nervous system: Anxiety, confusion, depression, disorientation, dizziness, hallucinations, headache, insomnia, memory loss, nervousness, nightmares, somnolence

Dermatologic: Alopecia, angioedema, pseudopemphigoid, psoriasiform rash, psoriasis exacerbation, rash, urticaria

Endocrine & metabolic: Hypoglycemia masked, libido decreased

Gastrointestinal: Anorexia, diarrhea, dyspepsia, nausea, xerostomia

Genitourinary: Impotence, retoperitoneal fibrosis

Hematologic: Claudication

Neuromuscular & skeletal: Myasthenia gravis exacerbation, paresthesia

Ocular: Blepharitis, blurred vision, cataract, choroidal detachment (following filtration surgery), conjunctival injection, conjunctivitis, corneal sensitivity decreased, cystoid macular edema, diplopia, dry eyes, foreign body sensation, hyperemia, itching, keratitis, ocular discharge, ocular pain, ptosis, tearing, visual acuity decreased refractive changes, visual disturbances

Otic: Tinnitus

Respiratory: Bronchospasm, cough, dyspnea, nasal congestion, pulmonary edema, respiratory failure

Miscellaneous: Allergic reactions, cold hands/feet, Peyronie's disease, systemic lupus erythematosus

General Dosage Range Ophthalmic:

Gel-forming solution: *Children and Adults:* Instill 1 drop (0.25% or 0.5%) once daily

Solution: *Children and Adults:* Initial: Instill 1 drop (0.25%) twice daily; Maintenance: Instill 1 drop (0.25% or 0.5%) 1-2 times daily (maximum: 2 drops/day [0.5%])

Mechanism of Action Blocks both beta$_1$- and beta$_2$-adrenergic receptors, reduces intraocular pressure by reducing aqueous humor production or possibly outflow; reduces blood pressure by blocking adrenergic receptors and decreasing sympathetic outflow, produces a negative chronotropic and inotropic activity through an unknown mechanism

Pharmacodynamics/Kinetics

Onset of Action Intraocular pressure reduction: 30 minutes; Peak effect: 1-2 hours

Duration of Action 24 hours

Pregnancy Risk Factor C

Pregnancy Considerations Adverse events were not observed in animal reproduction studies; therefore, the manufacturer classifies timolol ophthalmic as pregnancy category C. Timolol crosses the placenta. Decreased fetal heart rate has been observed following maternal use of oral and ophthalmic timolol during pregnancy. In a cohort study, an increased risk of cardiovascular defects was observed following maternal use of beta-blockers during pregnancy. Intrauterine growth restriction (IUGR), small placentas, as well as fetal/neonatal bradycardia, hypoglycemia, and/or respiratory depression have been observed following *in utero* exposure to beta-blockers as a class. Adequate facilities for monitoring infants at birth should be available. Untreated chronic maternal hypertension and pre-eclampsia are also associated with adverse events in the fetus, infant, and mother. If timolol is required for the treatment of glaucoma during pregnancy, the minimum effective dose should be used in combination with punctual occlusion to decrease exposure to the fetus. Also refer to the Timolol (Systemic) monograph for additional information.

Tinidazole (tye NI da zole)

Brand Names: U.S. Tindamax®

Pharmacologic Category Amebicide; Antibiotic, Miscellaneous; Antiprotozoal, Nitroimidazole

Use Treatment of trichomoniasis caused by *T. vaginalis*; treatment of giardiasis caused by *G. duodenalis* (*G. lamblia*); treatment of intestinal amebiasis and amebic liver abscess caused by *E. histolytica*; treatment of bacterial vaginosis caused by *Bacteroides* spp, *Gardnerella vaginalis*, and *Prevotella* spp in nonpregnant females

Local Anesthetic/Vasoconstrictor Precautions No information available to require special precautions

Effects on Dental Treatment Key adverse event(s) related to dental treatment: Xerostomia and changes in salivation (normal salivary flow resumes upon discontinuation), metallic/bitter taste, oral candidiasis, tongue discoloration, stomatitis, furry tongue. See Dental Comment.

Effects on Bleeding No information available to require special precautions

Adverse Effects

1% to 10%:

Central nervous system: Fatigue/malaise (1% to 2%), dizziness (≤1%), headache (≤1%)

Endocrine & metabolic: Menorrhagia (>2%)

Gastrointestinal: Metallic/bitter taste (4% to 6%), nausea (3% to 5%), anorexia (2% to 3%), appetite decreased (>2%), flatulence (>2%), dyspepsia/cramps/epigastric discomfort (1% to 2%), vomiting (1% to 2%), constipation (≤1%)

Genitourinary: *Candida* vaginitis (5%), painful urination (>2%), pelvic pain (>2%), urine abnormality (>2%), vaginal odor (>2%), vulvovaginal discomfort (>2%)

Neuromuscular & skeletal: Weakness (1% to 2%)

Renal: Urinary tract infection (>2%)

Respiratory: Upper respiratory tract infection (>2%)

Frequency not defined:

Cardiovascular: Flushing, palpitation

Central nervous system: Ataxia, coma (rare), confusion (rare), depression (rare), drowsiness, fever, giddiness, insomnia, seizure, vertigo

Dermatologic: Angioedema, pruritus, rash, urticaria

Gastrointestinal: Abdominal pain, diarrhea, furry tongue (rare), oral candidiasis, salivation, stomatitis, thirst, tongue discoloration, xerostomia

Genitourinary: Urine darkened, vaginal discharge increased

Hematologic: Leukopenia (transient), neutropenia (transient), thrombocytopenia (reversible; rare)

Hepatic: Transaminases increased

Neuromuscular & skeletal: Arthralgia, arthritis, myalgia, peripheral neuropathy (transient, includes numbness and paresthesia)

Respiratory: Bronchospasm (rare), dyspnea (rare), pharyngitis (rare)

Miscellaneous: Burning sensation, *Candida* overgrowth, diaphoresis

General Dosage Range Oral:

Children >3 years: 50 mg/kg/day (maximum: 2 g/day)

Adults: 1-2 g/day

Mechanism of Action After diffusing into the organism, it is proposed that tinidazole causes cytotoxicity by damaging DNA and preventing further DNA synthesis.

Pharmacodynamics/Kinetics

Half-life Elimination 13 hours

Time to Peak 1.6 hours

Pregnancy Risk Factor C

Pregnancy Considerations Adverse events have been observed in some animal reproduction studies. Carcinogenicity studies have not been completed with tinidazole; however, metronidazole has a similar chemical structure and has caused carcinogenic effects in rats and mice. Tinidazole crosses the human placenta and enters the fetal circulation. Use of tinidazole is contraindicated during the first trimester of pregnancy.

Dental Comment Although this drug is a member of the metronidazole family, there is no specific dental indication for its use. Just as with metronidazole, alcohol in any form is contraindicated while the patient is on this medication because of the danger of a disulfiram-type reaction.

Tinzaparin (tin ZA pa rin)

Related Information

Cardiovascular Diseases *on page 1492*

Brand Names: Canada Innohep®

Pharmacologic Category Low Molecular Weight Heparin

Use Treatment of deep vein thrombosis (DVT) and/or pulmonary embolism (PE) (except in patients with severe hemodynamic instability); prevention of venous thromboembolism (VTE) following orthopedic surgery or following general surgery in patients at high risk of VTE; prevention of clotting in indwelling intravenous lines and extracorporeal circuit during hemodialysis (in patients without high bleeding risk)

Local Anesthetic/Vasoconstrictor Precautions No information available to require special precautions

Effects on Dental Treatment Key adverse event(s) related to dental treatment: Bleeding is the major adverse effect of tinzaparin. See Effects on Bleeding.

Effects on Bleeding As with all anticoagulants, bleeding is the major adverse effect of tinzaparin. Hemorrhage may occur at virtually any site; risk is dependent on multiple variables including the intensity of anticoagulation and patient susceptibility. At the recommended doses, LMWHS do not significantly influence platelet aggregation or affect global clotting time (ie, PT or aPTT). Medical consult is suggested.

Adverse Effects As with all anticoagulants, bleeding is the major adverse effect of tinzaparin. Hemorrhage may occur at virtually any site. Risk is dependent on multiple variables. **Note:** Incidence not always reported.

>10%:

Hepatic: ALT increased (≤13%)

Local: Injection site hematoma

1% to 10%:

Cardiovascular: Chest pain (2%), angina pectoris (≥1%), arrhythmia (≥1%), coronary thrombosis/MI (≥1%), dependent edema (≥1%), thromboembolism (≥1%)

Central nervous system: Fever (2%), headache (2%), pain (2%)

Dermatologic: Bullous eruption (≥1%), erythematous rash (≥1%), maculopapular rash (≥1%), skin necrosis (≥1%)

Gastrointestinal: Nausea (2%), abdominal pain (1%), constipation (1%), diarrhea (1%), vomiting (1%)

Genitourinary: Urinary tract infection (4%)

Hematologic: Bleeding events (major events including intracranial, retroperitoneal, or bleeding into a major prosthetic joint: ≤3%; hemorrhage site not specified (2%); other bleeding events reported at an incidence of ≥1% include anorectal bleeding, GI hemorrhage, hemarthrosis, hematemesis, hematuria, hemopericardium, injection site bleeding, melena, purpura, intra-abdominal bleeding, vaginal bleeding, wound hemorrhage), granulocytopenia (≥1%), thrombocytopenia (≥1%)

Hepatic: AST increased (9%)

Local: Injection site cellulitis (≥1%)

Neuromuscular & skeletal: Back pain (2%)

Respiratory: Epistaxis (2%), dyspnea (1%)

Miscellaneous: Allergic reaction (≥1%), neoplasm (≥1%)

General Dosage Range Dosage adjustment recommended in renal impairment and extended (>4 hours) hemodialysis sessions.

I.V. or added to hemodialysis circuit: *Adults:* 2250-4500 anti-Xa units

SubQ: *Adults:* 50 anti-Xa units/kg or 3500 anti-Xa units/kg preoperatively; 75-3500 anti-Xa units/kg once daily (maximum: 18,000 anti-Xa units daily)

Mechanism of Action Tinzaparin is a low molecular weight heparin (average molecular weight ranges between 5500 and 7500 daltons, distributed as <2000 daltons [<10%], 2000-8000 daltons [60% to 72%], and >8000 daltons [22% to 36%]) that binds antithrombin III, enhancing the inhibition of several clotting factors, particularly factor Xa. Tinzaparin anti-Xa activity (70-120 units/mg) is greater than anti-IIa activity (~55 units/mg) and it has a higher ratio of antifactor Xa to antifactor IIa activity compared to unfractionated heparin. Low molecular weight heparins have a small effect on the activated partial thromboplastin time.

Pharmacodynamics/Kinetics

Onset of Action 2-3 hours

Duration of Action Detectable anti-Xa activity persists for 24 hours

Half-life Elimination 82 minutes; prolonged in renal impairment

Time to Peak 4-6 hours

Pregnancy Considerations Teratogenic events were not observed in animal reproduction studies. Tinzaparin does not cross the human placenta. A pharmacokinetic study in pregnant women found no dose adjustment was needed during pregnancy. Vaginal bleeding was reported in ~10% of pregnant patients during tinzaparin therapy. LMWH is recommended over unfractionated heparin for the treatment of acute venous thromboembolism (VTE) in pregnant women. LMWH is also recommended over unfractionated heparin for VTE prophylaxis in pregnant women with certain risk factors. LMWH should be discontinued prior to induction of labor or a planned cesarean delivery. When choosing therapy, fetal outcomes (ie, pregnancy loss, malformations), maternal outcomes (ie, VTE, hemorrhage), burden of therapy, and maternal preference should be considered (Guyatt, 2012). Contains benzyl alcohol; use with caution in pregnant women due to association with gasping syndrome in premature infants.

Tioconazole (tye oh KONE a zole)

Brand Names: U.S. 1-Day™ [OTC]; Vagistat®-1 [OTC]
Pharmacologic Category Antifungal Agent, Vaginal
Use Local treatment of vulvovaginal candidiasis
Local Anesthetic/Vasoconstrictor Precautions No information available to require special precautions
Effects on Dental Treatment No significant effects or complications reported
Effects on Bleeding No information available to require special precautions
Adverse Effects Frequency not defined.
Central nervous system: Headache
Gastrointestinal: Abdominal pain
Dermatologic: Burning, desquamation
Genitourinary: Discharge, dyspareunia, dysuria, irritation, itching, nocturia, vaginal pain, vaginitis, vulvar swelling
General Dosage Range Intravaginal: *Adults:* Insert 1 applicatorful prior to bedtime, as a single dose
Mechanism of Action A 1-substituted imidazole derivative with a broad antifungal spectrum against a wide variety of dermatophytes and yeasts, including *Trichophyton mentagrophytes*, *T. rubrum*, *T. erinacei*, *T. tonsurans*, *Microsporum canis*, *Microsporum gypseum*, and *Candida albicans*. Both agents appear to be similarly effective against *Epidermophyton floccosum*.
Pharmacodynamics/Kinetics
Onset of Action Some improvement: Within 24 hours; Complete relief: Within 7 days
Pregnancy Considerations May damage rubber or latex condoms or diaphragms; separate use by 3 days.

Tiopronin (tye oh PROE nin)

Brand Names: U.S. Thiola®
Pharmacologic Category Urinary Tract Product
Use Prevention of kidney stone (cystine) formation in patients with severe homozygous cystinuria who have urinary cystine >500 mg/day who are resistant to treatment with high fluid intake, alkali and diet modification, or who have had adverse reactions to penicillamine
Local Anesthetic/Vasoconstrictor Precautions No information available to require special precautions
Effects on Dental Treatment No significant effects or complications reported

Effects on Bleeding No information available to require special precautions
Adverse Effects Frequency not defined.
Central nervous system: Chills, fatigue, fever
Dermatologic: Bruising, pemphigus, pruritus, rash, skin friability/wrinkling, urticaria, warts
Gastrointestinal: Abdominal pain, anorexia, bloating, diarrhea, flatulence, loss of taste perception, nausea, oral ulceration, vomiting
Hematologic: Anemia, bleeding, eosinophilia, leukopenia, thrombocytopenia
Hepatic: Jaundice, liver function tests abnormal
Neuromuscular & skeletal: Arthralgia, myalgia, myasthenia gravis, weakness
Renal: Goodpasture's syndrome, hematuria, nephrotic syndrome, proteinuria
Respiratory: Bronchiolitis, dyspnea, hemoptysis, laryngeal edema, pharyngitis, pulmonary infiltrates, respiratory distress
Miscellaneous: Elastosis perforans serpiginosa, hypersensitivity, loss of smell, lupus-like syndrome, lymphadenopathy, positive ANA test
General Dosage Range Oral:
Children ≥9 years: Initial: 15 mg/kg/day in 3 divided doses
Adults: Initial: 800 mg/day in 3 divided doses; average dose: 1000 mg/day
Mechanism of Action As an active reducing agent, tiopronin undergoes thiol-disulfide exchange with cystine to form tiopronin-cystine disulfide, which is more water soluble than cystine. As a result, the amount of sparingly soluble cystine in the urine is decreased and the formation of cystine calculi is reduced.
Pregnancy Risk Factor C
Pregnancy Considerations Teratogenic effects, including skeletal defects and cleft palates, have been observed following penicillamine exposure in animal reproduction studies. Birth defects, including congenital cutix laxa and associated defects, have been reported in infants following penicillamine exposure during pregnancy. Similar effects may be expected with tiopronin; however, animal studies have not shown these same findings. Use is contraindicated during pregnancy; use only if the possible benefits to the mother outweigh the potential risks to the fetus.

Tiotropium (ty oh TRO pee um)

Related Information
Respiratory Diseases *on page 1514*
Brand Names: U.S. Spiriva® HandiHaler®
Brand Names: Canada Spiriva®
Pharmacologic Category Anticholinergic Agent; Anticholinergic Agent, Long-Acting
Use Maintenance treatment of bronchospasm associated with COPD (including bronchitis and emphysema); reduction of COPD exacerbations
Local Anesthetic/Vasoconstrictor Precautions No information available to require special precautions
Effects on Dental Treatment Key adverse event(s) related to dental treatment: Xerostomia (normal salivary flow resumes upon discontinuation) and ulcerative stomatitis.
Effects on Bleeding No information available to require special precautions

◄ **Adverse Effects**
>10%:
Gastrointestinal: Xerostomia (5% to 16%)
Respiratory: Upper respiratory tract infection (41%), pharyngitis (9% to 13%), sinusitis (7% to 11%)
1% to 10%:
Cardiovascular: Chest pain (1% to 7%), edema (dependent, 5%)
Central nervous system: Headache (6%), insomnia (4%), depression (1% to 4%), dysphonia (1% to 3%)
Dermatologic: Rash (4%)
Endocrine & metabolic: Hypercholesterolemia (1% to 3%), hyperglycemia (1% to 3%)
Gastrointestinal: Dyspepsia (6%), abdominal pain (5%), constipation (1% to 5%), vomiting (4%), gastroesophageal reflux (1% to 3%), stomatitis (including ulcerative; 1% to 3%)
Genitourinary: Urinary tract infection (7%)
Neuromuscular & skeletal: Arthralgia (4%), myalgia (4%), arthritis (≥3%), leg pain (1% to 3%), paresthesia (1% to 3%), skeletal pain (1% to 3%)
Ocular: Cataract (1% to 3%)
Respiratory: Rhinitis (6%), epistaxis (4%), cough (≥3%), laryngitis (1% to 3%)
Miscellaneous: Infection (4%), moniliasis (4%), flu-like syndrome (≥3%), allergic reaction (1% to 3%), herpes zoster (1% to 3%)
General Dosage Range Inhalation: *Adults:* Contents of 1 capsule (18 mcg) once daily
Mechanism of Action Competitively and reversibly inhibits the action of acetylcholine at type 3 muscarinic (M_3) receptors in bronchial smooth muscle causing bronchodilation
Pharmacodynamics/Kinetics
Half-life Elimination 5-6 days
Time to Peak Plasma: 5 minutes (following inhalation)
Pregnancy Risk Factor C
Pregnancy Considerations Adverse events (fetal loss, decreased birth weights, delayed sexual maturation) were observed in some animal studies. There are no adequate and well-controlled studies in pregnant women. Use only when expected benefit to mother outweighs potential risk to the fetus.

Tipranavir (tip RA na veer)

Related Information
HIV Infection and AIDS *on page 1520*
Brand Names: U.S. Aptivus®
Brand Names: Canada Aptivus®
Pharmacologic Category Antiretroviral Agent, Protease Inhibitor
Use Treatment of HIV-1 infections in combination with ritonavir and other antiretroviral agents; limited to highly treatment-experienced or multiprotease inhibitor-resistant patients.
Local Anesthetic/Vasoconstrictor Precautions No information available to require special precautions
Effects on Dental Treatment No significant effects or complications reported
Effects on Bleeding Increased bleeding has been noted with protease inhibitors in patients with hemophilia A or B. No information available to require routine special precautions relative to hemostasis in other patients.
Adverse Effects
>10%:
Dermatologic: Rash (children 21%; adults 3% to 10%)

Endocrine & metabolic: Hypertriglyceridemia (>400 mg/dL: 61%), hypercholesterolemia (>300 mg/dL: 22%)
Gastrointestinal: Diarrhea (15%)
Hepatic: Transaminases increased (>2.5 x ULN: 26% to 32%; grade 3/4: 10% to 20%)
Neuromuscular & skeletal: CPK increased (grade 3/4: children 11%)
2% to 10%:
Central nervous system: Fever (6% to 8%), fatigue (6%), headache (5%)
Endocrine & metabolic: Dehydration (2%)
Gastrointestinal: Nausea (5% to 9%), amylase increased (grade 3: 6% to 8%), vomiting (6%), abdominal pain (4%), diarrhea (children 4%), weight loss (3%)
Hematologic: Bleeding (children 8%), WBC decreased (grades 3: 5%), anemia (3%), neutropenia (2%)
Hepatic: ALT increased (2%, grades 3/4: 10%), AST increased (grades 3/4: 6%), GGT increased (2%)
Neuromuscular & skeletal: Myalgia (2%)
Respiratory: Cough (children 6%), dyspnea (2%), epistaxis (children 4%)
General Dosage Range Dosage adjustment recommended in patients on concomitant therapy
Oral:
Children ≥2 years: 12-14 mg/kg or 290-375 mg/m^2 (maximum: 500 mg/dose) twice daily
Adults: 500 mg twice daily
Mechanism of Action Binds to the site of HIV-1 protease activity and inhibits cleavage of viral Gag-Pol polyprotein precursors into individual functional proteins required for infectious HIV. This results in the formation of immature, noninfectious viral particles.
Pharmacodynamics/Kinetics
Half-life Elimination Children 2-<6 years of age: ~8 hours, 6-<12 years of age: ~7 hours, 12-18 years: ~5 hours; Adults: 6 hours
Time to Peak 3 hours
Pregnancy Risk Factor C
Pregnancy Considerations Teratogenic effects were not observed in animal reproduction studies; fetotoxicity was observed with some doses. Tipranavir crosses the human placenta. The DHHS Perinatal HIV Guidelines note there are insufficient data to recommend use during pregnancy; however, if used, tipranavir must be given with low-dose ritonavir boosting. A small increased risk of preterm birth has been associated with maternal use of protease inhibitor-based combination antiretroviral (ARV) therapy during pregnancy; however, the benefits of use generally outweigh this risk and protease inhibitors (PIs) should not be withheld if otherwise recommended. Hyperglycemia, new onset of diabetes mellitus, or diabetic ketoacidosis have been reported with PIs; it is not clear if pregnancy increases this risk.

Regardless of CD4 count or HIV RNA copy number, all HIV-infected pregnant women should receive a combination antepartum ARV drug regimen; this includes women who require therapy for their own health, as well as women who do not yet require therapy for their own health. ARV therapy should be started as soon as possible if required for the woman's health. Although earlier initiation may be more effective in reducing the perinatal transmission of HIV, also consider maternal conditions (eg, nausea and vomiting) and the potential risks of first trimester fetal exposure for specific agents. Plasma HIV RNA levels should be assessed at ~34-36 weeks gestation in order to help determine mode of delivery. If ARV therapy must be interrupted for <24 hours during the peripartum period, stop then restart all medications simultaneously in order to decrease the chance of developing resistance. Long-term follow-up is recommended for all infants exposed to ARV medications.

Healthcare providers are encouraged to enroll pregnant women exposed to antiretroviral medications in the Antiretroviral Pregnancy Registry (1-800-258-4263 or www.APRegistry.com). Healthcare providers caring for HIV-infected women and their infants may contact the National Perinatal HIV Hotline (888-448-8765) for clinical consultation (DHHS [perinatal], 2012).

Women receiving estrogen (as hormonal contraception or replacement therapy) may have an increased incidence of rash.

Tirofiban (tye roe FYE ban)

Related Information
Cardiovascular Diseases *on page 1492*
Brand Names: U.S. Aggrastat®
Brand Names: Canada Aggrastat®
Pharmacologic Category Antiplatelet Agent, Glycoprotein IIb/IIIa Inhibitor
Use Treatment of acute coronary syndrome (ie, unstable angina/non-ST-elevation myocardial infarction [UA/NSTEMI]) in combination with heparin
Unlabeled Use To support PCI (administered at the time of PCI) for ST-elevation myocardial infarction (STEMI), UA/NSTEMI, and stable ischemic heart disease (ie, elective PCI)
Local Anesthetic/Vasoconstrictor Precautions No information available to require special precautions
Effects on Dental Treatment Key adverse event(s) related to dental treatment: Bleeding is a potential adverse effect of tirofiban. See Effects on Bleeding.
Effects on Bleeding As with all anticoagulants, bleeding is a potential adverse effect of tirofiban during dental surgery; risk is dependent on multiple variables, including the intensity of anticoagulation and patient susceptibility. Medical consult is suggested. It is unlikely that ambulatory patients presenting for dental treatment will be taking intravenous anticoagulant therapy.
Adverse Effects Bleeding is the major drug-related adverse effect. Patients received background treatment with aspirin and heparin. Major bleeding was reported in 1.4% to 2.2%; minor bleeding in 10.5% to 12%; transfusion was required in 4% to 4.3%.
>1% (nonbleeding adverse events):
Cardiovascular: Coronary artery dissection (5%), bradycardia (4%), edema (2%)
Central nervous system: Dizziness (3%), vasovagal reaction (2%), fever (>1%), headache (>1%)
Gastrointestinal: Nausea (>1%)
Genitourinary: Pelvic pain (6%)
Hematologic: Thrombocytopenia: <90,000/mm^3 (1.5%), <50,000/mm^3 (0.3%)
Neuromuscular & skeletal: Leg pain (3%)
Miscellaneous: Diaphoresis (2%)
General Dosage Range Dosage adjustment recommended in patients with renal impairment
I.V.: *Adults:* Initial: 0.4 mcg/kg/minute for 30 minutes; Maintenance infusion: 0.1 mcg/kg/minute

Mechanism of Action A reversible antagonist of fibrinogen binding to the GP IIb/IIIa receptor, the major platelet surface receptor involved in platelet aggregation. When administered intravenously, it inhibits *ex vivo* platelet aggregation in a dose- and concentration-dependent manner. When given according to the recommended regimen, >90% inhibition is attained by the end of the 30-minute infusion. Platelet aggregation inhibition is reversible following cessation of the infusion.
Pharmacodynamics/Kinetics
Half-life Elimination 2 hours
Pregnancy Risk Factor B
Pregnancy Considerations Adverse events have not been observed in animal reproduction studies. Information related to use in pregnancy is limited; successful use during pregnancy has been described in a case report (Boztosun, 2008).

TiZANidine (tye ZAN i deen)

Brand Names: U.S. Zanaflex Capsules®; Zanaflex®
Brand Names: Canada Apo-Tizanidine®; Gen-Tizanidine; Mylan-Tizanidine; Zanaflex®
Generic Availability (U.S.) Yes
Pharmacologic Category Alpha$_2$-Adrenergic Agonist
Use Skeletal muscle relaxant used for treatment of muscle spasticity
Unlabeled Use Tension headaches, acute low back pain
Local Anesthetic/Vasoconstrictor Precautions No information available to require special precautions
Effects on Dental Treatment Key adverse event(s) related to dental treatment: Significant xerostomia (normal salivary flow resumes upon discontinuation).
Effects on Bleeding No information available to require special precautions
Adverse Effects Frequency percentages below reported during multiple-dose studies, unless specified otherwise.
>10%:
Cardiovascular: Hypotension (16% to 33%)
Central nervous system: Somnolence (48%), dizziness (16%)
Gastrointestinal: Xerostomia (49%)
Neuromuscular & skeletal: Weakness (41%)
1% to 10%:
Cardiovascular: Bradycardia (2% to 10%)
Central nervous system: Nervousness (3%), speech disorder (3%), visual hallucinations/delusions (3%), anxiety (1%), depression (1%), fever (1%)
Dermatologic: Rash (1%), skin ulcer (1%)
Gastrointestinal: Constipation (4%), vomiting (3%), abdominal pain (1%), diarrhea (1%), dyspepsia (1%)
Genitourinary: UTI (10%), urinary frequency (3%)
Hepatic: Liver enzymes increased (3% to 5%)
Neuromuscular & skeletal: Dyskinesia (3%), back pain (1%), myasthenia (1%), paresthesia (1%)
Ocular: Blurred vision (3%)
Respiratory: Pharyngitis (3%), rhinitis (3%)
Miscellaneous: Infection (6%), flu-like syndrome (3%), diaphoresis (1%)
Dosage Oral:
Adults: Initial: 4 mg up to 3 times daily (at 6- to 8-hour intervals); may titrate to optimal effect in 2-4 mg increments as needed to a maximum of 3 doses in 24 hours (at 6- to 8-hour intervals); maximum: 36 mg daily.
Note: Limited experience with single doses >8 mg and daily doses >24 mg.

◄ Elderly: Refer to adult dosing. Use with caution; clearance is decreased.

Dosing adjustment in renal impairment:
Cl_{cr} ≥25 mL/minute: No dosage adjustment provided in manufacturer's labeling; however, caution may be needed as creatinine clearance decreases.
Cl_{cr} <25 mL/minute: Use with caution; clearance reduced >50%. During initial dose titration, use reduced doses. If higher doses are necessary, increase dose instead of increasing dosing frequency.

Dosing adjustment in hepatic impairment: Avoid use in hepatic impairment; if used, lowest possible dose should be used initially with close monitoring for adverse effects (eg, hypotension).

Mechanism of Action An $alpha_2$-adrenergic agonist agent which decreases excitatory input to alpha motor neurons; an imidazole derivative chemically-related to clonidine, is a centrally acting muscle relaxant with $alpha_2$-adrenergic agonist properties; acts on the level of the spinal cord

Contraindications Hypersensitivity to tizanidine or any component of the formulation; concomitant therapy with ciprofloxacin or fluvoxamine (potent CYP1A2 inhibitors)

Warnings/Precautions Significant hypotension (possibly with bradycardia or orthostatic hypotension) and sedation may occur; use caution in patients with cardiac disease or those at risk for severe hypotensive (eg, patients taking concurrent medications which may predispose to hypotension/bradycardia) or sedative effects (patients must be cautioned about performing tasks which require mental alertness [eg, operating machinery or driving]). Should not be used with other $alpha_2$-adrenergic agonists. Avoid concomitant administration with CYP1A2 inhibitors; increased tizanidine levels/effects (severe hypotension and sedation) may occur. Concomitant use of ciprofloxacin or fluvoxamine is contraindicated. These effects may also be increased with concomitant administration with other CNS depressants and/or antihypertensives; use caution. In general, avoid concomitant use of oral contraceptives with tizanidine; clearance of tizanidine may be decreased by 50%; if taken concomitantly, decrease initial tizanidine dose and titration rate. Elderly patients are at risk due to decreased clearance, particulary in elderly patients with renal insufficiency (Cl_{cr} <25 mL/minute) compared to healthy elderly subjects; this may lead to an increased risk of adverse effects and/or a longer duration of effects. Use caution in any patient with renal impairment. Clearance decreased significantly in patients with severe impairment (Cl_{cr}<25 mL/minute); dose reductions recommended. Use with extreme caution or avoid in hepatic impairment due to extensive hepatic metabolism and potential hepatotoxicity; AST/ALT elevations (>3 times ULN) and rarely hepatic failure have occurred; monitoring recommended.

May be inappropriate in older adults depending on comorbidities (eg, dementia, delirium) due to its potent anticholinergic effects (Beers Criteria).

Use has been associated with visual hallucinations or delusions, generally in first 6 weeks of therapy; use caution in patients with psychiatric disorders. Withdrawal resulting in rebound hypertension, tachycardia, and hypertonia may occur upon discontinuation; doses should be decreased slowly, particularly in patients receiving high doses for prolonged periods. Pharmacokinetics and bioequivalence between capsules and tablets altered by nonfasting vs fasting conditions (capsules and tablets are bioequivalent under fasting conditions,

but not under nonfasting conditions). Limited data exist for chronic use of single doses >8 mg and multiple doses >24 mg/day.

Drug Interactions
Metabolism/Transport Effects Substrate of CYP1A2 (major); **Note:** Assignment of Major/Minor substrate status based on clinically relevant drug interaction potential

Avoid Concomitant Use
Avoid concomitant use of TiZANidine with any of the following: Azelastine (Nasal); Ciprofloxacin (Systemic); FluvoxaMINE; Iobenguane I 123; Paraldehyde

Increased Effect/Toxicity
TiZANidine may increase the levels/effects of: ACE Inhibitors; Alcohol (Ethyl); Azelastine (Nasal); Beta-Blockers; Buprenorphine; CNS Depressants; Highest Risk QTc-Prolonging Agents; Hypotensive Agents; Lisinopril; Methotrimeprazine; Metyrosine; Moderate Risk QTc-Prolonging Agents; Paraldehyde; Pramipexole; ROPINIRole; Rotigotine; Selective Serotonin Reuptake Inhibitors; Zolpidem

The levels/effects of TiZANidine may be increased by: Abiraterone Acetate; Beta-Blockers; Ciprofloxacin (Systemic); Contraceptives (Estrogens); CYP1A2 Inhibitors (Moderate); CYP1A2 Inhibitors (Strong); Deferasirox; Droperidol; FluvoxaMINE; HydrOXYzine; Magnesium Sulfate; MAO Inhibitors; Methotrimeprazine; Mifepristone; Perampanel; Sodium Oxybate

Decreased Effect
TiZANidine may decrease the levels/effects of: Iobenguane I 123

The levels/effects of TiZANidine may be decreased by: Antidepressants (Alpha2-Antagonist); Serotonin/Norepinephrine Reuptake Inhibitors; Tricyclic Antidepressants

Ethanol/Nutrition/Herb Interactions
Ethanol: May increase CNS depression; monitor for increased effects with coadministration. Caution patients about effects.
Food: The tablet and capsule dosage forms are not bioequivalent when administered with food. Food increases both the time to peak concentration and the extent of absorption for both the tablet and capsule. However, maximal concentrations of tizanidine achieved when administered with food were increased by 30% for the tablet, but decreased by 20% for the capsule. Under fed conditions, the capsule is approximately 80% bioavailable relative to the tablet.
Herb/Nutraceutical: Avoid valerian, St John's wort, kava kava, gotu kola (may increase CNS depression). Avoid black cohosh, California poppy, coleus, golden seal, hawthorn, mistletoe, periwinkle, quinine, shepherd's purse (may increase hypotensive effects).

Dietary Considerations Administration with food compared to administration in the fasting state results in clinically-significant differences in absorption and other pharmacokinetic parameters. Patients should be consistent and should not switch administration of the tablets or the capsules between the fasting and nonfasting state. In addition, switching between the capsules and the tablets in the fed state will also result in significant differences. Opening capsule contents to sprinkle on applesauce compared to swallowing intact capsules whole will also result in significant absorption differences. Patients should be consistent with regards to administration.

Pharmacodynamics/Kinetics
Onset of Action Single dose (8 mg): Peak effect: 1-2 hours

Duration of Action Single dose (8 mg): 3-6 hours

Half-life Elimination 2.5 hours

Time to Peak
Fasting state: Capsule, tablet: 1 hour
Fed state: Capsule: 3-4 hours, Tablet: 1.5 hours

Pregnancy Risk Factor C

Pregnancy Considerations Adverse events were observed in some animal reproduction studies.

Lactation Excretion in breast milk unknown

Breast-Feeding Considerations Excretion in breast milk is unknown, but expected due to lipid solubility.

Dosage Forms
Capsule, oral: 2 mg, 4 mg, 6 mg
Zanaflex Capsules®: 2 mg, 4 mg, 6 mg
Tablet, oral: 2 mg, 4 mg
Zanaflex®: 4 mg

Tobramycin (Systemic, Oral Inhalation)
(toe bra MYE sin)

Brand Names: U.S. TOBI®

Brand Names: Canada TOBI®; TOBI® Podhaler®; Tobramycin Injection, USP

Pharmacologic Category Antibiotic, Aminoglycoside

Use Treatment of documented or suspected infections caused by susceptible gram-negative bacilli, including *Pseudomonas aeruginosa*. Tobramycin solution for inhalation and powder for inhalation (Canadian availability; not available in the U.S.) are indicated for the management of cystic fibrosis patients with *Pseudomonas aeruginosa*.

Local Anesthetic/Vasoconstrictor Precautions No information available to require special precautions

Effects on Dental Treatment No significant effects or complications reported

Effects on Bleeding No information available to require special precautions

Adverse Effects

Injection: Frequency not defined:
Central nervous system: Confusion, disorientation, dizziness, fever, headache, lethargy, vertigo
Dermatologic: Exfoliative dermatitis, itching, rash, urticaria
Endocrine & metabolic: Serum calcium, magnesium, potassium, and/or sodium decreased
Gastrointestinal: Diarrhea, nausea, vomiting
Hematologic: Anemia, eosinophilia, granulocytopenia, leukocytosis, leukopenia, thrombocytopenia
Hepatic: ALT increased, AST increased, bilirubin increased, LDH increased
Local: Pain at the injection site
Otic: Hearing loss, tinnitus, ototoxicity (auditory), ototoxicity (vestibular), roaring in the ears
Renal: BUN increased, cylindruria, serum creatinine increased, oliguria, proteinuria

Inhalation (as reported for solution for inhalation unless otherwise noted):
>10%:
Gastrointestinal: Sputum discoloration (21%)
Respiratory: FEV_1 decreased (2% to 31%), cough (22% [powder for inhalation]), rales (19%), voice alteration (6% to 13%)
1% to 10%:
Cardiovascular: Chest discomfort (3% [powder for inhalation])
Central nervous system: Malaise (6%), pyrexia (1% [powder for inhalation])

Gastrointestinal: Abnormal taste (5% [powder for inhalation]), diarrhea (2%), xerostomia (2% [powder for inhalation])
Hematologic: RBC sedimentation rate increased (8%), eosinophilia (2%)
Otic: Tinnitus (3%)
Respiratory: Wheezing (5%), dyspnea (4% [powder for inhalation]), oropharyngeal pain (4% [powder for inhalation]), bronchitis (3%), epistaxis (3%), pharyngolaryngeal pain (3%), throat irritation (3% [powder for inhalation]), pulmonary function decreased (2% to 16%), rhinitis (2%), tonsillitis (2%), bronchospasm (1% [powder for inhalation]), upper respiratory tract infection (1% [powder for inhalation])
Miscellaneous: Immunoglobulins increased (2%)
Respiratory: Dyspnea (4% [powder for inhalation]), oropharyngeal pain (4% [powder for inhalation]), throat irritation (3% [powder for inhalation]), FEV decreased (2% [powder for inhalation]), pulmonary function decreased (2% [powder for inhalation]), bronchospasm (1% [powder for inhalation]), upper respiratory tract infection (1% [powder for inhalation])

General Dosage Range Dosage adjustment recommended for the I.M. and I.V. routes in patients with renal impairment

I.M.:
Infants and Children <5 years: 2.5 mg/kg every 8 hours
Children ≥5 years: 2-3.3 mg/kg every 6-8 hours
Adults: 1-2.5 mg/kg every 8-12 hours (1 mg/kg used for synergy) **or** 4-7 mg/kg/day as a single daily dose
Elderly: 1.5-5 mg/kg/day in 1-2 divided doses

I.V.:
Infants and Children <5 years: 2.5 mg/kg every 8 hours
Children ≥5 years: 2-3.3 mg/kg every 6-8 hours
Adults: 1-2.5 mg/kg every 8-12 hours (1 mg/kg/dose used for synergy) **or** 4-7 mg/kg/day as a single daily dose
Elderly: 1.5-5 mg/kg/day in 1-2 divided doses **or** 5-7 mg/kg given every 24, 36, or 48 hours based on Cl_{cr}

Inhalation: *Children ≥6 years and Adults:* 300 mg every 12 hours [Bethkis®, TOBI®]

Mechanism of Action Interferes with bacterial protein synthesis by binding to 30S and 50S ribosomal subunits, resulting in a defective bacterial cell membrane

Pharmacodynamics/Kinetics

Half-life Elimination
Neonates: ≤1200 g: 11 hours; >1200 g: 2-9 hours
Adults: I.V.: 2-3 hours; directly dependent upon glomerular filtration rate; Inhalation: ~4 hours
Adults with impaired renal function: 5-70 hours

Time to Peak Serum: I.M.: 30-60 minutes; I.V.: ~30 minutes

Pregnancy Risk Factor D

Pregnancy Considerations [U.S. Boxed Warning]: Aminoglycosides may cause fetal harm if administered to a pregnant woman. There are several reports of total irreversible bilateral congenital deafness in children whose mothers received another aminoglycoside (streptomycin) during pregnancy; therefore, tobramycin is classified as pregnancy category D. Tobramycin crosses the placenta and produces detectable serum levels in the fetus. Although serious side effects to the fetus have not been reported following maternal use of tobramycin, a potential for harm exists.

Due to pregnancy-induced physiologic changes, some pharmacokinetic parameters of tobramycin may be altered. Pregnant women have an average-to-larger volume of distribution which may result in lower serum peak levels than for the same dose in nonpregnant women. Serum half-life is also shorter.

Product Availability

Bethkis®: FDA approved October 2012; availability is expected during the second or third quarter of 2013.

Bethkis® inhalation solution (300 mg/4 mL) is approved for the management of cystic fibrosis patients (≥6 years) with *Pseudomonas aeruginosa*.

TOBI® Podhaler™: FDA approved March 2013; availability anticipated in the second quarter of 2013. Consult prescribing information for additional information.

Tobramycin and Dexamethasone
(toe bra MYE sin & deks a METH a sone)

Brand Names: U.S. TobraDex®; TobraDex® ST
Brand Names: Canada Tobradex®
Pharmacologic Category Antibiotic/Corticosteroid, Ophthalmic
Use Treatment of external ocular infection caused by susceptible gram-negative bacteria and steroid responsive inflammatory conditions of the palpebral and bulbar conjunctiva, cornea, and anterior segment of the globe
Local Anesthetic/Vasoconstrictor Precautions No information available to require special precautions
Effects on Dental Treatment No significant effects or complications reported
Effects on Bleeding No information available to require special precautions
Adverse Effects Frequency not always defined:
Dermatologic: Allergic contact dermatitis, delayed wound healing
Ocular: Conjunctival erythema (<4%), lid itching (<4%), lid swelling (<4%), cataract formation, glaucoma, intraocular pressure increased, keratitis, lacrimation, optic nerve damage, secondary infection
General Dosage Range Ophthalmic: *Children ≥2 years and Adults:* Ointment: Apply ~1/2" ribbon up to 3-4 times/day; Suspension: Instill 1-2 drops every every 4-6 hours, may increase to 1-2 drops every 2 hours for 24-48 hours
Mechanism of Action See individual agents.
Pregnancy Risk Factor C
Pregnancy Considerations See individual agents.

Tocilizumab (toe si LIZ oo mab)

Related Information
Rheumatoid Arthritis, Osteoarthritis, and Osteoporosis on page 1526
Brand Names: U.S. Actemra®
Brand Names: Canada Actemra®
Pharmacologic Category Antirheumatic, Disease Modifying; Interleukin-6 Receptor Antagonist
Use Treatment of moderately- to severely-active rheumatoid arthritis in adult patients who have had an inadequate response to one or more disease-modifying antirheumatic drugs (DMARDs) (as monotherapy or in combination with methotrexate or other nonbiological DMARDs); treatment of active systemic juvenile idiopathic arthritis (SJIA) (as monotherapy or in combination with methotrexate)
Local Anesthetic/Vasoconstrictor Precautions No information available to require special precautions

Effects on Dental Treatment Key adverse event(s) related to dental treatment: Mouth ulcerations and stomatitis
Effects on Bleeding No information available to require special precautions
Adverse Effects Incidence as reported for monotherapy, except where noted. Combination therapy refers to use in rheumatoid arthritis with nonbiological DMARDs or use in SJIA in trials where most patients (~70%) were taking methotrexate at baseline.
>10%: Hepatic: ALT increased (≤36%; grades 3/4: <1%), AST increased (≤22%; grades 3/4: <1%)
1% to 10%:
Cardiovascular: Hypertension (1% to 6%), peripheral edema (<2%)
Central nervous system: Headache (1% to 7%), dizziness (3%)
Dermatologic: Rash (2%), skin reaction (combination therapy; 1% [includes pruritus, urticaria])
Endocrine & metabolic: LDL cholesterol increased (>1.5-2 x ULN; combination therapy; children 2%), total cholesterol increased (>1.5-2 x ULN; combination therapy; children 2%), hypothyroidism (<2%)
Gastrointestinal: Diarrhea (children ≤5%), abdominal pain (2%), mouth ulceration (2%), gastric ulcer (<2%), stomatitis (<2%), weight gain (<2%), gastritis (1%)
Hematologic: Neutropenia (combination therapy; grade 3: 2% to 7%; grade 4: <1%), thrombocytopenia (combination therapy; 1% to 2%), leukopenia (<2%)
Hepatic: Bilirubin increased (<2%)
Local: Infusion-related reactions (combination therapy; 4% to 16%)
Ocular: Conjunctivitis (<2%)
Renal: Nephrolithiasis (<2%)
Respiratory: Upper respiratory tract infection (7%), nasopharyngitis (7%), bronchitis (3%), cough (<2%), dyspnea (<2%)
Miscellaneous: Anti-tocilizumab antibody formation (2%), herpes simplex (<2%)
General Dosage Range Dosage adjustment recommended in patients who develop toxicities
I.V.:
Children ≥2 years and <30 kg: 12 mg/kg every 2 weeks
Children ≥2 years and ≥30 kg: 8 mg/kg every 2 weeks
Adults: 4-8 mg/kg every 4 weeks (maximum dose: 800 mg)
Mechanism of Action Antagonist of the interleukin-6 (IL-6) receptor. Endogenous IL-6 is induced by inflammatory stimuli and mediates a variety of immunological responses. Inhibition of IL-6 receptors by tocilizumab leads to a reduction in cytokine and acute phase reactant production.
Pharmacodynamics/Kinetics
Half-life Elimination Terminal, single dose: 6.3 days (concentration-dependent; may be increased up to 23 days [children] or 13 days [adults] at steady state)
Pregnancy Risk Factor C
Pregnancy Considerations No evidence of impaired fertility, teratogenic, or dysmorphogenic effects in animal models; an increased incidence of abortion and embryo-fetal death has been observed in animal reproduction studies. Use during pregnancy only if clearly needed. A pregnancy registry has been established to monitor outcomes of women exposed to tocilizumab during pregnancy (877-311-8972).

Tofacitinib (toe fa SYE ti nib)

Related Information
Rheumatoid Arthritis, Osteoarthritis, and Osteoporosis *on page 1526*
Brand Names: U.S. Xeljanz®
Pharmacologic Category Antirheumatic Miscellaneous; Antirheumatic, Disease Modifying; Janus Associated Kinase Inhibitor
Use Treatment of moderately- to severely-active rheumatoid arthritis (as monotherapy or in combination with methotrexate or other nonbiologic disease-modifying antirheumatic drugs [DMARDs]) in patients who have had an inadequate response to, or are intolerant of, methotrexate
Local Anesthetic/Vasoconstrictor Precautions No information available to require special precautions
Effects on Dental Treatment No significant effects or complications reported
Effects on Bleeding Active therapy with tofacitinib may result in significant myelosuppression; medical consult is suggested.
Adverse Effects
Percentages noted include the highest frequency regardless of dosage. Frequencies may vary for specific doses; consult prescribing information.
>10%: Miscellaneous: Infections (20%)
1% to 10%:
   Cardiovascular: Hypertension (2%)
   Central nervous system: Headache (4%)
   Gastrointestinal: Diarrhea (4%)
   Genitourinary: Urinary tract infection (2%)
   Hepatic: ALT increased (>3 x upper limit of normal; 1%)
   Renal: Serum creatinine increased (<2%)
   Respiratory: Upper respiratory tract infections (5%), nasopharyngitis (4%)
   Miscellaneous: Serious infections (2%)
<1%: Abdominal pain, anemia, arthralgia, cough, dehydration, dyspepsia, dyspnea, erythema, fatigue, gastritis, hepatic steatosis, insomnia, joint swelling, lymphocytopenia, malignancies, musculoskeletal pain, nausea, neutropenia, paresthesia, peripheral edema, pruritus, pyrexia, rash, sinus congestion, tendonitis, tuberculosis, vomiting
Postmarketing and/or case reports: Drug-induced liver injury
General Dosage Range Dosage adjustment recommended in patients with renal impairment, hepatic impairment, on concomitant therapy, and who develop toxicities.
Oral: *Adults:* 5 mg twice daily
Mechanism of Action Tofacitinib inhibits Janus kinase (JAK) enzymes, which are intracellular enzymes involved in stimulating hematopoiesis and immune cell function through a signaling pathway. In response to extracellular cytokine or growth factor signaling, JAKs activate signal transducers and activators of transcription (STATs), which regulate gene expression and intracellular activity. Inhibition of JAKs prevents cytokine- or growth factor-mediated gene expression and intracellular activity of immune cells, reduces circulating CD16/56+ natural killer cells, serum IgG, IgM, IgA, and C-reactive protein, and increases B cells.
Pharmacodynamics/Kinetics
Half-life Elimination ~3 hours
Time to Peak 0.5-1 hour
Pregnancy Risk Factor C

Pregnancy Considerations Adverse events have been observed in animal reproduction studies. Healthcare providers are encouraged to enroll women exposed to tofacitinib during pregnancy in the Xeljanz® Pregnancy Registry (877-311-8972); patients may also enroll themselves.
Prescribing and Access Restrictions Available through specialty/network pharmacies. Further information may be obtained from the manufacturer, Pfizer Inc, at 1-855-493-5526 or at http://www.xeljanz.com/.

TOLAZamide (tole AZ a mide)

Related Information
Endocrine Disorders and Pregnancy *on page 1517*
Pharmacologic Category Antidiabetic Agent, Sulfonylurea
Use Adjunct to diet for the management of mild-to-moderately severe, stable, type 2 diabetes mellitus (noninsulin dependent, NIDDM)
Local Anesthetic/Vasoconstrictor Precautions No information available to require special precautions
Effects on Dental Treatment Use salicylates with caution in patients taking tolazamide due to potential increased hypoglycemia; NSAIDs such as ibuprofen and naproxen may be safely used. Tolazamide-dependent patients with diabetes (noninsulin dependent, type 2) should be appointed for dental treatment in morning in order to minimize chance of stress-induced hypoglycemia.
Effects on Bleeding No information available to require special precautions
Adverse Effects Frequency not defined.
   Central nervous system: Dizziness, fatigue, headache, malaise, vertigo
   Dermatologic: Maculopapular eruptions, morbilliform eruptions, photosensitivity, pruritus, rash, urticaria
   Endocrine & metabolic: Disulfiram-like reaction, hypoglycemia, hyponatremia, SIADH
   Gastrointestinal: Anorexia, constipation, diarrhea, epigastric fullness, heartburn, nausea, vomiting
   Hematologic: Agranulocytosis, aplastic anemia, hemolytic anemia, leukopenia, pancytopenia, porphyria cutanea tarda, thrombocytopenia
   Hepatic: Cholestatic jaundice, hepatic porphyria
   Neuromuscular & skeletal: Weakness
   Renal: Diuretic effect
General Dosage Range Oral: *Adults:* Initial: 100-250 mg/day with first main meal of day; Maintenance: 100-1000 mg/day in 1-2 (doses >500 mg) divided doses (maximum: 1 g/day)
Mechanism of Action Stimulates insulin release from the pancreatic beta cells; reduces glucose output from the liver; insulin sensitivity is increased at peripheral target sites
Pharmacodynamics/Kinetics
Onset of Action Hypoglycemic effect: 20 minutes; Peak hypoglycemic effect: 4-6 hours
Duration of Action 10-24 hours
Half-life Elimination 7 hours
Time to Peak Serum: 3-4 hours
Pregnancy Risk Factor C
Pregnancy Considerations Adverse events have been observed in animal studies; therefore, tolazamide is classified as pregnancy category C. Severe hypoglycemia lasting 4-10 days has been noted in infants born to mothers taking a sulfonylurea at the time of delivery. Maternal hyperglycemia can be associated with adverse effects in the fetus, including macrosomia, neonatal

hyperglycemia and hyperbilirubinemia; the risk of congenital malformations is increased when the Hb A_{1c} is above the normal range. Diabetes can also be associated with adverse effects in the mother. Poorly-treated diabetes may cause end-organ damage that may in turn negatively affect obstetric outcomes. Physiologic glucose levels should be maintained prior to and during pregnancy to decrease the risk of adverse events in the mother and the fetus. Until additional safety and efficacy data are obtained, the use of oral agents is generally not recommended as routine management of GDM or type 2 diabetes mellitus during pregnancy. The manufacturer recommends if tolazamide is used during pregnancy, it should be discontinued at least 2 weeks before the expected delivery date. Insulin is the drug of choice for the control of diabetes mellitus during pregnancy.

TOLBUTamide (tole BYOO ta mide)

Related Information
Endocrine Disorders and Pregnancy *on page 1517*
Brand Names: Canada Apo-Tolbutamide®
Pharmacologic Category Antidiabetic Agent, Sulfonylurea
Use Adjunct to diet for the management of type 2 diabetes mellitus (noninsulin dependent, NIDDM)
Local Anesthetic/Vasoconstrictor Precautions No information available to require special precautions
Effects on Dental Treatment Key adverse event(s) related to dental treatment: Taste alteration.

Use salicylates with caution in patients taking tolazamide due to potential increased hypoglycemia; NSAIDs such as ibuprofen and naproxen may be safely used. Tolbutamide-dependent patients with diabetes (noninsulin dependent, type 2) should be appointed for dental treatment in morning in order to minimize chance of stress-induced hypoglycemia.

Effects on Bleeding No information available to require special precautions
Adverse Effects Frequency not defined.
Central nervous system: Headache
Dermatologic: Erythema, maculopapular rash, morbilliform rash, pruritus, urticaria, photosensitivity
Endocrine & metabolic: Disulfiram-like reactions, hypoglycemia, hyponatremia, SIADH
Gastrointestinal: Epigastric fullness, heartburn, nausea, taste alteration
Hematologic: Agranulocytosis, aplastic anemia, hemolytic anemia, leukopenia, pancytopenia, thrombocytopenia
Hepatic: Cholestatic jaundice, hepatic porphyria, porphyria cutanea tarda
Miscellaneous: Hypersensitivity reaction
General Dosage Range Oral:
Adults: Initial: 1-2 g/day as a single dose or divided doses; Maintenance: 0.25-3 g/day as a single dose or divided doses
Elderly: Initial: 0.25 g 1-3 times/day; Maintenance: 0.5-2 g/day in 1-3 divided doses (maximum: 3 g/day)
Mechanism of Action Stimulates insulin release from the pancreatic beta cells; reduces glucose output from the liver; insulin sensitivity is increased at peripheral target sites, suppression of glucagon may also contribute
Pharmacodynamics/Kinetics
Onset of Action 1 hour
Duration of Action Oral: 6-24 hours

Half-life Elimination 4.5-6.5 hours (range: 4-25 hours)
Time to Peak Serum: 3-4 hours
Pregnancy Risk Factor C
Pregnancy Considerations Adverse events have been observed in animal studies; therefore, tolbutamide is classified as pregnancy category C. Tolbutamide crosses the placenta and levels can be measured in the serum of newborn infants following maternal use during pregnancy. Teratogenic effects have been noted in some case reports. Prolonged hyperinsulinemic hypoglycemia has been reported in an infant following maternal use of tolbutamide and severe hypoglycemia lasting 4-10 days has been noted in infants born to mothers taking a sulfonylurea at the time of delivery. Maternal hyperglycemia can be associated with adverse effects in the fetus, including macrosomia, neonatal hyperglycemia, and hyperbilirubinemia; the risk of congenital malformations is increased when the Hb A_{1c} is above the normal range. Diabetes can also be associated with adverse effects in the mother. Poorly-treated diabetes may cause end-organ damage that may in turn negatively affect obstetric outcomes. Physiologic glucose levels should be maintained prior to and during pregnancy to decrease the risk of adverse events in the mother and the fetus. Until additional safety and efficacy data are obtained, the use of oral agents is generally not recommended as routine management of GDM or type 2 diabetes mellitus during pregnancy. The manufacturer recommends if tolbutamide is used during pregnancy, it should be discontinued at least 2 weeks before the expected delivery date. Insulin is the drug of choice for the control of diabetes mellitus during pregnancy.

Tolcapone (TOLE ka pone)

Brand Names: U.S. Tasmar®
Pharmacologic Category Anti-Parkinson's Agent, COMT Inhibitor
Use Adjunct to levodopa and carbidopa for the treatment of signs and symptoms of idiopathic Parkinson's disease in patients with motor fluctuations not responsive to other therapies
Local Anesthetic/Vasoconstrictor Precautions No information available to require special precautions
Effects on Dental Treatment Key adverse event(s) related to dental treatment: Significant xerostomia (normal salivary flow resumes upon discontinuation) and tooth disorder.
Dopaminergic therapy in Parkinson's disease (ie, treatment with levodopa) is associated with orthostatic hypotension. Tolcapone enhances levodopa bioavailability and may increase the occurrence of hypotension/syncope in the dental patient. The patient should be carefully assisted from the chair and observed for signs of orthostatic hypotension.
Effects on Bleeding No information available to require special precautions
Adverse Effects
>10%:
Cardiovascular: Orthostatic hypotension (17%)
Central nervous system: Somnolence (14% to 32%), sleep disorder (24% to 25%), hallucinations (8% to 24%), excessive dreaming (16% to 21%), dizziness (6% to 13%), headache (10% to 11%), confusion (10% to 11%)
Gastrointestinal: Nausea (28% to 50%), diarrhea (16% to 34%; approximately 3% to 4% severe), anorexia (19% to 23%)

Neuromuscular & skeletal: Dyskinesia (42% to 51%), dystonia (19% to 22%), muscle cramps (17% to 18%)

1% to 10%:

Cardiovascular: Syncope (4% to 5%), chest pain (1% to 3%), hypotension (2%), palpitation

Central nervous system: Fatigue (3% to 7%), loss of balance (2% to 3%), agitation (1%), euphoria (1%), hyperactivity (1%), malaise (1%), panic reaction (1%), irritability (1%), mental deficiency (1%), fever (1%), depression, hypoesthesia, tremor, speech disorder, vertigo, emotional lability, hyperkinesia

Dermatologic: Alopecia (1%), bleeding (1%), tumor (1%), rash

Gastrointestinal: Vomiting (8% to 10%), constipation (6% to 8%), xerostomia (5% to 6%), abdominal pain (5% to 6%), dyspepsia (3% to 4%), flatulence (2% to 4%)

Genitourinary: UTI (5%), hematuria (4% to 5%), urine discoloration (2% to 3%), urination disorder (1% to 2%), uterine tumor (1%), incontinence, impotence

Hepatic: Transaminases increased (1% to 3%; 3 times ULN, usually with first 6 months of therapy)

Neuromuscular & skeletal: Paresthesia (1% to 3%), hyper-/hypokinesia (1% to 3%), arthritis (1% to 2%), neck pain (2%), stiffness (2%), myalgia, rhabdomyolysis

Ocular: Cataract (1%), eye inflammation (1%)

Otic: Tinnitus

Respiratory: Upper respiratory infection (5% to 7%), dyspnea (3%), sinus congestion (1% to 2%), bronchitis, pharyngitis

Miscellaneous: Diaphoresis (4% to 7%), influenza (3% to 4%), burning (1% to 2%), flank pain, injury, infection

General Dosage Range Oral: *Adults:* Initial: 100 mg 3 times/day; Maintenance: 100-200 mg 3 times/day

Mechanism of Action Tolcapone is a selective and reversible inhibitor of catechol-o-methyltransferase (COMT). In the presence of a decarboxylase inhibitor (eg, carbidopa), COMT is the major degradation pathway for levodopa. Inhibition of COMT leads to more sustained plasma levels of levodopa and enhanced central dopaminergic activity.

Pharmacodynamics/Kinetics

Half-life Elimination 2-3 hours

Time to Peak ~2 hours

Pregnancy Risk Factor C

Pregnancy Considerations Tolcapone may be teratogenic based on animal studies. There are no adequate and well-controlled studies in pregnant women. Use only if benefit outweighs risk.

Prescribing and Access Restrictions A patient signed consent form acknowledging the risks of hepatic injury should be obtained by the treating physician.

Tolmetin (TOLE met in)

Related Information

Rheumatoid Arthritis, Osteoarthritis, and Osteoporosis *on page 1526*

Temporomandibular Dysfunction (TMD), Chronic Pain, and Fibromyalgia *on page 1590*

Generic Availability (U.S.) Yes

Pharmacologic Category Nonsteroidal Anti-inflammatory Drug (NSAID), Oral

Use Treatment of rheumatoid arthritis and osteoarthritis, juvenile idiopathic arthritis (JIA)

Local Anesthetic/Vasoconstrictor Precautions No information available to require special precautions

Effects on Dental Treatment The dentist should be aware of the potential of abnormal coagulation. Caution should also be exercised in the use of NSAIDs in patients already on anticoagulant therapy with drugs such as warfarin (Coumadin®). See Effects on Bleeding.

Effects on Bleeding Nonselective NSAIDs, such as tolmetin, inhibit platelet aggregation and prolong bleeding time in some patients. Unlike aspirin, the NSAID effect on platelet function is quantitatively less, of shorter duration, and reversible. Normal platelet function should occur in ~5 elimination half-lives or in <10 hours after discontinuation of tolmetin. Concomitant use of other NSAIDs should be avoided.

Adverse Effects

>10%: Gastrointestinal: Nausea (11%)

1% to 10%:

Cardiovascular: Edema (3% to 9%), hypertension (3% to 9%), chest pain (1% to 3%)

Central nervous system: Dizziness (3% to 9%), headache (3% to 9%), depression (1% to 3%), drowsiness (1% to 3%)

Dermatologic: Skin irritation (1% to 3%)

Endocrine & metabolic: Weight gain/loss (3% to 9%)

Gastrointestinal: Abdominal pain (3% to 9%), diarrhea (3% to 9%), dyspepsia (3% to 9%), flatulence (3% to 9%), gastrointestinal distress (3% to 9%), vomiting (3% to 9%), constipation (1% to 3%), gastritis (1% to 3%), peptic ulcer (1% to 3%)

Genitourinary: Urinary tract infection (1% to 3%)

Hematologic: Hemoglobin/hematocrit decreased (transient; 1% to 3%)

Neuromuscular & skeletal: Weakness (3% to 9%)

Ocular: Visual disturbances (1% to 3%)

Otic: Tinnitus (1% to 3%)

Renal: BUN increased (1% to 3%)

Dosage Oral:

Children ≥2 years:

Juvenile idiopathic arthritis (JIA): Initial: 20 mg/kg/day in 3-4 divided doses, then 15-30 mg/kg/day in 3-4 divided doses (maximum dose: 30 mg/kg/day)

Analgesic (unlabeled use): 5-7 mg/kg/dose every 6-8 hours

Adults: RA, osteoarthritis: 400 mg 3 times/day; usual dose: 600 mg to 1.8 g/day; maximum: 1.8 g/day

Mechanism of Action Reversibly inhibits cyclooxygenase-1 and 2 (COX-1 and 2) enzymes, which results in decreased formation of prostaglandin precursors; has antipyretic, analgesic, and anti-inflammatory properties.

Other proposed mechanisms not fully elucidated (and possibly contributing to the anti-inflammatory effect to varying degrees) include inhibiting chemotaxis, altering lymphocyte activity, inhibiting neutrophil aggregation/activation, and decreasing proinflammatory cytokine levels.

Contraindications Hypersensitivity to tolmetin, aspirin, other NSAIDs, or any component of the formulation; perioperative pain in the setting of coronary artery bypass graft (CABG) surgery

Warnings/Precautions [U.S. Boxed Warning]: NSAIDs are associated with an increased risk of adverse cardiovascular thrombotic events, including MI and stroke. Risk may be increased with duration of use or pre-existing cardiovascular risk factors or disease. Carefully evaluate individual cardiovascular risk profiles prior to prescribing. May cause new-onset hypertension or worsening of existing hypertension. Use caution with fluid retention. Avoid use in heart failure. Concurrent administration of ibuprofen, and potentially ▶

other nonselective NSAIDs, may interfere with aspirin's cardioprotective effect. **[U.S. Boxed Warning]: Use is contraindicated for treatment of perioperative pain in the setting of coronary artery bypass graft (CABG) surgery.** Risk of MI and stroke may be increased with use following CABG surgery.

Platelet adhesion and aggregation may be decreased; may prolong bleeding time; patients with coagulation disorders or who are receiving anticoagulants should be monitored closely. Anemia may occur; patients on long-term NSAID therapy should be monitored for anemia. Rarely, NSAID use may cause severe blood dyscrasias (eg, agranulocytosis, aplastic anemia, thrombocytopenia).

NSAID use may compromise existing renal function; dose-dependent decreases in prostaglandin synthesis may result from NSAID use, reducing renal blood flow which may cause renal decompensation. NSAID use may increase the risk for hyperkalemia. Patients with impaired renal function, dehydration, heart failure, liver dysfunction, those taking diuretics, and ACE inhibitors, and the elderly are at greater risk of renal toxicity and hyperkalemia. Rehydrate patient before starting therapy; monitor renal function closely. Not recommended for use in patients with advanced renal disease. Long-term NSAID use may result in renal papillary necrosis. Acute interstitial nephritis and nephritic syndrome have been reported with tolmetin.

In the elderly, avoid chronic use (unless alternative agents ineffective and patient can receive concomitant gastroprotective agent); nonselective oral NSAID use is associated with an increased risk of GI bleeding and peptic ulcer disease in older adults in high risk category (eg, >75 years or age or receiving concomitant oral/parenteral corticosteroids, anticoagulants, or antiplatelet agents) (Beers Criteria).

[U.S. Boxed Warning]: NSAIDs may increase risk of gastrointestinal irritation, inflammation, ulceration, bleeding, and perforation. These events may occur at any time during therapy and without warning. Use caution with a history of GI disease (bleeding or ulcers), concurrent therapy with aspirin, anticoagulants and/or corticosteroids, smoking, use of alcohol, the elderly or debilitated patients. When used concomitantly with ≤325 mg of aspirin, a substantial increase in the risk of gastrointestinal complications (eg, ulcer) occurs; concomitant gastroprotective therapy (eg, proton pump inhibitors) is recommended (Bhatt, 2008).

Use the lowest effective dose for the shortest duration of time, consistent with individual patient goals, to reduce risk of cardiovascular or GI adverse events. Alternate therapies should be considered for patients at high risk.

NSAIDs may cause serious skin adverse events including exfoliative dermatitis, Stevens-Johnson syndrome (SJS) and toxic epidermal necrolysis (TEN); discontinue use at first sign of skin rash or hypersensitivity. Anaphylactoid reactions may occur, even without prior exposure; patients with "aspirin triad" (bronchial asthma, aspirin intolerance, rhinitis) may be at increased risk. Do not use in patients who experience bronchospasm, asthma, rhinitis, or urticaria with NSAID or aspirin therapy.

Use with caution in patients with decreased hepatic function. Closely monitor patients with any abnormal LFT. Severe hepatic reactions (eg, fulminant hepatitis, liver failure) have occurred with NSAID use, rarely; discontinue if signs or symptoms of liver disease develop, or if systemic manifestations occur.

NSAIDS may cause drowsiness, dizziness, blurred vision, and other neurologic effects which may impair physical or mental abilities; patients must be cautioned about performing tasks which require mental alertness (eg, operating machinery or driving). Discontinue use with blurred or diminished vision and perform ophthalmologic exam. Monitor vision with long-term therapy.

The elderly are at increased risk for adverse effects (especially peptic ulceration, CNS effects, renal toxicity) from NSAIDs even at low doses.

Withhold for at least 4-6 half-lives prior to surgical or dental procedures.

Drug Interactions

Metabolism/Transport Effects None known.

Avoid Concomitant Use

Avoid concomitant use of Tolmetin with any of the following: Floctafenine; Ketorolac (Nasal); Ketorolac (Systemic); NSAID (COX-2 Inhibitor); Omacetaxine

Increased Effect/Toxicity

Tolmetin may increase the levels/effects of: Agents with Antiplatelet Properties; Aliskiren; Aminoglycosides; Anticoagulants; Bisphosphonate Derivatives; Collagenase (Systemic); CycloSPORINE (Systemic); Dabigatran Etexilate; Deferasirox; Desmopressin; Digoxin; Drotrecogin Alfa (Activated); Eplerenone; Haloperidol; Ibritumomab; Lithium; Methotrexate; Nonsteroidal Anti-Inflammatory Agents; NSAID (COX-2 Inhibitor); Omacetaxine; PEMEtrexed; Porfimer; Potassium-Sparing Diuretics; PRALAtrexate; Quinolone Antibiotics; Rivaroxaban; Salicylates; Thrombolytic Agents; Tositumomab and Iodine I 131 Tositumomab; Vancomycin; Vitamin K Antagonists

The levels/effects of Tolmetin may be increased by: ACE Inhibitors; Angiotensin II Receptor Blockers; Antidepressants (Tricyclic, Tertiary Amine); Corticosteroids (Systemic); CycloSPORINE (Systemic); Dasatinib; Floctafenine; Glucosamine; Herbs (Anticoagulant/Antiplatelet Properties); Ketorolac (Nasal); Ketorolac (Systemic); Multivitamins/Minerals (with ADEK, Folate, Iron); Omega-3 Fatty Acids; Pentosan Polysulfate Sodium; Pentoxifylline; Probenecid; Prostacyclin Analogues; Selective Serotonin Reuptake Inhibitors; Serotonin/Norepinephrine Reuptake Inhibitors; Sodium Phosphates; Tipranavir; Treprostinil; Vitamin E

Decreased Effect

Tolmetin may decrease the levels/effects of: ACE Inhibitors; Agents with Antiplatelet Properties; Aliskiren; Angiotensin II Receptor Blockers; Beta-Blockers; Eplerenone; HydrALAZINE; Loop Diuretics; Potassium-Sparing Diuretics; Salicylates; Selective Serotonin Reuptake Inhibitors; Thiazide Diuretics

The levels/effects of Tolmetin may be decreased by: Bile Acid Sequestrants; Salicylates

Ethanol/Nutrition/Herb Interactions

Ethanol: Avoid ethanol (may enhance gastric mucosal irritation).

Food: Tolmetin peak serum concentrations may be decreased if taken with food or milk.

Herb/Nutraceutical: Avoid alfalfa, anise, bilberry, bladderwrack, bromelain, cat's claw, celery, chamomile, coleus, cordyceps, dong quai, evening primrose, fenugreek, feverfew, fenugreek, garlic, ginger, ginkgo biloba, ginseng (American, Panax, Siberian), grapeseed, green tea, guggul, horse chestnut seed, horseradish, licorice, prickly ash, red clover, reishi, SAMe (S-adenosylmethionine), sweet clover, turmeric, white willow (all have additional antiplatelet activity).

Dietary Considerations May be taken with antacids to minimize stomach upset. Administration with food or milk decreases bioavailability by 16%. Some products may contain sodium.

Pharmacodynamics/Kinetics
Onset of Action Analgesic: 1-2 hours; Anti-inflammatory: Days to weeks
Half-life Elimination Biphasic: Rapid: 1-2 hours; Slow: 5 hours
Time to Peak Serum: 30-60 minutes
Pregnancy Risk Factor C
Pregnancy Considerations Adverse events were not observed in the initial animal reproduction studies; therefore, the manufacturer classifies tolmetin as pregnancy category C. NSAID exposure during the first trimester is not strongly associated with congenital malformations; however, cardiovascular anomalies and cleft palate have been observed following NSAID exposure in some studies. The use of an NSAID close to conception may be associated with an increased risk of miscarriage. Nonteratogenic effects have been observed following NSAID administration during the third trimester including myocardial degenerative changes, prenatal constriction of the ductus arteriosus, fetal tricuspid regurgitation, failure of the ductus arteriosus to close postnatally; renal dysfunction or failure, oligohydramnios; gastrointestinal bleeding or perforation, increased risk of necrotizing enterocolitis; intracranial bleeding (including intraventricular hemorrhage), platelet dysfunction with resultant bleeding; pulmonary hypertension. Because they may cause premature closure of the ductus arteriosus, use of NSAIDs late in pregnancy should be avoided (use after 31 or 32 weeks gestation is not recommended by some clinicians). The chronic use of NSAIDs in women of reproductive age may be associated with infertility that is reversible upon discontinuation of the medication.

Lactation Enters breast milk/not recommended (AAP rates "compatible"; AAP 2001 update pending)
Breast-Feeding Considerations Tolmetin is found in breast milk and breast-feeding is not recommended by the manufacturer.

Dosage Forms
Capsule, oral: 400 mg
Tablet, oral: 200 mg, 600 mg

Tolnaftate (tole NAF tate)

Brand Names: U.S. Blis-To-Sol® [OTC]; Mycocide® NS [OTC]; Podactin Powder [OTC]; Tinactin® Antifungal Deodorant [OTC]; Tinactin® Antifungal Jock Itch [OTC]; Tinactin® Antifungal [OTC]; Tinaderm [OTC]; Ting® Cream [OTC]; Ting® Spray Liquid [OTC]
Brand Names: Canada Pitrex
Pharmacologic Category Antifungal Agent, Topical
Use Treatment of tinea pedis, tinea cruris, tinea corporis
Local Anesthetic/Vasoconstrictor Precautions No information available to require special precautions
Effects on Dental Treatment No significant effects or complications reported

Effects on Bleeding No information available to require special precautions
Adverse Effects Frequency not defined.
Dermatologic: Contact dermatitis, pruritus
Local: Irritation, stinging
General Dosage Range Topical: *Children ≥2 years and Adults:* Apply to affected areas 2 times/day
Mechanism of Action Distorts the hyphae and stunts mycelial growth in susceptible fungi
Pharmacodynamics/Kinetics
Onset of Action 24-72 hours

Tolterodine (tole TER oh deen)

Brand Names: U.S. Detrol®; Detrol® LA
Brand Names: Canada Detrol®; Detrol® LA; Unidet®
Generic Availability (U.S.) Yes: Tablet
Pharmacologic Category Anticholinergic Agent
Use Treatment of patients with an overactive bladder with symptoms of urinary frequency, urgency, or urge incontinence
Local Anesthetic/Vasoconstrictor Precautions No information available to require special precautions
Effects on Dental Treatment The anticholinergic effects of tolterodine are selective for the urinary bladder rather than salivary glands; xerostomia and changes in salivation (normal salivary flow resumes upon discontinuation).
Effects on Bleeding No information available to require special precautions
Adverse Effects As reported with immediate release tablet, unless otherwise specified
>10%: Gastrointestinal: Dry mouth (35%; extended release capsules 23%)
1% to 10%:
Cardiovascular: Chest pain (2%)
Central nervous system: Headache (7%; extended release capsules 6%), dizziness (5%; extended release capsules 2%), fatigue (4%; extended release capsules 2%), somnolence (3%; extended release capsules 3%), anxiety (extended release capsules 1%)
Dermatologic: Dry skin (1%)
Gastrointestinal: Constipation (7%; extended release capsules 6%), abdominal pain (5%; extended release capsules 4%), diarrhea (4%), dyspepsia (4%; extended release capsules 3%), weight gain (1%)
Genitourinary: Dysuria (2%; extended release capsules 1%)
Neuromuscular & skeletal: Arthralgia (2%)
Ocular: Dry eyes (3%; extended release capsules 3%), abnormal vision (2%; extended release capsules 1%)
Respiratory: Bronchitis (2%), sinusitis (extended release capsules 2%)
Miscellaneous: Flu-like syndrome (3%), infection (1%)
Dosage
Oral: Adults: Treatment of overactive bladder:
Immediate release tablet: 2 mg twice daily; the dose may be lowered to 1 mg twice daily based on individual response and tolerability
Dosing adjustment in patients concurrently taking strong CYP3A4 inhibitors (eg, ketoconazole, clarithromycin, ritonavir): 1 mg twice daily
Extended release capsule: 4 mg once daily; dose may be lowered to 2 mg once daily based on individual response and tolerability
Dosing adjustment in patients concurrently taking strong CYP3A4 inhibitors (eg, ketoconazole, clarithromycin, ritonavir): 2 mg once daily

Elderly: Safety and efficacy in patients >64 years was found to be similar to that in younger patients; no dosage adjustment is needed based on age

Dosing adjustment in renal impairment:
Immediate release tablet: Significantly reduced renal function (studies conducted in patients with Cl_{cr} 10-30 mL/minute): 1 mg twice daily; use with caution
Extended release capsule:
Cl_{cr} 10-30 mL/minute: 2 mg once daily
Cl_{cr} <10 mL/minute: Use is not recommended; has not been studied.

Dosing adjustment in hepatic impairment:
Immediate release tablet: Significantly reduced hepatic function: 1 mg twice daily; use with caution
Extended release capsule:
Mild-to-moderate impairment (Child-Pugh class A or B): 2 mg once daily
Severe impairment (Child-Pugh class C): Use is not recommended; has not been studied.

Mechanism of Action Tolterodine is a competitive antagonist of muscarinic receptors. In animal models, tolterodine demonstrates selectivity for urinary bladder receptors over salivary receptors. Urinary bladder contraction is mediated by muscarinic receptors. Tolterodine increases residual urine volume and decreases detrusor muscle pressure.

Contraindications Hypersensitivity to tolterodine or fesoterodine (both are metabolized to 5-hydroxymethyl tolterodine) or any component of the formulation; urinary retention; gastric retention; uncontrolled narrow-angle glaucoma

Warnings/Precautions Cases of angioedema have been reported; some cases have occurred after a single dose. Discontinue immediately if angioedema and associated difficulty breathing, airway obstruction, or hypotension develop. May cause drowsiness, dizziness, and/or blurred vision, which may impair physical or mental abilities; patients must be cautioned about performing tasks which require mental alertness (eg, operating machinery or driving). Consider dose reduction or discontinuation if CNS effects occur. Use with caution in patients with bladder flow obstruction, may increase the risk of urinary retention. Use with caution in patients with gastrointestinal obstructive disorders (ie, pyloric stenosis), may increase the risk of gastric retention. Use with caution in patients with myasthenia gravis and controlled (treated) narrow-angle glaucoma; metabolized in the liver and excreted in the urine and feces, dosage adjustment is required for patients with renal or hepatic impairment. Tolterodine has been associated with QT_c prolongation at high (supratherapeutic) doses. The manufacturer recommends caution in patients with congenital prolonged QT or in patients receiving concurrent therapy with QT_c-prolonging drugs (class Ia or III antiarrhythmics). However, the mean change in QT_c even at supratherapeutic dosages was less than 15 msec. Individuals who are CYP2D6 poor metabolizers or in the presence of inhibitors of CYP2D6 and CYP3A4 may be more likely to exhibit prolongation. Dosage adjustment is recommended in patients receiving CYP3A4 inhibitors (a lower dose of tolterodine is recommended). This medication is associated with potent anticholinergic properties which may be inappropriate in older adults depending on comorbidities (eg, dementia, delirium) (Beers Criteria).

Drug Interactions
Metabolism/Transport Effects Substrate of CYP2C19 (minor), CYP2C9 (minor), CYP2D6 (major), CYP3A4 (major); **Note:** Assignment of Major/Minor substrate status based on clinically relevant drug interaction potential

Avoid Concomitant Use
Avoid concomitant use of Tolterodine with any of the following: Aclidinium; Ipratropium (Oral Inhalation); Potassium Chloride; Tiotropium

Increased Effect/Toxicity
Tolterodine may increase the levels/effects of: AbobotulinumtoxinA; Anticholinergics; Cannabinoids; Mirabegron; OnabotulinumtoxinA; Potassium Chloride; RimabotulinumtoxinB; Tiotropium; Topiramate; Warfarin

The levels/effects of Tolterodine may be increased by: Abiraterone Acetate; Aclidinium; Antifungal Agents (Azole Derivatives, Systemic); CYP2D6 Inhibitors (Moderate); CYP2D6 Inhibitors (Strong); CYP3A4 Inhibitors (Moderate); CYP3A4 Inhibitors (Strong); Dasatinib; Fluconazole; Ipratropium (Oral Inhalation); Ivacaftor; Mifepristone; Pramlintide; VinBLAStine

Decreased Effect
Tolterodine may decrease the levels/effects of: Acetylcholinesterase Inhibitors (Central); Secretin

The levels/effects of Tolterodine may be decreased by: Acetylcholinesterase Inhibitors (Central); CYP3A4 Inducers (Strong); Deferasirox; Herbs (CYP3A4 Inducers); Peginterferon Alfa-2b; Tocilizumab

Ethanol/Nutrition/Herb Interactions
Food: Increases bioavailability (~53% increase) of tolterodine tablets (dose adjustment not necessary); does not affect the pharmacokinetics of tolterodine extended release capsules. As a CYP3A4 inhibitor, grapefruit juice may increase the serum level and/or toxicity of tolterodine, but unlikely secondary to high oral bioavailability.
Herb/Nutraceutical: St John's wort (*Hypericum*) appears to induce CYP3A enzymes.

Pharmacodynamics/Kinetics
Half-life Elimination
Immediate release tablet: Extensive metabolizers: ~2 hours; Poor metabolizers: ~10 hours
Extended release capsule: Extensive metabolizers: ~7 hours; Poor metabolizers: ~18 hours
Time to Peak Immediate release tablet: 1-2 hours; Extended release capsule: 2-6 hours

Pregnancy Risk Factor C
Pregnancy Considerations Teratogenic effects were observed in some animal reproduction studies.
Lactation Excretion in breast milk unknown/not recommended

Dosage Forms
Capsule, extended release, oral:
Detrol® LA: 2 mg, 4 mg
Tablet, oral: 1 mg, 2 mg
Detrol®: 1 mg, 2 mg

Tolvaptan (tol VAP tan)

Brand Names: U.S. Samsca™
Brand Names: Canada Samsca™
Pharmacologic Category Vasopressin Antagonist

Use Treatment of clinically significant hypervolemic or euvolemic hyponatremia (associated with heart failure, cirrhosis, or SIADH) with either a serum sodium <125 mEq/L or less marked hyponatremia that is symptomatic and resistant to fluid restriction

Local Anesthetic/Vasoconstrictor Precautions No information available to require special precautions

Effects on Dental Treatment No significant effects or complications reported

Effects on Bleeding No information available to require special precautions

Adverse Effects

>10%:

Gastrointestinal: Nausea (21%), xerostomia (7% to 13%)

Renal: Pollakiuria (4% to 11%), polyuria (4% to 11%)

Miscellaneous: Thirst (12% to 16%)

2% to 10%:

Central nervous system: Fever (4%)

Endocrine & metabolic: Hyperglycemia (6%), hypernatremia (<2%)

Gastrointestinal: GI bleeding (cirrhosis patients 10%), constipation (7%), anorexia (4%)

Neuromuscular & skeletal: Weakness (9%)

General Dosage Range Oral: *Adults:* 15-60 mg once daily

Mechanism of Action An arginine vasopressin (AVP) receptor antagonist with affinity for AVP receptor subtypes V_2 and V_{1a} in a ratio of 29:1. Antagonism of the V_2 receptor by tolvaptan promotes the excretion of free water (without loss of serum electrolytes) resulting in net fluid loss, increased urine output, decreased urine osmolality, and subsequent restoration of normal serum sodium levels.

Pharmacodynamics/Kinetics

Onset of Action 2-4 hour; Peak effect: 4-8 hours

Duration of Action 60% peak serum sodium elevation is retained at 24 hours; urinary excretion of free water is no longer elevated

Half-life Elimination 5-12 hours; dominant half-life <12 hours

Time to Peak Plasma: 2-4 hours

Pregnancy Risk Factor C

Pregnancy Considerations Adverse events were observed in animal reproduction studies.

Topiramate (toe PYRE a mate)

Brand Names: U.S. Topamax®

Brand Names: Canada Apo-Topiramate®; CO Topiramate; Dom-Topiramate; Mint-Topiramate; Mylan-Topiramate; Novo-Topiramate; PHL-Topiramate; PMS-Topiramate; PRO-Topiramate; ratio-Topiramate; Sandoz-Topiramate; Topamax®; ZYM-Topiramate

Generic Availability (U.S.) Yes

Pharmacologic Category Anticonvulsant, Miscellaneous

Use Monotherapy or adjunctive therapy for partial onset seizures and primary generalized tonic-clonic seizures; adjunctive treatment of seizures associated with Lennox-Gastaut syndrome; prophylaxis of migraine headache

Unlabeled Use Diabetic neuropathy, infantile spasms, neuropathic pain; prophylaxis of cluster headache

Local Anesthetic/Vasoconstrictor Precautions No information available to require special precautions

Effects on Dental Treatment Key adverse event(s) related to dental treatment: Gingivitis, dysphagia, glossitis, gum hyperplasia, and xerostomia (normal salivary flow resumes upon discontinuation).

Effects on Bleeding No information available to require special precautions

Adverse Effects Adverse events are reported for placebo-controlled trials of adjunctive therapy in adult and pediatric patients. Unless otherwise noted, the percentages refer to incidence in epilepsy trials. **Note:** A wide range of dosages were studied; incidence of adverse events was frequently lower in the pediatric population studied.

>10%:

Central nervous system: Somnolence (15% to 29%), dizziness (4% to 25%; dose dependent), fatigue (9% to 16%; dose-dependent), nervousness (9% to 18%), ataxia (6% to 16%), psychomotor slowing (3% to 13%; dose dependent), speech problems (2% to 13%), memory difficulties (2% to 12%), behavior problems (children 11%), confusion (4% to 11%)

Endocrine & metabolic: Serum bicarbonate decreased (dose related: 7% to 67%; marked reductions [to <17 mEq/L] 1% to 11%)

Gastrointestinal: Anorexia (4% to 24%; dose dependent), nausea (6% to 10%; migraine trial: 9% to 14%)

Neuromuscular & skeletal: Paresthesia (1% to 11%; migraine trial: 35% to 51%)

Ocular: Abnormal vision (2% to 13%)

Respiratory: Upper respiratory infection (migraine trial: 12% to 14%)

Miscellaneous: Injury (14%)

1% to 10%:

Cardiovascular: Chest pain (2% to 4%), edema (2%), hypertension (1% to 2%), bradycardia (1%), pallor (1%), syncope (1%)

Central nervous system: Difficulty concentrating (5% to 10%), aggressive reactions (2% to 9%), depression (5% to 9%; dose dependent, insomnia (4% to 8%), mood problems (≤6%), abnormal coordination (4%), agitation (3%), cognitive problems (3%), emotional lability (3%), anxiety (2% to 3%; dose dependent), hypoesthesia (2%; migraine trial: 6% to 8%), stupor (2%), vertigo (2%), fever (migraine trial: 1% to 2%), apathy (1%), hallucination (1%), neurosis (1%), psychosis (1%), seizure (1%), suicide attempt (1%)

Dermatologic: Pruritus (migraine trial: 2% to 4%), skin disorder (2% to 3%), alopecia (2%), dermatitis (2%), hypertrichosis (2%), rash erythematous (1% to 2%), eczema (1%), seborrhea (1%), skin discoloration (1%)

Endocrine & metabolic: Breast pain (4%), hot flashes (1% to 2%), libido decreased (<1% to 2%), menstrual irregularities (1% to 2%), hypoglycemia (1%), metabolic acidosis (hyperchloremia, nonanion gap)

Gastrointestinal: Weight loss (4% to 9%), dyspepsia (2% to 7%), abdominal pain (5% to 6%), salivation increased (6%), constipation (4% to 5%), gastroenteritis (2% to 3%), vomiting (migraine trial: 1% to 3%), diarrhea (2%; migraine trial: 9% to 11%), dysgeusia (2%; migraine trial: 8% to 15%), xerostomia (2%), loss of taste (migraine trial: ≤2%), appetite increased (1%), dysphagia (1%), fecal incontinence (1%), flatulence (1%), GERD (1%), gingivitis (1%), glossitis (1%), gum hyperplasia (1%), weight gain (1%)

Genitourinary: Incontinence (2% to 4%), UTI (2%), premature ejaculation (migraine trial: ≤3%), cystitis (2%), leukorrhea (2%), impotence (1%), nocturia (1%)

Hematologic: Purpura (8%), leukopenia (2%), anemia (1%), hematoma (1%), prothrombin time increased (1%), thrombocytopenia (1%)

Neuromuscular & skeletal: Tremor (3% to 9%), gait abnormal (3% to 8%), arthralgia (migraine trial: 1% to 7%), weakness (6%), hyperkinesia (5%), back pain (1% to 5%), involuntary muscle contractions (2%; migraine trial: 2% to 4%), leg cramps (2%), leg pain (2%), myalgia (2%), hyporeflexia (2%), rigors (1%), skeletal pain (1%)

Ocular: Diplopia (1% to 10%), nystagmus (10%), conjunctivitis (1%), lacrimation abnormal (1%), myopia (1%)

Otic: Hearing decreased (2%), tinnitus (2%), otitis media (migraine trial: 1% to 2%)

Renal: Hematuria (2%), renal calculus (migraine trial ≤2%)

Respiratory: Rhinitis (4% to 7%), pharyngitis (6%), sinusitis (5%; migraine trial: 6% to 10%), pneumonia (5%), epistaxis (2% to 4%), cough (migraine trial: 2% to 4%), bronchitis (migraine trial: 3%), dyspnea (migraine trial: 1% to 3%)

Miscellaneous: Viral infection (2% to 7%: migraine trial: 3% to 4%), flu-like syndrome (3%), allergy (2%), infection (2%), thirst (2%), body odor (1%), diaphoresis (1%), moniliasis (1%)

Dosage Oral: **Note:** Do not abruptly discontinue therapy; taper dosage gradually to prevent rebound effects. (In clinical trials, adult doses were withdrawn by decreasing in weekly intervals of 50-100 mg/day gradually over 2-8 weeks for seizure treatment, and by decreasing in weekly intervals by 25-50 mg/day for migraine prophylaxis.)

Epilepsy, monotherapy:
Children 2-9 years: Partial onset seizure and primary generalized tonic-clonic seizure:
Initial: 25 mg once daily (in evening); may increase to 25 mg twice daily in week 2; thereafter, may increase by 25-50 mg/day at weekly intervals over 5-7 weeks up to the following minimum recommended maintenance dose:
≤11 kg: 150 mg/day in 2 divided doses
12-22 kg: 200 mg/day in 2 divided doses
23-31 kg: 200 mg/day in 2 divided doses
32-38 kg: 250 mg/day in 2 divided doses
≥39 kg: 250 mg/day in 2 divided doses

Maximum maintenance dose: If additional seizure control is needed and therapy is tolerated, may further increase by 25-50 mg/day at weekly intervals up to the following maximum recommended maintenance dose:
≤11 kg: 250 mg/day in 2 divided doses
12-22 kg: 300 mg/day in 2 divided doses
23-31 kg: 350 mg/day in 2 divided doses
32-38 kg: 350 mg/day in 2 divided doses
≥39 kg: 400 mg/day in 2 divided doses

Children ≥10 years and Adults: Partial onset seizure and primary generalized tonic-clonic seizure: Initial: 25 mg twice daily; may increase weekly by 50 mg/day up to 100 mg twice daily (week 4 dose); thereafter, may further increase weekly by 100 mg/day up to the recommended maximum of 200 mg twice daily.

Canadian labeling: Children ≥6 years and Adults: Initial: 25 mg once daily (in evening); may increase to 25 mg twice daily in weeks 2 or 3, and up to 50 mg twice daily by weeks 3 or 4; may further increase weekly in increments of 50 mg/day up to recommended maximum of 200 mg twice daily.

Epilepsy, adjunctive therapy:
Children 2-16 years:
Partial onset seizure or seizure associated with Lennox-Gastaut syndrome: Initial: 25 mg (1-3 mg/kg/day) once daily (in evening); may increase every 1-2 weeks in increments of 1-3 mg/kg/day up to the recommended maximum of 5-9 mg/kg/day in 2 divided doses

Primary generalized tonic-clonic seizure: Use initial dose listed above for partial onset seizures, but use slower initial titration rate; titrate to the recommended maintenance dose of 6 mg/kg/day by the end of 8 weeks

Canadian labeling: Initial: 25 mg (1-3 mg/kg/day) once daily (in evening); may increase every 1-2 weeks in increments of 1-3 mg/kg/day up to the recommended maximum of 5-9 mg/kg/day in 2 divided doses

Adolescents ≥17 years and Adults:
Partial onset seizure: Initial: 25 mg once or twice daily for 1 week; may increase weekly by 25-50 mg/day until response; usual maintenance dose: 100-200 mg twice daily. Doses >1600 mg/day have not been studied.

Primary generalized tonic-clonic seizure: Use initial dose as listed above for partial onset seizures, but use slower initial titration rate; titrate upwards to recommended dose by the end of 8 weeks; usual maintenance dose: 200 mg twice daily. Doses >1600 mg/day have not been studied.

Canadian labeling: Initial: 25 mg once or twice daily; may increase weekly by 50 mg/day up to the recommended dose of 100-200 mg twice daily (maximum recommended dose: 800 mg/day; doses >400 mg/day have shown no additional benefit)

Migraine prophylaxis: Adults: Initial: 25 mg once daily (in evening); may increase weekly by 25 mg/day, up to the recommended dose of 100 mg/day given in 2 divided doses. Doses >100 mg/day have shown no additional benefit.

Cluster headache prophylaxis (unlabeled use): Adults: Initial: 25 mg/day, titrated at weekly intervals in 25 mg increments, up to 200 mg/day (Pascual, 2007)

Diabetic neuropathy (unlabeled use): Adults: Initial: 25 mg/day, titrated at weekly intervals in 25-50 mg increments to target dose of 400 mg daily in 2 divided doses (Raskin, 2004; Thienel, 2004)

Dosing adjustment in renal impairment: Cl_{cr} <70 mL/minute/1.73 m^2: Administer 50% dose and titrate more slowly

Hemodialysis: Supplemental dose may be needed during hemodialysis

Dosing adjustment in hepatic impairment: Clearance may be reduced; however the manufacturer's labeling provides no specific dosing recommendations

Mechanism of Action Anticonvulsant activity may be due to a combination of potential mechanisms: Blocks neuronal voltage-dependent sodium channels, enhances GABA(A) activity, antagonizes AMPA/kainate glutamate receptors, and weakly inhibits carbonic anhydrase.

Contraindications There are no contraindications listed in the manufacturer's labeling.

Canadian labeling (not in U.S. labeling): Hypersensitivity to topiramate or any component of the formulation or container; pregnancy and women in childbearing years not using effective contraception (migraine prophylaxis only)

Warnings/Precautions Antiepileptics are associated with an increased risk of suicidal behavior/thoughts with use (regardless of indication); patients should be monitored for signs/symptoms of depression, suicidal tendencies, and other unusual behavior changes during therapy and instructed to inform their healthcare provider immediately if symptoms occur. Use with caution in patients with hepatic, respiratory, or renal impairment. Topiramate may decrease serum bicarbonate concentrations (up to 67% of patients); treatment-emergent metabolic acidosis is less common. Risk may be increased in patients with a predisposing condition (organ dysfunction, ketogenic diet, or concurrent treatment with other drugs which may cause acidosis). Metabolic acidosis may occur at dosages as low as 50 mg/day. Monitor serum bicarbonate as well as potential complications of chronic acidosis (nephrolithiasis, osteomalacia, and reduced growth rates in children). Kidney stones have been reported in both children and adults; the risk of kidney stones is about 2-4 times that of the untreated population; the risk of this event may be reduced by increasing fluid intake.

Cognitive dysfunction, psychiatric disturbances (mood disorders), and sedation (somnolence or fatigue) may occur with topiramate use; incidence may be related to rapid titration and higher doses. Patients must be cautioned about performing tasks which require mental alertness (eg, operating machinery or driving). Topiramate may also cause paresthesia, dizziness, and ataxia. Topiramate has been associated with acute myopia and secondary angle-closure glaucoma in adults and children, typically within 1 month of initiation; discontinue in patients with acute onset of decreased visual acuity or ocular pain. Hyperammonemia with or without encephalopathy may occur with or without concomitant valproate administration; valproic acid dose-dependency was observed in limited pediatric studies; use with caution in patients with inborn errors of metabolism or decreased hepatic mitochondrial activity. Hypothermia (core body temperature <35°C [95°F]) has been reported with concomitant use of topiramate and valproic acid; may occur with or without associated hyperammonemia and may develop after topiramate initiation or dosage increase; discontinuation of topiramate or valproic acid may be necessary. Topiramate may be associated (rarely) with severe oligohydrosis and hyperthermia, most frequently in children; use caution and monitor closely during strenuous exercise, during exposure to high environmental temperature, or in patients receiving receiving other carbonic anhydrase inhibitors and drugs with anticholinergic activity. Concurrent use of topiramate and hydrochlorothiazide may increase the risk for hypokalemia; monitor potassium closely.

Avoid abrupt withdrawal of topiramate therapy, it should be withdrawn/tapered slowly to minimize the potential of increased seizure frequency. Doses were also gradually withdrawn in migraine prophylaxis studies. Effects with other sedative drugs or ethanol may be potentiated. Safety and efficacy have not been established in children <2 years of age for treatment of seizures. In pediatric patients, weight loss may occur most often early in therapy; in clinical trials of at least 1 year, the majority of patients with weight loss had a resumption of weight gain within the study period. Safety and efficacy have not been established in children for migraine prophylaxis.

Drug Interactions

Metabolism/Transport Effects Inhibits CYP2C19 (weak); **Induces** CYP3A4 (weak/moderate)

Avoid Concomitant Use

Avoid concomitant use of Topiramate with any of the following: Axitinib; Azelastine (Nasal); Carbonic Anhydrase Inhibitors; Paraldehyde

Increased Effect/Toxicity

Topiramate may increase the levels/effects of: Alcohol (Ethyl); Alpha-/Beta-Agonists; Amphetamines; Anticonvulsants (Barbiturate); Anticonvulsants (Hydantoin); Azelastine (Nasal); Buprenorphine; Carbonic Anhydrase Inhibitors; CNS Depressants; Flecainide; Fosphenytoin; Lithium; Memantine; MetFORMIN; Methotrimeprazine; Metyrosine; Mirtazapine; Paraldehyde; Phenytoin; Pramipexole; Primidone; QuiNIDine; ROPINIRole; Rotigotine; Selective Serotonin Reuptake Inhibitors; Valproic Acid; Zolpidem

The levels/effects of Topiramate may be increased by: Anticholinergic Agents; Divalproex; Droperidol; HydrOXYzine; Loop Diuretics; Magnesium Sulfate; Methotrimeprazine; Perampanel; Salicylates; Sodium Oxybate; Thiazide Diuretics

Decreased Effect

Topiramate may decrease the levels/effects of: ARIPiprazole; Axitinib; Contraceptives (Estrogens); Contraceptives (Progestins); Methenamine; Primidone; Saxagliptin

The levels/effects of Topiramate may be decreased by: CarBAMazepine; Fosphenytoin; Ketorolac (Nasal); Ketorolac (Systemic); Mefloquine; Phenytoin

Ethanol/Nutrition/Herb Interactions

Ethanol: May increase CNS depression; monitor for increased effects with coadministration. Caution patients about effects.

Food: Ketogenic diet may increase the possibility of acidosis and/or kidney stones.

Herb/Nutraceutical: Avoid evening primrose (seizure threshold decreased).

Pharmacodynamics/Kinetics

Half-life Elimination Mean: Adults: Normal renal function: 21 hours; shorter in pediatric patients; clearance is 50% higher in pediatric patients; Elderly: ~24 hours

Time to Peak Serum: ~1-4 hours

Pregnancy Risk Factor D

Pregnancy Considerations Topiramate was found to be teratogenic in animal studies. Based on limited data, topiramate was found to cross the placenta. An increase risk of oral clefts (cleft lip and/or palate) has been observed following first trimester exposure. Data, from the North American Antiepileptic Drug (NAAED) Pregnancy Registry, reported that the prevalence of oral clefts was 1.4% for infants exposed to topiramate during the first trimester of pregnancy, versus 0.38% to 0.55% for infants exposed to other antiepileptic drugs and 0.07% with no exposure. Hypospadias and other congenital anomalies have also been reported. Although not evaluated during pregnancy, metabolic acidosis may be induced by topiramate. In general, metabolic acidosis during pregnancy may result in adverse effects and fetal death. Pregnant women and their newborns should be monitored for metabolic acidosis. Maternal serum concentrations may decrease during the second and third trimesters of pregnancy therefore therapeutic drug monitoring should be considered in pregnant women who require therapy.

Patients exposed to topiramate during pregnancy are encouraged to enroll themselves into the AED Pregnancy Registry by calling 1-888-233-2334. Additional information is available at www.aedpregnancyregistry.org.

Lactation Enters breast milk/use caution

Breast-Feeding Considerations Based on limited data, topiramate was found in breast milk. Infant plasma concentrations of topiramate have been reported as 10% to 20% of the maternal plasma concentration.

Dosage Forms

Capsule, sprinkle, oral: 15 mg, 25 mg
Topamax®: 15 mg, 25 mg
Tablet, oral: 25 mg, 50 mg, 100 mg, 200 mg
Topamax®: 25 mg, 50 mg, 100 mg, 200 mg

Topotecan (toe poe TEE kan)

Brand Names: U.S. Hycamtin®

Brand Names: Canada Hycamtin®; Topotecan For Injection; Topotecan Hydrochloride For Injection

Pharmacologic Category Antineoplastic Agent, Camptothecin; Antineoplastic Agent, Natural Source (Plant) Derivative; Antineoplastic Agent, Topoisomerase I Inhibitor

Use Treatment of metastatic ovarian cancer, relapsed or refractory small cell lung cancer, recurrent or resistant (stage IVB) cervical cancer (in combination with cisplatin)

Unlabeled Use Treatment of central nervous system lesions (metastatic from lung cancer), central nervous system lymphoma (primary), Ewing's sarcoma, merkel cell cancer, osteosarcoma, rhabdomyosarcoma (pediatrics), neuroblastoma (pediatrics)

Local Anesthetic/Vasoconstrictor Precautions No information available to require special precautions

Effects on Dental Treatment Key adverse event(s) related to dental treatment: Stomatitis.

Effects on Bleeding Chemotherapy may result in significant myelosuppression, potentially including significant thrombocytopenia (grade 4: 6% to 27%, nadir 15 days, duration 3-5 days) and altered hemostasis. In patients who are under active treatment with these agents, medical consult is suggested.

Adverse Effects

>10%:

Central nervous system: Fatigue (6% to 29%), fever (5% to 28%), pain (5% to 23%), headache (18%)

Dermatologic: Alopecia (10% to 49%), rash (16%)

Gastrointestinal: Nausea (8% to 64%), vomiting (10% to 45%), diarrhea (6% to 32%; Oral: grade 3: 4%; grade 4: ≤1%; onset: 9 days), constipation (5% to 29%), abdominal pain (5% to 22%), anorexia (7% to 19%), stomatitis (18%)

Hematologic: Anemia (89% to 98%; grade 4: 7% to 37%; nadir: 15 days), neutropenia (83% to 97%; grade 4: 32% to 80%; nadir 12-15 days; duration: 7 days), leukopenia (86% to 97%; grade 4: 15% to 32%), thrombocytopenia (69% to 81%; grade 4: 6% to 27%; nadir: 15 days; duration: 3-5 days), neutropenic fever/sepsis (2% to 43%)

Neuromuscular & skeletal: Weakness (3% to 25%)

Respiratory: Dyspnea (6% to 22%), cough (15%)

Miscellaneous: Infection (≤17%)

1% to 10%:

Gastrointestinal: Obstruction (5%)

Hepatic: Liver enzymes increased (transient; 8%; grades 3/4: 4%), bilirubin increased (grades 3/4: <2%)

Neuromuscular & skeletal: Paresthesia (7%)

Respiratory: Pneumonia (8%)

Miscellaneous: Sepsis (grades 3/4: 5%)

General Dosage Range Dosage adjustment recommended in patients with renal impairment or who develop toxicities

Oral: *Adults:* 2.3 mg/m²/day for 5 days; repeated every 21 days

I.V.: *Adults:* IVPB: 1.5 mg/m²/day for 5 days; repeated every 21 days **or** 0.75 mg/m²/day for 3 days; repeated every 21 days

Mechanism of Action Binds to topoisomerase I and stabilizes the cleavable complex so that religation of the cleaved DNA strand cannot occur. This results in the accumulation of cleavable complexes and single-strand DNA breaks. Topotecan acts in S phase of the cell cycle.

Pharmacodynamics/Kinetics

Half-life Elimination I.V.: 2-3 hours; renal impairment: 5 hours; Oral: 3-6 hours

Time to Peak Oral: 1-2 hours; delayed with high-fat meal (1.5-4 hours)

Pregnancy Risk Factor D

Pregnancy Considerations Animal reproduction studies found embryotoxicity, fetotoxicity, reduced fetal body weight, and teratogenicity including eye, brain, skull, and vertebrae malformations. May cause fetal harm in pregnant women. Women of childbearing potential should use effective contraception to prevent pregnancy during treatment.

Toremifene (tore EM i feen)

Related Information

Clinical Risk Related to Drugs Prolonging QT Interval *on page 1510*

Brand Names: U.S. Fareston®

Brand Names: Canada Fareston®

Pharmacologic Category Antineoplastic Agent, Estrogen Receptor Antagonist; Selective Estrogen Receptor Modulator (SERM)

Use Treatment of metastatic breast cancer in postmenopausal women with estrogen receptor positive or estrogen receptor status unknown

Unlabeled Use Treatment of soft tissue sarcoma (desmoid tumors)

Local Anesthetic/Vasoconstrictor Precautions Toremifene is one of the drugs confirmed to prolong the QT interval and is accepted as having a risk of causing torsade de pointes. The risk of drug-induced torsade de pointes is extremely low when a single QT interval prolonging drug is prescribed. In terms of epinephrine, it is not known what effect vasoconstrictors in the local anesthetic regimen will have in patients with a known history of congenital prolonged QT interval or in patients taking any medication that prolongs the QT interval. Until more information is obtained, it is suggested that the clinician consult with the physician prior to the use of a vasoconstrictor in suspected patients, and that the vasoconstrictor (epinephrine, mepivacaine and levonordefrin [Carbocaine® 2% with Neo-Cobefrin®]) be used with caution.

Effects on Dental Treatment No significant effects or complications reported

Effects on Bleeding Although significant myelosuppression with associated altered hemostasis has been reported for many chemotherapeutic agents, myelosuppression is not common with toremifene and no specific precautions appear to be necessary.

Adverse Effects

>10%:
Endocrine & metabolic: Hot flashes (35%)
Gastrointestinal: Nausea (14%)
Genitourinary: Vaginal discharge (13%)
Hepatic: Alkaline phosphatase increased (8% to 19%),
AST increased (5% to 19%)
Miscellaneous: Diaphoresis (20%)

1% to 10%:
Cardiovascular: Edema (5%), arrhythmia (≤2%), CVA/
TIA (≤2%), thrombosis (≤2%), cardiac failure (≤1%),
MI (≤1%)
Central nervous system: Dizziness (9%)
Endocrine & metabolic: Hypercalcemia (≤3%)
Gastrointestinal: Vomiting (4%)
Genitourinary: Vaginal bleeding (2%)
Hepatic: Bilirubin increased (1% to 2%)
Local: Thrombophlebitis (≤2%)
Ocular: Cataracts (≤10%), xerophthalmia (≤9%), visual
field abnormal (≤4%), corneal keratopathy (≤2%),
glaucoma (≤2%), vision abnormal/diplopia (≤2%)
Respiratory: Pulmonary embolism (≤2%)

General Dosage Range Oral: *Adults:* 60 mg once
daily

Mechanism of Action Nonsteroidal, triphenylethylene
derivative with potent antiestrogenic properties (also has
estrogenic effects). Competitively binds to estrogen
receptors on tumors and other tissue targets, producing
a nuclear complex that decreases DNA synthesis and
inhibits estrogen effects. Competes with estrogen for
binding sites in breast and other tissues; cells accumulate in the G_0 and G_1 phases; therefore, toremifene is
cytostatic rather than cytocidal.

Pharmacodynamics/Kinetics

Half-life Elimination Toremifene: ~5 days; N-deme-
thyltoremifene: 6 days

Time to Peak Serum: ≤3 hours

Pregnancy Risk Factor D

Pregnancy Considerations Animal studies have
demonstrated embryotoxicity and fetal adverse effects.
There are no adequate and well-controlled studies in
pregnant women. Only approved for use in postmenopausal women. May cause fetal harm if administered
during pregnancy.

Dental Comment Toremifene is known to prolong the
QT interval. The QT interval is measured as the time and
distance between the Q point of the QRS complex and
the end of the T wave in the ECG tracing. After adjustment for heart rate, the QT interval is defined as
prolonged if it is more than 450 msec in men and 460
msec in women. A long QT syndrome was first
described in the 1950s and 60s as a congenital syndrome involving QT interval prolongation and syncope
and sudden death. Some of the congenital long QT
syndromes were characterized by a peculiar electrocardiographic appearance of the QRS complex involving a premature atria beat followed by a pause, then a
subsequent sinus beat showing marked QT prolongation and deformity. This type of cardiac arrhythmia was
originally termed "torsade de pointes" (translated from
the French as "twisting of the points"). Toremifene is
considered as having a risk of causing torsade de
pointes. Since it is not known what effect vasoconstrictors in the local anesthetic regimen will have in patients
with a known history of congenital prolonged QT interval
or in patients taking any medication that prolongs the QT
interval, a medical consult is suggested.

Torsemide (TORE se mide)

Related Information
Cardiovascular Diseases *on page 1492*
Brand Names: U.S. Demadex®
Pharmacologic Category Diuretic, Loop
Use Management of edema associated with heart failure
and hepatic or renal disease (including chronic renal
failure); treatment of hypertension
Local Anesthetic/Vasoconstrictor Precautions No
information available to require special precautions
Effects on Dental Treatment No significant effects or
complications reported
Effects on Bleeding No information available to
require special precautions
Adverse Effects 1% to 10%:
Cardiovascular: ECG abnormality (2%), chest pain (1%)
Central nervous system: Nervousness (1%)
Gastrointestinal: Constipation (2%), diarrhea (2%), dys-
pepsia (2%), nausea (2%), sore throat (2%)
Genitourinary: Excessive urination (7%)
Neuromuscular & skeletal: Arthralgia (2%), myalgia
(2%), weakness (2%)
Respiratory: Rhinitis (3%), cough (2%)
General Dosage Range
I.V.: *Adults:* 10-200 mg once daily
Oral: *Adults:* 5-200 mg once daily (maximum:
200 mg/day)
Mechanism of Action Inhibits reabsorption of sodium
and chloride in the ascending loop of Henle and distal
renal tubule, interfering with the chloride-binding cotran-
sport system, thus causing increased excretion of water,
sodium, chloride, magnesium, and calcium; does not
alter GFR, renal plasma flow, or acid-base balance
Pharmacodynamics/Kinetics
Onset of Action Diuresis: Oral: Within 1 hour; Peak
effect: Diuresis: Oral: 1-2 hours; Antihypertensive:
Oral: 4-6 weeks (up to 12 weeks)
Duration of Action Diuresis: Oral: ~6-8 hours
Half-life Elimination ~3.5 hours; Cirrhosis: 7-8 hours
Time to Peak Plasma: Oral: 1 hour; delayed ~30
minutes when administered with food
Pregnancy Risk Factor B
Pregnancy Considerations A decrease in fetal
weight, an increase in fetal resorption, and delayed fetal
ossification has occurred in animal studies.

Trace Elements (trase EL e ments)

Related Information
Iodine *on page 755*
Selenium *on page 1229*
Brand Names: U.S. Multitrace®-4; Multitrace®-4 Con-
centrate; Multitrace®-4 Neonatal; Multitrace®-4 Pedia-
tric; Multitrace®-5; Multitrace®-5 Concentrate; Trace
Elements 4 Pediatric
Pharmacologic Category Trace Element, Parenteral
Use Prevention and correction of trace metal deficiencies
Local Anesthetic/Vasoconstrictor Precautions No
information available to require special precautions
Effects on Dental Treatment No significant effects or
complications reported
Effects on Bleeding No information available to
require special precautions
General Dosage Range I.V.: *Infants, Children, and
Adults:* Dosage varies greatly depending on indication
Pregnancy Risk Factor C

Pregnancy Considerations Refer to individual elements for requirements in pregnancy.

TraMADol (TRA ma dole)

Related Sample Prescriptions
Moderate/Moderately Severe Oral Pain *on page 1606*
Brand Names: U.S. ConZip™; Rybix™ ODT; Ryzolt™; Ultram®; Ultram® ER
Brand Names: Canada Durela™; Ralivia™; Tridural™; Ultram®; Zytram® XL
Generic Availability (U.S.) Yes: Excludes tablet (orally disintegrating)
Pharmacologic Category Analgesic, Opioid
Dental Use Relief of moderate to moderately-severe dental pain
Use Relief of moderate to moderately-severe pain
Extended release formulations are indicated for patients requiring around-the-clock management of moderate to moderately-severe pain for an extended period of time
Local Anesthetic/Vasoconstrictor Precautions No information available to require special precautions
Effects on Dental Treatment Key adverse event(s) related to dental treatment: Xerostomia and changes in salivation (normal salivary flow resumes upon discontinuation). See Dental Comment.
Effects on Bleeding No information available to require special precautions
Adverse Effects
>10%:
Cardiovascular: Flushing (8% to 16%)
Central nervous system: Dizziness (10% to 33%), headache (4% to 32%), somnolence (7% to 25%), insomnia (2% to 11%)
Dermatologic: Pruritus (3% to 12%)
Gastrointestinal: Constipation (9% to 46%), nausea (15% to 40%), vomiting (5% to 17%), dyspepsia (1% to 13%)
Neuromuscular & skeletal: Weakness (4% to 12%)
1% to 10%:
Cardiovascular: Orthostatic hypotension (2% to 5%), chest pain (1% to <5%), hypertension (1% to <5%), peripheral edema (1% to <5%), vasodilation (1% to <5%)
Central nervous system: Agitation (1% to <5%), anxiety (1% to <5%), apathy (1% to <5%), chills (1% to <5%), confusion (1% to <5%), coordination impaired (1% to <5%), depersonalization (1% to <5%), depression (1% to <5%), euphoria (1% to <5%), fever (1% to <5%), hypoesthesia (1% to <5%), lethargy (1% to <5%), nervousness (1% to <5%), pain (1% to <5%), pyrexia (1% to <5%), restlessness (1% to <5%), malaise (<1% to <5%), fatigue (2%), vertigo (2%)
Dermatologic: Dermatitis (1% to <5%), rash (1% to <5%)
Endocrine & metabolic: Hot flashes (2% to 9%), hyperglycemia (1% to <5%), menopausal symptoms (1% to <5%)
Gastrointestinal: Diarrhea (5% to 10%), xerostomia (3% to 13%), anorexia (1% to 6%), abdominal pain (1% to <5%), appetite decreased (1% to <5%), weight loss (1% to <5%), flatulence (<1% to <5%)
Genitourinary: Pelvic pain (1% to <5%), prostatic disorder (1% to <5%), urine abnormalities (1% to <5%), urinary tract infection (1% to <5%), urinary frequency (<1% to <5%), urinary retention (<1% to <5%)

Neuromuscular & skeletal: Arthralgia (1% to 5%), back pain (1% to <5%), creatine phosphokinase increased (1% to <5%), myalgia (1% to <5%), hypertonia (1% to <5%), neck pain (1% to <5%), rigors (1% to <5%), paresthesia (1% to <5%), tremor (1% to <5%)
Ocular: Blurred vision (1% to <5%), miosis (1% to <5%)
Respiratory: Bronchitis (1% to <5%), congestion (nasal/sinus) (1% to <5%), cough (1% to <5%), dyspnea (1% to <5%), nasopharyngitis (1% to <5%), pharyngitis (1% to <5%), rhinitis (1% to <5%), rhinorrhea (1% to <5%), sinusitis (1% to <5%), sneezing (1% to <5%), sore throat (1% to <5%), upper respiratory infection (1% to <5%)
Miscellaneous: Diaphoresis (2% to 9%), flu-like syndrome (1% to <5%), withdrawal syndrome (1% to <5%), shivering (<1% to <5%)
A withdrawal syndrome may include anxiety, diarrhea, hallucinations (rare), nausea, pain, piloerection, rigors, sweating, and tremor. Uncommon discontinuation symptoms may include severe anxiety, panic attacks, or paresthesia.
Dental Usual Dosage Moderate-to-severe chronic pain: Oral:
Adults:
Immediate release formulation: 50-100 mg every 4-6 hours (not to exceed 400 mg/day)
For patients not requiring rapid onset of effect, tolerability may be improved by starting dose at 25 mg/day and titrating dose by 25 mg every 3 days, until reaching 25 mg 4 times/day. The total daily dose may then be increased by 50 mg every 3 days as tolerated, to reach dose of 50 mg 4 times/day. After titration, 50-100 mg may be given every 4-6 hours as needed up to a maximum 400 mg/day.
Extended release formulations:
Ultram® ER:
Patients not currently on immediate-release: 100 mg once daily; titrate every 5 days (maximum: 300 mg/day)
Patients currently on immediate-release: Calculate 24-hour immediate release total and initiate total daily dose (round dose to the next lowest 100 mg increment); titrate (maximum: 300 mg/day)
Ralivia™ (Canadian labeling, not available in U.S.): 100 mg once daily; titrate every 5 days as needed based on clinical response and severity of pain (maximum: 300 mg/day)
Ryzolt™:
Patients not currently on immediate-release: 100 mg once daily; titrate every 2-3 days by 100 mg/day increments; usual daily dose: 200-300 mg/day (maximum: 300 mg/day)
Patients currently on immediate-release: Calculate 24 hour immediate release total dose and initiate total extended release daily dose (round dose to the next lowest 100 mg increment); titrate (maximum: 300 mg/day)
Tridural™ (Canadian labeling, not available in U.S.): 100 mg once daily; titrate by 100 mg/day every 2 days as needed based on clinical response and severity of pain (maximum: 300 mg/day)
Zytram® XL (Canadian labeling, not available in U.S.): 150 mg once daily; if pain relief is not achieved may titrate by increasing dosage incrementally, with sufficient time to evaluate effect of increased dosage; generally not more often than every 7 days (maximum: 400 mg/day)

Elderly >75 years:

Immediate release: 50 mg every 6 hours (not to exceed 300 mg/day); see dosing adjustments for renal and hepatic impairment.

Extended release formulation: Use with great caution. See adult dosing.

Dosage Oral: Moderate-to-severe pain:

Children ≥17 years and Adults:

Immediate release: 50-100 mg every 4-6 hours (not to exceed 400 mg/day).For patients not requiring rapid onset of effect, tolerability may be improved by starting dose at 25 mg/day and titrating dose by 25 mg every 3 days, until reaching 25 mg 4 times/day. The total daily dose may then be increased by 50 mg every 3 days as tolerated, to reach dose of 50 mg 4 times/day. After titration, 50-100 mg may be given every 4-6 hours as needed up to a maximum 400 mg/day.

Orally-disintegrating tablet (Rybix™ ODT): 50-100 mg every 4-6 hours (not to exceed 400 mg/day); for patients not requiring rapid onset of effect, tolerability may be improved by starting dose at 50 mg/day and titrating dose by 50 mg every 3 days, until reaching 50 mg 4 times/day. After titration, 50-100 mg may be given every 4-6 hours as needed up to a maximum 400 mg/day.

Adults: Extended release:

U.S. labeling: ConZip™, Ryzolt™, Ultram® ER:

Patients not currently on immediate-release tramadol: 100 mg once daily; titrate every 5 days (ConZip™, Ultram® ER) or every 2-3 days (Ryzolt™); maximum dose: 300 mg daily

Patients currently on immediate-release tramadol: Calculate 24-hour immediate release total dose and initiate total extended release daily dose (round dose to the next lowest 100 mg increment); titrate as tolerated to desired effect (maximum: 300 mg daily)

Canadian labeling: **Note:** Patients currently on immediate-release tramadol: When switching to extended release, initiate at the same or lowest nearest total daily tramadol dose. Not to exceed recommended maximum daily dosing.

Durela™, Ralivia™, Tridural™: Patients not currently on immediate-release tramadol or opioids: Initial: 100 mg once daily; titrate every 5 days (Durela™, Ralivia™) or every 2 days (Tridural™) as needed based on clinical response and severity of pain (maximum: 300 mg daily)

Zytram® XL: Patients not currently on immediate-release tramadol or opioids: 150 mg once daily; if pain relief is not achieved may titrate by increasing dosage incrementally, with sufficient time to evaluate effect of increased dosage; generally not more often than every 7 days (maximum: 400 mg daily)

Elderly >65 years: Use caution and initiate at the lower end of the dosing range

Elderly >75 years:

Immediate release: Do not exceed 300 mg/day; see dosing adjustments for renal and hepatic impairment.

Extended release: Use with great caution. See adult, renal, and hepatic dosing.

Dosage adjustment in renal impairment:

Immediate release: Cl_{cr} <30 mL/minute: Administer 50-100 mg dose every 12 hours (maximum: 200 mg daily)

Extended release: Should not be used in patients with Cl_{cr} <30 mL/minute

Dosage adjustment in hepatic impairment:

Immediate release: Cirrhosis: Recommended dose: 50 mg every 12 hours

Extended release: Should not be used in patients with severe (Child-Pugh class C) hepatic dysfunction; Ryzolt™ should not be used in any degree of hepatic impairment

Mechanism of Action Tramadol and its active metabolite (M1) binds to μ-opiate receptors in the CNS causing inhibition of ascending pain pathways, altering the perception of and response to pain; also inhibits the reuptake of norepinephrine and serotonin, which also modifies the ascending pain pathway

Contraindications Hypersensitivity to tramadol, opioids, or any component of the formulation

Additional contraindications for Ultram®, Rybix™ ODT, and Ultram® ER: Any situation where opioids are contraindicated, including acute intoxication with alcohol, hypnotics, centrally-acting analgesics, opioids, or psychotropic drugs

Additional contraindications for ConZip™, Ryzolt™: Severe/acute bronchial asthma, hypercapnia, or significant respiratory depression in the absence of appropriately monitored setting and/or resuscitative equipment

Canadian product labeling:

Tramadol is contraindicated during or within 14 days following MAO inhibitor therapy

Extended release formulations: Additional contraindications:

Ralivia™, Tridural™: Severe (Cl_{cr} <30 mL/minute) renal dysfunction, severe (Child-Pugh class C) hepatic dysfunction

Durela™ and Zytram® XL: Severe (Cl_{cr} <30 mL/minute) renal dysfunction, severe (Child-Pugh class C) hepatic dysfunction; known or suspected mechanical GI obstruction or any disease/condition that affects bowel transit; mild, intermittent or short-duration pain that can be managed with other pain medication; management of peri-operative pain; obstructive airway, acute respiratory depression, cor pulmonale, delirium tremens, seizure disorder, severe CNS depression, increased cerebrospinal or intracranial pressure, head injury, breast-feeding, pregnancy; use during labor and delivery

Warnings/Precautions Rare but serious anaphylactoid reactions (including fatalities) often following initial dosing have been reported. Pruritus, hives, bronchospasm, angioedema, toxic epidermal necrolysis (TEN) and Stevens-Johnson syndrome also have been reported with use. Previous anaphylactoid reactions to opioids may increase risks for similar reactions to tramadol. Caution patients to swallow extended release tablets whole. Rapid release and absorption of tramadol from extended release tablets that are broken, crushed, or chewed may lead to a potentially lethal overdose. May cause CNS depression, which may impair physical or mental abilities; patients must be cautioned about performing tasks which require mental alertness (eg, operating machinery or driving). May cause CNS depression and/or respiratory depression, particularly when combined with other CNS depressants. Use with caution and reduce dosage when administered to patients receiving other CNS depressants. An increased risk of seizures may occur in patients receiving serotonin reuptake inhibitors (SSRIs or anorectics), tricyclic antidepressants or other cyclic compounds (including cyclobenzaprine, promethazine), neuroleptics, drugs which may lower seizure threshold, or drugs which impair metabolism of tramadol (ie, CYP2D6 and 3A4 inhibitors). Patients with a history of seizures, or with a risk of seizures (head trauma, metabolic disorders, CNS infection, or malignancy, or during ethanol/drug withdrawal) are also at increased risk. Avoid use, if possible, with serotonergic agents such as TCAs, MAO inhibitors (use with extreme caution; contraindicated in Canadian product labeling), triptans, venlafaxine, trazodone, lithium, sibutramine, meperidine, dextromethorphan, St John's wort, SNRIs, and SSRIs; use caution with drugs which impair metabolism of tramadol (ie, CYP2D6 and 3A4 inhibitors); concomitant may increase the risk of serotonin syndrome.

Elderly (particularly >75 years of age), debilitated patients and patients with chronic respiratory disorders may be at greater risk of adverse events. Use with caution in patients with increased intracranial pressure or head injury. Avoid use in patients who are suicidal or addiction prone; use with caution in patients taking tranquilizers and/or antidepressants, or those with an emotional disturbance including depression. Healthcare provider should be alert to problems of abuse, misuse, and diversion. Use caution in heavy alcohol users. Use caution in treatment of acute abdominal conditions; may mask pain. Use tramadol with caution and reduce dosage in patients with liver disease or renal dysfunction. Avoid using extended release tablets in severe hepatic impairment. Do not use Ryzolt™ in any degree of hepatic impairment. Tolerance or drug dependence may result from extended use (withdrawal symptoms have been reported); abrupt discontinuation should be avoided. Tapering of dose at the time of discontinuation limits the risk of withdrawal symptoms. Some products may contain phenylalanine.

Drug Interactions
Metabolism/Transport Effects Substrate of CYP2B6 (minor), CYP2D6 (major), CYP3A4 (major); **Note:** Assignment of Major/Minor substrate status based on clinically relevant drug interaction potential

Avoid Concomitant Use
Avoid concomitant use of TraMADol with any of the following: Azelastine (Nasal); CarBAMazepine; Conivaptan; Paraldehyde

Increased Effect/Toxicity
TraMADol may increase the levels/effects of: Alcohol (Ethyl); Alvimopan; Azelastine (Nasal); CarBAMazepine; CNS Depressants; Desmopressin; MAO Inhibitors; Metoclopramide; Metyrosine; Paraldehyde; Pramipexole; ROPINIRole; Rotigotine; Selective Serotonin Reuptake Inhibitors; Serotonin Modulators; Thiazide Diuretics; Vitamin K Antagonists; Zolpidem

The levels/effects of TraMADol may be increased by: Amphetamines; Antipsychotic Agents (Phenothiazines); Antipsychotics; Conivaptan; Cyclobenzaprine; CYP3A4 Inhibitors (Moderate); CYP3A4 Inhibitors (Strong); Dasatinib; HydrOXYzine; Ivacaftor; Magnesium Sulfate; Mifepristone; Perampanel; Selective Serotonin Reuptake Inhibitors; Sodium Oxybate; Succinylcholine; Tricyclic Antidepressants

Decreased Effect
TraMADol may decrease the levels/effects of: CarBAMazepine; Pegvisomant

The levels/effects of TraMADol may be decreased by: Ammonium Chloride; Antiemetics (5HT3 Antagonists); CarBAMazepine; CYP2D6 Inhibitors (Moderate); CYP2D6 Inhibitors (Strong); CYP3A4 Inducers (Strong); Deferasirox; Mixed Agonist / Antagonist Opioids; Tocilizumab

Ethanol/Nutrition/Herb Interactions
Ethanol: May increase CNS depression; monitor for increased effects with coadministration. Caution patients about effects.
Food:
Immediate release tablet: Rate and extent of absorption were not significantly affected.
Extended release:
ConZip™: Rate and extent of absorption were unaffected.
Ryzolt™: Increased C_{max}; no effect on AUC.
Ultram® ER: High-fat meal reduced C_{max} and AUC, and increased T_{max} by 3 hours.
Orally disintegrating tablet: Food delays the time to peak serum concentration by 30 minutes; extent of absorption was not significantly affected.
Herb/Nutraceutical: Avoid valerian, St John's wort, kava kava, gotu kola (may increase CNS depression).

Dietary Considerations Some products may contain phenylalanine.

Pharmacodynamics/Kinetics
Onset of Action Immediate release: ~1 hour
Duration of Action 9 hours
Half-life Elimination Tramadol: ~6-8 hours; Active metabolite: 7-9 hours; prolonged in elderly, hepatic or renal impairment; Zytram® XL: Apparent half-life: ~16 hours; Durela™, Ralivia™, Ryzolt™, Tridural™: ~5-9 hours
Time to Peak Immediate release: ~2 hours; Extended release: ConZip™: ~10-12 hours, Ryzolt™, Tridural™: ~4 hours; Durela™, Ultram® ER: ~12 hours

Pregnancy Risk Factor C
Pregnancy Considerations Adverse events were observed in animal studies. Tramadol has been shown to cross the human placenta when administered during labor. Postmarketing reports following tramadol use during pregnancy include neonatal seizures, withdrawal syndrome, fetal death, and stillbirth. Not recommended for use during labor and delivery.

Lactation Enters breast milk/not recommended
Breast-Feeding Considerations Sixteen hours following a single 100 mg I.V. dose, the amount of tramadol found in breast milk was 0.1% of the maternal dose. Use is not recommended by the manufacturer for postdelivery analgesia in nursing mothers.

Dosage Forms
Capsule, variable release, oral: 150 mg [37.5 mg (immediate release) and 112.5 mg (extended release)]
ConZip™: 100 mg [25 mg (immediate release) and 75 mg (extended release)]
ConZip™: 200 mg [50 mg (immediate release) and 150 mg (extended release)]
ConZip™: 300 mg [50 mg (immediate release) and 250 mg (extended release)]
Tablet, oral: 50 mg
Ultram®: 50 mg
Tablet, extended release, oral: 100 mg, 200 mg, 300 mg
Ryzolt™: 100 mg, 200 mg, 300 mg
Ultram® ER: 100 mg, 200 mg, 300 mg
Tablet, orally disintegrating, oral:
Rybix™ ODT: 50 mg
Dosage Forms: Canada
Tablet, extended release:
Durela™, Ralivia™, Tridural™: 100 mg, 200 mg, 300 mg
Zytram® XL: 75 mg, 100 mg, 150 mg, 200 mg, 300 mg, 400 mg

Dental Comment Literature reports suggest that the efficacy of tramadol in oral surgery pain is equivalent to the combination of aspirin and codeine. One study (Olson, 1990) showed acetaminophen and dextropropoxyphene combination to be superior to tramadol and another study showed tramadol to be superior to acetaminophen and dextropropoxyphene combination. Tramadol appears to be at least equal to if not better than codeine alone. Seizures have been reported with the use of tramadol.

References

Collins M, Young I, Sweeney P, et al, "The Effect of Tramadol on Dento-Alveolar Surgical Pain," *Br J Oral Maxillofac Surg*, 1997, 35 (1):54-8.

Doroschak AM, Bowles WR, and Hargreaves KM, "Evaluation of the Combination of Flurbiprofen and Tramadol for Management of Endodontic Pain," *J Endod*, 1999, 25(10):660-3.

Lewis KS and Han NH, "Tramadol: A New Centrally Acting Analgesic," *Am J Health Syst Pharm*, 1997, 54(6):643-52.

Moore PA, "Pain Management in Dental Practice: Tramadol vs. Codeine Combinations," *J Am Dent Assoc*, 1999, 130(7):1075-9.

Moore PA, Crout RJ, Jackson DL, et al, "Tramadol Hydrochloride: Analgesic Efficacy Compared With Codeine, Aspirin With Codeine, and Placebo After Dental Extraction," *J Clin Pharmacol*, 1998, 38 (6):554-60.

Olson NZ, Sunshine A, O'Neill, et al, *Tramadol Hydrochloride: Oral Efficacy in Postoperative Pain*, American Pain Society 9th Annual Scientific Meeting, St Louis, MO, October, 1990.

Sunshine A, Olson NZ, Zighelboim I, et al, "Analgesic Oral Efficacy of Tramadol Hydrochloride in Postoperative Pain," *Clin Pharmacol Ther*, 1992, 51(6):740-6.

Wynn RL, "Tramadol (Ultram) - A New Kind of Analgesic," *Gen Dent*, 1996, 44(3):216-8,220.

Trandolapril (tran DOE la pril)

Related Information

Cardiovascular Diseases *on page 1492*

Brand Names: U.S. Mavik®

Brand Names: Canada Mavik®

Pharmacologic Category Angiotensin-Converting Enzyme (ACE) Inhibitor

Use Treatment of hypertension alone or in combination with other antihypertensive agents; treatment of heart failure (HF) or left ventricular (LV) dysfunction after myocardial infarction (MI)

Unlabeled Use To delay the progression of nephropathy and reduce risks of cardiovascular events in hypertensive patients with type 1 or 2 diabetes mellitus

Local Anesthetic/Vasoconstrictor Precautions No information available to require special precautions

Effects on Dental Treatment No significant effects or complications reported

Effects on Bleeding No information available to require special precautions

Adverse Effects Note: Frequency ranges include data from hypertension and heart failure trials. Higher rates of adverse reactions have generally been noted in patients with CHF. However, the frequency of adverse effects associated with placebo is also increased in this population.

>1%:

Cardiovascular: Hypotension (<1% to 11%), syncope (6%), bradycardia (<1% to 5%), cardiogenic shock (4%), intermittent claudication (4%)

Central nervous system: Dizziness (1% to 23%), stroke (3%)

Endocrine & metabolic: Uric acid increased (15%), hyperkalemia (5%), hypocalcemia (5%)

Gastrointestinal: Gastritis (4%), diarrhea (1%)

Neuromuscular & skeletal: Myalgia (5%), weakness (3%)

Renal: BUN increased (9%), serum creatinine increased (1% to 5%)

Respiratory: Cough (2% to 35%)

Worsening of renal function may occur in patients with bilateral renal artery stenosis or hypovolemia. In addition, a syndrome which may include fever, myalgia, arthralgia, interstitial nephritis, vasculitis, rash, eosinophilia and positive ANA, and elevated ESR has been reported with ACE inhibitors. Eosinophilic pneumonitis has also been reported with other ACE inhibitors.

General Dosage Range Dosage adjustment recommended in patients with hepatic or renal impairment

Oral: *Adults:* Initial: 1-2 mg once daily; Maintenance: 1-4 mg once daily

Mechanism of Action Trandolapril is an ACE inhibitor which prevents the formation of angiotensin II from angiotensin I. Trandolapril must undergo enzymatic hydrolysis, mainly in liver, to its biologically active metabolite, trandolaprilat. A CNS mechanism may also be involved in the hypotensive effect as angiotensin II increases adrenergic outflow from the CNS. Vasoactive kallikrein's may be decreased in conversion to active hormones by ACE inhibitors, thus reducing blood pressure.

Pharmacodynamics/Kinetics

Onset of Action 1-2 hours; Peak effect: Reduction in blood pressure: 6 hours

Duration of Action Prolonged; 72 hours after single dose

Half-life Elimination Trandolapril: 6 hours; Trandolaprilat: Effective: 22.5 hours

Time to Peak Parent: 1 hour; Active metabolite trandolaprilat: 4-10 hours

Pregnancy Risk Factor D

Pregnancy Considerations [U.S. Boxed Warning]: Drugs that act on the renin-angiotensin system can cause injury and death to the developing fetus. Discontinue as soon as possible once pregnancy is detected. Teratogenic effects may occur following maternal use during pregnancy. Drugs that act on the renin-angiotensin system are associated with oligohydramnios. Oligohydramnios, due to decreased fetal renal function, may lead to fetal lung hypoplasia and skeletal malformations. Their use in pregnancy is also associated with anuria, hypotension, renal failure, skull hypoplasia, and death in the fetus/neonate. Chronic maternal hypertension itself is also associated with adverse events in the fetus/infant. ACE inhibitors are not recommended during pregnancy to treat maternal hypertension or heart failure. Use of an ACE inhibitor should also be avoided in any woman of reproductive age. Women who are planning a pregnancy should be considered for other medication options if an ACE inhibitor is currently prescribed or the ACE inhibitor should be discontinued as soon as possible once pregnancy is detected. The exposed fetus should be monitored for fetal growth, amniotic fluid volume, and organ formation. Infants exposed to an ACE inhibitor *in utero* should be monitored for hyperkalemia, hypotension, and oliguria.

Trandolapril and Verapamil
(tran DOE la pril & ver AP a mil)

Related Information

Trandolapril *on page 1349*

Verapamil *on page 1397*

Brand Names: U.S. Tarka®

Brand Names: Canada Tarka®

Pharmacologic Category Angiotensin-Converting Enzyme (ACE) Inhibitor; Calcium Channel Blocker

Use Treatment of hypertension; however, not indicated for initial treatment of hypertension

Local Anesthetic/Vasoconstrictor Precautions No information available to require special precautions

Effects on Dental Treatment No significant effects or complications reported

Effects on Bleeding No information available to require special precautions

Adverse Effects See individual agents.

General Dosage Range Dosage adjustment recommended in patients with hepatic or renal impairment

Oral: *Adults:* Trandolapril 1-4 mg and verapamil 180-240 mg once daily

Pregnancy Risk Factor D

Pregnancy Considerations [U.S. Boxed Warning]: Drugs that act on the renin-angiotensin system can cause injury and death to the developing fetus. Discontinue as soon as possible once pregnancy is detected. Also see individual agents.

Tranexamic Acid (tran eks AM ik AS id)

Related Information

Antiplatelet and Anticoagulation Considerations in Dentistry *on page 1503*

Brand Names: U.S. Cyklokapron®; Lysteda™

Brand Names: Canada Cyklokapron®; Tranexamic Acid Injection BP

Pharmacologic Category Antifibrinolytic Agent; Antihemophilic Agent; Hemostatic Agent; Lysine Analog

Use

Solution for injection: Short-term use (2-8 days) in hemophilia patients to reduce or prevent hemorrhage and reduce need for replacement therapy during and following tooth extraction

Tablet: Treatment of cyclic heavy menstrual bleeding

Unlabeled Use Trauma-associated hemorrhage; treatment of traumatic hyphema; topical treatment (mouth rinse) of bleeding associated with dental procedures in patients on oral anticoagulant therapy; prevention of perioperative bleeding associated with cardiac surgery; prevention of bleeding associated with craniosynostosis surgery, extracorporeal membrane oxygenation (ECMO), orthognathic surgery, spinal surgery (eg, spinal fusion), total knee replacement surgery, or transurethral prostatectomy; reduction of blood loss associated with cesarean delivery; hereditary angioedema (long-term prophylaxis)

Local Anesthetic/Vasoconstrictor Precautions No information available to require special precautions

Effects on Dental Treatment No significant effects or complications reported. See Effects on Bleeding and Dental Comment.

Effects on Bleeding General dental procedures and simple restorative procedures are not associated with bleeding; therefore, there is no contraindication to general dental treatment for most patients with bleeding disorders. However, after dental extractions and other dental surgeries including deep scaling, block anesthesia, and large fillings, in patients with hemophilia, antifibrinolytic drugs such as tranexamic acid are useful in controlling bleeding. A carefully coordinated strategy between the dental and medical team may be required to ensure adequate procedures for hemostasis. As preparation for selected dental procedures tranexamic acid may be required.

Immediately before dental extraction in hemophilic patients, administer 10 mg/kg tranexamic acid I.V. together with replacement therapy.

Adverse Effects

Injection: Frequency not defined:
Cardiovascular: Hypotension (with rapid I.V. injection)
Central nervous system: Giddiness
Dermatologic: Allergic dermatitis
Endocrine & metabolic: Unusual menstrual discomfort
Gastrointestinal: Diarrhea, nausea, vomiting
Ocular: Blurred vision

Oral:
>10%:
Central nervous system: Headache (50%)
Gastrointestinal: Abdominal pain (20%)
Neuromuscular & skeletal: Back pain (21%), muscle pain (11%)
Respiratory: Nasal/sinus symptoms (25%)
1% to 10%:
Central nervous system: Fatigue (5%)
Hematologic: Anemia (6%)
Neuromuscular & skeletal: Arthralgia (7%), muscle cramps/spasms (7%)

General Dosage Range Dosage adjustment recommended in patients with renal impairment

I.V.: *Children and Adults:* Initial: 10 mg/kg as a single dose; Maintenance: 10 mg/kg/dose 3-4 times/day

Oral: *Adults:* 1300 mg 3 times daily (3900 mg/day)

Mechanism of Action Forms a reversible complex that displaces plasminogen from fibrin resulting in inhibition of fibrinolysis; it also inhibits the proteolytic activity of plasmin

With reduction in plasmin activity, tranexamic acid also reduces activation of complement and consumption of C1 esterase inhibitor (C1-INH), thereby decreasing inflammation associated with hereditary angioedema.

Pharmacodynamics/Kinetics

Half-life Elimination ~2-11 hours

Time to Peak Oral: ~3 hours

Pregnancy Risk Factor B

Pregnancy Considerations Adverse events were not observed in animal reproduction studies. There are no adequate and well-controlled studies in pregnant women. Tranexamic acid crosses the placenta and concentrations within cord blood are similar to maternal concentrations. Use only if the potential benefit justifies the potential risk to the fetus. Lysteda™ is not indicated for use in pregnant women.

Dental Comment Antifibrinolytic drugs are useful for the control of bleeding after dental extractions in patients with hemophilia because the oral mucosa and saliva are rich in plasminogen activators.

Tranylcypromine (tran il SIP roe meen)

Related Information

Vasoconstrictor Interactions With Antidepressants *on page 1650*

Brand Names: U.S. Parnate®

Brand Names: Canada Parnate®

Pharmacologic Category Antidepressant, Monoamine Oxidase Inhibitor

Use Treatment of major depressive episode without melancholia

Local Anesthetic/Vasoconstrictor Precautions Attempts should be made to avoid use of vasoconstrictor due to possibility of hypertensive episodes with monoamine oxidase inhibitors

Effects on Dental Treatment Key adverse event(s) related to dental treatment: Orthostatic hypotension. Avoid use as an analgesic due to toxic reactions with MAO inhibitors. Xerostomia (normal salivary flow resumes upon discontinuation).

Effects on Bleeding No information available to require special precautions

Adverse Effects Frequency not defined.

Cardiovascular: Edema, orthostatic hypotension, palpitation, tachycardia

Central nervous system: Agitation, anxiety, chills, dizziness, drowsiness, headache, insomnia, mania, restlessness

Dermatologic: Alopecia (rare), rash (rare), urticaria

Endocrine & metabolic: Sexual dysfunction (anorgasmia, ejaculatory disturbances, impotence); SIADH

Gastrointestinal: Abdominal pain, anorexia, constipation, diarrhea, nausea, xerostomia

Genitourinary: Urinary retention

Hematologic: Agranulocytosis, anemia, leukopenia, thrombocytopenia

Hepatic: Hepatitis (rare)

Neuromuscular & skeletal: Muscle spasm, myoclonus, numbness, paresthesia, tremor, weakness

Ocular: Blurred vision

Otic: Tinnitus

Miscellaneous: Diaphoresis

General Dosage Range Oral: *Adults:* 10-30 mg twice daily (maximum: 60 mg/day)

Mechanism of Action Tranylcypromine is a nonhydrazine monoamine oxidase inhibitor. It increases endogenous concentrations of epinephrine, norepinephrine, dopamine, and serotonin through inhibition of the enzyme (monoamine oxidase) responsible for the breakdown of these neurotransmitters.

Pharmacodynamics/Kinetics

Onset of Action Therapeutic: 2 days to 3 weeks continued dosing

Duration of Action MAO inhibition may persist for up to 10 days following discontinuation.

Half-life Elimination 90-190 minutes

Time to Peak Serum: ~2 hours

Pregnancy Considerations Adverse events were observed in animal reproduction studies.

Trastuzumab (tras TU zoo mab)

Brand Names: U.S. Herceptin®

Brand Names: Canada Herceptin®

Pharmacologic Category Antineoplastic Agent, Anti-HER2; Antineoplastic Agent, Monoclonal Antibody; Monoclonal Antibody

Use Treatment (adjuvant) of HER2 overexpressing breast cancer as part of a combination regimen with doxorubicin, cyclophosphamide, and either paclitaxel or docetaxel; in combination with docetaxel and carboplatin; as a single agent following anthracycline-based combination treatment; treatment of HER2 overexpressing metastatic breast cancer in combination with paclitaxel as first-line treatment or as a single agent in patients who have received prior chemotherapy regimens for treatment of metastatic disease; treatment of HER2 overexpressing metastatic gastric or gastroesophageal junction adenocarcinoma in combination with cisplatin and either capecitabine or fluorouracil in patients who have not received prior treatment for metastatic disease

Unlabeled Use Treatment of HER2-positive metastatic breast cancer (in combination with pertuzumab and docetaxel) in patients who have not received prior anti-HER2 therapy or chemotherapy to treat metastatic disease; treatment of HER2 overexpressing metastatic breast cancer (in combination with lapatinib) which had progressed on prior trastuzumab containing therapy

Local Anesthetic/Vasoconstrictor Precautions No information available to require special precautions

Effects on Dental Treatment No significant effects or complications reported

Effects on Bleeding Although significant myelosuppression with associated altered hemostasis has been reported for many chemotherapeutic agents, myelosuppression is not common with trastuzumab and no specific precautions appear to necessary.

Adverse Effects Note: Percentages reported with single-agent therapy.

>10%:

Cardiovascular: LVEF decreased (4% to 22%)

Central nervous system: Pain (47%), fever (6% to 36%), chills (5% to 32%), headache (10% to 26%), insomnia (14%), dizziness (4% to 13%)

Dermatologic: Rash (4% to 18%)

Gastrointestinal: Nausea (6% to 33%), diarrhea (7% to 25%), vomiting (4% to 23%), abdominal pain (2% to 22%), anorexia (14%)

Neuromuscular & skeletal: Weakness (4% to 42%), back pain (5% to 22%)

Respiratory: Cough (5% to 26%), dyspnea (3% to 22%), rhinitis (2% to 14%), pharyngitis (12%)

Miscellaneous: Infusion reaction (21% to 40%, chills and fever most common; severe: 1%), infection (20%)

1% to 10%:

Cardiovascular: Peripheral edema (5% to 10%), edema (8%), HF (2% to 7%; severe: <1%), tachycardia (5%), hypertension (4%), arrhythmia (3%), palpitation (3%)

Central nervous system: Depression (6%)

Dermatologic: Acne (2%), nail disorder (2%), pruritus (2%)

Gastrointestinal: Constipation (2%), dyspepsia (2%)

Genitourinary: Urinary tract infection (3% to 5%)

Hematologic: Anemia (4%), leukopenia (3%)

Neuromuscular & skeletal: Paresthesia (2% to 9%), bone pain (3% to 7%), arthralgia (6% to 8%), myalgia (4%), muscle spasm (3%), peripheral neuritis (2%), neuropathy (1%)

Respiratory: Sinusitis (2% to 9%), nasopharyngitis (8%), upper respiratory infection (3%), epistaxis (2%), pharyngolaryngeal pain (2%)

Miscellaneous: Flu-like syndrome (2% to 10%), accidental injury (6%), influenza (4%), allergic reaction (3%), herpes simplex (2%)

General Dosage Range Dosage adjustment recommended in patients who develop toxicities

I.V.: *Adults:* Loading dose: 4 mg/kg; Maintenance: 2 mg/kg once weekly **or** Loading dose: 8 mg/kg; Maintenance: 6 mg/kg every 3 weeks

Mechanism of Action Trastuzumab is a monoclonal antibody which binds to the extracellular domain of the human epidermal growth factor receptor 2 protein (HER-2); it mediates antibody-dependent cellular cytotoxicity by inhibiting proliferation of cells which overexpress HER-2 protein.

Pharmacodynamics/Kinetics
Half-life Elimination Weekly dosing: Mean: 6 days (range: 1-32 days); every 3 week regimen: Mean: 16 days (range: 11-23 days)
Pregnancy Risk Factor D
Pregnancy Considerations Reproductive studies in cynomolgus monkeys showed no evidence of impaired fertility or fetal harm. However, trastuzumab inhibits HER2 protein, which has a role in embryonic development. **[U.S. Boxed Warning]: Trastuzumab exposure during pregnancy may result in oligohydramnios and oligohydramnios sequence (pulmonary hypoplasia, skeletal malformations and neonatal death).** Oligohydramnios (reversible in some cases) has been reported with trastuzumab use alone or with combination chemotherapy. If trastuzumab exposure occurs during pregnancy, monitor for oligohydramnios. Effective contraception is recommended during and for 6 months after treatment for women of childbearing potential. Women exposed to trastuzumab during pregnancy are encouraged to enroll in MotHER (the Herceptin Pregnancy Registry; 1-800-690-6720).

The National Comprehensive Cancer Network (NCCN) breast cancer guidelines (v.1.2013) consider pregnancy a contraindication to trastuzumab treatment and recommend (if indicated) administering trastuzumab in the postpartum period.

Travoprost (TRA voe prost)

Brand Names: U.S. Travatan Z®
Brand Names: Canada Travatan Z®
Pharmacologic Category Ophthalmic Agent, Antiglaucoma; Prostaglandin, Ophthalmic
Use Reduction of elevated intraocular pressure in patients with open-angle glaucoma or ocular hypertension
Local Anesthetic/Vasoconstrictor Precautions No significant effects or complications reported
Effects on Dental Treatment No information available to require special precautions
Effects on Bleeding No information available to require special precautions
Adverse Effects
>10%: Ocular: Hyperemia (30% to 50%)
1% to 10%:
Cardiovascular: Angina pectoris (1% to 5%), bradycardia (1% to 5%), hyper-/hypotension (1% to 5%)
Central nervous system: Anxiety (1% to 5%), depression (1% to 5%), headache (1% to 5%), pain (1% to 5%)
Endocrine & metabolic: Hypercholesterolemia (1% to 5%)
Gastrointestinal: Dyspepsia (1% to 5%), gastrointestinal symptoms (1% to 5%)
Genitourinary: Prostate disorder (1% to 5%), urinary incontinence (1% to 5%), urinary tract infection (1% to 5%)
Miscellaneous: Allergic reaction (1% to 5%), flu-like syndrome (1% to 5%), infection (1% to 5%)
Neuromuscular & skeletal: Arthritis (1% to 5%), back pain (1% to 5%), chest pain (1% to 5%)
Ocular: Decreased visual acuity (5% to 10%), eye discomfort (5% to 10%), foreign body sensation (5% to 10%), pain (5% to 10%), pruritus (5% to 10%), abnormal vision (1% to 4%), blepharitis (1% to 4%), blurred vision (1% to 4%), cataract (1% to 4%),

conjunctivitis (1% to 4%), corneal staining (1% to 4%), dry eye (1% to 4%), eyelash darkening (1% to 4%), eyelash growth increased (1% to 4%), inflammation (1% to 4%), iris discoloration (1% to 4%), keratitis (1% to 4%), lid margin crusting (1% to 4%), periorbital skin discoloration (darkening) (1% to 4%), photophobia (1% to 4%), subconjunctival hemorrhage (1% to 4%), tearing (1% to 4%)
Respiratory: Bronchitis (1% to 5%), sinusitis (1% to 5%)

General Dosage Range Ophthalmic: *Adolescents ≥16 years and Adults:* Instill 1 drop into affected eye(s) once daily
Mechanism of Action A selective FP prostanoid receptor agonist which lowers intraocular pressure by increasing trabecular meshwork and outflow
Pharmacodynamics/Kinetics
Onset of Action ~2 hours; Peak effect: 12 hours
Half-life Elimination 45 minutes (range:17-86 minutes)
Pregnancy Risk Factor C
Pregnancy Considerations Adverse events were observed in animal reproduction studies when administered intravenously at doses greater than the recommended human dose. Following ophthalmic administration, systemic absorption is minimal; systemic absorption would be required in order for travoprost to cross the placenta and reach the fetus. If ophthalmic agents are needed during pregnancy, the minimum effective dose should be used in combination with punctual occlusion to decrease potential exposure to the fetus (Samples, 1988).

TraZODone (TRAZ oh done)

Related Information
Clinical Risk Related to Drugs Prolonging QT Interval *on page 1510*
Management of the Patient With Anxiety or Depression *on page 1594*
Vasoconstrictor Interactions With Antidepressants *on page 1650*
Brand Names: U.S. Oleptro™
Brand Names: Canada Apo-Trazodone D®; Apo-Trazodone®; Dom-Trazodone; Mylan-Trazodone; Novo-Trazodone; Nu-Trazodone; Nu-Trazodone D; Oleptro™; PHL-Trazodone; PMS-Trazodone; ratio-Trazodone; Teva-Trazodone; Trazorel®; ZYM-Trazodone
Generic Availability (U.S.) Yes: Excludes extended release tablet
Pharmacologic Category Antidepressant, Serotonin Reuptake Inhibitor/Antagonist
Use Treatment of major depressive disorder
Unlabeled Use Potential augmenting agent for antidepressants, hypnotic
Local Anesthetic/Vasoconstrictor Precautions Trazodone inhibits reuptake of both serotonin and norepinephrine and also blocks some serotonin receptors. No precautions with vasoconstrictors appear to be necessary.

Trazodone is one of the drugs confirmed to prolong the QT interval and is accepted as having a risk of causing torsade de pointes. The risk of drug-induced torsade de pointes is extremely low when a single QT interval prolonging drug is prescribed. In terms of epinephrine, it is not known what effect vasoconstrictors in the local anesthetic regimen will have in patients with a known history of congenital prolonged QT interval or in patients taking any medication that prolongs the QT interval. Until more information is obtained, it is suggested that the clinician consult with the physician prior to the use of a vasoconstrictor in suspected patients, and that the vasoconstrictor (epinephrine, mepivacaine and levonordefrin [Carbocaine® 2% with Neo-Cobefrin®]) be used with caution.

Effects on Dental Treatment Key adverse event(s) related to dental treatment: Significant xerostomia (normal salivary flow resumes upon discontinuation).

Effects on Bleeding No information available to require special precautions

Adverse Effects

>10%:

Central nervous system: Sedation (≤46%), headache (10% to 33%), dizziness (20% to 28%), fatigue (6% to 15%)

Gastrointestinal: Xerostomia (15% to 34%), nausea (10% to 21%)

Ocular: Blurred vision (5% to 15%)

1% to 10%:

Cardiovascular: Edema (3% to 7%), hypotension (≤7%), syncope (≤5%), hypertension (1% to 2%)

Central nervous system: Confusion (5% to 6%), incoordination (2% to 5%), concentration decreased (1% to 3%), disorientation (≤2%), memory impairment (≤1%), agitation, migraine

Endocrine & metabolic: Libido decreased (1% to 2%)

Gastrointestinal: Diarrhea (5% to 9%), constipation (7% to 8%), abdominal pain, abnormal taste, flatulence, vomiting, weight gain/loss

Genitourinary: Ejaculation disorder (2%), urinary urgency

Neuromuscular & skeletal: Back pain (≤5%), tremor (1% to 5%), paresthesia (≤1%), myalgia

Ocular: Visual disturbance

Respiratory: Nasal congestion (3% to 6%), dyspnea

Miscellaneous: Night sweats

Dosage Oral: Therapeutic effects may take up to 6 weeks to occur; therapy is normally maintained for 6-12 months after optimum response is reached to prevent recurrence of depression

Children 6-12 years: Depression (unlabeled use): Initial: 1.5-2 mg/kg/day in divided doses; increase gradually every 3-4 days as needed; maximum: 6 mg/kg/day in 3 divided doses

Adolescents: Depression (unlabeled use): Initial: 25-50 mg/day; increase to 100-150 mg/day in divided doses

Adults:

Depression: Initial: 150 mg/day in 3 divided doses (may increase by 50 mg/day every 3-7 days); maximum dose: 600 mg/day

Extended release formulation: Initial: 150 mg once daily at bedtime (may increase by 75 mg/day every 3 days); maximum dose: 375 mg/day; once adequate response obtained, gradually reduce with adjustment based on therapeutic response

Note: Therapeutic effects may take up to 6 weeks. Therapy is normally maintained for 6-12 months after optimum response is reached to prevent recurrence of depression.

Sedation/hypnotic (unlabeled use): 25-50 mg at bedtime (often in combination with daytime SSRIs); may increase up to 200 mg at bedtime

Elderly: 25-50 mg at bedtime with 25-50 mg/day dose increase every 3 days for inpatients and weekly for outpatients, if tolerated; usual dose: 75-150 mg/day

MAO inhibitor recommendations:

Switching to or from an MAO inhibitor intended to treat psychiatric disorders:

Allow 14 days to elapse between discontinuing an MAO inhibitor intended to treat psychiatric disorders and initiation of trazodone.

Allow 14 days to elapse between discontinuing trazodone and initiation of an MAO inhibitor intended to treat psychiatric disorders.

Use with other MAO inhibitors (linezolid or I.V. methylene blue):

Do not initiate trazodone in patients receiving linezolid or I.V. methylene blue; consider other interventions for psychiatric condition.

If urgent treatment with linezolid or I.V. methylene blue is required in a patient already receiving trazodone and potential benefits outweigh potential risks, discontinue trazodone promptly and administer linezolid or I.V. methylene blue. Monitor for serotonin syndrome for 2 weeks or until 24 hours after the last dose of linezolid or I.V. methylene blue, whichever comes first. May resume trazodone 24 hours after the last dose of linezolid or I.V. methylene blue.

Mechanism of Action Inhibits reuptake of serotonin, causes adrenoreceptor subsensitivity, and induces significant changes in 5-HT presynaptic receptor adrenoreceptors. Trazodone also significantly blocks histamine (H_1) and alpha$_1$-adrenergic receptors.

Contraindications Hypersensitivity to trazodone or any component of the formulation; use of MAO inhibitors intended to treat psychiatric disorders (concurrently or within 14 days of discontinuing either trazodone or the MAO inhibitor); initiation of trazodone in a patient receiving linezolid or intravenous methylene blue

Warnings/Precautions [U.S. Boxed Warning]: Antidepressants increase the risk of suicidal thinking and behavior in children, adolescents, and young adults (18-24 years of age) with major depressive disorder (MDD) and other psychiatric disorders; consider risk prior to prescribing. Short-term studies did not show an increased risk in patients >24 years of age and showed a decreased risk in patients ≥65 years of age. Closely monitor for clinical worsening, suicidality, or unusual changes in behavior; the patient's family or caregiver should be instructed to closely observe the patient and communicate condition with healthcare provider. A medication guide should be dispensed with each prescription. **Trazodone is not FDA approved for use in children.**

The possibility of a suicide attempt is inherent in major depression and may persist until remission occurs. Monitor for worsening of depression or suicidality, especially during initiation of therapy (generally first 1-2 months) or with dose increases or decreases. Use caution in high-risk patients. Worsening depression and severe abrupt suicidality that are not part of the presenting symptoms may require discontinuation or modification of drug therapy. The patient's family or caregiver should be alerted to monitor patients for the emergence of suicidality and associated behaviors (such as agitation, irritability, hostility, impulsivity, and hypomania) and call healthcare provider.

May worsen psychosis in some patients or precipitate a shift to mania or hypomania in patients with bipolar disorder. Patients presenting with depressive symptoms should be screened for bipolar disorder. Monotherapy in patients with bipolar disorder should be avoided. **Trazodone is not FDA approved for the treatment of bipolar depression.**

Priapism, including cases resulting in permanent dysfunction, has occurred with the use of trazodone. Instruct patient to seek medical assistance for erection lasting >4 hours; use with caution in patients who have conditions which may predispose them to priapism (eg, sickle cell anemia, multiple myeloma, leukemia). Not recommended for use in a patient during the acute recovery phase of MI. The risks of sedation, postural hypotension, and/or syncope are high relative to other antidepressants. Trazodone frequently causes sedation, which may result in impaired performance of tasks requiring alertness (eg, operating machinery or driving).

Use with caution in patients with a history of cardiovascular disease (including previous MI, stroke, tachycardia, or conduction abnormalities). Although the risk of conduction abnormalities with this agent is low relative to other antidepressants, QT prolongation (with or without torsade de pointes), ventricular tachycardia, and other arrhythmias have been observed with the use of trazodone (reports limited to immediate-release formulation); use with caution in patients with pre-existing cardiac disease. May impair platelet aggregation resulting in increased risk of bleeding events (eg, epistaxis, life threatening bleeding).

Potentially life-threatening serotonin syndrome (SS) has occurred with serotonergic agents (eg, SSRIs, SNRIs), particularly when used in combination with other serotonergic agents (eg, triptans, TCAs, fentanyl, lithium, tramadol, buspirone, St John's wort, tryptophan) or agents that impair metabolism of serotonin (eg, MOA inhibitors intended to treat psychiatric disorders, other MAO inhibitors [ie, linezolid and intravenous methylene blue]). Discontinue treatment (and any concomitant serotonergic agent) immediately if signs/symptoms arise.

Serotonin syndrome (SS)/neuroleptic malignant syndrome (NMS)-like reactions may occur with trazodone when used alone, particularly if used with other serotonergic agents (eg, serotonin/norepinephrine reuptake inhibitors [SNRIs], selective serotonin reuptake inhibitors [SSRIs], or triptans), drugs that impair serotonin metabolism (eg, MAO inhibitors), or antidopaminergic agents (eg, antipsychotics). If concurrent use is clinically warranted, carefully observe patient during treatment initiation and dose increases. Do not use concurrently with serotonin precursors (eg, tryptophan).

Therapy should not be abruptly discontinued in patients receiving high doses for prolonged periods; gradually reduce dosage prior to complete discontinuation to avoid withdrawal symptoms (eg, anxiety, agitation, sleep disturbance). Use caution in patients with a previous seizure disorder or condition predisposing to seizures such as brain damage, or alcoholism. Use with caution in patients with hepatic or renal dysfunction and in elderly patients. May cause SIADH and hyponatremia, predominantly in the elderly; volume depletion and/or concurrent use of diuretics likely increases risk. Potentially significant interactions may exist, requiring dose or frequency adjustment, additional monitoring, and/or selection of alternative therapy. Consult drug interactions database for more detailed information.

Drug Interactions

Metabolism/Transport Effects Substrate of CYP2D6 (minor), CYP3A4 (major); **Note:** Assignment of Major/Minor substrate status based on clinically relevant drug interaction potential; **Inhibits** CYP3A4 (weak); **Induces** P-glycoprotein

Avoid Concomitant Use

Avoid concomitant use of TraZODone with any of the following: Conivaptan; Dabigatran Etexilate; Highest Risk QTc-Prolonging Agents; Ivabradine; Linezolid; MAO Inhibitors; Methylene Blue; Mifepristone; Pomalidomide; Saquinavir; VinCRIStine (Liposomal)

Increased Effect/Toxicity

TraZODone may increase the levels/effects of: Antipsychotic Agents (Phenothiazines); Fosphenytoin; Highest Risk QTc-Prolonging Agents; Lomitapide; Methylene Blue; Metoclopramide; Moderate Risk QTc-Prolonging Agents; Phenytoin; Serotonin Modulators

The levels/effects of TraZODone may be increased by: Antipsychotic Agents (Phenothiazines); Antipsychotics; Atazanavir; Boceprevir; BusPIRone; Cobicistat; Conivaptan; CYP3A4 Inhibitors (Moderate); CYP3A4 Inhibitors (Strong); Darunavir; Dasatinib; Fosamprenavir; Indinavir; Ivabradine; Ivacaftor; Linezolid; Lopinavir; MAO Inhibitors; Mifepristone; Nelfinavir; QTc-Prolonging Agents (Indeterminate Risk and Risk Modifying); Saquinavir; Selective Serotonin Reuptake Inhibitors; Telaprevir; Tipranavir; Venlafaxine

Decreased Effect

TraZODone may decrease the levels/effects of: Dabigatran Etexilate; Linagliptin; P-glycoprotein/ABCB1 Substrates; Pomalidomide; VinCRIStine (Liposomal); Warfarin

The levels/effects of TraZODone may be decreased by: CYP3A4 Inducers (Strong); Deferasirox; Fosphenytoin; Peginterferon Alfa-2b; Phenytoin; Tocilizumab

Ethanol/Nutrition/Herb Interactions

Ethanol: May increase CNS depression; monitor for increased effects with coadministration. Caution patients about effects.

Food: Time to peak serum levels may be increased if immediate release trazodone is taken with food.

Herb/Nutraceutical: Avoid valerian, St John's wort, tryptophan, SAMe, kava kava (may increase risk of serotonin syndrome and/or excessive sedation).

Pharmacodynamics/Kinetics

Onset of Action Therapeutic (antidepressant): Up to 6 weeks; sleep aid: 1-3 hours

Half-life Elimination 7-10 hours

Time to Peak

Immediate release: 30-100 minutes; delayed with food (up to 2.5 hours)

Extended release: 9 hours; not significantly affected by food

Pregnancy Risk Factor C

Pregnancy Considerations Adverse effects were observed in some animal reproduction studies. When trazodone is taken during pregnancy, an increased risk of major malformations has not been observed in the limited number of pregnancies studied (Einarson, 2003; Einarson, 2009). The long-term effects of *in utero* trazodone exposure on infant development and behavior are not known.

The ACOG recommends that therapy with antidepressants during pregnancy be individualized; treatment of depression during pregnancy should incorporate the clinical expertise of the mental health clinician, obstetrician, primary healthcare provider, and pediatrician. According to the American Psychiatric Association (APA), the risks of medication treatment should be weighed against other treatment options and untreated depression. Consideration should be given to using agents with safety data in pregnancy. For women who discontinue antidepressant medications during pregnancy and who may be at high risk for postpartum depression, the medications can be restarted following delivery. Treatment algorithms have been developed by the ACOG and the APA for the management of depression in women prior to conception and during pregnancy (ACOG, 2008; APA, 2010; Yonkers, 2009).

Lactation Enters breast milk/use caution (AAP rates "of concern"; AAP 2001 update pending)

Breast-Feeding Considerations Trazodone is excreted into breast milk; breast milk concentrations peak ~2 hours following administration. It is not known if the trazodone metabolite is found in breast milk (Verbeeck, 1986). The long-term effects on neurobehavior have not been studied. The manufacturer recommends that caution be exercised when administering trazodone to nursing women.

Dosage Forms
Tablet, oral: 50 mg, 100 mg, 150 mg, 300 mg
Tablet, extended release, oral:
Oleptro™: 150 mg, 300 mg

Dental Comment Trazodone is known to prolong the QT interval. The QT interval is measured as the time and distance between the Q point of the QRS complex and the end of the T wave in the ECG tracing. After adjustment for heart rate, the QT interval is defined as prolonged if it is more than 450 msec in men and 460 msec in women. A long QT syndrome was first described in the 1950s and 60s as a congenital syndrome involving QT interval prolongation and syncope and sudden death. Some of the congenital long QT syndromes were characterized by a peculiar electrocardiographic appearance of the QRS complex involving a premature atria beat followed by a pause, then a subsequent sinus beat showing marked QT prolongation and deformity. This type of cardiac arrhythmia was originally termed "torsade de pointes" (translated from the French as "twisting of the points"). Trazodone is considered as having a risk of causing torsade de pointes. Since it is not known what effect vasoconstrictors in the local anesthetic regimen will have in patients with a known history of congenital prolonged QT interval or in patients taking any medication that prolongs the QT interval, a medical consult is suggested.

Treprostinil (tre PROST in il)

Brand Names: U.S. Remodulin®; Tyvaso™
Brand Names: Canada Remodulin®
Pharmacologic Category Prostacyclin; Prostaglandin; Vasodilator
Use
Injection: Treatment of pulmonary arterial hypertension (PAH) (WHO Group I) in patients with NYHA Class II-IV symptoms to decrease exercise-associated symptoms; to diminish clinical deterioration when transitioning from epoprostenol (I.V.)

Inhalation: Treatment of pulmonary arterial hypertension (PAH) (WHO Group I) in patients with NYHA Class III symptoms to improve exercise ability. **Note:** Nearly all controlled clinical trial experience has been with concomitant bosentan or sildenafil.

Local Anesthetic/Vasoconstrictor Precautions No information available to require special precautions

Effects on Dental Treatment No significant effects or complications reported. Treprostinil may enhance the risk of bleeding associated with other antiplatelet agents (aspirin or NSAIDs).

Effects on Bleeding Treprostinil is an inhibitor of platelet aggregation and may prolong bleeding times.
Adverse Effects
>10%:
Cardiovascular: Flushing (11%; inhalation: 15%)
Central nervous system: Headache (27% to 41%)
Dermatologic: Rash (14%)
Gastrointestinal: Diarrhea (25%), nausea (19% to 22%)
Local: Infusion site pain (SubQ: 85%; may improve after several months of therapy), infusion site reaction (SubQ: 83%)
Neuromuscular & skeletal: Jaw pain (13%)
Respiratory: Cough (inhalation: 54%), throat irritation/pharyngolaryngeal pain (inhalation: 25%)
1% to 10%:
Cardiovascular: Edema (9%), syncope (inhalation: 6%), hypotension (4%)
Central nervous system: Dizziness (9%)
Dermatologic: Pruritus (8%)
Respiratory: Epistaxis (inhalation), hemoptysis, pneumonia, wheezing (inhalation)

General Dosage Range Dosage adjustment recommended for the I.V. infusion and SubQ routes in patients with hepatic impairment
Inhalation: *Adults:* Initial: 18 mcg (or 3 inhalations) every 4 hours 4 times/day; Maintenance: Maximum dose: 54 mcg (or 9 inhalations) 4 times/day
I.V. Infusion, SubQ: *Adults:* Initial: 0.625-1.25 ng/kg/minute; Maintenance: 1.25-40 ng/kg/minute

Mechanism of Action Treprostinil is a direct vasodilator of both pulmonary and systemic arterial vascular beds; also inhibits platelet aggregation.
Pharmacodynamics/Kinetics
Half-life Elimination Terminal: ~4 hours
Pregnancy Risk Factor B
Pregnancy Considerations Some skeletal malformations and maternal toxicity noted in animal studies. There are no adequate and well-controlled studies in pregnant women. Use with caution and only if clearly needed.

Tretinoin (Systemic) (TRET i noyn)

Brand Names: Canada Vesanoid®
Pharmacologic Category Antineoplastic Agent, Miscellaneous; Retinoic Acid Derivative
Use Induction of remission in patients with acute promyelocytic leukemia (APL), French American British (FAB) classification M3 (including the M3 variant) characterized by t(15;17) translocation and/or PML/RARα gene presence
Unlabeled Use Post consolidation and maintenance therapy in APL; combination therapy (with arsenic trioxide) for remission induction in APL
Local Anesthetic/Vasoconstrictor Precautions No information available to require special precautions
Effects on Dental Treatment Key adverse event(s) related to dental treatment: Xerostomia (normal salivary flow resumes upon discontinuation).
Effects on Bleeding Although significant myelosuppression with associated altered hemostasis has been reported for many chemotherapeutic agents, myelosuppression is not common with tretinoin and no specific precautions appear to necessary.
Adverse Effects Most patients will experience drug-related toxicity, especially headache, fever, weakness and fatigue. These are seldom permanent or irreversible and do not typically require therapy interruption.

>10%:

Cardiovascular: Peripheral edema (52%), chest discomfort (32%), edema (29%), arrhythmias (23%), flushing (23%), hypotension (14%), hypertension (11%)

Central nervous system: Headache (86%), fever (83%), malaise (66%), pain (37%), dizziness (20%), anxiety (17%), depression (14%), insomnia (14%), confusion (11%)

Dermatologic: Skin/mucous membrane dryness (77%), rash (54%), pruritus (20%), alopecia (14%), skin changes (14%)

Endocrine & metabolic: Hypercholesterolemia and/or hypertriglyceridemia (≤60%)

Gastrointestinal: Nausea/vomiting (57%), GI hemorrhage (34%), abdominal pain (31%), mucositis (26%), diarrhea (23%), weight gain (23%), anorexia (17%), constipation (17%), weight loss (17%), dyspepsia (14%), abdominal distention (11%)

Hematologic: Hemorrhage (60%), leukocytosis (40%), disseminated intravascular coagulation (DIC) (26%)

Hepatic: Liver function tests increased (50% to 60%)

Local: Phlebitis (11%)

Neuromuscular & skeletal: Bone pain (77%), paresthesia (17%), myalgia (14%)

Ocular: Ocular disorder (17%), visual disturbances (17%)

Otic: Earache/ear fullness (23%)

Renal: Renal insufficiency (11%)

Respiratory: Upper respiratory tract disorders (63%), dyspnea (60%), respiratory insufficiency (26%), pleural effusion (20%), expiratory wheezing (14%), pneumonia (14%), rales (14%)

Miscellaneous: Shivering (63%), infections (58%), retinoic acid-acute promyelocytic leukemia syndrome differentiation syndrome (≤25%), diaphoresis (20%)

1% to 10%:

Cardiovascular: Cerebral hemorrhage (9%), cardiac failure (6%), facial edema (6%), pallor (6%), cardiac arrest (3%), cardiomyopathy (3%), heart enlarged (3%), heart murmur (3%), ischemia (3%), MI (3%), myocarditis (3%), pericarditis (3%), stroke (3%)

Central nervous system: Agitation (9%), intracranial hypertension (9%), hallucination (6%), aphasia (3%), cerebellar edema (3%), CNS depression (3%), coma (3%), dementia (3%), encephalopathy (3%), facial paralysis (3%), forgetfulness (3%), hypotaxia (3%), hypothermia (3%), light reflex absent (3%), seizure (3%), slow speech (3%), somnolence (3%), spinal cord disorder (3%), unconsciousness (3%)

Dermatologic: Cellulitis (8%)

Endocrine & metabolic: Fluid imbalance (6%), acidosis (3%)

Gastrointestinal: Hepatosplenomegaly (9%), ulcer (3%)

Genitourinary: Dysuria (9%), micturition frequency (3%), prostate enlarged (3%)

Hepatic: Ascites (3%), hepatitis (3%)

Neuromuscular & skeletal: Flank pain (9%), abnormal gait (3%), asterixis (3%), bone inflammation (3%), dysarthria (3%), hemiplegia (3%), hyporeflexia (3%), leg weakness (3%), tremor (3%)

Ocular: Visual acuity change (6%), agnosia (3%), visual field deficit (3%)

Otic: Hearing loss (6%)

Renal: Acute renal failure (3%), renal tubular necrosis (3%)

Respiratory: Lower respiratory tract disorders (9%), pulmonary infiltration (6%), bronchial asthma (3%), larynx edema (3%), pulmonary hypertension (3%)

Miscellaneous: Lymph disorder (6%)

General Dosage Range Dosage adjustment recommended in patients who develop toxicities

Oral: *Children and Adults:* Induction: 45 mg/m^2/day in 2 divided doses (maximum duration of treatment: 90 days)

Mechanism of Action Tretinoin appears to bind one or more nuclear receptors and decreases proliferation and induces differentiation of APL cells; initially produces maturation of primitive promyelocytes and repopulates the marrow and peripheral blood with normal hematopoietic cells to achieve complete remission

Pharmacodynamics/Kinetics

Half-life Elimination Terminal: Parent drug: 0.5-2 hours

Time to Peak Serum: 1-2 hours

Pregnancy Risk Factor D

Pregnancy Considerations [U.S. Boxed Warning]: High risk of teratogenicity; if treatment with tretinoin is required in women of childbearing potential, two reliable forms of contraception should be used during and for 1 month after treatment. Within 1 week prior to starting therapy, serum or urine pregnancy test (sensitivity 50 mIU/mL) should be collected. If possible, delay therapy until results are available. Repeat pregnancy testing and contraception counseling monthly throughout the period of treatment. An increase in fetal resorptions and a decrease in live fetuses were observed in all animal reproduction studies; teratogenic effects have also been observed. Use in humans is limited, however, major fetal abnormalities and spontaneous abortions have been reported with other retinoids. If the clinical condition of a patient presenting with APL during pregnancy warrants immediate treatment, tretinoin use should be avoided in the first trimester; treatment with tretinoin may be considered in the second and third trimester with careful fetal cardiac monitoring.

Tretinoin (Topical) (TRET i noyn)

Brand Names: U.S. Atralin™; Avita®; Refissa®; Renova®; Retin-A Micro®; Retin-A®; Tretin-X®

Brand Names: Canada Rejuva-A®; Renova®; Retin-A Micro®; Retin-A®; Retinova®; Stieva-A; Vitamin A Acid

Pharmacologic Category Acne Products; Retinoic Acid Derivative; Topical Skin Product, Acne

Use Treatment of acne vulgaris; photodamaged skin; palliation of fine wrinkles, mottled hyperpigmentation, and tactile roughness of facial skin as part of a comprehensive skin care and sun avoidance program

Unlabeled Use Some skin cancers

Local Anesthetic/Vasoconstrictor Precautions No information available to require special precautions

Effects on Dental Treatment No significant effects or complications reported

Effects on Bleeding No information available to require special precautions

Adverse Effects

>10%: Dermatologic: Excessive dryness, erythema, scaling of the skin, pruritus

1% to 10%:
Dermatologic: Hyperpigmentation or hypopigmentation, photosensitivity, initial acne flare-up
Local: Edema, blistering, stinging

General Dosage Range Topical: *Children >12 years and Adults:* Apply once daily **or** every other day

Mechanism of Action Keratinocytes in the sebaceous follicle become less adherent which allows for easy removal; inhibits microcomedone formation and eliminates lesions already present

Pregnancy Risk Factor C

Pregnancy Considerations Oral tretinoin is teratogenic and fetotoxic in rats at doses 1000 and 500 times the topical human dose, respectively. Tretinoin does not appear to be teratogenic when used topically since it is rapidly metabolized by the skin; however, there are rare reports of fetal defects. Use for acne only if benefit to mother outweighs potential risk to fetus. During pregnancy, do not use for palliation of fine wrinkles, mottled hyperpigmentation, and tactile roughness of facial skin.

Triamcinolone (Systemic) (trye am SIN oh lone)

Related Information
Respiratory Diseases *on page 1514*
Brand Names: U.S. Aristospan®; Kenalog®-10; Kenalog®-40
Brand Names: Canada Aristospan®
Generic Availability (U.S.) No
Pharmacologic Category Corticosteroid, Systemic
Dental Use Adjunctive treatment and temporary relief of symptoms associated with oral inflammatory lesions and ulcerative lesions resulting from trauma

Use
Intra-articular (soft tissue): Acute gouty arthritis, acute/subacute bursitis, acute tenosynovitis, epicondylitis, rheumatoid arthritis, synovitis of osteoarthritis
Intralesional: Alopecia areata, discoid lupus erythematosus, keloids, granuloma annulare lesions (localized hypertrophic, infiltrated, or inflammatory), lichen planus plaques, lichen simplex chronicus plaques, psoriatic plaques, necrobiosis lipoidica diabeticorum, cystic tumors of aponeurosis or tendon (ganglia)
Systemic: Adrenocortical insufficiency, dermatologic diseases, endocrine disorders, gastrointestinal diseases, hematologic and neoplastic disorders, nervous system disorders, nephrotic syndrome, rheumatic disorders, allergic states, respiratory diseases, systemic lupus erythematosus (SLE), and other diseases requiring anti-inflammatory or immunosuppressive effects

Local Anesthetic/Vasoconstrictor Precautions No information available to require special precautions

Effects on Dental Treatment Key adverse event(s) related to dental treatment: Ulcerative esophagitis, perioral dermatitis, atrophy of oral mucosa, burning, irritation, and oral monilia (oral inhaler).

Effects on Bleeding No information available to require special precautions

Adverse Effects Frequency not defined; reactions reported with corticosteroid therapy in general:
Cardiovascular: Arrhythmia, bradycardia, cardiac arrest, cardiac enlargement, CHF, circulatory collapse, edema, hypertension, hypertrophic cardiomyopathy (premature infants), myocardial rupture (following recent MI), syncope, tachycardia, thromboembolism, vasculitis

Central nervous system: Arachnoiditis (I.T.), depression, emotional instability, euphoria, headache, insomnia, intracranial pressure increased, malaise, meningitis (I.T.), mood changes, neuritis, neuropathy, personality change, pseudotumor cerebri (with discontinuation), seizure, spinal cord infarction, stroke, vertigo
Dermatologic: Abscess (sterile), acne, allergic dermatitis, angioedema, atrophy (cutaneous/subcutaneous), bruising, dry skin, erythema, hair thinning, hirsutism, hyper-/hypopigmentation, hypertrichosis, impaired wound healing, lupus erythematosus-like lesions, petechiae, purpura, rash, skin test suppression, striae, thin skin
Endocrine & metabolic: Carbohydrate intolerance, Cushingoid state, diabetes mellitus, fluid retention, glucose intolerance, growth suppression (children), hypokalemia, hypokalemic alkalosis, menstrual irregularities, negative nitrogen balance, sodium retention, sperm motility altered
Gastrointestinal: Abdominal distention, appetite increased, GI hemorrhage, GI perforation, nausea, pancreatitis, peptic ulcer, ulcerative esophagitis, weight gain
Hepatic: Hepatomegaly, liver function tests increased
Local: Thrombophlebitis
Neuromuscular & skeletal: Aseptic necrosis of femoral and humeral heads, calcinosis, Charcot-like arthropathy, fractures, joint tissue damage, muscle mass loss, myopathy, osteoporosis, parasthesia, paraplegia, quadriplegia, tendon rupture, vertebral compression fractures, weakness
Ocular: Cataracts, cortical blindness, exophthalmos, glaucoma, ocular pressure increased, papilledema
Renal: Glycosuria
Respiratory: Pulmonary edema
Miscellaneous: Abnormal fat deposits, anaphylactoid reaction, anaphylaxis, diaphoresis, hiccups, infection, moon face

Dosage The lowest possible dose should be used to control the condition; when dose reduction is possible, the dose should be reduced gradually.

Injection:
Acetonide:
Intra-articular, intrabursal, tendon sheaths: Adults: Initial: Smaller joints: 2.5-5 mg, larger joints: 5-15 mg; may require up to 10 mg for small joints and up to 40 mg for large joints; maximum dose/treatment (several joints at one time): 20-80 mg
Intradermal: Adults: Initial: 1 mg
I.M.: Range: 2.5-100 mg/day
Children: Initial: 0.11-1.6 mg/kg/day in 3-4 divided doses
Children 6-12 years: Initial: 40 mg
Children >12 years and Adults: Initial: 60 mg
Hay fever/pollen asthma: 40-100 mg as a single injection/season
Multiple sclerosis (acute exacerbation): 160 mg daily for 1 week, followed by 64 mg every other day for 1 month
Hexacetonide: Adults:
Intralesional, sublesional: Up to 0.5 mg/square inch of affected skin; range: 2-48 mg/day

Intra-articular: Average dose: 2-20 mg; smaller joints: 2-6 mg; larger joints: 10-20 mg. Frequency of injection into a single joint is every 3-4 weeks as necessary; to avoid possible joint destruction use as infrequently as possible.

Triamcinolone Dosing

	Acetonide	Hexacetonide
Intrasynovial	5-40 mg	
Intralesional	1-30 mg (usually 1 mg per injection site); 10 mg/mL suspension usually used	Up to 0.5 mg/sq inch affected area
Sublesional	1-30 mg	
Systemic I.M.	2.5-60 mg/dose (usual adult dose: 60 mg; may repeat with 20-100 mg dose when symptoms recur)	
Intra-articular	2.5-40 mg	2-20 mg average
large joints	5-15 mg	10-20 mg
small joints	2.5-5 mg	2-6 mg
Tendon sheaths	2.5-10 mg	
Intradermal	1 mg/site	

Mechanism of Action Decreases inflammation by suppression of migration of polymorphonuclear leukocytes and reversal of increased capillary permeability; suppresses the immune system by reducing activity and volume of the lymphatic system; suppresses adrenal function at high doses

Contraindications Hypersensitivity to triamcinolone or any component of the formulation; systemic fungal infections; cerebral malaria; idiopathic thrombocytopenic purpura (I.M. injection)

Warnings/Precautions May cause hypercorticism or suppression of hypothalamic-pituitary-adrenal (HPA) axis, particularly in younger children or in patients receiving high doses for prolonged periods. HPA axis suppression may lead to adrenal crisis. Withdrawal and discontinuation of a corticosteroid should be done slowly and carefully.

Acute myopathy has been reported with high-dose corticosteroids, usually in patients with neuromuscular transmission disorders; may involve ocular and/or respiratory muscles; monitor creatine kinase; recovery may be delayed. Corticosteroid use may cause psychiatric disturbances, including depression, euphoria, insomnia, mood swings, and personality changes. Pre-existing psychiatric conditions may be exacerbated by corticosteroid use. Prolonged use of corticosteroids may also increase the incidence of secondary infection, mask acute infection (including fungal infections), prolong or exacerbate viral infections, or limit response to vaccines. Exposure to chickenpox should be avoided; corticosteroids should not be used to treat ocular herpes simplex. Corticosteroids should not be used for cerebral malaria or viral hepatitis. Close observation is required in patients with latent tuberculosis and/or TB reactivity; restrict use in active TB (only in conjunction with antituberculosis treatment). Use with caution in patients with threadworm infection; may cause serious hyperinfection. Prolonged treatment with corticosteroids has been associated with the development of Kaposi's sarcoma (case reports); if noted, discontinuation of therapy should be considered. Avoid use in head injury patients.

Use with caution in patients with thyroid disease, hepatic impairment, renal impairment, cardiovascular disease, diabetes, myasthenia gravis, patients at risk for osteoporosis, patients at risk for seizures, or GI diseases (diverticulitis, peptic ulcer, ulcerative colitis) due to perforation risk. Avoid use in head injury patients. Use caution following acute MI (corticosteroids have been associated with myocardial rupture). Because of the risk of adverse effects, systemic corticosteroids should be used cautiously in the elderly in the smallest possible effective dose for the shortest duration. Patients should not be immunized with live, viral vaccines while receiving immunosuppressive doses of corticosteroids. The ability to respond to dead viral vaccines is unknown.

Withdraw therapy with gradual tapering of dose. There have been reports of systemic corticosteroid withdrawal symptoms (eg, joint/muscle pain, lassitude, depression) when withdrawing oral inhalation therapy. Injection suspension contains benzyl alcohol; benzyl alcohol has been associated with the "gasping syndrome" in neonates and low-birth-weight infants. Administer products only via recommended route (depending on product used). Do **not** administer any triamcinolone product via the epidural or intrathecal route; serious adverse events, including fatalities, have been reported.

Drug Interactions

Metabolism/Transport Effects Substrate of CYP3A4 (minor); **Note:** Assignment of Major/Minor substrate status based on clinically relevant drug interaction potential

Avoid Concomitant Use

Avoid concomitant use of Triamcinolone (Systemic) with any of the following: Aldesleukin; BCG; Mifepristone; Natalizumab; Pimecrolimus; Tacrolimus (Topical); Tofacitinib

Increased Effect/Toxicity

Triamcinolone (Systemic) may increase the levels/effects of: Acetylcholinesterase Inhibitors; Amphotericin B; Deferasirox; Leflunomide; Loop Diuretics; Natalizumab; NSAID (COX-2 Inhibitor); NSAID (Nonselective); Thiazide Diuretics; Tofacitinib; Vaccines (Live); Warfarin

The levels/effects of Triamcinolone (Systemic) may be increased by: Antifungal Agents (Azole Derivatives, Systemic); Aprepitant; Calcium Channel Blockers (Nondihydropyridine); Denosumab; Estrogen Derivatives; Fluconazole; Fosaprepitant; Indacaterol; Macrolide Antibiotics; Mifepristone; Neuromuscular-Blocking Agents (Nondepolarizing); Pimecrolimus; Quinolone Antibiotics; Ritonavir; Roflumilast; Salicylates; Tacrolimus (Topical); Telaprevir; Trastuzumab

Decreased Effect

Triamcinolone (Systemic) may decrease the levels/effects of: Aldesleukin; Antidiabetic Agents; BCG; Calcitriol; Coccidioidin Skin Test; Corticorelin; Hyaluronidase; Isoniazid; Salicylates; Sipuleucel-T; Telaprevir; Vaccines (Inactivated)

The levels/effects of Triamcinolone (Systemic) may be decreased by: Aminoglutethimide; Barbiturates; Echinacea; Mifepristone; Mitotane; Primidone; Rifamycin Derivatives

Dietary Considerations Ensure adequate intake of calcium and vitamins (or consider supplementation) in patients on medium-to-high doses of systemic corticosteroids.

Pharmacodynamics/Kinetics

Half-life Elimination Biologic: 18-36 hours

Time to Peak I.M.: 8-10 hours

Pregnancy Risk Factor C

Pregnancy Considerations Triamcinolone was shown to be teratogenic in animal reproduction studies. Some studies have shown an association between first trimester corticosteroid use and oral clefts; adverse events in the fetus/neonate have been noted in case reports following large doses of systemic corticosteroids during pregnancy.

Lactation Excretion in breast milk unknown/use caution

Breast-Feeding Considerations Corticosteroids are excreted in human milk; information specific to triamcinolone has not been located.

Dosage Forms

Injection, suspension:

Aristospan®: 5 mg/mL (5 mL); 20 mg/mL (1 mL, 5 mL)

Kenalog®-10: 10 mg/mL (5 mL)

Kenalog®-40: 40 mg/mL (1 mL, 5 mL, 10 mL)

Triamcinolone (Nasal) (trye am SIN oh lone)

Brand Names: U.S. Nasacort® AQ

Brand Names: Canada Nasacort® AQ; Trinasal®

Pharmacologic Category Corticosteroid, Nasal

Use Management of seasonal and perennial allergic rhinitis

Unlabeled Use Adjunct to antibiotics in empiric treatment of acute bacterial rhinosinusitis (ABRS) (Chow, 2012)

Local Anesthetic/Vasoconstrictor Precautions No information available to require special precautions

Effects on Dental Treatment No significant effects or complications reported

Effects on Bleeding No information available to require special precautions

Adverse Effects

>10%:

Central nervous system: Headache (2% to 51%)

Respiratory: Pharyngitis (5% to 25%)

1% to 10%:

Cardiovascular: Facial edema (1% to 3%)

Central nervous system: Pain (1% to 3%)

Dermatologic: Photosensitivity (1% to 3%), rash (1% to 3%)

Endocrine & metabolic: Dysmenorrhea (≥2%)

Gastrointestinal: Taste perversion (5% to 8%), dyspepsia (3% to 5%), abdominal pain (1% to 5%), nausea (2% to 3%), diarrhea (1% to 3%), oral moniliasis (1% to 3%), toothache (1% to 3%), vomiting (1% to 3%), weight gain (1% to 3%), xerostomia (1% to 3%)

Genitourinary: Cystitis (1% to 3%), urinary tract infection (1% to 3%), vaginal moniliasis (1% to 3%)

Local: Nasal burning (≥2%; transient), nasal stinging (≥2%; transient)

Neuromuscular & skeletal: Back pain (2% to 8%), bursitis (1% to 3%), myalgia (1% to 3%), tenosynovitis (1% to 3%)

Ocular: Conjunctivitis (1% to 4%)

Otic: Otitis media (≥2%)

Respiratory: Sinusitis (2% to 9%), cough (≤8%), epistaxis (≤5%), bronchitis (children 3%), chest congestion (1% to 3%), asthma (≥2%), rhinitis (≥2%)

Miscellaneous: Flu-like syndrome (2% to 59%), voice alteration (1% to 3%), allergic reaction (≥2%), infection (≥2%)

General Dosage Range Inhalation:

Nasal inhaler:

Children 6-11 years: 220 mcg/day as 2 sprays in each nostril once daily

Children ≥12 years and Adults: 220-440 mcg/day as 2-4 sprays in each nostril 1-4 times/day

Nasal spray:

Children 2-5 years: 110 mcg/day as 1 spray in each nostril once daily (maximum: 110 mcg/day)

Children 6-11 years: Initial: 110 mcg/day as 1 spray in each nostril once daily; Maintenance: 110-220 mcg/day as 1-2 sprays in each nostril

Children ≥12 years and Adults: 110-220 mcg/day as 1-2 sprays in each nostril once daily

Mechanism of Action Suppresses the immune system by reducing activity and volume of the lymphatic system

Pharmacodynamics/Kinetics

Half-life Elimination Biologic: 18-36 hours

Pregnancy Risk Factor C

Pregnancy Considerations Triamcinolone was shown to be teratogenic in animal reproduction studies. Some studies have shown an association between first trimester corticosteroid use and oral clefts; adverse events in the fetus/neonate have been noted in case reports following large doses of systemic corticosteroids during pregnancy. Inhaled corticosteroids are recommended for the treatment of allergic rhinitis during pregnancy.

Triamcinolone (Topical) (trye am SIN oh lone)

Related Information

Ulcerative, Erosive, and Painful Oral Mucosal Disorders *on page 1578*

Related Sample Prescriptions

Mild Lichen Planus *on page 1618*

Recurrent Aphthous Stomatitis *on page 1618*

Brand Names: U.S. Kenalog®; Oralone®; Pediaderm™ TA; Trianex™; Triderm®; Zytopic™

Brand Names: Canada Kenalog®; Oracort; Triaderm

Generic Availability (U.S.) Yes: Excludes spray

Pharmacologic Category Corticosteroid, Topical

Dental Use Oral topical: Adjunctive treatment and temporary relief of symptoms associated with oral inflammatory lesions and ulcerative lesions resulting from trauma

Use

Oral topical: Adjunctive treatment and temporary relief of symptoms associated with oral inflammatory lesions and ulcerative lesions resulting from trauma

Topical: Inflammatory dermatoses responsive to steroids

Local Anesthetic/Vasoconstrictor Precautions No information available to require special precautions

Effects on Dental Treatment Key adverse event(s) related to dental treatment: Ulcerative esophagitis, perioral dermatitis, atrophy of oral mucosa, burning, and irritation.

Effects on Bleeding No information available to require special precautions

Adverse Effects Frequency not defined.

Dermatologic: Acneiform eruptions, allergic contact dermatitis, dryness, folliculitis, hypertrichosis, hypopigmentation, miliaria, perioral dermatitis, pruritus, skin atrophy, skin infection (secondary), skin maceration, striae

Endocrine: HPA axis suppression; metabolic effects (hyperglycemia, hypokalemia)

Local: Burning, irritation

◀ **Dental Usual Dosage** Oral inflammatory lesions/ ulcers: Adults: Oral topical: Press a small dab (about ¼ inch) to the lesion until a thin film develops; a larger quantity may be required for coverage of some lesions. For optimal results, use only enough to coat the lesion with a thin film; do not rub in.

Dosage

Oral topical: Oral inflammatory lesions/ulcers: Press a small dab (about ¼ inch) to the lesion until a thin film develops. A larger quantity may be required for coverage of some lesions. For optimal results use only enough to coat the lesion with a thin film; do not rub in.

Topical:

Cream, Ointment:

0.025% or 0.05%: Apply thin film to affected areas 2-4 times/day

0.1% or 0.5%: Apply thin film to affected areas 2-3 times/day

Spray: Apply to affected area 3-4 times/day

Mechanism of Action Decreases inflammation by suppression of migration of polymorphonuclear leukocytes and reversal of increased capillary permeability; suppresses the immune system by reducing activity and volume of the lymphatic system

Contraindications Hypersensitivity to triamcinolone or any component of the formulation; fungal, viral, or bacterial infections of the mouth or throat (oral topical formulation)

Warnings/Precautions Topical corticosteroids may be absorbed percutaneously. Absorption may cause manifestations of Cushing's syndrome, hyperglycemia, or glycosuria. Absorption is increased by the use of occlusive dressings, application to denuded skin, or application to large surface areas. Do not use occlusive dressings on weeping or exudative lesions and general caution with occlusive dressings should be observed; discontinue if skin irritation or contact dermatitis should occur; do not use in patients with decreased skin circulation. May cause hypercorticism or suppression of hypothalamic-pituitary-adrenal (HPA) axis, particularly in younger children or in patients receiving high doses for prolonged periods. HPA axis suppression may lead to adrenal crisis.

Prolonged use may result in fungal or bacterial superinfection; discontinue if dermatological infection persists despite appropriate antimicrobial therapy. Topical use has been associated with local sensitization (redness, irritation); discontinue if sensitization is noted. When used as a topical agent in the oral cavity, if significant regeneration or repair of oral tissues has not occurred in seven days, re-evaluation of the etiology of the oral lesion is advised.

Because of the risk of adverse effects associated with systemic absorption, topical corticosteroids should be used cautiously in the elderly in the smallest possible effective dose for the shortest duration. Children may absorb proportionally larger amounts after topical application and may be more prone to systemic effects. HPA axis suppression, intracranial hypertension, and Cushing's syndrome have been reported in children receiving topical corticosteroids. Prolonged use may affect growth velocity; growth should be routinely monitored in pediatric patients.

Drug Interactions

Metabolism/Transport Effects None known.

Avoid Concomitant Use

Avoid concomitant use of Triamcinolone (Topical) with any of the following: Aldesleukin

Increased Effect/Toxicity

Triamcinolone (Topical) may increase the levels/effects of: Deferasirox

The levels/effects of Triamcinolone (Topical) may be increased by: Telaprevir

Decreased Effect

Triamcinolone (Topical) may decrease the levels/ effects of: Aldesleukin; Corticorelin; Hyaluronidase; Telaprevir

Pharmacodynamics/Kinetics

Half-life Elimination Biologic: 18-36 hours

Pregnancy Risk Factor C

Pregnancy Considerations Corticosteroids were found to be teratogenic following topical application in animal reproduction studies. In general, the use of topical corticosteroids during pregnancy is not considered to have significant risk, however, intrauterine growth retardation in the infant has been reported (rare). The use of large amounts or for prolonged periods of time should be avoided.

Lactation Excretion in breast milk unknown/use caution

Breast-Feeding Considerations Corticosteroids are excreted in human milk; information specific to triamcinolone has not been located. The amount of triamcinolone absorbed systemically following topical administration is variable. Hypertension in the nursing infant has been reported following corticosteroid ointment applied to the nipples. Use with caution.

Dosage Forms

Aerosol, spray, topical:

Kenalog®: 0.2 mg/2-second spray (63 g, 100 g)

Cream, topical: 0.025% (15 g, 80 g, 454 g); 0.1% (15 g, 30 g, 80 g, 454 g, 2240 g, 2270 g); 0.5% (15 g)

Pediaderm™ TA: 0.1% (30 g)

Triderm®: 0.1% (30 g, 85 g)

Zytopic™: 0.1% (85 g)

Lotion, topical: 0.025% (60 mL); 0.1% (60 mL); 0.1%

Ointment, topical: 0.025% (15 g, 80 g, 454 g); 0.05% (430 g); 0.1% (15 g, 80 g, 454 g); 0.5% (15 g)

Trianex™: 0.05% (17 g, 85 g)

Paste, oral topical: 0.1% (5 g)

Oralone®: 0.1% (5 g)

Triamterene (trye AM ter een)

Related Information

Cardiovascular Diseases on page 1492

Brand Names: U.S. Dyrenium®

Pharmacologic Category Diuretic, Potassium-Sparing

Use Alone or in combination with other diuretics in treatment of edema and hypertension; decreases potassium excretion caused by kaliuretic diuretics

Local Anesthetic/Vasoconstrictor Precautions No information available to require special precautions

Effects on Dental Treatment No significant effects or complications reported

Effects on Bleeding No information available to require special precautions

Adverse Effects 1% to 10%:

Cardiovascular: Hypotension, edema, CHF, bradycardia

Central nervous system: Dizziness, headache, fatigue

Gastrointestinal: Constipation, nausea

Respiratory: Dyspnea

General Dosage Range Oral: Adults: 50-300 mg/day in 1-2 divided doses (maximum: 300 mg/day)

Mechanism of Action Blocks epithelial sodium channels in the late distal convoluted tubule (DCT) and collecting duct which inhibits sodium reabsorption from the lumen. This effectively reduces intracellular sodium, decreasing the function of Na+/K+ ATPase, leading to potassium retention and decreased calcium, magnesium, and hydrogen excretion. As sodium uptake capacity in the DCT/collecting duct is limited, the natriuretic, diuretic, and antihypertensive effects are generally considered weak.

Pharmacodynamics/Kinetics

Onset of Action Diuresis: 2-4 hours

Duration of Action 7-9 hours

Pregnancy Risk Factor C

Pregnancy Considerations No data available. Generally, use of diuretics during pregnancy is avoided due to risk of decreased placental perfusion.

Triazolam (trye AY zoe lam)

Related Information

Management of the Patient With Anxiety or Depression *on page 1594*

Related Sample Prescriptions

Sedation (Prior to Dental Treatment) *on page 1621*

Brand Names: U.S. Halcion®

Brand Names: Canada Apo-Triazo®; Gen-Triazolam; Halcion®; Mylan-Triazolam

Generic Availability (U.S.) Yes

Pharmacologic Category Benzodiazepine

Dental Use Oral premedication before dental procedures

Use Short-term (generally 7-10 days) treatment of insomnia

Unlabeled Use Oral sedation prior to outpatient dental procedures

Local Anesthetic/Vasoconstrictor Precautions No information available to require special precautions

Effects on Dental Treatment No significant effects or complications reported (see Dental Comment)

Effects on Bleeding No information available to require special precautions

Adverse Effects

>10%: Central nervous system: Drowsiness (14%)

1% to 10%:

Central nervous system: Headache (10%), dizziness (8%), ataxia (5%), lightheadedness (5%), nervousness (5%)

Gastrointestinal: Nausea (5%), vomiting (5%)

Dental Usual Dosage Preprocedure sedation (unlabeled use): Adults: Oral: 0.25 mg 1 hour before procedure; 0.125 mg used for elderly patients or patients sensitive to sedative effects of medications (Dionne, 2006)

Dosage

Insomnia (short-term use): Oral:

Adults: Usual dose: 0.25 mg at bedtime; 0.125 mg at bedtime may be sufficient in some patients, such as those with low body weight; maximum dose: 0.5 mg daily

Elderly and/or debilitated patients: Initial: 0.125 mg at bedtime; maximum dose: 0.25 mg daily

Dental preprocedure oral sedation (unlabeled use): Adults: 0.25 mg 1 hour before procedure; 0.125 mg used for elderly patients or patients sensitive to sedative effects (Dionne, 2006)

Dosing adjustment in renal impairment: No dosage adjustment provided in manufacturer's labeling; however, caution is recommended

Dosing adjustment in hepatic impairment: No dosage adjustment provided in manufacturer's labeling; however, use caution or avoid due to extensive hepatic metabolism

Mechanism of Action Binds to stereospecific benzodiazepine receptors on the postsynaptic GABA neuron at several sites within the central nervous system, including the limbic system, reticular formation. Enhancement of the inhibitory effect of GABA on neuronal excitability results by increased neuronal membrane permeability to chloride ions. This shift in chloride ions results in hyperpolarization (a less excitable state) and stabilization.

Contraindications Hypersensitivity to triazolam, other benzodiazepines, or any component of the formulation; concurrent therapy with itraconazole, ketoconazole, or nefazodone; pregnancy

Warnings/Precautions As a hypnotic, should be used only after evaluation of potential causes of sleep disturbance. Failure of sleep disturbance to resolve after 7-10 days may indicate psychiatric or medical illness. A worsening of insomnia or the emergence of new abnormalities of thought or behavior may represent unrecognized psychiatric or medical illness and requires immediate and careful evaluation. Prescription should be written for a maximum of 7-10 days and should not be prescribed in quantities exceeding a 1-month supply. Abrupt discontinuation after sustained use (generally >10 days) may cause withdrawal symptoms.

An increase in daytime anxiety may occur after as few as 10 days of continuous use, which may be related to withdrawal reaction in some patients. Anterograde amnesia may occur at a higher rate with triazolam than with other benzodiazepines. Use with caution in elderly or debilitated patients, patients with hepatic disease (including alcoholics), or renal impairment. Use with caution in patients with respiratory disease or impaired gag reflex. Avoid use in patients with sleep apnea.

In older adults, benzodiazepines increase the risk of impaired cognition, delirium, falls, fractures, and motor vehicle accidents. Due to increased sensitivity in this age group, avoid use for treatment of insomnia, agitation, or delirium. (Beers Criteria). Pharmacokinetics of triazolam are altered in older adults compared to younger adults (higher C_{max}, increased AUC, decreased clearance); the elderly also experience greater sedation and increased psychomotor impairment (Greenblatt, 1991).

In debilitated patients, benzodiazepines increase the risk for oversedation, impaired coordination, and dizziness with use.

Causes CNS depression (dose-related) resulting in sedation, dizziness, confusion, or ataxia which may impair physical and mental capabilities. Patients must be cautioned about performing tasks which require mental alertness (eg, operating machinery or driving). Use with caution in patients receiving other CNS depressants or psychoactive agents. Postmarketing studies have indicated that the use of hypnotic/sedative agents for sleep has been associated with hypersensitivity reactions including anaphylaxis as well as angioedema. An increased risk for hazardous sleep-related activities such as sleep-driving; cooking and eating food, and making phone calls while asleep have also been noted. Patients will often not remember doing these

◄ activities. Effects with other sedative drugs or ethanol may be potentiated. Benzodiazepines have been associated with falls and traumatic injury and should be used with extreme caution in patients who are at risk of these events (especially the elderly).

Avoid use with potent CYP3A4 inhibitors, as they may significantly decrease the clearance of triazolam. Use caution in patients with suicidal risk. Use with caution in patients with a history of drug dependence. Benzodiazepines have been associated with dependence and acute withdrawal symptoms on discontinuation or reduction in dose. Acute withdrawal, including seizures, may be precipitated after administration of flumazenil to patients receiving long-term benzodiazepine therapy.

Paradoxical reactions, including hyperactive or aggressive behavior have been reported with benzodiazepines, particularly in adolescent/pediatric or psychiatric patients. Evaluate any new changes in behavior. Does not have analgesic, antidepressant, or antipsychotic properties.

Drug Interactions

Metabolism/Transport Effects Substrate of CYP3A4 (major); **Note:** Assignment of Major/Minor substrate status based on clinically relevant drug interaction potential; **Inhibits** CYP2C8 (weak), CYP2C9 (weak)

Avoid Concomitant Use

Avoid concomitant use of Triazolam with any of the following: Azelastine (Nasal); Boceprevir; Cobicistat; Conivaptan; Efavirenz; OLANZapine; Paraldehyde; Protease Inhibitors; Sodium Oxybate; Telaprevir

Increased Effect/Toxicity

Triazolam may increase the levels/effects of: Alcohol (Ethyl); Azelastine (Nasal); Buprenorphine; CloZAPine; CNS Depressants; Fosphenytoin; Methotrimeprazine; Metyrosine; Mirtazapine; Paraldehyde; Phenytoin; Pramipexole; ROPINIRole; Rotigotine; Selective Serotonin Reuptake Inhibitors; Sodium Oxybate; Zolpidem

The levels/effects of Triazolam may be increased by: Antifungal Agents (Azole Derivatives, Systemic); Aprepitant; Boceprevir; Calcium Channel Blockers (Nondihydropyridine); Cimetidine; Cobicistat; Conivaptan; Contraceptives (Estrogens); Contraceptives (Progestins); CYP3A4 Inhibitors (Moderate); CYP3A4 Inhibitors (Strong); Dasatinib; Droperidol; Efavirenz; Fosaprepitant; Grapefruit Juice; HydrOXYzine; Isoniazid; Ivacaftor; Macrolide Antibiotics; Magnesium Sulfate; Methotrimeprazine; Mifepristone; OLANZapine; Perampanel; Protease Inhibitors; Proton Pump Inhibitors; Selective Serotonin Reuptake Inhibitors; Telaprevir

Decreased Effect

The levels/effects of Triazolam may be decreased by: CarBAMazepine; CYP3A4 Inducers (Strong); Deferasirox; Rifamycin Derivatives; St Johns Wort; Theophylline Derivatives; Tocilizumab; Yohimbine

Ethanol/Nutrition/Herb Interactions

Ethanol: Ethanol may increase CNS depression. Management: Limit or avoid ethanol consumption.

Food: Food may decrease the rate of absorption. Benzodiazepine serum concentrations may be increased by grapefruit juice. Management: Limit or avoid grapefruit juice.

Herb/Nutraceutical: St John's wort may decrease levels/effects of benzodiazepines. Other herbal medications may increase CNS depression. Management: Avoid St John's wort, valerian, kava kava, and gotu kola.

Pharmacodynamics/Kinetics

Onset of Action Hypnotic: 15-30 minutes

Half-life Elimination 1.5-5.5 hours

Time to Peak Oral: Within 2 hours

Pregnancy Risk Factor X

Pregnancy Considerations Triazolam was found to cross the placenta in animals. A case report describes placental transfer of triazolam following a maternal overdose. Teratogenic effects have been observed with some benzodiazepines; however, additional studies are needed. The incidence of premature birth and low birth weights may be increased following maternal use of benzodiazepines; hypoglycemia and respiratory problems in the neonate may occur following exposure late in pregnancy. Neonatal withdrawal symptoms may occur within days to weeks after birth and "floppy infant syndrome" (which also includes withdrawal symptoms) have been reported with some benzodiazepines. Use of triazolam is contraindicated in pregnant women.

Lactation Excretion in breast milk unknown/not recommended

Breast-Feeding Considerations Drowsiness, lethargy, or weight loss in nursing infants have been observed in case reports following maternal use of some benzodiazepines.

Controlled Substance C-IV

Dosage Forms

Tablet, oral: 0.125 mg, 0.25 mg

Halcion®: 0.25 mg

Dental Comment Triazolam (0.25 mg) 1 hour prior to dental procedure has been used as an oral preop sedative.

Triazolam is a benzodiazepine and is being used in dentistry as a preprocedural oral sedative. There has been recent interest in its use as an orally titratable sedative to render anxious patients at ease during difficult dental procedures. This technique has been referred to as enteral conscious sedation (ECS) and oral conscious sedation (OCS).

Triazolam has the shortest half-life of all the orally administered benzodiazepines. Although midazolam is shorter, it is used parenterally, not orally. The relatively fast onset of action (15-30 minutes) of triazolam offers an advantage in its use as an oral sedative. The clinician is reminded that no kinetic data has been reported with multiple titration doses of triazolam, a technique often used in the ECS/OCS regimen.

References

Berthold CW, Dionne RA, and Corey SE, "Comparison of Sublingually and Orally Administered Triazolam for Premedication Before Oral Surgery," *Oral Surg Oral Med Oral Pathol Oral Radiol Endod*, 1997, 84(2):119-24.

Berthold CW, Schneider A, and Dionne RA, "Using Triazolam to Reduce Dental Anxiety," *J Am Dent Assoc*, 1993, 124(11):58-64.

Dionne R, "Oral Sedation," *Compend Contin Educ Dent*, 1998, 19 (9):868-70.

Flanagan D, "Oral Triazolam Sedation in Implant Dentistry," *J Oral Implantol*, 2004, 30(2):93-7.

Goodchild JH, Feck AS, and Silverman MD, "Anxiolysis in General Dental Practice," *Dent Today*, 2003, 22(3):106-11.

Kaufman E, Hargreaves KM, and Dionne RA, "Comparison of Oral Triazolam and Nitrous Oxide With Placebo and Intravenous Diazepam for Outpatient Premedication," *Oral Surg Oral Med Oral Pathol*, 1993, 75(2):156-64.

Kurzrock M, "Triazolam and Dental Anxiety," *J Am Dent Assoc*, 1994, 125(4):358, 360.

Lieblich SE and Horswell B, "Attenuation of Anxiety in Ambulatory Oral Surgery Patients With Oral Triazolam," *J Oral Maxillofac Surg*, 1991, 49(8):792-7.

Matear DW and Clarke D, "Considerations for the Use of Oral Sedation in the Institutionalized Geriatric Patient During Dental Interventions: A Review of the Literature," *Spec Care Dentist*, 1999, 19(2):56-63.

Milgrom P, Quarnstrom FC, Longley A, et al, "The Efficacy and Memory Effects of Oral Triazolam Premedication in Highly Anxious Dental Patients," *Anesth Prog*, 1994, 41(3):70-6.

Quarnstrom F, "Should Dentists Do Oral Sedation?" *Dent Today*, 2004, 23(3):16-8.

Trichloroacetic Acid (trye klor oh a SEE tik AS id)

Brand Names: U.S. Tri-Chlor®

Pharmacologic Category Keratolytic Agent

Use Chemical used in compounding agents for the treatment of warts, skin resurfacing (chemical peels)

Local Anesthetic/Vasoconstrictor Precautions No information available to require special precautions

Effects on Dental Treatment No significant effects or complications reported

Effects on Bleeding No information available to require special precautions

Pregnancy Considerations Effective for treatment when used topically for the treatment of genital condylomas in pregnant women (Schwartz, 1988).

Triclosan and Fluoride (trye KLOE san & FLOR ide)

Related Information

Dentifrices With Antigingivitis Agents *on page 1646*

Dentifrices: No Sodium Lauryl Sulfate (SLS) *on page 1643*

Fluoride *on page 606*

Periodontal Diseases *on page 1570*

Brand Names: U.S. Colgate Total®

Generic Availability (U.S.) No

Pharmacologic Category Antibacterial, Dental; Mineral, Oral (Topical)

Dental Use Anticavity, antigingivitis, antiplaque toothpaste

Use Used exclusively in dental applications for the prevention of cavities, plaque, and gingivitis

Local Anesthetic/Vasoconstrictor Precautions No information available to require special precautions

Effects on Dental Treatment No significant effects or complications reported (see Dental Comment)

Effects on Bleeding No information available to require special precautions

Dental Usual Dosage Prevention of dental caries and gingivitis: Adults: Oral: Brush teeth thoroughly after each meal or at least twice daily

Dosage Oral: Children ≥6 years and Adults: Brush teeth thoroughly after each meal or at least twice daily

Mechanism of Action Triclosan is an antibacterial agent which helps to prevent gingivitis with regular use. Fluoride promotes remineralization of decalcified enamel, inhibits the cariogenic microbial process in dental plaque, and increases tooth resistance to acid dissolution

Warnings/Precautions Antigingivitis and antiplaque effects have not been determined in children <6 years of age. If an amount greater than used for brushing is swallowed, seek professional assistance of contact a poison control center immediately

Drug Interactions

Metabolism/Transport Effects None known.

Avoid Concomitant Use There are no known interactions where it is recommended to avoid concomitant use.

Increased Effect/Toxicity There are no known significant interactions involving an increase in effect.

Decreased Effect There are no known significant interactions involving a decrease in effect.

Pregnancy Considerations Refer to fluoride monograph.

Breast-Feeding Considerations Refer to fluoride monograph.

Dosage Forms

Gel, oral [toothpaste]:
Colgate Total®: Triclosan 0.30% and fluoride 0.24% (119 g, 170 g, 221 g)

Paste, oral [toothpaste]:
Colgate Total®: Triclosan 0.30% and fluoride 0.24% (119 g, 170 g, 221 g)

Dental Comment It has been shown that stannous fluoride and triclosan when formulated into a toothpaste vehicle provide plaque inhibitory effects. To provide a longer retention time of the triclosan in plaque, a polymer has been added to the toothpaste vehicle. The polymer is known as PVM/MA which stands for polyvinylmethyl ether/maleic acid copolymer, and is listed as an inactive ingredient (PVM/MA Copolymer) on the manufacturer's label. Studies have reported that the retention of triclosan in plaque (exceeding the minimal inhibitory concentration) after polymer application was 14 hours after brushing. Ongoing studies are evaluating the effects of triclosan/copolymer on alveolar bone loss. Rosling et al. have reported that the daily use of Colgate Total® reduced (1) the frequency of deep periodontal pockets and (2) the number of sites that exhibited additional probing attachment and bone loss.

References

Binney A, Addy M, Owens J, et al, "A Comparison of Triclosan and Stannous Fluoride Toothpastes for Inhibition of Plaque Regrowth. A Crossover Study Designed to Access Carry Over," *J Clin Periodontol*, 1997, 24(3):166-70.

Ellwood RP, Worthington HV, Blinkhorn AS, et al, "Effect of a Triclosan/Copolymer Dentifrice on the Incidence of Periodontal Attachment Loss in Adolescents," *J Clin Periodontol*, 1998, 25(5):363-7.

Mandel ID, "The New Toothpastes," *J Calif Dent Assoc*, 1998, 26 (3):186-90.

Rosling B, Wannfors B, Volpe AR, et al, "The Use of a Triclosan/Copolymer Dentifrice May Retard the Progression of Periodontitis," *J Clin Periodontol*, 1997, 24(12):873-80.

Trifluoperazine (trye floo oh PER a zeen)

Brand Names: Canada Apo-Trifluoperazine®; Novo-Trifluzine; PMS-Trifluoperazine; Terfluzine

Pharmacologic Category Antipsychotic Agent, Typical, Phenothiazine

Use Treatment of schizophrenia; short-term treatment of generalized nonpsychotic anxiety

Unlabeled Use Management of psychotic disorders; behavioral symptoms associated with dementia behavior (elderly); psychosis/agitation related to Alzheimer's dementia

Local Anesthetic/Vasoconstrictor Precautions Most pharmacology textbooks state that in presence of phenothiazines, systemic doses of epinephrine paradoxically decrease the blood pressure. This is the so called "epinephrine reversal" phenomenon. This has never been observed when epinephrine is given by infiltration as part of the anesthesia procedure.

Effects on Dental Treatment Key adverse event(s) related to dental treatment: Significant hypotension may occur, especially when the drug is administered parenterally; orthostatic hypotension is due to alpha-receptor blockade, the elderly are at greater risk for orthostatic hypotension. Xerostomia (normal salivary flow resumes upon discontinuation).

Tardive dyskinesia: Prevalence rate may be 40% in elderly; development of the syndrome and the irreversible nature are proportional to duration and total cumulative dose over time. Extrapyramidal reactions are more common in elderly with up to 50% developing these reactions after 60 years of age. Drug-induced Parkinson's syndrome occurs often; akathisia is the most common extrapyramidal reaction in elderly.

Effects on Bleeding No information available to require special precautions

Adverse Effects Frequency not defined.

Cardiovascular: Cardiac arrest, hypotension, orthostatic hypotension

Central nervous system: Dizziness; extrapyramidal symptoms (akathisia, dystonias, pseudoparkinsonism, tardive dyskinesia); headache, impairment of temperature regulation, lowering of seizure threshold, neuroleptic malignant syndrome (NMS)

Dermatologic: Discoloration of skin (blue-gray), increased sensitivity to sun, photosensitivity, rash

Endocrine & metabolic: Breast pain, galactorrhea, gynecomastia, hyperglycemia, hypoglycemia, lactation, libido (changes in), menstrual cycle (changes in)

Gastrointestinal: Constipation, nausea, stomach pain, vomiting, weight gain, xerostomia

Genitourinary: Difficulty in urination, ejaculatory disturbances, priapism, urinary retention

Hematologic: Agranulocytosis, aplastic anemia, eosinophilia, hemolytic anemia, leukopenia, pancytopenia, thrombocytopenic purpura

Hepatic: Cholestatic jaundice, hepatotoxicity

Neuromuscular & skeletal: Tremor

Ocular: Cornea and lens changes, pigmentary retinopathy

Respiratory: Nasal congestion

General Dosage Range Oral:

Children 6-12 years: Initial: 1 mg 1-2 times/day; Maintenance: 1-15 mg/day in 1-2 divided doses (maximum: 15 mg/day)

Adults: Inpatient: Initial: 2-5 mg twice daily; Maintenance: 15-40 mg/day in 2 divided doses (maximum: 40 mg/day); Outpatient: Initial: 1-3 mg twice daily (maximum: 40 mg/day)

Mechanism of Action Trifluoperazine is a piperazine phenothiazine antipsychotic which blocks postsynaptic mesolimbic dopaminergic receptors in the brain; exhibits alpha-adrenergic blocking effect and depresses the release of hypothalamic and hypophyseal hormones

Pharmacodynamics/Kinetics

Half-life Elimination >24 hours with chronic use

Pregnancy Considerations Adverse events were not observed in animal reproduction studies, except when using doses that were also maternally toxic. Jaundice or hyper-/hyporeflexia have been reported in newborn infants following maternal use of phenothiazines. Antipsychotic use during the third trimester of pregnancy has a risk for abnormal muscle movements (extrapyramidal symptoms [EPS]) and withdrawal symptoms in newborns following delivery. Symptoms in the newborn may include agitation, feeding disorder, hypertonia, hypotonia, respiratory distress, somnolence, and tremor; these effects may be self-limiting or require hospitalization.

Trifluridine (trye FLURE i deen)

Related Information

Systemic Viral Diseases *on page 1537*

Brand Names: U.S. Viroptic®

Brand Names: Canada Sandoz-Trifluridine; Viroptic®

Pharmacologic Category Antiviral Agent, Ophthalmic

Use Treatment of primary keratoconjunctivitis and recurrent epithelial keratitis caused by herpes simplex virus types I and II

Local Anesthetic/Vasoconstrictor Precautions No information available to require special precautions

Effects on Dental Treatment No significant effects or complications reported

Effects on Bleeding No information available to require special precautions

Adverse Effects Ocular: Burning or stinging (5%), palpebral edema (3%), epithelial keratopathy, hyperemia, hypersensitivity reactions, irritation, keratitis sicca, ocular pressure increased, stromal edema, superficial punctate keratopathy

General Dosage Range Ophthalmic: *Children ≥6 years, Adolescents, and Adults:* Initial: Instill 1 drop into affected eye(s) every 2 hours while awake (maximum: 9 drops daily); After re-epithelialization of corneal ulcer: 1 drop every 4 hours (maximum: 21 days of treatment)

Mechanism of Action Interferes with viral replication by inhibiting thymidylate synthetase and incorporating into viral DNA in place of thymidine.

Pharmacodynamics/Kinetics

Half-life Elimination 12 minutes

Pregnancy Risk Factor C

Pregnancy Considerations Adverse effects were not observed during animal reproduction studies of the ophthalmic solution.

Trihexyphenidyl (trye heks ee FEN i dil)

Brand Names: Canada PMS-Trihexyphenidyl; Trihexyphen; Trihexyphenidyl

Generic Availability (U.S.) Yes

Pharmacologic Category Anti-Parkinson's Agent, Anticholinergic; Anticholinergic Agent

Use Adjunctive treatment of Parkinson's disease; treatment of drug-induced extrapyramidal symptoms

Local Anesthetic/Vasoconstrictor Precautions No information available to require special precautions

Effects on Dental Treatment Key adverse event(s) related to dental treatment: Xerostomia, dry throat (normal salivary flow resumes upon discontinuation). Prolonged xerostomia may contribute to discomfort and dental disease (ie, caries, periodontal disease, and oral candidiasis).

Effects on Bleeding No information available to require special precautions

Adverse Effects Frequency not defined.

Cardiovascular: Tachycardia

Central nervous system: Agitation, confusion, delusions, dizziness, drowsiness, euphoria, hallucinations, headache, nervousness, paranoia, psychiatric disturbances

Dermatologic: Rash

Gastrointestinal: Constipation, dilatation of colon, ileus, nausea, parotitis, vomiting, xerostomia

Genitourinary: Urinary retention

Neuromuscular & skeletal: Weakness

Ocular: Blurred vision, glaucoma, intraocular pressure increased, mydriasis

Dosage Oral:

Adults:

Parkinson's disease: Initial: 1 mg/day, increase by 2 mg increments at intervals of 3-5 days; usual dose: 6-10 mg/day in 3-4 divided doses; doses of 12-15 mg/day may be required

Drug-induced EPS: Initial: 1 mg/day; increase as necessary to usual range: 5-15 mg/day in 3-4 divided doses

Use in combination with levodopa: Usual range: 3-6 mg/day in divided doses

Elderly: Parkinson's disease: Refer to adult dosing. **Note:** Conservative initial doses and gradual titration is especially important in patients >60 years of age.

Mechanism of Action Exerts a direct inhibitory effect on the parasympathetic nervous system. It also has a relaxing effect on smooth musculature; exerted both directly on the muscle itself and indirectly through parasympathetic nervous system (inhibitory effect)

Contraindications There are no contraindications listed within the manufacturer's labeling.

Warnings/Precautions Use with caution in hot weather or during exercise, especially when administered concomitantly with other atropine-like drugs to chronically-ill patients, alcoholics, patients with CNS disease, or persons doing manual labor in a hot environment. Use with caution in patients with cardiovascular disease (including hypertension), glaucoma, prostatic hyperplasia or any tendency toward urinary retention, liver or kidney disorders, and obstructive disease of the GI tract. May exacerbate mental symptoms when used to treat extrapyramidal symptoms. When given in large doses or to susceptible patients, may cause weakness. May impair physical or mental abilities; patients must be cautioned about performing tasks which require mental alertness (eg, operating machinery or driving). Does not improve symptoms of tardive dyskinesias. Avoid use in older adults; not recommended for prevention of extrapyramidal symptoms with antipsychotics; alternative agents preferred in the treatment of Parkinson disease. May be inappropriate in older adults depending on comorbidities(eg, dementia, delirium) due to its potent anticholinergic effects (Beers Criteria).

Drug Interactions

Metabolism/Transport Effects None known.

Avoid Concomitant Use

Avoid concomitant use of Trihexyphenidyl with any of the following: Aclidinium; Ipratropium (Oral Inhalation); Potassium Chloride; Tiotropium

Increased Effect/Toxicity

Trihexyphenidyl may increase the levels/effects of: AbobotulinumtoxinA; Anticholinergics; Cannabinoids; Mirabegron; OnabotulinumtoxinA; Potassium Chloride; RimabotulinumtoxinB; Tiotropium; Topiramate

The levels/effects of Trihexyphenidyl may be increased by: Aclidinium; Ipratropium (Oral Inhalation); Pramlintide

Decreased Effect

Trihexyphenidyl may decrease the levels/effects of: Acetylcholinesterase Inhibitors (Central); Secretin

The levels/effects of Trihexyphenidyl may be decreased by: Acetylcholinesterase Inhibitors (Central)

Ethanol/Nutrition/Herb Interactions Ethanol: Avoid ethanol (may increase CNS depression).

Dietary Considerations May be taken before or after meals; tolerated best if given with food.

Pharmacodynamics/Kinetics

Half-life Elimination 33 hours

Time to Peak Serum: 1.3 hours

Pregnancy Risk Factor C

Pregnancy Considerations Animal reproduction studies have not been conducted. One case report did not show evidence of adverse events after trihexyphenidyl administration during pregnancy (Robottom, 2011).

Lactation Excretion in breast milk unknown/use caution

Breast-Feeding Considerations Anticholinergic agents may suppress lactation.

Dosage Forms

Elixir, oral: 2 mg/5 mL (473 mL)

Tablet, oral: 2 mg, 5 mg

Trimethobenzamide (trye meth oh BEN za mide)

Brand Names: U.S. Tigan®

Brand Names: Canada Tigan®

Pharmacologic Category Antiemetic

Use Treatment of postoperative nausea and vomiting; treatment of nausea associated with gastroenteritis

Local Anesthetic/Vasoconstrictor Precautions No information available to require special precautions

Effects on Dental Treatment No significant effects or complications reported

Effects on Bleeding No information available to require special precautions

Adverse Effects Frequency not defined.

Cardiovascular: Hypotension (I.V. administration)

Central nervous system: Coma, depression, disorientation, dizziness, drowsiness, EPS, headache, Parkinson-like symptoms, seizure

Dermatologic: Allergic-type skin reactions

Gastrointestinal: Diarrhea

Hematologic: Blood dyscrasias

Hepatic: Jaundice

Local: Injection site burning, pain, redness, stinging, or swelling

Neuromuscular & skeletal: Muscle cramps, opisthotonos

Ocular: Blurred vision

Miscellaneous: Hypersensitivity reactions

General Dosage Range

I.M.: *Adults:* 200 mg 3-4 times/day **or** 200 mg as a single dose, repeat 1 hour later

Oral: *Children >40 kg and Adults:* 300 mg 3-4 times/day

Mechanism of Action Acts centrally to inhibit the medullary chemoreceptor trigger zone by blocking emetic impulses to the vomiting center

Pharmacodynamics/Kinetics

Onset of Action Antiemetic: Oral: 10-40 minutes; I.M.: 15-35 minutes

Duration of Action 3-4 hours

Half-life Elimination 7-9 hours

Time to Peak Oral: ~45 minutes; I.M.: ~30 minutes

Pregnancy Considerations Teratogenic effects were not observed in animal studies. Safety and efficacy have not been established in pregnant patients. Trimethobenzamide has been used to treat nausea and vomiting of pregnancy.

Dental Comment Consider trimethobenzamide as a safer alternative to phenothiazines (ie, promethazine) to prevent nausea and vomiting or treat mild nausea and vomiting.

Trimethoprim (trye METH oh prim)

Brand Names: U.S. Primsol®

Brand Names: Canada Apo-Trimethoprim®

Pharmacologic Category Antibiotic, Miscellaneous

◄ **Use** Treatment of urinary tract infections due to susceptible strains of *E. coli, P. mirabilis, K. pneumoniae, Enterobacter* spp and coagulase-negative *Staphylococcus* including *S. saprophyticus*; acute otitis media due to susceptible strains of *S. pneumoniae* and *H. influenzae* in children

Unlabeled Use Alternative agent for *Pneumocystis jirovecii* pneumonia (in combination with dapsone)

Local Anesthetic/Vasoconstrictor Precautions No information available to require special precautions

Effects on Dental Treatment Key adverse event(s) related to dental treatment: Glossitis.

Effects on Bleeding Trimethoprim has been shown to induce acute thrombocytopenic purpura, as a consequence of immune-mediated platelet destruction. Platelet numbers as low as <5 x 10^9 /L have been observed with normal white blood cell counts. A review of clinical case reports indicates the thrombocytopenic purpura risk typically occurs when trimethoprim is coadministered with sulfamethoxazole. Clinicians should be aware of this adverse effect and closely observe patients for cutaneous manifestations and bleeding attributable to thrombocytopenia in order to withdraw the drug promptly.

Adverse Effects Frequency not defined.

Central nervous system: Aseptic meningitis (rare), fever

Dermatologic: Maculopapular rash (3% to 7% at 200 mg/day; incidence higher with larger daily doses), erythema multiforme (rare), exfoliative dermatitis (rare), pruritus (common), phototoxic skin eruptions, Stevens-Johnson syndrome (rare), toxic epidermal necrolysis (rare)

Endocrine & metabolic: Hyperkalemia, hyponatremia

Gastrointestinal: Epigastric distress, glossitis, nausea, vomiting

Hematologic: Leukopenia, megaloblastic anemia, methemoglobinemia, neutropenia, thrombocytopenia

Hepatic: Cholestatic jaundice (rare), liver enzymes increased

Renal: BUN and creatinine increased

Miscellaneous: Anaphylaxis, hypersensitivity reactions

General Dosage Range Dosage adjustment recommended in patients with renal impairment

Oral:

Children ≥2 months: 4-12 mg/kg/day in divided doses every 12 hours

Adults: 100 mg once daily **or** 100 mg every 12 hours **or** 200 mg every 24 hours; up to 15mg/kg/day

Mechanism of Action Inhibits folic acid reduction to tetrahydrofolate, and thereby inhibits microbial growth

Pharmacodynamics/Kinetics

Half-life Elimination 8-14 hours; prolonged with renal impairment

Time to Peak Serum: 1-4 hours

Pregnancy Risk Factor C

Pregnancy Considerations Because adverse effects have been observed in animals, trimethoprim is classified pregnancy category C. Trimethoprim crosses the placenta and can be detected in the fetal serum and amniotic fluid. Due to trimethoprim's potential effect on folic acid metabolism, TMP should only be used during pregnancy if the benefit justifies the potential risk. The use of dihydrofolate reductase inhibitors, including trimethoprim, during pregnancy may increase the risk of congenital anomalies including cardiovascular defects, oral clefts, urinary tract anomalies, and neural tube defects. Folic acid supplementation may decrease this risk. The majority of studies evaluating the effects of trimethoprim administration in pregnancy have been conducted with sulfamethoxazole/trimethoprim.

Trimethoprim in combination with sulfamethoxazole is used in pregnancy for various indications (see the Sulfamethoxazole and Trimethoprim monograph for details).

Trimethoprim and Polymyxin B
(trye METH oh prim & pol i MIKS in bee)

Related Information

Polymyxin B *on page 1112*

Trimethoprim *on page 1365*

Brand Names: U.S. Polytrim®

Brand Names: Canada PMS-Polytrimethoprim; Polytrim™

Pharmacologic Category Antibiotic, Ophthalmic

Use Treatment of surface ocular bacterial conjunctivitis and blepharoconjunctivitis

Local Anesthetic/Vasoconstrictor Precautions No information available to require special precautions

Effects on Dental Treatment No significant effects or complications reported

Effects on Bleeding Trimethoprim has been shown to induce acute thrombocytopenic purpura, as a consequence of immune-mediated platelet destruction. Platelet numbers as low as <5 x 10^9 /L have been observed with normal white blood cell counts. A review of clinical case reports indicates the thrombocytopenic purpura risk typically occurs when trimethoprim is coadministered with sulfamethoxazole. Clinicians should be aware of this adverse effect and closely observe patients for cutaneous manifestations and bleeding attributable to thrombocytopenia in order to withdraw the drug promptly.

Adverse Effects Frequency not defined: Ocular: Burning, itching, edema, rash, redness increased, stinging, tearing

General Dosage Range Ophthalmic: *Children ≥2 months and Adults:* Instill 1 drop in affected eye(s) every 3 hours (maximum: 6 doses per day) for 7-10 days

Pregnancy Risk Factor C

Pregnancy Considerations Teratogenic events have been observed with trimethoprim in animal studies; animal reproduction studies have not been conducted with polymyxin B. Trimethoprim/polymyxin B is classified as pregnancy category C. Due to trimethoprim's potential effect on folic acid metabolism, trimethoprim should only be used during pregnancy if the benefit justifies the potential risk. See individual agents.

Trimipramine (trye MI pra meen)

Related Information

Vasoconstrictor Interactions With Antidepressants *on page 1650*

Brand Names: U.S. Surmontil®

Brand Names: Canada Apo-Trimip®; Nu-Trimipramine; Rhotrimine®; Surmontil®

Pharmacologic Category Antidepressant, Tricyclic (Tertiary Amine)

Use Treatment of depression

Local Anesthetic/Vasoconstrictor Precautions

Use with caution; epinephrine and levonordefrin have been shown to have an increased pressor response in combination with TCAs. Trimipramine is one of the drugs confirmed to prolong the QT interval and is accepted as having a risk of causing torsade de pointes. The risk of drug-induced torsade de pointes is extremely low when a single QT interval prolonging drug is prescribed. In terms of epinephrine, it is not known what effect vasoconstrictors in the local anesthetic regimen will have in patients with a known history of congenital prolonged QT interval or in patients taking any medication that prolongs the QT interval. Until more information is obtained, it is suggested that the clinician consult with the physician prior to the use of a vasoconstrictor in suspected patients, and that the vasoconstrictor (epinephrine, mepivacaine and levonordefrin [Carbocaine® 2% with Neo-Cobefrin®]) be used with caution.

Effects on Dental Treatment Key adverse event(s) related to dental treatment: Xerostomia (normal salivary flow resumes upon discontinuation) and unpleasant taste. Long-term treatment with TCAs, such as trimipramine, increases the risk of caries by reducing salivation and salivary buffer capacity.

Effects on Bleeding No information available to require special precautions

Adverse Effects Frequency not defined.

Cardiovascular: Arrhythmias, facial edema, flushing, heart block, hyper-/hypotension, MI, palpitation, stroke, tachycardia

Central nervous system: Agitation, anxiety, confusion, delusions, disorientation, dizziness, drowsiness, EEG abnormalities, exacerbation of psychosis, fatigue, hallucinations, headache, hypomania, insomnia, nightmares, restlessness, seizure

Dermatologic: Alopecia, itching, petechiae, photosensitivity, rash, urticaria

Endocrine & metabolic: Breast enlargement, galactorrhea, gynecomastia, hyper-/hypoglycemia, libido (changes in), parotid swelling, syndrome of inappropriate ADH secretion (SIADH)

Gastrointestinal: Abdominal cramps, anorexia, black tongue, constipation, diarrhea, epigastric distress, nausea, paralytic ileus, stomatitis, tongue edema, unpleasant taste, tongue edema, vomiting, weight gain/loss, xerostomia

Genitourinary: Delayed/difficult urination, impotence, polyuria, testicular edema, urinary retention

Hematologic: Agranulocytosis, eosinophilia, purpura, thrombocytopenia

Hepatic: Cholestatic jaundice, liver enzymes increased

Neuromuscular & skeletal: Ataxia, extrapyramidal symptoms, incoordination, numbness, paresthesia, peripheral neuropathy, tingling, tremor, weakness

Ocular: Blurred vision, disturbances in accommodation, mydriasis

Otic: Tinnitus

Miscellaneous: Diaphoresis, withdrawal syndrome

General Dosage Range

Oral:

Adolescents: Initial: 50 mg/day (maximum: 100 mg/day)

Adults: 50-200 mg at bedtime (maximum: 200 mg/day [outpatient] or 300 mg/day [inpatient])

Elderly: 50-100 mg at bedtime (maximum: 100 mg/day)

Mechanism of Action Increases the synaptic concentration of serotonin and/or norepinephrine in the central nervous system by inhibition of their reuptake by the presynaptic neuronal membrane

Pharmacodynamics/Kinetics

Half-life Elimination 16-40 hours

Pregnancy Risk Factor C

Pregnancy Considerations Adverse events have been observed in animal reproduction studies.

Dental Comment Trimipramine is known to prolong the QT interval. The QT interval is measured as the time and distance between the Q point of the QRS complex and the end of the T wave in the ECG tracing. After adjustment for heart rate, the QT interval is defined as prolonged if it is more than 450 msec in men and 460 msec in women. A long QT syndrome was first described in the 1950s and 60s as a congenital syndrome involving QT interval prolongation and syncope and sudden death. Some of the congenital long QT syndromes were characterized by a peculiar electrocardiographic appearance of the QRS complex involving a premature atria beat followed by a pause, then a subsequent sinus beat showing marked QT prolongation and deformity. This type of cardiac arrhythmia was originally termed "torsade de pointes" (translated from the French for "twisting of the points"). Trimipramine is considered as having a risk of causing torsade de pointes. Since it is not known what effect vasoconstrictors in the local anesthetic regimen will have in patients with a known history of congenital prolonged QT interval or in patients taking any medication that prolongs the QT interval, a medical consult is suggested.

Triprolidine and Pseudoephedrine
(trye PROE li deen & soo doe e FED rin)

Related Information

Pseudoephedrine *on page 1159*

Brand Names: U.S. Aprodine [OTC]; Pediatex® TD; Silafed [OTC]

Brand Names: Canada Actifed®

Pharmacologic Category Alkylamine Derivative; Alpha/Beta Agonist; Decongestant; Histamine H_1 Antagonist; Histamine H_1 Antagonist, First Generation

Use Temporary relief of nasal congestion, decongest sinus openings, running nose, sneezing, itching of nose or throat and itchy, watery eyes due to common cold, hay fever, or other upper respiratory allergies

Local Anesthetic/Vasoconstrictor Precautions Use with caution since pseudoephedrine is a sympathomimetic amine which could interact with epinephrine to cause a pressor response

Effects on Dental Treatment Key adverse event(s) related to dental treatment: Pseudoephedrine: Xerostomia (normal salivary flow resumes upon discontinuation). Chronic use of antihistamines will inhibit salivary flow, particularly in elderly patients; this may contribute to periodontal disease and oral discomfort.

Effects on Bleeding No information available to require special precautions

Adverse Effects Frequency not defined.

Cardiovascular: Tachycardia

Central nervous system: Dizziness, drowsiness, fatigue, headache, insomnia, nervousness, transient stimulation

Gastrointestinal: Abdominal pain, appetite increase, diarrhea, nausea, weight gain, xerostomia

Genitourinary: Dysuria

Neuromuscular & skeletal: Arthralgia, weakness

Respiratory: Pharyngitis, thickening of bronchial secretions

Miscellaneous: Diaphoresis

General Dosage Range Oral: *Children ≥6 years and Adults:* Dosage varies greatly depending on product

Mechanism of Action Refer to Pseudoephedrine monograph.

Triprolidine is a member of the propylamine (alkylamine) chemical class of H_1-antagonist antihistamines. As such, it is considered to be relatively less sedating than traditional antihistamines of the ethanolamine, phenothiazine, and ethylenediamine classes of antihistamines. Triprolidine has a shorter half-life and duration of action than most of the other alkylamine antihistamines. Like all H_1-antagonist antihistamines, the mechanism of action of triprolidine is believed to involve competitive blockade of H_1-receptor sites resulting in the inability of histamine to combine with its receptor sites and exert its usual effects on target cells. Antihistamines do not interrupt any effects of histamine which have already occurred. Therefore, these agents are used more successfully in the prevention rather than the treatment of histamine-induced reactions.

Pharmacodynamics/Kinetics

Half-life Elimination Triprolidine: ~2 hours (Simons, 1986)

Time to Peak Serum: Triprolidine: ~2 hours (Simons, 1986)

Pregnancy Considerations Maternal antihistamine use has generally not resulted in an increased risk of birth defects; however, information related to triprolidine is limited. Refer to the pseudoephedrine monograph for information related to decongestants.

Triprolidine, Pseudoephedrine, and Codeine (trye PROE li deen, soo doe e FED rin, & KOE deen)

Related Information

Codeine on page 344
Pseudoephedrine on page 1159

Brand Names: Canada CoActifed®; Covan®; ratio-Cotridin

Pharmacologic Category Alkylamine Derivative; Alpha/Beta Agonist; Analgesic, Opioid; Antitussive; Decongestant; Histamine H_1 Antagonist; Histamine H_1 Antagonist, First Generation

Use Symptomatic relief of upper respiratory symptoms and cough

Local Anesthetic/Vasoconstrictor Precautions Use with caution since pseudoephedrine is a sympathomimetic amine which could interact with epinephrine to cause a pressor response

Effects on Dental Treatment Key adverse event(s) related to dental treatment: Pseudoephedrine: Xerostomia (normal salivary flow resumes upon discontinuation) and taste disturbance.

Effects on Bleeding No information available to require special precautions

Adverse Effects Frequency not defined.

Cardiovascular: Hypotension
Central nervous system: Agitation, dizziness, drowsiness, dysphoria, euphoria, hallucination, headache, ICP increased, lightheadedness, sedation, seizure
Dermatologic: Pruritus, rash
Gastrointestinal: Constipation, nausea, vomiting, anorexia, xerostomia, taste disturbance, biliary tract spasm
Genitourinary: Urinary retention, urinary tract spasm
Neuromuscular & skeletal: Muscle tremor, paresthesia, muscular rigidity (rare)
Ocular: Blurred vision, nystagmus
Respiratory: Respiratory depression
Miscellaneous: Diaphoresis, physical or psychological dependence with continued use, withdrawal syndrome

General Dosage Range Oral:

Children 2-6 years: 2.5 mL 4 times/day
Children 7-12 years: 5 mL 4 times/day or 1/2 tablet 4 times/day
Children >12 years and Adults: 10 mL 4 times/day or 1 tablet 4 times/day

---

Pregnancy Considerations See individual agents.
Product Availability Not available in U.S.
Controlled Substance CDSA-I

Triptorelin (trip toe REL in)

Brand Names: U.S. Trelstar®
Brand Names: Canada Decapeptyl®; Trelstar®
Pharmacologic Category Gonadotropin Releasing Hormone Agonist
Use Palliative treatment of advanced prostate cancer

Decapeptyl® (Canadian labeling; not available in U.S.): Adjunctive therapy in women undergoing controlled ovarian hyperstimulation for assisted reproductive technologies (ART)

Unlabeled Use Treatment of endometriosis, in vitro fertilization, precocious puberty, uterine sarcoma; treatment of paraphilia/hypersexuality

Local Anesthetic/Vasoconstrictor Precautions No information available to require special precautions

Effects on Dental Treatment No significant effects or complications reported

Effects on Bleeding Although significant myelosuppression with associated altered hemostasis has been reported for many chemotherapeutic agents, myelosuppression is not common with triptorelin and no specific precautions appear to be necessary.

Adverse Effects Prostate cancer: As reported with all strengths; frequency of effect may vary by strength:

>10%:
Endocrine & metabolic: Hot flashes (59% to 73%), glucose increased, testosterone levels increased (peak: days 2-4; decline to low levels by weeks 3-4)
Hematologic: Hemoglobin decreased, RBC count decreased
Hepatic: Alkaline phosphatase increased (2% to >10%), ALT increased, AST increased
Neuromuscular & skeletal: Skeletal pain (12% to 13%)
Renal: BUN increased

1% to 10%:
Cardiovascular: Leg edema (6%), hypertension (1% to 4%), chest pain (2%), edema (2%), peripheral edema (≤1%)
Central nervous system: Headache (2% to 7%), pain (2% to 3%), dizziness (1% to 3%), fatigue (2%), insomnia (1% to 2%), emotional lability (1%)
Dermatologic: Rash (2%), pruritus (1%)
Endocrine & metabolic: Breast pain (2%), gynecomastia (2%), libido decreased (2%)
Gastrointestinal: Nausea (3%), anorexia (2%), constipation (2%), dyspepsia (2%), vomiting (2%), abdominal pain (1%), diarrhea (1%)
Genitourinary: Erectile dysfunction (10%), testicular atrophy (8%), impotence (2% to 7%), dysuria (5%), urinary retention (≤1%), urinary tract infection (≤1%)
Hematologic: Anemia (1%)
Local: Injection site pain (4%)
Neuromuscular & skeletal: Leg pain (2% to 5%), back pain (1% to 3%), leg cramps (2%), arthralgia (1% to 2%), extremity pain (1%), myalgia (1%), weakness (1%)
Ocular: Conjunctivitis (1%), eye pain (1%)
Respiratory: Cough (2%), dyspnea (1%), pharyngitis (1%)

Reproductive studies:
>10%:
Central nervous system: Headache (4% to 27%)
Gastrointestinal: Abdominal pain (9% to 15%)

Genitourinary: Vaginal hemorrhage (2% to 24%)
Local: Injection site inflammation (10% to 12%)
1% to 10%:
Cardiovascular: Flushing (4%)
Central nervous system: Dizziness (4% to 5%), fatigue (3% to 4%), malaise (2%)
Endocrine & metabolic: Spontaneous abortion (7%), dysmenorrhea (2% to 6%), OHSS (3%), hot flashes (2%), ovarian cyst (1%)
Gastrointestinal: Nausea (3% to 10%), vomiting (3%), abdominal distension (2%), diarrhea (2%)
Genitourinary: Pelvic pain (6%), adnexa uteri pain (2%), leukorrhea (2%)
Local: Injection site pain (4% to 7%), injection site bruising (3%), injection site reaction (2% to 3%)
Neuromuscular & skeletal: Postprocedural pain (4%), back pain (3%), postoperative pain (3%)
Respiratory: Upper respiratory tract infection (4%), pharyngitis (3%), dyspnea (2%), rhinitis (2%)
Miscellaneous: Influenza-like symptoms (3%)

General Dosage Range I.M.: *Adults:* 3.75 mg once every 4 weeks **or** 11.25 mg once every 12 weeks **or** 22.5 mg once every 24 weeks

Mechanism of Action Causes suppression of ovarian and testicular steroidogenesis due to decreased levels of LH and FSH with subsequent decrease in testosterone (male) and estrogen (female) levels. After chronic and continuous administration, usually 2-4 weeks after initiation, a sustained decrease in LH and FSH secretion occurs. When used for ART, prevents premature LH surge in women undergoing controlled ovarian hyperstimulation.

Pharmacodynamics/Kinetics
Half-life Elimination 2.8 ± 1.2 hours
Moderate-to-severe renal impairment: 6.5-7.7 hours
Hepatic impairment: 7.6 hours
Time to Peak 1-3 hours
Pregnancy Risk Factor X
Pregnancy Considerations Use is contraindicated in pregnant women. When used for ART, pregnancy must be ruled out prior to therapy and nonhormonal contraception should be used until menses occurs. Due to the short half-life of triptorelin (formulations used for ART), it is not expected to be present in the maternal serum at the time of embryo transfer. In case reports, spontaneous abortion, congenital anomalies, and other adverse events have been reported following triptorelin (Decapeptyl®) exposure during pregnancy.

Trolamine (TROLE a meen)

Brand Names: U.S. Aspercreme® [OTC]; Flex-Power [OTC]; Mobisyl® [OTC]; Myoflex® [OTC]; Sportscreme® [OTC]
Brand Names: Canada Antiphlogistine Rub A-535 No Odour; Myoflex®
Pharmacologic Category Analgesic, Topical; Salicylate; Topical Skin Product
Use Relief of pain of muscular aches, rheumatism, neuralgia, sprains, arthritis on intact skin
Local Anesthetic/Vasoconstrictor Precautions No information available to require special precautions
Effects on Dental Treatment No significant effects or complications reported
Effects on Bleeding No information available to require special precautions

Adverse Effects 1% to 10%:
Central nervous system: Confusion, drowsiness
Gastrointestinal: Nausea, vomiting, diarrhea
Respiratory: Hyperventilation
General Dosage Range Topical: *Children ≥12 years and Adults:* Apply to affected area as needed up to 3-4 times/day
Pregnancy Considerations Systemic absorption of salicylate occurs following topical administration of trolamine (Rabinowitz, 1984).

Tromethamine (troe METH a meen)

Brand Names: U.S. THAM®
Pharmacologic Category Alkalinizing Agent, Parenteral
Use Correction of metabolic acidosis associated with cardiac bypass surgery or cardiac arrest; to correct excess acidity of stored blood that is preserved with acid citrate dextrose (ACD); indicated in infants needing alkalinization after receiving maximum sodium bicarbonate (8-10 mEq/kg/24 hours)
Local Anesthetic/Vasoconstrictor Precautions No information available to require special precautions
Effects on Dental Treatment No significant effects or complications reported
Effects on Bleeding No information available to require special precautions
Adverse Effects Frequency not defined.
Cardiovascular: Hypervolemia, venospasm
Endocrine & metabolic: Hyperkalemia, hypoglycemia (usually doses >500 mg/kg administered over <1 hour)
Hepatic: Hepatic necrosis (resulted during delivery via umbilical venous catheter)
Local: Necrosis with extravasation, phlebitis, tissue irritation
Respiratory: Apnea, pulmonary edema, respiratory depression
General Dosage Range
I.V.:
Infants: Initial: Approximately 1 mL/kg for each pH unit below 7.4; additional doses determined by changes in PaO_2, pH, and pCO_2
Adults: 3.6-10.8 g (111-333 mL) **or** 9 mL/kg (maximum: 500 mg/kg) **or** 15-77 mL added to each 500 mL of blood
Intraventricular: *Adults:* 3.6-10.8 g (111-333 mL) **or** 9 mL/kg (maximum: 500 mg/kg) **or** 15-77 mL added to each 500 mL of blood
Mechanism of Action Acts as a proton acceptor, which combines with hydrogen ions, liberating bicarbonate buffer, to correct acidosis. It buffers both metabolic and respiratory acids, limiting carbon dioxide generation. Also an osmotic diuretic.
Pharmacodynamics/Kinetics
Half-life Elimination 5.6 hours
Pregnancy Risk Factor C
Pregnancy Considerations Animal studies have not been conducted. There are no adequate and well-controlled studies in pregnant women. Use only if potential benefit outweighs possible risk to the fetus.

Tropicamide (troe PIK a mide)

Brand Names: U.S. Mydriacyl®; Tropicacyl®
Brand Names: Canada Diotrope®; Mydriacyl®
Pharmacologic Category Ophthalmic Agent, Mydriatic

Use Short-acting mydriatic used in diagnostic procedures; as well as preoperatively and postoperatively; treatment of some cases of acute iritis, iridocyclitis, and keratitis

Local Anesthetic/Vasoconstrictor Precautions No information available to require special precautions

Effects on Dental Treatment Key adverse event(s) related to dental treatment: Dryness of mouth.

Effects on Bleeding No information available to require special precautions

Adverse Effects Frequency not defined.

Cardiovascular: Edema, tachycardia, vascular congestion

Central nervous system: Headache, parasympathetic stimulations, somnolence

Dermatologic: Eczematoid dermatitis

Gastrointestinal: Dryness of mouth

Local: Transient stinging

Ocular: Blurred vision, follicular conjunctivitis, increased intraocular pressure, photophobia with or without corneal staining

General Dosage Range Ophthalmic: *Children and Adults:* 0.5%: Instill 1-2 drops 15-20 minutes before exam, may repeat; 1%: Instill 1-2 drops, may repeat in 5 minutes

Mechanism of Action Prevents the sphincter muscle of the iris and the muscle of the ciliary body from responding to cholinergic stimulation

Pharmacodynamics/Kinetics

Onset of Action Mydriasis: ~20-40 minutes; Cycloplegia: ~30 minutes

Duration of Action Mydriasis: ~6-7 hours; Cycloplegia: <6 hours

Pregnancy Risk Factor C

Pregnancy Considerations Animal reproduction studies have not been conducted.

Trospium (TROSE pee um)

Brand Names: U.S. Sanctura®; Sanctura® XR

Brand Names: Canada Sanctura® XR; Trosec

Pharmacologic Category Anticholinergic Agent

Use Treatment of overactive bladder with symptoms of urgency, incontinence, and urinary frequency

Local Anesthetic/Vasoconstrictor Precautions No information available to require special precautions

Effects on Dental Treatment Key adverse event(s) related to dental treatment: Significant xerostomia and changes in salivation (normal salivary flow resumes upon discontinuation).

Effects on Bleeding No information available to require special precautions

Adverse Effects

>10%: Gastrointestinal: Xerostomia (9% to 22%)

1% to 10%:

Cardiovascular: Tachycardia (<2%)

Central nervous system: Headache (4% to 7%), fatigue (2%)

Dermatologic: Rash (<2%), dry skin

Gastrointestinal: Constipation (9% to 10%), abdominal pain (1% to 3%), dyspepsia (1% to 2%), flatulence (1% to 2%), nausea (1%), abdominal distention (<2%), taste abnormal, vomiting

Genitourinary: Urinary tract infection (1% to 7%), urinary retention (≤1%)

Ocular: Dry eyes (1% to 2%), blurred vision (1%)

Respiratory: Nasopharyngitis (3%), nasal dryness (1%)

Miscellaneous: Influenza (2%)

General Dosage Range Dosage adjustment recommended in patients with renal impairment

Oral:

Adults <75 years: Immediate release: 20 mg twice daily; Extended release: 60 mg once daily

Elderly ≥75 years: Immediate release: Initial: 20 mg; Extended release: 60 mg once daily

Mechanism of Action Trospium antagonizes the effects of acetylcholine on muscarinic receptors in cholinergically innervated organs. It reduces the smooth muscle tone of the bladder.

Pharmacodynamics/Kinetics

Half-life Elimination Immediate release formulation: 20 hours

Severe renal insufficiency (Cl_{cr} <30 mL/minute): ~33 hours; extended release formulation: ~35 hours

Time to Peak 5-6 hours

Pregnancy Risk Factor C

Pregnancy Considerations Adverse events were observed in animal studies. There are no adequate or well-controlled studies in pregnant women; use only if clearly needed.

Trypsin, Balsam Peru, and Castor Oil
(TRIP sin, BAL sam pe RUE, & KAS tor oyl)

Related Information

Castor Oil *on page 260*

Brand Names: U.S. Granulex®; TBC; Vasolex™; Xenaderm®

Pharmacologic Category Protectant, Topical

Use

Granulex®: Treatment of decubitus ulcers, varicose ulcers, debridement of eschar, dehiscent wounds and sunburn; promote wound healing; reduce odor from necrotic wounds

Vasolex™, Xenaderm ®: Treatment of decubitus ulcers, varicose ulcers, and dehiscent wounds; promote wound healing; reduce odor from necrotic wounds

Local Anesthetic/Vasoconstrictor Precautions No information available to require special precautions

Effects on Dental Treatment No significant effects or complications reported

Effects on Bleeding No information available to require special precautions

Adverse Effects Frequency not defined: Local: Temporary stinging at application site

General Dosage Range Topical: *Adults:* Apply a minimum of twice daily or as often as necessary

Mechanism of Action Trypsin may be used to debride necrotic tissue; balsam peru stimulates circulation at the wound site and may be mildly bactericidal; castor oil improves epithelialization, acts as a protectant covering and helps reduce pain

---

Tuberculin Tests (too BER kyoo lin tests)

Brand Names: U.S. Aplisol®; Tubersol®

Pharmacologic Category Diagnostic Agent

Use Skin test in diagnosis of tuberculosis

Local Anesthetic/Vasoconstrictor Precautions No information available to require special precautions

Effects on Dental Treatment No significant effects or complications reported

Effects on Bleeding No information available to require special precautions

Adverse Effects Suspected adverse reactions should be reported to the Food and Drug Administration (FDA) MedWatch Program at 1-800-332-1088

Frequency not defined:
Dermatologic: Rash
Local: Injection site reactions: Bleeding, bruising, discomfort, erythematous reaction, hematoma, necrosis, pain, pruritus, redness, scarring, ulceration, vesiculation
Miscellaneous: Anaphylaxis

General Dosage Range Intradermal: *Children and Adults:* 0.1 mL

Mechanism of Action Tuberculosis results in individuals becoming sensitized to certain antigenic components of the *M. tuberculosis* organism. Culture extracts called tuberculins are contained in tuberculin skin test preparations. Upon intracutaneous injection of these culture extracts, a classic delayed (cellular) hypersensitivity reaction occurs. This reaction is characteristic of a delayed course (peak occurs >24 hours after injection, induration of the skin secondary to cell infiltration, and occasional vesiculation and necrosis). Delayed hypersensitivity reactions to tuberculin may indicate infection with a variety of nontuberculosis mycobacteria, or vaccination with the live attenuated mycobacterial strain of *M. bovis* vaccine, BCG, in addition to previous natural infection with *M. tuberculosis.*

Pharmacodynamics/Kinetics
Onset of Action Delayed hypersensitivity reactions: 5-6 hours; Peak effect: 48-72 hours
Duration of Action Reactions subside over a few days

Pregnancy Risk Factor C

Pregnancy Considerations Reproduction studies have not been conducted. Pregnancy is not a contraindication to testing.

Typhoid and Hepatitis A Vaccine
(TYE foid & hep a TYE tis aye vak SEEN)

Brand Names: Canada ViVAXIM®
Pharmacologic Category Vaccine, Inactivated (Bacterial); Vaccine, Inactivated (Viral)
Use Active immunization against typhoid fever caused by *Salmonella typhi* and against disease caused by hepatitis A virus (HAV)

National Advisory Committee on Immunizations (NACI) does not recommend use for routine vaccination but does recommend that immunization be considered in the following groups:
- Travelers to areas with a prolonged risk (>4 weeks) of exposure to *S. typhi* or travelers to areas with endemic hepatitis A
- Persons with intimate exposure to a *S. typhi* carrier or who are residing in communities with high endemic rates of hepatitis A virus or at risk of outbreaks
- Laboratory technicians with frequent exposure to *S. typhi* or individuals involved in hepatitis A research or production of hepatitis A vaccine
- Travelers with achlorhydria or hypochlorhydria
- Military personnel, relief workers, or others relocated to areas with high rates of hepatitis A infection
- Persons with lifestyle risks for hepatitis A infection (eg, drug abusers, homosexual men), chronic liver disease, receiving hepatotoxic medication or with disease(s) which may necessitate use of hepatotoxic medications
- Persons with hemophilia A or B treated with plasma-derived clotting factors
- Zookeepers, veterinarians, and researchers who handle nonhuman primates

Local Anesthetic/Vasoconstrictor Precautions No information available to require special precautions
Effects on Dental Treatment No significant effects or complications reported
Effects on Bleeding No information available to require special precautions
Adverse Effects In Canada, adverse reactions may be reported to local provincial/territorial health agencies or to the Vaccine Safety Section at Public Health Agency of Canada (1-866-844-0018).
>10%:
Central nervous system: Headache (15%)
Local: Injection site: Pain (90%), induration/edema (28%), erythema (10%)
Neuromuscular & skeletal: Weakness (17%), myalgia (16%)
1% to 10%:
Central nervous system: Fever (5%), malaise (3%), dizziness (1%)
Gastrointestinal: Diarrhea (3%), nausea (3%)

General Dosage Range I.M.: *Children ≥16 years and Adults:* 1 mL given at least 2 weeks prior to expected exposure; may administer 1 mL booster dose 3 years after previous dose when necessary

Mechanism of Action Provides active immunization against typhoid fever through production of antibodies (predominantly IgG) and against hepatitis A infection through production of antihepatitis A virus antibodies.

Pharmacodynamics/Kinetics
Onset of Action Seroprotection rate at 14 days: Hepatitis A: ~96%, typhoid: ~89%; Seroprotection at 28 days: Hepatitis A: ~100%, typhoid: ~90%
Duration of Action Kinetic models suggest antihepatitis A antibodies may persist ≥20 years (NACI, 2006); Typhoid: 3 years

Pregnancy Considerations Reproduction studies have not been conducted. The Canadian labeling does not recommend use in pregnant women. Although the safety of vaccination during pregnancy has not been determined, the theoretical risk to the infant is expected to be low. Inactivated vaccines have not been shown to cause increased risks to the fetus (Canadian NACI, 2006; CDC, 2011).

Product Availability Not available in the U.S.

Typhoid Vaccine (TYE foid vak SEEN)

Brand Names: U.S. Typhim Vi®; Vivotif®
Brand Names: Canada Typherix®; Typhim Vi®; Vivotif®
Pharmacologic Category Vaccine, Inactivated (Bacterial); Vaccine, Live (Bacterial)
Use Active immunization against typhoid fever caused by *Salmonella typhi*
Not for routine vaccination. In the United States and Canada, use should be limited to:
– Travelers to areas with a prolonged risk of exposure to *S. typhi*
– Persons with intimate exposure to a *S. typhi* carrier
– Laboratory technicians with exposure to *S. typhi*
– Travelers with achlorhydria or hypochlorhydria (Canadian recommendation)

Local Anesthetic/Vasoconstrictor Precautions No information available to require special precautions
Effects on Dental Treatment No significant effects or complications reported
Effects on Bleeding No information available to require special precautions

◄ **Adverse Effects** In the U.S., all serious adverse reactions must be reported to the Department of Health and Human Services (DHHS) Vaccine Adverse Event Reporting System (VAERS) 1-800-822-7967 or online at https://vaers.hhs.gov/esub/index. In Canada, adverse reactions may be reported to local provincial/territorial health agencies or to the Vaccine Safety Section at Public Health Agency of Canada (1-866-844-0018).

Injection (incidence may vary based on age and/or product used):
>10%:
Central nervous system: Fever (undefined; 2% to 32%), malaise (4% to 24%), headache (16% to 20%)
Local: Injection site: Tenderness (97% to 98%), pain (27% to 41%), soreness (up to 16%), induration (5% to 15%)
Neuromuscular & skeletal: General aches (1% to 13%)
1% to 10%:
Central nervous system: Fever ≥100°F (2%), >102°F (2%)
Dermatologic: Pruritus (up to 8%)
Gastrointestinal: Nausea (up to 8%), vomiting (2%)
Local: Injection site: Erythema (up to 5%), swelling (up to 4%)
Neuromuscular & skeletal: Myalgia (3% to 7%)
Oral:
1% to 10%:
Central nervous system: Headache (5%), fever (3%)
Dermatologic: Rash (1%)
Gastrointestinal: Abdominal pain (6%), nausea (6%), diarrhea (3%), vomiting (2%)
Postmarketing and/or case reports: Anaphylactic reaction, demyelinating disease, myalgia, pain, RA, urticaria, sepsis, weakness

General Dosage Range
I.M.: *Children ≥2 years and Adults:* 0.5 mL given at least 2 weeks prior to expected exposure; may repeat every 2 years
Oral: *Children ≥6 years and Adults:* 1 capsule on alternate days for a total of 4 doses; may repeat full course every 5 years
Mechanism of Action Virulent strains of *Salmonella typhi* cause disease by penetrating the intestinal mucosa and entering the systemic circulation via the lymphatic vasculature. One possible mechanism of conferring immunity may be the provocation of a local immune response in the intestinal tract induced by oral ingesting of a live strain with subsequent aborted infection. The ability of *Salmonella typhi* to produce clinical disease (and to elicit an immune response) is dependent on the bacteria having a complete lipopolysaccharide. The live attenuate Ty21a strain lacks the enzyme UDP-4-galactose epimerase so that lipopolysaccharide is only synthesized under conditions that induce bacterial autolysis. Thus, the strain remains avirulent despite the production of sufficient lipopolysaccharide to evoke a protective immune response. Despite low levels of lipopolysaccharide synthesis, cells lyse before gaining a virulent phenotype due to the intracellular accumulation of metabolic intermediates.
Pharmacodynamics/Kinetics
Onset of Action Immunity to *Salmonella typhi*: Oral: ~1 week
Duration of Action Immunity: Oral: ~4-7 years; Parenteral: Typhim Vi®: >17-21 months, Typherix®: ~3 years

Pregnancy Risk Factor C
Pregnancy Considerations Reproduction studies have not been conducted. The manufacturer of the Typhim Vi® injection suggests delaying vaccination until the 2nd or 3rd trimester if possible. Untreated typhoid fever may lead to miscarriage or vertical intrauterine transmission causing neonatal typhoid (rare).

Ulipristal (ue li PRIS tal)

Brand Names: U.S. ella®
Pharmacologic Category Contraceptive; Progestin Receptor Modulator
Use Emergency contraception following unprotected intercourse or possible contraceptive failure
Local Anesthetic/Vasoconstrictor Precautions No information available to require special precautions
Effects on Dental Treatment No significant effects or complications reported
Effects on Bleeding No information available to require special precautions
Adverse Effects
>10%:
Central nervous system: Headache (18% to 19%)
Endocrine & metabolic: Menstruation occurring ≥7 days later than expected (19%), dysmenorrhea (7% to 13%)
Gastrointestinal: Abdominal pain (8% to 15%), nausea (12% to 13%)
1% to 10%:
Central nervous system: Fatigue (6%), dizziness (5%)
Endocrine & metabolic: Intermenstrual bleeding (9%), menstruation occurring ≥7 days earlier than expected (7%)
General Dosage Range Oral: *Adults:* 1 tablet (30 mg) as a single dose
Mechanism of Action Prevents progestin from binding to the progesterone receptor. Ulipristal postpones follicular rupture when administered prior to ovulation, thereby inhibiting or delaying ovulation. May also alter the normal endometrium, impairing implantation.
Pharmacodynamics/Kinetics
Half-life Elimination Ulipristal: ~32 hours; Monodemethylated metabolite: ~27 hours
Time to Peak Serum: 1 hour (ulipristal and monodemethylated metabolite)
Pregnancy Risk Factor X
Pregnancy Considerations Embryofetal loss was observed following administration of ulipristal to pregnant rats and rabbits during the period of organogenesis at doses that were 1/3 and 1/2 the human dose (based on BSA), respectively. Teratogenic effects were not observed in surviving fetuses. Pregnancy terminations were also observed in pregnant monkeys following administration of ulipristal during the first trimester in doses ~3 times the human dose (based on BSA). Exclude pregnancy prior to therapy; not indicated for terminating an existing pregnancy. A rapid return of fertility is expected following use for emergency contraception; routine contraceptive measures should be initiated or continued following use to ensure ongoing prevention of pregnancy. Barrier contraception is recommended immediately following emergency contraception and throughout the same menstrual cycle; efficacy of hormonal contraceptives may be decreased.

Undecylenic Acid and Derivatives
(un de sil EN ik AS id & dah RIV ah tivs)

Brand Names: U.S. Fungi-Nail® [OTC]
Pharmacologic Category Antifungal Agent, Topical
Use Treatment of athlete's foot (tinea pedis); ringworm (except nails and scalp)
Local Anesthetic/Vasoconstrictor Precautions No information available to require special precautions
Effects on Dental Treatment No significant effects or complications reported
Effects on Bleeding No information available to require special precautions
General Dosage Range Topical: *Children ≥2 years and Adults:* Apply twice daily to affected area

Unoprostone (yoo noe PROS tone)

Brand Names: U.S. Rescula®
Pharmacologic Category Ophthalmic Agent, Anti-glaucoma; Prostaglandin, Ophthalmic
Use To lower intraocular pressure (IOP) in patients with open-angle glaucoma or ocular hypertension
Local Anesthetic/Vasoconstrictor Precautions No information available to require special precautions
Effects on Dental Treatment No significant effects or complications reported
Effects on Bleeding No information available to require special precautions
Adverse Effects
>10%: Ocular: Burning/stinging (10% to 25%), dry eyes (10% to 25%), injection (10% to 25%), ophthalmic itching (10% to 25%), increased length of eyelashes (≥1 mm) at 12 months (10% to 14%)
1% to 10%:
Cardiovascular: Hypertension
Central nervous system: Dizziness, headache, insomnia, pain
Endocrine & metabolic: Diabetes mellitus
Neuromuscular & skeletal: Back pain
Ocular: Abnormal vision (5% to 10%), eyelid disorder (5% to 10%), foreign body sensation (5% to 10%), lacrimation disorder (5% to 10%), decreased length of eyelashes (7%), blepharitis, cataract, conjunctivitis, corneal lesion, eye discharge, eye hemorrhage, eye pain, irritation, keratitis, photophobia, vitreous disorder
Respiratory: Bronchitis, cough increased, pharyngitis, rhinitis, sinusitis
Miscellaneous: Flu-like syndrome (6%), accidental injury, allergic reaction
General Dosage Range Ophthalmic: *Adults:* Instill 1 drop into affected eye(s) twice daily
Mechanism of Action The exact mechanism of action is unknown; however, unoprostone likely decreases IOP by increasing the outflow of aqueous humor. Cardiovascular and pulmonary function were not affected in clinical studies. IOP was decreased by 3-4 mm Hg in patients with a mean baseline IOP of 23 mm Hg.
Pharmacodynamics/Kinetics
Half-life Elimination 14 minutes
Pregnancy Risk Factor C
Pregnancy Considerations In animal reproduction studies, adverse events were observed when administered subcutaneously at doses greater than the recommended human dose. Following ophthalmic administration, systemic absorption is minimal; systemic absorption would be required in order for unoprostone to cross the placenta and reach the fetus. If ophthalmic agents are needed during pregnancy, the minimum effective dose should be used in combination with punctual occlusion to decrease potential exposure to the fetus (Samples, 1988).

Urea (yoor EE a)

Brand Names: U.S. Aluvea™; Aqua Care® [OTC]; Aquaphilic® with Carbamide [OTC]; BP 50%; Carmol® 10 [OTC]; Carmol® 20 [OTC]; Carmol® 40; Carmol® Deep Cleansing [OTC]; DPM™ [OTC]; Gordon's® Urea [OTC]; Gormel® Ten [OTC]; Gormel® [OTC]; Hydro 35™; Hydro 40™; Kerafoam®; Kerafoam® 42; Keralac™; Keralac™ Nailstik; Kerol™; Kerol™ AD; Kerol™ Redi-Cloths; Kerol™ ZX; Lanaphilic® with Urea [OTC]; Nutraplus® [OTC]; Quinnostik; Rea Lo® 30 [OTC]; Rea Lo® 40; Remeven™; RevitaDERM® 40; Ultra Mide 25® [OTC]; Umecta PD™; Umecta®; Umecta® Nail Film; Uramaxin®; Uramaxin® GT; Uramaxin® GT Kit; Ureacin-10® [OTC]; Ureacin-20® [OTC]; X-Viate™
Brand Names: Canada UltraMide 25™; Uremol®; Urisec®
Pharmacologic Category Diuretic, Osmotic; Keratolytic Agent; Topical Skin Product
Use Keratolytic agent to soften nails or skin; OTC: Moisturizer for dry, rough skin
Local Anesthetic/Vasoconstrictor Precautions No information available to require special precautions
Effects on Dental Treatment No significant effects or complications reported
Effects on Bleeding No information available to require special precautions
Adverse Effects Frequency not defined: Local: Transient stinging, local irritation
General Dosage Range Topical: *Adults:* Apply 1-3 times/day
Mechanism of Action Urea softens hyperkeratotic areas by dissolving the intracellular matrix, resulting in loosening the horny layer of the skin, or softening and debridement of the nail plate
Pregnancy Risk Factor B/C (manufacturer specific)
Pregnancy Considerations Reproduction studies have not been conducted with all products. When conducted, adverse events were not observed in animal studies.

Urea and Hydrocortisone
(yoor EE a & hye droe KOR ti sone)

Related Information
Hydrocortisone (Topical) *on page 699*
Urea *on page 1373*
Brand Names: U.S. Carmol-HC®
Brand Names: Canada Ti-U-Lac® H; Uremol® HC
Pharmacologic Category Corticosteroid, Topical
Use Inflammation of corticosteroid-responsive dermatoses
Local Anesthetic/Vasoconstrictor Precautions No information available to require special precautions
Effects on Dental Treatment No significant effects or complications reported
Effects on Bleeding No information available to require special precautions
General Dosage Range Topical: *Children and Adults:* Apply thin film and rub in well 2-4 times/day
Pregnancy Risk Factor C

◀ **Pregnancy Considerations** Teratogenic effects have been observed in animals administered potent topical corticosteroids. Topical products are not recommended for extensive use, in large quantities, or for long periods of time in pregnant women.

Urofollitropin (yoor oh fol li TROE pin)

Brand Names: U.S. Bravelle®
Brand Names: Canada Bravelle®; Fertinorm® H.P.
Pharmacologic Category Gonadotropin; Ovulation Stimulator
Use Ovulation induction in patients who previously received pituitary suppression; development of multiple follicles with Assisted Reproductive Technologies (ART)
Local Anesthetic/Vasoconstrictor Precautions No information available to require special precautions
Effects on Dental Treatment No significant effects or complications reported
Effects on Bleeding Medical consult is suggested.
Adverse Effects Percentage may vary by indication, route of administration.
>10%:
  Central nervous system: Headache
  Endocrine & metabolic: Ovarian enlargement, ovarian hyperstimulation syndrome
  Gastrointestinal: Abdominal cramps
1% to 10%:
  Cardiovascular: Hypertension
  Central nervous system: Depression, emotional lability, fever, pain
  Dermatologic: Acne, exfoliative dermatitis, rash
  Endocrine & metabolic: Breast tenderness, hot flashes, ovarian disorder (pain, cyst)
  Gastrointestinal: Abdomen enlarged, abdominal pain, constipation, diarrhea, dehydration, nausea, vomiting, weight gain
  Genitourinary: Cervical disorder, urinary tract infection, pelvic pain/cramps, uterine spasms, vaginal discharge, vaginal hemorrhage, vaginal spotting
  Local: Injection site reaction
  Neuromuscular & skeletal: Neck pain
  Respiratory: Respiratory disorder, sinusitis
  Miscellaneous: Infection, post retrieval pain
General Dosage Range
  I.M.: *Adults (females):* Initial: 150 units once daily for 5 days; Maintenance: Up to 450 units/day (maximum: 12 days therapy)
  SubQ: *Adults (females):* Initial: 150-225 units once daily for 5 days; Maintenance: Up to 450 units/day (maximum: 12 days therapy)
Mechanism of Action Urofollitropin is a preparation of highly purified follicle-stimulating hormone (FSH) extracted from the urine of postmenopausal women. Follitropins stimulate ovarian follicular growth in women who do not have primary ovarian failure. FSH is required for normal follicular growth, maturation, gonadal steroid production, and spermatogenesis.
Pharmacodynamics/Kinetics
  Half-life Elimination
    I.M.: 37 hours, 15 hours following multiple doses
    SubQ: 32 hours, 21 hours following multiple doses
  Time to Peak
    I.M.: 17 hours, 11 hours following multiple doses
    SubQ: 21 hours, 10 hours following multiple doses
Pregnancy Risk Factor X

Pregnancy Considerations Ectopic pregnancy, congenital abnormalities, spontaneous abortion, and multiple births have been reported. The incidence of congenital abnormality may be slightly higher after ART than with spontaneous conception; higher incidence may be related to parenteral characteristics (maternal age, sperm characteristics).

Ursodiol (ur soe DYE ol)

Brand Names: U.S. Actigall®; Urso 250®; Urso Forte®
Brand Names: Canada Dom-Ursodiol C; PHL-Ursodiol C; PMS-Ursodiol C; Urso®; Urso® DS
Pharmacologic Category Gallstone Dissolution Agent
Use
  Actigall®: Gallbladder stone dissolution; prevention of gallstones in obese patients experiencing rapid weight loss
  Urso®, Urso Forte®: Primary biliary cirrhosis
Local Anesthetic/Vasoconstrictor Precautions No information available to require special precautions
Effects on Dental Treatment No significant effects or complications reported
Effects on Bleeding Medical consult is suggested.
Adverse Effects
>10%:
  Central nervous system: Headache (up to 25%), dizziness (17%)
  Gastrointestinal: Diarrhea (up to 27%), constipation (up to 26%), dyspepsia (17%), nausea (up to 17%), vomiting (up to 14%)
  Neuromuscular & skeletal: Back pain (up to 12%)
  Respiratory: Upper respiratory tract infection (up to 16%)
1% to 10%:
  Dermatologic: Alopecia (5%), rash (3%)
  Endocrine & metabolic: Hyperglycemia (1%)
  Gastrointestinal: Flatulence (up to 8%), peptic ulcer (1%)
  Genitourinary: Urinary tract infection (7%)
  Hematologic: Leukopenia (3%), thrombocytopenia (1%)
  Hepatic: Cholecystitis (5%)
  Neuromuscular & skeletal: Arthritis (6%), myalgia (6%)
  Renal: Serum creatinine increased (1%)
  Respiratory: Pharyngitis (up to 8%), bronchitis (7%), cough (7%)
  Miscellaneous: Viral infection (9%), flu-like syndrome (7%), allergy (5%)
General Dosage Range Oral: *Adults:* 8-15 mg/kg/day in 2-4 divided doses **or** 300 mg twice daily
Mechanism of Action Decreases the cholesterol content of bile and bile stones by reducing the secretion of cholesterol from the liver and the fractional reabsorption of cholesterol by the intestines. Mechanism of action in primary biliary cirrhosis is not clearly defined.
Pregnancy Risk Factor B
Pregnancy Considerations Adverse events have not been observed in animal reproduction studies. Ursodiol (ursodeoxycholic acid) is the treatment of choice for intrahepatic cholestasis of pregnancy (Kremer, 2011).

Ustekinumab (yoo stek in YOO mab)

Brand Names: U.S. Stelara™
Brand Names: Canada Stelara™
Pharmacologic Category Antipsoriatic Agent; Interleukin-12 Inhibitor; Interleukin-23 Inhibitor; Monoclonal Antibody

Use Treatment of moderate-to-severe plaque psoriasis

Local Anesthetic/Vasoconstrictor Precautions No information available to require special precautions

Effects on Dental Treatment No significant effects or complications reported

Effects on Bleeding No information available to require special precautions

Adverse Effects

>10%: Miscellaneous: Infection (27% to 61%)

1% to 10%:

Central nervous system: Headache (5%), fatigue (3%), dizziness (1% to 2%), depression (1%)

Dermatologic: Pruritus (1% to 2%)

Local: Injection site erythema (1% to 2%)

Neuromuscular & skeletal: Back pain (1% to 2%)

Respiratory: Pharyngolaryngeal pain (1% to 2%)

Miscellaneous: Antibody formation (3% to 5%)

General Dosage Range Oral: *Adults:* ≤100 kg: 45 mg at 0 and 4 weeks, and then every 12 weeks; >100 kg: 45 mg or 90 mg at 0 and 4 weeks, and then every 12 weeks

Mechanism of Action Ustekinumab is a human monoclonal antibody that binds to and interferes with the proinflammatory cytokines, interleukin (IL)-12 and IL-23. Biological effects of IL-12 and IL-23 include natural killer (NK) cell activation, CD4+ T-cell differentiation and activation. Ustekinumab also interferes with the expression of monocyte chemotactic protein-1 (MCP-1), tumor necrosis factor-alpha (TNF-α), interferon-inducible protein-10 (IP-10), and interleukin-8 (IL-8). Significant clinical improvement in psoriasis patients is seen in association with reduction of these proinflammatory signalers.

Pharmacodynamics/Kinetics

Half-life Elimination 10-126 days

Time to Peak Plasma: 45 mg: 13.5 days; 90 mg: 7 days

Pregnancy Risk Factor B

Pregnancy Considerations Reproduction studies have not been conducted in pregnant women. Use during pregnancy only if clearly needed.

Vaccinia Immune Globulin (Intravenous)
(vax IN ee a i MYUN GLOB yoo lin IN tra VEE nus)

Brand Names: U.S. CNJ-016®

Pharmacologic Category Blood Product Derivative; Immune Globulin

Use Treatment of infectious complications of smallpox (vaccinia virus) vaccination, such as eczema vaccinatum, progressive vaccinia, and severe generalized vaccinia; treatment of vaccinia infections in individuals with concurrent skin conditions or accidental virus exposure to eyes (except vaccinia keratitis), mouth, or other areas where viral infection would pose significant risk

CDC guidelines for use:

Use is recommended for:

- Inadvertent inoculation (considering severity, toxicity of affected person, and pain)
- Eczema vaccinatum
- Generalized vaccinia (severe form or if underlying illness is present)
- Progressive vaccinia

Use may be considered for:

- Severe ocular complications except isolated keratitis

Use is not recommended for:

- Inadvertent inoculation that is not severe
- Mild or limited generalized vaccinia
- Nonspecific rashes, erythema multiforme, or Stevens-Johnson syndrome
- Postvaccinial encephalitis or encephalomyelitis

Local Anesthetic/Vasoconstrictor Precautions No information available to require special precautions

Effects on Dental Treatment No significant effects or complications reported

Effects on Bleeding No information available to require special precautions

Adverse Effects Note: Actual frequency varies by dose and rate of infusion

Cardiovascular: Peripheral edema

Central nervous system: Cold or hot feeling, dizziness, fatigue, headache, pain, pallor, pyrexia

Dermatologic: Erythema

Gastrointestinal: Appetite decreased, nausea, vomiting

Local: Injection site reaction

Neuromuscular & skeletal: Back pain, paraesthesia, muscle spasm, rigors, tremor, weakness

Miscellaneous: Diaphoresis

General Dosage Range I.V.: *Adults:* Initial: 6000 units/kg; may repeat 6000-9000 units/kg if needed (maximum: 24,000 units/kg)

Mechanism of Action Antibodies obtained from pooled human plasma of individuals immunized with the smallpox vaccine provide passive immunity

Pharmacodynamics/Kinetics

Half-life Elimination 30 days (range: 13-67 days)

Time to Peak Plasma: ≤2 hours

Pregnancy Risk Factor C

Pregnancy Considerations Animal reproduction studies have not been conducted. Immune globulins cross the placenta in increased amounts after 30 weeks gestation. There are no adequate and well-controlled studies in pregnant women. Vaccinia immune globulin is currently not recommended for use in persons with contraindications to smallpox vaccine; inadvertent exposure to smallpox vaccine in high risk populations (eg pregnant women) should be reported to the CDC so that standardized treatment may be provided.

Prescribing and Access Restrictions Vaccinia immune globulin is not available for general public use. All supplies are currently owned by the federal government for inclusion in the Strategic National Stockpile. The CDC Smallpox Adverse Events Clinical Consultation team will coordinate shipment. The State Health Department should be contacted first concerning severe or unexpected adverse events from smallpox vaccination.

ValACYclovir (val ay SYE kloe veer)

Related Information

Acyclovir (Systemic) *on page 45*

Systemic Viral Diseases *on page 1537*

Viral Infections *on page 1575*

Related Sample Prescriptions

Herpes Simplex (Recurrent) *on page 1616*

Shingles (Varicella-Zoster Virus) *on page 1616*

Brand Names: U.S. Valtrex®

Brand Names: Canada Apo-Valacyclovir®; CO Valacyclovir; DOM-Valacyclovir; Mylan-Valacyclovir; PHL-Valacyclovir; PMS-Valacyclovir; PRO-Valacyclovir; Riva-Valacyclovir; Valtrex®

Generic Availability (U.S.) Yes

◀ **Pharmacologic Category** Antiviral Agent; Antiviral Agent, Oral

Dental Use Treatment of herpes labialis (cold sores)

Use Treatment of herpes zoster (shingles) in immunocompetent patients; treatment of first-episode and recurrent genital herpes; suppression of recurrent genital herpes and reduction of transmission of genital herpes in immunocompetent patients; suppression of genital herpes in HIV-infected individuals; treatment of herpes labialis (cold sores); chickenpox in immunocompetent children

Unlabeled Use Prophylaxis of cancer-related HSV, VZV, and CMV infections; treatment of cancer-related HSV, VZV infection

Local Anesthetic/Vasoconstrictor Precautions No information available to require special precautions

Effects on Dental Treatment No significant effects or complications reported

Effects on Bleeding Medical consult is suggested.

Adverse Effects

>10%:
Central nervous system: Headache (13% to 38%)
Gastrointestinal: Nausea (5% to 15%), abdominal pain (1% to 11%)
Hematologic: Neutropenia (≤18%)
Hepatic: ALT increased (≤14%), AST increased (2% to 16%)
Respiratory: Nasopharyngitis (≤16%)

1% to 10%:
Central nervous system: Fatigue (≤8%), depression (≤7%), fever (children 4%), dizziness (2% to 4%)
Dermatologic: Rash (≤8%)
Endocrine: Dysmenorrhea (≤1% to 8%), dehydration (children 2%)
Gastrointestinal: Vomiting (<1% to 6%), diarrhea (children 5%; adults <1%)
Hematologic: Thrombocytopenia (≤3%)
Hepatic: Alkaline phosphatase increased (≤4%)
Neuromuscular & skeletal: Arthralgia (<1 to 6%)
Respiratory: Rhinorrhea (children 2%)
Miscellaneous: Herpes simplex (children 2%)

Dental Usual Dosage

Herpes labialis (cold sores): Adolescents and Adults: Oral: 2 g twice daily for 1 day (separate doses by ~12 hours)

Dosage Oral:

Children 2 to <18 years: Chickenpox: 20 mg/kg/dose 3 times/day for 5 days (maximum: 1 g 3 times/day)

Children ≥12 and Adults: Herpes labialis (cold sores): 2 g twice daily for 1 day (separate doses by ~12 hours)

Adults:

CMV prophylaxis in allogeneic HSCT recipients (unlabeled use): 2 g 4 times/day

Herpes zoster (shingles): 1 g 3 times/day for 7 days

HSV, VZV in cancer patients (unlabeled use): Prophylaxis: 500 mg 2-3 times/day; Treatment: 1 g 3 times/day

Genital herpes:

Initial episode: 1 g twice daily for 10 days

Recurrent episode: 500 mg twice daily for 3 days

Reduction of transmission: 500 mg once daily (source partner)

Suppressive therapy:

Immunocompetent patients: 1 g once daily (500 mg once daily in patients with <9 recurrences per year)

HIV-infected patients (CD4 ≥100 cells/mm³): 500 mg twice daily

Dosing adjustment in renal impairment:

Herpes zoster: Adults:

U.S. labeling:

Cl$_{cr}$ 30-49 mL/minute: 1 g every 12 hours
Cl$_{cr}$ 10-29 mL/minute: 1 g every 24 hours
Cl$_{cr}$ <10 mL/minute: 500 mg every 24 hours

Canadian labeling:

Cl$_{cr}$ >30 mL/minute: No dosage adjustment required
Cl$_{cr}$ 15-30 mL/minute: 1 g every 12 hours
Cl$_{cr}$ <15 mL/minute: 1 g every 24 hours

Genital herpes: Adults:

U.S. labeling:

Initial episode:

Cl$_{cr}$ 10-29 mL/minute: 1 g every 24 hours
Cl$_{cr}$ <10 mL/minute: 500 mg every 24 hours

Recurrent episode: Cl$_{cr}$ <29 mL/minute: 500 mg every 24 hours

Suppressive therapy: Cl$_{cr}$ <29 mL/minute:

For usual dose of 1 g every 24 hours, decrease dose to 500 mg every 24 hours

For usual dose of 500 mg every 24 hours, decrease dose to 500 mg every 48 hours

HIV-infected patients: 500 mg every 24 hours

Canadian labeling:

Initial episode:

Cl$_{cr}$ 15-30 mL/minute: 1 g every 24 hours
Cl$_{cr}$ <15 mL/minute: 500 mg every 24 hours

Recurrent episode:

Cl$_{cr}$ 15-30 mL/minute: 500 mg every 12 hours
Cl$_{cr}$ <15 mL/minute: 500 mg every 24 hours

Suppressive therapy:

Cl$_{cr}$ 15-30 mL/minute: 500 mg every 24 hours
Cl$_{cr}$ <15 mL/minute:

Immunocompetent or HIV-infected patients: 500 mg every 24 hours

Immunocompetent patients and ≤9 recurrences/year: 500 mg every 48 hours

Herpes labialis: Adolescents and Adults (U.S. labeling) or Adults (Canadian labeling):

Cl$_{cr}$ 30-49 mL/minute: 1 g every 12 hours for 2 doses
Cl$_{cr}$ 10-29 mL/minute: 500 mg every 12 hours for 2 doses
Cl$_{cr}$ <10 mL/minute: 500 mg as a single dose

Hemodialysis: Dialyzable (~33% removed during 4-hour session); administer dose postdialysis

Chronic ambulatory peritoneal dialysis/continuous arteriovenous hemofiltration dialysis: Pharmacokinetic parameters are similar to those in patients with ESRD; supplemental dose not needed following dialysis

Dosing adjustment in hepatic impairment: No adjustment required.

Mechanism of Action Valacyclovir is rapidly and nearly completely converted to acyclovir by intestinal and hepatic metabolism. Acyclovir is converted to acyclovir monophosphate by virus-specific thymidine kinase then further converted to acyclovir triphosphate by other cellular enzymes. Acyclovir triphosphate inhibits DNA synthesis and viral replication by competing with deoxyguanosine triphosphate for viral DNA polymerase and being incorporated into viral DNA.

Contraindications Hypersensitivity to valacyclovir, acyclovir, or any component of the formulation

Warnings/Precautions Thrombotic thrombocytopenic purpura/hemolytic uremic syndrome has occurred in immunocompromised patients (at doses of 8 g/day). Safety and efficacy have not been established for treatment/suppression of recurrent genital herpes or disseminated herpes in patients with profound immunosuppression (eg, advanced HIV with CD4 <100 cells/mm³). CNS adverse effects (including agitation, hallucinations, confusion, delirium, seizures, and encephalopathy) have been reported. Use caution in patients with renal impairment, the elderly, and/or those receiving nephrotoxic agents. Acute renal failure has been observed in patients with renal dysfunction; dose adjustment may be required. Decreased precipitation in renal tubules may occur leading to urinary precipitation; adequately hydrate patient. For cold sores, treatment should begin at with earliest symptom (tingling, itching, burning). For genital herpes, treatment should begin as soon as possible after the first signs and symptoms (within 72 hours of onset of first diagnosis or within 24 hours of onset of recurrent episodes). For herpes zoster, treatment should begin within 72 hours of onset of rash. For chickenpox, treatment should begin with earliest sign or symptom. Use with caution in the elderly; CNS effects have been reported. Safety and efficacy have not been established in patients <2 years of age.

Drug Interactions
Metabolism/Transport Effects None known.
Avoid Concomitant Use
Avoid concomitant use of ValACYclovir with any of the following: Zoster Vaccine
Increased Effect/Toxicity
ValACYclovir may increase the levels/effects of: Mycophenolate; Tenofovir; Zidovudine

The levels/effects of ValACYclovir may be increased by: Mycophenolate
Decreased Effect
ValACYclovir may decrease the levels/effects of: Zoster Vaccine

Dietary Considerations May be taken with or without food.

Pharmacodynamics/Kinetics
Half-life Elimination Normal renal function: Adults: 2.5-3.3 hours (acyclovir), ~30 minutes (valacyclovir); End-stage renal disease: 14-20 hours (acyclovir); During hemodialysis: 4 hours

Pregnancy Risk Factor B

Pregnancy Considerations Teratogenic events were not observed in animal studies. Data from a pregnancy registry has shown no increased rate of birth defects than that of the general population; however, the registry is small and use during pregnancy is only warranted if the potential benefit to the mother justifies the risk of the fetus.

Lactation Enters breast milk/use caution

Breast-Feeding Considerations Peak concentrations in breast milk range from 0.5-2.3 times the corresponding maternal acyclovir serum concentration. This is expected to provide a nursing infant with a dose of acyclovir equivalent to ~0.6 mg/kg/day following ingestion of valacyclovir 500 mg twice daily by the mother. Use with caution while breast-feeding.

Dosage Forms
Caplet, oral: 500 mg, 1 g
Valtrex®: 500 mg, 1 g
Tablet, oral: 500 mg, 1 g

ValGANciclovir (val gan SYE kloh veer)

Related Information
Ganciclovir (Systemic) *on page 647*
Systemic Viral Diseases *on page 1537*
Brand Names: U.S. Valcyte®
Brand Names: Canada Valcyte®
Pharmacologic Category Antiviral Agent

Use Treatment of cytomegalovirus (CMV) retinitis in patients with acquired immunodeficiency syndrome (AIDS); prevention of CMV disease in high-risk patients (donor CMV positive/recipient CMV negative) undergoing kidney, heart, or kidney/pancreas transplantation

Local Anesthetic/Vasoconstrictor Precautions No information available to require special precautions

Effects on Dental Treatment No significant effects or complications reported

Effects on Bleeding Medical consult is suggested.

Adverse Effects
>10%:
Cardiovascular: Hypertension (12% to 18%)
Central nervous system: Fever (9% to 31%), headache (6% to 22%), insomnia (6% to 20%)
Gastrointestinal: Diarrhea (16% to 41%), nausea (8% to 30%), vomiting (3% to 21%), abdominal pain (15%), constipation
Hematologic: Anemia (≤31%), thrombocytopenia (≤22%), neutropenia (3% to 19%)
Neuromuscular & skeletal: Tremor (12% to 28%)
Ocular: Retinal detachment (15%)
Renal: Serum creatinine increased (S_{cr} >1.5-2.5 mg/dL: 12% to 50%; S_{cr} >2.5: 3% to 17%)
Respiratory: Cough, upper respiratory tract infection
5% to 10%: Central nervous system: Peripheral neuropathy (9%), paresthesia (8%)
<5%:
Cardiovascular: Edema, hypotension, peripheral edema
Central nervous system: Agitation, confusion, depression, dizziness, fatigue, hallucination, pain, psychosis, seizure
Dermatologic: Acne, dermatitis, pruritus
Endocrine & metabolic: Dehydration, hyperglycemia, hyper-/hypokalemia, hypocalcemia, hypomagnesemia, hypophosphatemia
Gastrointestinal: Abdominal distention/pain, appetite (decreased), dyspepsia
Genitourinary: Urinary tract infection
Hematologic: Aplastic anemia, bleeding (potentially life-threatening due to thrombocytopenia), bone marrow depression, pancytopenia
Hepatic: Ascites
Neuromuscular & skeletal: Arthralgia, back pain, limb pain, muscle cramps, weakness
Renal: Creatinine clearance (decreased), dysuria, renal impairment
Respiratory: Dyspnea, nasopharyngitis, pharyngitis, pleural effusion, rhinorrhea
Miscellaneous: Allergic reaction, local and systemic infection (including sepsis)

General Dosage Range Dosage adjustment recommended in patients with renal impairment
Oral:
Children 4 months to 16 years: Dose (mg) = 7 x body surface area x creatinine clearance once daily
Children >16 years and Adults: 900 mg 1-2 times/day

Mechanism of Action Valganciclovir is rapidly converted to ganciclovir in the body. The bioavailability of ganciclovir from valganciclovir is increased 10-fold compared to oral ganciclovir. A dose of 900 mg achieved systemic exposure of ganciclovir comparable to that achieved with the recommended doses of intravenous ganciclovir of 5 mg/kg. Ganciclovir is phosphorylated to a substrate which competitively inhibits the binding of deoxyguanosine triphosphate to DNA polymerase resulting in inhibition of viral DNA synthesis.

◀ **Pharmacodynamics/Kinetics**
Half-life Elimination Ganciclovir: 4.08 hours, prolonged with renal impairment; Severe renal impairment: Up to 68 hours
Time to Peak Ganciclovir: 1-3 hours
Pregnancy Risk Factor C
Pregnancy Considerations Valganciclovir is converted to ganciclovir and shares its reproductive toxicity. **[U.S. Boxed Warning]: Ganciclovir may be teratogenic and cause aspermatogenesis.** Based on animal data, temporary or permanent impairment of fertility may occur in males and females. Ganciclovir is also teratogenic in animals. Females should use effective contraception during treatment and for 30 days after; males should use barrier contraception during treatment and for 90 days after.

Valproic Acid and Derivatives
(val PROE ik AS id & dah RIV ah tives)

Brand Names: U.S. Depacon®; Depakene®; Depakote®; Depakote® ER; Depakote® Sprinkle; Stavzor™
Brand Names: Canada Apo-Divalproex®; Apo-Valproic®; Depakene®; Dom-Divalproex; Epival®; Mylan-Divalproex; Mylan-Valproic; Novo-Divalproex; Nu-Divalproex; PHL-Divalproex; PHL-Valproic Acid; PHL-Valproic Acid E.C.; PMS-Divalproex; PMS-Valproic Acid; PMS-Valproic Acid E.C.; ratio-Valproic; ratio-Valproic ECC; Rhoxal-valproic; Sandoz-Valproic
Generic Availability (U.S.) Yes: Excludes delayed release capsule
Pharmacologic Category Anticonvulsant, Miscellaneous; Antimanic Agent; Histone Deacetylase Inhibitor
Use
Oral, I.V.: Monotherapy and adjunctive therapy in the treatment of patients with complex partial seizures; monotherapy and adjunctive therapy of simple and complex absence seizures; adjunctive therapy in patients with multiple seizure types that include absence seizures
Additional indications: Depakote®, Depakote® ER, Stavzor™: Mania associated with bipolar disorder; migraine prophylaxis
Unlabeled Use Refractory status epilepticus, diabetic neuropathy
Local Anesthetic/Vasoconstrictor Precautions No information available to require special precautions
Effects on Dental Treatment Key adverse event(s) related to dental treatment: Periodontal abscess and taste perversion.
Effects on Bleeding Has been associated with dose-related thrombocytopenia. Normal coagulation may generally be expected unless thrombocytopenia is present and severe.
Adverse Effects
>10%:
Central nervous system: Headache (≤31%), somnolence (≤30%), dizziness (12% to 25%), insomnia (>1% to 15%), nervousness (>1% to 11%), pain (1% to 11%)
Dermatologic: Alopecia (>1% to 24%)
Gastrointestinal: Nausea (15% to 48%), vomiting (7% to 27%), diarrhea (7% to 23%), abdominal pain (7% to 23%), dyspepsia (7% to 23%), anorexia (>1% to 12%)
Hematologic: Thrombocytopenia (1% to 24%; dose related)
Neuromuscular & skeletal: Tremor (≤57%), weakness (6% to 27%)

Ocular: Diplopia (>1% to 16%), amblyopia/blurred vision (≤12%)
Miscellaneous: Infection (≤20%), flu-like syndrome (12%)
1% to 10%:
Cardiovascular: Peripheral edema (>1% to 8%), chest pain (>1% to <5%), edema (>1% to <5%), facial edema (>1% to <5%), hypertension (>1% to <5%), hypotension (>1% to <5%), orthostatic hypotension (>1% to <5%), palpitation (>1% to <5%), tachycardia (>1% to <5%), vasodilation (>1% to <5%), arrhythmia (>1% to <5%)
Central nervous system: Ataxia (>1% to 8%), amnesia (>1% to 7%), emotional lability (>1% to 6%), fever (>1% to 6%), abnormal thinking (≤6%), depression (>1% to 5%), abnormal dreams (>1% to <5%), agitation (>1% to <5%), anxiety (>1% to <5%), catatonia (>1% to <5%), chills (>1% to <5%), confusion (>1% to <5%), coordination abnormal (>1% to <5%), hallucination (>1% to <5%), malaise (>1% to <5%), personality disorder (>1% to <5%), speech disorder (>1% to <5%), tardive dyskinesia (>1% to <5%), vertigo (>1% to <5%), euphoria (1%), hypoesthesia (1%)
Dermatologic: Rash (>1% to 6%), bruising (>1% to 5%), discoid lupus erythematosus (>1% to <5%), dry skin (>1% to <5%), furunculosis (>1% to <5%), petechia (>1% to <5%), pruritus (>1% to <5), seborrhea (>1% to <5%)
Endocrine & metabolic: Amenorrhea (>1% to <5%), dysmenorrhea (>1% to <5%), metrorrhagia (>1% to <5%), hypoproteinemia
Gastrointestinal: Weight gain (4% to 9%), weight loss (6%), appetite increased (≤6%), constipation (>1% to 5%), xerostomia (>1% to 5%), eructation (>1% to <5%), fecal incontinence (>1% to <5%), flatulence (>1% to <5%), gastroenteritis (>1% to <5%), glossitis (>1% to <5%), hematemesis (>1% to <5%), pancreatitis (>1% to <5%), periodontal abscess (>1% to <5%), stomatitis (>1% to <5%), taste perversion (>1% to <5%), dysphagia, gum hemorrhage, mouth ulceration
Genitourinary: Cystitis (>1% to 5%), dysuria (>1% to 5%), urinary frequency (>1% to <5%), urinary incontinence (>1% to <5%), vaginal hemorrhage (>1% to 5%), vaginitis (>1% to <5%)
Hepatic: ALT increased (>1% to <5%), AST increased (>1% to <5%)
Local: Injection site pain (3%), injection site reaction (2%), injection site inflammation (1%)
Neuromuscular & skeletal: Back pain (≤8%), abnormal gait (>1% to <5%), arthralgia (>1% to <5%), arthrosis (>1% to <5%), dysarthria (>1% to <5%), hypertonia (>1% to <5%), hypokinesia (>1% to <5%), leg cramps (>1% to <5%), myalgia (>1% to <5%), myasthenia (>1% to <5%), neck pain (>1% to <5%), neck rigidity (>1% to <5%), paresthesia (>1% to <5%), reflex increased (>1% to <5%), twitching (>1% to <5%)
Ocular: Nystagmus (1% to 8%), dry eyes (>1% to 5%), eye pain (>1% to 5%), abnormal vision (>1% to <5%), conjunctivitis (>1% to <5%)
Otic: Tinnitus (1% to 7%), ear pain (>1% to 5%), deafness (>1% to <5%), otitis media (>1% to <5%)
Respiratory: Pharyngitis (2% to 8%), bronchitis (5%), rhinitis (>1% to 5%), dyspnea (1% to 5%), cough (>1% to <5%), epistaxis (>1% to <5%), pneumonia (>1% to <5%), sinusitis (>1% to <5%)
Miscellaneous: Diaphoresis (1%), hiccups

Dosage

Seizure disorders: Note: Administer doses >250 mg daily in divided doses.

Oral:

Simple and complex absence seizures: Children and Adults: Initial: 15 mg/kg/day; increase by 5-10 mg/kg/day at weekly intervals until therapeutic levels are achieved; maximum: 60 mg/kg/day. Larger maintenance doses may be required in younger children.

Complex partial seizures: Children ≥10 years and Adults: Initial: 10-15 mg/kg/day; increase by 5-10 mg/kg/day at weekly intervals until therapeutic levels are achieved; maximum: 60 mg/kg/day. Larger maintenance doses may be required in younger children.

Note: Regular release and delayed release formulations are usually given in 2-4 divided doses per day; extended release formulation (Depakote® ER) is usually given once daily. Depakote® ER is not recommended for use in children <10 years of age. In patients previously maintained on regular release valproic acid therapy (Depakene®) who convert to delayed release valproate tablets or capsules (Depakote®, Stavzor™), the same daily dose and frequency as the regular release should be used; once therapy is stabilized, the frequency of Depakote® or Stavzor™ may be adjusted to 2-3 times daily.

Conversion to Depakote® ER from a stable dose of Depakote®: Children ≥10 years and Adults: May require an increase in the total daily dose between 8% and 20% to maintain similar serum concentrations.

Conversion to monotherapy from adjunctive therapy: The concomitant antiepileptic drug (AED) can be decreased by ~25% every 2 weeks; dosage reduction of the concomitant AED may begin when valproate therapy is initiated or 1-2 weeks following valproate initiation.

I.V.: Total daily I.V. dose should be equivalent to the total daily dose of the oral valproate product; administer dose as a 60-minute infusion (≤20 mg/minute) with the same frequency as oral products; switch patient to oral products as soon as possible. Alternatively, rapid infusions of 1.5-6 mg/kg/minute have been used in clinical trials to quickly achieve therapeutic concentrations, and were generally well tolerated (Ramsay, 2003; Wheless, 2004; Venkataraman, 1999). One study reported undiluted valproic acid administered at ≤10 mg/kg/minute (dose of ≤30 mg/kg) was well tolerated (Limdi, 2007).

Rectal (unlabeled route): Children: Dilute syrup 1:1 with water for use as a retention enema; acute and maintenance dose: 6-15 mg/kg/dose (Graves, 1987)

Status epilepticus, refractory (unlabeled use): Adults: I.V.: Loading dose: 15-20 mg/kg administered at 20 mg/minute; maintenance dose: I.V. infusion: 1-5 mg/kg/hour (Gaitanis, 2003). Alternatively, median loading dose of 25-30 mg/kg (maximum dose: 45 mg/kg) administered at ≤6 mg/kg/minute have also been reported (Limdi, 2005; Misra, 2006; Sinha, 2000).

Mania: Adults: Oral:

Depakote® tablet, Stavzor™: Initial: 750 mg/day in divided doses; dose should be adjusted as rapidly as possible to desired clinical effect; maximum recommended dosage: 60 mg/kg/day

Depakote® ER: Initial: 25 mg/kg/day given once daily; dose should be adjusted as rapidly as possible to desired clinical effect; maximum recommended dose: 60 mg/kg/day.

Migraine prophylaxis: Oral:

Children ≥12 years (Stavzor™): 250 mg twice daily; adjust dose based on patient response, up to 1000 mg/day

Children ≥16 years and Adults (Depakote® tablet): 250 mg twice daily; adjust dose based on patient response, up to 1000 mg/day

Adults (Depakote® ER): 500 mg once daily for 7 days, then increase to 1000 mg once daily; adjust dose based on patient response; usual dosage range 500-1000 mg/day

Diabetic neuropathy (unlabeled use): Adults: Oral: 500-1200 mg/day (Bril, 2011)

Elderly: Oral, I.V.: Lower initial doses are recommended due to decreased elimination and increased incidences of somnolence in the elderly; no specific dosage recommendations are provided by the manufacturer. Upward titration should be done slowly and with close monitoring for adverse events (eg, sedation, dehydration, decreased nutritional intake). Safety and efficacy for use in patients >65 years have not been studied for migraine prophylaxis.

Dosing adjustment in renal impairment: Mild-to-severe impairment: No dosage adjustment necessary; however, due to decreased protein binding in renal impairment, monitoring only total valproate concentrations may be misleading.

Dosing adjustment/comments in hepatic impairment:

Mild-to-moderate impairment: Not recommended for use in hepatic disease; clearance is decreased with liver impairment. Hepatic disease is also associated with decreased albumin concentrations and 2- to 2.6-fold increase in the unbound fraction. Free concentrations of valproate may be elevated while total concentrations appear normal, therefore, monitoring only total valproate concentrations may be misleading.

Severe impairment: Use is contraindicated.

Mechanism of Action Causes increased availability of gamma-aminobutyric acid (GABA), an inhibitory neurotransmitter, to brain neurons or may enhance the action of GABA or mimic its action at postsynaptic receptor sites

Contraindications Hypersensitivity to valproic acid, divalproex, derivatives, or any component of the formulation; hepatic disease or significant impairment; urea cycle disorders

Warnings/Precautions Hazardous agent; use appropriate precautions for handling and disposal (NIOSH, 2012). **[U.S. Boxed Warning]: Hepatic failure resulting in fatalities has occurred in patients; children <2 years of age are at considerable risk.** Other risk factors include organic brain disease, mental retardation with severe seizure disorders, congenital metabolic disorders, and patients on multiple anticonvulsants. Hepatotoxicity has usually been reported within 6 months of therapy initiation. Monitor patients closely for appearance of malaise, weakness, facial edema, anorexia, jaundice, and vomiting; discontinue immediately with signs/symptom of significant or suspected impairment. Liver function tests should be performed at baseline and at regular intervals after initiation of therapy, especially within the first 6 months. Hepatic dysfunction may progress despite discontinuing treatment. Should only be used as monotherapy and with extreme caution in children <2 years of age and/or patients at high risk for hepatotoxicity. Contraindicated with significant hepatic impairment.

◀ **[U.S. Boxed Warning]: Cases of life-threatening pancreatitis, occurring at the start of therapy or following years of use, have been reported in adults and children.** Some cases have been hemorrhagic with rapid progression of initial symptoms to death. Promptly evaluate symptoms of abdominal pain, nausea, vomiting, and/or anorexia; should generally be discontinued if pancreatitis is diagnosed.

[U.S. Boxed Warning]: May cause teratogenic effects such as neural tube defects (eg, spina bifida). Use in women of childbearing potential requires that benefits of use in mother be weighed against the potential risk to fetus, especially when used for conditions not associated with permanent injury or risk of death (eg, migraine).

May cause severe thrombocytopenia, inhibition of platelet aggregation, and bleeding. Hypersensitivity reactions affecting multiple organs have been reported in association with valproate use; may include dermatologic and/or hematologic changes (eosinophilia, neutropenia, thrombocytopenia) or symptoms of organ dysfunction.

Hyperammonemia and/or encephalopathy, sometimes fatal, have been reported following the initiation of valproate therapy and may be present with normal transaminase levels. Ammonia levels should be measured in patients who develop unexplained lethargy and vomiting, changes in mental status, or in patients who present with hypothermia (unintentional drop in core body temperature to <35°C/95°F). Discontinue therapy if ammonia levels are increased and evaluate for possible urea cycle disorder (UCD); contraindicated in patients with UCD. Evaluation of UCD should be considered for the following patients prior to the start of therapy: History of unexplained encephalopathy or coma; encephalopathy associated with protein load; pregnancy or postpartum encephalopathy; unexplained mental retardation; history of elevated plasma ammonia or glutamine; history of cyclical vomiting and lethargy; episodic extreme irritability, ataxia; low BUN or protein avoidance; family history of UCD or unexplained infant deaths (particularly male); or signs or symptoms of UCD (hyperammonemia, encephalopathy, respiratory alkalosis). Hypothermia has been reported with valproate therapy; hypothermia may or may not be associated with hyperammonemia; may also occur with concomitant topiramate therapy following topiramate initiation or dosage increase.

In vitro studies have suggested valproate stimulates the replication of HIV and CMV viruses under experimental conditions. The clinical consequence of this is unknown, but should be considered when monitoring affected patients.

Antiepileptics are associated with an increased risk of suicidal behavior/thoughts with use (regardless of indication); patients should be monitored for signs/symptoms of depression, suicidal tendencies, and other unusual behavior changes during therapy and instructed to inform their healthcare provider immediately if symptoms occur.

Intravenous valproate is not recommended for post-traumatic seizure prophylaxis in patients with acute head trauma; study results for this indication suggested increased mortality with I.V. valproate use compared to I.V. phenytoin. Anticonvulsants should not be discontinued abruptly because of the possibility of increasing seizure frequency; valproate should be withdrawn gradually to minimize the potential of increased seizure frequency, unless safety concerns require a more rapid withdrawal. Concomitant use with carbapenem antibiotics may reduce valproic acid levels to subtherapeutic levels; monitor levels frequently and consider alternate therapy if levels drop significantly or lack of seizure control occurs. Patients treated for bipolar disorder should be monitored closely for clinical worsening or suicidality; prescriptions should be written for the smallest quantity consistent with good patient care.

CNS depression may occur with valproate use. Patients must be cautioned about performing tasks which require mental alertness (operating machinery or driving). Effects with other sedative drugs or ethanol may be potentiated. Use with caution in the elderly as the elderly may be more sensitive to sedating effects and dehydration; in some elderly patients with somnolence, concomitant decreases in nutritional intake and weight loss were observed. Reduce initial dosages in elderly and closely monitor fluid status, nutritional intake, somnolence, and other adverse events.

Medication residue in stool has been reported (rarely) with oral Depakote® (divalproex sodium) formulations; some reports have occurred in patients with shortened GI transit times (eg, diarrhea) or anatomic GI disorders (eg, ileostomy, colostomy). In patients reporting medication residue in stool, it is recommended to monitor valproate level and clinical condition.

Drug Interactions

Metabolism/Transport Effects For valproic acid:
Substrate (minor) of CYP2A6, 2B6, 2C9, 2C19, 2E1;
Inhibits CYP2C9 (weak), 2C19 (weak), 2D6 (weak), 3A4 (weak); **Induces** CYP2A6 (weak)

Avoid Concomitant Use
Avoid concomitant use of Valproic Acid with any of the following: Cosyntropin

Increased Effect/Toxicity
Valproic Acid may increase the levels/effects of: Barbiturates; Ethosuximide; LamoTRIgine; LORazepam; Paliperidone; Primidone; RisperiDONE; Rufinamide; Temozolomide; Tricyclic Antidepressants; Vorinostat; Zidovudine

The levels/effects of Valproic Acid may be increased by: ChlorproMAZINE; Cosyntropin; Felbamate; GuanFACINE; Salicylates; Topiramate

Decreased Effect
Valproic Acid may decrease the levels/effects of: CarBAMazepine; Fosphenytoin; OXcarbazepine; Phenytoin

The levels/effects of Valproic Acid may be decreased by: Barbiturates; CarBAMazepine; Carbapenems; Ethosuximide; Fosphenytoin; Methylfolate; Phenytoin; Primidone; Protease Inhibitors; Rifampin

Ethanol/Nutrition/Herb Interactions
Ethanol: Avoid ethanol (may increase CNS depression).
Food: Food may delay but does not affect the extent of absorption.

Pharmacodynamics/Kinetics
Half-life Elimination Increased in neonates, elderly and those with liver disease; Children >2 months: 7-13 hours; Adults: 9-16 hours
Time to Peak
Oral: Depakote® tablet: ~4 hours; Depakote® ER: 4-17 hours; Stavzor™: 2 hours
Rectal (unlabeled route): 1-3 hours (Graves, 1987)
Pregnancy Risk Factor D

Pregnancy Considerations [U.S. Boxed Warning]: May cause teratogenic effects such as neural tube defects (eg, spina bifida). Teratogenic effects have been reported in animals and humans. Valproic acid crosses the placenta. Neural tube, cardiac, facial (characteristic pattern of dysmorphic facial features), skeletal, multiple other defects reported. Epilepsy itself, number of medications, genetic factors, or a combination of these probably influence the teratogenicity of anticonvulsant therapy. Information from the North American Antiepileptic Drug Pregnancy Registry notes a fourfold increase in congenital malformations with exposure to valproic acid monotherapy during the 1st trimester of pregnancy when compared to monotherapy with other antiepileptic drugs (AED). The risk of neural tube defects is ~1% to 2% (general population risk estimated to be 0.14% to 0.2%). The effect of folic acid supplementation to decrease this risk is unknown, however, folic acid supplementation is recommended for all women contemplating pregnancy. An information sheet describing the teratogenic potential is available from the manufacturer.

Nonteratogenic effects have also been reported. Afibrinogenemia leading to fatal hemorrhage and hepatotoxicity have been noted in case reports of infants following *in utero* exposure to valproic acid. Developmental delay, autism and/or autism spectrum disorder have also been reported. In a prospective cohort study conducted in the U.S. and the United Kingdom, a lower Differential Ability Scale ([D.A.S.]; a battery of tests which measure cognitive development in children) score was observed in children 3 years of age with prenatal exposure to valproate compared to children with prenatal exposure to other antiepileptics (lamotrigine, carbamazepine, or phenytoin). Use in women of childbearing potential requires that benefits of use in mother be weighed against the potential risk to fetus, especially when used for conditions not associated with permanent injury or risk of death (eg, migraine).

Patients exposed to valproic acid during pregnancy are encouraged to enroll themselves into the AED Pregnancy Registry by calling 1-888-233-2334. Additional information is available at www.aedpregnancyregistry.org.

Lactation Enters breast milk/not recommended (AAP considers "compatible"; AAP 2001 update pending)

Breast-Feeding Considerations Breast milk concentrations of valproic acid have been reported as 1% to 10% of maternal concentration. The weight-adjusted dose to the infant has been calculated to be ~4%.

Dosage Forms Strength expressed as valproic acid.

Capsule, softgel, oral: 250 mg
Depakene®: 250 mg
Capsule, softgel, delayed release, oral:
Stavzor™: 125 mg, 250 mg, 500 mg
Capsule, sprinkles, oral: 125 mg
Depakote® Sprinkle: 125 mg
Injection, solution [preservative free]: 100 mg/mL (5 mL)
Depacon®: 100 mg/mL (5 mL)
Solution, oral: 250 mg/5 mL
Syrup, oral: 250 mg/5 mL
Depakene®: 250 mg/5 mL
Tablet, delayed release, oral: 125 mg, 250 mg, 500 mg
Depakote®: 125 mg, 250 mg, 500 mg
Tablet, extended release, oral: 250 mg, 500 mg
Depakote® ER: 250 mg, 500 mg

Valrubicin (val ROO bi sin)

Brand Names: U.S. Valstar®
Brand Names: Canada Valtaxin®
Pharmacologic Category Antineoplastic Agent, Anthracycline
Use Intravesical treatment of BCG-refractory bladder carcinoma *in situ*
Local Anesthetic/Vasoconstrictor Precautions No information available to require special precautions
Effects on Dental Treatment No significant effects or complications reported
Effects on Bleeding This chemotherapy is administered locally and hematologic toxicity is not experienced.
Adverse Effects Note: In general, local adverse reactions occur during or shortly after instillation and resolve within 1-7 days.
>10%: Genitourinary: Bladder irritation (88%), urinary frequency (61%), urinary urgency (57%), dysuria (56%), bladder spasm (31%), hematuria (29%; gross: 1%), bladder pain (28%), urinary incontinence (22%), cystitis (15%), urinary tract infection (15%), urine red-tinged
1% to 10%:
Cardiovascular: Chest pain (3%), vasodilation (2%), peripheral edema (1%)
Central nervous system: Headache (4%), malaise (4%), dizziness (3%), fever (2%)
Dermatologic: Rash (3%)
Endocrine & metabolic: Hyperglycemia (1%)
Gastrointestinal: Abdominal pain (5%), nausea (5%), diarrhea (3%), vomiting (2%), flatulence (1%)
Genitourinary: Nocturia (7%), burning symptoms (5%), urinary retention (4%), urethral pain (3%), pelvic pain (1%), hematuria (microscopic) (3%)
Hematologic: Anemia (2%)
Neuromuscular & skeletal: Weakness (4%), back pain (3%), myalgia (1%)
Respiratory: Pneumonia (1%)
General Dosage Range Dosage adjustment recommended in patients who develop toxicities
Intravesical: *Adults:* 800 mg once weekly for 6 weeks
Mechanism of Action Blocks function of DNA topoisomerase II; inhibits DNA synthesis, causes extensive chromosomal damage, and arrests cell development (G_2 phase); unlike other anthracyclines, does not appear to intercalate DNA; readily penetrates cells.
Pregnancy Risk Factor C
Pregnancy Considerations Embryotoxicity and teratogenic effects were observed in animal reproduction studies. Systemic exposure (eg, with bladder perforation) during human pregnancy may result in fetal harm. Women of childbearing potential should avoid becoming pregnant during treatment. All patients of reproductive age should use an effective method of contraception during the treatment period.

Valsartan (val SAR tan)

Related Information
Cardiovascular Diseases *on page 1492*
Brand Names: U.S. Diovan®
Brand Names: Canada CO Valsartan; Diovan®; Ran-Valsartan; Sandoz-Valsartan; Teva-Valsartan
Generic Availability (U.S.) No
Pharmacologic Category Angiotensin II Receptor Blocker

Use Alone or in combination with other antihypertensive agents in the treatment of essential hypertension; reduction of cardiovascular mortality in patients with left ventricular dysfunction postmyocardial infarction; treatment of heart failure (NYHA Class II-IV)

Local Anesthetic/Vasoconstrictor Precautions No information available to require special precautions

Effects on Dental Treatment No significant effects or complications reported

Effects on Bleeding No information available to require special precautions

Adverse Effects

>10%:

Central nervous system: Dizziness (heart failure trials 17%)

Renal: BUN increased >50% (heart failure trials 17%)

1% to 10%:

Cardiovascular: Hypotension (heart failure trials 7%; MI trial 1%), orthostatic hypotension (heart failure trials 2%), syncope (up to >1%)

Central nervous system: Dizziness (hypertension trial 2% to 8%), fatigue (heart failure trials 3%; hypertension trial 2%), postural dizziness (heart failure trials 2%), headache (heart failure trials >1%), vertigo (up to >1%)

Endocrine & metabolic: Serum potassium increased by >20% (4% to 10%), hyperkalemia (heart failure trials 2%)

Gastrointestinal: Diarrhea (heart failure trials 5%), abdominal pain (2%), nausea (heart failure trials >1%), upper abdominal pain (heart failure trials >1%)

Hematologic: Neutropenia (2%)

Neuromuscular & skeletal: Arthralgia (heart failure trials 3%), back pain (up to 3%)

Ocular: Blurred vision (heart failure trials >1%)

Renal: Creatinine doubled (MI trial 4%), creatinine increased >50% (heart failure trials 4%), renal dysfunction (up to >1%)

Respiratory: Cough (1% to 3%)

Miscellaneous: Viral infection (3%)

Dosage Oral:

Hypertension:

Children 6-16 years: Initial: 1.3 mg/kg once daily (maximum: 40 mg/day); dose may be increased to achieve desired effect; doses >2.7 mg/kg (maximum: 160 mg) have not been studied

Adults: Initial: 80 mg or 160 mg once daily (in patients who are not volume depleted); dose may be increased to achieve desired effect; maximum recommended dose: 320 mg daily

Heart failure: Adults: Initial: 40 mg twice daily; titrate dose to 80-160 mg twice daily, as tolerated; maximum daily dose: 320 mg

Left ventricular dysfunction after MI: Adults: Initial: 20 mg twice daily; titrate dose to target of 160 mg twice daily as tolerated; may initiate ≥12 hours following MI

Dosing adjustment in renal impairment:

Cl_{cr} ≥30 mL/minute: No dosage adjustment necessary.

Cl_{cr} <30 mL/minute: No dosage adjustment provided in manufacturer's labeling; safety and efficacy have not been established.

Dialysis: Not significantly removed

Dosing adjustment in hepatic impairment:

Mild-to-moderate impairment: No dosage adjustment necessary; use caution in patients with liver disease. Patients with mild-to-moderate chronic disease have twice the exposure as healthy volunteers.

Severe impairment: No dosage adjustment provided in manufacturer's labeling; has not been studied

Mechanism of Action Valsartan produces direct antagonism of the angiotensin II (AT2) receptors, unlike the ACE inhibitors. It displaces angiotensin II from the AT1 receptor and produces its blood pressure-lowering effects by antagonizing AT1-induced vasoconstriction, aldosterone release, catecholamine release, arginine vasopressin release, water intake, and hypertrophic responses. This action results in more efficient blockade of the cardiovascular effects of angiotensin II and fewer side effects than the ACE inhibitors.

Contraindications Hypersensitivity to valsartan or any component of the formulation; concomitant use with aliskiren in patients with diabetes mellitus

Warnings/Precautions [U.S. Boxed Warning]: Drugs that act on the renin-angiotensin system can cause injury and death to the developing fetus. Discontinue as soon as possible once pregnancy is detected. May cause hyperkalemia; avoid potassium supplementation unless specifically required by healthcare provider. During the initiation of therapy, hypotension may occur, particularly in patients with heart failure or post-MI patients. Use extreme caution with concurrent administration of potassium-sparing diuretics or potassium supplements, in patients with mild-to-moderate hepatic dysfunction (adjust dose), in those who may be sodium/water depleted (eg, on high-dose diuretics), and in the elderly; correct depletion first.

Use caution with unstented unilateral/bilateral renal artery stenosis. When unstented bilateral renal artery stenosis is present, use is generally avoided due to the elevated risk of deterioration in renal function unless possible benefits outweigh risks. Use with caution with preexisting renal insufficiency; significant aortic/mitral stenosis. May be associated with deterioration of renal function and/or increases in serum creatinine, particularly in patients with low renal blood flow (eg, renal artery stenosis, heart failure) whose glomerular filtration rate (GFR) is dependent on efferent arteriolar vasoconstriction by angiotensin II. Use caution in patients with severe renal impairment or significant hepatic dysfunction. Monitor renal function closely in patients with severe heart failure; changes in renal function should be anticipated and dosage adjustments of valsartan or concomitant medications may be needed. Concomitant use of an angiotensin-converting enzyme (ACE) inhibitor or renin inhibitor (eg, aliskiren) is associated with an increased risk of hypotension, hyperkalemia, and renal dysfunction; concomitant use with aliskiren should be avoided in patients with GFR <60 mL/minute and is contraindicated in patients with diabetes mellitus (regardless of GFR). In Canada, use is not approved in patients <18 years of age.

Drug Interactions

Metabolism/Transport Effects Substrate of SLCO1B1; **Inhibits** CYP2C9 (weak)

Avoid Concomitant Use There are no known interactions where it is recommended to avoid concomitant use.

Increased Effect/Toxicity

Valsartan may increase the levels/effects of: ACE Inhibitors; Amifostine; Antihypertensives; CycloSPORINE (Systemic); Hydrochlorothiazide; Hypotensive Agents; Lithium; Nonsteroidal Anti-Inflammatory Agents; Potassium-Sparing Diuretics; RiTUXimab; Sodium Phosphates

The levels/effects of Valsartan may be increased by: Alfuzosin; Aliskiren; Canagliflozin; Diazoxide; Eltrombopag; Eplerenone; Herbs (Hypotensive Properties); Hydrochlorothiazide; MAO Inhibitors; Pentoxifylline; Phosphodiesterase 5 Inhibitors; Potassium Salts; Prostacyclin Analogues; Tolvaptan; Trimethoprim

Decreased Effect

The levels/effects of Valsartan may be decreased by: Herbs (Hypertensive Properties); Methylphenidate; Nonsteroidal Anti-Inflammatory Agents; Yohimbine

Ethanol/Nutrition/Herb Interactions

Food: Decreases the peak plasma concentration and extent of absorption by 50% and 40%, respectively. Potassium supplements and/or potassium-containing salts may cause or worsen hyperkalemia. Management: Take consistently with regard to food. Consult prescriber before consuming a potassium-rich diet, potassium supplements, or salt substitutes.

Herb/Nutraceutical: Some herbal medications may worsen hypertension (eg, licorice); others may increase the antihypertensive effect of valsartan (eg, shepherd's purse). Management: Avoid bayberry, blue cohosh, cayenne, ephedra, ginger, ginseng (American), kola, licorice, and yohimbe. Avoid black cohosh, California poppy, coleus, golden seal, hawthorn, mistletoe, periwinkle, quinine, and shepherd's purse.

Dietary Considerations Avoid salt substitutes which contain potassium. May be taken with or without food.

Pharmacodynamics/Kinetics

Onset of Action ~2 hours

Duration of Action 24 hours

Half-life Elimination ~6 hours

Time to Peak Serum: 2-4 hours

Pregnancy Risk Factor D

Pregnancy Considerations [U.S. Boxed Warning]: Drugs that act on the renin-angiotensin system can cause injury and death to the developing fetus. Discontinue as soon as possible once pregnancy is detected. The use of drugs which act on the renin-angiotensin system are associated with oligohydramnios. Oligohydramnios, due to decreased fetal renal function, may lead to fetal lung hypoplasia and skeletal malformations. Use is also associated with anuria, hypotension, renal failure, skull hypoplasia, and death in the fetus/neonate. The exposed fetus should be monitored for fetal growth, amniotic fluid volume, and organ formation. Infants exposed *in utero* should be monitored for hyperkalemia, hypotension, and oliguria.

Lactation Excretion in breast milk unknown/not recommended

Breast-Feeding Considerations It is not known if valsartan is found in breast milk; the manufacturer recommends discontinuing the drug or discontinuing nursing based on the importance of the drug to the mother.

Dosage Forms

Tablet, oral:

Diovan®: 40 mg, 80 mg, 160 mg, 320 mg

Valsartan and Hydrochlorothiazide

(val SAR tan & hye droe klor oh THYE a zide)

Related Information

Hydrochlorothiazide *on page 687*

Valsartan *on page 1381*

Brand Names: U.S. Diovan HCT®

Brand Names: Canada Diovan HCT®; Sandoz Valsartan HCT; Teva-Valsartan HCTZ; Valsartan-HCTZ

Pharmacologic Category Angiotensin II Receptor Blocker; Diuretic, Thiazide

Use Treatment of hypertension

Local Anesthetic/Vasoconstrictor Precautions No information available to require special precautions

Effects on Dental Treatment No significant effects or complications reported

Effects on Bleeding No information available to require special precautions

Adverse Effects Percentages reported with combination product; other reactions have been reported (see individual agents for additional information)

>10%: Renal: BUN increased (15%)

1% to 10%:

Cardiovascular: Hypotension (1%)

Central nervous system: Dizziness (6%; dose related)

Endocrine & metabolic: Hypokalemia (3%)

Renal: Creatinine increased (2%)

Respiratory: Nasopharyngitis (2%)

General Dosage Range Oral: *Adults:* Valsartan 80-320 mg and hydrochlorothiazide 12.5-25 mg once daily (maximum: 25 mg/day [hydrochlorothiazide]; 320 mg/day [valsartan])

Mechanism of Action Valsartan produces direct antagonism of the angiotensin II (AT2) receptors, unlike the ACE inhibitors. It displaces angiotensin II from the AT1 receptor and produces its blood pressure-lowering effects by antagonizing AT1-induced vasoconstriction, aldosterone release, catecholamine release, arginine vasopressin release, water intake, and hypertrophic responses. This action results in more efficient blockade of the cardiovascular effects of angiotensin II and fewer side effects than the ACE inhibitors.

Hydrochlorothiazide inhibits sodium reabsorption in the distal tubules causing increased excretion of sodium and water as well as potassium and hydrogen ions

Pregnancy Risk Factor D

Pregnancy Considerations [U.S. Boxed Warning]: Drugs that act on the renin-angiotensin system can cause injury and death to the developing fetus. Discontinue as soon as possible once pregnancy is detected. Also see individual agents.

Vancomycin (van koe MYE sin)

Brand Names: U.S. Vancocin®

Brand Names: Canada PMS-Vancomycin; Sterile Vancomycin Hydrochloride, USP; Val-Vancomycin; Vancocin®; Vancomycin Hydrochloride for Injection, USP

Generic Availability (U.S.) Yes

Pharmacologic Category Glycopeptide

Use

I.V.: Treatment of patients with infections caused by staphylococcal species and streptococcal species

Oral: Treatment of *C. difficile*-associated diarrhea and treatment of enterocolitis caused by *Staphylococcus aureus* (including methicillin-resistant strains)

Unlabeled Use Bacterial endophthalmitis; treatment of infections caused by gram-positive organisms in patients who have serious allergies to beta-lactam agents; treatment of beta-lactam resistant gram-positive infections; surgical prophylaxis; treatment of prosthetic joint infection; group B streptococcus maternal use for neonatal prophylaxis

Local Anesthetic/Vasoconstrictor Precautions No information available to require special precautions

◀ **Effects on Dental Treatment** Key adverse event(s) related to dental treatment: Bitter taste. "Red man syndrome", characterized by skin rash and hypotension, is not an allergic reaction but rather is associated with too rapid infusion of the drug. To alleviate or prevent the reaction, infuse vancomycin at a rate of ≥30 minutes for each 500 mg of drug being administered (eg, 1 g over ≥60 minutes); 1.5 g over ≥90 minutes.

Effects on Bleeding Vancomycin has been demonstrated to induce immune thrombocytopenia, causing a significant drop in platelet count following a short (ie, 12-15 hours) period of time after treatment. Both IgG and IgM vancomycin-dependent platelets have been identified post vancomycin administration. Discontinuation has shown to be an effective remedy, as platelet levels return to the pre-exposure counts within 4 days of drug withdrawal.

Adverse Effects
Injection:
>10%:
Cardiovascular: Hypotension accompanied by flushing
Dermatologic: Erythematous rash on face and upper body (red neck or red man syndrome - infusion rate related)
1% to 10%:
Central nervous system: Chills, drug fever
Dermatologic: Rash
Hematologic: Eosinophilia, reversible neutropenia
Local: Phlebitis

Oral:
>10%: Gastrointestinal: Abdominal pain, bad taste (with oral solution), nausea
1% to 10%:
Cardiovascular: Peripheral edema
Central nervous system: Fatigue, fever, headache
Gastrointestinal: Diarrhea, flatulence, vomiting
Genitourinary: Urinary tract infection
Neuromuscular & skeletal: Back pain

Dental Usual Dosage
Prophylaxis against infective endocarditis: I.V.:

Infants >1 month and Children:
Dental, oral, or upper respiratory tract surgery: 20 mg/kg 1 hour prior to the procedure. **Note:** American Heart Association (AHA) guidelines now recommend prophylaxis only in patients undergoing invasive procedures and in whom underlying cardiac conditions may predispose to a higher risk of adverse outcomes should infection occur.
GI/GU procedure: 20 mg/kg plus gentamicin 2 mg/kg 1 hour prior to surgery. **Note:** As of April 2007, routine prophylaxis no longer recommended by the AHA.
Adults:
Dental, oral, or upper respiratory tract surgery: 1 g 1 hour before surgery. **Note:** AHA guidelines now recommend prophylaxis only in patients undergoing invasive procedures and in whom underlying cardiac conditions may predispose to a higher risk of adverse outcomes should infection occur
GI/GU procedure: 1 g plus 1.5 mg/kg gentamicin 1 hour prior to surgery. **Note:** As of April 2007, routine prophylaxis no longer recommended by the AHA.

Dosage
Usual dosage range:
Infants >1 month and Children: I.V.: 10-15 mg/kg every 6 hours
Adults: Initial intravenous dosing should be based on actual body weight; subsequent dosing adjusted based on serum trough vancomycin concentrations.

I.V.: 2000-3000 mg/day (or 30-60 mg/kg/day) in divided doses every 8-12 hours (Rybak, 2009); **Note:** Dose requires adjustment in renal impairment
Oral: 500-2000 mg/day in divided doses every 6 hours

Indication-specific dosing:
Catheter-related infections: Adults: Antibiotic lock technique (Mermel, 2009): 2 mg/mL ± 10 units heparin/mL **or** 2.5 mg/mL ± 2500 **or** 5000 units heparin/mL **or** 5 mg/mL ± 5000 units heparin/mL (preferred regimen); instill into catheter port with a volume sufficient to fill the catheter (2-5 mL). **Note:** May use SWFI/NS or D$_5$W as diluents. Do not mix with any other solutions. Dwell times generally should not exceed 48 hours before renewal of lock solution. Remove lock solution prior to catheter use, then replace.

C. difficile -associated diarrhea (CDAD):
Infants >1 month and Children: Oral: 40 mg/kg/day in 3-4 divided doses for 7-10 days (maximum: 2000 mg/day)
Adults:
Oral:
Manufacturer recommendations: 125 mg 4 times/day for 10 days
IDSA guideline recommendations: Severe infection: 125 mg every 6 hours for 10-14 days; Severe, complicated infection: 500 mg every 6 hours with or without concurrent I.V. metronidazole. May consider vancomycin retention enema (in patients with complete ileus) (Cohen, 2010).
Rectal (unlabeled route): Retention enema (in patients with complete ileus): SHEA/IDSA guideline recommendations: Severe, complicated infection in patients with ileus: 500 mg every 6 hours (in 100 mL 0.9% sodium chloride) with oral vancomycin with or without concurrent I.V. metronidazole (Cohen, 2010)

Complicated infections in seriously-ill patients: Adults: I.V.: Loading dose: 25-30 mg/kg (based on actual body weight) may be used to rapidly achieve target concentration; then 15-20 mg/kg/dose every 8-12 hours (Rybak, 2009)

Enterocolitis (S. aureus):
Infants >1 months and Children: Oral: 40 mg/kg/day in 3-4 divided doses for 7-10 days (maximum: 2000 mg/day)
Adults: Oral: 500-2000 mg/day in 3-4 divided doses for 7-10 days (usual dose: 125-500 mg every 6 hours)

Group B streptococcus (neonatal prophylaxis): Adults: I.V.: 1000 mg every 12 hours until delivery. **Note:** reserved for penicillin allergic patients at high risk for anaphylaxis if organism is resistant to clindamycin or where no susceptibility data are available (CDC, 2010).

Meningitis:
Infants >1 month and Children:
I.V.: 15 mg/kg every 6 hours (Tunkel, 2004)
Intrathecal, intraventricular (unlabeled route): 5-20 mg/day (Tunkel, 2004)
Children: Alternate regimen: S. aureus (methicillin-resistant) (unlabeled use; Liu, 2011): I.V.: 15 mg/kg/dose every 6 hours for 2 weeks (some experts combine with rifampin)
Adults:
I.V.: 30-60 mg/kg/day in divided doses every 8-12 hours (Rybak, 2009) **or** 500-750 mg every 6 hours. **Note:** For PCN-resistant Streptococcus pneumoniae (MIC ≥2 mcg/mL), combine with a third-generation cephalosporin.

Alternate regimen: *S. aureus* (methicillin-resistant) (unlabeled use; Liu, 2011): 15-20 mg/kg/dose every 8-12 hours for 2 weeks (some experts combine with rifampin)

Intrathecal, intraventricular (unlabeled route): 5-20 mg/day

Pneumonia:

Community-acquired pneumonia (CAP):

Infants >3 months and Children (IDSA/PIDS, 2011): I.V.: **Note:** In children ≥5 years, a macrolide antibiotic should be added if atypical pneumonia cannot be ruled out.

Group A *Streptococcus* (alternative to ampicillin or penicillin in beta-lactam allergic patients): 40-60 mg/kg/day divided every 6-8 hours

Presumed bacterial (in addition to recommended antibiotic therapy), *S. pneumoniae*, moderate-to-severe infection (MICs to penicillin ≤2.0 mcg/mL) (alternative to ampicillin or penicillin): 40-60 mg/kg/day divided every 6-8 hours

S. aureus (methicillin-susceptible) (alternative to cefazolin/oxacillin): 40-60 mg/kg/day divided every 6-8 hours

S. aureus, moderate-to-severe infection (methicillin-resistant +/- clindamycin susceptible) (preferred): 40-60 mg/kg/day divided every 6-8 hours **or** dosing to achieve AUC/MIC >400

Alternate regimen: 60 mg/kg/day divided every 6 hours for 7-21 days, depending on severity (Liu, 2011)

S. pneumoniae, moderate-to-severe infection (MICs to penicillin ≥4.0 mcg/mL) (alternative to ceftriaxone in beta-lactam allergic patients): 40-60 mg/kg/day divided every 6-8 hours

Adults: *S. aureus* (methicillin-resistant): I.V.: 45-60 mg/kg/day divided every 8-12 hours (maximum: 2000 mg/dose) for 7-21 days depending on severity (Liu, 2011)

Healthcare-associated pneumonia (HAP): *S. aureus* (methicillin-resistant): I.V.:

Infants and Children: 60 mg/kg/day divided every 6 hours for 7-21 days depending on severity (Liu, 2011)

Adults: 45-60 mg/kg/day divided every 8-12 hours (maximum: 2000 mg/dose) for 7-21 days depending on severity (American Thoracic Society [ATS], 2005; Liu, 2011; Rybak 2009)

Prophylaxis against infective endocarditis: I.V.:

Children:

Dental, oral, or upper respiratory tract surgery: 20 mg/kg/dose administered 1 hour prior to the procedure. **Note:** American Heart Association (AHA) guidelines recommend prophylaxis only in patients undergoing invasive procedures and in whom underlying cardiac conditions may predispose to a higher risk of adverse outcomes should infection occur.

GI/GU procedure: 20 mg/kg (plus gentamicin 1.5 mg/kg) administered 1 hour prior to surgery. **Note:** Routine prophylaxis no longer recommended by the AHA.

Adults:

Dental, oral, or upper respiratory tract surgery: 1000 mg 1 hour before surgery. **Note:** AHA guidelines now recommend prophylaxis only in patients undergoing invasive procedures and in whom underlying cardiac conditions may predispose to a higher risk of adverse outcomes should infection occur.

GI/GU procedure: 1000 mg plus 1.5 mg/kg gentamicin 1 hour prior to surgery. **Note:** As of April 2007, routine prophylaxis no longer recommended by the AHA.

Susceptible gram-positive infections (MIC ≤1 mcg/mL; Rybak, 2009): I.V.:

Infants >1 month and Children: 10 mg/kg/dose every 6 hours (manufacturer recommendations) **or** 15 mg/kg/dose (maximum: 2000 mg/dose) every 6 hours (Liu, 2011)

Adults: 15-20 mg/kg/dose (usual: 750-1500 mg) every 8-12 hours

Note: If MIC ≥2 mcg/mL, alternative therapies are recommended.

Bacteremia (*S. aureus* [methicillin-resistant]) (unlabeled use; Liu, 2011): I.V.:

Children: 15 mg/kg/dose every 6 hours for 2-6 weeks depending on severity

Adults: 15-20 mg/kg/dose every 8-12 hours for 2-6 weeks depending on severity

Brain abscess, subdural empyema, spinal epidural abscess (*S. aureus* [methicillin-resistant]) (unlabeled use; Liu, 2011): I.V.:

Children: 15 mg/kg/dose every 6 hours for 4-6 weeks (some experts combine with rifampin)

Adults: 15-20 mg/kg/dose every 8-12 hours for 4-6 weeks (some experts combine with rifampin)

Endocarditis:

Native valve (*Enterococcus*, vancomycin MIC ≤4 mg/L) (unlabeled use; Gould, 2012): I.V.: Adults: 1000 mg every 12 hours for 4-6 weeks (combine with gentamicin for 4-6 weeks)

Native valve (*S. aureus* [methicillin-resistant]) (unlabeled use; Liu, 2011): I.V.:

Children: 15 mg/kg/dose every 6 hours for 6 weeks

Adults: 15-20 mg/kg/dose every 8-12 hours for 6 weeks (European guidelines support the entire duration of therapy to be 4 weeks and in combination with rifampin [Gould, 2012])

Native or prosthetic valve (streptococcal [penicillin MIC >0.5 mg/L or patient intolerant to penicillin]) (unlabeled use; Gould, 2012): I.V.: Adults: 1000 mg every 12 hours for 4-6 weeks (combine with gentamicin for at least the first 2 weeks); **Note:** The longer duration of treatment (ie, 6 weeks) should be used for patients with prosthetic valve endocarditis.

Prosthetic valve (*Enterococcus*, vancomycin MIC ≤4 mg/L) (unlabeled use; Gould, 2012): I.V.: Adults: 1000 mg every 12 hours for 6 weeks (combine with gentamicin for 4-6 weeks)

Prosthetic valve (*S. aureus* [methicillin-resistant]) (unlabeled use; Liu, 2011): I.V.:

Children: 15 mg/kg/dose every 6 hours for at least 6 weeks

Adults: 15-20 mg/kg/dose every 8-12 hours for at least 6 weeks (combine with rifampin for the entire duration of therapy and gentamicin for the first 2 weeks)

Endophthalmitis (unlabeled use): Adults: Intravitreal: Usual dose: 1 mg/0.1 mL NS instilled into vitreum; may repeat administration if necessary in 3-4 days, usually in combination with ceftazidime or an aminoglycoside. **Note:** Some clinicians have recommended using a lower dose of 0.2 mg/0.1 mL, based on concerns for retinotoxicity.

◄ **Osteomyelitis (S. aureus [methicillin-resistant])**
(unlabeled use; Liu, 2011): I.V.:
Children: 15 mg/kg/dose every 6 hours for 4-6 weeks
Adults: 15-20 mg/kg/dose every 8-12 hours for a minimum of 8 weeks (some experts combine with rifampin)

Prosthetic joint infection (unlabeled use; Osman, 2013): I.V.: Adults:
Enterococcus spp (penicillin-susceptible or –resistant), *Propionibacterium acnes,* streptococci (beta-hemolytic): 15 mg/kg every 12 hours for 4-6 weeks, followed by an oral antibiotic suppressive regimen
Note: For penicillin-susceptible or -resistant *Enterococcus* spp, consider addition of an aminoglycoside; in penicillin-susceptible *Enterococcus,* beta-hemolytic streptococcus or *Propionibacterium acnes* infections, only use vancomycin if patient has penicillin allergy.
Staphylococci (oxacillin-susceptible or –resistant):15 mg/kg every 12 hours for 2-6 weeks in combination with rifampin followed by oral antibiotic treatment and suppressive regimens

Septic arthritis (S. aureus [methicillin-resistant])
(unlabeled use; Liu, 2011): I.V.:
Children: 15 mg/kg/dose every 6 hours for minimum of 3-4 weeks
Adults: 15-20 mg/kg/dose every 8-12 hours for 3-4 weeks

Septic thrombosis of cavernous or dural venous sinus (S. aureus [methicillin-resistant]) (unlabeled use; Liu, 2011): I.V.:
Children: 15 mg/kg/dose every 6 hours for 4-6 weeks (some experts combine with rifampin)
Adults: 15-20 mg/kg/dose every 8-12 hours for 4-6 weeks (some experts combine with rifampin)

Skin and skin structure infections, complicated (S. aureus [methicillin-resistant]) (unlabeled use; Liu, 2011): I.V.:
Children: 15 mg/kg/dose every 6 hours for 7-14 days
Adults: 15-20 mg/kg/dose every 8-12 hours for 7-14 days

Surgical prophylaxis (unlabeled use): I.V.: Adults:
1000 mg or 10-15 mg/kg over 60 minutes (longer infusion time if dose >1000 mg) (Bratzler, 2004)
The Society of Thoracic Surgeons recommends 1000-1500 mg or 15 mg/kg over 60 minutes with completion within 1 hour of skin incision. Although not well established, a second dose of 7.5 mg/kg may be considered during cardiopulmonary bypass (Engelman, 2007).

Dosing interval in renal impairment (vancomycin levels should be monitored in patients with any renal impairment): I.V.:
Cl_{cr} >50 mL/minute: Start with 15-20 mg/kg/dose (usual: 750-1500 mg) every 8-12 hours
Cl_{cr} 20-49 mL/minute: Start with 15-20 mg/kg/dose (usual: 750-1500 mg) every 24 hours
Cl_{cr} <20 mL/minute: Will need longer intervals; determine by serum concentration monitoring
Note: In the critically-ill patient with renal insufficiency, the initial loading dose (25-30 mg/kg) should not be reduced. However, subsequent dosage adjustments should be made based on renal function and trough serum concentrations.
Poorly dialyzable by intermittent hemodialysis (0% to 5%); however, use of high-flux membranes and continuous renal replacement therapy (CRRT) increases vancomycin clearance, and generally requires replacement dosing.

Intermittent hemodialysis (IHD) (administer after hemodialysis on dialysis days): Following loading dose of 15-25 mg/kg, give either 500-1000 mg **or** 5-10 mg/kg after each dialysis session. (Heintz, 2009). **Note:** Dosing dependent on the assumption of 3 times/week, complete IHD sessions.
Redosing based on pre-HD concentrations:
<10 mg/L: Administer 1000 mg after HD
10-25 mg/L: Administer 500-750 mg after HD
>25 mg/L: Hold vancomycin
Redosing based on post-HD concentrations:
<10-15 mg/L: Administer 500-1000 mg
Peritoneal dialysis (PD):
Administration via PD fluid: 15-30 mg/L (15-30 mcg/mL) of PD fluid
Systemic: Loading dose of 1000 mg, followed by 500-1000 mg every 48-72 hours with close monitoring of levels
Continuous renal replacement therapy (CRRT) (Heintz, 2009; Trotman, 2005): Drug clearance is highly dependent on the method of renal replacement, filter type, and flow rate. Appropriate dosing requires close monitoring of pharmacologic response, signs of adverse reactions due to drug accumulation, as well as drug concentrations in relation to target trough (if appropriate). The following are general recommendations only (based on dialysate flow/ultrafiltration rates of 1-2 L/hour and minimal residual renal function) and should not supersede clinical judgment:
CVVH: Loading dose of 15-25 mg/kg, followed by either 1000 mg every 48 hours **or** 10-15 mg/kg every 24-48 hours
CVVHD: Loading dose of 15-25 mg/kg, followed by either 1000 mg every 24 hours **or** 10-15 mg/kg every 24 hours
CVVHDF: Loading dose of 15-25 mg/kg, followed by either 1000 mg every 24 hours **or** 7.5-10 mg/kg every 12 hours
Note: Consider redosing patients receiving CRRT for vancomycin concentrations <10-15 mg/L.

Dosage adjustment in hepatic impairment: Degrees of hepatic dysfunction do not affect the pharmacokinetics of vancomycin (Marti, 1996).
Oral: No adjustment provided in the manufacturer's labeling.

Mechanism of Action Inhibits bacterial cell wall synthesis by blocking glycopeptide polymerization through binding tightly to D-alanyl-D-alanine portion of cell wall precursor

Contraindications Hypersensitivity to vancomycin or any component of the formulation

Warnings/Precautions May cause nephrotoxicity although limited data suggest direct causal relationship; usual risk factors include pre-existing renal impairment, concomitant nephrotoxic medications, advanced age, and dehydration (nephrotoxicity has also been reported following treatment with oral vancomycin, typically in patients >65 years of age). If multiple sequential (≥2) serum creatinine concentrations demonstrate an increase of 0.5 mg/dL or ≥50% increase from baseline (whichever is greater) in the absence of an alternative explanation, the patient should be identified as having vancomycin-induced nephrotoxicity (Rybak, 2009). Discontinue treatment if signs of nephrotoxicity occur; renal damage is usually reversible.

May cause neurotoxicity; usual risk factors include pre-existing renal impairment, concomitant neuro-/nephrotoxic medications, advanced age, and dehydration. Ototoxicity, although rarely associated with monotherapy, is proportional to the amount of drug given and the duration of treatment. Tinnitus or vertigo may be indications of vestibular injury and impending bilateral irreversible damage. Discontinue treatment if signs of ototoxicity occur. Prolonged therapy (>1 week) or total doses exceeding 25 g may increase the risk of neutropenia; prompt reversal of neutropenia is expected after discontinuation of therapy. Prolonged use may result in fungal or bacterial superinfection, including *C. difficile*-associated diarrhea (CDAD) and pseudomembranous colitis; CDAD has been observed >2 months postantibiotic treatment. Use with caution in patients with renal impairment or those receiving other nephrotoxic or ototoxic drugs; dosage modification required in patients with impaired renal function (especially elderly). Accumulation may occur after multiple oral doses of vancomycin in patients with renal impairment; consider monitoring trough concentrations in this circumstance.

Rapid I.V. administration may result in hypotension, flushing, erythema, urticaria, and/or pruritus. Oral vancomycin is only indicated for the treatment of pseudomembranous colitis due to *C. difficile* and enterocolitis due to *S. aureus* and is not effective for systemic infections; parenteral vancomycin is not effective for the treatment of colitis due to *C. difficile* and enterocolitis due to *S. aureus*. Clinically significant serum concentrations have been reported in patients with inflammatory disorders of the intestinal mucosa who have taken oral vancomycin (multiple doses) for the treatment of *C. difficile*-associated diarrhea. Although use may be warranted, the risk for adverse reactions may be higher in this situation; consider monitoring serum trough concentrations, especially with renal insufficiency, severe colitis, concurrent rectal vancomycin administration, and/or concomitant I.V. aminoglycosides. The IDSA suggests that it is appropriate to obtain trough concentrations when a patient is receiving long courses of ≥2 g/day (Cohen, 2010). **Note:** The Infectious Disease Society of America (IDSA) recommends the use of oral metronidazole for initial treatment of mild-to-moderate *C. difficile* infection and the use of oral vancomycin for initial treatment of severe *C. difficile* infection (Cohen, 2010).

Drug Interactions

Metabolism/Transport Effects None known.

Avoid Concomitant Use

Avoid concomitant use of Vancomycin with any of the following: BCG; Gallium Nitrate

Increased Effect/Toxicity

Vancomycin may increase the levels/effects of: Aminoglycosides; Colistimethate; Gallium Nitrate; Neuromuscular-Blocking Agents

The levels/effects of Vancomycin may be increased by: Nonsteroidal Anti-Inflammatory Agents

Decreased Effect

Vancomycin may decrease the levels/effects of: BCG; Sodium Picosulfate; Typhoid Vaccine

The levels/effects of Vancomycin may be decreased by: Bile Acid Sequestrants

Dietary Considerations May be taken with food.

Pharmacodynamics/Kinetics

Half-life Elimination Biphasic: Terminal:

Newborns: 6-10 hours

Infants and Children 3 months to 4 years: 4 hours

Children >3 years: 2.2-3 hours

Adults: 5-11 hours; significantly prolonged with renal impairment

End-stage renal disease: 200-250 hours

Time to Peak Serum: I.V.: Immediately after completion of infusion

Pregnancy Risk Factor B (oral); C (injection)

Pregnancy Considerations Adverse events have not been observed in animal reproduction studies. Vancomycin crosses the placenta and may result in therapeutic fetal concentrations. Adverse fetal effects, including hearing loss or nephrotoxicity, have not been reported following maternal use during pregnancy. A case report has been published of a vancomycin dose rapidly administered over ~3 minutes leading to maternal hypotension and fetal bradycardia.

The pharmacokinetics of vancomycin may be altered during pregnancy and pregnant patients may need a higher dose of vancomycin. Maternal half-life is unchanged, but the volume of distribution and the total plasma clearance are increased. Individualization of therapy through serum concentration monitoring may be warranted. Vancomycin is recommended as an alternative agent to prevent the transmission of group B streptococcal (GBS) disease from mothers to newborns.

Lactation Enters breast milk/not recommended

Breast-Feeding Considerations Vancomycin is excreted in human milk following I.V. administration. If given orally to the mother, the minimal systemic absorption of the dose would limit the amount available to pass into the milk. Breast-feeding is not recommended by the manufacturer. Nondose-related effects could include modification of bowel flora.

Dosage Forms

Capsule, oral: 125 mg, 250 mg

Vancocin®: 125 mg, 250 mg

Infusion, premixed iso-osmotic dextrose solution: 500 mg (100 mL); 750 mg (150 mL); 1 g (200 mL)

Injection, powder for reconstitution: 500 mg, 750 mg, 1 g, 5 g, 10 g

---

Vandetanib (van DET a nib)

Related Information

Clinical Risk Related to Drugs Prolonging QT Interval *on page 1510*

Brand Names: U.S. Caprelsa®

Brand Names: Canada Caprelsa®

Pharmacologic Category Antineoplastic Agent, Tyrosine Kinase Inhibitor; Epidermal Growth Factor Receptor (EGFR) Inhibitor; Vascular Endothelial Growth Factor (VEGF) Inhibitor

Use Treatment of metastatic or unresectable locally advanced medullary thyroid cancer (symptomatic or progressive)

Local Anesthetic/Vasoconstrictor Precautions Hypertension can occur with the use of this drug, particularly early in the treatment course. Monitor for hypertension prior to using local anesthetic with vasoconstrictor; medical consult if necessary.

Vandetanib is one of the drugs confirmed to prolong the QT interval and is accepted as having a risk of causing torsade de pointes. The risk of drug-induced torsade de pointes is extremely low when a single QT interval prolonging drug is prescribed. In terms of epinephrine, it is not known what effect vasoconstrictors in the local anesthetic regimen will have in patients with a known history of congenital prolonged QT interval or in patients taking any medication that prolongs the QT interval. Until more information is obtained, it is suggested that the clinician consult with the physician prior to the use of a vasoconstrictor in suspected patients, and that the vasoconstrictor (epinephrine, mepivacaine and levonordefrin [Carbocaine® 2% with Neo-Cobefrin®]) be used with caution.

Effects on Dental Treatment Key adverse event(s) related to dental treatment: Xerostomia (normal salivary flow resumes upon discontinuation), mucositis/stomatitis, taste perversion, and oral pain.

Effects on Bleeding Chemotherapy may result in significant myelosuppression, potentially including significant reduction in platelet counts (thrombocytopenia: 9%) and altered hemostasis. In patients who are under active treatment with these agents, medical consult is suggested.

Adverse Effects

>10%:

Cardiovascular: Hypertension (33%; grades 3/4: 9%), QT prolongation (14%; grades 3/4: 8%)

Central nervous system: Headache (26%), fatigue (24%), insomnia (13%)

Dermatologic: Rash (53%; grades 3/4: 5%), dermatitis acneiform/acne (35%; grades 3/4: 1%), dry skin (15%), photosensitivity (13%), pruritus (11%)

Endocrine & metabolic: Hypocalcemia (11% to 57%), hypoglycemia (24%)

Gastrointestinal: Diarrhea/colitis (57%; grades 3/4: 11%), nausea (33%), abdominal pain (21%), appetite decreased (21%), vomiting (15%), dyspepsia (11%)

Hematologic: Leukopenia (19%), anemia (13%; grades 3/4: <1%), hemorrhage (13% to 14%)

Hepatic: ALT increased (51%), bilirubin increased (13%)

Neuromuscular & skeletal: Weakness (15%)

Ocular: Corneal abnormalities (corneal edema, corneal opacity, corneal dystrophy, corneal pigmentation, keratopathy, arcus lipoides, corneal deposits, acquired corneal dystrophy: 13%)

Renal: Creatinine increased (16%)

Respiratory: Upper respiratory tract infection (23%), cough (11%), nasopharyngitis (11%)

1% to 10%:

Cardiovascular: Cardiac failure (2%)

Central nervous system: Depression (10%)

Dermatologic: Nail disorder (inflammation, tenderness, paronychia: 9%), alopecia (8%)

Endocrine & metabolic: Hypercalcemia (7%), hypomagnesemia (7%), hyperkalemia (6%), hypokalemia (6%), hyperglycemia (5%), hypermagnesemia (3%)

Gastrointestinal: Weight loss (10%), xerostomia (9%), abnormal taste (8%)

Hematologic: Neutropenia (10%; grades 3/4: <1%), thrombocytopenia (9%)

Neuromuscular & skeletal: Muscle spasms (6%)

Ocular: Blurred vision (9%)

Renal: Proteinuria (10%)

Respiratory: Aspiration pneumonia (2%), respiratory arrest (2%), respiratory failure (2%)

Miscellaneous: Sepsis (2%)

Mechanism of Action Multikinase inhibitor; inhibits tyrosine kinases including epidermal growth factor reception (EGFR), vascular endothelial growth factor (VEGF), rearranged during transfection (RET), protein tyrosine kinase 6 (BRK), TIE2, EPH kinase receptors and SRC kinase receptors, selectively blocking intracellular signaling, angiogenesis and cellular proliferation

Pharmacodynamics/Kinetics

Half-life Elimination 19 days

Time to Peak 6 hours (range: 4-10 hours)

Pregnancy Risk Factor D

Pregnancy Considerations Animal reproduction studies have demonstrated teratogenic effects and fetal loss. Because vandetanib inhibits angiogenesis, a critical component of fetal development, adverse effects on pregnancy would be expected. Women of childbearing potential should be advised to avoid pregnancy during and for 4 months following treatment with vandetanib. Canadian labeling recommends that nonsterile males employ reliable contraceptive methods (barrier method in conjunction with spermicide) during and for 2 months after vandetanib treatment.

Prescribing and Access Restrictions As a requirement of the REMS program, access to vandetanib is restricted. Vandetanib is approved for marketing under a Food and Drug Administration (FDA) approved, risk management program, and through a restricted distribution program, the Vandetanib REMS Program (1-800-236-9933). Prescribers and pharmacies must be certified with the program to prescribe or dispense vandetanib.

In Canada, vandetanib is available only through the CAPRELSA Restricted Distribution Program. Prescribers and pharmacies must be certified with the program to prescribe or dispense vandetanib. Further information may be obtained at 1-800-668-6000.

Dental Comment Vandetanib is known to prolong the QT interval. The QT interval is measured as the time and distance between the Q point of the QRS complex and the end of the T wave in the ECG tracing. After adjustment for heart rate, the QT interval is defined as prolonged if it is more than 450 msec in men and 460 msec in women. A long QT syndrome was first described in the 1950s and 60s as a congenital syndrome involving QT interval prolongation and syncope and sudden death. Some of the congenital long QT syndromes were characterized by a peculiar electrocardiographic appearance of the QRS complex involving a premature atria beat followed by a pause, then a subsequent sinus beat showing marked QT prolongation and deformity. This type of cardiac arrhythmia was originally termed "torsade de pointes" (translated from the French as "twisting of the points"). Vandetanib is considered as having a risk of causing torsade de pointes. Since it is not known what effect vasoconstrictors in the local anesthetic regimen will have in patients with a known history of congenital prolonged QT interval or in patients taking any medication that prolongs the QT interval, a medical consult is suggested.

Vardenafil (var DEN a fil)

Brand Names: U.S. Levitra®; Staxyn™

Brand Names: Canada Levitra®; Staxyn™

Generic Availability (U.S.) No

Pharmacologic Category Phosphodiesterase-5 Enzyme Inhibitor

Use Treatment of erectile dysfunction (ED)

Local Anesthetic/Vasoconstrictor Precautions No information available to require special precautions

Effects on Dental Treatment No significant effects or complications reported

Effects on Bleeding No information available to require special precautions

Adverse Effects

>10%:

Cardiovascular: Flushing (8% to 11%)

Central nervous system: Headache (14% to 15%)

2% to 10%:
Central nervous system: Dizziness (2%)
Gastrointestinal: Dyspepsia (3% to 4%), nausea (2%)
Neuromuscular & skeletal: Back pain (2%), CPK increased (2%)
Respiratory: Rhinitis (9%), nasal congestion (3%), sinusitis (3%)
Miscellaneous: Flu-like syndrome (3%)

Dosage Note: Oral disintegrating tablets should not be used interchangeably with film-coated tablets; patients requiring a dose other than 10 mg should use the film-coated tablets.

Oral: Erectile dysfunction:
Adults:
Film-coated tablet (Levitra®): 10 mg 60 minutes prior to sexual activity; dosing range: 5-20 mg; to be given as one single dose and not given more than once daily
Oral disintegrating tablet (Staxyn™): 10 mg 60 minutes prior to sexual activity; maximum: 10 mg/day
Elderly ≥65 years: Initial: 5 mg 60 minutes prior to sexual activity; to be given as one single dose and not given more than once daily

Dosing adjustment with concomitant medications:
Alpha-blocker (dose should be stable at time of vardenafil initiation):
Film-coated tablet (Levitra®): Initial vardenafil dose: 5 mg/24 hours; if an alpha-blocker is added to vardenafil therapy, it should be initiated at the smallest possible dose and titrated carefully.
Oral disintegrating tablet (Staxyn™): Do not use to initiate therapy. Initial therapy should be with film-coated tablets at lower doses. Patients who have previously used film-coated tablets may be switched to oral disintegrating tablets as recommended by healthcare provider.

Film-coated tablet (Levitra®):
Atazanavir: Maximum vardenafil dose: 2.5 mg/24 hours
Clarithromycin: Maximum vardenafil dose: 2.5 mg/24 hours
Darunavir: Maximum vardenafil dose: 2.5 mg/72 hours
Erythromycin: Maximum vardenafil dose: 5 mg/24 hours
Fosamprenavir: Maximum vardenafil dose: 2.5 mg/24 hours
Fosamprenavir/ritonavir: Maximum vardenafil dose: 2.5 mg/72 hours
Indinavir: Maximum vardenafil dose: 2.5 mg/24 hours
Itraconazole:
200 mg/day: Maximum vardenafil dose: 5 mg/24 hours
400 mg/day: Maximum vardenafil dose: 2.5 mg/24 hours
Ketoconazole:
200 mg/day: Maximum vardenafil dose: 5 mg/24 hours
400 mg/day: Maximum vardenafil dose: 2.5 mg/24 hours
Lopinavir/ritonavir: Maximum vardenafil dose: 2.5 mg/72 hours
Nelfinavir: Maximum vardenafil dose: 2.5 mg/24 hours
Ritonavir: Maximum vardenafil dose: 2.5 mg/72 hours
Saquinavir: Maximum vardenafil dose: 2.5 mg/24 hours
Tipranavir: Maximum vardenafil dose: 2.5 mg/72 hours
Oral disintegrating tablet (Staxyn™): Concurrent use not recommended with potent or moderate CYP3A4 inhibitors (atazanavir, clarithromycin, erythromycin, indinavir, itraconazole, ketoconazole, ritonavir, saquinavir)

Dosage adjustment in renal impairment: Dose adjustment not needed for mild, moderate, or severe impairment; use not recommended in patients on hemodialysis

Dosage adjustment in hepatic impairment:
Child-Pugh class A: No adjustment required
Child-Pugh class B:
Film-coated tablet (Levitra®): Initial: 5 mg 60 minutes prior to sexual activity (maximum dose: 10 mg); to be given as one single dose and not given more than once daily
Oral disintegrating tablet (Staxyn™): Use not recommended
Child-Pugh class C: Has not been studied; use is not recommended by the manufacturer

Mechanism of Action Does not directly cause penile erections, but affects the response to sexual stimulation. The physiologic mechanism of erection of the penis involves release of nitric oxide (NO) in the corpus cavernosum during sexual stimulation. NO then activates the enzyme guanylate cyclase, which results in increased levels of cyclic guanosine monophosphate (cGMP), producing smooth muscle relaxation and inflow of blood to the corpus cavernosum. Vardenafil enhances the effect of NO by inhibiting phosphodiesterase type 5 (PDE-5), which is responsible for degradation of cGMP in the corpus cavernosum; when sexual stimulation causes local release of NO, inhibition of PDE-5 by vardenafil causes increased levels of cGMP in the corpus cavernosum, resulting in smooth muscle relaxation and inflow of blood to the corpus cavernosum; at recommended doses, it has no effect in the absence of sexual stimulation.

Contraindications Hypersensitivity to vardenafil or any component of the formulation; concurrent (regular or intermittent) use of organic nitrates in any form (eg, nitroglycerin, isosorbide dinitrate)

Warnings/Precautions There is a degree of cardiac risk associated with sexual activity; therefore, physicians may wish to consider the patient's cardiovascular status prior to initiating any treatment for erectile dysfunction. Use caution in patients with anatomical deformation of the penis (angulation, cavernosal fibrosis, or Peyronie's disease) and in patients who have conditions which may predispose them to priapism (sickle cell anemia, multiple myeloma, leukemia). Instruct patients to seek immediate medical attention if erection persists >4 hours.

Use is not recommended in patients with hypotension (<90/50 mm Hg); uncontrolled hypertension (>170/100 mm Hg); unstable angina or angina during intercourse; life-threatening arrhythmias, stroke, or MI within the last 6 months; cardiac failure or coronary artery disease causing unstable angina. Safety and efficacy have not been studied in these patients. Use caution in patients with left ventricular outflow obstruction (eg, aortic stenosis). Use caution with alpha-blockers, effective CYP3A4 inhibitors, the elderly, or those with hepatic impairment (Child-Pugh class B); dosage adjustment is needed. Concurrent use with alpha-adrenergic antagonist therapy may cause symptomatic hypotension; patients should be hemodynamically stable prior to initiating tadalafil therapy at the lowest possible dose. Avoid or limit concurrent substantial alcohol consumption as this may increase the risk of symptomatic hypotension.

Rare cases of nonarteritic ischemic optic neuropathy (NAION) have been reported; risk may be increased with history of vision loss. Other risk factors for NAION include heart disease, diabetes, hypertension, smoking, age >50 years, or history of certain eye problems. Sudden decrease or loss of hearing has been reported rarely; hearing changes may be accompanied by tinnitus and dizziness.

Safety and efficacy have not been studied in patients with the following conditions, therefore, use in these patients is not recommended at this time: Congenital QT prolongation, patients taking medications known to prolong the QT interval (avoid use in patients taking Class Ia or III antiarrhythmics); severe hepatic impairment (Child-Pugh class C); end-stage renal disease requiring dialysis; retinitis pigmentosa or other degenerative retinal disorders. The safety and efficacy of vardenafil with other treatments for erectile dysfunction have not been studied and are not recommended as combination therapy. Concomitant use with all forms of nitrates is contraindicated. If nitrate administration is medically necessary, it is not known when nitrates can be safely administered following the use of vardenafil; the ACC/AHA 2007 guidelines support administration of nitrates only if 24 hours have elapsed. Potential underlying causes of erectile dysfunction should be evaluated prior to treatment. Some products may contain phylalanine. Some products may contain sorbitol; do not use in patients with fructose intolerance.

Drug Interactions

Metabolism/Transport Effects Substrate of CYP3A4 (major); **Note:** Assignment of Major/Minor substrate status based on clinically relevant drug interaction potential

Avoid Concomitant Use

Avoid concomitant use of Vardenafil with any of the following: Alprostadil; Amyl Nitrite; Cobicistat; Phosphodiesterase 5 Inhibitors; Vasodilators (Organic Nitrates)

Increased Effect/Toxicity

Vardenafil may increase the levels/effects of: Alpha1-Blockers; Alprostadil; Amyl Nitrite; Antihypertensives; Bosentan; Highest Risk QTc-Prolonging Agents; Moderate Risk QTc-Prolonging Agents; Phosphodiesterase 5 Inhibitors; Vasodilators (Organic Nitrates)

The levels/effects of Vardenafil may be increased by: Alcohol (Ethyl); Boceprevir; Clarithromycin; Cobicistat; CYP3A4 Inhibitors (Moderate); CYP3A4 Inhibitors (Strong); Dasatinib; Erythromycin (Systemic); Fluconazole; Itraconazole; Ivacaftor; Ketoconazole (Systemic); Lorcaserin; Mifepristone; Posaconazole; Protease Inhibitors; Sapropterin; Telaprevir; Voriconazole

Decreased Effect

The levels/effects of Vardenafil may be decreased by: Bosentan; Etravirine

Ethanol/Nutrition/Herb Interactions Ethanol: Substantial consumption of ethanol may increase the risk of hypotension and orthostasis. Lower ethanol consumption has not been associated with significant changes in blood pressure or increase in orthostatic symptoms. Management: Avoid or limit ethanol consumption.

Food: High-fat meals decrease maximum serum concentration 18% to 50%. Serum concentrations/toxicity may be increased with grapefruit juice. Management: Do not take with a high-fat meal. Avoid grapefruit juice.

Dietary Considerations May take with or without food. Avoid grapefruit juice. Some products may contain phenylalanine. Some products may contain sorbitol; do not use in patients with fructose intolerance.

Pharmacodynamics/Kinetics

Onset of Action ~60 minutes

Half-life Elimination Terminal: Vardenafil and metabolite: 3-6 hours

Time to Peak Plasma: 0.5-2 hours

Pregnancy Risk Factor B

Pregnancy Considerations Teratogenic effects were not observed in animal studies; however, vardenafil is not indicated for use in women. No effects on sperm motility or morphology were observed in healthy males.

Lactation Excretion in breast milk unknown/not indicated for use in women.

Dosage Forms

Tablet, oral:

Levitra®: 2.5 mg, 5 mg, 10 mg, 20 mg

Tablet, orally disintegrating, oral:

Staxyn™: 10 mg

Varenicline (var e NI kleen)

Brand Names: U.S. Chantix®

Brand Names: Canada Champix®

Generic Availability (U.S.) No

Pharmacologic Category Partial Nicotine Agonist; Smoking Cessation Aid

Use Smoking cessation: Aid to smoking cessation treatment

Local Anesthetic/Vasoconstrictor Precautions No information available to require special precautions

Effects on Dental Treatment Key adverse event(s) related to dental treatment: Xerostomia (normal salivary flow resumes upon discontinuation).

Effects on Bleeding No information available to require special precautions

Adverse Effects

>10%:

Central nervous system: Headache (15% to 19%), insomnia (10% to 19%), abnormal dreams (9% to 13%), suicidal ideation (11%)

Gastrointestinal: Nausea (16% to 40%), vomiting (≤5% to 11%)

1% to 10%:

Cardiovascular: Angina pectoris (4%), peripheral edema (2%), myocardial infarction (1%)

Central nervous system: Malaise (≤7%), sleep disorder (≤5%), drowsiness (3%), lethargy (1% to 2%), nightmares (1% to 2%)

Dermatologic: Skin rash (≤3%)

Gastrointestinal: Flatulence (6% to 9%), constipation (5% to 8%), dysgeusia (5% to 8%), abdominal pain (≤7%), xerostomia (≤6%), dyspepsia (5%), increased appetite (3% to 4%), anorexia (≤2%), gastroesophageal reflux disease (1%)

Respiratory: Upper respiratory tract infection (5% to 7%), dyspnea (≤2%), rhinorrhea (≤1%)

Dosage Oral: Adults:

Initial:

Days 1-3: 0.5 mg once daily

Days 4-7: 0.5 mg twice daily

Maintenance (≥ Day 8):

U.S. labeling: 1 mg twice daily for 11 weeks

Canadian labeling: 0.5-1 mg twice daily for 11 weeks

Note: Start 1 week before target quit date. Alternatively, patients may consider setting a quit date up to 35 days after initiation of varenicline and then quit smoking between 8-35 days of treatment (some data suggest that an extended pretreatment regimen may result in higher abstinence rates [Hajek, 2011]). If patient successfully quits smoking at the end of the 12 weeks, may continue for another 12 weeks to help maintain success. If not successful in first 12 weeks, then stop medication and reassess factors contributing to failure.

Dosage adjustment for toxicity: Patients who cannot tolerate adverse events may require temporary (or permanent) reduction in dose. Lower dose for a period of time, then may increase dose again or remain on lower dose.

Dosage adjustment in renal impairment:

Cl_{cr} ≥30 mL/minute: No dosage adjustment necessary.

Cl_{cr} <30 mL/minute: Initial: 0.5 mg once daily; maximum dose: 0.5 mg twice daily

End-stage renal disease (ESRD) (receiving hemodialysis): Maximum dose: 0.5 mg once daily

Dosage adjustment in hepatic impairment: No dosage adjustment necessary.

Mechanism of Action Partial neuronal $α_4$ $β_2$ nicotinic receptor agonist; prevents nicotine stimulation of mesolimbic dopamine system associated with nicotine addiction. Also binds to $5\text{-}HT_3$ receptor (significance not determined) with moderate affinity. Varenicline stimulates dopamine activity but to a much smaller degree than nicotine does, resulting in decreased craving and withdrawal symptoms.

Contraindications Serious hypersensitivity or skin reactions to varenicline or any component of the formulation

Warnings/Precautions [U.S. Boxed Warning]: Serious neuropsychiatric events (including depression, suicidal thoughts, and suicide) have been reported with use; some cases may have been complicated by symptoms of nicotine withdrawal following smoking cessation. Smoking cessation (with or without treatment) is associated with nicotine withdrawal symptoms and the exacerbation of underlying psychiatric illness; however, some of the behavioral disturbances were reported in treated patients who continued to smoke. Neuropsychiatric symptoms (eg, mood disturbances, psychosis, hostility) have occurred in patients with and without pre-existing psychiatric disease; many cases resolved following therapy discontinuation although in some cases, symptoms persisted. Ethanol consumption may increase the risk of psychiatric adverse events. Monitor all patients for behavioral changes and psychiatric symptoms (eg, agitation, depression, suicidal behavior, suicidal ideation); inform patients to discontinue treatment and contact their healthcare provider immediately if they experience any behavioral and/or mood changes. **[U.S. Boxed Warning]: Before prescribing, the risks of serious neuropsychiatric events must be weighed against the immediate and long term benefits of smoking abstinence for each patient.**

Hypersensitivity reactions (including angioedema) and rare cases of serious skin reactions (including Stevens-Johnson syndrome and erythema multiforme) have been reported. Patients should be instructed to discontinue use and contact healthcare provider if signs/symptoms occur. Treatment may increase risk of cardiovascular events. A meta-analysis of 15 clinical trials, including a placebo-controlled trial in patients with stable cardiovascular disease, showed an increased incidence of major cardiovascular events (combined outcome of cardiovascular-related death, nonfatal MI, nonfatal stroke) in patients using varenicline compared with placebo. Cardiovascular events were uncommon in both the varenicline and placebo groups. These findings did not reach statistical significance, although data was consistent. Events occurred primarily in patients with known cardiovascular disease. The meta-analysis also showed a lower incidence of all-cause and cardiovascular mortality in varenicline-treated patients, although this was not statistically significant either. Dose-dependent nausea may occur; both transient and persistent nausea has been reported. Dosage reduction may be considered for intolerable nausea. May cause CNS depression, which may impair physical or mental abilities; patients must be cautioned about performing tasks which require mental alertness (eg, operating machinery or driving). There have been postmarketing reports of traffic accidents, near-miss incidents in traffic, or other accidental injuries in patients taking varenicline.

Use caution in renal dysfunction; dosage adjustment required. Safety and efficacy of varenicline with other smoking cessation therapies have not been established; increased adverse events when used concurrently with nicotine replacement therapy.

Drug Interactions

Metabolism/Transport Effects None known.

Avoid Concomitant Use There are no known interactions where it is recommended to avoid concomitant use.

Increased Effect/Toxicity

The levels/effects of Varenicline may be increased by: Alcohol (Ethyl); H2-Antagonists; Quinolone Antibiotics; Trimethoprim

Decreased Effect There are no known significant interactions involving a decrease in effect.

Ethanol/Nutrition/Herb Interactions Ethanol: May increase the risk of psychiatric adverse events. Caution patients about the potential effects of ethanol consumption during therapy.

Dietary Considerations Should be given with food and a full glass of water to decrease gastric upset.

Pharmacodynamics/Kinetics

Half-life Elimination ~24 hours

Time to Peak Plasma: ~3-4 hours

Pregnancy Risk Factor C

Pregnancy Considerations Teratogenic effects were not observed in animal studies; however, decreased fertility, decreased fetal weight, and increased auditory startle response were observed in the offspring. There are no adequate or well-controlled studies in pregnant women. Use only if benefit outweighs the potential risk to fetus.

Lactation Excretion in breast milk unknown/not recommended

Breast-Feeding Considerations It is not known if varenicline is excreted in breast milk. Due to the potential for serious adverse reactions in the nursing infant, breast-feeding is not recommended.

Dosage Forms

Combination package, oral:

Chantix®: Tablet: 0.5 mg (11s) [white tablets] and Tablet: 1 mg (42s) [light blue tablets]

Tablet, oral:

Chantix®: 0.5 mg, 1 mg

Varicella-Zoster Immune Globulin (Human)
(var i SEL a- ZOS ter i MYUN GLOB yoo lin HYU man)

Brand Names: U.S. Varizig®
Brand Names: Canada VariZIG™
Pharmacologic Category Blood Product Derivative; Immune Globulin
Use
U.S. labeling: Postexposure prophylaxis of varicella in high-risk individuals. High-risk groups include:
- Immunocompromised children and adults
- Newborns of mothers with varicella shortly before or after delivery
- Premature infants
- Neonates and infants <1 year of age
- Adults without evidence of immunity
- Pregnant women

Canadian labeling: In pregnant women, for the prevention or reduction in severity of maternal infection within 4 days of exposure to the varicella zoster virus.

The Advisory Committee on Immunization Practices (ACIP) recommends varicella-zoster immune globulin (VZIG) for the passive immunization of patients who are at a greater risk of complications following significant exposure to varicella and do not have evidence of immunity (postexposure prophylaxis). Guidelines restrict administration to those patients meeting the following criteria (CDC, 2007):
- Immunocompromised patients without evidence of immunity, including those with neoplastic disease (eg, leukemia or lymphoma); primary or acquired immunodeficiency; immunosuppressive therapy (including steroid therapy equivalent to prednisone ≥2 mg/kg or 20 mg/day)
- Newborn of mother who had onset of varicella (chickenpox) within 5 days before delivery or within 48 hours after delivery
- Premature infants (≥28 weeks gestation) who were exposed during the neonatal period and whose mother has no evidence of immunity
- Premature infants (<28 weeks gestation or ≤1000 g) regardless of maternal history and who were exposed during the neonatal period
- Pregnant women without evidence of immunity who have been exposed

Significant exposure includes:
Continuous household contact
Face-to-face indoor contact (>5 minutes or >1 hour depending on reference)
Hospital contact (sharing a room with an infectious patient or face-to-face contact with an infectious staff member or patient)

Local Anesthetic/Vasoconstrictor Precautions No information available to require special precautions
Effects on Dental Treatment No significant effects or complications reported
Effects on Bleeding No information available to require special precautions
Adverse Effects
U.S. labeling:
1% to 10%:
Central nervous system: Headache (4%), chills (2%), fatigue (2%)
Local: Injection site pain (9%)

Canadian labeling:
>10%:
Central nervous system: Headache (7% to 11%)
Local: Injection site pain (17% to 47%)
1% to 10%:
Cardiovascular: Flushing (≤2%)
Central nervous system: Dizziness (≤5%), fever (≤5%), pain (≤5%), chills (≤2%), fatigue (≤2%), insomnia (≤2%)
Dermatologic: Rash (≤5%), dermatitis (≤2%), erythematous rash (≤2%)
Gastrointestinal: Nausea (2% to 5%), dysgeusia (≤2%)
Local: Injection site bruising, itching, or tenderness (≤2%)
Neuromuscular & skeletal: Neck pain (≤5%), myalgia (≤2%)
General Dosage Range I.M.: *Children and Adults:* Dose is based on body weight. Minimum dose: 62.5 units; maximum dose: 625 units.
Mechanism of Action Antibodies obtained from pooled human plasma of individuals with high titers of varicella-zoster provide passive immunity.
Pharmacodynamics/Kinetics
Duration of Action ≥6 weeks
Half-life Elimination I.V.: 18-24 days; I.M.: 24-30 days
Time to Peak I.V.: <3 hours; I.M.: 2-7 days
Pregnancy Risk Factor C
Pregnancy Considerations Animal reproduction studies have not been conducted. Endogenous immune globulins cross the placenta. Clinical use of other immunoglobulins suggest that there are no adverse effects on the fetus. Women who do not have evidence of immunity to varicella may be at increased risk of complications if infected during pregnancy. Varicella infection in the mother can also lead to intrauterine infection in the fetus. VZIG is primarily used to prevent maternal complications, not fetal infection (CDC, 2007).

Vasopressin (vay soe PRES in)

Brand Names: U.S. Pitressin®
Brand Names: Canada Pressyn®; Pressyn® AR
Pharmacologic Category Antidiuretic Hormone Analog; Hormone, Posterior Pituitary
Use Treatment of central diabetes insipidus; differential diagnosis of diabetes insipidus
Unlabeled Use ACLS guidelines: Pulseless arrest (ventricular tachycardia [VT]/ventricular fibrillation [VF]; asystole/pulseless electrical activity [PEA]); cardiac arrest secondary to anaphylaxis (unresponsive to epinephrine)

Adjunct in the treatment of GI hemorrhage and esophageal varices; adjunct in the treatment of vasodilatory shock (septic shock); donor management in brain-dead patients (hormone replacement therapy)
Local Anesthetic/Vasoconstrictor Precautions No information available to require special precautions
Effects on Dental Treatment No significant effects or complications reported
Effects on Bleeding No information available to require special precautions
Adverse Effects Frequency not defined.
Cardiovascular: Arrhythmia, asystole (>0.04 units/minute), blood pressure increased, cardiac output decreased (>0.04 units/minute), chest pain, MI, vasoconstriction (with higher doses), venous thrombosis
Central nervous system: Pounding in the head, fever, vertigo

Dermatologic: Ischemic skin lesions, circumoral pallor, urticaria

Gastrointestinal: Abdominal cramps, flatulence, mesenteric ischemia, nausea, vomiting

Genitourinary: Uterine contraction

Neuromuscular & skeletal: Tremor

Respiratory: Bronchial constriction

Miscellaneous: Diaphoresis

General Dosage Range I.M., SubQ:
Children: 2.5-10 units 2-4 times/day as needed
Adults: 5-10 units 2-4 times/day as needed

Mechanism of Action Increases cyclic adenosine monophosphate (cAMP) which increases water permeability at the renal tubule resulting in decreased urine volume and increased osmolality; causes peristalsis by directly stimulating the smooth muscle in the GI tract; direct vasoconstrictor without inotropic or chronotropic effects

Pharmacodynamics/Kinetics
Onset of Action Nasal: 1 hour

Duration of Action Nasal: 3-8 hours; I.M., SubQ: 2-8 hours

Half-life Elimination Nasal: 15 minutes; Parenteral: 10-20 minutes

Pregnancy Risk Factor C

Pregnancy Considerations Animal reproduction studies have not been conducted. Vasopressin and desmopressin have been used safely during pregnancy based on case reports.

Velaglucerase Alfa (vel a GLOO ser ase AL fa)

Brand Names: U.S. VPRIV™
Brand Names: Canada VPRIV™
Pharmacologic Category Enzyme
Use Long-term enzyme replacement therapy for patients with type 1 Gaucher's disease
Local Anesthetic/Vasoconstrictor Precautions No information available to require special precautions
Effects on Dental Treatment No significant effects or complications reported
Effects on Bleeding No information available to require special precautions
Adverse Effects
>10%:
  Central nervous system: Headache (30% to 35%), fatigue (13%), fever (13% to 22%; more common in children), dizziness (8% to 22%)
  Gastrointestinal: Abdominal pain (15% to 19%)
  Hematologic: aPPT prolonged (5% to 11%; more common in children)
  Respiratory: Upper respiratory tract infections (30% to 32%; more common in children)
  Miscellaneous: Infusion-related reactions (23% to 52%)
1% to 10%:
  Cardiovascular: Flushing (>2%), hyper-/hypotension (>2%), tachycardia (>2%)
  Dermatologic: Rash (>2%; more common in children), urticaria (>2%)
  Gastrointestinal: Nausea (6% to 10%)
  Miscellaneous: Hypersensitivity reactions

General Dosage Range I.V.: *Children ≥4 years and Adults:* 15-60 units/kg every other week

Mechanism of Action Velaglucerase alfa, an analogue of endogenous glucocerebrosidase, contains the native human enzyme sequence. In patients with type 1 Gaucher's disease, glucocerebrosidase deficiency results in accumulation of glucocerebroside in

macrophages, thereby causing the associated signs and symptoms. Velaglucerase alfa is used to diminish hepatosplenomegaly and improve anemia, thrombocytopenia, and bone disease.

Pharmacodynamics/Kinetics
Half-life Elimination 11-12 minutes
Pregnancy Risk Factor B
Pregnancy Considerations Teratogenic effects were not observed in animal studies when administered at ~2-4 times the human dose based on body surface area. There are no adequate and well-controlled studies in pregnant women. Use only if clearly indicated.

Vemurafenib (vem ue RAF e nib)

Related Information
Clinical Risk Related to Drugs Prolonging QT Interval *on page 1510*
Brand Names: U.S. Zelboraf™
Brand Names: Canada Zelboraf™
Pharmacologic Category Antineoplastic Agent, BRAF Kinase Inhibitor
Use
U.S. labeling: Treatment of unresectable or metastatic melanoma in patients with a BRAF^{V600E} mutation (as detected by an FDA-approved test); **Note:** Not recommended in patients with wild-type BRAF melanoma.
Canadian labeling: Treatment of unresectable or metastatic melanoma in patients with a BRAF^{V600} mutation (as identified by a validated test)
Unlabeled Use Treatment of metastatic melanoma in patients with a BRAF^{V600K} mutation

Local Anesthetic/Vasoconstrictor Precautions Vemurafenib is one of the drugs confirmed to prolong the QT interval and is accepted as having a risk of causing torsade de pointes. The risk of drug-induced torsade de pointes is extremely low when a single QT interval prolonging drug is prescribed. In terms of epinephrine, it is not known what effect vasoconstrictors in the local anesthetic regimen will have in patients with a known history of congenital prolonged QT interval or in patients taking any medication that prolongs the QT interval. Until more information is obtained, it is suggested that the clinician consult with the physician prior to the use of a vasoconstrictor in suspected patients, and that the vasoconstrictor (epinephrine, mepivacaine, and levonordefrin [Carbocaine® 2% with Neo-Cobefrin®]) be used with caution.

Effects on Dental Treatment Key adverse event(s) related to dental treatment: Taste alteration has been reported

Effects on Bleeding Does not cause significant hematologic toxicity.

Adverse Effects
>10%:
  Cardiovascular: Peripheral edema (17% to 23%)
  Central nervous system: Fatigue (38% to 54%), headache (23% to 27%), fever (17% to 19%)
  Dermatologic: Rash (37% to 52%; grade 3: 7% to 8%), photosensitivity (33% to 49%; grade 3: 3%), alopecia (36% to 45%), pruritus (23% to 30%), skin papilloma (21% to 30%), hyperkeratosis (24% to 28%), cutaneous squamous cell carcinoma (24%; grade 3: 22% to 24%), maculopapular rash (9% to 21%), dry skin (16% to 19%), actinic keratosis (8% to 17%), seborrheic keratosis (10% to 14%), sunburn (10% to 14%), erythema (8% to 14%), papular rash (5% to 13%)

Gastrointestinal: Nausea (35% to 37%; grade 3: 2%), diarrhea (28% to 29%; grade 3: <1%), vomiting (18% to 26%; grade 3: 1% to 2%), appetite decreased (18% to 21%), constipation (12% to 16%), taste alteration (11% to 14%)

Hepatic: GGT increased (5% to 15%)

Neuromuscular & skeletal: Arthralgia (53% to 67%), myalgia (13% to 24%), limb pain (9% to 18%), back pain (8% to 11%), musculoskeletal pain (8% to 11%), weakness (2% to 11%)

Respiratory: Cough (8% to 12%)

≤10% and/or case reports:

Cardiovascular: Atrial fibrillation, hypotension, QT prolongation, vasculitis

Central nervous system: Dizziness, nerve paralysis (VII)

Dermatologic: Basal cell carcinoma, erythema nodosum, folliculitis, keratosis pilaris, melanoma (new primary), palmar-plantar erythrodysesthesia, Stevens-Johnson syndrome, toxic epidermal necrolysis

Gastrointestinal: Weight loss

Hepatic: Alkaline phosphatase increased, ALT increase, AST increased, bilirubin increased

Neuromuscular & skeletal: Arthritis, peripheral neuropathy

Ocular: Blurred vision, iritis, photophobia, retinal vein occlusion, uveitis

Renal: Creatinine increased

Miscellaneous: Anaphylaxis, hypersensitivity

General Dosage Range Dosage adjustment recommended in patients who develop toxicities.

Oral: *Adults:* 960 mg twice daily

Mechanism of Action BRAF kinase inhibitor (potent) which inhibits tumor growth in melanomas by inhibiting kinase activity of certain mutated forms of BRAF, including BRAF with V600E mutation, thereby blocking cellular proliferation in melanoma cells with the mutation. Does not have activity against cells with wild-type BRAF. BRAF^{V600E} activating mutations present in ~50% of melanomas; V600E mutation involves the substitution of glutamic acid for valine at amino acid 600. The cobas® 4800 BRAF V600 mutation test is approved to detect BRAF^{V600E} mutation.

Pharmacodynamics/Kinetics

Half-life Elimination 57 hours (range: 30-120 hours)

Time to Peak ~3 hours

Pregnancy Risk Factor D

Pregnancy Considerations Adverse effects were not demonstrated in animal reproduction studies. Based on the mechanism of action, vemurafenib may cause fetal harm if administered during pregnancy or in patients who become pregnant during treatment. Women of childbearing potential and men of reproductive potential should use adequate contraception methods during and for at least 2 months after treatment (Canadian labeling recommends during and for at least 6 months after treatment).

Prescribing and Access Restrictions Available through specialty pharmacies. Further information may be obtained from the manufacturer, Genentech, at 1-888-249-4918, or at http://www.zelboraf.com.

Dental Comment Vemurafenib is known to prolong the QT interval. The QT interval is measured as the time and distance between the Q point of the QRS complex and the end of the T wave in the ECG tracing. After adjustment for heart rate, the QT interval is defined as prolonged if it is more than 450 msec in men and 460 msec in women. A long QT syndrome was first described in the 1950s and 60s as a congenital syndrome involving QT interval prolongation and syncope and sudden death. Some of the congenital long QT syndromes were characterized by a peculiar electrocardiographic appearance of the QRS complex involving a premature atria beat followed by a pause, then a subsequent sinus beat showing marked QT prolongation and deformity. This type of cardiac arrhythmia was originally termed "torsade de pointes" (translated from the French as "twisting of the points"). Vemurafenib is considered as having a risk of causing torsade de pointes. Since it is not known what effect vasoconstrictors in the local anesthetic regimen will have in patients with a known history of congenital prolonged QT interval or in patients taking any medication that prolongs the QT interval, a medical consult is suggested.

Venlafaxine (ven la FAX een)

Related Information

Vasoconstrictor Interactions With Antidepressants *on page 1650*

Brand Names: U.S. Effexor XR®

Brand Names: Canada CO Venlafaxine XR; Effexor XR®; GD-Venlafaxine XR; Mylan-Venlafaxine XR; PMS-Venlafaxine XR; Ran-Venlafaxine XR; ratio-Venlafaxine XR; Riva-Venlafaxine XR; Sandoz-Venlafaxine XR; Teva-Venlafaxine XR; Venlafaxine XR

Generic Availability (U.S.) Yes

Pharmacologic Category Antidepressant, Serotonin/Norepinephrine Reuptake Inhibitor

Use Treatment of major depressive disorder, generalized anxiety disorder (GAD), social anxiety disorder (social phobia), panic disorder

Unlabeled Use Obsessive-compulsive disorder (OCD); hot flashes; neuropathic pain (including diabetic neuropathy); attention-deficit/hyperactivity disorder (ADHD); post-traumatic stress disorder (PTSD); migraine prophylaxis

Local Anesthetic/Vasoconstrictor Precautions Although venlafaxine is not a tricyclic antidepressant, it does block norepinephrine reuptake within CNS synapses as part of its mechanisms. It has been suggested that vasoconstrictor be administered with caution and to monitor vital signs in dental patients taking antidepressants that affect norepinephrine in this way. This is particularly important in patients taking venlafaxine, which has been noted to produce a sustained increase in diastolic blood pressure and heart rate as a side effect.

Effects on Dental Treatment Key adverse event(s) related to dental treatment: Significant xerostomia (normal salivary flow resumes upon discontinuation); may contribute to oral discomfort, especially in the elderly; taste perversion. See Effects on Bleeding.

Effects on Bleeding May impair platelet aggregation resulting in increased risk of bleeding events, particularly if used concomitantly with aspirin, NSAIDs, warfarin, or other anticoagulants. Bleeding related to SSRI use has been reported to range from relatively minor bruising and epistaxis to life-threatening hemorrhage. Routine interruption of therapy for most dental procedures is not warranted. In medically complicated patients or extensive oral surgery, the decision to interrupt therapy must be based on the risk to benefit in an individual patient and a medical consult is suggested. If therapy is continued without interruption, the clinician should anticipate the potential for a prolonged bleeding time.

Adverse Effects Note: Actual frequency may be dependent upon formulation and/or indication

>10%:

Central nervous system: Headache (25% to 38%), somnolence (12% to 26%), dizziness (11% to 24%), insomnia (15% to 24%), nervousness (6% to 21%), anxiety (2% to 11%),

Gastrointestinal: Nausea (21% to 58%), xerostomia (12% to 22%), anorexia (8% to 17%), constipation (8% to 15%)

Genitourinary: Abnormal ejaculation/orgasm (2% to 19%)

Neuromuscular & skeletal: Weakness (8% to 19%)

Miscellaneous: Diaphoresis (7% to 19%)

1% to 10%:

Cardiovascular: Vasodilation (2% to 6%), hypertension (dose related; 3% in patients receiving <100 mg/day, up to 13% in patients receiving >300 mg/day), palpitation (3%), tachycardia (2%), chest pain (2%), orthostatic hypotension (1%), edema

Central nervous system: Yawning (3% to 8%), abnormal dreams (3% to 7%), chills (2% to 7%), agitation (2% to 5%), confusion (2%), abnormal thinking (2%), depersonalization (1%), depression (1% to 3%), fever, migraine, amnesia, hypoesthesia, vertigo

Dermatologic: Rash (3%), pruritus (1%), bruising

Endocrine & metabolic: Libido decreased (2% to 8%), hypercholesterolemia (5%), triglycerides increased

Gastrointestinal: Abdominal pain (8%), diarrhea (8%), vomiting (3% to 8%), dyspepsia (5% to 7%), weight loss (1% to 6%), flatulence (3% to 4%), taste perversion (2%), appetite increased, belching, weight gain

Genitourinary: Impotence (4% to 6%), urinary frequency (3%), urination impaired (2%), urinary retention (1%), metrorrhagia, prostatic disorder, vaginitis

Neuromuscular & skeletal: Tremor (1% to 10%), hypertonia (3%), paresthesia (2% to 3%), twitching (1% to 3%), arthralgia, neck pain, trismus

Ocular: Accommodation abnormal (6% to 9%), abnormal or blurred vision (4% to 6%), mydriasis (2%)

Otic: Tinnitus (2%)

Renal: Albuminuria

Respiratory: Pharyngitis (7%), sinusitis (2%), bronchitis, cough increased, dyspnea

Miscellaneous: Infection (6%), flu-like syndrome (2%), trauma (2%)

Dosage Oral:

Children and Adolescents:

Attention-deficit/hyperactivity disorder (unlabeled use; Olvera, 1996): Initial: 12.5 mg/day

Children <40 kg: Increase by 12.5 mg/week to maximum of 50 mg/day in 2 divided doses

Children ≥40 kg: Increase by 25 mg/week to maximum of 75 mg/day in 3 divided doses

Mean dose: 60 mg or 1.4 mg/kg administered in 2-3 divided doses

Adults:

Depression:

Immediate-release tablets: Initial: 75 mg/day, administered in 2 or 3 divided doses; may increase in ≤75 mg/day increments at intervals of ≥4 days as tolerated (maximum daily dose: 225-375 mg)

Extended-release capsules or tablets: Initial: 37.5-75 mg once daily; in patients who are initiated at 37.5 mg once daily, may increase to 75 mg once daily after 4-7 days; dose may then be increased by ≤75 mg/day increments at intervals of ≥4 days as tolerated (maximum daily dose: 225 mg)

Generalized anxiety disorder: Extended-release capsules: Initial: 37.5-75 mg once daily; in patients who are initiated at 37.5 mg once daily, may increase to 75 mg once daily after 4-7 days; may then be increased by ≤75 mg/day increments at intervals of ≥4 days as tolerated (maximum daily dose: 225 mg)

Panic disorder: Extended-release capsules: Initial: 37.5 mg once daily for 1 week; may increase to 75 mg once daily after 7 days, may then be increased by ≤75 mg/day increments at intervals of ≥7 days (maximum daily dose: 225 mg).

Social anxiety disorder: Extended-release capsules or tablets: 75 mg once daily (maximum daily dose: 75 mg); no evidence that doses >75 mg/day offer any additional benefit

Obsessive-compulsive disorder (unlabeled use): Titrate to usual dosage range of 150-300 mg/day; however, doses up to 375 mg/day have been used; response may be seen in 4 weeks (Phelps, 2005)

Neuropathic pain (unlabeled use): Dosages evaluated varied considerably based on etiology of chronic pain, but efficacy has been shown for many conditions in the range of 75-225 mg/day; onset of relief may occur in 1-2 weeks, or take up to 6 weeks for full benefit (Grothe, 2004).

Diabetic neuropathy (unlabeled use): 75-225 mg/day (Bril, 2011)

Hot flashes (unlabeled use): Doses of 37.5-75 mg/day have demonstrated significant improvement of vasomotor symptoms after 4-8 weeks of treatment; in one study, doses >75 mg/day offered no additional benefit (Evans, 2005; Loprinzi, 2000); however, higher doses (225 mg/day) may be beneficial in patients with perimenopausal depression

Attention-deficit disorder (unlabeled use): Initial: Doses vary between 18.75 to 75 mg/day; may increase after 4 weeks to 150 mg/day; if tolerated, doses up to 225 mg/day have been used (Maidment, 2003)

Post-traumatic stress disorder (PTSD) (unlabeled use): Extended release formulation: 37.5-300 mg/day (Bandelow, 2008; Benedek, 2009)

Note: When discontinuing this medication after more than 1 week of treatment, it is generally recommended that the dose be tapered. If venlafaxine is used for 6 weeks or longer, the dose should be tapered over 2 weeks when discontinuing its use.

Elderly: Refer to adult dosing. No specific recommendations for elderly, but may be best to start lower at 25-50 mg twice daily and increase as tolerated by 25 mg/dose. Extended-release formulation: 37.5 mg once daily, increase by 37.5 mg every 4-7 days as tolerated

MAO inhibitor recommendations:

Switching to or from an MAO inhibitor intended to treat psychiatric disorders:

Allow 14 days to elapse between discontinuing an MAO inhibitor intended to treat psychiatric disorders and initiation of venlafaxine.

Allow 7 days to elapse between discontinuing venlafaxine and initiation of an MAO inhibitor intended to treat psychiatric disorders.

Use with other MAO inhibitors (linezolid or I.V. methylene blue):

Do not initiate venlafaxine in patients receiving linezolid or I.V. methylene blue; consider other interventions for psychiatric condition.

If urgent treatment with linezolid or I.V. methylene blue is required in a patient already receiving venlafaxine and potential benefits outweigh potential risks, discontinue venlafaxine promptly and administer linezolid or I.V. methylene blue. Monitor for SS for 7 days or until 24 hours after the last dose of linezolid or I.V. methylene blue, whichever comes first. May resume venlafaxine 24 hours after the last dose of linezolid or I.V. methylene blue.

Dosing adjustment in renal impairment:
GFR: 10-70 mL/minute: Reduce total daily dose by 25% to 50%
Hemodialysis: Reduce total daily dose by 50%
Dosing adjustment in hepatic impairment: Mild-to-moderate hepatic impairment: Reduce total daily dose by 50%; further reductions may be necessary in some patients

Mechanism of Action Venlafaxine and its active metabolite, O-desmethylvenlafaxine (ODV), are potent inhibitors of neuronal serotonin and norepinephrine reuptake and weak inhibitors of dopamine reuptake. Venlafaxine and ODV have no significant activity for muscarinic cholinergic, H_1-histaminergic, or alpha$_2$-adrenergic receptors. Venlafaxine and ODV do not possess MAO-inhibitory activity.

Contraindications Hypersensitivity to venlafaxine or any component of the formulation; use of MAO inhibitors intended to treat psychiatric disorders (concurrently or within 14 days of discontinuing the MAO inhibitor); initiation of MAO inhibitor intended to treat psychiatric disorders within 7 days of discontinuing venlafaxine; initiation of venlafaxine in a patient receiving linezolid or intravenous methylene blue

Warnings/Precautions [U.S. Boxed Warning]: Antidepressants increase the risk of suicidal thinking and behavior in children, adolescents, and young adults (18-24 years of age) with major depressive disorder (MDD) and other psychiatric disorders; consider risk prior to prescribing. Short-term studies did not show an increased risk in patients >24 years of age and showed a decreased risk in patients ≥65 years. Closely monitor for clinical worsening, suicidality, or unusual changes in behavior; the patient's family or caregiver should be instructed to closely observe the patient and communicate condition with healthcare provider. Reduced growth rate has been observed with venlafaxine therapy in children. A medication guide should be dispensed with each prescription. **Venlafaxine is not FDA approved for use in children.**

The possibility of a suicide attempt is inherent in major depression and may persist until remission occurs. Monitor for worsening of depression or suicidality, especially during initiation of therapy (generally first 1-2 months) or with dose increases or decreases. Use caution in high-risk patients. Worsening depression and severe abrupt suicidality that are not part of the presenting symptoms may require discontinuation or modification of drug therapy. The patient's family or caregiver should be alerted to monitor patients for the emergence of suicidality and associated behaviors (such as agitation, irritability, hostility, impulsivity, and hypomania) and call healthcare provider.

May worsen psychosis in some patients or precipitate a shift to mania or hypomania in patients with bipolar disorder. Patients presenting with depressive symptoms should be screened for bipolar disorder. Monotherapy in patients with bipolar disorder should be avoided. **Venlafaxine is not FDA approved for the treatment of bipolar depression.**

Potentially life-threatening serotonin syndrome (SS) has occurred with serotonergic agents (eg, SSRIs, SNRIs), particularly when used in combination with other serotonergic agents (eg, triptans, TCAs, fentanyl, lithium, tramadol, buspirone, St John's wort, tryptophan) or agents that impair metabolism of serotonin (eg, MOA inhibitors intended to treat psychiatric disorders, other MAO inhibitors [ie, linezolid and intravenous methylene blue]). Discontinue treatment (and any concomitant serotonergic agent) immediately if signs/symptoms arise.

May cause sustained increase in blood pressure or tachycardia; dose related and increases are generally modest (12-15 mm Hg diastolic). Control pre-existing hypertension prior to initiation of venlafaxine. Use caution in patients with recent history of MI, unstable heart disease, or hyperthyroidism; may cause increase in anxiety, nervousness, insomnia; may cause weight loss (use with caution in patients where weight loss is undesirable); may cause increases in serum cholesterol. Use caution with hepatic or renal impairment; dosage adjustments recommended. May cause hyponatremia/SIADH (elderly at increased risk); volume depletion (diuretics may increase risk).

Bleeding related to SSRI or SNRI use has been reported to range from relatively minor bruising and epistaxis to life-threatening hemorrhage. Interstitial lung disease and eosinophilic pneumonia have been rarely reported; may present as progressive dyspnea, cough, and/or chest pain. Prompt evaluation and possible discontinuation of therapy may be necessary. Venlafaxine may increase the risks associated with electroconvulsive therapy. Use cautiously in patients with a history of seizures. The risks of cognitive or motor impairment, as well as the potential for anticholinergic effects are very low. May cause or exacerbate sexual dysfunction.

Use caution in elderly patients; may cause or exacerbate syndrome of inappropriate antidiuretic hormone secretion or hyponatremia; monitor sodium closely with initiation or dosage adjustments in older adults (Beers Criteria).

Abrupt discontinuation or dosage reduction after extended (≥6 weeks) therapy may lead to agitation, dysphoria, nervousness, anxiety, and other symptoms. When discontinuing therapy, dosage should be tapered gradually over at least a 2-week period. If intolerable symptoms occur following a decrease in dosage or upon discontinuation of therapy, then resuming the previous dose with a more gradual taper should be considered. Use caution in patients with increased intraocular pressure or at risk of acute narrow-angle glaucoma. Potentially significant interactions may exist, requiring dose or frequency adjustment, additional monitoring, and/or selection of alternative therapy. Consult drug interactions database for more detailed information.

Drug Interactions

Metabolism/Transport Effects Substrate of CYP2C19 (minor), CYP2C9 (minor), CYP2D6 (major), CYP3A4 (major); **Note:** Assignment of Major/Minor substrate status based on clinically relevant drug interaction potential; **Inhibits** CYP2B6 (weak), CYP2D6 (weak), CYP3A4 (weak)

Avoid Concomitant Use
Avoid concomitant use of Venlafaxine with any of the following: Conivaptan; Iobenguane I 123; Linezolid; MAO Inhibitors; Methylene Blue

Increased Effect/Toxicity

Venlafaxine may increase the levels/effects of: Alpha-/ Beta-Agonists; Aspirin; Highest Risk QTc-Prolonging Agents; Lomitapide; Methylene Blue; Moderate Risk QTc-Prolonging Agents; NSAID (Nonselective); Serotonin Modulators; TraZODone; Vitamin K Antagonists

The levels/effects of Venlafaxine may be increased by: Abiraterone Acetate; Alcohol (Ethyl); Antipsychotics; Conivaptan; CYP2D6 Inhibitors (Moderate); CYP2D6 Inhibitors (Strong); CYP3A4 Inhibitors (Moderate); CYP3A4 Inhibitors (Strong); Darunavir; Dasatinib; Ivacaftor; Linezolid; MAO Inhibitors; Metoclopramide; Mifepristone; Propafenone; Voriconazole

Decreased Effect

Venlafaxine may decrease the levels/effects of: Alpha2-Agonists; Indinavir; Iobenguane I 123; Ioflupane I 123

The levels/effects of Venlafaxine may be decreased by: CYP3A4 Inducers (Strong); Deferasirox; Peginterferon Alfa-2b; Tocilizumab

Ethanol/Nutrition/Herb Interactions

Ethanol: May increase CNS depression; monitor for increased effects with coadministration. Caution patients about effects.

Herb/Nutraceutical: Avoid valerian, St John's wort, SAMe, kava kava, tryptophan (may increase risk of serotonin syndrome and/or excessive sedation).

Dietary Considerations Should be taken with food.

Pharmacodynamics/Kinetics

Half-life Elimination Venlafaxine: 5 ± 2 hours; ODV: 11 ± 2 hours; prolonged with cirrhosis (venlafaxine: ~30%, ODV: ~60%), renal impairment (venlafaxine: ~50%, ODV: ~40%), and during dialysis (venlafaxine: ~180%, ODV: ~142%)

Time to Peak

Immediate release: Venlafaxine: 2 hours, ODV: 3 hours

Extended release: Venlafaxine: 5.5 hours, ODV: 9 hours

Pregnancy Risk Factor C

Pregnancy Considerations Adverse events have been observed in some animal reproduction studies. Venlafaxine and its active metabolite ODV cross the human placenta. An increased risk of teratogenic effects following venlafaxine exposure during pregnancy has not been observed, based on available data. The risk of spontaneous abortion may be increased. Neonatal seizures and neonatal abstinence syndrome have been noted in case reports following maternal use of venlafaxine during pregnancy. Nonteratogenic effects in the newborn following SSRI/SNRI exposure late in the third trimester include respiratory distress, cyanosis, apnea, seizures, temperature instability, feeding difficulty, vomiting, hypoglycemia, hyper- or hypotonia, hyper-reflexia, jitteriness, irritability, constant crying, and tremor. Symptoms may be due to the toxicity of the SNRI or a discontinuation syndrome and may be consistent with serotonin syndrome associated with treatment. The long-term effects of *in utero* SNRI/SSRI exposure on infant development and behavior are not known.

Due to pregnancy-induced physiologic changes, some pharmacokinetic parameters of venlafaxine may be altered. Women should be monitored for decreased efficacy. The ACOG recommends that therapy with SSRIs or SNRIs during pregnancy be individualized; treatment of depression during pregnancy should incorporate the clinical expertise of the mental health clinician, obstetrician, primary healthcare provider, and pediatrician. According to the American Psychiatric Association (APA), the risks of medication treatment should be weighed against other treatment options and untreated depression. For women who discontinue antidepressant medications during pregnancy and who may be at high risk for postpartum depression, the medications can be restarted following delivery. Treatment algorithms have been developed by the ACOG and the APA for the management of depression in women prior to conception and during pregnancy.

Lactation Enters breast milk/not recommended

Breast-Feeding Considerations Venlafaxine and ODV are found in breast milk and the serum of nursing infants. Adverse events have not been observed; however, it is recommended to monitor the infant for adverse events if the decision to breast-feed has been made. The long-term effects on neurobehavior have not been studied, thus one should prescribe venlafaxine to a mother who is breast-feeding only when the benefits outweigh the potential risks. The manufacturer does not recommend breast-feeding during therapy.

Dosage Forms

Capsule, extended release, oral: 37.5 mg, 75 mg, 150 mg

Effexor XR®: 37.5 mg, 75 mg, 150 mg

Tablet, oral: 25 mg, 37.5 mg, 50 mg, 75 mg, 100 mg

Tablet, extended release, oral: 37.5 mg, 75 mg, 150 mg, 225 mg

---

Verapamil (ver AP a mil)

Related Information

Calcium Channel Blockers and Gingival Hyperplasia *on page 1640*

Cardiovascular Diseases *on page 1492*

Brand Names: U.S. Calan®; Calan® SR; Covera-HS® [DSC]; Isoptin® SR; Verelan®; Verelan® PM

Brand Names: Canada Apo-Verap®; Apo-Verap® SR; Covera-HS®; Covera®; Dom-Verapamil SR; Isoptin® SR; Mylan-Verapamil; Mylan-Verapamil SR; Novo-Veramil; Novo-Veramil SR; Nu-Verap; Nu-Verap SR; PHL-Verapamil SR; PMS-Verapamil SR; PRO-Verapamil SR; Riva-Verapamil SR; Verapamil Hydrochloride Injection, USP; Verapamil SR; Verelan®

Generic Availability (U.S.) Yes: Excludes caplet (sustained release) and tablet (extended release, controlled onset)

Pharmacologic Category Antianginal Agent; Antiarrhythmic Agent, Class IV; Calcium Channel Blocker; Calcium Channel Blocker, Nondihydropyridine

Use

Oral: Treatment of hypertension; angina pectoris (vasospastic, chronic stable, unstable) (Calan®, Covera-HS®); supraventricular tachyarrhythmia (PSVT, atrial fibrillation/flutter [rate control])

I.V.: Supraventricular tachyarrhythmia (PSVT, atrial fibrillation/flutter [rate control])

Unlabeled Use Hypertrophic cardiomyopathy; bipolar disorder (manic manifestations)

Local Anesthetic/Vasoconstrictor Precautions No information available to require special precautions

Effects on Dental Treatment Key adverse event(s) related to dental treatment: Gingival hyperplasia. Calcium channel blockers (CCB) have been reported to cause gingival hyperplasia (GH). Verapamil-induced GH has appeared 11 months or more after subjects took daily doses of 240-360 mg. The severity of hyperplastic syndrome does not seem to be dose dependent. Gingivectomy is only successful if CCB therapy is discontinued. GH regresses markedly 1 week after CCB discontinuance with all symptoms resolving in 2 months. If a patient must continue CCB therapy, begin a program of professional cleaning and patient plaque control to minimize severity and growth rate of gingival tissue.

Effects on Bleeding No information available to require special precautions

Adverse Effects

>10%:

Central nervous system: Headache (1% to 12%)

Gastrointestinal: Gingival hyperplasia (≤19%), constipation (7% to 12%)

1% to 10%:

Cardiovascular: Peripheral edema (1% to 4%), hypotension (3%), CHF/pulmonary edema (2%), AV block (1% to 2%), bradycardia (HR <50 bpm: 1%), flushing (1%)

Central nervous system: Fatigue (2% to 5%), dizziness (1% to 5%), lethargy (3%), pain (2%), sleep disturbance (1%)

Dermatologic: Rash (1% to 2%)

Gastrointestinal: Dyspepsia (3%), nausea (1% to 3%), diarrhea (2%)

Hepatic: Liver enzymes increased (1%)

Neuromuscular & skeletal: Myalgia (1%), paresthesia (1%)

Respiratory: Dyspnea (1%)

Miscellaneous: Flu-like syndrome (4%)

Dosage

Children: **Note:** Verapamil is no longer included in the Pediatric Advanced Life Support (PALS) tachyarrhythmia algorithm.

Children: 1-15 years: SVT: I.V.: 0.1-0.3 mg/kg/dose over 2 minutes; maximum: 5 mg/dose, may repeat dose in 30 minutes if inadequate response; maximum for second dose: 10 mg

Adults:

SVT (ACLS, 2010): I.V.: 2.5-5 mg over 2 minutes; second dose of 5-10 mg (~0.15 mg/kg) may be given 15-30 minutes after the initial dose if patient tolerates, but does not respond to initial dose; maximum total dose: 20-30 mg

Angina: Oral: **Note:** When switching from immediate-release to extended/sustained release formulations, the total daily dose remains the same unless formulation strength does not allow for equal conversion.

Immediate release: Initial: 80-120 mg 3 times/day (elderly or small stature: 40 mg 3 times/day); Usual dose range (Gibbons, 2003): 80-160 mg 3 times/day

Extended release (Covera-HS®): Initial: 180 mg once daily at bedtime; if inadequate response, may increase dose at weekly intervals to 240 mg once daily, then 360 mg once daily, then 480 mg once daily; maximum dose: 480 mg/day

Chronic atrial fibrillation (rate-control), PSVT prophylaxis: Oral: Immediate release: 240-480 mg/day in 3-4 divided doses; Usual dose range (Fuster, 2006): 120-360 mg/day in divided doses

Hypertension: Oral: **Note:** When switching from immediate-release to extended/sustained release formulations, the total daily dose remains the same unless formulation strength does not allow for equal conversion.

Immediate release: 80 mg 3 times/day; usual dose range (JNC 7): 80-320 mg/day in 2 divided doses

Sustained release: Usual dose range (JNC 7): 120-480 mg/day in 1-2 divided doses; **Note:** There is no evidence of additional benefit with doses >360 mg/day.

Calan® SR, Isoptin® SR: Initial: 180 mg once daily in the morning (elderly or small stature: 120 mg/day); if inadequate response, may increase dose at weekly intervals to 240 mg once daily, then 180 mg twice daily (or 240 mg in the morning followed by 120 mg in the evening); maximum dose: 240 mg twice daily.

Verelan®: Initial: 180 mg once daily in the morning (elderly or small stature: 120 mg/day); if inadequate response, may increase dose at weekly intervals to 240 mg once daily, then 360 mg once daily, then 480 mg once daily; maximum dose: 480 mg/day

Extended release: Usual dose range (JNC 7): 120-360 mg once daily (once-daily dosing is recommended at bedtime)

Covera-HS®: Initial: 180 mg once daily at bedtime; if inadequate response, may increase dose at weekly intervals to 240 mg once daily, then 360 mg once daily, then 480 mg once daily; maximum dose: 480 mg/day

Verelan® PM: Initial: 200 mg once daily at bedtime (elderly or small stature: 100 mg/day); if inadequate response, may increase dose at weekly intervals to 300 mg once daily, then 400 mg once daily; maximum dose: 400 mg/day

Elderly: Hypertension: Oral: **Note:** When switching from immediate release to extended or sustained release formulations, the total daily dose remains the same unless formulation strength does not allow for equal conversion.

Manufacturer's recommendations:

Immediate release: Initial: 40 mg 3 times daily

Sustained release: Calan® SR, Isoptin® SR,Verelan®: Initial: 120 mg once daily in the morning

Extended release:

Covera-HS®: Initial: 180 mg once daily at bedtime

Verelan® PM: Initial: 100 mg once daily at bedtime

ACCF/AHA Expert Consensus recommendations: Consider lower initial doses and titrating to response (Aronow, 2011)

Dosing adjustment in renal impairment: Manufacturer recommends caution and additional ECG monitoring in patients with renal insufficiency. The manufacturer of Verelan PM® recommends an initial dose of 100 mg/day at bedtime. **Note:** A multiple dose study in adults suggests reduced renal clearance of verapamil and its metabolite (norverapamil) with advanced renal failure (Storstein, 1984). Additionally, several clinical papers report adverse effects of verapamil in patients with chronic renal failure receiving recommended doses of verapamil (Pritza, 1991; Váquez, 1996). In contrast, a number of single dose studies show no difference in verapamil (or norverapamil metabolite) disposition between chronic renal failure and control patients (Beyerlein, 1990; Hanyok, 1988; Mooy, 1985; Zachariah, 1991).

Dialysis: Not removed by hemodialysis (Mooy, 1985); supplemental dose is not necessary.

Dosing adjustment/comments in hepatic disease: In cirrhosis, reduce dose to 20% and 50% of normal for oral and intravenous administration, respectively, and monitor ECG (Somogyi, 1981). The manufacturer of Verelan PM® recommends an initial adult dose of 100 mg/day at bedtime. The manufacturers of Calan®, Calan® SR, Covera-HS®, Isoptin® SR, and Verelan® recommend giving 30% of the normal dose to patients with severe hepatic impairment.

Mechanism of Action Inhibits calcium ion from entering the "slow channels" or select voltage-sensitive areas of vascular smooth muscle and myocardium during depolarization; produces relaxation of coronary vascular smooth muscle and coronary vasodilation; increases myocardial oxygen delivery in patients with vasospastic angina; slows automaticity and conduction of AV node.

Contraindications Hypersensitivity to verapamil or any component of the formulation; severe left ventricular dysfunction; hypotension (systolic pressure <90 mm Hg) or cardiogenic shock; sick sinus syndrome (except in patients with a functioning artificial ventricular pacemaker); second- or third-degree AV block (except in patients with a functioning artificial ventricular pacemaker); atrial flutter or fibrillation and an accessory bypass tract (Wolff-Parkinson-White [WPW] syndrome, Lown-Ganong-Levine syndrome)

I.V.: Additional contraindications include concurrent use of I.V. beta-blocking agents; ventricular tachycardia

Warnings/Precautions Avoid use in heart failure; can exacerbate condition; use is contraindicated in severe left ventricular dysfunction. Symptomatic hypotension with or without syncope can rarely occur; blood pressure must be lowered at a rate appropriate for the patient's clinical condition. Rare increases in hepatic enzymes can be observed. Can cause first-degree AV block or sinus bradycardia; use is contraindicated in patients with sick sinus syndrome, second- or third-degree AV block (except in patients with a functioning artificial pacemaker), or an accessory bypass tract (eg, WPW syndrome). Other conduction abnormalities are rare. Considered contraindicated in patients with wide complex tachycardias unless known to be supraventricular in origin; severe hypotension likely to occur upon administration (ACLS, 2010). Use caution when using verapamil together with a beta-blocker. Administration of I.V. verapamil and an I.V. beta-blocker within a few hours of each other may result in asystole and should be avoided; simultaneous administration is contraindicated. Use with other agents known to reduce SA node function and/or AV nodal conduction (eg, digoxin) or reduce sympathetic outflow (eg, clonidine) may increase the risk of serious bradycardia. Verapamil significantly increases digoxin serum concentrations; adjust digoxin dose. Use with caution in patients with HCM with outflow tract obstruction (especially those with high gradients, advanced heart failure, or sinus bradycardia); may be used in patients who cannot tolerate beta-blockade. Verapamil should not be used in those with systemic hypotension or severe dyspnea at rest (Gersh, 2011; Nishimura, 2004).

Decreased neuromuscular transmission has been reported with verapamil; use with caution in patients with attenuated neuromuscular transmission (Duchenne's muscular dystrophy, myasthenia gravis); dosage reduction may be required. Use with caution in renal impairment; monitor hemodynamics and possibly ECG if severe impairment, particularly if concomitant hepatic impairment. Use with caution in patients with hepatic impairment; dosage reduction may be required; monitor hemodynamics and possibly ECG if severe impairment. May prolong recovery from nondepolarizing neuromuscular-blocking agents. Use Covera-HS® (extended-release delivery system) with caution in patients with severe GI narrowing. In patients with extremely short GI transit times (eg, <7 hours), dosage adjustment may be required; inadequate pharmacokinetic data. I.V. use for SVT for is not recommended in infants; use with caution in children as myocardial depression/hypotension may occur.

Drug Interactions

Metabolism/Transport Effects Substrate of CYP1A2 (minor), CYP2B6 (minor), CYP2C9 (minor), CYP2E1 (minor), CYP3A4 (major), P-glycoprotein; **Note:** Assignment of Major/Minor substrate status based on clinically relevant drug interaction potential; **Inhibits** CYP1A2 (weak), CYP2C9 (weak), CYP2D6 (weak), CYP3A4 (moderate), P-glycoprotein

Avoid Concomitant Use

Avoid concomitant use of Verapamil with any of the following: Bosutinib; Conivaptan; Dantrolene; Disopyramide; Dofetilide; Ivabradine; Lomitapide; Pimozide; Pomalidomide; Tolvaptan; Topotecan; VinCRIStine (Liposomal)

Increased Effect/Toxicity

Verapamil may increase the levels/effects of: Alcohol (Ethyl); Aliskiren; Amifostine; Amiodarone; Antihypertensives; ARIPiprazole; AtorvaSTATin; Atosiban; Avanafil; Benzodiazepines (metabolized by oxidation); Beta-Blockers; Bosutinib; Budesonide (Systemic, Oral Inhalation); BusPIRone; Calcium Channel Blockers (Dihydropyridine); CarBAMazepine; Cardiac Glycosides; Colchicine; Corticosteroids (Systemic); CycloSPORINE (Systemic); CYP3A4 Substrates; Dabigatran Etexilate; Disopyramide; Dofetilide; Dronedarone; Eletriptan; Eplerenone; Everolimus; Fexofenadine; Fingolimod; Flecainide; Fosphenytoin; Halofantrine; Hypotensive Agents; Ivabradine; Ivacaftor; Lithium; Lomitapide; Lovastatin; Lurasidone; Magnesium Salts; Midodrine; Neuromuscular-Blocking Agents (Nondepolarizing); Nitroprusside; P-glycoprotein/ABCB1 Substrates; Phenytoin; Pimecrolimus; Pimozide; Pomalidomide; Propafenone; Prucalopride; QuiNIDine; Ranolazine; Red Yeast Rice; RisperiDONE; RiTUXimab; Rivaroxaban; Salicylates; Salmeterol; Saxagliptin; Simvastatin; Tacrolimus (Systemic); Tacrolimus (Topical); Tolvaptan; Topotecan; Vilazodone; VinCRIStine (Liposomal); Zuclopenthixol

The levels/effects of Verapamil may be increased by: Alpha1-Blockers; Anilidopiperidine Opioids; Antifungal Agents (Azole Derivatives, Systemic); AtorvaSTATin; Calcium Channel Blockers (Dihydropyridine); Cimetidine; CloNIDine; Conivaptan; CycloSPORINE (Systemic); CYP3A4 Inhibitors (Moderate); CYP3A4 Inhibitors (Strong); Dantrolene; Dasatinib; Diazoxide; Dronedarone; Fluconazole; Grapefruit Juice; Herbs (Hypotensive Properties); Ivabradine; Ivacaftor; Macrolide Antibiotics; Magnesium Salts; MAO Inhibitors; Mifepristone; Pentoxifylline; P-glycoprotein/ABCB1 Inhibitors; Phosphodiesterase 5 Inhibitors; Prostacyclin Analogues; Protease Inhibitors; QuiNIDine; Telithromycin

Decreased Effect

Verapamil may decrease the levels/effects of: Clopidogrel; Ifosfamide

The levels/effects of Verapamil may be decreased by: Barbiturates; Calcium Salts; CarBAMazepine; CYP3A4 Inducers (Strong); Deferasirox; Herbs (CYP3A4 Inducers); Herbs (Hypertensive Properties); Methylphenidate; Nafcillin; P-glycoprotein/ABCB1 Inducers; Rifamycin Derivatives; Tocilizumab; Yohimbine

Ethanol/Nutrition/Herb Interactions

Ethanol: Ethanol may increase ethanol levels. Management: Avoid or limit ethanol.

Food: Grapefruit juice may increase the serum concentration of verapamil. Management: Avoid grapefruit juice or use with caution and monitor for effects. Calan® SR and Isoptin® SR products should be taken with food or milk; other formulations may be administered without regard to meals.

Herb/Nutraceutical: St John's wort may decrease levels of verapamil. Some herbal medications have hypertensive properties (eg, licorice); others may increase or decrease the antihypertensive effect of verapamil. Management: Avoid St John's wort, bayberry, blue cohosh, cayenne, ephedra, ginger, ginseng (American), kola, licorice, and yohimbe. Avoid black cohosh, California poppy, coleus, golden seal, hawthorn, mistletoe, periwinkle, quinine, and shepherd's purse.

Dietary Considerations Calan® SR and Isoptin® SR products may be taken with food or milk, other formulations may be administered without regard to meals; sprinkling contents of Verelan® or Verelan® PM capsule onto applesauce does not affect oral absorption.

Pharmacodynamics/Kinetics

Onset of Action Oral (immediate release tablets): Peak effect: 1-2 hours; I.V.: Peak effect: 1-5 minutes

Duration of Action Oral: Immediate release tablets: 6-8 hours; I.V.: 10-20 minutes

Half-life Elimination Infants: 4.4-6.9 hours; Adults: Single dose: 3-7 hours, Multiple doses: 4.5-12 hours; severe hepatic impairment: 14-16 hours

Time to Peak Serum: Oral:

Immediate release: 1-2 hours

Extended release (Covera-HS®, Verelan PM®): ~11 hours, drug release delayed ~4-5 hours

Sustained release: 5.21 hours (Calan® SR, Isoptin® SR); 7-9 hours (Verelan®)

Pregnancy Risk Factor C

Pregnancy Considerations In some animal reproduction studies verapamil has been shown to cause fetal harm; adverse maternal effects were also observed. Verapamil crosses the placenta. Although verapamil is not considered a major human teratogen, use during pregnancy may cause adverse fetal effects (bradycardia, heart block, hypotension).

Lactation Enters breast milk/not recommended (AAP considers "compatible"; AAP 2001 update pending)

Breast-Feeding Considerations Crosses into breast milk; manufacturer recommends to discontinue breast-feeding while taking verapamil.

Dosage Forms

Caplet, sustained release, oral:

Calan® SR: 120 mg, 180 mg, 240 mg

Capsule, extended release, oral: 120 mg, 180 mg, 240 mg

Capsule, extended release, controlled onset, oral: 100 mg, 200 mg, 300 mg

Verelan® PM: 100 mg, 200 mg, 300 mg

Capsule, sustained release, oral: 120 mg, 180 mg, 240 mg, 360 mg

Verelan®: 120 mg, 180 mg, 240 mg, 360 mg

Injection, solution: 2.5 mg/mL (2 mL, 4 mL)

Tablet, oral: 40 mg, 80 mg, 120 mg

Calan®: 80 mg, 120 mg

Tablet, extended release, oral: 120 mg, 180 mg, 240 mg

Tablet, sustained release, oral: 120 mg, 180 mg, 240 mg

Isoptin® SR: 120 mg, 180 mg

Verteporfin (ver te POR fin)

Brand Names: U.S. Visudyne®

Brand Names: Canada Visudyne®

Pharmacologic Category Ophthalmic Agent

Use Treatment of predominantly classic subfoveal choroidal neovascularization due to age-related macular degeneration, presumed ocular histoplasmosis, or pathologic myopia

Unlabeled Use Predominantly **occult** subfoveal choroidal neovascularization

Local Anesthetic/Vasoconstrictor Precautions No information available to require special precautions

Effects on Dental Treatment No significant effects or complications reported

Effects on Bleeding No information available to require special precautions

Adverse Effects

>10%:

Local: Injection site reactions (including injection site discoloration, edema, extravasation, hemorrhage, inflammation, pain, and rash)

Ocular: Blurred vision, flashes of light, visual acuity decreased, visual field defects (including scotoma)

1% to 10%:

Cardiovascular: Atrial fibrillation, hypertension, peripheral vascular disorder, varicose veins

Central nervous system: Fever, hypoesthesia, sleep disturbance, vertigo

Dermatologic: Eczema, photosensitivity

Gastrointestinal: Constipation, gastrointestinal cancers, nausea

Genitourinary: Prostatic disorder

Hematologic: Anemia, leukocytosis, leukopenia

Hepatic: Liver function tests increased

Neuromuscular & skeletal: Arthralgia, arthrosis, back pain (primarily during infusion), myasthenia, weakness

Ocular: Diplopia, lacrimation disorder

Treatment site: Blepharitis, cataracts, conjunctivitis/conjunctival injection, dry eyes, ocular itching, severe vision loss with or without subretinal/retinal or vitreous hemorrhage (decrease in 4 lines or more within 7 days of treatment [1% to 5%])

Otic: Hearing loss

Renal: Albuminuria, creatinine increased

Respiratory: Cough, pharyngitis, pneumonia

Miscellaneous: Flu-like syndrome

General Dosage Range I.V.: *Adults:* 6 mg/m^2 body surface area

Mechanism of Action Following intravenous administration, verteporfin is transported by lipoproteins to the neovascular endothelium in the affected eye(s), including choroidal neovasculature and the retina. Verteporfin then needs to be activated by nonthermal red light, which results in local damage to the endothelium, leading to temporary choroidal vessel occlusion.

Pharmacodynamics/Kinetics

Half-life Elimination Terminal: 5-6 hours, biexponential

Pregnancy Risk Factor C

Pregnancy Considerations Teratogenic effects were observed in some animal reproduction studies.

Vigabatrin (vye GA ba trin)

Brand Names: U.S. Sabril®

Brand Names: Canada Sabril®

Pharmacologic Category Anticonvulsant, Miscellaneous

Use Treatment of infantile spasms; refractory complex partial seizures not controlled by usual treatments

Canadian labeling: Additional uses (not in U.S. labeling): Active management of partial or secondary generalized seizures not controlled by usual treatments

Local Anesthetic/Vasoconstrictor Precautions No information available to require special precautions

Effects on Dental Treatment No significant effects or complications reported

Effects on Bleeding No information available to require special precautions

Adverse Effects Note: Adult and pediatric information presented combined unless significantly different.

>10%:

Central nervous system: Somnolence (adults 22% to 24%; infants 17% to 45%), headache (33%), fever (adults 4% to 5%; infants 19% to 29%), fatigue (23% to 28%), dizziness (21% to 24%), irritability (adults 10%; infants 16% to 23%), sedation (adults 2% to 4%; infants 17% to 19%), insomnia (infants 10% to 12%)

Dermatologic: Rash (infants 8% to 11%)

Gastrointestinal: Vomiting (adults 7%; infants 14% to 20%), constipation (adults 6% to 8%; infants 12% to 14%), diarrhea (10% to 13%)

Neuromuscular & skeletal: Tremor (14% to 15%)

Ocular: Visual field constriction (≥30%), nystagmus (13% to 15%), blurred vision (11% to 13%)

Otic: Otitis media (infants 10% to 44%)

Respiratory: Upper respiratory tract infection (adults 7% to 9%; infants 46% to 51%), bronchitis (infants 30%), pharyngitis (13% to 14%), pneumonia (infants 11% to 13%), nasal congestion (infants 4% to 13%)

Miscellaneous: Viral infection (infants 19% to 20%)

1% to 10%:

Cardiovascular: Peripheral edema (2% to 5%), edema (1%)

Central nervous system: Memory impairment (7% to 10%), coordination impaired (7% to 9%), disturbance in attention (5% to 9%), depression (4% to 7%), lethargy (4% to 7%), seizure (infants 4% to 7%), confusion (4% to 6%), hypotonia (infants 4% to 6%), status epilepticus (2% to 6%), sensory disturbance (4% to 5%), anxiety (4%), hypoesthesia (3% to 4%), abnormal behavior (3%), abnormal thinking (3%), aggression (2%), postictal state (2%), vertigo (2%)

Dermatologic: Contusion (3% to 4%)

Endocrine & metabolic: Dysmenorrhea (7% to 9%), fluid retention (2%)

Gastrointestinal: Nausea (9% to 10%), appetite decreased (infants 7% to 9%), weight gain (6% to 8%), viral gastroenteritis (infants 5% to 6%), abdominal pain (3% to 5%), dyspepsia (4%), abdominal distention (2%), appetite increased (2%), hemorrhoidal symptoms (2%)

Genitourinary: Urinary tract infection (4% to 6%)

Neuromuscular & skeletal: Arthralgia (8% to 10%), pain in extremity (5% to 6%), back pain (4% to 6%), hyporeflexia (4% to 5%), paresthesia (5%), weakness (5%), hyper-reflexia (4%), myalgia (3%), muscle spasms (2% to 3%), dysarthria (2%), joint swelling (2%), shoulder pain (2%)

Ocular: Diplopia (3% to 7%), strabismus (5%), conjunctivitis (2% to 5%), eye strain (2%)

Otic: Tinnitus (2%)

Respiratory: Pharyngolaryngeal pain (7% to 9%), sinusitis (infants 5% to 9%), cough (2% to 8%), sinus headache (4% to 6%), dyspnea (2%)

Miscellaneous: Candidiasis (infants 3% to 8%), influenza (3% to 5%), croup (infants 1% to 5%), thirst (2%)

General Dosage Range Dosage adjustment recommended in patients with renal impairment

Oral:

Infants: 50-150 mg/kg/day in 2 divided doses

Adults: 1-3 g/day in 2 divided doses

Mechanism of Action Irreversibly inhibits gamma-aminobutyric acid transaminase (GABA-T), increasing the levels of the inhibitory compound gamma amino butyric acid (GABA) within the brain. Duration of effect is dependent upon rate of GABA-T resynthesis.

Pharmacodynamics/Kinetics

Duration of Action Resynthesis of GABA-T dependent: Variable (not strictly correlated to serum concentrations)

Half-life Elimination Infants: 5.7 hours; Adults: 7.5 hours; Elderly: 12-13 hours

Time to Peak Infants: 2.5 hours; Children: 1 hour; Adults: 1 hour

Pregnancy Risk Factor C

Pregnancy Considerations Adverse events were observed in animal reproduction studies. Vigabatrin crosses the placenta in humans (Tran, 1998). Birth defects have been reported following use in pregnancy and include: cardiac defects, limb defects, male genital malformations, fetal anticonvulsant syndrome, renal and ear abnormalities. Time of exposure or maternal dosage was not reported and information is not available relating to the incidence or types of these outcomes in comparison to the general epilepsy population. Visual field examinations have been conducted following in utero exposure in a limited number of children tested at ≥6 years of age; no visual field loss was observed in 4 children and results were inconclusive in 2 others (Lawthorn, 2009; Sorri 2005). Use during pregnancy is contraindicated in Canadian product labeling.

Patients exposed to vigabatrin during pregnancy are encouraged to enroll themselves into the NAAED Pregnancy Registry by calling 1-888-233-2334. Additional information is available at www.aedpregnancyregistry.org.

Prescribing and Access Restrictions As a requirement of the REMS program, access to this medication is restricted. Vigabatrin is only available in the U.S. under a special restricted distribution program (SHARE). Under the SHARE program, only prescribers and pharmacies registered with the program are able to prescribe and distribute vigabatrin. Vigabatrin may only be dispensed to patients who are enrolled in and meet all conditions of SHARE. Contact the SHARE program at 1-888-45-SHARE.

Vilazodone (vil AZ oh done)

Related Information

Vasoconstrictor Interactions With Antidepressants *on page 1650*

Brand Names: U.S. Viibryd™

Pharmacologic Category Antidepressant, Selective Serotonin Reuptake Inhibitor/5-HT$_{1A}$ Receptor Partial Agonist

Use Treatment of major depressive disorder

◀ **Local Anesthetic/Vasoconstrictor Precautions** Although caution should be used in patients taking tricyclic antidepressants, no interactions have been reported with vasoconstrictors and vilazodone, a non-tricyclic antidepressant which acts to increase serotonin; no precautions appear to be needed

Effects on Dental Treatment Key adverse event(s) related to dental treatment: Xerostomia (normal salivary flow resumes upon discontinuation) and abnormal taste. See Effects on Bleeding.

Effects on Bleeding May impair platelet aggregation resulting in increased risk of bleeding events, particularly if used concomitantly with aspirin, NSAIDs, warfarin, or other anticoagulants. Bleeding related to SSRI use has been reported to range from relatively minor bruising and epistaxis to life-threatening hemorrhage. Routine interruption of therapy for most dental procedures is not warranted. In medically complicated patients or extensive oral surgery, the decision to interrupt therapy must be based on the risk to benefit in an individual patient and a medical consult is suggested. If therapy is continued without interruption, the clinician should anticipate the potential for a prolonged bleeding time.

Adverse Effects
>10%:
  Gastrointestinal: Diarrhea (28%), nausea (23%)
1% to 10%:
  Cardiovascular: Palpitation (2%)
  Central nervous system: Dizziness (9%), insomnia (6%), dreams abnormal (4%), fatigue (4%), restlessness (3%), somnolence (3%), migraine (≥1%), sedation (≥1%)
  Dermatologic: Hyperhidrosis (≥1%)
  Endocrine & metabolic: Libido decreased (3% to 5%), orgasm abnormal (2% to 4%), sexual dysfunction (≤2%)
  Gastrointestinal: Xerostomia (8%), vomiting (5%), dyspepsia (3%), flatulence (3%), gastroenteritis (3%), appetite increased (2%), appetite decreased (≥1%)
  Genitourinary: Ejaculation delayed (2%), erectile dysfunction (2%)
  Neuromuscular & skeletal: Arthralgia (3%), paresthesia (3%), jittery (2%), tremor (2%)
  Ocular: Blurred vision (≥1%), dry eyes (≥1%)
  Miscellaneous: Night sweats (≥1%)

General Dosage Range Dosage adjustment recommended in patients on concomitant therapy
Oral: *Adults:* 10-40 mg once daily
Mechanism of Action Vilazodone inhibits CNS neuron serotonin uptake; minimal or no effect on reuptake of norepinephrine or dopamine. It also binds selectively with high affinity to 5-HT$_{1A}$ receptors and is a 5-HT$_{1A}$ receptor partial agonist. 5-HT$_{1A}$ receptor activity may be altered in depression and anxiety.

Pharmacodynamics/Kinetics
Half-life Elimination Terminal: ~25 hours
Time to Peak Serum: 4-5 hours
Pregnancy Risk Factor C
Pregnancy Considerations Adverse events have been observed in animal reproduction studies. An increased risk of teratogenic effects may be associated with maternal use of other SSRIs. However, available information is conflicting and information specific to the use of vilazodone has not been located. Nonteratogenic effects in the newborn following SSRI/SNRI exposure late in the third trimester include respiratory distress, cyanosis, apnea, seizures, temperature instability, feeding difficulty, vomiting, hypoglycemia, hypo- or hypertonia, hyper-reflexia, jitteriness, irritability, constant crying, and tremor. Symptoms may be due to the toxicity of the SSRIs/SNRIs or a discontinuation syndrome and may be consistent with serotonin syndrome associated with SSRI treatment. Persistent pulmonary hypertension of the newborn (PPHN) has also been reported with SSRI exposure. The long-term effects of *in utero* SSRI exposure on infant development and behavior are not known.

The ACOG recommends that therapy with SSRIs or SNRIs during pregnancy be individualized; treatment of depression during pregnancy should incorporate the clinical expertise of the mental health clinician, obstetrician, primary healthcare provider, and pediatrician. According to the American Psychiatric Association (APA), the risks of medication treatment should be weighed against other treatment options and untreated depression. For women who discontinue antidepressant medications during pregnancy and who may be at high risk for postpartum depression, the medications can be restarted following delivery. Treatment algorithms have been developed by the ACOG and the APA for the management of depression in women prior to conception and during pregnancy. Consideration should be given to using an agent with some safety information in pregnant women.

VinBLAStine (vin BLAS teen)

Brand Names: Canada Vinblastine Sulphate Injection
Pharmacologic Category Antineoplastic Agent, Natural Source (Plant) Derivative; Antineoplastic Agent, Vinca Alkaloid
Use Treatment of Hodgkin's and non-Hodgkin's lymphoma; testicular cancer; breast cancer; mycosis fungoides; Kaposi's sarcoma; histiocytosis (Letterer-Siwe disease); choriocarcinoma
Unlabeled Use Treatment of bladder cancer, melanoma, nonsmall cell lung cancer (NSCLC), ovarian cancer, soft tissue sarcoma (desmoid tumors)
Local Anesthetic/Vasoconstrictor Precautions No information available to require special precautions
Effects on Dental Treatment Key adverse event(s) related to dental treatment: Stomatitis, metallic taste, and jaw pain.
Effects on Bleeding Chemotherapy may result in significant myelosuppression, potentially including significant reduction in platelet counts and altered hemostasis. In patients who are under active treatment with these agents, medical consult is suggested.
Adverse Effects Frequency not defined.
Common:
  Cardiovascular: Hypertension
  Central nervous system: Malaise
  Dermatologic: Alopecia
  Gastrointestinal: Constipation
  Hematologic: Myelosuppression, leukopenia/granulocytopenia (nadir: 5-10 days; recovery: 7-14 days; dose-limiting toxicity)
  Neuromuscular & skeletal: Bone pain, jaw pain, tumor pain
Less common:
  Cardiovascular: Angina, cerebrovascular accident, coronary ischemia, ECG abnormalities, limb ischemia, MI, myocardial ischemia, Raynaud's phenomenon
  Central nervous system: Depression, dizziness, headache, neurotoxicity (duration: >24 hours), seizure, vertigo

Dermatologic: Dermatitis, photosensitivity (rare), rash, skin blistering

Endocrine & metabolic: Aspermia, hyperuricemia, SIADH

Gastrointestinal: Abdominal pain, anorexia, diarrhea, gastrointestinal bleeding, hemorrhagic enterocolitis, ileus, metallic taste, nausea (mild), paralytic ileus, rectal bleeding, stomatitis, toxic megacolon, vomiting (mild)

Genitourinary: Urinary retention

Hematologic: Anemia, thrombocytopenia (recovery within a few days), thrombotic thrombocytopenic purpura

Local: Cellulitis (with extravasation), irritation, phlebitis (with extravasation), radiation recall

Neuromuscular & skeletal: Deep tendon reflex loss, myalgia, paresthesia, peripheral neuritis, weakness

Ocular: Nystagmus

Otic: Auditory damage, deafness, vestibular damage

Renal: Hemolytic uremic syndrome

Respiratory: Bronchospasm, dyspnea, pharyngitis

General Dosage Range Dosage adjustment recommended in patients with hepatic impairment

I.V.:

Children: Initial dose: 3-6.5 mg/m^2 every 7 days as needed

Adults: Initial: 3.7 mg/m^2; adjust dose every 7 days; Second dose: 5.5 mg/m^2; Third dose: 7.4 mg/m^2; Fourth dose: 9.25 mg/m^2; Fifth dose: 11.1 mg/m^2; Usual range: 5.5-7.4 mg/m^2 every 7 days; Maximum dose: 18.5 mg/m^2

Mechanism of Action Vinblastine binds to tubulin and inhibits microtubule formation, therefore, arresting the cell at metaphase by disrupting the formation of the mitotic spindle; it is specific for the M and S phases. Vinblastine may also interfere with nucleic acid and protein synthesis by blocking glutamic acid utilization.

Pharmacodynamics/Kinetics

Half-life Elimination Biphasic: Initial: 4 minutes; Terminal: 25 hours

Pregnancy Risk Factor D

Pregnancy Considerations Animal studies have demonstrated resorption and teratogenic effects. There are no adequate and well-controlled studies in pregnant women. Women of childbearing potential should avoid becoming pregnant during vinblastine treatment. Aspermia has been reported in males who have received treatment with vinblastine.

VinCRIStine (vin KRIS teen)

Brand Names: U.S. Vincasar PFS®

Brand Names: Canada Vincristine Sulfate Injection

Pharmacologic Category Antineoplastic Agent, Natural Source (Plant) Derivative; Antineoplastic Agent, Vinca Alkaloid

Use Treatment of acute lymphocytic leukemia (ALL), Hodgkin lymphoma, non-Hodgkin lymphomas, Wilms' tumor, neuroblastoma, rhabdomyosarcoma

Unlabeled Use Treatment of central nervous system tumors, chronic lymphocytic leukemia (CLL), Ewing's sarcoma, gestational trophoblastic tumors (high-risk), multiple myeloma, ovarian germ cell tumors, retinoblastoma, small cell lung cancer (SCLC); thymoma (advanced)

Local Anesthetic/Vasoconstrictor Precautions No information available to require special precautions

Effects on Dental Treatment Key adverse event(s) related to dental treatment: Oral ulceration, metallic taste, orthostatic hypotension or hypertension.

Effects on Bleeding Although significant myelosuppression with associated altered hemostasis has been reported for many chemotherapeutic agents, myelosuppression is not common with vincristine and no specific precautions appear to necessary.

Adverse Effects Frequency not defined.

Cardiovascular: Edema, hyper-/hypotension, MI, myocardial ischemia

Central nervous system: Ataxia, coma, cranial nerve dysfunction (auditory damage, extraocular muscle impairment, laryngeal muscle impairment, paralysis, paresis, vestibular damage, vocal cord paralysis), dizziness, fever, headache, neurotoxicity (dose-related), neuropathic pain (common), seizure, vertigo

Dermatologic toxicity: Alopecia (common), rash

Endocrine & metabolic: Hyperuricemia, parotid pain, SIADH (rare)

Gastrointestinal: Abdominal cramps, abdominal pain, anorexia, constipation (common), diarrhea, intestinal necrosis, intestinal perforation, nausea, oral ulcers, paralytic ileus, vomiting, weight loss

Genitourinary: Bladder atony, dysuria, polyuria, urinary retention

Hematologic: Anemia (mild), leukopenia (mild), thrombocytopenia (mild), thrombotic thrombocytopenic purpura

Hepatic: Hepatic sinusoidal obstruction syndrome (SOS; veno-occlusive liver disease)

Local: Phlebitis, tissue irritation/necrosis (if infiltrated)

Neuromuscular & skeletal: Back pain, bone pain, deep tendon reflex loss, difficulty walking, foot drop, gait changes, jaw pain, limb pain, motor difficulties, muscle wasting, myalgia, paralysis, paresthesia, peripheral neuropathy (common), sensorimotor dysfunction, sensory loss

Ocular: Cortical blindness (transient), nystagmus, optic atrophy with blindness

Otic: Deafness

Renal: Acute uric acid nephropathy, hemolytic uremic syndrome

Respiratory: Bronchospasm, dyspnea, pharyngeal pain

Miscellaneous: Allergic reactions (rare), anaphylaxis (rare), hypersensitivity (rare)

General Dosage Range Dosage adjustment recommended in patients with hepatic impairment

I.V.:

Children ≤10 kg: 0.05 mg/kg once weekly (maximum: 2 mg/dose)

Children >10 kg: 1.5-2 mg/m^2/dose (maximum: 2 mg/dose)

Adults: 1.4 mg/m^2/dose (maximum: 2 mg/dose)

Mechanism of Action Binds to tubulin and inhibits microtubule formation, therefore, arresting the cell at metaphase by disrupting the formation of the mitotic spindle; it is specific for the M and S phases. Vincristine may also interfere with nucleic acid and protein synthesis by blocking glutamic acid utilization.

Pharmacodynamics/Kinetics

Half-life Elimination Terminal: 85 hours (range: 19-155 hours)

Pregnancy Risk Factor D

Pregnancy Considerations Animal reproduction studies have demonstrated teratogenicity and fetal loss. May cause fetal harm if administered during pregnancy. Women of childbearing potential should avoid becoming pregnant during treatment.

VinCRIStine (Liposomal)
(vin KRIS teen lye po SO mal)

Pharmacologic Category Antineoplastic Agent, Natural Source (Plant) Derivative; Antineoplastic Agent, Vinca Alkaloid

Use Treatment of relapsed Philadelphia chromosome-negative (Ph-) acute lymphoblastic leukemia (ALL) in adult patients whose disease has progressed after two or more antileukemic therapies

Local Anesthetic/Vasoconstrictor Precautions No information available to require special precautions

Effects on Dental Treatment No significant effects or complications reported

Effects on Bleeding Although significant myelosuppression with associated altered hemostasis has been reported for many chemotherapeutic agents, myelosuppression is not common with vincristine and no specific precautions appear to be necessary.

Adverse Effects
>10%:
Central nervous system: Fever (43%), fatigue (41%), insomnia (32%)
Gastrointestinal: Constipation (57%), nausea (52%), diarrhea (37%), appetite decreased (33%)
Hematologic: Neutropenic fever (38%; grades 3/4: 31%), anemia (34%; grades 3/4: 17%), neutropenia (grades 3/4: 18%), thrombocytopenia (grades 3/4: 17%)
Hepatic: AST increased (grades 3/4: 6% to 11%)
Neuromuscular & skeletal: Peripheral neuropathy (39%; grades 3/4: 17%)
1% to 10%:
Cardiovascular: Cardiac arrest (grades 3/4: 6%), hypotension (grades 3/4: 6%)
Central nervous system: Pain (grades 3/4: 8%), mental status changes (grades 3/4: 4%)
Gastrointestinal: Abdominal pain (grades 3/4: 8%), ileus (grades 3/4: 6%)
Neuromuscular & skeletal: Weakness (grades 3/4: 5%), muscle weakness (grades 3/4: 1%)
Respiratory: Pneumonia (grades 3/4: 8%), respiratory distress (grades 3/4: 6%), respiratory failure (grades 3/4: 5%)
Miscellaneous: Septic shock (grades 3/4: 6%), staphylococcal bacteremia (grades 3/4: 6%)

General Dosage Range Dosage adjustment recommended in patients with hepatic impairment or who develop toxicities.
I.V.: *Adults:* 2.25 mg/m^2 once every 7 days

Mechanism of Action Vincristine is a cell cycle specific agent which binds to tubulin, leading to microtubule depolymerization and cellular apoptosis. The liposomal formulation increases the half-life, allowing for enhanced cytotoxic activity in tumor cells.

Pharmacodynamics/Kinetics
Half-life Elimination 45 hours (urinary half-life); dependent on rate of vincristine release from sphingosome (Bedikian, 2006)

Pregnancy Risk Factor D

Pregnancy Considerations Adverse events (fetal malformations, decreased fetal weight, and fetal loss) were observed in animal reproduction studies at doses less than the recommended human dose. Given the mechanism of action, adverse fetal events would be expected to occur with use in pregnant women. Women of childbearing potential should avoid becoming pregnant during therapy.

Product Availability Marqibo®: FDA approved August 9, 2012; availability is currently undetermined. Consult prescribing information for additional information.

Vinorelbine (vi NOR el been)

Brand Names: U.S. Navelbine®
Brand Names: Canada Navelbine®; Vinorelbine Injection, USP; Vinorelbine Tartrate for Injection
Pharmacologic Category Antineoplastic Agent, Natural Source (Plant) Derivative; Antineoplastic Agent, Vinca Alkaloid

Use Treatment of nonsmall cell lung cancer (NSCLC)

Unlabeled Use Treatment of breast cancer (metastatic), cervical cancer (persistent or recurrent), Hodgkin lymphoma (relapsed or refractory), ovarian cancer (relapsed), malignant pleural mesothelioma, salivary gland cancer, small cell lung cancer, and soft tissue sarcoma (advanced)

Local Anesthetic/Vasoconstrictor Precautions No information available to require special precautions

Effects on Dental Treatment No significant effects or complications reported

Effects on Bleeding Chemotherapy may result in significant myelosuppression, potentially including significant reduction in platelet counts and altered hemostasis. In patients who are under active treatment with these agents, medical consult is suggested.

Adverse Effects Note: Reported with single-agent therapy.
>10%:
Central nervous system: Fatigue (27%)
Dermatologic: Alopecia (12% to 30%)
Gastrointestinal: Nausea (31% to 44%; grade 3: 1% to 2%), constipation (35%; grade 3: 3%), vomiting (20% to 31%; grade 3: 1% to 2%), diarrhea (12% to 17%)
Hematologic: Leukopenia (83% to 92%; grade 4: 6% to 15%), granulocytopenia (90%; grade 4: 36%; nadir: 7-10 days; recovery 14-21 days), neutropenia (85%; grade 4: 28%), anemia (83%; grades 3/4: 9%)
Hepatic: AST increased (67%; grade 3: 5%; grade 4: 1%), total bilirubin increased (5% to 13%; grade 3: 4%; grade 4: 3%)
Local: Injection site reaction (22% to 28%; includes erythema, vein discoloration), injection site pain (16%)
Neuromuscular & skeletal: Weakness (36%), peripheral neuropathy (25%; grade 3: 1%; grade 4: <1%)
Renal: Creatinine increased (13%)
1% to 10%:
Cardiovascular: Chest pain (5%)
Dermatologic: Rash (<5%)
Gastrointestinal: Paralytic ileus (1%)
Hematologic: Neutropenic fever/sepsis (8%; grade 4: 4%), thrombocytopenia (3% to 5%; grades 3/4: 1%)
Local: Phlebitis (7% to 10%)
Neuromuscular & skeletal: Loss of deep tendon reflexes (<5%), myalgia (<5%), arthralgia (<5%), jaw pain (<5%)
Otic: Ototoxicity (≤1%)
Respiratory: Dyspnea (7%)

General Dosage Range Dosage adjustment recommended in patients with hepatic or renal impairment or who develop toxicities
I.V.: *Adults:* 25-30 mg/m^2 every 7 days

Mechanism of Action Semisynthetic vinca alkaloid which binds to tubulin and inhibits microtubule formation, therefore, arresting the cell at metaphase by disrupting the formation of the mitotic spindle; it is specific for the M and S phases. Vinorelbine may also interfere with nucleic acid and protein synthesis by blocking glutamic acid utilization.

Pharmacodynamics/Kinetics

Half-life Elimination Triphasic: Terminal: 28-44 hours

Pregnancy Risk Factor D

Pregnancy Considerations Animal reproduction studies have demonstrated embryotoxicity, fetotoxicity, decreased fetal weight, and delayed ossification. May cause fetal harm if administered during pregnancy. Women of childbearing potential should avoid becoming pregnant during vinorelbine treatment.

Vismodegib (vis moe DEG ib)

Brand Names: U.S. Erivedge™

Pharmacologic Category Antineoplastic Agent, Hedgehog Pathway Inhibitor

Use Treatment of metastatic basal cell carcinoma, or locally-advanced basal cell carcinoma that has recurred following surgery or in patients who are not candidates for surgery, and not candidates for radiation therapy

Local Anesthetic/Vasoconstrictor Precautions No information available to require special precautions

Effects on Dental Treatment Key adverse event(s) related to dental treatment: Abnormal taste and loss of taste perception have been reported

Effects on Bleeding No information available to require special precautions

Adverse Effects

>10%:

Central nervous system: Fatigue (40%)

Dermatologic: Alopecia (64%)

Endocrine & metabolic: Amenorrhea (30%)

Gastrointestinal: Abnormal taste (55%), weight loss (45%), nausea (30%), diarrhea (29%), appetite decreased (25%), constipation (21%), vomiting (14%), loss of taste perception (11%)

Neuromuscular & skeletal: Muscle spasm (72%), arthralgia (16%)

1% to 10%:

Endocrine & metabolic: Hyponatremia (grade 3: 4%), hypokalemia (grade 3: 1%)

Renal: Azotemia (grade 3: 2%)

General Dosage Range Oral: *Adults:* 150 mg once daily

Mechanism of Action Basal cell cancer is associated with mutations in Hedgehog pathway components. Hedgehog regulates cell growth and differentiation in embryogenesis; while generally not active in adult tissue, Hedgehog mutations associated with basal cell cancer can activate the pathway resulting in unrestricted proliferation of skin basal cells. Vismodegib is a selective Hedgehog pathway inhibitor which binds to and inhibits Smoothened homologue (SMO), the transmembrane protein involved in Hedgehog signal transduction.

Pharmacodynamics/Kinetics

Half-life Elimination Continuous daily dosing: ~4 days; Single dose: ~12 days

Time to Peak ~2.4 days (Graham, 2011)

Pregnancy Risk Factor D

Pregnancy Considerations [U.S. Boxed Warning]: May result in severe birth defects or embryo-fetal death. Teratogenic effects (severe midline defects, missing digits, and other irreversible malformations), embryotoxic, and fetotoxic events were observed in animal reproduction studies when administered in doses less than the normal human dose. Based on its mechanism of action adverse effects on pregnancy would be expected. **[U.S. Boxed Warning]: Verify pregnancy status prior to initiating treatment and advise patients (female and male) of the risk of birth defects, the need for contraception and risk of exposure through semen.** In females of childbearing potential, obtain pregnancy test within 7 days prior to treatment initiation; after the negative pregnancy test, initiate highly effective contraception prior to the first vismodegib dose and continue during and for 7 months after treatment. Males with female partners of childbearing potential should use condoms with spermicide (even after vasectomy) during and for 2 months after treatment. Women exposed to vismodegib during pregnancy (directly or via seminal fluid) are encouraged to participate in the Erivedge Pregnancy Pharmacovigilance program by contacting the Genentech Adverse Event Line (1-888-835-2555). Pregnancies occurring during or within 7 months after treatment should be reported to the Genentech Adverse Event Line.

Prescribing and Access Restrictions Available at specialty pharmacies through the Erivedge Access Solutions program. Further information may be obtained from the manufacturer, Genentech, at 1-888-249-4918, or at www.ErivedgeAccessSolutions.com

---

Vitamin A (VYE ta min aye)

Brand Names: U.S. A-25 [OTC]; A-Natural [OTC]; A-Natural-25 [OTC]; Aquasol A®

Pharmacologic Category Vitamin, Fat Soluble

Use Treatment and prevention of vitamin A deficiency; parenteral (I.M.) route is indicated when oral administration is not feasible or when absorption is insufficient (malabsorption syndrome); dietary supplement (OTC)

Unlabeled Use Treatment of xerophthalmia caused by vitamin A deficiency; supplement to prevent complications in children with measles in certain settings

Local Anesthetic/Vasoconstrictor Precautions No information available to require special precautions

Effects on Dental Treatment No significant effects or complications reported

Effects on Bleeding No information available to require special precautions

Adverse Effects Frequency not defined: Miscellaneous: Allergic reactions (rare), anaphylactic shock (following I.V. administration)

General Dosage Range I.M., Oral: *Children and Adults:* Dosage varies greatly depending on indication

Mechanism of Action Vitamin A is a fat soluble vitamin needed for visual adaptation to darkness, maintenance of epithelial cells, immune function and embryonic development.

Pregnancy Risk Factor X

Pregnancy Considerations Adverse events have been observed in animal reproduction studies. In humans, the critical period of exposure is the first trimester of pregnancy. Excess vitamin A during pregnancy may cause craniofacial malformations, as well as CNS, heart, and thymus abnormalities. Maternal vitamin A deficiency also causes adverse effects in the fetus, and vitamin A requirements are increased in pregnant ▶

women (IOM, 2000). The manufacturer notes that the safety of doses >6000 units/day in pregnant women has not been established and doses greater than the RDA are contraindicated in pregnant women or those who may become pregnant. High doses are used in some areas of the world for supplementation where deficiency is a public health problem (eg, to prevent night blindness); however, single doses >25,000 units should be avoided within 60 days of conception. High-dose supplementation is otherwise not recommended as part of routine antenatal care (WHO, 2011c).

Vitamin A and Vitamin D (Systemic)
(VYE ta min aye & VYE ta min dee)

Related Information
Vitamin A on page 1405
Brand Names: U.S. A&D Jr. [OTC]; D-Natural-5 [OTC]
Pharmacologic Category Vitamin, Fat Soluble
Use Dietary supplement
Local Anesthetic/Vasoconstrictor Precautions No information available to require special precautions
Effects on Dental Treatment No significant effects or complications reported
Effects on Bleeding No information available to require special precautions
Adverse Effects Refer to individual vitamins for additional information.
General Dosage Range Oral: *Adults:* One tablet or capsule once daily.
Pregnancy Considerations Refer to individual vitamins for additional information and specific requirements during pregnancy.

Vitamin A and Vitamin D (Topical)
(VYE ta min aye & VYE ta min dee)

Brand Names: U.S. A+D® Original [OTC]; Baza® Clear [OTC]; Sween Cream® [OTC]
Pharmacologic Category Topical Skin Product
Use Temporary relief of discomfort due to chapped skin or lips, cuts and scrapes, diaper rash, or minor burns
Local Anesthetic/Vasoconstrictor Precautions No information available to require special precautions
Effects on Dental Treatment No significant effects or complications reported
Effects on Bleeding No information available to require special precautions
Adverse Effects Frequency not defined: Local: Irritation
General Dosage Range Topical: *Children and Adults:* Apply to affected areas as needed.

Vitamin B Complex Combinations
(VYE ta min bee KOM pleks kom bi NAY shuns)

Pharmacologic Category Vitamin
Use Dietary supplement
Local Anesthetic/Vasoconstrictor Precautions No information available to require special precautions
Effects on Dental Treatment No significant effects or complications reported
Effects on Bleeding No information available to require special precautions
General Dosage Range
Oral: *Adults:* Dosage varies greatly depending on product

Pregnancy Considerations Water soluble vitamins cross the placenta (IOM, 1998). Refer to individual vitamins for additional information and specific requirements during pregnancy.

Vitamin E (VYE ta min ee)

Brand Names: U.S. Alph-E [OTC]; Alph-E-Mixed [OTC]; Aqua Gem-E™ [OTC]; Aquasol E® [OTC]; d-Alpha Gems™ [OTC]; E-Gems® Elite [OTC]; E-Gems® Plus [OTC]; E-Gems® [OTC]; E-Gem® Lip Care [OTC]; E-Gem® [OTC]; Ester-E™ [OTC]; Gamma E-Gems® [OTC]; Gamma-E PLUS [OTC]; High Gamma Vitamin E Complete™ [OTC]; Key-E® Kaps [OTC]; Key-E® Powder [OTC]; Key-E® [OTC]
Pharmacologic Category Vitamin, Fat Soluble
Use Dietary supplement
Local Anesthetic/Vasoconstrictor Precautions No information available to require special precautions
Effects on Dental Treatment No significant effects or complications reported
Effects on Bleeding No information available to require special precautions
Adverse Effects Frequency not defined.
  Central nervous system: Fatigue, headache
  Dermatologic: Contact dermatitis with topical preparation, rash
  Endocrine & metabolic: Creatinuria, gonadal dysfunction, hypercholesterolemia, hypertriglyceridemia, serum thyroxine decreased, serum triiodothyronine decreased
  Gastrointestinal: Diarrhea, intestinal cramps, nausea, necrotizing enterocolitis (infants)
  Neuromuscular & skeletal: CPK increased, weakness
  Ocular: Blurred vision
  Renal: Serum creatinine increased
General Dosage Range
  Oral:
    Infants 1-6 months: Adequate intake: 4 mg
    Infants 7-12 months: Adequate intake: 5 mg
    Children 1-3 years: RDA: 6 mg; upper limit of intake should not exceed 200 mg/day
    Children 4-8 years: RDA: 7 mg; upper limit of intake should not exceed 300 mg/day
    Children 9-13 years: RDA: 11 mg; upper limit of intake should not exceed 600 mg/day
    Children 14-18 years: RDA: 15 mg; upper limit of intake should not exceed 800 mg/day
    Adults: RDA: 15 mg; upper limit of intake should not exceed 1000 mg/day
    Pregnant female:
      ≤18 years: RDA: 15 mg; upper level of intake should not exceed 800 mg/day
      19-50 years: RDA: 15 mg; upper level of intake should not exceed 1000 mg/day
    Lactating female:
      ≤18 years: RDA: 19 mg; upper level of intake should not exceed 800 mg/day
      19-50 years: RDA: 19 mg; upper level of intake should not exceed 1000 mg/day
    Topical: *Adults:* Apply a thin layer over affected area.
Mechanism of Action Prevents oxidation of vitamin A and C; protects polyunsaturated fatty acids in membranes from attack by free radicals and protects red blood cells against hemolysis

Pregnancy Considerations Vitamin E crosses the placenta. Maternal serum concentrations of α tocopherol increase with lipid concentrations as pregnancy progresses; however, placental transfer remains constant. Additional supplementation is not needed in pregnant women without deficiency (IOM, 2000).

Vitamins (Fluoride) (VYE ta mins, FLOOR ide)

Brand Names: U.S. Poly-Vi-Flor®; Poly-Vi-Flor® With Iron; Soluvite-F; Tri-Vi-Flor®; Tri-Vi-Flor® with Iron; Vi-Daylin®/F + Iron [DSC]; Vi-Daylin®/F ADC [DSC]; Vi-Daylin®/F ADC + Iron [DSC]; Vi-Daylin®/F [DSC]

Pharmacologic Category Vitamin

Use Prevention/treatment of vitamin deficiency; products containing fluoride are used to prevent dental caries; labeled for OTC use as a dietary supplement

Local Anesthetic/Vasoconstrictor Precautions No information available to require special precautions

Effects on Dental Treatment No significant effects or complications reported

Dosage Daily dose varies by product; refer to package insert for specific product labeling

Contraindications Hypersensitivity to any component of the formulation; pre-existing hypervitaminosis

Warnings/Precautions Not all products can be used in children of all age groups; consult specific product labeling prior to use. Do not exceed recommended doses. Use caution with severe renal or hepatic dysfunction or failure. **[U.S. Boxed Warning]: Products may contain iron. Severe iron toxicity may occur in overdose, particularly when ingested by children; iron is a leading cause of fatal poisoning in children; store out of children's reach and in child-resistant containers.**

Dietary Considerations May take with food to decrease stomach upset.

Dosage Forms Content varies depending on product used. For more detailed information on ingredients in these and other multivitamins, please refer to package labeling.

Dental Comment Chronic overdose of fluoride may result in mottling of tooth enamel and osseous changes.

Vitamins (Multiple/Oral)
(VYE ta mins, MUL ti pul/OR al)

Brand Names: U.S. Androvite® [OTC]; CalciFolic-D™; Centamin [OTC]; Centrum Cardio® [OTC]; Centrum Performance® [OTC]; Centrum® Silver® Ultra Men's [OTC]; Centrum® Silver® Ultra Women's [OTC]; Centrum® Silver® [OTC]; Centrum® Ultra Men's [OTC]; Centrum® Ultra Women's [OTC]; Centrum® [OTC]; Diatx®Zn; Drinkables® Fruits and Vegetables [OTC]; Drinkables® MultiVitamins [OTC]; Encora®; Foltrin®; Freedavite [OTC]; Geri-Freeda [OTC]; Geriation [OTC]; Geritol Complete® [OTC]; Geritol Extend® [OTC]; Geritol® Tonic [OTC]; Glutofac®-MX; Gynovite® Plus [OTC]; Hemocyte Plus®; Hi-Kovite [OTC]; Iberet®-500 [OTC] [DSC]; Monocaps [OTC]; Myadec® [OTC]; Nutrimin-Plus [OTC]; Ocuvite® Adult 50+ [OTC]; Ocuvite® Extra® [OTC]; Ocuvite® Lutein [OTC]; Ocuvite® [OTC]; One A Day® Cholesterol Plus [OTC]; One A Day® Energy [OTC]; One A Day® Essential [OTC]; One A Day® Maximum [OTC]; One A Day® Men's 50+ Advantage [OTC]; One A Day® Men's Health Formula [OTC]; One A Day® Teen Advantage for Her [OTC]; One A Day® Teen Advantage for Him [OTC]; One A Day® Weight Smart® Advanced [OTC]; One A Day® Women's 50+ Advantage [OTC]; One A Day® Women's Active Mind & Body [OTC]; One A Day® Women's [OTC]; Optivite® P.M.T. [OTC]; PreserVision® AREDS [OTC]; PreserVision® Lutein [OTC]; Quintabs [OTC]; Quintabs-M Iron-Free [OTC]; Quintabs-M [OTC]; Renax®; Renax® 5.5; Replace Without Iron [OTC]; Replace [OTC]; Repliva 21/7®; SourceCF®; Strovite®; Strovite® Advance; Strovite® Forte; Strovite® Plus; T-Vites [OTC]; Ultra Freeda A-Free [OTC]; Ultra Freeda Iron-Free [OTC]; Ultra Freeda With Iron [OTC]; Viactiv® Calcium Flavor Glides™ [OTC]; Viactiv® Flavor Glides [OTC]; Viactiv® for Teens [OTC]; Viactiv® With Calcium [OTC]; Viactiv® [OTC]; Vitafol®; Xtramins [OTC]; Yelets [OTC]

Pharmacologic Category Vitamin

Use Prevention/treatment of vitamin and mineral deficiencies; labeled for OTC use as a dietary supplement

Local Anesthetic/Vasoconstrictor Precautions No information available to require special precautions

Effects on Dental Treatment No significant effects or complications reported

Effects on Bleeding No information available to require special precautions

Adverse Effects See individual vitamin monographs.

General Dosage Range Oral: *Adults:* 1 tablet/capsule or 5-15 mL once daily

Pregnancy Considerations Refer to individual vitamin monographs for requirements during pregnancy.

Voriconazole (vor i KOE na zole)

Related Information

Clinical Risk Related to Drugs Prolonging QT Interval *on page 1510*

Fungal Infections *on page 1573*

Brand Names: U.S. VFEND®

Brand Names: Canada VFEND®

Generic Availability (U.S.) Yes: Excludes powder for suspension

Pharmacologic Category Antifungal Agent, Oral; Antifungal Agent, Parenteral

Use Treatment of invasive aspergillosis; treatment of esophageal candidiasis; treatment of candidemia (in non-neutropenic patients); treatment of disseminated *Candida* infections of the skin and viscera; treatment of serious fungal infections caused by *Scedosporium apiospermum* and *Fusarium* spp (including *Fusarium solani*) in patients intolerant of, or refractory to, other therapy

Unlabeled Use Fungal infection prophylaxis in intermediate or high risk neutropenic cancer patients with myelodysplastic syndrome (MDS) or acute myelogenous leukemia (AML), neutropenic allogeneic hematopoietic stem cell recipients, and patients with significant graft-versus-host disease; empiric antifungal therapy (second-line) for persistent neutropenic fever; empiric treatment of fungal meningitis or osteoarticular infections

Local Anesthetic/Vasoconstrictor Precautions Voriconazole is one of the drugs confirmed to prolong the QT interval and is accepted as having a risk of causing torsade de pointes. The risk of drug-induced torsade de pointes is extremely low when a single QT interval prolonging drug is prescribed. In terms of epinephrine, it is not known what effect vasoconstrictors in the local anesthetic regimen will have in patients with a known history of congenital prolonged QT interval or in patients taking any medication that prolongs the QT interval. Until more information is obtained, it is suggested that the clinician consult with the physician prior to the use of a vasoconstrictor in suspected patients, and that the vasoconstrictor (epinephrine, mepivacaine and levonordefrin [Carbocaine® 2% with Neo-Cobefrin®]) be used with caution.

Effects on Dental Treatment Key adverse event(s) related to dental treatment: Xerostomia (normal salivary flow resumes upon discontinuation).

Effects on Bleeding No information available to require special precautions

Adverse Effects

>10%:

Central nervous system: Hallucinations (4% to 12%; auditory and/or visual and likely serum concentration-dependent)

Ocular: Visual changes (dose related; photophobia, color changes, increased or decreased visual acuity, or blurred vision occur in ~21%)

Renal: Creatinine increased (1% to 21%)

2% to 10%:

Cardiovascular: Tachycardia (≤2%)

Central nervous system: Fever (≤6%), chills (≤4%), headache (≤3%)

Dermatologic: Rash (≤7%)

Endocrine & metabolic: Hypokalemia (≤2%)

Gastrointestinal: Nausea (1% to 5%), vomiting (1% to 4%)

Hepatic: Alkaline phosphatase increased (4% to 5%), AST increased (2% to 4%), ALT increased (2% to 3%), cholestatic jaundice (1% to 2%)

Ocular: Photophobia (2% to 3%)

Dosage

Usual dosage ranges:

Children <12 years: Dosage not established

Children ≥12 years and Adults:

Oral: 100-300 mg every 12 hours

I.V.: 6 mg/kg every 12 hours for 2 doses; followed by maintenance dose of 4 mg/kg every 12 hours

Indication-specific dosing:

Children >2 to <12 years:

Aspergillosis, invasive including disseminated and extrapulmonary infection in HIV-exposed/-positive patients: (unlabeled; CDC, 2009):

Oral: Loading dose: 8 mg/kg/dose (maximum: 400 mg/dose) every 12 hours for 2 doses on day 1, followed by maintenance dose of 7 mg/kg/dose (maximum: 200 mg/dose) every 12 hours for ≥12 weeks

I.V.: Loading dose: 6-8 mg/kg/dose (maximum: 400 mg/dose) every 12 hours for 2 doses on day 1, followed by maintenance dose of 7 mg/kg/dose (maximum: 200 mg/dose) every 12 hours for ≥12 weeks

Children ≥12 years and Adults:

Aspergillosis, invasive, including disseminated and extrapulmonary infection: Duration of therapy should be a minimum of 6-12 weeks or throughout period of immunosuppression (Walsh, 2008):

I.V.: Initial: Loading dose: 6 mg/kg every 12 hours for 2 doses; followed by maintenance dose of 4 mg/kg every 12 hours

Oral: Maintenance dose:

Manufacturer's recommendations:

Patients <40 kg: 100 mg every 12 hours; maximum: 300 mg/day

Patients ≥40 kg: 200 mg every 12 hours; maximum: 600 mg/day

IDSA recommendations (Walsh, 2008): May consider oral therapy in place of I.V. with dosing of 4 mg/kg (rounded up to convenient tablet dosage form) every 12 hours; however, I.V. administration is preferred in serious infections since comparative efficacy with the oral formulation has not been established.

Scedosporiosis, fusariosis:

I.V.: Initial: Loading dose: 6 mg/kg every 12 hours for 2 doses; followed by maintenance dose of 4 mg/kg every 12 hours

Oral: Maintenance dose:

Patients <40 kg: 100 mg every 12 hours; maximum: 300 mg/day

Patients ≥40 kg: 200 mg every 12 hours; maximum: 600 mg/day

Candidemia and other deep tissue *Candida* infections: Treatment should continue for a minimum of 14 days following resolution of symptoms or following last positive culture, whichever is longer.

I.V.: Initial: Loading dose 6 mg/kg every 12 hours for 2 doses; followed by maintenance dose of 3-4 mg/kg every 12 hours

Oral:

Manufacturer's recommendations: Maintenance dose:

Patients <40 kg: 100 mg every 12 hours; maximum: 300 mg/day

Patients ≥40 kg: 200 mg every 12 hours; maximum: 600 mg/day

IDSA recommendations (Pappas, 2009): Initial: Loading dose: 400 mg every 12 hours for 2 doses; followed by 200 mg every 12 hours

Endophthalmitis, fungal (unlabeled use; Pappas, 2009): I.V.: 6 mg/kg every 12 hours for 2 doses, then 3-4 mg/kg every 12 hours

Esophageal candidiasis: Oral: Treatment should continue for a minimum of 14 days, and for at least 7 days following resolution of symptoms:

Patients <40 kg: 100 mg every 12 hours; maximum: 300 mg/day

Patients ≥40 kg: 200 mg every 12 hours; maximum: 600 mg/day

Meningitis (secondary to contaminated [eg, *Exserohilum rostratum*] steroid products) (unlabeled use) (CDC [parameningeal], 2012; Kauffman, 2012): Note: Consult an infectious disease specialist and current CDC guidelines for specific treatment recommendations. Therapy duration is ≥3 months; trough serum concentrations must be maintained between 2-5 mcg/mL.

I.V.: 6 mg/kg every 12 hours. If patient does not improve or has severe disease, consider adding amphotericin B (liposomal)

Oral (only in mild disease in adherent patients whose trough concentrations/response to therapy can be closely monitored): 6 mg/kg every 12 hours (CDC [parameningeal], 2012)

Osteoarticular infection involving the spine, discitis, epidural abscess or vertebral osteomyelitis (secondary to contaminated [eg, *Exserohilum rostratum*] steroid products) (unlabeled use) (CDC [osteoarticular], 2012; Kauffmann, 2012): I.V.: 6 mg/kg every 12 hours for ≥3 months. **Note:** Consult an infectious disease specialist and current CDC guidelines for specific treatment recommendations. Trough serum concentrations must be maintained between 2-5 mcg/mL. If patient has severe disease, consider adding amphotericin B (liposomal). Patients may be switched to oral therapy if condition has improved or stabilized.

Osteoarticular infection not involving the spine (secondary to contaminated [eg, *Exserohilum rostratum*] steroid products) (unlabeled use) (CDC [osteoarticular], 2012; Kauffman, 2012): Note: Consult an infectious disease specialist and current CDC guidelines for specific treatment recommendations. Therapy duration is ≥3 months. Trough serum concentrations must be maintained between 2-5 mcg/mL.

I.V.: 6 mg/kg every 12 hours for 2 doses, then 4 mg/kg every 12 hours. If patient has severe disease, consider adding amphotericin B (liposomal)

Oral (only in mild disease in adherent patients whose trough concentrations/response to therapy can be closely monitored): 6 mg/kg every 12 hours for 2 doses, then 4 mg/kg every 12 hours

Dosage adjustment in patients unable to tolerate treatment:

I.V.: Dose may be reduced to 3-4 mg/kg every 12 hours, depending upon condition

Oral: Dose may be reduced in 50 mg decrements to a minimum dosage of 200 mg every 12 hours in patients weighing ≥40 kg (100 mg every 12 hours in patients <40 kg)

Dosage adjustment in patients receiving concomitant CYP450 enzyme inducers or substrates:

Efavirenz: Oral: Increase maintenance dose of voriconazole to 400 mg every 12 hours and reduce efavirenz dose to 300 mg once daily; upon discontinuation of voriconazole, return to the initial dose of efavirenz

Phenytoin:

I.V.: Increase voriconazole maintenance dosage to 5 mg/kg every 12 hours

Oral: Increase voriconazole dose to 400 mg every 12 hours in patients ≥40 kg (200 mg every 12 hours in patients <40 kg)

Dosage adjustment in renal impairment: In patients with Cl$_{cr}$ <50 mL/minute, accumulation of the intravenous vehicle (cyclodextrin) occurs. After initial I.V. loading dose, oral voriconazole should be administered to these patients, unless an assessment of the benefit:risk to the patient justifies the use of I.V. voriconazole. Monitor serum creatinine and change to oral voriconazole therapy when possible.

Oral: Poorly dialyzed; no supplemental dose or dosage adjustment necessary, including patients on intermittent hemodialysis, peritoneal dialysis, or continuous renal replacement therapy (eg, CVVHD).

Note: I.V. dosing **NOT** recommended since cyclodextrin vehicle is cleared at half the rate of voriconazole and may accumulate.

Dosage adjustment in hepatic impairment:

Mild-to-moderate hepatic dysfunction (Child-Pugh class A or B): Following standard loading dose, reduce maintenance dosage by 50%

Severe hepatic impairment: Should only be used if benefit outweighs risk; monitor closely for toxicity

Mechanism of Action Interferes with fungal cytochrome P450 activity (selectively inhibits 14-alpha-lanosterol demethylation), decreasing ergosterol synthesis (principal sterol in fungal cell membrane) and inhibiting fungal cell membrane formation.

Contraindications Hypersensitivity to voriconazole or any component of the formulation (cross-reaction with other azole antifungal agents may occur but has not been established, use caution); coadministration of CYP3A4 substrates which may lead to QT$_c$ prolongation (cisapride, pimozide, or quinidine); coadministration with

barbiturates (long acting), carbamazepine, efavirenz (with standard [eg, not adjusted] voriconazole and efavirenz doses), ergot derivatives, rifampin, rifabutin, ritonavir (≥800 mg/day), sirolimus, St John's wort

Warnings/Precautions Visual changes, including blurred vision, changes in visual acuity, color perception, and photophobia, are commonly associated with treatment; postmarketing cases of optic neuritis and papilledema (lasting >1 month) have also been reported. Patients should be warned to avoid tasks which depend on vision, including operating machinery or driving. Changes are reversible on discontinuation following brief exposure/treatment regimens (≤28 days).

Serious hepatic reactions (including hepatitis, cholestasis, and fulminant hepatic failure) have occurred during treatment, primarily in patients with serious concomitant medical conditions. However, hepatotoxicity has occurred in patients with no identifiable risk factors. Use caution in patients with pre-existing hepatic impairment (dose adjustment or discontinuation may be required).

Voriconazole tablets contain lactose; avoid administration in hereditary galactose intolerance, Lapp lactase deficiency, or glucose-galactose malabsorption. Suspension contains sucrose; use caution with fructose intolerance, sucrase-isomaltase deficiency, or glucose-galactose malabsorption. Avoid/limit use of intravenous formulation in patients with renal impairment; intravenous formulation contains excipient cyclodextrin (sulfobutyl ether beta-cyclodextrin), which may accumulate in renal insufficiency. Acute renal failure has been observed in severely ill patients; use with caution in patients receiving concomitant nephrotoxic medications. Anaphylactoid-type infusion-related reactions may occur with intravenous dosing. Consider discontinuation of infusion if reaction is severe.

Use caution in patients taking strong cytochrome P450 inducers, CYP2C9 inhibitors, and major 3A4 substrates (see Drug Interactions); consider alternative agents that avoid or lessen the potential for CYP-mediated interactions. QT interval prolongation has been associated with voriconazole use; rare cases of arrhythmia (including torsade de pointes), cardiac arrest, and sudden death have been reported, usually in seriously ill patients with comorbidities and/or risk factors (eg, prior cardiotoxic chemotherapy, cardiomyopathy, electrolyte imbalance, or concomitant QT$_c$-prolonging drugs). Use with caution in these patient populations; correct electrolyte abnormalities (eg, hypokalemia, hypomagnesemia, hypocalcemia) prior to initiating therapy. Do not infuse concomitantly with blood products or short-term concentrated electrolyte solutions, even if the two infusions are running in separate intravenous lines (or cannulas).

Rare cases of malignancy (melanoma, squamous cell carcinoma) have been reported in patients (mostly immunocompromised) with prior onset of severe photosensitivity reactions and exposure to long-term voriconazole therapy. Other serious exfoliative cutaneous reactions, including Stevens-Johnson syndrome, have also been reported. Patient should avoid strong, direct exposure to sunlight; may cause photosensitivity, especially with long-term use. Discontinue use in patients who develop an exfoliative cutaneous reaction or a skin lesion consistent with squamous cell carcinoma or melanoma. Periodic total body skin examinations should be performed, particularly with prolonged use.

Monitor pancreatic function in patients (children and adults) at risk for acute pancreatitis (eg, recent chemotherapy or hematopoietic stem cell transplantation); there have been postmarketing reports of pancreatitis in children.

Drug Interactions

Metabolism/Transport Effects Substrate of CYP2C19 (major), CYP2C9 (major), CYP3A4 (minor); **Note:** Assignment of Major/Minor substrate status based on clinically relevant drug interaction potential; **Inhibits** CYP2C19 (moderate), CYP2C9 (moderate), CYP3A4 (strong)

Avoid Concomitant Use

Avoid concomitant use of Voriconazole with any of the following: Ado-Trastuzumab Emtansine; Alfuzosin; Apixaban; Astemizole; Atazanavir; Avanafil; Axitinib; Barbiturates; Bosutinib; Cabozantinib; CarBAMazepine; Cisapride; Clopidogrel; Conivaptan; Crizotinib; Darunavir; Dihydroergotamine; Dofetilide; Dronedarone; Eletriptan; Eplerenone; Ergoloid Mesylates; Ergonovine; Ergotamine; Everolimus; Fluconazole; Fluticasone (Oral Inhalation); Halofantrine; Highest Risk QTc-Prolonging Agents; Ivabradine; Lapatinib; Lomitapide; Lopinavir; Lovastatin; Lurasidone; Methylergonovine; Mifepristone; Nilotinib; Nisoldipine; Pimozide; Pomalidomide; QuiNIDine; Ranolazine; Red Yeast Rice; Regorafenib; Rifamycin Derivatives; Ritonavir; Rivaroxaban; RomiDEPsin; Salmeterol; Silodosin; Simvastatin; Sirolimus; St Johns Wort; Tamsulosin; Terfenadine; Ticagrelor; Tolvaptan; Toremifene; VinCRIStine (Liposomal)

Increased Effect/Toxicity

Voriconazole may increase the levels/effects of: Ado-Trastuzumab Emtansine; Alfentanil; Alfuzosin; Almotriptan; Alosetron; Antineoplastic Agents (Vinca Alkaloids); Apixaban; Aprepitant; ARIPiprazole; Astemizole; AtorvaSTATin; Avanafil; Axitinib; Bedaquiline; Benzodiazepines (metabolized by oxidation); Boceprevir; Bortezomib; Bosentan; Bosutinib; Brentuximab Vedotin; Brinzolamide; Budesonide (Nasal); Budesonide (Systemic, Oral Inhalation); BusPIRone; Busulfan; Cabozantinib; Calcium Channel Blockers; Carvedilol; Cilostazol; Cinacalcet; Cisapride; Cobicistat; Colchicine; Conivaptan; Contraceptives (Estrogens); Contraceptives (Progestins); Corticosteroids (Orally Inhaled); Corticosteroids (Systemic); Crizotinib; CycloSPORINE (Systemic); CYP2C19 Substrates; CYP2C9 Substrates; CYP3A4 Substrates; Diclofenac (Systemic); Diclofenac (Topical); Dienogest; Dihydroergotamine; DOCEtaxel; Dofetilide; Dronedarone; Dutasteride; Eletriptan; Elvitegravir; Enzalutamide; Eplerenone; Ergoloid Mesylates; Ergonovine; Ergotamine; Erlotinib; Eszopiclone; Etravirine; Everolimus; FentaNYL; Fesoterodine; Fluticasone (Nasal); Fluticasone (Oral Inhalation); Fosamprenavir; Fosaprepitant; Fosphenytoin; Gefitinib; GuanFACINE; Halofantrine; Highest Risk QTc-Prolonging Agents; Ibuprofen; Iloperidone; Imatinib; Irinotecan; Ivabradine; Ivacaftor; Ixabepilone; Lapatinib; Lomitapide; Losartan; Lovastatin; Lumefantrine; Lurasidone; Macrolide Antibiotics; Maraviroc; Meloxicam; Methadone; Methylergonovine; MethylPREDNISolone; Mifepristone; Moderate Risk QTc-Prolonging Agents; Nelfinavir; Nilotinib; Nisoldipine; Ospemifene; OxyCODONE; Paricalcitol; Pazopanib; Phenytoin; Pimecrolimus; Pimozide; Pomalidomide; Ponatinib; Propafenone; Proton Pump Inhibitors; QuiNIDine; Ramelteon; Ranolazine; Red Yeast Rice; Regorafenib; Repaglinide; Reverse Transcriptase Inhibitors (Non-Nucleoside); Rifamycin Derivatives; Rivaroxaban; RomiDEPsin; Ruxolitinib;

Salmeterol; Saxagliptin; Sildenafil; Silodosin; Simvastatin; Sirolimus; Solifenacin; SORAfenib; Sulfonylureas; SUNItinib; Tacrolimus (Systemic); Tacrolimus (Topical); Tadalafil; Tamsulosin; Telaprevir; Terfenadine; Ticagrelor; Tofacitinib; Tolterodine; Tolvaptan; Toremifene; Vardenafil; Vemurafenib; Venlafaxine; Vilazodone; VinCRIStine (Liposomal); Vitamin K Antagonists; Ziprasidone; Zolpidem; Zuclopenthixol

The levels/effects of Voriconazole may be increased by: Atazanavir; Boceprevir; Chloramphenicol; Cobicistat; Contraceptives (Estrogens); Contraceptives (Progestins); CYP2C19 Inhibitors (Moderate); CYP2C19 Inhibitors (Strong); CYP2C9 Inhibitors (Moderate); CYP2C9 Inhibitors (Strong); Etravirine; Fluconazole; Fosamprenavir; Grapefruit Juice; Ivabradine; Macrolide Antibiotics; Mifepristone; Proton Pump Inhibitors; QTc-Prolonging Agents (Indeterminate Risk and Risk Modifying); Telaprevir

Decreased Effect

Voriconazole may decrease the levels/effects of: Amphotericin B; Atazanavir; Clopidogrel; Ifosfamide; Prasugrel; Saccharomyces boulardii; Ticagrelor

The levels/effects of Voriconazole may be decreased by: Atazanavir; Barbiturates; CarBAMazepine; CYP2C19 Inducers (Strong); CYP2C9 Inducers (Strong); Darunavir; Didanosine; Etravirine; Fosphenytoin; Lopinavir; Peginterferon Alfa-2b; Phenytoin; Reverse Transcriptase Inhibitors (Non-Nucleoside); Rifamycin Derivatives; Ritonavir; St Johns Wort; Sucralfate; Telaprevir

Ethanol/Nutrition/Herb Interactions

Food: Food may decrease voriconazole absorption. Grapefruit juice may decrease voriconazole levels. Management: Oral voriconazole should be taken 1 hour before or 1 hour after a meal. Avoid grapefruit juice. Maintain adequate hydration unless instructed to restrict fluid intake.

Herb/Nutraceutical: St John's wort may decrease voriconazole levels. Management: Concurrent use of St John's wort with voriconazole is contraindicated.

Dietary Considerations Oral: Should be taken 1 hour before or 1 hour after a meal. Voriconazole tablets contain lactose; avoid administration in hereditary galactose intolerance, Lapp lactase deficiency, or glucosegalactose malabsorption. Suspension contains sucrose; use caution with fructose intolerance, sucrose-isomaltase deficiency, or glucose-galactose malabsorption.

Pharmacodynamics/Kinetics

Half-life Elimination Variable, dose dependent

Time to Peak Oral: 1-2 hours; 0.5 hours (crushed tablet)

Pregnancy Risk Factor D

Pregnancy Considerations Voriconazole can cause fetal harm when administered to a pregnant woman. Voriconazole was teratogenic and embryotoxic in animal studies, and lowered plasma estradiol in animal models. Women of childbearing potential should use effective contraception during treatment. Should be used in pregnant woman only if benefit to mother justifies potential risk to the fetus.

Lactation Excretion in breast milk unknown/not recommended

Breast-Feeding Considerations Excretion in breast milk has not been investigated; avoid breast-feeding until additional data are available.

Dosage Forms

Injection, powder for reconstitution: 200 mg
VFEND®: 200 mg

Powder for suspension, oral:
VFEND®: 40 mg/mL (70 mL)
Tablet, oral: 50 mg, 200 mg
VFEND®: 50 mg, 200 mg

Dental Comment Voriconazole is known to prolong the QT interval. The QT interval is measured as the time and distance between the Q point of the QRS complex and the end of the T wave in the ECG tracing. After adjustment for heart rate, the QT interval is defined as prolonged if it is more than 450 msec in men and 460 msec in women. A long QT syndrome was first described in the 1950s and 60s as a congenital syndrome involving QT interval prolongation and syncope and sudden death. Some of the congenital long QT syndromes were characterized by a peculiar electrocardiographic appearance of the QRS complex involving a premature atria beat followed by a pause, then a subsequent sinus beat showing marked QT prolongation and deformity. This type of cardiac arrhythmia was originally termed "torsade de pointes" (translated from the French as "twisting of the points"). Voriconazole is considered as having a risk of causing torsade de pointes. Since it is not known what effect vasoconstrictors in the local anesthetic regimen will have in patients with a known history of congenital prolonged QT interval or in patients taking any medication that prolongs the QT interval, a medical consult is suggested.

Vorinostat (vor IN oh stat)

Brand Names: U.S. Zolinza®
Brand Names: Canada Zolinza®
Pharmacologic Category Antineoplastic Agent, Histone Deacetylase Inhibitor
Use Treatment of cutaneous manifestations of progressive, persistent, or recurrent cutaneous T-cell lymphoma (CTCL)
Local Anesthetic/Vasoconstrictor Precautions No information available to require special precautions
Effects on Dental Treatment Key adverse event(s) related to dental treatment: High incidence of xerostomia (normal salivary flow resumes upon discontinuation) and taste perversion.
Effects on Bleeding Chemotherapy may result in significant myelosuppression, potentially including significant reduction in platelet counts (thrombocytopenia grades 3/4: 6%) and altered hemostasis. In patients who are under active treatment with these agents, medical consult is suggested.
Adverse Effects
>10%:
Cardiovascular: Peripheral edema (13%)
Central nervous system: Fatigue (52%), chills (16%), dizziness (15%), headache (12%), fever (11%)
Dermatologic: Alopecia (19%), pruritus (12%)
Endocrine & metabolic: Hyperglycemia (8% to 69%; grade 3: 5%), dehydration (1% to 16%)
Gastrointestinal: Diarrhea (52%), nausea (41%), taste alteration (28%), anorexia (24%), weight loss (21%), xerostomia (16%), constipation (15%), vomiting (15%), appetite decreased (14%)
Hematologic: Thrombocytopenia (26%; grades 3/4: 6%), anemia (14%; grades 3/4: 2%)
Neuromuscular & skeletal: Muscle spasm (20%)
Renal: Proteinuria (51%), creatinine increased (16% to 47%)
Respiratory: Cough (11%), upper respiratory infection (11%)

1% to 10%:
Cardiovascular: QT_c prolongation (3% to 4%)
Dermatologic: Squamous cell carcinoma (4%)
Respiratory: Pulmonary embolism (5%)
General Dosage Range Dosage adjustment recommended in patients who develop toxicities and those with hepatic impairment
Oral: *Adults:* 400 mg once daily
Mechanism of Action Inhibition of histone deacetylase enzymes, HDAC1, HDAC2, HDAC3, and HDAC6, which catalyze acetyl group removal from protein lysine residues (including histones and transcription factors). Inhibition of histone deacetylase results in accumulation of acetyl groups, which alters chromatin structure and transcription factor activation; cell growth is terminated and apoptosis occurs.
Pharmacodynamics/Kinetics
Half-life Elimination ~2 hours
Time to Peak Plasma: With high-fat meal: ~4 hours (range: 2-10 hours)
Pregnancy Risk Factor D
Pregnancy Considerations Animal reproduction studies have demonstrated adverse fetal effects, including fetal loss, decreased fetal weight, and skeletal malformation. Inform patient of potential hazard if used during pregnancy or if pregnancy occurs during treatment.

Dental Comment This drug is known to prolong the QT interval. The QT interval is measured as the time and distance between the Q point of the QRS complex and the end of the T wave in the ECG tracing. After adjustment for heart rate, the QT interval is defined as prolonged if it is more than 450 msec in men and 460 msec in women. A long QT syndrome was first described in the 1950s and 60s as a congenital syndrome involving QT interval prolongation and syncope and sudden death. Some of the congenital long QT syndromes were characterized by a peculiar electrocardiographic appearance of the QRS complex involving a premature atria beat followed by a pause, then a subsequent sinus beat showing marked QT prolongation and deformity. This type of cardiac arrhythmia was originally termed "torsade de pointes" (translated from the French as "twisting of the points").

Prolongation of the QT interval is thought to result from delayed ventricular repolarization. The repolarization process within the myocardial cell is due to the efflux of intracellular potassium. The channels associated with this current can be blocked by many drugs and predispose the electrical propagation cycle to torsade de pointes.

Vorinostat is one of the drugs confirmed to prolong the QT interval and is accepted as having a risk of causing torsade de pointes. The risk of drug-induced torsade de pointes is extremely low when a single QT interval prolonging drug is prescribed. In terms of epinephrine, it is not known what effect vasoconstrictors in the local anesthetic regimen will have in patients with a known history of congenital prolonged QT interval or in patients taking any medication that prolongs the QT interval. Until more information is obtained, it is suggested that the clinician consult with the physician prior to the use of a vasoconstrictor in suspected patients, and that the vasoconstrictor (epinephrine, levonordefrin [Neo-Cobefrin®]) be used with caution.

Warfarin (WAR far in)

Related Information

Antiplatelet and Anticoagulation Considerations in Dentistry *on page 1503*

Cardiovascular Diseases *on page 1492*

Brand Names: U.S. Coumadin®; Jantoven®

Brand Names: Canada Apo-Warfarin®; Coumadin®; Mylan-Warfarin; Novo-Warfarin; Taro-Warfarin

Generic Availability (U.S.) Yes: Tablet

Pharmacologic Category Anticoagulant, Coumarin Derivative; Vitamin K Antagonist

Use Prophylaxis and treatment of thromboembolic disorders (eg, venous, pulmonary) and embolic complications arising from atrial fibrillation or cardiac valve replacement; adjunct to reduce risk of systemic embolism (eg, recurrent MI, stroke) after myocardial infarction

Unlabeled Use Prevention of recurrent transient ischemic attacks

Local Anesthetic/Vasoconstrictor Precautions No information available to require special precautions

Effects on Dental Treatment Key adverse event(s) related to dental treatment: Mouth ulcers and taste disturbance.

Signs of warfarin overdose may first appear as bleeding from gingival tissue. See Effects on Bleeding.

Effects on Bleeding A recent study assessed the amount of bleeding during a single tooth extraction in patients who remained on warfarin during the procedure versus those who discontinued warfarin (Karsli, 2011). All patients had coronary artery disease. There was no significant difference in bleeding with or without warfarin. The mean blood loss was 2486 ± 1408 g in the warfarin group, compared to 1736 ± 876 g in the patients who stopped warfarin. The mean INR value in the warfarin group was 2.6 ± 0.7. Hemostasis was successfully established locally by packing the extraction sockets with oxidized cellulose (Surgicel®) and suturing with 3-0 silk sutures.

As with all anticoagulants, bleeding is a potential adverse effect of warfarin during dental surgery; risk is dependent on multiple variables, including the intensity of anticoagulation and patient susceptibility. Consultation with prescribing physician is advisable prior to surgery to determine temporary dose reduction or withdrawal of medication.

A retrospective study evaluating over 38,000 patients ≥65 years of age showed exposure to any antibiotic agent was associated with at least a 2-fold increased risk of bleeding that required hospitalization among continuous warfarin users (Baillargeon, 2012). All five antibiotic drug classes examined (macrolides, quinolones, cotrimoxazole, penicillins, and cephalosporins) were associated with an increased risk of bleeding. Exposure to an azole antifungal (fluconazole, ketoconazole, or miconazole) while on warfarin was associated with a 4-fold increased risk of bleeding.

Adverse Effects Bleeding is the major adverse effect of warfarin. Hemorrhage may occur at virtually any site. Risk is dependent on multiple variables, including the intensity of anticoagulation and patient susceptibility.

Cardiovascular: Vasculitis

Central nervous system: Signs/symptoms of bleeding (eg, dizziness, fatigue, fever, headache, lethargy, malaise, pain)

Dermatologic: Alopecia, bullous eruptions, dermatitis, rash, pruritus, urticaria

Gastrointestinal: Abdominal pain, diarrhea, flatulence, gastrointestinal bleeding, nausea, taste disturbance, vomiting

Genitourinary: Hematuria

Hematologic: Anemia, retroperitoneal hematoma, unrecognized bleeding sites (eg, colon cancer) may be uncovered by anticoagulation

Hepatic: Hepatitis (including cholestatic hepatitis), transaminases increased

Neuromuscular & skeletal: Osteoporosis (potential association with long-term use), paralysis, paresthesia, weakness

Respiratory: Respiratory tract bleeding, tracheobronchial calcification

Miscellaneous: Anaphylactic reaction, hypersensitivity/allergic reactions, skin necrosis, gangrene, "purple toes" syndrome

Dosage Note: Labeling identifies genetic factors which may increase patient sensitivity to warfarin. Specifically, genetic variations in the proteins CYP2C9 and VKORC1, responsible for warfarin's primary metabolism and pharmacodynamic activity, respectively, have been identified as predisposing factors associated with decreased dose requirement and increased bleeding risk. Genotyping tests are available, and may provide guidance on initiation of anticoagulant therapy. The American College of Chest Physicians recommends against the use of routine pharmacogenomic testing to guide dosing (Guyatt, 2012).

Oral:

Infants and Children (unlabeled use): Initial loading dose (if baseline INR is 1-1.3): 0.2 mg/kg (maximum: 10 mg/dose); adjust dose based on INR (reported ranges to maintain INR of 2-3: 0.09-0.33 mg/kg/day). Infants <12 months of age may require doses at or near the high end of this range; consistent anticoagulation may be difficult to maintain in children <5 years of age (Monagle, 2012).

Adults: Initial dosing must be individualized. Consider the patient (hepatic function, cardiac function, age, nutritional status, concurrent therapy, risk of bleeding) in addition to prior dose response (if available) and the clinical situation. Start 2-5 mg once daily for 2 days **or** for healthy individuals, 10 mg once daily for 2 days; lower doses (eg, 5 mg once daily) recommended for patients with confirmed HIT once platelet recovery has occurred (Guyatt, 2012). In patients with acute venous thromboembolism, initiation may begin on the first or second day of low molecular weight heparin or unfractionated heparin therapy (Guyatt, 2012). Adjust dose according to INR results; usual maintenance dose ranges from 2-10 mg daily (individual patients may require loading and maintenance doses outside these general guidelines).

Note: Lower starting doses may be required for patients with hepatic impairment, poor nutrition, CHF, elderly, high risk of bleeding, or patients who are debilitated, or those with reduced function genomic variants of the catabolic enzymes CYP2C9 (*2 or *3 alleles) or VKORC1 (-1639 polymorphism); see table. Higher initial doses may be reasonable in selected patients (ie, receiving enzyme-inducing agents and with low risk of bleeding).

Range[1] of Expected Therapeutic Maintenance Dose Based on CYP2C9[2] and VKORC1[3] Genotypes

VKORC1	CYP2C9					
	*1/*1	*1/*2	*1/*3	*2/*2	*2/*3	*3/*3
GG	5-7 mg	5-7 mg	3-4 mg	3-4 mg	3-4 mg	0.5-2 mg
AG	5-7 mg	3-4 mg	3-4 mg	3-4 mg	0.5-2 mg	0.5-2 mg
AA	3-4 mg	3-4 mg	0.5-2 mg	0.5-2 mg	0.5-2 mg	0.5-2 mg

Note: Must also take into account other patient related factors when determining initial dose (eg, age, body weight, concomitant medications, comorbidities). The American College of Chest Physicians recommends against the use of routine pharmacogenomic testing to guide dosing (Guyatt, 2012).

[1]Ranges derived from multiple published clinical studies.

[2]Patients with CYP2C9 *1/*3, *2/*2, *2/*3, and *3/*3 alleles may take up to 4 weeks to achieve maximum INR with a given dose regimen.

[3]VKORC1 -1639G>A (rs 9923231) variant is used in this table; other VKORC1 variants may also be important determinants of dose.

I.V.: Adults: 2-5 mg/day administered as a slow bolus injection

Dosing adjustment in renal disease: No adjustment required, however, patients with renal failure have an increased risk of bleeding complications. Monitor closely.

Dosing adjustment in hepatic disease: Monitor effect at usual doses; the response to oral anticoagulants may be markedly enhanced in obstructive jaundice (due to reduced vitamin K absorption) and also in hepatitis and cirrhosis (due to decreased production of vitamin K-dependent clotting factors); INR should be closely monitored

Mechanism of Action Hepatic synthesis of coagulation factors II, VII, IX, and X, as well as proteins C and S, requires the presence of vitamin K. These clotting factors are biologically activated by the addition of carboxyl groups to key glutamic acid residues within the proteins' structure. In the process, "active" vitamin K is oxidatively converted to an "inactive" form, which is then subsequently reactivated by vitamin K epoxide reductase complex 1 (VKORC1). Warfarin competitively inhibits the subunit 1 of the multi-unit VKOR complex, thus depleting functional vitamin K reserves and hence reduces synthesis of active clotting factors.

Contraindications Hypersensitivity to warfarin or any component of the formulation; hemorrhagic tendencies (eg, patients bleeding from the GI, respiratory, or GU tract; cerebral aneurysm; cerebrovascular hemorrhage; dissecting aortic aneurysm; spinal puncture and other diagnostic or therapeutic procedures with potential for significant bleeding; history of bleeding diathesis); recent or potential surgery of the eye or CNS; major regional lumbar block anesthesia or traumatic surgery resulting in large, open surfaces; blood dyscrasias; severe uncontrolled or malignant hypertension; pericarditis or pericardial effusion; bacterial endocarditis; unsupervised patients with conditions associated with a high potential for noncompliance; eclampsia/pre-eclampsia, threatened abortion, pregnancy (except in women with mechanical heart valves at high risk for thromboembolism)

Warnings/Precautions Hazardous agent - use appropriate precautions for handling and disposal (EPA, P-listed [>0.3%]; U-listed [<0.3%]). Use care in the selection of patients appropriate for this treatment. Ensure patient cooperation especially from the alcoholic, illicit drug user, demented, or psychotic patient; ability to comply with routine laboratory monitoring is essential. Use with caution in trauma, acute infection, moderate-severe renal insufficiency, prolonged dietary insufficiencies, moderate-severe hypertension, polycythemia vera, vasculitis, open wound, active TB, any disruption in normal GI flora, history of PUD, anaphylactic disorders, indwelling catheters, severe diabetes, and menstruating and postpartum women. Use with caution in patients with thyroid disease; warfarin responsiveness may increase (Ageno, 2012). Use with caution in protein C deficiency. Use with caution in patients with heparin-induced thrombocytopenia and DVT. Warfarin monotherapy is contraindicated in the initial treatment of active HIT. Reduced liver function, regardless of etiology, may impair synthesis of coagulation factors leading to increased warfarin sensitivity.

[U.S. Boxed Warning]: May cause major or fatal bleeding. Risk factors for bleeding include high intensity anticoagulation (INR >4), age (>65 years), variable INRs, history of GI bleeding, hypertension, cerebrovascular disease, serious heart disease, anemia, malignancy, trauma, renal insufficiency, drug-drug interactions, long duration of therapy, or known genetic deficiency in CYP2C9 activity. Patient must be instructed to report bleeding, accidents, or falls. Unrecognized bleeding sites (eg, colon cancer) may be uncovered by anticoagulation. Patient must also report any new or discontinued medications, herbal or alternative products used, or significant changes in smoking or dietary habits. Necrosis or gangrene of the skin and other tissue can occur, usually in conjunction with protein C or S deficiency. Consider alternative therapies if anticoagulation is necessary. Warfarin therapy may release atheromatous plaque emboli; symptoms depend on site of embolization, most commonly kidneys, pancreas, liver, and spleen. In some cases may lead to necrosis or death. "Purple toes syndrome," due to cholesterol microembolization, may rarely occur. The elderly may be more sensitive to anticoagulant therapy.

Presence of the CYP2C9*2 or *3 allele and/or polymorphism of the vitamin K oxidoreductase (VKORC1) gene may increase the risk of bleeding. Lower doses may be required in these patients; genetic testing may help determine appropriate dosing.

When temporary interruption is necessary before surgery, discontinue for approximately 5 days before surgery; when there is adequate hemostasis, may reinstitute warfarin therapy ~12-24 hours after surgery (evening of or next morning). Decision to safely continue warfarin therapy through the procedure and whether or not bridging of anticoagulation is necessary is dependent upon risk of perioperative bleeding and risk of thromboembolism, respectively. If risk of thromboembolism is elevated, consider bridging warfarin therapy with an alternative anticoagulant (eg, unfractionated heparin, LMWH) (Guyatt, 2012).

Drug Interactions

Metabolism/Transport Effects Substrate of
CYP1A2 (minor), CYP2C19 (minor), CYP2C9 (major), CYP3A4 (minor); **Note:** Assignment of Major/Minor substrate status based on clinically relevant drug interaction potential; **Inhibits** CYP2C19 (weak), CYP2C9 (weak)

Avoid Concomitant Use
Avoid concomitant use of Warfarin with any of the following: Apixaban; Dabigatran Etexilate; Enzalutamide; Rivaroxaban; Tamoxifen

Increased Effect/Toxicity
Warfarin may increase the levels/effects of: Anticoagulants; Collagenase (Systemic); Deferasirox; Drotrecogin Alfa (Activated); Ethotoin; Fosphenytoin; Phenytoin; Regorafenib; Rivaroxaban; Sulfonylureas

The levels/effects of Warfarin may be increased by: Acetaminophen; Agents with Antiplatelet Properties; Allopurinol; Amiodarone; Androgens; Antineoplastic Agents; Apixaban; Atazanavir; Bicalutamide; Boceprevir; Capecitabine; Cephalosporins; Chloral Hydrate; Chloramphenicol; Cimetidine; Clopidogrel; Cloxacillin; Cobicistat; Corticosteroids (Systemic); Cranberry; CYP2C9 Inhibitors (Moderate); CYP2C9 Inhibitors (Strong); Dabigatran Etexilate; Desvenlafaxine; Dexmethylphenidate; Disulfiram; Dronedarone; Efavirenz; Erythromycin (Ophthalmic); Esomeprazole; Ethacrynic Acid; Ethotoin; Etoposide; Exenatide; Fenofibrate; Fenofibric Acid; Fenugreek; Fibric Acid Derivatives; Fluconazole; Fluorouracil (Systemic); Fluorouracil (Topical); Fosamprenavir; Fosphenytoin; Gefitinib; Ginkgo Biloba; Glucagon; Green Tea; Herbs (Anticoagulant/Antiplatelet Properties); HMG-CoA Reductase Inhibitors; Ifosfamide; Imatinib; Itraconazole; Ivermectin (Systemic); Ketoconazole (Systemic); Lansoprazole; Leflunomide; Lomitapide; Macrolide Antibiotics; Methylphenidate; MetroNIDAZOLE (Systemic); Miconazole (Topical); Mifepristone; Milnacipran; Mirtazapine; Multivitamins/Minerals (with ADEK, Folate, Iron); Nelfinavir; Neomycin; NSAID (COX-2 Inhibitor); NSAID (Nonselective); Omega-3 Fatty Acids; Omeprazole; Orlistat; Penicillins; Pentosan Polysulfate Sodium; Pentoxifylline; Phenytoin; Posaconazole; Propafenone; Prostacyclin Analogues; QuiNIDine; QuiNINE; Quinolone Antibiotics; Ranitidine; RomiDEPsin; Salicylates; Saquinavir; Selective Serotonin Reuptake Inhibitors; Sitaxentan; SORAfenib; Sulfinpyrazone [Off Market]; Sulfonamide Derivatives; Sulfonylureas; Tamoxifen; Telaprevir; Tetracycline Derivatives; Thrombolytic Agents; Thyroid Products; Tigecycline; Tipranavir; Tolterodine; Toremifene; Torsemide; TraMADol; Tricyclic Antidepressants; Venlafaxine; Vitamin E; Voriconazole; Vorinostat; Zafirlukast; Zileuton

Decreased Effect
The levels/effects of Warfarin may be decreased by: Adalimumab; Aminoglutethimide; Antineoplastic Agents; Antithyroid Agents; Aprepitant; AzaTHIOprine; Barbiturates; Bile Acid Sequestrants; Boceprevir; Bosentan; CarBAMazepine; Cloxacillin; Coenzyme Q-10; Contraceptives (Estrogens); Contraceptives (Progestins); CYP2C9 Inducers (Strong); Darunavir; Dicloxacillin; Efavirenz; Elvitegravir; Enzalutamide; Fosaprepitant; Ginseng (American); Glutethimide; Green Tea; Griseofulvin; Lopinavir; Mercaptopurine; Multivitamins/Minerals (with ADEK, Folate, Iron); Nafcillin; Nelfinavir; Peginterferon Alfa-2b; Phytonadione; Rifamycin Derivatives; Ritonavir; St Johns Wort; Sucralfate; Telaprevir; Teriflunomide; TraZODone

Ethanol/Nutrition/Herb Interactions
Ethanol: Acute ethanol ingestion (binge drinking) decreases the metabolism of warfarin and increases PT/INR. Chronic daily ethanol use increases the metabolism of warfarin and decreases PT/INR. Management: Avoid ethanol.

Food: The anticoagulant effects of warfarin may be decreased if taken with foods rich in vitamin K. Vitamin E may increase warfarin effect. Cranberry juice may increase warfarin effect. Management: Maintain a consistent diet; consult prescriber before making changes in diet. Take warfarin at the same time each day.

Herb/Nutraceutical: Some herbal medications (eg, St John's wort) may decrease warfarin levels and effects; many others can add additional antiplatelet activity to warfarin therapy. Management: Avoid ginseng (American), coenzyme Q_{10}, and St John's wort. Avoid cranberry, fenugreek, ginkgo biloba, glucosamine, alfalfa, anise, bilberry, bladderwrack, bromelain, cat's claw, celery, chamomile, coleus, cordyceps, dong quai, evening primrose oil, fenugreek, feverfew, garlic, ginger, ginkgo biloba, ginseng (Panax), ginseng (Siberian), grapeseed, green tea, guggul, horse chestnut seed, horseradish, licorice, omega-3-acids, prickly ash, red clover, reishi, SAMe (s-adenosylmethionine), sweet clover, turmeric, and white willow.

Dietary Considerations Foods high in vitamin K (eg, beef liver, pork liver, green tea, and leafy green vegetables) inhibit anticoagulant effect. Do not change dietary habits once stabilized on warfarin therapy. A balanced diet with a consistent intake of vitamin K is essential. Avoid large amounts of alfalfa, asparagus, broccoli, Brussels sprouts, cabbage, cauliflower, green teas, kale, lettuce, spinach, turnip greens, and watercress; decreased efficacy of warfarin. It is recommended that the diet contain a CONSISTENT vitamin K content of 70-140 mcg/day. Check with healthcare provider before changing diet.

Pharmacodynamics/Kinetics
Onset of Action Anticoagulation: Oral: 24-72 hours; Peak effect: Full therapeutic effect: 5-7 days; INR may increase in 36-72 hours

Duration of Action 2-5 days

Half-life Elimination 20-60 hours; Mean: 40 hours; highly variable among individuals

Time to Peak Oral: ~4 hours

Pregnancy Risk Factor D (women with mechanical heart valves)/X (other indications)

Pregnancy Considerations Warfarin crosses the placenta; concentrations in the fetal plasma are similar to maternal values. Teratogenic effects have been reported following first trimester exposure and may include coumarin embryopathy (nasal hypoplasia and/or stippled epiphyses; limb hypoplasia may also be present). Adverse CNS events to the fetus have also been observed following exposure during any trimester and may include CNS abnormalities (including ventral midline dysplasia, dorsal midline dysplasia). Spontaneous abortion, fetal hemorrhage, and fetal death may also occur. Use is contraindicated during pregnancy (or in women of reproductive potential) except in women with mechanical heart valves who are at high risk for thromboembolism; use is also contraindicated in women with threatened abortion, eclampsia, or preeclampsia. Frequent pregnancy tests are recommended for women who are planning to become pregnant and adjusted-dose heparin or low molecular weight heparin (LMWH) should be substituted as soon as pregnancy is confirmed or adjusted-dose heparin or LMWH should be used instead of warfarin prior to conception.

In pregnant women with high-risk mechanical heart valves, the benefits of warfarin therapy should be discussed with the risks of available treatments; when possible avoid warfarin use during the first trimester and close to delivery. Adjusted-dose LMWH or adjusted-dose heparin may be used throughout pregnancy or until week 13 of gestation when therapy can be changed to warfarin. LMWH or heparin should be resumed close to delivery. In women who are at a very high risk for thromboembolism (older generation prothesis in mitral position or history of thromboembolism), warfarin can be used throughout pregnancy and replaced with LMWH or heparin near term; the use of low-dose aspirin is also recommended. Women who require long-term anticoagulation with warfarin and who are considering pregnancy, LMWH substitution should be done prior to conception when possible. When choosing therapy, fetal outcomes (ie, pregnancy loss, malformations), maternal outcomes (ie, VTE, hemorrhage), burden of therapy, and maternal preference should be considered (Bates, 2012).

Lactation Does not enter breast milk/use caution (AAP rates "compatible"; AAP 2001 update pending)

Breast-Feeding Considerations Breast-feeding women may be treated with warfarin. Based on available data, warfarin does not pass into breast milk. Women who are breast-feeding should be carefully monitored to avoid excessive anticoagulation. According to the American College of Chest Physicians (ACCP), warfarin may be used in lactating women who wish to breast-feed their infants (Bates, 2012). Monitor nursing infants for bruising or bleeding (per manufacturer).

Dosage Forms

Injection, powder for reconstitution:
Coumadin®: 5 mg
Tablet, oral: 1 mg, 2 mg, 2.5 mg, 3 mg, 4 mg, 5 mg, 6 mg, 7.5 mg, 10 mg
Coumadin®: 1 mg, 2 mg, 2.5 mg, 3 mg, 4 mg, 5 mg, 6 mg, 7.5 mg, 10 mg
Jantoven®: 1 mg, 2 mg, 2.5 mg, 3 mg, 4 mg, 5 mg, 6 mg, 7.5 mg, 10 mg

References

Baillargeon J, Holmes HM, Lin YL, et al, "Concurrent Use of Warfarin and Antibiotics and the Risk of Bleeding in Older Adults," Am J Med, 2012, 125(2):183-9.
Jeske AH, Suchko GD, ADA Council on Scientific Affairs and Division of Science, et al, "Lack of a Scientific Basis for Routine Discontinuation of Oral Anticoagulation Therapy Before Dental Treatment," J Am Dent Assoc, 2003, 134(11):1492-7.
Karsli ED, Erdogan Ö, Esen E, et al, "Comparison of the Effects of Warfarin and Heparin on Bleeding Caused by Dental Extraction: A Clinical Study," J Oral Maxillofac Surg, 2011, 69(10):2500-7.
Little JW, Miller CS, Henry RG, et al, "Antithrombotic Agents: Implications in Dentistry," Oral Surg Oral Med Oral Pathol Oral Radiol Endod, 2002, 93(5):544-51.
Scully C and Wolff A, "Oral Surgery in Patients on Anticoagulant Therapy," Oral Surg Oral Med Oral Pathol Oral Radiol Endod, 2002, 94(1):57-64.

Wheat Dextrin (weet DEKS trin)

Brand Names: U.S. Benefiber® Plus Calcium [OTC]; Benefiber® [OTC]
Pharmacologic Category Fiber Supplement; Laxative, Bulk-Producing
Use OTC labeling: Dietary fiber supplement
Unlabeled Use Treatment of constipation; aid to enhance LDL lowering to reduce the risk of coronary heart disease
Local Anesthetic/Vasoconstrictor Precautions No information available to require special precautions
Effects on Dental Treatment No significant effects or complications reported

Effects on Bleeding No information available to require special precautions
Adverse Effects Frequency not defined: Gastrointestinal: Bloating, flatulence, GI discomfort
General Dosage Range Oral: *Children and Adults:* Dosage varies greatly depending on product
Mechanism of Action Wheat dextrin is a soluble fiber. It absorbs water in the intestine to form a viscous liquid which promotes peristalsis and reduces transit time.

Zafirlukast (za FIR loo kast)

Related Information
Respiratory Diseases *on page 1514*
Brand Names: U.S. Accolate®
Brand Names: Canada Accolate®
Generic Availability (U.S.) Yes
Pharmacologic Category Leukotriene-Receptor Antagonist
Use Prophylaxis and chronic treatment of asthma
Local Anesthetic/Vasoconstrictor Precautions No information available to require special precautions
Effects on Dental Treatment No significant effects or complications reported
Effects on Bleeding No information available to require special precautions
Adverse Effects Incidence reported in children ≥12 years and adults unless otherwise specified.
>10%: Central nervous system: Headache (13%; children 5-11 years: 5%)
1% to 10%:
Central nervous system: Dizziness (2%), pain (2%), fever (2%)
Gastrointestinal: Nausea (3%), diarrhea (3%), abdominal pain (2%; children 5-11 years: 3%), vomiting (2%), dyspepsia (1%)
Hepatic: ALT increased (2%)
Neuromuscular & skeletal: Back pain (2%), myalgia (2%), weakness (2%)
Miscellaneous: Infection (4%)
Dosage Oral:
U.S. labeling:
Children 5-11 years: 10 mg twice daily
Children ≥12 years and Adults: 20 mg twice daily
Canadian labeling: Children ≥12 years and Adults: 20 mg twice daily
Elderly: Refer to adult dosing.

Dosage adjustment in renal impairment: No dosage adjustment necessary.
Dosage adjustment in hepatic impairment: Use is contraindicated.
Mechanism of Action Zafirlukast is a selectively and competitive leukotriene-receptor antagonist (LTRA) of leukotriene D4 and E4 (LTD4 and LTE4), components of slow-reacting substance of anaphylaxis (SRSA). Cysteinyl leukotriene production and receptor occupation have been correlated with the pathophysiology of asthma, including airway edema, smooth muscle constriction, and altered cellular activity associated with the inflammatory process, which contribute to the signs and symptoms of asthma.
Contraindications Hypersensitivity to zafirlukast or any component of the formulation; hepatic impairment (including hepatic cirrhosis)

Canadian labeling: Additional contraindications (not in U.S. labeling): Patients in whom zafirlukast was discontinued due to treatment related hepatotoxicity

Warnings/Precautions Zafirlukast is not approved for use in the reversal of bronchospasm in acute asthma attacks, including status asthmaticus. Therapy with zafirlukast can be continued during acute exacerbations of asthma.

Hepatic adverse events (including hepatitis, hyperbilirubinemia, and hepatic failure) have been reported; female patients may be at greater risk. Periodic testing of liver function may be considered (early detection coupled with therapy discontinuation is generally believed to improve the likelihood of recovery). Advise patients to be alert for and to immediately report symptoms (eg, anorexia, right upper quadrant abdominal pain, nausea). If hepatic dysfunction is suspected (due to clinical signs/symptoms), discontinue use immediately and measure liver function tests (particularly ALT); resolution observed in most but not all cases upon discontinuation of therapy. Do not resume or restart if hepatic function studies indicate dysfunction. Use in patients with hepatic impairment (including hepatic cirrhosis) is contraindicated. Postmarketing reports of behavioral changes (ie, depression, insomnia) have been noted. Instruct patients to report neuropsychiatric symptoms/events during therapy.

Monitor INR closely with concomitant warfarin use. Rare cases of eosinophilic vasculitis (Churg-Strauss) have been reported in patients receiving zafirlukast (usually, but not always, associated with reduction in concurrent steroid dosage). No causal relationship established. Monitor for eosinophilic vasculitis, rash, pulmonary symptoms, cardiac symptoms, or neuropathy.

Clearance is decreased in elderly patients; C_{max} and AUC are increased approximately two- to threefold in adults ≥65 years compared to younger adults; however, no dosage adjustments are recommended in this age group. An increased proportion of zafirlukast patients >55 years of age reported infections as compared to placebo-treated patients. These infections were mostly mild or moderate in intensity and predominantly affected the respiratory tract. Infections occurred equally in both sexes, were dose-proportional to total milligrams of zafirlukast exposure, and were associated with coadministration of inhaled corticosteroids.

Drug Interactions

Metabolism/Transport Effects Substrate of CYP2C9 (major); **Note:** Assignment of Major/Minor substrate status based on clinically relevant drug interaction potential; **Inhibits** CYP1A2 (weak), CYP2C19 (weak), CYP2C8 (weak), CYP2C9 (moderate), CYP2D6 (weak), CYP3A4 (weak)

Avoid Concomitant Use
Avoid concomitant use of Zafirlukast with any of the following: Pimozide

Increased Effect/Toxicity
Zafirlukast may increase the levels/effects of: ARIPiprazole; Carvedilol; CYP2C9 Substrates; Lomitapide; Pimozide; Theophylline Derivatives; Vitamin K Antagonists

The levels/effects of Zafirlukast may be increased by: CYP2C9 Inhibitors (Moderate); CYP2C9 Inhibitors (Strong); Mifepristone

Decreased Effect
The levels/effects of Zafirlukast may be decreased by: CYP2C9 Inducers (Strong); Erythromycin (Systemic); Peginterferon Alfa-2b; Theophylline Derivatives

Ethanol/Nutrition/Herb Interactions Food: Food decreases bioavailability of zafirlukast by 40%. Management: Take on an empty stomach 1 hour before or 2 hours after meals.

Dietary Considerations Should be taken on an empty stomach (1 hour before or 2 hours after meals).

Pharmacodynamics/Kinetics
Half-life Elimination ~10 hours
Time to Peak Serum: 3 hours

Pregnancy Risk Factor B

Pregnancy Considerations Teratogenic effects have not been observed in animal reproduction studies. Based on available information, zafirlukast may be considered for use in women who had a favorable response prior to becoming pregnant; however, it is not a preferred option in new patients (NAEPP, 2004).

Lactation Enters breast milk/not recommended

Breast-Feeding Considerations Zafirlukast is excreted into breast milk; breast-feeding is not recommended by the manufacturer.

Dosage Forms
Tablet, oral: 10 mg, 20 mg
Accolate®: 10 mg, 20 mg

Zaleplon (ZAL e plon)

Brand Names: U.S. Sonata®
Generic Availability (U.S.) Yes
Pharmacologic Category Hypnotic, Miscellaneous
Use Short-term (7-10 days) treatment of insomnia (has been demonstrated to be effective for up to 5 weeks in controlled trial)

Local Anesthetic/Vasoconstrictor Precautions No information available to require special precautions

Effects on Dental Treatment Key adverse event(s) related to dental treatment: Xerostomia (normal salivary flow resumes upon discontinuation).

Effects on Bleeding No information available to require special precautions

Adverse Effects
>10%: Central nervous system: Headache (30% to 42%)
1% to 10%:
Cardiovascular: Chest pain (≥1%), peripheral edema (≤1%)
Central nervous system: Dizziness (7% to 9%), somnolence (5% to 6%), amnesia (2% to 4%), depersonalization (<1% to 2%), hypoesthesia (<1% to 2%), malaise (<1% to 2%), abnormal thinking (≥1%), anxiety (≥1%), depression (≥1%), fever (≥1%), migraine (≥1%), nervousness (≥1%), confusion (≤1%), hallucination (≤1%), vertigo (≤1%)
Dermatologic: Pruritus (≥1%), rash (≥1%), photosensitivity reaction (≤1%)
Endocrine & metabolic: Dysmenorrhea (3% to 4%)
Gastrointestinal: Nausea (6% to 8%), abdominal pain (6%), anorexia (<1% to 2%), constipation (≥1%), dyspepsia (≥1%), taste perversion (≥1%), xerostomia (≥1%), colitis (up to 1%)
Neuromuscular & skeletal: Weakness (5% to 7%), paresthesia (3%), tremor (2%), arthralgia (≥1%), arthritis (≥1%), back pain (≥1%), myalgia (≥1%), hypertonia (1%)
Ocular: Eye pain (3% to 4%), abnormal vision (<1% to 2%), conjunctivitis (≥1%)
Otic: Hyperacusis (1% to 2%), ear pain (≤1%)
Respiratory: Bronchitis (≥1%), epistaxis (≤1%)
Miscellaneous: Parosmia (<1% to 2%)

Dosage Oral:

Adults: 10 mg at bedtime (range: 5-20 mg); has been used for up to 5 weeks of treatment in controlled trial setting

Elderly: 5 mg at bedtime; maximum: 10 mg/day

Dosage adjustment in renal impairment: No adjustment for mild-to-moderate renal impairment; use in severe renal impairment has not been adequately studied

Dosage adjustment in hepatic impairment: Mild-to-moderate impairment: 5 mg; not recommended for use in patients with severe hepatic impairment

Mechanism of Action Zaleplon is unrelated to benzodiazepines, barbiturates, or other hypnotics. However, it interacts with the benzodiazepine GABA receptor complex. Nonclinical studies have shown that it binds selectively to the brain omega-1 receptor situated on the alpha subunit of the GABA-A receptor complex.

Contraindications Hypersensitivity to zaleplon or any component of the formulation

Warnings/Precautions Symptomatic treatment of insomnia should be initiated only after careful evaluation of potential causes of sleep disturbance. Failure of sleep disturbance to resolve after 7-10 days may indicate psychiatric and/or medical illness.

Use with caution in patients with depression, particularly if suicidal risk may be present. Use with caution in patients with a history of drug dependence. Abrupt discontinuance may lead to withdrawal symptoms. Hypnotics/sedatives have been associated with abnormal thinking and behavior changes including decreased inhibition, aggression, bizarre behavior, agitation, hallucinations, and depersonalization. These changes may occur unpredictably and may indicate previously unrecognized psychiatric disorders; evaluate appropriately. May impair physical and mental capabilities. Patients must be cautioned about performing tasks which require mental alertness (operating machinery or driving). Use with caution in patients receiving other CNS depressants or psychoactive medications. Effects with other sedative drugs or ethanol may be potentiated. Postmarketing studies have indicated that the use of hypnotic/sedative agents for sleep has been associated with hypersensitivity reactions including anaphylaxis as well as angioedema. An increased risk for hazardous sleep-related activities such as sleep-driving, cooking and eating food, and making phone calls while asleep have been noted; amnesia may also occur. Evaluation is recommended in patients who report any sleep-related episodes.

Avoid chronic use (>90 days) in older adults; adverse events, including delirium, falls, fractures, has been observed with nonbenzodiazepine hypnotic use in the elderly similar to events observed with benzodiazepines. Data suggests improvements in sleep duration and latency are minimal (Beers Criteria).

Use with caution in the elderly, those with compromised respiratory function, or hepatic impairment (dosage adjustment recommended in mild-to-moderate hepatic impairment; use is not recommended in patients with severe impairment). Because of the rapid onset of action, zaleplon should be administered immediately prior to bedtime or after the patient has gone to bed and is having difficulty falling asleep. Capsules contain tartrazine (FDC yellow #5); avoid in patients with sensitivity (caution in patients with asthma).

Drug Interactions

Metabolism/Transport Effects Substrate of CYP3A4 (minor); **Note:** Assignment of Major/Minor substrate status based on clinically relevant drug interaction potential

Avoid Concomitant Use

Avoid concomitant use of Zaleplon with any of the following: Azelastine (Nasal); Paraldehyde; Sodium Oxybate

Increased Effect/Toxicity

Zaleplon may increase the levels/effects of: Alcohol (Ethyl); Azelastine (Nasal); Buprenorphine; CNS Depressants; Methotrimeprazine; Metyrosine; Mirtazapine; Paraldehyde; Pramipexole; ROPINIRole; Rotigotine; Selective Serotonin Reuptake Inhibitors; Sodium Oxybate; Zolpidem

The levels/effects of Zaleplon may be increased by: Cimetidine; Droperidol; HydrOXYzine; Magnesium Sulfate; Methotrimeprazine; Perampanel

Decreased Effect

The levels/effects of Zaleplon may be decreased by: Flumazenil; Rifamycin Derivatives

Ethanol/Nutrition/Herb Interactions

Ethanol: Ethanol may increase CNS depression. Management: Avoid or limit use of ethanol and monitor for increased effects.

Food: High-fat meals prolong absorption; delay T_{max} by 2 hours, and reduce C_{max} by 35%. Management: Avoid taking after a high-fat meal.

Herb/Nutraceutical: St John's wort may decrease zaleplon levels. Some herbal medications may increase CNS depression. Management: Avoid St John's wort, valerian, kava kava, and gotu kola.

Dietary Considerations Avoid taking with or after a heavy, high-fat meal; reduces absorption.

Pharmacodynamics/Kinetics

Onset of Action Rapid

Half-life Elimination 1 hour

Time to Peak Serum: 1 hour

Pregnancy Risk Factor C

Pregnancy Considerations Teratogenic effects were not observed in animal reproduction studies. Adverse effects, including stillbirth, postnatal mortality, and decreased growth and physical development, were observed near the end of gestation. A small study of pregnant women did not show an increased risk of teratogenic effects when used early in pregnancy (Wiker, 2011). Use during pregnancy is not recommended by the manufacturer.

Lactation Enters breast milk/not recommended

Breast-Feeding Considerations Zaleplon is excreted in human milk with the highest concentration ~1 hour after administration; therefore, the manufacturer does not recommended use while breast-feeding.

Controlled Substance C-IV

Dosage Forms

Capsule, oral: 5 mg, 10 mg

Sonata®: 5 mg, 10 mg

Zanamivir (za NA mi veer)

Related Information

Systemic Viral Diseases on page 1537

Brand Names: U.S. Relenza®

Brand Names: Canada Relenza®

Pharmacologic Category Antiviral Agent; Neuraminidase Inhibitor

Use Treatment of uncomplicated acute illness due to influenza virus A and B in patients who have been symptomatic for no more than 2 days; prophylaxis against influenza virus A and B

The Advisory Committee on Immunization Practices (ACIP) recommends that **treatment** be considered for the following:
• Persons with severe, complicated or progressive illness
• Hospitalized persons
• Persons at higher risk for influenza complications:
  - Children <2 years of age (highest risk in children <6 months of age)
  - Adults ≥65 years of age
  - Persons with chronic disorders of the pulmonary (including asthma) or cardiovascular systems (except hypertension)
  - Persons with chronic metabolic diseases (including diabetes mellitus), hepatic disease, renal dysfunction, hematologic disorders (including sickle cell disease), or immunosuppression (including immunosuppression caused by medications or HIV)
  - Persons with neurologic/neuromuscular conditions (including conditions such as spinal cord injuries, seizure disorders, cerebral palsy, stroke, mental retardation, moderate to severe developmental delay, or muscular dystrophy) which may compromise respiratory function, the handling of respiratory secretions, or that can increase the risk of aspiration
  - Pregnant or postpartum women (≤2 weeks after delivery)
  - Persons <19 years of age on long-term aspirin therapy
  - American Indians and Alaskan Natives
  - Persons who are morbidly obese (BMI ≥40)
  - Residents of nursing homes or other chronic care facilities
• Use may also be considered for previously healthy, nonhigh-risk outpatients with confirmed or suspected influenza based on clinical judgment when treatment can be started within 48 hours of illness onset.

The ACIP recommends that **prophylaxis** be considered for the following:
• Postexposure prophylaxis may be considered for family or close contacts of suspected or confirmed cases, who are at higher risk of influenza complications, and who have not been vaccinated against the circulating strain at the time of the exposure.
• Postexposure prophylaxis may be considered for unvaccinated healthcare workers who had occupational exposure without protective equipment.
• Pre-exposure prophylaxis should only be used for persons at very high risk of influenza complications who cannot be otherwise protected at times of high risk for exposure.
• Prophylaxis should also be administered to all eligible residents of institutions that house patients at high risk when needed to control outbreaks.

Local Anesthetic/Vasoconstrictor Precautions No information available to require special precautions

Effects on Dental Treatment No significant effects or complications reported

Effects on Bleeding No information available to require special precautions

Adverse Effects Most adverse reactions occurred at a frequency which was less than or equal to the control (lactose vehicle).

>10%:
Central nervous system: Headache (prophylaxis 13% to 24%; treatment 2%)
Gastrointestinal: Throat/tonsil discomfort/pain (prophylaxis 8% to 19%)
Respiratory: Nasal signs and symptoms (prophylaxis 12% to 20%; treatment 2%), cough (prophylaxis 7% to 17%; treatment ≤2%)
Miscellaneous: Viral infection (prophylaxis 3% to 13%)
1% to 10%:
Central nervous system: Fever/chills (prophylaxis 5% to 9%; treatment <1.5%), fatigue (prophylaxis 5% to 8%; treatment <1.5%), malaise (prophylaxis 5% to 8%; treatment <1.5%), dizziness (treatment 1% to 2%)
Dermatologic: Urticaria (treatment <1.5%)
Gastrointestinal: Anorexia/appetite decreased (prophylaxis 2% to 4%), appetite increased (prophylaxis 2% to 4%), nausea (prophylaxis 1% to 2%; treatment ≤3%), diarrhea (prophylaxis 2%; treatment 2% to 3%), vomiting (prophylaxis 1% to 2%; treatment 1% to 2%), abdominal pain (treatment <1.5%)
Neuromuscular & skeletal: Muscle pain (prophylaxis 3% to 8%), musculoskeletal pain (prophylaxis 6%), arthralgia/articular rheumatism (prophylaxis 2%), arthralgia (treatment <1.5%), myalgia (treatment <1.5%)
Respiratory: Infection (ear/nose/throat; prophylaxis 2%; treatment 1% to 5%), sinusitis (treatment 3%), bronchitis (treatment 2%), nasal inflammation (prophylaxis 1%)

General Dosage Range Oral inhalation:
Children ≥5 years: Prophylaxis: 10 mg once daily
Children ≥7 years: Treatment: 10 mg twice daily
Adolescents and Adults: Prophylaxis: 10 mg once to twice daily; Treatment: 10 mg twice daily

Mechanism of Action Zanamivir inhibits influenza virus neuraminidase enzymes, potentially altering virus particle aggregation and release.

Pharmacodynamics/Kinetics

Half-life Elimination Serum: 2.5-5.1 hours; Mild-to-moderate renal impairment: 4.7 hours; Severe renal impairment: 18.5 hours

Time to Peak 1-2 hours

Pregnancy Risk Factor C

Pregnancy Considerations Adverse events were not observed in animal reproduction studies. Influenza infection may be more severe in pregnant women. Untreated influenza infection is associated with an increased risk of adverse events to the fetus and an increased risk of complications or death to the mother. Oseltamivir and zanamivir are currently recommended for the treatment or prophylaxis of influenza in pregnant women and women up to 2 weeks postpartum. Oseltamivir and zanamivir are currently recommended as an adjunct to vaccination and should not be used as a substitute for vaccination in pregnant women (consult current CDC guidelines).

Prescribing and Access Restrictions Zanamivir *aqueous solution* intended for nebulization or intravenous (I.V.) administration is **not** currently approved for use. Data on safety and efficacy via these routes of administration are limited. However, limited supplies of zanamivir aqueous solution may be made available through the Zanamivir Compassionate Use Program for qualifying patients for the treatment of serious influenza illness. For information, contact the GlaxoSmithKline Clinical Support Help Desk at 1-866-341-9160 or gskclinicalsupportHD@gsk.com.

1

Ziconotide (zi KOE no tide)

Brand Names: U.S. Prialt®

Pharmacologic Category Analgesic, Nonopioid; Calcium Channel Blocker, N-Type

Use Management of severe chronic pain in patients requiring intrathecal (I.T.) therapy and who are intolerant or refractory to other therapies

Local Anesthetic/Vasoconstrictor Precautions No information available to require special precautions

Effects on Dental Treatment Key adverse event(s) related to dental treatment: Xerostomia (normal salivary flow resumes upon discontinuation) and taste perversion.

Effects on Bleeding No information available to require special precautions

Adverse Effects

>10%:

Central nervous system: Dizziness (46%), confusion (15% to 33%), memory impairment (7% to 22%), somnolence (17%), ataxia (14%), speech disorder (14%), headache (13%), aphasia (12%), hallucination (12%; including auditory and visual)

Gastrointestinal: Nausea (40%), diarrhea (18%), vomiting (16%)

Neuromuscular & skeletal: Creatine kinase increased (40%; ≥3 times ULN: 11%), weakness (18%), gait disturbances (14%)

Ocular: Blurred vision (12%)

2% to 10%:

Cardiovascular: Hypotension, orthostatic hypotension, peripheral edema

Central nervous system: Abnormal thinking (8%), amnesia (8%), anxiety (8%), vertigo (7%), insomnia (6%), fever (5%), paranoid reaction (3%), delirium (2%), hostility (2%), stupor (2%), agitation, attention disturbance, balance impaired, burning sensation, coordination abnormal, depression, disorientation, fatigue, fever, hypoesthesia, irritability, lethargy, mental impairment, mood disorder, nervousness, pain, sedation

Dermatologic: Pruritus (7%)

Gastrointestinal: Anorexia (6%), taste perversion (5%), abdominal pain, appetite decreased, constipation, xerostomia

Genitourinary: Urinary retention (9%), dysuria, urinary hesitance

Neuromuscular & skeletal: Dysarthria (7%), paresthesia (7%), rigors (7%), tremor (7%), muscle spasm (6%), limb pain (5%), areflexia, muscle cramp, muscle weakness, myalgia

Ocular: Nystagmus (8%), diplopia, visual disturbance

Respiratory: Sinusitis (5%)

Miscellaneous: Diaphoresis (5%)

General Dosage Range Dosage adjustment recommended in patients who develop toxicities

I.T.: *Adults:* Initial dose: ≤2.4 mcg/day (0.1 mcg/hour); Maintenance range: 2.4-19.2 mcg/day (0.1-0.8 mcg/hour) (maximum: 19.2 mcg/day [0.8 mcg/hour])

Mechanism of Action Ziconotide selectively binds to N-type voltage-sensitive calcium channels located on the nociceptive afferent nerves of the dorsal horn in the spinal cord. This binding is thought to block N-type calcium channels, leading to a blockade of excitatory neurotransmitter release and reducing sensitivity to painful stimuli.

Pharmacodynamics/Kinetics

Half-life Elimination I.V.: 1-1.6 hours (plasma); I.T.: 2.9-6.5 hours (CSF)

Pregnancy Risk Factor C

Pregnancy Considerations Teratogenic effects were not observed in animal studies, but increased postimplantation pup loss was reported. Maternal toxicity was also noted. There are no adequate and well-controlled studies in pregnant women.

Zidovudine (zye DOE vyoo deen)

Related Information

HIV Infection and AIDS *on page 1520*

Brand Names: U.S. Retrovir®

Brand Names: Canada Apo-Zidovudine®; AZT™; Novo-AZT; Retrovir®; Retrovir® (AZT™)

Pharmacologic Category Antiretroviral Agent, Reverse Transcriptase Inhibitor (Nucleoside)

Use Treatment of HIV infection in combination with at least two other antiretroviral agents; prevention of maternal/fetal HIV transmission

Unlabeled Use Postexposure prophylaxis for HIV exposure as part of a multidrug regimen

Local Anesthetic/Vasoconstrictor Precautions No information available to require special precautions

Effects on Dental Treatment Key adverse event(s) related to dental treatment: Taste perversion, oral mucosa pigmentation, dysphagia, and mouth ulcer.

Effects on Bleeding No information available to require special precautions relative to hemostasis.

Adverse Effects Note: Percentages noted with adults unless otherwise stated.

>10%:

Central nervous system: Headache (63%), malaise (53%), fever (children 25%)

Dermatologic: Rash (children 12%)

Gastrointestinal: Nausea (adults 51%; children 8%), anorexia (20%), vomiting (adults 17%; children 8%)

Hematologic: Macrocytosis (children >50%), anemia (neonates 22%; children 4%; adults 1%; onset 2-4 weeks)

Hepatic: Hepatomegaly (children 11%)

Respiratory: Cough (children 15%)

1% to 10%:

Cardiovascular: ECG abnormality (children <6%), edema (children <6%), heart failure (children <6%), left ventricular dilation (children <6%)

Central nervous system: Irritability (children <6%), nervousness (children <6%), chills (≥5%), fatigue (≥5%), insomnia (≥5%)

Gastrointestinal: Diarrhea (children 8%), constipation (6%), weight loss (children <6%), abdominal cramps (≥5%), abdominal pain (≥5%), dyspepsia (≥5%)

Genitourinary: Hematuria (children <6%)

Hematologic: Neutropenia (children 8%), granulocytopenia (2%; onset 6-8 weeks), thrombocytopenia (children 1%)

Hepatic: Transaminases increased (1% to 3%)

Neuromuscular & skeletal: Weakness (9%), arthralgia (≥5%), musculoskeletal pain (≥5%), myalgia (≥5%), neuropathy (≥5%)

Otic: Discharge/erythema/pain/swelling (7%)

General Dosage Range Dosage adjustment recommended in patients with renal impairment or who develop toxicities

I.V.:

Infants <30 weeks gestation at birth: 1.5 mg/kg/dose every 12 hours; at 4 weeks of age advance to 2.3 mg/kg/dose every 12 hours

Infants ≥30 weeks and <35 weeks gestation at birth: 1.5 mg/kg/dose every 12 hours; at 15 days of age, advance to 2.3 mg/kg/dose every 12 hours
Infants ≥35 weeks: 3 mg/kg/dose every 12 hour
Children 6 weeks to <12 years: 120 mg/m²/dose every 6 hours **or** 20 mg/m²/hour as a continuous infusion
Children ≥12 years and Adults: 1 mg/kg/dose every 4 hours around-the-clock **or** 2 mg/kg bolus followed by 1 mg/kg/hour continuous infusion during labor and delivery

Oral:

Infants <30 weeks gestation at birth: 2 mg/kg/dose every 12 hours; at 4 weeks of age advance to 3 mg/kg/dose every 12 hours
Infants ≥30 weeks and <35 weeks gestation at birth: 2 mg/kg/dose every 12 hours; at 15 days of age, advance to 3 mg/kg/dose every 12 hours
Infants ≥35 weeks: 4 mg/kg/dose twice daily
Children 4 weeks to <18 years: 240 mg/m² every 12 hours (maximum: 300 mg every 12 hours) **or** 160 mg/m²/dose every 8 hours (maximum: 200 mg every 8 hours)

4 to <9 kg: 12 mg/kg/dose twice daily **or** 8 mg/kg/dose 3 times/day
≥9 to <30 kg: 9 mg/kg/dose twice daily **or** 6 mg/kg/dose 3 times/day
≥30 kg and Adults: 300 mg twice daily **or** 200 mg 3 times/day

Mechanism of Action Zidovudine is a thymidine analog which interferes with the HIV viral RNA-dependent DNA polymerase resulting in inhibition of viral replication; nucleoside reverse transcriptase inhibitor

Pharmacodynamics/Kinetics

Half-life Elimination Terminal: 0.5-3 hours
Time to Peak Serum: 30-90 minutes

Pregnancy Risk Factor C

Pregnancy Considerations Adverse events have been observed in some animal reproduction studies. Zidovudine crosses the placenta and the placenta also metabolizes zidovudine to the active metabolite. No increased risk of overall birth defects has been observed following first trimester exposure according to data collected by the antiretroviral pregnancy registry. The pharmacokinetics of zidovudine are not significantly altered in pregnancy and dosing adjustment is not needed. The DHHS Perinatal HIV Guidelines consider zidovudine the preferred NRTI for use in combination regimens during pregnancy. The use of zidovudine has been shown to reduce the maternal-fetal transmission of HIV by ~70%. Zidovudine should be administered I.V. near delivery regardless of antepartum regimen or mode of delivery in women with HIV RNA >400 copies/mL or unknown HIV RNA status. In HIV-infected mothers not previously on antiretroviral therapy, and who do not need therapy for their own health, treatment may be delayed until after the first trimester; however, earlier initiation of therapy may be more effective in reducing perinatal transmission.

Cases of lactic acidosis/hepatic steatosis syndrome related to mitochondrial toxicity have been reported in pregnant women with prolonged use of nucleoside analogues. It is not known if pregnancy itself potentiates this known side effect; however, women may be at increased risk of lactic acidosis and liver damage. In addition, these adverse events are similar to other rare but life-threatening syndromes which occur during pregnancy (eg HELLP syndrome). Hepatic enzymes and electrolytes should be monitored in women receiving nucleoside analogues and clinicians should watch for early signs of the syndrome. In addition, mitochondrial dysfunction may develop in infants following *in utero* exposure.

Regardless of CD4 count or HIV RNA copy number, all HIV-infected pregnant women should receive a combination antepartum antiretroviral (ARV) drug regimen; this includes women who require therapy for their own health, as well as women who do not yet require therapy for their own health. ARV therapy should be started as soon as possible if required for the woman's health. health. Although earlier initiation may be more effective in reducing the perinatal transmission of HIV), also consider maternal conditions (eg, nausea and vomiting) and the potential risks of first trimester fetal exposure for specific agents. Plasma HIV RNA levels should be assessed at ~34-36 weeks gestation in order to help determine mode of delivery. If ARV therapy must be interrupted for <24 hours during the peripartum period, stop then restart all medications simultaneously in order to decrease the chance of developing resistance. Long-term follow-up is recommended for all infants exposed to ARV medications.

Healthcare providers are encouraged to enroll pregnant women exposed to antiretroviral medications in the Antiretroviral Pregnancy Registry (1-800-258-4263 or www.APRegistry.com). Healthcare providers caring for HIV-infected women and their infants may contact the National Perinatal HIV Hotline (888-448-8765) for clinical consultation (DHHS [perinatal], 2012).

Zileuton (zye LOO ton)

Related Information
Respiratory Diseases *on page 1514*
Brand Names: U.S. Zyflo CR®; Zyflo®
Pharmacologic Category 5-Lipoxygenase Inhibitor
Use Prophylaxis and chronic treatment of asthma
Local Anesthetic/Vasoconstrictor Precautions No information available to require special precautions
Effects on Dental Treatment No significant effects or complications reported
Effects on Bleeding No information available to require special precautions

Adverse Effects
>10%: Central nervous system: Headache (23% to 25%)
1% to 10%:
Cardiovascular: Chest pain
Central nervous system: Pain (8%), dizziness, fever, insomnia, malaise, nervousness, somnolence
Dermatologic: Pruritus, rash
Gastrointestinal: Dyspepsia (8%), diarrhea (5%), nausea (5% to 6%), abdominal pain (5%), constipation, flatulence, vomiting
Genitourinary: Urinary tract infection, vaginitis
Hematologic: Leukopenia (1% to 3%)
Hepatic: ALT increased (≥3 x ULN: 2% to 5%), hepatotoxicity
Neuromuscular & skeletal: Myalgia (7%), weakness (4%), arthralgia, hypertonia, neck pain/rigidity
Ocular: Conjunctivitis
Respiratory: Upper respiratory tract infection (9%), sinusitis (7%), pharyngolaryngeal pain (5%)
Miscellaneous: Hypersensitivity reactions, lymphadenopathy

General Dosage Range Oral:
Extended release: *Children ≥12 years and Adults:* 1200 mg twice daily
Immediate release: *Children ≥12 years and Adults:* 600 mg 4 times/day
Mechanism of Action Specific 5-lipoxygenase inhibitor which inhibits leukotriene formation. Leukotrienes augment neutrophil and eosinophil migration, neutrophil and monocyte aggregation, leukocyte adhesion, increased capillary permeability, and smooth muscle contraction (which contribute to inflammation, edema, mucous secretion, and bronchoconstriction in the airway of the asthmatic.)
Pharmacodynamics/Kinetics
Half-life Elimination ~3 hours
Time to Peak Immediate release: 1.7 hours
Pregnancy Risk Factor C
Pregnancy Considerations Adverse events were observed in animal reproduction studies. If a leukotriene modifier is needed during pregnancy, other agents are preferred (ACOG, 2008).

Zinc Acetate (zink AS e tate)

Brand Names: U.S. Galzin®
Pharmacologic Category Trace Element
Use Maintenance treatment of Wilson's disease following initial chelation therapy
Local Anesthetic/Vasoconstrictor Precautions No information available to require special precautions
Effects on Dental Treatment No significant effects or complications reported
Effects on Bleeding No information available to require special precautions
Adverse Effects Frequency not defined.
Central nervous system: Neurologic deterioration (uncommon)
Endocrine & metabolic: Amylase increased, lipase increased
Gastrointestinal: Gastric irritation
Hepatic: Alkaline phosphatase increased, hepatic function decreased (rare)
General Dosage Range Oral:
Children ≥10 years and Adults (pregnant females): 75-150 mg/day in 3 divided doses
Adults (males and nonpregnant females): 150 mg/day in 3 divided doses
Mechanism of Action Zinc induces production of the copper binding protein metallothionein in enterocytes. Copper binding within enterocytes results in an impairment of the intestinal absorption of dietary copper and reabsorption of endogenously secreted copper in saliva, bile, gastric acid. Following enterocyte desquamation, bound copper is eliminated in the feces.
Pharmacodynamics/Kinetics
Onset of Action Slow
Half-life Elimination Inhibition of copper uptake: ~11 days following cessation of therapy
Pregnancy Risk Factor A
Pregnancy Considerations The risk of fetal harm appears remote with use of zinc acetate during pregnancy. An increased risk of fetal abnormalities has not been observed in pregnant women receiving zinc acetate (regardless of trimester).

Zinc Chloride (zink KLOR ide)

Pharmacologic Category Trace Element

Use Cofactor for replacement therapy to different enzymes; helps maintain normal growth rates, normal skin hydration, and senses of taste and smell
Local Anesthetic/Vasoconstrictor Precautions No information available to require special precautions
Effects on Dental Treatment No significant effects or complications reported
Effects on Bleeding No information available to require special precautions
General Dosage Range I.V.:
Premature infants <1500 g up to 3 kg: 300 mcg/kg/day
Infants (full term) and Children ≤5 years: 100 mcg/kg/day to I.V. fluid
Adults: 2-6 mg/day, up to 12.2 mg/L TPN **or** 17.1 mg/kg of stool or ileostomy output
Pregnancy Risk Factor C
Pregnancy Considerations Zinc crosses the placenta and can be measured in the cord blood and placenta. Fetal concentrations are regulated by the placenta (de Moraes, 2011).

Zinc Gelatin (zink JEL ah tin)

Brand Names: U.S. Gelucast®
Pharmacologic Category Topical Skin Product
Use As a protectant and to support varicosities and similar lesions of the lower limbs
Local Anesthetic/Vasoconstrictor Precautions No information available to require special precautions
Effects on Dental Treatment No significant effects or complications reported
Effects on Bleeding No information available to require special precautions
Adverse Effects 1% to 10%: Local: Irritation
General Dosage Range Topical: *Adults:* Apply externally as an occlusive boot

Zinc Oxide (zink OKS ide)

Brand Names: U.S. Ammens® Original Medicated [OTC]; Ammens® Shower Fresh [OTC]; Balmex® [OTC]; Boudreaux's® Butt Paste [OTC]; Critic-Aid Skin Care® [OTC]; Desitin® Creamy [OTC]; Desitin® [OTC]
Brand Names: Canada Zincofax®
Pharmacologic Category Topical Skin Product
Use Protective coating for mild skin irritations and abrasions; soothing and protective ointment to promote healing of chapped skin, diaper rash
Local Anesthetic/Vasoconstrictor Precautions No information available to require special precautions
Effects on Dental Treatment No significant effects or complications reported
Effects on Bleeding No information available to require special precautions
Adverse Effects 1% to 10%: Local: Skin sensitivity, irritation
General Dosage Range Topical: *Children and Adults:* Apply as required to affected areas several times daily
Mechanism of Action Mild astringent with weak antiseptic properties
Pregnancy Considerations Zinc oxide is not expected to be absorbed systemically following topical administration to healthy skin (Newman, 2009). Systemic absorption would be required in order for zinc oxide to cross the placenta and reach the fetus.

Zinc Sulfate (zink SUL fate)

Brand Names: U.S. Orazinc® 110 [OTC]; Orazinc® 220 [OTC]; Zinc 15 [OTC]; Zincate® [DSC]
Brand Names: Canada Anuzinc; Rivasol
Pharmacologic Category Trace Element
Use Zinc supplement (oral and parenteral); may improve wound healing in those who are deficient
Local Anesthetic/Vasoconstrictor Precautions No information available to require special precautions
Effects on Dental Treatment No significant effects or complications reported
Effects on Bleeding No information available to require special precautions
Adverse Effects Frequency not defined.
Central nervous system: Dizziness, headache
Gastrointestinal: Abdominal cramps, diarrhea, nausea, vomiting
General Dosage Range
I.V.:
Premature infants (<1500 g up to 3 kg): 300 mcg/kg/day
Infants (full term) and Children ≤5 years: 100 mcg/kg/day
Adults: 2.5-6 mg/day **or** 12.2 mg/L of TPN **or** 17.1 mg/kg of stool or ileostomy output
Oral: *Children and Adults:* Dosage varies depending on product labeling
Pregnancy Risk Factor C
Pregnancy Considerations Zinc crosses the placenta and can be measured in the cord blood and placenta. Fetal concentrations are regulated by the placenta (de Moraes, 2011).

Ziprasidone (zi PRAS i done)

Related Information
Clinical Risk Related to Drugs Prolonging QT Interval *on page 1510*
Brand Names: U.S. Geodon®
Brand Names: Canada Zeldox®
Pharmacologic Category Antipsychotic Agent, Atypical
Use Treatment of schizophrenia; treatment of acute manic or mixed episodes associated with bipolar disorder with or without psychosis; maintenance treatment of bipolar disorder as an adjunct to lithium or valproate; acute agitation in patients with schizophrenia
Unlabeled Use Tourette's syndrome; psychosis/agitation related to Alzheimer's dementia
Local Anesthetic/Vasoconstrictor Precautions Ziprasidone is one of the drugs confirmed to prolong the QT interval and is accepted as having a risk of causing torsade de pointes. The risk of drug-induced torsade de pointes is extremely low when a single QT interval prolonging drug is prescribed. In terms of epinephrine, it is not known what effect vasoconstrictors in the local anesthetic regimen will have in patients with a known history of congenital prolonged QT interval or in patients taking any medication that prolongs the QT interval. Until more information is obtained, it is suggested that the clinician consult with the physician prior to the use of a vasoconstrictor in suspected patients, and that the vasoconstrictor (epinephrine, mepivacaine and levonordefrin [Carbocaine® 2% with Neo-Cobefrin®]) be used with caution.

Effects on Dental Treatment Key adverse event(s) related to dental treatment: Xerostomia and changes in salivation (normal salivary flow resumes upon discontinuation), orthostatic hypotension, tongue edema, dysphagia, and tooth disorder.
Effects on Bleeding No information available to require special precautions
Adverse Effects Note: Although minor QT$_c$ prolongation (mean: 10 msec at 160 mg/day) may occur more frequently (incidence not specified), clinically-relevant prolongation (>500 msec) was rare (0.06%) and less than placebo (0.23%).

>10%:
Central nervous system: Extrapyramidal symptoms (2% to 31%), somnolence (8% to 31%), headache (3% to 18%), dizziness (3% to 16%)
Gastrointestinal: Nausea (4% to 12%)
1% to 10%:
Cardiovascular: Orthostatic hypotension (5%), chest pain (3%), hypertension (2% to 3%), tachycardia (2%), bradycardia (≤2%), facial edema (1%), vasodilation (≤1%)
Central nervous system: Akathisia (2% to 10%), anxiety (2% to 5%), insomnia (3%), agitation (2%), speech disorder (2%), personality disorder (2%), akinesia (≥1%), amnesia (≥1%), ataxia (≥1%), confusion (≥1%), coordination abnormal (≥1%), delirium (≥1%), dystonia (≥1%), hostility (≥1%), oculogyric crisis (≥1%), vertigo (≥1%), chills (1%), fever (1%), hypothermia (1%), psychosis (1%)
Dermatologic: Rash (4% to 5%), fungal dermatitis (2%), photosensitivity reaction (1%)
Endocrine & metabolic: Dysmenorrhea (2%)
Gastrointestinal: Weight gain (6% to 10%), constipation (2% to 9%), dyspepsia (1% to 8%), diarrhea (3% to 5%), vomiting (3% to 5%), xerostomia (1% to 5%), salivation increased (4%), tongue edema (≤3%), anorexia (2%), abdominal pain (≤2%), dysphagia (≤2%), rectal hemorrhage (≤2%), buccoglossal syndrome (≥1%)
Genitourinary: Priapism (1%)
Local: Injection site pain (7% to 9%)
Neuromuscular & skeletal: Weakness (2% to 6%), hypoesthesia (2%), myalgia (2%), paresthesia (2%), abnormal gait (≥1%), choreoathetosis (≥1%), dysarthria (≥1%), dyskinesia (≥1%), hyper-/hypokinesia (≥1%), hypotonia (≥1%), neuropathy (≥1%), tremor (≥1%), twitching (≥1%), back pain (1%), cogwheel rigidity (1%), hypertonia (1%)
Ocular: Vision abnormal (3% to 6%), diplopia (≥1%)
Respiratory: Infection (8%), rhinitis (1% to 4%), cough (3%), pharyngitis (3%), dyspnea (2%)
Miscellaneous: Diaphoresis (2%), furunculosis (2%), withdrawal syndrome (≥1%), flank pain (1%), flu-like syndrome (1%)
General Dosage Range
I.M.: *Adults:* 10 mg every 2 hours **or** 20 mg every 4 hours (maximum: 40 mg/day)
Oral: *Adults:* Initial: 20-40 mg twice daily; Maintenance: 20-80 mg twice daily (maximum: 200 mg/day)
Mechanism of Action Ziprasidone is a benzylisothiazolylpiperazine antipsychotic. The exact mechanism of action is unknown. However, *in vitro* radioligand studies show that ziprasidone has high affinity for D$_2$, D$_3$, 5-HT$_{2A}$, 5-HT$_{1A}$, 5-HT$_{2C}$, 5-HT$_{1D}$, and alpha$_1$-adrenergic; moderate affinity for histamine H$_1$ receptors; and no appreciable affinity for alpha$_2$-adrenergic receptors, beta-adrenergic, 5-HT$_3$, 5-HT$_4$, cholinergic, mu, sigma, or benzodiazepine receptors. Ziprasidone functions as

an antagonist at the D_2, $5\text{-}HT_{2A}$, and $5\text{-}HT_{1D}$ receptors and as an agonist at the $5\text{-}HT_{1A}$ receptor. Ziprasidone moderately inhibits the reuptake of serotonin and nor-epinephrine.

Pharmacodynamics/Kinetics
Half-life Elimination 2-7 hours
Time to Peak Oral: 6-8 hours; I.M.: ≤60 minutes
Pregnancy Risk Factor C
Pregnancy Considerations Developmental toxicity demonstrated in animals. Antipsychotic use during the third trimester of pregnancy has a risk for abnormal muscle movements (extrapyramidal symptoms [EPS]) and withdrawal symptoms in newborns following delivery. Symptoms in the newborn may include agitation, feeding disorder, hypertonia, hypotonia, respiratory distress, somnolence, and tremor; these effects may be self-limiting or require hospitalization. There are no adequate and well-controlled studies in pregnant women. Use only if potential benefit justifies risk to the fetus. Healthcare providers are encouraged to enroll women 18-45 years of age exposed to ziprasidone during pregnancy in the Atypical Antipsychotics Pregnancy Registry (1-866-961-2388 or http://www.-womensmentalhealth.org/pregnancyregistry).

Dental Comment Ziprasidone is known to prolong the QT interval. The QT interval is measured as the time and distance between the Q point of the QRS complex and the end of the T wave in the ECG tracing. After adjustment for heart rate, the QT interval is defined as prolonged if it is more than 450 msec in men and 460 msec in women. A long QT syndrome was first described in the 1950s and 60s as a congenital syndrome involving QT interval prolongation and syncope and sudden death. Some of the congenital long QT syndromes were characterized by a peculiar electrocardiographic appearance of the QRS complex involving a premature atria beat followed by a pause, then a subsequent sinus beat showing marked QT prolongation and deformity. This type of cardiac arrhythmia was originally termed "torsade de pointes" (translated from the French as "twisting of the points"). Ziprasidone is considered as having a risk of causing torsade de pointes. Since it is not known what effect vasoconstrictors in the local anesthetic regimen will have in patients with a known history of congenital prolonged QT interval or in patients taking any medication that prolongs the QT interval, a medical consult is suggested.

Ziv-Aflibercept (Systemic) (ziv a FLIB er sept)

Brand Names: U.S. Zaltrap®
Pharmacologic Category Antineoplastic Agent; Vascular Endothelial Growth Factor (VEGF) Inhibitor
Use Treatment of metastatic colorectal cancer (in combination with fluorouracil, leucovorin, and irinotecan [FOLFIRI]) in patients who are resistant to or have progressed on an oxaliplatin-based regimen
Local Anesthetic/Vasoconstrictor Precautions Use vasoconstrictor with caution; patients may experience significant hypertension when taking Ziv-Aflibercept (Systemic)
Effects on Dental Treatment Key adverse event(s) related to dental treatment: Stomatitis has been reported in ≤50% of patients
Effects on Bleeding The risk of hemorrhage is increased; GI tract bleeding has been reported
Adverse Effects Note: Reactions reported in combination therapy with fluorouracil, leucovorin, and irinotecan (FOLFIRI).

>10%:
Cardiovascular: Hypertension (41%; grades 3/4: 19%)
Central nervous system: Fatigue (48%), dysphonia (25%), headache (22%)
Dermatologic: Palmar-plantar erythrodysesthesia (11%)
Gastrointestinal: Diarrhea (69%), stomatitis (50%), appetite decreased (32%), weight loss (32%), abdominal pain (27%), upper abdominal pain (11%)
Hematologic: Leukopenia (78%; grades 3/4: 16%), neutropenia (67%; grades 3/4: 37%), thrombocytopenia (48%; grades 3/4: 3%), bleeding (38%; grades 3/4: 3%)
Hepatic: AST increased (62%), ALT increased (50%)
Neuromuscular & skeletal: Weakness (18%)
Renal: Proteinuria (62%; grades 3/4: 8%), creatinine increased (23%)
Respiratory: Epistaxis (28%), dyspnea (12%)
Miscellaneous: Infection (46%)
1% to 10%:
Cardiovascular: Venous thromboembolic events (9%), arterial thromboembolic events (3%; grades 3/4: 2%)
Central nervous system: Reversible posterior encephalopathy syndrome (RPLS) (1%)
Dermatologic: Hyperpigmentation (8%)
Endocrine & metabolic: Dehydration (9%)
Gastrointestinal: Hemorrhoids (6%), proctalgia (5%), rectal hemorrhage (5%), gastrointestinal perforation (1%)
Genitourinary: Urinary tract infection (9%)
Hematologic: Neutropenic fever (grades 3/4: 4%), neutropenic infection/sepsis (grades 3/4: 2%)
Renal: Nephrotic syndrome (1%)
Respiratory: Oropharyngeal pain (8%), rhinorrhea (6%), pulmonary embolism (5%)
Miscellaneous: Antibody formation (3%), fistula formation (2%; grades 3/4: <1%)
General Dosage Range Dosage adjustment recommended in patients who develop toxicities.
I.V.: *Adults:* 4 mg/kg every 2 weeks
Mechanism of Action Also known as VEGF-trap, ziv-aflibercept is a recombinant fusion protein which is comprised of portions of binding domains for vascular endothelial growth factor (VEGF) receptors 1 and 2, attached to the Fc portion of human IgG1. Ziv-aflibercept acts as a decoy receptor for VEGF-A, VEGF-B, and placental growth factor (PIGF) which prevent VEGF receptor binding/activation to their receptors (an action critical to angiogenesis), thus leading to antiangiogenesis and tumor regression.
Pharmacodynamics/Kinetics
Half-life Elimination ~6 days (range: 4-7 days)
Pregnancy Risk Factor C
Pregnancy Considerations Adverse events were observed in animal reproduction studies with doses providing systemic exposure equivalent to ~30% of a human dose. The incidence of fetal malformations increased with increasing doses. Patients (male and female) should use effective contraception during therapy and for at least 3 months following treatment.

Zoledronic Acid (zoe le DRON ik AS id)

Related Information
Rheumatoid Arthritis, Osteoarthritis, and Osteoporosis *on page 1526*
Brand Names: U.S. Reclast®; Zometa®
Brand Names: Canada Aclasta®; Zometa®
Generic Availability (U.S.) Yes

◀ **Pharmacologic Category** Bisphosphonate Derivative
Use

Oncology-related uses: Treatment of hypercalcemia of
malignancy (albumin-corrected serum calcium
>12 mg/dL); treatment of multiple myeloma; treatment
of bone metastases of solid tumors

Nononcology uses: Treatment of Paget's disease of
bone; treatment of osteoporosis in postmenopausal
women (to reduce the incidence of fractures or to
reduce the incidence of new clinical fractures in
patients with low-trauma hip fracture); prevention of
osteoporosis in postmenopausal women, treatment of
osteoporosis in men (to increase bone mass); treatment and prevention of glucocorticoid-induced osteoporosis (in patients initiating or continuing prednisone
≥7.5 mg/day [or equivalent] and expected to remain on
glucocorticoids for at least 12 months)

Unlabeled Use Prevention of bone loss associated with
aromatase inhibitor therapy in postmenopausal women
with breast cancer; prevention of bone loss associated
with androgen deprivation therapy in prostate cancer

Local Anesthetic/Vasoconstrictor Precautions No
information available to require special precautions

Effects on Dental Treatment Key adverse event(s)
related to dental treatment: Mucositis, dysphagia, stomatitis, and sore throat.

Osteonecrosis of the jaw (ONJ), generally associated
with local infection and/or tooth extraction and often
with delayed healing, has been reported in patients
taking bisphosphonates. Symptoms included nonhealing extraction socket or an exposed jawbone. Most
reported cases of bisphosphonate-associated osteonecrosis have been in cancer patients treated with
intravenous bisphosphonates. However, some have
occurred in patients with postmenopausal osteoporosis taking oral bisphosphonates. Dental surgery, particularly tooth extraction, may increase the risk for
ONJ. Patients who develop ONJ while on bisphosphonate therapy should receive care by an oral surgeon.
See Dental Comment.

Effects on Bleeding Zoledronic acid has been shown
to induce thrombotic thrombocytopenia purpura-hemolytic uremic syndrome (TTP-HUS). In a clinical report,
zoledronic acid therapy caused acute anemia and
thrombocytopenia, with reticulocyte count at 6% and
bilirubin at 1.6 mg/dL, with few fragmented erythrocytes.
Treatment for this thrombocytopenia complication is
discontinuation of the drug and plasma exchange therapy to increase platelet count.

Adverse Effects Note: An acute reaction (eg, arthralgia, fever, flu-like symptoms, myalgia) may occur within
the first 3 days following infusion in up to 44% of
patients; usually resolves within 3-4 days of onset,
although may take up to 14 days to resolve. The
incidence may be decreased with acetaminophen (prior
to infusion and for 72 hours postinfusion).

Oncology indications:

>10%:

Cardiovascular: Leg edema (5% to 21%), hypotension (11%)

Central nervous system: Fatigue (39%), fever (32% to
44%), headache (5% to 19%), dizziness (18%),
insomnia (15% to 16%), anxiety (11% to 14%),
depression (14%), agitation (13%), confusion (7% to
13%), hypoesthesia (12%)

Dermatologic: Alopecia (12%), dermatitis (11%)

Endocrine & metabolic: Dehydration (5% to 14%),
hypophosphatemia (13%), hypokalemia (12%), hypomagnesemia (11%)

Gastrointestinal: Nausea (29% to 46%), vomiting (14%
to 32%), constipation (27% to 31%), diarrhea (17% to
24%), anorexia (9% to 22%), abdominal pain (14% to
16%), weight loss (16%), appetite decreased (13%)

Genitourinary: Urinary tract infection (12% to 14%)

Hematologic: Anemia (22% to 33%), neutropenia (12%)

Neuromuscular & skeletal: Bone pain (55%), weakness (5% to 24%), myalgia (23%), arthralgia (5% to
21%), back pain (15%), paresthesia (15%), limb pain
(14%), skeletal pain (12%), rigors (11%)

Renal: Renal deterioration (8% to 17%; up to 40% in
patients with abnormal baseline creatinine)

Respiratory: Dyspnea (22% to 27%), cough (12%
to 22%)

Miscellaneous: Cancer progression (16% to 20%),
moniliasis (12%)

1% to 10%:

Cardiovascular: Chest pain (5% to 10%)

Central nervous system: Somnolence (5% to 10%)

Endocrine & metabolic: Hypocalcemia (5% to 10%;
grades 3/4: ≤1%), hypermagnesemia (grade 3: 2%)

Gastrointestinal: Dyspepsia (10%), dysphagia (5% to
10%), mucositis (5% to 10%), stomatitis (8%), sore
throat (8%)

Hematologic: Granulocytopenia (5% to 10%), pancytopenia (5% to 10%), thrombocytopenia (5% to 10%)

Renal: Serum creatinine increased (grades 3/4: ≤2%)

Respiratory: Upper respiratory tract infection (10%)

Miscellaneous: Infection (nonspecific; 5% to 10%)

Nononcology indications:

>10%:

Cardiovascular: Hypertension (5% to 13%)

Central nervous system: Pain (2% to 24%), fever (9%
to 22%), headache (4% to 20%), chills (2% to 18%),
fatigue (2% to 18%)

Endocrine & metabolic: Hypocalcemia (≤3%; Paget's
disease 21%)

Gastrointestinal: Nausea (5% to 18%)

Neuromuscular & skeletal: Arthralgia (9% to 27%),
myalgia (5% to 23%), back pain (4% to 18%), limb
pain (3% to 16%), musculoskeletal pain (≤12%)

Miscellaneous: Acute phase reaction (4% to 25%), flu-
like syndrome (1% to 11%)

1% to 10%:

Cardiovascular: Chest pain (1% to 8%), peripheral
edema (3% to 6%), atrial fibrillation (1% to 3%),
palpitation (≤3%)

Central nervous system: Dizziness (2% to 9%),
malaise (1% to 7%), hypoesthesia (≤6%), lethargy
(3% to 5%), vertigo (1% to 4%), hyperthermia (≤2%)

Dermatologic: Rash (2% to 3%), hyperhidrosis (≤3%)

Gastrointestinal: Abdominal pain (1% to 9%), diarrhea
(5% to 8%), vomiting (2% to 8%), constipation (6% to
7%), dyspepsia (2% to 7%), abdominal discomfort/
distension (1% to 2%), anorexia (1% to 2%)

Neuromuscular & skeletal: Bone pain (3% to 9%),
arthritis (2% to 9%), rigors (8%), shoulder pain
(≤7%), neck pain (1% to 7%), weakness (2% to
6%), muscle spasm (2% to 6%), stiffness (1% to
5%), jaw pain (2% to 4%), joint swelling (≤3%),
paresthesia (2%)

Ocular: Eye pain (≤2%)

Renal: Serum creatinine increased (2%)

Respiratory: Dyspnea (5% to 7%)

Miscellaneous: C-reactive protein increased (≤5%)

Dosage I.V.: Adults: **Note:** Acetaminophen administration after the infusion may reduce symptoms of acute-phase reactions. Patients treated for multiple myeloma, osteoporosis, and Paget's disease should receive a daily calcium supplement and multivitamin containing vitamin D (if dietary intake is inadequate).

Hypercalcemia of malignancy (albumin-corrected serum calcium ≥12 mg/dL) (Zometa®): 4 mg (maximum) given as a single dose. Wait at least 7 days before considering retreatment.

Multiple myeloma or metastatic bone lesions from solid tumors (Zometa®): 4 mg every 3-4 weeks

Osteoporosis, glucocorticoid-induced, treatment and prevention (Reclast®, Aclasta® [Canadian availability]): 5 mg once a year

Osteoporosis, prevention:

Reclast®: 5 mg once every 2 years

Aclasta® (Canadian availability): 5 mg as a single (one-time) dose

Osteoporosis, treatment (Reclast®, Aclasta® [Canadian availability]): 5 mg once a year

Paget's disease:

Reclast®: 5 mg as a single dose. **Note:** Data concerning retreatment is not available; retreatment may be considered for relapse (increase in alkaline phosphatase) if appropriate, for inadequate response, or in patients who are symptomatic.

Aclasta® (Canadian availability): 5 mg as a single (one-time) dose

Prevention of aromatase inhibitor-induced bone loss in breast cancer (unlabeled use): 4 mg every 6 months for 5 years (Brufsky, 2012)

Prevention of androgen deprivation-induced bone loss in nonmetastatic prostate cancer (unlabeled use): 4 mg every 3 months for 1 year (Smith, 2003) or 4 mg every 12 months (Michaelson, 2007)

Dosage adjustment in renal impairment (at treatment initiation): Note: Calculate the creatinine clearance using the Cockcroft-Gault formula.

Nononcology uses:

Cl_{cr} ≥35 mL/minute: No dosage adjustment required.

Cl_{cr} <35 mL/minute: Use is contraindicated.

Oncology uses:

Multiple myeloma and bone metastases:

Cl_{cr} >60 mL/minute: 4 mg (no dosage adjustment necessary)

Cl_{cr} 50-60 mL/minute: Reduce dose to 3.5 mg

Cl_{cr} 40-49 mL/minute: Reduce dose to 3.3 mg

Cl_{cr} 30-39 mL/minute: Reduce dose to 3 mg

Cl_{cr} <30 mL/minute: Use is not recommended.

Hypercalcemia of malignancy:

Mild-to-moderate impairment: No dosage adjustment necessary.

Severe impairment (serum creatinine >4.5 mg/dL):

U.S. labeling: Evaluate risk versus benefit

Canadian labeling: Use is not recommended.

Dosage adjustment for renal toxicity (during treatment):

Hypercalcemia of malignancy: Evidence of renal deterioration: Evaluate risk versus benefit.

Multiple myeloma and bone metastases: Evidence of renal deterioration: Withhold dose until renal function returns to within 10% of baseline; renal deterioration defined as follows:

Normal baseline creatinine: Increase of 0.5 mg/dL

Abnormal baseline creatinine: Increase of 1 mg/dL

Reinitiate therapy at the same dose administered prior to treatment interruption.

Multiple myeloma: Albuminuria >500 mg/24 hours (unexplained): Withhold dose until return to baseline, then re-evaluate every 3-4 weeks; consider reinitiating with a longer infusion time of at least 30 minutes (Kyle, 2007).

Dosage adjustment in hepatic impairment: No dosage adjustment provided in the manufacturer's labeling (has not been studied).

Mechanism of Action A bisphosphonate which inhibits bone resorption via actions on osteoclasts or on osteoclast precursors; inhibits osteoclastic activity and skeletal calcium release induced by tumors. Decreases serum calcium and phosphorus, and increases their elimination. In osteoporosis, zoledronic acid inhibits osteoclast-mediated resorption, therefore reducing bone turnover.

Contraindications

U.S. labeling:

All indications: Hypersensitivity to zoledronic acid or any component of the formulatio

Nononcology uses: Additional contraindications: Hypocalcemia; use in patients with creatinine clearance (Cl_{cr}) <35 mL/minute and use in patients with evidence of acute renal impairment due to an increased risk of renal failure

Canadian labeling:

All indications: Hypersensitivity to zoledronic acid or other bisphosphonates, or any component of the formulation; pregnancy, breast-feeding

Nononcology uses: Additional contraindications: Uncorrected hypocalcemia at the time of infusion, use in patients with Cl_{cr} <35 mL/minute and use in patients with evidence of acute renal impairment due to an increased risk of renal failure

Warnings/Precautions Hazardous agent - use appropriate precautions for handling and disposal (NIOSH, 2012). Osteonecrosis of the jaw (ONJ) has been reported in patients receiving bisphosphonates. Risk factors include invasive dental procedures (eg, tooth extraction, dental implants, boney surgery); a diagnosis of cancer, with concomitant chemotherapy, radiotherapy, or corticosteroids; poor oral hygiene, ill-fitting dentures; and comorbid disorders (anemia, coagulopathy, infection, pre-existing dental disease). Most reported cases occurred after I.V. bisphosphonate therapy; however, cases have been reported following oral therapy. A dental exam and preventative dentistry should be performed prior to placing patients with risk factors on chronic bisphosphonate therapy. The manufacturer's labeling states that there are no data to suggest whether discontinuing bisphosphonates in patients requiring invasive dental procedures reduces the risk of ONJ. However, other experts suggest that there is no evidence that discontinuing therapy reduces the risk of developing ONJ (Assael, 2009). The benefit/risk must be assessed by the treating physician and/or dentist/surgeon prior to any invasive dental procedure. Patients developing ONJ while on bisphosphonates should receive care by an oral surgeon.

Atypical, low energy, or low trauma femur fractures have been reported in patients receiving bisphosphonates for treatment/prevention of osteoporosis. The fractures include subtrochanteric femur (bone just below the hip joint) and diaphyseal femur (long segment of the thigh bone). Some patients experience prodromal pain weeks or months before the fracture occurs. It is unclear if bisphosphonate therapy is the cause for these fractures; atypical femur fractures have also been reported in patients not taking bisphosphonates, and in patients receiving glucocorticoids. Patients receiving long-term (>3-5 years) bisphosphonate therapy may be at an increased risk. Patients presenting with thigh or groin pain with a history of receiving bisphosphonates should be evaluated for femur fracture. Consider interrupting bisphosphonate therapy in patients who develop a femoral shaft fracture; assess for fracture in the contralateral limb.

Infrequently, severe (and occasionally debilitating) musculoskeletal (bone, joint, and/or muscle) pain have been reported during bisphosphonate treatment. The onset of pain ranged from a single day to several months. Consider discontinuing therapy in patients who experience severe symptoms; symptoms usually resolve upon discontinuation. Some patients experienced recurrence when rechallenged with same drug or another bisphosphonate; avoid use in patients with a history of these symptoms in association with bisphosphonate therapy.

May cause a significant risk of hypocalcemia in patients with Paget's disease, in whom the pretreatment rate of bone turnover may be greatly elevated. Hypocalcemia must be corrected before initiation of therapy in patients with Paget's disease and osteoporosis. Ensure adequate calcium and vitamin D intake during therapy. Use caution in patients with disturbances of calcium and mineral metabolism (eg, hypoparathyroidism, thyroid/parathyroid, surgery, malabsorption syndromes, excision of small intestine).

Nononcology indications: Use is contraindicated in patients with Cl$_{cr}$ <35 mL/minute and in patients with evidence of acute renal impairment due to an increased risk of renal failure. Re-evaluate the need for continued therapy for the treatment of osteoporosis periodically; the optimal duration of treatment has not yet been determined.

Oncology indications: Use caution in mild-to-moderate renal dysfunction; dosage adjustment required. In cancer patients, renal toxicity has been reported with doses >4 mg or infusions administered over 15 minutes. Risk factors for renal deterioration include pre-existing renal insufficiency and repeated doses of zoledronic acid and other bisphosphonates. Dehydration and the use of other nephrotoxic drugs which may contribute to renal deterioration should be identified and managed. Use is not recommended in patients with severe renal impairment (serum creatinine >3 mg/dL or Cl$_{cr}$ <30 mL/minute) and bone metastases (limited data); use in patients with hypercalcemia of malignancy and severe renal impairment (serum creatinine >4.5 mg/dL for hypercalcemia of malignancy) should only be done if the benefits outweigh the risks. Diuretics should not be used before correcting hypovolemia. Renal deterioration, resulting in renal failure and dialysis has occurred in patients treated with zoledronic acid after single and multiple infusions at recommended doses of 4 mg over 15 minutes. Assess renal function prior to treatment and withhold for renal deterioration [increase in serum creatinine of 0.5 mg/dL (if baseline level normal) or increase of 1 mg/dL (if baseline level abnormal)]; treatment should be withheld until renal function returns to within 10% of baseline.

According to the American Society of Clinical Oncology (ASCO) guidelines for bisphosphonates in multiple myeloma, treatment with zoledronic acid is not recommended for asymptomatic (smoldering) or indolent myeloma or with solitary plasmacytoma (Kyle, 2007). The National Comprehensive Cancer Network® (NCCN) multiple myeloma guidelines (v.1.2013) also do not recommend the use of bisphosphonates in stage 1 or smoldering disease, unless part of a clinical trial.

Adequate hydration is required during treatment (urine output ~2 L/day); avoid overhydration, especially in patients with heart failure. Pre-existing renal compromise, severe dehydration, and concurrent use with diuretics or other nephrotoxic drugs may increase the risk for renal impairment. Single and multiple infusions in patients with both normal and impaired renal function have been associated with renal deterioration, resulting in renal failure and dialysis or death (rare). Patients with underlying moderate-to-severe renal impairment, increased age, concurrent use of nephrotoxic or diuretic medications, or severe dehydration prior to or after zoledronic acid administration may have an increased risk of acute renal impairment or renal failure. Others with increased risk include patients with renal impairment or dehydration secondary to fever, sepsis, gastrointestinal losses, or diuretic use. If history or physical exam suggests dehydration, treatment should not be given until the patient is normovolemic. Creatinine clearance (using actual body weight) should be calculated with the Cockcroft-Gault formula prior to each administration. Transient increases in serum creatinine may be more pronounced in patients with impaired renal function; consider monitoring creatinine clearance in at-risk patients taking other renally-eliminated drugs.

Use caution in patients with aspirin-sensitive asthma (may cause bronchoconstriction) and the elderly. Rare cases of urticaria and angioedema and very rare cases of anaphylactic reactions/shock have been reported. Women of childbearing age should be advised against becoming pregnant. Not approved for use in children. Do not administer Zometa® and Reclast® to the same patient for different indications.

Drug Interactions

Metabolism/Transport Effects None known.

Avoid Concomitant Use There are no known interactions where it is recommended to avoid concomitant use.

Increased Effect/Toxicity

Zoledronic Acid may increase the levels/effects of: Deferasirox; Phosphate Supplements; SUNItinib

The levels/effects of Zoledronic Acid may be increased by: Aminoglycosides; Nonsteroidal Anti-Inflammatory Agents; Thalidomide

Decreased Effect

The levels/effects of Zoledronic Acid may be decreased by: Proton Pump Inhibitors

Dietary Considerations

Multiple myeloma or metastatic bone lesions from solid tumors: Take daily calcium supplement (500 mg) and daily multivitamin (with 400 units vitamin D).

Osteoporosis: Ensure adequate calcium and vitamin D supplementation; general requirements are calcium 1200 mg/day and vitamin D 800-1000 units/day.

Paget's disease: Take elemental calcium 1500 mg/day (750 mg twice daily or 500 mg 3 times/day) and vitamin D 800 units/day, particularly during the first 2 weeks after administration.

Pharmacodynamics/Kinetics

Half-life Elimination Triphasic; Terminal: 146 hours

Pregnancy Risk Factor D

Pregnancy Considerations Animal reproduction studies resulted in embryotoxicity and losses. Zoledronic acid should not be used during pregnancy; may cause fetal harm if administered to a pregnant woman.

Bisphosphonates are incorporated into the bone matrix and gradually released over time. Theoretically, there may be a risk of fetal harm when pregnancy follows the completion of therapy. Based on limited case reports with pamidronate, serum calcium levels in the newborn may be altered if administered during pregnancy.

Lactation Excretion in breast milk unknown/not recommended

Breast-Feeding Considerations Because it binds to bone long term, zoledronic acid use is not recommended in nursing women.

Dosage Forms
Infusion, premixed:
Reclast®: 5 mg (100 mL)
Zometa®: 4 mg (100 mL)
Injection, solution: 4 mg/5 mL (5 mL)
Zometa®: 4 mg/5 mL (5 mL)
Dosage Forms: Canada
Infusion, solution [premixed]:
Aclasta®: 5 mg (100 mL)

Dental Comment Zoledronic acid (Reclast®) is administered once annually for the treatment of osteoporosis. A single, large prospective, placebo-controlled study established its efficacy for this indication through 3 years of treatment (Black, 2007). Two cases of ONJ were reported, one each in the treatment and control groups, suggesting a low risk of ONJ with this treatment protocol through 3 years.

The American Association of Oral and Maxillofacial Surgeons position paper on bisphosphonate-related osteonecrosis of the jaws, 2009 update, stated that I.V. bisphosphonate exposure in the setting of managing malignancy remains the major risk factor for the development of ONJ. After reviewing case series, case-controlled studies, and cohort studies, the estimates of the cumulative incidence of I.V. bisphosphonate-associated ONJ ranges from 0.8% to 12%.

Two reports have attempted to assess more accurately the percent of cancer patients developing ONJ after bisphosphonate treatment. Maerevoet et al, reported that among 194 patients treated with Zometa® every 3-4 weeks, nine developed ONJ. Before receiving Zometa®, six had received Aredia® 90 mg every 3-4 weeks. The median duration of treatment with Aredia® was 39 months and for Zometa® 18 months. The incidence of ONJ in these patients was calculated to be 4.6%. Durie et al, described the results of a survey by the International Myeloma Foundation in 2004 to assess the risk factors of ONJ. Out of 1203 respondents, 904 had myeloma and 299 had breast cancer. Of the myeloma patients, 62 developed ONJ and 54 had suspicious findings. Of the breast cancer patients, 13 had ONJ and 23 had suspicious findings. The total number of cases of either ONJ or suspicious findings was 152. ONJ developed in 10% of 211 patients receiving Zometa® compared to 4% of 413 receiving Aredia®. The mean time to onset of ONJ among patients taking Zometa® was 18 months; the mean time to onset after Aredia® was 6 years. It should be noted that an early report by authors from Novartis Pharmaceuticals Corporation stressed that Aredia® and Zometa® had been used in 2.5 million patients world wide and reports of ONJ during their extensive use had been rare (Tarassoff, 2003). In addition, these authors stated that review of the reported cases revealed multiple risk factors for avascular necrosis. McMahon et al, followed up with a report that, along with other factors, bisphosphonates are additional stressors of bone health that can tip the balance to osteonecrosis. They suggested that the prevention of ONJ should be stressed such as the elimination of chronic dental infections prior to chemotherapy and bisphosphonate use in cancer patients.

According to the 2011 report by the American Dental Association (ADA), the incidence of BP-associated ONJ remains low and the benefits of using oral bisphosphonates significantly outweighs the risk of developing BP-associated ONJ for treatment and prevention of osteoporosis and cancer treatment (Hellstein, 2011). The full 47 page report can be accessed at http://www.ada.org/sections/professionalResources/pdfs/topics_AR-ONJ_report.pdf.

The ADA review of 2011 stated the incidence of oral BP-associated ONJ was one case for every 1000 individuals exposed to oral bisphosphonates (0.1%) (Hellstein, 2011).

References

Black DM, Delmas PD, Eastell R, et al, "Once-Yearly Zoledronic Acid for Treatment of Postmenopausal Osteoporosis," New Engl J Med, 2007, 356(18):1809-22.

Durie BG, Katz M, and Crowley J, "Osteonecrosis of the Jaw and Bisphosphonates," N Engl J Med, 2005, 353(1):99-102.

Hellstein JW, Adler RA, Edwards B, et al, "Managing the Care of Patients Receiving Antiresorptive Therapy for Prevention and Treatment of Osteoporosis: Executive Summary of Recommendations From the American Dental Association Council on Scientific Affairs," J Am Dent Assoc, 2011, 142(11):1243-51.

Hellstein JW, Adler RA, Edwards B, et al, "Managing the Care of Patients Receiving Antiresorptive Therapy for Prevention and Treatment of Osteoporosis: Recommendations From the American Dental Association Council on Scientific Affairs," 2011, Available at http://www.ada.org/sections/professionalResources/pdfs/topics_ARONJ_report.pdf. Accessed February 2013.

Maerevoet M, Martin C, and Duck L, "Osteonecrosis of the Jaw and Bisphosphonates," N Engl J Med, 2005, 353(1):99-102.

McMahon RE, Bouquot JE, Glueck CJ, et al, "Osteonecrosis: A Multifactorial Etiology," J Oral Maxillofac Surg, 2004, 62(7):904-5.

Ruggiero SL, Dodson TB, Assael LA, et al, "American Association of Oral and Maxillofacial Surgeons Position Paper on Bisphosphonate-Related Osteonecrosis of the Jaws-2009 Update," J Oral Maxillofac Surg, 2009, 67(5 Suppl):2-12.

Ruggiero S, Gralow J, Marx RE, et al, "Practical Guidelines for the Prevention, Diagnosis, and Treatment of Osteonecrosis of the Jaw in Patients With Cancer," J Clin Oncol, 2006, 2(1):7-14.

Tarassoff P and Csermak K, "Avascular Necrosis of the Jaws: Risk Factors in Metastatic Cancer Patients," J Oral Maxillofac Surg, 2003, 61(10):1238-9.

ZOLMitriptan (zohl mi TRIP tan)

Related Information
Temporomandibular Dysfunction (TMD), Chronic Pain, and Fibromyalgia on page 1590
Brand Names: U.S. Zomig-ZMT®; Zomig®
Brand Names: Canada Mylan-Zolmitriptan; PMS-Zolmitriptan; PMS-Zolmitriptan ODT; Sandoz-Zolmitriptan; Sandoz-Zolmitriptan ODT; Teva-Zolmitriptan; Teva-Zolmitriptan OD; Zolmitriptan ODT; Zomig®; Zomig® Nasal Spray; Zomig® Rapimelt
Pharmacologic Category Antimigraine Agent; Serotonin 5-HT$_{1B, 1D}$ Receptor Agonist
Use Acute treatment of migraine with or without aura
Unlabeled Use Short-term prevention of menstrual migraines
Local Anesthetic/Vasoconstrictor Precautions No information available to require special precautions
Effects on Dental Treatment Key adverse event(s) related to dental treatment: Xerostomia (normal salivary flow resumes upon discontinuation) and dysphagia.
Effects on Bleeding No information available to require special precautions
Adverse Effects
>10%: Gastrointestinal: Abnormal taste (21%)
1% to 10%:
Cardiovascular: Chest pain/tightness (1% to 4%), palpitation (≤2%)

Central nervous system: Dizziness (6% to 10%), somnolence (4% to 8%), pain (2% to 4%), vertigo (≤2%), headache (1% to <2%), insomnia (1% to <2%)

Gastrointestinal: Nausea (6% to 9%), xerostomia (2% to 5%), dyspepsia (2% to 3%), dysphagia (≤2%), abdominal pain (1% to <2%), vomiting (1% to <2%)

Local: Application site irritation/soreness (nasal spray 3%)

Neuromuscular & skeletal: Paresthesia (5% to 10%), weakness (5% to 9%), warm/cold sensation (5% to 7%), hypoesthesia (1% to 5%), myalgia (1% to 2%), myasthenia (≤2%)

Respiratory: Nasal discomfort (nasal spray 3%), throat pressure/tightness (1% to 2%)

Miscellaneous: Neck/throat/jaw pain (4% to 10%), pressure/tightness/heaviness (2% to 5%), diaphoresis (≤3%), allergic reaction (≤1%)

General Dosage Range Dosage adjustment recommended in patients with hepatic impairment

Nasal inhalation: *Adults:* 5 mg (1 spray) at the onset of migraine headache; may repeat in 2 hours if no relief (maximum: 10 mg [2 sprays] daily)

Oral: *Adults:* 1.25-2.5 mg at the onset of migraine headache; may repeat in 2 hours if no relief (maximum: 10 mg daily)

Mechanism of Action Selective agonist for serotonin (5-HT$_{1B}$ and 5-HT$_{1D}$ receptors) in cranial arteries and sensory nerves of the trigeminal system; causes vasoconstriction and reduces inflammation associated with antidromic neuronal transmission correlating with relief of migraine

Pharmacodynamics/Kinetics

Onset of Action 0.5-1 hour

Half-life Elimination 2.8-3.7 hours

Time to Peak Serum: Tablet: 1.5 hours; Orally-disintegrating tablet and nasal spray: 3 hours

Pregnancy Risk Factor C

Pregnancy Considerations There are no adequate and well-controlled studies using zolmitriptan in pregnant women. Use only if potential benefit to the mother outweighs the potential risk to the fetus. In animal studies, administration was associated with embryolethality, fetal abnormalities, and pup mortality.

Zolpidem (zole PI dem)

Brand Names: U.S. Ambien CR®; Ambien®; Edluar™; Intermezzo®; Zolpimist®

Brand Names: Canada Sublinox™

Generic Availability (U.S.) Yes: Excludes oral spray, sublingual tablet

Pharmacologic Category Hypnotic, Miscellaneous

Use

Ambien®, Edluar™, Zolpimist®: Short-term treatment of insomnia (with difficulty of sleep onset)

Ambien CR®: Treatment of insomnia (with difficulty of sleep onset and/or sleep maintenance)

Intermezzo®: "As needed" treatment of middle-of-the-night insomnia with ≥4 hours of sleep time remaining.

Sublinox™ (Canadian availability; not available in U.S.): Short-term treatment of insomnia (with difficulty of sleep onset, frequent awakenings, and/or early awakenings)

Local Anesthetic/Vasoconstrictor Precautions No information available to require special precautions

Effects on Dental Treatment Key adverse event(s) related to dental treatment: Xerostomia (normal salivary flow resumes upon discontinuation).

Effects on Bleeding No information available to require special precautions

Adverse Effects Actual frequency may be dosage form, dose, and/or age dependent

>10%: Central nervous system: Headache (3% to 19%), somnolence (6% to 15%), dizziness (1% to 12%)

1% to 10%:

Cardiovascular: Blood pressure increased, chest discomfort/pain, palpitation

Central nervous system: Abnormal dreams, anxiety, apathy, amnesia, ataxia, attention disturbance, body temperature increased, burning sensation, confusion, depersonalization, depression, disinhibition, disorientation, drowsiness, drugged feeling, euphoria, fatigue, fever, hallucinations, hypoesthesia, insomnia, lethargy, lightheadedness, memory disorder, mood swings, sleep disorder, stress

Dermatologic: Rash, urticaria, wrinkling

Endocrine & metabolic: Menorrhagia

Gastrointestinal: Abdominal discomfort, abdominal pain, abdominal tenderness, appetite disorder, constipation, diarrhea, dyspepsia, flatulence, gastroenteritis, gastroesophageal reflux, hiccup, nausea, vomiting, xerostomia

Genitourinary: Urinary tract infection, vulvovaginal dryness

Neuromuscular & skeletal: Arthralgia, back pain, balance disorder, involuntary muscle contractions, myalgia, neck pain, paresthesia, psychomotor retardation, tremor, weakness

Ocular: Asthenopia, blurred vision, depth perception altered, diplopia, red eye, visual disturbance

Otic: Labyrinthitis, tinnitus, vertigo

Renal: Dysuria

Respiratory: Pharyngitis, sinusitis, throat irritation, upper respiratory tract infection

Miscellaneous: Allergy, binge eating, flu-like syndrome

Dosage Oral:

Adults: **Note:** The lowest effective dose should be used; higher doses may be more likely to impair next morning activities.

Immediate release tablet, spray: 5 mg (females) or 5-10 mg (males) immediately before bedtime; maximum dose: 10 mg daily

Extended release tablet: 6.25 mg (females) or 6.25-12.5 mg (males) immediately before bedtime

Sublingual tablet:

Edluar™: 5 mg (females) or 5-10 mg (males) immediately before bedtime; maximum dose: 10 mg daily

Sublinox™ (Canadian availability; not available in U.S.): 10 mg immediately before bedtime; maximum dose: 10 mg daily

Intermezzo®: **Note:** Take only if ≥4 hours left before waking

Females: 1.75 mg once per night as needed (maximum: 1.75 mg/night)

Males: 3.5 mg once per night as needed (maximum: 3.5 mg/night)

Dosage adjustment with concomitant CNS depressants: Females and males: 1.75 mg once per night as needed; dose adjustment of concomitant CNS depressant(s) may be necessary.

Elderly:

Immediate release tablet, spray: 5 mg immediately before bedtime

Sublingual tablet:
U.S. labeling:
Edluar™: 5 mg immediately before bedtime
Intermezzo®: Females and males: 1.75 mg once per night as needed (maximum: 1.75 mg/night). **Note:** Take only if ≥4 hours left before waking.
Canadian labeling (Sublinox™): Not recommended; tablet cannot not be split for a reduced dose.
Extended release tablet: 6.25 mg immediately before bedtime

Dosing adjustment in renal impairment: No dosage adjustment provided in manufacturer's labeling; however, some zolpidem labeling recommends monitoring patients with renal impairment closely.
Hemodialysis: Not dialyzable
Dosing adjustment in hepatic impairment:
U.S. labeling:
Immediate release tablet, spray: 5 mg immediately before bedtime
Extended release tablet: 6.25 mg immediately before bedtime
Sublingual tablet:
Edluar™: 5 mg immediately before bedtime
Intermezzo®: Females and males: 1.75 mg once per night as needed. **Note:** Take only if ≥4 hours left before waking.
Canadian labeling: Sublingual tablet: Sublinox®:
Mild-to-moderate impairment: Use is not recommended; tablet cannot be split for reduced dose.
Severe impairment: Use is contraindicated.

Mechanism of Action Zolpidem, an imidazopyridine hypnotic that is structurally dissimilar to benzodiazepines, enhances the activity of the inhibitory neurotransmitter, γ-aminobutyric acid (GABA), via selective agonism at the benzodiazepine-1 (BZ_1) receptor; the result is increased chloride conductance, neuronal hyperpolarization, inhibition of the action potential, and a decrease in neuronal excitability leading to sedative and hypnotic effects. Because of its selectivity for the BZ_1 receptor site over the BZ_2 receptor site, zolpidem exhibits minimal anxiolytic, myorelaxant, and anticonvulsant properties (effects largely attributed to agonism at the BZ_2 receptor site).

Contraindications Hypersensitivity to zolpidem or any component of the formulation

Canadian labeling: Additional contraindications (not in U.S. labeling): Significant obstructive sleep apnea syndrome and acute and/or severe impairment of respiratory function; myasthenia gravis; severe hepatic impairment; personal or family history of sleepwalking

Warnings/Precautions Should be used only after evaluation of potential causes of sleep disturbance. Failure of sleep disturbance to resolve after 7-10 days may indicate psychiatric or medical illness. Hypnotics/sedatives have been associated with abnormal thinking and behavior changes including decreased inhibition, aggression, bizarre behavior, agitation, hallucinations, and depersonalization. These changes may occur unpredictably and may indicate previously unrecognized psychiatric disorders; evaluate appropriately. Sedative/hypnotics may produce withdrawal symptoms following abrupt discontinuation. Use with caution in patients with depression; worsening of depression, including suicide or suicidal ideation has been reported with the use of hypnotics. Intentional overdose may be an issue in this population. The minimum dose that will effectively treat the individual patient should be used. Prescriptions should be written for the smallest quantity consistent with good patient care. Causes CNS depression, which may impair physical and mental capabilities. Zolpidem should only be administered when the patient is able to stay in bed a full night (7-8 hours) before being active again. Effects with other sedative drugs or ethanol may be potentiated. Canadian labeling does not recommend concomitant use with alcohol.

Use caution in patients with myasthenia gravis (contraindicated in the Canadian labeling). Avoid use in patients with sleep apnea or a history of sedative-hypnotic abuse. Postmarketing studies have indicated that the use of hypnotic/sedative agents for sleep has been associated with hypersensitivity reactions including anaphylaxis as well as angioedema. An increased risk for hazardous sleep-related activities such as sleep-driving; cooking and eating food, and making phone calls while asleep have also been noted; amnesia may also occur. Discontinue treatment in patients who report any sleep-related episodes. Canadian labeling recommends avoiding use in patients with disorders (eg, restless legs syndrome, periodic limb movement disorder, sleep apnea) that may disrupt sleep and cause frequent awakenings, potentially increasing the risk of complex sleep-related behaviors.

Use caution with respiratory disease (Canadian labeling contraindicates use with acute and/or severe impairment of respiratory function). Use caution with hepatic impairment (Canadian labeling contraindicates use in severe impairment); dose adjustment required. Because of the rapid onset of action, administer immediately prior to bedtime or after the patient has gone to bed and is having difficulty falling asleep.

Use caution in the elderly; dose adjustment recommended. Closely monitor elderly or debilitated patients for impaired cognitive and/or motor performance, confusion, and potential for falling. Avoid chronic use (>90 days) in older adults; adverse events, including delirium, falls, fractures, have been observed with nonbenzodiazepine hypnotic use in the elderly similar to events observed with benzodiazepines. Data suggests improvements in sleep duration and latency are minimal (Beers Criteria).

Dosage adjustment is recommended for females receiving Intermezzo®; pharmacokinetic studies involving sublingual zolpidem (Intermezzo®) showed a significant increase in maximum concentration and exposure in females compared to males at the same dose. When studied for the unapproved use of insomnia associated with ADHD in children, a higher incidence (~7%) of hallucinations was reported. In addition, sleep latency did not decrease compared to placebo. Zolpidem is **not** FDA- or Health Canada-approved for use in pediatric patients.

Drug Interactions

Metabolism/Transport Effects Substrate of CYP1A2 (minor), CYP2C19 (minor), CYP2C9 (minor), CYP2D6 (minor), CYP3A4 (major); **Note:** Assignment of Major/Minor substrate status based on clinically relevant drug interaction potential

Avoid Concomitant Use

Avoid concomitant use of Zolpidem with any of the following: Azelastine (Nasal); Conivaptan; Paraldehyde; Sodium Oxybate

Increased Effect/Toxicity

Zolpidem may increase the levels/effects of: Alcohol (Ethyl); Azelastine (Nasal); Buprenorphine; CarBAMazepine; Methotrimeprazine; Metyrosine; Mirtazapine; Paraldehyde; Pramipexole; ROPINIRole; Rotigotine; Selective Serotonin Reuptake Inhibitors; Sodium Oxybate

The levels/effects of Zolpidem may be increased by: Antifungal Agents (Azole Derivatives, Systemic); CNS Depressants; Conivaptan; CYP3A4 Inhibitors (Moderate); CYP3A4 Inhibitors (Strong); Dasatinib; Droperidol; Fluconazole; FluvoxaMINE; HydrOXYzine; Ivacaftor; Magnesium Sulfate; Methotrimeprazine; Mifepristone; Perampanel

Decreased Effect

The levels/effects of Zolpidem may be decreased by: CarBAMazepine; CYP3A4 Inducers (Strong); Deferasirox; Flumazenil; Herbs (CYP3A4 Inducers); Peginterferon Alfa-2b; Rifamycin Derivatives; Telaprevir; Tocilizumab

Ethanol/Nutrition/Herb Interactions

Ethanol: May enhance the adverse/toxic effects of zolpidem. Management: Avoid use of ethanol.

Food: Maximum plasma concentration and bioavailability are decreased with food; time to peak plasma concentration is increased; half-life remains unchanged. Grapefruit juice may decrease the metabolism of zolpidem. Management: Avoid grapefruit juice.

Herb/Nutraceutical: St John's wort may decrease the levels/effects of zolpidem. Some herbal medications should be avoided due to the risk of increased CNS depression. Management: Avoid concomitant use of St John's wort. Avoid valerian, kava kava, and gotu kola.

Dietary Considerations

For faster sleep onset, do not administer with (or immediately after) a meal.

Pharmacodynamics/Kinetics

Onset of Action Immediate release: 30 minutes

Duration of Action Immediate release: 6-8 hours

Half-life Elimination

Immediate release, Extended release: ~2.5 hours (range: 1.4-4.5 hours); Cirrhosis: Up to 9.9 hours; Elderly: Prolonged up to 32%

Spray: ~3 hours (range: 1.7-8.4)

Sublingual tablet (Edluar™, Intermezzo®): ~3 hours (range: 1.4-6.7 hours)

Time to Peak

Immediate release: 1.6 hours; 2.2 hours with food

Extended release: 1.5 hours; 4 hours with food

Spray: ~0.9 hours

Sublingual tablet: Edluar™: ~1.4 hours, ~1.8 hours with food; Intermezzo®: 0.6-1.3 hours, ~3 hours with food

Pregnancy Risk Factor C

Pregnancy Considerations Teratogenic effects were not observed in animal studies. Adverse effects were noted in animal reproduction studies at doses 20-100 times the maximum recommended human dose. Severe neonatal respiratory depression has been reported when zolpidem was used at the end of pregnancy, especially when used concurrently with other CNS depressants. Studies of prenatal exposure to zolpidem have not been conducted in children. Children born of mothers taking sedative/hypnotics may be at risk for withdrawal; neonatal flaccidity has been reported in infants following maternal use of sedative/hypnotics during pregnancy. Use during pregnancy only if the benefits justify the risk to the fetus.

Lactation Enters breast milk/use caution (AAP rates "compatible"; AAP 2001 update pending)

Controlled Substance C-IV

Dosage Forms

Solution, oral:

Zolpimist®: 5 mg/actuation (8.2 g)

Tablet, oral: 5 mg, 10 mg

Ambien®: 5 mg, 10 mg

Tablet, sublingual:

Edluar™: 5 mg, 10 mg

Intermezzo®: 1.75 mg, 3.5 mg

Tablet, extended release, oral: 6.25 mg, 12.5 mg

Ambien CR®: 6.25 mg, 12.5 mg

Dosage Forms: Canada

Tablet, sublingual:

Sublinox™: 10 mg

Zonisamide (zoe NIS a mide)

Brand Names: U.S. Zonegran®

Pharmacologic Category Anticonvulsant, Miscellaneous

Use Adjunct treatment of partial seizures in children >16 years of age and adults with epilepsy

Unlabeled Use Bipolar disorder

Local Anesthetic/Vasoconstrictor Precautions No information available to require special precautions

Effects on Dental Treatment Key adverse event(s) related to dental treatment: Xerostomia (normal salivary flow resumes upon discontinuation) and abnormal taste.

Effects on Bleeding No information available to require special precautions

Adverse Effects Frequencies noted in patients receiving other anticonvulsants:

>10%:

Central nervous system: Somnolence (17%), dizziness (13%)

Gastrointestinal: Anorexia (13%)

1% to 10%:

Central nervous system: Headache (10%), agitation/irritability (9%), fatigue (8%), tiredness (7%), ataxia (6%), confusion (6%), concentration decreased (6%), memory impairment (6%), depression (6%), insomnia (6%), speech disorders (5%), mental slowing (4%), anxiety (3%), nervousness (2%), schizophrenic/schizophreniform behavior (2%), difficulty in verbal expression (2%), status epilepticus (1%), seizure (1%), hyperesthesia (1%), incoordination (1%)

Dermatologic: Rash (3%), bruising (2%), pruritus (1%)

Gastrointestinal: Nausea (9%), abdominal pain (6%), diarrhea (5%), dyspepsia (3%), weight loss (3%), constipation (2%), taste perversion (2%), xerostomia (2%), vomiting (1%)

Neuromuscular & skeletal: Paresthesia (4%), abnormal gait (1%), tremor (1%), weakness (1%)

Ocular: Diplopia (6%), nystagmus (4%), amblyopia (1%)

Otic: Tinnitus (1%)

Renal: Kidney stones (4%, children 3% to 8%)

Respiratory: Rhinitis (2%), pharyngitis (1%), increased cough (1%)

Miscellaneous: Flu-like syndrome (4%) accidental injury (1%)

General Dosage Range Oral: *Children >16 years and Adults:* Initial: 100 mg/day; Maintenance: 100-600 mg/day (maximum: 600 mg/day)

Mechanism of Action The exact mechanism of action is not known. May stabilize neuronal membranes and suppress neuronal hypersynchronization through action at sodium and calcium channels. Does not affect GABA activity.

Pharmacodynamics/Kinetics
Half-life Elimination Plasma: ~63 hours
Time to Peak 2-6 hours
Pregnancy Risk Factor C
Pregnancy Considerations Teratogenic effects were observed in animal reproduction studies; therefore, zonisamide is classified as pregnancy category C. Zonisamide crosses the placenta and can be detected in the newborn following delivery. Although adverse fetal events have been reported, the risk of teratogenic effects following maternal use of zonisamide in not clearly defined. Other agents may be preferred until additional data is available. Newborns should be monitored for transient metabolic acidosis after birth. Zonisamide clearance may increase in the second trimester of pregnancy, requiring dosage adjustment. Women of childbearing potential are advised to use effective contraception during therapy.

Patients exposed to zonisamide during pregnancy are encouraged to enroll themselves into the AED Pregnancy Registry by calling 1-888-233-2334. Additional information is available at http://www.aedpregnancy-registry.org.

Zopiclone (ZOE pi clone)

Brand Names: Canada Apo-Zopiclone®; CO Zopiclone; Dom-Zopiclone; Imovane®; Mylan-Zopiclone; Novo-Zopiclone; Nu-Zopiclone; PHL-Zopiclone; PMS-Zopiclone; PRO-Zopiclone; RAN™-Zopiclone; ratio-Zopiclone; Rhovane®; Riva-Zopiclone; Sandoz-Zopiclone
Pharmacologic Category Hypnotic, Miscellaneous
Use Short-term and symptomatic relief of insomnia
Local Anesthetic/Vasoconstrictor Precautions No information available to require special precautions
Effects on Dental Treatment Key adverse event(s) related to dental treatment: Coated tongue, dry mouth, halitosis, taste alteration (bitter taste, common).
Effects on Bleeding No information available to require special precautions
Adverse Effects Frequency not defined.
Cardiovascular: Palpitations
Central nervous system: Aggressiveness, agitation, anterograde amnesia, anger, anxiety, chills, complex sleep-related behaviors, confusion, depression, difficulty awakening, dizziness, drowsiness, euphoria, hallucinations, headache, hostility, irritability, memory impairment, nervousness, nightmares, somnolence, speech abnormalities
Dermatological: Angioedema, pruritus, rash, spots on skin
Endocrine & metabolic: Libido decreased
Gastrointestinal: Anorexia, appetite increased, constipation, coated tongue, diarrhea, dry mouth, dyspepsia, halitosis, nausea, taste alteration (bitter taste), vomiting, weight loss
Hepatic: Alkaline phosphatase increased, ALT increased, AST increased
Neuromuscular & skeletal: Coordination impaired, hypotonia, limb heaviness, muscle spasms, paresthesia, tremor, weakness
Ocular: Amblyopia
Respiratory: Dyspnea
Miscellaneous: Anaphylaxis, diaphoresis
General Dosage Range Dosage adjustment recommended in patients with hepatic and renal impairment, elderly and debilitated patients, and patients with chronic respiratory insufficiency.

Oral:
Adults: 3.75-7.5 mg once daily at bedtime
Elderly: Initial: 3.75 mg once daily at bedtime
Mechanism of Action Zopiclone is a cyclopyrrolone derivative and has a pharmacological profile similar to benzodiazepines. Zopiclone reduces sleep latency, increases duration of sleep, and decreases the number of nocturnal awakenings.
Pharmacodynamics/Kinetics
Half-life Elimination ~5 hours; Elderly: ~7 hours; Hepatic impairment: ~12 hours
Time to Peak Serum: <2 hours; Hepatic impairment: 3.5 hours
Pregnancy Considerations There is insufficient data on safety in pregnancy; however, benzodiazepines may cause congenital malformations during the 1st trimester and neonatal CNS depression during the last few weeks of pregnancy; it is expected zopiclone may do the same. Use is not recommended during pregnancy.
Product Availability Not available in U.S.

Zoster Vaccine (ZOS ter vak SEEN)

Related Information
Systemic Viral Diseases *on page 1537*
Brand Names: U.S. Zostavax®
Brand Names: Canada Zostavax®
Pharmacologic Category Vaccine, Live (Viral)
Use Prevention of herpes zoster (shingles) in patients ≥50 years of age
The Advisory Committee on Immunization Practices (ACIP) recommends routine vaccination of **all patients ≥60 years of age, including** patients who report a previous episode of zoster; patients with chronic medical conditions (eg, chronic renal failure, diabetes mellitus, rheumatoid arthritis, chronic pulmonary disease) unless those conditions are contraindications; and residents of nursing homes and other long-term care facilities without contraindications (CDC, 2008).
Although not specifically recommended for their profession, healthcare providers within the recommended age group should also receive the zoster vaccine (CDC, 2013).
Local Anesthetic/Vasoconstrictor Precautions No information available to require special precautions
Effects on Dental Treatment No significant effects or complications reported
Effects on Bleeding No information available to require special precautions
Adverse Effects All serious adverse reactions must be reported to the U.S. Department of Health and Human Services (DHHS) Vaccine Adverse Event Reporting System (VAERS) 1-800-822-7967 or online at https://vaers.hhs.gov/esub/index.
>10%: Local: Injection site reaction (48% to 64%; includes erythema, tenderness, pain, swelling, hematoma, pruritus, and/or warmth)
1% to 10% (**Note:** Rates similar to placebo):
Central nervous system: Fever (2%), headache (1% to 9%)
Dermatologic: Skin disorder (1%)
Gastrointestinal: Diarrhea (2%)
Neuromuscular & skeletal: Weakness (1%)
Respiratory: Respiratory tract infection (2%), rhinitis (1%)
Miscellaneous: Flu-like syndrome (2%)
General Dosage Range SubQ: *Adults ≥50 years:* 0.65 mL as a single dose

Mechanism of Action As a live, attenuated vaccine (Oka/Merck strain of varicella-zoster virus), zoster virus vaccine stimulates active immunity to disease caused by the varicella-zoster virus. Administration has been demonstrated to protect against the development of herpes zoster, with the highest efficacy in patients 60-69 years of age. It may also reduce the severity of complications, including postherpetic neuralgia, in patients who develop zoster following vaccination.

Pharmacodynamics/Kinetics

Onset of Action Seroconversion: ~6 weeks

Duration of Action Not established; protection has been demonstrated for at least 4 years

Pregnancy Considerations Use during pregnancy is contraindicated. Women should avoid becoming pregnant for 3 months after vaccination (4 weeks per CDC). Risk to the fetus following exposure to wild-type varicella zoster virus is small and risk following exposure from the attenuated vaccine is probably even less. Inadvertent exposure to the vaccine during pregnancy should be reported to Merck's National Service Center (800-986-8999).

Zucapsaicin (zu kap SAY sin)

Brand Names: Canada ZUACTA™

Pharmacologic Category Analgesic, Topical; Topical Skin Product; Transient Receptor Potential Vanilloid 1 (TRPV1) Agonist

Use In conjunction with an oral NSAID or COX-2 inhibitor for short-term (≤3 months) treatment of severe pain associated with osteoarthritis of the knee that is not controlled by NSAID or COX-2 inhibitor monotherapy

Local Anesthetic/Vasoconstrictor Precautions No information available to require special precautions

Effects on Dental Treatment The safety and efficacy of zucapsaicin have only been assessed in treating pain associated with osteoarthritis of the knee; its use as a topical application in treating pain of the temporomandibular joint in the patient with temporomandibular dysfunction has not been studied and is not recommended (see Warnings/Precautions)

Effects on Bleeding No information available to require special precautions

Adverse Effects

>10%: Local: Application site: Burning (22% to 35%)

1% to 10%:
Dermatologic: Burning sensation (2%)
Local: Application site: Warming (4% to 6%), reaction (4%), anesthesia (3%), irritation (1%), pruritus (1%), rash (1%)
Neuromuscular & skeletal: Arthralgia (1%)
Ocular: Eye irritation (1%)
Respiratory: Cough (2%), sneezing (1%)

Dosage Topical: Adults: Apply a pea-sized amount to each of 3 locations around affected knee 3 times/day; allow at least 4 hours between applications (maximum: 3 applications/day). **Note:** Should be used concomitantly with an oral NSAID or COX-2 inhibitor.

Mechanism of Action Actions are thought to be similar to other capsaicinoids, such as capsaicin, which is a transient receptor potential vanilloid 1 receptor (TRPV1) agonist, that activates TRPV1 ligand-gated cation channels on nociceptive nerve fibers, resulting in depolarization, initiation of action potential, and pain signal transmission to the spinal cord; capsaicin exposure results in subsequent desensitization of the sensory axons, depletion of proinflammatory neuropeptides (eg, calcitonin gene-related peptide, substance P) and inhibition of pain transmission initiation. In arthritis, capsaicin induces release of substance P, the principal chemomediator of pain impulses from the periphery to the CNS, from peripheral sensory neurons; after repeated application, capsaicin depletes the neuron of substance P and prevents reaccumulation. The functional link between substance P and the capsaicin receptor, TRPV1, is not well understood.

Contraindications Hypersensitivity to zucapsaicin or any component of the formulation; application to broken or irritated skin or areas with a compromised skin barrier

Warnings/Precautions May induce cough; do not apply to the face. Wash hands thoroughly after each application. Avoid contact with eyes, lips, or genital areas. Avoid application of other topical products to zucapsaicin treated areas. Safety and efficacy have only been assessed in treating pain associated with osteoarthritis of the knee; use in other arthritic conditions (eg, rheumatoid arthritis, psoriatic arthritis), musculoskeletal disorders (eg, fibromyalgia), or severe neurologic or vascular disease has not been studied and is not recommended.

Drug Interactions

Metabolism/Transport Effects None known.

Avoid Concomitant Use There are no known interactions where it is recommended to avoid concomitant use.

Increased Effect/Toxicity There are no known significant interactions involving an increase in effect.

Decreased Effect There are no known significant interactions involving a decrease in effect.

Pregnancy Considerations Animal studies have not demonstrated adverse effects. Use has not been studied in pregnant women. Systemic absorption, following topical administration, has not been observed in healthy patients. Systemic absorption would be required in order for zucapsaicin to cross the placenta and reach the fetus.

Lactation Excretion in human breast milk is unknown/ use caution

Product Availability Not available in the U.S.

Dosage Forms: Canada

Cream, topical:
Zuacta™: 0.075% (30 g, 60 g)

ALPHABETICAL LISTING OF
NATURAL PRODUCTS

Acacia Gum

Clinical Overview

Use

Acacia gum has been used in pharmaceuticals as a demulcent. It is used topically for healing wounds and has been shown to inhibit the growth of periodontic bacteria and the early deposition of plaque.

Dosing

Gum acacia is usually used to modify the physical properties of foods. It was used in a clinical study of cholesterol reduction at a dose of 15 g per day.

Contraindications

Contraindications have not yet been identified.

Pregnancy/Lactation

Information regarding safety and efficacy in pregnancy and lactation is lacking.

Interactions

None well documented.

Adverse Reactions

Ingestion may raise serum cholesterol. Various forms of acacia gum can cause allergic reactions, including respiratory problems and skin lesions.

Toxicology

Acacia is essentially nontoxic when ingested.

Local Anesthetic/Vasoconstrictor Precautions No information available to require special precautions
Effects on Bleeding None reported

Acai

Clinical Overview

Use

Antioxidant and anti-inflammatory activity of acai has been documented. Folk medicinal uses include treatment of fever, pain, and flu. The fruit's dark green oil has been used as an antidiarrheal agent. However, there is a lack of clinical information to recommend acai for any use.

Dosing

Numerous dosage forms are available including juices, powders, capsules, liquids, creams, and lotions. Capsule dosage guidelines are typically 1,000 mg once or twice daily with food. Follow manufacturers' suggested regimen.

Contraindications

Avoid use if hypersensitivity to any acai palm components exists.

Pregnancy/Lactation

Information regarding safety and efficacy in pregnancy and lactation is lacking.

Interactions

None well documented.

Adverse Reactions

No data.

Toxicology

No data.

Local Anesthetic/Vasoconstrictor Precautions No information available to require special precautions
Effects on Bleeding None reported

Agrimony

Clinical Overview

Use

Agrimony is used as a tea and gargle for sore throat, and externally as a mild antiseptic and astringent.

Dosing

There is no published clinical evidence for a safe or effective dose; however, the German Komission E recommended a daily dose of 3 g of the herb for internal use. Agrimony also is used as a poultice from a 10% decoction of the herb.

Contraindications

Contraindications have not yet been identified.

Pregnancy/Lactation

Information regarding safety and efficacy in pregnancy and lactation is lacking.

Interactions

None well documented.

Adverse Reactions

Agrimony reportedly can produce photodermatitis.

Toxicology

No data.

Local Anesthetic/Vasoconstrictor Precautions No information available to require special precautions
Effects on Bleeding None reported

Alfalfa

Clinical Overview

Use

There is no evidence supporting the use of various parts of the alfalfa plant for diuretic, anti-inflammatory, antidiabetic, or antiulcer purposes. Results from 1 small human study showed that the plant might reduce cholesterol levels.

Dosing

Alfalfa seeds are used commonly as a supplement to lower cholesterol at doses of 0.75 to 3 g/day; however, clinical trials have not been performed to validate this dosage.

Contraindications

The FDA issued an advisory indicating that children, the elderly, and people with compromised immune systems should avoid eating alfalfa sprouts because of frequent bacterial contamination.

Pregnancy/Lactation

Documented adverse effects. May cause uterine stimulation. Avoid use.

Interactions

The vitamin K found in alfalfa can antagonize the anticoagulant effect of warfarin, resulting in decreased anticoagulant activity and lowered prothrombin time. Based on the potential immunostimulating effect of alfalfa, it has been theorized that alfalfa may interfere with the immunosuppressive action of corticosteroids (eg, prednisone) or cyclosporine.

Adverse Reactions

Alfalfa ingestion, especially of the seeds, has been associated with various deleterious effects, and alfalfa seeds and fresh sprouts can be contaminated with bacteria such as S. enterica and E. coli. The FDA issued an advisory indicating that children, the elderly, and people with compromised immune systems should avoid eating alfalfa sprouts. Ingestion of dried alfalfa preparations is generally without important side effects in healthy adults.

Toxicology

Alfalfa tablets have been associated with the reactivation of SLE in at least 2 patients. Changes in intestinal cellular morphology were noted in rats fed alfalfa.

Local Anesthetic/Vasoconstrictor Precautions No information available to require special precautions

Effects on Bleeding As a single agent, alfalfa has no effect on bleeding. Due to the vitamin K content found in alfalfa, it has the potential to reduce the anticoagulant effect of warfarin.

Almond

Clinical Overview

Use

Almonds are used as a dietary source of protein, unsaturated fats, minerals, micronutrients, phytochemicals, alpha-tocopheral, and fiber, as well as in confectioneries. The efficacy of almonds in altering the lipid profile is weakly supported by the literature; larger, more robust clinical trials of longer duration are required. The almond derivative laetrile/amygdalin has been used as an alternative cancer treatment, but there is no clinical evidence to support this use. Laetrile is banned by the US Food and Drug Administration (FDA) and in Europe for use in cancer therapy.

Dosing

Trials of almond dietary supplementation in adults have used 25 to 168 g of almonds per day. The American Heart Association (AHA) recommends the daily intake of nuts (28.35 to 56.7 g) as part of a healthy diet. There is no widely accepted standard for laetrile/amygdalin dosing due to the potential for toxicity and no evidence for efficacy.

Contraindications

Allergy to almonds or its products.

Pregnancy/Lactation

Consumption of bitter almond or laetrile is not recommended in pregnant or breast-feeding women because of insufficient data and a theoretical risk of birth defects. Consumption of sweet almond has generally recognized as safe (GRAS) status when used as food. Avoid dosages above those found in food because safety is unproven.

Interactions

None well documented.

Adverse Reactions

Adverse reactions similar to those of cyanide poisoning have been reported.

Toxicology

Cyanide poisoning and death have resulted from laetrile and bitter almond consumption.

Local Anesthetic/Vasoconstrictor Precautions No information available to require special precautions

Effects on Bleeding None reported

Aloe

Clinical Overview

Use

Topical aloe appears to inhibit infection and promote healing of minor burns and wounds, frostbite, as well as in skin affected by diseases such as psoriasis and seborrheic dermatitis, although studies have had conflicting results. Dried aloe latex should be ingested with caution as a drastic cathartic, but its use is not recommended. In 2002, the US Food and Drug Administration required all over-the-counter aloe laxative products to be removed from the US market or reformulated because manufacturers have not provided the necessary safety data.

Dosing

As a gel, A. vera may be applied externally. The resin product is cathartic and not recommended for internal use.

Contraindications

Ingestion is contraindicated in pregnant and breast-feeding women, children younger than 12 years of age, patients with inflammatory bowel disease, and elderly patients with suspected intestinal obstruction.

Pregnancy/Lactation

Documented adverse effects with ingestion; do not use. Cathartic, reputed abortifacient.

Interactions

Potential interactions between ingested aloe resin and the following medications have been identified: digoxin, furosemide, thiazide diuretics, sevoflurane stimulant laxatives, and antidiabetic agents.

Adverse Reactions

There has been 1 report that aloe gel as standard wound therapy delayed healing. The gel may cause burning sensations in dermabraded skin, and redness and itching also can occur. Use caution with cosmetic products containing A. vera gel. A case of acute hepatitis induced by aloe vera ingestion has been reported.

Toxicology

The resin product is cathartic at doses of 250 mg and is not recommended for internal use.

Local Anesthetic/Vasoconstrictor Precautions No information available to require special precautions.

Effects on Bleeding None reported

Alpha-Lipoic Acid

Clinical Overview

Use

Alpha-lipoic acid (ALA) has been used as an antioxidant for the treatment of diabetes and HIV. It also has been used for cancer, liver ailments, and various other conditions.

Dosing

Oral dosage of alpha-lipoic acid given in numerous clinical studies ranges from 300 to 1,800 mg daily. It also is given intravenously at similar daily dosages.

Contraindications

Contraindications have not yet been determined.

Pregnancy/Lactation

Information regarding safety and efficacy in pregnancy and lactation is lacking.

Interactions

None well documented.

Adverse Reactions

No adverse reactions have been reported.

Toxicology

No data.

Local Anesthetic/Vasoconstrictor Precautions No information available to require special precautions

Effects on Bleeding None reported

Andrographis

Clinical Overview

Use

Kalmegh has been used for liver complaints and fever, and as an anti-inflammatory and immunostimulant. In clinical trials, Andrographis extract has been studied for use as an immunostimulant in upper respiratory tract infections and HIV infection. The potential of andrographolide as an anticancer agent is being investigated. However, clinical evidence to support the use of Kalmegh for any indication is lacking.

Dosing

The usual daily dose of andrographolides for common cold, sinusitis, and tonsillitis is 60 mg. Doses of 10 mg/kg resulted in the discontinuation of a clinical trial because of adverse reactions. Clinical trials in children with upper respiratory tract infection reported the use of andrographolide 30 mg daily for 10 days.

Contraindications

Contraindications have not been identified.

Pregnancy/Lactation

Documented adverse reactions. Abortifacient. Avoid use.

Interactions

None well documented.

Adverse Reactions

Headache, fatigue, rash, bitter/metallic taste, diarrhea, pruritus, and decreased sex drive were reported in 1 clinical trial. One HIV-positive participant experienced an anaphylactic reaction. Doses used in this trial were 10 mg/kg body weight.

Toxicology

Data are limited. Male reproductive adverse reaction studies have been equivocal.

Local Anesthetic/Vasoconstrictor Precautions No information available to require special precautions

Effects on Bleeding None reported

Angelica

Clinical Overview

Use

Often used as a flavoring or scent, angelica has been used medicinally to stimulate gastric secretion, treat flatulence, and topically treat rheumatic and skin disorders; however, there is little documentation to support these uses.

Dosing

Angelica root typically is given at doses of 3 to 6 g/day of the crude root.

Contraindications

The leaf and seed of angelica are unapproved.

Pregnancy/Lactation

Documented adverse effects. Emmenagogue effects. Avoid use.

Interactions

Avoid using angelica root concurrently with warfarin.

Adverse Reactions

Furanocoumarins in the plant may cause photodermatitis.

Toxicology

Poisoning has been reported with high doses of angelica oils.

Local Anesthetic/Vasoconstrictor Precautions No information available to require special precautions

Effects on Bleeding Angelica root has the potential to increase the risk of bleeding or potentiate the effects of warfarin.

Anise

Clinical Overview

Use

Anise has been used as a flavoring in alcohols, liqueurs, dairy products, gelatins, puddings, meats, and candies, and as a scent in perfumes, soaps, and sachets. The oil has been used to treat lice, scabies, and psoriasis. Anise frequently is used as a carminative and expectorant. Anise also is used to decrease bloating and settle the digestive tract in children. In

high doses, it is used as an antispasmodic and an antiseptic and for the treatment of cough, asthma, and bronchitis. However, research reveals no clinical data regarding the use of anise for any of these applications.

Dosing

There are no recent clinical studies to guide use of anise; however, typical use in dyspepsia is 0.5 to 3 g of seed, or 0.1 to 0.3 mL of the essential oil.

Contraindications

Anise is not recommended for use in pregnancy.

Pregnancy/Lactation

Aniseed is a reputed abortifacient. Excessive use is not recommended in pregnancy.

Interactions

None well documented.

Adverse Reactions

Anise may cause allergic reactions of the skin, respiratory tract, and gastrointestinal tract.

Toxicology

Ingestion of the oil may result in pulmonary edema, vomiting, and seizures.

Local Anesthetic/Vasoconstrictor Precautions No information available to require special precautions

Effects on Bleeding None reported

Arnica

Clinical Overview

Use

Arnica and its extracts have been widely used in folk and homeopathic medicine as a treatment for acne, boils, bruises, rashes, sprains, pains, and other wounds. Overall, there does not appear to be sufficient evidence to support the use of arnica as an anti-inflammatory or analgesic agent, or to prevent bruising; however, heterogeneity of doses and delivery forms (as well as indications) in available clinical studies makes generalizations difficult.

Dosing

Arnica should not be administered orally or applied to broken skin where absorption can occur. No consensus exists on topical dosing, and evidence from clinical trials is lacking to support therapeutic dosing. In *homeopathic* use, less concentrated strengths such as 200 C, 1 M (1,000 C), and 10 M (10,000 C) (C = centisimal dilution [1 part in 100]; M = millesimal dilution [1 part in 1,000]), are recommended for use pre- and postsurgically; clinical evidence is lacking to support therapeutic dosing.

Contraindications

Contraindications have not been identified.

Pregnancy/Lactation

Uterine stimulant action. Avoid use.

Interactions

None well documented.

Adverse Reactions

Homeopathic doses of arnica are unlikely to exert any adverse reactions because of the minimal amount ingested. Arnica irritates mucous membranes and causes stomach pain, diarrhea, and vomiting. Allergy and contact dermatitis have been reported.

Toxicology

The plant is poisonous and ingestion can cause gastroenteritis, dyspnea, cardiac arrest, and death.

Local Anesthetic/Vasoconstrictor Precautions May cause serious interactions with anesthetic drugs

Effects on Bleeding May see increased bleeding due to inhibition of platelet aggregation

Artichoke

Clinical Overview

Use

Artichoke has been used for its antioxidant and GI soothing effects. It also may have cytoprotective actions in the liver and hypocholesterolemic effects.

Dosing

Artichoke leaf extract at 1.5 g/day was found to lower serum cholesterol and triglycerides in a postmarketing survey study.

Contraindications

Contraindications to the use of artichoke include allergy to Asteraceae family plants and any bile duct obstruction.

Pregnancy/Lactation

Generally recognized as safe or used as food. Avoid dosages above those found in food because safety and efficacy are unproven.

Interactions

None well documented.

Adverse Reactions

Artichoke can cause allergic reactions in sensitive individuals, most commonly dermatitis.

Toxicology

Lack of toxicity data suggests limiting use during pregnancy and lactation.

Local Anesthetic/Vasoconstrictor Precautions No information available to require special precautions

Effects on Bleeding None reported

Ashwagandha

Clinical Overview

Use

Ashwagandha has been used as an adaptogen, diuretic, and sedative and is available in the United States as a dietary supplement. Trials supporting its clinical use are limited; however, many in vitro and animal experiments suggest effects on the immune and CNS systems, as well as in the pathogenesis of cancer and inflammatory conditions.

Dosing

Dosing information is limited. W. somnifera root powder has generally been used at dosages of 450 mg to 2 g in combination with other preparations.

Contraindications

Contraindications have not been identified.

Pregnancy/Lactation

Abortifacient properties have been reported for ashwagandha. Avoid use.

Interactions

None well documented.

Adverse Reactions

Limited clinical trials are available and case reports are lacking.

Toxicology

Acute toxicity of W. somnifera is modest; at reasonable doses, ashwagandha is nontoxic.

Local Anesthetic/Vasoconstrictor Precautions No information available to require special precautions

Effects on Bleeding None reported

Asparagus

Clinical Overview

Use

Asparagus stalks are commonly eaten as a vegetable. Roots, seeds, and extracts have been used as a treatment for various illnesses and as a diuretic, despite the lack of clinical evidence. Other species, such as Asparagus racemosus, are used in traditional Chinese and Ayurvedic medicine systems.

Dosing

There is insufficient clinical evidence to guide the dosage of asparagus. A maximum of 2.4 g daily of dried asparagus root in divided doses contained in a combination preparation with parsley has been evaluated for antihypertensive effect; however, adverse reactions led to significant participant withdrawal from the study.

Contraindications

Contraindications have not yet been identified.

Pregnancy/Lactation

Generally recognized as safe when used as food. Avoid dosages above those found in food because safety and efficacy are unknown.

Interactions

None well documented.

Adverse Reactions

Symptoms of allergy, including rhinitis, occupational asthma, oral allergic syndrome, allergic contact dermatitis, and anaphylaxis, are well documented. Exacerbation of gout with excessive consumption has been reported.

Toxicology

Information is lacking.

Local Anesthetic/Vasoconstrictor Precautions No information available to require special precautions

Effects on Bleeding None reported

Astragalus

Clinical Overview

Use

Astragalus root may have use in the restoration of immune function after cancer chemotherapy and for the treatment of HIV infection. However, there are no clinical trials to support any of these uses.

Dosing

There is no recent clinical evidence to guide dosage of astragalus products; however, typical recommendations are 2 to 6 g daily of the powdered root.

Contraindications

Contraindications have not yet been identified.

Pregnancy/Lactation

Information regarding safety and efficacy in pregnancy and lactation is lacking.

Interactions

None well documented.

Adverse Reactions

Astragalus extract was mutagenic in the Ames test for possible carcinogens.

Toxicology

No data.

Local Anesthetic/Vasoconstrictor Precautions No information available to require special precautions

Effects on Bleeding Astragalus may increase the risk of bleeding.

Barberry

Clinical Overview

Use
The fruits have been used in jams, jellies, and juices. Plant alkaloids have been found to be antibacterial, antifungal, anti-inflammatory, antioxidant, and antidiarrheal. Berberine is a uterine stimulant.

Dosing
Barberry berries and root bark have been used as a source of berberine. Daily doses of 2 g of the berries have been used, but there are no clinical studies to substantiate barberry's varied uses.

Contraindications
Barberry is contraindicated in patients with hypersensitivity to M. aquifolium.

Pregnancy/Lactation
Documented adverse effects (including uterine stimulant effects). Avoid use.

Interactions
None well documented.

Adverse Reactions
Hypersensitivity reactions (eg, burning, itching, redness) have occurred in some patients using topical dosage forms.

Toxicology
Symptoms of poisoning are characterized by lethargy, stupor and daze, vomiting and diarrhea, and nephritis. Barberry is contraindicated during lactation and pregnancy.

Local Anesthetic/Vasoconstrictor Precautions No information available to require special precautions
Effects on Bleeding None reported

Bee Pollen

Clinical Overview

Use
Although bee pollen is nutritionally rich, claims that it enhances everyday and athletic performance have not been reliably verified. It has been traditionally used for a variety of purposes, including relief of constipation; treatment of prostatic conditions, such as prostatitis, benign prostatic hyperplasia, and prostate cancer; wound healing; and for its proposed antioxidant action. It also has been promoted as an energy booster, immune system strengthener, and vitality enhancer. Bee pollen has been used to prevent hay fever, but there is a risk of severe allergic reaction with this practice. It may also relieve premenstrual syndrome and climacteric symptoms associated with menopause.

Dosing
The best recommended dose of bee pollen is unknown. Doses vary among products because tablets contain differing amounts of bee pollen. Manufacturers' recommendations may provide more guidance.

Contraindications
None well documented.

Pregnancy/Lactation
Clinical data regarding safety and efficacy in pregnancy and lactation are lacking. However, use in pregnant rats resulted in fetuses with higher birth weights and decreased death rates, suggesting that bee pollen may be an effective prenatal nutrient.

Interactions
None well documented.

Adverse Reactions
Ingestion produces allergic reactions in sensitive individuals. Attempts to hyposensitize patients by administering bee pollen may produce severe anaphylaxis and other acute or chronic responses. Although rare, bee pollen can cause serious, sometimes fatal, adverse reactions. Some case reports of acute hepatitis and photosensitivity following ingestion of bee pollen have been reported.

Toxicology
Research reveals little or no information regarding toxicity with the use of this product.

Local Anesthetic/Vasoconstrictor Precautions No information available to require special precautions
Effects on Bleeding None reported

Beta Sitosterol

Clinical Overview

Use
Cholesterol lowering and symptom improvement in mild to moderate benign prostatic hypertrophy. Possible role in the control of chronic inflammatory conditions.

Dosing
Beta sitosterol is incorporated in margarine, yogurt, or other foods to give a daily intake of 1.5 to 3 g.

Contraindications
Contraindications have not yet been identified.

Pregnancy/Lactation
Information regarding safety and efficacy in pregnancy and lactation is lacking.

Interactions
None well documented.

Adverse Reactions
No major adverse effects at recommended dose. Reduced absorption of carotenes and vitamin E may occur.

Toxicology
No data.

Local Anesthetic/Vasoconstrictor Precautions No information available to require special precautions
Effects on Bleeding None reported

Bilberry

Clinical Overview

Use
Dried bilberry tea is used internally to treat nonspecific diarrhea and topically to treat inflamed mouth and throat mucosa. Bilberry extracts may improve visual acuity and ability to adjust to changing light. Derivatives demonstrate vasoprotective, antiedema, and gastroprotective effects.

Dosing
Typical bilberry products are standardized to 25% anthocyanoside content. One recent study administered 160 mg of the extract tid to improve night vision.

Contraindications
Contraindications have not yet been identified.

Pregnancy/Lactation
Generally recognized as safe or used as food. Avoid dosages above those found in food because safety and efficacy are unproven.

Interactions
None well documented.

Adverse Reactions
No data.

Toxicology

The effects of ingesting large doses of bilberry are not known.

Local Anesthetic/Vasoconstrictor Precautions No information available to require special precautions

Effects on Bleeding May increase risk of bleeding by inhibiting platelet aggregation

Bitter Melon

Clinical Overview

Use

There is insufficient evidence from quality clinical trials to recommend the use of bitter melon as a therapeutic option in type 2 diabetes.

Dosing

Bitter melon juice has been recommended for diabetes at daily doses of 50 to 100 mL; 900 mg of fruit given 3 times/day has also been given for the same indication. There is insufficient clinical trial evidence to substantiate these doses.

Contraindications

Patients deficient in glucose-6-phosphate dehydrogenase should avoid consumption of bitter melon preparations due to the presence of vicine in the seeds.

Pregnancy/Lactation

Documented adverse reactions include emmenagogue and abortifacient effects. Avoid use.

Interactions

None well documented.

Adverse Reactions

Bitter melon generally causes few adverse reactions. GI effects (eg, abdominal pain, diarrhea) and headache have been reported in clinical trials. Case reports exist of hypoglycemic coma and atrial fibrillation associated with bitter melon intake. Increases in liver enzymes have been observed experimentally, but without histological changes. Bitter melon should be used with caution in patients with impaired hepatic function.

Toxicology

The red arils around bitter melon seeds are toxic to children.

Local Anesthetic/Vasoconstrictor Precautions No information available to require special precautions

Effects on Bleeding None reported

Bitter Orange

Clinical Overview

Use

Pharmacological actions for C. aurantium include the following: antispasmodic, sedative, tranquilizer, cholagogue, demulcent, eupeptic, tonic, and vascular stimulant; as an anti-inflammatory, antibacterial, and antifungal agent; and for reducing cholesterol; however, clinical data is limited. Most medical literature focuses on the safety and efficacy of its use in over-the-counter weight-loss supplement formulations. Studies examining this use have used small sample sizes and often focus on combination products.

Dosing

Follow manufacturer's dosage guidelines because synephrine content may vary in supplement formulation. There is evidence of effective weight loss at a synephrine dose of 32 mg/day in treating obesity.

Contraindications

Because of the potential for additive effects, synephrine use is best avoided in patients with hypertension, tachyarrhythmia, or narrow angle glaucoma.

Pregnancy/Lactation

Avoid use due to lack of clinical data regarding safety and efficacy during pregnancy and lactation.

Interactions

Bitter orange may inhibit intestinal CYP3A4 and intestinal efflux and may interact with numerous drugs, including anxiolytics, antidepressants, antiviral agents, calcium channel blockers, dextromethorphan, GI prokinetic agents, vasoconstrictors, and weight-loss formulas.

Adverse Reactions

There are numerous case reports of adverse cardiac reactions associated with C. aurantium extract use.

Toxicology

Medical literature primarily documents cardiovascular toxicity, especially due to the stimulant amines synephrine, octopamine, and N-methyltyramine, which may cause vasoconstriction as well as increased heart rate and blood pressure.

Local Anesthetic/Vasoconstrictor Precautions Synephrine, the main chemical constituent in the fruit, is a sympathomimetic amine having properties of vasoconstriction and tachycardia. Use vasoconstrictor with caution; synephrine may interact with epinephrine and levonordefrin to cause a pressor response.

Effects on Bleeding None reported

Bittersweet Nightshade

Clinical Overview

Use

Bittersweet nightshade has been used as a traditional external remedy for skin abrasions and inflammation. The stems were approved by the German Commission E for external use as supportive therapy in chronic eczema (see Toxicology).

Dosing

Traditional use of the stem has been at a dosage of 1 to 3 g/day, usually given as a decoction or infusion in 250 mL of water.

Contraindications

Contraindications have not yet been identified.

Pregnancy/Lactation

Documented teratogenic effects of the glycoalkaloids in animals. Avoid use.

Interactions

None well documented.

Adverse Reactions

No data.

Toxicology

The plant is toxic. Ingestion of unripened berries should be considered a medical emergency. Symptoms may be delayed for several hours.

Local Anesthetic/Vasoconstrictor Precautions No information available to require special precautions

Effects on Bleeding None reported

Black Cohosh

Clinical Overview

Use

Black cohosh has been used to help manage some symptoms of menopause and as an alternative to hormone replacement therapy (HRT). It may be useful ▶

◀ for treatment of hypercholesteremia or peripheral arterial disease. Clinical studies do not support these uses.

Dosing

On the basis of clinical studies, the currently recommended daily dose of black cohosh is a 40% to 60% ethanol or isopropanol extract of 40 to 80 mg herbal drug that is standardized to contain 1 mg of triterpene 27-deoxyactein per 20 mg tablet. Counsel patients that therapeutic effects generally begin after 2 weeks, with maximum effects usually observed within 8 weeks.

Contraindications

Patients with aspirin sensitivity because it contains salicylates.

Pregnancy/Lactation

Black cohosh is contraindicated in pregnancy and may cause premature birth in large doses. Avoid black cohosh during lactation.

Interactions

None well documented.

Adverse Reactions

There is a low incidence of adverse reactions.

Toxicology

Overdose of black cohosh may cause nausea, vomiting, dizziness, nervous system and visual disturbances, reduced pulse rate, and increased perspiration. Case reports primarily document hepatic toxicity; however, cardiovascular and circulatory disorders and 1 case of convulsions have been documented.

Local Anesthetic/Vasoconstrictor Precautions No information available to require special precautions

Effects on Bleeding None reported

Black Currant

Clinical Overview

Use

From the limited data, black currant oil and juice extracts appear useful as an antioxidant source and in treating rheumatoid arthritis and night and fatigue-related visual impairment; the oil and juice extracts also exhibit limited antimicrobial and anticancer properties.

Dosing

No trials have been conducted to establish appropriate dosage.

Contraindications

Contraindications have not been identified.

Pregnancy/Lactation

Information regarding safety and efficacy in pregnancy and lactation is lacking.

Interactions

None well documented.

Adverse Reactions

No adverse reactions have been reported. Although no direct evidence is available, use caution in epileptic patients because of reports of lowered seizure threshold with evening primrose oil.

Toxicology

No toxicity, carcinogenicity, or teratogenicity has been reported.

Local Anesthetic/Vasoconstrictor Precautions No information available to require special precautions

Effects on Bleeding None reported

Black Walnut

Clinical Overview

Use

Black walnut has many traditional uses; however, there are no human trials to support these effects. Black walnuts are a good dietary source of essential fatty acids.

Dosing

No clinical trials are available to support dosage recommendations.

Contraindications

None well documented.

Pregnancy/Lactation

Avoid use. Documented adverse reactions (mutagenic properties).

Interactions

None well documented.

Adverse Reactions

Allergic reactions have occurred.

Toxicology

The quinones juglone and plumbagin found in black walnut are regarded as toxins.

Local Anesthetic/Vasoconstrictor Precautions No information available to require special precautions

Effects on Bleeding None reported

Blessed Thistle

Clinical Overview

Use

Blessed thistle is used to stimulate secretion of gastric juices and saliva, to increase appetite and facilitate digestion, and to stimulate the flow of bile. It has been used as a minor component of the alternative cancer remedy Flor-Essence and has antibacterial and antifungal activity. Other pharmacologic activities for blessed thistle include blockade of gonadotropin and anti-inflammatory properties. However, there are no reported human clinical trials for any of these uses.

Dosing

There are no clinical studies to justify dosing of blessed thistle. Traditionally, 4 to 6 g of blessed thistle is used daily.

Contraindications

Because of its irritating effect, blessed thistle is contraindicated in gastric ulcer or in inflammatory bowel conditions such as Crohn disease.

Pregnancy/Lactation

Blessed thistle should not be used in pregnancy. No evidence exists to support the efficacy of its common use to promote lactation.

Interactions

None well documented.

Adverse Reactions

People sensitive to the sesquiterpene lactones of other asteraceous plants should use blessed thistle with caution. Blessed thistle extract was strongly sensitizing in a study of 12 species in the family Asteraceae.

Toxicology

At high single doses (5 to 6 g) blessed thistle is known to be emetic.

Local Anesthetic/Vasoconstrictor Precautions No information available to require special precautions

Effects on Bleeding None reported

Blue Cohosh

Clinical Overview

Use

Blue cohosh has been used to induce uterine contractions. It is widely advertised on the internet but is dangerous (see Toxicology and Adverse Reactions).

Dosing

Blue cohosh has traditionally been used at doses of 0.5 to 3 g/day; however, its potential for teratogenicity makes it unsuitable for women who are or may become pregnant. Because its principal indications are for gynecological disorders, avoid its use.

Contraindications

Contraindications have not yet been identified.

Pregnancy/Lactation

Documented adverse effects (including GI symptoms, contraction of uterine muscle, arterial constriction, inhibition of embryo implantation, and abortifacient effects). Avoid use.

Interactions

None well documented.

Adverse Reactions

Because blue cohosh can be toxic to humans and fetuses, there is little or no information about adverse reactions. Its toxicity appears to outweigh any medical benefit.

Toxicology

Blue cohosh root is potentially toxic to humans and fetuses.

Local Anesthetic/Vasoconstrictor Precautions No information available to require special precautions

Effects on Bleeding None reported

Boldo

Clinical Overview

Use

Boldo has been shown to possess cytoprotective and anti-inflammatory actions and to improve GI disorders; however, there is limited data to support these uses.

Dosing

Boldo extract was studied at a dose of 2.5 g daily for its effect on intestinal transit time. Classical use of boldo leaves was at a dose of 0.5 g.

Contraindications

Patients with kidney disorders, liver disease, gallstones, and other medical illnesses should not use this herbal.

Pregnancy/Lactation

Documented adverse effects from the irritant oil. Avoid use.

Interactions

Boldo ingestion may enhance the anticoagulant effect of warfarin, increasing the risk of bleeding. Patients taking warfarin should consult their health care provider before taking boldo or other herbal products.

Adverse Reactions

Boldo is known to be a CNS stimulant.

Toxicology

Serious health hazards exist with internal use. Patients with kidney disorders, liver disease, gallstones, and other medical illnesses should not use this herbal. Large doses cause paralysis and death.

Local Anesthetic/Vasoconstrictor Precautions No information available to require special precautions

Effects on Bleeding As a single agent, boldo has no effect on bleeding. Boldo may enhance the anticoagulant effects of warfarin when taken simultaneously. This effect has not been confirmed.

Boneset

Clinical Overview

Use

Boneset has chiefly been used to treat fevers.

Dosing

There is no recent clinical evidence to guide dosage of boneset. Traditional use was at a dose of 2 g of leaves and flowers. Internal use should be tempered by the occurrence of hepatotoxic pyrrolizidine alkaloids in this plant.

Contraindications

Contraindications have not yet been identified.

Pregnancy/Lactation

Documented adverse effects, including cytotoxic constituents. Avoid use.

Interactions

None well documented.

Adverse Reactions

The FDA has classified boneset as an "Herb of Undefined Safety."

Toxicology

The ingestion of large amounts of teas or extracts may result in severe diarrhea. The identification of pyrrolizidine alkaloids in related Eupatorium species is cause for concern until detailed phytochemical investigations are carried out on boneset. This class of alkaloids is known to cause hepatic impairment after long-term ingestion. While direct evidence for a hepatotoxic effect from boneset does not exist, there is sufficient evidence to indicate that any plant containing unsaturated pyrrolizidine alkaloids should not be ingested.

Local Anesthetic/Vasoconstrictor Precautions No information available to require special precautions

Effects on Bleeding None reported

Borage

Clinical Overview

Use

Borage has been used in European herbal medicine since the Middle Ages, alone and in combination with fish oil in rheumatoid arthritis, atopic eczema, and osteoporosis, although limited clinical evidence is available to support these uses.

Dosing

Borage seed oil 1 to 3 g/day has been given in clinical trials (1 g/day has been used in children and up to 3 g/day in adults). The content of gamma-linolenic acid is between 20% and 26% of the oil.

Contraindications

Contraindications have not been identified.

Pregnancy/Lactation

Documented adverse effects (pyrrolizidine alkaloids). Avoid use.

Interactions

None well documented.

Adverse Reactions

No adverse effects have been reported. Although no direct evidence is available, caution is advised in patients with epilepsy because of reports of lowered seizure threshold with evening primrose oil.

Toxicology

The presence of unsaturated pyrrolizidine alkaloids in leaves, flowers, and seeds of borage suggests a potential for hepatotoxicity, although the total plant alkaloid content is low.

Local Anesthetic/Vasoconstrictor Precautions No information available to require special precautions
Effects on Bleeding None reported

Boron

Clinical Overview
Use

Boric acid is a topical astringent, mild disinfectant and eye wash. Sprinkled in crevices and corners, boric acid powder controls rodents and insects. Sodium borate is used in cold creams, eye washes and mouth rinses. Boron compounds are used to enhance the cell selectivity of radiation therapy.

Dosing

Boron has been studied in several clinical studies at a wide range of doses. Daily dosage of 2.5 to 6 mg as boron has been administered for osteoarthritis and strength conditioning. Intravaginal boric acid (600 mg daily) was administered for vulvovaginal candidiasis. A single dose of 102.6 mg sodium tetraborate was studied for its effects on factor VIIa.

Contraindications

Contraindications have not yet been identified.

Pregnancy/Lactation

Information regarding safety and efficacy in pregnancy and lactation is lacking.

Interactions

None well documented.

Adverse Reactions

There is little or no clinical data about the adverse effects of boron; boron compounds can be toxic to humans.

Toxicology

While boric acid, borates, and other compounds containing boron are used medicinally, they are potentially toxic if ingested or absorbed through nonintact skin.

Local Anesthetic/Vasoconstrictor Precautions No information available to require special precautions
Effects on Bleeding None reported

Bovine Colostrum

Clinical Overview
Use

Bovine colostrum has been used to treat diarrhea, to improve GI health, to boost the immune system.

Dosing

Bovine colostrum is a difficult preparation to standardize because its antibody content may vary widely. Some clinical studies have been performed with hyperimmune colostrum, which may have a specific antibody titer; however, most products do not meet this criterion. Studies administering 25 to 125 mL of liquid formulations or 10 to 20 g of dry powder have been reported.

Contraindications

Contraindications have not yet been identified.

Pregnancy/Lactation

Information regarding safety and efficacy in pregnancy and lactation is lacking.

Interactions

None well documented.

Adverse Reactions

Bovine colostrum is well tolerated. A few symptoms, including mild nausea and flatulence have been reported.

Toxicology

Bovine colostrum appears to be safe and effective. There is no data in the literature concerning any toxicities.

Local Anesthetic/Vasoconstrictor Precautions No information available to require special precautions
Effects on Bleeding None reported

Brahmi

Clinical Overview
Use

Brahmi is used as a nerve tonic and an aid to learning.

Dosing

A single clinical trial of brahmi's effects on cognition reported a daily dose of 300 mg of extract.

Contraindications

Contraindications have not yet been identified.

Pregnancy/Lactation

Information regarding safety and efficacy in pregnancy and lactation is lacking.

Interactions

None well documented.

Adverse Reactions

Brahmi appears to be free of reported adverse reactions. Brahmi has CNS effects, but no serious sedation.

Toxicology

Research reveals little or no information regarding toxicology with the use of this product.

Local Anesthetic/Vasoconstrictor Precautions No information available to require special precautions
Effects on Bleeding None reported

Brewer's yeast

Clinical Overview
Use

Brewer's yeast is traditionally used as a source of vitamin B, selenium, and chromium, especially by vegetarians. Clinical trials have evaluated yeast for a role in immunomodulation, respiratory infections, prevention of postsurgical infections (as beta-glucan), and as a source of dietary fiber to improve the lipid profile. However, there is a lack of quality trials.

Dosing

Upper respiratory tract infections: S. cerevisiae 500 mg daily has been used in clinical trials over 12 weeks to treat respiratory infections and allergic rhinitis.

Laxative: 6 to 50 g of fresh baker's yeast over 3 days was used in a study for the treatment of cancer-related constipation.

Acute diarrhea: 500 mg daily of brewer's yeast is recommended in the German Commission E Monographs.

Contraindications

Crohn disease; concomitant monoamine oxidase inhibitor (MAOI) therapy.

Pregnancy/Lactation

Information regarding safety and efficacy in pregnancy and lactation is lacking.

Interactions

Brewer's yeast contains tyramine. Avoid concurrent use with MAOIs.

Adverse Reactions

Mild GI symptoms, including flatulence.

Toxicology

Information is limited. Baker's yeast has Food and Drug Administration (FDA) GRAS (generally recognized as safe) status.

Local Anesthetic/Vasoconstrictor Precautions No information available to require special precautions

Effects on Bleeding None reported

Buchu

Clinical Overview

Use

Buchu has been used to treat inflammation and kidney and urinary tract infections; as a diuretic and as a stomach tonic. Other uses include carminative action and treatment of cystitis, urethritis, prostatitis and gout. It has also been used for leukorrhea and yeast infections.

Dosing

There is no recent clinical evidence to guide dosage of buchu. Classical doses were from 1 to 2 g of the leaves daily.

Contraindications

Contraindications have not yet been identified.

Pregnancy/Lactation

Documented adverse effects, including uterine stimulant effects. Avoid use.

Interactions

None well documented.

Adverse Reactions

Buchu can cause stomach and kidney irritation and can be an abortifacient. It can also induce increased menstrual flow. Buchu is not recommended during pregnancy.

Toxicology

Poisoning has not been reported. Buchu contains the hepatotoxin pulegone, also known to be present in pennyroyal.

Local Anesthetic/Vasoconstrictor Precautions No information available to require special precautions

Effects on Bleeding None reported

Bupleurum

Clinical Overview

Use

Bupleurum is being investigated for its antipyretic, immunomodulatory, GI tract, and hepatoprotective effects, as well as its potential in the prevention and treatment of cancers. Clinical trials are generally lacking.

Dosing

No clinical trials exist.

Contraindications

Contraindications have not been identified.

Pregnancy/Lactation

Information regarding safety and efficacy in pregnancy and lactation is lacking.

Interactions

None well documented.

Adverse Reactions

Mild lassitude, sedation, and drowsiness. Large doses may increase flatulence and bowel movements. Allergy to injected bupleurum has been reported.

Toxicology

The toxicity profile appears to be low; however, information is limited.

Local Anesthetic/Vasoconstrictor Precautions No information available to require special precautions

Effects on Bleeding None reported

Bur Marigold

Clinical Overview

Use

Several Bidens species have been, and continue to be, used extensively in folk medicine.

Dosing

There is no clinical evidence to guide dosage of bur marigold.

Contraindications

Contraindications have not been identified.

Pregnancy/Lactation

Information regarding safety and efficacy during pregnancy and lactation is lacking.

Interactions

None well documented.

Adverse Reactions

Cross-hypersensitivity to other members of the Asteraceae family is possible. Cell-mediated airway inflammation is possible for people with allergies and/or asthma.

Toxicology

Little information is available.

Local Anesthetic/Vasoconstrictor Precautions No information available to require special precautions

Effects on Bleeding None reported

Butcher's Broom

Clinical Overview

Use

Butcher's broom has been used in many forms as a laxative, diuretic, treatment for circulatory disease, and cytotoxic agent, although limited results from clinical trials are available.

Dosing

Butchers broom has been used in clinical trials for chronic venous insufficiency standardized to 7 to 11 mg of ruscogenin. Hesperidin methyl chalcone has also been used as a marker for standardization in the product Cyclo 3 Fort. Extracts have been dosed at 16 mg daily for chronic phlebopathy, while a topical cream formulation was used to apply 64 to 96 mg of extract daily.

Contraindications

Contraindications have not yet been identified.

Pregnancy/Lactation

Information regarding safety and efficacy in pregnancy and lactation is lacking. Avoid use.

Interactions

None well documented.

Adverse Reactions

No adverse reactions have been reported.

Toxicology

Not known to be toxic.

Local Anesthetic/Vasoconstrictor Precautions No information available to require special precautions

Effects on Bleeding None reported

Calendula

Clinical Overview

Use
Potential uses include treatment of radiation therapy-associated dermatitis and other inflammatory skin conditions. Few clinical trials are available to support traditional uses.

Dosing
Clinical trials are lacking. Commercial topical preparations are available.

Contraindications
Contraindications have not been identified.

Pregnancy/Lactation
Limited evidence is available to guide usage in pregnancy.

Interactions
None well documented.

Adverse Reactions
Allergic reactions, contact sensitization, and one case of anaphylaxis have been reported.

Toxicology
The plant appears to have a low potential for toxicity.

Local Anesthetic/Vasoconstrictor Precautions No information available to require special precautions
Effects on Bleeding None reported

Capsicum Peppers

Clinical Overview

Use
Many varieties are eaten as vegetables, condiments, and spices. The component capsaicin is an irritant and analgesic used in self-defense sprays, and in a variety of conditions associated with pain. Other studies have evaluated a role in weight loss, GI conditions, postoperative nausea, and rhinitis, although limited information is available.

Dosing
For external uses, capsaicin and Capsicum creams are available in several strengths, from 0.025% to 0.075% capsaicin. Clinical trials are lacking to guide dosage for other uses.

Contraindications
None clearly established.

Pregnancy/Lactation
Generally recognized as safe (GRAS) when used as food. Safety and efficacy for dosages above those in foods are unproven and should be avoided. Studies in animals have shown both positive and negative effects.

Interactions
Use of capsaicin by patients receiving captopril or other angiotensin-converting enzyme (ACE) inhibitors may cause or exacerbate ACE inhibitor-induced cough. Nonheme iron absorption may be inhibited by concomitant chili consumption.

Adverse Reactions
Topical, mucosal, and GI irritations are common. Allergies and cross-sensitization to other allergens have been reported.

Toxicology
Toxicity is evidenced in animal experiments in higher dosages. Controversy exists regarding capsaicin's mutagenicity and tumorigenicity. Toxicity from long-term exposure to chili powder has not been found, and the use of defense sprays likewise has not resulted in reports of toxicity.

Local Anesthetic/Vasoconstrictor Precautions No information available to require special precautions
Effects on Bleeding May have some antiplatelet effects

Cascara

Clinical Overview

Use
Limited clinical studies exist for cascara aside from those of its laxative effects. Attention has shifted to studying the effects of its constituent emodin, particularly with regard to possible therapeutic applications in the treatment of cancer.

Dosing
Cascara sagrada over-the-counter (OTC) laxative products were declared no longer safe and effective by the US Food and Drug Administration (FDA) in 2002. Typical doses of cascara are 1 g of bark, 2 to 6 mL of fluid extract or 325 mg of dried extract.

Contraindications
Cascara is contraindicated in ileus of any origin and in inflammatory diseases of the colon, including ulcerative colitis, irritable bowel syndrome (IBS), and Crohn disease.

Pregnancy/Lactation
Documented emmenagogue and abortifacient effects. Avoid use. Anthranoid metabolites may be excreted in breast milk.

Interactions
None well documented.

Adverse Reactions
Extended use may cause chronic diarrhea and consequent electrolyte imbalance.

Toxicology
Overdose of anthraquinone laxatives results in intestinal pain and severe diarrhea with consequent electrolyte imbalance and dehydration. No causal relationship between long-term use of cascara and colorectal cancer has been established. The carcinogenicity of emodin has been studied with equivocal results.

Local Anesthetic/Vasoconstrictor Precautions No information available to require special precautions
Effects on Bleeding None reported

Catnip

Clinical Overview

Use
There is little clinical data to support any use of catnip in humans, except as an insect repellant.

Dosing
There is no clinical evidence to guide dosage of catnip. Traditional doses for sedation require 4 g of dried herb, usually given as a tea. A 15% lotion of the essential oil has been used as an insect repellant.

Contraindications
None well documented.

Pregnancy/Lactation
Documented adverse effects when consumed (eg, emmenagogue and abortifacient effects). Avoid use.

Interactions
None well documented.

Adverse Reactions
Headache and malaise have been reported.

Toxicology
Information is lacking.

Local Anesthetic/Vasoconstrictor Precautions No
information available to require special precautions
Effects on Bleeding None reported

Cat's Claw

Clinical Overview
Use
Despite multiple purported effects, controlled clinical
trials are lacking. Suggested anti-inflammatory, anticancer, and immunostimulant properties are largely
based on in vitro and limited animal studies.

Dosing
One gram of root bark given 2 to 3 times daily is a
typical dose, while 20 to 30 mg of a root bark extract
has been recommended. Clinical trials are generally
lacking to support appropriate dosages. A standardized extract containing 8% to 10% carboxy alkyl
esters and less than 0.5% oxindole alkaloids has been
used in clinical studies in doses of 250 to 300 mg.

Contraindications
Cat's claw products should be avoided before and after
surgery, as well as by those using immunosuppressant
therapy and in children due to lack of safety data.

Pregnancy/Lactation
Information regarding safety and efficacy during pregnancy and lactation is lacking.

Interactions
Case reports are generally lacking; however, there is a
reported interaction with protease inhibitors.

Adverse Reactions
Although reports of adverse effects are rare, GI complaints (nausea, diarrhea, stomach discomfort), renal
effects, neuropathy, and an increased risk of bleeding
with anticoagulant therapy are possible.

Toxicology
Historical ethnomedicinal evidence and current use by
consumers suggest low toxicity; however, toxicological
studies are limited.

Local Anesthetic/Vasoconstrictor Precautions No
information available to require special precautions
Effects on Bleeding May cause increased bleeding
due to inhibition of platelet aggregation

Chamomile

Clinical Overview
Use
Chamomile is used topically in skin and mucous membrane inflammations and skin diseases. It can be
inhaled for respiratory tract inflammations or irritations;
used in baths as irrigation for anogenital inflammation;
and used internally for GI spasms and inflammatory
diseases. However, clinical trials supporting any use of
chamomile are limited.

Dosing
Chamomile has been used as a tea for various conditions and as a topical cream. Typical oral doses are 9
to 15 g/day. Gargles made from 8 g chamomile flowers
in 1,000 mL of water have been used in clinical trials.

Contraindications
The use of chamomile-containing preparations is contraindicated in persons with hypersensitivity to ragweed pollens.

Pregnancy/Lactation
Unreferenced adverse reactions have been cited.
Avoid use during pregnancy. No clinical data are
available on use during lactation.

Interactions
Possible interactions have been reported with warfarin
or cyclosporine. Because warfarin and cyclosporine
have a narrow therapeutic index, patients taking either
of these medications in other than modest amounts
should avoid concurrent use of chamomile.

Adverse Reactions
Use of the tea and essential oil has resulted in
anaphylaxis, contact dermatitis, and other severe
hypersensitivity reactions. Cross-reactivity to asters,
chrysanthemums, ragweed, and other members of
the Asteraceae family exists.

Toxicology
Animal studies report low toxicity with oral ingestion of
chamomile.

Local Anesthetic/Vasoconstrictor Precautions No
information available to require special precautions
Effects on Bleeding None reported

Chaparral

Clinical Overview
Use
Chaparral has been traditionally used for the treatment
of cancer, acne, rheumatism, and diabetes. It has also
been promoted for its antioxidant effects by inhibiting
free radicals. Chaparral has also been used as a blood
purifier and a weight loss agent. However, clinical trials
are lacking to support any of these uses.

Dosing
Because chaparral has been documented as hepatotoxic at doses of crude herb from 1.5 to 3.5 g/day, its
use is discouraged.

Contraindications
Chaparral was removed from the US Food and Drug
Administration's Generally Recognized as Safe
(GRAS) list in 1968. Increased risk for hepatotoxicity
is expected in patients with hepatic dysfunction. Chaparral is not recommended for use in patients with
renal dysfunction due to a risk for accumulation of
chaparral and toxicity.

Pregnancy/Lactation
Documented adverse effects (uterine activity, hepatotoxic). Avoid use.

Interactions
None well documented.

Adverse Reactions
The creosote bush can induce contact dermatitis.

Toxicology
Chaparral may cause liver damage, stimulate some
malignancies, and cause contact dermatitis.

Local Anesthetic/Vasoconstrictor Precautions No
information available to require special precautions
Effects on Bleeding Nordihydroguaiaretic acid
(NDGA), believed to be responsible for the biological
activity of chaparral, is a platelet aggregation inhibitor;
there is potential for an increased risk of bleeding in
patients undergoing invasive dental procedures, particularly in patients taking concomitant anticoagulants,
antiplatelet drugs, or any drugs or herbals with antiplatelet properties.

Chaste Tree

Clinical Overview
Use
Chaste tree extract has been used to manage symptoms related to premenstrual syndrome (PMS) and
cyclic mastalgia and may be a suitable alternative to

standard pharmacological management. Although the Complete German Commission E Monographs supports its use for PMS and cyclic mastalgia, there are limited clinical trials to support these uses. Limited evidence exists for its use in menopause.

Dosing
Daily doses of chaste tree fruit extract are typically 20 to 40 mg.

Contraindications
Patients who have an allergy to or are hypersensitive to V. agnus-castus or patients who are pregnant or breast-feeding should avoid use. Safe use in children has not been established.

Pregnancy/Lactation
Information regarding safety and efficacy in pregnancy and lactation is lacking. However, chaste tree may have estrogenic, progesterogenic, and/or uterine stimulant activity and should be avoided in pregnancy and while breast-feeding.

Interactions
None well documented.

Adverse Reactions
Generally regarded as safe; mild and reversible adverse effects include GI reactions, itching, rash, headache, fatigue, acne, and menstrual disturbances.

Toxicology
Information is limited and safety has not been determined in children.

Local Anesthetic/Vasoconstrictor Precautions No information available to require special precautions
Effects on Bleeding None reported

Chinese Cucumber

Clinical Overview
Use
Chinese cucumber has been used to induce abortion. It possesses antitumor activity and has been used to treat invasive moles. Chinese cucumber is being studied as a treatment for the management of AIDS infections.

Dosing
There is no recent published clinical evidence to guide dosage of Chinese cucumber. It is most commonly administered as part of a polyherbal preparation in TCM.

Contraindications
Contraindications have not yet been identified.

Pregnancy/Lactation
Documented adverse effects. Avoid use.

Interactions
None well documented.

Adverse Reactions
Side effects include hormone changes, allergic reaction, fluid in the lungs or brain, bleeding in the brain, heart damage, seizures, and fever.

Toxicology
Extracts of the Chinese cucumber are extremely toxic (death has occurred), particularly with parenteral use.

Local Anesthetic/Vasoconstrictor Precautions No information available to require special precautions
Effects on Bleeding None reported

Chinese Foxglove

Clinical Overview
Use
Rehmannia rhizome extracts are used extensively in traditional Chinese medicine. Clinical trials to support

documented uses are lacking, and because the preparation is often used in combination with other agents, it is difficult to attribute any benefits to the plant. Catalpol, a chemical constituent of the root, is being evaluated for its potential in treating CNS diseases and its effects on aging.

Dosing
None validated by clinical data. Common prescription products range from Rehmannia root 55 to 350 mg extract in polyherbal mixtures.

Contraindications
Chronic liver disease and GI disease, including diarrhea.

Pregnancy/Lactation
Avoid use. Rehmannia has been used traditionally as an emmenagogue.

Interactions
None well documented.

Adverse Reactions
Minor and transient adverse reactions have been reported and include GI discomfort (eg, mild nausea, loose bowels, flatulence), allergy, headache, dizziness, heart palpitations, fatigue, and vertigo.

Toxicology
None well documented.

Local Anesthetic/Vasoconstrictor Precautions No information available to require special precautions
Effects on Bleeding None reported

Chitosan

Clinical Overview
Use
There is some evidence of the effect of chitosan on lowering cholesterol and body weight, but the effect is unlikely to be of clinical importance. To some extent, chitosan is used in the emergency setting to control bleeding. Chitosan has been used in various drug delivery systems. Antimicrobial and other effects are being evaluated for use in dentistry.

Dosing
Chitosan has been administered at wide-ranging doses in clinical studies. In studies evaluating weight loss, 2.4 g/day is commonly used.

Contraindications
None well established.

Pregnancy/Lactation
Information regarding safety and efficacy in pregnancy and lactation is lacking.

Interactions
Data are limited. Potentiation of the anticoagulant effect of warfarin was reported in a patient receiving chitosan 2.4 g/day.

Adverse Reactions
The potential for allergy exists in individuals allergic to shellfish. Clinical trials report few adverse events, generally limited to flatulence and constipation.

Toxicology
Chitosan's toxicity profile is relatively low.

Local Anesthetic/Vasoconstrictor Precautions No information available to require special precautions
Effects on Bleeding None reported

Chondroitin

Clinical Overview
Use
Chondroitin sulfate has been studied for the treatment of arthritis; however, information on its effectiveness is

conflicting. It is commonly given in combination with other agents, such as glucosamine sulfate or glucosamine hydrochloride. It has also been studied for use in drug delivery, antithrombotic and extravasation therapy, and treatment of dry eyes and interstitial cystitis.

Dosing
Chondroitin sulfate has been administered orally for treatment of arthritis at a dosage of 800 to 1,200 mg/day. Positive results often require several months to manifest, and a posttreatment effect has been observed. Animal studies have suggested that the bioavailability of chondroitin sulfate may be increased when given multiple times a day.

Contraindications
Contraindications have not been identified.

Pregnancy/Lactation
Information regarding safety and efficacy in pregnancy and lactation is lacking.

Interactions
An increase in the international normalized ratio (INR) may occur in patients taking anticoagulants, such as warfarin (eg, Coumadin), with either chondroitin alone or in combination with glucosamine.

Adverse Reactions
Potential adverse reactions associated with chondroitin sulfate include alopecia, constipation, diarrhea, epigastralgia, extrasystoles, eyelid edema, lower limb edema, and skin symptoms. Chondroitin sulfate may also exacerbate asthma.

Toxicology
There is little information regarding the long-term effects of chondroitin. Most reports conclude that it is safe.

Local Anesthetic/Vasoconstrictor Precautions No information available to require special precautions
Effects on Bleeding None reported

Chromium

Clinical Overview
Use
Chromium supplementation has been studied for a variety of indications, especially diabetes and weight loss, but clinical studies have shown inconsistent results. The role of supplemental chromium remains controversial.

Dosing
The currently accepted value for chromium dietary intake is 25 mcg/day for women and 35 mcg/day for men. Daily dosages used in clinical trials for periods of up to 9 months range as follows: brewer's yeast up to 400 mcg/day; chromium chloride 50 to 600 mcg/day; chromium nicotinate 200 to 800 mcg/day; chromium picolinate 60 to 1,000 mcg/day. The potential for genotoxic effects exists at higher dosages.

Contraindications
None well documented. Renal failure may be considered a relative contraindication.

Pregnancy/Lactation
Information regarding safety and efficacy in pregnancy and lactation is lacking. Limited animal experimentation showed skeletal and neurological defects in the offspring of mice fed chromium picolinate.

Interactions
None well documented.

Adverse Reactions
Ingestion or exposure to certain forms of chromium may cause or contribute to GI irritation and ulcers, dermatitis, hemorrhage, circulatory shock, and renal tubule damage.

Toxicology
No risk of genotoxicity at low dosages over the short-term exists for chromium as a dietary supplement. However, at higher dosages, such as those used in trials evaluating the efficacy of chromium in glycemic control, concern exists for potential genotoxic effects.

Local Anesthetic/Vasoconstrictor Precautions No information available to require special precautions
Effects on Bleeding None reported

Clove

Clinical Overview
Use
Clove has historically been used for its antiseptic and analgesic effects. Clove and clove oils are used safely in foods, beverages, and toothpastes. Clove oil cream has been used in the treatment of anal fissures and an extract has exhibited aphrodisiac action in rats; however, there are limited studies supporting clinical applications for clove oil.

Dosing
There are limited studies to support therapeutic dosing for clove oil.

Contraindications
Contraindications have not been identified.

Pregnancy/Lactation
Information regarding safety and efficacy in pregnancy and lactation is lacking.

Interactions
None well documented.

Adverse Reactions
Contact dermatitis has been noted.

Toxicology
Toxicity has been observed following ingestion of the oil, but is rare and poorly documented.

Local Anesthetic/Vasoconstrictor Precautions No information available to require special precautions
Effects on Bleeding Clove has been reported to have antiplatelet effects; however, case reports and clinical data are lacking. Presently, there is no information available to require special precautions.

Cocoa

Clinical Overview
Use
Cocoa solid, cocoa butter, and chocolate are all rich sources of antioxidants. Epidemiological studies show an inverse association between the consumption of cocoa and the risk of cardiovascular disease. The likely mechanisms are antioxidant activity; improvement in endothelial function, vascular function, and insulin sensitivity; as well as attenuation of platelet reactivity and reduction in blood pressure.

Dosing
No specific dosing recommendations can be made. Further studies characterizing the polyphenol content of cocoa products and method of measurement are needed. In one study, an inverse relationship was demonstrated between cocoa intake and blood pressure, as well as a 15-year cardiovascular and all-cause mortality; the median cocoa intake among users was 2.11 g/day.

Contraindications
None known.

Pregnancy/Lactation
Generally recognized as safe (GRAS) when used in moderate amounts or in amounts used in foods. Avoid dosages greater than those found in food because safety and efficacy are unproven. Caffeine content should be restricted during pregnancy.

Interactions
None well documented.

Adverse Reactions
Children consuming large amounts of chocolate and caffeinated beverages may exhibit tics or restlessness. Ingredients in chocolate may precipitate migraine headaches, and cocoa products may be allergenic.

Toxicology
Cocoa is nontoxic when ingested in typical confectionery amounts.

Local Anesthetic/Vasoconstrictor Precautions No information available to require special precautions

Effects on Bleeding None reported

Comfrey

Clinical Overview
Use
Therapeutic use of comfrey is limited because of its toxicity. A limited number of clinical trials show short-term efficacy of topically applied, alkaloid-free comfrey preparations in skin abrasions and inflammatory conditions. Although not examined in clinical trials, comfrey may possess antifungal and anticancer activity.

Dosing
Oral use of comfrey is not supported because of potential hepatotoxicity. Additionally, because externally applied alkaloids are well absorbed and detected in the urine, topical use of comfrey should not exceed an alkaloid exposure of 100 mcg/day. Limited trials have evaluated the efficacy of alkaloid-free preparations for topical use; however, these studies do not report on hepatic laboratory indices of study participants.

Contraindications
Comfrey is not recommended for internal use because of the hepatotoxic pyrrolizidine alkaloid content. Patients with hypersensitivity or allergic reactions to the plant should avoid external use. Use is contraindicated during pregnancy and lactation, in infants, and in patients with liver or kidney disease.

Pregnancy/Lactation
Contraindicated because of documented adverse effects. Pyrrolizidine alkaloids have abortifacient effects and increase the risk of fatal hepatic veno-occlusive disease. Animal experiments have detected alkaloids in breast milk.

Interactions
None well documented.

Adverse Reactions
Neither internal nor extensive topical use of comfrey is recommended because of numerous reports of liver toxicity (see Toxicology). Case reports show hepatic veno-occlusive disease and pulmonary hypertension related to comfrey use. Infants are more susceptible to pyrrolizidine-related, veno-occlusive disease; therefore, the use of comfrey in this population is contraindicated.

Toxicology
The Food and Drug Administration (FDA) released an advisory in July 2001 recommending that comfrey products be removed from the market because of cases of hepatic veno-occlusive disease. Comfrey is generally considered unsafe, with numerous toxicological effects in animals and humans.

Local Anesthetic/Vasoconstrictor Precautions No information available to require special precautions

Effects on Bleeding None reported

Cordyceps

Clinical Overview
Use
Well-controlled clinical trials are lacking.

Dosing
Dosing supported by product quality data is unavailable, and many herbal supplements on the market contain varying undefined levels of this product. Cordyceps 3 to 6 g/day has been used in patients with chronic renal failure for periods ranging from days to years.

Contraindications
Contraindications have not been identified.

Pregnancy/Lactation
Information regarding safety and efficacy in pregnancy and lactation is lacking.

Interactions
None well documented.

Adverse Reactions
Mild GI discomfort, including diarrhea, dry mouth, and nausea, has been reported.

Toxicology
Cordyceps is generally considered safe.

Local Anesthetic/Vasoconstrictor Precautions No information available to require special precautions

Effects on Bleeding Cordyceps has been reported to have antiplatelet effects; however, case reports and clinical data are lacking. Presently, there is no information available to require special precautions.

Cranberry

Clinical Overview
Use
Some evidence exists for the use of cranberry in preventing, but not treating, urinary tract infections (UTIs). Other possible uses for cranberry, with limited evidence, include reduction of the risk of cardiovascular disease and cancer.

Dosing
Cranberry juice, juice concentrate, and dried extract have been studied in UTIs; however, consistency in dosage regimens is lacking. Doses of juice cocktail (25% pure cranberry juice) have ranged from 120 to 1,000 mL/day in divided doses. Concentrated cranberry extract in the form of tablets and capsules is available and 600 to more than 1,200 mg/day in divided doses have been used in studies in UTIs.

Contraindications
Predisposition to or history of nephrolithiasis (kidney stones).

Pregnancy/Lactation
Information is limited; however, when ingested at normal food consumption amounts, cranberry is considered relatively safe in pregnancy. Safety during lactation is unknown.

Interactions

An interaction between cranberry and warfarin has been suggested based on case reports; however, evidence for a causal relationship is lacking from clinical trials.

Adverse Reactions

The berries and juice have few adverse reactions associated with their consumption. Large daily doses may produce GI symptoms, such as diarrhea. Concentrated cranberry tablets may predispose patients to nephrolithiasis. Cranberry juice should not be used to clear enteral feeding tubes.

Toxicology

Information is lacking.

Local Anesthetic/Vasoconstrictor Precautions No information available to require special precautions

Effects on Bleeding None reported

Creatine

Clinical Overview

Use

Creatine has enhanced performance in short-duration, high-intensity exercise in limited trials. Creatine supplementation has been extensively studied in myopathies and neurodegenerative disorders, but with limited efficacy. Further trials are ongoing.

Dosing

Dosage regimens in clinical trials vary from 2 to 20 g daily, and from 1 to 6 weeks and longer.

Contraindications

Patients with a history of renal impairment or those taking nephrotoxic agents should avoid concomitant creatine supplementation or be monitored closely if supplementation is necessary.

Pregnancy/Lactation

Information regarding safety and efficacy in pregnancy and lactation is lacking.

Interactions

None well documented.

Adverse Reactions

Few adverse reactions have been reported in clinical studies among patients with neurological or muscle disorders, or in healthy individuals

Concerns regarding renal and hepatic toxicity exist; unequivocal proof of safety is lacking and caution is warranted.

Case reports of adverse reactions among athletes include dehydration, electrolyte imbalance, and muscle cramping. Minor GI upset (diarrhea, GI pain, nausea), dizziness, and short-term loss in body mass have also been reported. The safety of creatine in children has not been established.

Toxicology

Information is limited; however, the French Agency for Food, Environmental and Occupational Health & Safety (ANSES) has warned of the potential for production of cytotoxic compounds, especially at high dosages.

Local Anesthetic/Vasoconstrictor Precautions No information available to require special precautions

Effects on Bleeding None reported

Cumin

Clinical Overview

Use

Cumin seeds are used in cooking and the oil is used to flavor food and scent cosmetics. Components may have antioxidant, anticancer, hypoglycemic, antiepileptic, antiosteoporotic, ophthalmic, antibacterial, and larvicidal effects; however, there is no clinical evidence to support these claims. Cumin is generally recognized as safe for human consumption as a spice and flavoring.

Dosing

There are no recent clinical studies of cumin that provide a basis for dosage recommendations.

Contraindications

Contraindications have not yet been identified.

Pregnancy/Lactation

Information regarding safety and efficacy in pregnancy and lactation is lacking.

Interactions

None well documented.

Adverse Reactions

The oil may have photosensitizing effects. Cumin may also cause hypoglycemia.

Toxicology

No data are available.

Local Anesthetic/Vasoconstrictor Precautions No information available to require special precautions

Effects on Bleeding A study published in 1989 showed that cumin inhibits human platelet aggregation in *in vitro* testing; the clinical significance of this effect is unknown at this time.

Damiana

Clinical Overview

Use

Damiana is reportedly an aphrodisiac and hallucinogen.

Dosing

There are no recent clinical studies of damiana that provide a basis for dosage recommendations, though it has been studied in combination with other agents. Classical dosage of the leaf was 2 g.

Contraindications

Contraindications have not yet been identified.

Pregnancy/Lactation

Documented adverse effects include cyanogenetic glycosides and risk of cyanide toxicity in high doses. Avoid use.

Interactions

None well documented.

Adverse Reactions

Significant adverse effects have not been reported.

Toxicology

Research reveals little or no information regarding toxicology with the use of this product.

Local Anesthetic/Vasoconstrictor Precautions No information available to require special precautions

Effects on Bleeding None reported

Dandelion

Clinical Overview

Use

Dandelion has been used for its nutritional value in addition to other uses including diuresis, regulation of blood glucose, liver and gall bladder disorders, appetite stimulation, and for dyspeptic complaints.

Dosing

Dandelion root has been used as a tonic for digestive complaints in doses of 9 to 12 g/day, prepared as a tea.

Contraindications

Contraindications have not yet been identified.

Pregnancy/Lactation

Generally recognized as safe or used as food. Safety and efficacy for dosages above those in foods unproven and should be avoided.

Interactions

None well documented.

Adverse Reactions

Contact dermatitis and gastric discomfort have been reported.

Toxicology

Dandelion may be potentially toxic because of the high concentration of potassium, magnesium, and other minerals.

Local Anesthetic/Vasoconstrictor Precautions No information available to require special precautions

Effects on Bleeding None reported

Danshen

Clinical Overview

Use

Danshen has been used extensively in Chinese medicine for many years. Limited studies have shown efficacy in coronary artery disease and acute ischemic stroke, but the quality of methodology limits the validity of the findings.

Dosing

Active components in commercially available preparations vary greatly. Commonly cited dosages include the following: 10 "dripping" pills taken 3 times a day (oral or sublingual), 3 Fu Fang Dan Shen tablets taken orally 3 times a day, or danshen 20 mg/kg capsules. Doses of 100 mg/kg as a bolus injection have been used in children.

Contraindications

Data are lacking.

Pregnancy/Lactation

Information regarding safety and efficacy in pregnancy and lactation is lacking.

Interactions

Danshen may interfere with laboratory digoxin plasma levels and increase the anticoagulant effect of warfarin. It may reduce midazolam plasma concentrations, decreasing the pharmacologic effects, and inhibits numerous cytochrome P450 (CYP-450) enzymes in vitro.

Adverse Reactions

Adverse reactions appear to be limited to allergy, dizziness, headache, mild GI symptoms, and reversible thrombocytopenia.

Toxicology

Information is limited.

Local Anesthetic/Vasoconstrictor Precautions No information available to require special precautions

Effects on Bleeding Danshen has been shown to inhibit platelet aggregation *in vitro* in animals and is suggested to inhibit platelet aggregation in humans; the clinical significance of this effect is unknown at this time. Case reports described increased anticoagulation in patients taking warfarin, but this appears to be a result of a pharmacokinetic/pharmacodynamic interaction rather than any anticoagulation activity on the part of danshen.

Dehydroepiandrosterone

Clinical Overview

Use

Adequately powered, long-term clinical trials are lacking to support a place in therapy for dehydroepiandrosterone (DHEA) and dehydroepiandrosterone sulfate (DHEAS) supplementation (henceforth, jointly referred to as DHEA/S). Reviews of clinical trials found no convincing evidence to support a place in therapy for postmenopausal symptoms in women, in improving cognitive function or physical strength in elderly patients, in hyperlipidemia or insulin resistance, or in schizophrenia or cancer. Some evidence exists to support the use of DHEA/S supplementation in women with diminished ovarian reserves, in subpopulations of elderly women with osteoporosis, and in mild systemic lupus erythematosus.

Dosing

Orally administered DHEA has a less than 10% bioavailability and is converted into inactive DHEAS, which can then act as a reservoir for the body to utilize. Daily dosing of DHEA 25 mg has been suggested in postmenopausal women because this dose minimizes the adverse androgenic effects; however, only studies in which at least 50 mg/day were used demonstrated positive outcomes. Dosages used in clinical studies of assisted reproduction were in the range of 50 to 75 mg/day (in divided doses). In adrenal insufficiency, DHEA 50 mg/day for 3 months is considered a replacement dose, while 200 mg/day achieves supraphysiological circulating levels and would thus be considered a pharmacological dose.

Contraindications

Contraindications have not been identified. Use of DHEA or DHEAS is not recommended in breast or prostate cancer.

Pregnancy/Lactation

Information regarding safety and efficacy in pregnancy and lactation is lacking. DHEA supplementation has been evaluated to improve oocyte production in infertility.

Interactions

None well documented.

Adverse Reactions

Studies in adrenal insufficiency suggest DHEA is generally well tolerated. However, data from long-term studies are lacking. Observed adverse effects include acne, hirsutism, and decreased high-density lipoprotein (HDL) levels.

Toxicology

Information in humans is limited. DHEA has been shown to be carcinogenic as well as protective against certain cancers in rodents.

Local Anesthetic/Vasoconstrictor Precautions No information available to require special precautions

Effects on Bleeding None reported

Devil's Claw

Clinical Overview

Use

Devil's claw is a folk remedy used for an extensive range of diseases, including arthritis and rheumatism. Clinical trials are generally supportive of its use as an anti-inflammatory and analgesic in low back pain and osteoarthritis.

Dosing

Devil's claw has been studied for low back pain, muscle pain, and osteoarthritis using daily doses of crude tuber up to 9 g, 1 to 3 g of extract, or harpagoside 50 to 100 mg.

Contraindications

Because of the bitterness of the preparation and consequent increase in gastric secretion, devil's claw is contraindicated in patients with gastric or duodenal ulcers.

Pregnancy/Lactation

Documented oxytoxic adverse effects. Avoid use.

Interactions

None well documented.

Adverse Reactions

Rare, generally consisting of headache, tinnitus, or anorexia.

Toxicology

Clinically important toxicity has not been observed in limited, short-term use.

Local Anesthetic/Vasoconstrictor Precautions No information available to require special precautions

Effects on Bleeding Purpura has occurred in a patient taking warfarin and Devil's Claw concurrently, suggesting over anticoagulation.

Dong Quai

Clinical Overview

Use

Dong quai is used in combination with other plant extracts in Chinese traditional medicine as an analgesic for rheumatism, an allergy suppressant, and in the treatment of menstrual disorders. Dong quai and its chemical constituents possess antiasthmatic, antispasmodic, anti-inflammatory, and anticoagulant properties. Clinical trials supporting traditional uses are limited. It has also been used to flavor liqueurs and confections.

Dosing

Several forms of the plant exist and dosages vary widely: crude root extract by decoction ranges from 3 to 15 g/day; while in combination, preparations 75 mg to 500 mg may be taken up to 6 times a day.

Contraindications

Relative contraindications in patients receiving warfarin, heparin, or other anticoagulant/antiplatelet therapy, in those with breast cancer, or in the first trimester of pregnancy.

Pregnancy/Lactation

Avoid use. Uterine stimulant and relaxant activity have been reported with A. sinensis, while a related species, Angelica archangelica L., was a reported abortifacient and affected the menstrual cycle.

Interactions

Warfarin, heparin, and other antiplatelet therapy due to anticoagulant/antiplatelet action of A. sinensis.

Adverse Reactions

Case reports exist of fever, gynaecomastia, and bleeding with concurrent warfarin use. A risk of photosensitization exists.

Toxicology

Data are limited. Chemical constituents have demonstrated cytotoxic properties.

Local Anesthetic/Vasoconstrictor Precautions No information available to require special precautions

Effects on Bleeding May inhibit platelet aggregation and therefore increase bleeding

Du Zhong

Clinical Overview

Use

The medical literature includes numerous studies on the use of *Eucommia ulmoides* (du zhong) for treating diabetes, inflammation, and obesity. One clinical study exists for its use in treating hypertension.

Dosing

E. ulmoides is commercially available as a combination product or alone as a capsule, tablet, powder, or tea, primarily for treating hypertension. *Tablets*: 3 to 5 (100 mg) tablets 3 times per day with warm water after meals. One clinical study used a 500 mg standardized extract 3 times daily for 8 weeks.

Contraindications

Avoid use in patients who are hypersensitive to any components of *E. ulmoides*. The herb may be contraindicated in patients diagnosed with estrogen-dependent cancers.

Pregnancy/Lactation

Information regarding safety and efficacy in pregnancy and lactation is lacking.

Interactions

None well documented.

Adverse Reactions

One clinical study of *E. ulmoides* documented moderately severe headache, dizziness, edema, and onset of a cold.

Toxicology

No information in humans is available.

Local Anesthetic/Vasoconstrictor Precautions No information available to require special precautions

Effects on Bleeding No information available to require special precautions

Echinacea

Clinical Overview

Use

There is limited evidence that echinacea is effective in shortening the duration of symptoms of upper respiratory tract infections, but a lack of effectiveness for its use in prevention. Echinacea is hypothesized to be an immunomodulator. There is also interest in its potential use in cancer therapy, but clinical trials are lacking. The variation in available commercial products and lack of consistency in clinical trials make specific recommendations difficult.

Dosing

Many commercial preparations are available containing components derived from different plant parts as well as from different species and varieties. Recommended dosing (all administered 3 times daily) include the following: 300 mg dry powdered extract (standardized to 3.5% echinacoside), 0.25 to 1.25 mL liquid extract (1:1 in 45% alcohol), 1 to 2 mL tincture (1:5 in 45% alcohol), 2 to 3 mL expressed juice of E. purpurea, and 0.5 to 1 g dried root or tea. Echinacea use for more than 8 weeks at a time should be avoided because of the potential for immune suppression. Intravenous (IV) use is not recommended.

Contraindications

Known hypersensitivity to plants of the Asteraceae/Compositae family; any condition in which immune stimulation or suppression would be considered disadvantageous.

Pregnancy/Lactation

Limited clinical evidence, expert opinion, and long-term traditional use suggest that oral echinacea is safe for use during pregnancy at normal dosages. Direct evidence for safety during lactation is lacking. Use with caution.

Interactions

Specific case reports of interactions are lacking, and limited, conflicting data regarding effects on the cytochrome P450 (CYP-450) enzyme system have been published.

Adverse Reactions

Adverse reactions are rare. In clinical trials, adverse reactions caused by echinacea were generally not statistically significant compared with placebo. The most commonly reported reactions were allergy, GI upset, and rash. Individuals with allergy to ragweed or related allergens should use echinacea with caution. A case report of leukopenia, possibly caused by long-term use of echinacea, has been published. Potential immune suppression with long-term use has been suggested.

Toxicology

Little is known about the toxicity of echinacea. Animal studies generally indicate low toxicity.

Local Anesthetic/Vasoconstrictor Precautions No information available to require special precautions

Effects on Bleeding None reported

Elderberry

Clinical Overview

Use

Limited clinical trials have been conducted. Elderberry extracts may have some value in the treatment of influenza and appear to have antioxidant potential.

Dosing

The bioavailability of active constituents in elderberry extracts is considered to be poor. Trials are lacking to provide dosing information. For the treatment of influenza, 15 mL of syrup taken 4 times per day for 5 days has been used in clinical trials.

Contraindications

Contraindications have not been identified.

Pregnancy/Lactation

Information regarding safety and efficacy in pregnancy and lactation is lacking.

Interactions

None well documented.

Adverse Reactions

Consumption of uncooked berries may result in vomiting and diarrhea. Commercial preparations generally do not cause adverse reactions at the recommended dosage. Type 1 allergy to elderberry (positive skin prick tests) has been recorded.

Toxicology

Poisonous alkaloids, lectins, and cyanogenic glycosides are present in some plant parts. Short-term use of elderberry extract preparations appears to be relatively safe; however, long-term toxicological studies are lacking.

Local Anesthetic/Vasoconstrictor Precautions No information available to require special precautions

Effects on Bleeding None reported

Ephedra

Clinical Overview

Use

The whole Ephedra sinica plant has traditionally been used to treat symptoms of bronchial asthma, colds, influenza, allergies, and hives in teas or tinctures. Because of adverse events and lack of efficacy, use is not recommended for weight loss or increased athletic performance. Ephedra-containing supplements are banned for sale in the United States.

Dosing

Ephedra-containing dietary supplements are currently banned in the United States. Dosages of ephedra more than 32 mg/day have resulted in adverse reactions.

Contraindications

Cardiovascular and cerebrovascular adverse events have been documented in case reports.

Pregnancy/Lactation

Documented adverse reactions. Avoid use.

Interactions

Interactions are likely to be similar to those established for synthetic ephedrine and include monoamine oxidase inhibitors (MAOIs), the anesthetic propofol, cholinergic agents such as tricyclic antidepressants, caffeine, theophylline, and steroids such as dexamethasone.

Adverse Reactions

Reported adverse reactions include arrhythmia and sudden death, myocardial infarction, stroke, psychiatric symptoms, autonomic hyperactivity, seizures, and ischemic colitis and gastric mucosal injury.

Toxicology

Toxicological data are limited. Periconceptional use of ephedra-containing products has been associated with an increased adjusted odds ratio for anencephaly.

Local Anesthetic/Vasoconstrictor Precautions Use vasoconstrictor with caution since ephedrine may enhance cardiostimulation and vasopressor effects of sympathomimetics such as epinephrine and levonordefrin.

Effects on Bleeding None reported

Evening Primrose Oil

Clinical Overview

Use

Evidence suggests that evening primrose oil may be effective for treating rheumatoid arthritis and diabetic neuropathy, but is lacking to support its place in the treatment of atopic dermatitis, menopausal vasomotor symptoms, mastalgia, or multiple sclerosis.

Dosing

Evening primrose oil has been administered orally in clinical trials at doses between 6 and 8 g/day in adults and 2 and 4 g/day in children. The typical content of gamma-linolenic acid (GLA) in the oil is 8% to 10%.

Contraindications

No contraindications have been identified.

Pregnancy/Lactation

Information regarding safety and efficacy in pregnancy and lactation is lacking. A case report exists of transient petechiae in a newborn following oral and intravaginal use of evening primrose oil for cervical ripening for a week prior to the infant's birth. Both linoleic and GLA are normally present in breast milk, and it is reasonable to assume that evening primrose oil may be taken while breast-feeding.

Interactions

A case report exists of an interaction between evening primrose oil and lopinavir in which lopinavir plasma concentrations were elevated to toxic levels.

Adverse Reactions

Evening primrose oil was previously suspected to lower the seizure threshold in schizophrenic patients; however, this is now disputed.

Toxicology

No toxicity, carcinogenicity, or teratogenicity have been reported.

Local Anesthetic/Vasoconstrictor Precautions No information available to require special precautions

Effects on Bleeding Contains gamma-linolenic acid which can inhibit platelet aggregation and prolong bleeding.

Eyebright

Clinical Overview

Use

Eyebright preparations have been used to treat a variety of complaints, especially inflammatory eye disease.

Dosing

There are no recent clinical studies of eyebright to provide a basis for dosage recommendations. The herb is typically applied topically.

Contraindications

No longer considered safe.

Pregnancy/Lactation

Information regarding safety and efficacy in pregnancy and lactation is lacking. Avoid use.

Interactions

None well documented.

Adverse Reactions

The range of adverse effects is considered to outweigh the dubious benefits.

Toxicology

Research reveals little or no information regarding toxicology with the use of this product.

Local Anesthetic/Vasoconstrictor Precautions No information available to require special precautions

Effects on Bleeding None reported

Fennel

Clinical Overview

Use

Fennel has been used as a flavoring agent, a scent, and an insect repellent, as well as an herbal remedy for poisoning and GI conditions. It has also been used as a stimulant to promote lactation and menstruation. However, clinical evidence to support the use of fennel for any indication is lacking.

Dosing

Fennel seed and fennel seed oil have been used as stimulant and carminative agents in doses of 5 to 7 g and 0.1 to 0.6 mL, respectively.

Contraindications

Contraindications have not been identified.

Pregnancy/Lactation

There are documented adverse reactions and emmenagogue effects. Avoid use.

Interactions

One study suggested that the fennel constituent 5-methoxypsoralen has the ability to inhibit cytochrome

P450 3A4. Therefore, fennel should be used cautiously with medications requiring this isoenzyme as a substrate.

Adverse Reactions

Fennel may cause photodermatitis, contact dermatitis, and cross reactions. The oil may induce reactions, such as hallucinations and seizures. Four case reports of premature thelarche (breast development) in girls have been reported with the use of fennel. Poison hemlock may be mistaken for fennel.

Toxicology

Fennel oil is genotoxic in the Bacillus subtilis DNA repair test. Estragole, present in the volatile oil, has caused tumors in animals.

Local Anesthetic/Vasoconstrictor Precautions No information available to require special precautions

Effects on Bleeding May see increased bleeding

Fenugreek

Clinical Overview

Use

Clinical data from very small studies suggest the use of fenugreek for cholesterol lowering. It is used as a flavoring in Indian and Asian cookery, and in folk medicine for the treatment of boils, cellulitis, and tuberculosis, and for its anti-inflammatory and diuretic effects.

Dosing

Studies investigating the use of fenugreek in diabetes and cholesterol lowering have used 5 g/day of seeds or 1 g of a hydroalcoholic extract.

Contraindications

Contraindications have not yet been identified.

Pregnancy/Lactation

Avoid use in pregnancy as fenugreek has documented uterine stimulant effects. It has been used to stimulate milk production in nursing mothers. Excretion into milk has not been studied.

Interactions

The effects of anticoagulant drugs such as warfarin may be potentiated. Patients taking anticoagulants should consult their health care provider before taking fenugreek; dosage adjustments may be necessary.

Adverse Reactions

Dyspepsia and mild abdominal distention have been reported in studies using large doses of the seeds. Culinary quantities are essentially devoid of adverse effects; however, a case of hypersensitivity to fenugreek in curry powder has been reported.

Toxicology

The acute toxicity from large doses of fenugreek has not been characterized. Hypoglycemia is a potential danger.

Local Anesthetic/Vasoconstrictor Precautions No information available to require special precautions

Effects on Bleeding As a single agent, fenugreek has no effect on bleeding. Fenugreek may enhance the anticoagulant effects of warfarin when taken simultaneously. This effect has not been confirmed.

Feverfew

Clinical Overview

Use

Feverfew is primarily known for use in prophylactic treatment of migraine headaches and associated nausea and vomiting; however, evidence to support this use is inconclusive. Feverfew has numerous other pharmacological actions, including inhibition of prostaglandin synthesis, blockage of platelet granule secretion, effects on smooth muscle, antitumor activity, inhibition of serotonin release, inhibition of histamine release, and mast cell inhibition, but information from clinical trials is limited.

Dosing

Feverfew is generally given for migraine headaches at a daily dosage of 50 to 150 mg of dried leaves, 2.5 fresh leaves with or after food, or 5 to 20 drops of a 1:5, 25% ethanol tincture. Though optimal doses of feverfew have not been established, an adult dosage of parentholide 0.2 to 0.6 mg/day is recommended for the prevention of migraine. However, parthenolide has not been confirmed as a major active principle for migraine. Numerous feverfew products are commercially available; most are standardized to parthenolide 0.7% in tablet or capsule dosage forms.

Contraindications

Feverfew is contraindicated in patients allergic to other members of the Asteraceae family, such as aster, chamomile, chrysanthemum, ragweed, sunflower, tansy, and yarrow. Due to its potential antiplatelet effects, it is not recommended for use in patients undergoing surgery. Patients with blood-clotting disorders should consult their health care provider prior to using products containing feverfew.

Pregnancy/Lactation

Avoid use because of documented adverse effects. Pregnant women should not use the plant because the leaves possess emmenagogue activity (ejection of the placenta and fetal membranes) and may induce abortion. It is not recommended for breast-feeding mothers or for use in children younger than 2 years of age.

Interactions

None well documented.

Adverse Reactions

Patients withdrawn from feverfew may experience ill effects often known as "postfeverfew" syndrome. Handling fresh feverfew leaves may cause allergic contact dermatitis. Swelling of the lips, tongue, and oral mucosa, in addition to mouth ulceration, have been reported with feverfew use. GI effects, such as abdominal pain, nausea, vomiting, diarrhea, indigestion, and flatulence, may also occur.

Toxicology

No studies of chronic toxicity have been performed on the plant. The safety of long-term use has not been established.

Local Anesthetic/Vasoconstrictor Precautions No information available to require special precautions

Effects on Bleeding May see increased bleeding due to inhibition of platelet aggregation

Flax

Clinical Overview

Use

Flaxseed and flaxseed oil contain various essential fatty acids but are particularly rich in alpha linolenic acid (ALA). Flaxseed (but not flaxseed oil) also has a high fiber content that may have health benefits similar to those of other high-fiber products and phytoestrogens. Historically, linseed oil, derived from flaxseed, has been used as a topical demulcent and emollient, as a laxative, and as a treatment for coughs, colds, and urinary tract infections. Interest in flaxseed centers on atherosclerosis, cancer, diabetes, and to a lesser

extent, menopause, attention deficit hyperactivity disorder, bipolar disorder, and systemic lupus erythematosus (SLE).

Dosing

Flaxseed (whole or ground) has been used in clinical trials at doses from 5 to 50 g/day or 60 mL flaxseed oil daily, and has been used in children at doses equivalent to 400 mg of ALA in divided doses.

Eight grams of ground flaxseed (or 2.5 g of flaxseed oil) per day provides a daily intake of 1.1 g of ALA for women and 1.6 g for men.

Contraindications

Contraindicated in patients with known hypersensitivity to flaxseed.

Pregnancy/Lactation

The use of flaxseed and flaxseed oil during pregnancy and lactation is not recommended.

Interactions

None well documented.

Adverse Reactions

Flaxseed and flaxseed oil appear to be well tolerated, with few adverse reactions reported except allergy.

Toxicology

The US Food and Drug Administration has not granted GRAS (Generally Recognized as Safe) status to flaxseed or flaxseed oil. The safety of ingested amounts greater than 50 g/day of flaxseed is not established.

Local Anesthetic/Vasoconstrictor Precautions No information available to require special precautions

Effects on Bleeding None reported

Forskolin

Clinical Overview

Use

Forskolin has multiple sites of action and should be used with caution. Forskolin derivatives have been developed for use in cardiovascular conditions. Quality clinical trials are lacking to substantiate claims made of the weight loss properties of forskolin, and clinical studies conducted with oral and inhaled forskolin in patients with asthma are limited.

Dosing

Asthma: Oral forskolin has been studied using 10 mg daily over 2 to 6 months.

Obesity: 250 mg of a 10% forskolin extract twice daily for 12 weeks has been studied.

Contraindications

Case reports are lacking.

Pregnancy/Lactation

Information regarding safety and efficacy in pregnancy and lactation is lacking. P. barbatus has been traditionally used as an emmenagogue and oral contraceptive.

Interactions

None well documented.

Adverse Reactions

Clinical trial data are generally lacking. Adverse events reported with the use of colforsin (a forskolin derivative) include tachycardia and arrhythmias. Forskolin should be avoided in patients with polycystic kidney disease.

Toxicology

Information is limited. Embryo-related toxicity has been reported.

Local Anesthetic/Vasoconstrictor Precautions No information available to require special precautions

Effects on Bleeding Forskolin has been shown *in vitro* to inhibit platelet aggregation. Clinical relevance of this effect is unknown. There are no current published reports of any anticoagulant effect in patients taking Forskolin.

Forsythia

Clinical Overview

Use

Forsythia has been used for treatment of bacterial infections and upper respiratory tract infections, although the clinical evidence supporting its use is limited.

Dosing

There are no recent clinical studies of forsythia to provide a basis for dosage recommendations.

Contraindications

Contraindications have not yet been identified.

Pregnancy/Lactation

Documented adverse effects. Uterine stimulant, emmenagogue. Avoid use.

Interactions

None well documented.

Adverse Reactions

Forsythia is contraindicated in pregnancy.

Toxicology

Forsythia has minimal potential for toxicity.

Local Anesthetic/Vasoconstrictor Precautions No information available to require special precautions

Effects on Bleeding None reported

Frankincense, Indian

Clinical Overview

Use

The extract of Indian frankincense tree has anti-inflammatory activity. Boswellic acids may play a role in preventing formation of anaphylatoxins during severe acute allergic reactions.

Dosing

An extract of frankincense (H15) was studied in arthritis at a dose of 3.6 g daily. The gum resin of frankincense has been used at a daily dose of 900 mg for bronchial asthma.

Contraindications

Contraindications have not yet been identified.

Pregnancy/Lactation

Information regarding safety and efficacy in pregnancy and lactation is lacking.

Interactions

None well documented.

Adverse Reactions

Although data are limited, no side effects have been reported that necessitated stopping treatment.

Toxicology

No data.

Local Anesthetic/Vasoconstrictor Precautions No information available to require special precautions

Effects on Bleeding None reported

Fruit Acids

Clinical Overview

Use

Fruit acids have been used to treat a range of dermatological conditions, including acne, photoaging, dry skin, psoriasis, actinic keratosis, and melasma.

Additionally, they have been investigated as a treatment for fibromyalgia.

Dosing

For dry skin disorders, alpha hydroxy acid 8% to 10% cream or lotion is applied 2 to 3 times daily to the affected area. If the dry skin persists after 2 weeks, the concentration can be increased by 2% to 4%. Once the skin appears healthy, the frequency can be reduced to every 2 to 3 days. For fibromyalgia, clinical data suggest the use of 3 Super Malic tablets (each containing malic acid 200 mg) twice daily. Dosing for chemical peels involving glycolic acid will depend on a variety of factors, including the condition being treated, patient expectations, patient age, cumulative sun exposure, skin type, area being treated, peeling agent used, concentration of peel agent, frequency of application, quantity applied, and length of time applied. Typically, on the first visit, glycolic acid is applied for approximately 2 to 3 minutes to determine sensitivity and provide guidance for future length of exposure. Intervals between peels are generally 2 to 4 weeks, and 6 to 8 peels are required for most patients.

Contraindications

Hypersensitive individuals and those with irritated skin should use alpha hydroxy acids cautiously. Patients who have undergone recent cosmetic surgeries, patients with open wounds, and those who have used isotretinoin therapy within the last 6 to 12 months should not receive alpha hydroxy acid peels. In patients who have a history of recurrent or active herpes simplex lesions, treatment with an oral antiviral agent should occur before undergoing chemical peels.

Pregnancy/Lactation

Information regarding safety and efficacy in pregnancy and lactation is lacking.

Interactions

Use of isotretinoin causes a reduction in the number and size of pilosebaceous units in the skin and may cause a delay in wound healing and increase the risk of scarring. It is advised that patients wait at least 6 to 12 months after receiving isotretinoin to begin chemical peels. Antimetabolites and corticosteroids may delay wound healing in patients using chemical peels. Use of hormone replacement therapy and oral contraceptives may cause postinflammatory hyperpigmentation in some patients using chemical peels. Following a chemical peel with glycolic acid, there may be an increase in risk of photosensitivity in patients using photosensitizing agents, such as tetracyclines and other photosensitizing agents.

Adverse Reactions

Dryness, scaling, burning, erythema, and similar effects may occur in sensitive individuals or with prolonged use.

Toxicology

In rats, long-term ingestion of malic acid was found to reduce body weight gains and feed consumption when given for a period of 2 years.

Local Anesthetic/Vasoconstrictor Precautions No information available to require special precautions

Effects on Bleeding None reported

Garcinia (hydroxycitric acid)

Clinical Overview

Use

The medical literature primarily documents weight loss and lipid-lowering activity for the plant. However, trials supporting its use are limited.

Dosing

The dosages of G. cambogia extract in clinical trials ranged from 1,500 to 4,667 mg/day (25 to 78 mg/kg/day). The equivalent hydroxycitric acid (HCA) dose in the trials ranged from 900 to 2,800 mg/day (15 to 47 mg/kg/day). G. cambogia is available in capsule or tablet form with a maximum dose of 1,500 mg/day.

Contraindications

Avoid use if there is a known allergy or hypersensitivity to any components of G. cambogia.

Pregnancy/Lactation

Information regarding safety and efficacy in pregnancy and lactation is lacking.

Interactions

The herb has documented drug interactions.

Adverse Reactions

At least 15 clinical studies involving approximately 900 patients document very mild adverse reactions. Most adverse reactions included headache, dizziness, dry mouth, and GI complaints such as nausea and diarrhea.

Toxicology

Toxicology studies resulted in no toxicity or deaths in animals at dosages of HCA 5,000 mg/kg, equivalent to 350 g or 233 times the maximum dosage of 1.5 g/day of HCA. In patients taking certain combination weight-loss supplements containing G. cambogia, severe or even fatal hepatotoxicity may occur.

Local Anesthetic/Vasoconstrictor Precautions No information available to require special precautions

Effects on Bleeding None reported

Garlic

Clinical Overview

Use

Evidence suggests that garlic may produce modest but not clinically significant effects in the treatment of dyslipidemia and hypertension. Traditionally, it has been used for its antiseptic and antibacterial properties, as well as for treating the common cold, upper respiratory tract infections, mild bronchitis, and rhinitis, and to relieve cough and congestion. Other potential uses include treatment of atherosclerosis, benign prostatic hyperplasia, diabetes, gastrointestinal (GI) disorders, and stomach and colon cancer; however, evidence is lacking.

Dosing

The following doses are recommended: 2 to 5 g of fresh raw garlic; 0.4 to 1.2 g of dried garlic powder; 2 to 5 mg garlic oil; 300 to 1,000 mg of garlic extract (as solid material). Other preparations should correspond to 4 to 12 mg of alliin or approximately 2 to 5 mg of allicin, an active constituent of garlic. However, dosage is complicated by the volatility and instability of important constituents in various products (eg, aged extracts, deodorized garlic, distilled oils). Administer garlic preparations with food to minimize GI upset. Because garlic is widely consumed, dosage will remain a matter of personal tolerance.

Contraindications

Contraindicated if known allergy to garlic and its constituents.

Pregnancy/Lactation

Garlic may be used safely in pregnancy and breast-feeding. However, consumption by breast-feeding mothers may impact the infant's behavior during breast-feeding, causing prolonged attachment to the breast and increased sucking. There have been documented emmenagogue effects.

Interactions

Garlic may reduce saquinavir plasma concentrations. Caution patients taking saquinavir to limit ingestion of garlic and to avoid taking garlic supplements without consulting their health care provider. Based on available reports, no special precautions are necessary in patients eating garlic and taking warfarin. However, because warfarin has a narrow therapeutic index, caution patients against use of alternative medicines without consulting their health care provider and to report any signs of bleeding. Based on an initial study, garlic does not appear to interact with alprazolam, dextromethorphan, docetaxel, or ritonavir.

Adverse Reactions

Body odor and malodorous breath are the most common complaints after ingesting garlic preparations. Mild GI adverse reactions (eg, bloating, flatulence, nausea) have been commonly reported with use. Ingestion of a single 25 mL dose of fresh garlic extract has caused burning of the mouth, esophagus, and stomach; nausea; sweating; and light-headedness. The safety of repeated doses of this amount has not been defined. Alterations in coagulation have also been reported. Ingestion of large amounts may increase the risk of postoperative and spontaneous bleeding. Ingestion as a food or supplement or topical use may cause allergic reactions (contact dermatitis, anaphylaxis, angioedema, generalized urticaria, pemphigus, and photoallergy). Topical exposure to crushed, uncooked garlic cloves for 3 to 5 minutes has resulted in toxic contact dermatitis. Repeated exposure to garlic dust can induce asthmatic reactions.

Toxicology

Research reveals little or no information regarding the toxicology of garlic.

Local Anesthetic/Vasoconstrictor Precautions No information available to require special precautions

Effects on Bleeding Causes platelet dysfunction and prolonged bleeding time

Gelsemium

Clinical Overview

Use

Gelsemium has been traditionally used to treat pain and respiratory ailments.

Dosing

There are no recent clinical studies of gelsemium to provide a basis for dosage recommendations. Classical use of this herb indicated 30 mg of the rhizome. Current use is primarily homeopathic.

Contraindications

No longer considered safe.

Pregnancy/Lactation

Documented adverse effects. Avoid use.

Interactions

None well documented.

Adverse Reactions

Research reveals little or no information regarding adverse reactions with the use of this product.

Toxicology

All parts of the gelsemium are toxic and can cause death when ingested.

Local Anesthetic/Vasoconstrictor Precautions No information available to require special precautions

Effects on Bleeding None reported

Ginger

Clinical Overview

Use

There are many traditional uses for ginger, but more recent interest in the use of ginger centers on the prevention and management of nausea. Ginger may play a role in osteoarthritic pain and cancer. However, there is limited clinical information to support these uses.

Dosing

Ginger has been used in clinical trials in doses of 250 mg to 1 g, 3 to 4 times daily.

Contraindications

Contraindications have not been identified.

Pregnancy/Lactation

Despite trials conducted to determine its effectiveness in pregnancy-related nausea, reasons for caution exist. Avoid use until safety is established.

Interactions

None well documented.

Adverse Reactions

The United States Food and Drug Administration (FDA) considers ginger to be a safe food supplement ("generally recognized as safe"). Large doses carry the potential for adverse reactions. Mild GI effects (eg, heartburn, diarrhea, mouth irritation) have been reported. Case reports of arrhythmia and immunoglobulin E (IgE) allergic reaction are documented.

Toxicology

Toxicologic information regarding use in humans is lacking.

Local Anesthetic/Vasoconstrictor Precautions No information available to require special precautions

Effects on Bleeding No information available to require special precautions

Ginkgo biloba

Clinical Overview

Use

Ginkgo has been studied extensively in diverse medical conditions. Evidence is lacking to support a protective role in cardiovascular conditions and stroke, and a definitive place in therapy for dementia and schizophrenia, although promising, is yet to be established. The findings from 2 large trials are pivotal in evaluating the efficacy of G. biloba extracts.

Dosing

Standardized ginkgo leaf extracts, such as EGb 761 (Tebonin forte, Schwabe), have been used in clinical trials for cognitive and circulatory disorders at daily doses of 120 to 240 mg of extract.

Contraindications

Absolute contraindications have not been established.

Pregnancy/Lactation

Evidence is lacking on the safety of ginkgo; preparations should not be used during pregnancy and lactation.

Interactions

Ginkgo interacts with the human cytochrome P450 (CYP-450) system and its isoenzymes, which may affect the metabolism of various drugs. Case reports of various interactions exist; however, consistent data are limited.

Adverse Reactions

Severe adverse reactions are rare; possible reactions include headache, dizziness, heart palpitations, and GI and dermatologic reactions. Ginkgo pollen can be strongly allergenic. Contact with the fleshy fruit pulp may cause allergic dermatitis similar to poison ivy.

Toxicology

A toxic syndrome has been recognized in Asian children who have ingested ginkgo seeds.

Local Anesthetic/Vasoconstrictor Precautions No information available to require special precautions

Effects on Bleeding Spontaneous bleeding is a concerning side effect. Significant peri- and postoperative bleeding have been reported. Chronic use inhibits platelet aggregation and prolongs bleeding.

Ginseng

Clinical Overview

Use

Ginseng root is widely used for its adaptogenic, immunomodulatory, antineoplastic, cardiovascular, CNS, endocrine, and ergogenic effects, but these uses have not been confirmed by clinical trials.

Dosing

According to the Complete German Commission E Monographs, crude preparations of dried root powder 1 to 2 g can be taken daily for up to 3 months. In numerous clinical trials, the dosage of crude root has ranged from 0.5 to 3 g/day and the dose of extracts has generally ranged from 100 to 400 mg.

Contraindications

Contraindications have not been established aside from known hypersensitivity.

Pregnancy/Lactation

Information regarding safety and efficacy in pregnancy and lactation is lacking.

Interactions

Limited evidence exists for any established interactions, with most data derived from laboratory studies and healthy volunteers. Very few case reports exist; however, exercise caution when using the following medicines: antidiabetic drugs/insulin, antipsychotic drugs, caffeine and other stimulants, furosemide, imatinib, monoamine oxidase inhibitors (MAOIs), and nifedipine. Interactions with warfarin and antiviral drugs are conflicting.

Adverse Reactions

It is estimated that more than 6 million people ingest ginseng regularly in the United States. There have been few reports of severe reactions and a very low incidence of adverse events has been reported in clinical trials. Hypersensitivity and anaphylaxis have been reported. Inappropriate use of P. ginseng or ginseng abuse syndrome includes symptoms such as hypertension, diarrhea, sleeplessness, mastalgia, skin rash, confusion, and depression.

Toxicology

None known.

Local Anesthetic/Vasoconstrictor Precautions Has potential to interact with epinephrine and levonordefrin to result in increased BP; use vasoconstrictor with caution

Effects on Bleeding May prolong thrombin time (TT) and activated partial thromboplastin time (aPTT).

Glucosamine

Clinical Overview

Use
Glucosamine is being investigated extensively for its action in osteoarthritis. However, there is a lack of consensus in clinical trials regarding its efficacy.

Dosing
In clinical studies of arthritis, glucosamine dosage has typically been 1.5 g/day, as a single dose or in divided doses.

Contraindications
No absolute contraindications have been identified.

Pregnancy/Lactation
Information regarding safety and efficacy in pregnancy and lactation is lacking.

Interactions
None well documented.

Adverse Reactions
Glucosamine is generally considered safe. Use caution when administering to persons with poorly controlled diabetes.

Toxicology
Mutagenicity studies are limited and conflicting.

Local Anesthetic/Vasoconstrictor Precautions No information available to require special precautions

Effects on Bleeding None reported

Goat's Rue

Clinical Overview

Use
Goat's rue derivatives have been associated with reductions in blood sugar levels, but more study is needed. Goat's rue is also a well-known diuretic and increases breast milk production. Other effects include use as a tonic, liver-protectant, and as a platelet aggregation inhibitor.

Dosing
There are no recent clinical studies of goat's rue herb to provide a basis for dosage recommendations. Classical use of the herb was 2 g in an infusion.

Contraindications
Contraindications have not yet been identified.

Pregnancy/Lactation
Information regarding safety and efficacy in pregnancy and lactation is lacking.

Interactions
Possible interactions may exist with other hypoglycemic medications. Goat's rue may interfere with absorption of iron and other minerals.

Adverse Reactions
Discontinue use if symptoms such as headache, jitteriness, or weakness occur. The safety of the plant has not been proven in pregnancy or breastfeeding. Goat's rue may interfere with the absorption of iron and other minerals.

Toxicology
In humans, danger of intoxication has been observed with other guanidine derivatives.

Local Anesthetic/Vasoconstrictor Precautions No information available to require special precautions

Effects on Bleeding None reported

Goji Berry

Clinical Overview

Use
Limited quality clinical trials exist to support therapeutic claims. In vitro and animal experiments suggest antioxidant, hypoglycemic, immune-enhancing, and neuro-, hepato-, and ophthalmic-protective effects.

Dosing
Data are lacking to guide dosage in the clinical setting.

Contraindications
Contraindications have not been identified.

Pregnancy/Lactation
Information regarding safety and efficacy in pregnancy and lactation is lacking.

Interactions
Case reports of interactions with warfarin exist.

Adverse Reactions
Clinical trials report few or no adverse reactions. Information is limited.

Toxicology
Information is lacking.

Local Anesthetic/Vasoconstrictor Precautions No information available to require special precautions

Effects on Bleeding None reported

Goldenseal

Clinical Overview

Use
Goldenseal may be of use in topical infections and is used as an eyewash, but clinical trials are lacking to support its effectiveness. Goldenseal has been included in cold and flu preparations for its anticatarrhal effects, but little evidence supports this use and its effects are debatable. The berberine extract of goldenseal has been used to treat diarrhea. Cardiovascular effects are not clearly defined.

Dosing
Few well-controlled clinical trials are available to guide dosage. Recommended dosages vary considerably: 250 mg to 1 g 3 times daily; some product labeling suggests dosages as high as 3,420 mg/day. Ten to 30 drops of the extract 2 to 4 times a day have been recommended for influenza.

Contraindications
None well defined.

Pregnancy/Lactation
Documented uterine stimulant. Avoid use.

Interactions
Goldenseal may affect the CYP-450 system; however, the clinical importance of this interaction is not clear.

Adverse Reactions
Adverse reactions with usual doses are rare. Berberine may displace bilirubin. Very high doses of goldenseal may rarely induce nausea, anxiety, depression, seizures, or paralysis.

Toxicology
Research reveals little or no information regarding toxicology with the use of this product. Berberine may exhibit phototoxic ocular effects. The sodium-sparing diuretic effect of goldenseal resulted in a case report of reversible hypernatremia in a child.

Local Anesthetic/Vasoconstrictor Precautions No information available to require special precautions

Effects on Bleeding None reported

Gossypol

Clinical Overview

Use

According to Chinese studies, gossypol is effective as a nonhormonal male contraceptive; however, it has been documented to have irreversible effects on male fertility. It is being studied for clinical applications in cancer therapy.

Dosing

Antifertility: Trials have used 5 to 10 mg daily for 2 to 3 months to achieve azoospermia, with a lower maintenance dose for up to 2 years.

Cancer: Maximum tolerated dosages appear to be 40 mg of gossypol (as AT-101) per day.

Contraindications

None well documented.

Pregnancy/Lactation

Documented abortifacient effects. Avoid use.

Interactions

None well documented.

Adverse Reactions

Nausea, emesis, anorexia, diarrhea, altered taste sensation, small intestine obstruction, and fatigue have been recorded in clinical trials. The irreversible effects of gossypol on male fertility have been well documented, as has the incidence of hypokalemia.

Toxicology

Gossypol is potentially toxic.

Local Anesthetic/Vasoconstrictor Precautions No information available to require special precautions
Effects on Bleeding None reported

Gotu Kola

Clinical Overview

Use

Gotu kola has been traditionally used as treatment for a variety of conditions and as an aphrodisiac. There is potential efficacy in treating wounds, varicose veins, skin disorders, venous insufficiency, and to enhance memory, although there is little clinical information to support these claims.

Dosing

Dosages of gotu kola in crude form range from 1.5 to 4 g/day. Various extracts standardized to asiaticoside content also are available and have been studied in clinical trials in venous insufficiency and wound healing at doses of 30 to 90 mg/day. Wound-healing studies have involved topical application of a hydrogel ointment containing a titrated extract of C. asiatica (TECA). Commercial manufacturers have numerous dosage regimens listed for gotu kola.

Contraindications

Avoid use if hypersensitive to any of the ingredients of C. asiatica or gotu kola.

Pregnancy/Lactation

Avoid use during pregnancy and lactation, because gotu kola may have emmenagogue effects.

Interactions

None well documented.

Adverse Reactions

Contact dermatitis is documented in some clinical trials.

Toxicology

Three cases of hepatotoxicity have been reported with patients using C. asiatica for 20 to 60 days.

Local Anesthetic/Vasoconstrictor Precautions No information available to require special precautions
Effects on Bleeding None reported

Grapefruit

Clinical Overview

Use

Clinical trials are generally lacking for therapeutic applications. Grapefruit or its juice have potential in influencing weight loss and promoting cholesterol reduction, and have demonstrated antibacterial activity in the urinary tract.

Dosing

Quality clinical trials upon which to base therapeutic dosing recommendations are limited. Improved lipid profiles were achieved with consumption of 1 grapefruit daily for 30 days. Grapefruit juice 8 oz (237 mL), or half of a fresh grapefruit, 3 times a day before each meal for 12 weeks resulted in weight loss in a clinical trial evaluating the effect on metabolic syndrome.

Contraindications

None well defined. In patients with major myocardial structural disorders, pink grapefruit should probably be avoided due to proarrhythmic effects. The potential for drug interaction with grapefruit should be considered in cases where an increase or decrease of the available drug is clinically important.

Pregnancy/Lactation

GRAS (generally recognized as safe) for use as food. Safety and efficacy for dosages above those in foods are unproven.

Interactions

Grapefruit juice has been reported to interact with numerous drugs; however, case reports of significant interactions are rare. Interactions between grapefruit and cyclosporine and some, but not all, calcium channel antagonists and HMG-CoA reductase inhibitors are considered relevant. However, the potential for an interaction with grapefruit should be considered in cases where an increase or decrease of the available drug is clinically important.

Adverse Reactions

Reports of adverse reactions to grapefruit consumption are limited and are largely related to drug interactions. Case reports exist of allergy to pectin and pectin-induced asthma.

Toxicology

Toxicological studies on whole grapefruit are lacking. A meta-analysis of 3 landmark studies evaluating the association of grapefruit consumption and risk of breast cancer found no increased risk. The constituent d-limonene in grapefruit has GRAS status. Grapefruit seed extract has been shown to be toxic to human skin fibroblast cells.

Local Anesthetic/Vasoconstrictor Precautions No information available to require special precautions
Effects on Bleeding None reported

Grape Seed

Clinical Overview

Use

Grape seed is known for its antioxidant properties. Limited studies suggest possible cardiovascular, chemopreventive, and cytoprotective effects.

Dosing

Extracts of grape seeds containing mostly proantho-cyanidin have been studied for antioxidant and cardi-ovascular properties, as well as for venous insufficiency and ophthalmologic disorders at doses of 50 to 300 mg/day. A maximum of 900 mg/day has been used.

Contraindications

Contraindicated in patients with known hypersensitivity to grape seed.

Pregnancy/Lactation

Information regarding safety and efficacy in pregnancy and lactation is lacking.

Interactions

Caution is advised when administering supplements containing grape seed polyphenols concomitantly with vitamin C to hypertensive patients because increases in blood pressure may occur.

Adverse Reactions

None well documented. It is contraindicated in patients with known hypersensitivity to grape seed. Gastralgia, headache, and an allergic reaction have been reported in the literature. Additional clinical studies are recommended.

Toxicology

No toxicity in humans has been reported.

Local Anesthetic/Vasoconstrictor Precautions No information available to require special precautions

Effects on Bleeding None reported

Green Tea

Clinical Overview

Use

Tea is traditionally consumed as a beverage. Evidence from clinical trials suggests that green tea plays a role in metabolic syndrome because it may have an impact on body weight, glucose homeostasis, and other cardiovascular risk factors. It has yet to be determined whether green tea is an agent in cancer prevention; however, a role in the prevention of stroke has been suggested. Topical applications have been studied for protection from ultraviolet (UV) damage, and a commercial preparation has been approved for use in the treatment of anogenital warts.

Dosing A daily intake of 3 to 5 cups/day (1,200 mL) of green tea will provide at least 250 mg/day of catechins. Green tea extract should not be taken on an empty stomach due to the potential for hepatotoxicity from excessive levels of epigallocatechin gallate.

Anogenital warts: topical application of sinecatechins 3 times a day for a maximum of 6 weeks.

Cardiovascular effect: 400 to 716 mg/day of catechins have been used in trials in divided dosages.

Diabetes: Dosages of epigallocatechin gallate range from 84 to 386 mg/day in trials evaluating glucose homeostasis.

Obesity: Dosage ranges used in trials include 270 to 800 mg/day of epigallocatechin gallate, or 125 to 625 mg/day of catechins.

Contraindications

Contraindications have not been identified; however, use caution when hepatic failure is present.

Pregnancy/Lactation

The US Food and Drug Administration (FDA) advises those who are or may become pregnant to avoid caffeine.

Interactions

Vitamin K present in green tea may antagonize the anticoagulant effect of warfarin. Green tea consumption reduces the bioavailability of folic acid and may interfere with the absorption of iron.

Adverse Reactions

There are no reports of clinical toxicity from daily tea consumption as a beverage. Adverse events include headache, dizziness, and GI symptoms. Hepatotoxicity, including 1 fatality, has been associated with high plasma levels of epigallocatechin gallate or its metabolites.

Toxicology

Multidose pharmacokinetic studies suggest a daily dosage of 800 mg/day of epigallocatechin gallate capsules for up to 4 weeks to be safe and well tolerated. High-dose oral green tea extract and catechins were hepatotoxic in rats.

Local Anesthetic/Vasoconstrictor Precautions No information available to require special precautions

Effects on Bleeding Caffeine in green tea may have antiplatelet effects

Guggul

Clinical Overview

Use

Guggul has been used in the traditional Ayurvedic medical system for centuries and has been studied extensively in India. Commercial products are promoted for use in hyperlipidemia; however, clinical studies do not substantiate this claim. Anti-inflammatory and cardiovascular effects are being evaluated, as well as use in cancer, obesity, and diabetes.

Dosing

Clinical trials are lacking to provide dosage guidelines; however, in a US clinical trial of hyperlipidemia, 75 to 150 mg of standardized guggulsterones were administered daily. In a study evaluating the anti-inflammatory effect of guggul, 500 mg of gum guggul was taken 3 times per day.

Contraindications

None identified. Caution may be warranted in patients previously experiencing adverse effects to statins.

Pregnancy/Lactation

Information regarding safety and efficacy in pregnancy and lactation is lacking.

Interactions

None well documented.

Adverse Reactions

Although generally accepted as relatively safe, case reports of adverse events exist. Moderate to severe generalized acute eczematous reactions to oral guggul have been reported, and caution may be warranted. A case report exists of rhabdomyolysis possibly caused by guggul consumption.

Toxicology

Research reveals little information regarding toxicology with the use of guggul.

Local Anesthetic/Vasoconstrictor Precautions No information available to require special precautions

Effects on Bleeding None reported

Gymnema

Clinical Overview

Use

The plant has been used in traditional medicine, most notably to control blood glucose. Use as a lipid-lowering agent, for weight loss, and for the inhibition of caries have also been investigated, primarily in rodent studies. However, little to no clinical information is available to support the use of gymnema for any indication.

Dosing

Limited controlled studies exist. Clinical studies investigating antidiabetic effects have typically used 200 or 400 mg extract daily standardized to contain 25% gymnemic acids.

Contraindications

None established.

Pregnancy/Lactation

Information regarding safety and efficacy in pregnancy and lactation is lacking.

Interactions

None well documented.

Adverse Reactions

A case report of hepatotoxicity exists.

Toxicology

Information is lacking.

Local Anesthetic/Vasoconstrictor Precautions No information available to require special precautions

Effects on Bleeding None reported

Hawthorn

Clinical Overview

Use

Hawthorn may have a role as adjunctive therapy in mild heart failure and exhibits some advantages over digoxin. In more severe cases of congestive heart failure (CHF), its place in therapy is less clear. Studies in animals suggest that hawthorn extracts exert effects on the CNS, including anxiolytic and analgesic action; however, clinical studies are limited. Although limited clinical studies have shown improvement in hyperlipidemia with hawthorn extracts, specific, well-designed trials are needed before hawthorn extracts can be recommended.

Dosing

Trials have evaluated dosages ranging from 160 to 1,800 mg/day standardized extracts (mostly WS 1442) in divided doses over 3 to 24 weeks. A minimum effective dose for adjunctive therapy in mild CHF is suggested to be standardized extract 300 mg daily, and maximum benefit appears after 6 to 8 weeks of therapy. Clinical trials conducted in patients with class II and III CHF found hawthorn extract 900 mg daily to be safe, but not superior to placebo.

Contraindications

Known allergy to members of the rose family.

Pregnancy/Lactation

In the absence of clear data, hawthorn extracts should be avoided in pregnancy and during lactation. Animal studies, however, have not shown any adverse effect on embryonic development.

Interactions

None well documented.

Adverse Reactions

Serious adverse reactions are rarely reported. Mild to moderate dizziness, headache, rash, palpitations, and nausea and other GI symptoms have been reported.

Toxicology

Hawthorn is reportedly toxic in high doses; low doses of hawthorn usually lack adverse effects. No increase in the frequency of fetal malformations or teratogenicity has been found in animal studies.

Local Anesthetic/Vasoconstrictor Precautions No information available to require special precautions

Effects on Bleeding None reported

Holy Basil

Clinical Overview

Use

Clinical trials are lacking. In animal and in vitro experiments, effects of holy basil are largely attributed to antioxidant activity. Hypoglycemic activity and protective effects against noise stress have been studied, but clinical trials are lacking.

Dosing

Information is lacking. One clinical trial for hypoglycemic effect used 2.5 g leaves as dried powder in 200 mL water daily for 2 months.

Contraindications

None established.

Pregnancy/Lactation

Information regarding safety and efficacy in pregnancy and lactation is lacking.

Interactions

None well documented.

Adverse Reactions

Information is lacking.

Toxicology

Information is limited. Reversible inhibition of spermatogenesis, and decreased total sperm count and motility have been demonstrated in mice.

Local Anesthetic/Vasoconstrictor Precautions No information available to require special precautions

Effects on Bleeding None reported

Hops

Clinical Overview

Use

Hops have been used for flavoring; hops and lupulin have been used as a digestive aid, for mild sedation, diuresis, and treating menstrual problems, but no clinical studies are available to confirm these uses.

Dosing

Hops has been used as a mild sedative or sleep aid, with the dried strobile given in doses of 1.5 to 2 g. An extract combination with valerian, Ze 91019 (ReDormin, Ivel) has been studied at a hops dose of 60 mg for insomnia.

Contraindications

Contraindications have not yet been identified.

Pregnancy/Lactation

Information regarding safety and efficacy in pregnancy and lactation is lacking.

Interactions

None well documented.

Adverse Reactions

There are no reported side effects when used in moderation.

Toxicology

Malignant hyperthermic reactions have been observed in dogs that consumed boiled hops residues. A wide safety margin for humans has been extrapolated from animal experiments.

Local Anesthetic/Vasoconstrictor Precautions No information available to require special precautions

Effects on Bleeding None reported

Horehound

Clinical Overview

Use

Horehound has been used as a flavoring, expectorant, vasodilator, diaphoretic, diuretic and treatment for intestinal parasites. It reportedly has hypoglycemic effects and influences bile secretion.

Dosing

Horehound is given for digestive complaints as a crude herb at a daily dose of 4.5 g and as a pressed juice of the herb at 30 to 60 mL.

Contraindications

Contraindications have not yet been identified.

Pregnancy/Lactation

Information regarding safety and efficacy in pregnancy and lactation is lacking. Avoid use. Horehound has emmenagogue and abortifacient effects.

Interactions

None well documented.

Adverse Reactions

Large doses may induce cardiac irregularities.

Toxicology

Marrubiin has an LD_{50} of 370 mg/kg when administered orally to rats.

Local Anesthetic/Vasoconstrictor Precautions No information available to require special precautions

Effects on Bleeding None reported

Horse Chestnut

Clinical Overview

Use

Oral horse chestnut seed extract is effective in the short-term treatment of mild to moderate long-term venous insufficiency. Other investigations focus on the role of the major component aescin in antiobesity and anti-inflammatory effects, as well as potential cancer treatment. Aescin gel has been evaluated for use in bruising.

Dosing

Aescin 20 to 120 mg taken orally has been used for venous insufficiency and is available in tablet form. Oral tinctures and topical gels containing aescin 2% are also available.

Contraindications

Renal or hepatic impairment may be relative contraindications to the use of aescin or horse chestnut derivatives.

Pregnancy/Lactation

Avoid use. Information regarding safety and efficacy in pregnancy and lactation is lacking.

Interactions

None well documented.

Adverse Reactions

The most commonly cited adverse effects include nausea and stomach discomfort, which may be minimized by the use of film-coated tablets. Other mild and infrequent complaints include headache, dizziness,

and pruritus. Rare cases of allergy and anaphylaxis have been reported.

Toxicology

All parts of plants in the Aesculus family are potentially toxic, especially the seeds (nuts). Horse chestnut has been classified by the Food and Drug Administration (FDA) as an unsafe herb.

Local Anesthetic/Vasoconstrictor Precautions No information available to require special precautions

Effects on Bleeding Contains esculin which has antithrombotic effects and may increase the risk of bleeding or bruising.

Horseradish

Clinical Overview

Use

Horseradish has been used internally as a condiment, GI stimulant, diuretic, and a vermifuge, and externally for sciatica and facial neuralgia. However, there are no clinical trials to support any therapeutic use for horseradish. Animal data suggest potential antibacterial and hypotensive effects.

Dosing

Traditional use for colds and respiratory infections was 20 g/day of fresh root. Externally, preparations with 2% mustard oil have been used.

Contraindications

Contraindicated in patients with GI ulcers and in those with kidney impairment. Not recommended for children younger than 4 years of age.

Pregnancy/Lactation

Documented adverse effects. Avoid use. Use should be avoided during pregnancy and lactation because the allylisothiocyanates are toxic mucosal irritants. Horseradish has abortifacient effects.

Interactions

None well documented.

Adverse Reactions

Irritant effects on GI mucosa. External use may cause erythematous rash. Horseradish is part of the cabbage and mustard family; therefore, it may suppress thyroid function. The isothiocyanates may irritate mucous membranes on contact or if inhaled.

Toxicology

Ingestion of large amounts can cause bloody vomiting and diarrhea.

Local Anesthetic/Vasoconstrictor Precautions No information available to require special precautions

Effects on Bleeding None reported

Horsetail

Clinical Overview

Use

Horsetail has been used as a diuretic, in the treatment of kidney and bladder ailments, as an astringent to stop bleeding and stimulate healing, as an antitubercular drug, and as a cosmetic component, although there is a lack of clinical trials.

Dosing

A water extract of horsetail was used in a clinical study as a hypoglycemic in type 2 diabetes at 0.33 g/kg via the oral route.

Contraindications

No longer considered safe for use.

Pregnancy/Lactation

Information regarding safety and efficacy in pregnancy and lactation is lacking. Avoid use.

Interactions

None well documented.

Adverse Reactions

No data.

Toxicology

Horsetail is of undefined safety and may be toxic, especially to children. Avoid use during pregnancy.

Local Anesthetic/Vasoconstrictor Precautions No information available to require special precautions

Effects on Bleeding None reported

5-HTP

Clinical Overview

Use

Clinical trials of 5-HTP conducted in various conditions have resulted in limited evidence suggesting a place in therapy for anxiety, depression, and neurological conditions in which a serotonin deficiency is a contributory factor. 5-HTP may also be an effective appetite suppressant, but further clinical trials are needed.

Dosing

Recent clinical trials do not provide adequate dosing guidelines. Studies in depression have used 5-HTP 200 to 300 mg/day given in 3 to 4 divided doses to prevent possible nausea.

Contraindications

The potential for serotonin syndrome exists with concomitant use of selective serotonin reuptake inhibitors (SSRIs) or monoamine oxidase inhibitors (MAOIs).

Pregnancy/Lactation

Information regarding safety and efficacy in pregnancy and lactation is lacking.

Interactions

The potential for serotonin syndrome exists with concomitant use of SSRIs or MAOIs. 5-HTP augments the effect of citalopram and clomipramine, while carbidopa increases the bioavailability of 5-HTP.

Adverse Reactions

Nausea and vomiting are the most common dose-related adverse events. Diarrhea, abdominal pain, mild headache, and sleepiness have also been reported.

Toxicology

There is little information on the toxicology of 5-HTP. A possible association with fatal eosinophilia-myalgia syndrome in the 1980s and 1990s has now been attributed to contaminated L-tryptophan.

Local Anesthetic/Vasoconstrictor Precautions No information available to require special precautions

Effects on Bleeding None reported

Human Chorionic Gonadotropin

Clinical Overview

Use

Existing evidence does not support the use of human chorionic gonadotropin (hCG) in weight reduction, and the use of hCG for this purpose is not supported by the American Medical Association (AMA) or the American Society of Bariatric Physicians. Homeopathic preparations of hCG do not contain significant amount of the active ingredient, and clinical trials have not been conducted to provide evidence for effect.

Dosing

Recommendations for dosing for indications other than those approved for hCG cannot be made because evidence to support efficacy is lacking.

Contraindications

Precocious puberty, prostatic carcinoma or other androgen-dependent neoplasia, prior allergic reaction to chorionic gonadotropin, and pregnancy.

Pregnancy/Lactation

hCG is contraindicated in pregnant women. Avoid use in lactation.

Interactions

None well documented.

Adverse Reactions

Arterial thromboembolism, headache, irritability and other CNS symptoms, genitourinary effects, and hypersensitivity have been reported.

Toxicology

Defects of forelimbs and the CNS, as well as alterations in sex ratio, have been reported in mice on combined gonadotropin and hCG regimens. No mutagenic effect has been clearly established in humans.

Local Anesthetic/Vasoconstrictor Precautions No information available to require special precautions

Effects on Bleeding None reported

Huperzine A

Clinical Overview

Use

Historically, club moss has been used for the treatment of bruises, strains, swelling, rheumatism, and colds, to relax muscles and tendons, and to improve blood circulation. Because of its anticholinesterase activity, huperzine A, a constituent of the whole plant, has been studied for potential use in treating Alzheimer disease and other CNS disorders; however, there is still insufficient evidence to support its routine use.

Dosing

Huperzine A has been studied at oral dosages of 0.2 to 0.4 mg/day for Alzheimer disease.

Contraindications

Contraindications have not been identified.

Pregnancy/Lactation

Information regarding safety and efficacy in pregnancy and lactation is lacking.

Interactions

None well documented.

Adverse Reactions

In clinical trials, cholinergic adverse reactions have been noted, including hyperactivity, nasal obstruction, nausea, vomiting, diarrhea, insomnia, anxiety, dizziness, thirst, and constipation. One trial reported abnormalities in electrocardiogram (ECG) patterns (cardiac ischemia and arrhythmia).

Toxicology

Symptoms of acute toxicity are similar to those of other cholinergic inhibitors and include muscular tremor, drooling, tears, increased bronchial secretions, and incontinence. No mutagenicity or teratogenicity were found in rodent studies.

Local Anesthetic/Vasoconstrictor Precautions No information available to require special precautions

Effects on Bleeding None reported

Hyssop

Clinical Overview

Use

Hyssop is used as flavoring, fragrance, insecticide, insect repellent and cough and cold treatment.

Dosing

There is no clinical evidence for hyssop upon which dosing recommendations can be based.

Contraindications

Contraindications have not yet been identified.

Pregnancy/Lactation

Documented adverse effects. Avoid use. Hyssop has emmenagogue and abortifacient effects.

Interactions

None well documented.

Adverse Reactions

No data.

Toxicology

The essential oils have produced fatal convulsions in rats.

Local Anesthetic/Vasoconstrictor Precautions No information available to require special precautions

Effects on Bleeding None reported

Iboga

Clinical Overview

Use

Iboga is used ritually as an hallucinogen. Studies suggest that ibogaine, one of the iboga alkaloids, has potential in the treatment of addiction to several substances. Use of iboga is illegal in the United States.

Dosing

Ibogaine has been used in single doses of 500 to 800 mg in the treatment of drug addiction; strict medical supervision is essential.

Contraindications

Several deaths have been associated with the use of ibogaine; use of the agent without the supervision of an experienced physician is contraindicated.

Pregnancy/Lactation

Information regarding the safety and efficacy in pregnancy and lactation is lacking. Avoid use.

Interactions

None well documented.

Adverse Reactions

Ataxia, bradycardia, hypotension, mild tremor, and nausea have been reported.

Toxicology

Large doses of iboga can induce convulsions, paralysis, and death from respiratory failure. Dose-dependent brain damage has been observed in rodents.

Local Anesthetic/Vasoconstrictor Precautions No information available to require special precautions

Effects on Bleeding None reported

Ipecac

Clinical Overview

Use

Ipecac has been used as an emetic and treatment for dysentery. It has amebicidal components. It currently is not recommended as an emetic for childhood poisonings. Activated charcoal now is the treatment of choice. Always consult a health care professional or poison control center when an accidental poisoning occurs.

Dosing

Ipecac syrup, which contains total alkaloids123 to 157 mg per 100 mL, has been used to induce vomiting. The usual dose range for the syrup is 10 to 30 mL, yielding a dose of alkaloids of 12 to 48 mg. Do not confuse the syrup with the fluid extract of ipecac, which is 14 times stronger. Cumulative toxicity requires administration of emetine for amebic dysentery in low doses for a short time with intervals of several weeks before further treatment.

Contraindications

Do not administer ipecac when a patient has a decreased level of consciousness or has ingested either a corrosive substance or hydrocarbon with a high aspiration potential.

Pregnancy/Lactation

Documented adverse effects include uterine stimulation. Avoid use.

Interactions

None well documented.

Adverse Reactions

Repeated exposure to powdered ipecac may cause rhinitis or asthma. Emetine can irritate skin if applied topically. Diarrhea, lethargy, drowsiness, and prolonged vomiting may occur.

Toxicology

Ipecac extracts may be highly toxic; do not confuse with syrup of ipecac. Emetine is a cardiotoxin and has been associated with serious cardiotoxicity.

Local Anesthetic/Vasoconstrictor Precautions No information available to require special precautions

Effects on Bleeding None reported

Jiaogulan

Clinical Overview

Use

Limited clinical studies have been conducted to support therapeutic applications. Jiaogulan may play a role in the management of type 2 diabetes, fatty liver disease, immune response (such as asthma), and cancer. *G. pentaphyllum* extracts may also have a place in beneficial antioxidant therapy.

Dosing

Clinical information is lacking. Jiaogulan tea (aqueous extract) 6 g/day, in divided doses twice a day 30 minutes before meals, has been studied in 2 clinical trials in patients with type 2 diabetes.

Contraindications

Contraindications have not yet been identified.

Pregnancy/Lactation

Information regarding safety and efficacy in pregnancy and lactation is lacking.

Interactions

None well documented.

Adverse Reactions

Severe nausea and increased bowel movements are possible.

Toxicology

No data available for human toxicity.

Local Anesthetic/Vasoconstrictor Precautions No information available to require special precautions

Effects on Bleeding None reported

Jojoba

Clinical Overview

Use

The toxicity of the constituent simmondsin in jojoba seed meal and some oil components limits the likelihood of clinical applications. Jojoba oil is commonly used in dermatological preparations.

Dosing

There is no clinical evidence to guide dosage of jojoba or its oil; it is primarily used as a vehicle for oxidation-sensitive substances in ointments.

Contraindications

Although absolute contraindications have not been identified, jojoba should not be ingested by humans due to potential toxicity.

Pregnancy/Lactation

Information regarding safety and efficacy in pregnancy and lactation is lacking. Adverse toxicological studies in rodents and birds exist.

Interactions

None well documented.

Adverse Reactions

Case reports of contact dermatitis, confirmed by skin patch tests, exist for jojoba oil.

Toxicology

Constituents of jojoba are toxic. Studies demonstrate hematological toxicity, histological abnormalities, and other adverse effects.

Local Anesthetic/Vasoconstrictor Precautions No information available to require special precautions

Effects on Bleeding None reported

Juniper

Clinical Overview

Use

Juniper berries have long been used as a flavoring for beverages and as a seasoning for cooking. It is also used as a diuretic and in the management of bronchitis and arthritis. Use is limited to low concentrations.

Dosing

There are no recent clinical studies of juniper; however, classical use of the oil called for dosage of 0.1 mL or 20 to 100 mg of the essential oil, or 2 to 10 g of the berry, for dyspepsia, and as a diuretic or emmenagogue.

Contraindications

Juniper is contraindicated in those patients with reduced renal function.

Pregnancy/Lactation

Documented adverse effects include allergenic, catharsis in large doses, diuretic, and increases uterine tone (ie, possible anti-implantation, abortifacient, and emmenagogue effects). Avoid use.

Interactions

None well documented.

Adverse Reactions

Skin and respiratory allergic reactions may occur.

Toxicology

Topically applied juniper can cause potentially carcinogenic DNA damage and, in large doses, convulsions and renal damage. Juniper should not be ingested by pregnant women.

Local Anesthetic/Vasoconstrictor Precautions No information available to require special precautions

Effects on Bleeding None reported

Kava

Clinical Overview

Use

A number of meta-analyses and systematic reviews of kava use in anxiety have found in favor of kava over placebo, but results are not consistent. Kava has also been studied for effects on cognitive function and for potential cancer applications. However, concerns over hepatotoxicity have limited clinical studies.

Dosing

A maximum daily dose of kavalactones 250 mg is suggested to avoid potential hepatotoxicity. Studies in children are lacking, and use is not recommended.

Contraindications

Kava and kava-containing products are not recommended for use in children or in patients with hepatic disease. Kava should be used cautiously in patients with renal or liver disease, blood disorders, Parkinson disease, or depression.

Pregnancy/Lactation

Documented adverse effects. Avoid use.

Interactions

Kava extracts have been shown to interfere with cytochrome P450 (CYP-450) enzymes; however, specific reports on the metabolism of pharmaceuticals are sparse. Case reports exist on interactions with alprazolam, alcohol, barbiturates, and levodopa. Concomitant administration of kava with haloperidol, risperidone, and metoclopramide, among other drugs, may be associated with adverse reactions.

Adverse Reactions

Heavy kava use may cause a scaly skin rash. A variety of adverse reactions, including visual disturbances, urinary retention, GI discomfort, exacerbation of Parkinson disease, extrapyramidal effects, and rhabdomyolysis, have been reported.

Toxicology

Rare cases of severe liver toxicity have been reported.

Local Anesthetic/Vasoconstrictor Precautions No information available to require special precautions

Effects on Bleeding None reported

Kudzu

Clinical Overview

Use

Current interest in kudzu centers on its use as therapy for alcoholism, although sufficient and consistent clinical trials are lacking. Estrogenic activity of kudzu is also being investigated, although clinical trials are limited.

Dosing

Kudzu extract 3 g daily with 25% isoflavone content has been studied in adult heavy drinkers. In another study, 2.4 g kudzu root was given daily.

Contraindications

Contraindications have not yet been identified.

Pregnancy/Lactation

Information regarding safety in pregnancy and lactation is lacking.

Interactions

None well documented.

Adverse Reactions

A few case reports of allergy exist.

Toxicology

Limited data available.

Local Anesthetic/Vasoconstrictor Precautions No information available to require special precautions

Effects on Bleeding None reported

Lady's Mantle

Clinical Overview

Use

Lady's mantle has been used topically and internally, as a treatment for wounds, gastrointestinal complaints, and female ailments. Its tannin content appears to justify astringent and antidiarrheal uses. It may protect ▶

conjunctive and elastic tissues and possibly be useful as an antioxidant.

Dosing

There is no clinical evidence to support specific dosage recommendations for lady's mantle. Classical use of the herb for treatment of diarrhea was 5 to 10 g of herb daily.

Contraindications

Contraindications have not yet been identified.

Pregnancy/Lactation

Information regarding safety and efficacy in pregnancy and lactation is lacking.

Interactions

None well documented.

Adverse Reactions

None known for low doses.

Toxicology

No significant toxicology data available.

Local Anesthetic/Vasoconstrictor Precautions No information available to require special precautions

Effects on Bleeding None reported

Laminaria

Clinical Overview

Use

Laminaria has been used traditionally as a hygroscopic cervical dilator and inducer of labor, and commercial products are available for this purpose. The basal parts of the blades of Laminaria japonica and Laminaria angustata have been used as a hypotensive agent (ne-kombu) in Japanese folk medicine.

Dosing

Clinical trials are lacking to provide dosing information for uses other than mechanical cervical dilation.

Contraindications

Use is contraindicated during pregnancy.

Pregnancy/Lactation

Laminaria dilators have been used to dilate the cervix and to induce labor in abortions. Information on the use of laminaria for other purposes during pregnancy is lacking. Avoid use.

Interactions

None well documented.

Adverse Reactions

There is a risk of laminaria dilators becoming trapped and fragmenting.

Toxicology

Information is lacking.

Local Anesthetic/Vasoconstrictor Precautions No information available to require special precautions

Effects on Bleeding None reported

L-arginine

Clinical Overview

Use

L-arginine is a nonessential amino acid that may play an important role in the treatment of cardiovascular disease due to its antiatherogenic, anti-ischemic, anti-platelet, and antithrombotic properties. It has been promoted as a growth stimulant and as a treatment for erectile dysfunction in men.

Dosing

L-arginine has been studied at oral doses of 6 to 30 g/day for a variety of conditions. Parenteral, enteral, intramural, and topical formulations have been used.

Contraindications

Absolute contraindications have not yet been identified. L-arginine is not recommended in patients following an acute myocardial infarction.

Pregnancy/Lactation

Specific information regarding safety and efficacy in pregnancy and lactation is lacking, although several trials have been conducted in pregnant women without notable ill effects.

Interactions

L-arginine has unpredictable effects on insulin and cholesterol-lowering agents. L-arginine may potentiate the effects of isosorbide mononitrate and other nitric oxide donors, such as glyceryl trinitrate and sodium nitroprusside.

Adverse Reactions

L-arginine has few reported adverse reactions. Nausea and diarrhea have been reported infrequently. Bitter taste may occur with higher doses. Due to its vasodilatory effects, hypotension may occur. Intravenous (IV) preparations containing L-arginine hydrochloride have a high chloride content that may increase the risk for metabolic acidosis in patients with electrolyte imbalances. Hyperkalemia and elevations in serum urea nitrogen (BUN) levels may occur in patients with renal and/or hepatic impairment.

Toxicology

High concentrations of nitric oxide are considered toxic to brain tissue.

Local Anesthetic/Vasoconstrictor Precautions No information available to require special precautions

Effects on Bleeding None reported

Lavender

Clinical Overview

Use

Lavender has been used for restlessness, insomnia, anxiety, diabetes, GI distress, perineal discomfort following childbirth, chemoprevention, as an insect repellant, and as a food flavoring agent. However, there are limited clinical trials to support any therapeutic use for lavender.

Dosing

Aromatherapy for a bath: 6 drops (120 mg) added to 20 L of bath water or 20 to 100 g of the dried herb in 20 L of bath water.

Inhalational aromatherapy: 2 to 4 drops in 2 to 3 cups (480 to 720 mL) of boiling water or used in an aromatic diffuser and inhaled.

Massage: 1 to 4 drops/Tbsp (15 mL) of base or carrier oil may be used or it may be mixed with other oils.

Tea: 1 to 2 tsp (5 to 10 mL) of lavender per cup (240 mL) of water.

Oil for ingestion: 1 to 4 drops (20 mg to 80 mg), often given on a sugar cube.

Contraindications

Cautious use or avoidance is warranted in patients with known allergy/hypersensitivity to lavender.

Pregnancy/Lactation

Information regarding safety and efficacy in pregnancy and lactation is lacking. Lavender may possess emmenagogue properties, and excessive internal use should be avoided in pregnancy.

Interactions

CNS depressants and anticonvulsants may increase or potentiate narcotic and sedative effects when given in combination with lavender-containing products. Anticoagulants may increase the risk of bleeding when given concomitantly with lavender. Lavender may also cause additive cholesterol-lowering effects when given along with other drugs that lower cholesterol (eg, statins, nicotinic acid, fibric acid derivatives).

Adverse Reactions

Lavender may cause allergic contact dermatitis and photosensitization. Large oral doses have been associated with nausea, vomiting, and anorexia. Additionally, 3 case reports suggest a possible association between topical application of lavender and tea tree oils and prepubertal gynecomastia.

Toxicology

A case report describes an accidental ingestion of lavandin resulting in central nervous system depression in an 18-month-old child. The child's neurological state normalized within 6 hours of ingestion.

Local Anesthetic/Vasoconstrictor Precautions No information available to require special precautions
Effects on Bleeding None reported

Lecithin

Clinical Overview

Use

Lecithin is used for its emulsifying properties in the food, pharmaceutical, and cosmetic industries. Pharmacological use of lecithin includes treatment for hypercholesterolemia, neurologic disorders, and liver ailments. It has also been used to modify the immune system by activating specific and nonspecific defense systems.

Dosing

Studies of lecithin in cognitive impairment have used a wide variety of doses, from 1 to 35 g daily. A systematic review has been published.

Contraindications

Contraindications have not yet been identified.

Pregnancy/Lactation

Information regarding safety and efficacy in pregnancy and lactation is lacking.

Interactions

None well documented.

Adverse Reactions

Adverse effects are usually not associated with lecithin. However, there have been reports of anorexia, nausea, increased salivation, other GI effects, and hepatitis.

Toxicology

Research reveals little or no information regarding toxicology with the use of this product.

Local Anesthetic/Vasoconstrictor Precautions No information available to require special precautions
Effects on Bleeding None reported

Lemon Balm

Clinical Overview

Use

Primary interest in lemon balm surrounds its effects on the central nervous system. One small study demonstrated decreased stress and agitation in patients with dementia and Alzheimer disease. Lemon balm cream has shown some efficacy in herpes virus lesions in a few small placebo-controlled trials.

Dosing

Crude lemon balm herb is typically dosed at 1.5 to 4.5 g/day. Doses of 600 to 1,600 mg extract have been studied in trials. A standardized preparation of lemon balm (80 mg) and valerian extract (160 mg) has been

given 2 or 3 times/day as a sleep aid, and has also been studied in children. A 1% extract cream has been studied as a topical agent for treatment of herpes virus lesions.

Contraindications

Contraindications have not yet been identified.

Pregnancy/Lactation

Information regarding safety and efficacy in pregnancy and lactation is lacking.

Interactions

None well documented.

Adverse Reactions

Clinical trials generally report no adverse reactions.

Toxicology

Research reveals little or no information regarding toxicology with the use of this product.

Local Anesthetic/Vasoconstrictor Precautions No information available to require special precautions
Effects on Bleeding None reported

Lemongrass

Clinical Overview

Use

Lemongrass is used as a fragrance and flavoring and for a wide variety of ailments in folk medicine. However, clinical trials are lacking to support these uses. Limited studies have demonstrated antifungal and insecticide efficacy, as well as potential anticarcinogenic activity, while suggested hypotensive and hypoglycemic actions have not been confirmed.

Dosing

Information from clinical trials is lacking.

Contraindications

Contraindications have not yet been identified.

Pregnancy/Lactation

Information regarding safety and efficacy in pregnancy and lactation is lacking. Avoid use.

Interactions

None well documented.

Adverse Reactions

Rare cases of hypersensitivity have been reported. Toxic alveolitis has been associated with inhalation of the oil.

Toxicology

Lemongrass is considered to be of low toxicity at low doses.

Local Anesthetic/Vasoconstrictor Precautions No information available to require special precautions
Effects on Bleeding None reported

Licorice

Clinical Overview

Use

Used historically for GI complaints, licorice is primarily used as a flavoring agent in the tobacco and candy industries and to some extent in the pharmaceutical and beverage industries today. The chemical compounds found in licorice have been investigated as cancer therapy as well as for their antiviral activity.

Dosing

Licorice root has been used in daily doses from 2 to 15 g for ulcer and gastritis. Higher doses given for extended periods of time may pose a risk of hyperkalemia. The acceptable daily intake (ADI) for glycyrrhizin is suggested to be 0.2 mg/kg/day.

Contraindications

Contraindications have not yet been identified.

Pregnancy/Lactation

Use during pregnancy should be avoided. Licorice exhibits estrogenic activity and has reputed abortifacient effects. There is no clinical evidence to support the use of licorice tea as a galactogogue.

Interactions

Glycyrrhizin in licorice may alter prednisolone plasma concentrations and may increase the risk of digitalis toxicity.

Adverse Reactions

At lower dosages or normal consumption levels, few adverse reactions are evident. Ocular effects and hypersensitivity have been described. Hypertension and hypokalemia are recognized effects of excessive licorice consumption.

Toxicology

Toxicity from excessive licorice ingestion is well established. Mutagenicity and teratogenicity studies have generally shown no ill effects.

Local Anesthetic/Vasoconstrictor Precautions No information available to require special precautions

Effects on Bleeding None reported

Lobelia

Clinical Overview

Use

Lobelia inflata and its major alkaloid, lobeline, have been used in smoking cessation programs and have been proposed for treatment of other drug dependencies; however, there is only modest evidence for efficacy.

Dosing

Clinical studies of lobeline for smoking withdrawal used doses of 5 mg twice daily, with 0.5 mg lozenges used in addition when there was an urge to smoke. The useful dose of lobeline is very close to the toxic dose. In use of the whole plant, minor variations in alkaloid content could increase the potential for toxicity.

Contraindications

Contraindications have not yet been identified.

Pregnancy/Lactation

Documented adverse effects include loss of uterine tone. Avoid use.

Interactions

None well documented.

Adverse Reactions

Lobelia and lobeline are capable of inducing nausea, vomiting, and dizziness at high doses (8 mg lobeline sulfate).

Toxicology

The therapeutic dose of lobeline is very close to the toxic dose.

Local Anesthetic/Vasoconstrictor Precautions No information available to require special precautions

Effects on Bleeding None reported

Lycopene

Clinical Overview

Use

The scientific literature documents the antioxidant activity of lycopene and its use in cancer prevention and cardiovascular disease.

Dosing

Lycopene administered as a pure compound has been studied in clinical trials at dosages of 13 to 75 mg/day. Lycopene is mostly available in capsule and softgel form, with dosage guidelines from manufacturers ranging from 10 to 30 mg taken twice daily with meals. Lycopene is also incorporated in multivitamin and multimineral products.

Contraindications

Avoid with hypersensitivity to lycopene or to any of its food sources, especially tomatoes. Tomato-based products are acidic and may irritate stomach ulcers.

Pregnancy/Lactation

Information regarding safety and efficacy during pregnancy and lactation is lacking. The amount of lycopene in foods is assumed to be safe. Tomato consumption does increase lycopene concentrations in the breast milk and plasma of lactating women.

Interactions

Lycopene interacts with some cancer chemotherapy agents, as well as with ciprofloxacin and olestra.

Adverse Reactions

In general, tomato-based products and lycopene supplements are generally well tolerated. The scientific literature documents some GI complaints, such as diarrhea, dyspepsia, gas, nausea, and vomiting. One trial documented a cancer-related hemorrhage in a patient taking lycopene, although causality is unclear.

Toxicology

No toxic effects were observed in rats treated with lycopene 2,000 mg/kg/day for 28 days, an intake similar to approximately 200 mg of lycopene per kg of body weight per day in humans. Another 13-week toxicity study generated similar results.

Local Anesthetic/Vasoconstrictor Precautions No information available to require special precautions

Effects on Bleeding None reported

Maitake

Clinical Overview

Use

Maitake has been used for its antiviral action and to treat diabetes, high blood pressure, cholesterol, and obesity. Maitake has been studied to a limited extent for treating cancer; however, the information available is not sufficient to recommend it for this use.

Dosing

Disease-prevention doses of commercial preparations range from 12 to 25 mg of the extract and 200 to 250 mg or 500 to 2,500 mg of whole powder daily. A trial among HIV-positive patients used doses of 6 g/day whole powder or 20 mg purified extract with 4 g whole maitake powder.

Contraindications

Contraindications have not been identified.

Pregnancy/Lactation

Information regarding safety and efficacy during pregnancy and lactation is lacking.

Interactions

None well documented.

Adverse Reactions

Information is limited.

Toxicology

Information is limited.

Local Anesthetic/Vasoconstrictor Precautions No information available to require special precautions

Effects on Bleeding None reported

Marijuana

Clinical Overview

Use

The use of medical marijuana for the management of chemotherapy-induced nausea, glaucoma, spasticity in multiple sclerosis, and neuropathic pain has been clinically demonstrated to some extent. The likelihood of undesirable adverse reactions limits its applications, and therapeutic use may be limited to either concomitant therapy or when conventional therapy has failed.

Dosing

Clinical studies use a wide range of preparations and usually allow dosage titration for effect, making standard dosage recommendations difficult. A large, multicenter trial used initial doses of 5 mg of oral delta-9-tetrahydrocannabinol (THC) daily, self-titrated up to 25 mg THC daily for up to 52 weeks in multiple sclerosis. Estimates of relative efficacy for THC compared with codeine for pain are 10 mg THC to 60 mg codeine.

Contraindications

Contraindications have not been identified. The benefits versus risks of the use of cannabis extracts should be carefully weighed in individuals with psychosocial disorders.

Pregnancy/Lactation

Information regarding safety and efficacy of medicinal marijuana in pregnancy and lactation is lacking. Avoid use. In retrospective studies, marijuana use has had a modest effect on fetal growth. THC crosses the placental barrier and is excreted in breast milk.

Interactions

None well documented. Potentiation of analgesic medicines can be expected.

Adverse Reactions

The use of medical marijuana or cannabinoid preparations is mainly considered safe and devoid of major adverse reactions. Impairments in cognitive and motor function may limit it use.

Toxicology

Marijuana has a strong potential for abuse and is classified as a schedule I drug. No consensus exists as to the risk of lung cancer from smoked medical marijuana, or the risk of psychotic events from oral cannabinoid consumption. All risk factors should be considered in the context of applications for medical marijuana in intractable diseases. Long-term toxicity due to nonmedical (recreational) cannabis includes increased risk of psychotic, respiratory, and cardiovascular events, as well as cancer.

Local Anesthetic/Vasoconstrictor Precautions No information available to require special precautions

Effects on Bleeding None reported

Maritime Pine

Clinical Overview

Use

Pine bark extract demonstrates antioxidant and anti-inflammatory actions and has been studied for a wide range of clinical conditions, including chronic venous insufficiency, cardiovascular conditions, and erectile dysfunction. However, many clinical studies have been limited in size, with nonrandomized or open-label designs conducted by a limited pool of researchers.

Dosing

Doses of pine bark extract have been studied in clinical trials, most commonly at 150 mg of Pycnogenol per day.

Contraindications

Contraindications have not been identified.

Pregnancy/Lactation

Information regarding safety and efficacy during pregnancy and lactation is lacking.

Interactions

None well documented.

Adverse Reactions

Pine bark extract is generally well tolerated, with minor gastric discomfort, dizziness, nausea, and headache occasionally noted. Clinical studies using Pycnogenol report no clinically important adverse events.

Toxicology

Pine bark extract is generally recognized as safe (GRAS), based on data from clinical trials. Limited toxicological data are available.

Local Anesthetic/Vasoconstrictor Precautions No information available to require special precautions

Effects on Bleeding May see increased bleeding due to inhibition of platelet aggregation

Marsh Mallow

Clinical Overview

Use

Althea mucilage has been used to soothe dermal irritations, sore throats, and coughs. It appears to have bactericidal and anti-inflammatory properties.

Dosing

There is no recent clinical evidence to guide dosage of marsh mallow. Classical daily doses of the root or leaf in cough and bronchitis were 6 g.

Contraindications

Contraindications have not yet been identified.

Pregnancy/Lactation

Information regarding safety and efficacy in pregnancy and lactation is lacking.

Interactions

None well documented.

Adverse Reactions

Research reveals little or no information regarding adverse reactions with the use of this product.

Toxicology

Althea extracts generally have not been associated with toxicity.

Local Anesthetic/Vasoconstrictor Precautions No information available to require special precautions

Effects on Bleeding None reported

Mastic

Clinical Overview

Use

The pharmacology and medicinal use of mastic is diverse. The resin has been used in cancer, infection, surgical wound adhesion, and ulcers. Studies also document its use as an antioxidant and an insecticide, and for treatment of high cholesterol, Crohn disease, diabetes, and hypertension. However, clinical trials to support these uses are limited.

Dosing

Mastic resin has been studied as a treatment for ulcers at a dosage of 1 g daily. Various commercial products are available including Mastika, which contains mastic gum 250 mg in capsule form. The manufacturer's dosage guidelines are 4 capsules by mouth before bed or on an empty stomach for 4 weeks, followed by a maintenance dosage of 2 capsules daily to maintain GI health.

Contraindications
Avoid use with hypersensitivity to any ingredients of mastic gum as well as with pollen hypersensitivity.

Pregnancy/Lactation
Information regarding safety and efficacy in pregnancy and lactation is lacking.

Interactions
None well documented.

Adverse Reactions
Most adverse reactions are associated with hypersensitivity to the plant or to allergic reactions.

Toxicology
Most toxicity involves allergic reactions.

Local Anesthetic/Vasoconstrictor Precautions No information available to require special precautions

Effects on Bleeding None reported

Meadowsweet

Clinical Overview
Use
Meadowsweet has been used for colds, respiratory problems, acid indigestion, peptic ulcers, arthritis and rheumatism, skin diseases, and diarrhea.

Dosing
Doses of 2.5 to 3.5 g/day of flower and 4 to 5 g of herb are considered conventional; however, no clinical trials support the safety or efficacy of these dosages. A tea may be prepared from 4 to 6 g of the dried herb and taken 3 times daily.

Contraindications
Patients with salicylate or sulfite sensitivity. Use with caution in patients with asthma.

Pregnancy/Lactation
Documented adverse effects. Uteroactivity from meadowsweet has been observed in vitro; avoid administration during pregnancy and lactation.

Interactions
Because meadowsweet contains salicylates, it may increase the risk of bleeding when given concomitantly with antiplatelet or anticoagulant drugs, with nonsteroidal anti-inflammatory drugs (NSAIDs), or with any alternative medicines with antiplatelet properties.

Adverse Reactions
Meadowsweet may cause GI bleeding.

Toxicology
Few toxic events have been reported.

Local Anesthetic/Vasoconstrictor Precautions No information available to require special precautions

Effects on Bleeding Limited evidence suggests an anticoagulant effect *in vitro* and *in vivo* by meadowsweet flowers and seeds. Clinical relevance of this effect is unknown. There are no current published reports of any anticoagulant effect in patients taking meadowsweet.

Melatonin

Clinical Overview
Use
A large amount of clinical trial data exists to support melatonin's role in reducing sleep onset latency in many sleep-related disorders in both adults and children. Evidence is less clear for improvements in sleep duration or quality. Clinical trial data suggest that melatonin may increase survival rates in solid tumor

cancers and decrease the adverse effects of chemotherapy. Increased healing rates in gastric and duodenal ulcers have been found in a small number of studies when melatonin was used as adjunctive therapy. Treatment of infertility, hypertension, anxiety, headache, and tinnitus has also been studied.

Dosing
Adjunctive therapy in cancer: Dosages of up to 20 mg/day have been used in trials.

Insomnia: 3 to 5 mg daily in the evening over 4 weeks. Independent studies have not yet clarified the efficacy of sustained-release preparations.

Jet lag: In general, lower doses (0.5 to 2 mg) preflight and higher doses (5 mg) postflight over a period of up to 4 days appear to be adequate.

Pediatric: Melatonin 2 to 5 mg has been used in children

Contraindications
Until it is studied more thoroughly, melatonin is contraindicated for patients with an autoimmune disease.

Pregnancy/Lactation
Information regarding safety and efficacy in pregnancy and lactation is lacking.

Interactions
Melatonin has been used in many conditions as an adjunct to standard therapy with few reports of interactions. Caffeine and fluvoxamine may increase the effects of melatonin. Exogenous melatonin may potentiate the effects of warfarin.

Adverse Reactions
Possible adverse effects include dizziness, enuresis, excessive daytime somnolence, headache, nausea, and transient depression. Drowsiness may be experienced within 30 minutes after taking melatonin and may persist for approximately 1 hour; as a result, melatonin may affect driving ability.

Toxicology
Studies are limited. There is little or no evidence of major toxicities with melatonin, even at high doses.

Local Anesthetic/Vasoconstrictor Precautions No information available to require special precautions

Effects on Bleeding None reported

Methylsulfonylmethane (MSM)

Clinical Overview
Use
MSM is commonly used for osteoarthritis, but may also benefit in alleviating GI upset, musculoskeletal pain, and allergies; boosting the immune system; and fighting antimicrobial infection. Clinical trials are needed to verify these potential uses.

Dosing
MSM commonly is given as 2 to 6 g/day in 2 to 3 divided doses for arthritis and other joint conditions.

Contraindications
Contraindications have not been identified.

Pregnancy/Lactation
Information regarding safety and efficacy in pregnancy and lactation in humans is lacking.

Interactions
None well documented.

Adverse Reactions
No conclusive data on adverse reactions with MSM have been reported.

Toxicology
No toxicity was noted in animal studies.

Local Anesthetic/Vasoconstrictor Precautions No information available to require special precautions
Effects on Bleeding None reported

Milk Thistle

Clinical Overview

Use
Adequate evidence from prospective clinical trial data for milk thistle is lacking. However, studies suggest potential clinical applications for silymarin, a flavonoid extract of milk thistle, in treating alcohol-related hepatitis, toxicity due to Amanita mushroom poisoning, diabetes, and cancer.

Dosing
Consumption of the oral form of milk thistle (standardized to 70% to 80% silymarin) at 420 mg/day in divided doses is considered safe for up to 41 months, based on clinical trial data. High-dose milk thistle has been used within the confines of clinical trials.

Contraindications
Allergy to any plant in the Asteraceae family.

Pregnancy/Lactation
Information is limited. Use in pregnant and breast-feeding women has been reported in limited clinical studies without apparent ill-effect; however, until further data are available, avoid the use of milk thistle in pregnant or breast-feeding women.

Interactions
Despite widespread usage of milk thistle, case reports of clinically important interactions are lacking. Exercise caution when using milk thistle at higher dosages or concomitantly with drugs of a narrow therapeutic index. Milk thistle decreases indinavir trough plasma concentrations.

Adverse Reactions
In most clinical trials, the incidence of adverse reactions was approximately equal in milk thistle and placebo groups. No serious adverse events have been reported at recommended dosages. The most common effects occurring after oral ingestion included brief GI disturbances.

Toxicology
There are no milk thistle toxicities documented in humans, and toxicity appears to be low in laboratory animals.

Local Anesthetic/Vasoconstrictor Precautions No information available to require special precautions
Effects on Bleeding None reported

Mistletoe

Clinical Overview

Use
Mistletoe has been used to treat cancer, although there is a lack of quality clinical trials and no evidence of an effect. Further study is needed. In folk medicine, it has been used for its cardiovascular properties. Clinical efficacy has not been established. Injectable mistletoe extract is widely used in Europe but is not licensed for use in the United States.

Dosing
Crude mistletoe fruit or herb is used to make a tea to treat hypertension at a dosage of 10 g/day. There are a number of proprietary extracts containing low levels of mistletoe lectin-I (ML-I) used as adjuvant cancer therapies. These extracts usually are given by intravenous (IV) or subcutaneous injection at dosages of 0.1 to 30 mg several times per week. Mistletoe preparations, produced according to anthroposophical methods, are given in incrementally increasing dosages depending on the patient's general condition and response to the injection. Use in pediatric patients has been reported. The pharmacokinetics in healthy adults has been determined.

Contraindications
Data are limited. Use of mistletoe extracts in patients with primary or secondary brain tumors, leukemia, or malignant lymphoma is contraindicated.

Pregnancy/Lactation
Mistletoe contains toxic constituents. Avoid use during pregnancy or lactation.

Interactions
None well documented.

Adverse Reactions
Local reactions following injection include redness, itching, inflammation, and induration at the injection site. Systemic reactions include mild fever or flu-like symptoms. Anaphylaxis has been reported.

Toxicology
Poison centers report toxicity of the whole plant, but especially mistletoe berries. The use of preparations standardized to small doses of ML-I or depleted of lectins may reduce toxicity.

Local Anesthetic/Vasoconstrictor Precautions No information available to require special precautions
Effects on Bleeding None reported

Muira Puama

Clinical Overview

Use
P. olacoides is used as a tonic for neuromuscular problems. A root decoction is used externally in massages and baths for paralysis and beriberi. Oral use of tea made from the roots for sexual impotence, rheumatism, and GI problems has been noted. Muira puama is currently promoted as a male aphrodisiac or as a treatment for impotence.

Dosing
Muira puama leaves, stem, and roots typically are used at a dose of 0.5 to 1.5 g/day, although there are no clinical studies supporting this dose.

Contraindications
Contraindications have not yet been identified.

Pregnancy/Lactation
Information regarding safety and efficacy in pregnancy and lactation is lacking.

Interactions
None well documented.

Adverse Reactions
Research reveals little or no information about adverse reactions of muira puama.

Toxicology
Muira puama does not appear to have the serious side effect potential of yohimbine.

Local Anesthetic/Vasoconstrictor Precautions No information available to require special precautions
Effects on Bleeding None reported

Mullein

Clinical Overview

Use
Mullein has expectorant and cough suppressant properties that make it useful for symptomatic treatment of sore throat and cough. Antiviral activity of mullein has

been reported against herpes simplex type I virus and influenza A and B strains.

Dosing

There is no recent clinical evidence to support specific dosage of mullein; however, classical use of the herb was at 3 to 4 g daily.

Contraindications

Contraindications have not yet been identified.

Pregnancy/Lactation

Information regarding safety and efficacy in pregnancy and lactation is lacking.

Interactions

None well documented.

Adverse Reactions

No adverse effects have been reported.

Toxicology

Research reveals no reports of serious toxicities with mullein.

Local Anesthetic/Vasoconstrictor Precautions No information available to require special precautions

Effects on Bleeding None reported

Nettles

Clinical Overview

Use

The primary use of nettles is in the management of symptoms due to benign prostatic hyperplasia (BPH). However, limited clinical trials are available. Nettles are also used in arthritis and allergic rhinitis. A role in diabetes is being investigated in animals.

Dosing

Freeze-dried nettle leaf 600 mg has been used in a clinical trial for allergic rhinitis. Clinical trials for BPH have used aqueous extracts of U. dioica root 360 mg daily over 6 months and methanol root extract 600 to 1,200 mg daily for 6 to 9 weeks.

Contraindications

Due to the effects on androgen and estrogen metabolism, nettle preparations are contraindicated in pregnancy and lactation and should not be used in children younger than 12 years.

Pregnancy/Lactation

Documented adverse effects. Avoid use.

Interactions

None well documented.

Adverse Reactions

Nettles are known primarily for their ability to induce topical irritation following contact with exposed skin. The acute urticaria is caused by the release of histamine, serotonin, and choline from the hairs and spines of the leaves and stem and generally resolves spontaneously. Radix urticae extracts and other nettle preparations are generally well tolerated, with minor and transient gastric effects, including diarrhea, gastric pain, and nausea reported.

Toxicology

The acute oral toxicity of nettle preparations is considered to be very low. Mutagenicity and carcinogenicity studies were negative for the aqueous extract.

Local Anesthetic/Vasoconstrictor Precautions No information available to require special precautions

Effects on Bleeding None reported

Nutmeg

Clinical Overview

Use

Nutmeg and mace, widely accepted as flavoring agents, have been used in higher doses for their aphrodisiac and psychoactive properties.

Dosing

There are no clinical trials to support therapeutic dosing. Consumption of nutmeg at 1 to 2 mg/kg body weight was reported to induce CNS effects. Toxic overdose occurred at a 5 g dose.

Contraindications

Contraindications have not been identified. The excessive use of nutmeg or mace is not recommended in people with psychiatric conditions.

Pregnancy/Lactation

Generally recognized as safe when used in food as a flavoring agent. Safety for doses above those found in foods is unproven; avoid because of possible abortifacient effects.

Interactions

None well documented.

Adverse Reactions

Allergy, contact dermatitis, and asthma have been reported.

Toxicology

CNS excitation with anxiety/fear, cutaneous flushing, decreased salivation, GI symptoms, and tachycardia. Acute psychosis and anticholinergic-like episodes have been documented; death has rarely been reported following the ingestion of large doses of nutmeg.

Local Anesthetic/Vasoconstrictor Precautions No information available to require special precautions

Effects on Bleeding None reported

Octacosanol

Clinical Overview

Use

Octacosanol is being investigated as a herpes antiviral and as a treatment for inflammatory diseases of the skin. It may be helpful with Parkinson disease and ALS, but more studies are needed. Octacosanol administration also has conferred enhanced physical endurance in some studies.

Dosing

Octacosanol (policosanol) has been studied at doses from 10 to 20 mg daily in cholesterol reduction and heart disease.

Contraindications

Contraindications have not yet been identified.

Pregnancy/Lactation

Information regarding safety and efficacy in pregnancy and lactation is lacking.

Interactions

None well documented.

Adverse Reactions

There have been no reported side effects with the use of octacosanol except for a suggestion of interaction with levodopa/carbidopa in Parkinson disease patients.

Toxicology

There are no data on the long-term toxicity of products containing octacosanol.

Local Anesthetic/Vasoconstrictor Precautions No information available to require special precautions

Effects on Bleeding None reported

Oleander

Clinical Overview

Use

Oleander has been used in the treatment of cardiac illness, asthma, diabetes mellitus, corns, scabies, cancer, and epilepsy. However, in none of these conditions is there good evidence for use.

Dosing

There is no clinical evidence to support specific doses of oleander. Extreme caution should be used because of its acute cardiotoxicity.

Contraindications

No longer considered safe.

Pregnancy/Lactation

Information regarding safety and efficacy in pregnancy and lactation is lacking. Avoid use.

Interactions

None well documented.

Adverse Reactions

Phytodermatitis caused by contact with oleander has been reported frequently.

Toxicology

Oleander is extremely toxic. Major toxicity includes disturbances in heart rhythm and death. Other signs of toxicity include pain in the oral cavity, nausea, emesis, abdominal pain, cramping, and diarrhea.

Local Anesthetic/Vasoconstrictor Precautions No information available to require special precautions

Effects on Bleeding None reported

Olive Leaf

Clinical Overview

Use

Interest in olive leaf use centers on antioxidant and antiviral activity, but clinical trials are lacking.

Dosing

There is no basis for dosage recommendations.

Contraindications

Contraindications have not been identified.

Pregnancy/Lactation

Information regarding safety and efficacy during pregnancy and lactation is lacking.

Interactions

None well documented.

Adverse Reactions

None well documented. Diabetic patients should be supervised carefully because of potential hypoglycemic effects.

Toxicology

The potential toxicity of olive leaf is not well documented.

Local Anesthetic/Vasoconstrictor Precautions No information available to require special precautions

Effects on Bleeding None reported

Onion

Clinical Overview

Use

Onion has potential in treating cardiovascular disease, hyperglycemia, and stomach cancer, although few quality clinical trials are available to support these uses. Topical preparations have been evaluated for the prevention of surgical scarring with varying results.

Dosing

Clinical trials are lacking to provide dosage recommendations. Average daily doses of 50 g of fresh onion, 50 g of fresh onion juice, or 20 g of dried onion have been suggested. Topical onion extract gels have been used in studies evaluating the effect on scarring and are generally applied 3 times daily.

Contraindications

Contraindications have not been identified.

Pregnancy/Lactation

Generally recognized as safe when used as food. Avoid dosages above those found in foods because safety is unproven.

Interactions

None well documented.

Adverse Reactions

Few reported.

Toxicology

Information is limited.

Local Anesthetic/Vasoconstrictor Precautions No information available to require special precautions

Effects on Bleeding None reported

Pantothenic Acid

Clinical Overview

Use

Vitamin B-5 may be beneficial in lipid, ophthalmic, and skin disorders. It also has possible radioprotective and adaptogen effects.

Dosing

Pantothenic acid is available in capsule, liquid, and tablet dosage forms from numerous commercial manufacturers. Clinical studies have used pantethine 600 to 1,200 mg per day for hyperlipidemias; however, most commercial Web sites document a typical dose of 300 mg 3 times a day. The US recommended daily allowance (RDA) for pantothenic acid in nutritional supplements and foods is 1 to 7 mg/day.

Contraindications

Avoid use if hypersensitive to pantothenic acid.

Pregnancy/Lactation

US Food and Drug Administration Pregnancy category A (Controlled studies show no risk. Adequate, well-controlled studies in pregnant women have failed to demonstrate risk to the fetus). Pantothenic acid is classified as category C (Risk cannot be ruled out. Human studies are lacking, and animal studies are either positive for fetal risk or lacking. However, potential benefits may justify the potential risks.) when dosed above the recommended dietary allowance. During pregnancy and lactation, the daily maximum dosages are 6 and 7 mg/day of pantothenic acid, respectively.

Interactions

None well documented.

Adverse Reactions

In high doses, pantothenic acid may inhibit the absorption of biotin produced by the microflora in the large intestine. Diarrhea may occur with large doses of pantothenic acid. Allergic contact dermatitis has been reported with topical use of dexpanthenol. A meta-analysis from 1966 to 2002 recorded an adverse reaction rate of 1.4 per 100 subjects. The majority of these reactions were mild GI complaints.

Toxicology

Overall, pantothenic acid is considered to be safe.

Local Anesthetic/Vasoconstrictor Precautions No information available to require special precautions
Effects on Bleeding None reported

Papaya

Clinical Overview

Use

In some developing countries, the traditional use of papaya is being investigated as an alternative to standard treatments for a range of ailments. C. papaya has a wide range of purported medicinal properties including antiseptic, antimicrobial, antiparasitic, anti-inflammatory, antihypertensive, diuretic, antihyperlipidemic, antidiabetic, and contraceptive activity. While there are only limited data to support most of these uses, there is some evidence for use in healing decubitus ulcers and other wounds and in treating intestinal worms in humans.

Dosing

A commercially produced debriding ointment is available by prescription in the United States. Each 1 g contains 8.3×10^5 USP units papain and 100 mg of urea. There are very little data available to make specific recommendations regarding systemic doses of papaya. One study used a 4 g dose of air-dried papaya seeds in 20 mL of honey to treat helminthiasis. In the United States, the fruit is generally recognized as safe (GRAS status) when used as a food.

Contraindications

Papaya may cause severe allergic reactions and is therefore contraindicated in sensitive people.

Pregnancy/Lactation

Possibly unsafe depending on the part of the plant being used and dose administered. Avoid use.

Interactions

None documented.

Adverse Reactions

Papaya may cause severe allergic reactions in sensitive people. Topically, papaya latex can be a severe irritant and vesicant. Papaya juice and papaya seeds are unlikely to cause adverse effects when taken orally; however, papaya leaves at high doses may cause gastric irritation.

Toxicology

There are parts of the plant (eg, seeds) that contain benzyl isothiocyanate, which may cause toxicity at high doses.

Local Anesthetic/Vasoconstrictor Precautions No information available to require special precautions
Effects on Bleeding None reported

Parsley

Clinical Overview

Use

Parsley, in addition to being a source of certain vitamins and minerals, has been used in the treatment of prostate, liver and spleen diseases, as well as anemia, arthritis, and microbial infections. It has also been found useful as a diuretic and laxative. However, there have been no clinical trials to confirm these uses.

Dosing

Parsley has been used at daily doses of 6 g, however, no clinical studies have been found that support this dose. The essential oil should not be used because of toxicity.

Contraindications

Contraindications have not yet been identified.

Pregnancy/Lactation

Generally recognized as safe or used as food. Safety and efficacy for dosages above those in foods are unproven and should be avoided. Emmenagogue and abortifacient effects in higher doses.

Interactions

None well documented.

Adverse Reactions

Adverse effects from the ingestion of parsley oil include headache, giddiness, loss of balance, convulsions, and renal damage.

Toxicology

While no major toxicities have been reported with the use of parsley, pregnant women should not take parsley because of possible uterotonic effects.

Local Anesthetic/Vasoconstrictor Precautions No information available to require special precautions
Effects on Bleeding None reported

Passion Flower

Clinical Overview

Use

Passion flower has been used to treat sleep disorders and historically in homeopathic medicine to treat pain, insomnia related to neurasthenia or hysteria, and nervous exhaustion.

Dosing

No clinical trials of passion flower as a single agent have been reported; however, a daily dose of 4 to 8 g is typical.

Contraindications

Contraindications have not yet been identified.

Pregnancy/Lactation

Documented adverse effects. Avoid use. Passion flower is a known uterine stimulant.

Interactions

None well documented.

Adverse Reactions

Though no adverse effects of passion flower have been reported, large doses may result in CNS depression.

Toxicology

No major clinical trials have been conducted to assess the plant's toxicity.

Local Anesthetic/Vasoconstrictor Precautions No information available to require special precautions
Effects on Bleeding None reported

Pectin

Clinical Overview

Use

Pectin has been used in antidiarrheal products and to lower blood lipoprotein levels. Pectin also has been investigated for its ability to reduce the consequence of exposure to radiation and to inhibit prostate cancer growth, but more study is needed.

Dosing

Pectin and/or modified pectin have been used in clinical studies in doses of 10 to 20 g daily.

Contraindications

Contraindications have not yet been identified.

Pregnancy/Lactation

Information regarding safety and efficacy in pregnancy and lactation is lacking.

Interactions

Coadministration of pectin with beta-carotene–containing foods or supplements can reduce beta-carotene blood levels by more than 50%. Concomitant use of pectin and lovastatin, and other HMG-CoA reductase inhibitors may decrease absorption of the HMG-CoA reductase inhibitor.

Adverse Reactions

Pectin is generally well tolerated when ingested. Occupational asthma has been associated with the inhalation of pectin dust, along with cross-sensitivity to cashew and pistachio nuts.

Toxicology

No major toxicities have been reported with the use of pectin.

Local Anesthetic/Vasoconstrictor Precautions No information available to require special precautions
Effects on Bleeding None reported

Peppermint

Clinical Overview

Use

In addition to use as a seasoning and flavoring, peppermint is used to treat irritable bowel syndrome (IBS) and other GI conditions. Menthol is available in numerous commercial preparations used to treat respiratory tract infections and topically for its cooling and warming action to relieve pain. However, there is limited clinical information supporting its use for these conditions.

Dosing

Peppermint oil has been used as a carminative at doses of 0.1 to 0.24 mL. Up to 1,200 mg of the oil in enteric-coated tablets has been used to treat IBS. Peppermint oil (40 mL) has been added to barium suspensions and also administered intraluminally (8 mL) during colonoscopy.

Contraindications

Peppermint oil should not be administered to patients with gastroesophageal reflux or active gastric ulcers because the oil decreases esophageal sphincter pressure. Peppermint oil should not be applied to the face, especially under the nose of a child or infant. Enteric-coated preparations are not recommended for use in children younger than 8 years.

Pregnancy/Lactation

Documented adverse reactions. Avoid use because of emmenagogue effects.

Interactions

Peppermint oil may influence metabolism of certain drugs, including felodipine and simvastatin, via inhibition of the cytochrome P450 (CYP-450) enzyme system, increasing pharmacologic and adverse reactions. Absorption of caffeine may be delayed by menthol. Decreased cyclosporine levels have been reported with consumption of a tea containing peppermint and 8 other herbs.

Adverse Reactions

Peppermint oil may cause allergic reactions characterized by contact dermatitis, flushing, and headache and may worsen the symptoms of heartburn, hiatus hernias, and stomach ulcers.

Toxicology

Peppermint is GRAS (generally recognized as safe) in amounts used in seasoning or flavoring, although medicinal uses of the plant can cause adverse reactions. (See Adverse Reactions.)

Local Anesthetic/Vasoconstrictor Precautions No information available to require special precautions
Effects on Bleeding None reported

Periwinkle

Clinical Overview

Use

Periwinkle alkaloids have been used in the treatment of leukemia, Hodgkin's disease, malignant lymphomas, neuroblastoma, Wilms tumor, Kaposi's sarcoma, mycosis fungoides, to improve cerebral blood flow, and treat high blood pressure.

Dosing

There is no recent clinical evidence to support specific doses of periwinkle herb. The pure alkaloids vincristine and vinblastine are used in cancer therapy at single weekly IV doses of 0.05 to 0.15 mg/kg and 0.1 to 0.2 mg/kg respectively.

Contraindications

Contraindications have not yet been identified.

Pregnancy/Lactation

Information regarding safety and efficacy in pregnancy and lactation is lacking. Avoid use.

Interactions

None well documented.

Adverse Reactions

Do not self-administer the plant periwinkle. Physicians will inform patients using pharmaceutical forms of periwinkle of possible adverse reactions.

Toxicology

Periwinkle is potentially toxic and has been known to cause acute dyspnea.

Local Anesthetic/Vasoconstrictor Precautions No information available to require special precautions
Effects on Bleeding None reported

Peru Balsam

Clinical Overview

Use

Peru balsam has been used in the treatment of dry socket in dentistry, topically as a treatment for wounds and ulcers, and in suppositories for hemorrhoids. However, there are only older, small case studies to support this use. The material is not used internally.

Dosing

Peru balsam has been used topically in 5% to 20% formulations for wounds and burns. Case reports and small clinical studies report the efficacy of balsam combined with other ingredients in the management of certain wounds; however, there are no recent, well-controlled clinical studies to support appropriate dosing.

Contraindications

Contraindications have not been identified.

Pregnancy/Lactation

Information regarding safety and efficacy in pregnancy and lactation is lacking. Systemic toxicity following application of Peru balsam to the nipples of breastfeeding mothers has been reported.

Interactions

None well documented.

Adverse Reactions

Peru balsam is an allergen.

Toxicology

Information is lacking.

◀ No
information available to require special precautions
Effects on Bleeding None reported

Pineapple

Clinical Overview

Use

Few well-controlled clinical trials have been published
to support the wide range of therapeutic claims for
bromelain, a crude, aqueous extract of pineapple.
Evidence exists primarily for the use of bromelain in
debridement of burns and as an anti-inflammatory
agent.

Dosing

Two slices of pineapple contain approximately 100 mg
of ascorbic acid (vitamin C). The usual dosage of
bromelain is 40 mg taken 3 or 4 times daily. Pineapple
products are available commercially in liquid, tablet,
and capsule doseforms. Most products contain bromelain 500 mg; manufacturers suggest a dose of 500 to
1,000 mg daily.

Contraindications

Hypersensitivity to any of the components in pineapple. Cross-reaction with honeybee venom, olive tree
pollen, celery, cypress pollen, bromelain, and papain
have been reported.

Pregnancy/Lactation

Information regarding safety and efficacy in pregnancy
and lactation is lacking. Data is lacking to support the
historical use of pineapple as an emmenagogue and
abortifacient.

Interactions

Potentiation of amoxicillin and tetracycline because of
increased volume of distribution by bromelain has
been documented.

Adverse Reactions

The juice from unripe pineapples can act as a violent
purgative. Bromelain ingestion is associated with a low
incidence of adverse reactions, including diarrhea,
menorrhagia, nausea, skin rash, and vomiting. Angular
stomatitis/cheilitis can result from eating large amounts
of the fruit.

Toxicology

Bromelain has very low toxicity.

No
information available to require special precautions
Effects on Bleeding May cause increased bleeding
due to inhibition of platelet aggregation

Plantain

Clinical Overview

Use

The psyllium in plantain has been used as GI therapy,
to treat hyperlipidemia for anticancer effects, respiratory treatment, and other uses.

Dosing

Plantain leaves have been given as a tea for cold and
cough at 3 to 6 g/day.

Contraindications

Contraindications have not yet been identified.

Pregnancy/Lactation

Documented adverse effects. Avoid use. Uterine activity, laxative.

Interactions

Patients taking lithium or carbamazepine should avoid
coadministration of plantain. Caution patients receiving
lithium or carbamazepine to consult their health care
provider before using herbal products.

Adverse Reactions

Adverse events include anaphylaxis, chest congestion,
sneezing and watery eyes, occupational asthma, and
a situation involving the occurrence of a giant phyto-
bezoar composed of psyllium seed husks.

Toxicology

The pollen contains allergenic glycoproteins that react
with concanavalin A, as well as components that bind
IgE. IgE antibodies have been demonstrated. The IgE-
mediated sensitization has contributes to seasonal
allergy.

No
information available to require special precautions
Effects on Bleeding None reported

Poinsettia

Clinical Overview

Use

Poinsettias are used as Christmas ornamentation; their
latex for a dipilatory; and for other uses such as pain
relief, antibacterial and emetic. Folk uses include
remedies for skin, warts, and toothache.

Dosing

There is no recent clinical evidence to support specific
dosage of poinsettia in a therapeutic context. Its
reputed toxicity gives reason for caution.

Contraindications

Contraindications have not yet been identified.

Pregnancy/Lactation

Information regarding safety and efficacy in pregnancy
and lactation is lacking.

Interactions

None well documented.

Adverse Reactions

There is little published evidence to suggest that the
plant poses a great toxicologic danger; however, the
following side effects have occurred: Nausea, vomiting, local mucosa irritation, GI tract distress, skin
irritation, eye inflammation, and temporary blindness.

Toxicology

Many published reports have warned of the toxicity of
this plant; however, there appears to be little factual
evidence for this claim. These reports seem to stem
from one poorly documented case of a known fatality,
but several authors have concluded that the report was
based more on hearsay than fact.

No
information available to require special precautions
Effects on Bleeding None reported

Pokeweed

Clinical Overview

Use

Young pokeweed leaves and berries may be eaten as
food, but only after being cooked properly by boiling in
several changes of water.

Dosing

At doses of 1 g, dried pokeweed root is emetic and
purgative. At lower doses of 60 to 100 mg/day, the root
and berries have been used to treat rheumatism and
for immune stimulation; however, there are no clinical
trials that support these uses or doses.

Contraindications

Contraindications have not yet been identified.

Pregnancy/Lactation

Documented adverse effects. Avoid use. Uterine stimulant with toxic constituents; is reputed to affect menstrual cycle.

Interactions

None well documented.

Adverse Reactions

GI distress, possibly leading to severe toxicities (see Toxicology).

Toxicology

Ingestion of poisonous parts of the plant may cause severe stomach cramping, nausea with persistent diarrhea and vomiting, slow and difficult breathing, weakness, spasms, hypotension, severe convulsions, and death.

Local Anesthetic/Vasoconstrictor Precautions No information available to require special precautions

Effects on Bleeding None reported

Policosanol

Clinical Overview

Use

Cholesterol-lowering effects previously attributed to policosanol have not been validated by more recent trials. Policosanol has been studied in platelet aggregation and intermittent claudication, but data are insufficient to support this use.

Dosing

Policosanol is typically initiated at 5 mg/day and titrated up to 20 mg/day for hypercholesterolemia.

Contraindications

Contraindications have not been identified.

Pregnancy/Lactation

Information regarding safety and efficacy in pregnancy and lactation is lacking. Studies in rats and mice demonstrated no adverse effects on fertility, reproduction, teratogenesis, or development at doses equivalent to 1,500 times the normal human dose of 20 mg/kg/day.

Interactions

Because of policosanol's possible effects on platelet aggregation, caution is warranted if policosanol is used concurrently with anticoagulants (eg, warfarin) or antiplatelet agents (eg, aspirin, clopidogrel, prasugrel). In a study in healthy men, policosanol did not affect the pharmacokinetics of warfarin.

Adverse Reactions

Animal and human studies have demonstrated few adverse reactions from policosanol.

Toxicology

Limited animal and human studies have found policosanol to be safe.

Local Anesthetic/Vasoconstrictor Precautions No information available to require special precautions

Effects on Bleeding May see increased bleeding due to inhibition of platelet aggregation

Prickly Pear

Clinical Overview

Use

Prickly pear is widely cultivated and commercially used in juices, jellies, candies, teas, and alcoholic drinks. American Indians used prickly pear juice to treat burns, and prickly pear has a long history in traditional Mexican folk medicine for treating diabetes. Its use in treating diabetes, lipid disorders, inflammation, and ulcers, as well as its other pharmacologic effects, have

been documented. However, there is limited clinical information to support these uses.

Dosing

Prickly pear is commercially available in numerous doseforms, including capsules, tablets, powders, and juices, and as food. Follow manufacturers' suggested guidelines if using commercial products. Typical dosage regimens are two 250 mg capsules by mouth 3 times a day or every 8 hours.

Contraindications

Hypersensitivity to any components of prickly pear.

Pregnancy/Lactation

Avoid use during pregnancy and lactation because of the lack of clinical studies.

Interactions

None well documented.

Adverse Reactions

Dermatitis is the most common adverse reaction to prickly pear.

Toxicology

Little information is available.

Local Anesthetic/Vasoconstrictor Precautions No information available to require special precautions

Effects on Bleeding None reported

Pygeum

Clinical Overview

Use

Pygeum has been used to improve symptoms of benign prostatic hypertrophy and to improve sexual function. Usual dosage is 100 mg/day in 6- to 8-week cycles.

Dosing

Pygeum is available as the standardized preparations Tadenan and Pigenil. It has been studied in clinical trials for benign prostatic hypertrophy at daily doses of 25 to 200 mg.

Contraindications

Contraindications have not yet been identified.

Pregnancy/Lactation

Information regarding safety and efficacy in pregnancy and lactation is lacking.

Interactions

None well documented.

Adverse Reactions

GI irritation has been reported with the use of pygeum.

Toxicology

In human trials, a low incidence of toxicity has been demonstrated.

Local Anesthetic/Vasoconstrictor Precautions No information available to require special precautions

Effects on Bleeding None reported

Quassia

Clinical Overview

Use

Quassia has a variety of uses, including treatment for measles, diarrhea, fever, and lice. Quassia has antibacterial, antifungal, antifertility, antitumor, antileukemic, and insecticidal actions as well. However, efficacy in clinical trials has not been proven.

Dosing

Quassia wood has been used as a bitter tonic, with a typical oral dose of 500 mg. No studies have been performed to support this dose. Several recent studies of topical quassia tincture for head lice have been reported.

Contraindications

Contraindications have not yet been identified.

Pregnancy/Lactation

Documented adverse reactions. Avoid use.

Interactions

None well documented.

Adverse Reactions

Quassia is used in a number of food products and is considered safe by the FDA. If taken in large doses, this product can irritate the GI tract and cause vomiting. It is not recommended for pregnant women.

Toxicology

Quassia is listed as generally regarded as safe (GRAS) by the FDA. Parenteral administration of quassin is toxic, leading to cardiac irregularities, tremors, and paralysis.

Local Anesthetic/Vasoconstrictor Precautions No information available to require special precautions

Effects on Bleeding None reported

Queen's Delight

Clinical Overview

Use

With the exception of prostratin, the other Stillingia factors are likely to be tumor promoters and to possess the typical pleiotropic effects possessed by most other phorbol esters.

Dosing

There is no clinical evidence to support specific dosage recommendations for queen's delight. Classical use of queen's delight called for 2 g of the root, however the documented presence of irritant and tumor-promoting phorbol esters in this plant contraindicates therapeutic use.

Contraindications

No longer considered safe.

Pregnancy/Lactation

Documented adverse effects. Not to be used while nursing. Avoid use.

Interactions

None well documented.

Adverse Reactions

Do not ingest or use topically in human medicine. Observe particular caution with the fresh root, which appears to be more toxic than the dried product. Stillingia root is a purgative and irritant product that should be avoided because of a high likelihood of tumor promotion and documented severe irritancy to skin.

Toxicology

There are reports of sheep poisoned by Stillingia in Florida. Because of the reported phorbol esters, this plant should not be ingested or used topically in human medicine. Observe particular caution with the fresh root, which appears to be more toxic than the dried product.

Local Anesthetic/Vasoconstrictor Precautions No information available to require special precautions

Effects on Bleeding None reported

Raspberry

Clinical Overview

Use

Raspberry leaves may be helpful for diarrhea or as a mouthwash because of their astringent action. They have been used historically in painful or profuse menstruation and to regulate labor pains in childbirth, but there is little evidence to support this use.

Dosing

Typical doses of raspberry leaf as a tea are 1.5 to 2.4 g/day. A clinical trial has been conducted to define its safety in labor.

Contraindications

Contraindications have not yet been identified.

Pregnancy/Lactation

Documented adverse effects (including antigonatographic activity and stimulation of contraction in strips of pregnant human uterus). Avoid use.

Interactions

None well documented.

Adverse Reactions

Research reveals little or no information regarding adverse reactions with the use of this product.

Toxicology

There is no evidence that raspberry leaf tea is toxic.

Local Anesthetic/Vasoconstrictor Precautions No information available to require special precautions

Effects on Bleeding None reported

Red Clover

Clinical Overview

Use

Red clover flowers have been used traditionally as a sedative, to purify the blood, and to treat respiratory conditions; topical preparations have been used for psoriasis, eczema, and rashes, and to accelerate wound healing. More recently, clinical trials have been conducted examining red clover's use in the treatment of menopausal symptoms, but with minimal to no possible effects. A few additional studies have shown positive effects on cardiovascular health and bone density, although they have included only a small number of subjects.

Dosing

The traditional dose of red clover blossoms for sedation is 4 g. Red clover is now used primarily as a source of isoflavones. The usual dose is 40 to 80 mg/day of standardized isoflavones, typically containing biochanin A, formononetin, genistein, and daidzein. Several commercial preparations are available.

Contraindications

Contraindicated in patients with a history of breast cancer and during pregnancy or lactation.

Pregnancy/Lactation

Red clover has estrogenic activity. Avoid use.

Interactions

Isoflavonoids may interfere with hormonal agents; avoid use with oral contraceptives, estrogen, or progesterone therapies.

Adverse Reactions

Few adverse reactions have been reported in doses used in clinical trials. High doses of isoflavones have been associated with loss of appetite, pedal edema, and abdominal tenderness.

Toxicology

The phytoestrogens in red clover may be expected to act through estrogenic mechanisms with the associated risk of estrogen-like adverse effects, including increased incidence of endometrial, ovarian, and breast cancers.

Local Anesthetic/Vasoconstrictor Precautions No information available to require special precautions
Effects on Bleeding Red clover contains coumarins; it may enhance the anticoagulant effects of warfarin when taken simultaneously. This effect has not been confirmed.

Red Yeast Rice

Clinical Overview
Use
M. purpureus is a natural source of mevinolin, the active ingredient of lovastatin, and therefore has beneficial effects in the treatment of hyperlipidemia. However, it should not be used in place of lovastatin and regular medical care because there are no studies that directly compare red yeast rice to a statin. Some evidence also exists for its antibacterial and anticancer effects, as well as its activity on glycemic metabolism.

Dosing
Red yeast rice is available commercially, primarily as a 600 mg capsule. Most manufacturers suggest a dosage of 2 capsules twice a day by mouth for a total of 2,400 mg/day. Commercial OTC products often contain coenzyme Q_{10} to supplement the low levels of this enzyme found in patients with statin myopathy. Past clinical trials have used dosages of 2,400 mg/day.

Contraindications
Hypersensitivity to any components of red yeast rice. Anaphylactic reactions in certain patient populations are documented. Red yeast rice depletes tissue of coenzyme Q_{10}, which may increase the risk of statin-induced myopathy. Therefore patients with muscle damage caused by statins should avoid use of red yeast rice.

Pregnancy/Lactation
Avoid use during pregnancy and lactation. The major ingredient in red yeast rice is monacolin K, which is also known as mevinolin or lovastatin and has statin-like activity. Statins are potential teratogens based on theoretical considerations and in small case studies. CNS and limb defects have been reported in newborns exposed to statins in utero.

Interactions
Avoid using red yeast rice with cholesterol-lowering (statin) medications, cyclosporine, or grapefruit juice due to additive effects, which can increase risk of liver damage and rhabdomyolysis.

Adverse Reactions
Meta-analysis of the efficacy of 3 red yeast rice preparations (Cholestin, Xuezhikang, and Zhibituo) from 93 randomized trials (9,625 patients) documented no serious adverse reactions. The most common adverse reactions included dizziness, decreased appetite, nausea, stomachache, abdominal distension, and diarrhea. A small number of patients suffered from increased serum blood urea nitrogen (BUN) and alanine aminotransferase (ALT) levels.

Toxicology
The nephrotoxic mycotoxin citrinin has been isolated from some strains of M. purpureus and Monascus ruber. No severe toxicities at high doses have been reported. Not recommended for use in patients with liver disease.

Local Anesthetic/Vasoconstrictor Precautions No information available to require special precautions
Effects on Bleeding None reported

Reishi Mushroom

Clinical Overview
Use
The polysaccharide content of reishi mushroom is responsible for possible anticancer and immunostimulatory effects. Reishi may also provide hepatoprotective action, antiviral activity, and beneficial effect on the cardiovascular system, rheumatoid arthritis, chronic fatigue syndrome, and diabetes. Few clinical trials have been conducted.

Dosing
The Pharmacopoeia of the People's Republic of China recommends 6 to 12 g reishi extract daily. Ganopoly (a Ganoderma lucidum polysaccharide extract) in doses up to 5.4 g daily (equivalent to 81 g of the fruiting body) for 12 weeks has been used in a few clinical trials.

Contraindications
Contraindications have not been identified.

Pregnancy/Lactation
Information regarding safety and efficacy in pregnancy and lactation is lacking.

Interactions
None well documented.

Adverse Reactions
Adverse reactions are mild and may include dizziness, GI upset, and skin irritation.

Toxicology
There are few reports of toxicity with the use of reishi mushroom.

Local Anesthetic/Vasoconstrictor Precautions No information available to require special precautions
Effects on Bleeding Reishi mushroom may have an antiplatelet effect. Clinical significance of this property is unknown.

Rhubarb

Clinical Overview
Use
Rhubarb is extensively used in traditional Chinese medicine. Rhubarb has been studied for the management of GI and renal function disorders, and for the treatment of hyperlipidemia and cancer. However, sound clinical evidence for its use is lacking.

Dosing
Dried rhubarb extract 20 to 50 mg/kg daily has been used in clinical trials.

Contraindications
Contraindications have not been identified.

Pregnancy/Lactation
Avoid dosages higher than those found in food because safety and efficacy are unproven.

Interactions
Interaction with cardiac glycosides (digoxin) and a reduction in the absorption of orally administered drugs have been noted when rhubarb is taken in large quantities.

Adverse Reactions
A few reactions, primarily GI effects, have been reported in clinical trials.

Toxicology
The leaf blades (but not the stalks) of rhubarb contain enough oxalic acid to cause poisoning. Acute renal failure has been associated with long-term anthraquinone use.

◀ Local Anesthetic/Vasoconstrictor Precautions No information available to require special precautions
Effects on Bleeding None reported

Rose Hips

Clinical Overview

Use

Rose hips provide vitamin C supplements. Rose hips have been used for diuretic actions, to reduce thirst, to alleviate gastric inflammation, and to flavor teas and jams.

Dosing

There is no recent clinical evidence upon which dosage recommandations can be based. Classical use of rose petals was 3 to 6 g daily.

Contraindications

Contraindications have not yet been identified.

Pregnancy/Lactation

Information regarding safety and efficacy in pregnancy and lactation is lacking.

Interactions

None well documented.

Adverse Reactions

There have been no reported side effects except in those exposed to rose hips dust who have developed severe respiratory allergies.

Toxicology

No data.

Local Anesthetic/Vasoconstrictor Precautions No information available to require special precautions
Effects on Bleeding None reported

Royal Jelly

Clinical Overview

Use

Royal jelly has been studied for a variety of actions, including antimicrobial, antitumor, antihypertensive, and immunoregulatory activity. Additionally, effects on lipid profile, insulin-like action, and neurological and estrogenic effects have been demonstrated. However, clinical trials are lacking.

Dosing

Clinical trials are generally lacking in dosage recommendation. Small clinical trials have used 6 to 10 g royal jelly per day for 14 to 28 days in trials evaluating the effect on the lipid profile.

Contraindications

Contraindications have not been identified. Allergy to bee venom is considered a relative contraindication.

Pregnancy/Lactation

Information regarding safety and efficacy in pregnancy and lactation is lacking. Royal jelly possesses some estrogenic activity.

Interactions

Case reports of hematuria due to potentiation of warfarin have been documented.

Adverse Reactions

In many allergy patients, skin tests were positive for royal jelly. There have been case reports of allergy, acute exacerbation of asthma, anaphylaxis, and death.

Toxicology

Data are limited.

Local Anesthetic/Vasoconstrictor Precautions No information available to require special precautions
Effects on Bleeding None reported

Rue

Clinical Overview

Use

Rue extract is potentially useful as a potassium channel blocker. It has been used to treat many neuromuscular problems and to stimulate the onset of menstruation. Because rue has an antispasmodic effect at relatively low doses, it should be taken with caution. However, considering rue's potential for severe adverse effects, clinical trials are limited.

Dosing

There is no recent clinical evidence to support dosing recommendations for rue. Traditional use calls for 0.5 to 1 g of the herb daily or 65 mg of the essential oil. In larger doses, rue is an emmenagogue, an aphrodisiac, and an abortifacient, and should be considered dangerous.

Contraindications

Contraindications have not yet been identified.

Pregnancy/Lactation

Documented adverse effects, including emmenagogue and abortifacient effects. Avoid use.

Interactions

None well documented.

Adverse Reactions

Rue extracts are mutagenic and furocoumarins have been associated with photosensitization. If ingested, rue oil may result in kidney damage and hepatic degeneration. Large doses can cause violent gastric pain, vomiting, and systemic complications, including death. Because of possible abortifacient effects, the plant should never be ingested by women of childbearing potential. Toxic hepatitis due to Ruta has been reported.

Toxicology

Rue should only be taken with extreme caution. A case report describes multiorgan toxicity in a 78-year-old woman ingesting R. graveolens for cardiovascular protection. After 3 days of use, the patient entered the emergency department with bradycardia, acute renal failure with hyperkalemia necessitating hemodialysis, and coagulopathy.

Local Anesthetic/Vasoconstrictor Precautions No information available to require special precautions
Effects on Bleeding None reported

Safflower

Clinical Overview

Use

Safflower has been used as a laxative and as a dietary supplement to modify lipid profiles and treat fevers. However, clinical trials are lacking.

Dosing

Foods are commonly cooked in safflower oil. There are few clinical trials to support dosage; however, 10 g of oil per day has been used as placebo.

Contraindications

Contraindications have not yet been identified.

Pregnancy/Lactation

Information is limited. Abortifacient and emmenagogue effects have been suggested.

Interactions

None well documented.

Adverse Reactions

Allergy to the flowers has been reported. Safflower oil used in clinical trials as a control appears to be generally well tolerated.

Toxicology

Research reveals little or no information regarding toxicity with the use of safflower oil.

Local Anesthetic/Vasoconstrictor Precautions No information available to require special precautions

Effects on Bleeding None reported

Salvia divinorum

Clinical Overview
Use

Salvia divinorum is a hallucinogen and is illegal in some jurisdictions. Check individual state legislation.

Dosing

200 to 500 mcg of salvinorin A, or several leaves, smoked or absorbed perorally, is sufficient to cause hallucinations.

Contraindications

S. divinorum should not be used in people with any mental disease.

Pregnancy/Lactation

Use during pregnancy or lactation is not recommended.

Interactions

None well documented.

Adverse Reactions

None systematically reported.

Toxicology

No toxicity was observed in a 2-week study in mice.

Local Anesthetic/Vasoconstrictor Precautions No information available to require special precautions

Effects on Bleeding None reported

SAMe

Clinical Overview
Use

SAMe has been studied for the treatment of depressive disorders, osteoarthritis, and liver disorders.

Dosing

Depression: 200 mg to 1,600 mg/day.
Liver disease: 800 to 1,000 mg/day.
Osteoarthritis: 1,200 mg/day initially, then maintenance 400 mg/day.

Contraindications

SAMe should not be used in patients with bipolar depression because of reports of increased anxiety and mania.

Pregnancy/Lactation

Trials conducted in pregnant women documented no harmful effects.

Interactions

None well documented.

Adverse Reactions

Available data indicate nausea, diarrhea, constipation, mild insomnia, dizziness, and sweating to be the most commonly reported adverse reactions of SAMe. Data from long-term use of SAMe are lacking.

Toxicology

Toxicological studies concluded that SAMe is safe even at the highest doses.

Local Anesthetic/Vasoconstrictor Precautions No information available to require special precautions

Effects on Bleeding None reported

Sarsaparilla

Clinical Overview
Use

Sarsaparilla has been used for treating syphilis, leprosy, psoriasis, and other ailments.

Dosing

Typical doses of sarsaparilla for a variety of uses range from 0.3 to 2 g/day of the powdered root.

Contraindications

Contraindications have not yet been identified.

Pregnancy/Lactation

Information regarding safety and efficacy in pregnancy and lactation is lacking.

Interactions

None well documented.

Adverse Reactions

No major contraindications, warnings or side effects have been documented; avoid excessive ingestion. In unusually high doses, the plant possibly could be harmful, including GI irritation.

Toxicology

Research reveals little or no information regarding toxicology with the use of sarsaparilla.

Local Anesthetic/Vasoconstrictor Precautions No information available to require special precautions

Effects on Bleeding None reported

Sassafras

Clinical Overview
Use

Sassafras has been used historically for a variety of illnesses, and is now banned in the US, even for use as a flavoring or fragrance.

Dosing

Sassafras root bark has been used as an aromatic and carminative at doses of 10 g; however, the carcinogenicity of its constituent safrole has limited its use.

Contraindications

No longer considered safe.

Pregnancy/Lactation

Documented emmenagogue, abortifacient effects. Avoid use.

Interactions

None well documented.

Adverse Reactions

Besides being a cancer-causing agent, sassafras can induce vomiting, stupor and hallucinations. It can also cause abortion, diaphoresis, and dermatitis.

Toxicology

Sassafras oil and safrole have been banned for use as flavors and food additives by the FDA because of their carcinogenic potential.

Local Anesthetic/Vasoconstrictor Precautions No information available to require special precautions

Effects on Bleeding None reported

Saw Palmetto

Clinical Overview
Use

Saw palmetto has been used to treat symptoms of benign prostatic hyperplasia (BPH), but evidence from quality clinical trials and a meta-analysis does not support this use. Data suggesting a positive effect on erectile dysfunction are limited, and results from studies evaluating the effect of saw palmetto on outcomes of transurethral resection of the prostate surgery are equivocal. Some effects on in vitro prostate cancer cells have been described; however, clinical trials are lacking.

Dosing

Benign prostatic hyperplasia: 320 mg/day standardized extract.

Contraindications

Contraindications have not been identified. Use in children younger than 12 years is not recommended.

Pregnancy/Lactation

Information regarding safety and efficacy in pregnancy and lactation is lacking. Effects on androgen and estrogen metabolism have been identified, as well as a lack of rationale for its use in pregnancy, and suggest that saw palmetto should not be used.

Interactions

Case reports of interactions are lacking. Caution may be warranted with concomitant coagulation therapy.

Adverse Reactions

Results from clinical trials note that saw palmetto products are generally well tolerated, with occasional reports of adverse GI effects and headache.

Toxicology

Information is limited.

Local Anesthetic/Vasoconstrictor Precautions No information available to require special precautions
Effects on Bleeding None reported

Schisandra

Clinical Overview
Use

Schisandra has been used as a tonic and restorative, as well as for liver protection, nervous system effects, respiratory treatment, and GI therapy. However, there are limited clinical trials to support these uses.

Dosing

Schisandra fruit is used as an adaptogen at dosages of 1.5 to 6 g/day. A standardized extract containing 3.4% schisandrin has been used in a clinical trial for improved athletic performance at 91 mg/day of extract. Examples of various doses used in Russia include the following: *Tinctura Fructum*: Schisandrae prepared with air-dried fruits and 95% ethanol given as 20 to 30 drops twice daily; *Tinctura Seminum*: Schizandrae prepared with dried seeds and 95% ethanol given as 20 to 30 drops twice daily; *Infusion Fructum*: Schizandrae prepared with air-dried fruits and water (1:20 w/v) given as 150 mL twice daily; *Fructum Schizandrae*: contains air-dried fruits given at a dose of 0.5 to 1.5 g twice daily; *Schizandra seed powder*: given as 0.5 to 1.5 g twice daily before lunch and dinner over 20 to 30 days; *Schizandra seed extract*: prepared with air-dried seed and 95% ethanol given as a single dose of 0.05 or 0.2 mL/kg.

Contraindications

Contraindications have not been identified.

Pregnancy/Lactation

Information regarding safety and efficacy in pregnancy and lactation is lacking. Various compounds from the stem of Schisandra propinqua were found to be cytotoxic against rat luteal cells and human decidual cells in vitro.

Interactions

Because of its documented effects on hepatic and gastric enzyme activity, particularly CYP3A, it is possible that schisandra may interfere with the metabolism of coadministered drugs (eg, midazolam). Findings

from a study of healthy volunteers suggest patients receiving schisandra while concomitantly taking drugs that are P-glycoprotein (P-gp) substrates (eg, tacrolimus) may require a dosage adjustment.

Adverse Reactions

Research does not report any incidence of adverse effects.

Toxicology

The minimal toxic dose when given orally to mice is 3.6 g/kg. The acute toxicity was studied in mice, and following intraperitoneal administration, no effects on blood pressure, breath, or motility were noted; however, high doses caused convulsions (median effective dose $[ED_{50}]$ = 175 mg/kg) and paresis (ED_{50} = 370 mg/kg).

Local Anesthetic/Vasoconstrictor Precautions No information available to require special precautions
Effects on Bleeding None reported

Scullcap

Clinical Overview
Use

Scullcap traditionally has been used as a sedative for nervousness and anxiety, although there is little to no data to support any of these uses.

Dosing Limit doses of American skullcap to no more than the package recommendation. Typical doses (see individual product information):
Dried herb: 1 to 2 grams 3 times/day.
Tea: 240 mL 3 times/day (Pour 250 mL of boiling water over 5 to 10 mL of the dried herb and steep for 10 to 15 minutes).
Tincture: 2 to 4 mL 3 times/day.

Contraindications

Contraindications have not yet been identified.

Pregnancy/Lactation

Documented adverse effects in pregnancy. Avoid use. May inhibit pituitary and chorionic gonadotropins, as well as prolactin.

Interactions

None well documented, though it may exaggerate the effects of other drugs that cause drowsiness.

Adverse Reactions

If taken according to the manufacturer's directions, scullcap does not seem to exhibit any adverse effects.

Toxicology

An overdose of the tincture causes giddiness, stupor, confusion, twitching of the limbs, intermission of the pulse, and other symptoms similar to epilepsy.

Local Anesthetic/Vasoconstrictor Precautions No information available to require special precautions
Effects on Bleeding None reported

Sea Buckthorn

Clinical Overview
Use

Numerous pharmacological effects are documented in the scientific literature, including antimicrobial, antiulcerogenic, antioxidant, anticancer, radioprotective activity, platelet aggregation, liver injury, cardiovascular risk factors, and effects on skin and mucosa.

Dosing

Five to 45 g of seed oil and 300 mL/day of juice have been studied in clinical trials.

Contraindications

None well documented.

Pregnancy/Lactation

Avoid use during pregnancy and lactation because clinical trial data are lacking.

Interactions

Sea buckthorn oil reportedly induces the cytogenetic activity of cyclophosphamide and farmorubicin.

Adverse Reactions

None well documented.

Toxicology

Sea buckthorn has been used as a food in Asia and in Europe. Toxicological studies in animals suggest seed oil and oil from the fruit's soft parts are safe. Acute and chronic toxicity of blood, liver, and heart as well as mutagenicity and teratogenicity of sea buckthorn oils have been studied.

Local Anesthetic/Vasoconstrictor Precautions No information available to require special precautions

Effects on Bleeding Sea buckthorn inhibits platelet aggregation *in vitro*. One clinical report showed an inhibition of platelet aggregation in 12 healthy volunteers with daily ingestion of sea buckthorn berry oil. The clinician should anticipate that ingestion of sea buckthorn may pose some increased risk of bleeding.

Seaweed

Clinical Overview

Use

Clinical trials are generally lacking to support definitive therapeutic recommendations for seaweeds. However, seaweeds are an important nutritional source of minerals and elements and are low in sodium. Applications may exist for use in cardiovascular conditions due to potential in cholesterol reduction and appetite suppression. Alginates extracted from seaweed have been used in wound dressings.

Dosing

Clinical trials have used an oral dosage range of 4 to 12 g seaweed daily for up to 2 months.

Contraindications

Contraindications have not been identified.

Pregnancy/Lactation

Information regarding safety and efficacy in pregnancy and lactation is lacking.

Interactions

Patients taking warfarin and consuming a large quantity of food containing seaweed may experience a change in international normalized ratio (INR) because of seaweed's high vitamin K content.

Adverse Reactions

Contact dermatitis, goiter, and, occasionally, GI effects may occur.

Toxicology

Excessive intake of dried seaweed may result in increased serum thyroid-stimulating hormone (TSH). There have been case reports of carotenodermia (yellowing of the skin) with excessive seaweed consumption.

Local Anesthetic/Vasoconstrictor Precautions No information available to require special precautions

Effects on Bleeding May see increased bleeding due to anticoagulant effects.

Shark Derivatives

Clinical Overview

Use

The shark cartilage was thought to be a cancer control agent, but no studies have proven this theory.

Squalamine has been used as a potent antibiotic with fungicidal and antiprotozoal activity.

Dosing

A standardized shark cartilage product has been marketed under the name Neovastat (AE-941). Clinical trials in cancer angiogenesis have used doses of 60 to 240 mL daily, while another trial of a liquid shark cartilage product used only 7 to 21 mL daily.

Contraindications

Contraindications have not yet been identified.

Pregnancy/Lactation

Information regarding safety and efficacy in pregnancy and lactation is lacking.

Interactions

None well documented.

Adverse Reactions

Research reveals little or no information regarding adverse reactions with the use of shark derivatives.

Toxicology

Research reveals little or no information regarding toxicology with the use of shark derivatives.

Local Anesthetic/Vasoconstrictor Precautions No information available to require special precautions

Effects on Bleeding None reported

Shark Liver Oil

Clinical Overview

Use

Shark liver oil (SLO) has been used to help treat cancer, skin conditions, and respiratory ailments, as well as to reduce recurrent aphthous stomatitis and prevent radiation sickness. However, limited clinical data are available. Alkylglycerols have been studied as an immune system stimulant. Animal data suggest SLO may improve fertility.

Dosing

SLO marketed under the name isolutrol has been studied in a clinical trial of acne at a topical concentration of 0.15 g per 100 mL.

Contraindications

Contraindications have not been identified.

Pregnancy/Lactation

Information regarding safety and efficacy in pregnancy and lactation is lacking.

Interactions

None well documented.

Adverse Reactions

Few toxic effects have been reported. SLO supplements may have an unpleasant taste and/or odor. There have been reports of SLO-induced pneumonia in humans and pigs.

Toxicology

No adverse reactions or effects on mortality were noted in rats receiving short- and long-term doses of a supercritical fluid extract of SLO at doses 100 to 200 times that of normal human consumption. In Sweden, a SLO product (Ecomer) was prohibited for use by the National Board of Health and Welfare because of suspected adverse effects.

Local Anesthetic/Vasoconstrictor Precautions No information available to require special precautions

Effects on Bleeding None reported

Slippery Elm

Clinical Overview

Use

Slippery elm has been used as an emollient and in lozenges. It protects irritated skin and intestinal membranes in such conditions as gout, rheumatism, cold sores, wounds, abscesses, ulcers, and toothaches.

Dosing

Slippery elm inner bark has been used for treatment of ulcers at doses of 1.5 to 3 g/day. It is commonly decocted with ethyl alcohol. No formal clinical studies support this dosage.

Contraindications

Contraindications have not yet been identified.

Pregnancy/Lactation

Documented abortifacient effects. Avoid use.

Interactions

None well documented.

Adverse Reactions

Extracts from slippery elm have caused contact dermatitis, and the pollen has been reported to be allergenic.

Toxicology

The FDA has declared slippery elm to be a safe and effective oral demulcent.

Local Anesthetic/Vasoconstrictor Precautions No information available to require special precautions
Effects on Bleeding None reported

Soy

Clinical Overview

Use

Soy is commonly used as a source of fiber, protein, and minerals. A number of meta-analyses are now available; however, evidence is lacking to support a definitive place in therapy for menopausal symptoms, osteoporosis, diabetes, or heart disease. Epidemiologic data suggest an association with a lower incidence of certain cancers with higher intake of dietary soy.

Dosing

A large number of clinical trials have been conducted for conditions (eg, menopause, osteoporosis, breast cancer, cardiovascular diseases) using daily doses of isoflavones from 40 to 120 mg.

Contraindications

Contraindications have not been identified.

Pregnancy/Lactation

Generally recognized as safe (GRAS) when used as food. Avoid dosages above those found in food because safety and efficacy are unproven.

Interactions

None well documented. A decrease in the anticoagulated effect of warfarin has been reported in 1 patient.

Adverse Reactions

Soybeans and their products are generally well tolerated. Minor GI disturbances have been reported. The National Toxicology Program (US Department of Health and Human Services) has concluded that there is minimal concern for developmental effects in infants fed soy infant formula.

Toxicology

Evidence exists from animal studies on the adverse effects of the isoflavone genistein on the developing female reproductive tract.

Local Anesthetic/Vasoconstrictor Precautions No information available to require special precautions
Effects on Bleeding None reported

Spirulina

Clinical Overview

Use

Spirulina is sold in the United States as a health food or supplement. Diverse claims exist for its immunostimulatory, hypolipidemic, antiviral, and anticancer effects; however, there is limited evidence to support these indications.

Dosing

Doses in clinical studies have ranged from 1 to 10 g/day.

Contraindications

Phenylketonuria; however, this has not been substantiated.

Pregnancy/Lactation

Information regarding safety and efficacy in pregnancy and lactation is lacking. Because of possible mercury and other heavy metal contamination, spirulina should be avoided during pregnancy.

Interactions

None well documented.

Adverse Reactions

Few reports of adverse reactions are available. However, spirulina-associated hepatotoxicity and reactions from heavy metal contamination are possible.

Toxicology

Spirulina is considered nontoxic to humans at usual levels of consumption; however, information is limited.

Local Anesthetic/Vasoconstrictor Precautions No information available to require special precautions
Effects on Bleeding None reported

Stevia

Clinical Overview

Use

Stevia leaf is used as a sweetening agent and contains several sweet glycosides. The glycoside rebaudioside A is used in commercially available products in the United States and has not shown any pharmacologic effects. Stevioside and stevia preparations have shown conflicting data, indicating possible effects as hypotensive and hypoglycemic agents and possible bactericidal properties.

Dosing

Stevia leaf is used for sweetening foods.

Contraindications

Contraindications have not yet been identified.

Pregnancy/Lactation

Information regarding safety and efficacy in pregnancy and lactation is lacking.

Interactions

None well documented.

Adverse Reactions

No major contraindications, warnings, or adverse reactions have been documented.

Toxicology

Stevioside, a main glycoside of stevia, was found to be nontoxic in acute toxicity studies in a variety of laboratory animals.

Local Anesthetic/Vasoconstrictor Precautions No information available to require special precautions
Effects on Bleeding None reported

St. John's Wort

Clinical Overview

Use

Meta-analyses of quality clinical trials support Hypericum 's place in the treatment of depression. Effectiveness is comparable with standard antidepressants, while adverse events are lower than with conventional antidepressants. Interactions with other drugs and quality control issues may limit use. Other areas of therapeutic research for St. John's wort include smoking cessation, premenstrual symptoms, somatoform disorder, and attention deficit hyperactivity disorder, as well as its possible role in treating cancer and HIV.

Dosing

Preparations vary greatly in chemical content and quality, and may be standardized to quantity of hyperforin (commonly 3% to 5%) or hypericin (commonly 0.3%). Clinical trials evaluating the efficacy of St. John's wort in depression have commonly used 900 mg of extract daily in 3 divided doses, both in short-term treatment and for ongoing therapy, for periods of up to 1 year (range, 600 to 1,200 mg/day).

Contraindications

Use with cyclosporine, tacrolimus, irinotecan, and imatinib mesylate, as well as protease inhibitors and nonnucleoside reverse transcriptase inhibitors in HIV treatment, is contraindicated.

Pregnancy/Lactation

Avoid use. The use of St. John's wort in perinatal depression has been considered; however, insufficient data on efficacy or safety exist to support its use. St. John's wort should be avoided during pregnancy and lactation until further long-term studies demonstrate a lack of toxicity in the developing fetus and breastfeeding newborn.

Interactions

St. John's wort has been reported to interact with numerous drugs. Drugs with a narrow therapeutic window should be monitored closely. Patients should be cautioned on the potential for interactions and the need to consult their health care provider before taking St. John's wort with prescription or nonprescription drugs. Drugs that are most prominently affected, and therefore for which concomitant use with St. John's wort should be avoided, include protease inhibitors (eg, saquinavir) and nonnucleoside reverse transcriptase inhibitors (eg, nevirapine) used in HIV, and cyclosporine, tacrolimus, irinotecan, and imatinib mesylate. Ethinyl estradiol is metabolized by CYP3A4; therefore, a high possibility of interaction exists. The risk of developing serotonin syndrome and other CNS adverse reactions cannot be ruled out; extreme caution is needed with combinations of psychotropic medications. Reviews of interactions with St. John's wort are available.

Adverse Reactions

Adverse reactions are usually mild. Potential adverse reactions include dry mouth, dizziness, constipation, and other GI symptoms, and confusion. Photosensitization also may occur. In clinical trials, adverse reactions and discontinuation with St. John's wort were usually less than those observed with standard antidepressants. Other possible rare adverse reactions include induction of mania and effects on male and female reproductive capabilities.

Toxicology

Limited information on genotoxicity exists. Potent inhibition of sperm motility was observed in vitro. A case report exists of an overdose of St. John's wort in a 16-year-old patient consuming 15 tablets (300 mcg strength) per day for 2 weeks, requiring management in an intensive care unit.

Local Anesthetic/Vasoconstrictor Precautions No information available to require special precautions

Effects on Bleeding None reported

Syrian Rue

Clinical Overview

Use

In several countries the plant has been traditionally used as an hallucinogen in ceremonies, and has found its way into modern day recreational use. Although in vitro and animal experiments suggest a role as an antimicrobial, vasorelaxant, antidepressant, analgesic, or cytotoxic agent, clinical studies are lacking to support any therapeutic application.

Dosing

Clinical applications are lacking to provide therapeutic dosages. Consumption of decoctions made from 100 to 150 g of seeds has resulted in toxic effects.

Contraindications

Harmala alkaloids (specifically harmine and harmaline) are reversible monoamine oxidase inhibitors (MAOI), thus concomitant use with MAOI medicines and tyramine-containing foods is not advised.

Pregnancy/Lactation

Documented adverse reactions. Avoid use.

Interactions

None well documented.

Adverse Reactions

Case reports of toxicity include nausea and vomiting, visual and auditory hallucinations, confusion, agitation, locomotor ataxia, tremors and convulsions, and life-threatening respiratory depression and coma. Severe gastrointestinal distress, vomiting blood, gastric ulceration, and convulsions have also been reported, as well as bradycardia and low blood pressure. Symptoms are generally of short duration (a few hours) and supportive therapy is recommended.

Toxicology

Information is limited. Elevated renal and liver function tests have been reported.

Local Anesthetic/Vasoconstrictor Precautions Long-term use of syrian rue has been associated with hypertension, tachycardia, tachypnea, and heart block. Use vasoconstrictor with caution in order to minimize risk of hypertension or tachycardia.

Effects on Bleeding None reported

Tea Tree Oil

Clinical Overview

Use

Despite an abundance of commercial preparations promoted for antimicrobial use, sound clinical trials are limited. Trials have been conducted in conditions including nail infections, athlete's foot, fungal skin infections, acne, and methicillin-resistant Staphylococcus aureus. Case reports exist for use in other conditions.

Dosing

Decolonization of methicillin-resistant S. aureus: Tea tree oil as a nasal cream (4% to 10%) applied 3 times a day for 5 days and 5% body wash for 5 days. Acne vulgaris: 5% tea tree oil gel applied for 20 minutes twice daily, then washed off. Onchomycosis (fungal nail infections): 100% tea tree oil applied for 6 months. Tinea pedis (athlete's foot): 25% to 50% tea tree oil for 4 weeks.

Contraindications

Oral ingestion is contraindicated.

Pregnancy/Lactation

Information regarding safety and efficacy in pregnancy and lactation is lacking.

Interactions

None well documented.

Adverse Reactions

Case reports exist of dermatitis associated with topical tea tree oil.

Toxicology

Tea tree oil is toxic when ingested orally. Some case studies of accidental and intentional poisoning exist; however, no deaths have been reported to the American Association of Poison Control Centers through 2006. Mutagenicity of tea tree oil appears to be low; however, chemical constituents have been shown to be cytotoxic and embryotoxic.

Local Anesthetic/Vasoconstrictor Precautions No information available to require special precautions
Effects on Bleeding None reported

Thunder God Vine

Clinical Overview
Use

Thunder god vine has been evaluated for use primarily in rheumatoid arthritis (RA); however, its adverse event profile and limited quality trials restrict any recommendations for clinical use. Antifertility properties in men have been described, while amenorrhea was observed in women.

Dosing

In RA trials, 60 mg/day of T2 (a chloroform-methanol extract of Tripterygium wilfordii) for 12 weeks has been evaluated, as well as ethanol/ethyl alcohol root extract 180 to 360 mg/day. Several long-term studies have evaluated the use of 1 mg/kg/day of T2 for up to 5 years; however, adequate safety data during the same time period are limited.

Contraindications

Contraindications have not been determined. Due to immune suppression, thunder god vine preparations should not be used in immune-compromised patients.

Pregnancy/Lactation

Avoid use. Embryotoxicity has been demonstrated in mice.

Interactions

None well documented.

Adverse Reactions

Clinically important adverse events have been reported in clinical trials. GI upset, male and female infertility, and immune suppression are common side effects of thunder god vine.

Toxicology

Information is limited. Embryotoxicity was demonstrated in mice, including neural effects, absence of limb buds, and ophthalmic-related effects.

Local Anesthetic/Vasoconstrictor Precautions No information available to require special precautions
Effects on Bleeding None reported

Thyme

Clinical Overview
Use

Thyme has primarily culinary uses. Thyme extracts and thymol have been used in cough mixtures and mouthwashes, as well as for skin conditions, especially fungal infections. Clinical trials are lacking to support these uses.

Dosing

Studies are lacking to guide clinical dosages.

Contraindications

Information is lacking.

Pregnancy/Lactation

Information regarding safety and efficacy in pregnancy and lactation is lacking.

Interactions

None well documented.

Adverse Reactions

Contact dermatitis and systemic allergy have been reported.

Toxicology

Information is lacking.

Local Anesthetic/Vasoconstrictor Precautions No information available to require special precautions
Effects on Bleeding An extract from thyme has been shown to have antiplatelet aggregating activity. The clinical significance of this effect is unknown.

Tolu Balsam

Clinical Overview
Use

Tolu balsam is best known for its fragrance and use as flavoring in pharmaceutical products, although it also has mild antiseptic and expectorant properties. There are no clinical data to support its use in any condition.

Dosing

There is no recent clinical evidence to support specific dosing of tolu balsam. Traditional dosage of the herb for colds has been 0.6 g daily.

Contraindications

Contraindications have not yet been determined.

Pregnancy/Lactation

Information regarding safety and efficacy in pregnancy and lactation is lacking.

Interactions

None well documented.

Adverse Reactions

Allergic reactions have been reported.

Toxicology

Information is lacking.

Local Anesthetic/Vasoconstrictor Precautions No information available to require special precautions
Effects on Bleeding None reported

Turmeric

Clinical Overview
Use

Use of curcumin (tumeric) as a pharmacologic agent is limited due to its low systemic bioavailability following oral dosing. Curcumin is used as a spice in curry powders and mustard. It is marketed with claims of potent antioxidant activity, improving bone and joint health, and reducing inflammation, but clinical trials are limited. Its efficacy in treating numerous cancers has been investigated.

Dosing

Curcumin is primarily available in capsule form from commercial manufacturers. The most common regimen is one to three 500 mg capsules daily with or without food. Powdered turmeric root has traditionally been used as a stimulant and carminative at dosages of 0.5 to 3 g/day. Dosages of 3 to 6 g/day have been investigated for protective effects against ulcers. Daily oral doses of curcumin 3,600 mg have been typically used in clinical trials, but dosages of up to curcumin 8 g/day have also been used. Higher doses are associated with adverse GI effects.

Contraindications

Avoid use if hypersensitive to any of the components of curcumin. Avoid use during pregnancy and lactation due to emmenagogue and uterine stimulant effects. The herb should not be used in patients with gall stones or bile duct or passage obstruction.

Pregnancy/Lactation

Avoid use. Documented emmenagogue and abortifacient effects.

Interactions

None well documented.

Adverse Reactions

Clinical trials report few adverse reactions. Rare cases of contact dermatitis and anaphylaxis have been reported.

Toxicology

Limited clinical data are available. The oral median lethal dose (LD_{50}) of curcumin in rats and mice was higher than 2,000 mg/kg body weight.

Local Anesthetic/Vasoconstrictor Precautions No information available to require special precautions

Effects on Bleeding May see increased bleeding due to inhibition of platelet aggregation

---

Ubiquinone

Clinical Overview

Use

Ubiquinone may have applications in cardiovascular disease, especially congestive heart failure (CHF), although there is a lack of consensus. Studies in neurological disorders are less promising. Limited clinical trials have been conducted to support its widespread use for other conditions.

Dosing

Cardiovascular and neurologic trials predominantly use ubiquinone dosages of 300 mg/day or idebenone dosages of 5 mg/kg/day. Higher dosages of ubiquinone (up to 3,000 mg/day) have been used. Pharmacokinetic studies suggest split dosing is superior to single daily dosing.

Contraindications

Absolute contraindications have not been identified.

Pregnancy/Lactation

Information regarding safety and efficacy in pregnancy and lactation is lacking.

Interactions

Findings are conflicting. Case reports show ubiquinone decreases the anticoagulant effect of warfarin; however, a randomized clinical trial found no effect on the international normalized ratio (INR).

Adverse Reactions

Adverse effects are rare and include diarrhea, GI discomfort, headache, loss of appetite, and nausea. Allergic reactions have been reported.

Toxicology

An observed intake safety level of 1,200 mg/day is based on clinical data; however, dosages exceeding this amount have been used with no apparent adverse effect. No accumulation in plasma or tissue following cessation of coenzyme Q10 consumption has been noted.

Local Anesthetic/Vasoconstrictor Precautions No information available to require special precautions

Effects on Bleeding May increase the risk of bleeding

Uva Ursi

Clinical Overview

Use

Uva ursi has been used to treat urinary tract infections; as a diuretic; to treat induced contact dermatitis, allergic reaction-type hypersensitivity, and arthritis in conjuction with prednisolone and dexamethasone. However, research reveals very limited clinical data regarding the use of uva ursi to treat any condition.

Dosing

While there is no recently published clinical evidence to support specific dosage, uva ursi has been used for urinary tract infections at doses of up to 10 g of leaf daily, equivalent to 400 to 840 mg arbutin.

Contraindications

Ingestion of uva ursi in large doses has resulted in ringing of the ears, nausea, vomiting, cyanosis, convulsions, collapse, and death.

Pregnancy/Lactation

The published report of the Expert Advisory Committee in Herbs and Botanical Preparations to the Canadian Health Protection Branch (January 1986) recommended that food preparations containing uva ursi provide labeling contraindicating their use during pregnancy and lactation because large doses of uva ursi are oxytocic. Avoid use.

Interactions

None well documented.

Adverse Reactions

Ingestion of uva ursi in large doses has resulted in ringing of the ears, nausea, vomiting, cyanosis, convulsions, collapse, and death. The product may also impart a green color to the urine and cause gastric discomfort.

Toxicology

Ingestion of 1 g of hydroquinone resulted in ringing of the ears, nausea, vomiting, cyanosis, convulsions and collapse. Death followed the ingestion of 5 g of hydroquinone. These symptoms are rare; most commercial products have less than 1 g of crude uva ursi per dose.

Local Anesthetic/Vasoconstrictor Precautions No information available to require special precautions

Effects on Bleeding None reported

Valerian

Clinical Overview

Use

The evidence to support the common use of valerian in insomnia remains weak. However, as valerian preparations seem to have a wide margin of safety, further trials for insomnia and anxiety may be warranted.

Dosing

Anxiety: Valeprotriates 150 mg/day in 3 divided doses for 4 weeks has been used in a clinical trial. Other trials used the dried herb 0.5 to 2 g, extract 0.5 to 2 mL, and valerian tincture 2 to 4 mL for anxiety. Insomnia: Valerian extract 400 to 600 mg/day taken 1 hour before bedtime for 2 to 4 weeks has been used in clinical trials. Single-dose studies have consistently found no effect for single doses of valerian in insomnia.

Contraindications

Contraindications have not been identified.

Pregnancy/Lactation

Information regarding safety and efficacy in pregnancy and lactation is lacking.

Interactions

None well documented.

Adverse Reactions

In general, clinical studies have found valerian to have a wide margin of safety, be devoid of adverse effects, and have fewer adverse reactions than positive control drugs, such as diazepam. Headache and diarrhea have been reported in clinical trials, but hangover is seldom reported.

Toxicology

Valerian has been classified as GRAS (generally recognized as safe) in the United States for food use; extracts and the root oil are used as flavorings in foods and beverages. The observed in vitro cytotoxicity of valepotriate compounds may not be relevant in vivo because of limited absorption.

Local Anesthetic/Vasoconstrictor Precautions No information available to require special precautions

Effects on Bleeding None reported

Vinpocetine

Clinical Overview

Use

The scientific literature contains numerous studies and investigations on the pharmacological and biochemical actions of vinpocetine, including antioxidant effects, menopause, antiulcer activity, and phosphodiesterase-1 inhibition. Vinpocetine is best known for its neuroprotective effects. However, there are limited clinical studies to support the use of vinpocetine for many of these potential uses.

Dosing

Follow suggested manufacturers' product guidelines. Most clinical studies used vinpocetine 10 mg 3 times daily, orally or parenterally.

Contraindications

The drug should not be used in patients with severe, general, cerebral hypertensive crises, or in elderly or senile patients with acute cardio-cerebral or cerebro-cardiac syndrome, postinfarction cardiosclerosis, or marked disorders of heart rhythm.

Pregnancy/Lactation

Avoid use during pregnancy and lactation because of lack of clinical studies.

Interactions

Caution is warranted in patients on blood-thinning medications because vinpocetine decreases platelet aggregation. In 1 study, bioavailability increased 60% to 100% when vinpocetine was taken with food.

Adverse Reactions

One review article documents patients reporting flushing, rashes, and minor GI problems.

Toxicology

None well documented in the scientific literature.

Local Anesthetic/Vasoconstrictor Precautions No information available to require special precautions

Effects on Bleeding Vinpocetine has the potential to increase the risk of bleeding or potentiate the effects of warfarin. Clinical relevance of this effect is unknown.

Vitamin D

Clinical Overview

Use

Vitamin D, long recognized as playing a role in bone and calcium homeostasis, is being investigated for use in cardiovascular disease, cancer, diabetes, infections, multiple sclerosis, psoriasis, respiratory health, and other conditions. More clinical trials are needed.

Dosing

The American Academy of Pediatrics recommends 400 units/day of vitamin D in infants and adolescents. Clinical data are not yet sufficiently robust to make definitive recommendations for therapeutic dosages of vitamin D; however, in the elderly, 700 to 1,000 units/day have been shown to reduce the risk of falls.

Contraindications

Contraindications have not been identified.

Pregnancy/Lactation

Routine use of supplemental vitamin D during pregnancy is not supported by safety evidence. However, adequate maternal intake of vitamin D-containing foods during lactation ensures that breast-fed infants receive sufficient vitamin D.

Interactions

The use of statins has been shown to increase serum vitamin D levels. Corticosteriods decrease the metabolism of vitamin D and orlistat reduces its absorption; phenobarbital and phenytoin increase the hepatic metabolism of vitamin D.

Adverse Reactions

High doses of vitamin D have rarely produced adverse events in clinical trials.

Toxicology

Toxicity due to vitamin D is considered to manifest at serum levels greater than 150 ng/mL of 25-hydroxyvitamin D. Symptoms of hypervitaminosis D include fatigue, nausea, vomiting, and weakness associated with hypercalcemia.

Local Anesthetic/Vasoconstrictor Precautions No information available to require special precautions

Effects on Bleeding None reported

Wild Yam

Clinical Overview

Use

Clinical trials are generally lacking for topical formulations of Dioscorea for menopausal symptoms. Chinese yam polysaccharides have been evaluated in laboratory studies for potential as prebiotics, with varying results. Dioscorea oppositifolia tubers have been used as a saliva substitute.

Dosing

There are inadequate clinical trials on which to base dosing guidelines.

Contraindications

Contraindications have not been identified.

Pregnancy/Lactation

Information regarding safety and efficacy in pregnancy and lactation is lacking.

Interactions

None well documented.

Adverse Reactions

A clinical study evaluating the daily consumption of wild yam reported no adverse events. Topical preparations of wild yam extract are relatively free from adverse effects. Based on a single study in rats, oral D. villosa should be avoided in people with compromised renal function.

Toxicology

Topical D. villosa (with an upper limit of 3.5% diosgenin) was not found to be systemically toxic or genotoxic.

Local Anesthetic/Vasoconstrictor Precautions No information available to require special precautions

Effects on Bleeding None reported

Willow Bark

Clinical Overview
Use

Willow bark can be an effective analgesic if the salicylate content is adequate. Anticancer, antioxidant, and anti-inflammatory activity has been documented in limited trials. Clinical trials have shown that willow has moderate efficacy in treating lower back pain but very little efficacy in treating arthritic conditions.

Dosing

Willow is available in several dosage forms, including tablets, capsules, powder, and liquid. Willow bark has been used for analgesia at daily doses of 1 to 3 g of bark, corresponding to salicin 60 to 120 mg. A clinical study of patients with lower back pain used willow bark at a dose of salicin 120 to 240 mg/day. A proprietary extract of willow bark, Assalix, was standardized to contain 15% salicin. The pharmacokinetics of salicylic acid delivered from willow bark have been studied, and plasma half-life is approximately 2.5 hours. Another pharmacokinetic study of salicylic acid from salicin found peak levels within 2 hours after oral administration.

Contraindications

Patients with known hypersensitivity to aspirin should avoid any willow-containing product. This caution also applies to patients with asthma, impaired thrombocyte function, vitamin K antagonistic treatment, diabetes, gout, kidney or liver conditions, peptic ulcer disease, and in any other medical conditions in which aspirin is contraindicated.

Pregnancy/Lactation

Avoid use because of the lack of information regarding safety and efficacy during pregnancy and lactation.

Interactions

In general, drug interactions associated with salicylates may apply to willow-containing products. Therefore, avoid use with alcohol, barbiturates, sedatives, and other salicylate-containing products because of additive irritant effects and adverse reactions on the GI tract and blood platelets. Willow may also interact with oral anticoagulants (eg, warfarin), seizure medications (eg, phenytoin, valproate acid), and other medications (eg, methotrexate).

Adverse Reactions

Reports from clinical trials primarily document GI discomfort, such as nausea and stomachache, as well as dizziness and rash. An anaphylactic reaction to willow bark has been reported.

Toxicology

There is little or no toxicity information on the use of willow bark. However, the same toxicity associated with salicylates applies to willow. Patients should monitor for blood in stools, tinnitus, nausea or vomiting, and stomach or kidney irritation.

Local Anesthetic/Vasoconstrictor Precautions No information available to require special precautions

Effects on Bleeding Salicylate derivatives of willow bark had little effect on platelet aggregation when compared with a daily cardioprotective dose of acetylsalicylate 100 mg. The total serum salicylate concentration of salicin, one of the principle salicylates of willow, was bioequivalent to acetylsalicylate 50 mg. There are no reports of bleeding caused by willow bark.

Wormwood

Clinical Overview
Use

Wormwood was traditionally used to treat worm infestations, although there is no clinical data supporting this use. Anti-inflammatory, antipyretic, and chemotherapeutic activity is documented in nonhuman studies. Information regarding the plant's use in Crohn disease is limited. Wormwood is also used as a flavoring agent.

Dosing

Wormwood is commercially available as an essential oil, as well as in capsule, tablet, tincture, and aqueous extract dosage forms. However, there is no recent clinical evidence to support dose recommendations for wormwood. Traditional use for treating dyspepsia was dosed at 3 to 5 g daily as an infusion or 2 to 3 g daily as the herb.

Contraindications

Avoid use with hypersensitivity to any of the components of wormwood, particularly the essential oil. It may be contraindicated in patients with an underlying defect with hepatic heme synthesis (thujone is a porphyrogenic terpenoid).

Pregnancy/Lactation

Documented abortifacient and emmenagogue effects. Avoid use.

Interactions

None well documented.

Adverse Reactions

Thujone produces a state of excitement and is a powerful convulsant. Ingestion of wormwood may result in absinthism, a syndrome characterized by digestive disorders, thirst, restlessness, vertigo, trembling of the limbs, numbness of the extremities, loss of intellect, delirium, paralysis, and death.

Toxicology

Wormwood is classified as an unsafe herb by the Food and Drug Administration (FDA) because of the neurotoxic potential of thujone and its derivatives. The safety of wormwood is poorly documented despite its long history as a food additive. Convulsions, dermatitis, and renal failure have been documented.

Local Anesthetic/Vasoconstrictor Precautions No information available to require special precautions

Effects on Bleeding None reported

Xylitol

Clinical Overview
Use

Medical literature documents the use of xylitol in medical conditions and applications, including acute otitis media, dental caries, intravenous (IV) nutrition, and osteoporosis, although limited clinical trials exist.

Dosing

Dosage regimens vary. In one study to prevent ear infections in children, the daily dose varied from 8.4 g in chewing gum to 10 g in syrup. Xylitol oral solution at dosages of 5 g orally 3 times a day and 7.5 g orally once a day was well tolerated in young children. Xylitol chewing gum was effective in reducing dental caries when divided into at least 3 consumption periods per day for a total dose of 6 to 10 g.

Contraindications

Avoid use if allergic to xylitol. Hypersensitivity reactions are documented.

Pregnancy/Lactation

Pregnancy: Category B. Xylitol is considered safe in pregnancy and during breast-feeding, according to the US Food and Drug Administration (FDA). The use of xylitol chewing gum in mothers lowered maternal oral bacterial load and reduced transmission of mutans streptococci to infants late in pregnancy and during the postpartum period.

Interactions

None well documented.

Adverse Reactions

The main adverse effects reported from oral xylitol use at a dosage exceeding 40 to 50 g/day included nausea, bloating, borborygmi (rumbling sounds of gas moving through the intestine), colic, diarrhea, and increased total bowel movement frequency.

Toxicology

Xylitol is generally nontoxic based on various clinical studies and its historical use in foods, pharmaceuticals, and nutraceuticals. Animal studies also confirm its overall safety profile. Renocerebral oxalosis with renal failure is documented with large doses of IV administered xylitol.

Local Anesthetic/Vasoconstrictor Precautions No information available to require special precautions
Effects on Bleeding None reported

Yarrow

Clinical Overview

Use

Research reveals no clinical data regarding the use of yarrow to treat any condition. However, yarrow has been used to induce sweating and to stop wound bleeding. It has also been reported to reduce heavy menstrual bleeding and pain. It has been used to relieve GI ailments, for cerebral and coronary thromboses, to lower high blood pressure, to improve circulation, and to tone varicose veins. It has antimicrobial actions, is a natural source for food flavoring, and is used in alcoholic beverages and bitters.

Dosing

A typical dose of yarrow herb is 4.5 g/day for inflammatory conditions. However, there are no modern clinical studies to validate this dose.

Contraindications

Yarrow is contraindicated in individuals with an existing hypersensitivity to any member of the Asteraceae family. Use in epileptic patients is contraindicated.

Pregnancy/Lactation

Documented adverse effects (eg, emmenagogue, abortifacient). Avoid use of yarrow's volatile oil during pregnancy.

Interactions

None well documented.

Adverse Reactions

Contact dermatitis is the most commonly reported side effect.

Toxicology

Yarrow is generally not considered toxic.

Local Anesthetic/Vasoconstrictor Precautions No information available to require special precautions
Effects on Bleeding None reported

Yohimbe

Clinical Overview

Use

Yohimbine has been used primarily in the treatment of sexual dysfunction, weight (body fat) loss, and xerostomia (dry mouth). It has also been used in studies investigating autonomic failure and orthostatic hypotension.

Dosing

Yohimbine 6 mg given 3 times a day has been used in xerostomia trials. A mean dose of 0.4 mg/kg body weight or 30 mg daily, and a maximum of 50 mg, has been used in erectile dysfunction studies. In studies investigating effects on body mass, yohimbine 20 mg daily has been used.

Contraindications

This drug should not be used in the presence of renal or hepatic function impairment.

Pregnancy/Lactation

Do not use during pregnancy or lactation.

Interactions

None well documented.

Adverse Reactions

Clinical trials report few serious adverse reactions. There are case reports of rash, lupus-like syndrome, bronchospasm, severe hypotension, dysrhythmia, heart failure, and death. Increased anxiety, irritability, and excitability have also been reported. Animal studies suggest yohimbine may increase motor activity and seizures at higher dosages. Yohimbe may precipitate psychoses in predisposed individuals.

Toxicology

No data.

Local Anesthetic/Vasoconstrictor Precautions Has potential to interact with epinephrine and levonordefrin to result in increased BP; use vasoconstrictor with caution
Effects on Bleeding None reported

ORAL MEDICINE TOPICS

PART I:

DENTAL MANAGEMENT
AND THERAPEUTIC CONSIDERATIONS
IN MEDICALLY-COMPROMISED PATIENTS

This first part of the chapter focuses on common medical conditions and their associated drug therapies with which the dentist must be familiar. Patient profiles with commonly associated drug regimens are described.

TABLE OF CONTENTS

CARDIOVASCULAR DISEASES

Cardiovascular disease is the most prevalent human disease affecting over 60 million Americans, accounting for >50% of all deaths in the United States. Surgical and pharmacological therapies have resulted in many cardiovascular patients living healthy and profitable lives. Consequently, patients presenting to the dental office may require treatment planning modifications related to the medical management of their cardiovascular disease. For the purposes of this text, we will cover coronary artery disease (CAD) including angina pectoris, myocardial infarction, cardiac arrhythmias, heart failure, and hypertension.

CARDIOVASCULAR DRUGS: DENTAL CONSIDERATIONS

Some of the drug listings are redundant because the drugs are used to treat more than one cardiovascular disorder. As a convenience to the reader, each table has been constructed as a stand alone listing of drugs for the given disorder.

CORONARY ARTERY DISEASE

Any long-term decrease in the delivery of oxygen to the heart muscle can lead to the condition ischemic heart disease. Often arteriosclerosis and atherosclerosis result in a narrowing of the coronary vessels' lumina and are the most common causes of vascular ischemic heart disease. Other causes such as previous infarct, mitral valve regurgitation, and ruptured septa may also lead to ischemia in the heart muscle. The two most common major conditions that result from ischemic heart disease are angina pectoris and myocardial infarction. Sudden death can likewise result from ischemia.

To the physician, the most common presenting sign or symptom of ischemic heart disease is chest pain. This chest pain can be of a transient nature as in angina pectoris or the result of a myocardial infarction. This is a more typical presentation in men; women may have more subtle signs of fatigue and general malaise. It is now believed that sudden death represents a separate occurrence that essentially involves the development of a lethal cardiac arrhythmia or coronary artery spasm leading to an acute shutdown of the heart muscle blood supply. Risk factors in patients for coronary atherosclerosis include age (males ≥45, females ≥55 years), family history of premature development, hypertension, hypercholesterolemia, low HDL, cigarette smoking, and diabetes mellitus.

CAD is the cause of about half of all deaths in the United States. CAD has been shown to be correlated with the levels of plasma cholesterol and/or triacylglycerol-containing lipoprotein particles. Primary prevention focuses on averting the development of CAD. In contrast, secondary prevention of CAD focuses on therapies to reduce morbidity and mortality in patients with clinically documented CAD.

Lipid-lowering and cardioprotective drugs provide significant risk-reducing benefits in the secondary prevention of CAD. By reducing the levels of total and low density cholesterol through the inhibition of hydroxymethylglutaryl-coenzyme A (HMG-CoA) reductase, statin drugs significantly improve survival. Cardioprotective drug therapy includes antiplatelet/antico-agulant agents to inhibit platelet adhesion; aggregation and blood coagulation; beta-blockers to lower heart rate, contractility and blood pressure; and the angiotensin-converting enzyme (ACE) inhibitors to lower peripheral resistance and workload. For a listing of lipid lowering drugs, see Table 1.

Table 1. Drugs Used in the Treatment of Hyperlipidemia
Reduction of Total and Low-Density Cholesterol Levels

HMG-CoA Reductase Inhibitors
- Fluvastatin on page 622
- Lovastatin on page 846
- Pitavastatin on page 1106
- Pravastatin on page 1128
- Rosuvastatin on page 1215
- Simvastatin on page 1236
- Atorvastatin on page 145

Fibrate Group
- Fenofibrate on page 571
- Fenofibric Acid on page 574
- Gemfibrozil on page 651

Bile Acid Sequestrants
- Cholestyramine Resin on page 298
- Colesevelam on page 347
- Colestipol on page 348

Nicotinic Acid
- Niacin on page 972

Cholesterol Absorption Inhibitor
- Ezetimibe on page 562

Antilipemic Agent, Microsomal Triglyceride Transfer Protein (MTP) Inhibitor
- Lomitapide on page 835

Miscellaneous
- Omega-3-Acid Ethyl Esters on page 1008

ANGINA PECTORIS (Emphasis on Unstable Angina)

Numerous physiologic triggers can initiate the rupture of plaque in coronary blood vessels. Rupture leads to the activation, adhesion and aggregation of platelets, and the activation of the clotting cascade, resulting in the formation of occlusive thrombus. If this process leads to the complete occlusion of the artery, acute myocardial infarction with ST-segment elevation occurs. Alternatively, if the process leads to severe stenosis and the artery remains patent, unstable angina can occur. Triggers which induce unstable angina include physical exertion, mechanical stress due to an increase in cardiac contractility, pulse rate, blood pressure, and vasoconstriction.

Recently unstable angina/non-ST-elevation MI guidelines have been updated by the American College of Cardiology Foundation and the American Heart Association (Jneid, 2012). These guidelines may be helpful in outlining treatment strategies.

Pharmacologic therapy to treat unstable angina includes antiplatelet drugs, antithrombin therapy, and conventional antianginal therapy with beta-blockers (or calcium channel blockers) and nitrates. These drug groups and selected agents are listed in Table 2 and see Antiplatelet and Anticoagulation Considerations in Dentistry on page 1503.

Conventional Antianginal Therapy: Beta-Blockers, Nitrates, Calcium Channel Blockers

The pharmacotherapeutic strategy in treating angina is directed at improving myocardial oxygen supply and/or decreasing myocardial oxygen demand. Myocardial oxygen supply can be increased through enhancing coronary blood flow. Myocardial oxygen demand can be reduced by decreasing heart rate, contractility, and myocardial wall tension. Preload, afterload, and myocardial wall thickness are determinants of myocardial wall tension.

Organic Nitrates

Organic nitrates benefit angina by enhancing coronary blood flow via vasodilation of both large epicardial vessels and neighboring collateral vessels and decreasing myocardial oxygen demand by dilating veins and reducing preload. In order to be effective for the chronic prevention of angina, organic nitrates need to be dosed in a manner that does not induce nitrate tolerance.

Beta-Blockers

Beta-blockers are beneficial in treating angina since they decrease heart rate and contractility. Beta-blockers without intrinsic sympathomimetic activity (ISA) are preferred and those with ISA generally should be avoided when treating angina (such beta-blockers may actually increase myocardial workload). Beta-blockers are useful in the treatment of stable and unstable angina; but, since they can induce coronary vasospasm, they should be avoided in patients with variant angina.

Beta-blockers are the preferred initial choice, often used in conjunction with an organic nitrate to more positively address the hemodynamic imbalances causing the angina. If the patient cannot tolerate the beta-blocker or if the beta-blocker therapy is contraindicated, a calcium channel blocker with or without an organic nitrate can be considered. If dual combination therapy is ineffective, a calcium channel blocker may be added. Since the combination of a beta-blocker and either verapamil or diltiazem frequently induces undesirable bradycardia, a dihydropyridine is often selected in combination with a beta-blocker, unless the patient is experiencing unstable angina. Caution should be used when using beta-blockers in patients with difficult-to-control diabetes mellitus, bronchospastic disease, or peripheral vascular disease. The medications may be dosed as high as possible without inducing symptomatic bradycardia, hypotension, and/or heart blocks. Some patients on beta-blockers will experience fatigue and other adverse effects related to the central nervous system. Abrupt withdrawal of beta-blockers in patients with angina has been known to cause a rebound effect.

Calcium Channel Blockers

Three "types" of agents comprise calcium channel blockers: Diltiazem, verapamil, and the dihydropyridine family. These agents are useful in treating stable and unstable angina and are the drugs of choice in treating variant angina. All three agents increase coronary blood flow. Verapamil and diltiazem reduce contractility, heart rate, and, to some extent, afterload (thus reducing wall tension). Dihydropyridines (eg, nifedipine) are potent afterload reducers and have no impact on reducing heart rate. In fact, dihydropyridines may actually increase heart rate in patients not on a beta-blocker and may increase ischemia in patients experiencing unstable angina.

Stable and Unstable Angina

Since stable and unstable angina are nearly always related to coronary artery disease, patients should be placed on aspirin and an angiotensin-converting enzyme inhibitor (especially if the patient has heart failure) in addition to antianginal therapy. Clopidogrel or prasugrel may be considered if the patient is allergic to aspirin. If applicable, weight reduction, smoking cessation, and following an appropriate low-cholesterol, low-fat diet should be encouraged as well as an effort to reduce other CAD risk factors. The lipid profile of these patients should be determined and, if needed, treated aggressively - LDL-C <70 mg/dL.

Patients with cardiac stents who have not completed their full course of dual antiplatelet therapy should not have their antiplatelet agents discontinued even if only briefly. Premature interruption of therapy may result in stent thrombosis with subsequent MI. Discussion with the patient's cardiologist is required especially if urgent dental procedures are necessary.

◀ **Dental Management**

The dental management of the patient with angina pectoris may include sedation techniques for complicated procedures (see the Sedation section in Management of the Patient With Anxiety or Depression on page 1594), to limit the extent of procedures, and to limit the use of local anesthesia containing 1:100,000 epinephrine to two carpules. Anesthesia without a vasoconstrictor might also be selected. The appropriate use of a vasoconstrictor in anesthesia, however, should be weighed against the necessity to maximize anesthesia. Complete history, appropriate referral, and consultation with the patient's physician should be done for patients who are known to be at risk for angina pectoris.

MYOCARDIAL INFARCTION

Myocardial infarction is the leading cause of death in the United States. It is an acute irreversible ischemic event that produces an area of myocardial necrosis in the heart tissue. If a patient has a previous history of myocardial infarction, he/she may be taking a variety of drugs (ie, antihypertensives, lipid lowering drugs, ACE inhibitors, and antianginal medications) to not only prevent a second infarct, but to treat the long-term effects associated ischemic heart disease. Postmyocardial infarction patients are often taking anticoagulants, such as warfarin, and antiplatelet agents, such as aspirin, clopidogrel, or prasugrel. Consultation with the prescribing physician by the dentist is necessary prior to invasive procedures. Temporary dose reduction may allow the dentist to proceed with very invasive procedures. Most procedures, however, can be accomplished without changing the anticoagulant or antiplatelet therapy at all, using local hemostasis techniques and thereby keeping the thromboembolic risk to a minimum.

Aspirin on page 135
Warfarin on page 1412

Thrombolytic drugs, which might dissolve hemostatic plugs, may also be given on a short-term basis immediately following an infarct and include:

Alteplase on page 71
Reteplase on page 1189
Tenecteplase on page 1298

Alteplase (tissue plasminogen activator [TPA]) is also currently in use for acute myocardial infarction. Following myocardial infarction and rehabilitation, outpatients may be placed on antiplatelet agents, anticoagulants (such as Coumadin®), diuretics, beta-adrenergic blockers, ACE inhibitors or angiotensin receptor blockers, lipid-lowering therapies, and possibly aldosterone inhibitors if significant heart failure is associated with the MI. Depending on the presence or absence of continued angina pectoris, patients may also be taking nitrates, beta-blockers, or calcium channel blockers as indicated for treatment of angina.

Beta-Adrenergic Blocking Agents Categorized According to Specific Properties

Alpha-Adrenergic Blocking Activity

Carvedilol on page 257
Labetalol on page 788

Intrinsic Sympathomimetic Activity

Acebutolol on page 26
Pindolol on page 1095

Long Duration of Action and Fewer CNS Effects

Atenolol on page 141
Betaxolol (Systemic) on page 187
Nadolol on page 950

Beta$_1$-Receptor Selectivity

Atenolol on page 141
Betaxolol (Systemic) on page 187
Metoprolol on page 908
Nebivolol on page 963

Nonselective (blocks both beta$_1$- and beta$_2$-receptors)

Nadolol on page 950
Propranolol on page 1153
Timolol (Systemic) on page 1326

ARRHYTHMIAS

Abnormal cardiac rhythm can develop spontaneously and survivors of a myocardial infarction are often left with an arrhythmia. An arrhythmia is any alteration or disturbance in the normal rate, rhythm, or conduction through the cardiac tissue. Abnormalities in rhythm can occur in either the atria or the ventricles. Various valvular deformities, drug effects, and chemical derangements can initiate arrhythmias. These arrhythmias can be a slowing of the heart rate (<60 beats/minute) as defined in bradycardia or tachycardia resulting in a rapid heart beat (usually >150 beats/minute). The dentist will encounter a variety of treatments for management of arrhythmias. Usually, underlying causes such as reduced cardiac output, hypertension, and irregular ventricular beats will require treatment. Pacemaker therapy is also sometimes used. Indwelling pacemakers may require supplementation with antibiotics, and consultation with the physician is certainly appropriate.

Beta-blockers are often used to slow cardiac rate and diazepam may be helpful when anxiety is a contributing factor in arrhythmia. When atrial flutter and atrial fibrillation are diagnosed, drug therapy is usually required.

Digoxin on page 423

Atrial fibrillation (AF) is an arrhythmia characterized by multiple electrical activations in the atria resulting in scattered and disorganized depolarization and repolarization of the myocardium. Atrial contraction can lead to an irregular and rapid rate of ventricular contraction. The prevalence of AF within the US population ranges between 1% and 4%, with the incidence increasing with age. It is often associated with rheumatic valvular disease and nonvalvular conditions including coronary artery disease, heart failure, and hypertension. Coronary artery disease is present in about one-half of the patients with AF. Atrial fibrillation is a major risk factor for systemic and cerebral embolism. It is thought that thrombi develop as a result of stasis in the dilated left atrium and are dislodged by sudden changes in cardiac rhythm. About 10% of all strokes in patients >60 years of age are caused by AF.

The cornerstones of drug therapy for atrial fibrillation are the restoration and maintenance of a normal sinus rhythm through the use of antiarrhythmic drugs, ventricular rate control through the use of beta-blockers, digitalis drugs or calcium channel blockers, and stroke prevention through the use of anticoagulants.

Antiarrhythmic Drugs

Cardiac rhythm is conducted through the sinoatrial (SA) and atrioventricular (AV) nodes, bundle branches, and Purkinje fibers. Electrical impulses are transmitted within this system by the opening and closing of sodium and potassium channels. Antiarrhythmic drugs are classified by which primary channel they act upon, a classification known as Vaughan Williams. The Class I agents act primarily on sodium channels, and the Class III agents act on potassium channels. In addition, there are subclassifications within the Class I agents according to effects of the drug on conduction and refractoriness within the Purkinje and ventricular tissues. Class IA agents show moderate depression of conduction and prolongation of repolarization.

Atrial Fibrillation: Restoring and Maintaining Normal Sinus Rhythm

Pharmacologic cardioversion may be attempted in hemodynamically stable patients whose ventricular rate is controlled. If a patient has been in atrial fibrillation for >48 hours, anticoagulation should be considered prior to cardioversion. Drugs more commonly used for pharmacologic cardioversion include amiodarone, dofetilide, dronedarone, propafenone, or sotalol, depending upon patient's specific characteristics (eg, heart failure).

Ventricular Rate Control

It is accepted practice to treat patients with medication when the resting ventricular rate is >110 beats/minute. Digoxin, calcium channel blockers, and beta-adrenergic blockers are used in the regulation of ventricular rate. Digoxin increases the vagal tone to the AV node, calcium channel blockers slow the AV nodal conduction, and the beta-adrenergic blocking drugs decrease the sympathetic activation of the AV nodal conduction.

Anticoagulants Useful in Arrhythmias

Warfarin (Coumadin®) elicits its anticoagulant effect by interfering with the hepatic synthesis of vitamin K-dependent coagulation factors II, VII, IX, and X. Although warfarin appears to be somewhat effective after myocardial infarction in preventing death or recurrent myocardial infarction, its effectiveness in the treatment of acute coronary syndrome is questionable. Combination therapy with aspirin and heparin, followed by warfarin, has resulted in reduced incidence of recurrent angina, myocardial infarction, death, or all three at 14 days, compared to aspirin alone. In contrast, another study failed to show any additional benefit in the treatment of acute coronary syndrome using a combination of aspirin and warfarin, compared to aspirin alone (Douketis, 2012).

Recently, the FDA approved Dabigatran (Pradaxa®) for the prevention of stroke and systemic embolism in patients with atrial fibrillation. Dabigatran is the first FDA-approved replacement available for warfarin. Dabigatran is an anticoagulant that acts by inhibiting thrombin, an enzyme in the blood that is involved in blood clotting. Thrombin (serine protease) enables the conversion of fibrinogen to fibrin during the coagulation cascade, preventing the development of thrombus. The recommended oral dose is 150 mg twice daily for patients with a creatinine clearance >30 mL/minute. For patients with a creatinine clearance 15-30 mL/minute, the recommended oral dose is 75 mg twice daily.

◄ Dental clinicians should consider consultation with the patient's healthcare provider prior to invasive therapies. However, recent reviews have argued that inappropriate adjustments in anticoagulation therapy places the patient at far greater risk of stroke than hemorrhage during most dental procedures (Douketis, 2012; Jeske, 2003). Therefore, scientific evidence does not support changing regimens of anticoagulation therapy in most instances.

Table 2. Drugs Used to Manage Unstable Angina

Antiplatelet Drugs

Aspirin on page 135

Cilostazol on page 304

Clopidogrel on page 335

Prasugrel on page 1126

Ticagrelor on page 1322

Glycoprotein IIb/IIIa Receptor Antagonists

Abciximab on page 24

Eptifibatide on page 490

Tirofiban on page 1331

Antithrombin Drugs

Indirect Thrombin Inhibitors

Heparin (unfractionated) on page 679

Low molecular weight heparins

Dalteparin on page 373

Enoxaparin on page 479

Nadroparin on page 951

Tinzaparin on page 1328

Direct Thrombin Inhibitors

Argatroban on page 121

Lepirudin on page 801

Bivalirudin on page 194

Desirudin on page 392

REFERENCES

American Diabetes Association, "Standards of Medical Care in Diabetes-2012," *Diabetes Care*, 2012, 35(Suppl 1):11-63.

Anderson JL, Adams CD, Antman EM, et al, "2011 ACCF/AHA Focused Update Incorporated Into the ACC/AHA 2007 Guidelines for the Management of Patients With Unstable Angina/Non-ST-Elevation Myocardial Infarction: A Report of the American College of Cardiology Foundation/American Heart Association Task Force on Practice Guidelines," *Circulation*, 2011, 123(18):e426-579.

Brunzell JD, Davidson M, Furberg CD, et al, "Lipoprotein Management in Patients With Cardiometabolic Risk: Consensus Statement From the American Diabetes Association and the American College of Cardiology Foundation," *Diabetes Care*, 2008, 31(4):811-22.

Douketis JD, "Contra: "Bridging Anticoagulation Is Needed During Warfarin Interruption When Patients Require Elective Surgery"," *Thromb Haemost*, 2012, 108(2):210-2.

Fihn SD, Gardin JM, Abrams J, et al, "2012 ACCF/AHA/ACP/AATS/PCNA/SCAI/STS Guideline for the Diagnosis and Management of Patients With Stable Ischemic Heart Disease: A Report of the American College of Cardiology Foundation/American Heart Association Task Force on Practice Guidelines, and the American College of Physicians, American Association for Thoracic Surgery, Preventive Cardiovascular Nurses Association, Society for Cardiovascular Angiography and Interventions, and Society of Thoracic Surgeons," *Circulation*, 2012, 126(25):e354-471.

Heart Failure Society of America, Lindenfeld J, Albert NM, et al, "HFSA 2010 Comprehensive Heart Failure Practice Guideline," *J Card Fail*, 2010, 16 (6):e1-194.

Hunt SA, Abraham WT, Chin MH, et al, "2009 Focused Update Incorporated Into the ACC/AHA 2005 Guidelines for the Diagnosis and Management of Heart Failure in Adults: A Report of the American College of Cardiology Foundation/American Heart Association Task Force on Practice Guidelines Developed in Collaboration With the International Society for Heart and Lung Transplantation," *J Am Coll Cardiol*, 2009, 53(15):e1-e90.

Jeske AH, Suchko GD, ADA Council on Scientific Affairs and Division of Science, et al, "Lack of a Scientific Basis for Routine Discontinuation of Oral Anticoagulation Therapy Before Dental Treatment," *J Am Dent Assoc*, 2003, 134(11):1492-7.

Jneid H, Anderson JL, Wright RS, et al, "2012 ACCF/AHA Focused Update of the Guideline for the Management of Patients With Unstable Angina/Non-ST-Elevation Myocardial Infarction (Updating the 2007 Guideline and Replacing the 2011 Focused Update): A Report of the American College of Cardiology Foundation/American Heart Association Task Force on Practice Guidelines," *Circulation*, 2012, 126(7):875-910.

Kushner FG, Hand M, Smith SC Jr, et al, "2009 Focused Updates: ACC/AHA Guidelines for the Management of Patients With ST-Elevation Myocardial Infarction (Updating the 2004 Guideline and 2007 Focused Update) and ACC/AHA/SCAI Guidelines on Percutaneous Coronary Intervention (Updating the 2005 Guideline and 2007 Focused Update) a Report of the American College of Cardiology Foundation/American Heart Association Task Force on Practice Guidelines," *J Am Coll Cardiol*, 2009, 54(23):2205-41.

O'Gara PT, Kushner FG, Ascheim DD, et al, "2013 ACCF/AHA Guideline for the Management of ST-Elevation Myocardial Infarction: A Report of the American College of Cardiology Foundation/American Heart Association Task Force on Practice Guidelines," *Circulation*, 2013, 127(4):e362-425.

Skanes AC, Healey JS, Cairns JA, et al, "Focused 2012 Update of the Canadian Cardiovascular Society Atrial Fibrillation Guidelines: Recommendations for Stroke Prevention and Rate/Rhythm Control," *Can J Cardiol*, 2012, 28(2):125-36.

Smith SC Jr, Benjamin EJ, Bonow RO, et al, "AHA/ACCF Secondary Prevention and Risk Reduction Therapy for Patients With Coronary and Other Atherosclerotic Vascular Disease: 2011 Update: A Guideline From the American Heart Association and American College of Cardiology Foundation," *Circulation*, 2011, 124(22):2458-73.

Wann LS, Curtis AB, January CT, et al, "2011 ACCF/AHA/HRS Focused Update on the Management of Patients With Atrial Fibrillation (Updating the 2006 Guideline): A Report of the American College of Cardiology Foundation/American Heart Association Task Force on Practice Guidelines," *Circulation*, 2011, 123(1):104-23.

HEART FAILURE

Heart failure is a condition in which the heart is unable to pump sufficient blood to meet the needs of the body. It is caused by an impaired ability of the cardiac muscle to contract or by an increased workload imposed on the heart. Most frequently, the underlying cause of heart failure is coronary artery disease. Other contributory causes include hypertension, diabetes, idiopathic dilated cardiomyopathy, and valvular heart disease. It is estimated that heart failure affects approximately 5 million Americans. The New York Heart Association functional classification is regarded as the standard measure to describe the severity of a patient's symptom. Class I is characterized by having no limitation of physical activity. There is no dyspnea, fatigue, palpitations, or angina with ordinary physical activity. There is no objective evidence of cardiovascular dysfunction. Class II includes those patients having slight limitation of physical activity. These patients experience fatigue, palpitations, dyspnea, or angina with ordinary physical activity, but are comfortable at rest. There is evidence of minimal cardiovascular dysfunction. Class III is characterized by marked limitation of activity. Less-than-ordinary physical activity causes fatigue, palpitations, dyspnea, or angina, but patients are comfortable at rest. There is objective evidence of moderately severe cardiovascular dysfunction. Class IV is characterized by the inability to carry out any physical activity without discomfort. Symptoms of heart failure may be present even at rest, and any physical activity undertaken increases discomfort. There is objective evidence of severe cardiovascular dysfunction. Drug classes and the specific agents used to treat heart failure are listed in Table 3.

Table 3. Drugs Used in the Treatment of Heart Failure

Angiotensin-Converting Enzyme (ACE) Inhibitors[1]

Benazepril on page 173

Captopril on page 242

Enalapril on page 475

Fosinopril on page 634

Lisinopril on page 830

Moexipril on page 933

Perindopril Erbumine on page 1076

Quinapril on page 1169

Ramipril on page 1179

Trandolapril on page 1349

Angiotensin II Receptor Blockers

Candesartan on page 237

Losartan on page 843

Valsartan on page 1381

Diuretics

Thiazides

Hydrochlorothiazide on page 687

Loop Diuretics

Bumetanide on page 208

Furosemide on page 640

Torsemide on page 1345

Aldosterone Blocker (Selective)

Eplerenone on page 487

Spironolactone on page 1254

Digitalis Glycosides

Digoxin on page 423

Beta-Adrenergic Receptor Blockers

Bisoprolol on page 193

Carvedilol on page 257

Metoprolol on page 908

Supplemental Agents

Direct-Acting Vasodilators

HydrALAZINE on page 686

Isosorbide Dinitrate on page 767

Isosorbide Mononitrate on page 769

Nitroglycerin on page 986

[1]Regarded as the cornerstone of heart failure treatment and should be used routinely and early in all patients.

Drug Classes and Specific Agents Used to Treat Heart Failure

Angiotensin-converting enzyme (ACE) inhibitors reduce left ventricular volume and filling pressure while decreasing total peripheral resistance. They improve cardiac output (modestly) and natriuresis. ACE inhibitors are usually used in all patients with heart failure if no contraindication or intolerance exists. This group of drugs is considered the cornerstone of treatment and is used routinely and early if pharmacologic treatment is indicated. Angiotensin receptor blockers may be used if a patient cannot tolerate an ACE inhibitor or in rare instances used with an ACE inhibitor when persistent symptoms or progressive worsening occurs despite optimal ACE inhibitor and beta-blocker therapy.

Beta-adrenergic receptor blocking drugs (beta-blockers), specifically carvedilol, bisoprolol, and metoprolol extended release, are used in the treatment of heart failure because of their beneficial effect in reducing mortality.

Diuretics increase sodium chloride and water excretion resulting in reduction of preload, thus relieving the symptoms of pulmonary congestion associated with heart failure. They may also reduce myocardial oxygen demand. The thiazides, loop diuretics, and potassium-sparing agents are all useful in reducing preload by way of their diuretic actions.

Digitalis glycosides have been used in the treatment of heart failure for more than 200 years. Digitalis drugs increase cardiac output by a direct positive inotropic action on the myocardium. This increased cardiac output results in decreased venous pressure, reduced heart size, and diminished compensatory tachycardia.

Other drugs used in the treatment of heart failure include aldosterone blockers and direct-acting vasodilators. Direct-acting vasodilators (hydralazine, isosorbide) may be used in place of an ACE inhibitor or angiotensin receptor blocker. The direct-acting vasodilators reduce excessive vasoconstriction and reduce workload of the failing heart. Aldosterone blockers may be used in severe forms of heart failure to enhance survival; close attention to introduction and monitoring is essential to prevent hyperkalemia.

HYPERTENSION

In the United States, almost 50 million adults, 25-74 years of age, have hypertension. Hypertension is defined as systolic blood pressure ≥140 mm Hg, and/or diastolic pressure >90 mm Hg. People with blood pressure above normal are considered at increased risk of developing damage to the heart, kidney, brain, and eyes, resulting in premature morbidity and mortality.

The Joint National Committee on Prevention, Detection, Evaluation, and Treatment of High Blood Pressure, released its 7th Report in the summer of 2003. The highlights of the report are that several of the categories have been renamed to connote changes in philosophy towards earlier treatment and intervention for patients with elevated blood pressure.

Also, there is an increased importance in the elevation of systolic blood pressure for people >50 years of age. The category of high normal blood pressure has now been replaced with the term prehypertension for those patients with systolic blood pressure of 120-139 mm Hg and for those with diastolic blood pressure of 80-89 mm Hg. The remaining stages of hypertension have been broken into simply two categories: Stage 1 and Stage 2. Stage 1 diastolic pressure is 90-99 mm Hg and systolic pressure is 140-159 mm Hg, whereas in Stage 2, diastolic pressure >100 mm Hg or systolic pressure >160 mm Hg are the respective cut-off for treatment decisions. This greatly simplifies the classification of blood pressure.

In addition, the 7th Joint National Committee Report highlights the importance of lifestyle modifications in controlling blood pressure along with pharmacologic intervention. Thiazide diuretics have been considered one of the most important treatments in uncomplicated hypertension and their benefits of lowering blood pressure have been greatly emphasized. The role of dentistry in detection, as well as assisting in compliance for patients, has been clearly emphasized in this report.

The suggested initial goals of drug therapy are the maintenance of an arterial pressure of ≤140/90 mm Hg with concurrent control of other modifiable cardiovascular risk factors. Further reduction to 130/85 mm Hg should be pursued if cardiovascular and cerebrovascular function is not compromised. The Hypertension Optimal Treatment (HOT) randomized trial using patients 50-80 years of age found that the lowest incidence of major cardiovascular events and the lowest risk of cardiovascular mortality occurred at a mean diastolic blood pressure of 82.6 and 86.5 mm Hg, respectively. The target blood pressure for patients with diabetes or chronic kidney disease is <130/90 mm Hg.

Table 4. Classification of Blood Pressure for Adults ≥18 Years of Age

BP Classification	Systolic BP (mm Hg)		Diastolic BP (mm Hg)
Normotensive	<120	and	<80
Prehypertension[1]	120-139	or	80-89
Stage 1 hypertension[2]	140-159	or	90-99
Stage 2 hypertension[3]	≥160	or	≥100

[1]Not taking antihypertensive drugs and not acutely ill. When systolic and diastolic blood pressures fall into different categories, the higher category should be selected to classify the individual's blood pressure status. In addition to classifying stages of hypertension on the basis of average blood pressure levels, clinicians should specify presence or absence of target organ disease and additional risk factors. The specificity is important for risk classification and treatment.

[2]Optimal blood pressure with respect to cardiovascular risk is below 120/80 mm Hg. However, unusually low readings should be evaluated for clinical significance.

[3]Based on the average of two or more readings taken at each of two or more visits after an initial screening.

Adapted from Chobanian AV, Bakris GL, Black HR, et al, "Joint National Committee on Prevention, Detection, Evaluation, and Treatment of High Blood Pressure. National Heart, Lung, and Blood Institute; National High Blood Pressure Education Program Coordinating Committee. Seventh Report of the Joint National Committee on Prevention, Detection, Evaluation, and Treatment of High Blood Pressure," *Hypertension*, 2003, 42(6):1206-52.

Table 5. Lifestyle Modifications to Manage Hypertension[1-3]

Modification	Recommendation	Approximate Systolic Reduction (Range)
Weight reduction	Maintain normal body weight (body mass index 18.5-24.9 kg/m^2)	5-20 mm of Hg/10 kg weight loss[4]
Adopt DASH[5] eating plan	Consume a diet rich in fruits, vegetables, and low fat dairy products with a reduced content of saturated and total fat	8-14 mm Hg[6]
Dietary sodium reduction	Reduce dietary sodium intake to ≤100 mmol/day (2.4 g sodium or 6 g sodium chloride)	2-8 mm Hg[7]
Physical activity	Engage in regular aerobic physical activity such as brisk walking (≥30 minutes/day, most days of the week)	4-9 mm Hg[8]
Moderation of alcohol consumption	Limit consumption to ≤2 drinks (1 oz or 30 mL ethanol); (eg, 24 oz beer, 10 oz wine, or 3 oz 80-proof whiskey) per day in most men and to ≤1 drink/day in women and lighter weight people	2-4 mm Hg[9]

[1]Adapted from U.S. Department of Health and Human Services; National Institutes of Health; National Heart, Lung, and Blood Institute; National High Blood Pressure Education Program

[2]Overall cardiovascular risk education can be achieved by cessation of smoking

[3]The effects of implementing these modifications are dose- and time-dependent and could be greater for some people.

[4]The trials of Hypertension Prevention Collaborative Research Group; He and colleagues

[5]DASH: Dietary Approaches to Stop Hypertension

[6]Sacks and colleagues; Vollmer and colleagues

[7]Sacks and colleagues; Vollmer and colleagues; Chobanian and Hill

[8]Kelley and Kelley; Whelton and colleagues

[9]Xin and colleagues

Classes of Drugs Used in the Treatment of Hypertension

Diuretics
Beta-adrenergic receptor blocking agents (beta-blockers)
Alpha$_1$-adrenergic receptor blocking agents (alpha$_1$-blockers)
Agents which have both alpha- and beta-adrenergic blocking properties (alpha-/beta-blockers)
Angiotensin-converting enzyme (ACE) inhibitors
Angiotensin II receptor blockers
Calcium channel blocking agents
Supplemental agents such as centrally-acting alpha$_2$-adrenergic receptor agonists and direct-acting peripheral vaso-dilators.
Renin inhibitors
Selective aldosterone blockers

Table 6 lists the drug categories and representative agents used to treat hypertension. Combination drugs are now available to supply several classes of these drugs.

Table 6. Drug Categories and Representative Agents Used in the Treatment of Hypertension[1]

Diuretics

Thiazide Types

Loops

Potassium-Sparing

Table 6. Drug Categories and Representative Agents Used in the Treatment of Hypertension[1] *(continued)*

Beta-Blockers

Cardioselective

Atenolol on page 141

Betaxolol (Systemic) on page 187

Bisoprolol on page 193

Metoprolol on page 908

Nebivolol on page 963

Noncardioselective

Nadolol on page 950

Propranolol on page 1153

Timolol (Systemic) on page 1326

Alpha₁-Blocker

Doxazosin on page 449

Prazosin on page 1130

Terazosin on page 1300

Alpha-/Beta-Blocker

Carvedilol on page 257

Labetalol on page 788

Angiotensin-Converting Enzyme (ACE) Inhibitors

Benazepril on page 173

Captopril on page 242

Enalapril on page 475

Fosinopril on page 634

Lisinopril on page 830

Moexipril on page 933

Perindopril Erbumine on page 1076

Quinapril on page 1169

Ramipril on page 1179

Trandolapril on page 1349

Angiotensin II Receptor Blockers

Azilsartan on page 157

Candesartan on page 237

Eprosartan on page 489

Irbesartan on page 762

Losartan on page 843

Olmesartan on page 1004

Telmisartan on page 1293

Valsartan on page 1381

Renin Inhibitor

Aliskiren on page 63

Calcium Channel Blockers

AmLODIPine on page 88

Diltiazem on page 429

Felodipine on page 571

Isradipine on page 771

NiCARdipine on page 976

NIFEdipine on page 979

Nisoldipine on page 983

Verapamil on page 1397

Supplemental Agents

Centrally-acting Alpha₂-Agonist

CloNIDine on page 332

GuanFACINE on page 676

Methyldopa on page 897

Direct-Acting Peripheral Vasodilator

HydrALAZINE on page 686

Minoxidil (Systemic) on page 927

Current Thinking Regarding Antihypertensive Drug Selection

Medications in the first eight categories in Table 6 were held to be equally effective in two large-scale studies reported in the *New England Journal of Medicine* and the *Journal of the American Medical Association*, and that any of the medications could be used initially for monotherapy. According to the Seventh Report of the Joint National Committee on Prevention, Detection, Evaluation, and Treatment of High Blood Pressure (JNC 7), diuretics or beta-blockers are recommended as initial therapy for uncomplicated hypertension. If a diuretic is selected as initial therapy, a thiazide diuretic is preferred in patients with normal renal function. If necessary, potassium replacement or concurrent treatment with a potassium-sparing agent may prevent hypokalemia. Loop diuretics are used in patients with impaired renal function or who cannot tolerate thiazides. Diuretics are well-tolerated and inexpensive. They are considered the drugs of choice for treating isolated systolic hypertension in the elderly.

Beta-blockers are the agents of choice in patients with coronary artery disease or supraventricular arrhythmia, and in young patients with hyperdynamic circulation. Beta-blockers are alternatives for initial therapy and are more effective in Caucasian patients than in African-American patients. Beta-blockers are not considered first choice drugs in elderly patients with uncomplicated hypertension. The beta-blocking drug carvedilol also selectively blocks alpha$_1$ receptors and has been shown to reduce mortality in hypertensive patients.

Alpha$_1$-adrenergic blocking agents can be used as initial therapy in patients with benign prostatic hypertrophy (BPH).

ACE inhibitors are the preferred drugs for patients with coexisting heart failure. They are useful as initial therapy in hypertensive patients with kidney damage or diabetes mellitus with proteinuria, and in Caucasian patients. No clinically relevant differences have been found among the available ACE inhibitors. The ACE inhibitors are well-tolerated by young, physically active patients and the elderly. The most common adverse effect of the ACE inhibitors is dry cough. Angiotensin II receptor blockers produce hemodynamic effects similar to ACE inhibitors while avoiding dry cough. These agents are similar to the ACE inhibitors in potency and are useful for initial therapy.

Calcium channel blocking agents are effective as initial therapy in both African-American and Caucasian patients, and are well-tolerated by the elderly. These agents inhibit entry of calcium ion into cardiac cells and smooth muscle cells of the coronary and systemic vasculature. Nifedipine (Procardia®) and amlodipine (Norvasc®) are more potent as peripheral vasodilators than diltiazem (Cardizem®).

Supplemental antihypertensive agents include the centrally-acting alpha$_2$ agonists and direct-acting vasodilators. These agents are less commonly prescribed for initial therapy because of the impressive effectiveness of the other drug groups. Clonidine (Catapres®) lowers blood pressure by activating inhibitory alpha$_2$ receptors in the CNS, thus reducing sympathetic outflow. It lowers both supine and standing blood pressure by reducing total peripheral resistance.

The most common oral side effects of the management of the hypertensive patient are related to the antihypertensive drug therapy. A dry, sore mouth can be caused by diuretics and centrally-acting adrenergic inhibitors. Occasionally, lichenoid reactions can occur in patients taking methyldopa. The thiazides are occasionally also implicated. Lupus-like face rashes can be seen in patients taking calcium channel blockers as well.

REFERENCES

Hunt SA, Abraham WT, Chin MH, et al, "2009 Focused Update Incorporated into the ACC/AHA 2005 Guidelines for the Diagnosis and Management of Heart Failure in Adults: A Report of the American College of Cardiology Foundation/American Heart Association Task Force on Practice Guidelines Developed in Collaboration With the International Society for Heart and Lung Transplantation," *J Am Coll Cardiol*, 2009, 53(15):e1-e90.
Lindenfeld J, Albert NM, Boehmer JP, et al, "HFSA 2010 Comprehensive Heart Failure Practice Guideline," *J Card Fail*, 2010, 16(6):e1-194.
Pickering TG, Hall JE, Appel LJ, et al, "Recommendations for Blood Pressure Measurement in Humans and Experimental Animals: Part 1: Blood Pressure Measurement in Humans: A Statement for Professionals From the Subcommittee of Professional and Public Education of the American Heart Association Council on High Blood Pressure Research," *Circulation*, 2005, 111(5):697-716.

CARDIOVASCULAR DISEASE IN WOMEN

American Heart Association Guidelines for Reducing Cardiovascular Risk in Women

Most cardiovascular disease (CVD) in women is preventable, according to the American Heart Association (AHA). In 1999, the AHA published a set of guidelines based on a 1997 review of the literature that described risk factor management and occurrence of CVD in women. The American College of Cardiology has a new guideline for the prevention of cardiovascular disease in women (Mosca, 2011).

Cardiovascular disease is the largest single cause of death among women worldwide and accounts for one-third of all deaths. New reports have shown that in the United States, more women than men die every year of CVD.

In general the women who are at risk of CVD are those that have more than one major risk factor for CVD including:

- Cigarette smoking
- Poor diet
- Physical inactivity
- Obesity
- Family history of CVD at <55 years of age in male relative and <65 years of age in female relative
- Hypertension
- Dyslipidemia
- Evidence of subclinical vascular disease (eg, coronary calcification)
- Metabolic syndrome

- Poor exercise capacity on treadmill test
- Abnormal heart rate recovery after stopping exercise

Specific Recommendations

Aspirin:

Aspirin use in high risk women

As a preventive drug intervention in women, aspirin therapy at a dose of 75-162 mg/day should be used in high risk women unless contraindicated. High risk women were defined as those with established coronary artery disease, cerebrovascular disease, or peripheral artery disease.

Aspirin use for other at risk or healthy women

In women ≥65 years of age, consider aspirin therapy 81 mg/day if blood pressure is controlled and benefit for ischemic stroke and myocardial infarction (MI) prevention is likely to outweigh the risk of gastrointestinal bleeding and hemorrhagic stroke. However, the new guidelines suggested that the routine use of aspirin in healthy women <65 years of age is not recommended to prevent MI. It was noted in these new guidelines that previous guidelines by the AHA did not recommend aspirin at all in lower risk or healthy women.

Smoking Cessation: The guidelines suggest smokers try behavioral modification programs, counseling, nicotine replacement therapy, or prescription smoking cessation medications such as bupropion (Zyban®). Also, women should avoid environmental tobacco smoke.

Exercise: Women should accumulate a minimum of 30 minutes of moderate-intensity physical activity on most, and preferably all, days of the week.

Obesity and Exercise: Women who need to lose weight or sustain weight loss should accumulate a minimum of 60-90 minutes of moderate-intensity physical activity, such as brisk walking, on most days of the week.

Dietary Intake: Consume a diet rich in fruits and vegetables. Choose whole grain, high fiber foods. Consume fish, especially oily fish such as mackerel or salmon, at least twice a week. Limit intake of dietary saturated fat to <10% of caloric intake, cholesterol intake to <300 mg/day, sodium intake to no more than 1 teaspoonful daily, and consumption of trans-fatty acids to <1% of caloric intake.

Alcohol Consumption: Limit to no more than one drink per day. A drink is equivalent to a 12 ounce bottle of beer, a 5 ounce glass of wine, or a 1.5 ounce shot of 80 proof spirit. It does not matter what form of alcohol is consumed. In contrast to the recommendations by the AHA for moderate alcohol intake as part of the updated guidelines for heart disease prevention in women, a recent report showed that alcohol consumption increases the risk of breast cancer. One to two drinks per day increased the risk of breast cancer by 10% and excessive drinking defined as three or more drinks per day increased the risk by 30%. The researchers examined data from 70,033 women who gave health information during medical examinations during 1978-1985. In 2004, follow ups indicated that 2829 of the women in the study were diagnosed with breast cancer. The study examined alcohol preferences, frequency of drinking one type of alcohol, and overall alcohol consumption. High consumption of any alcohol was linked with a significant increased risk of being diagnosed with breast cancer.

Omega-3 Fatty Acids: As an adjunct to diet, omega-3 fatty acids in capsule form (approximately 850-1000 mg of EPA [eicosapentaenoic acid] and DHA [docosahexaenoic acid]) should be considered in those with coronary heart disease and for treatment of women with high triglyceride levels.

In addition, the new guidelines suggested that the following interventions were not useful and may be harmful for CVD or MI in women.

Menopausal Therapy: Hormone replacement therapy, such as Premarin® and Prempro™, and selective estrogen-receptor modulators (SERMs), such as raloxifene (Evista®), should not be used for the primary prevention or secondary prevention of CVD.

Antioxidant Supplements: Antioxidant vitamin supplements such as vitamin E, C, or beta-carotene should not be used for the primary or secondary prevention of CVD.

Folic Acid: Folic acid, with or without vitamin B_6 and B_{12} supplementation, should not be used for the primary or secondary prevention of CVD.

REFERENCES

Mosca L, Benjamin EJ, Berra K, et al, "Effectiveness-Based Guidelines for the Prevention of Cardiovascular Disease in Women-2011 Update: A Guideline From the American Heart Association," *J Am Coll Cardiol*, 2011, 57(12):1404-23. Available at http://content.onlinejacc.org/cgi/reprint-framed/57/12/1404

Mosca L, Linfante AH, Benjamin EJ, et al, "National Study of Physician Awareness and Adherence to Cardiovascular Disease Prevention Guidelines," *Circulation*, 2005, 111(4):499-510.

ANTIPLATELET AND ANTICOAGULATION CONSIDERATIONS IN DENTISTRY

Over the last 30 years, there has been an increasing use of drugs that relate to the clotting mechanisms in patients. These drugs have included the widespread use of aspirin, as well as an increasing use of anticoagulants found in warfarin and synthetic drugs that also have anticoagulation effects. Many patients with ischemic heart disease, atherosclerosis, atrial fibrillation, and in patients at high risk for stroke, we find the increased use of these anticoagulants. Large numbers of these patients are receiving oral anticoagulation therapy as outpatients. The dental clinician is often faced with the decision as to how to manage these patients prior to dental procedures. Key factors regarding the patient receiving any form of anticoagulation therapy include:

- Is the surgery urgent or elective?
- Can the procedure be done safely without discontinuing the drug?
- Does the patient understand the nature of the dental procedure and the risks associated with continuing or discontinuing the drug?
- What degree of risk are the patient and the provider willing to accept?
- Is the patient on a single antiplatelet drug or on combination therapy with another drug?
- What is the thromboembolic risk for this patient?
- What is the bleeding risk of the dental procedure planned?
- If an invasive procedure is planned in the face of a high thromboembolic risk, what is the managing physician's opinion on altering the dosage of anticoagulation therapy?

Often, in order to determine these factors, consultation with a patient's physician is necessary. However, recent reviews have argued that inappropriate adjustments in anticoagulation therapy create far greater risk for the patient than the risk of hemorrhage during most dental procedures (Jeske, 2003 and others in the reference list). Therefore, the scientific evidence does not support changing regimens of anticoagulation therapy in most instances. This decision can only be determined by weighing the factors described above and discussing the situation with the patient's physician.

Antiplatelet Drugs Used in Cardiovascular Diseases

Aspirin reduces platelet aggregation by blocking platelet cyclo-oxygenase through irreversible acetylation. This action prevents the formation of thromboxane A_2. A number of studies have confirmed that aspirin reduces the risk of death from cardiac causes and fatal and nonfatal myocardial infarction by ~50% to 70% in patients presenting with unstable angina (see Aspirin Alert Update for Dentistry at the end of this chapter).

Clopidogrel inhibits platelet aggregation by affecting the ADP-dependent activation of the glycoprotein IIb/IIIa complex. Clopidogrel is chemically related to ticlopidine but has fewer side effects.

Prasugrel is a prodrug and has no biological activity but is metabolized in the body to an active molecule exhibiting antiplatelet action. The active compound irreversibly blocks P2Y12 component of adenosine diphosphate (ADP) receptors on the platelet for their lifespan, inhibiting activation and decreasing subsequent platelet aggregation. Normal platelet aggregation returns only when new platelets are produced (5-9 days after discontinuation of prasugrel).

Platelet Glycoprotein IIb / IIIa Receptor Antagonists

Antagonists of glycoprotein IIb/IIIa, a receptor on the platelet for adhesive proteins, inhibit the final common pathway involved in adhesion, activation, and aggregation. Presently, there exist three classes of inhibitors. One class is murine-human chimeric antibodies of which abciximab is the prototype. The other two classes are the synthetic peptide forms (eg, eptifibatide) and the synthetic nonpeptide forms (eg, tirofiban). These agents, in combination with heparin and aspirin, have been used to treat unstable angina, significantly reducing the incidence of death or myocardial infarction.

Antithrombin Drugs

Unfractionated heparin, in combination with aspirin, is used to treat unstable angina. Unfractionated heparin consists of polysaccharide chains which bind to antithrombin III, causing a conformational change that accelerates the inhibition of thrombin and factor Xa. Unfractionated heparin is therefore an indirect thrombin inhibitor. Unfractionated heparin can only be administered intravenously. Low-molecular-weight heparins (LMWH) have a more predictable pharmacokinetic profile than unfractionated heparin and can be administered subcutaneously. These heparins have a mechanism of action and use similar to unfractionated heparin.

The direct antithrombins decrease thrombin activity in a manner independent of any actions on antithrombin III. Two such direct antithrombins are lepirudin (also known as recombinant hirudin) and argatroban. These agents are highly specific. They bind directly to thrombin (circulating and clot bound) and inhibit thrombogenic activity. Direct antithrombins are used for the prevention or reduction of ischemic complications associated with unstable angina.

Warfarin (Coumadin®) elicits its anticoagulant effect by interfering with the hepatic synthesis of vitamin K-dependent coagulation factors II, VII, IX, and X. Although warfarin appears to be somewhat effective after myocardial infarction in preventing death or recurrent myocardial infarction, its effectiveness in the treatment of acute coronary syndrome is questionable. Combination therapy with aspirin and heparin, followed by warfarin, has resulted in reduced incidence of recurrent angina, myocardial infarction, death, or all three at 14 days as compared with aspirin alone. In contrast, another study failed to show any additional benefit in the treatment of acute coronary syndrome using a combination of aspirin and warfarin compared to aspirin alone.

Recently, the FDA approved Dabigatran (Pradaxa®) for the prevention of stroke and systemic embolism in patients with atrial fibrillation. Dabigatran is the first FDA-approved replacement available for warfarin. Dabigatran is an anticoagulant that acts by inhibiting thrombin, an enzyme in the blood that is involved in blood clotting. Thrombin (serine protease) enables the conversion of fibrinogen to fibrin during the coagulation cascade preventing the development of thrombus. The recommended oral dose is 150 mg twice daily for patients with a creatinine clearance >30 mL/minute. For patients with a creatinine clearance 15-30 mL/minute, the recommended oral dose is 75 mg twice daily.

It is quite common for a patient to be taking both warfarin and low-molecular-weight heparins, such as Dalteparin (Fragmin®) or Enoxaparin (Lovenox®). Low-molecular-weight heparins begin working right away, while warfarin does not. In fact, in the short period of time when a patient first begins taking warfarin, the drug may actually increase the risk of clots. Therefore, warfarin and low-molecular-weight heparins are often taken together. The low-molecular-weight heparins prevent clots while the warfarin begins working. The low-molecular-weight heparins can be stopped once the INR is in the appropriate range.

A similar situation sometimes occurs in patients who have been taking warfarin for awhile. If a PT/INR test shows that the patient is at a high risk for clots, a healthcare provider may recommend using low-molecular-weight heparins as a "bridge therapy" while the warfarin dose is being adjusted. The aPTT is the appropriate test to evaluate the effects of heparin. Bridging guidelines and their application in dental surgery must be discussed with the healthcare provider on a case-by-case basis.

Dental clinicians should consider consultation with patient's healthcare provider prior to invasive therapies. However, recent reviews have argued that inappropriate adjustments in anticoagulation therapy places the patient at far greater risk of stroke than hemorrhage during most dental procedures (Douketis, 2012; Jeske, 2003). Therefore, scientific evidence does not support changing regimens of anticoagulation therapy in most instances.

Evaluating Antiplatelet Response

Partial thromboplastin time and bleeding time (IVY) are appropriate measures for platelet dysfunction. Aspirin, Clopidogrel (Plavix®), Prasugrel (Effient®), and other drugs, such as ticlopidine (Ticlid®) are considered antiplatelet drugs, whereas oral Coumadin® is considered an oral anticoagulant. Aspirin works by inhibiting cyclo-oxygenase which is an enzyme involved in the platelet system associated with clot formation. As little as one aspirin (300 mg dose) can result in an alteration in this enzyme pathway. Although aspirin is cleared from the circulation very quickly (within 15-30 minutes), the effect on the life of the platelet may last up to 7-10 days. Most routine dental procedures can be accomplished with no change in these medications using aggressive local hemostasis efforts and prudent treatment planning.

Evaluating Coumadin® Response

The effects of Coumadin® on the coagulation within patients occur by way of the vitamin K-dependent clotting mechanism and are generally monitored by measuring the prothrombin time known as the PT. Often, to prevent venous thrombosis, a patient will be maintained at approximately 2.5 times their normal prothrombin time. Other anticoagulant goals, such as prevention of arterial thromboembolism as in patients with artificial heart valves, may require 2.5-3.5 times the normal prothrombin time. It is important for the clinician to obtain the International Normalized Ratio (INR) for the patient. This ratio is calculated by dividing the patient's PT by the mean normal PT for the laboratory, which is determined by using the International Sensitivity Index (ISI) to adjust for the lab's reagents.

The response to oral anticoagulants varies greatly in patients and should be monitored regularly. The dental clinician planning an invasive procedure should consider not only what the patient can tell them from a historical point-of-view, but also when the last monitoring test was performed. In general, all dental procedures can be performed in patients that are 3 times normal or less. Most researchers further suggest that even less than 4 times normal pose little risk in most dental patients and procedures, but these values may be misleading unless the INR is also determined at a time close to the actual planned dental procedure. When in doubt, the prudent dental clinician will consult with the patient's physician and obtain current prothrombin time and INR in order to evaluate fully and plan for his patients.

At recommended therapeutic doses, dabigatran (Pradaxa™) prolongs the activated partial thromboplastin time (aPTT). For an oral dose of 150 mg twice daily, the median peak aPTT is approximately twice that of control values. Twelve hours after the last dose, the median aPTT is 1.5 times the control values. The INR test is relatively insensitive to the activity of dabigatran and may not be elevated in patients on this medication.

Regarding dental management patients that are already taking warfarin, the use of analgesics is implicated as a potential source of drug interaction. Hayek, in *JAMA*, found that patients taking warfarin had dangerously elevated INRs and were taking acetaminophen (not necessarily with their physician's recommendation). Additional factors independently influence the INR, as well as a potential interaction with acetaminophen. Effects on the INR are greatest in patients taking acetaminophen at high doses over a protracted time period. Short-term pain management with acetaminophen poses little risk. Other factors influencing INR include advanced malignancy, patients who did not take their warfarin properly (therefore, took more than was necessary), changes in oral intake of liquids or solids, acute diarrhea leading to dehydration, alcohol consumption, and vitamin K intake.

The mechanisms of these augmenting factors for enhancement of the INR are that the cytochrome P450 system is also affected by changes in metabolism associated with these factors. For instance, the metabolism of alcohol in the liver alters its ability to manage the CYP450 enzyme system necessary for warfarin; therefore, enhancing its presence and potentially increasing the half-life of warfarin. As oral intake of nutrients declines in patients with either diarrhea or reduced intake of liquids and/or solids, absorption of vitamin K is reduced and the vitamin K-dependent system of metabolism of warfarin changes, therefore increases warfarin blood levels. These factors, along with the liver metabolism of acetaminophen, have resulted in the increased concern that patients, who may be taking acetaminophen as an analgesic or for other reasons, may be at risk for enhancing or elevating, inadvertently, their anticoagulation effect of warfarin. The dentist should be aware of these potential interactions in prescribing any drug containing acetaminophen or in recommending that a patient use an analgesic for relief of even mild pain on a prolonged basis.

Acetaminophen on page 27

It should also be noted that as we learn more about herbal and nutritional supplements, we will find that some of these products have affects on coagulation. Patients sometimes do not include this information in their normal history and it is important for the practitioner to delve into all types of over-the-counter, as well as prescription drugs, that the patient may be taking.

Although not used specifically for this purpose, numerous herbal medicines and natural dietary supplements have been associated with inhibition of platelet aggregation or other anticoagulation effects, and therefore may lead to increased bleeding during invasive dental procedures. Current reports include bilberry, bromelain, cat's claw, devil's claw, dong quai, evening primrose, feverfew, garlic (irreversible inhibition), ginger (only at very high doses), ginkgo biloba, ginseng, grape seed, green tea, horse chestnut, and turmeric.

ASPIRIN ALERT UPDATE FOR DENTISTRY

There are three special alerts provided by the FDA of clinical importance relative to the aspirin patient:

Special Alert 1: Sudden aspirin discontinuation may elevate the risk of myocardial infarction

It was reported in 2004 by Collett et al, that patients with acute coronary syndrome (ACS) who discontinued aspirin use had worse short-term outcomes than individuals not previously on aspirin therapy. Fischer et al, have also reported similar findings and have suggested that discontinuation of aspirin by daily aspirin users may increase the risk of myocardial infarction. A Harvard Health Letter in 2005 also stated that quitting aspirin "cold turkey" could be dangerous and studies have linked aspirin withdrawal to heart attacks.

A more recent review updated the risks associated with discontinuing aspirin antiplatelet therapy and the bleeding risks associated with continuing aspirin during surgical procedures (Lordkipanidze, 2009). The article review confirmed the possibility of a pharmacological rebound phenomenon which could lead to adverse ischemic events and supports the warning against premature discontinuation of aspirin issued previously. An analysis of data obtained from 50,279 patients, reported that the increased risk of major adverse cardiac events attributed to aspirin withdrawal/nonadherence was approximately threefold (Biondi-Zoccai, 2006).

Special Alert 2: Ibuprofen may interfere with aspirin's cardioprotection

In a statement released on September 8, 2006, the Food and Drug Administration (FDA) notified consumers and healthcare professionals that the administration of ibuprofen for pain relief to patients taking aspirin for cardioprotection may interfere with aspirin's cardiovascular benefits. The report stated that ibuprofen can interfere with the antiplatelet effect of low-dose aspirin (81 mg daily). This could result in diminished effectiveness of aspirin as used for cardioprotection and stroke prevention. The FDA added that although ibuprofen and aspirin can be taken together, it is recommended that consumers talk with their healthcare providers for additional information.

Special Alert 3: Strong advisory warning against the discontinuation of dual aspirin and clopidogrel (Plavix®) antiplatelet therapy in patients with coronary artery stents

Aspirin and clopidogrel (Plavix®) in combination is the primary prevention strategy against stent thrombosis after placement of drug-eluting metal stents in coronary patients (Grines, 2007). Premature discontinuation of this drug combination strongly increases the risk of a catastrophic event of stent thrombosis leading to myocardial infarction and/or death (Grines, 2007). The AHA stresses a 12-month therapy of aspirin and Plavix® combination after placement of a drug-eluting stent in order to prevent thrombosis at the stent site. The AHA also stresses educating both the patient and the healthcare provider about the hazards of premature antiplatelet drug discontinuation. Any elective surgery should be postponed for 1 year after stent implantation, and if surgery must be performed, consideration should be given to continuing the antiplatelet therapy during the perioperative period in high risk patients with drug-eluting stents.

The recommendations from the AHA advisory panel were summarized for the dental professional according to the following:

Dental professionals and other healthcare providers who perform invasive or surgical procedures and are concerned about periprocedural and postoperative bleeding must be made aware of the potential catastrophic risks of premature discontinuation of dual antiplatelet (aspirin and Plavix®) therapy. The dental professional should contact the patient's cardiologist if issues regarding the patient's antiplatelet therapy are unclear, in order to discuss optimal patient management strategy.

Elective procedures for which there is significant risk of perioperative or postoperative bleeding should be deferred until patients have completed an appropriate course of dual antiplatelet therapy. The course of this therapy is suggested as 12 months after drug-eluting stent implantation if patient is not at high risk of bleeding.

◀ **Agents Useful to Aid in Hemostasis During or Prior to Perioperative Bleeding**

Hemostatic agents inhibit the activation of plasminogen to plasmin, producing antifibrinolytic activity. These agents have been used systemically and locally for treatment and prevention of various bleeding disorders. The oral mucosa tissues are rich in plasminogen activators, making hemostatic agents potentially effective for controlling oral bleeding. Although many hemostatic agents are available, only tranexamic acid and epsilon aminocaproic acid can be prepared and used as mouthwashes. Tranexamic acid is available as an intravenous injection (100 mg/mL). Aminocaproic acid is available as a 500 mg tablet, an injectable solution (250 mg/mL), and a raspberry-flavored oral syrup (250 mg/mL). A potentially critical difference between these drugs is that tranexamic acid is 6-10 times more potent that aminocaproic acid, as show in both *in vitro* and *in vivo* assays. Neither agent is commercially available as a mouthwash. The EACA oral syrup is most readily usable as a mouthwash; however, due to cost the tablet is usually compounded to form a mouthwash. In addition, the solution for injection may be diluted with sterile water and used as a mouthwash. To ensure stability and sterility, this is commonly prepared the day of surgery. The adverse effects of these agents are dose dependent and generally manifest as nausea, vomiting, abdominal pain, and diarrhea. Theoretically, adverse effects are more likely to occur with systemic use than with local use.

Oral Anticoagulant Comparison Chart

Medication	Mechanism of Action	Metabolism	Monitoring Parameters	Pharmacotherapy Pearls	Reversal Strategies[1]	Preoperative/Preprocedure Management (General Guide)
Warfarin	Inhibits formation of vitamin K-dependent clotting factors II, VII, IX, X, and proteins C and S	• CYP2C9 • CYP1A2 • CYP3A4 • CYP2C19	• PT/INR (individualized; depends on INR stability)	• CYP1A2, 3A4, 2C9, and 2C19 drug interactions and vitamin K-containing food interactions • Full therapeutic effect usually seen within 5-7 days • Half-life is ~40 hours	• Vitamin K (route and dose will depend on clinical situation and INR) • For major bleeding (at any INR): Consider PCC with vitamin K ± FFP	• Hold at least 5 days before surgery, depending on urgency of surgery/procedure; may administer low-dose I.V. or oral vitamin K
Dabigatran (Pradaxa®)	Directly inhibits thrombin	• Hepatic glucuronidation • P-gp substrate	• Routine lab monitoring not required; aPTT, ECT (if available), TT (most sensitive) may be used to detect presence of dabigatran • Renal function	• Compliance issues (BID dosing) • Specific conversions to/from warfarin, parenteral anticoagulants • Renal dosing adjustment required; per ACCP, contraindicated with Cl$_{Cr}$ ≤30 mL/minute • Use with caution in patients ≥80 years of age • Dose reduction or avoidance required if used with dronedarone, ketoconazole, P-gp inhibitors • P-gp drug interactions • Half-life is 12-17 hours; considerably prolonged with severe renal impairment	• No specific antidote; for major bleeding, may consider activated PCC (ie, FEIBA NF), recombinant factor VIIa[2], or concentrates of factors II, IX, or X[3] • Use of 4-factor PCC is **not** effective • Dabigatran is ~60% dialyzable • Activated charcoal may be used if ingestion occurred <2 hours prior to presentation	• Cl$_{Cr}$ ≥50 mL/minute: Hold 1-2 days before surgery • Cl$_{Cr}$ <50 mL/minute: Hold 3-5 days before surgery • May consider holding for >5 days in patients undergoing major surgery, spinal puncture, or insertion of a spinal or epidural catheter or port
Rivaroxaban (Xarelto®)	Directly inhibits factor Xa	• CYP3A4 • CYP3A5 • CYP2J2 • P-gp substrate	• Routine lab monitoring not required; may use PT to detect presence of rivaroxaban • Renal and hepatic function	• Administer doses ≥15 mg/day with food • Dosing frequency depends on indication • Specific conversions to/from warfarin, parenteral anticoagulants • Renal dosing adjustment required • Avoid in moderate or severe hepatic impairment • CYP3A4 and P-gp drug interactions • Half-life is 5-9 hours; slightly prolonged with renal impairment	• No specific antidote; for major bleeding, may consider PCC, activated PCC (ie, FEIBA NF), or recombinant factor VIIa[2] • Rivaroxaban is **not** dialyzable	• Hold at least 24 hours before surgery; longer duration of treatment cessation may be necessary based on individual patient situation and physician clinical judgment
Apixaban (Eliquis®)	Directly inhibits factor Xa	• CYP3A4 • P-gp substrate	• Routine lab monitoring not required; PT, INR, and aPTT may be used to detect presence of apixaban	• Compliance issues (BID dosing) • Specific conversions to/from warfarin, parenteral anticoagulants • Renal dosing adjustment required; the AHA/ASA recommends to avoid use with Cl$_{Cr}$ <25 mL/minute • Not recommended in patients with severe liver impairment • CYP3A4 and P-gp drug interactions • Half-life is ~8-15 hours; slightly prolonged with renal impairment	• No specific antidote; for major bleeding, may consider PCC, activated PCC (ie, FEIBA NF), or recombinant factor VIIa[2] • Apixaban is **not** dialyzable • Activated charcoal may be used if ingestion occurred within 2-6 hours of presentation	• Hold at least 24-48 hours, depending on risk or location of bleeding, before elective surgery or invasive procedures.

Abbreviations: ACCP = American College of Chest Physicians, AHA/ASA = American Heart Association/American Stroke Association, aPTT = activated partial thromboplastin time, BID = twice daily, ECT = ecarin clotting time, FFP = fresh frozen plasma, INR = international normalized ratio, PCC = prothrombin complex concentrate, P-gp = P-glycoprotein, PT = prothrombin time, TT = thrombin time

Note: Recommendations listed reflect only the U.S. labeling or U.S. clinical practice guidelines.

[1]Management of anticoagulant-associated bleeding requires careful consideration of the indication for anticoagulant therapy and bleeding extent (eg, epistaxis vs intracranial hemorrhage); minor bleeding may only require local hemostasis.

[2]The use of rFVIIa in healthy subjects treated with another direct thrombin inhibitor, melagatran (not FDA-approved), did not reverse the anticoagulant effects of melagatran.

[3]The evidence in support of these reversal strategies is limited; an exception to this may be the use of 4-factor PCC for rivaroxaban reversal; however, only 3-factor PCCs are available in the U.S. (Bebulin® VH and Profilnine® SD).

Furie KL, Goldstein LB, Albers GW, et al, "Oral Antithrombotic Agents for the Prevention of Stroke in Nonvalvular Atrial Fibrillation: A Science Advisory for Healthcare Professionals From the American Heart Association/American Stroke Association," *Stroke*, 2012, 43(12):3442-53.
Guyatt GH, Akl EA, Crowther M, et al, "Executive Summary: Antithrombotic Therapy and Prevention of Thrombosis, 9th ed: American College of Chest Physicians Evidence-Based Clinical Practice Guidelines," *Chest*, 2012, 141(2 Suppl):7S-47S.
Kaatz S, Kouides PA, Garcia DA, et al, "Guidance on the Emergent Reversal of Oral Thrombin and Factor Xa Inhibitors," *Am J Hematol*, 2012, 87(Suppl 1):S141-5.
Levi M, Eerenberg E, and Kamphuisen PW, "Bleeding Risk and Reversal Strategies for Old and New Anticoagulants and Antiplatelet Agents," *J Thromb Haemost*, 2011, 9(9):1705-12.
Poulsen BK, Grove EL, and Husted SE, "New Oral Anticoagulants: A Review of the Literature With Particular Emphasis on Patients With Impaired Renal Function," *Drugs*, 2012, 72(13):1739-53.
Wolzt M, Levi M, Sarich TC, et al, "Effect of Recombinant Factor VIIa on Melagatran-Induced Inhibition of Thrombin Generation and Platelet Activation in Healthy Volunteers," *Thromb Haemost*, 2004, 91 (6):1090-6.

Oral Antiplatelet Comparison Chart

Medication	Mechanism of Action	Reversible Platelet Inhibition	Prodrug	Metabolism	Pharmacotherapy Pearls	Reversal Strategies[1]	Preoperative/Preprocedure Management (General Guide)
Aspirin	Inhibits cyclooxygenase-1 and 2	No	No	• CYP2C9	• Chronic NSAID use can compromise antiplatelet effects • Monitor for GI ulceration	• No specific antidote • Consider platelet transfusion ± DDAVP • Normal platelet function returns within 7-10 days after discontinuation	• Hold 7-10 days before surgery • May be continued through surgery for CABG or noncardiac surgery in patients with high cardiac risk
Cilostazol (Pletal®)	Inhibits platelet phosphodiesterase III	Yes	No	• CYP3A4 • CYP2C19 • CYP1A2 • CYP2D6	• Administer before or 2 hours after meals • Contraindicated in patients with heart failure of any severity • CYP3A4 and 2C19 drug interactions	• No specific antidote • Normal platelet function returns within 4 days after discontinuation	• Hold 2-3 days before surgery
Clopidogrel (Plavix®)	Inhibits P2Y$_{12}$ component of ADP receptors	No	Yes	• CYP2C19 • CYP3A4	• CYP2C19 inhibitors may reduce concentrations of active metabolite • CYP2C19 polymorphisms may affect clopidogrel efficacy	• No specific antidote • Consider platelet transfusion ± DDAVP • Normal platelet function returns within 7-10 days after discontinuation	• Hold 5-10 days before surgery[2]
Ticlopidine	Inhibits P2Y$_{12}$ component of ADP receptors	No	Yes	• CYP3A4	• Black Box warning on hematologic toxicities (aplastic anemia, TTP) • Frequent CBC monitoring required • BID dosing	• No specific antidote • Consider platelet transfusion ± DDAVP • Normal platelet function returns within 5-10 days after discontinuation	• Hold 10-14 days before surgery
Prasugrel (Effient®)	Inhibits P2Y$_{12}$ component of ADP receptors	No	Yes	• CYP3A4 • CYP2B6	• Reduce maintenance dose to 5 mg in patients <60 kg • Contraindicated in patients with history of stroke, TIA • Not recommended in patients ≥75 years of age	• No specific antidote • Consider platelet transfusion ± DDAVP • Normal platelet function returns within 5-9 days after discontinuation	• Hold 5-7 days before surgery[2]
Ticagrelor (Brilinta™)	Inhibits P2Y$_{12}$ component of ADP receptors	Yes	No	• CYP3A4 • CYP3A5	• Used in combination with aspirin; daily maintenance aspirin dose should not exceed 81 mg • CYP3A4 drug interactions • BID dosing • Monitor closely for dyspnea, bradyarrhythmia (including ventricular pauses)	• No specific antidote • Consider aminocaproic acid, tranexamic acid, recombinant factor VIIa • Normal platelet function returns within 3-5 days after discontinuation	• Hold at least 5 days before surgery[2]

[1]Management of antiplatelet-associated bleeding requires careful consideration of the indication for antiplatelet therapy and bleeding extent (eg, epistaxis vs intracranial hemorrhage); minor bleeding may only require local hemostasis.

[2]When urgent CABG is necessary, the ACCF/AHA CABG guidelines recommend discontinuation for at least 24 hours prior to surgery (Hillis, 2011).

Hillis LD, Smith PK, Anderson JL, et al. "2011 ACCF/AHA Guideline for Coronary Artery Bypass Graft Surgery: Executive Summary: A Report of the American College of Cardiology Foundation/American Heart Association Task Force on Practice Guidelines," *Circulation*, 2011, 124(23):2610-42.

Levi M, Eerenberg E, and Kamphuisen PW, "Bleeding Risk and Reversal Strategies for Old and New Anticoagulants and Antiplatelet Agents," *J Thromb Haemost*, 2011, 9(9):1705-12.

Patrono C, Andreotti F, Arnesen H, et al, "Antiplatelet Agents for the Treatment and Prevention of Atherothrombosis," *Eur Heart J*, 2011, 32(23):2922-32.

REFERENCES

"Aspirin: Quitting Cold Turkey Could Be Dangerous. Studies Have Linked Aspirin Withdrawal to Heart Attacks," *Harv Health Lett*, 2005, 30(12):6.

Biondi-Zoccai GG, Lotrionte M, Agostoni P, et al, "A Systematic Review and Meta-Analysis on the Hazards of Discontinuing or Not Adhering to Aspirin Among 50,279 Patients at Risk for Coronary Artery Disease," *Eur Heart J*, 2006, 27(22):2667-74.

Brennan MT, Wynn RL, and Miller CS, "Aspirin and Bleeding in Dentistry: An Update and Recommendations," *Oral Surg Oral Med Oral Pathol Oral Radiol Endod*, 2007, 104(3):316-23.

Connolly SJ, Ezekowitz MD, Yusuf S, et al, "Dabigatran Versus Warfarin in Patients With Atrial Fibrillation," *N Engl J Med*, 2009, 361(12):1139-51.

Douketis JD, Spyropoulos AC, Spencer FA, et al, "Perioperative Management of Antithrombotic Therapy: Antithrombotic Therapy and Prevention of Thrombosis, 9th ed: American College of Chest Physicians Evidence-Based Clinical Practice Guidelines," *Chest*, 2012, 141(2 Suppl):e326S-50S.

du Breuil AL and Umland EM, "Outpatient Management of Anticoagulation Therapy," *Am Fam Physician*, 2007, 75(7):1031-42.

Eisenberg MJ, Richard PR, Libersan D, et al, "Safety of Short-Term Discontinuation of Antiplatelet Therapy in Patients With Drug-Eluting Stents," *Circulation*, 2009, 119(12):1634-42.

FDA, "Ibuprofen and Aspirin Taken Together." Available at http://www.fda.gov/Safety/MedWatch/SafetyInformation/SafetyAlertsforHumanMedical-Products/ucm150611.htm

Jeske AH, Suchko GD, ADA Council on Scientific Affairs and Division of Science, et al, "Lack of a Scientific Basis for Routine Discontinuation of Oral Anticoagulation Therapy Before Dental Treatment," *J Am Dent Assoc*, 2003, 134(11):1492-7.

Lockhart PB, Gibson J, Pond SH, et al, "Dental Management Considerations for the Patient With an Acquired Coagulopathy. Part 2: Coagulopathies From Drugs," *Br Dent J*, 2003, 195(9):495-501.

Lordkipanidzé M, Diodati JG, and Pharand C, "Possibility of a Rebound Phenomenon Following Antiplatelet Therapy Withdrawal: A Look at the Clinical and Pharmacological Evidence," *Pharmacol Ther*, 2009, 123(2):178-86.

"Managing Anticoagulation in the Perioperative Period: ACCP Guidelines," 9th ed, 2012.

CLINICAL RISK RELATED TO DRUGS PROLONGING QT INTERVAL

The QT interval is measured as the time and distance between the Q point of the QRS complex and the end of the T wave in the ECG tracing. After adjustment for heart rate, the QT interval is defined as prolonged if it is more than 450 msec in men and 460 msec in women. A long QT syndrome was first described in the 1950s and 60s as a congenital syndrome involving QT interval prolongation, syncope, and sudden death. Some of the congenital long QT syndromes were characterized by a peculiar electrocardiographic appearance of the QRS complex involving a premature atria beat, followed by a pause, then a subsequent sinus beat showing marked QT prolongation and deformity. This type of cardiac arrhythmia was originally termed "torsade de pointes" (translated from the French as "twisting of the points").

Prolongation of the QT interval is thought to result from delayed ventricular repolarization. The repolarization process within the myocardial cell is due to the efflux of intracellular potassium. The channels associated with this current can be blocked by many drugs and predispose the electrical propagation cycle to torsade de pointes.

Erythromycin, a drug often associated as a dental antibiotic, is considered to have a risk of causing torsade de pointes. Drug-induced torsade de pointes, a specific type of ventricular arrhythmia associated with prolongation of the QT interval, is a well understood form of drug toxicity. The evidence for risk of this event varies among the many drugs associated with torsade de pointes and with the patients' characteristics. The risk of drug-induced torsade de pointes is extremely low when a single QT interval prolonging drug is prescribed. It is not known what effect vasoconstrictors in the local anesthetic regimen will have in patients with a known history of congenital prolonged QT interval or in patients taking any medication that prolongs the QT interval. Until more information is obtained, it is suggested that the clinician consult with the physician prior to the use of a vasoconstrictor in suspected patients, and that the vasoconstrictor (epinephrine, levonordefrin [Neo-Cobefrin®]) be used with caution. Other drugs commonly used in oral diseases that have been associated with significant QT interval changes include fluconazole, azithromycin, and levofloxacin, each having variable risk. This past May (2012), the FDA notified healthcare providers that it is aware of the study published in the *New England Journal of Medicine* (May 17) reporting a small increase in cardiovascular deaths and in the risk of death from any cause in patients treated with a 5 day course of azithromycin (Zithromax®) compared to patients treated with amoxicillin, ciprofloxacin, or no drug. The FDA is reviewing the results from this study and will communicate any new information on azithromycin and this study or the potential risk of QT interval prolongation after the agency has completed its review.

Patients taking azithromycin should not stop taking their medicine without talking to their healthcare provider. Healthcare providers should be aware of the potential for QT interval prolongation and heart arrhythmias when prescribing or administering any macrolide antibiotic.

Thioridazine is another drug confirmed to prolong the QT interval and is accepted as having a risk of causing torsade de pointes. The risk of drug-induced torsade de pointes is extremely low when a single QT interval prolonging drug is prescribed. In terms of epinephrine, it is not known what effect vasoconstrictors in the local anesthetic regimen will have in patients with a known history of congenital prolonged QT interval or in patients taking any medication that prolongs the QT interval. Until more information is obtained, it is suggested that the clinician consult with the physician prior to the use of a vasoconstrictor in suspected patients, and that the vasoconstrictor (epinephrine, levonordefrin [Neo-Cobefrin®]) be used with caution.

Drugs Generally Accepted as Having a Risk of Causing Torsade de Pointes

Generic Name	Brand Name	Use
Alfuzosin	Uroxatral®	Alpha$_1$ Blocker
Amiodarone	Cordarone®	Antiarrhythmic
Arsenic Trioxide	Trisenox®	Antileukemic agent
Artemether and Lumefantrine	Coartem®	Antimalarial Agent
Asenapine	Saphris®	Antipsychotic
Azithromycin (Systemic)	**Zithromax®**	**Antibiotic**
Bedaquiline	-	Antitubercular Agent
Chloroquine	Aralen®	Antimalarial
ChlorproMAZINE	-	Antipsychotic
Citalopram	CeleXA®	Antidepressant
Clarithromycin	**Biaxin®**	**Antibiotic**
Crizotinib	Xalkori®	Antineoplastic
Disopyramide	Norpace®	Antiarrhythmic
Dofetilide	Tikosyn®	Antiarrhythmic
Dolasetron	Anzemet®	Antiemetic
Dronedarone	Multaq®	Antiarrhythmic
Droperidol	-	Antiemetic
Erythromycin (Systemic)	**Various brand names available**	**Antibiotic**
Escitalopram	Lexapro®	Antidepressant

Drugs Generally Accepted as Having a Risk of Causing Torsade de Pointes (continued)

Generic Name	Brand Name	Use
Flecainide	Tambocor™	Antiarrhythmic
Fluconazole	**Diflucan®**	**Antifungal**
FLUoxetine	PROzac®	Antidepressant
Gemifloxacin	Factive®	Antibiotic
Granisetron	Granisol™, Sancuso®	Antiemetic
Haloperidol	Haldol®	Antipsychotic
Ibutilide	Corvert®	Antiarrhythmic
Iloperidone	Fanapt®	Antipsychotic
Lapatinib	Tykerb®	Antineoplastic
Levofloxacin (Systemic)	**Levaquin®**	**Antibiotic**
Methadone	Various brand names available	Analgesic, Opioid
Mifepristone	Korlym™, Mifeprex®	Abortifacient, Cortisol Receptor Blocker
Moxifloxacin (Systemic)	**Avelox®**	**Antibiotic**
Nilotinib	Tasigna®	Antineoplastic
Ofloxacin (Systemic)	-	Antibiotic
Ondansetron	Zofran®, Zofran® ODT, Zuplenz®	Antiemetic
Paliperidone	Invega®, Invega® Sustenna®	Antipsychotic
Pasireotide	Signifor®	Somatostatin Analog
Pazopanib	Votrient™	Antineoplastic Agent, Tyrosine Kinase Inhibitor
Pentamidine	NebuPent®	Antibiotic
Pimozide	Orap®	Antipsychotic
Procainamide	Procanbid®	Antiarrhythmic
Propafenone	Rythmol®, Rythmol® SR	Antiarrhythmic
Rilpivirine	Edurant®	Antiretroviral Agent
QUEtiapine	SEROquel®	Antipsychotic
QuiNIDine	-	Antiarrhythmic
QuiNINE	Qualaquin®	Antimalarial Agent
Ranolazine	Ranexa®	Antianginal
RisperiDONE	RisperDAL®	Antipsychotic
RomiDEPsin	Istodax®	Antineoplastic Agent, Histone Deacetylase Inhibitor
Saquinavir	Invirase®	Antiretroviral Agent
Sotalol	Betapace®	Antiarrhythmic
SUNItinib	Sutent®	Antineoplastic
Telithromycin	**Ketek®**	**Antibiotic**
Tetrabenazine	Xenazine®	Huntington's Disease
Thioridazine	-	Antipsychotic
Toremifene	Fareston®	Antineoplastic
TraZODone	Oleptro™	Antidepressant
Vandetanib	-	Medullary thyroid cancer (symptomatic or progressive)
Vemurafenib	Zelboraf™	Antineoplastic
Voriconazole	**VFEND®**	**Antifungal**
Ziprasidone	Geodon®	Antipsychotic
Zuclopenthixol	Clopixol®	Antipsychotic

Note: Dental drugs are identified by bold print. This is not a comprehensive list; additional resources should be consulted.

GASTROINTESTINAL DISORDERS

The oral cavity and related structures comprise the first part of the gastrointestinal tract. Diseases affecting the oral cavity are often reflected in GI disturbances. In addition, the oral cavity may indeed reflect diseases of the GI tract, including ulcers, polyps, and liver and gallbladder diseases. The first oral condition that may reflect or be reflected in GI disturbances is taste. Typically, complaints of taste abnormalities are presented to the dentist. The sweet, saline, sour, and bitter taste sensations all vary in quality and intensity and are affected by the olfactory system. Often, anemic conditions are reflected in changes in the tongue, also resulting in potential taste aberrations.

Gastric and duodenal ulcers represent the primary diseases that can be reflected in the oral cavity. Gastroesophageal reflux disease (GERD), also known as gastroesophageal reflux disease (GORD), gastric reflux disease, or acid reflux disease, is a chronic symptom of mucosal damage caused by stomach acid coming up from the stomach into the esophagus. GERD is caused by changes in the barrier between the stomach and the esophagus, including abnormal relaxation of the lower esophageal sphincter, which normally holds the top of the stomach closed, impaired expulsion of gastric reflux from the esophagus, or a hiatal hernia. These changes may be permanent or temporary.

Another kind of acid reflux, which can cause respiratory and laryngeal signs and symptoms, is called extraesophageal reflux disease (EERD). Unlike GERD, EERD is unlikely to produce heartburn, and is sometimes called "silent reflux." Crohn's disease and ulcerative colitis have also been associated with these conditions and should be ruled out in a differential diagnostic work-up. Chronic recurring oral ulcerations are sometimes associated with Crohn's disease and this association should be considered in patients with a history of both conditions.

Gastric reflux and problems with food metabolism often present as acid erosions to the teeth and occasionally as changes in the mucosal surface as well, resulting in chronic oral ulcerations. In some studies, this has also been associated with burning mouth syndrome. Patients may be identified, upon diagnosis, as harboring the organism *Helicobacter pylori*. Treatment with antibiotics can oftentimes aid in correcting the ulcerative disease.

PROTON PUMP AND GASTRIC ACID SECRETION INHIBITORS

Dexlansoprazole on page 400
Esomeprazole on page 502
Lansoprazole on page 794
Lansoprazole, Amoxicillin, and Clarithromycin on page 796
Omeprazole on page 1009
Omeprazole and Sodium Bicarbonate on page 1011
Pantoprazole on page 1046
RABEprazole on page 1174

HISTAMINE H$_2$ ANTAGONIST

Cimetidine on page 305
Famotidine on page 568
Nizatidine on page 989
Ranitidine on page 1182

The oral aspects of gastrointestinal disease are often nonspecific and are related to the patient's gastric reflux problems. Intestinal polyps occasionally present as part of the "Peutz-Jeghers Syndrome," resulting in pigmented areas of the perioral region that resemble freckles. The astute dentist will need to differentiate these from melanin pigmentation, while at the same time encouraging the patient to seek evaluation for an intestinal disorder.

Diseases of the liver and gallbladder system are complex. Most of the disorders of interest to the dentist are covered in the section on Systemic Viral Diseases on page 1537. All of the new drugs, including interferons, are mentioned in this section.

Multiple Drug Regimens for the Treatment of *H. pylori* Infection in Adult Patients

Medication Regimen	Dosages	Duration of Therapy
First-Line Therapy (Option 1)		
H₂-Receptor antagonist (H$_2$RA) **or** proton pump inhibitor (PPI)	Standard dose of H$_2$RA or PPI[1]	10-14 days
plus		
Bismuth subsalicylate on page 192	525 mg 4 times/day	10-14 days
plus		
MetroNIDAZOLE on page 911	250 mg 4 times/day	10-14 days
plus		
Tetracycline on page 1308	500 mg 4 times/day	10-14 days
First-Line Therapy (Option 2)		
PPI	Standard dose[1]	10-14 days
plus		
Clarithromycin on page 316	500 mg 2 times/day	10-14 days
plus		
Amoxicillin on page 96	1000 mg 2 times/day	10-14 days
First-Line Therapy (Option 3)		
PPI	Standard dose[1]	10-14 days
plus		
Clarithromycin on page 316	500 mg 2 times/day	10-14 days
plus		
MetroNIDAZOLE on page 911	500 mg 2 times/day	10-14 days
Salvage Therapy for Persistent Infection (Option 1)		
PPI (once daily), bismuth, metroNIDAZOLE, and tetracycline (4 times/day) for 7-14 days		
Salvage Therapy for Persistent Infection (Option 2)		
PPI (standard dose[1]), levofloxacin 500 mg (once daily), and amoxicillin 1000 mg (2 times/day) for 10 days		

[1]Standard proton pump inhibitor dose: Esomeprazole = 40 mg once daily, lansoprazole = 30 mg 2 times/day, omeprazole = 20 mg 2 times/day, RABEprazole = 20 mg 2 times/day

REFERENCES

Chey WD, Wong BC, and Practice Parameters Committee of the American College of Gastroenterology, "American College of Gastroenterology Guideline on the Management of *Helicobacter pylori* Infection," *Am J Gastroenterol*, 2007, 102(8):1808-25.

Cobrin GM and Abreu MT, "Defects in Mucosal Immunity Leading to Crohn's Disease," *Immunol Rev*, 2005, 206:277-95.

Daley TD and Armstrong JE, "Oral Manifestations of Gastrointestinal Diseases," *Can J Gastroenterol*, 2007, 21(4):241-4.

Permin H and Andersen LP, "Inflammation, Immunity, and Vaccines for *Helicobacter* Infection," *Helicobacter*, 2005, 10(Suppl 1):21-5.

Saad RJ, Schoenfeld P, Kim HM, et al, "Levofloxacin-Based Triple Therapy Versus Bismuth-Based Quadruple Therapy for Persistent *Helicobacter pylori* Infection: A Meta-Analysis," *Am J Gastroenterol*, 2006, 101(3):488-96.

Schreiber S, Rosenstiel P, Albrecht M, et al, "Genetics of Crohn Disease, an Archetypal Inflammatory Barrier Disease," *Nat Rev Genet*, 2005, 6 (5):376-88.

Tummala S, Keates S, and Kelly CP, "Update on the Immunologic Basis of *Helicobacter pylori* Gastritis," *Curr Opin Gastroenterol*, 2004, 20(6):592-7.

Yuan Y, Padol IT, and Hunt RH, "Peptic Ulcer Disease Today," *Nat Clin Pract Gastroenterol Hepatol*, 2006, 3(2):80-9.

RESPIRATORY DISEASES

Diseases of the respiratory system put dental patients at increased risk in the dental office because of their decreased pulmonary reserve, the medications they may be taking, drug interactions between these medications, medications the dentist may prescribe, and in some patients with infectious respiratory diseases, a risk of disease transmission.

The respiratory system consists of the nasal cavity, the nasopharynx, the trachea, and the components of the lung including, the bronchi, the bronchioles, and the alveoli. The diseases that affect the lungs and the respiratory system can be separated by location of affected tissue. Diseases that affect the lower respiratory tract are often chronic, although infections can also occur. Three major diseases that affect the lower respiratory tract are often encountered in the medical history for dental patients. These include chronic bronchitis, emphysema, and asthma. Diseases that affect the upper respiratory tract are usually of the infectious nature and include sinusitis and the common cold. The upper respiratory tract infections may also include a wide variety of nonspecific infections, most of which are also caused by viruses. Influenza produces upper respiratory type symptoms and is often caused by orthomyxoviruses. Herpangina is caused by the Coxsackie type viruses and results in upper respiratory infections in addition to pharyngitis or sore throat. One serious condition, known as croup, has been associated with *Haemophilus influenzae* infections. Other more serious infections might include respiratory syncytial virus, adenoviruses, and parainfluenza viruses.

The respiratory symptoms that are often encountered in both upper respiratory and lower respiratory disorders include cough, dyspnea (difficulty in breathing), the production of sputum, hemoptysis (coughing up blood), a wheeze, and occasionally chest pain. One additional symptom, orthopnea (difficulty in breathing when lying down), is often used by the dentist to assist in evaluating the patient with the condition pulmonary edema. This condition results from either respiratory disease or congestive heart failure.

No effective drug treatments are available for the management of many of the upper respiratory tract viral infections. However, amantadine (Symmetrel®) is a synthetic drug given orally (200 mg/day) and has been found to be effective against some strains of influenza. Treatment other than for influenza includes supportive care products, available over-the-counter. These might include antihistamines for symptomatic relief of the upper respiratory congestion, antibiotics to combat secondary bacterial infections, and in severe cases, fluids, when patients have become dehydrated during the illness (see Pharmacologic Category Index for selection). The treatment of herpangina may include management of the painful ulcerations of the oropharynx. The dentist may become involved in managing these lesions in a similar way to those seen in other acute viral infections (see Systemic Viral Diseases on page 1537).

SINUSITIS

Sinusitis represents an upper respiratory condition that often comes under the purview of the practicing dentist. Acute sinusitis is characterized by nasal obstruction, fever, chills, and midface head pain. Oftentimes there is only evidence of inflammation rather than true infection. This condition may be discovered as part of a differential workup for other facial or dental pain since the symptoms are often referred to teeth adjacent to the affected sinus. Chronic sinusitis may likewise produce similar dental symptoms. Dental drugs of choice may include ephedrine or nasal drops, antihistamines, and analgesics. When infection accompanies the inflammation of sinusitis, antibiotics may be required. Most commonly, broad spectrum antibiotics such as ampicillin are prescribed. These are often combined with antral lavage to re-establish drainage from the sinus area. Surgical intervention, such as a Caldwell-Luc procedure opening into the sinus, is rarely necessary and many of the second generation antibiotics, such as cephalosporins, are used successfully in treating the acute and chronic sinusitis patient (see Antibiotic Prophylaxis on page 1542).

LOWER RESPIRATORY DISEASES

Lower respiratory tract diseases, including asthma, chronic bronchitis, and emphysema are often identified in dental patients. Asthma is an intermittent respiratory disorder that produces recurrent bronchial smooth muscle spasm, inflammation of the bronchial mucosa, and hypersecretion of mucus. The incidence of childhood asthma appears to be increasing and may be related to the presence of pollutants such as sulfur dioxide and indoor cigarette smoke. The end result is widespread narrowing of the airways and decreased ventilation with increased airway resistance, especially to expiration. Asthmatic patients often suffer asthmatic attacks when stimulated by respiratory tract infections, exercise, and cold air. Medications such as aspirin and some NSAIDs, as well as cholinergic and beta-adrenergic blocking drugs, can also trigger asthmatic attacks in addition to chemicals, smoke, and emotional anxiety.

The classic chronic obstructive pulmonary diseases (COPD) of chronic bronchitis and emphysema are both characterized by chronic airflow obstructions during normal ventilation efforts. They often occur in combination in the same patient and their treatment is similar. One common finding is that the patient is often a smoker. The dentist can play a role in reinforcement of smoking cessation in patients with chronic respiratory diseases.

Treatments include a variety of drugs depending on the severity of the symptoms and the respiratory compromise upon full respiratory evaluation. Patients who are having acute and chronic obstructive pulmonary attacks may be susceptible to infection and antibiotics such as penicillin, ampicillin, tetracycline, or sulfamethoxazole-trimethoprim are often used to eradicate susceptible infective organisms. Corticosteroids, as well as a wide variety of respiratory stimulants, are available in inhalant and/or oral forms. In patients using inhalant medication, oral candidiasis is occasionally encountered. Aclidinium bromide (Tudorza™ Pressair™) has been approved for the long-term maintenance treatment of bronchospasm (narrowing of the airways in the lung) associated with chronic obstructive pulmonary disease (COPD), including chronic bronchitis and emphysema. Aclidinium bromide is a long-acting anticholinergic and, as such, becomes the second approved inhaled long-acting muscarinic antagonist (LAMA), along with tiotropium. Both drugs produce bronchodilation by inhibiting acetylcholine's effect on the muscarinic M3 receptor in the airway smooth mucus. Both drugs are inhaled as dry powders.

Analgesics
Antibiotics
Antihistamines
Decongestants

SPECIFIC DRUGS USED IN THE TREATMENT OF CHRONIC RESPIRATORY CONDITIONS

Beta$_2$-Selective Agonists

Albuterol on page 54
Arformoterol on page   121
Formoterol on page 629
Indacaterol on page 732
Levalbuterol on page 805
Metaproterenol on page 881
Pirbuterol on page 1103
Salmeterol on page 1221

Methylxanthines

Aminophylline on page 79
Theophylline on page 1315

Mast Cell Stabilizer

Cromolyn (Systemic, Oral Inhalation) on page 356
Ketotifen (Systemic) on page 787

Corticosteroids

Beclomethasone (Oral Inhalation) on page 168
Budesonide (Systemic, Oral Inhalation) on page 203
Ciclesonide (Oral Inhalation) on page 301
Dexamethasone (Systemic) on page 397
Flunisolide (Oral Inhalation) on page 603
Fluticasone (Oral Inhalation) on page 617
MethylPREDNISolone on page 903
Mometasone (Oral Inhalation) on page 934
PredniSONE on page 1133

Anticholinergics

Aclidinium on page 44
Ipratropium (Oral Inhalation) on page 760
Tiotropium on page 1329

Leukotriene Receptor Antagonists

Montelukast on page 937
Zafirlukast on page 1415

5-Lipoxygenase Inhibitors

Zileuton on page 1420

Monoclonal Antibody, Antiasthmatic

Omalizumab on page 1007

Other respiratory diseases include tuberculosis and sarcoidosis which are considered to be restrictive granulomatous respiratory diseases. Sarcoidosis is a relatively rare acquired systemic granulomatous disease affecting multiple organs and tissues. The respiratory system is most commonly affected, with approximately 90% of patients presenting pulmonary findings during the course of their disease. Cutaneous manifestations occur in ~25% of cases but are more common in chronic forms. Head and neck lesions of sarcoidosis are manifested in 10% to 15% of patients. In the maxillofacial region, the salivary glands are frequently involved, with xerostomia and bilateral parotid swelling present. Lesions that occur in the soft tissues of the oral cavity and/or in the jaws are not common but may be the initial presenting findings of sarcoidosis. The diagnosis of sarcoidosis is established by biopsy and the histopathological evidence of typical noncaseating granulomas. These findings are usually supported by elevated serum angiotensin converting enzyme (ACE) levels. Any patient with cutaneous sarcoidosis should be evaluated for the possibility of systemic disease. Testing should include a complete physical exam, chest x-ray, pulmonary function test, electrocardiogram, tuberculin skin testing, a urinalysis, and several blood studies.

Sarcoidosis is a condition that at one time was thought to be similar to tuberculosis; however, it is a multisystem disorder of unknown origin which has a characteristic lymphocytic and mononuclear phagocytic accumulation in epithelioid granulomas within the lung. It occurs worldwide but shows a slight increased prevalence in temperate climates. The treatment of sarcoidosis is usually one that corresponds to its usually benign course; however, many patients are placed on corticosteroids at the level of 40-60 mg of prednisone daily. This treatment is continued for a protracted period of time. As in any disease requiring steroid therapy, consideration of adrenal suppression is necessary. Alteration of steroid dosage prior to stressful dental procedures may be necessary, usually increasing the steroid dosage prior to and during the stressful procedures and then gradually returning the patient to the original dosage over several days. Many dentists prefer to use the Medrol® Dosepak™; however, consultation with the patient's physician regarding dose selection is always advised. Even in the absence of evidence of adrenal suppression, consultation with the prescribing physician for appropriate dosing and timing of procedures is advisable.

PredniSONE on page 1133

Relative Potency of Endogenous and Synthetic Corticosteroids

Agent	Equivalent Dose (mg)
Short-Acting (8-12 h)	
Cortisol	20
Cortisone acetate	25
Intermediate-Acting (18-36 h)	
PrednisoLONE	5
PredniSONE	5
MethylPREDNISolone	4
Triamcinolone	4
Long-Acting (36-54 h)	
Betamethasone	0.75
Dexamethasone	0.75

Potential drug interactions for the respiratory disease patient exist. Check a patient's medical regimen to identify any potential interactions that may affect dental prescribing or a planned dental procedure. An acute sensitivity to aspirin-containing drugs and some of the nonsteroidal anti-inflammatory drugs is a threat for the asthmatic patient. Benzodiazepines may require adjustments, especially if respiratory reserve is limited. Patients that are taking steroid preparations as part of their respiratory therapy may require alteration in dosing prior to stressful dental procedures.

REFERENCES AND SELECTED READINGS

de Almeida FR, Lowe AA, Tsuiki S, et al, "Long-Term Compliance and Side Effects of Oral Appliances Used for the Treatment of Snoring and Obstructive Sleep Apnea Syndrome," *J Clin Sleep Med*, 2005, 1(2):143-52.

Dincer HE and O'Neill W, "Deleterious Effects of Sleep-Disordered Breathing on the Heart and Vascular System," *Respiration*, 2006, 73(1):124-30.

Ferguson KA, Cartwright R, Rogers R, et al, "Oral Appliances for Snoring and Obstructive Sleep Apnea: A Review," *Sleep*, 2006, 29(2):244-62.

Gay P, Weaver T, Loube D, et al, "Evaluation of Positive Airway Pressure Treatment for Sleep Related Breathing Disorders in Adults," *Sleep*, 2006, 29(3):381-401.

Global Initiative for COPD Science Committee, "Global Strategy for Diagnosis, Management, and Prevention of COPD," 2011. Available at http://www.goldcopd.org/guidelines-global-strategy-for-diagnosis-management.html

Global Initiative for COPD Science Committee, "Global Strategy for Diagnosis, Management, and Prevention of COPD," 2013. Available at http://www.goldcopd.org/guidelines-global-strategy-for-diagnosis-management.html

Hu S, Pallonen U, McAlister AL, et al, "Knowing How to Help Tobacco Users. Dentists' Familiarity and Compliance With the Clinical Practice Guideline," *J Am Dent Assoc*, 2006, 137(2):170-9.

Kowalczyk JP, Ricotti CA, de Araujo T, et al, "'Strawberry Gums' in Sarcoidosis," *J Am Acad Dermatol*, 2008, 59(5 Suppl):S118-20.

Lodha S, Sanchez M, and Prystowsky S, "Sarcoidosis of the Skin: A Review for the Pulmonologist," *Chest*, 2009, 136(2):583-96.

Schwab R, Kuna S, and Remmers JE, "Anatomy and Physiology of Upper Airway Obstruction," *Principles and Practice of Sleep Medicine*, 4th ed, Kryger MH, Roth T, and Dement WC, Philadelphia, PA: Elsevier, 2005, 983-1000.

Suresh L and Radfar L, "Oral Sarcoidosis: A Review of Literature," *Oral Dis*, 2005, 11(3):138-45.

The International Classification of Sleep Disorders: Diagnostic and Coding Manual, 2nd ed, Westchester, IL: American Academy of Sleep Medicine, 2005.

ENDOCRINE DISORDERS AND PREGNANCY

The human endocrine system manages metabolism and homeostasis. Numerous glandular tissues produce hormones that act in broad reactions with tissues throughout the body. Cells in various organ systems may be sensitive to the hormone, or they release, in reaction to the hormone, a second hormone that acts directly on another organ. Diseases of the endocrine system may have importance in dentistry. For the purposes of this section, we will limit our discussion to diseases of the thyroid tissues, diabetes mellitus, conditions requiring the administration of synthetic hormones, and pregnancy.

THYROID

Thyroid diseases can be classified into conditions that cause the thyroid to be overactive (hyperthyroidism) and those that cause the thyroid to be underactive (hypothyroidism). Clinical signs and symptoms associated with hyperthyroidism may include goiter, heat intolerance, tremor, weight loss, diarrhea, and hyperactivity. Thyroid hormone production can be tested by TSH levels and additional screens may include radioactive iodine uptake or a pre-T_4 (tetraiodothyronine, thyroxine) assay or iodine index or total serum T_3 (triiodothyronine). The results of thyroid function tests may be altered by ingestion of antithyroid drugs such as propylthiouracil, estrogen-containing drugs, and organic and inorganic iodides. When a diagnosis of hyperthyroidism has been made, treatment usually begins with antithyroid drugs which may include propranolol coupled with radioactive iodides, as well as surgical procedures, to reduce thyroid tissue. Generally, the beta-blockers are used to control cardiovascular effects of excessive T_4. Propylthiouracil or methimazole are the most common antithyroid drugs used. The dentist should be aware that epinephrine is definitely contraindicated in patients with uncontrolled hyper-thyroidism.

Diseases and conditions associated with hypothyroidism may include bradycardia, drowsiness, cold intolerance, thick dry skin, and constipation. Generally, hypothyroidism is treated with replacement thyroid hormone until a euthyroid state is achieved. Various preparations are available, the most common is levothyroxine and is generally the drug of choice for thyroid replacement therapy.

Drugs to Treat Hypothyroidism

Levothyroxine on page 814
Liothyronine on page 828
Liotrix on page 828
Thyroid, Desiccated on page 1320

Drugs to Treat Hyperthyroidism

Methimazole on page 887
Potassium Iodide on page 1121
Propranolol on page 1153
Propylthiouracil on page 1157
Sodium Iodide I^{131} on page 1246

DIABETES

Diabetes mellitus refers to a condition of prolonged hyperglycemia associated with either abnormal production or lack of production of insulin. Commonly known as Type 1 diabetes, insulin-dependent diabetes (IDDM) is a condition where there are absent or deficient levels of circulating insulin therefore triggering tissue reactions associated with prolonged hyperglycemia. The kidney's attempt to excrete the excess glucose and the organs that do not receive adequate glucose essentially are damaged. Small vessels and arterial vessels in the eye, kidney, and brain are usually at the greatest risk. Generally, blood sugar levels between 70-120 mg/dL are considered to be normal. Inadequate insulin levels allow glucose to rise to greater than the renal threshold which is 180 mg/dL, and such elevations prolonged lead to organ damage.

The goals of treatment of the diabetic are to maintain metabolic control of the blood glucose levels and to reduce the morbid effects of periodic hyperglycemia. Insulin therapy is the primary mechanism to attain management of consistent insulin levels. Insulin preparations are categorized according to their duration of action. Generally, intermediate-acting insulin and long-acting insulin can be used in combination with short-acting or rapid-acting insulins to maintain levels consistent throughout the day.

In Type 2 or noninsulin-dependent diabetes (NIDDM), the receptor for insulin in the tissues is generally down regulated; therefore, the glucose is not utilized at an appropriate rate. There is perhaps a stronger genetic basis for noninsulin-dependent diabetes than for Type 1. Treatment of the diabetes Type 2 patient is generally directed toward early nonpharmacologic intervention, mainly weight reduction, moderate exercise, and lower plasma-glucose concentrations. Oral hypoglycemic agents as seen in the following list are often used to maintain blood sugar levels. Thirty percent of Type 2 diabetics require insulin, as well as oral hypoglycemics, in order to manage their diabetes. Generally, the two classes of oral hypoglycemics are the sulfonylureas and the biguanides. The sulfonylureas are prescribed more frequently. They stimulate beta cell production of insulin, increase glucose utilization, and tend to normalize glucose metabolism in the liver. The uncontrolled diabetic may represent a challenge to the dental practitioner.

Glycosylated hemoglobin or glycol-hemoglobin assays have emerged as a "gold standard" by which glycemic control is measured in diabetic patients. The test does not rely on the patient's ability to monitor their daily blood glucose levels and is not influenced by acute changes in blood glucose or by the interval since the last meal. Glycohemoglobin is formed when glucose reacts with hemoglobin A in the blood and is composed of several fractions. Numerous assay methods have been developed, however, they vary in their precision. Dental clinicians are advised to be aware of the laboratory's particular standardization procedures when requesting glycosylated hemoglobin values. One major advantage of the glycosylated hemoglobin assay is that it provides an overview of the level of glucose in the life span of the red blood cell population in the patient, and therefore is a measure of overall glycemic control for the previous six to twelve weeks. Thus, clinicians use glycosylated hemoglobin values to determine whether their patient is under good control, on average. These assays have less value in medication dosing decisions. Blood glucose monitoring methods are actually better in that respect. The values of glycosylated hemoglobin are expressed as a percentage of the total hemoglobin in the red blood cell population and a normal value is considered to be <6%. The goal is generally for diabetic patients to remain at <7% and values >8% would constitute a worrisome signal. Medical conditions such as anemias or any red blood cell disease, numerous levels of myelosuppression, or pregnancy can artificially lower glycosylated hemoglobin values.

Rapid-Acting Insulins

Insulin Lispro (HumaLOG®) on page 745
Insulin Aspart (NovoLOG®) on page 742
Insulin Glulisine (Apidra®) on page 744

Short-Acting Insulin

Insulin Regular on page 748

Intermediate-Acting Insulin

Insulin NPH on page 747

Intermediate- to Long-Acting Insulin

Insulin Detemir on page 743

Long-Acting Insulin

Insulin Glargine on page 744

Oral Hypoglycemic Agents

Acarbose on page 26
ChlorproPAMIDE on page 296
Exenatide on page 562
Glimepiride on page 658
GlipiZIDE on page 659
GlyBURIDE on page 664
Linagliptin on page 826
Liraglutide on page 829
MetFORMIN on page 882
Miglitol on page 921
Nateglinide on page 963
Pioglitazone on page 1096
Pramlintide on page 1125
Repaglinide on page 1187
Rosiglitazone on page 1212
Saxagliptin on page 1225
SitaGLIPtin on page 1242
TOLAZamide on page 1335
TOLBUTamide on page 1336

Neuropathic pain can be a significant problem in the management of diabetes. Recently, Tapentadol (Nucynta® ER) received approval for use in the management of neuropathic pain in patients with diabetic peripheral neuropathy (DPN). Tapentadol is a dual-acting agent that combines a strong opioid agonist action together with inhibition of norepinephrine and serotonin reuptake. Essentially, it functions in a similar way to combining a schedule II opioid (ie, morphine, oxycodone) with a tricyclic or SNRI antidepressant. Serotonin and especially norepinephrine are important for reducing pain signal transmission in the spinal cord as part of the descending pathways for pain modulation. Opioids also produce spinal analgesia, directly on spinal cord neurons, but also by stimulating the activity of the descending pathways (primarily serotonin). Neuropathic pain is a complex disorder that usually affects ascending pathways initially, but, over time, descending pain pathways can also become damaged or less efficient in pain modulation. Other oral manifestations of uncontrolled diabetes require aggressive dental management and might include abnormal neutrophil function, resulting in a poor response to periodontal pathogens. Increased risk of gingivitis and periodontitis in these patients is common. Candidiasis is also a frequent occurrence. Denture-sore mouth may be more common. Poor wound-healing following extractions may be one of the complications encountered.

HORMONAL THERAPY

Two uses of hormonal supplementation include oral contraceptives and estrogen replacement therapy. Drugs used for contraception interfere with fertility by inhibiting release of follicle stimulating hormone, luteinizing hormone, and by preventing ovulation. There are few oral side effects; however, moderate gingivitis, similar to that seen during pregnancy, has been reported.

Drugs commonly encountered include:

Estradiol and Dienogest on page 506
Estradiol and Norethindrone on page 507
Estradiol and Norgestimate on page 508
Ethinyl Estradiol and Drospirenone on page 523
Ethinyl Estradiol and Ethynodiol Diacetate on page 526
Ethinyl Estradiol and Etonogestrel on page 528
Ethinyl Estradiol and Levonorgestrel on page 531
Ethinyl Estradiol and Norethindrone on page 538
Ethinyl Estradiol and Norgestimate on page 543
Ethinyl Estradiol and Norgestrel on page 546
Ethinyl Estradiol, Drospirenone, and Levomefolate on page 549
MedroxyPROGESTERone on page 861
Norethindrone on page 990
Norethindrone and Mestranol on page 990

Estrogens or derivatives are usually prescribed as replacement therapy following menopause or cyclic irregularities and to inhibit osteoporosis. The following list of drugs may interact with antidepressants and barbiturates. New tissue-specific estrogens like Evista® may help with the problem of osteoporosis.

Estradiol (Systemic) on page 505
Estradiol and Levonorgestrel on page 507
Estrogens (Conjugated/Equine, Systemic) on page 511
Estrogens (Conjugated A/Synthetic) on page 509
Estrogens (Conjugated B/Synthetic) on page 510
Estrogens (Esterified) on page 514
Estrogens (Conjugated/Equine) and Medroxyprogesterone on page 513
Estrogens (Esterified) and Methyltestosterone on page 515
Estropipate on page 515
Raloxifene on page 1177

PREGNANCY

Normal endocrine and physiologic functions are altered during pregnancy. Endogenous estrogens and progesterone increase and placental hormones are secreted. Thyroid stimulating hormone and growth hormone also increase. Cardiovascular changes can result and increased blood volume can lead to blood pressure elevations and transient heart murmurs. Generally, in a normal pregnancy, oral gingival changes will be limited to gingivitis. Alteration of treatment plans might include limiting administration of all drugs to emergency procedures only during the first and third trimesters and medical consultation regarding the patients' status for all elective procedures. Limiting dental care throughout pregnancy to preventive procedures is reasonable. The effects on dental treatment of the "morning after pill" (Plan B® and PREVEN®) and the abortifacient, mifepristone on page 920, have not been documented at this time. Consultation with the patient's internist and obstetrician for evaluation of medication safety in pregnancy is advised.

Hypertensive Disorders and Pregnancy

Hypertensive disorders, including chronic or pre-existing hypertension and the development of hypertension during pregnancy, occur in 12% to 22% of pregnant women. Oral health professionals should consult with patient's prenatal care provider before initiating dental procedures due to increased bleeding with uncontrolled severe hypertension (blood pressure values ≥160/110 mm Hg).

Diabetes and Pregnancy

Gestational diabetes occurs in 2% to 5% of pregnant women in the U.S. It is usually diagnosed after 24 weeks of gestation. Any inflammatory process, including acute and chronic periodontal infection, may make diabetes control more difficult. Poorly controlled diabetes is associated with adverse pregnancy outcomes, such as pre-eclampsia, congenital anomalies, and large-for-gestational-age newborns. Meticulous control to avoid or minimize dental infection is important for pregnant women with diabetes. Regulating all sources of acute or chronic inflammation helps manage diabetes.

REFERENCES AND SELECTED READINGS

American Diabetes Association, "Standards of Medical Care in Diabetes-2013," *Diabetes Care*, 2013, 36(Suppl 1):S11-66.
Carlos-Fabue L, Jimenez-Soriano Y, and Sarrion-Perez MG, "Dental Management of Patients With Endocrine Disorders," *J Clin Exp Dent*, 2010, 196–203.
De Groot L, Abalovich M, Alexander EK, et al, "Management of Thyroid Dysfunction During Pregnancy and Postpartum: An Endocrine Society Clinical Practice Guideline," *J Clin Endocrinol Metab*, 2012, 97(8):2543-65.
Handelsman Y, Mechanick JI, Blonde L, et al, "American Association of Clinical Endocrinologists Medical Guidelines for Clinical Practice for Developing a Diabetes Mellitus Comprehensive Care Plan," *Endocr Pract*, 2011, 17(Suppl 2):1-53.
Huber MA and Terézhalmy GT, "Risk Stratification and Dental Management of the Patient With Thyroid Dysfunction," *Quintessence Int*, 2008, 39 (2):139-50.
Michalowicz BS, DiAngelis AJ, Novak MJ, et al, "Examining the Safety of Dental Treatment in Pregnant Women," *J Am Dent Assoc*, 2008, 139 (6):685-95.
Michalowicz BS, Hodges JS, DiAngelis AJ, et al, "Treatment of Periodontal Disease and the Risk of Preterm Birth," *N Engl J Med*, 2006, 355 (18):1885-94.
Nathan DM, Buse JB, Davidson MB, "Medical Management of Hyperglycemia in Type 2 Diabetes: A Consensus Algorithm for the Initiation and Adjustment of Therapy: A Consensus Statement of the American Diabetes Association and the European Association for the Study of Diabetes," *Diabetes Care*, 2009, 32(1):193-203.
Rodbard HW, Jellinger PS, Davidson JA, "Statement by an American Association of Clinical Endocrinologists/American College of Endocrinology Consensus Panel on Type 2 Diabetes Mellitus: An Algorithm for Glycemic Control," *Endocr Pract*, 2009, 15(6):540-59.
Stagnaro-Green A, Abalovich M, Alexander E, "Guidelines of the American Thyroid Association for the Diagnosis and Management of Thyroid Disease During Pregnancy and Postpartum," *Thyroid*, 2011, 21(10):1081-125.

HIV INFECTION AND AIDS

Human immunodeficiency virus (HIV) represents agents HIV-1 and HIV-2 that produce a devastating systemic disease. The virus causes disease by leading to elevated risk of infections in patients and, from our experience over the last 18 years, there clearly are oral manifestations associated with these patients. Also, there has been a revolution in infection control in our dental offices over the last two decades due to our expanding knowledge of this infectious agent. Infection control practices have been elevated to include all of the infectious agents with which dentists often come into contact. These might include, in addition to HIV, hepatitis viruses (of which the serotypes include A, B, C, D, E, F, and G), the herpes viruses (see Systemic Viral Diseases on page 1537); STDs such as syphilis, gonorrhea, and papillomavirus (see Sexually-Transmitted Diseases on page 1536).

Acquired immunodeficiency syndrome (AIDS) has been recognized since early 1981 as a unique clinical syndrome manifest by opportunistic infections or by neoplasms complicating the underlying defect in the cellular immune system. These defects are now known to be brought on by infection and pathogenesis with human immunodeficiency virus 1 or 2 (HIV-1 is the predominant serotype identified). The major cellular defect brought on by infection with HIV is a depletion of T-cells, primarily the subtype, T-helper cells, known as CD4+ cells. When the CD4 cell count falls below 200 cells/μL, patients are at high risk for life-threatening AIDS-defining opportunistic infections (eg, *Pneumocystis jiroveci* pneumonia, *Toxoplasma gondii* encephalitis, disseminated *Mycobacterium avium* complex disease, tuberculosis, bacterial pneumonia). Over these years, our knowledge regarding HIV infection and the oral manifestations often associated with patients with HIV or AIDS, has increased dramatically. Populations of individuals known to be at high risk of HIV transmission include homosexuals, intravenous drug abuse patients, transfusion recipients, patients with other sexually transmitted diseases, and patients practicing promiscuous sex.

The definitions of AIDS have also evolved over this period of time. The natural history of HIV infection along with some of the oral manifestations can be reviewed in Table 1. The risk of developing these opportunistic infections increases as the patient progresses to AIDS.

Table 1. Natural History of HIV Infection/Oral Manifestations

Time From Transmission (Average)	Observation	CD4 Cell Count
0	Viral transmissions	Normal: 1000 ($\pm$500/mm^3)
2-4 weeks	Self-limited infectious mononucleosis-like illness with fever, rash, leukopenia, mucocutaneous ulcerations (mouth, genitals, etc), thrush	Transient decrease
6-12 weeks	Seroconversion (rarely requires ≥3 months for seroconversion)	Normal
0-8 years	Healthy/asymptomatic HIV infection; peripheral/persistent generalized lymphadenopathy; HPV, thrush, OHL; RAU, periodontal diseases, salivary gland diseases; dermatitis	≥500/mm^3 gradual reduction with average decrease of 50-80/mm^3/year
4-8 years	Early symptomatic HIV infection previously called (AIDS-related complex): Thrush, vaginal candidiasis (persistent, frequent and/or severe), cervical dysplasia/CA Hodgkin's lymphoma, B-cell lymphoma, oral hairy leukoplakia, salivary gland diseases, ITP, xerostomia, dermatitis, shingles; RAU, herpes simplex, HPV, bacterial infections, periodontal diseases, molluscum contagiosum, other physical symptoms: fever, weight loss, fatigue	≥300-500/mm^3
6-10 years	AIDS: Wasting syndrome, *Candida* esophagitis, Kaposi's sarcoma, HIV-associated dementia, disseminated *M. avium*, Hodgkin's or B-cell lymphoma, herpes simplex >30 days; PCP; cryptococcal meningitis, other systemic fungal infections; CMV	<200/mm^3

Natural history indicates course of HIV infection in absence of antiretroviral treatment. Adapted from Bartlett JG, "A Guide to HIV Care from the AIDS Care Program of the Johns Hopkins Medical Institutions," 2nd ed.

PCP = *Pneumocystis carinii* pneumonia, ITP = idiopathic thrombocytopenia purpura, HPV = human papilloma virus, OHL = oral hairy leukoplakia, RAU = recurrent aphthous ulcer

Patients with HIV infection and/or AIDS are seen in dental offices throughout the country. In general, it is the dentist's obligation to treat HIV individuals including patients of record and other patients who may seek treatment when the office is accepting new patients. These patients are protected under the Americans with Disabilities Act and the dentist has an obligation as described. Two excellent publications, one by the American Dental Association and the other by the American Academy of Oral Medicine, outline the dentist's responsibility as well as a very detailed explanation of dental management protocols for HIV patients. These protocols, however, are evolving just as our knowledge of HIV has evolved. New drugs and their interactions present the dentist with continuous need for updates regarding the appropriate management of HIV patients. Diagnostic tests, including determining viral load in combination with the CD4 status, now are used to modify a patient's treatment in ways that allow them to remain relatively illness-free for longer periods of time. This places more of a responsibility on the dental practice team to be aware of drug changes, of new drugs, and of the appropriate oral management in such patients.

Our knowledge of AIDS allows us to properly treat these patients while protecting ourselves, our staff, and other patients in the office. All types of infectious disease require consistent practices in our dental offices known as Standard/Universal Precautions. These agents include sexually transmitted disease agents, the highly virulent hepatitis viruses, and the less virulent but always worrisome HIV. In general, an office that is practicing standard/universal precautions is one that is considered safe for patients and staff. Throughout this spectrum, HIV is placed somewhere in the middle, in terms of infection risk in the dental office. Other sexually transmitted diseases and infectious diseases such as tuberculosis represent a greater threat to the dentist than HIV itself. However, due to the grave danger of HIV infection, many of our precautions have been instituted to assist the dentist in protecting himself, his staff, and other patients in situations where the office may be involved in treating a patient that is HIV positive.

As in the management of all medically-compromised patients, the appropriate care of HIV patients begins with a complete and thorough history. This history must allow the dentist to identify risk factors in the development of HIV as well as identify those patients known to be HIV positive. Knowledge of all medications prescribed to patients at risk is also important.

The current antiretroviral therapy used to treat patients with HIV infection and/or AIDS includes three primary classifications of drugs. These are the nucleoside analogs, protease inhibitors, and the non-nucleoside/nucleotide analogs (analogs refers to chemicals that can substitute competitively for naturally produced cell components as found in DNA, RNA, or proteins). The newest drugs include several nucleoside analogs, abacavir (Ziagen®), sub protease inhibitors, amprenavir, several non-nucleoside analogs, efavirenz (Sustiva®), and adefovir, as well as the latest combination drugs, such as elvitegravir, cobicistat, emtricitabine, and tenofovir (Stribild™; formerly Quad). Finding the perfect "cocktail" of anti-HIV medications still eludes clinicians. This is partly due to the fact that therapies are still too novel and the patient's years too few to study. Numerous studies have indicated that combinations of drugs are far better than individual drug therapy. Several of these studies have looked at two drug combinations, particularly between nucleoside analogs in combination with protease inhibitors. The newer drugs (non-nucleoside analogs) have added the possibility of a triple "cocktail". Recently several studies indicated that this three-drug combination may be the best in managing HIV infection.

When HIV was first discovered, the efforts for monitoring HIV infection focused on the CD4 blood levels and the ratios between the helper cells, suppressor cells within the patient's immune system. These markers were used to indicate success or failure of drug therapies as patients moved through HIV pathogenesis toward AIDS. More recently, however, the advent of protease inhibitors has allowed clinicians to monitor the actual presence of viral RNA within the patient and the term viral load has become the focus of therapy monitoring. The availability of better therapies and our rapidly expanding knowledge of molecular biology of the HIV virus have created new opportunities to control the AIDS epidemic. Cases can be monitored closely looking at the number of copy units or virions within the patient's bloodstream as an indication in combination with other infections and/or declining or increasing CD4 numbers to establish prognostic values for the patient's success. Long-term survival of patients infected with HIV has been accomplished by monitoring and adjusting therapy to these numbers.

Comprehensive coordinated approaches, that have been advocated by researchers, have sought to establish national standards for HIV reporting, greater access to effective newly approved medications, improved access to individual physicians treating HIV patients, and continued protection of patient's privacy. These goals allow the reporting of studies that suggest that combination therapies, some of which have been tried in less controlled individual patient treatments, may prove useful in larger populations of HIV-infected individuals. As these studies are reported, the dental clinician should be aware that patients' drug therapies change rapidly, various combinations may be tried, and the side effects and interactions as described in the chapter on drug interactions and the CYP system will also emerge. The dentist must be aware of these potential interactions with seemingly innocuous drugs such as clarithromycin, erythromycin, and some of the sedative drugs that a dentist may utilize in their practice as well as some of the analgesics. These drug interactions may be the most important part of monitoring that the dentist provides in helping to manage a situation. Some of the antiviral drugs more commonly used for HIV, AIDS, Asymptomatic, CD4 <500, and the newer drugs (ie, protease inhibitors, nucleoside analogs, and non-nucleoside nucleotide analogs) are listed in Table 2.

Table 2. Examples of Drugs

Nucleoside Analogs	Protease Inhibitors	Non-nucleoside Analogs	Nucleotide Analogs	Fusion Protein Inhibitor	Integrase Inhibitor
Zidovudine	Saquinavir	Nevirapine	Adefovir	Enfuvirtide	Raltegravir
(Retrovir®, AZT, SDV)	(Invirase®)	(Viramune®)	(Hepsera™)	(Fuzeon®)	(Isentress®)
Didanosine	Ritonavir	Delavirdine	Tenofovir	Maraviroc	
(Videx®, ddi)	(Norvir®)	(Rescriptor®)	(Viread®)	(Selzentry®)	
Zalcitabine	Indinavir	Efavirenz			
(Hivid® [DSC], ddc)	(Crixivan®)	(Sustiva®)			
Stavudine	Nelfinavir				
(Zerit®, d4T)	(Viracept®)				
LamiVUDine	Fosamprenavir				
(Epivir®)	(Lexiva™)				
Abacavir	Atazanavir				
(Ziagen®)	(Reyataz®)				
Emtricitabine	Darunavir				
(Emtriva®)	(Prezista®)				
Entecavir	Tipranavir				
(Baraclude®)	(Aptivus®)				
Telbivudine					
(Tyzeka®)					

The presence of other infections is an important part of the health history. Appropriate medical consultation may be mandated after a health history in order to accomplish a complete evaluation of the patients at risk. Uniformity in the taking of a history from a patient is the dentist's best plan for all patients so that no selectivity or discrimination can be implicated.

An appropriate review of symptoms may also identify oral and systemic conditions that may be present in aggressive HIV disease. Medical physical examination may reveal pre-existing or developing intra- or extra-oral signs/symptoms of progressive disease. Aggressive herpes simplex, herpes zoster, papillomavirus, Kaposi's sarcoma or lymphoma are among the disorders that might be identified. In addition to these, intra-oral examination may raise suspicion regarding fungal infections, angular cheilitis, squamous cell carcinoma, and recurrent aphthous ulcers. The dentist should be vigilant in all patients regardless of HIV risk.

It will always be up to the dental practitioner to determine whether testing for HIV should be recommended following the history and physical examination of a new patient. Because of the severe psychological implications of learning of HIV positivity for a patient, the dentist should be aware that there are appropriate referral sites where psychological counseling and appropriate discrete testing for the patient is available. The dentist's office should have these sites available for referral should the patient be interested. Candid discussions, however, with the patient regarding risk factors and/or other signs or symptoms in their history and physical condition that may indicate a higher HIV risk than the normal population, should be an area the dentist feels comfortable in broaching with any new patient. Oftentimes, it is appropriate to recommend testing for other infectious diseases should risk factors be present. For example, testing for hepatitis B may be appropriate for the patient and along with this the dentist could recommend that the patient consider HIV testing. Because of the legal issues involved, anonymity for HIV testing may be appropriate and it is always up to the patient to follow the doctor's recommendations.

When a patient has either given a positive history of knowing that they are HIV positive or it has been determined after referral for consultation, the dentist should be aware of the AIDS-defining illnesses. Of course, current medical status and drug therapy that the patient may be undergoing is of equal importance. The dentist, through medical consultation and regular follow-up with the patient's physician, should be made aware of the CD4 count (Table 3), the viral load, and the drugs that the patient is taking. The presence of other AIDS-defining illnesses as well as complications, such as higher risk of endocarditis and the risk of other systemic infections such as tuberculosis, are extremely important for the dentist. These may make an impact on the dental treatment plan in terms of the selection of preprocedural antibiotics or the use of oral medications to treat opportunistic infections in or around the oral cavity.

Table 3. CD4+ Lymphocyte Count and Percentage as Related to the Risk of Opportunistic Infection

CD4+ Cells/mm^3	CD4+ Percentage[1]	Risk of Opportunistic Infection
>600	32-60	No increased risk
400-500	<29	Initial immune suppression
200-400	14-28	Appearance of opportunistic infections, some may be major
<200	<14	Severe immune suppression. AIDS diagnosis. Major opportunistic infections. Although variable, prognosis for surviving greater than 3 years is poor
<50	—	Although variable, prognosis for surviving greater than 1 year is poor

[1]Several studies have suggested that the CD4+ percentage demonstrates less variability between measurements, as compared to the absolute CD4+ cell count. CD4+ percentages may therefore give a clearer impression of the course of disease.

Adapted from Glick M and Silverman S, "Dental Management of HIV-Infected Patients," *J Am Dent Assoc* (Supplement to Reviewers), 1995.

AIDS-defining illnesses, such as oral-pharyngeal candidiasis, herpes infections lasting >30 days, recurrent pneumonia, or lymphoma are clearly important to the dentist. Chemotherapy that might be being given to the patient for treatment for any or all of these disorders can have implications in terms of the patient's response to simple dental procedures.

Drug therapies have become complex in the treatment of HIV/AIDS. Because of the moderate successes with protease inhibitors and the drug combination therapies, more patients are living longer and receiving more dental care throughout their lives. Drug therapies are often tailored to the current CD4 count in combination with the viral load. In general, patients with high CD4 counts are usually at lower risk for complications in the dental office than patients with low CD4 counts. However, the presence of a high viral load with or without a stable CD4 count may be indicative or a more rapid progression of the HIV/AIDS disease process than had previously been thought. Patients with a high viral load and a declining CD4 count are considered to have the greatest risk and the poorest prognosis of all the groups.

In HIV infections, a new drug known as raltegravir is an integrase inhibitor which works by interrupting HIV integration into the host cell DNA. In addition, in 2007, a new class of anti-HIV drugs was introduced, these are the chemokine receptor 5 antagonists or the CCR5 receptor blockers. The drug of interest for this class is maraviroc. This antiviral drug has shown great promise as an adjuvant therapy along with other anti-HIV drugs.

Other organ damage, such as liver compromise potentially leading to bleeding disorders, can be found as the disease progresses to AIDS. Liver dysfunction may be related to pre-existing hepatic diseases due to previous infection with a hepatitis virus such as hepatitis B or other drug toxicities associated with the treatment of AIDS. The dentist must have available current prothrombin and partial thromboplastin times (PT and PTT) in order to accurately evaluate any risk of bleeding abnormality. Platelet count and liver function studies are also important. Potential drug interactions include some antibiotics, as well as any anticoagulating drugs, which may be contraindicated in such patients. It may be necessary to avoid NSAIDs, as well as aspirin. (See Drug Interactions: Metabolism/Transport Effects on page 1637).

The use of preprocedural antibiotics is another issue in the HIV patient. As the absolute neutrophil count declines during the progression of AIDS, the use of antibiotics as a preprocedural step prior to dental care may be necessary. If protracted treatment plans are necessary, the dentist should receive updated information as the patient receives such from their physician. It is always important that the dentist have current CD4 counts, viral load assay, as well as liver function studies,

AST and ALT, and bleeding indicators including platelet count, PT, and PTT. If any other existing conditions such as cardiac involvement or joint prostheses are involved, antibiotic coverage may also be necessary. However, these determinations are no different than in the non-HIV population and this subject is covered in Antibiotic Prophylaxis - Preprocedural Guidelines for Dental Patients on page 1542. Use the table of Normal Blood Values on page 1639 as a general guideline for provision of dental care.

The consideration of current blood values is important in long-term care of any medically compromised patient and in particular the HIV-positive patient. Preventive dental care is likewise valuable in these patients, however, the dentist's approach should be no different than as with all patients. See Table 4 for oral lesions commonly associated with HIV disease and a brief description of their usual treatment (see Part II of this Oral Medicine chapter for more detailed descriptions of these common oral lesions).

The clinician should be aware that several of the protease inhibitors have now been associated with drug interactions. Some of these drug interactions include therapies that the dentist may be utilizing. The basis for these drug interactions with protease inhibitors is the inhibition of cytochrome P450 isoforms, which are important in normal liver function and metabolism of drugs. A detailed description of the mechanisms of inhibition can be found in Drug Interactions: Metabolism/ Transport Effects on page 1637, as well as a table illustrating some known drug interactions with antiviral therapy and drugs commonly prescribed in the dental office. The metabolism of these drugs could be affected by the patient's antiviral therapy.

Every dental office should have in place protocols for standard/universal precautions during patient care and for emergency procedures in case of occupational exposure to blood-borne pathogens.

Table 4. Oral Lesions Commonly Seen in HIV/AIDS

Condition	Management
Oral candidiasis	See Fungal Infections on page 1573
Angular cheilitis	
Oral hairy leukoplakia	See Systemic Viral Diseases on page 1537
Periodontal diseases	See Bacterial Infections on page 1562
Linear gingivitis	
Ulcerative periodontitis	
Herpes simplex	See Systemic Viral Diseases on page 1537
Herpes zoster	
Chronic aphthous ulceration	Palliation/Thalidomide (Thalomid®)
Salivary gland disease	Referral
Human papillomavirus	Laser/Surgical excision
Kaposi's sarcoma	See Antibiotic Prophylaxis on page 1542; Biopsy/Laser
Non-Hodgkin's lymphoma	Biopsy/Referral
Tuberculosis	Referral

Several new classes of drugs have been developed as antiretroviral drug classifications in the management of HIV infection. These are fusion inhibitors, CCR5 receptor blockers, and integrase inhibitors. The prototype fusion inhibitor is enfuvirtide (Fuzeon®). There are no significant drug interactions; however, there are numerous side effects and toxicities including Guillain-Barré syndrome, as well as taste aberrations with this drug. The prototype CCR5 receptor blocker is maraviroc (Selzentry®) and the integrase inhibitor is raltegravir (Isentress®) both with no specific oral side effects.

First FDA-Approved Medication to Reduce HIV Risk

The FDA has approved a new indication for the existing drug emtricitabine and tenofovir (Truvada®) as a once daily dose used in combination with safer sex practices to reduce the risk of sexually-acquired HIV infection in high-risk adults not currently infected with HIV. The drug, first approved for treating HIV infection in 2004, is a combination of the cytosine analogue nucleoside reverse transcriptase inhibitor emtricitabine and the nucleotide reverse transcriptase inhibitor tenofovir, an analog of adenosine 5'-monophosphate. Each drug interferes with HIV viral RNA-dependent DNA polymerase, resulting in inhibition of viral replication. In two large clinical trials, daily use of Truvada® was shown to significantly reduce the risk of contracting HIV. In a study sponsored by the National Institutes of Health (NIH) of about 2500 HIV-negative gay and bisexual men and transgender women, Truvada® reduced the risk of infection by ~42%. In a study sponsored by the University of Washington, risk was reduced by 75% in about 4800 heterosexual couples in which one partner was HIV-positive and the other was not.

It is important that patients recognize that Truvada® is not a substitute for safer sex practices. The drug is meant to be used as an adjunct to a comprehensive HIV prevention plan that includes consistent and correct condom use, risk reduction counseling, regular HIV testing, and treatment of any other sexually-transmitted infections. Healthcare providers must stress that healthy patients adhere to the pill's daily-dose regimen, which is necessary for it to work, and not discontinue other prevention measures, such as condom use. Truvada® must be taken every day in order to help prevent HIV infection. One fear is that high-risk patients will not take this medication correctly, become infected, and develop a drug-resistant strain of HIV infection that may be more difficult to treat. These patients may then spread the infection to others, believing they are still HIV-negative.

Common side effects of Truvada® include gastrointestinal problems (eg, nausea, abdominal pain, decreased appetite, weight loss, cramping, diarrhea). Joint or muscle pain, pain or tingling in the hands or feet, headache, dizziness, and fatigue are also possible. Obviously, such side effects can compromise daily compliance. Serious side effects may include fatal lactic acidosis and liver disease, as well as muscle weakness, blood disorders, renal failure, and pancreatitis.

The approval of this new indication is not without controversy. The AIDS Healthcare Foundation, a global AIDS organization that provides medical care and services to HIV-infected people, called the FDA's approval of Truvada® for HIV prevention "reckless" and criticized the agency for not requiring proof of a negative HIV test in users. In March, the group had filed a petition with the agency urging it to reject Truvada®'s application, citing concerns about drug side effects, the nearly $14,000 annual cost of the drug and the difficulty of sticking with a daily pill regimen.

FDA Approves HIV Home Test Kit

With the CDC estimating that of the 1.2 million people living with HIV in this country, one-fifth or ~240,000 are unaware of their status. Furthermore, there are ~50,000 new cases of HIV infection added to that number annually. Because of these statistics, many people are unaware they are HIV positive may be transmitting the virus unknowingly. Testing helps slow new infections. In that regard, the FDA approved the first over-the-counter HIV test kit that allows people to test for HIV infection in the privacy of their own homes. The OraQuick® In-Home HIV Test detects the presence of antibodies to human immunodeficiency virus type 1 (HIV-1) and type 2 (HIV-2). In essence, the kit is an OTC version of a test used in the clinical setting that was approved by the FDA in 2004. The idea is not for the home test kit to replace medical testing but to provide another route for people to find out their HIV status. In this test, the user takes an oral swab and places it in a specially prepared vial that comes with the kit. The result is ready in 20-40 minutes. However, the newly approved OTC kit is not as reliable as being tested by a trained clinician.

The FDA stressed in its approval announcement that the test is not 100% accurate in identifying people with the virus. A trial conducted by test maker OraSure showed OraQuick® detected HIV in those carrying the virus only 92% of the time, though it was 99.9% accurate in ruling out HIV in patients not carrying the virus. That means the test could miss one in 12 HIV-infected people (false-negative) who use it but would incorrectly identify only one patient as having HIV for every 5000 HIV-negative people tested (false-positive). As with other HIV tests performed by trained personnel, a positive result does not necessarily mean that the user is definitely infected with HIV, but that they should then go and be tested in a medical setting to confirm the result. Similarly, a negative result does not necessarily mean the user is definitely not infected, particularly if they may have picked up the virus in the previous 2-3 months and have not yet seroconverted.

FREQUENTLY ASKED QUESTIONS

How does one get AIDS, aside from having unprotected sex?

Our current knowledge about the immunodeficiency virus is that it is carried via semen, contaminated needles, blood products, transfusion products not tested, and potentially in other fluids of the body. Patients at highest risk include I.V. drug-abusers, those receiving multiple transfusions with blood that has not been screened for HIV, or patients practicing unprotected sex with multiple partners, where the history of the partner may not be as clear as the patient would like.

Are patients safe from AIDS or HIV infection when they present to the dentist office?

Our current knowledge indicates that the answer is an unequivocal "yes". The patient is protected because dental offices are practicing standard/universal precautions, using antimicrobial handwashing agents, gloves, face masks, eye protection, special clothing, aerosol control, and instrument soaking and autoclaving. All of these procedures stop potential transmission to a new patient, as well as, allow for easy disposal of contaminated office supplies for elimination of microbes by an antimicrobial technique, should they be contaminated through treatment of another patient. These precautions are mandated by OSHA requirements.

What is the most common opportunistic infection that HIV-positive patients suffer that may be important in dentistry?

The most common opportunistic infection important to dentistry is oral candidiasis. This disease can present as white plaques, red areas, or angular cheilitis occurring at the corners of the mouth. Management of such lesions is appropriate by the dentist and is described in this handbook (see Fungal Infections on page 1573). Other oral complications include HIV-associated periodontal disease, as well as the other conditions outlined in Table 4. Of great concern to the dentist is the risk of tuberculosis. In many HIV-positive patients, tuberculosis has become a serious, life-threatening opportunistic infection. The dentist should be aware that appropriate referral for anyone showing such respiratory signs and symptoms would be prudent.

Can one patient infect another through unprotected sex if the other patient has tested negative for HIV?

Yes, there is always the possibility that a sexual partner may be in the early window of time when plasma viremia is not at a detectable level. The antibody response to plasma viremia may be slightly delayed and diagnostic testing may not indicate HIV positivity. This window of time represents a period when the patient may be infectious but not show up yet on normal diagnostic testing.

Can HIV be passed by oral fluids?

As our knowledge about HIV has evolved, we have thought that HIV is inactivated in saliva by an agent possibly associated with secretory leukocyte protease inhibitors known as SLPI. There is, however, a current resurgence in our interest in oral transmission because some research indicates that in moderate to advanced periodontal lesions or other oral lesions where there is tissue damage, the presence of a serous exudate may increase the risk of transmission. The dentist should be aware of this ongoing research and attempt to renew knowledge regularly so that any future breakthroughs will be noted.

REFERENCES AND SELECTED READINGS

Barouch DH, Baden LR, and Dolin R, "Human Immunodeficiency Virus Vaccines," *Principles and Practice of Infectious Disease*, 6th ed, Mandell GL, Bennett JE, and Dolin R, eds, Philadelphia, PA: Churchhill Livingstone, 2005, 1707-17.

DHHS Panel on Antiretroviral Guidelines for Adults and Adolescents, "Guidelines for the Use of Antiretroviral Agents in HIV-1-Infected Adults and Adolescents, Department of Health and Human Services," February 12, 2013, 1-267. Available at http://aidsinfo.nih.gov/contentfiles/lvguidelines/adultandadolescentgl.pdf

DHHS Panel on Antiretroviral Therapy and Medical Management of HIV-Infected Children, "Guidelines for the Use of Antiretroviral Agents in Pediatric HIV Infection, Department of Health and Human Services," August 11, 2011, 1-268. Available at http://www.aidsinfo.nih.gov

DHHS Panel on Treatment of HIV-Infected Pregnant Women and Prevention of Perinatal Transmission, "Recommendations for Use of Antiretroviral Drugs in Pregnant HIV-1-Infected Women for Maternal Health and Interventions to Reduce Perinatal HIV Transmission in the United States," July 31, 2012. Available at http://aidsinfo.nih.gov/contentfiles/lvguidelines/perinatalgl.pdf

Merson MH, "The HIV-AIDS Pandemic at 25-The Global Response," *N Engl J Med*, 2006, 354(23):2414-7.

Sax PE and Walker BD, "Immunology Related to AIDS," *Cecil Textbook of Medicine*, 22nd ed, Goldman L and Ausiello D, eds, Philadelphia, PA: Saunders, 2004, 2137-8.

Workowski KA, Berman S, and Centers for Disease Control and Prevention (CDC), "Sexually Transmitted Diseases Treatment Guidelines, 2010," *MMWR Recomm Rep*, 2010, 59(RR-12):1-110. Available at http://www.cdc.gov/std/treatment/2010/STD-Treatment-2010-RR5912.pdf

RHEUMATOID ARTHRITIS, OSTEOARTHRITIS, AND OSTEOPOROSIS

RA AND OSTEOARTHRITIS MANAGEMENT

Arthritis and its variations represent the most common chronic musculoskeletal disorders of man. The conditions can essentially be divided into rheumatoid, osteoarthritic, and polyarthritic presentations. Differences in age of onset and joint involvement exist and it is now currently believed that the diagnosis of each may be less clear than previously thought. These degenerative and autoinflammatory diseases have now been shown to affect young and old alike. Criteria for a diagnosis of rheumatoid arthritis include a positive serologic test for rheumatoid factor, subcutaneous nodules, affected joints on opposite sides of the body, and clear radiographic changes. The hematologic picture includes moderate normocytic hypochromic anemia, mild leukocytosis, and mild thrombocytopenia. During acute inflammatory periods, C-reactive protein and tumor-necrosis-factor alpha (TNF-alpha) are elevated and IgG and IgM (rheumatoid factors) can be detected. Osteoarthritis is a degenerative disease of the joints and lacks these diagnostic features.

Other systemic conditions, such as gout, psoriasis, systemic lupus erythematosus and Sjögren's syndrome, are often found simultaneously with some of the arthritic conditions. The treatment of arthritis includes the use of slow-acting and rapid-acting anti-inflammatory agents ranging from the gold salts to aspirin (see following listings). Long-term usage of these drugs can lead to numerous adverse effects including bone marrow suppression, platelet suppression, and oral ulcerations. The dentist should be aware that steroids (usually prednisone) are often prescribed together with the listed drugs and are often used in dosages sufficient to induce adrenal suppression. Adjustment of dosing prior to invasive dental procedures may be indicated along with consultation with the managing physician. Alteration of steroid dosage, usually increasing the steroid dosage prior to and during the stressful procedures and then gradually returning the patient to the original dosage over several days. Even in the absence of evidence of adrenal suppression, consultation with the prescribing physician for appropriate dosing and timing of procedures is advisable.

Antirheumatic, Disease Modifying

Gold Salts

Metabolic Inhibitor

Nonsteroidal Anti-inflammatory Agents

COX-2 Inhibitor NSAID

Celecoxib on page 275

Combination NSAID Product to Prevent GI Distress

Diclofenac and Misoprostol on page 417
Naproxen and Esomeprazole on page 961

Acetylated Salicylates

Aspirin on page 135

Other

Hydroxychloroquine on page 703
PredniSONE on page 1133

OSTEOPOROSIS MANAGEMENT

Prevalence

Osteoporosis effects 25 million Americans of which 80% are women; 27% of American women >80 years of age have osteopenia and 70% of American women >80 years of age have osteoporosis.

Consequences of Osteoporosis

1.3 million bone fractures annually (low impact/nontraumatic) and pain, pulmonary insufficiency, decreased quality of life, and economic costs; >250,000 hip fractures per year with a 20% mortality rate.

Risk Factors of Osteoporosis

Advanced age, female gender, chronic renal disease, hyperparathyroidism, Cushing's disease, hypogonadism/anorexia, hyperprolactinemia, cancer, large and prolonged dose heparin or glucocorticoids, anticonvulsants, hyperthyroidism (current or history, or excessive thyroid supplements), sedentary lifestyle, excessive exercise, early menopause, oophorectomy without hormone replacement, excessive aluminum-containing antacids, smoking, and methotrexate have all been at some time associated with risk of osteoporosis.

Diagnosis/Monitoring of Osteoporosis

DXA bone density, history of fracture (low impact or nontraumatic), compressed vertebrae, decreased height, hump-back appearance. Osteomark® urine assay measures bone breakdown fragments and may help assess therapy response earlier than DXA but diagnostic value is uncertain as Osteomark® does not reveal extent of bone loss. The clinician is referred to Osteonecrosis of the Jaw on page 1529 since the bisphosphonates are associated with this adverse event and its incidence associated with bisphosphonates for osteoporosis management is greater than previously estimated.

Prevention of Osteoporosis

1. Adequate dietary calcium (eg, dairy products)

2. Vitamin D (eg, fortified dairy products, cod, fatty fish)

3. Weight-bearing exercise (eg, walking) as tolerated

4. Fall prevention (eg, visual/hearing checks, minimizing pharmacologic agents that contribute to fall risk, checking environment for safety hazards)

5. Avoidance of tobacco use and excessive alcohol intake

6. Calcium: Adequate intake of at least 1200 mg **elemental** calcium daily in the form of dietary calcium or calcium supplementation, particularly women ≥50 years of age. Intakes exceeding 1200-1500 mg offer limited additional benefit and may increase the risk for cardiovascular disease or kidney stones. To minimize constipation add fiber and start with 500 mg/day for several months, then increase to 500 mg twice daily taken at different times than fiber. Chewable and liquid products are available. Calcium carbonate is given with food to enhance bioavailability. Calcium citrate may be given without regards to meals.

   • Contraindications: Hypercalcemia, ventricular fibrillation

   • Side effects: Constipation, anorexia

   • Drug interactions: Fiber, tetracycline, iron supplement, minerals

7. Vitamin D Supplement: Adequate intake of at least 800-1000 int. units of vitamin D for adults ≥50 years of age. Measuring serum vitamin D concentrations may be warranted, particularly in those at greatest risk for deficiency, to allow for the administration of vitamin D replacement. **Note:** Certain patients at risk for vitamin D deficiency (eg, elderly, diseases associated with malabsorption, chronic renal insufficiency) may require higher intakes. Some elderly, especially with significant renal or liver disease cannot metabolize (activate) vitamin D and require calcitriol 0.25 mcg orally twice daily or adjusted per serum calcium level, the active form of vitamin D.

   • Contraindications: Hypercalcemia (weakness, headache, drowsiness, nausea, diarrhea), hypercalciuria and renal stones

- Side effects (uncommon): Hypercalcemia (see above)
- Monitor 24-hour urine and serum calcium if using >1000 units/day

8. Bisphosphonates: Osteoporosis prevention: Postmenopausal Females:

- Alendronate: Oral: 5 mg once daily **or** 35 mg once weekly
- Ibandronate: Oral: 2.5 mg once daily **or** 150 mg once per month
- Risedronate: Oral: 5 mg once daily **or** 35 mg once weekly **or** one 75 mg tablet once daily on two consecutive days per month (total: 2 tablets/month) or 150 mg once per month
- Zoledronic acid (Reclast®): I.V.: 5 mg infused over at least 15 minutes every 2 years

9. Glucocorticoid-induced osteoporosis prevention: Males and Females:

- Alendronate: Oral: 5-10 mg once daily
- Risedronate: Oral: 5 mg once daily
- Zoledronic acid (Reclast®): I.V.: 5 mg every 12 months

10. Estrogen agonist/antagonist (previously known as selective estrogen receptor modulators):

- Postmenopausal Females: Raloxifene: Oral: 60 mg once daily; may be taken any time of the day without regard to meals but should be stopped 72 hours prior to or during immobilization due to risk of thromboembolic events.

11. Parathyroid hormone: Initial administration of teriparatide should occur under circumstances in which the patient may sit or lie down, in the event of orthostasis

- Glucocorticoid-induced osteoporosis prevention: Males and Females: Teriparatide: SubQ: 20 mcg once daily

12. Estrogens/hormone therapy: Should not be considered first agents for preventing osteoporosis due to increased risk of breast cancer, heart disease, stroke, and deep-vein thrombosis (DVT) found in the Women's Health Initiative study. Estrogens, as well as various combination therapies, including ethinyl estradiol and norethindrone (femhrt®) and estradiol and norgestimate (Prefest™), have been approved for the prevention of osteoporosis. The FDA recommends that approved nonestrogen treatments should be considered before the use of estrogen/hormone therapy for the sole purpose of prevention of osteoporosis. **Note:** In women with an intact uterus, administer estrogen with oral progesterone; unopposed estrogen can cause endometrial cancer.

13. Bone-modifying agent: Osteoporosis in postmenopausal female: Denosumab: SubQ: 60 mg once every 6 months. Also used to treat bone loss caused by specific cancers or treatments of specific cancers.

Treatment of Osteoporosis

1. Calcium, vitamin D, exercise, and estrogen: As above

2. Bisphosphonates: Oral bisphosphonates should be administered ≥30 minutes before first food or drink (except water) with 6-8 ounces tap water (**not** mineral water) and patients should remain upright (or raise head of bed to at least a 30° angle) to avoid ulcerative esophagitis. Consult individual monographs for details regarding use, precautions, dosing, and administration.

3. Fall prevention: Minimize psychoactive and cardiovascular drugs (monitor BP for orthostasis), give diuretics early in the day, environmental safety check.

	% Elemental Calcium	Elemental Calcium
Calcium gluconate (various)	9	500 mg = 45 mg
Calcium glubionate (Calcionate)	6.5	1.8 g = 115 g/5 mL
Calcium lactate (various)	13	325 mg = 42.25 mg
Calcium citrate (Citracal®)	21	950 mg = 200 mg
Effervescent tabs (Citracal Liquitab®)		2376 mg = 500 mg
Calcium acetate (Phos-Lo®)		667 mg = 169 mg
Calcium phosphate, tribasic (Posture®)	39	1565.2 mg = 600 mg
Calcium carbonate Tums®	40	1.2 g = 500 mg
Oral suspension		1.25 g/5 mL = 500 mg
Caltrate® 600		1.5 g = 600 mg

REFERENCES AND SELECTED READINGS

National Osteoporosis Foundation, "Clinician's Guide to Prevention and Treatment of Osteoporosis," Washington, DC, 2010. Available at http://www.nof.org/files/nof/public/content/file/344/upload/159.pdf
Singh JA, Furst DE, Bharat A, et al, "2012 Update of the 2008 American College of Rheumatology Recommendations for the Use of Disease-Modifying Antirheumatic Drugs and Biologic Agents in the Treatment of Rheumatoid Arthritis," *Arthritis Care Res (Hoboken)*, 2012, 64(5):625-39.

OSTEONECROSIS OF THE JAW

Osteonecrosis of the jaw (ONJ), which is relevant to the discussion of osteoporosis as well as Management of Patients Undergoing Cancer Therapy, on page 1596 is an uncommon condition that results in exposure of bone in the oral cavity. Other signs and symptoms may be associated with changes in bone metabolism and/or poor wound healing, but the condition can also develop spontaneously, such as along the mylohyoid ridge, away from teeth, or any site where acute or chronic trauma could have occurred.

Cases of ONJ began to emerge in approximately 2003 and were linked primarily with patients with cancer and those receiving the drugs zoledronic acid (Zometa®) and/or pamidronate (Aredia®) which are bisphosphonates administered by an intravenous route. Patients receiving a third intravenous bisphosphonate, clodronate (Bonefos®), appeared initially to develop this adverse reaction less frequently. Data has continued to emerge related to oral bisphosphonates and the risk of ONJ in patients who are receiving a significantly lower dosage of bisphosphonate via the oral route. Also refer to Management of Patients Undergoing Cancer Therapy on page 1596. The American Dental Association recently updated and clarified their guidelines (Hellstein, 2011). Some researchers are using the term antiresorptive osteonecrosis of the jaw (ARONJ) to report that other drugs, primarily denosumab, which is not a bisphosphonate, also is associated with exposed bone and delayed wound healing in the oral cavity. In this handbook, the acronym ONJ will continue to be used.

Bone disease occurs in many patients with cancer, particularly those with multiple myeloma and metastatic lesions associated with breast cancer, prostate cancer, and other cancers. These changes are often associated with pain and pathologic fractures. This bone destruction often results from changes in the osteoclast and osteoblast activities related to bone remodeling and healing following trauma. Bisphosphonates act at sites of active bone remodeling, changing the activity of the cells necessary for osteoclastic activity. There are no data that indicate that bisphosphonates directly change mineralization of the bone; however, these drugs do result in changes in the vascularity of the bone and cell activity.

Of the 2408 cases of bisphosphonate (BP)-associated ONJ published since 2003, BP therapy was used to treat malignancies in 89% and nonmalignant conditions in 11% (Filleul, 2010). Tooth extraction preceded 67% of the reported cases and 35% of these patients' cases resolved. The specific BP used was provided in 1694 of the cases. Eighty-eight percent of the patients received intravenous BP therapy, primarily zoledronic acid, and 12% received oral treatment, primarily alendronate (Fosamax®) (Filleul, 2010).

Orally Administered Bisphosphonates
Alendronate (Fosamax®) on page 59
Clodronate (Clasteon®) (Canada only) on page 327
Etidronate (Didronel®) on page 553
Ibandronate (Boniva®) on page 708
Risedronate (Actonel®) on page 1198
Tiludronate (Skelid®) on page 1325

The risk of developing ONJ in patients taking bisphosphonates or denosumab remains low with a prevalence of ~0.1% (1:1000) (Hellstein, 2011). The study also suggests that the benefits of using oral bisphosphonates to prevent osteoporosis significantly outweighs the risk of developing BP-associated ONJ, which can occur spontaneously. There are no diagnostic techniques to determine which patients are at increased risk of developing ONJ, though the risk is increased with procedures that increase bone trauma, particularly tooth extractions. Other factors that have been associated with increased risk are patients who are >65 years of age, periodontitis, use of bisphosphonates for >2 years, smoking, wearing dentures, and diabetes. The study makes the following recommendations in patients taking bisphosphonates or denosumab based on type of dental care (Hellstein, 2011):

- **General dentistry:** Inform patients of the risk of developing ONJ, but treatment should continue as planned.

- **Oral and maxillofacial surgery:** Inform patients of the risk of developing ONJ and discuss alternative treatment plans, including endodontic treatment, followed by removal of the clinical crown, allowing the roots to exfoliate rather than tooth extraction. Before and after any surgical procedures involving bone, patients should rinse with chlorhexidine twice daily for 4-8 weeks after surgery. In addition, antibiotic prophylaxis starting one day before the procedure and for 3-7 days after may be effective in preventing ONJ.

- **Restorative dentistry and prosthodontics:** There is no evidence that malocclusion or masticatory forces increase the risk of developing ONJ. Treatment should continue as planned.

- **Orthodontics:** Reports have shown an increase in tooth movement in patients taking bisphosphonates; patients should be advised of this potential complication; the duration of orthodontic treatment may be prolonged and uniform tooth movement may be compromised.

- **Implant placement and maintenance:** Bisphosphonate treatment does not impact implant placement or maintenance, except in extensive cases; treatment should continue as planned.

- **Management of periodontal disease:** Patients who have active periodontal disease should receive appropriate forms of nonsurgical therapy. There is no evidence that periodontal procedures, such as guided tissue regeneration or bone replacement grafts, increase the risk of developing ONJ.

- **Endodontics:** Endodontic treatment is preferable to surgical manipulation if the tooth is salvageable. Limited evidence shows that periapical healing after endodontic therapy is similar regardless of bisphosphonate use.

◀ **FREQUENTLY ASKED QUESTIONS**

According to the latest literature, what is the incidence of ONJ in oral bisphosphonates users?

Presently, the current estimates of the frequency of occurrence of ONJ in oral bisphosphonate users are the following: Merck drug company, the manufacturer of Fosamax® calculated the incidence of ONJ to be 0.7 cases per 100,000 person-years of exposure to oral bisphosphonates. The Medical Consultants of Consumer Reports On-Health Bulletin reported an incidence of one case for every 20,000 users of oral bisphosphonates (0.005%). A recent report from Australia estimated that the frequency of ONJ in osteoporotic patients mainly on weekly oral alendronate (Fosamax®) ranged from a minimum of 1 in 8470 to a maximum of 1 in 2260 (0.01% to 0.04%) patients. If extractions were performed, the frequency increased to 0.09% to 0.34%. The risk of developing ONJ in patients taking bisphosphonates or denosumab remains low with a prevalence of ~0.1% (1:1000) (Hellstein, 2011).

What numbers can practitioners use to tell the dental patient their risk of developing ONJ with oral bisphosphonates?

The recommendations from the Expert Panel of the American Dental Association suggest that the patient be informed that there is a very low risk of developing ONJ. The true risk posed by oral bisphosphonates remains uncertain, but appears to be very small. All the data seem to point to a risk of ~0.1% of total users and that the risk increases with dental extractions to ~0.3%. The risks of developing ONJ can be minimized but never totally eliminated. Good oral hygiene along with regular dental care is the best way to lower the risk of developing ONJ. The current data on incidence of ONJ in patients taking oral bisphosphonates is retrospective information derived primarily from surveys and the number of reported cases in patients taking the drugs. More meaningful assessment of incidence of ONJ in the population at risk must come from prospective cohort investigations.

Is the risk of acquiring osteonecrosis of the jaw bone diminished with the use of other oral bisphosphonates compared to Fosamax®?

In addition to alendronate (Fosamax®), cases of ONJ, albeit rare, have been reported in patients taking either risedronate (Actonel®) or ibandronate (Boniva®). Among the class of oral bisphosphonates, more cases have been associated with Fosamax® than with Actonel® or Boniva®. Also, there is no evidence to suggest that the risk of ONJ is less when taking monthly doses of Boniva®. Zoledronic acid under the band name of Reclast® has recently been approved as a once-annual, 15-minute intravenous infusion of a dose of 5 mg to prevent osteoporosis. This dosing was associated with a significant improvement in bone mineral density and bone metabolism markers. It is unknown whether this dosing schedule places the patient at risk for ONJ; however, data do show a higher risk of serious atrial fibrillation in patients receiving Reclast® compared to patients receiving placebo.

Will Fosamax® or the other oral bisphosphonates continue to be the standard treatment for osteoporosis?

Yes. The oral bisphosphonates continue to be the most effective class of drugs in reducing the risk of osteoporotic fractures and are the first-line therapy in the treatment of osteoporosis. Fosamax® has been shown to prevent bone loss at the spine and hip in postmenopausal women and to reduce fractures by ~50%. Risedronate (Actonel®) produced a 30% reduction in hip fractures. Fosamax® continues to be in the top 50 of the most widely prescribed drugs in the U.S.

Do we know the pathogenesis of ONJ?

This question has not been answered and information is only speculative at this time. Osteoporosis can occur due to age-related changes in the number of osteoclasts and bone resorption sites. This overwhelms the production of new bone by osteoblasts and a decrease in bone mass occurs. By inhibiting osteoclastic activity, the oral bisphosphonates seemingly arrest the osteoporotic syndrome. In the process, however, the maxilla and mandible, upon continued exposure to the bisphosphonates, exhibit delayed wound healing following injury from mechanical forces or invasive surgery, such as tooth extraction. This coupled with the antiangiogenic effect (ie, a reduction in bone blood supply by the bisphosphonates) may contribute to jaw bone necrosis. Ruggiero and Drew have suggested that a preferential deposition of the bisphosphonates in the mandible and maxilla may contribute to the necrosis appearing within the jaw rather than within bones outside the craniofacial skeleton.

What are the factors that increase the risk of ONJ in oral bisphosphonate users?

Patients with a history of periodontal disease and dental abscesses are at increased risk of developing ONJ if taking oral bisphosphonates. Also, dentoalveolar trauma will increase the risk. The use of chronic steroids such as prednisone has been identified as a risk factor. Other factors are periodontitis, smoking, wearing dentures, diabetes, and the duration of exposure and age, with longer treatment regimens and age >65 years associated with a greater risk of developing the disease (Hellstein, 2011). Patients identified with jaw bone necrosis typically were exposed to oral bisphosphonates for 2 years or longer.

What are the symptoms that an oral bisphosphonates patient would experience which could indicate necrotic jaw bone?

Tooth mobility, mucosal swelling, and/or ulceration. Clinical symptoms would include a nonhealing extraction site, exposed bone surrounded by inflamed soft tissue, and purulent discharge at site of exposed bone. Exposed bone is usually more prevalent in areas such as the tori and the mylohyoid ridge.

What kind of dental procedures can be performed in oral bisphosphonate users with no increase in risk for ONJ?

According to the American Dental Association, all routine procedures can be carried out. Routine dental treatment should not be modified on the basis of oral bisphosphonate use. However, the presence of risk factors, such as steroid use, >65 years of age, or prolonged exposure to oral bisphosphonates, may require consultation with an expert in metabolic bone disease prior to routine dental treatment.

Is dentoalveolar surgery contraindicated in Fosamax® users?

According to both Ruggiero et al, and Marx et al, no alteration or delay in planned surgery is typically necessary in patients taking an oral bisphosphonate for <3 years and having no other risk factors for ONJ. In asymptomatic patients receiving oral bisphosphonate therapy, dentoalveolar surgery is not contraindicated. Also surgery common to periodontists and other dental providers need not be delayed.

In addition, Marx suggested that if dental implants are placed, informed consent should be obtained related to the potential for implant failure and possible ONJ if the patient continues to take an oral bisphosphonate.

Is a so-called "drug holiday" an effective way to reduce the risks of ONJ?

Although a "drug holiday" would seem logical and has been suggested by some groups, there is no statistically significant evidence indicating in the cancer patient population that this is beneficial in reducing ONJ risk and in fact may be detrimental if the chance of a skeletal related event increases. The data in oral bisphosphonates use are even less compelling since the incidence is so low to begin with that subjective drug holidays can not be documented with any degree of confidence. As mentioned earlier, for individuals who have taken a bisphosphonate for <3 years and have no other risk factors for ONJ, no alteration or delay in the planned surgery is recommended, but the caveat is that the risk remains unknown.

In patients about to begin oral bisphosphonate therapy, should the bisphosphonate be delayed until dental health is optimized?

No. It does not appear necessary for patients to initiate prophylactic dental treatment prior to initiating oral bisphosphonate therapy for osteoporosis. It would be prudent, however, to encourage these patients to maintain an optimal level of dental health.

Is diagnostic imaging useful in assessing oral bisphosphonate individuals at risk for ONJ?

Imaging modalities have proved helpful in determining the extent of existing necrotic process, but have not been able to demonstrate any efficacy in assessing patients at risk for ONJ. It has been reported that panoramic and periapical radiographs probably will not reveal significant changes in early stages of osteonecrosis and they are poor screening tools for prediction. Computerized tomography (CT) scan also has not proved helpful with early identification of osteonecrosis in asymptomatic patients.

Do the Fosamax®-type drugs increase the risk of ONJ in patients receiving dental implants?

A conclusive cause and effect relationship between bisphosphonate therapy and ONJ still has not been established. Evidence does suggest, however, that such an association may exist, particularly with intravenous bisphosphonate use in cancer patients. Oral bisphosphonates are widely used for the treatment of osteoporosis. It is estimated that 22-30 million prescriptions were written for alendronate (Fosamax®), the most widely used oral bisphosphonate in the United States, between May 2003 and April 2004. For many years, dental implants have been placed in many patients taking oral bisphosphonates. Prior to the reports on the risk of bisphosphonate-associated ONJ, these patients were treated without any modification of the surgically placed implant procedure. Recently, however, guidelines from the American Dental Association (ADA) and the American Association of Oral and Maxillofacial Surgeons (AAOMS) have suggested a cautious approach to implant surgery and extractions for patients receiving bisphosphonate therapy.

Regarding dental implants, the ADA report cautions practitioners that patients may be at increased risk of developing osteonecrosis of the jaw bone when extensive implant placement or guided bone regeneration is necessary.

If dental implants are to be placed, the AAOMS Task Force suggested contacting the physician who prescribed the oral bisphosphonate prior to surgery to suggest an alternate dosing schedule, a drug holiday (discontinuance of the drug for a short time period), or an alternative to bisphosphonate therapy. It is important to remember that any beneficial or detrimental effects of these drug holidays have not been prospectively studied.

In addition, Marx has suggested the following precautions. Dental implant, if elected, can be placed in the patient about to begin oral bisphosphonate therapy. However, informed consent concerning the potential for implant loss and/or exposed bone related to the bisphosphonates should be obtained as the patient continues bisphosphonate therapy and exceeds 3 years of continuous use. For individuals who have taken an oral bisphosphonate for <3 years and have no clinical or radiographic risk factors, no alteration or delay is necessary for planned dental surgeries. If dental implants are placed, inform consent should be obtained related to the potential for implant failure and possible ONJ if the patient continues to take the bisphosphonate.

For patients who have taken an oral bisphosphonates for >3 years, it is advised that the prescribing physician be contacted and a recommendation made to discontinue the oral bisphosphonate for 3 months prior to the procedure and refrain from reinstating use until 3 months after the procedure.

One report from the UK suggested an even more conservative approach. Scully et al, suggested that where possible, extractions should be avoided in patients receiving oral bisphosphonates and it is best to avoid all elective surgery in these patients including endosseous implant placement or treatment should be performed well in advance prior to bisphosphonate therapy. If surgery is performed on patients taking bisphosphonates, they must be counseled about the risk.

A new report showed that implant surgery on patients receiving Fosamax®-type drugs did not result in bisphosphonate-associated ONJ. This study, out of the Dentistry/Oral Surgery Group at Montefiore Medical Center, Albert Einstein College of Medicine, reported that of 115 patients taking oral bisphosphonates, none showed evidence or had symptoms of osteonecrosis after implant placement. This report had findings similar to a previous report by Dr Jeffcoat, who showed success in implant placement and no signs of necrosis in patients taking oral bisphosphonates.

The Montefiore study, by Grant et al, used a survey to collect information from patients who had received dental implants and were taking oral bisphosphonates. The study, reported in the *Journal of Oral and Maxillofacial Surgery*, identified 1319 female patients >40 years of age who had implant surgery between January 1998 and December 2006. A survey was mailed to each of these individuals asking about current and past use of oral bisphosphonates. Of the 1319 surveys mailed out, 458 (35%) were returned. From those returned, 115 individuals reported taking oral bisphosphonates before or after implant surgery. None reported receiving intravenous bisphosphonates. In this population, it was then determined that a total of 468 implants had been placed in the 115 individuals. This population that responded to the survey was then compared to a random sample of individuals who did not respond with regard to age and number of implants. It was found that only five among 100 nonresponders to the survey had a history of bisphosphonate use compared to the 115 of the 458 responders. The remaining 343 patients indicated that they had not received bisphosphonate therapy. From the pool of 458 responders, there were 1450 implants placed in these patients and 1436 had integrated successfully. Implant success was defined using criteria which included the absence of symptoms such as pain, infection, paresthesia, or neuropathies and that the dental implant should provide functional service for 5 years in 75% of the cases.

The results were the following:

1. None of the 458 responders to the survey reported symptoms of bisphosphonate-associated ONJ.

2. Since 115 of the 458 responders indicated they were treated with bisphosphonates, it was assumed that none of the 115 responders treated with bisphosphonates had ONJ.

3. Out of the pool of 115 patients, there was a total of 468 implants placed. It was found that 466 of those implants were in function and were considered successful. Only two implants failed. In one case of failure, the patient had taken oral bisphosphonates for 3 years prior to implant placement but no longer was taking any drug at the time of implant placement or thereafter. The investigators removed and replaced the implant and it was still in function for more than 4 years. In the second case, the patient had been taking bisphosphonates for more than 8 years and the failure occurred in one implant out of a total of 13 in place. The failed implant was removed, not replaced, and the area healed uneventfully.

4. There were no reports of ONJ from any of the 861 patients who did not return the survey.

This report from Montefiore is consistent with that of the findings of Jeffcoat. She also reported success in implant placement and no signs of necrosis in patients taking oral bisphosphonates. Her method was a single blind controlled study using 50 postmenopausal female dental implant patients. Twenty-five had taken oral bisphosphonates for 1-4 years and the other 25 patients did not take oral bisphosphonates prior to or during the study. In the bisphosphonate group, there was a total of 102 implants that were placed and in the nondrug group, there were 108 implants that were placed. After 3 years, there was 100% success rate with no evidence of infection, pain, or necrosis in patients receiving bisphosphonates. There was 99.2% success rate in the group not taking oral bisphosphonates.

A further review of the literature found only two cases of dental implant failure associated with oral bisphosphonate use. One was a case report from 1995 that suggested that failure of five implants was caused by bisphosphonate therapy. In that case, five implants were placed and successfully integrated in the mandible. The patient then began bisphosphonate therapy 28 months after implant placement and after 4 months, a panoramic radiograph revealed osteolysis around all implants and all five were removed one month later.

In the report by Wang et al, a patient developed a significant bone defect with necrosis after proper implant placement. The patient was a 65-year old female who had taken Fosamax® for 10 years. She received five implants in the mandible. Ten days after surgery, healing appeared to be progression uneventfully. Four weeks later upon evaluation, bone defects were observed and noted around two of the implants. The defects were repaired with mineralized human cancellous bone mixed with tetracycline and covered with collagen membrane. Eventually after some further antibiotics and chlorhexidine daily rinsing, complete uneventful healing occurred.

Is the CTX bone marker useful to assess the risk of ONJ in oral bisphosphonate users?

CTX is an acronym for C-terminal telopeptide. During bone resorption, the dominant type 1 collagen is degraded and, during this collagen breakdown, the telopeptide (CTX) is released. Thus, serum levels of CTX can be used as an indicator of bone breakdown/resorption. The CTX blood test, as a risk marker for ONJ, first proposed by Marx in 2007, was used in an Australian study to determine its effectiveness in the prevention and management of ONJ in patient taking bisphosphonates. Essentially, this test was found to be able to identify groups of those individuals in the "risk zone" for developing ONJ, which was defined as a blood level of 150 picograms/mL (pg/mL) to 200 picograms/mL (pg/mL). It was, however, not found to be predictive of the development of ONJ in any individual patient. The CTX test requires a 1 mL sample of whole blood drawn in the morning in fasted individuals. Marx used Quest Diagnostics Nichols East Lab in San Juan Capistrano California to perform the analysis on the samples. Values lower than 100 pg/mL were correlated with a high risk of ONJ; values between 100 pg/mL and 150 pg/mL correlated to a moderate risk and values >150 pg/mL associated with minimal or no risk. According to Ruggiero and Drew, low bone turnover in the jaw due to osteoclastic inhibition by bisphosphonates results in the inability of the bone to repair local microdamage from normal mechanical loading or injury. This ultimately results in bone necrosis. Thus, individuals with low CTX values while taking bisphosphonates are assumed to have jaw bones which may not be able to normally repair themselves and these individuals would have a relatively higher risk of developing ONJ compared to individuals having higher CTX serum values.

Rigorous prospective studies on greater numbers of individuals are required before the use of the CTX serum test could be suggested with any confidence. In 2011, the American Dental Association (ADA) reaffirmed its earlier position that CTX cannot be recommended as a predictive tool for ONJ risk assessment.

Are there other bone markers that may be useful?

Researchers have been seeking screening tools to predict and allow prevention of ONJ. A recent study by the Memorial Sloan-Kettering Cancer Center of New York investigated specific bone turnover markers as predictive models to assess risks of ONJ in patients exposed to bisphosphonates (Morris, 2012). This retrospective study showed that N-telopeptide of type-I collagen (NTX) and bone-specific alkaline phosphatase (BAP) did not predict for the development of ONJ. No significant trend for either biomarker was detected. Thus, to date, there is insufficient evidence to recommend the use of serum tests as predictors of ONJ.

Do the new anti-RANK-L drugs such as denosumab (Prolia™, Xgeva®) increase the risk of ONJ?

ONJ has been reported in clinical studies in patients receiving denosumab at FDA-approved doses for osteoporosis. In clinical studies, patients with advanced cancer treated with 120 mg denosumab administered monthly, have reported a 2% incidence of ONJ. Known risk factors for ONJ include a diagnosis of cancer with bone lesions, concomitant therapies (eg, chemotherapy, antiangiogenic biologics, corticosteroids, radiotherapy to the head and neck), poor oral hygiene, dental extractions, comorbid disorders (eg, pre-existing dental disease, anaemia, coagulopathy, infection) and previous treatment with bisphosphonates.

A dental examination with appropriate preventive dentistry should be considered prior to initiating denosumab treatment in patients with concomitant risk factors. These patients should avoid invasive dental procedures if possible during treatment with denosumab. Patients should maintain good oral hygiene during treatment. For patients who develop ONJ while on denosumab therapy, dental surgery may exacerbate the condition. Use clinical judgement and guide the management plan of each patient based on individual risk:benefit evaluation.

Denosumab on page 389

CLINICAL DENTAL MANAGEMENT CONSIDERATIONS

Suggested Preventive Dentistry Before Initiating Chemotherapy, Immunotherapy, or Antiresorptive Therapy

- Remove abscessed and nonrestorable teeth and teeth with severe periodontal disease involvement
- Remove teeth with poor long-term prognosis
- Functionally rehabilitate salvageable dentition, including endodontic therapy
- Perform dental prophylaxis, caries control, and stabilizing restorative dental care
- Examine dentures to ensure proper fit (dentures should be removed at night)
- Educate patients on oral self-care hygiene

Patients at Risk of ONJ Due to Antiresorptive Therapy (Without Any Signs of ONJ):

Invasive dental procedures should be avoided in patients receiving intravenous bisphosphonate therapy. These procedures should also be performed ideally prior to a patient starting bisphosphonate I.V. therapy. The treating physician should guide the management plan of each patient based on individual benefit:risk assessment and communication with the dentist. For patients requiring dental procedures, there are no prospective data available to suggest whether discontinuation of bisphosphonate treatment reduces the risk of ONJ.

There are five primary actions in this management plan:

1. Patients should be educated on maintaining excellent oral hygiene to reduce the risk of need for invasive procedures in the future.
2. Patients should check and adjust removable appliances such as prostheses to avoid soft tissue injury.
3. Routine cleaning should be performed with care, attempting to reduce any soft tissue injury; however, since hygiene is important, the normal recall planning and treatment should continue.
4. Dental infection should be managed aggressively and nonsurgically when possible. Alternatives such as endodontic therapy or over extraction may be advisable.
5. Endodontic therapy is preferable to extractions; treatment with endodontics followed by coronal amputation and root canal therapy on the retained roots may be necessary.

If a Patient Develops Osteonecrosis of the Jaw: Consultations between oral surgeons/dental oncologists and the treating physician are strongly recommended:

- A nonsurgical approach is recommended to prevent further osseous injury.
- Only minimal bony debridement to reduce sharp and rough surfaces to prevent further trauma to adjacent or opposing tissues is recommended.
- A removable appliance or protective stent may be used to protect exposed bone or adjacent tissues.

- Before discontinuing bisphosphonate therapy, patient should be evaluated for potential risk of further osteonecrosis versus the risk of skeletal complications.

- Hyperbaric oxygen therapy is not recommended.

- Biopsy is not recommended unless metastasis to the jaw is suspected.

- Cultures should be taken for directed antimicrobial therapy.

- Prophylactic antibiotic therapy may be considered for pain and disease control.

SAMPLE PRESCRIPTIONS FOR PROPHYLACTIC ANTIBIOTIC THERAPY

Rx:
Amoxicillin 875 mg tablets
Disp: 60 tablets
Sig: Take 1 tablet twice daily

Note: Alternatively, 500 mg tablet 3 times daily can be prescribed and may be continued for >1 month. Patients should be cautioned regarding gastrointestinal side effects with long-term use of any antibiotic. Probiotics may help but evidence is conflicted on true efficacy.

Rx:
Clindamycin (Systemic) 300 mg capsules
Disp: 40 capsules
Sig: Take 1 capsule 3 or 4 times/day for 7-10 days

Note: Prescription usually selected for patients allergic to penicillin; may be prescribed for 3 or 4 times/day. This prescription can be continued for >1 month; however, risk of *Clostridium difficile* colitis increases. Patients should be cautioned to take clindamycin with food and monitor for gastrointestinal side effects with long-term use. Probiotics may help but evidence is conflicted on true efficacy.

Rx:
Chlorhexidine Oral Rinse
Disp: 1 bottle
Sig: Rinse with 20 cc twice daily for 30 seconds and expectorate

ONJ Diagnosis and Definition

- Intraoral pain is variable

- Complaint of roughness along the teeth or ridge

- History of dental procedures eg, extractions, but may occur on tissues

- Complaint of ill-fitting denture(s)

- Diagnosis made clinically with presence of exposed bone in maxillofacial region (>8 weeks duration [with no history of radiation therapy])

- If the presence of exposed bone in maxillofacial region is noted but is <8 weeks duration (with no history of radiation therapy), the clinician must consider a differential diagnosis of:

  - Spontaneous lingual mandibular sequestration with ulceration

  - Trauma

  - Advanced periodontal disease with dehiscence

  - Local malignancy

  - Metastatic cancer

REFERENCES AND SELECTED READINGS

Advisory Task Force on Bisphosphonate-Related Osteonecrosis of the Jaws, American Association of Oral and Maxillofacial Surgeons, "American Association of Oral and Maxillofacial Surgeons Position Paper on Bisphosphonate-Related Osteonecrosis of the Jaws," *J Oral Maxillofac Surg*, 2007, 65(3):369-76.

Aghaloo TL, Felsenfeld AL, and Tetradis S, "Osteonecrosis of the Jaw in a Patient on Denosumab," *J Oral Maxillofac Surg*, 2010, 68(5):959-63.

Almubarak H, Jones A, Chaisuparat R, et al, "Zoledronic Acid Directly Suppresses Cell Proliferation and Induces Apoptosis in Highly Tumorigenic Prostate and Breast Cancers," *J Carcinog*, 2011, 10:2.

American Dental Association Council on Scientific Affairs, "Dental Management of Patients Receiving Oral Bisphosphonate Therapy: Expert Panel Recommendations," *J Am Dent Assoc*, 2006, 137(8):1144-50.

Badros A, Weikel D, Salama A, et al, "Osteonecrosis of the Jaw in Multiple Myeloma Patients: Clinical Features and Risk Factors," *J Clin Oncol*, 2006, 24(6):945-52.

Filleul O, Crompot E, and Saussez S, "Bisphosphonate-Induced Osteonecrosis of the Jaw: A Review of 2,400 Patient Cases," *J Cancer Res Clin Oncol*, 2010, 136(8):1117-24.

Grant BT, Amenedo C, Freeman K, et al, "Outcomes of Placing Dental Implants in Patients Taking Oral Bisphosphonates: A Review of 115 Cases," *J Oral Maxillofac Surg*, 2008, 66(2):223-30.

Hellstein JW, Adler RA, Edwards B, et al, "Managing the Care of Patients Receiving Antiresorptive Therapy for Prevention and Treatment of Osteoporosis: Executive Summary of Recommendations From the American Dental Association Council on Scientific Affairs," *J Am Dent Assoc*, 2011, 142(11):1243-51. Available at http://www.ada.org/sections/professionalResources/pdfs/topics_ARONJ_report.pdf. Accessed Nov. 25, 2011.

Kyrgidis A and Toulis KA, "Denosumab-Related Osteonecrosis of the Jaws," *Osteoporos Int*, 2011, 22(1):369-70.

Marx RE, Cillo JE Jr, and Ulloa JJ, "Oral Bisphosphonate-Induced Osteonecrosis: Risk Factors, Prediction of Risk Using Serum CTX Testing, Prevention, and Treatment," *J Oral Maxillofac Surg*, 2007, 65(12):2397-410.

Marx RE, *Oral and Intravenous Bisphosphonate-Induced Osteonecrosis of the Jaws: History, Etiology, Prevention and Treatment*, Chicago, IL: Quintessence Publishing Company, 2007, 87-91.

Marx RE, Sawatari Y, Fortin M, et al, "Bisphosphonate-Induced Exposed Bone (Osteonecrosis/Osteopetrosis) of the Jaws: Risk Factors, Recognition, Prevention, and Treatment," *J Oral Maxillofac Surg*, 2005, 63(11):1567-75.

Mavrokokki T, Cheng A, Stein B, et al, "Nature and Frequency of Bisphosphonate-Associated Osteonecrosis of the Jaws in Australia," *J Oral Maxillofac Surg*, 2007, 65(3):415-23.

Migliorati CA, Casiglia J, Epstein J, et al, "Managing the Care of Patients With Bisphosphonate-Associated Osteonecrosis: An American Academy of Oral Medicine Position Paper," *J Am Dent Assoc*, 2005, 136(12):1658-68.

Morris PG, Fazio M, Farooki A, et al, "Serum N-Telopeptide and Bone-Specific Alkaline Phosphatase Levels in Patients With Osteonecrosis of the Jaw Receiving Bisphosphonates for Bone Metastases," *J Oral Maxillofac Surg*, 2012, 70(12):2768-75.

Ruggiero S, Gralow J, Marx RE, "Practical Guidelines for the Prevention, Diagnosis, and Treatment of Osteonecrosis of the Jaw in Patients With Cancer," *J Oncol Pract*, 2006, 2(1):7-14.

Ruggiero SL and Drew SJ, "Osteonecrosis of the Jaws and Bisphosphonate Therapy," *J Dent Res*, 2007, 86(11):1013-21.

Ruggiero SL, Dodson TB, Assael LA, et al, "American Association of Oral and Maxillofacial Surgeons Position Paper on Bisphosphonate-Related Osteonecrosis of the Jaw – 2009 Update," *Aust Endod J*, 2009, 35(3):119-30.

Ruggiero SL, Fantasia J, and Carlson E, "Bisphosphonate-Related Osteonecrosis of the Jaw: Background and Guidelines for Diagnosis, Staging and Management," *Oral Surg Oral Med Oral Pathol Oral Radiol Endod*, 2006, 102(4):433-41.

Ruggiero SL, Mehrotra B, Rosenberg TJ, et al, "Osteonecrosis of the Jaws Associated With the Use of Bisphosphonates: A Review of 63 Cases," *J Oral Maxillofac Surg*, 2004, 62(5):527-34.

Scheper MA, Badros A, Chaisuparat R, et al, "Effect of Zoledronic Acid on Oral Fibroblasts and Epithelial Cells: A Potential Mechanism of Bisphosphonate-Associated Osteonecrosis," *Br J Haematol*, 2009, 144(5):667-76.

Scheper MA, Badros A, Salama AR, et al, "A Novel Bioassay Model to Determine Clinically Significant Bisphosphonate Levels," *Support Care Cancer*, 2009, 17(12):1553-7.

Scheper M, Chaisuparat R, Cullen K, et al, "A Novel Soft-Tissue *in vitro* Model for Bisphosphonate-Associated Osteonecrosis," *Fibrogenesis Tissue Repair*, 2010, 3:6.

Scully C, Madrid C, and Bagan J, "Dental Endosseous Implants in Patients on Bisphosphonate Therapy," *Implant Dent*, 2006, 15(3):212-8.

Taylor KH, Middlefell LS, and Mizen KD, "Osteonecrosis of the Jaws Induced by Anti-RANK Ligand Therapy," *Br J Oral Maxillofac Surg*, 2010, 48(3):221-3.

Wang HL, Weber D, and McCauley LK, "Effect of Long-Term Oral Bisphosphonates on Implant Wound Healing: Literature Review and a Case Report," *J Periodontol*, 2007, 78(3):584-94.

SEXUALLY-TRANSMITTED DISEASES

Sexually transmitted diseases (STDs) represent a group of infectious diseases that include bacterial, fungal, and viral etiologies. Several related infections are covered elsewhere. Several viral STDs can be effectively prevented through vaccination with widely available vaccines, including hepatitis A, hepatitis B, and human papilloma virus vaccines. Human papilloma virus is widespread and serotypes 16 and 18 have been associated with cervical cancer. Although most types that cause oral HPV lesions are not of these serotypes, the clinician should recommend appropriate surgical removal of all such lesions. Lesions in the posterior oral pharyngeal region are of particular concern. Pre-exposure vaccination is one of the most effective methods for preventing transmission of some STDs. Quadrivalent HPV vaccine (Gardasil®) and the bivalent HPV vaccine (Cervarix®) are available for females 9-26 years of age to prevent cervical precancer and cancer. Routine vaccination for females 11-12 years of age is recommended with either vaccine. A catch-up vaccination for females 13-26 years of age is also recommended. Gardasil® can be administered to males 9-26 years of age to prevent genital warts. Details regarding HPV vaccination are available at www.cdc.gov/std/hpv. Vaccines for other STDs (eg, HIV and herpes simplex virus) are under development or undergoing clinical trials. Vaccines are not available for bacterial or fungal STDs.

The management of a patient with an STD begins with identification. Paramount to the correct management of patients with a history of gonorrhea or syphilis is when the condition was diagnosed, how and with what agent it was treated, did the condition recur, and are there any residual signs and symptoms potentially indicating active or recurrent disease. With standard/universal precautions, the patient with *Neisseria gonorrhoea* or *Treponema pallidum* infection poses little threat to the dentist; however, diagnosis of oral lesions may be problematic. Gonococcal pharyngitis, primary syphilitic lesions (chancre), secondary syphilitic lesions (mucous patch), and tertiary lesions (gumma) may be identified by the dentist. All patients who have gonorrhea should also be tested for other STDs, including chlamydia, syphilis, and HIV. Most gonococcal infections of the pharynx are asymptomatic and can be relatively common in some populations. Gonococcal infections of the pharynx are more difficult to eradicate than urogenital and anorectal infections. Few antimicrobial regimens, including those involving oral cephalosporins, can reliably cure >90% of gonococcal pharyngeal infections. Chlamydial coinfection of the pharynx is unusual; however, because coinfection at genital sites sometimes occurs, treatment for both gonorrhea and chlamydia is recommended.

Gonorrhea is the second most commonly reported bacterial STD. The majority of urethral infections caused by *N. gonorrhoeae* among men produce symptoms that cause them to seek curative treatment soon enough to prevent serious sequelae, but treatment may not be soon enough to prevent transmission to others. Among women, gonococcal infections may not produce recognizable symptoms until complications (eg, pelvic inflammatory disease [PID]) have occurred. PID can result in tubal scarring that can lead to infertility or ectopic pregnancy. Treatment of uncomplicated gonococcal infections of the cervix, urethra, and rectum include ceftriaxone, cefixime, azithromycin, and doxycycline.

Chlamydial genital infection is the most frequently reported infectious disease in the United States and is found more commonly in patients ≤25 years of age. Several important sequelae can result from *C. trachomatous* infection in women including PID, infertility, and ectopic pregnancy. Chlamydia treatment should be provided promptly for all patients testing positive for infection. Coinfection with *C. trachomatous* frequently occurs among patients who have gonococcal infection; therefore, concurrent treatment for both infections is recommended. Chlamydial infections can be treated with azithromycin or doxycycline. Alternative treatments include erythromycin, levofloxacin, or ofloxacin (systemic). If treating gonorrhea concurrently, would not consider use of a fluoroquinolone as resistance is high.

DRUGS USED IN TREATMENT OF CHLAMYDIA, GONORRHEA/SYPHILIS INCLUDE:

Azithromycin (Systemic) on page 158
Cefixime on page 266
CefTRIAXone on page 273
Doxycycline on page 456
Penicillin G Benzathine on page 1065
Penicillin G (Parenteral/Aqueous) on page 1065

The drugs listed above are often used alone or in stepped regimens, particularly when there is concomitant *Chlamydia* infection or when there is evidence of disseminated disease. The proper treatment for syphilis depends on the state of the disease.

REFERENCES AND SELECTED READINGS

Centers for Disease Control and Prevention (CDC), "Update to CDC's Sexually Transmitted Diseases Treatment Guidelines, 2006: Fluoroquinolones No Longer Recommended for Treatment of Gonococcal Infections," *MMWR Morb Mortal Wkly Rep*, 2007, 56(14):332-6.
Centers for Disease Control and Prevention (CDC), "Update to CDC's Sexually Transmitted Diseases Treatment Guidelines, 2010: Oral Cephalosporins No Longer a Recommended Treatment for Gonococcal Infections," *MMWR Morb Mortal Wkly Rep*, 2012, 61(31):590-4.
Little JW, "Syphilis: An Update," *Oral Surg Oral Med Oral Pathol Oral Radiol Endod*, 2005, 100(1):3-9.
Miller WC and Zenilman JM, "Epidemiology of Chlamydial Infection, Gonorrhea, and Trichomoniasis in the United States-2005," *Infect Dis Clin North Am*, 2005, 19(2):281-96.
Workowski KA, Berman S, and Centers for Disease Control and Prevention (CDC), "Sexually Transmitted Diseases Treatment Guidelines, 2010," *MMWR Recomm Rep*, 2010, 59(RR-12):1-110. Available at http://www.cdc.gov/std/treatment/2010/STD-Treatment-2010-RR5912.pdf

SYSTEMIC VIRAL DISEASES

HEPATITIS

The hepatitis viruses are a group of DNA and RNA viruses that produce symptoms associated with inflammation of the liver. Currently, hepatitis A through G have been identified by immunological testing; however, hepatitis A through E have received most attention in terms of disease identification. Recently, there has been increased interest in hepatitis viruses F and G, particularly as related to healthcare professionals. Our knowledge is expanding rapidly in this area and the clinician should be alert to changes in the literature that might update their knowledge. Hepatitis F, for instance, remains a diagnosis of exclusion, effectively being non-A, B, C, D, E, or G. Hepatitis G has serologic testing available; however, it is not commercially at this time. Research evaluations of various antibody and RT-PCR tests for hepatitis G are under development at this time.

Signs and symptoms of viral hepatitis in general are quite variable. Patients infected may range from asymptomatic to experiencing flu-like symptoms only. In addition, fever, nausea, joint muscle pain, jaundice, and hepatomegaly along with abdominal pain can result from infection with one of the hepatitis viruses. The virus also can create an acute or chronic infection. Usually following these early symptoms or the asymptomatic period, the patient may recover or may go on to develop chronic liver dysfunction. Liver dysfunction may be represented primarily by changes in liver function tests known as LFTs and these primarily include aspartate aminotransferase known as AST and alanine aminotransferase known as ALT. In addition, for A, B, C, D, and E, there are serologic tests for either antigen, antibody, or both. Of hepatitis A through G, five forms have both acute and chronic forms whereas A and E appear to only create acute disease. There are differences in the way clinicians may approach a known postexposure to one of the hepatitis viruses. In many instances, gamma globulin may be used; however, the indications for gamma globulin as a drug limit their use to several of the viruses only. The dental clinician should be aware that the gastroenterologist may choose to give gamma globulin off-label.

Hepatitis A

Hepatitis A virus is an enteric virus that is a member of the Picornavirus family along with Coxsackie viruses and poliovirus. Previously known as infectious hepatitis, hepatitis A has been detected in humans for centuries. It causes acute hepatitis, often transmitted by oral-fecal contamination and having an incubation period of approximately 30 days. Typically, constitutional symptoms are present and jaundice may occur. Drug therapy that the dentist may encounter in a patient being treated for hepatitis A would primarily include immunoglobulin. Hepatitis A vaccine (inactivated) is an FDA-approved vaccine indicated in the prevention of contracting hepatitis A in exposed or high-risk individuals. Candidates at high-risk for HAV infection include persons traveling internationally to highly endemic areas, individuals with chronic liver disease, individuals engaging in high-risk sexual behavior, illicit drug users, persons with high-risk occupational exposure, hemophiliacs or other persons receiving blood products, and pediatric populations. Hepatitis A, caused by infection with HAV, has an incubation period of ~28 days (range: 15-50 days). HAV replicates in the liver and is shed in high concentrations in feces from 2 weeks before to 1 week after the onset of clinical illness. HAV infection produces a self-limited disease that does not result in chronic infection or chronic liver disease; however, 10% to 15% of patients experience relapse symptoms during the 6 months after acute illness. Patients with acute hepatitis A usually require only supportive care with no restrictions in diet or activity. Hospitalization may be necessary for patients who become dehydrated due to nausea and vomiting, but is critical for patients with signs or symptoms of acute liver failure. Medications that may cause liver damage or are metabolized by the liver should be used with caution among patients with hepatitis A.

Two products are available for the prevention of HAV infection: Hepatitis A vaccine and immune globulin (IG) for I.M. administration. Patients recently exposed (within 14 days and prior to development of illness) to HAV and have not received a hepatitis A vaccine should be administered a single dose of the vaccine or IG ([GamaSTAN™ S/D] 0.02 mL/kg) as soon as possible.

Hepatitis B

Hepatitis B virus is previously known as serum hepatitis and has particular trophism for liver cells. Hepatitis B virus causes both acute and chronic disease in susceptible patients. The incubation period is often long and the diagnosis might be made by serologic markers even in the absence of symptoms.

Hepatitis B is caused by infection with the hepatitis B virus (HBV). The incubation period from the time of exposure to onset of symptoms is 6 weeks to 6 months. The highest concentrations of HBV are found in blood with lower concentrations found in other body fluids.

HBV infection can be self-limited or chronic. In adults, only ~1/2 of newly acquired HBV infections are symptomatic and ~1% of reported cases result in acute liver failure. HBV is efficiently transmitted by percutaneous or mucous membrane exposure to blood or body fluids that contain blood. Preventing disease after exposure in a person without previous hepatitis B vaccine protection is important. Passive-active postexposure prophylaxis (PEP) occurs with administration of hepatitis B immune globulin and hepatitis B vaccine.

◀ **Hepatitis C**

The hepatitis C virus (HCV) is an RNA virus. HCV is a major cause of both acute and chronic hepatitis. Persons become infected mainly through parenteral exposure to infected material by blood transfusions or injections with nonsterile needles. Persons who inject illegal drugs and healthcare workers who are at risk for needlestick and other exposures are at highest risk for HCV infection. Another major risk factor for HCV is high-risk sexual behavior. Cutaneous symptoms or findings relevant to HCV infection manifest in 20% to 40% of patients presenting to dermatologists and in a significant percentage (15% to 20%) of general patients. HCV is suggested and must appear in the differential diagnosis of these patients to avoid missing this important but occult factor in clinical disease in the appropriate setting. HCV has been considered in the differential diagnosis for the causes of oral lichen planus; however, no concrete relationship has been established.

Extrahepatic manifestations of hepatitis C virus are numerous. The most prevalent and most closely linked with HCV is essential mixed cryoglobulins with dermatologic, neurologic, renal, and rheumatologic complications. A less definite relationship to HCV is observed with systemic vasculitis, porphyria cutanea tarda, and the sicca syndromes, which could also affect the oral cavity. HCV is a major public health problem because it causes chronic hepatitis, cirrhosis, and hepatocellular carcinoma (HCC).

Treatment of acute hepatitis C infection is initially supportive with monitoring to assess the need for antiviral therapy. Treatment regimens are typically based upon hepatitis C genome, whether the patient is treatment-naïve, has cirrhosis, or has other comorbid conditions, such as HIV.

No vaccine is available for hepatitis C and prophylaxis with immune globulin is not effective in preventing HCV infection after exposure. Testing to determine whether HCV infection has developed is recommended for healthcare workers after percutaneous or perimucosal exposure to HCV-positive blood.

Hepatitis D

Hepatitis D, previously known as the delta agent, is a virus that is incomplete in that it requires previous infection with hepatitis B in order to be manifested. Antiviral therapy is not indicated for an acute infection.

Hepatitis E

Hepatitis E virus is an RNA virus that represents a proportion of the previously classified non-A/non-B diagnoses. There is currently no antiviral therapy against hepatitis E.

Hepatitis F

Hepatitis F remains a diagnosis of exclusion. There are no known immunological tests available for identification of hepatitis F at present and currently the Centers for Disease Control have not come out with specific guidelines or recommendations. It is thought that hepatitis F is a blood-borne virus and it has been used as a diagnosis in several cases of post-transfusion hepatitis.

Hepatitis G

Hepatitis G virus (HGV) is the newest hepatitis and is also assumed to be a blood-borne virus. Similar in family to hepatitis C, it is thought to occur concomitantly with hepatitis C and appears to be even more prevalent in some blood donors than hepatitis C. Occupational transmission of HGV is currently under study (see the references for updated information) and currently there are no specific CDC recommendations for postexposure to an HGV individual as the testing for identification remains experimental.

For further information, refer to the following:

Types of Hepatitis Virus

Features	A	B	C	D	E	F	G
Incubation Period	2-6 wks	8-24 wks	2-52 wks	3-13 wks	3-6 wks	Unknown	Unknown
Onset	Abrupt	Insidious	Insidious	Abrupt	Abrupt	Insidious	Insidious
Symptoms							
Jaundice	Adults: 70% to 80%; Children: 10%	25%	25%	Varies	Unknown	Unknown	Unknown
Asymptomatic patients	Adults: 50%; Children: Most	~75%	~75%	Rare	Rare	Common	Common
Routes of Transmission							
Fecal/Oral	Yes	No	No	No	Yes	Unknown	Unknown
Parenteral	Rare	Yes	Yes	Yes	No		
Sexual	No	Yes	Possible	Yes	No		
Perinatal	No	Yes	Possible	Possible	No		
Water/Food	Yes	No	No	No	Yes		
Sequelae (% of patients)							
Chronic state	No	Adults: 6% to 10%; Children: 25% to 50%; Infants: 70% to 90%	>75%	10% to 15%	No	Unknown	Likely
Case-Fatality Rate	0.6%	1.4%	1% to 2%	30%	1% to 2% Pregnant women: 20%	Unknown	Unknown

Pre-exposure Risk Factors for Hepatitis B

Healthcare factors:

Healthcare workers[1]

Special patient groups (eg, adolescents, infants born to HB$_s$Ag–positive mothers, military personnel, etc)

Hemodialysis patients[2]

Recipients of certain blood products[3]

Lifestyle factors:

Homosexual and bisexual men

I.V. drug-abusers

Heterosexually active persons with multiple sexual partners or recently acquired sexually transmitted diseases

Environmental factors:

Household and sexual contacts of HBV carriers

Prison inmates

Clients and staff of institutions for the mentally handicapped

Residents, immigrants, and refugees from areas with endemic HBV infection

International travelers at increased risk of acquiring HBV infection

[1]The risk of hepatitis B virus (HBV) infection for healthcare workers varies both between hospitals and within hospitals. Hepatitis B vaccination is recommended for all healthcare workers with blood exposure.

[2]Hemodialysis patients often respond poorly to hepatitis B vaccination; higher vaccine doses or increased number of doses are required. A special formulation of one vaccine is now available for such persons (Recombivax HB®, 40 mcg/mL). The anti-HB$_s$ (antibody to hepatitis B surface antigen) response of such persons should be tested after they are vaccinated, and those who have not responded should be revaccinated with 1-3 additional doses.

Patients with chronic renal disease should be vaccinated as early as possible, ideally before they require hemodialysis. In addition, their anti-HB$_s$ levels should be monitored at 6- to 12-month intervals to assess the need for revaccination.

[3]Patients with hemophilia should be immunized SubQ, not I.M.

PRE-EXPOSURE VACCINATION

Pre-exposure vaccination is one of the most effective methods for preventing transmission of some STDs. Two human papillomavirus (HPV) vaccines are available for females 9-26 years of age to prevent cervical precancer and cancer, quadrivalent HPV vaccine (Gardasil®) and the bivalent HPV vaccine (Cervarix®). Routine vaccination for females 11-12 years of age is recommended with either vaccine. Gardasil® is recommended for males 9-26 years of age to prevent genital warts, anal cancer, and anal intraepithelial neoplasm. Details regarding HPV vaccination are available at www.cdc.gov/std/hpv.

Hepatitis B vaccination is recommended for all unvaccinated and uninfected patients being evaluated for an STD. In addition, hepatitis A and B vaccines are recommended for men who have sex with men and injection drug users; each of these vaccines should also be administered to HIV-infected patients not yet infected with one or both types of hepatitis virus. Details regarding hepatitis A and B vaccination are available at http://www.cdc.gov/hepatitis.

HERPES

The herpes viruses not only represent a topic of specific interest to the dentist due to oral manifestations, but are widespread as systemic infections. Herpes simplex virus is also of interest because of its central nervous system infections and its relationship as one of the viral infections commonly found in AIDS patients. Oral herpes infections will be covered elsewhere. Current recommended drug therapy includes acyclovir, valacyclovir, or famciclovir. Epstein-Barr virus is a member of the herpesvirus family and produces syndromes important in dentistry, including infectious mononucleosis with the commonly found oral pharyngitis and petechial hemorrhages, as well as being the causative agent of Burkitt's lymphoma. The relationship between Epstein-Barr virus to oral hairy leukoplakia in AIDS patients has not been shown to be one of cause and effect; however, the presence of Epstein-Barr in these lesions is consistent. Currently, there is no accepted treatment for Epstein-Barr virus, although acyclovir has been shown in *in vitro* studies to have some efficacy.

Varicella-zoster virus is another member of the herpesvirus family and is the causative agent of two clinical entities, chickenpox and shingles, or herpes zoster. Oral manifestations of both chickenpox and herpes zoster include vesicular eruptions often leading to confluent mucosal ulcerations. Although the thoracic region is a common site for shingles, the face and/or oral cavity are not rare areas affected. The dentist should be concerned if lesions are confined to one side of the face or oral cavity. Rapid intervention can result in significant reduction in the pain and eruptions of an adult zoster infection. Acyclovir, valacyclovir, or famciclovir are the drugs of choice for treatment of herpes zoster infections.

The vaccine for shingles (Zostavax®) is recommended for use in persons ≥60 years of age to prevent shingles. The older a person is, the more severe the effects of shingles typically are. The shingles vaccine is specifically designed to protect people against shingles and will **not** protect people against other forms of herpes, such as genital herpes. The shingles vaccine is **not** recommended to treat active shingles or postherpetic neuralgia (pain after the rash is gone) once it develops. At this time, the CDC does recommend that healthcare providers within the recommended age group (≥50 years of age) receive the zoster vaccine.

There are other herpes viruses that produce disease in man and animals. These viruses have no specific treatment; therefore, incidence is thought to be less common than those mentioned and the specific treatment is not determined at present. The role of some of these viruses in concomitant infection with the HIV and other coinfection viruses is still under study.

REFERENCES

ACIP Adult Immunization Work Group, Bridges CB, Woods L, et al, "Advisory Committee on Immunization Practices (ACIP) Recommended Immunization Schedule for Adults Aged 19 Years and Older-United States, 2013," *MMWR Surveill Summ*, 2013, 62(Suppl 1):9-19.

Advisory Committee on Immunization Practices (ACIP) Centers for Disease Control and Prevention (CDC), "Update: Prevention of Hepatitis A After Exposure to Hepatitis A Virus and in International Travelers. Updated Recommendations of the Advisory Committee on Immunization Practices (ACIP)," *MMWR Morb Mortal Wkly Rep*, 2007, 56(41):1080-4.

Advisory Committee on Immunization Practices (ACIP), "Prevention of Hepatitis A Through Active or Passive Immunization: Recommendations of the Advisory Committee on Immunization Practices (ACIP)," *MMWR Recomm Rep*, 2006, 55(RR-7):1-23.

Centers for Disease Control and Prevention (CDC), "Recommendations of the Advisory Committee on Immunization Practices (ACIP): General Recommendations on Immunization," *MMWR Recomm Rep*, 2011, 60(2):1-64.

Centers for Disease Control and Prevention (CDC), "Update on Herpes Zoster Vaccine: Licensure for Persons Aged 50 Through 59 Years," *MMWR Morb Mortal Wkly Rep*, 2011, 60(44):1528.

Corey L, Wald A, Patel R, et al, "Once-Daily Valacyclovir to Reduce the Risk of Transmission of Genital Herpes," *N Engl J Med*, 2004, 350(1):11-20.

Ghany MG, Nelson DR, Strader DB, et al, "An Update on Treatment of Genotype 1 Chronic Hepatitis C Virus Infection: 2011 Practice Guideline by the American Association for the Study of Liver Diseases," *Hepatology*, 2011, 54(4):1433-44.

Ghany MG, Strader DB, Thomas DL, et al, "Diagnosis, Management, and Treatment of Hepatitis C: An Update," *Hepatology*, 2009, 49(4):1335-74.

Kaplan JE, Benson C, Holmes KH, et al, "Guidelines for Prevention and Treatment of Opportunistic Infections in HIV-Infected Adults and Adolescents: Recommendations From CDC, the National Institutes of Health, and the HIV Medicine Association of the Infectious Diseases Society of America," *MMWR Recomm Rep*, 2009, 58(RR-4):1-207.

Mast EE, Margolis HS, Fiore AE, et al, "A Comprehensive Immunization Strategy to Eliminate Transmission of Hepatitis B Virus Infection in the United States: Recommendations of the Advisory Committee on Immunization Practices (ACIP) Part 1: Immunization of Infants, Children, and Adolescents," *MMWR Recomm Rep*, 2005, 54(RR-16):1-31.

Miller CS, Avdiushko SA, Kryscio RJ, et al, "Effect of Prophylactic Valacyclovir on the Presence of Human Herpesvirus DNA in Saliva of Healthy Individuals After Dental Treatment," *J Clin Microbiol* , 2005, 43(5):2173-80.

Mofenson LM, Brady MT, Danner SP, et al, "Guidelines for the Prevention and Treatment of Opportunistic Infections Among HIV-Exposed and HIV-Infected Children: Recommendations From CDC, the National Institutes of Health, the HIV Medicine Association of The Infectious Diseases Society of America, the Pediatric Infectious Diseases Society, and the American Academy of Pediatrics," *MMWR Recomm Rep*, 2009, 58(RR-11):1-166.

Niro GA, Gioffreda D, and Fontana R, "Hepatitis Delta Virus Infection: Open Issues," *Dig Liver Dis*, 2011, 43(Suppl 1):S19-24.

Pascarella S and Negro F, "Hepatitis D Virus: An Update," *Liver Int*, 2011, 31(1):7-21.

Sherman KE, "Hepatitis E Virus Infection: More Common Than Previously Realized?" *Gastroenterol Hepatol (N Y)*, 2011, 7(11):759-61.

Teshale EH and Hu DJ, "Hepatitis E: Epidemiology and Prevention," *World J Hepatol*, 2011, 3(12):285-91.

Triantos C, Kalafateli M, Nikolopoulou V, et al, "Meta-Analysis: Antiviral Treatment for Hepatitis D," *Aliment Pharmacol Ther*, 2012, 35(6):663-73.

Workowski KA, Berman S, and Centers for Disease Control and Prevention (CDC), "Sexually Transmitted Diseases Treatment Guidelines, 2010," *MMWR Recomm Rep*, 2010, 59(RR-12):1-110. Available at http://www.cdc.gov/std/treatment/2010/STD-Treatment-2010-RR5912.pdf

ANTIBIOTIC PROPHYLAXIS

PREPROCEDURAL GUIDELINES FOR DENTAL PATIENTS

INTRODUCTION

In dental practice, antibiotic prophylaxis has been identified for certain at-risk patients to prevent infective endocarditis, orthopedic implant infection, or contamination through the surgical site. The guidelines are generally provided through a joint effort of medical and dental organizations and are reviewed and rewritten periodically based upon clinical and scientific evidence. In this section, these guidelines are reviewed.

PREVENTION OF INFECTIVE ENDOCARDITIS

In 2007, the American Heart Association (AHA), in conjunction with the American Dental Association (ADA) and other experts in both medicine and dentistry, following an extensive evidence-based literature review, provided the most recent guidelines regarding the use of antibiotic prophylaxis to prevent infective endocarditis (IE) related to dental procedures. Since the mid-1950s, it has been recommended that patients at risk for IE from a variety of medical conditions should be premedicated with antibiotics prior to dental and other procedures. Earlier changes in the guidelines (1984, 1990, 1997) focused on the recommended antibiotics, dose, and dosing frequency. While indicating a minor modification of recommended antibiotics, the most recent change (2007) focused primarily on the patients for whom prophylaxis is recommended.

Infective endocarditis is the consequence of a sequence of events. This sequence is initiated by the formation of nonbacterial thrombotic endocarditis (NBTE) on the surface of a cardiac valve or elsewhere that endothelial damage occurs within the heart. Turbulent blood flow produced by congenital or acquired heart disease, including flow from high- to low-flow chambers and flow across a narrowed orifice, traumatizes the endothelium. This predisposes for deposition of platelets and fibrin on the endothelial surface and results in NBTE. If bacteremia then occurs following invasion of the bloodstream with a microbial species that has the pathogenic potential to colonize this site, IE can occur. Mucosal surfaces are populated by dense endogenous microflora. Trauma to a mucosal surface releases many different microbial species transiently into the blood stream. Transient bacteremia caused by oral microflora occurs commonly with dental extractions or other dental procedures or with routine daily activities. The frequency and intensity of the resulting bacteremias are related to the nature and magnitude of the trauma, density of the microbial flora, and degree of inflammation or infection at the site. The microbial species entering circulation depends on the unique endogenous microflora that colonize the traumatized site. The ability of the bacteria in the blood stream to adhere to specific NBTE sites determines the anatomic localization of the infection. Mediators of bacterial adherence serve as virulence factors. Common oral flora, including viridans group Streptococci and Staphylococci have cellular components that serve as adhesions to the NBTE and these adhesions are immunogenic. Microorganisms adherent to the vegetation stimulate further deposition of fibrin and platelets on their surface. The buried microorganisms multiply as rapidly as bacteria in broth cultures to reach maximal densities within a short time on the left side of the heart, apparently uninhibited by host defenses in left-sided lesions. Right-sided vegetations have lower bacterial densities due to host defense, such as PMN activity or platelet-derived antibacterial proteins. More than 90% of microorganisms in mature valvular vegetations are metabolically inactive and are therefore less responsive to the bacterial effects of antibiotics.

Viridans group Streptococci are normal oral tract flora and cause more than 50% of cases of community-acquired native valve IE that is not associated with I.V. drug use. As early as 1935, a report indicated that 11% of patients with poor oral hygiene had positive blood cultures, yet 61% of patients experienced bacteremia with dental extractions. Historically, the additional assumptions associated with antibiotic prophylaxis for IE are that these microorganisms are susceptible to antibiotics recommended for prophylaxis, that antibiotic prophylaxis prevents experimental endocarditis in animals, that a temporal relationship exists between dental procedures and the onset of symptoms of IE, that the risk of adverse drugs reactions is low, and that morbidity and mortality of IE are high.

A primary determinant of the changes for the 2007 guidelines are that the estimated absolute risk for IE from a dental procedure in patients with underlying cardiac conditions increases from 1:1.1 million for mitral valve prolapsed (MVP) to 1:475,000 for congenital heart disease (CHD). The absolute risk increases further for rheumatic heart disease (RHD) (1:142,000), prosthetic valve (1:114,000), and previous IE (1:95,000). Cardiac conditions with predisposition for IE show similar trends. Additionally, mortality associated with prosthetic valve endocarditis (PVE) is >20% and PVE increases the risk of heart failure.

As a result, antibiotic prophylaxis with certain dental procedures is recommended for patients at highest risk of IE due to specific cardiac conditions:

- Prosthetic cardiac valve

- A prior incidence of IE

- Heart transplant patients who develop cardiac valvulopathy

- Patients with CHD are required prophylaxis with the following conditions:

  - Unrepaired cyanotic CHD, including palliative shunts and conduits

  - Completely repaired CHD with prosthetic material or device during the first 6 months after the surgical or catheter intervention procedure

  - Repaired CHD with residual defects at the site or adjacent to the site of a prosthetic patch (which inhibits endothelialization)

These patients with high-risk cardiac conditions are recommended for prophylaxis for all dental procedures involving manipulation of gingival tissue or the periapical region of teeth or perforation of the oral mucosa.

Dental procedures that do not require prophylaxis include:

- Routine anesthetic injection into noninfected tissue

- Taking dental radiographs

- Placement of removable prosthodontic or orthodontic appliances

- Adjustment of orthodontic appliances

- Placement of orthodontic brackets

- Shedding of deciduous teeth

- Bleeding from trauma to the lips or oral mucosa

ANTIBIOTIC SELECTION

For examples of sample prescriptions see Infective Endocarditis (Prevention) on page 1604. Dentists should be vigilant in reviewing literature for updates.

Table 1 provides the recommended antibiotics and doses. Specific dosage forms available for each antibiotic can be found in the drug monographs. Extended or delayed release dosage formulations should not be used for antibiotic prophylaxis because they will not produce high immediate peak concentrations.

For those patients able to take oral antibiotics and those not allergic to beta-lactam antibiotics (penicillins, cephalosporins, monobactams, and carbapenems), the antibiotic of choice is amoxicillin, an amino penicillin. Aminopenicillins have an extended spectrum of antibacterial action compared to penicillin VK-treating gram-positive aerobes, such as staph and strep, but also some gram-aerobes, such as *Haemophilus* influenza. Aminopenicillins are more stable in the gastrointestinal tract, allowing them to be taken with food or beverages, providing higher plasma concentrations following oral administration.

For individuals unable to take oral medications and not allergic to beta-lactam antibiotics, intramuscular (I.M.) or intravenous (I.V.) ampicillin, also an aminopenicillin, is recommended.

Table 1. Prophylactic Regimens for Infective Endocarditis for Dental Procedures

Situation	Drug	Single Dosage 30-60 minutes prior to procedure
Oral	Amoxicillin on page 96	Children: 50 mg/kg Adults: 2 g
Unable to take oral medications	Ampicillin on page 106 or	Children: 50 mg/kg I.M. or I.V. Adults: 2 g I.M. or I.V.
	CeFAZolin on page 262 or CefTRIAXone on page 273	Children: 50 mg/kg I.M. or I.V. Adults: 1 g I.M. or I.V.
Allergic to penicillins or ampicillin (oral)	Cephalexin on page 279[1,2] or	Children: 50 mg/kg Adults: 2 g
	Clindamycin (Systemic) on page 320 or	Children: 20 mg/kg Adults: 600 mg
	Azithromycin (Systemic) on page 158 or Clarithromycin on page 316	Children: 15 mg/kg Adults: 500 mg
Allergic to penicillins or ampicillin and unable to take oral medications	CeFAZolin on page 262 or CefTRIAXone on page 273[2]	Children: 50 mg/kg I.M. or I.V. Adults: 1 g I.M. or I.V.
	Clindamycin (Systemic) on page 320	Children: 20 mg/kg I.M. or I.V. Adults: 600 mg I.M. or I.V.

Note: Intramuscular injections should be avoided in patients receiving anticoagulant therapy.

[1]Can use first- or second-generation oral cephalosporins in equivalent doses.

[2]Cephalosporins should not be used in individuals with immediate-type hypersensitivity reaction (urticaria, angioedema, or anaphylaxis) to penicillins.

Individuals who are allergic to the penicillins, such as amoxicillin or ampicillin, should be treated with an alternate antibiotic. The 2007 guidelines suggest a number of alternate agents, including clindamycin, cephalosporins, azithromycin, and clarithromycin. Patients who do not have a Type I (immediate) allergic (hypersensitivity) reaction to penicillins (urticaria, bronchospasm, angioedema, anaphylaxis) may receive a first or second generation cephalosporin. Oral first generation cephalosporins include cephalexin (Keflex®) and cefadroxil (Duricef®). First generation cephalosporins have an anti-bacterial spectrum of activity similar to amoxicillin and ampicillin. Oral second generation cephalosporins include cefaclor (Ceclor®), cefprozil, or cefuroxime axetil (Ceftin®). Second generation cephalosporins have an antibacterial spectrum of activity broader than aminopenicillins and first generation cephalosporins and similar to amoxicillin with clavulanic acid. For patients unable to take oral cephalosporins, the first generation cephalosporin cefazolin (Ancef®) is recommended for I.M. or I.V. administration. A third generation cephalosporin, ceftriaxone (Rocephin®), is also listed as a parenteral option. Third generation cephalosporins have a broader antibacterial spectrum of activity than first and second generation cephalosporins should generally be reserved for more serious gram infections or for gram-positive infections not responsive to first-line therapy.

Penicillin and cephalosporin antibiotics have a bactericidal mechanism of action by inhibiting synthesis of the bacterial cell wall. They are most effective in bacteria that are actively growing and reproducing. The most common adverse reaction is a Type I or immediate hypersensitivity reaction which generally produces urticaria, bronchospasm, angioedema, or anaphylaxis. Because both penicillins and cephalosporins are beta-lactam antibiotics, patients with Type I immediate hypersensitivity reactions can be cross-allergic.

Clindamycin (Cleocin®) is a lincosamide antibiotic effective against gram-positive aerobes and many anaerobic bacteria. Clindamycin is an option both orally or I.M. or I.V. for patients with any penicillin allergy. Clindamycin is a bacteriostatic antibiotic that inhibits bacterial protein synthesis. Adverse effects of clindamycin after a single dose are rare. Although it is estimated that 1% of patients taking clindamycin will develop symptoms of pseudomembranous colitis, these symptoms usually develop after 9-14 days of clindamycin therapy. These symptoms are rare and only one case has been reported in a patient taking an acute dose for the prevention of endocarditis.

Azithromycin (Zithromax®) and clarithromycin (Biaxin®) are members of the class of antibiotics known as macrolides. The pharmacology of these drugs has been reviewed previously in *General Dentistry*. Erythromycins have been available for use in dentistry and medicine since the mid-1950s. Azithromycin and clarithromycin represent the first additions to this class in more than 40 years. The adult prophylactic dose for either drug is 500 mg 30-60 minutes before the procedure with no follow-up dose. The pediatric prophylactic dose of azithromycin and clarithromycin is 15 mg/kg orally 30-60 minutes before the procedure. Although the erythromycin family of drugs is known to inhibit the hepatic metabolism of theophylline and carbamazepine to enhance their effects, azithromycin has not been shown to affect the liver metabolism of these drugs.

Azithromycin is well absorbed from the gastrointestinal tract and is extensively taken up from circulation into tissues with a slow release from those tissues. It reaches peak serum levels in 2-4 hours and serum half-life is 68 hours. Zithromax® is supplied as 250 mg, 500 mg, and 600 mg tablets. It is also available for oral suspension at concentrations of 100 mg/5 mL, 200 mg/5 mL, and single-dose packets containing 1 g. In May 2012, the FDA notified healthcare providers that they are reviewing the results of an azithromycin study published in the *New England Journal of Medicine*. This study reported a small increase in cardiovascular deaths and in the risk of death from any cause in persons treated with a 5-day course of azithromycin (Zithromax®) compared to persons treated with amoxicillin, ciprofloxacin, or no medication. The FDA will communicate any new information on azithromycin and this study or the potential risk of QT interval prolongation after the agency has completed its review. Patients taking azithromycin should not stop taking their medicine without talking to their healthcare provider. Healthcare providers should be aware of the potential for QT interval prolongation and heart arrhythmias when prescribing or administering any macrolide antibiotic.

Clarithromycin (Biaxin®) achieves peak plasma concentrations in 3 hours and maintains effective serum concentrations over a 12-hour period. Reports indicate that it probably interacts with theophylline and carbamazepine by elevating the plasma concentrations of the two drugs. Biaxin® is supplied as 250 mg and 500 mg tablets and 500 mg extended release tablets. It is also available as granules for oral suspension at concentrations of 125 mg/5 mL and 250 mg/5 mL.

Clinical Considerations for Dentistry

See Figure 1.

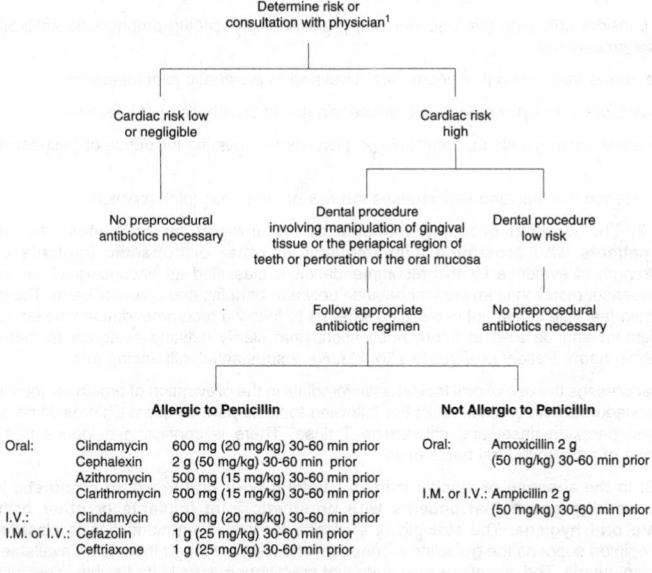

Figure 1
Preprocedural Dental Action Plan for Patients With a History
Indicative of Elevated Endocarditis Risk

Dosages for children are in parentheses and should never exceed adult dose. Cephalosporins should be avoided in patients with previous Type I hypersensitivity reactions to penicillin due to some evidence of cross-allergenicity.

[1]For Emergency Dental Care, the clinician should attempt phone consultation. If unable to contact patient's physician or determine risk, the patient should be treated as though there is a high risk of cardiac complication and follow the algorithm.

An antibiotic for prophylaxis should be administered in a single dose before the procedure. If the dosage of antibiotic is inadvertently not administered before the procedure, the dosage may be administered up to 2 hours after the procedure. However, administration of the dosage after the procedure should be considered only when the patient did not receive the preprocedural dose.

PREPROCEDURAL ANTIBIOTICS FOR PROSTHETIC IMPLANTS

A significant number of dental patients have had total joint replacements or other implanted prosthetic devices. Prior to performing dental procedures that might induce bacteremia, the dentist has historically been advised to consider the use of antibiotic prophylaxis in these patients. In December 2012, the American Academy of Orthopedic Surgeons (AAOS) and the ADA released an Evidence-Based Guideline and Evidence Report entitled "Prevention of Orthopaedic Implant Infection in Patients Undergoing Dental Procedures". The report concludes that the groups found insufficient evidence to recommend the routine use of antibiotics for joint replacement patients. They advised that there is no direct evidence that routine dental procedures cause prosthetic joint infections. **Although, many patients will no longer need antibiotic prophylaxis, consultation with the individuals' healthcare providers is recommended.**

These new guidelines update the previous ones from February 2009 ("Antibiotic Prophylaxis for Bacteremia in Patients With Joint Replacements Information Statement) that were revised in June 2010. The previous guidelines recommended providing antibiotic prophylaxis for all joint prosthetic patients. These new guidelines are based on clinical research which examined a large group of patients, all having a prosthetic hip or knee and half with an infected prosthetic joint. The research showed that invasive dental procedures, with or without antibiotics, did not increase the odds of developing a prosthetic joint infection. These new guidelines include three recommendations, along with "strength of evidence" ratings as the basis for the recommendation. The guidelines are available at http://www.ada.org/sections/professionalResources/pdfs/PUDP_guideline.pdf.

◀ **Recommendation 1: The practitioner might consider discontinuing the practice of routinely prescribing prophylactic antibiotics for patients with hip and knee prosthetic implants undergoing dental procedures.** The strength of evidence for this recommendation is classified as "limited", meaning that the quality of the supporting evidence that exists is unconvincing or that well-conducted studies show little clear advantage to one approach versus another. The guidelines also state that practitioners should be cautious in deciding whether to follow a recommendation classified as "limited" and should exercise judgment and be alert for emerging publications that report more extensive evidence. Patient preference should have a substantial influencing role.

Recommendation 1 is supported by the highest grade of evidence of the three recommendations. Its key points are:

1. Practitioners consider changing the long standing practice of prescribing prophylactic antibiotics for patients who undergo dental procedures.

2. The evidence shows that dental procedures are unrelated to prosthetic joint infections.

3. Subsequent antibiotic prophylaxis does not reduce the risk of prosthetic joint infections.

4. High-strength evidence suggests that antibiotic prophylaxis reduces the incidence of post-dental procedure-related bacteremia.

5. There is no evidence that bacteremia increases the risk of prosthetic joint infections.

Recommendation 2: The working group was unable to recommend for or against the use of topical oral antimicrobials in patients with prosthetic joint implants or other orthopaedic implants undergoing dental procedures. The strength of evidence for this recommendation is classified as "inconclusive", meaning that there is a lack of compelling evidence, resulting in an unclear balance between benefits and potential harm. The guidelines also state that practitioners should feel little constraint in deciding whether to follow a recommendation labeled as "inconclusive" and should exercise judgment and be alert to future publications that clarify existing evidence for determining balance of benefits versus potential harm. Patient preference should have a substantial influencing role.

Recommendation 2 addresses the use of oral topical antimicrobials in the prevention of prosthetic joint infections in patients undergoing dental procedures. The guidelines list the following topicals as examples: Chlorhexidine oral rinse, povidone-iodine rinse, hydrogen peroxide rinse, and chloramine T rinse. There is conflicting evidence that these agents may decrease the incidence of postprocedural bacteremia.

Recommendation 3: In the absence of reliable evidence linking poor oral health to prosthetic joint infection, it is the opinion of the working group that patients with prosthetic joint implants or other orthopaedic implants maintain appropriate oral hygiene. The strength of evidence for this recommendation is classified as "consensus", meaning that expert opinion supports the guideline recommendation, even though there is no available empirical evidence that meets the inclusion criteria. The guidelines also state that practitioners should be flexible in deciding whether to follow a recommendation classified as "consensus", although they may set boundaries on alternatives. Patient preference should have a substantial influencing role.

Recommendation 3 addresses the maintenance of good oral hygiene and is the only consensus recommendation in the new guidelines. In concordance with consensus recommendations, oral hygiene measures are low-cost, provide potential benefit, are consistent with current practice, and are in accordance with good oral health.

These major changes in the guidelines were based primarily on a detailed review of clinical studies. The first report is from the Mayo Clinic published in January 2010, which described a large case-control study which examined the association between dental procedures, with or without antibiotic prophylaxis, and prosthetic joint infections. The study found no increased risk of prosthetic joint infections after dental procedures. The study also found that antibiotic prophylaxis was not associated with any reduction in risk of infection. The study data indicated that there is no need for antibiotic prophylaxis in patients with total hip or knee replacements and undergoing dental procedures.

This Mayo Clinic study was designed to determine whether dental procedures with and without antibiotic prophylaxis are risk factors for prosthetic hip or knee infection. It was designed as a prospective, case-controlled study in a single institution, conducted from 2001-2006. The full report can be found in the January 1, 2010, issue of the Clinical Infectious Diseases journal. Dental records were obtained from each patient's dentist. Dental procedures were categorized into low-risk and high-risk procedures. Low-risk procedures included restorative dentistry, dental filling, endodontic treatment, and fluoride treatment. High-risk procedures included dental hygiene, mouth surgery, periodontal treatment, dental extraction, and therapy for dental abscess. Hip or knee infections were determined using routine microbiological techniques that isolated the bacterial flora.

There was no increased risk of prosthetic hip or knee infection for patients undergoing a high-risk or low-risk dental procedure who were not administered antibiotic prophylaxis. Also, for the subjects who took antibiotics, the study found no significant differences between the risk of prosthetic joint infections, regardless of the use of antibiotic prophylaxis.

Results summary:

1. There was no increased risk of prosthetic hip or knee infection for patients undergoing a high-risk or low-risk dental procedure who were not administered antibiotic prophylaxis compared with the risk for patients not undergoing a dental procedure.

2. Antibiotic prophylaxis in high-risk or low-risk dental procedures did not decrease the risk of subsequent total hip or knee infection.

The recommendations from these 2012 guidelines increase the importance for dentists when planning invasive oral procedures to consult with the patient's orthopedic surgeon to determine the risk associated with infection and the need for antibiotics.

Table 2. Patients With Medical Conditions Suggesting a Need for Medical Consultation to Determine Potential Risk of Joint Infection

All patients with prosthetic joint replacement
Immunocompromised/immunosuppressed patients
Inflammatory arthropathies (eg, rheumatoid arthritis, systemic lupus erythematosus)
Drug-induced immunosuppression
Radiation-induced immunosuppression
Patients with comorbidity (eg, diabetes, obesity, HIV, and smoking)
Previous prosthetic infections
Malnourishment
Hemophilia
HIV infection
Type 1 diabetes mellitus (insulin dependent, IDDM)
Malignancy
Megaprosthesis

Source: January 2013 AAOS Information Statement. Available at http://www.aaos.org/about/papers/advistmt/1033.asp. Original source: American Dental Association; American Academy of Orthopedic Surgeons, "Antibiotic Prophylaxis for Dental Patients With Total Joint Replacements," *J Am Dent Assoc*, 2003, 134(7):895-9.

Even in these patients, the new guidelines should be considered and a medical consultation with the physician will determine whether or not to use antibiotics because late infections of implanted prosthetic devices have rarely been associated with microbial organisms of oral origin. Also, since late infections in such patients are often not reported, data is lacking to substantiate or refute this potential.

ANTIBIOTIC REGIMENS

The new guidelines should be carefully reviewed for any patient to prevent prosthetic joint late infections. Decisions must be made on a case-by-case basis. If using preprocedural antibiotics are found to be appropriate after careful consideration, the antibiotic prophylaxis regimens, as suggested by the advisory panel, are listed in Table 3. These regimens are not exactly the same as those listed in Table 1 (for prevention of endocarditis) and must be reviewed carefully to avoid confusion. Cephalexin or amoxicillin may be used in patients not allergic to penicillin. The selected antibiotic is given as a single 2 g dose 1 hour before the procedure. A follow-up dose is not recommended. Cephalexin (Keflex®) and amoxicillin were described earlier in this section.

Parenteral cefazolin (Ancef®) or ampicillin is the recommended antibiotic for patients unable to take oral medications (see Table 3 for doses). Cefazolin is a first-generation cephalosporin, effective against anaerobes and aerobic gram-positive bacteria. Ampicillin is an aminopenicillin (described earlier). For patients allergic to penicillin, clindamycin is the recommended antibiotic of choice. Clindamycin is active against aerobic and anaerobic streptococci, most staphylococci, the *Bacteroides*, and the *Actinomyces* families of bacteria. The recommended oral and parenteral doses of clindamycin in the joint prosthetic patient are listed in Table 3 below.

Table 3. Antibiotic Regimens for Patients With Prosthetic Implants

Patients not allergic to penicillin:	Cephalexin or amoxicillin:	2 g orally 1 hour prior to the procedure
Patients not allergic to penicillin and unable to take oral medications:	CeFAZolin:	1 g I.M. or I.V. 1 hour prior to the procedure
	or Ampicillin:	2 g I.M. or I.V. 1 hour prior to the procedure
Patients allergic to penicillin:	Clindamycin (Systemic):	600 mg orally 1 hour prior to dental procedure
Patients allergic to penicillin and unable to take oral medications:	Clindamycin (Systemic):	600 mg I.V. 1 hour prior to the procedure

Please review the new guidelines for prevention of prosthetic joint late infections. Decisions must be made on a case-by-case basis. If using preprocedural antibiotics are found to be appropriate after careful consideration, the example prescriptions in the section entitled **Prosthetic Joint Late Infections (Prevention)** apply.

Cephalexin on page 279
Clindamycin (Systemic) on page 320

As more evidence and data are collected, these recommendations may be revised; however, it is thought to be prudent for the dental clinician to fully evaluate all patients with respect to history and/or physical findings and a medical consultation prior to determining the risk.

In patients in whom concern exists over joint complications and a medical consultation cannot be immediately obtained, the patient should be treated as though antibiotic coverage is necessary until such time that an appropriate consultation can be completed.

◀ FREQUENTLY ASKED QUESTIONS FOR INFECTIVE ENDOCARDITIS (IE) AND PROSTHETIC IMPLANTS

When should we start following the new prevention of IE guidelines?

Immediately, since the previous update was from June 2010.

What should we do for patients who have been premedicated for IE in the past but are no longer recommended for prophylaxis?

If the patient does not fall into one of the highest risk groups, premedication should not be used.

Should I just premedicate to be safe?

No, the new guidelines are based on evidence which documents that the risk of adverse side effects from the antibiotics (allergy, GI upset, development of microbial resistance, etc) outweigh the benefits in many patients who previously received SBE/IE prophylaxis. The new Guidelines clearly recommend the use of prophylactic antibiotics only for those at the highest risk.

What if a patient did not meet the new high-risk criteria outlined in the new Guidelines and the patient's physician still recommends IE prophylaxis?

Please contact the physician to see if there are compelling medical reasons for continuing IE prophylaxis.

*What if a patient who has received IE prophylaxis in the past for a condition that is now deemed as **not** being high risk for IE prophylaxis still insists on being premedicated?*

Recommend that the patient contacts the physician to see if there are compelling medical reasons for continuing IE prophylaxis.

If the patient is presently taking antibiotics for some other ailment, is prophylaxis still necessary?

If a patient is already taking antibiotics for another condition, prophylaxis (when deemed necessary under the new guidelines) should be accomplished with a drug recommendation from another class. For example, in the patient who is not allergic to penicillin and is taking a macrolide antibiotic for a medical condition, amoxicillin would be the drug of choice for prophylaxis. Also, in the penicillin-allergic patient taking clindamycin, prophylaxis would best be accomplished with azithromycin or clarithromycin.

Can clindamycin be used safely in patients with gastrointestinal disorders?

If a patient has a history of inflammatory bowel disease and is allergic to penicillin, azithromycin or clarithromycin might be selected over clindamycin. In patients with a negative history of inflammatory bowel disease, clindamycin has not been shown to induce colitis following a single-dose administration.

What should I do if medical consultation results in a recommendation that differs from the published guidelines endorsed by the American Dental Association?

The dentist is ultimately responsible for treatment recommendations. Ideally, by communicating with the physician, a consensus can be achieved that is either in agreement with the guidelines or is based on other established medical reasoning.

Is there cross-allergenicity between the cephalosporins and penicillin?

The incidence of cross-allergenicity is 5% to 8% in the overall population. If a patient has demonstrated a Type I hypersensitivity reaction to penicillin, including urticaria, bronchospasm, angioedema, or anaphylaxis, then this incidence increases to 20%.

Is there definitely an interaction between contraception agents and antibiotics?

There are well-founded interactions between contraceptives and antibiotics. The best instructions that a patient could be given by his/her dentist are that should an antibiotic be necessary, and the dentist is aware that the patient is on contraceptives, and if the patient is using chemical contraceptives, the patient should seriously consider additional means of contraception during the antibiotic management.

Are PROBIOTICS important in patients receiving long-term or repeated care with antibiotics?

There is always concern regarding disruption of healthy microflora of the gastrointestinal system when antibiotics are prescribed for an extended period of time or on closely repeated occasions. GI symptoms often occur and do not represent any direct drug allergy or toxicity but rather are the effects of this gut flora alteration.

Cultures of direct-fed microorganisms or probiotics are able to multiply in the intestinal tract to create a balance of microflora. Some lactobacillus species used in probiotic applications include *L. acidophilus*, *L. casei*, *L. reuteri*, *L. rhamnosus*, and *Bifidobacterium bifidum*. These and other organisms form a symbiotic or mutual relationship with their host. Each species develops a resistance to the disease-causing potential of such organisms and form mutual beneficial relationships with these organisms. The familiar *L. acidophilus* produces lactic acid, reduces gut pH, and acts as a colonizer. Some forms of antibiotics, such as cephalosporins, clindamycin, or fluoroquinolones, induce colitis, an inflammation of the large intestine, in some individuals. This type of colitis is caused by a toxin produced by the bacteria *Clostridium difficile*, which is resistant to many antibiotics and proliferates in the intestines when other normal bacterial flora in the intestine are altered by the antibiotics.

It is usually recommended to take probiotics at least 3 hours apart from antibiotics. Taking both at the same time defeats the purpose as the friendly bacteria will be totally destroyed by the drug. During antibiotic therapy, a good dose of viable probiotic cells is 6-25 billion colony-forming units per day. Probiotics are also being studied as adjunctive therapy to periodontal treatment and treatment of other bacterial infections.

Has there been any change in the guidelines for prophylaxis for patients with prosthetic joint replacements?

Yes, the 2012 guidelines recommend that practitioners might consider discontinuing the practice of routinely prescribing prophylactic antibiotics for patients with hip and knee prosthetic joint implants undergoing dental procedures. As more evidence and data are collected, these recommendations may be revised; however, to be prudent, the dental clinician should fully evaluate all patients with respect to history and/or physical findings and perform a medical consultation prior to determining the risk. If concern over joint complications exists and a medical consultation cannot be immediately obtained, the dentist should treat the patient as though antibiotic coverage is necessary until an appropriate consultation can be completed.

REFERENCES

American Academy of Orthopaedic Surgeons and American Association of Orthopaedic Surgeons, "Statement Release for New 2012 Clinical Practice Guideline - New Guideline Includes Shared Decision-Making Tool, Implications for Practice," 2013. Available at http://www6.aaos.org/news/PDFopen/PDFopen.cfm?page_url=http://www.aaos.org/news/aaosnow/jan13/cover1.asp

Baddour LM, Bettmann MA, Bolger AF, et al, "Nonvalvular Cardiovascular Device-Related Infections," *Circulation*, 2003, 108(16):2015-31.

Bashore TM, Cabell C, and Fowler V Jr, "Update on Infective Endocarditis," *Curr Probl Cardiol*, 2006, 31(4):274-352.

Brennan MT, Kent ML, Fox PC, et al, "The Impact of Oral Disease and Nonsurgical Treatment on Bacteremia in Children," *J Am Dent Assoc*, 2007, 138 (1):80-5.

Burton JP, Chilcott CN, Moore CJ, et al, "A Preliminary Study of the Effect of Probiotic *Streptococcus salivarius* K12 on Oral Malodour Parameters," *J Appl Microbiol*, 2006, 100(4):754-64.

Duval X, Alla F, Hoen B, et al, "Estimated Risk of Endocarditis in Adults With Predisposing Cardiac Conditions Undergoing Dental Procedures With or Without Antibiotic Prophylaxis," *Clin Infect Dis*, 2006, 42(12):e102-7.

Gould FK, Elliott TS, Foweraker J, et al, "Guidelines for the Prevention of Endocarditis: Report of the Working Party of the British Society for Antimicrobial Chemotherapy," *J Antimicrob Chemother*, 2006, 57(6):1035-42.

Karchmer AW, "Infective Endocarditis," *Braunwald's Heart Disease: A Textbook Of Cardiovascular Medicine*, 7th ed, Zipes D, Libby P, and Bonow RO, eds, Philadelphia, PA: WB Saunders Co, 2005, 1633-58.

Krasse P, Carlsson B, Dahl C, et al, "Decreased Gum Bleeding and Reduced Gingivitis by the Probiotic *Lactobacillus reuteri*," *Swed Dent J*, 2006, 30 (2):55-60.

Meurman JH and Stamatova I, "Probiotics: Contributions to Oral Health," *Oral Dis*, 2007, 13(5):443-5.

Napeñas JJ, Lockhart PB, and Epstein JB, "Comment on the 2009 American Academy of Orthopaedic Surgeons' Information Statement on Antibiotic Prophylaxis for Bacteremia in Patients With Joint Replacements," *J Can Dent Assoc*, 2009, 75(6):447-9.

Teughels W, Van Essche M, Sliepen I, et al, "Probiotics and Oral Healthcare," *Periodontol 2000*, 2008, 48:111-47.

Twetman S and Stecksén-Blicks C, "Probiotics and Oral Health Effects in Children," *Int J Paediatr Dent*, 2008, 18(1):3-10.

Wilson W, Taubert KA, Gewitz M, et al, "Prevention of Infective Endocarditis: Guidelines From the American Heart Association: A Guideline From the American Heart Association Rheumatic Fever, Endocarditis, and Kawasaki Disease Committee, Council on Cardiovascular Disease in the Young, and the Council on Clinical Cardiology, Council on Cardiovascular Surgery and Anesthesia, and the Quality of Care and Outcomes Research Interdisciplinary Working Group," *Circulation*, 2007, 116(15):1736-54.

MANAGEMENT OF THE CHEMICALLY DEPENDENT PATIENT

INTRODUCTION

As long as history has been recorded, man has used drugs to alter mood, thought, and feeling. The financial and emotional cost to society due to the abuse and addiction of these substances is staggering. Some reports place the cost to society of alcoholism and alcohol abuse as high as $185 billion dollars annually. Increased on-the-job accidents, absenteeism, welfare costs, and alcohol-related auto fatalities contribute to this cost.

In 1986, the American Dental Association (ADA) passed a policy statement recognizing chemical dependency as a disease. In recognizing this disease, the Association mandated that dentists have a responsibility to include questions relating to a history of chemical dependency, or more broadly, substance abuse in their health history questionnaire. This policy statement included patients who are actively abusing drugs as well as patients who are in recovery. An affirmative response was an alert to the dentist and dental team to use caution with certain medications and that the treatment plan may have to be altered. This policy statement was revised in 1989 and 1991 with minor changes. In October 2005 at the annual ADA session, the House of Delegates passed several resolutions encompassing the use of opioids in management of dental pain, alcohol, and other substance use by pregnant and postpartum patients, and guidelines related to alcohol, nicotine, and/or drug use by child or adolescent patients. The House of Delegates in 2005 reaffirmed the disease concept of alcoholism and other substance use disorders and provided a more current statement on provision of dental treatment for patients with substance use disorders. For an in-depth review of these resolutions, refer to www.ada.org. At the minimum, the patient's past medical history questionnaire should include a question asking if there is a history of chemical dependency and if so, how long they have been in recovery. The dental office should have a list available of local resources for drug counseling in the event the patient admits drug use and seeks some help.

This chapter reviews substances of abuse, where they come from, signs and symptoms of the substance abuser, and some of the dental implications of treating patients actively using or in recovery from these substances. There are many books and articles devoted to this topic that provide greater detail. The intent of this chapter is to provide an overview of some of the most prevalent drugs, how abuse of these substances by patients may influence dental treatment, and how to recognize some signs and symptoms of substance abuse and withdrawal.

Substances of abuse originate from many sources. They may be naturally occurring, semisynthetic, synthetic, over-the-counter, or prescription drugs. There is a paucity of information in the dental literature correlating substance abuse with dental manifestations for a simple reason. Most substance abusers do not seek routine dental care because obtaining their drug of choice is their top priority. Most often they will be episodic patients. In fact, that is one of the cardinal signs of addiction, a preoccupation with obtaining the drug or sex or gambling or whatever the addiction. Again, it is not the intent of this chapter to explore addiction or abuse in detail. The reader is referred to several comprehensive texts on this disease.

As a general rule, the stimulant (uppers) abusing dental patient will not be going to the dentist while under the influence of the drug because the upper will increase their already existing anxiety. It is more likely that a patient will use or abuse a depressant (downer) substance to self-medicate anxiety. This is important to the dentist because uppers such as cocaine, methamphetamine, and ecstasy are sympathomimetics and in combination with vasoconstrictor could result in a hypertensive crisis (stroke). **Plain local anesthetic without vasoconstrictor is not contraindicated in that patient.** Patients who self-medicate with depressant drugs such as alcohol, opiates, barbiturates, or marijuana are generally more compliant while in the dental chair, and the drug combination does not pose a serious threat.

ALCOHOL

Ethyl alcohol (referred to as alcohol) is the most abused drug in the United States today and the number one most abused drug by dentists. As mentioned above, the cost to society for the treatment of alcoholism and alcohol abuse is billions of dollars annually. Alcohol is a depressant drug (downer) and not a stimulant as many people (particularly the adolescent population) believe. Its effect on the central nervous system is dose-dependent and correlated with the rising blood alcohol concentration rather than the falling concentration. Cognitive ability, reaction time, memory, psychomotor, and perceptual ability are impaired to varying degrees.

The majority of consumed alcohol is absorbed from the small intestine and is, therefore, affected by the gastric emptying time and the consumption of food. Alcohol is metabolized by the liver and excess consumption of alcohol can result in hepatic damage that may affect the patient's ability to metabolize medications. Doses of medications that are metabolized by the liver, such as acetaminophen, may have to be reduced when treating a patient with confirmed hepatic damage from alcohol or other substance abuse. Alcohol readily crosses the placental barrier and has the potential of producing fetal alcohol syndrome (FAS) resulting in mental retardation, supernumerary teeth, and facial deformities to name a few. There are many resources that provide greater detail about this preventable syndrome and the reader is referred to those sources.

Excessive alcohol use has been associated with an increased incidence of periodontal disease, poor wound healing, chronic orofacial infections, iatrogenic injury, and an increased incidence of oral cancer. Since alcohol is a depressant drug, any medication that causes respiratory depression should be prescribed or administered with caution or not at all. Patients who present to the dental office and are obviously intoxicated should not be provided dental treatment. The major concern with the intoxicated patient is a failure to follow directions while in the chair, and the inability to follow postoperative instructions. An additional concern is the aggressive, combative behavior exhibited by some that are intoxicated.

Signs and Symptoms of Alcohol Use or Abuse	
Lethargic, slow to respond	Odor on breath and/or clothes
Slurred speech	Inability to respond to commands
Telangiectasia	Psychomotor impairment

MARIJUANA

The most abused illegal drug by high school students today is marijuana. Marijuana is a plant that grows throughout the world, but is particularly suited for a warm, humid environment. There are three species of plants but the two most frequently cited are *Cannabis sativa* and *Cannabis indica*. All species possess a female and male plant. Although approximately 450 chemicals have been isolated from the plant, the major psychoactive ingredient is delta-9-tetrahydrocannabinol (THC). Of these 450 chemicals, there are approximately 23 psychoactive chemicals, THC being the most abundant. The highest concentration of THC is found in the bud of the female plant (hashish). The concentration of THC varies according to growing conditions and the part of the plant but has increased from approximately 2% to 3% in marijuana sold in the 1950s to approximately 40% sold on the streets today. Marijuana can be smoked in cigarettes (joints), pipes, water pipes (bongs), or baked in brownies, cakes, etc, and then ingested. However, smoking marijuana is more efficient and the "high" has a quicker onset. Marijuana is a Schedule I drug but has been promoted as medicinal for the treatment of glaucoma (according to the Glaucoma Research Foundation, "the number of significant side effects generated by long-term oral use of marijuana or long-term inhalation of marijuana smoke make marijuana a poor choice in the treatment of glaucoma, a chronic disease requiring proven and effective treatment"), for increasing appetite in patients who have HIV disease, to prevent the nausea associated with cancer chemotherapy, and as an analgesic for chronic pain. In response to this request, the FDA approved dronabinol (Marinol®), a synthetic THC, and placed this drug in Schedule III to be prescribed by physicians for the indicated medical conditions. The synthetic THC does not produce a "high" and in fact is not well-absorbed from the gastrointestinal tract. Currently, there are 18 states and the District of Columbia that have passed legislation for marijuana to be used for medical purposes. Additionally, 11 states have pending legislation for medical marijuana. The laws passed or pending by these states differ in the allowable quantity of usable marijuana, as well as the quantity of plants possessed. The medical indications for the use of marijuana have been expanded to include multiple sclerosis-induced spasticity, including the neuropathic pain associated with this condition. Washington and Colorado, have passed legislation to allow marijuana use for recreational purposes in spite of the DEA classification as a Schedule I Controlled Substance which states possession, distribution, and manufacturing of marijuana is a violation. The Department of Justice has not issued a statement regarding the resolution of this conflict between the states and the federal government.

An individual under the influence of marijuana may exhibit no signs or symptoms of intoxication. The pharmacologic effects are dose-dependent and depend to a large extent on the set and setting of the intoxicated individual. As the dose of THC increases, the person experiences euphoria or a state of well-being, often referred to as "mellowing out". Everything becomes comical, problems disappear, and their appetite for snack foods increases. This is called the "munchies". Additionally, marijuana produces time and spatial distortion, which contribute, as the dose increases, to a dysphoria characterized by paranoia and fear. Although there has never been a death reported from marijuana overdose, certainly the higher doses may produce such bizarre circumstances as to increase the chances of accidental death. THC is fat soluble. Daily consumption of marijuana will result in THC being stored in body fat which will result in detectable amounts of THC being found in the urine for as long as 60 days in some cases.

Synthetic Cannabinoids: These chemicals are synthetic versions of delta 9-tetrahydrocannabinol (THC), the major psychoactive ingredient in marijuana. They are reported to be 200-800 times more potent than THC. The effects of these chemicals are similar to marijuana: Increased heart rate, increased blood pressure, paranoia, agitation, giddiness, and increased appetite. Synthetic cannabinoids are advertised as being undetectable in urine drug tests for THC; however, this is untrue. The chemicals can be detected by urinalysis, but it takes a very sophisticated system for detection, testing is expensive, and most laboratories do not routinely test for synthetic cannabinoids.

Internet sales of the chemicals have been connected to sources in China, Pakistan, and India. Once the chemicals have been purchased, the final product can be assembled in the United States. It is sold in small packets labeled as incense, which contain dried herbal materials that are sprayed with the synthetic cannabinoids. The product is typically smoked, and has various street names such as "Spice Diamond," "Dream," "Essence," and "K-2." Packets vary in cost from $20 to $50 and weigh 100-300 mg.

These "designer" drugs are intended to circumvent the Controlled Substances Act of 1970. The problem for law enforcement is that underground chemists continue to modify chemicals into new ones that are not illegal to possess or use. On March 1, 2011, the U.S. Drug Enforcement Administration (DEA) placed five synthetic cannabinoids on the Controlled Substances list in Schedule I. Officially, the chemicals are designated as: JWH 018, JWH 073, JWH 200, CP 47, 497, and cannabicyclohexanol.

Because of anxiety associated with dental visits, marijuana would be the most likely drug, after alcohol, to be used when coming to the dental office. But, unlike alcohol, marijuana may not produce any detectable odor on the breath nor signs of intoxication. Fortunately, local anesthetics, analgesics, and antibiotics used by the general dentist do not interact with marijuana. The major concern with the marijuana-intoxicated patient, similar to the alcohol-intoxicated patient, is a failure to follow directions while in the chair, and the inability to follow postoperative instructions.

Signs and Symptoms of Marijuana Use	
Blood shot eyes	Odor on breath and clothes
Lethargic, slow to respond	Inability to respond to commands
Slurred speech	Memory impairment

OPIATES

The opiates are most often called narcotics. The word "narcosis" means sleep. These drugs are referred to on the street as "downers", the most common being heroin. Heroin is the diacetyl derivative of morphine which is extracted from opium. Although commercial production of morphine involves extraction from the dried opium plant which grows in many parts of the world, some areas still harvest opium by making slits in the unripened seed pod. The pod secretes a white, viscous material which upon contact with the air turns a blackish-brown color. It is this off-white material that is called opium. The opium is then dried and smoked or processed to yield morphine and codeine. Actually, the raw opium contains several chemicals that are used medicinally or commercially. Much (approximately 50%) of morphine is converted chemically into heroin which finds its way into the United States and then on the street. Heroin is a Schedule I drug and has no acceptable use in the United States today. In fact, possession is a violation of the Controlled Substances Act of 1970. The majority of the heroin found on the streets in the United States is from Colombia, South America (65%) and can be as pure as 50% to 60%. Approximately 30% of the heroin in the United States originates in Mexico and the remainder is produced in the "Golden Triangle" (Burma [Myanmar], Laos, and Thailand).

The heroin user goes through many phases once the drug has been administered. When administered intravenously, the user initially feels a "rush" often described as an "orgasmic rush". This initial feeling is most likely due to the release of histamine resulting in cutaneous vasodilation, itching, and a flushed appearance. Shortly after this "rush" the user becomes euphoric. This euphoric stage often called "stoned" or being "high" lasts approximately 3-4 hours. During this stage, the user is lethargic, slow to react to stimuli, speech is slurred, pain reaction threshold is elevated, exhibits xerostomia, experiences slowed heart rate, and his/hers pupils may be constricted. Following the "high", the abuser is "straight" for about 2 hours, with no tell-tale signs of abuse. Approximately 6-8 hours following the last injection of heroin, the user begins to experience a runny nose, lacrimation, and abdominal muscle cramps as the withdrawal from the drug begins. During this stage and the one that follows, the person may become agitated as he/she develops anxiety about where the next "hit" will come from. The withdrawal signs and symptoms become more intense. For the next 3 days, the abuser begins to sweat profusely in combination with cutaneous vasoconstriction. The skin becomes cold and clammy, hence the term "cold turkey". Tachycardia, pupillary dilation, diarrhea, and salivation occur for 3 days following the last injection. Withdrawal signs and symptoms may last longer than the average of 3 days or they may be more abrupt.

Many patients who have been abusing opiates will exhibit multiple carious lesions, particularly class V lesions. This increased caries rate is probably a result of the heroin-induced xerostomia, high intake of sweets, and lack of daily oral hygiene. Patients who are recovering from heroin or any opiate addiction should not be given any kind of opiate analgesic, whether it is for sedation or as a postoperative analgesic because of the increased chance of relapse. Nonsteroidal anti-inflammatory drugs (NSAIDs) should be used to control any postoperative discomfort. Patients who admit to a past history of intravenous heroin use, or any intravenous drug for that matter, are at higher risk for subacute bacterial endocarditis (SBE), HIV disease, and hepatitis, with the exception of postoperative analgesia should present no special problem for dental care.

Signs and Symptoms of Narcotic Use	
Pin point pupils	Glazed eyes
Lethargic, slow to respond	Inability to respond to commands
Slurred speech	Xerostomia

METHAMPHETAMINE

Methamphetamine has been available clinically for 45 years as a medication to curb appetite. Today it is one of the most widely abused drugs on the street. Methamphetamine can be smoked in the form of "ice", snorted, injected, or consumed orally. The onset of action varies with the route of administration, smoking providing the most rapid onset of action. Clandestine methamphetamine is usually synthesized from pseudoephedrine or ephedrine. The methamphetamine molecule can exist in either the "D" isomer or the "L" isomer. The latter isomer has its greatest effect on the cardiovascular system and, in fact, is available commercially over-the-counter as a nasal decongestant. The "D" isomer has its principle effects on the central nervous system as a stimulant (upper) and can not be converted from the "L" form. It is a sympathomimetic and as such raises blood pressure. This effect on the autonomic nervous system results in increased basal metabolic rate (BMR) and increased body temperature, resulting in the "sweats". Methamphetamine users crave sweets possibly as a source of energy to fuel the increased BMR. As a consequence of the increased sweating the individual becomes dehydrated and thirsty. The sympathetic stimulation produces thick, ropey saliva. This lack of saliva, increased consumption of sweets in the form of soda pop, and lack of routine dental care no doubt is the primary cause of "meth mouth". Initially the meth user experiences a feeling of exhilaration, alertness, and incredible energy. With successive uses, tolerance occurs and the user abuses increasing amounts of methamphetamine looking for the same high they experienced on the first time. They never quite attain it. This has been referred to on the street as "chasing the monkey". As a substitute, the user continues their high for several hours or days in some cases. This is called bingeing. A binge may last for 5 or 6 days. The user becomes very paranoid, develops psychotic episodes, and has the potential of becoming violent. stereotypical behavior develops such as rocking back and forth in a chair, picking their fingernails, or other behavior. During this stage the user begins "tweaking", using small amounts to stay high, and begins to hallucinate.

Characteristically, they will describe the feeling that bugs are crawling under their skin and they scratch their arms, face, and any other exposed part of their body. The street term for this hallucination is called "coke bugs". Usually, the user will collapse from the physical exhaustion. Withdrawal can take weeks after the last use. As mentioned above, vasoconstrictor is contraindicated if there has been methamphetamine use within the last 24 hours.

Methamphetamine Signs and Symptoms in the Dental Office	
Dilated pupils	Jittery, irritable behavior
Rapid speech	Unable to sit still, twitching
Tremendous anxiety	Difficult to anesthetize

BENZODIAZEPINES AND OTHER NONALCOHOL SEDATIVES

These drugs are used mainly for treatment of anxiety disorders and, in some instances, insomnia. These drugs are commonly abused, either by themselves or as adjunct to the opiates. They have the ability to produce a strong physical dependency on the use of the medication. As tolerance builds up to the drug, the physical dependency increases dramatically. Unlike street drugs, where addiction is a primary consideration, the overuse of benzodiazepine lies in their ability to induce physical dependency. When these drugs are taken for several weeks, there is relatively little tolerance induced. However, after several months, the proportion of patients who become tolerant increases and reducing the dose or stopping the medication produces severe withdrawal symptoms often resulting in death.

It is extremely difficult for the physician to distinguish between the withdrawal symptoms and the reappearance of the myriad anxiety symptoms that cause the drug to be prescribed initially. Many patients increase their dose over time because tolerance develops to at least the sedative effects of the drug. The antianxiety benefits of the benzodiazepines continue to occur long after tolerance to the sedating effects. Patients often take these drugs for many years with relatively few ill effects other than the risk of withdrawal. The dentist should be keenly aware of the signs and symptoms and the historical pattern in patients taking benzodiazepines. On the street, the abuser will often mix a benzodiazepine with an opioid to enhance the opioid-induced euphoria.

NICOTINE

Cigarette (nicotine) addiction is influenced by multiple variables. Nicotine itself produces reinforcement; users compare nicotine to stimulants such as cocaine or amphetamine, although its effects are of lower magnitude.

Nicotine is absorbed readily through the skin, mucous membranes, and of course, through the lungs. The pulmonary route produces discernible central nervous system effects in as little as 7 seconds. Thus, each puff produces some discrete reinforcement. With 10 puffs per cigarette, the 1 pack per day smoker reinforces the habit 200 times daily. The timing, setting, situation, and preparation all become associated repetitively with the effects of nicotine.

Nicotine has both stimulant and depressant actions. The smoker feels alert, yet there is some muscle relaxation. Nicotine activates the nucleus accumbens reward system in the brain. Increased extracellular dopamine has been found in this region after nicotine injections in rats. Nicotine affects other systems as well, including the release of endogenous opioids and glucocorticoids.

Nicotine Withdrawal Syndrome Signs and Symptoms	
Irritability, impatience, hostility	Restlessness
Anxiety	Decreased heart rate
Dysphoric or depressed mood	Increased appetite or weight gain
Difficulty concentrating	

SMOKING CESSATION PRODUCTS

Several years ago, the journal, *Science*, stated that approximately 80% of smokers say they want to quit, but each year <1 in 10 actually succeed. Nicotine transdermal delivery preparations (or nicotine patches) were approved by the U.S. Food and Drug Administration in 1992 as aids to smoking cessation for the relief of nicotine withdrawal symptoms. Four preparations were approved simultaneously: Habitrol®, Nicoderm®, Nicotrol®, and ProStep®. These products differ in how much nicotine is released and whether they provide a 24- or 16-hour release time.

Studies are still being reported on the effectiveness of nicotine patches on tobacco cessation. Most previous studies had good entry criteria including definition of the Fagerstrom score. Dr Fred Cowan of Oregon Health Sciences University described these Fagerstrom criteria in a previous report on nicotine substitutes in AGD *Impact*. Abstinence of smoking cessation has usually been assessed by self-report, measurement of carbon monoxide in breath, and plasma or urine nicotine products.

In numerous protocols, percentages of study subjects who abstained from smoking after 3-10 weeks of patch treatment with nicotine compared to placebo, have never exceeded 40%. After the initial assessment, six studies continued to follow the study subjects through 24-52 weeks of patch treatment. The results were even poorer with <25% sustained success. A review of these and additional studies, reveals some general conclusions regarding the effectiveness of nicotine patches in tobacco cessation. In every study, many smokers abstained after treatment with placebo patches; nicotine treatment was initially more effective than placebo; and improved abstinence rates were more marked in the short term (10 weeks) than in the long term (52 weeks). Subjects undergoing tobacco cessation trials tended to gain weight irrespective of whether placebo or nicotine patches were worn. Patients often favor the nicotine polacrilex gum (Nicorette®) which releases nicotine into the blood stream via the oral mucosa.

Data are now available from tobacco cessation studies carried out in general medical practices. The effectiveness of nicotine patch substitution under these conditions is similar to the results described previous. Most patch systems and gum are now available as over-the-counter products; only Habitrol® remains prescription. bupropion (Zyban®) is another approach to the treatment of tobacco cessation. This drug is a norepinephrine/serotonin/dopamine reuptake inhibitor and its action directly affects the craving for tobacco. Another new product just introduced is varenicline (Chantix®). This product targets certain nicotine receptors to prevent nicotine access and diminishes the mesolimbic dopamine reward associated with nicotine use. The reader is referred to more comprehensive information about these products and the treatment of tobacco cessation. In addition, the reader should familiarize themselves with the supportive ADA posture on the role of the dental team in tobacco cessation treatment.

COCAINE

Cocaine, referred to on the street as "snow", "nose candy", "girl", and many other euphemisms, has created an epidemic. This drug is like no other local anesthetic. Known for about the last 2000 years, cocaine has been used and abused by politicians, scientists, farmers, warriors, and of course, on the street. Cocaine is derived from the leaves of a plant called *Erythroxylon* coca which grows in South America. Ninety percent of the world's supply of cocaine originates in Peru, Bolivia, and Colombia. At last estimate, the United States consumes 75% of the world's supply. The plant grows to a height of approximately 4 feet and produces a red berry. Farmers go through the fields stripping the leaves from the plant three times a year. During the working day, the farmers chew the coca leaves to suppress appetite and fight the fatigue of working the fields. The leaves are transported to a laboratory site where the cocaine is extracted by a process called maceration. It takes approximately 7-8 pounds of leaves to produce 1 ounce of cocaine.

On the streets of the United States, cocaine can be found in two forms - one is the hydrochloride salt which can be "snorted" or dissolved in water and injected intravenously, the other is the free base form which can be smoked and is sometimes referred to as "crack", "rock", or "free base". It is called crack because it cracks or pops when large pieces are smoked. It is called rock because it is hard and difficult to break into smaller pieces. The most popular method of administration of cocaine is "snorting" in which small amounts of cocaine hydrochloride are divided into segments or "lines" and any straw-like device can be used to inhale one or more lines of the cocaine into the nose. Although cocaine does not reach the lungs, enough cocaine is absorbed through nasal mucosa to provide a "high" within 3-5 minutes. Rock or crack, on the other hand, is heated and inhaled from any device available. This form of cocaine does reach the lungs and provides a much faster onset of action as well as a more intense stimulation. There are dangers to the user with any form of cocaine. Undoubtedly, the most dangerous form is the intravenous route.

Signs and Symptoms of Cocaine Use	
Dilated pupils	Tremors
Jitteriness	Talkative
Irritability	Increased blood pressure

The cocaine user, regardless of how the cocaine was administered, presents a potential life-threatening situation in the dental operatory. The patient under the influence of cocaine could be compared to a car going 100 miles per hour. Blood pressure is elevated and heart rate is likely increased. Use of a local anesthetic with epinephrine in such a patient may result in a medical emergency. Such patients can be identified by jitteriness, irritability, talkativeness, tremors, and short abrupt speech patterns. These same signs and symptoms may also be seen in a normal dental patient with preoperative dental anxiety; therefore, the dentist must be particularly alert to identify the potential cocaine abuser. If a patient is suspected, they should never be given a local anesthetic with vasoconstrictor for fear of exacerbating cocaine-induced sympathetic response. Life-threatening episodes of cardiac arrhythmias and hypertensive crises have been reported when local anesthetic with vasoconstrictor was administered to a patient under the influence of cocaine. No local anesthetic used by any dentist can interfere with, nor test positive for cocaine in any urine testing screen. Therefore, the dentist need not be concerned with any false drug use accusations associated with dental anesthesia.

CLUB DRUGS

Perceptual distortions that include hallucinations, illusions, and disorders of thinking such as paranoia can be produced by toxic doses of many drugs. These phenomena also may be seen during toxic withdrawal from sedatives such as alcohol. There are, however, certain drugs that have as their primary effect the production of perception, thought, or mood disturbances at low doses with minimal effects on memory and orientation. These are commonly called *hallucinogenic drugs*, but their use does not always result in frank hallucinations.

Ecstasy (MDMA) and Phenylethylamines (MDA): MDA and MDMA have stimulant, as well as, psychedelic effects and produce degeneration of serotonergic nerve cells and axons. While nerve degeneration has not been well-demonstrated in human beings, the potential remains. Thus, there is possible neurotoxicity with overuse of these drugs. Ecstasy became popular during the 1980s on college campuses and it is still recommended by some psychotherapists as an aid to the process of therapy, although very little controlled data is available. Acute effects are dose-dependent and include dry mouth, jaw clinching, muscle aches, and tachycardia. At higher doses, effects include agitation, hyperthermia, panic attacks, and visual hallucinations. Frequent, repeated use of psychedelic drugs is unusual and, therefore, tolerance is not commonly seen. However, tolerance does develop to the behavioral effects of various psychedelic drugs, and after numerous doses, the tendency towards behavioral tolerance can be observed.

Lysergic Acid Diethylamide (LSD): LSD is the most potent hallucinogenic drug and produces significant psychedelic effects with a total dose of as little as 25-50 mcg. This drug is over 3000 times more potent than mescaline. It is sold on the illicit market in a variety of forms, as a tablet, capsule, sugar cube, or on blotting paper, a popular contemporary system involving postage stamp-sized papers impregnated with varying doses of LSD (50-300 mcg). A majority of street samples sold as LSD actually do contain LSD, while mushrooms and other botanicals sold as sources of psilocybin and other psychedelics have a low probability of containing the advertised hallucinogenics. Adverse effects which may affect treatment include visual and auditory hallucinations, tachycardia, psychosis, fear, tremors, delirium, hyperglycemia, fever, sweating, flushing, euphoria, hypertonia, nausea, vomiting, coma, seizures, tachypnea, and respiratory arrest.

Bath Salts (synthetic cathinones): This potentially deadly street drug acquired the name bath salts, because it is packaged in containers that resemble the scented soaps that can be added to bath water. The term "bath salt" is a generic term which originally described three distinct synthetic chemicals: Mephedrone; 3,4-methylenedioxypyrovalerone (MDPV); and methylone. As of October 21, 2011, these substances were designated as Schedule I Controlled Substances by the U.S. Drug Enforcement Administration (DEA). This action makes possession or selling of these chemicals illegal in the United States. These chemicals are synthetic forms of cathinone which is derived from the shrub Catha edulis (khat). There are several street terms for these crystalline chemicals; some of the more popular are "Ivory Wave," "Red Dove," "Vanilla Sky," and "White Lightning." The packages are usually labeled "Not Intended for Human Consumption," but users may snort, swallow, or inject the contents. A package may weigh from 300-500 mg and can cost approximately $25 to $40 on the street.

The effects of the chemicals in "bath salts" have been described as a combination of cocaine, ecstasy, and methamphet-amine. Psychological effects include insomnia, suicidal ideation, paranoia, agitation, and seizures. The user describes heightened awareness, euphoria, and enhanced sexual ability. Since these medications are sympathomimetics, vaso-constrictors should **not** be used in individuals suspected to be under the influence of "bath salts."

INHALANTS

Anesthetic gases such as nitrous oxide or halothane are sometimes used as intoxicants by medical personnel. Nitrous oxide also is abused by food service employees because it is supplied for use as a propellant in disposable aluminum mini tanks for whipping cream canisters. Nitrous oxide produces euphoria and analgesia and then loss of consciousness. Compulsive use and chronic toxicity rarely are reported, but there are obvious risks of overdose associated with the abuse of this anesthetic. Chronic use has been reported to cause peripheral neuropathy. Glue, correction fluid, gasoline, aerosol key board cleaners, model paint, in fact, any volatile substance has the potential to cause a "high" and like all of the above can become very addictive and deadly.

The dental team should be alert to the signs and symptoms of drug abuse and withdrawal. Further reading is recommended.

ORAL MEDICINE TOPICS

PART II:

DENTAL MANAGEMENT AND THERAPEUTIC CONSIDERATIONS IN PATIENTS WITH SPECIFIC ORAL CONDITIONS AND OTHER MEDICINE TOPICS

The second part of the chapter focuses on therapies the dentist may choose to prescribe for patients suffering from oral disease or who are in need of special care. Some overlap between these sections has resulted from systemic conditions that have oral manifestations and vice-versa. Cross-references to the descriptions and the monographs for individual drugs described elsewhere in this handbook allow for easy retrieval of information. Example prescriptions of selected drug therapies for each condition are presented so that the clinician can evaluate alternate approaches to treatment, since there is seldom a single drug of choice.

Drug prescriptions shown represent prototype drugs and popular prescriptions and are examples only. The pharmacologic category index is available for cross-referencing if alternatives and additional drugs are sought.

TABLE OF CONTENTS

ORAL PAIN

PAIN PREVENTION

For the dental patient, the prevention of pain aids in relieving anxiety and reduces the probability of stress during dental care. For the practitioner, dental procedures can be accomplished more efficiently in a "painless" situation. Appropriate selection and use of local anesthetics is one of the foundations for success in this arena. Local anesthetics listed below include drugs for the most commonly confronted dental procedures. Ester anesthetics are no longer available in dose form for dental injections, and historically had a higher incidence of allergic manifestations due to the formation of the metabolic byproduct, para-aminobenzoic acid. Articaine, which has an ester side chain, is rapidly metabolized to a non-PABA acid and functions as an amide and has a low allergic potential. The amides, in general, have a nearly negligible incidence of true allergic reactions, and only one well-documented case of amide allergy has been reported by Seng, et al. Although injectable diphenhydramine (Benadryl®) has been used in an attempt to provide anesthesia in patients allergic to all the local anesthetics, it is no longer recommended in this context. The vehicle for injectable diphenhydramine can cause tissue necrosis.

Local Anesthetics

Articaine and Epinephrine on page 128
Bupivacaine on page 209
Bupivacaine and Epinephrine on page 209
Chloroprocaine on page 290
Lidocaine and Epinephrine on page 820
Lidocaine (Systemic) on page 816
Mepivacaine Dental Anesthetic on page 874
Mepivacaine and Levonordefrin on page 876
Prilocaine on page 1139
Prilocaine and Epinephrine on page 1140
Ropivacaine on page 1211
Tetracaine (Topical) on page 1307

The selection of a vasoconstrictor with the local anesthetic must be based on the length of the procedure to be performed, the patient's medical status (epinephrine is contraindicated in patients with uncontrolled hyperthyroidism), and the need for hemorrhage control. The following table lists some of the common drugs with their duration of action. The long-acting amide injectable, Ropivacaine (Naropin®) may be useful for postoperative pain management.

Dental Anesthetics (Average Duration by Route)

Product	Infiltration	Inferior Alveolar Block
Articaine HCl 4% and epinephrine 1:100,000	60 minutes	~60 minutes
Articaine HCl 4% and epinephrine 1:200,000	40 minutes	50 minutes
Carbocaine® HCl 2% with Neo-Cobefrin® 1:20,000 (mepivacaine HCl and levonordefrin)	50 minutes	60-75 minutes
Carbocaine® Plain 3%	20 minutes	40 minutes
Citanest® Plain 4% (prilocaine)	20 minutes	2.5 hours
Citanest® Forte with epinephrine 1:200,000 (prilocaine with epinephrine)	2.25 hours	3 hours
Lidocaine HCl 2% and epinephrine 1:100,000	60 minutes	90 minutes
Marcaine® HCl 0.5% with epinephrine 1:200,000 (bupivacaine and epinephrine)	60 minutes	5-7 hours
Vivacaine™ 0.5% with epinephrine 1:200,000 (bupivacaine and epinephrine)	60 minutes	5-7 hours

The use of articaine 4% with epinephrine 1:100,000 solution for mandibular blocks has been associated occasionally with paresthesia (*J Am Dent Assoc*, 2001, 132(2):177-85).

The use of preinjection topical anesthetics can assist in pain prevention (see also Viral Infections on page 1575 and Ulcerative, Erosive, and Painful Oral Mucosal Disorders on page 1578). It should be noted that the FDA recently warned healthcare professionals regarding potential risks associated with unsupervised patient cutaneous use of topical anesthetic products. Life-threatening adverse events such as arrhythmias, seizures, coma, and respiratory complications have been reported. Thus, healthcare professionals are advised to prescribe FDA-approved topical anesthetics in the lowest concentration consistent with pain relief goals. It is not known if oral mucosa misuse may pose the same risk factors.

Clinicians are also using a eutectic mixture of 2.5% lidocaine with 2.5% prilocaine in a periodontal gel form in adults who require localized anesthesia in periodontal pockets during scaling and/or root planing. However, the same mixture available as a skin patch (EMLA®) from Astra is not currently approved for oral use.

OraVerse™ (phentolamine mesylate) injection is a local anesthetic reversal agent that accelerates the return to normal sensation and function following restorative and periodontal maintenance procedures. OraVerse™ is indicated for the reversal of soft tissue anesthesia (ie, anesthesia of the lip, tongue, and the associated functional deficits resulting from an intraoral submucosal injection of a local anesthetic containing a vasoconstrictor). OraVerse™ is not recommended for use in children <6 years of age or weighing <15 kg (33 lbs).

Phentolamine (OraVerse™), as used in its original context as a medical hypotensive agent, could be expected to cause significant hypotension and reflex tachycardia when used as the anesthetic reversal agent in children. Studies have shown, however, that neither of these reactions occurred in the children receiving the drug. According to the authors of the study, there was an impressive benefit:risk ratio suggesting a safe approach in accelerating recovery from soft tissue anesthesia in children (Tavares, et al, *JADA*, 2008, 139(8):1095-1104). There were no serious adverse events observed. The adverse reactions were observed from study populations of 484 adults and 152 children. It should be anticipated that more adverse effects could occur as OraVerse™ is used in a larger number of patients. The clinical studies used a maximum of 2 cartridges of OraVerse™ (0.8 mg phentolamine). There is no information published on effects that occur with higher doses of OraVerse™. Phentolamine is a very powerful alpha-adrenergic receptor blocker which can cause cardiovascular effects if inadvertently injected in high doses. The manufacturer advises to adhere to the recommended dosing for the OraVerse™ formulation. The dosing for OraVerse™ is based on the number of cartridges of local anesthetic with vasoconstrictor administered, with 1 cartridge of OraVerse™ containing 0.4 mg of phentolamine and 2 cartridges containing 0.8 mg phentolamine. Dosing is as a 1:1 cartridge ratio to local anesthetic using the same injection site and administration technique as that used for the local anesthetic.

Benzocaine on page 176
Lidocaine (Systemic) on page 816
Phentolamine on page 1086
Tetracaine (Topical) on page 1307

PAIN MANAGEMENT

The patient with existing acute or chronic oral pain requires appropriate treatment and sensitivity on the part of the dentist, all for the purpose of achieving relief from the oral source of pain. Pain can be divided into mild, moderate, and severe levels and requires a subjective assessment by the dentist based on knowledge of the dental procedures to be performed, the presenting signs and symptoms of the patient, and the realization that most dental procedures are invasive often leading to pain once the patient has left the dental office. The practitioner must be aware that the treatment of the source of the pain is usually the best management. If infection is present, treatment of the infection will directly alleviate the patient's discomfort. However, a patient who is not in pain tends to heal better and it is wise to adequately cover the patient for any residual or recurrent discomfort suffered. Likewise, many of the procedures that the dentist performs have pain associated with them. Much of this pain occurs after leaving the dentist office due to an inflammatory process or a healing process that has been initiated. It is difficult to assign specific pain levels (mild, moderate, or severe) for specific procedures; however, the dentist should use his or her prescribing capacity judiciously so that overmedication is avoided.

The potential interaction between acetaminophen and warfarin has been recently raised in the literature. The cytochrome P450 system of drug metabolism for these vitamin K-dependent metabolic pathways has raised the possibility that prolonged use of acetaminophen may inadvertently enhance, to dangerous levels, the anticoagulation effect of warfarin. As monitored by the INR, the effects of these drugs may be one and one-half to two times greater than as expected from the warfarin dosage alone. This potential interaction could be of importance in selecting an analgesic/antipyretic drug for the dental patient.

The following categories of drugs and appropriate example prescriptions for each can be found in the example prescriptions quick reference section, following the chapters. These include management of mild pain with aspirin products, acetaminophen, and some of the nonsteroidal noninflammatory agents (eg, ibuprofen). Management of moderate pain includes codeine, Toradol®, Vicodin®, Vicodin ES®, Opana®; and Motrin® in the 800 mg dosage. Etodolac is approved as an NSAID for mild-to-moderate acute and chronic pain, as well as, for pain of osteo and rheumatoid arthritis. Severe pain may require treatment with Percodan® or Percocet®. A new drug, tapentadol is similar to tramadol in its actions and was approved in November 2008 for moderate-to-severe acute pain. Tapentadol is classified as a narcotic analgesic having a unique ability to bind to μ-opiate receptors and inhibit the reuptake of norepinephrine. It shares many properties of traditional narcotic drugs including addiction liability. A report by Kleinert et al, showed that a single dose of tapentadol ≥75 mg effectively reduced moderate-to-severe postoperative dental pain in a dose related fashion and was well tolerated compared to 60 mg morphine. Their study showed that tapentadol was a highly effective, central-acting analgesic with a favorable side effect profile with rapid onset of action (Kleinert, 2008). All prescription pain preparations should be closely monitored for efficacy and discontinued if the pain persists or requires a higher level formulation. Combination drugs such as the recently released Combunox™ containing 5 mg of oxycodone and 400 mg of ibuprofen have proven usefulness in acute moderately severe to severe pain management.

The chronic pain patient represents a particular challenge for the practitioner. Some additional drugs that may be useful in managing the patient with chronic pain of neuropathic origin are covered in the temporomandibular dysfunction section. It is always incumbent on the practitioner to reevaluate the diagnosis, source of pain, and treatment, whenever prolonged use of analgesics (narcotic or non-narcotic) is contemplated. Drugs such as Dilaudid® are not recommended for management of dental pain in most states.

Recently, the FDA has formally requested manufacturers to limit the amount of acetaminophen in prescription combination products to no more than 325 mg in each tablet or capsule. Manufacturers have until January 2014 to limit the amount of acetaminophen in their oral prescription drug products. The FDA is also requiring manufacturers to update labeling of all prescription combination acetaminophen products to warn of the potential risk for severe liver injury. The over-the-counter acetaminophen products are not affected by this ruling. Some manufacturers have already reduced acetaminophen amounts to 300-325 mg per tablet in combination prescription products. Examples include hydrocodone and acetaminophen products such as Norco®, Vicodin®, and Xodol®.

Overdose from prescription combination products containing acetaminophen account for nearly half of all cases of acetaminophen-related liver failure in the United States. Many cases result in liver transplant or death. There is no immediate danger to patients taking these combination pain medications. Patients should continue to take them as directed by healthcare provider. The risk of liver injury primarily occurs when patients take multiple products containing acetaminophen at one time and exceed the current maximum adult dose of 4000 mg within a 24-hour period. For more information and a complete list of affected products see www.fda.gov/Drugs/DrugSafety/InformationbyDrugClass/ucm239874.htm

Narcotic analgesics can be used on a short-term basis or intermittently in combination with non-narcotic therapy in the chronic pain patient. Judicious prescribing, monitoring, and maintenance by the practitioner are imperative, particularly whenever considering the use of a narcotic analgesic due to the abuse and addiction liabilities. For all prescribers of extended release and long-acting opioid analgesics, patient information as noted below is required.

DOs and DON'Ts of Extended Release/Long-Acting Opioid Analgesics

DO:

- Read the **Medication Guide**
- Take your medicine exactly as prescribed
- Store your medicine away from children and in a safe place
- Check with pharmacy about disposal of unused medicine.
- Call your healthcare provider for medical advice about side effects. You may report side effects to the FDA at (800) FDA-1088

Call 911 or your local emergency service right away if:

- You take too much medicine
- You have trouble breathing or shortness of breath
- A child has taken this medicine

Talk to your healthcare provider:

- If the dose you are taking does not control your pain
- About any side effects you may be having
- About all the medicines you take, including over-the-counter medicines, vitamins, and dietary supplements

DON'T:

- **Do not** give your medicine to others
- **Do not** take medicine unless it was prescribed for you
- **Do not** stop taking your medicine without talking to your healthcare provider
- **Do not** break, chew, crush, dissolve, or inject your medicine. If you cannot swallow your medicine whole, talk to your healthcare provider
- **Do not** drink alcohol while taking this medicine

MILD PAIN

Acetaminophen on page 27
Aspirin (various products) on page 135
Diflunisal on page 421
Etodolac on page 554
Ibuprofen on page 711
Ketoprofen on page 781
Naproxen on page 958

MODERATE/MODERATELY SEVERE PAIN

Dihydrocodeine, Aspirin, and Caffeine on page 426
Hydrocodone and Acetaminophen on page 689
Hydrocodone and Ibuprofen on page 693
Acetaminophen and Tramadol on page 35
Ibuprofen (various products) on page 711
Ketorolac (Systemic) on page 783
Oxymorphone on page 1037
Tapentadol on page 1283

An additional class of NSAIDs has been approved and indicated in the treatment of arthritis, COX-2 inhibitors. Celecoxib (Celebrex®) has been approved for use in oral pain management.

The following is a guideline to use when prescribing codeine with either aspirin or acetaminophen (Tylenol®):

Codeine No. 2 = codeine 15 mg
Codeine No. 3 = codeine 30 mg
Codeine No. 4 = codeine 60 mg

Example: ASA No. 3 = aspirin 325 mg + codeine 30 mg

HYDROCODONE PRODUCTS

Available hydrocodone oral products are listed in the following table and are scheduled as C-III controlled substances, indicating that prescriptions may either be oral or written. Thus, the prescriber may call in a prescription to the pharmacy for any of these hydrocodone products. All the formulations are combined with acetaminophen except for Vicoprofen®, which contains ibuprofen. Most of these brand name drugs are available generically and the pharmacist will dispense the generic equivalent if available, unless the prescriber indicates otherwise.

HYDROCODONE ANALGESIC COMBINATION ORAL PRODUCTS (All Products DEA Schedule C-III)

Hydrocodone is available under numerous brand names with varying dosages and in combination with aspirin or ibuprofen.					
Hydrocodone Bitartrate	Acetaminophen (APAP[1])	Other	Brand Name	Generic Available	Form
5 mg	300 mg	–	Vicodin®	Yes	Tablet
7.5 mg	300 mg	–	Vicodin ES®	Yes	Tablet
7.5 mg	325 mg	–	Norco®	Yes	Tablet
10 mg	325 mg	–	Norco®	Yes	Tablet
10 mg	300 mg	–	Vicodin HP®	Yes	Tablet
7.5 mg/15 mL	325 mg/15 mL	–	-	Yes	Elixir
7.5 mg	–	Ibuprofen 200 mg	Vicoprofen®	Yes	Tablet
5 mg	–	Ibuprofen 200 mg	Ibudone®; Reprexain™	Yes	Tablet

Note: Although there are products still available with >325 mg of acetaminophen per dosage form, the deadline for reduction of acetaminophen is January 2014.

[1]APAP is the common acronym for acetaminophen and is the abbreviation of the chemical name N-acetyl-para-aminophenol.

SEVERE PAIN

HYDROmorphone on page 701
OxyCODONE on page 1028
Oxycodone and Acetaminophen on page 1030
Oxycodone and Aspirin on page 1032
Oxycodone and Ibuprofen on page 1034

Oxycodone is available in a variety of dosages and combinations under numerous brand names.

SAMPLE PRESCRIPTIONS

Rx:
Ibuprofen 800 mg tablets
Disp: 16 tablets
Sig: Take 1 tablet 3 times/day as needed for pain

Note: For severe pain, can be given up to 4 times/day. Also available as 600 mg tablets

Rx:
Norco® 10 mg
Disp: 16 tablets
Sig: Take 1 or 2 tablets every 4 hours as needed for pain; not to exceed 8 tablets in 24 hours

Note: Restrictions: C-III; no refills
Ingredients: Hydrocodone 10 mg and acetaminophen 325 mg; available as generic equivalent

For additional sample prescriptions see Oral Pain on page 1606

BACTERIAL INFECTIONS

Dental infection can occur for any number of reasons, primarily involving pulpal and periodontal infections. Secondary infections of the soft tissues as well as sinus infections pose special treatment challenges. The drugs of choice in treating most oral infections have been selected because of their efficacy in providing adequate blood levels for delivery to the oral tissues and their proven usefulness in managing dental infections. Penicillin remains the primary drug for treatment of dental infections of pulpal origin. The management of soft tissue infections may require the use of additional drugs.

OROFACIAL INFECTIONS

The basis of all infections is the successful multiplication of a microbial pathogen on or within a host. The pathogen is usually defined as any microorganism that has the capacity to cause disease. If the pathogen is bacterial in nature, antibiotic therapy is often indicated.

DIFFERENTIAL DIAGNOSIS OF ODONTOGENIC INFECTIONS

In choosing the appropriate antibiotic for therapy of a given infection, a number of important factors must be considered. First, the identity of the organism must be known. In odontogenic infections involving dental or periodontal structures, this is seldom the case. Secondly, accurate information regarding antibiotic susceptibility is required. Again, unless the organism has been identified, this is not possible. And thirdly, host factors must be taken into account, in terms of ability to absorb an antibiotic, to achieve appropriate host response. When clinical evidence of cellulitis or odontogenic infection is found and the cardinal signs of swelling, inflammation, pain, and perhaps fever are present, the selection by the clinician of the appropriate antibiotic agent may lead to eradication.

CAUSES OF ODONTOGENIC INFECTIONS

Most acute orofacial infections are of odontogenic origin. Dental caries, resulting in infection of dental pulp, is the leading cause of odontogenic infection.

The major causative organisms involved in dental caries have been identified as members of the viridans (alpha-hemolytic) streptococci and include *Streptococcus mutans, Streptococcus sobrinus,* and *Streptococcus milleri.* Once the bacteria have breached the enamel they invade the dentin and eventually the dental pulp. An inflammatory reaction occurs in the pulp tissue resulting in necrosis and a lower tissue oxidation-reduction potential. At this point, the bacterial flora changes from predominantly aerobic to a more obligate anaerobic flora. The anaerobic gram-positive cocci *(Peptostreptococcus* species), and the anaerobic gram-negative rods, including *Bacteroides, Prevotella, Porphyromonas,* and *Fusobacterium* are most frequently present. An abscess usually forms at the apex of the involved tooth resulting in destruction of bone. Depending on the effectiveness of the host resistance and the virulence of the bacteria, the infection may spread through the marrow spaces, perforate the cortical plate, and enter the surrounding soft tissues.

The other major source of odontogenic infection arises from the anaerobic bacterial flora that inhabits the periodontal and supporting structures of the teeth. The most important potential pathogenic anaerobes within these structures are *Actinobacillus actinomycetemcomitans, Prevotella intermedius, Porphyromonas gingivalis, Fusobacterium nucleatum,* and *Eikenella corrodens.*

Most odontogenic infections (70%) have mixed aerobic and anaerobic flora. Pure aerobic infections are much less common and comprise ~5% incidence. Pure anaerobic infections make up the remaining 25% of odontogenic infections. Clinical correlates suggest that early odontogenic infections are characterized by rapid spreading and cellulitis with the absence of abscess formation. The bacteria are predominantly aerobic with gram-positive, alpha-hemolytic streptococci *(S. viridans)* the predominant pathogen. As the infection matures and becomes more severe, the microbial flora becomes a mix of aerobes and anaerobes. The anaerobes present are determined by the characteristic flora associated with the site of origin, whether it is pulpal or periodontal. Finally, as the infectious process becomes controlled by host defenses, the flora becomes primarily anaerobic. For example, Lewis and MacFarlane found a predominance of facultative oral streptococci in the early infections (<3 days of symptoms) with the later predominance of obligate anaerobes.

In a review of severe odontogenic infections, it was reported that Brook, et al, observed that 50% of odontogenic deep facial space infections yielded anaerobic bacteria only. Also, 44% of these infections yielded a mix of aerobic and anaerobic flora. The results of a study published in 1998 by Sakamoto, et al, were also described in the review. The study confirmed that odontogenic infections usually result from a synergistic interaction among several bacterial species and usually consist of an oral streptococcus and an oral anaerobic gram-negative rod. Sakamoto and his group reported a high level of the *Streptococcus milleri* group of aerobic gram-positive cocci, and high levels of oral anaerobes, including the *Peptostreptococcus* species and the *Prevotella, Porphyromonas,* and *Fusobacterium* species.

Oral streptococci, especially of the *Streptococcus milleri* group, can invade soft tissues initially, thus preparing an environment conducive to growth of anaerobic bacteria. Obligate oral anaerobes are dependent on nutrients synthesized by the aerobes. Thus the anaerobes appear approximately 3 days after onset of symptoms. Early infections are thus caused primarily by the aerobic streptococci (exquisitely sensitive to penicillin) and late infections are caused by the anaerobes (frequently resistant to penicillin).

It appears logical, as Flynn has noted, to separate infections presenting early in their course from those presenting later when selecting empiric antibiotics of choice for odontogenic infections.

If the patient is not allergic to penicillin, penicillin VK still remains the empiric antibiotic of first choice to treat mild or early odontogenic infections (see Table 1). In patients allergic to penicillin, clindamycin clearly remains the alternative antibiotic for treatment of mild or early infections. Secondary alternative antibiotics still recognized as useful in these conditions are cephalexin (Keflex®), or other first generation cephalosporins available in oral dose forms. The first generation cephalosporins can be used in both penicillin-allergic and nonallergic patients, providing that the penicillin allergy is not the anaphylactoid type.

PENICILLIN VK

The spectrum of antibacterial action of penicillin VK is consistent with most of the organisms identified in odontogenic infections (see Table 2). Penicillin VK is a beta-lactam antibiotic, as are all the penicillins and cephalosporins, and is bactericidal against gram-positive cocci and the major pathogens of mixed anaerobic infections. It elicits virtually no adverse effects in the absence of allergy and is relatively low in cost. Adverse drug reactions occurring in >10% of patients include mild diarrhea, nausea, and oral candidiasis. To treat odontogenic infections and other orofacial infections, the usual dose for adults and children >12 years of age is 500 mg every 6 hours for at least 7 days (see Table 4). The daily dose for children ≤12 years of age is 25-50 mg/kg of body weight in divided doses every 6-8 hours (see Table 4). The patient must be instructed to take the penicillin continuously for the duration of therapy.

After oral dosing, penicillin VK achieves peak serum levels within 1 hour. Penicillin VK may be given with meals; however, blood concentrations may be slightly higher when penicillin is given on an empty stomach. The preferred dosing is 1 hour before meals or 2 hours after meals to ensure maximum serum levels. Penicillin VK diffuses into most body tissues, including oral tissues, soon after dosing. Hepatic metabolism accounts for <30% of the elimination of penicillins. Elimination is primarily renal. The nonmetabolized penicillin is excreted largely unchanged in the urine by glomerular filtration and active tubular secretion. Penicillins cross the placenta and are distributed in breast milk. Penicillin VK, like all beta-lactam antibiotics, causes death of bacteria by inhibiting synthesis of the bacterial cell wall during cell division. This action is dependent on the ability of penicillins to reach and bind to penicillin-binding proteins (PBPs) located on the inner membrane of the bacterial cell wall. PBPs (which include transpeptidases, carboxypeptidases, and endopeptidases) are enzymes that are involved in the terminal stages of assembling and reshaping the bacterial cell wall during growth. Penicillins and beta-lactams bind to and inactivate PBPs resulting in lysis of the cell due to weakening of the cell wall.

Penicillin VK is considered a "narrow spectrum" antibiotic. This class of antibiotics produces less alteration of normal microflora thereby reducing the incidence of superinfection. Also, its bactericidal action will reduce the numbers of microorganisms resulting in less reliance on host-phagocyte mechanisms for eradication of the pathogen.

Among patients, 0.7% to 10% are allergic to penicillins. There is no evidence that any single penicillin derivative differs from others in terms of incidence or severity when administered orally. About 85% of allergic reactions associated with penicillin VK are delayed and take >2 days to develop. This allergic response manifests as skin rashes characterized as erythema and bullous eruptions. This type of allergic reaction is mild, reversible, and usually responds to concurrent antihistamine therapy, such as diphenhydramine (Benadryl®). Severe reactions of angioedema have occurred, characterized by marked swelling of the lips, tongue, face, and periorbital tissues. Patients with a history of penicillin allergy must never be given penicillin VK for treatment of infections. The alternative antibiotic is clindamycin. If the allergy is the delayed type and not the anaphylactoid type, a first generation cephalosporin may be used as an alternate antibiotic.

CLINDAMYCIN

In the event of penicillin allergy, clindamycin is clearly an alternative of choice in treating mild or early odontogenic infections (see Table 1). It is highly effective against almost all oral pathogens. Clindamycin is active against most aerobic gram-positive cocci, including staphylococci, S. pneumoniae, other streptococci, and anaerobic gram-negative and gram-positive organisms, including bacteroides (see Table 3). Clindamycin is not effective against mycoplasma or gram-negative aerobes. It inhibits protein synthesis in bacteria through binding to the 50 S subunit of bacterial ribosomes. Clindamycin has bacteriostatic actions at low concentrations, but is known to elicit bactericidal effects against susceptible bacteria at higher concentrations of drug at the site of infection.

The usual adult oral dose of clindamycin to treat orofacial infections of odontogenic origin is 150-450 mg every 6 hours for 7-10 days. The usual daily oral dose for children is 8-25 mg/kg in 3-4 equally divided doses (see Table 4).

Following oral administration of a 150 mg or a 300 mg dose on an empty stomach, 90% of the dose is rapidly absorbed into the bloodstream and peak serum concentrations are attained in 45-60 minutes. Administration with food does not markedly impair absorption into the bloodstream. Clindamycin serum levels exceed the minimum inhibitory concentration for bacterial growth for at least 6 hours after the recommended doses. The serum half-life is 2-3 hours. Clindamycin is distributed effectively to most body tissues, including saliva and bone. Its small molecular weight enables it to more readily enter bacterial cytoplasm and to penetrate bone. It is partially metabolized in the liver to active and inactive metabolites and is excreted in the urine, bile, and feces.

Adverse effects caused by clindamycin can include abdominal pain, nausea, vomiting, and diarrhea. Hypersensitivity reactions are rare, but have resulted in skin rash. Approximately 1% of clindamycin users develop pseudomembranous colitis characterized by severe diarrhea, abdominal cramps, and excretion of blood or mucus in the stools. The mechanism is disruption of normal bacterial flora of the colon, which leads to colonization of the bacterium Clostridium difficile. This bacterium releases endotoxins that cause mucosal damage and inflammation. Symptoms usually develop 2-9 days after initiation of therapy, but may not occur until several weeks after taking the drug. If significant diarrhea develops, clindamycin therapy should be discontinued immediately. Theoretically, any antibiotic can cause antibiotic-associated colitis and clindamycin probably has an undeserved reputation associated with this condition.

Sandor, et al, also notes that odontogenic infections are typically polymicrobial and that anaerobes outnumber aerobes by at least four-fold. The penicillins have historically been used as the first-line therapy in these cases, but increasing rates of resistance have lowered their usefulness. Bacterial resistance to penicillins is predominantly achieved through production of beta-lactamases. Clindamycin, because of its relatively broad spectrum of activity and resistance to beta-lactamase degradation, is an attractive first-line therapy in treatment of odontogenic infections. Recently, researchers have ▶

◀ established a causal link between exposure to antibiotics and antibiotic resistance and they also have established evidence that the development of resistance to one class of antibiotic may confer persistent increased resistance to other antibiotic classes.

FIRST GENERATION CEPHALOSPORINS

Antibiotics of this class, which are available in oral dosage forms, include cefadroxil (Duricef®) and cephalexin (Keflex®). The first generation cephalosporins are alternates to penicillin VK in the treatment of odontogenic infections based on bactericidal effectiveness against the oral streptococci. These drugs are most active against gram-positive cocci, but are not very active against many anaerobes. First generation cephalosporins are indicated as alternatives in early infections because they are effective in killing the aerobes. First generation cephalosporins are active against gram-positive staphylococci and streptococci, but not enterococci. They are active against many gram-negative aerobic bacilli, including *E. coli, Klebsiella,* and *Proteus mirabilis.* They are inactive against methicillin-resistant *S. aureus* and penicillin-resistant *S. pneumoniae.* The gram-negative aerobic cocci, *Moraxella catarrhalis,* portrays variable sensitivity to first generation cephalosporins.

Cephalexin (Keflex®) is the first generation cephalosporin often used to treat odontogenic infections. The usual adult dose is 250-1000 mg every 6 hours with a maximum of 4 g/day. Children's dose is 25-50 mg/kg/day in divided doses every 6 hours; for severe infections: 50-100 mg/kg/day in divided doses every 6 hours with a maximum dose of 3 g/day (see Table 4).

Cephalexin (Keflex®) causes diarrhea in about 1% to 10% of patients. About 90% of the cephalexin is excreted unchanged in urine.

SECOND GENERATION CEPHALOSPORINS

The second generation cephalosporins such as cefaclor (Ceclor®) have better activity against some of the anaerobes including some *Bacteroides, Peptococcus,* and *Peptostreptococcus* species. Cefaclor (Ceclor®) and cefuroxime (Ceftin®) have been used to treat early stage infections. These antibiotics have the advantage of twice-a-day dosing. The usual oral adult dose of cefaclor is 250-500 mg every 8 hours (or daily dose can be given in 2 divided doses) for at least 7 days. Children's dose is 20-40 mg/kg/day divided every 8-12 hours with a maximum dose of 2 g/day. The usual adult oral dose of cefuroxime is 250-500 mg twice daily. Children's dose is 20 mg/kg/day (maximum: 500 mg/day) in 2 divided doses.

The cephalosporins inhibit bacterial cell wall synthesis by binding to one or more of the penicillin-binding proteins (PBPs), which in turn inhibit the final transpeptidation step of peptidoglycan synthesis in bacterial cell walls, thus inhibiting cell wall biosynthesis. Bacteria eventually lyse due to ongoing activity of cell wall autolytic enzymes while cell wall assembly is arrested.

BACTERIAL RESISTANCE TO ANTIBIOTICS

If a patient with an early stage odontogenic infection does not respond to penicillin VK within 24-36 hours, it is evidence of the presence of resistant bacteria. Bacterial resistance to the penicillins is predominantly achieved through the production of beta-lactamase. A switch to beta-lactamase-stable antibiotics should be made. For example, Kuriyama, et al, reported that past beta-lactam administration increases the emergence of beta-lactamase-producing bacteria and that beta-lactamase-stable antibiotics should be prescribed to patients with unresolved infections who have received beta-lactams. These include either clindamycin or amoxicillin/clavulanic acid (Augmentin®). Doses are listed in Table 4.

In the past, all *S. viridans* species were uniformly susceptible to beta-lactam antibiotics. However, over the years, there has been a significant increase in resistant strains. Resistance may also be due to alteration of penicillin-binding proteins. Consequently, drugs which combine a beta-lactam antibiotic with a beta-lactamase inhibitor, such as amoxicillin/clavulanic acid (Augmentin®), may no longer be more effective than the penicillin VK alone. In these situations, clindamycin is the recommended alternate antibiotic.

Evidence suggests that empirical use of penicillin VK as the first-line drug in treating early odontogenic infections is still the best way to ensure the minimal production of resistant bacteria to other classes of antibiotics, since any overuse of clindamycin or amoxicillin/clavulanic acid (Augmentin®) is minimized in these situations. There is concern that overuse of clindamycin could contribute to development of clindamycin-resistant pathogens.

In late odontogenic infections, it is suggested that clindamycin be considered the first-line antibiotic to treat these infections. The dose of clindamycin would be the same as that used to treat early infections (see Table 4). In these infections, anaerobic bacteria usually predominate. Since penicillin spectrum includes anaerobes, penicillin VK is also useful as an empiric drug of first choice in these infections. It has been reported, however, that the penicillin resistance rate among patients with serious and late infections is in the 35% to 50% range. Therefore, if penicillin is the drug of first choice and the patient does not respond within 24-36 hours, a resistant pathogen should be suspected and a switch to clindamycin be made. Clindamycin, because of its relatively broad spectrum of activity and resistance to beta-lactamase degradation, is an attractive first-line therapy in the treatment of these infections. Another alternative is to add a second drug to the penicillin (eg, metronidazole [Flagyl®]). Consequently, for those infections not responding to treatment with penicillin, the addition of a second drug (eg, metronidazole), not a beta-lactam or macrolide, is likely to be more effective. Bacterial resistance to metronidazole is very rare. The metronidazole dose is listed in Table 4.

Nonionized metronidazole is readily taken up by anaerobic organisms. Its selectivity for anaerobic bacteria is a result of the ability of these organisms to reduce metronidazole to its active form within the bacterial cell. The electron transport proteins necessary for this reaction are found only in anaerobic bacteria. Reduced metronidazole then disrupts DNA's helical structure, thereby inhibiting bacterial nucleic acid synthesis leading to death of the organism. Consequently, metronidazole is not effective against gram-positive aerobic cocci and most *Actinomyces, Lactobacillus,* and *Propionibacterium* species.

Since most odontogenic infections are mixed aerobic and anaerobic, metronidazole should rarely be used as a single agent but it can be useful when combined with penicillins. Alternatively, one can switch to a beta-lactamase resistant drug (eg, amoxicillin/clavulanic acid [Augmentin®]). The beta-lactamase resistant penicillins including methicillin, oxacillin, cloxacillin, dicloxacillin, and nafcillin, are only effective against gram-positive cocci and have no activity against anaerobes, hence, should not be used to treat the late stage odontogenic infections.

RESISTANCE IN ODONTOGENIC INFECTIONS

Recently, there has been an alarming increase in the incidence of resistant bacterial isolates in odontogenic infections. Many anaerobic bacteria have developed resistance to beta-lactam antibiotics via production of beta-lactamase enzymes. These include several species of *Prevotella, Porphyromonas, Fusobacterium nucleatum,* and *Campylobacter gracilis.* *Fusobacterium,* especially in combination with *S. viridans* species, has been associated with severe odontogenic infections. Often, they are resistant to macrolides. Clindamycin is the empiric drug of first choice in these patients.

SEVERE INFECTIONS

In patients hospitalized for severe odontogenic infections, I.V. antibiotics are indicated and clindamycin is the clear empiric antibiotic of choice. Alternative antibiotics include an I.V. combination of penicillin and metronidazole or I.V. ampicillin-sulbactam (Unasyn®). Clindamycin, I.V. cephalosporins (if penicillin allergy is not the anaphylactoid type), and ciprofloxacin have been used in patients allergic to penicillins. Flynn notes that *Eikenella corrodens,* an occasional oral pathogen, is resistant to clindamycin. Ciprofloxacin is an excellent antibiotic for this organism.

ERYTHROMYCIN, CLARITHROMYCIN, AND AZITHROMYCIN

In the past, erythromycins were considered highly effective antibiotics for treating odontogenic infections, especially in penicillin allergy. At the present time, however, the current high resistance rates of both oral streptococci and oral anaerobes have rendered the entire macrolide family of antibiotics obsolete for odontogenic infections. Montgomery has noted that resistance develops rapidly to macrolides and there may be cross-resistance between erythromycin and newer macrolides, particularly among streptococci and staphylococci. Hardee has stated that erythromycin is no longer very useful because of resistant pathogens. The antibacterial spectrum of the erythromycin family is similar to penicillin VK. Erythromycins are effective against streptococcus, staphylococcus, and gram-negative aerobes, such as *H. influenzae, M. catarrhalis, N. gonorrhoeae, Bordetella pertussis,* and *Legionella pneumophilia.* Erythromycins are considered narrow spectrum antibiotics.

Both azithromycin and clarithromycin have been used to treat acute odontogenic infections. This is because of the following spectrum of actions: Clarithromycin shows good activity against many gram-positive and gram-negative aerobic and anaerobic organisms. It is active against methicillin-sensitive *S. aureus* and most streptococcus species. *S. aureus* strains resistant to erythromycin are resistant to clarithromycin. Clarithromycin is active against *H. influenzae.* It is similar to erythromycin in effectiveness against anaerobic gram-positive cocci and *Bacteroides sp.* Clarithromycin has been suggested as an alternative antibiotic if the prescriber wants to give an antibiotic from the macrolide family (see Table 3). The recommended oral adult dose is 500 mg twice daily for 7 days.

Azithromycin is active against staphylococci, including *S. aureus* and *S. epidermitis,* as well as streptococci, such as *S. pyogenes* and *S. pneumoniae.* Erythromycin-resistant strains of staphylococcus, enterococcus, and streptococcus, including methicillin-resistant *S. aureus,* are also resistant to azithromycin. It has excellent activity against *H. influenzae.* Inhibition of anaerobes, such as *Clostridium perfringens,* is better with azithromycin than with erythromycin. Inhibition of *Bacteroides fragilis* and other bacteroides species by azithromycin is comparable to erythromycin. Both azithromycin and clarithromycin are presently recommended as alternatives in the prophylactic regimen for prevention of bacterial endocarditis. This past May, the FDA notified healthcare professionals that it is aware of the study published in the *New England Journal of Medicine* (Ray, 2012) reporting a small increase in cardiovascular deaths and in the risk of death from any cause in persons treated with a 5-day course of azithromycin (Zithromax®) compared to persons treated with amoxicillin, ciprofloxacin, or no drug. The FDA is reviewing the results from this study and will communicate any new information on azithromycin and this study or the potential risk of QT interval prolongation after the agency has completed its review.

Patients taking azithromycin should not stop taking their medicine without talking to their healthcare provider. Healthcare providers should be aware of the potential for QT interval prolongation and heart arrhythmias when prescribing or administering any macrolide antibiotic.

AMOXICILLIN

Some clinicians select amoxicillin over penicillin VK as the penicillin of choice to empirically treat odontogenic infections. Except for coverage of *Haemophilus influenzae* in acute sinus and otitis media infections, amoxicillin does not offer any advantage over penicillin VK for treatment of odontogenic infections. It is less effective than penicillin VK for aerobic gram-positive cocci, and similar to penicillin for coverage of anaerobes. Although it does provide coverage against gram-negative enteric bacteria, this is not needed to treat odontogenic infections, except in immunosuppressed patients where these organisms may be present. If one adheres to the principle of using the most effective narrow spectrum antibiotic, amoxicillin should not be favored over penicillin VK.

Note: The ADA Council on Scientific Affairs has published a review on the subject of antibiotic interaction with oral contraceptives in which a clear statement of the dental professional's responsibility was made. In essence, it was concluded that in any situation where a dentist is planning to prescribe a course of antibiotics, alternative/additional means of contraception should be recommended to the oral contraceptive users. Specifically, patients should be told about the potential for antibiotics to lower the usefulness of oral contraceptives and advised to consult their physician about nonhormonal contraceptive techniques while continuing their oral contraceptive regimen. Even though there is minimal scientific data supporting this position, the risk of possible unwanted pregnancies warrants this simple approach for professionals licensed to prescribe antibiotics *(JADA, 2002, 133:880)*.

The following tables have been adapted from Wynn RL, Bergman SA, Meiller TF, et al, "Antibiotics in Treating Orofacial Infections of Odontogenic Origin," *Gen Dent*, 2001, 47(3):238-52.

Table 1. Empiric Antibiotics of Choice for Odontogenic Infections

Type of Infection	Antibiotic of Choice
Early (first 3 days of symptoms)	Penicillin VK, amoxicillin Clindamycin Cephalexin (or other first generation cephalosporin)[1]
No improvement in 24-36 hours	Beta-lactamase-stable antibiotic: Clindamycin or amoxicillin / clavulanic acid
Penicillin allergy	Clindamycin Cephalexin (if penicillin allergy is not anaphylactoid type) Clarithromycin (Biaxin®)[2]
Late (>3 days)	Clindamycin Penicillin VK-metroNIDAZOLE, amoxicillin-metroNIDAZOLE
Penicillin allergy	Clindamycin

[1]For better patient compliance, second generation cephalosporins (cefaclor; cefuroxime) at twice daily dosing have been used; see text.

[2]A macrolide useful in patients allergic to penicillin, given as twice daily dosing for better patient compliance; see text.

Table 2. Penicillin VK: Antibacterial Spectrum

Gram-Positive Cocci	Oral Anaerobes
Streptococci	*Bacteroides*
Nonresistant staphylococci[1]	*Porphyromonas*
Pneumococci	*Prevotella*
	Peptococci
Gram-Negative Cocci	*Peptostreptococci*
Neisseria meningitides	*Actinomyces*
Neisseria gonorrhoeae	*Veillonella*
	Eubacterium
Gram-Positive Rods	*Eikenella*
Bacillus	*Capnocytophaga*
Corynebacterium	*Campylobacter*
Clostridium	*Fusobacterium*
	Others

[1]Nonresistant staphylococcus represents a small portion of community-acquired strains of *S. aureus* (5% to 15%). Most strains of *S. aureus* and *S. epidermitis* produce beta-lactamases, which destroy penicillins.

Table 3. Clindamycin: Antibacterial Spectrum[1]

Gram-Positive Cocci	Anaerobes[2]
Streptococci[3]	**Gram-Negative Bacilli**
S. aureus[4]	Bacteroides species including B. fragilis
Penicillinase and nonpenicillinase-producing staphylococcus	B. melaninogenicus Fusobacterium species
S. epidermitis	**Gram-Positive Nonspore-Forming Bacilli**
Pneumococci	Propionibacterium
	Eubacterium
	Actinomyces species
	Gram-Positive Cocci
	Peptococcus
	Peptostreptococcus
	Microaerophilic streptococci

[1] *In vitro* activity against isolates; information from manufacturer's package insert

[2] *Clostridia* are more resistant than most anaerobes to clindamycin. Most *Clostridium perfringens* are susceptible but *C. sporogens* and *C. tertium* are frequently resistant.

[3] Except S. faecalis

[4] Some staph strains originally resistant to erythromycin rapidly develop resistance to clindamycin.

Table 4. Oral Dose Ranges of Antibiotics Useful in Treating Odontogenic Infections[1]

Antibiotic	Clinicians must select specific dose and regimen from ranges available to be prescribed based on clinical judgment	
	Dosage	
	Children	Adults
Penicillin VK	≤12 years: 25-50 mg/kg body weight in equally divided doses q6-8h for at least 7 days; maximum dose: 3 g/day	>12 years: 500 mg q6h for at least 7 days
Clindamycin	8-25 mg/kg in 3-4 equally divided doses	150-450 mg q6h for at least 7 days; maximum dose: 1.8 g/day
Cephalexin (Keflex®)	25-50 mg/kg/d in divided doses q6h severe infection: 50-100 mg/kg/d in divided doses q6h; maximum dose: 3 g/24 h	250-1000 mg q6h; maximum dose: 4 g/day
Amoxicillin	<40 kg: 20-40 mg (amoxicillin)/kg/d in divided doses q8h >40 kg: 250-500 mg q8h or 875 mg q12h for at least 7 days; maximum dose 2 g/day	>40 kg: 250-500 mg q8h or 875 mg q12h for at least 7 days; maximum dose: 2 g/day
Amoxicillin/clavulanic acid (Augmentin®)	<40 kg: 20-40 mg (amoxicillin)/kg/d in divided doses q8h >40 kg: 250-500 mg q8h or 875 mg q12h for at least 7 days; maximum dose 2 g/day	>40 kg: 250-500 mg q8h or 875 mg q12h for at least 7 days; maximum dose: 2 g/day
MetroNIDAZOLE (Flagyl®)		500 mg q6-8h for 7-10 days; maximum dose: 4 g/day

[1] For doses of other antibiotics, see monographs

SAMPLE PRESCRIPTIONS

Rx:
Penicillin V potassium 500 mg
Disp: 40 tablets
Sig: Take 1 tablet 4 times/day for 7-10 days (consider a loading dose of 1 g for acute infection)

Rx:
Clindamycin 300 mg
Disp: 40 capsules
Sig: Take 1 capsule 4 times/day for 7-10 days

Note: Prescription usually selected for patients allergic to penicillin; may be prescribed for 3 or 4 times/day. This prescription can be continued for treatment of some infections >1 month; however, risk of *Clostridium difficile* infection increases with long-term clindamycin use. Patient should be cautioned to take clindamycin with food and contact healthcare provider if diarrhea develops even after antibiotic course is completed. Probiotics may help but evidence is conflicted on true efficacy.

◀ **Rx:**
Amoxicillin 500 mg
Disp: 30 capsules or tablets
Sig: Take 1 capsule or tablet 3 times/day for 7-10 days

For additional sample prescriptions see Bacterial Infections and Periodontal Diseases on page 1609

SINUSITIS TREATMENT

Sinusitis represents a common condition which may present with confounding dental complaints. Sinusitis (or rhinosinusitis) is an inflammation of the mucous membrane that lines the paranasal sinuses. It is classified into several categories:

- Acute rhinosinusitis: A new episode that may last ≤4 weeks

- Recurrent acute rhinosinusitis: ≥4 separate episodes of acute sinusitis that occur within 1 year

- Chronic rhinosinusitis: Signs and symptoms last for >12 weeks

All of these types of sinusitis have similar symptoms and are often difficult to distinguish. Acute sinusitis is very common. It has been estimated that 90% of adults have had sinusitis at some point in their lives.

Treatment is sometimes instituted by the dentist, but due to the often chronic and recurrent nature of sinusitis, early involvement of an otolaryngologist is advised. Most sinusitis is brought on by a nasopharyngeal viral infection best treated by sinus lavage, but some infections may require antibiotics of varying spectrum as well as requiring the management of sinus congestion. Although amoxicillin is usually adequate, many otolaryngologists initially prescribe Augmentin®. Second-generation cephalosporins and clarithromycin are sometimes used, depending on the chronicity of the problem.

For examples of sample prescriptions see Sinus Infection Treatment on page 1611

LYME DISEASE

Lyme disease is a challenging infectious, toxic disease that may exhibit many different symptoms. The clinical picture of Lyme disease can be similar to fibromyalgia, including chronic fatigue, joint pain (arthralgia), or muscle, fibrous tissue, and tendon pain. Lyme disease can also manifest primarily as a neurological disorder, including fatigue and other neurological symptoms. Early, aggressive, and comprehensive treatment improves the prognosis tremendously.

Chronic Persistent Infection

Some symptoms and signs of Lyme disease may not appear until weeks, months, or years after a tick bite. This typically involves intermittent episodes of joint pain or numerous neurological symptoms such as meningitis, Bell's palsy, dysfunction of cardiac rhythm, and migratory pain to joints, tendons, muscle, and bone. Arthritis is most likely to appear as brief bouts of pain and swelling, usually in one or more large joints; however, any combination of symptoms can be present.

In a minority of individuals (~11%), development of chronic Lyme arthritis may lead to erosion of cartilage and/or bone. Other clinical manifestations associated with chronic Lyme arthritis include neurologic complications, such as disturbances in memory, mood, or sleep patterns, and sensations of numbness and tingling.

Oral symptoms can occur as a mimic to atypical facial pain, burning mouth, or other orofacial symptoms with little or no organic basis identified. Although symptoms similar to fibromyalgia are common, the two conditions are not currently thought to be directly connected.

Diagnosis of Lyme Disease

Lyme disease is diagnosed based on history, clinical symptoms, and response to therapy. No test can conclusively rule out lyme disease since routine laboratory tests are usually normal. Liver enzymes may be slightly elevated. The erythrocyte sediment rate (ESR) is most often normal, distinguishing Lyme disease from some of the purely inflammatory disorders such as rheumatoid arthritis or lupus; however, overlap between Lyme disease and autoimmune diseases frequently occurs. A prompt biopsy of the erythema migrans rash can confirm *Borrelia burgdorferi* in the culture. Serological (blood) tests currently available for Lyme disease caused by *B. burgdorferi* include, the immunologically based ELISA and Western blot assays. Clinically, over 75% of patients with Lyme disease are negative by ELISA but positive by Western blot, adding to the complexity of diagnosis (Honegr, 2001).

Treatment

Antibiotics are the foundation of Lyme disease therapy. Oral therapy with doxycycline, cefuroxime, or amoxicillin is appropriate for early cases of Lyme disease. Parenteral therapy, usually I.V. administration, may be used for patients with neurologic involvement, severe arthritis, or any life-threatening manifestation of Lyme disease, such as complete heart block.

Treatment of 2-4 weeks is usually effective if initiated at the first appearance of a erythema migrans rash. In patients with symptoms present for more than 6 months, the treatment course may need to be more prolonged or a retreatment course of varying length may be needed. Consult the American Lyme Disease Foundation for treatment suggestions (available at http://www.aldf.com/raad.shtml).

FREQUENTLY ASKED QUESTIONS

What is the best antibiotic modality for treating dental infections?

Penicillin is still the drug of choice for treatment of infections in and around the oral cavity. Phenoxymethyl penicillin (Pen VK) long has been the most commonly selected antibiotic. In penicillin-allergic individuals, clindamycin may be an appropriate consideration, prescribing 300 mg as a loading dose followed by 150 mg 4 times/day would be an appropriate regimen for a dental infection. In general, if there is no response to Pen VK, then Augmentin® may be a good alternative in the nonpenicillin-allergic patient because of its slightly altered spectrum. Recommendations would include that the patient should take the drug with food.

Is there cross-allergenicity between the cephalosporins and penicillin?

The incidence of cross-allergenicity is 5% to 8% in the overall population. If a patient has demonstrated a Type I hypersensitivity reaction to penicillin, namely urticaria or anaphylaxis, then this incidence would increase to 20%.

Is there definitely an interaction between contraception agents and antibiotics?

There are well founded interactions between contraceptives and antibiotics. The best instructions that a patient could be given by their dentist are that should an antibiotic be necessary and the dentist is aware that the patient is on contraceptives, and if the patient is using chemical contraceptives, the patient should seriously consider additional means of contraception during the antibiotic management.

Are antibiotics necessary in diabetic mellitus patients?

In the management of diabetes, control of the diabetic status is the key factor relative to all morbidity issues. If a patient is well controlled, then antibiotics will likely not be necessary. However, in patients where the control is questionable or where they have recently been given a different drug regimen for their diabetes or if they are being titrated to an appropriate level of either insulin or oral hypoglycemic agents during these periods of time, the dentist might consider preprocedural antibiotics to be efficacious.

Do nonsteroidal anti-inflammatory drugs interfere with blood pressure medication?

At the current time there is no clear evidence that NSAIDs interfere with any of the blood pressure medications that are currently in usage.

REFERENCES AND SELECTED READINGS

Flynn TR, "The Swollen Face. Severe Odontogenic Infections," *Emerg Med Clin North Am*, 2000, 18(3):481-519.
Flynn TR, "What are the Antibiotics of Choice for Odontogenic Infections, and How Long Should the Treatment Course Last?" *Oral Maxillofac Surg Clin North Am*, 2011, 23(4):519-36.
Hardee WM, "Tried-and-True Medication," *Practical Endodontics*, 1997, 7(5):38.
Hayward G, Heneghan C, Perera R, et al, "Intranasal Corticosteroids in Management of Acute Sinusitis: A Systematic Review and Meta-Analysis," *Ann Fam Med*, 2012, 10(3):241-9.
Honegr K, Hulínská D, Dostál V, et al, "Persistence of *Borrelia burgdorferi* Sensu Lato in Patients With *Lyme borreliosis*," *Epidemiol Mikrobiol Imunol*, 2001, 50(1):10-6.
Kuriyama T, Nakagawa K, Karasawa T, et al, "Past Administration of Beta-lactam Antibiotics and Increase in the Emergence of Beta-lactamase-producing Bacteria in Patients With Orofacial Odontogenic Infections," *Oral Surg Oral Med Oral Path Oral Radiol Endod*, 2000, 89(2):186-92.
Lewis MA, Parkhurst CL, Douglas CW, et al, "Prevalence of Penicillin Resistant Bacteria in Acute Suppurative Oral Infection," *J Antimicrob Chemother*, 1995, 35(6):785-91.
Mayer G, "Antibiotics - Protein Synthesis, Nucleic Acid Synthesis and Metabolism," *Medical Microbiology*, 6th ed, Murray PR, Rosenthal KS, and Pfaller MA, eds, Elseiver, 2010, Chapter 20.
Montgomery EH, "Antimicrobial Agents in the Prevention and Treatment of Infection," *Pharmacology and Therapeutics for Dentistry*, 4th ed, Yagiela JA, Neidle EA, Dowd FJ, eds, St. Louis, MO: Mosby-Year Book, Inc, 1998, 637.
Petri WA, "Penicillins, Cephalosporins, and Other β-Lactam Antibiotics," *Goodman and Gilman's the Pharmacological Basis of Therapeutics*, 11th ed, Brunton LL, Lazo JS, and Parker KL, eds, New York, NY: McGraw Hill, 2006, 1127-54.
Ray WA, Murray KT, Hall K, et al, "Azithromycin and the Risk of Cardiovascular Death," *N Engl J Med*, 2012, 366:1881-90.
Rosenfeld RM, Andes D, Bhattacharyya N, et al, "Clinical Practice Guideline: Adult Sinusitis," *Otolaryngol Head Neck Surg*, 2007, 137(3 Suppl):S1-31.
Smith SR, Montgomery LG, and Williams JW Jr, "Treatment of Mild to Moderate Sinusitis," *Arch Intern Med*, 2012, 172(6):510-3.
Wormser GP, Dattwyler RJ, Shapiro ED, et al, "The Clinical Assessment, Treatment, and Prevention of Lyme Disease, Human Granulocytic Anaplasmosis, and Babesiosis: Clinical Practice Guidelines by the Infectious Diseases Society of America," *Clin Infect Dis*, 2006, 43(9):1089-134.
Zalmanovici A and Yaphe J, "Intranasal Steroids for Acute Sinusitis," *Cochrane Database Syst Rev*, 2009, (4):CD005149.

PERIODONTAL DISEASES

Periodontal diseases are common to mankind affecting, according to some epidemiologic studies, greater than 80% of the worldwide population. The conditions refer primarily to diseases that are caused by accumulations of dental plaque and the subsequent immune response of the host to the bacteria and toxins present in this plaque. Although most of the organisms that have been implicated in advanced periodontal diseases are anaerobic in nature, some aerobes contribute by either coaggregation with the anaerobic species or direct involvement with specific disease types.

As a group of diseases, the soft tissues are affected, supporting the teeth (ie, gingiva) leading to the term gingivitis or inflammation of gingival structures and those conditions that affect the bone and ligament supporting the teeth (ie, periodontitis) result from the infection and/or inflammation of these structures. Diseases of the periodontia can be further subdivided into various types including chronic periodontitis (localized and generalized, mainly in adults), aggressive periodontitis (localized and generalized, including previously classified), early onset periodontitis, prepubertal periodontitis, and rapidly progressing periodontitis. In addition, periodontitis as a manifestation of systemic diseases (hematologic, genetic disorders, not otherwise specified) as well as a necrotizing type due to specific conditions associated with predisposing immunodeficiency disease, such as those found in HIV-infected patients, create further subclassifications of the periodontal diseases, some of which are covered in those chapters associated with those conditions.

It is well accepted control of most periodontal diseases requires, at the very minimum, appropriate mechanical cleansing of the dentition and the supporting structures by the patient. These efforts include brushing, some type of interdental cleaning, preferably with either floss or other aids, as well as appropriate sulcular cleaning usually with a brush.

Following appropriate dental treatment by the general dental practitioner and/or the periodontist, aids to these efforts by the patient might include the use of chemical agents to assist in the control of the periodontal diseases, or to prevent periodontal diseases. There are many available chemical agents on the market, only some of which are approved by the American Dental Association (ADA). Several have been tested utilizing guidelines published in 1986 by the ADA for assessment of agents that claim efficacy in the management of periodontal diseases. These chemical agents, including chlorhexidine (Peridex®, PerioGard®), a quaternary compound, are bisbiguanides. Chlorhexidine, in various concentrations, has shown efficacy in reducing plaque and gingivitis in patients with short-term utilization. Some side effects include staining of the dentition, which is reversible by dental prophylaxis. Chlorhexidine demonstrates the concept of substantivity, indicating that after its use, it has a continued effect in reducing the ability of plaque to form. It has been shown to be useful in a variety of periodontal conditions including acute necrotizing ulcerative gingivitis and healing studies. Some disturbances in taste and accumulation of calculus have been reported; however, chlorhexidine is the most applicable chemical agent of the bisbiguanides that has been studied to date.

Other chemical agents available as mouthwashes include the phenol compound Listerine Antiseptic®. These compounds are primarily restricted to prototype agents; the first to be approved by the ADA being Listerine Antiseptic®. Listerine Antiseptic® has been shown to be effective against plaque and gingivitis in long-term studies and comparable to chlorhexidine in these long-term investigations. However, chlorhexidine performs better than Listerine Antiseptic® in short-term investigations. Triclosan, the chemical agent found in the toothpaste Total®, has been recently approved by the FDA and is an aid in the prevention of gingivitis. Antiplaque activity of triclosan is enhanced with the addition of zinc citrate and there are no serious side effects to the use of triclosan in the dose found in the dentifrice. Sanguinarine is a principle herbal extract used for antiplaque activity. It is an alkaloid from the plant *Sanguinaria canadensis* and has some antimicrobial properties perhaps due to its enzyme activity although a relationship was found between epithelial mucosa premalignant changes and sanguinarine use in mouth rinse. Zinc citrate and zinc chloride have often been added to toothpastes as well as enzymes such as mucinase, mutanase, and dextrinase which have demonstrated varying results in studies. Some commercial anionic surfactants are available on the market, which include amino alcohols and the agent Plax® which essentially is comprised of sodium thiosulfate as a surfactant. Recent studies have shown Plax® to have some efficacy when it is added to triclosan.

Long-term use of prescription medications, including antibiotics, is seldom recommended and is not in any way a substitute for general dental/periodontal therapies. As adjunctive therapy, however, benefit has been shown and the new formulations of doxycycline (Periostat® [available in Canada] and Atridox®), are recommended for long-term or repetitive treatments. It should be noted that the manufacturer's claims indicate that Periostat® functions as a collagenase inhibitor not as an antibiotic at recommended low doses for long-term therapy. Atridox® functions as an antibiotic and is not recommended for constant long-term therapy, but rather in repetitive applications as necessary. Prescription medications used in efforts to treat periodontal diseases have historically included the use of antibiotics such as tetracycline although complications with use with young patients (ie, teeth intrinsic staining) have often precluded their prescription. Doxycycline is often preferred to tetracycline in low doses. This broad-spectrum bacteriostatic agent has shown efficacy against a wide variety of bacterial organisms found in periodontal disease. Minocycline slow-release (Arestin™) has recently been approved.

The drug metronidazole is a nitroimidazole, an agent that was originally used in treatment of protozoan infections and some anaerobic bacteria. It is bactericidal and has a good absorption and distribution throughout the body. The studies using metronidazole have suggested that it has a variety of uses in periodontal treatment and can be used as adjunct in both acute necrotizing ulcerative gingivitis and has specific efficacy against spirochetes, bacteria, and some *Porphyromonas* species. Metronidazole has also been useful alone or with clavulanic acid when combined with amoxicillin for management of acute periodontal infections and in cases of gingival hyperplasia. Recently, it has been used in combination with amoxicillin alone or with clavulanic acid in the management of osteomyelitis associated with bisphosphonate use.

Clindamycin is a derivative of vancomycin and has been useful in treatment of suppurative periodontal lesions. Long-term use is precluded by its complicating toxicities associated with colitis and gastrointestinal problems; however, recent studies have shown that a variety of antibiotics can result in colitis, thus, clindamycin should not be singled out as the sole or main culprit of this reported complication.

When severe gingival inflammation appears to be refractory to routine periodontal therapies the clinician should consider a biopsy since autoimmune conditions that comprise desquamative gingivitis diseases must be considered.

Research has also shown that various combination therapies of metronidazole and tetracycline for localized aggressive periodontitis and metronidazole with amoxicillin for rapidly progressive disease can be useful. The use of other prescription drugs including nonsteroidal anti-inflammatory, as well as other antibacterial agents, have been under study. Effects on prostaglandins of NSAIDs may indirectly slow periodontal disease progression. New research is currently underway in this regard. Perhaps, in combination therapy with some of the antibiotics, these drugs may assist in reducing the patient's immune response or inflammatory response to the presence of disease-causing bacteria.

Of greatest interest has been the improvement in technology for delivery of chemical agents to the periodontally-diseased site. These systems include biodegradable gelatins and biodegradable chips that can be placed under the gingiva and deliver antibacterial agents directly to the site as an adjunct to periodontal treatment. The initial therapy of mechanical debridement by the periodontal therapist is essential prior to using any chemical agent, and the dentist should be aware that the development of newer agents does not substitute for appropriate periodontal therapy and maintenance. The trade names of the gelatin chips and subgingival delivery systems include Periochip®, Atridox®, and Periostat® (available in Canada).

In addition to the periodontal therapy, consideration of the patient's pre-existing or developing medical conditions are important in the management of the periodontal patient. Several diseases illustrate these points most acutely. The reader is referred to the chapters on Diabetes, Cardiovascular Disease, Pregnancy, Respiratory Disease, HIV, and Cancer Chemotherapy. It has long been accepted that uncontrolled diabetes mellitus may predispose to periodontal lesions. Now, under current investigation is the hypothesis that pre-existing periodontal diseases may make it more difficult for a diabetic patient to come under control. In addition, the inflammatory response and immune challenge that is ongoing in periodontal disease appears to be implicated in the development of coronary artery disease as well as an increased risk of myocardial infarction and/or stroke. The accumulation of intra-arterial plaques appears enhanced by the presence of the inflammatory response often seen systemically in patients suffering with periodontal disease. In addition, the clinician is referred to the section on preprocedural antibiotics in the text for a consideration of antibiotic usage in patients that may be at risk for infective endocarditis. Other conditions including pregnancy and respiratory diseases such as COPD, HIV, and cancer therapy must be considered in the overall view of periodontal diseases. The reader is referred to the sections within the text.

TISSUE REGENERATION

Periodontal therapies rely on disease control and the success of surgery followed by medicinal therapeutics to stabilize and manage patients with advanced periodontal diseases. Efforts in tissue regeneration have largely consisted of free gingival graft procedures, transplanting host tissue from one site to another, or placing lyophilized bone into defects. Recently, the FDA approved a new living cell construct, called GINTUIT™, that is made up of an allogeneic cellularized scaffold (McGuire, 2011). GINTUIT™ is intended for use as keratinized tissue to be added to surgical sites to enhance the success and stability of attached gingival surgery and implant placement. Use of this product would not require a donor site surgery, such as a free gingival graft procedure, which may reduce pain and the risk of postoperative infection. It is not known if this product offers long-term improvement in outcomes of periodontal surgery over conventional techniques and materials.

REFERENCE
McGuire MK, Scheyer ET, Nevins ML, et al, "Living Cellular Construct for Increasing the Width of Keratinized Gingiva: Results From a Randomized, Within-Patient, Controlled Trial," *J Periodontol*, 2011, 82(10):1414-23.

NECROTIZING ULCERATING PERIODONTITIS (HIV Periodontal Disease)

Initial Treatment *(In-Office)*

Gentle debridement
Note: Ensure patient has no iodine allergies

Betadine® rinse on page 1123

At-Home Treatment

Listerine® antiseptic rinse (20 mL for 30 seconds twice daily)
Peridex® rinse on page 288
MetroNIDAZOLE (Systemic) (Flagyl®) 7-10 days on page 911

◀ # Follow-Up Therapy

Proper dental cleaning, including scaling and root planing (repeat as needed)
Continue Peridex® and Listerine® rinse (indefinitely)
Amoxicillin on page 96
Chlorhexidine Gluconate on page 288
Ciprofloxacin (Systemic) on page 306
Clindamycin (Systemic) on page 320
Doxycycline Hyclate Periodontal Extended-Release Liquid on page 460
Listerine Antiseptic® on page 943
MetroNIDAZOLE (Systemic) on page 911
Minocycline Hydrochloride (Periodontal) on page 927
NSAIDs see Oral Pain section on page 1558
Tetracycline on page 1308
Triclosan and Fluoride on page 1363

For examples of sample prescriptions seeBacterial Infections and Periodontal Diseases on page 1609

Pharmacologic Management of Periodontal Diseases

Antibiotic	Adult Dosage
Azithromycin	500 mg once daily for 4-7 days
Ciprofloxacin (Systemic)	500 mg bid for 8 days
Clindamycin (Systemic)	300 mg tid for 8 days
Doxycycline or minocycline	100-200 mg once daily for 21 days
MetroNIDAZOLE (Systemic)	500 mg tid for 8 days
Metronidazole + amoxicillin	250 mg tid for 8 days of each drug
Metronidazole + ciprofloxacin (systemic)	500 mg bid for 8 days of each drug

Adapted from: Recommendations from the American Academy of Periodontology. Available at: www.perio.org.

FUNGAL INFECTIONS

Oral fungal infections can result from alteration in oral flora, immunosuppression, and underlying systemic diseases that may allow the overgrowth of these opportunistic organisms. These systemic conditions might include infection with the human immunodeficiency virus (and its treatments), diabetes mellitus, long-term xerostomia, adrenal suppression, anemia, and chemotherapy-induced myelosuppression for the management of cancer. Long-term administration of antibiotics such as doripenem used to treat advanced systemic infections, has been implicated in elevating the risk of fungal infections. Also, the use of oral inhalers that include steroids, such as Advair Diskus®, have been implicated in the enhancing of the risk of fungal overgrowth. Clinical presentation might include pseudomembranous, erythematous, and hyperkeratotic forms. Fungus has also been implicated in denture stomatitis, angular cheilitis, and symptomatic geographic tongue (erythema migrans). Patients being treated for fungal skin infections or common oral conditions (eg, angular cheilitis) may also be using topical antifungal preparations coupled with a steroid, such as triamcinolone. *Candida albicans* is the fungal species most commonly isolated from the oral cavity, but other species can be found, some of which are azole resistant, such as *Candida glabrata*.

Nystatin (Mycostatin®) is effective topically in the treatment of candidal infections of the skin and mucous membrane. The drug is extremely well tolerated and appears to be nonsensitizing although gastrointestinal upset and nausea are fairly common side effects. Clotrimazole troches are also useful as a topical therapy. Due to the significant sugar content in nystatin, patients with salivary gland hypofunction should be prescribed an alternative medication, such as clotrimazole, in order to lessen the caries risk. Clotrimazole is also available as an over-the-counter product in vaginal suppository formulations. In persons with denture stomatitis in which *Candida albicans* plays at least a contributory role, it is important to soak the prosthesis (laden with organisms) overnight in a nystatin liquid suspension besides treatment of the affected oral mucosa. Nystatin ointment can be placed in the denture during the daytime much like a denture adhesive. Antifungal medication should be continued for at least 14 days in order to prevent relapse and the patient must be re-evaluated. Predisposing systemic factors must be reconsidered if the oral fungal infection persists. Topical applications rely on contact of the drug with the organism within the lesions; therefore, 4-5 times daily with a dissolving troche or a nystatin rinse is appropriate. Chronically recurring oral mucosal fungal infections are often seen in patients who use systemic steroids or steroid inhalers for respiratory disease, such as asthma or COPD. Dental prosthesis wearers also often experience recurrent fungal colonization coupled with denture stomatitis. These predisposing conditions may be more resistant to antifungal therapy, possibly requiring a combination of topical and systemic drugs.

Several drugs of different classes can be used in treating systemic and localized fungal infections including, amphotericin B, anidulafungin, caspofungin, ciclopirox olamine, clotrimazole, fluconazole, itraconazole, ketoconazole, micafungin, miconazole, naftifine hydrochloride, nystatin, oxiconazole, posaconazole, and voriconazole.

MANAGEMENT OF FUNGAL INFECTIONS REQUIRING SYSTEMIC MEDICATION

If the patient is refractory to topical treatment, consideration of a systemic route usually includes fluconazole (Diflucan®) or ketoconazole. Also, when the patient cannot tolerate topical therapy, these choices are effective, well-tolerated, systematic drugs for mucocutaneous candidiasis. Concern over liver function and possible drug interactions must be considered.

In patients who appear to be refractory to ketoconazole, itraconazole, or fluconazole related to the treatment of oropharyngeal candidiasis, posaconazole has been approved for usage. Anidulafungin (Eraxis™), caspofungin (Cancidas®), micafungin (Mycamine®), or voriconazole (VFEND®) are also indicated for treatment of serious fungal infections in patients intolerant of, or refractory to, other therapy.

Amphotericin B (Conventional) on page 102
Anidulafungin on page 113
Caspofungin on page 259
Clotrimazole (Oral) on page 339
Fluconazole on page 595
Ketoconazole (Systemic) on page 779
Ketoconazole (Topical) on page 780
Micafungin on page 914
Nystatin (Oral) on page 995
Nystatin (Topical) on page 995
Nystatin and Triamcinolone on page 996
Posaconazole on page 1116
Voriconazole on page 1407

Note: Consider Peridex® oral rinse or Listerine® antiseptic oral rinse for long-term control in immunosuppressed patients.

SAMPLE PRESCRIPTIONS FOR SYSTEMIC TREATMENT

Rx:
Diflucan® 100 mg tablets
Disp: 16 tablets
Sig: Take 2 tablets day 1, then 1 tablet/day until gone

Note: Sometimes a shorter course is adequate; however, oral infections commonly are more difficult to eradicate often a 21-day (3-week) course, or and even a second course, may be necessary.

Ingredient: Fluconazole

◀ **Rx:**
Ketoconazole (Systemic) 200 mg
Disp: 14 tablets
Sig: Take 1 tablet daily, with a meal, for 2 weeks

Note: May cause irreversible liver damage; liver function should be monitored with long-term use (ie, >3 weeks)

Ingredient: Ketoconazole

SAMPLE PRESCRIPTIONS FOR TOPICAL TREATMENT

Rx:
Nystatin 100,000 units/mL oral suspension
Disp: 300 mL
Sig: Rinse with 1 teaspoon (5 mL) for 2 minutes 4-5 times/day and expectorate

Rx:
Mycelex® 10 mg troches
Disp: 70 troches
Sig: Dissolve 1 troche in mouth 4-5 times/day until gone; leave any prostheses out during treatment and soak prosthesis
  in nystatin liquid suspension overnight

Ingredient: Clotrimazole (Oral)

For additional sample prescriptions see Fungal Infections on page 1614

MANAGEMENT OF ANGULAR CHEILITIS

Angular cheilitis may represent the clinical manifestation of a multitude of etiologic factors. Cheilitis-like lesions may result from local habits, from a decrease in the intermaxillary space, or from nutritional deficiency. More commonly, angular cheilitis represents a mixed infection coupled with an inflammatory response involving *Candida albicans* and other organisms (most frequently *Staphylococcus aureus*). The drug of choice is now formulated to contain nystatin and triamcinolone (formerly known as Mycolog® and Mycolog® II) and the effect is excellent. In addition, an off-label use of iodoquinol and hydrocortisone has also been reported to be effective in the treatment of angular cheilitis.

VIRAL INFECTIONS

Oropharyngeal viral infections are most commonly caused by herpes simplex viruses and Coxsackie viruses. Infections of the oropharynx and upper respiratory infections are commonly caused by the Coxsackie group A viruses. Oral cavity proper soft tissue viral infections, on the other hand, are most often caused by the herpes simplex viruses. Herpes zoster or varicella-zoster virus, which is one of the herpes family of viruses, can likewise cause similar viral eruptions involving the oral mucosa. Oral manifestations of mononucleosis caused by Epstein-Barr virus (another Herpes family virus) can lead to petechiae on the soft palate during mononucleosis but usually do not require direct therapy but resolve as the systemic condition improves. When EBV causes hairy leukoplakia in HIV/AIDS patients, the lesions usually respond to the anti-retroviral therapies. Human *Papillomavirus* is causative in a number of oral lesions, the most common of which are *Condyloma acuminatum* and Verruca vulgaris. Within the past few years, certain subtypes of human *Papillomavirus* already proven to cause uterine cervical carcinoma are suspected of also being responsible for some posterior oral cavity squamous cell carcinomas.

The diagnosis of an acute viral infection begins by ruling out bacterial etiology and having an awareness of the presenting signs and symptoms associated with viral infection. Acute onset and vesicular eruption on the soft tissues generally favors a diagnosis of viral infection. Unfortunately, vesicles do not remain for a great length of time in the oral cavity; therefore, the short-lived vesicles rupture leaving ulcerated bases as the only indication of their presence. These ulcers are generally small in size and only when left unmanaged, coalesce to form larger, irregular ulcerations. Distinction must be made between the commonly recurring intraoral atraumatic ulcers (aphthous ulcerations) which do not have a viral etiology and the lesions associated with intraoral recurrent herpes since their effective treatment is distinctly different.

The management of an oral viral infection may be palliative for the most part; however, with the advent of improved antiviral prescription medications there now exists a family of drugs that can assist in managing primary and secondary infection. Aldara® has been approved for treatment of genital warts (superficial basal cell carcinomas and actinic keratosis); oral mucosa use is still under study.

It should be noted that herpes can present as a primary infection (gingivostomatitis or pharyngo stomatitis), recurrent lip lesions (herpes labialis of the skin and adjacent vermilion border), and intraoral ulcers (recurrent intraoral herpes), involving the oral and perioral tissues. Primary infection is a systemic infection that leads to acute gingivostomatitis that may involve all moveable and nonmovable sites of the oral cavity (buccal mucosa, lips, tongue, floor of the mouth, palate, and the gingiva). Treatment of primary infections utilizes prescription antivirals such as acyclovir in combination with supportive care. Topical anesthetics, such as lidocaine 1% or dyclonine HCl 1%, used in combination with Benadryl® 0.5% in a saline vehicle was found to be an effective oral rinse in the symptomatic treatment of primary herpetic gingivostomatitis. Other agents for symptomatic and supportive treatment include commercially available elixir of Benadryl®, Xylocaine® viscous, Orajel® (OTC), and antibiotics to prevent secondary infections. Systemic supportive therapy should include forced fluids, high concentration protein, vitamin and mineral food supplements, and rest.

Antivirals

Abreva® (OTC) on page 443
Acyclovir (Systemic) on page 45
Acyclovir (Topical) on page 47
Famciclovir on page 566
Imiquimod on page 725
L-Lysine on page 834
Nelfinavir on page 967
Penciclovir on page 1063
ValACYclovir on page 1375

Supportive Therapy

DiphenhydrAMINE (Systemic) on page 433
Lidocaine (Topical) on page 818

Prevention of Secondary Bacterial Infection

Penicillin V Potassium on page 1066

SUPPORTIVE CARE FOR PAIN AND PREVENTION OF SECONDARY INFECTION

Primary infections often become secondarily infected with bacteria, requiring antibiotics. Dietary supplement may be necessary. Options are presented due to variability in patient compliance and response.

RECURRENT HERPETIC INFECTIONS

Following the primary herpetic infection, the herpesvirus remains latent until such time as it has the opportunity to recur. The etiology of this latent period and the degree of viral shedding present during latency is currently under study; however, it is thought that some trigger in the mucosa or the skin causes the virus to begin to replicate. This process may involve Langerhans cells which are immunocompetent antigen-presenting cells resident in all epidermal and epithelial surfaces. The virus replication then leads to physical movement of the virus along the sensory axon leading to eruptions in innervated tissues surrounding the mouth or within. The most common form of recurrence is the lip lesion or herpes labialis; however, intraoral recurrent herpes also occurs with some frequency (attached gingival and hard palate preferentially).

Prevention of recurrences has been attempted with lysine (OTC) 500-1000 mg/day and acyclovir but response has been variable. Herpes zoster outbreaks can also involve the oral and facial tissues, although this is less common. The zoster vaccine (Zostavax®) is approved for individuals >50 years of age and may protect against VZV outbreaks. Valacyclovir or famciclovir are the drugs of choice in the event of a shingles outbreak. Of the two medications, famciclovir is reported to be more effective against postherpetic neuralgia. Valacyclovir HCl in 500 mg and 1 g tablets has recently been approved by the FDA for first time generic formulations.

Water-soluble bioflavonoid-ascorbic acid complex, now available as Peridin-C®, may be helpful in reducing the signs and symptoms associated with recurrent herpes simplex virus infections. As with all agents used, the therapy is more effective when instituted in the early prodromal stage of the disease process.

PREVENTATIVE SAMPLE PRESCRIPTIONS

Rx:
L-Lysine (OTC) 500 mg
Sig: Take 2 tablets/day as preventive; increase to 4 tablets/day if prodrome or recurrence begins

Rx:
Citrus bioflavonoids and ascorbic acid tablets 400 mg (Peridin-C®)
Disp: 10 tablets
Sig: Take 2 tablets at once, then 1 tablet 3 times/day for 3 days

Where a recurrence is usually precipitated by exposure to sunlight, the lesion may be prevented by the application to the area of a sunscreen, with a high skin protection factor (SPF) in the range of ≥25.

SUPPORTIVE CARE FOR PAIN AND MAINTENANCE OF NUTRITION DURING ORAL VIRAL INFECTIONS

Rx:
Benadryl® liquid 12.5 mg/5 mL
Disp: 4 oz bottle
Sig: Rinse with 1-2 teaspoonfuls every 2 hours and expectorate

Note: Benadryl® is available as a generic diphenhydramine liquid.

Rx:
Benadryl® liquid 12.5 mg/5 mL (mix 50/50) with Kaopectate®
Disp: 8 oz total
Sig: Rinse with 1-2 teaspoonfuls every 2 hours and expectorate.

Note: Maalox® can be used in place of Kaopectate® if constipation is a problem. Benadryl® is available as a generic diphenhydramine liquid.

Rx:
Xylocaine® viscous 2%
Disp: 450 mL bottle
Sig: Swish with 1 tablespoon 4 times/day and spit out

Ingredient: Lidocaine (Topical)

Rx:
Meritene®
Disp: 1 lb can (plain, chocolate, eggnog flavors)
Sig: Take 3 servings daily; prepare as indicated on can

Ingredient: Protein-vitamin-mineral food supplement

PRESCRIPTIVE TREATMENT

Acyclovir (Zovirax®) possesses antiviral activity against herpes simplex types 1 and 2. Historically, ophthalmic ointments were used topically to treat recurrent mucosal and skin lesions. These do not penetrate well on the skin lesions, thereby providing questionable relief of symptoms. If recommended, use should be closely monitored. Penciclovir, an active metabolite of famciclovir, has been specifically approved in a cream for treatment of recurrent herpes lesions. Valacyclovir and famciclovir have also been approved for treatment of herpes labialis (see monograph for dosing).

The FDA has also approved acyclovir cream 5% for treatment of herpes labialis in adults and adolescents. Other over-the-counter preparations include 2% tetracaine gel and L-lysine 500 mg tablets.

SAMPLE PRESCRIPTIONS

Rx:
Zovirax® 200 mg capsules
Disp: 50 or 60 capsules
Sig: Take 1 capsule 5 times/day for 10 days or 2 capsules 3 times/day for 10 days

Ingredient: Acyclovir (Systemic)

Rx:
Valtrex® 500 mg caplets
Disp: 42 caplets
Sig: Take 2 caplets 3 times/day for 7 days without regard to meals

Ingredient: ValACYclovir

Rx:
Famvir® 500 mg tablets
Disp: 3 tablets
Sig: Take 1500 mg as a single dose

Ingredient: Famciclovir; available as generic equivalent

Rx:
Denavir® topical cream 1%
Disp: 1.5 g tube
Sig: Apply locally as directed to lesion every 2 hours during waking hours (begin when symptoms first occur)

Ingredient: Penciclovir

For additional sample prescriptions see Viral Infections on page 1616

ULCERATIVE, EROSIVE, AND PAINFUL ORAL MUCOSAL DISORDERS

RECURRENT APHTHOUS STOMATITIS - MINOR, MAJOR, AND HERPETIFORM TYPES

Recurrent aphthous stomatitis is an extremely common mucosal disease. Although it is not considered a classic autoimmune disorder, the conditions that have been termed minor, major, and herpetiform types have in common a cellular-mediated event with underlying T-cells activation. This cytotoxicity leads to a destruction of the mucosal surface and is mediated by inflammatory cytokines throughout the oral tissues. The term herpetiform ulcerations is a misnomer and implies a herpes-type appearance to the ulcers when they are present. This is as far as the connection goes since there has never been a viral or bacterial etiology cited for any of the aphthous forms of ulcerations. The different subsets of patients have different triggering factors (eg, stress, hormonal, fluctuations and minor chemical irritations) and thus no one product or treatment technique is universally effective in all patients.

For minor or major aphthous ulcers that severely affect daily living and quality of life, corticosteroids seem to be the mainstay drug. It is believed that the immunomodulating effect of a short-term regimen of corticosteroids in an immunocompetent sufferer is effective without creating the well-known side effects of long-term or high-dose corticosteroid therapy. Sufferers of the herpetiform type of aphthae, in which as many as a hundred small ulcers appear per outbreak, may also obtain relief from an oral suspension corticosteroid, although management may be more protracted.

Triamcinolone dental paste (Oralone®) is indicated for the temporary relief of minor symptoms associated with infrequent recurrences of minor aphthous lesions and ulcerative lesions resulting from trauma. Some clinicians prescribe a soothing rinse containing corticosteroid (eg, dexamethasone), an antifungal agent (eg, nystatin), a topical anesthetic (eg, viscous lidocaine), an antihistamine (eg, diphenhydramine), an antimicrobial/antibiotic (chlorhexidine), and/or coating agent such as attapulgite creating a so-called "magic elixir." The most popular combination contains 1.5 g tetracycline; 60 mg hydrocortisone; nystatin 6 million international units and an equal volume elixir of Benadryl® and has been called Mary's Magic potion. Numerous other "Magic Mouthwash" mixtures have been formulated by clinicians, but there are insufficient data to provide evidence for selection of any of these combinations over others. All of the combinations do, however, have reasonable anecdotal evidence of palliative effects.

More severe forms of recurrent aphthous stomatitis may be treated with topical corticosteroids of higher strength (eg, fluocinonide, clobetasol) alone or mixed with Orabase®. An oral suspension of tetracycline may be prescribed for avoidance of secondary infection. Tetracycline use is contraindicated during pregnancy, infancy, and childhood to the age of 8 years due to intrinsic staining of teeth. *Lactobacillus acidophilus* preparations (Bacid®, Lactinex™) are occasionally effective for reducing the frequency and severity of the minor lesions.

With professional oversight, a cauterizing agent, such as Debacterol® may markedly decrease the pain associated with the aphthous ulcer. Clinician and patient must be extremely careful in using cauterizing agents within the oral cavity. Patients with long-standing history of recurrent aphthous stomatitis should be evaluated for iron, folic acid, and vitamin B_{12} deficiencies as well as hematological assessments for anemia. One subset of recurrent aphthous stomatitis sufferers markedly improve when tooth dentifrices lacking sodium lauryl sulfate are used.

A noncorticosteroid prescription medication, 5% Aphthasol® paste, has been approved for recurrent aphthous stomatitis and published studies indicate it hastens the healing of these lesions by more than a day. In patients with medical contraindications for corticosteroid use and when Aphthasol® has not been effective, alternatives (eg, colchicine, dapsone, immune globulin [intravenous], methotrexate, misoprostol, mycophenolate mofetil, pentoxifylline, tacrolimus, and tretinoin) have had anecdotal reports of effectiveness. These alternative drugs should only be considered in consultation with the patient's physician.

Regular use of Listerine® antiseptic has been shown in clinical trials to reduce the severity, duration, and frequency of aphthous stomatitis. An antimicrobial such as chlorhexidine oral rinses (20 mL for 30 seconds 2-3 times/day) has also demonstrated efficacy in reducing the duration of aphthae. With both of these products, however, patient intolerance of the burning from the alcohol content is of concern. The newer alcohol-free antimicrobial rinses have not been evaluated. Immunocompromised patients, such as those with AIDS, may have severe ulcer recurrences and thalidomide has been approved for these patients on an FDA orphan drug approved basis. See Periodontal Diseases on page 1570 for HIV-related periodontal considerations.

Two other conditions should be mentioned here since their diagnosis and management requires consideration of all of the ulcerative, erosive, and painful oral mucosal disorders. Necrotizing ulcerative gingivitis (NUG) is a condition that has been recognized for many years. The name historically included the term "acute," however, most investigators have discontinued this because there is not a chronic form of the disease and it is unnecessary to consider it as anything other than necrotizing gingivitis. The organism *Fusobacterium nucleatum* has been implicated with several other organisms particularly Spirochetes in this condition. The infections seem to occur primarily following periods of psychological stress and this is the most common unifying factor in patients who suffer with NUG. In addition, immunosuppression, smoking, and local trauma have also been implicated. Generally, the classical appearance of NUG includes punched-out interdental papillae that are inflamed and appear blunted, somewhat necrotic at their tips. A pseudomembrane often is present and a strong fetor oris is usually present. The patient sometimes has fever and malaise as well. The treatment is generally conservative using gentle debridement. There is some benefit in using antibiotics such metronidazole, tetracycline, or amoxicillin. Historically, some clinicians have also chosen to add a vitamin supplement, generally a vitamin B complex with vitamin C, to help with the mucosal healing.

Another condition occasionally encountered is plasma cell gingivitis, a diffuse but intense erythema of the gingival complex, including a rapid onset and soreness to the oral gingival tissues. The implicated etiologies in plasma cell gingivitis include various chewing gums, toothpastes with herbal additives, as well as spicy candies, mints, peppers, and other potential allergens. The treatment of plasma cell gingivitis is local use of topical steroids; although by removing the dietary stimulant, generally the condition will resolve spontaneously. If plasma cell gingivitis is being considered as a diagnosis, the autoimmune desquamative gingival diseases must also be considered, including lichen planus, mucous membrane pemphigoid, and pemphigus. A biopsy is usually necessary to determine a diagnosis.

MILD-TO-MODERATE FORMS OF ULCERATIONS AND EROSIONS

There are several over-the-counter preparations that may give the patient some or total relief, including Ulcerease®, BetaCell oral rinse®, Cankermelts-GX®, Gelclair® Bioadherent Oral Gel®, Orabase Sooth-N-Seal®, OraMoist™ Dry Mouth Patch, OraPatch®, Ricinol P.R.N.®, Zilactin® gel, Canker Cover®, Avamin™ Melts®, Benzoin tincture saturated swabsticks, and Orajel® Protective Mouth Sore Discs.

Aloclair (Ameseal™) is now available as a spray. It is marketed by OMNI Preventive Care as an oral lesion pain relief spray, useful for indications related to aphthous ulcerations and other mild-to-moderate oral erosions. Its prescription companion preparation Gelclair® has been suggested for use in the management of mucositis. Oralone® is a new formulation of triamcinolone acetonide dental paste which had previously been available as Kenalog in Orabase®.

A prescription viscous, mucoadhesive polymer rinse, MuGard™, provides a protective coating to the oral mucosa and can help protect against oral mucositis.

SYMPTOMATIC GEOGRAPHIC TONGUE (BENIGN MIGRATORY GLOSSITIS, ERYTHEMA MIGRANS)

Geographic tongue is a localized, transitory loss of the tongue's filiform papillae. Although disconcerting in appearance, it usually is asymptomatic; however, occasionally patients will report a burning sensation. Fungal colonization has been implicated in symptomatic geographic tongue and this condition needs to be ruled out as a contributing factor (see Fungal Infections on page 1573).

After infection has been ruled out, palliation for symptomatic geographic tongue can sometimes be achieved with an approach similar to managing minor oral ulcerations. Benadryl® elixir, a potent antihistamine, is used in the oral cavity primarily as a mild topical anesthetic agent for the symptomatic relief of certain allergic deficiencies which should be ruled out as possible etiologies for the oral condition under treatment. It is often used alone as well as in 50:50 solutions with agents such as Kaopectate® or Maalox® to assist in coating the oral mucosa. Benadryl® can also be used systemically in capsule form although the elixir mixed with a coating agent as above provides excellent palliation prior to meals. Frequently, Benadryl® alone or in combination with the above agents will be very effective in the relief of symptomatic geographic tongue.

Amlexanox on page 87
Attapulgite on page 151
Chlorhexidine Gluconate on page 288
Clobetasol on page 325
Debacterol® on page 1265
Dexamethasone (Systemic) on page 397
DiphenhydrAMINE (Systemic) on page 433
Fluocinonide ointment with Orabase on page 605
Lactobacillus on page 790
MetroNIDAZOLE (Systemic) on page 911
Mouthwash (Antiseptic) on page 943
PredniSONE on page 1133
Sulfonated Phenolics in Aqueous Solution on page 1265
Tetracaine (Topical) on page 1307
Tetracycline on page 1308
Thalidomide on page 1311
Triamcinolone (Topical) on page 1359

EROSIVE LICHEN PLANUS AND OTHER VESICULOEROSIVE DISEASES

Lichen planus is a chronic dermatologic disease that often affects the oral tissues. The name was first selected in 1869 because of the flat appearance of the white lesions on the oral mucosa. Lichen planus ranges from being totally asymptomatic to severely painful when present in its erosive forms. Reticular forms of lichen planus with no erosions show a white lacy pattern that has become pathognomic for the condition. The lesions on the skin often have a purplish hue and form slightly raised, pruritic papules, with an occasional white lacy or silvery appearance to the borders of the lesions. Patients do not need to have the skin lesions in order to suffer with oral lichen planus. The diagnosis of lichen planus is best performed by histopathology; however, often the pathognomic appearance and distribution of the lesions allows a presumptive diagnosis to be made from the clinical appearance. Generally the erosive forms of lichen planus require treatment based on the extent, severity, and pain level of the patient in question. Autoimmune desquamative gingival diseases, including pemphigoid and pemphigus, must also be considered. A biopsy is necessary to determine a diagnosis and systemic work-up for related disease effects must be completed in consultation with patient's physicians. Occasionally, an additional biopsy specimen is needed for diagnostic confirmation; the specimen is placed in Michel's transport media and then direct immunofluorescent studies are performed.

◀ Elixir of dexamethasone, a potent steroidal anti-inflammatory agent, is used topically (as a 2-minute rinse and expectorate) in the management of acute episodes of erosive lichen planus and other vesiculo-erosive disease processes such as benign mucous membrane pemphigoid and pemphigus vulgaris. Some patients will not achieve relief from topical agents and systemic delivery either by swish and swallow or tablets may be necessary. Prednisone corticosteroid tablet is a popular and often effective starting point with a regimen consisting of burst therapy (eg, 6-80 mg) for several days followed by 7-10 days of a maintenance and tapering dose.

Immunosuppressant agents, such as tacrolimus (Protopic®), hydroxychloroquine (Plaquenil®), and pimecrolimus (Elidel®), have shown some efficacy in off-label applications for severe cases. Prolonged use should be carried out in consult with the patient's physician and with a periodical Plaquenil®-related ophthalmologic examination. Continued supervision of the patient during treatment is essential and the dentist must be aware that treatment of any secondary infections such as fungal overgrowth may be essential in gaining control of the erosive lesions. Also, patients should be counseled that maximum benefit of the medication will be achieved when oral hygiene is maintained at excellent levels.

For examples of sample prescriptions see Ulcerative and Erosive Disorders on page 1618

BURNING MOUTH SYNDROME

Burning mouth syndrome (BMS) is a relatively common condition, of unknown etiology, and is a significant problem when it occurs, both in diagnosis and in management. Individuals often experience a burning or a scalding pain on the lips, tongue, and sometimes other parts of the oral cavity (eg, anterior hard palate). There are often no visible signs of irritation that the clinician can identify. The etiology of burning mouth syndrome remains unknown. The syndrome has been associated with everything ranging from vitamin deficiencies to the onset of menopause. It is estimated that nearly 5% of the population around the age of 60 may suffer with this condition. The symptoms often include burning mouth, dry mouth, a bitter or metallic taste, other taste alterations, changes in the patient's ability to eat, and onset of pain while attempting to sleep. Systemic conditions associated with BMS are abnormal hormonal fluctuations, diabetes, deficiencies in iron, zinc, and vitamins such as thiamine, B_{12}, niacin, complications associated with cancer therapy, and some patients report that the burning mouth syndrome symptoms occur after dental procedures.

The evaluation of a patient complaining of burning mouth begins with a detailed history/process of elimination and may lead to a biopsy to determine if any organic reason for the condition is identifiable. Dry mouth often accompanies burning mouth. The clinician should culture the tongue or oral mucosa to rule out oral fungal colonization. A normal hematologic work up will ensure that there is no developing diabetes, allergy, or abnormal liver or thyroid condition. The clinician should carefully examine all of the surfaces of the tissues to see if there are any abrasive components caused by rough teeth or prostheses. It is often necessary to have the patient evaluated by their primary care physician because of the common association of BMS with high stress situations, common in the process of aging. The condition has the features of a neuropathy and could be related to the production of toxic radicals that may be released at the cellular level during times of stress.

These widely divergent hypotheses related to the etiology of BMS have led to equally broad therapeutic suggestions. A variety of drugs have been suggested, including: Topical rinses and anesthetics for palliative management, clonazepam 0.25-3 mg/day, amitriptyline 25-100 mg/day, nortriptyline 10-50 mg/day, gabapentin 900-1500 mg/day, and doxepin cream, applied to the areas affected. Various studies indicate that alpha-lipoic acid in an initial dose of 600 mg may be used with a dose reduction to 200 mg after the initial 20 days. The rationale for attempting alpha-lipoic acid is the relationship between its antioxidant effects and the levels of glutathione and reduction of free radicals cellularly. In addition to alpha-lipoic acid, capsaicin has been used with some success. Capsaicin has been a prescription drug useful in arthritis care as a topical skin product. It has also been prescribed to assist with patients who have had shingles, post herpetic pain neuropathies associated with diabetes and other neuralgias. Its applications in oral use have been studied in very limited trials; however, it has recently been re-evaluated in a 0.75% topical application for use in BMS and oral mucositis. Curcumin, the active agent in turmeric, has been recommended to treat BMS, although placebo-controlled trials have not been completed to suggest any consistent response to these products. All of the medications suggested for managing burning mouth are off-label uses and there are limited data from placebo controlled clinical trials.

During a Cochrane analysis, nine clinical trials were reviewed. Of the nine trials, three interventions demonstrated reduction in BMS and all of these included varying effects of clonazepam and alpha-lipoic acid. Although the other trials considered randomized double-blind trials, study designs were small and lacked power to draw and define conclusions. There is little evidence to provide a clear standard of care for treating patients with burning mouth syndrome to date. The clinician must always be aware of this lack of conclusive evidence. These drugs should be selected and managed in collaboration with the patient's physician, particularly since many of these patients suffering with burning mouth syndrome have complicated medical histories including the use of additional medications that could be affected.

REFERENCES AND SELECTED READINGS

Aggarwal BB, Sundaram C, Malani N, et al, "Curcumin: The Indian Solid Gold," Adv Exp Med Biol, 2007, 595:1-75.
Baud CM, Colon LE, Gerberich J, et al, "Protection From Radiation-Induced Oral Mucositis by MuGard™ Oral Rinse A Clinical Study and in silico Analysis. Poster Presentation at the 18th International MASCC/ISOO Supportive Care in Cancer Symposium," 2006. Available at http://www.accesspharma.com/downloads/product-programs/MuGard-Poster.pdf
Buchanan J and Zakrzewska J, "Burning Mouth Syndrome," Clin Evid (online), March 14, 2008. Available at http://www.ncbi.nlm.nih.gov/pmc/articles/PMC2907957/pdf/2008-1301.pdf.
Chakrabarty AK, Mraz S, Geisse JK, et al, "Aphthous Ulcers Associated With Imiquimod and the Treatment of Actinic Cheilitis," J Am Acad Dermatol, 2005, 52(2 Suppl 1):35-7.
Donovan JC, Hayes RC, Burgess K, et al, "Refractory Erosive Oral Lichen Planus Associated With Hepatitis C: Response to Topical Tacrolimus Ointment," J Cutan Med Surg, 2005, 9(2):43-6.
Femiano F, Gombos F, and Scully C, "Burning Mouth Syndrome: Open Trial of Psychotherapy Alone, Medication With Alpha-Lipoic Acid (Thioctic Acid), and Combination Therapy," Med Oral, 2004, 9(1):8-13.
Goel A, Kunnumakkara AB, and Aggarwal BB, "Curcumin as 'Curecumin': From Kitchen to Clinic," Biochem Pharmacol, 2008, 75(4):787-809.
Gremeau-Richard C, Woda A, Navez ML, et al, "Topical Clonazepam in Stomatodynia: A Randomised Placebo-Controlled Study," Pain, 2004, 108 (1-2):51-7.
Hatcher H, Planalp R, Cho J, et al, "Curcumin: From Ancient Medicine to Current Clinical Trials," Cell Mol Life Sci, 2008, 65(11):1631-52.
Heckmann SM, Heckmann JG, Ungethüm A, et al, "Gabapentin has Little or no Effect in the Treatment of Burning Mouth Syndrome - Results of an Open-Label Pilot Study," Eur J Neurol, 2006, 13(7):e6-7.

Kutluay SB, Doroghazi J, Roemer ME, et al, "Curcumin Inhibits Herpes Simplex Virus Immediate-Early Gene Expression by a Mechanism Independent of p300/CBP Histone Acetyltransferase Activity," *Virology*, 2008, 373(2):239-47.

Minguez Serra MP, Salort Llorca C, Silvestre Donat FJ, "Pharmacological Treatment of Burning Mouth Syndrome: A Review and Update," *Med Oral Patol Oral Cir Bucal*, 2007, 12(4):E299-304.

Olivier V, Lacour JP, Mousnier A, et al, "Treatment of Chronic Erosive Oral Lichen Planus With Low Concentrations of Topical Tacrolimus: An Open Prospective Study," *Arch Dermatol*, 2002, 138(10):1335-8.

Patton LL, Siegel MA, Benoliel R, et al, "Management of Burning Mouth Syndrome: Systematic Review and Management Recommendations," *Oral Surg Oral Med Oral Pathol Oral Radiol Endod*, 2007, 103(Suppl S39):e1-13.

Petruzzi M, Lauritano D, De Benedittis M, et al, "Systemic Capsaicin for Burning Mouth Syndrome: Short-Term Results of a Pilot Study," *J Oral Pathol Med*, 2004, 33(2):111-4.

Thomson MA, Hamburger J, Stewart DG, et al, "Treatment of Erosive Oral Lichen Planus With Topical Tacrolimus," *J Dermatolog Treat*, 2004, 15 (5):308-14.

Vidal MA, Martinez-Fernandez E, Martinez-Vazquez de Castro J, et al, "Diabetic Neuropathy: Effectiveness of Amitriptyline and Gabapentin," *Rev Soc Esp Dolor*, 2004, 11(8):38-52.

White TL, Kent PF, Kurtz DB, et al, "Effectiveness of Gabapentin for Treatment of Burning Mouth Syndrome," *Arch Otolaryngol Head Neck Surg*, 2004, 130(6):786-8.

Yeon KY, Kim SA, Kim YH, et al, "Curcumin Produces an Antihyperalgesic Effect Via Antagonism of TRPV1," *J Dent Res*, 2010, 89(2):170-4.

Zakrzewska JM, Forssell H, and Glenny AM, "Interventions for the Treatment of Burning Mouth Syndrome," *Cochrane Database Syst Rev*, 2005.

DENTIN HYPERSENSITIVITY, ACID EROSION, HIGH CARIES INDEX, MANAGEMENT OF ALVEOLAR OSTEITIS, AND XEROSTOMIA

DENTIN HYPERSENSITIVITY

Suggested steps in resolving dentin hypersensitivity when a thorough exam has ruled-out any other source for the problem:

Treatment Steps

- Home treatment with a desensitizing toothpaste containing potassium nitrate (used to brush teeth as well as a thin layer applied, each night for 2 weeks)
- If needed, in office potassium oxalate (Protect® by Butler) and/or in office fluoride iontophoresis
- If sensitivity is still not tolerable to the patient, consider pumice then dentin adhesive and unfilled resin or composite restoration overlaying a glass ionomer base
- The use of 5% sodium fluoride varnishes (Duraflor®) have been encouraged for the prevention of decay in persons of high-risk populations and also show some efficacy for reducing sensitivity following multiple applications.

Home Products (all contain nitrate as active ingredient):

Promise®
Denquel®
Sensodyne®
THERADENT™

Other major brand name companies have added ingredients to their dentifrice product lines that also make hypersensitivity claims.

ACID EROSION

Acid erosion is the loss of tooth enamel through prolonged exposure to acid rich foods, beverages, and even fruits. The problem has been raised primarily in pediatric patients and can be significant. Several oral care products claim surface remineralization efficacy and should be coupled with dietary counseling to achieve a desirable reduction in tooth damage.

ReNew® Remineralizing and Desensitizing Paste
Sensodyne® ProNamel™ for Children
Recaldent, found in GC America's Prospec™ MI Paste with Recaldent™ and Trident XTRA CARE™ chewing gum
Amorphous calcium phosphate (ACP) found in Arm & Hammer® Enamel Care® Toothpaste
Premier Dental's Enamel Pro™ polishing paste
SensiStat, found in Ortek Therapeutic's ProClude® and DenClude® products
NovaMin, a synthetic mineral composed of calcium, sodium, phosphorus, and silica

ANTICARIES AGENTS

Fluoride (Gel 0.4%, Rinse 0.05%) on page 606

New toothpastes with triclosan such as Colgate Total® show promise for combined treatment/prevention of caries, plaque, and gingivitis. The use of 5% sodium fluoride varnishes (Duraflor®) have been encouraged for the prevention of decay in persons of high-risk populations.

FLUORIDES

Used for the prevention of demineralization of the tooth structure secondary to xerostomia. For patients with long-term or permanent xerostomia, daily application is accomplished using custom applicator trays, such as omnivac. Patients with porcelain crowns should use a neutral pH fluoride (see Fluoride monograph on page 606). Final selection of a fluoride product and/or saliva replacement/stimulant product must be based on patient comfort, taste, and ultimately, compliance. Experience has demonstrated that, often times, patients must try various combinations to achieve the greatest effect and their highest comfort levels. The presence of mucositis during cancer management complicates the clinician's selection of products.

Over-the-Counter (OTC) Products

Form	Brand Name	Strength / Size
Gel, topical (stannous fluoride)	Gel-Kam® (cinnamon, fruit, mint flavors)	0.4% [0.1%] (65 g, 105 g, 122 g)
	Gel-Tin® (lime, grape, cinnamon, raspberry, mint, orange flavors)	0.4% [0.1%] (60 g, 120 g)
	Stop® (grape, cinnamon, bubblegum, piña colada, mint flavors)	0.4% [0.1%] (60 g, 120 g)
Rinse, topical (as sodium)	ACT®, Fluorigard®	0.05% [0.02%] (90 mL, 180 mL, 300 mL, 360 mL, 480 mL)
	Listermint® with Fluoride	0.02% [0.01%] (180 mL, 300 mL, 360 mL, 480 mL, 540 mL, 720 mL, 960 mL, 1740 mL)

Prescription Only (Rx) Products

Form	Brand Name	Strength / Size
Drops, oral (as sodium)		0.275 mg/drop [0.125 mg/drop]
	Fluoritab®, Flura-Drops®	0.55 mg/drop [0.25 mg/drop] (22.8 mL, 24 mL)
	Karidium®, Luride®	0.275 mg/drop [0.125 mg/drop] (30 mL, 60 mL)
	Pediaflor®	1.1 mg/mL [0.5 mg/mL] (50 mL)
Gel-Drops	Thera-Flur® (lime flavored), Thera-Flur-N®	1.1% [0.55%] (24 mL)
Gel, topical		
Acidulated phosphate fluoride	Minute-Gel® (spearmint, strawberry, grape, apple-cinnamon, cherry cola, bubblegum flavors)	1.23% (480 mL)
Sodium fluoride	Karigel® (orange flavor)	1.1% [0.5%]
	Karigel®-N	1.1% [0.5%]
	PreviDent® (mint, berry, cherry, fruit sherbet flavors)	1.1% [0.5%] (24 g, 30 g, 60 g, 120 g, 130 g, 250 g)
Lozenge (as sodium)	Flura-Loz® (raspberry flavor)	2.2 mg [1 mg]
Rinse, topical (as sodium)	Fluorinse®, Point-Two®	0.2% [0.09%] (240 mL, 480 mL, 3780 mL)
Solution, oral (as sodium)	Phos-Flur® (cherry, cinnamon, grape, wintergreen flavors)	0.44 mg/mL [0.2 mg/mL] (250 mL, 500 mL, 3780 mL)
Tablet (as sodium)		1.1 mg [0.5 mg]; 2.2 mg [1 mg]
	Fluor-A-Day®	0.55 mg [0.25 mg]
Chewable	Fluor-A-Day®, Fluoritab®, Luride® Lozi-Tab®, Pharmaflur®	1.1 mg [0.5 mg]
	Fluor-A-Day®, Fluoritab®, Karidium®, Luride® Lozi-Tab®, Luride®-SF Lozi-Tab®, Pharmaflur®	2.2 mg [1 mg]
Oral	Flura®, Karidium®	2.2 mg [1 mg]
Varnish	Duraflor®	5% [50 mg/mL] (10 mL)

Tables copied from Newland, JR, Meiller, TF, Wynn, RL, et al, *Oral Soft Tissue Diseases,* 5th ed, Hudson (Cleveland), OH: Lexi-Comp, Inc, 2011.

ANTIMICROBIAL ORAL RINSE

Chlorhexidine Gluconate (Peridex®) on page 288
Chlorhexidine Gluconate alcohol-free (CHX®) on page 288
Mouthwash (Antiseptic) (Listerine®) on page 943

For examples of sample prescriptions see Antimicrobial Rinses on page 1613

MANAGEMENT OF ALVEOLAR OSTEITIS

Alveolar osteitis, as compared to simple postoperative pain, occurs in about 2% to 5% of extractions. Factors affecting risk include the complexity of the extraction and other factors, such as smoking, excessive spitting, or poor wound care in the first 5-7 days after extraction. Wound healing is a complex process and can be affected by many factors. Alveolar osteitis is the most common healing disturbance of extraction sockets.

Several types of alveolar osteitis can result from disturbances in the healing process. The type that is commonly referred to as dry socket occurs when the initial blood clot that forms after tooth extraction is disturbed or lost during early healing. The healing tissue that normally replaces the blood clot (granulation tissue) fails to grow or is disrupted after beginning to grow, leading to alveolar osteitis. Alveolar osteitis is characterized by grayish slough, moderate to severe pain, and foul odor. The foul odor is a result of a breakdown of the blood clot by putrefaction, rather than by orderly retraction, leaving bare bone visible in the socket. Suppurative osteitis results when the disturbance of extraction socket wound healing is later (usually after day 14), results in infection, and exhibits a purulence in the extraction socket. Disruption of the clot can also result in necrotizing osteitis with bony sequestra.

Signs and Symptoms of Dry Socket or Postop Infection

1. Moderate to severe pain beginning 2-5 days after tooth extraction
2. Loss of the blood clot or visible bone in extraction site
3. Foul odor or unpleasant taste in mouth
4. Tenderness or swelling of lymph nodes around jaw
5. At the first signs of suppurative osteitis, antibiotics must be considered.

Treatments of Dry Socket

Irrigation and medicated dressings are primary ways to treat dry socket. Active ingredients in these sedative dressings usually include substances like soluble aspirin, zinc oxide, and eugenol made from oil of cloves. It is usually necessary to repeat treatment for 2-5 consecutive days, although it may take longer.

Resorbable dry socket products in the market include:

- Eugenol-soaked Gelfoam® can be a one-time treatment with as needed follow-up if necessary
- Alvogyl by Septodont is resorbable but cannot be used on patients having a history of allergic reactions to procaine-type anesthetics or iodine

Nonresorbable dry socket products: **Note:** Must be removed and some have radiopaque markers; thus, patient compliance to return daily must be considered.

- Sultan Dry Socket Paste or Dry Socket Remedy is placed on a gauze strip and packed into the socket, follow-up and removal is needed (guaiacol, balsam peru, eugenol, 1.6% chlorobutanol); used to treat alveolitis and provides instant pain relief. Paste is introduced into socket with flat-bladed instrument, tamped down to cover exposed bone, and allowed to remain in the socket for 3-5 days. This is nonresorbable but is claimed to wash out gradually as socket heals.
- Dressol-X™ by Rainbow is another nonresorbable packing material with radiopaque marker; it contains aspirin and must not be used on patients with ASA allergy or G6PD deficiency.

REFERENCES
Benko P, "Emergency Dental Procedures," In: Roberts J, et al, eds, *Clinical Procedures in Emergency Medicine*, 5th ed, Philadelphia, Pa.: Saunders Elsevier, 2009.

Cardoso CL, Rodrigues MT, Ferreira Júnior O, et al, "Clinical Concepts of Dry Socket," *J Oral Maxillofac Surg*, 2010, 68(8):1922-32.

Noroozi AR and Philbert RF, "Modern Concepts in Understanding and Management of the "Dry Socket" Syndrome: Comprehensive Review of the Literature," *Oral Surg Oral Med Oral Pathol Oral Radiol Endod*, 2009, 107(1):30-5.

MANAGEMENT OF SIALORRHEA

In patients suffering with medical conditions that result in hypersalivation, the dentist may determine that it is appropriate to use an atropine sulfate medication to achieve a dry field for dental procedures or to reduce excessive drooling. Currently there is one ADA approved medication sold under the name of Sal-Tropine™. Pro-Banthine® (propantheline bromide), an antimuscarinic used for excessive stomach acid production is advocated by some for off-label use. See Atropine on page 148

XEROSTOMIA

Xerostomia refers to the subjective sensation of a dry mouth while salivary gland hypofunction can be objectively measured. Numerous factors can play a role in the patient's perception of xerostomia. Changes in salivary function caused by drugs, surgical intervention, or treatment of cancer are among the leading causes of xerostomia. Other factors including aging, smoking, mouth breathing, and autoimmune disorders such as Sjögren's syndrome, can also be implicated in a patient's perception of xerostomia. Human immunodeficiency virus (HIV) may produce xerostomia when viral changes in salivary glands are present. Xerostomia often occurs in patients taking antianxiety and antidepressant medication and often accompanies burning mouth syndrome. Xerostomia affects women more frequently than men and is also more common in older individuals. Some alteration in salivary function naturally occurs with age, but it is extremely difficult to quantify the effects. Xerostomia and salivary gland hypofunction in the elderly population are contributory to deterioration in the quality of life.

Once a diagnosis of xerostomia or salivary gland hypofunction is made and possible causes confirmed, treatment for the condition usually involves management of the underlying disease and avoidance of unnecessary medications. In addition, good hydration is essential and water is the drink of choice. Also, the use of artificial saliva substitutes, selected chewing gums, and/or toothpastes formulated to treat xerostomia, is often warranted. In more difficult cases, such as patients receiving radiotherapy for cancer of the head and neck regions or patients with Sjögren's syndrome, systemic cholinergic stimulants may be administered if no contraindications exist. The clinician must also rule out and treat concomitant conditions such as fungal colonization and overgrowth which often occur subsequent to xerostomia.

XEROSTOMIA TREATMENTS

Because of the complex nature of xerostomia, management by the dental clinician is difficult. Treatment success is also difficult to assess and is often unsatisfactory. The salivary stimulants, pilocarpine and cevimeline, may aid in some conditions but are only approved for use as sialogogues in patients receiving radiotherapy and in Sjögren's patients, specifically as described above. Artificial salivas are available as over-the-counter products and represent the potential for continuous application by the patient to achieve comfort for their xerostomic condition. Coenzyme Q_{10} (ubiquinone) has recently been proven successful with increasing saliva (100 mg daily) (Ryo, 2011).

The role of the clinician in attempting treatment of dry mouth is to first achieve a differential diagnosis and to ensure that other conditions are not simultaneously present. For example, many patients suffer burning mouth syndrome or painful oral tissues with no obvious etiology accompanying dry mouth. Also, higher caries incidence may be associated with changes in salivary flow. As previously mentioned, Sjögren's syndrome represents an immune complex of disorders that can affect the eyes, oral tissues, and other organ systems. The reader is referred to current oral pathology or oral medicine textbooks for review of signs and symptoms of Sjögren's syndrome.

Treatment of cancer often leads to dry mouth. Surgical intervention removing salivary tissue due to the presence of a salivary gland tumor results in loss of salivary function. Also, many of the chemotherapeutic agents produce transitory changes in salivary flow, such that the patient may perceive a dry mouth during chemotherapy. Most notably related to salivary dysfunction is the use of radiation regimens to head and neck tissues. Tumors in or about salivary gland tissue, the oral cavity, and oropharynx are most notably sensitive to radiation therapy and subsequent dry mouth. In the head and neck, therapeutic radiation is commonly used in treatment of squamous cell carcinomas and lymphomas. The radiation level necessary to destroy malignant cells ranges from 40-70 Gy. Salivary tissue is extremely sensitive to radiation changes. Radiation dosages >30 Gy are sufficient to permanently change salivary function. In addition to the mucositis and subsequent secondary infection by fungal colonization or viral exacerbation, oral tissues can become exceptionally dry due to the effects of radiation on salivary glands. In fact, permanent damage to salivary gland tissue within the beam path produces significant levels of xerostomia in most patients. Some recovery may be noted by the patient. Most often, the effects are permanent and even progressive as the radiation dosage increases.

Artificial salivas do not produce any protectant or stimulation of the salivary gland. The use of pilocarpine and cevimeline as salivary stimulants in pre-emptive treatment, as well as postradiation treatment, have been shown to have some efficacy in management of dry mouth. The success rate, however, still is often unsatisfactory and post-treatment management by the dentist usually requires fluoride supplements to prevent radiation-induced caries due to dry mouth. Also, management of dry mouth through patient use of the artificial salivary gel, solutions and sprays, or other over-the-counter products for dry mouth (eg, chewing gum, toothpaste, mouthwash, swabsticks, sugar-free candy) is highly recommended. The use of pilocarpine or cevimeline should only be considered by the dentist in consultation with the managing physician. The oftentimes severe and widespread cholinergic side effects of pilocarpine and cevimeline mandate close monitoring of the patient and certain medical conditions contraindicated their use.

The use of artificial salivary substitutes is less problematic for the dentist. The dentist should, in considering selection of a drug, base his or her decision on patient compliance and comfort. Salivary substitutes presently on the market may have some benefit in terms of electrolyte balance and salivary consistency. However, the ultimate decision needs to be based on patients' taste, their willingness to use the medication ad libitum, and improvement in their comfort related to dry mouth. Many of the drugs are pH balanced to reduce additional risk of dental demineralization or caries. Oftentimes, the dentist must try numerous medications, one at a time, prior to finding one which gives the patient some comfort. Another gauge of acceptability is to investigate whether the artificial saliva substitute has the American Dental Association's seal of approval. Most of the currently accepted saliva substitute products have been evaluated by the ADA.

In general, considerations that the clinician might use in a prescribed regimen would be that saliva substitutes are meant to be used regularly throughout the day by the patient to achieve comfort during meals, reduce tissue abrasion, and prevent salivary stagnation on teeth. Other than these, there are no specific recommendations for patients. Recommendations by the dentist need to be tailored to the patient's acceptance. Salivary substitutes may provide an allergic potential in patients who are sensitive to some of the preservatives present in artificial saliva products. In addition to this allergic potential, there is a risk of microbial contamination by placement of the salivary substitute container in close contact with the oral cavity.

Patient education regarding the use of saliva substitutes is also part of the clinical approach. The patient with chronic xerostomia should be educated about regular professional care, high performance in dental hygiene, the need to re-evaluate oral soft tissue pathology, and any changes that might occur long term. In patients with severe xerostomia, artificial salivary medications should be given in combination with topical fluoride treatment programs designed by the dentist to reduce caries (see Saliva Substitute monograph on page 1220).

REFERENCES

Ryo K, Ito A, Takatori R, et al, "Effects of Coenzyme Q_{10} on Salivary Secretion," *Clin Biochem*, 2011, 44(8-9):669-74.

Products and Drugs to Treat Dry Mouth

Medication	Manufacturer and Phone Number	Product Type	Manufacturer's Description	Indication	Ingredients	Directions for Use	Form and Availability
				Artificial Salivas (OTC)			
Biotene® OralBalance® Mouth Moisturizing Gel	Laclede Professional Products, Inc (800) 922-5856	Gel	Sugar-free oral lubricant; relieves dry mouth symptoms up to 8 hours; soothes and protects oral tissue to promote healing; helps to inhibit harmful bacteria; improves retention under dentures	Relieves symptoms of dry mouth; burning, itching, cotton palate, sore tissue swallowing difficulties	Contains the "Biotene®" protective salivary enzyme system. Active: Glucose oxidase (2000 units), lactoperoxidase (3000 units), lysozyme (5 mg), lactoferrin (5 mg) Other: Hydrogenated starch, xylitol, hydroxyethyl cellulose, glycerate polyhydrate, aloe vera	Using a clean fingertip, apply a 1" ribbon of gel on tongue; add additional amount of gel on other dry; use as needed	1.4 oz tube; available at mass merchandise stores, food stores, and drugstores
BreathTech™ Plaque Fighter Mouth Spray	Omnii Oral Pharmaceuticals (800) 445-3386	Pump dispenser	Plaque inhibitor in vanilla-mint flavor for breath malodor or reduced salivary flow	Treats the discomfort of oral dryness	Microdent® patented plaque-inhibitor formula	Spray directly into mouth; spread over teeth and tissue with tongue	18 mL pump dispenser; order directly from manufacturer
Moi-Stir® Moistening Solution	Kingswood Laboratories, Inc (800) 968-7772	Pump spray	Saliva supplement for moistening of mouth and mucosal area	Nontherapeutic treatment of dry mouth; intended for comfort only	Water, sorbitol, sodium carboxymethylcellulose, methylparaben, propylparaben, potassium chloride, sodium chloride, flavoring	Spray directly into mouth as necessary to treat drying conditions	4 oz spray bottle; order directly from manufacturer or various distributors
MouthKote® Oral Moisturizer	Parnell Pharmaceuticals, Inc. (800) 457-4276	Aqueous solution	Pleasant lemon-lime-flavored oral moisturizer to lubricate and protect oral tissue	Treats the discomfort of oral dryness caused by medications, disease, surgery, irradiation, aging	Water, xylitol, sorbitol, yerba santa, citric acid, ascorbic acid, flavor, sodium benzoate, sodium saccharin	Swirl 1 or 2 teaspoonfuls in mouth for 8-10 seconds; swallow or spit out; shake well before using	2 oz and 8 oz bottles; available at drugstores or order directly from manufacturer
Oasis® Moisturizing Mouthwash	GlaxoSmithKline (800) 777-2500	Oral moisturizer, aqueous solution	Moisturizing mouthwash for a dry mouth indication	Moisturizes mouth and helps it from drying out	Active: Glycerin Other: Water, sorbitol, poloxamer 338, PEG-60 hydrogenated castor oil, cellulose gum, cetylpyridinium chloride, copovidone, disodium phosphate, flavor, methylparaben, propylparaben, sodium benzoate, sodium phosphate, sodium saccharin, xanthan gum, FD&C blue #1	Rinse for 30 seconds with 1 ounce of mouthwash first thing in the morning and before going to bed or as needed; do not swallow; use as part of an effective oral hygiene program	16 oz bottle
Optimoist™ Oral Moisturizer	Colgate Oral Pharmaceuticals (800) 225-3756	Oral moisturizer, aqueous solution	Pleasant tasting saliva substitute for instant relief of dry mouth and throat without demineralizing tooth enamel	Treats the discomfort of oral dryness	Deionized water, xylitol, calcium phosphate monobasic, citric acid, sodium hydroxide, sodium benzoate, flavoring, acesulfame potassium, hydroxyethylcellulose, polysorbate 20 and sodium monofluorophosphate (fluoride concentration is 2 parts per million)	Spray directly into mouth to relieve dry mouth discomfort; may be swallowed or expectorated; use as needed	2 oz and 12 oz bottles; available at mass merchandise stores, food stores, and drugstores
Salivart® Synthetic Saliva, Aqueous Solution	Gebauer Co (800) 321-9348	Aerosol aqueous spray	Oral moisturizer for patients with reduced salivary flow	Replacement therapy for patients complaining of xerostomia	Sodium carboxymethylcellulose, sorbitol, sodium chloride, potassium chloride, calcium chloride dihydrate, magnesium chloride hexahydrate, potassium phosphate dibasic, purified water, nitrogen (propellant)	Spray directly into mouth or throat for 1-2 seconds; use as needed	2.48 fl oz (75 g); available at most drugstores or directly from manufacturer

Products and Drugs to Treat Dry Mouth *continued*

Medication	Manufacturer and Phone Number	Product Type	Manufacturer's Description	Indication	Ingredients	Directions for Use	Form and Availability
Other Dry Mouth Products (OTC)							
Biotene® Dry Mouth Gum	Laclede Professional Products, Inc (800) 922-9348	Chewing gum	Sugar-free; helps stimulate saliva flow; fights cause/ effect of bad breath; reduces plaque	Treats oral dryness	Active: Lactoperoxidase (0.11 Units), glucose oxidase (0.15 Units). Other: Sorbitol, gum base, xylitol, hydrogenated glucose, potassium thiocyanate	Chew 1 or 2 pieces; use as needed	Each package contains 17 pieces; available at drugstores or directly from manufacturer
Biotene® Dry Mouth Toothpaste	Laclede Professional Products, Inc (800) 922-9348	Toothpaste	Reduces harmful bacteria which cause cavities, periodontal disease, and oral infections	Use in place of regular toothpaste for dry mouth	Active: Lactoperoxidase (15,000 Units), glucose oxidase (10,000 Units), lysozyme (16 mg), sodium monofluorophosphate. Other: Sorbitol, glycerin, calcium pyrophosphate, hydrated silica, xylitol, isoceteth-20, cellulose gum, flavoring, sodium benzoate, beta-d-glucose, potassium thiocyanate	Use in place of regular toothpaste; rinse toothbrush before applying; brush for 2 minutes; rinse lightly	4.5 oz tube; available at drugstores or directly from manufacturer
Biotene® Gentle Mouthwash	Laclede Professional Products, Inc (800) 922-9348	Mouthwash	Alcohol-free; strong antibacterial formula neutralizes mouth odors; soothes as it cleans to protect teeth and oral tissue	Treats dry mouth or oral irritations	Lysozyme, lactoferrin, glucose oxidase, lactoperoxidase	Use 15 mL (1 tablespoonful); swish thoroughly for 30 seconds and spit out; for dry throat, sip 1 tablespoonful of mouthwash 2-3 times/day	Available at drugstores or directly from manufacturer
Moi-Stir® Oral Swabsticks	Kingswood Laboratories, Inc (800) 968-7772	Swabsticks	Lubricates and moistens mouth and mucosal area	Lubricates and moistens mouth and mucosal area	Water, sorbitol, sodium carboxymethylcellulose, methylparaben, propylparaben, potassium chloride, sodium chloride, flavoring	Gently swab all intraoral surfaces of mouth, gums, tongue, palate, buccal mucosa, gingival, teeth, and lips where uncomfortable dryness exists	3 swabsticks/packet, 100 packets/case; order directly from manufacturer or from various distributors.
Oasis® Moisturizing Mouth Spray	GlaxoSmithKline (800) 777-2500	Oral moisturizer	Moisturizing mouth spray for a dry mouth indication	Moisturizes mouth and helps it from drying out	Active: Glycerin 35% (prediluted) Other: Cetylpyridinium chloride, copovidone, flavor, methylparaben, PEG-60 hydrogenated castor oil propylparaben, sodium benzoate, sodium saccharin, water, xanthan gum, xylitol	Use as required up to a maximum of 30 times (or 60 sprays a day; spray 1-2 times into the affected area of mouth; do not rinse out	1 oz bottle
XyliMelts® Discs	OraHealth (877) 672-6541	Time-release adhering discs	Lubricant	Treats dry mouth, reduces plaque	Xylitol 500 mg, cellulose gum	Use 2 discs as needed	120 tablets
Saliva Substitute (Rx)							
Aquoral™	Auriga Laboratories (877) 287-4428	Pump spray	Lipid-based solution designed to moisten and lubricate the oral cavity and counteract by formation of lipid film which limits loss of water and restores the viscoelasticity of the oral mucosa	Chronic and temporary xerostomia which may be the result of Sjögren's syndrome, oral inflammation, medication, chemo- or radiotherapy, and stress or aging. **Note:** Contraindicated if patient has a known history of hypersensitivity to any of its ingredients. No known interactions with medicinal or other products.	Oxidized glyceral triesters (TGO), silicon dioxide, aspartame, and artificial flavoring	Shake gently; 1 dose (2 sprays) into the mouth 3-4 times/day; spread product onto inflamed and/or dry areas of the mouth with the tongue.	1 bottle (40 mL = 400 sprays)
Cholinergic Salivary Stimulants (Rx)							
Cevimeline (Evoxac®)	Snow Brand Pharmaceuticals (800) 475-6473			Treats symptoms of dry mouth in patients with Sjögren's syndrome	Active: Cevimeline 30 mg Other: Lactose monohydrate, hydroxypropyl cellulose, magnesium stearate	1 capsule (30 mg) 3 times/ day	30 mg capsules
Pilocarpine (Salagen®)	MGI Pharmaceuticals, Inc (800) 562-5580			Treats xerostomia caused by radiation therapy in patients with head/neck cancer, Sjögren's syndrome	Active: Pilocarpine 5 mg Other: Carnauba wax, hydroxypropyl methylcellulose, iron oxide, microcrystalline cellulose, stearic acid, titanium dioxide	1-2 tablets (5 mg) 3-4 times/day, not to exceed 30 mg/day	5 mg tablets

◀ CHOLINERGIC SALIVARY STIMULANTS (PRESCRIPTION ONLY)

Pilocarpine (Systemic) (Salagen® on page 1092) and cevimeline (Evoxac® on page 284) are cholinergic drugs which stimulate salivary flow. They stimulate muscarinic-type acetylcholine receptors in salivary glands within the parasympathetic division of the autonomic nervous system, causing an increase in serous-type saliva. Thus, they are considered cholinergic, muscarinic-type (parasympathomimetic) drugs. Due to significant side effects caused by these drugs, they are available by prescription only.

Pilocarpine (Salagen®) is indicated for the treatment of xerostomia caused by radiation therapy in patients with head and neck cancer and xerostomia in patients suffering from Sjögren's syndrome. The usual adult dosage is 1-2 tablets (5 mg or 7.5 mg/tablet) 3-4 times/day, not to exceed 30 mg/day. Patients should be treated for a minimum of 90 days for optimum effect. The most frequent adverse side effect is perspiration, which occurs in about 30% of patients who use 5 mg 3 times/day. Other adverse effects (in about 10% of patients) are nausea, rhinitis, chills, frequent urination, dizziness, headache, lacrimation, and pharyngitis. Salagen® is contraindicated for patients with uncontrolled asthma and narrow-angle glaucoma.

Pilocarpine has been documented to overcome xerostomia from different causes. More recent studies confirm its effectiveness in improving salivary flow in patients undergoing irradiation therapy for head and neck cancer. A capstone study by Johnson, et al, reported the effects of pilocarpine in 208 irradiation patients at 39 different treatment sites. Salagen®, at a dose of 5 mg 3 times/day, improved salivation in 44% of patients, compared with 25% in the placebo group. They concluded that treatment with pilocarpine (Salagen®) produced the best overall outcome with respect to saliva production and relief of symptoms of xerostomia in patients undergoing irradiation therapy.

Additional studies have been published showing the effectiveness of pilocarpine (Salagen®) in stimulating salivary flow in patients suffering from Sjögren's syndrome and the FDA has approved the use of Salagen® for this indication.

Recent reports suggest that pre-emptive use of pilocarpine may be effective in protecting salivary glands during therapeutic irradiation; further studies are needed to confirm this. As of this publication date, the use of pilocarpine has not been approved to treat xerostomia induced by chronic medication. Pilocarpine could be used as a sialagogue for individuals with xerostomia induced by antidepressants and other medications. However, the potential for serious drug interactions is a concern and more studies are needed to clarify the safety and effectiveness of pilocarpine when given in the presence of other medications.

Cevimeline (Evoxac®) is indicated for treatment of symptoms of dry mouth in patients with Sjögren's syndrome. The usual dosage in adults is 1 capsule (30 mg) 3 times/day. Cevimeline (Evoxac®) is supplied in 30 mg capsules. Some adverse effects reported for Evoxac® include increased sweating (19%), nausea (14%), rhinitis (11%), sinusitis (12%), and upper respiratory infection (11%). Evoxac® is contraindicated for patients with uncontrolled asthma, narrow-angle glaucoma, acute iritis, and other conditions where miosis is undesirable. Cevimeline's half-life elimination is significantly slower than pilocarpine (0.76 hours versus 5 hours).

Other Drugs Implicated in Xerostomia

>10%	1% to 10%
ALPRAZolam	Acrivastine and Pseudoephedrine
Amitriptyline hydrochloride	Albuterol
Amoxapine	Almotriptan
Anisotropine methylbromide	Amantadine hydrochloride
AtoMOXetine	Amphetamine sulfate
Atropine sulfate	Anastrozole
Belladonna and Opium	Armodafinil
Benztropine mesylate	Astemizole (withdrawn from market)
Boceprevir	Azatadine maleate
BuPROPion	Beclomethasone dipropionate
ChlordiazePOXIDE	Bendamustine
Clomipramine hydrochloride	Bepridil hydrochloride
ClonazePAM	Bevacizumab
CloNIDine	Bitolterol mesylate
Clorazepate dipotassium	Brompheniramine maleate
Cyclobenzaprine	Carbinoxamine and Pseudoephedrine
Desipramine hydrochloride	Chlorpheniramine maleate
Desvenlafaxine	Clemastine fumarate
Diazepam	CloZAPine
Dicyclomine hydrochloride	Cromolyn sodium
Diphenoxylate and Atropine	Cyproheptadine hydrochloride
Doxepin hydrochloride	Dexchlorpheniramine maleate
DULoxetine	Dextroamphetamine sulfate
Ergotamine	DimenhyDRINATE
Estazolam	DiphenhydrAMINE hydrochloride

Other Drugs Implicated in Xerostomia *(continued)*

>10%	1% to 10%
Everolimus	Disopyramide phosphate
FlavoxATE	Doxazosin
Flurazepam hydrochloride	Dronabinol
Glycopyrrolate	EPHEDrine sulfate
Guanabenz acetate	Escitalopram
GuanFACINE hydrochloride	Flumazenil
Hyoscyamine sulfate	FluvoxaMINE
IncobotulinumtoxinA	Gabapentin
Interferon alfa-2a	GuaiFENesin and Codeine
Interferon alfa-2b	Guanadrel sulfate
Interferon alfa-N3	Guanethidine sulfate
Ipratropium bromide	HydrOXYzine
Isoproterenol	Hyoscyamine, Atropine, Scopolamine, and Phenobarbital
ISOtretinoin	Iloperidone
Loratadine	Imipramine
LORazepam	Isoetharine
Loxapine	LamoTRIgine
Maprotiline hydrochloride	Levocabastine hydrochloride
Methscopolamine bromide	Levodopa
Molindone hydrochloride	Levodopa and Carbidopa
Nabilone	Levorphanol tartrate
Nefazodone	Meclizine hydrochloride
Oxazepam	Meperidine hydrochloride
Oxybutynin chloride	Methadone hydrochloride
PARoxetine	Methamphetamine hydrochloride
Phenelzine sulfate	Methyldopa
Prochlorperazine	Metoclopramide
Propafenone hydrochloride	Milnacipran
Protriptyline hydrochloride	Morphine sulfate
Quazepam	Nortriptyline hydrochloride
Reserpine	Ondansetron
RimabotulinumtoxinB	OxyCODONE and Acetaminophen
Selegiline hydrochloride	OxyCODONE and Aspirin
Temazepam	Peginterferons
Thiethylperazine maleate	Pentazocine
Tiotropium	Phenylpropanolamine hydrochloride
TiZANidine	Prazosin hydrochloride
Trihexyphenidyl hydrochloride	Promethazine hydrochloride
Trimipramine maleate	Propoxyphene
Trospium	Pseudoephedrine
Venlafaxine	RisperiDONE
Zuclopenthixol	ROPINIRole
	Sertraline hydrochloride
	Tapentadol
	Terazosin
	Terbutaline sulfate
	Varenicline

TEMPOROMANDIBULAR DYSFUNCTION (TMD), CHRONIC PAIN, AND FIBROMYALGIA

Temporomandibular dysfunction comprises a broad spectrum of signs and symptoms. Although TMD presents in patterns, diagnosis is often difficult. Evaluation and treatment is time-intensive and no single therapy or drug regimen has been shown to be universally beneficial.

The thorough diagnostician should perform a screening examination for temporomandibular dysfunction on all patients. Ideally, a baseline maximum mandibular opening along with lateral and protrusive movement evaluation should be performed. Secondly, the joint area should be palpated and an adequate exam of the muscles of mastication and the muscles of the neck and shoulders should be made. These muscles include the elevators of the mandible (masseter, internal pterygoid, and temporalis); the depressors of the mandible (including the external pterygoid and digastric); extrusive muscles (including the temporalis and digastric), and protrusive muscles (including the external and internal pterygoids). These muscles also account for lateral movement of the mandible.

The clinician should also be alert to indicators of dysfunction, primarily a history of pain with jaw function, chronic history of joint noise (although this can often be misinterpreted), pain in the muscles of the neck, limited jaw movement, pain in the actual muscles of mastication, and headache or even earache. The signs and symptoms are extremely variable and the clinician should be alert for any or all of these areas of interest. Because of the complexity of both evaluation and diagnosis, the general dentist often finds it too time consuming to spend the countless hours evaluating and treating the temporomandibular dysfunction patient. Therefore, oral medicine specialists trained in temporomandibular evaluation and treatment often accept referrals for the management of these complicated patients. TMD often accompanies other chronic pain conditions, such as facial neuralgia, fibromyalgia, and chronic headache.

Chronic Headache

The lifetime prevalence of headache is >90% for chronic headache patients. Most patients who present with headache have one of three main headache syndromes: Migraine, cluster headache, or tension headache. However, headache and facial pain can have numerous other etiologies that are important for the clinician to consider (eg, pain associated with chronic sinusitis). Two main idiopathic disorders that cause headache and facial pain are midfacial segment pain and atypical facial pain. Midfacial segment pain is a form of tension-type headache of the midface. This pain consists of a symmetric pressure sensation in the nasion, nasal dorsum, periorbital, or malar region. Hyperesthesia of the skin and soft tissues is also found. Treatment consists of low-dose amitriptyline at 10 mg for 6 months and may take up to 6 weeks to show effect. Atypical facial pain is also known as persistent idiopathic facial pain and is constant, deep, and ill-defined, usually crossing recognized dermatomes. The distribution is often unilateral. It occurs most commonly in women older than 40 years of age. The pain may alter in location and psychological factors may play a role. The treatment is similar to that for midfacial segment pain.

Fibromyalgia (Fibromyositis; Fibrositis)

Fibromyalgia is a common syndrome in which a patient has long-term, body-wide pain and tenderness in the joints, muscles, tendons, and other soft tissues. Fibromyalgia has also been linked to fatigue, sleep problems, headaches, depression, and anxiety. The cause of fibromyalgia is unknown; however, suggested causes or triggers include physical or emotional trauma, abnormal pain response, sleep disturbances, or infection (ie, unidentified virus). Fibromyalgia is most common among women 20-50 years of age.

Conditions that have been associated with fibromyalgia or mimic its symptoms include chronic neck or back pain, chronic fatigue syndrome, depression, hypothyroidism, Lyme disease, sleep disorders, and atypical facial pain. Patients with fibromyalgia tend to wake up with body aches and stiffness. For some patients, pain improves during the day and gets worse at night, while others experience pain all day long. The pain may get worse with activity, cold or damp weather, anxiety, and stress. Fatigue, depressed mood, and sleep problems (sleep interruption is often reported) are seen in almost all patients with fibromyalgia.

A patient must have at least 3 months of widespread pain and tenderness in at least 11 of 18 areas to be diagnosed with fibromyalgia. These areas may include arms (elbows), buttocks, chest, knees, lower back, neck, rib cage, shoulders, or thighs. Blood and urine tests are usually normal; however, tests may be done to rule out other conditions that may have similar symptoms.

The goal of treatment is to help relieve pain and other symptoms and to help the patient cope with symptoms. The first type of treatment may involve physical therapy, exercise and fitness programs, or stress-relief methods (eg, light massage and relaxation techniques). If these treatments fail, an antidepressant or muscle relaxant may be prescribed. The goal of medication is to improve sleep and pain tolerance. All medications should be used along with exercise and behavior therapy. Duloxetine, pregabalin, and milnacipran are medications that are approved specifically for treating fibromyalgia. Other medications that have been suggested to treat this condition include anti-seizure drugs, other antidepressants, muscle relaxants, pain relievers, or sleeping aids. Severe cases of fibromyalgia may require a referral to a pain clinic.

Studies are currently being performed to determine the efficacy of chronic pain medications in the specific management of TMD.

The oral medicine specialist in TMD management, the physical therapist interested in head and neck pain, and the oral and maxillofacial surgeon will all work together with the referring general dentist to accomplish successful patient treatment. Table 1 lists the wide variety of treatment alternatives available to the team. Depending on the diagnosis, one or more of the therapies might be selected. For organic diseases of the joint not responding to nonsurgical approaches, a wide variety of surgical techniques are available (Table 2).

ACUTE TMD

Acute TMD oftentimes presents alone or as an episode during a chronic pattern of signs and symptoms. Trauma, such as a blow to the chin or the side of the face, can result in acute TMD. Occasionally, similar symptoms will follow a lengthy wide open mouth dental procedure.

The condition usually presents as continuous deep pain in the TMJ. If edema is present in the joint, the condyle sometimes can be displaced which will cause abnormal occlusion of the posterior teeth on the affected side. The diagnosis is usually based on the history and clinical presentation. Management of the patient includes:

1. Restriction of all mandibular movement to function in a pain-free range of motion

2. Soft diet

3. NSAIDs (eg, Anaprox® DS 1 tablet every 12 hours for 7-10 days)

4. Moist heat applications to the affected area for 15-20 minutes, 4-6 times/day

5. Consideration of a muscle relaxant, such as Methocarbamol (Robaxin®) on page 888, adult patient of average height/weight, two (500 mg) tablets at bedtime; daytime dose can be tailored to patient

Additional therapies could include referral to a physical therapist for ultrasound therapy 2-4 times/week and a single injection of steroid in the joint space. A team approach with an oral maxillofacial surgeon for this procedure may be helpful.

CHRONIC TMD

Following diagnosis which is often problematic, the most common therapeutic modalities include:

- Explaining the problem to the patient

- Recommending a soft diet:
  - Diet should consist of soft foods (eg, eggs, yogurt, casseroles, soup, ground meat).
  - Avoid chewing gum, salads, large sandwiches, and hard fruit.

- Reducing stress; moist heat application 4-6 times/day for 15-20 minutes coupled with a monitored exercise program will be beneficial. Usually, working with a physical therapist is ideal.

- Medications include analgesics, anti-inflammatories, tranquilizers, and muscle relaxants

MEDICATION OPTIONS

Most commonly used medication (NSAIDs)

Choline Magnesium Trisalicylate on page 299
Diclofenac (Systemic) on page 413
Diflunisal on page 421
Etodolac on page 554
Fenoprofen on page 576
Flurbiprofen (Systemic) on page 615
Ibuprofen on page 711
Indomethacin on page 735
Ketoprofen on page 781
Ketorolac (Systemic) on page 783
Magnesium Salicylate on page 853
Meclofenamate on page 859
Mefenamic Acid on page 862
Nabumetone on page 948
Naproxen on page 958
Oxaprozin on page 1022
Piroxicam on page 1104
Salsalate on page 1221
Sulindac on page 1266
Tolmetin on page 1337

Tranquilizers and muscle relaxants, when used appropriately, can provide excellent adjunctive therapy. These drugs should be primarily used for a short period of time to manage acute pain. In low dosages, amitriptyline is often used to treat chronic pain and occasionally migraine headache. Two drugs similar to the prototype drug, amitriptyline, have been approved for use in adults only, for treatment of acute migraine with or without aura: Almotriptan malate (Axert™ [tablets]; Pharmacia

Corp) and frovatriptan succinate (Frova™ [tablets]; Endo Pharmaceuticals). Other approved abortive (but not preventative) antimigraine triptan drugs include eletriptan (Relpax®), naratriptan (Amerge®), rizatriptan (Maxalt®), sumatriptan (Imitrex®), and zolmitriptan (Zomig®). Selective serotonin reuptake inhibitors (SSRIs) are sometimes used in the management of chronic neuropathic pain, particularly in patients not responding to amitriptyline. Gabapentin (Neurontin®) has been approved for chronic pain. Problems of inducing bruxism with SSRIs, however, have been reported and may preclude their use. Clinicians attempting to evaluate any patient with bruxism or involuntary muscle movement, who is simultaneously being treated with an SSRI, should be aware of this potential association.

See individual monographs for dosing instructions.

Common minor tranquilizers include:

ALPRAZolam on page 68
Diazepam on page 409
LORazepam on page 839

Chronic neuropathic pain management:

Amitriptyline on page 84
CarBAMazepine on page 244
Gabapentin on page 642

Acute migraine management:

Almotriptan on page 66
Eletriptan on page 471
Frovatriptan on page 638
Naratriptan on page 961
Rizatriptan on page 1207
SUMAtriptan on page 1268
ZOLMitriptan on page 1427

Common muscle relaxants include:

Chlorzoxazone on page 297
Cyclobenzaprine on page 358
Methocarbamol on page 888
Orphenadrine on page 1018

Note: Muscle relaxants and tranquilizers should generally be prescribed with an analgesic or NSAID to relieve pain as well.

Narcotic analgesics can be used on a short-term basis or intermittently in combination with non-narcotic therapy in the chronic pain patient. Judicious prescribing, monitoring, and maintenance by the practitioner is imperative whenever considering the use of narcotic analgesics due to the abuse and addiction liabilities.

Table 1. TMD – Nonsurgical Therapies

1. Moist heat and cold spray

2. Injections in muscle trigger areas (procaine)

3. Exercises (passive, active)

4. Medications

   a. Muscle relaxants

   b. Minerals (magnesium, glucosamine, chondroitin)

   c. Multiple vitamins (Ca, B_6, B_{12})

   d. NSAIDs, opioid combinations, antidepressants

5. Orthopedic craniomandibular repositioning appliance (splints)

6. Biofeedback, acupuncture

7. Physiotherapy: TMJ muscle therapy

8. Myofunctional therapy (occasionally)

9. TENS (transcutaneous electrical neural stimulation), Myo-Monitor (occasionally)

10. Dental therapy

    a. Equilibration (coronoplasty) (occasionally)

    b. Restoring occlusion to proper vertical dimension of maxilla to mandible by orthodontics, dental restorative procedures, orthognathic surgery, permanent splint, or any combination of these

Table 2. TMD – Surgical Therapies

1. Cortisone injection into joint (with local anesthetic)

2. Bony and/or fibrous ankylosis: Requires surgery (osteoarthrotomy with prosthetic appliance)

3. Chronic subluxation: Requires surgery, depending on problem (possibly eminectomy and/or prosthetic implant)

4. Osteoarthritis: Requires surgery (arthroscopy), depending on problem

    a. Arthroplasty

    b. Meniscectomy

    c. Arthroplasty with repair of disc

    d. Arthrocentesis

5. Rheumatoid arthritis

    a. Arthroplasty

    b. "Total" TMJ replacement

6. Tumors: Require osteoarthrotomy – removal of tumor and restoring of joint when possible

7. Chronic disc displacement: Arthroscopy with arthrocentesis; possible removal of bone from condyle

REFERENCES

Abeles M, Solitar BM, Pillinger MH, et al, "Update on Fibromyalgia Therapy," *Am J Med*, 2008, 121(7):555-61.

Häuser W, Bernardy K, Uçeyler N, et al, "Treatment of Fibromyalgia Syndrome With Antidepressants: A Meta-Analysis," *JAMA*, 2009, 301(2):198-209.

Wolfe F and Rasker JJ, "Fibromyalgia," *Kelley's Textbook of Rheumatology*, 8th ed, Firestein GS, Budd RC, Harris ED Jr, et al, eds, Philadelphia, PA: Saunders Elsevier, 2008, chap 38.

Wolfe F, Clauw DJ, Fitzcharles MA, et al, "The American College of Rheumatology Preliminary Diagnostic Criteria for Fibromyalgia and Measurement of Symptom Severity," *Arthritis Care Res (Hoboken)*, 2010, 62(5):600-10.

MANAGEMENT OF THE PATIENT WITH ANXIETY OR DEPRESSION

ANXIETY AND DEPRESSION

Over the past two decades, there has been a gradual, but steady, increase in the number of patients who are taking antianxiety and antidepressant medications. Much of this is driven by the emergence of new medications for management of these conditions and an increasing awareness on the part of medical clinicians in recognizing signs and symptoms of depression and anxiety. In addition, society has now accepted that the quality of life for these patients can be improved on an outpatient basis.

The dentist often encounters patients taking medications that have the potential to induce mild-to-moderate adverse oral side effects and may create additional risk based on the types of medication used in the dental practice. In addition to a wide variety of depression-indicated signs and symptoms, antidepressant medications are prescribed for psychiatric disorders, pain control, sleep deprivation, smoking cessation, substance abuse, and eating disorders. The side effects of these drugs primarily fall into several categories. Xerostomia or altered salivary flow has long been known as a side effect of tricyclic antidepressants. Newer antidepressants, although the effects may be lessened, also have similar side effects. Coupled with xerostomia is an increased risk of fungal infections and a significant association with burning mouth syndrome (BMS). The reader is referred to Fungal Infections on page   1573 and Ulcerative, Erosive, and Painful Oral Mucosal Disorders on page   1578 for management if an infection is suspected. In addition, some drugs, including the selective serotonin reuptake inhibitors (SSRIs), have effects on orthostatic hypotension and there have been rare reports of increased bruxism with chronic use of the drugs. Many of the antianxiety and antidepressant medications have shown some efficacy in the management of chronic pain and some have approval for use in atypical facial pain and temporomandibular dysfunction (TMD). Generally, the dosing for these chronic pain conditions is lower than the dosing for the management of depression or anxiety, but the approved dosing should always be verified before prescribing.

Another potential adverse reaction is cardiotoxicity associated with the use of combination drugs, including the antidepressant medication classes, and the use of a vasoconstrictor in local anesthetics. The reader is referred to Vasoconstrictor Interactions With Antidepressants on page   1650 in the appendix which discusses the classes of antidepressant and antianxiety medications and the potential risk of interactions with local anesthetics.

In reviewing the epidemiology of antidepressant and antianxiety medications, female subjects outnumber males by ~2.3:1 ratio with selective serotonin reuptake inhibitors being the most commonly prescribed medications. Tricyclic antidepressants, atypical third-generation antidepressants, and monoamine oxidase inhibitors are also used. Some of the drugs used for smoking cessation also fall into this atypical antidepressant class.

BIPOLAR DISORDER

Many advances have occurred in the treatment of bipolar illness and a number of drugs have been FDA-approved for use, including some of the atypical antipsychotics (eg, aripiprazole, olanzapine, risperidone, ziprasidone). Treatment options include mood stabilizers (eg, lithium, valproic acid, carbamazepine, oxcarbazepine), antidepressants, electroconvulsive therapy, and antipsychotics (adjunctive therapy). Most people with bipolar disorder take combinations of lithium, valproate, and carbamazepine to manage symptoms and prevent recurrence of bipolar episodes. These medications are often called mood stabilizers, to even out emotional highs and lows. These patients may also be prescribed other medications to treat the agitation, anxiety, and sleep disturbances that may accompany their illness. In patients with concomitant depression, antidepressants can help manage the feelings of sadness, guilt, worthlessness, or hopelessness. Dry mouth, constipation, and nausea are the most common side effects.

SEDATION

Anxiety constitutes the most frequently found psychiatric problem in the general population. Anxiety can range from a simple phobia to a severe debilitating disorder. Functional results of this anxiety can, therefore, range from simple avoidance of dental procedures to panic attacks when confronting stressful situations, such as seen in some patients regarding dental visits. Many patients claim to be anxious over dental care, when in reality, they simply have not been managed with modern techniques of local anesthesia, the availability of sedation, or the caring dental practitioner.

The dentist may detect anxiety in patients during the treatment planning and evaluation phases of care. The anxious person may appear overly alert, may lean forward in the dental chair during conversation, or may appear concerned over time, possibly using this as a guise to cut short the dental visit. Anxious persons may also show signs of being nervous by demonstrating sweating; muscle tension, including their temporomandibular musculature; or they may complain of being tired due to an inability to obtain an adequate night's sleep.

The management of these patients requires a methodical approach to relaxation, discussing their dental needs, and then planning, along with the patient, the best way to accomplish dental treatment in the presence of their fears, either real or imagined. Consideration may be given to sedation. This sedation can be oral or parenteral, or inhalation in the case of nitrous oxide. The dentist must be adequately trained in administering the sedative of choice, as well as in monitoring the patient during the sedated procedures. Numerous medications are available to achieve the level of sedation usually necessary in the dental office: Valium®, Ativan®, Xanax®, Vistaril®, Serax®, and BuSpar® represent a few. These oral sedatives can be given prior to dental visits as outlined in the following prescriptions. They have the advantage of allowing the patient a good night's sleep prior to the day of the procedure and provide on-the-spot sedation during the procedure. Nitrous oxide is an in-the-office administered sedative that is relatively safe, but requires additional training and carefully planned monitoring protocols of auxiliary personnel during inhalation. Both oral and inhalation techniques can be used to manage the anxious patient in the dental office.

It is recommended that patients not drive themselves to or from dental appointments following use of these medications. Also, these medications should not be prescribed during pregnancy. For pediatric patients, oral preprocedural sedatives include primarily hydroxyzine and liquid meperidine. Dosing suggestions are described in each of the respective monographs.

ALPRAZolam on page 68
BusPIRone on page 219
Diazepam on page 409
HydrOXYzine on page 706
LORazepam on page 839
Meperidine on page 871
Nitrous Oxide on page 988
Prochlorperazine on page 1144
Triazolam on page 1361

Note: Although various antidepressants have been used for preprocedure sedation, no specific regimens or protocols have been established. Guidelines for use are still under study.

Doxepin (Systemic) on page 451
FLUoxetine on page 608
FluvoxaMINE on page 623
PARoxetine on page 1051
Sertraline on page 1229
TraZODone on page 1352

For examples of sample prescriptions see Sedation (Prior to Dental Treatment) on page 1621

REFERENCES

Anttila S, Knuuttila M, Ylöstalo P, et al, "Symptoms of Depression and Anxiety in Relation to Dental Health Behavior and Self-Perceived Dental Treatment Need," *Eur J Oral Sci*, 2006, 114(2):109-14.
Armfield JM, Stewart JF, and Spencer AJ, "The Vicious Cycle of Dental Fear: Exploring the Interplay Between Oral Health, Service Utilization and Dental Fear," *BMC Oral Health*, 2007, 14;7:1.
Brodine AH and Hartshorn MA, "Recognition and Management of Somatoform Disorders," *J Prosthet Dent*, 2004, 91(3):268-73.
Coulson NS and Buchanan H, "Self-Reported Efficacy of an Online Dental Anxiety Support Group: A Pilot Study," *Community Dent Oral Epidemiol*, 2008, 36(1):43-6.
Keene JJ Jr, Galasko GT, and Land MF, "Antidepressant Use in Psychiatry and Medicine: Importance for Dental Practice," *J Am Dent Assoc*, 2003, 134(1):71-9.
Klingberg G and Broberg AG, "Dental Fear/Anxiety and Dental Behaviour Management Problems in Children and Adolescents: A Review of Prevalence and Concomitant Psychological Factors," *Int J Paediatr Dent*, 2007, 17(6):391-406.
Lundgren J, Carlsson SG, and Berggren U, "Relaxation Versus Cognitive Therapies for Dental Fear - A Psychophysiological Approach," *Health Psychol*, 2006, 25(3):267-73.
Merry SN, Hetrick SE, Cox GR, et al, "Cochrane Review: Psychological and Educational Interventions for Preventing Depression in Children and Adolescents," *Cochrane Database Syst Rev*, 2012, 7(5):1409-685.
Stenebrand A, Boman UW, and Hakeberg M, "Dental Anxiety and Symptoms of General Anxiety and Depression in 15-Year-Olds," *Int J Dent Hyg*, 2012 [epub ahead of print]

MANAGEMENT OF PATIENTS UNDERGOING CANCER THERAPY

CANCER PATIENT DENTAL PROTOCOL

The objective in treatment of a patient with cancer is eradication of the disease. Oral complications, such as mucosal ulceration, xerostomia, bleeding, and infections can cause significant morbidity and may compromise systemic treatment of the patient. With proper oral evaluation before systemic treatment, many of the complications can be minimized or prevented.

MUCOSITIS

Normal oral mucosa acts as a barrier against chemical and food irritants and oral micro-organisms. Disruption of the mucosal barrier can lead to secondary infection, increased pain, delayed healing, and decreased nutritional intake.

Mucositis is an inflammation of the mucous membranes; however, its pathogenesis is more complicated, resulting from cytokine signals that lead to surface cell necrosis and delayed new cell proliferation. It is a common reaction to chemotherapy and radiation therapy. It is first seen as an erythematous patch. The mucosal epithelium becomes thin as a result of the killing of the rapidly dividing basal layer mucosal cells. Seven to ten days after cytoreduction chemotherapy and between 1000 cGy and 3000 cGy of radiation to the head and neck, mucosal tissues begin to desquamate and eventually develop into frank ulcerations. The mucosal integrity is broken and is often secondarily infected by normal oral flora. The resultant ulcerations can also act as a portal of entry for pathogenic organisms into the patient's bloodstream and may lead to systemic infections. These ulcerations often force interruption of therapy. A specific type of ulcerative stomatitis is encountered in patients treated for cancer with mTOR inhibitors such as everolimus (Afinitor®). These ulcers resemble aphthous ulcers and occur on tissues that are freely movable (most commonly the tongue and lips). The lesions are self-limiting but can interrupt chemotherapy. The pathogenesis of the lesions is not well understood, but they appear to respond to steroid rinses.

Prevention of radiation mucositis is difficult. Stents can be constructed to prevent irradiation of uninvolved tissues. Most recently, intensity-modulated radiotherapy has been used as an advanced approach to 3D conformal radiotherapy; it optimizes the delivery of irradiation to irregularly shaped volumes and thus spares normal tissue while delivering an adequate dose to the tumor volumes. The use of multiple ports and fractionation of therapy into smaller doses over a longer period of time can also reduce the severity. Fractured restorations, sharp teeth, and ill-fitted prostheses can damage soft tissues and lead to additional interruption of mucosal barriers. Correction of these problems before radiation therapy can diminish these complications.

CHEMOTHERAPY

Chemotherapy for neoplasia also frequently results in oral complications. Infections and mucositis are the most common complications seen in patients receiving chemotherapy. Also occurring frequently are pain, altered nutrition, and xerostomia, which can significantly affect the quality of life.

Certain chemotherapeutic agents, such as melphalan, 5-fluorouracil, methotrexate, and doxorubicin, are more commonly associated with the development of oral mucositis. Treatment of oral mucositis is mainly palliative, but steps should be taken to minimize secondary pathogenic infections. Culture and sensitivity data should be obtained to select appropriate therapy for the bacterial, viral, or fungal organisms found.

RADIATION CARIES

Dental caries that sometimes follow radiation therapy is called radiation caries. It usually develops in the cervical smooth surface region of the teeth adjacent to the gingiva, often affecting many teeth. It is secondary to the irreversible damage done to the salivary glands and is initiated by dental plaque, but its rapid progress is due to changes in saliva. In addition to the diminution in the amount of saliva, both the salivary pH and buffering capacity are diminished, which decreases anticaries activity of saliva. Oral bacterial flora also change with xerostomia leading to the increase in caries activity. Typically patients that receive a cumulative radiation dose of 30 Gy or more will suffer significant loss of saliva production, some of which will be irreversible.

Osteonecrosis of the jaw (ONJ) is pertinent to cancer patient management and patients with osteoporosis, as well as antiresorptive agents used secondary to multiple myeloma and breast cancer to prevent metastases to the skeleton (see Osteonecrosis of the Jaw on page 1529).

PERIORAL PREMALIGNANT LESIONS

Dentists are often the first to recognize changes in the skin, lips, or oral mucosal tissues that represent potential premalignancies. The general dentist may refer such patients to an oral and maxillofacial surgeon, oral pathologist, or otolaryngologist for biopsy. There are numerous drugs under study to manage premalignancies by preventing the progression of lesions from dysplasia to frank cancer. On the skin, the condition actinic keratosis and on the lips, its perioral equivalent actinic cheilitis, create a diagnostic and management challenge for clinicians. Until now 5-fluorouracil preparations have been used with mixed success, but recently, Zyclara® (imiquimod) has been approved for actinic keratosis.

SALIVARY CHANGES

Chemotherapy is not thought to directly alter salivary flow, but alterations in taste and subjective sensations of dry mouth are relatively common complaints. Patients with mucositis and graft-vs-host disease following bone marrow or stem cell transplantation often demonstrate signs and symptoms of xerostomia. Radiation does directly affect salivary production. Radiation to the salivary glands produces fibrosis and alters the production of saliva. If all the major salivary glands are in the field, the decrease in saliva can be dramatic and the serous portion of the glands seems to be most severely affected. The saliva produced is increased in viscosity, which contributes to food retention, increased plaque formation, and difficulty swallowing. These xerostomia patients have difficulty in managing a normal diet. Normal saliva also has bacteriostatic properties that are diminished in these patients.

The dental management recommendations for patients undergoing chemotherapy, bone marrow transplantation, and/or radiation therapy for the treatment of cancer are based primarily on clinical observations. The following protocols will provide a conservative, consistent approach to the dental management of patients undergoing chemotherapy or bone marrow transplantation. Many of the cancer chemotherapy drugs produce oral side effects including mucositis, oral ulceration, dry mouth, acute infections, and taste aberrations. Cancer drugs include antibiotics, alkylating agents, antimetabolites, DNA inhibitors, hormones, and cytokines.

All patients undergoing chemotherapy or bone marrow transplantation for malignant disease should have the following baseline:

A. Panoramic radiograph

B. Dental consultation and examination

C. Dental prophylaxis and cleaning (if the neutrophil count is >1500/mm^3 and the platelet count is >50,000/mm^3)

- Prophylaxis and cleaning will be deferred if the patient's neutrophil count is <1500 and the platelet count is <50,000. Oral hygiene recommendations will be made. These levels are arbitrary guidelines and the dentist should consider the patient's oral condition and planned procedure relative to hemorrhage and level of bacteremia.

D. Oral Hygiene: Patients should be encouraged to follow normal hygiene procedures. Addition of a chlorhexidine mouth rinse such as Peridex® or PerioGard® on page 288 is usually helpful. If the patient develops oral mucositis, tolerance of such alcohol-based products may be limited. A nonalcohol-containing chlorhexidine mouth rinse CHX® is also available. Biotène® products including Oralbalance® are also useful since many patients report alteration of quality and quantity of saliva.

PREVENTION AND TREATMENT OF MUCOSITIS

A. If the patient develops mucositis, bacterial, viral, and fungal cultures should be obtained. There are no standard of care recommendations for prevention of oral mucositis. The intravenous biologic product keratinocyte growth factor, palifermin (Kepivance®) is approved to help reduce the chance that certain cancer patients, those with blood cancers undergoing chemotherapy, would develop mucositis. Most therapies are palliative only or help in reducing secondary infection. Sucralfate suspension in a pharmacy-prepared form or Carafate® suspension, as well as Benadryl® on page 433 or Xylocaine® viscous on page 818 solution can assist in helping the patient to tolerate food. In addition to the mucosal-coating drugs described below, various emollients and lubricants can be tried. A cost-effective approach is to rinse with a solution of 1/2 teaspoon of baking soda (and/or 1/2 teaspoon of table salt) in 1 cup of lukewarm water several times a day. Lastly, multiple studies have indicated that lower-level laser therapy can reduce the severity of chemotherapy and radiation-induced oral mucositis.

B. Aloclair® is now available as an oral lesion relief spray. It indicated for aphthous ulcerations and other mild-to-moderate oral erosions.

C. The oral barrier Gelclair® and the mucositis treatment aid Caphosol® are FDA approved for mucositis. Gargle and spit Gelclair® mixture of one single-use packet (15 mL) and water 3 times/day or as needed; follow mixing and administration instructions on packet.

D. Mix contents of 1 blue (A) and 1 clear (B) Caphosol® ampul in clean container, swish thoroughly with 1/2 of mixture (15 mL) for 1 minute and spit; repeat. Use immediately after mixing ampuls. Use 4 doses/day from the onset of high dose chemotherapy or radiation treatment. Patients may also require systemic and topical analgesics for pain relief depending on the presence of mucositis. Systemic treatments currently being used with variable success include antioxidants, immunomodulatory drugs, anticholinergic drugs, pentoxifylline, cytokines antiviral drugs, and glutamic acid; a topical analgesic commonly used is lidocaine. Positive fungal cultures may require a nystatin swish-and-swallow prescription or the selection of another antifungal agent (see Fungal Infections on page 1573).

E. The determination of performing dental procedures must be based on the goal of preventing infection during periods of neutropenia and reducing the risk of bleeding when platelet counts are low. Timing of procedures must be coordinated with the patient's hematologic status.

F. If oral surgery is required, at least 7-10 days of healing should be allowed before the anticipated date of bone marrow suppression (eg, ANC <1000/mm^3 and/or platelet count of ≥50,000/mm^3).

G. Daily use of topical fluorides is recommended for those who have received radiation therapy to the head and neck region involving salivary glands. Any patients with prolonged xerostomia subsequent to graft-vs-host disease and/or chemotherapy can also be considered for fluoride supplement. Use the fluoride-containing mouthwashes (Act®, Fluorigard®, etc) each night before going to sleep; swish, hold 1-2 minutes, spit out or use prescription fluorides (gels or rinses); apply daily for 1-4 minutes as directed; if mouth is sore (mucositis), use flavorless/colorless gels (Thera-Flur®, Gel-Kam®, or Prevident®). Custom trays for fluoride applications can be produced by the clinician for the patient's home use using heat-formed materials such as omnivac. Patients with porcelain crowns, resin, or glass ionomer restorations should use a neutral pH fluoride. Improvement in salivary flow following radiation therapy to the head and neck has been noted with prescription sialogogue Salagen® on page 1092 or Evoxac® on page 284. Salagen®, containing the nonselective analogue cholinergic agonist, pilocarpine, is currently the sole sialogogic agent approved by the FDA for radiation-induced xerostomia. Evoxac®, containing the quinuclidine analogue of acetylcholine, cevimeline, has been found safe and effective in treating xerostomia in patients with Sjögren's syndrome and may have merit for the treatment of radiation-induced xerostomia.

Benzonatate on page 179
Cevimeline on page 284
Chlorhexidine Gluconate on page 288
DiphenhydrAMINE (Systemic) on page 433
Gelclair® Bioadherent Oral Gel® on page 946
Lidocaine (Topical) on page 818
MuGard™ on page 946
Pilocarpine (Systemic) on page 1092
Povidone-Iodine (Topical) on page 1123
Sucralfate on page 1257

ORAL CARE PRODUCTS

Bacterial Plaque Control

Patients should use an extra soft bristle toothbrush and dental floss for removal of plaque. Sponge/foam sticks and lemon-glycerine swabs do not adequately remove bacterial plaque.

Cholinergic Agents

See Products for Xerostomia on page 1582

Used for the treatment of xerostomia caused by radiation therapy in patients with head and neck cancer and from Sjögren's syndrome

Cevimeline on page 284
Pilocarpine (Systemic) on page 1092

Fluorides

See Fluorides in the Dentin Hypersensitivity, High Caries Index, and Xerostomia section.

Used for the prevention of demineralization of the tooth structure secondary to xerostomia. For patients with long-term or permanent xerostomia, daily application is accomplished using custom gel applicator trays, such as omnivac. Patients with porcelain crowns should use a neutral pH fluoride (see Fluoride monograph on page 606). Final selection of a fluoride product and/or saliva replacement/stimulant product must be based on patient comfort, taste, and ultimately, compliance. Experience has demonstrated that, often times, patients must try various combinations to achieve the greatest effect and their highest comfort levels. The presence of mucositis during cancer management complicates the clinician's selection of products.

Saliva Substitutes

See Products for Xerostomia on page 1582
Saliva Substitute on page 1220

Oral and Lip Moisturizers/Lubricants

Note: Water-based gels should first be used to provide moisture to dry oral tissues.

Surgilube®
K-Y Jelly®
Oralbalance®
Mouth Moisturizer®
Caphosol®

PALLIATION OF PAIN

Note: Palliative pain preparations should be monitored for efficacy.

- For relief of pain associated with isolated mucositis or ulcerations, topical anesthetic and protective preparations may be used.
  - Orabase-B® with 20% benzocaine on page 176
  - Zilactin-B® gel with 10% benzocaine
- For generalized oral pain:
  - Chloraseptic Spray® (OTC) anesthetic spray without alcohol on page 1082
  - Ulcer-Ease® anesthetic/analgesic mouthrinse
  - BetaCell® oral rinse
  - Xylocaine® 2% viscous on page 818
    Note: May anesthetize swallowing mechanism and cause aspiration of food; caution patient against using too close to eating; lack of sensation may also allow patient to damage intact mucosa
  - Tantum Mouthrinse® (benzydamine hydrochloride); may be diluted as required
    Note: Available only in Canada and Europe

Patient-Prepared Palliative Mixtures

Coating agents:
Maalox® on page 74
Mylanta® on page 74
Kaopectate® on page 151

These products can be mixed with Benadryl® elixir (50:50):

DiphenhydrAMINE (Systemic) (Benadryl®) on page 433

Topical anesthetics (diphenhydramine chloride):
Benadryl® elixir or Benylin® cough syrup on page 433
Note: Choose product with lowest alcohol and sucrose content; ask pharmacist for assistance
Mucotrol gel wafer

Pharmacy Preparations

A pharmacist may also prepare the following solutions for relief of generalized oral pain:
Benadryl-Lidocaine Solution
Diphenhydramine injectable 1.5 mL (50 mg/mL) on page 433
Xylocaine® viscous 2% (45 mL) on page 818
Magnesium aluminum hydroxide solution (45 mL)
Swish and hold 1 teaspoonful in mouth for 30 seconds; do not use too close to eating

REFERENCES

Eisen T, Sternberg CN, Robert C, et al, "Targeted Therapies for Renal Cell Carcinoma: Review of Adverse Event Management Strategies," *J Natl Cancer Inst*, 2012, 104(2):93-113.
Pilotte AP, Hohos MB, Polson KM, et al, "Managing Stomatitis in Patients Treated With Mammalian Target of Rapamycin Inhibitors," *Clin J Oncol Nurs*, 2011, 15(5):E83-9.
Porta C, Osanto S, Ravaud A, et al, "Management of Adverse Events Associated With the Use of Everolimus in Patients With Advanced Renal Cell Carcinoma," *Eur J Cancer*, 2011, 47(9):1287-98.
Sonis S, Treister N, Chawla S, et al, "Preliminary Characterization of Oral Lesions Associated With Inhibitors of Mammalian Target of Rapamycin in Cancer Patients," *Cancer*, 2010, 116(1):210-5.

DENTIST'S ROLE IN RECOGNIZING DOMESTIC VIOLENCE, ABUSE, AND NEGLECT

Recognition of the signs and symptoms of domestic violence is an important topic for dental and medical professionals throughout the world. Unfortunately, statistics related to domestic abuse and/or neglect of women, children, and the elderly appear to be on the rise, perhaps, in part, due to increased recognition.

Statistics are indeed staggering; one in four women will experience domestic violence in her lifetime (CDC, 2008). In the United States, a woman, child, or elder is physically abused every 5-15 seconds. In fact, violence is cited as one of the common causes of emergency room admissions for women 15-44 years of age. Furthermore, 50,000 deaths occur annually, which are attributable to violence in the form of homicide or suicide.

The dentist's responsibilities and professional role in this arena are not clear in all states. The literature, however, is clear regarding how each professional has the responsibility to understand current state laws regarding the reporting of domestic violence, abuse of children or the elderly, and/or neglect. Many states have existing codes defining the role of the professional in these regards. Many other states, such as Maryland, have adopted continuing education requirements specific to the subject. The overall problem of domestic violence, including child abuse, neglect, and other forms of abuse, are indeed public health issues. Likewise, the costs (eg, medical, dental, psychiatric, hospital, and emergency care fees) are borne to a great extent by the community as well as the individual.

Domestic abuse is defined as "controlling behavior." Neglect can take on a myriad of presentations. Although this often includes physical injury, the primary focus of domestic abuse is one person being in control of another person, making that person do something against his/her will. Women are often abused both physically and mentally in relationships that have existed for many years. Children are often the focus of domestic violence; however, the pattern for an entire family's abuse may be present. Abuse comes in many forms and many victims do not even realize that abuse is occurring. Some victims simply "chalk it up" to things that happen within families. Abuse may include battery and physical assault, such as throwing objects, pushing, hitting, slapping, kicking, or attacking with a weapon; sexual assault including the abuser forcing sexual activities upon another; and psychological abuse, such as forcing a victim to perform degrading or humiliating acts, threatening harm to a female or male partner or child, or destroying valued possessions of another. Verbal abuse can also be included; however, psychological forms of abuse are very difficult to ascertain and signs and symptoms may be difficult to separate from other psychological traits. Abuse tends to have a cyclic pattern, often where a partner or the controlling individual is extremely friendly, intimate, and a good household member; however, due to unknown reasons, as tension develops, family violence often erupts. Once battering has begun, it often increases in frequency and in severity with time. Early recognition can often prevent serious effects; however, until physical violence becomes part of the domestic abuse situation, recognition is usually difficult.

It is estimated that nearly 65% of abuse cases (where physical injury is involved) include injury to the head, neck, or mouth; therefore, dental professionals are in a unique position to detect and perhaps, if appropriate in that state, report suspected abuse. In children, these percentages are even higher. Being wards of adults, children are vulnerable. Child abuse includes any act that is not accidental, endangering or impairing a child's safety or emotional health. Types of child abuse may include physical abuse, emotional abuse and neglect, including neglect of proper healthcare. Any child suspected of suffering from an emotional injury, including sexual abuse or neglect, should be brought to the attention of the social welfare system. Occasionally, "Munchausen syndrome," which is defined as the guardians fabricating or inducing illness in the child, may be observed. Intentional poisoning and safety neglect are also included in this syndrome.

From a medical point-of-view, neglect is much more difficult to determine than abuse. The role of the dentist may be to define the state of normal and customary pediatric or elderly patient health within a locality; however, due to parents and families moving about the country, sometimes one standard may not be appropriate for all locations. Several key behavioral indicators:

- child, adult, or elderly patient:
  - avoids eye contact
  - is wary of a guardian or spouse
  - demonstrates fear when touched
  - exhibits dramatic mood changes (eg, hostile or aggressive behavior)
- history or reports of suicide attempts or running away
- unexplained injuries or injuries inconsistent with explanation or delay in seeking treatment
- inappropriate use of prescription drugs (ie, responsible adult controls compliance of a child or elderly patient)
- individual decides to change practitioner when questioned too intensely

For the dentist, head-neck examination is important and includes gathering an overall visual impression of general cleanliness, dress, and stature and examining for any specific physical indicators such as bruises, welts, bite marks, abrasions, lacerations, or other injuries to the head or neck. Contusions or bruises represent the highest percentage of abuse injuries to the young child. The extremely young child or infant often suffers fractures, which fall to second place in terms of incidence as the child matures. In the adult, fractures are much less common. The dentist needs to document the location since this often represents the characteristic that may be difficult for the person to explain. Common areas for injuries include the bony eminences over the knees, shins, and elbows but could also be on the face, including the zygomatic arch and the chin. Burns are rarer, but represent one of the most serious types of injuries. Intraoral injuries, including trauma to the oral mucosa, tooth fractures, palatal lesions, ecchymoses, and fractures, represent serious evidence of domestic or child abuse. Physical indicators of sexual abuse may not be obvious to the dentist; however, bruising of the hard palate or other evidence of sexual dysfunction may sometimes be found.

The dentist has the responsibility to document, from a forensic point-of-view, the characteristics of abuse that are observed. As with all diagnostic considerations, the dentist must form a differential diagnosis to rule in or out oral and dental pathologies before suspecting abuse or neglect. History and probability are key to making these determinations. If necessary, evidence including impressions for bite marks or photographs to document unexplained injuries to the head, neck, and face may be necessary. The legal liability for the dentist is determined by the state laws governing the dental practice. The dental practitioner's failure to diagnose child abuse and neglect is another consideration which goes along with ethical and legal considerations. States are generally much clearer in the area of child abuse than they are regarding spousal or elderly abuse or overall domestic violence. The dentist has a responsibility to refer a patient for a second opinion, such as to their primary care pediatrician or internist, if there are concerns of abuse.

Under the Federal Child Abuse Prevention and Treatment Act (CAPTA) passed in 1974, all 50 states have passed laws mandating the reporting of child abuse and neglect. CAPTA provides a foundation for states by identifying a minimum set of acts or behaviors that characterize physical abuse, neglect, and sexual abuse. These laws vary from state to state. Each states responsible for the following:

- providing its own definition of child abuse and neglect

- describing the circumstances and conditions that obligate mandated individuals to report known or suspected child abuse

- providing definitions for juvenile/family courts when to take custody of the child

- specifying the forms of maltreatment that are criminally punishable

Unfortunately, there is little uniformity in the state laws regarding either the responsibility for reporting adult domestic violence or abuse or in protecting the healthcare professional by reporting, in good faith, abuse situations. When spousal or elderly abuse or other domestic violence is suspected, the definitions become even less clear. They are very similar in ambiguity to those that are faced by the professional regarding neglect as opposed to direct physical or mental abuse. The American Dental Association code is clear on principles and ethics regarding professional conduct regarding the responsibility for recognition of child abuse. They are much less clear on spousal or other abuse and it is likely that in the future, as some consistency is noted between and among the various state laws, the ADA Council will undoubtedly take a stronger position.

It is clearly up to the individual states to take the lead in establishing strict guidelines for recognition and reporting of domestic abuse, including protection under the "good faith" statutes for the practitioner. Rules and regulations regarding malicious reporting should also be better defined. The national position is difficult to define because of the extreme variation among states. Dentists are encouraged to use their best judgment in proceeding in any situation of suspected domestic abuse or neglect. They should primarily know their state laws and join in the discussion of the topic so that appropriate state actions and formation of legal codes can be undertaken. The current move by some states toward requiring continuing education on these subjects is an excellent sign that there is movement in a constructive direction.

REFERENCES

American Academy of Pediatric Dentistry, "Clinical Guideline on Oral and Dental Aspects of Child Abuse and Neglect," *Pediatr Dent*, 2004, 26(7 Suppl):63-6.

American Dental Association Council on Ethics, Bylaws and Judicial Affairs, "American Dental Association Principles of Ethics and Code of Professional Conduct, with Official Advisory Opinions," 2012. Available at http://www.ada.org/sections/about/pdfs/code_of_ethics_2012.pdf

Centers for Disease Control and Prevention (CDC), "Adverse Health Conditions and Health Risk Behaviors Associated With Intimate Partner Violence-United States, 2005," *MMWR Morb Mortal Wkly Rep*, 2008, 57(5):113-7.

Dubowitz H, Kim J, Black MM, et al, "Identifying Children at High Risk for a Child Maltreatment Report," *Child Abuse Negl*, 2011, 35(2):96-104.

Katner DR and Brown CE, "Mandatory Reporting of Oral Injuries Indicating Possible Child Abuse," *J Am Dent Assoc*, 2012, 143(10):1087-92.

Kellogg ND and American Academy of Pediatrics Committee on Child Abuse and Neglect, "Evaluation of Suspected Child Physical Abuse," *Pediatrics*, 2007, 119(6):1232-41.

Kenney JP, "Domestic Violence: A Complex Health Care Issue for Dentistry Today," *Forensic Sci Int*, 2006, 159(Suppl 1):S121–5.

Manea S, Favero GA, Stellini E, et al, "Dentists' Perceptions, Attitudes, Knowledge, and Experience About Child Abuse and Neglect in Northeast Italy," *J Clin Pediatr Dent*, 2007, 32(1):19-25.

Nelms AP, Gutmann ME, Solomon ES, et al, "What Victims of Domestic Violence Need From the Dental Profession," *J Dent Educ*, 2009, 73(4):490-8.

Stechey F, "P.A.N.D.A. A Dentist's Introduction to Recognizing Child Abuse," *Dental Practice Management*, 2001. Available at http://www.rcdso.org/life/ll_learning_pdf/DPM_PANDA.pdf

US Department of Health and Human Services, Administration for Children and Families, and Child Welfare Information Gateway, "Mandatory Reporters of Child Abuse and Neglect," 2012. Available at https://www.childwelfare.gov/systemwide/laws_policies/statutes/manda.pdf

Wiseman M, "The Role of the Dentist in Recognizing Elder Abuse," *J Can Dent Assoc*, 2008, 74(8):715-20.

ORAL MEDICINE TOPICS

PART III:

SAMPLE PRESCRIPTIONS

Drug prescriptions shown represent prototype drugs and popular prescriptions and are examples only. The pharmacologic category index is available for cross-referencing if alternatives and additional drugs are sought.

TABLE OF CONTENTS

INFECTIVE ENDOCARDITIS (PREVENTION)

General Prescription Comments

Prescriptions dispense amounts are for 3 visits. These numbers can be adjusted for each patient treatment plan.

Sample Prescriptions

Rx:
Amoxicillin 500 mg
Disp: 12 tablets
Sig: 4 tablets (2 g) 30-60 minutes prior to dental visit and repeat at each appointment

Rx:
Clindamycin (Systemic) 150 mg
Disp: 12 capsules
Sig: 4 capsules (600 mg) 30-60 minutes prior to dental visit and repeat at each appointment

Rx:
Cephalexin 500 mg
Disp: 12 tablets
Sig: 4 tablets (2 g) 30-60 minutes prior to dental visit and repeat at each appointment

Rx:
Azithromycin (Systemic) 500 mg
Disp: 3 tablets
Sig: 1 tablet 30-60 minutes prior to dental visit and repeat at each appointment

PROSTHETIC JOINT LATE INFECTIONS (PREVENTION)

General Prescription Comments

Please review the new guidelines for prevention of prosthetic joint late infections. Decisions must be made on a case-by-case basis. If after careful consideration preprocedural antibiotics are found to be appropriate, the following example prescriptions apply. Prescription dispensing amounts are for 3 visits. These numbers can be adjusted for each patient treatment plan. Clinicians will be advised if and when any changes in the guidelines are forthcoming.

Sample Prescriptions

Rx:
Amoxicillin 500 mg
Disp: 12 tablets
Sig: 4 tablets (2 g) 1 hour prior to dental visit and repeat at each appointment

Rx:
Clindamycin (Systemic) 150 mg
Disp: 12 capsules
Sig: 4 capsules (600 mg) 1 hour prior to dental visit and repeat at each appointment

Rx:
Cephalexin 500 mg
Disp: 12 tablets
Sig: 4 tablets (2 g) 1 hour prior to dental visit and repeat at each appointment

ORAL PAIN

Mild/Moderate Oral Pain

General Prescription Comments

Recently, the FDA has formally requested manufacturers to limit the amount of acetaminophen in prescription combination products (eg, Vicodin®, Lortab®) to no more than 325 mg per dosage unit. The FDA is also requiring manufacturers to update labeling of all prescription combination acetaminophen products to warn of the potential risk for severe liver injury (see Oral Pain on page 1558 for more information). Some manufacturers have already reduced acetaminophen amounts to 300-325 mg per tablet in combination prescription products. Examples include hydrocodone and acetaminophen products such as Norco®, Vicodin®, and Xodol®.

Note: Numerous brand name products for infants and children that contain ibuprofen or acetaminophen have been voluntarily recalled by manufacturers due to investigation by the FDA.

Closely monitor and re-evaluate response at least every 2 weeks. If response is inadequate, re-evaluate diagnosis, medication choice, and dosage.

Sample Prescriptions

Note: The following sample prescriptions are for adults.

Rx:
Acetaminophen 325 mg tablets
Disp: To be determined by practitioner
Sig: Take 2 tablets every 4 hours

Note: Products include Tylenol® and others.
Note: Acetaminophen can be given if patient has allergies, bleeding problems, or stomach upset secondary to aspirin or NSAIDs.

Rx:
Ibuprofen 200 mg tablets
Disp: To be determined by practitioner
Sig: Take 1-2 tablets every 4 hours

Note: Ibuprofen is an available OTC as Advil®, Motrin® IB, and many store brand generic names. NSAIDs should not be combined with aspirin. NSAIDs may increase post-treatment bleeding. Use with caution in patients receiving anti-coagulants or antiplatelet drugs.

Rx:
Naproxen sodium 220 mg tablets
Disp: To be determined by practitioner
Sig: Take 1-2 tablets every 8 hours

Note: Naproxen sodium is an available OTC as Aleve® and many store brand generic names.

Rx:
Ibuprofen 400 mg tablets
Disp: 20 tablets
Sig: Take 1 tablet every 4-6 hours as needed for pain

Note: Prescription strength ibuprofen is available as the brand name Motrin®.

Rx:
Dolobid® 500 mg tablets
Disp: 16 tablets
Sig: Take 2 tablets initially, then 1 tablet every 8-12 hours as needed for pain

Ingredient: Diflunisal

MODERATE/MODERATELY SEVERE ORAL PAIN

General Prescription Comments

Closely monitor and re-evaluate response at least every 2 weeks. If response is inadequate, re-evaluate diagnosis, medication choice, and dosage.

Sample Prescriptions

Rx:
Ibuprofen 800 mg tablets
Disp: 16 tablets
Sig: Take 1 tablet 3 times/day as needed for pain

Note: For severe pain can be given up to 4 times/day. Also available as 600 mg tablets.

Rx:
TraMADol 50 mg tablets
Disp: 36 tablets
Sig: Take 1-2 tablets every 4-6 hours as needed for pain (maximum: 400 mg/day)

Note: Also available as the brand name Ultram®.

Rx:
Ultracet® tablets
Disp: 36 tablets
Sig: Take 2 tablets every 4-6 hours as needed for pain, not to exceed 8 tablets in 24 hours

Ingredients: Acetaminophen 325 mg and Tramadol 37.5 mg

Rx:
Vicoprofen® tablets
Disp: 16 tablets
Sig: Take 1-2 tablets every 4-6 hours as needed for pain (maximum: 5 tablets/day)

Note: Restrictions: C-III; no refills
Ingredients: Hydrocodone 7.5 mg and ibuprofen 200 mg; available as generic equivalent

Rx:
Vicodin ES® tablets
Disp: 16 tablets
Sig: Take 1 tablet every 4-6 hours as needed for pain (maximum: 5 tablets/day)

Note: Restrictions: C-III; no refills
Ingredients: Hydrocodone bitartrate 7.5 mg and acetaminophen 300 mg; available as generic equivalent. Also available as Vicodin® tablets: Ingredients: Hydrocodone bitartrate 5 mg and acetaminophen 300 mg; take 1 tablet every 4 hours as needed for pain.

Rx:
Lortab® 5 mg
Disp: 16 tablets
Sig: Take 1 or 2 tablets every 4 hours as needed for pain; not to exceed 8 tablets in 24 hours

Note: Restrictions: C-III; no refills
Ingredients: Hydrocodone 5 mg and acetaminophen 500 mg; available as generic equivalent

Rx:
Norco® 10 mg
Disp: 16 tablets
Sig: Take 1 or 2 tablets every 4 hours as needed for pain; not to exceed 8 tablets in 24 hours

Note: Restrictions: C-III; no refills
Ingredients: Hydrocodone 10 mg and acetaminophen 325 mg; available as generic equivalent

Rx:
Tylenol® #3
Disp: 16 tablets
Sig: Take 1 tablet every 4 hours as needed for pain

Note: Restrictions: C-III; no refills
Ingredients: Codeine 30 mg and acetaminophen 300 mg; available as generic equivalent

Rx:
Naproxen 275 mg tablets
Disp: 16 tablets
Sig: Take 2 tablets initially, then one tablet 3 times/day as needed for pain

SEVERE ORAL PAIN

General Prescription Comments

Closely monitor and re-evaluate response at least every 2 weeks. If response is inadequate, re-evaluate diagnosis, medication choice, and dosage.

Liquid volumes are suggested for a typical 2-week course. Check with pharmacist for available sizes.

Cream and ointment tube sizes may vary based on availability. Refer to individual monograph or check with pharmacist for available sizes.

◀ Sample Prescriptions

Rx:
Percocet® tablets
Disp: 16 tablets
Sig: Take 1 tablet every 6 hours as needed for pain

Note: Restrictions: C-II; no refills
Ingredients: Oxycodone 5 mg and acetaminophen 325 mg; available as generic equivalent; triplicate prescription required in some states

Rx:
Oxycodone and Ibuprofen tablets
Disp: 16 tablets
Sig: Take 1 tablet every 6 hours as needed for pain

Note: Restrictions: C-II; no refills
Ingredients: Oxycodone 5 mg and ibuprofen 400 mg; triplicate prescription required in some states

BACTERIAL INFECTIONS AND PERIODONTAL DISEASES

General Prescription Comments

Sample prescription dosing is for adults. Closely monitor and re-evaluate response at least every 2 weeks. If response is inadequate, re-evaluate diagnosis, medication choice, and dosage.

Sample Prescriptions

Rx:
Penicillin V potassium 500 mg
Disp: 40 tablets
Sig: Take 1 tablet 4 times/day for 7-10 days (consider a loading dose of 1 g for acute infection)

Rx:
Clindamycin (Systemic) 150 mg
Disp: 40 capsules
Sig: Take 1 capsule 4 times/day for 7-10 days

Note: Prescription usually selected for patients allergic to penicillin; may be prescribed for 3 or 4 times/day

Rx:
Clindamycin (Systemic) 300 mg
Disp: 40 capsules
Sig: Take 1 capsule 4 times/day for 7-10 days

Note: Prescription usually selected for patients allergic to penicillin; may be prescribed for 3 or 4 times/day

Rx:
Azithromycin (Systemic) 250 mg
Disp: 1 Z-Pak®
Sig: 2 tablets day 1, then 1 tablet/day until gone

OTHER ANTIBIOTICS:

Rx:
Amoxicillin 250 mg
Disp: 30 capsules
Sig: Take 1 capsule 3 times/day for 7-10 days

Rx:
Amoxicillin 500 mg
Disp: 30 capsules or tablets
Sig: Take 1 capsule or tablet 3 times/day for 7-10 days

Rx:
Amoxicillin 875 mg
Disp: 20 tablets
Sig: Take 1 tablet twice daily

Rx:
Augmentin® 250 mg
Disp: 30 tablets
Sig: Take 1 tablet 3 times/day for 7-10 days

Rx:
Augmentin® 500 mg
Disp: 30 tablets
Sig: Take 1 tablet 3 times/day for 7-10 days

Rx:
Augmentin® 875 mg
Disp: 20 tablets
Sig: Take 1 tablet twice daily for 7-10 days

Rx:
Augmentin XR™ 1000 mg
Disp: 20 tablets
Sig: Take 2 tablets twice daily for 7-10 days

Rx:
Cephalexin 250 mg
Disp: 40 capsules
Sig: Take 1 capsule 4 times/day for 7-10 days

Rx:
MetroNIDAZOLE (Systemic) 500 mg
Disp: 40 tablets
Sig: Take 1 tablet 4 times/day for 7-10 days

Note: Usually used in combination with amoxicillin; may be prescribed for 3 or 4 times/day

Rx:
Erythromycin (Systemic) 250 mg
Disp: 40 tablets
Sig: Take 1 tablet 4 times/day for 7-10 days

Note: Prescription for patients allergic to penicillin

Rx:
Zithromax® TRI-PAK™ 500 mg
Disp: 1 PAK
Sig: Follow package insert directions until gone

Ingredient: Azithromycin (Systemic)

Rx:
Levaquin® 500 mg
Disp: 10 tablets
Sig: Take 1 tablet/day until gone

PERIODONTAL DISEASE

Note: Sample prescriptions based on dosing suggestions from the American Academy of Periodontology

Rx:
Azithromycin (Systemic) 500 mg tablets
Disp: Dispense a dose pack
Sig: Take 1 tablet daily for 4-7 days as directed

Rx:
Ciprofloxacin (Systemic) 500 mg tablets
Disp: 16 tablets
Sig: Take 1 tablet 2 times/day for 8 days

Rx:
Clindamycin (Systemic) 300 mg tablets
Disp: 24 tablets
Sig: Take 1 tablet 3 times/day for 8 days

Rx:
Doxycycline or Minocycline 100-200 mg tablets
Disp: 21 tablets of selected dose
Sig: Take 1 tablet daily for 21 days

Rx:
Doxycycline 100 mg tablets
Disp: 42 tablets
Sig: Take 1 tablet twice daily for 21 days

Note: Prescription used for Lyme disease: Early stage (erythema migrans)

Rx:
MetroNIDAZOLE (Systemic) 500 mg
Disp: 24 tablets
Sig: Take 1 tablet 3 times/day for 8 days

Rx:
MetroNIDAZOLE (Systemic) and Amoxicillin 250 mg or 500 mg tablets
Disp: 24 tablets of each drug
Sig: Take 1 tablet of each drug 3 times/day for 8 days

Rx:
MetroNIDAZOLE (Systemic) and Ciprofloxacin (Systemic) 500 mg tablets
Disp: 16 tablets of each drug
Sig: Take 1 tablet of each drug 2 times/day for 8 days

SINUS INFECTION TREATMENT

General Prescription Comments

Closely monitor and re-evaluate response at least every 2 weeks. If response is inadequate, re-evaluate diagnosis, medication choice, and dosage.

Sinus infections represent a common condition which may present with confounding dental complaints. Treatment is sometimes instituted by the dentist, but due to the often chronic and recurrent nature of sinus infections, early involvement of an otolaryngologist is advised. These infections may require antibiotics of varying spectrum, as well as requiring the management of sinus congestion. Although amoxicillin is usually adequate, many otolaryngologists initially prescribe Augmentin®. Second generation cephalosporins, azithromycin and clarithromycin are sometimes used depending on the chronicity of the problem.

Sample Prescriptions

Rx:

Afrin® nasal spray [OTC]
Disp: 15 mg
Sig: Spray once in each nostril every 6-8 hours for no more than 3 days

Ingredient: Oxymetazoline (Nasal)

Rx:

Sudafed® 60 mg tablets [OTC]
Disp: 30 tablets
Sig: Take 1 tablet every 4-6 hours as needed for congestion

Note: Some reports have suggested alterations in blood pressure with pseudoephedrine which can range from minor to significant. This should be considered prior to prescribing.
Ingredient: Pseudoephedrine

Rx:

Chlor-Trimeton® 4 mg [OTC]
Disp: 14 tablets
Sig: Take 1 tablet twice daily

Ingredient: Chlorpheniramine

ANTIBIOTICS:

Note: Antibiotics are not always required but may be useful in acute management of infection.

Rx:

Azithromycin (Systemic) 250 mg
Disp: 1 Z-Pak®
Sig: 2 tablets day 1, then 1 tablet/day until gone

Rx:

Amoxicillin 250 mg
Disp: 30 capsules
Sig: Take 1 capsule 3 times/day for 7-10 days

Rx:

Amoxicillin 500 mg
Disp: 30 capsules or tablets
Sig: Take 1 capsule or tablet 3 times/day for 7-10 days

Rx:

Amoxicillin 875 mg
Disp: 20 tablets
Sig: Take 1 tablet twice daily

Rx:

Augmentin® 250 mg
Disp: 30 tablets
Sig: Take 1 tablet 3 times/day for 7-10 days

Rx:

Augmentin® 500 mg
Disp: 30 tablets
Sig: Take 1 tablet 3 times/day for 7-10 days

Rx:
Augmentin® 875 mg
Disp: 20 tablets
Sig: Take 1 tablet twice daily for 7-10 days

Rx:
Augmentin XR™ 1000 mg
Disp: 20 tablets
Sig: Take 2 tablets twice daily for 7-10 days

ANTIMICROBIAL ORAL RINSE

General Prescription Comments

Closely monitor and re-evaluate response at least every 2 weeks. If response is inadequate, re-evaluate diagnosis, medication choice, and dosage.

Liquid volumes for antimicrobial rinses are suggested for a typical 1 month course. Check with pharmacist for available sizes.

Sample Prescriptions

Rx:

Chlorhexidine gluconate 0.12% oral rinse
Disp: 32 oz bottle
Sig: Rinse with ½ oz twice daily for 30 seconds and expectorate

Note: Chlorhexidine gluconate available as the following brands: Peridex®, PerioGard®; it is also available in an alcohol-free formulation in some pharmaceutical locations.

Rx:

Listerine® antiseptic mouthwash [OTC]
Disp: Bottle
Sig: 20 mL, swish for 30 seconds twice daily

Note: Various formulations, such as Cool Mint, are also available in an alcohol-free formulation.

FUNGAL INFECTIONS

FUNGAL INFECTIONS REQUIRING TOPICAL THERAPY

General Prescription Comments

Closely monitor and re-evaluate response at least every 2 weeks. If response is inadequate, re-evaluate diagnosis, medication choice, and dosage.

Liquid volumes are suggested for a typical 2-week course. Check with pharmacist for available sizes.

Cream and ointment tube may vary from 5 g, 15 g, 30 g, 45 g, or 60 g sizes, based on availability. Refer to individual monograph or check with pharmacist for available sizes.

Sample Prescriptions

Rx:
Nystatin (Oral) 100,000 units/mL oral suspension
Disp: 300 mL
Sig: Rinse with 1 teaspoon (5 mL) for 2 minutes 4-5 times/day and expectorate

Rx:
Nystatin (Topical) ointment
Disp: 15 g tube
Sig: Apply locally as directed with a thin coat to inner surface of denture and the affected area 4-5 times/day

Rx:
Mycelex® 10 mg troches
Disp: 70 troches
Sig: Dissolve 1 troche in mouth 4-5 times/day until gone; leave any prosthesis out during treatment and soak prosthesis in nystatin liquid suspension overnight

Ingredient: Clotrimazole (Oral)

Rx:
Nizoral® 2% cream
Disp: 15 g tube
Sig: Apply locally as directed with a thin coat to inner surface of denture and affected areas after meals

Ingredient: Ketoconazole (Topical)

FUNGAL INFECTIONS REQUIRING SYSTEMIC THERAPY

General Prescription Comments

Note: Decision to use systemic antifungals should be based on diagnostic culture results or positive smear.

Closely monitor and re-evaluate response at least every 2 weeks. If response is inadequate, re-evaluate diagnosis, medication choice, and dosage.

Sample Prescriptions

Rx:
Diflucan® 100 mg tablets
Disp: 14 tablets
Sig: Take 1 tablet/day until gone

Note: Sometimes a shorter course is adequate. However, oral infections are more commonly difficult to eradicate and often a 21-day course, or even a second course, may be necessary.

Ingredient: Fluconazole

Rx:
Nizoral® 200 mg tablets
Disp: 14 tablets
Sig: Take 1 tablet/day with a meal for 2 weeks

Note: May cause irreversible liver damage; liver function should be monitored with long-term use (ie, >3 weeks)

Ingredient: Ketoconazole (Systemic)

Rx:
Posaconazole 100 mg tablets
Disp: 14 tablets
Sig: Take 2 tablets the first day, followed by 1 tablet each day for 13 days

Note: Posaconazole has been recently approved for use in patients refractory to itraconazole or fluconazole

ANGULAR CHEILITIS

General Prescription Comments

Closely monitor and re-evaluate response at least every 2 weeks. If response is inadequate, re-evaluate diagnosis, medication choice, and dosage. Other associated etiologies for angular cheilitis must also be considered, such as loss of vertical dimension, trauma, and vitamin deficiencies.

Cream and ointment tube may vary from 15 g, 30 g, or 45 g sizes, based on availability. Refer to individual monograph or check with pharmacist for available sizes.

Sample Prescriptions

Rx:

Nystatin and Triamcinolone acetonide ointment
Disp: 30 g tube
Sig: Apply locally as directed to affected area 4 times/day for 10-14 days and then re-evaluate

Rx:

Iodoquinol and Hydrocortisone cream
Disp: 45 g tube
Sig: Apply locally as directed 3-4 times/day for 10 days to 2 weeks and then re-evaluate

VIRAL INFECTIONS

HERPES SIMPLEX (PRIMARY)

General Prescription Comments

Closely monitor and re-evaluate response at least every 2 weeks. If response is inadequate, re-evaluate diagnosis, medication choice, and dosage.

Sample Prescriptions

Rx:
Zovirax® 200 mg capsules
Disp: 50 or 60 capsules
Sig: Take 1 capsule 5 times/day for 10 days or 2 capsules 3 times/day for 10 days

Ingredient: Acyclovir (Systemic)

Rx:
Zovirax® ointment 5%
Disp: 15 g tube
Sig: Apply thin layer to lesions 6 times/day for 7 days.

Ingredient: Acyclovir (Topical)

HERPES SIMPLEX (RECURRENT)

General Prescription Comments

Closely monitor and re-evaluate response at least every 2 weeks. If response is inadequate, re-evaluate diagnosis, medication choice, and dosage.

Cream and ointment tube sizes may vary based on availability. Refer to individual monograph or check with pharmacist for available sizes.

Sample Prescriptions

Rx:
Denavir® topical cream 1%
Disp: 1.5 g tube
Sig: Apply locally as directed to lesion every 2 hours during waking hours (begin when prodromal symptoms first occur)

Ingredient: Penciclovir

Rx:
Famciclovir 500 mg tablets
Disp: 3 tablets
Sig: Take 3 tablets (1500 mg) as a single dose; therapy should be initiated at the first sign of any prodrome such as tingling, burning, or itching

Note: Dispense in multiples of 3 so that patient has drug on hand for any recurrences; available as generic equivalent

Rx:
ValACYclovir 500 mg
Disp: 8 caplets
Sig: 4 caplets twice daily for 1 day (separate doses by 12 hours); therapy should be initiated at the first sign of any prodrome such as tingling, burning, or itching

Rx:
Abreva® cream [OTC]
Disp: 2 g tube
Sig: Apply to lesion 5 times/day during waking hours for 4 days (begin when symptoms first occur)

Ingredient: Docosanol

Rx:
Zovirax® cream 5%
Disp: 2 g tube; 5 g tube
Sig: Apply 5 times/day for 4 days

Ingredient: Acyclovir (Topical)

Rx:
Betamethasone 0.1% ointment
Disp: 45 g tube
Sig: Apply a small quantity with a Q-tip locally as directed to affected area 3-4 times/day

Rx:
Decadron® elixir 0.5 mg/5 mL
Disp: 300 mL
Sig: Rinse with 1 teaspoon for 2 minutes 4 times/day and expectorate

Ingredient: Dexamethasone (Systemic)

Note: Depending on severity of ulceration, instructions can be tailored to include swallowing initial doses and then tapering to every other dose eventually over 4-7 days to no swallowing. See Erosive Lichen Planus, Other Biopsy-Proven Desquamative Oral Diseases, and Major Aphthae for more examples.

MILD LICHEN PLANUS

General Prescription Comments

Some intraoral uses are off-label. Write directions as "use locally as directed" and closely monitor and re-evaluate response at least every 2 weeks. If response is inadequate, re-evaluate diagnosis, medication choice, and dosage.

Cream and ointment tube sizes may vary based on availability. Refer to individual monograph or check with pharmacist for available sizes.

Sample Prescriptions

Rx:
Oralone® 0.1%
Disp: 5 g tube
Sig: Apply locally as directed by coating the lesion with a thin film after each meal and at bedtime

Ingredient: Triamcinolone (Topical) 0.1%

Rx:
Fluocinonide 0.05% gel
Disp: 45 g tube
Sig: Apply locally as directed to lesion 4 times/day

Rx:
Temovate® 0.05%
Disp: 45 g tube
Sig: Apply a small quantity with a Q-tip locally as directed to affected area 3-4 times/day

Ingredient: Clobetasol

Note: The pharmacist can compound potent steroids, such as clobetasol with Orabase®, to enhance adherence to oral tissues.

Rx:
Betamethasone 0.1% ointment
Disp: 45 g tube
Sig: Apply a small quantity with a Q-tip locally as directed to affected area 3-4 times/day

Rx:
Decadron® elixir 0.5 mg/5 mL
Disp: 300 mL
Sig: Rinse with 1 teaspoon for 2 minutes 4 times/day and expectorate

Ingredient: Dexamethasone (Systemic)

Note: Depending on severity of ulceration, instructions can be tailored to include swallowing initial doses and then tapering to every other dose eventually over 4-7 days to no swallowing. See Erosive Lichen Planus, Other Biopsy-Proven Desquamative Oral Diseases, and Major Aphthae for more examples.

EROSIVE LICHEN PLANUS, OTHER BIOPSY-PROVEN DESQUAMATIVE ORAL DISEASES, AND MAJOR APHTHAE

General Prescription Comments

Some intraoral uses are off-label. Write directions as "use locally as directed" and closely monitor and re-evaluate response at least every 2 weeks. If response is inadequate, re-evaluate diagnosis, medication choice, and dosage.

Liquid volumes are suggested for a typical 2-week course. Check with pharmacist for available sizes.

Cream and ointment tube sizes may vary based on availability. Refer to individual monograph or check with pharmacist for available sizes.

Note: Soft, thin, vacuum-formed trays can be made (similar to bleaching trays but extending slightly onto the gingiva) to deliver steroid ointments or creams to gingival lesions. Also, the pharmacist can compound potent steroids, such as clobetasol with Orabase®, to enhance adherence to oral tissues. For chronically recurring lesions, prednisone can be prescribed at 40 mg/day for week 1, 30 mg/day for week 2, continue tapering dose each week to 0. Occasionally, the clinician needs to tailor the regimen by using alternating doses every other day, such as 20 mg day 1, 10 mg day 2, then back to 20 mg. It is important to assess patient compliance when such a regimen is considered.

Sample Prescriptions

Rx:

Decadron® 0.5 mg/5 mL elixir
Disp: 400 mL bottle
Sig: For 3 days, rinse with 1 tablespoonful (15 mL) 4 times/day and swallow; then for 3 days, rinse with 1 teaspoonful (5 mL) 4 times/day and swallow; then for 3 days, rinse with 1 teaspoonful (5 mL) 4 times/day and swallow every other time. Then for 3 days rinse with 1 teaspoonful (5 mL) 4 times/day and expectorate. Continue the rinse and expectorate mode for 2 minutes but discontinue medication when mouth becomes completely comfortable.

Ingredient: Dexamethasone (Systemic); the practitioner can tailor this rinse, hold expectorate and/or swallow prescription to the severity and lesion location for each individual patient.

Rx:

Temovate® 0.05% cream
Disp: 15 g tube
Sig: Apply locally as directed 4-5 times/day

Ingredient: Clobetasol; high potency topical steroid

Rx:

PredniSONE 5 mg tablets
Disp: 40 tablets
Sig: Take 5 tablets in the morning for 5 days, then 5 tablets in the morning every other day until gone

Rx:

PredniSONE 10 mg tablets
Disp: 50 tablets
Sig: Take 4 tablets in the morning for 5 days, then decrease by 1 tablet on each successive series of 5 days.
Note: Longer durations of a regimen (eg, 7-10 days) can be tailored to the severity of the oral condition.

Rx:

Medrol® Dose Pak
Disp: 1 Pack
Sig: Follow package insert directions until gone

Ingredient: MethylPREDNISolone

SEDATION (PRIOR TO DENTAL TREATMENT)

General Prescription Comments

Sample prescription doses are for healthy adults. Use of these drugs and/or dosage may not be appropriate for children, elderly, and/or debilitated patients. Dental sedation should be used cautiously in these patients. Patients receiving sedative agents must be advised that they will need to have someone drive them to and from their appointment.

Sample Prescriptions for Adults

Rx:
Valium® 5 mg
Disp: 1 tablet
Sig: Take 1 tablet 1 hour before appointment

Note: Also available as 2 mg and 10 mg
Ingredient: Diazepam

Rx:
Ativan® 1 mg
Disp: 2 tablets
Sig: Take 2 tablets 1 hour before appointment

Note: Also available as 0.5 mg and 2 mg
Ingredient: LORazepam

Rx:
Xanax® 0.5 mg
Disp: 1 tablet
Sig: Take 1 tablet 1 hour before appointment

Ingredient: ALPRAZolam

Rx:
Vistaril® 25 mg
Disp: 2 capsules
Sig: Take 2 capsules 1 hour before appointment

Ingredient: HydrOXYzine

Rx:
Halcion® 0.25 mg
Disp: 1 tablet
Sig: Take 1 tablet 1 hour before appointment

Ingredient: Triazolam

APPENDIX TABLE OF CONTENTS

ABBREVIATIONS, ACRONYMS, AND SYMBOLS

Abbreviations Which May Be Used in This Reference

Abbreviation	Meaning
½NS	0.45% sodium chloride
5-HT	5-hydroxytryptamine
AAP	American Academy of Pediatrics
AAPC	antibiotic-associated pseudomembranous colitis
ABG	arterial blood gases
ABMT	autologous bone marrow transplant
ABW	adjusted body weight
AACT	American Academy of Clinical Toxicology
ACC	American College of Cardiology
ACE	angiotensin-converting enzyme
ACLS	advanced cardiac life support
ACOG	American College of Obstetricians and Gynecologists
ACTH	adrenocorticotrophic hormone
ADH	antidiuretic hormone
ADHD	attention-deficit/hyperactivity disorder
ADI	adequate daily intake
ADLs	activities of daily living
AED	antiepileptic drug
AHA	American Heart Association
AHCPR	Agency for Health Care Policy and Research
AIDS	acquired immunodeficiency syndrome
AIMS	Abnormal Involuntary Movement Scale
ALL	acute lymphoblastic leukemia
ALS	amyotrophic lateral sclerosis
ALT	alanine aminotransferase (formerly called SGPT)
AMA	American Medical Association
AML	acute myeloblastic leukemia
ANA	antinuclear antibodies
ANC	absolute neutrophil count
ANLL	acute nonlymphoblastic leukemia
aPTT	activated partial thromboplastin time
ARB	angiotensin receptor blocker
ARDS	acute respiratory distress syndrome
ASA-PS	American Society of Anesthesiologists – Physical Status P1: Normal, healthy patient P2: Patient having mild systemic disease P3: Patient having severe systemic disease P4: Patient having severe systemic disease which is a constant threat to life P5: Moribund patient; not expected to survive without the procedure P6: Patient declared brain-dead; organs being removed for donor purposes
AST	aspartate aminotransferase (formerly called SGOT)
ATP	adenosine triphosphate
AUC	area under the curve (area under the serum concentration-time curve)
A-V	atrial-ventricular
BDI	Beck Depression Inventory
BEC	blood ethanol concentration
BLS	basic life support
BMI	body mass index
BMT	bone marrow transplant
BP	blood pressure
BPD	bronchopulmonary disease or dysplasia
BPH	benign prostatic hyperplasia
BPRS	Brief Psychiatric Rating Scale
BSA	body surface area
BUN	blood urea nitrogen

Abbreviations Which May Be Used in This Reference (continued)

Abbreviation	Meaning
CABG	coronary artery bypass graft
CAD	coronary artery disease
CADD	computer ambulatory drug delivery
cAMP	cyclic adenosine monophosphate
CAN	Canadian
CAPD	continuous ambulatory peritoneal dialysis
CAS	chemical abstract service
CBC	complete blood count
CBT	cognitive behavioral therapy
Cl_{cr}	creatinine clearance
CDC	Centers for Disease Control and Prevention
CF	cystic fibrosis
CFC	chlorofluorocarbons
CGI	Clinical Global Impression
CHD	coronary heart disease
CHF	congestive heart failure; chronic heart failure
CI	cardiac index
CIE	chemotherapy-induced emesis
C-II	schedule two controlled substance
C-III	schedule three controlled substance
C-IV	schedule four controlled substance
C-V	schedule five controlled substance
CIV	continuous I.V. infusion
Cl_{cr}	creatinine clearance
CLL	chronic lymphocytic leukemia
C_{max}	maximum plasma concentration
C_{min}	minimum plasma concentration
CML	chronic myelogenous leukemia
CMV	cytomegalovirus
CNS	central nervous system or coagulase negative staphylococcus
COLD	chronic obstructive lung disease
COPD	chronic obstructive pulmonary disease
COX	cyclooxygenase
CPK	creatine phosphokinase
CPR	cardiopulmonary resuscitation
CRF	chronic renal failure
CRP	C-reactive protein
CRRT	continuous renal replacement therapy
CSF	cerebrospinal fluid
CSII	continuous subcutaneous insulin infusion
CT	computed tomography
CVA	cerebrovascular accident
CVP	central venous pressure
CVVH	continuous venovenous hemofiltration
CVVHD	continuous venovenous hemodialysis
CVVHDF	continuous venovenous hemodiafiltration
CYP	cytochrome
$D_5{}^{1}/_4NS$	dextrose 5% in sodium chloride 0.2%
$D_5{}^{1}/_2NS$	dextrose 5% in sodium chloride 0.45%
D_5LR	dextrose 5% in lactated Ringer's
D_5NS	dextrose 5% in sodium chloride 0.9%
D_5W	dextrose 5% in water
$D_{10}W$	dextrose 10% in water
DBP	diastolic blood pressure
DEHP	di(3-ethylhexyl)phthalate
DIC	disseminated intravascular coagulation
DL_{co}	pulmonary diffusion capacity for carbon monoxide

◀ **Abbreviations Which May Be Used in This Reference** *(continued)*

Abbreviation	Meaning
DM	diabetes mellitus
DMARD	disease modifying antirheumatic drug
DNA	deoxyribonucleic acid
DSC	discontinued
DSM-IV	Diagnostic and Statistical Manual
DVT	deep vein thrombosis
EBV	Epstein-Barr virus
ECG	electrocardiogram
ECHO	echocardiogram
ECMO	extracorporeal membrane oxygenation
ECT	electroconvulsive therapy
ED	emergency department
EEG	electroencephalogram
EF	ejection fraction
EG	ethylene glycol
EGA	estimated gestational age
EIA	enzyme immunoassay
ELBW	extremely low birth weight
ELISA	enzyme-linked immunosorbent assay
EPS	extrapyramidal side effects
ESR	erythrocyte sedimentation rate
ESRD	end stage renal disease
E.T.	endotracheal
EtOH	alcohol
FDA	Food and Drug Administration (United States)
FEV$_1$	forced expiratory volume exhaled after 1 second
FSH	follicle-stimulating hormone
FTT	failure to thrive
FVC	forced vital capacity
G-6-PD	glucose-6-phosphate dehydrogenase
GA	gestational age
GABA	gamma-aminobutyric acid
GAD	generalized anxiety disorder
GE	gastroesophageal
GERD	gastroesophageal reflux disease
GFR	glomerular filtration rate
GGT	gamma-glutamyltransferase
GI	gastrointestinal
GU	genitourinary
GVHD	graft versus host disease
HAM-A	Hamilton Anxiety Scale
HAM-D	Hamilton Depression Scale
HARS	HIV-associated adipose redistribution syndrome
Hct	hematocrit
HDL-C	high density lipoprotein cholesterol
HF	heart failure
HFA	hydrofluoroalkane
HFSA	Heart Failure Society of America
Hgb	hemoglobin
HIV	human immunodeficiency virus
HMG-CoA	3-hydroxy-3-methylglutaryl-coenzyme A
HOCM	hypertrophic obstructive cardiomyopathy
HPA	hypothalamic-pituitary-adrenal
HPLC	high performance liquid chromatography
HSV	herpes simplex virus
HTN	hypertension
HUS	hemolytic uremic syndrome

Abbreviations Which May Be Used in This Reference *(continued)*

Abbreviation	Meaning
IBD	inflammatory bowel disease
IBS	irritable bowel syndrome
IBW	ideal body weight
ICD	implantable cardioverter defibrillator
ICH	intracranial hemorrhage
ICP	intracranial pressure
IDDM	insulin-dependent diabetes mellitus
IDSA	Infectious Diseases Society of America
IgG	immune globulin G
IHSS	idiopathic hypertrophic subaortic stenosis
I.M.	intramuscular
ILCOR	International Liaison Committee on Resuscitation
INR	international normalized ration
Int. unit	international unit
I.O.	intraosseous
I & O	input and output
IOP	intraocular pressure
IQ	intelligence quotient
I.T.	intrathecal
ITP	idiopathic thrombocytopenic purpura
IUGR	intrauterine growth retardation
I.V.	intravenous
IVH	intraventricular hemorrhage
IVP	intravenous push
IVPB	intravenous piggyback
JIA	juvenile idiopathic arthritis
JNC	Joint National Committee
JRA	juvenile rheumatoid arthritis
kg	kilogram
KIU	kallikrein inhibitor unit
KOH	potassium hydroxide
LAMM	L-α-acetyl methadol
LDH	lactate dehydrogenase
LDL-C	low density lipoprotein cholesterol
LE	lupus erythematosus
LFT	liver function test
LGA	large for gestational age
LH	luteinizing hormone
LP	lumbar posture
LR	lactated Ringer's
LV	left ventricular
LVEF	left ventricular ejection fraction
LVH	left ventricular hypertrophy
MAC	*Mycobacterium avium* complex
MADRS	Montgomery Asbery Depression Rating Scale
MAO	monoamine oxidase
MAOIs	monamine oxidase inhibitors
MAP	mean arterial pressure
MDD	major depressive disorder
MDRD	modification of diet in renal disease
MDRSP	multidrug resistant *streptococcus pneumoniae*
MI	myocardial infarction
MMSE	mini mental status examination
MOPP	mustargen (mechlorethamine), Oncovin® (vincristine), procarbazine, and prednisone
M/P	milk to plasma ratio
MPS I	mucopolysaccharidosis I
MRHD	maximum recommended human dose

Abbreviations Which May Be Used in This Reference *(continued)*

Abbreviation	Meaning
MRI	magnetic resonance imaging
MRSA	methicillin-resistant *Staphylococcus aureus*
MUGA	multiple gated acquisition scan
NAEPP	National Asthma Education and Prevention Program
NAS	neonatal abstinence syndrome
NCI	National Cancer Institute
ND	nasoduodenal
NF	National Formulary
NFD	Nephrogenic fibrosing dermopathy
NG	nasogastric
NIDDM	noninsulin-dependent diabetes mellitus
NIH	National Institute of Health
NIOSH	National Institute for Occupational Safety and Health
NKA	no known allergies
NKDA	No known drug allergies
NMDA	n-methyl-d-aspartate
NMS	neuroleptic malignant syndrome
NNRTI	non-nucleoside reverse transcriptase inhibitor
NRTI	nucleoside reverse transcriptase inhibitor
NS	normal saline (0.9% sodium chloride)
NSAID	nonsteroidal anti-inflammatory drug
NSF	nephrogenic systemic fibrosis
NSTEMI	Non-ST-elevation myocardial infarction
NYHA	New York Heart Association
OA	osteoarthritis
OCD	obsessive-compulsive disorder
OHSS	ovarian hyperstimulation syndrome
O.R.	operating room
OTC	over-the-counter (nonprescription)
PABA	para-aminobenzoic acid
PACTG	Pediatric AIDS Clinical Trials Group
PALS	pediatric advanced life support
PAT	paroxysmal atrial tachycardia
PCA	patient-controlled analgesia
PCP	*Pneumocystis jiroveci* pneumonia (also called *Pneumocystis carinii* pneumonia)
PCWP	pulmonary capillary wedge pressure
PD	Parkinson's disease; peritoneal dialysis
PDA	patent ductus arteriosus
PDE-5	phosphodiesterase-5
PE	pulmonary embolism
PEG tube	percutaneous endoscopic gastrostomy tube
P-gp	P-glycoprotein
PHN	post-herpetic neuralgia
PICU	Pediatric Intensive Care Unit
PID	pelvic inflammatory disease
PIP	peak inspiratory pressure
PMA	postmenstrual age
PMDD	premenstrual dysphoric disorder
PNA	postnatal age
PONV	postoperative nausea and vomiting
PPHN	persistent pulmonary hypertension of the neonate
PPN	peripheral parenteral nutrition
PROM	premature rupture of membranes
PSVT	paroxysmal supraventricular tachycardia
PT	prothrombin time
PTH	parathyroid hormone
PTSD	post-traumatic stress disorder

Abbreviations Which May Be Used in This Reference *(continued)*

Abbreviation	Meaning
PTT	partial thromboplastin time
PUD	peptic ulcer disease
PVC	premature ventricular contraction
PVD	peripheral vascular disease
PVR	peripheral vascular resistance
QT_c	corrected QT interval
QT_cF	corrected QT interval by Fredricia's formula
RA	rheumatoid arthritis
RAP	right arterial pressure
RDA	recommended daily allowance
REM	rapid eye movement
REMS	risk evaluation and mitigation strategies
RIA	radioimmunoassay
RNA	ribonucleic acid
RPLS	reversible posterior leukoencephalopathy syndrome
RSV	respiratory syncytial virus
SA	sinoatrial
SAD	seasonal affective disorder
SAH	subarachnoid hemorrhage
SBE	subacute bacterial endocarditis
SBP	systolic blood pressure
S_{cr}	serum creatinine
SERM	selective estrogen receptor modulator
SGA	small for gestational age
SGOT	serum glutamic oxaloacetic aminotransferase
SGPT	serum glutamic pyruvate transaminase
SI	International System of Units or Systeme international d'Unites
SIADH	syndrome of inappropriate antidiuretic hormone secretion
SLE	systemic lupus erythematosus
SLEDD	sustained low-efficiency daily diafiltration
SNRI	serotonin norepinephrine reuptake inhibitor
SSKI	saturated solution of potassium iodide
SSRIs	selective serotonin reuptake inhibitors
STD	sexually transmitted disease
STEM I	ST-elevation myocardial infarction
SVR	systemic vascular resistance
SVT	supraventricular tachycardia
SWFI	sterile water for injection
SWI	sterile water for injection
$T_{1/2}$	half-life
T_3	triiodothyronine
T_4	thyroxine
TB	tuberculosis
TC	total cholesterol
TCA	tricyclic antidepressant
TD	tardive dyskinesia
TG	triglyceride
TIA	transient ischemic attack
TIBC	total iron binding capacity
TMA	thrombotic microangiopathy
T_{max}	time to maximum observed concentration, plasma
TNF	tumor necrosis factor
TPN	total parenteral nutrition
TSH	thyroid stimulating hormone
TT	thrombin time
TTP	thrombotic thrombocytopenic purpura
UA	urine analysis

Abbreviations Which May Be Used in This Reference *(continued)*

Abbreviation	Meaning
UC	ulcerative colitis
ULN	upper limits of normal
URI	upper respiratory infection
USAN	United States Adopted Names
USP	United States Pharmacopeia
UTI	urinary tract infection
UV	ultraviolet
V_d	volume of distribution
V_{dss}	volume of distribution at steady-state
VEGF	vascular endothelial growth factor
VF	ventricular fibrillation
VLBW	very low birth weight
VMA	vanillylmandelic acid
VT	ventricular tachycardia
VTE	venous thromboembolism
vWD	von Willebrand disease
VZV	varicella zoster virus
WHO	World Health Organization
w/v	weight for volume
w/w	weight for weight
YBOC	Yale Brown Obsessive-Compulsive Scale
YMRS	Young Mania Rating Scale

Common Weights, Measures, or Apothecary Abbreviations

Abbreviation	Meaning
<[1]	less than
>[1]	greater than
≤	less than or equal to
≥	greater than or equal to
ac	before meals or food
ad	to, up to
ad lib	at pleasure
AM	morning
AMA	against medical advice
amp	ampul
amt	amount
aq	water
aq. dest.	distilled water
ASAP	as soon as possible
a.u.[1]	each ear
bid	twice daily
bm	bowel movement
C	Celsius, centigrade
cal	calorie
cap	capsule
cc[1]	cubic centimeter
cm	centimeter
comp	compound
cont	continue
d	day
d/c[1]	discharge
dil	dilute
disp	dispense
div	divide
dtd	give of such a dose

Common Weights, Measures, or Apothecary Abbreviations (continued)

Abbreviation	Meaning
Dx	diagnosis
elix, el	elixir
emp	as directed
et	and
ex aq	in water
F	Fahrenheit
f, ft	make, let be made
g	gram
gr	grain
gtt	a drop
h	hour
hs[1]	at bedtime
kcal	kilocalorie
kg	kilogram
L	liter
liq	a liquor, solution
M	molar
mcg	microgram
m. dict	as directed
mEq	milliequivalent
mg	milligram
microL	microliter
min	minute
mL	milliliter
mm	millimeter
mM	millimole
mm Hg	millimeters of mercury
mo	month
mOsm	milliosmoles
ng	nanogram
nmol	nanomole
no.	number
noc	in the night
non rep	do not repeat, no refills
NPO	nothing by mouth
NV	nausea and vomiting
O, Oct	a pint
o.d.[1]	right eye
o.l.	left eye
o.s.[1]	left eye
o.u.[1]	each eye
pc, post cib	after meals
PM	afternoon or evening
P.O.	by mouth
P.R.	rectally
prn	as needed
pulv	a powder
q	every
qad	every other day
qd[1,2]	every day, daily
qh	every hour
qid	four times a day
qod[1,2]	every other day
qs	a sufficient quantity
qs ad	a sufficient quantity to make
Rx	take, a recipe
S.L.	sublingual

Common Weights, Measures, or Apothecary Abbreviations *(continued)*

Abbreviation	Meaning
stat	at once, immediately
SubQ	subcutaneous
supp	suppository
syr	syrup
tab	tablet
tal	such
tid	three times a day
tr, tinct	tincture
trit	triturate
tsp	teaspoon
u.d.	as directed
ung	ointment
v.o.	verbal order
w.a.	while awake
x3	3 times
x4	4 times
y	year

[1]ISMP error-prone abbreviation

[2]JCAHO Do Not Use list

Additional abbreviations used and defined within a specific monograph or text piece may only apply to that text.

REFERENCES

The Institute for Safe Medication Practices (ISMP) list of Error-Prone Abbreviations, Symbols, and Dose Designations. Available at http://www.ismp.org/Tools/errorproneabbreviations.pdf

The Joint Commission Official "Do Not Use" list. Available at http://www.jointcommission.org/facts_about_the_official_/

APOTHECARY/METRIC EQUIVALENTS

Apothecary-Metric Exact Equivalents

1 gram (g)	=	15.43 grains (gr)		0.1 mg	=	1/600 gr
1 milliliter (mL)	=	16.23 minims		0.12 mg	=	1/500 gr
1 minim	=	0.06 mL		0.15 mg	=	1/400 gr
1 gr	=	64.8 milligrams (mg)		0.2 mg	=	1/300 gr
1 fluid ounce (fl oz)	=	29.57 mL		0.3 mg	=	1/200 gr
1 pint (pt)	=	473.2 mL		0.4 mg	=	1/150 gr
1 ounce (oz)	=	28.35 g		0.5 mg	=	1/120 gr
1 pound (lb)	=	453.6 g		0.6 mg	=	1/100 gr
1 killogram (kg)	=	2.2 lb		0.8 mg	=	1/80 gr
1 quart (qt)	=	946.4 mL		1 mg	=	1/65 gr

Apothecary-Metric Approximate Equivalents[1]

Liquids			Solids		
1 teaspoonful	=	5 mL	1/4 grain	=	15 mg
1 tablespoonful	=	15 mL	1/2 grain	=	30 mg
			1 grain	=	60 mg
			1 1/2 grain	=	100 mg
			5 grains	=	300 mg
			10 grains	=	600 mg

[1]Use exact equivalents for compounding and calculations requiring a high degree of accuracy.

AVERAGE WEIGHTS AND SURFACE AREAS

Average Height, Weight, and Surface Area by Age and Gender

Age	Girls			Boys		
	Height (cm)	Weight (kg)	BSA (m²)	Height (cm)	Weight (kg)	BSA (m²)
Birth	49.5	3.4	0.22	50	3.6	0.22
3 mo	59	5.6	0.3	61	6	0.32
6 mo	65	7.2	0.36	67	7.9	0.38
9 mo	70	8.3	0.4	72	9.3	0.43
12 mo	74.5	9.5	0.44	75.5	10.3	0.46
15 mo	77	10.3	0.47	79	11.1	0.49
18 mo	80	11	0.49	82	11.7	0.52
21 mo	83	11.6	0.52	85	12.2	0.54
2 y	86	12	0.54	87.5	12.6	0.55
2.5 y	91	13	0.57	92	13.5	0.59
3 y	94.5	13.8	0.6	96	14.3	0.62
3.5 y	97	15	0.64	98	15	0.64
4 y	101	16	0.67	102	16	0.67
4.5 y	104	17	0.7	105	17	0.7
5 y	107.5	18	0.73	109	18.5	0.75
6 y	115	20	0.80	115	21	0.82
7 y	121.5	23	0.88	122	23	0.88
8 y	127.5	25.5	0.95	127.5	26	0.96
9 y	133	29	1.04	133.5	28.5	1.03
10 y	138	33	1.12	138.5	32	1.1
11 y	144	37	1.22	143.5	36	1.2
12 y	151	41.5	1.32	149	40.5	1.29
13 y	157	46	1.42	156	45.5	1.4
14 y	160.5	49.5	1.49	163.5	51	1.52
15 y	162	52	1.53	170	56	1.63
16 y	162.5	54	1.56	173.5	61	1.71
17 y	163	55	1.58	175	64.5	1.77
Adult[1]	163.5	58	1.62	177	83.5	2.03

Data extracted from the CDC growth charts based on the 50th percentile height and weight for a given age[2]

Body surface area calculation[3]: Square root of [(Ht x Wt) / 3600]

[1]McDowell MA, Fryar CD, Hirsch R, et al, "Anthropometric Reference Data for Children and Adults: U.S. Population, 1999-2002," *Adv Data*, 2005, (361):1-5.

[2]Centers for Disease Control and Prevention, "2000 CDC Growth Charts: United States". Available at http://www.cdc.gov/growthcharts. Accessed November 16, 2007.

[3]Mosteller RD, "Simplified Calculation of Body-Surface Area," *N Engl J Med*, 1987, 317(17):1098.

BODY SURFACE AREA OF CHILDREN AND ADULTS

Calculating Body Surface Area in Children

In a child of average size, find weight and corresponding surface area on the boxed scale to the left or use the nomogram to the right. Lay a straightedge on the correct height and weight points for the child, then read the intersecting point on the surface area scale. (**Note:** 2.2 lb = 1 kg)

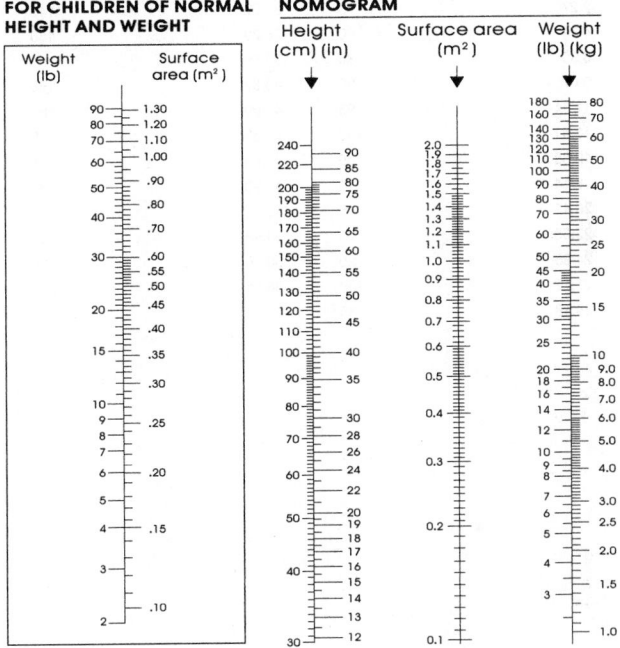

FOR CHILDREN OF NORMAL HEIGHT AND WEIGHT

NOMOGRAM

BODY SURFACE AREA FORMULA
(Adult and Pediatric)

$$BSA\ (m^2) = \sqrt{\frac{ht\ (in)\ x\ wt\ (lb)}{3131}} \quad \text{or, in metric: } BSA\ (m^2) = \sqrt{\frac{ht\ (cm)\ x\ wt\ (kg)}{3600}}$$

References

Lam TK and Leung DT, "More on Simplified Calculation of Body Surface Area," *N Engl J Med*, 1988, 318(17):1130 (letter).

Mosteller RD, "Simplified Calculation of Body Surface Area," *N Engl J Med*, 1987, 317(17):1098 (letter).

POUNDS/KILOGRAMS CONVERSION

1 pound = 0.45359 kilograms
1 kilogram = 2.2 pounds

lb	=	kg	lb	=	kg	lb	=	kg
1	=	0.45	70	=	31.75	140	=	63.50
5	=	2.27	75	=	34.02	145	=	65.77
10	=	4.54	80	=	36.29	150	=	68.04
15	=	6.80	85	=	38.56	155	=	70.31
20	=	9.07	90	=	40.82	160	=	72.58
25	=	11.34	95	=	43.09	165	=	74.84
30	=	13.61	100	=	45.36	170	=	77.11
35	=	15.88	105	=	47.63	175	=	79.38
40	=	18.14	110	=	49.90	180	=	81.65
45	=	20.41	115	=	52.16	185	=	83.92
50	=	22.68	120	=	54.43	190	=	86.18
55	=	24.95	125	=	56.70	195	=	88.45
60	=	27.22	130	=	58.91	200	=	90.72
65	=	29.48	135	=	61.24			

DRUG INTERACTIONS: METABOLISM/TRANSPORT EFFECTS

Most drugs are eliminated from the body, at least in part, by being chemically altered to less lipid-soluble products (ie, metabolized), and thus are more likely to be excreted via the kidneys or the bile. Phase I metabolism includes drug hydrolysis, oxidation, and reduction, and results in drugs that are more polar in their chemical structure, while Phase II metabolism involves the attachment of an additional molecule onto the drug (or partially metabolized drug) in order to create an inactive and/or more water soluble compound. Phase II processes include (primarily) glucuronidation, sulfation, glutathione conjugation, acetylation, and methylation.

Virtually any of the Phase I and II enzymes can be inhibited by some xenobiotic or drug. Some of the Phase I and II enzymes can be induced. Inhibition of the activity of metabolic enzymes will result in increased concentrations of the substrate (drug), whereas induction of the activity of metabolic enzymes will result in decreased concentrations of the substrate. For example, the well-documented enzyme-inducing effects of phenobarbital may include a combination of Phase I and II enzymes. Phase II glucuronidation may be increased via induced UDP-glucuronosyltransferase (UGT) activity, whereas Phase I oxidation may be increased via induced cytochrome P450 (CYP) activity. However, for most drugs, the primary route of metabolism (and the primary focus of drug-drug interaction) is Phase I oxidation, and specifically, metabolism.

CYP enzymes may be responsible for the metabolism (at least partial metabolism) of approximately 75% of all drugs, with the CYP3A subfamily responsible for nearly half of this activity. Found throughout plant, animal, and bacterial species, CYP enzymes represent a superfamily of xenobiotic metabolizing proteins. There have been several hundred CYP enzymes identified in nature, each of which has been assigned to a family (1, 2, 3, etc), subfamily (A, B, C, etc), and given a specific enzyme number (1, 2, 3, etc) according to the similarity in amino acid sequence that it shares with other enzymes. Of these many enzymes, only a few are found in humans, and even fewer appear to be involved in the metabolism of xenobiotics (eg, drugs). The key human enzyme subfamilies include CYP1A, CYP2A, CYP1B, CYP2B, CYP2C, CYP2D, CYP2E, and CYP3A.

CYP enzymes are found in the endoplasmic reticulum of cells in a variety of human tissues (eg, skin, kidneys, brain, lungs), but their predominant sites of concentration and activity are the liver and intestine. Though the abundance of CYP enzymes throughout the body is relatively equally distributed among the various subfamilies, the relative contribution to drug metabolism is (in decreasing order of magnitude) CYP3A4/5 (nearly 50%), CYP2D6 (nearly 25%), CYP2C8/9 (nearly 15%), then CYP1A1/2, CYP2C19, CYP2A6, CYP2E1, CYP1B1, and CYP2B6. Owing to their potential for numerous drug-drug interactions, those drugs that are identified in preclinical studies as substrates of CYP3A enzymes are often given a lower priority for continued research and development in favor of drugs that appear to be less affected by (or less likely to affect) this enzyme subfamily.

Each enzyme subfamily possesses unique selectivity toward potential substrates. For example, CYP1A1/2 preferentially binds medium-sized, planar, lipophilic molecules, while CYP2D6 preferentially binds molecules that possess a basic nitrogen atom. Some CYP subfamilies exhibit polymorphism (ie, multiple allelic variants that manifest differing catalytic properties). The best described polymorphisms involve CYP2C8/9, CYP2C19, and CYP2D6. Individuals possessing "wild type" gene alleles exhibit normal functioning CYP capacity. Others, however, possess allelic variants that leave the person with a subnormal level of catalytic potential (so called "poor metabolizers"). Poor metabolizers would be more likely to experience toxicity from drugs metabolized by the affected enzymes (or less effects if the enzyme is responsible for converting a prodrug to it's active form as in the case of codeine). The percentage of people classified as poor metabolizers varies by enzyme and population group. As an example, approximately 7% of Caucasians and only about 1% of Orientals appear to be CYP2D6 poor metabolizers.

CYP enzymes can be both inhibited and induced by other drugs, leading to increased or decreased serum concentrations (along with the associated effects), respectively. Induction occurs when a drug causes an increase in the amount of smooth endoplasmic reticulum, secondary to increasing the amount of the affected CYP enzymes in the tissues. This "revving up" of the CYP enzyme system may take several days to reach peak activity, and likewise, may take several days, even months, to return to normal following discontinuation of the inducing agent.

CYP inhibition occurs via several potential mechanisms. Most commonly, a CYP inhibitor competitively (and reversibly) binds to the active site on the enzyme, thus preventing the substrate from binding to the same site, and preventing the substrate from being metabolized. The affinity of an inhibitor for an enzyme may be expressed by an inhibition constant (Ki) or IC50 (defined as the concentration of the inhibitor required to cause 50% inhibition under a given set of conditions). In addition to reversible competition for an enzyme site, drugs may inhibit enzyme activity by binding to sites on the enzyme other than that to which the substrate would bind, and thereby cause a change in the functionality or physical structure of the enzyme. A drug may also bind to the enzyme in an irreversible (ie, "suicide") fashion. In such a case, it is not the concentration of drug at the enzyme site that is important (constantly binding and releasing), but the number of molecules available for binding (once bound, always bound).

Although an inhibitor or inducer may be known to affect a variety of CYP subfamilies, it may only inhibit one or two in a clinically important fashion. Likewise, although a substrate is known to be at least partially metabolized by a variety of CYP enzymes, only one or two enzymes may contribute significantly enough to its overall metabolism to warrant concern when used with potential inducers or inhibitors. Therefore, when attempting to predict the level of risk of using two drugs that may affect each other via altered CYP function, it is important to identify the relative effectiveness of the inhibiting/inducing drug on the CYP subfamilies that significantly contribute to the metabolism of the substrate. The contribution of a specific CYP pathway to substrate metabolism should be considered not only in light of other known CYP pathways, but also other nonoxidative pathways for substrate metabolism (eg, glucuronidation) and transporter proteins (eg, P-glycoprotein) that may affect the presentation of a substrate to a metabolic pathway.

SMOKING AND DRUG METABOLISM

A nonpharmaceutical interaction may be equally important because of its constant occurrence in users (tobacco). Smoking induces CYP1A2 activity, possibly causing a reduced effect of its substrates (eg, estradiol). Among postmenopausal women receiving 1 or 2 mg daily of oral estrogen, it has been found that the serum estradiol level in smokers was half that in nonsmokers. The effect was manifested by about a 50% reduction in breast tenderness in smokers. Thus, smoking may affect drugs metabolized by CYP1A2, with various consequences on target organs. A review of the literature suggests that at least a dozen drugs interact with cigarette smoke in a clinically significant manner. Polycyclic aromatic hydrocarbons (PAHs) are largely responsible for enhancing drug metabolism. Cigarette smoke induces an increase in the concentration of CYP1A2, the isoenzyme responsible for metabolism of theophylline. Theophylline is, therefore, eliminated more quickly in smokers than in nonsmokers. As a result of hepatic induction of CYP1A2, serum concentrations of theophylline have been shown to be reduced in smokers. Cigarette smoking may substantially reduce tacrine plasma concentrations. The manufacturer states that mean plasma tacrine concentrations in smokers are about one-third of the concentration in nonsmokers (presumably after multiple doses of tacrine).

Patients with insulin-dependent diabetes who smoke heavily may require a higher dosage of insulin than nonsmokers. Cigarette smoking may also reduce serum concentrations of flecainide. Although the mechanism of this interaction is unknown, enhanced hepatic metabolism is possible. Propoxyphene, a pain reliever, has been found to be less effective in smokers than in nonsmokers. The mechanism for the inefficacy of propoxyphene in smokers compared with nonsmokers may be enhanced biotransformation.

The norepinephrine and serotonin reuptake inhibitors, as a new class of smoking cessation drugs, have also received attention relative to metabolic interactions. *In vitro* studies indicate that bupropion (Zyban®) is primarily metabolized to hydroxybupropion by the CYP2B6 isoenzyme. Therefore, the potential exists for a drug interaction between Zyban® and drugs that affect the CYP2B6 isoenzyme metabolism [eg, orphenadrine (Norflex™) and cyclophosphamide (Cytoxan®)]. The hydroxybupropion metabolite of bupropion does not appear to be metabolized by the cytochrome P450 isoenzymes. No systemic data have been collected on the metabolism of Zyban® following concomitant administration with other drugs, or alternatively, the effect of concomitant administration of Zyban® on the metabolism of other drugs.

SUMMARY

Once a drug has been metabolized in the liver, it is eliminated through several different mechanisms. One is directly through bile, into the intestine, and eventually excreted in feces. More commonly, the metabolites and the original drug pass back into the liver from the general circulation and are carried to other organs and tissues. Eventually, these metabolites are excreted through the kidney. In the kidney, the drug and its metabolites may be filtered by the glomerulus or secreted by the renal tubules into the urine. From the kidney, some of the drug may be reabsorbed and pass back into the blood. The drug may also be carried to the lung. If the drug or its metabolite is volatile, it can pass from the blood into the alveolar air and be eliminated in the breath. To a minor extent, drugs and metabolites can be excreted by sweat and saliva. In nursing mothers, drugs are also excreted in mother's milk.

The clinical considerations of drug metabolism may affect which other drugs can and should be administered. Drug tolerance may be a consideration, in that larger doses of a drug may be necessary to obtain effect in patients in which the metabolism is extremely rapid. These interactions, via cytochrome P450 or its isoforms, can occasionally be used beneficially to increase/maintain blood levels of one drug by administering a second drug. Dental clinicians should attempt to stay current on this topic of drug interactions as knowledge evolves.

SELECTED READINGS

Bjarnason NH and Christiansen C, "The Influence of Thinness and Smoking on Bone Loss and Response to Hormone Replacement Therapy in Early Postmenopausal Women," *J Clin Endocrinol Metab*, 2000, 85(2):590-6.

Bjarnason NH, Jørgensen C, Kremmer H, et al, "Smoking Reduces Breast Tenderness During Oral Estrogen-Progestogen Therapy," *Climacteric*, 2004, 7(4):390-6.

Bjornsson TD, Callaghan JT, Einolf HJ, et al, "The Conduct of *in vitro* and *in vivo* Drug-Drug Interaction Studies: A PhRMA Perspective," *J Clin Pharmacol*, 2003, 43(5):443-69.

Drug-Drug Interactions, Rodrigues AD, ed, New York, NY: Marcel Dekker, Inc, 2002.

Hersh EV and Moore PA, "Drug Interactions in Dentistry: The Importance of Knowing Your CYP's," *J Am Dent Assoc*, 2004, 135(3):298-311.

Levy RH, Thummel KE, Trager WF, et al, eds, *Metabolic Drug Interactions*, Philadelphia, PA: Lippincott Williams & Wilkins, 2000.

Wilkinson GR, "Drug Metabolism and Variability Among Patients in Drug Response," *N Engl J Med*, 2005, 352(21):2211-21.

Wynn RL and Meiller TF, "CYP Enzymes and Adverse Drug Reactions," *Gen Dent*, 1998, 46(5):436-8.

Zhang Y and Benet LZ, "The Gut as a Barrier to Drug Absorption: Combined Role of Cytochrome P450 3A and P-Glycoprotein," *Clin Pharmacokinet*, 2001, 40(3):159-68.

SELECTED WEBSITES

http://www.bdbiosciences.com/
http://www.cypalleles.ki.se/
http://medicine.iupui.edu/clinpharm/ddis/
http://mhc.com/Cytochromes/

NORMAL BLOOD VALUES

Test	Range of Normal Values
Complete Blood Count (CBC)	
White blood cells	4,500-11,000
Red blood cells (male)	4.6-6.2 x 10^6 µL
Red blood cells (female)	4.2-5.4 x 10^6 µL
Platelets	150,000-450,000
Hematocrit (male)	40% to 54%
Hematocrit (female)	38% to 47%
Hemoglobin (male)	13.5-18 g/dL
Hemoglobin (female)	12-16 g/dL
Mean corpuscular volume (MCV)	80-96 µm^3
Mean corpuscular hemoglobin (MCH)	27-31 pg
Mean corpuscular hemoglobin concentration (MCHC)	32% to 36%
Differential White Blood Cell Count (%)	
Segmented neutrophils	56
Bands	3.0
Eosinophils	2.7
Basophils	0.3
Lymphocytes	34.0
Monocytes	4.0
Hemostasis	
Bleeding time (BT)	2-8 minutes
Prothrombin time (PT)	10-13 seconds
Activated partial thromboplastin time (aPTT)	25-35 seconds
Serum Chemistry	
Glucose (fasting)	70-110 mg/dL
Blood urea nitrogen (BUN)	8-23 mg/dL
Creatinine (male)	0.1-0.4 mg/dL
Creatinine (female)	0.2-0.7 mg/dL
Bilirubin, indirect (unconjugated)	0.3 mg/dL
Bilirubin, direct (conjugated)	0.1-1 mg/dL
Calcium	9.2-11 mg/dL
Magnesium	1.8-3 mg/dL
Phosphorus	2.3-4.7 mg/dL
Serum Electrolytes	
Sodium (Na$^+$)	136-142 mEq/L
Potassium (K$^+$)	3.8-5 mEq/L
Chloride (Cl$^-$)	95-103 mEq/L
Bicarbonate (HCO$_3^-$)	21-28 mmol/L
Serum Enzymes	
Alkaline phosphatase	20-130 IU/L
Alanine aminotransferase (ALT) (formerly called SGPT)	4-36 units/L
Aspartate aminotransferase (AST) (formerly called SGOT)	8-33 units/L
Amylase	16-120 Somogyi units/dL
Creatine kinase (CK) (male)	55-170 units/L
Creatine kinase (CK) (female)	30-135 units/L

CALCIUM CHANNEL BLOCKERS AND GINGIVAL HYPERPLASIA

The last published report on calcium channel blocker-induced gingival hyperplasia (GH) by this author was in 2009 (Wynn, 2009). This present update reviews the reports up through 2012, relative to the incidence of GH in patients taking calcium channel blockers (CCBs) and the mechanisms by which these drugs cause GH.

The first reported cases of gingival hyperplasia induced by nifedipine were reported by Ramon et al, in 1984 (Ramon, 1984). Since that report, additional reports and case studies have been published describing gingival hyperplasia caused by nifedipine and other calcium channel blockers. The following table lists the number of reported cases up through 2012. It lists the specific drug involved and the number of cases from 1995 to the present.

FDA Approval	General Preparation	Cases of Gingival Hyperplasia in Clinical Literature Through 1995	Cases Reported in Literature 1996-Present	Total Reported Cases
1982	Verapamil	7	9	16
1982	Diltiazem	20	33	53
1982	NIFEdipine	120	169	289
1989	NiCARdipine	0	0	0
1989	NiMODipine	0	0	0
1991	Isradipine	0	0	0
1992	AmLODIPine	0	33	33
1992	Felodipine	1	3	4
1993	Nisoldipine	0	0	0
2008	Nitrendipine[1]	1	0	1
	Clevidipine	0	0	0
	Pinaverium[1]	0	0	0

[1]Not approved in the United States

Calcium channel blockers are so named because of their effects on calcium at the cellular level. Contractile cells of the myocardium and smooth muscle cells of coronary and systemic arteries are influenced by the movement of calcium across their membranes. Part of this influence is in the regulation of contractile processes in these cells by way of movement of calcium ions through specific membrane channels. By blocking this channel movement of calcium, these drugs cause depression of the mechanical contraction of the myocardial cells, depression of electrical impulse formation and conduction velocity within the myocardium, and depression of smooth muscle contraction in coronary and systemic arteries. Thus, these drugs are useful in cardiovascular diseases, such as angina and hypertension, in which relaxation of these cells to cause vasodilatation is desired. These agents are sometimes referred to as calcium antagonists.

CLINICAL FINDINGS

Typical clinical findings of CCB-induced GH are hyperplastic gingiva around the maxillary and mandibular anterior teeth (Lederman, 1984). The hyperplastic gingiva usually originates in the interdental papilla, and in many areas, bleeding upon probing and small ulcerations are present. False periodontal pockets may be present with no evidence of bone loss. Histopathological analysis usually shows a thick layer of stratified squamous epithelium with parakeratosis and elongated rete pegs (Lederman, 1984; Lucas, 1985). In the submucosa, a proliferation of collagen fibers together with lymphocytic and plasma cell infiltration can be noticed (Lucas, 1985). The connective tissue usually shows large bundles of dense collagenous fibers with a moderate increase in fibroblasts. In addition, signs of inflammation are present with lymphocytes and plasma cells located perivascularly (Lucas, 1985).

MECHANISMS

Theories abound on the mechanism of CCB-induced gingival hyperplasia, but none have been proven. An early report using cell culture showed that the CCBs may lead to proliferation of selected fibroblasts, leading to an imbalance between regeneration and degeneration of those cells (Pernu, 1989). Brown et al, proposed that CCBs influence calcium/sodium flux in gingival fibroblast to result in decreased uptake of folic acid (Brown, 1990). The lack of intracellular folic acid then sets off a chain of events resulting in lack of production of active collagenases with no resultant catabolism of interstitial ground substance. The overabundance of ground substance manifests as gingival enlargement. Another theory suggests that these drugs elicit their effects indirectly through mediators which simulate proliferation and/or collagen synthesis by gingival fibroblasts (Giustiniani, 1987). Two of the mediators are reported to be Interleukin-2 from T cells and the testosterone metabolite 5-dihydrotestosterone (Nishikawa, 1991; Sooriyamoorthy, 1990). The report by Sooriyamoorthy et al, showed convincing evidence in controlled experiments that increased levels of 5-dihydrotestosterone occurred in gingival hyperplasia induced by nifedipine (Sooriyamoorthy, 1990). Their earlier work also showed that this testosterone metabolite had a stimulatory effect on the synthetic activity of fibroblasts (Sooriyamoorthy, 1988). In another theory, Nishikawa et al, suggests that alteration of the intracellular calcium level in gingival cells by nifedipine in combination with some local inflammatory factors is important in eliciting gingival hyperplasia (Nishikawa, 1991). Pre-existing gingival inflammation may be essential for onset of drug-induced gingival hyperplasia and that strict plaque control would be effective for preventing onset (Nishikawa, 1991). A more recent study using rats suggests that CCBs induce epithelial hyperplasia in gingival overgrowth not by an increase in keratinocyte proliferation, but by prolongation of cell life through reduction of apoptosis (controlled cell death) before epithelial hyperplasia is detected (Shimizu, 2002). Harel-Raviv et al, have argued that CCB-induced GH must be a calcium-dependent process because drugs, such as phenytoin and cyclosporin, which cause GH, also affect calcium ion cellular flux (Harel-Raviv, 1995). For example, phenytoin increases total intracellular calcium accumulation in gingival fibroblasts (Harel-Raviv, 1995).

INCIDENCE AND TREATMENT

The frequency and incidence of gingival hyperplasia caused by calcium channel blockers is difficult to assess. Literature numbers tell us that the effect by the calcium blockers is most prevalent with nifedipine (See table). The incidence of nifedipine-induced GH as currently reported are 28 cases out of 442 patients (6.3%), 11 cases out 29 patients (38%), and 79 cases out of 181 patients (44%) (Ellis, 1999; Nery, 1995; Steele, 1994). The other agents are diltiazem, 7 cases out of 33 patients (21%) and 4 cases out of 186 patients (2.2%), and amlodipine, 5 cases out of 150 patients (3.3%) and 3 cases out of 181 patients (1.7%) (Ellis, 1999; Jorgensen, 1997; Steele, 1994). For verapamil, the incidence has been reported as 5 cases out of 26 patients (19%) (Steele, 1994). A report from the Mayo clinic described the incidence of verapamil-induced GH as ranging between 4% to 19% (Meraw, 1998). Thus to summarize these values, nifedipine incidence ranged from 6.3% to 44%; diltiazem incidence ranged from 2.2% to 21%; amlodipine incidence ranged from 1.7% to 3.3%; and verapamil incidence ranged from 4% to 19%. In a more recent report, 20,636 patients taking a CCB or a non-CCB for treatment of various cardiovascular conditions were evaluated for incidence of gingival hyperplasia (Kaur, 2010). The report identified 103 patients with definite CCB-induced gingival hyperplasia. The number of CCB-identified cases included amlodipine (12), nifedipine (13), felodipine (1), verapamil (4), and diltiazem (8). Another three cases of GH associated with amlodipine were reported by Srivastava in 2010. Sanz 2012, reported that the current use of calcium channel blockers compared to no use of calcium channel blockers doubles the risk of gingival hyperplasia. Nifedipine use alone was shown to nearly triple the risk of gingival hyperplasia.

Treatment of CCB-induced GH includes the reinforcement and maintenance of good oral hygiene, along with frequent professional plaque removal (Camargo, 2000). The ideal treatment of choice; however, is the discontinuation of the suspected medication. Regression of GH has been demonstrated after discontinuation of the offending CCB (Meraw, 1998). In some situations, the use of another drug in the same class of medications has provided similar medical outcomes with reduced incidence of GH (Westbrook, 1997). If the nonsurgical approach is ineffective, then gingivectomy or periodontal flap procedures can reduce the enlarged gingival tissues (Camargo, 2000).

The following case report is an example of a three-step treatment approach to nifedipine-induced gingival overgrowth (Alandia-Roman, 2012). A 61 year old man had severe gingival overgrowth associated with nifedipine use for the management of hypertension. For step one, the treatment protocol was based on a consistent oral health hygiene program and nonsurgical techniques to reduce inflammation. Professional prophylaxis occurred over multiple visits. The patient also received printed and verbal information about oral hygiene and periodontal disease and was given toothbrushes, dental floss, therapeutic dentifrices, and mouthwashes formulated with 0.5% chloramine-T. Chlorhexidine was not used because of its tooth-staining properties. For the second step, the healthcare provider changed to a different antihypertension medication, in this case an angiotensin-converting enzyme inhibitor. The change in medication controlled the hypertension and the gingival overgrowth showed an expressive but not complete reduction in 4 weeks. Finally, surgical correction of the gingival overgrowth was still necessary and scalpel gingivectomy was conducted at six sites with one site treated per month for six months. Per the authors, the measures used to achieve a successful resolution were based on the most commonly cited and discussed techniques found in the literature.

REFERENCES

Alandia-Roman CC, Tirapelli C, Ribas P, et al, "Drug-Induced Gingival Overgrowth: A Case Report," *Gen Dent*, 2012, 60(4):312-5.
Brown RS, Sein P, Corio R, et al, "Nitrendipine-Induced Gingival Hyperplasia. First Case Report," *Oral Surg Oral Med Oral Pathol*, 1990, 70(5):593-6.
Camargo PM, Melnick PR, Pirih FQ, et al, "Treatment of Drug-Induced Gingival Enlargement: Aesthetic and Functional Considerations," *Periodontol 2000*, 2001, 27:131-8.
Ellis JS, Seymour RA, Steele JG, et al, "Prevalence of Gingival Overgrowth Induced by Calcium Channel Blockers: A Community-Based Study," *J Periodontol*, 1999, 70(1):63-7.
Giustiniani S, Robustelli della Cuna F, and Marieni M, "Hyperplastic Gingivitis During Diltiazem Therapy," *Int J Cardiol*, 1987, 15(2):247-9.
Harel-Raviv M, Eckler M, Lalani K, et al, "Nifedipine-Induced Gingival Hyperplasia. A Comprehensive Review and Analysis," *Oral Surg Oral Med Oral Pathol Oral Radiol Endod*, 1995, 79(6):715-22.
Jorgensen MG, "Prevalence of Amlodipine-Related Gingival Hyperplasia," *J Periodontol*, 1997, 68(7):676-8.
Kaur G, Verhamme KM, Dieleman JP, et al, "Association Between Calcium Channel Blockers and Gingival Hyperplasia, *J Clin Periodontol*, 2010, 37 (7):625-30.
Lederman D, Lumerman H, Reuben S, et al, "Gingival Hyperplasia Associated With Nifedipine Therapy. Report of a Case," *Oral Surg Oral Med Oral Pathol*, 1984, 57(6):620-2.
Lucas RM, Howell LP, and Wall BA, "Nifedipine-Induced Gingival Hyperplasia. A Histochemical and Ultrastructural Study," *J Periodontol*, 1985, 56 (4):211-5.
Meraw SJ and Sheridan PJ, "Medically Induced Gingival Hyperplasia," *Mayo Clin Proc*, 1998, 73(12):1196-9.
Nery EB, Edson RG, Lee KK, et al, "Prevalence of Nifedipine-Induced Gingival Hyperplasia," *J Periodontol*, 1995, 66(7):572-8.
Nishikawa S, Tada H, Hamasaki A, et al, "Nifedipine-Induced Gingival Hyperplasia: A Clinical and *in vitro* Study," *J Periodontol*, 1991, 62(1):30-5.
Pernu HE, Oikarinen K, Hietanen J, et al, "Verapamil-Induced Gingival Overgrowth: A Clinical, Histologic, and Biochemic Approach," *J Oral Pathol Med*, 1989, 18(7):422-5.
Ramon Y, Behar S, Kishon Y, et al, "Gingival Hyperplasia Caused by Nifedipine - A Preliminary Report," *Int J Cardiol*, 1984, 5(2):195-206.

Sanz M, "Current Use of Calcium Channel Blockers (CCBs) Is Associated With an Increased Risk of Gingival Hyperplasia," *J Evid Based Dent Pract*, 2012, 12(3 Suppl):147-8.

Shimizu Y, Kataoka M, Seto H, et al, "Nifedipine Induces Gingival Epithelial Hyperplasia in Rats Through Inhibition of Apoptosis," *J Periodontol*, 2002, 73(8):861-7.

Sooriyamoorthy M, Gower DB, and Eley BM, "Androgen Metabolism in Gingival Hyperplasia Induced by Nifedipine and Cyclosporin," *J Periodontal Res*, 1990, 25(1):25-30.

Sooriyamoorthy M, Harvey W, and Gower DB, "The Use of Human Gingival Fibroblasts in Culture for Studying the Effects of Phenytoin on Testosterone Metabolism," *Arch Oral Biol*, 1988, 33(5):353-9.

Srivastava AK, Kundu D, Bandyopadhyay P, et al, "Management of Amlodipine-Induced Gingival Enlargement: Series of Three Cases," *J Indian Soc Periodontol*, 2010, 14(4):279-81.

Steele RM, Schuna AA, and Schreiber RT, "Calcium Antagonist-Induced Gingival Hyperplasia," *Ann Intern Med*, 1994, 120(8):663-4.

Westbrook P, Bednarczyk EM, Carlson M, et al, "Regression of Nifedipine-Induced Gingival Hyperplasia Following Switch to a Same Class Calcium Channel Blocker, Isradipine," *J Periodontol*, 1997, 68(7):645-50.

Wynn RL, "Calcium Channel Blockers and Gingival Hyperplasia – An Update," *Gen Dent*, 2009, 57(2):105-7.

DENTIFRICES: NO SODIUM LAURYL SULFATE (SLS)

Brand Name	Abrasive Ingredient	Therapeutic Ingredient
Arm & Hammer Advance White™ Toothpaste for Sensitive Teeth	Hydrated silica	Sodium fluoride 0.24%, triclosan 0.3%
Other Ingredients: Sodium bicarbonate, cellulose gum, cocamidopropyl betaine, flavor, glycerin, sorbitol, titanium dioxide, water		
Baby Orajel® Tooth and Gum Cleanser (4–18 months of age)	None	None
Other Ingredients: Purified water, sorbitol, propylene glycol, glycerin, cellulose gum, poloxamer 407, flavor, simethicone, methylparaben, potassium sorbate, sodium saccharin, propylparaben, citric acid		
Biotene® Sensitive	Hydrated silica	Potassium nitrate 5% (antihypersensitivity), sodium monofluorophosphate 0.14% w/v fluoride ion (anticavity)
Other Ingredients: Acesulfame K, calcium lactate, calcium pyrophosphate, cellulose gum, flavor, beta-d-glucose, glycerin, isoceteth-20, potassium thiocyanate, sodium benzoate, sorbitol, xylitol, enzyme system (glucose oxidase, lactoferrin, lactoperoxidase, lysozyme)		
Burt's Bees® Natural Toothpaste(s)	Hydrated silica	Sodium monofluorophosphate 0.77% (0.14% w/v fluoride ion [anticavity])
Other Ingredients: Glycerin, xylitol, calcium sodium phosphosilicate, sodium cocoyl glutamate, titanium dioxide, *Vaccinium macrocarpon* (cranberry) fruit powder, *Chondrus crispus* (carrageenan), *Stevia rebaudiana* extract, xanthan gum, silica, flavor, lecithin, maltodextrin, natural flavor		
Dr. Collins Natural Toothpaste	Hydrated silica	Xylitol 25%
Other Ingredients: Dicalcium phosphate dihydrate, purified water, glycerin, cellulose gum, zinc citrate trihydrate, flavor, *Aloe barbadensis* leaf juice, *Magnolia officinalis* bark extract, *Lycium chinense* fruit extract (goji berry extract), *Punica granatum* (pomegranate) extract, *Melaleuca alternifolia* (tea tree) leaf oil, coenzyme Q_{10}, vitamin E acetate, *Stevia rebaudiana* leaf/stem extract, ascorbic acid, titanium dioxide, sodium methyl cocoyl taurate, propylene glycol, sodium hydroxide		
Orajel® Toddler Training Toothpaste(s)	None	None
Other Ingredients: Purified water, sorbitol, propylene glycol, glycerin, cellulose gum, poloxamer 407, flavor, simethicone, methylparaben, potassium sorbate, sodium saccharin, propylparaben, citric acid		
Sensodyne® Original	Hydrated silica	Potassium nitrate 5% (antihypersensitivity), sodium fluoride 0.13% w/v fluoride ion (anticavity)
Other Ingredients: Cellulose gum, D&C red no. 28, flavor, glycerin, silica, sodium methyl cocoyl taurate, sodium saccharin, sorbitol, titanium dioxide, trisodium phosphate, water		
Sensodyne® Iso-Active® Multi-Action Toothpaste	Hydrated silica	Potassium nitrate 5% (antihypersensitivity), sodium fluoride 0.15% w/v fluoride ion (anticavity)
Other Ingredients: Carrageenan gum, cocamidopropyl betaine, FD&C blue no. 1, flavor, glycerin, isopentane, PEG-6, sodium hydroxide, sodium methyl cocoyl taurate, sodium saccharin, sorbitol, water, xanthan gum		
Sensodyne® Iso-Active® Whitening Gel Toothpaste	Hydrated silica	Potassium nitrate 5% (antihypersensitivity), sodium fluoride 0.15% w/v fluoride ion (anticavity)
Other Ingredients: Water, glycerin, sorbitol, pentasodium triphosphate, PEG-8, isopentane, flavor, sodium methyl cocoyl taurate, cocamidopropyl betaine, xanthan gum, carrageenan, sodium hydroxide, sodium saccharin, sucralose, blue no. 1		

Brand Name	Abrasive Ingredient	Therapeutic Ingredient
Sensodyne® ProNamel® Iso-Active® Daily Protection	Hydrated silica	Potassium nitrate 5% (antihypersensitivity), sodium fluoride 0.15% w/v fluoride ion (anticavity)
	Other Ingredients: Water, sorbitol, glycerin, PEG-8, isopentane, flavor, cocamidopropyl betaine, sodium methyl cocoyl taurate, xanthan gum, carrageenan, sodium saccharin, sodium hydroxide, blue no. 1, yellow no. 10	
Sensodyne® ProNamel® Iso-Active® Gentle Whitening	Hydrated silica	Potassium nitrate 5% (antihypersensitivity), sodium fluoride 0.15% w/v fluoride ion (anticavity)
	Other Ingredients: Water, sorbitol, glycerin, PEG-8, isopentane, flavor, cocamidopropyl betaine, sodium methyl cocoyl taurate, xanthan gum, carrageenan, sodium saccharin, sodium hydroxide, blue no. 1	
Sensodyne® Extra Whitening	Hydrated silica	Potassium nitrate 5% (antihypersensitivity), sodium fluoride 0.15% w/v fluoride ion (anticavity)
	Other Ingredients: Water, sorbitol, glycerin, pentasodium triphosphate, PEG-8, flavor, titanium dioxide, cocamidopropyl betaine, sodium methyl cocoyl taurate, xanthan gum, sodium hydroxide, sodium saccharin, sucralose	
Sensodyne® Cool Gel	Hydrated silica	Potassium nitrate 5% (antihypersensitivity), sodium fluoride 0.15% w/v fluoride ion (anticavity)
	Other Ingredients: Water, sorbitol, glycerin, cocamidopropyl betaine, flavor, xanthan gum, titanium dioxide, sodium saccharin, sodium hydroxide, sucralose, blue no. 1	
Sensodyne® Fresh Impact	Hydrated silica	Potassium nitrate 5% (antihypersensitivity), sodium fluoride 0.15% w/v fluoride ion (anticavity)
	Other Ingredients: Water, sorbitol, glycerin, cocamidopropyl betaine, flavor, xanthan gum, titanium dioxide, sodium saccharin, sodium hydroxide, sucralose, blue no. 1	
Sensodyne® Full Protection Plus Whitening	Hydrated silica	Potassium nitrate 5% (antihypersensitivity), sodium fluoride 0.15% w/v fluoride ion (anticavity)
	Other Ingredients: Water, sorbitol, glycerin, pentasodium triphosphate, PEG-8, flavor, titanium dioxide, cocamidopropyl betaine, sodium methyl cocyl taurate, xanthan gum, sodium hydroxide, sodium saccharin, sucralose	
Sensodyne® Tartar Control Plus Whitening	Hydrated silica	Potassium nitrate 5% (antihypersensitivity), sodium fluoride 0.15% w/v fluoride ion (anticavity)
	Other Ingredients: Water, sorbitol, glycerin, pentasodium triphosphate, PEG-8, flavor, titanium dioxide, cocamidopropyl betaine, sodium methyl cocyl taurate, xanthan gum, sodium hydroxide, sodium saccharin, sucralose	
Sensodyne® ProNamel® Gentle Whitening Alpine Breeze	Hydrated silica	Potassium nitrate 5% (antihypersensitivity), sodium fluoride 0.15% w/v fluoride ion (anticavity)
	Other Ingredients: Water, sorbitol, glycerin, PEG-8, cocamidopropyl betaine, flavor, titanium dioxide, xanthan gum, sodium saccharin, sodium hydroxide	
Sensodyne® Fresh Mint	Hydrated silica	Potassium nitrate 5% (antihypersensitivity), sodium fluoride 0.15% w/v fluoride ion (anticavity)
	Other Ingredients: Water, sorbitol, glycerin, cocamidopropyl betaine, flavor, xanthan gum, titanium dioxide, sodium saccharin, sodium hydroxide, sucralose, yellow no. 10, blue no. 1	

(continued)

Brand Name	Abrasive Ingredient	Therapeutic Ingredient
Sensodyne® ProNamel® Mint Essence	Hydrated silica	Potassium nitrate 5% (antihypersensitivity), sodium fluoride 0.15% w/v fluoride ion (anticavity)
	Other Ingredients: Water, sorbitol, glycerin, PEG-8, cocamidopropyl betaine, flavor, xanthan gum, sodium saccharin, titanium dioxide, sodium hydroxide	
Sensodyne® ProNamel® Fresh Breath Fresh Wave	Hydrated silica	Potassium nitrate 5% (antihypersensitivity), sodium fluoride 0.15% w/v fluoride ion (anticavity)
	Other Ingredients: Water, sorbitol, glycerin, PEG-8, cocamidopropyl betaine, flavor, xanthan gum, sodium saccharin, titanium dioxide, sodium hydroxide	
Tom's™ of Maine Peppermint SLS Free Anticavity Plus Whitening Clean and Gentle	Hydrated silica	Sodium monofluorophosphate 0.76% (0.13% w/v fluoride ion [anticavity])
	Other Ingredients: Glycerin, water, calcium carbonate, *Aloe barbadensis* leaf juice (organic), xylitol, *Chondrus crispus* (carrageenan), *Acacia senegal* gum, glycyrrhizic acid, *Mentha piperita* (peppermint) oil	
Verve Ultra	Hydrated silica	Sodium fluoride 0.34%
	Other Ingredients: Purified water, glycerin, sorbitol, cellulose gum, flavor, sodium methyl cocoyl taurate, sodium benzoate, tocopheryl acetate (vitamin E), sodium saccharin, maritime pine extract (Pycnogenol®), FD&C blue no. 1, D&C yellow no. 10	

Note: It is thought that patients suffering from mucosal changes benefit from using dentifrices without a foaming agent, such as SLS. SLS has been removed from all Sensodyne® products.

DENTIFRICES WITH ANTIGINGIVITIS AGENTS

Brand Name	Abrasive Ingredient	Therapeutic Ingredient	Foaming Agent
Colgate® Total® Advanced Deep Clean Paste[1]	Hydrated silica	Sodium fluoride 0.24%, triclosan 0.3%	Sodium lauryl sulfate[2]
	Other Ingredients: Water, glycerin, sorbitol, PVM/MA copolymer, flavor, cellulose gum, sodium hydroxide, propylene glycol, carrageenan, sodium saccharin, titanium dioxide		
Colgate® Total® Advanced Fresh + Whitening Gel[1]	Hydrated silica, mica	Sodium fluoride 0.24%, triclosan 0.3%	Sodium lauryl sulfate[2]
	Other Ingredients: Water, glycerin, sorbitol, flavor, PVM/MA copolymer, cellulose gum, sodium hydroxide, propylene glycol, carrageenan, sodium saccharin, titanium dioxide, FD&C blue no. 1, D&C yellow no. 10		
Colgate® Total® Advanced Whitening Paste[1]	Hydrated silica	Sodium fluoride 0.24%, triclosan 0.3%	Sodium lauryl sulfate[2]
	Other Ingredients: Water, glycerin, sorbitol, PVM/MA copolymer, flavor, cellulose gum, sodium hydroxide, propylene glycol, carrageenan, sodium saccharin, titanium dioxide		
Colgate® Total® Advanced Whitening Gel[1]	Hydrated silica, mica	Sodium fluoride 0.24%, triclosan 0.3%	Sodium lauryl sulfate[2]
	Other Ingredients: Water, glycerin, sorbitol, flavor, PVM/MA copolymer, cellulose gum, sodium hydroxide, propylene glycol, carrageenan, sodium saccharin, titanium dioxide, FD&C blue no. 1, D&C yellow no. 10		
Colgate® Total® Gum Defense[1]	Hydrated silica	Sodium fluoride 0.24%, triclosan 0.3%	Sodium lauryl sulfate[2]
	Other Ingredients: Water, glycerin, sorbitol, PVM/MA copolymer, flavor, cellulose gum, sodium hydroxide, propylene glycol, carrageenan, sodium saccharin, titanium dioxide		
Colgate® Total® Enamel Strength[1]	Hydrated silica, mica	Sodium fluoride 0.24%, triclosan 0.3%	Sodium lauryl sulfate[2]
	Other Ingredients: Water, glycerin, sorbitol, flavor, PVM/MA copolymer, cellulose gum, sodium hydroxide, propylene glycol, carrageenan, sodium saccharin, titanium dioxide, FD&C blue no. 1, D&C yellow no. 10		
Colgate® Total® Clean Mint Paste[1]	Hydrated silica	Sodium fluoride 0.24%, triclosan 0.3%	Sodium lauryl sulfate[2]
	Other Ingredients: Water, glycerin, sorbitol, PVM/MA copolymer, flavor, cellulose gum, sodium hydroxide, propylene glycol, carrageenan, sodium saccharin, titanium dioxide		
Colgate® Total® Mint Stripe™ Gel[1]	Hydrated silica, mica	Sodium fluoride 0.24%, triclosan 0.3%	Sodium lauryl sulfate[2]
	Other Ingredients: Water, glycerin, sorbitol, flavor, PVM/MA copolymer, cellulose gum, sodium hydroxide, propylene glycol, carrageenan, sodium saccharin, titanium dioxide, FD&C blue no. 1, D&C yellow no. 10		
Colgate® Total® Whitening Paste[1]	Hydrated silica	Sodium fluoride 0.24%, triclosan 0.3%	Sodium lauryl sulfate[2]
	Other Ingredients: Water, glycerin, sorbitol, PVM/MA copolymer, flavor, cellulose gum, sodium hydroxide, propylene glycol, carrageenan, sodium saccharin, titanium dioxide		
Colgate® Total® Zx Pro-Shield Plus Sensitivity[1,3]	Hydrated silica, mica	Zinc citrate 2%, sodium monofluorophosphate 1.4%, potassium nitrate 5%	Sodium lauryl sulfate[2]
	Other Ingredients: Water, glycerin, sorbitol, PEG-12, tetrasodium pyrophosphate, PVM/MA copolymer, flavor, sodium saccharin, cellulose gum, sodium hydroxide, xanthan gum, polyethylene, titanium dioxide, FD&C blue no. 1, D&C yellow no. 10, FD&C blue no. 1 lake		
Crest® Pro-Health® Clean Mint[1]	Hydrated silica	Stannous fluoride 0.454%	Sodium lauryl sulfate[2]
	Other Ingredients: Glycerin, sodium hexametaphosphate, propylene glycol, PEG-6, water, zinc lactate, trisodium phosphate, flavor, sodium gluconate, carrageenan, sodium saccharin, polyethylene, xanthan gum, titanium dioxide, blue no. 1		
Crest® Pro-Health® Whitening[1]	Hydrated silica	Stannous fluoride 0.454%	Sodium lauryl sulfate[2]
	Other Ingredients: Glycerin, sodium hexametaphosphate, propylene glycol, PEG-6, water, zinc lactate, trisodium phosphate, flavor, sodium gluconate, carrageenan, sodium saccharin, polyethylene, xanthan gum, titanium dioxide, blue no. 1		
Crest® Pro-Health® Enamel Shield™	Hydrated silica	Stannous fluoride 0.454%	Sodium lauryl sulfate[2]
	Other Ingredients: Glycerin, sodium hexametaphosphate, propylene glycol, PEG-6, water, zinc lactate, trisodium phosphate, flavor, sodium gluconate, carrageenan, sodium saccharin, polyethylene, xanthan gum, blue no. 1 aluminum lake		
Crest® Pro-Health® Sensitive Shield™	Hydrated silica	Stannous fluoride 0.454%	Sodium lauryl sulfate[2]
	Other Ingredients: Glycerin, sodium hexametaphosphate, propylene glycol, PEG-6, water, zinc lactate, flavor, trisodium phosphate, sodium gluconate, carrageenan, sodium saccharin, polyethylene, xanthan gum, titanium dioxide, blue no. 1		

[1] Carries American Dental Association (ADA) Seal of Acceptance indicating safety and efficacy

[2] Sodium lauryl sulfate has been known to cause oral mucosal and skin changes

[3] This product also is listed in Calcium Phosphate Products on page 1649

Note: In addition to anticavity, these dentifrices have gained approval from the Food and Drug Administration to label the product as antigingivitis and antiplaque.

MOST PRESCRIBED DRUGS IN 2011

1. Hydrocodone and Acetaminophen
2. Levothyroxine
3. Lisinopril
4. Lipitor®
5. Simvastatin
6. Plavix®
7. Singulair®
8. Azithromycin
9. Crestor®
10. NexIUM®
11. Metoprolol
12. Synthroid®
13. Lexapro®
14. ProAir® HFA
15. Ibuprofen
16. TraZODone
17. Amoxicillin
18. Omeprazole
19. Advair Diskus®
20. Cymbalta®
21. TraMADol
22. Sulfamethoxazole and Trimethoprim
23. AmLODIPine
24. Fluticasone
25. Hydrochlorothiazide
26. Ventolin® HFA
27. Diovan®
28. Warfarin
29. Sertraline
30. ALPRAZolam
31. Pravastatin
32. Amoxicillin and Clavulanate
33. SEROquel®
34. Oxycodone and Acetaminophen
35. Zolpidem
36. MetFORMIN
37. PredniSONE
38. Fluconazole
39. ClonazePAM
40. Actos®
41. Gabapentin
42. Lantus®
43. Vitamin D
44. FLUoxetine
45. Furosemide
46. Citalopram
47. Ciprofloxacin (Systemic)
48. Atenolol
49. Meloxicam
50. LORazepam
51. CeleBREX®
52. Venlafaxine
53. Lyrica®
54. Nasonex®
55. Spiriva®
56. Cyclobenzaprin
57. Cephalexin
58. Abilify®
59. Carvedilol
60. Potassium Chloride
61. Viagra®
62. Vyvanse®
63. Zetia®
64. Albuterol
65. Namenda®
66. Januvia®
67. TriCor®
68. Diazepam
69. Loestrin® 24 Fe
70. Allopurinol
71. Cialis®
72. Alendronate
73. Losartan
74. Hydrochlorothiazide and Triamterene
75. Amitriptyline
76. OxyCODONE
77. Suboxone®
78. OxyCONTIN®
79. Niaspan®
80. Doxycycline
81. Digoxin
82. Vytorin®
83. Acetaminophen and Codeine
84. Triamcinolone
85. Premarin®
86. PARoxetine
87. Flovent® HFA

88. Promethazine
89. Carisoprodol
90. Klor-Con® M20
91. Benicar®
92. Lovastatin
93. Amphetamine
94. RisperiDONE
95. Levoxyl®
96. Naproxen
97. Lovaza®
98. Bystolic®
99. Penicillin V Potassium
100. Famotidine
101. MethylPREDNISolone
102. NuvaRing®
103. GlyBURIDE

104. Clindamycin
105. Folic Acid
106. Enalapril
107. Tamsulosin
108. Cheratussin® DAC
109. Levaquin®
110. TriNessa®
111. Ranitidine
112. GlipiZIDE
113. Tri-Sprintec®
114. Symbicort®
115. Lidoderm®
116. Pantoprazole
117. ZyPREXA®
118. Endocet®
119. Gianvi™

Based on units dispensed in U.S.

Source: Pharmacy Times, available at http://www.pharmacytimes.com/_media/_pdf/Top_200_Drugs_2011_Total_Rx.pdf

REMINERALIZATION AND DESENSITIZATION PRODUCTS

Brand Name	Category	Formula	Availability
Arm & Hammer™ Age Defying™ Toothpaste	Remineralization	ACP: <5% Sodium fluoride: 0.24%	OTC
Arm & Hammer™ Complete Care™ Plus Enamel Strengthening	Remineralization	ACP: <5% Sodium fluoride: 0.24%	OTC
Arm & Hammer™ Sensitive Freshening	Desensitization	Potassium nitrate[1]: 5% Sodium fluoride: 0.24%	OTC
Arm & Hammer™ Sensitive Multi-Protection	Desensitization	Potassium nitrate[1]: 5% Sodium fluoride: 0.24%	OTC
Arm & Hammer™ Sensitive Whitening	Desensitization Whitening	Potassium nitrate[1]: 5% Sodium fluoride: 0.24%	OTC
Burt's Bees® Natural Toothpastes	Remineralization	Sodium monofluorophosphate: 0.77% Calcium sodium phosphosilicate: % not indicated	OTC
Clinpro™ 5000	Remineralization	Sodium fluoride: 1.1% (5000 ppm fluoride ion) tri-calcium phosphate	OD, Rx
Colgate® Sensitive Pro-Relief™	Desensitization	Potassium nitrate[1]: 5% Sodium monofluorophosphate: 1.4%	OTC
Colgate® Sensitive Pro-Relief™ Desensitizing Paste	Desensitization	Calcium carbonate and arginine (Pro-Argin™ Technology[2])	OD (rotary cup paste used before and after scaling)
Colgate® Sensitive Pro-Relief™ Plus Whitening	Desensitization Whitening	Potassium nitrate[1]: 5% Sodium monofluorophosphate: 1.4%	OTC
Colgate® Sensitivity Pro-Relief™ Enamel Repair	Desensitization	Potassium nitrate[1]: 5% Sodium monofluorophosphate: 0.24%	OTC
Colgate® Total Zx Pro-Shield Plus Sensitivity	Anticavity Antigingivitis Antiplaque Desensitization	Potassium nitrate[1]: 5% Zinc citrate: 2% Sodium monofluorophosphate: 1.4%	OTC
DayWhite® ACP Gel	Desensitization Remineralization Whitening	ACP: 0.5% Hydrogen peroxide: 7.5%, 9.5%	OD
Dr. Collins Restore™ Toothpaste	Remineralization	Calcium sodium phosphosilicate (NovaMin® Technology[4])	Online, OD
MI Paste™	Desensitization Remineralization[3]	CPP-ACP (Recaldent™): 10%	OD, Rx
MI Paste Plus™	Desensitization Remineralization[3]	CPP-ACP (Recaldent™): 10% Sodium fluoride: 0.2%	OD, Rx
NiteWhite® ACP Gel	Desensitization Remineralization Whitening	ACP: 0.5% Carbamide peroxide: 10%, 16%, 22%	OD
Relief® ACP Oral Care Gel	Desensitization Remineralization	ACP: 0.375% Sodium fluoride: 0.22% Potassium nitrate[1]: 5%	OD, Rx
Topex® ReNew™ Toothpaste	Remineralization	Calcium sodium phosphosilicate (NovaMin® Technology[4]): 5% Neutral sodium fluoride: 1.1%	OD
Trident Xtra Care™ with Recaldent®	Remineralization	CPP-ACP (Recaldent™): 1% Xylitol	OTC

CPP-ACP = casein phosphopeptide-amorphous calcium phosphate; ACP component may contain properties that rebuild enamel and remineralize teeth; **OD** = office-dispensed; **Rx** = prescription only; **OTC** = over-the-counter; **ACP** = amorphous calcium phosphate; **ACP technology** = calcium ions, phosphate ions

[1]Potassium nitrate decreases sensitivity.

[2]Pro-Argin™ is proven to be effective in occluding tubules.

[3]Clinical cases available from GC America

[4]NovaMin® is a synthetic mineral composed of calcium, sodium, phosphorus, and silica.

VASOCONSTRICTOR INTERACTIONS WITH ANTIDEPRESSANTS

Antidepressant	Effects with Epinephrine, Levonordefrin	Contraindicated	Recommendation
Tricyclics			
Amitriptyline (Elavil® [DSC])	Epinephrine (Systemic, Oral Inhalation) = increased pressor response; cardiac dysrhythmias Levonordefrin = increased pressor response	No	Potentially dangerous; use minimal amounts with caution in local anesthetics
Amitriptyline and Chlordiazepoxide			
Amitriptyline and Perphenazine			
Amoxapine			
Clomipramine (Anafranil®)			
Desipramine (Norpramin®)			
Doxepin (Systemic) (Prudoxin™, SINEquan®, Zonalon®)			
Imipramine (Tofranil-PM®, Tofranil®)			
Nortriptyline (Pamelor®)			
Protriptyline (Vivactil®)			
Trimipramine (Surmontil®)			
Serotonin/Norepinephrine Reuptake Inhibitor			
Desvenlafaxine (Pristiq®)	No adverse interactions reported	No	Suggest caution since serotonin/norepinephrine reuptake inhibitors block norepinephrine reuptake in CNS
Milnacipran (Savella®)			
Venlafaxine (Effexor® XR, Effexor®)			
Serotonin-Only Reuptake Inhibitors			
Citalopram (CeleXA®)	No adverse interactions reported	No	No precautions appear to be necessary
Escitalopram (Lexapro™)			
FLUoxetine (PROzac® Weekly™, PROzac®, Sarafem™)			
FluvoxaMINE			
Olanzapine and Fluoxetine (Symbyax®)			
PARoxetine (Paxil CR®, Paxil®, Pexeva™)			
Sertraline (Zoloft®)			
Central Alpha-2 Antagonist			
Mirtazapine (Remeron SolTab®, Remeron®)	No adverse interactions reported	No	Suggest caution since mirtazapine increases release of norepinephrine
Dopamine Reuptake Inhibitor			
BuPROPion (Wellbutrin SR®, Wellbutrin XL®, Wellbutrin®, Zyban®)	No adverse interactions reported	No	Part of the mechanism of bupropion is to block norepinephrine reuptake within CNS; it has been suggested that vasoconstrictor be administered with caution
Others			
DULoxetine (Cymbalta®)	No adverse interactions reported	No	Part of the mechanism of duloxetine is to block norepinephrine reuptake within CNS; it has been suggested that vasoconstrictor be administered with caution
Maprotiline	Potential for increased pressor response	No	Blocks norepinephrine synaptic reuptake in the CNS; potentially dangerous; use minimal amounts with caution in local anesthetics

(continued)

Antidepressant	Effects with Epinephrine, Levonordefrin	Contraindicated	Recommendation
MAO Inhibitors			
Isocarboxazid (Marplan®)	No effects on blood pressure or heart rate reported; however, potential exists for slight increase in pressor response	No	Use vasoconstrictor with caution
Moclobemide			
Phenelzine (Nardil®)			
Tranylcypromine (Parnate®)			
Serotonin Reuptake Inhibitor/Serotonin Antagonist			
Nefazodone (Serzone® [DSC])	No adverse interactions reported	No	No precautions appear to be necessary
TraZODone (Desyrel®)			
Serotonin Reuptake Inhibitor/5-HT$_{1A}$ Receptor Partial Agonist			
Vilazodone (Viibryd™)	No adverse interactions reported	No	No precautions appear to be necessary

REFERENCES

Felpel LP, "Psychopharmacology: Antipsychotics and Antidepressants," *Pharmacology and Therapeutics for Dentistry*, 4th ed, Yagiela JA, Neidle EA, Dowd FJ, et al, eds, St. Louis, Missouri: Year Book, Inc, 1998, 162.

Naftalin LW and Yagiela JA, "Vasoconstrictors: Indications and Precautions," *Dent Clin North Am*, 2002, 46(4):733-46.

Wynn RL, "Antidepressant Medications," *Gen Dent*, 1992, 40(3):192-7.

Yagiela JA, "Adverse Drug Interactions in Dental Practice: Interactions Associated With Vasoconstrictors. Part V of a Series," *J Am Dent Assoc*, 1999, 130(5):701-9.

Yagiela JA, Duffin SR, and Hunt LM, "Drug Interactions and Vasoconstrictors Used in Local Anesthetic Solutions," *Oral Surg Oral Med Oral Pathol*, 1985, 59(6):565-71.

Yagiela JA, "Injectable and Topical Local Anesthetics," *ADA Guide to Dental Therapeutics*, 2nd ed, Chicago, IL: ADA Publishing, 2000, 1-16.

PHARMACOLOGIC CATEGORY INDEX

ALPHABETICAL INDEX

Segment

ALPHABETICAL INDEX

NOTES

NOTES

NOTES

NOTES

NOTES

NOTES

NOTES

NOTES

NOTES

NOTES